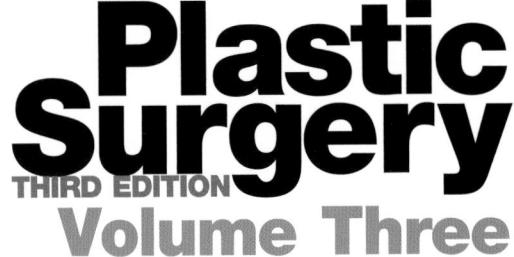

Plastic Surgery

THIRD EDITION

Volume Three

Craniofacial, Head and Neck Surgery
Pediatric Plastic Surgery

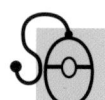

ExpertConsult.com

For additional online content visit expertconsult.com

Content Strategists: Sue Hodgson, Belinda Kuhn
Content Development Specialists: Alexandra Mortimer, Louise Cook, Poppy Garraway
Content Coordinators: Emma Cole, Trinity Hutton, Sam Crowe
Project Managers: Caroline Jones, Cheryl Brant
Design: Stewart Larking, Miles Hitchen
Illustration Manager: Jennifer Rose
Illustrator: Antbits
Marketing Manager: Helena Mutak
Technical Copyeditors: Darren Smith, Colin Woon
Video Reviewers: Leigh Jansen, James Saunders
Artwork Reviewer: Priya Chadha

Plastic Surgery

THIRD EDITION

Volume Three

Craniofacial, Head and Neck Surgery
Pediatric Plastic Surgery

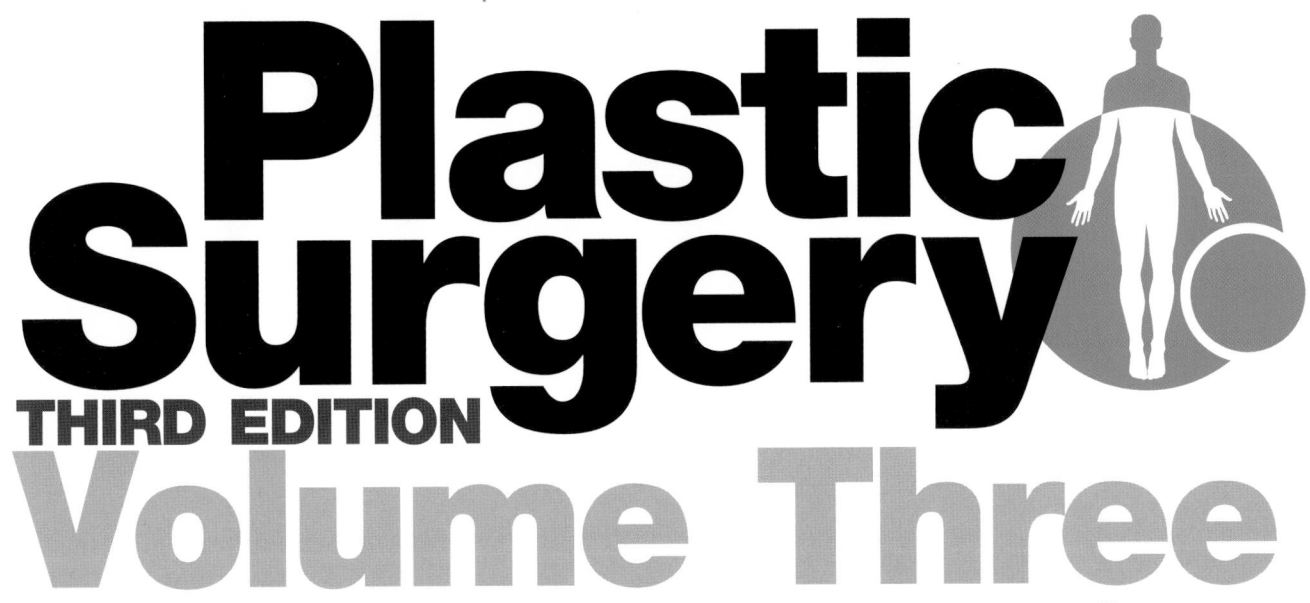

Editor in Chief:

Peter C. Neligan
MB, FRCS(I), FRCSC, FACS
Professor of Surgery
Department of Surgery, Division of Plastic Surgery
University of Washington
Seattle, WA, USA

Video Editor:

Allen L. Van Beek
MD, FACS
Adjunct Professor
University Minnesota School of Medicine
Division Plastic Surgery
Minneapolis, MN, USA

Craniofacial, Head and Neck Surgery
Volume Editor:

Eduardo D. Rodriguez
MD, DDS
Chief, Plastic Reconstructive and Maxillofacial
Surgery, R Adams Cowley Shock Trauma Center
Professor of Surgery
University of Maryland School of Medicine
Baltimore, MD, USA

Pediatric Plastic Surgery
Volume Editor:

Joseph E. Losee
MD, FACS, FAAP
Professor of Surgery and Pediatrics
Chief, Division Pediatric Plastic Surgery
Children's Hospital of Pittsburgh
University of Pittsburgh Medical Center
Pittsburgh, PA, USA

ELSEVIER
SAUNDERS

London, New York, Oxford, St Louis, Sydney, Toronto

ELSEVIER
SAUNDERS

SAUNDERS an imprint of Elsevier Inc

First edition 1990
Second edition 2006
Third edition 2013

Notices

Knowledge and best practice in this field are constantly changing. As new research and experience broaden our understanding, changes in research methods, professional practices, or medical treatment may become necessary.

Practitioners and researchers must always rely on their own experience and knowledge in evaluating and using any information, methods, compounds, or experiments described herein. In using such information or methods they should be mindful of their own safety and the safety of others, including parties for whom they have a professional responsibility.

With respect to any drug or pharmaceutical products identified, readers are advised to check the most current information provided (i) on procedures featured or (ii) by the manufacturer of each product to be administered, to verify the recommended dose or formula, the method and duration of administration, and contraindications. It is the responsibility of practitioners, relying on their own experience and knowledge of their patients, to make diagnoses, to determine dosages and the best treatment for each individual patient, and to take all appropriate safety precautions.

To the fullest extent of the law, neither the Publisher nor the authors, contributors, or editors, assume any liability for any injury and/or damage to persons or property as a matter of products liability, negligence or otherwise, or from any use or operation of any methods, products, instructions, or ideas contained in the material herein.

Volume 3 ISBN: 978-1-4557-1054-6
Volume 3 Ebook ISBN: 978-1-4557-4047-5
Volume set ISBN: 978-1-4377-1733-4

ELSEVIER your source for books, journals and multimedia in the health sciences
www.elsevierhealth.com

Working together to grow
libraries in developing countries

www.elsevier.com | www.bookaid.org | www.sabre.org

ELSEVIER   BOOK AID International   Sabre Foundation

The publisher's policy is to use paper manufactured from sustainable forests

Printed in China
Last digit is the print number: 9 8 7 6 5 4 3 2 1

Contents

Foreword by Joseph G. McCarthy   xvi
Preface to the Third Edition   xvii
List of Contributors   xviii
Acknowledgments   xl
Dedication   xli

Volume One: Principles
Geoffrey C. Gurtner

1 Plastic surgery and innovation in medicine   1
Peter C. Neligan

2 History of reconstructive and aesthetic surgery   11
Riccardo F. Mazzola and Isabella C. Mazzola

3 Psychological aspects of plastic surgery   30
Laurie A. Stevens and Mary H. McGrath

4 The role of ethics in plastic surgery   55
Phillip C. Haeck

5 Business principles for plastic surgeons   64
C. Scott Hultman

6 Medico-legal issues in plastic surgery   92
Neal R. Reisman

7 Photography in plastic surgery   104
Brian M. Kinney

8 Patient safety in plastic surgery   124
Bruce Halperin

9 Local anesthetics in plastic surgery   137
A. Aldo Mottura

10 Evidence-based medicine and health services
research in plastic surgery   150
*Carolyn L. Kerrigan, E. Dale Collins Vidal,
Andrea L. Pusic, Amy K. Alderman, and
Valerie Lemaine*

11 Genetics and prenatal diagnosis   176
*Daniel Nowinski, Elizabeth Kiwanuka, Florian Hackl,
Bohdan Pomahac, and Elof Eriksson*

12 Principles of cancer management   201
Tomer Avraham, Evan Matros, and Babak J. Mehrara

13 Stem cells and regenerative medicine   212
*Benjamin Levi, Derrick C. Wan, Victor W. Wong,
Geoffrey C. Gurtner, and Michael T. Longaker*

14 Wound healing   240
Chandan K. Sen and Sashwati Roy

15 Skin wound healing: Repair biology, wound,
and scar treatment   267
*Ursula Mirastschijski, Andreas Jokuszies, and
Peter M. Vogt*

16 Scar prevention, treatment, and revision   297
Peter Lorenz and A. Sina Bari

17 Skin graft   319
*Saja S. Scherer-Pietramaggiori, Giorgio Pietramaggiori,
and Dennis P. Orgill*

18 Tissue graft, tissue repair, and regeneration 339
Wei Liu and Yilin Cao

19 Tissue engineering   367
Andrea J. O'Connor and Wayne A. Morrison

20 Repair, grafting, and engineering of cartilage 397
Wei Liu and Yilin Cao

21 Repair and grafting of bone   425
Iris A. Seitz, Chad M. Teven, and Russell R. Reid

22 Repair and grafting of peripheral nerve   464
*Renata V. Weber, Kirsty U. Boyd, and
Susan E. Mackinnon*

23 Vascular territories   479
Steven F. Morris and G. Ian Taylor

24 Flap classification and applications   512
*Scott L. Hansen, David M. Young, Patrick Lang,
and Hani Sbitany*

25 Flap pathophysiology and pharmacology   573
Cho Y. Pang and Peter C. Neligan

26 Principles and techniques of microvascular
surgery   587
Fu-Chan Wei and Sherilyn Keng Lin Tay

27 Principles and applications of tissue
expansion   622
Malcolm W. Marks and Louis C. Argenta

28 Therapeutic radiation: Principles, effects,
and complications   654
Gabrielle M. Kane

29 Vascular anomalies   676
Arin K. Greene and John B. Mulliken

30 Benign and malignant nonmelanocytic
tumors of the skin and soft tissue   707
Rei Ogawa

31 Melanoma   743
Stephan Ariyan and Aaron Berger

32 Implants and biomaterials   786
Charles E. Butler and Timothy W. King

33 Facial prosthetics in plastic surgery   798
*Gordon H. Wilkes, Mohammed M. Al Kahtani, and
Johan F. Wolfaardt*

34 Transplantation in plastic surgery   814
*David W. Mathes, Peter E. M. Butler, and
W. P. Andrew Lee*

35 Technology innovation in plastic surgery:
A practical guide for the surgeon innovator   841
Leila Jazayeri and Geoffrey C. Gurtner

36 Robotics, simulation, and telemedicine in
plastic surgery   854
Joseph M. Rosen, Todd E. Burdette, Erin Donaldson,
Robyn Mosher, Lindsay B. Katona, and
Sarah A. Long

Volume Two: Aesthetic
Richard J. Warren

1 Managing the cosmetic patient   1
Michelle B. Locke and Foad Nahai

Section I: Aesthetic Surgery of the Face

2 Nonsurgical skin care and rejuvenation   13
Leslie Baumann

3 Botulinum toxin (BoNT-A)   30
Michael A.C. Kane

4 Soft-tissue fillers   44
Trevor M. Born, Lisa E. Airan, and Dimitrios Motakis

5 Facial skin resurfacing   60
Steven R. Cohen, Ryan C. Frank, and E. Victor Ross

6 Anatomy of the aging face   78
Bryan Mendelson and Chin-Ho Wong

7 Forehead rejuvenation   93
Richard J. Warren

8 Blepharoplasty   108
Julius Few Jr. and Marco Ellis

9 Secondary blepharoplasty: Techniques   138
Glenn W. Jelks, Elizabeth B. Jelks, Ernest S. Chiu,
and Douglas S. Steinbrech

10 Asian facial cosmetic surgery   163
Kyung S. Koh, Jong Woo Choi, and Clyde H. Ishii

11.1 Facelift: Principles   184
Richard J. Warren

11.2 Facelift: Introduction to deep tissue
techniques   208
Richard J. Warren

11.3 Facelift: Platysma-SMAS plication   216
Dai M. Davies and Miles G. Berry

11.4 Facelift: Facial rejuvenation with loop sutures,
the MACS lift and its derivatives   223
Mark Laurence Jewell

11.5 Facelift: Lateral SMASectomy   232
Daniel C. Baker

11.6 Facelift: The extended SMAS technique in
facial rejuvenation   238
James M. Stuzin

11.7 Facelift: SMAS with skin attached – the
"high SMAS" technique   257
Fritz E. Barton Jr.

11.8 Facelift: Subperiosteal facelift   266
Oscar M. Ramirez

12 Secondary deformities and the secondary
facelift   277
Timothy J. Marten and Dino Elyassnia

13 Neck rejuvenation   313
James E. Zins, Colin Myles Morrison, and
Claude-Jean Langevin

14 Structural fat grafting   327
Sydney R. Coleman and Alesia P. Saboeiro

15 Skeletal augmentation   339
Michael J. Yaremchuk

16 Anthropometry, cephalometry, and
orthognathic surgery   354
Daniel I. Taub, Jordan M.S. Jacobs, and
Jonathan S. Jacobs

17 Nasal analysis and anatomy   373
Joel E. Pessa and Rod J. Rohrich

18 Open technique rhinoplasty   387
Rod J. Rohrich and Jamil Ahmad

19 Closed technique rhinoplasty   413
Mark B. Constantian

20 Airway issues and the deviated nose   450
Bahman Guyuron and Bryan S. Armijo

21 Secondary rhinoplasty   466
Ronald P. Gruber, Simeon H. Wall Jr.,
David L. Kaufman, and David M. Kahn

22 Otoplasty   485
Charles H. Thorne

23 Hair restoration   494
Jack Fisher

Section II: General Aesthetic Surgery

24 Liposuction: A comprehensive review of
techniques and safety   507
Jeffrey M. Kenkel and Phillip J. Stephan

25 Abdominoplasty procedures   530
Dirk F. Richter and Alexander Stoff

26 Lipoabdominoplasty   559
Osvaldo Ribeiro Saldanha,
Sérgio Fernando Dantas de Azevedo,
Osvaldo Ribeiro Saldanha Filho,
Cristianna Bonneto Saldanha, and
Luis Humberto Uribe Morelli

27 Lower bodylifts   568
Al Aly, Khalid Al-Zahrani, and Albert Cram

28 Buttock augmentation   599
Terrence W. Bruner, José Abel de la Peña Salcedo,
Constantino G. Mendieta, and Thomas L. Roberts III

29 Upper limb contouring   617
Joseph F. Capella, Matthew J. Trovato, and
Scott Woehrle

30 Post-bariatric reconstruction   634
Jonathan W. Toy and J. Peter Rubin

31 Aesthetic genital surgery   655
Gary J. Alter

Volume Three: Craniofacial, Head and Neck Surgery and Pediatric Plastic Surgery

Part 1: Craniofacial, head and neck surgery: Eduardo D. Rodriguez

1 Anatomy of the head and neck   3
Ahmed M. Afifi and Risal Djohan

Section I: Craniofacial Trauma

2 Facial trauma: Soft tissue injuries   23
Reid V. Mueller

3 Facial fractures   49
Eduardo D. Rodriguez, Amir H. Dorafshar,
and Paul N. Manson

4 TMJ dysfunction and obstructive sleep apnea   89
Stephen A. Schendel and Brinda Thimmappa

Section II: Head and Neck Reconstruction

5 Scalp and forehead reconstruction   105
Mark D. Wells and Carla Skytta

6 Aesthetic nasal reconstruction   134
Frederick J. Menick

7 Reconstruction of the ear   187
Burton D. Brent

8 Acquired cranial and facial bone deformities   226
Renee M. Burke, Robert J. Morin,
and S. Anthony Wolfe

9 Midface reconstruction   243
Constance M. Chen, Joseph J. Disa,
and Peter G. Cordeiro

10 Cheek and lip reconstruction   254
Peter C. Neligan

11 Facial paralysis   278
Ronald M. Zuker, Eyal Gur, Gazi Hussain,
and Ralph T. Manktelow

12 Oral cavity, tongue, and mandibular
reconstructions   307
Ming-Huei Cheng and Jung-Ju Huang

13 Hypopharyngeal, esophageal, and neck
reconstruction   336
Peirong Yu

14 Salivary gland tumors   360
Stephan Ariyan, Deepak Narayan, and
Charlotte E. Ariyan

15 Tumors of the facial skeleton: Fibrous
dysplasia   380
You-Wei Cheong and Yu-Ray Chen

16 Tumors of the lips, oral cavity, oropharynx,
and mandible   398
John Joseph Coleman III and Anthony P. Tufaro

17 Carcinoma of the upper aerodigestive tract   420
Michael E. Kupferman, Justin M. Sacks,
and Edward I. Chang

18 Local flaps for facial coverage   440
Ian T. Jackson

19 Secondary facial reconstruction   461
Julian J. Pribaz and Rodney K. Chan

20 Facial transplant   473
Laurent Lantieri

21 Surgical management of migraine headaches   491
Bahman Guyuron and Ali Totonchi

Part 2: Pediatric plastic surgery: Joseph E. Losee

Section I: Clefts

22 Embryology of the craniofacial complex   503
Maryam Afshar, Samantha A. Brugmann,
and Jill A. Helms

23 Repair of unilateral cleft lip   517
Philip Kuo-Ting Chen, M. Samuel Noordhoff,
and Alex Kane

24 Repair of bilateral cleft lip   550
John B. Mulliken

25 Cleft palate   569
William Y. Hoffman

26 Alveolar clefts   584
Richard A. Hopper

27 Orthodontics in cleft lip and palate
management   595
Alvaro A. Figueroa and John W. Polley

28 Velopharyngeal dysfunction   614
Richard E. Kirschner and Adriane L. Baylis

29 Secondary deformities of the cleft lip, nose,
and palate   631
Evan M. Feldman, John C. Koshy, Larry H. Hollier Jr.,
and Samuel Stal

30 Cleft and craniofacial orthognathic surgery   655
Jesse A. Goldstein and Steven B. Baker

Section II: Craniofacial

31 Pediatric facial fractures   671
Joseph E. Losee and Darren M. Smith

32 Orbital hypertelorism   686
Eric Arnaud, Daniel Marchac, Federico Di Rocco,
and Dominique Renier

33 Craniofacial clefts   701
James P. Bradley and Henry K. Kawamoto Jr.

34 Nonsyndromic craniosynostosis   726
Derek M. Steinbacher and Scott P. Bartlett

35 Syndromic craniosynostosis   749
Jeffrey A. Fearon

36 Craniofacial microsomia   761
Joseph G. McCarthy, Barry H. Grayson,
Richard A. Hopper, and Oren M. Tepper

37 Hemifacial atrophy   792
Peter J. Taub, Lester Silver, and Kathryn S.Torok

38 Pierre Robin sequence   803
Christopher G. Zochowski and Arun K. Gosain

39 Treacher–Collins syndrome   828
Fernando Molina

Section III: Pediatrics

40 Congenital melanocytic nevi   837
Bruce S. Bauer and Neta Adler

41 Pediatric chest and trunk defects   855
*Lawrence J. Gottlieb, Russell R. Reid, and
Justine C. Lee*

42 Pediatric tumors   877
Sahil Kapur and Michael L. Bentz

43 Conjoined twins   893
Oksana Jackson, David W. Low and Don LaRossa

44 Reconstruction of urogenital defects:
Congenital   906
Mohan S. Gundeti and Michael C. Large

Volume Four: Lower Extremity, Trunk and Burns

David Song

Section I: Lower Extremity Surgery

1 Comprehensive lower extremity anatomy   1
Ginard I. Henry and Grant M. Kleiber

2 Management of lower extremity trauma   63
Shannon Colohan and Michel Saint-Cyr

3 Lymphatic reconstruction of the extremities   92
*Ruediger G. H. Baumeister, David W. Chang,
and Peter C. Neligan*

4 Lower extremity sarcoma reconstruction   101
Goetz A.Giessler and Michael Sauerbier

5 Reconstructive surgery: Lower extremity
coverage   127
Joon Pio Hong

6 Diagnosis and treatment of painful neuroma and
of nerve compression in the lower extremity   151
A. Lee Dellon

7 Skeletal reconstruction   174
Stephen J. Kovach and L. Scott Levin

8 Foot reconstruction   189
*Mark W. Clemens, Lawrence B. Colen,
and Christopher E. Attinger*

Section II: Trunk Surgery

9 Comprehensive trunk anatomy   220
Michael A. Howard and Sara R. Dickie

10 Reconstruction of the chest   239
David H. Song and Michelle C. Roughton

11 Reconstruction of the soft tissues of the back   256
Gregory A. Dumanian

12 Abdominal wall reconstruction   279
*Navin K. Singh, Marwan R. Khalifeh,
and Jonathan Bank*

13 Reconstruction of male genital defects   297
*Stan Monstrey, Peter Ceulemans, Nathalie Roche,
Philippe Houtmeyers, Nicolas Lumen, and Piet Hoebeke*

14 Reconstruction of acquired vaginal defects   326
Laura Snell, Peter G. Cordeiro, and Andrea L. Pusic

15 Surgery for gender identity disorder   336
Loren S. Schechter

16 Pressure sores   352
Robert Kwon and Jeffrey E. Janis

17 Perineal reconstruction   383
Hakim K. Said and Otway Louie

Section III: Burns Surgery

18 Acute management of burn/electrical injuries   393
Lars Steinstraesser and Sammy Al-Benna

19 Extremity burn reconstruction   435
*Lorenzo Borghese, Alessandro Masellis, and
Michele Masellis*

20 Cold and chemical injury to the upper
extremity   456
Dennis S. Kao and John Hijjawi

21 Management of facial burns   468
Robert J. Spence

22 Reconstructive burn surgery   500
Matthew B. Klein

23 Management of patients with exfoliative
disorders, epidermolysis bullosa, and TEN   511
Abdullah E. Kattan, Robert C. Cartotto, and Joel S. Fish

Volume Five: Breast

James C. Grotting

1 Anatomy for plastic surgery of the breast   1
Jorge I. de la Torre and Michael R. Davis

Section I: Cosmetic Surgery of the Breast

2 Breast augmentation   13
G. Patrick Maxwell and Allen Gabriel

3 Secondary breast augmentation   39
Mitchell H. Brown

4 Current concepts in revisionary breast surgery   67
G. Patrick Maxwell and Allen Gabriel

5 Endoscopic approaches to the breast   81
Neil A. Fine and Clark F. Schierle

6 Iatrogenic disorders following breast surgery   97
Walter Peters

7 Mastopexy   119
Kent K. Higdon and James C. Grotting

8.1 Reduction mammaplasty   152
Jack Fisher and Kent K. Higdon

8.2 Inferior pedicle breast reduction   165
Jack Fisher

8.3 Superior or medial pedicle   177
Frank Lista and Jamil Ahmad

8.4 Short scar periareolar inferior pedicle reduction
(SPAIR) mammaplasty   194
Dennis C. Hammond

8.5 The L short-scar mammaplasty   206
Armando Chiari Jr.

8.6 Periareolar technique with mesh support   216
Joao Carlos Sampaio Góes

8.7 Sculpted pillar vertical reduction mammaplasty   228
Kent K. Higdon and James C. Grotting

9 Revision surgery following breast reduction
and mastopexy   242
Kenneth C. Shestak

Section II: Reconstructive Surgery of the Breast

10 Breast cancer: Diagnosis therapy and
oncoplastic techniques   266
Elisabeth Beahm and Julie E. Lang

11 The oncoplastic approach to partial breast
reconstruction   296
Albert Losken

12 Patient-centered health communication   314
Gary L. Freed, Alice Andrews, and E. Dale Collins Vidal

13 Imaging in reconstructive breast surgery   326
Jaume Masia, Carmen Navarro, and Juan A. Clavero

14 Expander-implants breast reconstruction   336
*Maurizio B. Nava, Giuseppe Catanuto, Angela Pennati,
Valentina Visintini Cividin, and Andrea Spano*

15 Latissimus dorsi flap breast reconstruction   370
Scott L. Spear and Mark W. Clemens

16 The bilateral pedicled TRAM flap   393
*L. Franklyn Elliott, John D. Symbas, and
Hunter R. Moyer*

17 Free TRAM breast reconstruction   411
Joshua Fosnot and Joseph M. Serletti

18 The deep inferior epigastric artery perforator
(DIEAP) flap   435
*Phillip N. Blondeel, Colin M. Morrison, and
Robert J. Allen*

19 Alternative flaps for breast reconstruction   457
*Maria M. LoTempio, Robert J. Allen, and
Phillip N. Blondeel*

20 Omentum reconstruction of the breast   472
*Joao Carlos Sampaio Góes and Antonio Luiz
Vasconcellos Macedo*

21 Local flaps in partial breast reconstruction   482
Moustapha Hamdi and Eugenia J. Kyriopoulos

22 Reconstruction of the nipple-areola complex   499
Ketan M. Patel and Maurice Y. Nahabedian

23.1 Congenital anomalies of the breast   521
Egle Muti

23.2 Poland syndrome   548
Pietro Berrino and Valeria Berrino

24 Contouring of the arms, breast, upper trunk, and
male chest in the massive weight loss patient   558
Jonathan W. Toy and J. Peter Rubin

25 Fat grafting to the breast   582
Henry Wilson and Scott L. Spear

Volume Six: Hand and Upper Extremity

James Chang

Introduction: Plastic surgery contributions
to hand surgery   xxxvii
James Chang

Section I: Introduction and Principles

1 Anatomy and biomechanics of the hand   1
*James Chang, Francisco Valero-Cuevas,
Vincent R. Hentz, and Robert A. Chase*

2 Examination of the upper extremity   47
Ryosuke Kakinoki

3 Diagnostic imaging of the hand and wrist   68
Alphonsus K. Chong and David M.K. Tan

4 Anesthesia for upper extremity surgery   92
Jonay Hill, Vanila M. Singh and Subhro K. Sen

5 Principles of internal fixation as applied to
the hand and wrist   106
Jeffrey Yao and Christopher Cox

Section II: Acquired Traumatic Disorders

6 Nail and fingertip reconstruction   117
*Michael W. Neumeister, Elvin G. Zook,
Nicole Z. Sommer, and Theresa A. Hegge*

7 Hand fractures and joint injuries   138
Warren C. Hammert

8 Fractures and dislocations of the wrist and
distal radius   161
Kevin C. Chung and Steven C. Haase

9 Flexor tendon injury and reconstruction   178
Jin Bo Tang

10 Extensor tendon injuries   210
Kai Megerle and Günther Germann

11 Replantation and revascularization   228
William W. Dzwierzynski

12 Reconstructive surgery of the mutilated hand   250
William C. Pederson and Randolph Sherman

13 Thumb reconstruction: Nonmicrosurgical
techniques   282
Nicholas B. Vedder and Jeffrey B. Friedrich

14 Thumb and finger reconstruction: Microsurgical
techniques   295
Fu Chan Wei and Wee Leon Lam

Section III: Acquired Nontraumatic Disorders

15 Benign and malignant tumors of the hand   311
*Justin M. Sacks, Kodi K. Azari, Scott Oates,
and David W. Chang*

16 Infections of the hand   333
Sean M. Bidic and Tim Schaub

17 Management of Dupuytren's disease   346
Andrew J. Watt and Caroline Leclercq

18 Occupational hand disorders   363
Steven J. McCabe

19 Rheumatologic conditions of the hand
and wrist   371
Douglas M. Sammer and Kevin C. Chung

20 Osteoarthritis in the hand and wrist   411
*Brian T. Carlsen, Karim Bakri, Faisal M. Al-Mufarrej
and Steven L. Moran*

21 The stiff hand and the spastic hand   449
David T. Netscher

22 Ischemia of the hand   467
Hee Chang Ahn and Neil F. Jones

23 Complex regional pain syndrome in the upper
extremity   486
Ivica Ducic and John M. Felder III

24 Nerve entrapment syndromes   503
*Michael Bezuhly, James P. O'Brien and
Donald Lalonde*

Section IV: Congenital Disorders

25 Congenital hand I: Embryology, classification,
and principles   526
Michael Tonkin and Kerby Oberg

26 Congenital hand II: Disorders of formation
(transverse and longitudinal arrest)   548
Gill Smith and Paul Smith

27 Congenital hand III: Disorders of formation –
thumb hypoplasia   572
Joseph Upton III and Amir Taghinia

28 Congenital hand IV: Disorders of differentiation
and duplication   603
Steven E.R. Hovius

29 Congenital hand V: Disorders of overgrowth,
undergrowth, and generalized skeletal
deformities   634
*Leung Kim Hung, Ping Chung Leung, and
Takayuki Miura (Addendum by Michael Tonkin)*

30 Growth considerations in pediatric upper
extremity trauma and reconstruction   651
Marco Innocenti and Carla Baldrighi

31 Vascular anomalies of the upper extremity   667
Joseph Upton III

Section V: Paralytic Disorders

32 Peripheral nerve injuries of the upper
extremity   694
Simon Farnebo, Johan Thorfinn, and Lars B. Dahlin

33 Nerve transfers   719
Kirsty U. Boyd, Ida K. Fox, and Susan E. Mackinnon

34 Tendon transfers in the upper extremity   745
Neil F. Jones

35 Free-functioning muscle transfer in
the upper extremity   777
Isaac Harvey and Gregory H. Borschel

36 Brachial plexus injuries: Adult and pediatric 789
David Chwei-Chin Chuang

37 Restoration of upper extremity function in
tetraplegia   817
Catherine Curtin and Vincent R. Hentz

Section VI: Rehabilitation

38 Upper extremity composite allotransplantation 843
*Vijay S. Gorantla, Stefan S. Schneeberger,
and W.P. Andrew Lee*

39 Hand therapy   855
Christine B. Novak and Rebecca L. von der Heyde

40 Treatment of the upper extremity amputee   870
Gregory A. Dumanian and Todd A. Kuiken

Index to all volumes   *i1–i204*

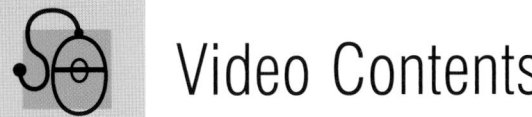

Video Contents

Volume One:

No Video

Volume Two:

Chapter 3: Botulinum Toxin

3.01 Botulinum toxin
Allen L. Van Beek

3.02 Botulinum toxin
Bahman Guyuron
From Plastic Surgery: Indications and Practice, Guyuron, 2009, with permission from Elsevier.

Chapter 4: Soft Tissue Fillers

4.01 Soft tissue fillers
Allen L. Van Beek

Chapter 5: Facial Skin Resurfacing

5.01 Chemical peel
Allen L. Van Beek

5.02 Facial resurfacing
Thomas E. Rohrer
From Plastic Surgery: Indications and Practice, Guyuron, 2009, with permission from Elsevier.

Chapter 7: Forehead Rejuvenation

7.01 Modified lateral brow lift
Richard J. Warren

Chapter 8: Blepharoplasty

8.01 Periorbital rejuvenation
Julius Few Jr. and Marco Ellis

Chapter 10: Asian Facial Cosmetic Surgery

10.01 Eyelidplasty: non-incisional method
10.02 Eyelidplasty: incisional method
Hong-Lim Choi and Tae-Joo Ahn

10.03 Secondary rhinoplasty: septal extension graft and costal cartilage strut fixed with K-wire
Jae-Hoon Kim

Chapter 11.01: Facelift Principles

11.01.01 Parotid masseteric fascia
11.01.02 Anterior incision
11.01.03 Posterior incision
11.01.04 Facelift skin flap
11.01.05 Facial fat injection
Richard J. Warren

Chapter 11.03: Platysma-SMAS Plication

11.03.01 Platysma SMAS plication
Dai M. Davies and Miles G. Berry

Chapter 11.04: Facial Rejuvenation with Loop Sutures; The Macs Lift And Its Derivatives

11.04.01 Loop sutures MACS facelift
Patrick L. Tonnard
From Aesthetic Plastic Surgery, Aston, 2009, with permission from Elsevier.

Chapter 11.06: The Extended SMAS Technique in Facial Rejuvenation

11.06.01 Extended SMAS technique in facial shaping
James M. Stuzin

Chapter 11.07: SMAS with Skin Attached: The High SMAS Technique

11.07.01 The high SMAS technique with septal reset
Fritz E. Barton, Jr.

Chapter 11.08 Subperiosteal Facelift

11.08.01 Facelift – Subperiosteal mid facelift endoscopic temporo-midface
Oscar M. Ramirez

Chapter 14: Structural Fat Grafting

14.01 Structural fat grafting of the face
Sydney R. Coleman and Alesia P. Saboeiro

Chapter 15: Skeletal Augmentation

15.01 Midface skeletal augmentation and rejuvenation
Michael J. Yaremchuk

Chapter 16: Anthropometry, Cephalometry, and Orthognathic Surgery

16.01 Anthropometry, cephalometry, and orthognathic surgery
Jonathon S. Jacobs, Jordan M. S. Jacobs, and Daniel I. Taub

Chapter 18: Open Technique Rhinoplasty

18.01 Open technique rhinopalsty
Allen L. Van Beek

Chapter 22: Otoplasty

22.01 Setback otoplasty
Leila Kasrai

Chapter 23: Hair Restoration

23.01 Donor closure tricophytic technique
From Procedures in Cosmetic Dermatology Series: Hair Transplantation, Haber and Stough, 2005, with permission from Elsevier.

23.02 Follicular unit hair transplantation
From Surgery of the Skin, 2nd edition, Robinson JK et al, 2010, with permission from Elsevier.

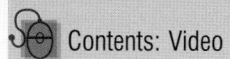
23.03 Follicular unit transplantation
From Procedures in Cosmetic Dermatology Series: Hair Transplantation, Haber and Stough, 2005, with permission from Elsevier.

23.04 FUE FOX procedure
From Procedures in Cosmetic Dermatology Series: Hair Transplantation, Haber and Stough, 2005, with permission from Elsevier.

23.05 FUE Harris safe system
From Procedures in Cosmetic Dermatology Series: Hair Transplantation, Haber and Stough, 2005, with permission from Elsevier.

23.06 Hair transplantation
From Surgery of the Skin, 2nd edition, Robinson JK et al, 2010, with permission from Elsevier.

23.07 Perpendicular angle grafting technique
23.08 Strip harvesting the haber spreader
23.09 Tension donor dissection
From Procedures in Cosmetic Dermatology Series: Hair Transplantation, Haber and Stough, 2005, with permission from Elsevier.

Chapter 24: Liposuction

24.01 Liposculpture
Fabio X. Nahas

From Plastic Surgery: Indications and Practice, Guyuron, 2009, with permission from Elsevier.

Chapter 25: Abdominoplasty

25.01 Abdominoplasty
Dirk F. Richter and Alexander Stoff

Chapter 26: Lipoabdominoplasty

26.01 Lipobdominoplasty (including secondary lipo)
Osvaldo Ribeiro Saldanha, Sérgio Fernando Dantas de Azevedo, Osvaldo Ribeiro Saldanha Filho, Cristianna Bonneto Saldanha, and Luis Humberto Uribe Morelli

Chapter 28: Buttock Augmentation

28.01 Buttock augmentation
Terrence W. Bruner, José Abel de la Peña Salcedo, Constantino G. Mendieta, and Thomas L. Roberts

Chapter 29: Upper Limb Contouring

29.01 Upper limb contouring
Joseph F. Capella, Matthew Trovato and Scott Woehrle

Chapter 30: Post Bariatric Surgery Reconstruction

30.01 Post bariatric reconstruction – bodylift procedure
J. Peter Rubin

Volume Three:

Chapter 6: Aesthetic reconstruction of the Nose

6.01 The 3-stage folded forehead flap for cover and lining
6.02 First stage transfer and intermediate operation
Frederick J. Menick

Chapter 7: Reconstruction of the Ear

7.01 Microtia: auricular reconstruction
Akira Yamada

From Plastic Surgery: Indications and Practice, Guyuron, 2009, with permission from Elsevier.

7.02 Reconstruction of acquired ear deformities
Sean G. Boutros

From Plastic Surgery: Indications and Practice, Guyuron, 2009, with permission from Elsevier.

Chapter 8: Acquired Cranial and Facial Bone Deformities

8.01 Removal of venous malformation enveloping intraconal optic nerve
S. Anthony Wolfe and Renee M. Burke

Chapter 11: Facial Paralysis

11.01 Facial paralysis
Eyal Gur

11.02 Facial paralysis
11.03 Cross face graft
11.04 Gracilis harvest
Peter C. Neligan

Chapter 12: Oral Cavity, Tongue, and Mandibular Reconstructions

12.01 Fibula osteoseptocutaneous flap for composite mandibular reconstruction
12.02 Ulnar forearm flap for buccal reconstruction
Ming-Huei Cheng and Jung-Ju Huang

Chapter 13: Hypopharyngeal, Esophageal, and Neck Reconstruction

13.01 Reconstruction of pharyngoesophageal defects with the anterolateral thigh flap
Peirong Yu

Chapter 18: Local Flaps for Facial Coverage

18.01 Facial artery perforator flap
18.02 Local flaps for facial coverage
Peter C. Neligan

Chapter 20: Facial Transplant

20.01 Facial transplant
Laurent Lantieri

Chapter 23: Repair of Unilateral Cleft Lip

23.01 Repair of unilateral cleft lip
Philip Kuo-Ting Chen, M. Samuel Noordhoff, Frank Chun-Shin, Chang and Fuan Chiang Chan

23.02 Unilateral cleft lip repair – anatomic subumit approximation technique
David M. Fisher

Chapter 24: Repair of Bilateral Cleft Lip

24.01 Repair of bilateral cleft lip
Barry H. Grayson

Chapter 28: Velopharyngeal Dysfunction

28.01 Velopharyngeal incompetence-1
28.02 Velopharyngeal incompetence-2
28.03 Velopharyngeal incompetence-3
Richard E. Kirschner and Adriane L. Baylis

Chapter 29: Secondary Deformities of the Cleft Lip, Nose, and Palate

29.01 Complete takedown
29.02 Abbé flap
Evan M. Feldman, John C. Koshy, Larry H. Hollier Jr. and Samuel Stal

29.03 Thick lip and buccal sulcus deformities
Evan M. Feldman and John C. Koshy

29.04 Alveolar bone grafting
29.05 Definitive rhinoplasty

Chapter 44: Reconstruction of Urogenital Defects: Congenital

44.01 First stage hypospadias repair with free inner preputial graft
44.02 Second stage hypospadias repair with tunica vaginalis flap
Mohan S. Gundeti and Michael C. Large

Volume Four:

Chapter 2: Management of Lower Extremity Trauma

2.01 Alternative flap harvest
Michel Saint-Cyr

Chapter 3: Lymphatic Reconstruction of the Extremities

3.01 Lymphatico-venous anastomosis
David W. Chang

3.02 Charles Procedure
Peter C. Neligan

Chapter 4: Lower Extremity Sarcoma Reconstruction

4.01 Management of lower extremity sarcoma reconstruction
Goetz A. Giessler and Michael Sauerbier

Chapter 6: Diagnosis and Treatment of Painful Neuroma and of Nerve Compression in the Lower Extremity

6.01 Diagnosis and treatment of painful neuroma and of nerve compression in the lower extremity 1
6.02 Diagnosis and treatment of painful neuroma and of nerve compression in the lower extremity 2
6.03 Diagnosis and treatment of painful neuroma and of nerve compression in the lower extremity 3
A. Lee Dellon

Chapter 10: Reconstruction of the Chest

10.01 Rigid fixation
David H. Song and Michelle C. Roughton

Chapter 12: Abdominal Wall Reconstruction

12.01 Component separation innovation
Peter C. Neligan

Chapter 13: Reconstruction of Male Genital Defects

13.01 Complete and partial penile reconstruction
Stan Monstrey, Peter Ceulemans, Nathalie Roche, Philippe Houtmeyers, Nicolas Lumen and Piet Hoebeke

Chapter 19: Extremity Burn Reconstruction

19.01 Extremity burn reconstruction
Lorenzo Borghese, Alessandro Masellis, and Michele Masellis

Chapter 21: Management of the Burned Face

21.01 Management of the burned face: full-thickness skin graft defatting technique
Robert J. Spence

Volume Five:

Chapter 4: Current Concepts in Revisionary Breast Surgery

4.01 Current concepts in revisionary breast surgery
Allen Gabriel

Chapter 5: Endoscopic Approaches to the Breast

5.01 Endoscopic transaxillary breast augmentation
5.02 Endoscopic approaches to the breast
Neil A. Fine

Chapter 7: Mastopexy

7.01 Circum areola mastopexy
Kenneth C. Shestak

Chapter 8.4: Short Scar Periareolar Inferior Pedicle Reduction (Spair) Mammaplasty

8.4.01 Spair technique
Dennis C. Hammond

Chapter 8.7: Sculpted Pillar Vertical Reduction Mammaplasty

8.7.01 Marking the sculpted pillar breast reduction
8.7.02 Breast reduction surgery
James C. Grotting

Chapter 10: Breast Cancer: Diagnosis Therapy and Oncoplastic Techniques

10.01 Breast cancer: diagnosis and therapy
Elizabeth Beahm and Julie E. Lang

Chapter 11: The Oncoplastic Approach to Partial Breast Reconstruction

11.01 Partial breast reconstruction using reduction mammaplasty
Maurice Y. Nahabedian

11.02 Partial breast reconstruction with a latissimus D
Neil A. Fine

11.03 Partial breast reconstruction with a pedicle TRAM
Maurice Y. Nahabedian

Chapter 14: Expander – Implant Reconstructions

14.01 Mastectomy and expander insertion: first stage
14.02 Mastectomy and expander insertion: second stage
Maurizio B. Nava, Giuseppe Catanuto, Angela Pennati, Valentina Visintini Cividin, and Andrea Spano

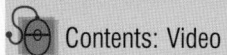

Chapter 15: Latissimus Dorsi Flap Breast Reconstruction

15.01 Latissimus dorsi flap tecnique
Scott L. Spear

Chapter 16: The Bilateral Pedicled TRAM Flap

16.01 Pedicle TRAM breast reconstruction
L. Franklyn Elliott and John D. Symbas

Chapter 17: Free TRAM Breast Reconstruction

17.01 The muscle sparing free TRAM flap
Joshua Fosnot, Joseph M. Serletti, and Jonas A Nelson

Chapter 18: The Deep Inferior Epigastric Artery Perforator (DIEAP) Flap

18.01 SIEA
Peter C. Neligan

18.02 DIEP flap breast reconstruction
Phillip N. Blondeel and Robert J. Allen

Chapter 19: Alternative Flaps for Breast Reconstruction

19.01 TUG
19.02 IGAP
19.03 SGAP
Peter C. Neligan

Chapter 23.1: Congenital Anomalies of the Breast

23.1.01 Congenital anomalies of the breast: An example of tuberous breast Type 1 corrected with glandular flap Type 1
Egle Muti

Chapter 24: Contouring of the Arms, Breast, Upper Trunk, and Male Chest in Massive Weight Loss Patient

24.01 Brachioplasty part 1: contouring of the arms
24.02 Brachioplasty part 2: contouring of the arms
J. Peter Rubin

24.03 Mastopexy
J. Peter Rubin

Volume Six:

Chapter 2: Examination of the Upper Extremity

2.01 Flexor profundus test in a normal long finger
2.02 Flexor sublimis test in a normal long finger
2.03 Extensor pollicis longus test in a normal person
2.04 Test for the extensor digitorum communis (EDC) muscle in a normal hand
2.05 Test for assessing thenar muscle function
2.06 The "cross fingers" sign
2.07 Static two point discrimination test (s-2PD test)
2.08 Moving 2PD test (m-2PD test) performed on the radial or ulnar aspect of the finger
2.09 Semmes-Weinstein monofilament test. The patient should sense the pressure produced by bending the filament
2.10 Allen's test in a normal person
2.11 Digital Allen's test
2.12 Scaphoid shift test

2.13 Dynamic tenodesis effect in a normal hand
2.14 The milking test of the fingers and thumb in a normal hand
2.15 Eichhoff test
2.16 Adson test
2.17 Roos test
Ryosuke Kakinoki

Chapter 3: Diagnostic Imaging of the Hand and Wrist

3.01 Scaphoid lunate dislocation
Alphonsus K. Chong and David M.K. Tan

Chapter 4: Anesthesia for Upper Extremity Surgery

4.01 Supraclavicular block
Subhro K. Sen

Chapter 5: Principles of Internal Fixation as Applied to the Hand and Wrist

5.01 Dynamic compression plating and lag screw technique
Christopher Cox

Chapter 8: Fractures and Dislocations of the Carpus and Distal Radius

8.01 Scaphoid fixation
Kevin C. Chung and Evan Kowalski

Chapter 9: Flexor Tendon Injury and Reconstruction

9.01 Zone II flexor tendon repair
Jin Bo Tang

Chapter 11: Replantation and Revascularization

11.01 Hand replantation
James Chang

Chapter 12: Reconstructive Surgery of the Mutilated Hand

12.01 Debridement technique
James Chang

Chapter 14: Thumb Reconstruction – Microsurgical Techniques

14.01 Trimmed great toe
14.02 Second toe for index finger
14.03 Combined second and third toe for metacarpal hand
Fu Chan Wei and Wee Leon Lam

Chapter 17: Management of Dupuytren's Disease

17.01 Dupuytren's disease dissection
Andrew J. Watt and Caroline Leclercq

Chapter 19: Rheumatologic Conditions of the Hand and Wrist

19.01 Extensor tendon rupture and end-side tendon transfer
James Chang

19.02 Silicone MCP arthroplasty
Kevin C. Chung and Evan Kowalski

Chapter 20: Management of Osteoarthritis in the Hand and Wrist

20.01 Ligament reconstruction tendon interposition arthroplasty of the thumb CMC joint
James W. Fletcher

Chapter 22: Ischemia of the Hand

22.01 Radial artery sympathectomy
22.02 Interposition arterial graft and sympathectomy
Hee Chang Ahn

Chapter 24: Nerve Entrapment Syndromes

24.01 Carpal tunnel and cubital tunnel releases in the same patient in one procedure with field sterility – Part 1: local anaesthetic injection for carpal tunnel
24.02 Part 2: local anaesthetic injection for cubital tunnel
24.03 Part 3: wide awake carpal tunnel surgery
24.04 Part 4: cubital tunnel surgery
Donald Lalonde and Michael Bezuhly

Chapter 27: Congenital Hand III: Disorders of Formation – Thumb Hypoplasia

27.01 Thumb hypoplasia
Joseph Upton III and Amir Taghinia

Chapter 29: Congenital Hand V: Disorders of Overgrowth, Undergrowth, and Generalized Skeletal Deformities

29.01 Addendum pediatric trigger thumb release
James Chang

Chapter 30: Growth Considerations in Pediatric Upper Extremity Trauma and Reconstruction

30.01 Epiphyseal transplant harvesting technique
Marco Innocenti and Carla Baldrighi

Chapter 31: Vascular Anomalies of the Upper Extremity

31.01 Excision of venous malformation
Joseph Upton III and Amir Taghinia

Chapter 32: Peripheral Nerve Injuries of the Upper Extremity

32.01 Suture repair of the cut digital nerve
32.02 Suture repair of the median nerve
Simon Farnebo and Johan Thorfinn

Chapter 33: Nerve Transfers

33.01 Scratch collapse test of ulnar nerve
33.02 Nerve transfers 2
33.03 Nerve transfers 3
Susan E. Mackinnon and Ida K. Fox

Chapter 34: Tendon Transfers in the Upper Extremity

34.01 EIP to EPL tendon transfer
Neil F. Jones, Gustavo Machado, and Surak Eo

Chapter 35: Free Functioning Muscle Transfer in the Upper Extremity

35.01 Gracilis functional muscle harvest
Gregory H. Borschel

Chapter 36: Brachial Plexus Injuries: Adult and Pediatric

36.01 Pediatric: shoulder correct and biceps-to-triceps transfer with preserving intact brachialis
36.02 Adult: results of one stage surgery for c5 rupture, c6-t1 root avulsion ten years after
David Chwei-Chin Chuang

Chapter 37: Restoration of Upper Extremity Function in Tetraplegia

37.01 1 Stage grasp IC 6 short term
37.02 2 Stage grasp release outcome
Catherine Curtin and Vincent R. Hentz

Chapter 38: Upper Extremity Composite Allotransplantation

38.01 Upper extremity composite tissue allotransplantation
W. P. Andrew Lee and Vijay S. Gorantla

Chapter 39: Hand Therapy

39.01 Goniometric measurement
39.02 Threshold testing
39.03 Fabrication of a synergistic splint
Rebecca L. Von Der Heyde

Chapter 40: Treatment of the Upper-Extremity Amputee

40.01 Targeted muscle reinnervation in the transhumeral amputee – surgical technique and guidelines for restoring intuitive neural control
Gregory A. Dumanian and Todd A. Kuiken

Foreword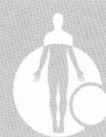

In many ways, a textbook defines a particular discipline, and this is especially true in the evolution of modern plastic surgery. The publication of Zeis's *Handbuch der Plastischen Chirurgie* in 1838 popularized the name of the specialty but von Graefe in his monograph *Rhinoplastik*, published in 1818, had first used the title "plastic". At the turn of the last century, Nélaton and Ombredanne compiled what was available in the nineteenth century literature and published in Paris a two volume text in 1904 and 1907. A pivotal book, published across the Atlantic, was that of Vilray Blair, entitled *Surgery and Diseases of the Jaws* (1912). It was, however, limited to a specific anatomic region of the human body, but it became an important handbook for the military surgeons of World War I. Gillies' classic *Plastic Surgery of the Face* (1920) was also limited to a single anatomic region and recapitulated his remarkable and pioneering World War I experience with reconstructive plastic surgery of the face. Davis' textbook, *Plastic Surgery: Its Principles and Practice* (1919), was probably the first comprehensive definition of this young specialty with its emphasis on plastic surgery as ranging from the "top of the head to the soles of the feet." Fomon's *The Surgery of Injury and Plastic Repair* (1939) reviewed all of the plastic surgery techniques available at that time, and it also served as a handbook for the military surgeons of World War II. Kazanjian and Converse's *The Surgical Treatment of Facial Injuries* (1949) was a review of the former's lifetime experience as a plastic surgeon, and the junior author's World War II experience. The comprehensive plastic surgery text entitled *Plastic and Reconstructive Surgery*, published in 1948 by Padgett and Stephenson, was modeled more on the 1919 Davis text.

The lineage of the Neligan text began with the publication of Converse's five volume *Reconstructive Plastic Surgery* in 1964. Unlike his co-authored book with Kazanjian 15 years earlier, Converse undertook a comprehensive view of plastic surgery as the specialty existed in mid-20th century. Chapters were also devoted to pertinent anatomy, research and the role of relevant specialties like anesthesiology and radiology. It immediately became the bible of the specialty. He followed up with a second edition published in 1977, and I was the Assistant Editor. The second edition had grown from five to seven volumes (3970 pages) because the specialty had also grown. I edited the 1990 edition which had grown to eight volumes and 5556 pages; the hand section was edited by J. William Littler and James W. May. I changed the name of the text from *Reconstructive Plastic Surgery* to *Plastic Surgery* because in my mind I could not fathom the distinction between both titles. To the mother of a child with cleft lip, the surgery is "cosmetic," and many of the facelift procedures at that time were truly reconstructive because of the multiple layers at which the facial soft tissues were being readjusted. The late Steve Mathes edited the 2006 edition in eight volumes. He changed the format somewhat and V.R. Hentz was the hand editor. At that time, the text had grown to more than 7000 pages.

The education of the plastic surgeon and the reference material that is critically needed are no longer limited to the printed page or what is described in modern parlance as "hard copy". Certainly, Gutenberg's invention of movable type printing around 1439 allowed publication and distribution of the classic texts of Vesalius (*Fabrica*, 1543) and Tagliacozzi (*De Curtorum Chirurgia Per Insitionem* (1597) and for many years, this was the only medium in which surgeons could be educated. However, by the nineteenth century, travel had become easier with the development of reliable railroads and oceangoing ships, and surgeons conscientiously visited different surgical centers and attended organized meetings. The American College of Surgeons after World War II pioneered the use of operating room movies, and this was followed by videos. The development of the internet has, however, placed almost all information at the fingertips of surgeons around the world with computer access. In turn, we now have virtual surgery education in which the student or surgeon sitting at a computer is interactive with a software program containing animations, intraoperative videos with sound overlay, and access to the world literature on a particular subject. We are rapidly progressing from the bound book of the Gutenberg era to the currently ubiquitous hand held device or tablet for the mastery of surgical/knowledge.

The Neligan text continues this grand tradition of surgical education by bringing the reader into the modern communications world. In line with advances of the electronic era, there is extra online content such as relevant history, complete reference lists and videos. The book is also available as an e-book. It has been a monumental task, consuming hours of work by the editor and all of its participants. The "text" still defines the specialty of plastic surgery. Moreover, it ensures that a new generation of plastic surgeons will have access to all that is known. They, in turn, will not only carry this information into the future but will also build on it. Kudos to Peter Neligan and his colleagues for continuing the chronicle of the plastic surgery saga that has been evolving over two millennia.

Joseph G. McCarthy, MD
2012

Preface

I have always loved textbooks. When I first started my training I was introduced to Converse's *Reconstructive Plastic Surgery*, then in its second edition. I was over-awed by the breadth of the specialty and the expertise contained within its pages. As a young plastic surgeon in practice I bought the first edition of this book, *Plastic Surgery*, edited by Dr. Joseph McCarthy and found it an invaluable resource to which I constantly referred. I was proud to be asked to contribute a chapter to the second edition, edited by Dr. Stephen Mathes and never thought that I would one day be given the responsibility for editing the next edition of the book. I consider this to be the definitive text on our specialty so I took that responsibility very seriously. The result is a very changed book from the previous edition, reflecting changes in the specialty, changes in presentation styles and changes in how textbooks are used.

In preparation for the task, I read the previous edition from cover to cover and tried to identify where major changes could occur. Inevitably in a text this size, there is some repetition and overlap. So the first job was to identify where the repetition and overlap occurred and try to eliminate it. This allowed me to condense some of the material and, along with some other changes, enabled me to reduce the number of volumes from 8 to 6. Reading the text led me to another realization. That is that the breadth of the specialty, impressive when I was first introduced to it, is even more impressive now, 30 years later and it continues to evolve. For this reason I quickly realized that in order to do this project justice, I could not do it on my own. My solution was to recruit volume editors for each of the major areas of practice as well as a video editor for the procedural videos. Drs. Gurtner, Warren, Rodriguez, Losee, Song, Grotting, Chang and Van Beek have done an outstanding job and this book truly represents a team effort.

Publishing is at a crossroads. The digital age has made information much more immediate, much more easy to access and much more flexible in how it is presented. We have tried to reflect that in this edition. The first big change is that everything is in color. All the illustrations have been re-drawn and the vast majority of patient photographs are in color. Chapters on anatomy have been highlighted with a red tone to make them easier to find as have pediatric chapters which have been highlighted in green. Reflecting on the way I personally use textbooks, I realized that while I like access to references, I rarely read the list of references at the end of a chapter. When I do though, I frequently pull some papers to read. So you will notice that we have kept the most important references in the printed text but we have moved the rest to the web. However, this has allowed us to greatly enhance the usefulness of the references. All the references are hyperlinked to PubMed and expertconsult facilitates a search across all volumes. Furthermore, while every chapter has a section devoted to the history of the topic, this is again something I like to be able to access but rarely have the leisure to read. That section in each of the chapters has also been moved to the web. This not only relieved the pressure on space in the printed text but also allowed us to give the authors more freedom in presenting the history of the topic. As well, there are extra illustrations in the web version that we simply could not accommodate in the printed version. The web edition of the book is therefore more complete than the printed version and owning the book, automatically gets one access to the web. A mouse icon has been added to the text to mark where further content is available online. In this digital age, video has become a very important way to impart knowledge. More than 160 procedural videos contributed by leading experts around the world accompany these volumes. These videos cover the full scope of our specialty. This text is also available as an e-Book.

This book then is very different from its predecessors. It is a reflection of a changing age in communication. However I will be extremely pleased if it fulfils its task of defining the current state of knowledge of the specialty as its predecessors did.

Peter C. Neligan, MB, FRCS(I), FRCSC, FACS
2012

List of Contributors

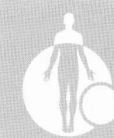

Neta Adler, MD
Senior Surgeon
Department of Plastic and Reconstructive
Surgery
Hadassah University Hospital
Jerusalem, Israel
*Volume 3, Chapter 40 Congenital melanocytic
nevi*

Ahmed M. Afifi, MD
Assistant Professor of Plastic Surgery
University of Winsconsin
Madison, WI, USA
Associate Professor of Plastic Surgery
Cairo University
Cairo, Egypt
*Volume 3, Chapter 1 Anatomy of the head and
neck*

Maryam Afshar, MD
Post Doctoral Fellow
Department of Surgery (Plastic and
Reconstructive Surgery)
Stanford University School of Medicine
Stanford, CA, USA
*Volume 3, Chapter 22 Embryology of the
craniofacial complex*

Jamil Ahmad, MD, FRCSC
Staff Plastic Surgeon
The Plastic Surgery Clinic
Mississauga, ON, Canada
*Volume 2, Chapter 18 Open technique
rhinoplasty*
*Volume 5, Chapter 8.3 Superior or medial
pedicle*

Hee Chang Ahn, MD, PhD
Professor
Department of Plastic and Reconstructive
Surgery
Hanyang University Hospital, School of
Medicine
Seoul, South Korea
Volume 6, Chapter 22 Ischemia of the hand
*Volume 6, Video 22.01 Radial artery periarterial
sympathectomy*
*Volume 6, Video 22.02 Ulnar artery periarterial
sympathectomy*
*Volume 6, Video 22.03 Digital artery periarterial
sympathectomy*

Tae-Joo Ahn, MD
Jeong-Won Aesthetic Plastic Surgical Clinic
Seoul, South Korea
*Volume 2, Video 10.01 Eyelidplasty non-
incisional method*
Volume 2, Video 10.02 Incisional method

Lisa E. Airan, MD
Assistant Clinical Professor
Department of Dermatology
Mount Sinai Hospital
Aesthetic Dermatologist
Private Practice
New York, NY, USA
Volume 2, Chapter 4 Soft-tissue fillers

Sammy Al-Benna, MD, PhD
Specialist in Plastic and Aesthetic Surgery
Department of Plastic Surgery
Burn Centre, Hand Centre, Operative
Reference Centre for Soft Tissue Sarcoma
BG University Hospital Bergmannsheil, Ruhr
University Bochum
Bochum, North Rhine-Westphalia, Germany
*Volume 4, Chapter 18 Acute management of
burn/electrical injuries*

Amy K. Alderman, MD, MPH
Private Practice
Atlanta, GA, USA
*Volume 1, Chapter 10 Evidence-based medicine
and health services research in plastic surgery*

Robert J. Allen, MD
Clinical Professor of Plastic Surgery
Department of Plastic Surgery
New York University Medical Centre
Charleston, SC, USA
*Volume 5, Chapter 18 The deep inferior
epigastric artery perforator (DIEAP) flap*
*Volume 5, Chapter 19 Alternative flaps for breast
reconstruction*
*Volume 5, Video 18.02 DIEP flap breast
reconstruction*

Mohammed M. Al Kahtani, MD, FRCSC
Clinical Fellow
Division of Plastic Surgery
Department of Surgery
University of Alberta
Edmonton, AB, Canada
*Volume 1, Chapter 33 Facial prosthetics in
plastic surgery*

Faisal Al-Mufarrej, MB, BCh
Chief Resident in Plastic Surgery
Division of Plastic Surgery
Department of Surgery
Mayo Clinic
Rochester, MN, USA
*Volume 6, Chapter 20 Osteoarthritis in the hand
and wrist*

Gary J. Alter, MD
Assistant Clinical Professor
Division of Plastic Surgery
University of Califronia at Los Angeles School
of Medicine
Los Angeles, CA, USA
Volume 2, Chapter 31 Aesthetic genital surgery

Al Aly, MD, FACS
Director of Aesthetic Surgery
Professor of Plastic Surgery
Aesthetic and Plastic Surgery Institute
University of California
Irvine, CA, USA
Volume 2, Chapter 27 Lower bodylifts

Khalid Al-Zahrani, MD, SSC-PLAST
Assistant Professor
Consultant Plastic Surgeon
King Khalid University Hospital
King Saud University
Riyadh, Saudi Arabia
Volume 2, Chapter 27 Lower bodylifts

Kenneth W. Anderson, MD
Marietta Facial Plastic Surgery & Aesthetics
Center
Mareitta, GA, USA
Volume 2, Video 23.04 FUE FOX procedure

Alice Andrews, PhD
Instructor
The Dartmouth Institute for Health Policy and
Clinical Practice
Lebanon, NH, USA
*Volume 5, Chapter 12 Patient-centered health
communication*

Louis C. Argenta, MD
Professor of Plastic and Reconstructive Surgery
Department of Plastic Surgery
Wake Forest Medical Center
Winston Salem, NC, USA
*Volume 1, Chapter 27 Principles and applications
of tissue expansion*

Charlotte E. Ariyan, MD, PhD
Surgical Oncologist
Gastric and Mixed Tumor Service
Memorial Sloan-Kettering Cancer Center
New York, NY, USA
Volume 3, Chapter 14 Salivary gland tumors

Stephan Ariyan, MD, MBA
Clinical Professor of Surgery
Plastic Surgery
Otolaryngology Yale University School of
Medicine Associate Chief
Department of Surgery
Yale New Haven Hospital Director
Yale Cancer Center Melanoma Program
New Haven, CT, USA
Volume 1, Chapter 31 Melanoma
Volume 3, Chapter 14 Salivary gland tumors

Bryan S. Armijo, MD
Plastic Surgery Chief Resident
Department of Plastic and Reconstructive
Surgery
Case Western Reserve/University Hospitals
Cleveland, OH, USA
*Volume 2, Chapter 20 Airway issues and the
deviated nose*

Eric Arnaud, MD
Chirurgie Plastique et Esthétique
Chirurgie Plastique Crânio-faciale
Unité de chirurgie crânio-faciale du
departement de neurochirurgie
Hôpital Necker Enfants Malades
Paris, France
Volume 3, Chapter 32 Orbital hypertelorism

Christopher E. Attinger, MD
Chief, Division of Wound Healing
Department of Plastic Surgery
Georgetown University Hospital
Georgetown, WA, USA
Volume 4, Chapter 8 Foot reconstruction

Tomer Avraham, MD
Resident, Plastic Surgery
Institute of Reconstructive Plastic Surgery
NYU Medical Center
New York, NY, USA
*Volume 1, Chapter 12 Principles of cancer
management*

Kodi K. Azari, MD, FACS
Associate Professor of Orthopaedic Surgery
Plastic Surgery Chief
Section of Reconstructive Transplantation
Department of Orthopaedic Surgery and
Surgery
David Geffen School of Medicine at UCLA
Los Angeles, CA, USA
*Volume 6, Chapter 15 Benign and malignant
tumors of the hand*

Sérgio Fernando Dantas de Azevedo, MD
Member
Brazilian Society of Plastic Surgery
Volunteer Professor of Plastic Surgery
Department of Plastic Surgery
Federal University of Pernambuco
Permambuco, Brazil
Volume 2, Chapter 26 Lipoabdominoplasty
*Volume 2, Video 26.01 Lipobdominoplasty
(including secondary lipo)*

Daniel C. Baker, MD
Professor of Surgery
Insitiue of Reconstructive Plastic Surgery
New York University Medical Center
Department of Plastic Surgery
New York, NY, USA
*Volume 2, Chapter 11.5 Facelift: Lateral
SMASectomy*

Steven B. Baker, MD, DDS, FACS
Associate Professor and Program Director
Co-director Inova Hospital for Children
Craniofacial Clinic
Department of Plastic Surgery
Georgetown University Hospital
Georgetown, WA, USA
*Volume 3, Chapter 30 Cleft and craniofacial
orthognathic surgery*

Karim Bakri, MD, MRCS
Chief Resident
Division of Plastic Surgery
Mayo Clinic
Rochester, MN, USA
*Volume 6, Chapter 20 Osteoarthritis in the hand
and wrist*

Carla Baldrighi, MD
Staff Surgeon
Reconstructive Microsurgery Unit
Azienda Ospedaliera Universitaria Careggi
Florence, Italy
*Volume 6, Chapter 30 Growth considerations in
pediatric upper extremity trauma and
reconstruction*
*Volume 6, Video 30.01 Epiphyseal transplant
harvesting technique*

Jonathan Bank, MD
Resident, Section of Plastic and Reconstructive
Surgery
Department of Surgery
Pritzker School of Medicine
University of Chicago Medical Center
Chicago, IL, USA
*Volume 4, Chapter 12 Abdominal wall
reconstruction*

A. Sina Bari, MD
Chief Resident
Division of Plastic and Reconstructive Surgery
Stanford University Hospital and Clinics
Stanford, CA, USA
*Volume 1, Chapter 16 Scar prevention,
treatment, and revision*

Scott P. Bartlett, MD
Professor of Surgery
Peter Randall Endowed Chair in Pediatric
Plastic Surgery
Childrens Hospital of Philadelphia, University of
Philadelphia
Philadelphia, PA, USA
*Volume 3, Chapter 34 Nonsyndromic
craniosynostosis*

Fritz E. Barton, Jr., MD
Clinical Professor
Department of Plastic Surgery
University of Texas Southwestern Medical
Center
Dallas, TX, USA
*Volume 2, Chapter 11.7 Facelift: SMAS with skin
attached – the "high SMAS" technique*
*Volume 2, Video 11.07.01 The High SMAS
technique with septal reset*

Bruce S. Bauer, MD, FACS, FAAP
Director of Pediatric Plastic Surgery, Clinical
Professor of Surgery
Northshore University Healthsystem
University of Chicago, Pritzker School of
Medicine, Highland Park Hospital
Chicago, IL, USA
*Volume 3, Chapter 40 Congenital melanocytic
nevi*

Ruediger G.H. Baumeister, MD, PhD
Professor of Surgery Emeritus
Consultant in Lymphology
Ludwig Maximilians University
Munich, Germany
*Volume 4, Chapter 3 Lymphatic reconstruction of
the extremities*

Leslie Baumann, MD
CEO
Baumann Cosmetic and Research Institute
Miami, FL, USA
*Volume 2, Chapter 2 Non surgical skin care and
rejuvenation*

Adriane L. Baylis, PhD
Speech Scientist
Section of Plastic and Reconstructive Surgery
Nationwide Children's Hospital
Columbus, OH, USA
*Volume 3, Chapter 28 Velopharyngeal
dysfunction*
*Volume 3, Video 28 Velopharyngeal
incompetence (1-3)*

Elisabeth Beahm, MD, FACS
Professor
Department of Plastic Surgery
University of Texas MD Anderson Cancer
Center
Houston, TX, USA
*Volume 5, Chapter 10 Breast cancer: Diagnosis
therapy and oncoplastic techniques*
*Volume 5, Video 10.01 Breast cancer: diagnosis
and therapy*

Michael L. Bentz, MD, FAAP, FACS
Professor of Surgery Pediatrics and
Neurosurgery Chairman
Chairman of Clinical Affairs
Department of Surgery
Division of Plastic Surgery Vice
University of Winconsin School of Medicine and
Public Health
Madison, WI, USA
Volume 3, Chapter 42 Pediatric tumors

Aaron Berger, MD, PhD
Resident
Division of Plastic Surgery, Department of
Surgery
Stanford University Medical Center
Palo Alto, CA, USA
Volume 1, Chapter 31 Melanoma

Pietro Berrino, MD
Teaching Professor
University of Milan
Director
Chirurgia Plastica Genova SRL
Genoa, Italy
Volume 5, Chapter 23 Poland's syndrome

Valeria Berrino, MS
In Training
Chirurgia Plastica Genova SRL
Genoa, Italy
Volume 5, Chapter 23 Poland's syndrome

Miles G. Berry, MS, FRCS(Plast)
Consultant Plastic and Aesthetic Surgeon
Institute of Cosmetic and Reconstructive
Surgery
London, UK
*Volume 2, Chapter 11.3 Facelift: Platysma-SMAS
plication*
*Volume 2, Video 11.03.01 Facelift – Platysma
SMAS plication*

Robert M. Bernstein, MD, FAAD
Associate Clinical Professor
Department of Dermatology
College of Physicians and Surgeons
Columbia University
Director
Private Practice
Bernstein Medical Center for Hair Restoration
New York, NY, USA
Volume 2, Video 23.04 FUE FOX procedure
*Volume 2, Video 23.02 Follicular unit hair
transplantation*

Michael Bezuhly, MD, MSc, SM, FRCSC
Assistant Professor
Department of Surgery, Division of Plastic and
Reconstructive Surgery
IWK Health Centre, Dalhousie University
Halifax, NS, Canada
*Volume 6, Chapter 23 Nerve entrapment
syndromes*
*Volume 6, Video 23.01-04 Carpal tunnel and
cubital tunnel releases in the same patient in one
procedure with field sterility – local anaesthetic
and surgery*

Sean M. Bidic, MD, MFA, FAAP, FACS
Private Practice
American Surgical Arts
Vineland, NJ, USA
Volume 6, Chapter 16 Infections of the hand

Phillip N. Blondeel, MD, PhD, FCCP
Professor of Plastic Surgery
Department of Plastic and Reconstructive
Surgery
University Hospital Gent
Gent, Belgium
*Volume 5, Chapter 18 The deep inferior
epigastric artery perforator (DIEAP) Flap*
*Volume 5, Chapter 19 Alternative flaps for breast
reconstruction*
*Volume 5, Video 18.02 DIEP flap breast
reconstruction*

Sean G. Boutros, MD
Assistant Professor of Surgery
Weill Cornell Medical College (Houston)
Clinical Instructor
University of Texas School of Medicine
(Houston)
Houston Plastic and Craniofacial Surgery
Houston, TX, USA
*Volume 3, Video 7.02 Reconstruction of
acquired ear deformities*

Lorenzo Borghese, MD
Plastic Surgeon
General Surgeon
Department of Plastic and Maxillo Facial
Surgery
Director of International Cooperation South
East Asia
Pediatric Hospital "Bambino Gesu'"
Rome, Italy
*Volume 4, Chapter 19 Extremity burn
reconstruction*
*Volume 4, Video 19.01 Extremity burn
reconstruction*

Trevor M. Born, MD, FRCSC
Lecturer
Division of Plastic and Reconstructive Surgery
The University of Toronto
Toronto, Ontario, Canada
Attending Physician
Lenox Hill Hospital
New York, NY, USA
Volume 2, Chapter 4 Soft-tissue fillers

Gregory H. Borschel, MD, FAAP, FACS
Assistant Professor
University of Toronto Division of Plastic and
Reconstructive Surgery
Assistant Professor
Institute of Biomaterials and Biomedical
Engineering
Associate Scientist
The SickKids Research Institute
The Hospital for Sick Children
Toronto, ON, Canada
*Volume 6, Chapter 35 Free functioning muscle
transfer in the upper extremity*

Kirsty U. Boyd, MD, FRCSC
Clinical Fellow – Hand Surgery
Department of Surgery – Division of Plastic
Surgery
Washington University School of Medicine
St. Louis, MO, USA
*Volume 1, Chapter 22 Repair and grafting of
peripheral nerve*
Volume 6, Chapter 33 Nerve transfers

James P. Bradley, MD
Professor of Plastic and Reconstructive Surgery
Department of Surgery
University of California, Los Angeles David
Geffen School of Medicine
Los Angeles, CA, USA
Volume 3, Chapter 33 Craniofacial clefts

Burton D. Brent, MD
Private Practice
Woodside, CA, USA
Volume 3, Chapter 7 Reconstruction of the ear

Mitchell H. Brown, MD, Med, FRCSC
Associate Professor of Plastic Surgery
Department of Surgery
University of Toronto
Toronto, ON, Canada
*Volume 5, Chapter 3 Secondary breast
augmentation*

Samantha A. Brugmann, PHD
Postdoctoral Fellow
Department of Surgery
Stanford University
Stanford, CA, USA
*Volume 3, Chapter 22 Embryology of the
craniofacial complex*

Terrence W. Bruner, MD, MBA
Private Practice
Greenville, SC, USA
Volume 2, Chapter 28 Buttock augmentation
Volume 2, Video 28.01 Buttock augmentation

Todd E. Burdette, MD
Staff Plastic Surgeon
Concord Plastic Surgery
Concord Hospital Medical Group
Concord, NH, USA
*Volume 1, Chapter 36 Robotics, simulation, and
telemedicine in plastic surgery*

Renee M. Burke, MD
Attending Plastic Surgeon
Department of Plastic Surgery
St. Alexius Medical Center
Hoffman Estates, IL, USA
*Volume 3, Chapter 8 Acquired cranial and facial
bone deformities*
*Volume 3, Video 8.01 Removal of venous
malformation enveloping intraconal optic nerve*

Charles E. Butler, MD, FACS
Professor, Department of Plastic Surgery
The University of Texas MD Anderson Cancer
Center
Houston, TX, USA
Volume 1, Chapter 32 Implants and biomaterials

**Peter E. M. Butler, MD, FRCSI, FRCS,
FRCS(Plast)**
Consultant Plastic Surgeon
Honorary Senior Lecturer
Royal Free Hospital
London, UK
*Volume 1, Chapter 34 Transplantation in plastic
surgery*

Yilin Cao, MD
Director, Department of Plastic and
Reconstructive Surgery
Shanghai 9th People's Hospital
Vice-Dean
Shanghai Jiao Tong University Medical School
Shanghai, The People's Republic of China
*Volume 1, Chapter 18 Tissue graft, tissue repair,
and regeneration*
*Volume 1, Chapter 20 Repair, grafting, and
engineering of cartilage*

Joseph F. Capella, MD, FACS
Chief, Post-Bariatric Body Contouring
Division of Plastic Surgery
Hackensack University Medical Center
Hackensack, NJ, USA
Volume 2, Chapter 29 Upper limb contouring
Volume 2, Video 29.01 Upper limb contouring

Brian T. Carlsen, MD
Assistant Professor of Plastic Surgery
Department of Surgery
Mayo Clinic
Rochester, MN, USA
*Volume 6, Chapter 20 Osteoarthritis in the hand
and wrist*

Robert C. Cartotto, MD, FRCS(C)
Attending Surgeon
Ross Tilley Burn Centre
Health Sciences Centre
Toronto, ON, Canada
*Volume 4, Chapter 23 Management of patients
with exfoliative disorders, epidermolysis bullosa,
and TEN*

Giuseppe Catanuto, MD, PhD
Research Fellow
The School of Oncological Reconstructive
Surgery
Milan, Italy
*Volume 5, Chapter 14 Expander/implant breast
reconstructions*
*Volume 5, Video 14.01 Mastectomy and
expander insertion: first stage*
*Volume 5, Video 14.02 Mastectomy and
expander insertion: second stage*

Peter Ceulemans, MD
Assistant Professor
Department of Plastic Surgery
Ghent University Hospital
Ghent, Belgium
*Volume 4, Chapter 13 Reconstruction of male
genital defects*

Rodney K. Chan, MD
Staff Plastic and Reconstructive Surgeon
Burn Center
United States Army Institute of Surgical
Research
Fort Sam
Houston, TX, USA
*Volume 3, Chapter 19 Secondary facial
reconstruction*

David W. Chang, MD, FACS
Professor
Department of Plastic Surgery
MD. Anderson Centre
Houston, TX, USA
*Volume 4, Chapter 3 Lymphatic reconstruction of
the extremities*
*Volume 4, Video 3.01 Lymphatico-venous
anastomosis*
*Volume 6, Chapter 15 Benign and malignant
tumors of the hand*

Edward I. Chang, MD
Assistant Professor
Department of Plastic Surgery
The University of Texas M.D. Anderson Cancer
Center
Houston, TX, USA
*Volume 3, Chapter 17 Carcinoma of the upper
aerodigestive tract*

James Chang, MD
Professor and Chief
Division of Plastic and Reconstructive Surgery
Stanford University Medical Center
Stanford, CA, USA
*Volume 6, Introduction: Plastic surgery
contributions to hand surgery*
*Volume 6, Chapter 1 Anatomy and biomechanics
of the hand*
Volume 6, Video 11.01 Hand replantation
Volume 6, Video 12.01 Debridement technique
*Volume 6, Video 19.01 Extensor tendon rupture
and end-side tendon transfer*
*Volume 6, Video 29.01 Addendum pediatric
trigger thumb release*

Robert A. Chase, MD
Holman Professor of Surgery – Emeritus
Stanford University Medical Center
Stanford, CA, USA
*Volume 6, Chapter 1 Anatomy and biomechanics
of the hand*

Constance M. Chen, MD, MPH
Plastic and Reconstructive Surgeon
Division of Plastic and Reconstructive Surgery
Lenox Hill Hospital
New York, NY, USA
Volume 3, Chapter 9 Midface reconstruction

Philip Kuo-Ting Chen, MD
Director
Department of Plastic and Reconstructive
Surgery
Chang Gung Memorial Hospital and Chang
Gung University
Taipei, Taiwan, The People's Republic of China
Volume 3, Chapter 23 Repair of unilateral cleft lip

Yu-Ray Chen, MD
Professor of Surgery
Department of Plastic and Reconstructive
Surgery
Chang Gung Memorial Hospital
Chang Gung University
Tao-Yuan, Taiwan, The People's Republic of
China
*Volume 3, Chapter 15 Tumors of the facial
skeleton: Fibrous dysplasia*

Ming-Huei Cheng, MD, MBA, FACS
Professor and Chief, Division of Reconstructive
Microsurgery
Department of Plastic and Reconstructive
Surgery
Chang Gung Memorial Hospital
Chang Gung Medical College
Chang Gung University
Taoyuan, Taiwan, The People's Republic of
China
*Volume 3, Chapter 12 Oral cavity, tongue, and
mandibular reconstructions*
*Volume 3, Video 12.02 Ulnar forearm flap for
buccal reconstruction*

You-Wei Cheong, MBBS, MS
Consultant Plastic Surgeon
Department of Surgery
Faculty of Medicine and Health Sciences,
University of Putra Malaysia
Selangor, Malaysia
*Volume 3, Chapter 15 Tumors of the facial
skeleton: Fibrous dysplasia*

Armando Chiari Jr., MD, PhD
Adjunct Professor
Department of Surgery
School of Medicine of the Federal University of
Minas Gerais
Belo Horzonti, Minas Gerais, Brazil
*Volume 5, Chapter 8.5 The L short scar
mammaplasty*

Ernest S. Chiu, MD, FACS
Associate Professor of Plastic Surgery
Department of Plastic Surgery
New York University
New York
USA
*Volume 2, Chapter 9 Secondary blepharoplasty:
Techniques*

Hong-Lim Choi, MD, PhD
Jeong-Won Aesthetic Plastic Surgical Clinic
Seoul, South Korea
*Volume 2, Video 10.01 Eyelidplasty non-
incisional method*
Volume 2, Video 10.02 Incisional method

Jong Woo Choi, MD, PhD
Associate Professor
Department of Plastic and Reconstructive
Surgery
Asan Medical Center
Ulsan University
College of Medicine
Seoul, South Korea
*Volume 2, Chapter 10 Asian facial cosmetic
surgery*

**Alphonsus K. Chong, MBBS, MRCS,
MMed(Orth), FAMS(Hand Surgery)**
Consultant Hand Surgeon
Department of Hand and Reconstructive
Microsurgery
National University Hospital
Assistant Professor
Department of Orthopaedic Surgery
Yong Loo Lin School of Medicine
National University of Singapore
Singapore
*Volume 6, Chapter 3 Diagnostic imaging of the
hand and wrist*
*Volume 6, Video 3.01 Diagnostic imaging of the
hand and wrist – Scaphoid lunate dislocation*

David Chwei-Chin Chuang, MD
Senior Consultant, Ex-President, Professor
Department of Plastic Surgery
Chang Gung University Hospital
Tao-Yuan, Taiwan, The People's Republic of
China
*Volume 6, Chapter 36 Brachial plexus injuries-
adult and pediatric*
*Volume 6, Video 36.01-02 Brachial plexus
injuries*

Kevin C. Chung, MD, MS
Charles B. G. de Nancrede, MD Professor
Section of Plastic Surgery, Department of
Surgery
Assistant Dean for Faculty Affairs
University of Michigan Medical School
Ann Arbor, MI, USA
*Volume 6, Chapter 8 Fractures and dislocations
of the carpus and distal radius*
*Volume 6, Chapter 19 Rheumatologic conditions
of the hand and wrist*
Volume 6, Video 8.01 Scaphoid fixation
*Volume 6, Video 19.01 Silicone MCP
arthroplasty*

Juan A. Clavero, MD, PhD
Radiologist Consultant
Radiology Department
Clínica Creu Blanca
Barcelona, Spain
*Volume 5, Chapter 13 Imaging in reconstructive
breast surgery*

Mark W. Clemens, MD
Assistant Professor
Department of Plastic Surgery
Anderson Cancer Center University of Texas
Houston, TX, USA
Volume 4, Chapter 8 Foot reconstruction
*Volume 5, Chapter 15 Latissimus dorsi flap
breast reconstruction*
*Volume 5, Video 15.01 Latissimus dorsi flap
technique*

Steven R. Cohen, MD
Senior Clinical Research Fellow, Clinical
Professor
Plastic Surgery
University of California
San Diego, CA
Director
Craniofacial Surgery
Rady Children's Hospital, Private Practice,
FACES+ Plastic Surgery, Skin and Laser Center
La Jolla, CA, USA
Volume 2, Chapter 5 Facial skin resurfacing

Sydney R. Coleman, MD
Clinical Assistant Professor
Department of Plastic Surgery
New York University Medical Center
New York, NY, USA
Volume 2, Chapter 14 Structural fat grafting
*Volume 2, Video 14.01 Structural fat grafting of
the face*

John Joseph Coleman III, MD
James E. Bennett Professor of Surgery,
Department of Dermatology and Cutaneuous
Surgery
University of Miami Miller School of Medicine
Miami, FA
Chief of Plastic Surgery
Department of Surgery
Indiana University School of Medicine
Indianapolis, IN, USA
*Volume 3, Chapter 16 Tumors of the lips, oral
cavity, oropharynx, and mandible*

Lawrence B. Colen, MD
Associate Professor of Surgery
Eastern Virginia Medical School
Norfolk, VA, USA
Volume 4, Chapter 8 Foot reconstruction

E. Dale Collins Vidal, MD, MS
Chief
Section of Plastic Surgery
Dartmouth-Hitchcock Medical Center
Professor of Surgery
Dartmouth Medical School
Director of the Center for Informed Choice
The Dartmouth Institute (TDI) for Health Policy
and Clinical Practice
Hanover, NH, USA
*Volume 1, Chapter 10 Evidence-based medicine
and health services research in plastic surgery*
*Volume 5, Chapter 12 Patient-centered health
communication*

Shannon Colohan, MD, FRCSC
Clinical Instructor, Plastic Surgery
Department of Plastic Surgery
University of Texas Southwestern Medical
Center
Dallas, TX, USA
*Volume 4, Chapter 2 Management of lower
extremity trauma*

Mark B. Constantian, MD, FACS
Active Staff
Saint Joseph Hospital
Nashua, NH (private practice)
Assistant Clinical Professor of Plastic Surgery
Division of Plastic Surgery
Department of Surgery
University of Wisconsin
Madison, WI, USA
*Volume 2, Chapter 19 Closed technique
rhinoplasty*

Peter G. Cordeiro, MD, FACS
Chief
Plastic and Reconstructive Surgery
Memorial Sloan-Kettering Cancer Center
Professor of Surgery
Weill Cornell Medical College
New York, NY, USA
Volume 3, Chapter 9 Midface reconstruction
*Volume 4, Chapter 14 Reconstruction of
acquired vaginal defects*

Christopher Cox, MD
Chief Resident
Department of Orthopaedic Surgery
Stanford University Medical School
Stanford, CA, USA
*Volume 6, Chapter 5 Principles of internal fixation
as applied to the hand and wrist*
*Volume 6, Video 5.01 Dynamic compression
plating and lag screw technique*

Albert Cram, MD
Professor Emeritus
University of Iowa
Iowa City Plastic Surgery
Coralville, IO, USA
Volume 2, Chapter 27 Lower bodylifts

Catherine Curtin, MD
Assistant Professor
Department of Surgery Division of Plastic
Stanford University
Stanford, CA, USA
*Volume 6, Chapter 37 Restoration of upper
extremity function*
*Volume 6, Video 37.01 1 Stage grasp IC 6 short
term*
*Volume 6, Video 37.02 2 Stage grasp release
outcome*

Lars B. Dahlin, MD, PhD
Professor and Consultant
Department of Clinical Sciences, Malmö-Hand
Surgery
University of Lund
Malmö, Sweden
*Volume 6, Chapter 32 Peripheral nerve injuries of
the upper extremity*
Volume 6, Video 32.01 Digital Nerve Suture
Volume 6, Video 32.02 Median Nerve Suture

Dai M. Davies, FRCS
Consultant and Institute Director
Institute of Cosmetic and Reconstructive
Surgery
London, UK
*Volume 2, Chapter 11.3 Facelift: Platysma-SMAS
plication*
*Volume 2, Video 11.03.01 Platysma SMAS
plication*

**Michael R. Davis, MD, FACS, LtCol,
USAF, MC**
Chief
Reconstructive Surgery and Regenerative
Medicine
Plastic and Reconstructive Surgeon
San Antonio Military Medical Center
Houston, TX, USA
*Volume 5, Chapter 1 Anatomy for plastic surgery
of the breast*

Jorge I. De La Torre, MD
Professor and Chief
Division of Plastic Surgery
University of Alabama at Birmingham
Birmingham, AL, USA
*Volume 5, Chapter 1 Anatomy for plastic surgery
of the breast*

A. Lee Dellon, MD, PhD
Professor of Plastic Surgery
Professor of Neurosurgery
Johns Hopkins University
Baltimore, MD, USA
*Volume 4, Chapter 6 Diagnosis and treatment of
painful neuroma and of nerve compression in the
lower extremity*
*Volume 4, Video 6.01 Diagnosis and treatment
of painful neuroma and of nerve compression in
the lower extremity*

Sara R. Dickie, MD
Resident, Section of Plastic and Reconstructive
Surgery
Department of Surgery
University of Chicago Medical Center
Chicago, IL, USA
*Volume 4, Chapter 9 Comprehensive trunk
anatomy*

Joseph J. Disa, MD, FACS
Attending Surgeon
Plastic and Reconstructive Surgery in the
Department of Surgery
Memorial Sloan Kettering Cancer Center
New York, NY, USA
Volume 3, Chapter 9 Midface reconstruction
*Volume 4, Chapter 14 Reconstruction of
acquired vaginal defects*

Risal Djohan, MD
Head of Regional Medical Practice
Department of Plastic Surgery
Cleveland Clinic
Cleveland, OH, USA
*Volume 3, Chapter 1 Anatomy of the head and
neck*

Erin Donaldson, MS
Instructor
Department of Otolaryngology
New York Medical College
Valhalla, NY, USA
*Volume 1, Chapter 36 Robotics, simulation, and
telemedicine in plastic surgery*

Amir H. Dorafshar, MBChB
Assistant Professor
Department of Plastic and Reconstructive
surgery
John Hopkins Medical Institute
John Hopkins Outpatient Center
Baltimore, MD, USA
Volume 3, Chapter 3 Facial fractures

Ivica Ducic, MD, PhD
Professor – Plastic Surgery
Director – Peripheral Nerve Surgery Institute
Department of Plastic Surgery
Georgetown University Hospital
Washington, DC, USA
*Volume 6, Chapter 23 Complex regional pain
syndrome in the upper extremity*

Gregory A. Dumanian, MD, FACS
Chief of Plastic Surgery
Division of Plastic Surgery, Department of
Surgery
Northwestern Feinberg School of Medicine
Chicago, IL, USA
*Volume 4, Chapter 11 Reconstruction of the soft
tissues of the back*
*Volume 6, Chapter 40 Treatment of the upper
extremity amputee*
*Volume 6, Video 40.01 Targeted muscle
reinnervation in the transhumeral amputee –
Surgical technique and guidelines for restoring
intuitive neural control*

William W. Dzwierzynski, MD
Professor and Program Director
Department of Plastic Surgery
Medical College of Wisconsin
Milwaukee, WI, USA
*Volume 6, Chapter 11 Replantation and
revascularization*

L. Franklyn Elliott, MD
Assistant Clinical Professor
Emory Section of Plastic Surgery
Emory University
Atlanta, GA, USA
*Volume 5, Chapter 16 The bilateral pedicled
TRAM flap*
*Volume 5, Video 16.01 Pedicle TRAM breast
reconstruction*

Marco Ellis, MD
Chief Resident
Division of Plastic Surgery
Northwestern Memorial Hospital
Northwestern University, Feinberg School of
Medicine
Chicago, IL, USA
Volume 2, Chapter 8 Blepharoplasty
Volume 2, Video 8.01 Periorbital rejuvenation

Dino Elyassnia, MD
Associate Plastic Surgeon
Marten Clinic of Plastic Surgery
San Francisco, CA, USA
*Volume 2, Chapter 12 Secondary deformities
and the secondary facelift*

Surak Eo, MD, PhD
Chief, Associate Professor
Plastic and Reconstructive Surgery
DongGuk University Medical Center
DongGuk University Graduate School of
Medicine
Gyeonggi-do, South Korea
*Volume 6, Video 34.01 EIP to EPL tendon
transfer*

Elof Eriksson, MD, PhD
Chief
Department of Plastic Surgery
Joseph E. Murray Professor of Plastic and
Reconstructive Surgery
Brigham and Women's Hospital
Boston, MA, USA
*Volume 1, Chapter 11 Genetics and prenatal
diagnosis*

Simon Farnebo, MD, PhD
Consultant Hand Surgeon
Department of Plastic Surgery, Hand Surgery
and Burns
Institution of Clinical and Experimental
Medicine, University of Linköping
Linköping, Sweden
*Volume 6, Chapter 32 Peripheral nerve injuries of
the upper extremity*
Volume 6, Video 32.01 Digital Nerve Suture
Volume 6, Video 32.02 Median Nerve Suture

Jeffrey A. Fearon, MD
Director
The Craniofacial Center
Medical City Children's Hospital
Dallas, TX, USA
Volume 3, Chapter 35 Syndromic craniosynostosis

John M. Felder III, MD
Resident Physician
Department of Plastic Surgery
Georgetown University Hospital
Washington, DC, USA
Volume 6, Chapter 23 Complex regional pain syndrome in the upper extremity

Evan M. Feldman, MD
Chief Resident
Division of Plastic Surgery
Baylor College of Medicine
Houston, TX, USA
Volume 3, Chapter 29 Secondary deformities of the cleft lip, nose, and palate
Volume 3, Video 29.01 Complete takedown
Volume 3, Video 29.02 Abbé flap
Volume 3, Video 29.03 Thick lip and buccal sulcus deformities
Volume 3, Video 29.04 Alveolar bone grafting
Volume 3, Video 29.05 Definitive rhinoplasty

Julius Few Jr., MD
Director
The Few Institute for Aesthetic Plastic Surgery
Clinical Associate
Division of Plastic Surgery
University of Chicago
Chicago, IL, USA
Volume 2, Chapter 8 Blepharoplasty
Volume 2, Video 8.01 Periorbital rejuvenation

Alvaro A. Figueroa, DDS, MS
Director
Rush Craniofacial Center
Rush University Medical Center
Chicago, IL, USA
Volume 3, Chapter 27 Orthodontics in cleft lip and palate management

Neil A. Fine, MD
Associate Professor of Clinical Surgery
Department of Surgery
Northwestern University
Chicago, IL, USA
Volume 5, Chapter 5 Endoscopic approaches to the breast
Volume 5, Video 5.01 Endoscopic transaxillary breast augmentation
Volume 5, Video 5.02 Endoscopic approaches to the breast
Volume 5, Video 11.02 Partial breast reconstruction with a latissimus D

Joel S. Fish, MD, MSc, FRCSC
Medical Director Burn Program
Department of Surgery, University of Toronto,
Division of Plastic and Reconstructive Surgery
Hospital for Sick Children
Toronto, ON, Canada
Volume 4, Chapter 23 Management of patients with exfoliative disorders, epidermolysis bullosa, and TEN

David M. Fisher, MB, BCh, FRCSC, FACS
Medical Director, Cleft Lip and Palate Program
Division of Plastic and Reconstructive Surgery
The Hospital for Sick Children
Toronto, ON, Canada
Volume 3, Video 23.02 Unilateral cleft lip repair – anatomic subumit approximation technique

Jack Fisher, MD
Department of Plastic Surgery
Vanderbilt University
Nashville, TN, USA
Volume 2, Chapter 23 Hair restoration
Volume 5, Chapter 8.1 Reduction mammaplasty
Volume 5, Chapter 8.2 Inferior pedicle breast reduction

James W. Fletcher, MD, FACS
Chief Hand Surgery
Department Plastic and Hand Surgery
Regions Hospital
Assistant Prof. U MN Dept of Surgery and Dept Orthopedics
St. Paul, MN, USA
Volume 6, Video 20.01 Ligament reconstruction tendon interposition arthroplasty of the thumb CMC joint

Joshua Fosnot, MD
Resident
Division of Plastic Surgery
The University of Pennsylvania Health System
Philadelphia, PA, USA
Volume 5, Chapter 17 Free TRAM breast reconstruction
Volume 5, Video 17.01 The muscle sparing free TRAM flap

Ida K. Fox, MD
Assistant Professor of Plastic Surgery
Department of Surgery
Washington University School of Medicine
Saint Louis, MO, USA
Volume 6, Chapter 33 Nerve transfers
Volume 6, Video 33.01 Nerve transfers

Ryan C. Frank, MD, FRCSC
Attending Surgeon
Plastic and Craniofacial Surgery
Alberta Children's Hospital
University of Calgary
Calgary, AB, Canada
Volume 2, Chapter 5 Facial skin resurfacing

Gary L. Freed, MD
Assistant Professor Plastic Surgery
Dartmouth-Hitchcock Medical Center
Lebanon, NH, USA
Volume 5, Chapter 12 Patient-centered health communication

Jeffrey B. Friedrich, MD
Assistant Professor of Surgery, Orthopedics and Urology (Adjunct)
Department of Surgery, Division of Plastic Surgery
University of Washington
Seattle, WA, USA
Volume 6, Chapter 13 Thumb reconstruction (non microsurgical)

Allen Gabriel, MD
Assitant Professor
Department of Plastic Surgery
Loma Linda University Medical Center
Chief of Plastic Surgery
Southwest Washington Medical Center
Vancouver, WA, USA
Volume 5, Chapter 2 Breast augmentation
Volume 5, Chapter 4 Current concepts in revisionary breast surgery
Volume 5, Video 4.01 Current concepts in revisionary breast surgery

Günter Germann, MD, PhD
Professor of Plastic Surgery
Clinic for Plastic and Reconstructive Surgery
Heidelberg University Hospital
Heidelberg, Germany
Volume 6, Chapter 10 Extensor tendon injuries and reconstruction

Goetz A. Giessler, MD, PhD
Plastic Surgeon, Hand Surgeon, Associate Professor of Plastic Surgery, Fellow of the European Board of Plastic Reconstructive and Aesthetic Surgery
BG Trauma Center Murnau
Murnau am Staffelsee, Germany
Volume 4, Chapter 4 Lower extremity sarcoma reconstruction
Volume 4, Video 4.01 Management of lower extremity sarcoma reconstruction

Jesse A. Goldstein, MD
Chief Resident
Department of Plastic Surgery
Georgetown University Hospital
Washington, DC, USA
Volume 3, Chapter 30 Cleft and craniofacial orthognathic surgery

Vijay S. Gorantla, MD, PhD
Associate Professor of Surgery
Department of Surgery, Division of Plastic and
Reconstructive Surgery
University of Pittsburgh Medical Center
Administrative Medical Director
Pittsburgh Reconstructive Transplantation
Program
Pittsburgh, PA, USA
*Volume 6, Chapter 38 Upper extremity
composite allotransplantation*
*Volume 6, Video 38.01 Upper extremity
composite allotransplantation*

Arun K. Gosain, MD
DeWayne Richey Professor and Vice Chair
Department of Plastic Surgery
University Hospitals Case Medical Center
Chief, Pediatric Plastic Surgery
Rainbow Babies and Children's Hospital
Cleveland, OH, USA
Volume 3, Chapter 38 Pierre Robin sequence

Lawrence J. Gottlieb, MD, FACS
Professor of Surgery
Director of Burn and Complex Wound Center
Director of Reconstructive Microsurgery
Fellowship
Section of Plastic and Reconstructive Surgery
Department of Surgery
University of Chicago
Chicago, IL, USA
*Volume 3, Chapter 41 Pediatric chest and trunk
defects*

Barry H. Grayson, DDS
Associate Professor of Surgery (Craniofacial
Orthodontics)
New York University Langone Medical Centre
Institute of Reconstructive Plastic Surgery
New York, NY, USA
Volume 3, Chapter 36 Craniofacial microsomia
Volume 3, Video 24.01 Repair of bilateral cleft lip

Arin K. Greene, MD, MMSc
Associate Professor of Surgery
Department of Plastic and Oral Surgery
Children's Hospital Boston
Harvard Medical School
Boston, MA, USA
Volume 1, Chapter 29 Vascular anomalies

James C. Grotting, MD, FACS
Clinical Professor of Plastic Surgery
University of Alabama at Birmingham;
The University of Wisconsin, Madison, WI;
Grotting and Cohn Plastic Surgery
Birmingham, AL, USA
Volume 5, Chapter 7 Mastopexy
Volume 5, Chapter 8.7 Sculpted pillar vertical
*Volume 5, Video 8.7.01 Marking the sculpted
pillar breast reduction*
Volume 5, Video 8.7.02 Breast reduction surgery

Ronald P. Gruber, MD
Associate Adjunct Clinical Professor
Division of Plastic and Reconstructive Surgery
Stanford University
Associate Clinical Professor
Division of Plastic and Reconstructive Surgery
University of California, San Francisco
San Francisco, CA, USA
Volume 2, Chapter 21 Secondary rhinoplasty

**Mohan S. Gundeti, MB, MCh, FEBU,
FRCS, FEAPU**
Associate Professor of Urology in Surgery and
Pediatrics, Director Pediatric Urology, Director
Centre for Pediatric Robotics and Minimal
Invasive Surgery
University of Chicago and Pritzker Medical
School Comer Children's Hospital
Chicago, IL, USA
*Volume 3, Chapter 44 Reconstruction of
urogenital defects: Congenital*
*Volume 3, Video 44.01 First stage hypospadias
repair with free inner preputial graft*
*Volume 3, Video 44.02 Second stage
hypospadias repair with tunica vaginalis flap*

Eyal Gur, MD
Head
Department of Plastic and Reconstructive
Surgery
The Tel Aviv Sourasky Medical Center
The Tel Aviv University School of Medicine
Tel Aviv, Israel
Volume 3, Chapter 11 Facial paralysis
Volume 3, Video 11.01 Facial paralysis

Geoffrey C. Gurtner, MD, FACS
Professor and Associate Chairman
Stanford University Department of Surgery
Stanford, CA, USA
*Volume 1, Chapter 13 Stem cells and
regenerative medecine*
*Volume 1, Chapter 35 Technology innovation in
plastic surgery*

Bahman Guyuron, MD
Kiehn-DesPrez Professor and Chairman
Department of Plastic Surgery
Case Western Reserve University School of
Medicine
Cleveland, OH, USA
*Volume 2, Chapter 20 Airway issues and the
deviated nose*
*Volume 3, Chapter 21 Surgical management of
migraine headaches*
Volume 2, Video 3.02 Botulinum toxin

Steven C. Haase, MD
Clinical Associate Professor
Department of Surgery, Section of Plastic
Surgery
University of Michigan Health
Ann Arbor, MI, USA
*Volume 6, Chapter 8 Fractures and dislocations
of the carpus and distal radius*

Robert S. Haber, MD, FAAD, FAAP
Assistant Professor, Dermatology and
Pediatrics
Case Western Reserve University School of
Medicine
Director
University Hair Transplant Center
Cleveland, OH, USA
*Volume 2, Video 23.08 Strip harvesting the
haber spreader*

Florian Hackl, MD
Research Fellow
Division of Plastic Surgery
Brigham and Women's Hospital
Harvard Medical School
Boston, MA, USA
*Volume 1, Chapter 11 Genetics and prenatal
diagnosis*

Phillip C. Haeck, MD
Private Practice
Seattle, WA, USA
*Volume 1, Chapter 4 The role of ethics in plastic
surgery*

Bruce Halperin, MD
Adjunct Associate Clinical Professor of
Anesthesia
Department of Anesthesia
Stanford University School of Medicine
Palo Alto, CA, USA
*Volume 1, Chapter 8 Patient safety in plastic
surgery*

Moustapha Hamdi, MD, PhD
Professor and Chairman of Plastic and
Reconstructive Surgery
Department of Plastic Surgery
Brussels University Hospital
Brussels, Belgium
*Volume 5, Chapter 21 Local flaps in partial
breast reconstruction*

Warren C. Hammert, MD
Associate Professor of Orthopaedic and
Plastic Surgery
Department of Orthopaedic Surgery
University of Rochester Medical Center
Rochester, NY, USA
*Volume 6, Chapter 7 Hand fractures and joint
injuries*

Dennis C. Hammond, MD
Clinical Assistant Professor
Department of Surgery
Michigan State University College of Human
Medicine
East Lansing
Associate Program Director
Plastic and Reconstructive Surgery
Grand Rapids Medical Education and Research
Center for Health Professions
Grand Rapids, MI, USA
*Volume 5, Chapter 8.4 Short scar periareolar
inferior pedicle reduction (SPAIR) mammaplasty*
Volume 5, Video 8.4.01 Spair technique

Scott L. Hansen, MD, FACS
Assistant Professor of Plastic and
Reconstructive Surgery
Chief, Hand and Microvascular Surgery
University of California, San Francisco
Chief, Plastic and Reconstructive Surgery
San Francisco General Hospital
San Francisco, CA, USA
*Volume 1, Chapter 24 Flap classification and
applications*

James A. Harris, MD
Cosmetic Surgeon
Private Practice
Hasson & Wong Aesthetic Surgery
Vancouver, BC, Canada
Volume 2, Video 23.05 FUE Harris safe system

Isaac Harvey, MD
Clinical Fellow
Department of Paediatric Plastic and
Reconstructive Surgery
Hospital for Sick Kids
Toronto, ON, Canada
*Volume 6, Chapter 35 Free functional muscle
transfers in the upper extremity*

Victor Hasson, MD
Cosmetic Surgeon
Private Practice
Hasson & Wong Aesthetic Surgery
Vancouver, BC, Canada
*Volume 2, Video 23.07 Perpendicular angle
grafting technique*

Theresa A Hegge, MD, MPH
Resident of Plastic Surgery
Division of Plastic Surgery
Southern Illinois University
Springfield, IL, USA
*Volume 6, Chapter 6 Nail and fingertip
reconstruction*

Jill A. Helms, DDS, PhD
Division of Plastic and Reconstructive Surgery
Department of Surgery
School of Medicine
Stanford University
Stanford, CA, USA
*Volume 3, Chapter 22 Embryology of the
craniofacial complex*

Ginard I. Henry, MD
Assistant Professor of Surgery
Section of Plastic Surgery
University of Chicago Medical Center
Chicago, IL, USA
*Volume 4, Chapter 1 Comprehensive lower
extremity anatomy, embryology, surgical exposure*

Vincent R. Hentz, MD
Emeritus Professor of Surgery and Orthopedic
Surgery (by courtesy)
Stanford University
Stanford, CA, USA
*Volume 6, Chapter 1 Anatomy and biomechanics
of the hand*
*Volume 6, Chapter 37 Restoration of upper
extremity function in tetraplegia*
*Volume 6, Video 37.01 1 Stage grasp IC 6 short
term*
*Volume 6, Video 37.02 2 Stage grasp release
outcome*

**Rebecca L. von der Heyde, PhD,
OTR/L, CHT**
Associate Professor
Program in Occupational Therapy
Maryville University
St. Louis, MO, USA
Volume 6, Chapter 39 Hand therapy
*Volume 6, Video 39.01 Hand therapy
Goniometric measurement*
Volume 6, Video 39.02 Threshold testing
*Volume 6, Video 39.03 Fabrication of a
synergistic splint*

Kent K. Higdon, MD
Former Aesthetic Fellow
Grotting and Cohn Plastic Surgery;
Current Assistant Professor
Vanderbilt University
Nashville, TN, USA
Volume 5, Chapter 7 Mastopexy
Volume 5, Chapter 8.1 Reduction mammaplasty
*Volume 5, Chapter 8.7 Sculpted pillar vertical
mammaplasty*

John Hijjawi, MD, FACS
Assistant Professor
Department of Plastic Surgery, Department of
General Surgery
Medical College of Wisconsin
Milwaukee, WI, USA
*Volume 4, Chapter 20 Cold and chemical injury
to the upper extremity*

Jonay Hill, MD
Clinical Assistant Professor
Anesthesiology Department
Anesthesia and Critical Care
Stanford University School of Medicine
Stanford, CA, USA
*Volume 6, Chapter 4 Anesthesia for upper
extremity surgery*

Piet Hoebeke, MD, PhD
Full Senior Professor of Paediatric Urology
Department of Urology
Ghent University Hospital
Ghent, Belgium
*Volume 4, Chapter 13 Reconstruction of male
genital defects*
*Volume 4, Video 13.01 Complete and partial
penile reconstruction*

William Y. Hoffman, MD
Professor and Chief
Division of Plastic and Reconstructive Surgery
University of California, San Francisco
San Francisco, CA, USA
Volume 3, Chapter 25 Cleft palate

Larry H. Hollier Jr., MD, FACS
Professor and Program Director
Division of Plastic Surgery
Baylor College of Medicine and Texas
Children's Hospital
Houston, TX, USA
*Volume 3, Chapter 29 Secondary deformities of
the cleft lip, nose, and palate*
Volume 3, Video 29.01 Complete takedown
Volume 3, Video 29.02 Abbé flap
*Volume 3, Video 29.03 Thick lip and buccal
sulcus deformities*
Volume 3, Video 29.04 Alveolar bone grafting
Volume 3, Video 29.05 Definitive rhinoplasty

Joon Pio Hong, MD, PhD, MMM
Chief and Associate Professor
Department of Plastic Surgery
Asian Medical Center University of Ulsan
School of Medicine
Seoul, Korea
*Volume 4, Chapter 5 Reconstructive surgery:
Lower extremity coverage*

Richard A. Hopper, MD, MS
Chief
Division of Pediatric Plastic Surgery
University of Washingtion
Surgical Director
Craniofacial Center
Seattle Childrens Hospital
Associate Professor
Division of Plastic Surgery
Seattle, WA, USA
Volume 3, Chapter 26 Alveolar clefts
Volume 3, Chapter 36 Craniofacial microsomia

Philippe Houtmeyers, MD
Resident
Plastic Surgery
Ghent University Hospital
Ghent, Belgium
*Volume 4, Chapter 13 Reconstruction of male
genital defects*
*Volume 4, Video 13.01 Complete and partial
penile reconstruction*

Steven E.R. Hovius, MD, PhD
Head
Department of Plastic, Reconstructive and
Hand Surgery
ErasmusmMC
University Medical Center
Rotterdam, The Netherlands
*Volume 6, Chapter 28 Congenital hand IV
disorders of differentiation and duplication*

Michael A. Howard, MD
Clinical Assistant Professor of Surgery
Division of Plastic Surgery
University of Chicago, Pritzker School of
Medicine
Northbrook, IL, USA
*Volume 4, Chapter 9 Comprehensive trunk
anatomy*

Jung-Ju Huang, MD
Assistant Professor
Division of Microsurgery
Plastic and Reconstructive Surgery
Chang Gung Memorial Hospital
Taoyuan, Taiwan, The People's Republic of
China
*Volume 3, Chapter 12 Oral cavity, tongue, and
mandibular reconstructions
Volume 3, Video 12.01 Fibula
osteoseptocutaneous flap for composite
mandibular reconstruction
Volume 3, Video 12.02 Ulnar forearm flap for
buccal reconstruction*

C. Scott Hultman, MD, MBA, FACS
Ethel and James Valone Distinguished
Professor of Surgery
Division of Plastic Surgery
University of North Carolina
Chapel Hill, NC, USA
*Volume 1, Chapter 5 Business principles for
plastic surgeons*

Leung-Kim Hung, MChOrtho (Liv)
Professor
Department of Orthopaedics and Traumatology
Faculty of Medicine
The Chinese University of Hong Kong
Hong Kong, The People's Republic of China
*Volume 6, Chapter 29 Congenital hand V
disorders of overgrowth, undergrowth, and
generalized skeletal deformities*

Gazi Hussain, MBBS, FRACS
Clinical Senior Lecturer
Macquarie Cosmetic and Plastic Surgery
Macquarie University
Sydney, Australia
Volume 3, Chapter 11 Facial paralysis

Marco Innocenti, MD
Director Reconstructive Microsurgery
Department of Oncology
Careggi University Hospital
Florence, Italy
*Volume 6, Chapter 30 Growth considerations in
pediatric upper extremity trauma and
reconstruction
Volume 6, Video 30.01 Epiphyseal transplant
harvesting technique*

Clyde H. Ishii, MD, FACS
Assistant Clinical Professor of Surgery
John A. Burns School of Medicine
Chief, Department of Plastic Surgery
Shriners Hospital
Honolulu Unit
Honolulu, HI, USA
*Volume 2, Chapter 10 Asian facial cosmetic
surgery*

Jonathan S. Jacobs, DMD, MD
Associate Professor of Clinical Plastic Surgery
Eastern Virginia Medical School
Norfolk, VA, USA
*Volume 2, Chapter 16 Anthropometry,
cephalometry, and orthognathic surgery
Volume 2, Video 16.01 Anthropometry,
cephalometry, and orthognathic surgery*

Jordan M.S. Jacobs, MD
Craniofacial Fellow
Department of Plastic Surgery
New York University Langone Medical Center
New York, NY, USA
*Volume 2, Chapter 16 Anthropometry,
cephalometry, and orthognathic surgery
Volume 2, Video 16.01 Anthropometry,
cephalometry, and orthognathic surgery*

**Ian T. Jackson, MD, DSc(Hon), FRCS,
FACS, FRACS (Hon)**
Emeritus Surgeon
Surgical Services Administration
William Beaumont Hospitals
Royal Oak, MI, USA
*Volume 3, Chapter 18 Local flaps for facial
coverage*

Oksana Jackson, MD
Assistant Professor of Surgery
Division of Plastic Surgery
University of Pennsylvania School of Medicine
Clinical Associate
The Children's Hospital of Philadelphia
Philadelphia, PA, USA
Volume 3, Chapter 43 Conjoined twins

Jeffrey E. Janis, MD, FACS
Associate Professor
Program Director
Department of Plastic Surgery
University of Texas Southwestern Medical
Center
Chief of Plastic Surgery
Chief of Wound Care
President-Elect
Medical Staff
Parkland Health and Hospital System
Dallas, TX, USA
Volume 4, Chapter 16 Pressure sores

Leila Jazayeri, MD
Resident
Stanford University Plastic and Reconstructive
Surgery
Stanford, CA, USA
*Volume 1, Chapter 35 Technology innovation in
plastic surgery*

Elizabeth B. Jelks, MD
Private Practice
Jelks Medical
New York, NY, USA
*Volume 2, Chapter 9 Secondary blepharoplasty:
Techniques*

Glenn W. Jelks, MD
Associate Professor
Department of Ophthalmology
Department of Plastic Surgery
New York University School of Medicine
New York, NY, USA
*Volume 2, Chapter 9 Secondary blepharoplasty:
Techniques*

Mark Laurence Jewell, MD
Assistant Clinical Professor of Plastic Surgery
Oregon Health Science University
Jewell Plastic Surgery Center
Eugene, OR, USA
*Volume 2, Chapter 11.4 Facelift: Facial
rejuvenation with loop sutures, the MACS lift and
its derivatives*

Andreas Jokuszies, MD
Consultant Plastic, Aesthetic and Hand
Surgeon
Department of Plastic, Hand and
Reconstructive Surgery
Hanover Medical School
Hanover, Germany
*Volume 1, Chapter 15 Skin wound healing:
Repair biology, wound, and scar treatment*

Neil F. Jones, MD, FRCS
Chief of Hand Surgery
University of California Medical Center
Professor of Orthopedic Surgery
Professor of Plastic and Reconstructive Surgery
University of California Irvine
Irvine, CA, USA
*Volume 6, Chapter 22 Ischemia of the hand
Volume 6, Chapter 34 Tendon transfers in the
upper extremity
Volume 6, Video 34.01 EIP to EPL tendon
transfer*

David M. Kahn, MD
Clinical Associate Professor of Plastic Surgery
Department of Surgery
Stanford University School of Medicine
Stanford, CA, USA
Volume 2, Chapter 21 Secondary rhinoplasty

Ryosuke Kakinoki, MD, PhD
Associate Professor
Chief of the Hand Surgery and Microsurgery
Unit
Department of Orthopedic Surgery and
Rehabilitation Medicine
Graduate School of Medicine
Kyoto University
Kyoto, Japan
*Volume 6, Chapter 2 Examination of the upper
extremity
Volume 2, Video 2.01-2.17 Examination of the
upper extremity*

Alex Kane, MD
Associate Professor of Surgery
Washington University School of Medicine
St. Louis, WO, USA
Volume 3, Chapter 23 Repair of unilateral cleft lip

Gabrielle M. Kane, MBBCh, EdD, FRCPC
Medical Director, Associate Professor
Department of Radiation Oncology
Associate Professor
Department of Medical Education and
Biomedical Informatics
University of Washington School of Medicine
Seattle, WA, USA
*Volume 1, Chapter 28 Therapeutic radiation:
Principles, effects, and complications*

Michael A. C. Kane, MD
Attending Surgeon Manhattan Eye, Ear and
Throat Institute
Department of Plastic Surgery
New York, NY, USA
Volume 2, Chapter 3 Botulinum toxin (BoNT-A)

Dennis S. Kao, MD
Hand Fellow
Department of Plastic Surgery
Medical College of Wisconsin
Milwaukee, WI, USA
*Volume 4, Chapter 20 Cold and chemical injury
to the upper extremity*

Sahil Kapur, MD
Resident, Plastic and Reconstructive Surgery
Department of Surgery, Division of Plastic and
Reconstructive Surgery
University of Wisconsin
Madison, WI, USA
Volume 3, Chapter 42 Pediatric tumors

Leila Kasrai, MD, MPH, FRCSC
Head, Division of Plastic Surgery
St Joseph's Hospital
Toronto, ON, Canada
Volume 2, Video 22.01 Setback otoplasty

Abdullah E. Kattan, MBBS, FRCS(C)
Clinical Fellow
Division of Plastic Surgery
Department of Surgery
University of Toronto
Toronto, ON, Canada
*Volume 4, Chapter 23 Management of patients
with exfoliative disorders, epidermolysis bullosa,
and TEN*

David L. Kaufman, MD, FACS
Private Practice Plastic Surgery
Aesthetic Artistry Surgical and Medical Center
Folsom, CA, USA
Volume 2, Chapter 21 Secondary rhinoplasty

Lindsay B. Katona, BA
Research Associate
Thayer School of Engineering
Dartmouth College
Hanover, NH, USA
*Volume 1, Chapter 36 Robotics, simulation, and
telemedicine in plastic surgery*

Henry K. Kawamoto, Jr., MD, DDS
Clinical Professor
Division of Plastic Surgery
University of California at Los Angeles
Los Angeles, CA, USA
Volume 3, Chapter 33 Craniofacial clefts

Jeffrey M. Kenkel, MD, FACS
Professor and Vice-Chairman
Rod J Rohrich MD Distinguished Professorship
in Wound Healing and Plastic Surgery
Department of Plastic Surgery
Southwestern Medical School
Director
Clinical Center for Cosmetic Laser Treatment
Dallas, TX, USA
*Volume 2, Chapter 24 Liposuction: A
comprehensive review of techniques and safety*

Carolyn L. Kerrigan, MD, MSc
Professor of Surgery
Section of Plastic Surgery
Dartmouth Hitchcock Medical Center
Lebanon, NH, USA
*Volume 1, Chapter 10 Evidence-based medicine
and health services research in plastic surgery*

Marwan R. Khalifeh, MD
Instructor of Plastic Surgery
Department of Plastic Surgery
Johns Hopkins University School of Medicine
Washington, DC, USA
*Volume 4, Chapter 12 Abdominal wall
reconstruction*

Jae-Hoon Kim, MD
April 31 Aesthetic Plastic Surgical Clinic
Seoul, South Korea
*Volume 2, Video 10.03 Secondary rhinoplasty:
septal extension graft and costal cartilage strut
fixed with K-wire*

**Timothy W. King, MD, PhD, MSBE,
FACS, FAAP**
Assistant Professor of Surgery and Pediatrics
Director of Research
Division of Plastic Surgery, Department of
Surgery
University of Wisconsin School of Medicine and
Public Health
Madison, WI, USA
Volume 1, Chapter 32 Implants and biomaterials

Brian M. Kinney, MD, FACS, MSME
Clinical Assistant Professor of Plastic Surgery
University of Southern California School of
Medicine
Los Angeles, CA, USA
*Volume 1, Chapter 7 Photography in plastic
surgery*

Richard E. Kirschner, MD
Chief, Section of Plastic and Reconstructive
Surgery
Director, Ambulatory Surgical Services
Director, Cleft Lip and Palate Center
Co-Director Nationwide Children's Hospital
Professor of Surgery and Pediatrics
Senior Vice Chair, Department of Plastic Surgery
The Ohio State University College of Medicine
Columbus, OH, USA
Volume 3, Chapter 28 Velopharyngeal dysfunction
*Volume 3, Video 28.01-28.03 Velopharyngeal
incompetence*

Elizabeth Kiwanuka, MD
Division of Plastic Surgery
Brigham and Women's Hospital
Harvard Medical School
Boston, MA, USA
*Volume 1, Chapter 11 Genetics and prenatal
diagnosis*

Grant M. Kleiber, MD
Plastic Surgery Resident
Section of Plastic and Reconstructive Surgery
University of Chicago Medical Center
Chicago, IL, USA
*Volume 4, Chapter 1 Comprehensive lower
extremity anatomy, embryology, surgical exposure*

Mathew B. Klein, MD, MS
David and Nancy Auth-Washington Research
Foundation Endowed Chair for Restorative
Burn Surgery
Division of Plastic Surgery
University of Washington
Program Director and Associate Professor
Division of Plastic Surgery
Harborview Medical Center
Seattle, WA, USA
Volume 4, Chapter 22 Reconstructive burn surgery

Kyung S Koh, MD, PhD
Professor of Plastic Surgery
Asan Medical Center, University of Ulsan
School of Medicine
Seoul, Korea
*Volume 2, Chapter 10 Asian facial cosmetic
surgery*

John C. Koshy, MD
Postdoctoral Research Fellow
Division of Plastic Surgery
Baylor College of Medicine
Houston, TX, USA
*Volume 3, Chapter 29 Secondary deformities of
the cleft lip, nose, and palate*
Volume 3, Video 29.01 Complete takedown
Volume 3, Video 29.02 Abbé flap
*Volume 3, Video 29.03 Thick lip and buccal
sulcus deformities*
Volume 3, Video 29.04 Alveolar bone grafting
Volume 3, Video 29.05 Definitive rhinoplasty

Evan Kowalski, BS
Section of Plastic Surgery
University of Michigan Health System
Ann Arbor, MI, USA
Volume 6, Video 19.02 Silicone MCP arthroplasty

Stephen J. Kovach, MD
Assistant Professor of Surgery
Division of Plastic and Reconstructive Surgery
University of Pennsylvannia Health System
Assistant Professor of Surgery
Department of Orthopaedic Surgery
University of Pennsylvannia Health System
Philadelphia, PA, USA
Volume 4, Chapter 7 Skeletal reconstruction

Steven J. Kronowitz, MD, FACS
Professor, Department of Plastic Surgery
MD Anderson Cancer Center
The University of Texas
Houston, TX, USA
Volume 1, Chapter 28 Therapeutic radiation principles, effects, and complications

Todd A. Kuiken, MD, PhD
Director
Center for Bionic Medicine
Rehabilitation Institute of Chicago
Professor
Department of PMandR
Fienberg School of Medicine
Northwestern University
Chicago, IL, USA
Volume 6, Chapter 40 Treatment of the upper extremity amputee
Volume 6, Video 40.01 Targeted muscle reinnervation in the transhumeral amputee

Michael E. Kupferman, MD
Assistant Professor
Department of Head and Neck Surgery
Division of Surgery
The University of Texas MD Anderson Cancer Center
Houston, TX, USA
Volume 3, Chapter 17 Carcinoma of the upper aerodigestive tract

Robert Kwon, MD
Plastic Surgeon
Regional Plastic Surgery Center
Richardson, TX, USA
Volume 4, Chapter 16 Pressure sores

Eugenia J. Kyriopoulos, MD, MSc, PhD, FEBOPRAS
Attending Plastic Surgeon
Department of Plastic Surgery and Burn Center
Athens General Hospital "G. Gennimatas"
Athens, Greece
Volume 5, Chapter 21 Local flaps in partial breast reconstruction

Donald Lalonde, BSC, MD, MSc, FRCSC
Professor Surgery
Division of Plastic Surgery
Saint John Campus of Dalhousie University
Saint John, NB, Canada
Volume 6, Chapter 24 Nerve entrapment syndromes
Volume 6, Video 24.01 Carpal tunnel and cubital tunnel releases

Wee Leon Lam, MB, ChB, M Phil, FRCS
Microsurgery Fellow
Department of Plastic and Reconstructive Surgery
Chang Gung Memorial Hospital
Taipei, Taiwan, The People's Republic of China
Volume 6, Chapter 14 Thumb and finger reconstruction – microsurgical techniques
Volume 6, Video 14.01 Trimmed great toe
Volume 6, Video 14.02 Second toe for index
Volume 6, Video 14.03 Combined second and third toe for metacarpal hand

Julie E. Lang, MD, FACS
Assistant Professor of Surgery
Department of surgery
Director of Breast Surgical Oncology
University of Arizona
Tucson, AZ, USA
Volume 5, Chapter 10 Breast cancer: Diagnosis therapy and oncoplastic techniques
Volume 5, Video 10.01 Breast cancer: diagnosis and therapy

Patrick Lang, MD
Plastic Surgery Resident
University of California
San Francisco, CA, USA
Volume 1, Chapter 24 Flap classification and applications

Claude-Jean Langevin, MD, DMD
Assistant Professor University of Central Florida
Department of Surgery MD Anderson Cancer Center
Plastic and Reconstructive Surgeon
University of Central Florida
Orlando, FL, USA
Volume 2, Chapter 13 Neck rejuvenation

Laurent Lantieri, MD
Department of Plastic Surgery
Hôpital Européen Georges Pompidou
Assistance Publique Hôpitaux de Paris
Paris Descartes University
Paris, France
Volume 3, Chapter 20 Facial transplant
Volume 3, Video 20.1 and 20.2 Facial transplant

Michael C. Large, MD
Urology Resident
Department of Surgery, Division of Urology
University of Chicago Hospitals
Chicago, IL, USA
Volume 3, Chapter 44 Reconstruction of urogenital defects: Congenital
Volume 3, Video 44.01 First stage hypospadias repair with free inner preputial graft
Volume 3, Video 44.02 Second stage hypospadias repair with tunica vaginalis flap

Don LaRossa, MD
Emeritus Professor of Surgery
Division of Plastic and Reconstructive Surgery
Perelman School of Medicine
University of Pennsylvania
Philadelphia, PA, USA
Volume 3, Chapter 43 Conjoined twins

Caroline Leclercq, MD
Consultant Hand Surgeon
Institut de la Main
Paris, France
Volume 6, Chapter 17 Management of Dupuytren's disease

Justine C. Lee, MD, PhD
Chief Resident
Section of Plastic and Reconstructive Surgery Department
University of Chicago Medical Center
Chicago, IL, USA
Volume 3, Chapter 41 Pediatric chest and trunk defects

W. P. Andrew Lee, MD
The Milton T. Edgerton, MD, Professor and Chairman
Department of Plastic and Reconstructive Surgery
Johns Hopkins University School of Medicine
Baltimore, MD, USA
Volume 1, Chapter 34 Transplantation in plastic surgery
Volume 6, Chapter 38 Upper extremity composite allotransplantation
Volume 6, Video 38.01 Upper extremity composite tissue allotransplantation

Valerie Lemaine, MD, MPH, FRCSC
Assistant Professor of Plastic Surgery
Department of Surgery
Division of Plastic Surgery
Mayo Clinic
Rochester, MN, USA
Volume 1, Chapter 10 Evidence-based medicine and health services research in plastic surgery

Ping-Chung Leung, SBS, OBE, JP, MBBS, MS, DSc, Hon DSocSc, FRACS, FRCS, FHKCOS, FHKAM (ORTH)
Professor Emeritus
Orthopaedics and Traumatology
The Chinese University of Hong Kong
Hong Kong, The People's Republic of China
Volume 6, Chapter 29 Congenital hand V disorders of overgrowth, undergrowth, and generalized skeletal deformities

Benjamin Levi, MD
Post Doctoral Research Fellow
Division of Plastic and Reconstructive Surgery
Stanford University
Stanford, CA
House Officer
Division of Plastic and Reconstructive Surgery
University of Michigan
Ann Arbor, MI, USA
Volume 1, Chapter 13 Stem cells and regenerative medicine

L. Scott Levin, MD, FACS
Chairman of Orthopedic Surgery
Department of Orthopaedic Surgery
University of Pennsylvania School of Medicine
Philadelphia, PA, USA
Volume 4, Chapter 7 Skeletal reconstruction

Bradley Limmer, MD
Assistant Clinical Professor
Department of Internal Medicine
Division of Dermatology
Associate Clinical Professor
Department of Plastic and Reconstructive
Surgery
Surgeon, Private Practice
Limmer Clinic
San Antonio, TX, USA
Volume 2, Video 23.02 Follicular unit hair
transplantation

Bobby L. Limmer, MD
Professor of Dermatology
University of Texas
Surgeon, Private Practice
Limmer Clinic
San Antonio, TX, USA
Volume 2, Video 23.02 Follicular unit hair
transplantation

Frank Lista, MD, FRCSC
Medical Director
Burn Program
The Plastic Surgery Clinic
Mississauga, ON, Canada
Volume 5, Chapter 8.3 Superior or medial
pedicle

Wei Liu, MD, PhD
Professor of Plastic Surgery
Associate Director of National Tissue
Engineering Research Center
Department of Plastic and Reconstructive
Surgery
Shanghai 9th People's Hospital
Shanghai Jiao Tong University School of
Medcine
Shanghai, The People's Republic of China
Volume 1, Chapter 18 Tissue graft, tissue repair,
and regeneration
Volume 1, Chapter 20 Repair, grafting, and
engineering of cartilage

Michelle B. Locke, MBChB, MD
Honourary Lecturer
University of Auckland Department of Surgery
Auckland City Hospital Support Building
Grafton, Auckland, New Zealand
Volume 2, Chapter 1 Managing the cosmetic
patient

Sarah A. Long, BA
Research Associate
Thayer School of Engineering
Dartmouth College
San Mateo, CA, USA
Volume 1, Chapter 36 Robotics, simulation, and
telemedicine in plastic surgery

Michael T. Longaker, MD, MBA, FACS
Deane P. and Louise Mitchell Professor and
Vice Chair
Department of Surgery
Stanford University
Stanford, CA, USA
Volume 1, Chapter 13 Stem cells and
regenerative medicine

Peter Lorenz, MD
Chief of Pediatric Plastic Surgery, Director
Craniofacial Surgery Fellowship
Department of Surgery, Division of Plastic
Surgery
Stanford University School of Medicine
Stanford, CA, USA
Volume 1, Chapter 16 Scar prevention,
treatment, and revision

Joseph E. Losee, MD, FACS, FAAP
Professor of Surgery and Pediatrics
Chief, Division Pediatric Plastic Surgery
Children's Hospital of Pittsburgh
University of Pittsburgh Medical Center
Pittsburgh, PA, USA
Volume 3, Chapter 31 Pediatric facial fractures

Albert Losken, MD, FACS
Associate Professor Program Director
Emory Division of Plastic and Reconstructive
Surgery
Emory University School of Medicine
Atlanta, GA, USA
Volume 5, Chapter 11 The oncoplastic approach
to partial breast reconstruction

Maria M. LoTempio, MD
Assistant Professor in Plastic Surgery
Medical University of South Carolina
Charleston, SC
Adjunct Assistant Professor in Plastic Surgery
New York Eye and Ear Infirmary
New York, NY, USA
Volume 5, Chapter 19 Alternative flaps for breast
reconstruction

Otway Louie, MD
Assistant Professor
Division of Plastic and Reconstructive Surgery
Department of Surgery
University of Washington Medical Center
Seattle, WA, USA
Volume 4, Chapter 17 Perineal reconstruction

David W. Low, MD
Professor of Surgery
Division of Plastic Surgery
University of Pennsylvania School of Medicine
Clinical Associate
The Children's Hospital of Philadelphia
Philadelphia, PA, USA
Volume 3, Chapter 43 Conjoined twins

Nicholas Lumen, MD, PhD
Assistant Professor of Urology
Urology
Ghent University Hospital
Ghent, Belgium
Volume 4, Chapter 13 Reconstruction of male
genital defects
Volume 4, Video 13.01 Complete and partial
penile reconstruction

Antonio Luiz de Vasconcellos Macedo, MD
General Surgery
Director of Robotic Surgery
President of Oncology
Board of Albert Einstein Hospital
Sao Paulo, Brazil
Volume 5, Chapter 20 Omentum reconstruction
of the breast

Gustavo R. Machado, MD
University of California Irvine Medical Center
Department of Orthopaedic Surgery, Orange,
CA, USA
Volume 6, Video 34.01 EIP to EPL tendon
transfer

Susan E. Mackinnon, MD
Sydney M. Shoenberg, Jr. and Robert H.
Shoenberg Professor
Department of Surgery, Division of Plastic and
Reconstructive Surgery
Washington University School of Medicine
St. Louis, MO, USA
Volume 1, Chapter 22 Repair and grafting of
peripheral nerve
Volume 6, Chapter 33 Nerve transfers
Volume 6, Video 33.01 Nerve transfers

Ralph T. Manktelow, BA, MD, FRCS(C)
Professor
Department of Surgery
University of Toronto
Toronto, ON, Canada
Volume 3, Chapter 11 Facial paralysis

Paul N. Manson, MD
Professor of Plastic Surgery
University of Maryland Shock Trauma Unit
University of Maryland and Johns Hopkins
Schools of Medicine
Baltimore, MD, USA
Volume 3, Chapter 3 Facial fractures

Daniel Marchac, MD
Professor
Plastic, Reconstructive and Aesthetic
College of Medicine of Paris Hospitals
Paris, France
Volume 3, Chapter 32 Orbital hypertelorism

Malcom W. Marks, MD
Professor and Chairman
Department of Plastic Surgery
Wake Forest University School of Medicine
Winston-Salem, NC, USA
Volume 1, Chapter 27 Principles and applications
of tissue expansion

Timothy J. Marten, MD, FACS
Founder and Director
Marten Clinic of Plastic Surgery
Medical Director
San Francisco Center for the Surgical Arts
San Francisco, CA, USA
Volume 2, Chapter 12 Secondary deformities
and the secondary facelift

Mario Marzola, MBBS
Private Practice
Norwood, SA, Australia
Volume 2, Video 23.01 Donor closure tricophytic technique

Alessandro Masellis, MD
Plastic Surgeon
Department of Plastic Surgery and Burn Therapy
Ospedale Civico ARNAS Palermo
Palermo, Italy
Volume 4, Chapter 19 Extremity burn reconstruction

Michele Masellis, MD, PhD
Plastic Surgeon
Former Chief
Professor Emeritus
Department of Plastic Surgery and Burn Unit
ARNAS Civico Hospital
Palermo, Italy
Volume 4, Chapter 19 Extremity burn reconstruction

Jaume Masia, MD, PhD
Professor and Chief
Plastic Surgery Department
Hospital de la Santa Creu i Sant Pau
Universidad Autónoma de Barcelona
Barcelona, Spain
Volume 5, Chapter 13 Imaging in reconstructive breast surgery

David W. Mathes, MD
Associate Professor of Surgery
Department of Surgery, Division of Plastic and Reconstructive Surgery
University of Washington School of Medicine
Chief of Plastic Surgery
Puget Sound Veterans Affairs Hospital
Seattle, WA, USA
Volume 1, Chapter 34 Transplantation in plastic surgery

Evan Matros, MD
Assistant Attending Surgeon
Department of Surgery
Memorial Sloan-Kettering Cancer Center
Assistant Professor of Surgery (Plastic)
Weill Cornell University Medical Center
New York, NY, USA
Volume 1, Chapter 12 Principles of cancer management

G. Patrick Maxwell, MD, FACS
Clinical Professor of Surgery
Department of Plastic Surgery
Loma Linda University Medical Center
Loma Linda, CA, USA
Volume 5, Chapter 2 Breast augmentation
Volume 5, Chapter 4 Current concepts in revisionary breast surgery

Isabella C. Mazzola
Milan, Italy
Volume 1, Chapter 2 History of reconstructive and aesthetic surgery

Riccardo F. Mazzola, MD
Professor of Plastic Surgery
Postgraduate School Plastic Surgery
Maxillo-Facial and Otolaryngolog
Department of Specialistic Surgical Science
School of Medicine
University of Milan
Milan, Italy
Volume 1, Chapter 2 History of reconstructive and aesthetic surgery

Steven J. McCabe, MD, MSc
Assistant Professor
Department of Bioinformatics and Biostatistics
University of Louisville School of Public Health and Information Sciences
Louisville, KY, USA
Volume 6, Chapter 18 Occupational hand disorders

Joseph G. McCarthy, MD
Lawrence D. Bell Professor of Plastic Surgery,
Director Institute of Reconstructive Plastic Surgery and Chair
Department of Plastic Surgery
New York University Langone Medical Center
New York, NY, USA
Volume 3, Chapter 36 Craniofacial microsomia

Mary H. McGrath, MD, MPH
Plastic Surgeon
Division of Plastic Surgery
University of California San Francisco
San Francisco, CA, USA
Volume 1, Chapter 3 Psychological aspects of plastic surgery

Kai Megerle, MD
Research Fellow
Division of Plastic and Reconstructive Surgery
Stanford Medical Center
Stanford, CA, USA
Volume 6, Chapter 10 Extensor tendon injuries

Babak J. Mehrara, MD, FACS
Associate Member, Associate Professor of Surgery (Plastic)
Memorial Sloan-Kettering Cancer Center
Weil Cornell University Medical Center
New York, NY, USA
Volume 1, Chapter 12 Principles of cancer management

Bryan Mendelson, FRCSE, FRACS, FACS
Private Plastic Surgeon
The Centre for Facial Plastic Surgery
Melbourne, Australia
Volume 2, Chapter 6 Anatomy of the aging face

Constantino G. Mendieta, MD, FACS
Private Practice
Miami, FL, USA
Volume 2, Chapter 28 Buttock augmentation
Volume 2, Video 28.01 Buttock augmentation

Frederick J. Menick, MD
Private Practitioner
Tucson, AZ, USA
Volume 3, Chapter 6 Aesthetic nasal reconstruction
Volume 3, Video 6.01 Aesthetic reconstruction of the nose – The 3-stage folded forehead flap for cover and lining,
Volume 3, Video 6.02 Aesthetic reconstruction of the nose-First stage transfer and intermediate operation

Ursula Mirastschijski, MD, PhD
Assistant Professor
Department of Plastic, Hand and Reconstructive Surgery, Burn Center Lower Saxony, Replantation Center
Hannover Medical School
Hannover, Germany
Volume 1, Chapter 15 Skin wound healing: Repair biology, wound, and scar treatment

Takayuki Miura, MD
Emeritus Professor of Orthopedic Surgery
Department of Orthopedic Surgery
Nagoya University School of Medicine
Nagoya, Japan
Volume 6, Chapter 29 Congenital hand V: Disorders of overgrowth, undergrowth, and generalized skeletal deformities

Fernando Molina, MD
Professor of Plastic, Aesthetic and Reconstructive Surgery
Reconstructive and Plastic Surgery
Hospital General "Dr. Manuel Gea Gonzalez"
Universidad Nacional Autonoma de Mexico
Mexico City, Mexico
Volume 3, Chapter 39 Treacher-Collins syndrome

Stan Monstrey, MD, PhD
Professor in Plastic Surgery
Department of Plastic Surgery
Ghent University Hospital
Ghent, Belgium
Volume 4, Chapter 13 Reconstruction of male genital defects
Volume 4, Video 13.01 Complete and partial penile reconstruction

Steven L. Moran, MD
Professor and Chair of Plastic Surgery
Division of Plastic Surgery, Division of Hand and Microsurgery
Professor of Orthopedics
Rochester, MN, USA
Volume 6, Chapter 20 Management of osteoarthritis of the hand and wrist

Luis Humberto Uribe Morelli, MD
Resident of Plastic Surgery
Unisanta Plastic Surgery Department
Sao Paulo, Brazil
Volume 2, Chapter 26 Lipoabdominoplasty
Volume 2, Video 26.01 Lipobdominoplasty
(including secondary lipo)

Robert J. Morin, MD
Plastic Surgeon and Craniofacial Surgeon
Department of Plastic Surgery
Hackensack University Medical Center
Hackensack, NJ
New York Eye and Ear Infirmary
New York, NY, USA
Volume 3, Chapter 8 Acquired cranial and facial bone deformities

Steven F. Morris, MD, MSc, FRCS(C)
Professor of Surgery
Professor of Anatomy and Neurobiology
Dalhousie University
Halifax, NS, Canada
Volume 1, Chapter 23 Vascular territories

Colin Myles Morrison, MSc (Hons), FRCSI (Plast)
Consultant Plastic Surgeon
Department of Plastic and Reconstructive Surgery
St. Vincent's University Hospital
Dublin, Ireland
Volume 2, Chapter 13 Neck rejuvenation
Volume 5, Chapter 18 The deep inferior epigastric artery perforator (DIEAP) flap

Wayne A. Morrison, MBBS, MD, FRACS
Director
O'Brien Institute
Professorial Fellow
Department of Surgery
St Vincent's Hospital
University of Melbourne
Plastic Surgeon
St Vincent's Hospital
Melbourne, Australia
Volume 1, Chapter 19 Tissue engineering

Robyn Mosher, MS
Medical Editor/Project Manager
Thayer School of Engineering (contract)
Dartmouth College
Norwich, VT, USA
Volume 1, Chapter 36 Robotics, simulation, and telemedicine in plastic surgery

Dimitrios Motakis, MD, PhD, FRCSC
Plastic and Reconstructive Surgeon
Private Practice
University Lecturer
Department of Surgery
University of Toronto
Toronto, ON, Canada
Volume 2, Chapter 4 Soft-tissue fillers

A. Aldo Mottura, MD, PhD
Associate Professor of Surgery
School of Medicine
National University of Córdoba
Cordoba, Argentina
Volume 1, Chapter 9 Local anesthetics in plastic surgery

Hunter R. Moyer, MD
Fellow
Department of Plastic and Reconstructive Surgery
Emory University, Atlanta, GA, USA
Volume 5, Chapter 16 The bilateral Pedicled TRAM flap

Gustavo Muchado, MD
Plastic surgeon
Division of Plastic and Reconstructive Surgery and Department of Orthopaedic Surgery
University of California Irvine Medical Center
Orange, CA, USA
Volume 6, Video 34.01 EIP to EPL tendon transfer

Reid V. Mueller, MD
Associate Professor
Division of Plastic and Reconstructive Surgery
Oregon Health and Science University
Portland, OR, USA
Volume 3, Chapter 2 Facial trauma: soft tissue injuries

John B. Mulliken, MD
Director, Craniofacial Centre
Department of Plastic and Oral Surgery
Children's Hospital
Boston, MA, USA
Volume 1, Chapter 29 Vascular anomalies
Volume 3, Chapter 24 Repair of bilateral cleft lip

Egle Muti, MD
Associate Professor of Plastic Reconstructive and Aesthetic Surgery
Department of Plastic Surgery
University of Turin School of Medicine
Turin, Italy
Volume 5, Chapter 23.1 Congenital anomalies of the breast
Volume 5, Video 23.01.01 Congenital anomalies of the breast: An example of tuberous breast type 1 corrected with glandular flap type 1

Maurice Y. Nahabedian, MD
Associate Professor Plastic Surgery
Department of Plastic Surgery
Georgetown University and Johns Hopkins University
Northwest, WA, USA
Volume 5, Chapter 22 Reconstruction of the nipple-areola complex
Volume 5, Video 11.01 Partial breast reconstruction using reduction mammaplasty
Volume 5, Video 11.03 Partial breast reconstruction with a pedicle TRAM

Foad Nahai, MD, FACS
Clinical Professor of Plastic Surgery
Department of Surgery
Emory University School of Medicine
Atlanta, GA, USA
Volume 2, Chapter 1 Managing the cosmetic patient

Fabio X. Nahas, MD, PhD
Associate Professor
Division of Plastic Surgery
Federal University of São Paulo
São Paulo, Brazil
Volume 2, Video 24.01 Liposculpture

Deepak Narayan, MS, FRCS (Eng), FRCS (Edin)
Associate Professor of Surgery
Yale University School of Medicine
Chief
Plastic Surgery
VA Medical Center
West Haven, CT, USA
Volume 3, Chapter 14 Salivary gland tumors

Maurizio B. Nava, MD
Chief of Plastic Surgery Unit
Istituto Nazionale dei Tumori
Milano, Italy
Volume 5, Chapter 14 Expander/implant reconstruction of the breast
Volume 5, Video 14.01 Mastectomy and expander insertion: first stage
Volume 5, Video 14.02 Mastectomy and expander insertion: second stage

Carmen Navarro, MD
Plastic Surgery Consultant
Plastic Surgery Department
Hospital de la Santa Creu i Sant Pau
Universidad Autónoma de Barcelona
Barcelona, Spain
Volume 5, Chapter 13 Imaging in reconstructive breast surgery

Peter C. Neligan, MB, FRCS(I), FRCSC, FACS
Professor of Surgery
Department of Surgery, Division of Plastic Surgery
University of Washington
Seattle, WA, USA
Volume 1, Chapter 1 Plastic surgery and innovation in medicine
Volume 1, Chapter 25 Flap pathophysiology and pharmacology
Volume 3, Chapter 10 Cheek and lip reconstruction
Volume 4, Chapter 3 Lymphatic reconstruction of the extremities
Volume 3, Video 11.01-03 (1) Facial paralysis (2) cross fact graft, (3) gracilis harvest
Volume 3, Video 18.01 Facial artery perforator flap
Volume 4, Video 3.02 Charles Procedure
Volume 5, Video 18.01 SIEA
Volume 5, Video 19.01-19.03 Alternative free flaps

Jonas A Nelson, MD
Integrated General/Plastic Surgery Resident
Department of Surgery
Division of Plastic Surgery
Perelman School of Medicine
University of Pennsylvania
Philadelphia, PA, USA
Volume 5, Video 17.01 The muscle sparing free TRAM flap

David T. Netscher, MD
Clinical Professor
Division of Plastic Surgery
Baylor College of Medicine
Houston, TX, USA
Volume 6, Chapter 21 The stiff hand and the spastic hand

Michael W. Neumeister, MD
Professor and Chairman
Division of Plastic Surgery
SIU School of Medicine
Springfield, IL, USA
Volume 6, Chapter 6 Nail and fingertip reconstruction

M. Samuel Noordhoff, MD, FACS
Emeritus Superintendent
Chang Gung Memorial Hospitals
Taipei, Taiwan, The People's Republic of China
Volume 3, Chapter 23 Repair of unilateral cleft lip

Christine B. Novak, PT, PhD
Research Associate
Hand Program, Division of Plastic and
Reconstructive Surgery
University Health Network, University of Toronto
Toronto, ON, Canada
Volume 6, Chapter 39 Hand therapy

Daniel Nowinski, MD, PhD
Director
Department of Plastic and Maxillofacial Surgery
Uppsala Craniofacial Center
Uppsala University Hospital
Uppsala, Sweden
Volume 1, Chapter 11 Genetics and prenatal diagnosis

Scott Oates, MD
Professor
Department of Plastic Surgery
The University of Texas MD Anderson Cancer
Center
Houston, TX, USA
Volume 6, Chapter 15 Benign and malignant tumors of the hand

Kerby Oberg, MD, PhD
Associate Professor
Department of Pathology and Human Anatomy
Loma Linda University School of Medicine
Loma Linda, CA, USA
Volume 6, Chapter 25 Congenital hand 1: embryology, classification, and principles

James P. O'Brien, MD, FRCSC
Associate Professor of Surgery
Dalhousie University
Halifax Nova Scotia
Clinical Associate Professor of Surgery
Memorial University
St. John's Newfoundland
Vice President Research
Innovation and Development
Horizon Health Network
New Brunswick, NB, Canada
Volume 6, Chapter 24 Nerve entrapment syndromes

Andrea J. O'Connor, BE(Hons), PhD
Associate Professor of Chemical and
Biomolecular Engineering
Department of Chemical and Biomolecular
Engineering
University of Melbourne
Melbourne, VIC, Australia
Volume 1, Chapter 19 Tissue engineering

Rei Ogawa, MD, PhD
Associate Professor
Department of Plastic
Reconstructive and Aesthetic Surgery Nippon
Medical School
Tokyo, Japan
Volume 1, Chapter 30 Benign and malignant nonmelanocytic tumors of the skin and soft tissue

Dennis P. Orgill, MD, PhD
Professor of Surgery
Division of Plastic Surgery, Brigham and
Women's Hospital
Harvard Medical School
Boston, MA, USA
Volume 1, Chapter 17 Skin graft

Cho Y. Pang, PhD
Senior Scientist
Research Institute
The Hospital for Sick Children
Professor
Departments of Surgery/Physiology
University of Toronto
Toronto, ON, Canada
Volume 1, Chapter 25 Flap pathophysiology and pharmacology

Ketan M. Patel, MD
Resident Physician
Department of Plastic Surgery
Georgetown University Hospital
Washington DC, USA
Volume 5, Chapter 22 Reconstruction of the nipple-areola complex

William C. Pederson, MD, FACS
President and Fellowship Director
The Hand Center of San Antonio
Adjunct Professor of Surgery
The University of Texas Health Science Center
at San Antonio
San Antonio, TX, USA
Volume 6, Chapter 12 Reconstructive surgery of the mutilated hand

José Abel de la Peña Salcedo, MD
Secretario Nacional
Federación Iberolatinoamericana de Cirugía
Plástica, Estética y Reconstructiva
Director del Instituto de Cirugia Plastica, S.C.
Hospital Angeles de las Lomas
Col.Valle de las Palmas
Huixquilucan, Edo de Mexico, Mexico
Volume 2, Chapter 28 Buttock augmentation
Volume 2, Video 28.01 Buttock augmentation

Angela Pennati, MD
Assistant Plastic Surgeon
Unit of Plastic Surgery
Istituto Nazionale dei Tumori
Milano, Italy
Volume 5, Chapter 14 Expander/implant breast reconstructions
Volume 5, Video 14.01 Mastectomy and expander insertion: first stage
Volume 5, Video 14.02 Mastectomy and expander insertion: second stage

Joel E. Pessa, MD
Clinical Associate Professor of Plastic Surgery
UTSW Medical School
Dallas, TX
Hand and Microsurgery Fellow
Christine M. Kleinert Hand and Microsurgery
Louisville, KY, USA
Volume 2, Chapter 17 Nasal analysis and anatomy

Walter Peters, MD, PhD, FRCSC
Professor of Surgery
Department of Plastic Surgery
University of Toronto
Toronto, ON, Canada
Volume 5, Chapter 6 Iatrogenic disorders following breast surgery

Giorgio Pietramaggiori, MD, PhD
Plastic Surgery Resident
Department of Plastic and Reconstructive
Surgery
University Hospital of Lausanne
Lausanne, Switzerland
Volume 1, Chapter 17 Skin graft

John W. Polley, MD
Professor and Chairman
Rush University Medical Center
Department of Plastic and Reconstructive
Surgery
John W. Curtin – Chair
Co-Director, Rush Craniofacial Center
Chicago, IL, USA
Volume 3, Chapter 27 Orthodontics in cleft lip and palate management

Bohdan Pomahac, MD
Assistant Professor
Harvard Medical School
Director
Plastic Surgery Transplantation
Medical Director
Burn Center
Division of Plastic Surgery
Brigham and Women's Hospital
Boston, MA, USA
Volume 1, Chapter 11 Genetics and prenatal diagnosis

Julian J. Pribaz, MD
Professor of Surgery Harvard Medical School
Division of Plastic Surgery
Brigham and Women's Hospital
Boston, MA, USA
Volume 3, Chapter 19 Secondary facial reconstruction

Andrea L. Pusic, MD, MHS, FRCSC
Associate Attending Surgeon
Department of Plastic and Reconstructive
Memorial Sloan-Kettering Cancer Center
New York, NY, USA
Volume 1, Chapter 10 Evidence-based medicine and health services research in plastic surgery
Volume 4, Chapter 14 Reconstruction of acquired vaginal defects

Oscar M. Ramirez, MD, FACS
Adjunct Clinical Faculty
Plastic Surgery Division
Cleveland Clinic Florida
Boca Raton, FL, USA
Volume 2, Chapter 11.8 Facelift: Subperiosteal facelift
Volume 2, Video 11.08.01 Facelift: Subperiosteal mid facelift endoscopic temporo-midface

William R. Rassman, MD
Director
Private Practice
New Hair Institution
Los Angeles, CA, USA
Volume 2, Video 23.04 FUE FOX procedure

Russell R. Reid, MD, PhD
Assistant Professor of Surgery, Bernard Sarnat Scholar
Section of Plastic and Reconstructive Surgery
University of Chicago
Chicago, IL, USA
Volume 1, Chapter 21 Repair and grafting of bone
Volume 3, Chapter 41 Pediatric chest and trunk defects

Neal R. Reisman, MD, JD
Chief of Plastic Surgery, Clinical Professor
Plastic Surgery
St. Luke's Episcopal Hospital
Baylor College of Medicine
Houston, TX, USA
Volume 1, Chapter 6 Medico-legal issues in plastic surgery

Dominique Renier, MD, PhD
Pediatric Neurosurgeon
Service de Neurochirurgie Pédiatrique
Hôpital Necker-Enfants Malades
Paris, France
Volume 3, Chapter 32 Orbital hypertelorism

Dirk F. Richter, MD, PhD
Clinical Director
Department of Plastic Surgery
Dreifaltigkeits-Hospital Wesseling
Wesseling, Germany
Volume 2, Chapter 25 Abdominoplasty procedures
Volume 2, Video 25.01 Abdominoplasty

Thomas L. Roberts III, FACS
Plastic Surgery Center of the Carolinas
Spartanburg, SC, USA
Volume 2, Chapter 28 Buttock augmentation
Volume 2, Video 28.01 Buttock augmentation

Federico Di Rocco, MD, PhD
Pediatric Neurosurgery
Hôpital Necker Enfants Malades
Paris, France
Volume 3, Chapter 32 Orbital hypertelorism

Natalie Roche, MD
Associate Professor
Department of Plastic Surgery
Ghent University Hospital
Ghent, Belgium
Volume 4, Chapter 13 Reconstruction of male genital defects
Volume 4, Video 13.01 Complete and partial penile reconstruction

Eduardo D. Rodriguez, MD, DDS
Chief, Plastic Reconstructive and Maxillofacial Surgery, R Adams Cowley Shock Trauma Center
Professor of Surgery
University of Maryland School of Medicine
Baltimore, MD, USA
Volume 3, Chapter 3 Facial fractures

Thomas E. Rohrer, MD
Director, Mohs Surgery
SkinCare Physicians of Chestnut Hill
Clinical Associate Professor
Department of Dermatology
Boston University
Boston, MA, USA
Volume 2, Video 5.02 Facial resurfacing

Rod J. Rohrich, MD, FACS
Professor and Chairman Crystal Charity Ball
Distinguished Chair in Plastic Surgery
Department of Plastic Surgery
Professor and Chairman Betty and Warren
Woodward Chair in Plastic and Reconstructive Surgery
University of Texas Southwestern Medical Center at Dallas
Dallas, TX, USA
Volume 2, Chapter 17 Nasal analysis and anatomy
Volume 2, Chapter 18 Open technique rhinoplasty

Joseph M. Rosen, MD
Professor of Surgery
Division of Plastic Surgery, Department of Surgery
Dartmouth-Hitchcock Medical Center
Lyme, NH, USA
Volume 1, Chapter 36 Robotics, simulation, and telemedicine in plastic surgery

E. Victor Ross, MD
Director of Laser and Cosmetic Dermatology
Scripps Clinic
San Diego, CA, USA
Volume 2, Chapter 5 Facial skin resurfacing

Michelle C. Roughton, MD
Chief Resident
Section of Plastic and Reconstructive Surgery
University of Chicago Medical Center
Chicago, IL, USA
Volume 4, Chapter 10 Reconstruction of the chest

Sashwati Roy, PhD
Associate Professor of Surgery
Department of Surgery
The Ohio State University Medical Center
Columbus, OH, USA
Volume 1, Chapter 14 Wound healing

J. Peter Rubin, MD, FACS
Chief of Plastic Surgery
Director, Life After Weight Loss Body Contouring Program
University of Pittsburgh
Pittsburgh, PA, USA
Volume 2, Chapter 30 Post-bariatric reconstruction
Volume 2, Video 30.01 Post bariatric reconstruction – bodylift procedure
Volume 5, Chapter 25 Contouring of the arms, breast, upper trunk, and male chest in the massive weight loss patient
Volume 5, Video 25.01 Brachioplasty part 1: contouring of the arms
Volume 5, Video 25.02 Bracioplasty part 2: contouring of the arms

Alesia P. Saboeiro, MD
Attending Physician
Private Practice
New York, NY, USA
Volume 2, Chapter 14 Structural fat grafting
*Volume 2, Video 14.01 Structural fat grafting of
the face*

Justin M. Sacks, MD
Assistant Professor
Department of Plastic and Reconstructive
Surgery
The Johns Hopkins University School of
Medicine
Baltimore, MD, USA
*Volume 3, Chapter 17 Carcinoma of the upper
aerodigestive tract*
*Volume 6, Chapter 15 Benign and malignant
tumors of the hand*

Hakim K. Said, MD
Assistant Professor of Surgery
Division of Plastic Surgery
University of Washington
Seattle, WA, USA
Volume 4, Chapter 17 Perineal reconstruction

Michel Saint-Cyr, MD, FRCSC
Associate Professor Plastic Surgery
Department of Plastic Surgery
University of Texas Southwestern Medical
Center
Dallas, TX, USA
*Volume 4, Chapter 2 Management of lower
extremity trauma*
Volume 4, Video 2.01 Alternative flap harvest

Cristianna Bonneto Saldanha, MD
Resident
General Surgery Department
Santa Casa of Santos Hospital
São Paulo, Brazil
Volume 2, Chapter 26 Lipoabdominoplasty
*Volume 2, Video 26.01 Lipobdominoplasty
(including secondary lipo)*

Osvaldo Ribeiro Saldanha, MD
Chairman of Plastic Surgery
Unisanta
Santos
Past President of the Brazilian Society of
Plastic Surgery (SBCP)
International Associate Editor of Plastic and
Reconstructive Surgery
São Paulo, Brazil
Volume 2, Chapter 26 Lipoabdominoplasty
*Volume 2, Video 26.01 Lipobdominoplasty
(including secondary lipo)*

Osvaldo Ribeiro Saldanha Filho, MD
São Paulo, Brazil
Volume 2, Chapter 26 Lipoabdominoplasty
*Volume 2, Video 26.01 Lipobdominoplasty
(including secondary lipo)*

Douglas M. Sammer, MD
Assistant Professor of Plastic Surgery
Department of Plastic Surgery
University of Texas Southwestern Medical
Center
Dallas, TX, USA
*Volume 6, Chapter 19 Rheumatologic conditions
of the hand and wrist*

Joao Carlos Sampaio Goes, MD, PhD
Director Instituto Brasileiro Controle Cancer
Chairman
Department Plastic Surgery and Mastology of
IBCC
Sao Paulo, Brazil
*Volume 5, Chapter 8.6 Periareolar technique with
mesh support*
*Volume 5, Chapter 20 Omentum reconstruction
of the breast*

Michael Sauerbier, MD, PhD
Chairman and Professor
Department for Plastic, Hand and
Reconstructive Surgery
Cooperation Hospital for Plastic Surgery of the
University Hospital Frankfurt
Academic Hospital University of Frankfurt a.
Main
Frankfurt, Germany
*Volume 4, Chapter 4 Lower extremity sarcoma
reconstruction*
*Volume 4, Video 4.01 Management of lower
extremity sarcoma reconstruction*

Hani Sbitany, MD
Plastic and Reconstructive Surgery
Assistant Professor of Surgery
University of California
San Francisco, CA, USA
*Volume 1, Chapter 24 Flap classification and
applications*

Tim Schaub, MD
Private Practice
Arizona Center for Hand Surgery, PC
Phoenix, AZ, USA
Volume 6, Chapter 16 Infections of the hand

Loren S. Schechter, MD, FACS
Assistant Professor of Surgery
Chief, Division of Plastic Surgery
Chicago Medical School
Chicago, IL, USA
*Volume 4, Chapter 15 Surgery for gender identity
disorder*

Stephen A. Schendel, MD
Professor Emeritus of Surgery and Clinical
Adjunct Professor of Neurosurgery
Department of Surgery and Neurosurgery
Stanford University Medical Center
Stanford, CA, USA
*Volume 3, Chapter 4 TMJ dysfunction and
obstructive sleep apnea*

Saja S. Scherer-Pietramaggiori, MD
Plastic Surgery Resident
Department of Plastic and Reconstructive
Surgery
University Hospital of Lausanne
Lausanne, Switzerland
Volume 1, Chapter 17 Skin graft

Clark F. Schierle, MD, PhD
Vice President
Aesthetic and Reconstructive Plastic Surgery
Northwestern Plastic Surgery Associates
Chicaho, IL, USA
*Volume 5, Chapter 5 Endoscopic approaches to
the breast*

Stefan S. Schneeberger, MD
Visiting Associate Professor of Surgery
Department of Plastic Surgery
Johns Hopkins Medical University
Baltimore, MD, USA
Associate Professor of Surgery
Center for Operative Medicine
Department for Viszeral
Transplant and Thoracic Surgery
Innsbruck Medical University
Innsbruck, Austria
*Volume 6, Chapter 38 Upper extremity
composite allotransplantation*

Iris A. Seitz, MD, PhD
Director of Research and International
Collaboration
University Plastic Surgery
Rosalind Franklin University
Clinical Instructor of Surgery
Chicago Medical School
University Plastic Surgery, affiliated with
Chicago Medical School, Rosalind Franklin
University
Morton Grove, IL, USA
*Volume 1, Chapter 21 Repair and grafting of
bone*

Chandan K. Sen, PhD, FACSM, FACN
Professor and Vice Chairman (Research) of
Surgery
Department of Surgery
The Ohio State University Medical Center
Associate Dean
Translational and Applied Research
College of Medicine
Executive Director
OSU Comprehensive Wound Center
Columbus, OH, USA
Volume 1, Chapter 14 Wound healing

Subhro K. Sen, MD
Clinical Assistant Professor
Division of Plastic and Reconstructive Surgery
Robert A. Chase Hand and Upper Limb
Center, Stanford University Medical Center
Palo Alto, CA, USA
Volume 1, Chapter 14 Wound healing
Volume 6, Chapter 4 Anesthesia for upper
extremity surgery
Volume 6, Video 4.01 Anesthesia for upper
extremity surgery

Joseph M. Serletti, MD, FACS
Henry Royster – William Maul Measey
Professor of Surgery and Chief
Division of Plastic Surgery
Vice Chair (Finance)
Department of Surgery
University of Pennsylvania
Philadelphia, PA, USA
Volume 5, Chapter 17 Free TRAM breast
reconstruction
Volume 5, Video 17.01 The muscle sparing free
TRAM flap

Randolph Sherman, MD
Vice Chair
Department of Surgery
Cedars-Sinai Medical Center
Los Angeles, CA, USA
Volume 6, Chapter 12 Reconstructive surgery of
the mutilated hand

Kenneth C. Shestak, MD
Professor of Plastic Surgery
Division of Plastic Surgery
University of Pittsburgh
Pittsburgh, PA, USA
Volume 5, Chapter 9 Revision surgery following
breast reduction and mastopexy
Volume 5, Video 7.01 Circum areola mastopexy

Lester Silver, MD, MS
Professor of Surgery
Department of Surgery/Division of Plastic
Surgery
Mount Sinai School of Medicine
New York, NY, USA
Volume 3, Chapter 37 Hemifacial atrophy

Navin K. Singh, MD, MSc
Assistant Professor of Plastic Surgery
Department of Plastic Surgery
Johns Hopkins University School of Medicine
Washington, DC, USA
Volume 4, Chapter 12 Abdominal wall
reconstruction

Vanila M. Singh, MD
Clinical Associate Professor
Stanford University Medical Center
Department of Anesthesiology and Pain
Management
Stanford, CA, USA
Volume 6, Chapter 4 Anesthesia for upper
extremity surgery

Carla Skytta, DO
Resident
Department of Surgery
Doctors Hospital
Columbus, OH, USA
Volume 3, Chapter 5 Scalp and forehead
reconstruction

Darren M. Smith, MD
Resident
Division of Plastic Surgery
University of Pittsburgh Medical Center
Pittsburgh, PA, USA
Volume 3, Chapter 31 Pediatric facial fractures

**Gill Smith, MB, BCh, FRCS(Ed),
FRCS(Plast)**
Consultant Hand, Plastic and Reconstructive
Surgeon
Great Ormond Street Hospital
London, UK
Volume 6, Chapter 26 Congenital hand II Failure
of formation (transverse and longitudinal arrest)

Paul Smith, MBBS, FRCS
Honorary Consultant Plastic Surgeon
Great Ormond Street Hospital London, UK
Volume 6, Chapter 26 Congenital hand II Failure
of formation (transverse and longitudinal arrest)

Laura Snell, MSc, MD, FRCSC
Assistant Professor
Division of Plastic Surgery
University of Toronto
Toronto, ON, Canada
Volume 4, Chapter 14 Reconstruction of
acquired vaginal defects

Nicole Z. Sommer, MD
Assistant Professor of Plastic Surgery
Southern Illinois University School of Medicine
Springfield, IL, USA
Volume 6, Chapter 6 Nail and fingertip
reconstruction

David H. Song, MD, MBA, FACS
Cynthia Chow Professor of Surgery
Chief, Section of Plastic and Reconstructive
Surgery
Vice-Chairman, Department of Surgery
The University of Chicago Medicine & Biological
Sciences
Chicago, IL, USA
Volume 4, Chapter 10 Reconstruction of the
chest

Andrea Spano, MD
Senior Assistant Plastic Surgeon
Unit of Plastic Surgery
Istituto Nazionale dei Tumori
Milano, Italy
Volume 5, Chapter 14 Expander/implant breast
reconstructions
Volume 5, Video 14.01 Mastectomy and
expander insertion: first stage
Volume 5, Video 14.02 Mastectomy and
expander insertion: second stage

Scott L. Spear, MD, FACS
Professor and Chairman
Department of Plastic Surgery
Georgetown University Hospital
Georgetown, WA, USA
Volume 5, Chapter 15 Latissimus dorsi flap
breast reconstruction
Volume 5, Chapter 26 Fat grafting to the breast
Volume 5, Video 15.01 Latissimus dorsi flap
technique

Robert J. Spence, MD
Director
National Burn Reconstruction Center
Good Samaritan Hospital
Baltimore, MD, USA
Volume 4, Chapter 21 Management of facial
burns
Volume 4, Video 21.01 Management of the
burned face intra-dermal skin closure
Volume 4, Video 21.02 Management of the
burned face full-thickness skin graft defatting
technique

Samuel Stal, MD, FACS
Professor and Chief
Division of Plastic Surgery, Baylor College of
Medicine and Texas Children's Hospital
Houston, TX, USA
Volume 3, Chapter 29 Secondary deformities of
the cleft lip, nose, and palate
Volume 3, Video 29.01 Complete takedown
Volume 3, Video 29.02 Abbé flap
Volume 3, Video 29.03 Thick lip and buccal
sulcus deformities
Volume 3, Video 29.04 Alveolar bone grafting
Volume 3, Video 29.05 Definitive rhinoplasty

Derek M. Steinbacher, MD, DMD
Assistant Professor
Plastic and Carniomaxillofacial Surgery
Yale University, School of Medicine
New Haven, CT, USA
Volume 3, Chapter 34 Nonsyndromic
craniosynostosis

Douglas S. Steinbrech, MD, FACS
Gotham Plastic Surgery
New York, NY, USA
Volume 2, Chapter 9 Secondary blepharoplasty:
Techniques

Lars Steinstraesser, MD
Heisenberg-Professor for Molecular Oncology
and Wound Healing
Department of Plastic and Reconstructive
Surgery, Burn Center
BG University Hospital Bergmannsheil, Ruhr
University
Bochum, North Rhine-Westphalia, Germany
Volume 4, Chapter 18 Acute management of
burn/electrical injuries

Phillip J. Stephan, MD
Clinical Instructor
Department of Plastic Surgery
University of Texas Southwestern
Wichita Falls, TX, USA
Volume 2, Chapter 24 Liposuction: A comprehensive review of techniques and safety

Laurie A. Stevens, MD
Associate Clinical Professor of Psychiatry
Columbia University College of Physicians and Surgeons
New York, NY, USA
Volume 1, Chapter 3 Psychological aspects of plastic surgery

Alexander Stoff, MD, PhD
Senior Fellow
Department of Plastic Surgery
Dreifaltigkeits-Hospital Wesseling
Wesseling, Germany
Volume 2, Chapter 25 Abdominoplasty procedures
Volume 2, Video 25.01 Abdominoplasty

Dowling B. Stough, MD
Medical Director
The Dermatology Clinic
Clinical Assistant Professor
Department of Dermatology
University of Arkansas for Medical Sciences
Little Rock, AR, USA
Volume 2, Video 23.09 Tension donor dissection

James M. Stuzin, MD
Associate Professor of Surgery (Plastic)
Voluntary
University of Miami Leonard M. Miller School of Medicine
Miami, FL, USA
Volume 2, Chapter 11.6 Facelift: The extended SMAS technique in facial rejuvenation
Volume 2, Video 11.06.01 Facelift – Extended SMAS technique in facial shaping

John D. Symbas, MD
Plastic and Reconstructive Surgeon
Private Practice
Marietta Plastic Surgery
Marietta, GA, USA
Volume 5, Chapter 16 The bilateral pedicled TRAM flap
Volume 5, Video 16.01 Pedicle TRAM breast reconstruction

Amir Taghinia, MD
Instructor in Surgery
Harvard Medical School
Staff Surgeon
Department of Plastic and Oral Surgery
Children's Hospital
Boston, MA, USA
Volume 6, Chapter 27 Congenital hand III disorders of formation – thumb hypoplasia
Volume 6, Video 27.01 Congenital hand III disorders of formation – thumb hypoplasia
Volume 6, Video 31.01 Vascular anomalies of the upper extremity

David M.K. Tan, MBBS
Consultant
Department of Hand and Reconstructive Microsurgery
National University Hospital
Yong Loo Lin School of Medicine
National University Singapore
Kent Ridge, Singapore
Volume 6, Chapter 3 Diagnostic imaging of the hand and wrist
Volume 6, Video 3.01 Diagnostic imaging of the hand and wrist – Scaphoid lunate dislocation

Jin Bo Tang, MD
Professor and Chair
Department of Hand Surgery
Chair
The Hand Surgery Research Center
Affiliated Hospital of Nantong University
Nantong, The People's Republic of China
Volume 6, Chapter 9 Flexor tendon injuries and reconstruction
Volume 6, Video 9.01 Flexor tendon injuries and reconstruction – Partial venting of the A2 pulley
Volume 6, Video 9.02 Flexor tendon injuries and reconstruction – Making a 6-strand repair
Volume 6, Video 9.03 Complete flexor-extension without bowstringing

Daniel I. Taub, DDS, MD
Assistant Professor
Oral and Maxillofacial Surgery
Thomas Jefferson University Hospital
Philadelphia, PA, USA
Volume 2, Chapter 16 Anthropometry, cephalometry, and orthognathic surgery
Volume 2, Video 16.01 Anthropometry, cephalometry, and orthognathic surgery

Peter J. Taub, MD, FACS, FAAP
Associate Professor, Surgery and Pediatrics
Division of Plastic and Reconstructive Surgery
Mount Sinai School of Medicine
New York, NY, USA
Volume 3, Chapter 37 Hemifacial atrophy

Sherilyn Keng Lin Tay, MBChB, MRCS, MSc
Microsurgical Fellow
Department of Plastic Surgery
Chang Gung Memorial Hospital
Taoyuan, Taiwan, The People's Republic of China
Specialist Registrar
Department of Reconstructive and Plastic Surgery
St George's Hospital
London, UK
Volume 1, Chapter 26 Principles and techniques of microvascular surgery

G. Ian Taylor, AO, MBBS, MD, MD (HonBrodeaux), FRACS, FRCS (Eng), FRCS (Hon Edinburgh), FRCSI (Hon), FRSC (Hon Canada), FACS (Hon)
Professor
Deparment of Plastic Surgery
Royal Melbourne Hospital
Professor
Department of Anatomy
University of Melbourne
Melbourne, Australia
Volume 1, Chapter 23 Vascular territories

Oren M. Tepper, MD
Assistant Professor
Plastic and Reconstructive Surgery
Montefiore Medical Center
Albert Einstein College of Medicine
New York, NY, USA
Volume 3, Chapter 36 Craniofacial microsomia

Chad M. Teven, BS
Research Associate
Section of Plastic and Reconstructive Surgery
University of Chicago
Chicago, IL, USA
Volume 1, Chapter 21 Repair and grafting of bone

Brinda Thimmappa, MD
Adjunct Assistant Professor
Department of Plastic and Reconstructive Surgery
Loma Linda Medical Center
Loma Linda, CA
Plastic Surgeon
Division of Plastic and Maxillofacial Surgery
Southwest Washington Medical Center
Vancouver, WA, USA
Volume 3, Chapter 4 TMJ dysfunction and obstructive sleep apnea

Johan Thorfinn, MD, PhD
Senior Consultant of Plastic Surgery, Burn Unit Co-Director
Department of Plastic Surgery, Hand Surgery, and Burns
Linköping University Hospital
Linköping, Sweden
Volume 6, Chapter 32 Peripheral nerve injuries of the upper extremity
Volume 6, Video 32.01-02 Peripheral nerve injuries (1) Digital Nerve Suture (2) Median Nerve Suture

Charles H. Thorne, MD
Associate Professor of Plastic Surgery
Department of Plastic Surgery
NYU School of Medicine
New York, NY, USA
Volume 2, Chapter 22 Otoplasty

Michael Tonkin, MBBS, MD, FRACS (Orth), FRCS Ed Orth
Professor of Hand Surgery
Department of Hand Surgery and Peripheral
Nerve Surgery
Royal North Shore Hospital
The Childrens Hospital at Westmead
University of Sydney Medical School
Sydney, Australia
*Volume 6, Chapter 25 Congenital hand 1
Principles, embryology, and classification*
*Volume 6, Chapter 29 Congenital hand V
Disorders of Overgrowth, Undergrowth, and
Generalized Skeletal Deformities (addendum)*

Patrick L Tonnard, MD
Coupure Centrum Voor Plastische Chirurgie
Ghent, Belgium
*Volume 2, Video 11.04.01 Loop sutures MACS
facelift*

Kathryn S. Torok, MD
Assistant Professor
Division of Pediatric Rheumatology
Department of Pediatrics
Univeristy of Pittsburgh School of Medicine
Childrens Hospital of Pittsburgh
Pittsburgh, PA, USA
Volume 3, Chapter 37 Hemifacial atrophy

Ali Totonchi, MD
Assistant Professor of Surgery
Division of Plastic Surgery
MetroHealth Medical Center
Case Western Reserve University
Cleveland, OH, USA
*Volume 3, Chapter 21 Surgical management of
migraine headaches*

Jonathan W. Toy, MD
Body Contouring Fellow
Division of Plastic and Reconstructive Surgery
University of Pittsburgh
University of Pittsburgh Medical Center Suite
Pittsburg, PA, USA
*Volume 2, Chapter 30 Post-bariatric
reconstruction*
*Volume 5, Chapter 25 Contouring of the arms,
breast, upper trunk, and male chest in the
massive weight loss patient*

Matthew J. Trovato, MD
Dallas Plastic Surgery Institute
Dallas, TX, USA
Volume 2, Chapter 29 Upper limb contouring
Volume 2, Video 29.01 Upper limb contouring

Anthony P. Tufaro, DDS, MD, FACS
Associate Professor of Surgery and Oncology
Departments of Plastic Surgery and Oncology
Johns Hopkins University
Baltimore, MD, USA
*Volume 3, Chapter 16 Tumors of the lips, oral
cavity, oropharynx, and mandible*

Joseph Upton III, MD
Clinical Professor of Surgery
Department of Plastic Surgery
Children's Hospital Boston
Shriner's Burn Hospital Boston
Beth Israel Deaconess Hospital
Harvard Medical School
Boston, MA, USA
*Volume 6, Chapter 27 Congenital hand III
disorders of formation – thumb hypoplasia*
*Volume 6, Chapter 31 Vascular anomalies of the
upper extremity*
*Volume 6, Video 27.01 Congenital hand III
disorders of formation – thumb hypoplasia*
*Volume 6, Video 31.01 Vascular anomalies of
the upper extremity*

Walter Unger, MD
Clinical Professor
Department of Dermatology
Mount Sinai School of Medicine
New York, NY
Associate Professor (Dermatology)
University of Toronto
Private Practice
New York, NY, USA
Toronto, ON, Canada
Volume 2, Video 23.06 Hair transplantation

Francisco Valero-Cuevas, PhD
Director
Brain-Body Dynamics Laboratory
Professor of Biomedical Engineering
Professor of Biokinesiology and Physical
Therapy
By courtesy Professor of Computer Science
and Aerospace and Mechanical Engineering
The University of Southern California
Los Angeles, CA, USA
*Volume 6, Chapter 1 Anatomy and biomechanics
of the hand*

Allen L. Van Beek, MD, FACS
Adjunct Professor
University Minnesota School of Medicine
Division Plastic Surgery
Minneapolis, MN, USA
Volume 2, Video 3.01 Botulinum toxin
Volume 2, Video 4.01 Soft tissue fillers
Volume 2, Video 5.01 Chemical peel
*Volume 2, Video 18.01 Open technique
rhinoplasty*

Nicholas B. Vedder
Professor of Surgery and Orthopaedics
Chief of Plastic Surgery Vice Chair, Department
of Surgery
University of Washington
Seattle, WA, USA
*Volume 6, Chapter 13 Thumb reconstruction:
non microsurgical techniques*

Valentina Visintini Cividin, MD
Assistant Plastic Surgeon
Unit of Plastic Surgery
Istituto Nazionale dei Tumori
Milano, Italy
*Volume 5, Chapter 14 Expander/implant
reconstruction of the breast*
*Volume 5, Video 14.01 Mastectomy and
expander insertion: first stage*
*Volume 5, Video 14.02 Mastectomy and
expander insertion: second stage*

Peter M. Vogt, MD, PhD
Professor and Chairman
Department of Plastic Hand and Reconstructive
Surgery
Hannover Medical School
Hannover, Germany
*Volume 1, Chapter 15 Skin wound healing:
Repair biology, wound, and scar treatment*

Richard J. Warren, MD, FRCSC
Clinical Professor
Division of Plastic Surgery
University of British Columbia
Vancouver, BC, Canada
Volume 2, Chapter 7 Forehead rejuvenation
Volume 2, Chapter 11.1 Facelift: Principles
*Volume 2, Chapter 11.2 Facelift: Introduction to
deep tissue techniques*
Volume 2, Video 7.01 Modified Lateral Brow Lift
*Volume 2, Video 11.1.01 Parotid masseteric
fascia*
Volume 2, Video 11.1.02 Anterior incision
Volume 2, Video 11.1.03 Posterior Incision
Volume 2, Video 11.1.04 Facelift skin flap
Volume 2, Video 11.1.05 Facial fat injection

Andrew J. Watt, MD
Plastic Surgeon
Department of Surgery
Division of Plastic and Reconstructive Surgery
Stanford University Medical Center
Stanford University Hospital and Clinics
Palo Alto, CA, USA
*Volume 6, Chapter 17 Management of
Dupuytren's disease*
*Volume 6, Video 17.01 Management of
Dupuytren's disease*

Simeon H. Wall, Jr., MD, FACS
Private Practice
The Wall Center for Plastic Surgery
Gratis Faculty
Division of Plastic Surgery
Department of Surgery
LSU Health Sciences Center at Shreveport
Shreveport, LA, USA
Volume 2, Chapter 21 Secondary rhinoplasty

Derrick C. Wan, MD
Assistant Professor
Department of Surgery
Stanford University School of Medicine
Stanford, CA, USA
*Volume 1, Chapter 13 Stem cells and
regenerative medicine*

Renata V. Weber, MD
Assistant Professor Surgery (Plastics)
Division of Plastic and Reconstructive Surgery
Albert Einstein College of Medicine
Bronx, NY, USA
*Volume 1, Chapter 22 Repair and grafting of
peripheral nerve*

Fu Chan Wei, MD
Professor
Department of Plastic Surgery
Chang Gung Memorial Hospital
Taoyuan, Taiwan, The People's Republic of
China
*Volume 1, Chapter 26 Principles and techniques
of microvascular surgery*
*Volume 6, Chapter 14 Thumb and finger
reconstruction – microsurgical techniques*
Volume 6, Video 14.01 Trimmed great toe
Volume 6, Video 14.02 Second toe for index
*Volume 6, Video 14.03 Combined second and
third toe for metacarpal hand*

Mark D. Wells, MD, FRCS, FACS
Clinical Assistant Professor of Surgery
The Ohio State University
Columbus, OH, USA
*Volume 3, Chapter 5 Scalp and forehead
reconstruction*

Gordon H. Wilkes, MD
Clinical Professor and Divisional Director
Division of Plastic Surgery
University of Alberta Faculty of Medicine
Alberta, AB, Canada
*Volume 1, Chapter 33 Facial prosthetics in
plastic surgery*

Henry Wilson, MD, FACS
Attending Plastic Surgeon
Private Practice
Plastic Surgery Associates
Lynchburg, VA, USA
Volume 5, Chapter 26 Fat grafting to the breast

Scott Woehrle, MS, BS
Physician Assistant
Department of Plastic Surgery
Jospeh Capella Plastic Surgery
Ramsey, NJ, USA
Volume 2, Chapter 29 Upper limb contouring
Volume 2, Video 29.01 Upper limb contouring

**Johan F. Wolfaardt, BDS, MDent
(Prosthodontics), PhD**
Professor
Division of Otolaryngology-Head and Neck
Surgery
Department of Surgery
Faculty of Medicine and Dentistry
Director of Clinics and International Relations
Institute for Reconstructive Sciences in
Medicine
University of Alberta
Covenant Health Group
Alberta Health Services
Alberta, AB, Canada
*Volume 1, Chapter 33 Facial prosthetics in
plastic surgery*

S. Anthony Wolfe, MD
Chief
Division of Plastic Surgery
Miami Children's Hospital
Miami, FL, USA
*Volume 3, Chapter 8 Acquired cranial and facial
bone deformities*
*Volume 3, Video 8.01 Removal of venous
malformation enveloping intraconal optic nerve*

**Chin-Ho Wong, MBBS, MRCS, MMed
(Surg), FAMS (Plast. Surg)**
Consultant
Department of Plastic Reconstructive and
Aesthetic Surgery
Singapore General Hospital
Singapore
Volume 2, Chapter 6 Anatomy of the aging face

Victor W. Wong, MD
Postdoctoral Research Fellow
Department of Surgery
Stanford University
Stanford, CA, USA
*Volume 1, Chapter 13 Stem cells and
regenerative medecine*

Jeffrey Yao, MD
Assistant Professor
Department of Orthopaedic Surgery
Stanford University Medical Center
Palo Alto, CA, USA
*Volume 6, Chapter 5 Principles of internal fixation
as applied to the hand and wrist*

Akira Yamada, MD
Assistant Professor
Department of Plastic and Reconstructive
Surgery
Osaka Medical College
Osaka, Japan
*Volume 3, Video 7.01 Microtia: auricular
reconstruction*

Michael J. Yaremchuk, MD, FACS
Chief of Craniofacial Surgery-Massachusetts
General Hospital
Program Director-Plastic Surgery Training
Program
Massachusetts General Hospital
Professor of Surgery
Harvard Medical School
Boston, MA, USA
Volume 2, Chapter 15 Skeletal augmentation
*Volume 2, Video 15.01 Midface skeletal
augmentation and rejuvenation*

David M. Young, MD
Professor of Plastic Surgery
Department of Surgery
University of California
San Francisco, CA, USA
*Volume 1, Chapter 24 Flap classification and
applications*

Peirong Yu, MD
Professor
Department of Plastic Surgery
The University of Texas M.D. Anderson Cancer
Center
Houston, TX, USA
*Volume 3, Chapter 13 Hypopharyngeal,
esophageal, and neck reconstruction*
*Volume 3, Video 13.01 Reconstruction of
pharyngoesophageal defects with the
anterolateral thigh flap*

James E. Zins, MD
Chairman
Department of Plastic Surgery
Dermatology and Plastic Surgery Institute
Cleveland Clinic
Cleveland, OH, USA
Volume 2, Chapter 13 Neck rejuvenation

Christopher G. Zochowski, MD
Chief Resident
Department of Plastic and Reconstructive
Surgery
Case Western Reserve University
Cleveland, OH, USA
Volume 3, Chapter 38 Pierre Robin sequence

Elvin G. Zook, MD
Professor Emeritus
Division of Plastic Surgery
Southern Illinois University School of Medicine
Springfield, IL, USA
*Volume 6, Chapter 6 Nail and fingertip
reconstruction*

**Ronald M. Zuker, MD, FRCSC, FACS,
FRCSEd(Hon)**
Staff Plastic Surgeon
The Hospital for Sick Children
Professor of Surgery
Department of Surgery
The University of Toronto
Toronto, ON, Canada
Volume 3, Chapter 11 Facial paralysis

Acknowledgments

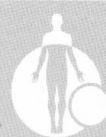

Editing a textbook such as this is an exciting, if daunting job. Only at the end of the project, over 4 years later, does one realize how much work it entailed and how many people helped make it happen. Sue Hodgson was the Commissioning Editor who trusted me to undertake this. Together, over several weekends in Seattle and countless e-mails and phone calls, we planned the format of this edition and laid the groundwork for a planning meeting in Chicago that included the volume editors and the Elsevier team with whom we have worked. I thank Drs. Gurtner, Warren, Rodriguez, Losee, Song, Grotting, Chang and Van Beek for tirelessly ensuring that each volume was as good as it could possibly be.

I had a weekly call with the Elsevier team as well as several visits to the offices in London. I will miss working with them. Louise Cook, Alexandra Mortimer and Poppy Garraway have been professional, thorough, and most of all, fun to work with. Emma Cole and Sam Crowe helped enormously with video content. Sadly, Sue Hodgson has left Elsevier, however Belinda Kuhn ably filled her shoes and ensured that we kept to our timeline, didn't lose momentum, and that the final product was something we would all be proud of.

Several residents helped, in focus groups to define format and style as well as specifically engaging in the editing process. I thank Darren Smith and Colin Woon for their help as technical copyeditors. Thanks to James Saunders and Leigh Jansen for reviewing video content and thanks also to Donnie Buck for all of his help with the electronic content. Of course we edited the book, we didn't write it. The writers were our contributing authors, all of whom engaged with enthusiasm. I thank them for defining Plastic Surgery, the book and the specialty.

Finally, I would like to thank my residents and fellows, who challenge me and make work fun. My partners in the Division of Plastic Surgery at the University of Washington, under the leadership of Nick Vedder, are a constant source of support and encouragement and I thank them. Finally, my family, Kate and David and most of all, my wife Gabrielle are unwavering in their love and support and I will never be able to thank them enough.

Peter C. Neligan, MB, FRCS(I), FRCSC, FACS
2012

Driven by constant innovation, the field of head, neck and craniofacial surgery has truly evolved and made noteworthy advances over the last several decades. The diverse expertise of the renowned contributors has provided the latest clinical evidence and surgical techniques to facilitate the decision-making process, which ultimately impacts the outcomes of patients with conditions involving congenital, oncologic, traumatic, and acquired deformities. This volume is a comprehensive resource for specialists of all levels. It has been a true privilege to work with such a distinguished faculty willing to share their vast experience and insights in their respective fields. It is with great admiration that I sincerely thank the contributors for their generous donation of time, commitment to excellence, dedication to education and advancement of the field.

Eduardo D. Rodriguez, MD, DDS
2012

As pediatric plastic surgery continues to evolve into a true subspecialty within plastic surgery, more young and promising surgeons dedicate their efforts to the unique care of children requiring these specialized services.

This volume represents the expertise of the pioneers and current leaders within pediatric plastic surgery. I am grateful for their dedication and efforts in making this text a reality and standard within the field. This work is dedicated to those children in my life – the many I regularly care for and who make going to the hospital each day never seem like "going to work"; and, to my son, Hudson Cladis Losee who has given me new perspective and a greater dimension to life.

Joseph E. Losee, MD, FACS, FAAP
2012

Dedicated to the memory of Stephen J. Mathes

PART 1

Craniofacial, head and neck surgery

Eduardo D. Rodriguez

Anatomy of the head and neck

Ahmed M. Afifi and Risal Djohan

SYNOPSIS

- The superficial fascial layer of the face and neck is formed of the superficial cervical fascia (enclosing the platysma), the superficial facial fascia (also referred to as the SMAS), the superficial temporal fascia (often called the temporoparietal fasica), and the galea.

- The deep fascial layer of the face and neck is formed of the deep cervical fascia (or the general investing fascia of the neck), the deep facial fascia (also known as the parotidomasseteric fascia), and the deep temporal fascia. The deep temporal fascia is continuous with the periosteum of the skull.

- The deep temporal fascia splits into two layers at the level of the superior orbital rim. The two layers insert into the superficial and deep surfaces of the zygomatic arch.

- The facial nerve is initially deep to the deep fascia, eventually penetrating it towards the superficial fascia. The fat and connective tissue filling the space between the superficial temporal fascia and the superficial layer of the deep temporal fascia is a subject of significant debate. Its importance stems from the temporal branch of the facial nerve crossing from deep to superficial in this layer.

- Most surgeons believe that it is the superficial temporal fat pad that fills this space. Others believe there is a distinct fascial layer in this region, named the parotidomasseteric fascia.

- The facial nerve is at significant risk of injury in the area right above the zygomatic arch.

- Pitanguy's line is an accurate description of the course of the largest and more significant branch of the temporal division of the facial nerve.

- The marginal mandibular nerve can be located above or below the level of the mandible. It is usually located between the platysma and the deep cervical fascia, and is always superficial to the facial vessels.

- There are multiple fat pads in the face. They can be superficial to the SMAS, between the SMAS and the deep fascia, or deep to the deep fascia.

- Knowledge of the sensory nerves is important, especially with our current understanding of their role in migraine headaches.

Aesthetic and reconstructive surgery of the head and neck depends on appreciating the three-dimensional anatomy and the functional and cosmetic methods of rearranging the different structures. This chapter is not intended to be a detailed description of the head and neck anatomy, which is beyond such a limited space. It rather offers a different perspective on the anatomy that is more relevant to the plastic surgeon, and highlights certain anatomical regions that have fundamental importance or are more controversial.

The fascial planes of the head and neck and the facial nerve

A peculiar feature of the anatomy of the head and neck is the concentric arrangement of the facial soft tissues in layers. These layers have different names and characteristics from one area of the head and neck to the other, but they maintain their continuity across boundaries *(Fig. 1.1)*. Unfortunately, inconsistent nomenclature has been used to describe these layers leading to significant confusion among readers. The facial nerve usually passes in defined planes in between these layers, crossing from one layer to the other only in specific well described zones. Knowledge of these planes and their relation to the facial nerve is vital if plastic surgeons are to safely access the soft tissues and bony structures of the head and neck.[1,2] In the following discussion, we will not only describe the anatomy and nomenclature of these layers as mostly agreed upon, but also try to elucidate the sources of deliberation and confusion in describing this crucial anatomy.[3]

The neck, cheek (lower face), temple and the scalp are arbitrarily divided by the lower border of the mandible, the zygomatic arch and the temporal line, respectively. In general, there are two layers of fascia, a superficial and deep, which cover these regions and extend over other structures, such as the eyelid and the nose *(Fig. 1.1)*.

The superficial layer of fascia is formed by the superficial cervical fascia (platysma), the superficial facial fascia (SMAS), the superficial temporal fascia (temporoparietal fascia) and

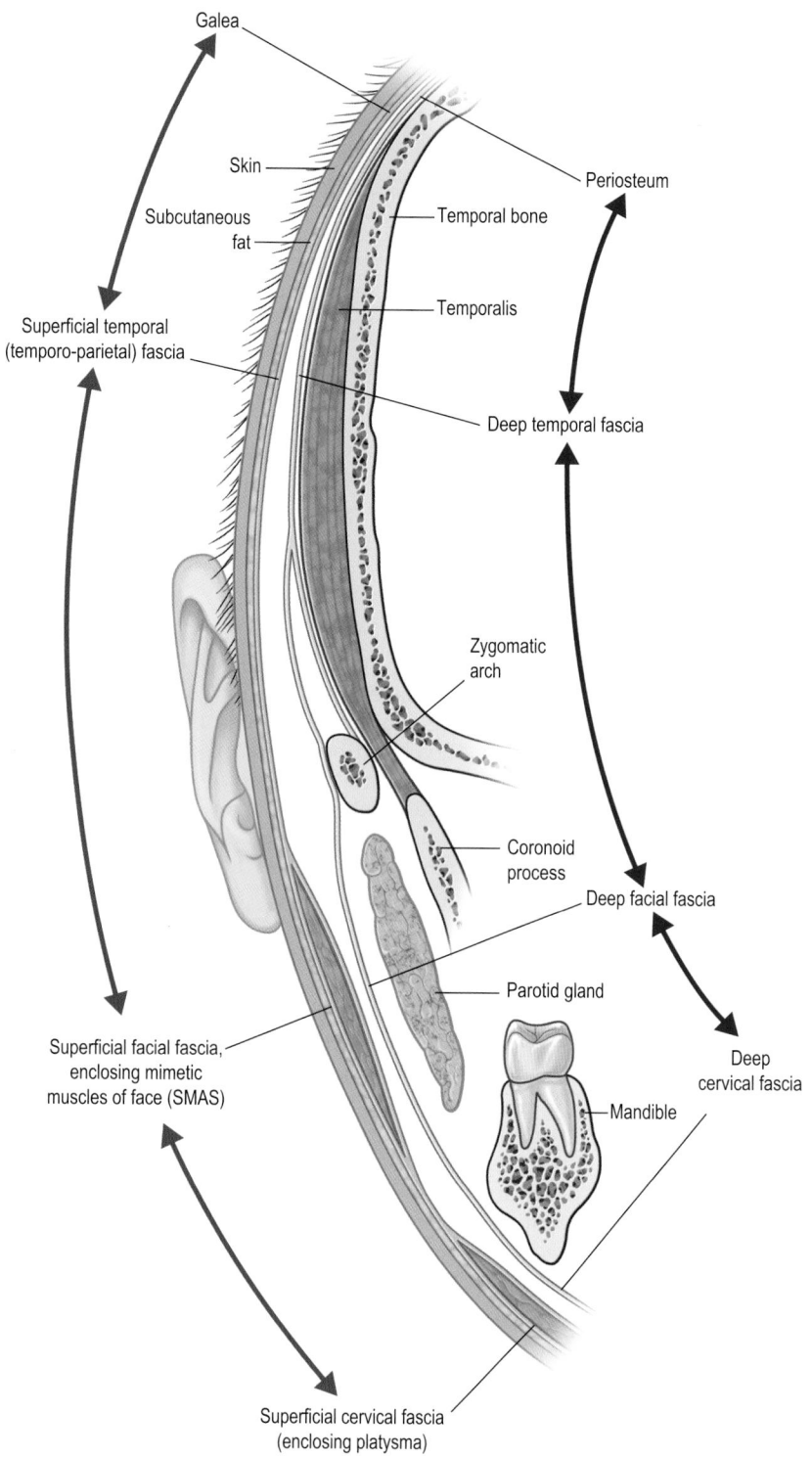

Galea

Skin

Subcutaneous
fat

Superficial temporal
(temporo-parietal) fascia

Temporal bone

Temporalis

Deep temporal fascia

Periosteum

Zygomatic
arch

Coronoid
process

Deep facial fascia

Parotid gland

Deep
cervical fascia

Superficial facial fascia,
enclosing mimetic
muscles of face (SMAS)

Mandible

Superficial cervical fascia
(enclosing platysma)

Fig. 1.1 The facial layers of the scalp, face, and neck.

the galea aponeurotica *(Figs 1.1, 1.2)*. To be more precise, this superficial fascia splits to enclose many of the facial muscles. This is a consistent pattern seen all over the head and neck region; e.g. the superficial cervical fascia splits into a deep and superficial layer to enclose the platysma, the superficial facial fascia splits to enclose the midfacial muscles, and the galea splits to enclose the frontalis. The two layers of the superficial fascia then rejoin at the other end of the muscle, before splitting again to enclose the next muscle and so on.

The deep layer of fascia is formed by the deep cervical fascia, the deep facial fascia (parotidomasseteric fascia), the deep temporal fascia and the periosteum. This layer is superficial to the muscles of mastication, the salivary glands and the main neurovascular structures *(Figs 1.1, 1.2)*. Over bony areas, such as the skull and the zygomatic arch, this deep fascia is inseparable from the periosteum.

The facial fat pads are localized collection of fat present deep to the superficial layer of fascia. These are separate

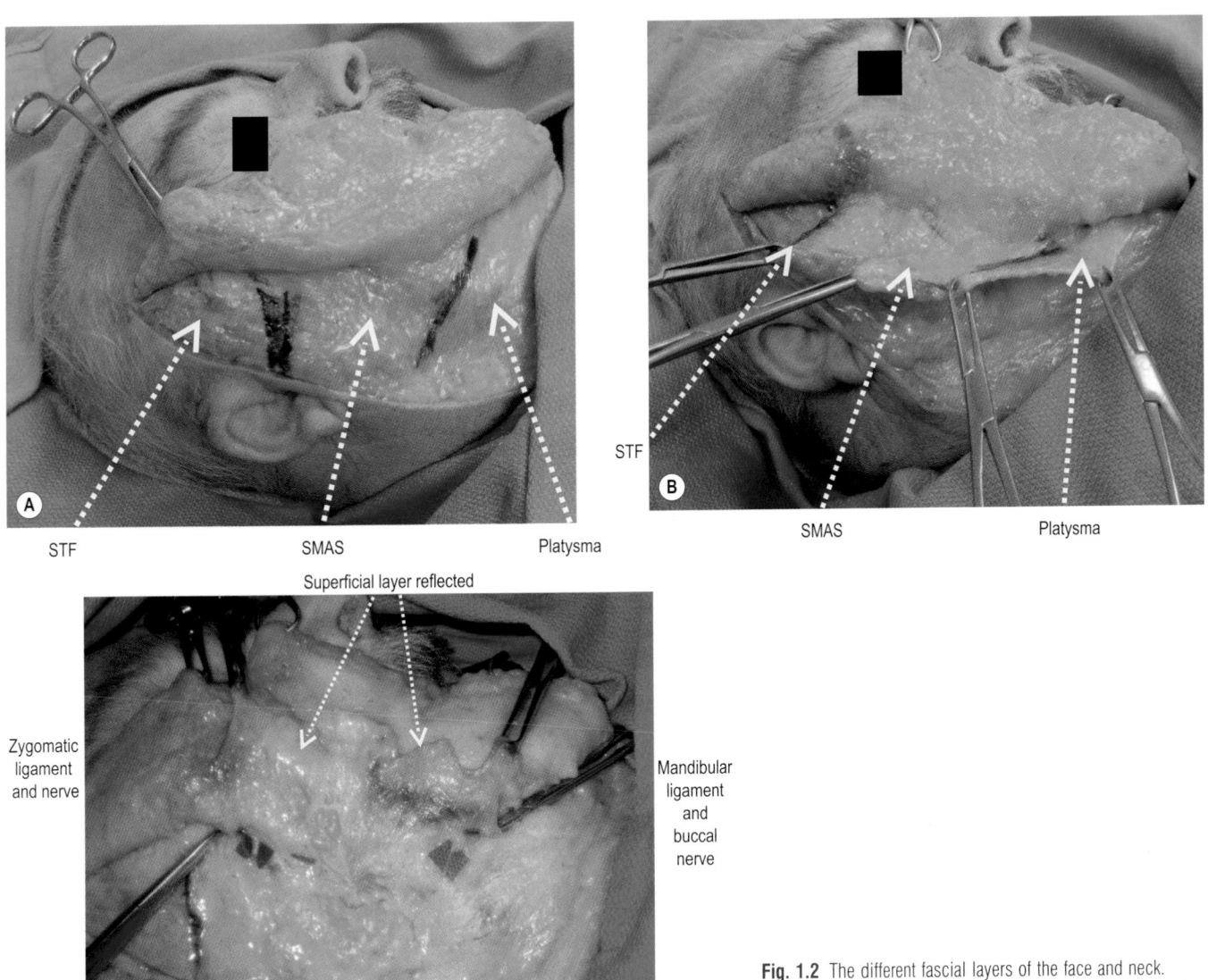

STF   SMAS   Platysma

Superficial layer reflected

STF

SMAS   Platysma

Zygomatic
ligament
and nerve

Mandibular
ligament
and
buccal
nerve

The nerves penetrate the deep fascia towards their
innervation of the SMAS and Platysma

Fig. 1.2 The different fascial layers of the face and neck.
(A) Dissection in the superficial plane, between the skin and
the superficial fascia. **(B)** Elevation of the superficial fascial
layer, formed of the superficial cervical fascia (platysma), the
superficial facial fascia (SMAS), and the superficial temporal fascia
(temproparietal fascia). **(C)** Note the proximity of the nerve (on the
blue background) to the zygomatic and mandibular ligaments (on
surgical the instrument).

anatomically and histologically from the subcutaneous fat present between the skin and the superficial fascia. These fat pads include the superficial temporal fat pad, the galeal fat pad, suborbicularis oculi fat pad (SOOF), the retro-orbicularis oculi fat pad (ROOF), and the preseptal fat of the eyelids. Deep to the deep fascia are several other fat pads; the deep temporal fat pads, the buccal fat pads, and the postseptal fat pads of the eyelids.[4]

The fascia in the face

The first layer the surgeon encounters in the face deep to the skin and its associated subcutaneous fat is the SMAS (Superficial Musculo-Aponeurotic System) *(Figs 1.1, 1.2)*.[5] The SMAS varies in thickness and composition between

individuals and from one area to another, and it can be fatty, fibrous, or muscular.[6] The muscles of facial expression, e.g. orbicularis oculi, oris, zygomaticus major and minor, frontalis, platysma are enclosed by (or form part of) the SMAS. The SMAS is often referred to as the superficial facial fascia. In reality, the superficial facial fascia covers the superficial and deep surfaces of the muscles. However, these layers are hard to separate intraoperatively (except in certain areas such as the neck). Dissection superficial to the superficial facial fascia (just under the skin) will generally avoid injury to the underlying facial nerve. However, such dissection can compromise the blood supply of the overlying skin flaps. Often, the surgeon can safely maintain this superficial fascia in the lower face and neck (whether it is the platysma or the SMAS) with the skin, allowing a secure double layer closure and maintaining skin vascularity (e.g. during a neck dissection). In the anterior (medial) face, the facial nerve branches become more superficial just under or within the SMAS layer.

The next layer in the face is the deep facial fascia, which is also known as the parotidomasseteric fascia *(Figs 1.1, 1.2)*. Over the parotid gland, this layer is adherent to the capsule of the gland. The facial nerve is initially (i.e. right after is exits the parotid gland) deep to the deep facial fascia. Most of the muscles of facial expression are superficial to the planes of the nerve. The nerve branches pierce the deep fascia to innervate the muscles from their deep surface, with the exception of the mentalis, levator anguli oris and the buccinators *(Fig. 1.2)*. These three muscles are deep to the facial nerve and are thus innervated on their superficial surface.

The fascia in the temporal region

The cheek and lower face are separated from the temporal region by the zygomatic arch. There are two layers of fascia in the temporal region (below the skull temporal lines); the superficial temporal fascia (also known as the temporoparietal fascia, TPF) and the deep temporal fascia *(Figs 1.3, 1.4A)*.[7-9] The deep temporal fascia lies on the superficial surface of the temporalis muscle. Between the superficial and deep temporal fascia is a loose areolar plane that is relatively avascular and easily dissected. However, the frontal branch of the facial nerve is within or directly beneath the superficial temporal fascia *(Fig. 1.4A)*.[5] Therefore, dissection in this plane should be strictly on the deep temporal fascia, which can be identified by its bright white color and sturdy texture. To ensure that the surgeon is in the right plane, he can attempt to grasp the areolar tissues over the deep temporal fascia using an Adson forceps; if in the right plane, one will not catch any tissue. Once deep enough and right on the deep temporal fascia, dissection can proceed quickly using a periosteal elevator hugging the tough deep temporal fascia *(Fig. 1.5)*.

In the region right above the zygomatic arch the space between the superficial TPF and the deep temporal fascia (sometimes referred to as the subaponeurotic space) and the fat/fascia it contains is both a debatable and an important subject *(Fig. 1.4)*. Its importance stems from the facial nerve crossing this space from deep to superficial right above the zygomatic arch. A third layer of fascia has been described in this space (between the superficial and deep layers), and is referred to as the parotido-temporal fascia, the subgaleal fascia, or the innominate fascia.[10,11] The term "fascial layer" is used loosely, as there is no general consensus as to how thick connective tissue must be before it can be considered a "fascial layer". What some authors refer to as "loose connective tissue" may be called a "fascial layer" or a "fat pad" by others. Our own cadaver dissection showed that this third fascial layer could often be identified. It extends for a short distance above and below the arch. Directly superficial to the arch, the facial nerve is deep to this layer, piercing it to become more superficial 1–2 cm cephalad to the arch (see below).

Above the zygomatic arch and at the same horizontal level as the superior orbital rim, the deep temporal fascia splits into two layers; the superficial layer of the deep temporal fascia (sometimes referred to as the middle temporal fascia, intermediate fascia, or the innominate fascia) and the deep layer of the deep temporal fascia *(Fig. 1.3)*.[7] The deep and superficial layers of the deep temporal fascia attach to the superficial

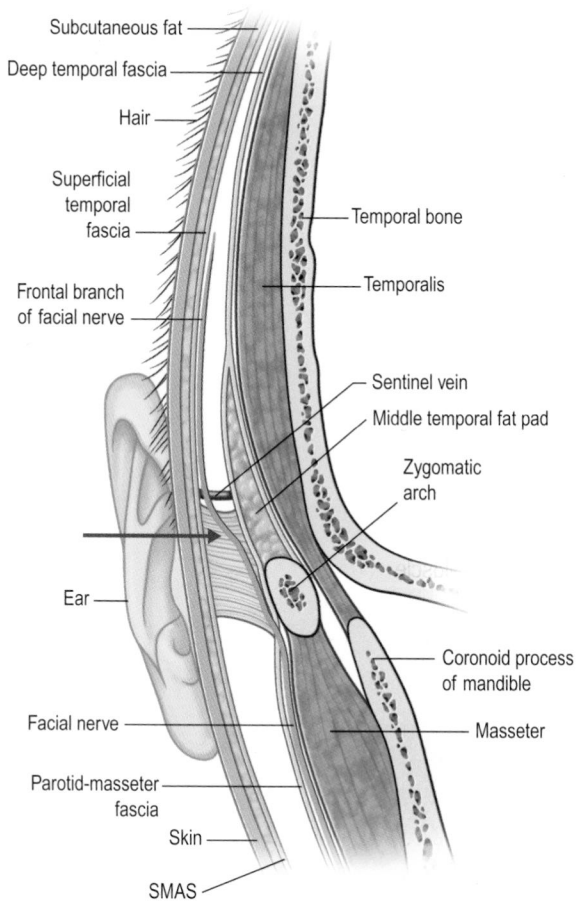

and deep surfaces of the zygomatic arch. There are three fat pads in this region.[7,12] The superficial fat pad is located between the superficial temporal fascia and superficial layer of the deep temporal fascia, and as described above, is analogous with the parotido-temporal fascia, subgaleal fascia, and/or the loose connective tissue between the superficial and deep temporal fascia. The middle fat pad is located directly above the zygomatic arch between the superficial and deep layers of the deep temporal fascia. Finally, the deep fat pad (also know as the buccal fat pad) is deep to the deep layer of the deep temporal fascia, superficial to the temporalis muscles and extends deep to the zygomatic arch. It is considered an extension of the buccal fat pad.

Most of the controversy in describing the fascial layers in the temporal region arises from confusing the *superficial temporal fascia* with the *superficial layer of the deep temporal fascia*. This is very significant since the facial nerve is deep to or within the former and superficial to the latter. The second baffling point is the location of the *deep* temporal fascia *superficial* to the temporalis muscle. There is another fascial layer on the deep surface of the muscle; this is not the deep temporal fascia and is of little significance from a surgical

Fig. 1.3 The facial layers of the temporal region. The fat/fascia in the subaponeurotic plane (arrow; between the the temporal fascia and deep temporal fascia) is intimately related to the facial nerve. Some authors believe that there is a separate fascial layer in this space referred to as the parotidomasseteric fascia.

Labels in figure:
Subcutaneous fat
Deep temporal fascia
Hair
Superficial temporal fascia
Frontal branch of facial nerve
Ear
Facial nerve
Parotid-masseter fascia
Skin
SMAS
Temporal bone
Temporalis
Sentinel vein
Middle temporal fat pad
Zygomatic arch
Coronoid process of mandible
Masseter

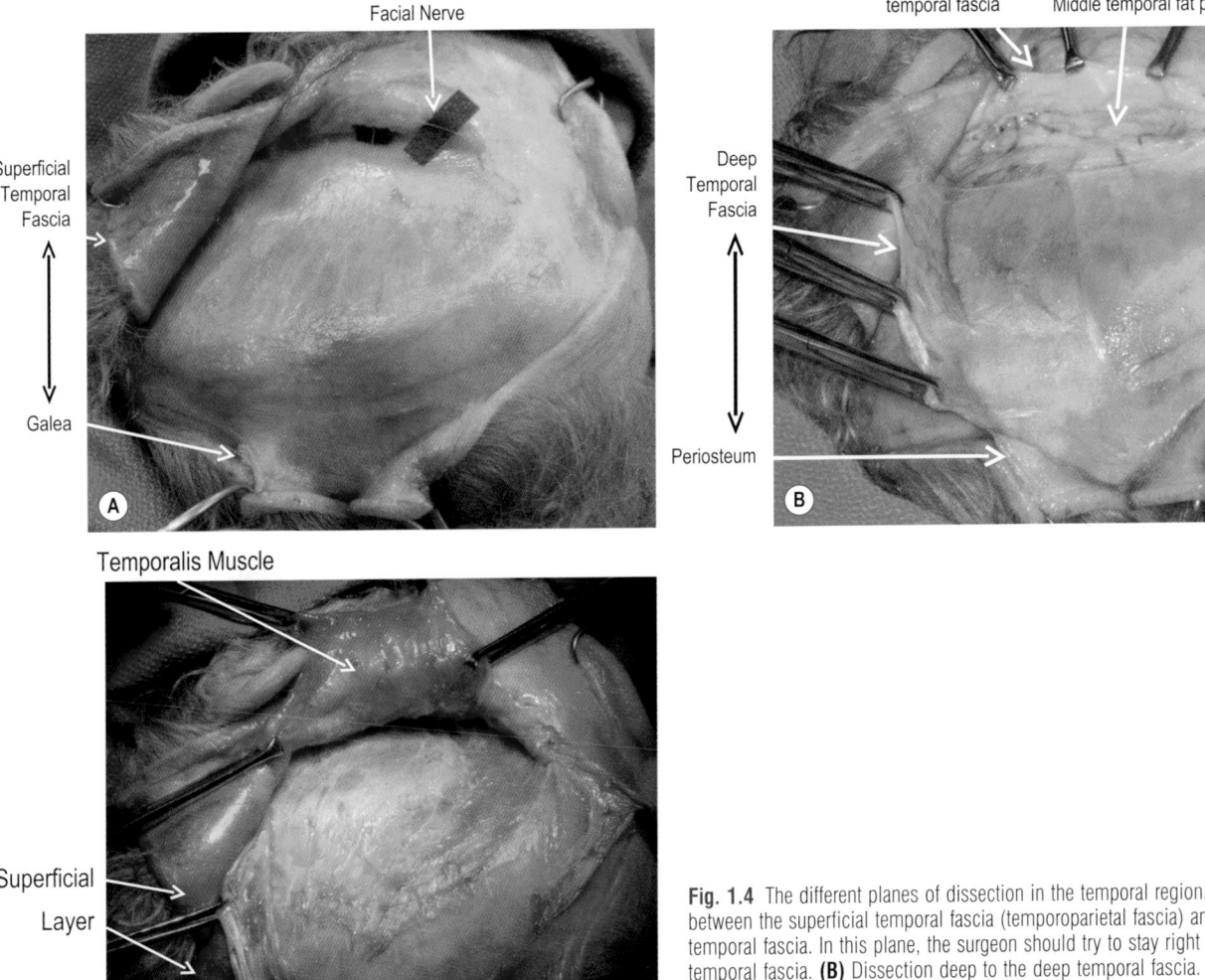

Fig. 1.4 The different planes of dissection in the temporal region. **(A)** Dissection between the superficial temporal fascia (temporoparietal fascia) and the deep temporal fascia. In this plane, the surgeon should try to stay right on the deep temporal fascia. **(B)** Dissection deep to the deep temporal fascia. This is a safe plan that will lead to the zygomatic arch. The facial nerve will be protected by the superficial layer of the deep temporal fascia. **(C)** Dissection deep the temporalis muscle. The muscle can be left as part of the skin flap. This is a safe and easy plan if no exposure of the arch is needed.

standpoint. The final controversy is what exactly is the *innominate* fascia? This term is often used to describe the superficial layer of the deep temporal fascia above the arch. Other surgeons reserve the term to the areolar tissue between the superficial layer of the deep temporal fascia and the superficial temporal fascia (i.e., the innominate fascia can be synonymous with the parotidotemporal fascia or subgaleal fascia or the superficial temporal fat pad).[13]

The plane of dissection in the temporal region depends on the goal of the surgery *(Fig. 1.4)*. In general, the surgeon should avoid the superficial temporal fascia as it harbors the frontal branch of the facial nerve. During surgery to expose the orbital rims and the forehead musculature, the dissection plane is between the superficial temporal fascia and deep temporal fascia *(Fig. 1.4A)*. To expose the arch, the superficial layer of the deep temporal fascia is divided and dissection proceeds between it and the middle fat pad (the superficial layer of deep temporal fascia will act as an extra layer protecting the nerve) *(Fig. 1.4B)*. Finally, when a coronal approach is used, but the arch does not need to be exposed, dissection can

proceed deep to the temporalis muscles, elevating them with the coronal flap *(Fig. 1.4B)*. Using this avascular plane avoids potential traction or injury to the frontal nerve, and ensures good aesthetic results as it prevents possible fat atrophy or retraction of the temporalis muscle.

While the fascial layers in the temporal region are well described, there is more debate and variability of the anatomy of the fascial layers and the facial nerve directly superficial to the arch.[12,14,15] The superficial facial fascia (SMAS) is continuous with the TPF, but it is not clear if the deep facial and deep temporal fasciae are continuous to each other or attach and arise from the periosteum of the arch separately. In addition, the thickness of the soft tissues from the periosteum to skin is minimal and the tissues are tightly adherent, making identification of the facial planes and the facial nerve hazardous in this region.[16] The frontal branch of the facial nerve pierces the deep temporal fascia to become more superficial near the vicinity of the upper border of the arch, and this area constitutes one of the danger zones of the face (see below).

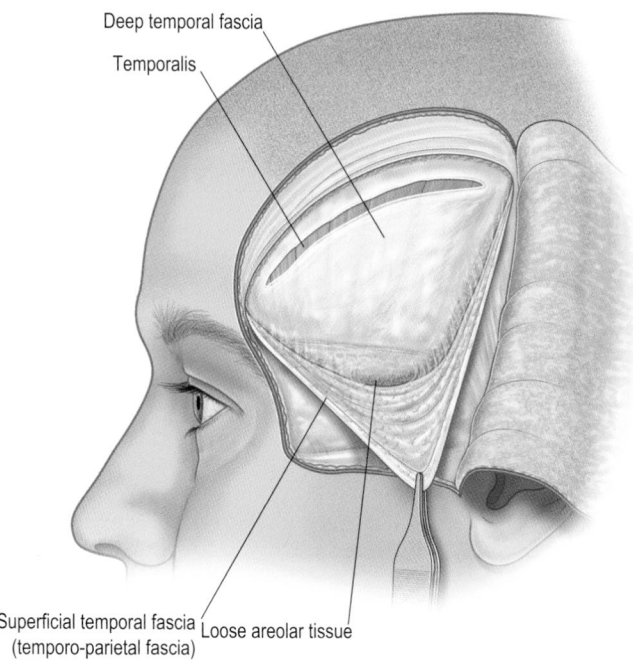

Fig. 1.5 Dissection in the temporal layer.

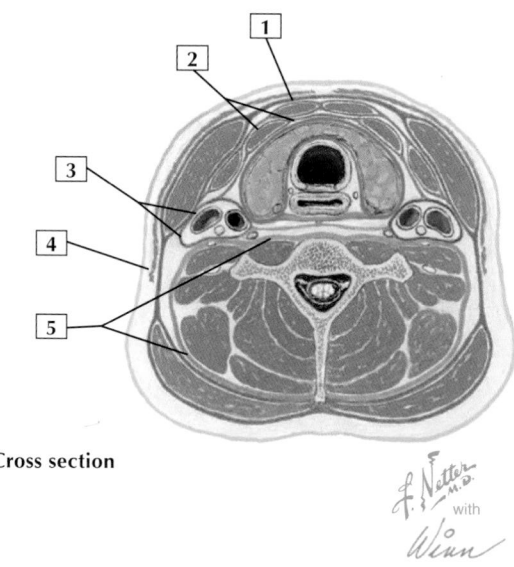

Cross section

Fig. 1.6 Fascial layers of the neck. 1, Investing layer of deep cervical fascia; 2, pretracheal fascia; 3, carotid sheath; 4, superficial fascia; 5, prevertebral fascia. (Reprinted with permission from www.netterimages.com ©Elsevier Inc. All rights reserved.)

The fascia in the neck

The nomenclature used to describe the different fascial layers in the neck also creates significant confusion. There are two different fascias in the neck: the superficial and the deep *(Figs 1.3, 1.6)*. The latter is composed of three different layers: (1) the superficial layer of the deep cervical fascia, also known the general investing layer of deep cervical fascia; (2) the middle layer, commonly named the pretracheal fascia; and (3) the deep layer, or the prevertebral fascia *(Figs 1.3, 1.6)*. The pretracheal fascia encircles the trachea, thyroid and the oesophagus, while the prevertebral fascia encloses the prevertebral muscles and forms the floor of the posterior triangle of the neck. For practical purposes, it is the superficial cervical fascia and the superficial layer of the deep cervical fascia that the plastic surgeon encounters.[17,18]

The superficial cervical fascia encloses the platysma muscle and is closely associated with the subcutaneous adipose tissue. The platysma muscle and its surrounding superficial cervical fascia represent the continuation of the SMAS into the neck. In general, when skin flaps are raised in the neck, the platysma muscle is maintained with the skin to enhance its blood supply (e.g. during neck dissections). However, in necklifts the skin is raised off the platysma to allow platysmal shaping and skin redraping. Tissue expanders placed in the neck could be placed either deep or superficial to the platysma. Placing them superficially will create thinner flaps that are more suitable for facial resurfacing, while placing them deeper allows a more secure coverage of the expander.[19,20]

The superficial layer of deep cervical fascia, or the general investing layer of deep cervical fascia, is what plastic surgeons commonly refer to simply as the "deep cervical fascia". It encircles the whole neck and has attachments to the spinous processes of the vertebrae and the ligamentum nuchae posteriorly. It splits to enclose the sternocleidomastoid and the trapezius muscles. It also splits to enclose the parotid and the submandibular glands. The deep facial fascia, or parotido-masseteric fascia, is therefore considered the continuation of the deep cervical fascia into the face.

Retaining ligaments and adhesions of the face

The ligaments of the face maintain the skin and soft tissues of the face in their normal positions, resisting gravitational changes. Knowledge of their anatomy is important for both the craniofacial and the aesthetic surgeon for several reasons. For the aesthetic surgeon, these ligaments play an important role in maintaining facial fat in its proper positions. For ideal aesthetic repositioning of the skin and soft tissues of the face, numerous surgeons recommend releasing the ligaments. For the craniofacial surgeon, the zones of adherence represent coalescence between different fascial layers, possibly luring the surgeon into an erroneous plane of dissection. In facial reconstruction or face transplants, reconstructing or maintaining these ligaments is important to prevent sagging of the soft tissues with its functional and aesthetic consequences.

Various terms have been used to describe these ligamentous attachments. Moss *et al.* classified them into ligaments (connecting deep fascia/periosteum to the dermis), adhesions (fibrous attachments between the deep and the superficial fascia), and septi (fibrous wall between layers).[21]

In the periorbital and temporal region, various ligaments and adhesions have been described with numerous names given to each *(Fig. 1.7)*. Along the skull temporal line lies temporal line of fusion, also know as the superior temporal septum.[21] This represents the coalition of the temporal fascia with the skull periosteum. These adhesions end as the

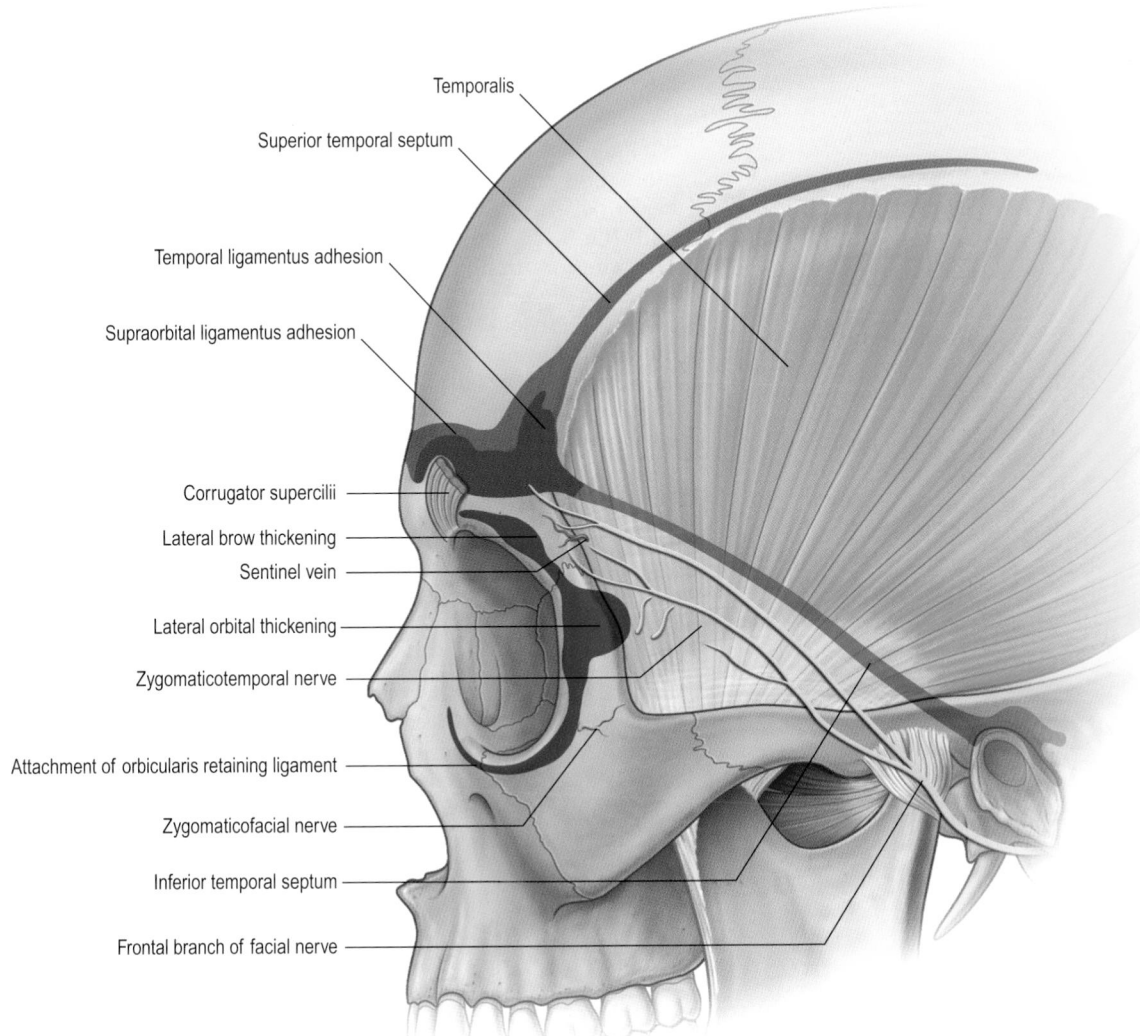

Temporalis

Superior temporal septum

Temporal ligamentus adhesion

Supraorbital ligamentus adhesion

Corrugator supercilii

Lateral brow thickening

Sentinel vein

Lateral orbital thickening

Zygomaticotemporal nerve

Attachment of orbicularis retaining ligament

Zygomaticofacial nerve

Inferior temporal septum

Frontal branch of facial nerve

Fig. 1.7 The ligaments of the periorbital region.

temporal ligamentous adhesions (TLA) at the lateral third of the eyebrow. The TLA measure approximately 20 mm in height and 15 mm in width, and begins 10 mm cephalad to the superior orbital rim. Both the temporal line of fusion and the TLA are sometimes referred to collectively as temporal adhesions. The inferior temporal septum extends posteriorly and inferiorly from the TLA on the surface of the deep temporal fascia towards the upper border of the zygoma. The supraorbital ligamentous adhesions extend from the TLA medially along the eyebrow.

The orbicularis retaining ligament (ORL) lies along the superior, lateral and inferior rims of the orbit, extending from the periosteum just outside the orbital rim to the deep surface of the orbicularis oculi muscle *(Fig. 1.8)*.[22,23] This ligament serves to anchor the orbicularis oculi muscle to the orbital rims. The orbicularis oculi muscle attaches directly to the bone from the anterior lacrimal crest to the level of the medial limbus. At this level the ORL replaces the bony origin of the muscle, continuing laterally around the orbit. Initially short, it reaches its maximum length centrally near the lateral limbus.[24] It then begins to diminish in length laterally, until

it finally blends with the lateral orbital thickening (LOT). The LOT is a condensation of the superficial and deep fascia on the frontal process of the zygoma and the adjacent deep temporal fascia. The ORL and the orbital septum both attach to the arcus marginalis, a thickening of the periosteum of the orbital rims.[23] The ORL is also referred to as the periorbital septum and, in its inferior portion, as the orbitomalar ligament. The ORL ligament attaches to the undersurface of the orbicularis oculi muscle at the junction of the pretarsal and orbital parts.

In the midface, the retaining ligaments have been divided into direct, or osteocutaneous ligaments, and indirect ligaments. Direct ligaments run directly from the periosteum to the dermis, and include the zygomatic and mandibular ligaments. Indirect ligaments represent a coalescence between the superficial and deep fascia, and include the parotid and the masseteric cutaneus ligaments *(Fig. 1.9,* and see *Fig. 1.2C)*. The retaining ligaments indirectly fix the mobile skin and its intimately related superficial fascia (SMAS), to the relatively immobile deep fascia and underlying structures (masseter and parotid).

muscle (namely the zygomaticus major, zygomaticus minor and the levator labii superioris). This fascial layer extends caudally over the muscles, gradually becoming thinner and allowing the muscle to be more discernible. The superior boundary of the prezygomatic space is the orbicularis retaining ligament, which separates it from the preseptal space. The more rigid inferior boundary is formed by the reflection of the fascia covering the floor as it curves superficially to blend with the fascia on the undersurface of the orbicularis oculi. This inferior boundary is further reinforced by the zygomatic retaining ligaments. Medially, the space is closed by the origins of the levator labii and the orbicular oculi muscle from the medial orbital rim. Finally, the lateral boundary is formed superiorly by the LOT over the frontal process of the zygoma and more inferiorly by the zygomatic ligaments.[32] The facial nerve branches cross in the roof of (i.e. superficial to) this space. The only structure traversing the pre zygomatic space is the zygomatico facial nerve, emerging from its foramen located just caudal to ORL.

The malar fat pad

This is a subcutaneous pad of fat superficial to the SMAS (which encloses the orbicularis oculi) in the cheek.[33] This pad is triangular in shape, with its base at the nasolabial crease and its apex more laterally towards the body of the zygoma. Elevation of the malar fat pad is important for facial rejuvenation and in facial palsy.

The buccal fat pad

The buccal fat pad is an underappreciated factor in post traumatic facial deformities and senile aging , and is frequently overlooked as a flap or graft donor site.[34,35] Senile laxity of the fascia allows the fat to prolapse laterally, contributing to the square appearance of the face.[36] With many traumatic injuries the fat herniates, either superficially, towards the oral mucosa, or even into the maxillary sinus.[24,37–39] This fat is anatomically and histologically distinct from the subcutaneous fat. It is voluminous in infants to prevent indrawing of the cheek during suckling, and gradually decreases in size with age.[40] It functions to fill the glide planes between the muscles of mastication.

It is usually described as being formed of a central body and four extensions, the buccal, pterygoid and superficial and deep temporal. The body is located on the periosteum of the posterior maxilla (surrounding the branches of the internal maxillary artery) overlying the buccinator muscle and extends forwards in the vestibule of the mouth to the level of the maxillary second molar. The buccal extension is the most superficial, extending along the anterior border of the masseter around the parotid duct. Both the body and the buccal extension are superficial to the buccinator and deep to the deep facial fascia (parotido-masseteric fascia), and are intimately related to the facial nerve branches and the parotid duct. The buccal extension is in the same plane as the facial artery, which marks its anterior boundary. The pterygoid extension passes backwards and downwards deep to the mandibular ramus to surround the pterygoid muscles. The

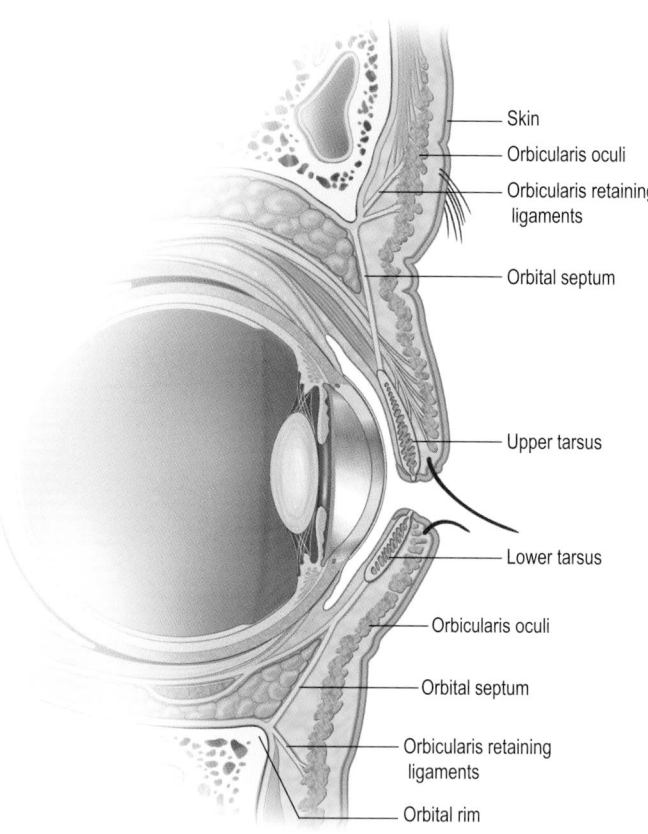

Skin
Orbicularis oculi
Orbicularis retaining ligaments
Orbital septum

Upper tarsus

Lower tarsus

Orbicularis oculi

Orbital septum

Orbicularis retaining ligaments

Orbital rim

Fig. 1.8 The orbicularis retaining ligaments.

The zygomatic and the masseteric ligaments together form and inverted L, with the angle of the L formed by the major zygomatic ligaments (*Fig. 1.9,* and see *Fig. 1.2C*). These ligaments are typically around 3 mm wide and are located 4.5 cm in front of the tragus and 5–9 mm behind the zygomaticus minor muscle.[25–28] Anterior to this main ligament are multiple other bundles that form the horizontal limb of the inverted L. The vertical limb of the L is formed by the masseteric ligaments, which are stronger near their upper end (at the zygomatic ligaments), and extend along the entire anterior border of the masseter as far as the mandibular border.[5,29] The parotid ligaments, also referred to as preauricular ligaments, represent another area of firm adherence between the superficial and deep fascia.[25,27,28] The mandibular ligaments originate from the parasymphysial region of the mandible around 1 cm above the lower mandibular border.[27,28] There are several descriptions of other retaining ligaments in the face, most notably the mandibular septum and the orbital retaining septum.[30,23]

The prezygomatic space

The prezygomatic space is a glide plane space overlying the body of the zygoma, deep to the orbicularis oculi and the suborbicularis fat (*Fig. 1.8*).[31] Its floor is formed by a fascial layer covering the body of the zygoma and the lip elevator

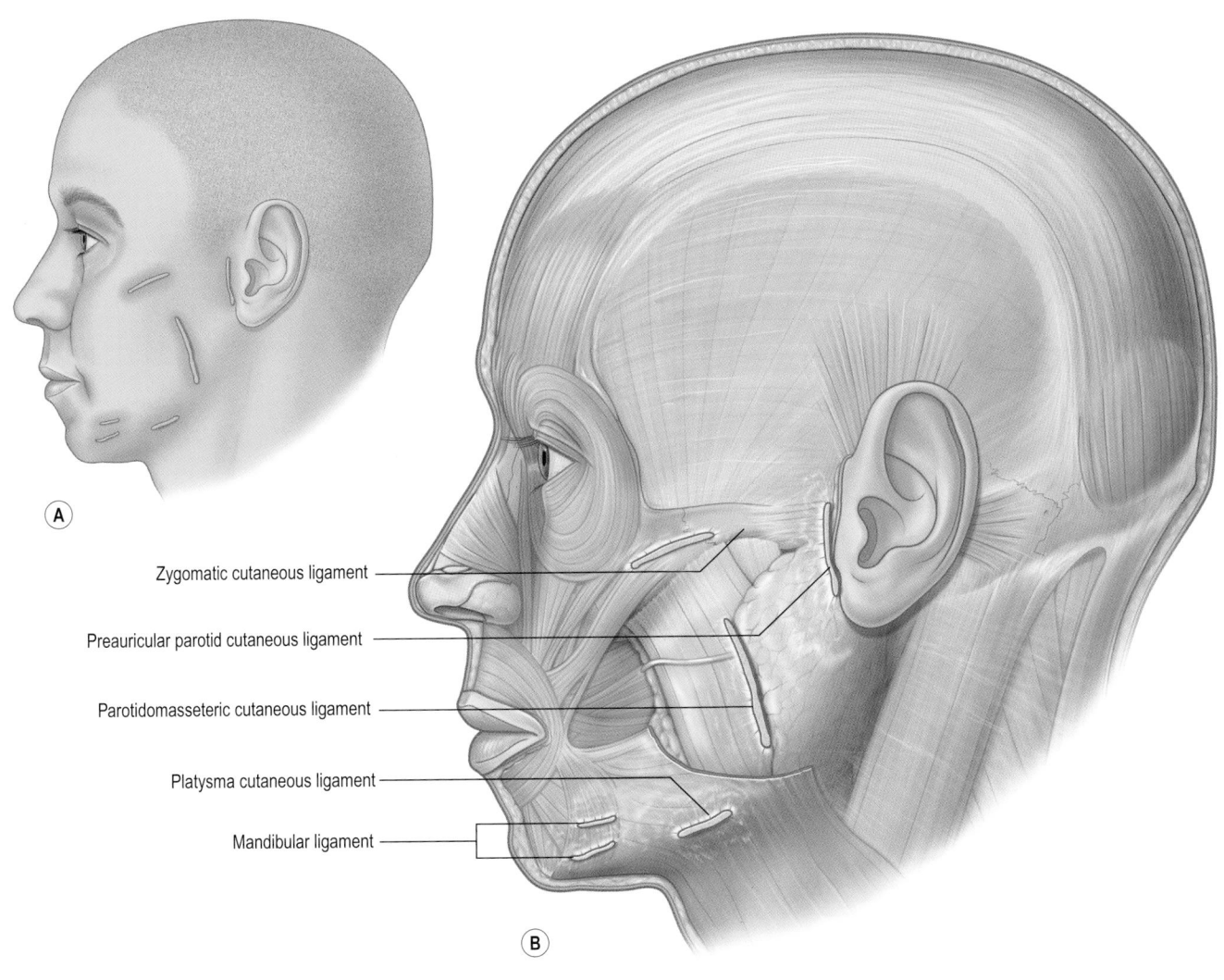

Zygomatic cutaneous ligament

Preauricular parotid cutaneous ligament

Parotidomasseteric cutaneous ligament

Platysma cutaneous ligament

Mandibular ligament

Ⓐ

Ⓑ

Fig. 1.9 The retaining ligaments of the face. (Reproduced with permission from Gray's Anatomy 40e, Standring S (ed), Churchill Livingstone, London, 2008.)

deep temporal extension passes superiorly between the temporalis and the zygomatic arch. The superficial temporal extension is actually totally separate from the main body, and lies between the two layers of the temporal fascia above the zygomatic arch.[41]

The facial nerve

During most facial plastic surgeries, whether congenital, reconstructive or aesthetic, there are one or more branches of the facial nerve that are at risk for injury. Although there is abundant literature on the anatomy of the facial nerve branches, the majority of publications describe two-dimensional anatomy, depicting the trajectory of the nerve and its surface anatomy in relation to anatomic landpoints (see *Fig. 1.3*).[9,16,42–49] However, it is the third dimension, the depth of the facial nerve in relation to the layers of the face that is most relevant to the practicing surgeon. In spite of the significant variability in the branching patterns, the facial nerve consistently passes in defined planes, crossing from one

plane to another in certain zones.[1] It is in these "danger zones" that dissection should be avoided or done carefully. In the rest of the face, the dissection can proceed relatively quickly by adhering to a certain plane, either superficial or deep to the plane of the nerve.

The facial nerve nucleus lies in the lower pons and is responsible for motor innervation to all the muscles derived from the second branchial arch. A few sensory fibers originating in the tractus solitarius join the facial nerve to supply the skin of the external acoustic meatus. The nerve emerges from the lower border of the pons, passes laterally in the cerebello pontine angle and enters the internal acoustic meatus. The facial nerve then traverses the temporal bone (being liable to injury in temporal bone fractures) to exit the skull through the stylomastoid foramen. Just after its exit it is enveloped by a thick layer of fascia that is continuous with the skull periosteum, and is surrounded by a small aggregation of fat and usually crossed by a small blood vessel. This makes its identification at this area a challenging task. Several methods for identification of the facial nerve trunk have been described:

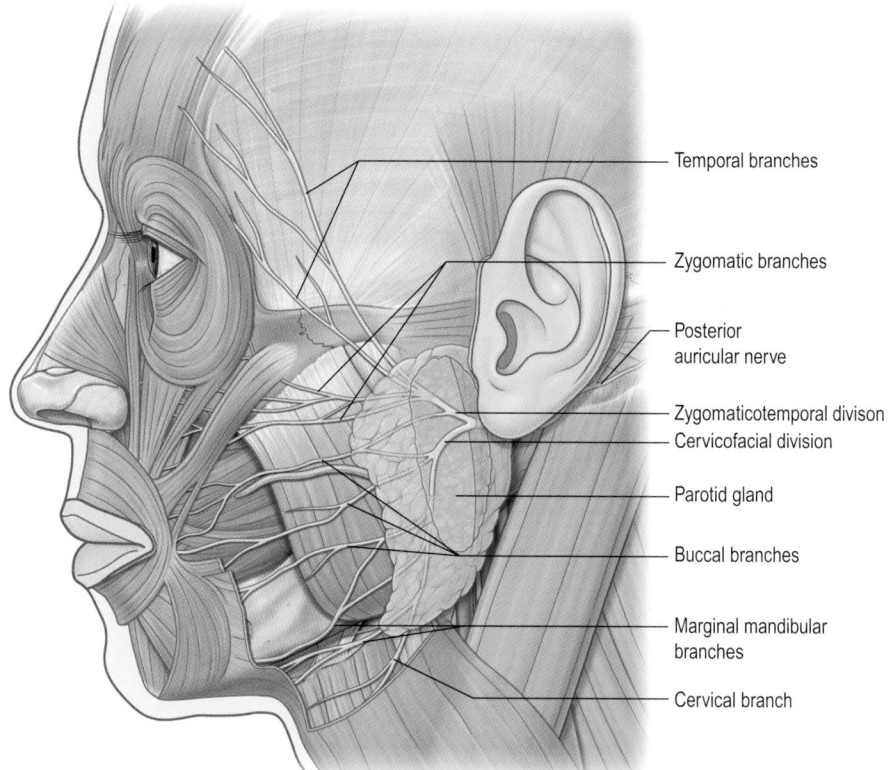

Temporal branches

Zygomatic branches

Posterior
auricular nerve

Zygomaticotemporal divison
Cervicofacial division

Parotid gland

Buccal branches

Marginal mandibular
branches

Cervical branch

Fig. 1.10 The facial nerve.

1. If the tragal cartilage is followed to its deep end, it
    terminates in a point. The nerve is 1 cm deep and
    inferior to this "tragal pointer". There is an avascular
    plane right on the anterior surface of the tragus that
    allows a safe and quick dissection to this tragal pointer.
2. By following the posterior belly of the digastric
    posteriorly, the nerve is found passing laterally
    immediately deep to the upper border of the posterior
    end of the muscle.
3. If the anterior border of the mastoid process is traced
    superiorly, if forms an angle with the tympanic bone.
    The nerve bisects the angle formed between these two
    bones (at the tympanomastoid suture).
4. By feeling the styloid process in between the mastoid
    bone and the posterior border of the mandible. The
    nerve is just lateral to this process.
5. By following the terminal branches of the nerve
    proximally.

    The nerve passes forwards and downwards to pierce the
parotid gland. In the parotid gland the nerve divides into the
zygomaticotemporal and the cervicofacial divisions, which in
turn divide into the five terminal branches of the facial nerve:
frontal, zygomatic, buccal, marginal mandibular, and cervical
(Fig. 1.10). However, the zygomatic and buccal branches show
significant variability in their location and branching patterns
as well as a significant overlap in the muscles they innervate
– they are sometimes grouped together and referred to as
"zygomaticobuccal". The temporal and the mandibular
branches are perhaps at the highest risk for iatrogenic injury,

especially that the muscles they innervate show little if any
cross innervation, making injury to these branches much more
noticeable.

Frontal (temporal) branch

This consists of 3–4 branches that innervate the orbicularis
oculi muscle, the corrugators and the frontalis muscle. Several
anatomic landmarks are used to describe their surface
anatomy. The most common description is Pitanguy's line;
extending from 0.5 cm below the tragus to a point 1 cm above
the lateral edge of the eyebrow (or 1 cm lateral to the lateral
canthus).[50,9] Ramirez described the nerve as crossing the zygomatic arch 4 cm behind the lateral canthus.[51] However, other
surgeons describe the area spanning the middle two thirds of
the arch as the territory of the nerve. Gosain *et al.* found
frontal nerve branches are found at the lower border of the
zygomatic arch between 10 mm anterior to external auditory
meatus and 19 mm posterior to the lateral orbital rim.[16] Finally,
Zani *et al.* in 300 cadaver dissections reported that the nerve
is in a region limited by two straight diverging lines; the first
line from the upper tragus border to the most cephalic wrinkle
of the frontal region, and the second line from the lower
tragus border to the most caudal wrinkle of the frontal region.[45]
Although there is no connection between the frontal nerve
and other branches of the facial nerve, there are connections
within the frontal branches themselves.[16] In addition, the
more posterior divisions of the frontal nerve may be less clinically significant than the anterior branches, the injury of
which will lead to noticeable brow deformities.[16] A line from

the tragus to 1 cm above the lateral eyebrow or 1.5 cm lateral to the lateral canthus seems to be a fairly accurate marking of the largest branch of the frontal nerve.

With this great variation in surface anatomy, it is the plane of the nerve (the depth) that is most important (see *Fig. 1.4*). After emerging from the parotid gland, the nerve is protected by the deep facial fascia (parotidomasseteric fascia) lying on the masseter muscle. In midfacial procedures (e.g. facelift), dissection is usually *superficial* to the deep facial fascia (which protects the nerve deep to it). In the temporal area, the nerve is on the undersurface of the superficial temporal fascia (see *Fig. 1.5A*). Here dissection is usually *deep* to the nerve, either directly superficial or deep to the deep temporal fascia (or the superficial layer of the deep temporal fascia). However, the crossing of the nerve from deep to superficial in the vicinity of the zygomatic arch is a matter of debate. This is largely because of the confusion regarding the anatomy of the fascia in relation to the arch. Directly over the arch, the facial layers are tightly adherent (with little thickness of tissues from the bone to the skin). While the SMAS is continuous with the temporoparietal fascia across the arch, it is not clear if the deep facial fascia is continuous with the deep temporal fascia or they are separate layers that adhere to the periosteum of the zygomatic arch.[7,8,52,53] At the lower border of the arch, the nerve is very close to the periosteum.[54–57] The nerve is still deep to the SMAS/TPF and deep to the areolar tissue between the TPF and the DTF (which as described above is sometimes considered as a separate layer of fascia called the parotido-temporal fascia). This deep location of the nerve allows safe transection of the SMAS at the level of the zygomatic arch in facelift surgeries.[58] The nerve passes from its deep location to the STF in the region right above the zygomatic arch.[13] In this area, the fascia layers are more tightly adherent, which is a warning sign that the facial nerve is in close proximity. Dissection in this transition zone, extending over the arch and the 2–3 cm above it, should be done carefully (see *Fig. 1.3*).

Zygomatic and buccal branches

These branches emerge from the parotid and diverge forwards lying over the masseter muscle under the parotidomasseteric (deep facial) fascia. The exact point where they pierce the deep fascia is variable, but is in the vicinity of the anterior border of the masseter. The upper branches to the midfacial muscle (zygomatic branches) pierce the deep fascia approximately 4 cm in front of the tragus in close proximity (around 1 cm inferior) to the zygomatic ligaments (see *Fig. 1.2C*). These branches soon innervate the zygomaticus major muscle through its deep surface. The buccal branches emerge from the parotid in the same plane as the parotid duct (deep to the parotidomasseteric fascia). They pierce the deep fascia at the anterior edge of the masseter, close to the masseteric cutaneous ligaments (see *Fig. 1.2C*). Together, the zygomatic and buccal branches supply the orbicularis oculi, midfacial muscle, orbicularis oris, and the buccinator. Unlike the marginal mandibular and the frontal divisions, there are a number of communicating branches between the buccal and zygomatic divisions, and injury to a single branch of these nerves is usually unnoticeable. Facial lacerations medial to the level of the lateral canthus are usually not amenable to exploration or repair of the facial nerve.

Marginal mandibular

The marginal mandibular nerve is one of the most commonly encountered branches of the facial nerve, and is in jeopardy in multiple operations, including neck dissections, submandibular sialadenectomy, and exposure of the mandible.[59] There are numerous descriptions and variations of both the trajectory of the nerve and its plane (i.e. depth), necessitating care in a wide are of dissection in the lower face and the submandibular triangle.[2,44,60–64] In addition, the nerve can vary between a single branch and up to 3 or 4 branches.[2,61,65,66]

After exiting the parotid gland near its lower border, the nerve loops downward, often below the mandibular border. Whether the nerve crosses the mandibular border into the submandibular triangle in all individuals is a matter of debate.[2,60,67] Although several cadaver studies found the nerve to be more commonly above the mandibular border, clinical experience has shown that it is frequently located in the submandibular triangle, up to 3 or even 4 cm below the mandible.[2,44,60,68–70] This might also vary with the position of the neck, and the surgeon must consider the wide variability of the nerve location in his dissection.[2] The nerve then passes upwards back into the face midway between the angle and mental protuberance. Once the nerve crosses the facial vessels, its major trunk is usually above the border of the mandible, although smaller branches may continue in the neck to supply the platysma.[2]

After exiting the parotid gland, the nerve is initially deep to the parotidomasseteric fascia. In the submandibular triangle, the nerve is usually described as lying between the platysma and the deep cervical fascia. However, it might occasionally be found deep to the deep fascia near the superficial surface of the submandibular gland. The nerve is deep to the platysma and superficial to the facial vessels throughout its course. As the nerve crosses into the lower face, the platysma thins and the nerve can be injured during a subcutaneous dissection.

The marginal mandibular nerve supplies the lower lip muscles, depressor anguli oris, mentalis, and the upper part of the platysma.[65,61] Injury to the marginal mandibular branch usually causes a recognizable deformity,[71–73] and several surgical maneuvers have been advocated to protect the nerve.[74,75] When exposing the mandible, the surgeon can identify the nerve in the usual subplatysmal location. However, it might be safer and faster to go to a deeper plane, elevating the deep fascia and/or the facial vessels and using them to protect the nerve. Dissection above the platysma laterally will also avoid nerve injury.

Cervical branch

The cervical branch of the facial nerve primarily supplies the platysma. It has received little attention in the literature, as injury of this nerve may pass unnoticed. However, such injury may cause weakness of the lower lip depressors, which is often confused with injury to the mandibular nerve (marginal mandibular nerve pseudoparalysis).[76,77] However, mentalis function differentiates the two conditions, as it is preserved in cases of cervical branch injury.

The cervical nerve exits the parotid gland and passes 1–15 mm behind the angle of the mandible. It then passes forwards, in the subplatysmal plane 1–4.5 cm below the border of the mandible.[78] The cervical nerve is often composed of more than one branch. It may communicate with the marginal mandibular nerve (which might explain the lower lip asymmetry after its injury), and consistently communicates with the transverse cervical nerve, although this latter communication is currently of little significance.[79,60]

Connection with sensory nerves

Several authors have noticed connections between the branches of the facial nerve with sensory nerves, including the infraorbital, mental nerves and transverse cervical nerves.[66,78,80,81] The exact clinical importance of this finding is yet to be seen. Interestingly, a face transplant recipient performed at the Cleveland Clinic developed 2-point discrimination in the cheek, although only the facial nerves (and not the sensory nerves) were repaired.[82]

The scalp

The five layers of the scalp are well known by the mnemonic SCALP:
- *Skin*
- *Connective tissue*
- *Galea Aponeurotica*
- *Loose areolar tissue*
- *Pericranium.*

The gale aponeurotica is also known as the epicranial aponeurosis and corresponds to the SMAS in the face. Peculiar to the scalp is the tight connection of the skin to the galea by a dense network of connective tissue fibers. This makes separation of the skin from the galea difficult (similar to the palm) and bloody. In addition, this connective tissue lace stents the vessels open which, combined with the scalp's rich vascularity, leads to profuse bleeding.

The galea is a dynamic structure, being controlled by the frontalis muscle anteriorly and the occipitalis posteriorly. The skin moves together with the galea due to their tight attachment. This is important in brow rejuvenation where weakening of the brow depressor muscles allows the epicranial aponeurosis to move backwards leading to elevation of the brow.

The loose areolar tissue between the galea and the periosteum is also referred to as the subgaleal fascia. This fascia is loose especially over the vertex of the scalp, allowing a quick dissection with minimal bleeding. It becomes more dense closer to the supra orbital rims. Most surgeons consider this layer as a potential dissection "plane" rather than a discrete "layer".[8,83] However, it has been shown to be a distinct layer that can be elevated independently as a vascularized flap.[84] This is especially possible closer to the zygomatic arch and the supraorbital rims where this layer is more substantial. It is formed histologically of multiple lamina, with most of the vasculature along the superficial and the deep lamina.[31,85,86]

The pericranium is simply the periosteum of the skull bones and is tightly adherent to normal sutures but easily dissected over the flat skull bones. It can be elevated as a separate flap for various uses, although once separated from the skull bones it significantly retracts.[87,88]

Five arteries supply the scalp. From the front, there is the supraorbital artery and the supratrochlear artery (branches of the ophthalmic artery from the internal carotid artery), the superficial temporal artery from the side, and the posterior auricular and the occipital arteries form the back (the latter three arteries arise from the external carotid artery). In general, these vessels run along the galea as they enter the periphery of the scalp. At this level, they give multiple perforating branches to the deeper subgaleal fascia. Closer to the vertex, most of the vessels become more superficial, anastomosing with the contralateral vessels. This explains why scalp flaps (formed of skin and galea with an intact subdermal plexus) can be safely extended across the midline, while pure galeal flaps cannot.[89]

The nerve supply of the anterior part of the scalp is by four branches of the trigeminal nerve: STN, SON, ZTN, and the auriculotemporal nerve. The posterior part of the scalp (roughly behind the level of the auricle) is supplied by four branches of the cervical nerves (C2 and C3): the great auricular nerve, the lesser occipital nerve, the greater occipital nerve, and the third occipital nerve.

The musculature

In general, the muscle of the forehead and eyebrow are arranged in three planes: the superficial plane right under the skin formed by the frontalis, procerus, the orbicularis oculi; the deep plane formed by the corrugators, and an intermediate plane formed by the depressor supercilii *(Fig. 1.11)*.

Frontalis, galeal fat pad, and the glide plane

The frontalis muscle originates from the galea aponeurosis and inserts distally (inferiorly) into the eyebrow skin interdigitating with the procerus, corrugator and the orbicularis oculi. Just above the nasion, both frontalis muscle are contiguous with each other. At a variable point (1.5–6 cm) above the level of the superior orbital rim, the muscles diverge, with the medial borders becoming connected by an extension of the galea aponeurotica.[90] This divergence point is higher in females. This is important when injecting botulinum toxin for treatment of forehead rhytides.

Deep to the frontalis at the level of the eyebrows is the galeal fat pad, a band of fibroadipose tissue that is frequently encountered in brow lift procedures.[91] This fat pad extends for 2–2.5 cm above the supraorbital rims being intimately related to the corrugator muscles. Between the galeal fat pad and the periosteum is the glide plane space, which allows mobility of the brow over the underlying bone. Similar to the SMAS in the face, the galea aponeurotica in the scalp seems to split to cover both deep and the superficial surfaces of the frontalis. At the level of the supraorbital rim, the fascia covering the deep surface of the frontalis becomes more adherent to the periosteum, sealing the galeal fat pad and the glide plane space above it from the eyelids. It is possible that the weakness of these attachments may be predisposed to brow ptosis, especially laterally.[92,93]

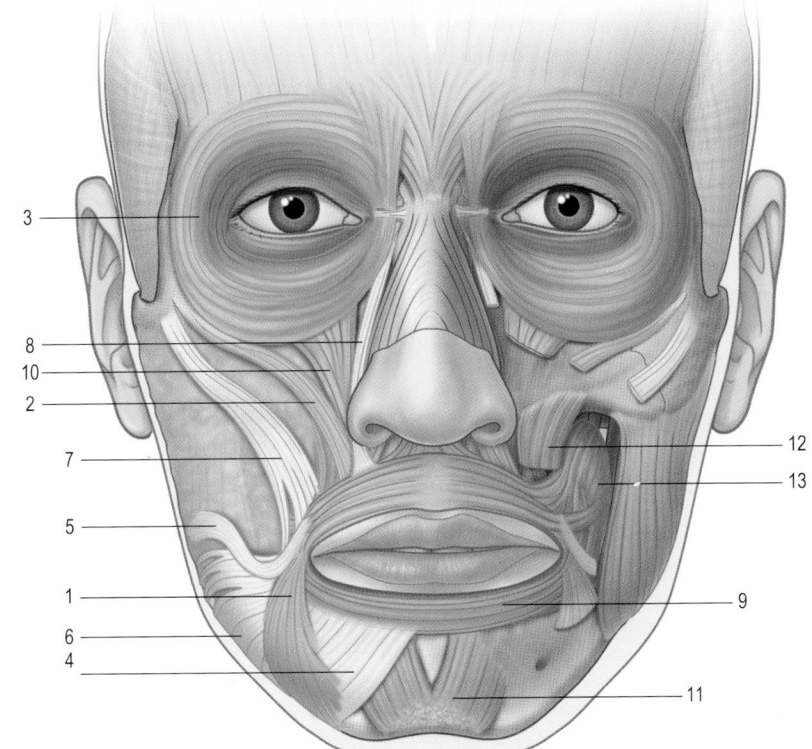

Layer 1
1. Depressor anguli oris
2. Zygomaticus minor
3. Orbicularis oculi

Layer 2
4. Depressor labii inferioris
5. Risorius
6. Platysma
7. Zygomaticus major
8. Levator labii superioris
   alaeque nasi

Layer 3
9. Orbicularis oris
10. Levator labii superioris

Layer 4
11. Mentalis
12. Levator anguli oris
13. Buccinator

Fig. 1.11 Muscles of facial expression.

Corrugators

The anatomy of the corrugators has gained significance recently, with the realization of its role in browlift, migraine surgery and treatment of forehead rhytides. This renewed interest has led to multiple anatomical studies that agree that the muscle is larger than originally described.[94,95] The muscle originates from the supraorbital ridge, and passes obliquely upwards and laterally to insert into the skin of the eyebrow. Usually described as being comprised of a transverse and an oblique head, Park et al. found that this distinction is not clear and described the muscle as being formed of three or four parallel muscle groups with loose areolar tissue in between.[94] Janis et al. similarly found that both heads are indistinguishable shortly after their origin.[95] In all cases, the muscle fibers blend together laterally, and become more superficial. Medial to the SON, the corrugator is clearly separated from the overlying frontalis/orbicularis oculi muscle. However, it becomes more superficial laterally near its insertion blending with the frontalis. This close interdigitation with the orbicularis explains the difference in description of the anatomy in this region between the different authors. Intraoperatively, the corrugator can be recognized by its parallel oblique fibers, darker color and deeper location, as opposed to the orbicularis oculi which is more superficial and inferior, is lighter in color, and has a circular orientation of the fibers.

The muscle origin is approximately 2.5 cm in width and 1 cm in height, starting a few millimeters lateral to midline and reaching almost to the level of the SON.[94] The muscle then passes laterally to insert in the skin of the eyebrow, reaching as far as the lateral third of the eyebrow. Janis et al. found that the lateral most extension of the muscle is 43 mm from the midline and 7 mm medial to the lateral orbital rim, while the most superior extension is 33 mm cephalad to the level of the nasion.

The nerve supply of the corrugator is probably from both the frontal (temporal) and the zygomatic divisions of the facial nerve.[66,70,96,97] The branch(es) from the frontal nerve enter the muscle from its lateral end, and hence the importance of complete muscle excision lateral to the SON so as not to leave intact innervated muscle. The zygomatic (or upper buccal) division sends a nerve that travels cranially along the side of the nose to innervate the nasalis followed by the procerus and the corrugator.[66,97]

Procerus

This small muscle arises from the nasal bone and the upper lateral cartilages and ascends superiorly to insert into the glabellar skin between the eyebrows and blending with frontalis along the medial ends of the eyebrow.[98] Contraction of the procerus produces transverse glabellar rhytids.

Depressor supercilii

This small muscle lies between the orbicularis oculi and the corrugators, although some authors consider it part of either muscle.[92,99–101] It arises from the frontal process of the maxilla 2–5 mm below the frontomaxillary suture, slightly posterior and superior to the posterior lacrimal crest.[99] Daniel and Landon described it as running vertically between the pale circular orbicularis oculi more superficially and the brownish transverse corrugator lying in a deeper plane.[100] It finally inserts into the dermis of the medial eyebrow.

Midfacial muscles

From lateral to medial, the zygomaticus major, zygomaticus minor, and the levator labii superioris originate from the anterior surface of the maxilla (*Fig. 1.11*). Their line of origin is a curved line, convex downwards, with the medial limit higher than the lateral end. These muscles form the floor of the prezygomatic space, and are covered by a fascial membrane that is more stout superiorly, being around 2–3 mm thick. This fascial membrane is identified by its pale color and coarse lobulation. The levator labii superioris origin reaches the inferior orbital rim while the zygomaticus major origin is separated from the inferior orbital rim by the front of the body of the zygoma. The three muscles insert into the substance of the upper lip.

The levator labii superioris alaeque nasi originates from the frontal process of the maxilla. Its fibers pass downwards and laterally to insert into the lower lateral cartilage of the nose and the upper lip.

The levator anguli oris arises from the maxilla below the orbital foramen lying deep to the lip elevators. It is one of the few facial muscles innervated on their superficial surface.

The depressor labii inferioris and the depressor anguli oris are continuous with the platysma and draw the lip downwards and laterally.

The mentalis is a thick small muscle that is important in exposure of the mandible and in chin surgery. It arises from the buccal surface of the mandible over the roots of the incisors and inserts into the chin. Repair of the mentalis is vital after buccal incisions to prevent chin ptosis.

Muscles of mastication

The four muscles of mastication, the temporalis, masseter, and lateral and medial pterygoids, are mostly present in the temporal and infratemporal fossae and control mandibular movement during speech and mastication. Being derivatives of the first pharyngeal arch, they are all supplied by the mandibular division of the trigeminal nerve.

The temporalis muscle

The temporalis arises from the bony floor of the temporal fossa, with attachments to the deep surface of the deep temporal fascia. It passes deep to the zygomatic arch to insert into the coronoid process of the mandible and the anterior border of the ramus of the mandible almost down to the third molar tooth. It receives its blood supply from the anterior and posterior deep temporal arteries, arising from the maxillary artery and supplying the muscle through its deep surface.[102] It receives secondary blood supply from the middle temporal artery, which arises from the superficial temporal artery near the zygomatic arch and travels along the deep temporal fascia.

Based on its dominant deep pedicle, the muscle's arc of rotation is at the zygomatic arch, and can be rotated as a flap for coverage of the orbit, upper cheek and ear.[103,104] The muscle is also frequently used for facial reanimation.

The masseter muscle

This strong muscle arises from the lower border and inner surface of the zygomatic arch by two heads: a superficial head from the anterior two-thirds of the arch and a deep head forms the posterior third. The superficial head descends downwards and backwards, while the deep head descends vertically downwards. Both heads then insert together at the lateral and inferior surfaces of the mandible.

The medial pterygoid muscle

The medial pterygoid muscle arises by two heads: a small superficial head from the maxillary tubercle behind the last molar and a deep large head from the medial surface of the medial pterygoid. Both heads run downwards and backwards to insert on the inner surface of the angle of the mandible. In mandibular fractures the action of this muscle is responsible for the upwards and forwards movement of the posterior segment.

The lateral pterygoid muscle

This muscle also has two heads, a smaller upper head from infratemporal surface and ridge of greater wing of sphenoid, and a lower larger head from the lateral surface of the lateral pterygoid plate. The fibers pass backwards to insert into the anterior surface of the neck of the mandible and the capsule of the temporomandibular joint. Some of the fibers pierce the capsule to attach to the intraarticular disc. In condylar fractures, this muscle is responsible for the displacement of the mandibular condyle, while in Le Fort fractures, the muscle pulls the maxillary segment downwards and backwards resulting in premature contact of the molar and an anterior open bite.

Actions of muscle of mastication

Together, these muscles control most of the movements of the mandible. Elevation of the mandible is achieved by the temporalis and the masseter, while the pterygoids protract the mandible and move it to the contralateral side.

The pterygomasseteric sling

The masseter and the medial pterygoid insert respectively into the lateral and medial surfaces of the lower edge of the mandible near the mandibular angle. These insertions are connected to each other by the pterygomasseteric sling, a fibrous raphe extending around the mandibular border and connecting both insertion.[105] Disruption of this raphe will lead to an unaesthetic upward retraction of the masseter, most visible on clinching the jaws.[106]

The aesthetic importance of the masseter and the temporalis muscle

Atrophy, hypertrophy, or displacement of either the masseter or the temporalis can be aesthetically bothersome. Masseter hypertrophy leads to an increased bigonial angle, although most cases of benign masseteric hypertrophy (BMH) are actually caused by a laterally positioned mandibular ramus and not by a true hypertrophy of the muscle. Deformities of the temporalis muscle are more common, and are usually iatrogenic due to improper resuspension of the origin of the muscle during a coronal incision leading to retraction of the muscle inferiorly. This leads to a visible bulge above the zygoma and a depression near the origin of the muscle. Repair of the atrophy or displacement of the masseter and the temporalis often involves the use of alloplastic implants, as the muscle cannot usually be stretched to their original lengths.

The sensory innervation

The anatomy of the sensory nerves and their relation to the surrounding muscles has gained significant importance with the recognition of their role in the aetiology of migraine headaches.[107,108] Knowledge of the anatomy of these nerves is also important both to avoid iatrogenic injury and for local anesthetic blocks.[109,110] In general, the face is supplied by the three divisions of the trigeminal nerve (through three branches from each division), with the scalp receiving additional supply from the cervical superficial spinal nerves (*Fig. 1.12* and see *Fig. 1.9*).

The frontal division of the trigeminal nerve supplies the upper eyelid, forehead and a large portion of the scalp through three branches; the supraorbital, supratrochlear, and the infratrochlear nerves (*Fig. 1.13A* and see *Fig. 1.12*). The first two are particularly important due to their role in triggering frontal migraine and the possibility of their injury during forehead and eyebrow rejuvenation.[108] In addition, successful anesthetic blocks of the SON can effectively anesthetize large areas of the scalp.

The SON exits the orbit through either a notch or foramen located at the level of the medial limbus.[111] There is significant variation in its exit point,[108,111–117] which can be a notch, a foramen, or a canal. This point of emergence is approximately 25–30 mm from the midline. It is usually a few millimeters above the orbital rim, but can be up to 19 mm above it.[112–115] The nerve then divides into a superficial (medial) and a deep (lateral) branch. The superficial division passes superficial to the frontalis to supply the forehead skin.[108] The larger deep division, which is more prone to iatrogenic injury, passes cephalad in a more lateral location. As its name suggests, it is in a deeper plane lying between the galea and the periosteum.[116,117] It passes upwards 1 cm medial to the temporal fusion line, and supplies sensation to the fronto-parietal scalp. Forehead dissection is safer in the subperiosteal plane as opposed to a subgaleal (subfrontalis) plane which places the deep branch of the SON in risk.[118]

The STN emerges from the medial orbit above the trochlea approximately 1 cm from the midline, and is usually composed of multiple branches. It supplies the central forehead. The ITN is a smaller nerve that supplies the medial eyelid and a small part of the medial upper nose.

The maxillary division contributes three branches to the sensory supply of the head; the zygomaticotemporal, zygomaticofacial, and the infraorbital nerve (*Fig. 1.13B*, and see *Fig. 1.12*). The ZTN pierces the temporalis muscle and emerges through the deep temporal fascia 17 mm lateral and 7 mm

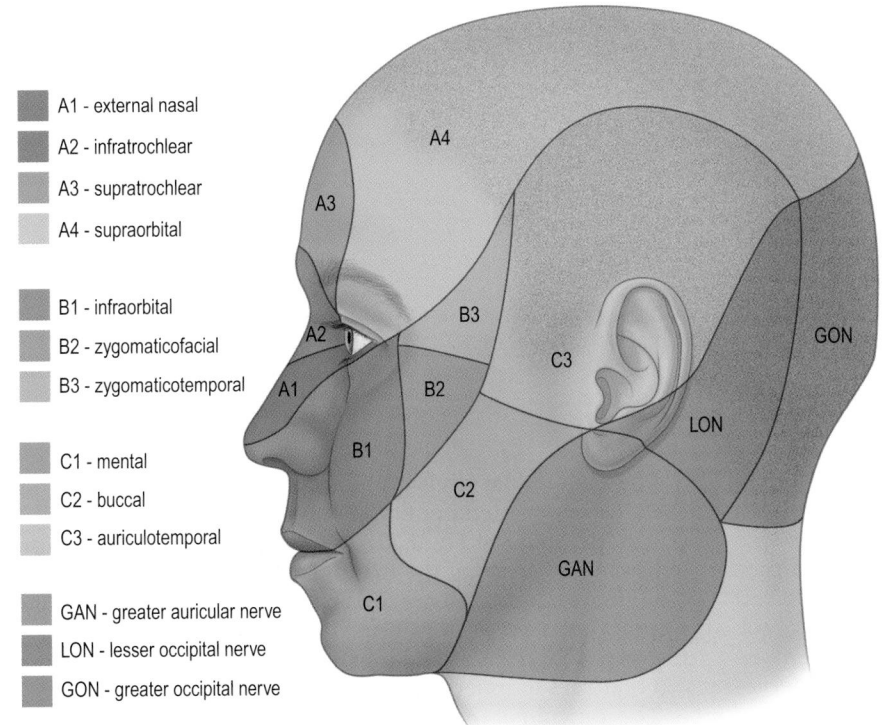

A1 - external nasal
A2 - infratrochlear
A3 - supratrochlear
A4 - supraorbital

B1 - infraorbital
B2 - zygomaticofacial
B3 - zygomaticotemporal

C1 - mental
C2 - buccal
C3 - auriculotemporal

GAN - greater auricular nerve
LON - lesser occipital nerve
GON - greater occipital nerve

Fig. 1.12 The sensory supply of the face.

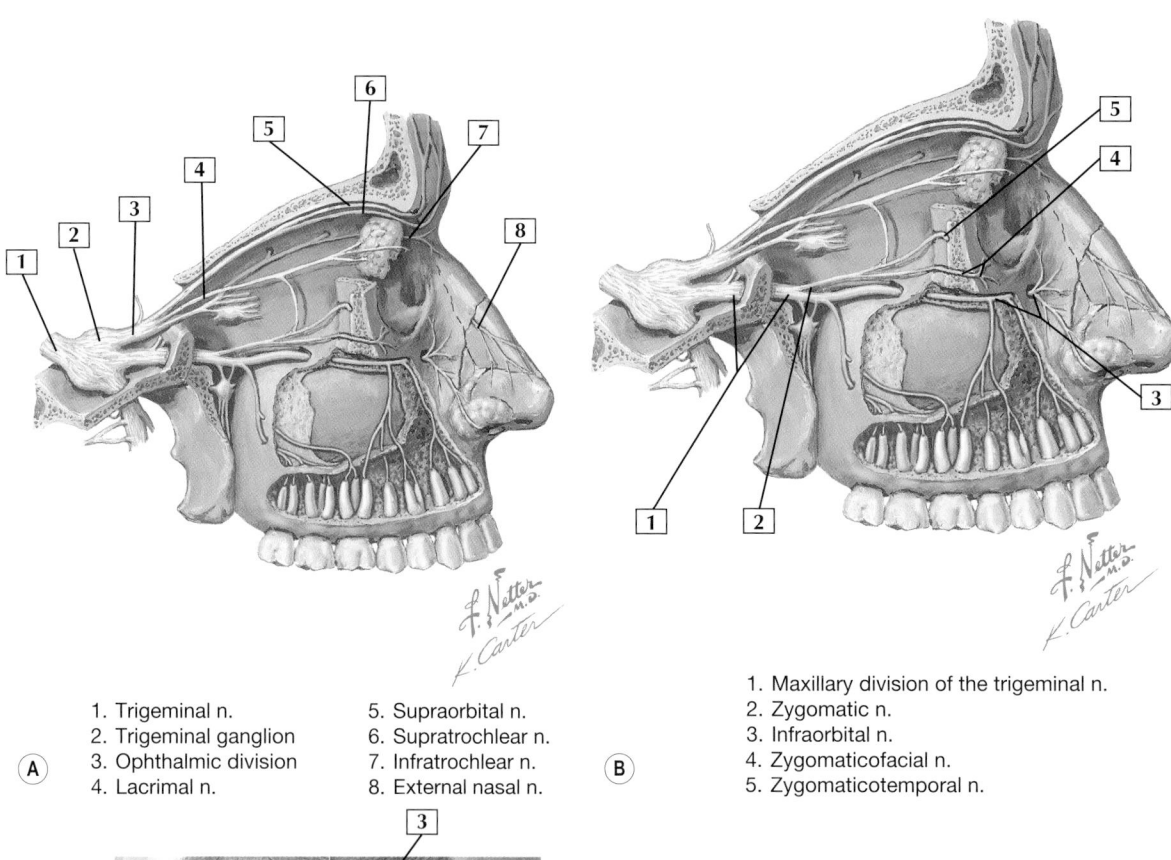

A
1. Trigeminal n.   5. Supraorbital n.
2. Trigeminal ganglion   6. Supratrochlear n.
3. Ophthalmic division   7. Infratrochlear n.
4. Lacrimal n.   8. External nasal n.

B
1. Maxillary division of the trigeminal n.
2. Zygomatic n.
3. Infraorbital n.
4. Zygomaticofacial n.
5. Zygomaticotemporal n.

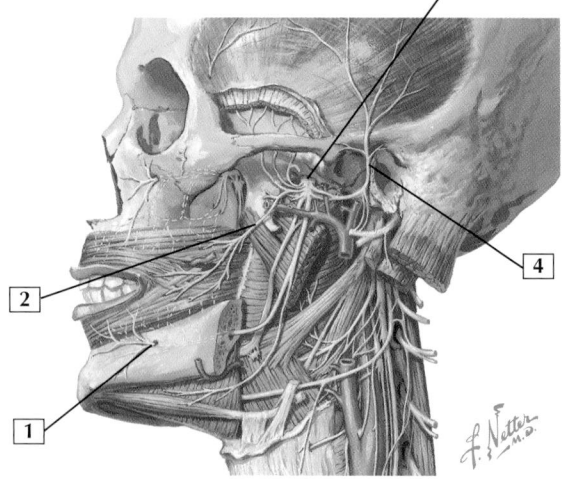

C   1. Mental n.   3. Mandibular division of the trigeminal n.
     2. Buccal n.   4. Auriculotemporal n.

Fig. 1.13 (A–C) The sensory nerves of the face. (Reprinted with permission from www.netterimages.com ©Elsevier Inc. All rights reserved.)

cephalad to the lateral canthus to supply the temporal fore-head.[119] It has also been incriminated as a cause of temporal migraine. The zygomaticofacial nerve exits the orbit through a foramen in the zygomatic bone to innervate the skin of the cheek below the zygoma. The infraorbital nerve is the direct continuation of the maxillary nerve and passes to the cheek through a foramen 1 cm below the infraorbital rim lying along in the same vertical plane with the SON and the mental nerves (roughly along the midpupillary line).[115] It supplies the skin of the cheek and the upper lid.

The mandibular division also gives three branches to the face: the auriculotemporal, the buccal and the mental nerves (*Fig. 1.13C*, and see *Fig. 1.12*). The mental nerve is at risk for injury in exposures of the mandible. It is the continuation of the inferior alveolar nerve, exiting the mandible through the mental foramen which is located in line with the mandibular first premolar (or first molar in children). It soon divides into 2–3 branches to innervate the lower lip and the chin.

The auriculotemporal nerve passes around the neck of the mandible and ascend over the posterior root of the zygomatic arch, giving a branch to supply the temporomandibular joint. As its names indicates, it supplies the auricle (and the external acoustic meatus and the tympanic membrane) and the skin of the temple. It also carries parasympathetic postganglionic fibers to the parotid gland, explaining its role in the development of Frey's syndrome (gustatory sweating). The best place for an auriculotemporal nerve block is 10–15 mm anterior to the upper origin of the helix.[112]

The buccal nerve runs in deep plane on the surface of the buccinators. It sends branches to the skin of the cheek before piercing the buccinator to supply the mucous membrane of the cheek.

Of all the cervical cutaneous nerves, the great auricular nerve has the most significance to the plastic surgeon.[120] It supplies the lower two-thirds of the lateral surface of the ear, the posterior and lower cheek, and the skin over the mastoid. It appears around the midpoint of the posterior border of the sternomastoid passing obliquely upwards towards the angle of the jaw. However, along the mid-belly of the muscle, it gently curves changing its direction towards the ear lobe. It passes either superficial or deep to the sternomastoid fascia.[121] It can be consistently found at a point on the mid-belly of the sternomastoid muscle 6.5 cm caudal to the bony external auditory meatus.[120]

Anatomy of the ear

The appearance of individual ear is unique. Its shape and contour follows the cartilaginous framework that is enveloped by a very thin skin and soft tissue. In general, there are three parts of external ear: helix-antihelical complex, conchal complex, and lobule. Each of these complexes has its own convoluted structures forming the surface anatomy with specific landmark nomenclature.[122]

These three divisions of ear are closely related to the embryological development process. The ear arises from the first and second branchial arches, also known as mandibular and hyoid. These arches then continued to develop into hillocks between the 3rd and 6th week of gestation. Located anteriorly, the first branchial arch forms into three hillocks: root of helix, tragus, and superior helix. The second branchial arch, which is located posteriorly, gives rise to the other three hillocks: antihelix, antitragus, and lobule. They become fully formed structures by the 4th month and continue to develop around the external meatus, which canalize by week 28. The middle ear arises from the first pharyngeal arch during the 4th week and forms into the incus and malleus. The stapes, on the other hand, is formed from the second arch.[122,123]

The component of soft tissue covering the framework comprised of vestigial intrinsic muscles of the ear, such as helicis major and minor, tragicus and antitragus, and the transverse and oblique muscles. Most of the extrinsic muscle covering are auricularis muscles (anterior, superior, and posterior). All of these structures are vascularized by the arborization of vessels from superficial temporal and posterior auricular arteries. The majority of the anterior surface of the ear is supplied by the latter through its perforating branches and over the helical rim. The branches of the superficial temporal artery only supply the superior helical rim and triangular fossa and scapha network. These vasculatures form

interconnecting system, which allow either of the system to support the ear.[122–124]

The sensory nerve supply of the ear is derived from combination of cranial and extracranial branches. The posterior ear and lobule are innervated by the greater auricular nerve (C2,C3) and the lesser occipital nerve (C2). The anterior ear and tragus are supplied by the trigeminal nerve (auriculotemporal branch of V3). The inferior ear and parts of the preauricular area are innervated by the greater auricular nerve (C2,3). The superior portion of ear and mastoid region are innervated by lesser occipital nerve (C2).

Anatomy of the eyelids

There is no consensus on the "ideal" aesthetic eyelids, with several factors such as age, ethnicity and surrounding skeletal structure causing wide variation in the normal eyelids.

In general, the palpebral fissure measures 29–32 mm horizontally and 9–12 mm vertically, with the lateral canthus 1–2 mm higher than the medial canthus. The upper eyelid usually covers the upper 1–2 mm of the iris (lying approximately halfway between the edge of the pupil and the limbus), while the lower eyelid rests at roughly the level of the inferior limbus. The highest point of the upper eyelids lies just nasal to the center of the pupil. Ensuring the eyelids lies at their normal position is important after periorbital surgery, especially if the canthal tendons are disrupted.

The eyelids can be separated into an anterior lamella, formed of skin and orbicularis oculi muscle, and a posterior lamella, formed by the tarsus and the conjunctiva (*Fig. 1.14*).

The skin of the eyelids is the thinnest skin of the body, mainly due to its thin dermis, and is relatively more elastic. As the skin crosses over the orbital rims, it abruptly thickens. Incisions in the eyelids usually heal rapidly and with minimal scarring.

The orbicularis oculi lies directly deep to the skin with minimal subcutaneous fat in between, and is divided into pretarsal, preseptal (both lying in the eyelid) and orbital (around the eyelids) portions. The pretarsal muscle arises medially by two heads that surround the lacrimal sac and attach to the anterior and posterior lacrimal crests. The deep head, also known as Horner's muscle, also attaches to the fascia over the lacrimal sac. This peculiar arrangement allows the muscle to play an important role in the lacrimal pump mechanism.[125] The preseptal orbicularis originates from the medial canthal ligament and inserts on the zygoma lateral to the orbital rim. The orbital part of the orbicularis muscle originates from the medial canthal ligament and the adjacent maxillary and frontal bones, and inserts with the preseptal portion into the lateral palpebral raphe (see below).

The tarsi provide support and rigidity to the eyelids. They are formed of collagen, aggregens and chondroitins. The upper tarsus measures 10–12 mm, while the lower tarsus measures 4–5 mm.[126] The edges of the tarsi are firmly attached to the eyelids margins, while the opposite edge is convex giving the tarsus a semilunar shape. The Meibomian glands are embedded within the tarsus, and their ducts orifices are located along the eyelid margin posterior to the eyelashes. Between the dust orifices and the lashes is the "gray line", which can be seen as a faint gray line or groove. This line

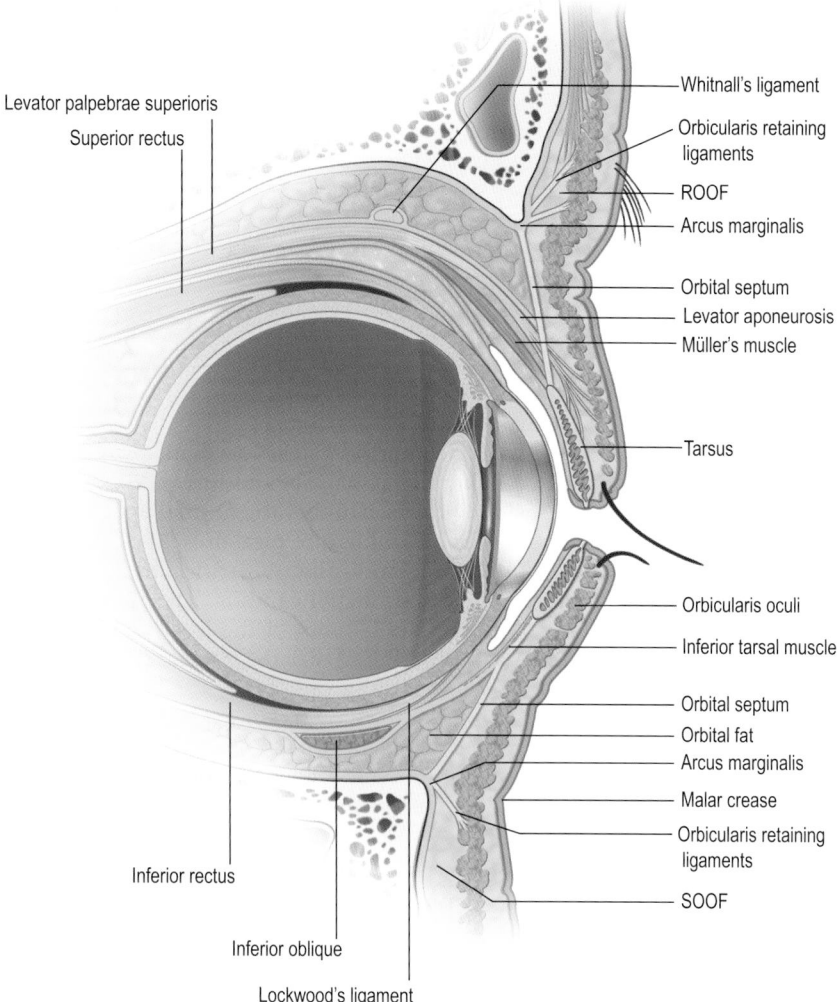

Levator palpebrae superioris
Superior rectus
Whitnall's ligament
Orbicularis retaining ligaments
ROOF
Arcus marginalis
Orbital septum
Levator aponeurosis
Müller's muscle
Tarsus
Orbicularis oculi
Inferior tarsal muscle
Orbital septum
Orbital fat
Arcus marginalis
Malar crease
Orbicularis retaining ligaments
SOOF
Inferior rectus
Inferior oblique
Lockwood's ligament

Fig. 1.14 Sagittal view through the eyelids.

corresponds to a terminal extension of the orbicularis muscle known as Riolan's muscle.[127] The gray line serves as an important landmark; this is the plane between the anterior and posterior lamella of the eyelids.

The orbital septum extends from the edges of the tarsi to the orbital rims, attaching to the edge of the rim except inferiorly, where it extends for 1–2 mm on the anterior surface of the inferior orbital rim, sharing a common origin with the orbicularis retaining ligament (see above). Directly deep to the septum is the orbital fat and the retractors of the upper and lower eyelids.

The levator palpebrae superioris is the important upper eyelid retractor; injury or weakness to this muscle leads to eyelid ptosis. Originating from the back of the orbit, its muscular fibers pass forwards above the superior rectus muscle. They then turn into the fibrous levator aponeurosis and curve inferiorly into the upper eyelid. This transition is encircled by the Whitnall's ligament. The Whitnall's ligament sends medial and lateral horns to attach to the zygomatic bone laterally and the medial canthal ligament and the posterior lacrimal crest medially. These attachments maintain the eyelids opposed to the eyeball with its movement. The levator aponeurosis inserts into the anterior surface of the tarsus, sending fibrous attachments thought the orbital septum and the orbicularis muscle

to skin to form the upper eyelid crease. The deep part of the elevator muscle is the Muller's muscle, which is sympathetically innervated.[128] In hyperthyroidism, sensitization of the Muller muscle leads to upper eyelid retraction and pseudo-proptosis. On the other hand, in Horner's syndrome loss of this muscle action leads to ptosis. Muller's muscle also sends a lateral extension surrounding the lacrimal gland and playing a role in tear excretion.[129]

The capsulopalpebral fascia assists in lower eyelid retraction and coordinates it with eyeball movement. It arises as an extension of the inferior rectus muscle and inserts into the lower edge of the lower tarsus and the adjacent orbital septum.[130] It might contain true muscle fibers, the inferior tarsus muscle, on its upper surface (similar to the Muller muscle in the upper eyelid).

The medial and lateral canthal ligaments are of significant importance due to their role in supporting and shaping the eyelids.[131,22] Unfortunately, there is significant confusion in terminology between the terms ligaments/tendons/and raphe when describing these structures.[131–133] Laterally, the tarsi are attached to the orbital rim by the superficial and deep parts of the lateral canthal ligament. The deeper stronger part attaches to Whitnall's tubercle, located on the deep surface of the lateral orbital wall 3 mm behind the rim.[134] The superficial part attaches to the anterior surface of the lateral orbital rim and the adjacent temporalis fascia and lateral orbital thickening. The orbicularis oculi muscles, superficial to the tarsi and the ligaments, curve around the eyelids and interlace together forming the lateral orbital raphe, which is superficial to the superficial part of the lateral canthal tendon.[133] Medially, the medial canthal ligaments arise from the medial edge of the upper and lower tarsus, and is similarly formed of anterior and posterior limbs that attach to the anterior and posterior limbs of the lacrimal crest.

Anatomy of the nose

The nose is strategically located in the central portion of the face with three-dimensional projection associated with complex and intricate anatomy. Nose anatomy can be divided into three parts: the outer skin and soft tissue envelope, bony and cartilaginous framework, and inner lining. The intricate relationship between first two components form contour reflections, which make up a unique individual nasal appearance varying from one to another.[135–137]

The skin and soft tissue covering of the nose is variable in its thickness, texture, and components. It is relatively thin in the cephalad two-thirds of the nose, especially at the osseo-cartilaginous junction (rhinion). The lower third portion of the nose covering has thicker skin and subcutaneous tissue with varying degree of sebaceous gland, contributing to the nasal tip morphology.[138] The nerves and vasculatures reside within this subcutaneous tissue. The nasalis muscle lies under the subcutaneous tissue, and partially covers the bone and cartilages.

The skeletal framework of the nose is structured by nasal bones and cartilages. They determine the individual nose configuration and shape. Starting from its most cephalad, the paired nasal bones bridge the frontal process of the maxilla, and frontal bones at the nasofrontal suture. The overlapping region between the inferior portion of the nasal bones with the superior portion of the upper lateral cartilages, is called the keystone area. The most caudal portion of the framework is supported by a uniquely shaped lower lateral (alar) cartilage. Inferior medial portion of this cartilage is called medial crus. As it ascends, it becomes middle or intermediate crus, and continues curving laterally to become lateral crus. The junction between the middle and lateral crus is called the dome, the most angulated portion of the structure and play an important role in forming tip definition of the nose. There are accessory cartilages, which are interspersed in the aponeurosis connecting the lateral crus and piriform aperture.[139–141]

The inner lining of the nose is mostly covered by thin mucosa, providing passage of the airway. Destruction or inappropriate reconstruction of this thin mucosal lining can cause a narrowing of the breathing pathway.

The surface anatomy of the nose follows the underlying structural anatomy of its framework in combination with the skin and soft tissue envelope. The most cephalad portion of the nose is called the root or radix of the nose. This continues caudally in the midline as a sloping downward segment called dorsum of the nose. The tip of the nose has several landmark anatomies. The region just above the tip of the nose is called the supra-tip region or break. It is the surface landmark above the dome (lateral genu) of the lower lateral cartilages. The dome of each lower lateral cartilages mark the tip defining points, and the region caudal to this points form infra-tip lobule and columella. The lateral curvature portion of the nose is called alar lobule, which forms the nostril opening. These surfaces form topographic subunits of the nose that are often used in recognizing the boundaries of light reflections bordering the anatomic landmarks: dorsum, sidewalls, nostril sills, nasal tip, soft triangles, and columella.[142]

The nose is vascularized by dual blood supply. Superiorly, the branches of the ophthalmic, anterior ethmoids, dorsal nasal, and external nasal arteries supply the proximal portion of the nose. The inferior region and tip of the nose is primarily supplied by branches of facial artery, which include superior labial and angular vessels.[143]

Access the complete reference list online at **http://www.expertconsult.com**

2. Baker DC, Conley J. Avoiding facial nerve injuries in rhytidectomy: Anatomical variations and pitfalls. *Plast Reconstr Surg*. 1979;64:781–795.

5. Stuzin JM, Baker TJ, Gordon HL. The relationship of the superficial and deep facial fascias: Relevance to rhytidectomy and aging. *Plast Reconstr Surg*. 1992; 89:441.

   The authors performed cadaveric dissections and made intraoperative observations to clarify the relationships between the muscles of facial expression, the facial nerve, and fascial planes. It is confirmed that the facial nerve branches in the cheek lay deep to the deep facial fascia.

16. Gosain AK, Sewall SR, Yousif NJ. The temporal branch of the facial nerve: how reliably can we predict its path? *Plast Reconstr Surg*. 1997;99:1224–1236.

21. Moss CJ, Mendelson BC, Taylor GI. Surgical anatomy of the ligamentous attachments in the temple and periorbital regions. *Plast Reconstr Surg*. 2000; 105(4):1475–1490.

   The authors report consistent deep attachments of the superficial fascia in the temporal and periorbital regions. The clinical relevance of predictable relationships between neurovascular structures and this connective tissue framework is discussed.

41. Stuzin JM, Wagstrom L, Kawamoto HK, et al. The anatomy and clinical applications of the buccal fat pad. *Plast Reconstr Surg*. 1990;85(1):29–37.

   The clinical importance of the buccal fat pad is discussed. Anatomical dissection and clinical experience inform recommendations for surgical modification of the structure to maximize aesthetic outcomes.

58. Barton FE Jr, Hunt J. The high-superficial musculoaponeurotic system technique in facial

rejuvenation: An update. *Plast Reconstr Surg.* 2003;112:1910–1917.

77. Ellenbogen R. Pseudo-paralysis of the mandibular branch of the facial nerve after platysmal face-lift operation. *Plast Reconstr Surg.* 1979;63:364–368.

    The clinical importance of injury to the cervical branch to the facial nerve is addressed. In platysmal facelifts, diminished modiolus retrusion may be secondary to an injury to the cervical, rather than the marginal mandibular, branch of the facial nerve.

88. Wolfe SA. The utility of pericranial flaps. *Ann Plast Surg.* 1978;1(2):147–153.

100. Daniel RK, Landon B. Endoscopic forehead lift: anatomic basis. *Aesthet Surg J.* 1997;17(2):97–104.

    Forehead anatomy as it relates to endoscopic rejuvenation is discussed.

107. Mosser SW, Guyuron B, Janis JE, et al. The anatomy of the greater occipital nerve: implications for the etiology of migraine headaches. *Plast Reconstr Surg.* 2004;113(2):693–700.

2

Facial trauma: Soft tissue injuries

Reid V. Mueller

SYNOPSIS

- Look for hidden injuries under the skin.
- Thoroughly cleanse to prevent dirt tattoo.
- Conservative debridement.
- Careful anatomic alignment and suture technique.

 Access the Historical Perspective section online at
http://www.expertconsult.com

Introduction

As humans, we live in a complex social structure that depends not only on the words we use for communication, but the emotive subtext of facial expression that imbues our words with greater meaning. Our faces are able to express a wondrous range of subtle emotions, and silent messages. Because the face is so important for negotiating the complex social interactions that are part of our everyday lives, the careful repair and restoration of function is an important task we must not engage in lightly. The achievements of those who have gone before us have given us the knowledge to repair the majority of soft tissue injuries to the face, provided we carefully consider the nature of the injury, and craft a well thought out reconstructive plan.

Soft tissue injuries are commonly encountered in the care of traumatized patients. Many of these injuries are simple superficial lacerations that require nothing more than a straightforward closure. Other seemly uncomplicated wounds harbor injuries to other structures. Recognition of the full nature of the injury, and a logical treatment plan will determine whether there will be future aesthetic or functional deformities. All wounds will benefit from cleansing, irrigation, conservative debridement and minimal tension closure. Some wounds will benefit from local or regional flaps for closure; and a few wounds will need tissue expansion, or free tissue transfer for complete restoration of function and appearance.

Basic science

The etiology of facial soft tissue trauma varies considerably depending upon age, sex, and geographic location. Many facial soft tissue injuries are relatively minor and are treated by the emergency department without a referral to a specialist. There are little data regarding the etiology of facial trauma that is subsequently referred to a specialist, but it is weighted towards more significant traumas such as road crashes and assaults. The location of facial soft tissue trauma tends to occur in certain areas of the head depending on the causative mechanism. When taking all etiologies of facial trauma into account, the distribution is concentrated in a "T-shaped" area that includes the forehead, nose, lips and chin. The lateral brows and occiput also have localized frequency increases.[4] These areas are more prone to injury because they primarily overlie bony prominences that are at risk from any blow to the face, whether that be an assault, fall, or accident (*Fig. 2.1*).

Global considerations

Almost all soft tissue injuries of the head involve the skin in some manner. The skin of the head shows more variety than any other area of the body in terms of thickness, elasticity, mobility and texture. Consider the profound differences between the thick, inelastic, hair-bearing skin of the scalp compared with the thin, elastic, mobile skin of the eyelids. Consider also, the transitions from external skin of the face to the orbital, nasal, and oral linings. Significant differences in the structure of the facial skin in different areas require different methods for the repair and reconstruction. In addition, many facial structures are layered with an outer skin layer, central cartilaginous support or muscular layer, and an inner mucosal lining or second skin layer (e.g., eyelids, nose, lips, ears).

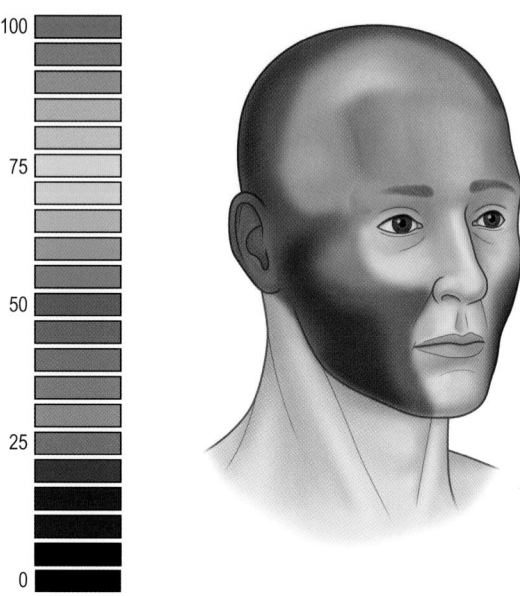

Fig. 2.1 A total of 700 facial soft tissue injuries segregated into the number of injuries for different facial areas, indicated by color. Note the "T" distribution across the forehead, nose, lips, and chin. Also note the concentration of injuries at the lateral brow. (Data from Hussain, K, Wijetunge, DB, Grubnic, S, *et al*. A comprehensive analysis of craniofacial trauma. J Trauma 1994;36(1):34.)

Anyone who has suffered a cut lip or scalp knows first hand that the face is well perfused. The dense interconnected network of collateral vessels in the face means that injured tissue with seemingly insufficient blood will in fact survive, whereas the same injury would result in tissue necrosis in another area of the body. The implication is that more (and potentially invaluable) tissue can be salvaged. This is especially important for areas with little or no excess tissue to sacrifice, or areas that are notoriously difficult to recreate later, for example, the oral commissure. When repairing the face, conservative debridement is usually preferable. If a segment of tissue appears only marginally viable, but is indispensable from a reconstructive standpoint, it should be loosely approximated and re-examined in 24–48 h. At that time, a line of demarcation will usually delineate what will survive and what will die. Nonviable tissue may then be debrided during a second look procedure.

Because the face is so well perfused its ability to resist infection is better than other areas of the body. Human bites to the hand treated without antibiotics have approximately a 47% risk of infection,[5] whereas if we inadvertently bite our cheeks, lips or tongue we almost never develop an infection. The lower risk of infection in the face has practical applications for management of facial soft tissue injuries. Many a medical student has been told that any wound that has been open for 6 hours cannot be closed primarily. This belief is based on tradition rather that good science. While there is no doubt that the longer a wound is open the more likely it is to become contaminated, there is no magical time cut-off for primary closure.[6] Because the face carries such profound cosmetic importance, the small increased risk of infection associated with delayed closure of a wound will be trumped by improved cosmesis associated with primary closure. This author recommends closure of facial wounds at the earliest time possible

that will not interfere with the management of other more serious injuries, but do not let time deter you from obtaining primary closure.

Diagnosis and patient presentation

Our attention is often captured by the obvious external manifestations of craniofacial soft tissue injuries because of the alteration in appearance, however, we should not be distracted from a methodical examination for other injuries. Seemly straightforward wounds often harbor injuries to the facial skeleton, teeth, nerves, parotid duct, eyes, or brain.

Evaluation for immediate life-threatening injuries

Evaluation of an injured patient should always start with establishment of an airway, ventilation, volume resuscitation, control of hemorrhage, and stabilization of other major injuries – the ABCs of an initial trauma assessment. While the plastic surgeon is rarely "on the front lines" of trauma care, neither can the plastic surgeon be complacent and assume that the emergency or trauma physician has completed a trauma assessment.

Once you are satisfied that there are no immediate life-threatening injuries, you should begin your examination. The assessment of facial injuries is guided by the nature of the mechanism of injury. A thermal burn will be approached very differently than a motor vehicle crash. The history of the injury, if known, will often provide some clue as to what other injuries one might expect to find. A child who falls against a coffee table is unlikely to have any associated fractures whereas a soccer player has a 17% chance of having an underlying fracture. Practitioners will have their own style of examination, but one should stick to a routine to decrease the likelihood of forgetting to check something. The author prefers to move from outside to inside, and top to bottom.

Systematic evaluation of the head and neck

Initial observation, inspection and palpation will generally provide most of the information a practitioner will need. Ideally, the examination should be done with adequate anesthesia and sterile technique, as well as good lighting, irrigation, and suction as needed.

Inspection of the skin will reveal abrasions, traumatic tattoos, simple or "clean" lacerations, complex or contusion type lacerations, bites, avulsions, or burns. A careful check for facial symmetry may reveal underlying bone injury. One should systematically palpate the skull, orbital rims, zygomatic arches, maxilla, and mandible feeling for asymmetry, bony step-off, crepitus or other evidence of underlying facial fracture. Palpation within the wound may identify palpable fractures or foreign bodies. Sensation of the face should be tested with a light touch, and motor activity of the facial nerve should be tested before the administration of local anesthetics. If local anesthetics are administered it is important that the time, location, and composition of the anesthetic is well documented in the chart so that subsequent examinations will not be confounded.

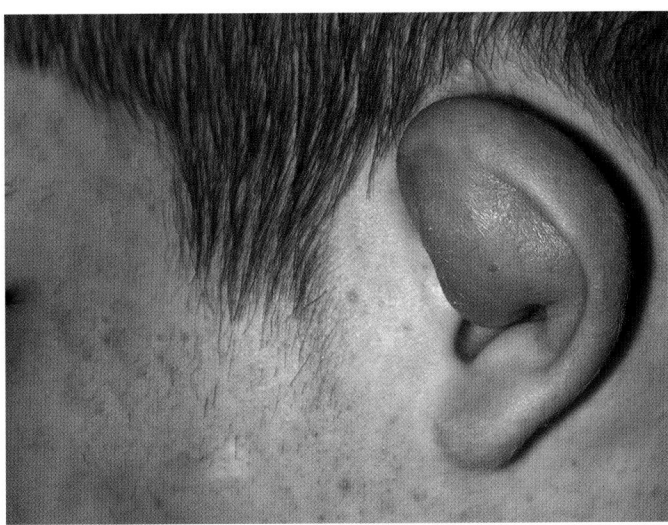

Fig. 2.2 An auricular hematoma after a wrestling injury. The collection of blood must be drained to prevent organization and calcification of the hematoma. Untreated hematomas will result in a "cauliflower ear".

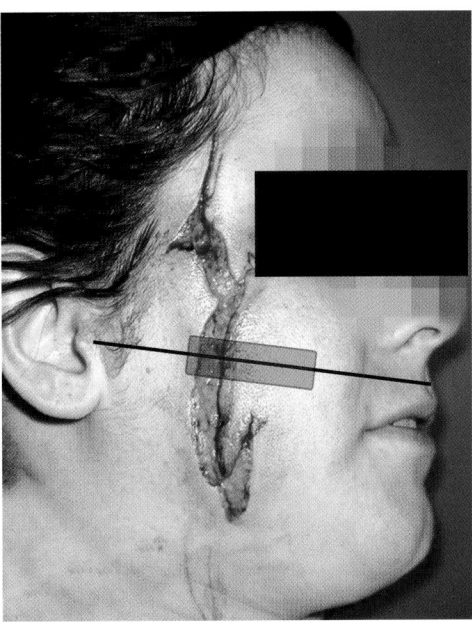

Fig. 2.3 The middle-third of a line between the tragus and the middle of the upper lip defines the course of the parotid duct. Evidence of injury to the zygomatic or buccal branches of the facial nerve or lacerations or the cheek near the area shaded in green should raise suspicion for parotid duct injury.

Eye examination

Trauma to the periorbital area or malar prominence should raise concern for associated orbital injury. Having the patient read or count fingers can be used to test gross visual acuity. The presence of a bony step-off, diplopia, restricted ocular movements, enophthalmos, or vertical dystopia may suggest an orbital blowout fracture. Traction on the eyelids can be used to test the integrity of the medial and lateral canthi. The canthi should have a snug and discernible endpoint when traction is applied. Rounding or laxity of the canthi suggests canthal injury or naso-orbital-ethmoidal (NOE) fracture. Any laceration near the medial third of the eye should raise suspicion of a canalicular injury. If there is any suspicion of globe injury, an immediate ophthalmology consultation is needed

Ear examination

The ears should be inspected for hematomas that will appear as a diffuse swelling under the skin of the auricle *(Fig. 2.2)*. Any lacerations should be noted. Otoscopy should be done to look for lacerations or the auditory canal, tympanic membrane injuries, or hemotympanum.

Nose examination

Inspect the nose for any asymmetry, or deviation to one side or the other. Palpate the nasal bones and cartilage for fracture or crepitus. Examine the internal nose with a speculum and good light to look for mucosal lacerations, exposed cartilage or bone, a deviated or buckled septum, or septal hematoma (a bluish boggy bulge of the septal mucosa).

Cheek examination

Any laceration of the cheek that is near any facial nerve branch or along the course of the parotid duct will need to be investigated. Asking the patient to raise their eyebrows, close their eyes tight, show their teeth or smile while looking for asymmetry or lack of movement will reveal any facial nerve injury. An imaginary line connecting the tragus to the central aspect of the philtrum defines the course of the parotid duct *(Fig. 2.3)*. The duct is at risk from any injury in the central third of this line. If you are unsure about a duct injury, Stensen's duct should be cannulated and fluid instilled to see if it leaks out of the wound.

Oral cavity and mouth

Inspect the oral cavity for loose or missing teeth. Any unaccounted for teeth may be loose in the wound, lost at the scene, or aspirated. If you cannot account for a missing tooth an X-ray of the head and chest should be done. The oral lining should be inspected for lacerations, and the occlusion should be checked. Palpation of the maxillary buttresses and mandible may reveal fractures. A sublingual hematoma suggests a mandible fracture.

Neck examination

The first priority when evaluating a soft tissue injury to the neck is evaluation of the airway. You should be concerned about the patient's airway if they have garbled speech, dysphonia, hoarseness, persistent oropharyngeal bleeding, or if they appear agitated or struggling for air.[7] Once the airway is secured, and the exam shows no compromise, the soft tissue injury should be examined with adequate light and suction to rule out penetration deep to the platysma. If the soft tissue injury penetrates through the platysma then the trauma surgeons must be consulted to evaluate a penetrating neck injury.

Diagnostic studies

Any diagnostic studies are directed towards defining injuries to underlying structures. Most soft tissue injuries in and of themselves do not need any special diagnostic studies, however the search for foreign bodies, missing teeth, or concomitant facial fractures should be followed-up with a radiographic evaluation.

Plain films

Plain films may be helpful in the evaluation of foreign bodies or to elucidate underlying facial fractures. In most institutions and imaging of facial trauma with plain films and largely been supplanted with computed tomography (CT).

CT

Maxillofacial CT is primarily used to evaluate brain injury and underlying facial fractures, and it may have some utility in identifying or locating foreign bodies within the soft tissues.

Consultation with other providers

Ophthalmology

Any patient with zygomaticomaxillary fractures, naso-orbital-ethmoidal fractures, orbital blowout fracture, canalicular injury, or suggestion of ocular injury should have an evaluation by an ophthalmologist.

Dental/OMFS

Dental injuries are commonly associated with facial soft tissue trauma and are rarely an emergency. A dentist should evaluate dental injuries, such as fractured or missing teeth, once the patient has recovered from their initial injury. If the patient has an avulsed tooth, an urgent consult should be called to replant the tooth if possible.

Treatment and surgical techniques

Anesthesia for treatment

Good anesthesia is often necessary for patient comfort and the cooperation that is needed to complete a comprehensive evaluation. Most soft tissue injuries of the head and neck can be managed with simple infiltration or regional anesthesia blocks. Patients who are uncooperative because of age, intoxication, or head injury may require general anesthesia. Patients with extensive injuries requiring more involved reconstruction, or who would require potentially toxic doses of local anesthetics will likewise require general anesthesia.

With the exception of cocaine, all of the local anesthetics cause some degree of vasodilatation. Epinephrine is commonly added to anesthetic solutions to counteract this effect, to cause vasoconstriction, to decrease bleeding, and to slow absorption and increase duration of action. Epinephrine should not be use in patients with pheochromocytoma, hyperthyroidism, severe hypertension, or severe peripheral vascular disease or patients taking propranolol. Every medical student has learned that epinephrine should never be injected in the "finger, toes, penis, nose, or ears." This admonition is based on anecdotal reports or simple assumptions. There is very little data to support the notion, and plastic surgeons routinely use epinephrine in the face including the ears and nose with very rare complications. Unfortunately, from a medico-legal standpoint it is probably best to avoid epinephrine in the above-mentioned areas unless clinical judgment determines that the very small risks of epinephrine are outweighed by the benefits.

Topical

Topical anesthetics are well established for the treatment of children with superficial facial wounds and to decrease the pain of injection. The most widely used topical agent is a 5% eutectic mixture of local anesthetics (EMLA) containing lidocaine and prilocaine.[8,9] EMLA has been shown to provide adequate anesthesia for split thickness skin grafting,[10] and minor surgical procedures such as excisional biopsy and electrosurgery.[11] Successful use of EMLA requires 60–90 min of application for adequate anesthesia. The most common mistake leading to failure is not allowing sufficient time for diffusion and anesthesia. Some areas such as the face with a thinner stratum corneum may have onset of anesthesia more quickly.

Local infiltration

Local anesthetics are appropriate for the repair of most simple facial soft tissue trauma. Intradermal or subdermal infiltration will provide rapid onset of anesthesia, and control of bleeding if epinephrine has been added. However, injection may distort some facial landmarks needed for alignment and accurate repair (such as the vermillion border of the lip) and therefore, anatomic landmarks should be noted and marked prior to injection.

Facial field block

Field block of the face can provide anesthesia of a larger area with less discomfort and fewer needle sticks for the patient. A field block may provide better patient tolerance of multiple painful injections of local anesthetic when a local infiltration of an epinephrine containing solution is needed. Field blocks are more challenging to perform, and take time to take effect. Impatient surgeons often fail to wait a sufficient amount of time (at least 10–15 min) for most blocks to take effect.

Forehead, anterior scalp to vertex, upper eyelids, glabella (supraorbital, supratrochlear, infratrochlear nerves)

Anatomy: The supraorbital nerve is located at the superior medial orbital rim about a finger-breadth medial to the midpupillary line. The supratrochlear nerve lies about 1.5 cm farther medially near the medial margin of the eyebrow. The infratrochlear is located superior to the medial canthus.

Method: Identify the supraorbital foramen or notch along the superior orbital rim and enter just lateral to that point. Direct the needle medially and advance to just medial of the medial canthus (about 2 cm). Inject 2 cc while withdrawing the needle *(Fig. 2.4)*.[12]

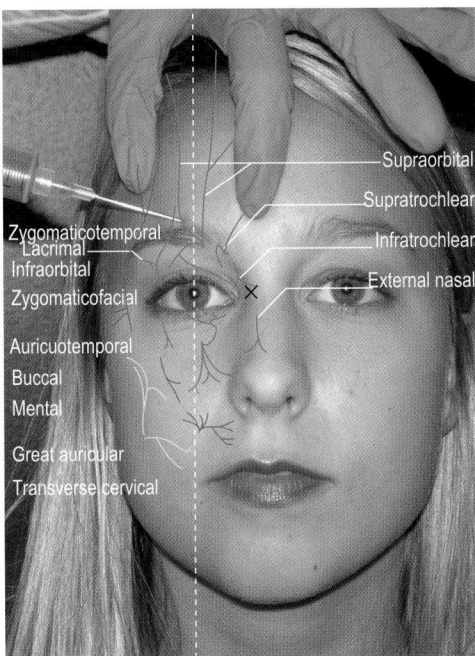

Fig. 2.4 The majority of the forehead, medial upper eyelid, and glabella can be anesthetized with a block of the ophthalmic division of the trigeminal nerve (CN V1). Identify the supraorbital notch by palpation and enter the skin just lateral to that point near the pupillary midline. Aim for a point just medial to the medial canthus (marked by an X) and advance the needle about 2 cm. Inject 2–3 cc while withdrawing the needle.

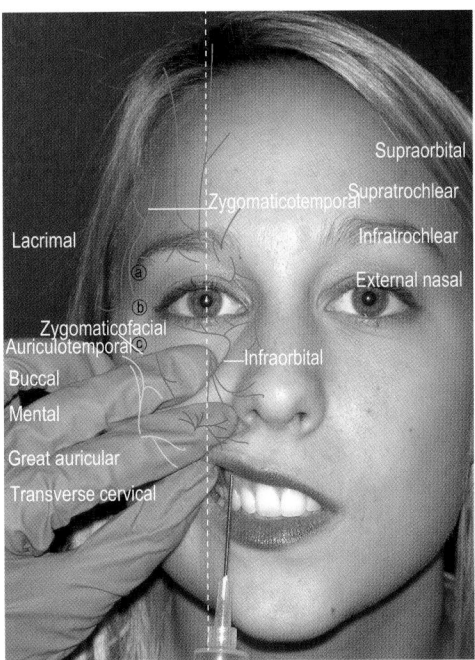

Fig. 2.5 The lower eyelid, medial cheek, and lower nose can be anesthetized with an infraorbital nerve block. The infraorbital foramen may be palpable about 1 cm below the orbital rim just medial to the mid-pupillary line (X). The intraoral approach is less painful and anxiety provoking for most patients. Place the long finger of the nondominant hand on the orbital rim at the infraorbital foramen. Grasp and retract the upper lip. Insert the needle in the superior gingival buccal sulcus above the canine tooth root and direct the needle towards your long finger and the foramen while injecting 2–3 cc.

Lateral nose, upper lip, upper teeth, lower eyelid, most of medial cheek (infraorbital nerve)

Anatomy: The infraorbital nerve exits the infraorbital foramen at a point that is medial of the mid-pupillary line and 6–10 mm below the inferior orbital rim.

Method: Identify the infraorbital foramen along the inferior orbital rim by palpation. An intraoral approach is better tolerated and less painful (*Fig. 2.5*). Place the long finger of the nondominant hand on the foramen and retract the upper lip with thumb and index finger. Insert the needle in the superior gingival buccal sulcus above the canine tooth root and direct the needle towards your long finger while injecting 2 cc. You may also inject percutaneously by identifying the infraorbital foramen about 1 cm below the orbital rim just medial to the mid-pupillary line. Enter perpendicular to the skin, advance the needle to the maxilla, and inject about 2 cc (*Fig. 2.6*).[12]

Lower lip and chin (mental nerve)

Anatomy: The mental nerve exits the mental foramen about 2 cm inferior to the alveolar ridge below the second premolar. The nerve can often be seen under the inferior gingival buccal mucosa when lower lip and cheek are retracted. It branches superiorly and medially to supply the lower lip and chin.

Method: The lower lip is retracted with the thumb and finger of the nondominant hand and the needle inserted at the apex of the second premolar. The needle is advanced 5–8 mm and 2 cc are injected (*Fig. 2.7*). When using the percutaneous approach, insert the needle at the mid-point of a line between the oral commissure and inferior mandibular border. Advance the needle to the mandible and inject 2 cc while slightly withdrawing the needle (*Fig. 2.8*).[12]

Posterior auricle, angle of the jaw, anterior neck (cervical plexus: great auricular, transverse cervical)

Anatomy: Both the great auricular nerve and transverse cervical nerves emerge from the midpoint of the posterior border of the sternocleidomastoid muscle at Erb's point. The great auricular nerve parallels the external jugular vein as it passes up towards the ear. The transverse cervical nerve is located about 1 cm farther inferiorly and passes parallel to the clavicle and then curves towards the chin. Both are in the superficial fascial of the sternocleidomastoid muscle.

Method: Locate Erb's point by having the patient flex against resistance. Mark the posterior border of the sternocleidomastoid muscle and locate the midpoint between clavicle and mastoid. Insert the needle about 1 cm superior to Erb's point and inject transversely across the surface of the muscle towards the anterior border. A second more vertically oriented injection may be needed to block the transverse cervical nerve.[12]

Ear (auriculotemporal nerve, great auricular nerve, lesser occipital nerve, and auditory branch of the vagus (Arnold's) nerve)

Most ear injuries will not require a total ear block and can be managed with local infiltration of anesthetic. While there is a theoretical concern of tissue necrosis when using epinephrine in any appendage (in medical school we learned "finger, toes,

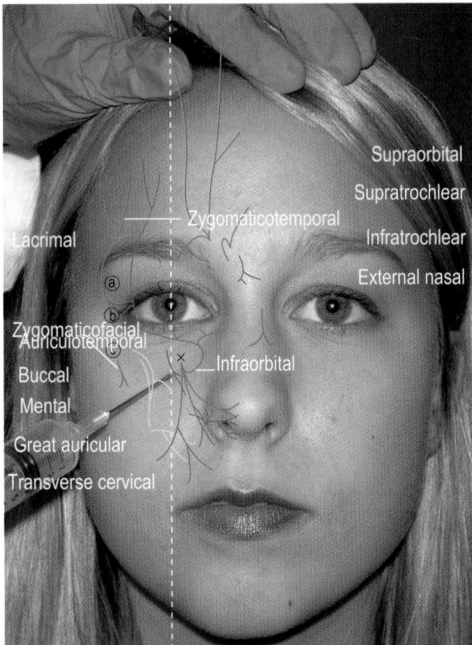

Fig. 2.6 The lower eyelid, medial cheek, and lower nose can be anesthetized with an infraorbital nerve block. The infraorbital foramen may be palpable about 1 cm below the orbital rim just medial to the mid-pupillary line (X). Enter the skin directly over the palpable or anticipated location of the infraorbital foramen and advance to the maxilla. Inject about 2 cc of anesthetic. Anesthesia of the anterior temple area can be achieved with a block of the zygomaticotemporal nerve. Enter just posterior to the lateral orbital rim at a level above the lateral canthus (marked a) and advance towards the chin to a point level with the lateral canthus (b). Inject 2–3 cc while withdrawing the needle. The zygomaticofacial nerve supplies the lateral malar prominence. To block this nerve enter at point one finger-breadth inferior and lateral to the intersection of the inferior and lateral orbital rim. Advance the needle to the zygoma and inject 1–2 cc.

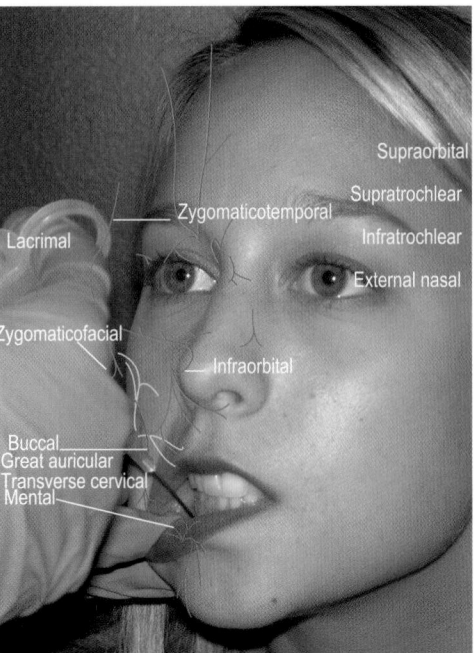

Fig. 2.7 The lower lip and chin can be anesthetized with a block of the mental nerve (CN V3). Retract the lower lip with the thumb and index finger of the nondominant hand. Many times the mental nerve is visible under the mandibular gingival buccal sulcus near the apex of the second premolar. Insert the needle at the apex of the second premolar and advance the needle 5–8 mm while injecting 2 cc.

penis, nose, and ears"), there is no good data to support this. Most plastic surgeons routinely use 1:100 000 epinephrine in the local anesthetics for ear infiltration. The advantages are prolonged duration of anesthesia and less bleeding. Complications attributed to the anesthetic infiltration are extremely rare.

Anatomy: The anterior half of the ear is supplied by the auriculotemporal nerve that branches from the mandibular division of the trigeminal nerve (CN V₃). The posterior half of the ear is innervated by the great auricular and lesser occipital nerves that are both branches from the cervical plexus (C2, C3). The auditory branch (Arnold's nerve) of the vagus nerve (CN X) supplies a portion of the concha and external auditory canal.

Method: Insert a 1.5 inch needle at the junction of the earlobe and head and advance subcutaneously towards the tragus while infiltrating 2–3 cc of anesthetic *(Fig. 2.9)*. Pull back the needle and redirect posteriorly along the posterior auricular sulcus again injecting 2–3 cc. Reinsert the needle at the superior junction of the ear and the head. Direct the needle along the preauricular sulcus towards the tragus and inject 2–3 cc. Pull back and redirect the needle along the posterior auricular sulcus while injecting. It may be necessary to insert the needle a third time along the posterior sulcus to complete a ring block. Care should be taken to avoid the temporal artery when directing the needle along the preauricular sulcus. If the artery is inadvertently punctured, apply pressure for 10 min to prevent formation of a hematoma.

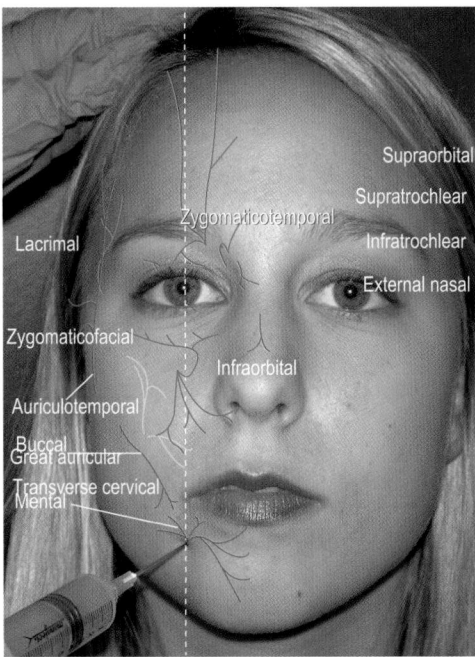

Fig. 2.8 The lower lip and chin can be anesthetized with a block of the mental nerve (CN V3). The mental foramen is located near the mid-point of a line from the oral commissure and the mandibular boarder. Enter the skin at this point and advance to the mandible. Inject 2–3 cc while slightly withdrawing the needle. The auriculotemporal nerve emerges deep and posterior to the temporomandibular joint and travels with the temporal vessels to supply the temporal scalp, lateral temple, and anterior auricle. Palpate the temporomandibular joint and base of the zygomatic arch. Enter the skin superior to the zygomatic arch just anterior to the auricle. Aspirate to ensure you are not within the temporal vessels and inject 2–3 cc.

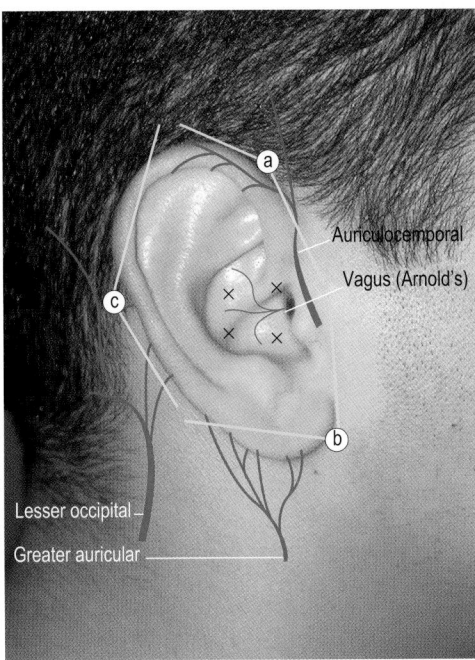

Fig. 2.9 The majority of the external ear can be anesthetized with a ring block. Insert a 1.5 inch needle at the superior junction of the ear and the head at (a). Direct the needle along the preauricular sulcus towards the tragus and inject 2–3 cc. Pull back and redirect the needle along the posterior auricular sulcus while injecting. Reinsert the needle at the junction of the earlobe and head, at (b), and advance subcutaneously towards the tragus while infiltrating 2–3 cc of anesthetic. Pull back the needle and redirect posteriorly along the posterior auricular sulcus again injecting 2–3 cc. It may be necessary to insert the needle a third time, at (c), along the posterior sulcus to complete a ring block. If anesthesia of the concha or external auditory canal is needed local infiltration (marked with Xs) will be required to anesthetize the auditory branch of the Vagus nerve (Arnold's nerve).

If anesthesia of the concha or external auditory canal is needed, local infiltration will be required to anesthetize the auditory branch of the Vagus nerve (Arnold's nerve).

General treatment considerations

The ultimate goal is to restore form and function with minimum morbidity. Function generally takes precedence over form, however the face plays a fundamental role in emotional expression and social interaction, and therefore the separation of facial appearance from function is impossible.

Irrigation and debridement

Once good anesthesia has been obtained, the wound should be cleansed of foreign matter and clearly nonviable tissue removed. This is the process of converting an untidy to a tidy wound. Clean lacerations from a sharp object will result in little collateral tissue damage or contamination, while a wound created by an impact with the asphalt will have significant foreign material and soft tissue damage. The process starts by irrigating the wound with a bulb syringe, or a 60 cc syringe with an 18-gauge angiocatheter attached to forcibly irrigate the wound. More contaminated wounds may benefit from pulse lavage systems.

After irrigation, hemostasis should be secured to give the surgeon a better opportunity to inspect the wound. The use of epinephrine in the local anesthetic will cause some degree of vasoconstriction and assist in this regard. Electrocautery should be applied at the lowest setting conducive to coagulation, and applied to specific vessels. Wholesale indiscriminate application of electrocautery causes unnecessary tissue necrosis. Use electrocautery cautiously when working in areas where important nerves might be located to avoid iatrogenic injury. Remember that nerves often are in proximity to vessels.

Limited sharp debridement should be used to remove clearly nonviable tissue. In areas where there is minimal tissue laxity, or irreplaceable structures (e.g., tip of nose, oral commissure) debridement should be kept to a minimum and later scar revision undertaken if needed. Areas such as the cheek or lip have significant tissue mobility debridement and will tolerate more aggressive debridement.

After the preliminary debridement and irrigation, a methodical search for foreign material should be undertaken. Small fragments of automobile glass become embedded through surprisingly small external wounds. They are usually evident on X-ray or CT scan or by careful palpation. Patients thrown from vehicles will often have dirt, pebbles, or plant material embedded in their wounds. Patients who have blast injuries from firearms or fireworks may have paper, wadding, or bullet fragments present. One should not undertake a major dissection for the sake of retrieving a bullet fragment, however one should make sure that other identifiable pieces of foreign matter are removed. Failure to do so may result in later infection.

Abrasions

Abrasions result from tangential trauma that removes the epithelium and a portion of the dermis leaving a partial thickness injury that is quite painful. This type of injury is often the result of sliding across pavement or dirt and therefore embeds small particulate debris within the dermis. If dirt and debris are not promptly removed the dermis and epithelium will grow over the particulates and create a traumatic tattoo that is very difficult to manage later. Topical anesthetics, if properly applied and given sufficient time for onset, can give good anesthesia for cleansing of simple abrasions. This can be accomplished with generous irrigation and cleansing with a surgical scrub brush (*Fig. 2.10*). If more involved debridement is needed general anesthesia is advisable.

Traumatic tattoo

There are two basic types of traumatic tattoo; those that result from blast injuries and those result from abrasive injuries. In either case various particles of dirt, asphalt, sand, carbon, tar, explosives, or other particulate matter is embedded into the dermis.

Abrasive traumatic tattoos are more common. Typically, a person is ejected from a vehicle, or thrown from a bicycle and subsequently grinds their face into the pavement. This causes a simultaneous traumatic dermabrasion of the epidermis and superficial dermis, and embedding of the pigment (dirt). If left untreated, the dermis and epidermis heal over the pigment resulting in a permanent tattoo (*Fig. 2.11*).

Blast type injuries seen in military casualties and civilian powder burns, as well as firework, and bomb mishaps produce numerous particles of dust, dirt, metal, combustion products,

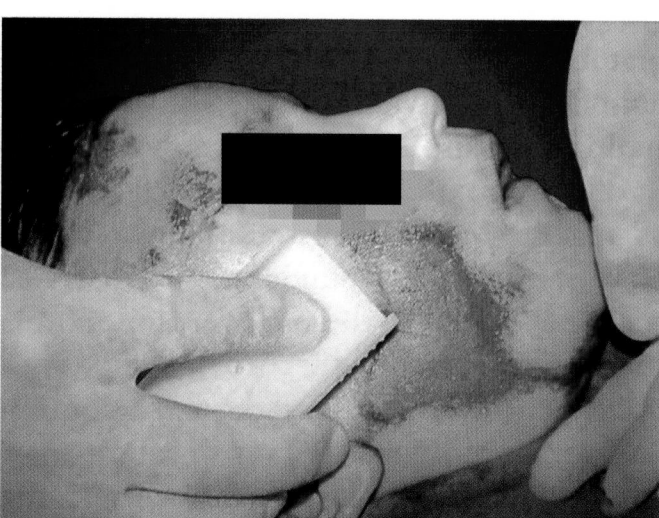

Fig. 2.10 Facial abrasions should be cleansed of any dirt and debris with generous irrigation and gentle scrubbing with a surgical scrub brush.

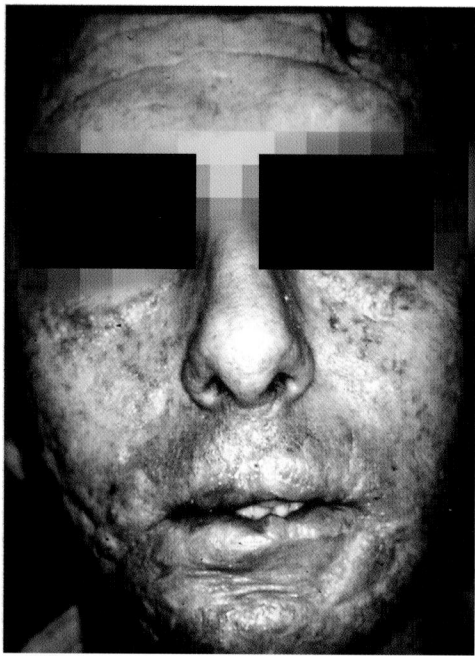

Fig. 2.11 This man has an established traumatic tattoo. The best opportunity to prevent such an outcome is meticulous debridement at the time of injury. Secondary treatment of traumatic tattoo is very difficult and includes dermabrasion, excision, and laser treatments.

un-ignited gunpowder, and other foreign materials that act like hundreds of small missiles, each penetrating the wound to various depths. The entry wounds collapse behind the particle, trapping them within the dermis.

Regardless of the mechanism of injury, prompt removal of the particulate matter results in a far better outcome than later removal. Once the skin has healed the opportunity to remove the particles with simple irrigation and scrubbing is lost. The initial treatment is vigorous scrubbing with a surgical scrub brush or gauze and copious irrigation.[13–17] Wounds treated within 24 hours show substantially better cosmetic outcome than those treated later,[15] however some improvement has been seen as late as 10 days.[18] Larger particles should be searched for and removed individually with fine forceps or needles, loupe magnification, and generous irrigation.[19] The tedious and time consuming nature of this procedure may require serial procedures over several days to complete, nonetheless meticulous debridement of the acute injury is the best opportunity for optimal outcome.

The treatment of a traumatic tattoo remains an unresolved problem in plastic surgery, and as such, there are multiplicities of techniques, none of which are perfect. Some of the treatment options include surgical excision and microsurgical planning,[20,21] dermabrasion,[22–25] salabrasion,[26] application of various solvents such as, diethyl ether,[16] cryosurgery, electrosurgery, and laser treatment with carbon dioxide, argon lasers,[13,14,16,27] Q-switched Nd:YAG laser,[28,29] erbium-YAG laser,[30] Q-switched alexandrite laser,[31,32] and Q-switched ruby laser.[33,34] The mechanism for laser removal is not entirely understood but is thought to involve the fragmentation of pigment particles, rupture of pigment containing cells, and subsequent phagocytosis of the tattoo pigment.[35,36] Laser therapy for pigment tattoos will require slightly higher fluencies than those used for removal of professional tattoos.[33]

A note of caution is in order when treating gunpowder traumatic tattoos. Several authors have noted ignition of retained gunpowder during laser tattoo removal,[29,37] resulting in spreading of the tattoo or creation of significant dermal pits. If initial laser treatment suggests the presence of un-ignited gunpowder in the dermis, laser removal should be discontinued in favor of other treatments such as dermabrasion or surgical micro-excision of the larger particles.

Simple lacerations

Sharp objects cutting the tissue usually cause simple or "clean" lacerations. Lacerations from window and automobile glass, or knife wounds are typical examples *(Fig. 2.12)*. Simple lacerations may be repaired primarily after irrigation and minimal debridement, even if the patient's condition has delayed closure for several days. When immediate closure is not feasible, the wound should be irrigated and kept moist with a saline and gauze dressing. Prior to repair, foreign bodies such as window glass should be removed. Wounds of this type usually require little or no debridement. A few well placed absorbable 4-0 or 5-0 sutures will help align the tissue and relieve tension on the skin closure. The temptation to place numerous dermal sutures should be avoided because excess suture material in the wound will only serve to incite inflammation and impair healing. The skin should be closed with 5-0 or 6-0 nylon interrupted or running sutures; alternatively, 5-0 nylon or monofilament absorbable running subcuticular pullout sutures can be placed. Any suture that traverses the epidermis should be removed from the face in 4–5 days. If sutures are left in place longer than this epithelization of the suture tracts will lead to permanent suture marks know as "railroad tracks". Sutures of the scalp may be left in place for 7–10 days. Pullout sutures should usually be removed following the same guidelines, however there less risk of permanent suture marks.

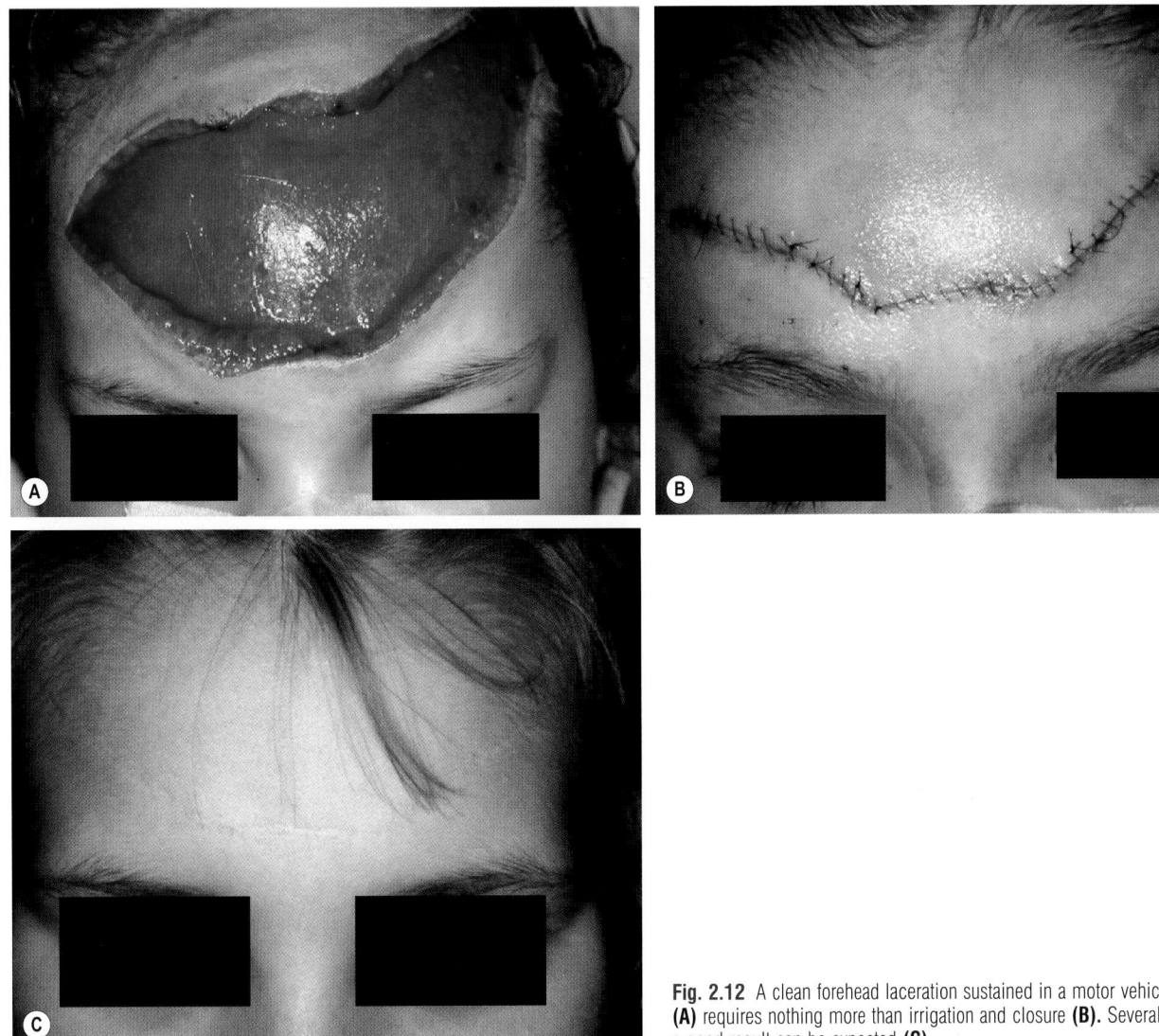

Fig. 2.12 A clean forehead laceration sustained in a motor vehicle crash. **(A)** requires nothing more than irrigation and closure **(B)**. Several months later, a good result can be expected **(C)**.

Complex lacerations

When soft tissue is compressed between a bony prominence and an object, it will burst or fracture resulting in a complex laceration pattern and significant contusion of the tissue. Typical examples of these types of lacerations are a brow laceration sustained when a toddler falls onto a coffee table, or an occupant is ejected from a vehicle in a crash striking an object *(Fig. 2.13)*. Many wounds on first impression suggest that there is significant tissue loss, however after irrigation, minimal debridement, and careful replacement of the tissue fragments piece by piece it becomes apparent that most of the tissue is present *(Fig. 2.14)*. Contused and clearly nonviable tissue should be debrided. Tissue that is contused, but has potential to survive should usually be returned to anatomic position. Elaborate repositioning of tissue with Z-plasties and the like should usually be reserved for secondary reconstructions after primary healing has finished. Limited undermining may be used to decrease tension and achieve closure, however wide undermining is rarely indicated. It is probably better to accept a modest area of secondary intention healing

and plan for later scar revision rather than risk tissue necrosis from overzealous undermining of already injured tissue.

Avulsions

Many wounds of the face suggest tissue loss upon initial inspection, but closer examination reveals that the tissue has simply retracted or folded over itself. Avulsive injuries that remain attached by a pedicle will often survive, and the likelihood of survival depends on the relative size of the pedicle to the segment of tissue it must nourish. Fortunately, the remarkably good perfusion of the face allows for survival of avulsed parts on surprisingly small pedicles. If there is any possibility that the avulsed tissue may survive it should be repaired and allowed to declare itself. If venous congestion develops it should be treated with medicinal leeches until the congestion resolves. Reconstruction of a failed reattachment can always be undertaken later, but a discarded part can never be replaced.

Many avulsed and amputated parts are amenable to replantation provided that the patient does not have underlying

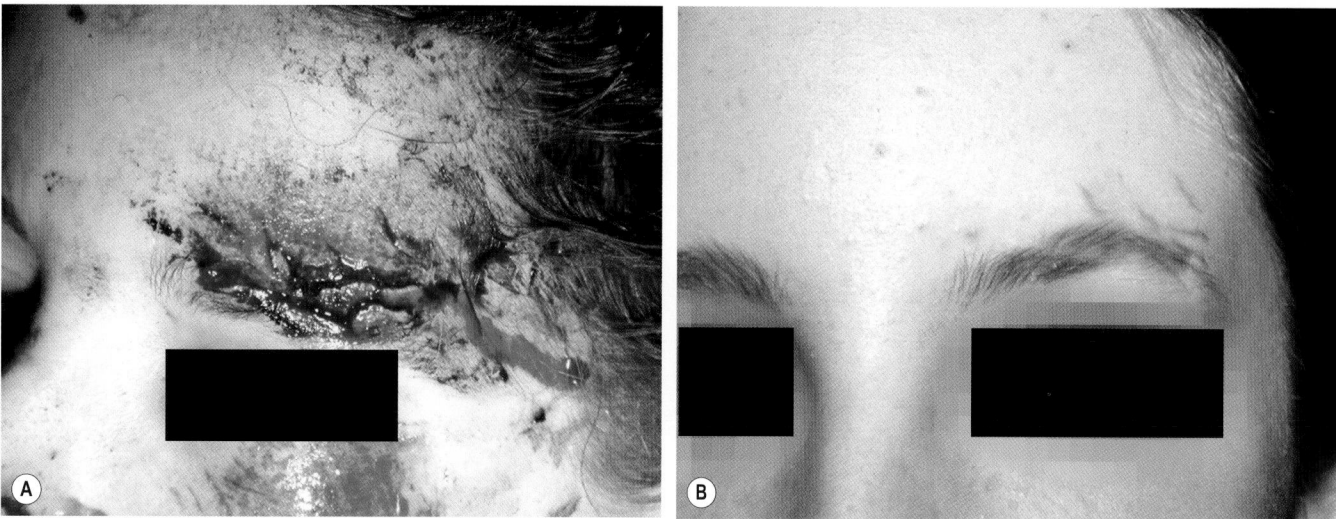

Fig. 2.13 Initial debridement of eyebrow lacerations should be minimal. Even badly contused tissue will survive and usually lead to a result better than any graft, flap, or hair transplantation.

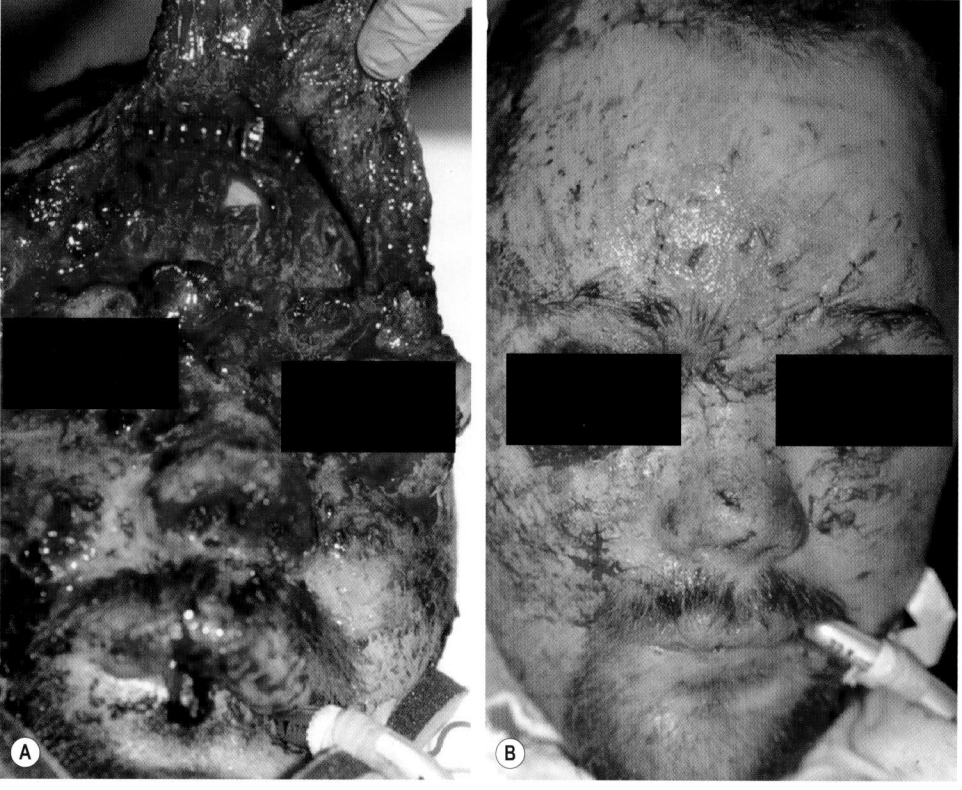

Fig. 2.14 Complex facial laceration after motor vehicle crash **(A)** that gives the impression of significant tissue loss. Irrigation, minimal debridement, and careful repositioning of the tissue fragments – "solving the jigsaw puzzle" – reveals that most of the tissue is present and usable **(B)**.

injuries or medical conditions that would preclude a lengthy operation. Examples of facial parts that have been successfully replanted include: scalp, nose, lip, ear, cheek. Vein grafts are often needed to complete the replantation, and venous congestion is a common complication that can be successfully manages with leeches or bleeding the part.

If tissue is truly missing such that primary repair cannot be accomplished then a more complex repair with an interpolation flap or other reconstruction may be needed. These specific techniques for specific areas are covered elsewhere.

Secondary intention healing

Some wounds with tissue loss may be best treated by secondary intention healing rather than a more complex reconstruction. The advantages of secondary intention treatment are that it is simple, it does not require an operation, the wound contraction can work to the patient's advantage, and in certain situations, the cosmetic result can rival other methods of closure. The best cosmetic results are obtained on concave surfaces of the *Nose, Eye, Ear* and *Temple* (NEET areas), and those on the convex surfaces of the *Nose*, *Oral* lips, *Cheeks* and chin, and *Helix* of the ear (NOCH areas) often heal with a poor quality scar. Most wounds can be dressed with a semi-occlusive dressing, or petrolatum ointment to prevent desiccation. Common complications include: pigmentation changes, unstable scar, excessive granulation, pain, dysesthesias, and wound contracture.[38,39]

Treatment of specific areas

Scalp

Most scalp injuries are the result of blunt force injuries sustained in road crashes, assaults, and falls. Motor vehicle crashes cause most of the avulsive injuries, while complete avulsion of the scalp happens in industrial or farm accidents when the hair becomes entangled around a rotating piece of machinery.

Scalp injuries can generally be evaluated with inspection and palpation of the scalp. One should determine if there is underlying unrecognized skull or frontal sinus fracture by palpation of the wound or X-ray examination.

The thickness of the skin of the scalp ranges from 3 to 8 mm making it some of the thickest on the body.[40] The galea is a strong relatively inelastic layer that is an important structure in repair of scalp wounds. It plays a role in protecting the skull and pericranium from superficial subcutaneous infections, provides a strength layer when suturing, and limits elastic deformation of the scalp often making closure more difficult.

The subgaleal fascia is a thin loose areolar connective tissue that lies between the galea and the pericranium and allows scalp mobility. The emissary veins cross this space as they drain the scalp into the intracranial venous sinuses. This is a potential site of ingress for bacteria contained within a subgaleal abscess leading to meningitis or septic venous sinus thrombosis although the incidence is very low.[41–44]

The treatment of other life-threatening injuries will take precedence over the scalp with the exception of bleeding. The adventitia of scalp arteries is intimately attached to the surrounding dense connective tissue, so that the cut ends of vessels do not collapse and tend to remain patent and bleeding. This coupled with the rich blood supply can make the scalp a source of significant and ongoing blood loss.[45] A pressure dressing or rapid mass closure will provide time for treatment of other more urgent injuries with deferred treatment of the scalp up to 24 h later.

Closed scalp injuries such as abrasions and contusions will heal without surgical intervention. Small scalp hematomas are common and do not need to be evacuated acutely. Large hematomas may benefit from evacuation after bleeding has stopped from tamponade and the patient is otherwise stabilized. Large undrained hematomas have the potential to organize into a fibrotic or calcified mass. This is of minimal consequence in the hair-bearing scalp, but may be a cosmetic deformity on the forehead.

Full-thickness scalp wounds with tissue loss may be treated with nonsurgical management as a bridge to later reconstruction. The bone or periosteum must be kept moist at all times, if there is to be any growth of granulation tissue over it or secondary intention healing. If the bone becomes desiccated, it will die. Once a bed of granulation tissue has formed, a skin graft may be applied, or allowed to epithelize from the margins of the wound. Often secondary intention healing will contract the wound such that later excision of the scar and associated alopecia will be easily achieved *(Fig. 2.15)*. Some have advocated a purse-string around the wound to expedite closure of the scalp wound.[46]

The wound should be thoroughly irrigated and hemostasis of major vessels should be completed with electrocautery or suture ligature. All foreign material such as dirt, glass, rocks, hair, plant matter, grease, and small bone fragments should be removed. The wound should be explored for any previously unrecognized skull fractures. There is seldom a need for radical debridement of the scalp due to the rich blood supply.

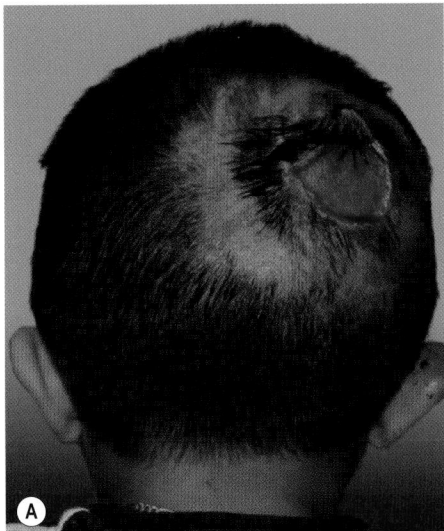 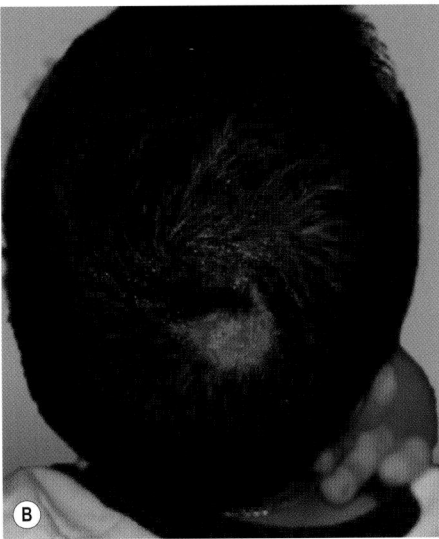 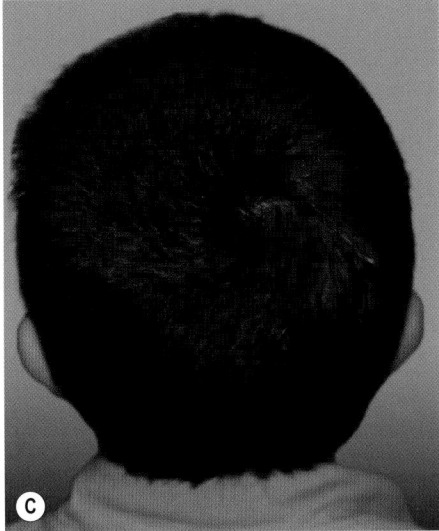

Fig. 2.15 A dog bite scalp avulsion with intact pericranium in a child **(A)**. After 1 month of secondary intention healing with bacitracin ointment and petrolatum gauze dressings the wound has contracted and epithelized markedly **(B)**. Several months later the wound was fully epithelized and a simple scar excision and primary closure achieved a good cosmetic result **(C)**.

Surprisingly large segments of scalp can survive on relatively small vascular pedicels and therefore it is often preferable to preserve any scalp tissue that has even a remote probability of survival. Shaving of the scalp in nonemergent neurosurgery has not been shown to be of any benefit in reducing wound infections.[47–50] It is reasonable to shave sufficient hair so that clear visualization of the injury is had. There is probably no benefit to shave the scalp for simple clean lacerations.

In general, scalp closure involves closure of the galea and subcutaneous tissue to control bleeding and provide strength, followed by skin closure. Absorbable 3-0 sutures are used for the galea and subcutaneous tissue in either a running or an interrupted manner. The skin can be closed with staples, or sutures. In children, a rapidly absorbable suture is often used to avoid the need for later removal.

Repair of the scalp will depend on the nature of the injury, whether there is tissue loss, and the condition of the underlying pericranium and bone. Simple cuts from sharp objects require nothing more than simple closure. Blows to the head from assaults, falls and road crashes often crush the soft tissue against the skull resulting in a jagged, bursting of the tissue. In these injuries, the initial impression may be that there has been tissue loss, but after careful inspection, and systematic replacement of tissue (solving the jigsaw puzzle) it becomes apparent that very little tissue is missing. The pieces should be reassembled and any areas of dubious survival should be given time to declare themselves. They often will survive.

Defects of 3 cm or less in diameter can usually be closed with wide undermining of the scalp at the subgaleal level.[51] The scalp is notoriously inelastic and will often require scoring of the galea with multiple incisions perpendicular to the desired direction of stretch. This is best done with electrocautery on low power, or a scalpel. Care should be taken to only cut through the galea leaving the subcutaneous tissue and vessels within unharmed (Fig. 2.16). Scalp defects too large for primary closure may be dressed with a damp dressing and closed with other standard scalp reconstruction techniques as described elsewhere in this volume.

Total scalp avulsion is best treated with microsurgical replantation whenever possible (Figs 2.17, 2.18). Avulsion injuries are most commonly caused when long hair becomes entangled around a rotating piece of industrial or agricultural machinery. The scalp detaches at the subgaleal plane with the skin tearing at the supraorbital, temporal, and auricular areas. Many authors have reported excellent results with scalp replantation, even when only one vein and artery were available for revascularization.[52–74] The scalp will tolerate up to 18 h of cold ischemia. Because the injuries are usually avulsive in nature, the veins and arteries needed for replantation have sustained significant intimal stretch injury. Because of this, vein grafts are frequently needed to bridge the zone of injury. Blood loss can be significant and blood transfusion is common. If possible, the venous anastomoses should be completed before the arteries to minimize unnecessary blood loss.[60] The scalp can survive on a single vessel, however other vessels should be repaired if possible.

Eyebrows

The eyebrows are nimble structures that are an important cosmetic part of the face, and serve as nonverbal organs of communication and facial expression.[75–78] Several notable anatomic considerations are important in the treatment of soft tissue injuries in this area. The most conspicuous aspect of the eyebrow is the pattern and direction of the associated hair follicles. The hair bulbs of the eyebrows extend deeply into the subcutaneous fat, placing them at risk if undermining is undertaken too superficially. The hairs grow from an inferior medial to superior lateral direction; therefore, incision placed along the inferior aspect of the brow may inadvertently transect hair bulbs lying inferior to the visual border of the brow. Any incision in the brow should be beveled along an axis parallel to the hair shafts to avoid injury to the hair bulbs or shafts.

Lacerations of the lateral brow area are common and place the temporal branch of the facial nerve at risk. The administration of local anesthetics will cause loss of temporal nerve function and mimic a nerve injury and therefore temporal branch injury should be tested before the administration of anesthetics. After adequate anesthesia and irrigation, the underlying structures should be inspected and palpated. In particular, the wound should be inspected for possible frontal sinus fracture, orbital rim fractures, and foreign bodies.

Reconstruction of the brow is difficult because the short thick hair of the brows and the unique orientation of the hair shafts are nearly impossible to accurately reproduce. Therefore, every effort should be made to preserve and repair the existing brow tissue with as little distortion as possible. After testing the integrity of the frontal branch of the facial nerve, local infiltration with local anesthetic will provide good anesthesia in most cases. Despite the fact the generations of medical students have heard that the brow should never be shaved for fear that it will not grow back, there is no scientific evidence to support this belief.[79] It is rarely necessary to shave the brow, and in fact shaving the brow may make proper alignment of the eyebrow repair more difficult. If the brow prevents proper visualization, it may be lightly clipped.

After irrigation, the underlying structures should be inspected and palpated. In particular, the wound should be inspected for possible frontal sinus fracture, orbital rim fractures, and foreign bodies. Debridement of the wound should be very conservative. Any tissue that has a potential to survive should be carefully sutured into position. If clearly nonvital tissue must be removed then the incision should be created parallel to the hair shafts to minimize damage to the underlying hair follicles. The closure should not be excessively tight, as constricting sutures may damage hair follicles and cause brow alopecia (Fig. 2.13).

Most brow wounds are simple lacerations, and as such may be simply closed by approximating the underlying muscular layer with fine resorbable suture and the skin with 5-0, or 6-0 nylon. Areas of full thickness brow loss (up to 1 cm) with little or no injury to the surrounding area can be repaired primarily with a number of local advancement flaps including a Burow's wedge advancement flap,[80] double-advancement flap,[81] and O-to-Z repair (Fig. 2.19).[82] Primary closure of larger defects may distort the remainder of the brow excessively. The medial half of the brow is thicker and cosmetically more prominent and therefore the illusion of symmetry is easier to preserve if the medial brow position is not disturbed. For this reason, it is generally better to advance the lateral brow medially to accommodate closure.[80] Small areas of tissue loss not

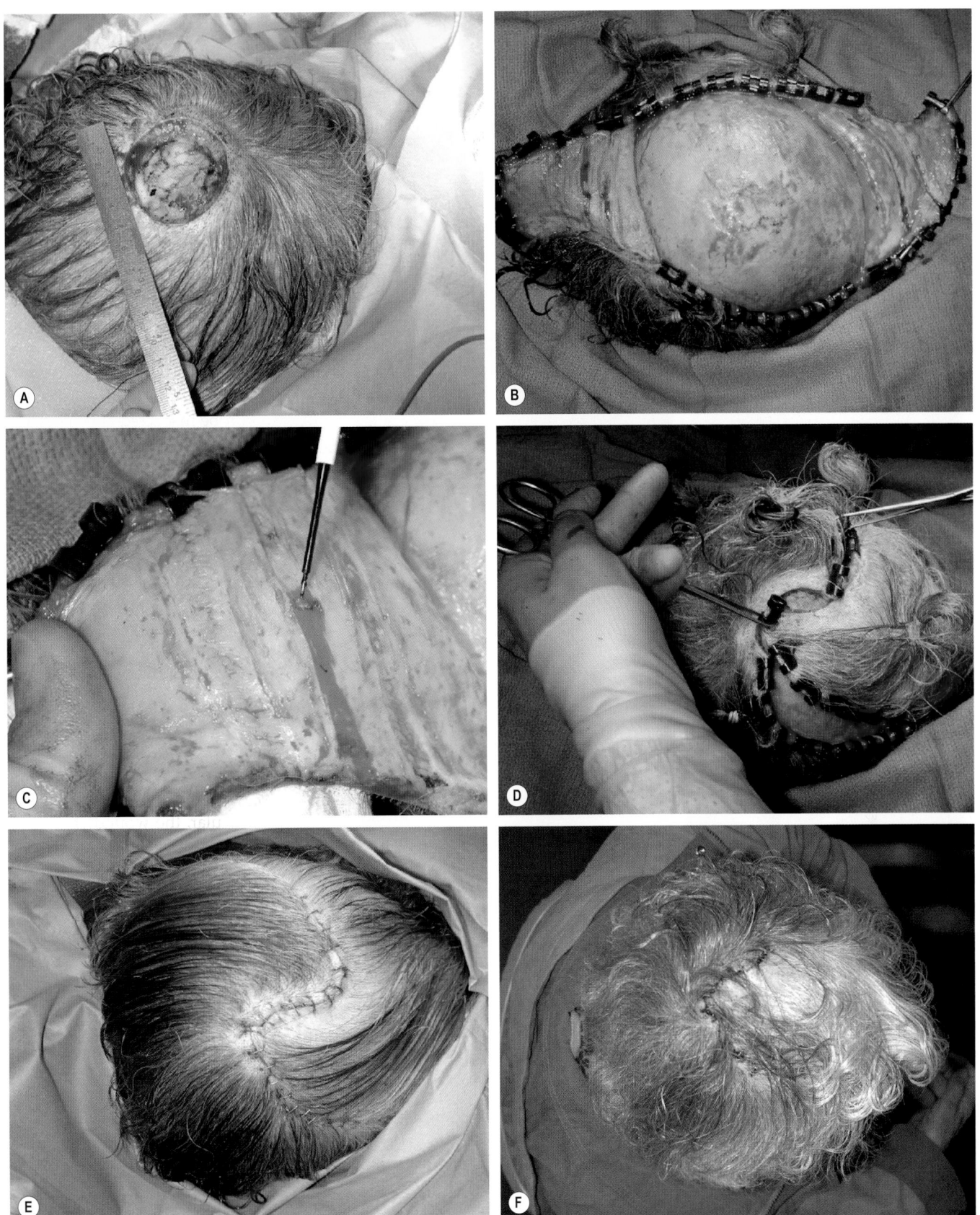

Fig. 2.16 Defects of the scalp for more than 2 cm **(A)** will often require creation of scalp flaps **(B)** for closure. Scoring the galea with electrocautery **(C)** or a scalpel will allow advancement of the flaps **(D)** and wound closure **(E)**. It is not necessary to shave any hair as a matter of routine when repairing scalp wound unless visualization is impaired. The scalp tends to heal well. Sutures are removed in about 14 days **(F)**.

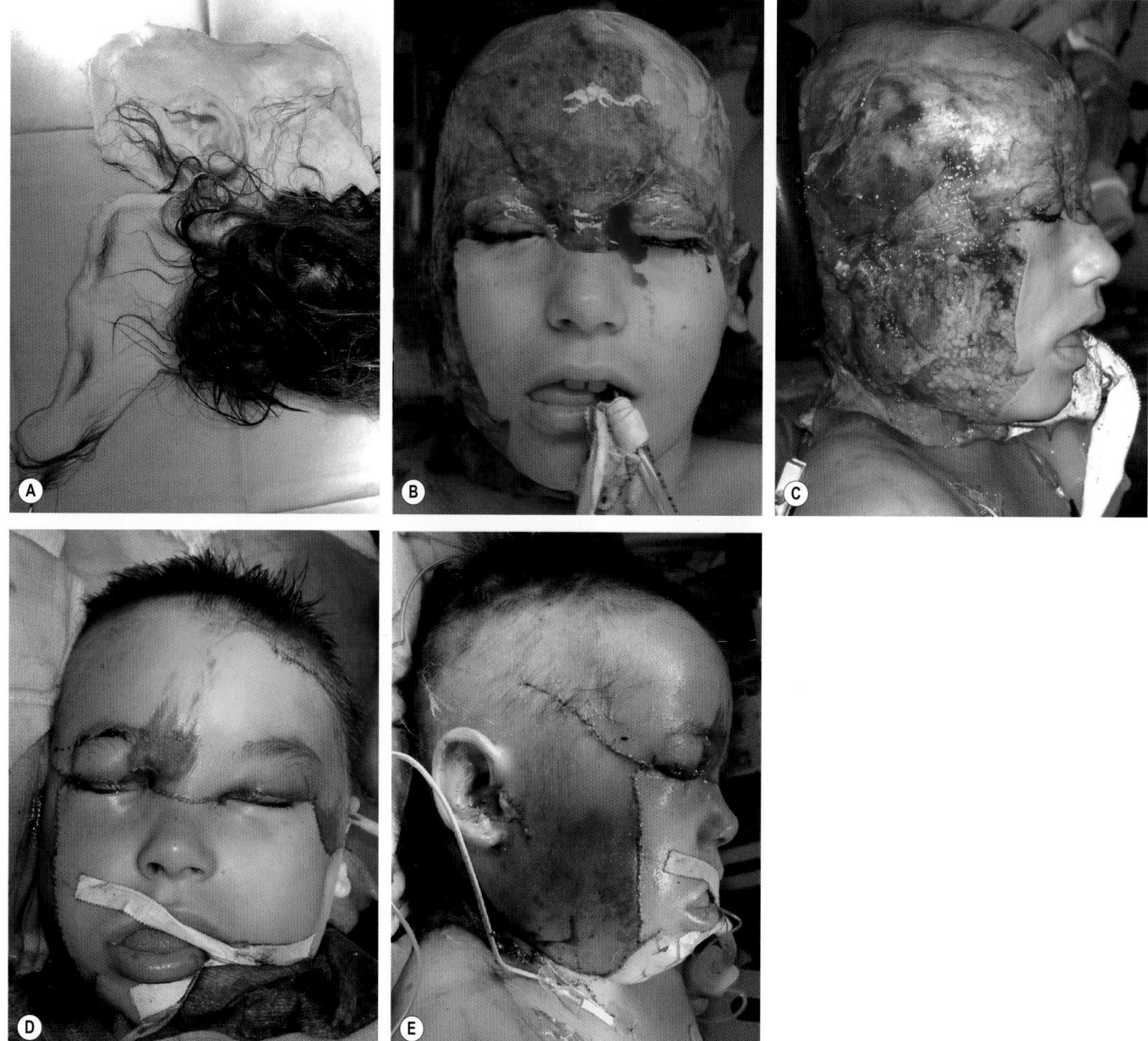

Fig. 2.17 A 15-year-old girl with a total scalp avulsion after her hair became entangled in a machine. **(A)** The avulsed scalp is shown at top. **(B,C)** The entire scalp, eyelids, right ear, face, and a portion of the neck were avulsed. Multiple vein grafts were needed for vascular anastomosis to the superficial temporal, supraorbital and facial vessels. Immediately after replantation **(D,E)** using multiple vein grafts. The right side of the face was congested and required leech therapy for 6 days.

amenable to primary closure should be allowed to heal by secondary intention. The resulting scar or deformity can be revised 6–12 months after the injury when the tissues have softened. Wound contracture, and the passage of time may allow for local flap reconstruction that was impossible initially. Larger defects may need to be reconstructed with a variety of scalp pedicel flaps[83–91] or individual hair follicle transplants.[92,93]

Local flap

A variety of local brow advancement flaps have been described for brow reconstruction of smaller defects. The cosmetic focus of the brow is in its medial half where the hair growth is thickest. When possible, it is usually preferable to advance the lateral brow medially, rather than advance the medial brow laterally, to close a defect. This is most important for defects of the medial brow. A Burrow's wedge advancement flap is suitable for these defects *(Fig. 2.19)*. When elevating the flap to be advanced, it is important that the dissection is of sufficient depth that the vulnerable hair follicles are not damaged. Defects of the lateral brow can be closed by advancing tissue from both directions with two advancement flaps (the so-called A-to-T closure), so long as there is no undue distortion of the medial brow.

The double advancement flap method that uses two rectangular flaps for closure affords similar capabilities as the

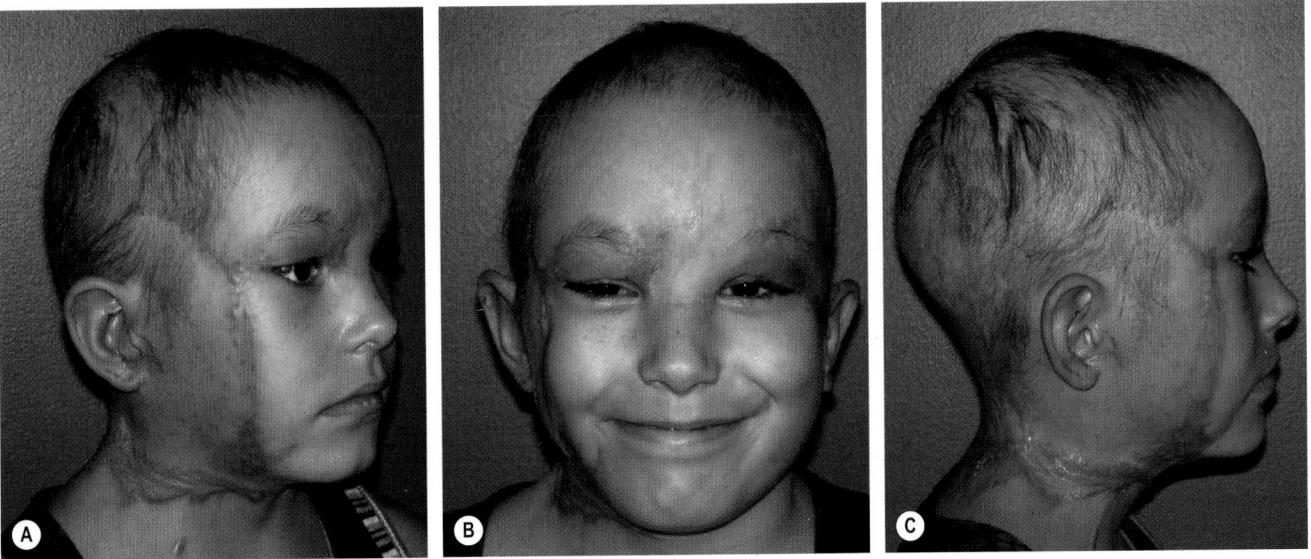

Fig. 2.18 At 2 months after replantation of scalp, eyelids, right face and ear. An area on the posterior neck needed skin grafting.

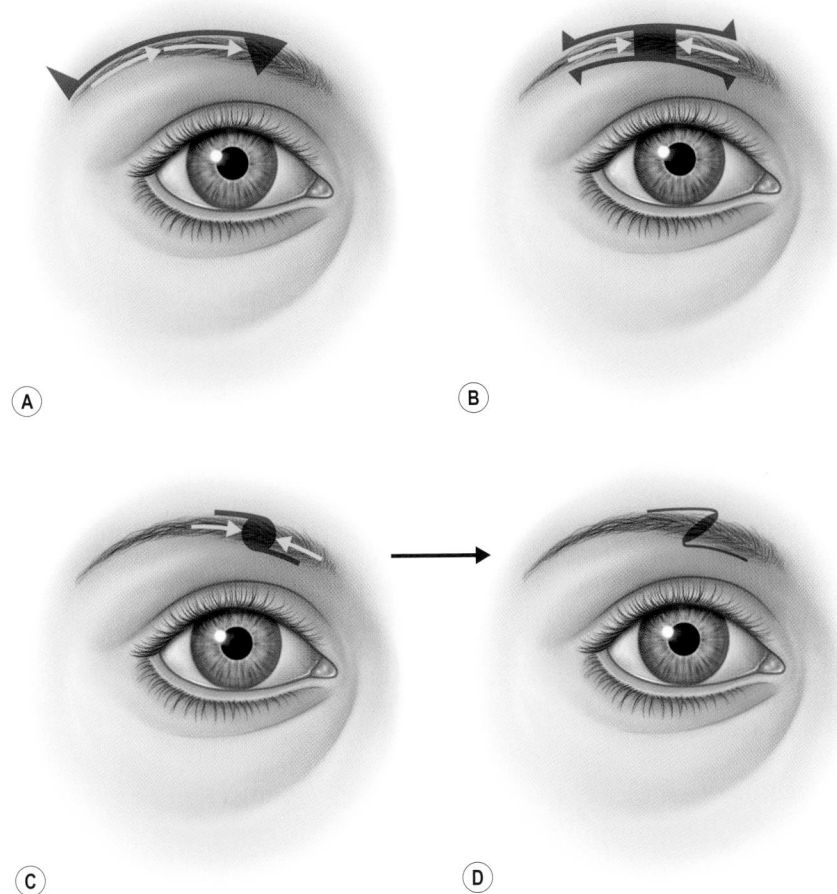

Fig. 2.19 A Burrow's wedge triangle closure **(A)** favors movement of the lateral brow medially. It affords easy alignment of the hair-bearing margin and a broad-based flap design. Two opposing rectangular flaps can be advanced with the aid of Burrow's wedge triangle excisions **(B).** This flap also provides easy alignment of the brow margins, but has a greater scar burden. The O-to-Z excision **(C)** and closure **(D)** results in some distortion of the eyebrow hair orientation.

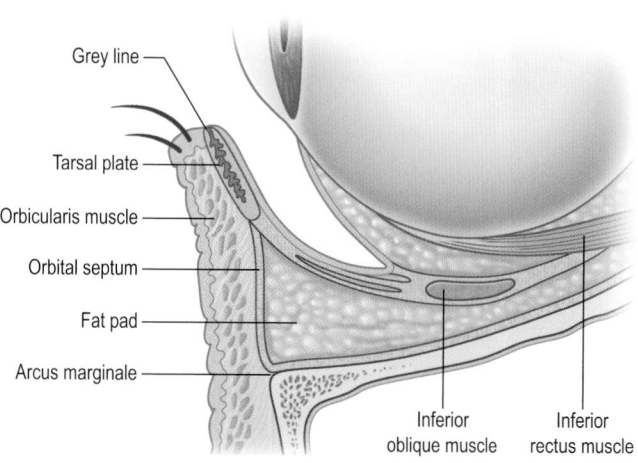

Fig. 2.20 Lower eyelid seen in cross-section shows the lamellar nature of the eyelids. Repair of full-thickness eyelid lacerations should include repair of the conjunctiva, tarsal plate, and skin. The lash line or gray line should be used as an anatomic landmark to ensure proper alignment of the lid margin during repair.

Burrow's wedge rotation flap but requires four incisions (*Fig. 2.19*). It is important that the margins of the hair-bearing skin are accurately aligned in much the same way as the vermillion border is aligned for lip lacerations. Inaccurate repair will result in an unsightly step-off. Both the Burrow's wedge rotation flap and the double advancement flap closures make alignment of the hair-bearing margin relatively easy.

Local graft

More significant brow defects will require more involved brow reconstruction with grafts and flaps. These techniques are discussed in Chapter 5.

Eyelids

Treatment of eyelid injuries is important to preserve the vital functions of the eyelids namely: protection of the globe, prevention of drying, and appearance.

The eyelids are composed of very thin skin, alveolar tissue, orbicularis oculi muscle, tarsus, septum orbitale, tarsal (meibomian) glands, and conjunctiva (*Fig. 2.20*). At the lid margin, the conjunctiva meets the skin at the grey line. Embedded within the margins of the lids are the hair follicles of the eyelashes. The tarsal plates are dense condensations of connective tissue that support and give form to the eyelids and assist in keeping the conjunctiva in apposition to the globe. It is important to remember that the eyelids are lamellar structures and in general each layer should be individually repair. A detailed discussion of eyelid anatomy can be found in Chapter 1.

The eyelids should be inspected for ptosis (suggesting levator apparatus injury), rounding of the canthi (suggesting canthus injury or NOE fracture). It may be helpful to tug on the lid with fingers or forceps to check the integrity of the canthi. A firm endpoint should be felt (try it on yourself). Epiphora may be a tip-off for canalicular injury. A search for concomitant globe, or facial fractures should be undertaken.

Any injury to the eyelids should raise suspicion to a globe injury. If there is any doubt about ocular injury, an ophthalmology consultation is needed.

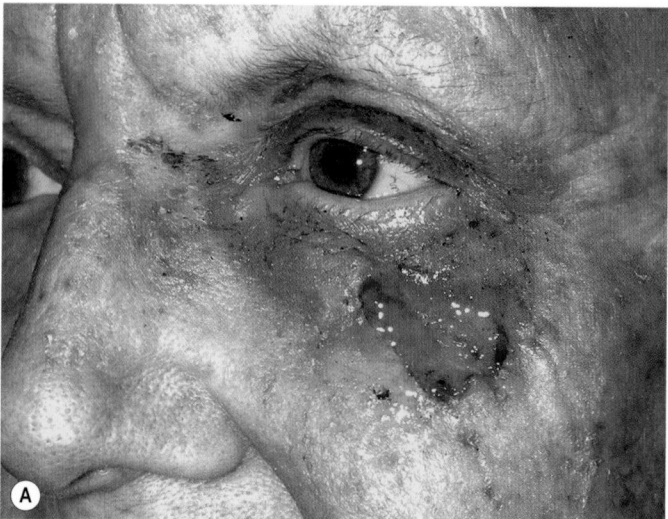

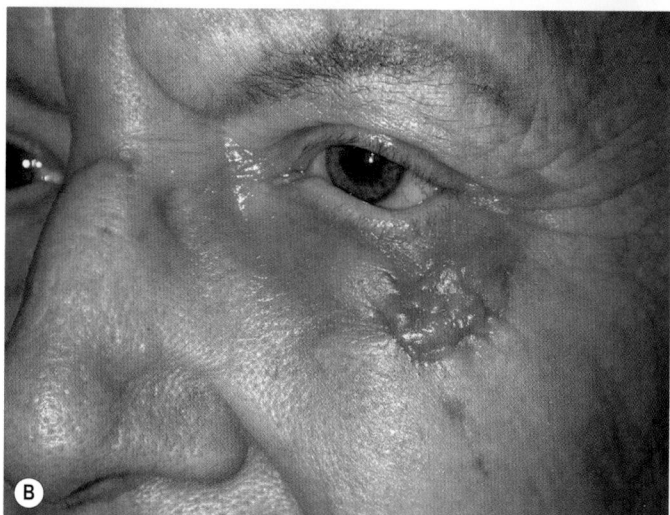

Fig. 2.21 A superficial cheek avulsion injury **(A)** was allowed to heal by secondary intention **(B)** resulting in a cicatricial ectropion. Any injury to the eyelids or on the upper cheek has the potential to distort the eyelid from the normal contractile forces of healing.

In general, nonsurgical treatment of eyelid injuries or neighboring areas with tissue loss is not advisable because the natural contraction of secondary intention healing may distort the lid, and result in lagophthalmos, ectropion, or distortion of the lid architecture (*Fig. 2.21*). Nonetheless, some wounds are amenable to nonsurgical treatment,[38,39,94] in particular wounds of the medial canthal area that do not involve the lid margin nor lacrimal apparatus tend to do well especially in the elderly who have greater intrinsic laxity of the skin. In most cases secondary intention nonsurgical treatment should be reserved for those cases where primary closure is not possible due to tissue loss, or where secondary intention healing is preferable to skin grafting or other reconstruction.

Simple lacerations of the eyelid that do not involve the lid margin or deeper structures may be minimally debrided and closed primarily. The eyelid is a layered structure and as such, full-thickness injuries should be repaired in layers. Usually, repair of the conjunctiva, tarsal plate, and skin is sufficient. Small injuries to the conjunctiva do not require closure, but

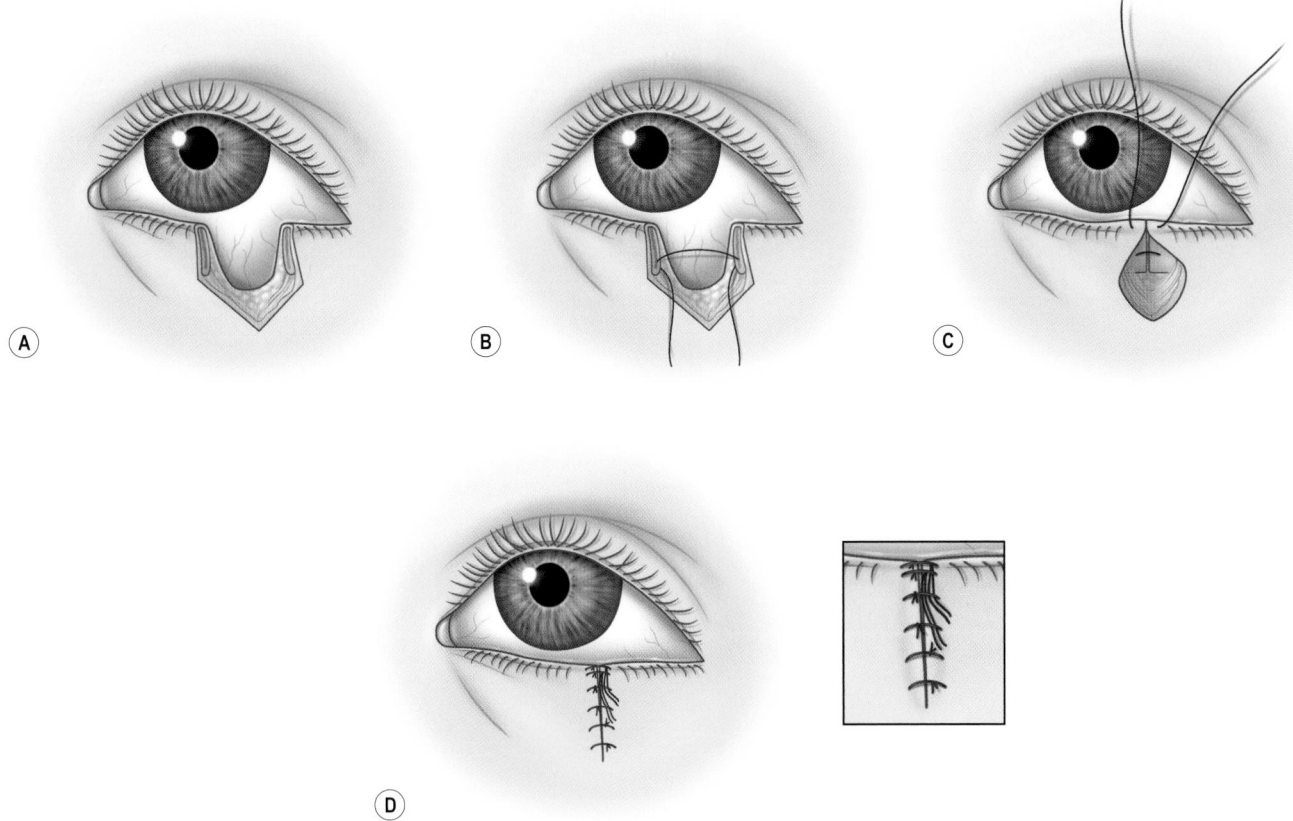

Fig. 2.22 A full-thickness eyelid injury involves skin, tarsal plate and conjunctiva **(A).** Repair starts with the conjunctiva and tarsal plate **(B),** a "key" suture is placed at the lash line to align the eyelid margin and prevent an unsightly step-off **(C).** The repair progresses from the lid margin outward. The ends of each suture are left long, such that they are captured under the subsequent sutures **(D and inset).** This prevents the loose suture ends from migrating up and irritating the eye.

larger lacerations should be repaired with 5-0 or 6-0 gut suture. The tarsal plate should be repaired with a 5-0 absorbable suture and the skin with 6-0 nylon.

Lacerations that involve the lid margin require careful closure to avoid lid notching and misalignment. The technique involves placement of several "key sutures" of 6-0 nylon at the lid margin to align the gray line and lash line. These sutures are not initially tied but used as traction and alignment sutures. The conjunctiva and tarsal plate are repaired and then the "key sutures" may be tied. The sutures are left long. Subsequent skin sutures are placed starting near the lid margin and working away. As each subsequent suture is place and tied and long ends of the sutures nearer the lid margin are tied under the subsequent sutures to prevent the loose ends from migrating towards the eye and irritating the cornea *(Fig. 2.22)*. Avulsive injuries to the lids that involve only skin may be treated with full thickness skin grafts from the postauricular region or contralateral upper eyelid. Lid switch pennant flaps are also an option. Injuries that involve full thickness loss of 25% of the lid may be debrided and closed primarily as any other full thickness laceration.[95] Loss of more that 25% of the lid will require more involved eyelid reconstruction covered in other chapters.

Any laceration to the medial third of the eyelids should raise suspicion for a canalicular injury *(Fig. 2.23)*. The canaliculus is a white tubular structure that is more easily seen with ×3 loop magnification. If the proximal end of the canaliculus cannot be found a lacrimal probe may be inserted into the puncta and passed distally out the cut end of the canaliculus. It is important to remember that the canaliculus travels perpendicular to the lid margin for 2 mm and then turns medially to parallel the lid margin.

The distal end of the inferior canaliculus may be located by placing a pool of saline in the eye while instilling air into the other (intact) canaliculus. Bubbles will reveal the location of the distal canalicular stump. Once identified, the canaliculus is repaired over a small double-ended silastic or polyethylene lacrimal stent with 8-0 absorbable sutures. The stent is left in place for 2–3 months. Unless the physician has specific experience with this procedure, a consultation with ophthalmology is indicated. Most patients with one intact canaliculus will not experience epiphora,[96,97] however if repair can be accomplished at the time of injury without jeopardizing the intact canaliculus, most authors would repair it. Good results are generally had with repair over a stent.[98,99]

Ears

Traumatic ear injuries may result from mechanical trauma such as motor vehicle crashes, boxing, wrestling, sports, industrial accidents, ear piercing, and animal or human bites.

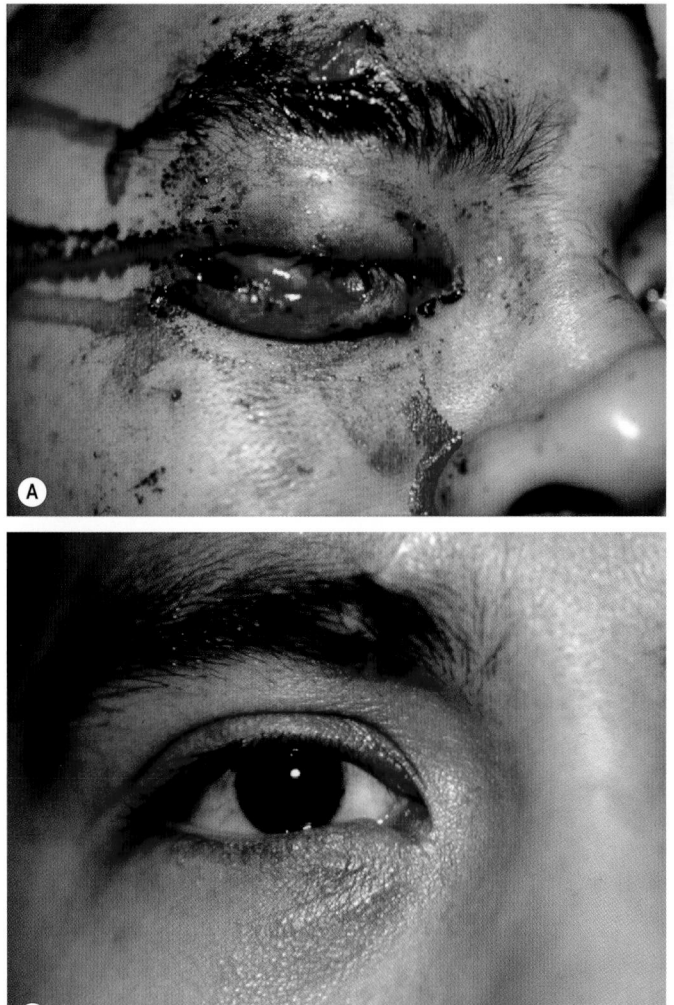

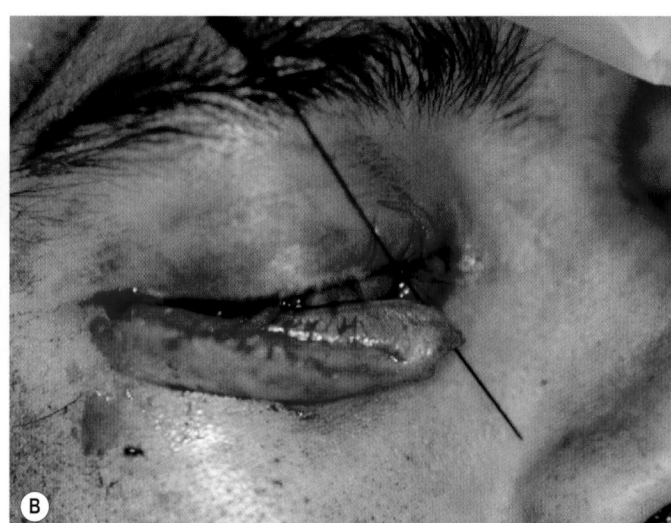

Fig. 2.23 A lower lid laceration involving the medial third of the lid **(A)**. A lacrimal probe is passed through the inferior puncta to identify the proximal end of the canaliculus **(B)**. The canaliculus was repaired over a Silastic stent after locating the distal canalicular duct, and the lid repaired in layers **(C)**.

Thermal burns to the ear are seen in over 90% of patients with other head and neck burns.[100] The ears are at particular risk because they are thin and are exposed on two sides.

Anatomy

The skin of the anterior ear is tightly adherent to the underlying auricular fibrocartilage that gives shape to the external ear. The posterior skin is somewhat thicker and more mobile. The anterior surface is rich in topography while the posterior surface is simple. As with most other areas of the face the blood supply is rich. A detailed discussion of ear anatomy can be found in Chapter 7.

A clinical examination is generally all that is required to diagnose and treat ear trauma. The pinna should be examined to determine if there has been any tissue loss or injury to the auricular cartilage. After blunt trauma or surgical procedure, patients may develop an auricular hematoma, which is an accumulation of blood under the perichondrium that can take several hours to develop. This presents as a painful swelling that obliterates the normal contours of the surface of the ear *(Fig. 2.2)*.

The goal of treatment is to restore cosmetic appearance of the ear, to maintain a superior auricular sulcus that can accommodate eyeglasses, and to minimize later complications from infection or fibrosis.

Hematoma

The most common complication of blunt trauma to the ear is the development of an auricular hematoma. Blunt trauma may cause a shearing force that separates the cartilage from the overlying soft tissue and perichondrium. Inevitably there is bleeding into the space that further separates the cartilage and perichondrium. The clinical appearance is of a convex ear with loss of the normal contours *(Fig. 2.2)*. If left untreated the blood will clot and eventually develop into a fibrotic mass that obliterates the normal ear topography. Over time (and with repeated injury), the fibrotic mass may develop into a calcified bumpy irregular mass leading to what is known as a "cauliflower ear". Ear cartilage is dependant upon the adjacent soft tissue for blood supply and therefore separation of the cartilage from the perichondrium places the cartilage at risk for necrosis and infection.

The treatment for an ear hematoma is evacuation of the hematoma, control of the bleeding, and pressure to prevent an accumulation of blood, and to encourage adherence of the soft tissues to the cartilage. Simple aspiration within a few hours of the injury may evacuate the blood, but without any other treatment hematoma or seroma will reaccumulate.[101,102] Some have advocated using a small liposuction cannula to more effectively evacuate the hematoma.[103] Aspiration with subsequent pressure dressing has been used effectively;[104,105] most authors recommend a surgical approach for more reliable removal of adherent fibrinous material that may delay healing of the soft tissue to the cartilage.[101,105–115]

Surgical drainage can be accomplished with an incision placed parallel to the antihelix and just inside of it where the scar can be hidden. The skin and perichondrial flap is gently elevated and a small suction used to evacuate the hematoma. If adherent fibrinous material remains, it should be removed with forceps. After the wound is irrigated, it should be inspected for bleeding that may require cautery for control. There are many different methods of pressure dressing. Some mold saline soaked cotton behind the ear, and then mold more cotton into the anterior contours of the ear.[107] A head wrap

dressing follows this. Others have used thermoplastic splints molded to the ear.[116] The author prefers to mold Xeroform® (petrolatum jelly, bismuth tribromophenate impregnated) gauze into the ear contours and secure the bolsters with several 3-0 nylon through-and-through mattress sutures (*Fig. 2.24*). A head wrap dressing is applied and the sutures and bolsters are removed in 1 week.

Lacerations

Simple lacerations should be irrigated and minimally debrided. Like other areas of the face, the blood supply of the ear is robust and will support large portions of the ear on small pedicles (*Fig. 2.25*). The cartilage is dependant on the perichondrium and soft tissue for its blood supply; as long as one surface of the cartilage is in contact with viable tissue, it should survive. Known landmarks such as the helical rim, or antihelix should be reapproximated with a few "key" sutures. The remainder of the repair is accomplished with 5-0 or 6-0 nylon skin sutures.[112] It is important that the closure be accurate with slight eversion of the wound edges, using vertical mattress sutures if needed. Any inversion will persist after healing and result in unsightly grooves across the ear.[117] It is usually not necessary to place sutures in the cartilage, and most authors prefer to rely on the soft tissue repair alone.[107,114,118–122] There is some concern that suturing the cartilage is detrimental,[123] leading to necrosis and increased risk of infection. If cartilage must be sutured, an absorbable 5-0 suture is best.[124]

There are no good data regarding the use of postoperative antibiotics following repair of ear lacerations, however, many authors recommend a period of prophylactic antibiotics to prevent suppurative chondritis, especially for lager injuries or those with degloved or poorly perfused cartilage.[125–131] There is no role for postoperative antibiotics after repair of simple lacerations of the ear.

Auditory canal stenosis

When an injury involves the external auditory canal, scarring and contracture may result in stenosis or occlusion of the canal. Canal injuries should be stented to prevent stenosis.[114] If a portion of the canal skin is avulsed out of the bony canal

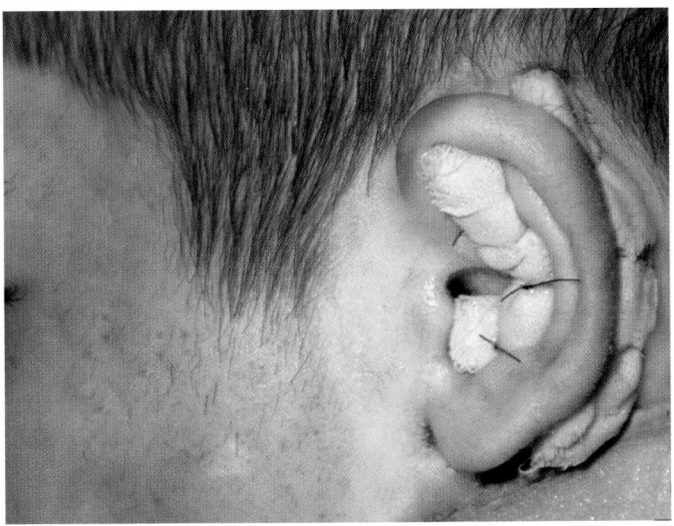

Fig. 2.24 After evacuation of an auricular hematoma a through and through tie-over bolster should be molded and secured to the ear to prevent reaccumulation of the hematoma.

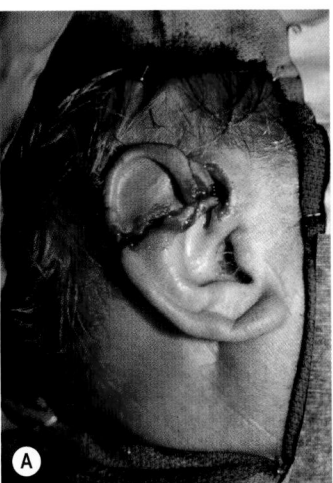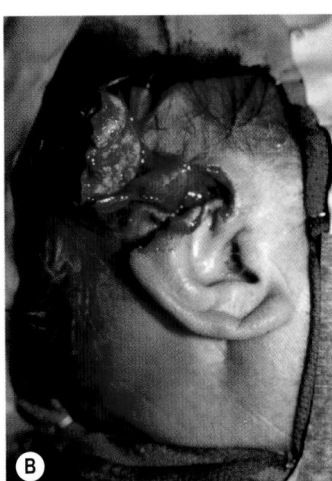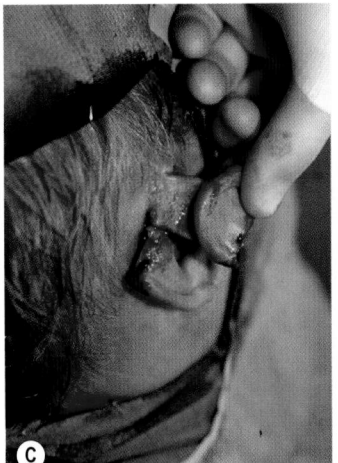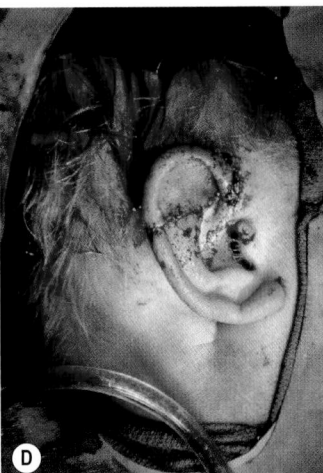

Fig. 2.25 An upper ear laceration from a motor vehicle crash **(A)** is attached by a posterior skin bridge **(B,C)**. The upper auricle survived on this pedicle because of the generous blood supply of the ear. The helical rim was sutured first for alignment and the remainder of the skin closed with 6-0 nylon **(D)**.

it may be repositioned and stented into place as a full-thickness skin graft.

Partial amputation with a wide pedicle

Figure 2.25 demonstrates a partial amputation with a wide pedicle relative to the amputated part. Because the pedicle is relatively large it should provide adequate perfusion and venous drainage of the part. The prognosis is excellent after conservative debridement and meticulous repair. Because there is no way to quantitatively asses for the adequacy of venous drainage the ear should be observed over the first 4–6 h for any signs of venous congestion if there is any suspicion that it may not be adequate. If venous congestion develops, leech therapy should be instituted.

Partial amputation with a narrow pedicle

When the amputated part is attached by a small pedicle you must consider the size of the pedicle relative to the amputated part and make a judgment about whether the pedicle can provide adequate perfusion to sustain the amputated part. An ear fragment that contains primarily soft tissue (e.g., the lobule) is more likely to survive than a similarly sized fragment that contains more cartilage.[107,132,133] Surprisingly, small pedicles can provide for good arterial inflow but the risk of venous congestion is much higher. The avulsed part must be observed over the first 4–6 h for venous congestion and if it develops, leech therapy should be instituted. In 5–7 days, or more, adequate venous drainage will reestablished itself. Ongoing blood loss during this time will require blood transfusion; typically 4–6 units. Prophylactic antibiotics to cover *Aeromonas hydrophilia* (a commensal organism in the leech gut) should be given.

If the pedicle is very narrow with inadequate or no perfusion, the avulsed part should be treated like a complete amputation (see below) or the perfusion should be augmented with local flaps.[122,134–141] Many varieties of local or regional flaps have been devised for ear salvage and all rely on opposing the flap to dermabraded dermis, or denuded cartilage. Some have advocated elevating a mastoid skin flap and applying the flap to a dermabraded portion on the lateral,[134] or medial[122] surface of the avulsed ear; while others have dermabraded the avulsed part and placed it into a subcutaneous retroauricular pocket. In 2–4 weeks, the ear is removed from the pocket and allowed to spontaneously epithelize.[114,123,140,142–144] These techniques are simple and provide a period of nutritive support until the wound heals and the ear becomes self-sustaining. It further maintains the delicate relationship between cartilage and dermis so important in maintaining the subtle folds and architecture that give an ear its shape.

Some authors have recommended similar techniques that remove the entire dermis and then cover denuded cartilage under retroauricular skin,[145] under a cervical flap,[146] or with a tunnel procedure.[147,148] Others have used a temporoparietal fascial flap to cover the denuded cartilage and then cover the temporoparietal fascial flap with a skin graft.[149] Another method involves removing the posterior skin from the avulsed part and fenestrating the remaining cartilage in several areas and then surfacing the posterior part with a mastoid skin flap.[150] The idea behind the cartilage fenestrations is to allow vascular in growth from the posterior to the anterior surface

and increase the likelihood of survival. One criticism of all of the methods that attempt to cover denuded cartilage is that the subtle architecture of the ears is often lost, resulting in a distorted thick formless disk.[132]

Complete amputation of all or part of the ear with the amputated part available

Amputated ear parts are difficult to reconstruct and the larger the defect the more challenging and time consuming the reconstruction. Reattaching amputated facial parts as composite grafts has a long history dating back at least to 1551.[151] Contemporary reports describe occasional successes and many failures.[126,132,140,150–153] A good outcome after simple reattachment of a composite graft is probably the exception rather than the rule. The final outcome is often marred by scar, hyper-pigmentation, partial loss and deformity.[114] Spira and Hardy[154] stated "if the amputated portion consists of anything more than the lobe or segment of helix, replacement is invariably doomed."

In an effort to salvage the cartilage, many authors have advocated burying the cartilage in a subcutaneous pocket in the abdomen[154–157] or under a postauricular flap.[145] Mladick improved upon these techniques by dermabrading the skin, rather than removing it, prior to placement in a subcutaneous pocket.[123,144,158,159] This has the advantage of preserving the intimate and delicate relationship between the dermis and cartilage that is so important for maintaining the subtle architecture of the ear.

Microsurgical replantation should be considered whenever feasible for patients who do not have concomitant trauma or medical conditions that would preclude a lengthy operation. The ear has fairly low metabolic demands, and as such, will tolerate prolonged periods of ischemia, with successful replantation reported after 33 hours of cold ischemia time.[160] After sharp injuries, the branches from superficial temporal artery or posterior auricular artery may be identifiable, and repairable. In some cases, a leash of superficial temporal artery may be brought down to the ear. In a similar manner, veins may be repaired primarily or with vein grafts. Nerves may be repaired if they can be identified; surprisingly however, a number of replanted ears without any nerve repair are reported to have had good sensation.[161] A protective dressing is placed that will allow for clinical monitoring for arterial or venous compromise.

Nose

The prominent position of the nose on the face places it at risk for frequent trauma. Many injuries result in nasal fractures without any soft tissue involvement. Nasal injuries in and of themselves are not life-threatening, however failure to treat nasal injuries appropriately at the time of injury may result in distorted appearance or nasal obstruction, whether due to loss of tissue, scarring, or misalignment of normal structures.

The nose is a layered structure that in simple terms can be thought of as an outer soft tissue envelope composed of skin, subcutaneous fat, and nasal muscles; a support structure composed of cartilage and bone to give the envelope shape and an internal mucosal lining that filters particulates, and exchanges heat and moisture. (A detailed discussion of nasal anatomy can be found in Chapter 1.)

When examining the nose, the three primary components (external covering, support structures, and lining) should be considered. The external soft tissue envelope can be quickly assed for lacerations, or tissue loss. The support structures of the nose can be assessed by observation for asymmetry, or deviation of the nasal dorsum. Fractures can usually be ascertained with palpation for bony step-off or crepitance. Significant nasal fractures are usually evident from clinic exam; X-rays rarely add significant information. If the lacerations are present, they will provide a window to the underlying structures of the nose. After adequate anesthesia and irrigation, any open wounds should be inspected for evidence of lacerated or fractures of the upper lateral or lower lateral cartilages.

Examination of the internal nose requires a nasal speculum, good lighting, and suction if there is active bleeding. The mucosa should be examined for any evidence of septal hematoma, mucosal laceration, or exposed or fractured septal cartilage. Septal hematoma will appear as a fusiform bluish boggy swelling of the septal mucosa. After adequate anesthesia and irrigation, the full nature of the injury to the support framework of the nose and lining can be appreciated.

Nasal fractures are common and should be suspected after blunt nasal trauma. Plain radiographs rarely add significant information to a thorough clinical exam in most isolated nasal injuries. If there is any suspicion of other facial fractures, or paranasal structures a facial CT scan should be acquired. The incidence of orbital injuries following major midfacial fractures has been reported to be as high as 59%.[162]

The goal is to restore normal nasal appearance without subsequent nasal obstruction. Less complex nasal injuries can be managed with local anesthesia, while major nasal injuries are best managed with general anesthesia. Laceration of the nose should be repaired primarily when possible. Smaller avulsive injuries of the cephalic third of the nose heal may be allowed to heal by secondary intention because of the mobility and laxity of the overlying skin in this area. Avulsive injuries to the remainder of the nose if allowed to heal by secondary intention will cause distortion of the nasal architecture due to contractile forces during healing.[94]

Abrasions

Nasal abrasions tend to heal rapidly and well due to the rich vascular supply and abundance of skin appendages that allow for rapid epithelization. The skin of the caudal half of the nose is rich in skin appendages that allow for rapid epithelization. Traumatic tattooing is not uncommon after nasal abrasions. Meticulous cleaning of the wound with pulse lavage, loop magnification to remove embedded particles, and very conservative debridement are needed. Occasionally, one is faced with the difficult decision to debride further, thereby creating a full thickness wound, or leaving some embedded material within the dermis. In general, when faced with such a decision it is best to stop the debridement and proceed with excision and reconstruction later if needed, for cosmesis.

A septal hematoma should be evacuated to prevent subsequent infection and septic necrosis of the septum, or organization of the clot into a calcified subperichondrial fibrotic mass. If a clot has yet to form within the hematoma, it is possible to aspirate with a large bore needle. Evacuation that is more reliable can be achieved with a small septal incision in the mucosa of the hematoma. The blood and clot is evacuated with a small suction and a through-and-through running 4-0 chromic gut quilting suture is placed across the septum to close the dead space and prevent re-accumulation of the blood.

Lacerations

In general, the repair of nasal trauma should begin with the nasal lining and then proceed from the inside out, repairing in turn: lining, framework, and finally skin.

Lining

The lining of the nose should be repaired with thin absorbable sutures such as 5-0 gut sutures. Because of the confined working space, a needle with a small radius of curvature will facilitate placement of the sutures. The knots should be placed facing into the nasal cavity. Small areas of exposed septal cartilage associated with septal fractures or mucosal lacerations will not pose a significant problem as long as intact mucosa is present on the other side. If lining is missing from both sides a mucosal flap should be created to cover at least one side.

Framework

Fractures of the septum should be reduced, and if the septum has become subluxed off the maxillary ridge, it should be reduced back towards the midline. Lacerations of the upper or lower lateral cartilages should be repaired anatomically if they are structurally significant. Usually 5-0 absorbable or clear nonabsorbable sutures should be used. Displaced bony fragments within the wound should be repositioned anatomically or removed if not needed to maintain the structure or shape of the nose. If loss of important support structures has occurred, then reconstruction of the nasal support must be undertaken within a few days. Delay will result in contraction and collapse of the soft tissues of the nose. Later, reconstruction is almost impossible. Reconstruction of this type will usually involve bone or cartilage grafts. If there is doubt about the viability of lining or coverage over the area where grafted cartilage or bone will be placed, then reconstruction should be delayed for a few days until the survival of the soft tissue coverage is no longer in doubt, or secondary soft tissue reconstruction can be accomplished.

Skin covering

After repair of the lining and framework the skin of the nose can be repaired. Key sutures should be placed at the nasal rim to ensure proper alignment prior to the remainder of the closure with 6-0 nylon sutures. The mobile skin of the cephalic nose is forgiving and can be undermined and mobilized to close small avulsive wounds.[163]

Avulsions

Avulsive injuries are frequently the result of automobile crashes, and animal or human bites. They usually involve only skin, but may involve portions of the underlying cartilage. One is frequently faced with the decision to proceed with nasal reconstruction with a local flap or temporary coverage with a skin graft. Smaller defects of the cephalic portion of the dorsum and sidewalls will heal by secondary intention without significant distortion of the anatomy. The skin of the

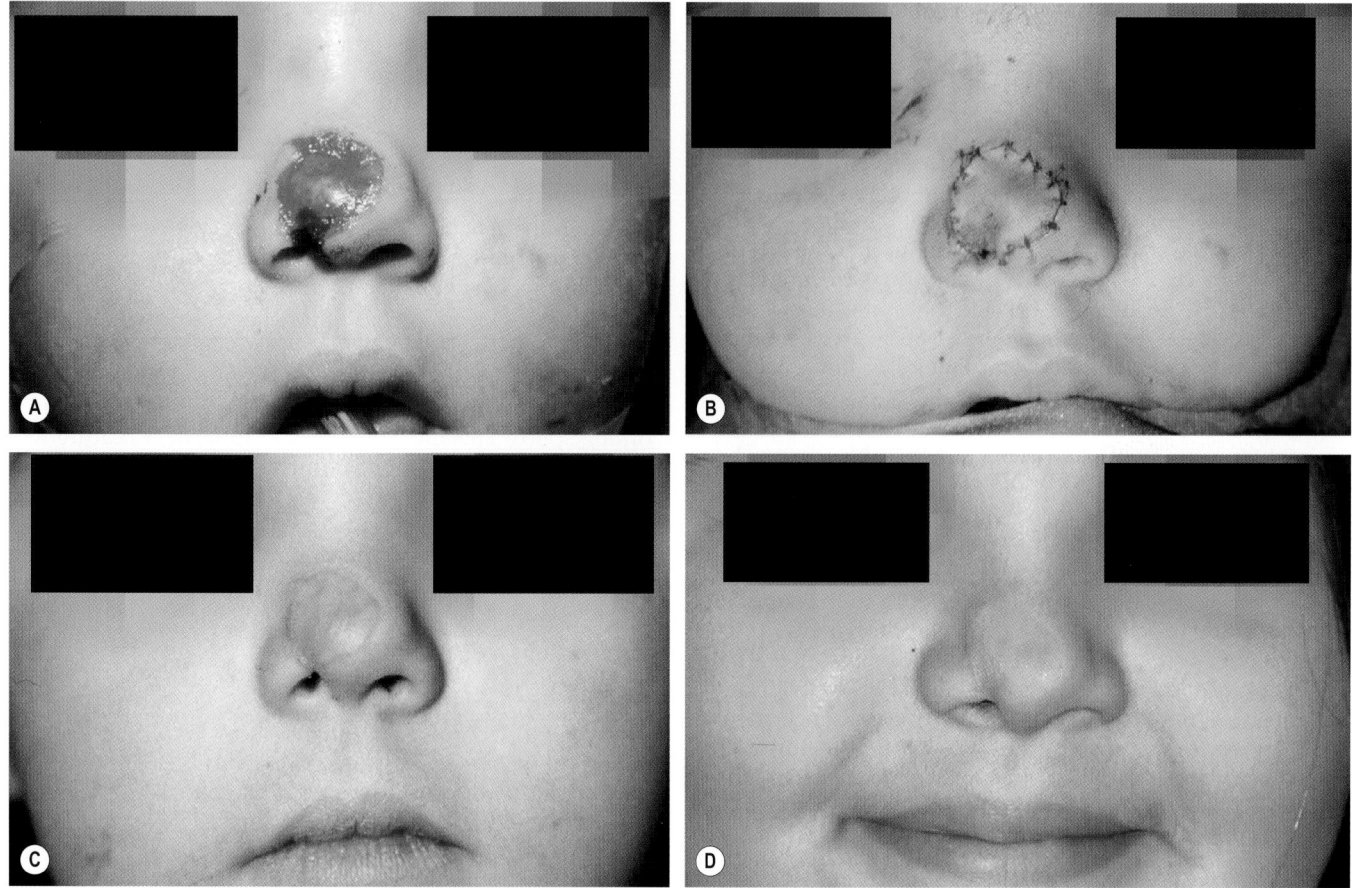

Fig. 2.26 A full-thickness dog bite avulsion injury to the nose **(A)** was treated with a full-thickness retro-auricular skin graft **(B)**. **(C)** At 6 weeks after grafting. **(D)** At 2 years later there is good contour and color match **(D)**.

caudal dorsum, tip, and ala is adherent and less mobile and will often defy primary closure. Secondary intention healing will result in contraction and distortion the nasal anatomy and are best treated with a retroauricular skin graft *(Fig. 2.26)*. Retroauricular full thickness skin grafts have excellent color and texture match. The healed skin graft limits most wound contraction. If secondary reconstruction is needed, the skin graft can be excised and a local flap reconstruction can be performed later.

Amputation

Small, amputated parts can be reattached as a composite graft,[164,165] however some authors warn of the risk of poor outcome and infection after reattachment of bite amputations.[163,166] Davis and Shaheen[167] have reported up to 50% failure of composite grafts, even under ideal conditions. They recommend that composite graft be attempted only when: the wound edges are cleanly cut; there is little risk of infection; the repair is not delayed; no part of the graft is more than 0.5 cm from viable cut edge of the wound, and when all bleeding is controlled. Others have advocated hyperbaric oxygen therapy[165] or cooling[168] to improve tissue survival. Microsurgical replantation may be possible with larger amputated nasal segments[169] or nose and lip composite replantation.[170]

Cheek

When repairing lacerations of the cheek, the primary concern is for injury to the underlying structures namely: facial nerve, facial muscles, parotid duct, and bone.

The blood supply of the cheek is derived primarily from the transverse facial and superficial temporal arteries. Generous collaterals and robust dermal plexus provide reliable perfusion after injury and reconstruction.

The facial nerve exits the stylomastoid foramen. It divides into five main branches within the substance of the parotid gland. The temporal and zygomatic branches run over the zygomatic arch, the buccal branch travels over the masseter along with the parotid duct. The mandibular branch usually loops below the inferior border of the mandible, but rarely more than 2 cm, and then rises above the mandibular border anterior to the facial artery and vein.[171–177] The zygomatic and buccal branches are at particular risk from cheek lacerations. The buccal branches usually have a number of interconnections and therefore a laceration of a single buccal branch may not be clinically apparent.

The parotid gland is a single-lobed gland with superficial and deep portions determined by their relation to the facial nerve running between them. The superficial part of the gland is lateral to the facial nerve and extends anteriorly to the border of the masseter. The parotid duct exits the

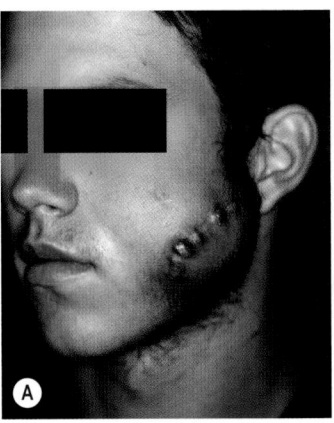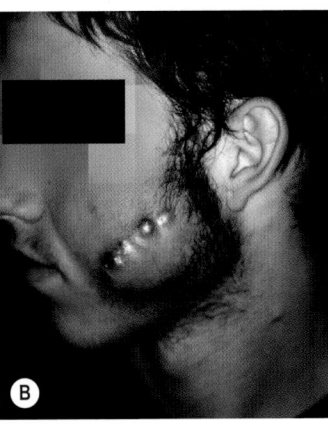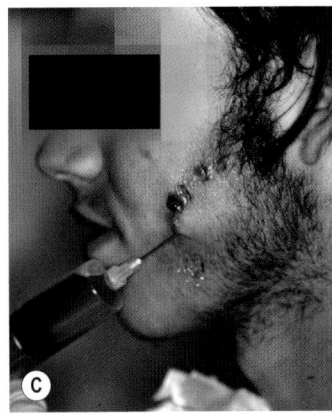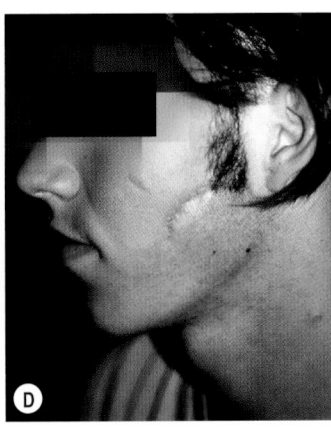

Fig. 2.27 A laceration of the cheek may injure the substance of the parotid gland resulting in an accumulation of saliva under the skin or a sialocele **(A,B)**. If recognized at the time of injury a drain may left in place and a pressure dressing applied. When a sialocele presents after initial repair serial aspirations **(C)** and a pressure dressing will resolve the problem **(D)**.

gland anteriorly and passes over the superficial portion of the masseter, penetrating the buccinator to enter the oral cavity opposite the upper second molar. The course of the parotid may be visualized on the external face by locating the middle-third of a line drawn from the tragus to the middle of the upper lip *(Fig. 2.3)*. The parotid duct travels adjacent to the buccal branches of the facial nerve. If buccal branch paralysis is noted in conjunction with a cheek laceration, then parotid duct injury should be suspected.

Clinical examination is directed towards identifying underlying injury to bone, facial nerve, or parotid duct. The function of facial nerve branches should be tested prior to administration of local anesthetics. Some patients will exhibit asymmetry in facial movement, simply due to pain and edema not related to any underlying facial nerve injury.

If parotid duct injury is suspected, a 22-gauge catheter may be inserted into Stensen's duct and a small quantity of saline or methylene blue solution can be injected. This can be facilitated with a lacrimal probe, however care must be taken not to injure the duct with overzealous probing. If egress of the fluid from the wound is noted, the diagnosis of parotid duct injury has been made.

Repair of parotid duct

Laceration to the parotid gland without duct injury may result in a sialocele but will rarely cause any long-term problems. If a gland injury is suspected, the overlying soft tissue should be repaired and a drain left in place. If a sialocele develops, serial aspirations and a pressure dressing should be sufficient *(Fig. 2.27)*.

Facial nerve injury

Facial nerve injuries should be primarily repaired. Surgical exploration and ×3 magnification with good lighting and hemostasis will assist in locating the cut ends of the nerve. Wounds with contused, stellate lacerations will provide greater challenges to finding the nerve ends. A nerve stimulator can be used to locate the distal nerve segments if within 48 hours of injury. After 48 hours, the distal nerve segments

will no longer conduct an impulse to the involved facial musculature rending the simulator useless. If the proximal ends of the facial nerves cannot be located, the uninjured proximal nerve trunk can be located and followed distally to the cut end of the nerve. The nerves should be repaired primarily with 9-0 nylon. If primary repair is not possible, nerve grafts should be placed, or the proximal and distal nerve ends should be tagged with nonabsorbable suture for easy location during later repair.

Mouth and oral cavity

The lips are the predominant feature of the lower-third of the face and are important for oral competence, articulation, expression of emotion, kissing, sucking, playing of various musical instruments, and as a symbol of beauty. In addition, the lips are important sensory organs that may provide pleasure and protect the oral cavity from ingestion of unacceptably hot or cold materials. The primary function of the lips is sphincteric and this is accomplished by the action of the orbicularis oris muscle. Other facial muscles are important for facial expression and clearing the gingival sulci but are not important in maintaining oral competence. The oral cavity should be carefully examined for dental, dentoalveolar, oral mucosal, tongue, and palate injuries.

Repair of the lip must provide for oral competence, adequate mouth opening, sensation, complete skin cover, oral lining, and the appearance of vermillion.[178] The restoration of the mental and nasolabial crease lines, philtral columns, and precisely aligned vermillion border are important cosmetic goals. The lip is a laminar structure composed of inner mucosal lining and, orbicularis oris muscle, and outer subcutaneous tissue and skin. Closure of lip lacerations should consider repair of each of these structures.

Smaller laceration of the cheek mucosa or gingiva will heal well without any repair. The exceptions are larger lacerations (>2 cm) where food may become entrapped in the laceration, and those that have flap of tissue that falls between the occlusal surfaces of the teeth. Small flaps of tissue that fall between the teeth should be debrided.[179]

The majority of lip lacerations can be managed in the outpatient setting after infiltration of local anesthetic with epinephrine. If the laceration involves the white roll or vermillion border, it may be useful to mark this important landmark with a needle dipped in methylene blue prior to infiltration with larger amounts of local anesthetic because subsequent vasoconstriction may obscure the vermillion border.

A good rule of thumb is to work from the inside of the mouth outwards. To this end, urgent dental or dentoalveolar injuries should be treated first, so that repaired soft tissue is not disrupted by retraction during repair of deeper structures. The wounds should be gently irrigated to remove any loose particles and debris. In most cases, normal saline applied with a 30 cc syringe and an 18-gauge angiocatheter will be sufficient. If there is evidence of broken teeth, and the fragments are not accounted for, a radiograph should be obtained to make sure the tooth fragments are not embedded within the soft tissues. Dead or clearly nonviable tissue should be debrided: once again, it should be emphasized that tissue of the face, and lips in particular, can survive on small pedicles that would be inadequate on any other part of the body. Fortunately, the lips have sufficient redundancy and elasticity that loss of up to 25–30% of the lip can be closed primarily. This also means that unlike many other areas of the face, more aggressive debridement may be undertaken.

The oral cavity

The tongue has a rich blood supply, and injuries to the tongue may cause significant blood loss. In addition, subsequent tongue swelling after larger injuries may cause oropharyngeal obstruction. Most tongue lacerations such as those associated with falls and seizures are small, linear, and superficial and do not require any treatment. Larger lacerations, or those that gape open, or continue to bleed should be repaired. The subsequent edema of the tongue may be profound and therefore the sutures should be loosely approximated to allow for some edema.

Repair of the tongue can be challenging for the patient and physician alike. Gaining the patients confidence is important if cooperation is to be had. Topical 4% lidocaine on gauze can be applied to an area of the tongue for 5 min and will provide some anesthesia that will allow for local infiltration of anesthetic or lingual nerve block. General anesthesia is frequently needed when repairing such lacerations in children. The laceration can be closed with an absorbable suture such as 4-0 or 5-0 chromic gut, or polyglycolic acid.

Oral mucosa repair

The buccal mucosa can be approximated in a single layered closure using interrupted 4-0 or 5-0 chromic gut or polyglycolic acid sutures. Only the minimal sutures should be placed. Occasionally, large flaps of degloved gingival will need repair. It can be difficult to suture these wounds because the gingival does not hold suture well. It can be helpful to attached these flaps of tissue with a suture passed around a nearby tooth.[179]

The lips

Poorly repaired lip lacerations can cause prominent cosmetic defects if not treated in a precise and proper manner. In particular, small misalignments of the white roll or vermillion border are conspicuous to even the casual observer.

Anesthesia of lip wounds is best accomplished with regional nerve blocks and minimal local infiltration. This will prevent distension and distortion of anatomic landmarks critical for accurate repair. An infraorbital nerve block is used for the upper lip and a mental nerve block for the lower.

When repairing simple superficial lip lacerations involving the vermillion border, the first suture should be placed at the vermillion border for alignment. The remainder of the laceration is then closed with 6-0 nonabsorbable sutures. If the laceration extends onto the moist portion of the lip, 5-0 or 6-0 gut sutures are preferred because they are softer when moist and therefore less bothersome for the patient.

Full thickness lip lacerations are repaired in three layers from the inside out. The oral mucosa is repaired first with absorbable suture such as 5-0 chromic or plain gut. If the oral mucosa and gingival has been avulsed from the alveolus, the soft tissue may be reattached by passing a suture from the soft tissue around the base of a neighboring tooth. In general, proceeding from buccal sulcus towards the lip makes the most sense. The muscle layer is approximated with 4-0 or 5-0 absorbable suture. Failure to approximate the orbicularis oris muscle or later dehiscence will result in an unsightly depression of the scar. It is best to include some of the fibrous tissue surrounding the muscle for more strength and placing these sutures. A key suture of 5-0 or 6-0 nylon is placed at the vermillion border and then the remainder of the external sutures are placed.

Avulsive wounds of the lip will often survive on surprisingly small pedicles. It is usually advisable to approximate even marginally viable tissue because of the possibility of survival (*Figs 2.28, 2.29*).

Neck

The most important consideration in soft tissue injuries of the neck is to exclude penetrating neck trauma deep to the platysma and compromise of the airway. Once those are excluded, closure of neck wounds is generally straightforward. Because the skin is mobile and has a fair amount of redundancy, neck lacerations can usually be closed primarily. Remember the course of the marginal mandibular branch deep to the platysma just below the mandibular border during the repair.

Conclusion

The repair of facial soft tissue injuries can be very satisfying for the patient and physician alike. Recognition and prompt treatment of underlying injuries will minimize complications for your patients. Meticulous cleansing of particulate matter will spare your patients a lifetime of facial discoloration from traumatic tattoo. Minimal debridement will salvage irreplaceable soft tissue structures. Careful approximation of important landmarks will minimize unsightly visual step-offs. And careful suture technique and timely suture removal will give your patient the best possible cosmetic outcome.

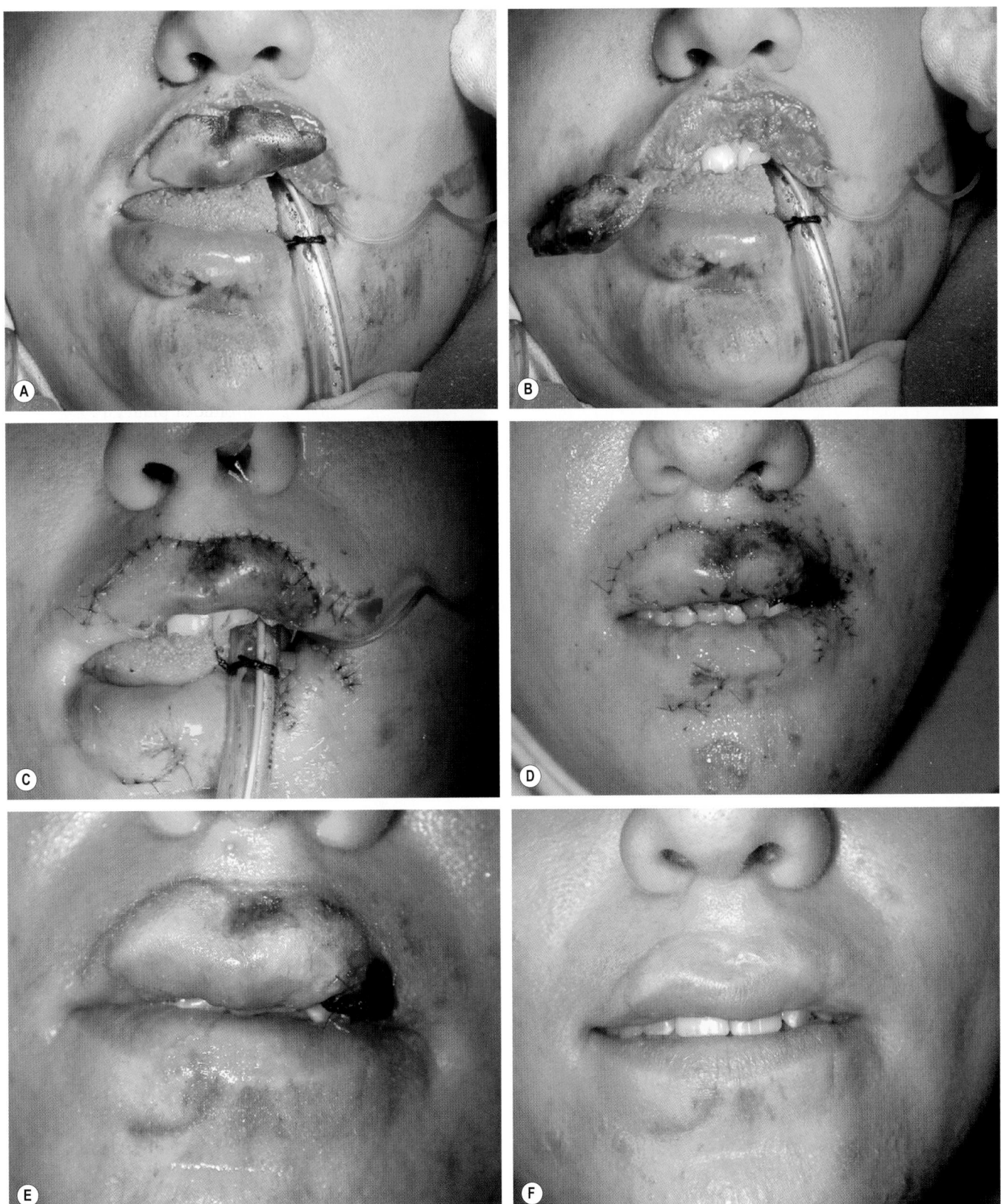

Fig. 2.28 An upper lip avulsion after a motor vehicle crash **(A)** is attached by a small lateral pedicle **(B)**. **(C)** After conservative debridement the landmarks were approximated and the wound closed. **(D)** An area of poor perfusion was present resulting in a small area of necrosis 4 days later. The necrotic area was allowed to head by secondary intention **(E)** and ultimately resulted in a healed wound **(F)**.

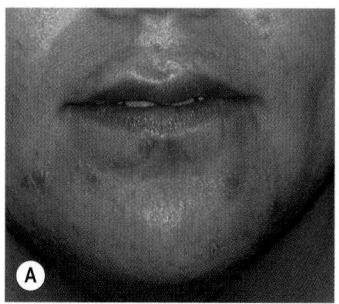 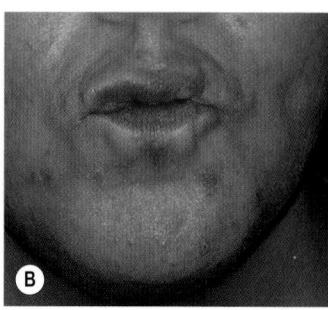 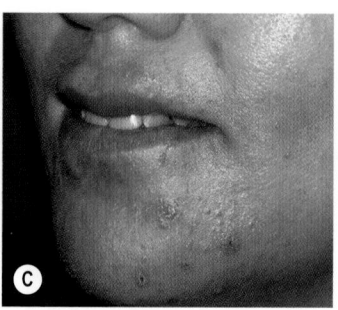 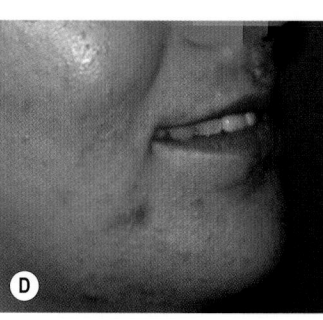

Fig. 2.29 At 3 months after repair of an avulsive lip wound **(A)** there is good orbicularis oris function and oral competence **(B)**, and an acceptable cosmetic result **(C,D)**.

Access the complete references list online at **http://www.expertconsult.com**

3. Chico-Ponce de Leon F, Ortiz-Monasterio F, et al. The dawn of plastic surgery in Mexico: XVIth century. *Plast Reconstr Surg.* 2003;111(6):2025–2031.

   This fascinating discussion on the state of plastic surgery in Mexico at the end of the Middle Ages and beginning of the Renaissance shows us that so much of what we view as "modern" plastic surgery and wound management was already standard teaching in the early 1500s in Mexico and Europe. The first American plastic surgeons in Mexico understood "the wounds of the face (have to be cured with extreme care because the face is a man's honor." They discuss correct suture placement, avoiding excess suture tension, and early suture removal for the best results. They also discuss nasal reconstruction with a cutaneous arm flap 18 years before Tagliacozzi. We are reminded that we stand on the shoulders of generations of surgeons who have come before us.

4. Hussain K, Wijetunge DB, Grubnic S, et al. A comprehensive analysis of craniofacial trauma. *J Trauma.* 1994;36(1):34–47.

   Craniofacial soft-tissue injuries occur most often on the forehead, nose, lips, and chin in a "T"-shaped zone. There is significant variability in the common causes of craniofacial trauma that can be stratified by sex and age. Falls are the most common cause in children and the elderly. Interpersonal violence and alcohol are associated with the majority of injuries in young men. Sports are a common cause of injury among youth. This article is a detailed review of craniofacial trauma patterns.

6. Leach J. Proper handling of soft tissue in the acute phase. *Facial Plast Surg.* 2001;17(4):227–238.

   An excellent overview of basic techniques for management of craniofacial soft tissue injuries, starting with initial evaluation, wound preparation and anesthetic techniques. The management of wound contamination, and steps to reduce the risk of infection are discussed. Planning of

difficult closures by respecting the resting skin tension lines is discussed. Wound undermining and specific suture techniques are discussed in detail.

12. Eaton JS, Grekin RC. Regional anesthesia of the face. *Dermatol Surg.* 2001;27(12):1006–1009.

    Successful regional blocks for facial trauma repair can often provide anesthesia for repair of larger facial wounds and provide initial anesthesia for later widespread infiltration of vasoconstricting agents. Successful regional anesthesia is based on a clear understanding of the anatomy. This article provides a detailed guide for success.

39. Zitelli JA. Secondary intention healing: an alternative to surgical repair. *Clin Dermatol.* 1984;2(3):92–106.

    This article reminds us that in cases of tissue loss secondary intention healing may produce acceptable outcomes in certain anatomic areas. The best cosmetic results are obtained on concave surfaces of the nose, eye, ear and temple (NEET areas), and those on the convex surfaces of the nose, oral lips, cheeks and chin, and helix of the ear (NOCH areas) often heal with a poor quality scar. Most wounds can be dressed with a semi-occlusive dressing, or petrolatum ointment to prevent desiccation. Common complications include: pigmentation changes, unstable scar, excessive granulation, pain, dysesthesias, and wound contracture.

51. Oishi SN, Luce EA. The difficult scalp and skull wound. *Clin Plast Surg.* 1995;22(1):51–59.

95. Beadles KA, Lessner AM. Management of traumatic eyelid lacerations. *Semin Ophthalmol.* 1994;9(3):145–151.

112. Punjabi AP, Haug RH, Jordan RB. Management of injuries to the auricle. *J Oral Maxillofac Surg.* 1997;55(7):732–739.

163. Stucker FJ, Hoasjoe DK. Soft tissue trauma over the nose. *Facial Plast Surg.* 1992;8(4):233–241.

179. Armstrong BD. Lacerations of the mouth. *Emerg Med Clin North Am.* 2000;18(3):471–480, vi.

3

Facial fractures

Eduardo D. Rodriguez, Amir H. Dorafshar, and Paul N. Manson

SYNOPSIS

- The teachings of John Converse, Nicholas Georgiade and Reed Dingman provided the benchmark for an entire generation of surgeons in facial injury repair.
- The treatment concepts discussed in this chapter were developed at the University of Maryland Shock Trauma Unit and ultimately employed at the International Center for Facial Injury Reconstruction at Johns Hopkins.
- The proportion of severe injuries seen at these centers is high.
- The treatment concepts, however, may be modified for common fractures and less significant injuries.
- Greater emphasis has been placed on minimizing operative techniques and limited exposures, whereas the decade of the eighties witnessed craniofacial principles of broad exposure and fixation at all buttresses for a particular fracture across all degrees of severity.
- Presently, the treatment of injuries is organized both by severity and anatomic area to permit the smallest exposure possible to achieve a good result (CT based facial fracture treatment).

 Access the Historical Perspective section and Fig. 3.1 online at **http://www.expertconsult.com**

Introduction

Over 4 million people are injured in automobile accidents in the United States yearly.[1] Statistics on the number of facial injuries vary widely based on social, economic and geographic differences. The causes of facial injuries in the United States include motor vehicle accidents, assaults, altercations, bicycle and motorcycle accidents, home and industrial accidents, domestic violence and athletic injuries. The automobile is frequently responsible for some of the most devastating facial injuries, and injuries to the head, face and cervical spine occur in over 50% of all victims. Seatbelts and airbags have reduced the severity and incidence of facial injury, but primary and secondary enforcement of the laws vary in effectiveness with ethnicity, education and geographic location.[2]

A unique aspect of facial injury treatment is that the aesthetic result may be the chief indication for treatment. In other cases, injuries may require surgery to restore function, but commonly, both goals are evident. Although there are few facial emergencies, the literature has under-emphasized the advantages of prompt definitive reconstruction and early operative intervention to achieve superior aesthetic and functional results. Economic, sociologic and psychologic factors operating in a competitive society make it imperative that an expedient and well-planned surgical correction be executed in order to return the patient to an active and productive life, while minimizing disability.

Initial assessment

Management begins with an initial physical examination and is followed by a radiologic evaluation accomplished with computerized tomographic (CT) scanning. CT scans must visualize soft tissue and bone. It is no longer feasible or economically justifiable to obtain plain radiographs with certain exceptions, such as the panorex mandible examination or dental films. The availability of regional Level I and II trauma centers has provided improved trauma care for severely or multiply-injured patients earlier and safer.

Timing of treatment

Timing is important in optimizing the management of facial injuries. Bone and soft tissue injuries in the facial area should be managed as soon as the patient's general condition permits. Time and time again it has been the authors' impression that early, skillful facial injury management decreases permanent facial disfigurement and limits serious functional disturbances.[3,4] This does not mean that one can be cavalier about deciding who might tolerate early operative intervention. Indeed, the skillful facial surgeon must have as complete a knowledge of their ancillary injuries as well as those of the face. Classically, facial soft tissue and bone injuries are not acute surgical emergencies, but both the ease of obtaining a good result and the quality of the result are better with early or immediate management. Less soft tissue stripping is required, bones are often easily replaced into their anatomic position and easier fracture repairs are performed. There are few patients, however, whose injuries cannot be definitively managed within a short time. Exceptions to acute treatment include patients with ongoing or significant blood loss (i.e., pelvic fractures), elevated intracranial pressures, coagulation problems, and abnormal pulmonary ventilation pressures. Under local anesthesia, however, lacerations are debrided and closed, IMF applied and grossly displaced fractures reduced. Many patients with mild brain injuries or multi-system traumas do not have criteria preventing operative management. These patients may receive facial injury management at the time that other injuries are being stabilized. Indeed it is not uncommon in the University of Maryland Shock Trauma Unit for several teams to operate on a patient at the same time in several anatomic areas.

Clinical examination of the face

A careful history and thorough clinical examination form the basis for the diagnosis of almost all facial injuries. Thorough examination of the face is indicated even if the patient has only minor wounds or abrasions. Abrasions, contusions and lacerations may be the most apparent symptom of an underlying fracture, which will surface later as a problem. A facial laceration may be the only sign of a penetrating injury to the eye, nose, ear or cranium. Lacerations may often be repaired during the treatment of other bodily injuries without the need for an additional operative session and should therefore not be deferred. Superficial lacerations or abrasions may leave disfiguring scars, despite their apparent inconsequential appearance if they are not adequately managed. Careful cleansing of all wounds, meticulous debridement, and a layered closure minimize conspicuous permanent deformity.

Blunt trauma craniofacial injuries

Bone injuries are suggested by soft tissue symptoms such as contusions, abrasions, ecchymosis, edema and distortion of the facial proportions. These symptoms prompt radiographic evaluation to confirm or exclude fractures. Subconjunctival hemorrhage with ecchymosis and edema of the orbit and a palpebral hematoma suggest a zygomatic or orbital fracture. Bilateral hematomas suggest Le Fort, nasal-ethmoid or anterior cranial fossa fractures. Ecchymotic, contused intra-oral tissue, loose teeth, and malocclusion suggest the possibility of a jaw fracture.

Facial bone fractures may be diagnosed on the basis of malocclusion or an open bite deformity due to fracture displacement involving the upper or the lower jaw. A fracture of the mandibular condyle for instance, may produce pain, deviation with motion to the side of the injury and inability to occlude the jaws properly. Pain with movement of the jaw (trismus) may result from a fracture of the zygoma or upper or lower jaw. Dystopia, enophthalmos, proptosis or diplopia

indicate zygomatic, orbital or maxillary fractures. A thorough palpation of all of the facial bones should be performed, systematically, checking for tenderness, crepitus or contour defects. An orderly examination of all facial structures should be accomplished, progressing from either superior to inferior or inferior to superior in a systematic fashion.

Symptoms and signs produced by facial injuries include: pain or localized tenderness; crepitation of bone movement; hypesthesia or anesthesia in the distribution of a sensory nerve; paralysis in the distribution of a motor nerve; malocclusion; visual acuity disturbance; diplopia; facial asymmetry; facial deformity; obstructed respiration; lacerations; bleeding and contusions. The clinical examination should begin with the evaluation for symmetry and deformity, inspecting the face comparing one side with the other. Palpation of all bony surfaces follows in an orderly manner. The forehead, orbital rims, nose, brows; zygomatic arches; malar eminence; and border of the mandible should be evaluated (Fig. 3.2). A thorough inspection of the intra-oral area should be made to detect lacerations, loose teeth or abnormalities of the dentition (Fig. 3.3). Palpation of the dental arches follows the inspection, noting mobility of dental-alveolar arch segments. The maxillary and mandibular dental arches are carefully visualized and palpated to detect an irregularity of the bone, loose teeth, intra-oral lacerations, bruising, hematoma, swelling, movement, tenderness or crepitus. An evaluation of sensory and motor nerve function in the facial area is performed. The presence of hypesthesia or anesthesia in the distribution of the supraorbital, infraorbital or mental nerves suggests a fracture along the bony path of these sensory nerves (cranial nerve V). Cutaneous branches of these nerves might have been interrupted by a facial laceration as well. ⊚ FIGS 3.2, 3.3 APPEAR ONLINE ONLY

Extraocular movements (cranial nerves III, IV and VI) and the muscles of facial expression (cranial nerve VII) are examined in the conscious, cooperative patient. Pupillary size and symmetry, speed of pupillary reaction, globe turgor, globe excursion, eyelid excursion, double vision and visual acuity and visual loss are noted. A funduscopic examination and measurements of globe pressure should be performed. The presence of a hyphema, corneal abrasion, visual field defect, visual loss, diplopia, decreased vision, or absent vision should be noted and appropriate consultation requested. A penetrating ocular injury or globe rupture should be suspected where any laceration in the eyelids or periorbital area is present. The presence of a periorbital hematoma with the eye swollen shut should not deter a clinician from examining the globe. It should be emphasized, however, that gentleness must be exercised to avoid extrusion of lens or vitreal contents through a globe laceration by vigorous manipulation. It is only by means of a thorough clinical examination that globe ruptures and penetrating globe injuries are not missed. The excursion and deviation of the jaws with motion, the presence of pain upon opening the jaw, the relationship of the teeth, the ability of the patient to bring the teeth into occlusion, the symmetry of the dental arches and the proper intercuspal dental relationship are important clues to the diagnosis of fractures involving the dentition. One finger in the ear canal and another over the condylar head can detect condylar movement, or crepitus either by patient movement or when the jaw is pulled forward (Fig. 3.4). The presence of a gingival laceration or a fractured or missing tooth or a split alveolus should imply the possibility of more significant maxillary or mandibular injuries, which must be confirmed by CT. Fractures of the mandible may be detected by pulling the jaw forward or by applying manual pressure on the anterior portion of the mandible while supporting the angle. Instability, crepitus and pain may be noted when this maneuver is performed. Edema and hemorrhage may mask the perception of facial asymmetry. Bleeding from laceration of vessels accompanying facial fractures may disguise a cerebrospinal fluid leak. Bleeding or fluid draining from the ear canal may indicate a laceration in the ear canal, a condylar dislocation, or a middle cranial fossa fracture with a CSF leak. Bleeding from the nose may indicate nasal or septal injuries, Le Fort, nasoethmoidal, or orbital fractures or anterior cranial fossa fractures. Mobility of the middle-third of the facial skeleton indicates a fracture of the Le Fort type (*Fig. 3.5*). Anterior or cribriform plate fractures or middle basilar skull fractures should be suspected when CSF rhinorrhea is present. Central nervous system injury is implied by paralysis of one or more of the cranial nerves, impaired consciousness, depressed sensorium, unequal pupillary size, extremity paralysis, abnormal neurological reflexes, convulsions, delirium, or irrational behavior. ⓔ FIG **3.4**, **3.5** APPEAR ONLINE ONLY

Computerized tomographic scans

The definitive radiographic evaluation is the craniofacial CT scan with axial, coronal and sagittal sections of bone and soft tissue windows.[5–7] However, the clinical examination remains the most sensitive detection of the character and functional implications of the facial injury.

CT evaluation of the face can define bone fractures, whereas, the soft tissue views allow for soft tissue definition of the area of the fracture. 3D CT Scans[8–10] allow comparison of symmetry and volume of the two sides of the facial bones. Specialized views, such as those of the orbital apex, allow for a special magnified visualization. Fractures missed in CT scans are those in which there is little or no bony displacement or films where reading occurs from soft tissue views or thicker cuts.

Upper facial fractures

Frontal bone and sinus injury patterns

The frontal sinuses are paired structures that have only an ethmoidal anlage at birth. They have no frontal bone component initially. They begin to be detected at 3 years of age, but significant pneumatic expansion does not begin to occur until approximately age 7 years. The full development of the frontal sinuses is complete by the age of 18–20.[11] The frontal sinuses are lined with respiratory epithelium, which consists of a ciliated membrane with mucus secreting glands. A blanket of mucin is essential for normal function and the cilia beat this mucin in the direction of the nasofrontal ducts. The exact function of the paranasal sinuses is still incompletely determined. When injured, they serve as a focus for infection, especially if duct function is impaired. Their structure, however, often protects the intracranial contents from injury by absorbing energy.

The predominant form of frontal sinus injury is fracture. Fracture involvement of the frontal sinus has been estimated to occur in 2–12% of all cranial fractures and severe fractures occur in 0.7–2% of patients with cranial or cerebral trauma.[11]

Approximately one-third of fractures involve the anterior table alone, and 60% involve the anterior table and posterior table and/or ducts. The remainder involves the posterior wall alone. Some 40% of frontal sinus fractures have an accompanying dural laceration.[11]

Clinical examination

Lacerations, bruises, hematomas, and contusions constitute the most frequent signs of frontal bone or sinus fractures. Skull fractures must be suspected if any of these signs are present. Anesthesia of the supraorbital nerve may be present. Cerebrospinal fluid rhinorrhea may occur. There may or may not be subconjunctival or periorbital ecchymoses with or without air in the orbit or intracranial cavity. In some cases, a depression may be observed over the frontal sinus, but swelling is usually predominant in the first few days after the injury, which may obscure the underlying bony deformity.

Small fractures of the frontal sinus may be difficult to detect, especially if they are nondisplaced. Therefore, occasionally the first presentation of a frontal sinus fracture may be an infection or symptom of frontal sinus obstruction, such as mucocele, or abscess formation.[12,13] Infection in the frontal sinus have the potential to cause significant morbidity due to its proximity to the brain location near the brain.[14] Infections include meningitis, extradural or intradural abscess, intracranial abscess, osteomyelitis of the frontal bone, or osteitis in devitalized bone fragments.[15–23]

Nasofrontal duct

The development of a frontal sinus mucocele is linked to obstruction of the nasofrontal duct,[1] which is involved with fractures in over nearly half of the cases of frontal sinus injury. The duct passes through the anterior ethmoidal air cells to exit adjacent to the ethmoidal infundibulum. Blockage of the nasofrontal duct prevents adequate drainage of the normal mucosal secretions and predisposes to the development of obstructive epithelial lined cysts or mucoceles. Mucoceles[24–26] may also develop when islands of mucosa are trapped by scar tissue within fracture lines and attempt to grow after the injury producing a mucus membrane lined cystic structure which is obstructed.

The sinus is completely obliterated only when the duct is also deprived of its lining and when the bone is burred, eliminating the foramina of Breschet,[27] in which it has been demonstrated that mucosal ingrowth occurs along veins in the walls of the sinuses.[28,29] Regrowth of mucosa can also occur from any portion of the frontal sinus, especially if incompletely debrided. The reported average interval between the primary injury and development of frontal sinus mucocele is 7.5 years.

Radiography

Frontal bone and sinus fractures are best demonstrated using CT Scans. Hematomas or air fluid levels in the frontal sinus may be visualized as well as potential injuries to the nasofrontal duct. Persisting air-fluid levels can imply the absence of duct function.

Surgical treatment

The best technique of exposure in major fractures involving the frontal bone is the coronal incision. This allows a combined intracranial and extracranial approach, making visualization of all areas possible, including repair of dural tears, debridement of any necrotic sections of frontal lobe, and repair of the bone structures.

Frontal sinus fractures should be characterized by describing both the anatomic location of the fractures and their displacement. The indications for surgical intervention in frontal sinus fractures include depression of the anterior table, radiographic demonstration of involvement of the nasofrontal duct with presumed future nonfunction, obstruction of the duct with persistent air fluid levels, mucocele formation, and fractures of the posterior table that are displaced and presumably have lacerated the dura.[30,31] Some authors recommend exploration of any posterior table fracture or any fracture in which an air fluid level is visible. Others have a more selective approach, exploring posterior wall fractures only if their displacement exceeds the width of the posterior table. This distance suggests simultaneous dural laceration. Simple linear fractures of the anterior and posterior sinus walls which are undisplaced are observed by many clinicians.

Any depressed frontal sinus fracture of the anterior wall potentially requires exploration and wall replacement in an anatomical position to prevent contour deformity. Most of these patients will have no compromise of nasofrontal duct function, however, some do and these should have the sinus defunctionalized. The anterior wall of the sinus may be explored by an appropriate local laceration or a coronal incision, or more recently endoscopically. Anterior wall fragments are elevated and plated into position. If it is desired that the nasofrontal duct[32–34] and sinus be obliterated because of involvement, the mucosa is thoroughly stripped, even into the recesses of the sinus, and the nasofrontal ducts occluded with well-designed "formed-to-fit" calvarial bone plugs *(Fig. 3.6)*. If most of the posterior bony wall is intact, the entire frontal sinus cavity may be filled either with fat or cancellous bone. The iliac crest provides a generous source of rich cancellous bone.[35] Alternatively, the cavity may be left vacant, a process called "osteoneogenesis". The cavity fills slowly with a combination of bone and fibrous tissue, but is more frequently

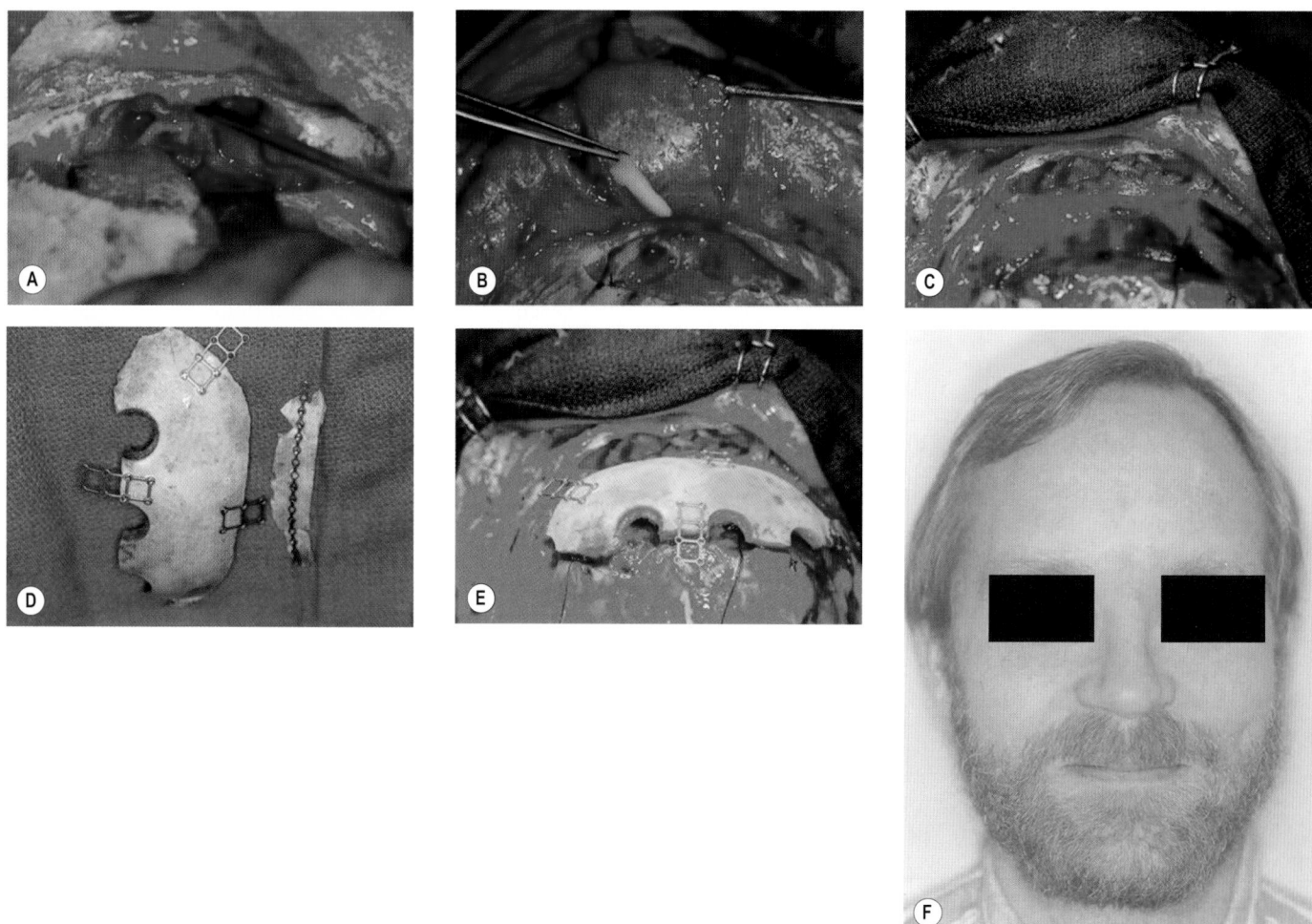

Fig. 3.6 (A) Nasofrontal duct. **(B)** Bone plug for nasofrontal duct and galeal flap. **(C)** Bone obliteration of frontal sinus. **(D)** "Back table" surgery for bone replacement. **(E)** Bone reconstruction and cranialization of the frontal sinus; intracranial neurosurgery. **(F)** Postoperative result.

infected in the authors' experience than sinuses treated with cavity filling.[36]

If the posterior table is missing, no grafting need be performed for localized defects, but it is emphasized that the floor of the anterior cranial fossa should be reconstructed with bone. In cranialization, the posterior wall of the frontal sinus is removed, effectively making the frontal sinus a part of the intracranial cavity. The "dead space" may be filled with cancellous bone[37] or left open. Any communication with the nose by the nasofrontal duct or with the ethmoid sinuses should be sealed with carefully designed bone grafts. The orbital roof should be reconstructed primarily by thin bone grafts placed external to the orbital cavity. An intracranial exposure is often required for this orbital roof reconstruction.

The use of a galeal flap[38,39] in the treatment of extensive frontal bone defects designed with a pedicle of the superficial temporal artery can be a useful method for vascularized soft tissue obliteration of frontal bone problems.

Complications

Complications of frontal bone and sinus fractures include:
- CSF fluid rhinorrhea
- Pneumocephalus and orbital emphysema
- Absence of orbital roof and pulsating exophthalmos
- Carotid-cavernous sinus fistula.

Orbital fractures

Orbital fractures may occur as isolated fractures of the internal orbit (also called "pure") or may involve both the internal orbit and the orbital rim (also called "impure") *(Fig. 3.7)*.[40–42]

Surgical anatomy of the orbit

In fracture treatment, the orbits are conceptualized in thirds progressing from anterior to posterior. Anteriorly, the orbital rims consist of thick bone. The middle-third of the orbit consists of thin bone and the bone structure thickens again in the posterior portion of the orbit. The orbital bone structure is thus analogous to a "shock-absorbing" device in which the middle portion of the orbit breaks first, followed by the rim.

The optic foramen is situated at the junction of the lateral and medial walls of the orbit posteriorly and is well above the horizontal plane of the orbital floor. The foramen is located 40–45 mm behind the inferior orbital rim.

Orbital physical examination

The examination should detect edema, corneal abrasion, laceration, contusion and hematoma. The simultaneous presence of a subconjunctival hematoma and a periorbital hematoma

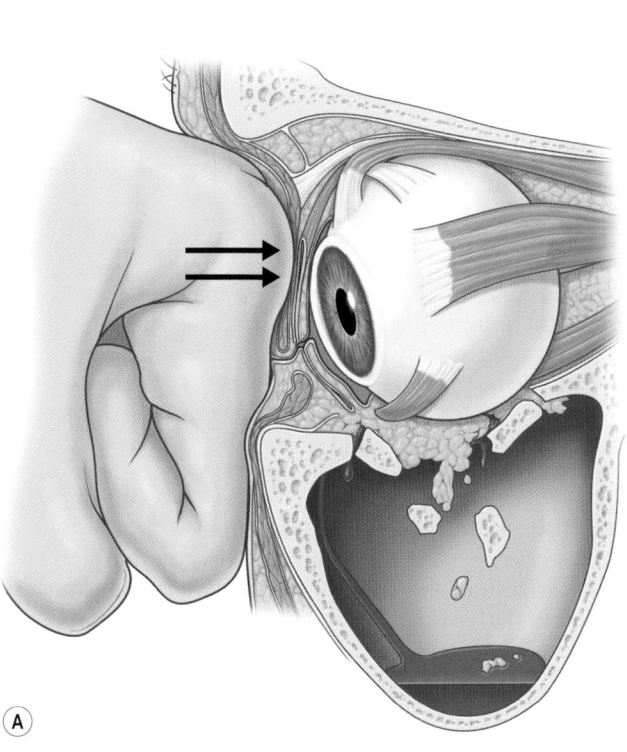

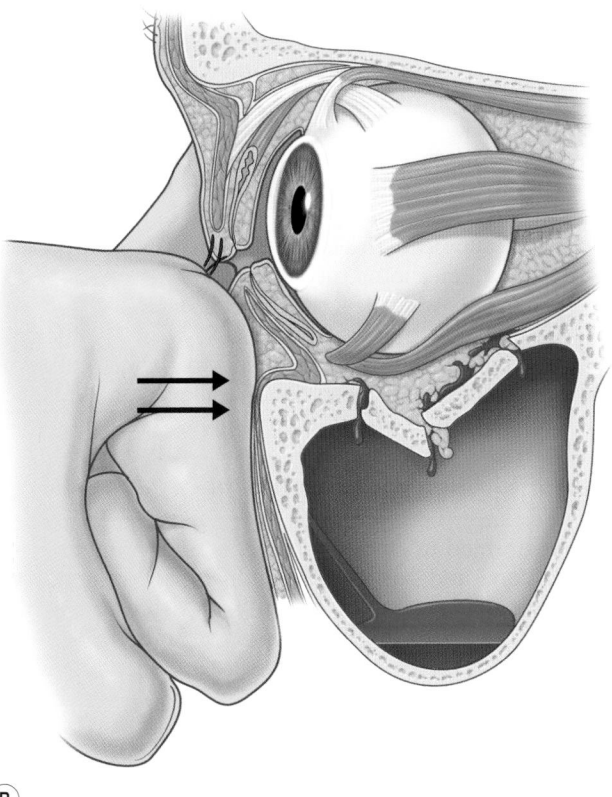

(A)   (B)

Fig. 3.7 (A) Mechanism of blow-out fracture from displacement of the globe itself into the orbital walls. The globe is displaced posteriorly, striking the orbital walls and forcing them outward, causing a "punched out" fracture the size of the globe. **(B)** "Force transmission" fracture of orbital floor.

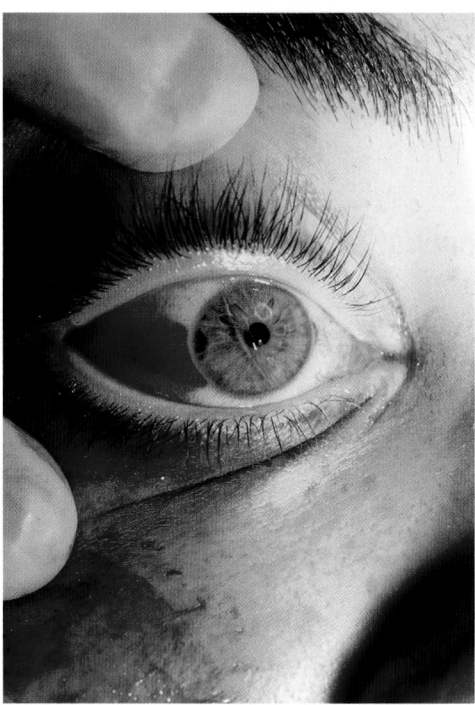

Fig. 3.8 The combination of a palpebral and subconjunctival hematoma is suggestive of a fracture somewhere within the orbit. There is frequently a zygomatic or orbital floor fracture present when these signs are confirmed.

confined to the distribution of the orbital septum is evidence of a facial fracture involving the orbit until proven otherwise by radiographs *(Fig. 3.8)*. The extraocular movements should note double vision or restricted globe movement. Visual acuity may be recorded by the patient's ability to read newsprint or an ophthalmic examination card such as the Rosenbaum® Pocket card. Visual field examinations should be performed. All patients must be frequently checked for light perception and pupillary afferent defects preoperatively and postoperatively. Globe pressure may be assessed by tonometry and should be less than 15 mm. The results of a fundus examination should be recorded. The presence of no light perception indicates optic nerve damage or globe rupture. Light perception without usable vision indicates optic nerve damage, retinal detachment, hyphema, vitreous hemorrhage or anterior or posterior chamber injuries. Globe and eye injuries require expert ophthalmologic consultation.

Radiographic evidence of fracture

CT scans performed in the axial, coronal and sagittal planes, using both bone and soft tissue windows, are essential to define the anatomy of the orbital walls and soft tissue contents, and the relation of the extraocular muscles to the fracture.

Indications for surgical treatment

The indications for surgical treatment include:
- Double vision caused by incarceration of muscle or the fine ligament system, documented by forced duction examination and suggested by CT scans.

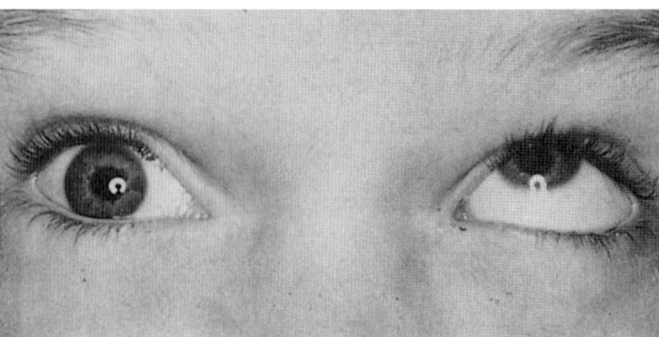

Fig. 3.9 Blow-out fracture in a child produced by a snowball. Note the nearly complete immobility of the ocular globe and the enophthalmos. Such severe loss of motion implies actual muscle incarceration, an injury that is more frequent in children than in adults. This fracture deserves *immediate* operation with release of the incarcerated extraocular muscle system. It is often accompanied by pain on attempted rotation of the globe and sometimes nausea and vomiting. These symptoms are unusual in orbital floor fractures without true muscle incarceration.

- Radiographic evidence of extensive fracture, such that enophthalmos would occur.
- Enophthalmos or exophthalmos (significant globe positional change) produced by an orbital volume change.
- Visual acuity deficit, increasing and not responsive to medical dose steroids, implying that optic canal decompression would be indicated.
- "Blow-in" orbital fractures that involve the medial or lateral walls of the orbit, and severely constrict orbital volume, creating increased intraorbital pressure.

Blow-out fractures of the floor of the orbit

A blow-out fracture is caused by the application of a traumatic force to the rim, globe or soft tissues of the orbit. Blow-out fractures are generally assumed to be accompanied by a sudden increase in intraorbital pressure.

Blow-out fractures in younger individuals

In children, the mechanism of entrapment is more frequently trapdoor than the "blow-out or punched out" fracture seen in adults. As opposed to incarceration of fat adjacent to the inferior rectus muscle, children more frequently "scissor" or capture the muscle directly in the fracture site. This may be suggested on physical examination with near immobility of the eye when upgaze is attempted on the affected side *(Fig. 3.9)*. Trapdoor fractures with actual muscle incarceration are an *urgent* situation that demands *immediate* release of the incarcerated muscle.[43–47] A number of authors have recently emphasized that a better prognosis is possible if the muscle is released early. The patient with true muscle entrapment may experience pain on attempted eye motion as well as nausea, vomiting, and an oculocardiac reflex,[48] which consists of nausea, bradycardia, and hypotension.

Surgical treatment

The surgical treatment of orbital fractures has three goals:
- Disengage entrapped structures and restore ocular rotatory function.

- Replace orbital contents into the usual confines of the normal bony orbital cavity, including restoration of both orbital *volume* and *shape*.
- Restore orbital cavity walls, which in effect replaces the tissues into their proper position and dictates the shape into which the soft tissue can scar.

The timing of surgical intervention

In isolated blow-out fractures, it is not necessary to operate immediately unless true muscle incarceration or severe restriction of limitation is present. In the presence of significant edema, retinal detachment or other significant globe injuries, such as hyphema, it is advisable to wait a number of days.

Significant orbital fractures are best treated by early surgical intervention. The authors firmly believe that the earlier significant orbital volume or muscle derangement can be corrected, the better the aesthetic and functional result.

Operative technique for orbital fractures

Endoscopic approaches for orbital floor fractures

Recently, endoscopic approaches through the maxillary sinus have permitted direct visualization of the orbital floor and manipulation of the soft tissue and floor repair with this approach, which avoids an eyelid incision *(Fig. 3.10)*.[49–52] ⊛ FIG **3.10** APPEARS ONLINE ONLY

Cutaneous exposures

A number of incisions have been employed to approach the orbital floor:

- Lower eyelid incision. These have the least incidence of lower eyelid ectropion of any lid incision location but tend to be the most noticeable and prone to lymphedema.[53–55]
- Subciliary skin muscle flap incision. This incision near the upper margin of the lid leaves the least conspicuous cutaneous scar.[56–58] However, they are prone to have the highest incidence of lid retraction.
- Transconjunctival incision. A preseptal or retroseptal dissection plane can be established.

Surgical treatment

Generally, a corneal protector is placed over the eye to protect the globe and cornea from instruments, retractors or rotating drills. The inferior rectus muscle, the orbital fat and any orbital soft tissue structures should be carefully dissected free from the areas of the blow-out fracture. Intact orbital floor must be located around all the edges of the displaced "blow-out" fracture. The floor must be explored sufficiently far back into the orbit that the posterior edge of the intact orbital floor beyond any defect can be identified. Many individuals call this "the ledge", and it may be the orbital process of the palatine bone. Placing a freer periosteal elevator into the maxillary sinus and feeling the back of the sinus can verify the position of "the ledge". The "ledge" is located just above the back of the maxillary sinus 35–38 mm behind the orbital rim.

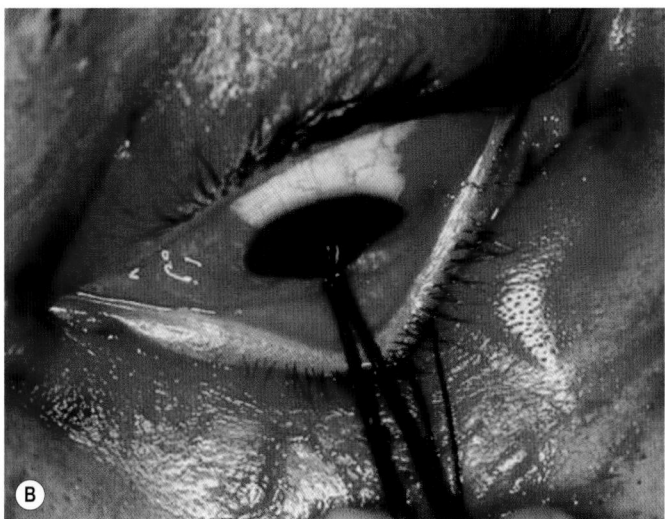

Fig. 3.11 The forced duction test. **(A)** Forceps grasp the ocular globe at the insertion of the inferior rectus muscle, which is approximately 7–10 mm from the limbus. **(B)** Clinical photograph. A drop of local anesthetic instilled into the conjunctival sac precedes the procedure.

Identification of the intact "ledge" may be verified on CT scan (best shown on sagittal images).[59,60] The "ledge" is the anatomical mark for which the implant material should be landed posteriorly to reestablish continuity of the orbital floor.

The forced duction test

Limitation of forced rotation of the eyeball is the *"forced duction"* test or the *"eyeball traction"* test *(Fig. 3.11)*. This test provides a means of differentiating entrapment of the extraocular muscles from weakness, paralysis or contusion. The forced duction test should be performed: (1) before dissection; (2) after dissection; (3) after the insertion of each material used to reconstruct the orbital wall; (4) just prior to closure of the incisions. It is vital that these measurements be compared. It is absolutely imperative that any reconstructive material does not interfere with globe movement in any way, and it is absolutely essential to prove this before any incisions are closed. A full range of all oculo-rotatory movements must accompany restoration of proper eye position.

Restoration of continuity of the orbital floor

The purpose of the orbital floor replacement, whether a bone graft or an inorganic implant, is to *reestablish the volume and the **shape** of the orbital cavity*. This replaces the orbital soft tissue contents and allows scar tissue to form in an anatomic position *(Fig. 3.12)*.

Bone grafts for orbital floor reconstruction

Split calvarial, iliac, or split rib bone grafts provide the ideal physiological substitute material for reconstruction of the internal orbital fractures.[61,62] It is not known whether bone grafts resist bacterial colonization better than inorganic implants, but that is the presumption. Bone grafts are presumed to survive at the 50–80% level.

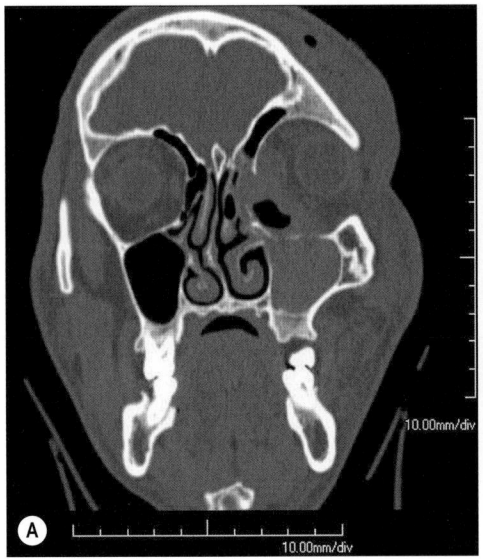
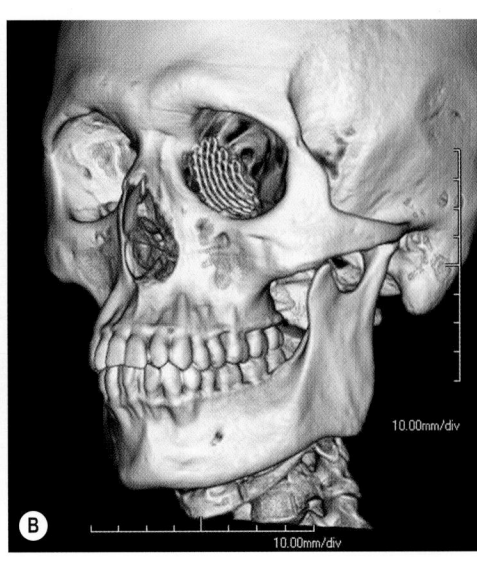

Fig. 3.12 Medial orbital wall fracture.
(A) Coronal CT scan image illustrating medial orbital wall fracture. **(B)** Postoperative three-dimensional CT scan demonstrating repair of medial orbital wall repair using titanium alloplastic mesh implant.

Inorganic implants

The inorganic implant offers the advantage of obtaining the material necessary for the reconstruction of the orbital floor without the need for a second operation for bone graft harvest. Inorganic implants are certainly satisfactory for limited size defect orbital fractures, and some authors utilize titanium mesh alone for large defects where stabilization of a bone graft becomes impractical. The incidence of late infection is certainly less than 1%, and displacement should not occur if the material has been properly anchored.

Postoperative care

All patients must be frequently checked for light perception preoperatively and postoperatively. Pupillary reactivity must be accessed before and after orbital surgery and at least twice daily for the first several days. Blindness has sometimes occurred more than 24 hours following orbital fracture treatment.

Complications of orbital fractures

Diplopia

Extraocular muscle imbalance and subjective diplopia are usually the result of muscle contusion, but can be the result of incarceration of either the muscle or the soft tissue adjacent to the muscles, or result of nerve damage to the third, fourth, and sixth cranial nerves.[63–65]

Enophthalmos

Enophthalmos,[66–70] the second major complication of a blowout fracture, has a number of causes. The major cause is enlargement of the orbital volume with herniation of the orbital soft tissue structures into an enlarged cavity. This allows soft tissue structural displacement with a remodeling of the shape of the soft tissue into a sphere. Another postulated mechanism of enophthalmos is the cicatricial retraction

of the globe. A popular theory was fat atrophy, but computerized volume studies shown prove that fat atrophy is only significant in 10% of orbital fractures.

Retrobulbar hematoma

In severe trauma, retrobulbar hematoma may displace the ocular globe. Retrobulbar hematoma is signaled by globe proptosis, congestion and prolapse of the edematous conjunctiva. Diagnosis is confirmed by a CT scan imaged with soft tissue windows and is treated by lateral canthotomy. It is usually not possible to drain retrobulbar hematomas as they are diffuse. They may not permit, if large in volume, primary restoration of the bony volume of the orbit and one may have to complete the internal portion of the orbital reconstruction several weeks later when the hemorrhage, swelling and congestion have subsided.

Ocular (globe) injuries and blindness

The incidence of ocular injuries following orbital fractures is between 14% and 30%.[71] The incidence depends on the scrutiny of the examination and the recognition of minor injuries, such as corneal abrasion. Ocular globe injury may vary in severity from a corneal abrasion to loss of vision to globe rupture, retinal detachment, vitreous hemorrhage, or a fracture involving the optic canal. Blindness, or loss of an eye, is remarkably infrequent, despite the severity of some of the injuries sustained because of the "shock absorber" type construction of the orbit. The incidence of blindness following facial fracture repair has been estimated to be about 0.2%.[72]

Implant migration, late hemorrhage around implants and implant fixation

Migration of an implant anteriorly may occur with extrusion if the implant is not secured to the orbital floor or to a plate that attaches to the rim. Spontaneous late proptosis can be caused by hemorrhage from long standing low grade infection around orbital implants or obstruction of the lacrimal system.[73]

Ptosis of the upper lid

True ptosis of the upper lid should be differentiated from "pseudoptosis" resulting from the downward displacement of the eyeball in enophthalmos. True ptosis results from loss of action of the levator palpebrae superioris. Ptosis in the presence of enophthalmos should not be treated until the globe position has been stabilized by enophthalmos correction.

Scleral show, ectropion and entropion: vertical shortening of the lower eyelid

Vertical shortening of the lower eyelid with exposure of the sclera below the limbus of the globe in the primary gaze (scleral show) may result from downward and backward displacement of the fractured inferior orbital rim. The septum and lower lid are "fixed length" structures and are therefore dragged downward by their tendency to adhere to the abnormally positioned orbital rim. Release of the septum orbitale attachment to the orbital rim and restoration of the position of the orbital rim by osteotomy may be required.

Lid lamellae and their relation to contracture

The problem should be defined as occurring in "anterior lid lamellae" (skin or orbicularis) or "posterior lid lamellae" (septum, lower lid retractors and conjunctiva) and a plan for operative intervention developed. Only in the actual performance of the operation can the surgeon define the true nature of the problem, release the adhesions and stabilize the lid with appropriate grafts. These procedures generally do not elevate the lower lid by more than 3 mm.

Infraorbital nerve anesthesia

Infraorbital nerve anesthesia is extremely disconcerting to patients who experience it, especially initially. The area of sensory loss usually extends from the lower lid to involve the medial cheek, the lateral portion of the nose, including the ala and the ipsilateral upper lip. The anterior maxillary teeth may be involved if the branch of the infraorbital nerve in the anterior maxillary wall is involved. Decompression of the infraorbital nerve from pressure of the bony fragments within the infraorbital canal may be indicated either acutely or late after fracture treatment especially if the zygoma demonstrates medial displacement into the infraorbital canal with impaction into the nerve.

The "superior orbital fissure" syndrome and the "orbital apex" syndrome

Significant fractures of the orbital roof extend posteriorly to involve the superior orbital fissure and optic foramen. Involvement of the structures of the superior orbital fissure produces a symptom complex known as the superior orbital fissure syndrome.[74,75] This consists of partial or complete involvement of the following structures: the two divisions of the cranial nerve III, superior and inferior, producing paralysis of the levator, superior rectus, inferior rectus, and inferior oblique muscles; cranial nerve IV causing paralysis of the superior oblique muscle; cranial nerve VI producing paralysis of the lateral rectus muscle; and the ophthalmic division of the trigeminal nerve (V) causing anesthesia in the brow, medial portion of the upper lid, medial upper nose, and ipsilateral forehead. All symptoms of the superior orbital fissure syndrome may be partial or complete in each of the nerves. When accompanied by visual acuity change or blindness, the injury implies concomitant involvement of the combined superior orbital fissure (CN III, IV, V & VI) and optic foramen (CN II). If involvement of both the optic nerve and superior orbital fissure occur, this symptom complex is called the orbital apex syndrome.[76]

Midfacial fractures

Nasal fractures

Types and locations of nasal fractures

Lateral forces,[77] account for the majority of nasal fractures and produce a wide variation of deformities, depending on the age of the patient, intensity and vector of force. Younger patients tend to have fracture dislocations of larger segments, whereas older patients with more dense, brittle bone often exhibit comminution. Kazanjian and Converse[78] and Murray and associates[79] confirmed that most nasal fractures occur in thin portions of the nasal bone. In the Kazanjian and Converse series, 80% of a series of 190 nasal fractures occurred at the junction of the thick and thin portions of the nasal bones. A direct force of moderate intensity from the lateral side may fracture only one nasal bone with displacement into the nasal cavity (plane I). When forces are of increased intensity, some displacement of the contralateral nasal bone occurs and the fracture may be incomplete or greensticked, requiring completion of the fracture to centralize the nasal processes (plane II). In more severe (plane III) frontal impact injuries, the frontal process of the maxilla may begin to fracture and may be depressed on one side. This depression first arises at the pyriform aperture and then involves the entire structure of the frontal process of the maxilla, and is in effect the beginning of a hemi-nasoethmoidal fracture, displaced inferiorly and posteriorly (plane III "lateral impact" fractures are identical to "Type I" hemi-nasoethmoidal fractures) (Fig. 3.13). These fractures are "greensticked" at the internal angular process of the frontal bone and most of the displacement is inferior. The sidewall of the nose drops on one side, the septum telescopes and displaces and the nasal airway is effectively closed on the ipsilateral side by the septum and sidewall displacing towards each other. In stronger blows, the septum begins to collapse from an anteroposterior perspective as the comminution increases. The medial displacement of the pyriform aperture into the nose effectively blocks the ipsilateral nasal airway. As anteroposterior blows result in decreased stability, the septum "telescopes" losing height and the nasal bridge drops. Violent blows result in multiple fractures of the nasal bones and frontal processes of the maxilla, lacrimal bone, septal cartilages and the ethmoidal areas, the nasoethmoidal orbital fracture.

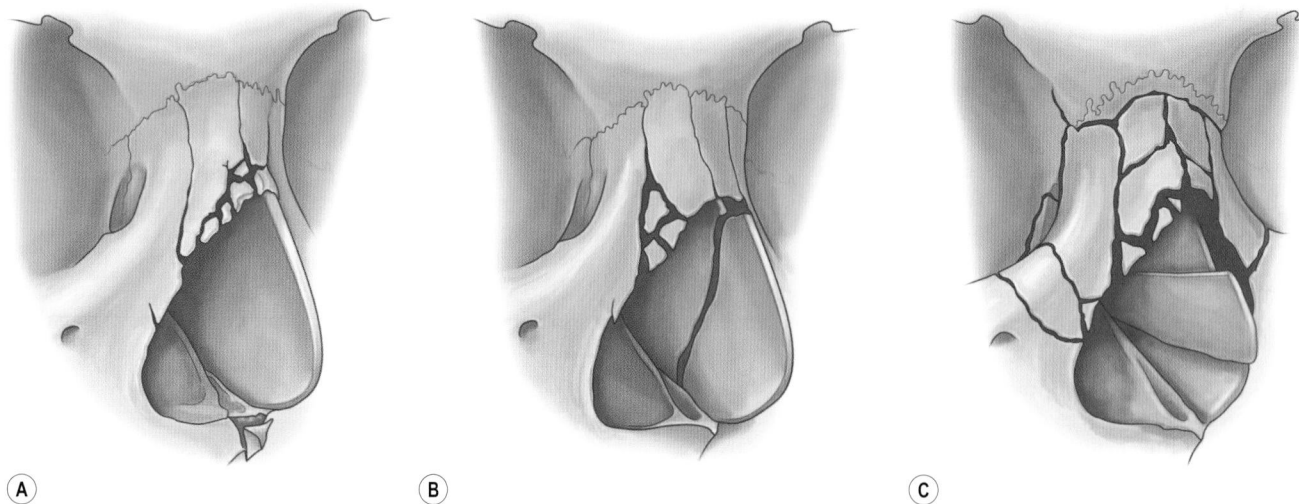

Fig. 3.13 Frontal impact nasal fractures are classified by degrees of displacement, as are lateral fractures. **(A)** Plane I frontal impact nasal fracture. Only the distal ends of the nasal bones and the septum are injured. **(B)** Plane II frontal impact nasal fracture. The injury is more extensive, involving the entire distal portion of the nasal bones and the frontal process of the maxilla at the piriform aperture. The septum is comminuted and begins to lose height. **(C)** Plane III frontal impact nasal fractures involve one or both frontal processes of the maxilla, and the fracture extends to the frontal bone. These fractures are in reality nasoethmoidal-orbital fractures because they involve the lower two-thirds of the medial orbital rim (central fragment of the nasoethmoidal-orbital fracture), as well as the bones of the nose.

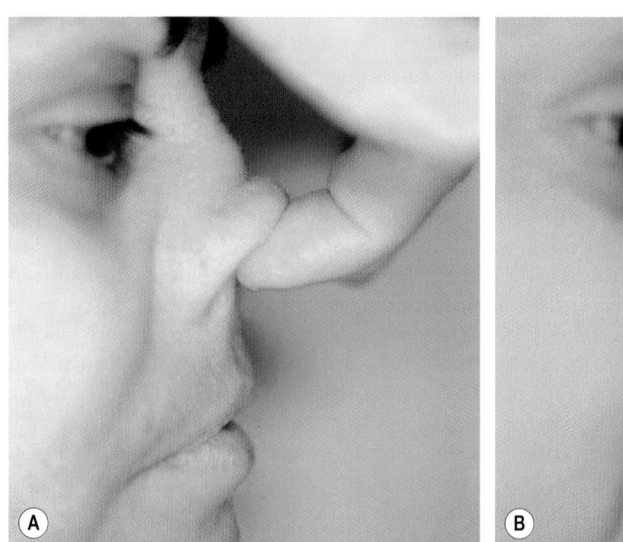
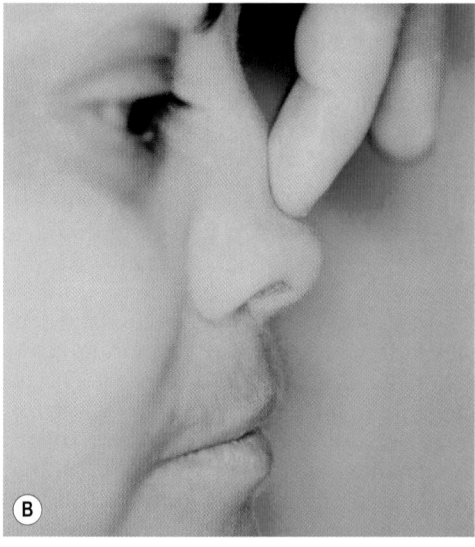

Fig. 3.14 Palpation of the columella **(A)** and dorsum **(B)** detects superior rotation of the septum and lack of dorsal support. There is an absence of columellar support and dorsal septal support.

Fractures and dislocations of the nasal septum

Fractures and dislocations of the septum may occur independently or concomitantly with fractures of the distal nasal bone framework. Most commonly, the two injuries occur together but frontal impact nasal fractures carry the worst prognosis regarding preservation of nasal height *(Fig. 3.14)*.[80] Because of the intimate association of the bones of the nose with the nasal cartilages and bony nasal septum, it is unusual to observe fractures of either structure without damage to the other. In particular, the caudal or cartilaginous portion of the septum is almost always injured in nasal fractures.[81]

The caudal portion of the septum has a degree of flexibility and bends to absorb moderate impact. The first stage of nasal septal injury is fracturing and bending, and the next stage involves overlap between fragments which reduces nasal

height. In mid level severity injuries, the septum fractures, often initially with a C-shaped or double transverse component in which the septum is fractured and dislocated out of the vomerine groove.[82]

Displacement of the fractured segment occurs with partial obstruction of the nasal airway. The cartilage may be fractured in any plane, but the most frequent location of the fracture is that described with horizontal and vertical components separating the anterior and posterior portions of the septum. As the cartilage heals, it can exhibit progressive deviation with warping forces due to the stresses created by the perichondrium.[83–86] Cartilage is thought to possess an inherent springiness, which internal stresses are released when tearing of the perichondrium on one side of the cartilage occurs. If the perichondrium and cartilage are torn, the septum deviates away from the torn area toward the intact perichondrial side.

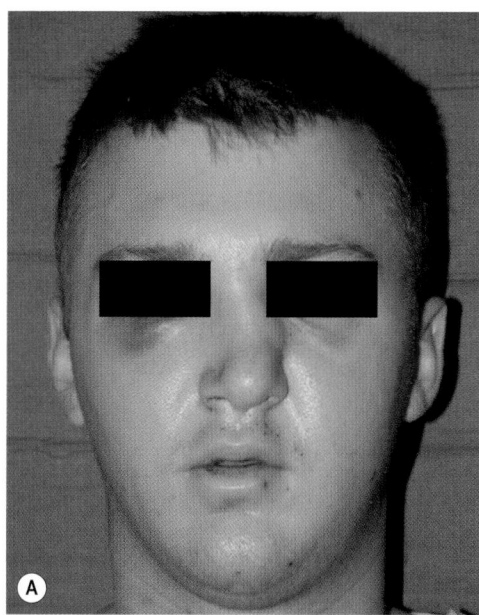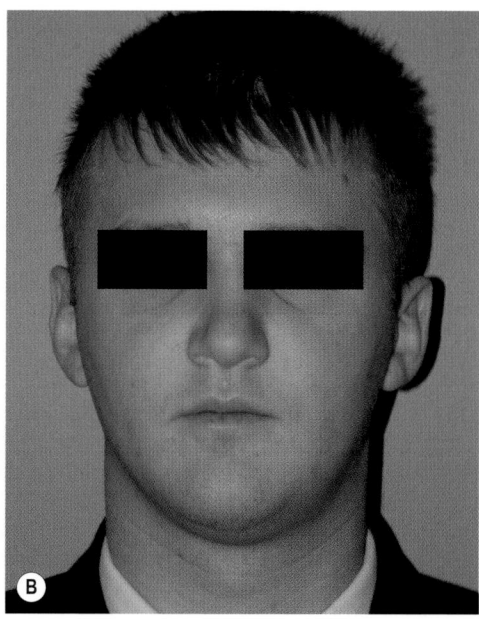

Fig. 3.16 (A) Preoperative and **(B)** postoperative images of a 20-year-old male who sustained a Le Fort II type injury during a wrestling match.

Severe fractures of the septum are additionally associated with "telescoping" displacement, resulting in a collapse with a "Z-shaped" overlapping and displacement of the septum.[87] The septum is shortened, giving rise to a retruded appearance in profile of the cartilage and also the columellar portion of the nose. Slight loss of the dorsal nasal height can give rise to a nasal hump, at the junction of the septum with the nasal bones.

The treatment of nasal fractures

Most nasal fractures are initially reduced by closed reduction *(Fig. 3.15)*. In more severe frontal impacts where loss of nasal height and length occurs, particularly in Plane II or nasoethmoidal orbital fractures, the use of open reduction and primary bone or cartilage grafting is beneficial to restore the support of the nose to its original volume, filling the original soft tissue envelope preventing soft tissue contracture *(Fig. 3.16)*.[88] It is helpful to perform a closed reduction before edema prevents accurate palpation and visual inspection to confirm the reduction. ⊛ FIG **3.15** APPEARS ONLINE ONLY

Open reduction and the use of supporting K wires

In severe nasal injury (i.e., plane II nasal injury), open reduction with bone or cartilage grafting to restore nasal height may be required. Semi-closed reductions[89] may be performed with limited incisions using small K wires to stabilize the nasal bones.[90,91] Internal splinting[92] may be required. Some nasal fractures are sufficiently dislocated that they can only be stabilized with an open rhinoplasty reduction.[93,94]

In practice, closed reduction of most nasal fractures is frequently deferred until the edema has partially subsided and the accuracy of the reduction may be confirmed by visual inspection and palpation.[95]

Treatment may be postponed for 5–7 days when required. After 2 weeks, it becomes more difficult to reduce a nasal fracture, as partial healing in malalignment has occurred and soft tissue contracture has occurred.

Treatment of fractures and dislocations of the septum

The nasal septum should be straightened and repositioned as soon after the injury as possible. When fractures of the nasal bones and septum occur simultaneously, it is important to ensure that at the time of reduction, the bone fragments can be freely deviated in all directions to ensure completion of the fractures. In terms of the nasal bones, they should be able to be deviated freely in both lateral directions to indicate satisfactory completion of any "greensticked" fractures. Incomplete fractures will cause the nasal bones to slowly "spring" back toward their original deviated position. When the reduction is incomplete, there is early recurrence of displacement. This is true for both the nasal bones and septum. When the nasal bones are reduced, the intimate relationship of the nasal bones with the upper and lower lateral cartilages tends to reduce the upper septal cartilage as well. Displacement of the cartilaginous septum out of the vomerine groove will not be reduced with nasal bone reduction alone. The correction of the position of the bony and cartilaginous septum must be completed with an Asch forceps, and the septal fragments maintained in position with an intranasal splint *(Fig. 3.15)*. In some cases, the septum should be reunited with the anterior nasal spine with a direct wire or suture.

When nasal fractures are treated more than 1 week after the injury, and especially after 2 weeks, it may not be possible to obtain the desired result with a single operation. Partial healing may make the reduction of the displaced or overlapped fragments difficult and less stable, and these patients often require a subsequent rhinoplasty with osteotomies.[96]

Although some individuals have performed open reductions routinely in nasal fractures, this amounts to resecting telescoped portions of the septum and creating additional osteotomies, and it is the author's opinion that such procedures are generally best performed secondarily when the initial swelling has disappeared and bone healing complete.

A more predictable result is usually obtained with secondary elective (late) rhinoplasty.

Acute open reductions of the septum usually are performed by removal of overlapped cartilage and therefore inevitably result in a loss of nasal height. All patients with nasal fractures should be warned that a late rhinoplasty may be indicated for correction of deviation of the nose, loss of or irregular nasal height or nasal airway obstruction.

Complications of nasal fractures

Untreated hematomas of the nasal septum may result in subperichondrial fibrosis and thickening with partial nasal airway obstruction. The septum in these cases may be as thick as 1 cm in areas, and may require thinning. In the case of repeated trauma, the cartilages of the septum may be largely replaced with calcified material. Submucous resection of thickened portions of the nasal septum may be required, and in many patients turbinate outfracture, or partial resection of enlarged turbinates may be advisable.

Synechiae may form between the septum and the turbinates in areas where soft tissue lacerations occur and the tissues are in contact.[97] These may be treated by division with placement of a splint or a nonadherent petrolatum impregnated gauze material between the cut surfaces for a period of 5 days. During this time, partial epithelialization begins.

Obstruction of the nasal vestibule may occur as a result of malunited fractures of the piriform margin, especially if displaced medially. It also occurs from telescoping and overlap of the nasal septum or lateral dislocation of the nasal septum into the airway. Soft tissue contracture and loss of vestibular lining produce narrowing, is difficult to correct without grafting material. Osteotomy of the bone fragments can correct displaced fractures; however, contracture due to loss of soft tissue may require excision of the scar and replacement with mucosal or composite grafts within the nasal vestibule or flap reconstruction.

Residual osteitis or infection of the bone or cartilage is occasionally seen in the compound fractures of the nose. These conditions are usually treated by repeated conservative debridements until the infected fragments are removed or sequestered. Debridement and antibiotic therapy constitute the preferred regimen of treatment. Secondary grafting may be performed where needed after an absence of infection and inflammation has persisted for 6 months. Chronic pain is infrequent, and usually affects the external nasal branches.[98]

Malunion of nasal fractures is common after closed reductions, since the exact anatomic position of the bone fragments can be difficult to detect by palpation alone, and the presence of closed splinting may not prevent subsequent deviation owing to the release of "interlocked stresses,"[99–101] following fracture of the cartilage. Any external or internal deformity of significance may require a corrective rhinoplasty.

Nasoethmoidal orbital fractures

Nasoethmoidal orbital fractures are severe fractures of the central one third of the upper midfacial skeleton. They comminute the nose, the medial orbital rims and the piriform aperture. Nasoethmoidal fractures are isolated in one-third and extended in two-thirds of cases to involve either the frontal bone, zygoma or maxilla. One-third are unilateral and two-thirds are bilateral injuries.

The central feature characterizing nasoethmoidal orbital fractures is the displacement of the section of the medial orbital rim carrying the attachment of the medial canthal ligament. Fractures that separate the frontal process of the maxilla and its canthal-bearing tendon allow canthal displacement.

Surgical pathology

The bones that form the skeletal framework of the nose are projected backwards between the orbits when subjected to strong traumatic forces. The bones involved are situated in the upper central portion of the middle third of the face anterior to the anatomic crossroads between the cranial, orbital, and nasal cavities. A typical cause of a nasoethmoidal orbital fracture is a blunt impact applied over the upper portion of the bridge of the nose caused by projection of the face against a blunt object such as a steering wheel or dashboard. The occupant of an automobile, for instance, is thrown forward, striking the nasofrontal area. A crushing injury with comminuted fractures is thus produced in the upper central midface. Bursting of the soft tissues, due to the severity of the impact and penetrating lacerations of the soft tissues resulting from projection of objects may transform the closed fractures into an open, and/or comminuted injury. If the impact force suffered by the strong nose and anterior frontal sinus is sufficient to cause backward displacement of these structures, no further resistance is offered by the delicate "matchbox-like" structures of the interorbital space; indeed, these structures "collapse and splinter like a pile of matchboxes struck by a hammer."[102]

Interorbital space

The term "*interorbital space*" designates an area between the orbits and below the floor of the anterior cranial fossa. The "interorbital space" contains two ethmoidal labyrinths, one on each side and consists of the ethmoidal cells, the superior and middle turbinates, and a median thicker plate of septal bone and the perpendicular plate of the ethmoid.

Traumatic telecanthus and hypertelorism

Traumatic telecanthus is an increase in the distance between the medial canthal ligaments in all but the first stage of nasoethmoidal orbital fractures, the patient has a characteristic appearance of telecanthus. The eyes may appear far apart, as in orbital hypertelorism.[103,104]

Traumatic orbital hypertelorism[105] (as opposed to telecanthus) is a deformity characterized by an increase in the distance between the orbits *and* the ocular globes.[106]

Clinical examination

The appearance of patients who suffer nasoethmoidal orbital fractures is typical. A significant frontal impact nasal fracture is generally present, with the nose flattened and appearing to have been pushed between the eyes. There is a loss of dorsal nasal prominence, and an obtuse angle is noted between the lip and columella. Finger pressure on the nose may document inadequate distal septal or proximal bony support. The medial

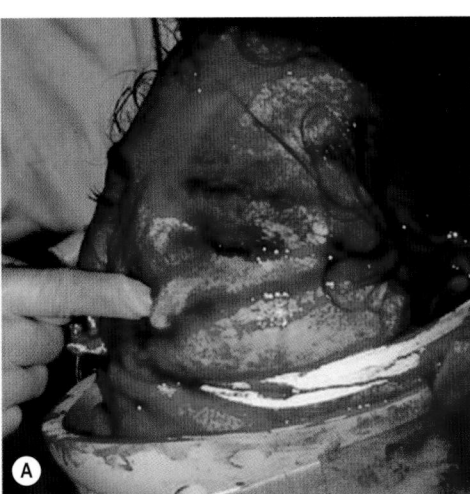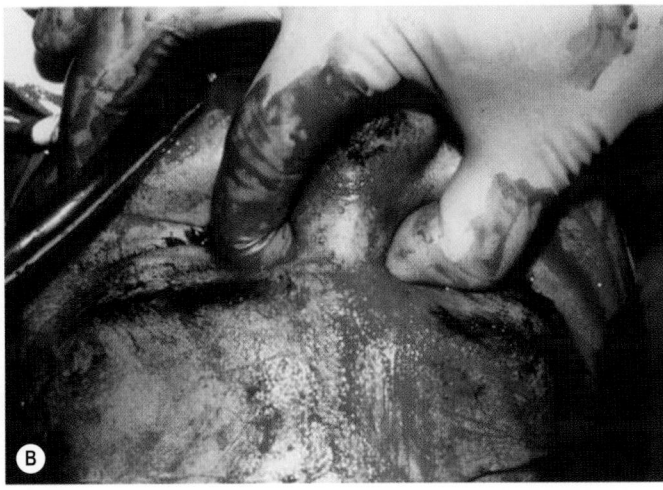

Fig. 3.17 **(A)** Finger pressure on the nasal dorsum and columella documents the lack of skeletal support in nasoethmoid fractures. **(B)** If the fingertips are pressed over the medial orbital rim (not the nasal bones), a click or movement confirms a mobile nasoethmoidal-orbital fracture.

canthal areas are swollen and distorted with palpebral and subconjunctival hematomas. Ecchymosis and subconjunctival hemorrhage are the usual findings. Directly over the medial canthal ligaments, crepitus or movement may be palpated with external pressure deeply over the canthal ligament (*Fig. 3.17*). A bimanual examination of the medial orbital rim is helpful if the diagnosis is uncertain. The bimanual examination is performed by placing a palpating finger deeply over the canthal ligament, and placing a clamp inside the nose with its tip directly under the finger. The frontal process of the maxilla may then, if fractured, be moved between the index finger and the clamp, indicating instability confirming both the diagnosis and the need for an open reduction. The clamp, if placed under the nasal bones (and not the medial orbital rim – medial canthal ligament attachment) can erroneously identify a nasal fracture as canthal instability.

Radiographs

CT scans are essential to document the injury. The diagnosis of a nasoethmoidal orbital fracture on radiographs requires at a minimum four fractures that isolate the frontal process of the maxilla from adjacent bones. These include: (1) fractures of the nose; (2) fractures of the junction of the frontal process of the maxilla with the frontal bone; (3) fractures of the medial orbit (ethmoidal area); and (4) fractures of the inferior orbital rim extending to involve the pyriform aperture and orbital floor. These fracture lines, therefore, define the "central fragment" of bone bearing the medial canthal ligament as "free", and, depending on periosteal integrity, the medial orbital rim could displace.

Classification of nasoethmoidal orbital fractures

Nasoethmoidal fractures are classified according to a pattern established by Markowitz and colleagues[107] types I–III, the bimanual examination and the CT scan.[108–110]

Type I is an incomplete fracture, mostly unilateral but occasionally bilateral, which is displaced only inferiorly at the infraorbital rim and piriform margin. Inferior alone approaches are necessary (*Fig. 3.18*). Bilateral nasoethmoidal orbital fractures can section the entire nasoethmoidal area as a single unit. These are not true nasoethmoidal orbital fractures, since telecanthus cannot occur. The entire central fragment is usually rotated and posteriorly displaced, and considerable canthal distortion occurs. Conceptually, these are treated with superior and inferior approaches as the fractures are complete at peripheral buttresses. These types of fractures do not require a canthal repositioning because the canthus is not unstable and remains attached to a large bone fragment.

Type II nasoethmoidal orbital fractures are comminuted nasoethmoidal fractures with the fractures remaining outside the canthal ligament insertion. The central fragment may be dealt with as a sizeable bone fragment and united to the canthal ligament-bearing fragment of the other side with a transnasal wire reduction. The remainder of the pieces of the nasoethmoidal orbital skeleton are reduced and then stabilized by junctional plate and screw fixation to the frontal bone, the infraorbital rim and to the Le Fort I level of the maxilla. They may be unilateral or bilateral (*Fig. 3.19*).

Type III nasoethmoidal orbital fractures either have avulsion of the canthal ligament (uncommon) or the fractures extend underneath the canthal ligament insertion. The fracture fragments are small enough that a reduction would require that the canthus be detached to accomplish the bone reduction. Therefore, canthal ligament reattachment is required, a separate step accomplished with a separate set of transnasal wires for both the bone of the medial orbital rim and the canthus. In general, the bony reduction of the intercanthal distance should be 5–7 mm per side less than the desired soft tissue distance (*Fig. 3.20*).

Treatment of nasoethmoidal orbital fractures

The technique of treatment in nasoethmoidal orbital fractures consists of a thorough exposure of the nasoorbital region by means of three incisions: a coronal (or an appropriate

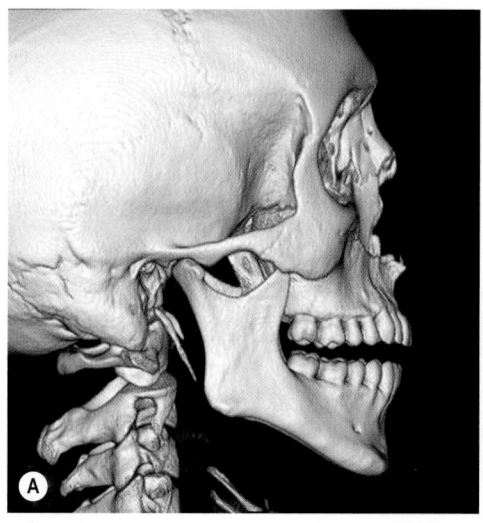
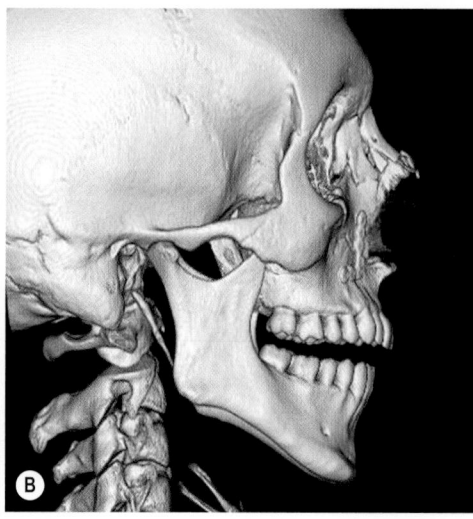

Fig. 3.18 (A,B) Lateral image of 3D craniofacial computer tomography scan of a type 1 naso-orbital ethmoidal fracture injury pattern pre- and post-open reduction and internal fixation of midface fractures using the inferior alone approach.

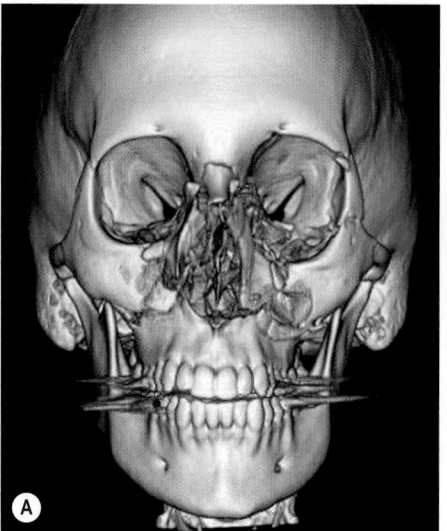
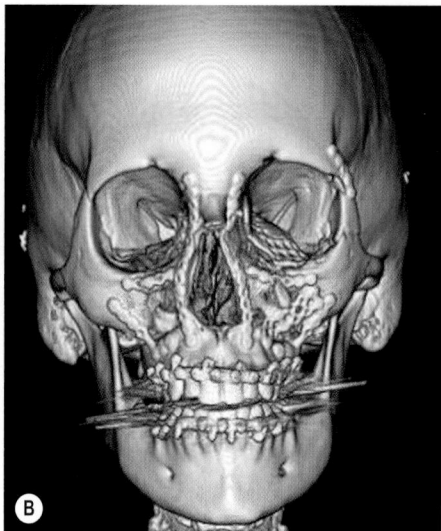
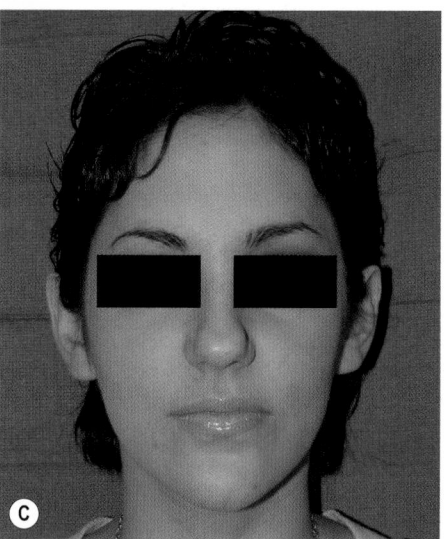

Fig. 3.19 (A) Frontal 3D craniofacial computer tomography scan of a type II naso-orbital ethmoidal fracture injury pattern in a 23-year-old female who sustained craniofacial injuries following being struck by a motor vehicle as a pedestrian. **(B)** Pre- and post-open reduction and internal fixation of midface fractures. **(C)** Postoperative frontal photograph view of patient approximately 12 months from surgery.

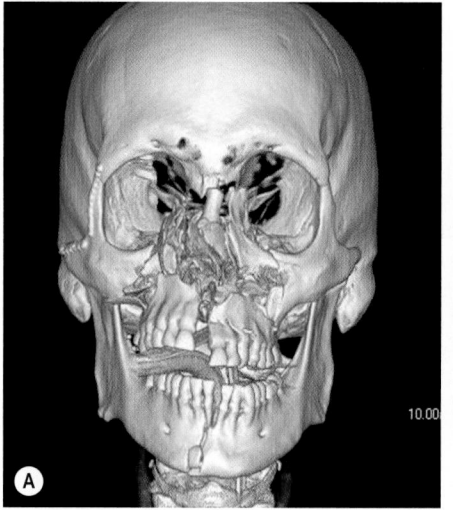
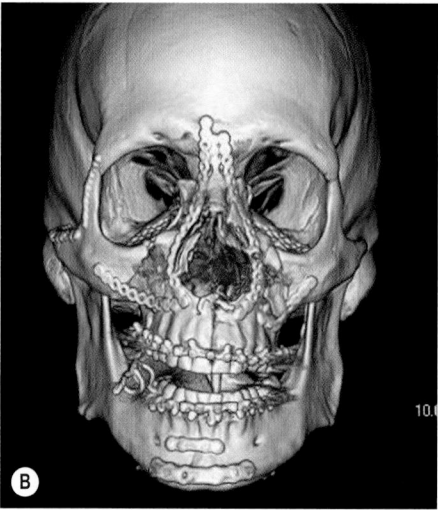
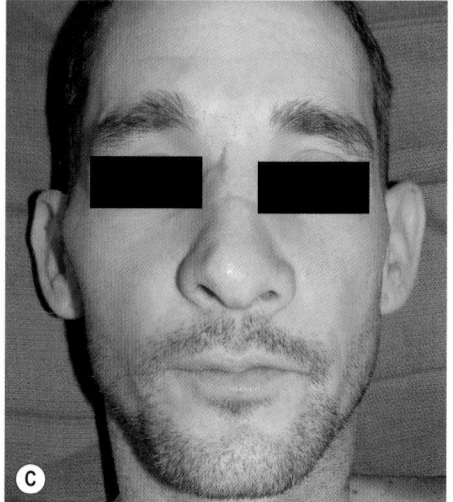

Fig. 3.20 (A) Frontal 3D craniofacial computer tomography scan of type III naso-orbital ethmoidal and a Le Fort II type injury pattern in a 33-year-old who sustained craniofacial injuries following being thrown off a motorcycle without a helmet. **(B)** Pre- and post-open reduction and internal fixation of midface and mandibular fractures. **(C)** Postoperative frontal photograph view of patient 6 months from surgery.

laceration or local incision), a lower eyelid incision, and a gingival buccal sulcus incision. In some cases, a laceration may be present over the forehead or nose, which provides sufficient access for a localized fracture to be treated. Nasal and forehead laceration are common, but often they are not quite long enough to provide sufficient exposure. Judgment must be exercised in the extension of these lacerations, as the scar deformity from extension is sometimes worse than making a separate coronal incision.

The primary principle underlying open treatment of nasoethmoidal orbital fractures involves the preservation of all fragments of bone and their accurate reassembly.[111] Despite the anatomic reassembly of the bone fragments of the nose, primary bone grafting is usually necessary to improve the true nasal height and to preserve the smooth contour of the dorsum of the nose. Occasionally, the bone onto which the canthal ligament is attached is so comminuted that a canthal detachment and reinsertion of the ligament into a structurally sound bone graft (a new "central fragment") is created.

The importance of the "central fragment" in nasoethmoid orbital fractures

In all cases of nasoethmoidal orbital fractures, one must identify and classify what is happening to the bone of the medial orbital rim, which bears the medial canthal attachment, as it has a direct relationship to the treatment techniques of the various fractures. Displacement of this medial canthal bone fragment is the *sine qua non* of the nasoethmoidal injury, and the correct definition and management of this fragment, the "central fragment", determines the outcome of the fracture.

The most essential feature of a nasoethmoidal reduction is the transnasal reduction of the medial orbital rims by a wire placed posterior and superior to the canthal ligament insertion. The medial orbital rim with its attached canthal-bearing segment is then dislocated anteriorly and laterally, brought clearly into view next to the nasal bones, where its superficial position facilitates drilling and wire passing of the "central" fragment. Nasal bone fragments can be temporarily dislocated or removed to permit better exposure of the medial orbital rim segments. Removing the nasal bones is especially helpful in passing a transnasal wire from the posterior and superior aspect of one "central" fragment (medial orbital rim canthal bearing bone fragment) to the other. Following the placement of two transnasal wires, one should pass one extra wire for soft tissue reapproximation to bone. The medial orbital rims are linked to adjacent nasal and frontal bone fragments. Junctional plate and screw fixation is employed after the initial interfragment wiring is tightened. It should be emphasized that the transnasal reduction wires must be passed posterior and superior to the lachrymal fossa in order to provide the proper direction of force to recreate the preinjury bony position of the central fragments. The transnasal reduction is not a "transnasal canthopexy", as it usually does not involve the canthal ligament. It is a reduction *only* of the "central bony fragment" of the nasoethmoidal orbital fracture.

Canthal reattachment

If the canthal ligament requires reattachment (the canthal tendon is rarely stripped from bone), the canthal tendon[112,113] may be grasped by one or two passes of 2-0 nonabsorbable suture adjacent to the medial commissure of the eyelids.[114,115] This area is accessed through a separate 3 mm external incision on the skin of the canthus oriented vertically or horizontally. Probes may be placed through the lachrymal system to avoid needle penetration of the lachrymal ducts. The lachrymal system may be intubated with disposable Quickert tubes where required. The 2-0 nonabsorbable suture is then passed into the internal aspect of the coronal incision by dissecting above the medial canthal ligament medially, and the suture connected to a separate set of #28 transnasal wires, one set for each canthal ligament, separate from those required for the bone reduction of the central fragment. The transnasal canthal ligament wires are tightened only as the last step of the reduction, after medial orbital and nasal bone grafting are completed and just before closure of the incision. Each set of canthal wires is tightened gently after a manual reduction of the canthus to the bone with forceps is performed, to reduce stress on the canthal sutures. The canthal reduction wire pairs are then twisted over a screw in the frontal bone.

Lacrimal system injury

Interruption of the continuity of the lacrimal apparatus demands specific action. Most lacrimal system obstruction occurs from bony malposition or damage to the lacrimal sac or duct.[116,117] The most effective treatment involves satisfactory precise repositioning of the fracture segments. If transection of the soft tissue portion of the canalicular lacrimal system has occurred, it should be repaired over fine tubes with magnification.[118]

Complications of nasoethmoidal orbital fractures

The early diagnosis and adequate treatment of nasoethmoidal orbital fractures achieves optimal aesthetic results with the least number of late complications. Depending on the quality of initial treatment and the results of healing, further reconstructive surgery may be required in some cases. Late complications, such as frontal sinus obstruction, occur in less than 5% of isolated nasoethmoidal orbital fractures.[119,120] Deformities and functional impairment are late complications can be minimized by early diagnosis and proper open reduction. The presence of a nasoethmoidal orbital fracture may be obscured by the swelling of other facial injuries and may escape detection. Only after several weeks nasal deformity and enophthalmos may become more evident.[121,122]

Fractures of the zygoma

The zygoma is a major buttress of the midfacial skeleton. It forms the malar eminence, giving prominence to the cheek, and forms the lateral and inferior portions of the orbit. The zygomatic bone has a quadrilateral shape with several processes that extend to reach the frontal bone, the maxilla, the temporal bone (zygomatic arch), and orbital processes (*Fig. 3.21*). The zygoma meets the maxilla medially at the inferior orbital rim and inferiorly at the maxillary alveolus. The zygomatic bone articulates with the external angular process of the frontal bone superiorly, and with the greater wing of the sphenoid in the lateral orbit. In the inferior orbit, it articulates with the maxilla. On the inner surface, beyond the orbital rim, it is concave and then convex and participates in the formation of the temporal fossa. The bone has its broadest and strongest attachment with the frontal bone and then with the maxilla. Thinner and weaker attachments occur with the sphenoid and through the zygomatic arch. The zygoma forms the greater portion of the lateral and inferior orbit including the anterior half of the lateral wall of the orbit. In most skulls, the zygoma forms the lateral and superior wall of the maxillary sinus. The bone furnishes attachments for the masseter, temporalis, zygomaticus major and minor, and the zygomatic head of the quadratus labii superiorus muscles. The zygomaticotemporal and zygomaticofacial nerves[123] pass through respectively, to innervate the soft tissues over the region of the zygomaticofrontal junction and malar eminence. ⊛ FIG **3.21** APPEARS ONLINE ONLY

Physical diagnosis and surgical pathology of zygoma fractures

Although the zygoma is a sturdy bone, it is frequently injured because of its prominent location. Moderately severe blows are absorbed by the bone and transferred to its buttresses. Severe blows may cause separation of the zygoma at its articulating surfaces and high energy injuries may cause shattering of the body of the zygoma, often through weak areas such as the zygomaticofacial foramen. As the zygoma is disrupted, it is usually displaced in a downward, medial, and posterior direction. The direction of displacement, however, varies with the direction of the injuring force and with the pull of the muscles, such as that of the masseter. The zygoma may be shattered, resulting in comminution not only of the body, but the zygoma's articulating attachments.

The zygoma is the principle buttressing bone between the maxilla and the cranium. Fractures usually involve the inferior orbital rim and result in hematoma which is limited by the orbital septum. Periorbital and subconjunctival hematomas are the most accurate physical signs of an orbital fracture associated with a zygoma fracture. Numbness of the infraorbital nerve is a common symptom as well. The infraorbital nerve runs in a groove in the posterior portion of the orbit and enters a canal in the anterior third of the orbit behind the infraorbital rim.[124] It may be crushed in a fracture, as the fracture occurs in the weak area of bone penetrated by the infraorbital foramen. Direct force to the lateral face may result in isolated fractures of the temporal extension of the zygoma (zygomatic arch), and the zygomatic process of the temporal bone. The zygomatic arch may be fractured in the absence of a fracture of the remainder of the zygoma and its articulations.

Medial displacement of an isolated arch fracture is usually observed, and if its displacement is sufficient, the arch itself may impinge against the temporalis muscle and coronoid process of the mandible resulting in restricted mandibular motion. Fractures in the posterior portion of the zygomatic arch may enter the glenoid fossa and produce stiffness or a change in occlusion because of the swelling in the joint or muscles. In high energy injuries or gunshots, fragments of bone can be driven through the temporal muscle and make

contact with the coronoid process and precipitate the formation of a fibrous or bony ankylosis, necessitating excision of the bone of the coronoid process and scar tissue as a secondary procedure.

Fracture dislocation of the zygoma with sufficient displacement to impinge on the coronoid process requires considerable backward dislocation of the malar eminence. About half of fracture dislocations of the zygoma result in separation at the zygomaticofrontal suture, which is palpable through the skin over the upper lateral margin of the orbit. Level discrepancies or step deformities at the infraorbital margin can usually be palpated in the presence of inferior and medial orbital rim displacement. The lateral and superior walls of the maxillary sinuses are involved in fractures of the zygoma, and the resulting tear of the maxillary sinus lining results in the accumulation of blood within the sinus with unilateral epistaxis. The lateral canthal attachment is directed towards Whitnall's tubercle located approximately 10 mm below the zygomaticofrontal suture. The ligament extends toward a shallow eminence on the internal aspect of the frontal process of the zygoma. When the zygoma is displaced inferiorly, the lateral attachment of the eyelids is also displaced inferiorly giving rise to an antimongoloid slant of the palpebral fissure. The globe follows the inferior displacement of the zygoma with a lower (inferior) position after fracture dislocation. Displacement of the orbital floor allows displacement of the rim. Dysfunction of the extraocular muscles may be noted as a result of the disruption of the floor and lateral portion of the orbit. The mechanism of diplopia is usually muscular contusion. Displacement of the globe and orbital contents may also occur as a result of downward displacement of Lockwood's suspensory ligament, which forms an inferior "sling" for the globe and orbital contents. Lockwood's ligament attaches to the lateral wall of the orbit adjacent to Whitnall's tubercle. Fragmentation of the bony orbital floor may disrupt the continuity of the suspensory ligaments of the globe and orbit, and orbital fat may be extruded from the intramuscular cone and herniate into the maxillary sinus, where it may become incarcerated or attached to sinus lining or bone segments by the development of adhesions. Double vision is usually transient in uncomplicated fractures of the zygoma which always involve the orbital floor. Diplopia may persist when the fracture is more extensive, especially if a fracture extends to comminute the inferior orbital floor. This diplopia may result from muscle contusion, incarceration of perimuscular soft tissue, or actual muscle incarceration or simply drooping of the muscular sling. The orbital portion of the fracture communicates with fractures of the inferior orbital rim. Frequently, one or two small maxillary fragments at the inferior orbital rim are fractured adjacent to its junction with the zygoma, and are called "butterfly fragments". These rim fractures result in considerable instability of the rim with inferior and posterior displacement. The orbital septum attaches to the orbital rim and is also displaced downward and backward creating a downward pull on the lower eyelid.

The infraorbital nerve travels obliquely from lateral to medial across the floor of the orbit.[125] In the posterior portion of the orbit, the nerve is in a groove and in the anterior portion of the orbit is located in a canal. Adjacent to the orbital rim, the canal turns downward and exits approximately 10 mm below the upper edge of the inferior orbital rim. The foramen is aligned parallel with the medial margin of the cornea when the eye is in straightforward gaze. The infraorbital nerve is often compressed by fractures, since the canal and groove represent a weak portion of the bone. Laceration of the nerve in the canal, when crushed by impaction of bone fragments may result in permanent anesthesia. The nerve is frequently contused, and although temporary symptoms of infraorbital nerve hypesthesia are present initially they usually partially resolve. After zygomatic fractures, sensory disturbances of a more minimal nature have been detected in up to 40% of patients.[126–130] Persistent total anesthesia following fracture may represent an indication for exploration and decompression of the infraorbital nerve with neurolysis, although the efficacy of the procedure has not been confirmed in large series.

Knight and North[131] proposed a classification in 1961 of fractures of zygoma, based on the direction of anatomic displacement and pattern created by the fracture. This classification, which was used for predicting the success of a closed reduction, is presented for acquaintance with classical knowledge about post reduction stability. The Knight and North classification, clarified by Yanagisawa,[132] identified fractures with complete dislocation of the zygomaticofrontal suture, and comminuted fractures with external rotation as unstable.

Presently, surgical practice is to explore the zygoma and the articular processes involved in complete fractures, in an effort to achieve direct anatomic alignment and provide fixation. In current practice, closed reductions are only employed in isolated zygomatic arch fractures. Limited reductions are very popular today, such as the use of the gingival buccal sulcus approach alone.[133,134] Such an approach is indicated in fractures which are "greensticked" at the Z-F suture, have a minimal or linear orbital floor component which would be reduced by the zygomatic reduction, and are displaced principally at the Z-M buttress at the maxillary alveolus. These limited reductions reduce the number of the incisions and thus the morbidity of open reduction, accounting for rapid and efficient procedures with reduced scarring and no eyelid morbidity.

Classification of zygoma fractures

Zygoma fractures may be classified into those that require an *anterior* treatment approach for treatment and those fewer fractures that require a simultaneous *anterior and posterior* approach.

Anterior approach

The anterior approach may be partial or complete and potentially involves up to three incisions: (1) access to the zygomaticofrontal suture; (2) access to the inferior orbital rim; and (3) access to the zygomaticomaxillary buttress, anterior maxilla and malar prominence. Sometimes (1) and (2) may be accomplished with the same incision, such as a subciliary incision with canthal detachment.

Many surgeons prefer not to detach the canthus because of the need to accurately replace it back on the frontal process.

Frequently, zygomatic fracture displacement is minimal and requires no treatment (25%). Most displaced zygomatic fractures are medially and posteriorly dislocated. In about 50–75% of those, an anterior gingival sulcus approach alone can be utilized.

"Minimalist" approach for fractures without zygomaticofrontal suture diastasis

In this approach, the gingivobuccal sulcus is opened and the anterior face of the maxilla and zygoma are degloved. The infraorbital rim and infraorbital nerve are visualized from an inferior direction. Palpation with a finger on the rim avoids entry of elevators into the orbit as the maxilla and zygoma are dissected. The infraorbital nerve is protected by the dissection and is immediately seen after detaching the levator anguli oris muscle. The zygoma may often be reduced by placing the tip of an elevator in the lateral aspect of the maxillary sinus directly underneath the malar eminence (not into the orbit!), and levering the body of the zygoma first outward and then forward. Alternately, a Carrol-Girard Screw (Walter Lorenz Co., Jacksonville, FL) can be placed in the malar eminence through a percutaneous incision, and manipulated (*Fig. 3.22*). Another reduction approach involves placing a "hook" elevator beneath the anterior zygomatic arch and malar eminence and raising both the arch and the body of the zygoma. In gingival buccal sulcus approaches, after the reduction maneuver has been completed, zygomatic stability depends upon a relatively intact, greensticked, zygomaticofrontal suture. The floor of the orbit can be inspected with an endoscope through the maxillary sinus. It is also possible to tell from a pre operative CT the degree of orbital floor comminution. Fractures with orbital floor comminution require a gingival approach and an inferior eyelid incision. ⊛ FIG **3.22** APPEARS ONLINE ONLY

Endoscopic confirmation of orbital floor integrity

In the endoscopic confirmation of orbital integrity, finger pressure on the globe "ballottes" the soft tissue and allows the perception of integrity of floor support to be determined by an endoscope placed in the maxillary sinus, visualizing the area of movement and degree of soft tissue prolapse. If there is significant motion over an area which exceeds a nickel in size, the orbital floor should be repaired endoscopically through the sinus. This may be accomplished with an alloplastic material such as Medpor®,[135–137] or by replacement of the orbital floor fracture fragments themselves, uniting them to intact bone with rigid fixation.

Fractures with Z-F suture diastasis

If the Z-F suture demonstrates diastasis, then an exposure of this suture needs to be accomplished for stabilization. This could be accomplished through the lateral portion of an upper blepharoplasty incision (<1 cm) which is made directly over the Z-F suture 8–10 mm above the lateral canthus). Palpating the frontal process of the zygoma between the thumb and index finger, the frontal process can be marked precisely in *eyelid* skin. The incision should be short and not progress laterally out of eyelid skin, as it will scar noticeably. Alternately, the Z-F suture may be approached through a brow laceration or by superior dissection from a subciliary or conjunctival

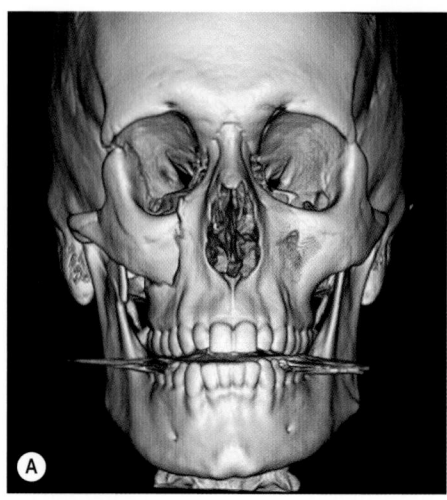 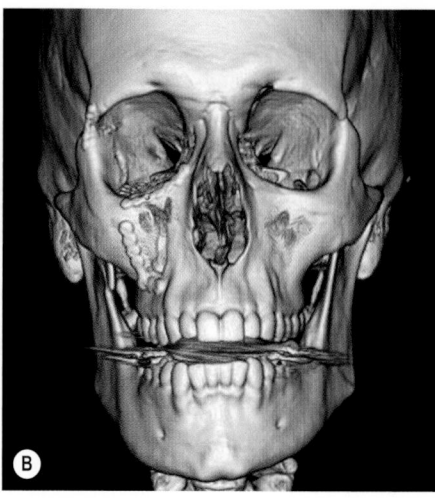 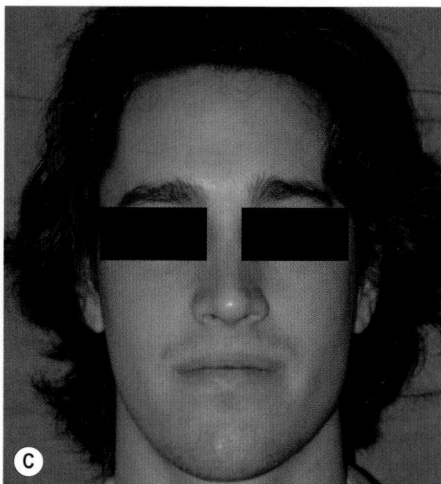

Fig. 3.23 (A,B) Frontal 3D craniofacial computer tomography scan of a right zygomaticomaxillary fracture in a 22-year-old male who sustained craniofacial injuries following a sports related injury, pre- and post-open reduction and internal fixation of the right zygomaticomaxillary complex and orbital floor fractures. **(C)** Postoperative frontal photograph view of patient 3 months following surgery.

lower lid incision by canthal detachment. Another approach is through the lateral conjunctiva.

The inferior portion of the orbit may be approached through a midtarsal, lower orbital rim, subciliary, or conjunctival incision. The conjunctival fornix incision produces the least cutaneous scarring but the exposure may be restricted by fat prolapse. The treatment of a zygoma fracture has recently become quite specific, and directed only at areas that require open reduction for confirmation of alignment or for fixation *(Fig. 3.23)*.

Posterior approach (coronal incisions)

Fractures with extreme posterior displacement, and those with lateral displacement of the zygomatic arch benefit from the addition of a coronal incision. The coronal incision allows exposure of the entire zygomatic arch and roof of the glenoid fossa for precise arch reconstruction. It also exposes the Z-F suture and the lateral orbital wall. Any sagittally oriented split of the glenoid fossa should be reduced first, following which reduction and fixation of the remainder of the zygomatic arch may be accomplished, confirming alignment in the lateral wall of the orbit and medial position of the arch. When the orbital process of the zygoma comes in line with the broad surface of the greater wing of the sphenoid, the arch is of the proper length and medial position (which guarantees the proper projection of the malar eminence). Medially displaced arch fractures, whether isolated or part of a more extensive zygomatic fracture, may be managed through Gilles or Dingman approaches, to be described later.

Treatment of fractures of the zygoma

Closed reduction

Formerly, closed reduction techniques were employed for most zygomatic fractures. The Knight and North classification,[138] were meant to identify those fractures which were stable following closed reduction. In practice, many fractures can be treated adequately with closed reduction, and especially where cost is an issue, this treatment would have to be considered. Those fractures amenable to closed reduction include medial displaced isolated arch fractures, and simple large segment or single piece zygoma fractures in which the displacement is medial and posterior, without comminution at the buttresses, and the fracture at the Z-F suture is incomplete. An elevator placed beneath the malar eminence allows the zygoma to be "popped" back into position. The stability of closed reduction depends on the integrity of periosteal attachments and principally "greensticking" at the Z-F suture. The force of contraction of the masseter muscle tends to create displacement.[139]

Zingg and colleagues achieved stability in closed reductions by impaction against adjacent articulating bones.[140,141] Displacement at the Z-F suture,[142] comminution of the inferior orbital rim or Z-M buttress, and lateral displacement of the arch and body are characteristics that were found to predict a poor result from closed reduction. Disappointment and frustration in the management of zygomatic fractures has been experienced after use of closed reduction. Complications include residual diplopia, malunion, and deformity, all of which indicate incomplete reduction or displacement following initial reduction. A more complete exposure of the fracture sites, including the zygomaticomaxillary buttress, has been recommended.[143–145] Their exposures provide the ability to visualize the anatomic accuracy of the reduction. In zygomatic fractures accompanied by Le Fort fractures, considerable lateral displacement of the zygoma is often observed with comminution of the arch. In cases of extreme posterior dislocation, exposure and anatomic reduction of the arch through a coronal incision restores proper anterior projection and alignment in the lateral orbit between the greater wing of the sphenoid and the orbital process of the zygoma.

Buttress articulations and alignment

Six points of alignment with adjacent bone may be confirmed with craniofacial exposure: Z-F suture, infraorbital rim, zygomaticomaxillary buttress, greater wing of the sphenoid, orbital floor, and zygomatic arch. The orbital floor may require reconstruction with bone or artificial materials such as Medpor or titanium. The inferior orbital fissure is an area where under correction of volume of the orbit is frequent, as are the inferiomedial buttress and the medial orbital wall.

Methods of reduction

Reduction through the maxillary sinus

Lothrop[146] employed a Caldwell-Luc maxillary antrostomy. The elevator contacts the posterior surface of the malar eminence. Upward, outward, and superiorly directed forces reduced the zygoma. A Carroll-Girard screw (Walter Lorenzo, Jacksonville, FL) may also be utilized percutaneously (Fig. 3.22), or from an intraoral approach.

Temporal approach

A temporal approach for the reduction of zygomatic fractures was described by Gilles and colleagues.[147] An incision is made behind the temporal hairline, and dissection accomplished to expose the temporalis muscle. An elevator was placed behind the zygomatic arch or under the malar eminence, depending on the areas of reduction required (Fig. 3.24). A small, 2 cm incision placed vertically within the temporal hair heals with an inconspicuous scar. The elevator must be placed deep to the deep temporal fascia, visualizing the temporalis muscle. The bone may be palpated with one hand to document the accuracy of reduction, while the other hand guides the elevator into position and corrects the displacement by force application. A folded towel placed in the temporal area protects the thin temporal bone from fracture. A gentle elevation often "clicks" the arch into position. Moving the elevator back and forth with repeated elevation movements may disrupt the periosteum holding the arch fragments together, and an open reduction would then be required. ⊚ FIG 3.24 APPEARS ONLINE ONLY

Dingman approach

An incision (or laceration) is used in the lateral brow approximately 1.5 cm in length. A periosteal elevator is passed through the incision behind the malar eminence and into the temporal fossa. The elevator is used to control the position of the zygoma, and to reduce it by upward, forward, and outward forces. After the reduction, the orbital floor can be explored and reduced.[148]

Fixation required to achieve stability

Several individuals have examined zygomatic stability following open reduction. Rinehart et al.[149] studied cadaver heads and used 1, 2, or 3 miniplates and accessed stability of noncomminuted zygoma fractures submitted to static and oscillating loads to simulate the effect of the masticatory apparatus on postoperative displacement. Neither single miniplate nor triple wire fixation was enough to stabilize the zygoma against simulated masseter forces, however 3 miniplates were sufficient which stabilized the Z-F, Z-M and infraorbital rim areas.

Del Santo and Ellis[150] felt that Rinehart and Marsh overestimated the postoperative forces that could be generated by the masseter muscle, and suggested that stability with less than 3 plates would be possible. Ellis's conclusions were based upon actual human measurements of bite forces after zygomatic fracture treatment.

Davidson and colleagues[151] studied combinations of wires and plates at the anterior fixation sites and determined that 3 point fixation was ideal at preventing displacement. Miniplates were recommended as at least one strong buttress as well as 2 and 3 point fixation. Plate bending and bone splitting at the screw or drill holes was the mechanism of failure.

Kasrai and collegues[152] studied the miniplate versus the bioresorbable systems. Titanium provided 39% of the strength of the nonfractured area and bioresorbable systems provided 13% of the intact breaking strength. Deformation or bending of miniplates was the primary mode of failure. Manson et al. and Solomon[153,154] performed experiments with stainless steel systems and found bone fractures were the primary mode of failure. This study implied that the titanium and resorbable systems are considerably less strong than the bone itself, but the stainless steel system compared favorably to the bone strength. Rohrich and Watumull[155] found plate fixation to be superior to wire fixation after a thorough study. They also found that fixed deformities were quite challenging to correct. O'Hara et al.[156] demonstrated that 2 and 3 point fixation with miniplates were superior to other methods of fixation. Rohner and colleagues[157] studied combinations of plate fixation and concluded that the addition of fixation within the lateral wall of the orbit was one of the most stable constructs. They demonstrated that titanium systems had one-third and bioresorbable <10% of the strength of the intact zygomatic complex. Plate bending was the cause of the failure of the titanium system, whereas plate and screw breakage was the cause of the failure in the resorbable system. Gosain et al.[158] demonstrated in parietal calvarial bone that in compression and distraction, titanium miniplates were considerably stronger than the bioresorbable systems. Therefore, there seems to be justification for using 3 plates, one each at the zygomaticofrontal suture, infraorbital rim and zygomaticomaxillary buttress. The upper 2 plates could be of the 1.3 mm system, and the lower plate of the 1.5 or 2.0 mm system.

"High energy" zygoma fractures

Violent injury to the zygoma results in shattering of the bone into multiple fragments. The method of management of complicated fractures must include a thorough visualization of the body, the frontal and maxillary processes of the zygoma and the zygomatic arch.[159,160] The zygomaticomaxillary buttress is restored by direct intraoral plate and screw fixation and wire reduction at the Z-F suture, infraorbital rim and perhaps the zygomatic arch for temporary positioning. An eyelid incision may provide exposure of the inferior rim and lateral wall. Wires allow minimal adjustments to improve reduction before application of rigid fixation. The entire lower and lateral zygoma may be exposed with an eyelid incision, dissecting the lateral canthal ligament off Whitnall's tubercle. The lateral aspect of the incision may therefore be retracted upward to expose the zygomaticofrontal suture. The lateral wall of the orbit is best inspected through a lower lid or coronal incision. The canthal ligament may be detached for

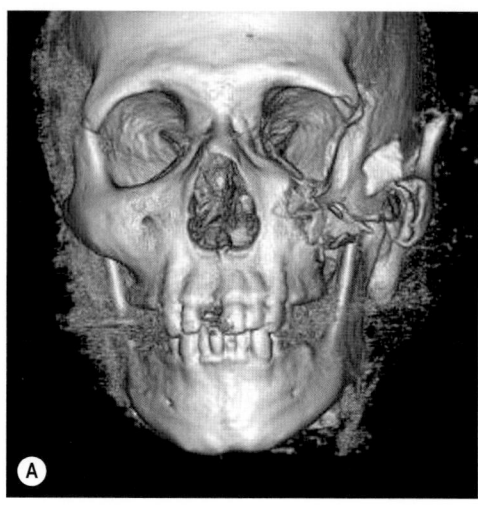 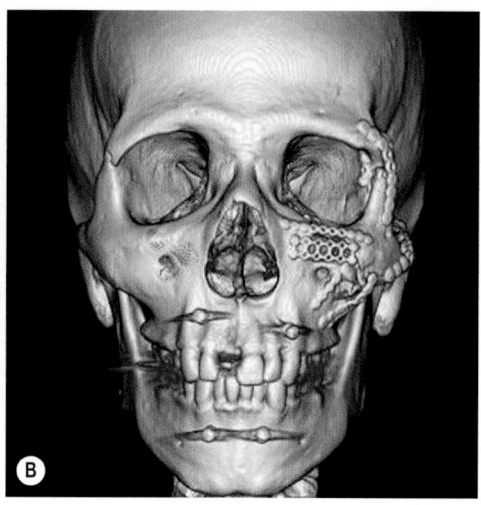

Fig. 3.25 (A) Frontal 3D craniofacial computer tomography scan of a Le Fort II type injury in a 33-year-old who sustained craniofacial injuries following a high speed motor vehicle collision. **(B)** Pre- and post-open reduction and internal fixation of the left orbital and zygomaticomaxillary complex.

exposure. In the lateral wall, one confirms alignment of the orbital process of the zygoma with the greater wing of the sphenoid *(Fig. 3.25)*.

The maxillary sinus approach, with and without endoscopic assistance

The maxillary sinus approach may include endoscopic visualization of the orbital floor and the sinus ostea. The orbital floor may be, replaced and stabilized with either small plates or by insertion of an alloplastic material. The sinus should have any blood or bone fragments removed and discarded. One should be able to irrigate freely into the nose through the sinus, confirming the integrity of the maxillary sinus ostea.

The intraoral approach

This approach is one of the most important approaches for reduction of zygomatic fractures. A gingivobuccal incision is made 1 cm above the attached gingiva, and then deepened through the buccinator straight to the anterior maxillary wall until the periosteum is identified. The periosteum is incised and reflected superiorly as a mucoperiosteal flap, exposing the entire anterior wall and lateral buttress of the maxilla and all of the anterior and lateral portions of the zygomaticomaxillary buttress. The dissection may be extended medially to the piriform aperture as required. The dissection then progresses superiorly and the entire malar eminence exposed. One should visualize the anterior edge of the masseter muscle inserting on the lower aspect of the malar prominence. The infraorbital foramen is reached after detaching the levator anguli oris muscle. The infraorbital foramen is seen just above this muscle, and the contents of the infraorbital canal protected by careful dissection. A Kelly clamp or elevator may then be placed through the anterior wall of the fractured maxillary sinus ("Caldwell-Luc") with the tip placed directly under the malar eminence. Gentle pressure is used to elevate the body of the zygoma anteriorly and laterally. An elevator may also be placed intraorally underneath the arch and medial arch fractures reduced. Impacted or partially healed fractures

may be dislodged by passing the osteotome through the line of the fracture, completing the fracture. The zygomaticomaxillary buttress may be reconstructed by using either temporary positioning wires or a loose reduction with a plate and a single screw in each fragment. A bone graft may be placed into any gap in the Z-M buttress or over the anterior wall of the maxillary sinus.

An L-shaped plate is generally used at the zygomaticomaxillary buttress, and its solid fixation depends on at least two stable screws beyond the areas of fracture in intact bone on each side. Fixation with a 1.5 or 2 mm system at the Le Fort I level is recommended. Tooth roots inferiorly should be avoided. In practice, screws which penetrate teeth have not had the frequency of adverse sequelae initially predicted. The "butterfly" buttress bone pieces may be screwed to the plate.

Since the zygoma conceptually requires three or four incisions for visualization of all of its buttress alignments, and since one can only look through one incision at a time, the use of temporary interfragment wire positioning for several of these fracture sites allows temporary control of displacement of the zygoma fracture while one is looking through the other fracture exposures. The technique allows more control of the displacement prior to rigid fixation.

In zygomatic fractures demonstrating only medial displacement, management with an anterior approach is satisfactory. A coronal incision is not required. The medially displaced zygomatic arch may be managed by a supplemental Gillestype approach used to perform a closed reduction of the arch segment. Anterior approaches permit the reduction of the anterior portion of the zygoma. Small plate and screws can then be used to span the fracture sites and provide positive fixation once the buttress alignment has been confirmed. Two screws per fragment in solid bone provide good immobilization. Often, a five-hole plate is selected for the Z-F suture with the central hole placed over the fracture site. Screws placed in comminuted bone do not provide secure fixation. In providing plate and screw fixation for a comminuted fracture of the orbital rim, the fragments may be removed, pieced together on a back table with a plate applied, and then the center fragments reinserted into the defect. Alternately, the defect can be spanned by a plate and then the intervening fragments individually screwed to the plate.

Compound comminuted fractures of the zygoma

Fractures of the zygoma may be compounded intraorally or extraorally when the force is severe enough to cause soft tissue wounds. A thorough inspection of the wound must be made to rule out the presence of foreign material, grass, debris, road dirt, and blood clots. Wood fragments are especially hazardous since they are colonized, driven in the soft tissue, and are not easily perceived at the time of wound inspection.

In isolated zygomatic arch fractures that demonstrate the tendency for medial displacement, some individuals use a protective splint, externally, to prevent displacement of the arch. If the reduction is performed carefully and precisely, the segments of the fractures are wedged, and the arch fracture will be stable without external support.

Delayed treatment of fractures of the zygoma

Repositioning after 2 weeks frequently requires osteotomy of the fracture sites to mobilize for reduction. After the bone has been mobilized, an inspection of each fracture site should be conducted to remove any area of fibrous ankylosis or any proliferative bone which was not present originally as its presence may prevent proper alignment. Plate and screw fixation then unites the segments. In fractures treated late, the masseter muscle may require division or mobilization from the inferior surface of the malar eminence and arch in order to allow the bone to be repositioned superiorly. The masseter muscle contracts in length in the case of the malreduced fracture, and it may not be able to be extended to length after several weeks have elapsed. Fractures treated delayed are more safely treated with osteotomy than mobilization by blunt forces. Mobilization of partially healed fractures may result in new fracture lines extending deep within the orbit, occasionally precipitating blindness. These forcible reduction techniques carry the risk of radiating fractures extending into the apex of the orbit, with cranial nerve injury.

Complications of zygomatic fractures

Bleeding and maxillary sinusitis

Bleeding into the maxillary sinus is usually of short duration. It may be necessary to irrigate blood clots from the antrum and to remove bone fragments, which sequester. Rarely, the ostea of the maxillary sinus will be occluded by the fractures, and require endoscopic sinus surgery. In those patients with preexisting sinus disease, acute exacerbation may be a complicating factor. Proper sinus drainage into the nose must be confirmed by free irrigation of saline into the nose at the time of Caldwell-Luc exposure. Otherwise, a persistent oral antral fistula may result in the sublabial area. Malfunction of the extraocular muscles occurs as a result of damage from fracture forces (contusion) or less frequently interference by segments of bone, orbital floor injury or fat or muscle entrapment. Several cases of blindness have occurred after malar fracture reduction.[161–163]

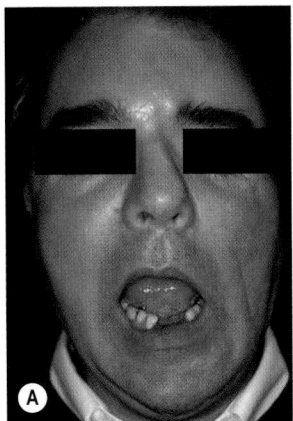 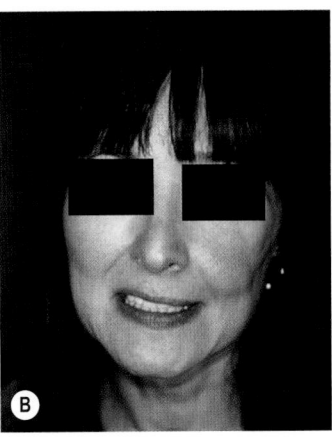

Fig. 3.26 (A) Soft tissue and bone deformity with enophthalmos, lateral canthal dystopia, ectropion, and soft tissue slippage in the midface. The lateral mandibular dentition is rotated lingually. **(B)** Enophthalmos, skeletonization of the orbital rim, scleral show, and retraction ("balling up") of midface soft tissue; slippage of the thick tissue off the malar eminence is caused by lack of soft tissue closure and lack of stabilization and fixation of the soft tissue onto the bone.

Late complications

Late complications of zygomatic fractures include nonunion, malunion, double vision, infraorbital nerve anesthesia or hypesthesia, and chronic maxillary sinusitis. Scarring may result from laceration or malpositioned incisions. Generally, ectropion and scleral show are mild, and resolve spontaneously. About 10% of patients having subciliary incisions of the lower eyelid develop a temporary ectropion. Gross downward dislocation of the zygoma results in diplopia and orbital dystopia *(Fig. 3.26)*. Usually, more than 5 mm of inferior globe dystopia is required to produce diplopia. Treatment[164,165] involves zygomatic mobilization by osteotomy with bone grafting to augment the malar eminence when malar projection is deficient. The position of the eye must be restored with intraorbital bone grafts or alloplastic material. Infection is not common, and usually responds to sinus or lacrimal drainage. Preexisting maxillary sinusitis or obstruction predisposes to infection, and the maxillary sinus should be cleared by endoscopic surgery before an elective osteotomy is performed.

Orbital complications

Orbital complications consist of diplopia, visual loss, globe injury, enophthalmos or exophthalmos, and lid malposition *(Fig. 3.26)*.

Impacted fractures of the zygomatic arch which abut the coronoid process may result in ankylosis. The gunshot wound is especially prone to this problem. If the zygomatic arch cannot be repositioned, coronoidectomy through an intraoral route usually frees the mandible from the ankylosis and permits normal function. It is important that the patient vigorously exercise to preserve and improve the range of motion obtained, which may take 6 months.

Numbness

Persistent anesthesia or hypesthesia in the distribution of the infraorbital nerve usually lasts only a short time. If total anesthesia exists for over 6 months, it is likely that the nerve is severely damaged or perhaps transected. If the nerve is impinged by bone fragments, especially in a medially and posteriorly impacted zygoma fracture, reduction or decompression of the infraorbital canal and neurolysis are indicated. Bone spurs, or constricting portions of the canal should be removed so that the nerve has an adequate opportunity for regeneration and relief of pressure. The nerve must be explored throughout the floor of the orbit so that it is free from any compression by bone fragments, scar tissue or callus. Anesthesia is annoying, especially immediately after the injury. Patients generally partially accommodate to the neurological deficit. Some spontaneous reinnervation may occur from adjacent facial regions as well as regrowth of axons through the infraorbital nerve. Usually some vague sensation is then present.

Oral-antral fistula

An oral-antral fistula requires debridement of bone or mucosa, confirmation of maxillary sinus drainage into the nose and closure with a transposition mucosal flap for cover. A 2-layer closure is required. A bone graft may be placed in between the layers of soft tissue. The buccal fat pad can be mobilized and sewn into the defect prior to the mucosa being sutured over it. Rarely, a distant flap is required for difficult persistent fistulae.

Plate complications

Complications include screw loosening or extrusion, plate exposure requiring removal and tooth root penetration by screws. Prominent plates over the zygomatic arch is directly due to associated soft tissue atrophy (temporalis) and to malreduction of the zygomatic arch laterally. Probably 10% of plates placed at the Le Fort I level need to be removed for exposure, non healing wound or cold sensitivity.

Midface buttresses

The midface is a system of sinus cavities where certain thicker areas (or buttresses) are present and provide considerable structural support. The important midface supporting skeleton consists of horizontal and vertical structural supports connected by thin plates of bone. The areas of structural support are the thicker pillars and must be anatomically reconstructed or repositioned to reestablish the preinjury facial bone architecture. The vertical supports consist of the nasal septum in the midline and the nasomaxillary, zygomaticomaxillary, and pterygoid buttresses anteriorly and laterally (*Fig. 3.27*). The nasomaxillary buttress extends along the pyriform aperture through the frontal process of the maxilla superiorly to the internal angular process of the frontal bone. The zygomaticomaxillary buttress extends through the bony mass of the body of the zygoma and through the frontal process of the zygoma to the external angular process of the frontal bone. Posteriorly, the pterygoid plates provide posterior stabilization of the vertical height of the midface and form the third or posterior maxillary buttress. The horizontal buttresses of the midface consist of the inferior orbital rims, the associated

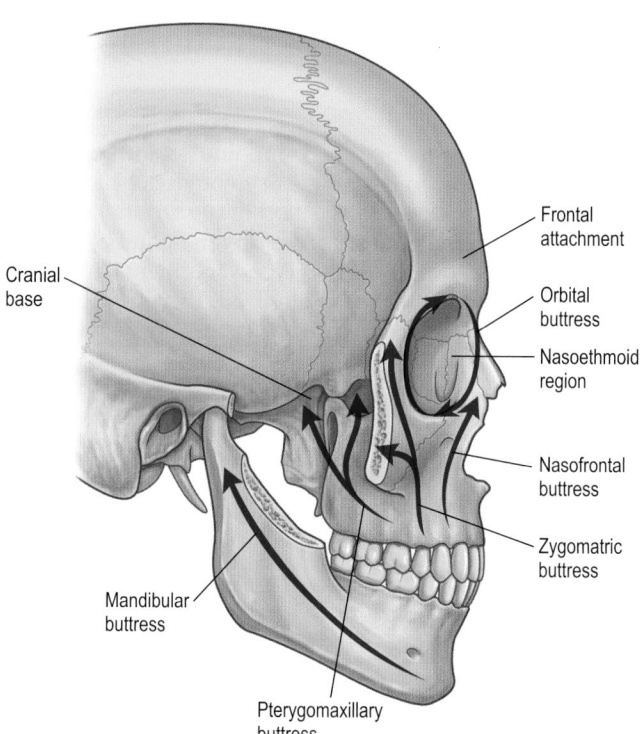

Fig. 3.27 The verticeal buttresses of the midfacial skeleton. Anteriorly, the nasofacial buttress skirts the piriform aperture inferiorly and composes the bone of the medial orbital rum superiorly to reach the frontal bone at its internal angular process. Laterally the zygomaticomaxillary buttress extends from the zygomatic process of the frontal bone through the lateral aspect of the zygoma to reach the maxillary alveolus. A component of the zygomaticomaxillary buttress extends laterally through the zygomatic arch to reach the temporal bone. Posteriorly, the pterygomaxillary buttress is seen. It extends from the posterior portion of the maxilla and the pterygoid fossa to reach the cranial base structures. The mandibular buttress forms a strong structural support for the lower midface in fracture treatment. This support for maxillary fracture reduction must conceptually be achieved by placement of both jaws in intermaxillary fixation. The other "transverse" maxillary buttresses include the palate, the inferior orbital rims, and the superior orbital rims. The superior orbital rims and lower sections of the frontal sinus are also known in the supraorbital regions as the frontal bar and are technically frontal bone and not part of the maxilla. (From Manson PN, Hoopes JE, Su CT. Structural pillars of the facial skeleton: an approach to the management of Le Fort fractures. Plast Reconstr Surg 1980;66:54.)

orbital floor, the zygomatic arch and the palate at the level of the maxillary alveolus.[166]

Clinical examination

Inspection

Epistaxis, bilateral ecchymosis (periorbital, subconjunctival, scleral) facial edema, and subcutaneous hematoma are suggestive of fractures involving the maxillary bone. The swelling is usually moderate to severe indicating the severity of the fracture. Malocclusion with an anterior open bite and rotation of the maxilla suggest a fracture of the maxilla. The maxillary segment is frequently displaced downward and posteriorly, resulting in a class III malocclusion and premature occlusion in the posterior dentition with an anterior open bite. On internal examination, there may be tearing of the soft tissues in the labial vestibule of the lip or the palate, findings that indicate the possibility of an alveolar or palate fracture. Hematomas may be present in the buccal or palatal mucosa. The face, after several days, may have an elongated, retruded appearance, the so-called "donkey-like faces" suggestive of a craniofacial disjunction. An increase in mid-facial length is seen.

Palpation

The bone should be palpated with the tips of the fingers both externally through the skin and internally intraorally. Bilateral palpation may reveal step deformities of the zygomaticomaxillary suture, indicating fractures of the inferior orbital rims. These findings suggest a pyramidal fracture of the maxilla or confirm the zygomatic component of a more complicated injury, such as a Le Fort III fracture. Intraoral palpation may reveal fractures of the anterior portion of the maxilla or fractured segments of the alveolar bone.

Digital manipulation

Manipulation of the maxilla may confirm movement in the entire middle third of the face, including the bridge of the nose. This movement is appreciated by holding the head securely with one hand and moving the maxilla with the other hand (*Fig. 3.5*). Crepitation may be heard when the maxilla is manipulated in loose fractures. The manipulation test for maxillary mobility is not entirely diagnostic because impacted or greenstick fractures may exhibit no movement but still possess bone displacement.

Malocclusion of the teeth

If the mandible is intact, malocclusion of the teeth is highly suggestive of a maxillary fracture. It is possible, however, that the malocclusion relates to a preinjury condition. A thorough study of the patient's dentition with reference to previous dental records and pictures is helpful.

Cerebral spinal rhinorrhea or otorrhea

Cerebral spinal fluid may leak from the anterior or middle cranial fossa in high Le Fort fractures and is then apparent in the nose or ear canal. A fluid leak signifies the presence of a dural fistula extending from the intracranial subarachnoid space through the skull and into the nose or ear.[167] Frequently the drainage is obscured by bloody secretions in the immediate post injury period.[168,169]

Radiological examination

Maxillary fractures are easily demonstrated in craniofacial CT scans, with the exception that fracture lines in minimally displaced fractures are more difficult to see. The presence of bilateral maxillary sinus opacity should always suggest the possibility of a maxillary fracture.

Treatment of maxillary fractures

Treatment of maxillary fractures is initially oriented toward the establishment of an airway, control of hemorrhage, closure of soft tissue lacerations and placement of the patient in intermaxillary fixation. The latter maneuver manually reduces the fracture, reduces movement and bleeding, and is the single most important treatment of a maxillary fracture.

Alveolar fractures

Simple fractures of the portions of the maxilla involving the alveolar process and the teeth can usually be digitally repositioned and held in reduction while an arch bar is applied to these teeth. The arch bar may be acrylated for stability, or an open reduction may utilize unicortical plates and screws to unite the alveolar fragment to the remainder of the maxilla. The position of the teeth may be maintained by ligating the teeth in the fractured segment to adjacent teeth with the use of an arch bar and interdental wiring technique. Fixation of the alveolar segment should be maintained for at least four to twelve weeks or until clinical immobility has been achieved.[170]

Le Fort classification of facial fractures

Le Fort (1901) completed experiments that determined the areas of structural weakness of the maxilla which he designated "lines of weakness". Between the lines of weakness were "areas of strength". This classification led to the Le Fort classification of maxillary fractures, which identifies the patterns of midfacial fractures (*Fig. 3.28*).[171] It should be emphasized that the usual Le Fort fracture consists of combinations of these patterns in that pure bilateral Le Fort I, Le Fort II, or Le Fort III fractures are less common than combination patterns.[172] The level of fracture is frequently different on one side from the other, and usually the fracture is more comminuted on the side of the injury.

Goals of Le Fort fracture treatment

Goals in the treatment of Le Fort fractures include:
- Restoration of midfacial height and projection
- Providing proper occlusion
- Restoring the integrity of the nose and orbit
- The structural supports between the areas of the buttress and maxillary alveolus must also be restored to provide for the proper soft tissue contour.

Transverse (Guerin) fractures or Le Fort I level fractures

Fractures which traverse the maxilla horizontally above the level of the apices of the maxillary teeth section the entire alveolar process of the maxilla, vault of the palate and the inferior ends of the pterygoid processes in a single block from the upper craniofacial skeleton. This type of injury is known as the Transverse, Le Fort I or Guerin fracture. This horizontal fracture extends transversely across the base of the maxillary sinuses and is almost always bilateral. The fracture level varies from just beneath the zygoma to just above the floor of the maxillary sinus and the inferior margin of the pyriform aperture (*Fig. 3.29*).

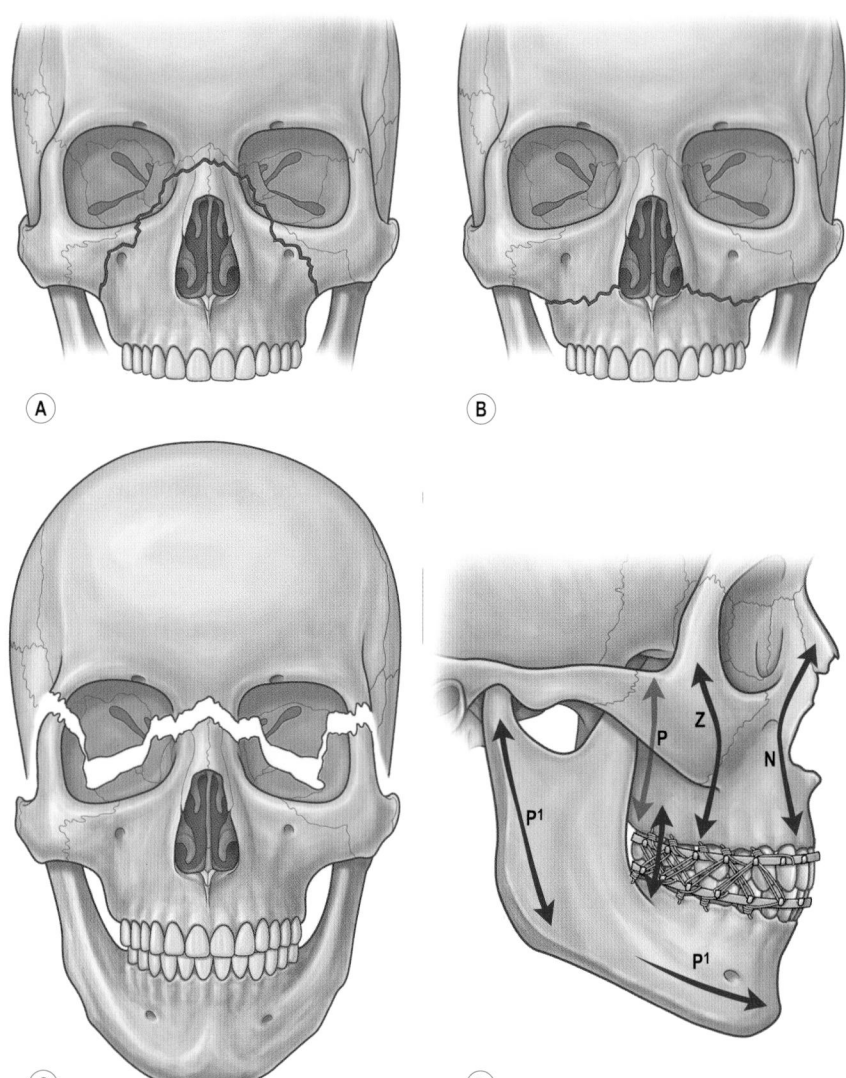

(A)

(B)

(C)

(D)

Fig. 3.28 The Le Fort classification of midfacial fractures. **(A)** The Le Fort I (horizontal or transverse) fracture of the maxilla, also known as Guerin fracture. **(B)** The Le Fort II (or pyramidal) fracture of the maxilla. In this fracture, the central maxilla is separated from the zygomatic areas. The fracture line may cross the nose through its cartilages or through the middle nasal bone area, or it may separate the nasal bones from the frontal bone through the junction of the nose and frontal sinus. **(C)** The Le Fort III fracture (or craniofacial disjunction). In this fracture, the entire facial bone mass is separated from the frontal bone by fracture lines traversing the zygoma nasoethmoid, and nasofrontal bone junctions. **(D)** Buttresses of the midface. N, nasofrontal buttress; Z, zygomatic buttress; P, pterygomaxillary buttress; P¹, posterior height and anteroposterior projection must be maintained in complicated fractures. This is especially true in Le Fort fractures accompanied by bilateral subcondylar fractures. (A–C from Kazanjian VH, Converse J. Surgical Treatment of Facial Injuries, 3rd edn. Baltimore MD: Williams & Wilkins; 1974.)

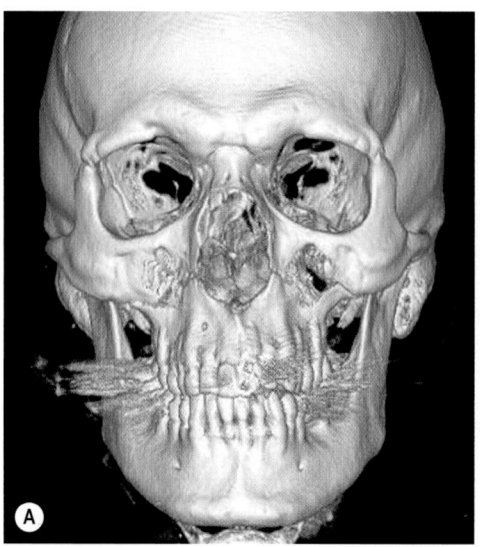

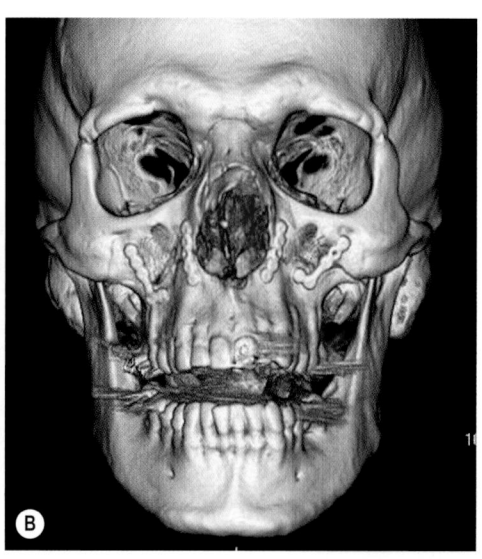

(A)

(B)

Fig. 3.29 Frontal 3D craniofacial computer tomography scan of a Le Fort I type injury pre- and post-open reduction and internal fixation.

Pyramidal fractures or Le Fort II level fractures

Blows to the central maxilla, especially those involving a frontal impact, frequently result in fractures with a pyramidally shaped central maxillary segment. This is a Le Fort II "central maxillary segment" and the fracture begins above the level of the apices of the maxillary teeth laterally and posteriorly in the zygomaticomaxillary buttress and extends through the pterygoid plates in the same fashion as the Le Fort I fracture. Fracture lines travel medially and superiorly to pass through the medial portion of the inferior orbital rim and extend across the nose to separate a pyramidally-shaped central maxillary segment from the superior cranial and midfacial structures. The fracture line centrally may traverse the nose high or low to separate superior cranial from midfacial structures *(Fig. 3.30)*.

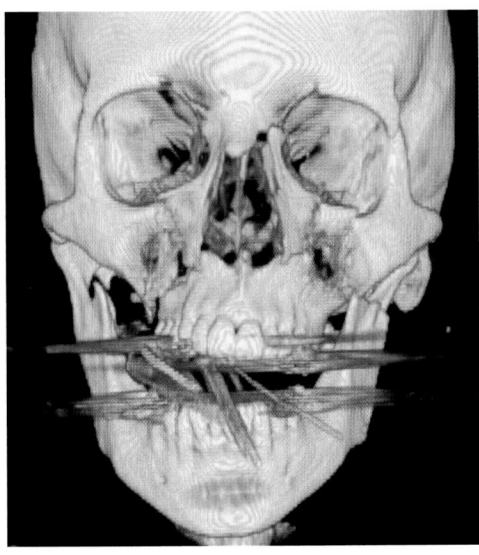

Fig. 3.30 Frontal 3D craniofacial computer tomography scan of a Le Fort II type injury pre- and post-open reduction and internal fixation.

Craniofacial dysjunction or Le Fort III fractures

Craniofacial dysjunction may occur when the fracture extends through the zygomaticofrontal suture and the nasal frontal suture and across the floor of the orbits to effectively separate all midfacial structures from the cranium. In these fractures, the maxilla is usually separated from the zygoma, but occasionally (5% of Le Fort III fractures) the entire midface may be a large single fragment, which is often only slightly displaced and immobile. These fractures are usually minimally displaced and present only with "black eyes" and with subtle occlusal problems. The Le Fort III segment may or may not be separated through the nasal structures. In these fractures, the entire midfacial skeleton is incompletely detached from the base of the skull and suspended by the soft tissues and "greensticked" fracture *(Fig. 3.31)*.[173]

Le Fort I level fractures

In fractures of the Le Fort I type, placing the patient in intermaxillary fixation may be all that is necessary in the case of a minimally mobile fracture. In most cases, however, the Le Fort I level should be opened through a gingival buccal sulcus incision and the fractures reduced and stabilized with plate and screw fixation at the bilateral nasomaxillary and zygomaticomaxillary buttresses. The primary consideration in Le Fort I fracture treatment is to reestablish a functional dental occlusion and this should be accomplished as soon as possible. Proper midfacial height and projection are achieved by open reduction.

Le Fort II level fractures

In the case of a simple Le Fort II level fracture, the patient is first placed in intermaxillary fixation. The fracture should be opened at the Le Fort I level through a gingival buccal sulcus incision and through both lower eyelids to provide reduction and fixation at the zygomaticomaxillary and nasomaxillary buttresses and at the inferior orbital rims. The need

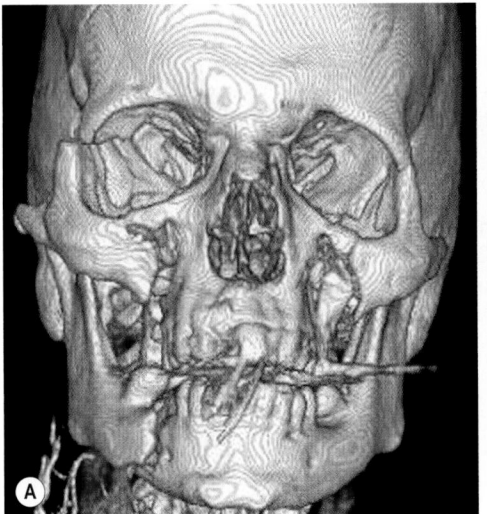
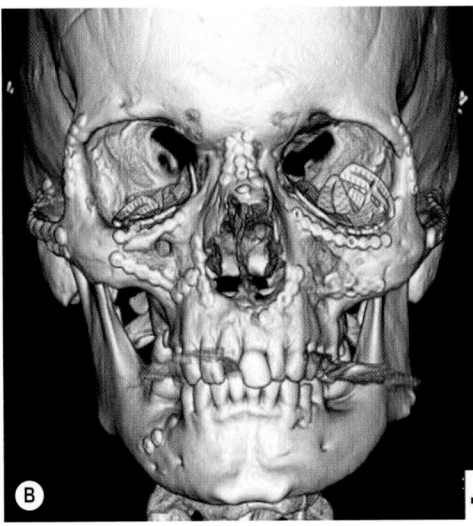

Fig. 3.31 Frontal 3D craniofacial computer tomography scan of a Le Fort III type injury pre- and post-open reduction and internal fixation.

for opening fractures crossing the nose must be assessed by the CT scan and the displacement at the nasofrontal junction.

Le Fort III fractures

Open reduction of Le Fort III fractures generally involves combining procedures at the Le Fort I, Le Fort II and zygomatic levels reduction in a single operation.

Postoperative care of maxillary fractures

The postoperative management of fractures of the maxilla consists of the usual general care of the facial fracture patient, including three times daily dental and oral hygiene, lip lubrication, mouthwashes, skin care and abrasion and laceration cleansing and lubrication with antibiotic ointments. Provision of adequate nutrition may be accomplished with a nasogastric tube or percutaneous gastrostomy. A liquid diet may be permitted with IMF, and a soft diet if the IMF is released.

Cleansing and aspiration of the nose and mouth is very important. The presence of a fever in patients with facial fractures should always prompt a sinus evaluation by radiographs if the fever cannot be explained by other sources. Any foul odor to the breath necessitates inspection, cleaning and/or a return to the operating room for irrigation and a thorough examination.

Complications of maxillary fractures

Airway

In almost all cases of extensive fractures, the airway is partially compromised by posterior displacement of the fracture fragments and by edema and swelling of the soft tissues in the nose, mouth, throat and floor of the mouth. In some patients, a nasopharyngeal airway may assist in establishing a route for ventilation. In other patients, intubation or tracheostomy may be indicated to provide a secure airway.

Bleeding

Hemorrhage may be managed by carefully identifying and ligating vessels in cutaneous lacerations, and by tamponade in closed midface injuries with anterior – posterior nasopharyngeal packing, manual reduction of the displaced maxilla and placing the teeth in intermaxillary fixation. Angiographic embolization and the combination of external carotid and superficial temporal artery ligation are usually unnecessary.

Infection

Maxillary fracture wounds are less complicated by infection than are mandibular fractures. Although, they are contaminated at the time of the injury, by entry into adjacent sinuses, fractures of the teeth and open intraoral wounds. Fractures passing through the sinuses do not usually result in infection unless there has been preexisting nasal or sinus disease, or in case of persistent obstruction of the sinus orifice by displaced bone fractures or blood clot. If the maxillary sinuses are obstructed, a nasal-antral window or preferably endoscopic drainage of the maxillary sinus by enlarging its orifice may be required.

CSF rhinorrhea

High Le Fort (II, III) level fractures may be associated with fractures of the cribriform area, which produce cerebrospinal fluid rhinorrhea and/or pneumocephalus. Antibiotic therapy may be utilized in these fractures at the discretion of the attending surgeon. Although antibiotic prophylaxis in CSF rhinorrhea has been quite widely employed, it is difficult to prove that antibiotics have substantially reduced the incidence of meningitis accompanying cerebrospinal fluid rhinorrhea when administered over a prolonged period. Blowing of the nose and placement of obstructing nasal packing should be avoided.

Blindness

Blindness is a rare complication of fractures of the orbit, and as such, may complicate fractures of the Le Fort II and III level. It is rare for the optic nerve to be severed by bone fragments. The most common etiology is a traumatic shock to the nerve or swelling of the nerve within the tight portion of the optic canal or interference with the capillary blood supply of the optic nerve by swelling and edema.

Late complications

Late complications of fractures of the maxilla include those referable to the orbit and zygoma, since these areas form a portion of the upper Le Fort (II and III) fractures. Specific complications referable to the maxilla include nonunion, malunion, plate exposure, lacrimal system obstruction, infraorbital and lip hypesthesia or anesthesia, and devitalization of teeth. There may be changes in facial appearance due to differences in midfacial height and projection, and differences in the transverse width of the face or dental arch.

Nonunion and bone grafting

True nonunion of the maxilla is rare and usually follows failure to provide even the most elementary type of intermaxillary fixation or open reduction. If nonunion occurs, the treatment consists of exposure of the fracture site, resection of the fibrous tissue in the fracture site, reduction of the displaced segments, removal of any proliferative bone edges, placement of bone grafts in all the existing gaps, and stabilization by plate and screw fixation.

Malunion

In multiple (complex) pan facial fractures, malunion may result from inadequate diagnosis, inadequate reduction or inadequate fixation. The period of intermaxillary fixation and observation may need to be longer when the injury is more comminuted.

Malocclusion

If malocclusion is detected, it may respond to elastic traction. Once partial healing has occurred, attempts to reestablish occlusion with elastics may simply extrude or loosen the teeth. Revision of the reduction after removal of the internal fixation devices or a new osteotomy may be necessary. When new (secondary) osteotomies are necessary, generally a Le Fort I osteotomy for repositioning of the tooth bearing segment of the maxilla is preferred as opposed to a higher level osteotomy. Occasionally, segmental osteotomies of the maxillary arch may be necessary to achieve optimal dental relationships.

Nasolacrimal duct injury

The nasolacrimal duct may be transected or obstructed by the fractures extending across the middle-third of the facial skeleton between the Le Fort I and Le Fort III levels. Anatomic repositioning of the fracture fragments of the medial portion of the maxilla and nasoethmoidal orbital area provides the best protection against obstruction. Obstruction of the lacrimal system produces dacryocystitis[174] and may require external drainage.

Lower facial fractures

Mandible fractures

Craniofacial fractures frequently involve the jaws. Fischer et al.[175] in 2001, looked at mandible fractures that were caused by motor vehicle collisions and found associated injuries in 99%. Fractures of the jaws invariably produce malocclusion. Knowledge of the dentition is thus an absolute prerequisite for the proper treatment of jaw fractures. Restoration of the occlusion usually indicates anatomic reduction and proper positioning of the jaws and facial bones.

Dental wiring and fixation techniques

Arch-bars

Prefabricated arch-bars are ligated to the external surface of the dental arch by passing 24 or 26 gauge steel wires around the arch-bar, and around the necks of the teeth. The wires are twisted tightly to individual teeth to hold the arch-bars in the form of the dental arch. If segments of teeth are missing, or if anterior support of the arch-bar is needed to balance the forces generated by elastic traction anteriorly, the arch-bar may be stabilized by additional wires passed to the skeleton (skeletal wires). Suspension wires may be passed through drill holes at the piriform margin or around screws. This is particularly applicable in children where the structure of the teeth tends to render arch-bars less stable. The mandibular arch-bar may also be stabilized by wires passed to a screw at the lower mandibular border, or by circummandibular wiring. It cannot be over emphasized that the stability and alignment of a fracture reduction depends greatly on the alignment of the teeth achieved by this initial application of arch-bars. Dental relationships are used to describe tooth movements and interdental relations. A malocclusion can sometimes be corrected by the simple use of orthodontic rubber bands. At the end of a course of fracture treatment, if there is mobility at the fracture site, fixation may be easily reestablished for a short period by reapplying IMF.

IMF screws

This is a rapid method of immobilizing the teeth in occlusion, given good dentition and uncomplicated fracture types. The number and position of the IMF screws is based on the fracture type, fracture location and surgeon preference. Screws must be positioned superior to the maxillary tooth roots and inferior to the mandibular tooth roots (*Fig. 3.32*).

The prominence, position, and anatomic configuration of the mandible are such that it is one of the most frequently injured facial bones. Following automobile accidents, the mandible is the most commonly encountered fracture seen at many major trauma centers. The mandible is a movable, predominantly U-shaped bone, consisting of horizontal and vertical segments. The horizontal segments consist of the body and the symphysis centrally. The vertical segments consist of the angles and rami, which articulate with the skull through the condyles and temporomandibular joints. The mandible is attached to other facial bones by muscles and ligaments and articulates with the maxilla through the occlusion of teeth.

The mandible is a strong bone, but has several weak areas that are prone to fracture. The body of the mandible is composed principally of dense cortical bone with a small substantia spongiosa, through which blood vessels, lymphatics, and nerves pass. The mandible is thin at the angles where the body joins with the ramus and can be further weakened by the presence of an unerupted third molar or a previous dental extraction.[176]

The mandible is also weak at the condylar neck, cuspid root (the longest root) and mental foramen, through which the mental nerve and vessels extend into the soft tissues of the lower lip. The weak areas for fractures are the subcondylar area, angle, distal body, and the mental foramen.[177-179] Timely loss of teeth results in atrophic changes of the alveolar bone

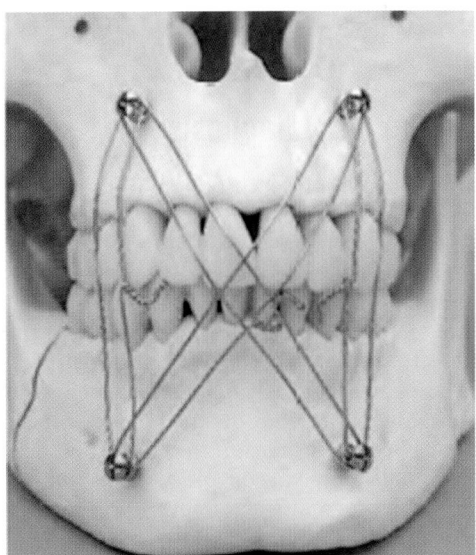

Fig. 3.32 The use of intermaxillary fixation screws for intermaxillary fixation. These devices do not provide the stability or flexibility obtained from arch bars and full intermaxillary fixation. Numbers of patients have been thought to be in good occlusion with this technique when actually they were in an open bite, were malreduced, and required osteotomy or fracture revision. Crossed wires may also be used to buttress the screw support obtained. (Courtesy of Synthes Maxillofacial, Paoli, PA.)

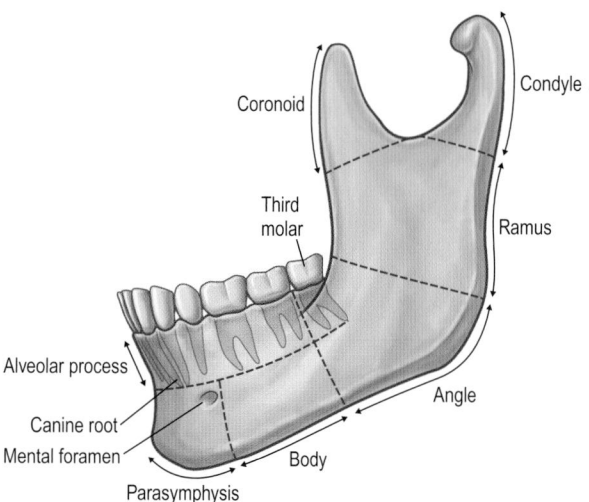

Fig. 3.33 Classification of mandibular fractures.

and alters the structural characteristics of the mandible. Fractures often occur through the edentulous areas rather than through the areas better supported by adequate tooth and alveolar bone structures.[180]

Mandibular movements are determined by the action of reciprocally placed muscles attached to the bone. When fractures occur, displacement of the segments is influenced by the pull of the muscles attaching to the segments. The direction of the fracture line may oppose forces created by these muscles.

Classification of mandibular fractures

Mandibular fractures are classified according to location (*Fig. 3.33*), condition of teeth, direction of fracture and favorability for treatment, presence of compound injury through the skin or mucosa, and anatomical fracture pattern.

Clinical examination and diagnosis

Pain and *tenderness* are usually present upon motion over the fracture and may be noted immediately as a result of injury. Fractures occurring along the course of the inferior alveolar nerve may produce *numbness* in the distribution of the nerve, which represents numbness of the ipsilateral lower lip (mental nerve) and ipsilateral teeth. The patient is unable to open the mouth or bring the teeth into proper occlusion (*trismus*). The patient may refuse to eat or to brush his teeth, which then causes discomfort and an abnormal, foul-smelling odor (*fetor oris*). Excessive saliva is often produced as a result of local irritation (*drooling*). Small gingival or mucosal *lacerations* between teeth indicate the possibility of a fracture. These gaps make the fracture compound into the mouth.

Diagnosis

Bimanual manipulation of the mandible causes *mobility* or *distraction* at the fracture site, especially when the fracture occurs in the body or parasymphysial area. One hand should stabilize the ramus, while the other manipulates the

symphysis or the body area. The fracture will be demonstrated by abnormal movement, and the condition and the symptom reinforced by the presence of discomfort. The mandible may be pulled forward with one hand while the other hand is placed one finger in the ear canal and one finger over the condylar process (*Fig. 3.4*). Abnormal *mobility* or *crepitus* indicates a fracture in the condylar/subcondylar area, or ligament laxity, indicating a temporal mandibular joint injury. The most reliable finding in the fractures of the mandible, in dentulous patients, is the presence of a *malocclusion*. Often, the most minute malocclusion caused by the fracture is quite obvious to the patient. The patient may be unable to move the jaw (*dysfunction*), and request liquid foods that require minimal jaw movement and mastication. Speech is difficult because of pain on motion of the mandible. *Crepitation* may be noticeable by manipulation of the fracture site. Often, the necessary manipulation produces such discomfort that it is not wise to demonstrate this physical sign. *Swelling* is usually quite obvious and frequently associated with ecchymosis and a hematoma. Often, an intraoral laceration is present over fractures in the horizontal portion of the mandible. There is frequently *deviation* to one side or the other; a finding that supports the diagnosis of a fracture. *Tenderness* over the fracture site is present, especially in the region of the temporomandibular joint. Such tenderness is highly suggestive of a fracture.

Muscles influencing mandibular movement

Muscle function is an important variable influencing the degree and direction of muscular displacement of the fractured mandible. Overcoming the forces of mandibular displacement is also important in designing reduction and fixation. The posterior group of muscles is commonly referred to as the "muscles of mastication" and includes the temporalis, masseter, and medial and lateral pterygoid muscles. The overall activity is to move the mandible in a general upward, forward, and medial direction.

The temporomandibular joint

The function and anatomy of this joint are important in considering injuries of the mandibular condyle. It is a ginglymodiarthrodial joint capable of a hinge-like action, as well as gliding and rotating action. The joint is composed of the articular head, condyle, and glenoid fossa. The glenoid fossa forms a portion of the floor of the middle cranial fossa. The articular surface of both the condyle and the temporal fossa is covered with a thin, smooth, layer of cartilage surrounded by connective tissue, which differentiates into an inner and outer layer. The inner layer or synovial membrane secretes a viscous fluid lubricant that minimizes friction and aids smooth joint functioning. The outer layer of the connective tissue is intimately associated with ligaments that surround the joint, and provides an enveloping capsule within which the articular surfaces function. The joint is separated into two distinct chambers, one above and the other below an articular disc composed of fibrocartilage known as the meniscus. Movement of the articular disc is controlled by the attachments of the lateral pterygoid muscle that insert, through the capsule of the joint, into the anterior disc and by the attachment of the disc to the posterior portion of the joint capsule. The hinge, rotating, and gliding movements of the temporomandibular joint are controlled by muscles attached to the mandible. The movement of the disc is regulated by its ligaments, and injuries to the ligaments result in abnormal disc motion, which produce clicking, rocking, and pain.

Fractures influencing displacement of fractured mandibular segments

The direction and extent of displacement depends on the site of the fracture, direction of the fracture and direction of muscle pull, direction and intensity of displacement forces, and presence or absence of teeth in the fragments. In fractures of the mandible, the segments may be displaced in the direction of the strongest muscular action.

Direction and angulation of the fracture line

Kelsey Frye and colleagues[181] described fractures as "favorable" or "unfavorable" according to their direction and bevel of displacement (Fig. 3.34). The muscular forces on some fracture fragments are opposed by the direction and bevel of the fracture line. Thus, in some fractures, the muscular force would pull the fragments into a position favorable for healing, whereas in other fractures, the muscular pull is unfavorable and separation of the fracture fragments occurs by action of the muscular forces. Mandibular fractures that are directed downward and forward are classified as horizontally favorable (HF) because the posterior group of muscles and the anterior group of muscles pull in antagonistic directions, favoring stability at the fracture site. Fractures running from above, downward, and posteriorly are classified as horizontally unfavorable (HU). The bevel of the fracture may also influence a displacement medially. If a fracture runs from

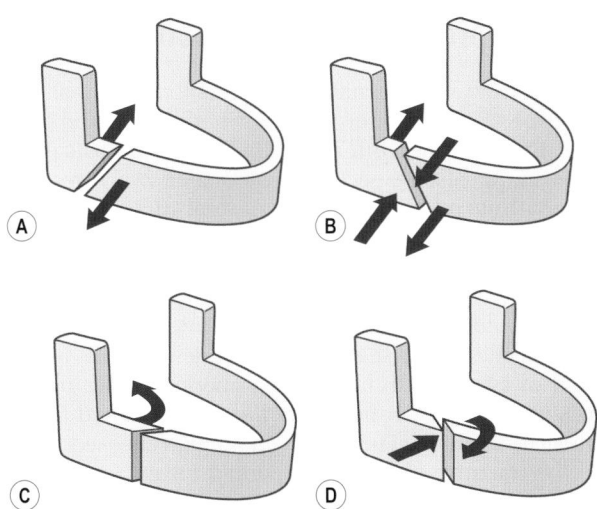

Fig. 3.34 (A,C) The direction and bevel of the fracture line does not resist displacement due to muscle action. The arrows indicate the direction of muscle pull. (B,D) The bevel and direction of the fracture line resist displacement and oppose muscle action. The direction of the muscle pull in fractures beveled in this direction would tend to impact the fractured bone ends. (After Fry WK, Shepherd PR, McLeod AC, et al. The Dental Treatment of Maxillofacial Injuries. Oxford: Blackwell Scientific; 1942.)

posteriorly forward and medially, displacement would take place in a medial direction because of the medial pull of the elevator muscles of mastication (vertically unfavorable, or VU). The fracture that passes from the lateral surface of the mandible posteriorly and medially is a favorable fracture because the muscle-pull tends to prevent displacement. It is called a vertically favorable fracture (VF).

The presence or absence of teeth in the fractured segments

Upper displacement of the posterior segment is prevented by occlusal contact of the lower against the upper teeth. The elevator muscles of the mandible pull the posterior segment forward. The anterior group of muscles depresses the anterior segments of the mandible, separating the teeth anterior to the fracture from the upper teeth. A single tooth in the posterior fragment may be extremely important, and should be retained, as the tooth acts as an occlusal stop and provides some stability for fracture alignment.[182,183]

Treatment principles of mandibular fractures

- Establish proper occlusion.
- Anatomically reduce the fractured bones into their normal position.
- Utilize fixation techniques that hold the fractured bone segments in occlusion and normal position until healing has occurred. Open reduction internal fixation (ORIF) can often permit limited function while healing is occurring.
- Control infection.

Methods of fixation vary with age, general health, surgical training, and facilities available for treatment. A satisfactory end-result may be accomplished by a number of methods. No method is without its specific requirements and approaches, and of course, advantages, disadvantages, cost, and complications.

Treatment of class I fractures

Class I fractures are those in which there are teeth on each side of the fracture. Although many of these fractures can be managed by intermaxillary fixation (IMF) alone in "favorable" fractures, if function is desired and post treatment displacement is to be prevented, (i.e., the mandible being used as a basis for Le Fort fracture treatment) internal fixation is also preferred. If IMF alone is to be used, the period of fixation should constitute 4–6 weeks.[184,185]

Many mandibular fractures, even if favorable, are best managed by ORIF. Miniplates may be used for non-comminuted, nonbone gap fractures where impaction of the bone bears a significant portion of the load of fracture stabilization.[186,187]

This technique prevents displacement and permits light function. ORIF is especially appealing to patients because the teeth do not need to remain wired, which permits intake of soft foods, oral hygiene and an early return to work. These desirable aspects might not justify open treatment, if external incisions are required which would produce permanent scars.[188]

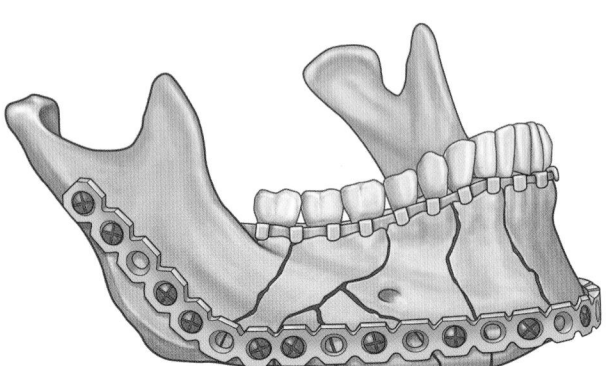

Fig. 3.35 Large reconstruction plate spans fractures of the entire body. (Courtesy of Synthes Maxillofacial, Paoli, PA.)

A soft diet, compared with liquid food required for a period of 4–6 weeks of IMF, is of temporary significance and should not influence the surgeon's treatment method, if a permanent scar would be necessary.

General principles of reduction and fixation

The principle underlying all mandibular fracture treatment is superior and inferior border stabilization. The general method of fracture fixation involves arch-bar placement and the use of a superior border unicortical noncompression miniplate. The inferior border is aligned and approximated by a stabilization plate. In severely displaced fractures, provisional stabilization with an inferior border wire assists the proper arch-bar application. The use of the "locking plate" minimizes the requirement for precise plate bending. Comminuted fractures *(Fig. 3.35)* require larger fixation plates, and are conceptually fractures with "bone loss", where the plate itself bears the entire load of fixation.

In general, fractures of the symphysis-parasymphysis area are broadly exposed with an intraoral degloving technique. Periosteal attachments should be retained where possible, as the periosteal blood supply is often the only remaining circulation (the medullary blood supply is generally injured by the fracture). Adequate exposure, especially for plate and screw fixation, demands wider soft tissue mobilization. Experience has shown that "free" bone fragments will generally survive if stabilization is sufficient and if they are covered by well-vascularized soft tissue. The periosteum, therefore, is not thought to be so important a blood supply that preservation is preferential to improper fracture reduction or inadequate fracture stabilization. A mentalis muscle stump on the bone should always be preserved and the muscle must be repaired during soft tissue closure. In general, both a muscular and mucosal closure of intraoral incisions is always preferred to mucosal closure alone.

Treatment of class II fractures

In class II fractures, teeth are present only one side of the fracture site and these fractures must have an open reduction. This type of fracture may occur in any portion of the horizontal mandible but frequently is at the angle. The type and strength of plate needed to control the nontoothbearing fragment and displacement of the fracture will vary according to the direction and bevel of the fracture and the position of the teeth and surrounding muscles. Generally, a larger inferior border plate with a smaller superior border plate is preferred with three screws placed in solid, nonfractured bone to each side of the fracture. The third screw represents "insurance" against one of the primary two screws becoming loose. One screw inserted in the compression mode may or may not be utilized. Compression screws impact the bone ends under pressure, but can unfavorably change the occlusion.

Comminuted fractures

Comminution negatively influences stability, and generally increases the degree of fracture displacement.[189] Three screws are utilized for fracture stabilization placed in nonfractured bone on each side of the fracture defect. ORIF is indicated for all class II fractures. Upper and lower border plates are preferred in the horizontal mandible and two plates also in the vertical mandible where possible.

Treatment of class III fractures

Class III fractures have no teeth on either side of the fracture. Nondisplaced, immobile fractures conceptually may be treated by a soft diet with close follow up. The majority of class III fractures however, should be managed with rigid fixation with superior and inferior border fixation. Precise positioning techniques are required in sequence in combined Le Fort and mandibular fractures, such as IMF, dentures or splints.

Extraoral approach to open reduction

The position of an external mandibular incision should always respect the location of the marginal mandibular branch of the facial nerve *(Fig. 3.36)*. The subperiosteal dissection technique also respects neurovascular structures such as the mental nerve. Careful subperiosteal dissection establishes the extent and pattern of the fracture, confirming the impression given from the CT. The fragments at the inferior border of the fracture are aligned with clamps. The occlusal reduction should be checked at this point, and loose arch bar wires on the minor segment are tightened. IMF is then confirmed or established. Usually, a superior border plate is now utilized at the upper border of the mandible and fixated with unicortical screws. The occlusion is again checked, alignment of the fractures re-confirmed, and a lower border plate and screws applied. A larger plate may be utilized. Generally, a large plate is initially "over bent" so that it stands 2–3 mm off the fracture site. Screw length may be determined by a depth gauge, and bicortical placement is preferred. If a larger plate is used, as the bicortical screws are tightened, the over-bent plate flattens itself against the outer border of the mandible and reduces the lingual cortex properly. If compression is desired only the *first two* screws (one on each side of the

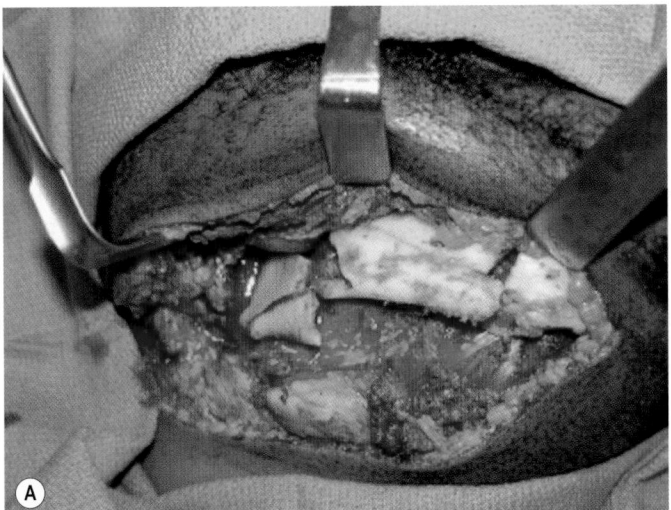
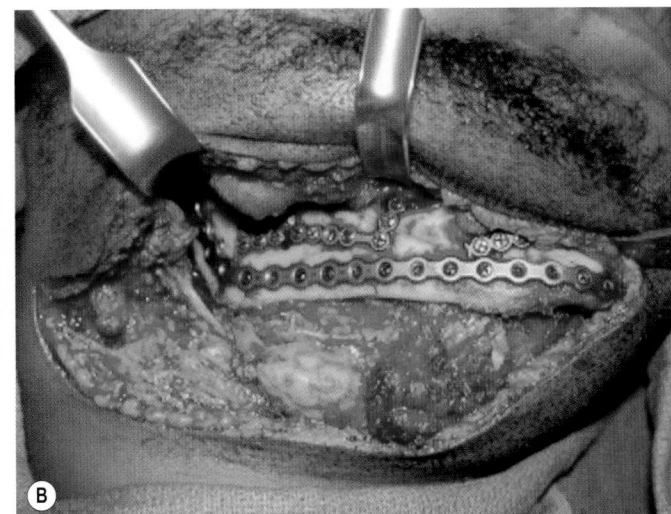
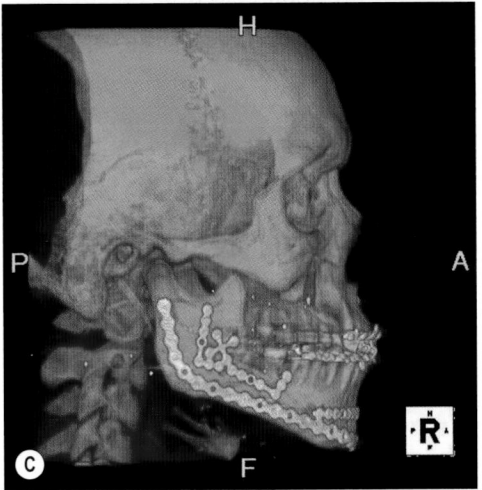

Fig. 3.36 Intraoperative photograph of comminuted mandibular fracture in a 23-year-old male following attempted homicidal gunshot wound to the face pre- and post-open reduction and internal fixation via the extra-oral approach using multiple miniplates. Lateral 3D craniofacial computer tomography postoperative scan following open reduction and internal fixation of comminuted mandibular fractures.

fracture) are inserted in compression mode; the remainder of the screw holes *must* be drilled in *neutral* mode. The compression mode is never used in "comminuted" or "bone defect" fractures. After the fixation is secure, any initial positioning wires are removed and the musculature repaired. Care must be taken in suture placement to avoid the marginal mandibular branch of the facial nerve, which is located up to 1–2 cm below the inferior edge of above the inferior mandible.[190] The platysma muscle and the skin are closed in layers, and a dependent drain placed. The cutaneous wound is closed in layers with subcuticular sutures to avoid suture marks.

Intraoral approach to open reduction

Any fracture in the horizontal or vertical mandible is usually amenable to an intraoral approach.[191–194] This is the preferred exposure for any symphysis or parasymphysis fracture, and for noncomminuted angle fractures. The body region is also able to be reduced but may require a percutaneous Trocar approach for drilling and screw placement. In the intraoral approach, the fracture site is exposed through an appropriately placed mucosal incision. The incision is generally brought about a centimeter out of the sulcus on the buccal

aspect of the mucosa, and mucosal and muscular layers separately incised.

Indications for ORIF of mandibular fractures

- Favorable or unfavorable class I fractures where stability is desired.
- Class II and class III fractures.
- Comminuted fractures.
- Displaced fractures and those subject to rotation.
- Edentulous fractures.
- The desire to avoid IMF in the postoperative period.
- Combined fractures of the upper and lower jaws.
- Uncooperative (head injured) patients.

The objectives are the reduction and fixation of the fractured segments to make a solid, one-piece mandible. The objective may also include the achievement of rigidity to obtain active and pain-free mobilization without jeopardizing the bone healing process or risk fracture displacement. This latter aim is achieved by accurate anatomic reduction with the patient in proper occlusion and secure soft tissue closure. The emphasis is therefore on simultaneous occlusal and basal bone repositioning and fixation (superior and inferior border).

The surgical technique must emphasize the protection of the soft tissue, and minimize the aesthetic deformity from incisions and exposures, and return the soft tissue to its normal position around the bone.

Selection of internal fixation devices for mandibular fractures

Edward Ellis, 3rd[195,196] clarified the issues regarding the selection of internal fixation devices for mandibular fractures. Normal bite forces must be initially countered by fixation devices; however, patients who have sustained mandible fractures do not generate normal bite forces for months after the injury. Rigid fixation is defined as internal fixation that is stable enough to prevent micromotion of the bony fragments under normal function. Most of the time, we do not achieve that; however, it has been recognized that rigidity of the bone fragments is not necessary for healing of the fracture to occur under functional loading. Ellis uses the term "functionally stable fixation" to apply to those forms of internal fixation recognized as not "rigid" but which satisfy the goals of maintaining fragment alignment, permitting healing during limited active use of the bone. Ellis also discusses the concepts of "load bearing" versus "load sharing" fixation. "Load bearing" fixation devices are of sufficient strength and rigidity that the devices bear the entire loads applied to the mandible during functional activities without impaction of the bone ends (i.e., 2.4 mm reconstruction plate). Load sharing is a form of internal fixation that is of insufficient stability to bear all the functional loads applied across the fracture (i.e., 2.0 mm miniplate). It relies on the impaction of the bone on each side of the fracture to bear the majority of the functional load. Compression plates have the ability to compress the fractured bony margins helping to bring them closer together and imparting additional stability by increasing the frictional interlocking between bone edges. While the functional load bearing factors are of advantage, if the plate is not perfectly applied there may be a geometric rearrangement of the fracture fragments over the first few weeks caused by the dissipation of the compression forces that can alter the occlusion. This is especially true in oblique fractures. Improper application of the compression plate may cause widening of the mandible if not properly overbent prior to application of the first two screws. In these cases, the lingual cortices may not contact even though the buccal cortices appear perfectly reduced. Slight over bending of the plate prevents this problem. Locking plate and screw systems function as "internal external fixators" achieving stability by locking the screw to the plate.[197]

The potential advantages of these fixation devices are that precise adaptation of the plate to the underlying bone is not necessary. As the screws are tightened they "lock" to the plate, thus stabilizing the segments without the need to compress the bone to the plate. This makes it impossible for the screw insertion to alter the reduction. This theoretically makes it less important to have good plate bending, as other plates must be perfectly adapted to the contour of the bone. Theoretically this hardware should be less prone to inflammatory complications from loosening of hardware since loose hardware propagates an inflammatory response and promotes infection.

Champy or miniplate system

Mandibular fixation by the use of smaller "miniplates," such as those advocated by Champy and colleagues in 1978[198,199] for mandibular fractures, speeded exposure and was more tolerant for mandibular shape and occlusion versus more rigid plates adaption as the screws were tightened. The malleable plates minimized malreductions from "plate bending errors" common to stiff larger plates. This technique did not result in maximum rigidity achieved with the large plates, but was generally sufficient for good immobilization without great movement at the fracture site for most fractures.[200]

As such, it was much more "user friendly" than more rigid systems and rose in popularity to surpass the use of rigid plate systems. Champy recommended two plates (upper and lower border) in the anterior (symphysis and parasymphysis) portion of the mandible, and a single plate along the superior border in the angle and upper border of the distal ramus (*Fig. 3.37*). The need for additional fixation must be assessed

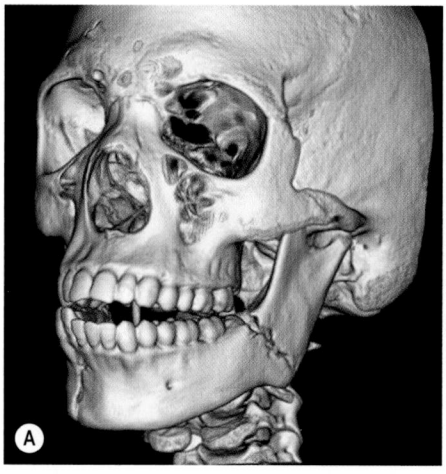
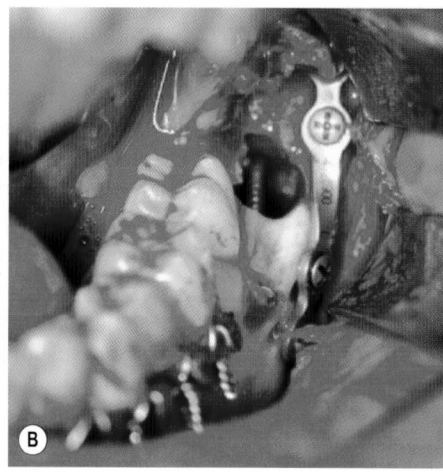
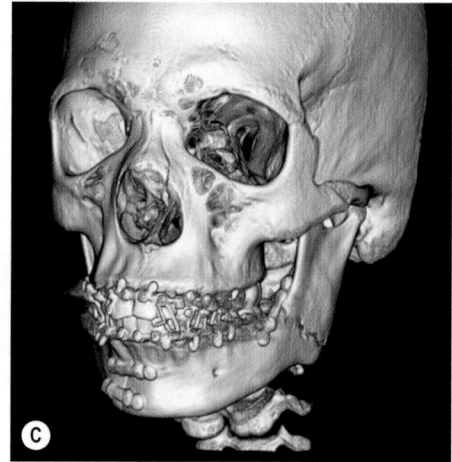

Fig. 3.37 (A) Three-quarter view of 3D craniofacial computer tomography preoperative scan on 16-year-old male who sustained a left mandibular angle fracture and right mandibular parasymphysial fracture following an altercation. **(B)** Intraoperative photograph of open reduction and internal fixation of left mandibular angle fracture using the Champy technique. **(C)** Three-quarter view of 3D craniofacial computer tomography postoperative scan.

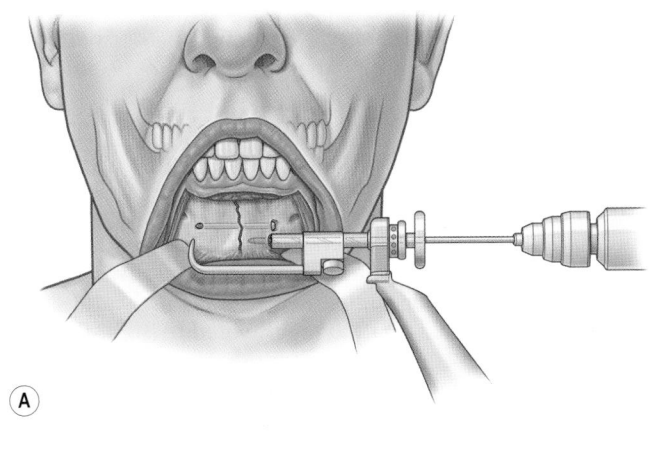

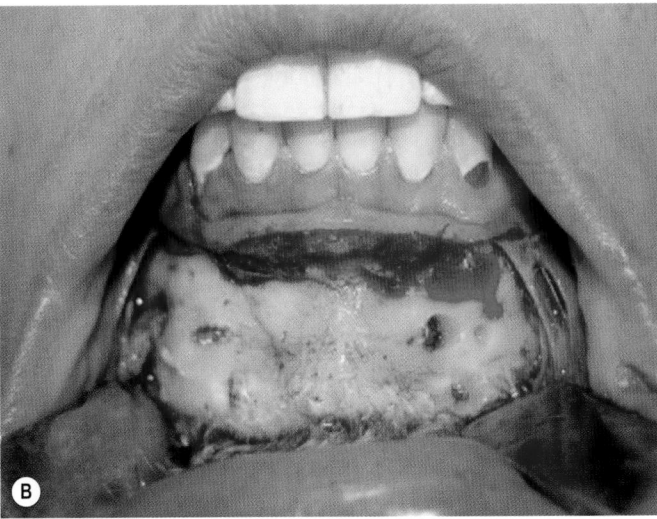

Fig. 3.38 (A) Placement of two horizontal lag screws to reduce and stabilize a parasymphysis fracture using a trocar device. (Courtesy of Synthes Maxillofacial, Paoli, PA.) **(B)** Intraoperative photograph of open reduction and internal fixation of mandibular symphyseal fracture using lag screws.

carefully, and this technique should be avoided in comminuted fractures and in the multiply-fractured mandible. The technique can only be used where the bone at the fracture site can be compressed by the plate to bear some of the "load" of the fracture across the impacted bone ends. The use of a brief initial period of rest in IMF (1 week) is used by some practitioners for soft tissue "rest" and provides an initial period of occlusion where less stress is placed on the fracture and more importantly the soft tissue.

Lag screw technique

This technique is indicated in noncomminuted parasymphysis or symphysis fractures,[201–203] where a long length of screw can be tolerated *(Fig. 3.38)*. Generally, these screw lengths require 35–45 mm anteriorly. A specific technique is utilized where the first cortex in the bone is over-drilled to the major diameter of the screw. The second segment of the screw path is drilled to the minor diameter of the screw. Only the screw head will engage bone in the first section of the path, and therefore, as the screw is tightened into the second section of the fracture, the screw head impacts the cortex toward the fracture site as it is tightened. Generally, two lag screws are recommended for each fracture to be stable, for if one becomes loose, the fracture would be unstable by virtue of the rotation. With only one screw, the fracture could still rotate around the single screw. A sleeve or drill guide is used to protect soft tissue. Oblique body or angle fractures may be lag screwed with 2–3 screws for stability. In screw placement, the angle between the bone and the direction of the screw should bisect a 90° angle from the bone in a plane parallel to the bone.

Third molars in mandibular angle fractures

Extraction of an impacted 3rd molar must be carefully considered and in some circumstances, where the 3rd molar is partially erupted and inflamed, it should be removed at the time of fracture treatment to avoid potential complications *(Fig. 3.39)*.[204]

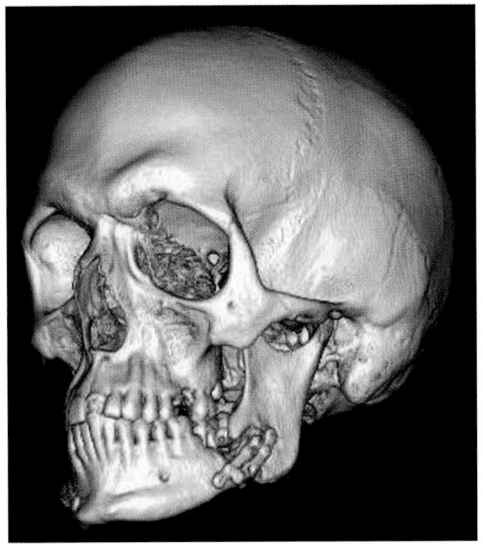

Fig. 3.39 Three-quarter view of 3D craniofacial computer tomography demonstrating malunion and continuity defect of left mandibular angle fracture with tooth in line of fracture.

Otherwise, it makes little sense to do osteotomies to remove a fully impacted 3rd molar, as further damage to the bone and mucosa in the area of the fracture may actually cause bone necrosis, further expose the fracture to the intraoral environment and contribute to bone instability and infection. Bony support of the fracture may be lost following extraction, and a linear fracture may be converted to a comminuted, less stable fracture by 3rd molar removal. The fracture site is often less vascularized following 3rd molar removal by virtue of periosteal stripping. Fully impacted 3rd molars can be electively removed when fracture healing is completed, unless the operative treatment of the fracture exposes the tooth or tooth removal is necessary to achieve alignment of the fracture.[205–207]

Antibiotic use

Intravenous administration of antibiotics at the time of the surgery is recommended.[208–210] This is especially helpful in patients undergoing delayed treatment, patients having long operations, patients with badly contused soft tissue where the fracture treatment is delayed and where the tissues are heavily contaminated, and where multiple intraoral lacerations are present. It is also indicated in patients who are medically compromised, have poor nutritional status or have systemic illness or local conditions of poor dental hygiene, periodontal or dental infections.

Antibiotic prophylaxis for mandibular fractures

Abubaker and Rollert[211] in 2001 published a prospective randomized double-blind study where they did not discern a benefit of postoperative oral antibiotics in uncomplicated mandible fractures. Their criteria for infection included purulent drainage from the fracture site, increased facial swelling beyond postoperative day 7, and fistula formation at the surgical site or fracture with drainage and fever associated with local evidence of infection, such as swelling, erythema and tenderness. Conceptually, mandible fractures involving tooth bearing regions of the angle and body can be classified as class III or contaminated wounds. Fractures whose treatment is delayed would be classed as class IV or infected wounds. The risk of potential infection in these wounds without the use of prophylactic antibiotics ranges from 22% to 50%. Many studies have indicated that the risk of infection should be as low as 10% with prophylactic antibiotics. In mandible fractures treated by experienced practitioners, the incidence of infection should be as low as 5% or 7%. Chole and Yuee[212] concluded that antibiotic prophylaxis was of value only in certain procedures. However, they noted that the majority of the studies surveyed were retrospective and the criteria used for diagnosis were subjective. Chole and Yuee reduced the incidence of infection from 42% to 8.9% in compound mandibular fractures by antibiotic use in facial fractures. Angle fractures have the most significant risk for infection and body fractures are second in overall frequency. Zallen and Curry[213] in an editorial discussing this recommend preoperative, intraoperative and postoperative antibiotics for 5 days.

Complications after fracture treatment

Malocclusion

Malocclusion is commonly the result of insufficient or inaccurate alignment in initial reduction that is especially common when IMF is poorly applied or loose. Other causes include inadequate final reduction, inadequate plate contour, or failure of fixation. Although subtle malocclusions may be corrected by grinding the occlusal facets of the teeth or orthodontics, any significant malocclusion requires refracture and/or osteotomy.

Hardware infection and migration

Loose hardware generally creates soft tissue irritation, producing a foreign body response and infection requiring hardware removal. Often, the fracture has healed and a repeat osteosynthesis is not necessary. Migration of loose hardware into soft tissue away from the fracture site occasionally occurs.[214]

Increased facial width and rotation of the mandible

Broadening of the distance between mandibular angles is produced by rotation of the lateral mandibular segments lingually at the occlusal surface of the teeth.[215] The distance between the mandibular angles increases as the mandible and lower face widen. This rotation (aggravated by tight IMF and the presence of subcondylar fractures) produces a malocclusion of the buccal cusps and a characteristic broadening and rounding of the face, which is aesthetically and functionally unacceptable. The lingual and palatal "open bite" is best observed in a dental model obtained after reduction looking internally at the posterior dentition. It may also be noticed on opening the mouth by observing the lingually oblique inclination of the lateral mandibular dentition. This complication cannot be treated by orthodontia, and requires refracture. The use of a long, strong, reconstruction plate to keep the mandibular angles rotated properly and the width narrow is required. In symphysis and parasymphysis fractures, the body and angle segments of the mandible must be held upright by the anteriorly placed plate.

Nonunion

Nonunion and pseudoarthrosis are uncommon after plate and screw fixation.[216–218] However, their presence may be masked by rigid fixation and surgeons should be aware of cases in which plate removal will unmask a poor union. This condition requires re-fixation of the fracture after a thorough debridement at the site of poor fracture healing. Revision of fixation and bone grafting of any fracture gap under a reconstruction plate is required.

Osteomyelitis

Soft tissue infection is common in mandibular fracture treatment, but true bone infection, osteomyelitis, is not. Local infection may almost always be managed with drainage and antibiotics. The fixation must be confirmed as adequate and intraoral closure inspected, and any instability in the fracture fixation noted and corrected. Less commonly, devitalized soft tissue and bone fragments that are dead or exposed must be debrided. Fracture stability must be maintained, and may need to be achieved by removal of current fixation devices and reapplication of longer, stronger reconstruction plates, whose screw fixation is outside the area of problem. In the uncommon persistent infection, the surgeon may wish to convert to external fixation, removing all internal fixation devices, but most cases may be stabilized with the repeat application of a reconstruction plate, which generally requires the use of a noncompression reconstruction plate with at least four screws on each side of the fracture located distinctly away from the fracture or infection site. No screws should be placed in an area of questionable bone. Serial debridement of devitalized bone and soft tissue may be required to confirm the absence of infection and adequacy of debridement. Secondary bone grafting should be conducted when the soft tissue and local area have been cleared of infection by debridement, drainage, antibiotics and dressing changes.

Condylar and subcondylar fractures

One must consider dislocation, angulation between the fragments, fracture override (which translates to ramus vertical length shortening) fracture angulation and bone gaps between the fragments. In children, growth considerations[219] create a capacity for both regeneration and remodeling, which is not present in later years.[220,221] Adults are capable only of partial restitutional remodeling.

High condylar (intracapsular) fractures (head and upper neck) are generally treated with closed reduction with a limited (2-week) period of postoperative IMF, followed by early "controlled" mobilization utilizing elastics for reestablishing occlusion in a rest position.[222] Most neck and low subcondylar fractures with good alignment, reasonable contact of the bone ends and preservation of ramus vertical height without condylar head dislocation may be treated by IMF for 4–6 weeks, with weekly or biweekly observation of the occlusion for at least 4 additional weeks after release of fixation in light function if fracture alignment is reasonable.[223,224] Some shortening of the ramus height is almost inevitable with a closed approach to condylar/subcondylar fracture treatment,[225–228] which may lead to a premature contact in the ipsilateral molar occlusion. Angulation between the fractured fragments in excess of 30° and fracture gap between the bone ends exceeding 4–5 mm, lateral override, and lack of contact of the ends of the fractured fragments should be a consideration justifying open reduction *(Fig. 3.40)*. Loss of ramus height is first heralded by a premature contact in the molar dentition on the fractured side, which produces a subtle open bite in the contralateral occlusion. ORIF of subcondylar fractures is preferred for any low, dislocated, fracture in conjunction with a multiply-fractured mandible, or a low fracture, which occurs simultaneous with Le Fort fractures, where the maxilla requires support from the intact mandible.[229]

Open treatment of a dislocated condylar head fracture brings with it the possibility of condylar head necrosis due to stripping of its blood supply, the possibility of damage to the temporal branch of the facial nerve if a pre-auricular incision is used, or the marginal mandibular branch if a lower (retromandibular or Risdon) incision is used.[230]

Edentulous mandible fractures

These fractures represent less than 5% of the mandibular fractures.[231-234] Fractures commonly occur through the most atrophic portions where the bone is thin and weak. The body is a common site for fracture, as compared to the angle and subcondylar region in dentulous patients.[235] Many fractures are bilateral or multiple, and displacement of a bilateral edentulous body fracture is often severe and a challenging condition to treat. The fractures in the horizontal mandible may be closed or open to the oral cavity. Closed fractures demonstrating minimal displacement may be treated with a soft diet and avoidance of dentures, however, in these cases, observation is critical to be sure that healing occurs within several weeks without further displacement. In practice, most fractures are better treated with a load-bearing plate. The edentulous mandible is characterized by the loss of the alveolar ridge and the teeth.[236] The bone atrophy may be minimal if there is sufficient height (>20 mm) of the mandibular body to ensure good bone healing. In cases with moderate atrophy, the height of the mandibular body ranges from 10–20 mm, and healing is usually satisfactory but not as certain if the height were >20 mm. Small plates with few screws often fail, as there is insufficient bone to provide buttressing support for the fracture treatment, and the plate must bear the entire load of the fracture. Large reconstruction ("locking") plates with three screws per side are recommended *(Fig. 3.41)*. In cases where the mandibular height is <10 mm (severe atrophy), one can assume that the patient has a disease of "poor bone healing". Complications following edentulous mandible fractures directly parallel the extent of mandibular atrophy. Obwegeser

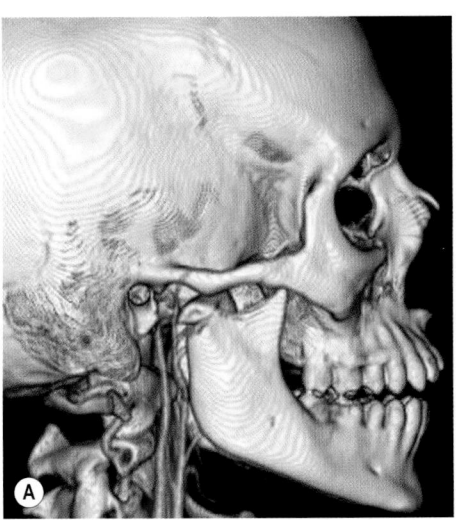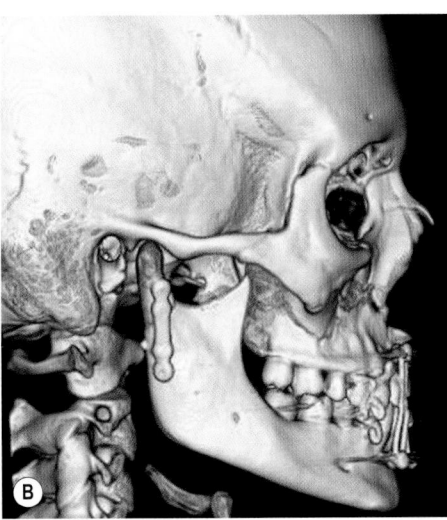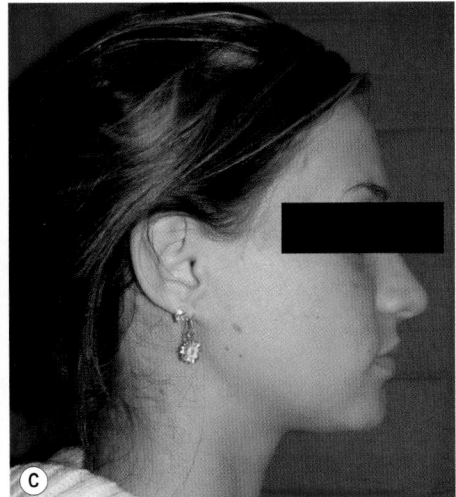

Fig. 3.40 (A,B) Lateral view of 3D craniofacial computer tomography on a 20-year-old female involved in a motor vehicle collision who sustained craniofacial injuries, pre- and post-open reduction and internal fixation of a right mandibular subcondylar fracture via a retromandibular extra-oral approach. Note that the patient also had a Le Fort II type fracture that was treated with closed reduction and interdental fixation. **(C)** Lateral profile view photograph of patient 1 year postoperatively.

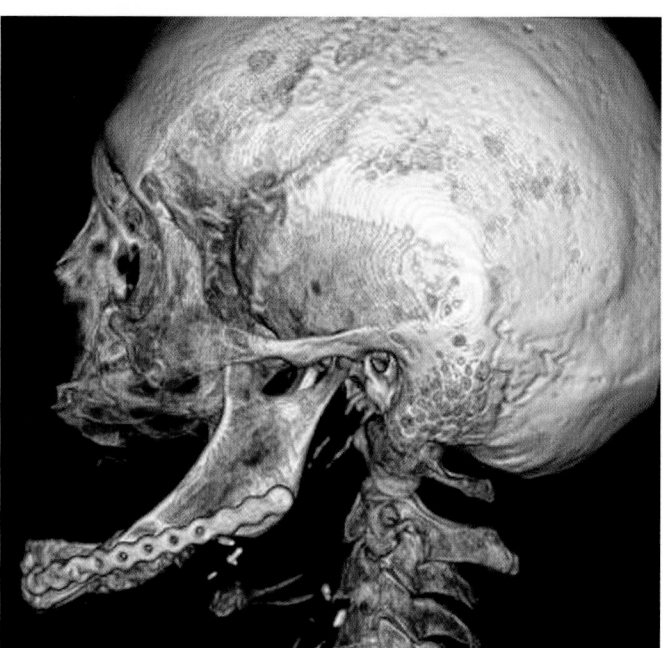

Fig. 3.41 Lateral view of 3D craniofacial computer tomography on a 64-year-old edentulous female, with a history of osteogenesis imperfecta who was referred for treatment of a malunion of a left mandibular fracture postoperative open reduction and internal fixation using a load bearing mandibular plate and iliac bone grafting via an extra-oral approach.

and Sailer,[237] in 1973 documented that 20% of the complications in edentulous mandible fractures were seen in the 10–20 mm mandibular height group, and 80% of the complications (i.e., poor or unsatisfactory bone union) were experienced in cases demonstrating a mandibular height <10 mm. Virtually no complications were seen in fractures exceeding 20 mm in height. This experience caused some authors[238,239] to recommend primary bone grafting, if there was no intraoral communication, for the severely atrophic edentulous mandible (≤10 mm in height) that required open reduction.[240]

It should be emphasized, however, that some severely atrophic mandible fractures may be treated without fixation (soft diet alone) if there is minimal instability and no displacement. In this treatment technique, the patient's dentures should be removed until healing has occurred.

The panfacial injury

Conceptually, panfacial fractures involve all three areas of the face: frontal bone, midface, and mandible. In practice, when two out of these three areas are involved, the term "panfacial fracture" has been applied.

The treatment of panfacial fractures

The optimal time for the easiest treatment of these injuries is within hours of the accident, before the development of massive edema and soft tissue rigidity that follow these injuries. This early treatment is only possible when other systems are not injured or are evaluated to exclude significant problems, managed and stabilized. However, no matter how severely the patient is injured, cutaneous wounds can be cleansed and closed, devitalized tissue removed, and the patient placed in intermaxillary fixation. This is the *minimum* urgent treatment of a significant maxillary or mandibular injury and may always be accomplished, despite the condition of the patient.

Presently, a one-stage restoration of the architecture of the craniofacial skeleton is the preferred method of treatment for severely comminuted, multiply-fractured facial bones.[241]

Open reduction of all fracture sites is performed with plate and screw fixation, supplementing bone defects with bone grafts. Although local incisions may be useful in selected cases, regional incisions such as the coronal, transconjunctival, upper and lower gingival buccal sulcus and the retromandibular incisions provide the complete exposure. In some cases, these exposures may be avoided because of the use of a suitable laceration.

In each subunit of the face, the important dimension to be considered first is facial width. In less severe fractures, correction of facial width is not challenging and an anterior alone approach is sufficient. Control of facial width in more severe injuries requires more complete dissection and alignment of each fracture component with all the peripheral and cranial base landmarks. Reconstructions which emphasize control of facial width are in fact the scheme which reciprocally restores facial projection.

The timing of soft tissue reduction is critical. Repositioning of the bone and replacement of the soft tissue must be accomplished *before* the soft tissue has developed significant memory (internal scarring) in the pattern of an abnormal bone configuration if a truly natural result is to be achieved. Soft tissue replacement requires: (1) layered closure; (2) reattachment of this closed soft tissue to the facial skeleton at several points, so that the tissue is first realigned and then repositioned onto an anatomically assembled craniofacial skeleton.

Order of procedure

Various sequences have been suggested such as "top to bottom", "bottom to top", "outside to inside", or "inside to outside". In reality, it does not make any difference what the order is, as long as the order makes sense and leads to a reproducible, anatomically accurate bone reconstruction, however, in our experience, it is more predictable to stabilize the occlusion in comminuted fractures by relating the maxilla to the mandible, than by relating the inferior maxilla to the superior maxilla.

Complications of panfacial fractures

Complications of panfacial fractures include complications referable to the bone and the soft tissue. The most common bony facial deformities following midface fracture treatment relate to lack of projection, enophthalmos, malocclusion, and increased facial width *(Fig. 3.42)*. Positional deformities seen in the frontal region that lead to midfacial subunit malposition are posterior and inferior positioning of the superior orbital rims and flattened frontal contour.

The most common soft tissue deformities are descent, diastasis, fat atrophy, ectropion, thickening and rigidity. Lack of periosteal closure over the zygomaticofrontal suture produces

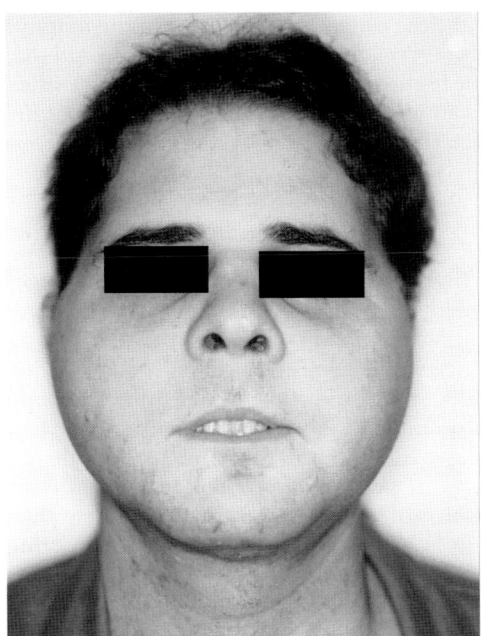

Fig. 3.42 Lack of restoration of the preinjury appearance, even if the underlying bone is finally replaced into its proper anatomic position, is the result of scarring within soft tissue. Examples of soft tissue rigidity accompanying malreduced fractures include the conditions of enophthalmos, medial canthal ligament malposition, short palpebral fissure, rounded canthus, and inferiorly displaced malar soft tissue pad. The lower lip has a disrupted mentalis attachment. Secondary management of any of these conditions is more challenging and less effective than is primary reconstruction. A unique opportunity thus exists in immediate fracture management to maintain expansion shape and position of the soft tissue envelope and to determine the geometry of soft tissue fibrosis by providing an anatomically aligned facial skeleton as support. Excellent restoration of appearance results from primary soft tissue positioning.

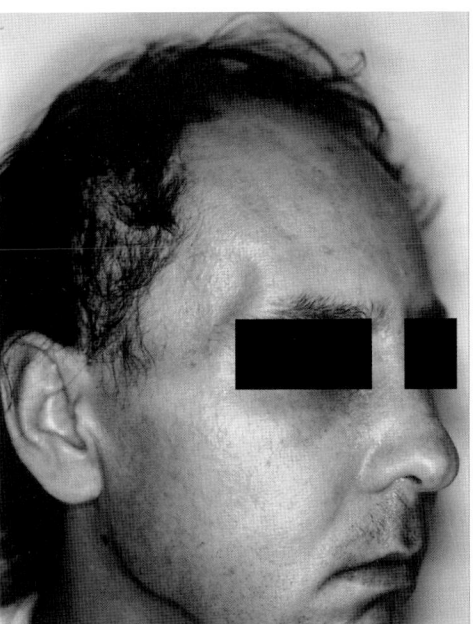

Fig. 3.43 "Skeletonization" of the frontal process of the zygoma from failure to close the temporal fascia to the orbital periosteum over the frontal process.

the appearance of temporal wasting because of the gap in the temporal aponeurosis and skeletalization of the frontal process of the zygoma *(Fig. 3.43)*. Incisions for arch exposure made higher in the posterior layer of the deep temporal fascia with dissection through the fat to reach the zygomatic arch produce fat atrophy by direct fat damage (interference with its middle temporal blood supply). Incisions in the deep temporal fascia just immediately above the arch minimize damage to this fat.

Postoperative care

Patients with large segment fractures may be adequately stabilized by plate and screw fixation to permit early release of intermaxillary fixation. Patients with comminuted midface or panfacial fractures are best served by varying periods of postoperative intermaxillary fixation in addition to plate and screw fixation. Intermaxillary fixation has more importance than has been emphasized in the recent literature. It is an unexcelled positioning and stabilizing device for the lower midface segment, both acutely at the initial reduction and postoperatively as required.

Gunshot wounds of the face

The treatment of gunshot and shotgun wounds of the face remains controversial, in that most authors advocate delayed reconstruction. Recently, immediate reconstruction,[242,243] and immediate soft tissue closure with "serial-second-look" procedures has become the standard of care.[244,245] The philosophy of delayed closure of these difficult wounds is no longer appropriate and delays effective rehabilitation of the affected individuals, some of whom represent suicide attempts.[246]

Recent experiences emphasize the safety and efficacy of immediate soft tissue closure and bone reconstruction in an anatomically correct position. These two principles prevent soft tissue shrinkage and loss of soft tissue position and provide improved functional and aesthetic results with shorter periods of disability and an improved potential for rehabilitation both functionally and aesthetically.

Ballistic injuries are classified into low, medium, and high-energy deposit injuries.[247,248] In formulating a treatment plan for ballistical injuries, it is helpful to identify the entrance and exit wounds, the presumed path of the bullet, and to appreciate the mass and velocity of the projectile, so that the extent of internal areas of tissue injury can be predicted. Conceptually, the separate categories of soft tissue and bone injury, and soft tissue loss and bone loss must all be individually assessed (four separate components) for each injury, and the areas of each recorded. The areas of injury and the areas of loss are each precisely outlined according to a facial pattern, which allows a treatment plan to be developed for early and intermediate treatment for the lower, middle and upper face.

Low velocity gunshot wounds

Low energy deposit ballistic weapons usually involve projectiles that have a limited mass and travel at speeds of <1000 feet per second. In general, low velocity gunshot wounds involve little soft tissue and bone loss and have limited associated soft tissue injury outside the exact path of the bullet. It is thus appropriate that they be treated with definitive stabilization of bone and primary soft tissue closure. Limited debridement of involved soft tissue is necessary. Small amounts of bone may need to be debrided or replaced with a primary bone graft, which can be performed primarily safely in the upper face. Because of the lack of significant associated soft tissue injury, little potential for progressive death or progressive necrosis of soft tissue exists, and these injuries may be treated as "facial fractures with overlying lacerations" both conceptually and practically.

Intermediate and high velocity ballistic injuries to the face

Shotgun pellets have a large mass and are considered intermediate energy deposit projectiles. They travel at speeds of approximately 1200 feet per second, and when grouped in a close distribution, at close range, is capable of causing massive injury. In civilian practice, many of these injuries represent shotgun wounds or high-energy rifle injuries, and they often result from suicide attempts or assaults. Close range shotgun wounds are characterized by extensive soft tissue and bone destruction.

Treatment

Intermediate and high velocity ballistic injuries to the face must be managed with a specific treatment plan that involves stabilization of existing bone and soft tissue in anatomic position, and maintenance of this bone and soft tissue stabilization throughout the period of soft tissue contracture and bone and soft tissue reconstruction. Wounds from intermediate and high-energy missiles usually demonstrate areas of both soft tissue and bone loss, as well as areas of soft tissue and bone injury. Usually, less loss of bone and soft tissue is present than is first suspected. It is important to reassemble the existing

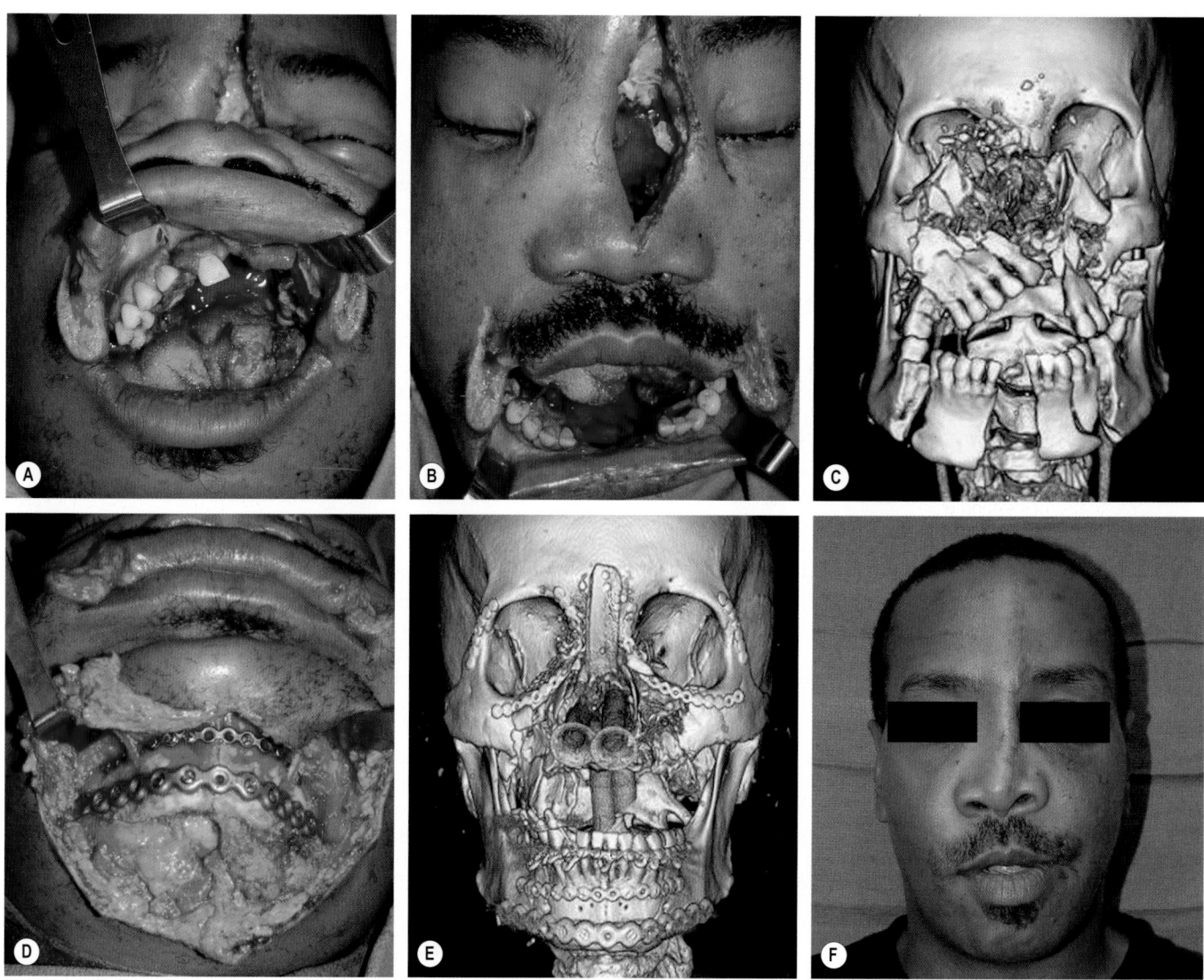

Fig. 3.44 (A,B) Frontal photographs of a 34-year-old male following a self-inflicted gunshot wound injury to the face demonstrating severe midfacial and mandibular fractures. **(C)** Intraoperative photographs following open reduction and internal fixation of mandibular fractures using a load bearing mandibular plate and a monocortical miniplate fixation via an extra-oral approach. **(D,E)** Frontal 3D craniofacial computer tomography scan of the patient pre- and post-open reduction and internal fixation of midfacial and mandibular fractures. **(F)** Postoperative photograph 1 year following surgery.

bone and soft tissue, and then at intervals to carryout serial surgical debridement "second look" procedures, which re-open the soft tissue to define additional areas of soft tissue necrosis, drain hematoma and/or developing fluid collections, and assure bone integrity. These "second look" procedures are imperative if primary reconstruction is attempted. Thus, the emphasis is on primary soft tissue, "skin to skin" or "skin to mucosa" closures, with stabilization of existing bone fragments in anatomical position. Re-exploration for additional debridement occurs at 48-hour intervals, or at an interval determined by the surgeon. These "second look" procedures are necessary and are continued until all soft tissue loss ceases and wound hematoma and fluid collections are controlled.

In each classification, a "zone of injury" is identified where fractures are present without significant bone or soft tissue loss. Fractures in the "zone of injury" are managed as routine facial fractures. When soft tissue and bone loss are present, it is important to stabilize existing bone in its anatomical position until soft tissue reconstruction can be completed. The soft tissue should be closed as far as possible to stretch and maintain length and shape of the soft tissue. In some cases, it may be possible to plan a more complex reconstruction of bone and soft tissue simultaneously by a composite free tissue transfer *(Fig. 3.44)*. The use of local tissue for soft tissue reconstruction, such as a local flap, ultimately provides the best cutaneous match and aesthetic result, but they may only be sufficient for the skin and require a deeper free flap reconstruction over which the cutaneous segment is stretched. These local flaps can be rotated over free tissue transfers to improve their color and contour match.

Bonus images for this chapter can be found online at http://www.expertconsult.com

Fig. 3.1 Cutaneous incisions (solid line) available for open reduction and internal fixation of facial fractures. The conjunctival approach (dotted line) also gives access to the orbital floor and anterior aspect of the maxilla, and exposure may be extended by a lateral canthotomy. Intraoral incisions (dotted line) are also indicated for the Le Fort I level of the maxilla and the anterior mandible. The lateral limb of an upper blepharoplasty incision is preferred for isolated zygomaticofrontal suture exposure if a coronal incision is not used.
A horizontal incision directly across the nasal radix is the one case in which a local incision can be tolerated over the nose. In many instances, a coronal incision is preferable unless the hair is short or the patient is balding.

Fig. 3.2 Palpation of the superior and inferior orbital rims. **(A)** The superior orbital rims are palpated with the pads of the fingertips. **(B)** Palpation of the inferior orbital rims. One should feel for discontinuity and level discrepancies in the bone of the rim and evaluate both the anterior and vertical position of the inferior orbital rims, comparing the prominence of the malar eminence of the two sides of the face.

Fig. 3.3 An intraoral examination demonstrates a fracture, a gingival laceration, and a gap in the dentition. These alveolar and gingival lacerations sometimes extend along the floor or roof of the mouth for a considerable distance.

Fig. 3.4 Condylar examination. The mandible is grasped with one hand, and the condyle area is bimanually palpated with one finger in the ear canal and one finger over the head of the condyle. Abnormal movement, or crepitation, indicates a condylar fracture. In the absence of a condylar fracture, a noncrepitant movement of the condylar head should occur synchronously with the anterior mandible. Disruption of the ligaments of the condyle will permit dislocations of the condylar head out of the fossa in the absence of fracture.

Fig. 3.5 With the head securely grasped, the midface is assessed for movement by grasping the dentition. Loose teeth, dentures, or bridgework should not be confused with mobility of the maxilla. Le Fort fractures demonstrate, as a rule, less mobility if they exist as large fragments, and especially if they are a "single fragment," than do lower Le Fort fractures. More comminuted Le Fort fractures demonstrate extreme mobility ("loose" maxillary fractures).

Fig. 3.10 Endoscopic approach through the maxillary sinus permits direct visualization of the orbital floor and manipulation of the soft tissue and floor repair.

Fig. 3.15 Reduction of a nasal fracture. **(A)** After vasoconstriction of the nasal mucous membrane with oxymetazoline-soaked cotton applicators, the nasal bones are "outfractured" with the handle of a #3 scalpel without the blade. **(B)** The septum is then straightened with an Asch forceps. Both the nasal bones and the septum should be able to be freely dislocated in each direction **(C)** if the fractures have been completed. If the incomplete fractures have been completed properly, the nasal bones may then be molded back into the midline and remain in reduction **(D)**. Care must be taken to avoid placing the reduction instruments into the intracranial space through a fracture or congenital defect in the cribriform plate. The cribriform plate (vertical level) may be detected with a cotton-tipped applicator by light palpation and its position noted and avoided with reduction maneuvers. **(E)** Steri-Strips and adhesive tape are applied to the nose, and a metal splint is applied over the tape. The tape keeps the edges of the metal splint from damaging the skin. A light packing material is placed inside the nose (such as Adaptic or Xeroform gauze) to minimize clot and hematoma in the distal portion of the nose.

Fig. 3.21 The zygoma and its articulating bones. (A) The zygoma articulates with the frontal, sphenoid, and temporal bones and the maxilla. The dotted area shows the portion of the zygoma and maxilla occupied by the maxillary sinus. (B) Lateral view of the zygoma. (From Kazanjian VH, Converse J. Surgical Treatment of Facial Injuries, 3rd edn. Baltimore MD: Williams & Wilkins; 1974.)

Fig. 3.22 **(A)** A Carroll-Girard screw may be placed through a small incision in the malar eminence into the body of the zygoma and the position of the zygomatic bone manipulated. **(B)** The screw is placed in position to align the rim.

Fig. 3.24 **(A)** Incision marked and checking position of elevator. **(B)** Elevator placed beneath deep temporal fascia superficial to muscle to reach depressed segment of arch, which is elevated in a smooth maneuver.

Access the complete reference list online at **http://www.expertconsult.com**

36. Rodriguez ED, Stanwix MG, Nam AJ, et al. Twenty-six-year experience treating frontal sinus fractures: a novel algorithm based on anatomical fracture pattern and failure of conventional techniques. *Plast Reconstr Surg.* 2008;122(6):1850–1866.

    Landmark article describing the longest experience with treating frontal sinus fractures and provides an algorithm for its treatment based on their outcomes, to minimize long-term complications.

104. Tessier P, Guiot G, Rougerie J, et al. Osteotomies cranio-naso-orbital-facials. *Hypertelorism Ann Chir Plast.* 1967;12:103.

    An article by the father of craniofacial surgery describing the possibilities of an intracranial approach for orbital reconstructive surgery.

107. Markowitz B, Manson P, Sargent, et al. Management of the medial canthal tendon in nasoethmoid orbital fractures: The importance of the central fragment in treatment and classification. *Plast Reconstr Surg.* 1991;87:843–853.

    Landmark article on the classification types of nasoethmoid-orbital region. Knowledge of this fracture pattern classification assists with the treatment of this complex surgical condition.

144. Gruss JS, MacKinnon SE, Kassel EE, et al. The role of primary bone grafting in complex craniomaxillofacial trauma. *Plast Reconstr Surg.* 1985;75:17.

145. Manson PN, Su CT, Hoopes JE. Structural pillars of the facial skeleton. *Plast Reconstr Surg.* 1980;66:54.

    Significant article describing the anatomical buttresses of the craniofacial skeleton that are required for reconstruction to maintain facial width and height.

171. Le Fort R. Etude experimentale sur les fractures de la machoire superieur. *Rev Chir Paris.* 1901;23:208, 360, 479.

    Original article describing the various fracture patterns associated with traumatic craniofacial injury. We associate the author's name to the different types of fracture patterns recognized.

190. Dingman RO, Grabb WC. Surgical anatomy of the mandibular ramus of the facial nerve based on the dissection of 100 facial halves. *Plast Reconstr Surg.* 1962;29:2166.

195. Ellis 3rd E. Treatment methods for fractures of the mandibular angle. *Int J Oral Maxillofac Surg.* 1999;28(4):243–252.

198. Champy M, Lodde JP, Schmidt R, et al. Mandibular osteosynthesis by miniature screwed plates via a buccal approach. *J Maxillofac Surg.* 1978;6:14.

243. Clark N, Birely B, Manson PN, et al. High-energy ballistic and avulsive facial injuries: Classification, patterns, and an algorithm for primary reconstruction. *Plast Reconstr Surg.* 1996;98:583–601.

4

TMJ dysfunction and obstructive sleep apnea

Stephen A. Schendel and Brinda Thimmappa

SYNOPSIS

- Tomography and magnetic resonance imaging (MRI) are used to evaluate the patient with temporomandibular joint (TMJ) pain if physical exam demonstrates limitation of movement.
- Occlusal splinting is the mainstay of management of patients with TMJ myofascial pain without abnormality of the joint.
- Surgical treatment of TMJ dysfunction often begins with arthroscopy, which allows joint examination, biopsy, and lavage.
- Diagnosis of obstructive sleep apnea (OSA) requires review of subjective symptoms and objective data, including polysomnogram (PSG).
- Surgical management of OSA consists of several phases based on the severity and location of anatomical obstruction.
- The last phase of surgical management consists of maxillomandibular advancement (MMA) by a LeFort I osteotomy and bilateral sagittal split osteotomy of the mandible. The success of this procedure has resulted in its increased use as the primary surgical management of OSA patients.

Access the Historical Perspective section online at
http://www.expertconsult.com

Temporomandibular joint dysfunction

Key points

- Temporomandibular pain may result from masticatory dysfunction, pain syndromes, or internal derangement of the joint.
- History and physical examination identify those individuals who require imaging work-up.
- Diet modification, nonsteroidal therapy, and occlusal splints are the first line of treatment.
- Surgical treatment is directed toward the underlying cause of joint derangement.

The prevalence of TMJ and muscle disorder-type pain in a recent survey of over 30 000 Americans was 4.6%.[1] Numerous studies have suggested an association of pain with gender, age, socioeconomic factors, or previous dental and orthodontic interventions. Persons with TMJ disorders can suffer from displacement of the articular disc, termed "internal derangement" of the TMJ.[2] However similar symptoms of pain and functional limitations of mouth opening may result from myofascial pain syndromes, congenital disorders, inflammatory conditions, and trauma. Medical and occlusal therapies control symptoms for many patients. For those who require surgical intervention, treatment options range from arthroscopy to joint replacement. An understanding of the normal function of the TMJ and the pathophysiology of its degenerative disorders are key to directing treatment.

Basic science/disease process

Anatomy

The mandibular bone allows for rotational and translational movement through the TMJ. The mandibular condyle articulates with the squamous portion of the temporal bone at the TMJ. The geniohyoid muscles insert on to the genial tubercles and, with the anterior belly of the digastric muscle, depress and retract the mandible. The muscles that elevate or protrude the mandible are the masseter, temporalis, medial, and lateral pterygoid muscles. The inferior portion of the lateral pterygoid muscle inserts on to the neck of the condyle, which helps protrude the mandible when contracting. The superior portion of the lateral pterygoid muscle inserts on the fibrous capsule and meniscus of the TMJ, stabilizing the meniscus during the movement of the mandible. All these muscles are innervated by cranial nerve V. The TMJ articular surfaces are lined with fibrocartilage, an avascular fibrous connective tissue that contains cartilage cells. This differs from other synovial joints that are lined with hyaline cartilage.

The articular disc is a dense fibrous connective tissue structure that separates the joint into two spaces.[14] The upper joint space volume of 1 mL extends from the glenoid fossa to the articular eminence. The lower joint space volume of 0.5 mL begins above the insertion of the lateral pterygoid muscle anteriorly and then spreads out over the condyle. The articular disc is an avascular, noninnervated fibrous sheet with some cartilaginous component. The pars gracilis is the thin central zone. The anterior band or pes meniscus is superiorly attached to the articular eminence and superior belly of the lateral pterygoid. Inferiorly, the anterior band attaches to the condyle by a synovial membrane along the attachment of the lateral pterygoid muscle. The posterior band is highly innervated and vascularized tissue, a bilaminar zone or retromeniscal pad. The upper layer of the bilaminar zone attaches to the tympanic plate of the temporal bone, while the lower runs from the posterior meniscus to the neck of the condyle. The disc is not attached to the capsule laterally or medially, but instead bound to the medial and lateral poles of the mandibular condyle.

Basic movements of the mandible are rotator or hinge movement, which consists of rotation around transverse axis that passes through condyles, and translator or sliding movement, which involves movement of mandible in anteroposterior and/or mediolateral direction. The rotatory movement of the mandible is completed in the inferior joint space (ginglymus), and translation is followed in the superior joint space (arthrodial). During mouth opening, translation moves the condyle and disc forward and downward along the articular eminence. These structures lie anterior to the greatest height of the eminence with maximal mouth opening. Closing returns the jaw to its occlusal position. Protrusion and retrusion of the mandible are mainly accomplished by translatory movements. The lateral ptyerygoids move the condyles and discs forward along the articular eminence, while the elevators and depressors stabilize the position of the jaw relative to the maxilla.

The retromeniscal or retrodiscal pad is believed to be the origin of pain in TMJ dysfunction. If there are abnormal loading forces on the joint surfaces as a result of disc disease, this can lead to TMJ disorders.[15] The fibrous joint capsule attaches to the condyle inferiorly and the zygomatic arch superiorly. It is reinforced anteriorly and laterally by the temporomandibular ligament. The auriculotemporal, masseteric, and deep temporal branches of the trigeminal nerve supply innervation to the TMJ.[16]

Myofascial problems

The cause of myofascial pain and dysfunction (MPD) is usually related to the masticatory muscles. MPD was first described by Laskin[17,18] and is characterized by a limited range of motion, aching pain, and severe tenderness on palpation of the muscles. Certain trigger points within the masticatory muscles refer the pain. The masseter muscle, producing an ache in the jaw, is the most common. Next most common is pain in the temporalis muscle, producing pain in the side of the head. The lateral pterygoid muscle can generate an earache or pain behind the eye. Medial pterygoid involvement causes pain on swallowing or stuffiness in the ear.

The limitation of mandibular movement in MPD usually correlates with the amount of pain. The etiology of MPD can be due to overclosure, occlusal prematurity, bruxism, and severe anxiety. Each of these leads to spasms of the masticatory muscles, focusing pain around the TMJ.

Inflammation

Posterior capsulitis involves the neurovascular bilaminar zone and the posterior capsular ligament. Such inflammation can be due to acute trauma, premature occlusal contact, or infection causing the retrodisc tissues to become edematous. Sprain of the capsular ligaments usually heals in several weeks. Chronic sprain can lead to stretching of the ligaments. Medical occlusal treatment usually addresses these conditions.

Osteoarthritis

Osteoarthritis is a chronic disease that characteristically affects the articular cartilage of synovial joints and is associated with remodeling of the underlying subchondral bone and the development of a secondary synovitis. It is the most common disease affecting the TMJ. It has a gradual onset. Usually, only one side is affected. Radiographically, sclerosis of the subchondral bone, osteophytic lipping, cyst formation, flattening of the condyle, and decreased height of the ramus are observed[19] (*Fig. 4.1*). Chronic anterior disc displacement is associated with posterior–superior condylar resorption, seen as flattening and loss of bone in this area. An open bite deformity and mandibular retrusion may result. Treatment frequently involves drug therapy, occlusal appliance therapy, physical therapy, and, when most severe, surgery.

Rheumatoid arthritis

Rheumatoid arthritis is a chronic inflammatory disease that primarily affects the periarticular structures, such as the synovial membrane, capsule, tendons, and ligaments. More than 50% of rheumatoid arthritis patients have involvement of the TMJ during the course of their disease.[20]

When the TMJ is involved, patients relate a dull aching pain in the preauricular area, muscle tenderness, poor range of jaw motion, clicking, and TMJ stiffness in the morning.

Progression of the disease includes condylar resorption and fibrous and bony ankylosis. The classic malocclusion is caused by loss of the height of the condyles. Juvenile rheumatoid arthritis affects patients before the age of 16 years. Up to 40% of children with juvenile rheumatoid arthritis have involvement of the TMJ.[21] Defective development of the mandible leads to micrognathia. MRI can delineate disc destruction, condylar bone erosion, and cartilaginous thinning. The radiographs of the TMJ include loss of joint space and condylar resorption with anterior subluxation of the condyle.

The treatment goals in rheumatoid arthritis are pain relief, reduction of inflammation, maintenance of function, and prevention of further deformity. This treatment may include drug therapy, occlusal appliance, physical therapy, and dental and surgical procedures of the TMJ and mandible. Most surgery is reserved for correction of joint ankylosis and severe malocclusion.

Condylar problems

Condylar fractures are discussed extensively in Chapter 2. A history of condylar fractures can lead to subsequent pain and limitation of the TMJ.

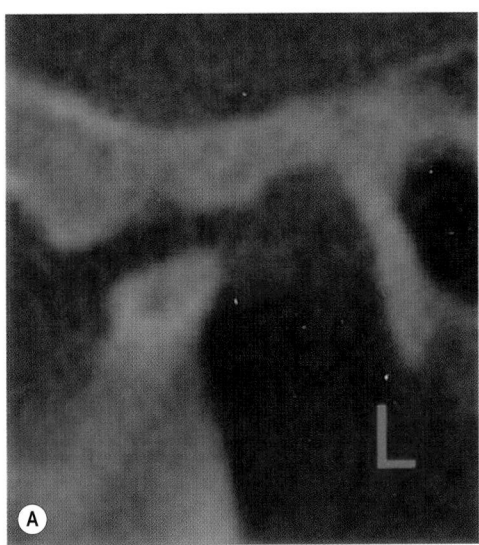
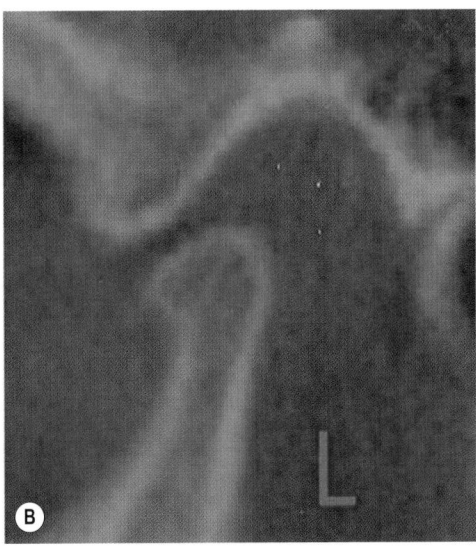

Fig. 4.1 (A) Tomography in the open-mouth position with severe osteoarthritic changes of the condylar head and near-total loss of the condyle. **(B)** The normal condyle in the same patient.

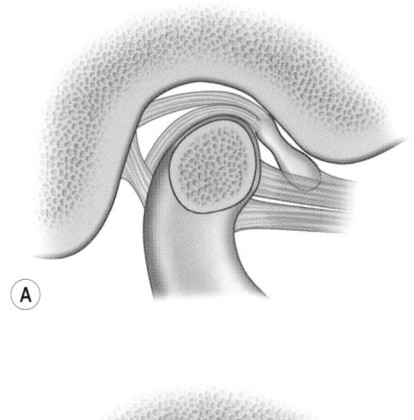
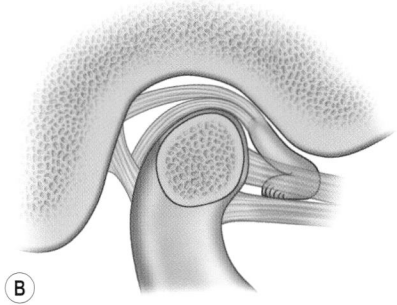
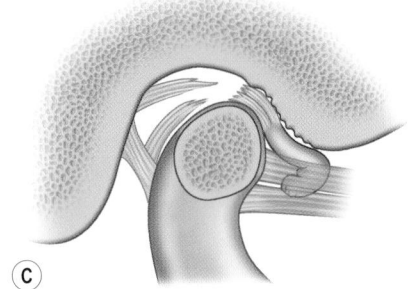
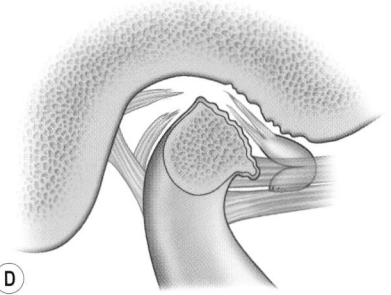

Fig. 4.2 Stages in the classic progression of internal derangement of the temporomandibular joint. **(A)** Internal joint derangement secondary to anterior disc displacement with reduction (intermittent locking may occur). **(B)** Anterior disc displacement without reduction. **(C)** Perforation of the bilaminar zone. **(D)** Osteoarthrosis.

Idiopathic condylar resorption can also occur in either juvenile or adult individuals. In both forms there is a diminished condylar head. In the juvenile form the exact cause is unknown and is multifactorial but leads to decreased mandibular growth and a class II malocclusion. The adult can follow orthognathic surgery to the mandible or disc displacement. Both types are self-limiting and are treated conservatively until the condition stabilizes. Surgery may then be indicated.[22,23]

Internal derangement

Wilkes established five stages of internal derangement based on clinical and imaging criteria.[24] In patients with early stage

I derangement, the patient complains of clicking in opening and closing of the jaw *(Fig. 4.2)*. On imaging, the disc is slightly displaced forward on opening, but it is "reduced," or returns to its normal position, at maximal opening. The oral excursion and lateral movements of the jaw should be within the normal range. The audible clicking sound is produced by reduction of the disc.

In stage II, the patient begins to complain of intermittent locking. Pain is common at this stage and localized over the TMJ. The disc may appear deformed, but generally still reduces with maximal opening. Osseous contour appears normal. In stage III, the patient has a chronic limitation of opening with frequent locking, headaches, and painful chewing. The mandible deviates to the affected side on opening and with protrusive movements. The internal derangement is anterior disc displacement.

Chronic internal derangement without disc reduction (stage IV) results in injury to the retrodiscal tissue. Pain may diminish because of fibrous changes occurring in the retrodiscal tissue.[25] Limited mouth opening is common here as the disc blocks full condylar translation. In stage V, remodeling of the temporal and condylar bone components occurs. This final common pathway of cartilage destruction and bone remodeling is shared with other conditions such as osteoarthritis. Yet there are few long-term longitudinal data to indicate the progression of disc displacement. A reducing disc disorder may be stable for years.[26]

The differential diagnoses associated with TMJ pain include numerous others. The work-up of this pain must exclude causes including inflammatory arthritis, connective tissue diseases, and tumors.

Diagnosis

History and physical examination

A patient may describe the pain originating from the TMJ, preauricular area, or surrounding masticatory muscles. Additionally the discomfort may radiate from the ear, teeth, or neck area. Often the onset of pain originating in the morning is due to nocturnal bruxism, grinding of teeth, in which constant pain after jaw function suggests intracapsular joint pathology. Patients with TMJ dysfunction relate a triad of preauricular pain, clicking or grinding noises from the TMJ, and poor mandibular movement. Some patients may describe noises in the joint associated with daily jaw movement. Such clicking may be benign solitary clicks, which occur in 40% of the normal population. When there is anterior subluxation of the disc with jaw opening, condylar contact results in a click. A reciprocal click occurs as the disc subluxes when the condyle repositions into the glenoid fossa. The abnormal joint surfaces lead to a grinding or crepitus from the joint. Closed lock is a sudden irreducible anterior subluxation of the disc, limiting mandibular motion. Other reasons for limited excursion of the jaw may be due to local muscular dysfuction, bony or fibrous ankylosis of the joint, and blocking of the coronoid process by the zygoma.

The examination of the patient with TMJ pain centers on the head, neck, and TMJ. The facial exam includes any soft-tissue aymmetry or skeletal deformities. Examination of the cranial nerves is performed to exclude any central nervous system disorders. The ear canals and tympanic membrane are examined to rule out primary benign or malignant diseases.

Similarly, the oral tissues are evaluated for mucosal lesions, swellings, periodontal disease, alveolar process abnormalities, and evidence of cheek or lip biting. The teeth are examined for caries, mobility of teeth, absent teeth, prosthetics, molar impactions, supraerupted teeth, malocclusion, and displacement of the mandible during contact of the teeth. The incisor relationship is important to delineate overbite, overjet, or open bite, all of which can contribute to the TMJ symptoms. Palpation of the area of the TMJ can detect clicking or crepitus. Joint sounds must be determined as popping, clicking (reciprocal or nonreciprocal), or crepitations.

Palpation of the TMJ can detect swelling, the presence of tenderness, and joint sounds. Auscultation can be more sensitive in determining the type of joint sounds. The masticatory and cervical muscles must also be excluded as areas of tenderness or spasm. The presence or absence of pain, intensity of pain, location of pain, and referred pain must be documented.

The TMJ range of motion should be measured. Any pain or deviation to the left or right on opening is noted. The normal interincisal opening distance is 40–50 mm, and the lateral jaw movement is at least 10 mm on each side of the incisor midline. Any restriction of the interincisal range of motion, lateral restriction, deviation on opening, and development of new anterior open bite can indicate the degree of joint involvement. At this point, diagnostic imaging is required.

Diagnostic imaging

A panoramic radiograph or transcranial radiographic view, commonly available in a dental office, can identify gross fractures, arthritic changes, bone cysts or tumors, or malformations.

Tomography provides sectional images in the sagittal or coronal views, usually taken in the open and closed positions. This modality demonstrates bone pathology and range of condylar motion but provides no information on soft-tissue disease. One study showed that up to 85% with TMJ disease patients had normal tomography.[27]

The evaluation of the TMJ soft tissue and disc was traditionally with contrast arthrography. Arthrography can be performed either as single-contrast lower compartment[2] or as dual-space contrast arthrotomography.[28] The information from TMJ arthrography is highly reliable in determining disc disease but has been replaced by the noninvasive modality MRI. It can also give information about the swelling and inflammation in the joint. In sagittal images, the disc is located anteriorly to the condyle in the closed-mouth position (*Figs 4.3 and 4.4*). Several MRI studies of adults have demonstrated disc displacement in 20–30% of asymptomatic volunteers;[29] however the type of disc displacement may be different. Affected patients with disc displacement demonstrated largely complete anterior or complete anterolateral displacement. MRI may also provide insight into the bone marrow abnormalities of the condyle. If the central area of the condyle has a low signal, this may suggest a pathologic condyle consistent with avascular necrosis.

CT scanning is useful to evaluate bone abnormalities, bony ankylosis, and acute traumatic injuries. Otherwise, CT of the disc is difficult. The advantages of MRI over CT include absence of ionizing radiation, fewer artifacts from dense bone and metal clips, imaging in multiple planes, and good detail of the soft tissues. Cone beam CT (CBCT) is increasingly available and offers lower radiation doses than standard CT. Panoramic and other dental modes of viewing are available with reconstruction software.

The first step in imaging a patient with TMJ pain and dysfunction is a plain film, including panographic film. The next modality should be CBCT of the joint in open and closed positions or an MRI, focusing on the soft tissue and disc.

Patient selection

Following investigation of TMJ pain and dysfunction, patients with pain disorders, sprains, inflammatory disorders, and

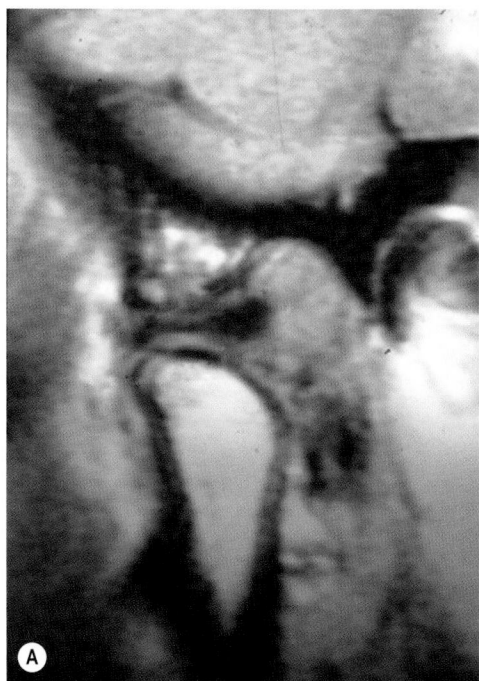
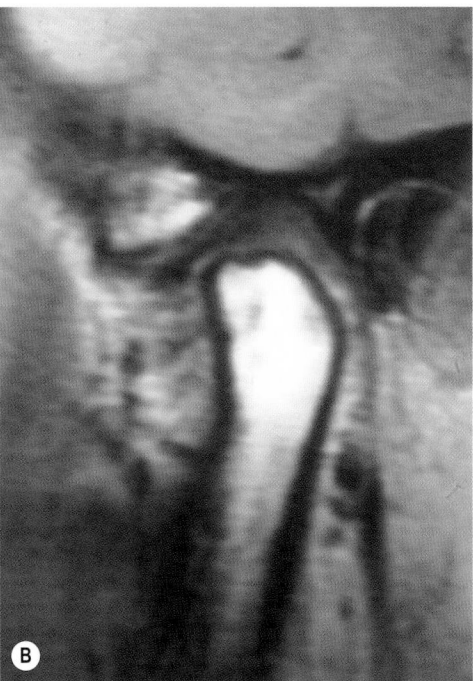

Fig. 4.3 Magnetic resonance imaging of the normal temporomandibular joint (TMJ). Sagittal proton density-weighted image of the TMJ in **(A)** open-mouth and **(B)** closed-mouth positions. Articular disc remains over the condylar head as it moves posterior along articular eminence.

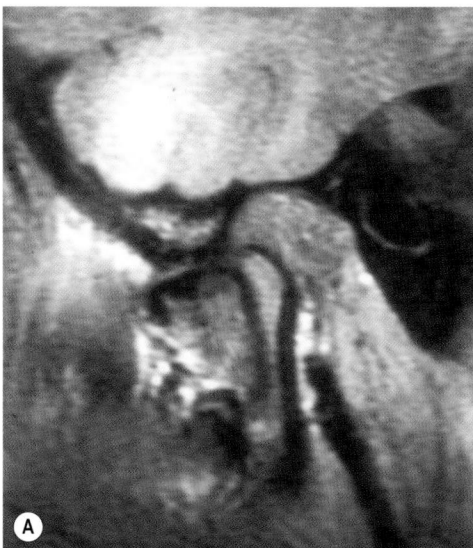
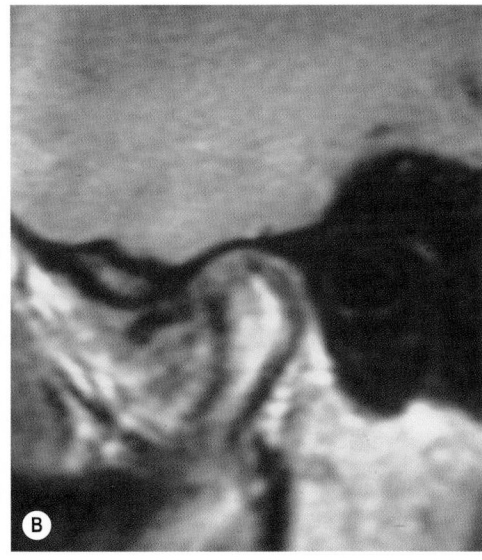

Fig. 4.4 Magnetic resonance imaging of anterior disc displacement. Sagittal proton density-weighted image of the temporomandibular joint in **(A)** open-mouth and **(B)** closed-mouth positions. Articular disc remains anteriorly displaced.

early stages of internal derangement are started on medical and occlusal management. If a patient fails noninvasive management, or presents at an advanced state of joint degeneration, surgical intervention is indicated. The type of surgical therapy is directed at the underlying cause of joint derangement.

Treatment

Noninvasive management

The goal of medical management is to break the cycle of pain and anxiety of myofascial dysfunction. Nonsteroidal anti-inflammatory agents are combined with a soft diet. Muscle relaxants, antidepressants, and local anesthetics for diagnostic blocks are adjunctive measures.[30] Recently the use of botulinum toxin in areas of muscle spasm has been reported.[31,32] The use of oral corticosteroids is effective for acute pain, but prolonged use will lead to osteoporosis, including of the TMJ. Intra-articular injections of corticosteroids are also effective for acute pain management and diagnosis, but repeated injections risk the destruction of articular cartilage. Physical therapy using modalities of heat, massage, ultrasound, transcutaneous electrical nerve stimulation, and biofeedback may also help in these patients.

Occlusal splints reduce the loading of the joint, muscle hyperactivity, and articular strain due to bruxism. The ease of insertion of the appliance and compliance of the patient affect the success of occlusal therapy. The various types of splints include the muscle relation appliance, anterior bite plate, pivot splint, and the soft appliance. Appliance therapy remains a common treatment of TMJ pain, though a review of studies has shown no definite benefit for its use, or for a specific type of splint.[33]

Surgical management

Acute dislocations result from the condyle extending anteriorly beyond the articular eminence. If spontaneous reduction does not occur, manual reduction with a muscle relaxant or anesthesia is often needed. The surgeon places downward force along the inferior border of the mandible while moving the jaw posteriorly to slide the condyle into the fossa.

Arthrocentesis and arthroscopy enable the surgeon to perform endoscopic joint examination, biopsy, and lavage. In addition to the arthroscope (1.8–2.6 mm in diameter), a high-intensity light source, video camera, and monitor are required. Measured landmarks for TMJ entry have been reported.[34] The point of entry is along a line from the tragus to the lateral canthus of the eye. The site is 10 mm anterior to the tragus and 2 mm inferior to the line. Using these landmarks will help to prevent complications involving the temporal branch of the facial nerve and the auriculotemporal branch of the trigeminal nerve. A needle is inserted at the posterior entry point to insufflate the TMJ with Ringer's lactate. After the superior compartment of the joint is distended, the arthroscope is gained through the same entry, or the single-portal technique (Fig. 4.5). A double-portal technique requires another cannula to be placed anteriorly so that the scope and the surgical instruments can be interchanged, alternating the inflow and outflow portals (Fig. 4.6). The synovial lining, articular cartilage, joint space, and integrity of disc are examined. Lysis of adhesions or removal of debris is achieved by intermittent

distension of the joint space by blocking the outflow needle and irrigating under pressure.[35] Although the lower joint space is not examined, the presence of a disc perforation would allow limited examination of this space and the condyle. Arthroscopic repositioning of the disc can be achieved by contracting the posterior disc attachments with laser, sclerosing agents, or suture.[36,37]

Arthotomy or open-joint surgery is most commonly approached from a preauricular approach. Maintaining dissection over the deep temporal fascia limits injury to the frontal branch of the facial nerve. Disc repositioning is performed if the disc is intact and can be moved without tension. Adhesions result from chronic disc displacement and require releasing incisions. If release is required medially, bleeding from the lateral pterygoid muscle or internal maxillary artery may be encountered. Removal of the diseased or deformed portion of the disc is completed if it cannot be repositioned. Autogenous materials such as temporalis muscle flaps, auricular cartilage, and dermal grafts have been used for disc replacement.[38] If the contour of the articular eminence contributes to interference of joint movement, this can be recontoured (Fig. 4.7). Exposure of bone marrow during recontouring does risk hetertopic bone formation.

Postoperative care

The patient maintains a soft diet for a few days following arthroscopy, and immediately begins range-of-motion

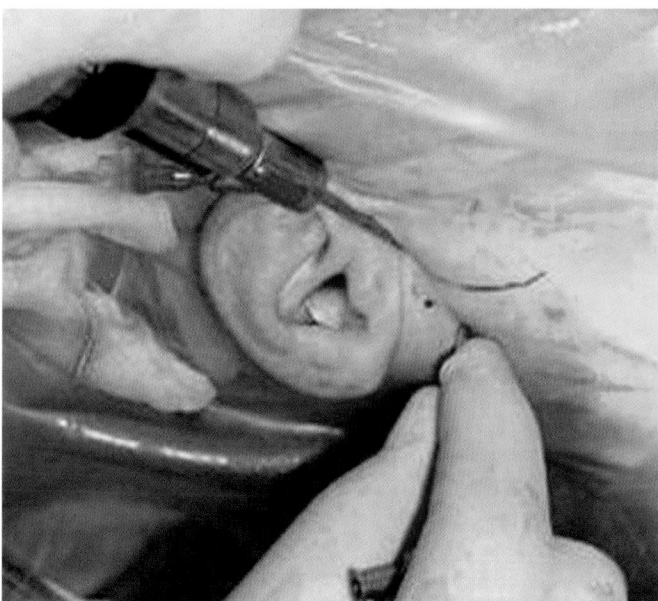

Fig. 4.5 Placement of arthroscope 10 mm anterior to tragus: single-portal technique. (Reproduced from Dolwick MF. Temporomandibular joint surgery for internal derangement. Dent Clin North Am 2007;51:195–208.)

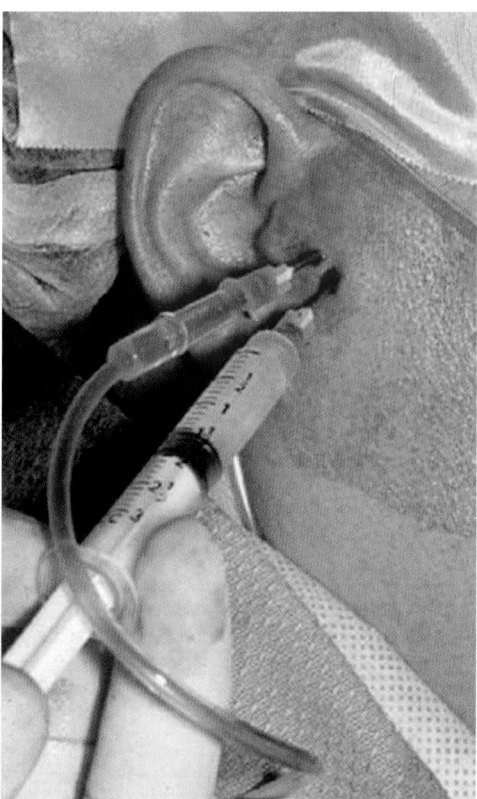

Fig. 4.6 Double-portal technique of arthroscopy. (Reproduced from Dolwick MF. Temporomandibular joint surgery for internal derangement. Dent Clin North Am 2007;51:195–208.)

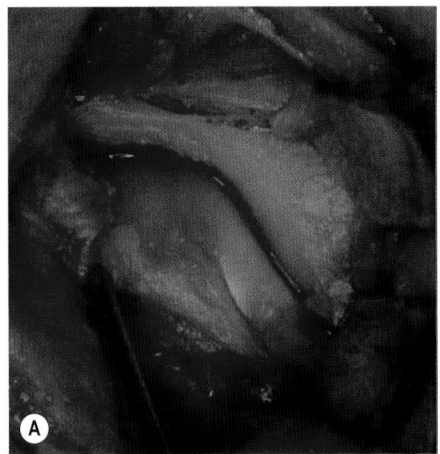 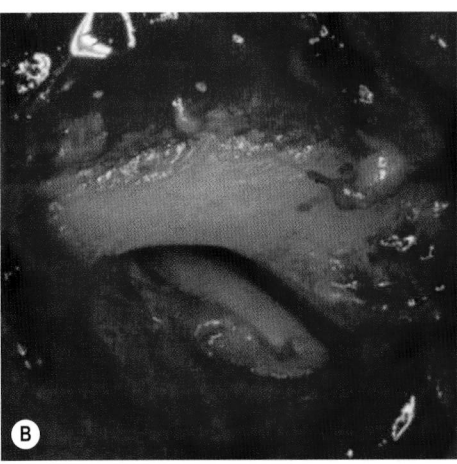

Fig. 4.7 (A) Exposed upper temporomandibular joint (TMJ) space showing articular eminence and displaced articular disc. **(B)** TMJ space after contouring of eminence and repositioning of disc. (Reproduced from Dolwick MF. Temporomandibular joint surgery for internal derangement. Dent Clin North Am 2007;51:195–208.)

exercises. Following open-joint surgery, swelling, numbness, and limited mouth opening or occlusal changes are common. Immediate start of exercises is essential and soft diet is maintained for 6 weeks.

Outcomes, prognosis, and complications

There are few prospective trials to guide surgical therapy.[39] Multiple retrospective studies have reported 70–90% success rates with arthrocentesis and arthroscopy,[40–42] with pain improvement maintained at long-term follow-up.[42] There are few reports of the long-term outcomes of arthroscopic repositioning of the disc,[36] but Zhang et al. have recently confirmed this in a large series as an effective technique using postoperative MRI.[37]

Disc repositioning has a similarly high success rate in the literature.[2,43] The main complication of open surgery is facial nerve injury. Complete paralysis is rare and temporary paralysis of the temporal branch is more common. This and the preauricular numbness generally resolve within 3 months. Aggressive range-of-motion exercises are necessary to prevent limited mouth opening. In a meta-analysis of surgical trials for TMJ disorders, all surgical modalities, including arthroscopic, disc repositioning, and discectomy improved pain and jaw motion.[44] No modality was superior to another, though few studies had directly comparable treatment groups. A multicenter prospective study of surgical treatments also demonstrated improvement in all groups, with no difference between surgical groups.[39]

Secondary procedures

TMJ reconstruction is reserved for individuals who have undergone multiple failed TMJ surgical procedures with severe disability, developed ankylosis of the joint, or have lost vertical mandibular height from bony resorption with resultant open-bite deformities.

Treatment of ankyloses includes condylectomy, gap arthroplasty, and interpositional arthroplasty. A gap arthroplasty involves removal of bone at or below the joint level without interposition of any material. Often there is a high recurrence rate of ankylosis. The interposition of alloplastic or

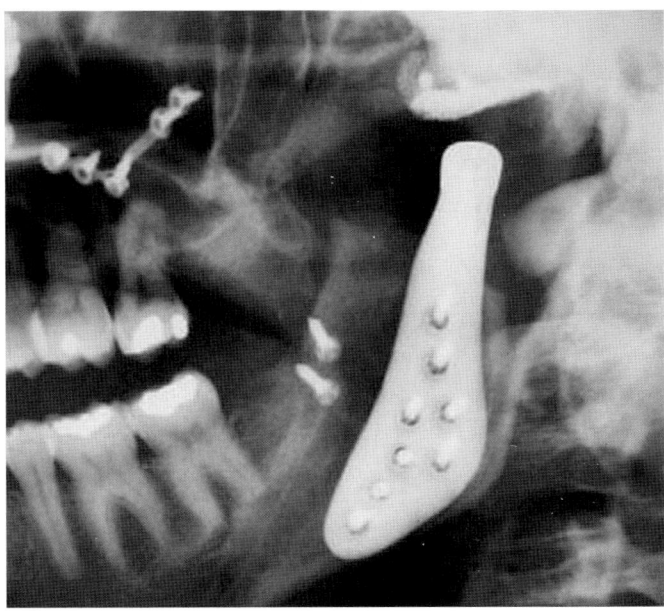

Fig. 4.8 Temporomandibular joint Concepts prosthesis. (Reproduced from Dolwick MF. Temporomandibular joint surgery for internal derangement. Dent Clin North Am 2007;51:195–208.)

autogenous materials is used to maintain vertical height and restore a functional joint. Autogenous materials used for replacement of the resected condyle include dermis, fat, fascia, and muscle.

Costochondral grafts have been utilized in the treatment of pediatric populations.[45] Autologous reconstruction is the preferred method in the growing patient given the growth potential of the graft. Over a lifetime, a prosthetic is also a risk of failure, infection, and replacement.

Alloplastic joints may be custom-fabricated with the aid of CT data *(Fig. 4.8)*. Placement requires preauricular and retromandibular incisions to access the TMJ and ramus *(Fig. 4.9)*. The condyle or ankylosed bone is removed, as well as the coronoid. Screw fixation of the implant ensures the stability necessary for osteointegration. A fat graft is generally placed surrounding the condyle. Improved pain and mouth opening have been reported.[46] Complications are similar to those in

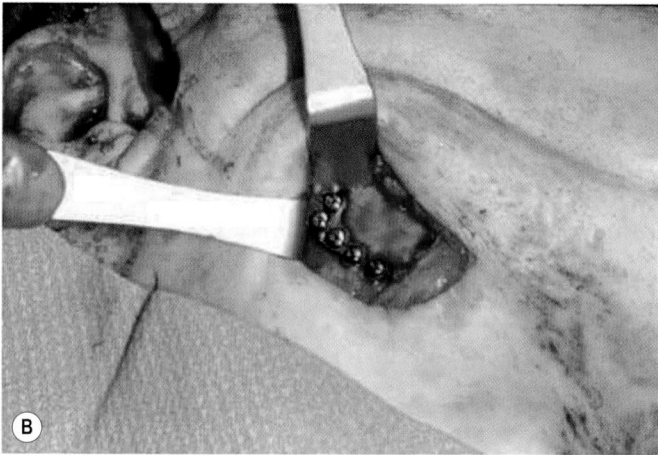

Fig. 4.9 Total joint prosthesis requires reconstruction of both **(A)** the glenoid fossa and **(B)** condylar elements.

other open arthrotomies, namely facial nerve injury. Foreign-body reaction and heterotopic bone formation were more common when fat grafts were not used.

Obstructive sleep apnea

Key points

- Obstruction occurs at three defined anatomic levels: nose, palate, and base of tongue.
- Continuous positive airway pressure (CPAP) is the first line of treatment in adult patients with OSA.
- MMA aims to enlarge the velo-oropharyngeal airway and associated soft tissue by skeletal advancement.

Central apneas are characterized by an absence or decrease in respiratory effort. In contrast, obstructive episodes are associated with an increased respiratory effort while airflow decreases. Hypopnea refers to a decrease in airflow by 30–50% from baseline. The apnea–hypopnea index (AHI) is the number of apnea–hypopnea episodes occurring during sleep in a given hour. An AHI of greater than 5 is diagnostic of OSA, and affects 24% of adult men and 9% of adult women.[47] Physiologic and psychological changes accompany the sleep disturbance, including cardiovascular disease, excessive daytime sleepiness, and decreased concentration and motor skills.

The primary medical treatment for adults is CPAP. Poor patient compliance is the main reason for failure of this therapy. Surgical treatment is directed at relieving airway obstruction at three defined levels: nose, palate, and base of tongue. Historically, primary surgical treatments offered included septoplasty, uvulopharyngoplasty (UVPP), and genioglossus advancement. Individuals who failed to improve with this first-stage surgical intervention underwent MMA. As evidence of the effectiveness of MMA accumulates, it is increasingly advocated as a first-line surgical treatment of OSA,[48–50] alone or in combination with other surgical interventions.

Basic science/disease process

OSA is associated with age and gender; however body mass is the most commonly associated epidemiologic factor. Dynamic upper airway imaging has demonstrated both a small airway and increased collapsibility of the airway with inspiration.[54] Airflow disturbances are produced at three main anatomical sites. A deviated septum, enlarged turbinates, or alar rim collapse may reduce nasal airflow. Reduced pharyngeal airway space is due to narrowing of the lateral pharyngeal walls. Tonsillar hypertrophy and laxity of the tonsillar pillars are causes. Finally relation of the genioglossus with sleep or macroglossia or retrognathia can also produce obstruction at the base of the tongue. Increased muscle tone during wakefulness compensates for the narrowed airway. During sleep, however, muscle relaxation allows the airway to collapse and resistance to airflow increases. Patients with a retropositioned mandible and/or maxilla are predisposed to narrowing of the airway. The result is apnea or hypopnea. Each obstructive episode is accompanied by cessations of respiration that induce partial arousals, re-establishing patency of the airway, and interfering with the shifts between sleep stages.

The association between OSA and cardiovascular disease has been demonstrated in many studies,[55–57] although the exact mechanism is not clear. Repeated desaturations and concomitant hypercapnia may stimulate sympathetic neural tone and vasoconstriction. The intermittent hypoxia may also stimulate inflammatory pathways which result in altered function of endothelium and leukocyte adhesion. Randomized prospective trials comparing the effect of therapeutic versus sham CPAP therapy in OSA patients found a decrease in systemic blood pressure only following therapeutic CPAP.[58,59] OSA has been shown to be an independent risk factor for the development of left ventricular hypertrophy[60] and stroke.[61]

Diagnosis/patient presentation

Diagnosis of OSA starts with a medical and sleep history. Sleep history elements include presence of snoring, witnessed apnea, daytime sleepiness, and the quantity and quality of sleep. Additional complaints may be related to quality of life, including morning headaches, memory loss, poor work performance, disrupted family relationships, and alterations in libido. The Epworth Sleepiness Scale (ESS) subjectively assesses the propensity to sleep in eight situations[62] *(Fig. 4.10)*. An evaluation of secondary conditions that may result from OSA, such as hypertension, stroke, and history of motor vehicle accidents, should also be obtained. ⊚ FIG **4.10** APPEARS ONLINE ONLY

Physical examination includes measurement of body mass index, blood pressure, and neck circumference. Inspection of nasal airway evaluates the patency of internal and external nasal valves, presence of septal deviation, and turbinate hypertrophy. Oral examination assesses size and character of tonsils, adenoids, lateral pharyngeal walls and palatal soft tissue. Malocclusions, retrognathia, and macroglossia are also noted on oral examination. Fiberoptic nasopharyngoscopy aids with examination of potential sites of obstruction that may be difficult to visualize directly, such as the base of tongue.

PSG establishes the diagnosis and documents the outcomes of surgical intervention. PSG records electroencephalogram, electro-oculogram, chin electromyogram, airflow, oxygen saturation, respiratory effort, and electrocardiogram. The frequency of obstructive events is reported as an AHI or respiratory disturbance index (RDI). An AHI of greater than 5 is diagnostic of OSA. Additional data obtained are percentage of time spent in each sleep stage and percentage of sleep time spent below threshold oxygen saturations. A full night study is recommended, and at least 240 minutes of total sleep time (TST) are required for a valid study. Split-night studies (one-half diagnostic, one-half therapeutic) apply CPAP for the second half of the night and may underestimate the severity of OSA. This result is common because the TST recorded occurs in the early portion of the night, while the deep stages of sleep occur more often in the second half of the night. A split-night study may be performed if the number of obstructive events is severe (AHI ≥40/hour over 2 hours).

A lateral cephalogram or CBCT scan is obtained in a natural head position with the mandible in centric relation and the soft tissues in repose. If radiographic and clinical examination of the soft tissues of the pharynx reveals a narrow airway, in conjunction with retrognathia of the maxilla and mandible, the patient should be considered a candidate for MMA. However MMA is also utilized in individuals with normal skeletal development, and cephalometric analysis[63,64] *(Fig. 4.11)* predicts movements of the maxilla and mandible that can be achieved to enlarge the pharyngeal airway while maintaining a normal facial balance. Three-dimensional CT and CBCT programs incorporate skeletal and soft-tissue analysis to aid in treatment planning. Airway analysis and dentofacial changes can be predicted and surgical outcomes assessed precisely with these programs.[65]

Patient selection

Surgical indications for OSA are significant OSA (AHI >15 or RDI >20) with associated symptoms of excessive daytime sleepiness, oxygen saturation of less than 90%, anatomic abnormalities of the upper airway, hypertension or arrhythmia, and failure of medical management because of nonacceptance of or poor adherence to therapy.[66]

Treatment/surgical technique

Surgical preparation

Laryngeal examination performed indirectly or fiberoptically allows both surgeon and anesthesiologist to assess the difficulties involved in intubation and extubation. If a tracheotomy is deemed necessary, it is recommended that it not be

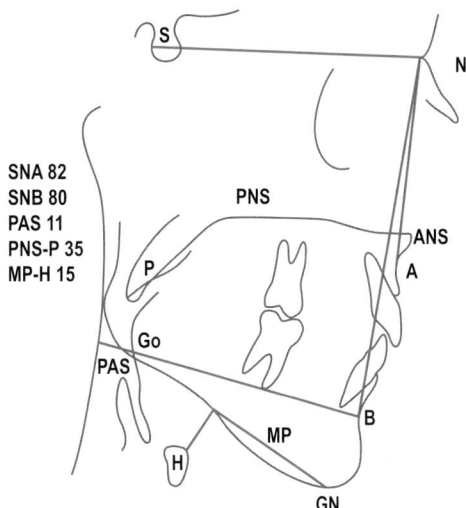

SNA 82
SNB 80
PAS 11
PNS-P 35
MP-H 15

Fig. 4.11 Lateral cephalometric measurements of interest in obstructive sleep apnea evaluation. Cephalometric analysis predicts movements of the maxilla and mandible that can enlarge the pharyngeal airway, maintaining normal facial balance. S, sella; N, nasion; ANS, anterior nasal spine; PNS, posterior nasal spine; Point A, deepest portion on the maxillary alveolar process; P, soft palate; Go, Gonion; Point B, deepest portion on the mandibular alveolar process; PAS, pharyngeal airway space; Gn, gnathion; MP, mandibular plane; H, hyoid.

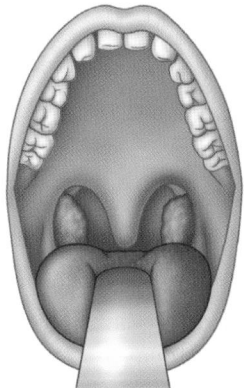
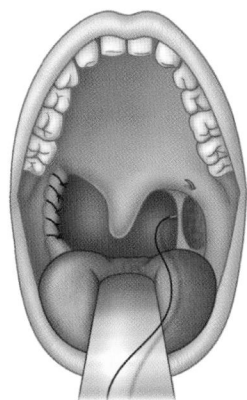
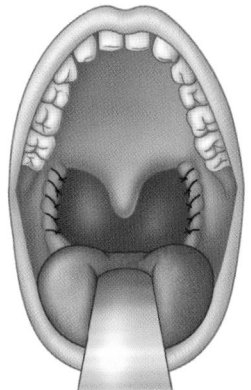

Fig. 4.12 Uvulopalatopharyngoplasty shortens the uvula, sutures the anterior to posterior tonsillar, and removes enlarged tonsils to address upper airway obstruction.

performed at the same time as a bimaxillary procedure. This may increase the risk of aspiration, especially in the setting of an already compromised airway. Naopharyngeal intubation is accomplished with a Ring Adair Elwyn tube which is fixed superiorly over the forehead and cranium. Because most MMA procedures are performed with cranial bone grafts, the tube is sutured to the scalp on the side from which the graft is taken. Procurement of the cranial graft is the first part of the procedure. Hypotensive anesthesia, with mean arterial pressure of approximately 70 mmHg, is necessary to reduce blood loss and improve visualization. Because hypotensive agents are needed, an arterial line and Foley catheter are customary. Judicious intravenous fluids are administered to limit edema. If bimaxillary advancement is planned, autologous or donor-directed blood is arranged.[67]

Nasal procedures

Nasal surgery aims to improve airway obstruction caused by bony, cartilaginous, or hypertrophied tissues. A patent nasal airway minimizes mouth breathing, which worsens upper-airway obstruction by forcing the mandible to rotate downward and backward and pushing the tongue into the posterior pharyngeal space. Septoplasty, alar rim reconstruction, and turbinectomy may be indicated. Radiofrequency treatments of the turbinate also effectively reduce hypertrophied mucosa. Nasal surgery alone seldom resolves moderate or severe OSA, but remains an essential part of OSA treatment. It may also improve the efficacy and tolerance of CPAP.

Uvulopalatopharyngoplasty

In UVPP, the uvula is excised and posterior pharyngeal pillars are trimmed *(Fig. 4.12)*. Tonsillectomy is performed at the same time if the tonsils are enlarged. Uvulopalatal flap is a modification of UVPP in which a limited excision of the uvula is performed and then retracted superiorly *(Fig. 4.13)*. This flap produces less scarring and is potentially reversible in the early postoperative period if nasopharyngeal incompetence is encountered. In mild to moderate OSA, UVPP achieves a 40–50% success rate, though this may diminish with time.[68] The risks of the procedure include velopharyngeal insufficiency, dysphagia, persistent dryness, and nasopharyngeal stenosis.[69,70]

Genioglossus advancement

The genioglossus muscle is attached to the lingual surface of the mandible at the geniotubercle and to the hyoid complex. Movement forward of either of these will advance the tongue base. A limited osteotomy of the mandibular symphysis is performed in genioglossus advancement. The bony segment, and the underlying attachment of the genioglossus, are pulled forward, rotated so that the bony ledges rest on the anterior mandible, and the segment is stabilized *(Fig. 4.14)*. This procedure is often performed at the time of UVPP or MMA, and is better tolerated than hyoid suspension. Fracture of the mandible, damage to tooth roots, avulsion of the muscle attachments, and permanent anesthesia are potential complications.[71]

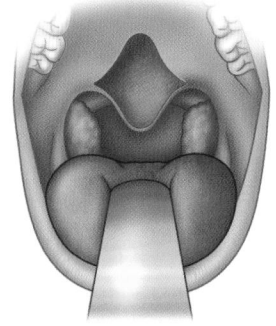
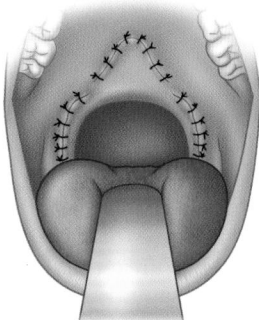

Fig. 4.13 The uvulopalatal flap places the uvula superior to the soft palate without removing it.

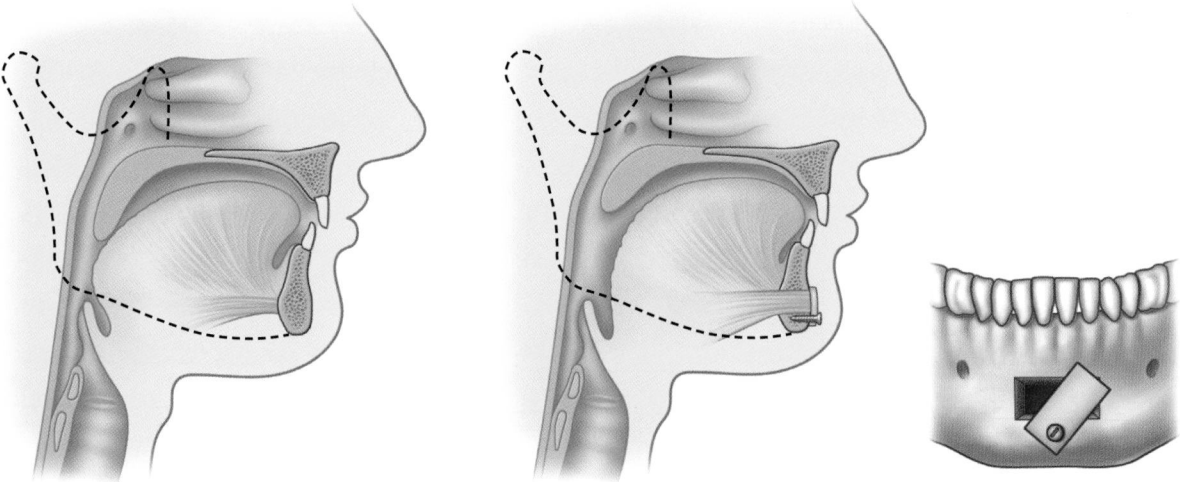

Fig. 4.14 Osteotomy of the mandibular symphysis allows advancement of the genioglossus muscle and tongue base. The advanced segment is stabilized with a screw.

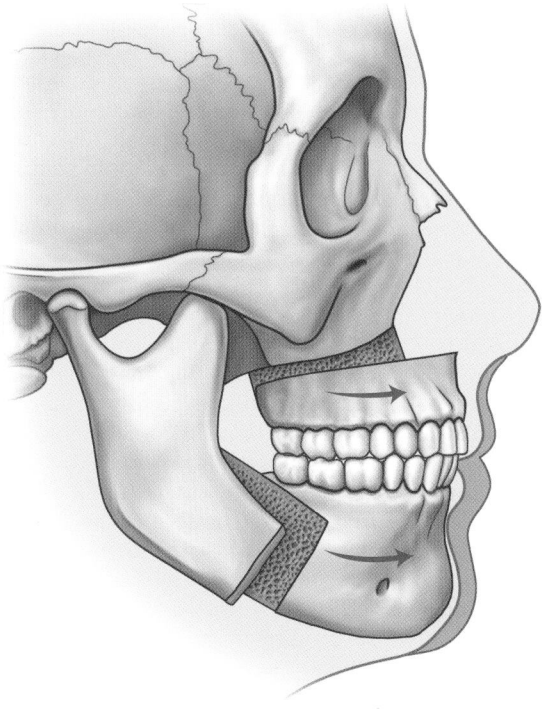

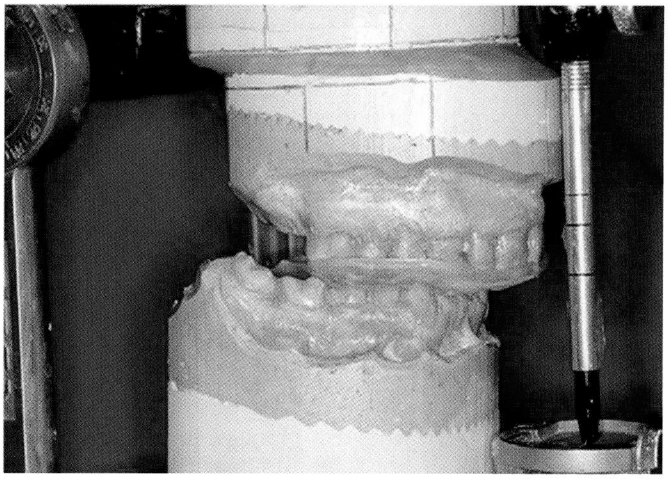

Fig. 4.16 Model surgery in preparation for maxillomandibular advancement, showing 10 mm maxillary advancement and interim splint. (Reproduced from Boyd SB. Management of obstructive sleep apnea by maxillomandibular advancement. Oral Maxillofacial Surg Clin North Am 2009;21:447–457.)

Fig. 4.15 LeFort I osteotomy of maxilla and sagittal split osteotomy of mandible utilized for maxillomandibular advancement.

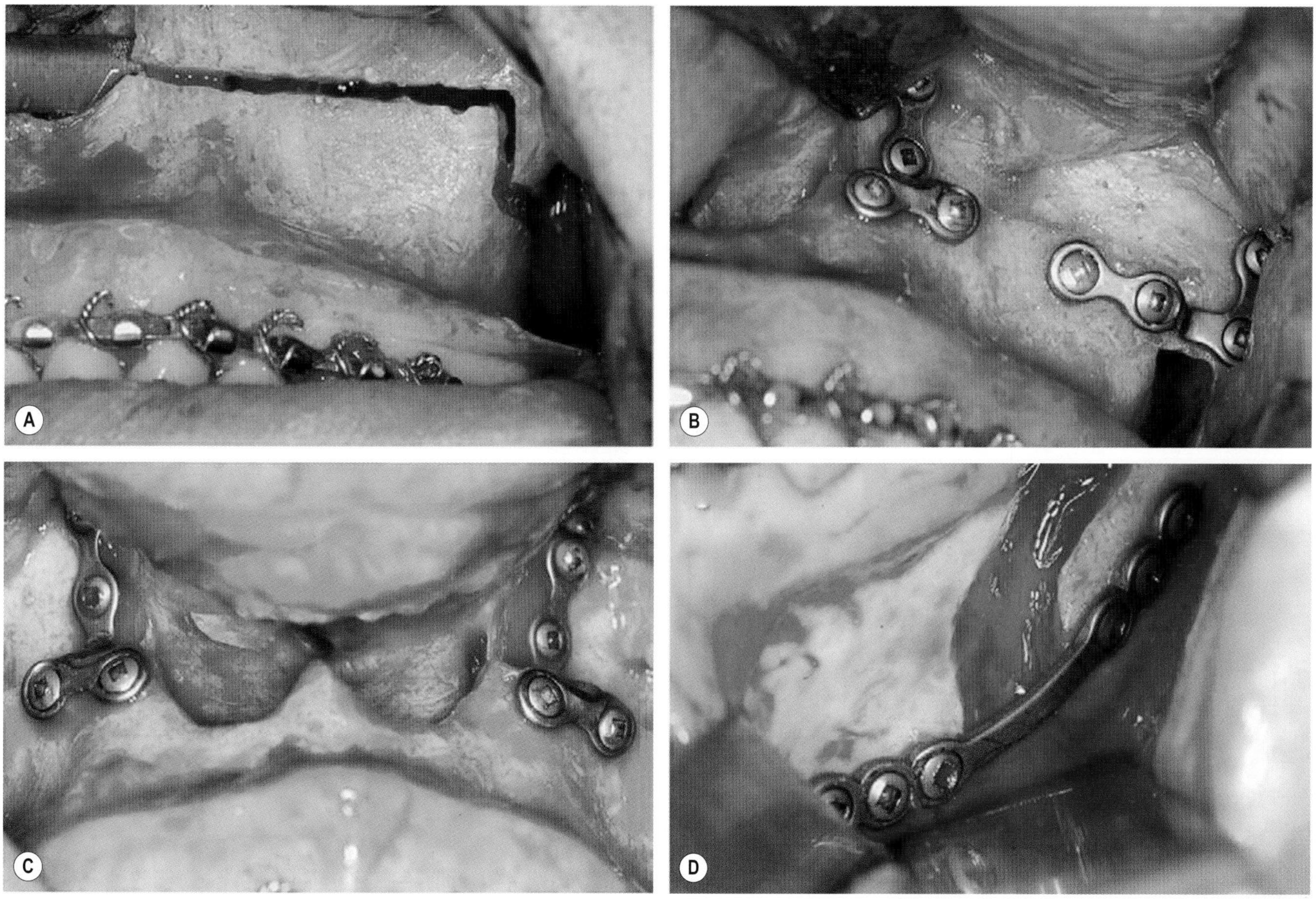

Fig. 4.17 Maxillomandibular advancement showing: **(A)** LeFort I osteotomy of maxilla; **(B)** placement of fixation at piriform rim and zygomaticomaxillary buttress; **(C)** piriform rim contouring and reduction of nasal spine; and **(D)** fixation of mandible at its inferior border to minimize risk to inferior alveolar nerve. (Reproduced from Boyd SB. Management of obstructive sleep apnea by maxillomandibular advancement. Oral Maxillofacial Surg Clin North Am 2009;21:447–457.)

Mandibulomaxillary advancement

MMA is achieved using a LeFort I maxillary osteotomy and a bilateral sagittal split osteotomy of the mandible *(Fig. 4.15)*. It enlarges the airway space by advancing the skeletal framework to which the pharyngeal soft tissue and tongue attach, resulting in reduced collapsibility during negative-pressure inspiration. Unless a class II or III malocclusion is also being corrected, synchronous advancement of the maxilla and mandible is performed to maintain preoperative occlusion. Ten millimeters of advancement is often necessary in OSA patients. Model surgery is performed to fabricate intermediate and occlusal splints, which are used intraoperatively to position the bone segments[72] *(Fig. 4.16)*.

The maxilla is approached first and a horizontal vestibular incision is made from the first molar on one side to the opposite first molar. Subperiosteal dissection exposes the anterior face of the maxilla back to the pterygoid process and the piriform rims anteriorly. The infraorbital nerve is visualized and attention made not to retract forcefully directly on the nerve. The anterior nasal spine is removed, and the nasal floor elevated; this includes separating the septum from the maxilla.

The pterygoid plates are fractured with curved osteotomes while the maxilla is still stable. Following osteotomy of the maxilla at least 5 mm above the apices of the teeth, the maxilla is downfractured *(Fig. 4.17A)*. The maxilla is mobilized with the aid of Rowe forceps. An interim splint facilitates accurate anteroposterior positioning of the maxilla and prevents midline discrepancies and sideways and vertical yaw of the jaw. Bone removal along the piriform aperture and maxillary sinus walls removes interferences to advancement. The anterior nasal spine is reduced to minimize overprojection and widening of the nasolabial soft tissues that may result from advancement *(Fig. 4.17C)*. The maxilla is rigidly fixed in the new position at the piriform rim and zygomaticomaxillary buttress *(Fig. 4.17B)*. The mandible is addressed next. An incision is made along the external oblique ridge from midramus height to lateral to the first molar. The tissues are then elevated at the subperiosteal level to expose the lateral border of the mandible and anterior aspect of the ramus only. The temporalis muscle must be stripped from the coronoid process high enough to access the medical ramus above the lingual canal. The medial ramus is then exposed to above and behind the lingual canal, which can easily be identified with a nerve

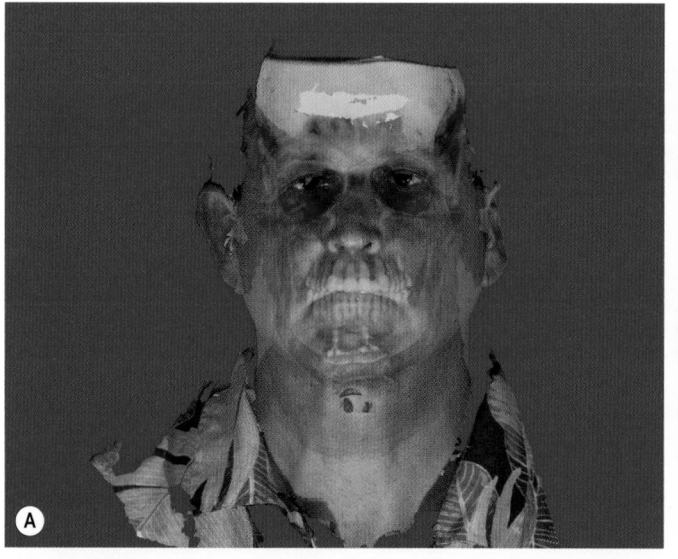

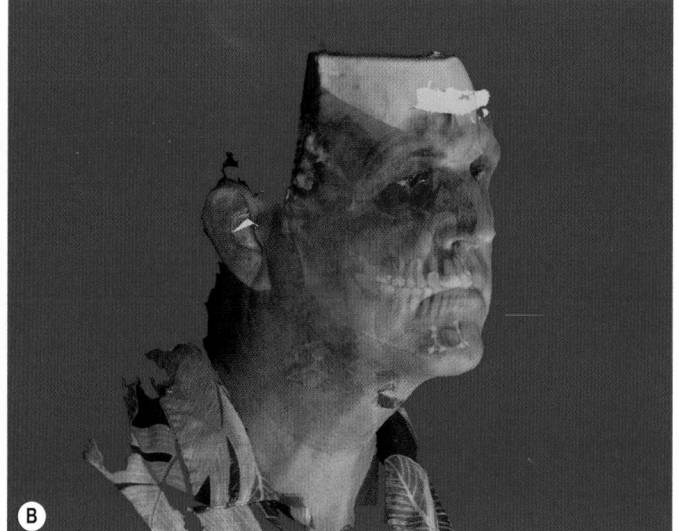

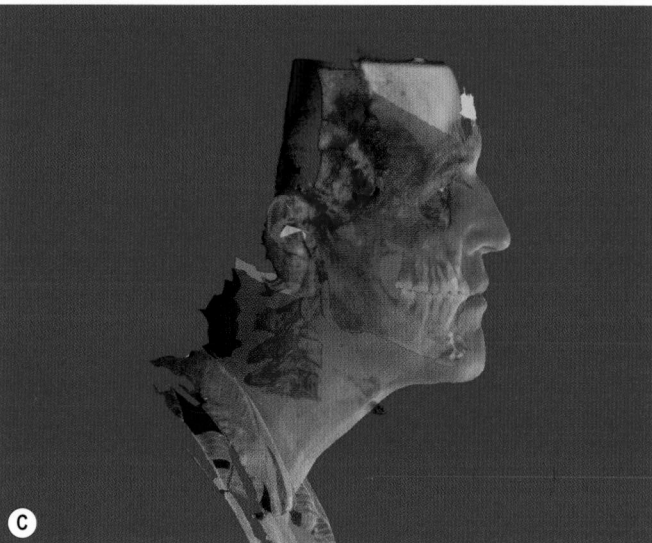

Fig. 4.18 Combined cone beam computed tomography and surface scan (Dolphin Imaging) of a 56-year-old male with continued severe obstructive sleep apnea post genioglossus advancement. Preoperative **(A)** frontal, **(B)** oblique, and **(C)** lateral images.

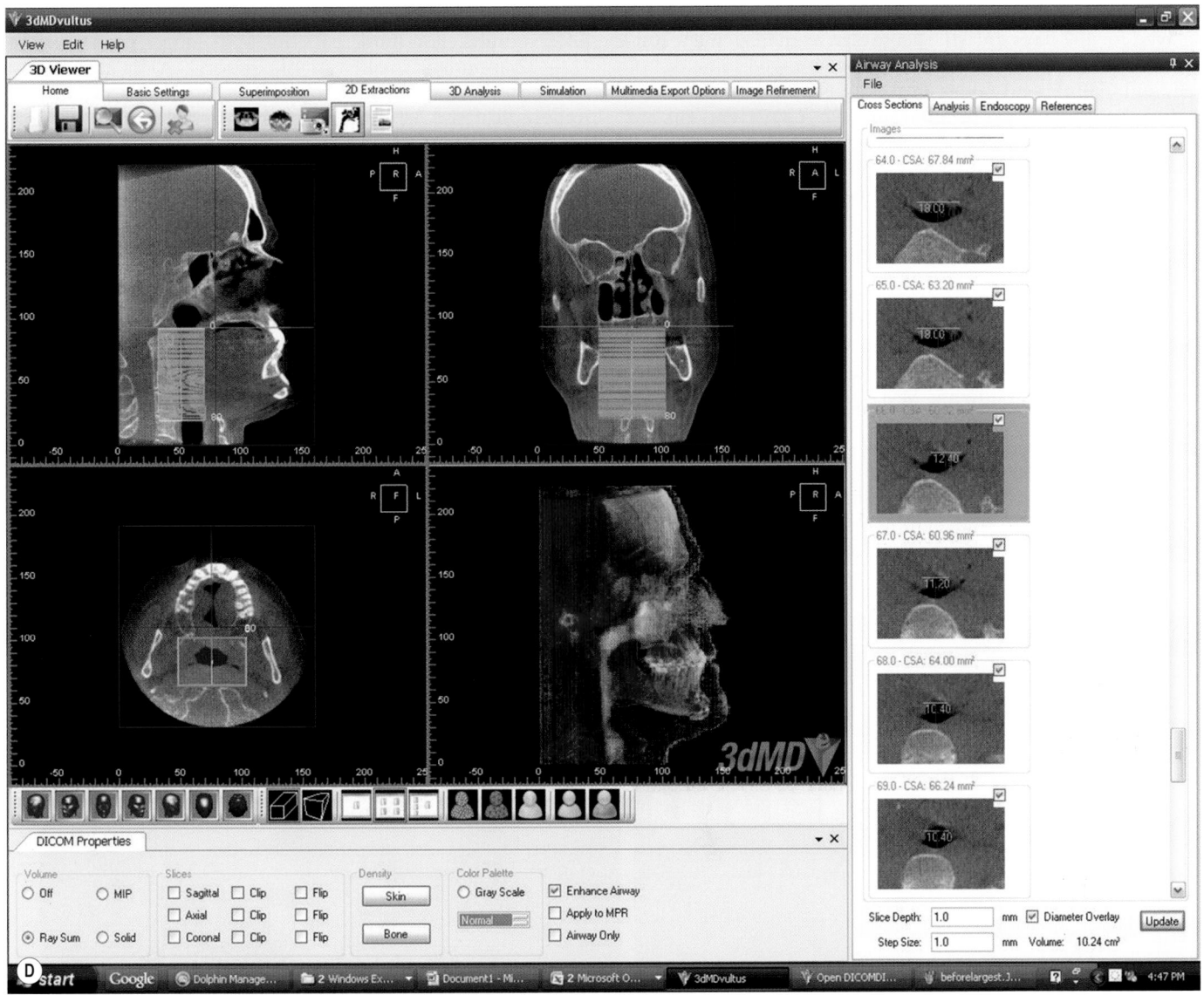

Fig. 4.18, cont'd (D) Cross-sectional airway size is calculated based on 1-mm images from hard palate to epiglottis. The location and area of the smallest airway size (60.32 cm²) are highlighted in pink.

hook and is always at the same level as the mandibular occlusal plane. An osteotomy is made 4–5 mm above the lingual canal with a saw or burr and carried along the anterior aspect of the ramus following the external oblique ridge. The osteotomy continues along the buccal mandible surface at the first molar or where the ridge turns down and the bone becomes thinner. A vertical osteotomy is then made inferiorly through the inferior border of the mandible, usually in the area of the antegonial notch. The split is then accomplished with osteotomes and spreaders. Careful attention must be made of the position of the inferior alveolar nerve during this process as it frequently can remain in the proximal fragment and must be gently teased out to prevent injury to it. The mandible is then brought into occlusion with the maxilla with the aid of an occlusal splint. The mandible is then plated or fixed with screws or a combination of the two. Bone grafts are now placed in the advancement gaps. The maxillary vestibular incision is closed with an alar cinch suture and a V-Y

advancement of the vestibular tissues. This prevents nasal widening and thinning of the lips.[73] The mandibular wound is closed in the standard fashion *(Figs 4.18 and 4.19)*.

Postoperative management

The postoperative management of a patient with OSA is more complicated than the typical orthognathic patient. At the time of extubation, the surgeon and anesthesiologist are present, and the necessary equipment for reintubation is immediately available. The patient is transferred to the intensive care unit for overnight monitoring. The use of a patient-controlled analgesia pump is not recommended because respiratory depression may occur even at low doses of narcotics in OSA patients. Pain is controlled with oral analgesics and intramuscular injections. The use of CPAP maintains the airway, controls edema, and may reduce patient anxiety. Interarch elastics are used to support the occlusion, but their placement may be delayed for 1–2 days until the acute airway management concerns have stabilized. The patient is encouraged to be out of bed, ambulating, and taking oral liquids on the first postoperative day. The typical hospital stay is 2–3 days. Patients are seen weekly until healed. CPAP use is continued until 1–2 weeks prior to follow-up PSG, which is completed at 3–6 months following surgery to evaluate treatment outcome objectively.

Outcome

Subjectively, MMA is associated with high patient satisfaction and improved symptoms of excessive daytime sleepiness.[74] The improvement in patient-reported symptoms and ESS scores was greater following MMA then with CPAP or soft palatal surgery.[51,74]

Riley et al. defined cure as achieving a postoperative AHI ≤20 and a least a 50% reduction of the AHI compared with preoperative values.[75] In addition, the lowest oxygen saturation should be ≥90% and symptoms of excessive daytime sleepiness resolved. They reported a success rate of 87% at 6–12 months. For those patients with long-term follow-up (12–132 months), quality of life reports, AHI, and lowest oxygen saturation benefits were maintained. Cephalometric data indicated a 34% relapse in the skeletal advancement at long-term follow-up. However the increase in airway space was not predictive of success, and the relapse at long-term follow-up did not affect clinical outcome.[76] Similar success is reported in the achievement and maintenance of normal sleep architecture at 6–12 weeks and 2 years,[48] and the ability to discontinue CPAP.[74] Cephalometric analysis and CT scans have demonstrated an increase in the airway size following MMA.[77] A meta-analysis of the outcome of MMA in treating OSA reported mean AHI decreased from 63.9/hour to 9.5/hour following surgery. The pooled surgical success and cure (defined as AHI <5) rates were 86% and 43.2% respectively. Younger age, lower preoperative weight, and greater degree of maxillary advancement were predictive of surgical success.[78]

Sensory loss and anesthesia of the lips and chin are the most common complications of MMA.[79] Nearly half of these patients recover normal sensation at an average of 18 months.

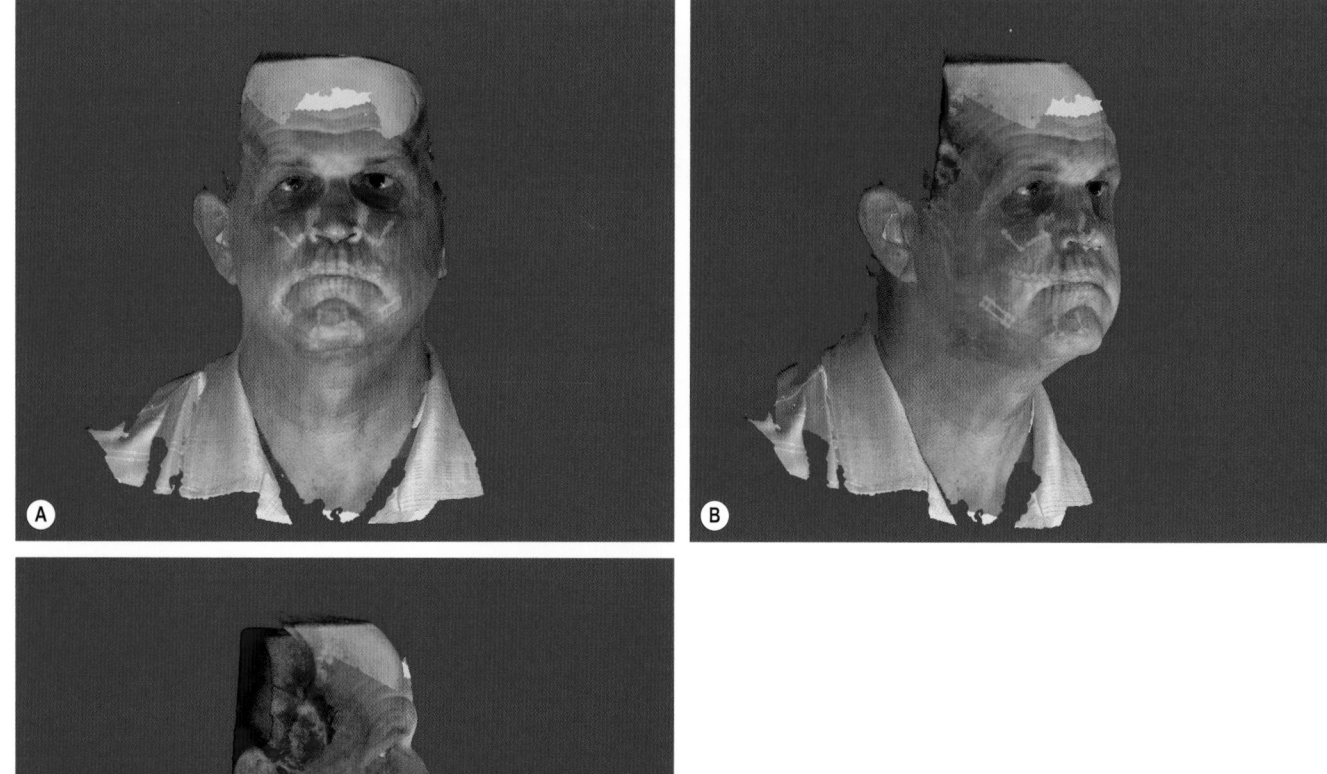

Fig. 4.19 Following maxillomandibular advancement, with 10-mm advancement of maxilla. Preoperative **(A)** frontal, **(B)** oblique, and **(C)** lateral images.

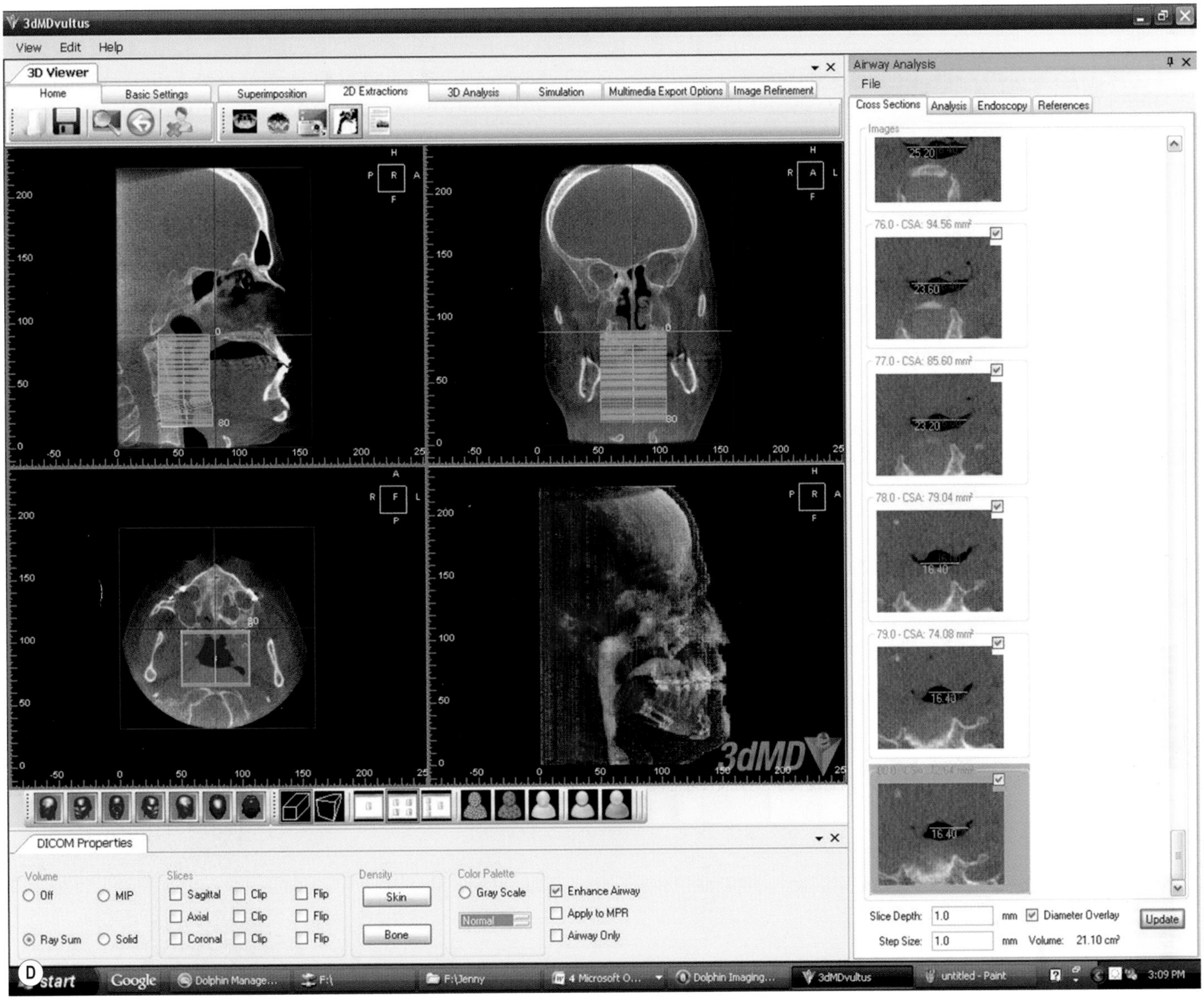

Fig. 4.19, cont'd (D) Smallest cross-sectional airway was 72.6 cm². Respiratory disturbance index improved from 62 to 5.

Additional complaints reported are TMJ pain or limited mouth opening.

MMA advances bones structures and facial soft tissues with a ratio from 0.6 to 0.9.[80,81] The majority of patients report facial changes following surgery.[79,82] Half of these patients find the changes favorable. Changes observed include upward rotation of the nasal tip, enlargement of the nostrils, and reduction in the height of the upper lip.[81]

Secondary procedures

In the larger advancements, distraction osteogenesis is utilized. The use of mandibular distraction for treatment of pediatric OSA is well established.[83–85] In adults, the senior author employs a 1-mm-a-day rate with no latency period. Distraction of the sagittal split segments or at the LeFort I level can be done with intraoral activation rods. Adjustment of the occlusion can be achieved with differential activation of distractors. Bone grafts are not required, and internal devices are available that do not require a subsequent surgery for removal.[86]

Transverse maxillary distraction has been described to alleviate the constricted nasal airway. In a small group of patients with mild OSA, surgically assisted transverse maxillary expansion was effective, with improvement in average AHI from 19 to 7.[87] As is true for other nasal procedures, correcting the nasal airway by itself is useful only in mild cases.

Bonus images for this chapter can be found online at

http://www.expertconsult.com

Fig. 4.10 Epworth Sleepiness Scale questionnaire.

Access the complete references list online at **http://www.expertconsult.com**

2. Farrar WB, McCarty WL. Inferior joint space athrography and characteristics of condylar paths in internal derangements of the TMJ. *J Prosthet Dent.* 1979;41:548–555.

   An early description of the anatomy of internal derangement of the articular disc. The authors report on the success of disc repositioning in over 300 patients.

24. Wilkes CH. Internal derangements of the temporomandibular joint: pathological variations. *Arch Otolaryngol Head Neck Surg.* 1989;115:469–477.

   A retrospective analysis of 740 joints with correlations drawn between clinical symptoms, radiographic, surgical, and pathologic findings.

35. Dolwick MF. Temporomandibular joint surgery for internal derangement. *Dent Clin North Am.* 2007;51:195–208.

   A succinct review of the diagnosis and treatment of TMJ disease related to disc derangement.

39. Hall HD, Indresano AT, Kirk WS, et al. Prospective muticenter comparison of 4 temporomandibular joint operations. *J Oral Maxillofac Surg.* 2005;63:1174–1179.

44. Reston JT, Turkelson CM. Meta-analysis of surgical treatments for temporomandibular articular disorders. *J Oral Maxillofac Surg.* 2003;61:3–10.

65. Schendel SA, Hatcher D. Automated 3-dimensional airway analysis from cone-beam computed tomography data. *J Oral Maxillofac Surg.* 2010;68:696–701.

67. Schendel SA, Powell NB. Surgical orthognathic management of sleep apnea. *J Craniofac Surg.* 2007;18:902–911.

72. Boyd SB. Management of obstructive sleep apnea by maxillomandibular advancement. *Oral Maxillofacial Surg Clin North Am.* 2009;21:447–457.

74. Goodday R. Diagnosis, treatment planning, and surgical correction of obstructive sleep apnea. *J Oral Maxillofac Surg.* 2009;67:2183–2196.

   The author's surgical planning and technique of maxillomandibular advancement are outlined with illustrative cases. Outcome data of sleep symptoms, appearance, and airway analysis are reviewed.

76. Li KK, Powel NB, Riley RW, et al. Long-term results of maxillomandibular advancement surgery. *Sleep Breath.* 2000;4:137–139.

   The follow-up of a previously reported cohort demonstrates long-term success in the majority of patients. Polysomnographic data are correlated with change in body mass index and cephalometric data.

5

Scalp and forehead reconstruction

Mark D. Wells and Carla Skytta

SYNOPSIS

- Anatomically the forehead and scalp have a complex three-dimensional anatomy that must be understood in order to perform reconstructive procedures successfully.
- The complex histology of the region allows for the development of a variety of unique congenital, traumatic, inflammatory, and neoplastic conditions.
- Reconstructive principles should be directed at replacing like tissue with similar tissue whenever possible. This is particularly important in the scalp given its unique hair-bearing characteristics.
- Incisions in the scalp should be made parallel to the direction of the hair follicles with minimal electrocautery to minimize scars and alopecia.
- The aesthetic subunit principles of the face should be considered when cosmetically critical areas of the forehead are reconstructed in order to prevent a "patchwork" effect.
- Care must be taken not to displace mobile structures such as brows or eyelids when developing a reconstructive plan.
- Reconstructive options include closure by secondary intention, vacuum-assisted closure (VAC) therapy, primary closure, tissue expansion, skin grafts, and a variety of local, regional, and distant flaps.

 Access the Historical Perspective section online at
http://www.expertconsult.com

Introduction

The exposed location of the scalp and forehead makes them susceptible to a wide variety of traumatic and environmental insults. The complex histology of the region allows for the development of a multitude of neoplastic and inflammatory conditions. The unique hair-bearing characteristics of the scalp and cosmetically sensitive region of the forehead impose unique reconstructive challenges.

Deformities can range from small defects that can be closed primarily to massive defects requiring free tissue transfer for closure.

A successful reconstructive plan requires a thorough understanding of the relevant anatomy, careful analysis of the defect, and knowledge of various reconstructive options. Each reconstructive plan must be carefully tailored to meet the unique requirements of the patient and associated wound characteristics.

In this chapter, we will focus on the anatomy relevant to the reconstructive surgeon. A review of disease processes unique to the forehead and scalp will be discussed. Finally, the wide variety of reconstructive options available to the treating surgeon will be outlined.

Basic science/disease process

Anatomy

Anatomically, the scalp and forehead extend from the supraorbital rims anteriorly to the nuchal line posteriorly. Laterally, it extends from the frontal process of the zygoma across the zygomatic arch to the prominence of the mastoid process.

The scalp consists of five layers which can easily be remembered by the mnemonic "SCALP," where S is skin, C is subcutaneous tissue, A is aponeurotic layer, L is loose areolar tissue, and P is pericranium *(Fig. 5.1)*.[6,7]

The outermost layer of the scalp consists of the skin and subcutaneous tissue. Contained within this layer are hair follicles, sweat glands, and fat. Connective tissue septa within the subcutaneous layer connect firmly to the underlying musculoaponeurotic layer.

Under the subcutaneous layer is the galea aponeurotica. This is a musculoaponeurotic layer that extends from the frontalis muscles anteriorly to the occipitalis muscle posteriorly. Laterally the galea continues as the temporoparietal fascia. This tissue is highly vascularized and has found great utility in reconstructive procedures about the head and neck.

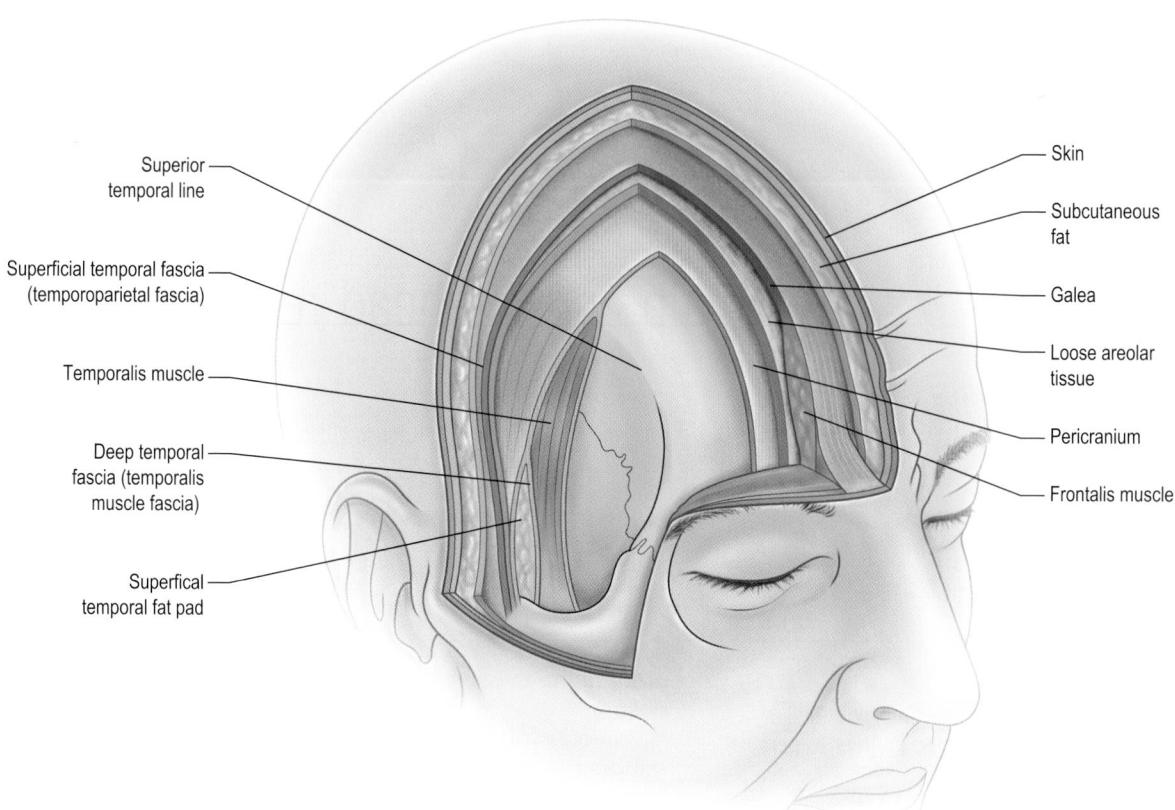

Superior temporal line

Superficial temporal fascia (temporoparietal fascia)

Temporalis muscle

Deep temporal fascia (temporalis muscle fascia)

Superfical temporal fat pad

Skin

Subcutaneous fat

Galea

Loose areolar tissue

Pericranium

Frontalis muscle

Fig. 5.1 Layers of the scalp: S, skin; C, subcutaneous tissue; A, aponeurotic layer; L, loose areolar tissue; and P, pericranium. (Reproduced from TerKonda RP, Sykes JM. Concepts of scalp and forehead reconstruction. *Otolaryngol Clin North Am.* 1997;30:519–539.)

Anteriorly, the galea extends into the face as the superficial musculoaponeurotic system, as outlined by Mitz and Peyronie[8] and later modified by Jost and Levet.[9]

The muscle component of this layer consists of the paired frontalis and occipitalis muscles as well as the auricular muscles laterally. The frontalis muscles originate from the galea and insert into the dermis at the level of the superciliary arch. Contraction of the frontalis causes elevation of the eyebrows and horizontal-oriented lines in the forehead. Anteriorly, the frontalis blends with the procerus, corrugator supercilii, and orbicularis oculi. The paired corrugator supercilii muscle arises from the frontal bone near the superomedial orbital rim. The muscle runs superolaterally through the fibers of orbicularis oculi and frontalis before inserting into the medial eyebrow skin. The corrugator muscle is a brow depressor, pulling the brow medially and inferiorly, producing vertical glabellar folds. The procerus muscle is a thin muscle that inserts into the glabella and lower mid-forehead. It is a brow depressor, forming horizontal nasal root creases. In the posterior scalp, paired occipitalis muscles take origin from the superior nuchal line and mastoid, inserting into the galea.

There are three auricular muscles on each side of the scalp: the anterior auricular, superior auricular, and posterior auricular muscles. They take origin from the temporalis fascia and the mastoid bone and insert into the perichondrium external ear *(Fig. 5.2)*.

The subgaleal fascia is a loose areolar layer beneath the galea. This tissue is thin over the vertex of the skull and becomes progressively thicker in the temporoparietal region. This layer is richly vascularized and can be elevated as an independent layer for reconstructive procedures.

The deepest layer of the scalp is the pericranium. This is the periosteal layer of the calvaria. It is a thick collagenous layer with a rich blood supply that is firmly attached to the skull in the region of the sutures. The use of pericranial flaps as a reconstructive option has been well described in the literature.

Anatomy of the temporal region

The temporoparietal region consists of four distinct fascial layers with anatomic significance. The most superficial layer is the superficial temporal fascia. This layer is a direct extension of the galea. It is closely applied to the overlying skin and subcutaneous tissue, making dissection difficult. Unless care is taken, it is easy to damage the overlying hair follicles, resulting in temporal alopecia *(Fig. 5.3)*.

Deep to the superficial temporal fascia is the subgaleal fascia. Contained within this easily dissected layer are the superficial temporal artery and the frontal branch of the facial nerve. Under the subgaleal fascia is the superficial temporal fat pad. Numerous large perforating veins course through this layer, making dissection somewhat difficult.

Beneath the superficial temporal fat pad is the deep temporal fascia. This is a thick fascial layer surrounding the temporalis muscle. Superiorly it fuses with the pericranium.

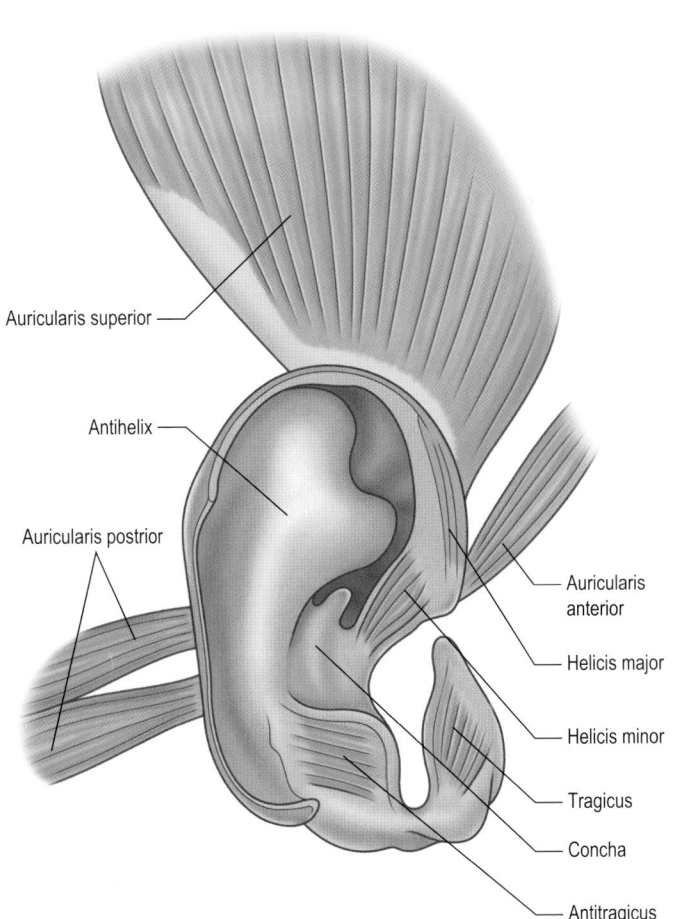

Fig. 5.2 Extrinsic muscles of the ear – anterior auricular, superior auricular, and posterior auricular muscles.

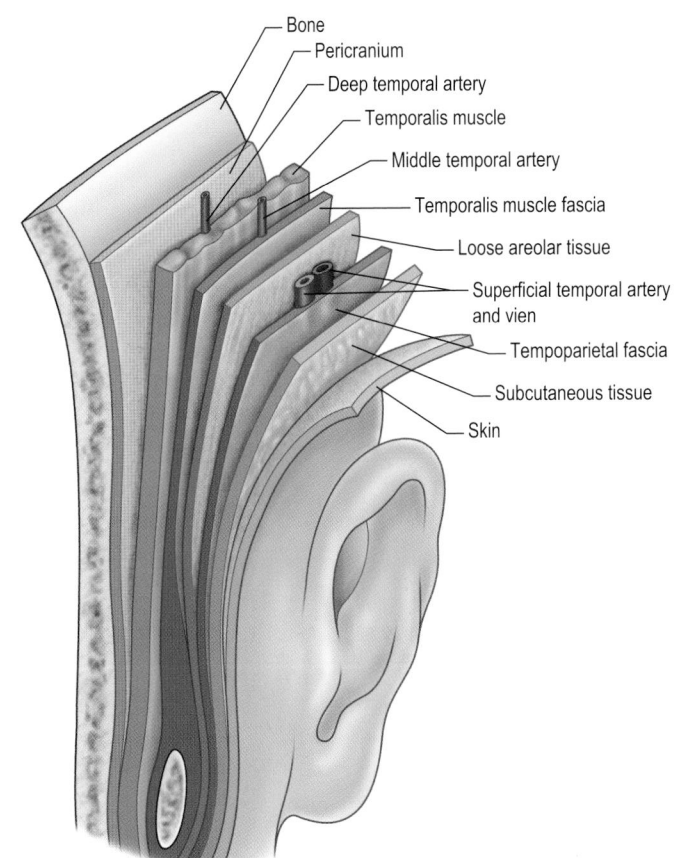

Fig. 5.3 Anatomy of the temporal region.

Inferiorly, it splits into two layers at the level of the frontozygomatic suture. The superficial portion of the deep temporal fascia attaches to the lateral border of the zygomatic arch. The deep layer fuses with the medial aspect of the arch. Reflection of the superficial portion of the deep temporal fascia with a bicoronal flap allows exposure of the craniofacial skeleton without injury to the frontal branch of the facial nerve as it passes over the arch of the zygoma.

Between the two layers of the deep temporal fascia lie temporalis muscle fibers and a thin layer of fat. This fat is continuous with the buccal fat pad of the midface. The temporalis muscle originates from the temporal fascia and inserts on to the coronoid process of the mandible. It is supplied by two deep temporal branches of the internal maxillary artery: the middle and deep temporal arteries.

Blood supply

The scalp and forehead have a rich vascular plexus supplied by branches of both the internal and external carotid arteries. The supraorbital and supratrochlear arteries are terminal branches of the internal carotid arteries, providing the blood supply to the forehead and anterior scalp. The superficial temporal artery, posterior auricular, and occipital arteries are branches of the external carotid artery. These vessels supply the lateral and posterior aspects of the scalp. The extensive

interconnection between each of the angiosomes allows replantation of the entire scalp based on a single donor vessel. The venous system parallels the arterial supply, eventually draining into the external and external jugular veins (*Fig. 5.4*).

Nerves

The frontal branch of the facial nerve supplies the motor innervation of the forehead. The nerve emerges from the parotid 2.5 cm anterior to the tragus. It ascends above the periosteum over the central portion of the zygomatic arch, passing 1.5 cm lateral to the orbital rim to innervate the frontalis muscles on their deep surfaces. It courses along the deep surface of the superficial temporal fascia, putting it at risk for injury with dissection into the temporal region (*Fig. 5.5*). The posterior auricular branch of the facial nerve supplies the occipitalis muscle. This branch originates with the facial nerve as it exits the stylomastoid foramen. The temporal muscles are supplied by the posterior and anterior deep temporal nerves, which are branches of the trigeminal nerve. This dichotomy of innervation is used successfully in developing reanimation procedures for patients with facial palsy.

The supratrochlear and supraorbital nerves, branches of the first division of the trigeminal nerve, provide sensation to the forehead and anterior scalp. The supratrochlear nerve exits the orbit between the pulley of the superior oblique and the supraorbital foramen. It ascends beneath the corrugator supercilii to supply the medial forehead, upper eyelid, and conjunctiva. The supraorbital nerve exits the frontal bone

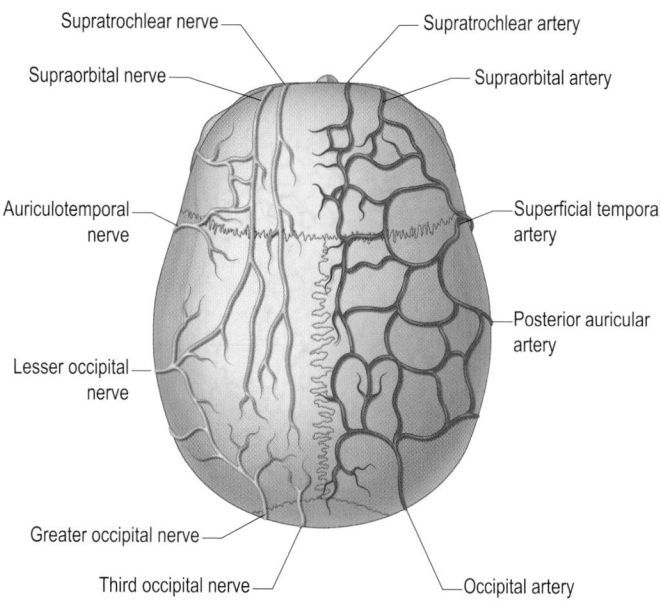

Fig. 5.4 Arterial and nervous supply of the scalp.

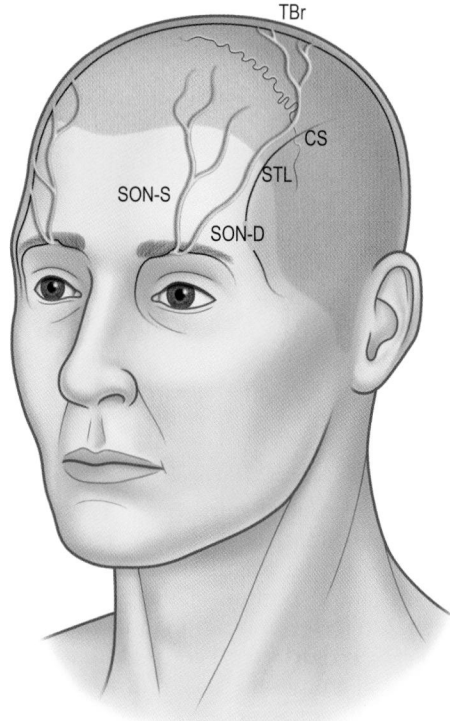

Fig. 5.6 The course of the deep branch of deep (SON-D) and superficial (SON-S) division of the supraorbital nerve. The deep branch superiorly or obliquely across the forehead between the galeal aponeurotica and the periosteum and by the midforehead level found between 0.5 and 1 cm medial to the superior temporal crest. It pierces the galea just before the coronal suture (CS). The superficial branch passes through the lower frontalis muscle to run over the surface of the muscle. TBr, terminal branch; STL, superior temporal line of the skull. (Reproduced from Knize DM. A study of the supraorbital nerve. *Plast Reconstr Surg.* 1995;96:564–569.)

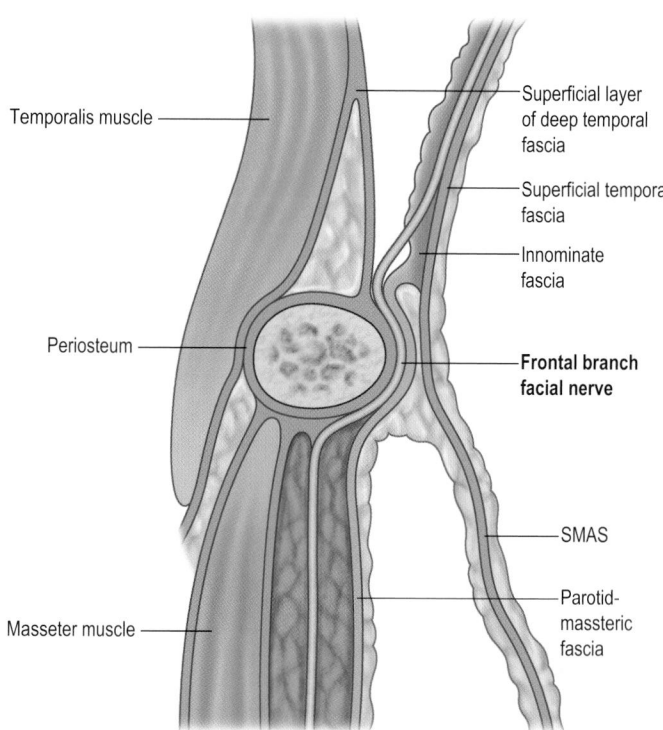

Fig. 5.5 Course of the frontal branch of the facial nerve. Left, histologic cross-section at the level of the zygomatic arch. Right, schematic illustration depicting the fascial planes of the cheek and temporal region. SMAS, superficial muscular aponeurotic system. (Reproduced from Agawal CA, Mendenahall SD, Foreman KB, et al. *Plast Reconstr Surg.* 2102;125:532–537.)

through the supraorbital foramen before dividing into two branches. The superficial branch of the supraorbital nerve courses over the surface of the frontalis muscle to provide sensation to the central forehead. The rest of the scalp and top of the head are innervated by the deep branch, which travels laterally between the periosteum and the galea. Knize[10] has described the anatomy of the deep branch of the supraorbital nerve. The deep branch runs in a 1-cm-wide band medial to the palpable temporal crest line to innervate the frontoparietal scalp *(Fig. 5.6)*.

The zygomaticotemporal nerve, a branch of the maxillary division of the trigeminal nerve, supplies the skin just lateral to the temporal crest. The auriculotemporal nerve, a branch from the third division of the trigeminal nerve, supplies the ear and lateral scalp.

The greater occipital nerve is a spinal nerve that arises between the first and second cervical vertebra along with the lesser occipital nerve. It emerges from the suboccipital triangle 3 cm below the occipital protuberance and 1.5 cm lateral to the midline to supply the posterior part of the scalp to the vertex.

Aesthetic units of the scalp and forehead

Gonzalez-Ulloa[11] first conceived the idea of aesthetic units of the face. Facial aesthetic units and subunits are visual anatomic boundaries formed by contour changes in facial topography. Making incisions along these boundaries or replacing entire subunits hides scars in the light reflections and shadows

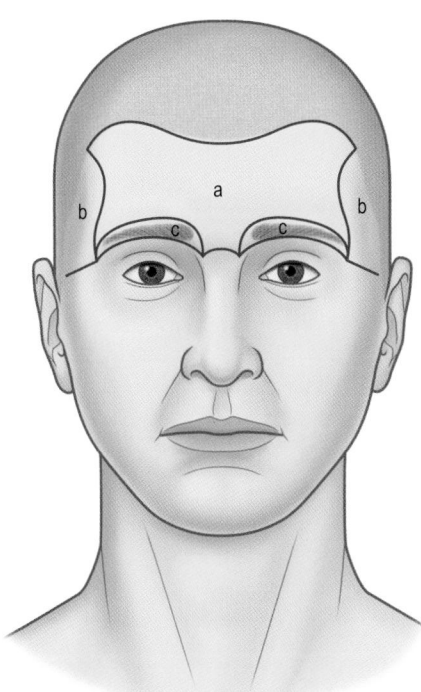

Fig. 5.7 Aesthetic units of the forehead region. a, central forehead unit; b, bilateral temporal units; c, two eyebrow units.

of the face. The aesthetic subunits of the face must be respected when planning reconstructive procedures of the head and neck.

The upper third of the face historically has been subdivided into five units: two temporal units posterior to the anterior temporal crest, a central forehead unit (*Fig. 5.7*), and two eyebrow units along the supraorbital rims. More recently, the forehead has been subdivided into paramedian, lateral, and lateral temporal subunits.[12] Care must be taken not to cause inadvertent displacement of mobile subunits such as the brow when operating on the forehead or scalp.

The hair-bearing scalp is its own aesthetic unit. Strict attention to the re-establishment of the temporal and anterior hairline can prevent unwanted secondary deformities.

Hair structure and cycle

Hair is the most visible feature of scalp anatomy. Hair has two separate structures: the follicle in the subcutaneous tissue and the shaft that we see. Of the human body's 5 million hair follicles, approximately 100 000 are present in the scalp.

Human hair is composed primarily of keratin. The visible hair shaft is dead. It is the proteinaceous end product of a living structure called the hair matrix contained within the subcutaneous tissue. Viable cells in the base of the matrix proliferate rapidly. Immediately above this area of cell division is the zone of keratinization. Cells in this zone undergo a process of dehydration and chemical change creating the dense, cohesive mass of keratinization forming the hair shaft. As new keratinized cells are added to the base of the hair shaft, the hair grows. Scalp hair grows 0.35 mm/day; however this can vary with age, nutrition, pregnancy, and environmental factors.

The follicle is an oval-shaped structure containing several different layers.[12] At the base of the follicle is the papilla. It contains capillary loops that perfuse the growing hair follicle. Hair growth requires diffusion of oxygen and nutrients from the vascular network of the papilla. The hair bulb caps the papilla to form a bulbous expansion that forms the hair shaft.

Under the influence of the dermal papilla, epidermal cell differentiation produces keratinized hair fibers. The matrix cells differentiate to form the hair cortex and surrounding hair cuticle. In the center of the hair shaft are large polygonal cells called the medulla. Cells that surround the hair shaft comprise the inner root sheath (IRS). The IRS consists of three distinct histological layers: the cuticle, Huxley layer, and Henley layer. Above the level of the attached sebaceous gland, the IRS breaks down to form on the hair cortex and surrounding cuticle to protrude above the epidermis.

The outer root sheath (ORS) is distinct from other epidermal components of the hair follicle, being continuous with the epidermis. In the "bulge" region of the hair follicle, an arrector pili muscle spans between the ORS and epidermis. Contraction of this muscle makes hair stand erect and produces "goosebumps" in the skin when subjected to cold. The "bulge" region is believed to be the storage area for hair follicle stems cells.

Also extending from the ORS is the sebaceous gland. It consists of specialized cells focused on the production of lipids. The products of the sebaceous gland are believed to break down the IRS. The ORS surrounds the hair fiber and IRS. Just above the bulb region containing the dermal papilla, the ORS tapers and ends. Thus, the ORS does not entirely cover the hair fiber and IRS.

There are two basic types of normal postnatal human hair. Vellus hair is fine, soft, short, hypopigmented, unmedullated, and almost invisible. It covers the forehead and bald scalp. Terminal hair of the scalp, beard, and eyebrows is relatively coarse, long, often medullated, and variably pigmented. Some vellus hairs become terminal hairs, as in beard development in adolescent males. Additionally, terminal hairs can become vellus hairs, as in androgenetic alopecia. Testosterone and dihydrotestosterone can reduce *in vitro* proliferation of dermal papilla cells and ORS keratinocytes from the frontoparietal scalp.

The matrix of all hair follicles undergoes cycles of growth and degeneration (*Fig. 5.8*). The hair cycle has three stages of growth: anagen (growing phase), catagen (involutional phase), and telogen (dormant phase). At any one time, 90–95% of hairs are in the anagen phase, 5–10% are in catagen, and 1–2% is in telogen. The growing phase of human hair lasts about 1000 days. Catagen occurs for 2–3 weeks and telogen for 2–3 months. Up to 100 telogen hairs are lost from the scalp per day, an amount approximating the number of hairs entering anagen per day.

Disorders of the scalp and forehead

Cicatricial alopecia

Cicatricial alopecia is characterized by scarring of the scalp with resultant hair loss. It is caused by a number of pathologic conditions.[13,14] The end result however is always the same: stem cell failure at the base of the follicle, inhibiting follicular

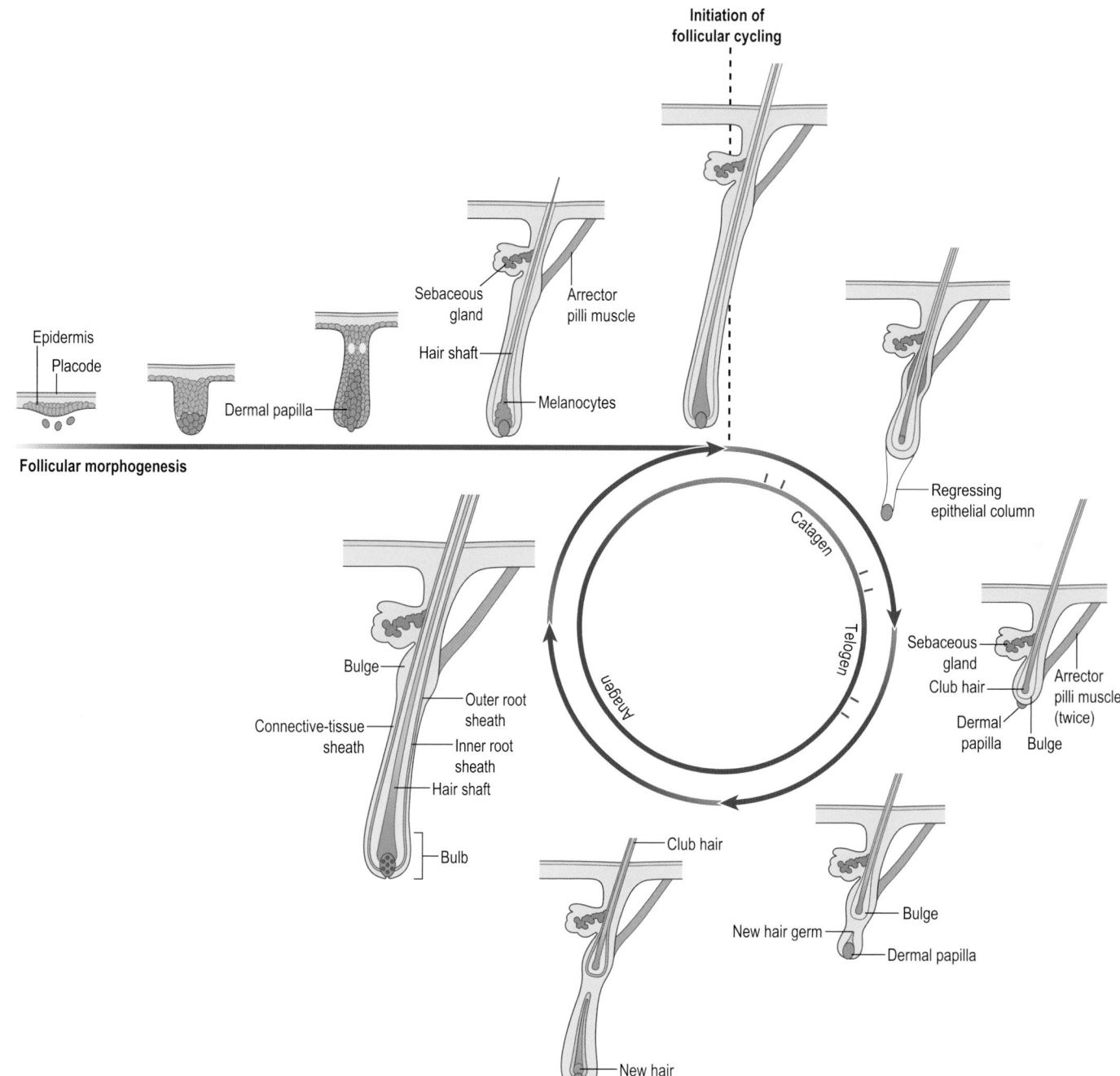

Fig. 5.8 The hair cycle. The stages of the hair cycle are illustrated beginning from the first postnatal anagen. Follicles progressing through a destructive phase (catagen) during which the lower two-thirds of the follicle undergoes degeneration. After the resting phase (telogen), stem cells become activated to form a new growing follicle (anagen). (Reproduced from Fuchs E. Scratching the surface of skin development. *Nature.* 2007;445:834–842.)

recovery from the telogen phase. It can be classified into five categories: congenital, autoimmune, neoplastic, infective, and acquired. A complete discussion regarding each of these conditions is not within the remit of this article, Highlighted conditions of special interest to the practicing surgeon will be discussed *(Table 5.1)*.

Aplasia cutis congenita (ACC)

This condition was first described in 1176. Since then, more than 500 patients with this condition have been described in

the literature. It is a rare congenital defect of the skin and subcutaneous tissue of the scalp. Less commonly, it can involve the periosteum, bone, and dura of the infant scalp.[12,13] The scalp is the most common location for ACC. It is involved in 65% of all patients presenting with the disease. At birth these defects are usually covered with a thin fragile transparent membrane *(Fig. 5.9)*. In older children, there is usually a hairless patch within the scalp resembling an atrophic scar. Less frequently, the lesions are found on the arms, knees, trunk, lower limbs, and face. Some patients with ACC also suffer from additional terminal transverse limb anomalies,

Table 5.1 Etiology of cicatricial alopecia

Congenital

a. Aplasia cutis congenita
b. Nevus sebaceous of Jadassohn
c. Nevoid basal cell nevus syndrome
d. Congenital melanoma
e. Dysplastic nevus syndrome
f. Giant hairy nevus
g. Xeroderma pigmentosa
h. En coup de sabre
i. Vascular malformations
j. Autoimmune
k. Scleroderma
l. Sarcoidosis
m. Chronic cutaneous lupus erythematosus
n. Lichen planopilaris
o. Cicatricial pemphigoid

Neoplastic

a. Malignant
   i. Basal cell carcinoma
   ii. Squamous cell
   iii. Malignant melanoma
   iv. Sarcoma
b. Benign
   i. Lipoma
   ii. Dermatofibroma
   iii. Keratoacanthoma
   iv. Neurofibroma
   v. Epidermal inclusion cyst
   vi. Trichoepithelioma
   vii. Hemangioma
   viii. Syringoma

Infective

a. Localized
   i. Bacterial
      1. Folliculitis decalvans
      2. Leprosy
   ii. Viral
   iii. Fungal
      1. Kerion
      2. Tinea capitis
b. Systemic

Acquired

a. Traumatic
   i. Physical
   ii. Burns
      1. Thermal
      2. Chemical
      3. Electrical
      4. Radiation

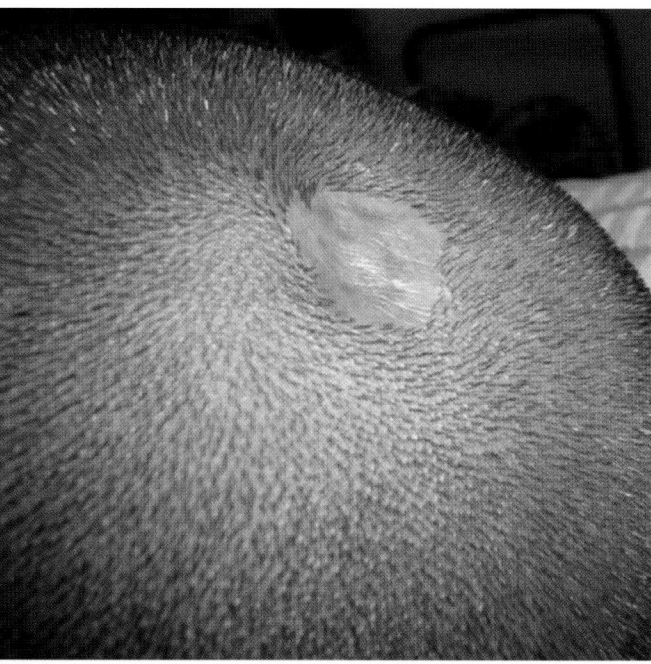

Fig. 5.9 Aplasia cutis congenita: a 10-year-old boy with thin atrophic scar of the scalp that was allowed to heal by secondary intention. (Copyright © The Regents of the University of California, Davis campus. Originally published in Dermatology Online Journal All rights reserved. Used with permission.)

appear to be sporadic; however an autosomal-dominant inheritance pattern has been described. Maternal exposure to methimazole and carbimazole may contribute to the development of ACC.

Wound treatment in patients with superficial ulceration is generally conservative with regular dressing changes. Larger defects, especially with underlying bone defects, are susceptible to infection, meningitis, sagittal sinus thrombosis, and hemorrhage. In these deeper lesions, dural reconstruction, cranioplasty, and flap reconstruction may prove life-saving.[15,16]

Nevus sebaceous of Jadassohn (sebaceous nevus)

Jadassohn first described nevus sebaceum in 1895.[17] It is a well-circumscribed yellow or orange lesion that occurs mainly on the face and scalp of infants. Of newborns, 0.3% are affected by nevus sebaceous. It occurs with equal frequency in males and females of all races. Clinically, the lesion presents as a solitary hairless patch noted at birth *(Fig. 5.10)*. At puberty, they can become raised, thickened, and nodular.[18]

Histologically, it is a hamartomatous lesion consisting of predominantly sebaceous glands, abortive hair follicles, and ectopic apocrine glands. The entity is important to recognize, because of its propensity for malignant degeneration. Malignant transformation occurs in 10–15% of lesions in some series.[19] The most common malignant neoplasm arising in this disorder is basal cell carcinoma. The most frequent benign tumor is trichoblastoma. Other benign and malignant tumors include syringocystadenoma papilliferum arising from the apocrine sweat glands, keratoacanthoma, apocrine cystadenoma, leiomyoma, and sebaceous cell carcinoma.

nail hypoplasia, omphalocele, cardiovascular and central nervous system abnormalities.

The etiology is unclear. Hypotheses include a malformation of the neural tube or mechanical disruption of the skin *in utero*. Vascular accident, direct pressure, and amnionic bands have been advanced as etiologic factors. Most of the cases

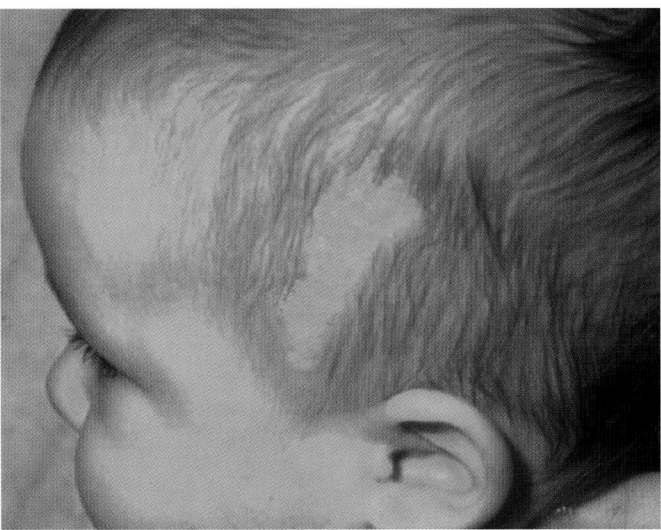

Fig. 5.10 Nevus sebaceous of Jadassohn. Note the orange hairless patch in this infant's scalp.

Table 5.2 Nevoid basal cell carcinoma syndrome (NBCCS)

Major criteria
More than 2 BCCs or BCC younger than 20 years of age
Odontogenic cysts of the jaw
Three or more palmar pits
Bilamellar calcification of the falx cerebri
Bifid, fused, or markedly splayed ribs
First-degree relative with NBCCS

Minor criteria
Macrocephaly
Congenital malformations such as cleft lip or palate, frontal bossing, coarse facies, and hypertelorism
Skeletal abnormalities such as Sprengel deformity, pectus deformity, or syndactyly of the digits
Radiologic abnormalities such as bridging of the sella turcica, vertebral anomalies, modeling defects of the hands and feet or flame-shaped lucencies of the hands and feet
Ovarian fibroma or medulloblastoma

BCC, basal cell carcinoma.

Rarely, malignant eccrine poroma and apocrine carcinomas have been reported.

Nevoid basal cell carcinoma syndrome (NBCCS)

This is an autosomal-dominant condition associated with the development of multiple basal cell carcinomas of the skin *(Fig. 5.11)*. First described by Gorlin and Goltz in 1960,[20] it is an inherited disorder involving defects within multiple organ systems including the skin, skeletal system, endocrine and nervous system. To be diagnosed with the disorder, patients must meet two major criteria or have one major and two minor criteria *(Table 5.2)*.[21,22]

The condition is caused by a mutation of the PTCH (patched) gene found on chromosome arm 9q. It has complete penetrance and variable expressivity. About a third of patients are new mutations.

Patients should be aware of the need for limiting ultraviolet exposure and the requirement for sunscreen. Basal cell carcinomas require frequent follow-up to achieve early diagnosis and treatment. Treatment of patients with NBCCS involves surveillance for the treatment of associated conditions (odontogenic cysts, ovarian fibromas, medulloblastoma) and treatment of multiple basal cell carcinomas. This often requires complex repairs, skin grafts, or flaps.

Xeroderma pigmentosum (XP)

XP is an autosomal-recessive disorder characterized by intolerance of the skin to ultraviolet light. It has a prevalence of 1/250 000 in the US.[23] Certain populations have a higher prevalence. For example, in Japan the prevalence is estimated at 1/40 000. The disease is due to the inability of the individuals affected with this disorder to repair damaged induced by sunlight to their DNA. Normally, damaged segments of DNA are excised and replaced with new sequences of bases. The most common defect in XP is an autosomal-recessive defect in which nucleotide excision repair (NER) enzymes are mutated, leading to a reduction in NER. Left unchecked, damage caused by ultraviolet light causes mutation in individual cell DNA. Seven XP repair genes, XPA through XPG, have been identified. These entities occur with varying frequencies, with XPA being the most common mutation. There is also an XP variant that has been described. The defect in this condition is not in NER, but is instead in postreplication repair. In XP variant, a mutation occurs in DNA polymerase *(Fig. 5.12)*.

There is no cure for XP. The DNA damage is cumulative and irreversible. As a result these patients develop multiple epithelial malignant neoplasms at an early age, most frequently in sun-exposed parts of the body. Tumors include squamous cell carcinoma, basal cell carcinomas, malignant melanoma, and fibrosarcoma. Two of the most common causes of death for XP patients are metastatic melanoma and squamous cell carcinoma.

Ocular problems occur in nearly 80% of patients with XP. These include photophobia, conjunctivitis, symblepharon, ectropion, and cutaneous malignancies.

Management is limited to avoidance of exposure to damaging ultraviolet radiation. This includes sunscreen, protective clothing, and sunglasses. Regular surveillance for treatment of neoplasms is very important. Gene therapy for XP is still in a theoretical and experimental stage. Various methods of correcting the defects in XP have been attempted using viral vectors carrying the gene replacement products.

Giant hair nevus – congenital nevomelanocytic nevus (CNN)

CNN, commonly called the congenital hairy nevus, is a pigmented surface lesion present at birth.[24,25] It is composed of neveomelancocytes, derivatives of melanoblasts. They are classified into three groups: small (<1.5 cm), medium (1.5–19.5 cm), and large (>20 cm in adolescents and adults or predicted to reach 20 cm by adulthood). CNN expands with

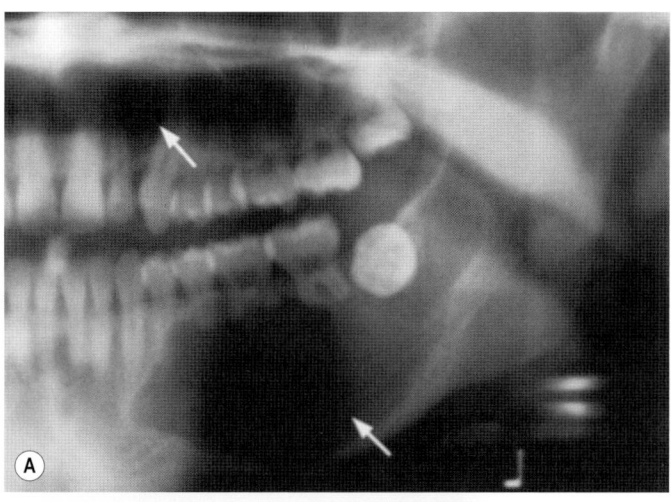

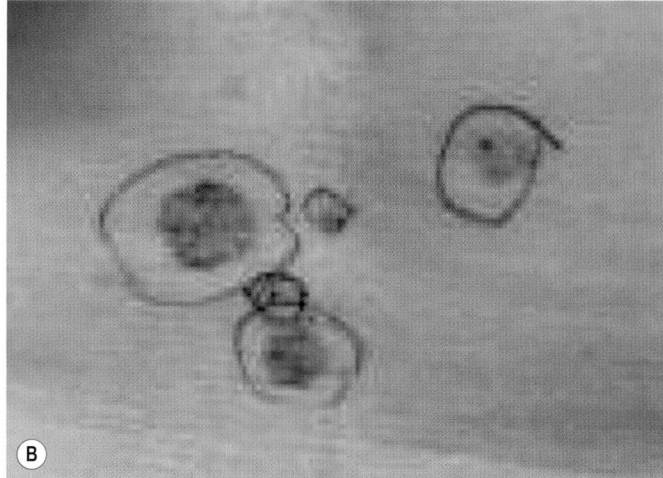

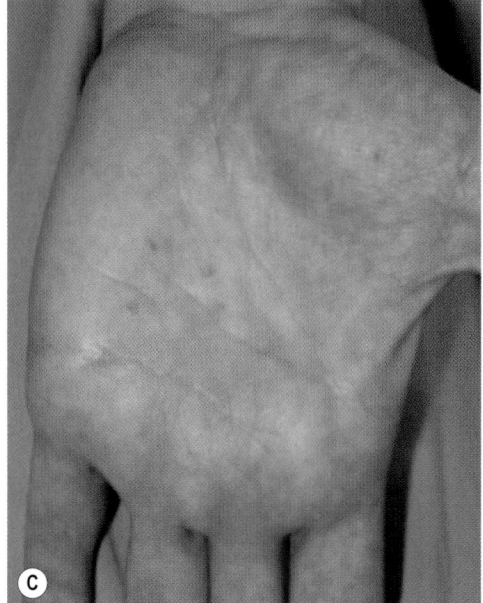

Fig. 5.11 Nevoid basal cell carcinoma syndrome: multiple basal cell carcinomas associated with palmar pits and jaw cysts.

growth of the child. The risk of melanoma development is proportional to the size of the congenital nevus *(Fig. 5.13)*.

The potential for large congenital nevi to become malignant has been variously debated in the literature. Lifetime rates have varied from 6 to 12%. In large nevi, 50% of malignancies develop by age 5, 60% by childhood, and 70% by puberty. Approximately 40% of malignant melanomas observed in children occur in large congenital nevi. Malignancy should be suspected with focal growth, pain, bleeding, ulceration, and significant pigmentary change.

Prophylactic excision remains the mainstay of treatment. Surgical removal has two goals: first, to improve the cosmetic appearance of the patient; and second, to reduce the likelihood of malignant transformation. Surgical treatment is typically begun at 6 months of age and usually requires a number of stages. Treatment consists of serial excision, skin grafting, tissue expansion, rotation flaps, and free tissue transfer. Cultured epidermal autografts and dermal regenerate templates have been used successfully after excision of giant hairy nevi.

Dysplastic nevus

Dysplastic nevi are compound nevus with cellular and architectural dysplasia. They can be flat or raised and vary in size, but are typically larger than normal compound nevus (5–15 mm) with lack of pigment uniformity. Atypical moles may appear anywhere on the body, but most frequently occur on the scalp, chest, back, and buttocks. They may occur in sun-exposed and sun-protected areas. Atypical moles can be inherited or sporadic. The prevalence of atypical moles in white populations has been reported to be as high as 10%. Familial atypical moles may be inherited as an autosomal-dominant trait. This familial form of dysplastic nevi is known as familial atypical mole and melanoma syndrome (FAMMM) *(Fig. 5.14)*.[26,27]

Melanoma can develop from atypical moles. The exact risk of an individual nevus transforming into a melanoma is thought to be 1 in 200000. Patients with numerous atypical moles are at higher risk of developing melanoma than those individuals with only a few atypical moles. The risk is more pronounced with a family history of melanoma. The lifetime risk of melanoma may approach 100% in individuals with FAMMM.

Patients with atypical nevi should undergo yearly cutaneous exam with serial color photography of suspicious lesions. Changing lesions or nevi suspicious for melanoma should be removed with narrow margins. Shave biopsy should be avoided in any pigmented lesion because it does not provide the necessary depth information. Wider excision may be indicated after interpretation of the lesion.

Linear scleroderma – en coup de sabre

En coup de sabre is a form of localized linear scleroderma that primarily affects the forehead of affected pediatric patients. It appears as an indented, vertical, colorless line of skin. Its

appearance to some resembles a deep saber wound. It is a rare disease of uncertain causation that is characterized by progressive craniofacial focal atrophy.[28] The active stage usually lasts 3–5 years. Involutionary atrophy of skin, muscle, and even bone may occur. Various ophthalmological and neurologic abnormalities have been observed in patients with linear scleroderma en coup de sabre, including seizures and cranial nerve palsies. The distinction between linear scleroderma en coup de sabre and Parry–Romberg syndrome is unclear. Parry–Romberg syndrome is characterized by a gradual

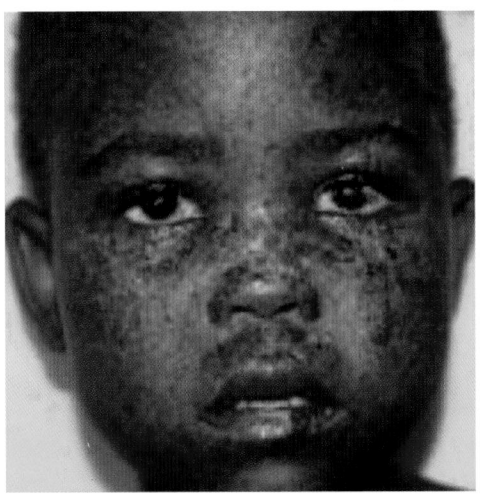

Fig. 5.12 Young patient with xeroderma pigmentosum. Note the freckling, crusts, and hypopigmentation in sun-exposed areas.

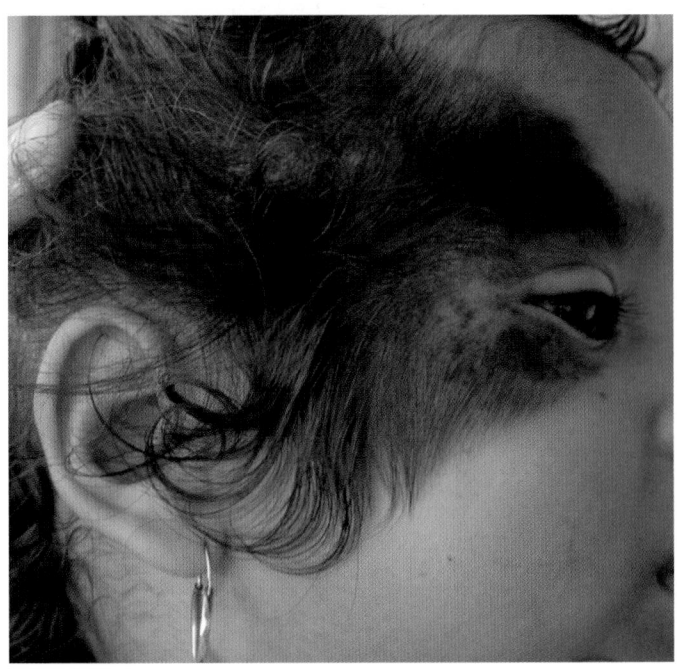

Fig. 5.13 Giant hairy nevus involving the forehead, temporal region, and eyelids of a young girl.

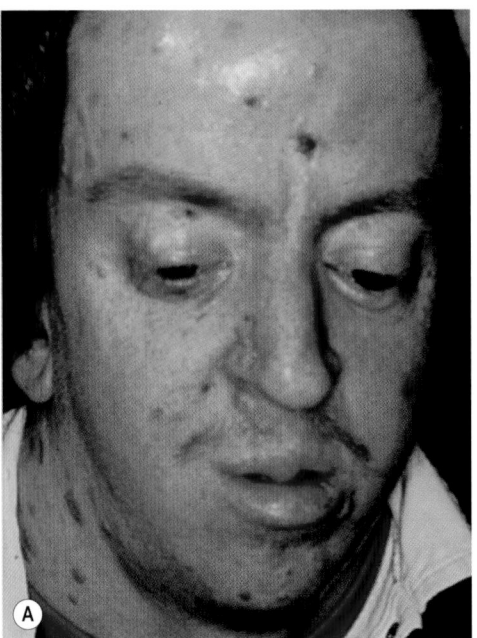

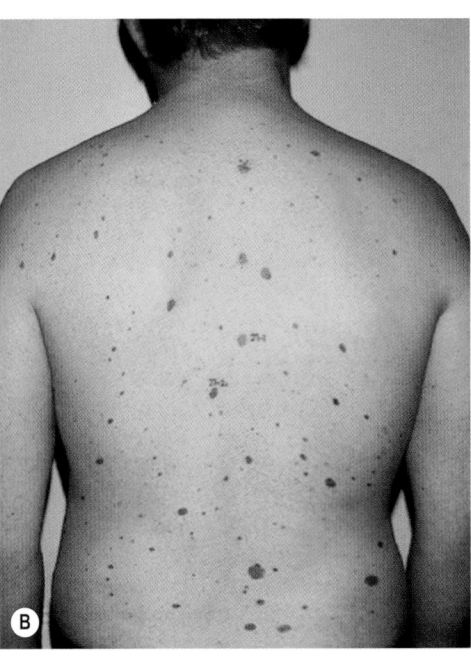

Fig. 5.14 (A, B) Familial atypical mole and melanoma syndrome (FAMM). Previously called dysplastic nevus syndrome, FAMM combines a family history of melanoma with multiple atypical nevi.

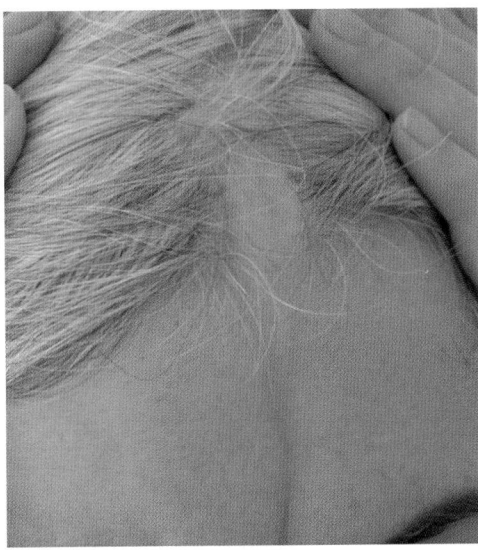

Fig. 5.15 Linear scleroderma – en coup de sabre. A 54-year-old woman with a 3-year history of progressive depigmentation and indentation of the forehead and scalp.

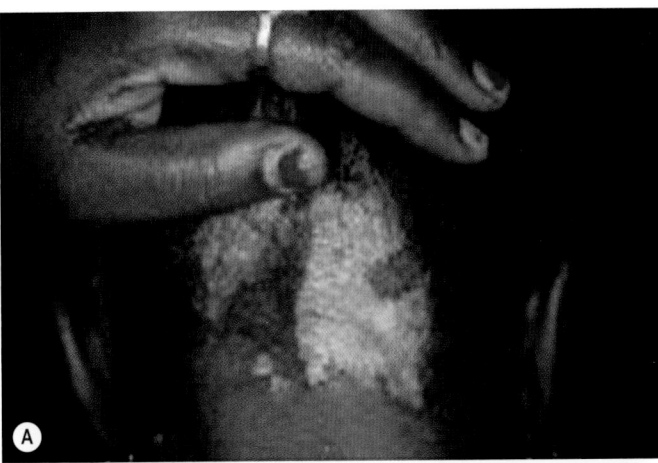

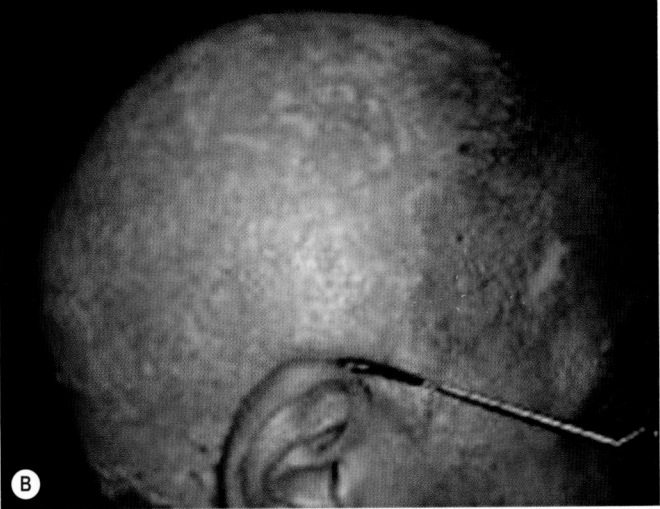

Fig. 5.16 (A, B) Discoid lupus erythematosus causing widespread scarring alopecia.

progressive facial hemiatrophy. In full-fledged cases, there is a significant deformity, with one side of the face smaller than the other. This is in sharp contrast to typical linear scleroderma en coup de sabre, where the abnormality is confined to the forehead *(Fig. 5.15)*.

The etiology is unknown. The most widely accepted theory is that the condition represents an autoimmune phenomenon directed at ectodermal derivatives of the forehead and scalp. Others invoke infective or genetic factors as possible mechanisms of action.

The management is unsatisfactory. Various therapeutic modalities (topical and pharmacologic agents, immunosuppression, and phototherapy) have been attempted, none with great success. Most require soft-tissue augmentation using microsurgical techniques once the condition has stabilized.[29]

Discoid lupus erythematosus (DLE)

DLE is a chronic skin condition that appears as a red inflamed patch with a scaling and crusting appearance. The center may appear lighter in color with a rim darker than the normal skin. There is a predilection for the face, scalp, and ears; however other regions of the body can be affected. When lesions occur in hairy areas such as the beard or scalp, permanent scarring and hair loss can occur *(Fig. 5.16)*.[30,31] DLE may occur in patients with systemic lupus erythematosus (SLE) and some patients (<5%) with DLE progress to SLE.

The pathophysiology of DLE is not well understood. It has been suggested that ultraviolet light induces the production of a heat shock protein. The protein then acts as a target for the host's T-cell-mediated immunity.

The condition is more common in African Americans than whites or Asians. It is more prevalent in woman than men. It most often affects patients between 20 and 40 years of age.

Therapy with sunscreens, topical steroids, topical calcineurin inhibitors, imiquimod, and antimalarial agents is usually effective. Occasionally immunosuppressives may be indicated. Surgical excision for burned-out areas of scarring has been attempted, occasionally followed by recurrence in the scar.

Cutaneous sarcoidosis

Sarcoidosis is a multisystem disease of unknown cause that may involve virtually any organ system. It is often called the great imitator. Cutaneous sarcoidosis has many morphologic presentations and often mimics other dermatologic diseases. Cutaneous involvement occurs in 20–35% of patients with systemic sarcoidosis but may also occur without systemic involvement.

Most authors divide lesions of cutaneous sarcoidosis into nonspecific and specific types based on the presence or absence of noncaseating granulomas on biopsy. In nonspecific lesions, no granulomas are found. Specific lesions display noncaseating granulomas.

Lupus pernio is one of the few cutaneous manifestations that are characteristic of sarcoidosis. Lesions appear as

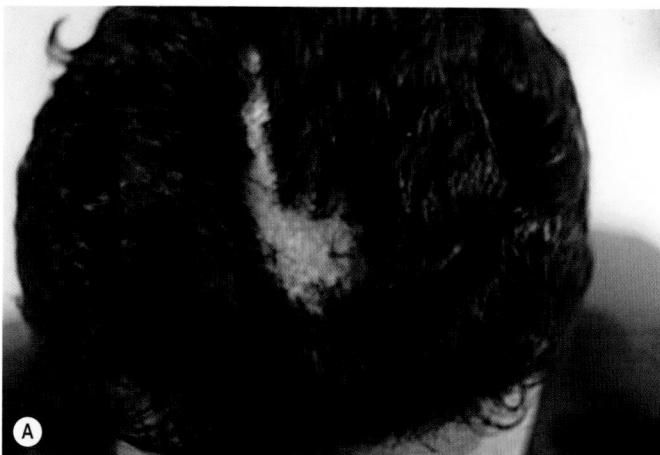

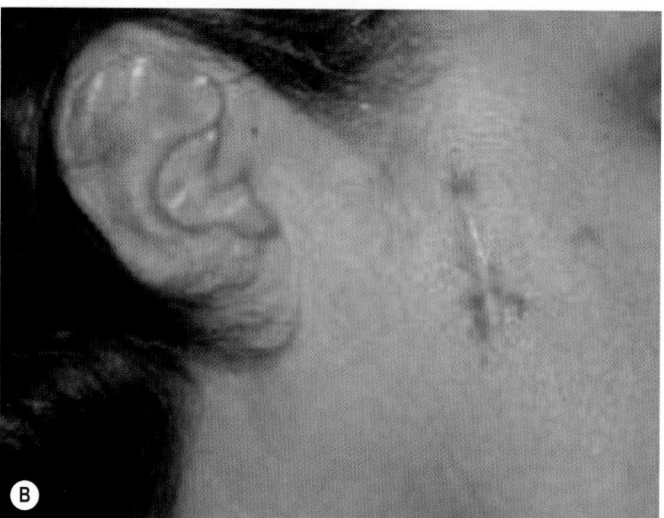

Fig. 5.17 **(A)** Cutaneous sarcoidosis of the scalp causing scarring alopecia. **(B)** A case of sarcoidosis occurring in a previous facial scar, so-called scar sarcoidosis.

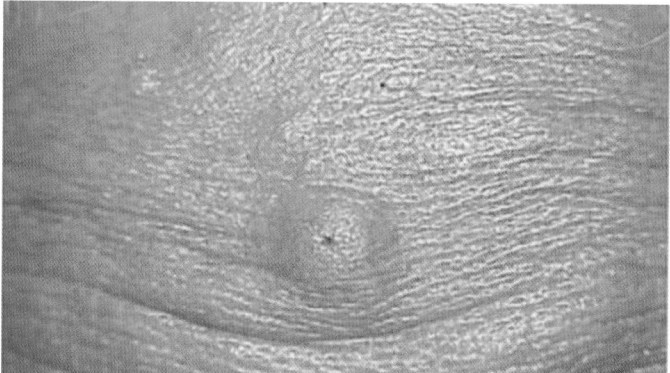

Fig. 5.18 Epidermoid cyst of the forehead.

indurated plaques that affect the midface, particularly the alar rim of the nose. Lesions of cutaneous sarcoidosis can also appear in pre-existing scars. This condition is called scar sarcoidosis. Therefore, sarcoidosis should be considered in the differential diagnosis of an enlarging, previously inactive scar. Often the lesion is mistaken for a keloid. Sarcoidosis of the scalp can result in scarring and nonscarring alopecia (*Fig. 5.17*). It is often mistaken for DLE, lichen planopilaris, and scleroderma. Local destruction and scarring of follicles in sarcoidosis may lead to permanent alopecia.[32,33]

Neoplasms

The differential diagnosis of a subcutaneous lesion of the scalp is legion. Most tumors of the scalp are benign. Primary malignant tumors of the scalp are most frequently epithelial in origin, although tumors from adnexal and connective tissue elements also occur. Approximately 2% of epithelial tumors of the skin are located in the scalp. Basal cell cancer predominates, followed by squamous cell tumors and malignant melanoma. Other primary tumors that may occur on the scalp are sarcomas (fibrosarcoma, dermatofibrosarcoma,

malignant fibrous histiocytoma, leiomyosarcoma, rhabdomyosarcoma), cutaneous T-cell lymphoma, and primary adnexal cancers. The scalp is a common repository for metastatic tumor, most likely because of its rich blood supply.

As with the majority of skin cancers, cumulative sun exposure and fair skin are risk factors. Approximately 65% of the tumors occur in men. The majority of skin cancers occur in hair-bearing skin rather than in bald areas, as one would intuitively expect. About half the tumors occur in the temporal regions, followed by the postauricular and occipital areas.

Lipoma

Lipomas are benign tumors composed of fatty tissue. They are the most common form of soft-tissue tumor in the body. Lipomas are commonly found in adults 40–60 years of age. Malignant transformation has not been convincingly demonstrated. There are several subtypes of lipomas. The superficial subcutaneous lipoma is the most common type, lying just below the surface of the skin. They occur most commonly on the trunk, thighs, and forearms. However, they may be found anywhere in the body where fat is located. Lipomas of the face and scalp are reported rarely, comprising less than 2% of lipomas.[34] They are often mistaken clinically for epidermal inclusion cysts. In addition to a subcutaneous position, lipomas have been described below the frontalis muscle and below the galea aponeurotica.

Epidermoid cyst

Epidermoid cysts represent the most common cutaneous cysts. While they may occur anywhere on the body, they occur most frequently on the face, scalp, neck, and trunk (*Fig. 5.18*). They result from the proliferation of epidermal cells within a circumscribed space of dermis. The source of the epidermis is nearly always the infundibulum of the hair follicle. The contents of the cyst evoke a strong inflammatory response. Epidermoid cysts are benign lesions; however on rare occasions they have been associated with malignancy.[35] Asymptomatic epidermoid cysts do not need to be treated. When inflamed or painful, simple excision with the cyst wall is indicated. If the entire cyst wall is not removed, the cyst will recur. Incision and drainage may be performed if a cyst is infected. Secondary cyst wall removal must be performed once the infection has resolved.

Trichoepithelioma

Trichoepithelioma is regarded as a poorly differentiated hamartoma of the hair germ cell line. They appear as rounded skin-colored nodules 2–8 mm in diameter. Over 50% of the lesions occur in the face and scalp *(Fig. 5.19)*. There is a familial form of the disease linked to the short arm of chromosome 9. Most trichoepitheliomas show slow growth. In cases of multiple trichoepitheliomas, the lesions may cause disfigurement. Solitary lesions can be excised. In the case of multiple tumors, this may not be possible. Split-thickness skin grafting,

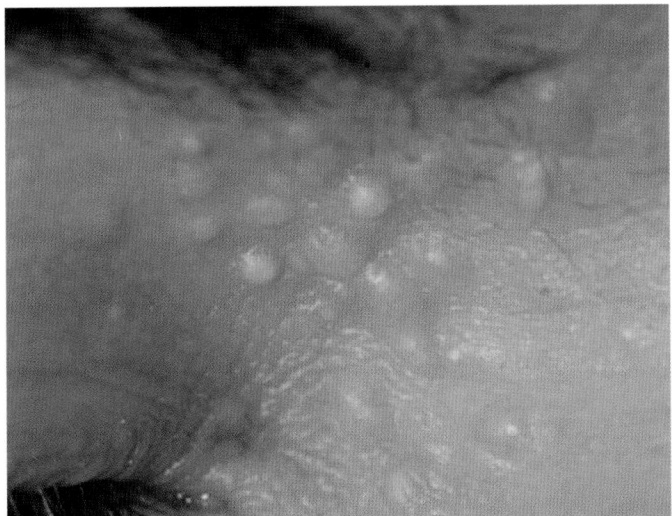

Fig. 5.19 Trichoepithelioma of the temporal region of a 4-year-old girl. It has the appearance of small rounded nodules.

dermabrasion, and laser ablation have been recommended. However, with the latter two techniques, regrowth of the papules may occur.

Syringoma

Syringoma is a benign skin tumor that is derived from eccrine sweat glands. The lesions usually appear during puberty or adult life and consist of small papules 1–3 mm in diameter *(Fig. 5.20)*. They are most common about the eyelids but can occur anywhere on the body.[36] When they occur on the scalp, they can form a type of scarring alopecia.

The main reason for treatment is cosmetic, particularly for syringomas of the face. A number of treatments have been recommended, including surgical excision, electrocautery, dermabrasion, trichloroacetic acid, and laser ablation. No comparative studies have been carried out to compare one treatment modality with another.

Basal cell carcinoma

As previously mentioned, basal cell carcinoma is the most common skin cancer of the head and neck. Basal cell carcinomas of the scalp are usually slowly progressive and rarely metastasize. Neglected tumors can continue to grow and lead to significant tissue destruction. Basal cell carcinomas occur most frequently in sun-exposed areas, including the scalp and forehead. Risk factors include sunlight exposure, light-colored skin, previous history of nonmelanoma skin cancer, ionizing radiation exposure, arsenic exposure, immunosuppression, and numerous genetic syndromes.

The tumor spreads radially for an extended period of time before developing a vertical phase. The scalp's thick dermis and galeal layer offer a natural barrier to vertical growth of cutaneous malignant neoplasms *(Fig. 5.21)*. Once penetrated, the areolar tissue in the subgaleal plane offers little resistance to lateral spread. The periosteum of the scalp and outer cortex of the skull also provide an effective barrier to tumor invasion.

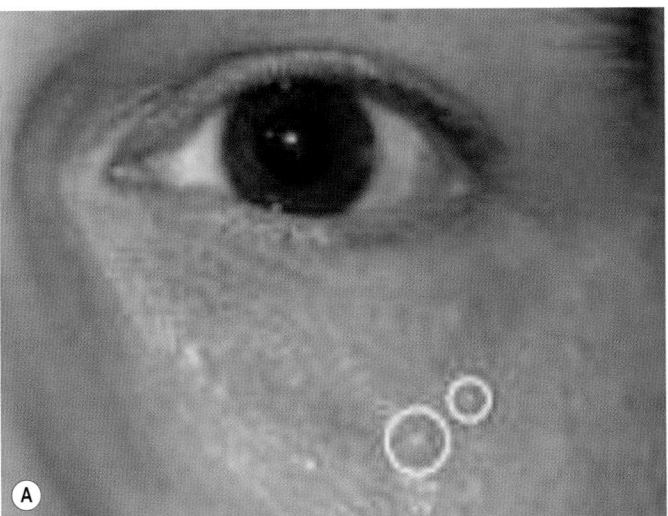
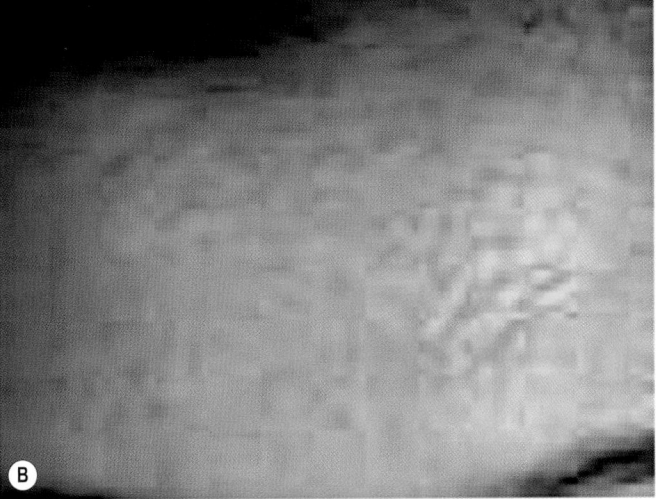

Fig. 5.20 (A, B) Syringomas are benign tumors of eccrine sweat glands. They occur most commonly on the eyelid, but can involve the forehead and scalp.

Once violated, however, tumor can spread in the diploic space and through perforating channels to the dura.[37–39]

The treatment of choice is generally surgical excision. Mohs micrographic surgery has been used on the scalp. Cure rates for basal cell carcinoma treated by this technique are 99%. This rate decreases with larger and deeper tumors. Indications for use of the technique include scar morpheiform or sclerosing basal cell carcinomas. Clinically suspected bone invasion is a contraindication to the technique.

Irradiation is usually less effective, particularly for large lesions. It may be indicated in debilitated patients who are poor operative candidates.

Cutaneous squamous cell carcinoma (cSCC)

Squamous cell carcinoma is the second most common type of skin cancer. It often presents as an ulcerative or fungating lesion of the scalp or forehead *(Fig. 5.22)*. The tumor occurs more often in men than women, at a 2:1 ratio. The incidence increases with age, peaking at 66 years. The incidence also increases with decreasing latitude. Risk factors are similar to those of basal cell carcinoma: light skin tone, ultraviolet exposure, indoor tanning, previous history of actinic keratosis, prior irradiation, immunosuppression, human immunodeficiency virus, human papillomavirus, coal tar and arsenic exposure. As previously described, a number of genetic syndromes are associated with the development of cSCC.

The pathogenesis of cSCC is unclear. More than 90% of patients diagnosed in the US demonstrate functional loss of the TP53 tumor suppressor gene. Ultraviolet radiation is thought to damage host DNA, resulting in a genetic mutation of TP53.[38]

Size is the most important determinant of outcome for patients with cSCC. Lesions greater than 2 cm have a higher rate of regional recurrence (15% versus 7%) and greater incidence of regional metastasis (30% versus 9%) than smaller lesions. Additionally, depth of invasion histologically is a critical variable.[40] Tumors with greater than 4 mm of depth of invasion have a 45% risk of metastatic spread. This compares to a 7% risk for cancers less than 3 mm in depth. Other poor prognostic variables include poor differentiation, perineural invasion, lymph vascular involvement, and an immunocompromised host.

Up to 14% of cSCCs exhibit perineural invasion. The most frequent cranial nerves involved by tumor are the facial and trigeminal nerve. Therefore every cSCC should undergo complete neurologic exam evaluating facial movement and sensation.

Regional lymph node metastases occur in 2–18% of patients with cSCC. The risk of metastasis correlates with tumor size and differentiation. The most frequently involved lymphatic basins are the parotid and upper cervical lymph nodes.[41] Fine-needle aspiration, computed tomography (CT) can and magnetic resonance imaging (MRI) can assist in determining the extent of metastatic disease.

Surgical excision and Mohs surgery are the primary modalities of treatment. Regional lymph node dissections are only indicated for clinically positive nodal disease or lymphatic basins that are positive after sentinel lymph node biopsy.

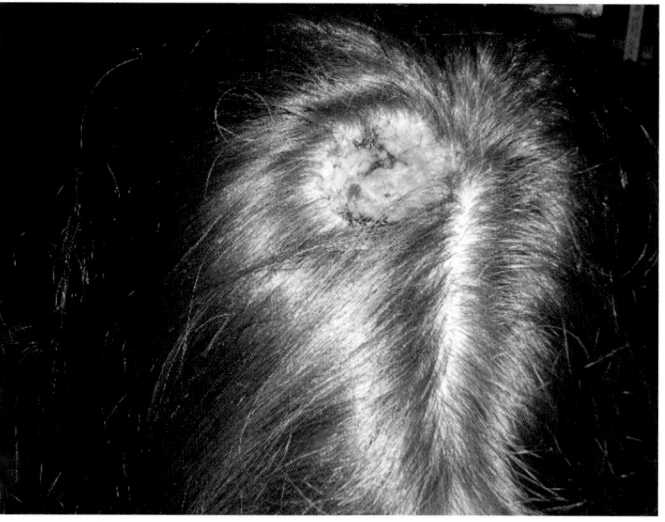

Fig. 5.21 Basal cell carcinoma of the scalp fixed to the underlying pericranium.

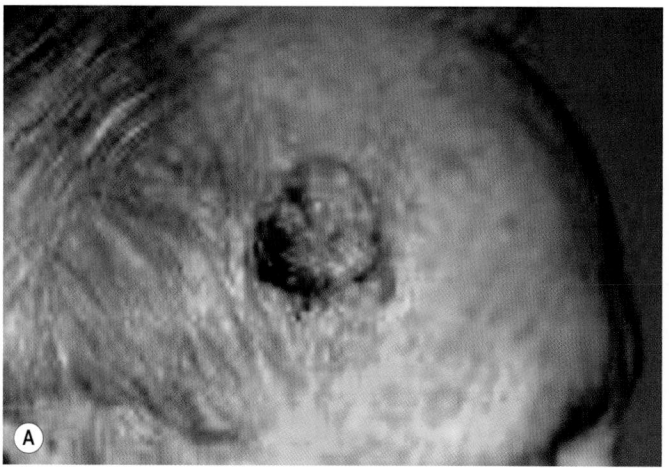
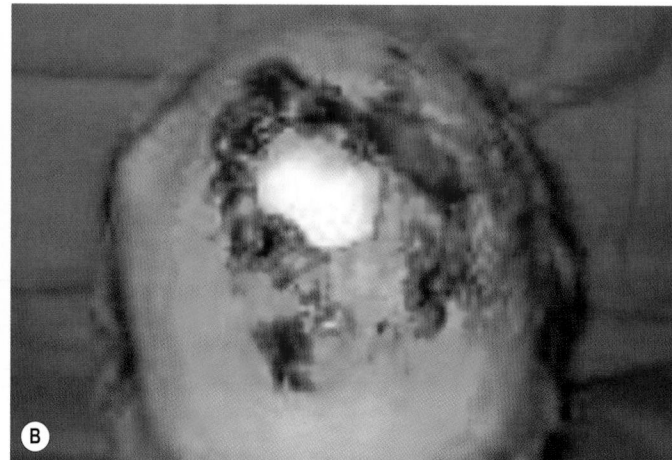

Fig. 5.22 (A, B) Squamous cell carcinoma of the temporal region and scalp.

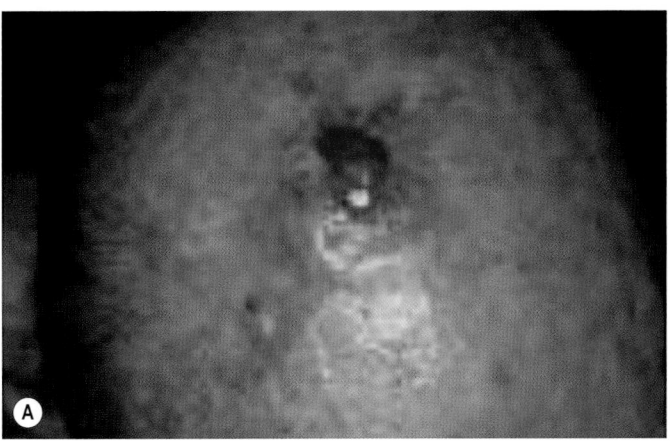
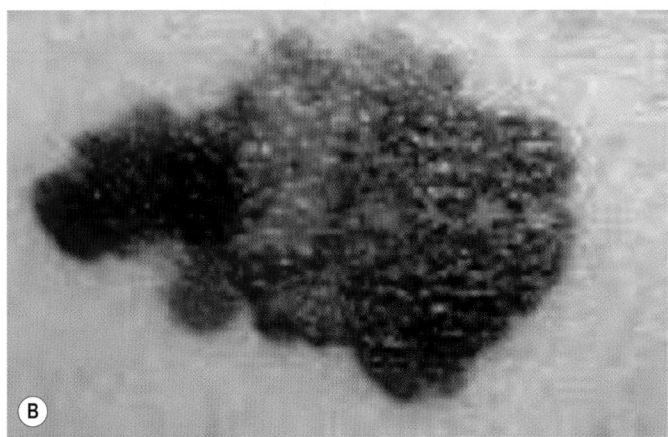

Fig. 5.23 (A) Malignant melanoma of the scalp. (B) A closer view of a superficial spreading melanoma of the forehead.

Radiation therapy is generally used as an adjunct to surgery to improve local regional control in high-risk lesions. As in basal cell carcinomas, it may be used primarily in high-risk individuals. Chemotherapy has not been especially useful for the treatment of cSCC.

Malignant melanoma

The incidence of melanoma has tripled in the white population during the last 20 years. Melanoma is currently the sixth most common cancer in the US. Risk factors include fair skin phenotype and the occurrence of blistering sunburns in childhood. Other factors include dysplastic nevi, large congenital nevi, previous melanoma, prior nonmelanoma skin cancers, male sex, age older than 50, XP or FAMM syndromes.

Malignant melanoma of the scalp and forehead is aggressive and often difficult to control (Fig. 5.23). The abundant vascular supply and rich lymphatic plexuses of the scalp allow early radial extension of the tumor.

Diagnosis is usually made with skin biopsy. If possible, an excisional biopsy should be performed with 1–3 mm of normal skin surrounding the lesion to provide accurate diagnosis and histologic staging. Superficial shave biopsies should be discouraged because partial removal of the primary melanoma may not provide an accurate measurement of tumor thickness.

Surgery is the primary mode of therapy for localized cutaneous melanoma. Surgical margins of 5 mm are currently recommended for melanoma in situ and margins of 1 cm for tumors up to 1 mm thick. For melanomas 1–4 mm in thickness, randomized trials have shown that 2-cm margins are appropriate, although thinner melanomas (1–2 mm) are effectively treated with 1-cm margins. For deep melanomas (>4 mm), excisional margins greater than 2 cm did not improve regional recurrence rates or improve overall survival. Therefore, 2-cm margins are recommended for this group of patients.[42,43]

Sentinel lymph node biopsy is generally indicated for pathologic staging of the regional nodal basins for primary tumors greater than or equal to 1 mm depth. Thinner melanomas might also be considered for sentinel lymph node biopsy if they contain high-risk histologic features (ulceration, extensive regression, high mitotic rate, angiolymphatic invasion). If sentinel lymph node biopsy is positive, elective lymph node dissection is warranted.

Interferon-α_{2b} is the only adjuvant therapy approved by the Food and Drug Administration for high-risk melanoma patients (stage IIB, IIC, and III). The potential benefits of high-dose interferon must be weighed against its substantial toxicity.

Infections

Systemic granulomatous diseases, such as leprosy, can result in permanent alopecia. Localized folliculitis and perifolliculitis can result in hair loss as well, sometimes permanent. Pyogenic infections like methicillin-resistant Staphylococcus aureus may cause abscess formation with secondary scarring. More advanced cases can result in necrotizing fasciitis of the scalp musculature. The outcome is often a significant soft-tissue deficit that must be reconstructed with complex reconstructive techniques. Viral diseases, such as herpes and varicella, have caused scalp scarring and hair loss. Fungal infections such as kerion and favus can result in cicatricial alopecia. Kerion is the result of the host's response to a fungal ringworm infection (dermatophytosis). A kerion appears as a thick mushy area of scalp. Its surface is often studded with pustules. It can break open and drain pus. If left untreated, a kerion can lead to permanent alopecia.[44] Favus is a chronic inflammatory dermatophytic infection usually caused by Trichophyton schoenleinii. In most patients favus is a severe form of tinea capitis. It is characterized by the development of a scutulum, a yellow cup-shaped crust that surrounds hair and pierces its center. Scutula form a dense plaque, each composed of mycelian and epidermal debris. Plaque removal leaves an erythematous moist base. Extensive hair loss and scarring can result.[45]

Physical trauma and burns

Scar may occur in the scalp from traumatic lacerations or avulsions. Postsurgical alopecia may result from surgical flaps or skin grafts applied for removal of benign or malignant neoplasms.

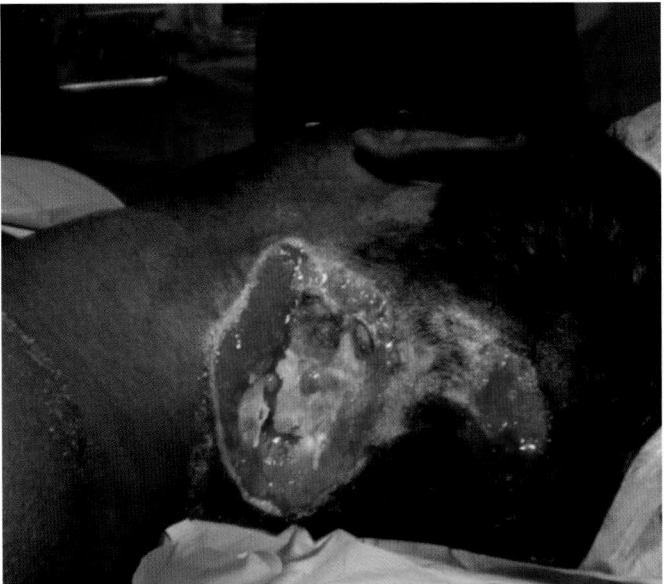

Fig. 5.24 Electrical burn to the occiput and neck.

Thermal injury to the scalp may result in large areas of skin loss and necrosis. Scald burns of hot water, coffee, and grease account for the majority of scalp injuries in children. Direct thermal injury by flame causes more scalp burns in adults. The depth of the burn determines the ultimate area of scalp loss. Second-degree burns may damage hair follicles, despite epidermal re-epithelialization. Deeper third-degree burns can destroy the subcutaneous layer, necessitating the use of skin grafts to effect closure. In fourth-degree injuries, the necrosis extends to the periosteum or bone. Avascularity of the wound dictates a more complex method of reconstruction.

Electrical burns of the scalp are less common than thermal injuries *(Fig. 5.24)*. Electrical wounds are more localized and often show deeper destruction. If the periosteum is intact, the wound can be debrided and skin grafts applied. For full-thickness injuries, bone debridement is required and the exposed dura covered with a flap. Secondary cranioplasty can be entertained once the patient has recovered and the wounds are stable.[46]

Contact of the scalp with toxic chemicals can result in tissue loss and alopecia. Industrial chemicals and occasionally concentrated cosmetic solutions for hair dying, bleaching, and straightening may damage the scalp and hair follicles.

Exposure to ionizing radiation can result in temporary or permanent alopecia. Heavily irradiated wounds are more susceptible to minor trauma and infections. Necrosis can extend down to the underlying calvaria and brain. In general, wide debridement of all nonviable tissue is recommended. These wounds are not favorable sites for local procedures such as direct closure, skin grafts, or local flaps because of the relative avascularity of the wounds. Free tissue transfer is generally selected to fight infection and to change the ischemic biology of the wound.[47] Luce and Hoopes[48] recommended preservation of the irradiated bone and coverage with well-vascularized tissue. If osteomyelitis is present, the bone is removed and the defect similarly resurfaced. Secondary cranioplasty is deferred for 3–6 months.

Diagnosis/patient presentation

A thorough history and physical exam are critical. This should include relevant medical factors such as a history of smoking, coronary artery disease, diabetes mellitus, immunosuppression, or radiation. The etiology of the defect is important. Malignant tumors may require a much wider and deeper resection than initially realized, affecting the extirpative and reconstructive plan. Obtaining previous operative reports allows the surgeon to anticipate scarred wound bed and limitation in the remaining blood supply.

Palpation of tumors for signs of local, regional, or distant metastatic disease is mandatory. Fixation of tumor to underlying bone is more readily determined by physical exam than adjunctive radiographic tests.

More than 60–70% of bone minerals must be lost before tumor invasion can be detected on plain films. Even axial CT scans cannot reliably demonstrate the presence or extent of tumor invasion into bone. Findings on CT scan are confirmed histologically in only 73% of patients.[5]

Bone scan or positron emission tomography scan may provide some benefit in selected patients. Unfortunately, the local inflammatory response to the adjacent cancer and the poor resolution combine to reduce the clinical utility of these studies. They are however useful in evaluation of distant metastatic disease, regional lymphatic metastasis, and recurrent disease.[49]

MRI may help detect cancer involving the marrow space because it does not rely on changes in bone density.[50] MRI occasionally helps in the preoperative planning of the extent of bone resection but may have an excessive rate of false-positive results.[51] Thus the decision to perform underlying bone excision relies heavily on physical examination and the surgeon's clinical judgment.

Incisional or excisional biopsies may be performed to aid in diagnosing benign and malignant disease. Sentinel lymph node mapping in the head and neck has been reported to be successful in 90–96% of patients.[52] The parotid gland takes up free technetium. High background counts over the parotid make probe-guided localization difficult.[53] The use of blue dye is invaluable in cases with suspected parotid lymph node drainage.

Patient selection

When contemplating forehead or scalp reconstruction, several factors should be considered when developing a treatment plan. These factors are summarized in *Table 5.3*, as modified from Temple and Ross's original publication.[54]

The size and depth of the defect are critical factors. If periosteum has been lost and there is bone exposure, flap reconstruction must be considered. If a bone defect is present, consideration should be given to cranioplasty. Bone reconstruction can be considered primarily or delayed if there is concern regarding the viability of the overlying soft tissues.

The viability of the skin surrounding the defect may affect the reconstructive plan. Prior irradiation or previous surgical scars may limit reconstructive options due to their effect on blood flow. With scalp flaps, the adage that bigger is better

Table 5.3 Consideration in defect analysis

Wound factors	Consideration
Location of the defect	Scalp Forehead Combined
Aesthetic subunits	Median/paramedian/lateral forehead Temporal/parietal/occipital scalp
Exposed structures	Subcutaneous Periosteum Bone Dura Alloplasts
Surrounding soft tissue	Hairline position Eyelids and brows Pattern of baldness Scars/previous procedures Burns Irradiation
Wound size	Small Medium Large
Contour	Dead space

often holds true. The relative inelasticity of the galea often necessitates larger flaps to distribute tension and to maximize the vascularity of the construct.

Like tissue should be replaced with like whenever possible, as espoused by Millard.[55] If hair-bearing scalp has been lost, it is best reconstructed with adjacent scalp tissue. Gonzalez-Ulloa's concept of aesthetic subunits of the face[11] should be considered when cosmetically critical areas of the forehead are reconstructed. Consideration should be given to excising entire subunits and repair of the defects in a unit. This allows the placement of incisions in cosmetically superior positions, avoiding a "patchwork" effect that results when only a portion of the subunit has been excised and repaired. Care must be taken not to displace mobile structures such as the brow or eyelid when developing a reconstructive plan. The hairline must be meticulously aligned to prevent cosmetically unacceptable step-offs. Small areas of alopecia along the hairline can often be repaired with micro-hair transplantation techniques.[56]

Treatment/surgical technique

Reconstructive options

Closure by secondary intention

Small, noncosmetically critical defects in the head and neck can be allowed to heal by secondary intention. Ideally, the defect is less than 1 cm in diameter and without bone exposure. Healing through secondary intention relies on cicatricial wound contracture and the need for vascularized tissue underlying the defect. Contracture of the wound can often make these defects difficult to perceive.

This method of reconstruction requires appropriate daily dressing changes and a compliant patient. A disadvantage to secondary-intention healing in the scalp is alopecia. It should be used with caution around mobile structures for fear of displacing cosmetic units.[57]

Vacuum-assisted closure

The VAC system is a noninvasive active therapy used to promote healing in difficult wounds that fail to respond to established treatment modalities. The system is based on the application of negative pressure to the surface of the wound. The device removes chronic edema and increases local blood flow, enhancing granulation formation and wound healing. Intermittent or cycled treatment appears more effective than continuous therapy. Wound bacterial counts are decreased with VAC use compared to control wounds (*Fig. 5.25*).[58]

It can be used until the wound has healed by secondary intention or combined with skin-grafting techniques. It is particularly useful in situations where the wound contours are irregular and fixation of the graft is difficult. The VAC holds the graft securely on to the wound bed, preventing pooling of tissue fluid that would otherwise prevent revascularization of the graft. Care should be taken when placing the VAC directly on viable periosteum. Use of pressures that exceed capillary closing pressure on noncomplaint bony surfaces can result in ischemic necrosis of the pericranium and graft loss.

Molnar *et al.*[59] described the use of the VAC in conjunction with skin grafts for full-thickness lesions of the scalp. They combined decortication of the outer surface of the skull with immediate skin grafting in four patients with successful graft take.

Primary closure

For larger defects (less than 3 cm) primary closure can be affected. Ideally, the incision should be in the line of resting tension to optimize the quality of the resultant scar. If tension is excessive, wide undermining and advancement are often possible. The rich blood supply of the scalp and face often allows closure under some tension without the development of wound necrosis. Some surgeons have advocated scoring the underlying galea as a method of decreasing tension on wound margins.[60] This technique may result in a significant decrease in blood supply to the overlying skin. Care must be taken to obtain meticulous hemostasis following galeotomy to prevent hematoma formation. Layered closure techniques, including closure of the galea, reduce wound closure tension. Wounds closed in this manner have a decreased incidence of alopecia and depressed widened scars.

Tissue expansion

Immediate intraoperative tissue expansion can be performed at the time of scalp excision. After placement of the device, three to four cycles of inflation and deflation of the expander for 3–5 minutes are performed. The expanding device is removed and primary wound closure is effected. Although the amount of tissue generated by this technique is small, it will

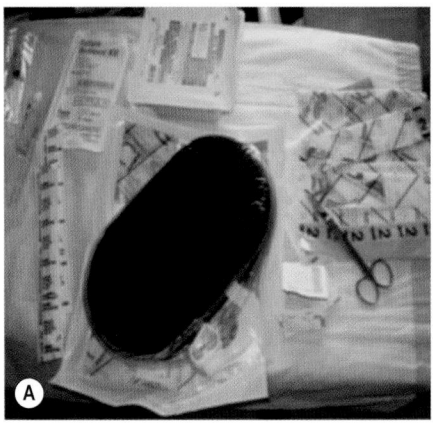 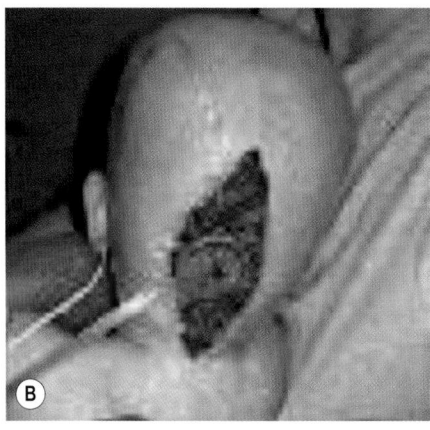 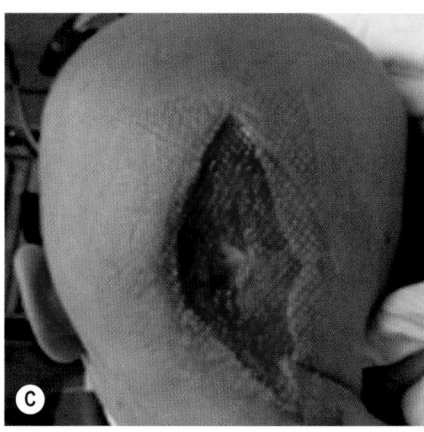

Fig. 5.25 (A, B) Sterile negative-pressure dressing applied to posterior scalp wound. **(C)** Note the stimulation of granulation tissue within the base of the wound after 1 week of treatment.

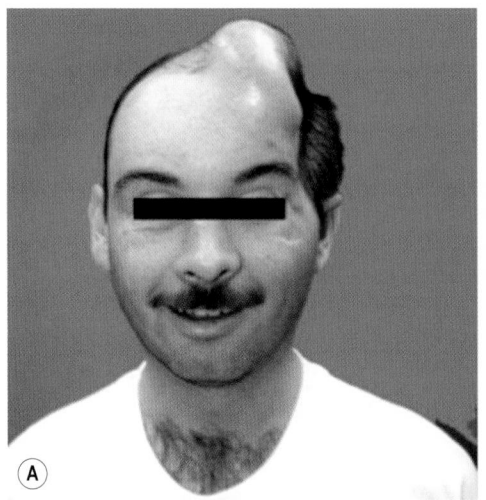 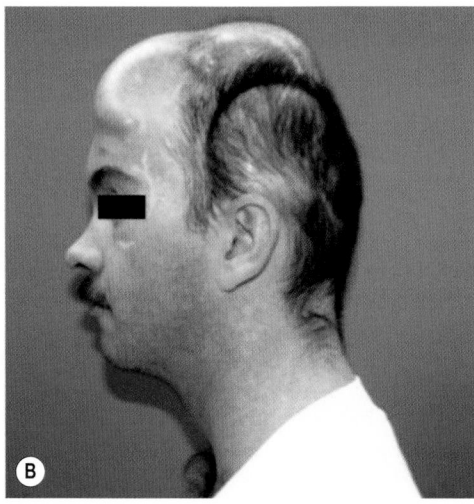

Fig. 5.26 (A, B) Insertion of tissue expanders to reconstruct a skin-grafted portion of the posterior scalp. Expansion allows the operator to replace missing tissue with tissue of a similar quality and thickness.

often allow the primary closure of a wound that might otherwise require a more complex modality to obtain closure.[61]

In staged tissue expansion techniques, an expandable silicone device is placed in a subcutaneous or subgaleal position connected to a one-way valve. Partial inflation of the expander is performed at the time of insertion to prevent seroma formation. Expansion begins at 2 weeks following placement. The device is expanded on a weekly or biweekly basis until the tissue requirements of the defect are met. Expansion should be continued until the expanded flap is approximately 20% larger than the size of the defect to account for the curvature of the skull and primary contracture of the flap during inset *(Fig. 5.26)*.[62]

Tissue expansion is a powerful tool because it allows the surgeon to replace like tissue with like. The technique increases the amount of locally available tissue, preserves sensation, and maintains hair follicles and adnexal structures. In addition, tissue expansion produces a delay phenomenon, increasing the vascularity of the expanded flap. Defects up to 50% of the scalp can be reconstructed. Expansion of adjacent scalp allows alopecic scalp to be replaced with similar tissue, albeit with a decreased follicular density. Similarly, expansion of the

forehead allows for the transfer of tissue with similar texture and blush characteristics.

The timing of expansion often depends on the etiology of the defect. If the lesion to be removed is benign it is often possible to expand adjacent to the lesion primarily. In traumatic wounds or in the face of malignancy, the wound is excised and temporarily closed with a skin graft or flap. Tissue expansion is initiated once there is stable coverage. Austad advocates against tissue expansion in acute injuries because of the risk of contamination and implant exposure.[63]

Care should be taken to mark out the vascular territories on the scalp, prior to the insertion of a tissue expander. Placement of the expander is not random. The proposed flap design should be mapped out prior to placement of the expanding device. This will maximize flap length and avoid scars that could jeopardize flap vascularity. Placement of the insertion incisions at the margin of the skin-grafted defect risks exposure of the expander. It is generally better to make distant radial incision at 90° relative to the expansion front to minimize the chance of expander exposure. Endoscopic assisted dissection aids in visualization of the pocket and ensures hemostasis.[64]

Intuitively, one might assume that the most efficient plan for coverage of a scalp defect would be the formation of an advancement flap from the expanded skin. However, Joss *et al.* noted that advancement flaps waste tissue at both ends of the flap. The tissue incorporated into these dog-ears can be more efficiently distributed over the defect by designing a rotation or transposition flap.[65]

One of the major disadvantages of tissue expansion is the length of time it takes to expand the adjacent tissue. Expansion periods of 2–3 months are not uncommon. During the period of expansion, distortion of the head and neck contour occurs, giving the patient an alien-like appearance. This distortion in body image can be quite unsettling if the patient is not forewarned. Another disadvantage is the requirement for two procedures, one to insert the expander and the second to remove the implant and develop flaps to rotate into the defect.

Tissue expansion of the scalp is not without problems. Complication rates as high as 48% have been described.[66] Common issues include hematoma, implant exposure, infection, flap necrosis, alopecia, and wide scars. Pressure from the expander can deform the cranial vault. This may require burring of the calvaria to improve contour. In children, these bony ridges often spontaneously resolve over several months.

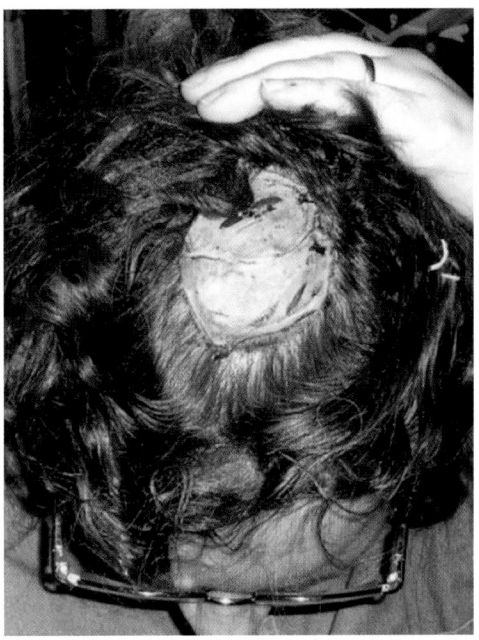

Fig. 5.27 Recent skin graft to the scalp on viable pericranium.

Skin graft

Primary split-thickness skin grafting may be used when the medical condition of the patient precludes larger, more complex procedures. It may be indicated after tumor resection when the risk of tumor recurrence is high. The thin nature of the graft makes monitoring for tumor recurrence an easier proposition than with thicker flap reconstructive techniques. Alternatively, grafting can be combined with staged procedures such as tissue expansion, to provide temporary wound coverage.

A necessary prerequisite for skin grafting is an adequately vascularized wound bed. Preservation of the cranial periosteum or the underlying subcutaneous tissue of the scalp allows for successful "take" of the graft *(Fig. 5.27)*. Exposure of the underlying bone generally requires resurfacing with a vascularized flap. Alternatively, multiple drill holes can be made in the outer cortex down to the diploic layer. The wound can be dressed or a wound VAC applied until granulation tissue is stimulated. Interval split-thickness skin grafting can be performed when the wound bed appears satisfactory. Long-term stability of this type of coverage tends to be problematic.[67]

The primary advantage of split-thickness skin grafting is technical simplicity. Disadvantages include mismatches of color, texture, and contour compared to the surrounding soft tissue. This is particularly evident in the scalp, where the price that is paid for a skin graft is a permanent area of alopecia. Additionally, skin graft may prove unstable in hostile wound environments, such as an irradiated wound.

Local flaps

For small to medium-sized defects of the scalp, local tissue rearrangement provides the bulk of the reconstructive armamentarium. These have included transposition, advancement, and rotation flaps.

The crane principle can treat avulsions of nonhair-bearing skin of the forehead. This technique involves rotating hair-bearing skin over an exposed bony defect in the forehead. The donor defect is covered with a temporary split-thickness skin graft. Several weeks later, the flap is elevated, leaving a layer of vascularized tissue over the donor defect. The previous split-thickness skin graft is excised and the hair-bearing flap is returned to its original anatomic position. The newly created vascularized bed is resurfaced with a full-thickness or thick split-thickness skin graft.[68]

Larger flaps with broad bases are generally preferable to smaller flaps in the scalp, given the thickness and relative noncompliance of the galea. If a named vessel (the superficial temporal, occipital, or supraorbital artery) can be included with the flap, the surviving length is often improved.[69] Small peripheral defects can often be closed with one flap. For larger defects of the vertex greater than 50 cm², multiple flaps are often needed to obtain closure. Orticochea published his four-flap scalp reconstructive technique based on known vascular territories of the scalp.[70] This was subsequently modified to a three-flap technique to maximize flap vascularity *(Fig. 5.28)*.[71] In this technique two flaps are used to reconstruct the defect, each based on the superficial temporal artery. A large posterior flap based on the occipital artery is used to close the donor defect. Defects as large as 30% of the cranium can be closed by this technique. Galeal scoring is a useful tactic to gain effective flap length and reduce tension. Care must be taken not to damage the subaponeurotic blood vessels when performing this maneuver.

For anterior hairline defect, the Juri flap[72] *(Fig. 5.29)* (temporoparieto-occipital flap) can be used. Although its initial application was cosmetic, it can be adapted to recreate anterior scalp defects following tumor resection. This hair-bearing flap is based on the parietal branch of the superficial temporal artery. To ensure survival of the tip of the flap, two preliminary delay procedures are carried out before

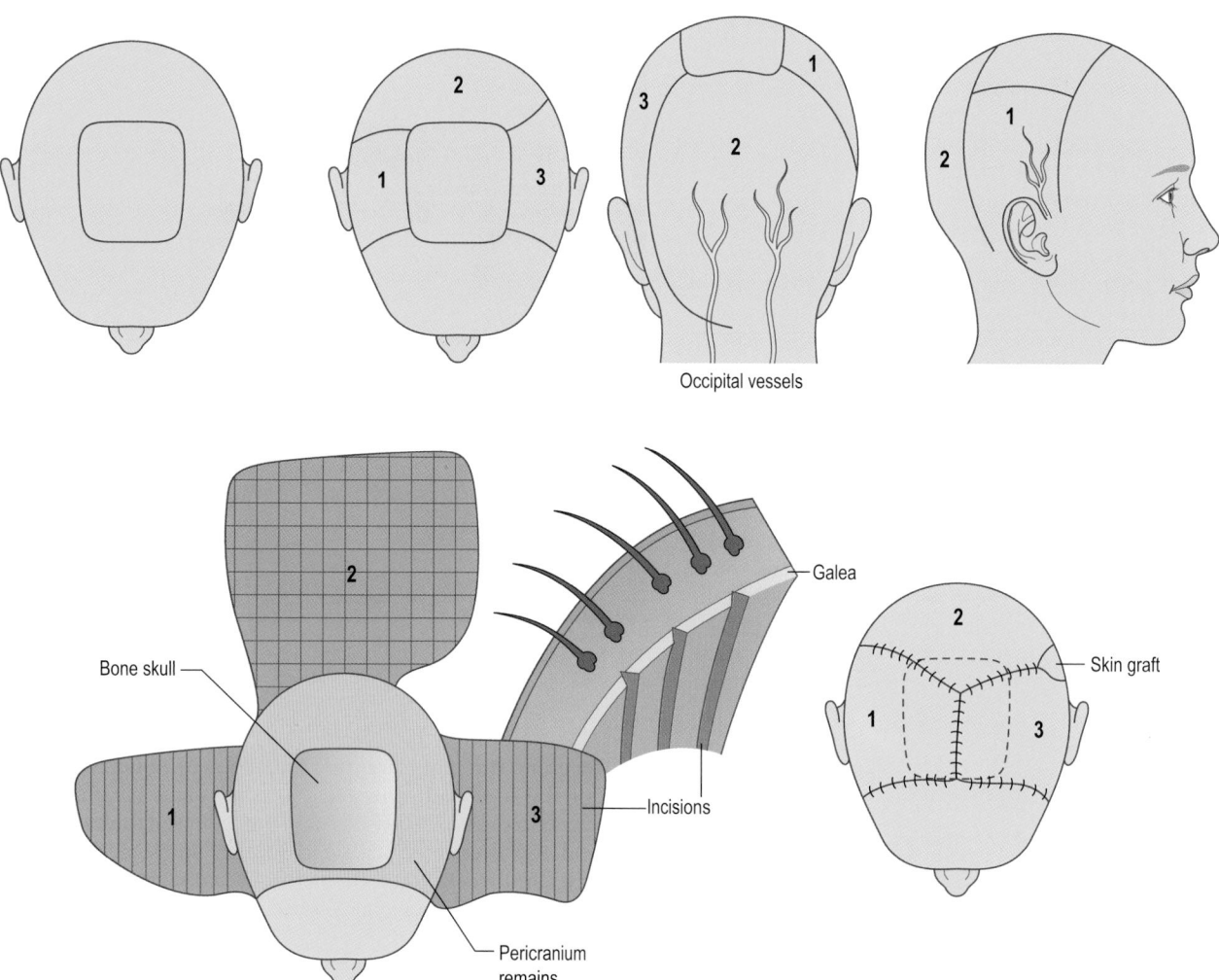

Fig. 5.28 Orticochea three-flap technique. Two flaps based on the superficial temporal artery are used to reconstruct the defect. A posterior-based flap based on the occipital vessels is used to fill the donor defect. (Reproduced from Arnold PG, Rangarathnam CS. Multiple flap scalp reconstruction: Orticochea revisited. *Plast Reconstr Surg.* 1982;69:607.)

transposition. Flaps as long as 28 cm based on a 4-cm pedicle have been described. Bilateral flaps can be performed for larger defects. The anterior scalp incision should be beveled to allow hair from the flap to grow up through the incision. This apparently softens the abrupt appearance of the anterior hairline. Nordström[73] was able to narrow the pedicle of the flap to 2 cm by including the vascular supply of the retroauricular artery with the superficial temporal artery. Disadvantages include the risk of flap necrosis, donor site alopecia, and the sharp frontal hairline. Additionally, the direction of hair growth of the flap is different from the surrounding frontal scalp. Instead of being oriented anteriorly, the flap hair is directed posteriorly. A patient may experience problems with hair styling as a result of this misdirection.

Scalp reduction techniques as popularized by Unger[74] can be used to reconstruct midline defect of the scalp. Wide undermining of bilateral temporal parietal flaps is performed superficial to the deep temporal fascia. Flap vascularity is provided by the superficial temporal artery. Repairing the galea layer in the midline minimizes stretch-back and slot formation *(Fig. 5.30).*

Multiple scalp flap designs have been described in the literature. The number of flaps appears to be directly proportional to the creativity of the surgeons designing them. These include rotation advancement flaps, pinwheel flaps, double opposing advancement flaps, large bipedicled fronto-occipital flaps, O to T, and Y to T flaps. Each has its own indications as well as advantages and disadvantages. Flap selection should be based on the location and size of the defect. Consideration should be given to the reliability of the flaps, donor site defect, and resultant scar pattern *(Fig. 5.31).*[55]

When a large scalp flap is rotated, the dissection should be subgaleal, preserving the underlying periosteum. The latter may prove to be an invaluable recipient bed for skin grafts if primary closure of the donor site is not possible. A large dog-ear is often formed at the point of rotation of the flap. The temptation to revise the dog-ear should be resisted. This maneuver will often narrow the vascular pedicle of the transposed flap, resulting in distal necrosis. A dog-ear will often flatten with time. If not, it can be revised at a later date. Excessive tension should be avoided because it will inhibit healing and increase the likelihood of necrosis of the tip of the flap.

Small transposition flaps, such as the Limberg and bilobe flap, have fewer applications in the scalp. Transposition flaps depend on local adjacent tissue laxity to close the donor site defect. This is not available in the scalp. Bilobe flaps work well in the temporal region because the donor site can be closed along the line of resting tension in the "crow's foot" area. Another useful flap for temporal reconstruction is the cervical facial advancement flap. Its greatest utility is in the elderly, because of the excess tissue present in the donor site. By mobilizing soft tissues from the check and neck,

the entire cosmetic unit of temporal region can be resurfaced *(Fig. 5.32)*.

A drain is used postoperatively to prevent fluid accumulation under the transposed flaps. Care should be taken not to apply a tight postoperative head dressing to the scalp, for fear of compromising flap circulation. If necessary, a temporary halo device can be affixed to the cranium to protect the flaps. By transferring the load to the halo ring, direct pressure on the flaps can be avoided while the patient is nursed in the recumbent position.

Component separation of the scalp has been described by a number of authors to close small defects of the scalp. The layers of the scalp are delaminated, providing vascularized tissue to cover adjacent areas of bone exposure. Examples include galeal frontalis flaps, osteogaleal flaps, and temporoparietal fascial flaps *(Fig. 5.33)*.

Galeal flaps have proven to be an extremely useful source of vascularized tissue in craniofacial surgery. The galeal flap is commonly based on a named scalp vessel or combination of vessels. Flap length can often cross the midline. It can be elevated with frontalis muscle of the forehead to reconstruct the anterior cranial base. Galeal flaps have the advantage of an excellent blood supply with minimal donor site morbidity. The thin supple nature of the flap allows them to conform to complex three-dimensional defects.[75]

The temporoparietal fascial flap has found its greatest utility in ear reconstruction. It can be lifted alone or with bone to repair a variety of craniofacial problems. The flap's vascular pedicle is based on the superficial temporal artery and vein. The artery bifurcates into an anterior and posterior branch to supply the majority of the parietal region of the skull. Care should be taken to avoid inclusion of the anterior branch in the flap design, as the frontal branch of the facial nerve runs in close proximity to this vessel. Injury can result in brow ptosis and unilateral forehead paralysis postoperatively. The plan of dissection between the overlying skin and the superficial temporal fascia is often difficult. Guiding the plan of dissection too superficially can result in damage to the overlying hair follicles. The consequence can be postoperative alopecia. Despite these disadvantages, the flap is useful in

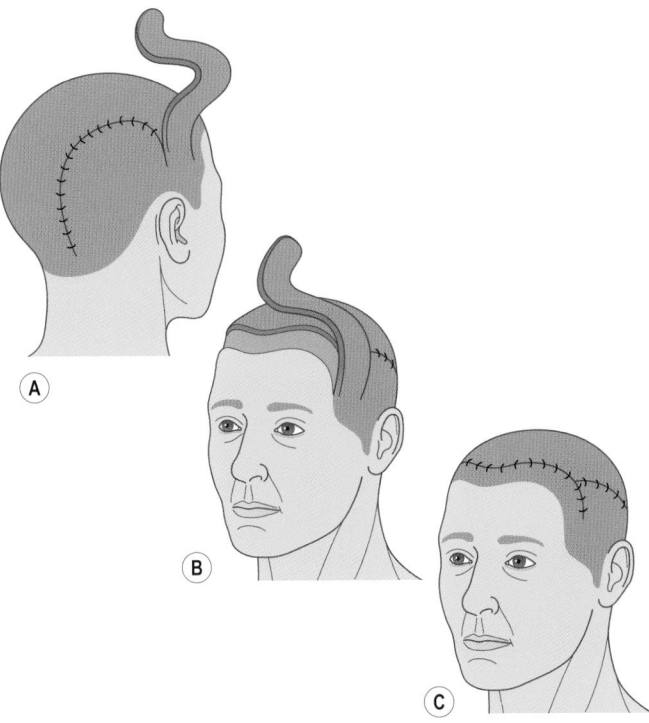

Fig. 5.29 The Juri flap. After two preliminary delay procedures **(A)**, a temporoparieto-occipital flap is elevated **(B)** and used to reconstruct defects in the anterior hairline **(C)**.

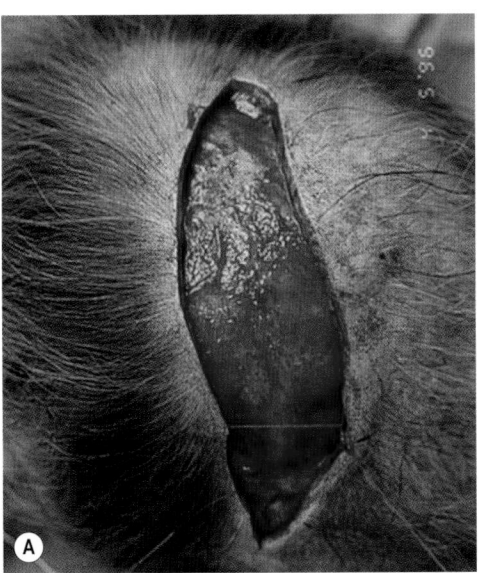
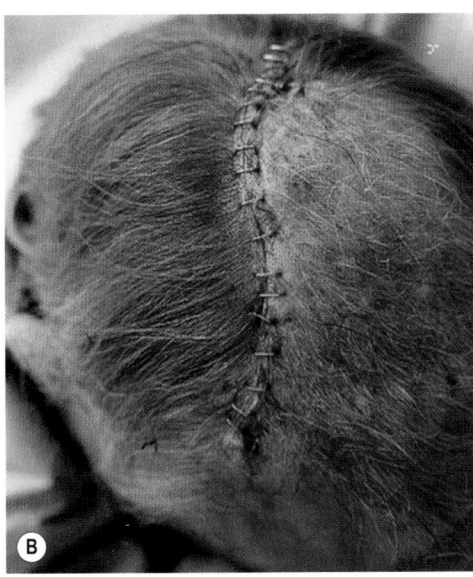

Fig. 5.30 Scalp reduction. **(A)** An elliptical midline excision has been completed. Wide undermining has been performed bilaterally. Flaps are advanced to the midline and the galea is closed to prevent stretch-back. **(B)** Final closure with staples.

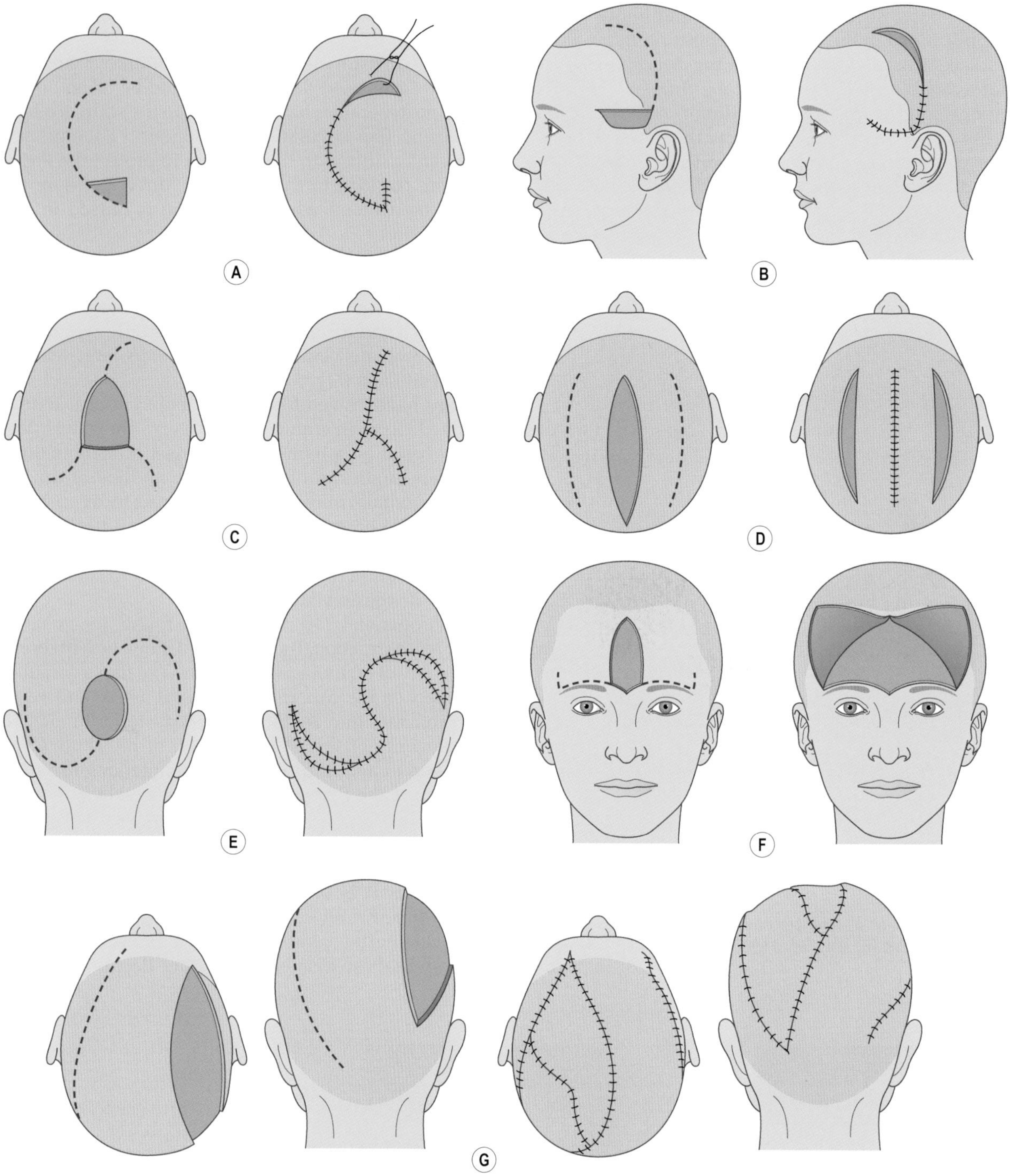

Fig. 5.31 Local scalp flaps. **(A, B)** scalp rotation flaps; **(C)** pinwheel flap; **(D)** bipedicle advancement flaps; **(E)** double opposing rotation flaps; **(F)** Y to T flap; **(G)** bipedicled fronto-occipital flap. (Reproduced from Marchac D. Deformities of the forehead, scalp, and cranial vault. In: McCarthy JG, ed. Plastic surgery. Philadelphia: WB Saunders, 1990:1538.)

reconstructive procedures. It has a reliable blood supply and an inconspicuous donor site. The flap is elastic and thin. It is able to conform snugly to a variety of defects.[76] When it is used with the underlying calvaria, it can provide a source of vascularized cranial bone for reconstruction about the orbit and facial skeleton.

The subgaleal fascia is an ultrathin vascularized structure between the overlying galea and the underlying periosteum

of the skull. This areolar layer receives its own blood flow from perforating vessels from the overlying galea. This delicate layer allows movement of the galea on top of the pericranium. On the superficial and deep surfaces of this tissue is an areolar layer consisting of blood vessels and nerves. Between these two structures is a central lamina of collagenous tissue. With some difficulty this layer can be dissected free between the galea and the periosteum. A cuff of galea is often

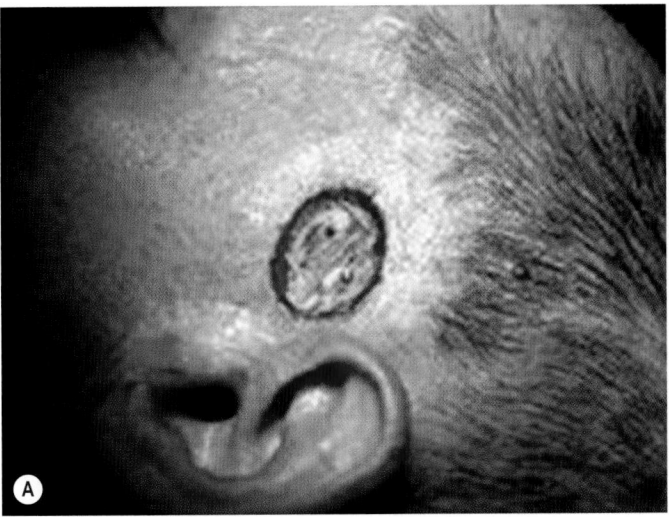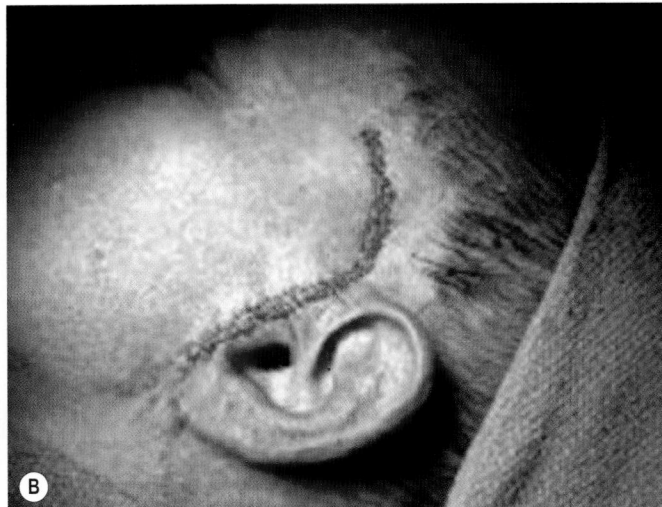

Fig. 5.32 (A, B) Cervical facial advancement flap for temporal defect.

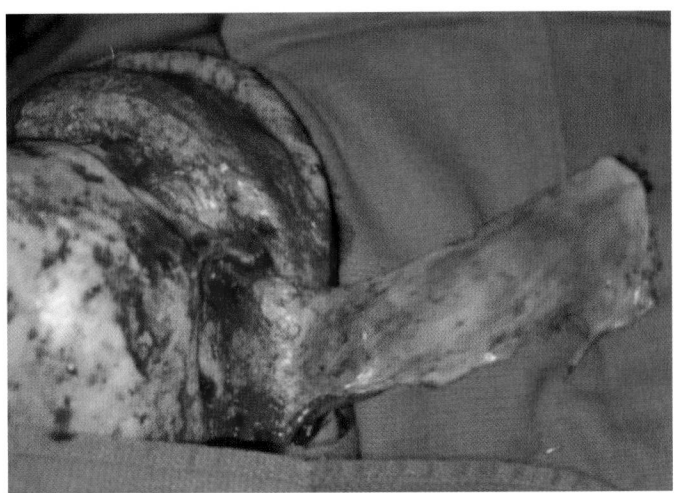

Fig. 5.33 Pericranial flap. The scalp layers can be delaminated to provide vascularized coverage over exposed bony surfaces. The temporalis fascia is a direct lateral extension of the scalp periosteum. It can be elevated with the temporalis muscle if required.

preserved at the perforating vessel to prevent inadvertent injury to the vascular pedicle. The delicate nature of this flap allows its coaptation to complex three-dimensional structures such as the ear.[77] Alternatively, it can be raised with the underlying periosteum as a turnover flap to provide vascularized coverage for denuded calvaria.

The temporalis fascia is a direct lateral extension of the scalp periosteum. This structure obtains its blood supply from the middle temporal artery, a branch of the superficial temporal artery. Thus, a composite flap of superficial temporal fascia and temporalis fascia can be isolated on the same vascular leash. By separating the two fascial structures, the overall surface area of the flap can be increased.[78]

The temporalis muscle takes origin from the temporalis fossa of the lateral portion of the skull. It passes under the zygomatic arch to insert on to the coronoid process of the mandible. It receives its blood supply from the paired deep

temporal arteries which are branches of the internal maxillary artery. The surface of the muscle will require grafting if it is used to reconstruct a cutaneous or intraoral surface. This is because there are no direct perforators from the muscle to the overlying skin. This muscle has found its greatest utility in orbital reconstruction.[79] However, by releasing the origin of the muscle, it can be rotated to fill defects that are more distant *(Fig. 5.34)*. Although the functional loss of one temporalis muscle is minimal, a cosmetically significant temporal hollow often remains after transfer of the muscle. This can often be camouflaged by insertion of one of the commercially available temporal implants.

Regional flaps

Regional flap options are somewhat limited in scalp and forehead reconstructions. None allows the reconstruction of vertex defects. They are indicated when local options are unavailable due to hostile wound conditions.

Perhaps the most useful regional flap for scalp reconstruction is the trapezius muscle flap. This muscle receives its blood supply from the transverse cervical, dorsal scapular, and occipital arteries. Two flaps have been described: a transverse flap base on the upper portion of the muscle and a vertical flap consisting of middle and inferior fibers of the trapezius. The transverse design may result in shoulder drop. It should be reserved for patients who have had previous sacrifice of their spinal accessory nerve. This flap is most useful for temporal and neck coverage. The vertical flap design has minimal functional consequences and is more useful for posterior scalp reconstruction. By designing a skin island between the spine and the scapula, defects of the occipital regions can be reached. The donor site can often be closed primarily *(Fig. 5.35)*.[80]

Both the pedicled and free variants of the latissimus dorsi flap have been used in scalp reconstruction. By passage of the muscle through the axilla, defects in the orbit and temporal bone can be repaired.[81] Risks of the flap include brachial plexus injury and axillary vessel injury. Larger defects are best treated with microsurgical transfer of the muscle.

The pectoralis major can reach the temporal and mastoid region with adequate mobilization. Inclusion of the rectus

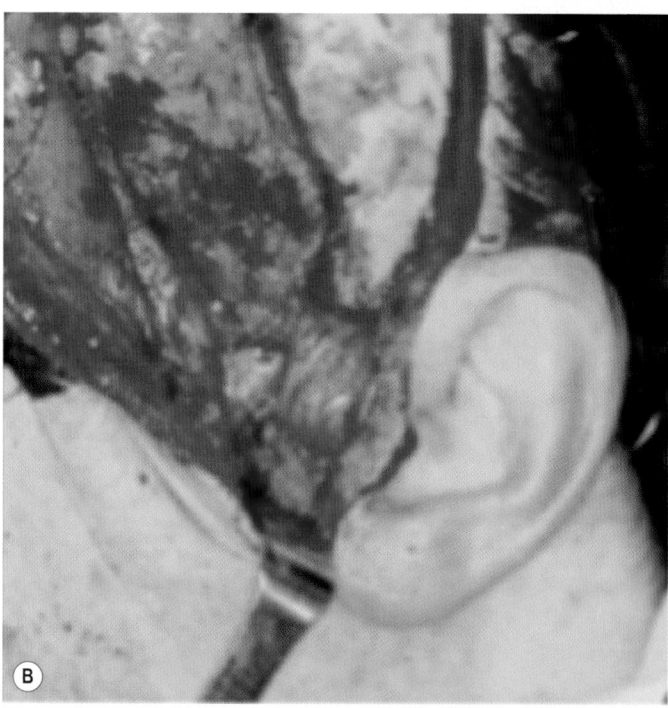

Fig. 5.34 (A, B) Temporalis muscle flap receives its blood supply from the paired deep temporal arteries. It is most useful for orbital and mid facial reconstruction. Release of the coronoid insertion allows it to be advanced to cover supraorbital rim defects.

fascia and transection of the clavicle can extend the arch of rotation of the muscle. Disadvantages include the thickness of the pedicle, poor skin color match, and the bulk of the skin island if included. Breast distortion may occur if the musculocutaneous option is used in women.

The splenius capitis muscle has been used to close small defects in the scalp. The muscle receives its blood supply from the occipital, transverse cervical, and vertebral arteries. By basing the muscle superiorly on the occipital artery, defects of the neck and occiput can be covered.[82]

Microsurgical reconstruction

Extensive and complex defects involving exposed vital structures are not amenable to local or regional techniques. In these difficult cases, free tissue transfer offers the best solution for coverage. Survival rates in excess of 95% have been described with low complication rates.

Both muscle and fasciocutaneous flaps are options for covering these difficult head and neck defects.[83] Each flap has its own proponents with unique advantages and disadvantages. Popular muscle flaps include the latissimus dorsi, serratus anterior, and the rectus abdominis. On the fasciocutaneous side, flap selection has included the radial forearm flap (*Fig. 5.36*), scapular flap, and anterior lateral thigh flap. Other flaps have been described, including omentum, prefabricated flaps, and hair-bearing flaps from identical twins.

Beasley *et al.*[84] have proposed a staging and treatment algorithm based on defect location, size, and characteristics of the adjacent wound environment. An unfavorable wound environment is one with heavy trauma, radiation, and previous

flap failure. This group recommends the scapular flap for forehead defect greater than 50 cm². If it extends to the scalp, a scapular or latissimus dorsi muscle with skin graft is advised. For large scalp defects between 200 and 600 cm², a single latissimus with skin graft is used. For massive defects larger than 600 cm² bilateral free latissimus flaps were performed.

These numbers are guidelines. Every patient must have an individual treatment plan. The decision about which type of free flap is indicated depends on multiple factors, including the size of the defect, location, wound conditions, tissue availability, and donor site morbidity as well as surgeon and patient's preference.

The head and neck region has an extensive bilateral vascular network, which is readily accessible for free tissue transfer.[85] The preferred recipient vessel in the upper third of the face is the superficial temporal artery and vein. If unavailable, lower branches of the external carotid system can be used (facial, superior thyroid, and transverse cervical) Branches of the internal and external jugular veins provide a wide variety of options for the venous anastomosis. The recipient vein should be prepared in close proximity to the recipient artery to prevent excessive separation of pedicle vessels. This design prevents kinking or pulling of the artery and vein in different directions with changes of head position. Long vein grafts should be avoided if possible, because the incidence of perioperative thrombosis of the flap is increased. Several salvage techniques have been described for microvascular access in the head and neck region. These include Corlett arteriovenous loops, cephalic vein transposition, thoracodorsal transposition, and the use of pedicle of the previous free flap.[86,87]

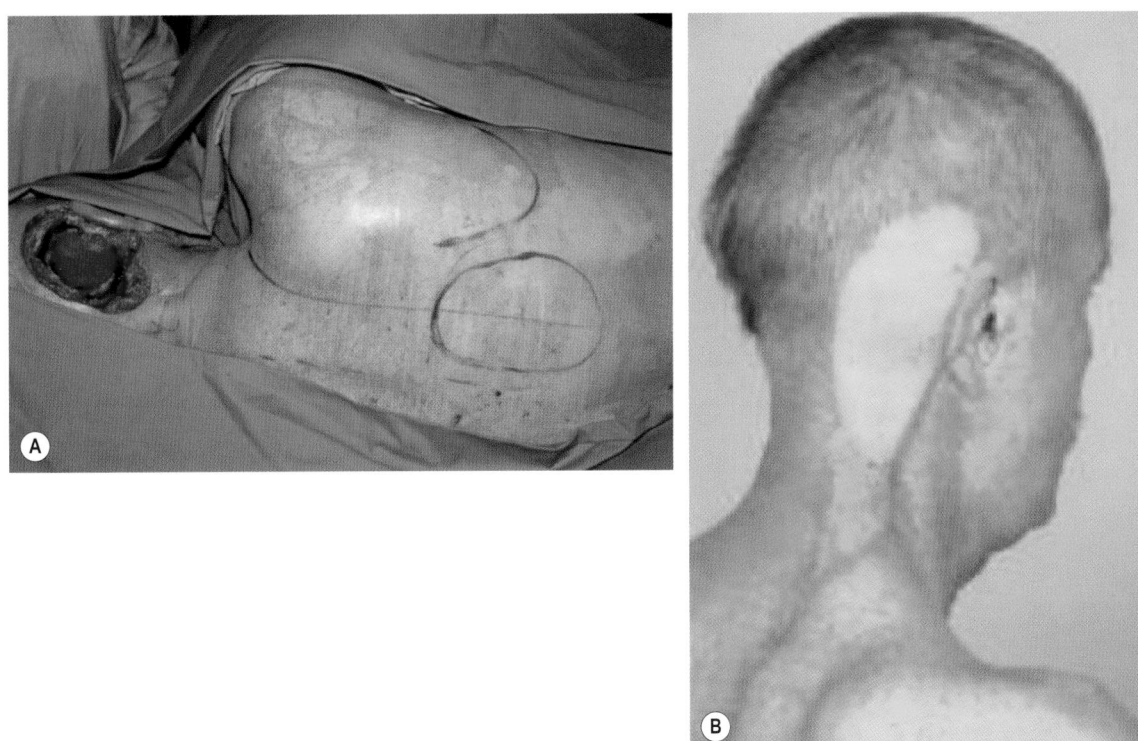

Fig. 5.35 (A, B) Vertical trapezius flap used to reconstruct recurrent squamous cell carcinoma of the occiput.

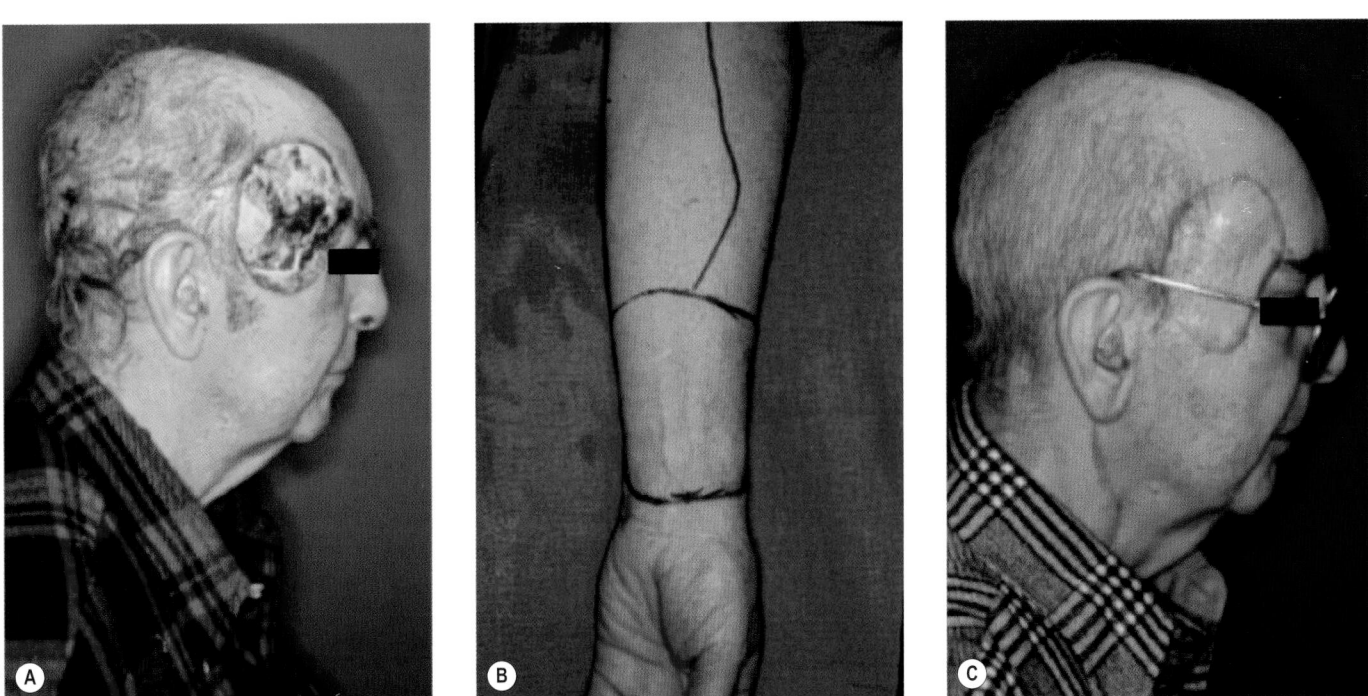

Fig. 5.36 (A–C) A 72-year-old man following Mohs resection of an invasive squamous cell carcinoma of the temporal region, reconstructed with a radial forearm fascial flap.

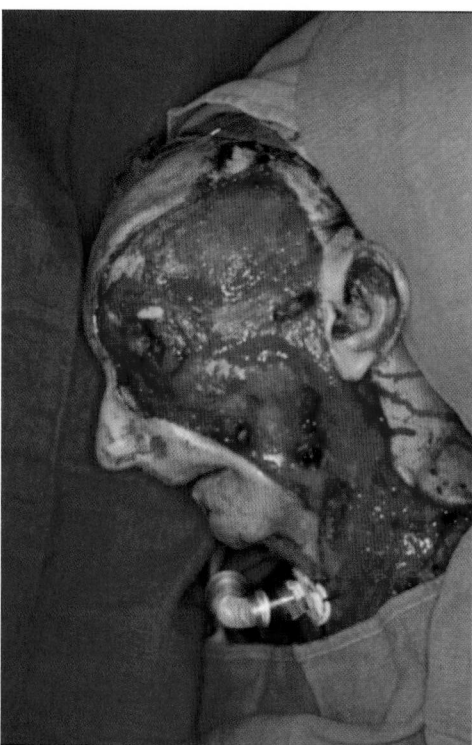

Fig. 5.37 Latissimus dorsi muscle flap with skin graft to resurface a necrotizing infection of the head and neck. Following serial debridement and enucleation of the left eye, coverage was affected with a combination of a free latissimus muscle flap and pectoralis muscle flap with skin graft.

The skin-grafted latissimus is the workhorse of scalp reconstruction *(Fig. 5.37)*. It has a long vascular pedicle and often allows primary anastomosis in the neck.[88] The intermuscular blood supply of the latissimus allows the muscle to be split into distinct muscle flaps for coverage of complex three-dimensional defects. If more tissue is required, the serratus muscle and scapular flap can be carried on the subscapular vascular pedicle. Although it can be raised as a myocutaneous flap, the thickness of the subcutaneous fat in most western populations precludes its use in scalp and forehead reconstruction. In general muscle flaps with skin grafts give a better long-term aesthetic result than similar-sized fasciocutaneous flaps and myocutaneous flaps. The skin paddles provided by myocutaneous and fasciocutaneous flaps produce constructs with poor color and texture matches in cutaneous head and neck reconstruction. Additionally, the bulk of these flaps result in a distortion of contour.

The aesthetic outcome of all free-flap reconstructions of the scalp is compromised when compared to the results achieved by local flaps. There are always areas of alopecia that detract from the result. Multiple methods have been described to improve the reconstruction, including serial excision, local flap transposition, tissue expansion, and follicular micrografting into skin-grafted muscle flaps.

Fasciocutaneous flaps work better to reconstruct forehead defects. The paucity of hair makes them less suitable for scalp reconstruction. The scapular, parascapular, radial forearm, and anterior lateral thigh free flaps are common options. The radial forearm flap has a thinner dermis than the back or thigh, making it more suitable for this purpose. However the donor site tissue is limited in size and the color match is poor.[89]

Since its description by Song *et al.*,[90] the anterolateral thigh flap has gained increasing popularity in reconstructive surgery. It has a long vascular pedicle with a suitable vessel diameter for microvascular anastomosis. Its cutaneous distribution is large with an acceptable donor site. There is some variation in vascular pedicle, but these have been well described in the literature. The thickness of the flap can be adjusted to individual needs during the primary surgery by removing the deep fascia and subcutaneous fat, except for a 2–3-cm area around the entry of the vascular pedicle, or including a cuff of muscle. Hair growth on hirsute flaps can be improved with laser hair removal as a secondary procedure.[91]

The omentum has been used to cover scalp defects. It is capable of covering large areas of the skull. Criticisms of the flap include lack of sufficient bulk to protect the brain and the morbidity associated with omental harvest.[92]

Free hair-bearing flaps have been described in the literature.[88] A temporo-occipital scalp flap can be elevated based on the superficial temporal artery and vein. The flap can be transplanted to the contralateral side and anastomosed to temporal vessels, providing coverage on the alopecic side. Advantages include a one-stage hair-bearing reconstruction with hair of normal direction and density. A preliminary tissue expansion phase can ensure that the donor site is closed primarily.

Potential disadvantages of microvascular reconstruction include the long duration of the procedure and the anesthetic risk for the patient. These procedures are technically demanding and risk flap failure. Additionally, costs, labor, and availability of microvascular surgeons may be hurdles to this type of reconstruction.

Scalp replantation

The first successful microsurgical replantation of the scalp was described in 1976. Since that time, replantation has been the treatment of complete and nearly complete avulsions of the scalp.[93] There is no other method of scalp reconstruction that can match the results of replantation. Avulsions usually result from entanglement of long hair in moving machinery. The cleavage is predictably subgaleal, starting in the supraorbital and neck areas because the frontalis and occipitalis muscles are less firmly attached. A portion of the ear, eyebrows, and upper nasal skin can be attached to the specimen. Blood loss is often extensive. Fluids and blood products should be replaced vigorously.

If the scalp is deemed replantable, two teams work simultaneously. One team identified recipient vessels and the other group searches for suitable vessels in the amputated part. Because of the avulsive nature of the injury, resection of damaged vessels and primary vein grafting are often required. To minimize the ischemic interval and to aid in the identification of suitable veins, the arterial repair is completed first *(Fig. 5.38)*. Most commonly, the superficial temporal artery has been used for microsurgical repair. One superficial temporal artery is capable of ensuring the survival of the entire scalp. The occipital, supraorbital, and postauricular vessels have also been used. Microvascular clamps should be placed on draining veins to prevent blood loss while the venous circulation is re-established. At least two venous repairs should be

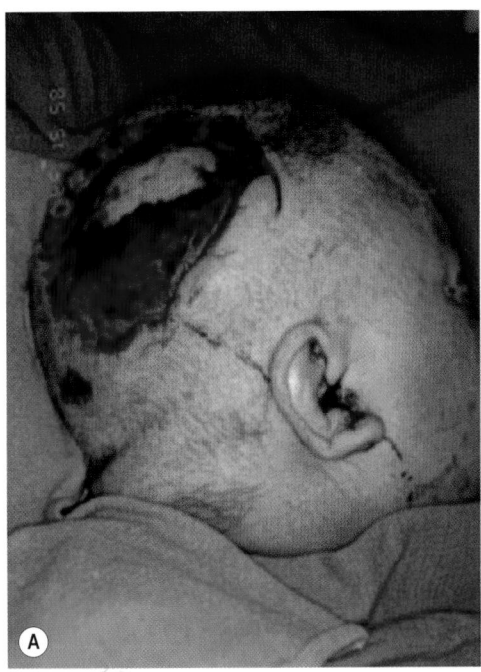 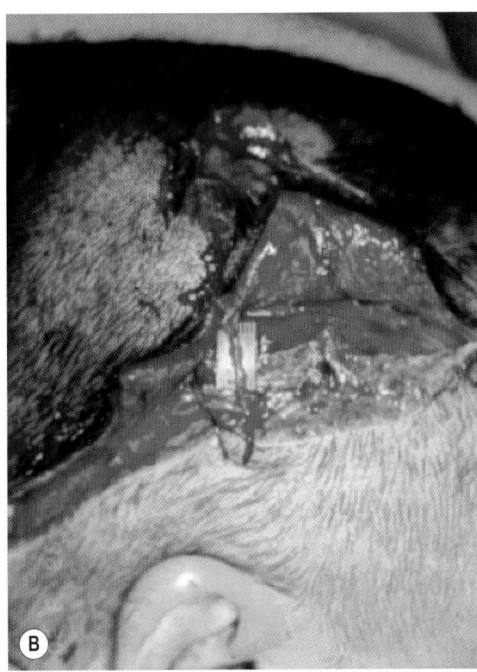

Fig. 5.38 (A, B) Replantation of avulsed scalp with bone exposure.

attempted to prevent flap congestion and subsequent venous insufficiency.

Contraindications to replantation of the scalp are few. These include hemodynamic instability of the patient and a severely macerated amputated part with multiple segmental injuries. Concomitant severe life-threatening injuries that prohibit a lengthy operation are obvious contraindications.

Facial transplantation

Composite tissue transplantation for complex facial deformities has generated tremendous interest over the recent years.[94] Since the first-reported partial face transplantation performed in France, seven procedures have been performed in three different countries. Significant controversy over the ethical, immunological, and psychological issues remains. Most of the transplants have been directed at replacing traumatically created mid facial defects, although one patient received reconstruction for a massive plexiform neurofibroma. It is not a stretch of the imagination that a similar technique could be applied to composite defects of the upper third of the face, given the success of replantation in the region. Many questions need to be answered: recipient selection, donor selection, and immunosuppression protocols. Only time and careful analysis will prove whether these microsurgical and transplant techniques will prove beneficial to patients with complex facial injuries.

Postoperative care

The postoperative regimen depends on the nature of the reconstructive procedure. Defects that are allowed to close by secondary intention often require several weeks of twice-daily dressing to undergo re-epithelialization.

If skin grafts are used, immobilization of the graft with tie-over dressing or wound VAC is performed for 5 days postoperatively. This is followed by nonadherent dressings for several weeks to ensure adherence of the graft.

Tissue expanders are generally drained for 3–5 days postoperatively. Expansion is initiated 2 weeks after the procedure at the time of suture removal. The expansion process is highly variable between different individuals. Much depends on the patient's pain tolerance and the compliance of the overlying tissues. For practical purposes, most patients are expanded on a weekly basis. Frequent small-volume inflations are better tolerated than infrequent large-volume boluses.

Regional skin, fascial, or muscle flaps are protected from direct pressure for 7–10 days following the procedure. In cooperative patients, simple positioning is often all that is required. In children or patients with associated head injuries where compliance is an issue, the application of a temporary halo device ensures that inadvertent pressure necrosis of the flap does not occur.[95]

In addition to avoidance of pressure, free tissue transfers and scalp replants require close monitoring to detect perioperative thrombosis. A variety of monitoring devices have been described, each with its own advantages and disadvantages.[96] At our institution we combine conventional monitoring techniques (clinical evaluation of color, capillary refill, and hand-held Doppler) with either an implantable Doppler system (Cook Medical) or tissue oximetry using near-infrared spectroscopy (ViOptix).

Outcome, prognosis, and complications

Potential complications

- Closure by secondary intention may not occur or create cosmetically unacceptable scars or alopecia. Revisional surgery using local flaps will often solve the problem. Care should be taken not to disturb adjacent mobile structures.

- VAC used in conjunction with skin-grafting techniques can destroy the underlying vascularized periosteal bed if excessive pressure is used with the device. Using lower pressures (10–25 mmHg) will usually prevent this complication.
- Wound dehiscence and infection can complicate any reconstructive procedure. This is usually managed by intraoperative debridement and regular dressing changes. When wound conditions improve, secondary closure over drains is often possible.
- Most complications occurring with tissue expansion are relatively minor and do not interfere with completion of the procedure. However, infection can occur. If significant pain, erythema, fever, and chills develop, the device should be removed, the wound irrigated, and the expanded tissue advanced over drains. Repeat attempts at expansion should be deferred for at least 3 months.
- Implant exposure can be prevented by adequate pocket dissection and conservative rates of expansion. If exposure occurs early, the device should be removed. If exposure is late in the expansion process it can continue with the application of antibiotic creams over the device. Careful monitoring for infectious complications is mandatory.
- Skin graft failure can occur if the graft is placed on an avascular bed or if a postoperative infection develops. Hematoma, seroma, and shear of the graft relative to the underlying bed can compromise graft take. Grafting should only be considered in well-vascularized infection-free beds. Proper immobilization of the graft and meticulous hemostasis are necessary prerequisites for a successful outcome.
- The most common complications following flap surgery include seroma, hematoma, necrosis, infection, and inadequate coverage of the defect. These are generally due to errors in judgment, technique, or patient management. Inadequate knowledge of the surgical anatomy or evaluation of the surgical defect can compromise the surgical result. Careful handling of tissues, protection of vascular pedicles, and meticulous hemostasis will generally prevent these complications.
- The failure rate for free tissue transfers in most centers is generally less than 5%. Complication rates are higher in head and neck free tissue transfers than for elective breast reconstruction. Prior irradiation, anesthesia time greater than 10 hours, age greater than 70, and pre-existing medical conditions increase the complication rate.[97] If vascular compromise is detected, an immediate return to the operating room is warranted. Salvage rates have varied between 54 and 100%, depending on the series.[98] The use of ancillary monitoring devices will allow for the detection of vascular compromise before it is clinically detectable, minimizing ischemia time and the development of a no-reflow state.

Secondary procedures

Patients may present with a myriad of secondary deformities following forehead or scalp reconstruction:

- Dog-ear deformities are common following scalp flap rotational procedures. Modifying these at the time of the initial procedure risks flap necrosis at the tip of the flap. Often, small dog-ears will settle with time, obviating the need for any further surgical procedures. If more substantial, revision should be delayed at least 6 weeks following the initial procedure.
- If split-thickness skin grafts are used to reconstruct cosmetically critical areas such as the forehead, the result can be mismatch of color and texture with the surrounding tissue elements. If relatively small, tissue expanders can be placed adjacent to the grafted area. Once expansion has occurred, the graft can be excised and resurfaced with the expanded flaps. If the area is larger, pre-expansion of neck full-thickness graft should be considered. Pre-expansion allows for primary closure of the donor site and resurfacing with a graft that has a better color match. Alternatively, a prefabricated free flap can be created incorporating the skin characteristics of the recipient site into the flap design.
- Widened scars may create concern for the patient. Often this is the result of closure under excessive tension. Re-excision with layered closure (including the galea) once scar maturation has occurred can often improve the cosmetic result. If scars are running across the resting lines of tension in cosmetically critical areas, consideration should be given to Z-plasty or W-plasty procedures.
- Alopecia may result from excessive tension, vascular insult to flaps, or skin grafts applied to the scalp. These can usually be dealt with by using a combination of local flaps and tissue expansion techniques.
- Mobile structures such as eyebrows and eyelids can be displaced following reconstructive procedures on the forehead creating asymmetries with the nonaffected side. While each case is unique, the use of local flaps, full-thickness skin grafts, or tissue expansion can often improve the final result.
- Hairlines can be displaced if flap planning is not optimal. The use of tissue expansion and fixation of the resultant flap to the underlying bone with bone anchors can restore symmetry and prevent secondary contracture.
- Patients who have been treated for malignant tumors of the scalp and forehead require careful monitoring in the postoperative period. Patients should be counseled on the need for regular follow-up and the possibility of further surgical intervention.
- Injuries or tumors in the temporal region can create frontal-branch injuries with resultant brow ptosis. These may require secondary brow suspension procedures to achieve symmetry at rest. Alternatively, Botox can be used to paralyze the unaffected side to achieve symmetry.
- Scalp trauma or tumor may destroy the underlying calvarium. Secondary cranioplasty procedures using alloplasts or autogenous bone can restore the integrity of the cranial vault. A necessary prerequisite is well-vascularized full-thickness coverage over the bony defect prior to any attempt at reconstruction.

6. Seitz IA, Gottlieb LJ. Reconstruction of scalp and forehead defects. *Clin Plast Surg.* 2009;36:355–377.

   Techniques in scalp and forehead reconstruction are detailed in this review.

7. TerKonda RP, Sykes JM. Concepts in scalp and forehead reconstruction. *Otolaryngol Clin North Am.* 1997;30:519–539.

   Anatomy and technical versatility are stressed in this primer on scalp reocnstruction. The roles of diverse methods in achieving optimal coverage are discussed.

54. Temple CL, Ross DC. Scalp and forehead reconstruction. *Clin Plast Surg.* 2005;32:377–390, vi–vii.

   The authors propose an algorithm for scalp reconstruction. Surgical antomy of the scalp is reviewed.

57. Angelos PC, Downs BW. Options for the management of forehead and scalp defects. *Facial Plast Surg Clin North Am.* 2009;17:379–393.

   This review covers methods in scalp wound management ranging from allowing for secondary healing to performing free tissue transfer.

69. Leedy JE, Janis JE, Rohrich RJ. Reconstruction of acquired scalp defects: an algorithmic approach. *Plast Reconstr Surg.* 2005;116:54e–72e.

   A multifaceted algorithm for scalp reconstruction is presented. The reconstructive surgeon is urged to achieve not only wound closure, but also an aesthetically optimal result.

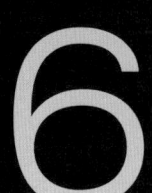

Aesthetic nasal reconstruction

Frederick J. Menick

SYNOPSIS

- The field of plastic surgery originated with the first early attempts to reconstruct the face, especially the nose.
- The face tells the world who we are and materially influences what we can become.
- The restoration of a normal appearance and an open airway to allow comfortable breathing remains the goal.
- Treatment choices will depend on an understanding of the deformity and wound healing, missing anatomic layers, available donor tissues, surgical planning, the surgeon's ability to modify them into "like" tissue, and the advantages, disadvantages, and limitations of the technique and its ability to achieve the desired outcome.

 Access the Historical Perspective section online at
http://www.expertconsult.com

Introduction

The primary functions of the nose are to look normal and allow easy nasal breathing.

The success of reconstruction will depend upon the site, size, and depth of the defect, donor availability and, most importantly, the surgeon's choices in material, method, and approach. An understanding of the deformity, both anatomically and aesthetically, and of wound healing and tissue transfer is required. The advantages, disadvantages, and limitations of each material, technique, and stage must be understood. What is missing must be replaced – missing external skin which matches adjacent facial skin in color and texture, a mi-layer support of soft tissue, bone, and cartilage, and internal lining. Covering skin must be thin, conforming, and vascular. Lining must be thin, supple, and vascular, neither occluding the airway nor distorting external nasal shape due to excessive bulk or stiffness. The rigid midlayer muscle must support, shape, and brace the repair against gravity, tension, and scar contraction to prevent collapse and distortion. The surgeon must choose tissues similar in kind to those which are missing. However, although donor tissues may have some characteristics which are similar to those that must be replaced, all tissues must be modified, thinned, and shaped to become truly "like" tissue. Flat forehead skin, ear, or rib cartilage, and traditional lining replacements have little similarity to the "normal" nose.

Basic science/disease process

Nasal deformity may follow congenital malformation, trauma (including burns), the sequela of skin cancer treatment by excision or radiation, infection, or immune disease.[25] Infection must be controlled, tumor eradicated, and immune disease in remission. Often reconstruction is delayed for weeks to years to allow wound stabilization and maturation and verification of disease control.

Staged excisions with delayed repair are especially advantageous in the more extensive cancer which requires more complex reconstruction. Ideally, the patient is seen prior to tumor excision. The diagnosis is verified, the likely extent of excision and reconstruction discussed, and the treatment options outlined. Preoperative medical clearance can be obtained, if necessary. Operative time is scheduled for the future. Excision is performed and a follow-up appointment made to evaluate the defect after tumor clearance. During the postexcisional consultation, the true extent of the defect is confirmed and anatomic and aesthetic losses are defined. Reconstruction follows within 48–72 hours. Because the extent of the defect has been defined prior to repair, the patient understands the requirements of reconstruction and becomes a cooperative, informed partner.

Such coordinated excision and repair provide an opportunity to think, plan, and discuss options with the patient in a leisurely manner, prior to entering the operating room. A surgical plan is developed preoperatively, decreasing patient and surgeon anxiety and ensuring the best result. Because tumor clearance has been confirmed prior to repair, the length of anesthesia and operative times are shortened. Most importantly, disruption of the operative schedule and intraoperative decision-making are minimized.

Diagnosis/patient presentation and patient selection

The preoperative consultation should clarify the diagnosis, define the anatomic and aesthetic deficiencies, ensure a healthy wound and patient, provide patient education, instill confidence and the patient's active participation, allow formulation of a surgical plan, and identify appropriate donor materials, methods, and staging. The patient's past medical history and physical examination are performed with special emphasis on the etiology of the nasal injury, disease remission, or cancer clearance. Facial photographs, combined with calibrated photographs and normative measurements of the human face, clarify anatomic losses, aesthetic injury, old scars, landmark malposition, and injury to available donor sites, and provide measurements which are useful intraoperatively. In complex three-dimensional injuries, a facial moulage of plaster of Paris is obtained preoperatively and a clay model of the desired result designed. This improves the surgeon's ability to visualize intellectually the dimension and contours which require replacement. Prior pathologic exams and old operative reports are examined. Facial X-rays, computed tomography (CT) scans, or magnetic resonance imaging (MRI) are occasionally employed to clarify bony and soft-tissue injury to the midface, when rebuilding composite defects of the nose and cheek.

Planning an aesthetic nasal reconstruction

The traditional approach

Traditionally,[22,25] surgeons sought to "fill the hole" and obtain a healed wound. The defect determined the repair. The design and dimension of a skin graft or flap were determined by the apparent, but often distorted, defect. Scars and additional donor injury were overriding concerns. A comprehensive plan to restore multiple, independent, three-dimensional facial features was rarely envisioned. The emphasis was on tissue transfer (skin graft or flap), blood supply, or the replacement of anatomic layers (cover, lining, support). Without primary support placement, unchecked forces of healing led to contracted scars, pincushioning, and airway collapse.

This traditional approach failed to appreciate the strong motivation of patients to look as they did before. It followed a "less is more" cautious approach with little expectation of restoring the normal.

False principles

Design the flap from a pattern of the defect

Traditionally, skin grafts or flaps are designed to replace the existing defect. But the defect does not reflect what is missing and what needs to be replaced. Fresh wounds are enlarged by edema, local anesthesia, tissue tension, and gravity. Old wounds may be contracted by secondary-intention healing or distorted by prior injury or past attempts at repair.

To repair the face successfully, the "true" tissue loss must be identified and replaced. The surgeon recreates the "true" defect and returns "the normal to its normal position." Then the defect is filled with exactly measured replacements.

Take extra tissue to be safe

Transferring extra tissue for "good measure" or out of fear for vascularity only complicates the reconstruction. If too much tissue is transferred, adjacent landmarks are displaced outward. Additional stages will be subsequently required to excise the extra bulk and restore unit outline.

Make the flap smaller to preserve the donor site

Sharing tissue from an area of excess to one of deficiency is a basic surgical tool. The surgeon must avoid the temptation to cheat the recipient site to preserve the donor site. Central features, such as the nose or lip, have an exact border outline and position. Missing tissues must be replaced in exact quantity to avoid distortion of the size, shape, and position of the nasal subunit by dragging the borders of the defect inward with tissue replacement which is too small.

Employ a tissue expander to conserve the donor site

The nose is an unforgiving facial feature, while the forehead is a forgiving one. Although useful if the hairline is exceptionally low or the forehead is scarred or previously harvested, the routine use of skin expansion is unnecessary. The nose comes first. The forehead donor is of secondary importance. Use an expander only if it will contribute to the overall nasal repair.

Never throw anything away

Surgeons are taught to preserve tissue. However, if skin is transferred to resurface only part of the facial feature, it may appear as a distracting patch, outlined by scars. It is often helpful to alter the defect and discard extra skin prior to repair, even if this makes the defect larger. Discardable tissues can be used for other purposes – as hingeover lining or subcutaneous bulk, or shifted to resurface an adjacent injury.

The presence and number of scars determine the final result: place incisions in existing scars, minimize scars, fear scars

A poor facial repair is identified by incorrect dimension, volume, position, and contour, not by the presence of scars. Scars are effectively camouflaged by positioning them in the joins between subunits.

Place a supportive framework and debulk excess tissue secondarily after the soft tissues have healed and matured

Traditionally, cover and lining have been replaced without support to avoid the risk of extrusion and infection. Occasionally, flimsy cartilage strips were placed within a prefabricated flap, which was lined with a skin graft. Months later, bone and cartilage grafts were placed as crude cantilevered grafts to lift the tip and dorsum. Unfortunately, unsupported soft tissues are rapidly distorted by gravity and tension and become fixed by scar. Late re-expansion with secondary cartilage grafts and soft-tissue "thinning" may not be successful.

One hole, one flap, and (often) one operation

It is difficult to reproduce the delicate three-dimensional character of multiple facial units with a single flap. A single flap takes a surgical shortcut and fails to supply enough skin to resurface three-dimensional contour. Myofibroblasts within the bed of scar under the healing flaps contract and draw the single flap into a dome-like pincushioned mass. For that reason, it is often preferable to repair individual facial units with separate grafts and flaps of exact dimension and skin quality.

The modern approach to nasal reconstruction

Aesthetic results depend upon the surgeon's and patient's choices.[22,25] The modern approach relies on the visualization of the "normal" and the determination of what is missing, both anatomically and aesthetically.[28] This regional unit approach emphasizes the judicious choice and modification of recipient and donor tissues to provide for the exact replacement of facial units. The principles of facial reconstruction have switched from traditional wound perspective (how big, how deep, anatomy, and flap blood supply) to a visual one. A healed wound, tissue survival, or the replacement of anatomic layers are necessary, but not sufficient, to restore a normal appearance and function. The mature surgeon, with training and experience, "sees the future." He or she conceptualizes what will work among available options, while visualizing the desired result. A plan is formulated, principles outlined, and techniques and methods chosen.

Fortunately, although each defect is different, all repairs are simplified because the "normal" is unchanging. Often, the contralateral normal remains as a visual standard for comparison. If not, the ideal is the guide. The "normal" nose is visually defined by its dimension, volume, position, projection, platform, symmetry, and expected skin quality, border outline, and three-dimensional contour. Major facial landmarks are described as regional units – adjacent topographic areas of characteristic quality, outline, and three-dimensional contour. A unit approach helps the surgeon conceptualize the goal, define the requirements of repair, balance options, and measure the success of the result. Goals, priorities, stages, materials, and method of tissue transfer are clearer with the ideal normal in mind (*Fig. 6.1* and *Table 6.1*).

In the latter half of the 20th century, Gonzalez-Ulloa *et al.*[29] divided the face into regions, based on skin thickness. Millard[30] envisioned major facial landmarks as "units" and recommended replacing them in their entirety with "like" tissue, of similar color and texture, to avoid a patch-like repair.

Burget and Menick[31] divided the nose into "subunits" based on skin quality, border outline, and three-dimensional contour.

The concept of peripheral and central facial units

The face can be divided into areas of characteristic skin quality, border outline, and three-dimensional contour. It can be divided into peripheral and central units. Practically speaking,

Table 6.1 Gillies' and Millard's "10 commandments" of plastic surgery

- Observation is the basis of diagnosis
- Diagnose before you treat
- Make a pattern of the defect and a plan
- Replace the normal in the normal position and retain it there
- Do something positive
- Treat the primary defect first. Do not let the secondary defect endanger the final result
- Borrow from Peter to pay Paul, if Peter can afford it
- Losses must be replaced in kind
- Never throw anything away, unless you are sure you don't want it
- Never let routine methods become your master
- Never do today what you can honorably put off until tomorrow. When in doubt, don't

(Reproduced from Gillies HD, Millard DR. The principles and art of plastic surgery. Boston: Little Brown, 1957.)

regional unit concepts provide a rational explanation for clinical observation and treatment recommendations.[22,25]

Peripheral units

The forehead and cheek are peripheral facial units. Like a "picture frame," they lie at the periphery of the face and receive secondary intention. Their surfaces are largely flat and expansive and their border outlines variable, according to hairline and eyebrow position. Because their borders are not visible in all views, their borders cannot be compared to the contralateral normal side for symmetry or outline.

So, because the character of peripheral units is less exact and constant, their repair is less demanding and of secondary importance. The principles of their repair differ from those applied to central facial units. The correct restoration of skin quality, not outline or three-dimensional contour, determines success.

Unlike a nasal wound, a moderate forehead defect can be allowed to heal secondarily. The resulting shiny, flat scar, supported by the underlying rigid bony platform of the skull, blends into the normal shiny, tight surface of the forehead without significant distortion or malposition of adjacent landmarks. Rarely, a skin graft may be used to replace the entire forehead unit or a lateral subunit, after discarding any residual skin within the unit. The uniform, shiny quality of the skin graft simulates the expected skin quality and contour of the entire unit or subunit, masking its peripheral scars along the hairline, brow, or contour lines between the lateral and central forehead subunits.

Most often, the lax and excess adjacent skin within the cheek is shared by resurfacing the defect with a nonsubunit rotation advancement flap. Enlarging the wound so that the entire forehead or cheek is recovered with one flap is impractical due to the paucity of available donor excess and the unreliability of flap blood supply. The subunit principle is rarely applied when resurfacing the cheek or forehead.

Central units

The central mid facial units of the nose, lip, and eyelids contribute more significantly to the overall visual facial gestalt and require a different reconstructive approach. The

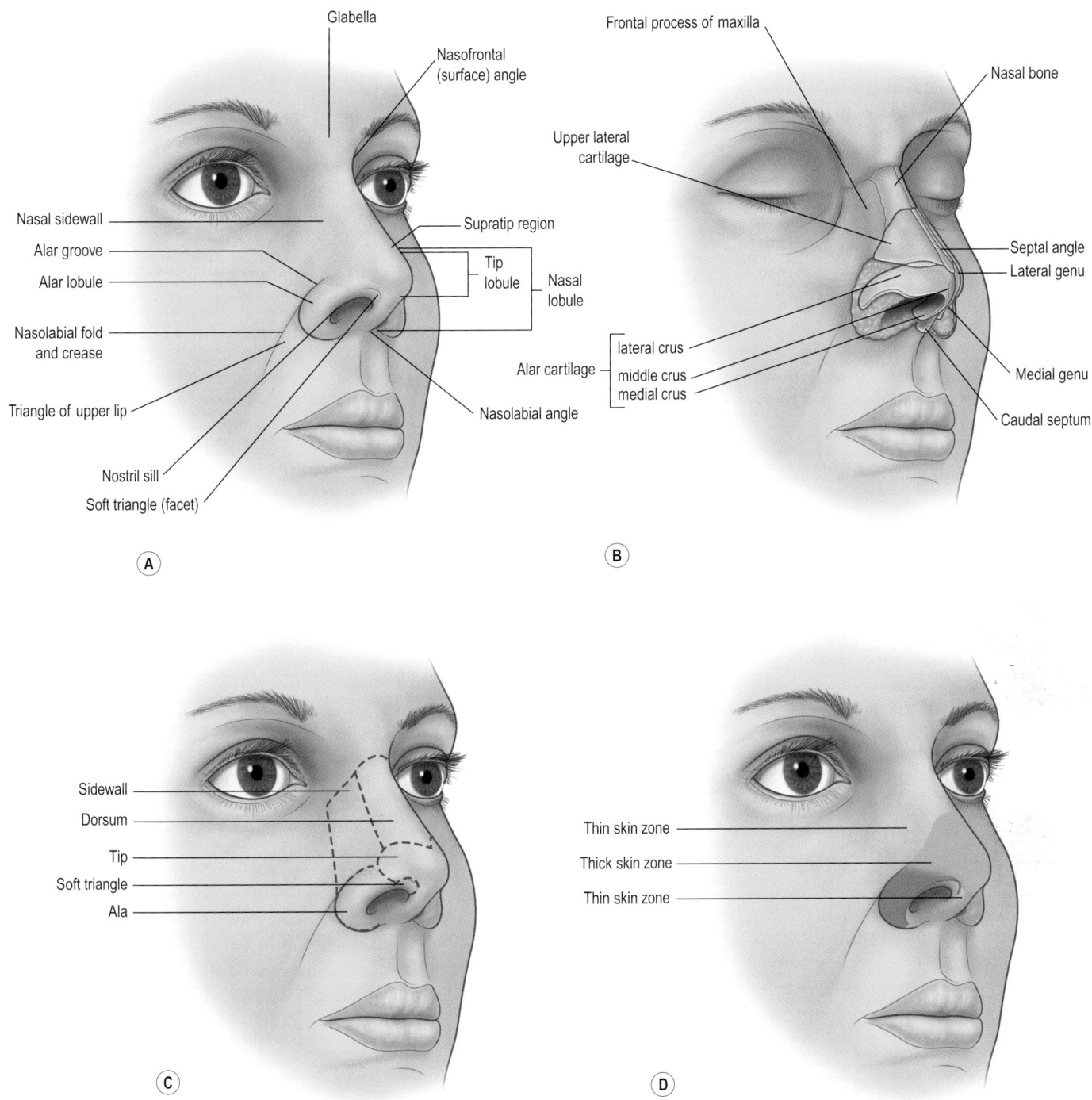

Fig. 6.1 (A–D) Anatomy, surface contour, and subunits.

principles of regional unit reconstruction apply primarily to repair central facial defects, not the peripheral units.

The nose has a fixed border outline, a three-dimensional shape, and contralateral symmetry that must be maintained. Although skin quality is important, landmark outline, contour, and symmetry are of greater importance. The central units are seen in primary gaze and demand the highest priority of repair.

Large nasal defects are reconstructed with regional transposition flaps of exact dimension and outline to avoid tension, collapse, or distortion of adjacent mobile landmarks. The dimension and outline of the wound may be altered by discarding additional residual normal skin within the subunit to resurface the defect as a unit. The external skin surface must be shaped in three dimensions with cartilage grafts for support and contour.

Principles of regional unit repair[25,28]

- Human beings wish to look normal.
- The normal is defined by three-dimensional contour, border outline, and skin quality which describe regional units. They do not correlate with wrinkle or resting skin tension lines.
- The nasal unit consists of the tip, dorsum, columella, and paired alae, sidewalls, and soft triangle subunits.
- Restore units, do not fill defects.
- If a defect, within part of a central unit, is filled without regard to the unit outline, the tissue replacement may appear as a distracting patch within the subunit. The reconstructive goal must restore the character of the unit, rather than simply fill the "hole."
- Alter the wound in site, size, outline, and depth. Discard adjacent normal tissue within convex nasal subunits to improve the result.

When part of a central convex nasal unit is missing, it is often useful to resurface the entire unit or subunit, rather than simply patch the defect. The wound's dimension, outline, or depth is altered. Residual tissue within the subunit may be discarded to enlarge the wound. Or the defect may be decreased in size by local advancement rotation flaps, or changed in border outline by a combination of excision and tissue rearrangement. Subunit resurfacing positions scars so that they are camouflaged within the joins between subunits. More importantly, myofibroblasts lie in the recipient bed under a transferred flap and contract, causing the transposed skin flap to raise above the level of adjacent skin. When an entire convex subunit is resurfaced, the pincushioned flap shrinkwraps around the underlying cartilage framework, augmenting, rather than distorting, the contour of a convex subunit.

The "subunit principle"[22,31]

If a defect of a central convex subunit, such as the tip or ala, is greater than 50% of the subunit, discard adjacent normal tissue within the subunit and resurface the entire subunit, rather than merely "patching the hole."

The consequences of the subunit principle are:

1. The defect may be enlarged and the donor requirement increased. A larger defect may preclude closure with local tissue and necessitate a regional flap repair.
2. The number of stages and the complexity of the repair may be increased.
3. The amount of cartilage material required to support the soft tissues may be increased.
4. Patient morbidity may increase if regional flaps or cartilage grafts are needed.

However, when applied appropriately, the final result may be significantly improved. It should be emphasized, however, that a good result does not depend on any one surgical maneuver. It reflects a series of choices, methods, and tissue manipulations that transfer a correctly thinned covering flap which blends into neighboring tissues, establishing a three-dimensional contour and replacing missing tissues in exact dimension and outline. Resurfacing a facial defect as a unit can be helpful, but it is only a single tool.

Use the contralateral normal or the ideal as a guide

The apparent defect may not reflect the actual tissue loss. Due to edema, tension, gravity, scar, or past repair, the wound may be larger, smaller, or altered in shape. The surgeon must use the contralateral normal – the opposite ala, hemitip or heminose, and hemilip subunit to design a foil template that reflects the size and shape of the missing subunit. If the contralateral normal is absent, a template can be designed from an ideal clay model, based on a moulage of the patient's face, or a template can be designed from another normal face.

Replace tissues in exact dimensions and outline

If a flap is larger than the defect, its bulk pushes adjacent landmarks outward, creating malposition and asymmetry. Excess skin also obscures the surface details created by the underlying support. If the flap is smaller than the defect, neighboring structures are pulled inward. The tension also collapses underlying cartilage grafts.

Exact three-dimensional patterns are designed to fit the needs of the "true" tissue defect, rather than a wound distorted by edema, tension, scar, or prior repair.

Employ templates

An exact foil template of the contralateral normal or ideal is used to design flaps and support grafts. Such templates determine the size of the flap, the shape of its border, or the position of facial landmarks (alar base, nasolabial fold, or alar crease).

Choose ideal donor materials and employ an ideal method of tissue transfer

Millard's admonition to use "like for like" applies.[30] Use lip for lip, cheek for cheek, and a forehead or nasolabial flap for nasal resurfacing. Distant tissues are employed for lining, to fill dead space, create a facial platform, or vascularize an ischemic, contaminated, or radiated wound. However, distant skin does not match the facial skin quality. Distant skin is not used to resurface the face. Regional skin should be used to replace facial skin.

Understand wound healing and tissue transfer

Traditionally, the method of tissue transfer is chosen based on the vascularity and depth of the defect. Skin grafts are employed to resurface well-vascularized superficial defects, when skin and a small amount of subcutaneous tissue are missing. Skin flaps are used to supply bulk to a deep defect or cover a poorly vascularized recipient site, a wound with exposed vital structures, or exposed or restored cartilage and bone. However, even though a donor skin may match the color and texture of the recipient site, the transient ischemia associated with skin graft "take" leads to unpredictable skin color and texture changes. Postoperatively, skin grafts are typically shiny, atrophic, and hypopigmented or hyperpigmented. However, full-thickness skin grafts may shrink modestly, but do not "trapdoor." In contrast, a flap, which maintains its own perfusion, retains the skin quality of its donor site. However, the scar between the flap and the recipient bed contracts, leading to pincushioning. The surface of flaps often develops a convex form as they contract. So skin grafts are best employed to resurface flat or concave recipient sites, such as the nasal sidewall, while skin flaps are most useful when resurfacing convex surfaces, such as the tip or ala, especially when an entire convex subunit is repaired as a unit or subunit. In this way, the surgeon harnesses wound healing and tissue transfer to his or her advantage.

Build on a stable platform

If a nasal injury extends on to the lip and cheek, the lip and cheek are repaired first. Unfortunately, the lip/cheek platform may shift postoperatively with resolution of edema, and late effects of gravity, tension, and scar contraction. The larger and deeper the defect, the greater the risk. If the lip/cheek platform is unstable and the nose is reconstructed at the same operative procedure, the nose may be dragged inferiorly and laterally over time.

Although a small superficial defect of the nose, cheek, and lip can often be rebuilt during a single-stage operation, large deep defects of the cheek and lip are more reliably reconstructed during a preliminary operation to establish a stable platform. Then the nose is built secondarily at a later stage.

Restore a subcutaneous framework of hard and soft tissue

A nose looks normal because it has a nasal shape. Primary and delayed primary support grafts must be placed to support, shape, and brace cover and lining against collapse and contraction. Cartilage must be placed along the nostril margin, even though the alar lobule and soft triangle normally contain no cartilage. Alar batten grafts brace the alar rim and prevent constriction inward, contraction outward, and airway collapse. Once soft tissues are contracted by scar, secondary placement of cartilage grafts is less effective. Precise soft-tissue excision can also add three-dimensional shape by improving overall nasal contour during each surgical stage.

Disregard old scars

To avoid additional incisional scars, bulky flaps are often "thinned" secondarily, during late revision by elevating the peripheral edges of the flap through its border scar. However, it is frequently preferable to disregard old scars and add additional incisions. Using accurate templates, based on the contralateral normal or ideal, the desired three-dimensional concavity of the alar crease or nasolabial fold is marked with ink. Once the ideal landmark position is incised and the wound edges on either side of the "new" incision are elevated, under direct vision, the underlying soft tissue is sculpted in three dimensions to create a flat sidewall, a round ala, and a full medial cheek. The overlying skin is then reapproximated to the newly contoured subcutaneous bed with quilting sutures. The wound is closed. Although a new incisional scar is created, it lies hidden in the border outline of the newly contoured subunits. Visually, the new scar is hidden if the contour depression and the old peripheral border scar become significantly less apparent because the nasal contour is correct.

Employ surgical staging to advantage

Each surgical staging is an opportunity to recreate the defect, return normal to normal, ensure viability, prepare excess tissue for other uses (hingeover lining flaps, soft-tissue bulk), surgically delay, prefabricate, transfer, and modify tissues by interval debulking or shaping, add or alter support grafts, improve imperfections, or treat complications or secondary priorities.

Consider a preliminary operation

A preliminary operation, prior to formal nasal reconstruction, can be helpful. Often, the extent of deformity is obscured by the effects of secondary healing or prior skin grafts or flaps. The defect is recreated and residual tissues returned to their normal position. Then the dimension and position of the defect can be better appreciated and the required tissue replacements more accurately defined. Although past history, physical examination, old operative reports, or radiographs may provide information, the extent of the true defect may only become apparent after recreating the defect.

Excision of scar or soft-tissue bulk can open an occluded airway, permitting its raw surfaces to be resurfaced with a skin graft or local flap. Residual local tissue or adjacent regional flaps can be positioned for later use or surgically delayed to maximize blood supply, especially when scar lies within the territory or injury to the flap's pedicle is suspected. Ischemic or chronically infected tissue may require debridement. Immature tissues are allowed to revascularize, soften, and stabilize. Defects of the lip and cheek may be repaired, establishing a stable platform on which to place the nose at a later date. If indicated, the wound can be biopsied to ensure complete clearance of tumor or immune disease remission.

When a defect is complex, the patient may be anxious and the surgeon uncertain of tissue needs or available options. The diagnosis may need clarification, the wound need preparation, or the problem need to be analyzed to prepare a comprehensive plan. Use time to advantage.

Classification of defects

The requirements and difficulty of repair are determined by the site, size, and depth of injury. Nasal defects are classified into small, superficial, large, deep, or composite defects.[22,25]

Small defect

A small defect is less than 1.5 cm in diameter. Although a skin graft can be employed to resurface larger defects, if the defect is larger than 1.5 cm local flaps are precluded because there is not enough residual skin to "share" over the entire nasal surface without excessive closure tension and landmark distortion.

Superficial defect

Superficial defects include skin and a small amount of underlying subcutaneous fat and nasalis muscle. Vascularized soft tissue remains in the depth of the wound which can revascularize a skin graft or be resurfaced with a flap. If the periosteum or perichondrium is missing, although a small defect may be allowed to heal secondarily, a skin graft is precluded and a vascularized flap will be required.

Adversely located defect

Adversely located defects are those whose position necessitates a regional flap for cover. If the defect is closer than 0.5–1 cm of the nostril margin, local flaps lead to tip and nostril distortion. Local flaps will not reach into the infratip lobule or columella. Regional flaps are used to repair these adversely located defects, even though the wound is not necessarily large.

Large defect

Large defects are greater than 1.5 cm in size. Insufficient skin remains over the residual nose to redistribute with a local flap. Skin must be added by transferring a skin graft or regional excess from the cheek or forehead.

Deep defect

Deep defects are those in which the underlying supportive framework or lining is missing and must be replaced to prevent soft-tissue and airway collapse, and landmark distortion.

This includes the ala, even though cartilage is not normally present. If a significant area of alar skin and its compact fibrofatty middle layer is excised, cartilage support must be placed.

But if a cartilage graft is needed, a skin graft or local flap cannot be employed. A skin graft will not "take" over bare cartilage grafts. And a local flap is precluded because delicate cartilage grafts collapse under the wound tension associated with local flaps which share residual tissue over the nasal surface. So, although a small rim defect can be closed with a composite skin graft, significant full-thickness defects require a vascularized regional flap for cover.

Composite defects

Composite defects[32] extend from the nose on to the adjacent cheek and upper lip. These nose, cheek, and lip units differ visually, anatomically, and functionally. The quality, outline, and contour are different for each facial unit. And the nose sits on the midface cheek and lip platform with characteristic projection, position, and angled relationships.

The degree of tissue loss varies from unit to unit and the need for cover, lining, support, and soft and hard tissue will be different.

For the surgeon, the simplest solution is to "fill the hole," replacing missing skin and soft tissue with a single flap. But it is difficult to reproduce the delicate three-dimensional character of a composite defect with a single flap. Geometrically, the shortest distance between two points is a straight line and a single flap often takes a "surgical shortcut" and fails to provide enough skin to restore three-dimensional contours. Scar contraction of a defect which includes multiple units draws a single flap into a domelike mass, outlined by patch-like peripheral scars. Using separate grafts or flaps for each facial unit better positions scars in the expected joins between landmarks and helps control flap pincushioning.

Treatment/surgical technique and postoperative care

Although "simple" at first glance, small and superficial defects are difficult to repair. Surgeons and patients fail to appreciate the complexity of nasal contour, the paucity of excess tissue, the difficulty of matching the remaining skin in color and texture, and the risk of distorting the residual mobile tip and nostril margins. Many options are available. The time, trouble,

morbidity, donor and recipient scars, number of stages, time to wound maturity, and cost must be balanced against the likelihood of secondary deformity.

Zones of nasal skin quality

The nose is covered by skin and an underlying layer of subcutaneous fat and nasalis muscle which lie over a rigid bony elastic framework of cartilage and fibrofatty support. However, the quality of the skin is not uniform, unless the skin is atrophic due to old age, sun injury, or radiation injury. In the normal nose, it can be divided into areas of thin smooth skin and thickly pitted skin. Note that the zones of skin quality do not correspond to the nasal units, which are defined by contour.

In the superior half of the nose, the skin of the dorsum and sidewalls is thin, smooth, pliable, and mobile. A modest excess of skin is present, which permits primary closure or a local flap to close small defects without distortion of adjacent mobile landmarks. A modest amount of skin can also be recruited from the cheek to close a small sidewall or alar defect. Although a simultaneous rhinoplasty, hoping to decrease the size of the nasal skeleton and relatively increase the available skin, has been recommended to ease the closure of small defects in a large nose, this is rarely helpful.

The inferior half of the nose is covered by a zone of tight skin, pitted with sebaceous glands, and adherent to the underlying deep structures. The thick skin zone begins in the alar grooves, crosses 5–10 mm above the supratip region, and extends inferiorly towards the caudal borders of the tip and alar subunits. About 2–3 mm above the alar margins and a few millimeters below the outermost point of the tip and on to the columella, the skin thins and loses its sebaceous quality. The lower half of the infratip lobule, including the soft triangle and columella, is covered by thin, but adherent, skin fixed to the underlying structures. The tip and alar margins are mobile and easily distorted by contracting scar or inaccurate tissue replacement.

Restoring nasal cover

Small, superficial defects

Healing by secondary intention

The body responds to injury by epithelialization, the formation of granulation tissue, and myofibroblast contraction. The process is simple, inexpensive, somewhat slow, but often satisfactory.

Healing by secondary intention is recommended for wounds created by a destructive process which precludes primary closure. These include electrodesiccation and curettage or those associated with wound dehiscence, infection, or necrosis. To avoid further injury due to desiccation or trauma, secondary healing is not employed if vital deep structures are exposed in the base of the wound.

No net gain in tissue occurs with secondary healing. Wound contraction progresses only to the degree that adjacent tissue can be pulled into the defect. The residual gap is filled with collagen covered with a shiny adherent thin layer of epidermis, containing few melanocytes or skin appendages. The result is a pale, shiny, flat, white scar. Secondary healing may be employed for defects which lie within a flat or concave nasal surface, at a distance from mobile landmarks, especially when they lie within sun or radiated injured skin where imperfections of skin quality due to spontaneous healing are less apparent.

A small superficial defect of the flat tight dorsum, sidewall, or deep alar crease may heal satisfactorily by secondary intention. However, imperfections in color or texture or contour depressions are visible in the thicker skin of the tip and ala. The mobile tip and nostril margins are also at risk for distortion due to scar contracture.

Despite limitations, almost any wound will heal spontaneously, if medical illness, cost, lifestyle, or lack of patient interest precludes a more formal repair. If the patient is unhappy, repair in the future.

Primary repair

Because a modest excess of skin is present in the more lax upper two-thirds of the nose, a primary repair may be possible if the defect is less than 5–6 mm. Because no extra skin is available in the thick adherent skin of the tip and ala, primary closure leads to landmark distortion and wide depressed scars.

Skin grafting

Skin grafts have many advantages.[22,25] No new scars are added to the nasal surface and the amount of locally available excess tissue is not a limiting factor. Skin grafts are typically harvested from preauricular, postauricular, or supraclavicular donor sites.

However, a skin graft must lie on a well-vascularized bed to ensure "take" and will not reliably survive when placed on denuded cartilage or a cartilage graft. Bare cartilage must be covered with a vascularized flap. A skin graft, placed over a narrow primary cartilage graft, may revascularize by the bridging phenomenon; however, this is a risky technique. The size of the cartilage graft must be limited. Complete or partial skin graft necrosis may occur.

The aesthetic result of skin graft is unpredictable. Because of the transient ischemia which accompanies skin graft transfer, the quality of donor skin deteriorates. Skin grafts often appear pale, smooth, and atrophic. Postauricular skin may remain red. Supraclavicular skin appears brown and shiny. The hairless patch between the tragus and sideburn provides a better match, especially when applied to the dorsum, sidewall, or columella.

The traditional full-thickness skin graft may blend satisfactorily into the relatively smooth atrophic upper nose within the thin skin of the dorsum and sidewall. However, traditional skin grafts, within the zone of thick skin zone of the tip and ala, often appear as depressed, shiny, off-colored patches, unless the skin of the recipient site is atrophic due to sun injury or radiation.

Preauricular and postauricular skin grafts

Hairless preauricular skin is a good donor site. A strip of skin 2–2.5 cm wide can be harvested. Larger grafts may transfer fine vellus hair in women or bearded skin in men. Postauricular skin can be harvested from the back of the ear and mastoid, across the postauricular crease. In unusual circumstances, the entire posterior surface of the ear can be taken and the donor site skin grafted with more distant skin.

Full-thickness forehead skin graft (Figs 6.2–6.6)

Although not traditionally transferred as a skin graft, forehead skin is useful for resurfacing small superficial defects, especially of the tip and ala. Forehead skin is acknowledged as the best match to replace nasal skin. Forehead skin and its underlying compact fibrofatty subcutaneous layer are thicker and stiffer than other donors. Significant amounts of soft tissue can be carried with the graft, permitting the replacement of the deeper soft tissues. Forehead skin grafts revascularize normally, with progressive changes in color from white to blue to pink. A good take is routinely expected. However, when failure seems imminent, the clinical evolution of the forehead skin graft is unique. Unlike grafts harvested from other sites, early separation does not occur. A hard and tightly adherent eschar develops and should be left undisturbed and not debrided. It may remain fixed to the underlying tissues for 4–6 weeks. After spontaneous separation, the surgeon often finds that the wound is healed, filled, and the aesthetic result is good. One to 1.5 cm of forehead skin is easily harvested below the frontal hairline with primary closure of the donor site. The scar is usually excellent and easily covered by hair. FIGS **6.4–6.6** APPEAR ONLINE ONLY

Skin graft technique

A skin graft must be placed on a vascular bed to ensure "take." It must be in direct contact and will not survive if tented across the defect or separated by hematoma or seroma. It must be immobile to allow the development of vascular connections to the recipient site.

Excessive coagulation of the recipient site is avoided, if possible. It is often helpful to delay skin grafting for 10–14 days to allow spontaneous separation of electrical burn eschar and the development of granulation tissue. The recipient site is protected from desiccation by daily cleansing with soap and water and multiple applications of antibiotic or petrolatum ointment to prevent drying out of the soft tissues, periosteum, or perichondrium. The skin graft is then applied as a delayed primary graft, avoiding exposure of the underlying cartilage during preparatory debridement.

A pattern is made of the defect prior to debridement. The margins and base of the wound are freshened to create a clean, sharp, right-angle skin edge and a vascular bed. Old scar, skin graft, or granulation tissue is removed. A pre- or postauricular skin graft is elevated in the subcutaneous layer and a forehead skin graft over the frontalis muscle. Fat is removed from the undersurface of the graft with curved scissors, but the graft is not necessarily thinned to dermis. The thickness of skin graft and its underlying fat should match the depth of recipient site. The graft is laid on the prepared bed, trimmed, and inset with a single layer of fine sutures, peripherally. Quilting sutures are placed through the skin graft and into the recipient bed to prevent lateral motion. A layer of antibiotic ointment and fine gauze is applied, followed by a soft foam bolus. Traditionally, individual bolus tie-over sutures are fixed to the wound edge and tied over the bolus dressing to each other. However, it is quicker and more efficient to tie a single 4-0 or 5-0 polypropylene suture about 5–10 mm from the wound edge and then criss-cross back and forth across the bolus in a running fashion. With each pass, the needle takes a bite of skin

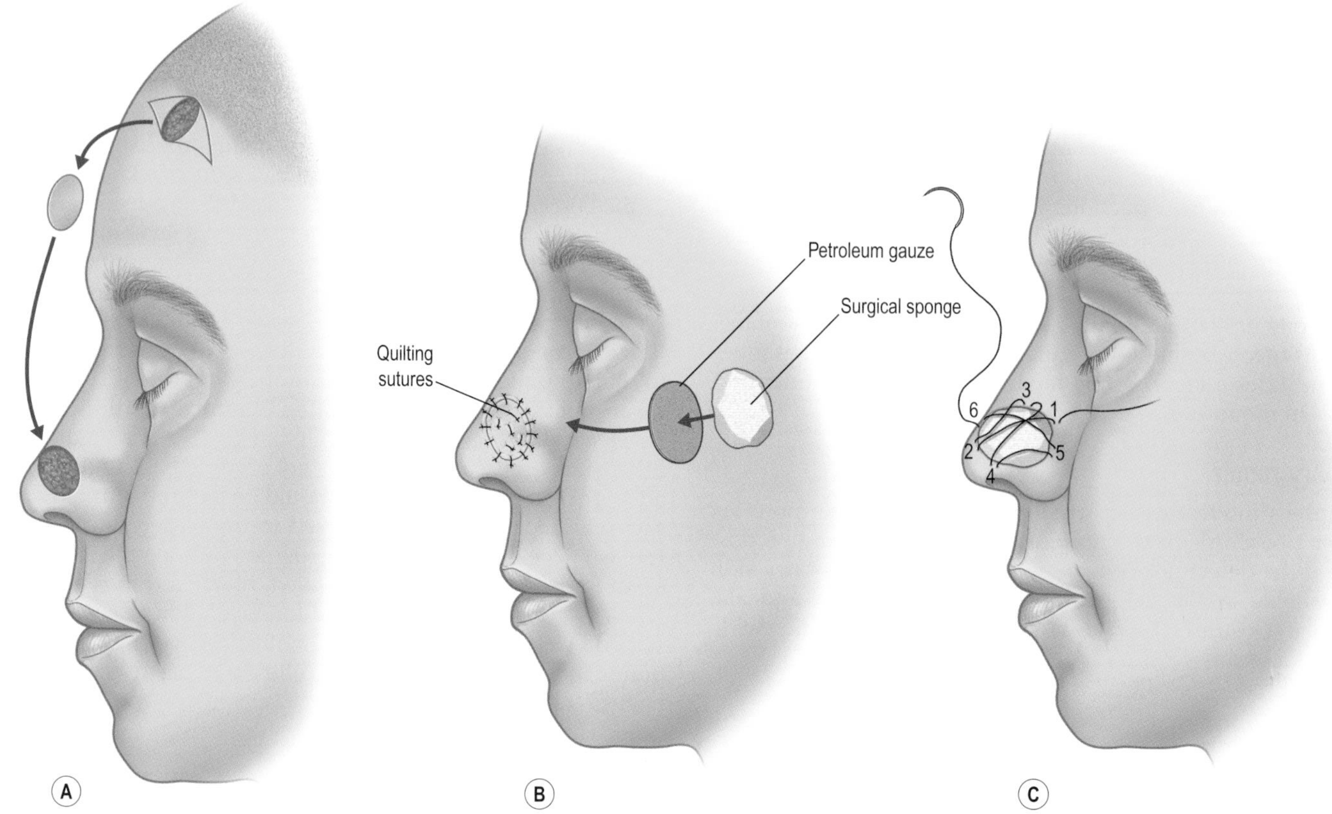

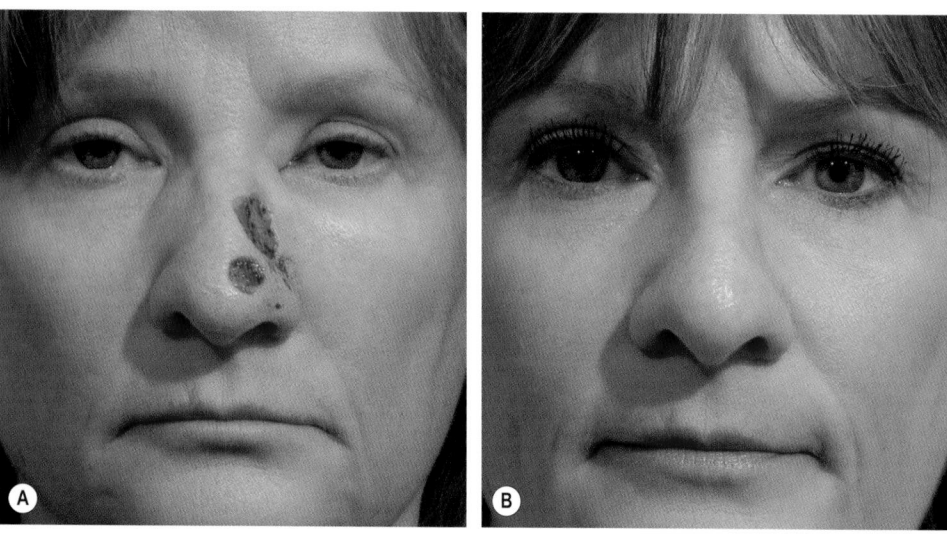

Fig. 6.2 (A–C) Forehead skin graft technique.

Fig. 6.3 (A) Before and **(B)** after full-thickness forehead skin graft to the nasal tip and preauricular skin graft to the left nasal sidewall to resurface small superficial defects within the dorsum, sidewall, and tip.

several millimeters away from the wound edge, finally tying the suture to itself. The surgeon only clips the suture in one or two areas to remove the dressing easily.

The stent dressing immobilizes the skin graft postoperatively and reinforces the quilting sutures. However, it is not a "pressure" dressing and should not be applied to stop bleeding or prevent hematoma. Initially, the skin graft appears white. Over several days, perfusion increases and the graft changes color from blue to visibly pink. Although the bolus

can be removed earlier, it is best left in place for 1 week. If the defect is repaired delicately with fine sutures and without tension, suture marks do not occur.

Local flaps

Unlike a skin graft, the quality of skin transferred as a vascularized flap maintains its original quality. So the color and texture of flaps are predictable. A skin flap is also thicker than a graft and may better supply missing subcutaneous bulk.

An excess of skin is present within the more mobile upper "thin" skin zones of the dorsum and sidewall and can be shared from an area of excess to one of deficiency. But there is no excess within the "thick" skin zone of the tip and ala.

Remember that local flaps add no new skin but simply share the available, but limited, excess within the upper nose to an area of deficiency. If the defect is larger than 1.5 cm, the remaining skin surface is insufficient to redistribute over the nasal skeleton without excess closure attention and distortion of mobile landmarks. Guidelines, applicable to almost all local nasal flaps, should be followed carefully. Local flaps are used for small superficial defects, greater than 5–10 mm from the nostril margins and above the tip defining points. Commonly described local flaps will not reach into the infratip area. Unfortunately, these rules are often broken, leading to nasal collapse, tip and alar margin malpositions. To avoid the morbidity or stages required by regional flaps, local flaps may be used inappropriately to resurface large defects or those near the tip or rim. In such instances, it would be better to allow the wound to heal secondarily or apply a skin graft.

The single-lobe transposition flap *(Fig. 6.7)*

A modest amount of excess mobile and lax skin is available within the superior nose. A single-lobe transposition flap, designed as a Banner or Romberg flap, is useful for small open defects.[33,34] These flaps transpose skin through an arc of 90°, taking excess from one axis to fill a deficiency in another. Because the skin in the superior nose is relatively mobile, available, and lies at a distance from the nostril margins, these small local flaps are unlikely to distort the tip or alar margin. However, if the flap donor scar crosses the bridge transversely, a depressed scar may become visible on profile view. Single-lobed flaps are not useful in the inflexible thick skin of the tip or ala, which shifts poorly. Deforming dog-ears or displacement of adjacent mobile landmarks are common.

The dorsal nasal flap

The dorsal nasal flap elevates skin, subcutaneous tissue, and muscle just above the perichondrium and periosteum and slides excess from the glabella towards the tip. The flap is best applied to defects within the dorsum and superior tip subunit.[35–37] It is vascularized from facial and angular vessels along the sidewall and medial canthus. Closure is facilitated by advancing cheek skin upward on to the nasal sidewall. The dorsal nasal flap can resurface the nasal tip and dorsum and parts of the ala or sidewall with local skin. Unfortunately, it slides thicker glabellar skin and soft tissue downward on to the nasal sidewall near the medial canthus where a mismatch in skin thickness may create an iatrogenic epicanthal fold. The depth of the radix may be obliterated, effacing the nasal root. Recent modifications have eliminated the glabellar extension. As the dorsal flap slides caudally, a dog-ear is excised inferiorly. Ideally, its borders are planned to lie along the dorsal sidewall junction. The inferior aspect of the flap's border may be visible as a depressed scar crossing the smooth surface of the tip unit. Like all local flaps, the larger the defect and the closer it lies to the nostril margin, the more likely the tip or rim will be distorted by tension or displaced by poor design.

The geometric bilobed flap

The bilobed flap is recommended for defects within the thick, stiff skin of the inferior nose.

The bilobed principle is applied.[38–40] Skin is shifted from an area of excess to an area of deficiency by designing the first lobe adjacent to the tip or alar defect. A second lobe, which lies at a distance in an area of tissue availability within the upper nose, is outlined in continuity. As the primary lobe shifts to repair the defect, the secondary lobe resurfaces the defect from the primary lobe. The tertiary defect from the second lobe is closed primarily, within the area of excess.

Traditionally, bilobed flaps were designed with 180° rotation. This created large dog-ears. The dog-ear excision narrowed the flap's vascular base, jeopardizing blood supply. McGregor and Soutar,[39] and later Zitelli,[40] developed a geometric design to decrease the flap's rotation to 90–100° and incorporated a dog-ear excision which did not diminish blood supply. It is useful for defects measuring 0.5–1.5 cm in the inferior nose.

The rotation-advancement flap can be oriented anywhere around the defect but the pedicle base must be positioned away from the nostril margin to prevent distortion. The second lobe must also lie within the loose excess skin of the upper sidewall or dorsum. It can be based medially or laterally. The pattern should not extend on to the cheek or lower lid.

Several rules apply:

1. The pivot point is established at a distance from the defect equal to one-half of the defect's diameter (or the radius of the defect). The flap is based laterally for tip defects and medially for defects of the alar lobule. The further the pivot point away from the defect, the larger the flap. Sharing the same pivot point, the circumferences of a larger outer and smaller inner concentric circle are drawn on to the nasal skin. The circumference of the outer circle is outlined at a distance three times the radius of the defect. The second smaller inner circle is marked to equal the distance from the pivot point to the center of the initial defect (the diameter of the defect). Because the nasal surface is round, not flat, a strip of foil or bent paper ruler, rather than a straight ruler, is used as a template which is rotated around the pivot point, like individual spokes of a wheel, until the circumference of both concentric circles is determined.

2. An exact pattern of the circular nasal defect is positioned immediately adjacent to the defect, along the outer concentric circle. The first lobe should replace the defect exactly, to prevent tip or alar rim distortion on closure. Because the second lobe lies within the more mobile skin of the upper nose, it can be designed slightly smaller than the defect. The secondary defect can be partially closed by recruitment of lax adjacent skin within the upper nose. A dog-ear excision, which extends lateral to the outer circle, is added to the second lobe.

A dog-ear excision is marked from the defect to the pivot point, creating space for the flap to rotate and advance. The flap rotates less than 100° with a wide base to maintain flap blood supply.

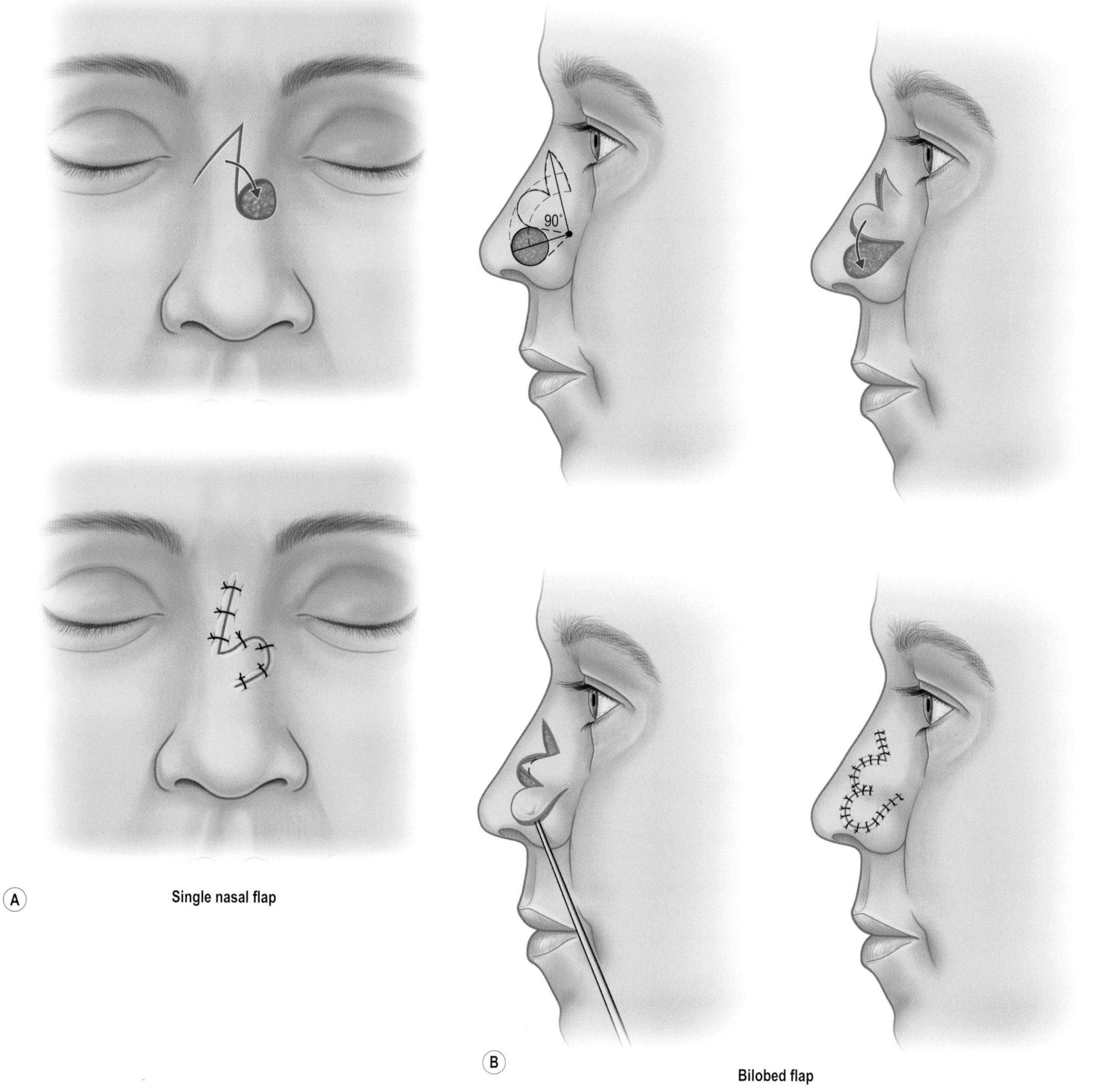

Fig. 6.7 The **(A)** single, **(B)** bilobed, and **(C)** dorsal nasal flaps.

3. The dog-ear extending from the defect of the pivot point is excised. The first and second lobes, including the distal dog-ear, are elevated above the periosteum. The flap includes skin, subcutaneous fat, and nasalis muscle. Residual normal nasal skin is undermined widely over the perichondrium and periosteum.

4. Significant pincushioning is infrequent with the bilobed flap, if it is carefully repaired, in layers. The tertiary defect, in the more mobile upper nose, is closed in layers. This pushes the flap inferiorly, preventing the tendency of the flap to return to its donor site. The primary lobe, after appropriate "thinning" so that its skin surface will match the level of the adjacent normal skin, is transferred to the primary defect. The secondary lobe is transposed to fill the gap created by the first. Each flap is fixed in place

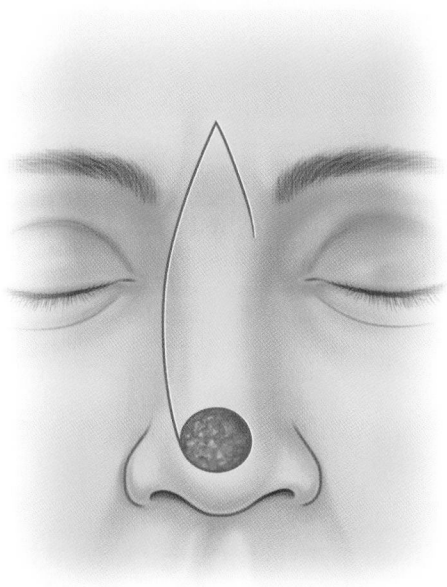

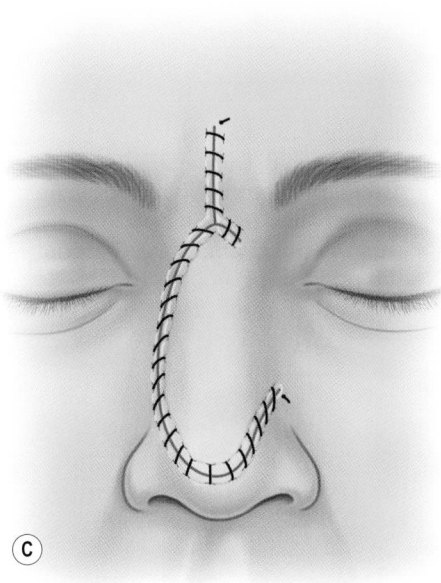

(c)

Fig. 6.7, cont'd

with sutures to approximate muscle, the subcuticular layer, and skin.

Unfortunately, even with careful intraoperative planning, postoperative tip or nostril distortion is common, especially when the defect lies within the tip or ala. Although planned as a single-stage repair, it is not uncommon to revise scars, recreate the obliterated alar crease, or reposition the nostril margin.

The geometric bilobed flap is effective. But it should be limited to defects of the tip which are less than or equal to

1.5 cm in diameter and which lie more than 1 cm away from the nostril margin. This precludes its use for significant alar defects. Despite the relatively small size of these defects, the technique is time-consuming, the dissection extensive, scars multiple, swelling significant, and distortions common.

The one-stage nasolabial flap *(Fig. 6.8)*

The one-stage nasolabial flap can resurface defects of the nasal sidewall and ala, up to 2 cm in size.[25] Excess skin of the medial cheek, lateral to the nasolabial fold, is transferred as a random-pattern extension of an advancing cheek flap. Unlike local flaps which redistribute residual nasal skin, this technique "adds" regional cheek skin to the nasal surface. This minimizes the risk of landmark distortion and permits the use of alar support grafts without fear of collapse due to excessive tension. FIG **6.8** APPEARS ONLINE ONLY

1. The sidewall and alar subunits are outlined in ink. Alar subunit excision is not performed but skin, which remains between the defect in the inferior nostril rim, can be excised, enlarging the defect inferiorly to the nostril margin. This positions the scar along the nostril border and improves the flap's blending with the recipient site. The underlying lining is braced with a septal or ear cartilage graft to prevent collapse or retraction of the nostril margin. The ends of the cartilage graft are buried, medially and laterally, in subcutaneous pockets along the rim and at the alar base, and fixed with percutaneous 5-0 polypropylene sutures. The cartilage graft is quilted to the underlying lining to fix the support graft and brace the nostril margin.

2. The nasolabial crease is marked and a pattern of the defect is positioned exactly adjacent to the nasolabial fold so that the late cheek scar lies exactly in the nasolabial crease. A dog-ear excision is marked inferiorly, distal to the template. Ensure that the sliding cheek advancement has adequate length to swing and correctly position the nasolabial extension on to the nasal defect. The most important flap dimension is width, which should equal the width of the defect. The distal margin of the flap will be trimmed during wound closure and does not need to be predetermined. The flap is elevated in continuity with the distal dog-ear. The superior lateral incision for the alar or sidewall flap extension should not extend higher than the alar remnant that must be "jumped over" to reach the recipient site. A higher incision is unnecessary and may impair blood supply.

3. The nasolabial skin extension and the cheek flap are undermined, with a few millimeters of subcutaneous fat, laterally for 3–5 cm. The cheek is advanced, fixing its underlying raw surface to the deep tissues along the nasal facial groove. This suture fixation advances the cheek flap, closes the donor defect, and restores the nasofacial sulcus. It eliminates lateral and vertical tension on the nasolabial extension, which travels with a cheek flap to resurface the primary defect. The vascularity of the random extension is good, but can be impaired by tension.

4. Excess subcutaneous fat is excised to match the thickness of the flap to the depth of the recipient bed.

Absorbable sutures can be placed to fix the deep surface of the flap gently to the underlying soft tissues at the ideal alar crease, if vascularity is maintained. If necessary, the crease can be recreated secondarily. The distal flap is gently laid over the inferior aspect of the nasal wound and trimmed to fit. The incisions are closed in layers.

Final scars blend within the sidewall or lie in the nasolabial fold. Pincushioning of this nonsubunit skin replacement can occur, but is minimized if the ala is supported and braced by primary cartilage grafts to control nostril margin shape and position.

The one-stage nasolabial flap is useful for defects of the sidewall and ala which are not effectively repaired with other local flaps. It can also be used to resurface the upper lip and nasal sill in a composite defect of the nose, lip, and cheek.[41-43] It is often combined with the Millard fat flip flap,[15,16] which hinges over excess subcutaneous fat, from the lateral cheek, to restore missing premaxillary soft-tissue bulk.

Large, deep, and adversely located defects

The superiorly based two-stage subunit nasolabial flap (Figs 6.9–6.11)

The two-stage nasolabial flap[22,44] transfers excess skin from the medial cheek, just lateral to the nasolabial fold, supplied by blood vessels which originate from the underlying facial and angular arteries, passing through the underlying

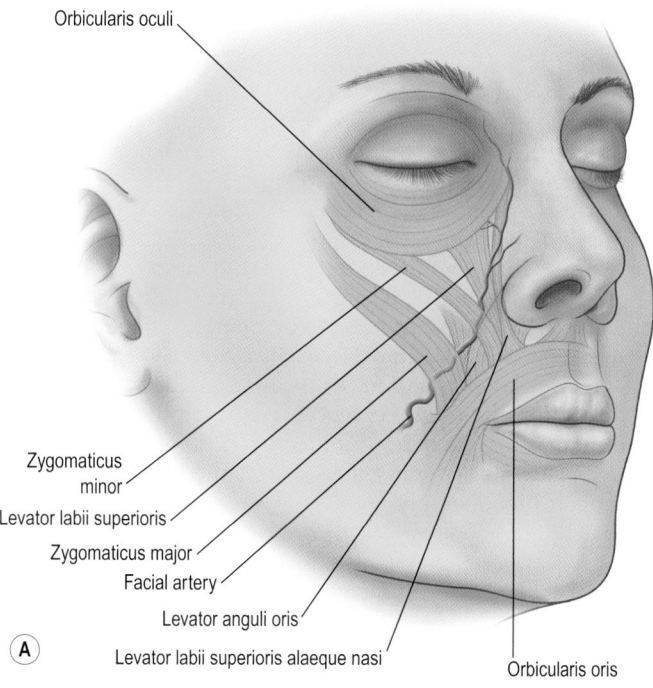

Orbicularis oculi
Zygomaticus minor
Levator labii superioris
Zygomaticus major
Facial artery
Levator anguli oris
(A)
Levator labii superioris alaeque nasi
Orbicularis oris

Fig. 6.9 (A, B) A two-stage nasolabial flap is employed to resurface the ala as a subunit. Residual normal skin is excised adjacent to the defect and the entire subunit is resurfaced as a subunit at the first stage. The superiorly based two-stage nasolabial flap is perfused by axial vessels which pass through the underlying facial musculature to vascularize the proximal flap base. Primary cartilage must be placed to support and brace the nostril margin. One month later, the proximal pedicle is divided, the alar inset completed after soft-tissue sculpturing, and the cheek donor site closed to position the donor scar exactly in the nasal labial fold.

subcutaneous tissue, above and below the levator labii muscle. Although the narrow skin pedicle contributes a modest random blood supply, the flap is a subcutaneously based island flap. If the underlying subcutaneous vascular base is intact, the flap is reliable even if skin lateral to the ala is scarred or has been excised. The subcutaneous pedicle permits easy transposition and the narrow skin component eliminates the superior dog-ear and its accompanying scar from extending on to the nasal sidewall on wound closure. The flap is designed with its medial border exactly along the nasolabial fold to place the final scar exactly in the nasolabial crease. In young patients or those with a poorly defined fold, the nasolabial crease may be indistinct and should be marked with ink preoperatively, before sedation or general anesthesia. FIGS **6.10, 6.11** APPEAR ONLINE ONLY

A two-stage nasolabial flap is best employed to resurface the convex ala as a subunit. Residual skin within the alar subunit is excised so that the entire subunit is resurfaced, rather than just patched.

Stage 1

The nasal subunits and nasolabial fold are marked with ink. An exact template is designed, based on the contralateral ala. The template is positioned adjacent to the nasolabial crease at the level of the oral commissure to ensure an adequate arc of rotation. The superior pedicle is tapered to a point lying just at the upper end of the nasolabial crease. A triangular dog-ear excision is designed distally exactly lateral to the nasolabial fold.

Residual skin within the alar subunit is discarded. The contralateral alar template is used to design a cartilage support graft – most often of conchal cartilage – with the correct dimension and nostril margin outline. The graft's medial and lateral ends are buried in subcutaneous pockets with percutaneous sutures within the soft triangle and the alar base. The graft is sutured to the underlying lining.

The skin flap is elevated from distal to proximal with 2–3 mm of fat.

The dissection is deepened superiorly, protecting the flap's base, which is incised in the subcutaneous fat more broadly than the proximal skin pedicle. Restricting subcutaneous fibrous bands are released. Undermining continues until the flap can be comfortably transferred to the defect. The cheek is advanced and the donor site closed in layers, after excision of the distal dog-ear. The flap is inset with a single layer of skin sutures. The exposed raw pedicle is covered with antibiotic ointment.

Stage 2

Three weeks later, the pedicle is divided. Skin is re-elevated with 2–3 mm of fat over the lateral aspect of the alar inset. Underlying subcutaneous fat and scar are excised, sculpting a convex alar contour and a defined alar crease. The flap is reapproximated to the recipient site. The superior aspect of nasolabial cheek scar is reopened, excess skin and soft tissue excised, and the cheek closed.

Practically speaking, the nasolabial flap has a limited role in nasal reconstruction. Because of the limited excess available in the medial cheek, there is only enough nasolabial tissue to resurface a defect of about 2 cm in width. Although this is a reliable flap, excessive undermining or tension may lead to

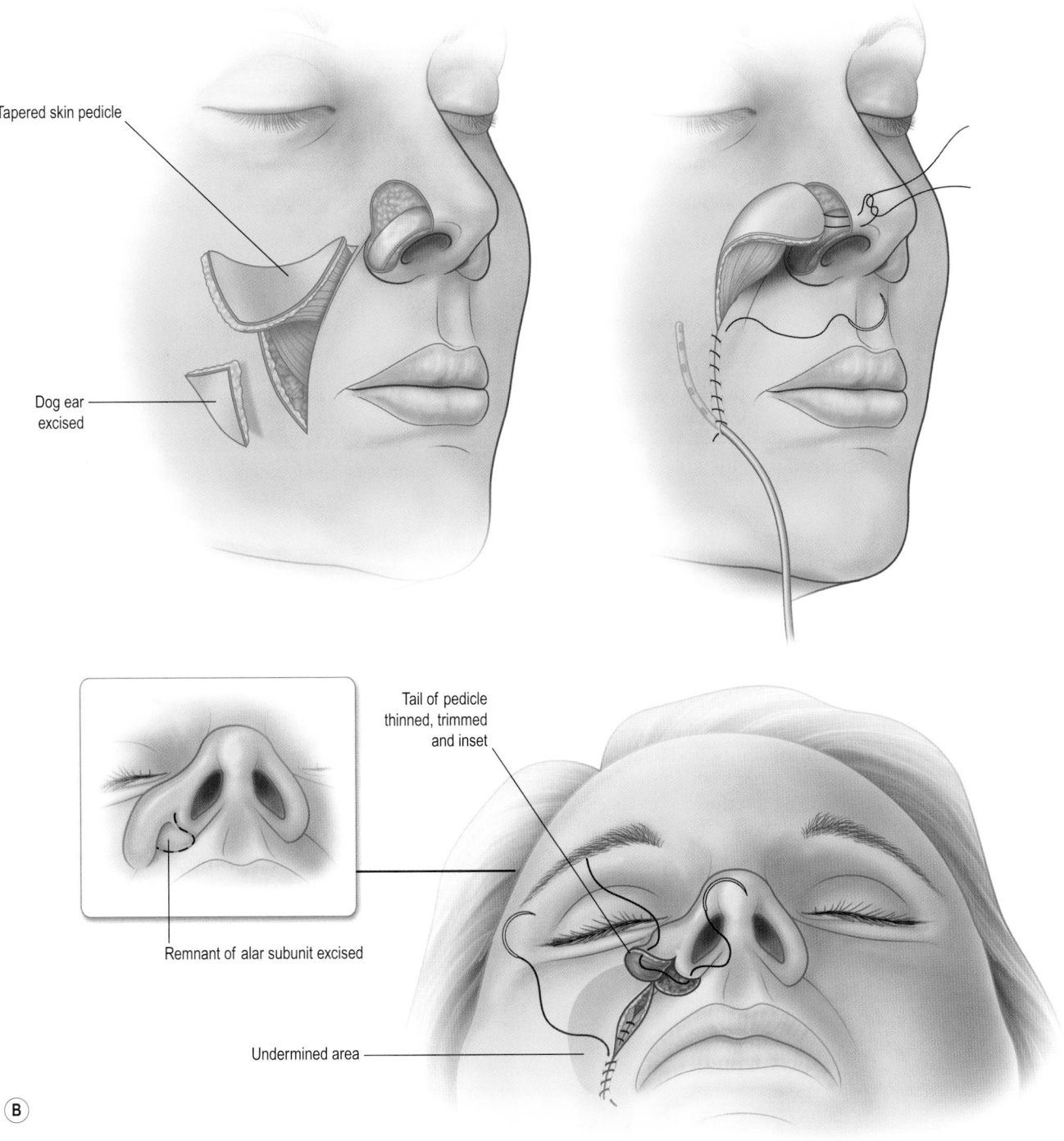

Tapered skin pedicle

Dog ear excised

Tail of pedicle thinned, trimmed and inset

Remnant of alar subunit excised

Undermined area

(B)

Fig. 6.9, cont'd

necrosis. It will not reliably revascularize a skin graft for lining or maintain its blood supply if folded for cover and lining. Its arc of rotation and reach are limited. It can be transposed to the ala, columella, or to resurface the upper lip but it will not safely reach the tip or dorsum. Although a nasolabial flap scar may be hidden in the nasolabial fold, the cheek becomes flattened and may necessitate a contralateral excision of medial cheek tissue to improve symmetry with the opposite cheek. A nasolabial flap routinely transfers beard in the male.

The two-stage nasolabial flap is employed to resurface the entire ala, as a subunit, or an alar defect which extends a few millimeters above the alar crease on to the nasal sidewall. Although the alar crease will be obliterated if the defect extends into the sidewall, a secondary operation can be performed to restore the alar crease. It can also resurface the columella or a nonnasal defect of the lip or the platform for the nasal base.

The forehead flap

The forehead with its superior color, texture, size, reach, vascularity, lining applications, and forgiving donor site is the first choice for most nasal repairs. It is multilaminar, composed of skin, subcutaneous fat, frontalis muscle, and a thin underlying areolar layer which separates it from frontal periosteum. Although forehead skin matches the nose in color, texture, and thickness, a forehead flap is thicker than nasal skin. Excess frontalis and subcutaneous fat must be removed to thin the flap to blend into the adjacent facial skin.

The forehead is perfused from the supraorbital, supratrochlear, the superficial temporal and posterior auricular arteries. Flaps can be based on each of these pedicles – the median forehead flap, the horizontal forehead flap, the up-and-down flap, or the scalping flap.

Today, the paramedian forehead flap is most often used. It transfers central forehead tissue on a unilateral vertical axial blood supply, based on the supratrochlear vessels. Its point of rotation is centered inferiorly towards the medial canthus. The anatomic studies of MacCarthy et al.[13] and Reece et al.[14] demonstrate that the paramedian forehead is perfused by a anastomotic arcade from the supratrochlear, supraorbital, infraorbital, dorsal nasal, and angular branches of the facial artery (*Fig. 6.12*).

The paramedian flap is the first choice for nasal resurfacing because of its vascularity, size, reach, reliability, and relatively minimal morbidity.[22,25,45,46] It takes skin from high on the forehead, under the hairline, with a narrow inferior pedicle base, within or inferior to the medial eyebrow. The inferior aspect of the donor site can be closed primarily. If a gap remains superiorly, it is allowed to heal secondarily. Wound contraction and re-epithelialization close any superior residual defect. Because the gap is away from the mobile brow, eyebrow distortion does not occur. Because the proximal pedicle is narrow, medialization of the eyebrow is not significant.

A paramedian forehead flap can resurface any nasal defect without significant donor deformity. Its pedicle is based on either the right or left supratrochlear vessels. A central nasal defect can be resurfaced on either pedicle, but a unilateral nasal defect is resurfaced with the ipsilateral pedicle to decrease the distance between its pivot point and the defect, unless precluded by an old scar within its territory. If the hairline is extremely low or the forehead scarred, pre-expansion may be considered, but is not routine.[47–50]

The two-stage forehead flap (*Figs 6.13–6.16*)

Anatomically, the supratrochlear vessels pass over the orbital rim, external to the periosteum, sandwiched between the corrugator and frontalis muscles. The vessels then travel vertically upward into the frontalis muscle. At the mid-forehead level, they pass through the muscle and lie in a superficial, subdermal position at the hairline. ⊕ FIGS **6.15, 6.16** APPEAR ONLINE ONLY

The flap can be transferred as an island flap,[51] in one stage, but excessive bulk of the pedicle, passing under tight glabellar skin, may jeopardize its blood supply or distort the nasal root. Most importantly, an aesthetic reconstruction can rarely be obtained in a single stage.

Traditionally, a forehead flap is transferred in two stages.[22] At the first stage, the flap is elevated over the periosteum. Frontalis muscle and subcutaneous fat are excised over the distal 1–2 cm. The distally thinned flap is transferred to the recipient site, perfused proximally through its thick proximal pedicle. During the second stage, 3 or 4 weeks later, when the distal flap has become vascularized by the recipient site, the pedicle is divided. The superior aspect is re-elevated, debulked, and the skin inset is completed.

Unfortunately, excision of muscle and subcutaneous fat, at the time of the initial transfer, removes its myocutaneous blood supply and may diminish vascularity. Although relatively safe, flap necrosis may occur in smokers, if the flap is under tension, or in patients undergoing major nasal repairs which require large flaps and wide initial soft-tissue thinning or flaps with multiple narrow extensions for the ala or columella. Most importantly, although tip and alar cartilage support may be placed at the first stage, the skin of the distal nose – the tip and ala – cannot be re-elevated. The most aesthetic part of the nose cannot be altered prior to pedicle division.

Although the two-stage forehead flap is routinely applied to heminasal and total nasal defects, aggressive operative debulking is required during both surgical stages. This puts the flap in some jeopardy, leading to occasional flap necrosis, especially in smokers. It is especially difficult to re-establish the subtle three-dimensional contours of multiple subunits when the defect is large or deep, requiring complex support and lining replacement.

The two-stage forehead flap may be best limited to small defects of the tip, dorsum, or ala that do not require delicate contour recreation, complex support grafts, or lining replacement.

Technique of the two-stage forehead flap

Stage 1: flap transfer

The nasal subunits are marked with ink and residual normal skin is excised within the convex tip subunit or ala (the subunit principle), but not within the flat dorsum or sidewall. Primary cartilage grafts are positioned, as necessary, over vascularized lining. An exact pattern of the defect, based on the contralateral normal or the ideal, is outlined, under the hairline, directly over the supratrochlear artery, which lies just lateral to the frown crease. It can be identified by Doppler. The proximal pedicle is drawn inferiorly, in continuity with the defect, through the medial brow. Pedicle width at the brow is about 1.2–1.5 cm. The reach of the flap is verified using a simple gauze measure, checking the distance from the pivot point below the eyebrow to the distal end of the flap on the forehead and most inferior aspect of the defect. The flap can be lengthened by extending the design into the hairline or, more often, the pedicle is extended inferiorly across the eyebrow towards the medial canthus.

Frontalis muscle and excess subcutaneous fat are excised within its distal 1.5–2 cm, producing a skin flap with 2–3 mm of fat distally which will be applied to the inferior aspect of the nasal defect. The dissection then passes under the frontalis

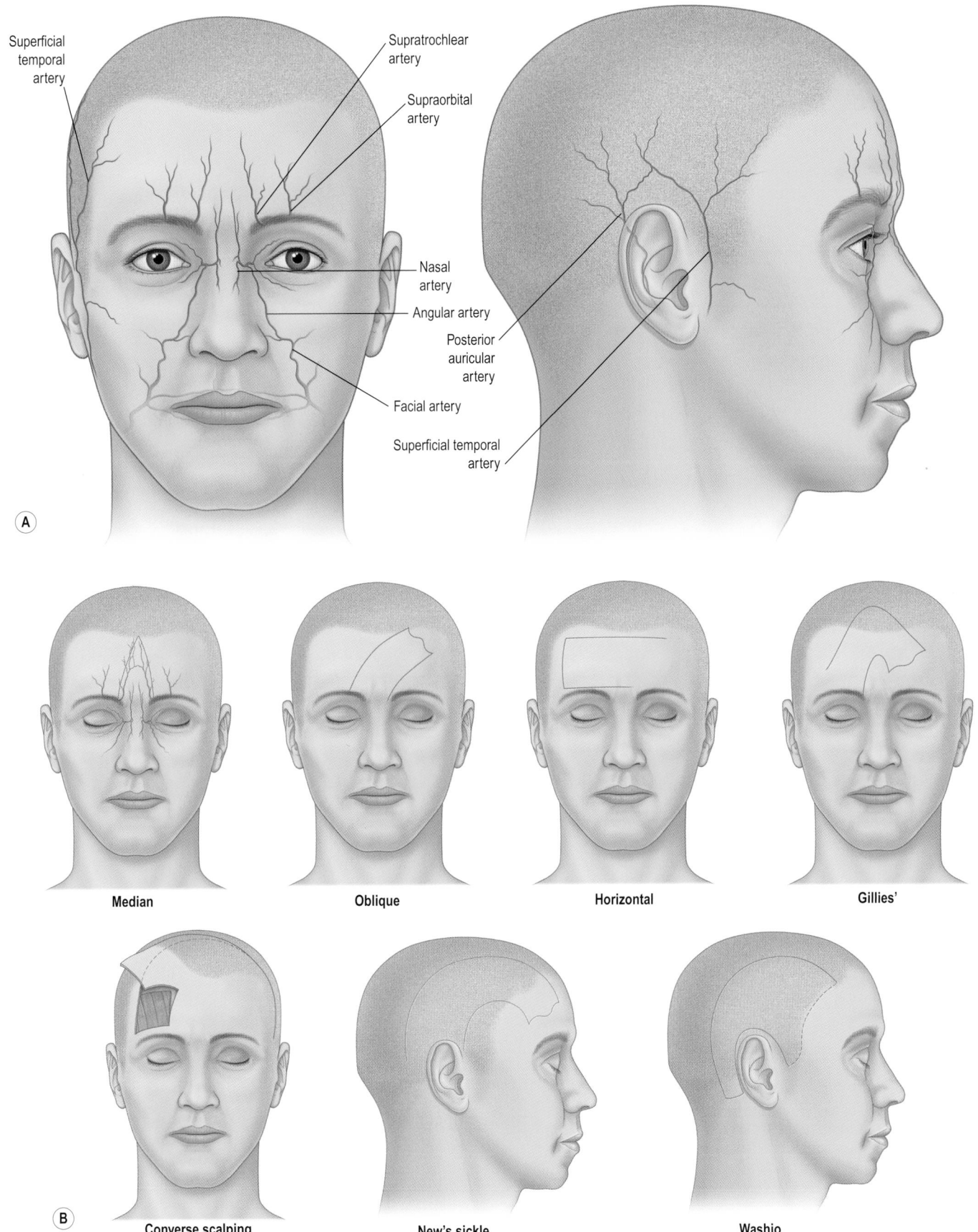

Fig. 6.12 (A) Forehead blood supply and **(B)** forehead flap designs. Forehead skin can be transferred on the many vessels which perfuse the scalp from its periphery.

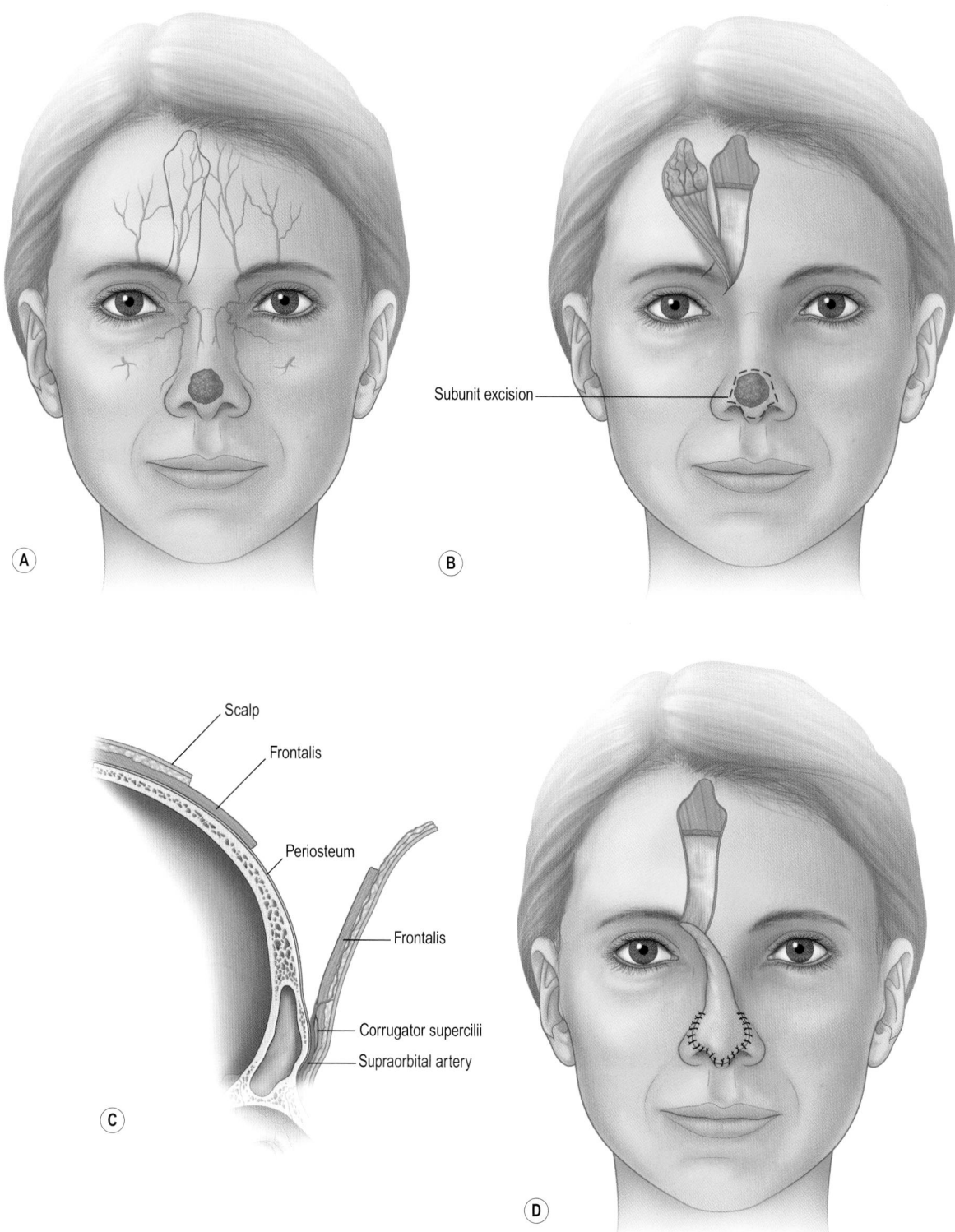

Fig. 6.13 (A–D) The two-stage paramedian forehead flap. A paramedian forehead flap is designed vertically over the axial supratrochlear vessels. Subcutaneous fat and frontalis are excised distally to thin the flap to nasal skin thinness.

and over the periosteum, through the medial brow until the flap reaches the defect without tension. It is sutured to the recipient site, from distal to proximal, with a single layer of fine suture. If the flap blanches, stop suturing and let the unsutured lateral flap edges heal secondarily to the recipient site. To avoid excessive oozing and crusting, the raw surface of the pedicle can be skin-grafted. The forehead is widely undermined into both temples and closed in layers. The scalp dog-ear is excised superiorly. Any gap, which remains under the hairline, is dressed with petrolatum gauze for 1 week and

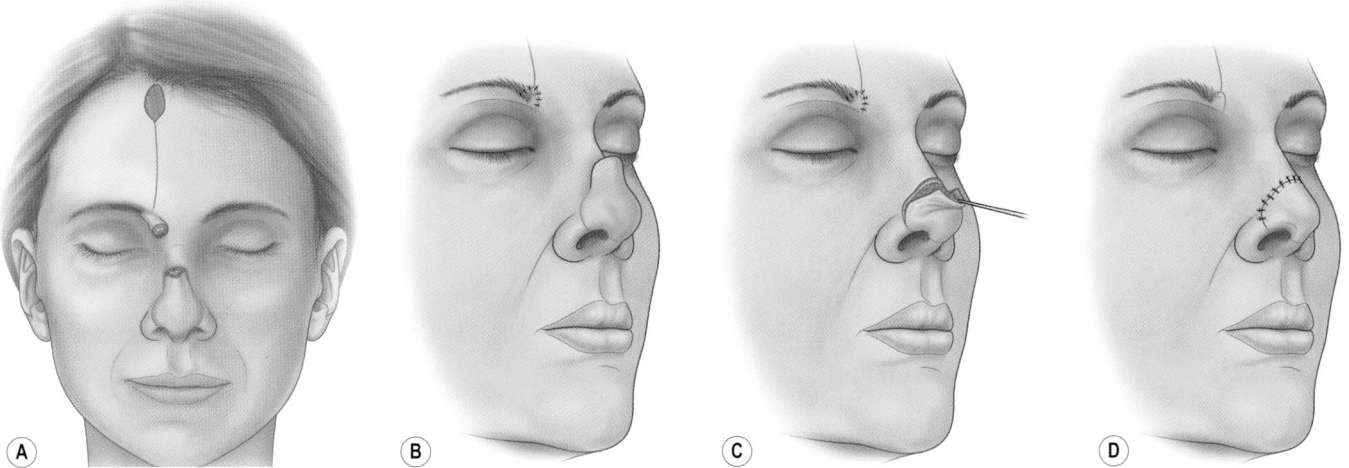

Fig. 6.14 (A–D) Forehead flap division – pedicle division is similar for both the two-stage and three-stage forehead flap. The pedicle was divided and excess subcutaneous tissue and skin excised from the proximal pedicle to allow its inset as a small anteverted "V" at the medial brow. The distal inset is partially elevated to remove excess soft-tissue bulk and smooth blending of forehead skin with nasal skin to resurface the nasal defect.

Table 6.2 The two-stage forehead flap is ideally suited for small defects
• Limited to one or two contiguous subunits • Requires modest cartilage replacement • Intact lining • Low ischemic risk – the nonsmoker, no prior forehead scarring, limited complex distal flap extensions

allowed to heal secondarily. The scar can be revised later, if needed.

Stage 2

The pedicle is divided 3–4 weeks later, the proximal aspect of the flap is re-elevated with 2–3 mm of fat, and the underlying excess soft tissue (fat, frontalis, and scar), which is adherent to recipient site, is excised, contouring the superior aspect of the defect. The flap remains well vascularized through its distal inset. The superior inset is completed. The proximal pedicle is untubed and returned to the medial brow as a small inverted "V," discarding any excess *(Table 6.2)*.

The three stage full-thickness forehead flap *(Fig. 6.17)*

Millard, in the 1970s,[30] and Burget, in the 1990s,[22,26] added an intermediate operation between transfer and division of the traditional two-stage forehead flap to improve vascular safety and permit more aggressive soft-tissue contouring. They thinned the flap distally at transfer but, 3 weeks later, elevated it from its bed over the mid-nose. The proximal pedicle remained intact while the distal inset was left attached over the tip, alar margins, and columella. Underlying fat and muscle over the dorsum and mid-vault were excised to improve mid-vault contour.

Although helpful, visualization of the middorsal excision was obstructed by the proximal pedicle and distal inset. Most importantly, once the flap was applied to the ala and tip at the first stage, further soft-tissue sculpting or cartilage modification of the distal nose could not be performed.

Menick,[25,52] in the late 1990s, modified the approach by transferring a full-thickness flap in three stages with an intermediate operation which permitted complete flap re-elevation and three-dimensional hard- and soft-tissue contouring over the entire nasal surface. The forehead is multilaminar and consists of skin, subcutaneous fat, and frontalis muscle. It is perfused with a myofascial, axial, and random blood supply. Initial distal thinning removes the myocutaneous component and creates a wounded deep soft tissue surface, more prone to contraction and less able to tolerate tension. However, if the flap is transferred with all its layers, maximal vascularity is maintained and the expected induration of wound healing does not occur, even months after transfer, as long as its subcutaneous plane is not injured or the frontalis excised. One month after transfer, its blood supply is augmented by surgical delay (its peripheral incision, elevation, and transfer). Forehead skin, with 2–3 mm of subcutaneous fat, can be completely elevated off the entire nasal inset, maintaining the proximal pedicle. The underlying excess of subcutaneous forehead fat and frontalis, previously positioned cartilage grafts, and lining are rigidly healed together. With complete visualization, the soft tissues are excised and cartilage grafts sculpted, repositioned, or augmented to refine three-dimensional contour. The thin supple forehead skin is then replaced to resurface the nose. Pedicle division is performed 1 month later.

Although this three-stage approach with a full-thickness flap adds an additional operation prior to pedicle division, it ensures a maximum blood supply at each stage, a thin uniform covering skin flap, unimpeded surgical exposure, controlled soft-tissue shaping and cartilage grafting over the entire nasal surface, prior to pedicle division. The surgeon can make intraoperative modifications during each stage and can perform a "revision" before the pedicle is divided. The aesthetic results are improved and the need for late formal revision is minimized.

The three-stage full-thickness forehead flap technique, with an intermediate operation, is applied to resurface partial-thickness or full-thickness nasal defects, regardless of defect size or depth. It is especially useful in smokers, when a scar

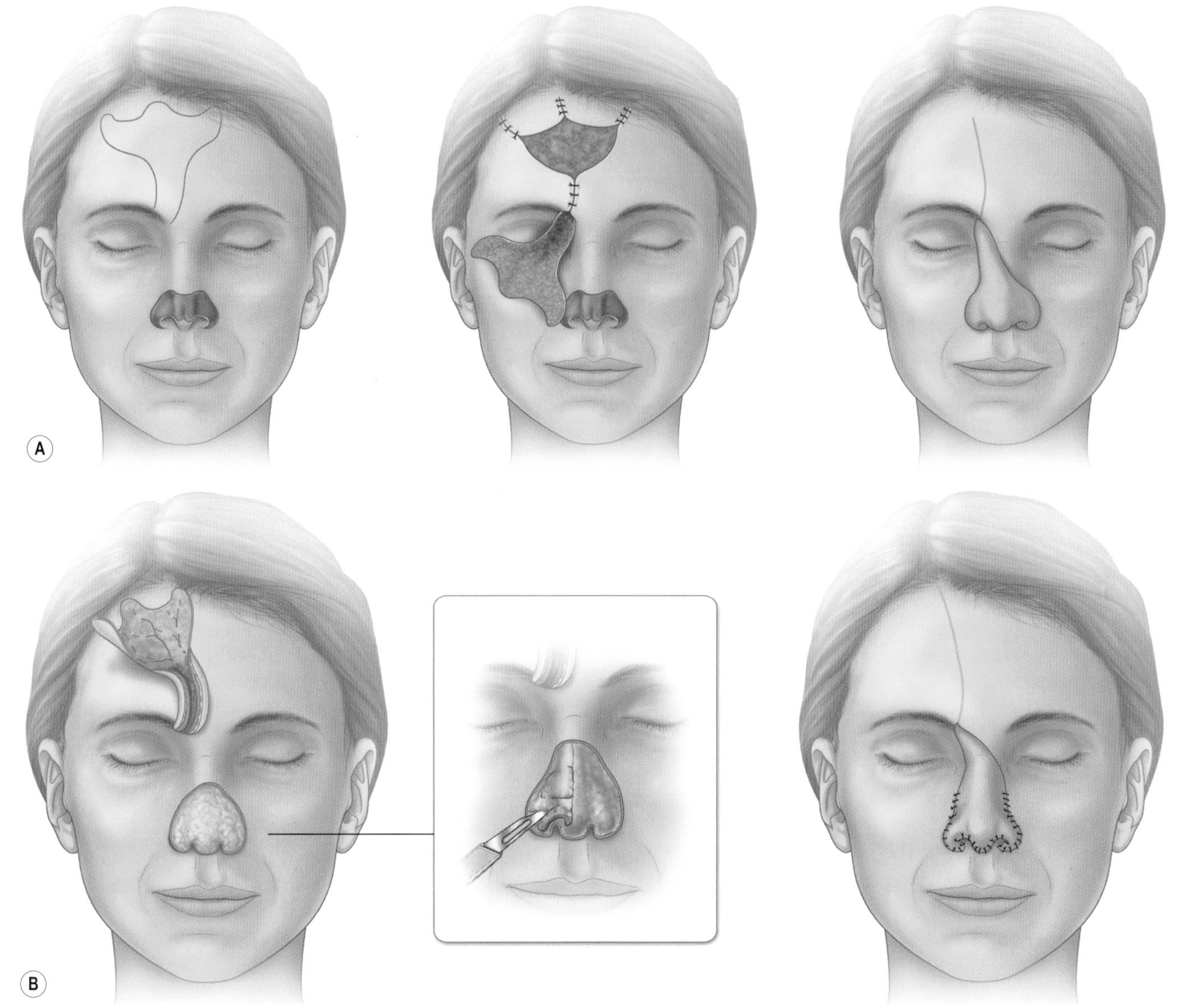

Fig. 6.17 **(A, B)** The three-stage paramedian full-thickness forehead flap. The forehead flap is elevated without distal thinning. It resurfaces a complex nasal defect with skin subcutaneous tissue and frontalis muscle. During the intermediate operation, 1 month later, the flap is re-elevated completely from the recipient site with 2–3 mm of subcutaneous fat. The excess underlying subcutaneous fat and frontalis muscle are excised to establish the correct three-dimensional contour. Cartilage grafts can be modified by sculpture, repositioning, or augmentation. The skin flap is then returned to the donor site. One month later (2 months after pedicle transfer), the pedicle is divided.

lies within the territory of the flap, or in large nasal defects that require wide thinning of the covering flap, especially with alar and columellar extensions. However, in small and superficial defects, such as an isolated alar or tip repair, initial distal and subsequent proximal debulking can safely resurface the nose in two stages.

Technique of a three-stage full-thickness forehead flap (Figs 6.18–6.27)

Stage 1

The regional units, old scars, and the location of planned vascular pedicles are marked with ink. Residual normal tissue within subunits is excised, when appropriate. An exact template of the nasal surface defect is positioned at the frontal

hairline over the supratrochlear pedicle and the more proximal pedicle, with a 1.2–1.5-cm base, is marked inferiorly through the medial brow. Primary cartilage grafts are placed, if vascularized intranasal lining is present or has been restored with intranasal flaps, hingeover flaps, a second flap, or a free flap. If the folded forehead flap or skin graft-lining techniques are planned to line a full-thickness defect, primary cartilage grafts are precluded during the first stage but can be positioned in a delayed primary fashion during intermediate operation.

The flap is elevated, with all its layers, above the periosteum. The pedicle is incised through the medial eyebrow towards the medial canthus until the distal flap reaches the defect without tension. Routinely, no frontalis or subcutaneous fat is excised. Frontalis can be trimmed along the nostril

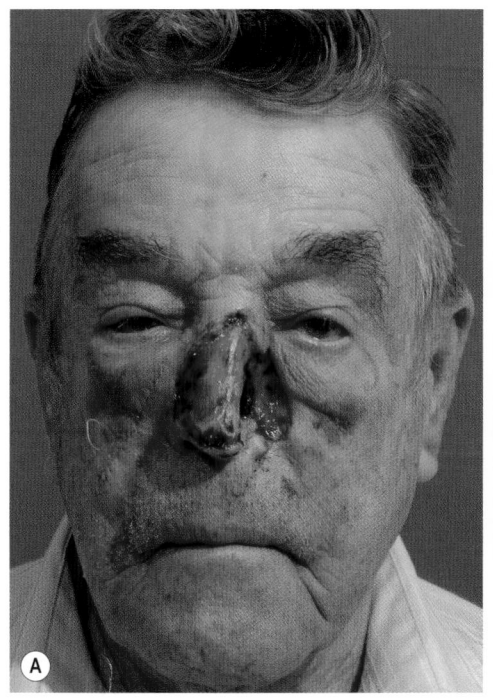

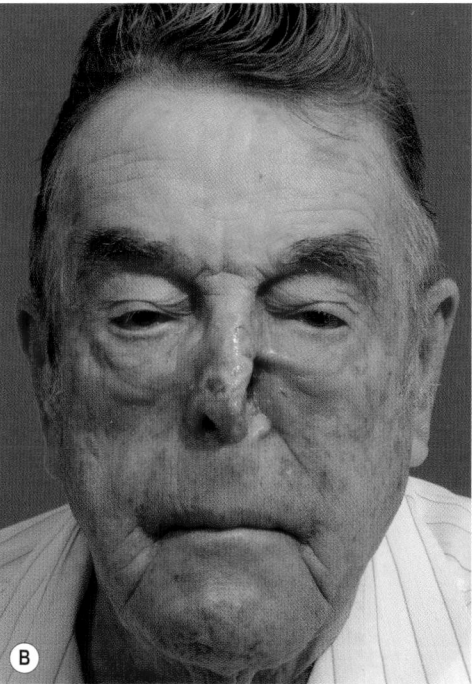

Fig. 6.18 (A, B) Reconstruction of a complex full-thickness nasal defect with a three-stage full-thickness forehead flap and intranasal lining flaps. A large, full-thickness defect is present after skin cancer excision. Skin is missing from the dorsum tip left sidewall and medial cheek. The tip cartilages and left upper lateral cartilage are missing. Lining for the left ala and sidewall is absent. The medial cheek defect was initially repaired with a fat flip flap and cheek advancement to allow reconstruction on the stable platform. This will be repaired with intranasal lining flaps and a three-stage full-thickness forehead flap.

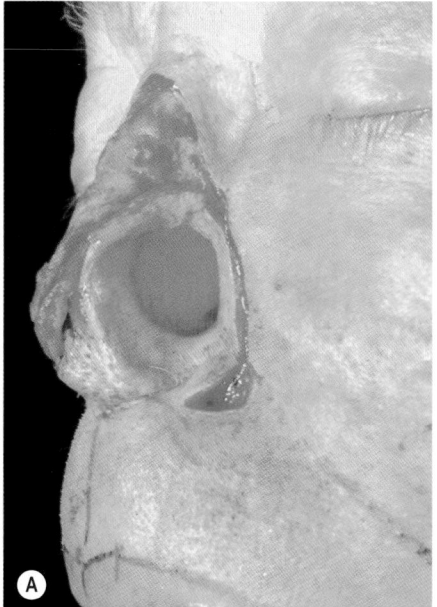

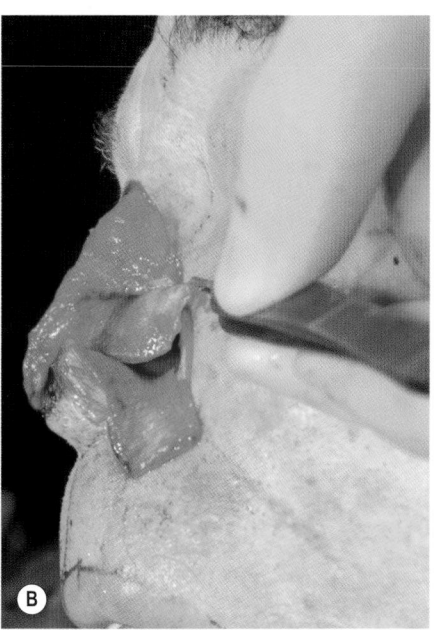

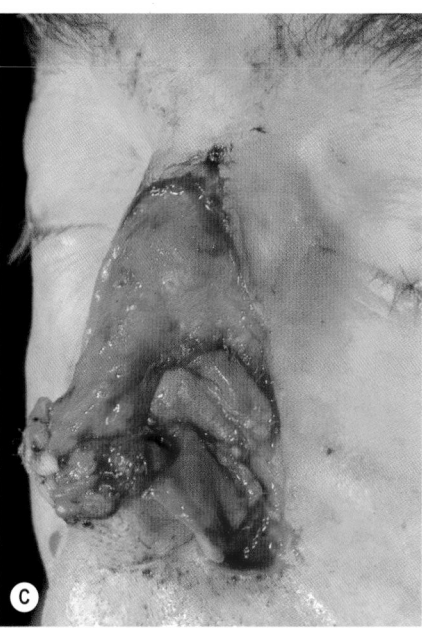

Fig. 6.19 (A–C) Six weeks later, the ipsilateral septal mucoperichondrium is elevated off the underlying septal cartilage and hinged downward and laterally on the septal branch of the left superior labial artery. Cartilage within the exposed septum is harvested, maintaining dorsal and caudal septal support. The contralateral septum is incised, maintaining a superior base perfused by the anterior ethmoidal arteries. Ipsilateral septal flap is fixed laterally to line the nostril margin and ala and the contralateral septal flap is transposed to provide lining of the nasal sidewall. Because the defect included part of the right ala, additional skin within the residual right ala was discarded to allow resurfacing of the nose as a subunit.

margin or distal ala to ease inset if the flap is unusually stiff. The flap is sutured to the recipient site in one layer. The forehead donor site is closed after wide undermining. A superior gap, which cannot be approximated, is allowed to heal secondarily.

Stage 2: the intermediate operation

Four weeks later, the forehead flap, now healed to the recipient bed, is physiologically delayed. The forehead skin is elevated with 2–3 mm of subcutaneous fat (nasal thinness) over the entire nasal inset. Axial subcutaneous vessels, lying

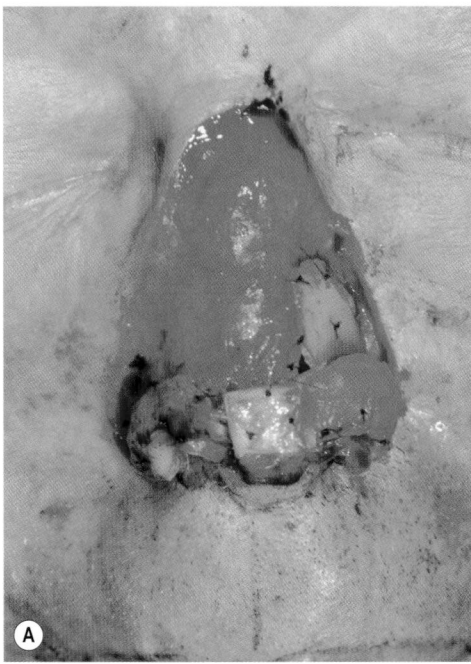 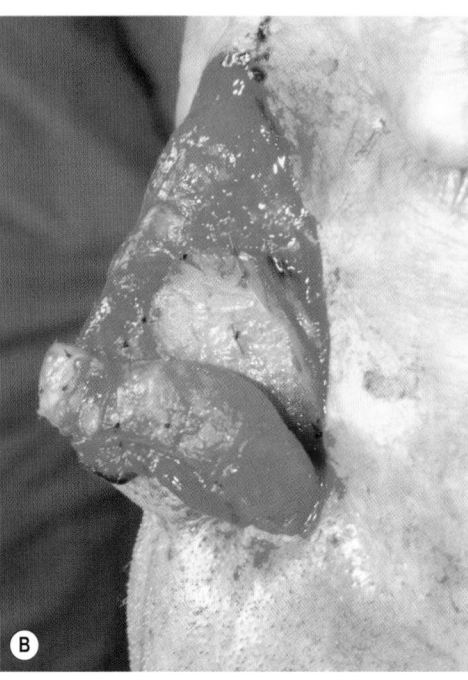

Fig. 6.20 (A, B) Primary ear and septal cartilage grafts are placed to shape, support, and brace the reconstruction. These grafts included a columellar strut, tip graft, bilateral alar margin grafts, and a sidewall brace.

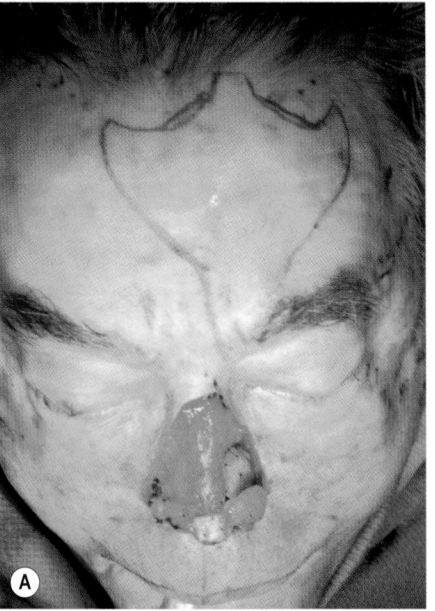 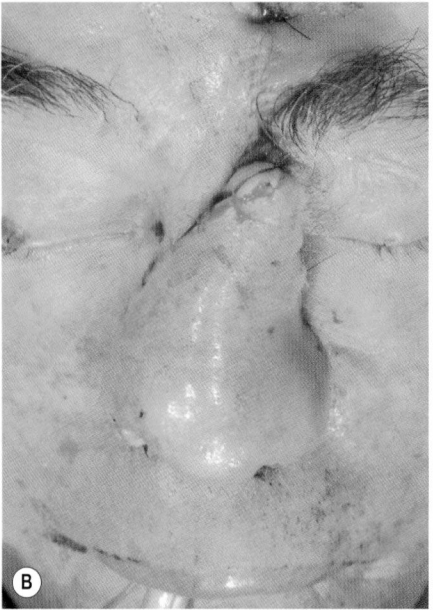 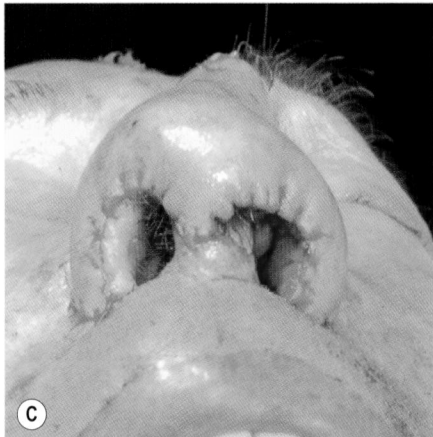

Fig. 6.21 (A–C) The nasal defect resurfaced as a nasal subunit with a full-thickness forehead flap.

in the subdermal superficial fat, are left adherent to the skin flap and are avoided. The flap is completely re-elevated and placed to the side of the face, maintaining the supratrochlear pedicle.

The underlying excess of subcutaneous fat and frontalis muscle, which remains adherent to the underlying support framework and lining, are healed together and form a living rigid structure that bleeds readily. With complete exposure, the entire exposed nasal subsurface is sculpted into a three-dimensional shape, highlighting the dorsal lines, alar crease, and tip contours. Previously placed primary cartilage

grafts can be remodeled by sculpting, repositioning, or augmentation. Delayed primary cartilage grafts are be placed over lining restored by the folded flap or skin graft techniques. The forehead skin flap is replaced on the recipient bed and fixed with quilting sutures to close the dead space and conform better to the underlying contour.

Although the forehead flap is routinely elevated over the entire inset, it can be left adherent to the columella and nostril margin to maintain a bipedicle blood supply, temporarily hanging from both the brow and the distal inset. This might be useful in a heavy smoker, when an old scar lies within the

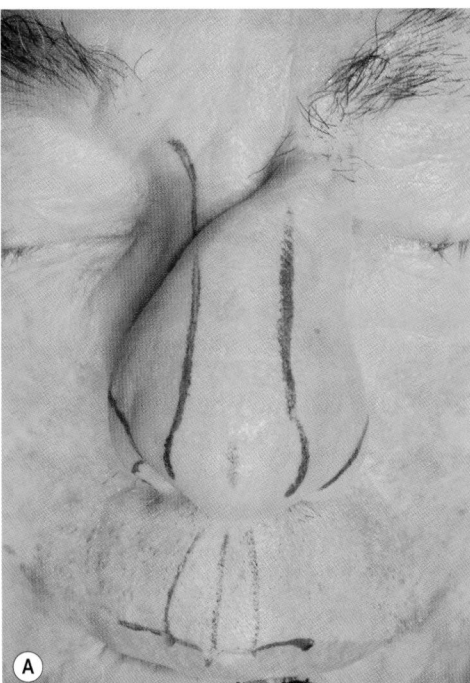
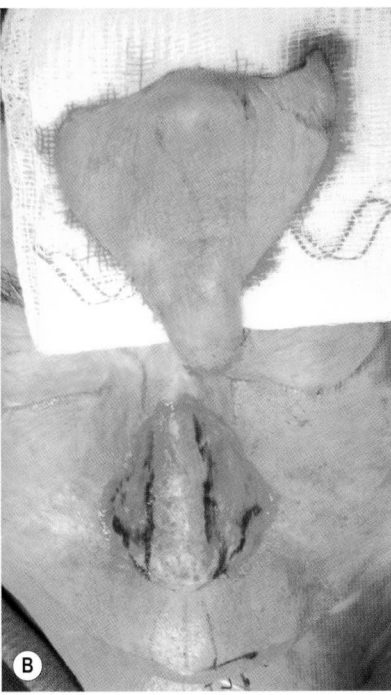

Fig. 6.22 (A, B) One month later, the repair is bulky and shapeless. The repair of the forehead flap is elevated completely with 2–3 mm of subcutaneous fat. Excess subcutaneous fat and frontalis are exposed.

Table 6.3 Indications for a full-thickness three-stage forehead flap

- Large or deep defect requiring extensive flap thinning or contour recreation
- Full-thickness defect
- Significant scarring within the flap territory
- Heavy smoker

flap's territory, when the flap contains unusually complex extensions, if the defect extends from the columella to high on the radix requiring debulking over an extremely large surface area, or if there is any concern for vascularity at initial transfer. This is rarely necessary. On very rare occasions, it may be helpful to perform two intermediate operations. The flap is re-elevated distally, maintaining the proximal inset into the nasal bridge, to supplement vascularity while the tip and columella are sculpted or delayed primary cartilage grafts placed. In a second intermediate operation, the flap is re-elevated over the mid-bridge and the nasal root, as a bipedicle, while maintaining the columella and rim inset. This approach is useful if there is significant scarring within the proximal flap and the surgeon has a concern for vascularity. The number of stages is unimportant, if the final result is good and complications are avoided.

Stage 3: pedicle division

Four weeks later (8 weeks after initial flap transfer), the pedicle is divided, the nasal inset completed, and the proximal pedicle returned to the brow as in the two-stage technique (*Table 6.3*).

Handling the forehead donor site

Foreheads vary in height and width, laxity, the presence of scars, prior injury, or past forehead flap harvest.

Primary closure of the forehead

The forehead is a forgiving donor site – expansive, highly vascular, self-healing, and lending itself to secondary revision. Preliminary surgical delay or expansion is usually unnecessary.

The paramedian forehead flap, based on the supratrochlear vessels, harvests skin under the hairline. Its narrow 1.2–1.5-cm pedicle width allows primary closure of the inferior forehead, leaving a single-line scar above the brow. The eyebrow is not distorted or medialized on return of the proximal pedicle base to the eyebrow. The forehead is closed under moderate tension using several key tacking sutures and a layered closure. The superior dog-ear is excised. If a gap remains superiorly, it is allowed to heal secondarily. A petrolatum bandage is applied to the raw periosteum and fixed temporarily with suture for 1 week. The open area heals by epithelialization and secondary contraction. The adjacent normal forehead stretches by autoexpansion. Frequently, at the time of pedicle division or during a revision, the area of secondary healing can be excised and the adjacent forehead readvanced. Occasionally, if the defect extends high on to the radix or extends laterally towards each medial canthus, the inferior forehead donor cannot be closed at the time of initial flap transfer. It is left open or temporarily skin-grafted. At pedicle division, the unused proximal pedicle is returned to the donor site, restoring the medial brow and resurfacing the inferior forehead defect. Any defect above is left to heal secondarily.

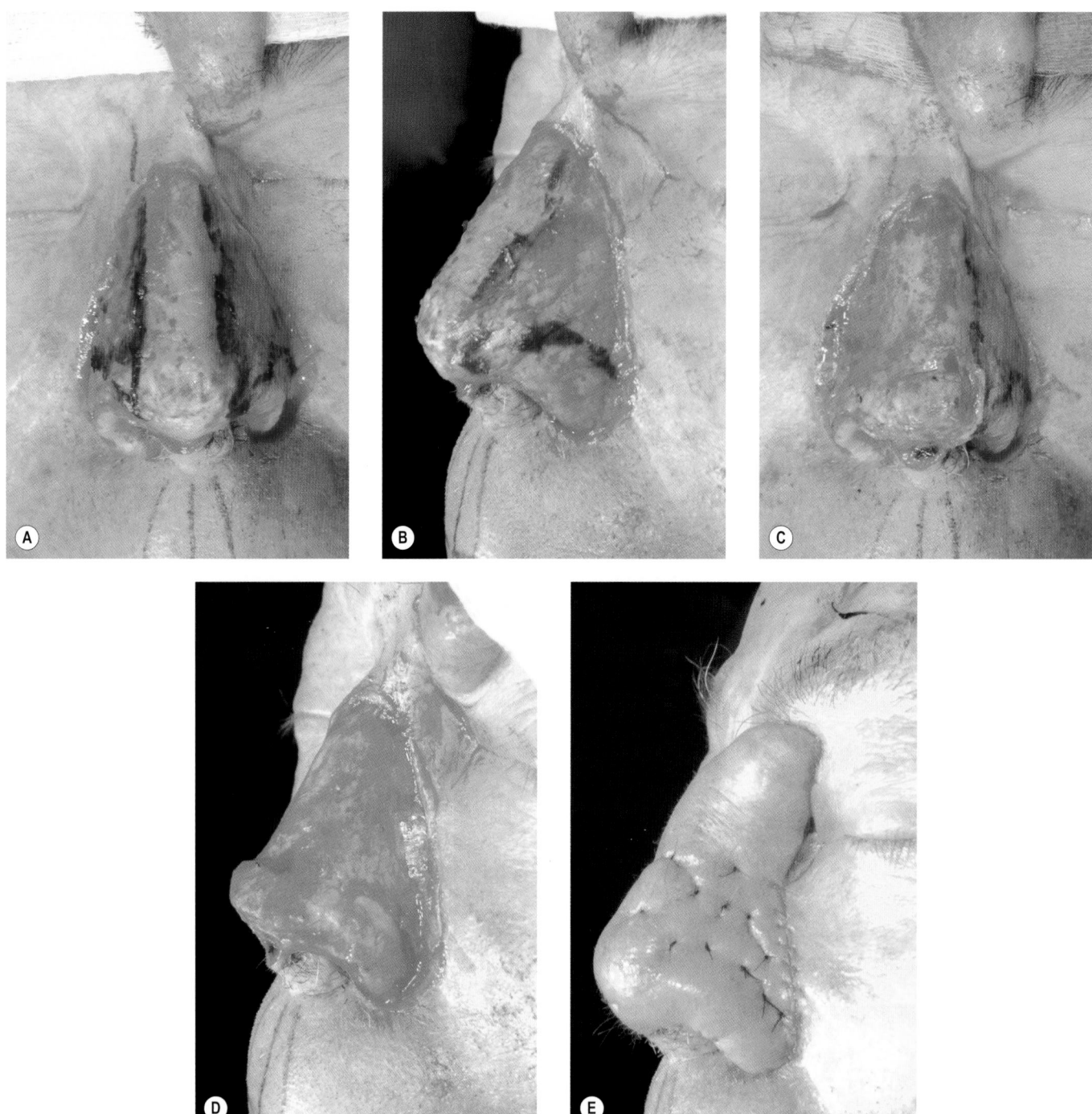

Fig. 6.23 (A–E) The regional contour units of the nose are marked with ink. Excess subcutaneous fat and frontalis are excised and the underlying primary cartilage grafts carved to create the ideal three-dimensional nasal contour. The "thin" forehead flap is returned to the recipient site, fixed with quilting and peripheral sutures.

Scars within the forehead territory

If a scar lies within the proposed flap territory, determine its site, direction, depth, and length.

A transverse scar puts the flap at greater risk. Old operative reports may clarify whether the injury extended only superficially, injuring only the random cutaneous blood supply, deeper through the frontalis, or directly to the vascular pedicle. Doppler examination of the supratrochlear vessels may confirm the presence of the supratrochlear artery.

If a scar within the flap's territory is short, vertical, superficial, or the supratrochlear vessels are verified by Doppler, it can be disregarded. Or the surgeon may avoid a scarred area completely by transferring skin from the opposite side of the forehead on the contralateral pedicle. The flap can be surgically delayed to augment its blood supply. The flap can be elevated as a full-thickness flap to maintain all vascular sources. An area of adjacent unscarred skin may be available for expansion, avoiding old scars. In rare instances, when both supratrochlear vessels have been ablated and the inferior

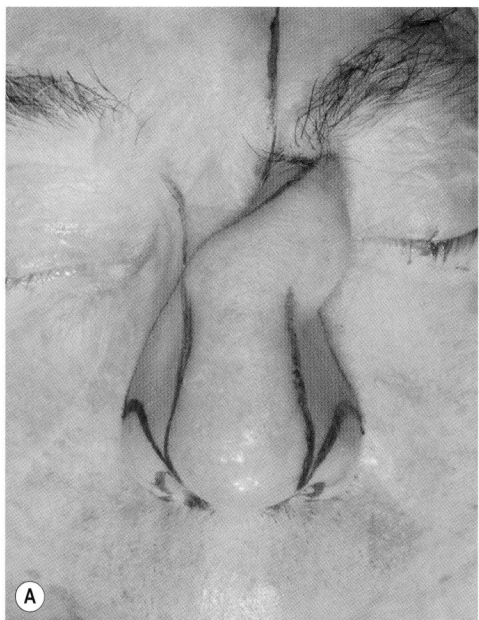
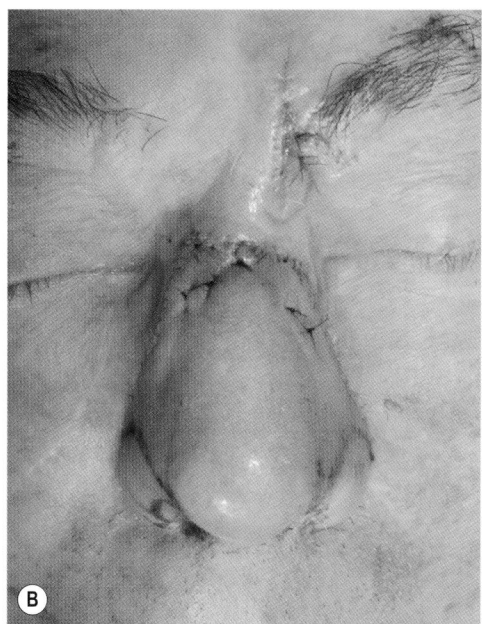

Fig. 6.24 (A, B) One month later, the pedicle was divided. The superior aspect of the nasal inset is sculpted after elevation of the forehead skin superficially. The proximal pedicle is inset as a small inverted "V."

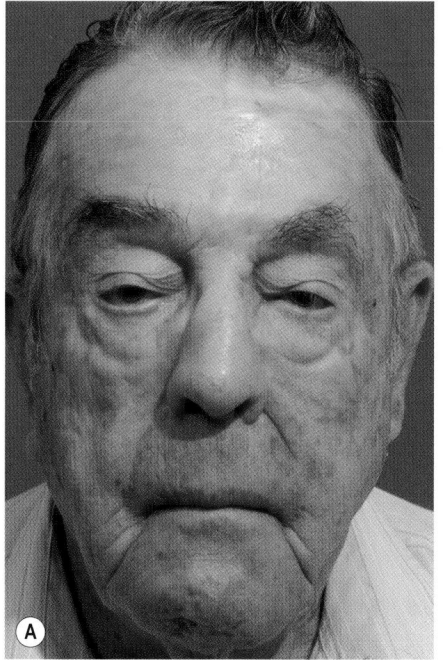
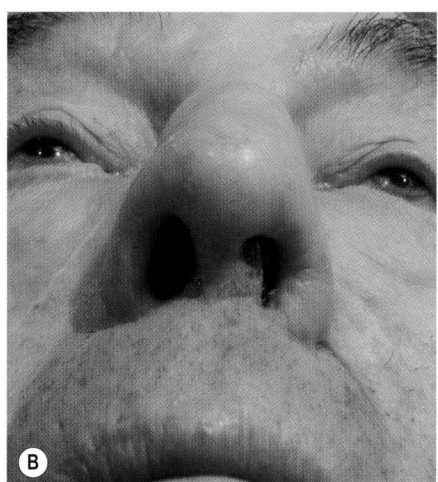
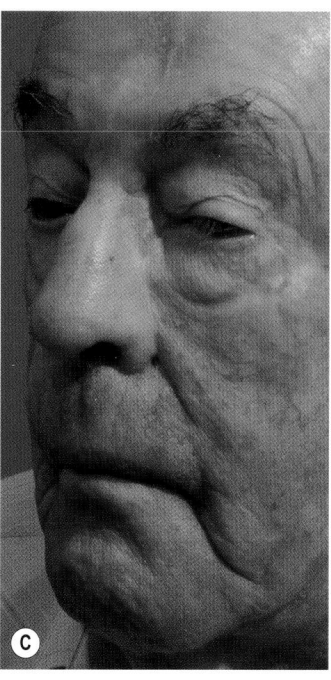

Fig. 6.25 (A–C) Postoperative result. No revision.

forehead is severely scarred, other uninjured forehead skin may be transferred on secondary vascular pedicles – a scalping or sickle flap.

Surgical delay of a forehead flap

Surgical delay of a forehead flap should be considered when:
- a significant old scar lies within the proposed flap territory
- the pedicle' s named blood supply has been injured
- unusually complex extensions of flap design are required (very uncommon)
- the patient is an end-stage smoker or has a history of high-voltage radiation
- a nonparamedian flap extends across one vascular territory into the territory of another flap (e.g., sickle flap). (The supratrochlear vessels reliably perfuse the forehead and scalp, allowing a paramedian flap to be designed in any size or length without delay)

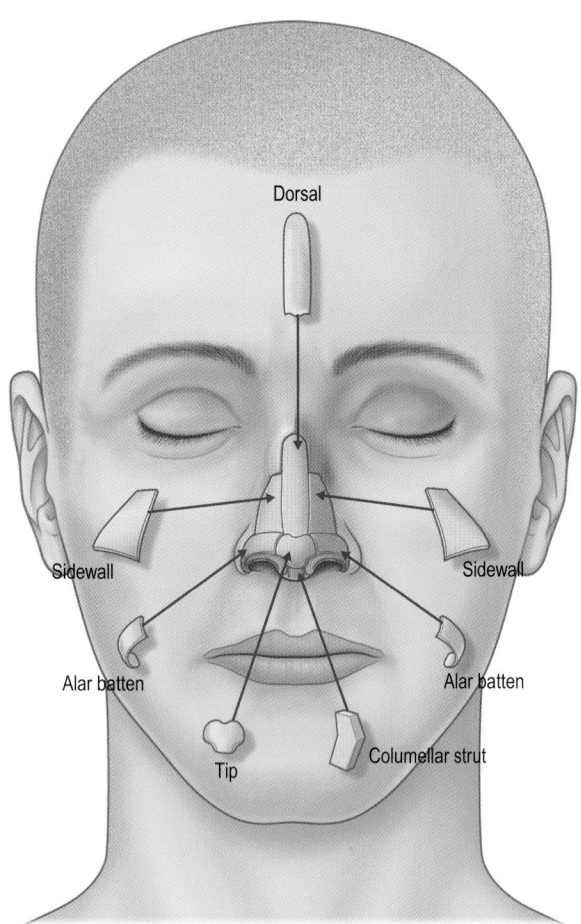

Fig. 6.26 Subunit support. Both cover and lining of the nasal reconstruction must be supported, shaped, and braced against wound contracture, tension, and gravity. The middle architectural layer of the nose must be replaced. Although there is no cartilage within the ala, the nostril margin must be supported during repair. If missing, dorsal, tip, ala, columella and sidewall grafts of bone or cartilage are designed in the shape and dimension of the normal. When placed under thin supple external skin, they will visually recreate normal surface contour while supporting and maintaining nostril position, shape, and airway.

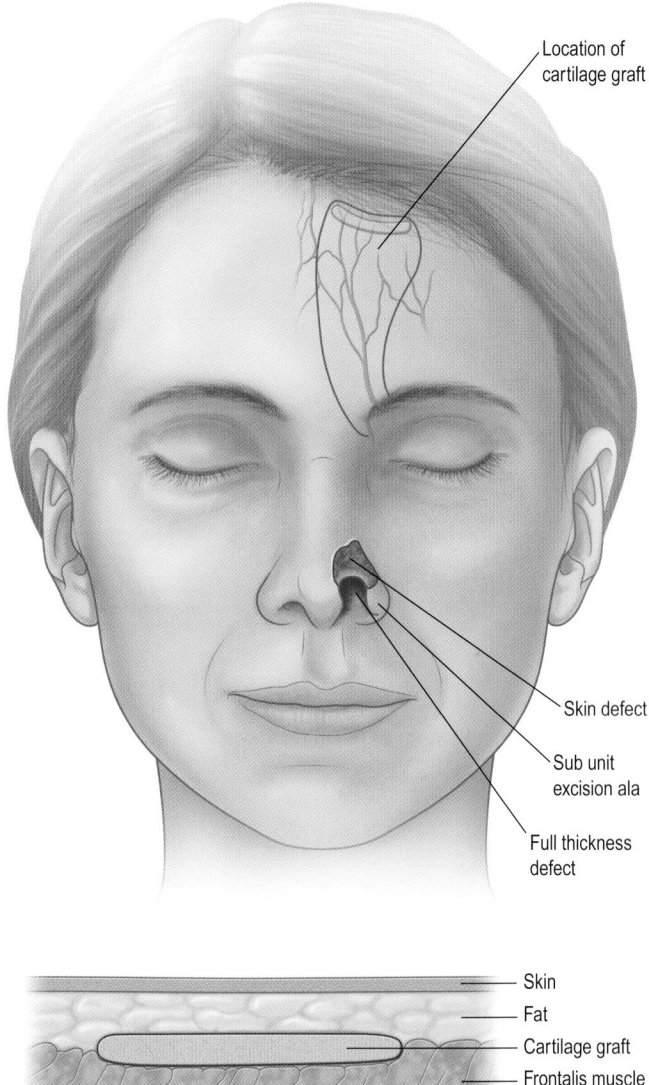

Fig. 6.27 Traditional nasal lining options: the **(A)** prelaminated, **(B)** hingeover, and **(C)** nasolabial flaps for lining.

- if the flap's vascularity is in doubt and a preliminary operation is required for other reasons (prefabrication of lining, delay of hingeover flaps).

However, unless needed, delay should be avoided. It adds additional stages and cost and prolongs the overall reconstruction. It can be difficult to determine precisely the requirements of the defect until the definitive repair. Once incised for delay, the dimension and outline of a delayed flap cannot be altered.

Technique of surgical delay

A template is positioned under the hairline and the proposed flap's outline is incised to periosteum. To ensure vascularity 2–4 mm of skin can be left temporarily intact at the columellar and alar tips. These skin bridges are divided subsequently. Because all significant contribution to forehead blood supply arises from peripheral axial vessels, elevation is unnecessary

and decreases flap pliability due to scarring of the flap's deep surface. Within 3–4 weeks, vessels at the flap's base enlarge and overall vascularity increases.

Expansion of the forehead

Pre-expansion, although not routinely helpful, can enlarge the available surface of the forehead for transfer to the nose.

Forehead expansion should be considered:

1. In an especially tight forehead with limited available skin due to scarring or prior forehead flap harvest. Expansion can increase the length and width of available skin within the proposed flap.

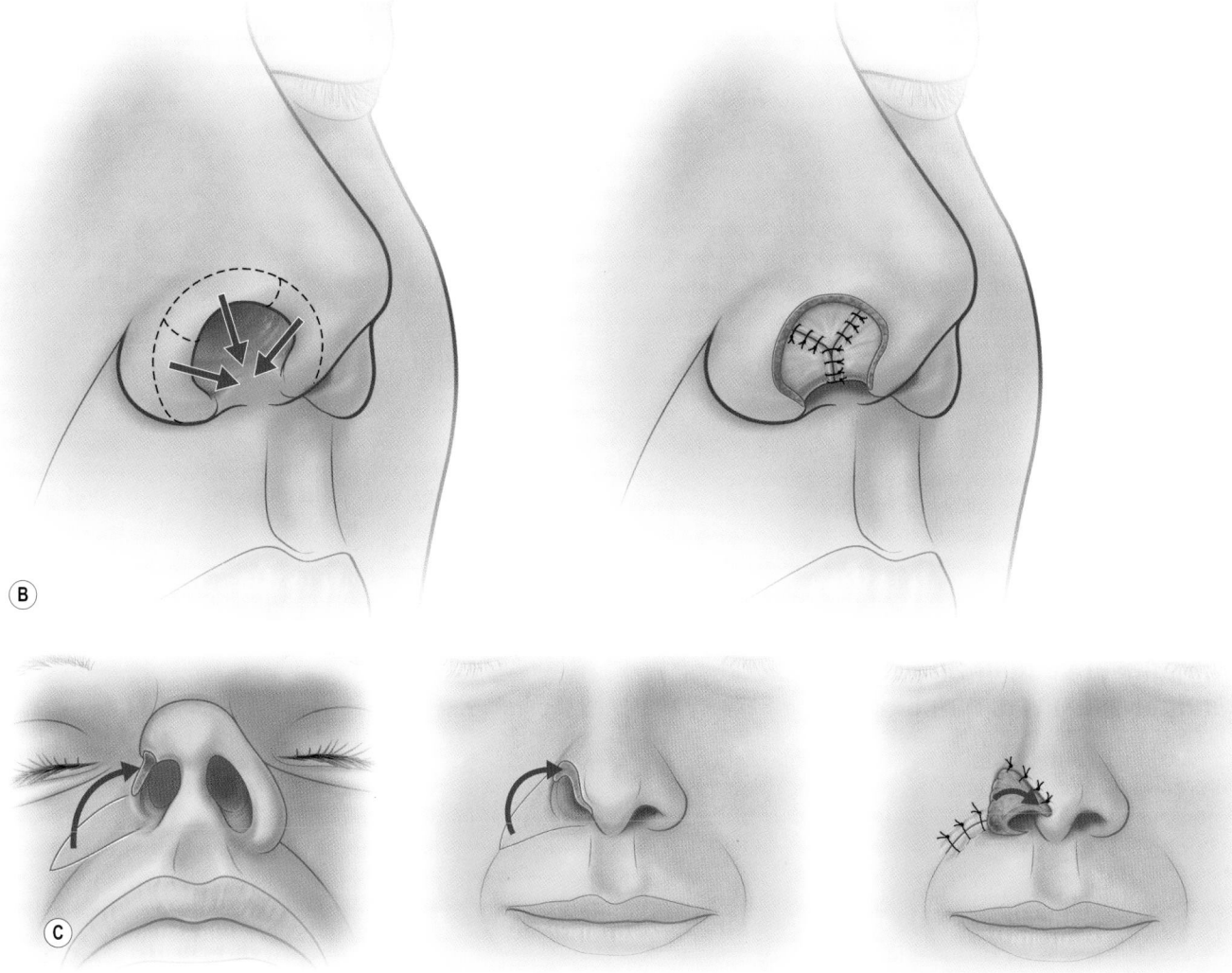

Fig. 6.27, cont'd

2. In the occasional, especially short forehead (less than 3–4 cm in height) to increase flap length and minimize hair transfer to the nose.

3. To expand the donor forehead adjacent to the proposed flap to facilitate closure of the forehead defect after transfer of a nonexpanded forehead flap.

However, there are many disadvantages to expansion – delay in repair, increased number of operative stages, added expense, more office visits, risk of infection and extrusion, and recoil. Expanded skin, if not rigidly braced with a hard-tissue support framework, contracts, leading to retraction and nasal shortening. Expansion does not clinically improve flap blood supply.

Expansion and delay

After expander placement and complete filling, the outline of the proposed forehead flap can be drawn over the dome of the filled expander. Its borders are incised, in stages, through the skin and subcutaneous tissue to the underlying

expander capsule to delay the flap. Subsequently, the flap is transposed and the expander removed.

Technique of forehead expansion

The site for expander placement is outlined in the pedicle's territory. A subfrontalis pocket is created through a distant radial incision within the scalp or through an old scar. After drain placement, the deflated expander is inserted and modestly filled with saline after closure of the scalp incision. Some weeks later, it is injected weekly over 6–10 weeks. Distance over the expander's dome is measured until the skin is adequate in length and width to resurface the defect. If the vascularity of the flap is in doubt due to past scars, the flap is surgically delayed, in stages, after expansion. At the time of transfer, a template is positioned over the expanded skin. The flap must be elevated across the supraorbital rim, transecting the capsule at the flap's base, to allow transposition and sufficient length. The capsule is excised. Elastic recoil occurs immediately on flap elevation and must be prevented with a strong nasal cartilage framework to avoid retraction and skin contraction.

Guidelines for harvesting multiple forehead flaps

Check the position and length of old scars. Determine the available forehead surface area and compare it to the recipient requirement. Consider use of the contralateral pedicle. Use a full-thickness forehead flap to increase vascular safety or delay across old scars. Consider tissue expansion of the flap. Consider using a nonparamedian forehead flap. Expand residual forehead to ease closure of the forehead donor.

If the donor site cannot be closed primarily under the hairline, allow the gap to heal secondarily. If the inferior forehead cannot be closed primarily due to the size and location of the nasal defect, return the unused proximal pedicle to the inferior forehead to facilitate its closure and the appearance of the eyebrow. In extreme cases, when the forehead has been extensively destroyed by previous injury or multiple flap harvest, excise scar and residual skin within the forehead and resurface the entire unit with a one-piece expanded, full-thickness supraclavicular skin graft.

Restoring nasal contour and support: recreating a subsurface architecture

Three-dimensional contour and landmark outline define a nose as "normal." Incorrect dimension, outline, position, projection, or symmetry describe the "abnormal." Most of these abnormalities reflect a poorly sized, misshapen, or malpositioned skeleton *(Fig. 6.26)*.

The middle plane of the nose, between cover and lining, is composed of two layers. Superficially lies a three-dimensional soft-tissue layer of variable thickness composed of fat, nasalis muscle, fibrous ligaments, and areolar tissue. More deeply lies a rigid cartilage and bone framework which includes the nasal bones, upper lateral cartilages, alar cartilages, the columella and septal partition, and the compact stiff fibrofatty tissue of the ala. External skin and internal lining impart only minimal stiffness and form to the nose. Bone, cartilage, and the compact fibrofatty soft tissue of the ala determine nasal contour.

It must be remembered that the nose sits on the lip and cheek platform of bone and soft tissue. The reconstructed nose must be positioned and projected in symmetry and proportion to other facial features. So if missing, the facial platform must be restored and the nose built on a stable base, prior to formal nasal reconstruction.

Hard-tissue support replacement

If missing, weakened, or distorted, the middle layer of soft and hard tissue must be restored. A complete cartilage and bone framework must extend from the nasal bone, above, to the base of the columella, inferiorly, and from one alar base and sidewall to the other, horizontally. Although the ala normally contains only soft tissue, cartilage support must be added to prevent collapse and retraction. Cartilage grafts support the nose and its airway, shape its external appearance, and brace the repair against gravity, tension, and wound contraction. Unlike the normal, the injured nose is subject to

Table 6.4 Functions of a hard-tissue framework
• Support cover and lining to create projection and prevent collapse
• Shape soft tissue
• Brace soft tissue to prevent retraction or contracture

edema, hematoma, tension, and fibrosis and is negatively influenced by unnaturally thick and stiff cover and lining replacements. The framework of the reconstructed nose must be stronger than that of a normal nose.[22,25,53–57]

Timing

Although support has been traditionally replaced secondarily during late revisions, it is difficult to mold cover and lining once contracted by scar. Ideally, if the underlying bone or cartilage structure is missing, primary and delayed primary support grafts are placed during flap transfer, the intermediate operation, or at the time of pedicle division.

Design

Each support graft is designed in the shape and dimension of the subunit that it will replace. A template of the contralateral normal or ideal is used to determine the appropriate length, width, and border outline of the cartilage grafts. The grafts are fashioned a few millimeters smaller in all dimensions so that, when seen through the thin supple cover, they re-establish the three-dimensional contour of the overlying subunit.

When a nonsubunit defect is resurfaced, only partial subunit cartilage replacement is necessary *(Table 6.4)*.

Materials

The tissue chosen to restore nasal support is of less importance than its shape. But materials must have the correct dimension, bulk, outline, contour, and rigidity to satisfy the needs of the defect.

Alloplasts are avoided in reconstructive rhinoplasty due to frequent infection and extrusion.

The septum can supply a modest amount (2–3 × 2–3 cm) of thin (2–3 mm), flat, moderately rigid cartilage. It is harvested through a single Killian incision or through a dorsal approach, as in an open rhinoplasty. Septal cartilage is especially useful as a single or layered onlay dorsal graft, a tip graft, a sidewall brace, or a columellar strut and can be bent and fixed with sutures to shape anatomic tip grafts or alar batten grafts.

Ear cartilage remains the workhorse of tip repair. The entire concha can be harvested with little deformity through an anterior or posterior approach. In most instances, the entire concha is removed and the ideal graft is designed with the precise dimension and contour needed to supply the defect, based on a template. Like septal and rib cartilage, ear cartilage can be shaped with horizontal mattress sutures to increase or decrease its convexity. Its cuplike shape can be incorporated into the curve of the alar batten graft or anatomic tip graft. It is more difficult to create a straight columellar, dorsal, or sidewall onlay graft from the ear.

Traditionally, rib cartilage is harvested from the synchondrosis of the sixth, seventh and eighth ribs, employing Gibson's principles of balanced carving. However, the floating ninth and 10th ribs are excellent donor sites due to their intrinsic length, width, and curvature. The rib is available for a tip graft, columellar strut, a dorsal graft, or alar batten. Osteocartilaginous grafts are especially useful for dorsal replacement. If the dorsal rib graft is 50% bone and 50% cartilage, the risk of late warping is minimized. Unfortunately, the rib donor site is more painful than other options.

Harvest

Based on a subunit template, the graft is examined to determine the ideal area which would best provide the appropriate contour and dimension. Then the exact graft is cut from the harvested material. Leftover graft is replaced in the donor site or banked within a soft-tissue pocket under scalp or chest skin.

Graft fixation

Primary and delayed primary grafts are positioned precisely and fixed with sutures to the residual normal skeleton, to each other, and to the underlying lining. Late secondary cartilage grafts can be placed in closed subcutaneous pockets, or after elevation of the flap through peripheral or direct incisions.

It is important to differentiate onlay grafts from cantilever dorsal grafts. If central support remains, an onlay graft in the shape and thickness needed to replace dorsal height is laid over the remaining solid base. If the septum is missing or collapsed, a rigid dorsal graft must be fixed, as a cantilever, with a screw or plate to the radix to support the dorsal profile. If residual septum remains within the piriform aperture, it may be rotated out of the nose as a septal composite flap, based on its septal vessels to provide central nasal support. An onlay dorsal graft is added to further shape further the dorsal subunit.

Soft-tissue support and contouring

Normal subcutaneous soft tissue adds shape, and a degree of strength, to all areas of the nose. It pads the underlying support and helps contour the external skin. Compact soft tissue is the primary support for ala and soft triangle, which normally contains no hard tissue.

Staged thinning of a full-thickness forehead flap, soft-tissue sculpturing during the intermediate operation, and contouring of the proximal inset at the time of pedicle division contribute significantly to three-dimensional contour.[25]

Restoring nasal lining

It is easy to fail to appreciate the importance of lining. If a raw area heals secondarily, the external shape of the nose becomes distorted by scar and the airway becomes contracted. Nearly as much skin is required to line a nose as is needed to cover its outer surface (*Fig. 6.27*).

It is useful to review all lining options systematically and to prepare a written list for each case to ensure that no method is overlooked.

Lining can be replaced by:

1. a composite skin graft
2. advancement of residual lining
3. prelamination of a forehead flap
4. folding of the distal forehead flap
5. a second flap (forehead, nasolabial, facial artery myomucosal flap, or any available discardable excess local tissue)
6. hingeover lining flaps
7. intranasal lining flaps
8. skin graft for lining
9. microvascular transfer of distant tissue.

Composite skin grafts

Composite skin grafts of skin and cartilage, taken from the ear, can repair skin and cartilage loss within the soft triangle and nostril margin or isolated defects of the nasal floor.[58,59] Most often, a two- or three-layered sandwich of skin, containing cartilage or fat, is taken from the helical root, helical rim, or lobule. They survive, if placed on a well-vascularized recipient, sutured with care, and immobilized. There are most reliable if less than 1.5 cm in size. Larger grafts have been recommended, with less predictable results. These larger grafts consist of large full-thickness skin grafts, which resurface an adjacent superficial defect and a modest distal composite extension for the full-thickness loss along the nostril margin.

The nasal defect and ear are examined. An exact template is created of the proper shape, size, and outline. The area which best matches the contour of the defect is identified. The graft is often harvested from the helical root. If significant coagulative injury is present, the wound is allowed to granulate for 7–14 days.

The defect is recreated and the graft applied to the clean wound. The repair is performed under local anesthesia, local anesthesia with sedation, or general anesthesia. The graft is harvested, avoiding pressure injury, and sutured to the recipient site in one layer. The ear defect is repaired by suturing the external skin of the helix to its medial surface or with a local preauricular or postauricular transposition flap, based on a superior or inferior pedicle.

Initially, these grafts appear white. Over 24–72 hours, they become progressively blue and subsequently pink, as vascularity improves. Ice-cold compresses to decrease the metabolic requirement of the graft in the first 48 hours have been recommended, although the clinical significance is questionable.

The "take," color, and texture of composite grafts are unpredictable. However, composite grafts are useful to repair small defects (0.5–1.0 cm) along the nostril margin or within the soft triangle due to their simplicity and adequate results. Their shiny atrophic appearance can match the "thin skin zone."

Advancement of residual lining

Occasionally, a surface defect along the nostril margin is accompanied by a modest lining loss. If minimal, residual vestibular lining can be freed superiorly from its overlying attachment to the alar cartilage and pulled inferiorly until it reaches the level of the ideal nostril margin. An advancement of 2–3 mm is maintained with a rigid primary cartilage graft to prevent retraction. The external skin loss is replaced with a vascularized cover flap.

The prelaminated forehead flap

In the prelaminated technique (formerly referred to as prefabrication), the nose is "built on the forehead."[60–62] During a preliminary operation, a full-thickness skin graft is placed on the deep areolar surface of the forehead's frontalis muscle to supply 1–1.5 cm of distal lining for the alar rims. The flap is elevated only enough to position the skin graft, which is immobilized with a small sponge bolus. A separate cartilage graft is buried in a subcutaneous pocket between the frontalis muscle and overlying skin to support the future distal nostril margin, placed through an incision along the lateral flap border. If desired, a composite graft from the ear or septum can be used in place of separate skin and cartilage grafts.

Once healed 6 weeks later, the composite forehead is transferred to provide cover, lining, and support as a single unit. Although prelamination adds a preliminary stage, the placement of skin and cartilage grafts and subsequent flap transfer and division are modest procedures and can be performed under light monitored sedation in a sick patient. Prelamination avoids extensive intranasal manipulation.

Traditionally, prelamination has been used to repair significant unilateral or bilateral full-thickness defects and has been combined with hingeover flaps, based on the scar along the border of an old full-thickness defect. The turned-over lining replaced the superior aspect of the defect while the distal aspect was lined with the prelaminated flap. Unfortunately, cartilage grafts, within a prelaminated flap, do not have a nasal shape and are fixed by the scar which forms around them as they heal on the forehead. The limited size, shape, and position of these cartilage strips provide only modest support to the nostril margin. Incompletely braced skin graft lining contracts, retracts the rim, and narrows the nostril aperture.

Prelamination of the forehead flap to repair a full-thickness defect has limited application but may be useful:
- for a small-to-moderate defect
- in elderly or debilitated patients to minimize anesthesia and morbidity
- in salvage cases, when other options are unavailable.

Hingeover lining flaps

When a full-thickness defect is created, whether sutured primarily or allowed to heal secondarily, residual cover and lining become contiguous along the defect margin. Six to 8 weeks later, external skin, an old skin graft applied to resurface an adjacent superficial skin loss, or scar adjacent to the healed margin can be hingeover, turning outside cover into inside lining.[15] Although the external skin deficiency is enlarged, the additional skin required to resurface the proximal nose is easily supplied by the proximal pedicle of the forehead flap used for cover.

Turnover flaps are vascularized across the scar at the wound margin. Because of their relative avascularity, they are unreliable if more than 1–1.5 cm in length. Hingeover scar is less likely to survive. Even a minor distal loss may lead to infection, especially if other cartilage grafts are simultaneously placed for support. To improve their limited vascularity, a preliminary delay, 3–4 weeks earlier, is recommended. The hingeover flap is incised, elevated inferiorly, and then returned to its bed to augment its blood supply physiologically. However, the usefulness of surgical delay, in this instance, is in doubt. It adds an additional surgical stage, delays the repair, increases fibrosis, and does not definitely improve survival.

Hingeover flaps are thick, stiff, and noncompliant. They are less easily shaped by primary cartilage grafts and their bulk may distort external nasal contour.

Indications for hingeover lining flaps

- Hingeover lining flaps are used to line small full-thickness defects after cover and lining have healed together along the wound margin.
- In salvage cases, all layers of the nose may be injured with nasal collapse and retraction. This is most commonly seen after multiple failed rhinoplasties, following intranasal lining necrosis with cartilage infection and collapse (as in the cocaine nose), or after prior failed reconstructions. In these instances, few lining options remain. Because scarred external skin will be replaced with a flap, it can be turned over to line the distorted distal margin, rather than being discarded.
- In pediatric nasal reconstruction: injury to the growth centers of the nose should be avoided until near-complete physical maturity. Hingeover flaps of residual skin, which border the margins of the defect, can provide lining, while avoiding additional intranasal injury in the child. Hingeover flaps remain a useful tool to line small full-thickness defects.
- Small defects can be repaired with composite skin grafts in children.

The disadvantages of hingeover flaps are:
- They are not applicable to the repair of a fresh nasal injury and require at least 6–8 weeks to allow the external and internal surface of the nose to heal and establish vascular connections across the scar.
- They are thick, stiff, and less able to be molded by cartilage grafts.
- If the initial defect encompassed most of the circumference of the airway, as the scar contracts, the airway becomes stenotic. Even though the reconstructed nostril margin may appear large after turning over external skin for lining, the internal stenosis cannot be opened initially without jeopardizing the vascular base of the hingeover flap. Late revision to open the constriction deep within the nose is difficult.

In such cases, open up the constriction initially, prior to the formal nasal repair. Once the airway is open, adjacent external skin is turned over for lining at a later operation. However, this further postpones formal nasal repair.

Use of a second flap for lining

If cover is missing, external skin can be replaced with a forehead flap. Absent lining can be replaced with a second flap, with a separate blood supply.

Although not commonly employed, a second vascularized flap for lining is useful when lining is required for a small isolated defect of the lateral alar base or when an isolated injury, due to cocaine, infection, or autoimmune disease, leads to nasal collapse, scar contraction, and foreshortening of the nose.

The nasolabial flap

Millard[15] popularized the use of random nasolabial flaps of cheek skin for lining. For large defects, which included the mid-vault and lower one-half of the nose, he hinged over residual skin from the upper nose to line the mid-vault and rolled over skin and fat within the nasolabial fold to line the distal aspect of the defect. For subtotal nasal defects, bilateral nasolabial flaps were turned inward, after surgical delay, to line each ala and one-half of the nasal vault, suturing the distal end of each nasolabial flap together centrally to supply columellar lining.

If employed to line a small defect of the lateral ala, no more than about 1.5 cm in length, they can survive, based only on scar about the pyriform aperture. Longer nasolabial lining flaps should include the angular and facial artery perforators at their base. Unfortunately, these flaps are thick and stiff and cannot be thinned at the time of transfer without jeopardizing blood supply. Primary cartilage grafts are often precluded by the excessive soft-tissue bulk and risk of necrosis with infection. Late revision is required to thin the nostril rims, open the airway, and contour the nasal surface. These flaps add scars to the central face and cannot be positioned exactly in the nasolabial fold. The technique is rarely used today.

A second forehead flap[25]

It is possible to line the nose with a second forehead flap based on the opposite supratrochlear or superficial temporal vessels. Whatever forehead skin that is necessary to rebuild a nose should be harvested. However, forehead skin is best used for cover. Injury to the remaining forehead skin should be avoided, if possible, to minimize scarring and permit harvesting of a second flap for a second nasal reconstruction needed in the future.

The facial artery myomucosal (FAMM) flap

The FAMM flap[63] is an axial oral musculomucosal flap, based on the facial artery which can line defects of the mouth and nose. It consists of intraoral mucosa, submucosa, a small amount of buccinator muscle, the deeper plexus of the orbicularis oris muscle, and the facial artery and its venous plexus. Based superiorly at the alar base and centered over the facial artery, oral mucosa and the overlying facial artery are raised, from distal to proximal, and passed into the nasal cavity at the alar base. The flap is 8–9 cm long and 1.5–2.0 cm in width and can line an isolated area of lining loss within the middle vault secondary to cocaine injury or Wegener's disease. Its primary advantages are its vascularity and ability to provide intranasal lining without adding visible scars to the external face. Bilateral flaps can be used.

Intranasal lining flaps

Intranasal stratified squamous and nasal mucoperichondrium are perfused by branches of the facial and angular arteries, the septal branch of the superior labial artery, or the anterior ethmoidal vessels.[64–70]

The lateral nose is perfused from branches of the facial and angular artery which supply the ipsilateral alar base and middle vault. The centrally placed septum is perfused inferiorly from bilateral septal branches of the superior labial arteries, which arise from the facial artery. The superior labial artery passes medially through the orbicularis oris muscle along the skin vermilion junction of the upper lip. It septal branch arises just lateral to the philtral column and moves vertically upward, lateral to the nasal spine, to supply the ipsilateral septal mucoperichondrium. The septal branch is located at the base of the columella within 1.0–1.2 cm of the nasal spine between the anterior plane of the upper lip and the inferior edge of the piriform aperture. Each side of the septal mucosa is perfused by its ipsilateral septal branch. The entire septum, containing septal cartilage and lined with bilateral mucoperichondrium, is vascularized by both superior labial vessels. The dorsal aspect of the septum is perfused by paired anterior ethmoidal vessels which pass from under the nasal bones to perfuse each side of the septal mucoperichondrium dorsally (Fig. 6.28).

Residual intranasal mucosal can be moved to line a deficiency based on the location and size of the defect and the pedicle position, dimension, and reach of each individual lining flap, as described by Burget and Menick.[22,25,71,72] These flaps may be unavailable if prior surgery or traumatic injury has interrupted their named vessels or their mucosal surfaces.

A bipedicle vestibular skin flap is employed if residual vestibular skin remains above a marginal defect. It is incised superiorly in the area of the intercartilaginous space, creating a bipedicle flap, based medially on the septum and laterally on the nasal floor. It is perfused, medially by the septal branch of the superior labial artery, and laterally by the branches of the facial angular artery. The flap is pulled inferiorly, like the hem of a skirt, to line the nostril rim. The superior defect, created by advancement of the bipedicle flap, is filled with an ipsilateral septal flap, a skin graft, or with a contralateral mucosoperichondrial flap.

Ipsilateral septal mucoperichondrial flaps, based on the right or left superior labial artery, can be elevated off septal cartilage and transposed laterally and inferiorly to line the vestibule and the lateral sidewall.

A contralateral mucoperichondrial flap, based on the dorsum of the septum and vascularized from branches of the ipsilateral ethmoidal vessels, can be hinged laterally to line the contralateral mid-vault. As originally described by de Quervain,[73] the ipsilateral septal mucosa was discarded, and a flap of cartilage and septal mucous membrane was swung laterally, through a large septal fistula. It is more practical to remove the septal cartilage, preserving a septal "L" strut, and pass the flap through a dorsal slit in the ipsilateral septal mucosa, preserving the opposite septal mucosa. The harvested septal cartilage is reapplied to support the mucosal repair after transfer, facilitating its design and positioning. This contralateral dorsal septal flap can line the mid-vault, an isolated defect of the mid-vault, the gap above a bipedicle vestibular flap, or above an ipsilateral septal flap transferred to line the inferior nose. But it is inadequate in size and reach to line the nostril margin or alar base, inferiorly.

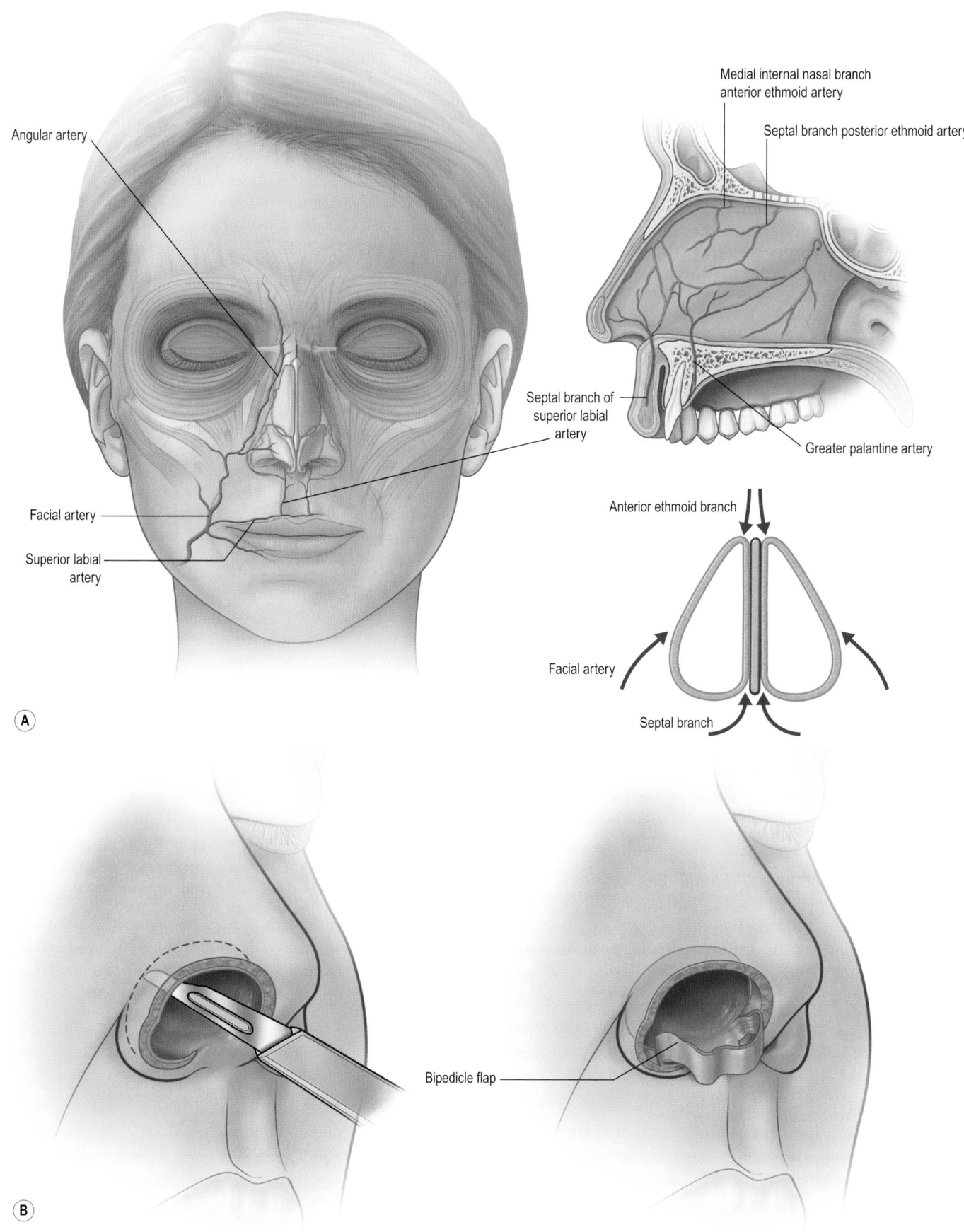

Angular artery

Medial internal nasal branch
anterior ethmoid artery

Septal branch posterior ethmoid artery

Septal branch of
superior labial
artery

Greater palantine artery

Facial artery

Superior labial
artery

Anterior ethmoid branch

Facial artery

Septal branch

A

Bipedicle flap

B

Fig. 6.28 (A–D) Blood supply and design of intranasal lining flaps.

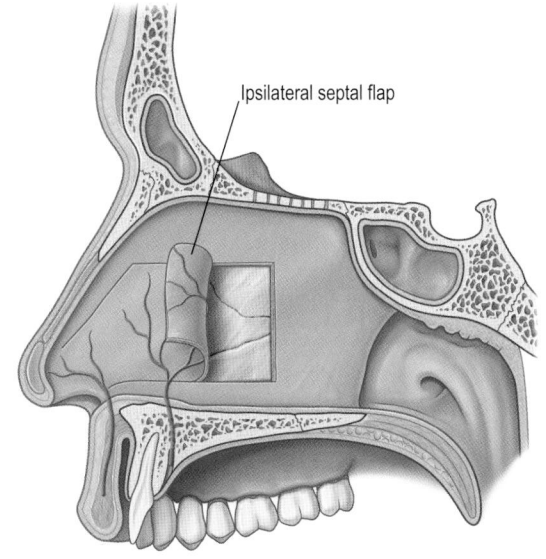

Ipsilateral septal flap

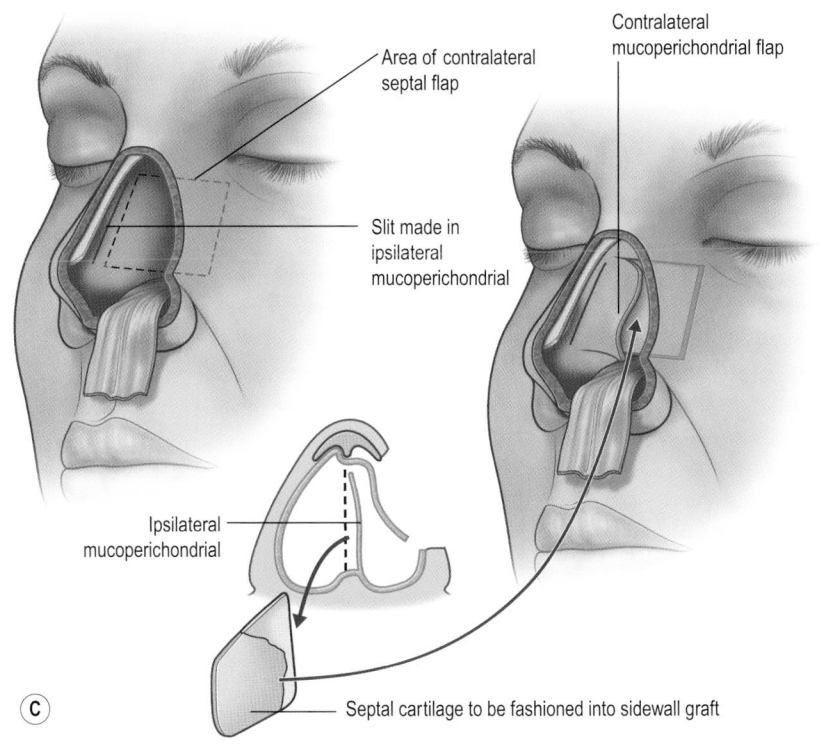

Area of contralateral septal flap

Contralateral mucoperichondrial flap

Slit made in ipsilateral mucoperichondrial

Ipsilateral mucoperichondrial

ⓒ

Septal cartilage to be fashioned into sidewall graft

Fig. 6.28, cont'd

The paired septal branches of the superior labial artery lie close together near the nasal spine. This allows the entire septum to be elevated as a composite septal flap on an inferior pedicle base. It is swung out of the pyriform aperture, transposing a "septal sandwich" of support and bilateral lining anterior to the plane of the face to restore basic central support and lining to both vestibules, columella, and the middle vault and dorsum. It is inadequate in length to reach the alar base and must be supplemented laterally, most often with flaps from the residual ala or nasolabial fold *(Table 6.5)*.

Although significant lining can be provided by intranasal lining flaps, they have no shape or structure and collapse into the nose. However, they are thin, pliable, and vascular, which permits the immediate restoration of support with primary cartilage grafts. This combination of intranasal lining flaps and primary cartilage grafts was a significant advance in nasal reconstruction. For the first time, reliable, thin, supple, vascularized lining was available which would not occlude the airway or distort the external shape. And primary cartilage grafts could be positioned to support, shape, and brace the soft tissues at the initial stage.

However, the limitations of intranasal lining flaps must be understood to ensure their proper application. Intranasal lining flaps are limited in dimension and availability due to

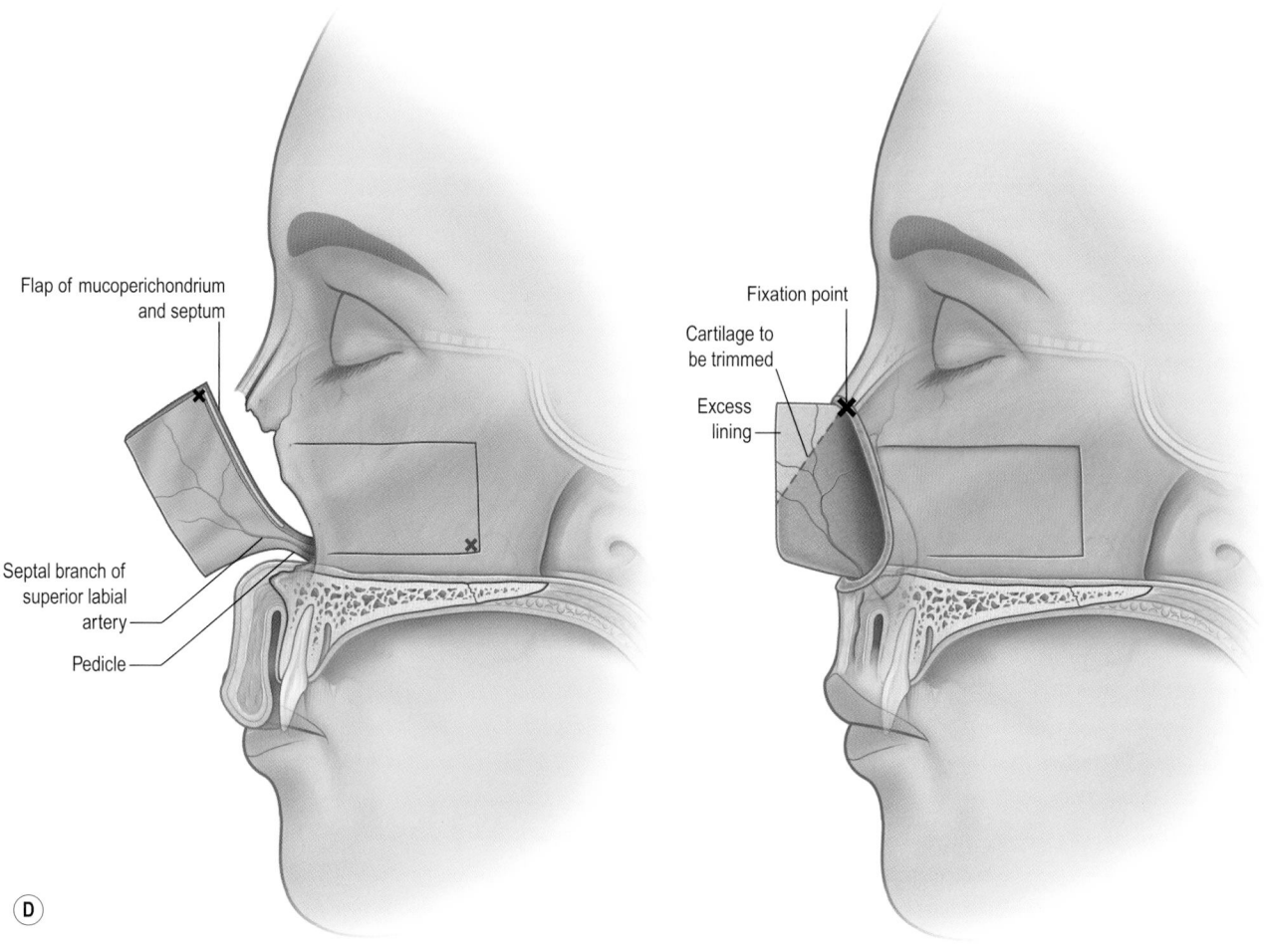

Flap of mucoperichondrium and septum

Septal branch of superior labial artery

Pedicle

Fixation point

Cartilage to be trimmed

Excess lining

(D)

Fig. 6.28, cont'd

their modest size, limited reach, or prior injury to their blood supply due to trauma or previous operation. Although highly vascular, that can be unpredictable in the smoker or in major repairs when multiple flaps are pushed to their limits to line large defects. A minor cartilage exposure may lead to serious infection and tissue loss.

Intranasal lining flaps are fragile and should be elevated subperichondrially to protect their blood supply. They must be supported and shaped by primary cartilage grafts. Their dissection is destructive to the nose and increases the overall morbidity of nasal repair due to temporary bleeding, crusting, and obstruction. Fortunately, the surgical fistula heals spontaneously around its border. The nose becomes self-cleansing. Whistling does not occur because of the fistula's large size.

In major repairs, intranasal flaps are relatively complex and time-consuming. The final result may be marred by late retraction, external distortion, or narrowing of the airway. The lack of rigidity and limited dimensions of intranasal lining flaps, the relatively unstable cartilage construction of multiple suture-fixated grafts, dead space, and scar contracture limit the final result. Late nostril stenosis may occur. However, intranasal lining flaps remain a valuable tool in the repair of isolated mid-vault or large unilateral full-thickness defects when other methods are less applicable.

Table 6.5 Intranasal lining flaps may be applied to varied defects, according to their location and dimension

1. Isolated unilateral defect of the mid-vault – contralateral septal mucosal flap
2. Unilateral defect of the lower one-third of the nose – bipedicle vestibular flap and ipsilateral septal flap
3. Unilateral defects up to one-half of the nose – bipedicle vestibular flap and contralateral septal flap
4. Unilateral defects of the vestibule, middle and upper vaults – ipsilateral and contralateral septal flaps
5. Central defect of the dorsum and tip – septal composite flap
6. Central defect combined with lateral alar lining loss – septal composite and turnover alar remnant or nasolabial flaps

Intranasal lining flap technique *(Figs 6.29–6.33)*

Isolated unilateral mid-vault lining loss

To repair the mid-vault, the contralateral septal mucoperichondrium is harvested through the full-thickness defect. Or if the ala remains intact but has been malpositioned superiorly by scar or prior excision, a full-thickness incision releases the remaining inferior nose in symmetry to the opposite normal side. The ipsilateral septal mucoperichondrium is incised transversely at the dorsum, exposing septal cartilage. The ipsilateral mucosa is elevated. Preserving 8–10 mm of superior dorsal support, the underlying septal cartilage is incised transversely in line with the anterior dorsal edge and septal cartilage is harvested for graft material. The contralateral mucosa is preserved and the anterior ethmoidal vessels are protected. A dorsally based flap of contralateral septal mucosa is incised, maintaining its dorsal blood supply. The contralateral flap is then passed through the ipsilateral dorsal slit and pulled laterally to the periphery of the mid-vault lining loss. The raw surface of ipsilateral flap, which now lies exposed with the contralateral airway, heals spontaneously. Harvested septal cartilage and bone are fashioned into a sidewall brace to support and shape the mid-vault and prevent the ala from retracting upward postoperatively. Missing external skin is advanced from the cheek or transposed from the forehead to resurface the external skin loss.

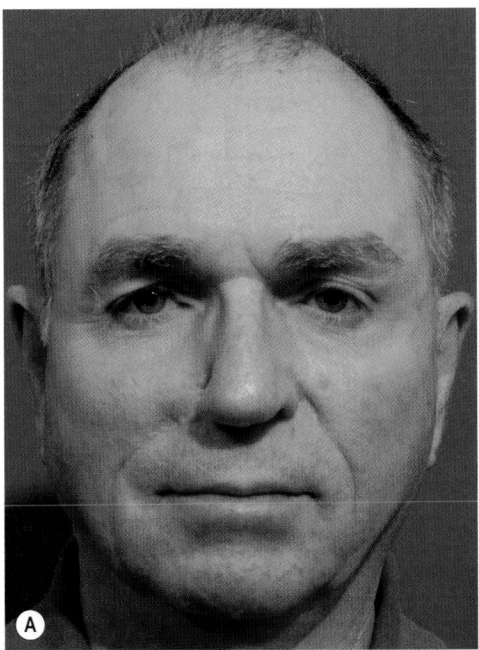
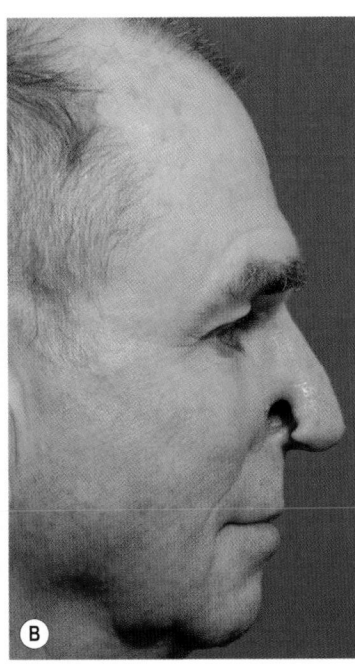

Fig. 6.29 **(A, B)** Full-thickness right ala and sidewall defect after preliminary operation to resurface the medial cheek and right upper lip with a fat flip flap and advancing cheek flap.

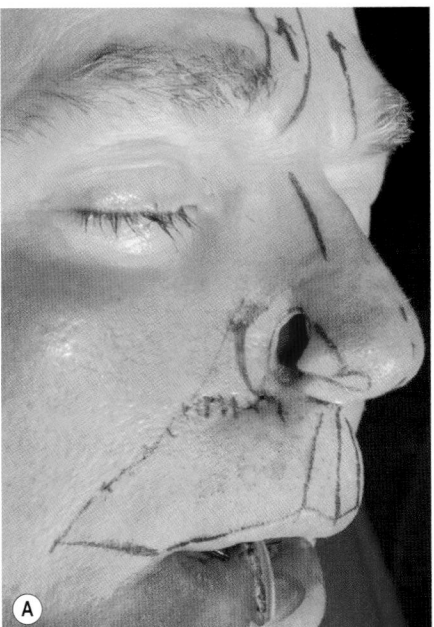
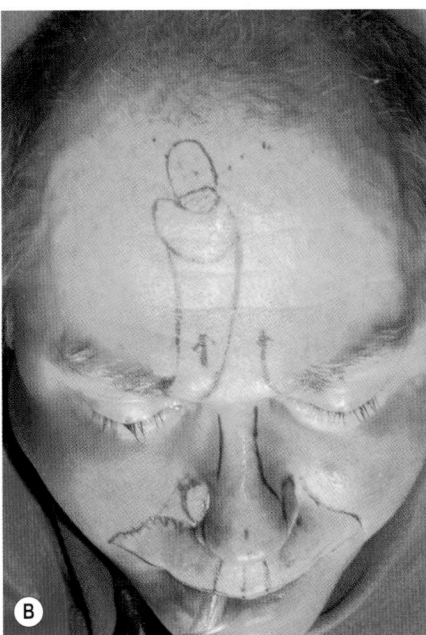
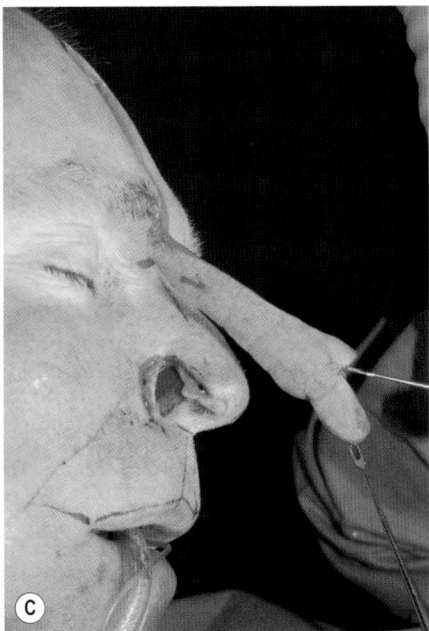

Fig. 6.30 **(A–C)** The regional units of the nose and the ideal alar base position are marked with ink based on the template of the contralateral normal upper lip. A full-thickness forehead flap is elevated with the distal extension for lining. The lining and skin deficiencies are based on exact templates.

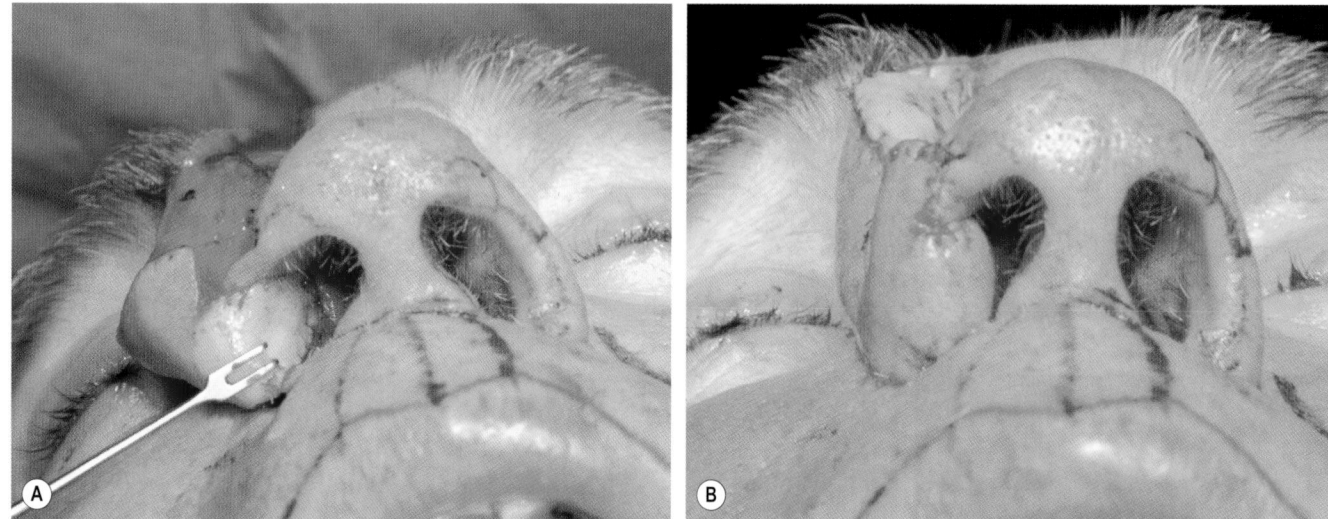

Fig. 6.31 (A, B) The distal extension of the full-thickness forehead flap is folded to replace missing nasal lining and the more proximal distal flap is turned back to resurface the defect. No primary cartilage grafts were placed.

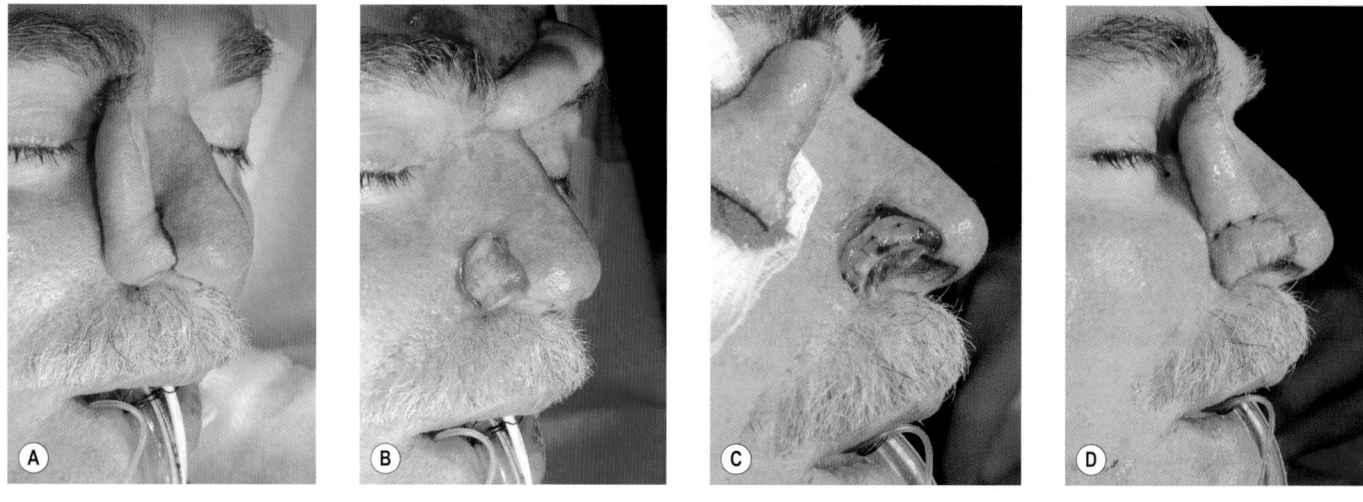

Fig. 6.32 (A–D) One month later, the reconstruction is bulky and unsupported. The ideal nostril margin is marked with ink and incised. The proximal forehead flap was elevated with 2–3 mm of subcutaneous fat. The folded double layer of fat and frontalis muscle is exposed. The excess is excised in the lining skin and supported and shaped with a delayed primary conchal cartilage graft. The thin forehead skin flap is returned to the defect and fixed with quilting sutures and peripheral sutures.

Unilateral lining loss

If the unilateral defect of the nostril margin is less than 1 cm in height, residual stratified squamous skin remains above the defect. A bipedicle flap of remnant vestibular skin, between the edge of the defect and the internal nasal valve, is moved caudally to line the nostril margin. The dry stratified squamous epithelium of the vestibular flap is less easily traumatized than septal mucosa, which can appear abnormally red postoperatively, secrete mucus, and bleed, if abraded. Medially, the flap is perfused through its connection to the ipsilateral septal lining at the septal angle. Laterally, it is vascularized by multiple branches of the facial angular arteries at the alar base.

A bipedicle flap, 8 mm wide, is designed within the existing lining, just above the defect. The incision of the flap's superior border (similar to the intercartilaginous incision of

an aesthetic rhinoplasty) is carried through the vestibular lining into the overlying soft tissues. The medial crus of the alar cartilage may need to be divided to mobilize the flap adequately. The flap is separated from the overlying subcutaneous tissues and hinged medially and laterally, as a bipedicle, to the level of the proposed nostril rim. The secondary defect, which remains above after advancement of the bipedicle flap, is filled with an ipsilateral septal flap. The ipsilateral septal flap, which measures up to 3 × 3 cm in width and length, passes towards the medial canthus about 6–8 mm below the dorsum and then travels posteriorly with a right angle to the nasal floor, proceeding anteriorly back towards the nasal spine. It is incised longitudinally with straight scissors. Its distal end is cut with a right-angle scissors. A 1.2-cm soft-tissue pedicle is maintained in the vicinity of the nasal spine to maintain the ipsilateral septal branch of the superior

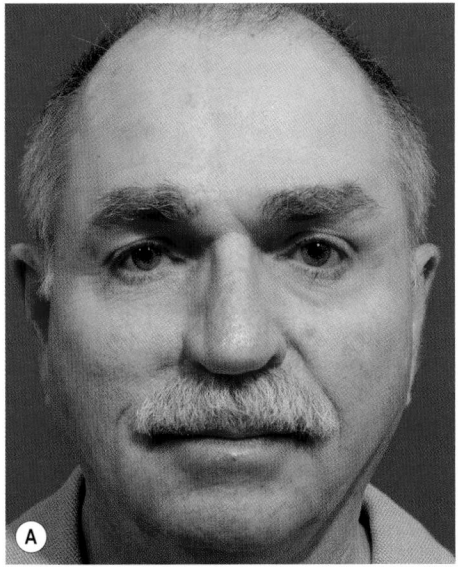
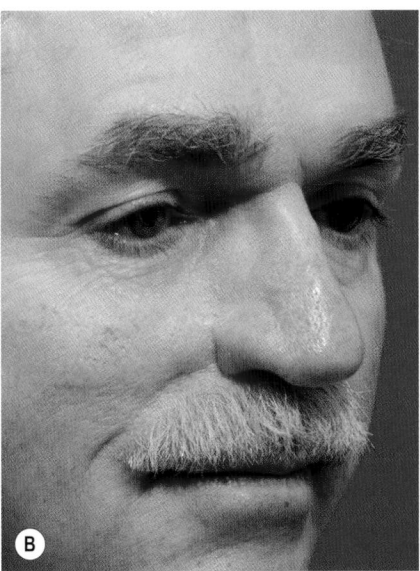
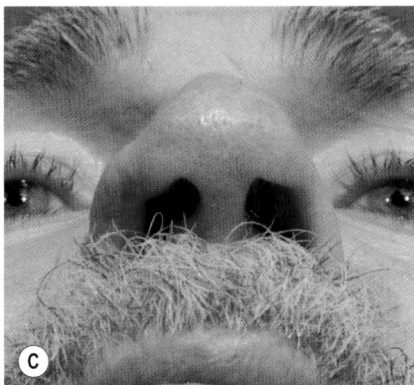

Fig. 6.33 (A–C) Postoperative result after pedicle division. No revision. The right alar crease could be refined by direct incision.

labial artery. The mucoperichondrium is elevated off the cartilage and bone of the septum and swung laterally. It is sutured to the superior aspect of the defect, laterally along the puriform aperture, and inferiorly to the bipedicle flap to create a complete lining sleeve for a unilateral nasal defect. The size of the flap is primarily limited by the surgeon's ability to incise within the confines of pyriform aperture. The flap can extend up to the medial canthus and inferiorly to the nasal floor. Leaving a strong septal "L," the central septal cartilage is harvested for graft material.

In larger defects, the secondary defect becomes too large to be replaced with an ipsilateral septal flap whose length is limited by the twist of its pedicle. The width of the flap may not be adequate to fill the height of the residual defect. In this instance, the contralateral septal flap is employed. First, the bipedicle flap of vestibular skin and mucosa is swung inferiorly. The ipsilateral septal mucosa is incised below the dorsum and elevated submucosally in line with the nasal bridge. The underlying septal cartilage is incised, protecting the contralateral mucosa. Septal cartilage is harvested, leaving a strong "L" strut. The dorsal mucosa is left intact while two parallel cuts are directed and then connected towards the floor of the nose. The flap is pulled to the ipsilateral mucosal slit to line the middle vault in the superior aspect of the vestibule while the bipedicle flap restores the nostril margin. The flaps are sutured to one another and supported by an alar batten and a sidewall brace of primary cartilage graft. The dorsally based, contralateral septal flap can be designed to extend on to the nasal floor, increasing its length, and allowing it to reach across the midline to the lateral aspect of the pyriform aperture. A wide flap can be designed along the entire dorsum to insure adequate vertical dimension to fill the height of the defect. However, the contralateral septal flap does not have length or width to reach inferiorly to the nostril rim. It is only useful for moderate mid-vault lateral nasal defects.

If the lining defect extends from the nostril margin to the nasal bones, an ipsilateral septal mucosal flap can be used to line the nostril margin inferiorly and a contralateral septal mucosal flap can be swung simultaneously to line the middle and upper vaults. This technique creates a permanent septal fistula, which is usually well tolerated. The mucoperichondrium is dissected off the entire ipsilateral septal, as in a submucous resection. The flap is swung laterally to expose septal bone and cartilage, which is harvested for graft material, maintaining an L-shaped strut of cartilage for dorsal and caudal support. Then a contralateral flap, based on the dorsum and anterior ethmoidal vessels, is incised, maintaining its dorsal pedicle and swung laterally to line the mid-vault. The ipsilateral septal flap is draped laterally towards the alar base to line the vestibule. The contralateral septal flap is passed through the septal fistula and sutured to the lateral edge of the nasal defect and then to the ipsilateral flap. The pedicle of the ipsilateral flap may partially obstruct the airway and need to be divided subsequently to open the airway.

Central lining loss

The high, converging medial and lateral walls of the upper and middle vaults may permit simple side-to-side approximation of lateral sidewall mucosa and medial septum if a modest central defect lies within the superior nose. This may lower the height of the nasal vault but may not significantly diminish nasal function. The height of the nasal bridge is restored with cartilage grafts.

Central nasal defects of the inferior nose are classified as subtotal (part of the projecting septum and bones at the radix are preserved) or total (loss of all soft tissue structures, anterior septum and nasal bones flush with the frontal bone of the maxilla). Fortunately, a large part of the anterior septum may remain projecting from the facial plane or lie hidden within the piriform aperture. This residual septum can be pulled out to provide lining for the projecting parts of the nose and its septal cartilage can be used as a foundation on which to rest a dorsal strut. The loss of the nasal bones is especially significant because they normally provide the fulcrum for a cantilevered dorsal support graft. In these instances, Millard perform a priliminay operation to reconstruct a bony base at the radix using local hingeover lining and a bone graft, covered initially by a median forehead flap. In other cases, he employed a superiorly based L-shaped full-thickness septal flap which was hinged out of the pyriform aperture to reestablish limited dorsal and caudal septal support and lining. Later, hinged over flaps of local tissue and bilateral nasolabial flaps were turned inward to line the mid-vault, ala and columella. A cantilever bone graft was anchored to the preplaced fulcrum to establish dorsal support, and a second forehead flap was used for cover. However, such traditional methods are unreliable due to vascularity, bulk, or inadequate support.

The septal composite flap, based on both superior labial arteries, mobilizes the entire septum out of the nasal cavity and projects it in front of the face. It positions a vertical sheet of bone and cartilage to support the dorsum of the nose. A dorsal costochondral rib graft can be placed on this hard tissue base and fixed to the residual nasal bones, or with a plate and screw, at the radix. The bilateral excess of septal mucosa is hinged laterally to provide lining for the lateral aspects of the defect. The full thickness of the septum is cut superiorly and inferiorly. Distally, it is transected with a right angle scissors. The mucosa is preserved in the region of the nasal spine and upper lip to preserve the right and left septal branches the superior labial arteries within a 1.2-cm soft-tissue pedicle. At the base of the flap, mucoperichondrial is separated on each side of the cartilaginous septum to remove a small wedge of bone and cartilage over the nasal spine. This allows the septal composite flap be drawn out of the pyriform aperture on a soft-tissue tether. The deep aspect of the flap is anchored to the stumps of the upper lateral cartilage or to the nasal bones with permanent suture or wire. The intranasal donor site is closed by mucosa to mucosa repair where possible. A large permanent septal fistula is created.

If the defect is limited to the upper or mid-vault, the composite flap restore the central bony platform while the mucosa of the right and left sides of the septum reflects laterally and is sutured to the lateral border of the defect to provide a complete vault lining. Primary subunit cartilage grafts are positioned to support and shape the covering forehead flap. In subtotal or total nasal reconstructions when the tip and ala are also missing, it is safer to mobilize and fix the septal composite flap to the radix or upper lateral cartilages. After insuring vascularity and healing to the residual nasal root, 6–8 weeks later, the exposed dorsal mucosal edge is split at its center and bilateral flaps are turned laterally. Superiorly, the septal mucosa is sufficient to line the upper and middle vaults however. More inferiorly, it will not reach the alar bases. It will not line the entire vestibule and ala, laterally. Additional alar lining must be supplied by hingeover flaps, turned up from a residual alar remnant or from a nasolabial flap. Presurgical delay of these local flaps may increase to their vascularity.

The modified folded forehead flap for lining (Figs 6.34–6.41)

Folding the distal end of the forehead flap on to itself to supply external cover and internal lining is a traditional method.[7] Unfortunately, it is difficult to position cartilage or bone grafts due to the bulk of soft tissues and limited exposure. The reconstructed nose is thick, shapeless and the airways are collapsed and occluded. However, the transfer of a full-thickness forehead flap in three operations with an intermediate stage between transfer and pedicle division has provided an opportunity to combine primary and delayed primary cartilage grafts and subcutaneous soft tissues sculpture with a modified folded approach. It has become a simple, efficient method, applicable to many lining defects. ☺ FIGS **6.36–6.41** APPEAR ONLINE ONLY

As described by Menick,[25,52,74,75] an extension of a full-thickness paramedian forehead flap, based on an exact template of the lining defect, is folded inward, Because the donor site lies within the area of forehead normally discarded as a dog-ear, there is minimal additional injury to the forehead. If the lining template must extend to the hairline, any transferred follicles simulate intranasal fibrous side and can be trimmed, postoperatively.

The flap, as a single cover and lining unit, is elevated from the distal to its proximal base, as a full-thickness flap. The

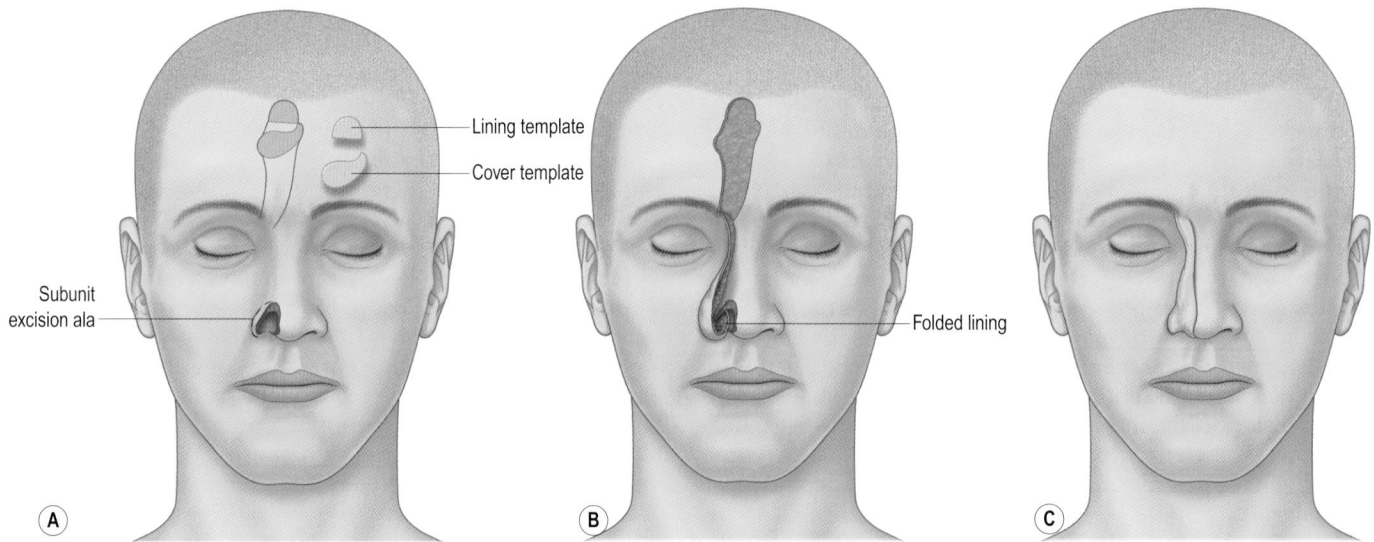

Fig. 6.34 (A–C) Folded forehead flap for lining – design and transfer. Based on exact patterns, a full-thickness forehead flap is elevated without thinning to supply external skin cover with the distal extension which will be folded inward to replace missing nasal lining. No primary cartilage grafts are placed.

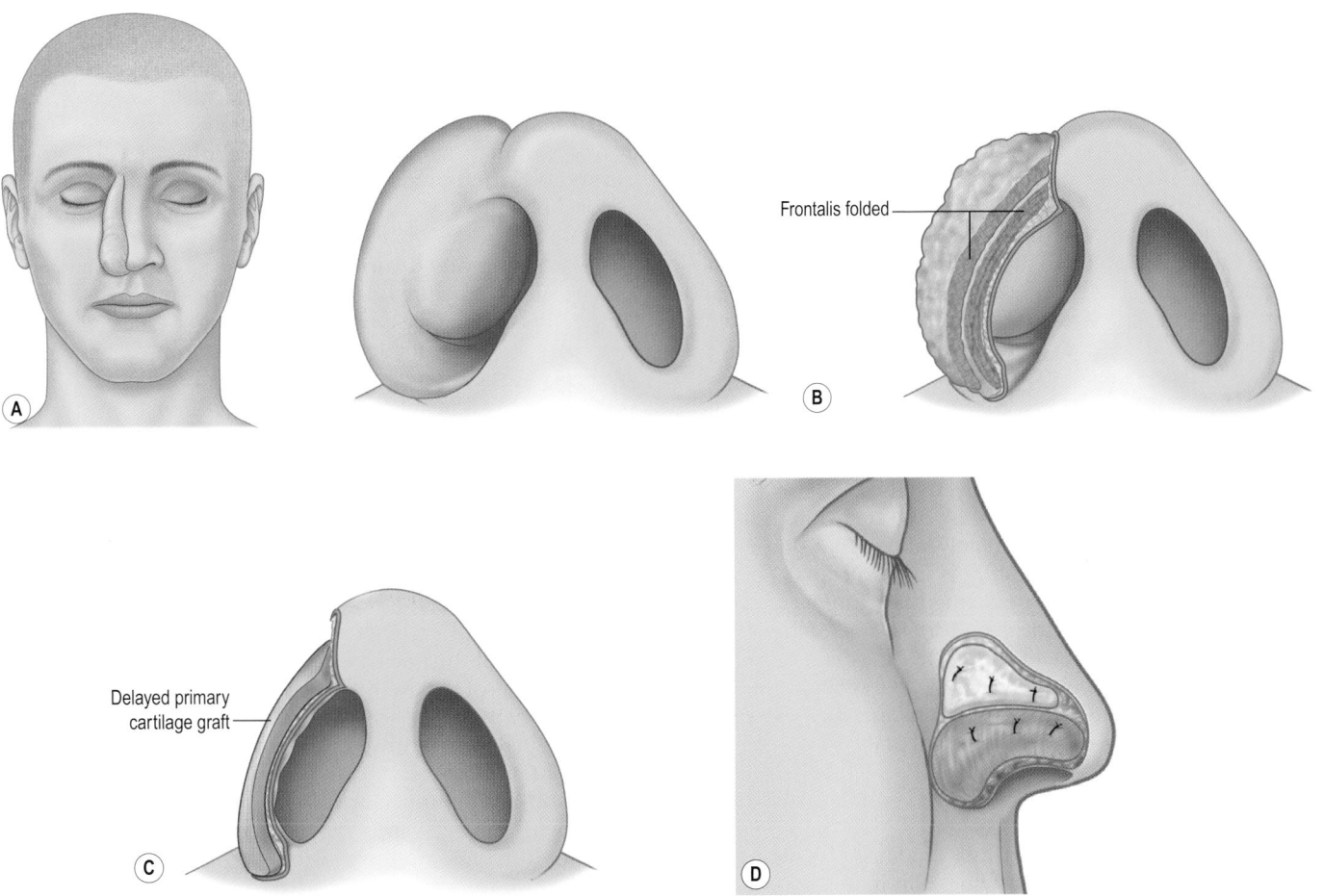

Fig. 6.35 (A–D) The intermediate operation of the modified folded forehead flap. One month later, the folded forehead flap lining extension is healed to the adjacent normal nasal lining and is no longer dependent on the forehead flap for its supratrochlear blood supply. The regional units of the nose and ideal alar margin are marked with ink. The forehead flap is incised between covering lining along the nostril margin and the covering flap is elevated with 23 mm of subcutaneous fat. This exposes the underlying unsupported subcutaneous fat and frontalis muscle which is excised from the underlying lining of folded forehead skin. A delayed primary cartilage graft is positioned to support the ala (and sidewall, if needed). The thin forehead flap is returned to the recipient site for nasal cover. One month later (2 months after the initial flap transfer), the proximal pedicle is divided.

distal lining extension (which can be partially thinned, if the full-thickness flap is especially stiff and difficult to turn inward) is folded inward and sutured to the residual mucosal lining of the defect. The more proximal aspect of the flap is folded back on to itself to provide nasal cover, creating a layer of external skin, subcutaneous fat, and frontalis muscle which provides nasal cover resting against an inner layer of frontalis muscle, subcutaneous fat and skin, which replaces the missing lining. No primary cartilage support is placed with the folded flap. However, primary cartilage grafts are placed in neighboring areas of more superficial injury with intact vascular lining.

At the second stage 4 weeks later, the proposed nostril margin is marked with ink, based on templates of the contralateral normal alar rim or the ideal. The nostril margin is incised, in the area of folding, separating the proximal covering skin from its distal lining extension. The proximal aspect of the covering flap is re-elevated with 2–3 mm of subcutaneous fat. Because the frontalis muscle was not excised or the subcutaneous plane of the flap injured during transfer, cover and lining skin remain soft, supple, and uncontracted. More

importantly, the folded distal extension, which was designed to line the nasal repair, is now healed and integrated into the residual normal lining. It is no longer dependent on the proximal forehead flap and its supratrochlear pedicle for blood supply. The underlying double layer of soft tissue – residual subcutaneous fat and frontalis is excised, exposing thin, supple and highly vascular lining. Delayed primary grafts are placed to create a complete subunit support framework. The thin, supple, unscarred skin of the proximal flap is returned to the recipient site. At the third stage, 4 weeks later (6–8 weeks after beginning the nasal repair), the pedicle is divided.

This modified folded forehead flap lining technique is reliable, efficient and effective in the repair of full-thickness unilateral and bilateral defects. It is employed to repair lining defects up to 3.0 cm in size and is useful for all small to moderate full-thickness defects. It avoids complex intranasal manipulation and minimizes the risk of postoperative bleeding or nasal obstruction, often associated with other techniques. The operative time is shortened, with less intranasal morbidity. If the defect extends from the ala on to the nasal floor, an additional distal extension can be added, at right angles to the alar lining extension, to line the ala and resurface the nostril sill. The vascularity of a full-thickness forehead flap is illustrated by the safety of such complex skin extensions.

Although all available lining options should be considered for any specific defect, the modified folded forehead lining technique has everyday application to complex nasal problems and should be a workhorse in nasal reconstruction. Due to its vascularity, it is especially useful in the smoker. Due to the shortened operative time and limited and intranasal manipulation, it is useful in the elderly or those with unassociated medical illness. When reopening a healed defect and returning normal to normal, it enhances the surgeon's ability to define the defect and immediately provide vascularized lining to fit the dimension, position and outline of the newly created defect, unlike prefabricated or hingeover flaps which require delay or intranasal lining flaps which may be precluded by injury to their vascular base or the position of the defect. It is a simple yet highly effective method.

Skin grafts have been used to line a two-stage forehead flap, at the time of transfer. Unfortunately, although a skin graft is thin and pliable, revascularization is unpredictable. To avoid this problem, most surgeons performed a preliminary prelamination (prefabrication) on the deep surface of a forehead flap 6 weeks before transfer. Later, once "take" was assured, the prelaminated forehead and underlying skin graft were transferred to the recipient site. Graft shrinkage, in these poorly supported noses, was accepted as a part of the technique.

Skin grafts for lining

Gillies developed a skin graft inlay method.[16] If lining and support were lost but the overlying skin remained intact (as in the syphilitic or leprotic saddle nose nose), scar was released on the undersurface of the external skin and a skin graft applied to the underlying raw surface. A permanent internal prosthesis, placed through a buccal fistula and fixed to dentures, splinted the graft to maintain airway patency and nasal shape.

More recently, Burget and Menick[22] tunneled a cartilage graft within the subcutaneous fat between the frontalis and the external skin of a paramedian forehead flap to repair modest nasal defects of the nostril margin and ala. The cartilage survived within the well vascularized soft tissue and supported the nostril margin. A full-thickness postauricular skin graft was sutured to the lining defect, raw surface outward. The deep surface of the frontalis muscle vascularized the underlying skin graft. The buried cartilage graft "stented" the skin grafted lining, much like Gillies' external splint.

In smaller unilateral defects, he combined a lining skin graft with an intranasal flap. When significant residual skin remained above the defect, a bipedicle flap of remnant vestibular skin, based on the septum medially and laterally at the alar base, was incised and transposed inferiorly to the level of the proposed alar margin. Because the marginal bipedicle flap had its own blood supply, a primary cartilage graft was fixed to its vascularized external surface. The secondary lining defect above the vestibular flap, was repaired with a full-thickness skin graft. No primary cartilage was placed in this area. A full-thickness forehead flap resurfaced the entire defect and revascularized the lining skin graft. 3–4 weeks later, after the skin graft lining was integrated and

vascularized from adjacent residual lining, the superior ala and sidewall were supported by a delayed primary cartilage graft at pedicle division. The forehead flap, maintaining a pedicle from the eyebrow to the distal flap inset along the nostril margin, could also be re-elevated over the mid-vault during an intermediate operation, to allow delayed primary support. Scarring in the vicinity of the internal valve, leading to nasal obstruction, occasionally followed and is difficult to correct.

These skin grafts retain most of their original dimensions. Some graft contracture does occur, causing minor distortions. Simplicity is a primary advantage, making it especially useful in an elderly or debilitated patient for whom more complex intranasal dissection should be avoided, when intranasal lining flaps are unavailable, or for the less demanding patient who desires a simple yet less delicate repair.

The three-stage full-thickness forehead flap has broadened the applications of skin grafts for lining, based on principles similar to those of the modified folded forehead flap technique.

As described by Menick,[25,76] a full-thickness forehead flap is highly vascular and a skin graft will routinely "take" on its deep raw surface. An exact pattern of the lining defect is outlined and a full-thickness postauricular skin graft is sutured to the margins of the lining defect. Primary cartilage grafts are precluded between the skin graft and the undersurface of the flap. Cartilage support can be placed over intact lining, adjacent to the full-thickness loss. Support grafts are not placed within soft-tissue tunnels within the forehead flap to avoid a thick nostril rim or the initiation of soft-tissue injury and scar. It is also difficult to design, position, or fix tunneled cartilage grafts. A full-thickness forehead flap resurfaces the nose. It provides a vascular bed for lining skin graft which is quilted to the overlying flap and is also splinted with a sponge bolus, placed with the nostril for 3–4 days to immobilize the repair and apply light pressure.

Four weeks later, the skin graft is healed to the adjacent normal residual lining and is no longer dependent on the covering flap for its blood supply. At the second stage, covering skin with 2–3 mm of subcutaneous fat is completely elevated from the nose. Excess subcutaneous fat and frontalis, which lay over the skin graft, are excised down to the newly reconstructed lining. The skin graft is thin, relatively supple, and vascularized by the adjacent residual lining. A delayed primary alar margin batten graft is fixed to support the nostril margin and a sidewall brace placed over the mid-vault to prevent upward retraction. The thin covering flap is replaced over the delayed primary cartilage grafts and the restored skin graft lining. Four weeks later (8 weeks after forehead flap transfer), the pedicle is divided.

Occasionally the skin graft fails. If so, the intermediate stage is delayed and the granulating bed of the undersurface of the forehead flap is sharply debrided and a second graft applied. The forehead flap does not need to be re-elevated. The skin graft is simply applied to its raw deep surface. Because frontalis muscle was not excised or the subcutaneous plane of the full-thickness forehead flap injured, fibrosis or contracture does not occur within the covering flap. Although an additional stage is required to replace the skin graft, the overall result is not impaired.

The modified skin graft for lining technique is reliable, efficient, and effective for the repair of small to moderate, full-thickness nasal defects. Scar contracture and secondary distortion are modest and a delicate alar rim can be created. The technique should be limited to lining defects at 0.5–1.5 cm in size. Skin graft "take" is routine, although a second graft may be required in 20–30% of cases. However, an initial skin graft loss delays pedicle division from the expected 8–12 weeks. The risk of poor skin graft take and contraction increases as the size of the lining defect increases. The method is especially useful in the elderly or debilitated patient with unassociated medical illness when the risk of temporary nasal obstruction caused by intranasal lining flaps should be minimized or when previous nasal injury precludes the use of intranasal lining flaps.

Overall, as in the folded-flap technique for lining, morbidity is minimal. Because equal or better results can be obtained with the folded forehead flap lining technique, without the risk of skin graft loss, it is preferred to the skin graft lining approach and can be applied to larger lining defects up to 3 cm. However, both methods are reliable, less complex, shorten operating time and are associated with minimal morbidity.

The modified skin graft technique has its most important application in salvage situations when lining is inadequate after forehead flap transfer by any lining technique. Rather than accept an inadequate airway, a lining skin graft can be applied prior to pedicle division to augment the lining surface dimension. If a full-thickness forehead flap has been employed initially, the flap is re-elevated during an intermediate operation, deficient lining at one or both alar bases is cut free. The lining gap is filled with a full-thickness skin graft. The full-thickness flap is reapplied without thinning to revascularize the skin graft. Once healed in place, the forehead flap is re-elevated thinly during a second intermediate operation, excess soft tissue excised, and delayed primary grafts placed to provide permanent support and shape over the augmented skin graft lining.

Microvascular lining with distant tissue

Especially "difficult" facial wounds are defined by their site, size, depth, and wound character (vascularity, contamination, radiation, immunosuppression and exposure of vital structures). Such complex, and often composite injuries to the adjacent cheek and lip, may make local tissues inadequate or unavailable for nasal repair and require the introduction of distant tissue, by microvascular transfer, to re-establish the midface platform or to supply nasal lining.[77,78] A regional forehead flap can provide covering skin, but distant tissue, transferred as a microvascular flap, will be needed for lining. The volume of missing tissues and the dimensions of the surface requirements must not be underestimated. Large amounts of healthy vascularized tissue will be needed to ensure primary healing.

A preliminary operation may be required to return normal to normal, establish a stable platform, or delay or reposition residual tissues, prior to the repair of the nose.

Principles of free flap nasal reconstruction

1. If missing, the midface platform must be reestablished during a preliminary operation prior to nasal reconstruction. When in doubt, reconstruct the lip and cheek first and rebuild the nose later. The nose must sit on the midface in the correct position and with the correct projection.

2. The septal partition is not restored to avoid excessive intranasal bulk and nasal obstruction. A septal fistula is accepted.

3. Columellar lining is provided only to provide a soft tissue pocket to position cartilage support and "back" the raw surface of the future covering forehead flap. The deeper septum is not restored.

4. The site and dimension of missing nasal lining must be identified. The vault spans from alar base to alar base and from the superior aspect of the defect to the base of the columella. If completely absent, this measures 7–8 cm transversely and 4 cm vertically from the nasal route to the tip with an additional 3 cm for the columella. Re-establishment of vault lining is straightforward because it must simply drape across a central support which prevents its collapse into the pyriform aperture. The columella must be long enough to project the nose and narrow enough to maintain patent airways. The nasal floor or sill is the skin platform on to which the nose must be placed. In many cases, the floor remains intact or has been previously restored during a preliminary operation to build the nasal platform. It may also be reconstructed at the time of free flap transfer with local tissue or with part of the free flap. A floor deficiency may be obvious after excision or trauma, especially if an open wound is present or, if , by history, the lip has suffered extensive injury. It is less apparent after injury due cocaine or other intranasal processes. Clinically, the upper lip is drawn back and up, identified by displacement and posterior angulation of the upper aspect of the lip. The tissue deficiency must be released and skin replaced under the future alar and columellar juice two.

5. The nasal reconstruction is planned in stages. Despite Gillies' admonition to employ "like" tissue, distant skin for lining, bulky rib grafts for support, or a thick, flat forehead flap for external cover are "unlike" the normal. The challenge is to modify these disparate donor materials into "nasal-like tissues" and integrate them together, restoring each anatomic layer to recreate a normal looking and functioning nose. The initial goal is to supply lining for the inner surface of the nose during a preliminary operation. This greatly simplifies the overall reconstruction. Once in place, the distant lining effectively turns a complex full thickness defect into a superficial one, requiring only support and cover which is addressed using traditional methods using local and regional tissue.

6. Distant tissue can close dead space, fill a cavity, protect vital structures, create a barrier between the central nervous system and the oral cavity, close a fistula, or build a stable platform. However, distant tissue always appears as a mismatched, discolored patch when it lies within residual normal facial skin. No free flap has a facial shape.

Microvascular distant flaps are used to provide nasal lining and vascularity. Excess is used to refill the wound and provide for other needs – soft-tissue cheek bulk, upper lip skin, nasal floor etc. Facial skin, transferred as a forehead flap with matching skin of correct color and texture, is used to resurface the nose.

The midfacial defect with an inadequate platform

Local or regional tissue are insufficient to restore such complex defects and distant tissue, most often harvested from the trunk, is necessary to provide sufficient soft tissue and skin – a scapular, parascapular, latissimus, or rectus flap. The immediate goal of surgery is to provide an excess of tissue with adequate bulk and projection, obliterating an open maxillary sinus, if necessary. Only the facial platform is restored initially. Both bone and soft tissue can be supplied. Nasal reconstruction is delayed until a stable platform is restored.

Restoring nasal lining with a free flap

If the midface platform is stable, the nasal repair can be initiated without delay. In smaller composite losses, minor lip and cheek defects may be replaced with local tissues or with extensions of the free lining flap.

Defects of the mid-vault alone

If the defect is limited to the nasal vault, only vault lining and preliminary central support are required at the first stage. Because of its thinness and long vascular pedicle, the radial forearm flap is preferred.

In general, if the nostril rims are intact and the defect includes only the mid-vault, the lining defect may be filled with a free flap, skin inward for lining. Its outer surface is skin grafted.

If the residual septum is intact with adequate height, it can temporarily support the lining flap until later definitive placement of additional cartilage grafts and a covering forehead flap.

If the normal nostril rim lining is missing, the flap is folded over on to itself along the future nostril margin. This allows placement of an autogenous dorsal cantilever bone graft for immediate central support. Subsequently during the definitive nasal repair, the external skin graft or folded skin are excised. A complete subunit support framework is placed and the nose is resurfaced with a forehead flap.

If the septum remains but has been partially resected, it can be swung out of the nasal cavity as an inferiorly based composite septal flap during a preliminary operation. Then the free flap is transferred for lining, once vascularity of the composite flap is assured.

If the majority of the septal partition is missing, it is not reconstructed. Local or distant tissue is too thick to replace the septum without creating airway obstruction. A permanent septal fistula is accepted. The surgeon only provides lining for the vault and backing for the columella.

Subtotal and total nasal defects – lining for the vault, columella, and nasal floor

Distant tissue has been transferred as cutaneous, composite helical, osteocutaneous, prelaminated, or prefabricated free flaps, with limited application and success.[61,62] The exception is the ground-breaking work of Burget and Walton[26,79] who employed multiple, longitudinally oriented forearm skin paddles to repair nasal defects. Two or three separate skin flaps were positioned, skin inward, to individually line the vault, columella, and nasal floor. Each paddle was vascularized by the underlying radial vessel, like a "string of beads." Their external raw surfaces were covered with full-thickness skin grafts, precluding primary soft-tissue support. Later, the individual skin paddles were sutured together, thinned, supported with cartilage grafts, and resurfaced with a distally thinned two-stage forehead flap. During a subsequent operation prior to pedicle division, forehead skin was elevated over the mid-vault and soft tissue was excised over the superior two-thirds of the nose, as described by Millard.[30] A second intermediate operation was performed to debulk the airways. Later, the pedicle was divided and a revision performed. Good results were obtained during six or more operations (Fig. 6.42).

However, limitations are apparent.[9] Elevating three separate paddles for the vault, columella, and nasal floor is technically tedious and leaves a short proximal vascular pedicle for anastomosis. Injury to the vascular pedicle during elevation, or kinking during positioning of these multiple paddles, could jeopardize blood flow. The vascular pedicle to each paddle is also exposed to injury during subsequent stages, which may compromise blood supply, already limited by the scars between the skin islands. This may be exemplified by their need for a second free flap to remedy columellar lining necrosis during revision. The cutaneous scars between each paddle may lead to skin contraction and limit the suppleness of the lining. Because primary support cannot be placed under the initial external skin grafts, soft-tissue collapse and skin shrinkage may occur. Most importantly, no excess tissue is available to salvage an imperfection in flap design or a complication.

The use of a two-stage forehead flap, with an intermediate operation, was originally suggested by Millard in 1974.[68] He combined traditional distal thinning of a forehead flap with an additional operation, prior to pedicle division. The forehead flap was elevated over the mid-vault as a bipedicle, maintaining the tip, alar and columellar inset. The superior two-thirds of the nose was reshaped. However, this forehead flap approach, which combines initial distal thinning of forehead flap and subsequent mid-vault elevation, has several disadvantages. Initial distal excision of frontalis muscle may decrease the overall blood supply to the forehead flap. It is more difficult to create a thin uniform skin flap when the forehead flap is thinned in stages. Precise contouring of the mid-vault is impeded by the bipedicle flap, which limits exposure. Most importantly, the contour of the distal inset – the most aesthetic part of the nose – is fixed. The shape of tip, ala, and columella cannot be altered after initial forehead flap transfer.

Menick and Salibian[27] have recently described a folded single-paddle forearm flap approach, combined with a three-stage full-thickness forehead flap for cover, which is a reliable efficient microvascular design, applicable to varied defects[14] (Figs 6.43–6.49).

Operation 1

A pattern of the lining defect is positioned on the forearm and face to verify the flap's size, outline, orientation, pedicle

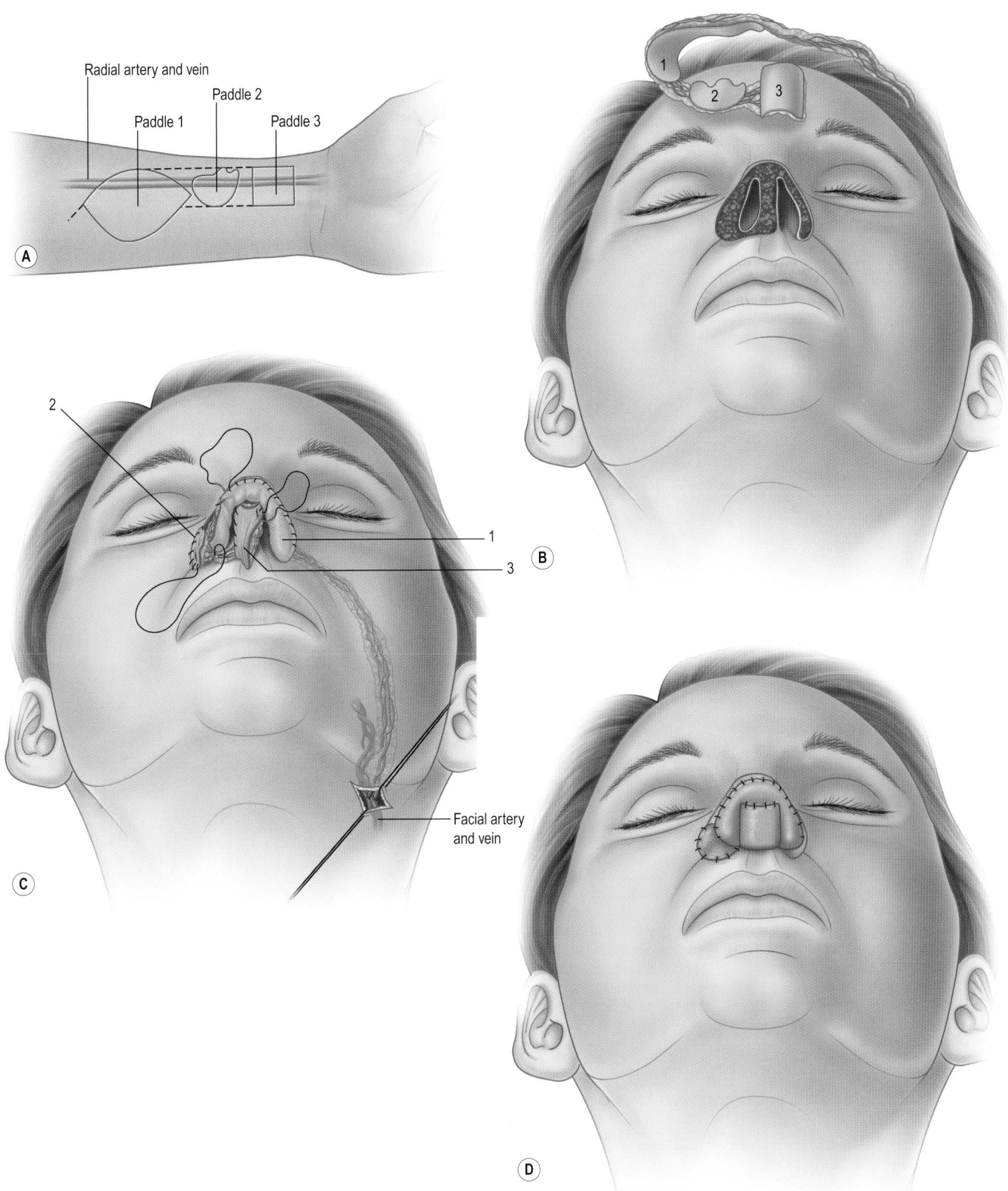

Fig. 6.42 (A–D) The Burget and Walton approach to microvascular nasal lining. Individual radial forearm flap paddle design to replace nasal vault, columellar, and nasal lining. Islands of skin, each perfused by the radial artery, are designed like a "string of beads" to supply lining for the nasal vault, columella, and nasal floor. Their unsupported external surfaces are temporarily covered with full-thickness skin grafts. Later, the skin grafts are excised, excess forearm subcutaneous fat excised, individual paddles sutured together to complete the lining, primary cartilage grafts placed, and the nose resurfaced with a distally thin forehead flap. During an intermediate operation, the flap is elevated over the mid-vault to allow local soft-tissue debulking, maintaining the proximal supratrochlear pedicle and the distal flap to the columellar tip and ala.

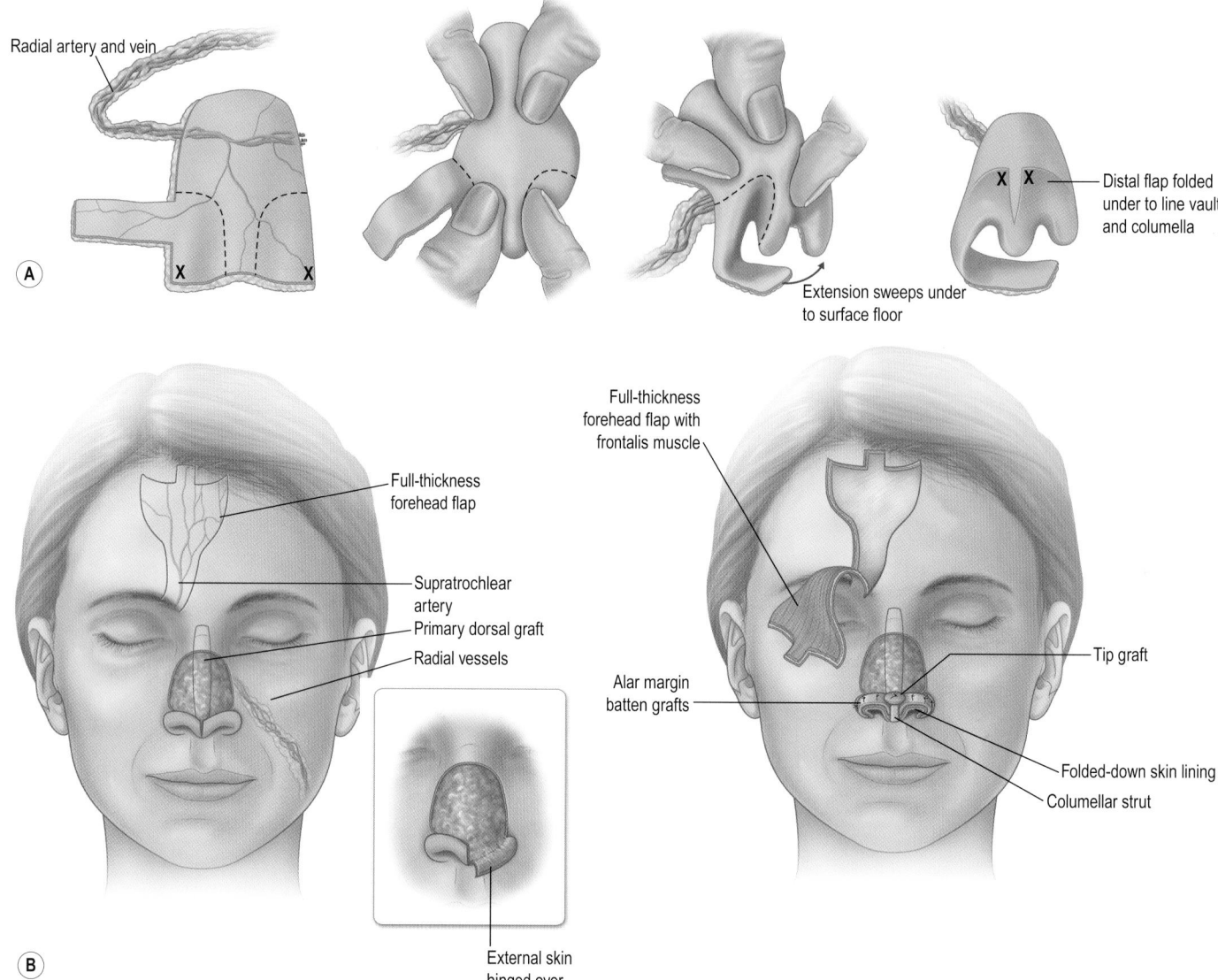

Fig. 6.43 (A, B) The Menick and Salibian approach to microvascular lining. Nasal lining is designed as a distal single-paddle radial forearm flap with an extension for the nasal floor. The flap is folded inward to line the columella and vault; the floor extension spontaneously rotates to resurface the nasal floor. More proximal skin is turned back to provide cover, creating a soft-tissue pocket which allows for placement of primary dorsal support at the initial stage. Later, external radial skin can be hinged inferiorly to permit adjustments in the nostril margin of the alar base position. Excess radial forearm subcutaneous tissue is excised, maintaining the radial artery pedicle intact. A complete subunit support framework is added to shape the columella, tip alar margins, and sidewalls. The repair is covered with a full-thickness forehead flap. During a subsequent intermediate operation the forehead skin is elevated completely, maintaining the supratrochlear pedicle. The underlying soft tissues are excised to sculpt a three-dimensional shape over the entire nasal surface and permit placement or adjustments of cartilage grafts. The "thinned" flap is returned to the contoured recipient site and the pedicle is divided later.

length, area of folding, and the position of the skin extension for the nasal floor.

A single, horizontally oriented paddle of forearm skin (8–10 cm in width and 6–8 cm in height) is outlined on the distal forearm, with or without a proximal extension for the nasal floor.

The flap can be raised as a skin flap, maintaining only fasciocutaneous connections over the radial vessels. However, it is safer to limit primary fascial excision to maintain maximum blood supply. The extension for the nasal floor is designed vertically, in continuity with the primary flap, just distal to the future site of infolding. This positions the extension to resurface the floor when the primary flap is turned inward for lining. Because the single skin paddle is placed distally on the forearm, a 12–15-cm arterial pedicle and a longer venous pedicle (extended through the communicating vein from the venae comitantes to the cephalic vein) are available. Large high-flow recipient vessels may be preferred and can be anastomosed to the first branch of the external carotid artery and the internal jugular vein or external jugular vein as recipients. The superficial temporal artery and external jugular vein or facial vessels are used in the short fat neck.

The thin, distal ulnar edge of the forearm flap is pinched together in the midline, with suture approximating its posterior raw surface to "manufacture" a skin columella which will

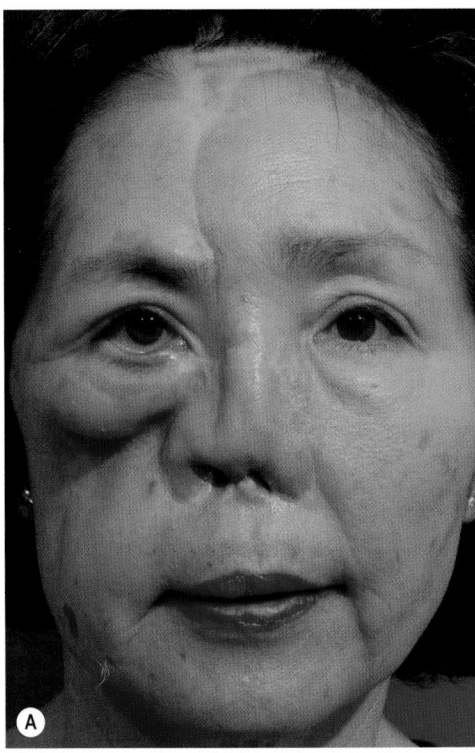
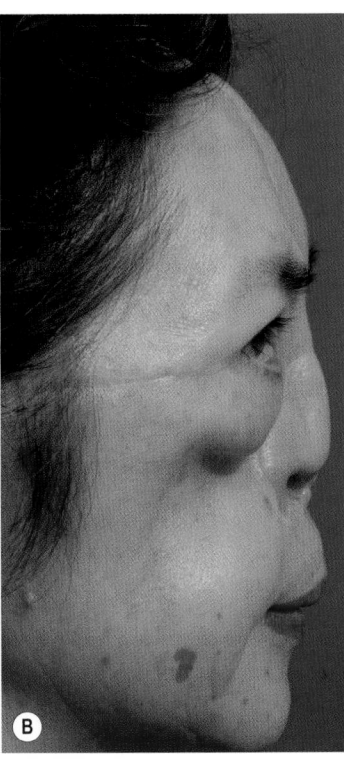

Fig. 6.44 (A, B) Deformity after excision of recurrent cancer. Past anterior maxillectomy, subtotal nasectomy, and reconstruction with inadequate local lining, support, and right paramedian forehead flap. The distal nose is covered with hair. The airways are occluded and the nasal shape is abnormal.

later provide a posterior backing for the columellar extension of the forehead flap. The septal partition is not restored.

The distal skin is folded under the more proximal skin flap to line both vaults. The lateral, distal tips of the flap are fixed to the midline of the lining defect and then sutured toward the alar bases, from medial to lateral, completing the inset. The height of the columella and dimension of the vault are adjusted, and slightly exaggerated, by altering the extent of infolding. As the flap folds inward to line the vault, the skin extension spontaneously rotates inward to resurface the floor. Tension, tight molding sutures, or aggressive thinning are avoided.

Proximal radial skin, with the vascular pedicle, is turned back over the infolded lining. This places the pedicle externally over the mid-vault, on the outer surface of the repair, out of the airway and away from the inferior one-third of the nose. The external skin is sutured to the periphery of the nasal defect to provide cover. A smooth, seamless, unscarred arching of the lining envelope recreates the nasal vault, columella, and nasal floor, as needed.

In subtotal and total defects requiring dorsal support, an osteocartilaginous rib graft is fixed primarily to the residual nasal bones or frontal bone within the soft-tissue pocket of external and internal forearm skin. Residual rib cartilage is "banked" on the chest.

The reconstructed columella is inset in the midline to the residual or resurfaced nasal floor.

Operation 2

Two months later, excess external skin can be discarded or hinged downward to adjust nasal length and modify the nostril rim and the alar base positions and symmetry. Inevitably, errors in flap design, malposition of the folded

nostril margin, alar base asymmetry, scar contracture, or any complication, such as rim necrosis or dehiscence, require correction. External forearm skin, with a few millimeters of subcutaneous fat, is elevated and turned over inferiorly. The hinged-over skin is trimmed to refine or reposition the nostril margins or alar bases, if needed. The external cutaneous surface of the columella is split in the midline. If lining for the columella was not included in the initial vault design or is unavailable due to tissue loss or wound separation with retraction, the external vault excess can be turned over to provide columellar or alar lining at this stage without delaying the repair or impairing the final result.

The vascular pedicle is not elevated and remains adherent to the underlying lining. The radial vessels, which perfused the folded flap through its external skin surface, are effectively "prelaminated" to the underlying lining. After elevation of external radial skin, the lining remains perfused through the radial pedicle and by its peripheral inset to the recipient site.

Excess subcutaneous fat and fascia, on the exposed surface of the underlying lining, are excised, protecting the radial vessels. This exposes thin, supple, scarless lining. Delayed primary rib support (a columellar strut, tip graft, alar battens, and sidewall cartilage grafts) is fixed to each other and to the previously positioned dorsal graft to complete the subunit support framework. The base of the columellar strut is sutured to the nasal spine through a buccal incision. A full-thickness forehead flap, with or without expansion and without distal thinning, is transferred for permanent nasal cover.

Operation 3

One month later, the forehead flap is physiologically delayed. Forehead skin with 2–3 mm of subcutaneous forehead fat is

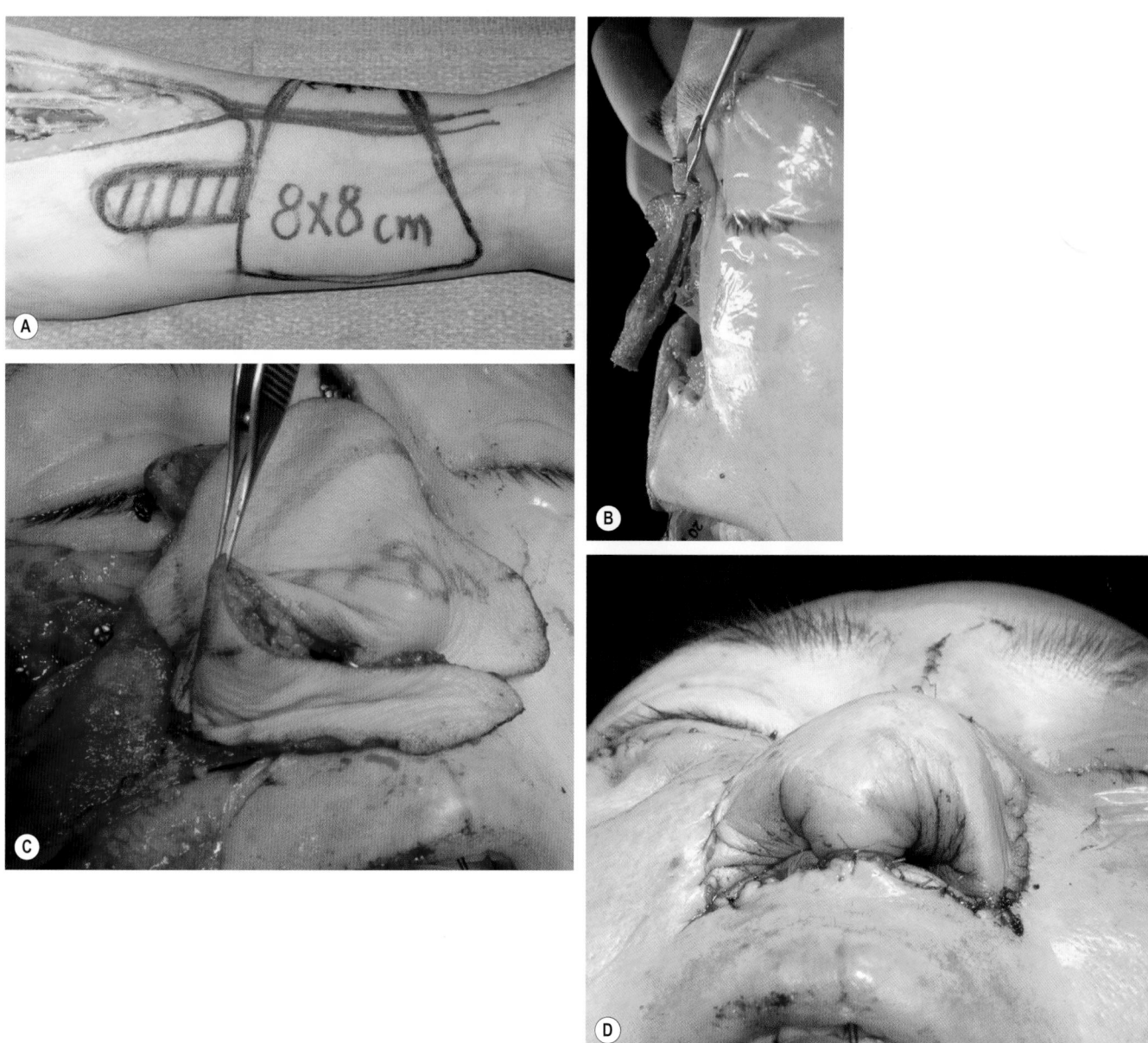

Fig. 6.45 (A–D) Distal radial forearm flap designed with an extension of the nasal floor. Its ulnar border is folded inward to create columella and pulled lining. The skin extension resurfaces the nasal floor. More proximal forearm skin and the radial vessels are turned back to provide temporary cover and permit placement of a primary dorsal osteocartilaginous graft.

completely elevated from the recipient site, maintaining an intact supratrochlear pedicle. With complete visualization, the underlying exposed subcutaneous fat and frontalis muscle are artistically excised over the entire nasal surface, including the tip and ala. Previously placed cartilage grafts are sculpted, repositioned, or augmented to shape an ideal three-dimensional support framework. Forehead skin, now with the thinness of nasal skin, is replaced on the recipient site.

Operation 4

One month later, the forehead pedicle is divided. Further debulking of the airway, by excising excess soft tissue between

the lining and cartilage grafts, can be performed through nostril marginal incisions at pedicle division or during a later revision.

Operation 5

Four months later, a revision is performed to improve the forehead scar, define the alar creases by direct incision, add a secondary tip graft, or trim the nostril margins or columella.

The result of any reconstruction will be determined by the choice of donor materials, methods of transfer, flap design, and the capacity to modify tissues to the needs of the defect. The ability to adjust the dimension and outline of each anatomic layer, correct imperfections, or salvage complications is

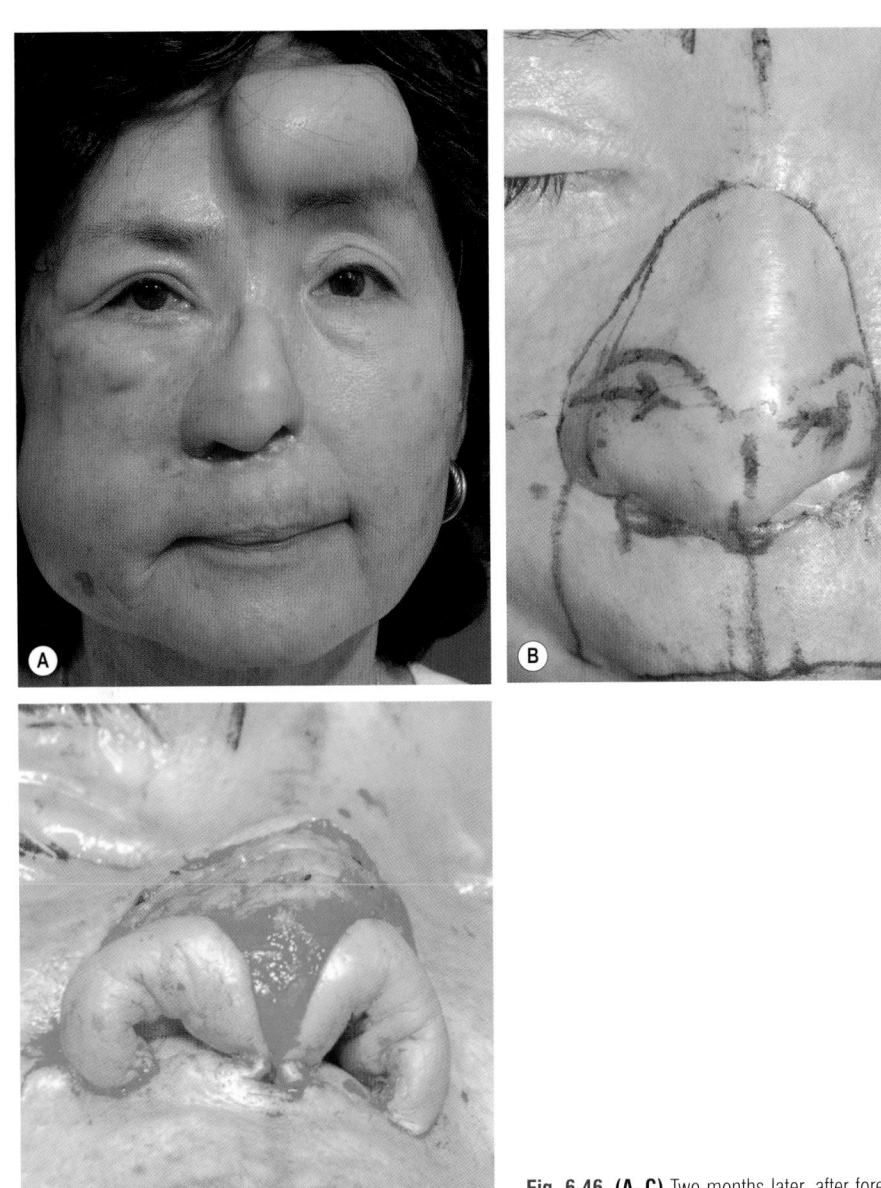

Fig. 6.46 (A–C) Two months later, after forehead expansion, external radial skin is hinged inferiorly. The reconstructed "columella" is split in the midline. The nostril margin and alar base insets are adjusted. The radial vessels are left adherent to the underlying folded lining. Excess forearm soft tissue is excised to trim the lining.

vital. This blending of distant folded radial forearm lining, timed rib grafts for support, and a regional three-stage full-thickness forehead flap for cover permits the integration of "unlike" tissues which can restore a nose which looks and functions normally. It is reliable, efficient, and reproducible. Good results – an attractive nose with patent airways – can be obtained in the repair of complex heminasal, subtotal, and total injuries.

Outcomes, prognosis, and complications

Complications are uncommon.[22,25,80,81] Fortunately, the abundant blood supply of the face mitigates against ischemia or infection. However, badly scarred tissues, a history of multiple past operations, prior alloplastic implant, or previous infection increases the risk.

If a complication ensues, the repair is almost always salvageable. However, a complication is of great concern due to the risk of loss of the invaluable building materials and the emotional stress on the patient and surgeon. Correction may prolong the reconstruction and increase the number of stages. The patient may have to live with undivided pedicle until the problem is resolved, the tissues have matured, and unplanned procedures are performed. This may require an early reoperation or a postponement of a previously scheduled operation. But the complication must be dealt with. Most importantly, save the repair. If not, limit the damage. Preserve viable donor materials for another day, at the very least. The rich vascularity of the soft tissues of a full-thickness forehead flap,

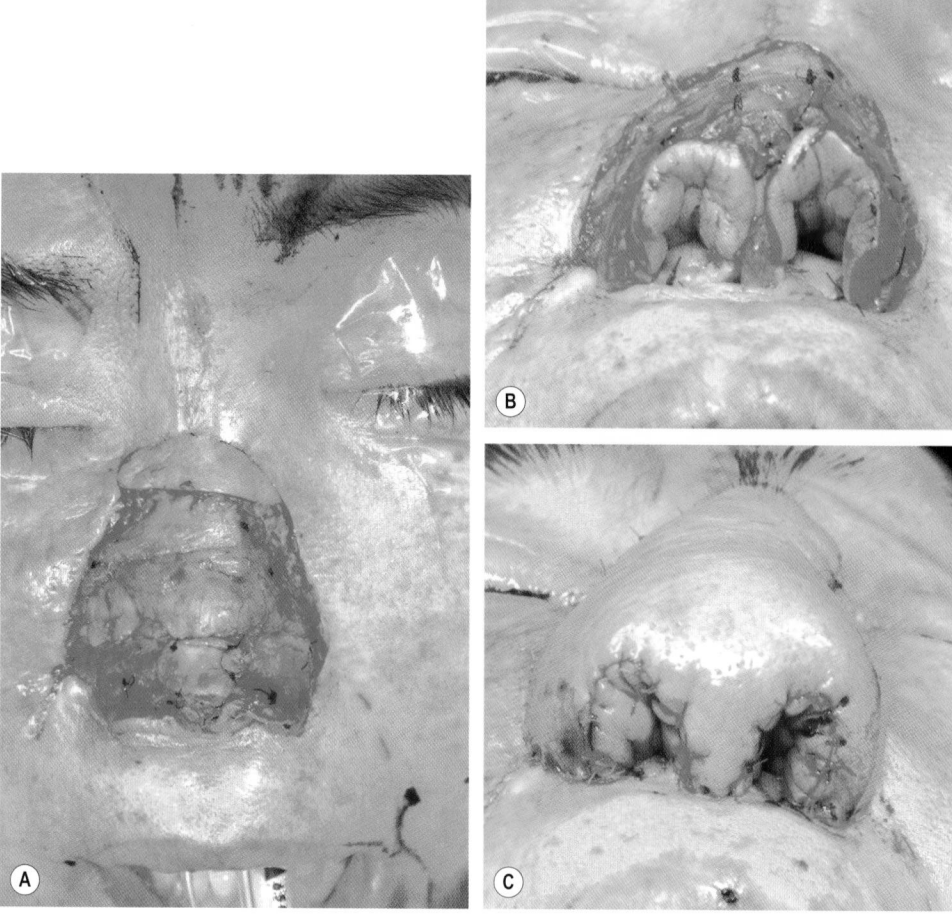

Fig. 6.47 (A–C) Subunit support is completed with a columellar strut, tip graft, and bilateral alar margin rib grafts. The repair is resurfaced with a full-thickness forehead flap.

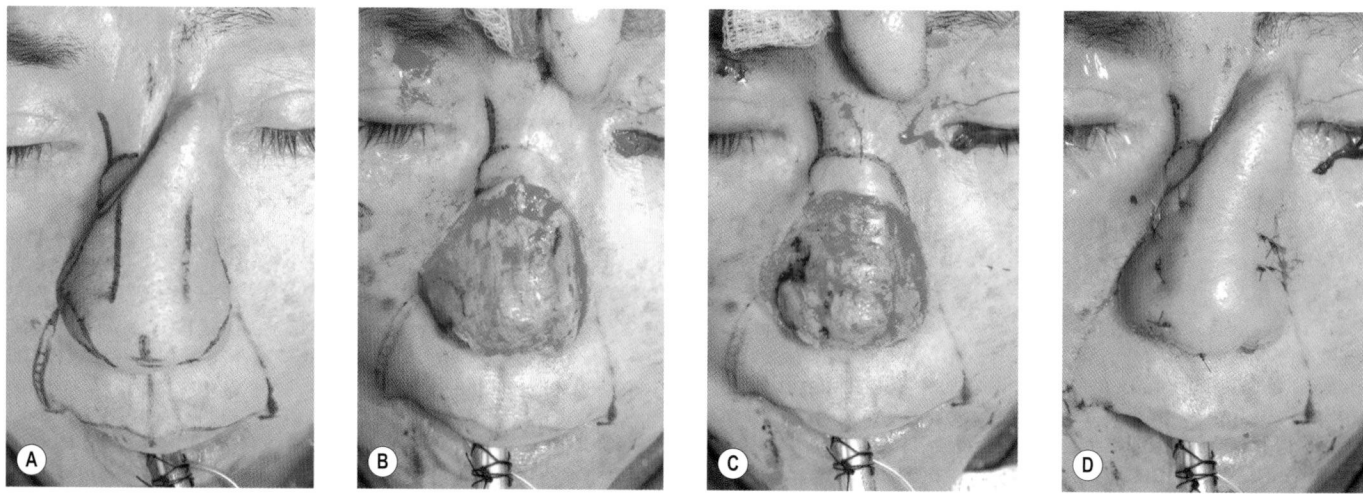

Fig. 6.48 (A–D) During the subsequent intermediate operation, forehead skin with 2–3 mm of subcutaneous fat is elevated over the entire nasal inset, maintaining the proximal supratrochlear pedicle. Underlying excess forehead subcutaneous fat and frontalis muscle are excised to sculpt a nasal shape. The "thin" forehead skin flap is returned to the recipient site.

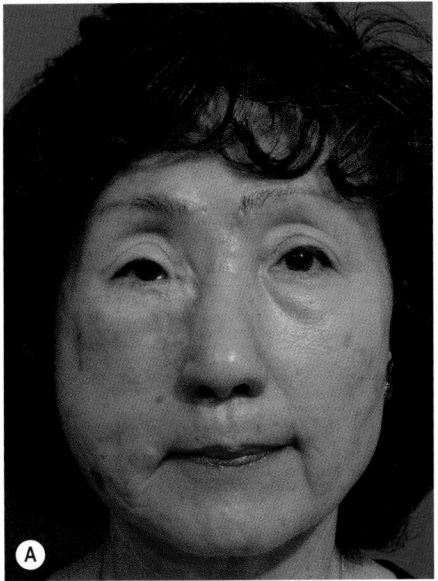
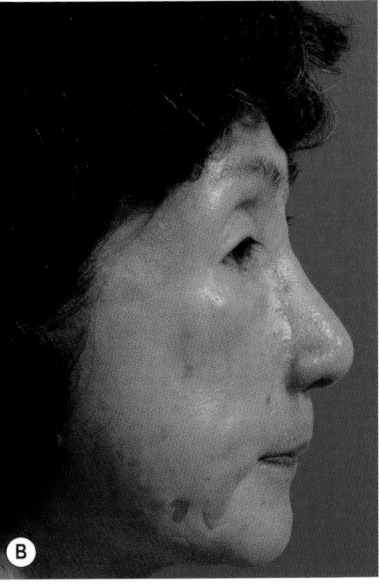
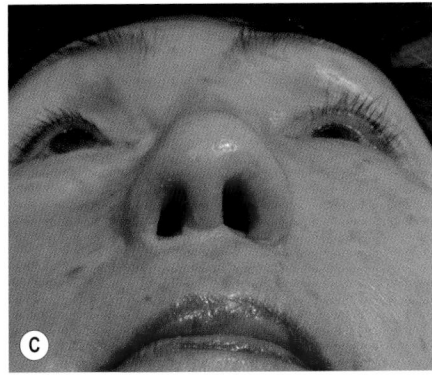

Fig. 6.49 (A–C) Postoperative result after pedicle division. The patient's cheek was recontoured with a de-epithelialized proximal fasciocutaneous radial extension, rib grafts, and a dermal fat graft.

transferred in three stages, may lessen the risk of complications and allow more reliable treatment.

Forehead flap necrosis is uncommon. It follows excessive wound closure due to inadequate dimension or aggressive suturing of the flap to the recipient site, failure to identify a significant old scar within the flap's territory, or injury to the vascular pedicle, overzealous thinning at transfer, or excessive re-elevation of the flap from the recipient site at pedicle division. To avoid underlying cartilage infection and progressive injury, early local debridement of a significant covering flap necrosis (more than a few millimeters) and immediate resurfacing with a second vascularized flap (often as a subunit) may be preferable to watchful waiting which will lead to severe soft-tissue distortion requiring a secondary reconstruction or chronic cartilage infection and progressive destruction.

Fulminant acute infection is extremely uncommon but may follow a failure in aseptic technique or lining necrosis. If limited necrosis of lining is identified prior to gross infection, early debridement of the necrotic lining, removal of overlying primary cartilage grafts, and skin grafting of the lining deficit are performed. The forehead flap is replaced. One month later, the skin graft is revascularized from adjacent lining and the forehead flap can be re-elevated and resupported with delayed primary grafts. If the infection is severe, aggressive debridement of infected and necrotic nasal tissues and return of the forehead flap to the donor site to preserve it for a later repair may be required.

Chronic cartilage infection presents as local redness with purulent discharge several weeks after surgery. It should be treated quickly with limited flap re-elevation and debridement if infected. It does not respond reliably to simple antibiotic coverage. Once controlled, secondary cartilage grafts are placed to resupport the deficient area 6–8 weeks later.

Watchful waiting for the resolution of tissue loss or infection, with or without antibiotic coverage, is rarely successful.

Secondary procedures

A complex nasal reconstruction will often require a revision to re-establish ideal nasal form and function. Exact templates, based on the contralateral normal or ideal, guide the revision, which is performed under general anesthesia, without local anesthesia, to avoid intraoperative distortion and blanching *(Figs 6.50–6.57)*. FIGS **6.54–6.57** APPEAR ONLINE ONLY

Revisions can be classified[25] as:

- minor: essential quality, outline, and contour have been restored with inadequate landmark definition
- major: failure of dimension, volume, contour, and symmetry or function
- redo: cover and lining are grossly deficient. Normal must be returned to normal and the repair redone with a second regional flap.

The minor revision

When the overall dimension and volume of the nose are correct, "finesse definition" can be achieved through direct incisions hidden in the joins between subunits, disregarding old scars. The alar crease or nasolabial fold are defined and secondary support placed. A minor revision can often be accomplished in one stage.

The nostril margins and columella may be thick and the airway stenotic. The nostril margin is incised, separating cover and lining. Lining is elevated thinly into the airway. Excess subcutaneous fat and scar are excised between the lining layer and the deep surface of previously positioned support grafts, debulking the airway. The lining is incised in the anterior vestibule and/or nasal floor at right angles to the nostril margin. Discardable excess, from the thick reconstructed alar rim and columella or from the lip, inferior to

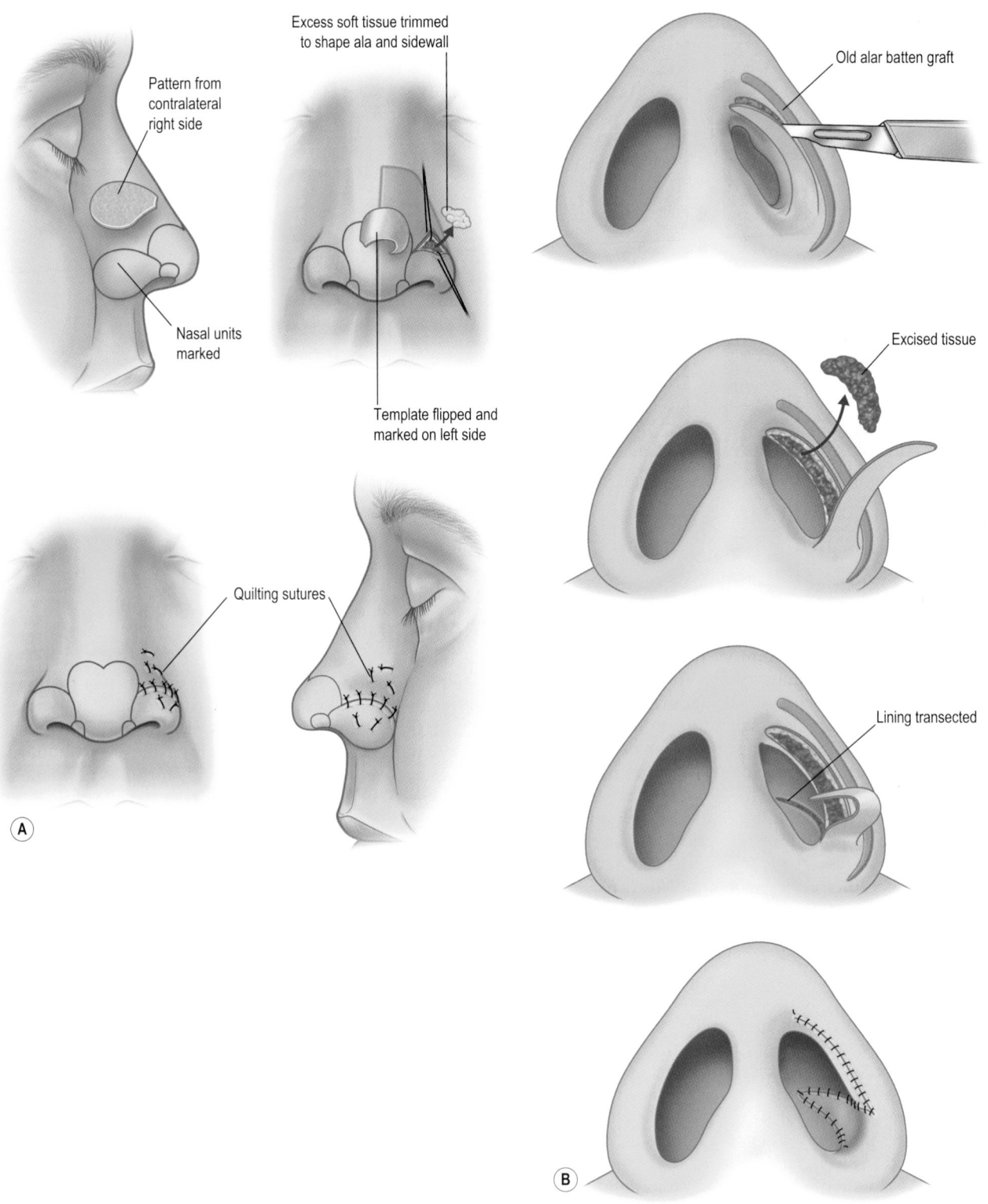

Fig. 6.50 (A, B) The contour and function of the reconstructed nose can be improved by secondary revision. Four to 6 months after reconstruction, soft tissues can be sculpted and secondary cartilage grafts placed. If the overall dimension, position, and volume of the nose are correct, the revision can be performed through direct incisions to re-establish fine landmarks. If not, the transferred flap is re-elevated along its periphery, based on its inset into the recipient site blood supply. Soft tissues are excised, secondary cartilage grafts added, and the flap returned to the recipient site. A secondary revision may be necessary to define the alar crease further. The alar crease is recreated by direct incision, based on the contralateral normal or on the ideal. Disregarding old scars, an incision is made at the ideal alar crease position, thin skin flaps are elevated superiorly and inferiorly a sculptured excision to restore the shape of the convex ala, a crisp alar crease, and a flat sidewall. A thick alar rim and a stenotic nostril can be improved. The ideal alar margin is incised and lining elevated thinly. Excessive subcutaneous bulk is excised between the lining and deep surface of the old alar margin support grafts to thin the lining and the nostril margin. The stenotic lining is incised at right angles to the nostril margin. Excess skin along the inferior edge of the nostril margin is transferred as a superiorly or inferiorly based skin flap to fill the lining gap and increase the dimension of the nostril.

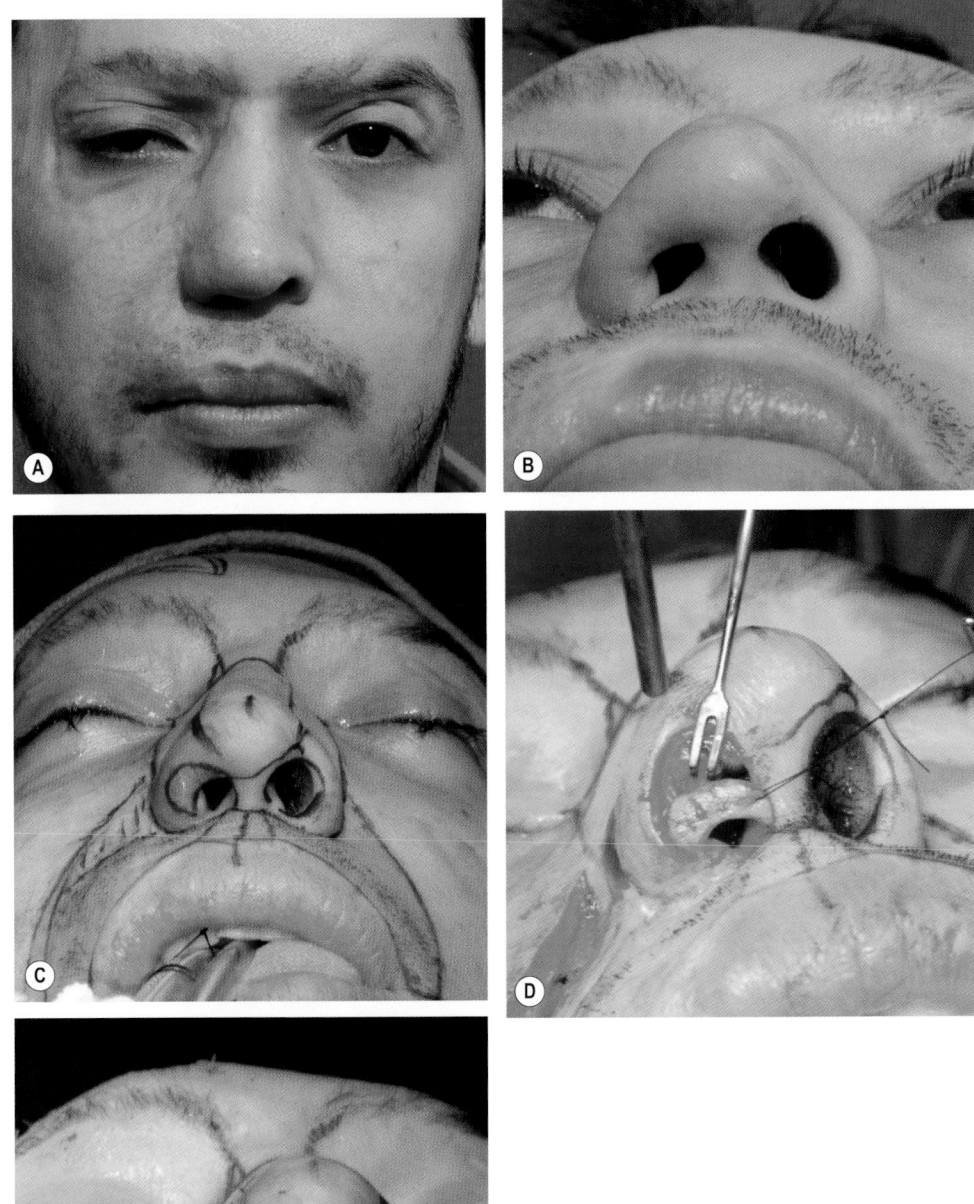

Fig. 6.51 (A–E) After complex facial fractures and soft-tissue avulsion of the forehead, cheek, and nose, a full-thickness defect of the right tip and ala was repaired with a cervical tube flap and cartilage grafts. The right alar rim is thick, the nostril small, the nostril margins asymmetric, and the alar crease and nasal labial fold absent. The ideal alar crease, nasal labial fold, and nostril are marked with ink based on pattern to the contralateral normal. The nostril margin is incised and the lining elevated thinly. Excess bulk is excised between the lining and the previously positioned alar margin support graft. The lining was transected laterally at the alar base and excess tissue within the thick nostril margin transposed with inferior base to fill a lining deficiency.

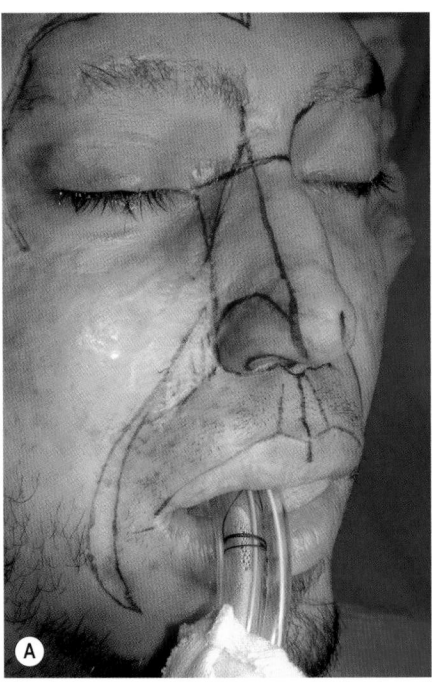
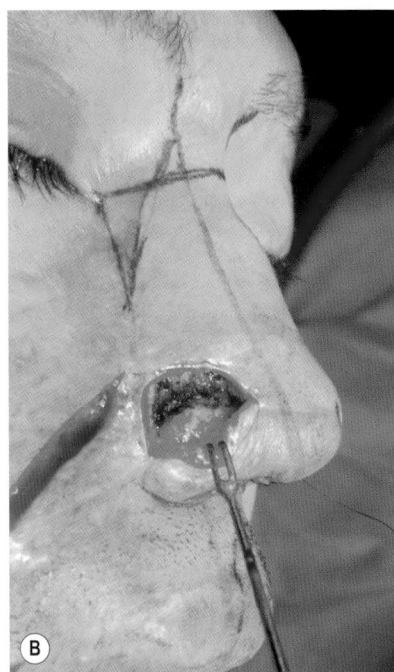
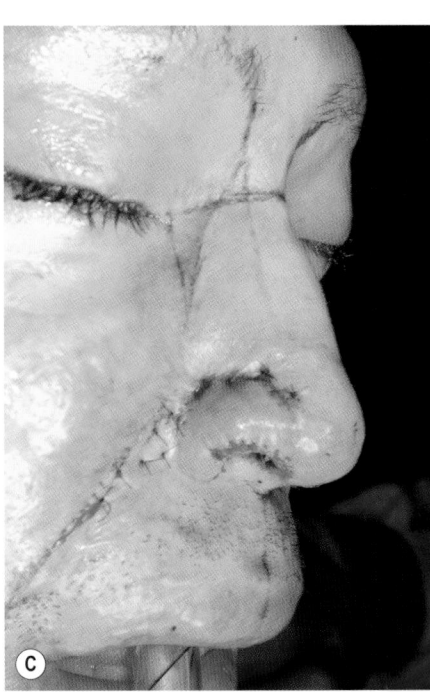

Fig. 6.52 (A–C) At the same time, direct incisions were made within the ideal alar crease and nasal labial fold based on pattern to the contralateral normal. Skin flaps were elevated and soft tissues excised to sculpt a round ala, flat sidewall, and flat hairless trigone of the upper lip.

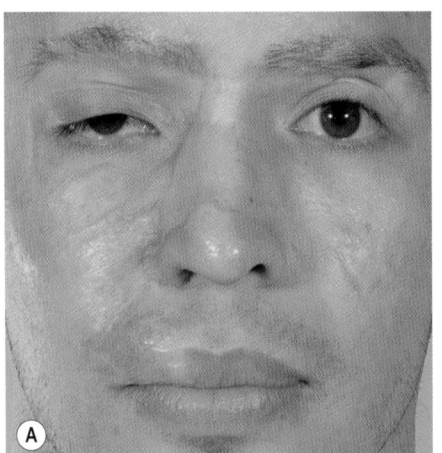
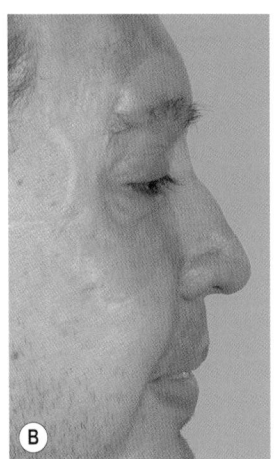
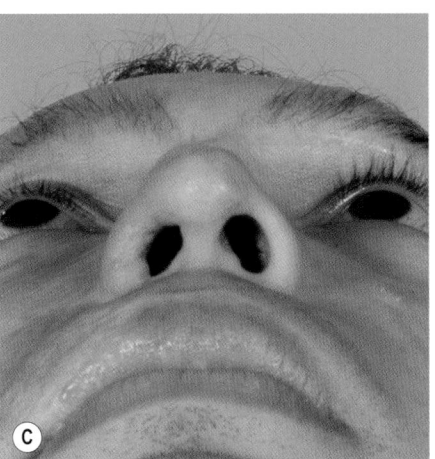

Fig. 6.53 (A–C) Postoperative result.

the nostril floor, is transposed, as small flaps, to fill the gap and augment the lining deficiency, opening the airway.

The major revision

When the nose is shapeless and bulky, "gross debulking" is approached through peripheral incisions around the border of the flap. The random blood supply of the old flap permits re-elevation of at least 80% of inset, permitting wide exposure. Underlying soft tissue and support are modified by sculpting excision and secondary cartilage grafting.

When all anatomical layers are scarred, the forehead flap is re-elevated with a few millimeters of subcutaneous fat. Scarred soft tissue and poorly designed support are completely excised. After excision of scar, the thinned cover and lining often re-expand and can be reshaped with a new, complete rigid support.

A second finesse revision, through direct incisions, will often be needed to improve landmark definition.

The redo

If tissues are grossly deficient, the repair must be redone, using a second regional flap. The defect is recreated, tissues are returned to their normal position, the deficiencies of cover, lining, and support identified, and the reconstructive plan reformulated for a successful repair, during a preliminary operation or at a later definitive secondary reconstruction.

Bonus images for this chapter can be found online at **http://www.expertconsult.com**

Fig. 6.4 (A, B) Intraoperative forehead and preauricular donor sites.

Fig. 6.5 (A) Oblique views of defect, **(B)** postoperative results and **(C)** donor sites.

Fig. 6.6 (A–D) Small superficial nasal tip defect resurfaced with full-thickness forehead skin graft.

Fig. 6.8 (A–G) Nasal defect after excision of basal cell carcinoma of the medial ala and tip resurfaced with one-stage nasolabial flap. No revision.

Fig. 6.10 (A–G) Subunit reconstruction of left ala with two-stage nasolabial flap. The subunits of the nose are marked with ink. A template of the right contralateral alar subunit will define the dimension and outline of the nasal labial flap and the primary cartilage graft. Residual skin within the left alar subunit is excised. A primary ear cartilage graft is fixed to support the alar lining. A subunit superiorly based axial nasolabial flap was elevated to resurface the alar subunit.

Fig. 6.11 (A–I) One month later, the pedicle is divided, the nasal inset is partially elevated, and the underlying excess soft-tissue bulk excised to create a convex alar contour and deep alar crease. Excess skin is excised and the flap inset completed. The cheek is closed to light exactly within the nasal labial fold. No revision.

Fig. 6.15 (A–G) Two-stage paramedian forehead flap resurfacing of the ala as a subunit. After Mohs excision of a basal cell carcinoma, greater than 50% of the left alar skin is missing. The nasal subunits are marked with ink. Excess skin within the alar subunit is discarded. The lining is supported with a primary ear cartilage graft. Because an old scar lies within the inferior left forehead, the contralateral right paramedian forehead flap is designed vertically over the supratrochlear vessels. It is thin distally and transferred to the defect.

Fig. 6.16 (A–F) One month later, the forehead pedicle was divided. Skin within the superior aspect of the recipient site is elevated thinly and the underlying cutaneous fat and primary cartilage graft excised to sculpt a convex ala and deep alar crease. Excess skin is excised and the inset is completed with quilting sutures and a single layer of fine peripheral sutures. No revision.

Fig. 6.36 (A–C) Full-thickness loss of the right ala and accompanying nostril floor.

Fig. 6.37 (A–D) The defect will be reconstructed as a subunit. Patterns are made of the left contralateral normal alar subunit end of the lining and floor defects. The lining defect pattern is added as an extension in the floor defect as an extension at right angle to the lining defect. This pattern will be employed to design a folded forehead flap which will supply a subunit external skin for the right ala, nonsubunit lining replacement and skin for the nostril floor.

Fig. 6.38 (A–E) A full-thickness forehead flap is designed to cover the right ala as a subunit with the distal extension to line the ala, and resurface the nasal floor. It is elevated and transposed.

Fig. 6.39 (A–D) One month later, the forehead flap is incised in the area of the future nostril margin and the proximal flap is elevated with 2–3 mm of subcutaneous fat. The folded forehead skin is healed to the adjacent nasal lining from which it receives its blood supply. It is no longer dependent on the supratrochlear vessels for survival. The folded frontalis and subcutaneous soft tissues are excised exposing thin supple vascular lining. A primary cartilage graft is placed to support and brace the alar rim.

Fig. 6.40 (A–D) The thin forehead flap is repositioned to resurface the ala as a subunit.

Fig. 6.41 (A–C) Postoperative result.

Fig. 6.54 (A–C) Bulky nonsubunit repair of the nasal tip with an unsupported two-stage forehead flap. The replacement of the proximal pedicle in the medial brow is pincushioned. The nasal tip is bulky and shapeless. The right nostril margin is collapsed. Soft tissues must be sculpted and resupported with secondary cartilage grafts to restore nasal shape and airway function.

Fig. 6.55 (A–E) The old forehead flap is elevated with 2–3 mm of subcutaneous fat, maintaining its vascularity on about 30% of its inset medially at the tip. Excess subcutaneous tissue is excised to decrease bulk and the nostril margin is supported with a conchal cartilage graft. The thin skin flap is returned to the contoured supported bed with quilting sutures and peripheral sutures. The "V" inset at the eyebrow was elevated and debulked.

Fig. 6.56 (A–C) Six weeks later, the right nostril margin is lower than the contralateral normal. Based on the pattern of the contralateral nose, the right nostril margin is trimmed to match.

Fig. 6.57 (A, B) Postoperative result. Although the scars are not positioned within the borders of subunit, the overall appearance is good because the volume, dimension, projection, position, quality, border outline, and three-dimensional contour are correct. The position of postoperative scars is relatively unimportant.

 Access the complete references list online at **http://www.expertconsult.com**

1. McDowell F. *The Source Book of Plastic Surgery*. Baltimore: Williams & Wilkins; 1977.

   Modern surgeons differ from their ancient predecessors because of the knowledge that developed over time. This book combines reproductions of the early literature in plastic surgery with biographies and modern commentary. The origins of skin grafting, rhinoplasty, cleft lip and palate, cross lip flaps, otoplasty, and facial fractures contributors are provided. Such a history provides perspective and insight.

8. Gillies HD. *Plastic surgery of the face*. London: Oxford Medical Publishers; 1920.

   Gillies, the modern father of plastic surgery, clearly describes his experience caring for the massive facial injuries which followed the trench warfare of World War I. The modern principles of facial reconstruction developed and are presented through clear case analysis with excellent photography. His results are superior. Historical but pertinent today.

15. Millard DR. *A rhinoplasty tetralogy*. Boston: Little Brown; 1996.

   Millard presents his 50-year experience during the second half of the 20th century. Difficult corrective, secondary, congenital and reconstructive nasal problems are presented to provide specific answers, guided by principle, and illustrate the innovative techniques which he developed over his lifetime.

16. Gillies HD, Millard DR. *The principles and art of plastic surgery*. Boston: Little Brown, 1957.

   Gillies and his student, Millard, present a comprehensive overview of principle and treatments between the two World Wars into the early 1950s. Core principles and ingenious solutions remain pertinent to any surgeon interested in facial reconstruction.

22. Burget G, Menick F. *Aesthetic reconstruction of the nose.* St. Louis, MO: Mosby, 1993.

   The first modern text dedicated to nasal reconstruction. The principles of facial repair are presented with indepth details of varied cases and solutions for small and superficial defects and large deep defects. The indications and use of local and regional flaps, intranasal lining, and primary support are illustrated. The treatment of complications and secondary late revision are detailed. This book is comprehensive, yet useful, as an atlas for the surgeon looking for a solution to a specific clinical problem.

23. Burget G, Menick F. Nasal support and lining: the marriage of beauty and blood supply. *Plast Reconstr Surg.* 1989;84:189.

   The use of thin supple intranasal lining, combined with primary cartilage grafts, and subunit resurfacing with a two-stage forehead flap revolutionized nasal reconstruction in the 1980s. This paper illustrates the technique with superb clinical case presentations.

25. Menick FJ. *Nasal reconstruction: art and practice.* London: Saunders-Elsevier; 2008.

   This text complements and expands the fundamental principles and approaches described in Burget and Menick's "Aesthetic Reconstruction of the Nose." Analysis, principles, materials and recently introduced techniques are presented to repair simple or the most complex defects with both traditional and more recently developed techniques. The use of the full-thickness forehead flap for nasal resurfacing of more difficult defects, the modified folded flap lining and skin graft lining techniques, the treatment of complications, and late surgical revision are presented in depth. The "table of cases"

   (a compendium of patient photographs repaired by case example within the text) provides a quick and easy reference to specific problems and their solutions to help readers find the information needed to treat their patient's presenting defect.

30. Millard DR. *Principalization of plastic surgery.* Boston: Little Brown; 1986.

   Millard outlines an approach to both cosmetic surgery and reconstruction based on principles. Every clinical problem or defect is different. Principles provide a tool to analyze the difficult problem and guide repair. Millard describes his approach, based on these principles, with wide and varied case examples that can be applied to clinical problems and how to live life, in general.

31. Burget GC, Menick FJ. Subunit principle in nasal reconstruction. *Plast Reconstr Surg.* 1985;76:239.

   The nose is divided into adjacent areas of characteristic surface quality, border outline, and three-dimensional contour. This paper introduced a subunit approach to nasal repair which positioned scars within the contours of the nasal surface and provided a rationale to harness wound healing by subunit resurfacing.

32. Menick FJ. Defects of the nose, lip, and cheek: rebuilding the composite defect. *Plast Reconstr Surg.* 2007;120:887.

   Composite defects of the midface are those which combine nasal, cheek, and lip. Their repair is especially difficult due to the complex aesthetics and tissue requirements. The basic principles of repair and current approaches are presented to satisfy the unique needs of these defects.

7

Reconstruction of the ear

Burton D. Brent

SYNOPSIS

- The commonest acquired ear deformity presenting for reconstruction is the partial ear defect.
- Apart from acquired ear deformities, microtia is one of the commonest and most complex conditions that present for reconstruction.
- Patients with microtia may have associated anomalies
- Reconstruction is usually a staged procedure.
- Creation of an adequate cartilage framework is key to the success of reconstruction.

 Access the Historical Perspective section online at
http://www.expertconsult.com

Introduction

Total auricular reconstruction with autogenous tissues is one of the greatest technical feats that a reconstructive surgeon may encounter. While an inherent understanding of sculpture and design influences surgical success, strict adherence to basic principles of plastic surgery and tissue transfer is of equal importance.

During the years, ear reconstruction has stimulated the imagination of many surgeons who have provided countless contributions. This chapter aims to document various techniques which have stood the test of time, and to provide the reader with guidelines for managing the microtic ear deformity.

Anatomy

The ear is difficult to reproduce surgically because it is comprised of a complexly convoluted frame of delicate elastic cartilage that is surrounded by a fine skin envelope. The denuded cartilage framework conforms almost exactly to the ear's surface contours except for its absence in the earlobe, which consists of a lobule of fibrofatty tissue rather than cartilage.

In most microtic vestiges, the presence of this lobule tissue is a valuable asset in the repair *(Fig. 7.1; see Fig. 7.13)*. When the lobule is lost in total ear avulsions, it is best recreated by shaping the bottom of the carved ear framework to resemble the lobe.

The ear's rich vascular supply comes from the superficial temporal and posterior auricular vessels, which can nourish a nearly avulsed ear even on surprisingly narrow tissue pedicles.

The sensory supply is chiefly derived from the inferiorly coursing greater auricular nerve. Upper portions of the ear are supplied by the lesser occipital and auriculotemporal nerves, whereas the conchal region is supplied by a vagal nerve branch.

Understanding this anatomy facilitates blocking the ear with local anesthetic solution. First, the greater auricular nerve is blocked by injecting a wheal underneath the lobule. After awaiting its effect, one continues injecting upward along the auriculocephalic sulcus, around the top of the ear and down to the tragus. Finally, the vagal branch can be numbed without discomfort by traversing the conchal cartilage with a needle placed through the already anesthetized auriculocephalic sulcus to raise a wheal of solution just behind the canal.

Practical embryology and understanding the middle-ear problem

At consultation, parents of a microtic infant are usually most concerned with the hearing problem. They either think that the child is completely deaf on the affected side or that hearing can be restored by merely opening a hole in the skin. As these are misconceptions, the physician can do much to alleviate parent's anxieties by fundamentally explaining ear embryology.

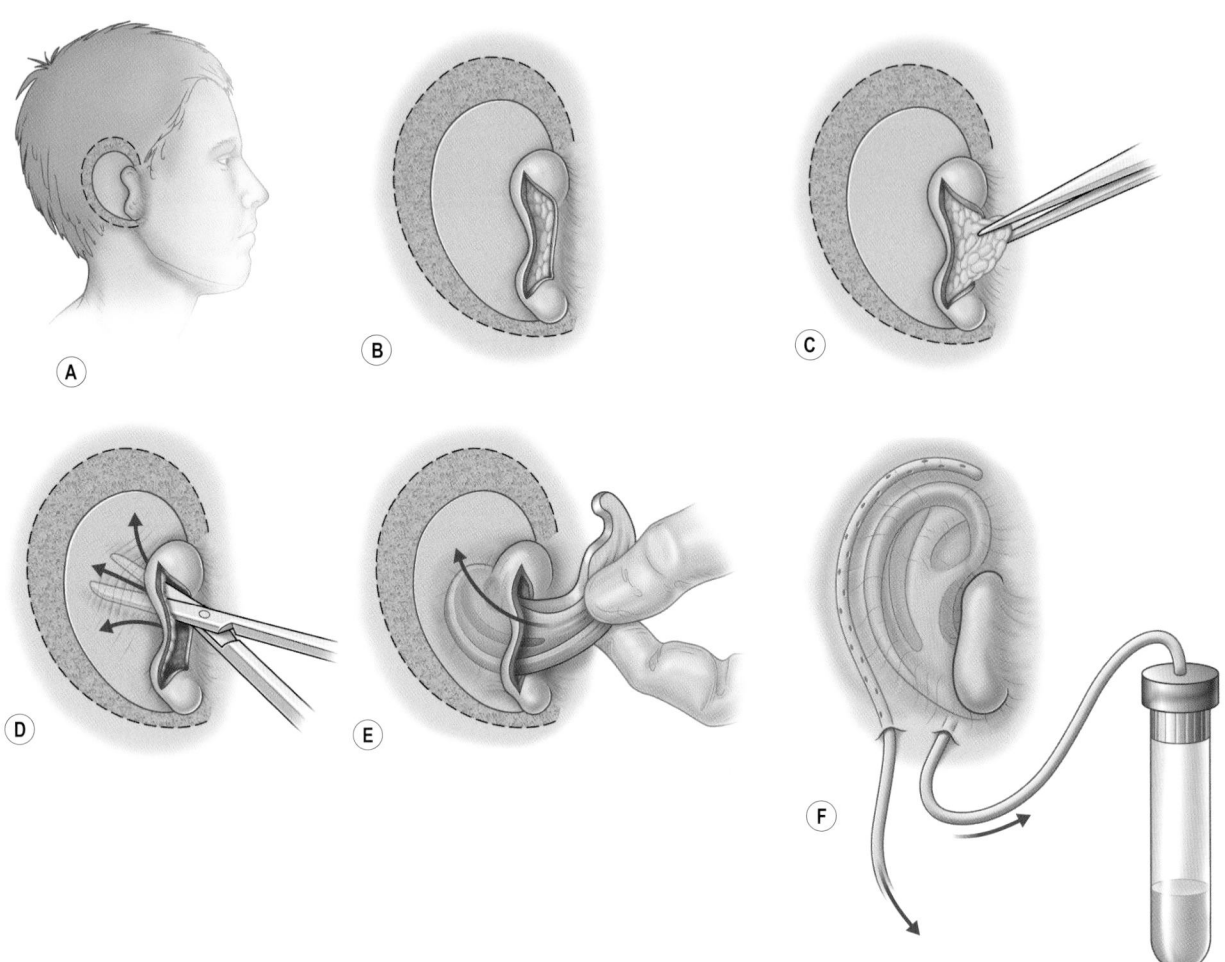

Fig. 7.1 (A–F) The cutaneous "pocket." The vestigial native cartilage is excised and then a skin pocket is created. To provide tension-free accommodation of the framework, the dissection is performed well beyond the proposed auricular position. Using two silicone catheters, the skin is coapted to the framework by means of vacuum tube suction.

As the human ear's receptive (inner) portion is derived from different embryologic tissue than the conductive (external and middle) portion, the inner ear is rarely involved in microtia and these patients have at least some hearing in the affected ear.

The problem is conduction. This is blocked by the malformed middle and external ear complex. Typically, these patients have a hearing threshold of 40–60 dB on the affected side. By comparison, normal function allows us to hear sounds between 0 and 20 dB.

Tissues of both the middle ear and external ear are derived chiefly from the first (mandibular) and second (hyoid) branchial arches. The auricle itself is formed from six "hillocks" of tissue that lie along these arches and can be first seen in the 5-week embryo[35–37] *(Fig. 7.2).* FIG **7.2** APPEARS ONLINE ONLY

The inner ear first appears at 3 weeks and is derived from tissues of distinctly separate ectodermal origin. Perhaps this explains why it is usually spared the developmental mishap that almost invariably involves the middle ear of microtic patients. Refinements in radiographic technique (polytomography and computed tomography scans) have only occasionally demonstrated dysplasia and hypoplasia of the inner ear.[38,39] Inner-ear abnormalities are found in approximately 10% of microtia and atresia cases, but the abnormalities are usually slight (e.g., a dilatation of the lateral semicircular

canal). Interestingly, in evaluating approximately 1500 microtic cases over a 25-year period, the author has seen only three patients who were totally deaf. Remarkably, these were unilateral microtias who had no family history of microtia. Because of their normal inner ear, even patients with bilateral microtia usually have serviceable hearing and use bone-conductive hearing aids to overcome the transmission block. If they are referred to an audiologist so that aids can be used as soon as possible, these patients usually develop normal speech. There is no point in waiting several months. Hearing aids should be applied within weeks of birth. Because these bone-conductive aids are cumbersome and label the child as "different" from his or her peers, it is optimal to correct the hearing deficit surgically to eliminate the aids. However, surgically correcting this conductive problem is difficult as the middle ear beneath the closed skin is not normal.

Exploration involves cautiously avoiding the facial nerve while drilling a canal through solid bone. The tympanum must usually be created with tissue grafts from the temporal fascia; the distorted or fused ossicles may be irreparable. As skin grafts do not take well on the drilled bony canal, chronic drainage is a frequent complication and meatal stenosis is common. Finally, unless the surgeon can close the functional difference between the repaired and normal ear to within 15–20 dB (an elusive feat in most surgeons' hands), binaural hearing will not be achieved. However, in the hands of a competent otologist with a large volume of experience, restoring middle-ear function surgically can be rewarding – even if only one ear is involved.[40,41]

As many microtia patients do well without middle-ear surgery – 8 out of 9 cases are unilateral and they are "born adjusted" to the monaural condition – most surgeons presently feel that potential gains from middle-ear surgery in unilateral microtia are outweighed by the potential risks and complications of the surgery and that this surgery should be reserved for bilateral cases.

When middle-ear surgery is contemplated, a team approach must be planned with an experienced otologist. In these cases, the auricular construction should precede the middle-ear surgery, as once an attempt is made to "open the ear" the virgin skin is scarred, which compromises a satisfactory auricular construction. On the horizon lie implantable acoustic devices, which may offer a solution for these patients. The bone-anchored hearing aid (BAHA) offers even better hearing than a bone-conductive hearing aid for patients who are not candidates for atresia surgery,[42,43] but does require two stages of surgery for optimal implantation of the metal posts in the skull.

Etiology

Incidence

According to an extensive study conducted by Grabb,[44] microtia occurs once in every 6000 births. The occurrence is estimated at 1 in 4000 in Japanese, and as high as one in 900–1200 births in Navajo Indians.[45]

Hereditary factors

In a study conducted by Rogers,[46] morphologic, anatomic, and genetic interrelationships were shown to exist between microtia, constricted, and protruding ears. In this thorough investigation, Rogers demonstrated that these deformities are interrelated and can be hereditary.

Preauricular pits and sinuses, and a combination of pits, preauricular appendages, cupping deformity, and deafness, are all hereditarily dominant.[1,47] Both dominant and recessive characteristics have been revealed in deafness associated with several auricular abnormalities.[48] Ear deformities frequently recur in families of mandibulofacial dysostosis (Treacher–Collins syndrome).[49] These are frequently constricted ear deformities, an abnormality that is known to be hereditary.[12,50–52] Hanhart found a severe form of microtia associated with a cleft or high palate in 10% of family members studied,[51] and Tanzer[53] found that approximately 25% of his 43 microtia patients had relatives with evidence of the first and second bronchial arch syndrome (craniofacial microsomia); microtia was present in four instances.

In 4.9% of the author's first 1000 microtia patients, family histories revealed that major auricular deformities occurred within the immediate family, i.e., parents, siblings, aunts, uncles, or grandparents.[23] When "distant" relatives were included, the percentage jumped up to 10.3%. In 6% of patients, preauricular skin tags or minor auricular defects were observed in the immediate family. This number also rose to 10.3% when all relatives were included. Immediate family members with normal auricles but underdeveloped jaws or facial nerves were seen in 1.2% of patients.[23]

In a thorough, intensive survey of 96 families of their 171 microtic patients, Takahashi and Maeda[54] ruled out chromosomal aberrations and concluded that inheritance must be multifactorial and that the recurrence risk is 5.7%. In previous studies, others have found multifactorial inheritance between 3 and 8% in first-degree relatives. If a couple has two children with microtia, the risk of recurrence in future offspring is thought to be as high as 15%.

Specific factors

McKenzie and Craig[55] and Poswillo[56] theorized that the cause of developmental auricular abnormalities is *in utero* tissue ischemia resulting from either an obliterated stapedial artery or a hemorrhage into the local tissues. This suggests that these deformities arise from a mishap during fetal development rather than from a hereditary source. Interestingly, the author has treated at least 15 microtia patients who have an affirmed identical twin with normal ears.[23] Only two sets of the author's identical twin patients have had concordance for outer-ear deformities; one set were identical mirror-image twins, and the other set both had right-sided microtia. Of interest in the latter set is that each of these male twins with right microtia also had signs and symptoms of pyloric stenosis within 2 days of each other and were operated on at 6 weeks of age *(Fig. 7.3)*. ⊕ FIG **7.3C and D** APPEARS ONLINE ONLY

The occurrence of deafness and occasional microtia resulting from rubella during the first trimester of pregnancy is well known. Also, certain drugs during this critical period may be causative; the author has seen at least 3 cases of microtia which resulted from the mother's ingestion of the tranquilizer, thalidomide.[57,58] Isotretinoin has also been cited as causing ear deformities when ingested during the first trimester.[59] In many instances mothers had been unaware of this problem and had used this drug to control acne. Other medications that reportedly cause microtia are clomiphene citrate[60] and retinoic acid.[61]

Diagnosis

Classification

Rogers noted that most types of auricular hypoplasia could be classified in a descending scale of severity.[46] This corresponds to Streeter's depiction of embryological patterns of auricular development.[37] Rogers divides developmental ear defects into four groups: (1) microtia; (2) lop ear, i.e., folding or deficiency of the superior helix and scapha; (3) "cup" or constricted ear, with a deep concha and deficiency of the superior helix and antihelical crura; and (4) the common prominent or protruding ear.

Using a system that correlates with embryological development, Tanzer classifies congenital ear defects according to the approach necessary for their surgical correction[62] *(Box 7.1 and Fig. 7.4)*.

Associated deformities

As discussed previously, embryological development dictates that the microtic ear is usually accompanied by middle-ear abnormalities. Full-blown, classic microtia is usually associated with canal atresia and ossicular abnormalities. The middle-ear deformity may range from diminished canal caliber and minor ossicular abnormalities to fused, hypoplastic ossicles and failure of mastoid cell pneumatization.

Because the auricle develops from tissues of the mandibular and hyoid branchial arches, it is not surprising that a significant percentage of microtic patients exhibit deficient facial components that originate from these embryological building blocks. These deformities are compiled under the heading of "craniofacial microsomia" (first and second branchial arch syndrome), and an obvious facial asymmetry was noted in 35% of the author's first 1000 microtia patients.[23] The most complete genetic expression of this condition includes defects of the external and middle ear; hypoplasia of the mandible, maxilla, zyogomatic, and temporal bones; macrostomia and lateral facial clefts; and atrophy of facial muscles and parotid gland.[44,63,64] Furthermore, Brent found that 15% of his 1000 patients had paresis of the facial nerve.[23] Dellon et al. have shown that the palatal muscles are rarely spared in this syndrome.[65]

Urogenital tract abnormalities are increased in the presence of microtia,[66] particularly when the patient is afflicted with other manifestations of the first and second branchial arch syndrome.[67] The associated deformities found in the author's first 1000 microtia patients are compiled in *Table 7.1*.

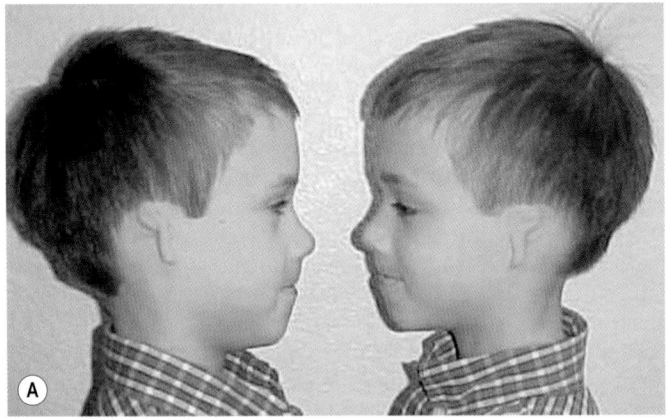

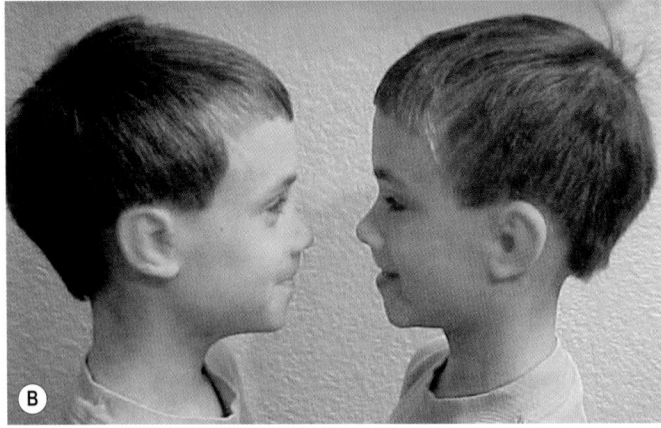

Fig. 7.3 Identical mirror-image twin 6-year old boys with microtia and author's repair with sculpted autogenous rib cartilage grafts. (Reproduced from Brent B. Repair of microtia with sculpted rib cartilage grafts in identical, mirror-image twins: a case study. *Ann Plast Surg.* 2011;66:62–64.)

Microtia

Clinical characteristics

Microtia varies from the complete absence of auricular tissues (anotia) to a somewhat normal but small ear with an atretic

---

BOX 7.1 Clinical classification of auricular defects (Tanzer)

I.   Anotia
II. Complete hypoplasia (microtia)
    A. With atresia of external auditory canal
    B. Without atresia of external auditory canal
III. Hypoplasia of middle third of auricle
IV. Hypoplasia of superior third of auricle
    A. Constricted (cup and lop) ear
    B. Cryptotia
    C. Hypoplasia of entire superior third
V.   Prominent ear

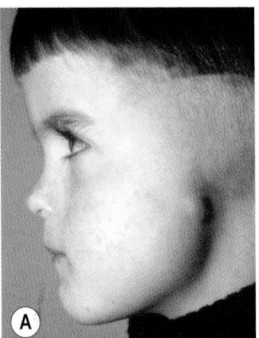 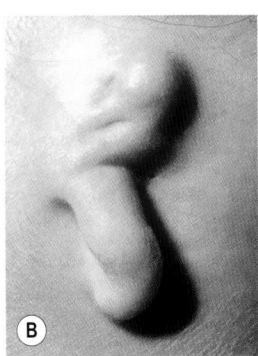 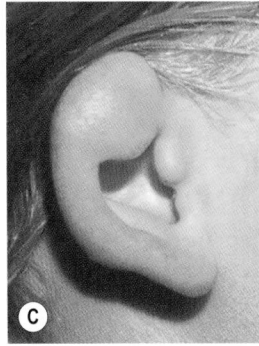 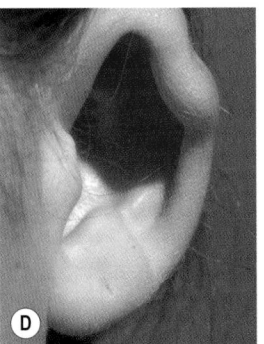 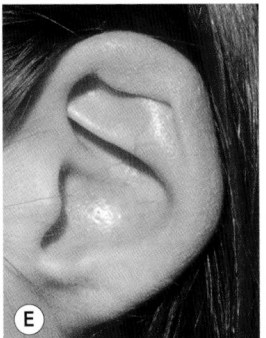

Fig. 7.4 Ear malformations, shown by severity. **(A)** Anotia. **(B)** Grade III microtia. **(C)** Moderate constriction. **(D)** Grade I constriction. **(E)** Lop ear.

Table 7.1 Microtia: case material (author's series of 1000 microtia patients)

	Cases	%	Total no. of ears		Cases	%
Right	582	58.2%	582	Males	631	63.1%
Left	324	32.4%	324	Females	369	36.9%
Bilateral	94	9.4%	188			
Total	1000	100.0%	1094	Total	1000	100.0%

BOX 7.2 **Associated deformities (author's series of 1000 microtia patients)**

Branchial arch deformities
 A. Obvious bony and soft-tissue deficit 36.5%
  Family perceives it as "significant" 49.4%
 B. Overt facial nerve weakness 15.2%
  Of these, more than one branch involved 42.6%
Macrostomia 2.5%
Cleft lip and/or palate 4.3%
Urogenital defects 4.0%
Cardiovascular malformations 2.5%
Miscellaneous deformities 1.7%

canal. Between these extremes there are an endless variety of vestiges, the most common being a vertically oriented sausage-shaped nubbin (*Figs 7.1, 7.5, and 7.6*). Microtia is nearly twice as frequent in males as in females, and the right–left–bilateral ratio is roughly 6:3:1 (*Box 7.2*).[23,29,68] FIGS **7.5 and 7.6** APPEAR ONLINE ONLY

In most instances, the microtic lobule is displaced superiorly to the level of the opposite, normal side, although incomplete ear migration occasionally leaves it in an inferior location. Approximately one-third to one-half the patients exhibit gross characteristics of craniofacial microsomia, although Converse and associates have demonstrated tomographically that skeletal deficiencies exist in all cases.[69,70] Whatever the deformity, the author has been impressed with its potential for psychological havoc amongst the entire family, varying from the patient's emotional insecurity to the parents' deep-seated guilt feelings.

General considerations

During the initial consultation, it is imperative to describe to the patient and/or his/her family realistically the technical limitations involved in surgically correcting microtia, and to outline alternative methods of managing each individual's particular deformity. Personally, the author strongly favors autogenous rib cartilage for auricular construction. Although its use necessitates an operation that includes chest surgery, it must be noted that, unlike a reconstruction utilizing alloplastic materials, a successful construction with autogenous tissue is less susceptible to trauma, and therefore eliminates a patient's overcautious concern during normal activities.

The age at which an auricular construction should begin is governed by both psychological and physical considerations.

Since the body image concept usually begins forming around the age of 4 or 5 years,[71] it would be ideal to begin construction before the child enters school, and before he/she is psychologically traumatized by his/her peers' cruel ridicule. However, surgery should be postponed until rib growth provides substantial cartilage to permit a quality framework fabrication.

In the author's experience with over 1700 microtia patients from age 1 month to 62 years, the patients and/or their families consistently stated that their psychological disturbances rarely began before age 7, and usually became overt from ages 7 to 10. The family is anxious to have the ear repaired as soon as possible, but it is important for the surgeon to wait until it is technically feasible. There usually is enough rib cartilage to serve as the sculpting medium by age 6 and many surgeons begin at that time. If the patient is small for his/her age and/or the opposite, normal ear is large, then it is prudent to postpone the surgery for several years. If not pressured by the family, the best age to begin is about 8 years, when the child is more aware of and concerned with the problem, usually wants it resolved as much as his/her family does, and is helpfully cooperative during the postoperative care phase.

At age 6, the normal ear has grown to within 6 or 7 mm of its full vertical height,[72] which permits construction of an ear that will have reasonably constant symmetry with the opposite normal ear. In his follow-up mail survey, Tanzer[16,73] found that an ear constructed from autogenous rib cartilage grows at the same rate as the normal ear, with the possible exception of patients operated at 6–7 years of age, where he noted that 50% of these ears lagged several millimeters behind in growth; the roles played in the growth of his patients' surgically constructed ears by soft tissues and by cartilage have not been determined. In evaluating my own patients[29] operated on between ages 5 and 10 with a minimum 5-year follow-up (76 patients), I found that 48.1% of the constructed ears grew at an even pace with the opposite, normal ear; 41.6% grew several millimeters larger; and 10.3% lagged several millimeters behind the normal side. From the limited number of long-term patients in this age group whom I have examined, I found that most constructed ears have grown, and many of these have not only kept up with the little residual growth in the opposite ear, but have slightly overgrown[29]. I found none to have shrunk, softened, or lost their detail .With all this in mind, I conclude that one should try to match the opposite side during the preoperative planning session, regardless of age. Certainly there is no reason to construct the ear larger, as some investigators have previously thought, and one might even consider making the framework several millimeters smaller in the youngest patients where normal, *in situ* costal cartilage can be expected to exceed normal auricular cartilage growth.

Author's method of repair

Staging the auricular construction

The cartilage graft is the "foundation" of an auricular construction and, as in constructing a house, it should be built and well established under ideal conditions before further stages or refinements are undertaken. By implanting the cartilage graft as the first surgical stage, one takes advantage of the optimal elasticity and circulation of an unviolated, virgin skin "pocket." For these reasons, I prefer to avoid initial lobule transposition or vestige division, since the resulting scars cannot help but inhibit the circulation and restrict the skin's elasticity. This, in turn, diminishes its ability to accommodate safely a three-dimensional cartilage graft. It seems easier both to judge the earlobe's placement and to "splice" the lobule correctly into position with reference to a well-established, underlying framework. Although Tanzer transposed the lobule simultaneously with implantation of the cartilage graft during the last three cases of his clinical practice[74] and Nagata routinely does this in his technique,[32] the author finds that there is far less risk of tissue necrosis and it is far more accurate to transpose the lobule as a secondary procedure[75–77] *(Fig. 7.7)*. The lobe can be safely transposed and simultaneously the ear can be elevated from the head with skin graft if the earlobe vestige is short, because its small wound closure will not compromise the ear's anterior circulation[23,29] *(Fig. 7.8)*.

⊛ FIG **7.8G and H** APPEARS ONLINE ONLY

During the third stage, the ear is separated from the head and surfaced on its underside with a skin graft to create an auriculocephalic sulcus.

Generally, the fourth stage combines tragus construction, conchal excavation, and simultaneous, contralateral otoplasty, if indicated to achieve optimal frontal symmetry. By combining these procedures, tissues that are normally discarded from an otoplasty can be advantageously employed as free grafts in the tragus construction.

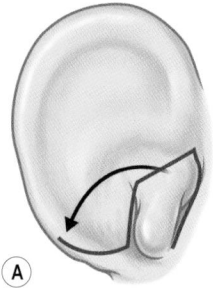
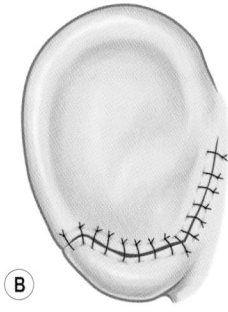

Fig. 7.7 Total ear construction, stage 2: lobule transposition. **(A)** Healed stage 1 repair and proposed lobule transposition. The appropriate lobule position will be de-epithelialized to receive the transposed earlobe. **(B)** Completed procedure. The lobule has been transposed as an inferiorly based flap.

Preoperative consultation

During the initial consultation, surgical expectations and psychological considerations should be discussed with the patient and family, emphasizing reconstruction.

Although costal cartilage can be carved to form a delicate framework, it must be remembered that the volume and projection of the furnished three-dimensional framework are limited by the two-dimensional skin flap under which the framework is placed. Furthermore, because the retroauricular-mastoid skin that covers the framework is somewhat thicker than normal, delicate anterolateral auricular skin, details of a carved framework tend to be blunted. It is important for these limitations to be stressed to the patient and family. In this way, unrealistic expectations as to what can or cannot be produced by surgery can be addressed.

The plastic surgeon's aim is to achieve accurate representation. That means creating an acceptable facsimile of an ear that is the proper size, in the proper position, and properly oriented to other facial features.

During the consultation, surgical discomforts and inconveniences should be described, including the expected chest pain, duration of dressings, and limited activities for 4–6 weeks. Finally, risks and possible complications of the surgery are discussed thoroughly. These include cartilage graft loss secondary to infection, skin flap necrosis, and hematoma. It should be stressed that with proper precautions, these risks are comparatively less severe than the emotional trauma created by an absent ear. After getting through the initial learning curve of my early years of practice, the ultimate complication rate has been well beneath 1% in the ears that I have constructed from autogenous rib cartilage grafts.

Planning, preparation, and correlation with the correction of other facial deficiencies

The result of a total ear reconstruction depends not only on a surgeon's meticulous surgical technique, but, even more importantly, on careful preoperative planning. It is essential to practice carving techniques on a volume of human cadaver cartilage prior to any live-patient application. Alternatively, ear framework carving can be demonstrated on large slices of potatoes; carrots serve well to practice forming a thin, flexible helix. An acrylic or plaster replica of a normal ear serves as an excellent model for practice carvings.

During the patient's second office consultation, preoperative study photographs are obtained, and an X-ray film or thin plastic film pattern is traced from the opposite, normal ear. This pattern is reversed, and a framework pattern is designed for the new ear. After sterilization, these patterns serve as guidelines for framework fabrication at the time of surgery.

The reconstructed ear's location is predetermined by first noting the topographical relationship of the opposite, normal ear with facial features and then duplicating its position at the proposed reconstruction site. First, the vestige's height is compared from the front view with that of the opposite, normal ear. From the side, it should be noted that the ear's axis is roughly parallel to the nasal profile[34,78] *(Fig. 7.9)*. Finally, one notes and records the distance between the lateral canthus and the normal ear's helical root. Typically, this distance is about 65–67 mm in a 6-year-old child.

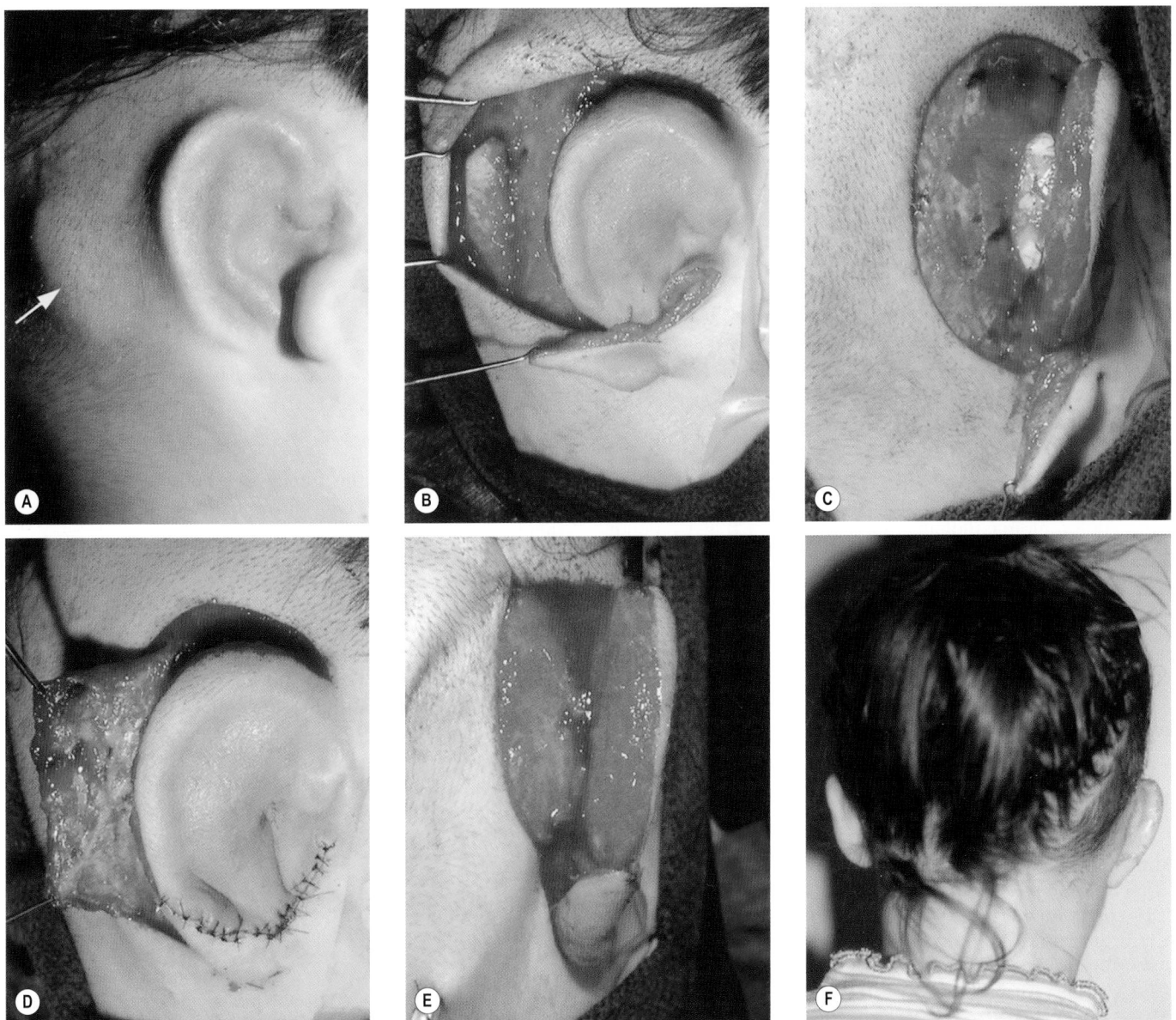

Fig. 7.8 Augmenting ear projection with a scalp-banked rib cartilage graft and fascial flap; simultaneous earlobe transposition. **(A)** Healed first-stage repair of a microtic ear. Note banked rib cartilage behind the ear framework (arrow). **(B)** Stage 2: retroauricular scalp undermined to retrieve banked cartilage; earlobe transposition begun. **(C)** Banked cartilage wedged behind the elevated ear to augment its projection; lobule suspended on the inferior pedicle. **(D)** Retroauricular fascial flap raised; earlobe transposition complete. **(E)** Fascial flap turned over the cartilage wedge to provide a nourishing cover for skin graft. **(F)** Complete skin graft "take" on the elevated ear. (Reproduced from Brent B. Technical advances in ear reconstruction with autogenous rib cartilage grafts: personal experience with 1200 cases. *Plast Reconstr Surg.* 1999;104:319.)

The ear's location is determined by first taping the reversed film pattern to the proposed construction site, and then adjusting its position until it is level to and symmetrical with the opposite normal ear. The pattern is traced on the head, noting the ear's axial relation to the nose, its distance from the lateral canthus, and its lobule's position, which is usually superiorly displaced. The ear's new position is straightforward and easy to plan in a pure microtia, but much more difficult when severe hemifacial microsomia exists. Not only are the heights of the facial halves asymmetrical, but the anteroposterior dimensions of the affected side are foreshortened as well. In these patients, the new ear's height is best determined by lining it up with the normal ear's upper pole

– its distance from the lateral canthus is somewhat arbitrary.

In pure microtia, the vestige-to-canthus distance mirrors the helical root-to-canthus distance of the opposite, normal side. However, in severe hemifacial microsomia patients, the vestige is much closer to the eye. If the new ear's anterior margin is placed at the vestige site, then the ear appears too close to the eye; if the measured distance of the normal side is used as a guide, then the ear looks too far back on the head. In these patients, I find it best to compromise by selecting a point halfway between these two positions.

When both auricular construction and bony repairs are planned, then careful, integrated timing is essential. Most

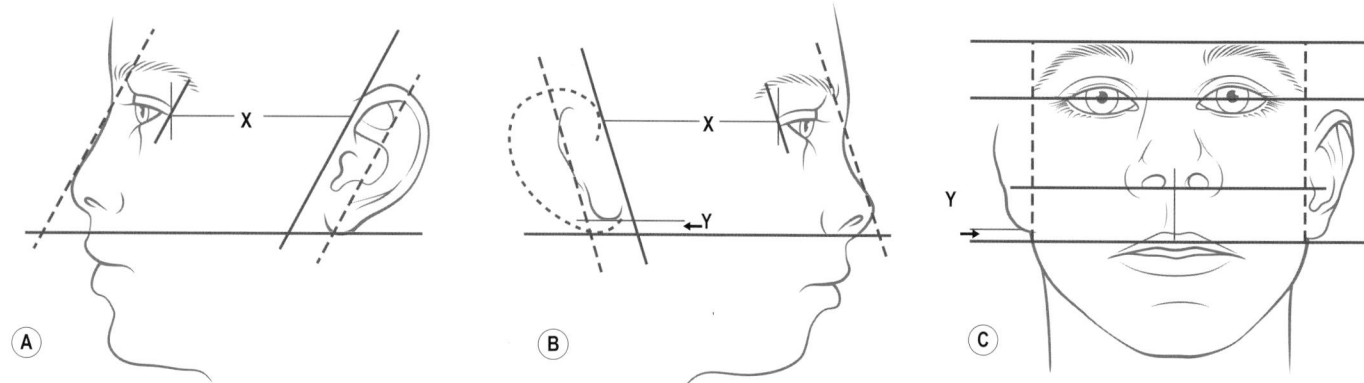

Fig. 7.9 (A–C) Preoperative determination of auricular location. The ear's axis is positioned to match the opposite side, roughly parallel to the nasal profile; the helical root is positioned equidistant from the lateral canthus. The reversed auricular pattern is traced 6 mm below the lobule, as determined by frontal measurement.

often the family pushes for the ear repair to begin first, which helpfully assures the auricular surgeon virginal, unscarred skin. The craniomaxillofacial surgeon argues that by going first s/he will correct the facial symmetry, thus making ear placement easier.[79] I find this unnecessary when the guidelines described above are followed.

If the bony work is done first, it is imperative that scars are peripheral to the proposed auricular site. When a coronal incision is used to approach the upper face or to harvest cranial bone grafts, special care must be taken that the scar does not precariously lie over the future region of the upper helix.

First stage of reconstruction

Almost invariably, the author's first-stage "foundation" in correcting microtia is fabricating and inserting the cartilaginous ear framework. As discussed previously, scars can be a significant handicap; the author rarely employs a preliminary procedure.

Obtaining the rib cartilage

Rib cartilages are obtained *en bloc* from the side contralateral to the ear being constructed, so as to utilize natural rib configuration. The rib cartilages are removed through a horizontal or slightly oblique incision which is made just above the costal margin. Following division of the external oblique and the rectus muscles, the film pattern is placed on the exposed cartilages to determine the necessary extent of rib resection.

The helical rim is fashioned separately with cartilage from the first free-floating rib *(Fig. 7.10)*. Excision of this cartilage facilitates access to the synchondrotic region of ribs 6 and 7, which supplies a sufficient block to carve the framework body. Extraperichondrial dissection is preferable in obtaining an unmarred specimen. I find that well-documented chest deformities[80,81] can be significantly decreased by preserving even a minimal rim of the upper margin of the sixth rib cartilage where the basic shape of the ear is obtained *(Fig. 7.10)*. This precautionary measure retains a tether to the sternum so that the rib does not flare outward to distort the chest as the child grows. If the synchondrotic region seems inadequate in width, one can compensate for framework width by bowing

the helix away from the framework body (the "expansile" design[82]), rather than violating the sixth-rib margin and sacrificing chest wall integrity.

In cases where the delicate pleura is entered during this dissection, there is no great reason for concern, as a leak in the lung has not been produced. However, when a pleural tear is discovered, a rubber catheter is inserted well into the chest through the pleural opening; then the chest wound is closed in layers by the assistant, while the surgeon fabricates the framework, thus conserving operative time. When skin closure is complete, the catheter is attached to suction, the lung is expanded with positive pressure by the anesthesiologist, and the surgeon rapidly withdraws the catheter. As a final precaution, the patient receives a portable upright chest X-ray in the operating room.

Framework fabrication

In fabricating an ear framework, the surgeon's aim is to exaggerate the helical rim and the details of the antihelical complex. This is achieved with scalpel blades and rounded woodcarving chisels. To minimize possible chondrocytic damage, the use of power tools for sculpting is strictly avoided – keep in mind that cartilage-sculpting differs from basic woodcarving in that a good long-term result ultimately depends upon living tissue.

The basic ear silhouette is carved from the previously obtained cartilage block *(Fig. 7.10)*. It is necessary to thin very little, if any, of the basic form for a small child's framework, but it is essential for framework fabrication in most older patients. When thinning is necessary, care should be taken to preserve the perichondrium on the lateral, outer aspect of the framework to facilitate its adherence and subsequent nourishment from surrounding tissues.

Because warping must be taken into consideration,[83] the cartilage is sculpted and thinned to cause a deliberate warping in a favorable direction. This allows one to produce the acute flexion necessary to create a helix, which is fastened to the framework body with horizontal mattress sutures; the knots are buried on the frame's undersurface. For this, I prefer 4-0 clear nylon suture material, which causes only few problems in contrast to the frequent extrusions encountered when using stainless-steel wire sutures for this purpose.

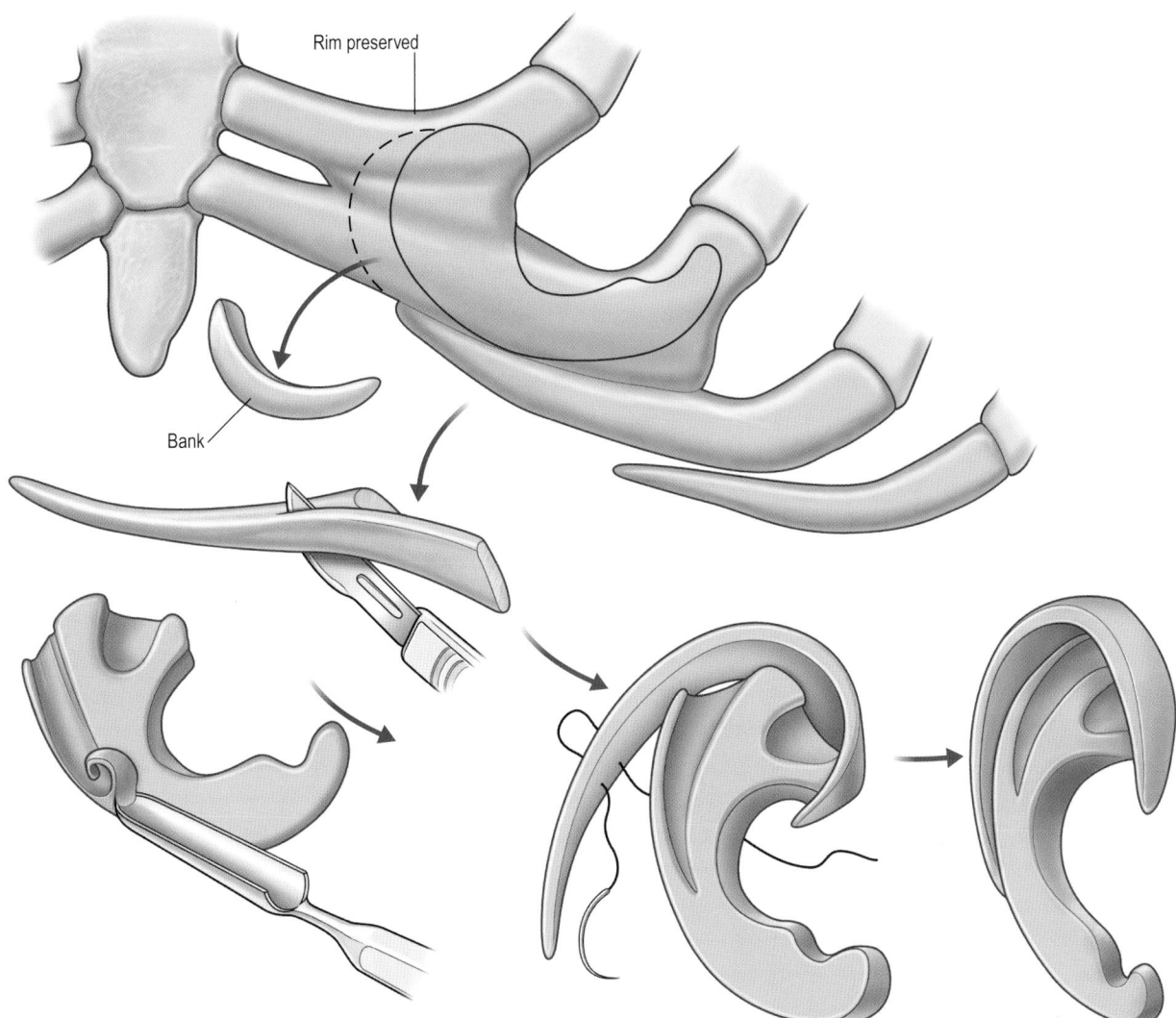

Fig. 7.10 Rib cartilage harvest for ear framework fabrication. Note that the upper border of the sixth cartilage is preserved; this will help prevent subsequent chest deformity as the child grows. The entire "floating cartilage" will be used to create the helix. To produce the acute flexion necessary to form the helix, the cartilage is deliberately warped in a favorable direction by thinning it on its outer, convex surface. The thinned helix is affixed to the main sculptural block with horizontal mattress sutures of 4-0 clear nylon; the knots are placed on the framework's undersurface.

Framework modifications in older patients

Adult rib cartilages are often fused into a solid block, which invites one to sculpt the ear framework in one piece – not unlike doing a wood carving *(Fig. 7.11)*. In my experience, this is advantageous because adult cartilage is often calcified; it is difficult, if not impossible, to create a separate helix that will bend without breaking. If a one-piece carving produces insufficient helical projection, the helix can be detached and slid up the framework body to augment the protrusion of the rim. This improved contour is maintained by reattaching the helix to the framework with several permanent sutures *(Fig. 7.12)*. ⊛ FIG 7.11 APPEARS ONLINE ONLY

Framework implantation

A cutaneous pocket is created with meticulous technique so as to provide an adequate recipient vascular covering for the framework. Through a small incision along the backside of the auricular vestige, a thin flap is raised by sharp dissection, taking care to preserve the subdermal vascular plexus. So as to evaluate the flap's vascular status and to assure accurate hemostasis, epinephrine-containing solutions are avoided. With great care, the skin is dissected from the gnarled, native cartilage remnant which then is excised and discarded. Finally, the pocket is completed by dissecting a centimeter or two peripherally to the projected framework markings *(Fig. 7.1)*.

Insertion of the framework into the cutaneous pocket takes up the valuable skin slack which was created when the native cartilage remnant was removed. The framework displaces this skin centrifugally in an advantageous posterosuperior direction so as to displace the hairline just behind the rim. This principle of anterior incision and centrifugal skin relaxation, introduced by Tanzer,[15] not only permits advantageous use of the hairless skin cover, but also preserves

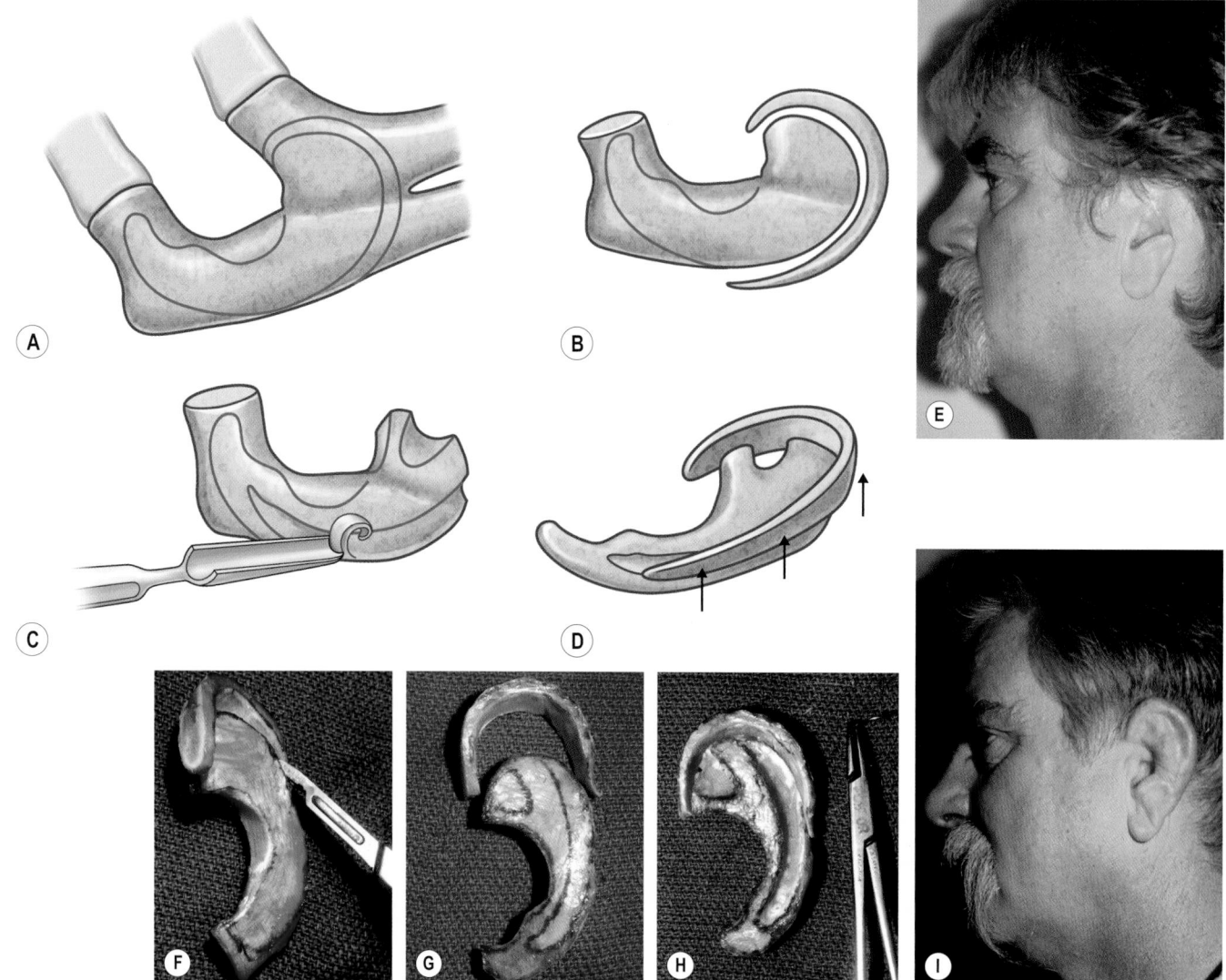

Fig. 7.12 Maximizing rim projection in adult patient with sliding helical advancement. **(A,B)** Harvesting fused rib cartilage block and separating the inflexible helical portion; **(C)** sculpting body of framework; **(D)** sliding and reattaching the helix to maximize its projection. **(E)** A 50-year-old man with ear loss from a dog bite. **(F–H)** Construction of the framework by use of the technique illustrated in the drawings. **(I)** The completed repair. This patient had his hairline "idealized" by laser treatment before the rib cartilage graft (see Fig. 7.20). (Reproduced from Brent B. Technical advances in ear reconstruction with autogenous rib cartilage grafts: personal experience with 1200 cases. *Plast Reconstr Surg*. 1999;104:319.)

circulation by avoiding incisions and scars along the helical border.

Although Tanzer initially suggested the use of bolster sutures to coapt the skin flap to underlying framework,[15,84] the author finds it far safer to do this with suction, which simultaneously prevents fluid collection and minimizes the risk of flap necrosis along the helical margin.

To attain skin coaptation via suction, silicone catheters are used with the needles inserted into rubber-topped vacuum tubes, the tubes being retained on a rack to observe changes in quantity and quality of drainage. Although a dressing is applied which accurately conforms to the convolutions of the newly created auricle, firm pressure is dangerous and unnecessary, and must be avoided. Hemostasis and skin coaptation are provided by the suction drain.[17,29,75,77]

Immediate postoperative care and management of complications

I pack the new ear's convolutions with Vaseline gauze and apply a bulky, noncompressive dressing. Since the vacuum system provides both skin coaptation and hemostasis, pressure is unnecessary and contraindicated. The first day, the tubes are changed by the ward nurses every few hours, then every 4–6 hours thereafter or when a tube is one-third full. I now discharge the patient the day after surgery and teach the parent to change the tubes (three times a day). The drains remain in place for several more days until the testtubes contain only drops of serosanguineous drainage. I routinely remove them at 5 days. By then the overlying skin is adherent to the framework and hematoma is no longer a threat; to leave them in longer seems unnecessary, particularly since the catheters could possibly serve as wicks to facilitate bacterial transport along the tubes.

Postoperatively, the ear is checked and the protective head dressing is changed several times, and discarded after about 11–12 days.

Attentive postoperative management is imperative for a successful ear reconstruction which remains unhampered by disastrous complications. The newly constructed auricle is scrutinized frequently and carefully for signs of infection or vascular compromise.

Usually, early infection manifests itself neither by auricular pain nor fever, but through local erythema, edema, subtle fluctuance, drainage, or a combination of the above. Hence, frequent observations and the immediate institution of aggressive therapy can deter an overwhelming infection.

Immediately upon suspecting an infection, an irrigation drain is introduced below the flap, and continuous antibiotic drip irrigation is begun. Appropriate adjustments are made in both the antibiotic drip irrigation and in the systemic therapy when sensitivities are available from the initial culture. Cronin[17] has salvaged Silastic-frame reconstructions impressively by this technique, and I had success in managing the rare infection in cartilage graft reconstructions when I was using bolster sutures during my first 15–20 cases. The problem of infections basically disappeared when I switched over to the suction drain system and I have not experienced one in an autogenous cartilage framework for nearly 30 years.

Skin flap necrosis results from excess tension in an inadequate-sized pocket, tight bolster sutures, or damage to the subdermal vascularity during the flap dissection. This complication is best avoided by meticulous technique; however, once skin necrosis becomes evident, appropriate steps must be taken without delay.

Although at times a small local flap may be required to cover exposed cartilage, small localized ulcerations may heal with good local wound care. This consists of continually keeping the wound covered with antibiotic ointment to prevent cartilage desiccation and using restraints to prevent the patient from lying on his/her ear during sleep.

However, major skin flap necrosis merits a more aggressive approach if the framework is to be salvaged. The necrotic skin is excised early, and the framework is covered by transposing a local skin flap or by using a small fascial flap and skin graft.

Postoperative activities and care

Once initially healed, no specific care is necessary for an ear constructed with autogenous tissues. To avoid flattening of the helical rim, the patient is instructed to sleep on the opposite side. A soft pillow assures protection if the patient turns over while sleeping.

Two weeks postoperatively the patient may return to school; however, running and sports are discouraged for an additional 3 weeks while the chest wound heals. This is the case in any major surgical procedure where wound strength is essential.

The ear itself withstands trauma well, since, like the opposite, normal ear, it houses a framework of autogenous cartilage. To date, the author has witnessed numerous reconstructed

ears undergo traumatic episodes, e.g., baseball and soccer blows, a bee sting, and a dog bite. They have all healed well.[29] For these reasons, the author recommends no conspicuous, protective headgear, except in sports such as football and wrestling, where such equipment is used routinely with normal ears.

Other stages of auricular construction

Major stages in auricular construction subsequent to the initial framework implantation are lobule rotation, separating the ear from the head with a skin graft, deepening of the concha, and formation of a tragus. These stages can be planned independently or in various combinations, depending on which best achieves the desired end result.

Rotation of the lobule

The author prefers to perform earlobe transposition as a secondary procedure, as it seems easier both to judge placement of the earlobe and to "splice" the lobule correctly into position with reference to a well-established, underlying framework. Although the author has occasionally transposed the lobule simultaneously with implantation of the cartilage graft, he has found it safer and far more accurate to transpose the lobule as a secondary procedure.

The "rotation" or repositioning of this normal but displaced structure is accomplished essentially by Z-plasty transposition of a narrow, inferiorly based triangular flap *(Fig. 7.13)*.

Nagata[32] and Firmin[85] transpose the earlobe and utilize skin from the lobule's posterior surface to line the framework's tragal strut during the first-stage surgery. This does produce an excellent tragal appearance, but the price paid is greater risk of skin necrosis, and earlobes which are at times compromised in appearance and often unable to accommodate earrings. This latter problem is no small issue for my young female patients, who often submit to surgery with eventual earlobe piercing as their highest priority.[23]

If the lobe vestige is short so that a substantial skin bridge can be preserved above it during its transposition, then the earlobe can safely be moved while simultaneously separating the auricle from the head to create the auriculocephalic sulcus[23,29] and preserve sufficient posterior earlobe skin to permit the use of earrings *(Fig. 7.8)*.

Tragal construction and conchal definition

One can form the tragus, excavate the concha, and mimic a canal in a single operation. This is accomplished by placing a thin elliptical-shaped chondrocutaneous composite graft beneath a J-shaped incision in the conchal region[75,77] *(Fig. 7.14)*. The main limb of the "J" is placed at the proposed posterior tragal margin; the crook of the "J" represents the intertragal notch. Extraneous soft tissues are excised beneath this tragal flap to deepen the concha; this excavated region looks quite like a meatus when the newly constructed tragus casts a shadow upon it.

It is advantageous to harvest the composite graft from the normal ear's anterolateral conchal surface due to its ideal

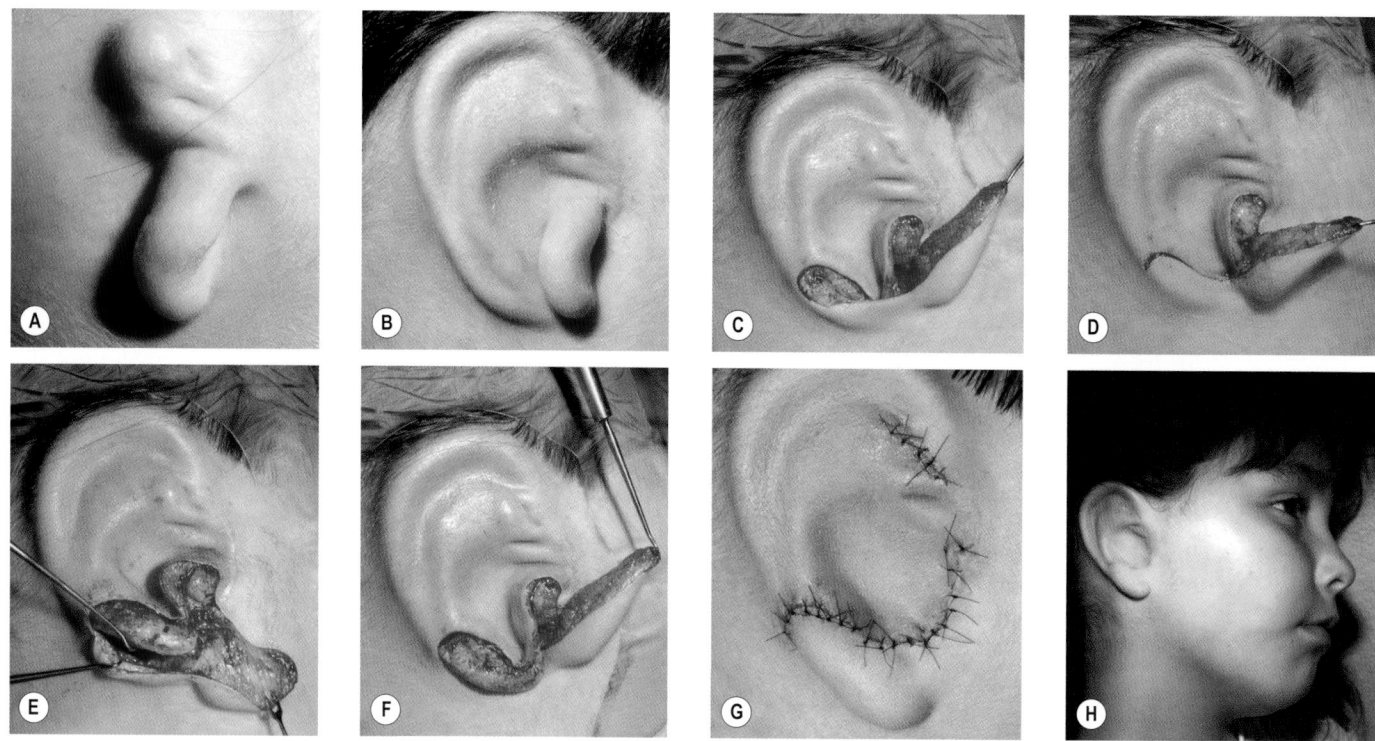

Fig. 7.13 Lobule transposition. **(A)** The microtic vestige. **(B)** The healed ear several months after framework insertion. **(C)** By incision around it, the lobule has been mobilized as an inferiorly based flap; an incision has been made at the proposed superior inset margin. **(D–F)** The skin overlying the lower ear region has been loosened and slid under the elevated framework's tip to surface the "floor" beneath it. Note that connective tissue has been carefully preserved over the cartilaginous tip. **(G)** The lobule has been filleted and wrapped around the framework tip in a two-layered wound closure; the former lobule site is closed, and the vestigial tissue is excised from the triangular fossa region. **(H)** The healed repair. (Reproduced from Brent B. Auricular repair with autogenous rib cartilage grafts: two decades of experience with 600 cases. *Plast Reconstr Surg.* 1992;90:355.)

shape and the paucity of subcutaneous tissue between the delicate anterolateral skin and adjacent cartilage. This technique is particularly ideal when a prominent concha exists in the normal donor ear, since closure of the donor site facilitates an otoplasty, which often is needed to gain frontal symmetry.

I also use an alternative method of creating the tragus as an integral strut of the original framework during its initial fabrication. I achieve this with a small piece of rib cartilage which is first fastened to the frame so as to create the antitragal eminence. The strut is thinned on one side, then curved around and affixed by its distal tip with a clear nylon suture which stretches across to the frame's crus helix. The result is a delicate tragus which flows naturally from the main framework through an arched intertragal notch *(Fig. 7.15)*. This method of tragus construction is particularly advantageous in bilateral microtia where there is no source for special composite tissue grafts. Nagata also creates the tragus with an extra cartilage piece attached to his main framework *(Fig. 7.16)*, and lines it with skin from the earlobe vestige during the first stage of surgery.

Another option for tragus construction in bilateral microtia is the modified Kirkham method, which consists of an anteriorly based conchal flap doubled on itself.[11]

Detaching the posterior auricular region

Auricular separation with skin grafting is done solely to eliminate the cryptotic appearance by defining the ear through creating a sulcus. This procedure will not project a framework which has been carved with insufficient depth.

The posterior auricular margin is defined by separating the ear from the head and covering its undersurface with a skin graft. In the past, I used a thick split graft but now strictly use full-thickness skin grafts. This stage of surgery should not be attempted until the edema has markedly subsided and the auricular details have become well defined. This surgery is initiated by making an incision several millimeters behind the rim, taking care to preserve a protective connective tissue layer on the cartilage framework. The retroauricular skin is then advanced into the newly created sulcus so that the only graft requirement is on the ear's undersurface. I harvest a full-thickness skin graft from the lower abdomen or groin crease and suture it to the wound with the sutures left long; these are tied over a bolster to tamponade the graft to the recipient bed *(Fig. 7.17)*. ⊗ FIG 7.17 APPEARS ONLINE ONLY

Greater projection of the auricle can be achieved by placing a wedge of rib cartilage behind the elevated ear, but this must be covered with a tissue flap in order for the skin graft to take over the cartilage. Nagata[32] accomplishes this with an axial flap of temporoparietal fascia *(Fig. 7.18)*. However, use of that fascial flap is not without a certain morbidity, and I feel that this fascia should be reserved for significant traumatic and secondary reconstruction cases where there is no other option for their solution.[29] Like Firmin[85] and Weerda,[86] I prefer to cover the cartilage wedge with a turnover "book flap" of occipitalis fascia from behind the ear[23] *(Fig. 7.8)*. When this

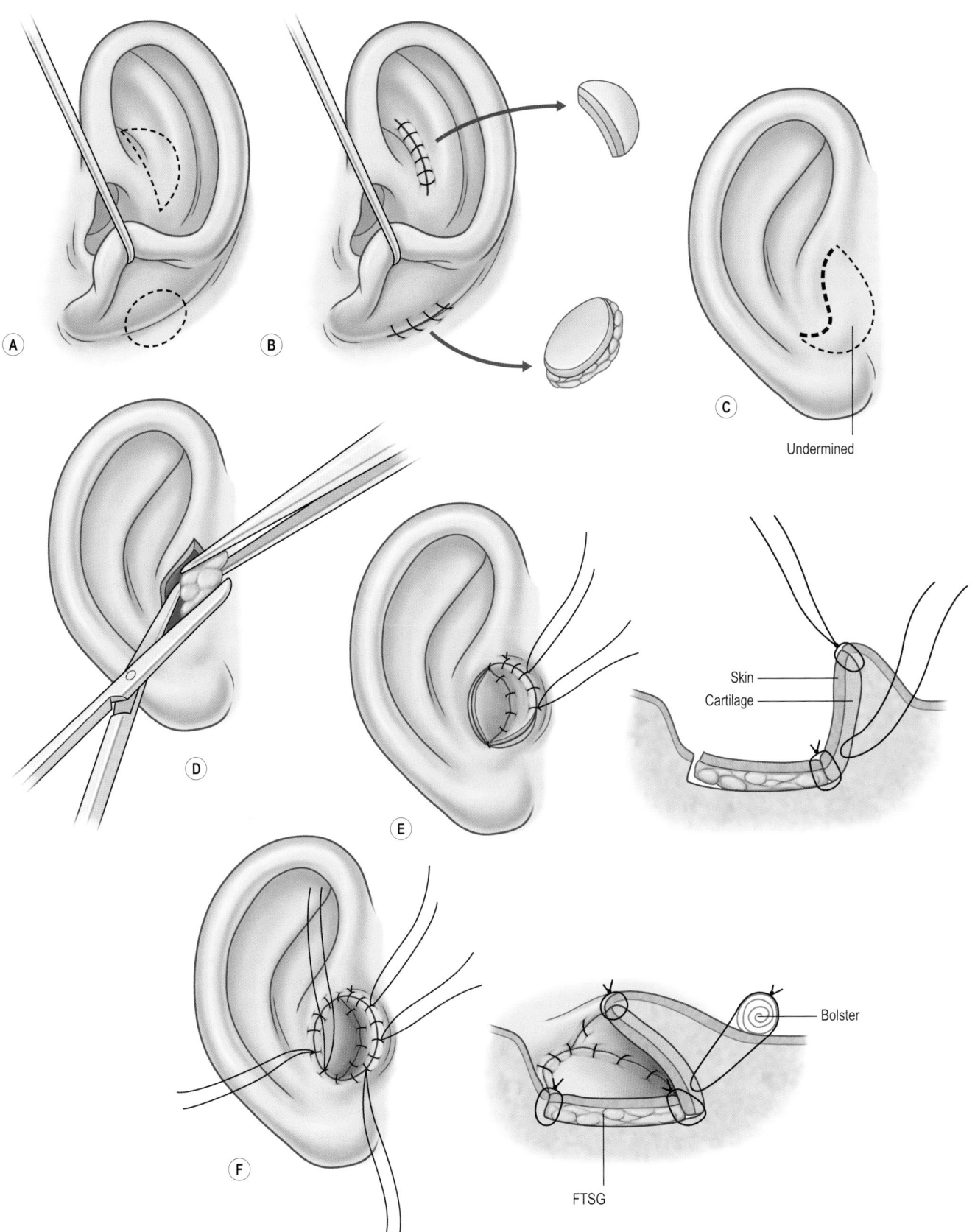

Fig. 7.14 (A–F) Stage 4, tragus construction and conchal excavation. Harvested from the opposite normal ear's conchal region, a chondrocutaneous composite graft is placed under a thin J-shaped flap to form the tragus. Before the floor of the tragal region is surfaced with a full-thickness skin graft (FTSG) harvested from behind the opposite earlobe, extraneous soft tissues are excised to deepen the region.

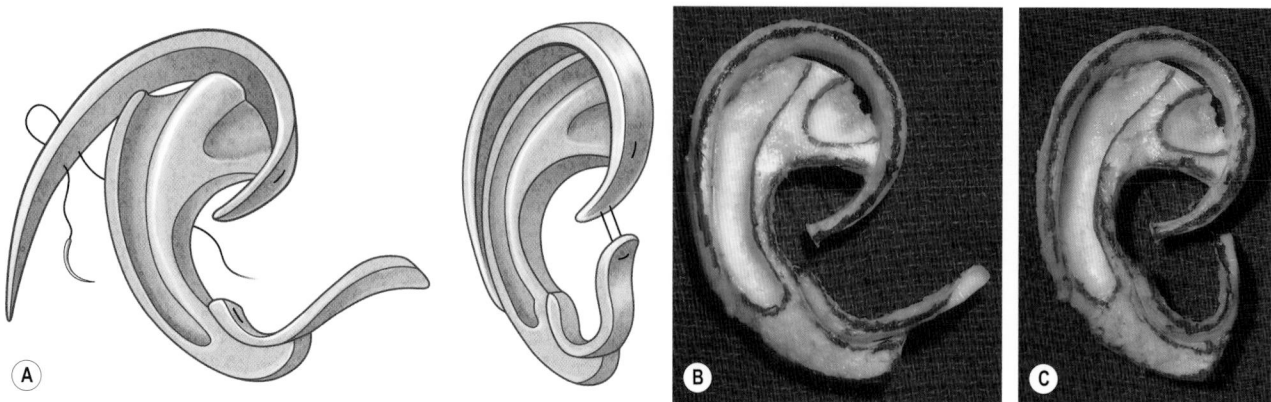

Fig. 7.15 Ear framework fabrication with integral tragal strut. **(A)** Construction of the frame. The floating cartilage creates a helix, and a second strut is arched around to form the antitragus, intertragal notch, and tragus. This arch is completed when the tip of the strut is affixed to the crus helix of the main frame with horizontal mattress suture of clear nylon. **(B, C)** Actual framework fabrication with the patient's rib cartilage. (Reproduced from Brent B. Technical advances in ear reconstruction with autogenous rib cartilage grafts: personal experience with 1200 cases. *Plast Reconstr Surg.* 1999;104:319.)

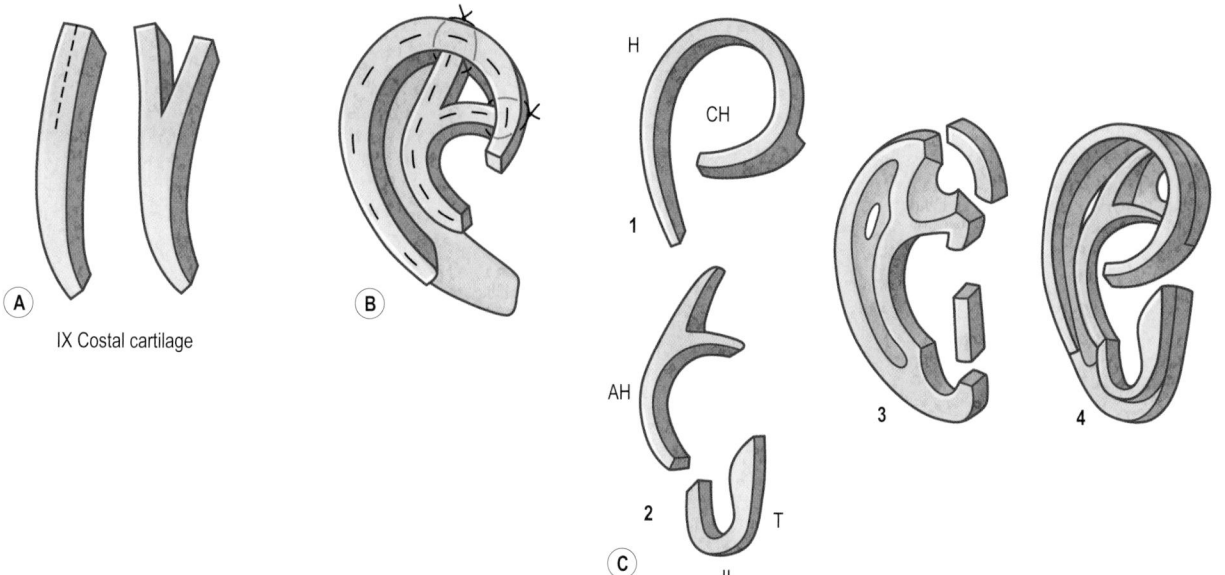

IX Costal cartilage

Fig. 7.16 Ear framework fabrication with appliqué of cartilage components. **(A, B)** Spina first applied a separate antihelical complex to the base block in 1971. (Redrawn from Spina V, Psillakis JM. Total reconstruction of the ear in congenital microtia. *Plast Reconstr Surg.* 1971;48:349.) **(C)** Nagata revived Spina's technique and added his own modifications. The numerous wire sutures used in this method lie precariously under the thin auricular skin. H, helix; CH, crus of helix; AH, antihelix; T, tragus. (Redrawn from Nagata S. Modification of the stages in total reconstruction of the auricle. *Plast Reconstr Surg.* 1994;93:221.) See text.

cartilage-wedging technique is used, there is no need to subject the patient to a second uncomfortable chest operation by harvesting rib cartilage anew, as does Nagata.[87] Instead, an extra piece of cartilage can be banked underneath the chest incision during the initial first-stage procedure. When the wedge is needed during the elevation procedure, it can be easily retrieved by incising through the original chest scar. Alternatively, I have also banked this cartilage wedge underneath the scalp, just posterior to the main pocket where the completed ear framework is placed[23] *(Fig. 7.8A)*. This site is particularly advantageous in that the nearby banked cartilage can more conveniently be retrieved when later lifting the new ear from the head; furthermore, this scalp site seemingly provides better nourishment for the banked cartilage than does the subcutaneous chest region.

When harvesting this cartilage wedge material during the first-stage procedure, the cartilage could be split *in situ*, which allows the surgeon to obtain a wider portion of cartilage to achieve maximum projection of the ear. This technique consists of shaving the outer cartilage from the rib and deliberately violates Gibson's balanced cross-sectional principles,[83] causing the cartilage wedge to warp into an ideal shape for the posterior conchal wall that it will form *(Fig. 7.19)*. This method of tissue harvest leaves the inner cartilage lamella intact, once again maximizing chest wall integrity and minimizing deformity. ⊛ FIG **7.19** APPEARS ONLINE ONLY

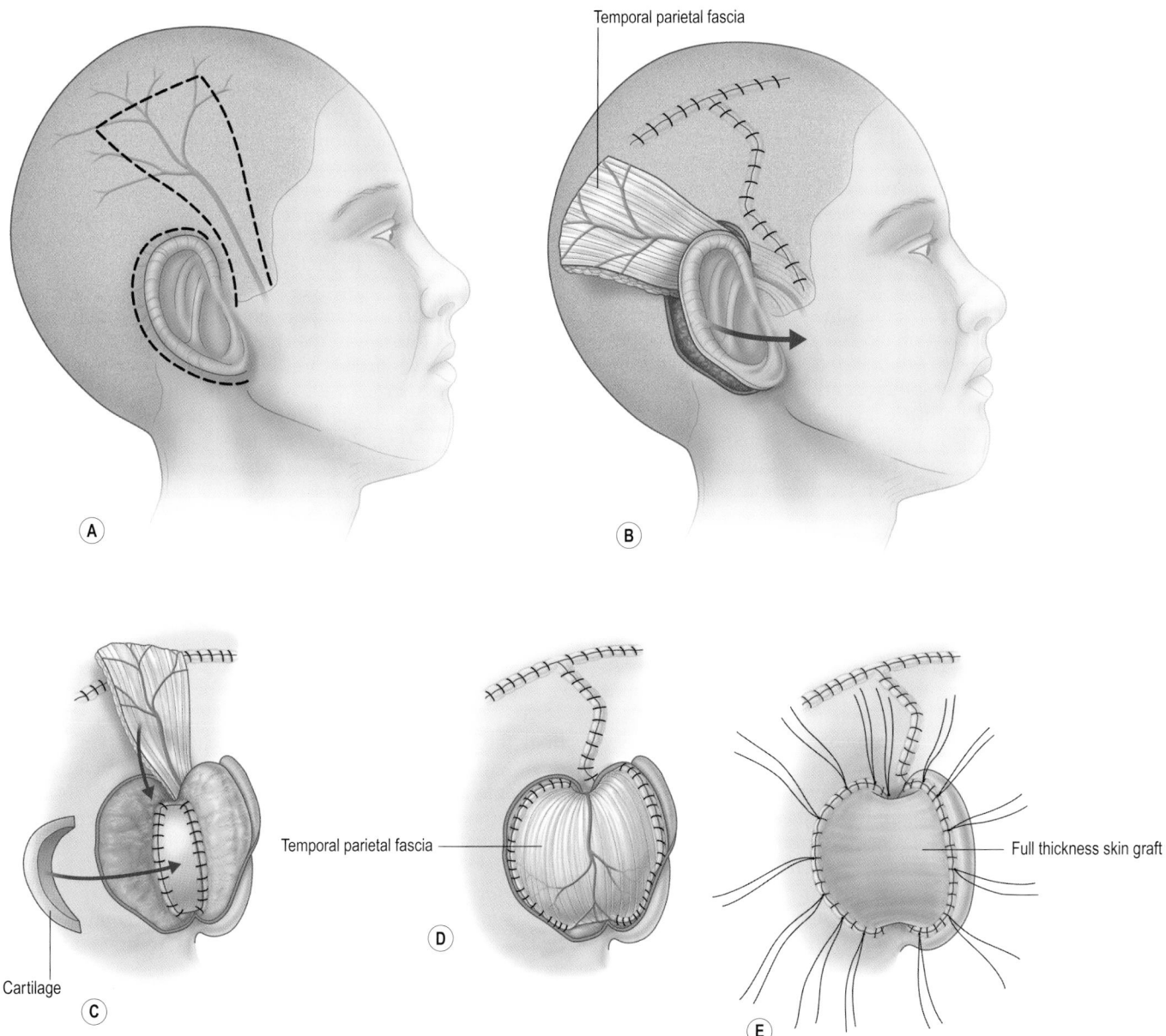

Fig. 7.18 (A–E) Separating and projecting the surgically constructed ear, Nagata technique. The surgically constructed ear is separated from the head at the second stage. Projection is supplemented by wedging a piece of rib cartilage (harvested anew from the chest), then covering it with a temporal vessel-containing fascial flap and skin graft.

Managing the hairline

Low hairline is one of the most common and troublesome problems in auricular construction. Because the normal hairline is usually lower than the apex of a normal ear, and sometimes considerably lower in microtia, inserting the framework beneath the periauricular skin often places hair on a portion of the new auricle. In trying to avoid hairy skin over the superior helix, the surgeon may be tempted to place the ear too low. Another complication arises when the framework is displaced anteriorly by the hairline, which acts as a constricting band at the juncture between the thin, hairless retroauricular skin and the thick scalp skin. This can be avoided by limiting the anterior dissection of the cutaneous pocket and by checking the framework's position before closing the incision.

Historically, Letterman and Harding[88] created a "scalp roll" and free skin graft to provide a hairless skin cover; however, this new cover lacks the elasticity of virgin skin. Instead, the author usually first implants the framework and later eradicates any undesirable hair. This can be done with electrolysis, laser, or by replacing the follicular skin with a graft.[29]

Prior to placing an ear framework, if one predicts a tight pocket and a hairline that will cover half the new ear, the surgeon may consider a primary fascial flap.[89]

Dealing with this unwanted hair depends on how much ear is involved. If hair is limited to the helix, then electrolysis or clipping is clearly the method of choice. If hair covers a third or more of the ear, I have often resurfaced the ear with a skin graft[29] (with or without a fascial flap). Regardless of hair quantity, it is ideal to eradicate the hair by nonsurgical means, which eliminates a "patchwork" appearance and preserves the normal aesthetic and protective qualities of the local skin. Such a depilatory method would be even better if it simultaneously thinned the follicle-containing scalp skin to provide the new ear with finer skin coverage. Perhaps in the future both of these goals will be achieved without surgery.

In recent years, lasers have become useful adjuncts for treating the skin and its appendages.[90] It has been found that treating axillary hidradinitis with the laser not only improves that condition by eliminating the apocrine sweat glands,[91] but by reducing the bulk these epidermal appendages constitute, the skin also becomes finer and softer (Sasaki, personal communication 1998). By virtue of the same principle, I am hopeful that significant reduction of the hair follicles may likewise alter the scalp skin so that when it does cover a portion of the ear framework, it will be somewhat thinner and finer, resulting in enhanced detail of the completed ear.

While still not consistently producing permanent results at this writing, laser treatment can favorably alter hair growth to make it both finer and slower. Furthermore, as contrasted to needle electrolysis, patients can tolerate laser treatment of much larger areas during a given session. The two schools of treatment concentrate on targeting the melanin (and thus the heavily pigmented follicles) within the depth of the dermis[92] versus targeting only the follicles by loading them with carbon particles via a gel transport medium and then focusing the laser on the carbon.[93,94] The trick is to deliver enough energy density through the laser to destroy the hair follicles without damaging the skin, which causes scarring and/or hypopigmentation. Presently, laser treatments decrease hair density and texture so that only a few "maintenance treatments" are needed per year. Laser technology continues to improve with such advances as better coolant techniques, which permit the safe delivery of a higher fluence of energy. Soon, it should consistently be possible to achieve permanent hair removal without injurious side-effects to the surrounding skin.[95] It is my vision to "pretreat" ear reconstruction patients with the laser and thus create the ideal hairline before initiating the surgical ear repair *(Fig. 7.20)*. To aid the laser technician (who often may be at a great distance from my practice), I create a template that makes it easy to locate the exact target area precisely during the serial treatments[23] *(Fig. 7.20)*.

Variations in total ear reconstruction technique

Over the years, numerous variations in technique have evolved and will continue to emerge. One of the current popular variations is the Nagata technique in which the ear reconstruction is accomplished in two stages.[32,87] In this method, the cartilage framework implantation, tragus construction, and lobule transposition are all performed in the first stage; the ear is separated from the head at the second stage with a block of cartilage (harvested by entering the chest for a second time) which is covered by a fascial flap and skin graft.

Although this eliminates several stages of surgery, all the soft-tissue manipulation in the initial stage significantly increases the risk of tissue necrosis. Though Nagata reports low complication rates, the complication rate with this procedure reported by others is as high as 14%[30] (by contrast, I have

experienced less than 0.25% complication rate during the past 1800 cases with my "less aggressive" reconstructive technique). This combination of procedures also sacrifices the earlobe quality by lining the tragus with the lobe's valuable backside skin. In my opinion, the final appearance and quality of the earlobe are far more important than creating a tragus during the initial first stage.

Because the Nagata technique produces the antihelical complex by wiring an extra piece of cartilage to the base block *(Fig. 7.10)*, the ears produced are thick and more rib cartilage is needed and excised from the chest with attendant chest wall donor deformity.[80,81] However Nagata has adopted his harvest technique, preserving the perichondrium – a technique that he reports as eliminating the chest wall deformity.[96,97]

The numerous wire sutures which are used to apply these two pieces together (as well as attaching the helix) are placed on the lateral cartilage surfaces and lie under the thin auricular integument *(Fig. 7.10)*, and thus bear risk of extrusion through the skin.[98] Tanzer reported wire extrusions in 20 of his 44 cases,[53] and he used one-quarter as many sutures per ear as does Nagata.

In order to achieve ear projection, the Nagata technique uses the superficial temporal vessel-containing fascial flap in every case *(Fig. 7.18)*, with its attendant scalp scar and its risk of hair thinning in the donor site.[29] Because Nagata enters the chest again (to obtain the cartilage wedge) during this procedure, the patient is subjected to a second uncomfortable operation.

The Nagata technique does produce greater projection than does the author's technique, in which frontal symmetry is dealt with during the tragus construction when the grafts for the tragus are harvested from the opposite ear *(Fig. 7.14)*. This allows the donor ear to be adjusted to the reconstructed ear and frontal symmetry achieved; by doing this as the final stage, the healed final position of the elevated ear has been set so the surgeon knows where to set the opposite ear during the tragus construction so that symmetry can be accomplished.

The Nagata technique has produced interesting and useful variations in ear reconstruction and continues to evolve.[30,85] Other variations will emerge as the quest for improved ear reconstruction continues. Walton and Beahm have published a balanced comparison of the Nagata and Brent techniques that the reader is encouraged to read.[99]

Secondary reconstruction

The difficulties in surgically constructing an ear are substantiated by the often disheartening result which emerges despite the surgeon's persistent efforts. Discouragingly, at times the end result bears no resemblance to an auricle, other than for its location. Furthermore, the scars which result from multiple procedures may extend the defect well beyond the original deformity. The impact of such failures is emotionally devastating to the patient and proportionately frustrating for the surgeon.

Tanzer[100] managed secondary reconstruction by first excising the scar and skin grafting the defect, and by then waiting for the graft to mature before implanting a new cartilage framework. However, this approach often is beset with compromises, in that skin-grafted tissues have limited

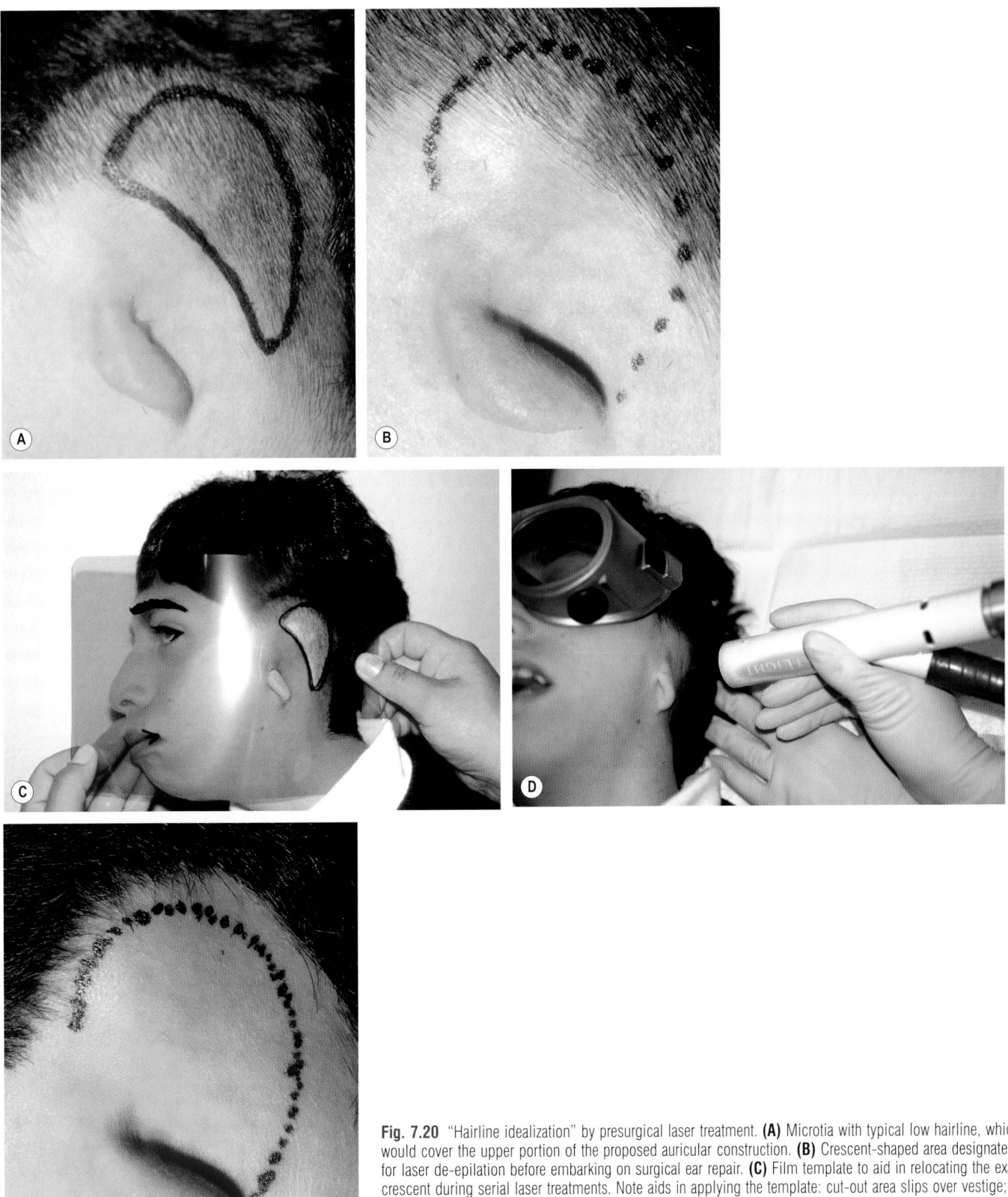

Fig. 7.20 "Hairline idealization" by presurgical laser treatment. **(A)** Microtia with typical low hairline, which would cover the upper portion of the proposed auricular construction. **(B)** Crescent-shaped area designated for laser de-epilation before embarking on surgical ear repair. **(C)** Film template to aid in relocating the exact crescent during serial laser treatments. Note aids in applying the template: cut-out area slips over vestige; eyebrow, lateral canthus, and oral commissure are marked on film. **(D)** The laser treatment in progress. **(E)** The same microtia after several laser treatments. The hairline is now ideal, and surgical construction of the ear will begin. (Reproduced from Brent B. Technical advances in ear reconstruction with autogenous rib cartilage grafts: personal experience with 1200 cases. *Plast Reconstr Surg.* 1999;104:319.)

elasticity as a cutaneous pocket, and a detailed framework with depth cannot be introduced without significant tension. Furthermore, deeply scarred tissue beds may be so severely damaged that this approach is not even possible, and, seemingly, the patient is left with no solution to the problem.

In an effort to resolve this skin coverage impasse, Brent and Byrd implemented a more optimal method for treating secondary ear reconstruction: excising of the entire auricular scar area, immediately placing a sculpted autogenous rib cartilage graft, and covering the latter with a temporoparietal fascial flap and skin graft[89] *(Fig. 7.6)*.

Bilateral microtia

Although relatively rare, bilateral microtia frequently afflicts patients with conditions such as Treacher–Collins–Franschetti syndrome, bilateral craniofacial microsomia, and other uncommon craniofacial malformations. The reconstructive principles for managing bilateral microtia are the same as for the unilateral deformity.

For optimal function and aesthetics in bilateral microtia, one must plan to integrate surgical procedures so that one does not compromise the other. In these cases, the auricular construction must precede the middle-ear surgery because once an attempt is made to "open" the ear, the chances of obtaining a satisfactory auricular repair are severely compromised because the invaluable virgin skin has been scarred.

In bilateral microtia, I cartilage-graft each side several months apart, because each hemithorax contains sufficient cartilage for only one good ear framework. Simultaneous bilateral reconstruction necessitates bilateral chest wounds with attendant splinting and respiratory distress. Furthermore, the first auricular repair might be jeopardized upon turning the head to do the second side. For these reasons, I prefer to do the first stage of each ear on separate occasions.

Several months after the second cartilage graft, both earlobes are transposed during a single procedure. Once this stage is healed, the ears are separated from the head with skin grafting. As a final touch, bilateral traguses can be constructed with modified Kirkham technique prior to pursuing the middle-ear surgery.

Nine of 10 patients with microtia have only unilateral involvement and most do well without middle-ear surgery, as they are born "adjusted" to their monaural condition.

To ensure that the gains of middle-ear surgery outweigh the risks and complications of the procedure itself, this surgery is reserved for cases in which there is high patient motivation and favorable radiologic evidence of middle-ear development. Then, it must be thoughtfully planned in a team approach[23] with an otologist who is competent and well experienced in atresia surgery.

In the team approach, the plastic surgeon initiates the procedure by lifting the ear from its bed while carefully preserving connective tissue on the framework's undersurface. Then the otologist proceeds, first drilling a bony canal, completing the ossiculoplasty, and then repairing the tympanum with a temporal fascial graft. Finally, the plastic surgeon resumes by excising soft tissues to exteriorize the meatus through the conchal region and harvesting a skin graft which the otologist uses to line the new canal and complete the repair *(Fig. 7.21)*.

Ⓔ FIG 7.21 APPEARS ONLINE ONLY

The constricted ear

Tanzer has applied "constricted ear" to a group of ear anomalies in which the encircling helix seems tight, as if constricted by a purse-string. Once loosely termed "cup" or "lop ears," these deformities collectively have helical and scaphal hooding and varying degrees of flattening of their antihelical complexes.

Although Tanzer gave these ears a numerical classification which corresponds to each deformity's severity,[62] in practical surgical terms it needs to be determined whether to repair the ear by reshaping the existing tissues or whether to supplement skin coverage and/or the supporting cartilage.

Constricted ear repairs must be individualized for each specific ear deformity. If helical lidding is the main defect and the height discrepancy is minimal, then the overhanging tissue can merely be excised. At times, the cartilage lid can be used as a "banner flap" to increase ear height *(Fig. 7.22)*. Moderate height discrepancies necessitate the augmentation of the cartilage height by modifying the ipsilateral ear cartilage[101,102] or employing contralateral conchal cartilage grafts.[76] The key to repairing these moderate deformities is to visualize the defective cartilage armature, which is only possible after the skin envelope has been "degloved" *(Figs 7.23 and 7.24)*.

When constriction is severe enough to produce a height difference of 1.5 cm, both skin and cartilage must be added, essentially to correct the deformity as if it were a formal microtia *(Fig. 7.25)*.

Cryptotia

Cryptotia is an unusual congenital deformity in which the upper pole of the ear cartilage is buried beneath the scalp *(Fig. 7.26)*. The superior auriculocephalic sulcus is absent, but can be demonstrated via gentle finger pressure. This has stimulated Japanese physicians to correct this deformity nonsurgically,[103] as it occurs in Japan as frequently as 1:400 births.[104]

This nonsurgical procedure is accomplished through applying an external conforming splint. If applied prior to 6 months of age, it may successfully mold a permanent retroauricular sulcus.[105] Tan *et al.*[106] have successfully applied such nonsurgical splinting techniques for constricted ears as well *(Fig. 7.27)*. Yotsuyanagi *et al.*[107] have successfully employed these nonsurgical methods to correct a variety of ear deformities in children older than neonates.

Surgical repairs entail the addition of skin to the deficient retroauricular sulcus via skin grafts and Z-plasties, V-Y advancement flaps,[108] or rotational flaps.[105] When a cartilage deformity accompanies the skin deficiency, then various remodeling techniques are needed to facilitate the repair.[104,109]

Prominent ear

Pathology

During the third month of gestation, the auricle's protrusion increases; by the end of the sixth month the helical margin curls, the antihelix forms its fold, and the antihelical crura

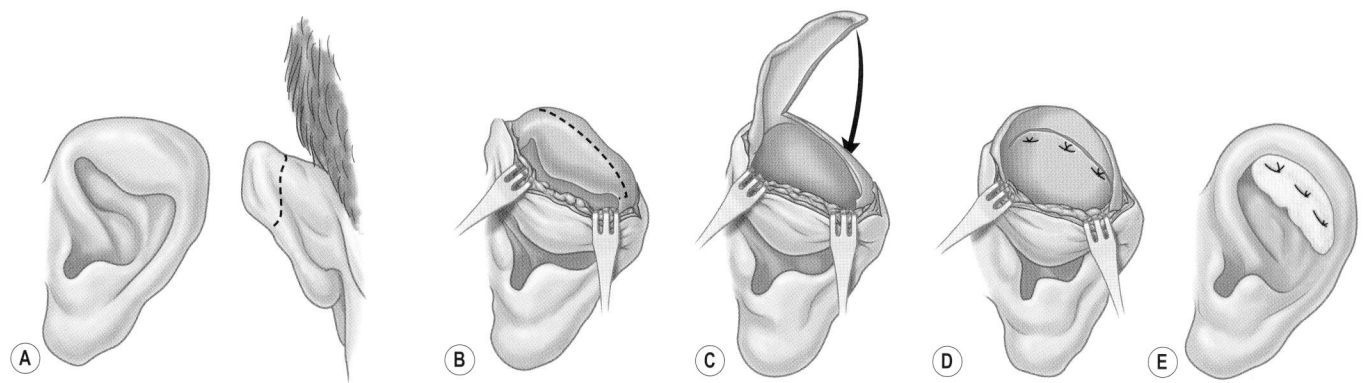

Fig. 7.22 Correction of grade I ear constriction. **(A)** The incision for exposure of the skeletal deformity. **(B)** The deformed cartilage has been filleted from its soft-tissue cover. The line of detachment of the angulated segment is marked. **(C)** The deformed cartilage is lifted on a medially based pedicle and rotated into an upright position. **(D)** The repositioned cartilage is sutured to the scapha. **(E)** The skin is redraped, and the helical sulcus is maintained by through-and-through sutures tied over gauze pledgets. (Reproduced from Tanzer RC, Edgerton MT, eds. *Symposium on reconstruction of the auricle*. St. Louis: CV Mosby, 1974:141.)

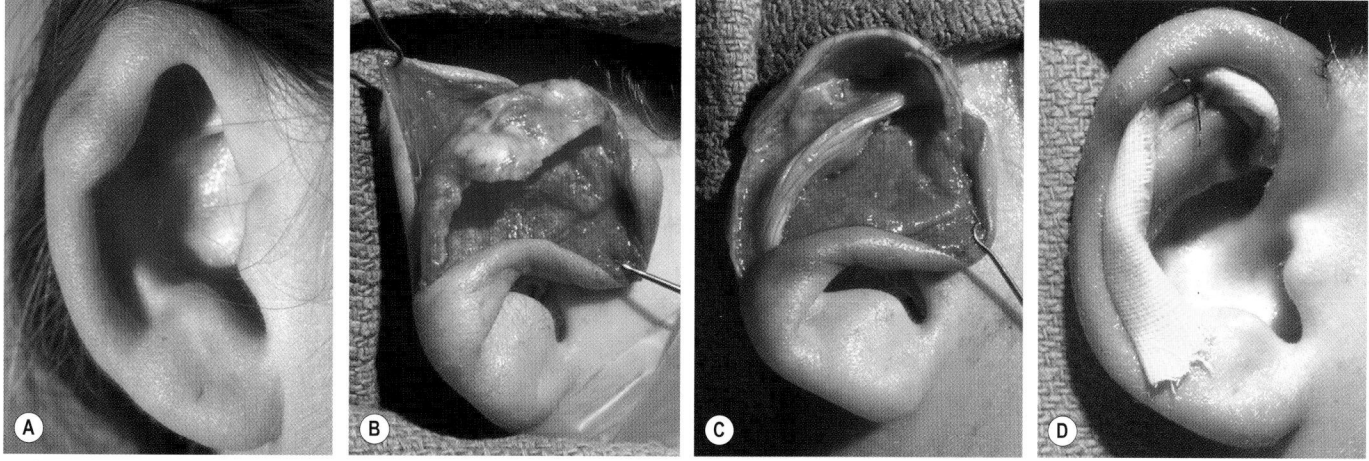

Fig. 7.23 Repair of a moderately constricted ear. **(A)** Preoperative appearance. **(B)** "Degloving" the ear to expose the distorted cartilage. **(C)** The cartilage is expanded, the antihelix is formed, and a contralateral conchal cartilage graft repairs the deficient upper third. **(D)** Skin redraped to complete the repair. See Figure 7.30B. (Reproduced from Brent B. The correction of microtia with autogenous cartilage grafts. II. Atypical and complex deformities. *Plast Reconstr Surg*. 1980;66:13.)

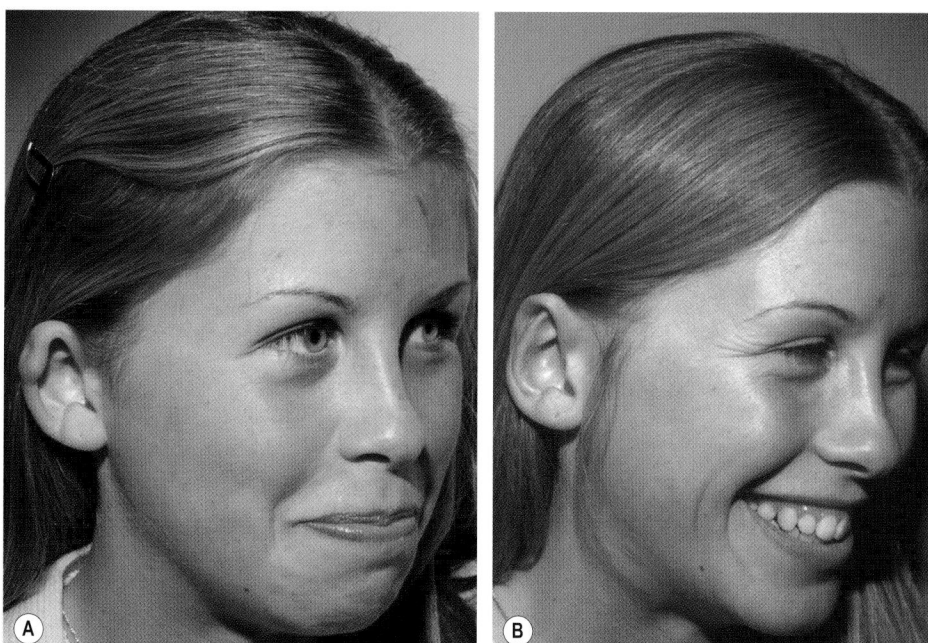

Fig. 7.24 Repair of a moderately constricted ear by the technique shown in Figure 7.23. (Reproduced from Brent B. The correction of microtia with autogenous cartilage grafts. II. Atypical and complex deformities. *Plast Reconstr Surg*. 1980;66:13.)

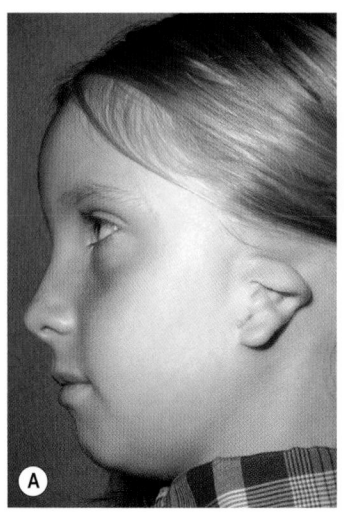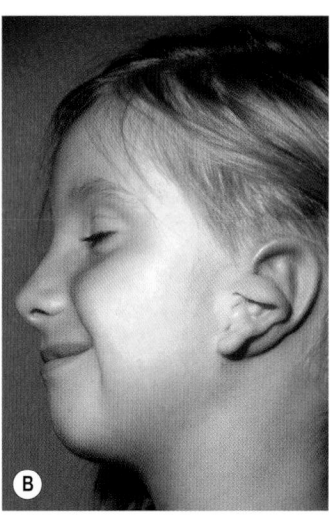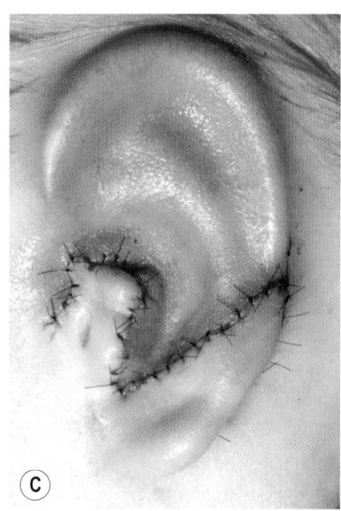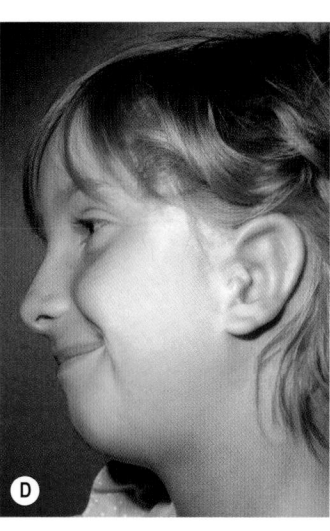

Fig. 7.25 Repair of severe ear constriction by the classic microtia technique. **(A)** A patient with a severely constricted ear. **(B)** Appearance after insertion of total ear framework of rib cartilage. **(C)** Use of the vestige to form the earlobe and tragus. **(D)** Final result after separation from the head with a skin graft. (Reproduced from Brent B. The correction of microtia with autogenous cartilage grafts. II. Atypical and complex deformities. *Plast Reconstr Surg.* 1980;66:13.)

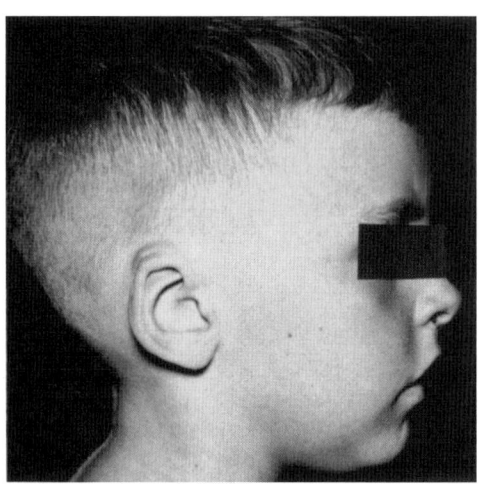

Fig. 7.26 Cryptotia.

appear. Anything that interferes with this process produces prominent ears.

The most common deformity arises from the antihelix's failing to fold. This widens the conchoscaphal angle as much as 150° or more *(Fig. 7.28)*, which flattens the superior crus and, in severe forms, the antihelical body and inferior crus. In extreme cases the helical roll may be absent, and this produces a flat, shell-like ear with no convolutions.

Producing protrusion of the ear's middle third, conchal widening may occur as an isolated deformity or may occur in conjunction with antihelical deformities, described above. This abnormality is usually bilateral and is frequently noted in siblings and parents.

Treatment

In repairing prominent ears, symmetry is most important and, paradoxically, may be more difficult to achieve in unilateral than in bilateral cases. The repaired ear convolutions should

appear smooth and unoperated. The most lateral point of the completed repair should be between 1.7 and 2.0 cm from the head, and the helix should be visible behind the antihelical body when the ears are seen from the frontal view.[110]

To attain these goals, a great number of techniques have been described, many of which produce acceptable results. However, the author recommends that surgeons should direct their efforts toward correcting the specific problem areas of each individual ear rather than following a routine "cookbook recipe."

If the upper third of the ear protrudes because of an absent or weak antihelix, then an exaggerated antihelix must be formed. If the middle third is too prominent, the concha must be recessed by either cartilage excision or suture fixation.[111] Finally, if the lobule protrudes, one must either resect or retroposition the cauda helicis' cartilaginous tail[112] and/or excise retrolobular skin.

Conchal alteration

Dieffenbach[3] is credited with the first otoplastic attempt in 1845. This consisted of excising skin from the auriculocephalic sulcus and then suturing conchal cartilage to the mastoid periosteum.

In addition to narrowing the auriculocephalic sulcus, Ely[4] (1881) and others excised a strip of conchal wall, a procedure that is attributed to Morestin in 1903.[113] This old method of tacking back the concha to mastoid periosteum has been revived throughout the years.[111,113–117]

Also, the wide concha can be corrected by excising a cartilaginous ellipse beneath the antihelical body. This may create a redundant skin fold which then may require excision.

Restoration of the antihelical fold

Luckett (1910) first conceptualized that prominent ears result from the antihelix's failure to fold. He restored this fold by excising a crescent of medial skin and cartilage.[118] The

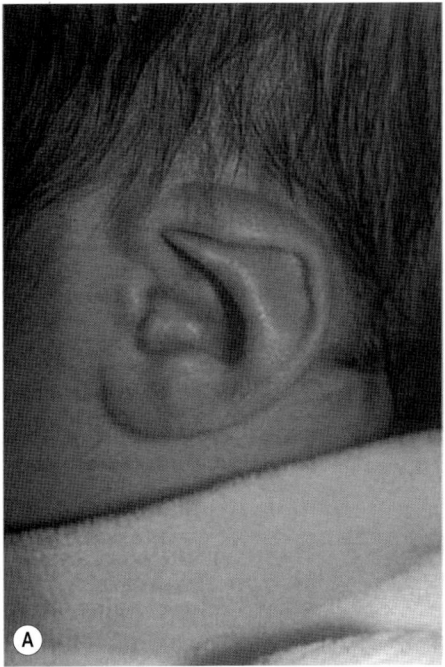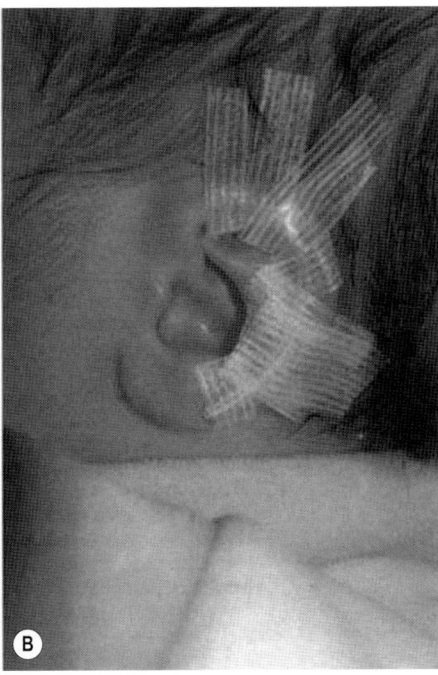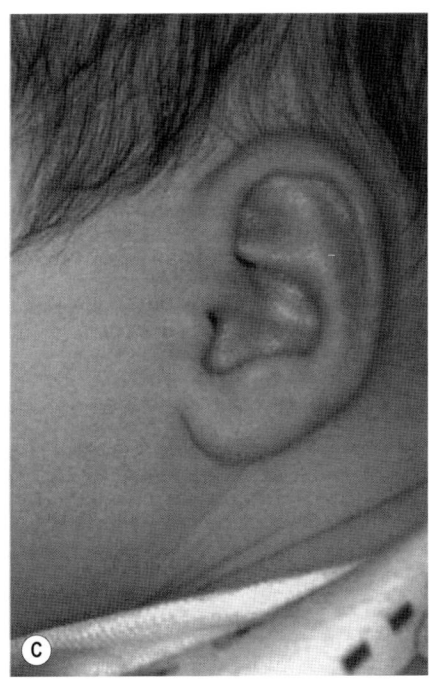

Fig. 7.27 (A) Neonate with lop ear. **(B)** Custom splint used to correct helical fold. **(C)** Follow-up photograph taken 2 months after completion of 10 weeks of splinting. (Reproduced from Tan ST, Abramson DL, MacDonald DM, et al. Molding therapy for infants with deformational auricular anomalies. *Ann Plast Surg.* 1997;38:263.)

majority of subsequent otoplasty procedures have focused upon creating a smoother antihelix than produced by employing Luckett's sharp cartilage-breaking technique.[110,119–121]

Altering the medial cartilage surface

In order to permit its smooth molding, the scaphal cartilage can be recontoured by a number of techniques. McEvitt[122] and Paletta et al.[115] weakened the scapha with multiple parallel cuts while Converse et al.,[123] used burr abrasion.

Becker,[124,125] Converse et al.,[123] and Tanzer[126] used parallel cuts and permanent sutures to form a smooth, cornucopia-like antihelix *(Fig. 7.29)*. Advantageously, this cartilage tube encases substantial scar to lock the cartilage into position and prevent recurrence of deformity. 🖥 FIG 7.29 APPEARS ONLINE ONLY

Reviving a long-forgotten suggestion of Morestin,[113] Mustardé[127,128] created the antihelix by inserting permanent mattress sutures through the cartilage without using any actual cartilage incisions. The author finds this technique particularly useful in the pliable ear cartilage of children. Surgeons who criticize this technique mention recurrence of the deformity, presumably because the sutures tear through the cartilage. This complication is largely avoided if one can get a substantial "bite" that encompasses both the cartilage and its overlying perichondrium. However, because the thin anterolateral auricular skin is adherent to the perichondrium with a concomitant paucity of subcutaneous tissue, it is difficult to make a good pass with the needle to achieve this objective because one tends to either "buttonhole" the skin above or lacerate the cartilage below. I circumvent this problem by hydrodissection with injectable saline. Just prior to each pass with a permanent suture, I facilitate the needle's safe passage through both cartilage and perichondrium by ballooning the skin away from the cartilage with saline forced through a short 30-gauge

needle *(Fig. 7.28A)*. To avoid dissipation of the fluid, I only inject right at the local site of each planned suture just prior to passing the needle *(Fig. 7.28E)* rather than ballooning up the skin over the entire auricular surface to be reconfigured. This has worked well in preventing recurrent deformities and produces a very natural-appearing antihelix *(Fig. 7.28G)*.

Altering the lateral cartilage surface

Exploiting cartilage's tendency to warp when one surface is cut,[83] Chongchet[129] scored the anterior scaphal cartilage with multiple cartilage cuts to roll it back and form an antihelix. While Chongchet did this under direct vision using a scalpel, Stenstrom[130] produced the same effect by using a short-tined rasp instrument to score the antihelical region "blindly" through a posterior stab incision near the cauda helicis. The lateral cartilage surface has also been morselized or abraded under direct vision through a lateral incision.[131]

Finally, Kaye advocates an otoplasty method which combines both lateral cartilage scoring and fixation with permanent sutures. He accomplishes both of these maneuvers through minimal incisions[132] *(Fig. 7.30)*. 🖥 FIG 7.30 APPEARS ONLINE ONLY

Acquired deformities

Video 2

Total auricular reconstruction in the acquired deformity presents special problems not encountered in microtia. These merit separate consideration.

The lack of skin coverage is much more critical than in microtia, since an existing meatus precludes use of the anterior incision, and extra skin, as usually gained via removing the crumpled microtic cartilage, is not available. This factor compounds the previously mentioned hairline problem. If the

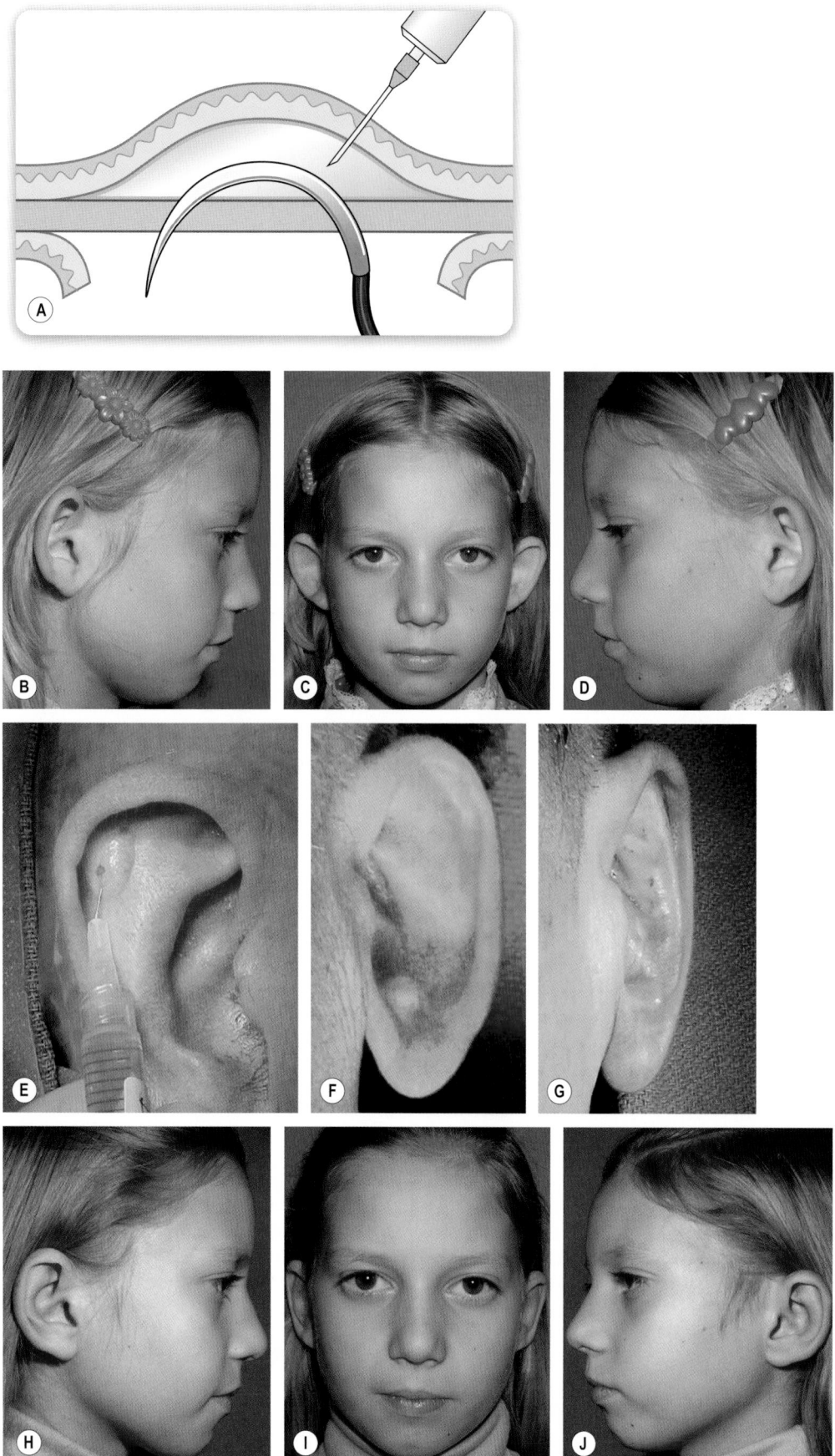

Fig. 7.28 Otoplasty by suture-only technique (Mustardé) facilitated by hydrodissection. **(A)** Facilitating needle passage by hydrodissection in otoplasty. Hydrodissection of skin with 30-gauge needle and saline allows for safe needle passage around cartilage and its perichondrium. **(B–D)** Ten-year-old girl with prominent ears. **(E)** Hydrodissecting away from the cartilage just prior to passing a Mustardé suture. Note the two blue skin marks which indicate proposed needle entrance and exit sites through cartilage below the hydrodissected skin. **(F)** Prominent ear with no antihelical definition. **(G)** Natural-appearing antihelix following Mustardé otoplasty facilitated by hydrodissection, immediately postoperative. **(H–J)** Result of the otoplasty. (Reproduced from Brent B. Hydrodissection as key to a natural-appearing otoplasty. *Plast Reconstr Surg.* 2008;122:1055.)

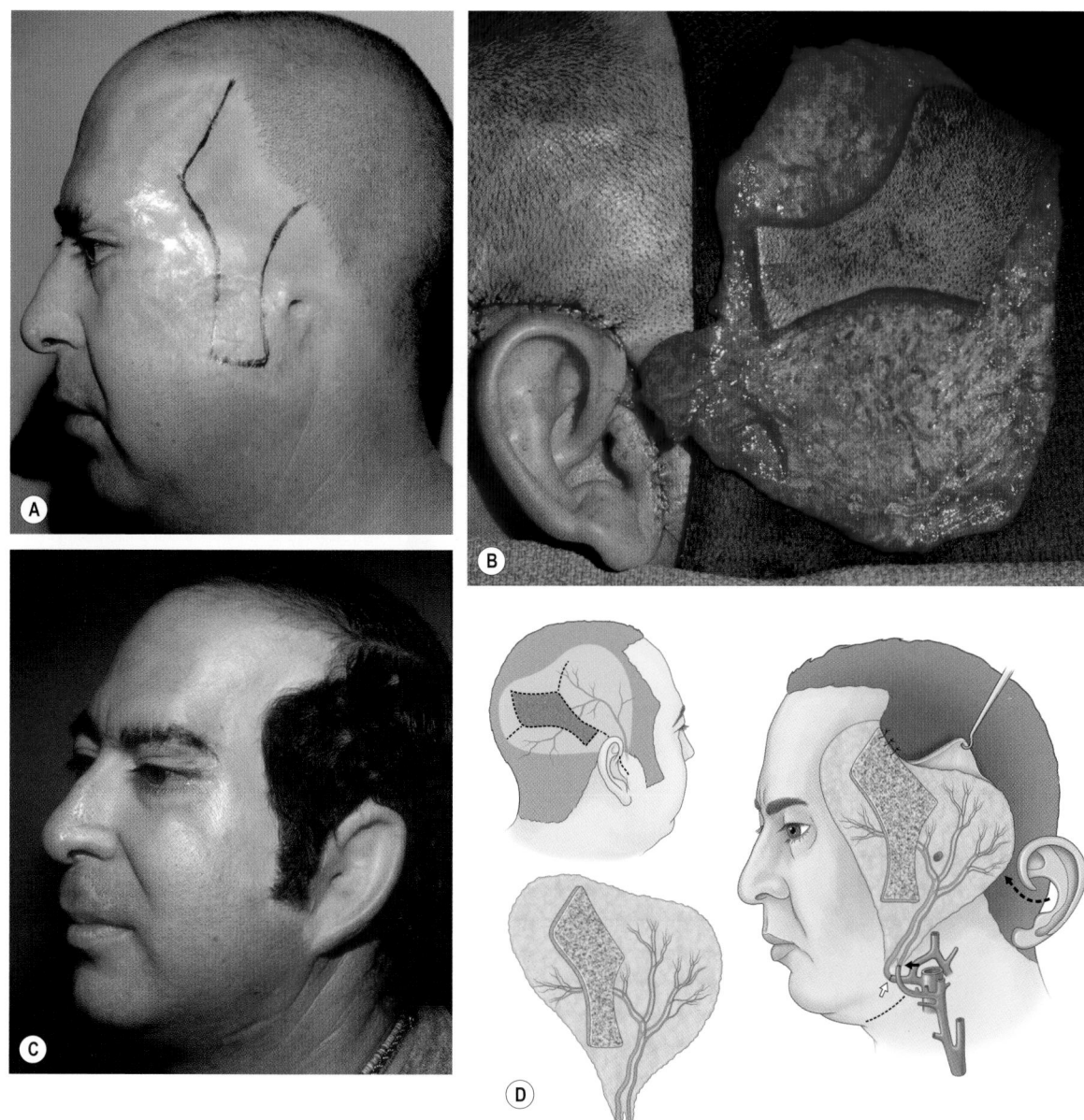

Fig. 7.31 Ear and temporal hairline restoration with rib cartilage graft covered by microsurgical transfer of contralateral fascial flap containing a scalp island. **(A)** Severe electrical burn injury. **(B)** The contralateral fascial flap with attached scalp island isolated on the temporal vessels. **(C)** Result of the repair. **(D)** The operative scheme. (Reproduced from Brent B. *The artistry of reconstructive surgery*. St. Louis: C.V. Mosby, 1987.)

existing skin can be used, then the cutaneous pocket is best developed by incisions above and/or below the proposed auricular site. If the local tissues are heavily scarred or restrict the surgeon from developing an ample skin pocket, then the repair must be supplemented with fascial flap coverage[89] *(Fig. 7.31)*. Skin expanders have also been employed to stretch the covering skin, but bear risks of extrusion and scar capsule formation.

Replantation of the amputated auricle

To the modern plastic surgeon, choosing a salvage procedure is influenced by the size of the amputated portion, the condition of the tissues of the amputated segment, and the condition of the stump and surrounding tissues, particularly in the

retroauricular area. A clean-cut amputation gives the surgeon a better chance for success. When the ear and its surrounding tissues are mangled and avulsed, and bone is exposed, the reconstruction is difficult, if not insurmountable. Small amputated segments are replaced as composite grafts with some hope of success. Larger amputated segments and subtotal amputation require further consideration.

Replantation of auricular tissue attached by a narrow pedicle

Because an ear is richly vascularized and has major vessels extending through its periphery, the partly avulsed auricular tissue can be successfully replaced, even though the remaining attachment is tenuous *(Fig. 7.32)*.

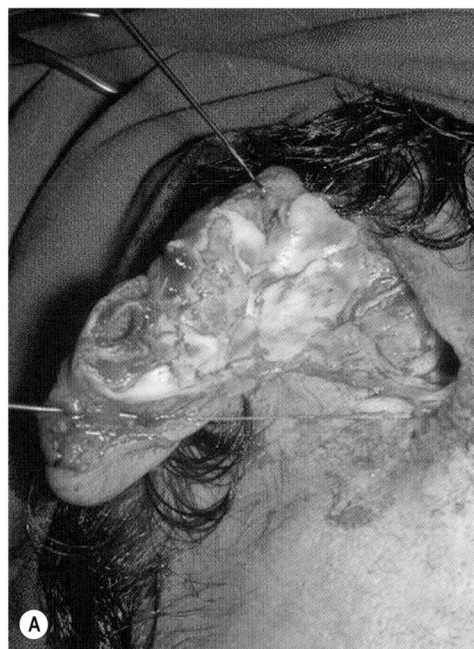 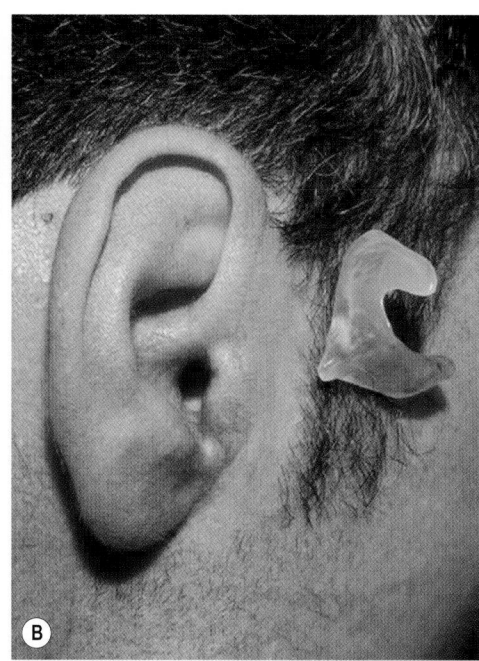

Fig. 7.32 Repair of a major auricular avulsion. **(A)** The avulsed ear remains attached by a narrow pedicle, which maintains its viability; the canal is transected. **(B)** Result after repair of the canal and maintenance of an acrylic mold for 4 months.

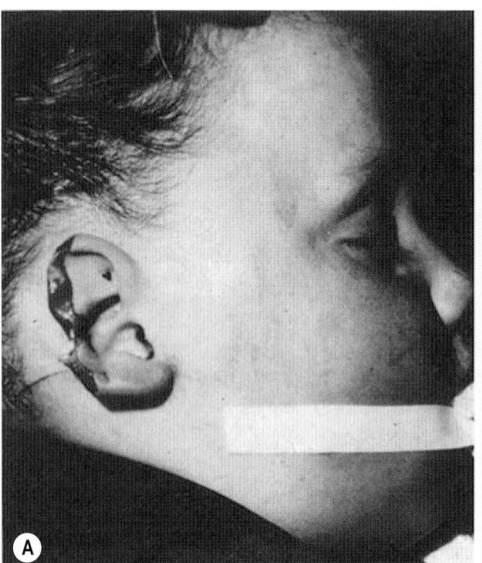 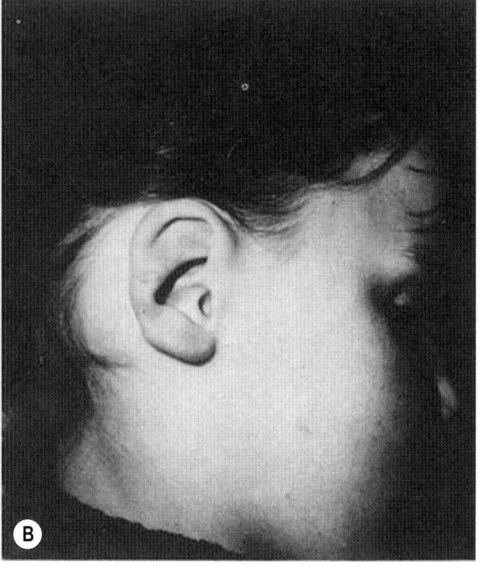

Fig. 7.33 Replantation of auricular tissue as a composite graft. **(A)** Loss of a portion of the scapha and helix resulting from a dog bite. **(B)** The amputated segment was retrieved and sutured in position as a composite graft, with this result 2 years later. (Patient of Dr. Andries Molenaar.) (Reproduced from Clemons JE, Connelly MV. Reattachment of a totally amputated auricle. *Arch Otolaryngol.* 1973;97:269.)

Replantation of auricular tissue as a composite graft

Even when the piece of auricle is quite large, the completely detached ear tissue may survive when replaced as a composite graft, although few successful cases have been reported in the plastic surgery literature[134–136] *(Fig. 7.33)*.

Replantation of auricular cartilage

Because a cartilaginous framework is difficult to reproduce, the salvage and use of denuded auricular cartilage

were recommended by numerous surgeons.[137–140] Various techniques have been employed to preserve cartilage from an avulsed ear. The skin may be removed and the cartilage buried in an abdominal pocket,[141] in a cervical pocket,[142] or placed under the skin of the retroauricular area.[143] The latter orthotopic cartilage replantation can be employed only if regional cutaneous tissues are in good condition.

Although logical, the author finds this procedure futile, as the flimsy ear cartilage almost invariably flattens beneath the snug, discrepant two-dimensional skin cover. Furthermore, when amputated ear cartilage has been "banked" in the retroauricular region, it hampers later reconstructive attempts by producing an irregular, amorphous structure which is adherent to the overlying regional skin.

Replantation of the dermabraded amputated auricle

Mladick *et al.*[144] and Mladick and Carraway[145] have advocated first dermabrading and then reattaching the amputated ear to its stump. The reattached ear is then buried in a subcutaneous postauricular pocket, which allows revascularization through the exposed dermis of the dermabraded auricle *(Fig. 7.34)*. Several weeks later, the ear is exteriorized by blunt dissection from its covering flap, which is allowed to slide behind the helical rim. At this time, the subcutaneous attachments of the medial auricular surface are left intact. The exposed raw auricular surface is dressed, and epithelialization begins within several days.

Rather than separate the medial auricular attachments from their bed several weeks later to allow spontaneous re-epithelialization as Mladick originally suggested, the author feels it is safer to wait several months before separating the ear frame from the head; at that time the new retroauricular sulcus could be skin-grafted as in a classic ear reconstruction.

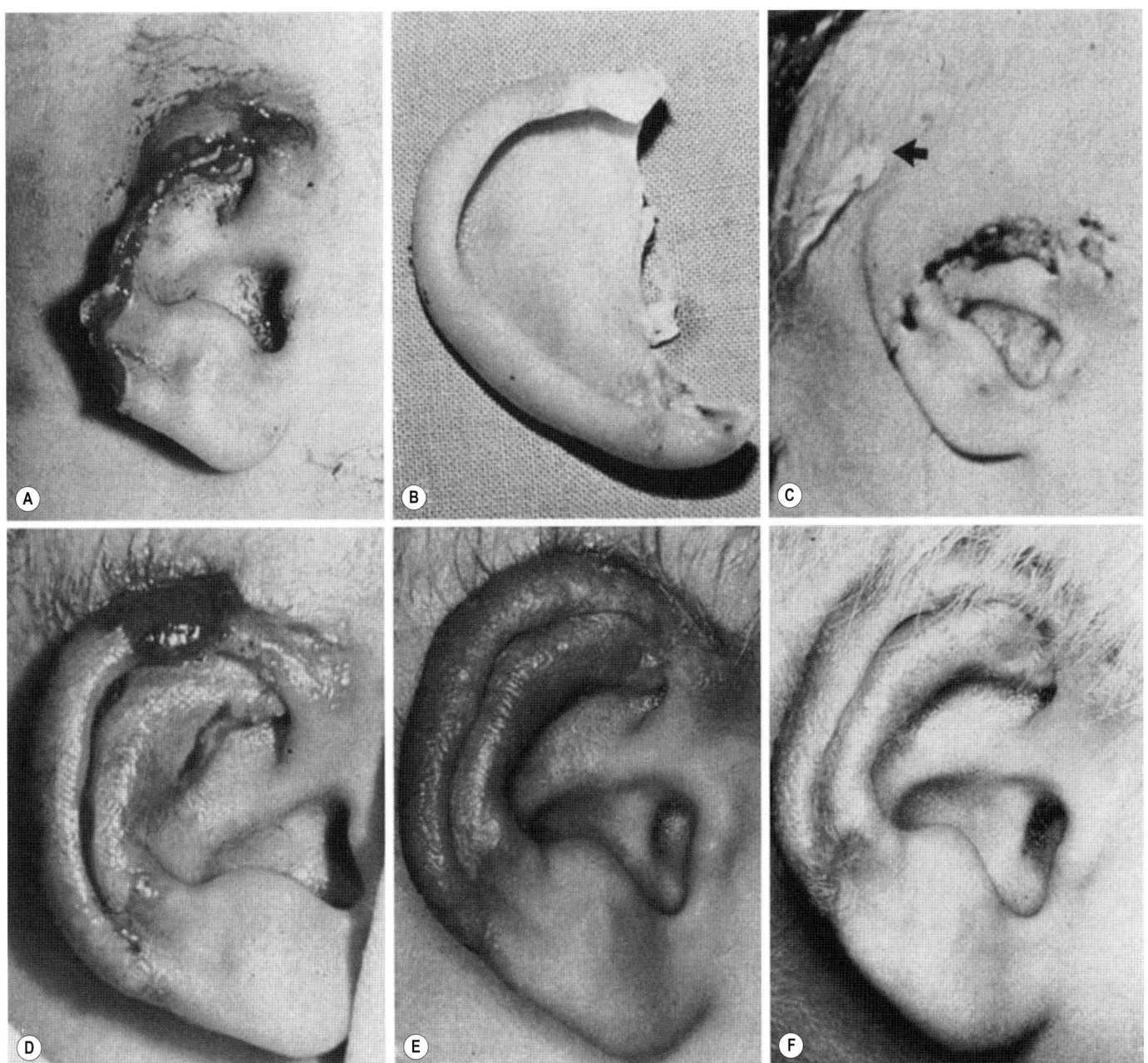

Fig. 7.34 Reattachment of the severed auricle by dermabrasion and subcutaneous "pocketing." **(A)** The amputated stump. **(B)** The severed part. **(C)** The dermabraded reattached part is buried in a postauricular pocket; a traction suture (arrow) from the helix flattens out the auricle to gain better apposition of the tissues. **(D)** The ear has been exteriorized and is almost completely epithelialized (see text for details); one granulating area is seen at the superior margin. **(E)** One month after injury, the ear has a red flush over the reattached segment. **(F)** Appearance at 5 months. (Reproduced from Mladick R, Carraway J. Ear reattachment by the modified pocket principle. *Plast Reconstr Surg.* 1973;51:584.Copyright © 1973, The Williams & Wilkins Company, Baltimore.)

Replantation of the amputated auricle upon removal of postauricular skin and fenestration of cartilage

Almost invariably, the replanting of large composite parts is doomed to fail,[146] unless the vascular recipient area is increased. Instead of employing dermabrasion to achieve this, Baudet *et al.*[147] removed the skin from the postauricular portion of the amputated part, fenestrated the cartilage, and placed the auricular segment into a raw area established by raising a flap of retroauricular mastoid skin *(Fig. 7.35)*. The cartilaginous windows allowed direct contact of the auricular skin with the recipient site, thus facilitating its revascularization. Although some distortion of the superior helical border occurred *(Fig. 7.36)*, the result was satisfactory.

Replanting the ear cartilage and immediately covering it with a fascial flap and skin graft

In selected cases where the wounds are clean, the scalp is intact, and the patient's general condition is stable, one might be tempted to remove the amputated ear's skin and cover the filleted cartilage immediately with a fascial flap and skin graft. Because I have routinely observed poor results in filleted ear cartilages which have been subcutaneously banked, I think that it would be preferable to utilize Baudet's fenestration technique initially, and to reserve the fascia for secondary reconstruction should this effort fail.

Microsurgical ear replantation

Although there have been several successful reports of microsurgically replanted ears,[148,149] this procedure tends to fail due to such small vessels within the amputated ear. Therefore, what initially appears to be a successful replant often fails as venous congestion ensues. However, such cases have been salvaged by applying leeches to the congested replant.[150]

With this in mind, the author feels that the anastomosis should be accomplished end-to-side in the temporal vessels rather than sacrificing them for an end-to-end repair, so as to preserve an axial pattern fascial flap for a future reconstruction should the replant fail.

Deformities without loss of auricular tissue

Irregularities in contour

The most common traumatic auricular deformities without tissue loss result from faulty approximation of full-thickness lacerations which manifest the helical border's distorting and notching.

Meticulously approximating sutures is essential when primarily repairing lacerations or when secondarily repairing maladjusted tissues. Z-plasties, stepping, halving, or dove-tailing cartilage edges and soft-tissue wounds are important measures in preventing recurrence of contour irregularities.

Otohematoma: "cauliflower ear"

Frequently found in pugilists, this deformity results from a direct blow or excessive traction which produces a hemorrhage. Blood collects between the perichondrium and cartilage, producing a fibrotic clot that thickens and obliterates the ear's convolutions. This is similar to the process which produces thickening of the septal cartilage, which is frequent in boxers and wrestlers.

Immediately after hematoma has occurred, the blood clots and serum must be drained. While mere needle aspiration is followed almost invariably by recurrent fluid collection, a small incision will permit evacuation of the hematoma under direct vision. The incision should be long enough to permit retraction, inspection, and the application of a large suction tip for the aspiration of blood clots. Conforming, compressive gauze bolsters are placed on either side of the auricle, and maintained for 7–10 days by horizontal mattress sutures (4-0 nylon) which traverse the bolsters as well as the ear *(Fig. 7.37)*.

Late treatment of the cauliflower-ear deformity consists of carving out the thickened tissue to improve the auricular contour. Exposure is obtained by raising a skin flap through carefully placed incisions. After completing the carving, similar dressings must be applied to assure coaptation of the soft tissues to the cartilaginous framework and to prevent hematoma.

Stenosis of the external auditory canal

The concha is elongated inward by the external auditory canal through an opening, the meatus, through which lacerations may extend and ultimately produce stenosis.

Whenever possible, circular lacerations must be carefully sutured, involving the canal and keeping the canal packed tightly during the healing period. A small prosthetic appliance should be prepared to keep the canal open. This is made by taking an impression with dental compound and creating a perforated mold of acrylic resin. The patient should wear this prosthetic support for 3 or 4 months until the tendency toward stenosis disappears *(Fig. 7.38)*.

Cicatricial stenosis of the external auditory meatus and canal is remedied by Z-plasties of the cicatricial bands.[151] In severe stenosis, when the meatus is closed and the canal is filled with scar tissue, the cicatricial tissue must be excised; the skin defect is repaired by means of the skin graft inlay technique, for which a full-thickness retroauricular graft is uniquely suitable.

To facilitate this grafting, two impressions of the canal are taken with dental compound. One impression serves to apply the graft firmly within the canal until the skin graft has taken; the other impression is duplicated in clear acrylic, and should be worn by the patient for a period of 3 or 4 months to counteract the tendency for secondary contraction of the graft and subsequent stenosis. A detail worth noting is to prepare the mold in such a manner that the mold's distal portion itself fills the concha; this precaution insures prosthesis stability.

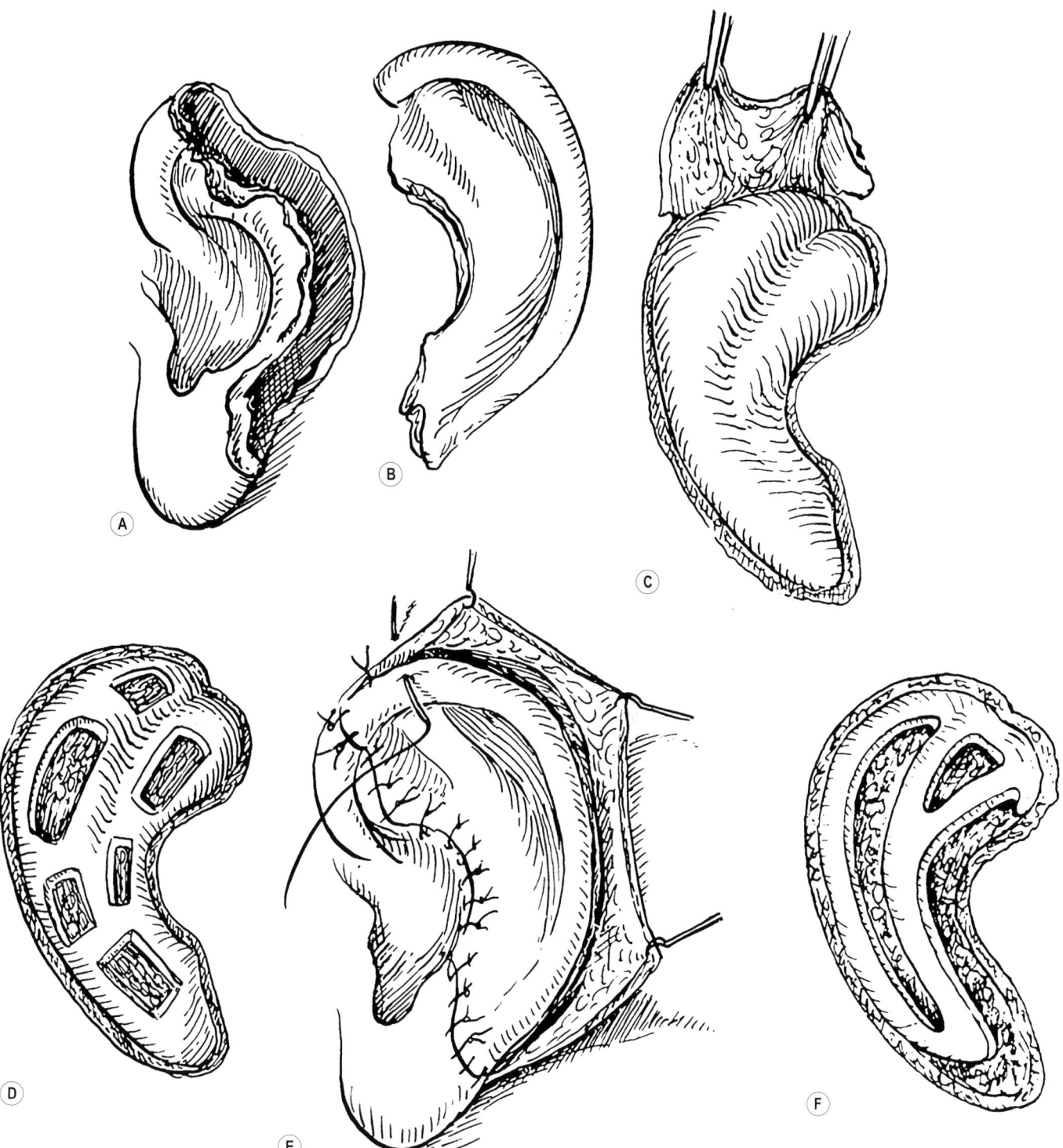

Fig. 7.35 Replantation of the amputated auricle after removal of the posteromedial auricular skin and fenestration of the cartilage. (After Baudet J, Tramond P, Goumain A. A propos d'un procédé original de réimplantation d'un pavillon de l'oreille totalement séparé. Ann Chir Plast 1972;17:67.). **(A and B)** The extent of the amputation. **(C)** Skin removed from the medial aspect of the amputated part. **(D)** Windows cut through the cartilage. **(E)** Reattachment of the amputated part; the denuded portion of the auricle is applied against the raw surface in the auriculomastoid area. **(F)** Technique of fenestration suggested by Brent to prevent the deformity seen in Figure 7.36.

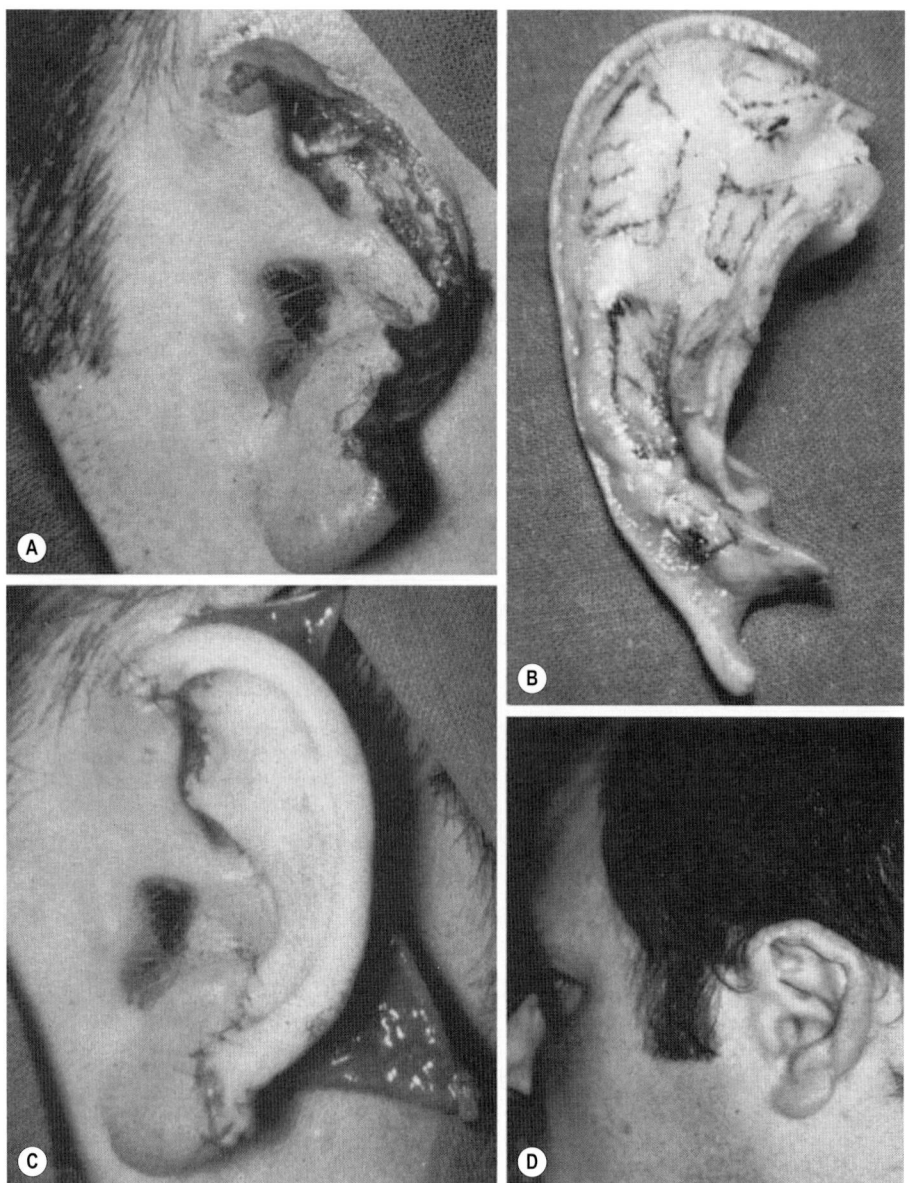

Fig. 7.36 Replantation of the amputated auricle after removal of the posteromedial auricular skin and fenestration of the cartilage. **(A)** Appearance of the stump of the amputated auricle. **(B)** The denuded medial aspect of the cartilage; the outlines of the windows to be cut through the cartilage are indicated. **(C)** The auricle immediately after reattachment. **(D)** Final appearance. (Courtesy of Dr. J. Baudet.)

Deformities with loss of auricular tissue

These deformities may result from loss of skin, cartilage, or full-thickness loss of auricular tissue.

Loss of auricular skin

Auricular trauma which results only in a skin loss is usually secondary to burns. Loss of retroauricular skin results in adhesions between the ear and the mastoid region, whereas skin loss from the anterolateral surface may cause forward folding of the ear. When a burn destroys the skin, the cartilage becomes involved also, the result being a full-thickness defect of the auricle (see vol. IV, Chapter 21 for early treatment of the burned ear). However, partial-thickness burns which are

adequately treated may heal with only varying degrees of contraction and thinning of the helical border.

Full-thickness defects of the auricle

For purposes of classification, full-thickness defects of the ear may be divided into six groups; (1) defects of the upper third; (2) defects of the middle third; (3) defects of the lower third; (4) partial loss; (5) total loss; and (6) loss of the lobule (or lobe) of the ear.

Major auricular loss following trauma

Loss of a major portion of the auricle or the entire ear may result from a razor slash, flying glass, a gunshot wound, flame or radiation burns, and human or dog bites. Complete traumatic loss of the auricle is an unusual occurrence, for a portion

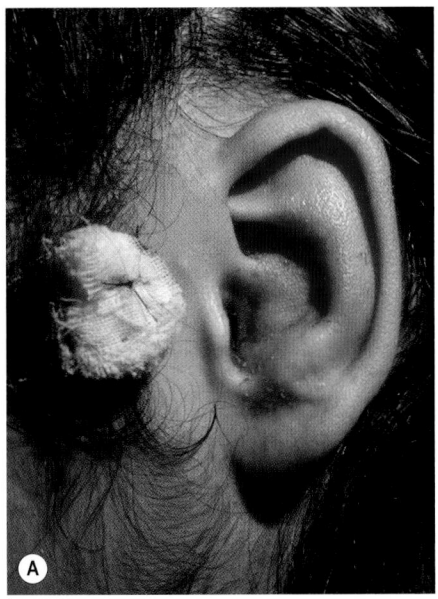 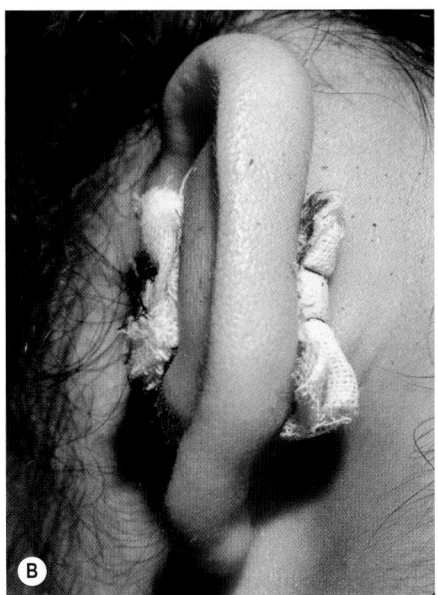 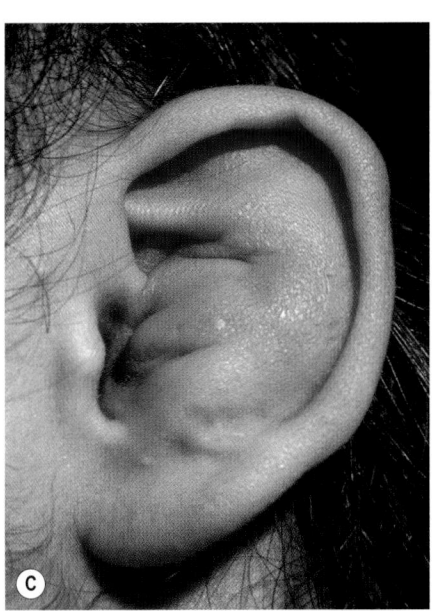

Fig. 7.37 Management of otohematoma. **(A)** Acute otohematoma. **(B)** Compressive dressing with through-and-through sutures. **(C)** Compressive bolsters removed at 10 days.

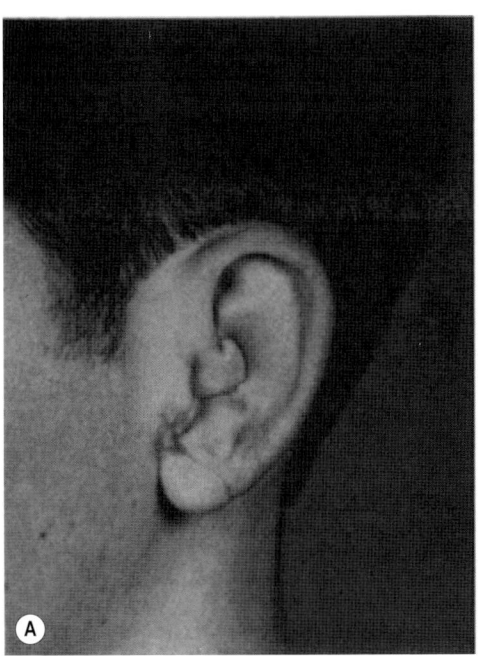 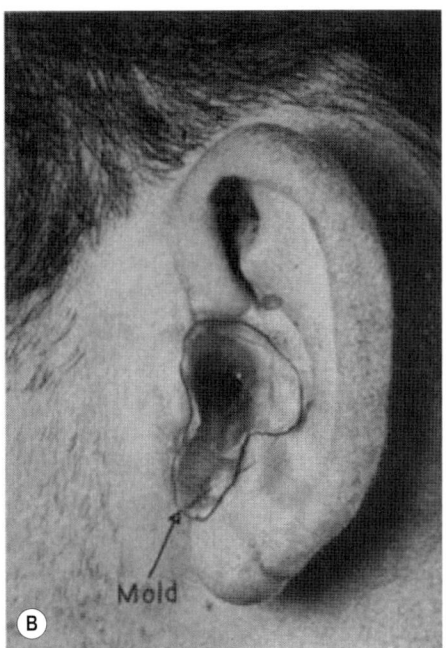 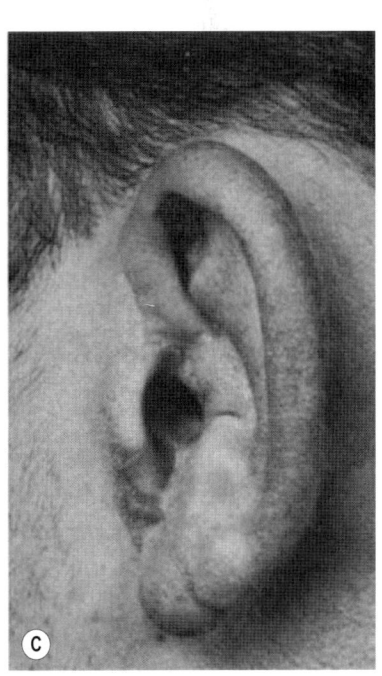

Fig. 7.38 Traumatic stenosis of the external auditory canal. **(A)** Stenosis of the external auditory canal resulting from laceration. **(B)** Acrylic mold worn after skin grafting. **(C)** Result obtained; the canal remains patent. (Reproduced from Converse JM. Reconstruction of the auricle. *Plast Reconstr Surg.* 1958;22:150.Copyright © 1958, Williams & Wilkins Company, Baltimore.)

of the concha and the external auditory canal are usually preserved even in cases of severe injury. When a large portion of the auricle or the entire ear has been destroyed, a number of obstacles must be surmounted in successive stages. These include: (1) a suitable skin covering devoid of hair follicles; (2) a framework of cartilage to maintain the upright position of the reconstructed auricle and to represent its characteristic convolutions; and (3) a covering of skin for the posteromedial aspect of the auricular framework after it is raised from the

mastoid area *(Fig. 7.39)*. Additional "retouching" procedures may be necessary to achieve a satisfactory repair of the reconstructed auricle.

The skin covering

The presence of supple and well-vascularized skin is a condition *sine qua non* for success in auricular reconstruction. The

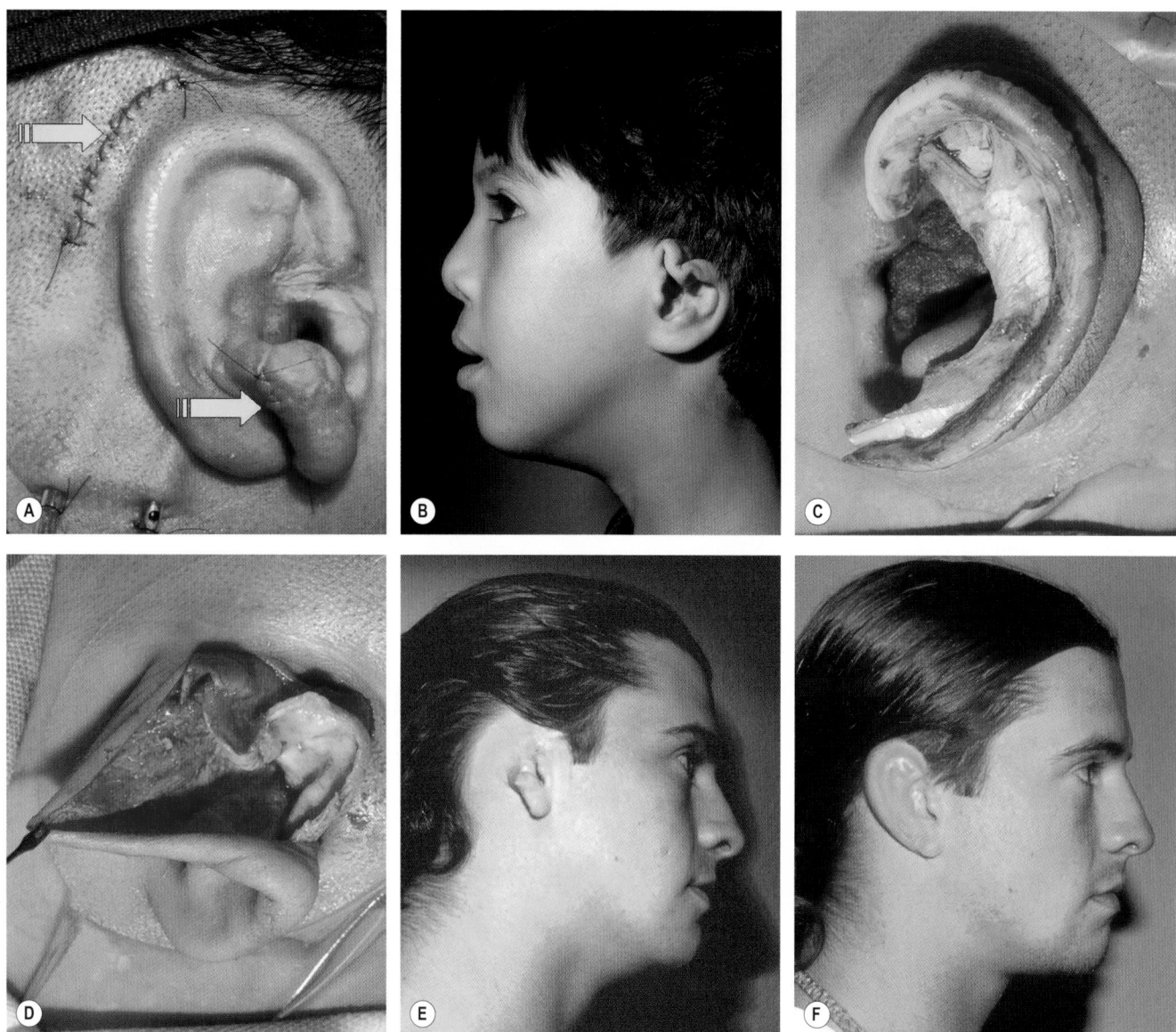

Fig. 7.39 Total ear reconstruction of acquired deformities with autogenous rib cartilage grafts. **(A)** Traumatic ear loss and its repair. Note incision sites (arrows) for developing cutaneous "pocket." **(B)** Crumpled ear secondary to infection that followed radical mastoidectomy. **(C, D)** Degloving of crumpled auricular cartilage and the sculpted rib cartilage framework to replace it. **(E, F)** Dog-bite ear avulsion and its repair.

quality of the residual local soft tissues varies in traumatic defects. When amputation of the auricle is by means of a clean-cut laceration, the local residual skin remains relatively unscarred, and thus may be utilized. Likewise, minimally scarred skin following healed partial-thickness burns may be of sufficiently good quality to avoid skin grafting. To the contrary, if the auricle has been avulsed, destroyed by a burn, or injured by a gunshot, the area may show multiple linear or surface scars, thus necessitating excision and replacement with a skin graft before the auricular reconstruction begins. Should this be necessary, a full-thickness graft from the contralateral retroauricular region is ideal for this purpose, although of course other donor areas can be considered. It is essential that the skin overlying a cartilage graft has an adequate blood supply, and is sufficiently loose to permit insertion of a good, three-dimensional framework. Therefore, the skin graft must be allowed to mature for a number of months before cartilage replacement.

At times, the local skin will be irreparably scarred or grafts will mature inadequately to permit framework placement without supplementing the soft-tissue cover. In these cases, a fascial flap must be employed.[89]

First, all heavy scars and unusable tissues are excised while taking great care to preserve the temporal vessels, which may be entangled in the traumatically scarred tissues. Then, rib cartilage is harvested and a framework is sculpted as for correcting a virgin microtia (*Figs 7.8–7.10*). Finally, the fascial flap is raised.

To realize how large a fascial flap is needed for adequate coverage, first assess the periauricular skin. At times, the scar excision will be so extensive that total fascial flap coverage of the framework is necessary. However, at other times the framework's lower portion can be "pocketed" beneath available skin, and therefore, only a variable portion of the upper framework will need fascial flap coverage.

In utilizing this fascial flap, one must be familiar with the course of the superficial temporal vessels. The artery remains beneath the subcutaneous tissue and within the temporoparietal fascia until a point approximately 12 cm above the anterosuperior auriculocephalic attachment. Here the artery emerges superficially and interlinks with the subdermal vascular plexus.[152] Consequently, this is the limit of fascial vascular domain, since continued distal dissection would interrupt the fascial circulation.

After first mapping the vessels with a Doppler, exposure to the fascia is gained via an incision that extends superiorly above the proposed auricular region. The dissection begins just deep to the hair follicles, and continues down to a plane where subcutaneous fat adheres to the temporoparietal fascia. As initial identification of this plane can be difficult, care must be taken to damage neither the follicles nor the underlying axial vessels. Although tedious, once the scalp dissection is accomplished, the inferiorly based temporoparietal fascial flap is raised easily from the underlying deep fascia which envelops the temporalis musculature.

Subsequently, the fascial flap is first draped over the framework (*Fig. 7.5*), and then coapted to it by means of suction via a small infusion catheter. Then the flap is affixed to the peripheral skin "vest-under-pants" fashion, so as to secure a tight closure. Finally, a patterned thick split skin graft is sutured on top of the fascia-covered framework. Then the new ear's convolutions are packed with Vaseline gauze; lastly, a head dressing is applied (*Fig. 7.31*).

Auricular prostheses

The auricular prosthesis should be reserved for instances in which surgical reconstruction is impractical or contraindicated.

For the most part, an auricular prosthesis has no practical value for children, and is worthwhile for older persons who have undergone ablative cancer surgery or who have extensive burns. Even so, many adults find them undesirable after a short trial experience, as there is always a constant fear of the prosthesis' becoming dislodged at embarrassing moments, and the psychological discomfort of wearing an "artificial part." The innovation of osseointegrated percutaneous implants have offered a solution to the retention of ear prostheses.[153]

Additional problems which arise from local skin irritation from the adhesive glue frequently necessitate discontinuance of the prosthesis for a period of time which, in turn, causes the patient further embarrassment. Furthermore, obvious color contrast calls attention to the prosthetic ear in climatic changes where the prosthetic part remains a constant color while the surrounding skin varies as the patient passes from indoor to outdoor environmental surroundings.

When an auricular prosthesis has been elected for the younger patient, a trial period should ensue, with the realization that surgical reconstruction may be desired later. It is wise to avoid preliminary excision of the microtic lobule or other remnants merely to "gain an improved surface for adherences of the prosthesis," as has been advocated. Should the patient desire surgical reconstruction later, which has often been my experience, then the missing lobule, shortage of skin, and existing scar become a significant handicap.

Partial auricular loss

Most auricular deformities encountered in everyday practice are acquired partial defects. They present the surgeon with an unlimited variety of unique problems whose reconstructions are influenced by the etiology, location, and nature of each residual deformity.

Utilization of residual tissues

In managing acute auricular trauma, initial meticulous reapproximation of tissues and appropriate wound care will greatly facilitate the reconstructive task ahead. Likewise the innovative utilization of residual local tissues in a posttraumatic deformity will greatly simplify the reconstruction and contribute to a pleasing outcome.

Structural support

Contralateral conchal cartilage

A variety of tissues are available to provide the structural support required for an auricular reconstruction. Although the quantity of cartilage needed to fabricate a total ear framework necessitates the use of costal cartilage, often one is not compelled to employ this tissue in a small, partial auricular reconstruction. Because it is possible to utilize an auricular cartilage graft, which is obtained most frequently from the contralateral concha, the correction of small partial losses is less extensive than the procedure to correct total auricular losses.

Auricular cartilage, used as an orthotopic graft in ear reconstruction, is superior to costal cartilage in that it provides a delicate, flexible, thin support.

The conchal cartilage graft can be obtained by a posteromedial incision, as described by Adams[2] and Gorney *et al.*,[34] or through an anterolateral approach, which the author uses more frequently. The latter, performed through an incision several millimeters inside the posterior conchal wall–inferior crus contour line, is a simple method of obtaining a precise graft with direct visual exposure.[155]

Ipsilateral conchal cartilage

In certain partial reconstructions, it is more advantageous to employ an ipsilateral rather than contralateral conchal cartilage graft. However, it is imperative that an intact antihelical strut be present to permit removal of an ipsilateral conchal cartilage graft without subsequent collapse and further deformity of the ear.

An ipsilateral conchal cartilage graft is particularly advantageous when a retroauricular flap is being raised to repair a major defect in the helical rim. Elevation of the flap provides the required conchal cartilage exposure without the need for an additional incision, and removal of this cartilage graft

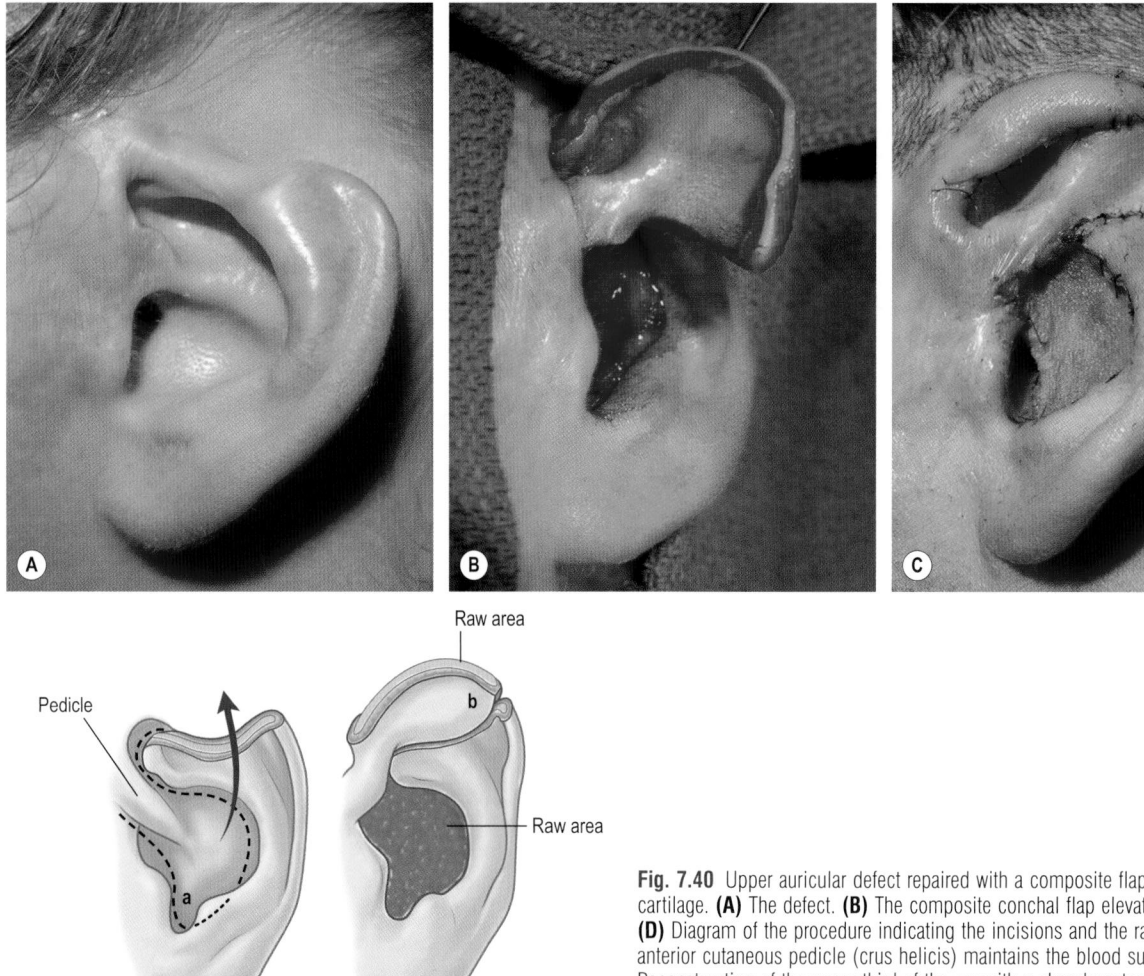

Fig. 7.40 Upper auricular defect repaired with a composite flap of conchal skin and cartilage. **(A)** The defect. **(B)** The composite conchal flap elevated. **(C)** The final appearance. **(D)** Diagram of the procedure indicating the incisions and the raw surfaces to be grafted. The anterior cutaneous pedicle (crus helicis) maintains the blood supply. (Modified from Davis J. Reconstruction of the upper third of the ear with a chondrocutaneous composite flap based on the crus helix. In: Tanzer RC, Edgerton MT, eds. *Symposium on reconstruction of the auricle*. St. Louis: CV Mosby; 1974:247.)

subsequently lowers the ear closer to the mastoid region. In effect, this produces a relative gain in length, thus enabling the flap to cover the cartilage graft once it is spliced on to the rim and eliminating the need for a skin graft in the flap's donor bed.

Furthermore, the ipsilateral concha may be used occasionally as a composite flap of skin and cartilage *(Fig. 7.40)*. This innovative technique, proposed by Davis,[33] is applicable to defects of the auricle's upper third, and again should be employed only when the antihelical support remains intact.

Composite grafts

Small to moderate-sized defects may be repaired with composite grafts from the unaffected ear, particularly if the latter is large and protruding.[154,156–158] A wedge-shaped composite graft of less than 1.5 cm in width is resected from the scapha and helix of the unaffected ear and transplanted to a clean-cut defect on the contralateral ear *(Fig. 7.41)*. The success rate of composite grafts can be enhanced by removing a portion of the skin and cartilage, thus converting part of the "wedge" to a full-thickness skin graft, which is readily vascularized by a recipient advancement flap mobilized from the loose

retroauricular skin.[159] A strut of the helical cartilage is preserved within the graft for contour and support *(Fig. 7.41)*. 🌐
FIG **7.41** APPEARS ONLINE ONLY

Despite a slight inclination toward shrinkage after transplantation, the composite graft offers a simple and expeditious reconstructive technique for partial auricular defects.

Specific regional defects

Helical rim

Acquired losses of the helical rim may vary from small defects to major portions of the helix. The former usually result from tumor excisions or from minor traumatic injuries, and are best closed by advancing the helix in both directions, as described by Antia and Buch.[160] The success of this excellent technique depends first upon totally freeing the entire helix from the scapha via an incision in the helical sulcus which extends through the cartilage but not through the skin on the ear's back surface. Secondly, the posteromedial auricular skin is undermined, dissecting just superficially to the

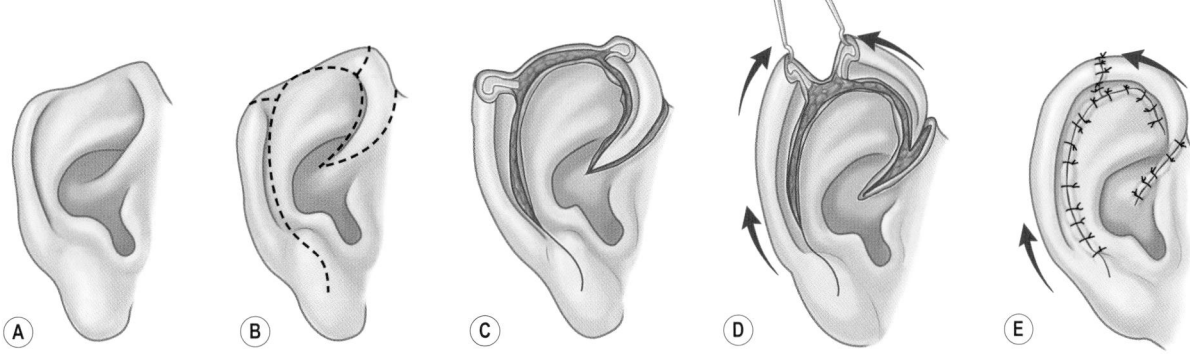

Fig. 7.42 Helical defect repaired by advancement of auricular skin cartilage. **(A)** Defect of the upper portion of the auricle. **(B)** Lines of incisions through skin and cartilage. **(C)** The incisions completed: note the downward extension into the earlobe. **(D)** The skin–cartilage flaps mobilized. **(E)** The repair completed. (Modified from Antia NH, Buch VI. Chondrocutaneous advancement of flap for the marginal defect of the ear. *Plast Reconstr Surg*. 1967;39:472.Copyright © 1967, The Williams & Wilkins Company, Baltimore.)

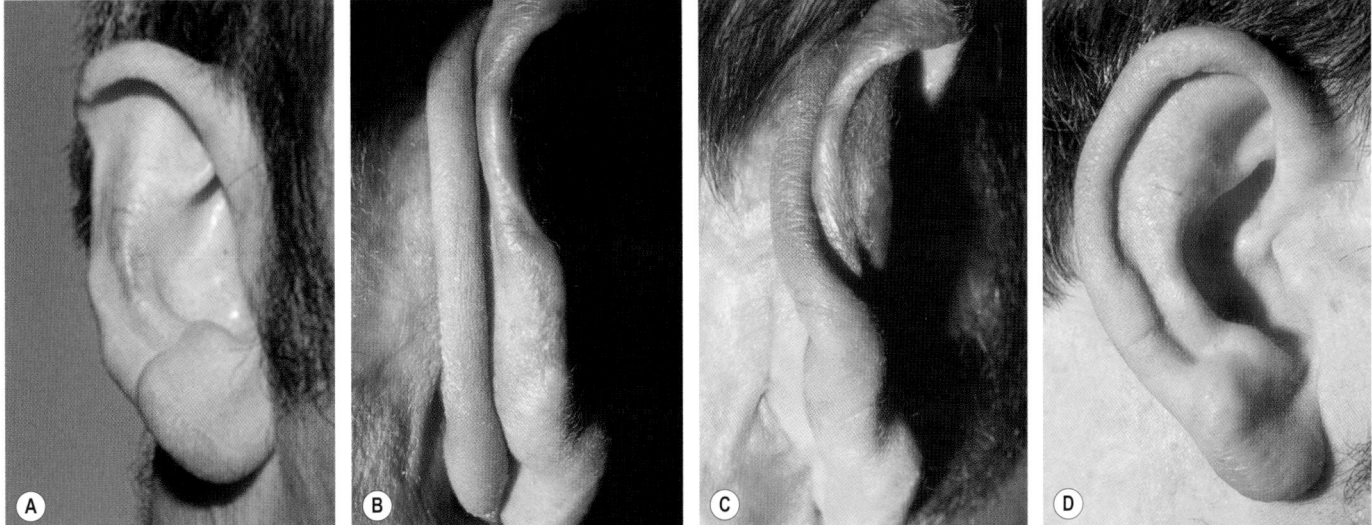

Fig. 7.44 Helical restoration with a fine-caliber tube flap. **(A)** Burn loss of helix. **(B)** Fine-caliber tube created with retroauricular skin. **(C)** Inferior portion of tube transferred to ear. **(D)** Inset of tube and completion of repair. (Reproduced from Brent B. The acquired auricular deformity: a systematic approach to its analysis and reconstruction. *Plast Reconstr Surg*. 1977;59:475.)

perichondrium until the entire helix is hanging as a chondrocutaneous component of the loosely mobilized skin *(Fig. 7.42C, D*. Extra length can be gained by a V-Y advancement of the crus helix, and surprisingly large defects can be closed without tension.

Although originally described for upper-third auricular defects[160] *(Fig. 7.43)*, the author has found that this technique is even more effective for middle-third defects. Reconstruction of larger helical defects requires a more sophisticated procedure which recreates the absent rim using an auricular cartilage graft covered by an adjacent flap, as previously described in the text. Although advancement flaps of local soft tissues have also been employed to provide helical contour, the author finds that these flaps often suffer a disappointing long-term result unless a strut of cartilage has been incorporated into the repair. ⊛ FIG **7.43** APPEARS ONLINE ONLY

Another sophisticated method of helical reconstruction is the use of thin-calibered tubes which can successfully create

a fine, realistic helical rim when meticulous technique is utilized in conjunction with careful case selection *(Fig. 7.44)*. Minor burns often destroy the helical rim yet leave the auriculocephalic sulcus skin intact, thus providing a superb site for tube construction,[161] and minimizing tube migration, risk of failure, and secondary deformity.

Upper-third auricular defects

Upper-third defects may be reconstructed by a number of methods. Usually, minor losses are confined to the rim and are repaired either by helical advancement, as previously described,[69] or by a readily accessible preauricular flap.

Intermediate losses of the upper third are repaired with a banner flap, as described by Crikelair,[162] which is based anterosuperiorly in the auriculocephalic sulcus. This flap should be used in conjunction with a small cartilage graft to assure a good long-term result.

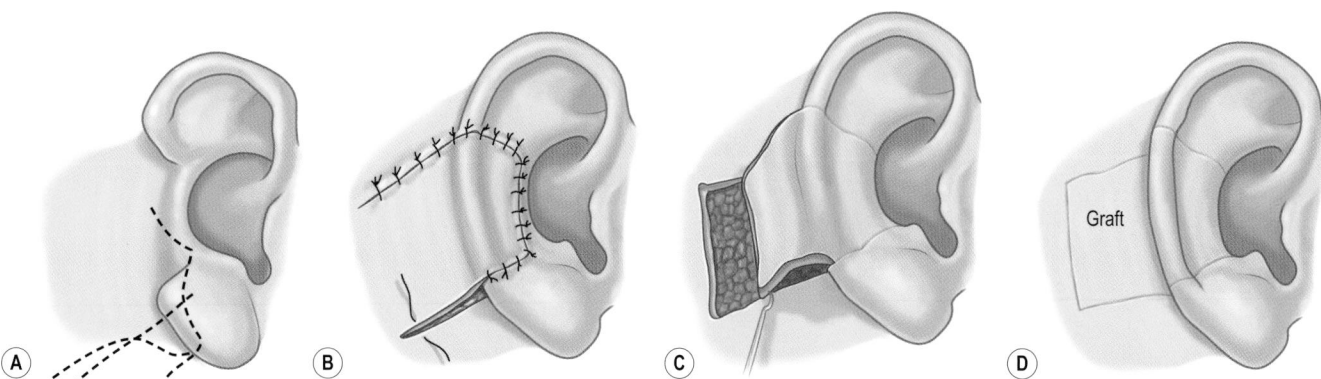

Fig. 7.45 Dieffenbach's technique for reconstruction of the middle third of the auricle, drawn from his description (1829–1834). **(A)** The defect and outline of the flap. **(B)** The flap advanced over the defect. **(C, D)** In a second stage, the base of the flap is divided and the flap is folded around the posteromedial aspect of the auricle. A skin graft covers the scalp donor site.

Major losses in the superior third can at times be successfully reconstructed with a contralateral conchal cartilage graft, as classically described by Adams.[154] In utilizing this technique, it is imperative that the cartilage graft be anchored to the cartilaginous remnant of the helical root by means of a suture placed through a small incision at that point. This prevents the cartilage graft from "drifting" and assures helical continuity.

Should the existing skin be unfavorable for the above technique, the entire concha may be rotated upward as a chondrocutaneous composite flap on a small anterior pedicle of the crus helix.[33] Technically, this is a demanding procedure, and is restricted to individual instances in which a large concha exists. Often, the best choice for support will be a nicely carved graft from the patient's rib cartilage.

Middle-third auricular defects

Major middle-third auricular defects are usually repaired with a cartilage graft which is either covered by an adjacent skin flap *(Fig. 7.45)*, or inserted via Converse's tunnel procedure[163] *(Fig. 7.46)*. Occasionally, conditions may favor a specially prepared composite graft, as described previously.

The tunnel procedure[163] is an effective technique for moderate-sized defects of the auricle *(Fig. 7.47)*, and in major defects it has the advantage of preserving the retroauricular sulcus. In employing this technique, the auricle is pressed against the mastoid area and an ink line drawn on the skin in this area, keeping the line parallel and adjacent to the edge of the auricular defect *(Fig. 7.48C)*. Incisions are made through the skin along the ink line, and also through the edge of the auricular defect *(Fig. 7.48D)*. The medial edge of the auricular incision is sutured to the anterior edge of the mastoid skin incision *(Fig. 7.48E, F)*. A cartilage graft is then placed in the soft-tissue bed and is joined to the edges of the auricular cartilage defect *(Fig. 7.48H)*. The mastoid skin, which has been undermined, is advanced to cover the cartilage graft, and the edge of this skin flap is sutured to the lateral edge of the auricular skin *(Fig. 7.48I)*. A healing and vascularization period of 3 or 4 months is permitted; during this period the cutaneous tunnel behind the auricle must be cleansed with cotton-tipped applicators. The auricle is detached in a second stage, and the resulting elliptical raw areas on the ear and mastoid region are grafted *(Figs 7.48J* and *7.49)*. ⊛ FIGS 7.47, 7.48, **7.49** APPEAR ONLINE ONLY

Middle-third auricular tumors are excised and closed either by wedge resection with accessory triangles, or by helical advancement, as previously described.

Lower-third auricular defects

Lower-third losses which encompass more than earlobe tissue are an especially complex challenge, and must include a cartilage graft to provide the support necessary to assure long-term contour.

Although Preaux[164] has described an impressive technique for repairing lower-third defects by means of a superiorly based flap doubled upon itself, the author finds that contour and support are created and maintained with less risk by primarily inserting a cartilage graft subcutaneously in the proposed site of reconstruction *(Fig. 7.50)*.

Acquired earlobe deformities

Traumatic clefts and keloids which result from ear piercing are the most common acquired defects of the earlobe. Cleft earlobes, usually occurring from the dramatic extraction of earrings, can be repaired by Pardue's ingenious adjacent flap which is rolled into the apex of the wedge repair, thus maintaining a tract lined with skin which permits further use of earrings[165] *(Fig. 7.49)*.

Another common occurrence in everyday practice is the earlobe keloid, which heretofore has been treated with varying degrees of success, with irradiation and steroid injections.[166,167] Because there is strong evidence that pressure plays an important role in keloid therapy,[168,169] a light pressure-spring earring device may be worth a trial in reducing postexcisional recurrence of earlobe keloids[170] *(Fig. 7.51)*. (The general management of keloid lesions and hypertrophic scars is discussed in vol. I, Chapter 16).

Construction of an earlobe is rarely required in congenital microtia, as the lobe is formed by the repositioning of auricular remnants. However, a portion or the entire lobe may be

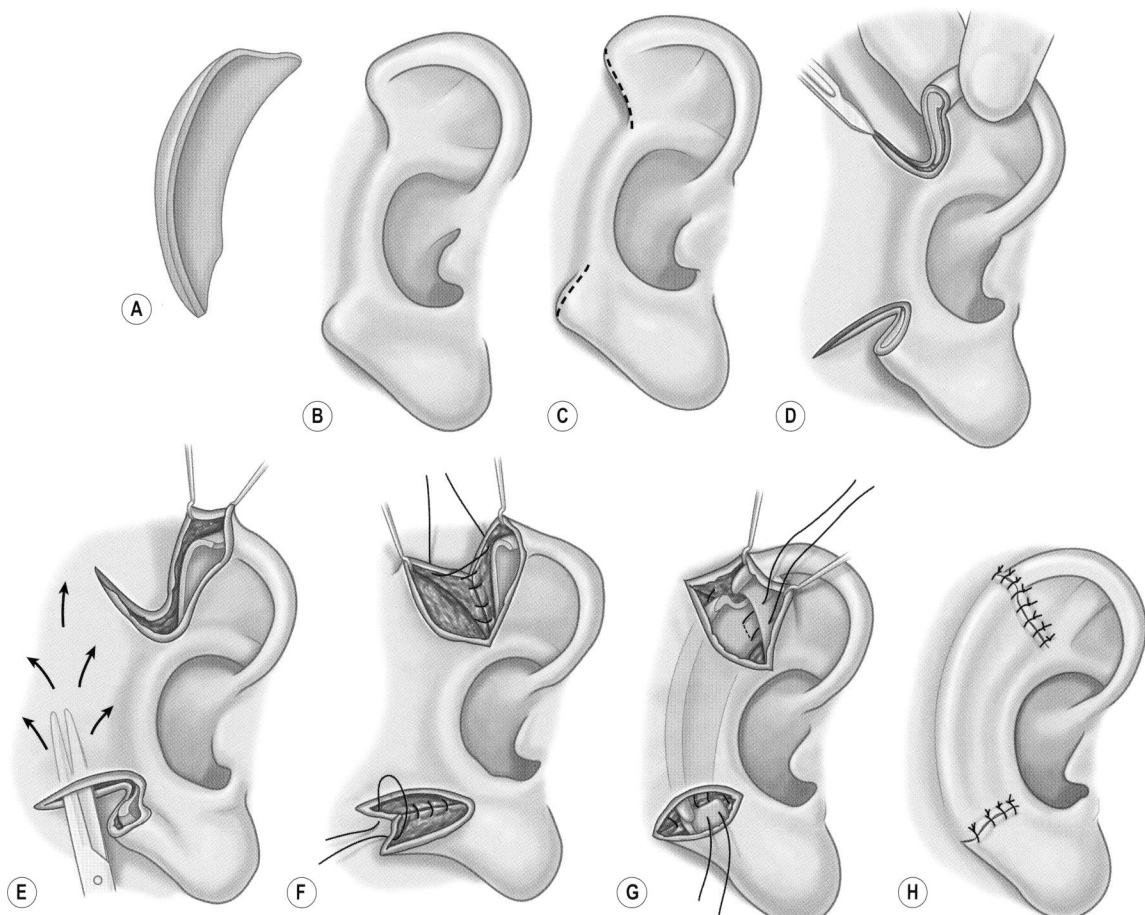

Fig. 7.46 Repair of a defect of the middle third of the auricle: the tunnel procedure. **(A)** Carved costal cartilage graft. **(B)** The defect. **(C)** Incisions through the margins of the defect. **(D)** Incisions through the edge of the defect are extended backward through the skin of the mastoid area. **(E)** The skin of the mastoid area is undermined between the two incisions. **(F)** The medial edge of the incision at the border of the auricular defect is sutured to the edge of the postauricular incision. A similar type of suture is placed at the lower edge of the defect. **(G)** The cartilage graft is placed under the skin of the mastoid area and anchored to the auricular cartilage with sutures. **(H)** Suture of the skin incision. (Reproduced from Converse JM. Reconstruction of the auricle. *Plast Reconstr Surg.* 1958;22:150, 230.Copyright © 1958, The Williams & Wilkins Company, Baltimore.)

missing in traumatic deformities of the ear, and a variety of techniques for its reconstruction have been proposed.

As early as 1907, effective techniques were introduced to repair earlobes with local flap tissues.[171] Since then, numerous methods have been developed[164,172–174] *(Figs 7.52–7.56).* ⊛ FIGS **7.52, 7.53, 7.54, 7.55, 7.56** APPEAR ONLINE ONLY

Tumors of the auricle

Benign tumors

Sebaceous cysts of the auricle are often treated improperly or neglected. Most often, they are found on the medial aspect of the ear, particularly in the lobe, and should be excised *in toto* during the quiescent period through the medial surface of the lobule to minimize deformity.

The most common auricular lesion is actinic keratosis, which occurs, as do carcinomas, in outdoor workers with fair complexions. Other benign auricular lesions, such as granuloma pyogenicum, beryllium granuloma, verruca contagiosa, verruca senilis, cylindroma, nevus, papilloma, lipoma, lymphangioma, leiomyoma, and chondroma, should be surgically excised.

Malignant tumors

Over 5% of skin cancers involve the auricle.[175] The vast majority of these are cutaneous, usually basal cell or squamous cell carcinomas. A lesser percentage are malignant melanoma.

When first seen, the cartilage is involved by direct extension in about one-third of the cutaneous carcinomas of the auricle. For this reason, and because cartilage is an excellent barrier to the tumor's spreading, many surgeons feel that the cartilage must be included in their surgical excision.[176]

The cervical lymph nodes are rarely involved in basal cell carcinoma of the auricle, but are involved in approximately one-third of all squamous cell carcinomas and malignant melanomas.

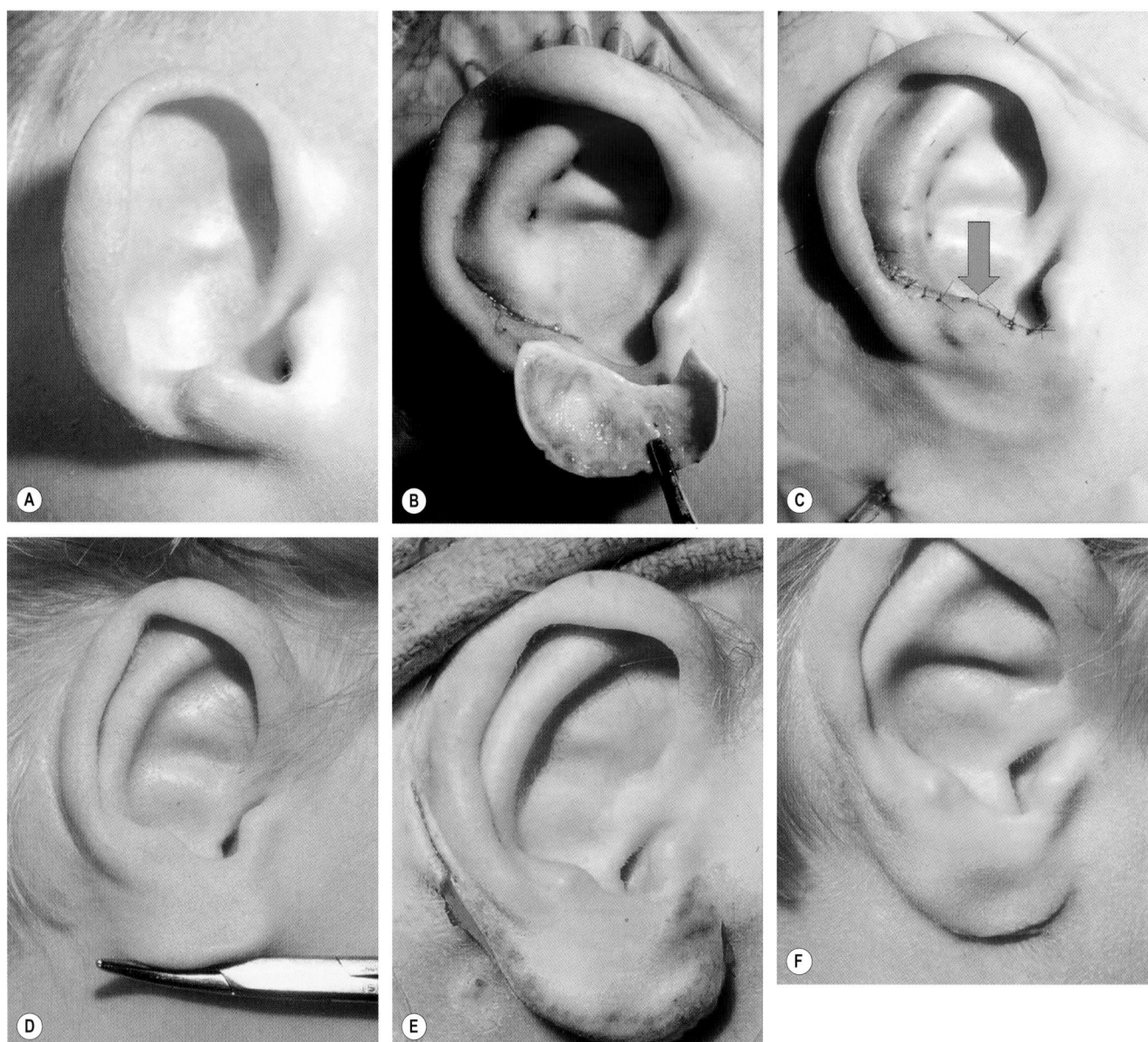

Fig. 7.50 Earlobe reconstruction with a conchal cartilage graft. **(A)** Congenital earlobe absence. **(B)** Conchal cartilage graft harvested from opposite ear. **(C)** Insertion of cartilage graft. Note access incision (arrow), and that an antihelical fold has been created with Mustardé sutures. The new "earlobe" outline can be seen beneath the skin and a suction drain is present. **(D)** Healed appearance; hemostat lifts tip of cartilage graft. **(E)** New earlobe has been surgically separated from head and awaits a skin graft. **(F)** Final result. (Reproduced from Brent B. *The artistry of reconstructive surgery*. St. Louis: C.V. Mosby, 1987.)

The majority of these malignant lesions are located on the helical rim, and can be eradicated with a wedge excision, or a helical advancement, as previously described. Many of the tumors located on the lateral and medial auricular surfaces can be treated adequately by excision and subsequent skin grafting, or by local flap coverage. Others require definitive reconstructive procedures previously detailed in this chapter. Radiation therapy is of no value in managing recurrences and metastases, and is poorly tolerated by the auricle.

When the cancer is large and includes cartilaginous invasion, the ear must be totally excised with surrounding soft tissue. Radical resection of the cervical lymph nodes in continuity with resection of the involved auricle should be performed. In patients with lymph node metastases, the ear and all cervical lymph nodes must be resected. Melanomas require early radical intervention. At times, the only hope of effecting a cure in auricular cancer includes resection of the temporal bone.[177–179]

Patients requiring total auricular ablation are usually older and generally are not candidates for total auricular reconstruction. Often, a prosthesis is preferred, but if total ear reconstruction is indicated, it is advisable that reconstruction is postponed until the threat of recurrence is well past.

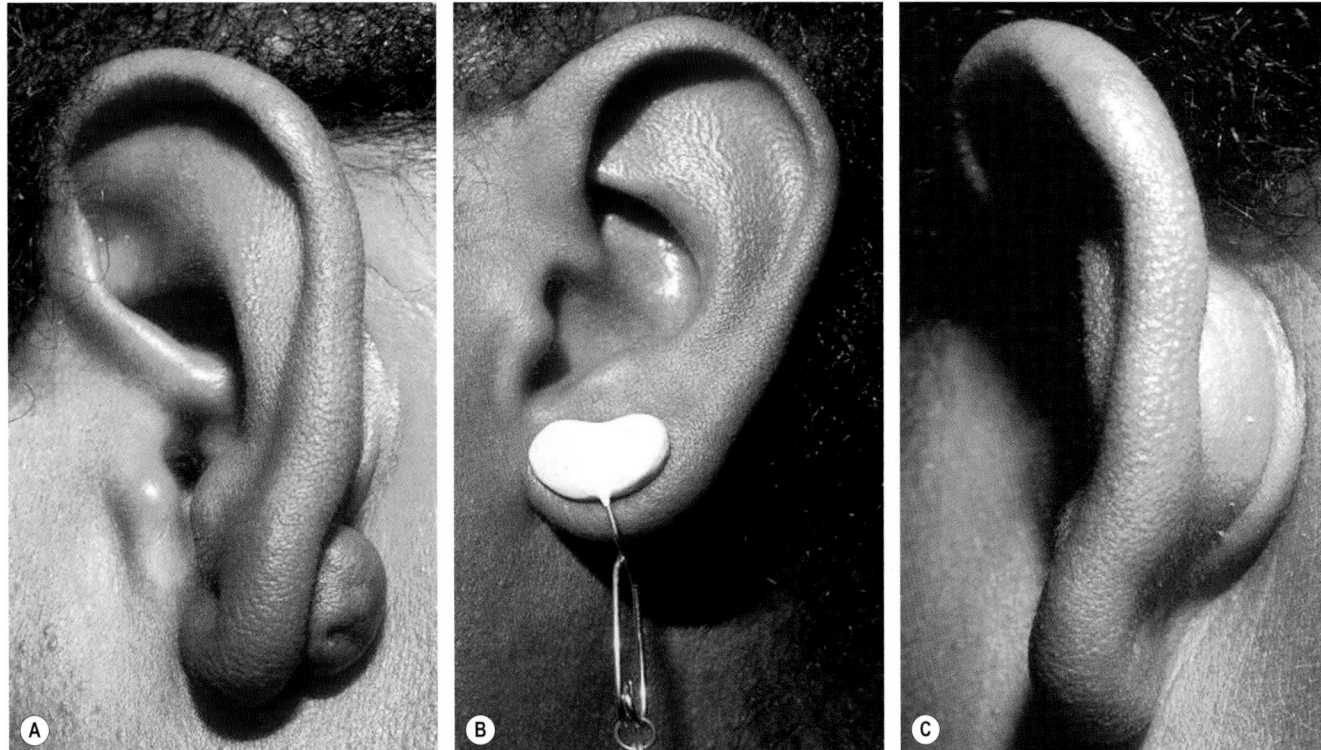

Fig. 7.51 Prevention of earlobe keloid recurrence with pressure therapy. **(A)** Earlobe keloid, resulting from piercing. **(B)** Use of spring-pressure earring after healing of surgical excision. **(C)** Successful suppression of keloid recurrence, 1 year postoperatively. (Reproduced from Brent B. The role of pressure therapy in management of earlobe keloids. *Ann Plast Surg.* 1978;1:579.)

Bonus images for this chapter can be found online at **http://www.expertconsult.com**

Fig. 7.2 Development of the auricle in a 5-week human embryo: 1–6, elevations (hillocks) on the mandibular and hyoid arches; ov, otic vesicle; af, auricular fold. (Modified from Arey LB. *Developmental anatomy*. 7th ed. Philadelphia: WB Saunders; 1974.)

Fig. 7.3 Identical mirror-image twin 6-year old boys with microtia and author's repair with sculpted autogenous rib cartilage grafts. (Reproduced from Brent B. Repair of microtia with sculpted rib cartilage grafts in identical, mirror-image twins: a case study. *Ann Plast Surg.* 2011;66:62–64.)

Fig. 7.4 (E) Lop ear.

Fig. 7.5 Ear reconstruction with autogenous rib cartilage surfaced by a skin graft-covered temporoparietal fascial flap. **(A)** A patient with a scarred auricular region. Doppler vessels, the flap extent, and the Y-shaped incision are indicated. **(B)** Scar excision, framework fabrication, and scalp dissection are begun. **(C)** Raising a fascial flap that contains the superficial temporal vessels. **(D)** Fascial flap draped over the ear framework. **(E)** Scalp wound sutured. **(F)** Skin graft applied over the fascia-covered ear framework. (Reproduced from Brent B, Byrd HS. Secondary ear reconstruction with cartilage grafts covered by axial, random, and free flaps of temporoparietal fascia. *Plast Reconstr Surg.* 1983;72:141.)

Fig. 7.6 Secondary ear reconstruction with a rib cartilage graft surfaced with a superficial temporoparietal fascial flap and skin graft. **(A)** A patient with a scarred auricular region after multiple failed procedures. **(B)** Result achieved in one surgical stage with rib cartilage graft and fascial flap by the techniques outlined in Figure 7.5.

Fig. 7.8 (G) Preoperative view of the patient. **(H)** Healed postoperative appearance.

Fig. 7.11 Framework modifications in the adult patient. When a solid, fused cartilage block is encountered, the framework is sculpted in one piece. **(A)** A 60-year-old man with traumatic total ear loss. **(B)** Cartilage block marked for carving. **(C)** Completed framework sculpted from the block. **(D, E)** Result achieved with a one-piece sculpture from a fused cartilage block, 1 year postoperatively. Simulation of the absent earlobe was achieved by sculpting its likeness in the framework's inferior pole. (Reproduced fom Brent B. Technical advances in ear reconstruction with autogenous rib cartilage grafts: personal experience with 1200 cases. *Plast Reconstr Surg.* 1999;104:319.)

Fig. 7.17 (A–D) Stage 3, separating the surgically constructed ear from the head with skin graft. An incision is made several millimeters peripheral to the surgically constructed ear, and the auricle is sharply elevated from its fascial bed. The scalp is advanced to the newly created sulcus both to decrease graft requirements and to hide the graft by limiting its placement mostly to the ear's undersurface. Long silk sutures are tied over a bolus dressing.

Fig. 7.19 Augmenting ear projection with split cartilage graft and retroauricular turnover fascial flap. **(A)** Broad cartilage wedge harvested by splitting rib cartilage. Chest wall integrity is maintained by preserving inner cartilage lamella; the harvested outer lamella predictably warps to shape the posterior conchal wall wedge favorably. **(B)** Splitting the rib cartilage *in situ*. **(C)** Outer cartilage lamella predictably begins to warp. **(D)** The harvested wedge. Note preserved inner cartilage lamella of the chest wall. **(E)** The curved cartilage graft is banked subcutaneously until needed for projecting the surgically constructed ear. Center, Scheme of separating the surgically constructed ear from the head **(F)**, placing the projection-maintaining cartilage wedge and **(G, H)** covering it with turnover flap of retroauricular fascia, then applying split-skin graft **(I)**. Projection of elevated ear augmented with the banked split-cartilage graft. Note how the purposeful warp has remained and produced an ideal shape for the new posterior conchal wall. This particular graft had been subcutaneously banked beneath the original chest incision. The fascial flap turned over the cartilage wedge, before skin graft is applied. The healed repair: note maintenance of projection and auriculocephalic sulcus. (Reproduced from Brent B. Technical advances in ear reconstruction with autogenous rib cartilage grafts: personal experience with 1200 cases. *Plast Reconstr Surg.* 1999;104:319.)

Fig. 7.21 Team approach to bilateral microtia. Above, left, Initial auricular repair, after framework placement and lobule transposition. Above, left center, Team approach to middle ear. The plastic surgeon lifts constructed auricle from bed, taking care to preserve connective tissue on cartilage framework; next, the otologic surgeon drills bony canal and completes middle-ear repair. Above, right center, The plastic surgeon then raises a conchal skin flap and removes intervening soft tissues to exteriorize canal. Above, right, With use of the flap to circumvent atresia by breaking up contractual forces, it is dropped into the introitus of the canal, which is skin-grafted to complete the repair. Alternatively, the skin flap could have been based anteriorly and doubled on itself for a Kirkham tragal construction. Below, center, Preoperative views of the same bilateral microtia patient. Below, left and right, Bilateral results of the external and middle-ear team repair. (Reproduced from Brent B. Auricular repair with autogenous rib cartilage grafts: two decades of experience with 600 cases. *Plast Reconstr Surg.* 1992;90:355.)

Fig. 7.29 Complete corrective otoplasty (Tanzer modification of Converse procedure).

Fig. 7.30 The Kaye method to correct flattening of the antihelix. **(A)** A subperichondrial tunnel is made on the lateral surface of the cartilage through a medial incision near the cauda helicis; a sharp-tined instrument produces curling by multiple vertical striations. **(B and C)** The proper amount of antihelical roll is maintained by several mattress sutures introduced through tiny incisions along the conchal crest and carried across the antihelical fold through holes in the skin. (Reproduced from Kaye BL. A simplified method for correcting the prominent ear. *Plast Reconstr Surg.* 1967;40:44. Copyright © 1967, The Williams & Wilkins Company, Baltimore.)

Fig. 7.41 Reconstruction of an auricular defect with a composite graft from the contralateral ear. Left: above, an auricular defect resulting from a human bite; center, appearance of the ear 3 years after reconstruction with a composite graft; below, appearance of the donor ear 14 days after the surgical procedure. Right, The sequence of repair, top to bottom: the donor ear is at the left, and the defective ear being reconstructed is on the right. (Reproduced from Nagel F. Reconstruction of a partial auricular loss. *Plast Reconstr Surg.* 1972;49:340. Copyright © 1972, The Williams & Wilkins Company, Baltimore.)

Fig. 7.43 (A) Traumatic defect of the superior helical region. **(B)** Repair by helical advancement. (Modified from Antia NH, Buch VI. Chondrocutaneous advancement of flap for the marginal defect of the ear. Plast Reconstr Surg 1967;39:472. Copyright © 1967, The Williams & Wilkins Company, Baltimore.)

Fig. 7.47 Partial auricular reconstruction with conchal cartilage graft, as illustrated in Figure 7.41. **(A)** Middle-third postsurgical defect. **(B)** Conchal cartilage graft from contralateral ear. **(C)** Result obtained by tunnel procedure of Converse. Secondary procedures will be necessary to release the ear and to improve helical contour. (Reproduced from Brent B. The versatile cartilage autograft: current trends in clinical transplantation. *Clin Plast Surg.* 1979;6:163.)

Fig. 7.48 Repair of a posterosuperior auricular defect by the tunnel procedure of Converse. **(A)** The portion of the ear to be restored.

(B) The auricle is pressed against the mastoid process. **(C)** An ink outline is traced on the skin overlying the mastoid process, parallel to the edge of the auricular defect. **(D)** Incisions are made along the edge of the defect and through the skin of the mastoid area. **(E)** Suture of the medial edge of the auricular incision to the anterior edge of the mastoid incision. **(F)** The suture has been completed. **(G)** Costal cartilage graft. **(H)** The costal cartilage graft has been embedded. **(I)** The skin of the mastoid area is advanced to cover the cartilage graft. **(J)** In a second stage, the auricle is separated from the mastoid area, and full-thickness retroauricular grafts from the contralateral ear cover the defects. (Reproduced from Converse JM. Reconstruction of the auricle. *Plast Reconstr Surg.* 1958;22:150, 230. Copyright © 1958, The Williams & Wilkins Company, Baltimore.)

Fig. 7.49 Repair of an earlobe cleft with preservation of the perforation for an earring. **(A)** A flap is prepared by a parallel incision on one side of the cleft; the other side is "freshened" by excision of the margin. **(B)** The flap is rolled in to provide a lining for preservation of the earring track. **(C)** Closure is completed; a small Z-plasty may be incorporated. (Modified from Pardue AM. Repair of torn earlobe with preservation of the perforation for an earring. *Plast Reconstr Surg.* 1973;51:472.)

Fig. 7.52 Reconstruction of the earlobe. **(A)** The curved line abc outlines the proposed earlobe as measured on the unaffected contralateral auricle. A vertical flap is outlined; line bd is equal in length to line ab, and cd is equal to ca. **(B)** Incisions are made through the outlined skin and subcutaneous tissue. **(C)** The vertical flap is raised from the underlying tissue as far upward as the horizontal line ac, and the apex of the flap is sutured to point a. **(D)** The operation completed. (Modified from Zenteno Alanis S. A new method for earlobe reconstruction. *Plast Reconstr Surg.* 1970;45:254.)

Fig. 7.53 Reconstruction of the earlobe by a two-flap technique (Converse). **(A)** The pattern of the planned earlobe. **(B)** The pattern has been placed on the posteromedial aspect of the auricle and an outline made. The outline of the second flap from the retroauricular area is also shown; note the line of the vertical incision for insertion of the lobe. **(C)** Each of the flaps is sutured to an edge of the vertical incision, thus anchoring the new earlobe. **(D)** The two flaps are sutured to each other. **(E)** The operation completed. (Reproduced from Kazanjian VH, Converse JM, eds. *Surgical treatment of facial injuries.* 3rd ed. Baltimore: Williams & Wilkins, 1974: 1292.)

Fig. 7.54 (A) Loss of the lower part of the auricle. **(B)** The result obtained with a flap based on the mastoid process and folded on itself. Note the scar of the approximated edges of the flap's donor site. (Courtesy of Dr. Cary L. Guy.)

Fig. 7.55 Construction of an earlobe with a reverse-contoured flap. **(A)** The earlobe deficiency. **(B)** An auriculomastoid flap outlined. **(C)** The elevated flap hanging as a curtain from the inferior auricular border. **(D)** The flap folded under and sutured and the mastoid defect closed. A small graft is placed over the auricular donor defect. **(E)** The completed earlobe, exaggerated by one-third to allow for shrinkage. (Reproduced from Brent B. Earlobe reconstruction with an auricular-mastoid flap. *Plast Reconstr Surg.* 1976;57:389. Copyright © 1976, The Williams & Wilkins Company, Baltimore.)

Fig. 7.56 Earlobe reconstruction. **(A)** The reverse contour pattern, in which ab is equal to ef, bc to ce, and ad to df. **(B)** Congenital deficiency of lobular tissue. **(C)** Completed construction by the technique illustrated in Figure 7.55. (Reproduced from Brent B. Earlobe reconstruction with an auricular-mastoid flap. *Plast Reconstr Surg.* 1976;57:389. Copyright © 1976, The Williams & Wilkins Company, Baltimore.)

Access the complete references list online at **http://www.expertconsult.com**

22. Reinisch RF, Lewin S. Ear reconstruction using a porous polyethylene framework and temporoparietal fascial flap. *Facial Plast Surg.* 2009;25:181.

30. Firmin F. Ear reconstruction in cases of typical microtia. Personal experience based on 352 microtic ear corrections. *Scan J Plast Reconstr Hand Surg.* 1998;32:35.

32. Nagata S. Modification of the stages in total reconstruction of the auricle. *PlastReconstr Surg.* 1994;93:221.

Total auricular reconstruction for microtia is dependent on the fabricated three-dimensional costal cartilage framework, with all the auricular features and the skin flaps formed and utilized to cover the three-dimensional framework, in which extreme caution is required. Furthermore, other factors, such as contraction of the skin graft, use of the remnant ear cartilage in construction of the tragus, and the number of surgeries required, all affect the final results of total auricular reconstruction for microtia, especially with reference to the contour of the constructed ear, morphologic locations of the auricular features, contraction, circulatory dysfunction, and resorption.

The grafting of the three-dimensional framework is the first stage of a two-stage surgical method for total auricular reconstruction without resorting to skin grafts, free composite grafts, and additional surgical procedures.

44. Grabb WC. The first and second branchial arch syndrome. *Plast Reconstr Surg.* 1965;36:485.

79. Lauritzen C, Munro IR, Ross RB. Classification and treatment of hemifacial microsomia. *Scand J Plast Reconstr Surg.* 1985;19:33.

96. Kawanabe Y, Nagata S. A new method of costal cartilage harvest for total auricular reconstruction: part I. Avoidance and prevention of intraoperative and postoperative complications and problems. *Plast Reconstr Surg.* 2006;117:2011–2018.

The authors developed a new method of costal cartilage harvest where the perichondrium is left completely intact at the donor site and the remaining costal cartilage after fabrication of the three-dimensional costal cartilage framework is returned to the perichondrial pocket to fill the dead space formed. By leaving the perichondrium completely intact, the most ideal environmental condition for regeneration of cartilage is attained.

The findings of the authors' study involving over 270 cases performed with the new method of costal cartilage harvest revealed that there were absolutely no postoperative chest wall deformities identified, and there was a significant decrease in intraoperative complications.

97. Kawanabe Y, Nagata S. A new method of costal cartilage harvest for total auricular reconstruction: part II. Evaluation and analysis of the regenerated costal cartilage. *Plast Reconstr Surg.* 2007;119:308–315.

The authors describe how regenerated cartilage can be used during the second-stage operation. Secondary auricular reconstruction was thought to be impossible because of the lack of costal cartilage for fabrication of a three-dimensional costal cartilage framework but this work proves that theory wrong.

99. Walton RL, Beahm EK. Auricular reconstruction for microtia: Part II. Surgical techniques. *Plast Reconstr Surg.* 2002;110:234–249; quiz 250–251, 387

Reconstruction of the microtic ear represents one of the most demanding challenges in reconstructive surgery. In this review the two most commonly used techniques for ear reconstruction, the Brent and Nagata techniques, are addressed in detail. Unique to this endeavor, the originator of each technique has been allowed to submit representative case material and to address the pros and cons of the other's technique. What follows is a detailed, insightful overview of microtia reconstruction, as a state of the art. The review then details commonly encountered problems in ear reconstruction and pertinent technical points. Finally, a glimpse into the future is offered with an accounting of the advances made in tissue engineering as this technology applies to auricular reconstruction.

159. Brent B. The acquired auricular deformity. A systemic approach to its analysis and reconstruction. *Plast Reconstr Surg.* 1977;59:475.

160. Antia NH, Buch VI. Chondrocutaneous advancement flap for the marginal defect of the ear. *Plast Reconstr Surg.* 1967;39:472.

This paper is the classic publication in which Antia and Buch describe their repair for marginal defects of the ear. Three cases of partial defect of the helix reconstructed by an advancement of the chondrocutaneous helical flap are presented. The operative technique employed in these cases is described. The principle underlying the operative procedure is that of advancement of the adjacent, intact helical margin as a flap based on a wide postauricular skin pedicle. The defect is in fact transferred to the extensile lobule. The reconstructed helix is more consistent with the architecture of the normal ear than when repair has been accomplished by some of the other methods proposed. Safety is combined with economy of tissue and time.

8

Acquired cranial and facial bone deformities

Renee M. Burke, Robert J. Morin, and S. Anthony Wolfe

SYNOPSIS

- Treatment of acquired cranial and facial bone deformities begins with a thorough physical examination prior to radiologic studies.
- Access incisions must allow visualization and exposure of the entire defect.
- Surgical treatment must follow Tessier's principles of subperiosteal exposure, judicious use of autogenous bone grafts, and rigid fixation.
- Alloplastic materials are to be avoided if possible.
- Late presentation of acquired deformities may require an osteotomy through the defect site prior to reduction.

Introduction

The various causes of acquired deformities of the facial skeleton include trauma, infection, and surgical or radiotherapeutic treatment of neoplasia. The surgical treatment of these acquired deformities has changed radically during the past three decades as a result of advances in the subspecialty of craniofacial surgery. Craniofacial surgery developed almost entirely from the work of Paul Tessier, who revolutionized facial skeletal surgery with his seminal work regarding treatment of congenital malformations, such as Crouzon disease,[1] Apert syndrome,[2] Treacher Collins–Franceschetti syndrome, vertical orbital dystopias, and orbital hypertelorism.[3–8] The basic principles Tessier stressed when operating on the facial skeleton include the following[9]:

Key points

- Complete subperiosteal exposure of the areas of interest through coronal, lower eyelid, or intraoral incisions.
- Repositioning misaligned segments of the craniofacial skeleton with rigid fixation and interposed autogenous bone grafts to provide consolidation of the structure.[10] Onlay "camouflage" grafts are to be avoided because

they do not provide a three-dimensional correction of the entire deformity.
- Utilizing only fresh, autogenous bone grafts, obtainable from the ribs, anterior and posterior ilium, tibia, and the skull.[11,12] There is little place for bone substitutes, whether alloplastic materials or cadaver bone, in craniofacial reconstruction.[13]
- If a structure is not present to be repositioned, it can be constructed in situ or constructed and then moved to the proper location.
- The once forbidden boundary zone between the cranial cavity and the midface can safely be transgressed if proper care is taken in its reconstruction. Regular and frequent collaboration between the plastic surgical and neurosurgical members of a craniofacial team decreases the risks associated with a transcranial approach.
- Other members of a craniofacial team, such as ophthalmologists and orthodontists, will need to be involved in the treatment of acquired deformities, just as for congenital malformations.

Basic science/disease process

Access incisions

Access to the facial skeleton is provided through coronal, lower eyelid, and intraoral incisions. The following paragraphs describe the proper techniques to be used when making these incisions.

Coronal incisions

Coronal incisions should be made at least 3 cm behind the anterior hairline, almost at the vertex. The incision is carried to a point just above the anterior attachment of the ear, where a small cutback of 8–10 mm is made in the direction of the immediate subciliary area[16] in order to avoid postoperative ectropion.

Intraoral incisions

Upper buccal sulcus incisions should have an adequate inferior mucosal cuff for subsequent closure. The infraorbital nerve should be protected and the buccal fat pad avoided during dissection. The entire mandible up to the sigmoid notch and inferior 1 cm of the coronoid process and condyle are accessible through a lower buccal sulcus incision.[17]

Bone grafts

The key element to success in repositioning or replacing portions of the facial skeleton lies in the liberal and exclusive use of fresh autogenous bone grafts. Cranial bone is the preferred donor site, given the ease of harvest and proximity to the operating field.

The preferred donor area for cranial grafts is the right parietal area in right-handed patients.[18] When large grafts are required, the craniotomy can be extended anteriorly beyond the coronal suture and posteriorly into the occipital region. If additional bone is required, the opposite parietal region may be utilized. The harvested bone should be slightly larger in dimension than the area to be corrected. Each graft can be split through the diploic space to give two segments of equal dimensions. The inner table is replaced in the donor area with one of the segments. A defect several millimeters in width will be present, varying with the thickness of the craniotome blade. This defect is placed posteriorly and filled in with small bone chips, slivers, and bone dust and covered with a pericranial flap.[19] The bone graft for the defect is tailored exactly to the defect. On occasion, it is good to enlarge the defect slightly by burring back to healthy bone. Fixation with wires, not miniplates, is preferred *(Fig. 8.2)*.

The exception to the rule of utilizing cranial bone as the primary donor site is iliac bone, with rib used only as a last resort. Iliac bone provides an excellent orbital floor because of the thin cortical floor with malleable cancellous bone that is rigid enough to support the globe. Also, iliac bone is an excellent choice when large amounts of cancellous bone are required, such as for obliterating a frontal sinus *(Fig. 8.3)*.

Soft-tissue cover

The success of free bone grafts depends on the intimate contact of well-vascularized soft tissues both above and below the grafts. This means that areas between bone grafts must be filled in with other graft material and hematoma formation prevented by fastidious hemostasis and adequate postoperative drainage. When soft tissues are inadequate because of the original trauma or radiotherapy, they must be replaced with good soft tissue before bone grafts can survive. Given adequate exposure, an acceptable amount of autogenous bone grafts, and the means to provide rigid fixation, the correction of deformities in various areas of the facial skeleton should proceed smoothly.

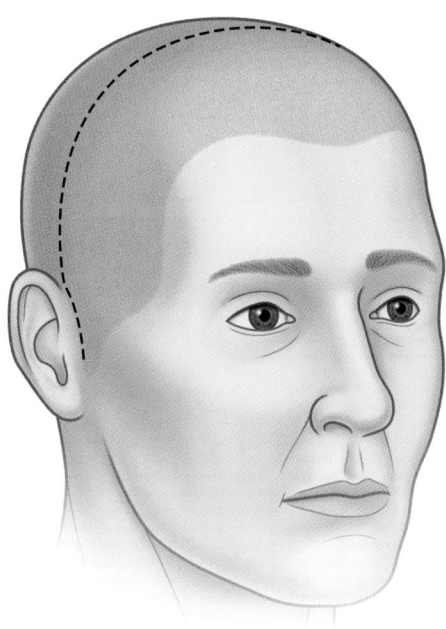

Fig. 8.1 Coronal incision.

lateral canthus, allowing the coronal flap to be turned forward without tension. Incisions close to or along the anterior hairline can be noticeable, and it may be difficult or impossible to improve these scars in areas of alopecia. The dissection is carried out in a supraperiosteal plane to the level of the supraorbital ridge, where it then becomes subperiosteal. The superficial temporal fascia (STF) is generally divided, exposing the deeper temporal fascia upon approaching the zygomatic arch and malar region. The temporalis muscle should be elevated separately from the scalp and resutured to the lateral orbital rim, anterior temporal crest, and posterior portion of the coronal incision, maintaining its original tension upon closure of the incision. The STF should also be resuspended at the time of closure. After the temporal muscle has been sutured back into position under proper tension, a suture is taken from near the lateral canthal raphe and passed through the temporal aponeurosis to reposition the lateral canthus properly *(Fig. 8.1)*.

Once a coronal incision has been made, the same incision should be used for any future surgeries, as a scalp with multiple scars may greatly complicate later reconstruction. Additionally, previously described incisions, such as the hemicoronal incision with an extension on to the forehead, are relics of the past and have no place in modern-day craniofacial surgery.

Lower eyelid incisions

The lower eyelid, inferior orbital rim, and orbital floor can be accessed through either the conjunctiva[14] or the lower eyelid.[15] If a cutaneous approach is used, it should be lower in the eyelid, beneath the tarsal plate, rather than in the

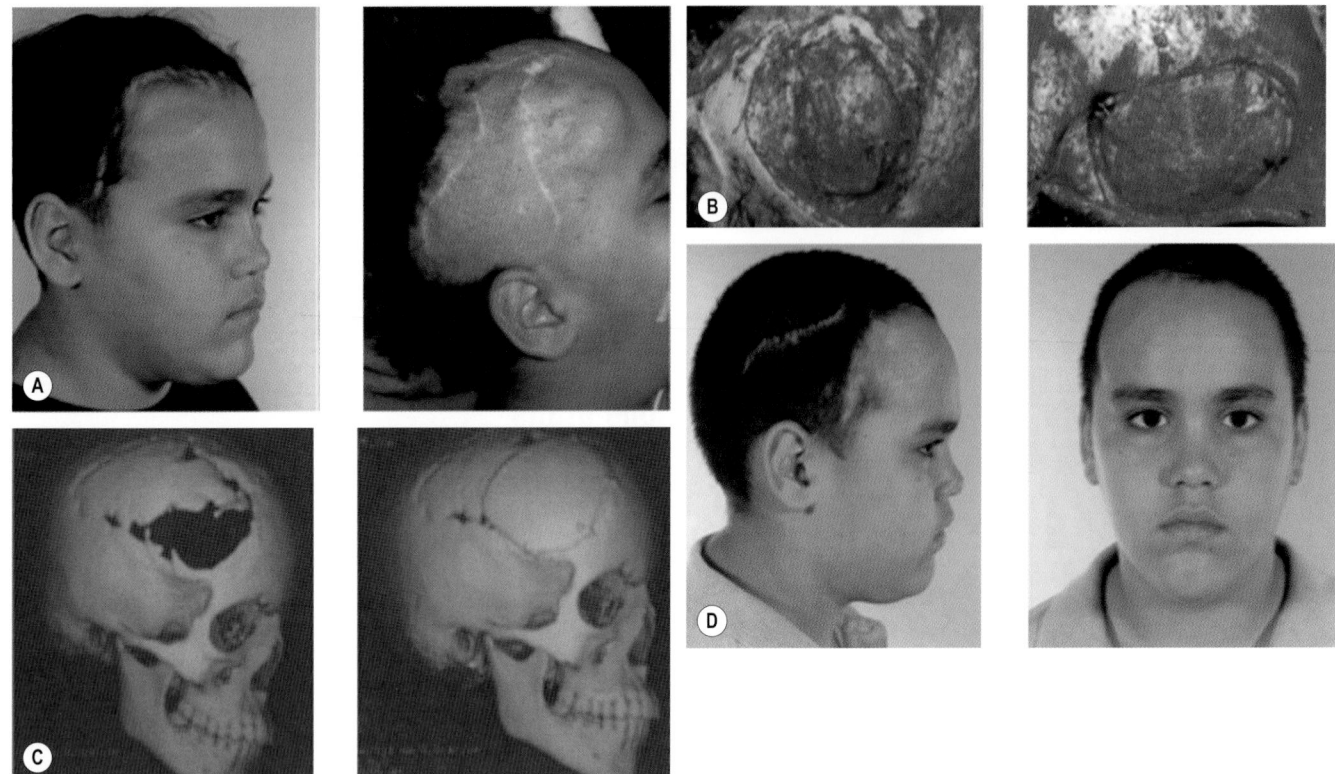

Fig. 8.2 This 12-year-old boy was in an automobile accident in Cuba and sustained an open right frontal fracture. The original laceration is apparently the sweeping scar from near the midpoint of the anterior hairline to a point above the right sideburn. A subsequent neurosurgical procedure was performed through an incision just along the right anterior hairline, and yet another procedure was performed through a more posterior incision **(A)**. Through one of these incisions, an attempt was made to correct the cranial defect with an alloplastic material that had to be removed because of infection. The cranial defect was approached through an anterior hairline incision that extended into a more posterior coronal incision on the left side. A left parietal craniotomy of a slightly larger dimension than the measurements of the right frontal cranial defect was performed, and the cranial flap was split (*ex vivo*) into two segments through the diploic space. The outer table segment was used for the frontal defect after precise trimming, and the inner table segment was placed back in the donor area **(B)**. **(C)** A postoperative three-dimensional computed tomography scan displays the precise repair of the cranial defect with the split calvarial graft. **(D)** Healing was uneventful. There are two important lessons to be learned from this patient. First, use a posterior coronal incision, and use it for all subsequent procedures. Second, use autogenous cranial bone for cranioplasties whenever possible.

Treatment/surgical technique

Treatment of specific defects

Acquired defects of the cranium and facial skeleton can be divided into two groups: those resulting from displaced fractures and those resulting from a loss of substance. We will discuss each specific area of the cranial and facial bone defects and their treatment.

Cranium

Cranial defects greater than half the thickness of the skull in patients older than 2 years of age should be repaired. In children younger than 2 years of age they often spontaneously ossify and do not require treatment. Cranial bone is the material of choice for most cranioplasties due both to the quality of bone and proximity to the field of operation.[20] In the authors' experience, the youngest patient with a cranial bone that can be successfully split *ex vivo* is between 3 and 4 years of age. Good results can also be obtained with split rib *(Fig. 8.4)*. Rib grafts can be used from the age of 4–5 years, depending on the size of the patient.

Alloplastic materials should not be used in children as a primary reconstructive option. If the cranial defect has been corrected with autogenous bone grafts and all reconstructive work is complete, for minor surface irregularities present after 1 year, small amounts of alloplastic material such as Norian, BoneSource, or hydroxyapatite may be utilized. In adults, small defects far from the frontal sinus may also be primarily corrected with these materials.

Near the frontal sinus, only autogenous bone should be used.[21] If there is a full-thickness cranial defect near the frontal sinus, the sinus should be cranialized; if the posterior wall of the sinus is intact and the nasofrontal duct appears to be blocked, all mucosa should be removed and the sinus filled with autogenous cancellous grafts *(Fig. 8.5)*.[22]

Nose

This region involves the nasal bones, cartilaginous and bony septum, and the upper lateral cartilages. Minimally displaced fractures can often be treated with closed reduction and placement of nasal splints *(Fig. 8.6)*. Comminuted fractures require an open rhinoplasty approach and usually require placement of an autogenous bone graft.[23–28] This approach makes it possible to separate the alar cartilages and then

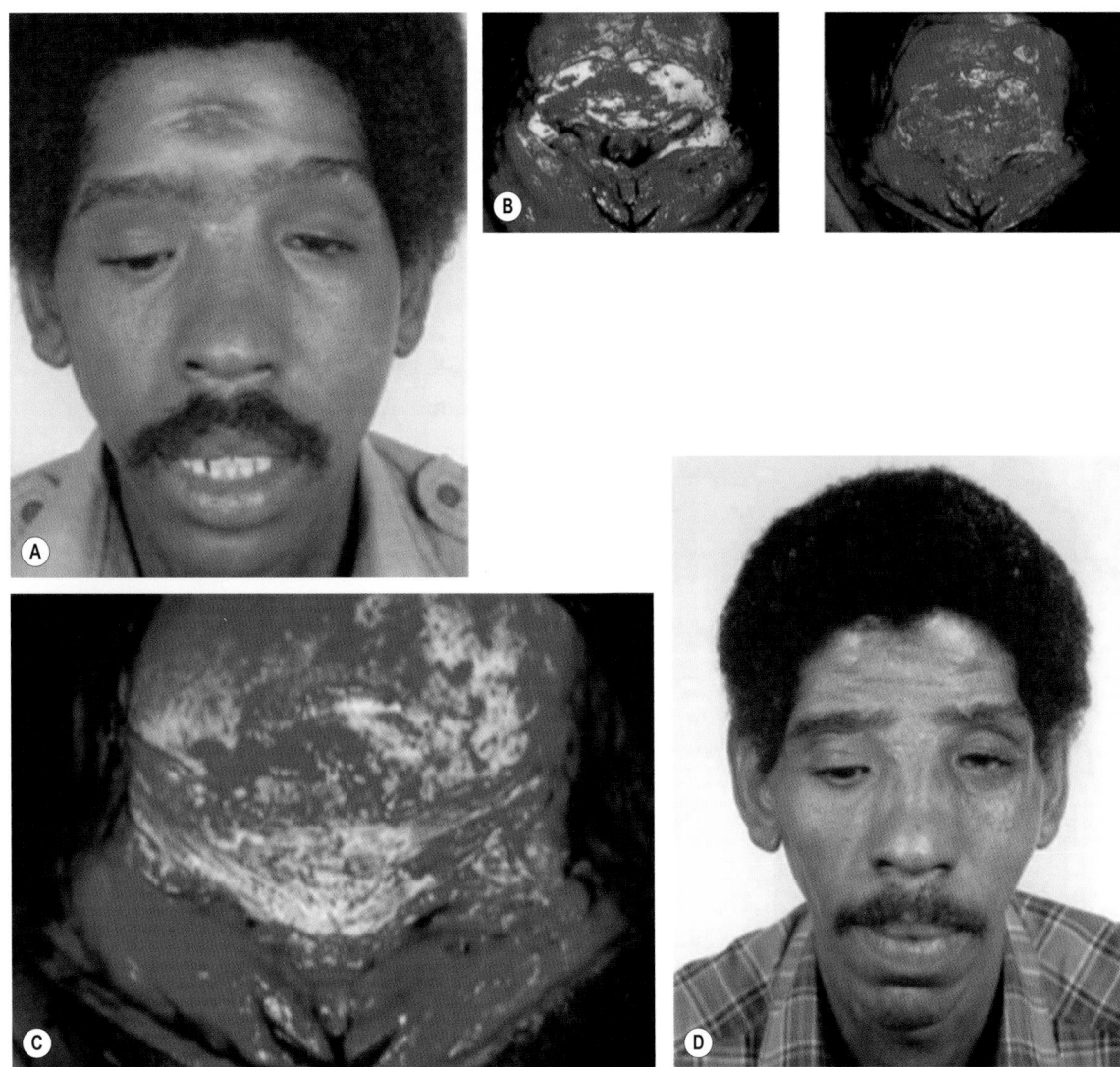

Fig. 8.3 This 25-year-old man had a chronic draining fistula communicating with a frontal sinus mucocele after treatment of fronto-orbital fractures elsewhere **(A)**. The fistula had been present for several years. The skin track was excised transversely and exposed through a coronal incision in the large frontal sinus extending almost from lateral orbital rim to lateral orbital rim. All mucosa was meticulously removed with a small burr, sharp periosteal elevators, and small curets **(B)**. The entire sinus cavity was then filled with fresh autogenous iliac cancellous bone **(C)** and covered with a pericranial flap. The wound healed without difficulty, and the patient is shown 6 years later **(D)** without having had any further surgery. Fresh, cancellous bone is the best material to use for obliteration of the frontal sinus, even with chronic infection, as was the situation here.

replace them over the nasal bone graft. Bone grafts for a depressed dorsum are simply placed into an appropriate pocket after dissection of the skin alone. In general, the bone graft is not rigidly fixed in place; care must be taken that the posterior portion of the bone graft is flat to avoid shifting of the graft. Making bilateral nasal vestibular incisions also helps provide an appropriate pocket so that the graft will remain in the center of the nose. If a graft does shift in the postoperative period, it can often be repositioned and maintained with a percutaneous K-wire, placed under local anesthesia, and maintained in position until consolidation of the bone graft occurs *(Fig. 8.7)*.

If substantial lengthening (>1 cm) of the nose is required, such as in Binder syndrome[29] or posttraumatic nasal foreshortening, dissection of the skin alone is not sufficient. The lining needs to be lengthened as well. Tessier *et al.* have shown

that considerable lengthening can be obtained, even in congenitally short noses, by dissecting the lining from beneath the nasal bones all the way back to the pharynx.[30] Another approach is purposely to section the lining (and bone) at the nasofrontal area, as in a Le Fort III osteotomy.[31]

The undersurface of the bone graft may be exposed to the nasal cavity, but healing proceeds uneventfully, as it does in a Le Fort III, over bone grafts exposed to the maxillary sinus, as with a Le Fort I, and over orbital floor bone grafts *(Fig. 8.8)*. This type of procedure would not be applicable to the contracted, foreshortened nose that is associated with sustained cocaine use. Here the lining is either altogether absent or chronically granulating and infected. Before a nasal bone graft can be added, nasal lining must be provided by bringing in tissue from other areas, such as nasolabial, forehead, or buccal sulcus flaps.[32]

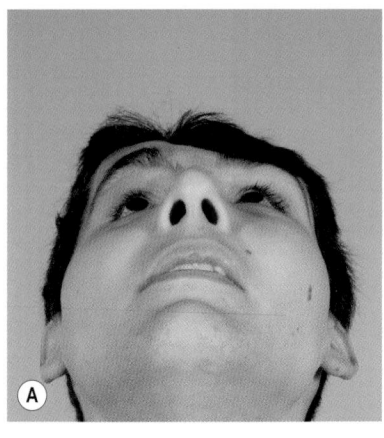
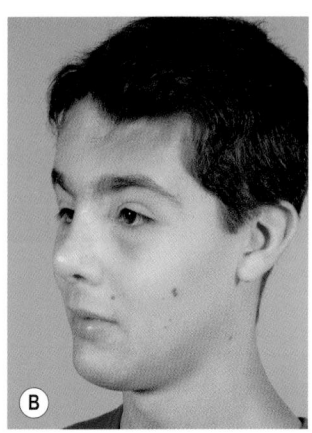
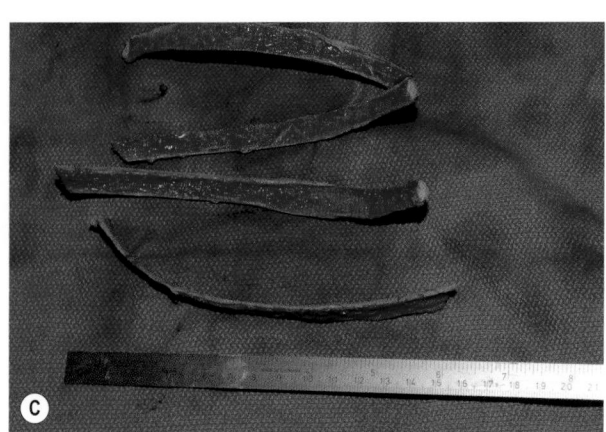
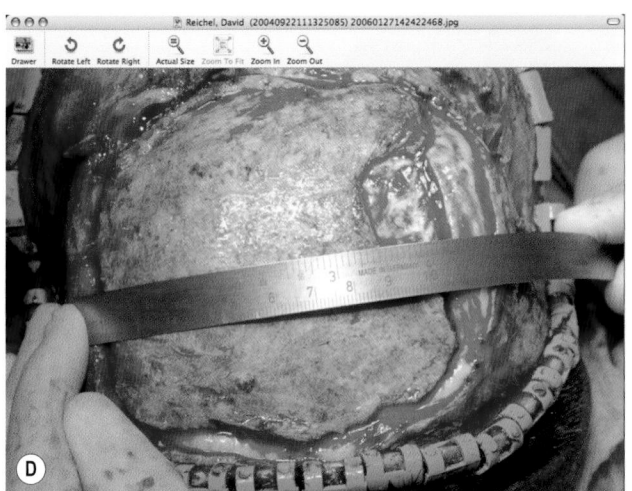
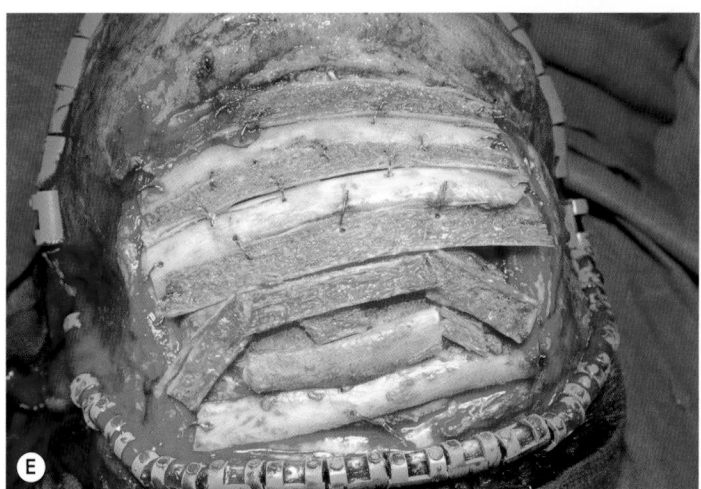
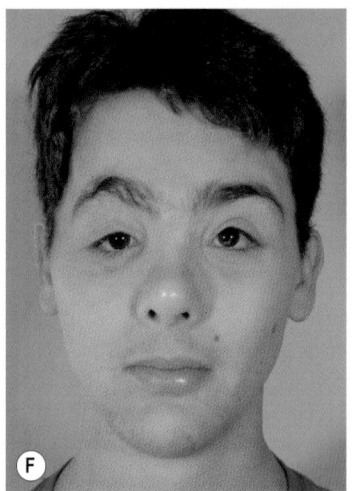
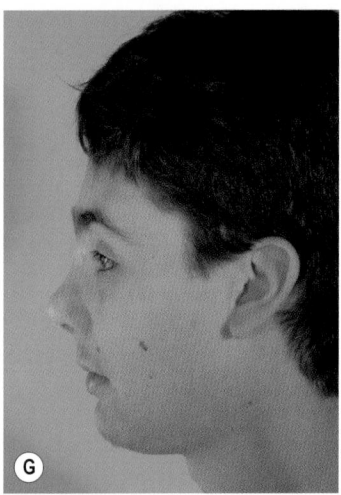

Fig. 8.4 This 22-year-old man had multiple facial and cranial fractures following a motor vehicle accident. He had a craniotomy for an acute epidural hematoma and subsequently developed a retrofrontal mucopyocele, necessitating removal of the infected frontal bone flap **(A, B)**. Six months later, the frontal defect was repaired with split-rib grafts **(C–E)**. He is shown 8 months after surgery with improved contour of the previous defect **(F, G)**.

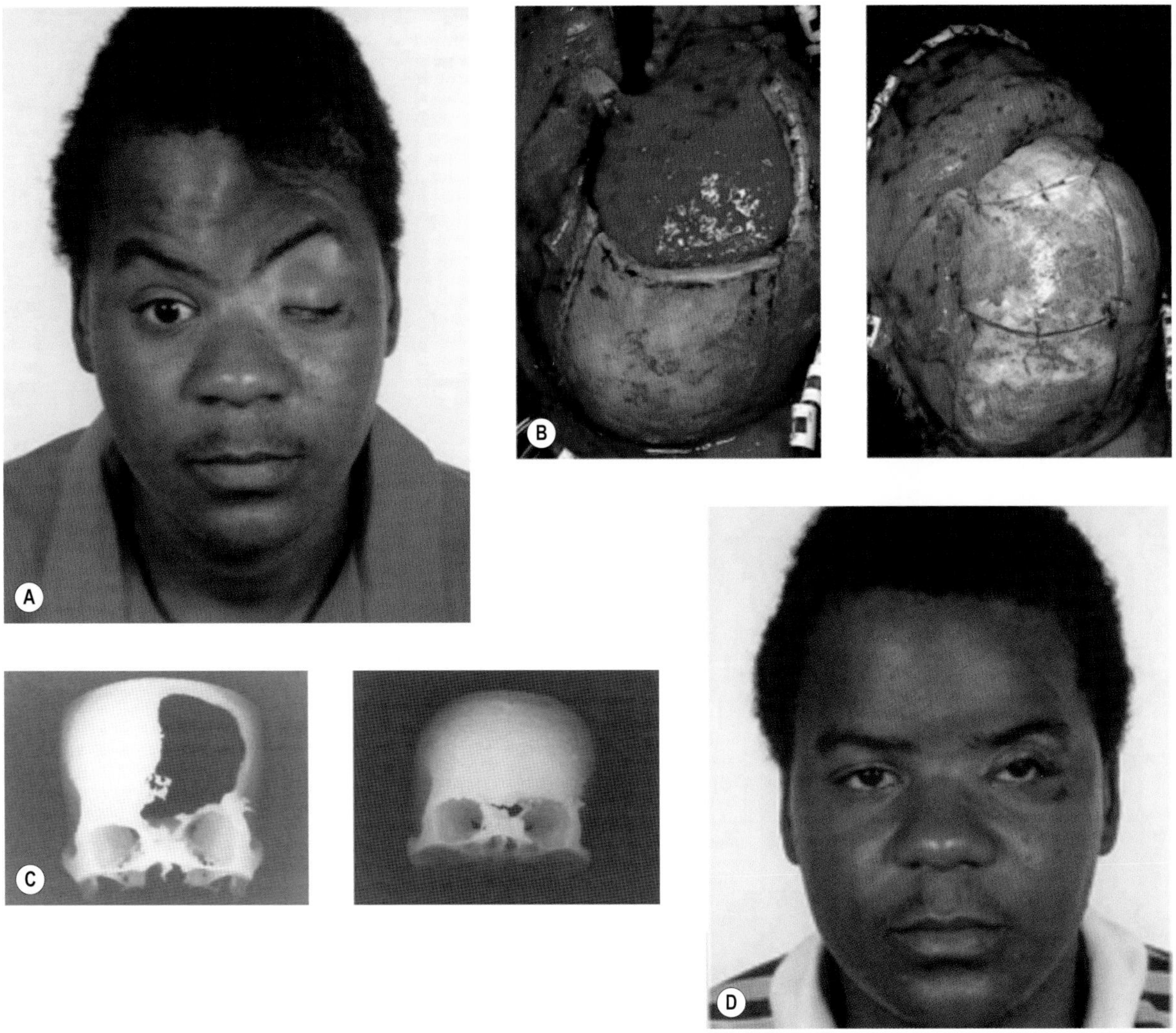

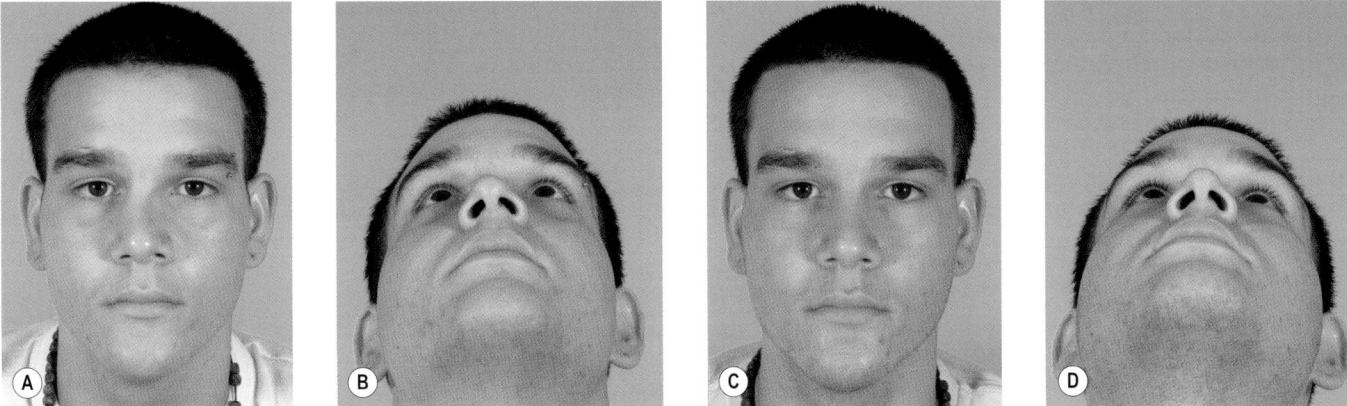

Fig. 8.5 This 23-year-old was shot through the right frontal region and has extensive debridement of the left frontal bone, supraorbital ridge, and orbital roof **(A, C).** He is shown after a split cranial bone cranioplasty **(B),** reconstruction of the orbital roof and supraorbital ridge, and subsequent ptosis correction by reattachment of the levator muscle to the tarsal plate **(D).**

Fig. 8.6 This 20-year-old male suffered an injury while playing football, resulting in a displaced nasal fracture with deviation of the nose and minimally depressed dorsum **(A, B).** He was treated with a closed reduction of the fracture. His 1-month postoperative photos show correction of the deformity **(C, D).**

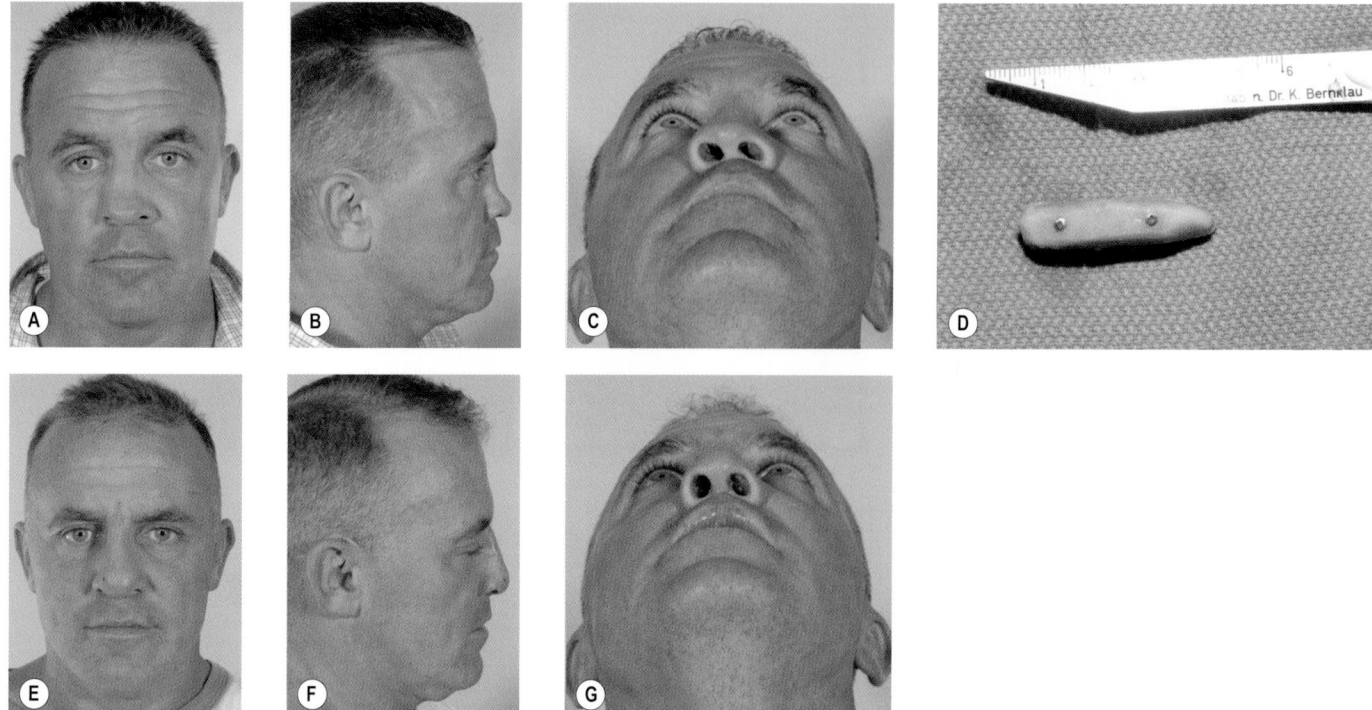

Fig. 8.7 This 42-year-old man presented 2 months after trauma to his nose resulting in a severe saddle-nose deformity, bilateral nasal bone fractures, and a significantly deviated septum, resulting in significant difficulty breathing through his nose **(A–C)**. He underwent cranial bone graft reconstruction of his dorsum **(D)** with columellar strut grafts, spreader grafts, and septoplasty. The patient is shown 1 month after surgery with resolution of both his functional and aesthetic concerns **(E–G)**.

Nasoethmoid area

Fractures in this region are often referred to as naso-orbital–ethmoid fractures, although the ethmoidal involvement, by definition, involves the orbit. Telecanthus, as a result of lateral displacement of the medial orbital walls and nasal foreshortening, is commonly seen after these fractures. One must resist the temptation to treat this conservatively with packing alone, as this pushes the structures further in, adding to the nasal foreshortening. A coronal incision should be used for adequate exposure unless a large facial laceration provides excellent exposure. Correction of telecanthus secondary to displaced bone fragments with the medial canthal tendons still attached can often be accomplished by anatomic reduction of the bone segments, without having to detach the tendons and perform a transnasal medial canthopexy.[33,34]

If the medial canthal tendon has been detached, a transnasal canthopexy must be performed. Some overcorrection of the medial wall segments is desirable, as in the correction of orbital hypertelorism. If there is significant loss of substance in the medial orbital wall, it may be necessary to perform a primary bone graft and medial canthopexy. The nasal dorsum will usually require a bone graft to repair the foreshortening resulting from the fracture *(Fig. 8.9)*.

Late reconstructions may pose an even greater challenge if the bones have consolidated in malposition. In such cases, the dissection must be extensive, often involving coronal, lower eyelid, and buccal sulcus incisions. The displaced segments must be delineated and osteotomized in order to return to their proper position. Plate and screw fixation is used to stabilize the segments.[35] A nasal bone graft is frequently necessary

for dorsal support and soft tissue may be needed to keep in conjunction with the principle of aesthetic subunits.

Orbitozygomatic region

Acute, isolated fractures of the zygomatic arch require an open approach if they cannot be reduced percutaneously. A coronal incision gives access for reduction and plating of the fracture or harvesting of bone grafts, if necessary.

Isolated orbital floor fractures are seen more commonly in younger patients, where the infraorbital rim is more elastic in comparison to adult patients *(Fig. 8.10)*. It appears that the causative force strikes the rim, which bends and then springs back to its original position. These actions can cause a fracture in the thin orbital floor. These injuries have the highest incidence of entrapment, diplopia, and inferior rectus damage which requires prompt intraoperative release.

Orbitozygomatic fractures vary considerably in their presentation, depending on the vector and force of the causative injury. Lesser injuries may result in nondisplaced fractures of the zygoma with minimal disruption of the orbital floor. In this instance, no treatment other than follow-up observation is necessary. If one has underappreciated the extent of the orbital floor fracture, late enophthalmos is a possible sequel[36]; however, one certainly does not have to operate on questionable fractures simply because of this possibility. Some advocated this approach when it was thought that enophthalmos could not be corrected.[37,38]

Greater forces cause greater disruption, and because of the elastic nature of bone, the extent of bone displacement during the injury may be much greater than the displacement seen

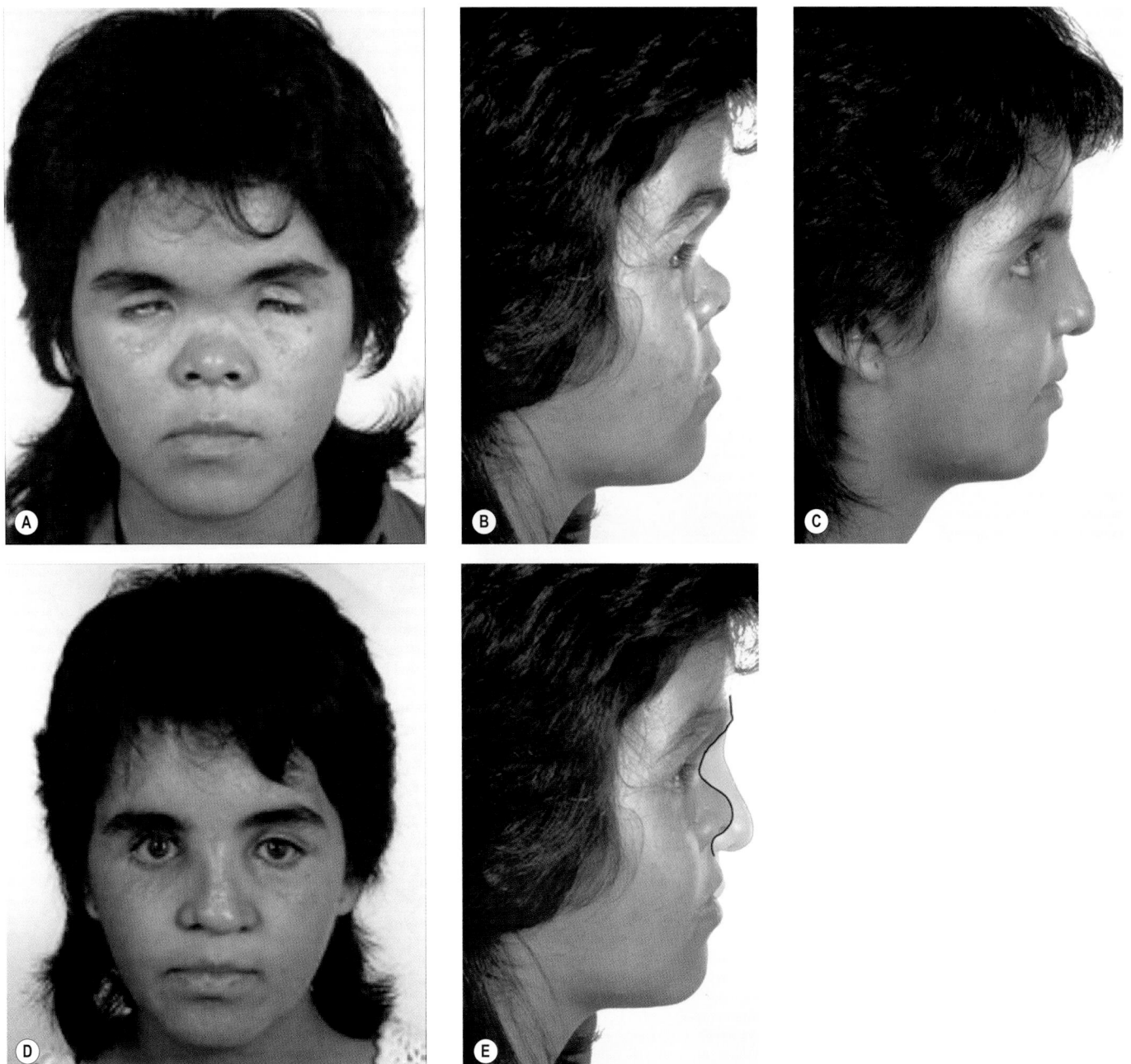

Fig. 8.8 This 17-year-old female was involved in a vehicular accident in South America. She was treated with wire traction from the zygomas to a head cap of some sort. Both globes were severely damaged, and she was blind **(A, B).** She is shown 6 months after a complete subperiosteal dissection of the orbital cavities and midface through coronal, intraorbital, and lower eyelid incisions, with mobilization of all malpositioned segments, extensive bone grafting with both iliac and cranial bone, and rigid fixation. The nasal lengthening was accomplished by sectioning of the contracted lining at the Le Fort III level and placement of an iliac bone graft in the created gap and as a dorsal graft along with a conchal cartilage graft to the nasal tip. This also corrected her class III malocclusion. In the postoperative photographs **(C, D),** she has ocular prostheses. The computer-generated overlay of her preoperative and postoperative photographs shows the degree of true nasal lengthening **(E).**

when the patient first presents. Again, late enophthalmos may develop if these injuries are not repaired properly *(Fig. 8.11).* If one puts the orbital framework into proper position with rigid fixation and repairs the internal orbital defects with autogenous bone grafts, enophthalmos will not result.

Reduction of an orbitozygomatic fracture in which the zygomatic body has been displaced away from the globe can usually be accomplished in the first week after the fracture simply by removing callus in the fracture lines and grasping solid segments of bone with bone clamps. When the zygoma

has been displaced by the injury toward the globe, proptosis or at least lack of enophthalmos may be present when the patient is first seen. In some instances it may not be possible to reduce the fracture. In these instances, one must be prepared to perform an osteotomy through the fracture lines in order to reduce the fracture adequately.

Most fractures that are seen after a delay of 3 weeks or more will have consolidated and will require refracture by osteotomy and repositioning. Coronal, lower eyelid, and buccal sulcus incisions are used in most of these patients to provide

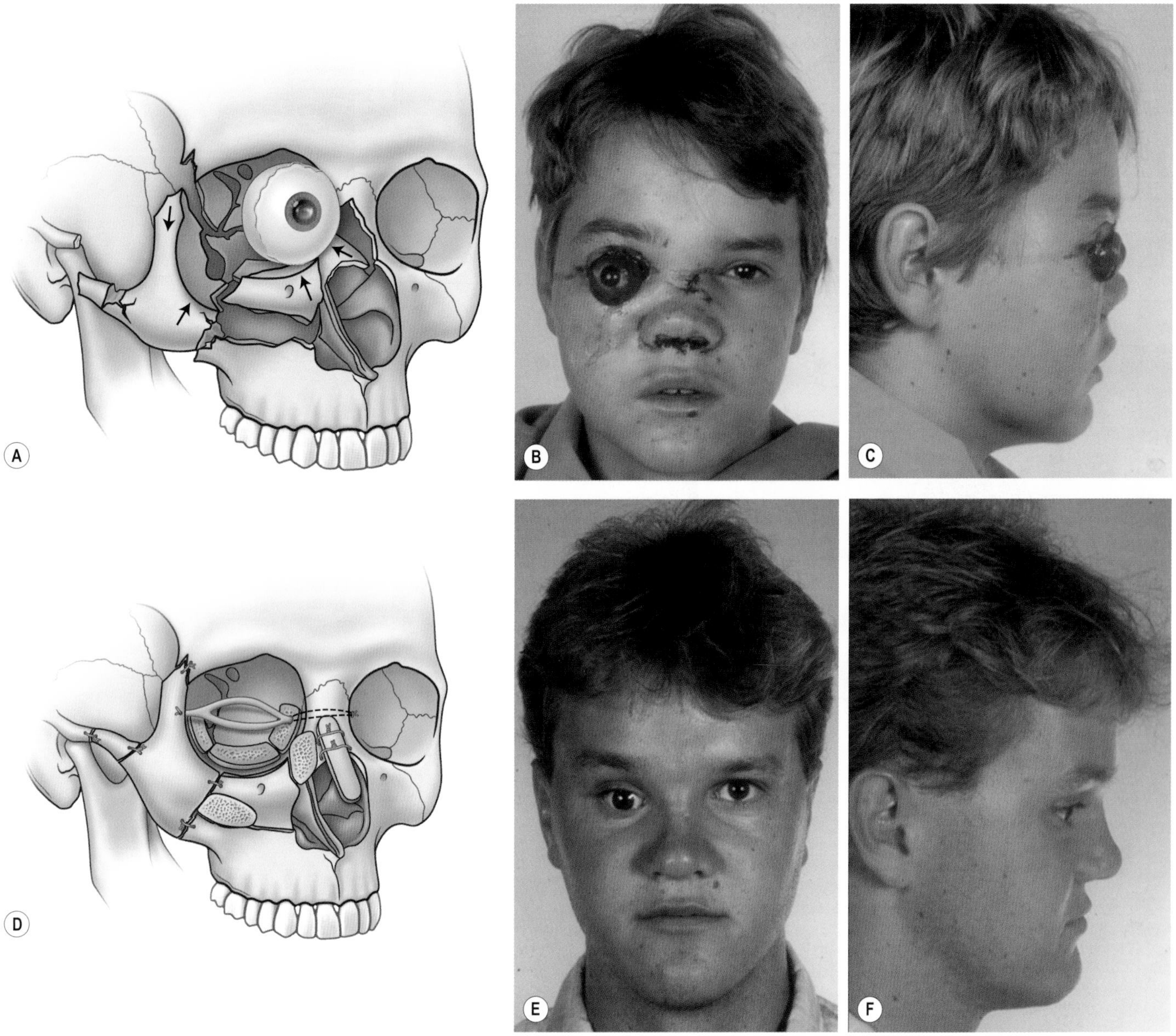

Fig. 8.9 This 13-year-old boy, living in Haiti, was struck by a pipe protruding from a car while he was on his bicycle. He presented 2 days after the injury with prolapse of the right globe and loss of vision, even though some extraocular motions were still present **(A-C)**. Additionally, avulsion of the right medial rectus was noted. Fractures of the right orbit and nasoethmoid region were present, as well as right telecanthus **(A)**. Treatment consisted of exposure of the fractures through coronal, right lower eyelid, and upper buccal sulcus incisions. Fractures were reduced and wire osteosynthesis placed. Replacement of the right globe into the orbital cavity required making multiple scoring incisions of the periorbitum. Iliac bone grafts to the nose, orbital floor, medial orbital wall, and anterior maxilla were placed, and a transnasal medial canthopexy through the medial orbital wall bone graft was performed **(D)**. He is shown 5 years postoperatively with a cosmetic cover shell over the right eye and good maintenance of nasal contour with the bone graft **(E, F)**.

good access for the osteotomies and also to allow the surgeon to appreciate the internal orbital anatomy fully, both of the medial orbital wall and of the lateral orbital wall. The sphenoidal portion of the lateral orbital wall should be perfectly aligned. A positioning wire is then placed through the frontozygomatic suture, and finally the inferior orbital rim is aligned. A wire is usually all that is needed for the frontozygomatic suture, and a small plate is placed to stabilize the inferior orbital rim. The zygomatic buttresses[39,40] should be checked through the upper sulcus incision and fixed in proper position with a larger plate. Finally, the zygomatic arch is plated, and one should have exposure of the normal side to check the exact shape of the normal zygomatic arch. If the arches are fractured on both sides, recall that they should be fairly straight, and not bowed, in order to provide proper projection of the midface.

Posttraumatic enophthalmos

Posttraumatic enophthalmos can result either from isolated defects of the orbital floor and medial orbital wall, in which

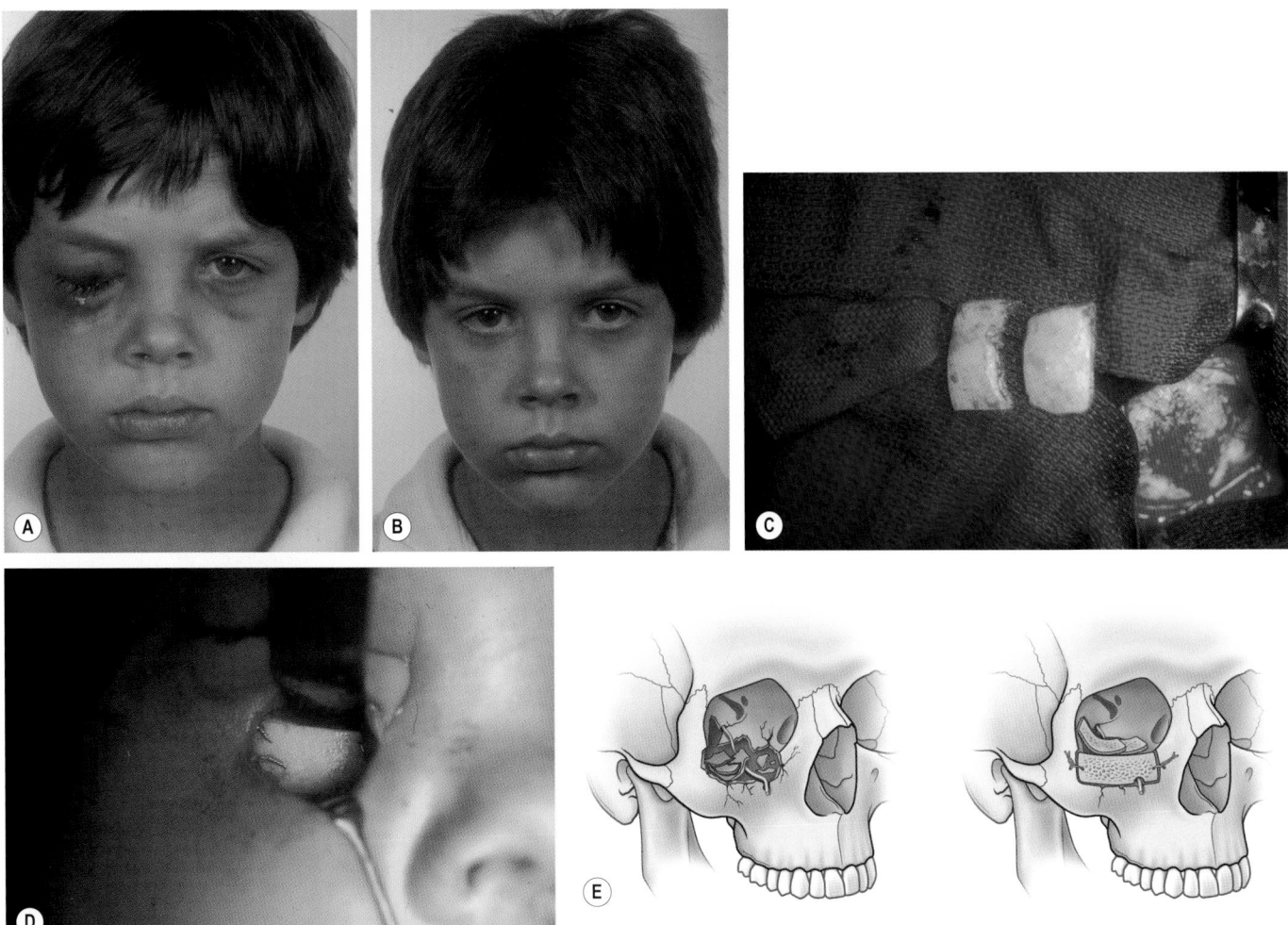

Fig. 8.10 This 9-year-old boy was kicked in the face by a horse. Ophthalmologic examination showed no damage to the eye itself. There was considerable ecchymosis and swelling of the eyelids, and, even with that, some enophthalmos was present **(A)**. There was a palpable depression of the infraorbital rim. A computed tomography scan showed comminution of the infraorbital rim and anterior maxilla with a large defect of the orbital floor. The malar bone, however, was not otherwise displaced. Treatment consisted of a lower lid incision, removal of multiple small comminuted bone fragments of the infraorbital rim, exploration of the orbital floor, with retrieval of orbital contents from the antrum, and placement of cranial bone grafts on the orbital floor and infraorbital rim/anterior maxilla **(C–E)**. His postoperative appearance at 1 year shows no evidence of enophthalmos **(B)**.

there is herniation of orbital contents into the maxillary and ethmoidal sinuses, or from displaced orbitozygomatic fractures, in which there is herniation of orbital contents into the paranasal sinuses.[41] If there is even a slight displacement of the zygoma from its proper position, it should be osteotomized and properly positioned. Autogenous bone grafts are used to replace missing or displaced portions of the internal orbit.[42–44] In the presence of a seeing eye, posttraumatic enophthalmos can be completely corrected in most instances if the bony orbit is completely reconstructed and all of the orbital contents returned to the orbital cavity.[45] Overcorrection by several millimeters in both the vertical and sagittal directions should be performed to compensate for operative swelling.

In patients with inadequate late correction of enophthalmos, even if it is mild, a coronal and sagittal computed tomographic (CT) scan will show a few areas where further bone grafting can provide a complete correction. When one is performing secondary bone grafting such as this, it is important to bear in mind that the orbital cavity may not have any areas

of egress because all of the communications into paranasal sinuses have been closed off with bone grafts. Bringing a small drain (such as a TLS drain) from the orbital floor out through the sideburn area will lessen the possibility of a volume and pressure increase due to hematoma *(Figs 8.12, 8.13)*.[46]

The irradiated orbit

Irradiation of the orbit in early childhood, such as for retinoblastoma, will result in a small orbit and often restriction of growth of the temporal fossa. If a seeing eye is still present, one can deal with the temporal fossa defect with a soft-tissue flap, most efficiently by composite tissue transplantation. The orbit itself should not be altered. If the eye is absent and the orbit small, an orbital expansion can be performed to give an orbit of normal dimensions.[47] This is followed by socket reconstruction and placement of an ocular prosthesis.

The overall approach for secondary correction of displaced facial bone segments is the same as for primary correction:

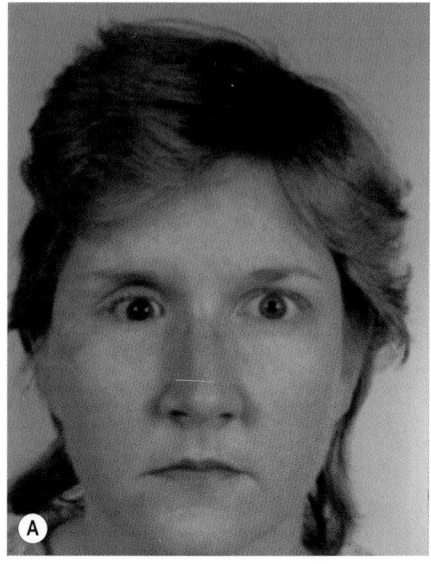
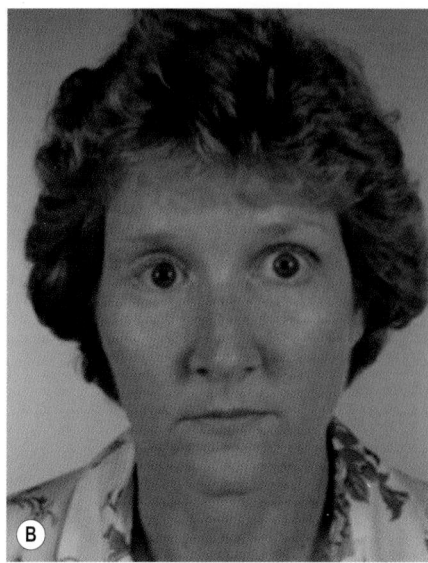
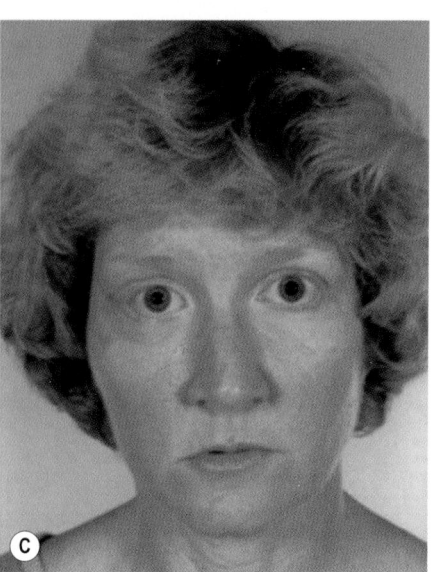

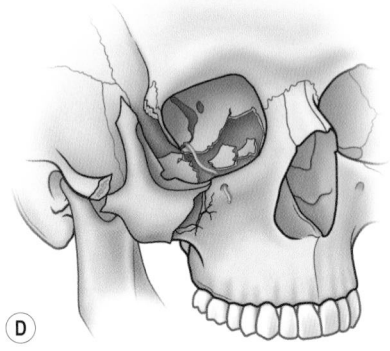
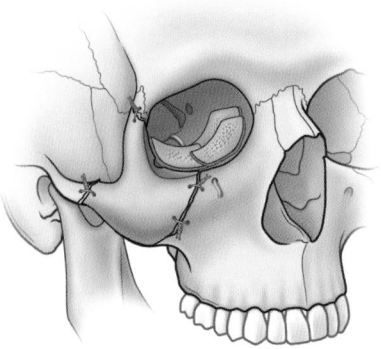

Fig. 8.11 This woman was 32 years old when an osteotomy and repositioning of the right zygoma were performed along with an iliac bone graft **(A).** An undercorrection was noted 6 years later **(B).** A computed tomographic evaluation showed a persistent small defect in the posteromedial orbital wall as well as an enlargement of the inferior orbital fissure; the addition of a small amount of cranial bone corrected the persistent enophthalmos completely, as seen in her photo 4 years after her second surgery **(C). (D)** Illustration showing the repositioning of the right zygoma.

obtain adequate exposure, place the segments into proper position, utilize rigid fixation, and liberally use autogenous bone grafts for any residual bone defects. The main difference is that the soft-tissue dissection is often much more difficult because of scarring and contraction of the soft-tissue envelope over the malpositioned facial bone segments. The buccal fat pad and other soft-tissue elements of the midface may have prolapsed into the maxillary sinus through defects in the anterior maxillary wall, and these must be completely retrieved. Autogenous bone grafts are used to recreate the anterior maxillary wall and to keep the soft tissues in their proper place.

As noted previously, the dissected midfacial tissues are suspended to the temporal aponeurosis, and a lateral canthopexy is performed.

Maxilla

When evaluating fractures of the maxilla, one must remember the importance of the maxillary buttresses, as described by Gruss and Mackinnon[48] and Manson *et al.*[40] These thickenings of bone conduct masticatory and other forces through the midface to the thicker bones of the skull and are divided into four categories:

1. Central: septo-vomerine-ethmoidal-frontal
2. Paracentral: maxillo-naso-frontal
3. Lateral: maxillo-malar-frontal
4. Posterior: maxillo-pterygoid.

When any of the maxillary buttresses is fractured transversely in only one place, but is otherwise intact, treatment consists of reducing the fracture to a proper occlusal relationship with the mandible, followed by rigid fixation across the fracture line. The use of intermaxillary fixation depends on the stability of the osteosynthesis. If the buttresses are comminuted with a loss of facial height, treatment must include reconstitution of the bony deficiencies with primary bone grafts. It is not uncommon for a Le Fort I fracture to be treated by intermaxillary fixation with a satisfactory occlusal result but a shortened midface. This occurs if the maxillary buttresses have all been fractured and the maxilla is jammed upward until bone contact occurs.[49] This deformity can be prevented if a primary reconstruction of the buttresses is carried out at the initial repair.[50,51]

If maxillary fractures have not been adequately reduced in the primary operation, they may require late treatment. This requires sectioning of the maxilla at the Le Fort I level, mobilization of the maxilla, and intermaxillary fixation. If

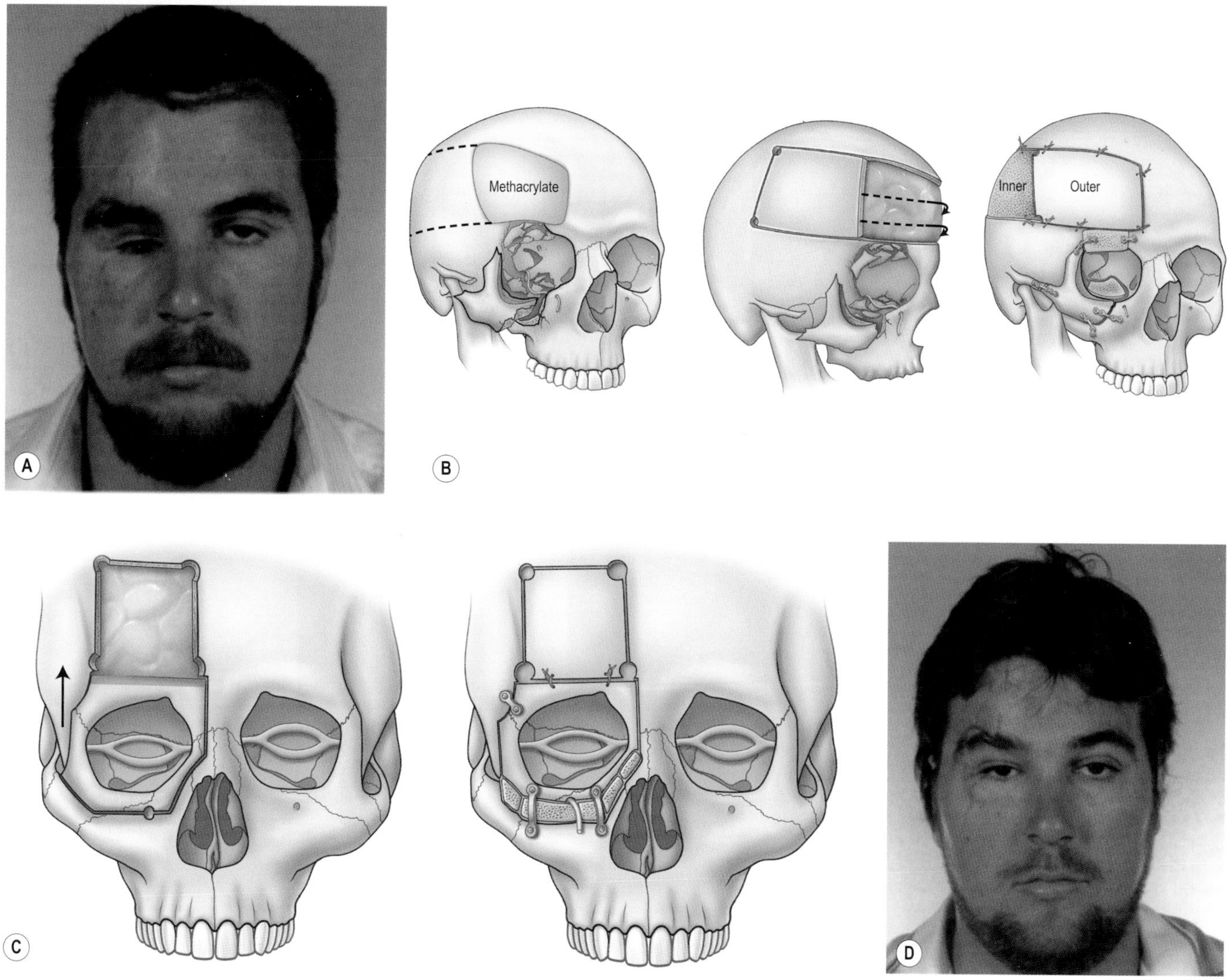

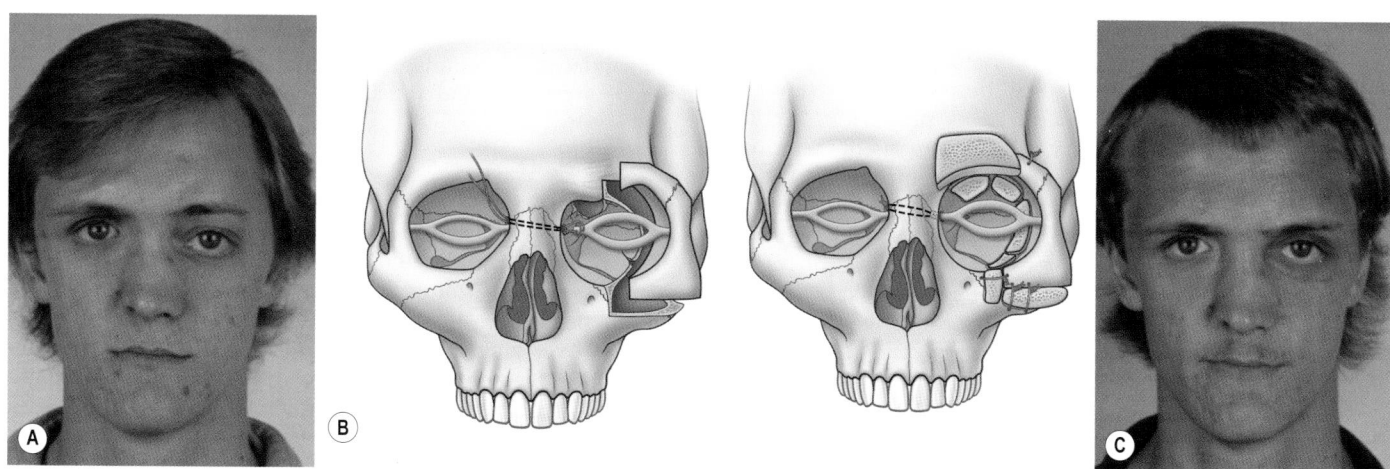

Fig. 8.12 This 23-year-old man had suffered major right orbitocranial fractures several years previously in a vehicular accident. A defect of most of the right frontal bone had been reconstructed with methyl methylmethacrylate. There was profound enophthalmos and hypoglobus of the right eye, which still retained some vision **(A).** In the initial operation, the alloplastic material was removed, and the frontal defect was reconstructed with split cranial bone **(B).** Major reconstructive orbital surgery is not recommended if there is any alloplastic material in the region of the periorbital sinuses. At the same time, refracture and repositioning of the right zygoma were performed along with cranial bone grafting of the medial orbital wall and orbital floor defects. This corrected the enophthalmos, but the patient was left with a considerable persistent hypoglobus. This was treated as a true vertical orbital dystopia, with an intracranial elevation of the entire – now intact – orbital cavity **(C).** The medial canthal tendon was left attached to bone and was elevated with the orbit. The patient is shown 3 years after the second operation **(D).**

Fig. 8.13 In this posttrauma patient, one can see a hypoglobus without enophthalmos **(A).** The orbital roof had been pushed into the orbital cavity, resulting in a slight proptosis. The globe was elevated by an osteotomy and repositioning of the zygoma, elevation of the orbital roof, and bone grafting of the orbital floor along with a transnasal medial canthopexy **(B).** The canthopexy shows that the canthal tendon is brought through a drill hole in the medial orbital wall just above and posterior to the lacrimal fossa and tied over a toggle on the contralateral side. He is shown operatively with correction of his hypoglobus **(C).**

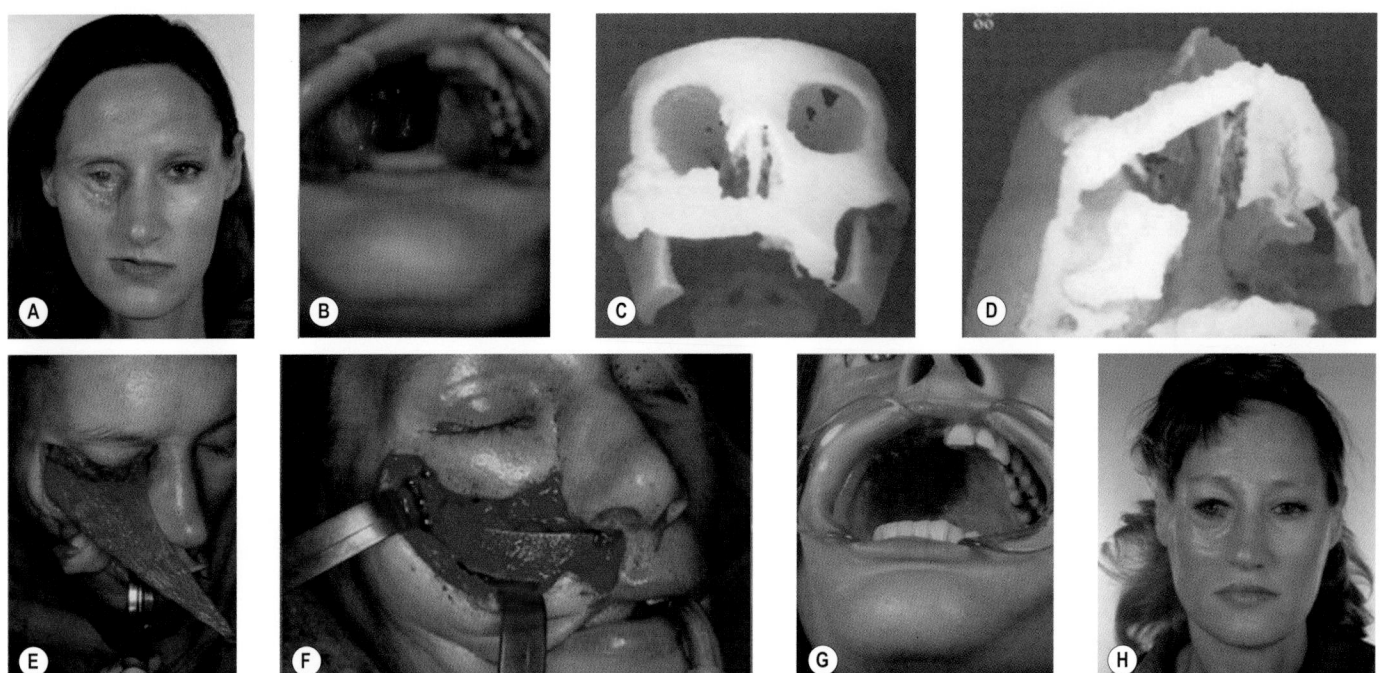

Fig. 8.14 This 29-year-old woman had undergone a hemimaxillectomy and postoperative irradiation for a neuroesthesioblastoma **(A)**. She was left with a large palatal defect **(B)**, as shown in her postresection computed tomography scans **(C,D)**. Shortly after the initial preoperative photograph was taken, her right eye spontaneously perforated and she underwent an evisceration (removal of all of the orbital contents down to periosteum). Reconstruction of her maxilla was performed using a temporalis muscle flap to close the palatal defect **(E)**. The radiation-damaged skin of the lower eyelid and cheek was resected and a skin graft placed over the temporalis muscle. At a subsequent operation, an iliac bone graft was placed from alveolar ridge to pterygoid region **(F)**, well nourished by the underlying temporalis muscle; the lower eyelid was reconstructed with a forehead flap. Osseointegrated implants have been placed in the maxillary bone graft, and this portion of her reconstruction has been completed **(G)**. A second forehead flap was required for the lower eyelid reconstruction and her final postoperative result is shown **(H)**.

the maxilla–mandible complex in intermaxillary fixation is allowed to find its own position in the lightly anesthetized, unparalyzed patient, this position represents the degree of lengthening desired. The two sides of the sectioned maxilla can now be plated in this position. Again, adequate amounts of autogenous bone grafts are essential to the consolidation of the maxilla in its new position.

Maxillary reconstruction

The same dissection previously described for traumatic deformities can be employed for either primary or secondary reconstruction of maxillary defects subsequent to removal of maxillary tumors, including use of the temporalis muscle.[52] In the initial coronal dissection, mobilization of the temporalis muscle is carried out to its posterior extent, which is often 5 cm or more posterior to the upper portion of the ear. The zygomatic arch is completely dissected, and the muscle is dissected from the lateral orbital wall deep into the temporal fossa. The zygomatic arch and a portion of the body of the zygoma are removed, and the muscle flap (which is usually about half of the muscle) is brought into the oral cavity after finger dissection enlarges the passage. A hemimaxillary defect can easily be closed with this muscle flap. The muscle does not need to be covered by mucosa or skin grafted because it is rapidly covered by mucosa naturally. An alveolar defect, either lateral or anterior, must be present to bring in the muscle flap easily. If the alveolar

ridge is intact, it is difficult to bring in a muscle flap because it involves making a hole through the anterior maxillary wall or bringing the muscle behind the maxillary tuberosity *(Fig. 8.14)*. For large central palatal defects that cannot be closed by local palatal flaps, a microsurgical solution is preferred. The flap of choice is the radial forearm flap.[53] After complete healing of the soft-tissue palatal repair, a bony alveolar ridge can be reconstructed with iliac bone grafts or microvascular osseous flaps (fibular or parascapular flaps are the most common).[54–56] After the bone repair is well consolidated, osseointegrated implants can be placed to accept a denture and finish the reconstruction.

Mandible

When evaluating a patient with a suspected mandibular fracture, the diagnosis can often be made by physical examination alone. Common findings include malocclusion, a step in the occlusal plane, a change in the axial inclination of the teeth, mental nerve paresthesias, ecchymosis or a tear in the buccal mucosa overlying the fracture, and localized pain on palpation and movement at the fracture site. To locate the fracture and any associated fractures precisely, a panorex or CT scan should be performed.[57]

Treatment of nondisplaced mandibular fractures in compliant patients may consist of a soft diet and careful observation alone with repeat radiological studies over 4–6 weeks. If the patient is noncompliant, he or she may be best served with 4–6 weeks of intermaxillary fixation.

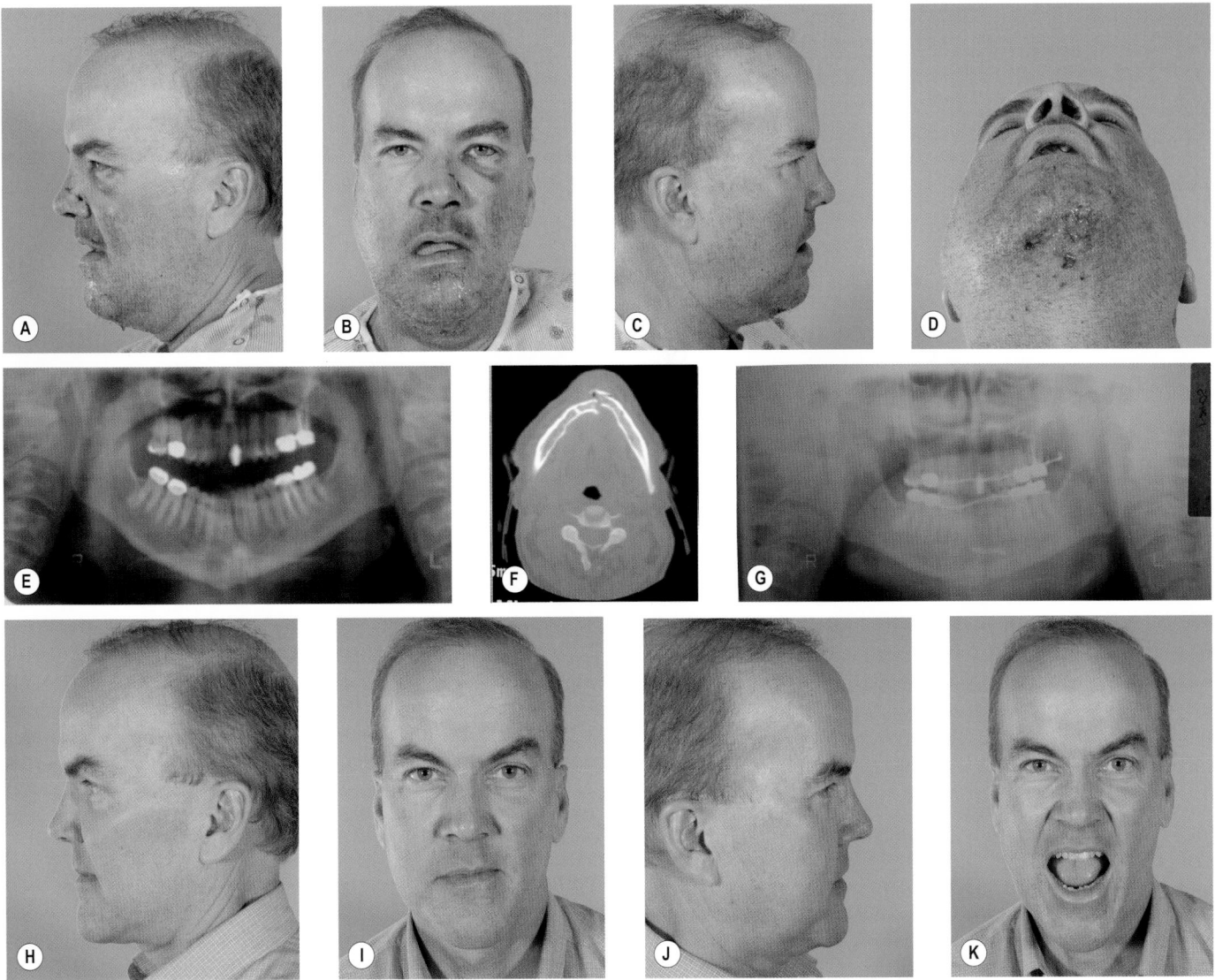

Fig. 8.15 This 51-year-old man fell from a height, resulting in left orbitozygomatic, mandibular symphysis, and right mandibular condyle fractures **(A–D)**. His panorex and computed tomography scan are shown, displaying his mandibular fractures **(E, F)**. He was treated with open reduction and rigid internal fixation with miniplates of the symphyseal fracture, reduction of the condylar fracture with intermaxillary fixation, and open reduction and rigid internal fixation of the left orbital zygomatic fracture with an iliac bone graft and miniplates. His postoperative panorex shows reduction of the fractures **(G)**. Intermaxillary fixation was removed after 2 weeks and the patient had normal facial height, class II occlusion, and excellent range of motion **(H–K)**.

Displaced fractures of the mandibular symphysis, body, or ascending angle are usually associated with malocclusion and require treatment with open reduction and internal fixation. In 1976, Spiessl[58] described the concept of the "tension band" in the treatment of displaced mandibular fractures. He described the use of one fixed point of osteosynthesis as a fulcrum in order to achieve greater compression of the bone fragments and therefore more stability and primary bone healing. Two levels of fixation, along the upper and lower border of the mandible, are required. In the nontooth-bearing regions (ascending ramus and angle), two plates may be used. In the tooth-bearing regions, an arch bar will provide stability for the upper border and a plate may be used along the lower border. In the symphysis and parasymphyseal regions, two plates can be placed in the space below the roots of the incisors and the lower border *(Fig. 8.15)*. Miniplates can be used

with this approach, unless there have been significant comminution and fragmentation of the mandible. In such cases, larger mandibular plates are required. When significant loss of mandibular substance occurs, a large reconstruction plate is necessary.

The edentulous state results in loss of alveolar bone, leaving a mandible that can be 1 cm or less in vertical height along the body. The thickness of the symphysis and structure of the vertical ramus change little, which accounts for the majority of fractures in edentulous mandibles occurring at the parasymphyseal area and body. These patients may have difficulty with fracture healing even with the use of rigid fixation, due to lack of bone stock. In select cases, primary bone grafting should be done to reinforce the fracture site.

Much debate remains as to the treatment of condylar fractures. In children under 12 years of age, no operative

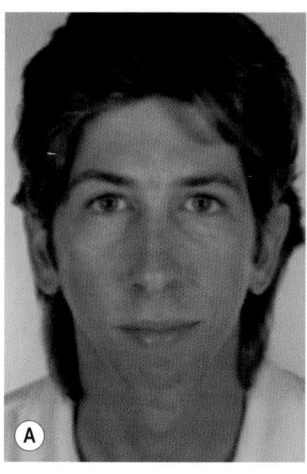 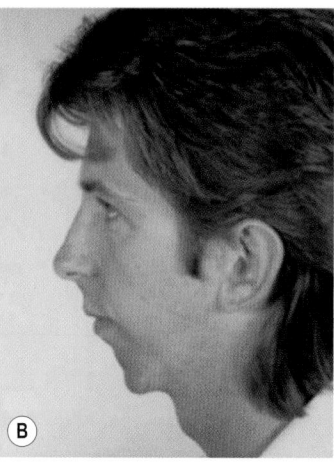 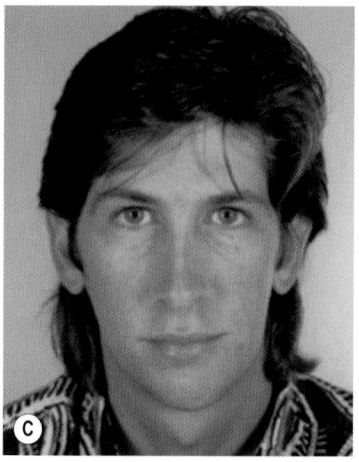 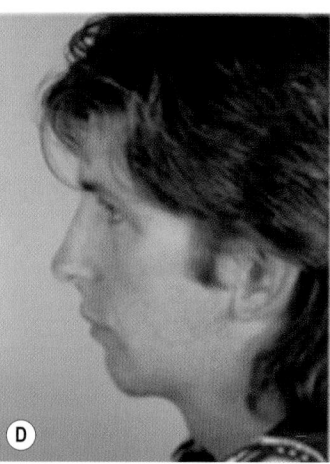

Fig. 8.16 This 30-year-old man had had five different chin implants **(A, B)**, the last one being a long "wrap-around" model placed below the lower border of his mandible. As with the others, he was displeased with the result of this one. He is shown after removal of the implant and a "jumping genioplasty" **(C, D)**. If he wished further projection of the chin, after an interval of 6 months or so, a sliding advancement genioplasty could be done through the previous genioplasty. Chin implants are appropriate for mild degrees of retrogenia, but severe retrogenia, chins requiring vertical or lateral alteration, and failures of previous chin implants should be treated with osseous genioplasties.

treatment is almost always indicated due to the tremendous potential of the condoyle to remodel and regenerate.[59,60] In teenagers and adults definite indications for operative treatment include the following: displacement of the condyle in the middle cranial fossa, bilateral fractures with an anterior open bite, multiple other maxillary and mandibular fractures where mandibular stability is important to maintaining facial height, and the situation in which the patient cannot be brought into occlusion with less invasive measures. If the patient has sustained a subcondylar fracture with the condyle in the glenoid fossa and no malocclusion, treatment consists of application of arch bars with elastics or wire fixation, soft diet, and occlusal splint for 4–6 weeks, followed by aggressive physical therapy. If, however, the condyle is out of the fossa, the debate continues as to whether open or closed treatment is best.

Mandibular reconstruction

In-continuity defects of the mandible less than 3–4 cm in length covered by healthy soft tissue can be corrected with free bone grafts[61,62] (iliac[63] and cranial[64] represent the bone grafts of choice) and rigid fixation with miniplates. An adequate amount should be present (20 mm or more) in the vertical dimension in tooth-bearing areas for placement of osseointegrated implants. If defects involve the alveolus alone, either in the maxilla or in the mandible, getting enough bone for implants to take as a free graft may be difficult. If enough bone is present to permit a horizontal osteotomy, distraction osteogenesis will provide the best result because the gingiva will come up with the distracted bone and one can easily overcorrect the bone defect. Overcorrection may cause premature contact at the apex of the (now overcorrected) deficiency, with overeruption of the posterior molar teeth.

Although in-continuity defects of the mandible longer than 5 cm can be dealt with by free nonvascularized bone grafts,[65] these larger defects are better corrected with microvascular transplantation of osseous flaps, particularly when the overlying soft tissues are less than optimal in condition or have been irradiated. The fibular free flap is ideal for longer defects because it can be repeatedly osteotomized and bent to any desired shape, and the iliac free flap is well suited for anterior defects. The lesser amount of bone available in the radial forearm and scapular free flaps makes them less desirable choices.

Chin

The most common reason for osseous procedures on the chin for acquired deformities has been an unfortunate outcome from a chin implant. Many of the patients have indeed had a number of chin implants, with removal, replacement, and often removal again, for reasons of infection and displacement.[66] Under these circumstances, an osseous genioplasty[67] should be performed,[68–70] rather than trying again with an alloplastic material. The capsule that forms around the implant should be removed to allow the osseous expansion to keep the soft-tissue envelope properly stretched. In some patients, a proper diagnosis had not been made in the first place, and the corrective procedure may need to provide proper correction of the original deformity, such as lengthening the chin for a congenital shortness *(Fig. 8.16)*. Rarely, if the chin has had many previous operations and there is not adequate bone stock for an osseous genioplasty, a microvascular osteocutaneous free flap may provide the only solution *(Fig. 8.17)*.

Postoperative care

With the exception of isolated orbital or nasal bone fractures, all patients will be placed on a liquid or soft diet for 2 weeks after surgery. Nasal splints can be removed after 1 week, and interdental fixation is usually removed within 4–6

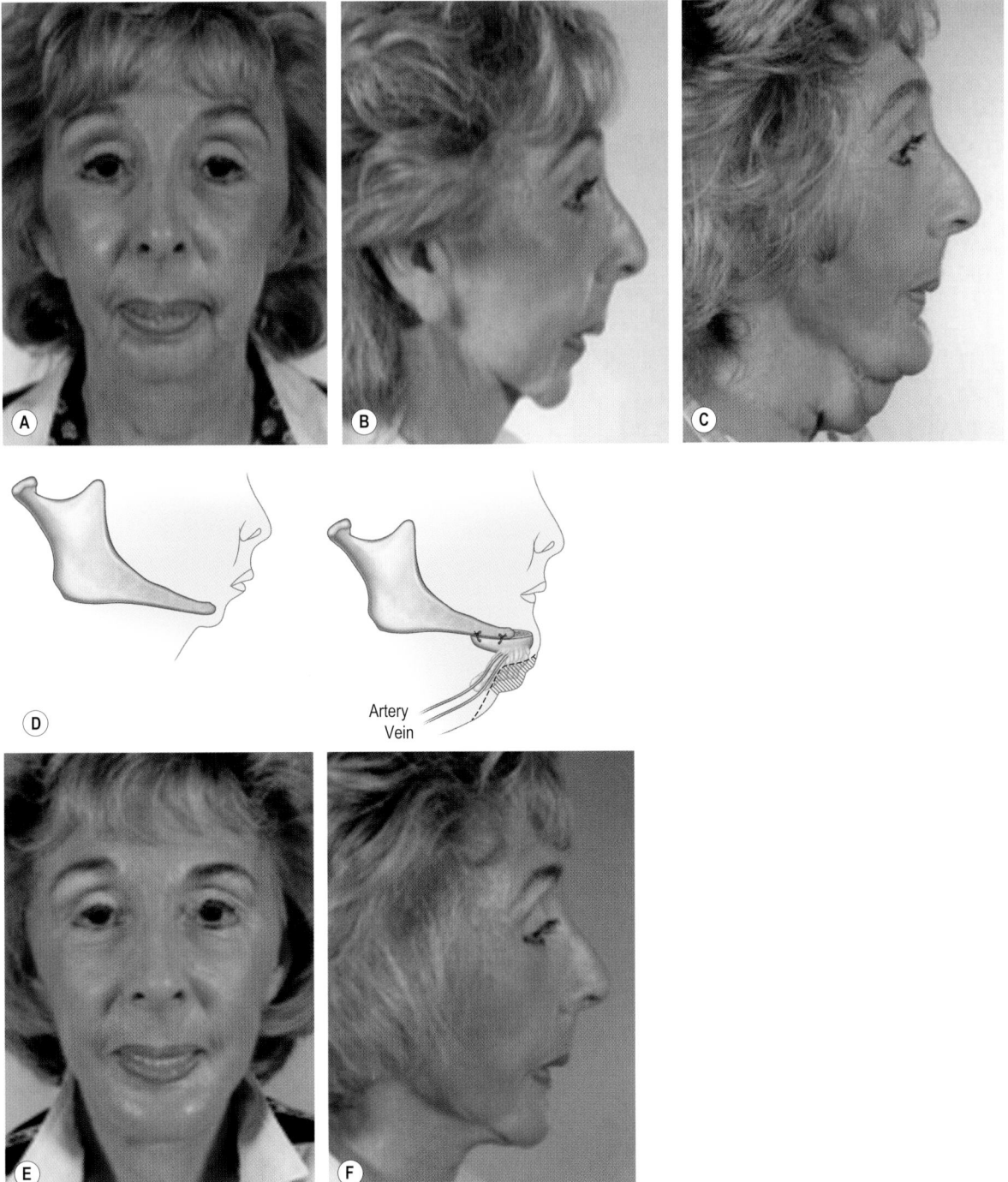

Artery
Vein

Fig. 8.17 This 67-year-old woman stated that she had undergone some sort of jaw injury as a child (perhaps condylar fractures) and had been treated, among others, by Dr. Robert Ivy in Philadelphia and Dr. Varaztad Kazanjian in Boston. In total, she had undergone more than 26 operations in attempts to construct a chin. Segments of block hydroxyapatite had been successfully placed along the mandibular body, but all of the chin implants had to be removed because of infection or intraoral exposure **(A, B)**. She had only a thin segment of bone connecting the parasymphyseal areas, and the intraoral soft tissues were thin and scarred; it was thought that they would not provide adequate coverage for any type of conventional genioplasty. After considerable explanation to the patient and her husband, the decision was made to go ahead with the only method that could most likely provide her with a chin: microsurgical reconstruction with use of an iliac osteocutaneous free flap. The U-shaped segment of iliac bone was attached to the inferior border of what remained of her native symphysis, and a skin paddle and soft-tissue attachments were transferred with the bone segment **(C)**. She is shown a month after the operation, with the skin paddle in place **(D)**, and a year after the original operation, following defatting of the pedicle and removal of the skin island **(E, F)**.

weeks. All suture material on the face should be removed within 7 days.

Outcomes, prognosis, and complications

It is advisable to obtain postoperative radiographic images to assess the adequacy of reduction achieved. If the fractures are not adequately reduced on imaging, the surgeon must plan to return the patient to the operating room for proper correction of the defects. Inadequacy of reduction of facial fractures can lead to enophthalmos, malocclusion, and loss of proper facial proportions.

Secondary procedures

If a secondary operation is required more than 1 week after the initial operation, it is best to perform osteotomies to recreate the defect. This is almost certainly to be followed by the use of bone grafts to restore facial harmony.

 Access the complete reference list online at **http://www.expertconsult.com**

9. Wolfe SA. The influence of Paul Tessier on our current treatment of facial trauma, both in primary care and in the management oflate sequelae. *Clin Plast Surg.* 1997;24:515–518.

   This article reviews the principles of facial skeletal surgery taught by Paul Tessier, the father of craniofacial surgery. His principles, such as obtaining complete subperiosteal exposure and the use of autogenous bone grafts, have withstood the test of time and remain critical for the education of all craniofacial surgeons.

11. Wolfe SA. Autogenous bone grafts versus alloplastic materials. In: Wolfe SA, Berkowitz S, eds. *Plastic Surgery of the Facial Skeleton.* Boston: Little, Brown; 1989:25–38.

14. Tessier P. The conjunctival approach to the orbital floor and maxilla in congenital malformation and trauma. *J Maxillofac Surg.* 1973;1:3.

31. Wolfe SA. Lengthening the nose: a lesson from craniofacial surgery applied to post-traumatic and congenital deformities. *Plast Reconstr Surg.* 1994;94:78.

   This article describes a variety of causes of nasal hypoplasias, from traumatic to congenital and the author's treatment strategies. The article stresses the liberal use of bone and cartilage grafts in rebuilding the nose.

32. Millard DR Jr. Reconstructive rhinoplasty. In: Millard DR Jr. *A Rhinoplasty Tetralogy.* Boston: Little, Brown; 1996:482–490.

36. Wolfe SA. Application of craniofacial surgical precepts in orbital reconstruction following trauma and tumor removal. *J Maxillofac Surg.* 1982;10:212.

   This article describes the principles of craniofacial surgery, as described by Paul Tessier, in working with the orbit and their application to management of the reconstructive or trauma patient. These include the use of subperiosteal exposure and liberal use of autogenous bone grafts when reconstruction of the floor is necessary to prevent enopthalmos.

40. Manson PN, Hoopes JE, Su CT. Structural pillars of the facial skeleton: an approach to the management of Le Fort fractures. *Plast Reconstr Surg.* 1980;66:54.

   This landmark article describes the facial buttresses and their relationship to facial structure. It describes the importance of these relationships in treating Le Fort fractures.

48. Gruss JS, Mackinnon SE. Complex maxillary fractures: role of buttress reconstruction and immediate bone grafts. *Plast Reconstr Surg.* 1986;78:9.

49. Wolfe SA, Baker S. Fractures of the Maxilla. In: Wolfe SA, Baker S, eds. *Operative Techniques in Plastic Surgery: Facial Fractures.* New York: Thieme Medical Publishers; 1993:61–71.

70. Cohen SR, Mardach OL, Kawamoto HK Jr. Chin disfigurement following removal of alloplastic chin implants. *Plast Reconstr Surg.* 1991;88:62, discussion 67.

   This article describes the risks involved with the use of alloplastic chin implants, particularly the associated changes in the mandible. It advocates the use of the osseous genioplasty.

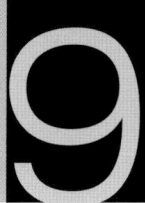

Midface reconstruction

Constance M. Chen, Joseph J. Disa, and Peter G. Cordeiro

SYNOPSIS

Reconstructive goals of midface defects:

- Wound closure.
- Restore barrier between sinonasal cavity and anterior cranial fossa.
- Separation oral and sinonasal cavities.
- Support orbital contents/maintenance of ocular globe position.
- Oral continence.
- Speech.
- Mastication.
- Avoidance ectropion.
- Maintenance patent nasal airway.
- Facial appearance: symmetry, contour, scars, eyelid position.

Access the Historical Perspective section online at
http://www.expertconsult.com

Introduction

Reconstruction of the midface is best approached through a clear understanding of the complex three-dimensional anatomy of the maxilla.[1] In the most basic terms, the maxilla may be thought of as a six-walled geometric box that includes the roof, which is made up by the orbital floor; the floor of the box, which is made up by each half of the anterior hard palate and alveolar ridge; and the medial wall of the box, which form the lateral walls of the nasal passage *(Fig. 9.1)*. The maxillary antrum is contained within the central portion of the maxilla. The cranial base overlies the posterior pterygoid region of the maxilla. The two horizontal and three vertical buttresses produce facial width, height, and projection. The overlying soft tissues, including the muscles of facial expression and mastication, insert on the maxilla and are responsible for individual facial appearance and function.

The goals of reconstruction are functional and aesthetic. Most extensive midface defects require free flaps for reconstruction, with the flap selection dependent on the amount of resected skin, soft tissue, and bone.[2–7] Small volume defects can be reconstructed with radial forearm fasciocutaneous or osseocutaneous flaps.[5,8] Large volume defects can be filled by a rectus abdominis myocutaneous flap.[7,9] Currently, complex structures such as lips, eyelids, and the nose should be reconstructed separately, usually with local flaps, without incorporating free tissue transfer.[10–14] By following an algorithm based on a clearly delineated classification system of midfacial defects, even patients with very large, complex defects can be restored to good function *(Fig. 9.2)*.[1,15]

The goal of midface reconstruction is not necessarily to reconstruct all the walls of the maxilla that have been resected. Rather, successful midface reconstruction should accomplish the following:

1. Close the wound
2. Obliterate the maxillectomy defect
3. Support the globe if preserved or fill the orbital cavity if the globe is exenterated
4. Maintain a barrier between the nasal sinuses and the anterior cranial fossa
5. Restore facial shape
6. Reconstruct the palate.

Basic science/disease process

Midface reconstruction related to oncologic surgery is most commonly needed after removal of a squamous cell carcinoma of the oral cavity or sinonasal mucosa. Removal of minor salivary tumors and adenocarcinoma, among others, can also result in defects requiring orbitomaxillary reconstruction. Midface reconstruction can also be required following high-energy trauma and often is concurrent with reconstruction of other craniofacial injuries.

Diagnosis/patient presentation

The algorithm we use to reconstruct complex midface defects is based on the extent to which the maxillary bone has been resected. Once the bony defect is assessed, we address the soft-tissue defects, including skin, muscle, palate, and mucosal lining of the cheek. Finally, important structures such as the palate, oral commissure, nasal airway, and eyelids are dealt with in an attempt to restore function.

Type I: limited maxillectomy defects

Type I, or partial, maxillectomy defects are those that involve one or two walls of the maxilla, most commonly the anterior and medial walls *(Fig. 9.3)*. Both the palate and the orbital floor are intact. The resection will often include the soft tissue and skin of the cheek, and even the lips, nose, and eyelids. Occasionally, the orbital rim will be resected and non-vascularized bone grafts will be necessary for reconstruction. Type I maxillectomy defects are small-volume deficiencies with large surface area requirements, often needing one or two skin islands. Our flap of choice is the radial forearm free flap, as it provides good external skin coverage and minimal bulk while allowing multiple skin islands that can be de-epithelialized to improve contour, wrap around bone grafts, and supply lining for the nasal cavity *(Fig. 9.4)*.

Type II: subtotal maxillectomy defects

Type II, or subtotal, maxillectomies are those that involve resection of the lower five walls of the maxilla, including the palate, but leaves the orbital floor intact *(Fig. 9.5)*. These defects may be further subdivided into type IIA defects, which include <50% of the transverse palate, or type IIB defects, which include >50% of the transverse palate and/or the anterior arch of the maxilla. Both type IIA and type IIB maxillectomy defects are moderate-volume deficiencies with large surface area requirements, which usually need one skin island.

For type IIA defects, which involve <50% of the transverse palate, reconstruction may proceed with either a microvascular free flap or a skin graft and an obturator, depending on patient and surgeon preference. If a free flap is selected to avoid the inconvenience and maintenance of a palatal obturator, our flap of choice is the radial forearm fasciocutaneous free flap *(Fig. 9.6)*. The skin inset is critical, and the skin paddle must be equal to or smaller than the original defect to

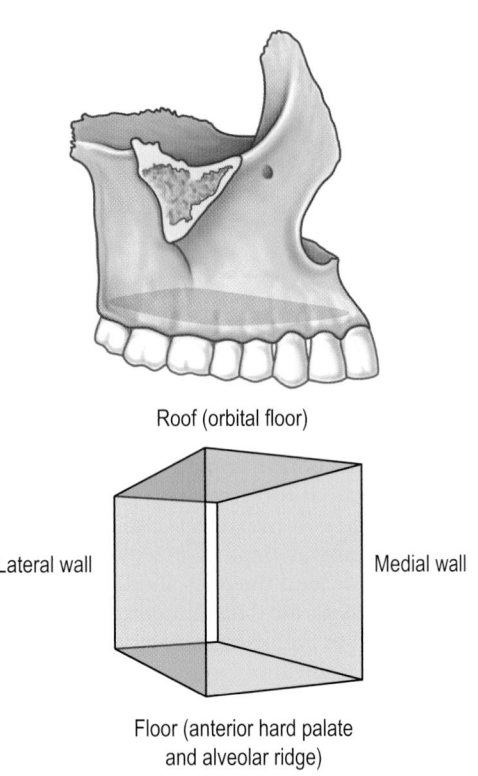

Roof (orbital floor)

Lateral wall

Medial wall

Floor (anterior hard palate and alveolar ridge)

Fig. 9.1 The maxilla may be thought of as a six-walled geometric box that includes the roof, which is made up by the orbital floor; the floor of the box, which is made up by each half of the anterior hard palate and alveolar ridge; and the medial wall of the box, which form the lateral walls of the nasal passage.

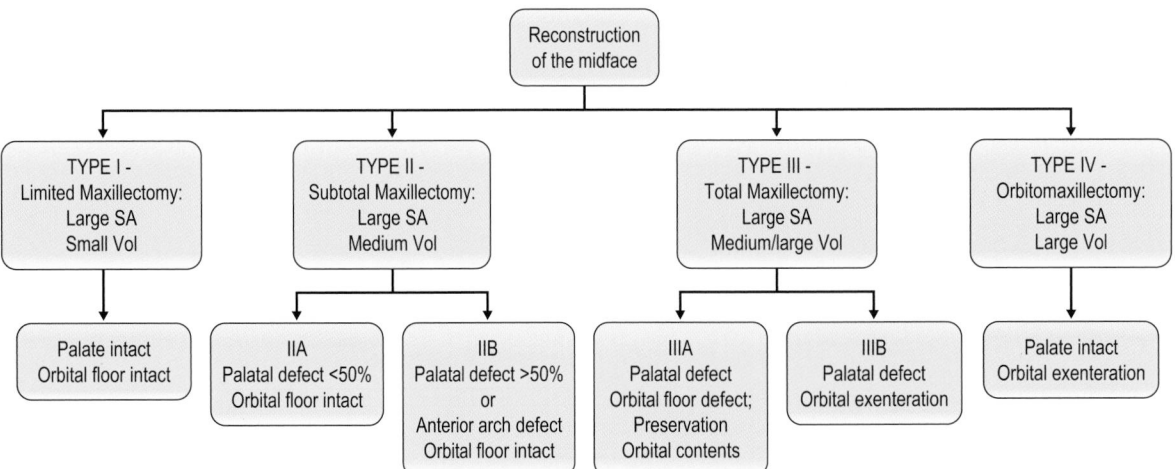

Fig. 9.2 By following an algorithm based on a clearly delineated classification system of midfacial defects, even patients with very large, complex defects can be restored to good function.

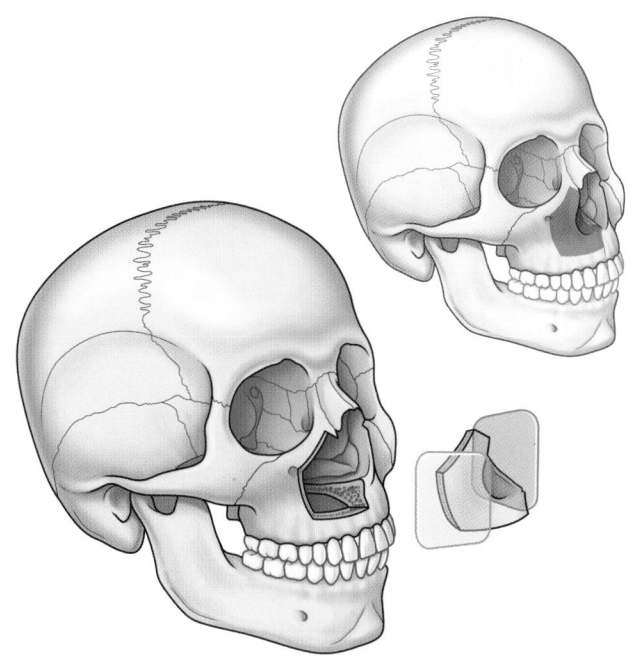

Fig. 9.3 Type I, or partial, maxillectomy defects are those that involve one or two walls of the maxilla, most commonly the anterior and medial walls.

keep the soft palate taut and recreate the buccal sulcus. Without a taut inset, the skin paddle can prolapse into the oral cavity. If adequate teeth or bone stock remain, dentures or even osseointegrated dental implants may be used.

For type IIB defects, which involve >50% of the transverse palate or a significant portion of the anterior arch, an osteocutaneous free flap is needed. These defects require bone for structural support as well as skin lining of the neopalate and nasal floor. A prosthesis is inadequate, because bone is needed to provide support to the upper lip. Our flap of choice is the radial forearm osteocutaneous "sandwich" flap *(Fig. 9.7)*.[8] The bone segment can be shaped to recreate the maxillary alveolar arch and support the upper lip, and the thin pliable skin can be wrapped around the bone like a sandwich to replace the lining of the palate and nose. If adequate bone is harvested, osseointegrated dental implants or conventional dentures may also be used to recreate teeth.

Type III: total maxillectomy defects

Type III defects are total maxillectomies that involve resection of all six walls of the maxilla. Type III defects can be further subdivided into resections that exclude (type IIIA) or include (type IIIB) the orbital contents. Both type IIIA and type IIIB

maxillectomy defects are moderate-to-large-volume deficiencies with large surface area requirements, which usually need at least one skin island.

For type IIIA defects, which involve resection of all six walls of the maxilla, including the palate and orbital floor, but preserves the orbital contents *(Fig. 9.8)*, a bone graft is needed to reconstruct the orbital floor and a free flap with one or more skin paddles is needed to recreate the palate, nasal lining and/or the cheek. The goals are to support the globe, obliterate any communication between the orbit and nasopharynx, and reconstruct the palatal surface. For bony support, we have used split calvarium, iliac crest or less commonly, split ribs, to reconstruct both the maxillary prominence and the orbital floor. For mucosal and skin lining, our flap of choice is the rectus abdominis myocutaneous flap, which may be wrapped around the bone graft to separate the orbital contents from the oral cavity *(Fig. 9.9A)*. The bulk of the rectus can also fill the dead space of the antrum and use of this can provide a water-tight closure of the palate. In patients who are not candidates for free tissue transfer, a temporalis flap may be used to cover the orbital floor bone graft and provide some volume to fill the midfacial defect *(Fig. 9.9B)*. Reconstruction with a temporalis flap, however, requires simultaneous use of a palatal obturator.

Type IIIA defect reconstructive goals:
- Support the globe
- Obliterate any communication between the orbit and nasopharynx
- Reconstruct the palatal surface.

The type IIIB defect, which involves resection of the entire maxilla including the orbital contents, is also known as an extended maxillectomy *(Fig. 9.10)*. The reconstructive goal of these extensive, large-volume defects is to close the palate, restore the nasal lining, and reconstruct the eyelids, cheek, and lip as necessary. If the anterior cranial base is exposed, the brain must also be covered. Our flap of choice is a rectus abdominis myocutaneous free flap with one or more skin islands used to recreate the palate, lateral nasal wall, and any cutaneous deficits *(Figs 9.11, 9.12)*. The latissimus dorsi flap may also provide adequate soft tissue bulk and pedicle length, but it is not as versatile with regard to providing multiple skin island coverage.

Type IV: orbitomaxillectomy defects

Type IV defects involve resection of the upper five walls of the maxilla and will usually include resection of the orbital contents, leaving the dura and brain exposed; the palate is usually left intact *(Fig. 9.13)*. These are large-volume defects with large surface area requirements. Our flap of choice is the rectus abdominis flap, with one or more skin islands used for external skin and/or nasal lining *(Fig. 9.14)*.

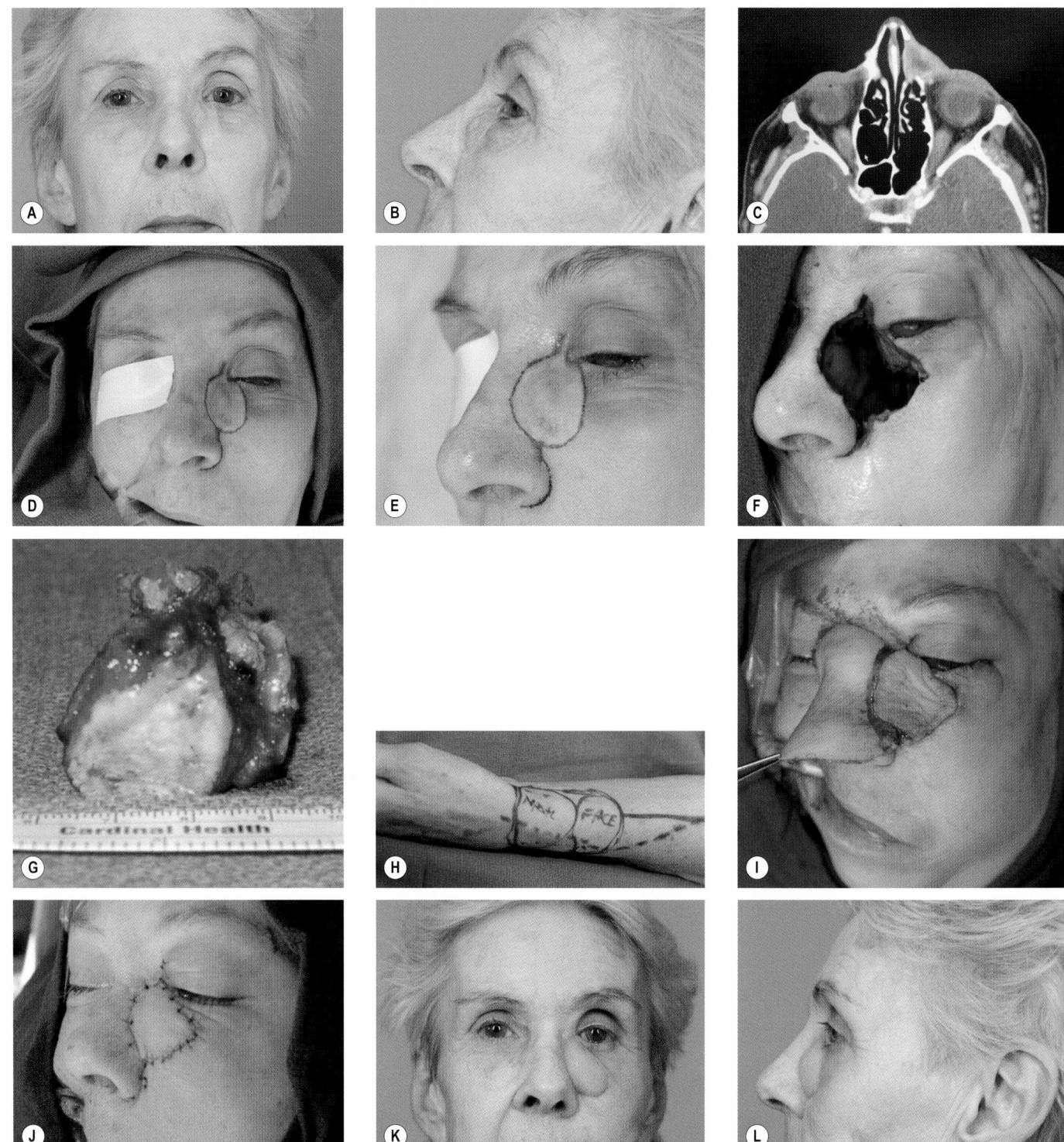

Fig. 9.4 For type I defects, our flap of choice is the radial forearm free flap, as it provides good external skin coverage and minimal bulk while allowing multiple skin islands that can be de-epithelialized to improve contour, wrap around bone grafts, and supply lining for the nasal cavity. **(A)** Type I maxillectomy defect prior to flap coverage – AP view. **(B)** Type I maxillectomy defect prior to flap coverage – lateral view. **(C)** Preoperative CT scan – axial view. **(D)** Preoperative marking – AP view. **(E)** Preoperative marking lateral view. **(F)** Type I defect – intraoperative view. **(G)** Type I defect – resection specimen. **(H)** Radial forearm free flap with two skin islands used to resurface medial nasal wall and anterior cheek. **(I)** Insetting radial forearm free flap with two skin islands for type I defect. **(J)** Radial forearm free flap inset into type I defect. **(K)** Type I defect – postoperative results after radial forearm free flap – AP view. **(L)** Type I defect – postoperative results after radial forearm free flap – lateral view.

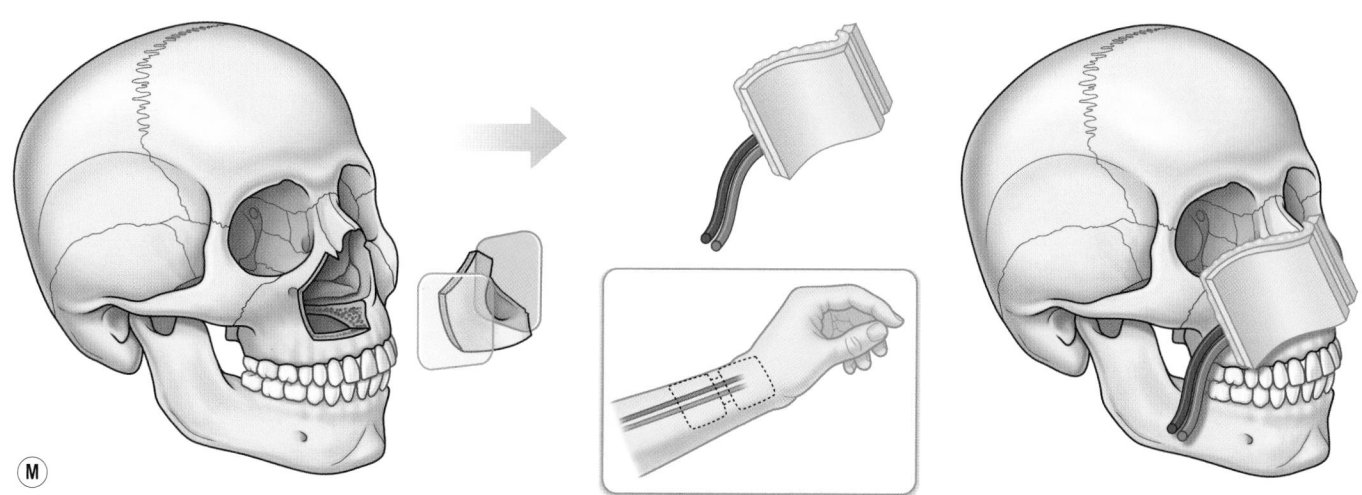

Fig. 9.4, cont'd (M) The radial forearm free flap, provides good external skin coverage and minimal bulk while allowing multiple skin islands that can be de-epithelialized to improve contour, wrap around bone grafts, and supply lining for the nasal cavity.

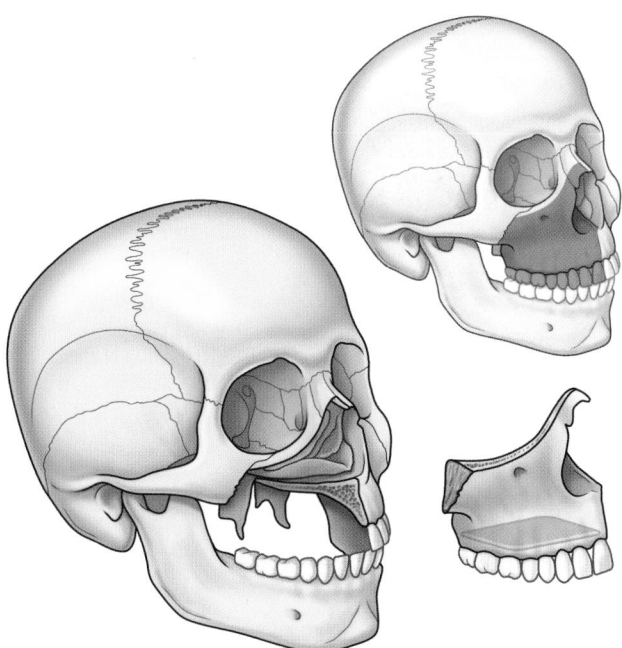

Fig. 9.5 Type II, or subtotal, maxillectomies are those that involve resection of the lower five walls of the maxilla, including the palate, but leaves the orbital floor intact.

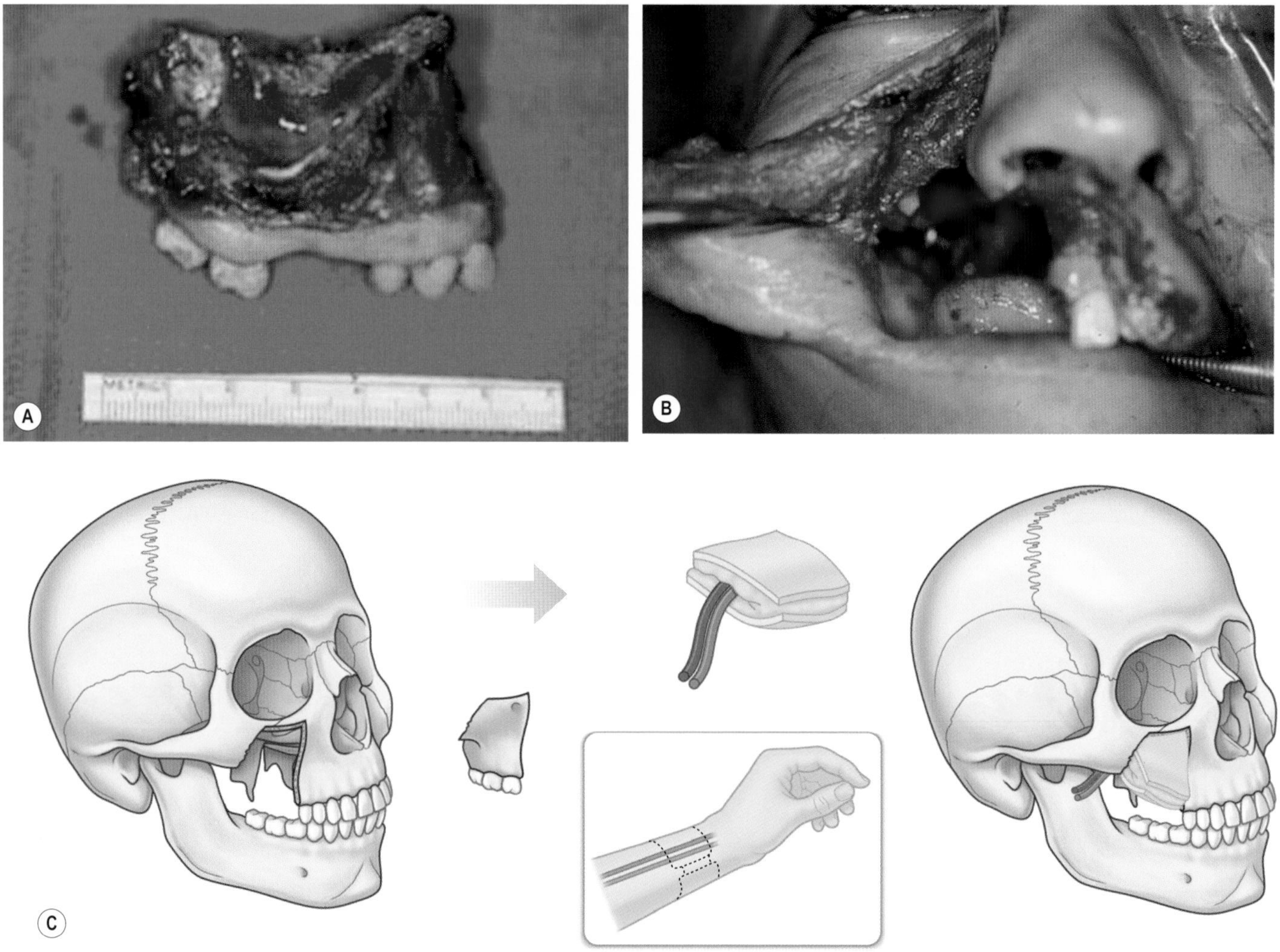

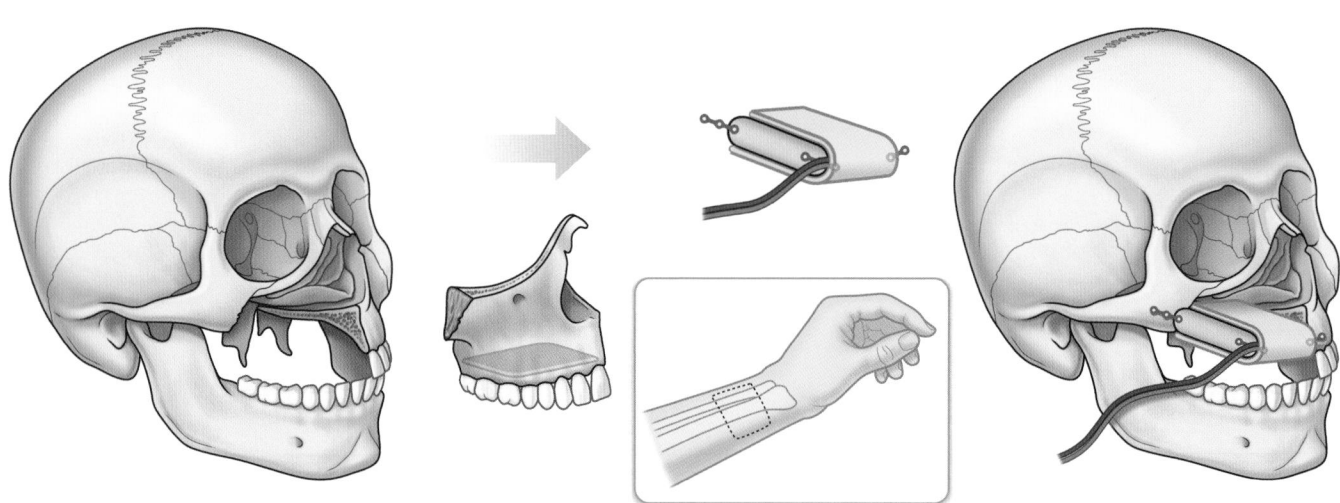

Fig. 9.6 (A) For Type IIA defects, which involve <50% of the transverse palate, reconstruction may proceed with either a microvascular free flap or a skin graft and an obturator, depending on patient and surgeon preference. If a free flap is selected to avoid the inconvenience and maintenance of a palatal obturator, our flap of choice is the radial forearm fasciocutaneous free flap. **(B)** Type II resection specimen and intraoperative defect. **(C)** Type II resection specimen and intraoperative defect.

Fig. 9.7 For type IIB defects, which involve >50% of the transverse palate or a significant portion of the anterior arch, an osteocutaneous free flap is needed. These defects require bone for structural support as well as skin lining of the neopalate and nasal floor. A prosthesis is inadequate, because bone is needed to provide support to the upper lip. Our flap of choice is the radial forearm osteocutaneous "sandwich" flap.

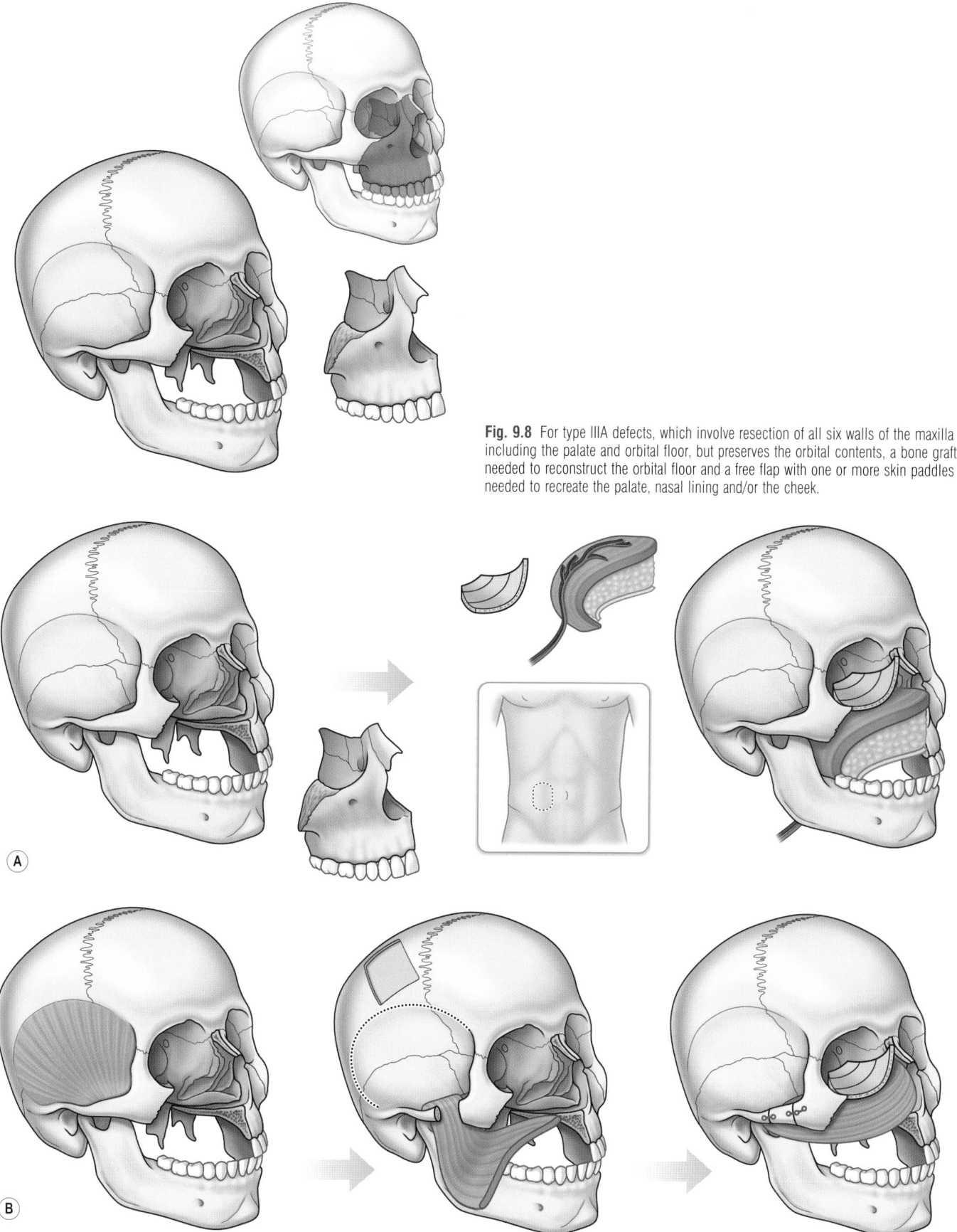

Fig. 9.8 For type IIIA defects, which involve resection of all six walls of the maxilla including the palate and orbital floor, but preserves the orbital contents, a bone graft is needed to reconstruct the orbital floor and a free flap with one or more skin paddles is needed to recreate the palate, nasal lining and/or the cheek.

(A)

(B)

Fig. 9.9 Type IIIA defect reconstructed with bone graft for floor of orbit. **(A)** Rectus abdominus free flap for closure of palate and coverage of bone graft. **(B)** Temporalis flap for coverage of bone graft.

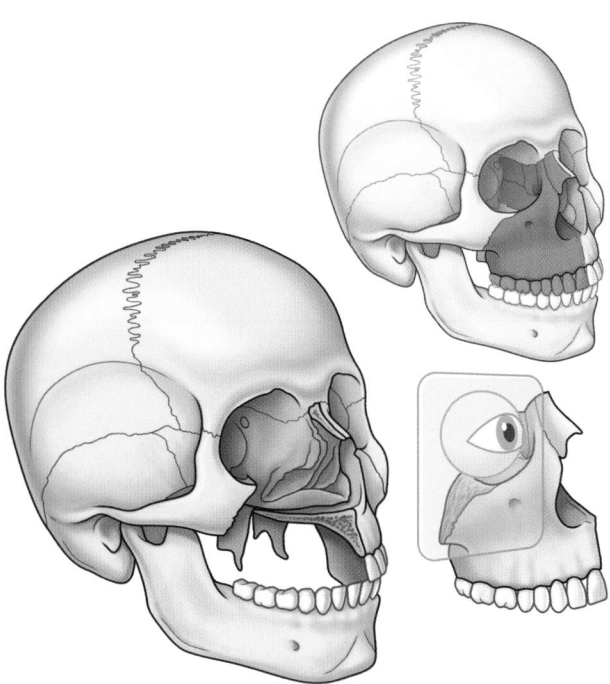

Fig. 9.10 The type IIIB defect, which involves resection of the entire maxilla including the orbital contents, is also known as an extended maxillectomy.

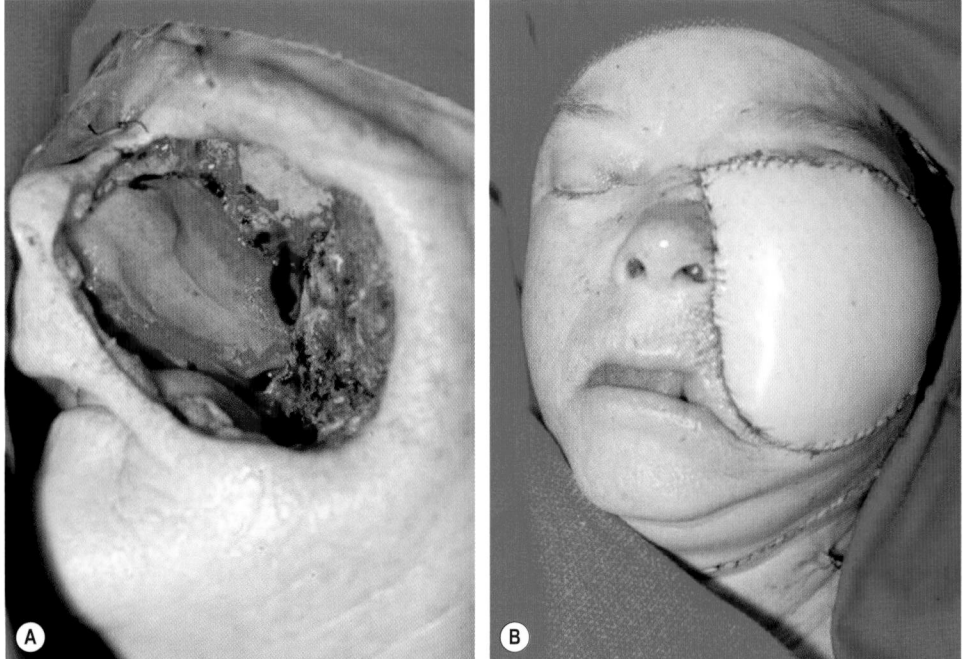

Fig. 9.11 Type IIIB defects involve resection of the upper five walls of the maxilla and will usually include resection of the orbital contents, leaving the dura and brain exposed. The palate is usually left intact. **(A)** Intraoperative photograph of type IIIB maxillectomy defect. **(B)** Postoperative photograph of type IIIB maxillectomy defect.

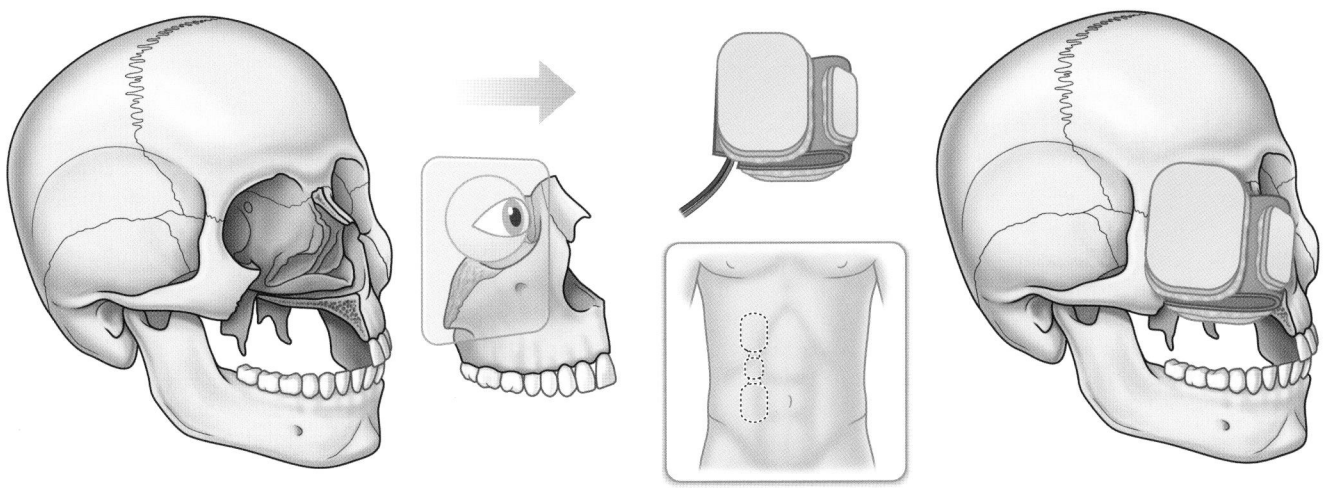

Fig. 9.12 For type IIIB defects, our flap of choice is a rectus abdominis myocutaneous free flap with one or more skin islands used to recreate the palate, lateral nasal wall, and any cutaneous deficits.

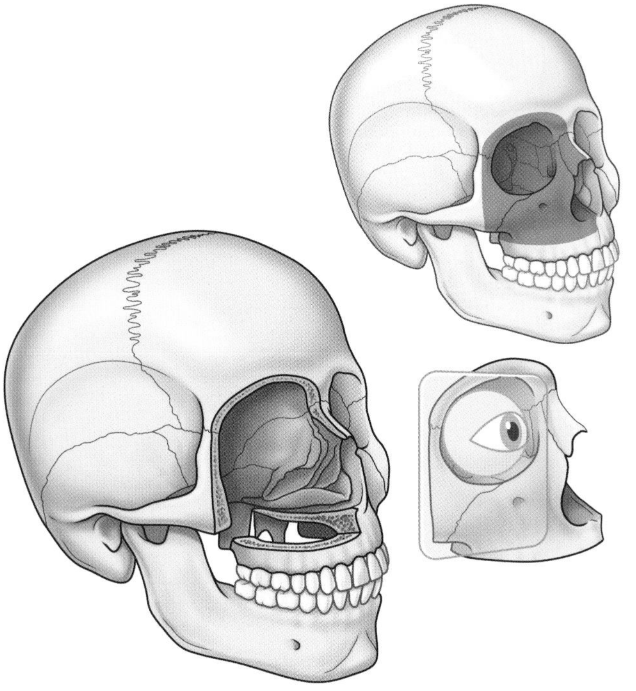

Fig. 9.13 A type IV or orbitomaxillectomy defect involves loss of the orbital contents and upper walls of the maxilla, leaving the palate intact.

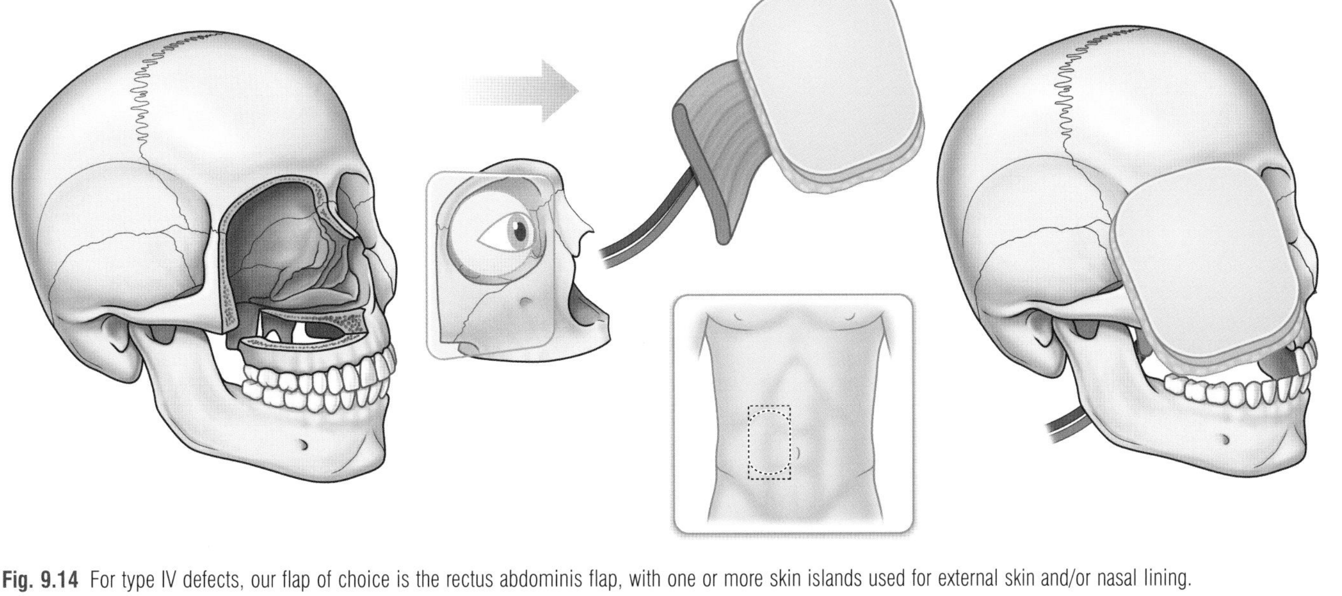

Fig. 9.14 For type IV defects, our flap of choice is the rectus abdominis flap, with one or more skin islands used for external skin and/or nasal lining.

Functional and aesthetic outcomes

Speech

In 44 patients who underwent resection of the palate, speech was rated as normal in 22 patients (50%), near normal in 15 patients (34.1%), intelligible in six patients (13.6%), and unintelligible in one patient (2.3%). Speech results by maxillectomy classification are presented in *Table 9.1*.

Diet

After midface reconstruction with palatal resection, 26 patients (52%) were able to eat an unrestricted diet, 21 patients (42%) could manage a soft diet, three patients (6%) were only able to tolerate liquids, and one patient (2%) required tube feeding *(Table 9.1)*.

Globe position and function

Of the 42 patients who underwent resection of the orbital floor with preservation of the orbital contents, 21 patients

Table 9.1 Functional and aesthetic outcomes

Maxillectomy defect	Type I (n = 20)	Type IIA (n = 8)	Type IIB (n = 8)	Type IIIA (n = 22)	Type IIIB (n = 23)	Type IV (n = 19)	Total (n = 100)
Speech	N/A = 18	N/A = 2	N/A = 3	N/A = 8	N/A = 8	N/A = 17	n = 44
Normal	2	3	2	8	5	2	22 (50%)
Near normal		2	1	5	7		15 (34.1%)
Intelligible		1	2	1	2		6 (13.6%)
Unintelligible					1		1 (2.3%)
Diet	N/A = 18	N/A = 1		N/A = 6	N/A = 7	N/A = 17	n = 50
Unrestricted	1	4	3	9	7	2	26 (52%)
Soft		3	4	7	7		21 (42%)
Liquids			1		2		3 (6%)
Feeding tube	1						1 (2%)
Eyeglobe position and function	N/A = 16	N/A = 8	N/A = 8	N/A = 4	N/A = 23	N/A = 19	n = 21
Normal	1			4			5 (23.8%)
Dystopia				1			1 (4.8%)
Diplopia				4			4 (19%)
Enophthalmos	1						1 (4.8%)
Ectropion	1			9			10 (47.6%)
Mild				4			4 (19%)
Moderate				3			3 (14.3%)
Severe	1			2			3 (14.3%)
Oral competence	N/A = 20	N/A = 6	N/A = 6	N/A = 21	N/A = 17	N/A = 18	n = 12
Yes		2	2	1	5	1	11 (91.7%)
No					1		1 (8.3%)
Microstomia	N/A = 20	N/A = 6	N/A = 6	N/A = 21	N/A = 21	N/A = 14	n = 12
Yes			1		1	1	3 (25%)
No		2	1	1	1	4	9 (75%)
Aesthetic result	N/A = 8	N/A = 1		N/A = 5	N/A = 9	N/A = 7	n = 70
Excellent	6	6	5	12	5	7	41 (58.6%)
Good	5	1	1	4	9	5	25 (35.7%)
Fair	1		2	1			4 (5.7%)
Poor							0 (0%)

were assessed. All patients maintained vision. Mild vertical dystopia developed in one patient (4.8%), but no treatment was necessary. Mild horizontal diplopia developed in four patients (19%), which did not cause functional problems. Enophthalmos developed in one patient (4.8%). Lower eyelid ectropion developed in 10 patients (47.6%), which was rated as mild in four patients (19%), moderate in three patients (14.3%), and severe in three patients (14.3%). None of the patients with ectropion underwent additional procedures *(Table 9.1)*.

Oral competence

Of the 12 patients who underwent resection and reconstruction of the oral commissure, 11 patients (91.7%) had good to excellent oral competence within 1 month postoperatively. After radiation therapy, three patients (25%) developed mild microstomia. No treatment was needed. Oral competence is described in *Table 9.1*.

Aesthetic results

Out of 70 patients who underwent evaluation of aesthetic outcomes, 41 patients had aesthetic results that were judged as excellent (58.6%), 25 patients had results judged as good (35.7%), and four patients had results judged as fair (5.7%). Although none of the patients were rated with poor results,

it was most difficult to obtain a positive aesthetic result in patients who underwent skin, eyelid, or lip resections. Aesthetic results by maxillectomy classification are detailed in *Table 9.1*.

Conclusions

Each type of maxillectomy defect has specific skin, soft tissue, and bony requirements. For complex maxillectomy defects, free-tissue transfer offers the most effective and reliable form of reconstruction. In particular, rectus abdominis and radial forearm free flaps in combination with immediate bone grafting or as osteocutaneous flaps consistently provide the best aesthetic and functional results. For small to medium volume defects with large surface area requirements, a radial forearm fasciocutaneous or osteocutaneous flap is best. For larger volume defects with medium to large surface area requirements, a rectus abdominis free flap works well. In total maxillectomy defects, soft tissue flaps can also be combined with bone grafts for orbital floor reconstruction.

By classifying midfacial defects based on the extent of maxilla that is resected, we have developed a concise algorithm for midface reconstruction. This algorithm is based on a clearly delineated anatomical classification of maxillectomy defects, and it results in a method of midface reconstruction that leads to consistently reliable and effective results.

Access the complete references list online at **http://www.expertconsult.com**

3. Wells MD, Luce EA. Reconstruction of midfacial defects after surgical resection of malignancies. *Clin Plast Surg.* 1995;22(1):79–89.

   Oncologic resections of the midface generate devastating deformities. Local reconstructions are preferred when sufficient support is available for osseointegrated implants; otherwise, osteocutaneous tissue transfer should be considered.

4. Foster RD, Anthony JP, Singer MI, et al. Reconstruction of complex midfacial defects. *Plast Reconstr Surg.* 1997;99(6):1555–1565.

   A series of 26 consecutive midface reconstructions over 5 years was assessed. An algorithm for free flap selection in this setting is advanced based on this experience.

6. Dalgorf D, Higgins K. Reconstruction of the midface and maxilla. *Curr Opin Otolaryngol Head Neck Surg.* 2008;16(4):303–311.

7. Zhang B, Li DZ, Xu ZG, et al. Deep inferior epigastric artery perforator free flaps in head and neck reconstruction. *Oral Oncol.* 2009;45(2):116–120.

   The DIEP flap is described as a reliable means of head and neck reconstruction with reduced donor site morbidity.

8. Cordeiro PG, Bacilious N, Schantz S, et al. The radial forearm osteocutaneous "sandwich" free flap for

reconstruction of the bilateral subtotal maxillectomy defect. *Ann Plast Surg.* 1998;40(4):397–402.

   Advantages of the osteocutaneous radial forearm free flap in maxillary reconstruction are discussed. "Sandwiching" the osseous component between the skin paddles provides for nasal and palatal lining as well as support for osteointegrated implants.

10. Cordeiro PG, Disa JJ. Challenges in midface reconstruction. *Semin Surg Oncol.* 2000;19(3):218–225.

12. Kusumoto K, Kakudo N, Ogawa Y. Success of the orbicularis oculi myocutaneous vertical V-Y advancement flap for upper eyelid reconstruction. *Plast Reconstr Surg.* 2009;123(1):423–424.

13. Herford AS, Cicciu M, Clark A. Traumatic eyelid defects: a review of reconstructive options. *J Oral Maxillofac Surg.* 2009;67(1):3–9.

15. Cordeiro PG, Santamaria E. A classification system and algorithm for reconstruction of maxillectomy and midfacial defects. *Plast Reconstr Surg.* 2000;105(7):2331–2346.

   Maxillary defects are classified, based on a series of 60 patients presenting for reconstruction after oncologic resection. Free flap selection is discussed in this context.

10

Cheek and lip reconstruction

Peter C. Neligan

SYNOPSIS

Lip reconstruction

- Accurate three-layered closure of lip defects is imperative to preserve function.
- Local tissue should be used whenever possible.
- Small defects can be closed by direct repair:
  - defects up to 25% of the width of the upper lip can be closed; and
  - defects up to 30% of the width of the lower lip can be closed.
- Intermediate defects are best reconstructed with local flaps.
- Total or sub-total lip defects are best reconstructed with free tissue.

Cheek reconstruction

- Local tissue should be used whenever possible.
- Local and regional flaps work well.
- Color match is important.
- For composite defects of lips and cheeks, each component defect can be reconstructed as a separate unit.

 Access the Historical Perspective section online at
http://www.expertconsult.com

Introduction

Because it represents the principal aesthetic feature of the lower face, subtle changes in the appearance of the vermillion border, labial commissures, or Cupid's bow are readily visible. For that reason, surgical resection of lip cancer, or trauma resulting in lip laceration or soft tissue loss, frequently result in alterations of normal lip appearance and function that can have a profound and lasting effect on the patient's self-image and quality of life. Neuromuscular injury or dysfunction can cause asymmetry at rest and particularly during facial expression. This can lead to distressing functional disability. Loss of

labial competence may be characterized by impairment in the ability to articulate, whistle, suck, kiss, and, probably most importantly, to control salivary secretions with consequent drooling. Surgeons have long appreciated the significance of lip function and aesthetics and many creative surgical techniques have been devised to reconstruct various lip defects. These techniques have evolved, and newer procedures have been developed that effectively address small to moderate defects. However, while many of the current techniques work well for small to moderate lip defects, the ultimate reconstructive approach for larger defects of the lip has remained elusive, and currently available methods provide results that are less than optimal.[1] While the lips have a very specific appearance and are such a prominent part of our physiognomy, the cheek, by comparison is, to a large extent, without a distinguishing feature. The nasolabial fold establishes the junction or interface between the cheek and lip and is an important part of the aesthetic appearance of the face. Symmetry of the nasolabial folds is also important in presenting a harmonious appearance to the face. While cheek reconstruction does not compare in intricacy and visual impact with lip, nasal, or eyelid reconstruction, symmetrical and balanced reconstruction is, nevertheless important. The slightly more lateral position of the cheek in the face allows for some leeway in our reconstructions. Both cheeks are never seen, in their entirety, together. This is in contrast, for example, to the lips where right and left sides are instantly comparable. As long as the nasolabial folds are symmetrical, a reasonably accurate replica of the intact contralateral cheek will result in a very satisfactory reconstruction, while a less than accurate lip reconstruction will provide a less than satisfactory result. The cheek consists of a soft tissue envelope of skin, subcutaneous tissue, muscle, and buccal mucosa draped over a bony framework, the most prominent part of which is the malar eminence. The parotid gland and duct as well as the facial nerve are embedded within this soft tissue. The texture of the cheek differs between male and female. In the female, it is smooth and soft. In the male, it is partially hair-bearing and less smooth. Probably the most important feature to consider when planning cheek reconstruction is skin color. While reconstructions in general terms are planned based on factors such as defect size and flap availability, in the head and neck in general and in the face in particular, we must also consider the fact that our reconstruction is going to be clearly visible. A cheek reconstruction can be marred, for example, if the skin color is strikingly different from the rest of the face. One final point is important to consider here; while we can think of the cheek as a separate aesthetic unit, reconstruction of the cheek will frequently impact on nearby units, e.g., the pull on the lower eyelid from a cheek advancement flap. Reconstruction of the underlying bony skeleton is obviously also an important part of cheek reconstruction. The integrity of the contour of the underlying bony skeleton is important in maintaining facial symmetry. Bony reconstruction of the cheek is seldom an isolated necessity, particularly in the context of tumor ablation and reconstruction. In this situation, we are generally dealing not only with the bony cheek but with the whole maxilla. This brings us into the area of orbital palatal and nasal reconstruction. A detailed description of maxillary reconstruction is beyond the scope of this chapter but it is important to realize that the two – cheek and maxilla – cannot always be separated.

Anatomic and functional considerations in lip reconstruction

The laminar structure of the lips consists of three layers: mucosa, muscle, and skin. Externally, the cutaneous portion of the lip surrounds and transitions into the mucosal lip. This transition between these two regions is characterized by the mucocutaneous ridge, or vermillion border. At the midline of the upper lip, there is a V-shaped indentation of the mucocutaneous ridge that is known as Cupid's bow. Above Cupid's bow, a vertical groove-shaped depression called the philtrum is bordered on either side by elevations known as philtral ridges or columns *(Fig. 10.1)*. The vermillion forms the major aesthetic feature of the upper and lower lips. The vermillion is composed of modified mucosa that lacks minor salivary glands. The characteristic color of the vermillion stems from a rich blood supply that underlies a very thin epithelial structure. The maxillary and mandibular divisions of the trigeminal nerve provide sensation to both upper and lower lips. The boundaries of the upper lip are defined by the base of the nose centrally and by the nasolabial folds laterally. The inferior margin of the lower lip is defined by the mental crease (labiomental crease) that separates the lip from the chin.[6] The upper and lower lips differ, in that the lower lip is composed of a single aesthetic unit while the upper lip has multiple subunits. According to Burget and Menick's description,[7] each side of the upper lip has two aesthetic subunits: the medial topographic subunit is one-half the philtrum, whereas the lateral subunit is bordered by the philtrum medially, the nostril sill and alar base superiorly, and the nasolabial fold laterally. Another way to think about the upper lip is that it is composed of three subunits, the philtrum centrally and the lateral lip elements on either side of the philtrum *(Fig. 10.1)*.[8]

The thickness of the lip largely results from the underlying orbicularis oris muscle, which forms a functional sphincteric ring and is essentially sandwiched between the skin on the outside, and the mucosa on the inside. The orbicularis oris has

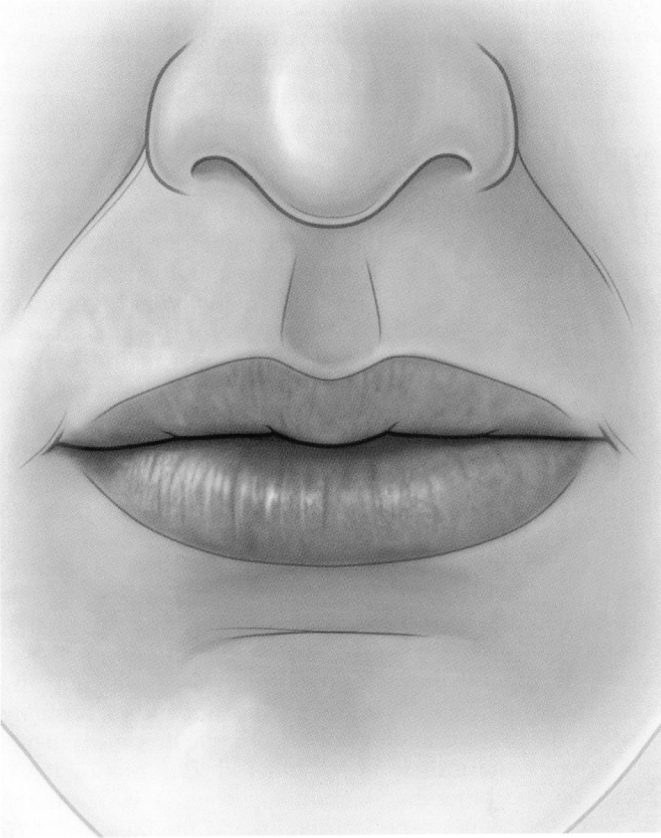

Fig. 10.1 The aesthetic landmarks of the lips are seen. The curve of the upper lip resembles a bow, known as cupids bow. The central concavity of the upper lip is the philtrum, bounded on either side by the convex philtral columns. The lateral elements of the upper lip are bounded by the philtral ridge medially, the nasal vestibule and alar base superiorly and the nasolabial fold laterally. The mental crease separates the lower lip from the aesthetic unit of the chin.

two functions that, at first might seem diametrically opposed but that, on reflection make sense. The superficial fibers of this muscle function to protrude the lips away from the facial plane, whereas the deep and oblique fibers approximate the lips to the alveolar arch.[9] The middle portion of the buccinator muscle extends anteriorly to the corner of the mouth and decussates so that the upper fibers of the mid-buccinator merge with the orbicularis fibers of the lower lip, and the lower fibers merge with the orbicularis fibers of the upper lip.[9] Several muscles elevate the lip. The two most important elevator muscles are the zygomaticus major and the levator anguli oris; the zygomaticus minor and the levator labii superioris also contribute to this function. The depressor muscles include the depressor anguli oris and the platysma, with minor contributions from the depressor labii inferioris. Variations in the contraction of all of these muscles result in the versatility of movement of this region and the myriad of shapes and expressions that contribute not only to facial aesthetics and animation but also to function. The modiolus is just lateral to the oral commissure. It is a 1 cm-thick fibrovascular region of muscle fiber intersection of the levator muscles and the depressor muscles that attach firmly to the dermis approximately 1.5 cm lateral to the oral commissure. The modiolus can be located by compressing the skin and mucosa of the commissure using bidigital palpation with the thumb and index finger.[10] The appearance of the labial commissures is significantly affected by movement of the modiolus on each side, which results from the summation of opposing contractile forces of the levator muscles (zygomaticus major and levator anguli oris) and the depressor muscles (depressor anguli oris and platysma).[11,12] Sometimes there is a dimple here. When present, the dimple results from a dermal insertion arising from the inferior muscle bundle of a bifid zygomaticus major muscle.[13,14] The elevators and depressors of the lips are innervated by the buccal and mandibular branches of the facial nerve, respectively. Disruption of the musculature that attaches to the modiolar region (or their neural supply) can alter the appearance of the labial commissure at rest and during function secondary to imbalanced muscular contraction. This gives a very abnormal appearance to the mouth and is one of the greatest complaints of patients with facial paralysis. Modiolar motion can be analyzed to measure the success of facial reanimation in these.[15]

The blood supply to the lips comes from the facial arteries, which give rise to the inferior and superior labial arteries. The variability of these vessels, both in terms of course as well of presence, has been shown by anatomic studies and dissections. The superior labial arteries from each side generally anastomose in the midportion of the upper lip, coursing between the mucosa and orbicularis muscle in some patients and through the muscle in the others.[16] The inferior labial artery, on the other hand, routinely courses between the mucosa of the inner aspect of the lip and the muscle.[16] Two separate cadaveric studies found that the inferior labial artery was absent on one side in 10% and 64%, respectively, of the cadavers evaluated.[16,17] The bilateral presence of inferior labial arteries was not always predictive of an end-to-end anastomosis between these vessels, and other arterial branches from the facial arteries were frequently identified (e.g., labiomental, sublabial arteries).[16,17] Even though the variable arterial distribution of this region could, at least in theory, affect the survival of reconstructive procedures involving the lip, local flap reconstruction has been performed for centuries with predictably excellent survival rates. Although the lips are an important aesthetic feature of the lower face, they also play an important role in facial expression. Oral competence is necessary for eating and drinking, and intact neuromuscular function is essential for speech articulation and other functions such as whistling and sucking. The lower lip functions as a dam that retains saliva and prevents drooling. The upper lip contributes to oral competence by providing opposition to the lower lip to effect closure.[18] Sensation allows the lips to monitor the texture and temperature of substances prior to oral intake.

Lip function

The lips are an important aesthetic feature of the lower face and any deformity of the lips is instantly recognizable. Even minor deformities are easily noticed. More important though are the functional characteristics of the lips. The lips play a very important part in speech articulation, as any of us who have tried to speak after extensive local anesthesia at the dentist can attest. Also the lips are vital for the maintenance of oral competence.[18] Sensation allows the lips to monitor the texture and temperature of substances prior to oral intake.

Patient selection and presentation

Goals of lip reconstruction

The goals of lip reconstruction *(Box 10.1)* are several. The most important of these is function. No matter how good a reconstructed lip looks, if it cannot maintain oral competence, the reconstruction is a failure. Maintenance of oral competence is vital. Similarly important is maintenance of an adequate oral aperture to facilitate oral hygiene and/or to accommodate removable dentures. The labial vestibule is an important feature of labial anatomy and its preservation or re-creation is important for oral hygiene, dental care and denture fitting. In order to achieve these functions, preservation of labial sensation is important and because of the vital role of the lips in facial aesthetics, maximization of cosmesis is one of the key goals of reconstruction.[19]

In situations where the orbicularis oris muscle has been disrupted, it is vitally important to restore continuity of that muscle if at all possible. Careful re-approximation of muscle edges with intact motor innervation usually results in complete restoration of dynamic orbicularis function. Although some authors contend that the upper lip functions primarily as a curtain that could be replaced with a static flap reconstruction, there is no doubt that a completely intact sphincter with active function and sensation yields the best functional result.[7,20] In cases where reconstruction of the sphincter is not feasible, an adynamic reconstruction must be pursued that provides some degree of oral competence. In repairing or reconstructing the lips, one of the main dangers is resulting microstomia. While patients can function reasonably well with a small degree of microstomia, it is very important to minimize it as may not only interfere with function but it can also hamper oral hygiene and patients should be counseled prior to surgery that denture insertion and removal may be difficult, or, quite simply, not possible. Decreases in the shape or depth of the labial vestibule can exacerbate oral incompetence and drooling, and may preclude patients from wearing a removable prosthesis. Preservation of labial sensation is vitally important to maximize oral competence and to fulfill its other sensory roles.

Because of the anatomic configuration of the upper lip and, specifically, because of its aesthetic subunit structure, reconstruction of the upper lip presents certain aesthetic challenges that are not of concern during lower lip reconstruction. Loss of the philtral ridges and Cupid's bow creates a noticeable cosmetic deformity that presents a significant reconstructive challenge. In profile, the upper lip should protrude in front of the lower lip, so a reconstruction that results in excisional

---

Box 10.1 **Goals of lip reconstruction**

- Preservation of function.
- Reconstitution of orbicularis oris.
- Three-layered closure.
- Accurate alignment of vermillion.
- Maintenance of relationship between upper and lower lips.
- Optimization of cosmesis.

tightness with reduction or elimination of this relationship is not only undesirable, but will certainly result in an inferior aesthetic outcome. In contrast, the lower lip is better able to withstand tissue loss without significant changes in its profile appearance, and can sustain a loss of one-third of its breadth before tightness or asymmetry begins to show.

Early lip reconstruction techniques focused primarily on primary closure of the surgical defect, whereas more contemporary techniques attempt to address the importance of an aesthetic, functional result. Reconstruction of the aesthetic subunits as described by Burget and Menick[7] is helpful, and aesthetic features such as Cupid's bow and the philtral columns must be carefully restored. Failure to restore these landmarks results in an abnormal appearance that is instantly detectable. One of the features that is readily picked up by the human eye is asymmetry. Surgery that results in asymmetry is typically more noticeable than symmetric alterations. As an example, rounding of both commissures is less obvious than rounding of one side. Whenever possible, the height, projection, and relationship between upper and lower lips should also be preserved or replicated. This is most easily achieved by using tissue from the adjacent or opposing lip.[21,22]

Patient selection is, arguably, less important than reconstructive choice. In the case of trauma, the damage is already done and the surgeon's task is to repair and reconstruct the lip so that it is as functional and aesthetically pleasing as possible. For patient's facing lip resection for disease, the task is no different, i.e., the surgeon must reconstruct the lip to be as functional and aesthetically pleasing as possible. However, in the latter case, the surgeon has the luxury of planning what reconstruction will best suit the patient. The choice depends on multiple factors, such as prognosis, general medical condition, availability of local tissue, history of prior radiation as well as co-morbidities. The lips are somewhat unique however, in that the need to reconstruct the lips is very different from, as an example, the need to reconstruct a breast. Oral competence is vital for normal eating, articulation and communication, so the option not to reconstruct the lip is really nonexistent. The algorithm presented later in this chapter (see *Fig. 10.17*, below) can be used as a guide in selecting the most appropriate procedure for a given defect.

Operative technique

Defect-specific reconstruction of the lip

Following injury to the lips or following surgical resection for disease, there are several options for reconstruction of the lips:[9,23] The first choice, of course, is to use the remaining lip segment and if the defect size allows, this is by far the best option. This choice assumes that there is enough lip to effect the repair while not creating microstomia. Another consideration is whether or not the defect is full thickness and whether all three elements, skin, muscle and mucosa, need to be replaced. Regardless of what the defect is, local tissue is the best option because it replaces what has been lost and is the perfect match in terms of color, thickness and composition. Defects of the upper lip of less than 25% can be closed by direct approximation. For the lower lip, a slightly larger defect, up to 30%, can be closed directly. Once again, care must be taken to ensure accurate closure of all layers. Repair

of the orbicularis oris and reconstitution of the circumoral sphincter is the most important aspect of a functional repair.

For through-and-through defects, if there is insufficient lip to effect a direct closure, the next choice becomes the opposite lip. Several lip-switch options are discussed below and fulfill the requirement of providing tissue of like composition and appearance. Sometimes, however, there simply is not enough lip tissue to achieve this, in which case it may become necessary to use tissue from the adjacent cheek, nasolabial region or neck. A very useful source of tissue that can be used to reconstruct the lip, particularly when a through-and-through reconstruction is not required, is to use tissue from the submental region. For extreme defects however, there is no other option but to use regional or distant or free flaps.

Defects of the vermillion

There are a few important points of which to be cognizant when repairing a lip. One is the appreciation of the fact that the human eye can detect asymmetry remarkably accurately. The lips are very symmetrical and the different elements of the lip blend with each other in a very pleasing and aesthetic way. The junction between vermillion and white lip, for example, is smooth and seamless. When the line of the vermillion is broken or when a segment of vermillion impinges on the white lip, the abnormality is immediately obvious. When dealing with lacerations, there is not a lot, in terms of repair options, that the surgeon can do. However, being precise in repair of the vermillion border and white lip roll will produce a scar that is imperceptible. When resecting a lesion that crossed the vermillion, however, there are some options. As surgeons, we know that scars contract and a straight-line scar that crosses the vermillion will not only contract but may possibly produce a visible deformity. In order to avoid this, breaking up the scar by incorporating a step in the excision may prevent this contraction, make the repair easier and minimize the risk of a visible scar *(Fig. 10.2)*.

Vermillionectomy is a procedure that is done to remove very superficial lesions in the vermillion, such as superficial squamous cell carcinoma, or to remove dysplastic tissue with malignant potential such as actinic cheilitis. Following vermillionectomy, a procedure that is also known as a lip-shave, reconstruction is achieved by advancing the buccal mucosa to cover the defect and to re-establish the mucocutaneous junction *(Fig. 10.3)*.[1] If there is any degree of tightness, back-cuts are made to facilitate further advancement of the mucosa. This type of vermillion reconstruction can sometimes result in excessive thinning of the lip from mucosal retraction or scar contraction, and decreased mucosal sensation.[6,24] However, in general, the results of lip shave are excellent. Other approaches to reconstruction of the vermillion include the mucosal V-Y advancement flap, the cross-lip mucosal flap, and transposition flaps harvested from the buccal mucosa or the ventral surface of the tongue.[6,25] Buccal mucosal flaps tend to be more erythematous than natural vermillion, resulting in a color mismatch with the remaining vermillion.[24] Mucosal tongue flaps require a second procedure 14–21 days later to release and inset the flap. A musculomucosal flap that includes buccal mucosa and buccinator muscle anteriorly pedicled on buccal branches of the facial artery and innervated sensory branches of the infraorbital nerve has been advocated as one option to

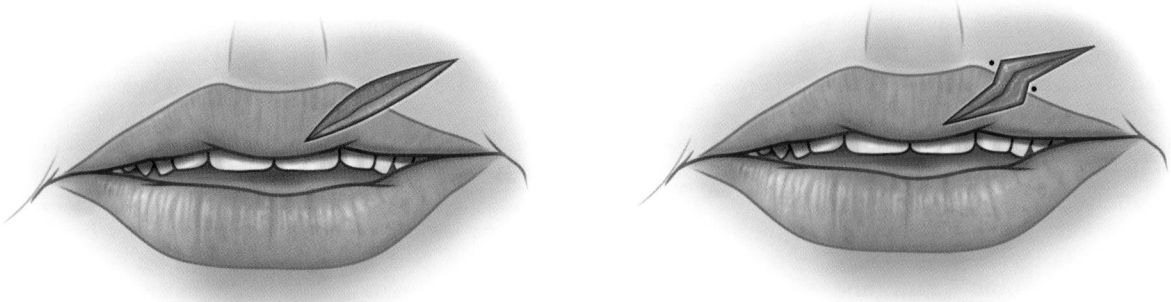

Fig. 10.2 Breaking up the linear scar by introducing a vertical element to an excision will allow for more precise closure as the vermillion borders can be accurately approximated (marked with dots). Furthermore, the resulting scar will not be linear and will therefore be less likely to contract.

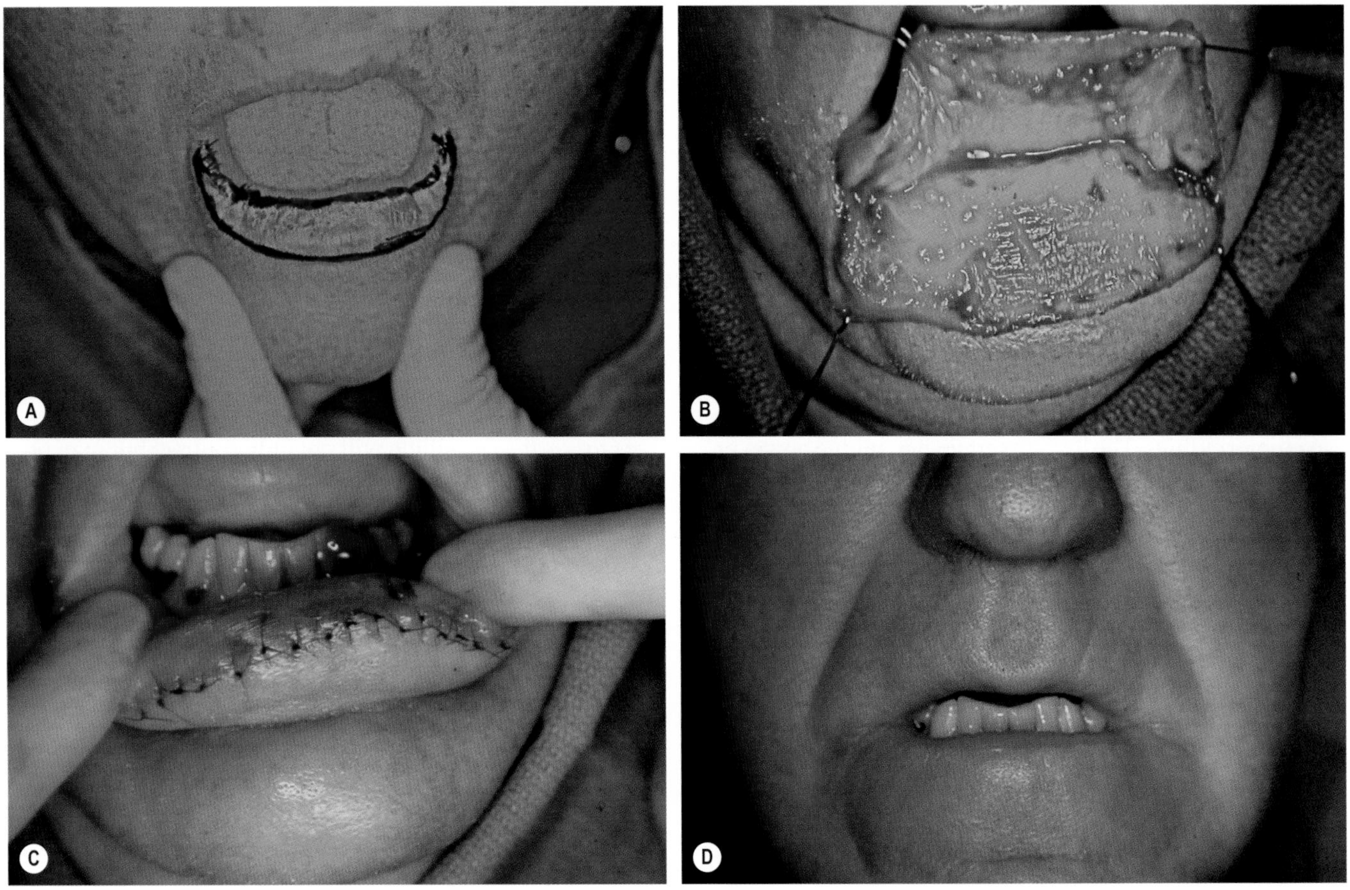

Fig. 10.3 (A) An area of vermillion is marked for excision. **(B)** The vermillion has been excised and a mucosal flap raised from the buccal mucosa. **(C)** The mucosal flap has been advanced and sutured to the white lip to recreate the mucocutaneous junction. **(D)** Postoperative appearance showing good restoration of vermillion.

remedy the loss of sensation in defects that also include loss of orbicularis muscle.[26]

Small full-thickness defects

Primary closure of defects that involve as much as one-quarter of the upper lip or one-third of the lower lip can be achieved *(Box 10.2)*.[18] A V-shaped wedge design usually permits closure of smaller defects, whereas a W-plasty placed at the base of the V facilitates the closure of larger defects. Furthermore, this modification will generally allow for the scar to be kept above the mental crease. This improves the cosmetic appearance of the repair, as it preserves the integrity of the chin aesthetic subunit *(Fig. 10.4)*. Wedge-shaped defects of the lateral lip should be more obliquely oriented so that the line of closure parallels the relaxed skin tension lines. If a W-plasty is incorporated into a lateral lip defect, the angle formed by the lateral V-shaped subunit of the W should be larger and more

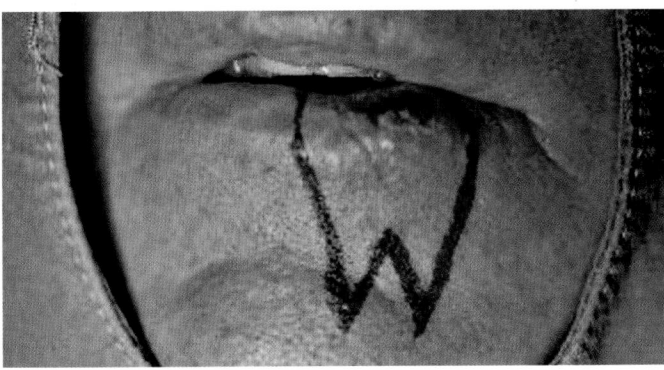

Fig. 10.4 Patient with a squamous cell carcinoma of the lower lip. A wedge excision has been planned and the patient is marked for a "W" excision in order to keep the scar above the mental crease and out of the aesthetic subunit of the chin.

Box 10.2 Wedge resection of the lip: technical tips

- Up to 25% of the upper lip can be resected and repaired directly.
- Up to 30% of the lower lip can be resected and repaired directly.
- Careful approximation of the muscle layer ensures a functional repair.
- Consider a W resection for larger wedges in order to keep the scar above the mental crease.

Box 10.3 Lip switch flaps: technical tips

- Width of the flap should be half the width of the defect.
- Height of the flap should be the same as height of the defect.
- Pedicle of Abbé flap should be placed at the midpoint of the defect.
- Pedicle division at 14–21 days.

---

obliquely oriented than the medial subunit to properly align the closure.[6,19] Careful attention to meticulous closure of all three layers will ensure optimal cosmesis and function. If actinic cheilitis of the adjacent lip is present, vermillionectomy can also be performed in combination with the wedge excision, using a labial mucosal advancement flap to recreate the vermillion border *(Fig. 10.5)*. This technique provides an elegant reconstruction of the vermillion, and the cosmetic outcome of this procedure is usually excellent. The aesthetic result following repair of a V-type excision is often less satisfactory in the upper lip, because the upper lip is able to withstand much less tissue loss before tightness becomes clinically apparent and the normal overhang of upper and lower lip is lost as a consequence of closure-induced tension. In addition, the anchorage of soft tissues around the pyriform aperture to the underlying bony skeleton limits compensatory movement of the remaining lip. This problem can be minimized by using a T excision, which facilitates advancement of the lateral lip elements. The symmetry of Cupid's bow is easily lost with even minor excision in the region of the philtrum. Webster's[27] technique of crescentic perialar cheek excision is an extension of the T-excision technique that increases upper lip movement without disturbing the lateral muscle function *(Fig. 10.6)*. If the defect is created lateral to the philtral columns, primary closure may produce deformity and notching. For this reason, it is occasionally preferable to use a lip-switch flap from the lower lip, even when the defect makes up less than 30% of the lip's width. This is particularly the case in younger patients whose tissues are less lax and where cosmesis is often of even greater importance.

Intermediate full-thickness defects

For all the reasons already described, local flaps are the best option for reconstructing larger defects involving up to two-thirds the width of either upper or lower lip. These flaps involve either a lip switching maneuver, rotation of tissue from one lip to another or recruitment and advancement of adjacent tissue, such as cheek tissue to achieve the reconstruction. Lip-switch (cross-lip) flaps are axial flaps based on the labial arteries *(Box 10.3)*. They replace tissue like with like, replacing the trilaminar defect in one lip with tri-laminar tissue from the other. The classic Abbé flap can reconstruct medial or lateral lip defects with a full-thickness composite flap that reconstructs all three layers and restores continuity of the vermillion.[28] Surgical technique is important and there are a few technical principles that are important to follow to achieve optimal results. The first is that the width of the flap does not need to be as big as the width of the defect. This technical trick allows for repair of the defect by taking advantage of the inherent elasticity of the lip tissues while, at the same time, reducing the amount of tissue that has to be sacrificed from the donor lip, thereby making closure of the secondary defect easier. So both lips end-up a little smaller but by taking some tissue from both lips, a better balance between the two lips is maintained. The second principle is that the height of the flap needs to match that of the defect. While one can get away with less width, less height will result in some element of notching and will produce a significantly inferior result. Finally, the position of the flap relative to the opposite lip is an important technical point to appreciate. This refers particularly to the Abbé flap and is important because the position of the flap determines the position of the pedicle. This is very important to appreciate. Essentially, the pedicle should be placed roughly at the mid-position of the defect. The reason for this is because of the fact that the flap will be half the width of the defect so that when the secondary defect is closed, the pedicle ends-up being in precise alignment with one end of the defect. This is best explained in *Figure 10.7*. Pedicle division is performed 14–21 days later as shown in *Figure 10.8*.

The Estlander flap is, in reality an Abbé flap that is brought around the commissure.[29] Once again, the width of the flap is usually one-half the width of the defect and is the same height as the defect. Using this technique, defects that involve the commissure and as much as 50% of the lower or upper lip can be adequately reconstructed with an acceptable functional and cosmetic result. However, in this case, since the flap is rotated, no pedicle division is necessary. One disadvantage is the blunting of the commissure that is seen. However, this rarely requires any correction *(Fig. 10.9)*. Several modifications of cross-lip flaps have also been described. Adhering to the aesthetic subunit principle, Burget and Menick,[7] for example, suggested that defects constituting more than half of a topographic subunit of the upper lip necessitate removal of the remaining portions of the subunit so that reconstruction of the entire subunit can be performed by using a foil template of the defect to design the Abbé flap in the lower lip.

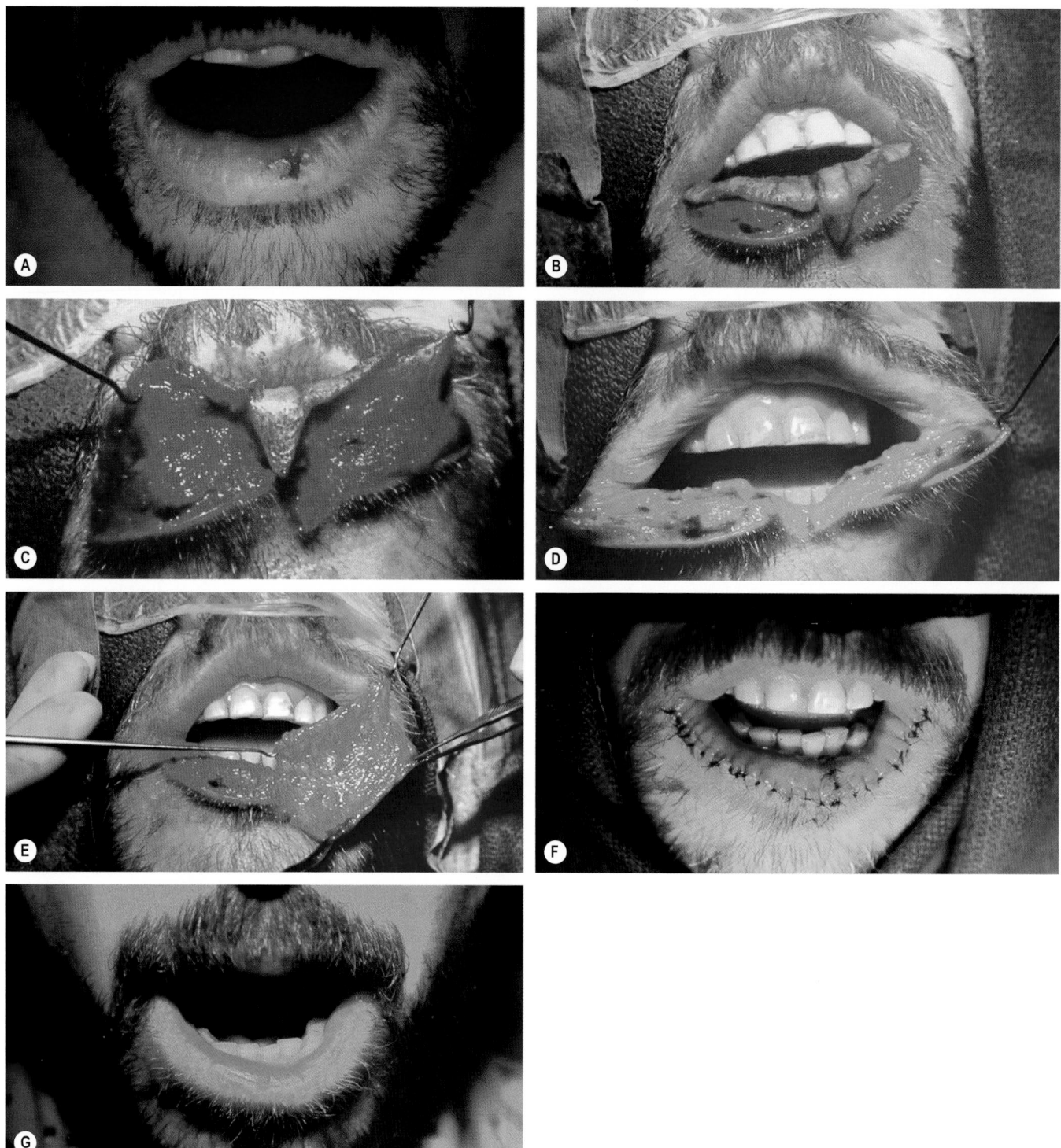

Fig. 10.5 (A) Patient with a small squamous cell carcinoma of the lip requiring wedge resection. The patient also has significant actinic cheilitis requiring a lip-shave. **(B)** Resection has begun and includes a central wedge of the lower lip in continuity with the vermillion. **(C)** Mucosal flaps have been elevated. **(D)** The surgical defect is seen. **(E)** The left mucosal flap is advanced. **(F)** Both mucosal flaps have been advanced, the wedge closed and the mucocutaneous junction re-established. **(G)** Postoperative appearance.

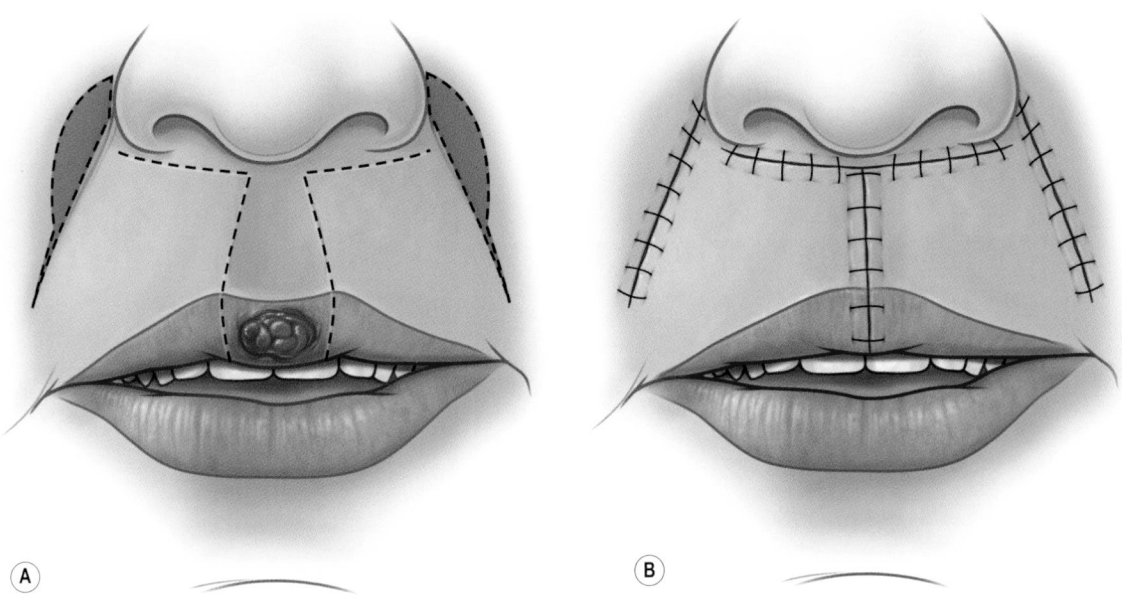

Fig. 10.6 **(A)** Resection of a central segment of the upper lip is shown. A "T" excision is performed with a Webster crescentic perialar excision allowing for advancement of the lip elements. **(B)** A schematic of the closure is shown.

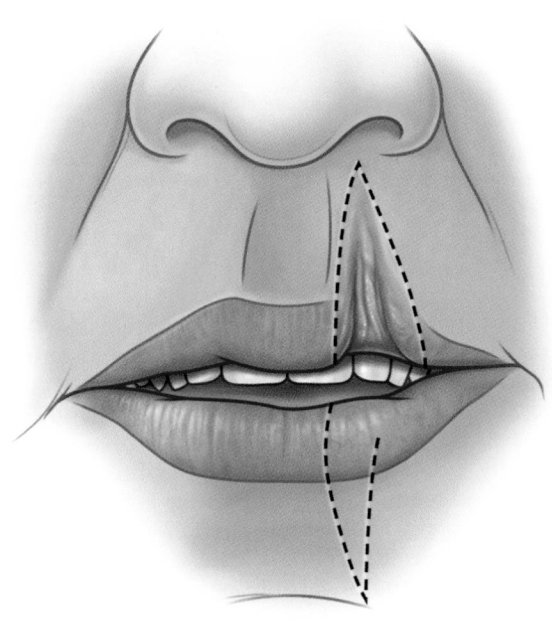

Fig. 10.7 [3] Schematic of an Abbé flap from the lower lip to the upper. Note that the width of the Abbé flap is half the width of the defect, while the height of the flap is the same as the height of the defect. The pedicle will be planned at a point opposite the mid-portion of the defect and will end-up at the medial end of the defect following rotation of the flap.

There are, however, several limitations to the cross-lip flaps. Even though the orbicularis muscle is reconstructed, and continuity of the circum-oral sphincter is re-established, disruption of the motor supply leads to varying degrees of abnormal lip motility. Where small flaps have been utilized, this may be barely if at all appreciable. However, where larger

reconstructions have been performed, the change in motility may be more obvious. A trap-door deformity or pin-cushioning occasionally develops at the recipient site, and the cross-lip flap tends to appear thicker than the adjacent lip. [6,7,24,28,29] The fan flap, initially described by Gillies and Millard [5] in 1957, is a modification of a technique described by von Bruns that utilized quadrilateral inferiorly based nasolabial flaps. [3] This flap rotates tissue around the commissure in the same fashion as an Estlander flap, but more tissue from the nasolabial region is included. [9] A vertical releasing incision is made in the donor lip. [6] A unilateral flap can be performed to reconstruct a lip defect, but bilateral fan flaps are more frequently employed to reconstruct total or sub-total defects *(Fig. 10.10)*. [9] Although defects involving up to 80% of the lip can be reconstructed with the Gillies fan flap, the biggest and least desirable sequel is significant microstomia as well as deficiency of the vermillion. Furthermore, denervation of the orbicularis oris can lead to oral incompetence. However, at least partial re-innervation seems to occur over a period of 12–18 months. [6,9,30] The circumoral advancement-rotation flap initially described by von Bruns in 1857 utilized full-thickness flaps that resulted in extensive denervation of the orbicularis muscle. [3] Although this technique effectively closed large composite defects of the lower lip, reconstruction was accomplished at the expense of sensation, motor function, and oral competence. These full-thickness flaps fell into disrepute until 1974, when Karapandzic [4] published a modification of von Bruns' technique. The incisional design of the Karapandzic flap, as it is now known, was identical to those advocated by von Bruns, but full-thickness flaps were not created, and the neurovascular supply to the lip was preserved via meticulous dissection *(Fig. 10.11)*. Although most authors report its use for the closure of lip defects that involve up to two-thirds of the lip, others state that the Karapandzic flap can successfully replace 80% of the total lip length. [1,6,9,22] However, reconstructing such a large defect with this technique can result in

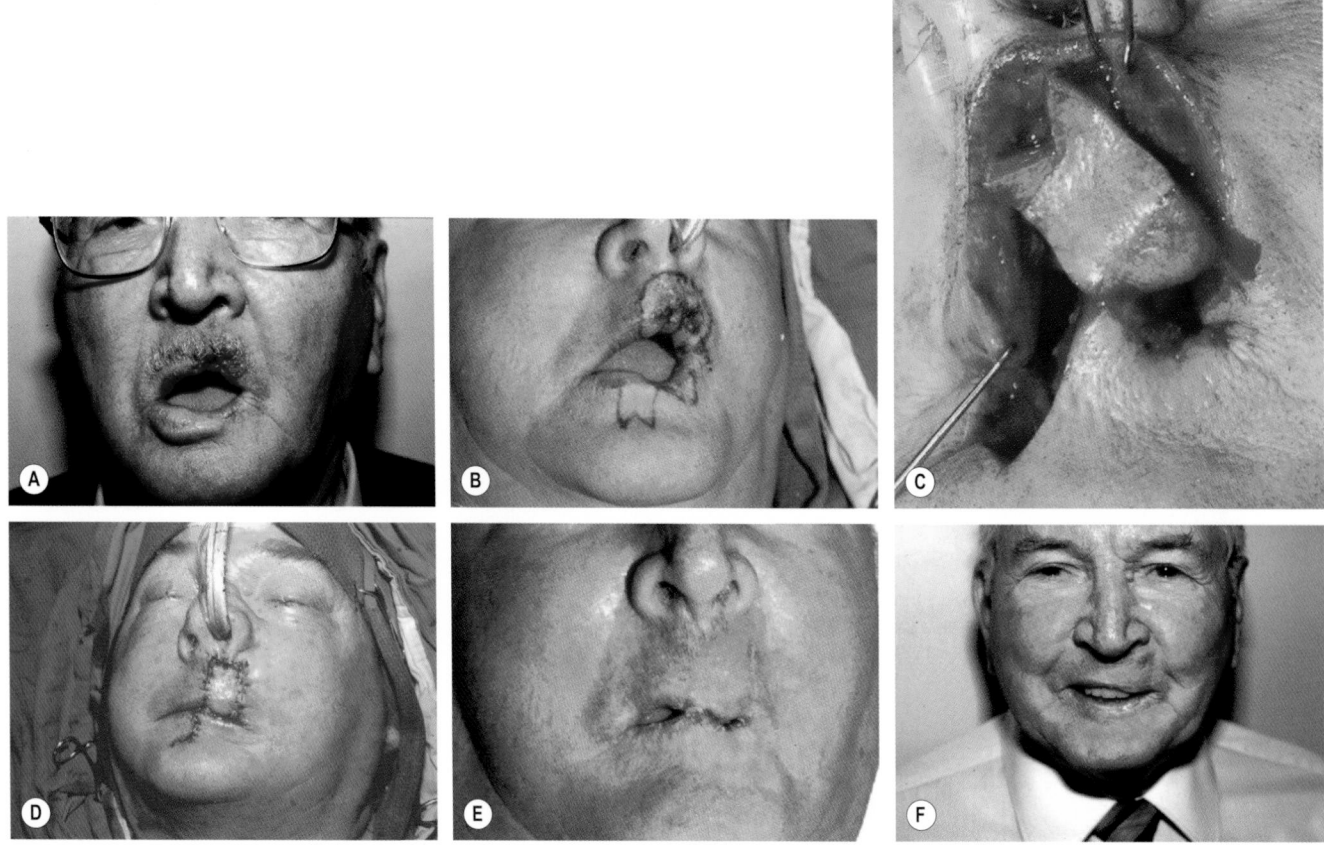

Fig. 10.8 (A) Patient with a squamous cell carcinoma of the left side of the upper lip. **(B)** The resection and the Abbé flap are marked. **(C)** The resection has been completed and the Abbé flap is being rotated from the lower lip. **(D)** Inset is complete and the pedicle remains attached, effectively securing the lower to the upper lip. **(E)** Patient was seen 3 weeks later at the time of pedicle division. The flap appears viable. **(F)** Postoperative appearance.

significant microstomia. This flap may be used to reconstruct defects of the upper or lower lip in the following manner: curvilinear circumoral incisions are extended bilaterally from the base of the defect, placing the incisions within the mental crease and the nasolabial creases. The incisions are designed to maintain a uniform thickness of the flap bilaterally. Because the nasolabial crease closely approximates the commissure, the incision should be placed slightly lateral to the nasolabial crease in this region, to maintain uniform thickness of the flap. If the defect is eccentrically located, the flap should be designed so that the contralateral lower lip is the longer limb of the flap. Careful dissection of the peripheral muscle fibers and concentric undermining allows advancement without any dissection of the mucosa. Preservation of the neurovascular bundles is imperative. A unilateral flap is adequate for smaller defects, whereas defects that constitute more than 50% of the lip require bilateral flaps. Function is restored because only the peripheral rim of orbicularis oris muscle is incised and the buccinator muscle is preserved. The Karapandzic flap results in blunting or rounding of both commissures, which is usually less noticeable than alteration of only one commissure. Some degree of microstomia is also inevitable, which may preclude the use of dentures. Because the combined width of the upper and lower lips is approximately 15 cm, reconstruction of a 5 cm defect results in a

rounded oral aperture with a circumference that is two-thirds of the original.[6,9,18,19] However, because of the superior and predictable functional and cosmetic results that can be achieved, the Karapandzic flap is possibly the flap of choice for most defects.

Frequently, a defect is too wide to close directly but is not wide enough to require a flap such as the Estlander or Abbé flap. Johanson *et al.*,[31,32] proposed the stair-step advancement flap for such a defect. Though ideally suited for smaller defects, this technique is capable of reconstructing defects extending to as much as two-thirds of the lower lip *(Fig. 10.12)*.[32] This technique involves the excision of 2–4 small rectangles arranged in a stair-step fashion that descend from medial to lateral at a 45° angle from either side of the base of the defect. When the defect is located laterally, the step incision is outlined exclusively on the remaining long side of the lip.[33] If the defect is located near the midline or its horizontal length exceeds 20 mm, the staircase pattern is marked on both sides of the lower lip. The first horizontal incision is made parallel to the vermillion border and is approximately half of the width of the resected region. Usually 2–4 additional steps are necessary in the vertical direction; the width of each step is approximately one-half of its height. Finally, a triangle is excised with its apex located inferiorly. Each of the rectangles and the triangle are excised through the full thickness of the

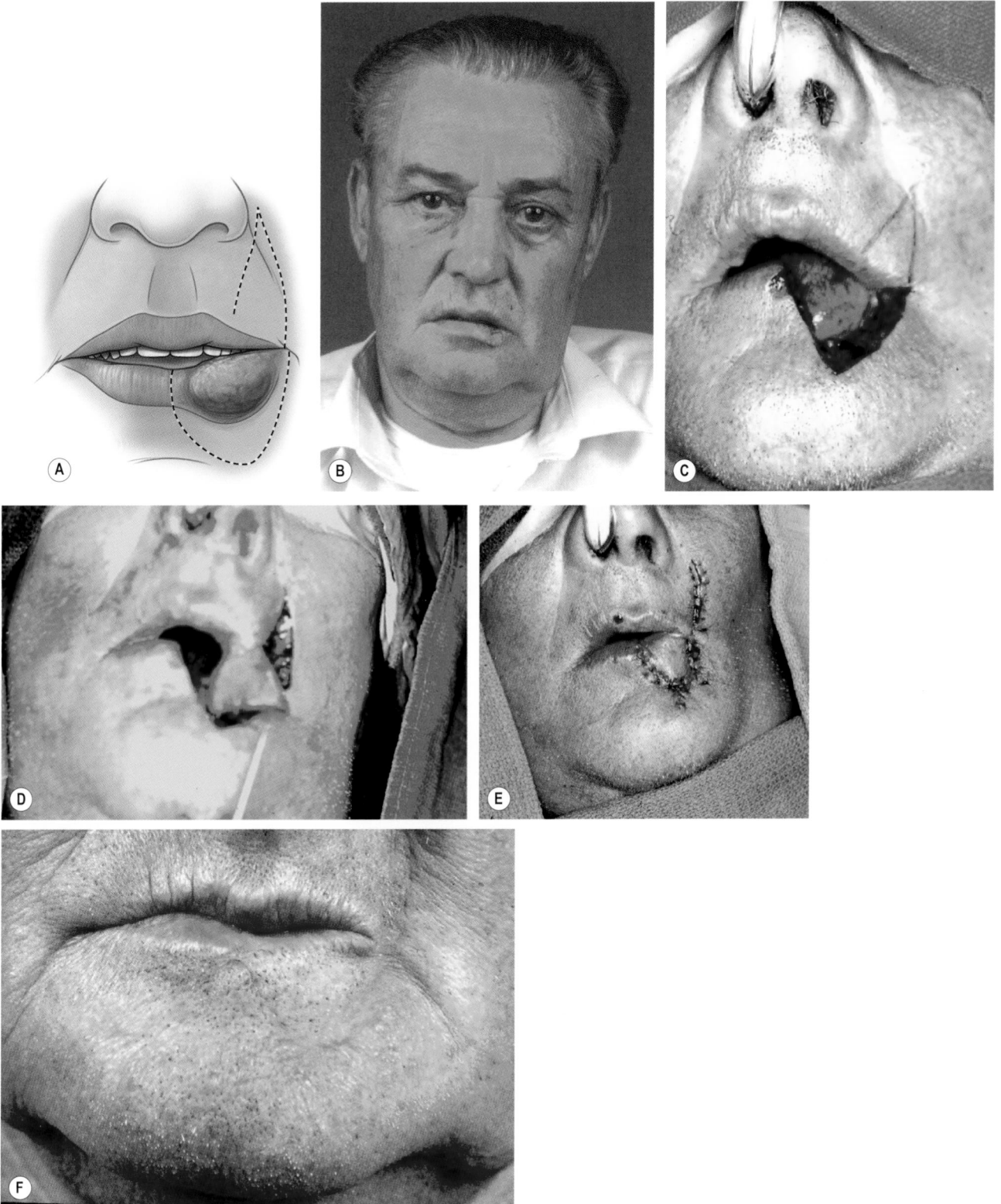

Fig. 10.9 **(A)** Schematic of Estlander flap designed to reconstruct a defect of the lower lip. **(B)** Patient with squamous cell carcinoma of the lower lip. **(C)** The lesion has been excised and the flap designed. Note the dimensions of the flap. The width is half that of the defect but the height is the same as the height of the defect. **(D)** The flap is being rotated into the defect. **(E)** Final inset of the flap and closure of the donor defect. **(F)** Final appearance. Note the slight blunting of the commissure.

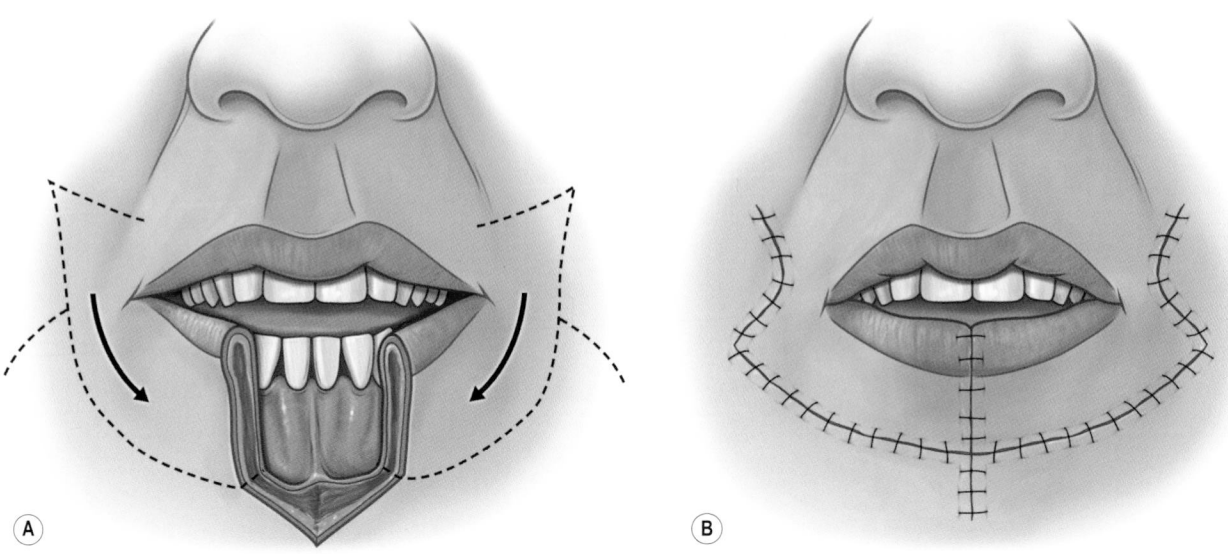

Fig. 10.10 A schematic of the Gillies fan flap is shown. Note the releasing incisions on the upper lip that allow the flap to rotate and advance.

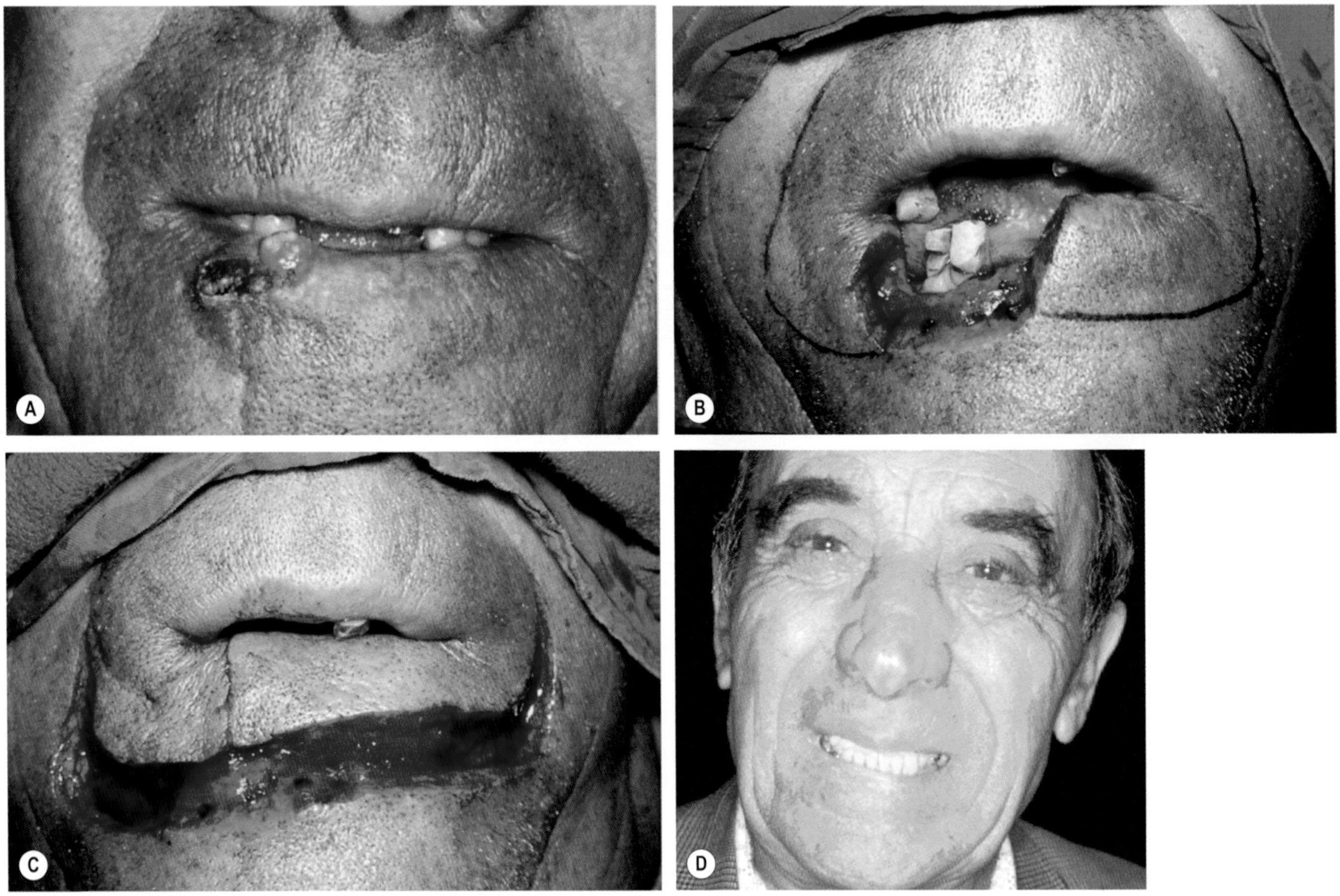

Fig. 10.11 **(A)** Patient with a squamous cell carcinoma of the lower lip. Note the scar from a previous wedge resection. **(B)** The resection has been completed and the markings made for a Karapandzic flap. **(C)** The flaps are rotated and advanced. Note that this is not a through-and-through dissection so that the motor and sensory nerves can be preserved. **(D)** Postoperative appearance showing good cosmesis and function.

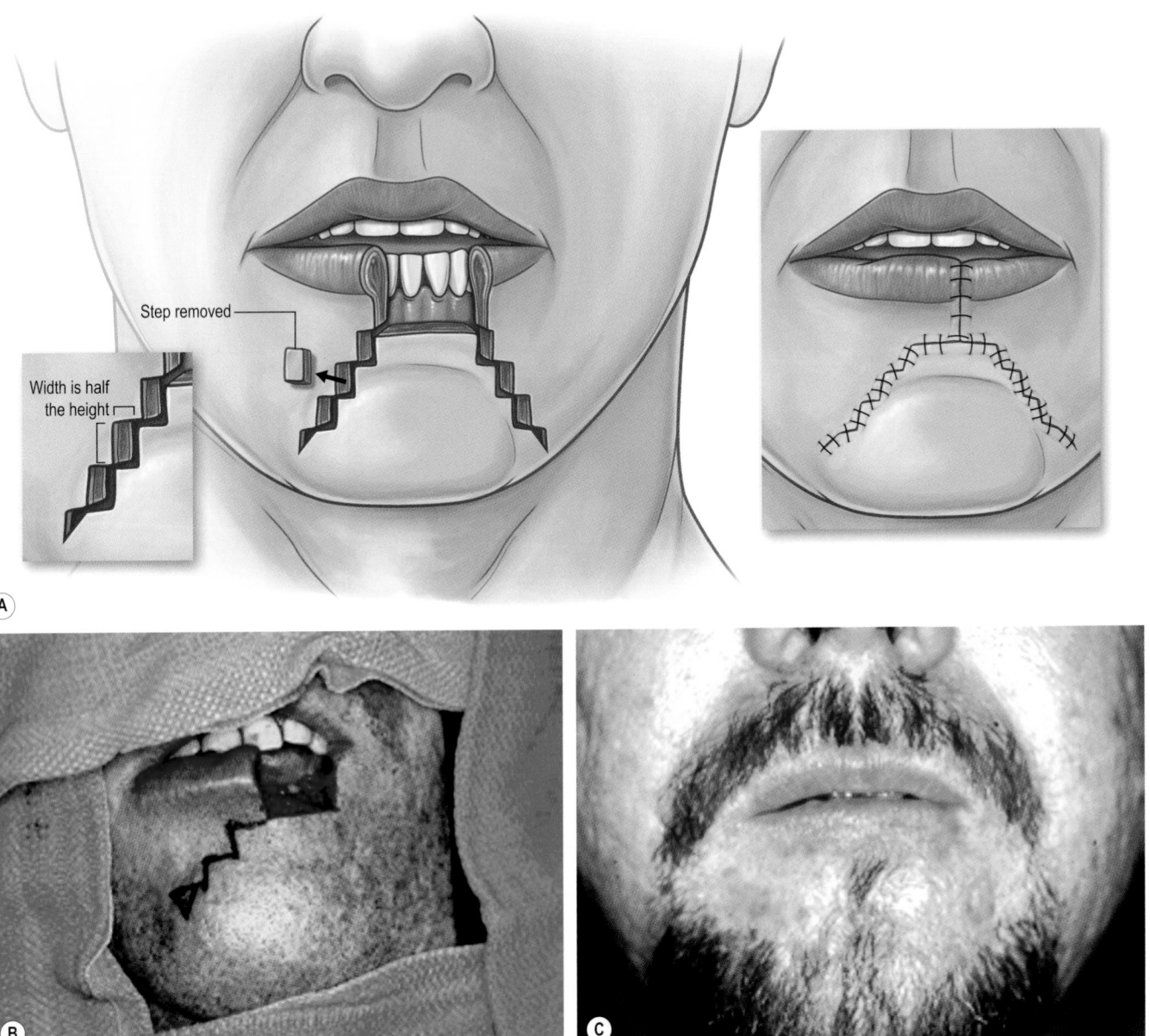

Fig. 10.12 (A) Schematic of a step flap reconstruction. Note that the steps are excised to allow the flaps to advance. Note also that the scar remains above the mental crease. **(B)** Patient following resection of a squamous cell carcinoma of the lower lip. Markings have been made for a unilateral step resection. **(C)** Postoperative appearance.

lower lip. This allows advancement of the flap in the direction of the defect with each succeeding higher step in the staircase, and the wound is closed in layers. By placing the step incisions outside of the mental crease, the aesthetic unit of the chin can be preserved *(Fig. 10.12)*. For this reason, the step technique is better than a wedge resection of similar size that would encroach on the chin subunit. The stair-step design allows for closure of the defect and minimizes contracture.

Large full-thickness defects

Defects that involve up to 80% of the total lip length may be reconstructed with bilateral Gillies fan flaps or the Karapandzic flap, as described above.[9] Reconstruction of total or near-total

defects constituting more than 80% of the lip typically leads to a poor aesthetic outcome and compromised oral competence. Because of denervation, the lip is largely adynamic. Dieffenbach (1845),[35] Bernard (1853), von Burow (1855) and von Bruns (1857)[3,9] all described techniques of cheek advancement from which the current reconstructive methods that employ horizontal cheek advancement flaps have evolved. Bernard and von Burow described the transposition of full-thickness flaps to reconstruct the upper or lower lip, reconstructing the vermillion with a mucosal advancement flap.[9] Transposition of these cutaneous flaps required the excision of four triangular regions of redundant cheek skin to reconstruct the upper lip, and the excision of three cutaneous triangles to reconstruct the lower lip. The reconstructive

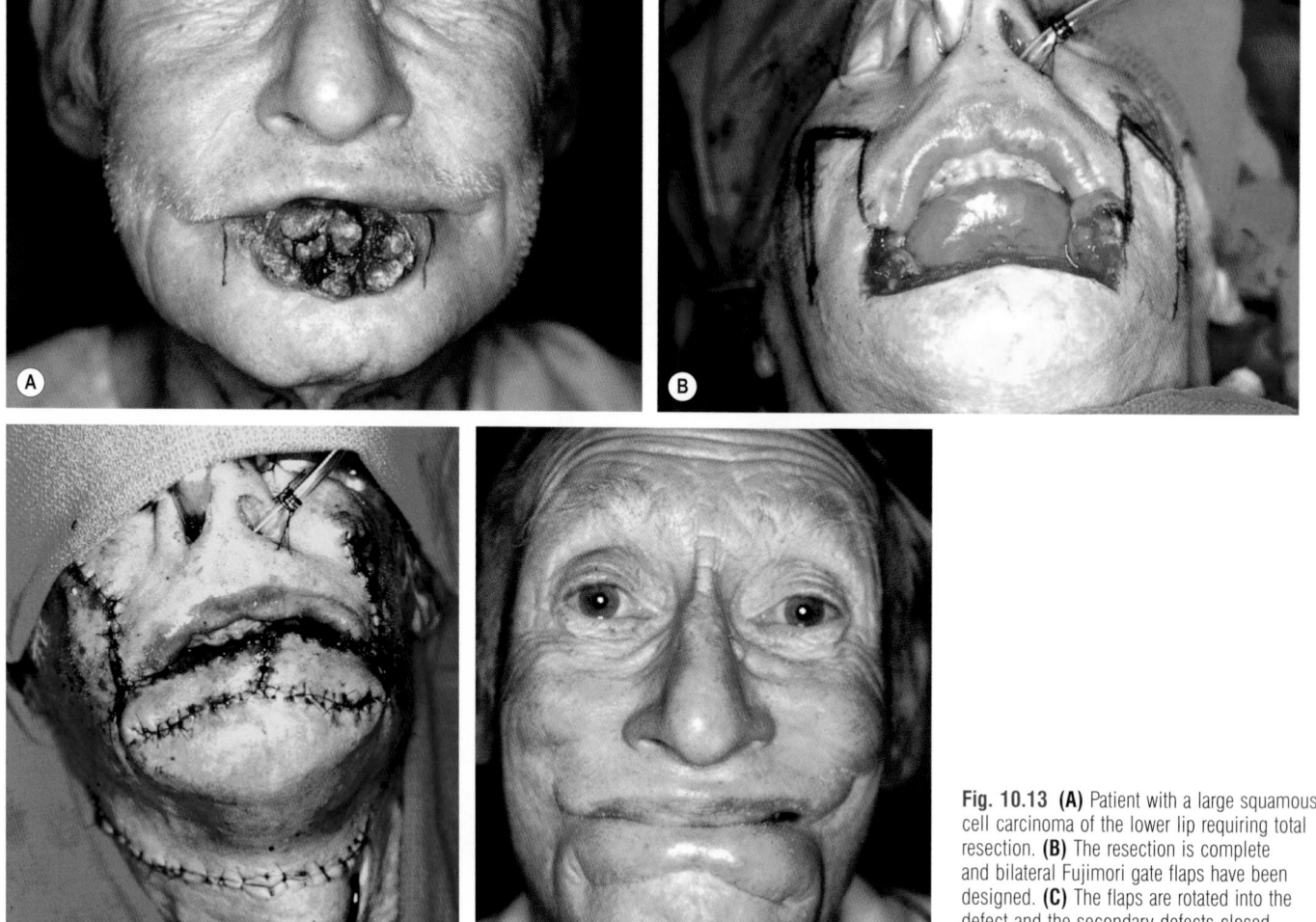

Fig. 10.13 (A) Patient with a large squamous cell carcinoma of the lower lip requiring total resection. **(B)** The resection is complete and bilateral Fujimori gate flaps have been designed. **(C)** The flaps are rotated into the defect and the secondary defects closed. **(D)** Postoperative appearance showing significant deformity of the lower face.

technique has become known as the "Bernard cheiloplasty" or the Bernard-Burow cheek advancement, and the triangular soft tissue excisions are referred to as "Burow's triangles."[6,27,34] Webster[27] suggested modifications of this technique that align the scars with the relaxed skin tension lines of the face. Although microstomia can be avoided with this approach, there is no functional orbicularis. Consequently, oral competence relies on the development of a tight adynamic lower lip. Prior to free tissue transfer, nasolabial flaps played a prominent role in total lip reconstruction. Dieffenbach[35] initially described the use of nasolabial flaps for upper lip reconstruction. The rectangular-shaped nasolabial flaps that von Bruns described in 1857 for lower lip defects were inferiorly-based.[3] The "gate flap" design, originally published by Fujimori[36] in 1980, rotates two nasolabial island flaps through 90°. These flaps are based on the angular artery *(Fig. 10.13)*. Although Fujimori's technique was fashioned for the lower lip, modifications of the gate flap have also been proposed for total upper lip reconstruction.[37] Reconstruction with any of these nasolabial flap designs are associated with suboptimal oral competence and aesthetics, and denervation of the flaps is inevitable. In an effort to address the limitations of local flaps for large lip defects, some surgeons have employed the use of multiple local flaps. Kroll[38] advocated reconstructing large

lower lip defects by re-establishing the oral sphincter with an extended Karapandzic flap, followed by two sequential Abbé flaps 3 weeks apart to augment the central lower lip and a commissure plasty to widen the oral aperture. The Abbé flaps were harvested from a philtral ridge so that the scar was relatively inconspicuous and any notching of the upper vermillion from scar contraction could be disguised as a peak in the Cupid's bow. Using this technique, Kroll noted that the transfer of redundant upper lip tissue improved the appearance and volume of the lower lip, particularly near the midline. In contrast, Williams and colleagues[21,22] reconstructed these defects by simultaneously performing a modified Bernard-Burow cheek advancement flap in combination with a medially based (Abbé) cross-lip flap. In contrast to Kroll's technique, they purport that less microstomia develops, and the orientation of the modiolus is not disturbed. Kroll's technique was described for lower lip defects, whereas Williams *et al.*'s approach can be used for upper and lower defects.

The radial forearm flap is the free tissue transfer technique that is most frequently employed for the reconstruction of total lower lip defects. Sakai *et al.*,[39] in 1989 reported the reconstruction of a lower lip defect with a composite radial forearm-palmaris longus tendon free flap. The forearm flap is folded over the tendon sling to resurface the internal and external surfaces of the lip and cheek. A microneural anastomosis between the lateral antebrachial cutaneous nerve and the cut end of the mental nerve can be performed to achieve sensory reinnervation.[40,41] A ventral tongue flap may be used to recreate the vermillion border, although a second procedure is necessary. Following flap reconstruction, medical tattooing can also be used to create the vermillion with acceptable cosmetic results.[42,43]

Though most commonly used for the lower lip, the radial forearm flap has also been used for total upper lip reconstruction.[43] Oral competence and aesthetics are optimized by placing the palmaris longus tendon under the appropriate degree of tension. Lip entropion can develop if the palmaris longus tendon is inset too tightly (bow-strung), and ectropion may develop if inadequate tension is placed on the tendon. Sakai et al.[44] sutured the palmaris tendon to the orbicularis oris muscle and dermis in the nasolabial region to suspend the reconstruction. Other surgeons have reported good outcomes by suturing the tendon to the periosteum of the malar eminence or to the orbicularis muscle of the upper lip near the philtral columns.[40,45] My personal technique is to weave the Palmaris sling through the remaining orbicularis muscle and then through itself.[46] Tension can be adjusted at the time of inset to optimize lip position. If adequate tension is placed on the tendon by the facial musculature at the modioli, the muscle action from the remaining facial muscles is transferred to the neolip, resulting in a more dynamic suspension. Using this technique, the tendon assumes some degree of dynamism because the orbicularis through which it is woven retains some function (*Fig. 10.14*).[46] Other surgeons have similarly chosen the modiolus as the preferred site of anchorage for the tendon.[47] The design of the radial forearm

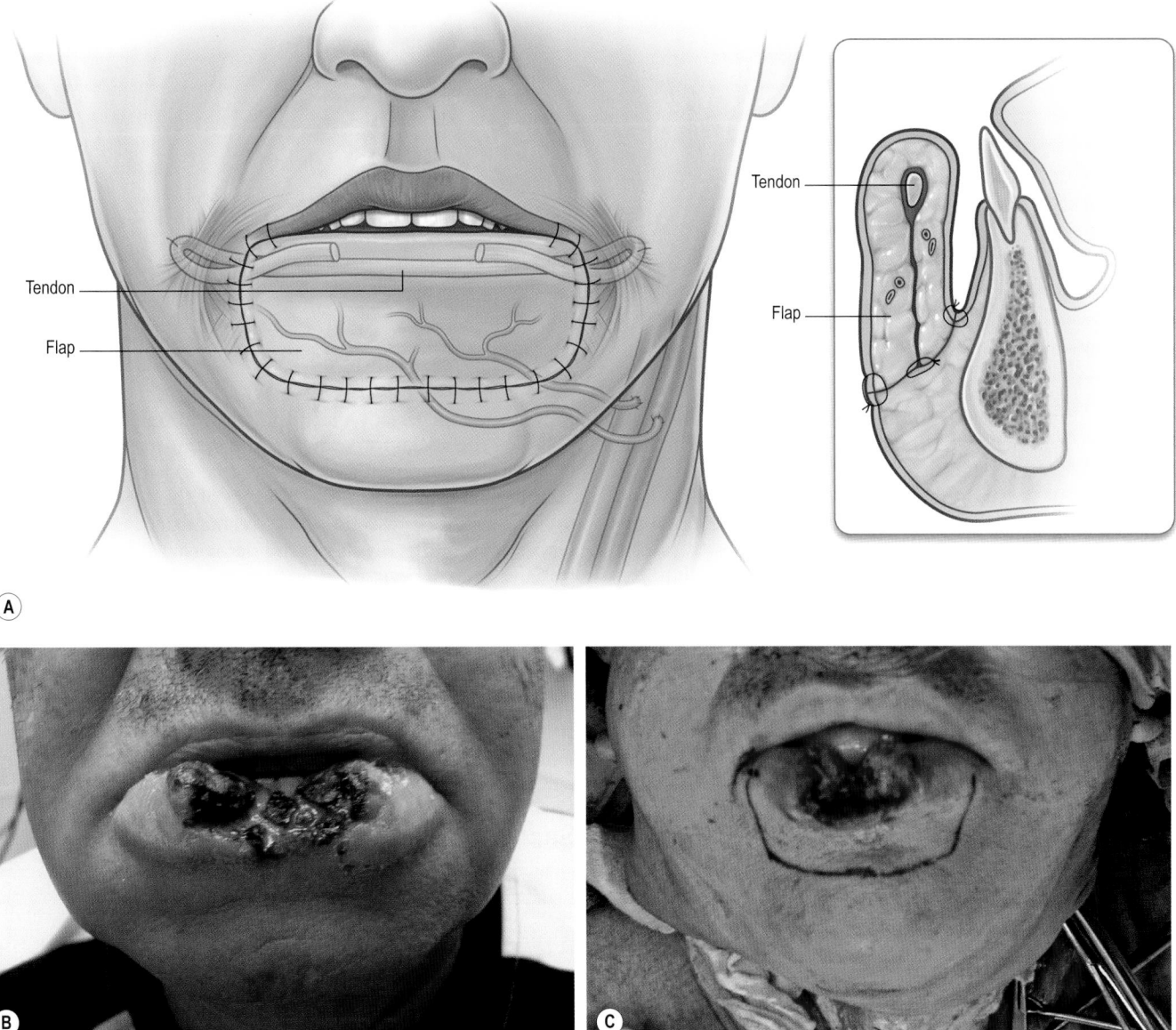

Fig. 10.14 (A) Schematic of palmaris/radial forearm flap reconstruction of the lower lip showing the Palmaris tendon woven through the remaining orbicularis muscle. **(B)** Patient shown with a large squamous cell carcinoma of the lower lip. **(C)** Resection of the lower lip planned.

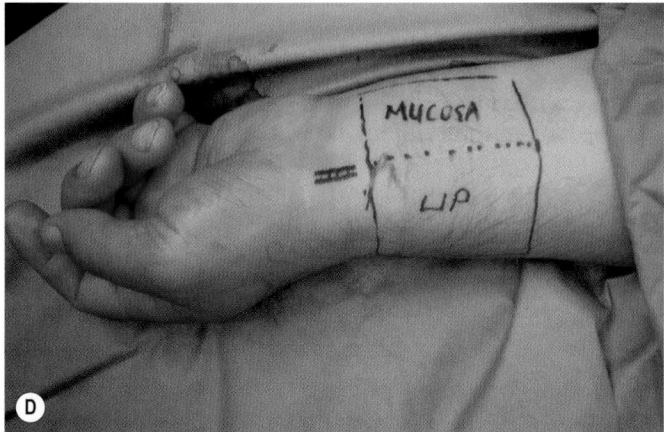

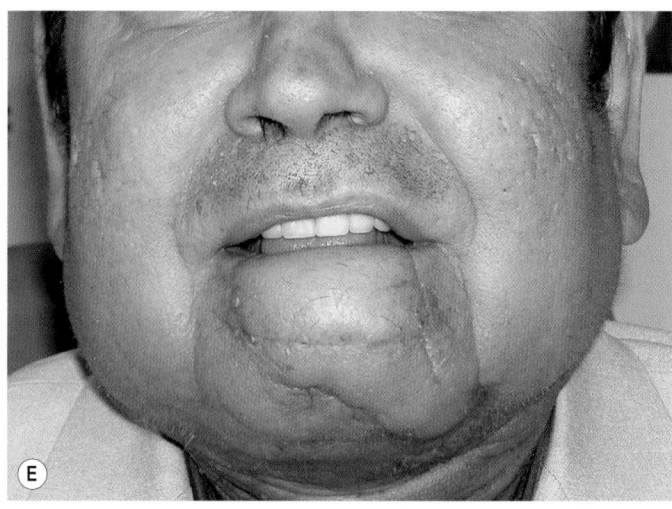

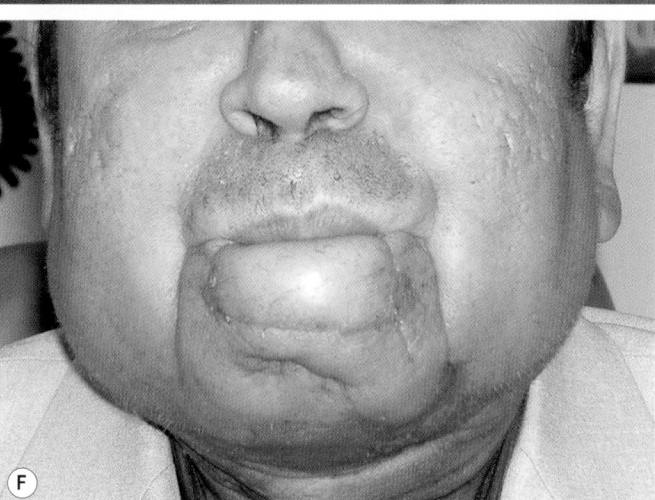

Fig. 10.14, cont'd **(D)** The planned radial forearm flap. Note the different dimensions of the skin and mucosal segments of the flap. **(E)** Postoperative appearance. **(F)** Note that the patient can purse his lips and has good oral competence.

free flap directly impacts the ultimate functional and aesthetic result. In our experience, optimal suspensory support for the tendon is achieved by slightly overcorrecting the tension. It is important to ensure that the pedicle is not compressed when the flap is folded over the tendon. Adequate suspension of the palmaris tendon will not eliminate lip ptosis and ectropion if the flap is too wide, so the flap should be narrower than the width of the defect (approx. 75%). Because the height of the skin excision and the mucosal resection usually differ, the skin and mucosal elements of the flap must be planned accordingly. Furthermore, fibrosis following surgery and radiation therapy tends to diminish the vertical height of the lip 6–12 months after reconstruction, so the vertical height of the reconstruction should be slightly greater than the height of the defect. It is also important to note that the height of the mucosal element of the lip will usually be shorter than the skin element. So these two elements of the defect need to be carefully measured so that the flap can be properly designed. The ultimate free flap reconstructive technique of the lip, which would also incorporate muscle between the inner and outer layers and restore the vermillion component, has not been described. Nevertheless, the composite radial forearm-palmaris longus tendon free flap has several advantages over pedicled flaps. This reconstruction allows for a single-stage procedure that results in complete skin coverage and intraoral lining. The large amount of skin that can be used with the radial forearm flap usually results in an adequate stomal size,

minimizing the risk of microstomia. Although the color match between the radial forearm flap and surrounding facial tissue is frequently suboptimal, acceptable cosmetic results are attainable by respecting the borders of the aesthetic subunits during surgical resection and reconstructive planning. In Japan, temporalis, masseter, and depressor anguli oris muscle transfers have been used in place of the palmaris longus tendon to achieve a more dynamic functional result when the lower lip is reconstructed with a radial forearm flap.[48–50] The functional outcomes with these reconstructive approaches have not been rigorously evaluated, and a prospective assessment of oral competence and dynamic function should be conducted to compare the outcomes following the use of palmaris longus tendon and muscle transfer techniques.

Secondary procedures

Secondary procedures may sometimes be necessary. Simple scar revision may be necessary in situations where scarring is very prominent or where scar contracture causes a visible or functional deformity. The standard principles of scar revision apply; Z-plasty or W-plasty for tight scars, skin grafts or further local flaps to release contractures. A skin graft may be necessary, for example, to correct an entropion or ectropion of the lip that is due to scar contracture. Occasionally, a denervated lower lip will become ptotic and some sort of

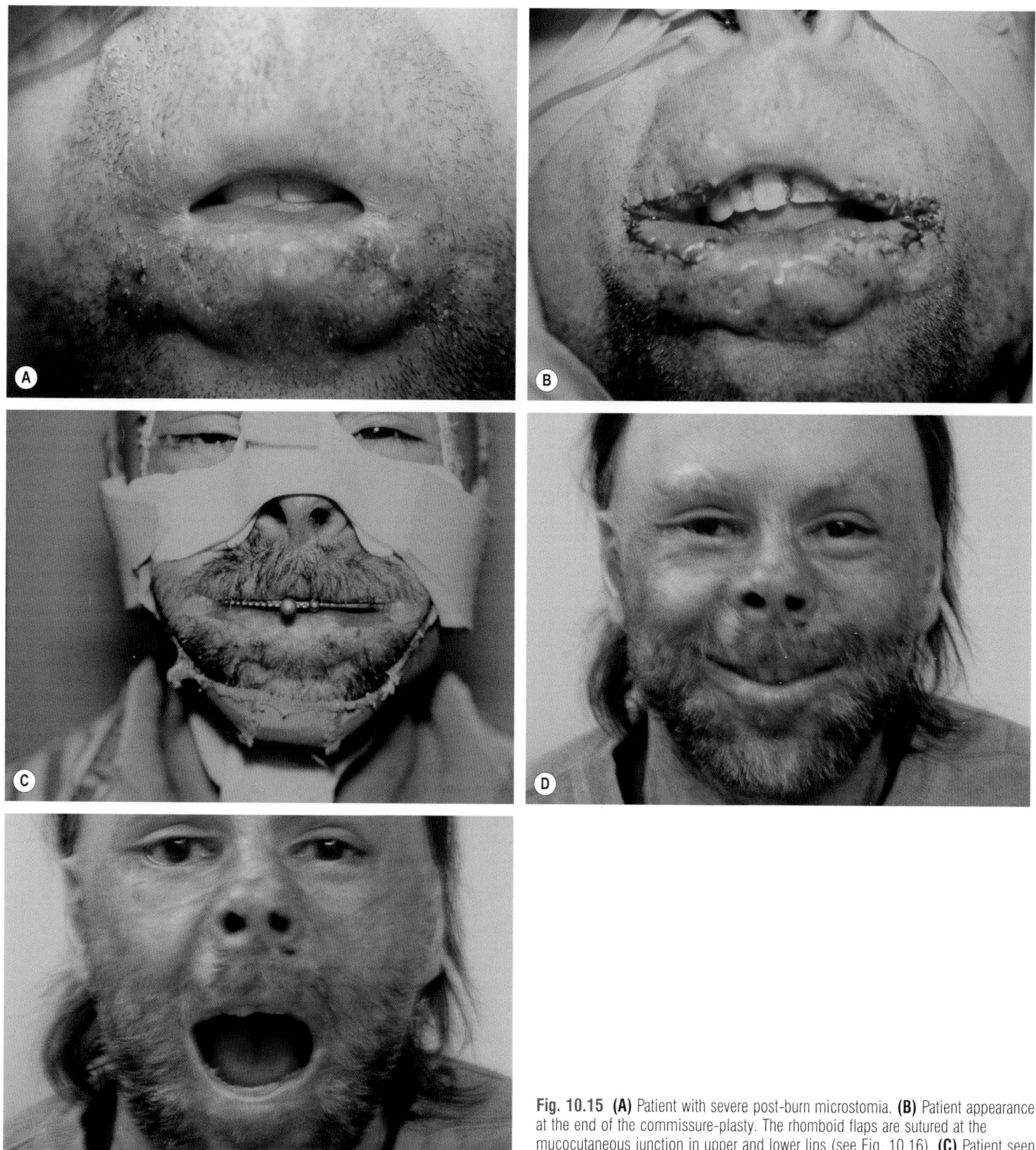

Fig. 10.15 **(A)** Patient with severe post-burn microstomia. **(B)** Patient appearance at the end of the commissure-plasty. The rhomboid flaps are sutured at the mucocutaneous junction in upper and lower lips (see Fig. 10.16). **(C)** Patient seen wearing his splint postoperatively. This patient wore his splint, except to eat, for 6 months. **(D,E)** At 10 year follow-up, showing maintenance of commissure position and excellent function.

lip shortening procedure may be necessary. These operations, however, are not routine and which procedure to do on which patient will depend very much on the specific problem. One operation that is somewhat standardized however, in secondary reconstruction, is the correction of microstomia.

Figure 10.15 shows a patient with post-burn microstomia corrected with bilateral commissure-plasty. This involves enlargement of the stomal opening by extending the commissure. The landmarks are the mid-pupillary lines. A vertical line dropped from the mid-pupil defines the normal position

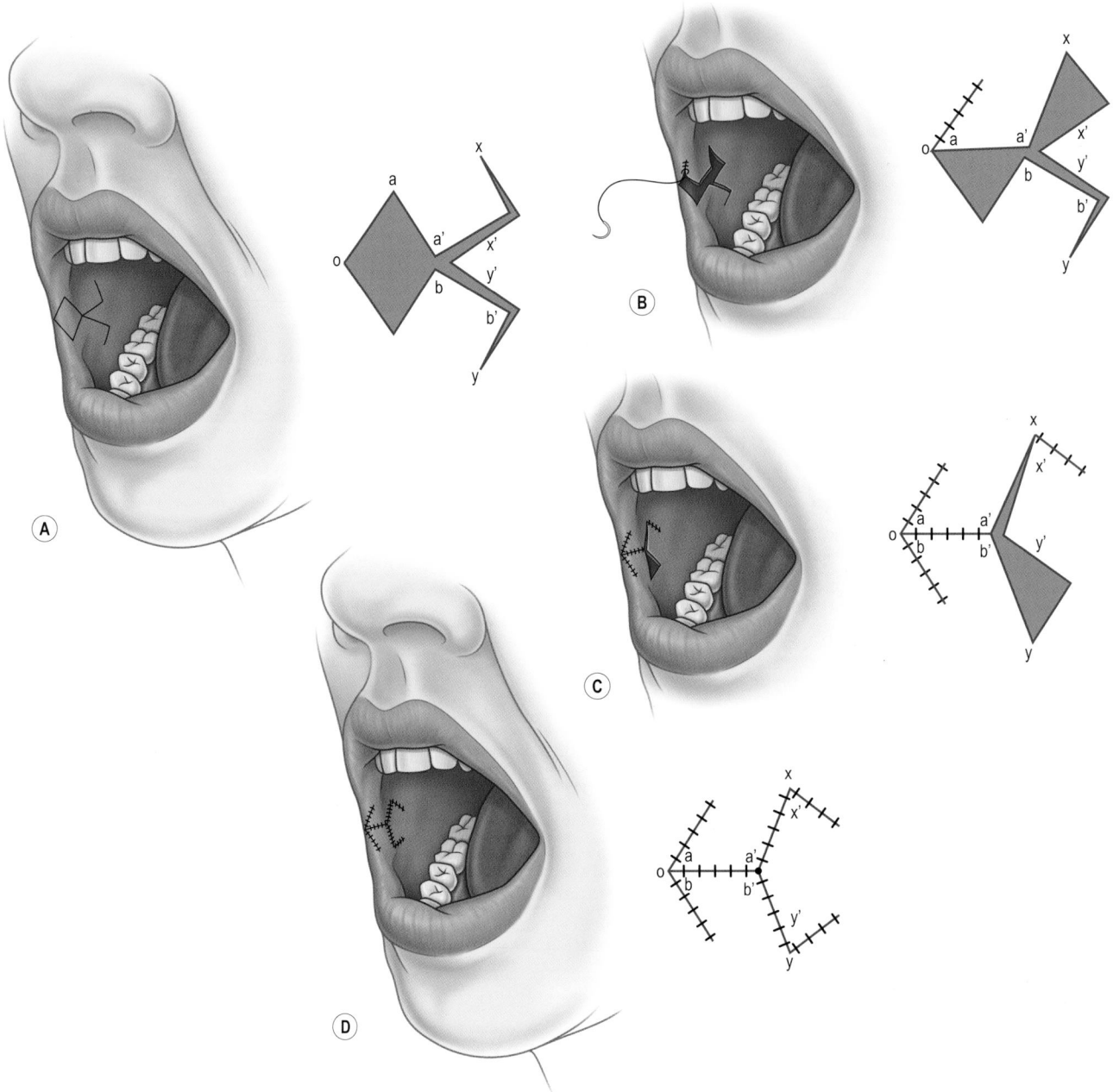

Fig. 10.16 (A) Schematic of split of commissure with rhomboid flaps marked above and below. **(B)** Flaps are raised. **(C)** Flaps are being rotated into the defect. **(D)** Flaps rotated into the defect, secondary defect closed by direct approximation.

of the commissure. To correct microstomia, a through and through incision is made from the commissure, horizontally to this line. The resulting raw areas are covered with mucosal rhomboid flaps *(Fig. 10.16)*. If the microstomia is caused by resection and reconstruction with, for example, Karapandzic flaps, this should correct the problem. However, if at all possible, the continuity of the sphincteric orbicularis oris muscle should be maintained. The boundaries of this muscle are hard to determine in these situations and it becomes a matter of judgment. In patients such as those depicted in *Figure 10.15*, the microstomia is caused by scar contracture, so that when

the microstomia is corrected it must be maintained by splinting.

Complications

Most of the complications encountered in lip reconstruction have already been alluded to earlier in this chapter. The standard complications that apply to any operation obviously apply in these repairs and the patient must be counseled about the possibility of postoperative wound infection, wound

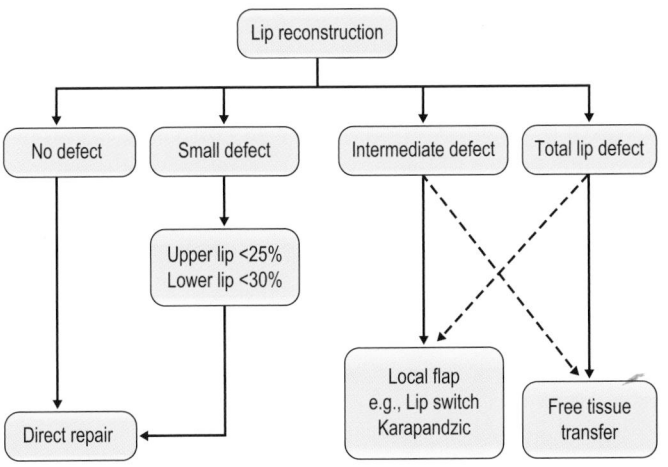

Fig. 10.17 An algorithmic approach to lip reconstruction.

dehiscence, bleeding, etc. With lip-switch procedures, and with the Abbé flap in particular, there is a risk of pedicle avulsion and it is important to ensure that the pedicle is not too radically skeletonized. Not only can an exposed pedicle be avulsed but it can thrombose or bleed. Fortunately, this complication is rare. With free flap lip reconstruction, the standard risks of microsurgical procedures apply and include partial and total flap loss, as well as the complications associated with flap harvest. However, the complications that are most predictable are those of microstomia, denervation, oral incontinence and aesthetic deformity. All of these have been discussed earlier in this chapter.

Postoperative care

The protocol for postoperative care depends on the procedure performed. Oral hygiene is important whatever the procedure, particularly if there are sutures intra-orally. For extensive reconstructions, the patient may need to be on a liquid or soft diet for several days after the procedure. Patients often find it more comfortable to suck a liquid diet through a straw initially. This is particularly the case for patients who have had an Abbé flap. Regardless of the complexity of the reconstruction, I will generally instruct patients to rinse with a mouthwash such as Peridex after eating, for 4 or 5 days after the procedure. Patients need to be instructed about dental hygiene. Using a toothbrush in the early postoperative period may not only be uncomfortable but may disrupt suture lines. So the postoperative regimen for each patient will depend on the procedure performed and may need to be individualized. *Figure 10.17* presents an algorithmic approach to lip reconstruction.

Cheek reconstruction

Operative technique: General principles

Local tissue works best in terms of replacing like with like in all parts of the body and especially in the very visible cheek. It provides tissue of like texture, of similar color and

with identical characteristics in terms of dermal appendages, hair growth, etc. Whenever possible, local tissue is the first choice in reconstructing the cheek. In situations where there is insufficient local tissue, tissue expansion may be an option, especially if the reconstructive indication is such that time can be spent setting the stage for the reconstruction. So, though it is not always an option, tissue expansion should be kept in the armamentarium when considering cheek reconstruction. The only indication to use distant tissue in cheek reconstruction is in the situation where there is insufficient local tissue.

Local flaps for cheek reconstruction

Several factors dictate the amount of local tissue available for cheek reconstruction. Defect size is obviously important. However, the age of the patient is also important. The greater skin laxity in an older patient will allow reconstructions to be performed that would be impossible, or certainly more complex, in a younger patient. Smaller cheek wounds can frequently be converted to an ellipse and closed directly. It is important to be cognizant of the relaxed skin tension lines and to keep all scars parallel to these lines if possible. In the elderly patient, these are usually easily visualized and incisions can be appropriately planned. All manner of local flaps can be used for defect closure and first principles apply: (1) Keep incisions parallel to relaxed skin tension lines and (2) avoid traction on vital structures that may cause secondary deformity. The perfect example in the context of cheek reconstruction is the lower eyelid. Even a relatively minor amount of traction on the lower eyelid can produce ectropion. Careful preoperative planning as well as attention to technical detail can help avoid problems such as this.

Cheek rotation advancement flap

Medially- or laterally-based cheek rotation advancement flaps are, by far, the most commonly used flaps in reconstructing cheek defects. Some basic principles apply and are important. There is some horizontal laxity in the cheek, particularly in older patients. However, the amount of laxity is limited. Therefore, the rotational element of the flap is very important. These flaps can be based anteriorly as described by Juri and Juri,[51,52] or posteriorly as described by Stark and Kaplan *(Fig. 10.18)*.[53] Basing the flap posteriorly *(Fig. 10.18B)* allows mobilization of the jowls so that this excess can be moved up onto the face. Basing the flap anteriorly *(Fig. 10.18A)* allows for mobilization of neck skin up onto the face. Extending the incision down onto the chest significantly increases the arc of the rotation of the flap *(Fig. 10.18A)*.[54,55] This incorporates a back-cut allows for better flap mobility of the flap as well as facilitating closure of the secondary defect.

The possibility of ectropion as a complication of a cheek rotation advancement flap is a very real one. This is because of the gravitational pull of the flap on the delicate lower eyelid. To avoid this, the flap should be suspended from the underlying bony skeleton either using periosteal sutures *(Fig. 10.19A)*[56] or with an anchoring device such as a Mitek anchor.[57] In this way, skin closure at the eyelid interface can be achieved completely without tension *(Fig. 10.19B)*. Particular care must be exercised in female patients to avoid advancing hair-bearing skin from the sideburn area onto the cheek. This can be avoided by placing the incision around the sideburn in these cases *(Fig. 10.18A)*. This can also facilitate closure so that the sideburn is not altered. As the flap is rotated, the resulting dog-ear is excised. It is usually possible to place this scar either in the nasolabial fold or parallel to it.

The submental artery flap

The submental flap is a very useful addition to our armamentarium for reconstructing defects of the cheek. As with the cheek rotation flap, it provides skin of similar texture and

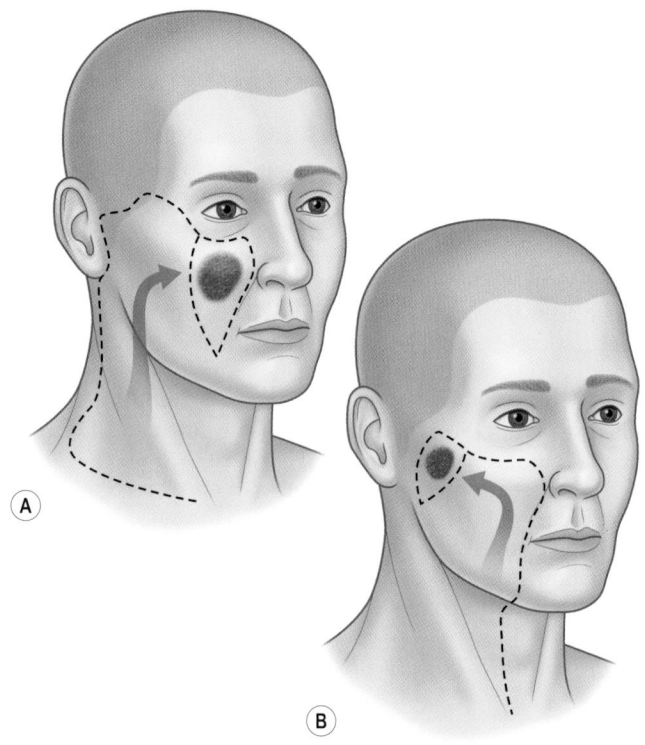

(A)

(B)

Fig. 10.18 (A) A medially-based cheek rotation flap. **(B)** A laterally-based cheek rotation flap.

color. Furthermore, the scar is very conveniently hidden under the chin, something that patients really appreciate. It can easily be tunneled up into the cheek. Be aware that this is beard-growing skin in the male. It is an excellent choice of flap for small to moderate sized defects *(Fig. 10.20)*. Based on the submental branch of the facial artery *(Fig. 10.21)*, the flap can be tunneled up into the cheek.[58] Increasing the arc of rotation can be achieved in two ways: antegrade or retrograde.[59] The facial artery gives off the submental branch before it continues up over the mandibular border to reach the face. If the facial artery is divided cephalad to the submental branch run-off, the facial artery can be dissected back towards its origin from the external carotid. Because of the tortuous nature of the facial artery as it crosses over the submandibular gland, this maneuver generally yields an extra couple of centimeters of pedicle length. Alternatively, the facial artery can be divided caudal to the submental branch. In this situation, the flap is perfused through retrograde flow from the facial artery. This reversed flow pattern of perfusion is adequate to sustain the flap.[59]

Free tissue transfer

For large defects, and in particular, for those large defects in which a cheek rotation flap may not be sufficient, an alternate source of tissue must be found. In this circumstance, a free flap may be required. Frequently, the defect is such that more than soft tissue reconstruction is required. While reconstruction of maxillectomy defects is not the subject of this chapter, it is important to be aware of the important issues that influence the choice of reconstruction in this clinical setting.

Soft tissue cheek reconstruction

Choosing the most appropriate free flap for cheek reconstruction is important for all the reasons already alluded to: color match, texture, thickness. The characteristics of the defect will dictate the required elements of the flap so that a through-and-though defect requires a more complex reconstruction than a simple skin-only defect. For through-and-through defects, an epithelial surface will be required for lining as well

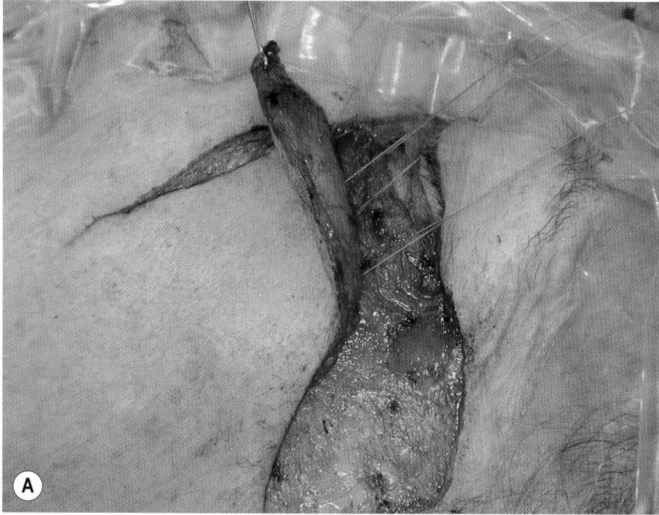

(A)

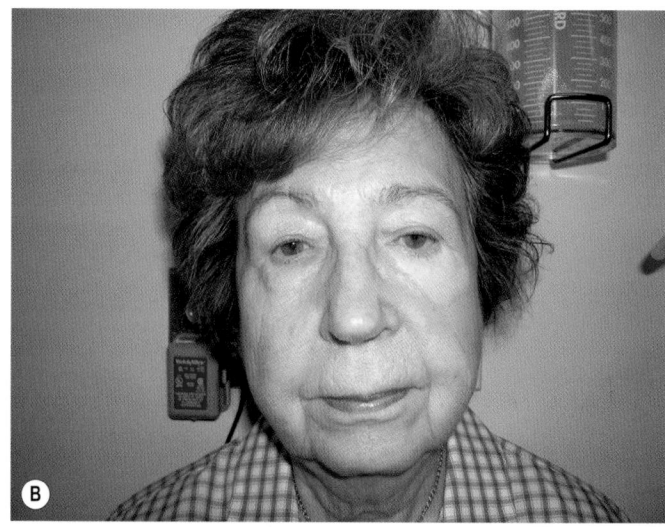

(B)

Fig. 10.19 (A) Sutures are placed through the periosteum of the inferior orbital rim to suspend a cheek rotation flap. **(B)** Patient's final appearance.

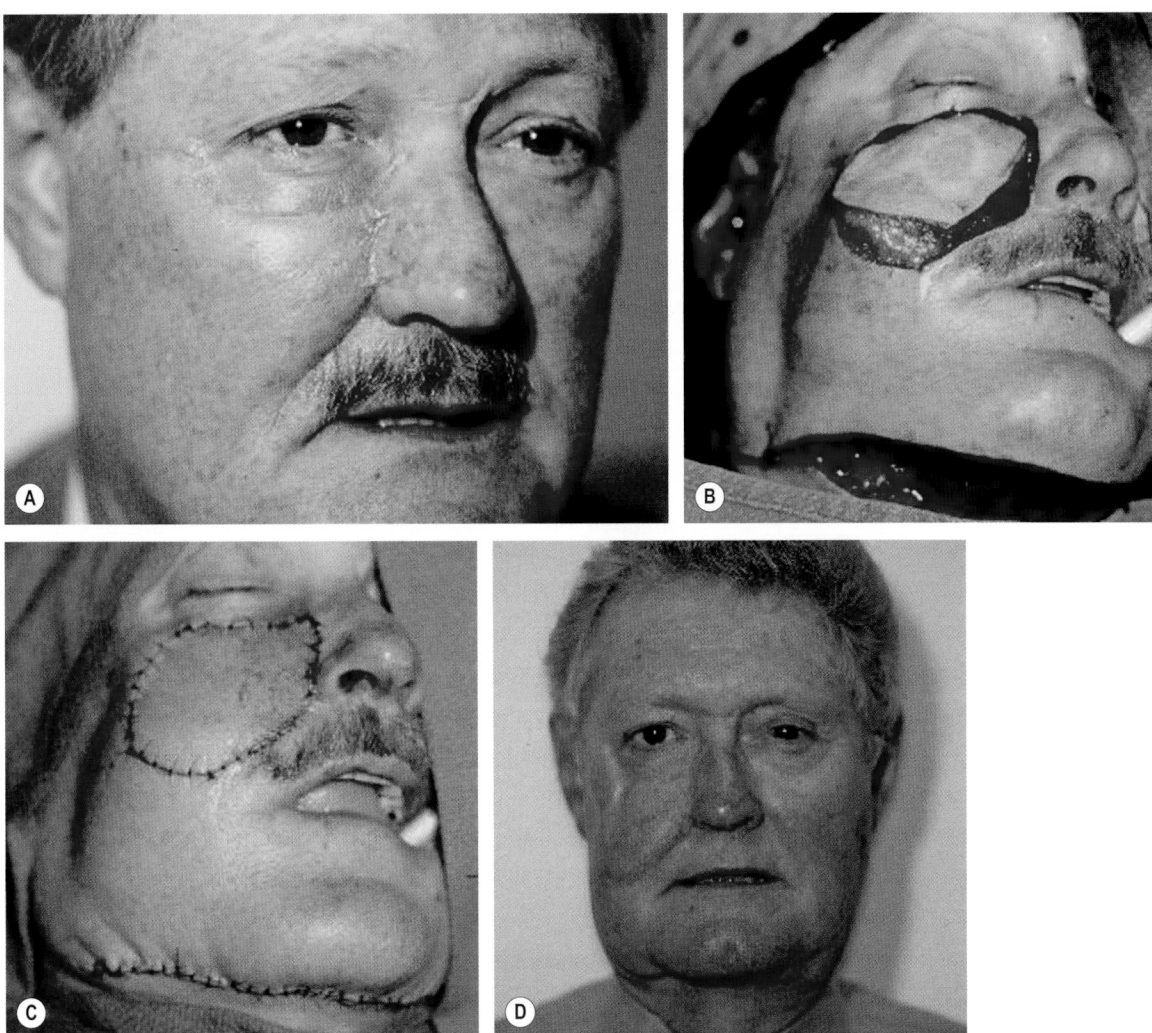

Fig. 10.20 **(A)** Patient with a recurrent morpheaform basal cell carcinoma of the right cheek. Patient has had a previous cheek rotation flap and the tissues are too tight to consider another cheek rotation. **(B)** A submental flap has been tunneled into the cheek to close the defect. **(C)** Appearance on insetting of the cheek and closure of the donor defect. **(D)** Patient's final appearance.

as cover. Bulk, while it is an issue, is not a major one, as the flap can be subsequently thinned if it is too thick. One of the most important issues in choosing a donor site is that of *color*. A good color match is, in many ways, the most important feature of the reconstruction. If the color match is good, many imperfections will not be noticed, whereas if the match is bad, the eye is drawn to the reconstruction and every imperfection will be noticed. Color match is, in part, also related to ethnicity. There is less difference in regional skin color in darker skinned patients. Studies have been carried out on patients with Fitzpatrick type II–III skin[60] showing which donor sites are best.[61,62] In most cases, flaps harvested from the upper trunk work best. In situations where color match is poor, the option of de-epithelialization and over-grafting with split thickness skin harvested from the scalp yields much improved results.[63,64]

Scapular and parascapular flaps

The skin territory of the scapular and parascapular flap is sufficiently large to allow for closure of the largest cheek

defect while at the same time closing the donor defect directly. Depending on the size of defect, the flap can be folded on itself in the case of through-and-through defects, to provide lining and cover *(Fig. 10.22)* or alternatively, scapular and parascapular flaps can be harvested on the transverse and descending branches of the circumflex scapular artery respectively, to provide lining and cover. This allows more leeway in terms of inset as both skin paddles can move independently of each other. The thoracodorsal perforator flap incorporates the same territory as the circumflex scapular system. *Figure 10.23* shows the relationship of the first dorsal perforator of the thoracodorsal system to the circumflex scapular artery. In some situations, it is nice to have an option in terms of pedicle placement and length. One of the biggest drawbacks of using scapular skin is the fact that flap harvest and ablation cannot be done simultaneously. Patient repositioning can be avoided by harvesting the parascapular skin territory and placing the patient on a beanbag in the semi-supine position with the arm free-draped. The scapula can also be taken with bone and this can be used effectively to reconstruct the bony contour of the cheek.

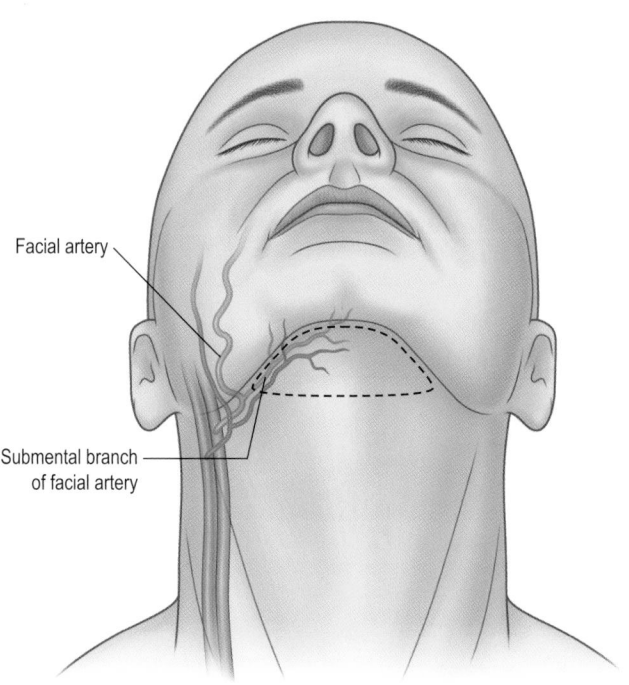

Facial artery

Submental branch
of facial artery

Fig. 10.21 Schematic diagram of the vascular supply of the submental flap. Note the separate vein draining the flap.

Anterolateral thigh flap

The anterolateral thigh flap is an alternative to the scapular/parascapular flap. Color match is not as good in lighter skinned patients. However, in darker skinned individuals the color difference is less marked. This flap has the advantage of facilitating a two team approach, allowing simultaneous flap harvest and tumor ablation. The anterolateral thigh flap provides adequate skin quantity and quality, though in a male, hairiness may be an issue. The flap can be harvested with or without fascia. Suprafascial dissection provides a thinner flap[65] which, in the context of cheek reconstruction, is optimal. In female patients, bulk may still be an issue as the thigh in older female patients may have a significant amount of subcutaneous fat. This fat can be safely trimmed without compromising flap vascularity.[66] The donor defect is very acceptable and in almost all cases can be closed directly. This flap can provide a very satisfactory solution for reconstruction of large cheek defects.

Other flaps

The radial forearm flap has also been used in cheek reconstruction. The thin nature of this flap makes it amenable to folding for through-and-through defects but my experience has been that even a folded radial forearm flap is too thin. The rectus abdominis myocutaneous flap has also been extensively used in this situation. While it provides adequate tissue, both color match and bulk may be unacceptable.

The facial nerve

A discussion on cheek reconstruction is not complete without considering the facial nerve. A full discussion on management of the facial nerve is beyond the scope of this chapter but it is important to consider the facial nerve in the context of cheek reconstruction. A decision frequently needs to be made with regard to facial nerve function in cases where the nerve is sacrificed. Options include primary nerve grafting, functional muscle transfer as well as static sling operations. The decision on which modality to use depends on several factors. For example, in an elderly patient with a poor prognosis, the chance of getting good function from primary nerve grafting is remote and a free functioning muscle transfer is not an option in this situation. However, the patient's quality of life will be significantly improved by use of static slings. Finally, contour is an important aspect of cheek reconstruction. Some ablative procedures, such as parotidectomy are associated with a postoperative contour defect that can be very disturbing for the patient. More radical ablations can include the whole of the parotid gland as well as the facial nerve. In these cases, a flap can be used to fill in the contour defect with excellent effect.

Composite defects

A chapter on lip and cheek reconstruction would also not be complete without a discussion of how to reconstruct defects that include both lip and cheek elements. *Figure 10.24* is a good illustration of such a defect that also raises the issue of facial nerve management. In this case, the defect included the upper lip, cheek, lower eyelid as well as facial nerve sacrifice. When considering such a defect, it is best to think of it in terms of the components that require reconstruction. In the case of the patient in *Figure 10.24*, the resection included upper lip, cheek and lower eyelid. The upper lip was reconstructed with an Estlander flap from the lower lip while the cheek was reconstructed with a scapular free flap. The eyelid reconstruction was deferred and the eye temporarily closed with a tarsorrhaphy. The eyelid was reconstructed later with a Hughes Tarso-conjunctival flap. Note also that a static plantaris tendon sling was used to position the new oral commissure. By breaking the defect into its separate components, the reconstruction was made much simpler.

Conclusion

Reconstruction of the lips following surgical resection should be guided by a defect-specific approach that strives to optimize oral competence and recreate natural-appearing lips. Each defect is unique. Therefore it is important to analyze each defect with respect to the tissue elements missing. Where at all possible, local tissue should be used for the reconstruction, as it gives the best aesthetic and functional result. A sensate dynamic flap that restores normal lip height, volume, and sphincteric function is preferred, and the aesthetic subunits of the lip should be respected. Limited defects can be reconstructed by using local flaps from the remaining labial tissue or the adjacent cheek, whereas larger

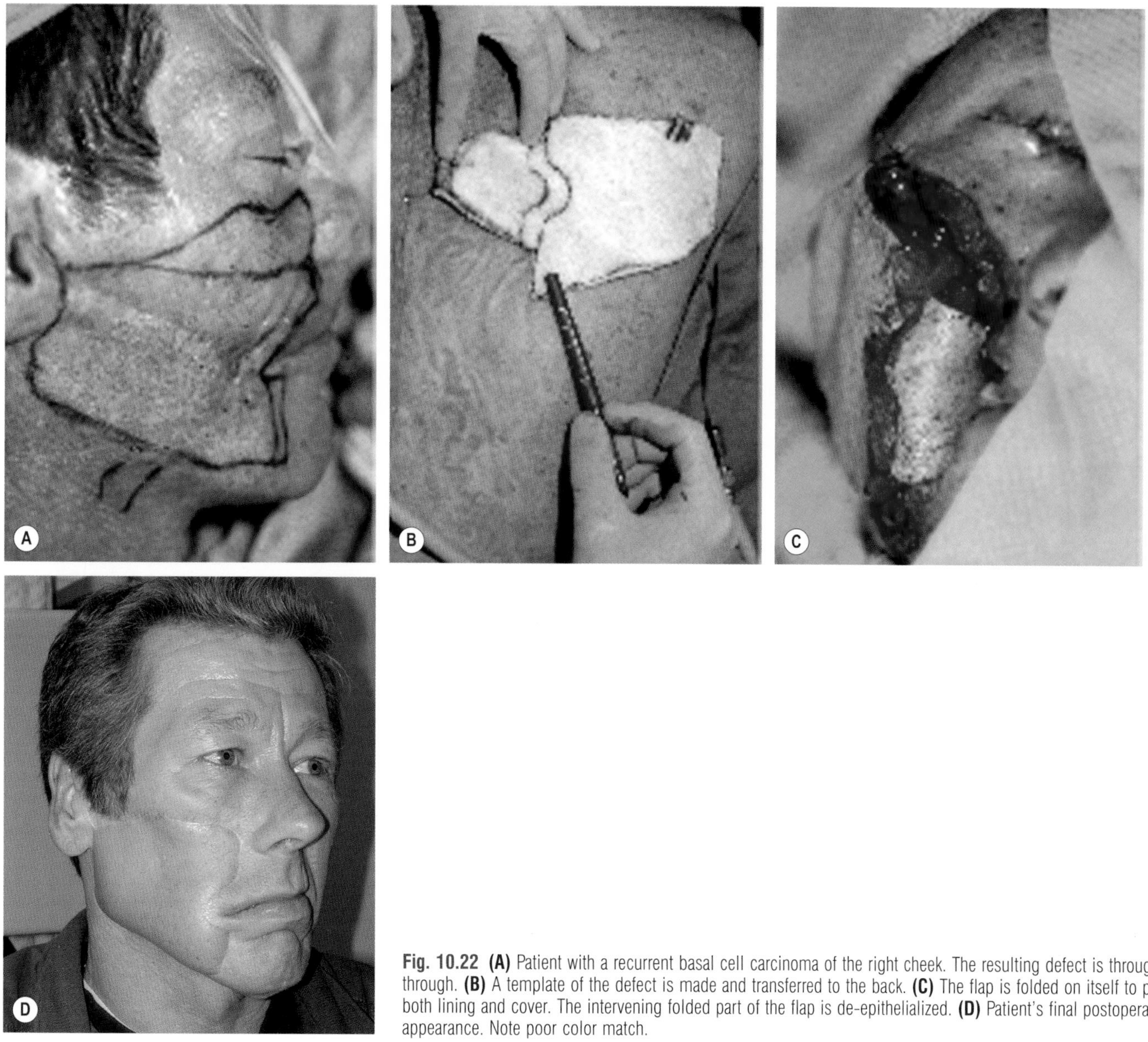

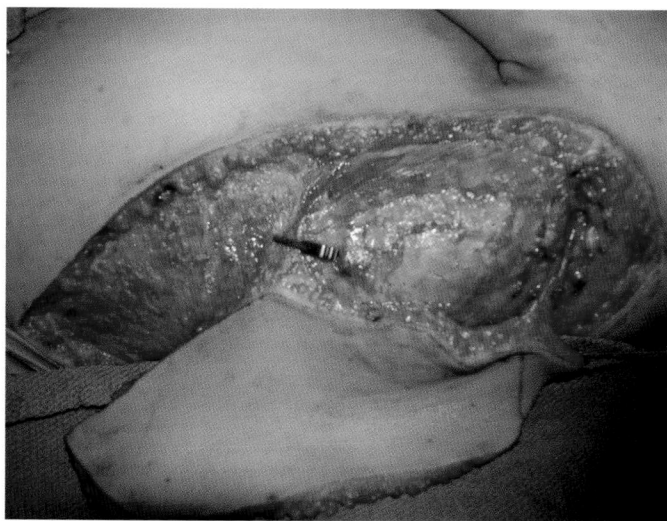

Fig. 10.22 (A) Patient with a recurrent basal cell carcinoma of the right cheek. The resulting defect is through and through. **(B)** A template of the defect is made and transferred to the back. **(C)** The flap is folded on itself to provide both lining and cover. The intervening folded part of the flap is de-epithelialized. **(D)** Patient's final postoperative appearance. Note poor color match.

Fig. 10.23 The blood supply of the parascapular region. Two pedicles are seen. On the right is the circumflex scapular artery. On the left with the vascular clamp, is the thoracodorsal perforator. Both these vessels supply the same region of skin.

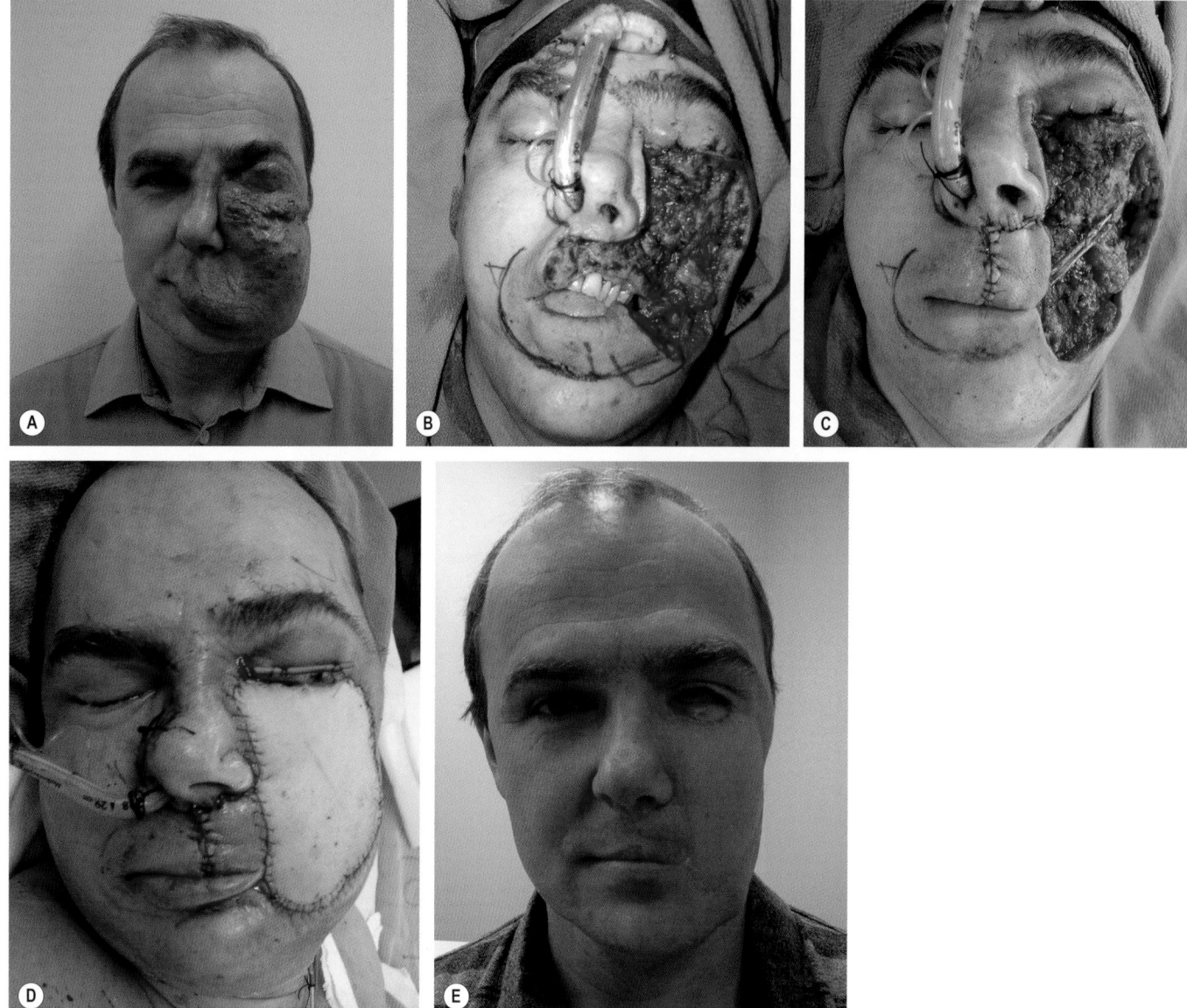

Fig. 10.24 **(A)** Patient with large venous malformation of the left cheek. **(B)** Resection includes upper lip, cheek and lower eyelid. **(C)** The lip is reconstructed with an Estlander flap from the lower lip. The eye is temporarily sutured closed and a plantaris tendon sling is used to position the oral commissure. **(D)** Patient's appearance at the time of final closure. **(E)** Final appearance following reconstruction of the lower eyelid.

defects may require free tissue transfer or multiple local reconstructive techniques. Because most traditional reconstructive techniques for extensive lip defects have a variety of inherent shortcomings, the most important of which is microstomia, improved outcomes should be sought by incorporating technical modifications or by employing novel surgical approaches such as the composite radial forearm-palmaris longus tendon free flap for the largest defects. The importance of restoring normal lip appearance and function following cancer resection is undeniable, and surgeons must be able to appreciate the nuances of surgical reconstruction that will make the greatest impact on the ultimate reconstructive outcome.

Reconstruction of the cheek should address issues of contour, color match as well as animation when indicated. Again, where possible, local tissue works best, as it replaces what has been lost with exactly similar tissue. Cheek rotation flaps, based whether medially or laterally, can be used to reconstruct large defects. Other local flaps, such as the submental flap, may also be useful. Where free tissue transfer is being used for reconstruction, the issue of color and texture match is more difficult to achieve.

Access the complete reference list online at **http://www.expertconsult.com**

1. Neligan PC. Strategies in lip reconstruction. *Clin Plast Surg.* 2009;36(3):477–485.

   Injury or surgical trauma can result in significant alterations of normal lip appearance and function that can profoundly impact the patient's self-image and quality of life. Neuromuscular injury can lead to asymmetry at rest and during facial animation, and distressing functional disabilities are common. Loss of labial competence may interfere with the ability to articulate, whistle, suck, kiss, and contain salivary secretions. For smaller defects, reconstruction can be very effective. Reconstructing an aesthetically pleasing and functional lip is more difficult with larger defects.

4. Karapandzic M. Reconstruction of lip defects by local arterial flaps. *Br J Plast Surg.* 1974;27(1):93–97.

18. Langstein H, Robb G. Lip and perioral reconstruction. *Clin Plast Surg.* 2005;32:431–445

20. Cordeiro PG, Santamaria E. Primary reconstruction of complex midfacial defects with combined lip-switch procedures and free flaps. *Plast Reconstr Surg.* 1999;103(7):1850–1856.

   Free flaps are generally the preferred method for reconstructing large defects of the midface, orbit, and maxilla that include the lip and oral commissure; commissuroplasty is traditionally performed at a second stage. Functional results of the oral sphincter using this reconstructive approach are, however, limited. This article presents a new approach to the reconstruction of massive defects of the lip and midface using a free flap in combination with a lip-switch flap. This was used in 10 patients. One-third to one-half of the upper lip was excised in seven patients, one-third of the lower lip was excised in one patient, and both the upper and lower lips were excised (one-third each) in two patients. All patients had maxillectomies, with or without mandibulectomies, in addition to full-thickness resections of the cheek. A switch flap from the opposite lip was used for reconstruction of the oral commissure and oral sphincter, and a rectus abdominis myocutaneous flap with two or three skin islands was used for reconstruction of the through-and-through defect in the midface. Free flap survival was 100%. All patients had good-to-excellent oral competence, and they were discharged without feeding tubes.

27. Webster J. Crescentic peri-alar cheek excision for upper lip flap advancement with a short history of upper lip repair. *Plast Reconstr Surg.* 1955;16:434–464.

28. Abbe R. A new plastic operation for the relief of deformity due to double harelip. *Plast Reconstr Surg.* 1968;42(5):481–483.

38. Kroll SS. Staged sequential flap reconstruction for large lower lip defects. *Plast Reconstr Surg.* 1991;88(4):620–627.

45. Jeng SF, Kuo YR, Wei FC, et al. Total lower lip reconstruction with a composite radial forearm-palmaris longus tendon flap: a clinical series. *Plast Reconstr Surg.* 2004;113(1):19–23.

   Large, full-thickness lip defects after head and neck surgery continue to be a challenge for reconstructive surgeons. The reconstructive aims are to restore the oral lining, the external cheek, oral competence, and function (i.e., articulation, speech, and mastication). These authors' refinement of the composite radial forearm-palmaris longus free flap technique meets these criteria and allows a functional reconstruction of extensive lip and cheek defects in one stage. A composite radial forearm flap including the palmaris longus tendon was designed. The skin flap for the reconstruction of the intraoral lining and the skin defect was folded over the palmaris longus tendon. Both ends of the vascularized tendon were laid through the bilateral modiolus and anchored with adequate tension to the intact orbicularis muscle of the upper lip. This procedure was used in 12 patients.

55. Shestak KC, Roth AG, Jones NF, et al. The cervicopectoral rotation flap – a valuable technique for facial reconstruction. *Br J Plast Surg.* 1993;46(5):375–377.

58. Curran AJ, Neligan P, Gullane PJ. Submental artery island flap. *Laryngoscope.* 1997;107(11 Pt 1):1545–1549.

11

Facial paralysis

Ronald M. Zuker, Eyal Gur, Gazi Hussain, and Ralph T. Manktelow

SYNOPSIS

- Assess clinical problem: functional, psychosocial, and aesthetic.
- Understand the etiology and natural history of disease processes associated with facial paralysis.
- Knowledge of anatomy is imperative for optimizing results.
- Formulate realistic, attainable, and practical management plan.
- Surgical management is multifocal and must be individualized for each patient.

Introduction

Facial paralysis is a complex multifaceted condition with profound functional deficiencies, devastating aesthetic effects, and tragic psychological consequences. It may be congenital or acquired, affect the old and the young, and vary from mild to severe. In this chapter we will focus on the clinical problem and the surgical solutions available today.

Historical perspective

Surgical correction of facial paralyses continues to evolve and improve. Early attempts were directed at static repositioning to address functional problems around the eye and mouth. Muscle transplants were initially nonvascularized grafts but function was impaired shortly thereafter with the muscle being revascularized and reinnervated. At first this was via ipsilateral nerves and later using contralateral nerves. For facial musculature that has the potential for reinnervation, nerve transfers were introduced as a very effective method of maintaining nerve function and muscle activation. Recent combinations of nerve transfers and muscle transplantation have been developed.

At present surgical methods to recover facial nerve function range from nerve repair, nerve grafting, and nerve transfer to static slings and muscle transfers and finally functioning muscle transplantation. A variety of combinations have also been introduced as this complex field continues to develop with newer and more effective treatment options.

Basic science

As a backdrop to the clinical management of facial paralysis, a detailed description of the anatomy of the facial nerve and the facial musculature follows:

The facial nerve

The extratemporal portion of the seventh cranial nerve begins at the stylomastoid foramen. It is in a deep position below the earlobe but becomes more superficial before it passes between the superficial and deep portions of the parotid gland. Here it divides into two main trunks which then further divide within the substance of the gland. In a series of anatomic dissections, Davis et al.[1] demonstrated several branching patterns of the facial nerve. Traditionally, it is taught that this results in five divisions of the facial nerve: frontotemporal, zygomatic, buccal, marginal mandibular, and cervical. In practice, however, there is no distinct separation between the zygomatic and buccal branches either in their location or in the muscles they innervate.

On leaving the parotid, the facial nerve may have 8–15 branches making up the five divisions. Distally, there is further arborization and interconnection of these branches (Fig. 11.1). The net effect is a great deal of functional overlap between the branches. For example, a single zygomaticobuccal branch may supply innervation to the orbicularis oculi as well as to the orbicularis oris.

The temporal division consists of three or four branches[2] that run obliquely along the undersurface of the temporoparietal fascia after crossing the zygomatriarch in a location 3–5 cm from the lateral orbital margin. The lower branches run along the undersurface of the superior portion of the orbicularis oculi for 3–4 mm before entering the muscle to

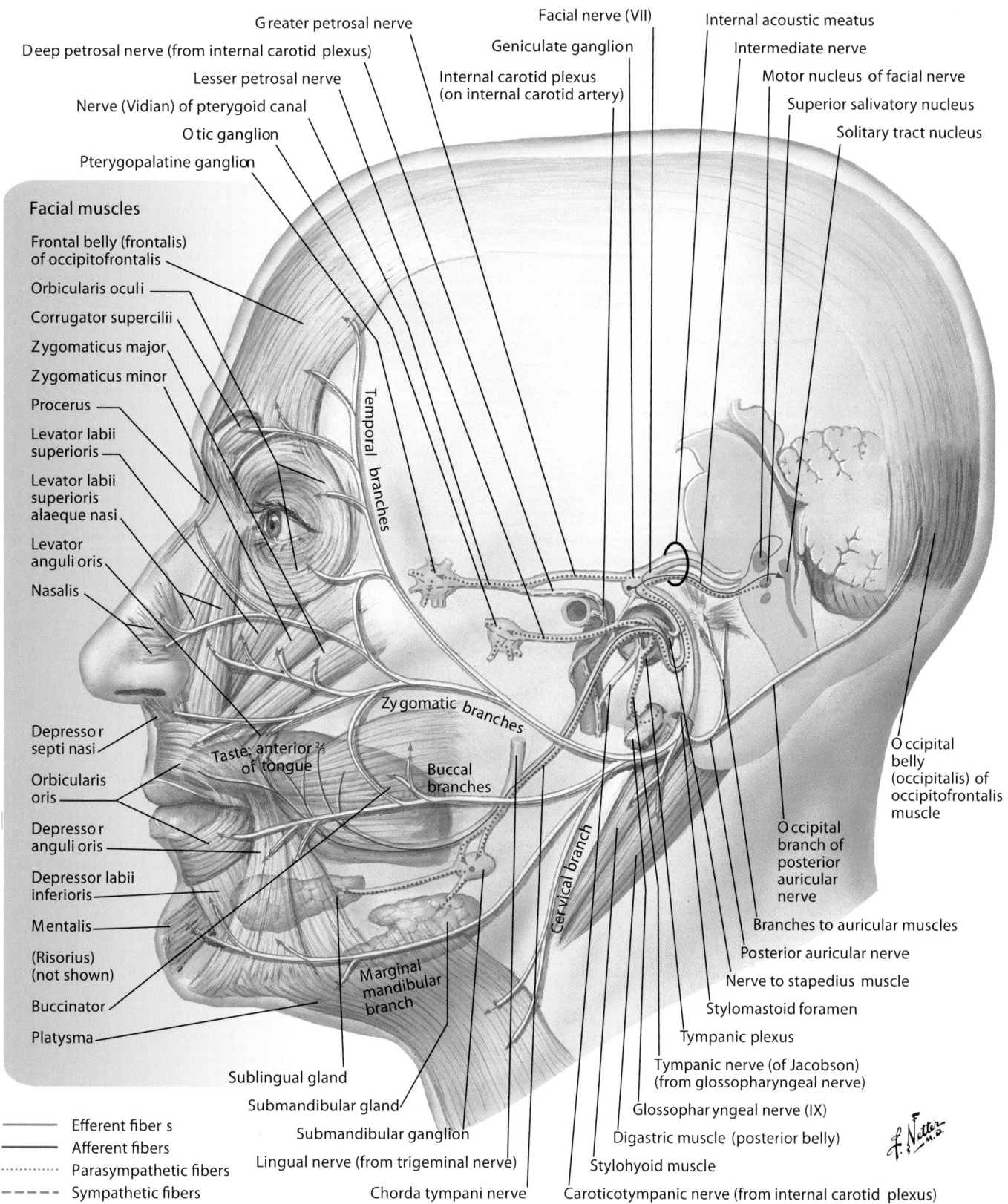

Greater petrosal nerve

Deep petrosal nerve (from internal carotid plexus)

Lesser petrosal nerve

Nerve (Vidian) of pterygoid canal

Otic ganglion

Pterygopalatine ganglion

Facial nerve (VII)

Geniculate ganglion

Internal carotid plexus
(on internal carotid artery)

Internal acoustic meatus

Intermediate nerve

Motor nucleus of facial nerve

Superior salivatory nucleus

Solitary tract nucleus

Facial muscles

Frontal belly (frontalis)
of occipitofrontalis

Orbicularis oculi

Corrugator supercilii

Zygomaticus major

Zygomaticus minor

Procerus

Levator labii
superioris

Levator labii
superioris
alaeque nasi

Levator
anguli oris

Nasalis

Temporal branches

Zygomatic branches

Taste: anterior ⅔
of tongue

Buccal
branches

Depressor
septi nasi

Orbicularis
oris

Depressor
anguli oris

Depressor labii
inferioris

Mentalis

(Risorius)
(not shown)

Buccinator

Platysma

Cervical branch

Marginal
mandibular
branch

Occipital
belly
(occipitalis) of
occipitofrontalis
muscle

Occipital
branch of
posterior
auricular
nerve

Branches to auricular muscles

Posterior auricular nerve

Nerve to stapedius muscle

Stylomastoid foramen

Tympanic plexus

Tympanic nerve (of Jacobson)
(from glossopharyngeal nerve)

Glossopharyngeal nerve (IX)

Digastric muscle (posterior belly)

Stylohyoid muscle

Caroticotympanic nerve (from internal carotid plexus)

Sublingual gland

Submandibular gland

Submandibular ganglion

Lingual nerve (from trigeminal nerve)

Chorda tympani nerve

——— Efferent fibers
——— Afferent fibers
············ Parasympathetic fibers
- - - - Sympathetic fibers

Fig. 11.1 A typical pattern of facial nerve branching. The main branch is divided into two components, each of which then branches in a random manner to all parts of the face. The extensive distal arborization and interconnections are apparent. (Reprinted with permission from www.netterimages.com ©Elsevier Inc. All rights reserved.)

innervate it.[3] According to Ishikawa,[2] the upper two branches entering the frontalis muscle at the level of the supraorbital ridge are usually located up to 3 cm above the lateral canthus. The nerves usually lie approximately 1.6 cm inferior to the frontal branch of the superficial temporal artery. Because there is relatively little adipose tissue at the lateral border of the frontalis, those nerves are virtually subcutaneous and susceptible to injury.

The zygomaticobuccal division consists of five to eight branches with significant overlap of muscle innervations such that one or more branches may be divided without causing weakness. These nerves supply innervations to the lip elevators as well as to the lower orbicularis oculi, orbicularis oris, and buccinators. Functional facial nerve mapping and cross-facial nerve grafting require the precise identification and stimulation of these zygomaticobuccal branches to isolate the exact branches responsible for smiling. These nerves lie deep near the parotid-masseteric fascia in the same plane as the parotid duct. There are sometimes connections between the lower branches and the marginal mandibular division.

The marginal mandibular division consists of one to three branches[4] whose course begins up to 2 cm below the ramus of the mandible and arcs upward to cross the mandible halfway between the angle and mental protuberance. It has been well documented[2,3,5] that these branches lie on the deep surface of the platysma and cross superficial to the facial vessels approximately 3.5 cm from the parotid edge. Nelson and Gingrass[5] described separate branches to the depressor angularis, depressor labii inferioris, and mentalis, and a variable superior ramus supplying the upper platysma and lower orbicularis oris.

The cervical division consists of one branch that leaves the parotid well below the angle of the mandible and runs on the deep surface of the platysma, which it innervates by entering the muscle at the junction of its cranial and middle thirds. This point of entry is 2 or 3 cm caudal to the platysma muscle branch of the facial vessel.[6]

Facial musculature

Facial musculature consists of 17 paired muscles and one unpaired sphincter muscle, the orbicularis oris (*Fig. 11.2*). The subtle movements that convey facial expression require coordination between all of these muscles.

The major muscles affecting the forehead and eyelids are the frontalis, corrugator, and orbicularis oculi. There are two main groups of muscles controlling the movement of the lips. The lip retractors include the levator labii superioris, levator anguli oris, zygomaticus major and minor for the upper lip, and depressor labii inferioris and depressor anguli oris for the lower lip. The antagonist of these lip-retracting muscles is the orbicularis oris, which is responsible for oral continence and some expressive movements of the lips.

Freilinger *et al.*[3] have demonstrated that the mimetic muscles are arranged in four layers. The depressor anguli oris, part of the zygomaticus minor, and the orbicularis oculi are the most superficial, whereas the buccinators, mentalis, and levator anguli oris make up the deepest layer. Except for the three deep muscles, all other facial muscles receive innervation from nerves entering their deep surfaces.

The muscles that are clinically important or most often require surgical management in patients with facial paralysis are the frontalis, orbicularis oculi, zygomaticus major, levator labii superioris, orbicularis oris, and depressor labii inferioris.

The frontalis muscle is a bilateral broad sheet-like muscle 5–6 cm in width and 1 mm thick.[4] The muscle takes origin from the galea aponeurotica at various levels near the coronal suture and inserts on to the superciliary ridge of the frontal bone and into fibers of the orbicularis oculi, procerus, and corrugators supercilii. It is firmly adherent to the skin through multiple fibrous septa but glides over the underlying periosteum. The two muscles fuse in the midline caudally; however, this is often a fibrous junction. Not only is the frontalis essential to elevate the brow, but also its tone at rest keeps the brow from descending. This tone is lost in the patient with facial paralysis, which allows the brow to fall and potentially obscure upward gaze.

The orbicularis oculi muscle acts as a sphincter to close the eyelids. Upper eyelid opening is performed by the levator palpebrae superioris muscle innervated by the third cranial nerve and the Müller muscle, which is a smooth fiber muscle innervated by the sympathetic nervous system. The orbicularis oculi muscle is one continuous muscle but has three subdivisions: pretarsal, covering the tarsal plate; preseptal portions, overlying the orbital septum; and the orbital, forming a ring over the orbital margin. The pretarsal and preseptal portions function together when a patient blinks, whereas the orbital portion is recruited during forceful eye closure and to lower the eyebrows. According to Jelks and Jelks,[7] the preseptal portion of the orbicularis oculi is under voluntary control, whereas the pretarsal provides reflex movement.

The pretarsal orbicularis oculi overlies the tarsal plate of the upper and lower eyelids. The tarsal plates are thin, elongated plates of connective tissue that support the eyelids. The superior tarsal plate is 8–10 mm in vertical height at its center but tapers medially and laterally, whereas the inferior tarsal plate is 3.8–4.5 mm in vertical height. The skin overlying the pretarsal orbicularis is the thinnest in the body and is adherent to the muscle over the tarsal plate. The skin is more lax and mobile over the preseptal and orbital regions. The eyelid skin also becomes thicker over the orbital part of the muscle. The preseptal orbicularis provides support to the orbital septa and is more mobile except at the medial and lateral canthi, where the muscle is firmly attached to the skin. The orbital portion of the orbicularis oculi extends in a wide circular fashion around the orbit. It originates medially from the superomedial orbital margin, the maxillary process of the frontal bone, the medial canthal tendon, the frontal process of the maxilla, and the inferomedial margin of the orbit. In the upper eyelid, the fibers sweep upward into the forehead and cover the frontalis and corrugators supercilii muscles; the fibers continue laterally to be superficial to the temporalis fascia.[8,9] Because this muscle is one of the superficial group of mimetic muscles,[10] in the lower eyelid the orbital portion lies over the origins of the zygomaticus major, levator labii superioris, levator labii superioris alaeque nasi, and part of the origin of the masseter muscle. There are multiple motor nerve branches that supply the upper and lower portions of the orbicularis oculi, and these enter the muscle just medial to its lateral edge.

Freilinger *et al.*[3] extensively studied the three major lip elevators, zygomaticus major, levator labii superioris, and

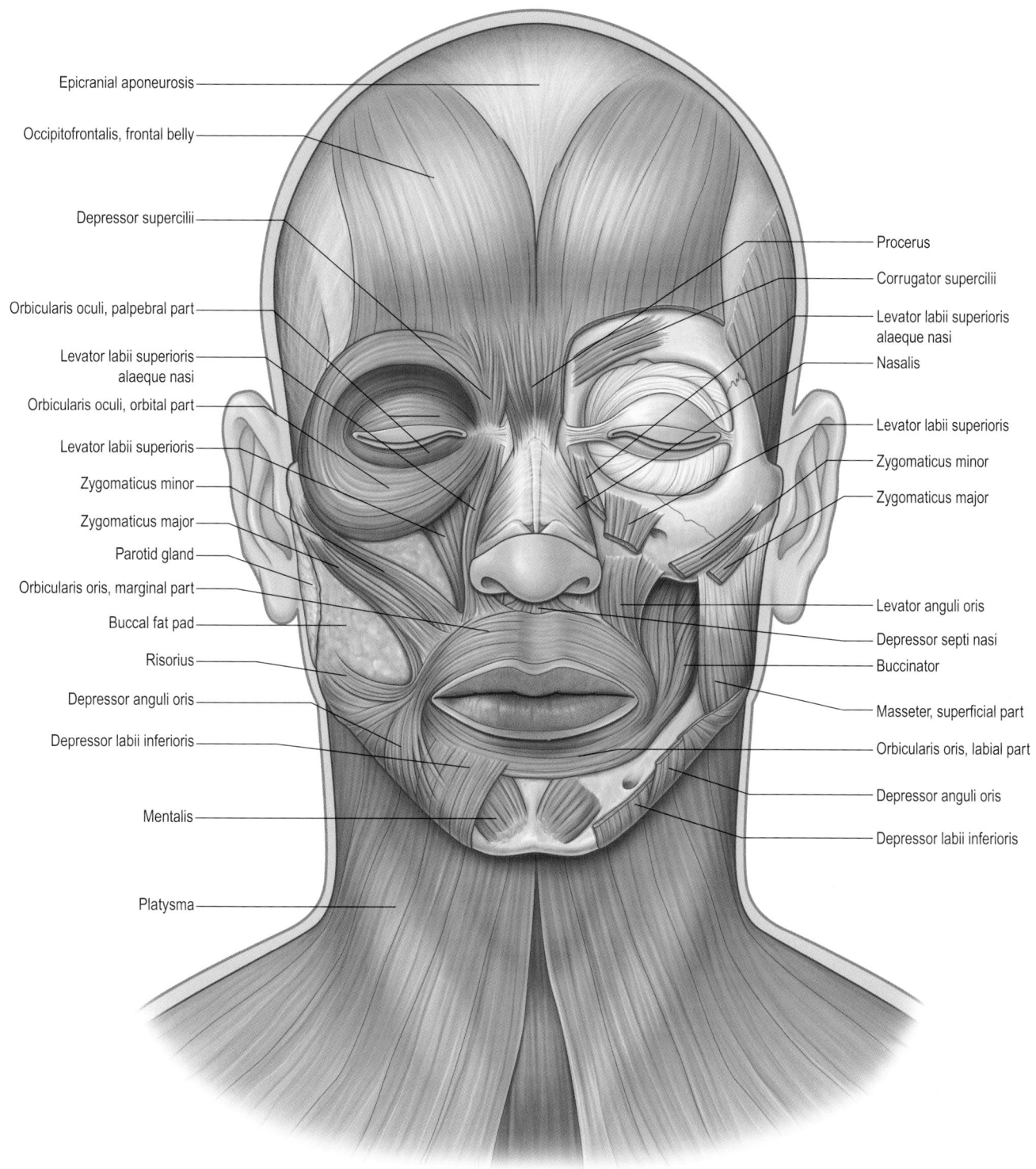

Epicranial aponeurosis

Occipitofrontalis, frontal belly

Depressor supercilii

Orbicularis oculi, palpebral part

Levator labii superioris
alaeque nasi

Orbicularis oculi, orbital part

Levator labii superioris

Zygomaticus minor

Zygomaticus major

Parotid gland

Orbicularis oris, marginal part

Buccal fat pad

Risorius

Depressor anguli oris

Depressor labii inferioris

Mentalis

Platysma

Procerus

Corrugator supercilii

Levator labii superioris
alaeque nasi

Nasalis

Levator labii superioris

Zygomaticus minor

Zygomaticus major

Levator anguli oris

Depressor septi nasi

Buccinator

Masseter, superficial part

Orbicularis oris, labial part

Depressor anguli oris

Depressor labii inferioris

Fig. 11.2 The muscles of facial expression are present in two layers. The buccinator, depressor labii inferioris, levator anguli oris, and corrugator are in the deeper layer.

levator anguli oris, and provided data on their length, width, and thickness *(Table 11.1)*.

The zygomaticus major takes origin from the lower lateral portion of the body of the zygoma; the orbicularis oculi and zygomaticus minor cover its upper part. Its course is along a line roughly from the helical root of the ear to the commissure

of the mouth, where it leads into the modiolus. The modiolus is the point of common attachment at which the fibers of the zygomaticus major and minor, orbicularis oris, buccinator, risorius, levator anguli oris, and depressor anguli oris come together. Deep fibers of the zygomaticus major are angled upward from the modiolus to fuse with the levator anguli

Table 11.1 Dimensions of the levators of the upper lip

Muscle	Length (mm)	Width (mm)	Thickness (mm)
Zygomaticus major	70	8	2
Levator labii superioris	34	25	1.8
Levator anguli oris	38	14	1.7

(Reproduced from Freilinger G, Gruber, Happak W, et al. Surgical anatomy of the mimic muscle system and the facial nerve: importance for reconstructive and aesthetic surgery. Plast Reconstr Surg 1987;80:686.)

oris, whereas caudal fibers continue into the depressor anguli oris. The main nerve to the zygomaticus major enters the deep surface of the upper third of the muscle.

The levator labii superioris originates along the lower portion of the orbital margin above the infraorbital foramen. The muscle courses inferiorly, partially inserting into the nasolabial crease. The lateral fibers pass inferiorly into the orbicularis oris, and the deepest fibers form part of the modiolus. The nerve to this muscle reaches it by first passing underneath the zygomaticus major muscle to supply the levator labii superioris on its deep surface.

The levator anguli oris is the third lip elevator. It takes origin from the maxilla below the infraorbital foramen and inserts into the modiolus. Because this muscle belongs to the deepest layer, it is innervated on its superficial surface by the same branch that supplies innervation to the buccinator.

Three muscles along with the zygomaticus minor serve to elevate the lip. The zygomaticus muscles move the commissure at an angle of approximately 45°, the levator anguli oris elevates the commissure vertically and medially, and the levator labii superioris elevates the lip vertically and laterally to expose the upper teeth.

The orbicularis oris is a complex muscle that functions as far more than a sphincter of the mouth; it serves to pucker and purse the lips. It makes up the bulk of the lip, as skin overlies it superficially and mucous membrane is attached on its deep surface. Philtral columns are formed by the insertion of the orbicularis, and a portion of levator labii superioris, into the skin.[11] The levator labii superioris fibers reach the philtral columns by coursing above the surface of the orbicularis oris to insert into the lower philtral columns and vermilion border as far medially as the peak of Cupid's bow. Anatomically and functionally, the orbicularis oris muscle consists of two parts, superficial and deep. The deep layers of the muscle encircle the orifice of the mouth and function as a constrictor. The superficial component also brings the lips together, but its fibers can contract independently to provide expression.[12]

The lower lip depressors consist of the depressor labii inferioris, also known as the quadratus labii inferioris, and the depressor anguli oris, also known as the triangularis *(Fig. 11.3)*. The mentalis, however, is not a lip depressor. Its indirect action on the lip is to elevate it.[8] The depressor labii inferioris arises from the lateral surface of the mandible, which is inferior and lateral to the mental foramen. It runs medially and superiorly to insert into the lower border of the orbicularis oris and its surface. Through fibrous septa, it attaches to the vermilion and the skin of the middle third of one side of the lip.[9] Its action is to draw the lower lip downward and laterally

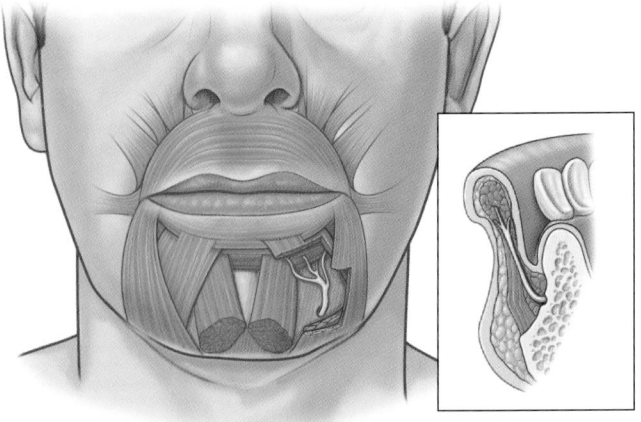

Fig. 11.3 The depressor anguli oris can be seen in the corner of the mouth. Muscle contraction pulls the corner of the mouth down as in the expression of sadness. The depressor labii inferioris goes into the orbicularis oris of the mid lateral portion of the lower lip and pulls the lip down. The muscle's function is apparent in an open-mouth smile showing the lower teeth. The mental nerve lies on the deep surface of the depressor labii inferioris.

and to evert the vermilion (e.g., as in showing the lower teeth). The depressor anguli oris arises from the mandible laterally and is superficial to the depressor labii inferioris. The medial fibers insert directly into the skin at the labiomandibular crease; the remainder blend into the modiolus.[13] It depresses the angle of the mouth (e.g., in frowning).

Diagnosis and patient presentation

Facial paralysis is a complex clinical problem with numerous consequences affecting the function, self-image, and social interactions of those afflicted and their families *(Fig 11.4)*. Function of the muscles vital for the protection of the eye, maintenance of the nasal airway, oral continence, and clear speech may be lost. These muscles support the face at rest and enable an individual to wink, pucker the lips, and express emotions of surprise, joy, anger, and sorrow.

Brow ptosis is more commonly a problem in the older patient. The weight of the forehead tissue may cause sagging of the eyebrow inferiorly over the superior orbital margin, which causes an asymmetric shape and obstructs the upward gaze. This may be complicated by overactivity of the contralateral frontalis muscle, which increases the discrepancy between eyebrow height. At rest, the depressed eyebrow gives the impression of unhappiness or excessive seriousness. With animation, the asymmetry of the brows and wrinkling of the forehead are accentuated.

The orbicularis oculi muscle is crucial for the protection of the eye. It enables eyelid closure and provides a physical barrier against wind and foreign matter. Repetitive blinking is also important for control of the even spread of tear film in a lateral to medial direction to prevent drying of the cornea. The effective drainage of tears is also dependent on a functioning orbicularis oculi muscle; its action on the lacrimal sac establishes a pump-like effect that facilitates the efficient clearance of tears.

When the eyelids are open, the distance between the upper and lower eyelid is 9–11 mm at its widest point. In the neutral gaze position, the upper eyelid covers 2–3 mm of the superior corneal limbus; the lower eyelid lies at the level of the inferior corneal limbus. Thus, there is normally no sclera showing.

With eye closure, the majority of movement occurs in the upper eyelid while the lower lid remains relatively static. However, with squinting or smiling, there is up to 2 mm of upward movement in the lower eyelid. The main function of

the inferior orbicularis oculi is the maintenance of lid margin contact with the globe and assistance with tear damage.

Patients with facial paralysis are troubled by significant discomfort in the eye because of corneal exposure and desiccation. This drying frequently produces a reflex tear flow. Excessive tears poorly managed by the paralyzed eyelids result in overflow. Therefore, patients with dry eyes often present with excessive tearing. This tearing problem can be distressing and is exacerbated by the downward inclination of the face (e.g., during reading).

The appearance of the paralyzed eye is also of concern to the patient. The eye has a widened palpebral aperture and is unable to convey expression. Thus, when the patient smiles, the paralyzed eyelids remain open instead of slightly closing. With the passage of time, the lower eyelid develops an ectropion, causing the inferior lacrimal punctum to pull away from the eye. An ectropion further exacerbates tearing and increases the risk of excessive corneal exposure.

The other major concern for patients with facial paralysis is the inability to control their lips. This affects the patient's ability to speak, eat, and drink properly. For example, many patients with facial paralysis have difficulty producing b and p sounds. Buccinator paralysis leads to problems in the control of food boluses. Food tends to pocket in the buccal sulcus of the paralyzed portion of the face; therefore, many patients chew only on the contralateral side. This type of paralysis also severely affects normal facial expressions. The main complaint heard from patients is their inability to smile. This should not be regarded as an aesthetic issue. It is a functional disability because it directly impairs communication. Paralysis of the orbicularis oris results in drooling and difficulty in controlling the mouth (e.g., drinking from a glass).

The emotional effects of facial paralysis cannot be underestimated. The unilaterally paralyzed face presents obvious asymmetry at rest, exacerbated by an attempt to smile **(Fig. 11.5)**. As a result, these patients avoid situations in which they are required to smile. They become characterized as serious

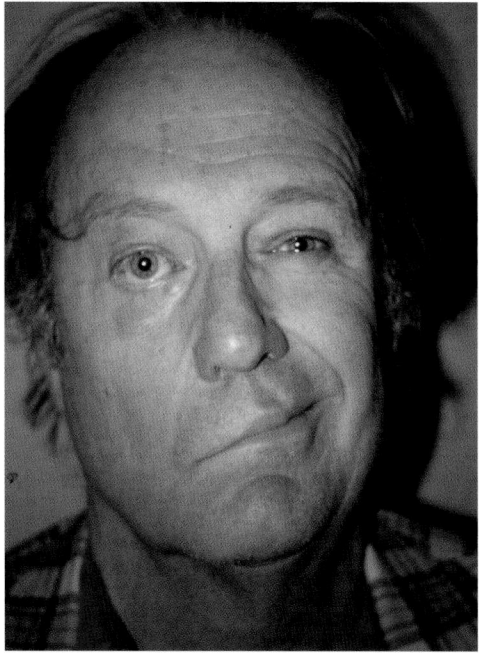

Fig. 11.4 Facial paralysis produces marked asymmetry at rest between the paralyzed side and the nonparalyzed side. The asymmetry is particularly severe in the older patient.

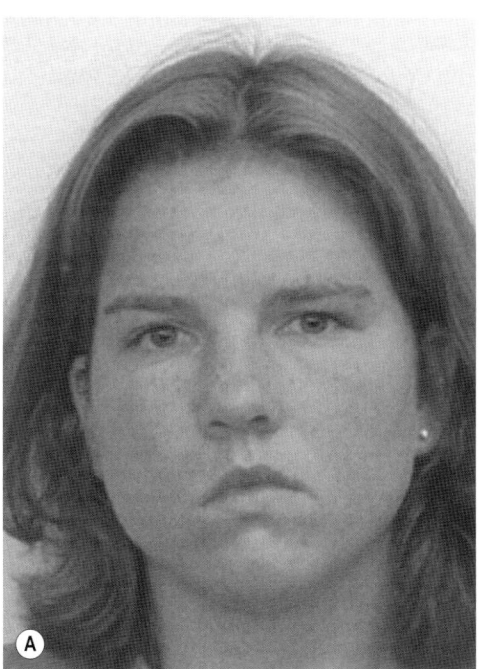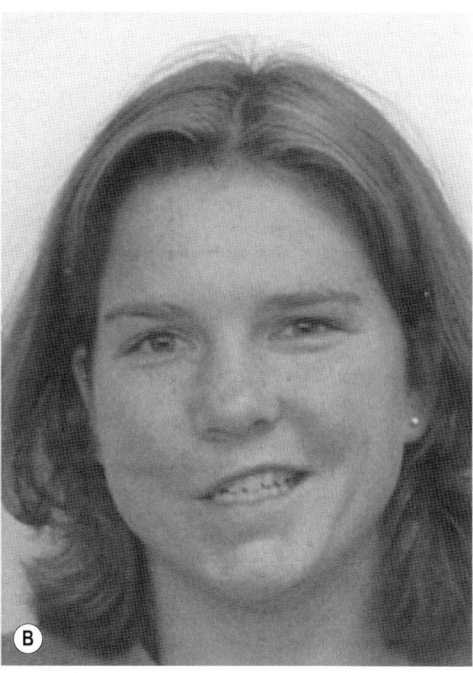

Fig. 11.5 (A) At rest, the right-sided partial facial paralysis in this young woman is minimally evident, as seen by a slight deviation of the mouth to her left and a slightly wider palpebral aperture in her right eye. **(B)** With smiling, the asymmetry becomes more apparent.

and unhappy, and their psychosocial functioning is frequently poor. A patient with bilateral facial paralysis has severe disability because his or her face cannot convey emotion.

Classification

In the formulation of a treatment plan, it is helpful to have a practical and clinically oriented classification. This will facilitate sound decision making and realistic surgical planning. Facial paralysis can take many forms. It can be classified anatomically and as congenital or acquired, and it can be broken down further into unilateral or bilateral categories.[14] In addition, the degree of muscle involvement varies from total to partial paralysis. More than 50% of patients with facial paralysis suffer from Bell's palsy and often recover fully.

Congenital facial paralysis is present at birth. This is the most common form of facial paralysis seen in a pediatric setting. It may be isolated with the involvement of the facial nerve and its musculature only, or it may be part of a syndrome.

It is estimated that facial paralysis occurs in 2.0% of live births.[15] In the majority of patients, it is believed to be the result of intrauterine pressure on the developing fetus from the sacral prominence. The facial nerve is superficial and easily compressed. This leads to the panfacial type and buccal branch variety of congenital facial paralysis. It is believed, however, that the mandibular branch component and syndromic forms of facial paralysis may have a different etiology. In the authors' experience, the cause of unilateral facial paralysis was congenital in two-thirds of patients encountered and acquired in one-third of patients. Acquired facial paralysis resulted from intracranial tumors in 50% of patients; and acquired facial paralysis from extracranial trauma. The majority of traumas were related to surgical procedures, most commonly cystic hygroma excision. In infants, the nerve is superficial at birth and can easily be traumatized through external compression or surgical misadventure. In contrast, the cause of facial paralysis for the majority of adults is acquired, from either intracranial lesions or inflammatory processes, such as Bell's palsy.

Congenital facial paralysis may be syndromic. The most common unilateral syndromic condition associated with facial paralysis is hemifacial microsomia. All tissues of the face can be affected to a variable degree, including the facial nerve musculature. The most common bilateral congenital facial paralysis is a result of Möbius syndrome. The functional effects of congenital facial paralysis tend to worsen gradually as the influence of gravity and aging prevails.

Bilateral facial paralysis may be the result of bilateral intracranial tumors or bilateral skull base trauma, but it is usually found to be the congenital bilateral facial paralysis or Möbius syndrome. Various cranial nerves accompany the seventh nerve's involvement, specifically the sixth, ninth, 10th, and 12th. Möbius syndrome is also associated with trunk and limb anomalies in about one-third of patients, the most common being talipes equinovarus and a variety of hand anomalies, including Poland syndrome. Cranial nerve involvement is usually bilateral and severe but often incomplete. There is frequently some residual function in the lower component of the face (the cervical and mandibular branch regions). The incidence of Möbius syndrome is estimated to be about 1 in 200 000 live births.

Acquired facial paralysis may also be unilateral or bilateral through local disruption of the nerve at various locations. Damage to the nerve may be intracranial in the nucleus or the peripheral nerve, extracranial in the peripheral nerve, or the result of damage to the muscle itself. Intracranial and extracranial neoplasms, Bell's palsy, and trauma are the most common causes seen in the adult setting. Although recovery is the rule in Bell's palsy, at least 10% of patients are left with some degree of paralysis. Bilateral acquired facial paralysis is usually the result of skull base fractures, intracranial lesions, usually in the brainstem, or intracranial surgery.

Throughout all of these areas, however, facial paralysis constitutes a spectrum of involvement. It may be complete or incomplete to varying degrees, obvious in some patients, and subtle in others *(Table 11.2)*.

Patient selection

Facial paralysis patients present with a broad spectrum of signs and symptoms. Thus treatment varies from individual to individual. A thorough history and examination will reveal the presence of a complete or partial seventh-nerve paralysis and, if the paralysis is partial, the specific muscles affected and the extent of the paralysis. Has there been any return of function? Is this improvement continuing or has it reached a plateau? The history must include any eye symptoms, such as dryness, excessive tearing, incomplete closure, discomfort when the patient is outdoors, and use of artificial tears. The patient should be questioned about the nasal airway, oral continence, speech, and level of psychosocial functioning and social interactions.

The patient's concerns and expectations must be sought. For some, attaining a symmetric appearance at rest is more important than achieving a smile. In comparison to the younger patient, the older patient is more likely to be worried about brow ptosis, ectropion, and drooping of the cheek.

The level of injury to the nerve, if it is not known, can be assessed clinically. Injury to the nerve within the bony canal may result in loss of ipsilateral taste appreciation, hyperacusis, and facial weakness because the chorda tympani and nerve to the stapedius may be injured at this level. Injury to the seventh cranial nerve near the geniculate ganglion will also result in decreased secretory function of the nose, mouth, and lacrimal gland.

Examination of the face begins with the brow. Its position at rest and with movement must be noted. The superior visual field may be diminished by the ptotic brow.

The eye must be thoroughly assessed. Visual acuity in each eye should be documented. The height of the palpebral aperture should be measured and compared with the nonparalyzed side. The degree of lagophthalmos and the presence of a Bell reflex will indicate the risk of corneal exposure. The lower eyelid position should be measured. Tone in the lower eyelid can be assessed by the use of the snap test. This is done by gently pulling the eyelid away from the globe and releasing it. The eyelid normally snaps back against the globe; however, this fails to occur in the patient with poor lid tone. The position of the inferior canalicular punctum should be assessed. Is it applied to the globe or is it rolled away and exposed? In addition, the patient should be examined for corneal irritation or ulceration.

Table 11.2 Classification of facial paralysis

Extracranial

Traumatic

Facial lacerations
Blunt forces
Penetrating wounds
Mandible fractures
Iatrogenic injuries
Newborn paralysis

Neoplastic

Parotid tumors
Tumors of the external canal and middle ear
Facial nerve neurinomas
Metastatic lesions

Congenital absence of facial musculature

Intratemporal

Traumatic

Fractures of petrous pyramid
Penetrating injuries
Iatrogenic injuries

Neoplastic

Glomus tumors
Cholesteatoma
Facial neurinomas
Squamous cell carcinomas
Rhabdomyosarcoma
Arachnoidal cysts
Metastatic

Infectious

Herpes zoster oticus
Acute otitis media
Malignant otitis externa

Idiopathic

Bell palsy
Melkersson–Rosenthal syndrome

Congenital: osteopertosis

Intracranial

Iatrogenic injury

Neoplastic – benign, malignant, primary, metastatic

Congenital

Absence of motor units

Syndromic

Hemifacial microsomia (unilateral)
Möbius syndrome (bilateral)

The nasal airway is examined next. Forced inspiration may reveal a collapsed nostril due to loss of muscle tone in the dilator naris and drooping of the cheek. An intranasal examination should also be done.

Examination of the mouth and surrounding structures documents the amount of philtral deviation, the presence or absence of a nasolabial fold, the amount of commissure depression and deviation, the degree to which the upper lip droops, and the presence of vermilion inversion. With animation, the amount of bilateral commissure movement is recorded; it is also noted how much of the upper incisors show when the patient is smiling. Speech should be assessed. An intraoral examination is performed to check dental hygiene and to look for evidence of cheek biting.

The presence of synkinesis, the simultaneous contraction of two or more groups of muscles that normally do not contract together,[16] should be documented. Synkinesis is thought to occur from a misdirected sprouting of axons. The most common types of synkinesis are eye closure with smiling,[17] brow wrinkling when the mouth is moved,[18] and mouth grimacing when the eyes are closed.

An assessment of the other cranial nerves, particularly the fifth, is also performed. Cranial nerve involvement may exacerbate the morbidity of facial nerve paralysis. These nerves should also be assessed as possible donor motor nerves.

Treatment: nonsurgical and surgical

Planning, priorities, and expectations

As has been stressed previously, treatment must be individualized. However, in general, the aims of treatment are to protect the eye, to provide symmetry at rest, and then to provide movement. The ultimate goal is to restore involuntary, independent, and spontaneous facial expression. The goals of treatment for the eye are to maintain vision, to provide protection, to maintain function of the eyelids, to improve cosmesis, and to enable the eye to express emotion. The goals for the mouth are to correct asymmetry, to provide oral continence, to improve speech, and to provide a balanced symmetric smile that the patient will use in social settings. Clearly, the accomplishment of all these gals is difficult, and they cannot be achieved completely.

The patient must be counseled as to what are real and achievable expectations. It is clearly impossible to restore intricate movements to all facial muscles, and the patient who is approximately informed is more likely to be satisfied with his or her outcome.

Nonsurgical management

Nonsurgical management of the patient with facial paralysis applies primarily to the eye and can frequently make the difference between a comfortable eye and a painful one. Nonsurgical maneuvers can protect the eye while surgery is being planned and are regularly used in concert with the surgical management of the eye. In some instances, surgery may be avoided. Nonsurgical management of the eye consists of protecting the eye and maintaining eye lubrication (*Table 11.3*).

Eye lubrication can be provided by a number of commercially available preparations. This includes clear watery drops containing either hydroxypropyl methylcellulose or polyvinyl alcohol along with other agents including preservatives. These drops function by absorbing into the cornea and lubricating it. Although the duration of action will vary, most are

Table 11.3 Nonsurgical maneuvers to protect the eye

Lid taping, particularly while sleeping
Soft contact lenses
Moisture chambers, which can be taped to the skin around the orbit
Modification of spectacles to provide a lateral shield
Forced blinking exercises in a patient with weak eye closure
Eye patches
Temporary tarsorrhaphy

Table 11.4 Most common surgical options for each region of the face

Brow (brow ptosis)

Direct brow lift (direct excision)
Coronal brow lift with static suspension
Endoscopic brow lift

Upper eyelid (lagophthalmos)

Gold weight
Temporalis transfer
Spring
Tarsorrhaphy

Lower eyelid (ectropion)

Tendon sling
Lateral canthoplasty
Horizontal lid shortening
Temporalis transfer
Cartilage graft

Nasal airway

Static sling
Alar base elevation
Septoplasty

Commissure and upper lip

Nerve transfer either directly or via nerve graft to reinnervate recently paralyzed muscles
Microneurovascular muscle transplantation with the use of ipsilateral seventh nerve, cross-facial nerve graft, or other cranial nerve for motor innervation
Temporalis transposition with or without masseter transposition
Static slings
Soft-tissue balancing procedures (rhytidectomy, mucosal excision or advancement)

Lower lip

Depressor labii inferioris resection (on normal side)
Muscle transfer (digastric, platysma)
Wedge excision

retained on the surface of the eye between 45 and 120 minutes.[19] Thus, to be most effective, they should be instilled frequently during the day. Thicker ointments containing petrolatum, mineral water, or lanolin alcohol are retained longer and can be used at night to protect and "seal" the eyelids during sleep. The patient who presents with excessive tearing may in fact have a dry eye and may benefit from the use of artificial tears. Corneal ulceration should be managed with prompt referral for ophthalmologic assessment.

In patients in whom there is incomplete facial nerve paralysis or recovering muscle activity after nerve injury, function may be improved with neuromuscular retraining supervised by an experienced therapist. This consists of various treatment modalities such as biofeedback, electromyography, and self-directed mirror exercises using slow, small, and symmetric movements.[20] Patients can often relearn some facial movements or strengthen movements that are weak.

Surgical management

Deciding on a surgical procedure can initially seem daunting. There are a number to choose from, and selecting the most appropriate reconstruction may be confusing. It is important to listen to each patient carefully to identify which aspects of the paralysis are most troublesome and to treat each region of the face separately. The age of the patient, duration of the facial paralysis, condition of the facial musculature and soft tissues, and status of the potential donor nerves and muscles will all influence treatment options. One must consider the patient's needs carefully and match the needs of the patient with the skill of the surgeon *(Table 11.4)*.

Brow

There are at least three approaches to a brow lift: direct excision of the tissue above the brow (direct brow lift), open brow lift performed through a coronal incision, and endoscopic brow lift. Unilateral frontalis paralysis may cause a difference in brow heights of up to 12 mm. A direct brow lift is best able to correct such a large discrepancy. Direct brow lift involves excision of a segment of skin and frontalis muscle just above and parallel to the eyebrow. If the incision is placed just along the first line of hair follicles, the resulting scar is usually less noticeable. Frontalis shortening by excision and repair provides a reliable correction, which minimally relaxes over time. However, overcorrection is still required. Slight overcorrection is particularly beneficial if the person's normal side of the forehead is quite active during facial expression. Branches of

the supraorbital nerve should be identified and preserved because they lie deep to the muscle *(Fig. 11.6)*.

Brow lift may be performed through a coronal incision with or without a fascial graft to suspend the brow from the temporalis fascia or medially on the frontal bone. Whereas the scar is concealed, this is a larger operation than a direct brow lift and may not achieve as adequate a lift.

The authors have had limited experience with endoscopically assisted brow lifts for facial paralysis. The amount of lift required in the patient with facial paralysis is usually more than can be achieved from a unilateral endoscopic brow lift. It is likely that, with time, there will be gradual drooping. Therefore, the longevity of results in patients with facial paralysis has yet to be demonstrated with this procedure, especially when a large unilateral lift is required.

Weakening of the contralateral normal frontalis muscle by transaction of the frontal nerve or resection of strips of muscle is occasionally useful to control wrinkle asymmetry.

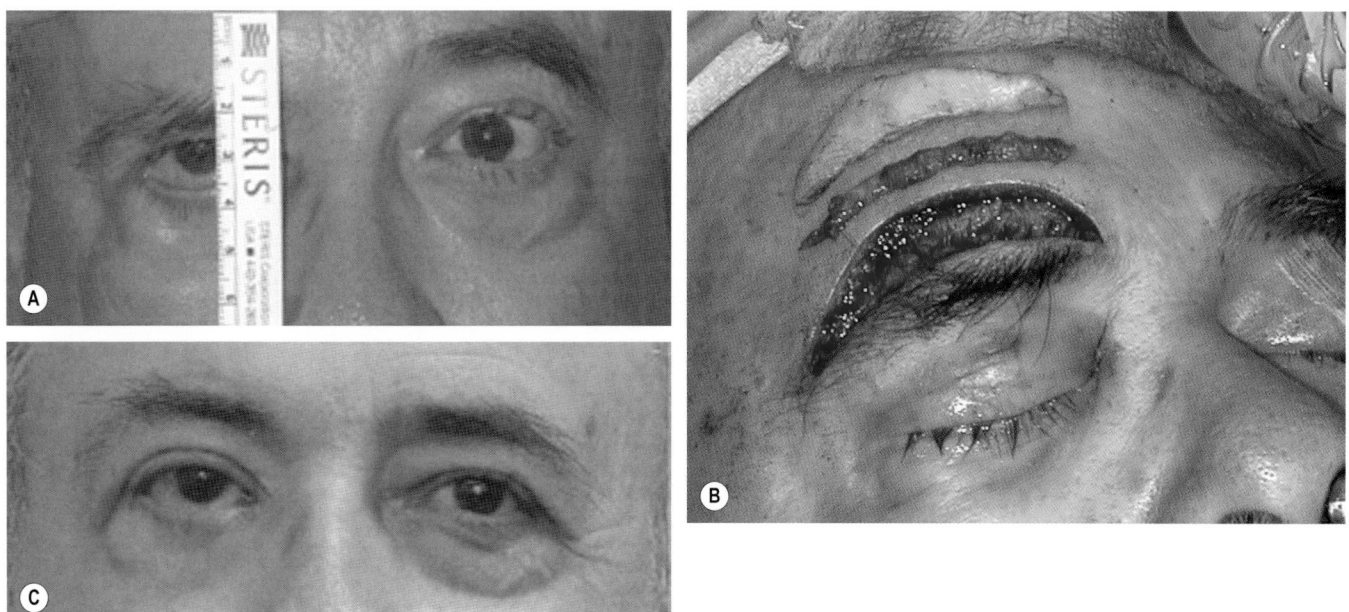

Fig. 11.6 (A) Assessment of the amount of brow depression on the paralyzed side compared with the normal eyebrow on the patient's left. **(B)** Excision of skin and a strip of frontalis muscle to correct brow ptosis. **(C)** Postoperative appearance.

Upper eyelid

Several techniques are available for the management of lagophthalmos. These are all directed at overcoming the unopposed action of the levator palpebrae superioris. Because of its relative technical ease and reversibility, lid loading with gold prosthesis is the most popular technique. The patient's eyelid configuration is important in determining whether the bulge of the gold weight will be visible when the eye is open. If the amount of exposed eyelid skin above the lashes is more than 5 mm when the eye is open, the gold weight is likely to be noticeable to the patient. If the distance is less than 5 mm, the gold weight will roll back and be covered by the supratarsal skinfold *(Fig. 11.7)*.

Because of its inertness, 24-carat gold is used; allergic reactions are rare, but if they occur, platinum weights are also available. Prostheses are available in weights ranging from 0.8 to 1.8 g. Adequate improvement in eye closure can be obtained with a weight of 0.8–1.2 g, giving the patient a comfortable eye without weight-related problems.[21] The appropriate weight is selected by taping trial prostheses to the upper eyelid over the tarsal plate with the patient awake. The lightest weight that will bring the upper eyelid within 2–4 mm of the lower lid and cover the cornea should be used. As long as the patient has an adequate Bell phenomenon, complete closure is not necessary. The prosthesis is fixed to the upper half of the tarsal plate by permanent sutures, which pass through the tarsal plate. Care should be taken not to interfere with the insertion of Müller muscle *(Fig. 11.8)*. With proper placement, the prosthesis should be hidden in the upper eyelid skin crease when the eye is open. The closure produced by the gold weight is slow, and the patient must be instructed to relax the levator muscle consciously for 1–2 seconds to allow the eyelid to descend *(Fig. 11.9)*. Complications include extrusion, excessive capsule formation by causing a visible

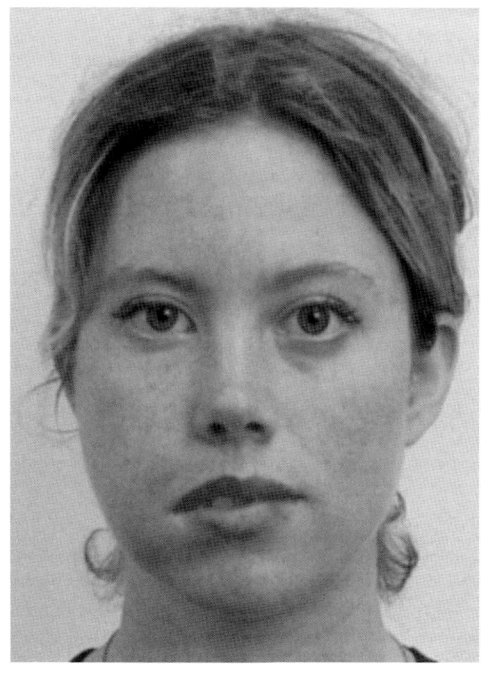

Fig. 11.7 Right facial paralysis in a young woman with total paralysis of the orbicularis oculi showing ideal eyelid configuration that allows gold weight insertion without visibility.

lump, and irritation of the eye by the weight. If these occur, the weight can easily be removed, replaced, or repositioned.

The authors have used the gold weight alone 27 times. The incidence of complications requiring removal of the weight was 2%, and 8% required revision of the weight. In 52% of patients, good symptomatic improvement was obtained. Of

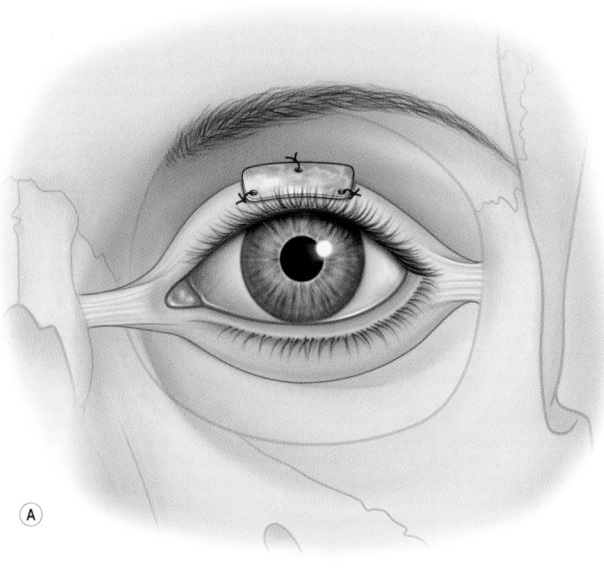

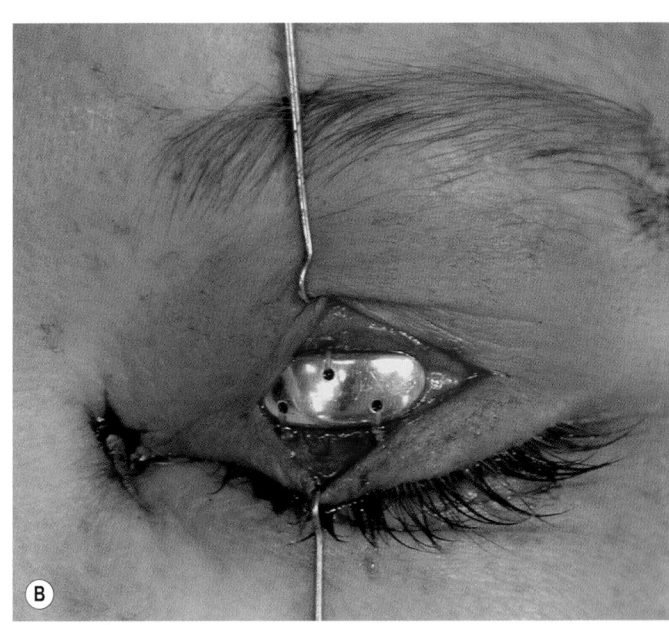

Fig. 11.8 (A) Placement of gold weight directly above the cornea on the upper half of the tarsal plate. **(B)** Gold weight sutured in place with the knots turned away from the skin.

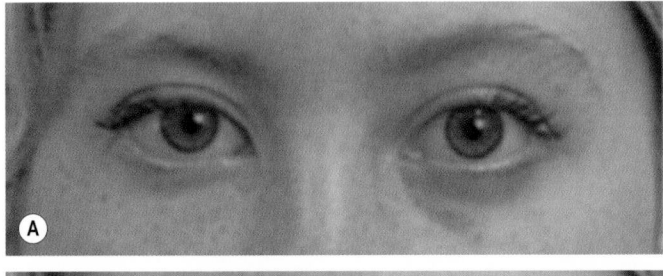

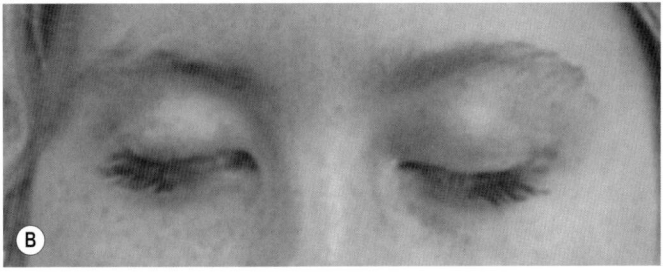

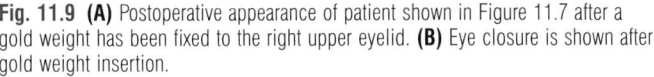

Fig. 11.9 (A) Postoperative appearance of patient shown in Figure 11.7 after a gold weight has been fixed to the right upper eyelid. **(B)** Eye closure is shown after gold weight insertion.

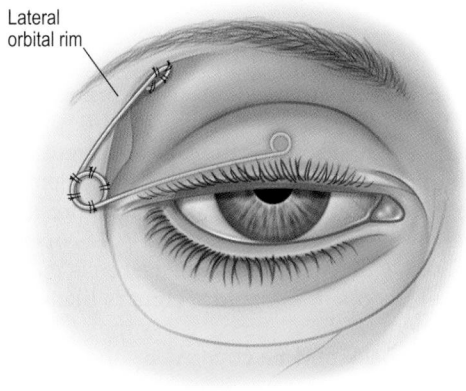

Fig. 11.10 Palpebral spring in right upper eyelid.

these patients, 64% subsequently required lower lid support with a static sling. As a result, it has become much more common to recommend both a gold weight and a lower-eyelid sling at the same operative sitting, which results in a 95% good improvement in symptoms.

An alternative procedure for the eyelid closure is the palpebral spring originally described by Morel-Fatio, which consists of a wire loop with two arms.[22] One arm is sutured along the lid margin, and the other arm is fixed to the inner aspect of the lateral orbital rim. When the eye is open, the two arms are brought close to each other; when the eyelid is relaxed, the "memory" of the wire loop moves the arms apart, causing closure of the eyelid *(Fig. 11.10)*.

The advantage of this procedure is that it is not dependent on gravity. However, problems with malpositioning of the spring, spring breakage or weakening, pseudoptosis due to excessive spring force, and skin erosion have prevented the widespread use of this procedure. It is certainly a more involved procedure than insertion of the gold weight, and results may be dependent on the surgeon's skill level.

For short-term use, there are implantable devices. These include magnetized rods inserted into the upper and lower eyelids and silicon bands sutured to the lateral and medial canthal ligaments.

Temporalis muscle transposition has the advantage of using autogenous tissue, thereby avoiding the use of foreign

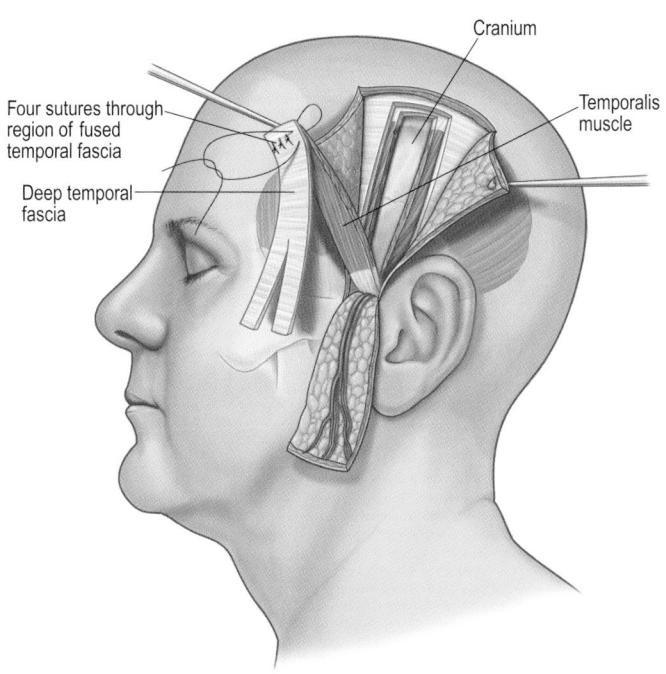

Fig. 11.11 Elevation of temporalis muscle for transfer to eye.

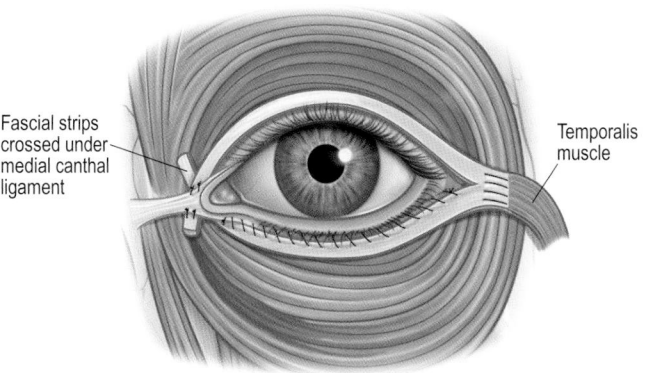

Fig. 11.12 Transplantation of temporalis muscle and fascia to upper and lower eyelids.

materials. First described by Gillies,[23] this procedure has since been modified by several authors.[24] A 1.5-cm-wide flap of temporalis muscle based inferiorly is raised along with the overlying temporalis fascia. Because both the blood supply and motor nerve innervation enter the muscle on its inferior deep surface, the flap remains functional. The fascia overlying the temporalis muscle is then detached. It is sutured firmly to the superior edge of the temporalis muscle that is about to be transposed *(Fig. 11.11)*. The flap is passed subcutaneously to the lateral canthus, where the fascial strips are tunneled along the upper and lower lid margins and sutured to the medial canthal ligament *(Fig. 11.12)*. With activation of the muscle, the fascial strips are pulled tight, causing eyelid closure. This technique has the advantage of addressing both upper eyelid closure and a static sling for the lower eyelid allows better eyelid closure. It is preferable to use a 2-mm strip of tendon; fascia appears to stretch, resulting in loss of effective eyelid movement. The disadvantages of this transfer are that, with muscle contraction, the lid aperture changes from an oval to a slit shape; there may be skin wrinkling over the lateral canthal region and an obvious muscle bulge over the lateral orbital margin. Movements of the eyelids during chewing may also be a disturbing feature for the patient. Nevertheless, this procedure usually provides an excellent static support, eye closure on command, and good lubrication of the eye through distribution of the tear film and consequent corneal protection. Microneurovascular muscle transplantation for orbicularis function is a relatively new procedure. Platysma transplantation procedures that involve revascularization with the superficial temporal artery and vein and reinnervation with a cross-facial nerve graft are tedious and complex and should be reserved for patients for whom simpler techniques have been unsuccessful. Transplantation of the

platysma may also produce some undesirable thickening of the eyelids.

Historically, lateral tarsorrhaphy has been one of the mainstay treatments for paralyzed eyelids. The McLaughlin lateral tarsorrhaphy[25] may provide a reasonably acceptable cosmetic result. However, horizontal lid length is decreased, which detracts from the aesthetic appeal and obstructs lateral vision. This procedure consists of resection of a segment of lateral skin, cilia, and orbicularis from the lower lid and a matching segment of conjunctiva and tarsus from the upper lid. The two raw surfaces are sutured together, preserving the upper eyelashes. At present, the main indication for lateral tarsorrhaphy is for the patient with an anesthetic cornea, severe corneal exposure, or failure of aesthetically more acceptable techniques.

Lower eyelid

The orbicularis oculi muscle, through its attachment to the canthal ligaments, holds the lower eyelid firmly against the globe and with contraction is able to raise the lid 2–3 mm. Ordinarily, the eyelid margin rests at the level if the limbus of the eye. With paralysis of the orbicularis, tone in the muscle is lost. Gravity causes the lower eyelid to stretch and sag, resulting in scleral show. Over time, the lid and inferior canalicular punctum roll away from the globe, resulting in an ectropion *(Fig. 11.13)*. Therefore, management is directed at resuspending the lid and reapposing the punctum to the globe.

Pronounced ectropion with lid eversion and more than 2–3 mm of sceral show is usually associated with symptoms of dryness and aesthetic concerns. This situation requires support of the entire length of the eyelid. This is best achieved with a static sling passed 1.5–2 mm inferior to the gray line of the eyelid and fixed both medially and laterally *(Fig. 11.14)*.[26] Tendon provides longer-lasting support with less stretching than the fascia lata. A 1.5-mm-wide strip of tendon (a part of either palmaris or plantaris) is sutured to the lateral orbital margin in the region above the zygomaticofrontal suture and tunneled subcutaneously along the lid anterior to the tarsal plate. Proper placement is crucial; too low a position will exacerbate the ectropion. In the elderly patient with

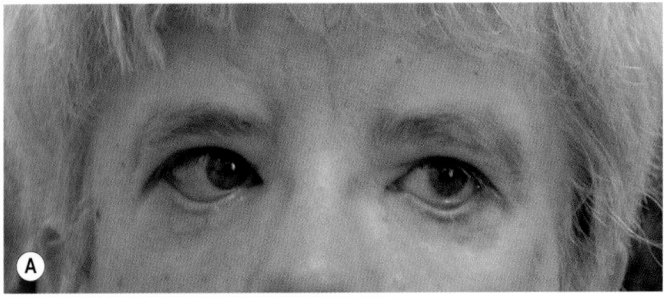
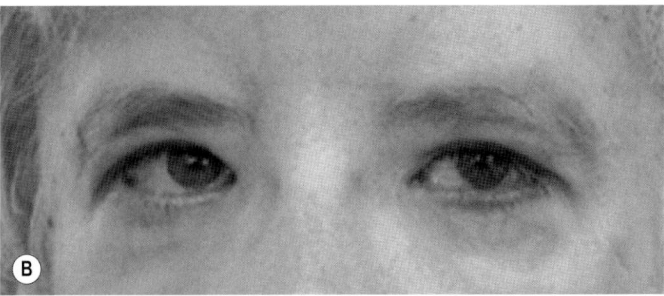

Fig. 11.13 (A) Marked bilateral ectropion in lower eyelids in a 52-year-old woman with Möbius syndrome. **(B)** Postoperative appearance after tendon sling insertion to lower eyelids.

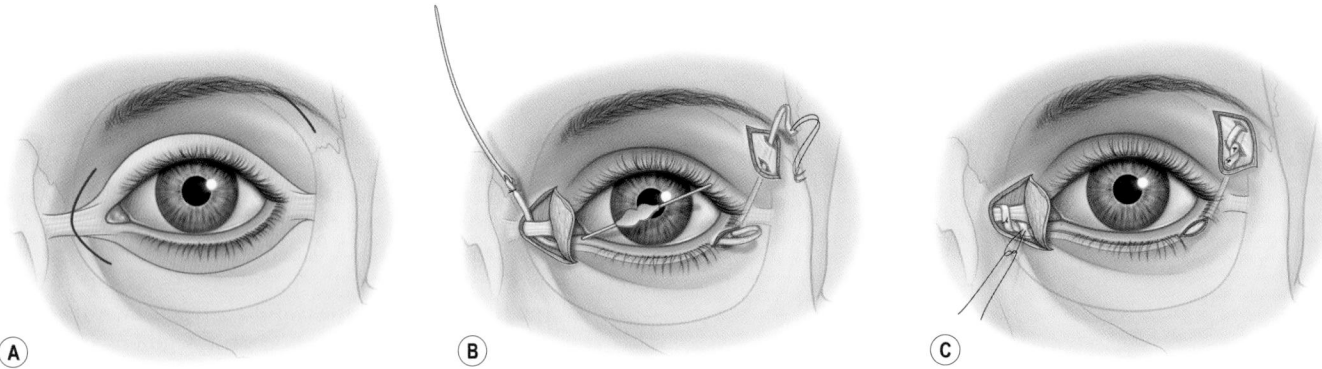

Fig. 11.14 (A) Incisions for insertion of static sling. **(B)** Static sling attachment to medial canthal ligament and periosteal strip on lateral orbital margin. **(C)** After fixation of sling.

particularly lax tissues, too superficial or high a placement may result in entropion. The sling is then passed around the anterior limb of the medial canthal ligament and sutured to itself. Subcutaneous tunneling of the tendon graft is facilitated by the use of a curved Keith needle. This procedure provides good support to the lower lid. It does not deform the eyelid, it is not apparent to an observer, and the effect appears to last well. If the sling is placed too loosely, it may be tightened at the lateral orbital margin.

Lateral examination of the eye and eyelid will determine its vector.[7] A negative vector occurs when the globe is anterior to the lid margin and the lid margin is anterior to the check prominence. In patients with a relatively proptotic eye, the lower eyelid sling will correct ectropion, but it may not decrease sclera show. In patients with a positive vector, in which the globe is posterior to the lid margin and the lid margin is posterior to the cheek prominence, the sling will be effective. However, lateral fixation of the tendon graft may need to be through a drill hole whereby the tendon is woven back to itself and sutured, 2–3 mm posterior to the lateral orbital margin, because fixation to the frontal periosteum may lift the lateral eyelid away from the globe.

The authors have used the lower lid sling on 25 occasions, and in combination with a gold weight to the upper lid, it results in 95% improvement in symptoms *(Fig. 11.13B)*. Two patients have had complications from the lower lid sling procedure, which required the sling to be tightened. One patient required revision because the sling exacerbated the ectropion,

and one required epilation of some lower eyelashes because of entropion. The lower lid tendon sling can be adjusted fairly readily if it is not in the correct position up to 1 week after placement.

Milder eyelid problems consisting of lower lid laxity and minimal scleral show may be treated with lateral canthoplasty. Jelks *et al.*[27] described various techniques of canthoplasty, such as the tarsal strip, dermal pennant, and inferior retinacular lateral canthoplasty. The canthal ligament must be reapproximated to the position of Whitnall tubercle, which is situated not only above the horizontal midpupillary line but also 2–3 mm posterior to the lateral orbital margin.

Horizontal lid shortening may be required to deal with redundant and stretched lower eyelid tissue. The Kuhnt-Szymanowski procedure involves the excision of a laterally placed triangular wedge of lower eyelid with its base being the lower lid margin. It can be modified not only to excise a wedge of tarsus and conjunctiva but also by resuspending the lid margin from the lateral canthus. However this tends to distort and expose the caruncle and does not provide a lasting correction.

Cartilage grafts to prop up the tarsal plate have also been used. By augmenting the middle lamella and suturing the cartilage to the inferior orbital margin, there will be less of a tendency for the lower eyelid to migrate inferiorly. However, results may be poor because the cartilage tends to rotate into a more horizontal position rather than a vertical one, producing a visible bulge and minimal eyelid support.

In patients with isolated medial ectropion that includes punctal eversion, the lower lid can be repositioned against the globe by direct excision of a tarsoconjunctival ellipse. This causes a vertical shortening of the inner aspect of the lower lid and helps reposition the punctum against the globe. Medial canthoplasty will also support the punctum.

Nasal airway

Paralysis of the nasalis and levator alaeque nasi combined with drooping and medial deviation of the paralyzed cheek leads to support loss of the nostril, collapse of the ala, and reduction of airflow. Nasal septal deviation, which occurs in patients with congenital facial paralysis, may further accentuate any breathing difficulties. In the patient who complains of significant symptoms, correction of airway collapse is best accomplished by elevation and lateral support of the alar base with the sling of tendon and by upper lip and cheek elevation procedures. Septoplasty may be indicated to provide an improvement in airway patency.

Upper lip and cheek: smile reconstruction

The majority of patients with facial paralysis who present for reconstruction do so for either correction of an asymmetric face at rest or reconstruction of a smile. However, significant functional problems are associated with paralysis of the oral musculature, including drooling and speech difficulties. The flaccid lip and cheek can also lead to difficulties with chewing food, cheek biting, and pocketing food in the buccal sulcus due to paralysis of the buccinator. However, the main emphasis of surgery is usually centered on reconstruction of a smile.

The surgeon and patient must have clearly defined goals. Some patients only request symmetry at rest and are not concerned about animation. For these patients, static slings and soft-tissue repositioning can be most helpful. However most patients would prefer a dynamic reconstruction.

Nerve transfers: principles and current use

Dynamic reanimation attempts to restore symmetry both at rest and while smiling. Three elements are required for the formation of a smile: neural input, a functional muscle innervated by the nerve, and proper muscle positioning. All three factor into the decision as to which would be the best for any given patient.

Reconstructive modalities for facial paralysis can be classified by two basic criteria. The first is whether reconstruction is based on the facial nerve or on a different cranial nerve,[28] and the second is whether the working muscle unit is the original facial musculature or a transferred muscle flap.[29] Reanimation based on the facial nerve can be on the ipsilateral or contralateral nerve depending on the presence of a functional and usable branch or stump. The duration of paralysis is the principal determinant for the need for muscle transfer or transplant. If duration is less than 12 months, the facial musculature is assumed to be able to be reinnervated. Muscles become irreversibly atrophic by 24 months, in which case muscle replacement is indicated. The effect of the facial musculature can be replaced by static procedures for balance or by dynamic procedures for animation. The combination of

regional muscle transfer and static positioning procedure has been recently described.[30]

Primary facial nerve repair is possible in cases of recent trauma to the facial nerve.[31] A sural cable nerve graft is used to interconnect ends when there is a gap between the ipsilateral proximal stump of facial nerve to the distal stumps of zygomaticobuccal facial branches.

When the ipsilateral proximal facial nerve stump is not usable (brain tumor, head trauma and fractures, Bell's palsy, or surgery) and the facial musculature can be reinnervated, connecting another cranial nerve such as the hypoglossal or the masseter (a branch of the trigeminal nerve) to the distal stump of a transected facial nerve is an option. Those procedures may give unnatural action to the paralyzed face, resulting in good muscle tone and symmetry at rest but an unsightly, unnatural mass movement with activation. This occurs when the patient is moving the tongue (hypoglossal transfer) or with mastication (masseter nerve transfer).

In cases of recent paralysis in which a functional facial nerve branch is available only on the contralateral face, a cross-face sural nerve graft is used to relay facial nerve across the face to the paralyzed facial musculature. Axons from the contralateral facial nerve regenerate through the sheath of the graft and innervate the muscle over 4–8 months. Since muscle atrophy can develop while the facial nerve regenerates, an ipsilateral motor nerve (either masseter or hypoglossal) can be transposed to serve as a temporary innervator or "babysitter," as proposed by Terzis[32,33] (*Fig. 11.15*). Thus muscle tone is preserved while spontaneous smiling will in due course be restored. At the first surgery two nerve grafts are connected

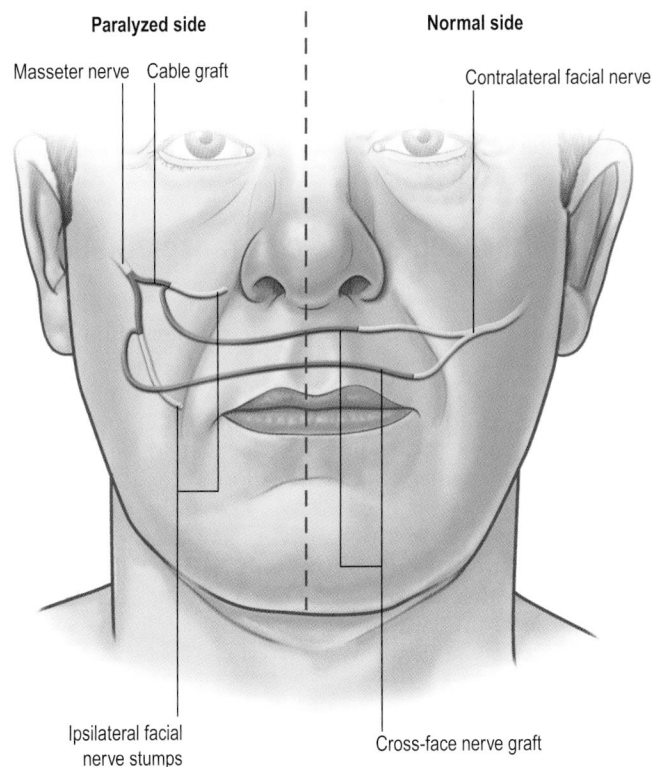

Fig. 11.15 Illustration of the "babysitter" procedure. P, paralyzed side; N, normal side; MN, masseter nerve; CNG, cross-face nerve graft; IFNS, ipsilateral facial nerve stumps; CFN, contralateral facial nerve.

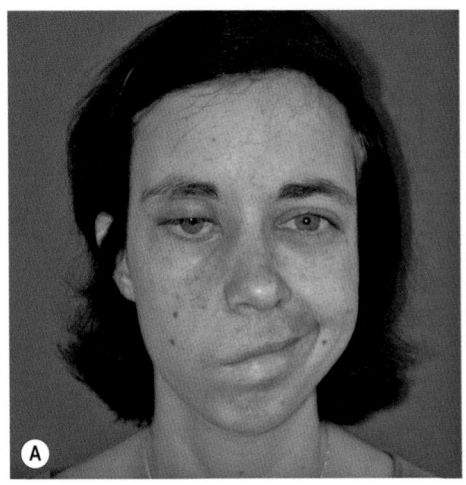
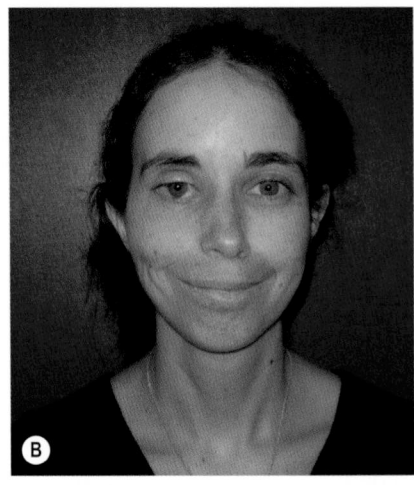
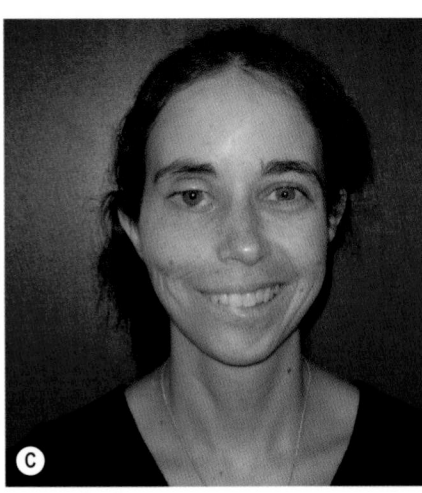

Fig. 11.16 (A) Preoperative photo prior to the "babysitter" procedure. **(B)** Closed-mouth smile after the "babysitter" procedure. **(C)** Open-mouth smile after the "babysitter" procedure.

to the upper and lower trunks of the normal contralateral facial nerve and are tunneled across the face through the upper lip. They are banked in the paralyzed, pretemporal region and marked by a 3/0 blue nylon suture. At that same procedure, a short nerve cable graft is used to connect the nerve to masseter or a part of the hypoglossal nerve to the distal stump of the affected facial nerve. Within 2–3 months, the paralyzed muscle will regain tone and then will begin to function in a mass pattern motion.

About 6–9 months after the initial procedure,[34] at the second surgery, the paralyzed side will be reoperated. The two cross-faced nerve grafts are identified, split into fascicles, and coapted to the facial nerve branches distal to the prior masseter-facial nerve repair. Within 3–6 months spontaneous facial nerve motion is initiated by the contralateral facial nerve *(Fig. 11.16)*; in time this will take control. If the masseter nerve action is still noticeable and unwanted, the masseter nerve can be transected.

Microneurovascular muscle transplantation

It is not possible to restore complete symmetry of all movements because of the complexity of muscle interaction and the number of facial muscles involved. There are 18 separate muscles of facial expression, and of these, five are elevators of the upper lip and two are depressors of the lower lip. A transplanted muscle can only be expected to produce one function and movement in one direction.

If the facial nerve is used to reinnervate the transplanted muscle, the smile with laughter will be spontaneous. When other nerves are used (e.g., the fifth, 11th, or 12th), teeth clenching or other movements are required to activate the smile, at least initially. With time, the smile movement will often become less of a conscious effort and more spontaneous.

The patient's sustainability for free muscle transplantation and reinnervation must be carefully assessed. This includes an assessment of the patient's ability to undergo a substantial operative procedure with general anesthesia as well as an evaluation of comorbidities that may affect the functioning of microneurovascular muscle transplantation. The patient

should also be counseled with regard to the time that it could take to achieve full movement, which is usually around 18 months. It is generally recognized that reinnervation does not often occur in older individuals. However, it is difficult to determine which patient should be classified as "older" because muscle reinnervation can occur at any age. However, it is the author's practice to be reluctant to perform functioning muscle transplantations on patients who are older than 65 years.

Smile analysis

Preoperative planning is crucial. It is recognized that the unopposed smile on the normal side in unilateral facial paralysis will be an exaggerated expression of the same movement after reconstruction of the paralyzed side. Therefore, careful analysis of the patient's smile on the nonparalyzed side will instruct the surgeon in establishing a symmetric smile. As Paletz *et al.*[35] have shown, individuals have various types of smiles. It is important to assess the direction of movement of the commissure and upper lip. How vertical is the movement? What is the strength of the smile and where around the mouth is the force most strongly focused? What is the position of the nasolabial fold with smiling? Is there a labial mental fold? Once these features have been determined, an estimate of the muscle's size, point of origin, tension, direction of movement, and placement can be planned *(Fig. 11.17)*.

Technique options

One-stage procedures for smile reconstruction with free muscle transplantations would seem to be the most appealing approach; however, for numerous reasons, they may not necessarily provide the best results *(Table 11.4)*. If the ipsilateral facial nerve trunk is available, it seems to be an ideal source of reinnervation for a muscle flap. However, the exact branches to the lip elevators may be difficult to determine. If incorrect innervation is used, muscle contraction may take place only when the patient performs some facial movement other than smiling, such as closing the eyes or puckering the lips.

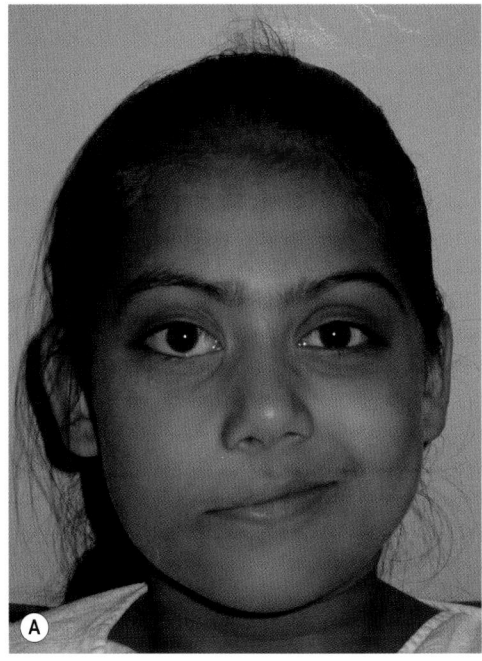
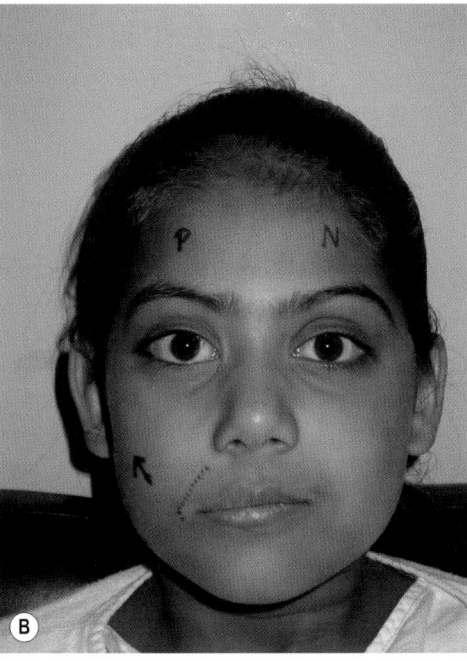

Fig. 11.17 **(A)** Patient shown smiling. Note direction of movement of the commissure and the mid upper lip on the normal left side, location of the fold in the nasolabial area, and shape of the upper and lower lip. **(B)** The nasolabial folds and directions of movement have been marked on the normal left side (N) and copied on the paralyzed side (P). The desired position of the muscle is outlined by two dotted lines across the cheek.

Single-stage muscle transplants with innervation from the contralateral facial nerve have been reported. This technique requires the use of a muscle with a long nerve segment, such as the latissimus dorsi or rectus abdominis.[36] However, even the gracilis[37] has been used. The nerve is tunneled across the lip and coapted to the facial nerve branches on the opposite side of the face. The advantages here are that the patient undergoes only one operation and there is only one site of coaptation for regenerating axons to cross. There does not appear to be any significant denervation atrophy of the muscle while it awaits reinnervation. However, although the muscle may function with facial movement, it may not contract when the patient smiles. This is because the facial nerve branches used are close to the mouth and are usually found through a nasolabial incision on the unaffected side. This approach does not allow thorough facial nerve mapping to be performed; thus, the most appropriate nerve branches may not be recruited. Also, this approach does not allow an assessment of what remaining branches have been left intact.

When there is neither an ipsilateral nor a contralateral facial nerve available to act as a donor, as in Möbius syndrome or other causes of bilateral facial paralysis, another cranial nerve must be used to reinnervate the muscle transplant. It is our practice to use the nerve to the masseter muscle.[37] Zuker et al.[37] have shown that in children this provides a symmetric smile with excellent muscle excursion. These patients may never achieve involuntary movement or a truly spontaneous smile. However, in many children and 50% of adults there appears to be some cortical "rewiring" such that these people are able to activate a smile without performing a biting motion and without conscious effort.

In treatment of younger patients with unilateral facial paralysis, we prefer to perform a two-stage reconstruction consisting of facial nerve mapping and cross-facial nerve grafting followed by a microneurovascular muscle transplantation.

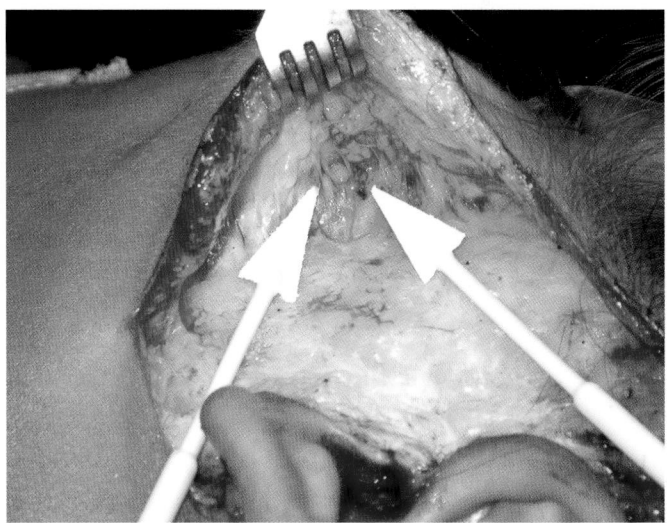

Fig. 11.18 The cross-facial nerve graft is inserted through a preauricular incision. The parotid gland can be seen immediately in front of the left ear, and branches of the facial nerve supplying the muscles of the mouth and eye are seen superficial to the background material.

Authors' preferred method: two-stage microneurovascular transplantation

Video 1

Cross-facial nerve graft

The first stage of this procedure involves a dissection of the facial nerve on the unaffected side through a preauricular incision with a submandibular extension *(Fig. 11.18)*. The zygomaticobuccal nerve branches medial to the parotid gland are meticulously identified and individually stimulated with a microbipolar electrical probe attached to a stimulator source that allows variable voltage and frequency control *(Fig. 11.19)*.

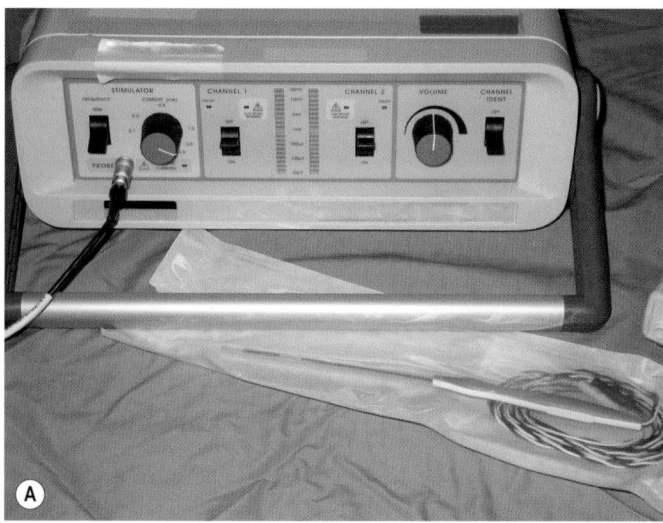
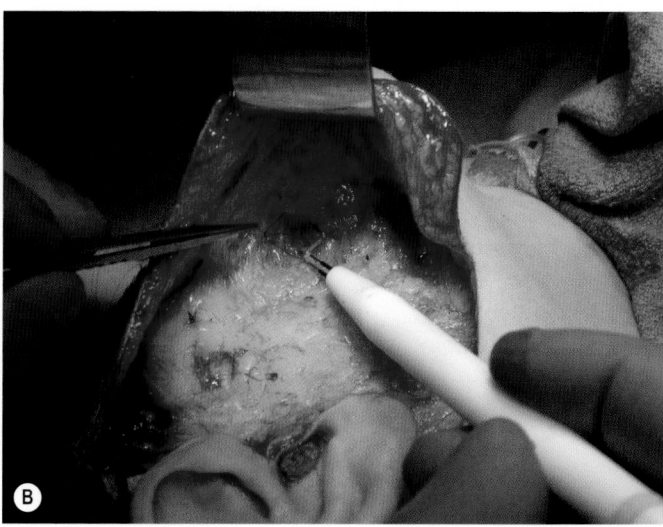

Fig. 11.19 **(A)** A portable electrical stimulator with variable voltage and frequency control is put in a sterile plastic bag placed close to the operating site so the surgeon can adjust the voltage as needed. **(B)** Bipolar electrical probe establishes an electrical current between the electrodes and a localized stimulus to a small area of tissue.

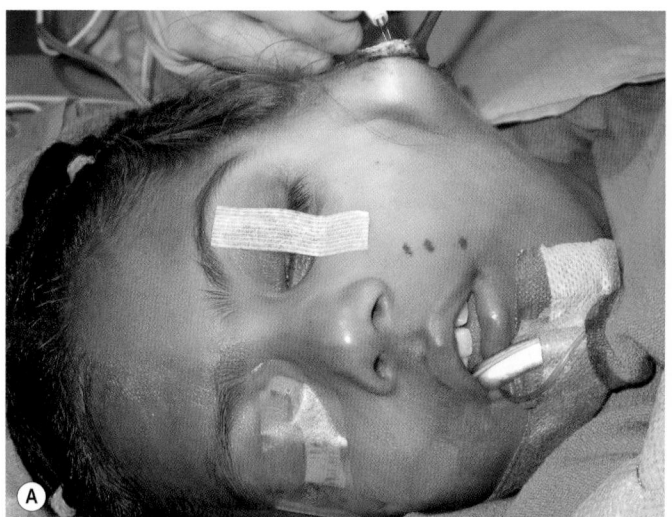
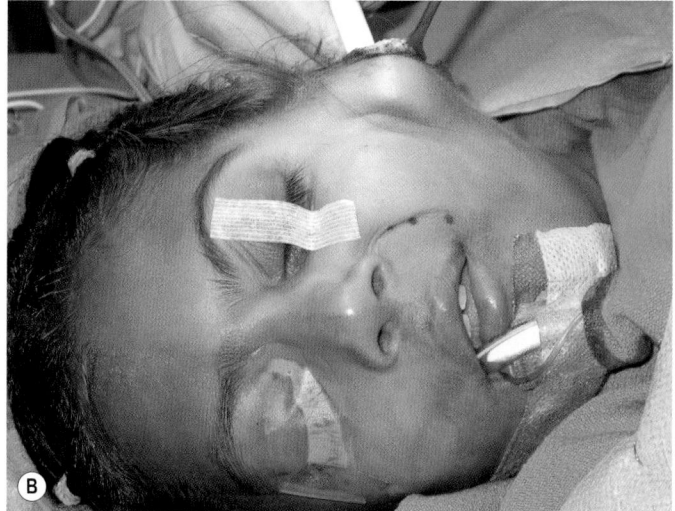

Fig. 11.20 **(A)** Patient with left facial paralysis under anesthesia. Facial nerve branches are prepared for functional nerve mapping of her right facial nerve. **(B)** Stimulation of a branch of the facial nerve to the zygomaticus major, an ideal branch for the coaptation to cross-facial nerve graft.

Disposable stimulators used to identify the presence of motor nerves do not provide reliable, controlled tetanic muscle contraction that will allow muscle palpation and clear visual identification of which muscle is being stimulated. Facial nerve mapping clearly identifies which nerve fibers stimulate the orbicularis oris and oculi muscles as well as the lip retractors. When stimulated, the facial nerve branches that produce a smile and no other movement are selected *(Fig. 11.20)*. It is sometimes difficult to find "smile" branches that do not contain some orbicularis oculi function. There are usually between two and four nerve branches that do not contain some orbicularis oculi function. There are usually between two and four nerve branches that activate the zygomaticus and levator labii superioris. This allows one or two branches to be used for the nerve graft coaptation while function of the normal facial muscles is preserved *(Fig. 11.21)*.

The sural nerve is the usual donor nerve. This is harvested with the use of a nerve stripper *(Fig. 11.22)*. Stripping of the nerve does not appear to affect its function as a graft.[38]

The proximal ends of the donor facial nerve branches are sutured to the distal end of the nerve graft such that regenerating axons will travel in a distal to proximal direction down the graft. The current practice is to use a short nerve graft, approximately 10 cm in length, and to bank the free end in the upper buccal sulcus. This should provide a well-innervated graft. In addition, the waiting period between the first and second stages is reduced with use of a short cross-facial nerve graft from 12 months to around 6 months. Patients who have had short nerve grafts achieve stronger muscle contraction than was previously obtained with traditional long cross-facial nerve grafts *(Table 11.5)*.

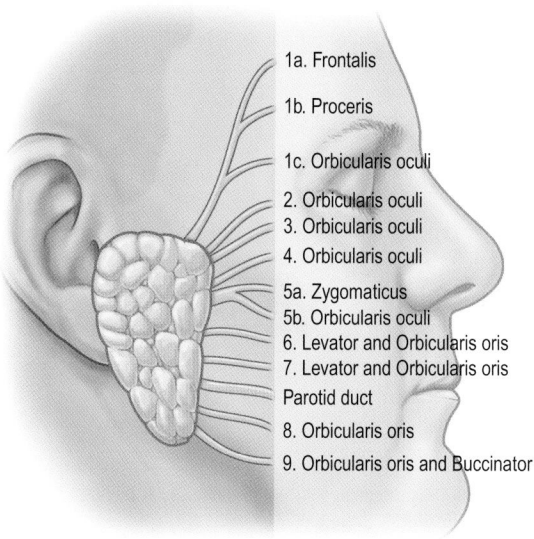

1a. Frontalis

1b. Proceris

1c. Orbicularis oculi

2. Orbicularis oculi
3. Orbicularis oculi
4. Orbicularis oculi
5a. Zygomaticus
5b. Orbicularis oculi
6. Levator and Orbicularis oris
7. Levator and Orbicularis oris
Parotid duct
8. Orbicularis oris
9. Orbicularis oris and Buccinator

Fig. 11.21 A functional nerve map is made of the branches of the facial nerve supplying the eye and mouth. The map identifies the muscles that contract when each branch is stimulated.

Table 11.5 Options for microneurovascular muscle transplantation	
One-stage	Muscle innervated by ipsilateral facial nerve (if available)
	Muscle with long nerve segment innervated by contralateral seventh-nerve branches
	Muscle innervated by masseter, hypoglossal, or accessory nerve
Two-stage	Cross-facial nerve graft followed by the muscle transplantation

Table 11.6 Muscles available for microneurovascular transplantation
Gracilis
Pectoralis minor
Rectus abdominis
Latissimus dorsi
Extensor carpi radialis brevis
Serratus anterior
Rectus femoris
Abductor hallucis

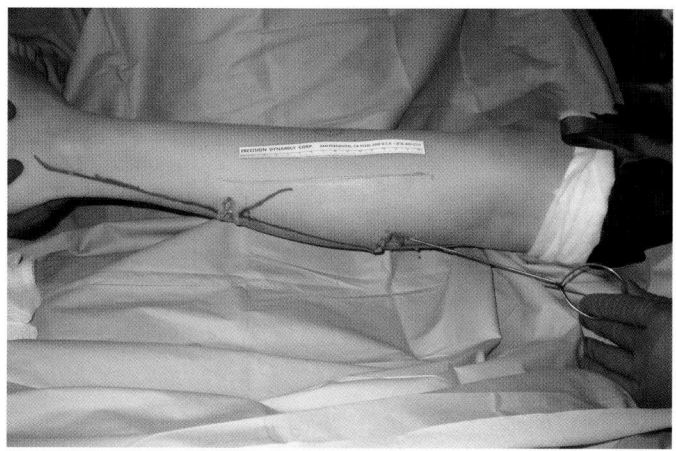

Fig. 11.22 A nerve stripper is used to harvest a segment of sural nerve. Through the posterior calf incision, the nerve is identified, dissected up to the popliteal, and cut. It is put in the stripper and the stripper passed to the midcalf. A second incision is made and the nerve is identified, cut, and withdrawn.

In addition to using a short nerve, one of the senior authors has been using the proximal end of the sural nerve as the cross-face nerve. The proximal segment from the popliteal fossa to the midcalf is thin, lacks branches, and is an excellent size match for both the selected branches of the seventh nerve and the motor nerve to gracilis.

Gracilis muscle transplantation

Many muscles are available for functioning muscle transplantation for lower facial reconstruction (*Table 11.6*). The muscle should be transplantable by vascular anastomoses and have a suitable motor nerve for nerve coaptation to the face. Initially, surgeons attempted to find a muscle that was exactly the right size for the face. However, a more suitable approach is to pare down a muscle to the desired size before

transplantation.[39] This concept allows the surgeon to use many different muscles and to customize the muscle to fit the functional requirements of the face. For example, a lightly structured face with only a partial paralysis will require a small piece of muscle. A large face with a strong movement of the mouth to the normal side and a total paralysis will require a large piece of muscle.

The gracilis muscle is suitable for facial paralysis reconstruction. The neurovascular pedicle is reliable and relatively easy to prepare. A segment of muscle can be cut to any desired size based on the neurovascular pedicle. This allows the surgeon to customize the muscle to the patient's facial requirements. There is no functional loss in the leg. Because the scar is in the medial aspect of the thigh, it is reasonably well hidden. However, the scar usually does spread. The thigh is far enough removed from the face that a simultaneous preparation of the muscle and the face is easily accomplished. The gracilis is the preferred muscle for transplantation because the anatomy is well known and the technique of preparing it for transplantation well described (*Figs 11.23–11.26*).[40]

The muscle is usually split longitudinally and the anterior portion of the muscle is used. The amount of muscle that is taken varies from 30% to 70% of the cross-section of the muscle, depending on the muscle size and needs of the face. The muscle can usually be split longitudinally without concern; however, on occasion, the vascular pedicle enters in the middle of the muscle on the deep surface. In this situation, it may be necessary to remove a portion of the anterior part of the muscle as well as the posterior to pare down the width of the muscle. After facial measurements are taken, a piece of muscle with a little extra length is removed. The end of the muscle that is to be inserted into the face is oversewn with mattress sutures, placing one more than the number of sutures inserted about the lips.

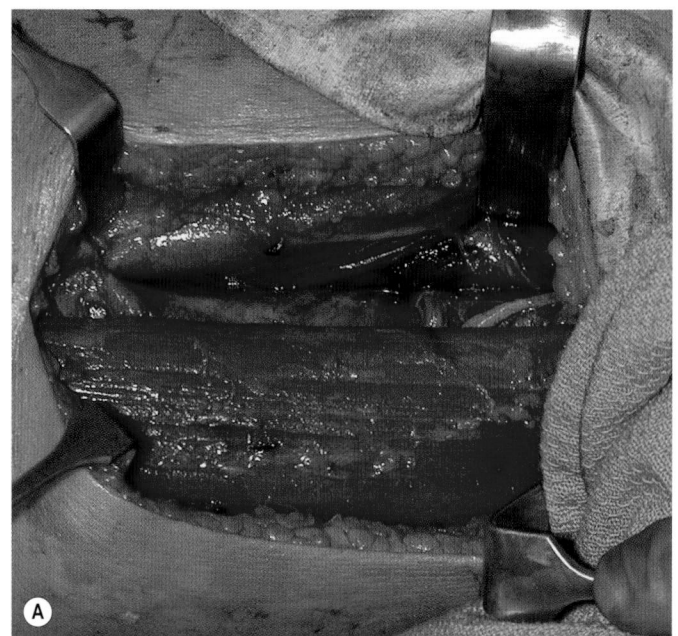

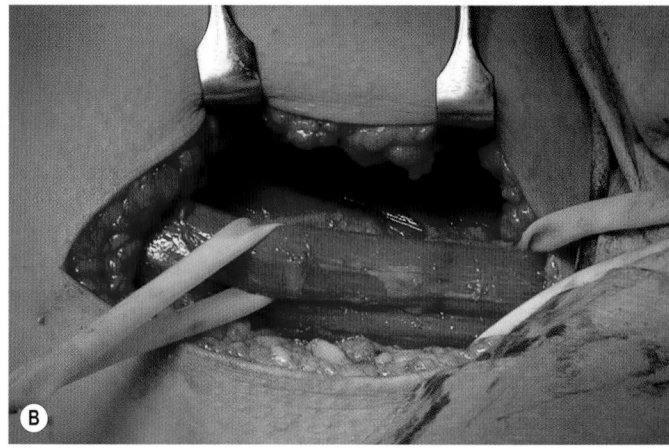

Fig. 11.23 (A) Preparation of gracilis muscle in right thigh. The motor nerve is seen in the right upper corner of the dissection adjacent to the vascular pedicle. **(B)** A longitudinal split of the anterior half of the gracilis muscle.

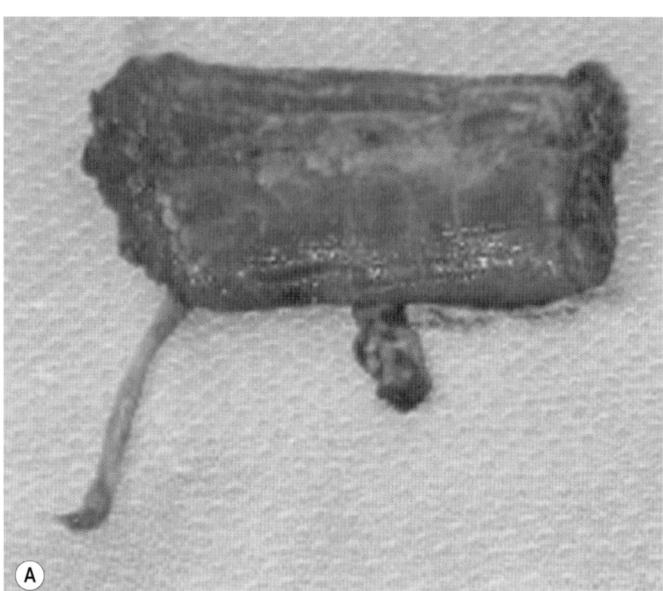

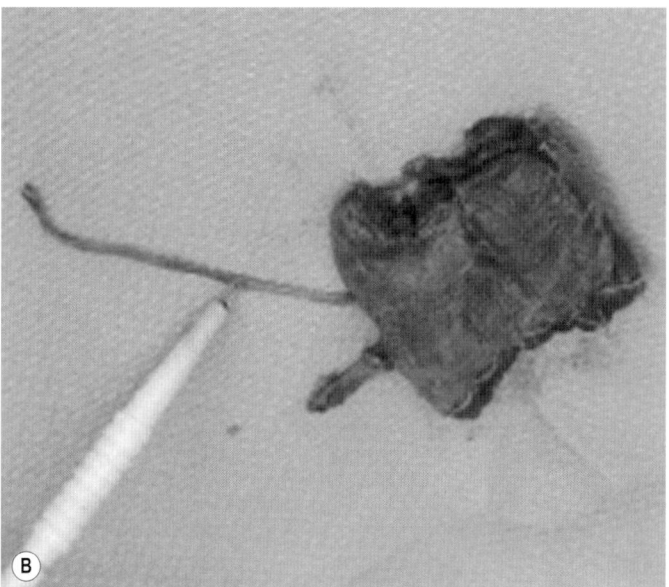

Fig. 11.24 (A) After removal of the segment of gracilis muscle, the motor nerve can be seen to the lower left and the pedicle inferiorly. The right-hand side demonstrates the distal end of the muscle, which has been oversewn with multiple mattress sutures. **(B)** Marked muscle shortening is possible in the gracilis muscle with motor stimulation.

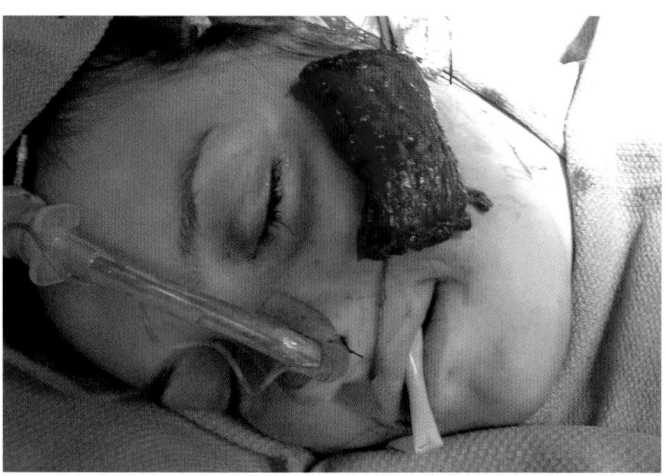

Fig. 11.25 The muscle has been removed and placed on the face to demonstrate its approximate position. The muscle's motor nerve is placed across the cheek in the position for coaptation to the cross-facial nerve graft in the upper buccal sulcus.

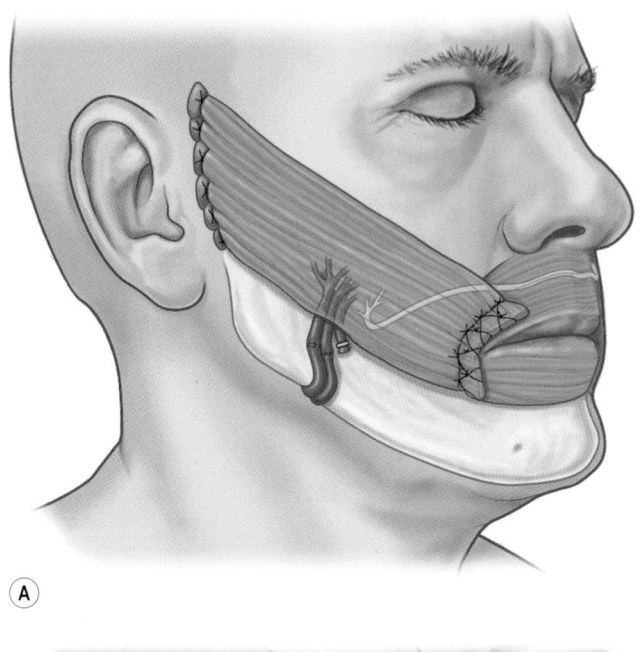

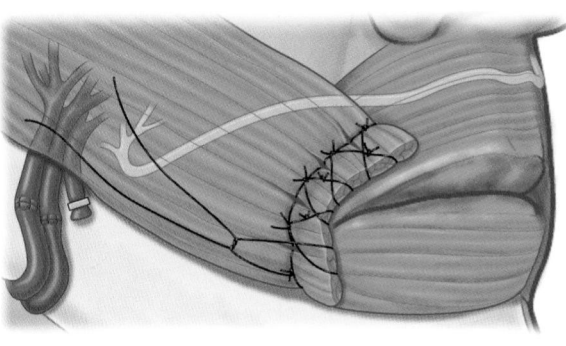

Fig. 11.26 (A) The muscle is placed in the face and revascularized by vascular anastomosis to the facial artery and the vein. Nerve coaptation to the cross-facial nerve graft is accomplished. The muscle is attached about the mouth and to the preauricular and superficial temporal fascia. **(B)** Insertion into the paralyzed orbicularis oris is accomplished with figure-of-eight sutures placed through the orbicularis oris and behind the mattress sutures at the end of the muscle. This ensures strong muscle fixation to the mouth, which should prevent dehiscence.

Attaching the muscle to the mouth is a critical part of the procedure *(Fig. 11.26)*. It is usually inserted into the fibers of the paralyzed orbicularis oris above and below the commissure and along the upper lip *(Fig. 11.27 A, B)*. Preoperative smile analysis determines the points of insertion. The preoperative smile analysis is also crucial for determining the origin of the muscle, which may be attached to the zygomatic body, arch, temporal fascia, or preauricular fascia. Intraoperative traction on the obicularis oris while the movement of the mouth is observed will verify the correct placement of the sutures. The correct tension is difficult to determine because the mechanical tension within the muscle, the degree of tone that the muscle develops, and the gravitational and muscle forces within the face will influence the eventual position *(Fig. 11.27C)*.

The vascular pedicle is usually anastomosed to the facial vessels; however, the facial vein may occasionally be absent.

There is invariably a large transverse facial vein that may be used instead. The superficial temporal vessels may also be used. The gracilis is positioned so that its hilum is close to the mouth and the motor nerve can be tunneled into the upper lip. The upper buccal sulcus incision is reopened, and the free end of the nerve graft is identified and coapted to the gracilis muscle motor nerve.

Movement does not usually occur until 6 months or more have elapsed, and maximal movement is usually gained by 18 months. At this stage, an assessment is made of the resting tension in the muscle and its excursion with smiling. It is not uncommon for the patient to require a third procedure to adjust the muscle (i.e., either tightening or loosening), and this can be combined with other touch-up procedures such as debulking or an adjustment of the insertion of origin.

With this procedure, patients usually gain around 50% as much movement on the paralyzed side as on the nonparalyzed side. This provides them with an excellent resting position and a pleasing smile that is totally spontaneous.

Muscle transplantation in the absence of seventh-nerve input

Video 4

The concept of muscle transplantation in the absence of seventh-nerve input can be applied to bilateral facial paralysis and Möbius syndrome. An effective motor nerve must be used to power the muscle. The use of the 12th and 11th nerve has been described, but preference is now given to the motor nerve to the masseter. This is a branch of the trigeminal (fifth nerve) and as such is almost always normal in patients who have bilateral facial paralysis, including Möbius syndrome. The nerve courses downward and anteriorly from the superoposterior border of the masseter in an oblique fashion. The nerve is always on the undersurface of the masseter muscle and enters this surface of the muscle belly approximately 2 cm below the zygomatic arch. The nerve courses through the muscle, giving off a variety of branches. Thus, the nerve can be traced distally, divided, and reflected proximally and superiorly to be in a position suitable for neural coaptation. The muscle transplant procedure is done much the same as described in the section on unilateral facial paralysis.

The origin and the insertion are the same, as is the revascularization process. The motor nerve to the transplanted muscle (segmented gracilis) is coapted to the motor nerve of the masseter. There is a remarkable similarity in size, and excellent reinnervation can be achieved. In fact, Bae *et al.*[41] have shown for patients with Möbius syndrome that the oral commissure movement accomplished by a gracilis transplant innervated by the masseter motor nerve comes within 2 mm of normal movement. There is approximately 15 mm of movement normally achieved at the oral commissure. With gracilis muscle transplantation innervated by the motor nerve to masseter, commissure movement of 13.8 mm on one side and 14.6 on the other side was achieved in 32 patients. With a cross-face nerve in a similar group of patients, only 7.9 mm of commissure movement was noted. The benefit of the cross-facial nerve graft, of course, is that it provides for spontaneity of activity, whereas the motor nerve to masseter does not and initially requires conscious activity. With a muscle that is innervated with cross-facial nerve graft, the patient develops spontaneous expression because the muscle is controlled by

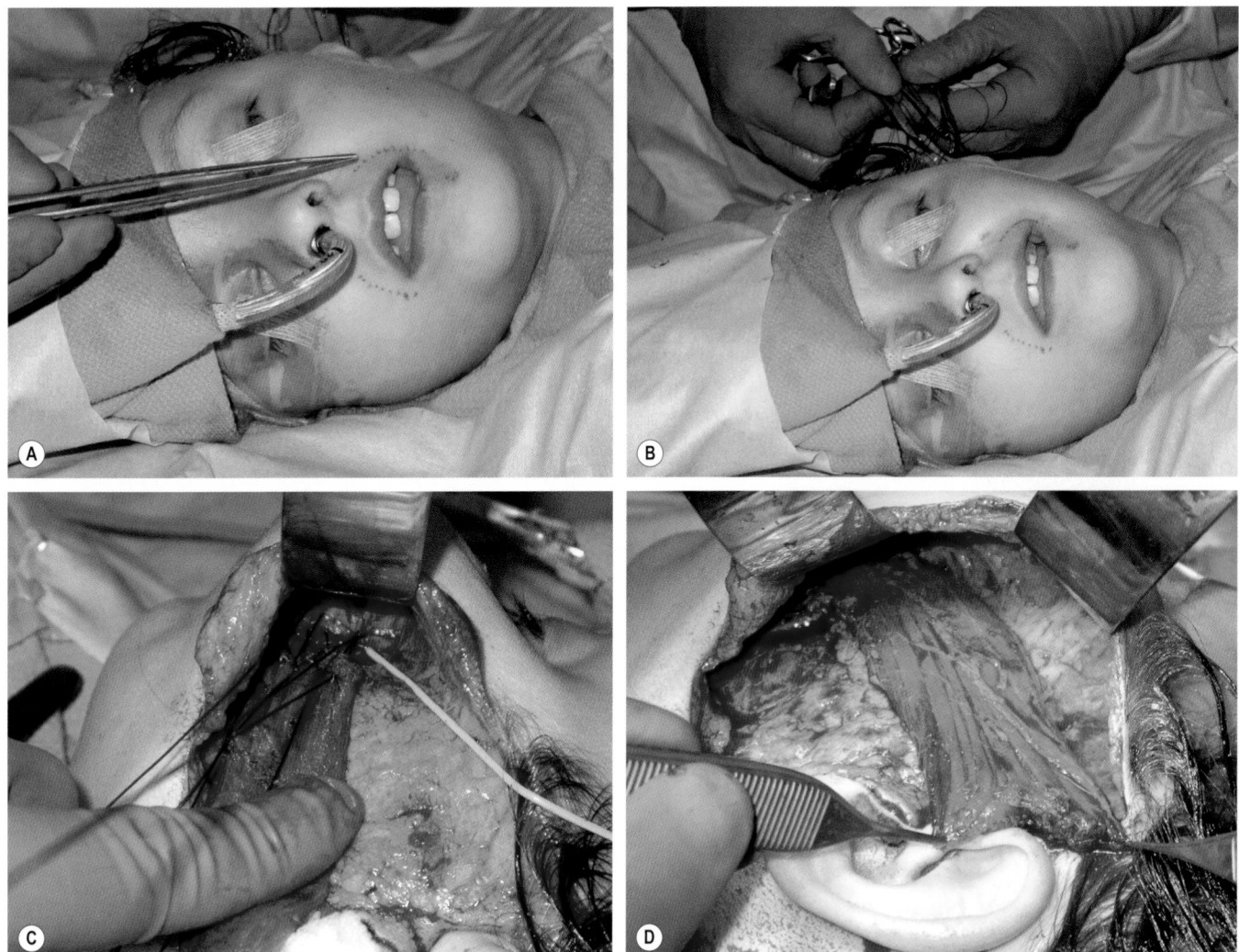

Fig. 11.27 (A) Anchoring sutures have been placed in the oral commissure and upper lip. The sutures can be seen at the top of the photograph. There is just enough traction to bring the commissure to an even position with the normal commissure on the right. **(B)** Traction is being placed on the anchoring sutures to the oral commissure and upper lip. A simulation of the smile that will occur can be seen. Our goal is to make this activity as close as possible to the normal side in vector and location of nasolabial crease formation. **(C)** The muscle is being inserted into the commissure and upper lip. The anchoring sutures are being placed behind the line of mattress sutures in the muscle so as to anchor the muscle securely, and avoid any postsurgical drift of the insertion. **(D)** The muscle has been secured to the oral commissure and upper lip, revascularized, and reinnervated. It is now placed under the appropriate tension and secured to the fascia in the temporal and preauricular region. The muscle is pulled out to length, and just enough tension to barely move the oral commissure is effected. With this, the location of the anchoring sutures to the temporal and preauricular fascia can be determined. The muscle is then secured in position, the wound thoroughly irrigated, and the flap closed over a Penrose drain.

the facial nerve on the normal side. However, when the masseter motor nerve is used, the smile movement must be learned as part of a conscious effort. Many patients are able to animate their face after some practice and biofeedback without moving their jaws and even without conscious effort. This is an area that is undergoing further study but we feel that there is a significant role for rehabilitative services after the muscles begin to contract.

Patients with Möbius syndrome are excellent candidates for this form of surgery as usually they have limited or no seventh-nerve activity and normal fifth-nerve activity so their masseter muscles are normal. We prefer to do each side separately spaced at least 2 months apart. The excursion of the muscle and resultant animation have been very satisfying. Innervation of the segmental gracilis muscle transplant by the motor nerve to masseter is now the preferred reconstruction

for these patients. It has proved to be extremely effective in helping improve lower lip incompetence and drooling as well as speech irregularities, especially those requiring bilabial sound production. Most importantly, however, it is effective in providing the patient with an acceptable level of smile animation that is not possible with other techniques *(Figs 11.28, 11.29)*.

Regional muscle transfer

Patients who are not suitable candidates for free muscle transplantation may be candidates for regional muscle transfer. These techniques, which have been in use for many decades, involve the transfer of either the temporalis or masseter muscle or both. Because these muscles are innervated by the trigeminal nerve to activate a smile, patients must initially

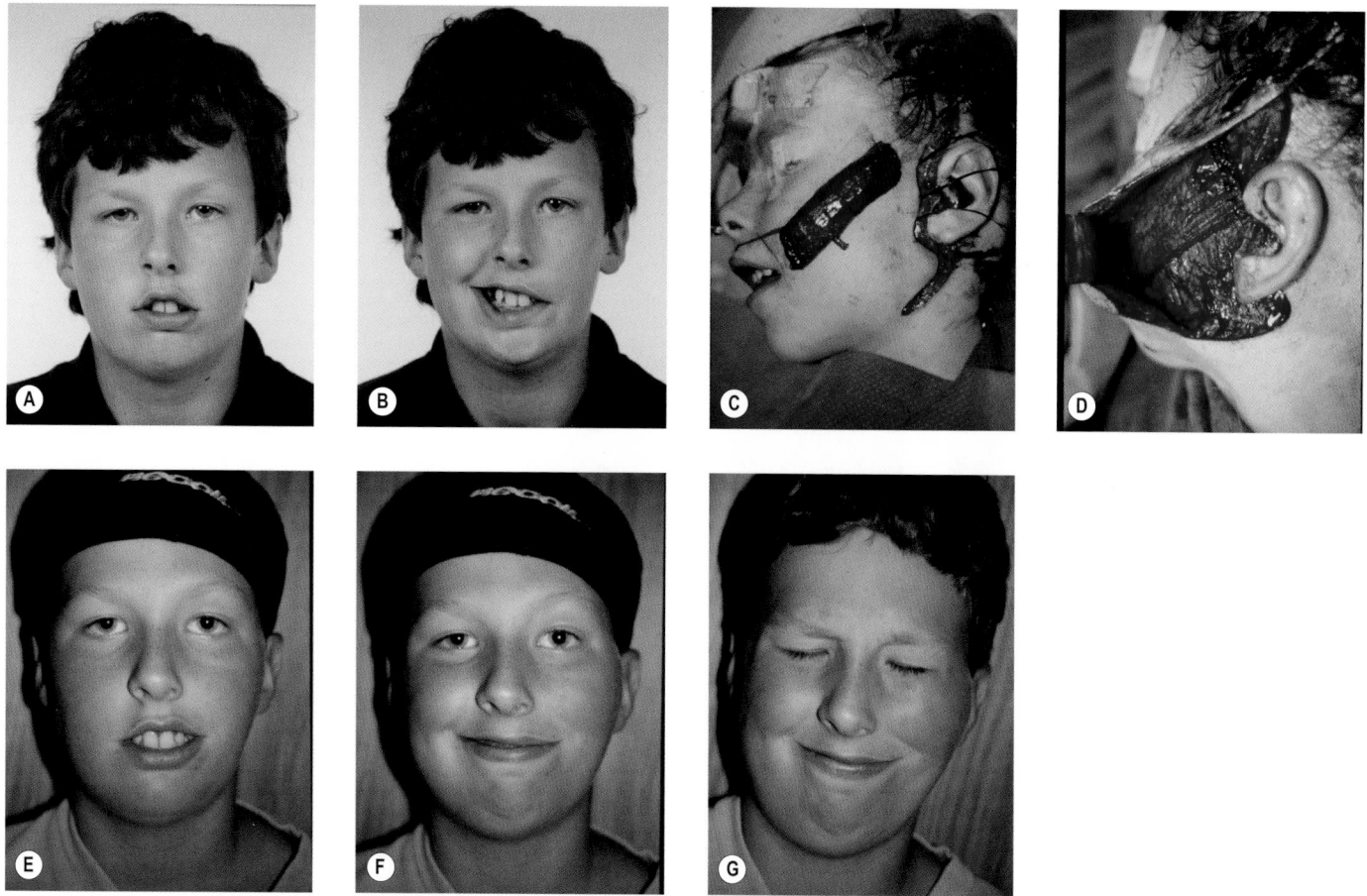

Fig. 11.28 **(A)** Preoperative view of child with congenital facial paralysis at rest. Note slight droop on affected side and shift of upper lip to normal side. **(B)** With smile. Note slight tension on affected side but no elevation. **(C)** Intraoperative view following cross-face nerve as segmental gracilis microneurovascular transport lies on check. Note vascular pedicle to be anastomosed to facial vessels and motor nerve to be coapted to cross-face nerve graft in upper buccal sulcus. **(D)** Intraoperative view. Microneurovascular transplant has been fixed at both ends, revascularized to the facial vessels, and reinnervated with previously placed cross-face nerve graft. **(E)** Postoperative view following cross-face nerve graft and microneurovascular muscle transplantation at rest. Note reasonable symmetry with no excess bulk. **(F)** With moderate smile. Note reasonable active movement with good commissure elevation and minimal bulk. **(G)** With full forced smile. Note good excursion and nice nasolabial crease formation.

clench the teeth. With practice they can activate the muscle without moving their jaws and some patients may achieve a degree of spontaneity.

The retrograde or turnover temporalis muscle transfer, as described by Gillies,[23] involves detaching the origin of the muscle from the temporal fossa and turning it over the zygomatic arch to extend to the oral commissure. Frequently, a fascial graft is required to achieve the necessary length to reach the mouth. This leaves a significant hollowing in the temporal region that can be filled with an implant. Baker and Conley[42] recommend leaving the anterior portion of the temporalis behind to partially camouflage the temporal hollowing. Another aesthetic disadvantage of the temporalis transfer is the bulge of the muscle present where it passes over the arch of the zygoma. To avoid these complications, McLaughlin[25] described an antegrade temporalis transfer. Through an intraoral, scalp, or nasolabial incision, the temporalis muscle is detached from the coronoid process of mandible and brought forward. Fascial grafts are used to reach the angle of the mouth.

Labbe and Huault modified this procedure to create a true myoplasty with a mobile insertion and fixed origin and

without the use of fascial grafts.[43] A further recent modification avoids undermining the anterior part of the temporalis muscle, thus simplifying the procedure and ensuring an enhanced blood supply. The coronoid is now osteotomized through the nasolabial incision, avoiding the transverse incision parallel to the zygoma arch and the osteotomy of the zygoma.[44] One of the key differences is that the temporalis insertion is tunneled through the buccal fat pad, thus aiding tendon gliding and consequently commissure excursion. It may be a good alternative in the older patient or when a muscle transplant is not possible.

The masseter muscle transplantation as described by Baker and Conley[42] involves transplanting the entire muscle or the anterior portion from its insertion on the mandible and inserting it around the mouth. Rubin[45] recommends separating the most anterior half of the muscle only and transposing it to the upper and lower lip. During the splitting dissection, the surgeon must be cautious not to injure the masseteric nerve, which enters the muscle on the deep surface superior to its midpoint.

Good static control of the mouth can be achieved with the masseter transplantations; however, it lacks sufficient force

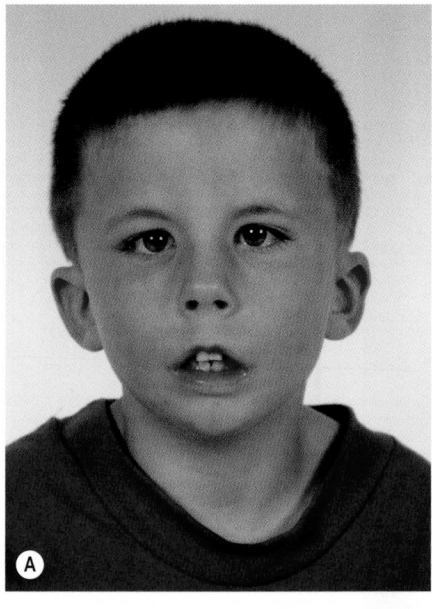
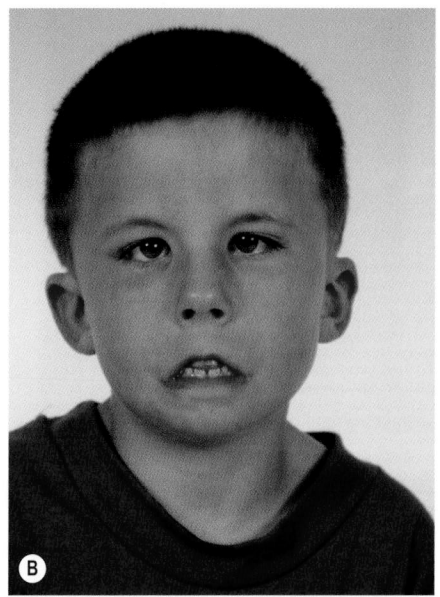
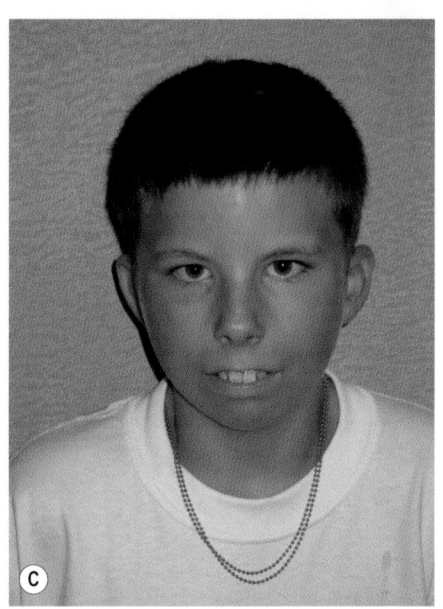
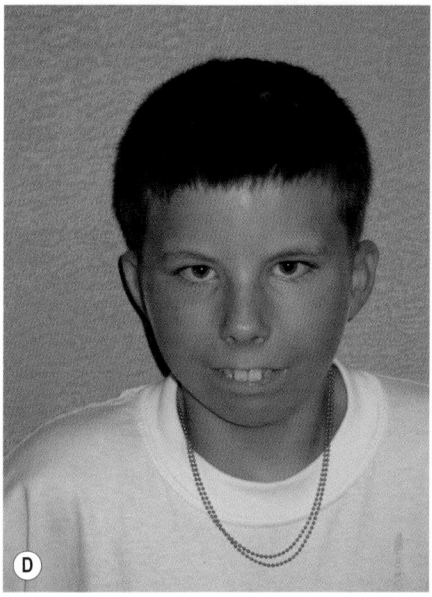
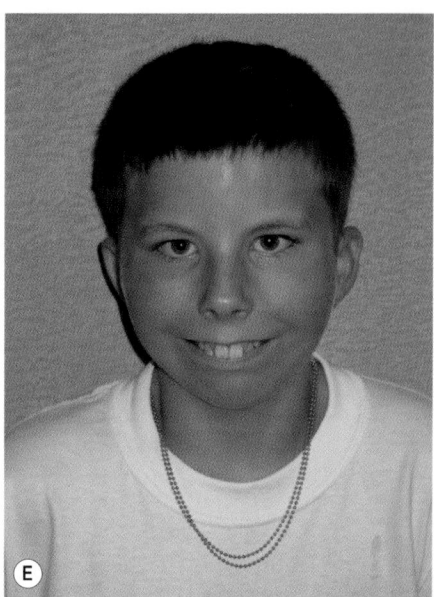

Fig. 11.29 (A) Preoperative view of child with Möbius syndrome at rest. **(B)** With attempted smile. Commissures actually turn down, giving a grimace appearance. **(C)** Postoperative view following segmental free gracilis microneurovascular muscle transplantation innervated by the motor nerve to masseter at rest. Note static support of oral commissures. **(D)** With small controlled smile. Note even elevation and tightening of oral commissures. **(E)** With full smile. Note fairly symmetrical commissure movement with nasolabial crease formation.

and excursion to produce a full smile, and the movement produced is too horizontal for most faces. Patients frequently have a hollow over the angle of the mandible.

Rubin[45] has advocated transplanting the temporalis and masseter muscles together *(Fig. 11.30)*. The temporalis provides motion to the upper lip and nasolabial fold; the masseter provides support to the corner of the mouth and lower lip.

Static slings

Static slings are used to achieve symmetry at rest without providing animation. They can be used alone or as an adjunct to dynamic procedures to provide immediate support. The

goal is to produce a facial position equal to or slightly overcorrected from the resting position on the normal side. The slings can be made of fascia (tensor fascia latae), tendon, or prosthetic material such as Gore-Tex®. In our experience, Gore-Tex® produces an undesirable inflammatory reaction. When fascia lata is taken from the thigh, it is preferable to repair the donor defect or an uncomfortable and unsightly muscle hernia may develop. The authors' preference, however, is to use tendon (palmaris longus, plantaris, or extensor digitorum longus) *(Fig. 11.31)*. Tendon can easily be harvested and woven through tissues. Curved, pointed forceps are useful for inserting the tendon through the tissues of the oral commissure and upper lip and the temporalis and zygomatic fascia. Exposure can be through a nasolabial combined with a preauricular approach or a preauricular approach alone.

When tension is applied to the grafts, the force should be distributed evenly around the mouth with a little overcorrection. This is done to compensate for the difference in facial tone when the patient is awake and for postoperative stretching. The graft is then attached to the temporal fascia or to the zygoma, depending on the desired direction of pull. Multiple grafts should be inserted, usually three, to provide an even lift to the corner of the mouth and upper lip *(Fig. 11.29)*. It is important to position the sling properly to achieve the correct elevation with regard to the upper lip and corner of the mouth *(Fig. 11.32)*. It is possible to insert the static sling too tightly,

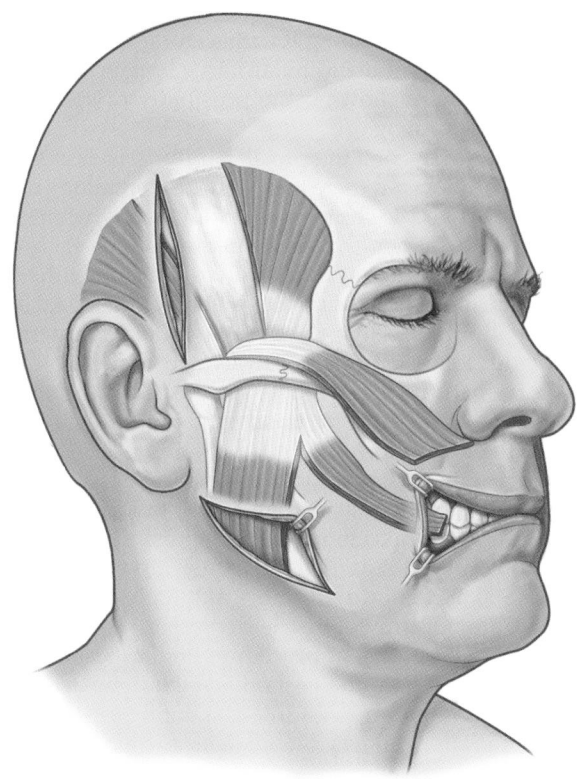

Fig. 11.30 Transplantation of both the temporalis and a portion of the masseter muscle to the periorbital region.

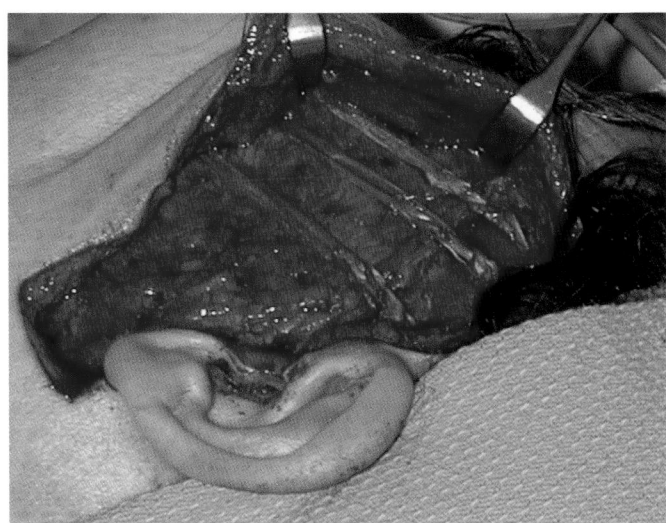

Fig. 11.31 Static slings of plantaris tendon in place to support the mouth and cheek.

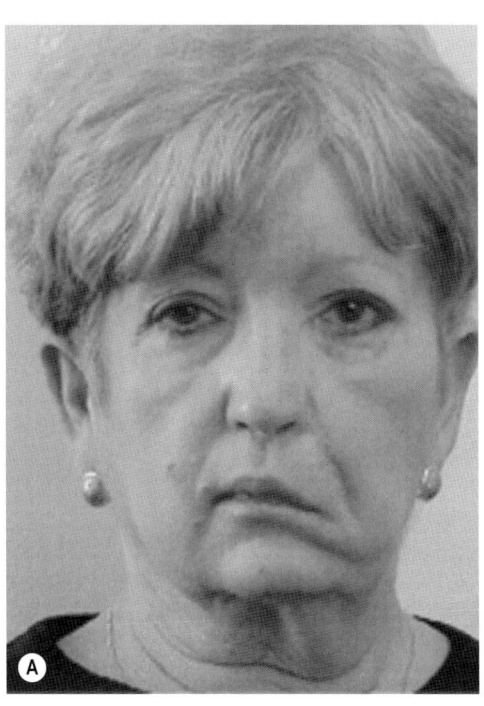

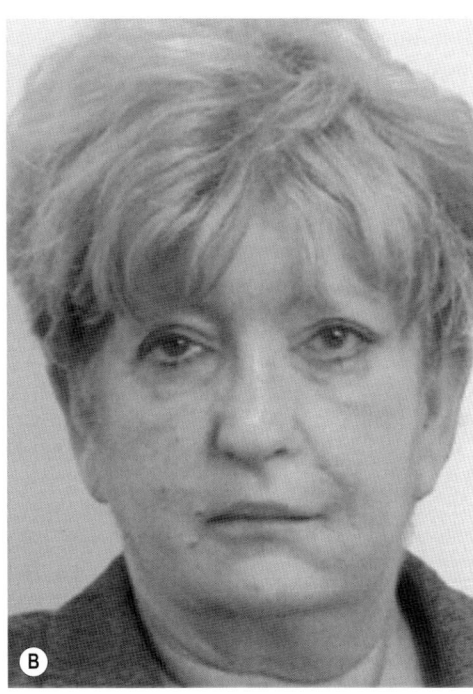

Fig. 11.32 **(A)** Preoperative view of an older patient at rest with marked facial asymmetry. Previous surgery elsewhere had placed a visible scar in the left nasolabial area. **(B)** Improvement in facial symmetry after insertion of static slings to the mouth.

particularly in the upper lip, which establishes a corridor through which air and liquid can escape.

Soft-tissue rebalancing

Soft-tissue procedures are useful adjuncts to both dynamic and static management. These procedures involve suspension and repositioning of the lax structures. This will include rhytidectomy with or without plication or suspension of the superficial musculoaponeurotic system; midface subperiosteal lifts may also be beneficial. Procedures on the nasolabial fold usually do not help define this important structure. Asymmetry of the upper lips may be corrected by mucosal excisions. These procedures, which may be minor, will often be of great benefit to patients.

Lower lip

The lower lip deformity caused by marginal mandibular nerve palsy may be part of a generalized facial paralysis or may occur in isolation as a congenital defect or secondary to trauma or surgery. It is a particular risk during rhytidectomy or parotid and upper neck surgery. The marginal mandibular nerve consists of one to three branches and supplies the depressor labii inferioris, depressor anguli oris, mentalis, and portions of the lower lip orbicularis oris. The orbicularis oris also receives innervation from buccal branches and the contralateral marginal mandibular nerves. The muscle function that is missed most by the patient is that of the depressor labii inferioris. Paralysis of this muscle results in the inability to depress, lateralize, and evert the lower lip. In the normal resting position, the deformity is not usually noticeable as the lips are closed and the depressors are relaxed. However, when the patient is talking, the paralyzed side is able to move inferiorly and away from the teeth. The deformity is most accentuated when the patient attempts a full smile, showing his or her teeth.

Problems with speech and eating may occur, but most patients are concerned primarily with the asymmetric appearance of the lower lip during speech and smiling. The inability to express rage and sorrow, which require a symmetric lower-lip depression, is also of concern.

Many techniques have been described for the correction of marginal mandibular nerve palsy, including operating on the affected side to try to animate it or operating on the unaffected side to minimize its function. Puckett *et al.*[46] described a technique of excising a wedge of skin and muscle but preserving orbicularis oris on the unaffected side. Glenn and Goode[47] described a full-thickness wedge resection of the paralyzed side of the lower lip. Edgerton[48] described transplantation of the anterior belly of the digastric muscle. The insertion of the digastric muscle to the mandible on the paralyzed side is divided and attached to a fascia lata graft that is then secured to the mucocutaneous border of the involved lip. Conley *et al.*[49] modified this technique by leaving the mandibular insertion intact but divided the tendon to the lateral aspect of the lower lip. As branches of the nerve to mylohyoid innervate the anterior belly of the digastrics, activation of the muscle requires a movement other than smiling. This is difficult to coordinate for most patients, and the result is that the digastric transplantation tends to act more as a passive restraint on the lower lip rather than as an active depressor.

Terzis and Kalantarin[6] have further modified the digastric transplantation by combining it with a cross-facial nerve graft coapted to a marginal mandibular nerve branch on the unaffected side, thereby allowing the possibility of spontaneous activation with smiling.

In patients in whom the facial paralysis is less than 24 months in duration and there is evidence of remaining depressor muscle after needle electromyography, Terzis recommends a mini hypoglossal nerve transplantation to the cervicofacial branch of the facial nerve. This involves division of the cervicofacial branch proximally and coaptation of the distal stump to a partially transected (20–30%) hypoglossal nerve. In patients with long-standing paralysis with a functional ipsilateral playsma muscle (i.e., an intact cervical division of the facial nerve), Terzis suggests transplantation of the platysma muscle to the lower lip.

The approach to depressor muscle paralysis has been to achieve symmetry both at rest and with expression by performing a selective myectomy of the depressor labii inferioris of the nonparalyzed side. This was first reported by Curtin *et al.*[50] in 1960 and later by Rubin,[45] although details of their techniques are not provided. The depressor resection can be performed as an outpatient procedure under local anesthetic and can be preceded by an injection of either long-acting local anesthetic or botulinum toxin into the depressor labii inferioris. This injection allows the patient a chance to decide whether to proceed with the muscle resection based on the loss of function of the depressor. As a result of this operation, the shape of the smile is altered on the normal side, and the lower lip is now symmetric with the opposite side (*Fig. 11.33*).

The depressor labii inferioris is marked preoperatively by asking the patient to show the teeth and palpating over the lower lip. The muscle can be felt as a band passing from the lateral aspect of the lower lip inferiorly and laterally to the chin. Through an intraoral buccal sulcus incision, the muscle is identified; it is partly hidden by the orbicularis oris, whose fibers must be elevated to reveal the more vertically and obliquely oriented fibers of the depressor labii inferioris, which measures approximately 1 cm in width. Care must be taken to preserve the branches of the mental nerve during the dissection (*Fig. 11.3*). Once the muscle has been identified, the central portion of the muscle belly is resected. Simple myotomy will not produce long-standing results, whereas results from myectomy have been permanent.

The authors have performed depressor labii inferioris resections on 27 patients, and these were reviewed with a follow-up questionnaire. Of these patients, 77% stated that their lower lip was more symmetric with smiling; half of these patients thought that their smile had changed from being significantly asymmetric to completely symmetric. Before the muscle resection, 53% of the patients were concerned about lower lip asymmetry in expressing other emotions, such as sorrow or anger. After the muscle resection, 80% of patients now thought that having a symmetric lower lip in expressing other emotions was more acceptable. Speech was unchanged in 73% of patients and improved in 27% after depressor labii inferioris resection. Some authors have suggested that depressor muscle resection will result in a deterioration of oral continence. However, in our series 89% of patients stated that oral continence was either unchanged or improved. Three patients reported a slight increase in drooling after depressor labii inferioris resection.

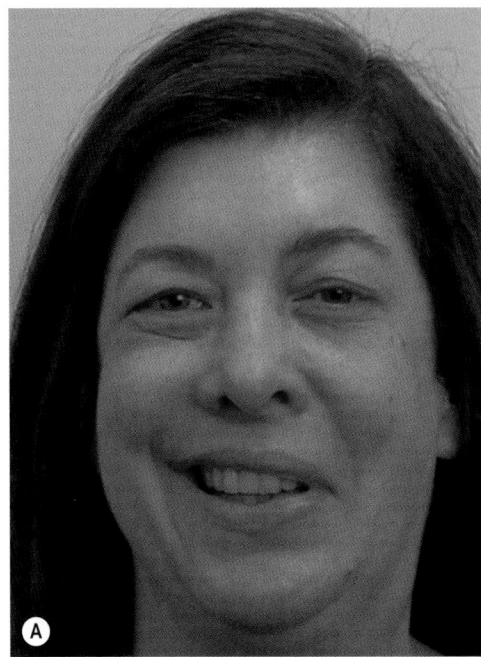 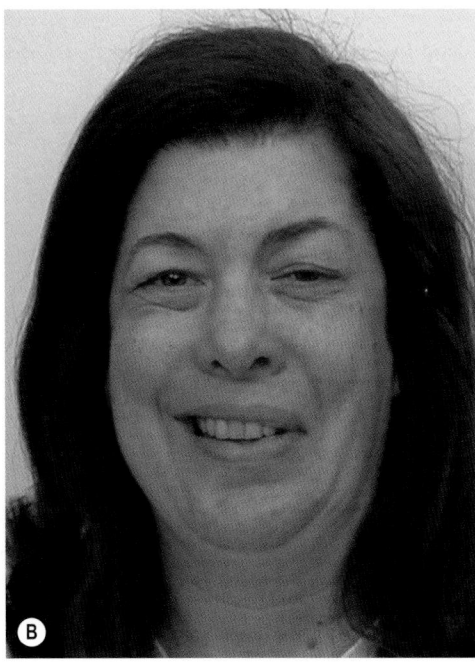

Fig. 11.33 Patient showing a "full dental" smile before depressor resection **(A)** and after depressor resection **(B)**, with marked improvement in symmetry of the lower lip.

Postoperative care

The postoperative care of all patients must be individualized as to their general medical health and postanesthetic management. However some generalizations can be made relative to specific procedures. Following muscle transplantation, it is important to maintain an adequate circulating blood volume, guarded mobilization to prevent hypotension, appropriate pain control, and perioperative antibiotics. We prefer to restrict nicotine and caffeine for 6 weeks as we feel they may cause vasoconstriction and increase the risk of vessel thrombosis. In *Table 11.7*, a typical postoperative order set is outlined following muscle transplantation to the face.

Outcomes, prognosis, and complications

As in all aspects of surgical intervention, the surgeon and patient must consider the risk-to-benefit ratio. In facial paralysis reconstruction, we cannot completely replicate normality. However we can improve the functional limitations imposed by the lack of corneal protection, the lack of oral competence with consequence leading to drooling, speech problems, and facial expression. Facial asymmetry can also lead to significant psychosocial problems. When the effects are subtle however, one must weigh the benefits to be obtained and this is often a function of how severe the paralysis is perceived by the patient and an assessment of this impact on the patient's general well-being. In the study by Bae *et al.*[41] it was found that the average commissure movement following cross-face nerve graft and muscle transplantation was about 75% of the normal side (12 versus 15 mm). Thus if an individual has 7–8 mm of movement, the two complex procedures would only potentially increase movement by 4–5 mm if all went

Table 11.7 Postoperative regimen following muscle transplantation

Fluids to soft diet as tolerated
Bed rest day 1 then up in chair with assistance and gradual guarded ambulation
Cefazolin in appropriate age-related dosage for 3 doses
Morphine PRN for 48 hours
Tylenol scheduled maximum dose for 3 days
No nicotine for 6 weeks
No caffeine for 6 weeks
No pressure on surgical site
Restrict sports or rough activities that may lead to trauma on surgical site for 6 weeks
After muscle begins to function, active exercises may be helpful with biofeedback to increase excursion, achieve symmetry, and facilitate spontaneity

well. This improvement may be worthwhile in some individuals but not in others. Each case must be assessed individually.

The potential complications are numerous but fortunately not very common. The early complications are bleeding, infection, and vascular compromise in a muscle transfer or transplant. The late complications are more common and much more difficult to deal with. They include firstly incorrect muscle positioning. This relates to the insertion at the oral commissure and upper lip which must be accurate and permanent, as previously outlined. The origin needs to be accurately placed, spread out to reduce bulk, and lead to the correct vector of the muscle being created. Secondly, great care needs to be taken to reduce bulk at the side of muscle placement. This will involve the use of only a small strip of muscle (5–15 grams in a 5-year-old child and up to 15–25 grams in an adult. In addition the muscle should be spread out at its origin. The removal of the buccal fat pad and a segment of the deep fat that will overlie the newly placed muscle may also aid in lessening the likelihood of excess bulk. Thirdly, the excursion of either a transferred muscle or transplanted muscle may not meet the expectations of the surgeon or the patient and be quite disappointing. We feel that excursion is related to the power of the motor nerve utilized and to the physical placement of the muscle as it must be under the appropriate tension to maximize excursion. A poorly functioning muscle may also be related to the vascularity of the muscle or the effects of a single or double nerve repair, although it may be related to a combination of the above factors. Unfortunately these insufficient excursion problems are not easy to correct and will be addressed in the next section.

Secondary procedures

Secondary procedures following muscle transfer or transplant are often palliative and not curative. The problems can be listed as incorrect muscle positioning, excess bulk at the side of the muscle, and poor excursion.

Muscle slippage at the insertion side is the most difficult to correct. Open reinsertion can be done but may leave the commissure too tight and the mouth distorted. This can be avoided by using a tendon graft to connect the displaced muscle to the oral commissure and upper lip. If the muscle is too tight it can be released at its origin and slid toward the mouth. However this may require a radical freeing of the muscle and put the neuromuscular pedicle at risk. If the vector is incorrect, it can be repositioned but only with great difficulty and again with significant risk to the pedicle. Whenever the position of the muscle is adjusted, one can expect a reduction in excursion. However this may be a reasonable price to pay to correct the distortions imposed by poorly positioned muscle.

Excess bulk at the side of the transferred or transplanted muscle can be addressed by defatting and shaving of the outer surface of the muscle. To facilitate this it is helpful to position the motor nerve on the deep surface of the muscle at the time of the muscle transplantation. This is particularly true when a cross-face nerve graft is used.

When the problem is poor excursion, the options are few. It may help to tighten the muscle if it has been inserted too loosely but care must be taken not to distort the mouth.

If this is not possible, then a thorough open discussion with the patient is required. Is there sufficient support or movement to alleviate the functional problems and position the mouth evenly at rest? How much movement with muscle activation is present? Is the patient content with the present situation, in view of the fact that improvement will not be easy or perhaps even possible?

If further surgery is requested after a full discussion and knowledge that improvement will be difficult, one must redo with transplantation of a second muscle. If the cause of the failure is not clear, it may be wise to use a motor nerve to power the new muscle that was not used before. This may be the motor nerve to masseter in the case of a failed cross-face nerve graft, muscle transplantation combination. The results of putting a muscle into scarred bed, and reusing the previous vessels and possibly nerve, will not be as likely for success as the primary procedure, but yet may be very helpful for selected patients.

Further considerations

Facial paralysis crosses many subspecialty lines. Limited eye closure, tear transport, and ectropion dictate the involvement of ophthalmologists as well as oculoplastic surgeons. Intranasal airflow may be limited and symptomatic, necessitating involvement of nasal surgeons often with otolaryngology background. Otolaryngologists may also be consulted for associated hearing loss, stapedial malfunction, or other components involving the middle ear. In certain patients, brainstem involvement may cause difficulty in dealing with oral secretions, aspirations, and swallowing. This may occur congenitally, such as in patients with Möbius syndrome, or it may be acquired, such as in patients with intracranial tumors. These situations may require the involvement of otolaryngologists.

There are other functional issues that may need to be addressed by subspecialists. For example, feeding may be a problem for infant or adult patients. Feeding experts from occupational therapy may be helpful in providing techniques for mechanical assistance. After surgical intervention, occupational therapy is also helpful in assisting with an exercise program to improve muscle excursion and symmetry of smile. Speech is often affected by facial paralysis. Speech therapy can help improve articulation errors and provide appropriate lip placement.

The psychosocial aspects of facial paralysis are enormous. Surgeons tend to focus on the physical, but it is extremely important to keep the entire patient in mind. A battery of psychosocial support personnel should be available to work with the surgeon for the overall benefit of the patient. This team should include social workers, clinical psychologists, developmental psychologists, and psychologists. It is important to sort out the various needs of the patient, not just from a physical standpoint but also from a psychosocial standpoint. Only then can true success in surgical management be achieved. A majority of patients with congenital facial paralysis have unilateral and isolated involvement. It is believed to be the result of a compression of the fetal face that limits facial nerve development. Consequently, there are no genetic implications. Parents have no predisposition for additional children with facial paralysis, nor does the patient have any greater increased likelihood of facial paralysis than that of the general population. The same can be said for patients with unilateral syndrome, which occurs with hemifacial microsomia, for example. This is thought to be acquired at an early stage of fetal development because of environmental factors. Thus, again, there are no genetic implications. The same is not true, however, for all patients with Möbius syndrome. Although most are thought to be sporadic, there has been a surge of interest in the genetics of the conditions.[51] Pedigrees have been described indicating that certain forms of Möbius syndrome are inherited by an autosomal-dominant gene with variable expressivity *(Fig. 11.34)*.

Incomplete penetration is also thought to account for the inconsistency of involvement. Certain chromosomes have also been identified in specific patients,[52] and a reciprocal translocation between the long arm of chromosome 13 and the

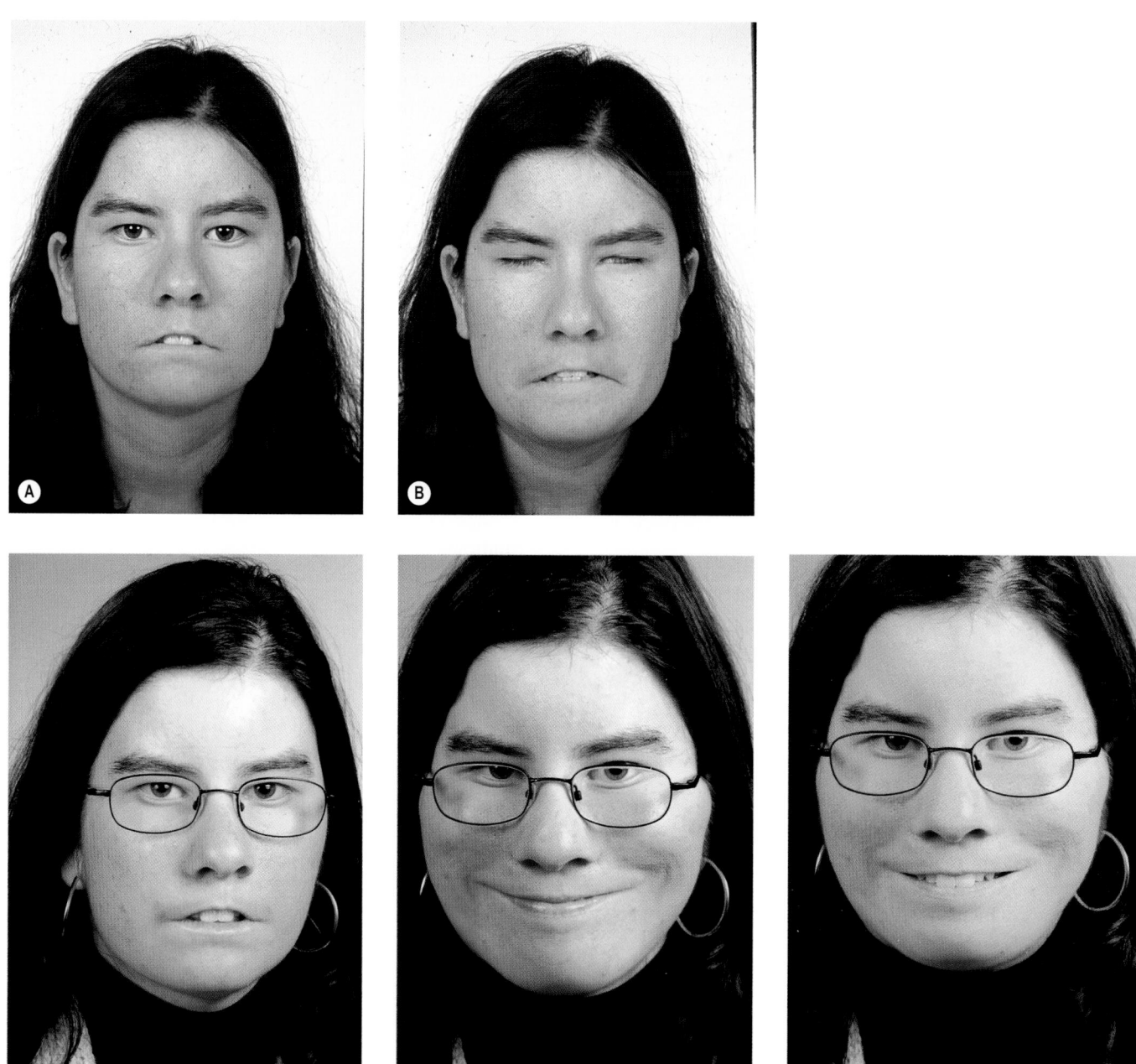

Fig. 11.34 **(A)** and **(B)** Preoperative views of a patient with Möbius syndrome at rest and with maximum animation. **(C)** Postoperative view of a patient after muscle transplantation to the lower face at rest. **(D)** Patient with closed-mouth smile. **(E)** Patient smiling and showing teeth.

short arm of chromosome 1 has been described.[53] A great deal of interest has been stimulated relative to the genetic aspects of Möbius syndrome and its relationship to other behavioral conditions. Research is under way in these areas and will undoubtedly shed light on inheritance features as well as the etiologic factors involved in Möbius syndrome.

Conclusions

Although significant progress has been made in the management of facial paralysis, much is yet to be done. Acceptable commissure movement can be achieved, but upper lip

elevation is far more difficult. The short distance of the muscle involved and the challenging access have proved difficult to overcome. However, new techniques are emerging, and work in this area continues.

Across any nerve repair, there is considerable loss of axonal continuity. Improved nerve coaptation techniques with the use of neurotrophic factors will undoubtedly be instrumental in providing further improvement. From a physical standpoint, does the length of the nerve graft affect recovery? Does its vascular nature or the technique of harvest result in alteration of function? Laboratory research in these areas is ongoing and could again provide some level of improvement in recovery. The placement, anchorage, and direction of movement of the muscle transplant are critical to success. Improvements have been made in these areas, but asymmetry continues to be a challenge. Further attention needs to be drawn to the direction of the smile and the positioning of the muscle relative to the oral commissure and nasolabial crease.

Fundamental to progress in any field is an assessment tool that is reliable, universally acceptable, and as simple as possible to use. In facial paralysis, it is necessary to measure muscle excursion, direction of movement, volume symmetries, and contour irregularities to assess the results of repair and reconstruction. For comparison of results from center to center, a common tool is needed. Also, to assess results from a psychosocial standpoint, a reliable common instrument of evaluation is needed if meaningful conclusions are to be drawn. Progress has been made on physical measurement and psychosocial profile tools,[54] and there is hope that these will be universally accepted and applied in the future.

In addition to these technical issues, concepts need to evolve with respect to new areas of development. Eye expression is an area that has not as yet been directed at commissure and upper lip elevation. Orbicularis oris function or reconstruction of the depressors has not been addressed. Finally, there is not as yet an effective method of managing synkinesis. This is an extremely disturbing phenomenon with psychosocial and functional implications. We are just beginning to see how Botox injection techniques can be effective in other areas of muscle overactivity, and perhaps some level of synkinesis control will evolve with this technique. Much is yet to be done for the patient with facial paralysis, and further research and development in this area will continue to yield improvements.

Access the complete references list online at **http://www.expertconsult.com**

In summary, facial paralysis reconstruction continues to be an exciting evolving area of surgical development.

9. Rubin L, ed. *The Paralyzed Face*. St. Louis: Mosby-Year Book; 1991.

   This is a classic text on facial expressions and how to produce them surgically. Although it predates current muscle transplantation techniques, it still offers the surgeon insight into smile analysis and surgical decision-making.

14. Westin LM, Zuker RM. A new classification system for facial paralysis in the clinical setting. *J Craniofac Surg.* 2003;14:672–679.

   This classification of facial paralysis was created as an aid to the clinician in understanding the breadth of this diverse condition. As such it can facilitate treatment planning.

16. May M. Microanatomy and pathophysiology of the facial nerve. In: May M, ed. *The facial nerve*. New York: Thieme; 1986:63.

   This classic text is a must for all students of facial paralysis. The concepts are still valid today and aid in treatment planning.

26. Carraway JH, Manktelow RT. Static sling reconstruction of the lower eyelid. *Operative Techniques Plast Reconstr Surg.* 1999;6:163.

   Eyelid surgery must be precise and well executed to be successful. This article describes in detail the technique and potential undesirable effects.

28. Manktelow RT, Tomat LR, Zuker RM, et al. Smile reconstruction in adults with free muscle transfer innervated by the masseter motor nerve: effectiveness and celebral adaptation. *Plast Reconstr Surg.* 2006;118: 885–899.

   In this paper, evidence is presented to suggest cerebral adaptation is a real entity in the adult population. It sets the stage for further exploration of this fascinating concept.

30. Michaelidou M, Chieh-Han J, Gerber H, et al. The combination of muscle transpositions and static procedures for reconstruction in the paralyzed face of the patient with limited life expectancy on who is not a candidate for free muscle transfer. *Plast Reconstr Surg.* 2009;123:121–129.

   This is an excellent article that provides the surgeon with practical alternatives to complex microsurgical procedures. They are particularly helpful when the patient is elderly or has a limited life expectancy but still would like a surgical correction to improve the quality of life that remains.

33. Terzis JK, Tzafetta K. The "babysitter" procedure: minihypoglossal to facial nerve transfer and cross-facial nerve grafting. *Plast Reconstr Surg.* 2009;123:865–876.

   This is the first article to resurrect the nerve transfer principle for facial paralysis. Use of the entire hypoglossal had serious and permanent negative effects on speech, food manipulation, and tongue bulk. This article addresses these issues and the partial use of the hypoglossal avoids these problems.

37. Zuker RM, Goldberg CS, Manktelow RT. Facial animation in children with Möbius syndrome after segmental gracilis muscle transplant. *Plast Reconstr Surg.* 2000;106:1.

   This article describes the problems of the Moebius syndrome from a reconstructive surgeon's viewpoint and suggests a surgical procedure for function and animation.

41. Bae Y, Zuker RM, Maktelow RM, et al. A comparison of commissure excursion following gracilis muscle transplantation for facial paralysis using a cross-face nerve graft versus the motor nerve to the masseter nerve. *Plast Reconstr Surg.* 2006;117:2407–2413.

   In this paper the strong input of the masseter motor nerve is shown to translate into increased commissure excursion.

43. Labbe D, Huault M. Lengthening temporalis myoplasty and lip reanimation. *Plast Reconstr Surg.* 2000;105: 1289–1297.

   This paper clearly outlines the technique of temporalis myoplasty that has evolved over the years. It has a role in a select group of patients.

12

Oral cavity, tongue, and mandibular reconstructions

Ming-Huei Cheng and Jung-Ju Huang

SYNOPSIS

- In head and neck reconstruction, a comprehensive review of the oral cavity, tongue and mandibular defects, the patient's disease status, and overall condition and prognosis are critical to achieving optimal reconstruction results while minimizing complications. Evaluation of the defect, including its size, shape, geometry, and relationship to the available recipient vessels, should be thorough, and a strategic approach to flap selection and design should be taken, in order to reconstruct the oral defect accurately and restore the patient to his/her preoperative functional and aesthetic status.

- There are several options to consider when performing a mandibular reconstruction, such as patient risk factors, defect characteristics, donor flap selection, and surgical technique. In mandibular reconstruction, the use of different tissue components to achieve composite reconstruction is essential for successful functional reconstruction. An understanding of the anatomical characteristics of the different osteocutaneous flaps available may increase the likelihood of selecting the appropriate donor flap for mandibular reconstruction.

- For reconstruction of type III mandibular defects, several options exist, including the use of a soft-tissue flap with a reconstruction plate, one osteocutaneous flap with one pedicled flap, double free flaps, chimeric flaps, a composite scapular flap, and an osteomyocutaneous peroneal artery combined (OPAC) flap. The evolution of the fibula flap from a bone-only flap to an osteocutaneous flap and an OPAC flap may increase the clinical application of this flap for type III mandibular defects. Due to the triangular profile of the fibula, the placement of plates and screws on the lateral aspect of the fibula reduces the incidence of injury to its pedicle and septocutaneous perforators.

 Access the Historical Perspective section online at
http://www.expertconsult.com

Introduction

Reconstruction of the oral cavity and mandible is complex and challenging with regard to both functional and aesthetic outcomes. An ideal reconstruction should mimic the missing tissue with regard to structure, geometry, and tissue character. For an oral cavity reconstruction without bony involvement, the ideal reconstruction involves a soft-tissue flap that is similar to the missing tissue in size, shape, and tissue quality.

The anatomy of the oral cavity is complicated, and each structure has a specific role in speech, swallowing, and facial expression. Furthermore, defects in one specific functional unit can also affect adjacent structures. Before reconstruction, a comprehensive assessment of the defect is required. Disease status and tumor staging may also affect postoperative treatment and outcome. A comprehensive understanding of the disease process also helps in selecting an optimal reconstructive method.

Reconstruction of the tongue is difficult due to its important role in articulation, deglutition, and airway protection.[1] Among westerners, the tongue is the most common site in the oral cavity for primary cancers. The incidence of tongue cancer remains as high as buccal cancer due to the popularity of habitual betel nut chewing, smoking, and alcohol consumption in Asian countries. Any reconstructive attempt has to restore bulk and mobility in order for the tongue to be functional.

Functionally, the mandible plays a key role in mastication, swallowing, speech, and smiling. Aesthetically, the mandible provides the shape, contour, and vertical height of the lower third of the face. Mandibular defects can result from resection of tumors, osteomyelitis or osteoradionecrotic lesions, or gunshot trauma. Soft-tissue involvement surrounding the mandible results in even larger and more complicated defects that require delicate shaping of the hard- and soft-tissue components of the flaps used for reconstruction. Wide excision of advanced oral tumors affecting the mandible can involve many adjacent structures, such as the oral lining, the tongue and floor of the mouth, the external skin of the cheek, the lower lip, the masseter muscle, the buccal fat pad, the parotid gland, and the partial maxilla. These composite defects complicate reconstruction.

The goals of composite mandibular reconstruction include restoration of the bony scaffold, adequate oral continence and deglutition, obliteration of dead space, and re-establishment of optimal cosmesis. Dead space created by the extirpation of masticator muscles, the buccal fat pad, and the parotid gland can lead to fluid accumulation and infection. When soft-tissue losses are not adequately replaced following tumor resection, this can lead to a sunken appearance from soft-tissue contracture, trismus, plate exposure, and impaired speech and swallowing function.[2] These conditions may be exacerbated by postoperative radiotherapy.

Basic anatomy/disease process

The oral cavity is bounded by the lip anteriorly, the oropharynx posteriorly, the hard palate superiorly, the tongue and mouth floor inferiorly, and the cheek laterally.The inner oral cavity is lined with buccal mucosa. Beneath the buccal mucosa are the muscles for facial expression, mouth movement, and maintenance of oral competence. Between the intraoral and cheek soft tissues are bony structures, including the mandible and maxilla, which form and maintain the structure of the lower face.

Approximately 86% of all oral tumors are squamous cell carcinomas, while other tumors, such as verrucous carcinoma, sarcoma, melanoma, or lymphoma, occur less frequently. The mean age-adjusted incidence of oral cavity and phalanx cancer is 11.9 per 100000 from 1975 to 2008 in the US; this value could be higher in specific areas where smoking and betel nut chewing are popular.[63] In 2008, it was estimated that head and neck cancers comprised 2–3% of all cancers and accounted for 1–2% of all cancer deaths in the US.[64,65] Most patients with head and neck cancer have metastatic disease at the time of diagnosis (with regional nodal involvement in 43% and distant metastasis in 10%). Moreover, patients with head and neck cancer often develop second primary tumors at an annual rate of 3–7%.[66,67] The male-to-female ratio is currently 3:1 for the incidence of oral cavity and pharyngeal cancers.[65]

Statistical analysis of a 10-year period revealed a trend toward earlier diagnosis of head and neck cancer. Surgical treatment with or without radiation and chemotherapy remains the standard of care.[68] Since the first introduction of the free intestinal flap in 1959[10] and the first fasciocutaneous free flap for head and neck reconstructions in 1976, free flap transfer has become the gold standard for reconstruction due to its high flap survival rate, improved cosmetic and functional results, and acceptable level of donor site morbidity.[12] These techniques also facilitate resection of even more advanced but localized tumors.[69,70]

Inadequate oral hygiene and contamination may increase the risk of infection and also compromise the survival of any inadequately vascularized tissue.[71] Irradiation produces detrimental acute and chronic effects not only in the periosteum and the marrow of the mandible but also in the oral mucosa and surrounding soft tissue.[72–75] With chronic hypoxia, cellular and vascular damage lead to skin atrophy and increase the susceptibility to wound breakdown and decrease healing potential following minor trauma. Vascular changes initially occur in the microcirculation; however, with progression, larger blood vessels can be affected as well. Many of these issues are addressed by the transplantation of well-vascularized tissue with bone and skin components.

Vascularized bone resists infection well, does not resorb, and is not dependent on the recipient bed vascularity for survival.[76]

Diagnosis/patient presentation

Currently, most patients with oral cancer still present with advanced-stage cancer.[77,78] Most patients complain about oral ulcers, sore throat, a tongue mass, and pain with swallowing. Cuffari *et al.* demonstrated that the type of pain reported is related to the TNM staging of the tongue and mouth floor.[79] A thorough physical examination, radiographic study of the tumor, and histology with TNM staging should be performed by both a surgical oncologist and a reconstructive surgeon prior to surgery. Any history of gunshot trauma, X-rays, and three-dimensional computed tomography (CT) scans of the defect should also be considered during preoperative planning. In addition to classical TNM staging,[80] gene expression[81,82] and profiling provide a subclassification based on DNA repair genes. This subclassification plays a role in predicting the clinical outcome after radiotherapy.[83] Liao *et al.* addressed that upregulation of centromere protein H is correlated with poor prognosis and progression in tongue cancer patients.[84] Chronic ulcer, leukoplakia, and tumor growth are regularly seen at specialized cancers.[85] Visual loss as an initial symptom of squamous cell carcinoma of the tongue was published by Foroozan.[86] It is important to keep in mind that rare constellations of symptoms may require differential diagnosis: a tumor or abscess of the tongue could also be a sign of atypical metastasis of lung cancer.[87,88] Recently, a rare schwannoma of the tongue was reported by Cohen and Wang.[89] Malignant fibrous histiocytoma of the tongue was reported by Rapidis *et al.*[90]

Patient selection and decision-making

Most buccal mucosa, tongue, or mandibular defects result from cancer ablation surgeries. Before reconstruction, a comprehensive assessment of the defects, the patient's general condition, and the availability of donor tissue should be performed. A thorough understanding of the missing tissue and its geometrical relation to each structure will elucidate the functional and aesthetic requirements of reconstruction and facilitate the selection of an optimal reconstructive method *(Tables 12.1–12.3)*. The surgeon's technique and decision-making ability as well as the patient's general status contribute to the quality of the reconstruction.

Patient factors *(Table 12.4)*

Many oral cavity cancer patients have a history of smoking and alcohol consumption, which increases the risk of perioperative pulmonary and overall complications. These factors also affect the microvascular anastomosis in a free flap transfer.[91,92] Diabetes mellitus is a risk factor for peripheral vasculopathy and is associated with a higher incidence of

Table 12.1 Comparisons of soft-tissue flaps for buccal mucosa and tongue reconstruction

Flap character / Flap type	Skin or mucosa	Flap dimension	Flap thickness	Pedicle size	Pedicle length	Dissection difficulty
Local/regional flap						
Nasolabial flap	++	+	++	–	–	–
Buccal fat pad flap	–	+	+	–	–	–
Facial artery musculomucosal flap	++	+	++	–	–	–
Submental flap	+++	+++	++	–	–	–
Deltopectoral flap	++	+++	+++	–	–	–
Pectoralis major myocutaneous flap	++++	++++	++++	–	–	–
Free flap						
Radial forearm flap	++++	++++	++	+++	++++	++++
Ulnar forearm flap	++++	++++	++	+++	++++	++++
Lateral arm flap	+++	++	++	++	+	+++
Rectus abdominis musculocutaneous flap	++++	+++	++++	++++	+++	++++
Anterolateral thigh fasciocutaneous flap	++++	++++	+++	++++	++++	+
Anterolateral thigh musculocutaneous flap	++++	++++	++++	++++	+++	+
Thoracodorsal artery perforator flap	++++	+++	+++	+++	+++	++
Medial sural artery perforator	++++	+++	++	+++	++++	++

Flap character rates as follows: ++++, excellent; +++, good; ++, fair; +, poor; –, not applicable. Dissection difficulty rates as follows: ++++, not difficult; +++, mild difficulty; ++, moderate difficulty; +, most difficult.

Table 12.2 Selection of soft-tissue flaps for buccal mucosa reconstruction

Defect character / Flap type	Small mucosa defect	Large mucosa defect	Mucosa trigon	Through and through	Mucosa and partial maxilla	Mucosa and marginal mandibulectomy
Local/regional flap						
Nasolabial flap	+	–	–	–	–	–
Buccal fat pad flap	++	++	–	–	–	–
Facial artery musculomucosal flap	++	–	–	–	–	–
Submental flap	++	++	–	–	–	–
Deltopectoral flap	–	+++	++	+++	++	+++
Pectoralis major myocutaneous flap	–	++++	++	+++	++	++++
Free flap						
Radial forearm flap	–	++++	++	+	+	+
Ulnar forearm flap	–	++++	++	+	+	+
Lateral arm flap	–	++	++	+	+	+
Rectus abdominis musculocutaneous flap	–	++	++	+++	++++	++++
Anterolateral thigh fasciocutaneous flap	–	+++	+++	+++	++	+++
Anterolateral thigh musculocutaneous flap	–	++	+++	++++	++++	++++
Thoracodorsal artery perforator flap	–	++++	++++	++	++	+++
Medial sural artery perforator	–	+++	++	+	+	+

Recommendation rates as follows: ++++, excellent; +++, good; ++, fair; +, poor; –, not applicable.

Table 12.3 Tongue defects and options available for reconstruction

	Tongue defect	Considerations	Preferred options	Alternatives
I	Hemi	Thin, pliable skin flap, motility	Radial forearm flap	Ulnar forearm flap Anterolateral thigh perforator flap
II	Subtotal			
IIa	Two-third	Bulky skin flap	Anterolateral thigh perforator flap	Rectus abdominis musculocutaneous flap
IIb	Three-quarter	Bulky musculocutaneous flap	Anterolateral thigh musculocutaneous flap	Rectus abdominis musculocutaneous flap
III	Total	Large musculocutaneous flap with adequate volume for swallowing	Pentagonal anterolateral thigh musculocutaneous flap	-

–, not applicable.

Table 12.4 Considerations in mandibular reconstruction

Considerations		Details
1	Patient's risk factors	Smoking, old age, diabetes, malnutrition, cardiovascular disease, liver cirrhosis, local advanced disease, distal metastasis, recurrent or second primary cancer, postoperative radiation
2	Defects	Length and location of bone defects Size, volume, and components of soft tissue Radiated skin and vessels, previous scarring, cosmesis
3	Recipient vessels	Ipsilateral or contralateral
4	Selection of donor flaps	See Table 12.6
5	Technique considerations	
	Plating	Reconstruction plate or miniplates, preoperative three-dimensional computed tomography plating before or after pedicle division Occlusion with intermaxillary wiring
	Osteotomy	Lengths and number of segments Before or after pedicle division
	Flap inset	Before versus after anastomosis Bone inset first, then mucosa or external skin
	Microsurgical anastomosis	Artery first or vein first
	Osseointegration	Immediate/delayed Number of dental implants

postoperative infection. A patient with end-stage renal disease undergoing a prolonged operation is at greater risk of developing postoperative fluid overload and other associated complications. Patients with Child's class B or C cirrhosis had more complications, including pulmonary complications, acute renal failure, and sepsis, than those with class A cirrhosis (80% versus 19.1%).[93] Advanced age is not a contraindication for extended-duration microsurgery. However, medical problems associated with chronological age, such as cardiopulmonary disease, atherosclerosis, and previous stroke, indicate a higher incidence of postoperative medical complications.[86] These advanced oromandibular cancer patients are often malnourished, which has an impact on normal wound healing, pulmonary function, and postoperative recovery.

Smoking should be ceased 2 weeks before a long operation to reduce pulmonary complications. For a malnourished patient, a short period of tube feeding before surgery can correct malnutrition status and improve wound healing and general recovery after surgery.

Defect factors (*Table 12.4*)

As dictated by the principle of reconstruction, it is necessary to replace tissue with like tissue. A complete assessment of the defect is just as important as a careful evaluation of the patient's medical history. However, when a severe medical comorbidity precludes advanced reconstruction, the surgeon should not hesitate to downgrade the reconstruction ladder. The assessment of the defects should include the size, volume, and components of the involved soft tissue, the length and location of the mandibular defect, the available recipient vessels, and the quality of the external skin.

The following are commonly applied reconstructive options.

Skin graft

Skin graft is a relatively easy procedure. However, its application in oral cavity reconstruction has largely been replaced by the use of pedicled and free flaps. The environment of the oral cavity is not conductive to survival of the skin graft. Furthermore, the progression of scar contracture from a skin graft often limits the mobility of the oral mucosa and tongue, which worsens the postoperative oral cavity function.[94]

Local/regional flap

Before the development of free-flap transfer, local and regional flaps were the treatment of choice. Today, the applications of pedicled flaps are limited for use in the reconstruction of small defects or in patients where free-flap transfer is not indicated (Tables 12.1–12.2).

Free tissue transfer

The advent of microsurgical free tissue transfer has significantly increased reconstructive alternatives through the ability to use larger flaps and the increased versatility to ensure a better fit of the defect. The use of free tissue transfer for composite reconstruction has allowed restoration of increasingly complex defects in a single stage with better functional and aesthetic outcomes.

Different decision-making processes for the most common oral conditions will be discussed below.

Decision making for buccal reconstruction (Table 12.2)

When the defect involves only the buccal mucosa, the reconstruction is relatively straightforward. The size of the defect should be measured with the mouth open at maximum. A mouth-opening retractor should be applied between the upper and lower teeth to facilitate adequate exposure. A sizeable flap is necessary to achieve satisfactory results; if the resurfacing is inadequate, an irreversible trismus will occur. A soft and pliable flap is generally the best choice for reconstruction. The pliability of the flap allows for better flap inset to fit the contour of the defect. Furthermore, it provides better functional restoration with regard to postoperative mouth movement, eating, speech, and facial expression (Figs 12.1–12.3).

When a buccal mucosa defect involves the buccal-gingival sulcus, the sulcus should be carefully recreated. The sulcus functions as a food reservoir during mastication and helps in directing the saliva and food toward the oropharynx during deglutition. In such cases, a slight folding of the flap is required to form the shape of the sulcus. It is also common that the inner surface of the lower and/or upper lip is involved (Figs 12.1 and 12.3). Although the wound between the edge of the

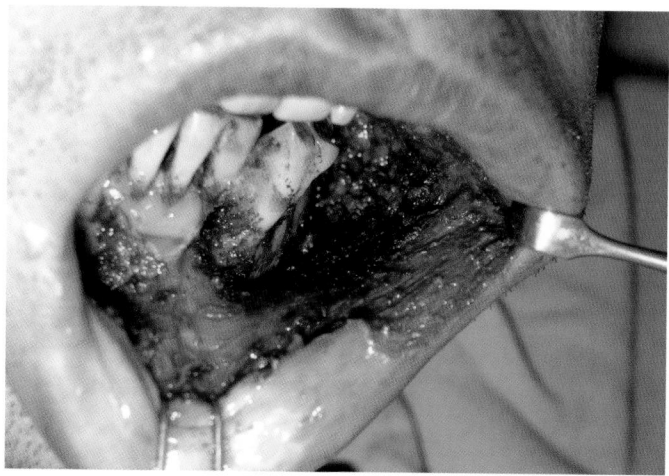

Fig. 12.1 A 40-year-old male patient was diagnosed with synchronous left buccal and lower lip squamous cell carcinoma. A defect measured 5.5 × 8 cm, extended from the inner surface of the left lower lip to the left buccal mucosa, and was left for reconstruction post wide tumor excision and neck lymph node dissection.

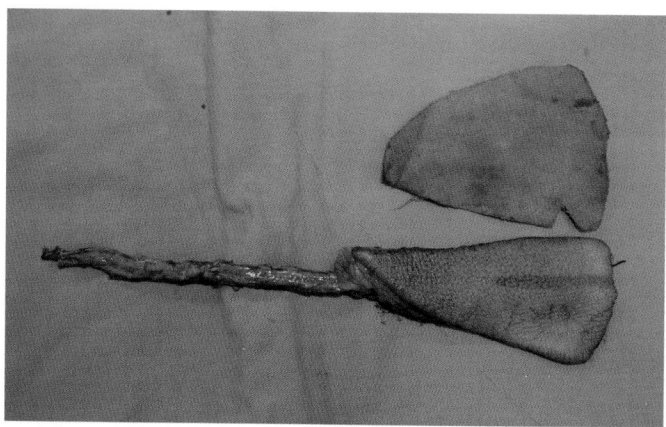

Fig. 12.2 A free radial forearm flap sized 6 × 9 cm was designed according to the tailored template and raised for reconstruction. The flap was then transferred to the defect, and the pedicle of the radial forearm flap was connected to the left facial artery and vein.

lip and the lower gum can usually be closed primarily, direct closure results in an unnatural appearance and poor postoperative function.

When the mucosa defect extends from the buccal mucosa to the trigone region, the mandible is often exposed. Such defects commonly involve the posterior tongue. Direct closure of partial wound may distort the natural anatomy of the tonsillar pillar and tethers the tongue. The tonsillar pillar separates the oro- and nasopharynx. An anatomical change can result in food regurgitation into the nasal cavity. Tongue tethering also limits function with regard to eating and speaking.

Flap selection for pure buccal mucosa reconstruction depends on the thickness of the flap required. According to the authors' experience, a free radial forearm or ulnar forearm flap is usually adequate (Figs 12.4–12.7). A relatively thin ALT perforator flap is required for a thicker defect. A medial sural artery perforator (MSAP) flap is a feasible alternative.[95]

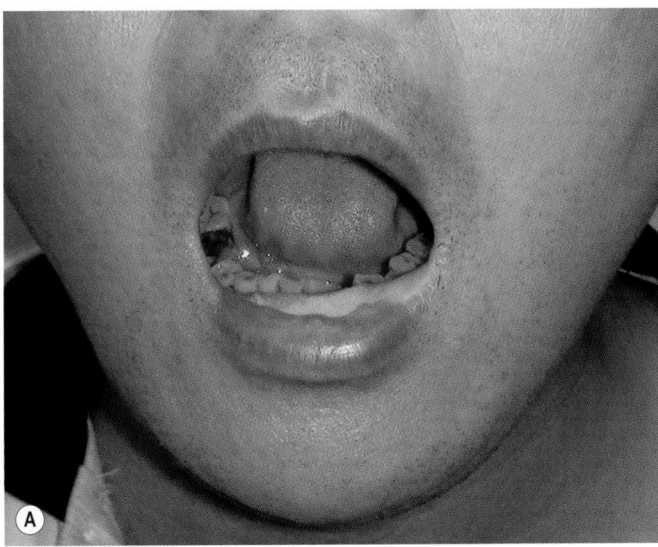
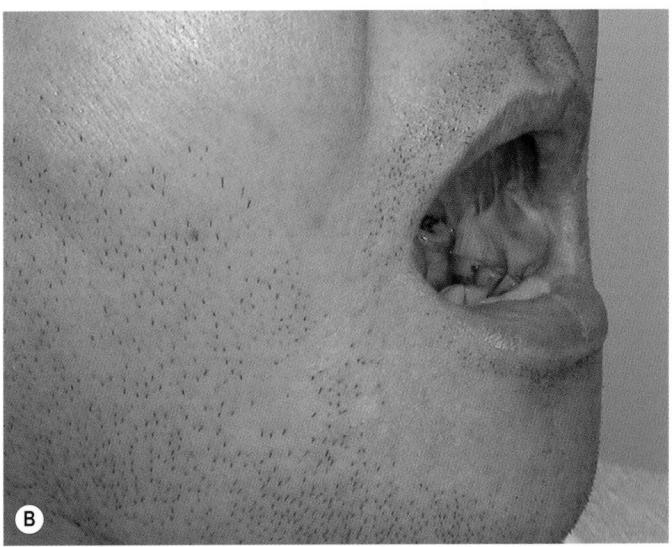

Fig. 12.3 (A, B) At a follow-up at 42 months, the patient was satisfied with both functional restoration and cosmesis.

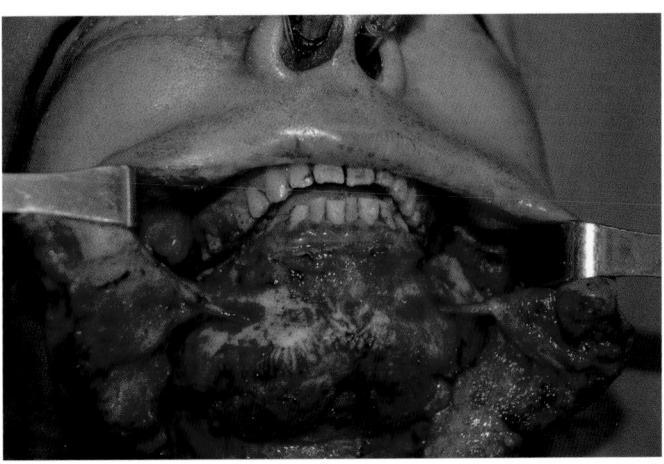

Fig. 12.4 A 36-year-old male patient suffered from bilateral buccal mucosa ulcerative tumors. Biopsy and image study revealed a squamous cell carcinoma (T2N1M0) in the right buccal mucosa and a verrucous carcinoma in the left buccal mucosa. Wide excisions of both tumors with bilateral neck dissection were planned. After tumor resections, there were two separate buccal mucosa defects.

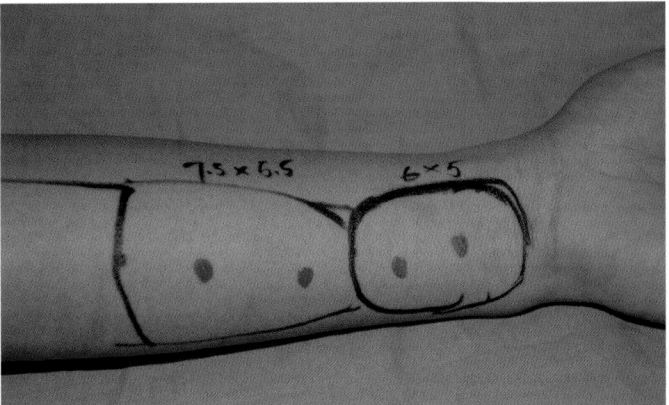

Fig. 12.5 Four septocutaneous perforators from the ulnar artery were identified with hand-held Doppler (red spots). Two skin paddles measuring 6 × 5 and 7.5 × 5.5 cm with independent perforators were designed in the same ulnar forearm.

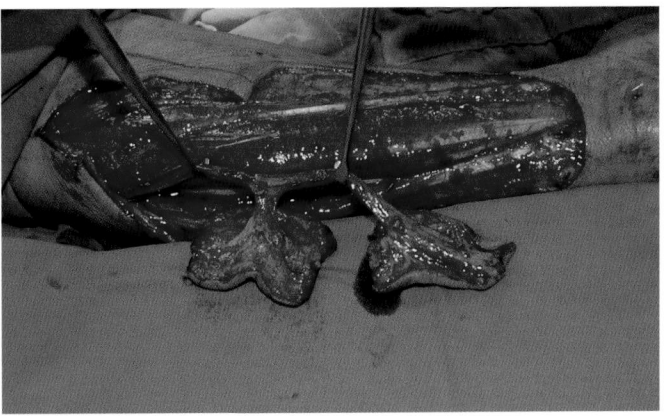

Fig. 12.6 After complete flap dissection, the skin paddle was split into two parts, which included two sizeable perforators. The pedicles were then divided one by one for flap transfer and vascular anastomosis.

In severe trauma or in advanced buccal cancer resection, the defect can extend from the mucosa to the external skin (through-and-through defect), often requiring a bulky myocutaneous flap or a thick fasciocutaneous flap with de-epithelialization. Alternatively, a chimeric flap design with two separate skin paddles for intraoral and cheek reconstructions can achieve good aesthetic results *(Figs 12.8–12.11)*. Each of the skin paddles can be customized according to the defect, preventing distortion of the mouth angle.

If the buccal mucosa resection is accompanied by marginal mandibulectomy, sufficient coverage of the exposed mandible bone is important. A redundant flap resurfacing in this area is important to prevent tethering of tongue movement after reconstruction. The reconstruction is necessary not only to resurface the defect but also to provide adequate bulk replacement of the resected teeth and alveolar bone for a more symmetrical facial contour. An ALT flap with or without vastus lateralis muscle is the preferred choice for reconstruction.

Sometimes an inferior maxillectomy is part of an advanced buccal mucosal tumor resection, which results in a dead space

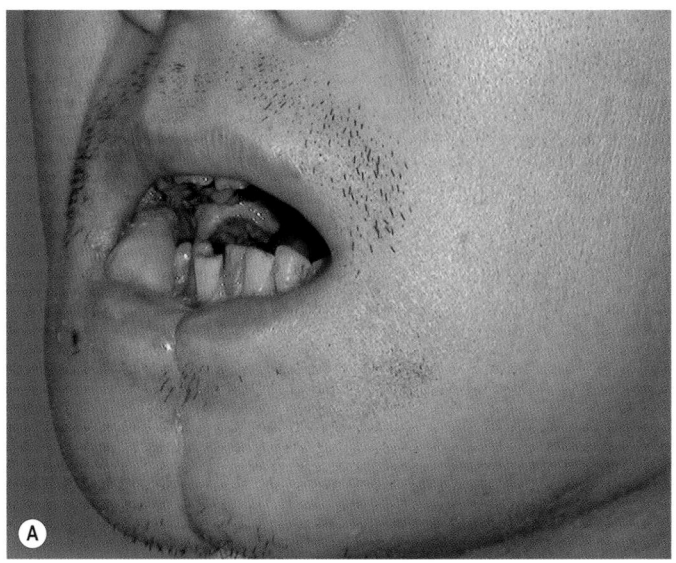
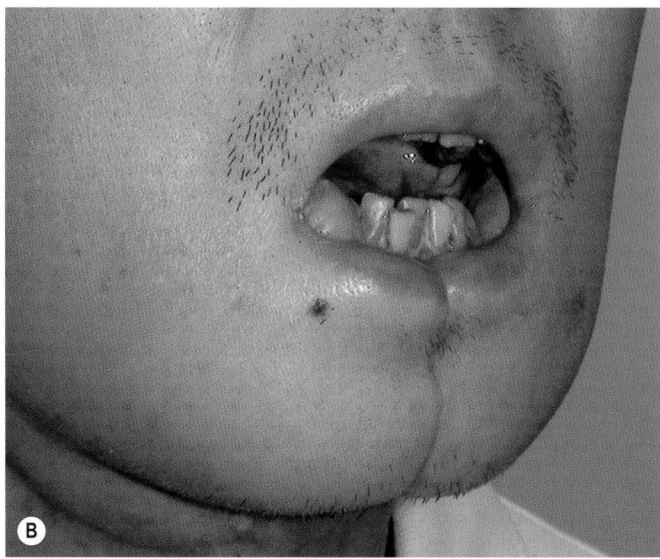

Fig. 12.7 (A, B) The distal smaller flap was transferred to the left buccal mucosa and, using the left facial vessels as the recipient site, the larger proximal flap was transferred to the right buccal mucosa and connected to the right superior thyroid vessels. After a follow-up of 4.5 months, the patient tolerated the postoperative course well and returned to normal life with improved oral function and symmetrical cheeks.

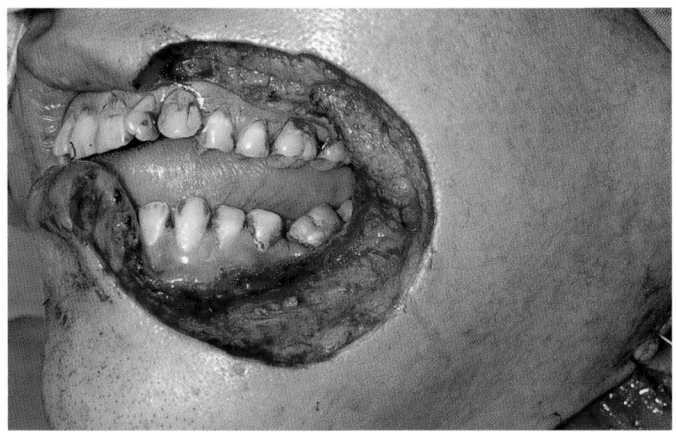

Fig. 12.8 This is a 35-year-old male who sustained left buccal squamous cell carcinoma (T4N2M0). A left buccal through-and-through defect involving the left oral commissure was noted after tumor resection.

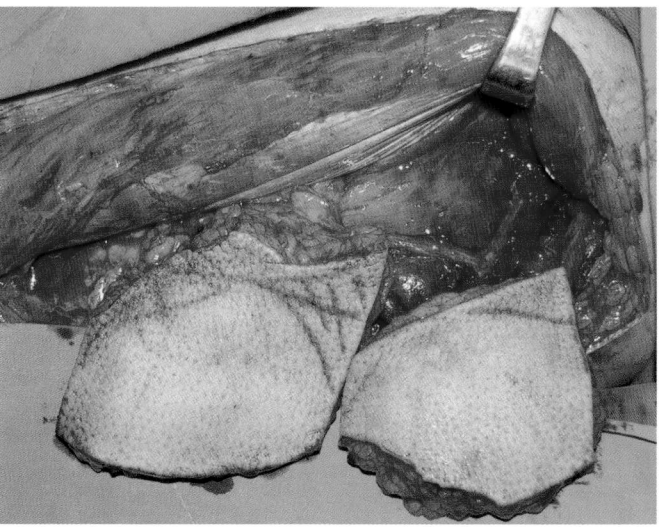

Fig. 12.9 Two separate skin paddles were obtained in a chimeric fashion with preoperative Doppler mapping to confirm the location of the perforators. The myocutaneous perforator of the distal skin island (left) originated from the descending branch of the lateral circumflex femoral artery, and the myocutaneous perforator of the proximal skin island (right) derived from the transverse branch. These two branches joined together as a single pair of pedicles for further microvascular anastomoses.

in the inferior maxillary area that requires soft-tissue obliteration to avoid fluid accumulation and postoperative infection. It is not uncommon that part of the soft or hard palate is involved in the resection. Few of the palatal wounds can be closed primarily; inadequate tissue resurfacing can result in oronasal fistula, which causes food regurgitation and hypernasality. For buccal defects involving an inferior maxilla, a myocutaneous flap usually provides sufficient muscle to obliterate the dead space as well as buccal and palatal resurfacing. An ALT flap with vastus lateralis muscle is used most frequently in the authors' experience. Alternatively, a free TRAM or VRAM flap can be used.

Table 12.1 summarizes the characteristics of each available flap and its clinical applications in buccal mucosa reconstruction. *Table 12.2* provides guidelines for flap selection for variable buccal defects.

Decision making for tongue reconstruction *(Table 12.3)*

Reconstruction of the tongue is a difficult procedure due to its central role in articulation, deglutition, and airway protection.[1] Several recent studies have used flap inset techniques to reconstruct a tongue with a three-dimensional shape closer to that of the actual tongue. Hsiao *et al.*[96] described a radial forearm flap design with a narrow waist to recreate the omega-shaped profile of the tongue in cross-section. Chepeha et al.[97] used a rectangular template, citing its simpler design and more dynamic reconstruction, as their method of choice. More recently, Davison et al.[98] used a combination of native tongue tip rotation and wedge de-epithelialization in the flap for optimizing tongue tip sensation and to reduce pooling on the mouth floor, respectively. Chiu and Burd[99] further expanded on this technique by describing their semicircular design with wedge de-epithelialization or resection to increase tongue elevation and deepening of the tongue floor at the mouth sulcus. Very little has been reported regarding the refinement of total tongue reconstruction, probably due to the mistaken notion that such reconstructions serve no purpose other than volume restoration.[100,101]

Most authors would classify tongue defects after tongue resection as hemiglossectomy, subtotal, and total glossectomy defects.[96,97,102–106] A goal-directed classification for tongue defects should not only provide descriptions but also facilitate precise judgment with therapeutic consequences. Cheng's modified classification (I, IIa, b, III) separates tongue defects into three major groups, which dictate the type of donor flap chosen *(Table 12.3)*.[107]

Current reconstructive options either maintain mobility or provide bulk. Flaps that maintain mobility include the infrahyoid myofascial flap,[108–110] MSAP flap,[111,112] radial forearm flap,[96,103,105,106,113–117] and ulnar forearm flap.[118] Flaps that provide bulk include the rectus abdominis myocutaneous flap,[119] latissimus dorsi myocutaneous flap,[100] PM myocutaneous flap,[5] and trapezius island flap.[6] The ALT flap has emerged in recent decades as a popular option for head and neck reconstruction due to its reliability, long pedicle, and acceptable donor morbidity. Due to its versatility, this flap has been used both to provide bulk and to ensure mobility.[97,103,106,114,120–130]

Most publications have reported only the use of a single flap to reconstruct a limited range of tongue defects,[100,101,116,118,125,131,132] while others compared two flaps but generally gave little or no information for why one flap was selected over another.[103,106,111,116]

For group I patients (defects ≤50%), a radial forearm flap is recommended because of its thinness, pliability, and long pedicle[96,115,116,128,131,133–136] *(Fig. 12.12)*; sometimes, the ALT perforator flap can be used instead in thin patients. Group II describes defects where up to 75% of the tongue is removed. In this classification system, a distinction is made between defects of 66% (IIa) and 75% (IIb). The additional division between groups IIa (66% resected) and IIb (75% resected) permits further refinements in flap selection. For group IIa patients (defects ≤66%), an ALT perforator flap is preferred over the radial forearm flap due to the larger flap size available, especially when encountering any accompanying mouth floor or buccal defects *(Fig. 12.13)*. For group IIb defects, the

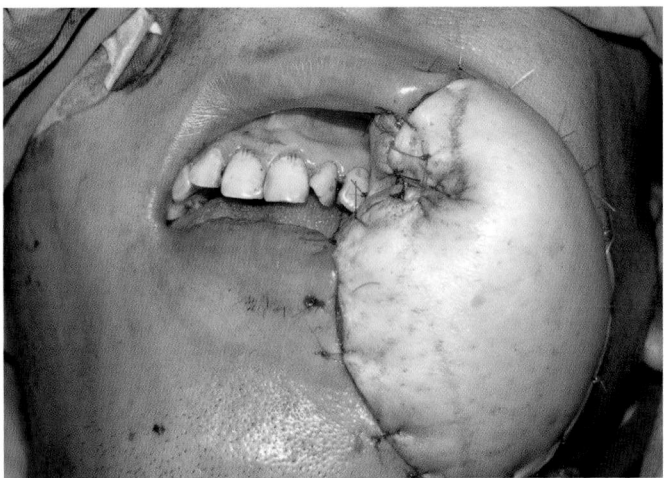

Fig. 12.10 The immediate postoperative appearance. Two skin paddles were transferred for the oral and cheek skin defects. The oral commissure was reconstructed by both skin paddles with some incompetence.

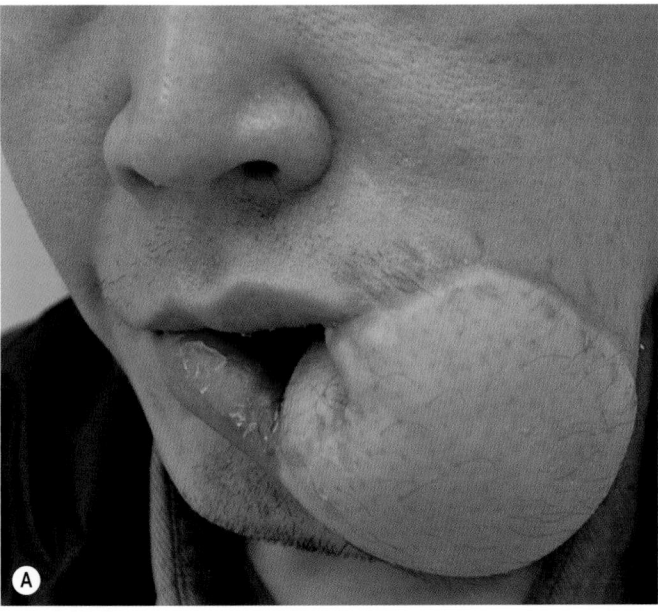
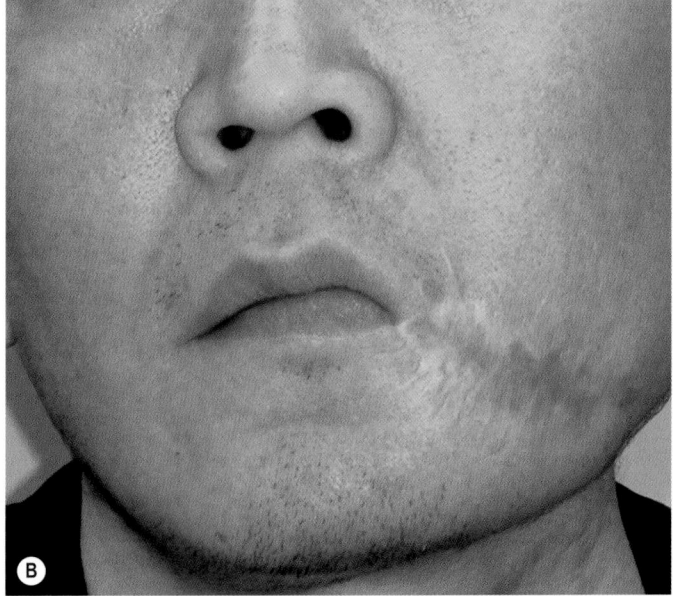

Fig. 12.11 (A) At 8-month follow-up, the reconstructed flap remained bulky. **(B)** At 18-month follow-up, the patient was disease-free and satisfied with the cosmetic outcome after several revisions, including a vermilion flap from the lower lip, V-Y advancement of the anterolateral thigh flap, flap debulking, and scar revision.

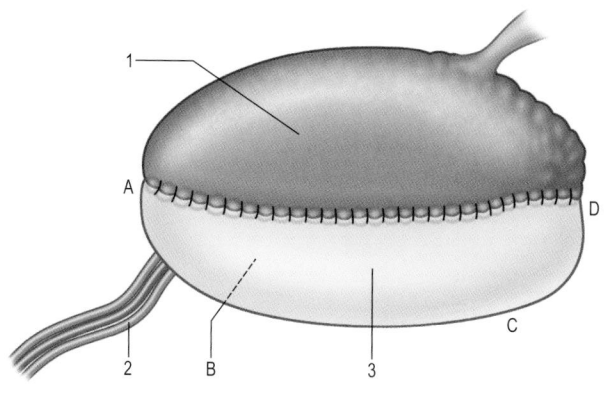

Fig. 12.12 The superior aspect of the tongue. Tongue defect type I (hemiglossectomy) is reconstructed with a thin pliable flap of rectangle shape *(Table 12.3)*. A, tongue tip; B, floor of mouth; C, trigone; D, base of tongue; 1, native tongue; 2, radial artery and comitant veins; 3, radial forearm flap.

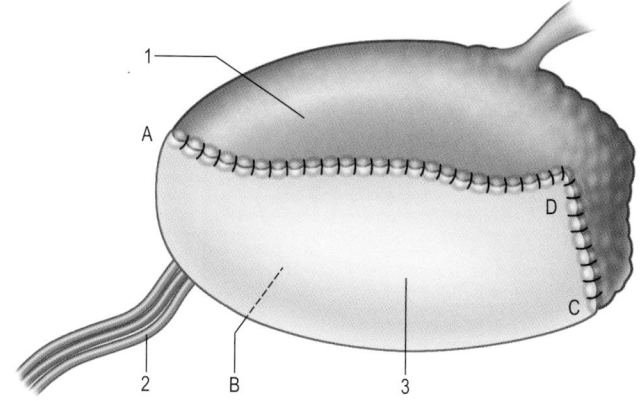

Fig. 12.13 Tongue defect type II (subtotal) is reconstructed with an anterolateral thigh fasciocutaneous or musculocutaneous flap *(Table 12.3)*. **A,** close to tongue tip; **B,** floor of mouth; **C,** trigone; **D,** base of tongue; 1, native tongue; 2, lateral circumflex femoral vessel; 3, anterolateral thigh fasciocutaneous or myocutaneous flap.

small amount of remaining tongue (about 25%) probably has no functional role, but it likely plays an important role in maintaining the anatomical integrity of the base of the tongue, the retromolar trigone, or one side of the pterygoid fossa, depending on its location *(Fig. 12.13 and Table 12.3)*. The thickness of the subcutaneous tissue in the ALT flap provides a better neotongue profile for defects crossing the midline in groups IIa and IIb.

In total glossectomy defect (group III), a specially designed pentagonal-shaped ALT myocutaneous flap facilitates better flap inset, provides adequate volume, and gives an aesthetically pleasing neotongue tip *(Fig. 12.14)*. The "V" shape of the pentagon posteriorly allows a greater sloping profile when viewed in cross-section as well as an increasing posterior-to-anterior tongue projection. Such a design yields a well-shaped tissue bulk that resembles a normal tongue more closely in its lateral and frontal views. The anterior "I" shape allows increased elevation and freeing of the neotongue tip and also creates a gingival sulcus that prevents saliva pooling and subsequent drooling. Most of these patients provide ratings of "good" and above for diet or cosmetic appearance following reconstruction using this method *(Figs 12.15–12.17)*.[107]

In both groups IIb and III, the ALT musculocutaneous flap rather than the fasciocutaneous flaps should be used for reconstruction to provide more bulk to augment the base of the tongue. The bulk at the base of the tongue is important to close off the oropharynx during swallowing with the assistance of the movement of hyoid bone. The rectus abdominis myocutaneous flap[119] and the latissimus dorsi myocutaneous flap[100,137] are alternative flap options for near-total or total tongue reconstruction, but with more significant donor site morbidity.

Decision making for mandibular reconstruction

Daniel categorized lower jaw defects as isolated, compound, composite, extensive composite, or *en bloc*.[138–140] Isolated

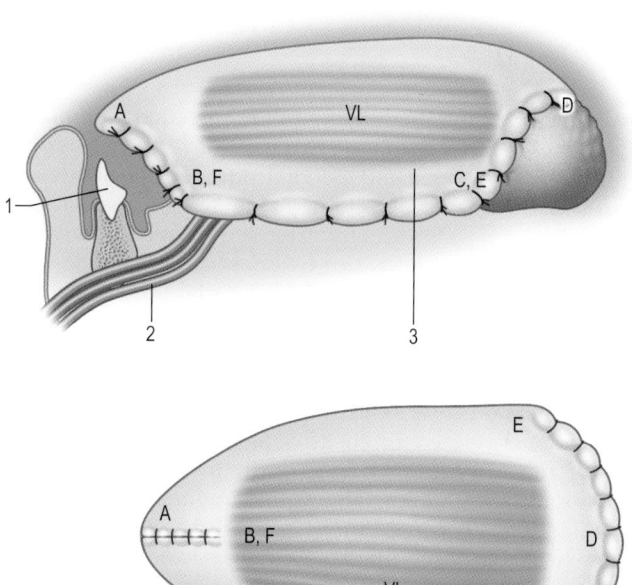

Fig. 12.14 A pentagonal anterolateral thigh musculocutaneous flap sized 10 × 15 cm with a segment of vastus lateralis is used to reconstruct a total tongue defect. The distance from B to F is 10 cm and from A to D is 15 cm. The vastus lateralis is 5 × 10 cm. B and F are sutured to form the floor of the mouth, and A becomes the tip of the neotongue. The margins between B and C and E and F are repaired to the gingival mucosa of the mandible. The distance between C, D, and E forms the base of the tongue and trigone. The pedicle is placed anteriorly to reach the recipient vessels in the neck. A, tongue tip; B and F, floor of mouth; C and E, trigone; D, base of tongue; VL, vastus lateralis muscle; 1, teeth; 2, lateral circumflex femoral vessel; 3, anterolateral thigh musculocutaneous flap.

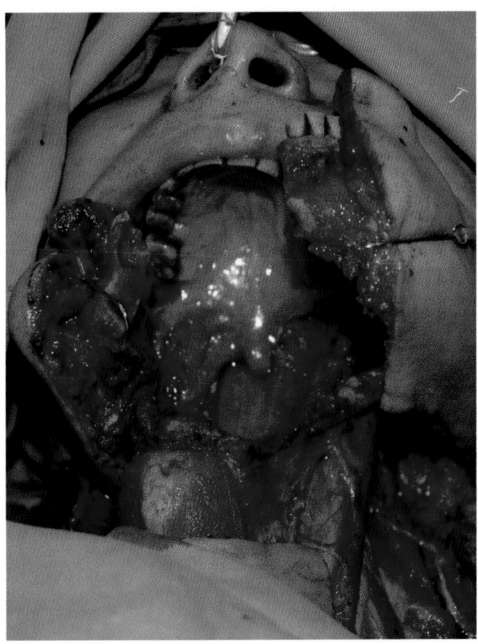

Fig. 12.15 A 41-year-old male patient with left tongue cancer (T4N0M0) underwent total glossectomy and bilateral modified radical neck dissection. The total tongue defect measured 9 × 14 cm.

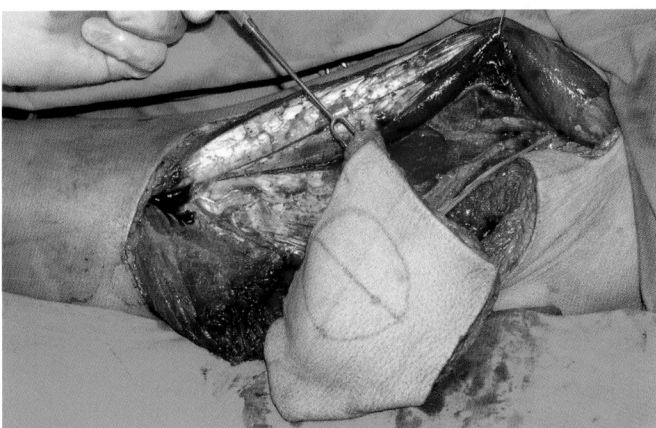

Fig. 12.16 A pentagonal anterolateral thigh musculocutaneous flap (10 × 15 cm) with a cuff of the vastus lateralis was harvested for total tongue reconstruction. The pedicle was 12 cm in length. Two myocutaneous perforators were included for the skin paddle perfusion. The recipient vessels were the left superior thyroid vessels.

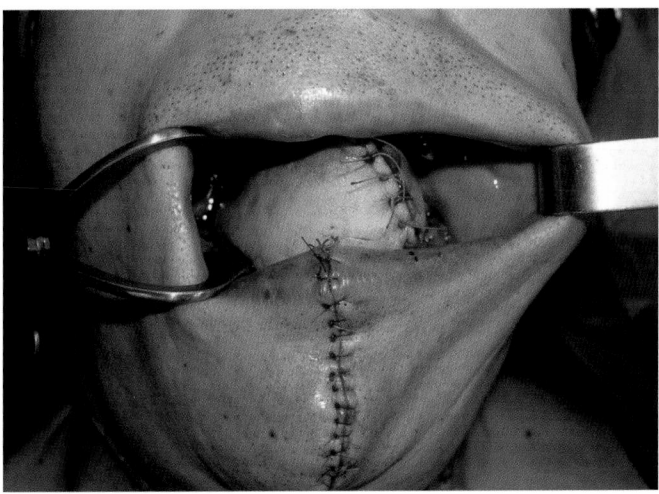

Fig. 12.17 The neotongue reconstructed by the pentagonal anterolateral thigh musculocutaneous flap with adequate bulkiness and projected tip.

defects include any single bone tissue resection; compound defects refer to those involving two tissue layers, such as bone and oral lining or bone and external skin. Composite defects indicate a three-layer-defect involving the mucosal lining, bone, and external skin; finally, extended composite or *en bloc* defects also include loss of soft tissue.[138,139]

Jewer *et al.* classified mandibular defects[141] of the bone as central, lateral, or hemimandibulectomy. The classification system was modified by Urken *et al.*[61] to consider associated soft-tissue defects and by Boyd *et al.*[142] to recognize subcategories such as mucosa, skin, or a combination of both. These classifications were comprehensive and based on the availability of reconstructive options. With the development of microsurgical techniques, and better understanding of the perforator flap concept, more reconstructive alternatives became available. A modified mandibular defect classification is recommended by the authors to define further the components involved in the mandibular defect. This is outlined in *Table 12.5*. The available classifications for mandibular defects, together with examples and possible reconstructive options, are compared and summarized in *Tables 12.6 and 12.7*.

Treatment/surgical technique

Part I: Soft-tissue flaps

Local flaps

Submental flap

The submental flap, as indicated by the name, is located in the submental area. Because of its location, it is a soft-tissue flap that can be transferred as a pedicled or free flap to the oral cavity.

The blood supply of the submental flap derives from the submental artery, which is a continuous branch of the facial artery, located 5–6.5 cm away from the origin of the facial artery. This branch penetrates deep to the submandibular gland through the mylohyoid muscle below the mandible angle, extending medially deep to the anterior belly of the digastric muscle. As the vessel travels along the mandible margin, it sends off cutaneous perforators through the platysma muscle to the skin. The anatomy is constant, and the flow it provides to the submental skin is reliable.[143,144]

Flap design is initiated by marking the inferior mandible border as the upper flap margin *(Fig. 12.18)*. The flap length extends from the ipsilateral mandible angle to the contralateral mandible angle. The flap width depends on the laxity of the skin: usually a width of 5 cm can be obtained. However, the flap can be even wider in older patients with loose skin. The flap can be elevated as an axial flap or a perforator flap. An easier surgical technique involves lifting the tissue as an

Table 12.5 Variable classifications of mandibular defects

Cheng's classification	Daniel's classification	Jewer's and Boyd's classification	Defects	Available managements	Examples
I-a	Isolated	Central (C)	Bone only	Plating, bone graft, bone flap	Benign tumor, trauma
I-b	Isolated	Lateral (L)	Bone only	Plating, bone graft, bone flap	Benign tumor, trauma
I-c	Isolated	Hemimandibulectomy (H)	Bone only	Plating, bone graft, bone flap	Benign tumor, trauma
II-a	Compound	HCL and mucosal (m)	Bone and intraoral mucosa	Osteocutaneous flap	Stage 3–4 oromandibular cancer
II-b	Compound	HCL and skin (s)	Bone and external skin	Osteocutaneous flap	Osteoradionecrosis of mandible
II-c	Compound	–	Bone, external skin and soft tissue*	Osteocutaneous flap, OPAC flap	Osteoradionecrosis of mandible
III-a	Composite	HCL with mucosa and skin (ms)	Composite three layers	Options in Table 12.7	Stage 4 oromandibular cancer, gunshot wound
III-b	Extensive composite	–	Composite three layers and partial tongue	Options in Table 12.7	Stage 4 oromandibular cancer, gunshot wound
III-c	Extensive composite	–	Composite three layers and partial maxilla	Options in Table 12.7	Stage 4 oromandibular cancer, gunshot wound

OPAC, osteomyocutaneous peroneal artery combined flap.
*Soft tissue: masseter muscle, parotid gland, and buccal fat pad. Four layers: mucosa, bone, soft tissue, and external skin.

Table 12.6 Comparisons of available osteocutaneous flaps

	Bone		Skin			Muscle availability	Pedicle length	Donor site morbidity	Disadvantages
	Height	Firmness	Length	Reliability	Pliability				
Fibula	++	++++	++++ (25 cm)	++++	++++	++++, soleus	+++	++++	Flap inset
Iliac	++++	++++	+++	+	+	–	+	++	Donor site morbidity, partial skin paddle loss
Scapula	+	+	++ (7 cm)	++++	+++	++++, latissimus dorsi	+++	+++	Intraoperative change of position
Radius	+	++	+ (10–12 cm)	++++	++++	-	++++	+	Radius fracture
Rib	++	++	++ (8–10 cm)	++	++	++, pectoralis major, serratus anterior	++	+++	Tenuous periosteal perfusion
Second metatarsal	+	++++	+ (6 cm)	++++	++++	–	+++	++	Donor site morbidity

++++, excellent; +++, good; ++, fair; +, poor, –, not applicable.

Table 12.7 Reconstructive options for mandibular defect type III in Cheng's classification

Cheng's classification	Defect	Option 1 Soft-tissue flap with reconstruction plate	Option 2 One free flap, one pedicled flap	Option 3 Double free flaps	Option 4 Chimeric LCFA flap	Option 5 Composite scapula flap	Option 6 Composite OPAC flap
IIIa	Bone	Reconstruction plate	Fibula	Fibula	Iliac	Scapula	Fibula
	Mucosa	ALT flap or RA flap	Fibula skin	Fibula skin	ALT flap	Scapula/parascapular skin	Fibula skin
	Soft tissue	Vastus lateralis, rectus abdominis	Pectoralis major, deltopectoral	Vastus lateralis, rectus abdominis	Vastus lateralis	LD	Soleus
	External skin	ALT flap or RA flap	Pectoralis major, deltopectoral	Radial forearm or ALT, RA	Groin skin	Scapula/parascapular skin	Fibula skin
IIIb	Tongue	ALT flap or RA flap	Fibula skin	Fibula skin	ALT flap	Scapula/parascapular skin	Fibula skin
IIIc	Maxilla	Vastus lateralis, rectus abdominis	Pectoralis major, deltopectoral	Vastus lateralis, rectus abdominis	Vastus lateralis	LD	Soleus

Soft-tissue flaps include: ALT, anterolateral thigh perforator (fasciocutaneous) or musculocutaneous flap; RA, rectus abdominis musculocutaneous flap; PM, pectoralis major musculocutaneous flap; LCFA, lateral circumflex femoral artery; OPAC, osteomyocutaneous peroneal artery combined flap; LD, latissimus dorsi.

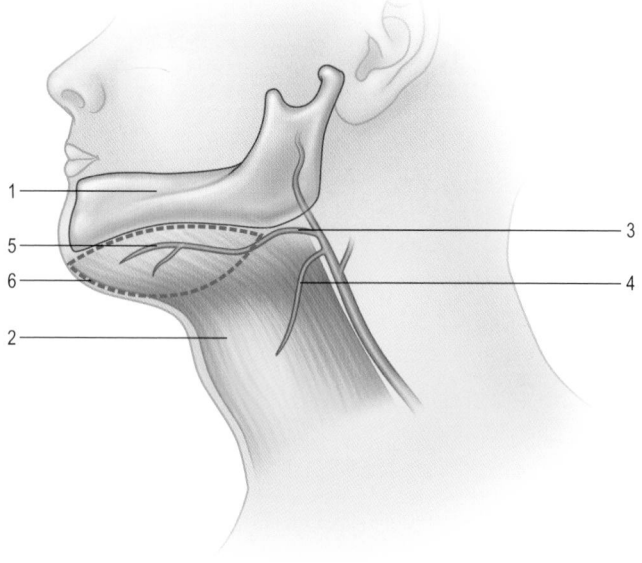

Fig. 12.18 Flap design of the submental flap. The submental flap is based on the submental artery (5), a branch of the facial artery (3). Flap elevation can be started from the inferior border of the mandible (1), between the ipsilateral and contralateral mandible angles. The pedicle runs under the platysma muscle (2) and anterior belly of the digastric muscle. It sends off cutaneous branches through the plastyma muscle. The flap is often elevated with the inclusion of the platysma muscle and the anterior belly of the digastric muscle for easy flap dissection. 1, mandible; 2, platysma muscle; 3, facial artery; 4, superior thyroid artery; 5, submental artery; 6, flap design.

axial flap without perforator dissection. In that case, an incision can be made in the inferior margin of the flap directly through the platysma muscle. Then, the dissection is carried out with division of the anterior belly of the digastric muscle, which is included in the flap to ensure inclusion of the submental perforator. When the pedicle is identified, its branches to the submandibular gland should be ligated carefully. Finally, when reaching the inferior border of the mandible, care should be taken not to injure the marginal mandibular nerve. The pedicle is then skeletonized and the flap is ready to be transferred. If the flap is going to be transferred as a free flap, dissection of the pedicle can be continued to the facial vessels to obtain a better size and length for anastomosis.[143–145]

The arc of the distal-based submental flap is suitable for rotating it to the lower third of the face and the entire oral cavity, making it a suitable pedicle flap for oral cavity reconstruction.[145,146] The only drawback is that many oral cavity reconstructions are performed during cancer ablation surgery, during which neck lymph node dissection is often required. After a neck lymph node dissection, the continuity of the submental skin and its main pedicle are usually disrupted **(Tables 12.1 and 12.2)**.

Regional flaps

Deltopectoral flap

The deltopectoral flap was popularized around 1965 by Bakamjian.[7] It is located in the anterior chest wall. Based on the internal mammary perforators in the second and third intercostal spaces, the flap extends from the central chest wall to the deltoid region.

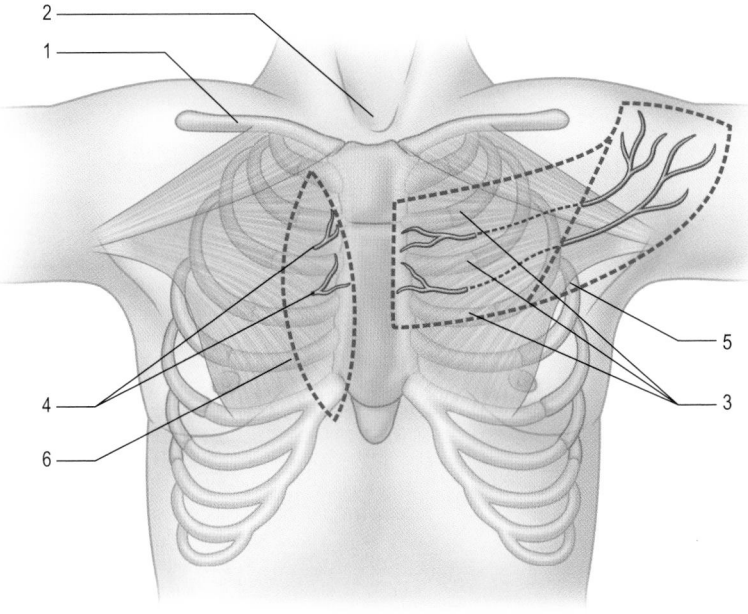

Fig. 12.19 Flap design of the deltopectoral flap. The deltopectoral flap is based on perforators from the internal mammary artery, usually perforators passing through the second and third intercostal spaces. (4) The flap is designed to originate lateral to the sternum and extend superiorly to reach the deltoid region. (5) However, the distal region of the flap is more likely a random flap. If a lengthy flap is required, a delay procedure is generally recommended. Traditionally, the flap is designed with the base left intact. With the technique of perforator flap dissection, the deltopectoral flap can also be modified to serve as an internal mammary arterial perforator flap (6) to allow more freedom in flap transposition so as to reach a more distant defect or to transfer the tissue as a free flap. 1, clavicle; 2, sternal notch; 3, second, third, and fourth ribs; 4, second and third internal mammary artery perforators; 5, deltopectoral flap design; 6, internal mammary artery perforator flap design.

The flap can be designed around the perforators, which can be located at the second and third intercostal spaces using a pencil Doppler. The flap base is situated in the anterior chest wall, and the flap extends superolaterally to the deltoid region. The exact flap required should be measured to ensure its ability to reach the defect. For an oral cavity reconstruction, a lengthier flap is usually required. However, the distal flap is a random flap with an uncertain blood supply. To obtain a longer flap, a prefabrication or a delayed procedure is usually required to reduce the risk of distal flap necrosis (*Fig. 12.19*).[147]

The disadvantages of the deltopectoral flap include the unattractive donor site scar, the requirement of a second surgery for flap division, and the possibility of a delayed procedure to lengthen the available flap. Today, the deltopectoral flap has been largely replaced by the PM myocutaneous flap (*Tables 12.1 and 12.2*).

Pectoralis major myocutaneous flap

Since its introduction by Ariyan in 1979, the PM flap has gained in popularity.[8] The PM flap has a reliable blood supply that provides a large skin paddle with sufficient bulk tissue for large-size reconstruction. This flap can reach the neck and lower third of the face, making it practical for intraoral and external cheek reconstruction. Today, the PM myocutaneous flap is useful for salvage procedures and in a vessel-depleted neck where a free flap transfer is not indicated.

The PM flap is a myocutaneous flap comprising the PM muscle and its overlying skin. The blood supply of the PM muscle mainly comes from the thoracoacromial artery and parasternal perforators. The lateral thoracic artery runs along the lateral edge of the PM muscle and sends off branches to augment the circulation of the PM muscle. The thoracoacromial artery runs inferiorly at the midpoint of the clavicle and this can be used as a pivot point when designing the flap (*Fig. 12.20*).

Because the skin paddle is located in the anterior chest wall, the cosmesis of the donor site is a major concern, especially in women. An alternative design is a nipple-sparing crescent-shaped skin paddle from the parasternal area to the inframammary region. However, care should be taken when designing the flap like this because the inframammary region is less reliable in terms of blood supply (*Fig. 12.20*).

Flap elevation can be started from a lateral incision to expose the lateral border of the PM. Dissection is then carried out under the PM muscle to include the thoracoacromial vessel. Once the muscle has been identified and the location of the vessel is confirmed, the medial border of skin edge can be incised. The muscle is then detached medially and laterally, and the flap is elevated toward the pedicle. The pedicle is divided after 2–3 weeks. The PM flap can also be elevated as an island flap after skeletonizing the pedicle. The muscle part of the flap can be buried under the neck skin, precluding the need for a second operation to divide the pedicle. The PM flap is a good alternative when a free-flap transfer is not possible for a buccal mucosa or tongue reconstruction (*Tables 12.1 and 12.2*).

Free fasciocutaneous or musculocutaneous flaps

Radial forearm flap

Introduced by Yang in 1981, the free radial forearm flap is currently one of the most commonly used flaps in head and neck reconstruction.[148] The radial forearm flap has become a popular flap due to its large skin paddle, lengthy and sizeable pedicle, and ease of flap harvest. Its thinness and pliability also make it the first choice in most reconstructions of thin buccal mucosa defects and small tongue defects (*Figs 12.1–12.3 and Tables 12.1–12.3*).[149]

A radial forearm flap is a type C fasciocutaneous flap derived from the radial artery. Before flap harvest, an Allen test should be performed to confirm the dominance of ulnar

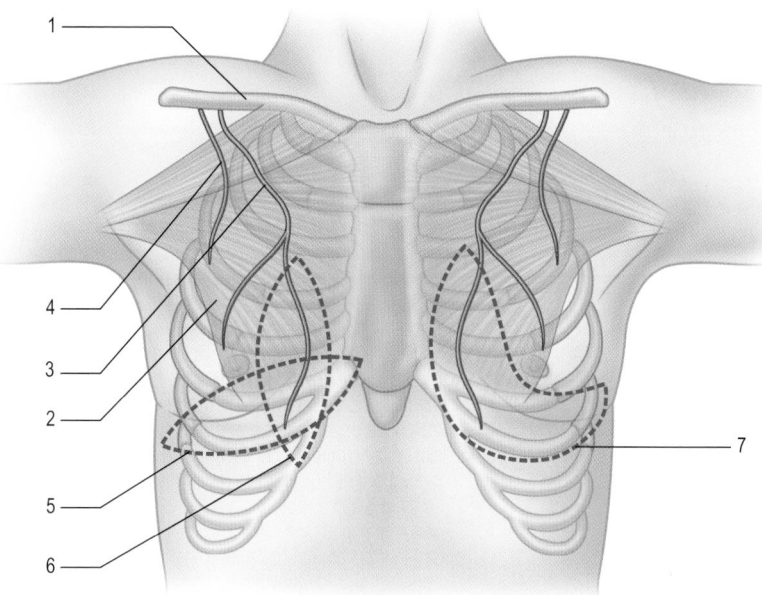

Fig. 12.20 Versatile flap design of the pectoralis major myocutaneous flap. The pectoralis muscle is a fan-shaped muscle originating in the 5, 6 and 7th ribs, clavicle (1) and sternum and inserting to the humerus. The blood supply of the pectoralis muscle derives mainly from the thoracoacromial artery (3) and the pectoral branch of the lateral thoracic artery (4). When the flap is elevated, it is usually based on the thoracoacrominal artery, which is more dominant and consistent. The flap can be designed with a skin paddle overlying the muscle. Considering the location of the defect and preservation of the nipple–areolar complex, especially in female patients, the skin paddle can be designed as a transverse (5), vertical (6), or crescent (7) shape. 1, clavicle; 2, pectoralis major muscle; 3, thoracoacromial artery; 4, pectoral branch of lateral thoracic artery; 5, transverse flap design; 6, vertical flap design; 7, crescent-shaped flap design.

artery. One or two of the concomitant veins are usually adequate for venous drainage.[150] Some authors would like to harvest the cephalic vein for another source of venous drainage. The cephalic vein is larger in diameter than the radial vein; therefore, venous anastomosis is easier. The flap is innervated by the lateral antebrachial cutaneous nerves, which can be incorporated if a sensate flap is desired.

Flap design is initiated by locating the radial artery by palpation. The borders of the skin paddle are designed with the radial artery axis centered, but not extending beyond the radial border of the forearm for better cosmesis. Under tourniquet, the flap dissection is carried out from the radial edge of the flap in the suprafascial plane.[151] A suprafascial dissection keeps the paratendons and superficial radial nerve intact, thus reducing the donor site morbidity.[152] After dividing the distal pedicle at the wrist, the dissection is then continued from distal to proximal by carefully preserving the deep fascia and conjoined tendon between the flexor carpi radialis and brachioradialis muscles. After flap dissection is finished, the tourniquet is released to perfuse the flap for 15 minutes. Circulation of the hand should be re-evaluated. Usually, sacrificing the radial artery does not cause any significant change in hand perfusion. However, an interposition vein graft for vascular reconstruction can be indicated if the distal fingers are not well perfused.[152]

The major drawbacks of the radial forearm flap are donor site morbidities and poor donor site cosmesis. Although the donor site morbidity can be reduced dramatically by a suprafascial dissection, the grafted donor site remains unsightly.

Ulnar forearm flap

Located in the ulnar aspect of the forearm, the ulnar forearm flap has similar advantages as the radial forearm flap with a relatively less noticeable donor site scar. Although the flap was introduced only 2 years after the radial forearm flap, it is used much less frequently than the radial forearm flap,

probably because dissection of the ulnar nerve is required during flap elevation.

The ulnar forearm flap is based on the ulnar vessels under the flexor carpi ulnaris (FCU) tendon. Similar to the radial forearm flap, this approach requires an Allen test to confirm the dominance of the radial artery before surgery. The ulnar artery and veins run underneath the FCU tendon and give several sizeable septocutaneous perforators to the skin paddle. As observed for the radial forearm flap, the venae comitantes are adequate for venous drainage. The basilic vein is available as a backup vein.

Flap design is started by marking the ulnar artery which is located underneath the FCU tendon. The skin paddle, based on septocutaneous perforators, is designed with the ulnar vessels centered. The flap dissection is performed under tourniquet. An incision is made in the radial border of the flap and a suprafascial dissection is then carried out until the tendons of the flexor digitorum superficialis are reached. Several septocutaneous perforators can be identified. The fascia is incised and the vascular pedicle is dissected out with the FCU tendon retracted. The entire skin flap can be nourished by these perforators, or split into two skin paddles based on separate perforators in a chimeric fashion (*Figs 12.4–12.7*). The flap design can be more versatile and sophisticated. After the ulnar vessels are dissected and separated away from the ulnar nerve, another skin incision is made on the ulnar side of the flap edge, and dissection is continued until the entire flap is elevated.

The ulnar forearm flap is an alternative to the radial forearm flap when the Allen test demonstrates codominant or dominant perfusion to the hand by the radial artery. The donor scar is also more favorable because of its location on the medial surface of the forearm. Although dissection of the ulnar nerve requires some technical training, flap dissection is straightforward and easy once the surgeon is familiar with the technique. It has been applied in oral cavity and tongue reconstruction, with favorable results *(Fig. 12.7)*. The authors recommend clinical application of this flap, especially in thin oral mucosa defects and type I tongue defects (hemiglossectomy) *(Tables 12.2 and 12.3)*.

Lateral arm flap

The blood supply of the lateral arm flap comes from the cutaneous branch of the posterior radial collateral artery, which is within the lateral intermuscular septum of the upper arm. The vascular pedicle provides four to seven branches to the overlying skin.[153]

The flap is designed by drawing a line between the deltoid tuberosity and the lateral epicondyle of the humerus. The septocutaneous perforators are located along the lower part of this line. After the flap is outlined, dissection from the posterior to the anterior aspect is performed to explore the intermuscular septum. Most of the perforators can thus be identified, and the main pedicle can be traced proximally.

The lateral arm flap was once commonly used in head and neck reconstruction. However, the vascular pedicle is short and the pedicle vessels are usually small. With the introduction of more soft-tissue flaps, the use of the lateral arm flap in oral cavity reconstruction has been substantially reduced.

Rectus abdominis musculocutaneous flap

The RAM flap can be designed transversely or vertically depending on the skin paddle required *(Fig. 12.21)*. By applying a perforator dissection technique, a free deep inferior epigastric perforator (DIEP) flap can be harvested from the same donor site without sacrificing the rectus abdominis muscle.

The RAM flap has two vascular supplies: the deep inferior epigastric vessel and the superior epigastric vessel. When transferred as a free flap, the flap is based on the deep inferior epigastric vessel to obtain a better blood supply. It is harvested from the inferior to superior direction once the vascular pedicle is identified.

The RAM flap has an adequate skin paddle flap bulk for reconstruction of large head and neck defects. It had been used commonly in buccal mucosa reconstruction (especially when marginal mandibulectomy is present) and in total tongue reconstruction. It is a reliable flap with a sizeable pedicle for the microanastomosis. The only drawback of this flap is the potential abdominal wall weakness after surgery. Careful repair of the fascia and use of mesh to repair large fascial defects can decrease the incidence of abdominal bulge or hernia postoperatively. The muscle sparing TRAM or VRAM flap can decrease the donor site morbidity.

Anterolateral thigh fasciocutaneous or musculocutaneous flap

The ALT flap was first introduced by Song *et al.* in 1984.[154] It gradually gained popularity when reconstructive surgeons found it to be a reliable flap with a long and sizeable pedicle that can be harvested with a large skin paddle, and additional muscle for the reconstruction of moderate to large oromandibular defects *(Fig. 12.8)*.[123]

The pedicle of the ALT flap is usually the descending branch of the lateral circumflex femoral artery *(Fig. 12.9)*. Sometimes, its perforators may come from the transverse or oblique branch of the lateral circumflex femoral vessels. The pedicle of the ALT flap runs in the muscle septum between

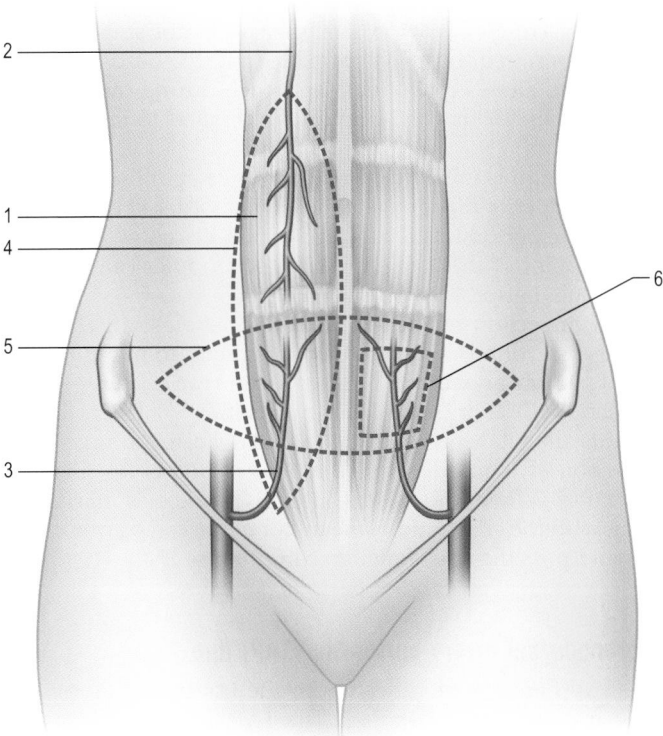

Fig. 12.21 Flap design of the rectus abdominis musculocutaneous (RAM) flap. The main pedicle of the rectus abdominis flap is the deep inferior epigastric artery (3) and vein, which run beneath the rectus abdominis muscle (1). The deep inferior epigastric artery connects to the superior epigastric artery above. Due to its more robust blood supply and sizeable pedicle diameter, the deep inferior epigastric artery was selected as the pedicle for free-flap transfer. It sends out branches through the rectus abdominis muscle to reach the fasciocutaneous flap and nourish the lower abdominal wall skin. The flap can be designed with the rectus abdominis muscle and its overlying skin in various positions. The skin can be designed vertically as a vertical rectus abdominis musculocutaneous (VRAM) flap (4) or transversely as a transverse rectus abdominis musculocutaneous (TRAM) flap (5). Through perforator dissection, the rectus abdominis muscle can be preserved *in situ* to obtain a deep inferior epigastric artery perforator (DIEP) flap (6). 1, rectus abdominis muscle; 2, superior epigastric artery; 3, deep inferior epigastric artery; 4, verticle rectus abdominis musculocutaneous flap design; 5, transverse rectus abdominis musculocutaneous flap design; 6, deep inferior epigastric artery perforator flap.

the vastus lateralis and rectus femoris muscles. A sizeable perforator can nourish a skin paddle that is 15 cm in diameter. The vastus lateralis muscle is nourished by the same pedicle and therefore can be harvested together with the ALT fasciocutaneous flap if a large flap volume is required. The transverse branch of the lateral circumflex femoral artery also nourishes the tensor fascia latae muscle and fascia. If fascia is required to serve as a sling, the tensor fascia latae can be included in the flap.[129]

The ALT flap usually contains more than one sizeable perforator and can also be designed as a chimeric flap to cover two or more separate defects.[129,130,155,156] This is useful when there are multiple buccal mucosal defects or when a through-and-through defect is presented *(Figs 12.8–12.11)*. The ALT flap can also be split into two small independent flaps to replace two defects simultaneously.[130,157]

The ALT flap has frequently been applied in head and neck reconstruction, especially when the soft-tissue defect is extremely large or when a forearm flap is not suitable. The distance between the lower extremity and the head and neck region also allows a two-team approach during the surgery. The thickness of the ALT flap can be thinned to improve its pliability.[129,158]

Flap design is initiated by marking a straight line from the anterior superior iliac spine to the lateral border of the patella. Most of the perforators are located within a circle of 3 cm from the midpoint of this axis. A hand-held Doppler can be used to map the perforators.

Flap dissection can be suprafascial or subfascial. The subfascial dissection is suggested for a beginner to minimize the risk of perforator damage. The perforators can either be septocutaneous (13%) or musculocutaneous (87%).[123] Unroofing of the musculocutaneous perforators and delicate intramuscular dissection of the perforators are the key points for this flap dissection. When the vastus lateralis muscle is harvested along with the skin paddle, the motor nerve can be preserved to avoid possible knee function compromise.[159,160]

Thoracodorsal artery perforator (TAP) flap

The TAP flap is a modification of the traditional latissimus dorsi myocutaneous flap.[161–163] The TAP flap has the advantages of having similar skin color to the facial skin and therefore can be used for facial resurfacing.

The musculocutaneous perforators of the TAP flap are derived from the medial or lateral branches of the thoracodorsal vessels. The perforators can be detected by a pencil Doppler either 4 cm below the scapular spine (medial branch), or 10 cm below the axilla and 2 cm medial to the posterior axillary line (lateral branch).

Flap dissection is initiated from the superior border of the flap with an incision directly above the latissimus dorsi muscle. After the perforator is identified, the intramuscular dissection is continued and the main pedicle is dissected. The inferior border of the flap is incised and the flap is elevated off the latissimus dorsi muscle.

The TAP flap has a reliable blood supply and leaves a hidden scar on the back. However, the need to change the patient's position during the operation can lengthen the operation time and decrease its clinical application.

Medial sural artery perforator (MSAP) flap

The MSAP flap was developed in 2001 by Cavadas et al. and is a relatively new flap used for head and neck reconstruction.[164] It is a modification of the gastrocnemius muscle flap, which was originally described for lower extremity reconstruction.[165]

Most of the sizeable perforators of the MSAP flap are located 8–12 cm inferior to the popliteal crease.[111]

Flap dissection is started by making the anterior incision and continued through a subfascial dissection to identify the perforators. The MSAP flap is a good alternative for most small buccal defects or moderate-sized buccal defects in obese patients where an ALT flap is too bulky to use (*Table 12.2*). The donor site can be closed primarily when the flap width is less than 5 cm. The major disadvantages include the visible

location of the donor site scar and the surgeon's uncomfortable posture during flap dissection with the patient's hip abduction and knee flexion.

Part II: Bone-carrying flaps

Pedicled osteocutaneous flaps

Pectoralis major osteomusculocutaneous flap

The traditional PM flap may include the fifth rib as a bony scaffold for mandibular reconstruction.[27,166] The blood supply of the fifth rib is supplied by the periosteal-muscular plexus which is small and not always reliable. The flap inset can be difficult. The strength of the fifth rib is not as good for hardware fixation or osseous integration as the fibula or the ilium. Risks of pneumothorax and hemothorax at the donor site are also possible.[167] The sternum may also be harvested with a PM flap for bony reconstruction of the mandible, but no long-term follow-up of this technique has been reported.[29,167]

Trapezius osteomusculocutaneous flap

The scapula spine can be harvested (up to 10 cm in length) with the pedicled trapezius muscle as an osteomusculocutaneous flap.[168–175] Although the technique for harvesting this flap is relatively straightforward, the restricted quality of the scapula bone and possible shoulder morbidity, especially as related to the acromion, may limit its use in mandibular reconstruction.

Temporalis osteomuscular flap

The vascularized cranial bone based on the superficial temporal artery has been used for mandibular reconstruction. It can be harvested as the outer cortex[176] or as a full-thickness[177] bone graft with the temporalis muscle. The temporalis osteomuscular flap that is harvested with the outer cortex usually has inadequate bone stock for hardware fixation and can easily fracture during shaping. Full-thickness calvarium is more durable but donor site cosmesis is a major concern.

Vascularized osteocutaneous flaps

Circumflex iliac osteocutaneous flap

The free circumflex iliac osteocutaneous flap was introduced by Taylor et al. in 1979.[178] The groin skin paddle can be elevated together with the iliac crest for mandibular reconstruction with a 94–95% success rate (*Fig. 12.22*).[141,179,180] The iliac osteocutaneous flap has the advantages of having a reliable vascular supply to the bone and providing good contour of the neomandible without the need for osteotomy due to the natural curve of the iliac crest. More recently, Dorafshar et al.[181] described the use of a split lateral iliac crest chimeric flap based on the lateral femoral circumflex vessels to provide vascularized bone and soft tissue for complex mandibular reconstruction. In spite of the successful outcome reported for mandibular reconstruction,[182–184] the bulky skin paddle and possible donor site morbidities, such as abdominal wall weakness, hernia, and contour deformity, remain a concern (*Tables 12.6 and 12.7*). Shenaq et al.[185] successfully harvested the inner cortex of the iliac as part of this flap to prevent complications at the donor site.

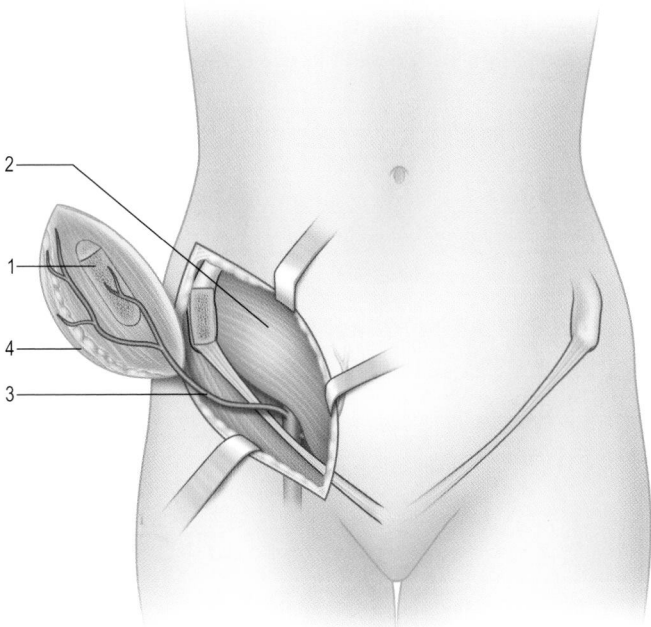

Fig. 12.22 The circumflex iliac osteocutaneous flap is based on the deep circumflex iliac artery. The shape of the iliac is good for the reconstruction of small or moderate-sized mandibular defects of type I-a to II-a. The perfusion of the groin skin paddle is not always reliable, and the bulkiness of the skin may make osseointegration of the implant difficult. 1, iliac bone; 2, external oblique muscle; 3, deep circumflex iliac artery; 4, flap design.

Scapular osteomusculocutaneous flap

The scapular osteomusculocutaneous flap includes the lateral border of the scapula, scapular and/or parascapular skin, and the latissimus dorsi muscle, based on the subscapular artery *(Fig. 12.23)*.[186] The scapular and parascapular skin flaps are valuable options for coverage of large complex oromandibular reconstruction.[187,188] The lateral border of the scapula is nourished by the circumflex scapular artery and can be harvested up to a length of 14 cm.[49] Some modifications of the osteocutaneous scapula flap harvest have been made, including the use of the medial border[189] of the scapula or a bipedicled structure.[190] However, the bone quality of the scapula is not as good as that of the ilium or the fibula. One of the major drawbacks is the intraoperative change in position, which requires additional operation time *(Tables 12.6 and 12.7)*.

Radius with radial forearm flap

The inner volar cortex of the distal radius can be harvested with the radial forearm flap as an osteocutaneous flap (10–12 cm in length) for mandibular reconstruction.[149,191–195] Postoperative full-length plaster cast for 3–4 weeks or the use of a dynamic compression plate for rigid fixation *(Table 12.6)* is necessary to prevent postoperative radius fracture.[193,196,197]

Fibula osteoseptocutaneous flap

Taylor *et al.* introduced the fibula osseous flap in 1975.[52] The free fibular OSC flap has undergone subsequent development and is now widely recognized as the reconstructive standard

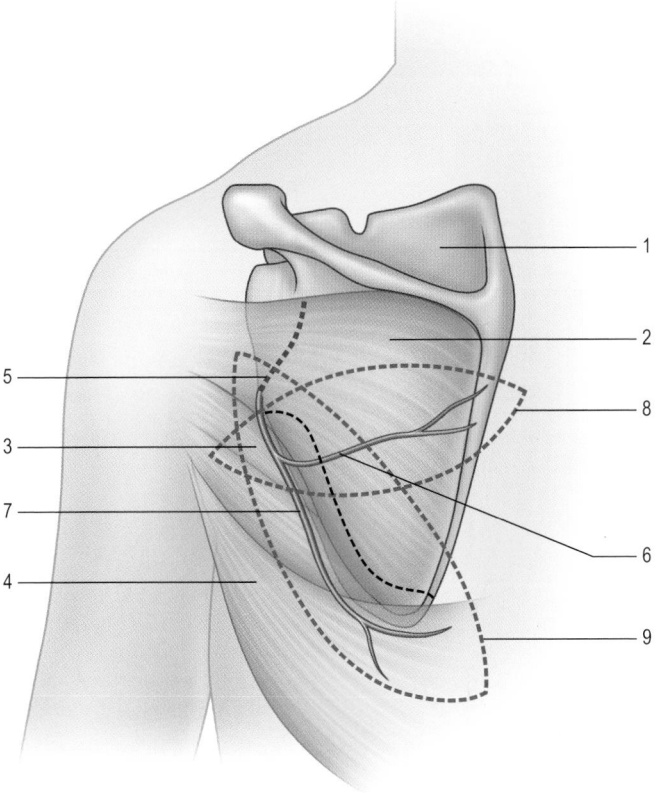

Fig. 12.23 The scapular osteomusculocutaneous flap can be created with three components, including the lateral border of the scapula, scapular and/or parascapular skin, and latissimus dorsi muscle, based on a single subscapular artery. The nourishment of the lateral border of the scapula by the circumflex scapular artery is reliable (at up to 14 cm in length). The versatility of skin territories with scapular and parascapular skin paddles renders this flap valuable for complex oromandibular reconstruction. 1, scapular bone; 2, scapular muscle; 3, teres minor muscle; 4, latissimus dorsi muscle; 5, subscapular artery; 6, scapular artery; 7, parascapular artery; 8, scapular flap design; 9, parascapular flap design.

for successful mandibular reconstruction.[53] Wei *et al.* demonstrated the reliability of harvesting the fibula bone flap along with a skin paddle based on identifiable septocutaneous perforators.[54] The skin paddle of the fibula flap provides pliable soft-tissue coverage for the underlying bone, mini or reconstruction plates, and osseointegrated dental implants.

Surgical technique: fibula osteoseptocutaneous flap for mandibular reconstruction (Tables 12.6–12.8)

Video 2

Assessment of mandibular defects and custom-made templates

Simple intermaxillary fixation is performed to obtain good dental occlusion. A reconstruction plate is molded and affixed to the two residual mandibular ends with at least two or three screws on each end. A paper ruler template is tailored and measured for the required fibula length, angle, and osteotomies. One or two sterile towels are used to map out the requirements for intraoral lining and external coverage. The

Table 12.8 Variable flap inset and available recipient vessels for mandibular reconstruction using fibula osteoseptocutaneous flap

Group	Code	Donor site: fibula	Recipient site: mandible	Fibula skin site transferred to	Recipient vessels: right	Recipient vessels: left	Note
1	LLI	Left	Left	Intraoral mucosa	FA, STA	STA	
2	LLC	Left	Left	External cheek skin		STA, STpA	
3	LRI	Left	Right	Intraoral mucosa	STA, STpA		Higher complication rate
4	LRC	Left	Right	External cheek skin	STA	FA, STA	
5	RLI	Right	Left	Intraoral mucosa		STA, STpA	Higher complication rate
6	RLC	Right	Left	External cheek skin	FA, STA	STA	
7	RRI	Right	Right	Intraoral mucosa	STA	FA, STA	
8	RRC	Right	Right	External cheek skin	STA, STpA		

FA, facial artery; STA, superior thyroid artery; STpA, superficial temporal artery.

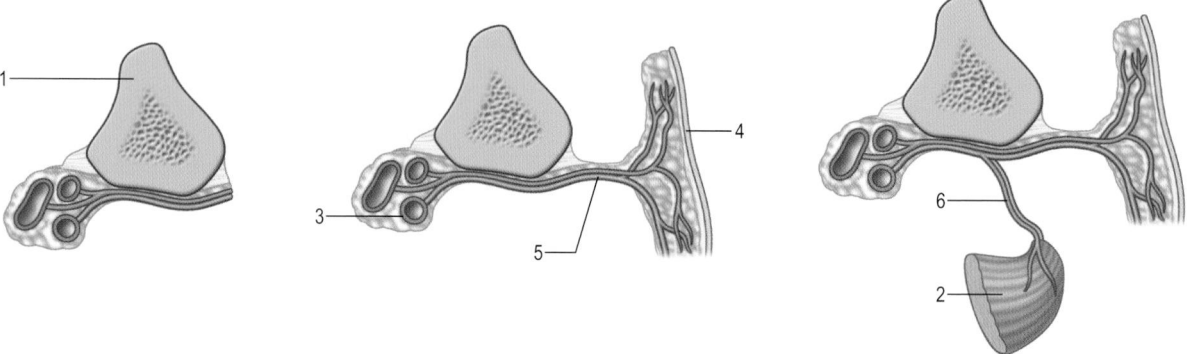

Fig. 12.24 The fibula flap evolves from a bone-only flap to an osteocutaneous flap with the inclusion of the septocutaneous perforator, to the osteomusculocutaneous flap with an additional and independent myocutaneous perforator for nourishing a segment of soleus muscle. 1, fibula bone; 2, soleus muscle; 3, peroneal vessels; 4, skin paddle; 5, septocutaneous perforator; 6, musculocutaneous perforator.

proposed pedicle orientation is also marked on each sterile drape template.[62]

Recipient site preparation

There are four possible arteries that can be used on either side of the neck: the facial artery, superior thyroid artery, superficial temporal artery, and the transverse cervical artery. The external carotid artery is seldom used in selected centers due to the risk of blowout. The recipient vessels may be damaged by the previous operative scar, radiated fibrosis, or certain types of neck dissection. The superficial temporal artery is usually spared by radiation therapy and is reliable as a recipient site.[198] The contralateral vessels in the neck are also good alternatives for secondary mandibular reconstruction.

Donor site selection

The fibula is a unique triangular bone, as seen in the cross-section (*Fig. 12.24*). The peroneal vessels, usually one artery and two concomitant veins, are located on the posteromedial aspect of the fibula, posterior to the fascia of the posterior tibialis, inside the flexor hallucis longus (FHL), and anterior to the posterior crucial septum. The skin paddle is based on osteocutaneous perforators, which run inside the posterior crucial septum (*Fig. 12.24*). The lateral surface is the safest and

preferred site for reconstruction plate fixation (*Fig. 12.24*). The septum should ideally be located posterosuperiorly to the reconstructed fibula and the plate to avoid any tethering of the perforators in the septum while insetting the skin paddle intraorally. Plate fixation on the anteromedial or posteromedial aspects of the fibula could result in the inadvertent shearing, entanglement, or outright disruption of either the vascular pedicle or the perforators. The use of the skin flap for either intraoral mucosal or cheek skin reconstruction will determine the final orientation of the bone inset and the orientation of the vascular pedicle. Therefore, the insetting of the bone to the plate has only two alternatives for a specific lateral mandibular defect, one as shown in *Figure 12.25* and the other rotated 180°, as in *Figure 12.32* (see below). If the fibula is turned upside down, the pedicle or perforators are easily injured or compressed by the plate and screws.

When the left fibula osteocutaneous flap is harvested for left mandibular reconstruction and the skin paddle is used for the intraoral lining (LLI group in *Table 12.8*), the pedicle is toward the right (*Fig. 12.25*). This pedicle can reach the ipsilateral superior thyroid artery, contralateral facial artery, or superior thyroid artery in the neck (*Figs 12.25–12.31 and Table 12.8*). When the left fibula osteocutaneous flap is used to reconstruct right composite mandibular defect, the flap must

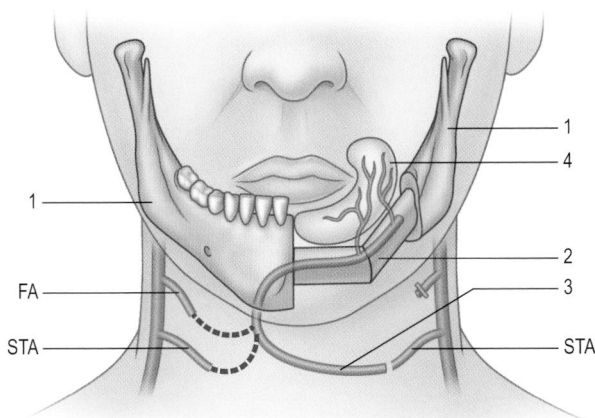

Fig. 12.25 The left fibula osteocutaneous flap is transferred to left mandibular defect type II-a (LLI group in Table 12.8). The lateral aspect of the fibula is used for fixation of the reconstruction plate and screws. The skin paddle is reconstructed for the intraoral lining. The pedicle of peroneal vessels is placed toward the right side to reach the recipient vessels of the ipsilateral superior thyroid artery, right facial artery, or right superior thyroid artery. 1, residual mandible bone; 2, fibula bone; 3, peroneal artery; 4, skin paddle of fibula flap; 5, recipient vessels – ipsilateral superior thyroid artery (STA), contralateral facial artery (FA), and STA.

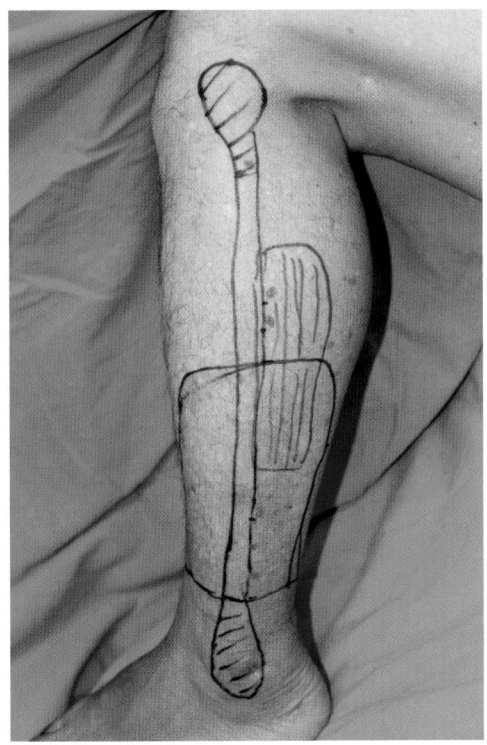

Fig. 12.27 An osteomyocutaneous peroneal artery combined flap was harvested with a skin paddle of 12 × 8 cm based on two septocutaneous perforators; 6 cm from both ends of the fibula were preserved. A soleus muscle cuff (10 × 5 cm) was planed to harvest based on a myocutaneous perforator located on the proximal third of the leg.

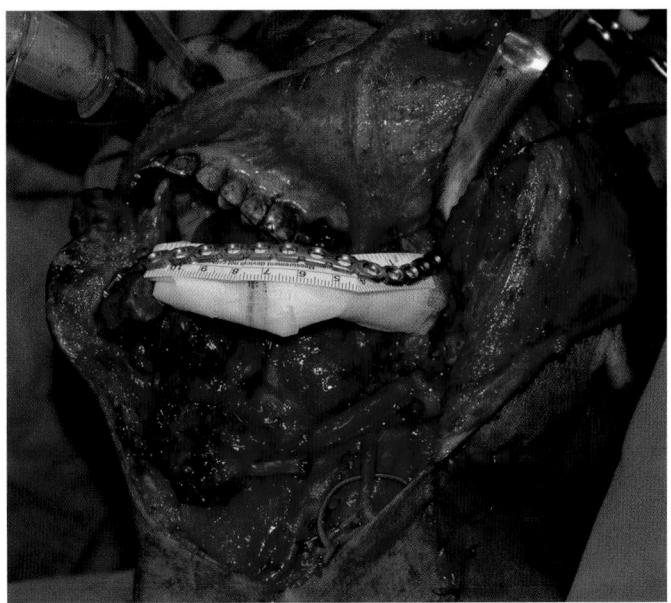

Fig. 12.26 A 70-year-old male patient with a lower gum squamous cell carcinoma (T4N0M0) underwent left segmental mandibulectomy and modified radical neck dissection. Mandibular defect type II-a included a bone defect of 9 cm in length; a buccal mucosal and adjunct soft-tissue defect measured 9 × 4 cm. A reconstruction plate was used to bridge the residual mandible ends after temporal intermaxillary wiring for occlusion. The plate was placed 1 cm higher than the lower margin of the native mandible for possible osseointegrating implantation. A paper ruler was used as a tailored template for measurement of the length, angle, and number of osteotomies.

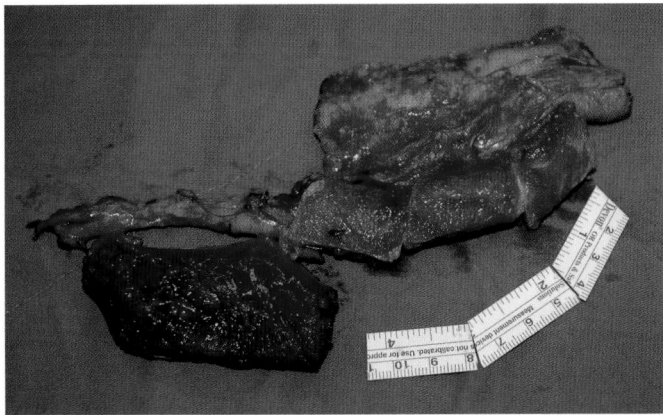

Fig. 12.28 The osteotomy was performed to obtain three bone segments (3.5, 4.5, and 3 cm in length, respectively) to simulate the tailored paper ruler templates on the back table. The pedicle located in the posteromedial aspect was skeletonized with a length of 10 cm toward the right side so as to reach the recipient vessels easily. The lateral aspect of the fibula is suitable for fixation of the reconstruction plate and screws without injury of the pedicle and septocutaneous perforators. A cuff of lateral soleus muscle, nourished by an independent myocutaneous perforator, 10 × 5 cm, was elevated.

be inset with the proximal fibula pointing posteriorly towards the mandibular ramus so that the skin paddle can be used to reconstruct the intraoral mucosal lining (LRI group in *Table 12.8*). In this configuration, the vascular pedicle will run inferiorly and posterolaterally to the fibula. To reach either the right superior thyroid artery or the right superficial temporal artery, the pedicle must make a sharp turn, which may make it susceptible to kinking (*Figs 12.32–12.36 and Table 12.8*). When the mandibular defect is extended to the ramus, the only available recipient vessel is the right superficial temporal artery, which has size discrepancy with the donor vessels and

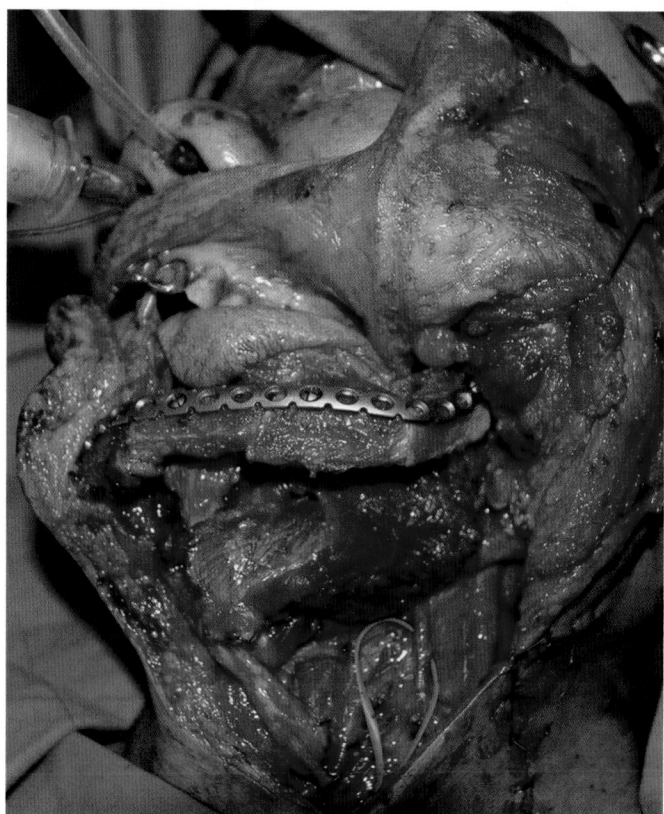

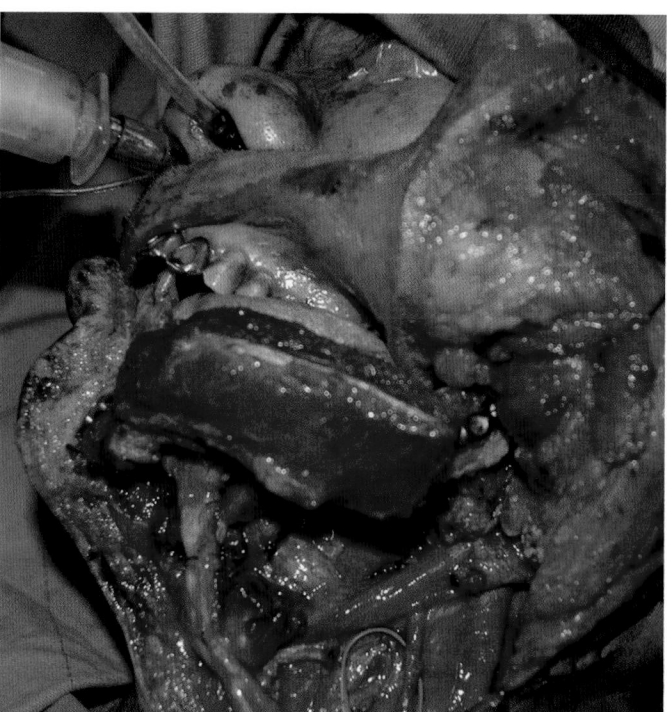

Fig. 12.30 The soleus muscle could be flipped over on top of the fibula and the reconstruction plate to prevent exposure of the reconstruction plate and potential osteoradionecrosis, as well as to provide better cheek contouring.

Fig. 12.29 The three fibula segments were fixed to the reconstruction plate with one screw for each. The pedicle was placed forward to right-sided and curved to reach the ipsilateral superior thyroid artery and facial vein (blue loop, facial vein).

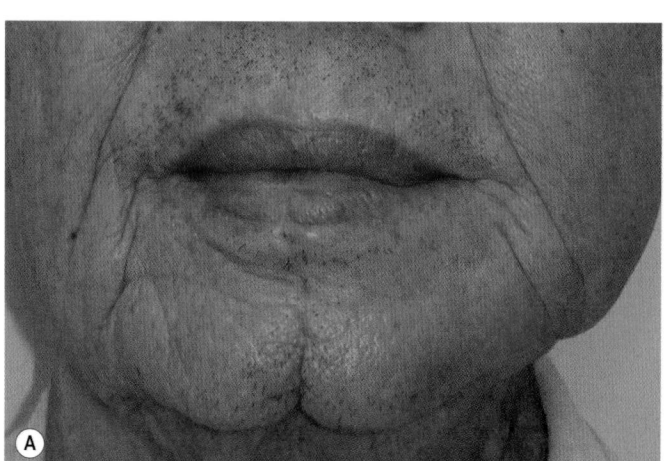

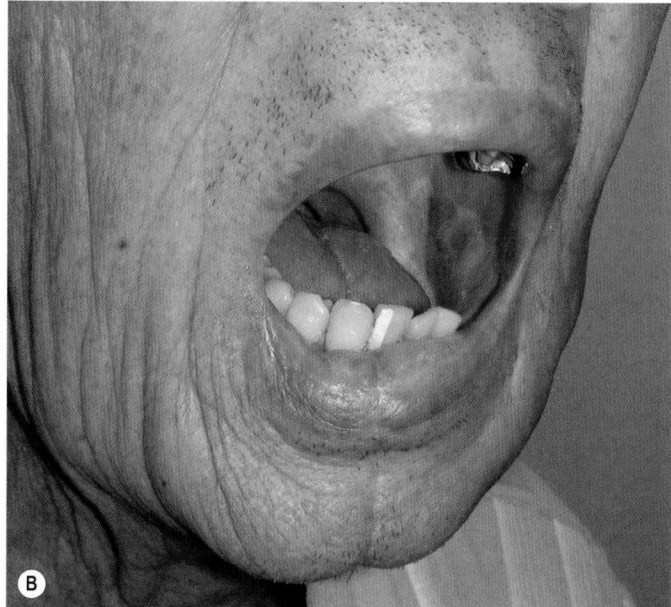

Fig. 12.31 At a follow-up of 24.4 months, the patient was satisfied with the functional and cosmetic outcomes. **(A)** Anteroposterior and **(B)** open-mouth views.

can easily kink, especially the venous anastomosis when the superificial temporal vein is flipped downward *(Fig. 12.32)*. Care must be taken to release the superficial temporal vein proximally from its attachments to the surrounding tissues in order to avoid any sharp turn in the vessel.

On the other hand, if the right fibula osteocutaneous flap is used for left mandibular reconstruction and the skin paddle is used for intraoral mucosa resurfacing (RLI group in *Table 12.8*), the vascular pedicle will be oriented inferiorly and posterolaterally to the fibula, making the left superior thyroid

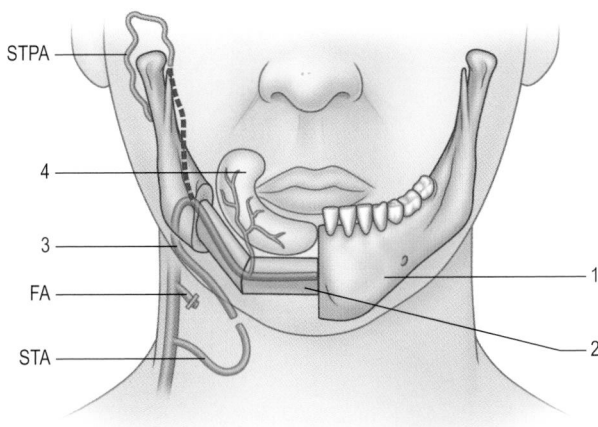

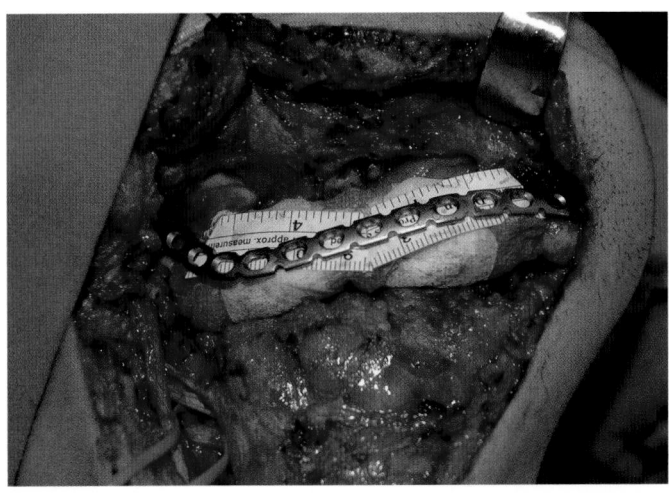

Fig. 12.32 The left fibula osteocutaneous flap is transferred to a right mandibular defect type II-a (LRI group in Table 12.8). The lateral aspect of the fibula is used for fixation of the reconstruction plate and screws. The skin paddle is reconstructed for the intraoral lining. The pedicle of peroneal vessels is placed laterally to reach the recipient vessels of the ipsilateral superior thyroid artery or the superiorly ipsilateral superficial temporal artery. 1, residual mandible bone; 2, fibula bone; 3, peroneal artery; 4, skin paddle of fibula flap; 5, recipient vessels – ipsilateral superior thyroid artery (STA) and superficial temporal artery (STpA); FA, facial artery.

Fig. 12.33 A 20-year-old male suffering from right ameloblastoma underwent wide excision and repeated nonvascularized iliac bone grafts with absorption. The residual iliac bone graft was debrided, and the buccal mucosal fibrosis was released. The bone defect measured 8 cm in length, as determined by a tailored paper ruler template.

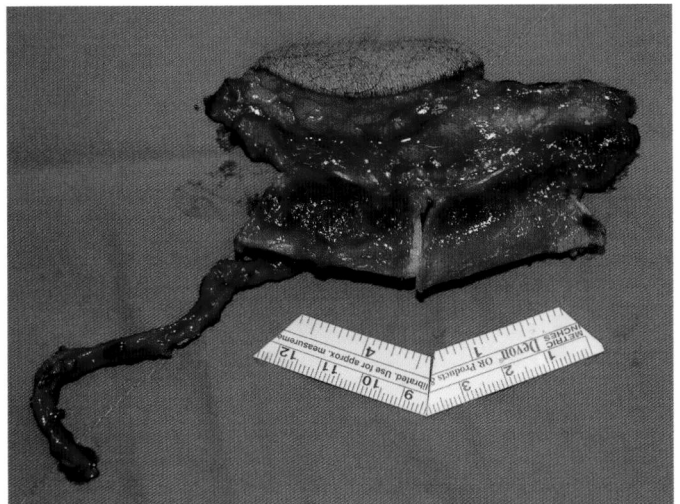

Fig. 12.34 A fibula osteocutaneous flap was elevated with a skin paddle of 8 × 2.5 cm. The osteotomy was performed with two segments of bone (each 4 cm in length) to simulate the tailored paper ruler templates on the back table. The pedicle was skeletonized with a length of 10 cm toward the right side to reach the recipient vessels easily. The lateral aspect of the fibula was prepared for fixation of the reconstruction plate and screws.

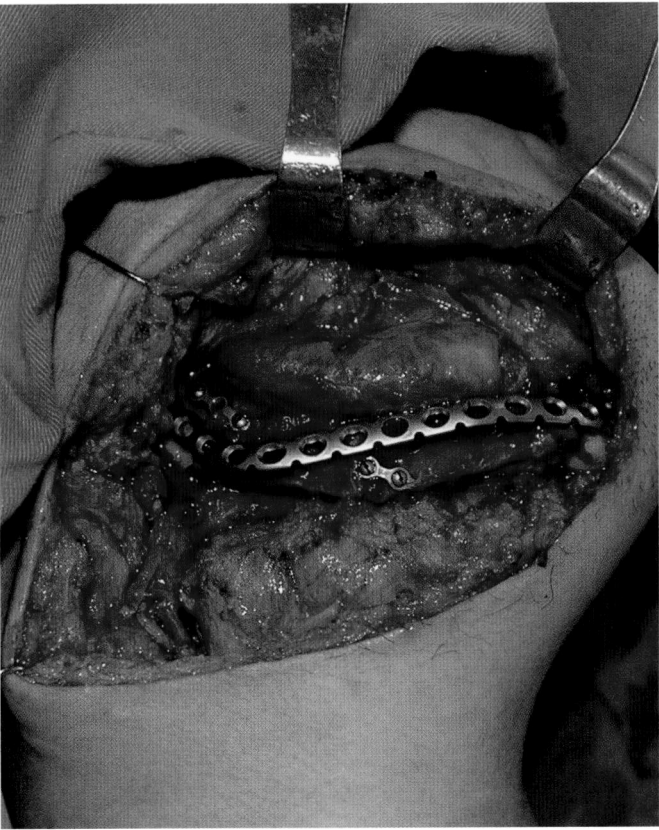

artery and superficial temporal artery the most reasonable recipient vessels *(Figs 12.37–12.41 and Table 12.8)*. If the right fibula OSC flap is used for right mandibular reconstruction and the skin paddle is used for intraoral lining, the anastomosis to the ipsilateral facial artery, superior thyroid artery, or contralateral superior thyroid artery gives the pedicle a gentle curvature that is unlikely to kink and occlude (RRI group in *Table 12.8*) *(Fig. 12.42)*. When the ipsilateral recipient vessels are not available, especially in patients who have undergone radiation therapy, the contralateral neck vessels are

Fig. 12.35 The fibula segments were fixed to the reconstruction plate; a miniplate was placed between two fibula bone segments. The skin paddle was inset as an intraoral lining.

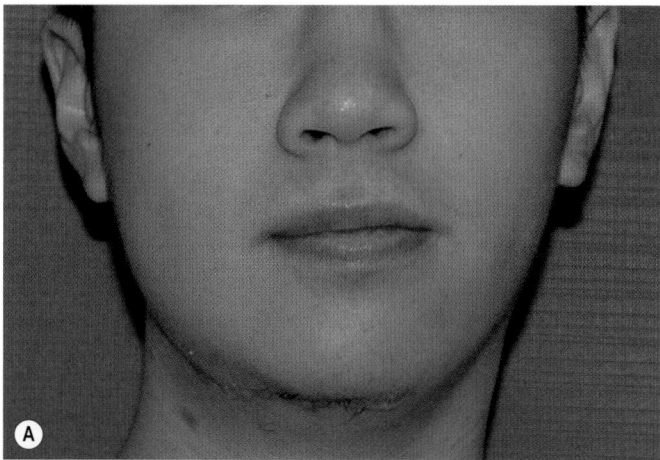

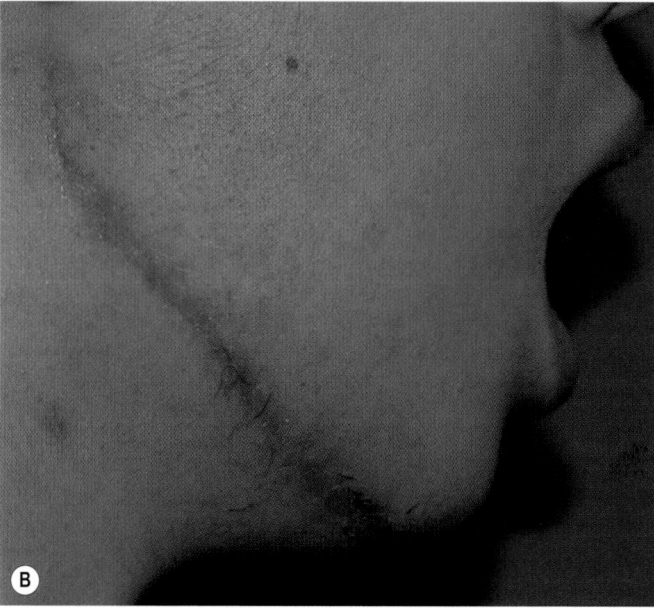

Fig. 12.36 (A, B) At an 18-month follow-up, the contour of the mandible was symmetrical.

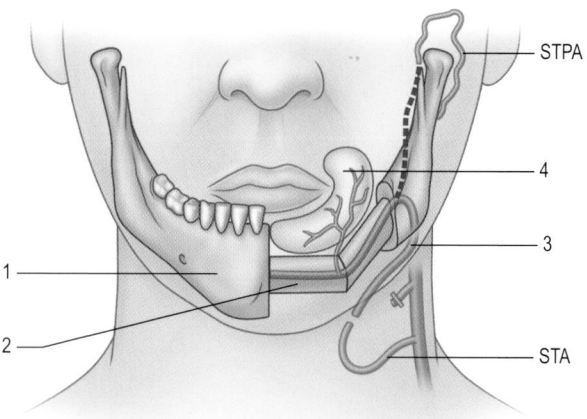

Fig. 12.37 The right fibula osteocutaneous flap is transferred to a left mandibular defect type II-a (RLI group in Table 12.8). The skin paddle is reconstructed for the intraoral lining. The pedicle of peroneal vessels is placed left-sided and laterally to the ipsilateral superior thyroid artery or superiorly to the ipsilateral superficial temporal artery. 1,. residual mandible bone; 2, fibula bone; 3, peroneal artery; 4, skin paddle of fibula flap; 5, recipient vessels – ipsilateral superior thyroid artery (STA) and superficial temporal artery (STpA).

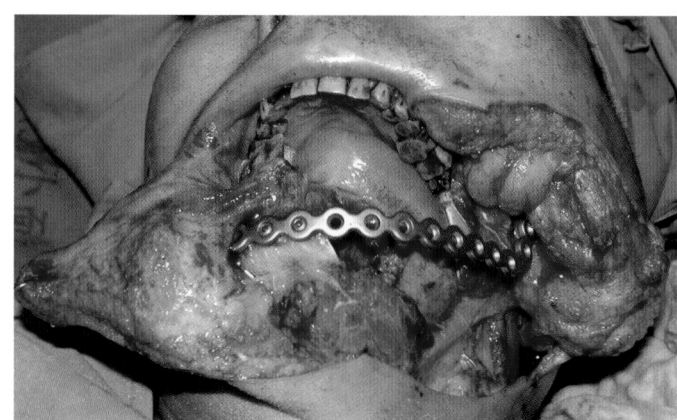

Fig. 12.38 A 55-year-old male patient sustained left buccal squamous cell carcinoma (T4N2M0), which was widely excised and resulted in a type II-a mandibular defect (RLI group in Table 12.8). A reconstruction plate was used for fixation of both ends of the native mandible after temporary intermaxillary wiring. The bone defect was measured 9 cm in length.

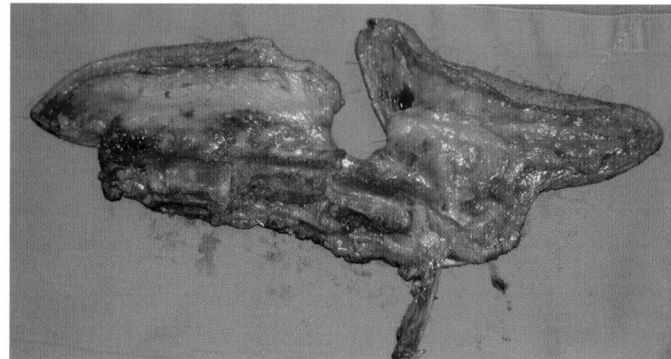

Fig. 12.39 The fibula was osteotomized into three segments, each 3 cm in length. The skin paddle was split into two parts, one 11 × 8 cm for the intraoral lining and the other 7 × 6 cm for the external cheek. The pedicle toward the left side was skeletonized to a length of 6 cm.

alternative recipient vessels *(Figs 12.42–12.46 and Table 12.8)*. The skeletonized pedicle is usually long and pliable enough to reach the contralateral side of the neck without difficulty.

Osteomyocutaneous peroneal artery combined flap harvest

The advantages of the fibula osteocutaneous flap are well established: adequate bone length and volume for extensive reconstruction and osseointegrated dental implant placement; a sturdy periosteal and endosteal blood supply allowing one or multiple osteotomies; a reliable skin paddle with adequate skin to resurface both intraoral and external skin defects; a distant donor site allowing for a two-team approach; and low donor site morbidity. Despite these benefits, one of the potential drawbacks of the osteocutaneous flap is the lack of available soft tissue for reconstructing extensive composite mandibular defect. Wide excision of intraoral tumors can result in defects involving the bone, oral lining, external skin, tongue, and masseter muscle. Despite an initial acceptable reconstruction, radiotherapy often leads to thinning of the

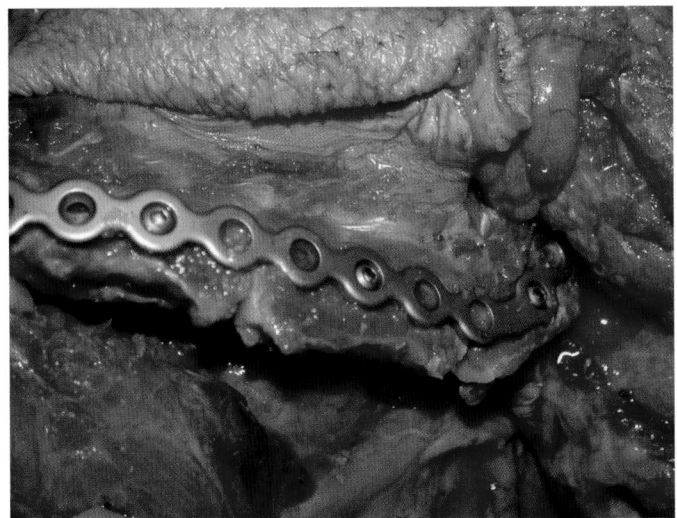

Fig. 12.40 Each fibula segment was fixed to the reconstruction plate with one screw with good bony contact and neomandible contour.

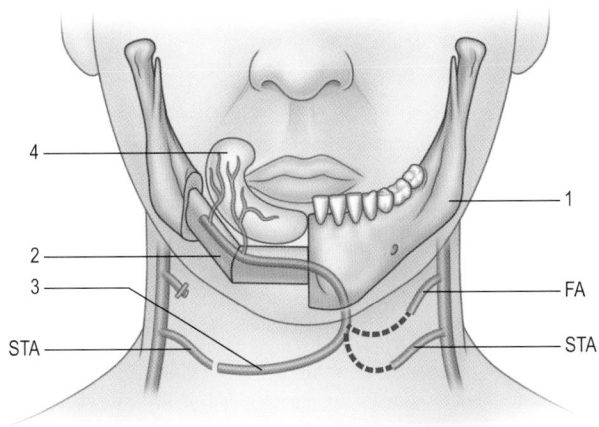

Fig. 12.42 The right fibula osteocutaneous flap is transferred to a right mandibular defect type II-a (RRI group in Table 12.8). The lateral aspect of the fibula is used for fixation of the reconstruction plate and screws. The skin paddle is reconstructed for the intraoral lining. The pedicle of peroneal vessels is placed toward the left side to reach the recipient vessels of the ipsilateral superior thyroid artery or contralateral facial or superior thyroid arteries. 1, residual mandible bone; 2, fibula bone; 3, peroneal artery. 4, skin paddle of fibula flap; 5, recipient vessels – ipsilateral superior thyroid artery (STA), contralateral facial artery, and superior thyroid artery.

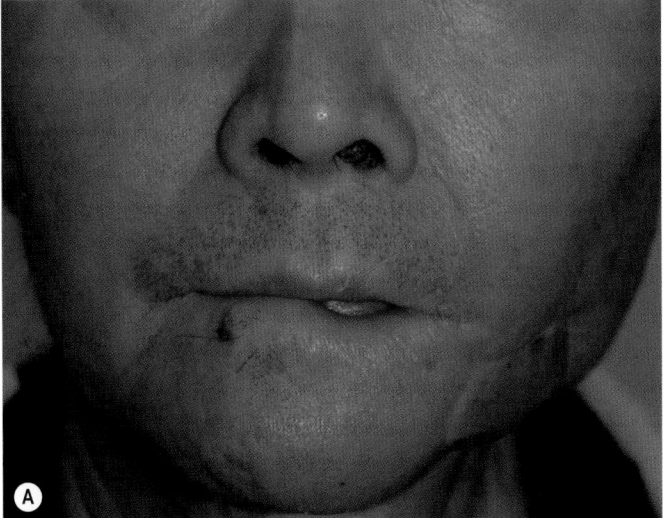

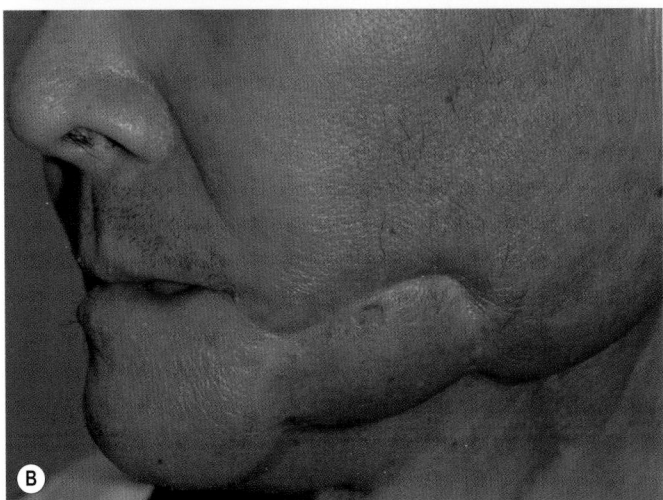

Fig. 12.41 The patient received postoperative radiation. **(A, B)** At a follow-up of 10 months, the patient was satisfied with the functional and cosmetic outcomes.

skin paddle and subsequent contraction, producing a loss of contour and hollowing of the cheek and neck area. Furthermore, wound-healing problems can lead to plate exposure and osteoradionecrosis.

To counteract these problems when using the fibula osteo-cutanoeus flap, two potential solutions exist. The first is to harvest a second flap (pedicled or free) to augment the soft-tissue or skin reconstruction, which may require a second pair of recipient vessels, and increase the operation time and potential complication rates. The other option is to increase the tissue that can potentially be harvested with a fibula flap in a single operative procedure by including a portion of the soleus muscle nourished by a separate myocutaenous

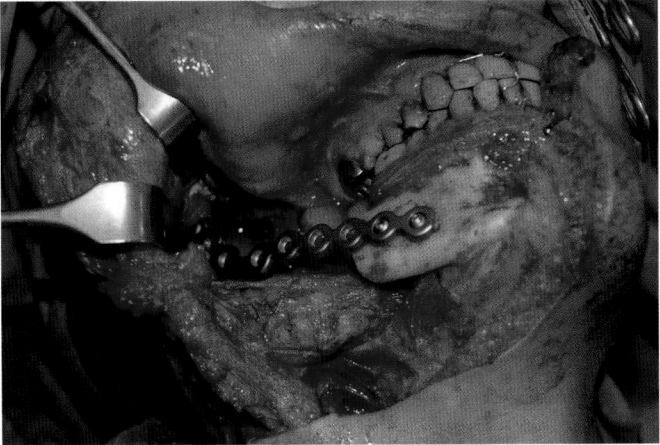

Fig. 12.43 A 35-year-old male with right ameloblastoma underwent wide excision, which resulted in a 6-cm mandibular defect type II-a. The residual mandible ends were bridged with a reconstruction plate and stabilized with temporary intermaxillary wiring.

perforator of the peroneal artery as the OPAC flap.[62,199] The OPAC flap has the advantages of requiring single-flap harvest with all components, a single donor site, and a single set of microanastomoses, leading to reduced operative time.

The harvest technique for the free fibula osteocutaneous flap was described by Wei and Cheng.[56,62,199] The fibula bone is marked on the skin. At both the proximal and distal ends 6 cm in length is preserved for knee and ankle stability (*Fig. 12.27*). The septocutaneous perforators to the skin, which are primarily located along the posterior margin of the fibula on the middle and lower third of the leg, are marked preoperatively by a hand-held Doppler. The skin island is centered over the septocutaneous perforators. The skin incision is made to the subcutaneous layer and kept above the fascia through the anterior approach. The flap is partially elevated, and the fascia is incised after passing through the anterior

cruciate ligament. The peroneus longus and brevis are elevated off the fibula periosteum. The anterior cruciate ligament is then divided. The periosteum of the fibula at both osteotomy sites is removed, and the bone is osteotomized by an electric saw. The fibula is then retracted posterolaterally to expose the extensor digitorum longus, brevis, and anterior tibialis muscles, which are all elevated off the periosteum. At this time, the posterior skin incision is made with meticulous care to keep the septocutaneous perforators intact inside the posterior cruciate septum. Distal ends of the peroneal vessels, which may be separated from the fibula bone, are ligated and divided. The pedicle is dissected out from the FHL. The FHL is detached with an index finger inserted between the FHL

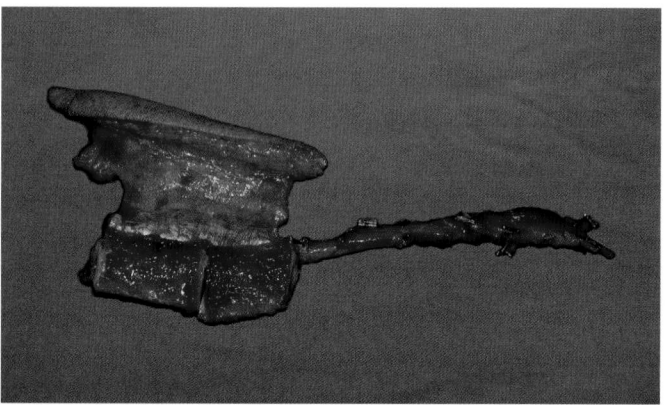

Fig. 12.44 A right fibula osteocutaneous flap was harvested with a 6 × 3 cm skin paddle. Two bone segments were obtained after osteotomies according to paper ruler templates (each 3 cm in length). Note that the pedicle was skeletonized and directed toward the left side.

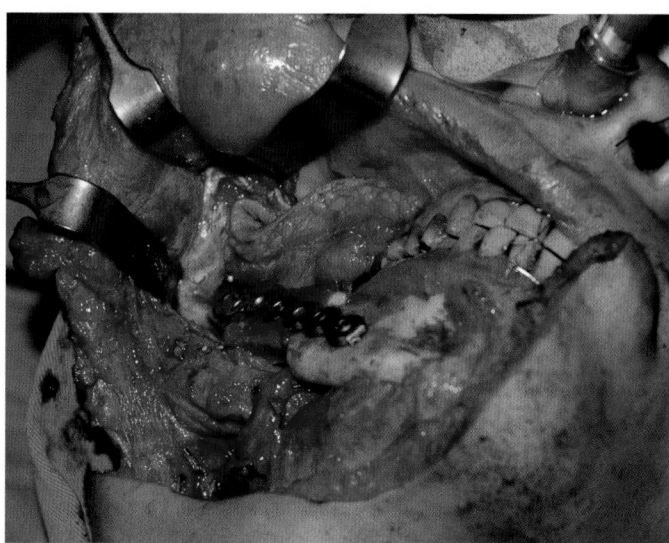

Fig. 12.45 The two fibula segments were fixed to the reconstruction plate. The pedicle was placed left-sided to reach the right superior thyroid artery and middle jugular vein.

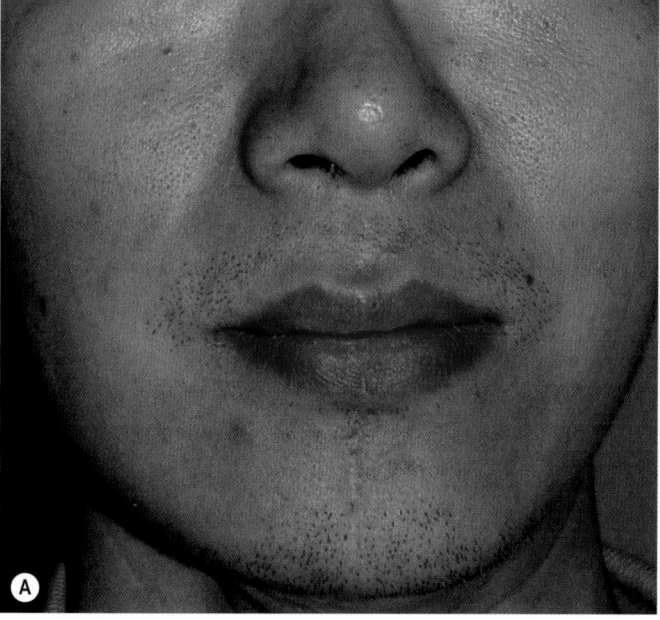

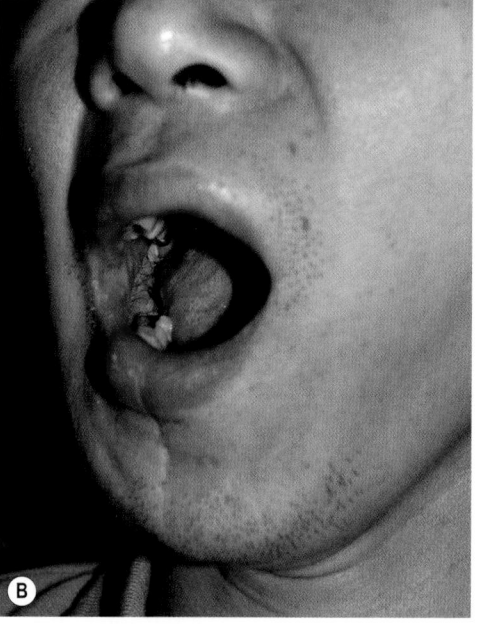

Fig. 12.46 (A, B) At a follow-up of 16 months, the patient was satisfied with both the functional and aesthetic outcomes.

and posterior cruciate septum, so as to protect the septocutaneous perforators. The residual posterior cruciate septum not containing the perforators is divided. The soleus muscle can be included with the musculocutaneous perforators frequently identified at the proximal third of the peroneal vessels.[62,199] The soleus muscle can be harvest 6 × 14 cm even up to half of soelus without significant donor site morbidity.

Osteotomies

After division of the proximal peroneal pedicle, further osteotomies are performed with an electric saw according to the tailored paper ruler templates displayed on the back table *(Figs 12.28 and 12.34)*. The skin paddle can be separated into two flaps if there are more than two septocutaneous perforators available *(Fig. 12.39)*. The pedicle is skeletonized with removal of unnecessary proximal periosteum and bone. Yagi *et al.* highlighted the importance of respecting the geometry of the fibula OSC flap to obtain good outcomes in mandibular reconstruction.[200] Some obstacles may appear during the shaping and insetting of a fibula OSC flap due to the limited mobility of each tissue component. It is important to protect the vascular pedicle and septocutaneous perforators to the skin paddle during the osteotomies to prevent injury to these structures. Furthermore, during insetting, if the septum and its perforators are stretched over the fibula and the plate to reach the defect, the vascularity of the skin paddle can be compromised. The minimal recommended bone segment length for osteotomy is 2.5 cm to include some perforators to nourish the periosteum. It has been suggested that there is decreased vascularity to the flap in the more distal segments of the multiple osteotomized bone, since the proximal segment supplied by a periosteal source as well as a nutrient artery, and the distal segments supplied only by a periosteal source. In addition, when plating is applied on top of the periosteum for fixation of the bone segments, there is a concern of possible decrease in periosteal vascular flow to the distal bone segments.

Flap inset

The OPAC or fibula OSC flap is inset from the osteotomized fibula segments that are contoured to fit the reconstruction plate. The authors recommend only a single screw fixation for each bone segment to minimize vascular compromise to the fibula *(Fig. 12.29)*. One skin paddle based on a septocutaneous perforator is inset for the intraoral lining, and a second skin paddle is based on a separate septocutaneous perforator of the same pedicle for the external cheek if needed.

For some patients, the soleus muscle of OPAC flap is placed on top of the fibula and reconstruction plate to improve cosmesis and prevent possible osteoradionecrosis and plate exposure after postoperative radiation *(Fig. 12.30)*.[62,199] It is recommended to keep the ischemia time for fibula osteocutaneous flaps to less than 5 hours to reduce the partial flap loss rate and other complication rates.[201]

In an attempt to simplify surgical planning, some surgeons prefer to use the contralateral leg as a donor site for mandibular defects because two teams may work simultaneously without any space conflict. The authors found that the left fibula osteocutaneous flap had a higher vascular complication rate when used for right mandibular reconstructions. This is likely due to the more restricted spatial relationship between the fibula flap inset and the available recipient vessels. An algorithm representing the different factors influencing the inset geometry should include the side from which the flap was harvested, the available recipient vessels, and the need for intraoral or external skin reconstruction. It is recommended to use an ipsilateral fibula osteocutaneous flap for mandibular reconstruction to decrease the risk of vascular complications. The ipsilateral superior thyroid artery, which is usually preserved by the surgical oncologist, is the preferred recipient vessel. The contralateral superior thyroid artery constitutes an equally viable alternative because up to 10–15 cm of the length of the peroneal artery can usually be harvested.

Plating

Intermaxillary fixation with screws or wires can both achieve good occlusion. A titanium reconstruction plate is used to bridge both residual mandibular ends, with at least two screws for each end *(Figs 12.26, 12.33, 12.38, and 12.43)*. A template using a paper ruler is made to match the contour of the plate. Care must be taken not to injure the pedicle or perforators during plating. Unicortical drilling and screw fixation should be performed under irrigation to prevent overheating injury of the reconstructed bone.[17,202,203] The plate can be positioned 1 cm higher than the lower margin of the native mandible to achieve adequate height for occlusion with osseointegrated implants *(Figs 12.26, 12.33, 12.38, and 12.43)*. If the height of the transplanted bone is insufficient, it is also possible to perform a "double-barrel" fibula flap for adequate and stable fixation of planned osseointegrated implants.[204–206] Recently, new techniques such as three-dimensional reconstruction images have been introduced to assist the surgeons with complex mandibular reconstruction.[206–208] Furthermore, rapid prototyping technologies can construct physical models from computer-aided designs via three-dimensional printers.[208] Vertical distraction osteogenesis is another option for increase of the reconstructed bone height *(Figs 12.47–12.50)*.[209]

Ischemia time

The ischemia time starts at the time of pedicle division and includes the osteotomy, the shaping and inset interval, and ends with the completion of the arterial anastomosis. The fibula flap ischemia time for mandibular reconstruction is dependent on several factors: the surgeon's experience; whether the sequence of fibula osteotomies and fixation takes place before or after pedicle division; whether the order of anastomosis is performed before or after flap insetting; and whether the artery or vein is anastomosed first. Partial flap loss has statistically been higher if the ischemia time is greater than 5 hours.[201] Fibula bone survival did not differ significantly with ischemia time.[201] Partial flap loss seems to be primarily a problem of the skin component of the fibula OSC flap, possibly due to kinking, twisting, or too much tension at the septocutaneous perforator during inseting and plating.

Temporomandibular joint reconstruction

Reconstruction of the temporomandibular joint usually yields unfavorable results. If the condyle is not reconstructed, movement of the mandible, which relies only on the contralateral temporomandibular joint, will eventually tilt, causing malocclusion and trismus. There are several alternatives to condyle reconstruction, such as: avascular bone graft, rounding off the end of the fibula, costochondral graft attached to the fibula end, or a titanium condyle prosthesis.[210] The condyle prosthesis has been associated with a higher rate of hardware exposure and even sensorineural hearing loss.[211] The fibula osteocutaneous flap had been reported for temporomandibular joint reconstruction with reasonable functional and cosmetic results.[212]

Dental rehabilitation: osseointegrated dental implants

Dental rehabilitation may enhance functional and cosmetic outcome after mandibular reconstruction. Two procedures are used: permanent prosthesis with osseointegrated dental implants and removable prosthesis. These procedures are usually performed by the oral surgeon and dentist. Briefly, the vestibuloplasty with split-thickness skin graft or palatal mucosal graft is performed first to obtain lingual and buccal sulci for a vestibule of 1.5 cm in depth. The reconstructed bone stock (10 × 6 mm) is required for the osseointegrated

implant. The bone is exposed after elevation of the periosteum and burred to yield a flat surface. Drilling is applied for insertion of the implant at a depth of 5 mm. For a permanent prosthesis, consolidation of the implant requires 3 months. Although the immediately osseointegrating implant was introduced by Chang for benign lesions,[204,213,214] delayed osseointegration is recommended for cancer patients who have undergone radiation.

Postoperative care

Patients are transferred to the intensive care unit for postoperative flap monitoring for 3–7 days depending on the patient's condition.

A tracheotomy or an endotracheal tube is required for ventilator support overnight and the patient is usually sedated on postoperative day 1. Restriction of neck motion is sometimes required to prevent traction or avulsion of the vascular anastomosis.

Prophylactic antibiotics for Gram-positive, Gram-negative, and anaerobic bacteria are given for 7 days. Due to

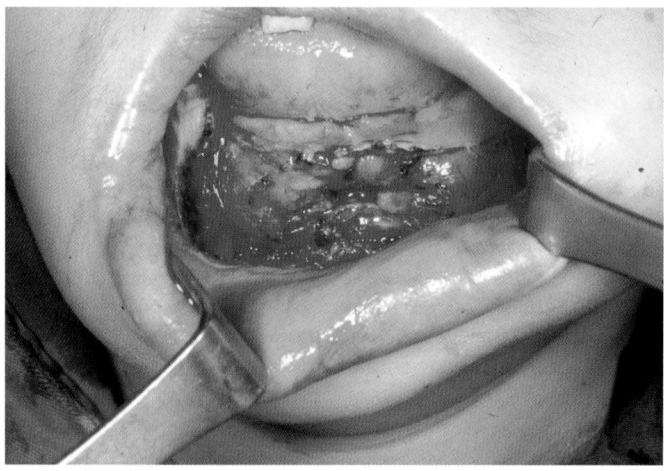

Fig. 12.47 A 26-year-old female suffered from lower gum ameloblastoma. The patient underwent wide excision through the intraoral approach. A mandibular defect type I-a measuring 7 cm was encountered.

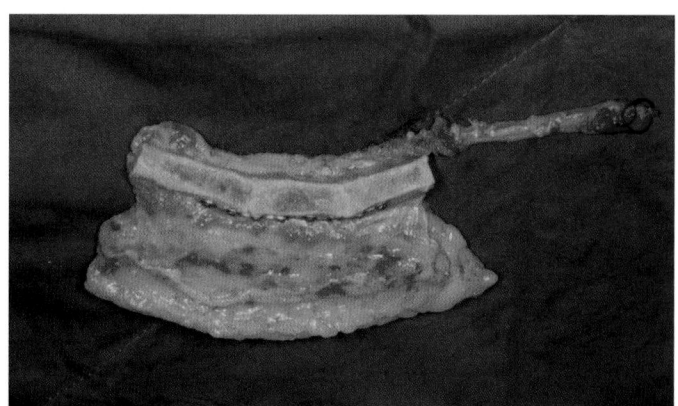

Fig. 12.48 A left fibula osteocutaneous flap of 12 × 5 cm was harvested. Three bone segments (2, 2.5, and 2.5 cm, respectively) were fixed with miniplates.

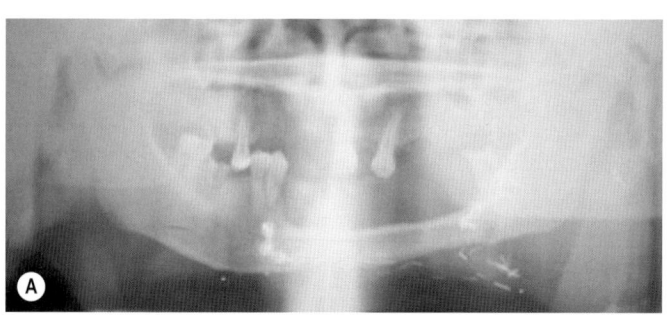

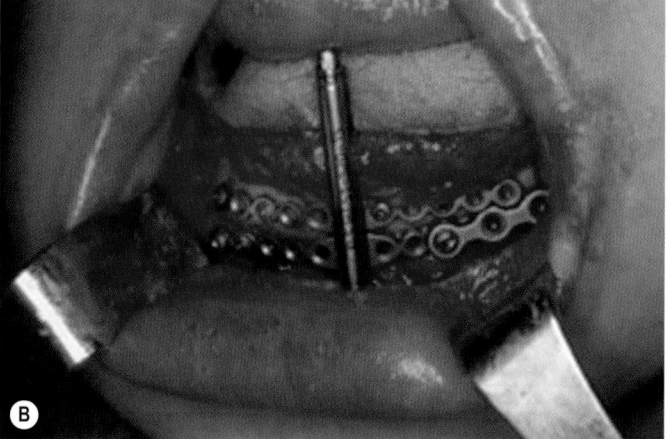

Fig. 12.49 Two years postoperatively, the patient requested a delayed osseointegrating implant with inadequate mandibular height. The subcutaneous fat was removed; the periosteum of the fibula was partially elevated. Longitudinal osteotomy of the fibula was performed, and the internal distraction device was applied to both bone segments for vertical distraction.

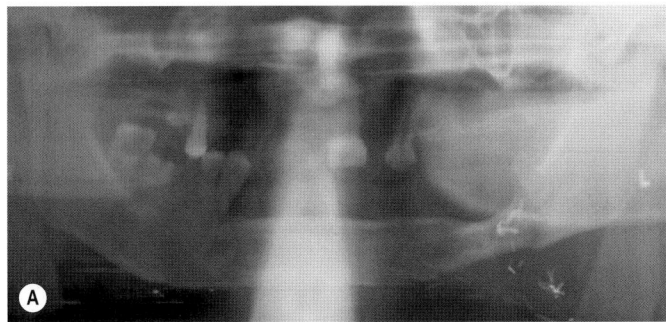

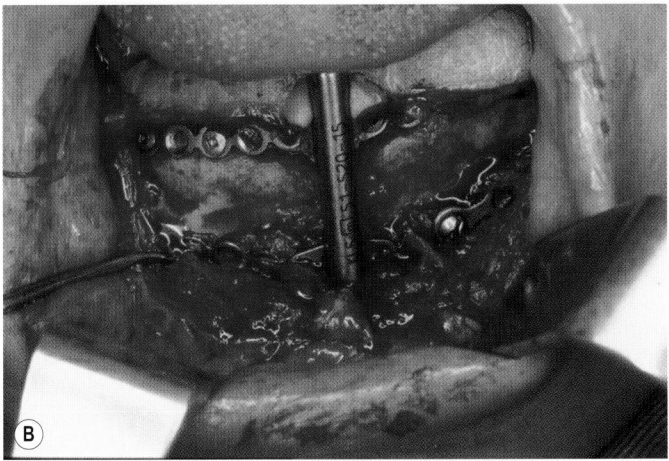

Fig. 12.50 (A, B) One week after the distraction device was stable, the distraction was increased by 0.5 mm every day until it reached 10.5 mm in height. The device was fixed for the consolidation period of 6 weeks. A vestibuloplasty was also performed for further prosthesis. The neomandibular 2.5 cm in height was adequate to hold the osseointegrating dental implant after the distraction osteogenesis.

the length of the operation, a prophylactic proton pump inhibitor is administered for 3 days to prevent stress ulcers. Relative overhydration is preferred, especially in young patients, to maintain adequate blood flow to the flap. Intake and output are carefully monitored. Enteral feeding is started as early as possible to ensure sufficient nutritional support. If enteral feeding is not possible or if nutritional status is already poor before surgery, short-term (3–5 days) partial parenteral nutritional support is recommended.

The flaps are monitored every hour for the first 24 hours and every 2 hours for the next 24 hours, and then every 4 hours starting from postoperative day 3 to the time of discharge. Physical examination of the flap (including color, temperature, capillary refill, and puncture test) is usually adequate. If there is a skin paddle on the outside of the oral cavity, a hand-held Doppler can be used to monitor vascular flow to the flap. Other devices, such as implantable Doppler, laser Doppler, or an O2C machine, can be used as alternatives.

Antithrombotic agents or vasodilation agents such as heparin, low-molecular-weight fraxiparin, promostan, or dextran are not routinely prescribed. Such drugs are only given if the pedicle has thrombosis or when the surgeons find it necessary.

Patients are given gentle and gradual rehabilitation with regard to mouth opening to prevent postoperative trismus by postoperative day 7.

Outcome, prognosis, and complications

Complications after a flap transfer to the oral cavity are not uncommon. Acute complications often relate to the surgery itself, while chronic complications may result from improper flap design and inset, poor patient self-care, or related to the cancer treatment, such as postoperative radiation therapy.

Complications post buccal and tongue reconstructions

Acute complications

The keys for high success rate of microsurgical free flap transfers include careful preoperative planning, delicate flap dissection, accurate microsurgical anastomosis, proper flap inset, and careful monitoring of the flap postoperatively. Early re-exploration and management of the complications are also very important. Acute complications include compromised flap circulation that requires re-exploration, poor wound healing, and wound infection.

The rate of re-exploration due to compromised flap circulation was reported in 5–25% of patients. However, the salvage rate for a compromised flap is highly dependent on the time of surgical intervention and the surgeon's experience.[215] Most cases of compromised vascular flow will manifest on the first postoperative day or within the first few days.[215] More than 50% of the vascular compromise cases presented signs of compromise as early as 4 hours postoperatively, and more than 80% of the cases within the first 24 hours.[216] With early intervention, the salvage rate of total flap loss can be greater than 80%. Vascular compromise can result from thrombosis due to poor microsurgical techniques. More frequently, however, it is related to improper flap inset, kinking or twisting of the vascular pedicle.

Wound infection is a common complication for head and neck reconstruction and accounts for up to 48% of all complications.[70,217] Effective drainage of the neck and obliteration of the dead space are important to decrease postoperative hematoma and subsequent infection.

Oral cavity cancer patients are usually malnourished, and this has a negative impact on wound healing. During surgery, a watertight closure is important to prevent saliva leakage from the oral cavity into the neck, which is one of the most common reasons for neck wound infection and delayed wound healing. Although the reported rate of an orocutaneous fistula after head and neck reconstruction is only 3%, its presence can threaten the viability of the flap.[218–221] Persistent exposure of the vascular pedicle to oral secretions and oral flora increases the incidence of infection and potential disruption of the anastomosis. This is the most common reason for delayed flap failure after wound infection. Enteral feeding as early as possible can help to reduce malnutrition and other related complications.

Chronic complications

Trismus is the most common long-term complication after oral cavity reconstruction, usually due to scar contracture, inadequate postoperative rehabilitation, and/or postoperative radiotherapy. The size of the free flap will usually shrink to a certain extent after surgery. This condition is exacerbated by radiotherapy. Progressive contraction of the flap can result in a sunken appearance, a condition typically seen in patients with through-and-through defects.

Orocutaneous fistulae with persistent saliva leakage from the oral cavity to the neck may result from poor intraoral wound healing, teeth necrosis, or osteoradionecrosis. Patients typically present with nonhealing intraoral and neck wounds with persistent discharge from the neck wound that does not improve despite aggressive wound care and antibiotics. Treatments should include enteral tube feeding and surgical debridement with flap coverage. Occasionally, the fistula is small and cannot be visually identified. A methylene blue-water test or a head and neck computed tomography scan can be performed to detect the fistulae.

Complications post mandibular reconstruction

Acute complications

Acute complications appear within 1 week postoperatively, including re-exploration, wound dehiscence, and partial skin paddle loss. Subacute complications occur between 1 week and 1 month postoperatively, consisting of infection, skin flap loss, wound dehiscence, donor site morbidity, and fibula bone loss. Chang reported a success rate of 98.2%, partial skin loss of 29%, and partial bone loss of 3% in a series of 116 mandibular reconstructions using fibula OSC flaps with a mean ischemia time of 3.6 hours.[209]

Chronic complications

Chronic complications beyond the 1-month period include infection, malocclusion, donor site morbidity, skin flap loss, or radiotherapy-related orocutaneous fistula or osteoradionecrosis. Osteoradionecrosis has been described as hypovascularity, hypocellularity, and local tissue hypoxia.[222] Radiation-related osteoradionecrosis, neck contractures, and wound-healing problems with subsequent plate exposure are frequent in patients undergoing fibula osteocutaneous flap for mandibular reconstruction.[223,224] Osteoradionecrosis due to obliteration of the inferior alveolar artery and radiated fibrosis of the periosteum was reported to occur in 0.8–37% of cases.[225] Osteoradionecrosis often involves the native residual mandible, especially in the buccal cortex.[226]

Once osteoradionecrosis develops, management should include wide excision of the radionecrotic bone, coverage with a muscle flap, or replacement with another osteocutaneous flap. Hyperbaric oxygen has been used in the treatment of osteoradionecrosis, without significant improvement. Its use is not indicated for cancer patients due to potential local recurrence.

One way of preventing osteoradionecrosis is having enough soft tissue and bone coverage in the irradiated field. The risks of osteoradionecrosis, trismus, and plate exposure were significantly lower in the OPAC flap with soleus (29%) than the traditional fibula osteocutaneous flap (53.1%)[227] (option 6 in **Table 12.7**). Additional soft-tissue coverage of the hardware and bone can also be provided to decrease these complications by means of double free flaps using one fibula osteocutaneous flap and one ALT myocutaneous flap (option 3 in **Table 12.7**).

Secondary procedures

Common reasons for secondary revisions following oral cavity reconstruction include functional correction and cosmetic improvement. When the tumor resection involves the angle of the mouth, oral incompetence is an issue. The revision improves the drooling, which is an inconvenience in daily life, as well as improving overall aesthetic appearance. If the upper and lower lips are largely preserved, a vermilion advancement flap can usually solve the problem **(Fig. 12.11)**. However, if the lips are inadequate for advancement, a tendon graft (usual the palmaris longus tendon) is required to serve as a sling to reconstruct and restore oral competency with cheek local flaps.

Scar release with Z-plasty is an easy and effective procedure to reduce scar contracture and to smooth out the flap edges. Another commonly encountered problem is an oversized flap or an inadequate flap volume, which results in an asymmetric lower third of the face. Flap reduction can be achieved by direct excision or liposuction. If inadequate flap volume is present, fat injection can be performed. In selected patients who present with severe soft-tissue insufficiency and bony structure exposure, a second free flap transfer is another option.[228]

Acknowledgment

The authors would like to thank Miffy Chia-yu Lin MSc, Shu-Wei Kao, Drs. Holger Engel, Dung Nguyen, and Wee Leon Lam for their assistances in the preparation of this manuscript, video clips, and figures.

Access the complete references list online at **http://www.expertconsult.com**

8. Ariyan S. The pectoralis major myocutaneous flap. A versatile flap for reconstruction in the head and neck. *Plast Reconstr Surg.* 1979;63:73–81.

49. Swartz WM, Banis JC, Newton ED, et al. The osteocutaneous scapular flap for mandibular and maxillary reconstruction. *Plast Reconstr Surg.* 1986;77:530–545.

50. Urken ML, Vickery C, Weinberg H, et al. The internal oblique-iliac crest osseomyocutaneous microvascular free flap in head and neck reconstruction. *J Reconstr Microsurg.* 1989;5:203–214; discussion 15–16.

54. Wei FC, Chen HC, Chuang CC, et al. Fibular osteoseptocutaneous flap: anatomic study and clinical application. *Plast Reconstr Surg.* 1986;78:191–200.
   This paper defined the septocutaneous perforators of the peroneal artery and developed the new concept and technique of elevation of the fibular osteoseptocutaneous flap.

This discovery expanded the applications of the fibula flap to complex composite tissue defect reconstruction, most notably in head and neck reconstruction.

55. Hidalgo DA. Fibula free flap: a new method of mandible reconstruction. *Plast Reconstr Surg.* 1989;84(1):71–79.

    This is a landmark paper that reported the first successful clinical series using the free fibula osseous flap for mandibular reconstruction. It revolutionized the surgical treatment of mandibular reconstruction. Hidalgo showed that the fibula osseous flap is a reliable flap that can give good reconstructive and aesthetic results, and can be harvested without significant donor site morbidity.

62. Cheng MH, Saint-Cyr M, Ali RS, et al. Osteomyocutaneous peroneal artery-based combined flap for reconstruction of composite and en bloc mandibular defects. *Head Neck.* 2009;31:361–370.

    The inclusion of the soleus muscle with the fibula septocutaneous flap based on separate musculocutaneous perforators defines the concept of a chimeric flap for head and neck reconstruction. This significant contribution allows for three-dimensional reconstruction of complex mandibular defects with better functional and aesthetic outcomes than previous reconstructive options.

107. Engel H, Huang JJ, Lin CY, et al. A Strategic Approach for Tongue Reconstruction to Achieve Predictable and Improved Functional and Aesthetic Outcomes. *Plast Reconstr Surg.* 2010;126:1967–1977.

    This paper provides a practical algorithm for the assessment and treatment options for tongue reconstruction. This is the first paper that comprehensively and logically outlines a decision-making tree to select the most appropriate flap for reconstruction, based on the size of the tongue defect and the involvement of the adjacent tissues. It also outlines the appropriate flap design to use for each type of tongue reconstruction to give predictable, evidence-based, good functional and aesthetic results.

141. Jewer DD, Boyd JB, Manktelow RT, et al. Orofacial and mandibular reconstruction with the iliac crest free flap: a review of 60 cases and a new method of classification. *Plast Reconstr Surg.* 1989;84:391–403; discussion 4–5.

148. Yang GF, Chen BJ, Gao YZ. The free forearm flap. *Chin Med J.* 1981;61:4.

154. Song YG, Chen GZ, Song YL. The free thigh flap: a new free flap concept based on the septocutaneous artery. *Br J Plast Surg.* 1984;37:149–159.

    Song et al. outlined the anatomical basis of the anterolateral thigh flap as a new donor site for a free flap or pedicled flap. This paper introduces the first perforator flap based on the lateral circumflex femoral vessels. This contribution is pivotal to the understanding and eventual development of other flaps based on the lateral thigh system. The anterolateral thigh flap and its various modifications have since became a workhorse flap in head and neck reconstruction.

13

Hypopharyngeal, esophageal, and neck reconstruction

Peirong Yu

SYNOPSIS

- Pharyngoesophageal defects are most commonly the result of a total laryngopharyngectomy for squamous cell carcinoma in the laryngeal region or hypopharynx. Other etiology includes benign strictures, pharyngocutaneous fistulas, and thyroid cancer involving the esophagus

- Radiotherapy has become the primary treatment for early stages of squamous cell carcinoma in these regions. Many pharyngoesophageal defects are the results of salvage laryngopharyngectomy following a radiation failure, making reconstruction more challenging. Pharyngoesophageal reconstruction requires great attention to detail, and there is no room for error. A small mistake can have a snowball effect and eventually lead to a disaster

- Commonly used flaps for pharyngoesophageal reconstruction include the jejunal flap, radial forearm flap, and the anterolateral thigh (ALT) flap. In recent years, the ALT flap has become the most popular flap for this type of reconstruction

- Major complications following pharyngoesophageal reconstruction include anastomotic strictures and fistulas. Great care should be taken to minimize these complications

- The ultimate goals of reconstruction are to provide alimentary continuity, protection of important structures such as the carotid artery, and restoration of functions such as speech and swallowing

- Most patients (greater than 90%) can eat an oral diet after reconstruction without the need for tube feeding

- Speech rehabilitation is typically provided with tracheoesophageal puncture (TEP) and fluent speech can be achieved in greater than 80% of patients. Speech quality is superior with a fasciocutaneous flap than an intestinal flap

- Many patients with pharyngoesophageal defects have a frozen neck due to previous radiotherapy and surgery, making reconstruction extremely difficult with high surgical risks. Careful planning, use of transverse cervical vessels as recipient vessels, and a two-skin island ALT flap to simultaneously resurface the neck for a through-and-through defect can simplify the procedure and reduce surgical risks.

 Access the Historical Perspective section online at
http://www.expertconsult.com

Introduction

Reconstruction of the hypopharynx and cervical esophagus is among the most challenging reconstructions today due to the complexity of reconstruction, previous radiation damage, important functional disabilities, and potential life-threatening complications such as carotid artery rupture. Therefore great care should be taken to plan the surgery carefully with more than one feasible option. One important aspect of surgical planning is to convert a complicated case into a more conventional or simple one to minimize surgical risks and maximize functional outcomes. The following key points should be kept in mind when reconstructing these defects:

- A noncircumferential esophageal defect should not be converted to a circumferential one as was commonly done when the jejunal flap was popular. Reconstruction of partial defects rarely results in anastomotic strictures.

- Distal flap-esophageal anastomosis should be spatulated to minimize stricture formation in circumferential defects.

- A layer of well-vascularized fascia of the ALT flap can be used to cover the suture lines, especially the distal anastomosis, to minimize the risk of anastomotic leakage and pharyngocutaneous fistula formation.

- Fasciocutaneous flaps provide better speech function than intestinal flaps.

- High-risk patients with significant comorbid diseases are relative contraindications for jejunal flap reconstruction. Fasciocutaneous flaps have much lower systemic morbidity.

- While bowel heals quickly when used for esophageal reconstruction, fasciocutaneous flaps may experience delayed healing when being soaked with saliva 24 hours a day, which may explain some delayed fistulas. Therefore delayed oral intake is recommended, particularly in radiated patients.

- Proper management of postoperative complications is important to prevent life-threatening sequelae and maximize function.

Basic science/anatomy

The pharynx is anatomically divided into the oropharynx, nasopharynx, and hypopharynx. The nasopharynx is essentially the structures around the nasal cavity above the soft palate. Its defects are usually the result of a maxillectomy and will be discussed elsewhere. The oropharynx is bounded by the nasopharynx superiorly, the oral cavity anteriorly, and the hypopharynx and larynx inferiorly. The superior border of the oropharynx is at the plane of the soft palate, and the inferior border is defined by the level of the hyoid bone. The main structures in the oropharynx are the base of tongue, tonsillar pillars, lateral and posterior oropharyngeal walls, and soft palate. Common oncologic defects in the oropharynx are the result of surgical resections of cancers in the base of tongue, which frequently extend to the lateral pharyngeal wall, or cancers in the tonsillar pillar extending to the soft palate. Cancers in the maxilla or parotid region with extension into the pterygoid or buccal spaces also require resection of the oropharynx, including the tonsillar pillars, lateral pharyngeal wall, soft and hard palate, and posterior mandible. The hypopharynx extends from the level of the hyoid bone to the lower border of the cricoid cartilage, which is congruous with the cervical esophagus below *(Fig. 13.1)*. This is a critical area that is responsible for airway protection and swallowing and speech functions. Common defects of the hypopharynx and cervical esophagus are the result of surgical resection of cancers in the hypopharynx and larynx, advanced thyroid cancers, radiation strictures, and chemical injuries. Isolated tumors in the cervical esophagus, although rare, may also require segmental esophagectomy and reconstruction *(Table 13.1)*. Pharyngoesophageal defects can be circumferential or partial *(Fig. 13.2)*.

Patient selection

Preoperative evaluation

Medical evaluation

Cardiovascular and pulmonary complications such as pneumonia, respiratory failure, prolonged ventilator support,

arrhythmia, myocardial infarction, pulmonary embolism, and stroke remain the most costly and debilitating medical complications after major head and neck surgery and microvascular reconstruction. Many patients with head and neck cancers have extended history of tobacco and alcohol abuse and many present at an advanced age. Therefore, a thorough medical evaluation before surgery is required. Patients with significant comorbid disease may tolerate the initial surgery but may not tolerate possible take-backs should vascular thromboses occur. Pulmonary function should be evaluated

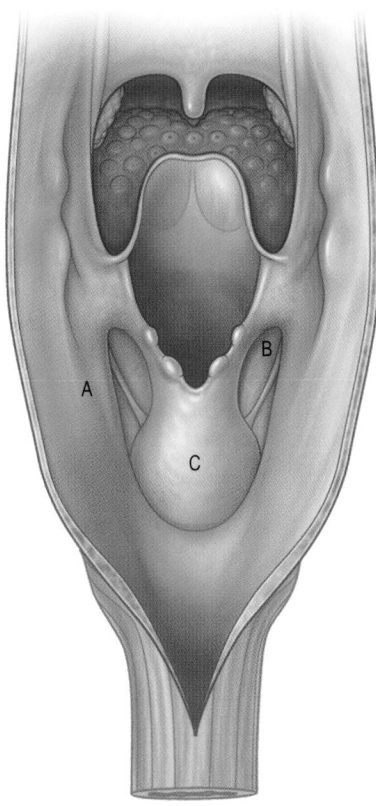

Fig. 13.1 The hypopharynx is located behind the larynx and in continuity with the oral pharynx superiorly and the cervical esophagus inferiorly. The hypopharynx is arbitrarily divided into three areas for purposes of tumor classification: the pharyngeal wall **(A)**, pyriform sinuses **(B)**, and postcricoid area **(C)**.

Table 13.1 Types of pharyngoesophageal defect requiring reconstruction

Pathology	Defect location	Type of defect
Primary SCC	Hypopharynx and cervical esophagus	Most commonly partial
Recurrent SCC	Hypopharynx and cervical esophagus	Most commonly circumferential
Advanced or recurrent thyroid cancer	Hypopharynx and cervical esophagus	Most commonly circumferential
Isolated esophageal tumors	Cervical esophagus with an intact larynx	Most commonly partial
Pharyngoesophageal or tracheoesophageal fistulas	Cervical esophagus or hypopharynx	Most commonly partial
Anastomotic strictures	Cervical esophagus	Most commonly circumferential
Radiation-induced strictures	Hypopharynx or cervical esophagus	Partial or circumferential, depending on the degree of stricture

SCC, squamous cell carcinoma.

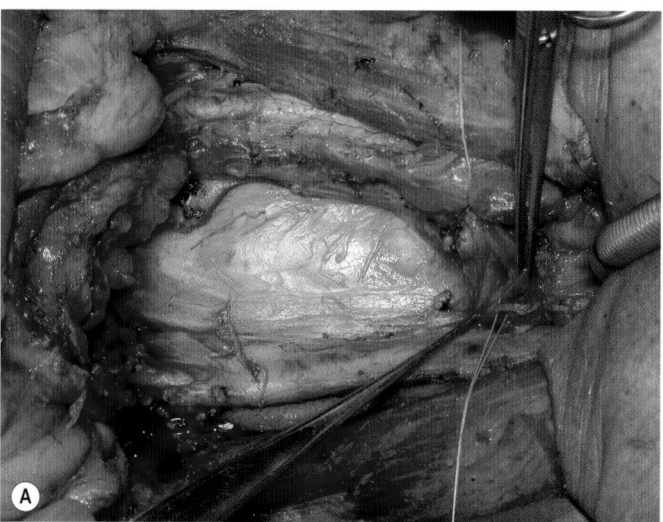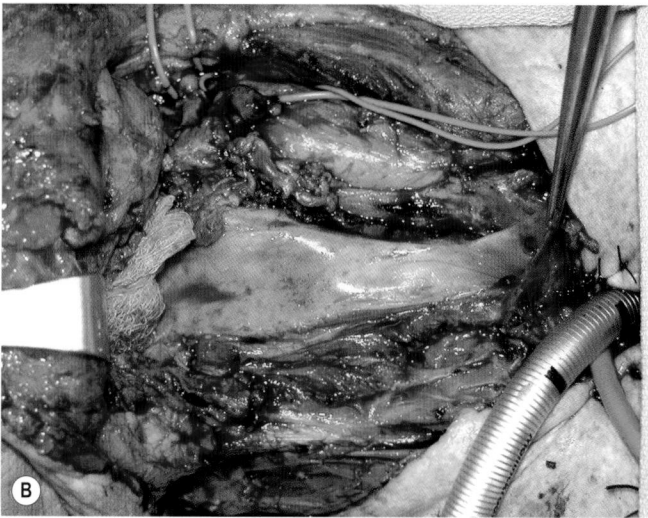

Fig. 13.2 Pharyngoesophageal defects can be circumferential **(A)** or partial **(B)**. In the former, the superior limit is the base of tongue and the inferior limit is the esophagus above the sternal notch. Posterior (deep) to the defect is the prevertebral fascia. In partial defects, there is usually 2 cm of posterior pharyngeal mucosa remaining.

in patients with chronic obstructive pulmonary disease, and cardiovascular workup should be performed as indicated. Carotid artery diseases are also common. History of cerebral vascular accidents should be noted and carotid artery imaging should be performed as indicated. Carefully reviewing head and neck computed tomography (CT) images with intravenous contrast can usually reveal the status of the carotid arteries and the availability of recipient vessels in the neck. Patients are encouraged at the time of presentation to stop smoking and drinking and are referred to smoking cessation clinics as needed.

History of radiotherapy and surgery

Radiotherapy has become the primary treatment for early stages of squamous cell carcinomas in the hypopharynx and larynx. Therefore, the majority of patients requiring pharyngoesophageal reconstruction are those of radiation failure. They also commonly have had neck dissection after radiotherapy. Thus, reconstructive surgeons now face more difficult cases with a history of radiotherapy and surgery. These defects are among the most difficult to repair in head and neck reconstruction. A thorough history of previous radiotherapy and surgery should be obtained to prepare better for a potentially complicated reconstruction. Preoperative CT images should be carefully reviewed to evaluate the availability of possible recipient vessels.

Donor site evaluation

Common donor sites such as the thigh, forearm, abdomen, and anterior chest should be evaluated for skin quality and thickness, history of surgery or trauma, and vascular disease. The subcutaneous tissue in the thigh in female patients is usually twice as thick as in male patients,[60] therefore, considerations should be given when choosing a flap. Allen's test is commonly used to assess the adequacy of hand perfusion through the ulnar artery when reconstruction with a radial forearm flap is planned. A bracelet with the words "NO IV"

is placed on the potential donor site arm, which is usually the one with the nondominant hand. Previous abdominal surgery and severe comorbid diseases are relative contraindications for a jejunal flap. Careful planning is essential for successful reconstruction. One should always have a "plan B" or even "plan C" for complex cases.

Pharyngoesophageal reconstruction requires great attention to detail, and there is no room for error. A small mistake can have a snowball effect and eventually lead to a series of problems and failure of reconstruction. Failure of reconstruction in the head and neck region may severely impair patients' function and quality of life. The patient and family should be made fully aware of potential functional deficits, including the possibility of long-term tube-feeding dependency, and the inability to speak. Complication rates with pharyngoesophageal reconstruction can be high and functional outcomes disappointing. Providing coverage alone is no longer adequate. Every effort should be made to maximize function, minimize donor site morbidities, and improve aesthetic results. In addition to being nonvocal following a total laryngopharyngectomy, postreconstruction complications such as pharyngocutaneous fistulas and anastomotic strictures may render patients dependent on tube feeding.

Choice of flaps

With the advances in microsurgery, free-flap reconstruction has largely replaced pedicled flaps for large head and neck oncological defects, especially those with prior radiotherapy, which renders pedicled flaps unreliable. The thoracic skin flap once used in the 1950s and the deltopectoral flap developed in the 1960s are no longer used for pharyngoesophageal reconstruction in modern-day practice. The only pedicled flap that still plays a role either as a primary reconstruction or as a salvage procedure is the pectoralis major flap which gained popularity in the early 1980s. Although it is easy to harvest, no microsurgical skills are required, and it may work well in experienced hands for partial pharyngoesophageal defects in male patients, the flap can be bulky, the skin paddle can be

Table 13.2 Advantages and disadvantages of commonly used flaps

	ALT	Jejunum	Radial forearm
Flap elevation	Moderately difficult	Moderately difficult	Easy
Flap reliability	Good	Good	Good
Flap thickness	Can be too thick	Good	Good
Primary healing	Good	Best	Good
Donor site morbidity	Low	High	Moderate
Recovery time	Quick	Can be slow	Quick
Fistula rates	Low	Low	Moderate
Stricture rates	Low	High	Moderate
TEP voice	Good	Poor	Good
Swallowing	Good	Good	Good
Use for circumferential defects	Yes	Yes	Second choice
Use for partial defects	Yes	No	Yes
Contraindications	Obesity, with a very thick thigh	Severe comorbidity, prior abdominal surgery	Thin patient with a small arm, radial dominance

ALT, anterolateral thigh flap; TEP, tracheoesophageal puncture.

unreliable especially in smokers, fistula rate can be high, and functional outcomes may not be as good. Common free-flap options include the radial forearm flap, the jejunal flap, and, more recently, the ALT flap. Although reliable and easy to harvest, the radial forearm flap traditionally has a reputation of having high fistula rates, especially delayed fistulas. The jejunal flap enjoyed its reliability and became the flap of choice for circumferential pharyngoesophageal defects in the early 1990s. The major disadvantage is the added abdominal surgery. Since the ALT flap was first used for pharyngoesophageal reconstruction at our institution in early 2002 by the author,[54] it quickly gained popularity and replaced both the radial forearm and jejunal flaps as the flap of choice for both partial and circumferential defects. The advantages and disadvantages of each flap are listed in *Table 13.2*. An algorithm for pharyngoesophageal reconstruction is outlined in *Figure 13.3*.

If the ALT flap is unavailable owing to a lack of perforators, the jejunal flap is the next choice for repair of circumferential defects in patients at low risk. In patients who are at high risk or obese or who have a history of abdominal/gastrointestinal surgeries and for partial defects, the radial forearm flap is the next choice. The pectoralis major flap can be used for partial defects in male patients, for salvage after failed free-flap reconstruction, or in very high-risk patients. In our recent experience of 119 pharyngoesophageal reconstructions,[59] the ALT flap was used in all but 5 patients. In these 5 patients, the ALT was deemed too thick or unavailable upon exploration.

If the patient is not considered a good candidate for reconstruction or does not wish to go through another major surgery after a failed reconstruction, a spit fistula is created in the upper neck to drain the saliva, the cervical esophagus is closed and covered with a pectoralis major muscle flap, and a permanent feeding gastrostomy or jejunostomy is performed.

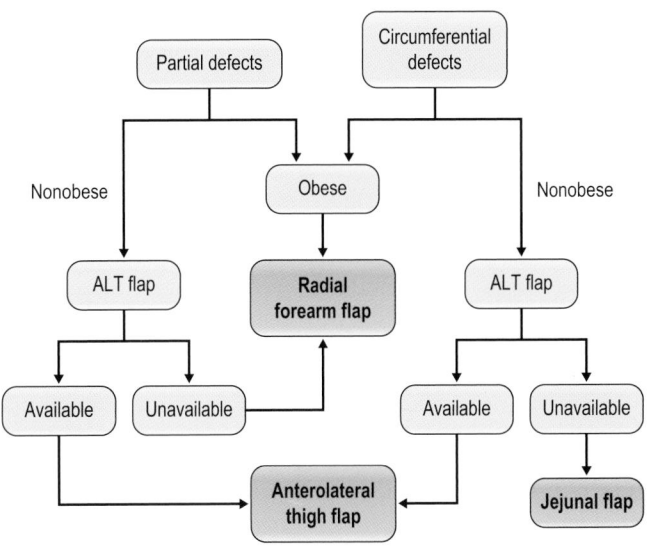

Fig. 13.3 An algorithm of flap selection for pharyngoesophageal reconstruction.

Surgical technique

Reconstruction with the anterolateral thigh flap

Video 1

Flap design and harvesting

Either thigh can be used to harvest the ALT flap. However, the right thigh is preferred for right-handed surgeons because it allows for easier dissection of the vascular pedicle. It is critical to keep the leg in a neutral position without rotations when designing the ALT flap. When a patient is under general anesthesia, the leg has a natural tendency to rotate outwards. Therefore, before prepping and draping, attention should be paid to avoiding such rotation, since it may cause misplacement of perforator locations and, ultimately, failure to capture the cutaneous perforators. An easy way to keep the legs from rotating outward is to wrap each foot with a towel and clip the towels together.

Once the legs are in the correct position, the anterior superior iliac spine and the superolateral corner of the patella are marked and a straight line is drawn connecting the two landmarks – the anteroposterior (A-P) line. The midpoint of the A-P line is then marked. There are usually one to three usable cutaneous perforators in the ALT flap territory. The middle perforator, perforator B, is located an average of 1.4 cm lateral to the midpoint of the A-P line.[60,61] Perforator A is located approximately 5 cm proximal to perforator B, and perforator C is 5 cm distal to perforator B *(Fig. 13.4)*. The flap design is centered on the presumed location of perforator B. Doppler examination can be used to help locate the cutaneous perforators. However, the accuracy is only fair. The false-positive rate can be high, and more than 25% of Doppler signals are more than 10 mm away from the actual location of the cutaneous perforator. The accuracy is particularly poor in obese patients.[61] We have found that localization of the perforators based on this "ABC" system is more accurate than hand-held Doppler examination.

Flap elevation is performed simultaneously with tumor ablation using a two-team approach. The reconstructed neoesophagus should have a diameter of 3 cm. Therefore, for circumferential defects, a flap 9.4 cm wide is needed to form a 3-cm-diameter $(3 \times \pi)$ tubed neoesophagus *(Fig. 13.5)*.[54] For partial defects, the width of the flap is calculated by subtracting the width of the remaining pharyngeal mucosa from 9.4 cm. For example, if the remaining mucosa is 2 cm wide, the needed flap width would be 7.4 cm. The flap length should be slightly longer than the actual defect but the two ends should be tapered and included in the flap design. Flap design is tentatively centered on the presumed perforator B location. A straight anterior incision approximately 15 cm long is made first across all three cutaneous perforators down to the fascia. This incision corresponds to the anterior midline of the thigh in most cases. A wider fascia is included for second-layer closure during flap insetting. Therefore, the fascial incision is made 1–2 cm more medially than the anterior skin incision *(Fig. 13.6)*. Subfascial dissection proceeds laterally until the

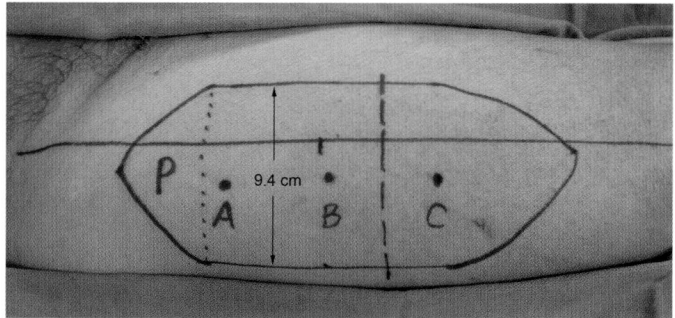

Fig. 13.5 The flap is designed to include two or three potential perforators so that a second skin paddle, usually based on perforator C, can be used for neck resurfacing or monitoring. A lip of the flap is extended proximally (P) to form an elongated oblique opening of the tube flap to accommodate the wider opening in the floor of the mouth.

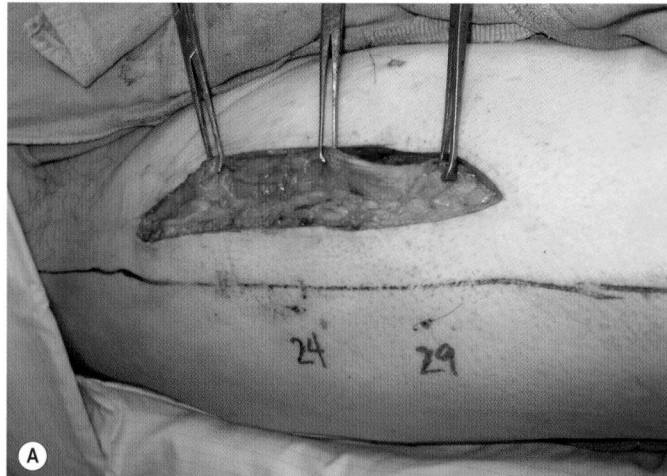

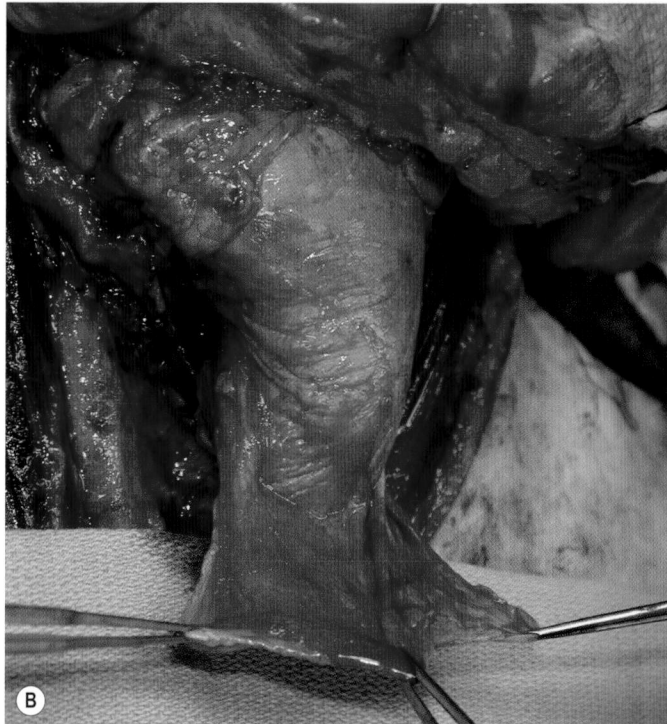

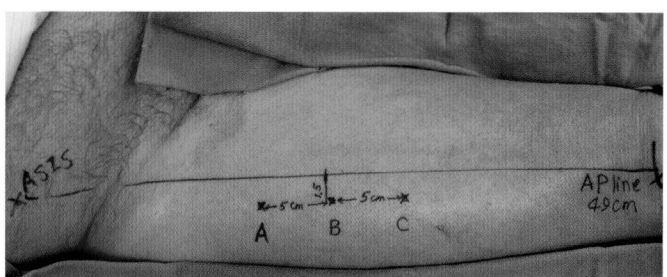

Fig. 13.4 Design of the anterolateral thigh flap for pharyngoesophageal reconstruction. The midpoint of the line connecting the anterior superior iliac spine and the superolateral corner of the patella (anteroposterior line) is marked. Perforator B is usually located 1.5 cm lateral to the midpoint. Perforators A and C are located 5 cm proximal and distal to perforator B, respectively. ASIS, anterior superior iliac spine; AP, anteroposterior.

Fig. 13.6 A wider fascia than skin is included in the anterolateral thigh flap **(A)** so that the fascia can be used to cover the suture line **(B)**.

cutaneous perforators are identified. The exact locations of the perforators are marked on the skin surface with a 5-0 polypropylene suture. The flap is then recentered, if necessary, on the basis of the actual perforator locations. To accommodate the wide opening in the pharyngeal inlet for the proximal anastomosis, an extended lip of skin is designed at the proximal end of the flap so that an elongated oblique opening can be created when the flap is tubed (*Figs 13.15* and *13.7*). Dissection of the perforators and the main pedicle can be performed through the anterior incision only. The remaining flap is incised only after the cutaneous perforators and the main vascular pedicle are located or dissected out. Two cutaneous perforators are included whenever possible so that the flap can be divided into two skin paddles (*Fig. 13.8*). The proximal one, usually based on perforator B or A, is used for reconstruction of the pharyngoesophageal defect, and the distal one, usually based on perforator C, is used for flap monitoring or for anterior neck and tracheal reconstruction (*Fig. 13.9*). If only one perforator is present and there is an anterior neck defect to be reconstructed, a segment or the superficial half of the vastus lateralis muscle is included in the ALT flap to support skin grafts to resurface the neck, eliminating the need for a second flap.[62] This layer of muscle is usually

no more than 1 cm thick, and usually a better option than a pectoralis major muscle flap (*Fig. 13.10*). The descending branch of the lateral circumflex femoral artery usually travels within the muscle, and the surgical plane of dissection is immediately deep to the descending branch, splitting the muscle.

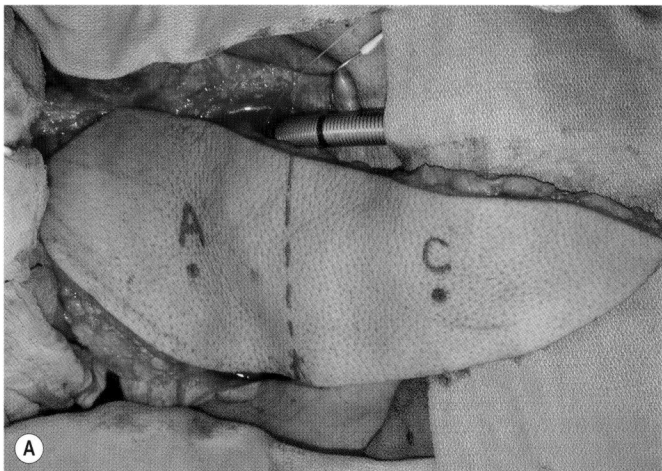

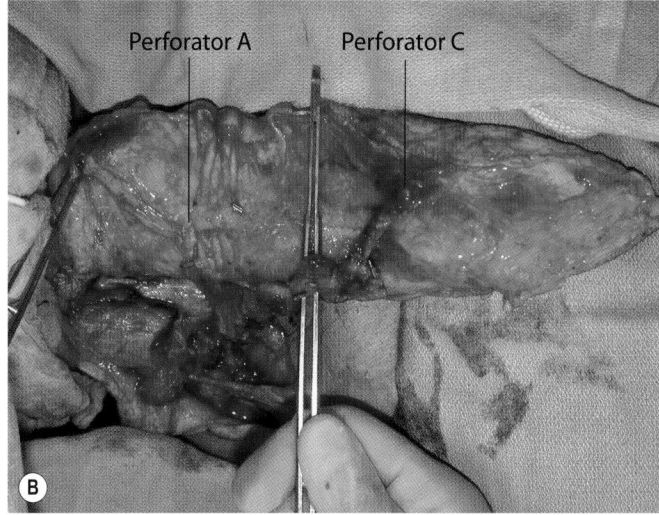

Fig. 13.8 (A) By including two perforators, the flap can be divided into two skin paddles based on separate cutaneous perforators A and C. **(B)** The forcep indicates where the division line is.

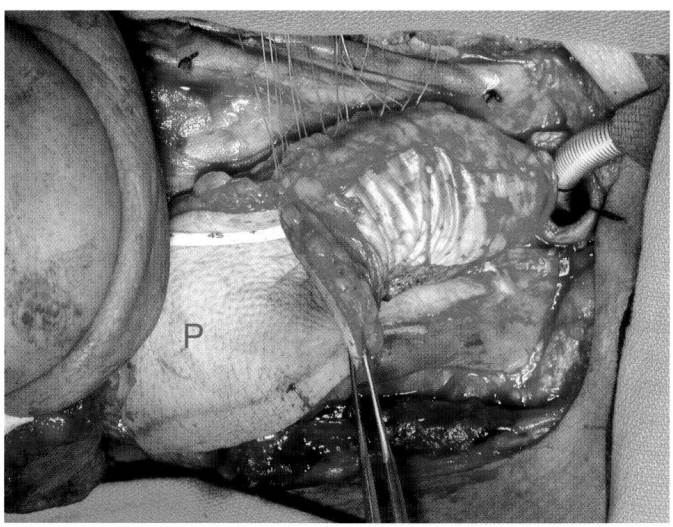

Fig. 13.7 The flap is tubed and a larger oblique opening at the proximal end of the tubed flap is formed by including the extended portion of the flap (P).

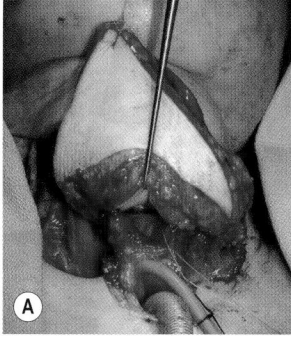
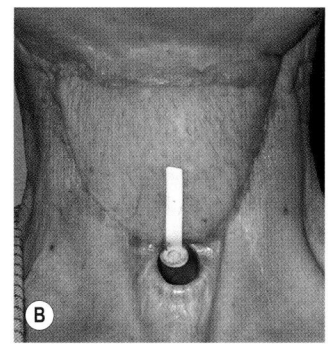
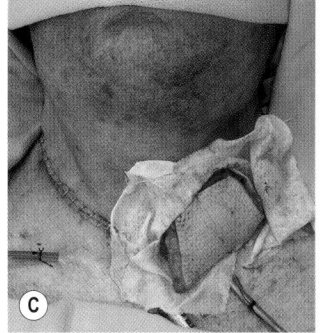
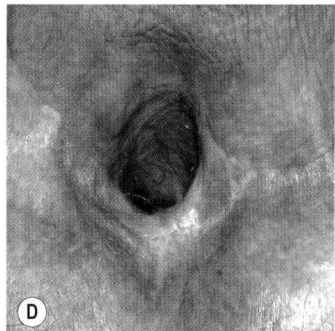

Fig. 13.9 The second skin paddle, based on perforator C, can be used for neck resurfacing **(A)**. This avoids the use of a second flap and adds minimal bulk in the neck so as not to obstruct the tracheostomy **(B)**. The second skin island can also be used solely as a monitoring segment **(C)**, and is removed before the patient is discharged from the hospital, or for posterior tracheal wall reconstruction. **(D)** Healed flap with hair growth.

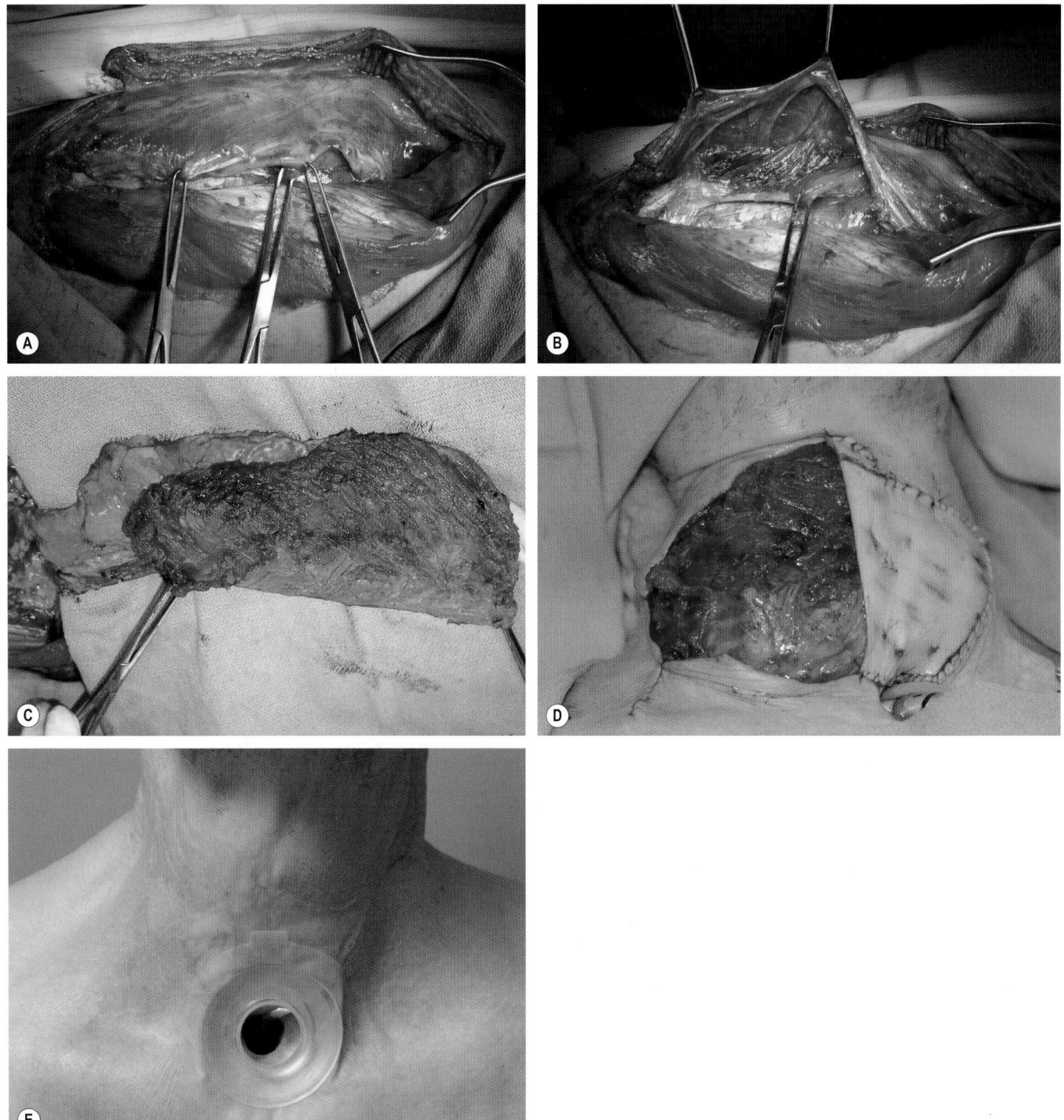

Fig. 13.10 When there is only one perforator present, the superficial half of the vastus lateralis muscle is included to support skin grafts. The descending branch travels alongside the medial edge of the vastus lateralis muscle **(A)**. The superficial half of the muscle is separated from the deep half immediately below the muscular branches **(B)**. A thin and broad muscle is thus obtained **(C)** to cover the neck defect with skin grafting **(D)**. Such a thin muscle produces minimal bulk so as not to obstruct the tracheostomy **(E)**.

Flap insetting

Partial or complete flap insetting is performed before vascular anastomosis to avoid accidental traction injury to the vascular pedicle. In most cases, the proximal anastomosis of the flap with the base of tongue and posterior pharyngeal mucosa is performed first *(Fig. 13.11)*. If the flap is longer than the defect,

the perforator of the flap should be placed near the center of the defect and extra flap trimmed if necessary. Although some surgeons prefer tubing the flap in the thigh before transfer, I find it is easier to perform the proximal anastomosis without tubing the flap first. I usually use a 3-0 polyglactin suture in a simple, interrupted fashion. The longitudinal seam is oriented posterolaterally at 4 or 8 o'clock *(Fig. 13.11)*. The

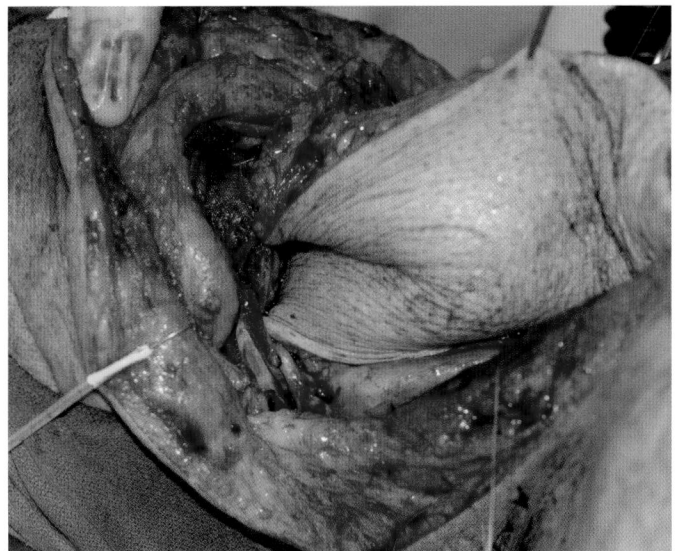

Fig. 13.11 The proximal anastomosis of the flap to base of tongue is usually performed first.

anastomosis starts with two corner sutures at 3 and 9 o'clock. The posterior wall is then completed, followed by the anterior wall. Large bites are recommended with inversion of the skin and mucosal edges into the lumen. Care should be taken to avoid catching the hypoglossal nerve when suturing the flap to the base of the tongue. Next, the longitudinal seam is completed towards the distal end of the flap, also with simple, interrupted sutures. For partial defects, the proximal end of the flap is sewn to the base of the tongue and the lateral edges to the remaining posterior pharyngeal wall mucosa *(Fig. 13.12)*.

The ALT flap in most patients is thicker than desired. The flap can be thinned by direct excision of subcutaneous fat at the periphery of the flap. In most cases, this is all that is needed for thinning. Peripheral thinning makes flap insetting much easier without jeopardizing the perfusion. When more aggressive thinning is needed, the perforators should be well visualized either with loupe magnification or under the microscope when they enter the flap and are traced within the subcutaneous tissue. The perforators usually divide into

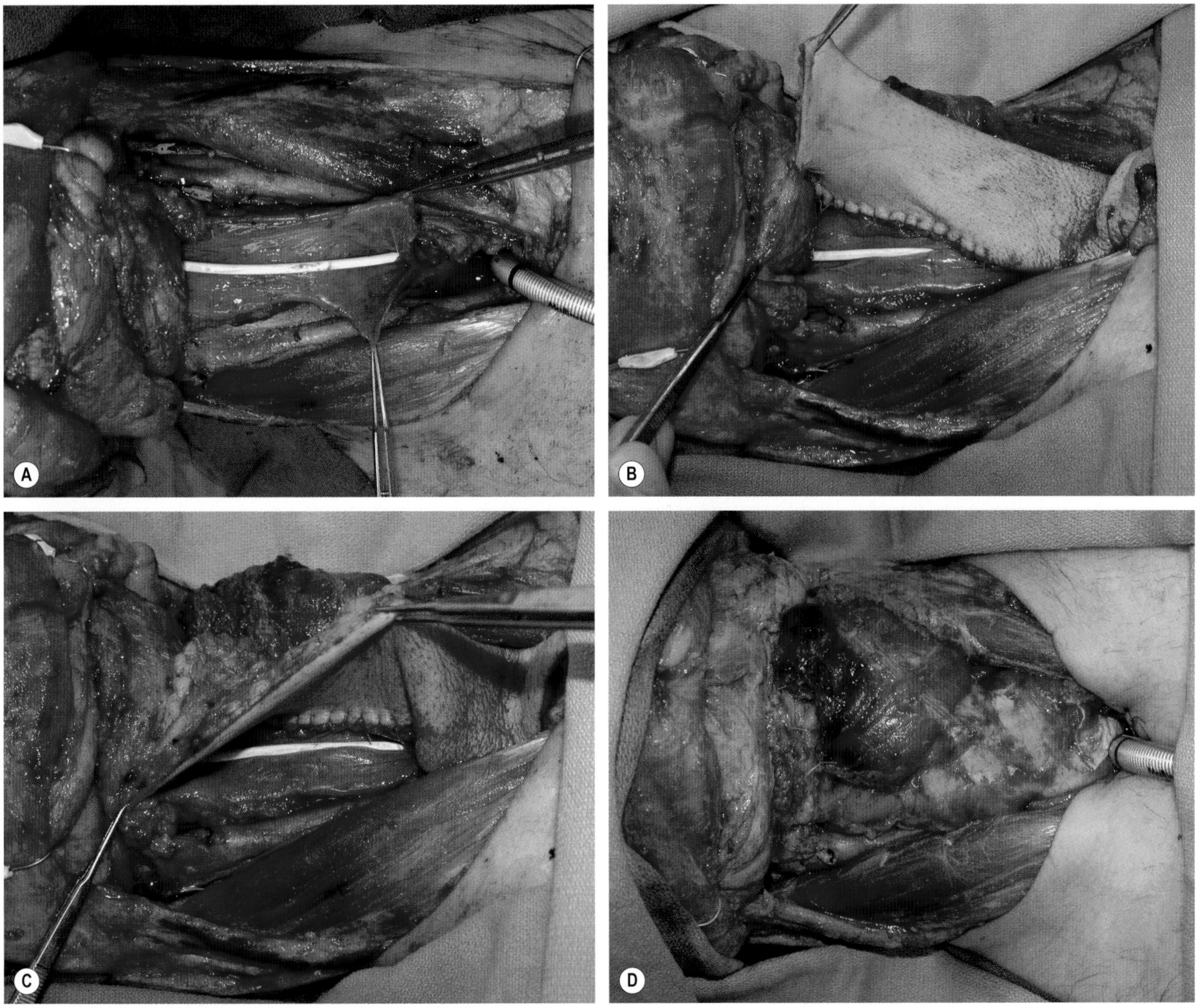

Fig. 13.12 For partial pharyngoesophageal defects **(A)**, the flap is sewn to the lateral edges of the posterior pharyngeal mucosa **(B, C)**. The fascia of the flap and a small segment of the vastus lateralis muscle can be used to cover the reconstruction **(D)**.

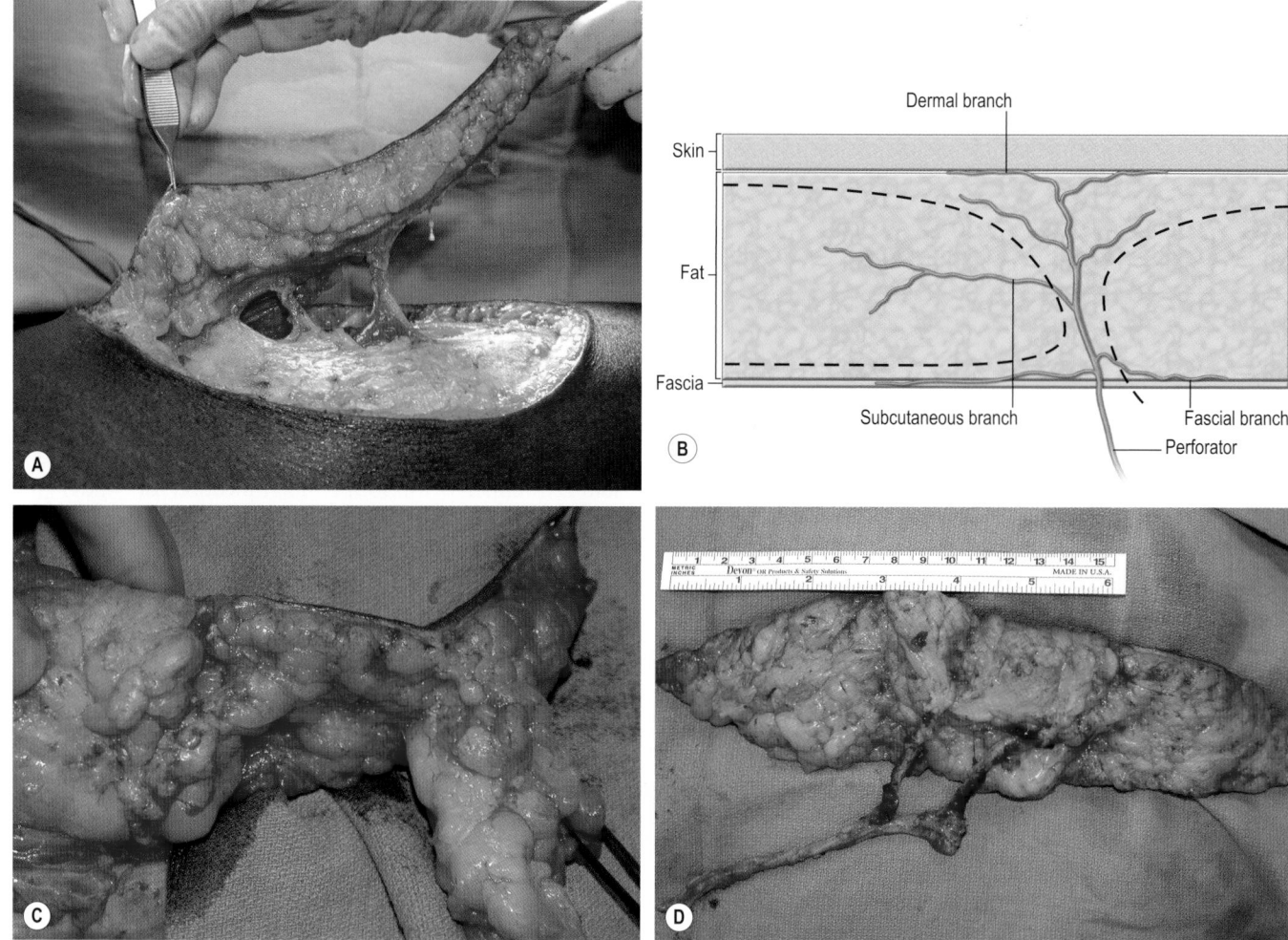

Fig. 13.13 Thinning of the anterolateral thigh flap. The proximal flap is thicker than the distal part **(A)**. Once entering the flap, the cutaneous perforator gives off several branches to the fascia, subcutaneous tissue, and subdermal plexus **(B)**. Flap thinning can be performed by direct excision of the subcutaneous fat away from the main perforator and the subdermal plexus (dotted lines). The fascia can be left intact if needed. Several millimeters of subcutaneous tissue are left below the dermis to protect the subdermal plexus **(C and D)**.

fascial branches, subcutaneous branches, and the main branch terminates in the subdermal plexus *(Fig. 13.13)*. These branches may take an oblique course within the subcutaneous tissue in a thick flap. Blindly trimming the fat around the main perforator may damage the branches within the flap and compromise the perfusion. Ample subcutaneous tissue should be left around the cutaneous perforators, and 2–3 mm of subcutaneous tissue is left on the dermis to protect the subdermal plexus *(Fig. 13.13)*.

Some surgeons advocate the use of the Montgomery salivary bypass tube in circumferential defects potentially to decrease the incidence of leak and stricture. The value, however, is unclear. In my experience, the indications for the use of the Montgomery tube include: a thick flap (narrow lumen), difficult flap insetting, very low location of the transected cervical esophageal end, small cervical esophagus, or poor tissue quality due to radiation injury. A 14-mm-diameter Montgomery salivary bypass tube is used. The tube is inserted through the mouth before the longitudinal seam of the flap is completed *(Fig. 13.14)*. The proximal flange of the bypass tube is placed above the proximal anastomosis and the

distal end in the esophagus below the distal anastomosis. A number 1 polypropylene suture is attached to the flange of the tube, brought out through the mouth, and taped to the cheek to prevent distal migration and facilitate easy removal of the tube. If a feeding tube has not yet been placed, a Dobhoff feeding tube is placed through the nose, the tubed flap, or inside the Montgomery salivary bypass tube, and the cervical esophagus to the stomach.

Next, the neck is repositioned from the hyperextended position to a neutral position by removing the shoulder roll. It is not necessary to flex the neck. The anterior wall of the cervical esophagus is split longitudinally for approximately 1.5 cm to spatulate the distal anastomosis *(Fig. 13.15)*. This is important to enlarge the distal anastomosis and minimize the risk of ring stricture. On the flap, a triangular lip is created and inserted into the longitudinal split of the esophagus to complete the spatulation *(Fig. 13.16)*. The tubed flap is slightly twisted so that the longitudinal seam at the distal anastomosis is facing posteriorly at 6 o'clock. Such positioning of the tubed flap places the perforator vessels anteriorly between 11 and 1 o'clock to avoid compression of the perforators against the

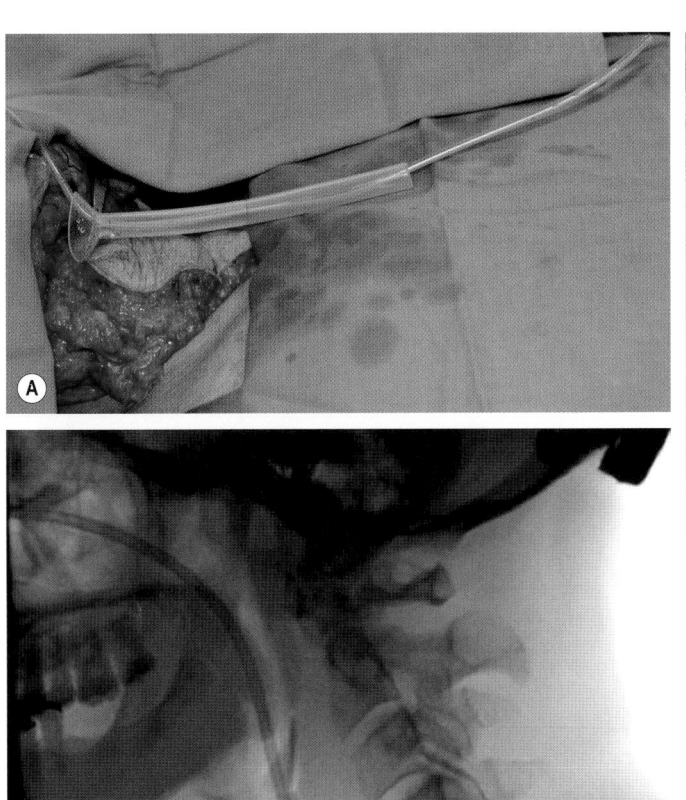

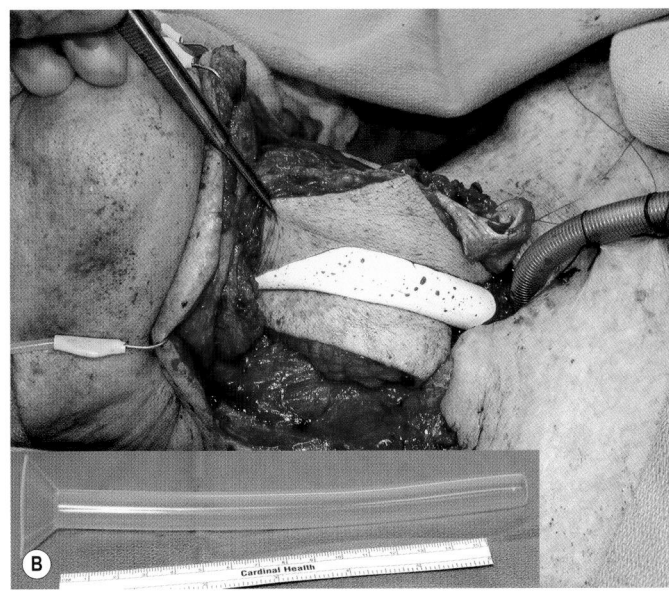

Fig. 13.14 (A, B) A Montgomery salivary bypass tube with a diameter of 14 mm can be used to stent the neopharynx temporarily for 2–6 weeks. **(C)** The flange of the tube at the proximal end sits above the neopharyngeal inlet.

prevertebral fascia *(Fig. 13.17)*. If necessary, the width of the flap is tapered to match the size of the cervical esophagus for the distal anastomosis. The flap is pulled straight to avoid redundancy but should not be stretched, as is commonly done with the jejunal flap, and anastomotic tension should be avoided. After completion of the distal anastomosis, the fascia of the flap is used to cover the suture lines *(Fig. 13.17)*.

The neck wound is then irrigated with an ample amount of warm normal saline (2 or 3 liters), taking care not to squirt the saline directly on the vascular pedicle to avoid vessel spasm. Meticulous hemostasis is essential to avoid a postoperative hematoma, which can compress the vascular pedicle. All areas should be carefully examined, even if they have already been examined by the ablative surgeons. A 15-Fr. Blake drain is placed on each side of the neck, lateral to the internal jugular vein. At this point, the neck is slightly flexed (take out the shoulder roll and flex the neck), and the vascular pedicle is examined again. Because the neck is usually hyperextended during surgery, flexing the neck to a normal position can significantly change the position of the vascular pedicle,

causing kinking or compression. The pedicle is repositioned as needed to avoid such problems. If the pedicle is long, a gentle loop of the pedicle can avoid kinking *(Fig. 13.18)*.

The second skin paddle is then turned outward to resurface the neck for flap monitoring or used to reconstruct the trachea or any neck skin defects *(Fig. 13.9)*. Externalizing a portion of the distal flap by de-epithelializing a strip of skin around the distal anastomosis *(Fig. 13.19)* is not recommended because it results in a high fistula rate.[54] To monitor a buried flap without an external skin island, an implantable Doppler probe (Cook-Swartz) can be secured to the vein and carefully fixed to the neck skin. Alternatively, a hand-held Doppler device can be used to monitor the perforator or the main vascular pedicle through the neck skin. Neither method is very reliable, however. The Cook-Swartz implantable Doppler has a high false-positive rate[63] because any movement of the neck, including coughing, can potentially dislodge the probe, resulting in an unnecessary surgical exploration. Also, tiny blood clots can lodge between the Doppler probe and the vessel wall, causing the disappearance of the Doppler signal. The

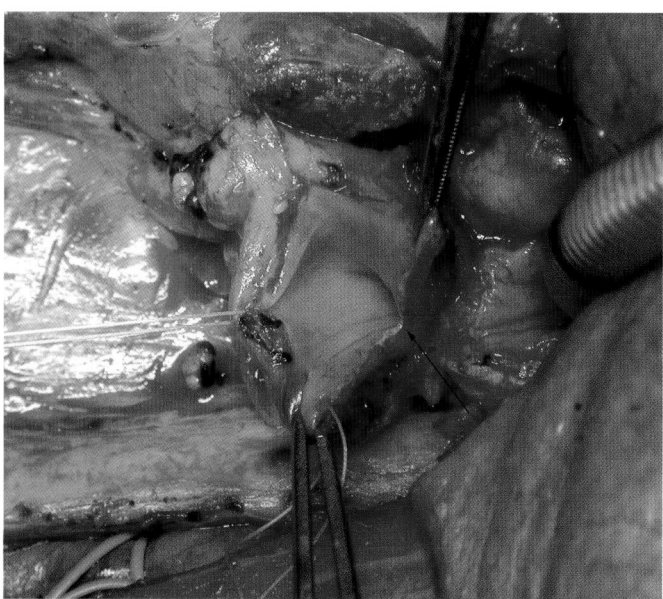

Fig. 13.15 The cervical esophageal end is incised longitudinally for about 1.5 cm to spatulate the anastomosis.

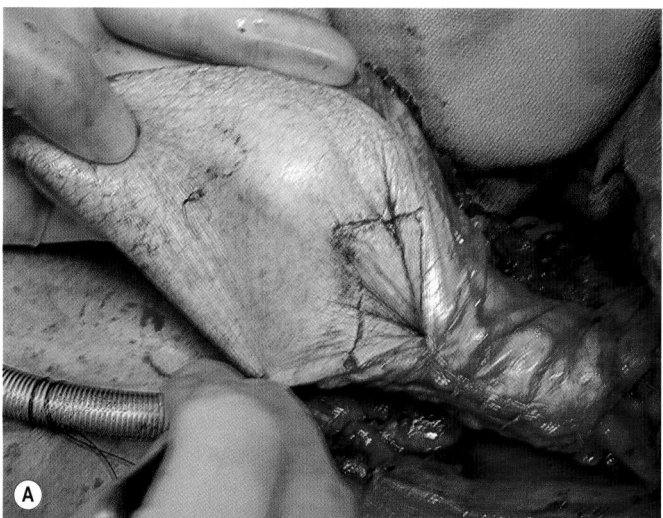

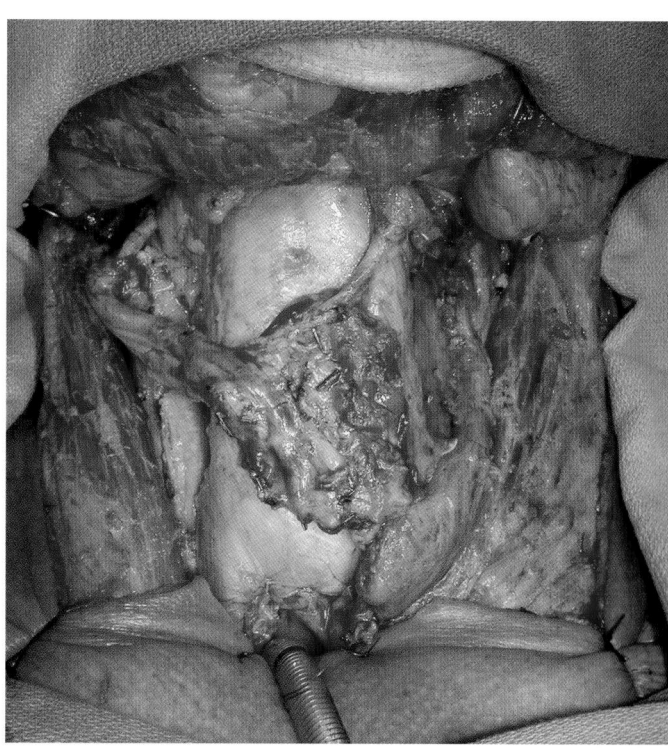

Fig. 13.17 The perforators are positioned anteriorly to avoid compression of the perforators between the flap and the prevertebral fascia. A wider fascia is designed to cover the suture lines as a second layer after flap insetting.

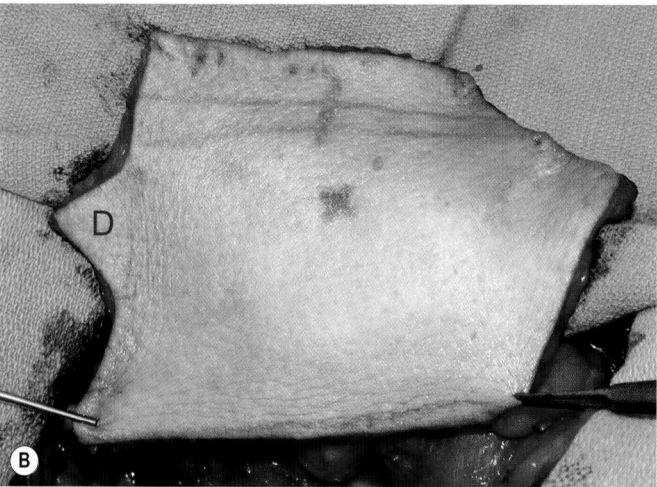

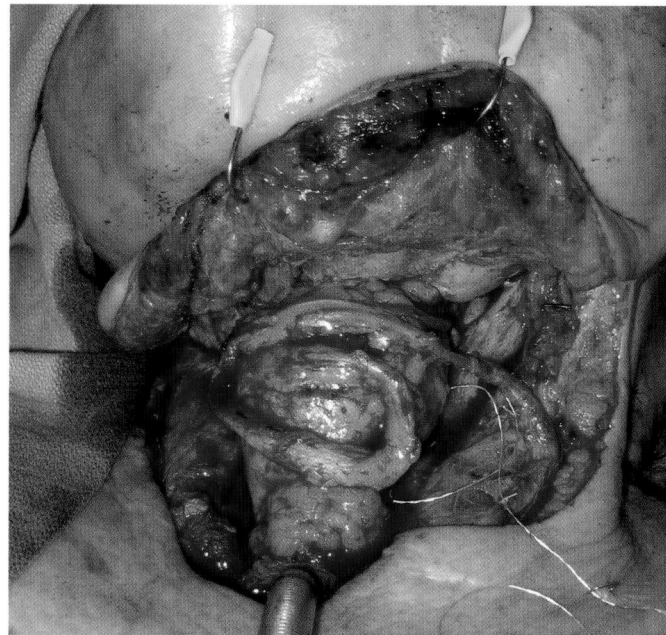

Fig. 13.18 When the vascular pedicle is long, it can be gently looped around to avoid sharp kinks.

Fig. 13.16 (A, B) A triangular lip of flap (marked D) is created so that it can be sutured to the spatulated cervical esophageal end.

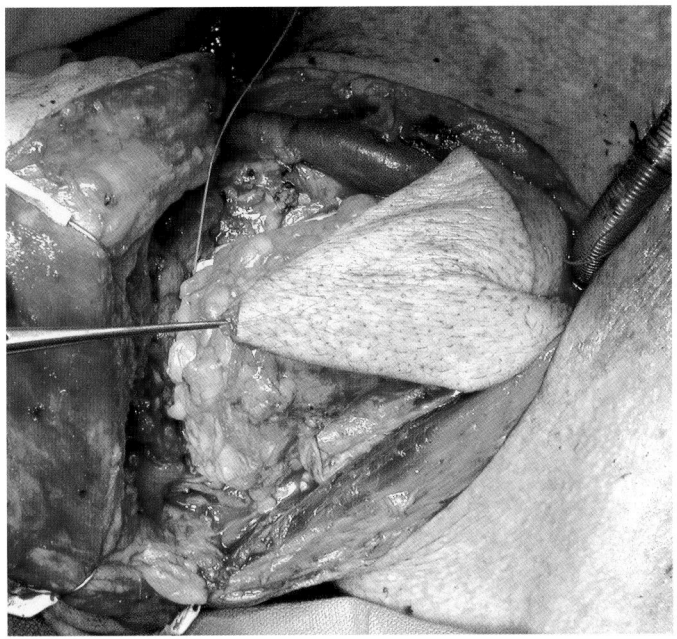

Fig. 13.19 De-epithelializing a strip of flap skin in order to externalize a portion of the flap should be avoided since it can lead to high fistula rates.

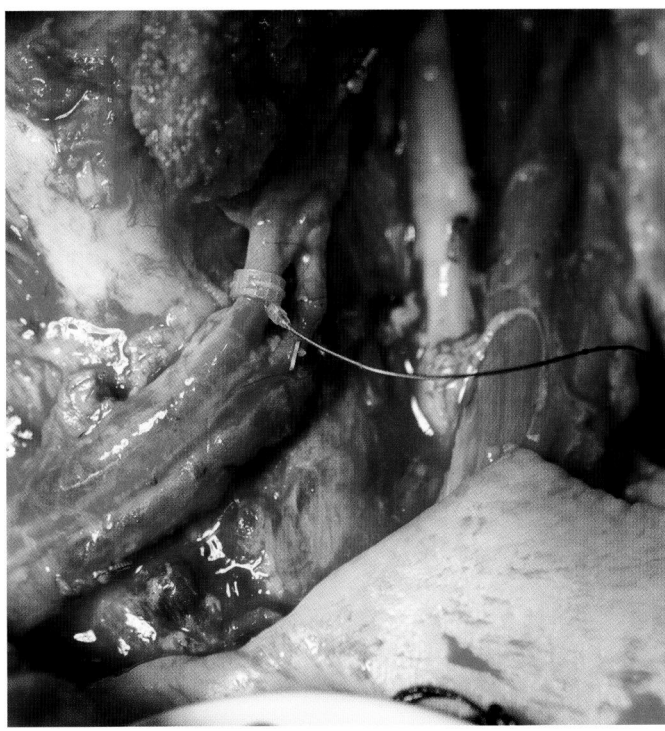

Fig. 13.20 The newly available flow coupler with a Doppler probe attached to the venous coupler can be used for monitoring buried flaps.

hand-held Doppler usually detects only the arterial signal, resulting in delayed exploration in the event of the more common venous failure. It is not uncommon still to have a Doppler signal with both devices when the flap has a venous thrombosis. Externalizing a small skin island based on a second cutaneous perforator is thus strongly recommended. If neck skin coverage is not needed, this second skin island can be brought out through the neck incision for monitoring purposes only *(Fig. 13.9C)* and removed 5–7 days later, before the patient is discharged from hospital. More recently, the flow coupler (Synovis Micro Companies Alliance, Birmingham, AL) became available to monitor buried flaps. The Doppler probe is attached to a venous coupler *(Fig. 13.20)*, thus reducing the chances of separation of the probe from the vessel wall, as commonly seen with the Cook-Swartz Doppler. However, its effectiveness is too new to conclude.

At the time of neck closure, the tracheostomy is sutured to the surrounding neck and anterior chest skin, and a number 8 Shiley tracheostomy tube is placed in the tracheostomy and secured to the chest skin. In patients with a short and thick neck, the superior flange of the Shiley tube is trimmed to avoid compressing the neck skin and the underlying flap *(Fig. 13.21)*. Skin necrosis and even fistulas can develop owing to such compression.

Reconstruction with the radial forearm flap

The radial forearm flap is the authors' second choice for primary pharyngoesophageal reconstruction following a laryngopharyngectomy. It is used in obese patients whose ALT flap is too thick. However, it is the first choice for treating pharyngocutaneous fistulas and strictures following a previous free-flap reconstruction (ALT or jejunum), as a very thin flap is preferred.

Flap design

The design of the radial forearm flap is similar to that of the ALT flap. The flap can be designed with an extended lip in the proximal forearm to accommodate the larger opening in the base of the tongue, as with the ALT flap. The circumference of the distal forearm at the wrist crease is 15–16 cm in average patients. For circumferential defects, the required flap width of 9.4 cm would require removal of nearly two-thirds of the forearm skin, creating an unsightly donor site scar. Pharyngoesophageal defects are usually no longer than 10 cm. In shorter defects, the flap can be rotated 90° from the conventional design orientation on the forearm to minimize donor site morbidity. For instance, for a 6-cm-long circumferential defect, the radial forearm flap would be 6 cm wide (lateral to medial) and 9.4 cm long (proximal to distal). When the flap is tubed, it is rolled from distal to proximal instead of from lateral to medial *(Fig. 13.22)*. Defects caused by persistent fistulas and strictures following free-flap reconstruction are usually only 3 or 4 cm long, but most likely circumferential. A radial forearm flap rotated 90° will only need to be 3 or 4 cm wide, thus significantly decreasing donor site morbidity.

Flap harvesting

Flap elevation is well described in the literature, with the following modifications. In most cases, the venae comitantes of the radial forearm flap are adequate for venous drainage without including the cephalic vein. However, the venae comitantes can be extremely small and inadequate in some patients. Therefore, the authors' approach is tentatively to

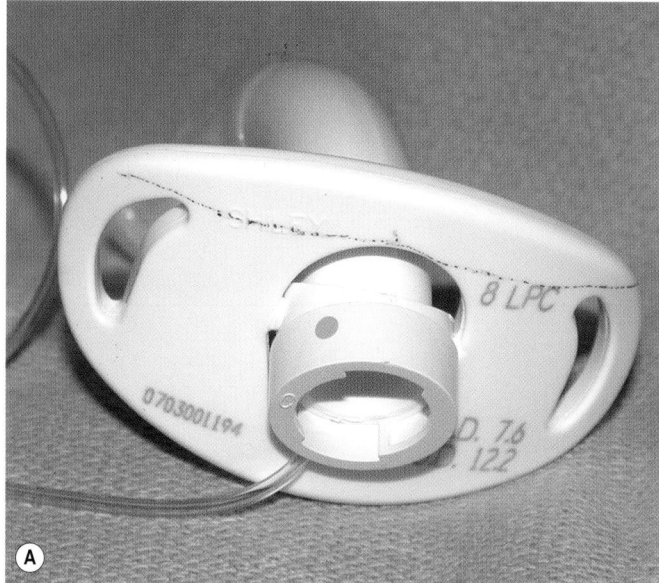

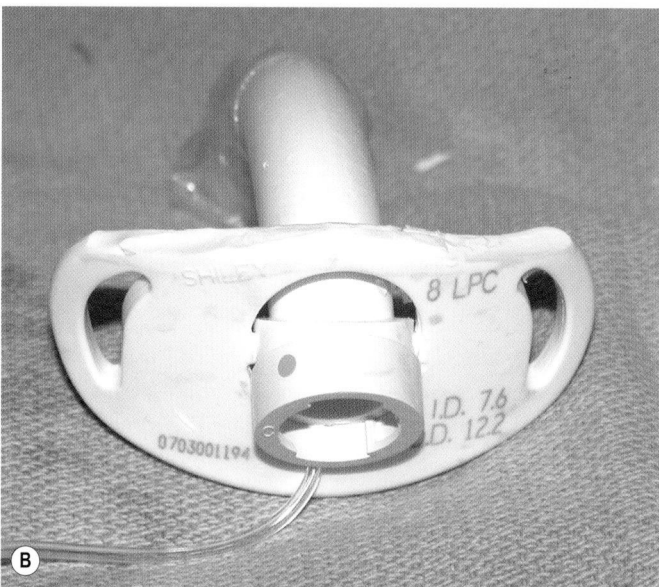

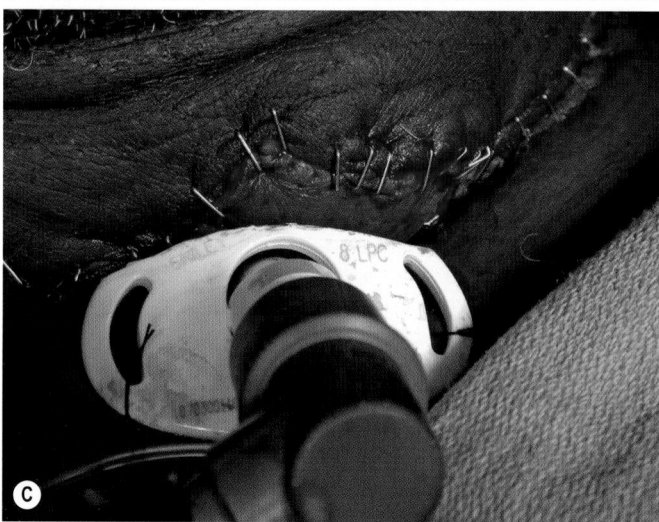

Fig. 13.21 The upper edge of the flange of the Shiley tracheostomy tube is trimmed to avoid compression of the flange against a bulky flap.

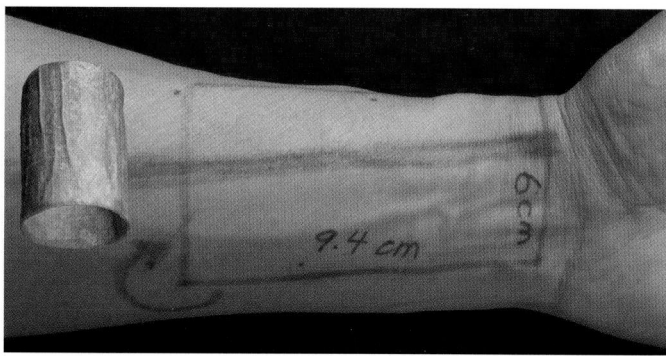

Fig. 13.22 For short circumferential pharyngoesophageal defects, the radial forearm flap is designed with the width of the flap as the length of the tubed neoesophagus to reduce donor site morbidity.

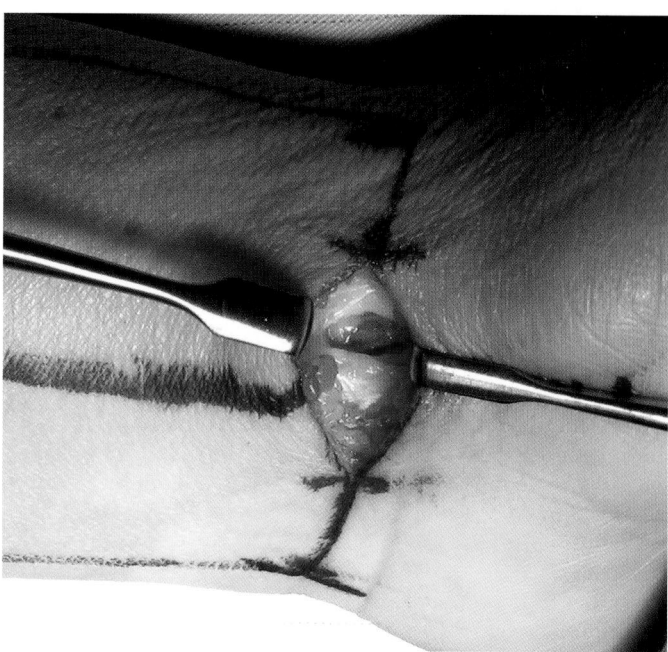

Fig. 13.23 A small exploratory incision was made first at the wrist crease to confirm the size of the venae comitantes of the radial forearm flap vascular pedicle. If both venae comitantes are less than 1 mm in diameter, the flap design is shifted more laterally to include the cephalic vein.

outline the flap centering on the radial vessels, and make a small transverse incision at the wrist crease to explore the venae comitantes first *(Fig. 13.23)*. If one of these veins is at least 1 mm in diameter, there is no need to use the cephalic vein. Otherwise, the flap design is shifted laterally to capture the cephalic vein. Suprafascial dissection is preferred,[64] and flap elevation is performed under tourniquet control. The venae comitantes are usually no bigger than 1.5 mm before they converge; therefore, the vein is usually taken above the convergence of the venae comitantes, where the diameter is greater than 2.5 mm in most cases. Once the flap and the vascular pedicle are completely dissected, the tourniquet is released to perfuse the flap and the hand for several minutes before dividing the pedicle.

A second skin island can also be fashioned with the radial forearm flap and externalized to resurface small neck skin defects *(Fig. 13.24)*.

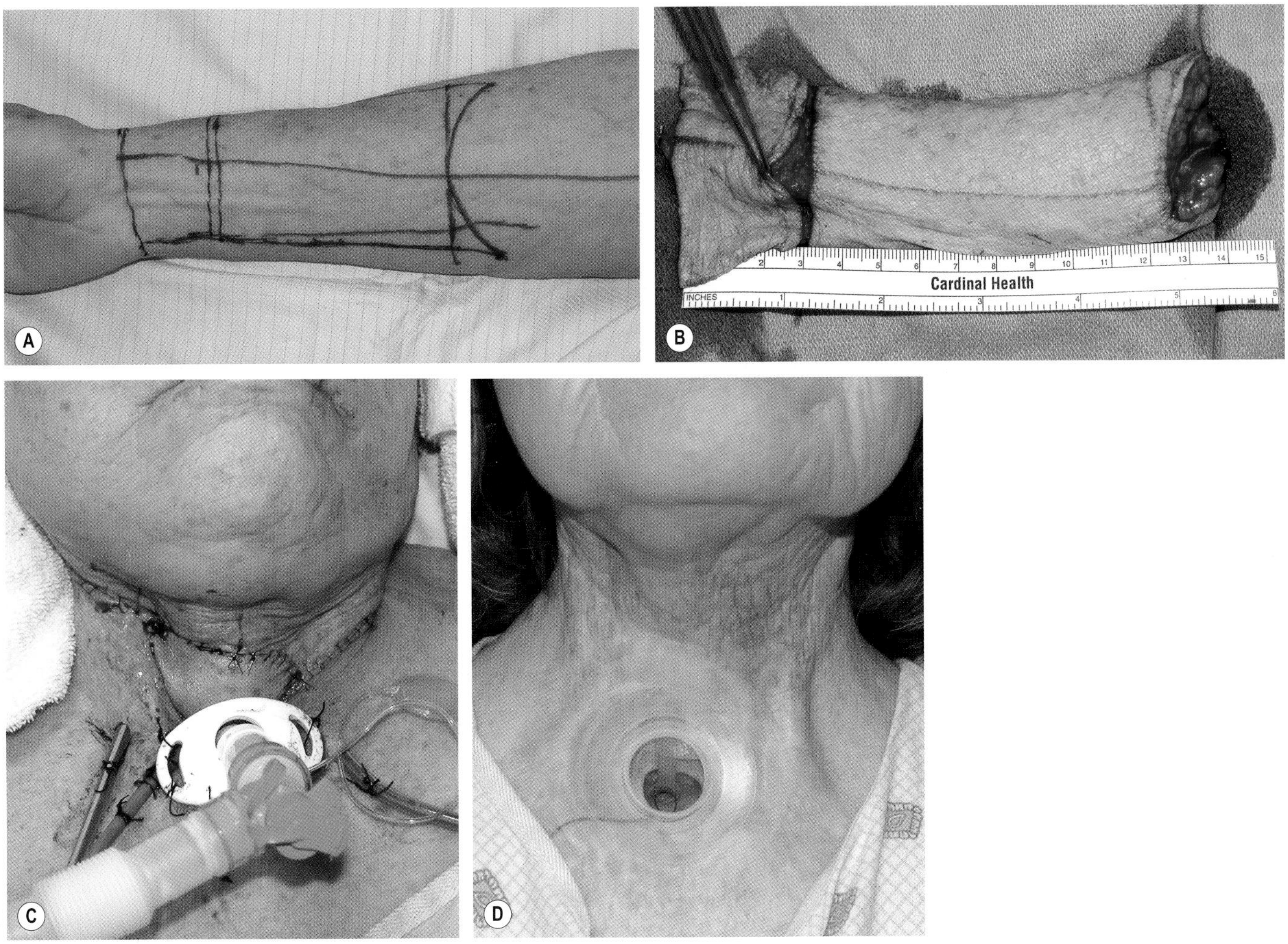

Fig. 13.24 (A, B) The radial forearm flap is designed to create a small second skin island at the distal end of the flap with the radial vessels in continuity. **(C)** The second skin island is externalized to repair a small neck skin defect. **(D)** Long-term results in the anterior neck are excellent.

Flap insetting is similar to that with the ALT flap. The radial forearm flap has a reputation of having high fistula rates, up to 50%, and having delayed fistulas. More recent reports have shown that the fistula rates are similar to those with the jejunal flap.[50–53] A fasciocutaneous flap may not heal as quickly as a jejunal flap once it is immersed in saliva 24 hours a day. It is conceivable that some areas of the flap edge may slough first, then heal secondarily. This may explain the high incidence of delayed fistula formation. If an oral diet is started early, for instance 7 days after surgery, as with the jejunal flap, fistulas will likely develop with the unhealed radial forearm flap.

Reconstruction with the jejunal flap

Flap harvesting

Through an upper midline abdominal incision, the mesentery arcade of the proximal jejunum is examined with fiberoptic backlighting to transilluminate the mesentery *(Fig. 13.25)*. The jejunal segment, usually based on the second mesenteric vessels from the ligament of Treitz, is chosen. Surgical

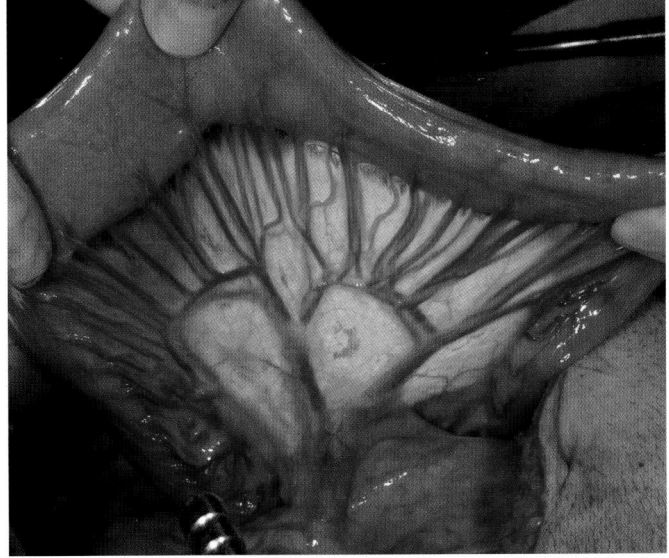

Fig. 13.25 During jejunal flap harvesting, the mesentery arcades of the jejunal flap are transilluminated with fiberoptic backlighting to facilitate vessel dissection.

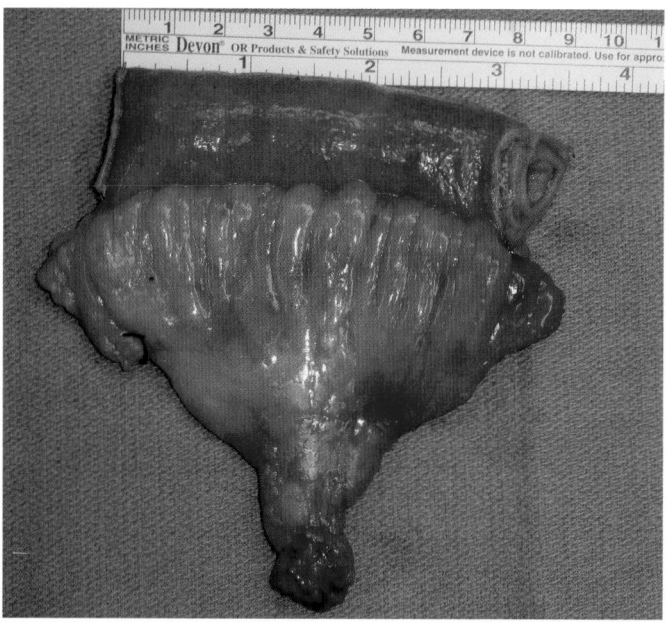

Fig. 13.26 A segment of jejunum is harvested for circumferential pharyngoesophageal reconstruction.

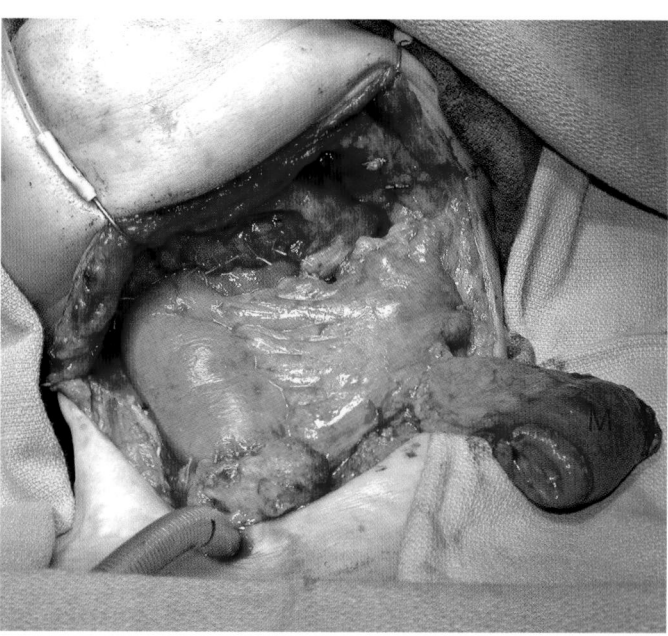

Fig. 13.27 During jejunal flap insetting, the proximal end of the jejunum was opened longitudinally to accommodate a wider opening at the base of the tongue. The flap is slightly stretched in a caudal direction to reduce redundancy.

dissection begins with isolation of the mesentery vessels to their origins at the superior mesenteric artery and vein. The mesentery between the adjacent arcade vessels is divided to the serosal border. The desired jejunal segment, usually about 10–15 cm long, is divided using a linear cutting stapler *(Fig. 13.26)*. The proximal end of the jejunal segment is marked with a serosal suture to maintain an isoperistaltic orientation during flap insetting. Once the recipient site is ready, the mesentery vessels are ligated and divided. The jejunum flap is removed and placed on a side table and its lumen is flushed with cold normal saline until clear.

Flap insetting

Because of the size discrepancy between the jejunum and the proximal pharyngeal defect, a 2–3-cm incision is made in the proximal end of the jejunum along the antimesenteric border to widen the jejunal end, creating a near end-to-side anastomosis *(Fig. 13.27)*. The proximal anastomosis is performed using interrupted 3-0 polyglactin sutures prior to revascularizing the flap. Some surgeons prefer a second-layer Lempert serosal closure. Attention should be paid to avoid the hypoglossal nerve at the base of the tongue during the second-layer closure. To avoid jejunal redundancy and elongation over time, which may cause dysphagia, the anastomoses are performed with the neck in a neutral position. The jejunal flap is slightly stretched in a caudal direction while marking the flap for the distal anastomosis.[65,66] The cervical esophagus is opened longitudinally to spatulate the distal anastomosis, as described above with the ALT flap. The distal anastomosis is performed using a single layer of interrupted 3-0 absorbable sutures.

A monitoring segment 3–4 cm long is created from the remaining jejunum based on branches of the pedicle vessels *(Figs 13.27 and 13.28)*. The monitoring segment is brought out through the lateral neck incision to avoid obstruction of the

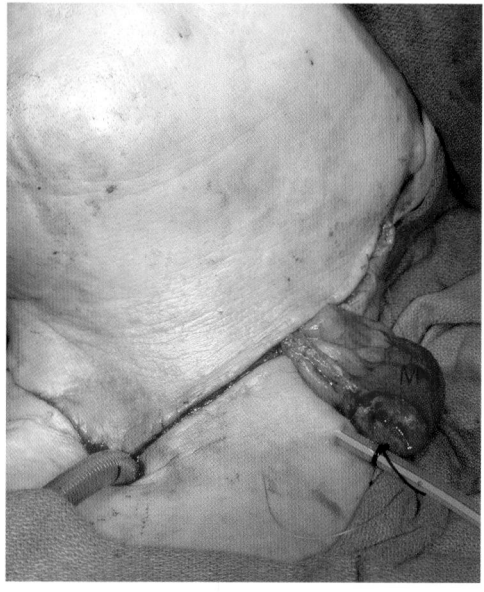

Fig. 13.28 A short-bowel segment is created and externalized as a monitoring segment, and is removed before the patient is discharged from the hospital.

tracheostomy and covered with petroleum jelly-impregnated gauze (Xeroform) to prevent desiccation. Both ends of the bowel segment are left open to avoid distension. The monitoring segment can also be completely open longitudinally. A 2-0 silk suture may be placed around the segment's small vascular pedicle at the skin level so that the pedicle can be easily tied off when it is time to remove the monitor segment. In the mean time, jejunal continuity in the abdomen is re-established, a feeding jejunostomy tube and a gastrostomy tube are inserted, and the abdomen is closed.

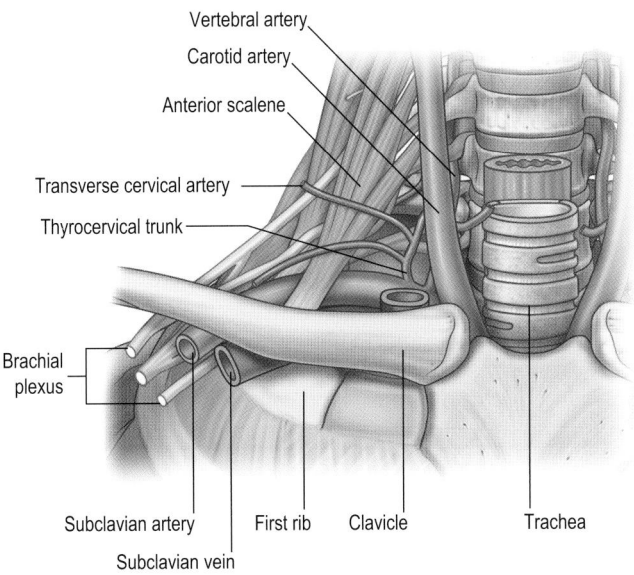

Fig. **13.29** Anatomy of the transverse cervical artery.

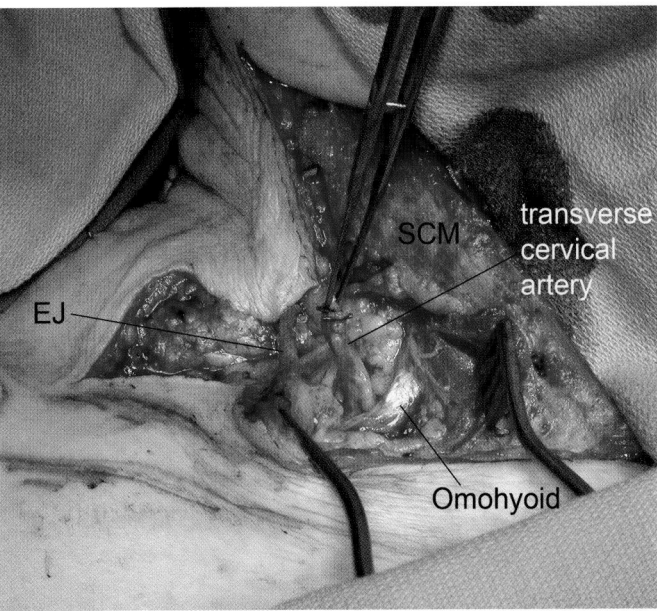

Fig. **13.30** The omohyoid muscle is a good landmark to locate the transverse cervical vessels. EJ, external jugular vein; SCM, sternocleidomastoid muscle.

Recipient vessel choices

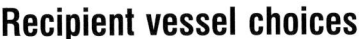

Branches of the external carotid artery and internal jugular vein are commonly used as recipient vessels if they are readily available. The lingual artery is my preferred recipient artery. The size match with the ALT flap pedicle artery is usually very good. The facial artery is the next choice. Sometimes the lingual and facial arteries share a common trunk which is larger in diameter. The superior thyroid artery is usually smaller than the lingual or facial artery, around 1.5 mm in most cases, thus less commonly used. The common facial vein stump off the internal jugular vein is my preferred recipient vein for end-to-end anastomosis with a vein coupler. End-to-side to the internal jugular vein itself is also commonly performed. In patients with previous neck dissection and radiotherapy, however, it can be challenging to find recipient vessels due to severe fibrosis in the neck. Dissection around the carotid artery in these patients may cause carotid artery rupture. Using the transverse cervical vessels may avoid difficult and risky dissection.[62]

In most cases, the transverse cervical artery arises from the thyrocervical trunk which originates from the subclavian artery *(Fig. 13.29)*. The transverse cervical artery then crosses anterior to the brachial plexus and middle scalene muscle on its way to the lateral border of the levator scapulae muscle. It travels behind the omohyoid and anterior scalene muscles. The omohyoid muscle immediately above the clavicle is a good landmark to locate the transverse cervical artery deep to it *(Fig. 13.30)*. The transverse cervical artery usually gives off a supraclavicular artery that supplies the overlying skin. This branch is the vascular pedicle of the supraclavicular flap. The main transverse cervical artery continues laterally and enters the trapezius muscle and nourishes this muscle. It is the vascular pedicle of the trapezius muscle or myocutaneous flap. Variations in the anatomy of the transverse cervical artery exist.[67–69] The transverse cervical artery may arise directly from the subclavian artery in 21% of the sides and from the internal mammary artery in 2% of the sides.[67] The

Table 13.3 **The presence and sizes of the transverse cervical vessels**

Neck	Right side[22]		Left side[11]	
	Artery	Vein	Artery	Vein
Absent	0	1	0	1
Removed	2	2	0	0
<2 mm	4	1	4	1
2–3 mm	16	12	7	6
>3 mm	0	6	0	3

transverse cervical artery has an external diameter between 2 and 3 mm after its take-off from the thyrocervical trunk but before the supraclavicular branch *(Table 13.3)*.[70] It never exceeds 3 mm in our experience. When the artery is less than 1.5 mm, it tends to have a vertical course down behind the clavicle rather than a transverse course, suggesting that it may arise from the subclavian or internal mammary artery rather than the thyrocervical trunk.

Although the transverse cervical artery always travels behind the omohyoid and anterior scalene muscles, the path of the transverse cervical vein is more variable.[71] The vein may run deep (75%) or superficial (25%) relative to the omohyoid muscle. The transverse cervical vein may drain into the external jugular vein or the subclavian vein. In our experience, the transverse cervical vein is usually available above the clavicle and has an adequate size regardless of where it drains *(Table 13.3)*. Only two veins (6%) were found to be less than 2 mm in diameter.[70] Overall, the transverse cervical vessels are available in 92% of patients and are very similar in size to those of the flap vascular pedicle.[70] The need to explore the

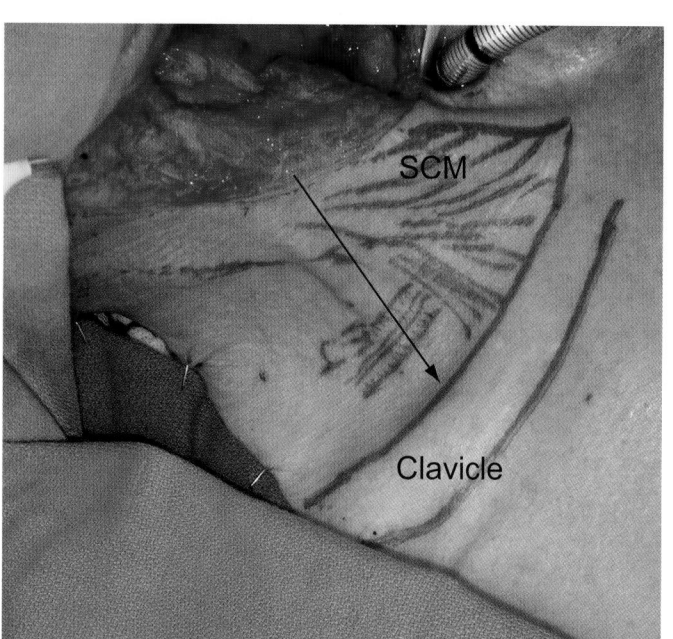

Fig. 13.31 To explore the transverse cervical vessels, an incision was made toward the mid-clavicle, lateral to the sternocleidomastoid muscle. EJ, external jugular vein; SCM, sternocleidomastoid muscle.

contralateral transverse cervical vessels due to absence or inadequacy is 23%.

The right side of the neck is preferred to avoid injury to the thoracic duct unless the surgical field is limited to the left side. With the visor neck incision typically performed by the tumor ablation team, the supraclavicular region (level V) is usually unexposed. Therefore, an additional incision needs to be made toward the mid-clavicle, perpendicular to the visor incision *(Fig. 13.31)*. The supraclavicular area/posterior triangle is usually spared during modern neck dissections and is infrequently heavily radiated. Therefore, exposure of the transverse cervical vessels in the supraclavicular area lateral to the sternocleidomastoid muscle is possible with little risk. On the left side of the neck, particular attention should be paid to avoiding injury to the thoracic duct. Dissection should start high, above the supraclavicular fat pad, and proceed deep to it. If the transverse cervical artery is deemed too small, the thyrocervical trunk is explored with dissection under the sternocleidomastoid muscle. The thyrocervical trunk is significantly larger than the transcervical artery, usually in the range of 2.5–3.5 mm. The external jugular vein usually joins the transverse cervical vein before entering the subclavian vein. This part of the external jugular vein is more deeply located and of good quality. If both veins are unavailable, such as in patients who have undergone a radical neck dissection, the internal jugular vein stump immediately above the subclavian vein is usually long enough for an end-to-side anastomosis.

When anastomoses to the transverse cervical vessels are done in the supraclavicular region, the vascular pedicle usually has a rather straight course, which minimizes kinking of the pedicle. It is also easier to position the microscope without the mandible in the way. For pharyngoesophageal reconstruction, the vascular pedicle of the flap will have a straight course if brought under the sternocleidomastoid muscle to reach the transverse cervical vessels. In patients with a frozen neck, however, the sternocleidomastoid muscle is usually severely fibrotic and contracted, and the muscle is no longer functional. It is advisable to divide the fibrotic band to release the contracture and to provide a flat surface for the vascular pedicle. It should be emphasized that the carotid artery is pulled toward the midline and is closed associated with the fibrotic sternocleidomastoid muscle in patients with a frozen neck. The fibrotic muscle should be divided close to the sternum and the clavicular head to avoid injury to the carotid artery. A handheld Doppler probe is helpful to locate the carotid artery since it is usually not palpable in these cases. In cases in which no tissue plane can be developed between the fibrotic sternocleidomastoid muscle and the carotid artery, the flap pedicle can simply be brought over the muscle to reach the transverse cervical vessels. In preparation for vascular anastomosis, the transverse cervical artery is trimmed as far as possible toward its origin to obtain better inflow.

Managing a frozen neck during pharyngoesophageal reconstruction

A frozen neck is usually defined as severe fibrosis in the neck without tissue planes. Frozen neck is the result of neck surgery (such as neck dissection) combined with radiotherapy. Longstanding pharyngocutaneous fistulas usually result in the worst cases of frozen neck. There are three major problems associated with managing a frozen neck during reconstruction: (1) risk of carotid artery rupture; (2) lack of recipient vessels; and (3) concomitant neck skin or tracheal defects. In a frozen neck, the carotid artery and internal jugular vein are usually encased in fibrotic tissue. Surgical dissection around these great vessels during fistula and scar tissue excision and preparation for recipient vessels can easily cause these already damaged vessels to rupture, resulting in high rates of morbidity and mortality. The best approach to avoiding carotid artery rupture is simply to "stay away from it." The author's preference is to use the transverse cervical vessels as recipient vessels. In this way, surgical dissection around the carotid artery and internal jugular vein can be avoided altogether if it is not required for oncologic reasons.

The use of the transverse cervical vessels solves the first two problems associated with a frozen neck. Successful management of the third problem, concomitant neck skin or tracheal defects, is also possible. Elevating an anterior neck skin flap from an area that has been previously irradiated and operated on often causes skin necrosis. Releasing the contractured neck and removing the scar tissue further creates a large neck skin defect. Therefore, a second flap is usually required to reconstruct the external defect when the jejunal flap or radial forearm flap is used for pharyngoesophageal reconstruction,[65,66,72] further complicating an already difficult case. The pedicled pectoralis major myocutaneous flap is probably the most frequently used flap for this purpose.[65,66] The main disadvantage of this flap is its bulk; even when the muscle alone is used, it often produces contour deformity in the neck and sometimes causes obstruction of the tracheostomy. Donor site morbidity with the pectoralis major flap is particularly undesirable in women. Although the deltopectoral flap is thinner, its use is limited by the need for skin grafting to the donor site, the unreliability of the distal portion of the flap, and sometimes, the need for flap delay.

The ALT flap provides simultaneous pharyngoesophageal reconstruction, neck resurfacing, and tracheostomy reconstruction. Seventy-eight percent of patients have more than one cutaneous perforator in the flap.[60,61] Therefore, the ALT flap can be divided into two independent skin islands based on separate perforators. One skin island is used for pharyngoesophageal reconstruction and the other for neck resurfacing. In cases where only one cutaneous perforator is present, various amounts of vastus lateralis muscle can be included in the flap to support skin grafting to resurface the neck *(Fig. 13.10)*. The muscle portion of the ALT flap can be separated from the fasciocutaneous portion with only the cutaneous perforator attached, providing more flexibility in flap insetting.

In summary, the use of the transverse cervical vessels and multi-island ALT flap can convert an extremely difficult case with a frozen neck into a relatively straightforward one, reducing surgical risks and donor site morbidities and improving quality of life.

Reconstruction of postlaryngectomy pharyngocutaneous fistulas

Since radiotherapy became the primary treatment for early stages of laryngeal and hypopharyngeal cancers,[73] physicians have faced a new problem in these patients: higher rates of pharyngocutaneous fistulas after salvage total laryngectomies for recurrent cancers. Local and regional recurrences following radiotherapy for laryngeal and hypopharyngeal cancers can exceed 30%, depending on tumor location and initial tumor stage.[74,75] Although the overall incidence of postlaryngectomy pharyngocutaneous fistulas has decreased significantly in the past decade, it remains very high in previously irradiated patients.[76–80] McCombe and Jones reported that the incidence increased from 4% to 39% when radiation was included in multimodal therapy.[77]

Once fistulas develop, the radiation effects are compounded by salivary contamination of the neck, leading to chronic inflammation and hypoxia of the neck skin and vasculature and putting the patient at risk for loss of neck skin and the remaining pharynx tracheostomy compromise, and even carotid artery rupture. Long-standing fistulas will inevitably promote scar formation, leading to pharyngeal stricture. These more severe cases create a very difficult challenge for even the most experienced reconstructive surgeon. Conservative management is usually ineffective, and outcomes with local and regional flaps are often disappointing. Therefore, many such patients are left unreconstructed.

Recent studies have shown that the mean overall survival of patients after salvage total laryngectomy was 7.2 years.[81] The mean 2-, 5-, and 10-year overall survival rates were around 70%, 55%, and 40%, respectively.[73,82,83] These data demonstrate that this patient population still has a reasonable survival expectation. Therefore, every effort should be made to restore function and improve quality of life. Major postoperative morbidities and death are mainly related to cardiopulmonary and cerebrovascular accidents, including carotid artery rupture.[80,83] The goals of surgical reconstruction should be to minimize surgical morbidity and mortality in addition to providing reliable reconstruction that achieves primary healing and a reasonable appearance and restores swallowing and speech functions.

Because all patients who have undergone total laryngectomy have also had radiotherapy, a frozen neck is always present *(Fig. 13.32A)*. Therefore, the strategies for reconstruction are the same as those for managing a frozen neck. During surgery, the fistula track and scar tissues are excised, without exposing the great vessels in the neck if they are cancer-free *(Fig. 13.32B)*. All patients have various degrees of pharyngeal stricture, particularly those with a long-standing fistula. The hypopharynx is opened superiorly to the base of the tongue, where the pharyngeal inlet is incised laterally and widened to approximately two to three fingers wide. This is important because primary closure of the pharynx following a total

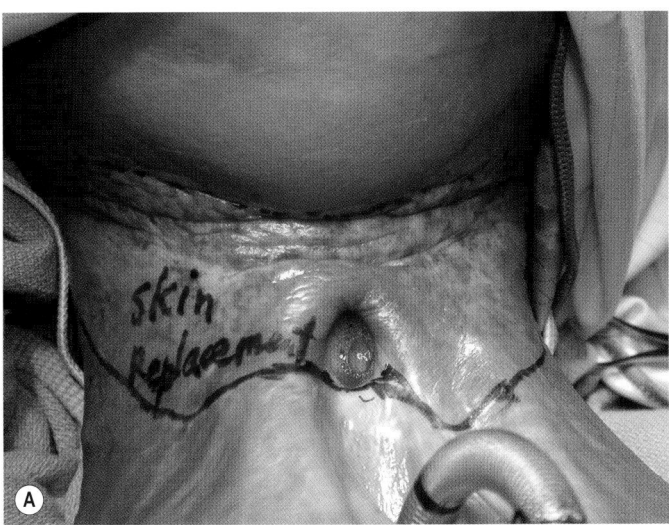
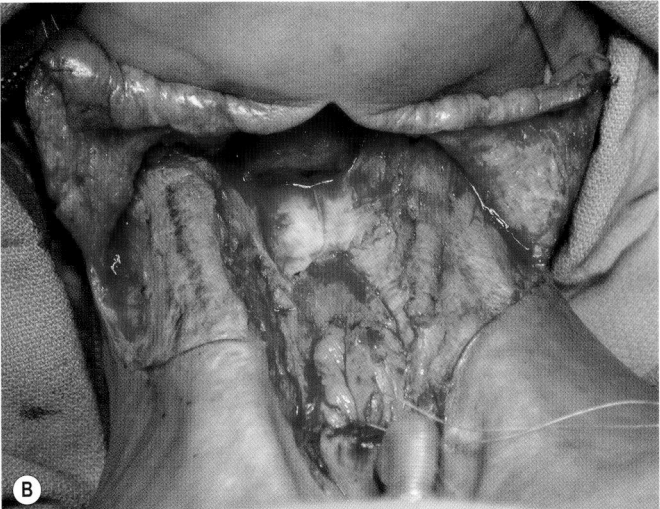

Fig. 13.32 A long-standing pharyngocutaneous fistula following a total laryngectomy and radiation therapy. Significant radiation burn and scarring in the neck are evident **(A)**. **(B)** In these patients without tumor recurrence, simply removing the scar tissue in the central neck without exposing the major vessels significantly reduces surgical risks.

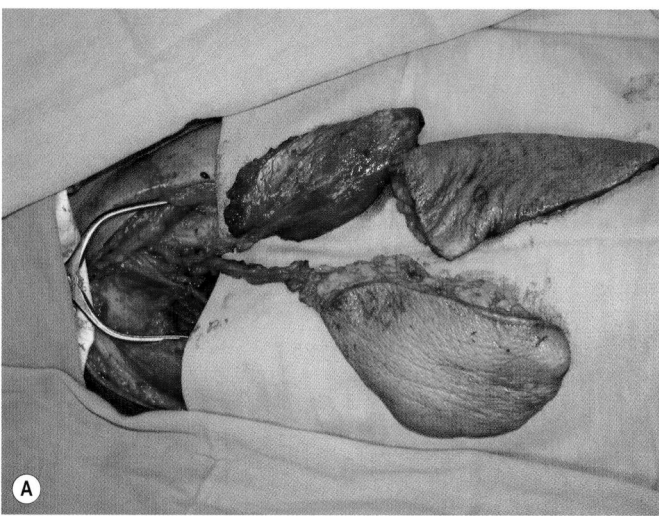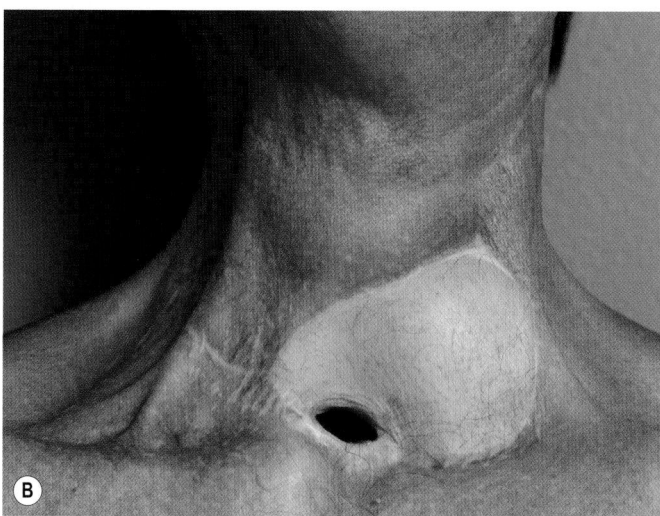

Fig. 13.33 Patients with pharyngocutaneous fistula often present with a through-and-through defect in the neck after fistula resection. A multi-island anterolateral thigh flap **(A)** can be used to simultaneously reconstruct the esophagus and resurface the neck **(B)**.

laryngectomy inevitably narrows the pharyngeal inlet. In patients with a relatively normal pharynx and cervical esophagus and no complications, a small degree of narrowing may not cause dysphagia. After pharyngoesophageal reconstruction, however, food transit through the reconstructed conduit is compromised no matter what type of flap is used. Any narrowing in the pharyngeal inlet or weakness of the base of the tongue thus further compounds the problem and causes dysphagia. Inferiorly, the posterior wall of the tracheostomy is carefully separated from the cervical esophagus just far enough, usually 1 cm, for the flap–esophageal anastomosis. Minimal dissection should be performed to avoid compromising blood supply to the remaining cervical esophagus and tracheal stoma. Meticulous tissue-handling techniques must be exercised in such difficult cases where there is no room for error. Once the pharyngoesophageal defect is recreated, the transverse cervical vessels are explored and a multi-island ALT flap is employed to reconstruct the defects, as described earlier *(Fig. 13.33)*.

Because of the lack of well-vascularized tissue in the neck in this patient population, pharyngocutaneous fistulas, unlike intraoral fistulas, do not respond to conservative management. We have seen that delayed repair of postlaryngectomy fistulas often results in a severe frozen neck and a circumferential pharyngoesophageal defect. Therefore, early surgical intervention to reconstruct the neck in these patients once large fistulas develop is strongly recommended.[84] Reconstructive surgery can be performed shortly after the development of the fistula (as early as 3 days later, if scheduling allows), before severe fibrosis sets in. Surgical dissection in the neck is therefore much easier than in patients with a longstanding fistula. Thorough debridement of infected and necrotic tissues and aggressive irrigation of the neck wound are mandatory in the reconstruction of defects caused by postlaryngectomy fistulas. Although the tissues are still somewhat edematous, anastomoses can be safely and reliably completed with proper tissue-handling techniques. The use of various amounts of the well-vascularized vastus lateralis muscle to repair neck defects may help to achieve primary healing.

Reconstruction of isolated cervical esophageal defects with an intact larynx

The vast majority of tumors arising in the cervical esophagus are malignant, and laryngectomy is required to achieve tumor-free margins and to prevent aspiration when the cricopharyngeus muscle is resected.[85] For benign tumors such as schwannomas and granular cell tumors, smaller margins are acceptable, but resection of a portion of the cricopharyngeus muscle increases the risk of reflux and aspiration. Therefore, the reconstruction of isolated cervical esophageal defects can be challenging. With an intact larynx and trachea, exposure of the cervical esophagus is limited, making reconstruction technically difficult. Given the small space around the esophagus, a free tissue transfer offers the best flexibility for insetting the flap; a thin flap is required for the same reason. The radial forearm flap is, therefore, the authors' flap of choice for both partial and circumferential defects. These defects are usually only a few centimeters long, so the radial forearm flap can be oriented 90° to the conventional flap design so that the width of the flap becomes the length of the neoesophagus. The longitudinal length of the flap is rolled along the vascular pedicle to form a tube *(Fig. 13.22)*.

Because defects of the cervical esophagus are usually located lower in the neck, the external carotid artery is often not exposed. Either the transverse cervical artery or the superior thyroid artery can be used as the recipient artery. The transverse cervical vein and the internal jugular vein are the common recipient veins. The vascular pedicle is often longer than needed and should be carefully looped to avoid kinking or twisting.

Postoperative care

General postoperative care

After microsurgical reconstruction of pharyngoesophageal defects, patients are usually kept in the surgical intensive care unit overnight, sedated, and placed on a ventilator which is usually weaned off in the next morning. Patients are transferred to a flap-monitoring floor by the afternoon. Elderly patients with limited cardiopulmonary reserve may be awakened at the end of surgery to avoid overnight sedation and ventilator support since sedation will most likely cause hypotension in these patients, requiring fluid resuscitation. They can easily suffer fluid overload, congestive heart failure, and respiratory failure. Delirium tremens prophylaxis should be given to patients who are known to be chronic alcohol users: this is common among patients with head and neck cancers. In patients with a history of alcohol abuse and narcotic dependence, postoperative confusion and agitation are common and may cause hypertension, hematoma, anastomotic breakdowns, and avulsion of the vascular pedicle. Therefore, prompt management of these issues by the critical care and neuropsychiatric staff is important.

Routine prophylaxis for deep-vein thrombosis starts in the operating room with stockings and sequential compression devices. Pharmacologic prophylaxis should be considered since most patients with head and neck cancer are at high risk. Anticoagulation after free-flap reconstruction is not routinely performed. In patients with postoperative vascular thrombosis requiring thrombectomy and difficult revisions of vascular anastomosis, an intravenous heparin bolus of 2500–3000 units is usually given intraoperatively at the time of take-back, followed by a low dose of heparin infusion, usually at 500 units per hour, for 3 days, then aspirin 325 mg/day for 1 week.

Tube feeding is started on postoperative day 1 after a fasciocutaneous flap reconstruction. Ambulation usually starts on postoperative day 2. Broad-spectrum antibiotics are usually continued for 3 days or longer, as indicated. Hourly flap check is performed for 2 days. In most cases, this can be reduced to every 2 hours for 2 days thereafter and then every 4 hours until discharge. Following a free jejunal flap reconstruction, the gastric tube is kept on low suction, and jejunal tube feeding is started once active bowel sounds return. The gastrostomy tube is placed on gravity and then clamped once bowel function returns fully, and output is diminished. Some patients may develop ileus for several days. It is important to monitor their gastrointestinal function carefully to avoid frequent vomiting, as this may disrupt the jejunopharyngeal anastomosis. The monitoring segment of the jejunum is usually removed before the patient is discharged from the hospital.

Oral diet

Oral feeding is withheld until a modified barium swallow (MBS) study is performed by the speech pathologists to evaluate the swallowing function and healing process (*Fig. 13.34*). Timing of MBS study is 1–6 weeks following reconstruction, depending on the type of flap used and prior radiotherapy (*Table 13.4*). MBS study is delayed for fasciocutaneous flaps due to the incidence of delayed fistula formation with the use of a fasciocutaneous flap for pharyngoesophageal

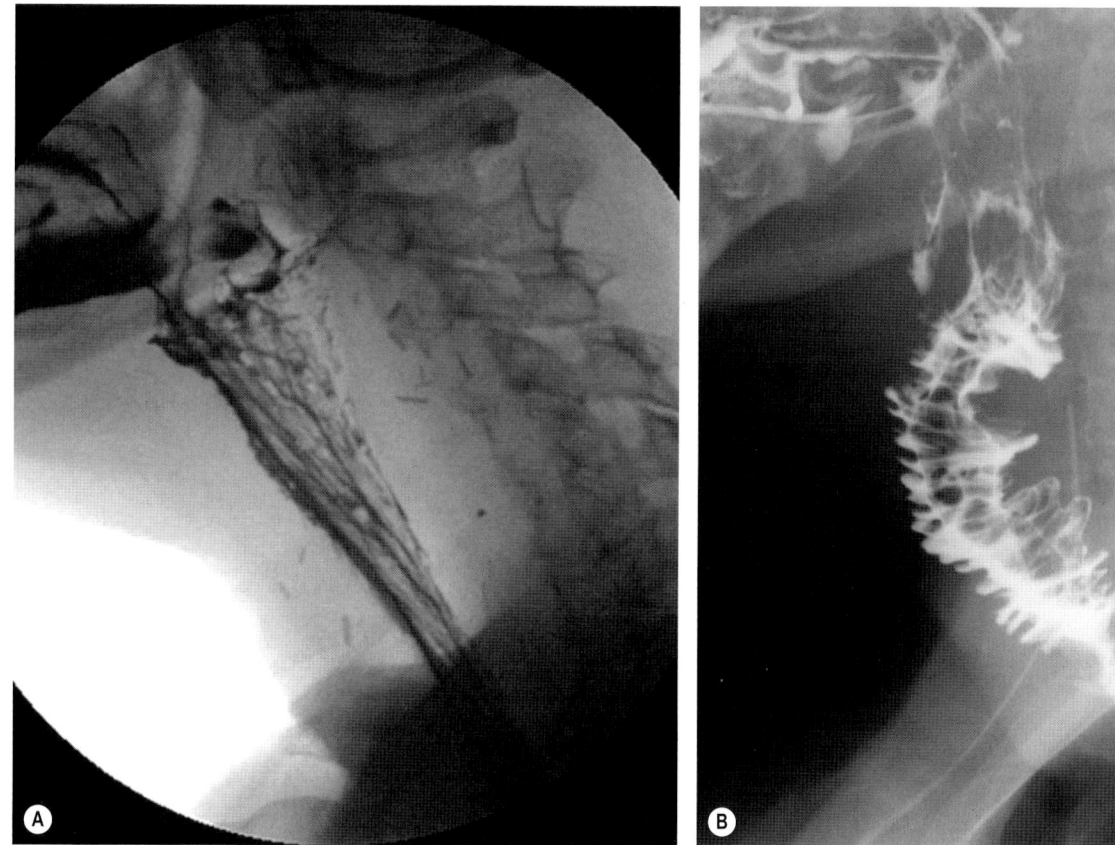

Fig. 13.34 A modified barium swallowing study following an anterolateral thigh **(A)** and jejunal flap **(B)** reconstruction demonstrated a patent neopharynx.

Table 13.4 Timing of postoperative modified barium swallowing study

Flaps	Prior radiation	No radiation
Jejunal flap	14 days	7 days
ALT flap	6 weeks	2 weeks
RFF	6 weeks	2 weeks

ALT, anterolateral thigh flap; RFF, radial forearm flap.

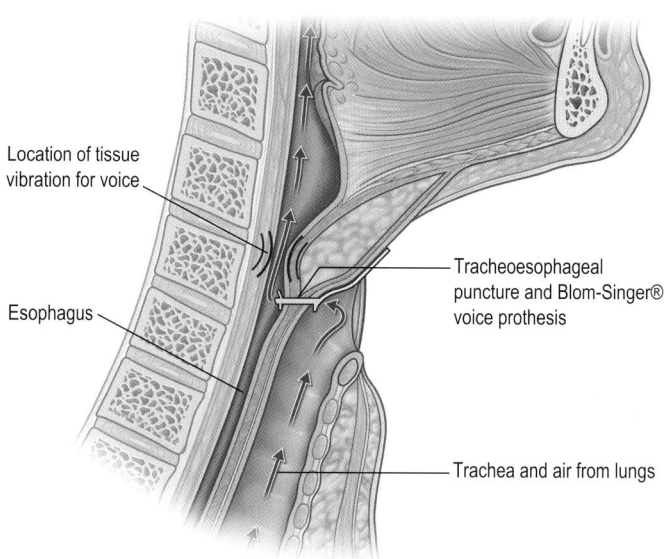

Fig. 13.35 A tracheoesophageal puncture is performed to create a communication between the trachea and neoesophagus for speech rehabilitation. A one-way valve voice prosthesis is placed in the puncture site so that the air generated from the lungs can be forced through the prosthesis to the neoesophagus, generating vibration and voice production. A skin flap vibrates better than an intestinal flap.

reconstruction.[53,54] If used with the reconstruction, the Montgomery salivary bypass tube is removed before the MBS study. In patients with no evidence of leaks or fistula, a liquid diet is started and then advanced to a soft diet 3 days later if no complications occurred. Diet can then be advanced to regular diet as tolerated. In patients with a leak or fistula, oral intake is withheld, tube feeds continued, and an MBS study is repeated in 2 weeks or longer, as clinically indicated. Most leaks heal spontaneously within 2 weeks.

Voice rehabilitation

TEP is the preferred method of voice rehabilitation. It is commonly used following a total laryngectomy without flap reconstruction. However, an increasing number of patients who undergo a flap reconstruction are being rehabilitated with TEP. TEP can be performed at the time of surgery (primary TEP) or several months after surgery with use of endoscopy (secondary TEP). Because of the higher failure rate of primary TEP with both the ALT and jejunal flaps,[59] secondary TEP, which is usually performed 4 or 5 months after reconstruction in patients without complications, is now preferred by the authors. Patient selection for primary TEP should be very carefully evaluated. Only those who have good quality of tissue and adequate length of cervical esophagus remaining, are compliant, have a good insufflation test, and more likely can manage the prosthesis postoperatively can be considered for primary TEP.

TEP is performed by puncturing the common wall between the esophagus and trachea 1.5 or 2 cm below the rim of the tracheostomy (Fig. 13.35). In patients with a very low resection of the cervical esophagus below the tracheostomy, the puncture needs to go through the flap and the posterior tracheal wall, which is slightly more difficult to do. Initially, a 14-Fr. red rubber catheter is inserted through the trachea to the esophagus and secured in place. The catheter is changed to a voice prosthesis 2–4 weeks later by speech pathologists. The patients are followed up regularly by speech pathologists to adjust the prosthesis. Complications include widening of the puncture site with leakage around the voice prosthesis, frequent mucus plugs inside the prosthesis, and fungal infections. The authors' experience suggests that TEP success rates and voice quality are significantly better with a fasciocutaneous flap than with a jejunal flap.[59,86] Because of mucus production, frequent redundancy, and softness of the bowel wall that prevents adequate vibration, the speech of patients with a jejunal flap is often wet and labored. Speech rehabilitation requires patient motivation and commitment. Careful patient selection is therefore important.

Outcomes and complications

Outcomes

In our recent experience with 114 consecutive ALT flaps used for pharyngoesophageal reconstruction,[59] mean intensive care unit stay was 1.9 ± 2.2 days, and mean hospital stay was 9.0 ± 4.7 days. Two patients experienced total flap loss and one patient had partial flap necrosis. Pharyngocutaneous fistulas and strictures occurred in 9% and 6% of patients, respectively. Ninety-one percent of patients tolerated an oral diet without the need for tube feeding. TEP was performed for speech rehabilitation in 51 patients. Eighty-one percent of patients with a secondary TEP achieved fluent speech versus 41% of patients with a primary TEP.

With the jejunal flap reconstruction, average hospital stay was 13 days and average intensive care unit stay was 3 days. The incidence of ileus and bowel obstruction was 9%, abdominal hernia, 6%, and anastomotic stricture, 19%. The fistula rate was lower (only 3%) when "inexperienced surgeons" were excluded from the series,[56] suggesting the importance of meticulous attention to technical details in such complex reconstructions. Unlike with the ALT flap, approximately half of the fistulas occur at the proximal anastomosis,[46,48] possibly owing to slight stretching of the thin walls of the jejunal flap during flap insetting.

Overall, 65% of patients tolerated an oral diet without supplemental tube feeding, and 23% were partially and 12% were totally tube-feeding-dependent. Fluent tracheoesophageal speech was achieved in 22% of patients who received a TEP. The quality of tracheoesophageal speech following jejunal flap reconstruction is usually characterized as "wet" compared with that following a fasciocutaneous flap reconstruction or a total laryngectomy without reconstruction.

Reported fistula rates with the radial forearm flap ranged from 17% to 40% and stricture rates were 17–50%.[50–53] Functional outcomes also vary considerably.

Managing postoperative complications

Pharyngocutaneous fistula

In the experience reported above, pharyngocutaneous fistulas occurred in 9% of patients with ALT flap reconstruction. Fistula rates are similar in partial and circumferential reconstructions. Proximal fistulas are rare with the ALT flap. It has been speculated that the longitudinal seam of a tubed fasciocutaneous flap or two longitudinal suture lines in a partial defect might have contributed to a higher incidence of fistula formation with the radial forearm flap. However, in the authors' experience, the fistula rate with the ALT flap is no higher than with the jejunal flap, and no fistulas have occurred through the longitudinal suture lines. Fistulas usually develop between 1 and 4 weeks postoperatively and manifest as leakage of saliva or liquids or, in some patients, as a neck infection. Therefore, any neck infection or abscess that occurs after a pharyngoesophageal reconstruction should raise suspicion for anastomotic leakage. Risk factors for fistula formation include improper suturing techniques, poor tissue quality at the anastomosis site, previous radiotherapy, and turbulent postoperative course. At the time of surgery, any questionable tissue in the proximal pharynx and cervical esophagus should be trimmed until only well-vascularized tissue is seen. The author uses single-layer, simple interrupted 3-0 Vicryl sutures for flap insetting, taking relatively big bites, inverting the skin/mucosa edges into the lumen, spacing each suture 5–7 mm apart, and avoiding tight knots.

Once a fistula is identified, oral intake is withheld and local wound care is initiated. Small fistulas, in the absence of tumor recurrence or distal obstruction, usually heal spontaneously within 2 weeks with conservative management. Therefore, an MBS is repeated 2 weeks later if the leakage has stopped. Larger fistulas or those with infection should be evaluated with CT to rule out abscess and assess the proximity of the fistula/abscess to the carotid artery. Any dead space or abscess around the carotid artery, especially in patients who have undergone previous radiotherapy or chemoradiation, should be thoroughly but carefully debrided without jeopardizing the carotid artery and filled with a muscle flap such as a pectoralis major muscle flap. This should be done as soon as possible to prevent rupture of the carotid artery. Attempting to repair the leak or dehiscence at this stage will not be successful and may cause more tissue damage. The muscle flap is adequate to obliterate the fistula track and will remucosalize quickly. It is extremely important not to delay the debridement when infection/abscess is identified. Early intervention may achieve rapid healing and prevent life-threatening complications.

With proper management, as described above, persistent fistulas are rare. However, if a fistula does persist, the patient should be evaluated for possible tumor recurrence and distal obstruction/stricture. Long-standing fistulas will eventually cause stricture due to scar tissue formation, which in return results in nonhealing of the fistula. In these cases, reconstruction with a radial forearm flap may be indicated in selected patients who are in good general health and have a good prognosis.

Anastomotic strictures

With the ALT flap, anastomotic strictures rarely occur at the proximal anastomosis site unless the flap was compromised at the time of reconstruction. Distal anastomotic strictures usually occur several months or years following reconstruction. Spatulation and the use of the Montgomery bypass tube may reduce the risk of stricture formation. In the authors' experience, strictures are most commonly seen in circumferential defect repair. Only one stricture occurred in a partial defect (*Fig. 13.36*). Therefore, removal of the narrow strip of the remaining posterior pharyngeal mucosa, thus converting a noncircumferential defect into a circumferential one, as frequently done when the jejunal flap was used, should be avoided. As mentioned earlier, the additional longitudinal suture lines do not seem to contribute to fistula formation.

If a patient develops dysphagia several months after reconstruction, anastomotic strictures should be suspected and an MBS study performed to confirm the diagnosis. In the past, surgical dilatation under general anesthesia was used to repair anastomotic strictures, and serious complications such as esophageal perforation occurred. In the past several years, endoscopic balloon dilatation has become the preferred treatment. This is usually done by a gastroenterologist. Repeated

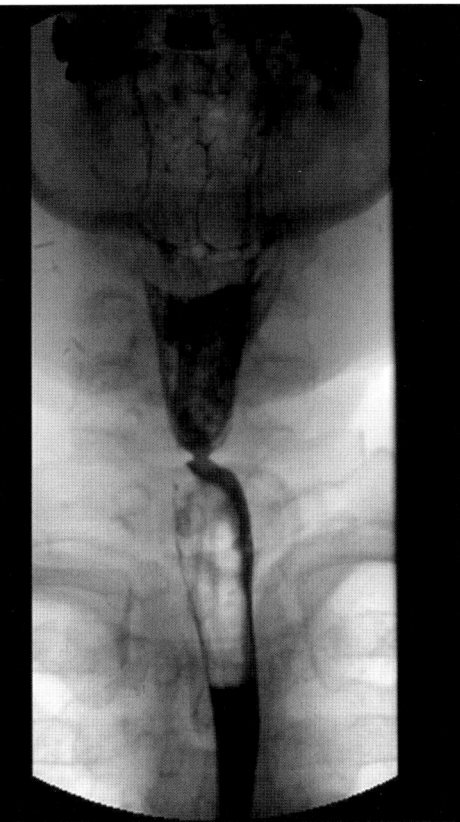

Fig. 13.36 A stricture at the distal anastomosis between the flap and the cervical esophagus. Endoscopic dilation is now the standard of care to manage strictures.

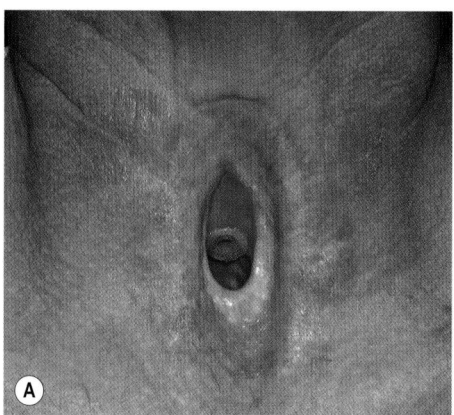
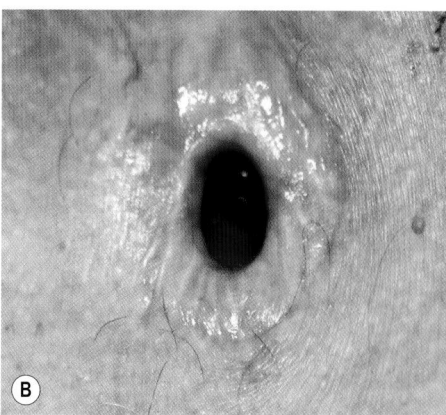
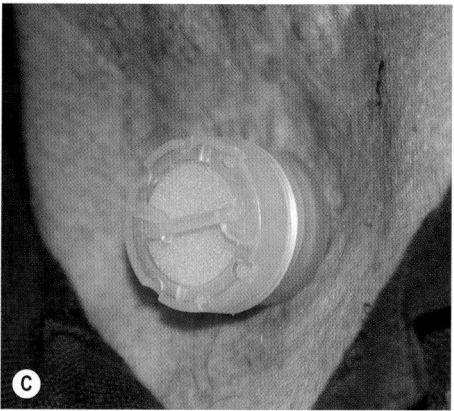

Fig. 13.37 Many patients with a tracheostomy lose the posterior ridge and thus lose the ability to retain the speech button **(A)**. A fascial graft can be placed subcutaneously around the tracheostomy to recreate the ridge **(B)** so that a hands-free button can be securely retained **(C)**. Patients can speak without needing to use their fingers to occlude the tracheostomy opening.

dilatations may be required in some patients. In refractory cases, surgical repair can be achieved with a radial forearm free flap.

Neck wound infection

Neck wound infection is the result of prolonged wound exposure and oral contamination during surgery. Many patients with head and neck cancer have poor oral hygiene. Prior chemoradiation therapy can also increase the risk of infection. Copious irrigation and obliteration of dead spaces are important to prevent postoperative wound infection, which often occurs 5–7 days following surgery. Once infection occurs, early drainage and thorough debridement and irrigation may enable primary wound closure over a drain. However, part of the wound should be left open for dressing changes if the wound is deemed compromised. Additional flaps are usually not needed to manage infection. Early recognition of wound infection and intervention is crucial to avoiding delays in adjuvant therapy, as postoperative radiotherapy usually starts 4–6 weeks after surgery. In patients with diabetes, manifestations of wound infection may be very subtle. They may not present fevers or erythema of the neck. An increase in white blood cell count and blood sugar level is an indication of wound infection. A CT scan can be performed to evaluate the neck when infection is suspected.

Secondary procedures

Commonly performed secondary procedures include debulking and tracheal stomaplasty.

Flap debulking

Occasionally the external skin paddle of the ALT flap is bulky, especially in obese patients. The bulkiness not only creates an aesthetic problem, it may also obstruct the tracheostomy opening. Therefore a debulking procedure is often performed to reduce the bulk. Suction-assisted lipectomy is very effective to reduce the subcutaneous fat. The redundant skin can then be excised surgically. Debulking procedures are usually performed 6–12 months after reconstruction. Postoperative radiotherapy may significantly shrink the flap. Debulking should be delayed for 1 year if the shrinkage is not enough.

Tracheal stomaplasty

A circular ridge around the tracheostomy is necessary to retain the speech button for TEP speech production. In many cases, however, the posterior stoma has no ridge to retain the button. A circular ridge can be recreated by subcutaneously placing a tendon or fascial graft such as a tensor fascia latae graft around the tracheostomy *(Fig. 13.37)*.

Access the complete references list online at **http://www.expertconsult.com**

37. Seidenberg B, Rosenak SS, Hurwitt ES, et al. Immediate reconstruction of the cervical esophagus by a revascularized isolated jejunal segment. *Ann Surg.* 1959;149:162–171.
    The authors report a series of free jejunal transfers for esophageal reconstruction in a canine model. Having refined the procedure in this preclinical model, they go on to describe the first application of their technique in a human patient.

43. Coleman JJ, Searles JM, Hester TR, et al. Ten years experience with the free jejunal autograft. *Am J Surg.* 1987;154:389–393.

This is a retrospective review of 96 jejunal free flaps. A critical assessment of outcomes and complications led to the conclusion that free jejunal transfer is a valuable reconstructive approach whose efficacy can be enhanced by careful patient selection.

46. Reece GP, Schusterman MA, Miller MJ, et al. Morbidity and functional outcome of free jejunal transfer reconstruction for circumferential defects of the pharynx and cervical esophagus. *Plast Reconstr Surg.* 1995; 96:1307.
    A series of 96 free jejunal transfers was assessed in the context of challenges to the procedure's efficacy and

compatibility with radiotherapy. The authors conclude that the jejunal free flap is reliable for pharyngoesophageal reconstruction and is tolerant of radiation.

50. Anthony JP, Singer MI, Mathes SJ. Pharyngoesophageal reconstruction using the tubed free radial forearm flap. *Clin Plast Surg.* 1994;21:137.

    The authors discuss their preference for the tubed free radial forearm flap in laryngopharyngectomy reconstruction. They note a higher leakage rate, but conclude the procedure's superior functional outcomes outweigh this risk.

54. Yu P, Robb GL. Pharyngoesophageal reconstruction with the anterolateral thigh flap: a clinical and functional outcomes study. *Plast Reconstr Surg.* 2005;116:1845–1855.

56. Yu P, Lewin JS, Reece GP, et al. Comparison of clinical and functional outcomes and hospital costs following pharyngoesophageal reconstruction with the anterolateral thigh free flap versus the jejunal flap. *Plast Reconstr Surg.* 2006;117:968–974.

59. Yu P, Hanasono MM, Skoracki RJ, et al. Pharyngoesophageal reconstruction with the anterolateral thigh flap after total laryngopharyngectomy. *Cancer.* 2010;116:1718–1724.

60. Yu P. Characteristics of the anterolateral thigh flap in a western population and its application in head and neck reconstruction. *Head Neck.* 2004;26:759–769.

    This is a retrospective review of 72 consecutive anterolateral thigh flaps. The authors identify consistent vascular patterns and conclude the procedure is an efficacious restorative modality in western patients as well as for those in Asia.

62. Yu P. One-stage reconstruction of complex pharyngoesophageal, tracheal, and anterior neck defects. *Plast Reconstr Surg.* 2005;116:949–956.

70. Yu P. The transverse cervical vessels as recipient vessels for previously treated head and neck cancer patients. *Plast Reconstr Surg.* 2005;115:1253–1258.

14

Salivary gland tumors

Stephan Ariyan, Deepak Narayan, and Charlotte E. Ariyan

SYNOPSIS

- Salivary gland tumors occur in the range of 1–3 per 100 000 in the US.[1]
- Diagnosis of an enlarged salivary gland may be difficult and requires methodical examination and appropriate testing.
- Salivary gland tumors can be classified by their cell type and behavior pattern.
- Treatment decisions are based on the lesion's natural history.
- Prognosis is variable and depends upon tumor type and stage at diagnosis.

Introduction

1. Most parotid tumors are benign, while submandibular and sublingual tumors are more likely to be malignant.

2. Fine-needle aspiration (FNA) is very useful in the preoperative diagnosis of the tumor masses.

3. Techetium scans are very effective in the diagnosis of Warthin's tumors.

4. High-grade mucoepidermoid and squamous cell carcinomas have a very high incidence of nodal metastases.

5. Knowledge of the anatomy and variations of the branches of the facial nerve is critical to the safe resection of the parotid gland.

Basic science/disease process

Anatomy

Salivary glands are arranged as lobules of both mucinous cells (producing mucus), serous cells (producing thin salivary fluid), or combinations of serous and mucinous cells. The serous cells are small and have basophilic cytoplasm, while mucinous cells are larger, oval, and have a larger eosinophilic cytoplasm.

Parotid gland

The parotid gland is the largest of the salivary glands and is located on the face between the zygomatic arch and the angle of the mandible *(Fig. 14.1)*. Histologically, the parotid is virtually totally serous glands *(Fig. 14.2A)*. Although the parotid has a dense sheath overlying its surface, which is derived from the submuscular aponeurotic system (SMAS), it is not an encapsulated gland. It has multiple small segments, growths, and islands of tissue that are found within the subcutaneous tissue of the face. Furthermore, the parotid gland is not segmented into "lobes." Rather it is a single-lobed, C-shaped gland wrapping itself from its location over the mandible, around the ascending ramus, and to a location deep to the ramus, which is called the "deeper segment" *(Fig. 14.3)*. The portion of the gland overlying the mandible is separated by the plane made by the branches of the facial nerve coursing within the gland, hence the "superficial segment" overlying the facial nerve.

The facial nerve exits the skull at the stylomastoid foramen, posterior to the styloid process, and gives off its first branch, the posterior auricular nerve. This nerve innervates the auricularis muscle (allowing some patients to wiggle their ears), and gives a branch to the posterior belly of the digastric muscle (the anterior belly is innervated by a branch of the trigeminal nerve), and another branch to the stylohyoid muscle. The remainder of the main trunk of the facial nerve penetrates the mass of the parotid gland to arborize into its five remaining branches *(Fig. 14.4)*:

1. temporal branch to the frontalis muscle
2. zygomatic branch to the orbicularis oculi muscle
3. buccal branch to the muscles of the cheek and upper lip
4. mandibular branch to the muscles of the lower lip and chin
5. cervical branch to the platysma muscle.

The main secretory duct of the gland, the Stensen's duct, courses through the structures of the cheek to empty into the oral cavity through its orifice in the buccal mucosa at the level of the crown of the upper first and second molar teeth *(Fig. 14.1)*. The course of this duct through the cheek is along an imaginary line drawn from the tragus to the curve of the lateral nares. Occasionally, a small "accessory" parotid gland may become enlarged, presenting as a small nubbin of tissue anterior to the parotid gland, and overlying the Stensen's duct of the parotid.

There are several lymph nodes associated with the external surface of the parotid gland, and some may be embedded within this surface tissue. Occasionally, a lymph node can be found in the segment deep to the facial nerve.

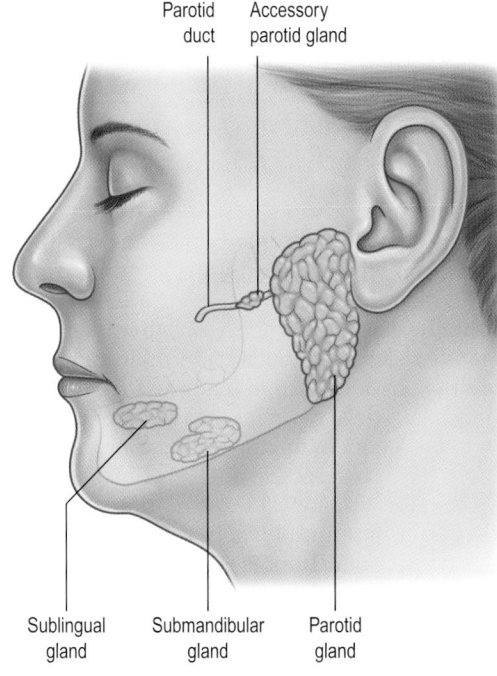

Fig. 14.1 The three paired salivary glands are located on the face. The parotid gland is above and behind the ascending ramus of the mandible; the submaxillary gland is under the body of the mandible, while the sublingual gland is under the mandible, deep to the floor of the mouth. A small accessory parotid gland may be located in front of the main parotid gland, overlying the parotid duct (Stensen's duct).

Submandibular gland

The submandibular glands (also called the submaxillary glands) lie bilaterally deep to the horizontal body of the mandible, and are about one-fourth to one-third the size of the parotid gland *(Fig. 14.1)*. They secrete saliva through the left and right Wharton's ducts, which course under the lateral floor of the mouth, each of which exits into the oral cavity just short of the midline along the root of the undersurface of the tongue. On histologic evaluation, the submandibular gland is composed of a mixture of serous and mucous glands *(Fig. 14.2B)*.

The mandibular branch of the facial nerve is found under the platysma muscle, coursing 1–2 cm below and parallel to the body of the mandible, and overlying the submandibular gland as it crosses the facial vessels. Usually, there is also a lymph node associated with the external surface of the submandibular gland.

Sublingual gland

This gland is the smallest of the salivary glands, and is frequently half the size of the submandibular gland. It is located under the mucosal surface of the lateral floor of the mouth, along the lingual surface of the mandible, located anterior to the submandibular gland. The gland has several secretory ducts that empty to the oral cavity through the oral mucosa, although on occasion they can become confluent and empty as a single duct into the Wharton's duct. Histologically, the sublingual glands are composed predominantly of mucous glands *(Fig. 14.2C)*.

Minor salivary glands

The oral cavity is also interspersed within a number of small aggregates of salivary tissue located in the palate, the lip, the buccal mucosa, or the oral mucosa.

Epidemiology

The incidence of salivary gland tumor in the US is in the range of 1–3 per 100 000 population.[1] This represents less than 3% of all tumors of the body, and the largest bulk of these salivary gland tumors are found in the parotid gland. In fact, the proportion of tumors of the parotid gland compared to the submandibular gland and sublingual gland are 100:10:1.[2]

While the vast majority of salivary gland tumors are found in the parotid gland, it is important to note that 80% are

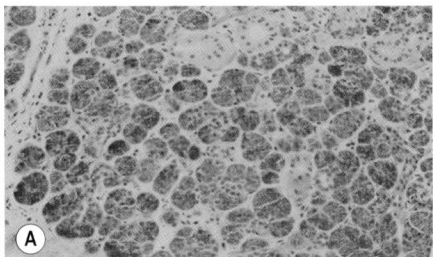
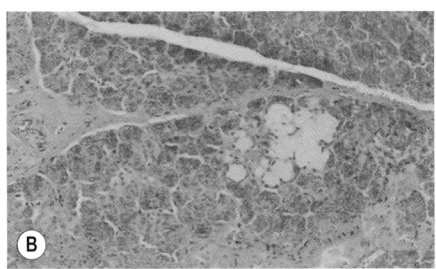
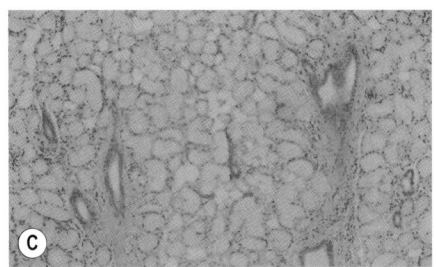

Fig. 14.2 The parotid gland is composed of essentially only serous glands **(A)**, the submandibular gland is a mixture of serous and mucous glands **(B)**, and the sublingual gland is virtually all mucous glands **(C)**.

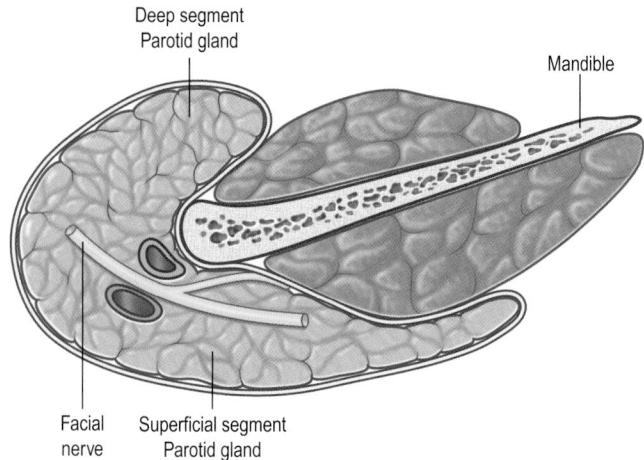

Fig. 14.3 The parotid gland is wrapped around the ascending ramus of the mandible with the deep segment, and the superficial segment overlying the facial nerve.

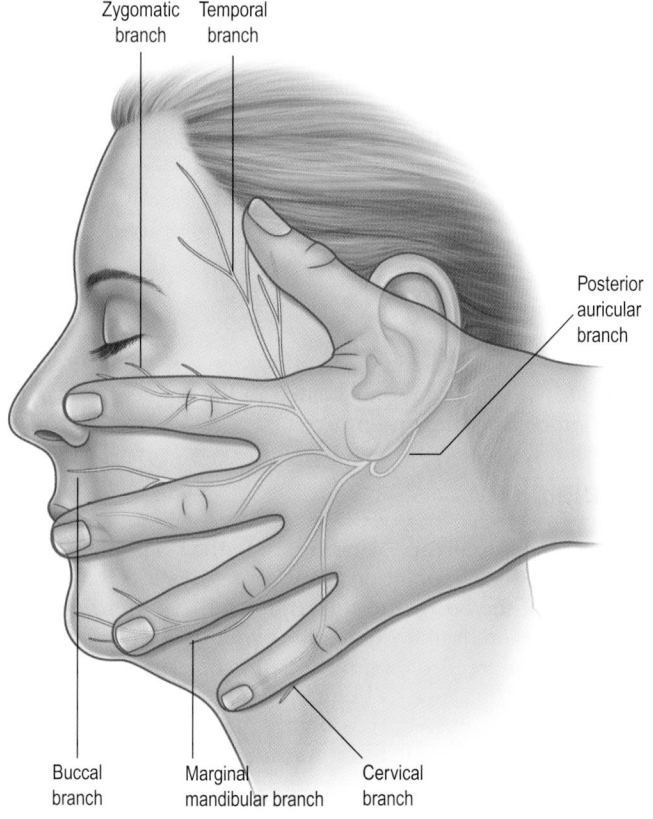

Fig. 14.4 The facial nerve exits the skull giving off one branch, the posterior auricular nerve to the auricularis muscle, and then proceeds to penetrate the parotid gland to give its next five branches. An easy way to remember these branches and their location is depicted by the five fingers of the hand superimposed on the face.

Table 14.1 **Tumors of the salivary glands**		
	Benign	**Malignant**
Parotid	80%	20%
Submaxillary	60%	40%
Sublingual	40%	60%
Minor salivary glands	20%	80%

that there is a high incidence of malignant tumors of the salivary glands among patients who had been exposed to previous radiation.[8]

An association between radiation exposure and salivary gland tumors was first identified in survivors of the atomic bomb in Hiroshima, Japan. One investigation selected 66 patients for a study to evaluate whether there was an increased incidence of malignant salivary gland tumors among individuals with exposure to radiation. Among the atomic bomb survivors, 52.8% (19/36) had malignant salivary gland tumors, while only 16.7% (5/30) of the nonexposed population developed malignant tumors.[9] A further analysis of this data determined that the risk was highest, but not limited to, mucoepidermoid tumors.[10] These reports have been followed by a more recent follow-up study of survivors evaluating dose of radiation exposure from the atomic bomb. In this study, there was an increase only in mucoepidermoid and Warthin's tumors among individuals with an increased radiation dose (estimated radiation dose according to the dosimetry system; high exposure relative risk 9.3 for mucoepidermoid cancer (11 cases) and relative risk 4.1 for Warthin's tumor (12 cases)).[11]

On the other hand, low-dose radiation has also been shown to be associated with subsequent malignant transformation of salivary gland tumors. A retrospective analysis of Israeli children who were treated with low-dose radiation for tinea capitis at the time of their immigration between 1949 and 1960 revealed an increase in parotid tumors (4/1000 in irradiated group versus 0/1000 in population control).[12] In another study, a population of patients receiving X-ray therapy for acne in Los Angeles revealed an increased incidence of malignant parotid tumors. Those patients who had received more than 15 such treatments had an 8.0 relative risk, and it is estimated that 28% of malignant tumors that occurred in Los Angeles from 1976 to 1984 were attributable to radiation.[13] All these reports suggest that there is a lag phase between the radiation exposure and the malignant transformation of the salivary and endocrine glands. In order to explore this further, a study of patients who had received head and neck irradiation to the tonsillar area and the nasopharynx demonstrated the interval between radiation exposure and tumor diagnosis was from 7 to 32 years.[14] For these reasons, it is essential that patients who have received radiation should be continually followed for the potential of developing subsequent salivary gland tumors.

Diagnosis/patient presentation

The interpretation of an enlarged salivary gland may prove to be a difficult clinical diagnosis. One of the reasons for this

benign.[3] On the other hand, 40% of tumors of the submandibular gland and 60% of tumors of the sublingual gland are found to be malignant[4] *(Table 14.1)*. While tumors of the minor salivary glands are uncommon, 60–80% are malignant.[5–7] No etiological factors have been found for the development of tumors of the salivary glands. However, it has been shown

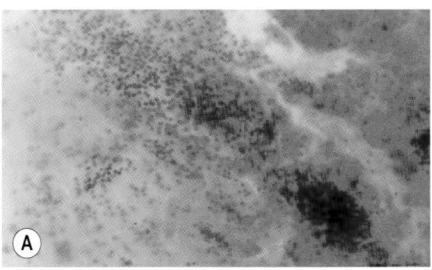 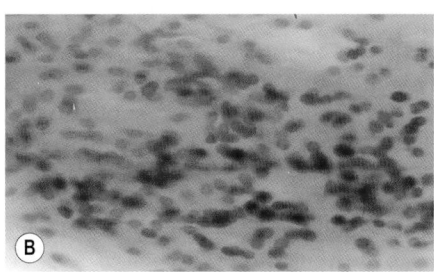 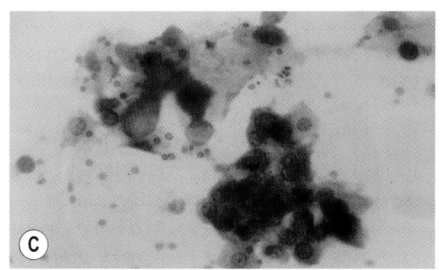

Fig. 14.5 Cytology of fine-needle aspiration specimens showing collections of serous cells mixed with mesenchymal stroma **(A)** representing pleomorphic adenoma. Malignant squamous cells **(B)** representing mucoepidermoid carcinoma. Lymphocytic collections **(C)** and salivary gland with cluster of lymphoid tissue representing Warthin's tumor.

is the fact that many benign enlargements are reactive inflammations, or salivary cysts. Nevertheless, each should be evaluated carefully and methodically with selected examination and tests.

Fine-needle aspiration

FNA biopsy of salivary gland tumors is an area of controversy since the presence of the tumor itself, in the view of many surgeons, should be indication enough to operate. Proponents of the technique argue that FNA is valuable in preoperatively counseling the patient about possible facial nerve sacrifice, prognosis, and the necessity for adjunctive procedures such as neck dissection if the tumor proves to be malignant (e.g., for high-grade mucoepidermoid carcinoma). Additionally, FNA may save the patient an unnecessary operation by differentiating a diagnosis of inflammatory versus neoplastic lesion, or by making a diagnosis of a Warthin's tumor in a patient who poses a poor surgical risk, enabling observation alone.

Germane to this discussion is the accuracy of FNA in the context of salivary gland tumors. The sensitivity and specificity of FNA for salivary gland tumors reported in the literature range from a high of 99% sensitivity and 100% specificity, as reported by Bhatia,[15] to a low of 90% sensitivity and 75% specificity, as reported by Cohen and colleagues.[16] In general, however, recent series document a trend towards a higher degree of sensitivity and specificity.[17,18] A higher degree of accuracy has been reported for benign tumors.[19–21]

The common diagnostic pitfalls involve distinction between benign oncocytic tumors and acinic cell carcinomas, pleomorphic adenomas and adenoid cystic carcinomas, high-grade mucoepidermoid carcinoma and metastatic squamous cell carcinoma, and finally low-grade mucoepidermoid carcinoma and Warthin's tumor *(Fig. 14.5)*. Mucoepidermoid carcinomas appear to be the most difficult to diagnose by FNA.[22] In an effort to improve diagnostic accuracy of aspirates, special immunohistochemical stains such as glial fibrillary acid protein for pleomorphic adenomas[23] and silver staining of nucleolar organizer region have been used.[24]

A diagnosis of lymphoma on FNA should necessitate an open biopsy or a superficial parotidectomy to evaluate nodal architecture and to obtain adequate tissue for immunohistochemical characterization in order to classify the lymphoma properly.

FNA is essentially free of complications. Hemorrhage and necrosis of the tumor following aspiration of a lymphoma[21]

and a Warthin's tumor[25] have been reported, but such occurrences are exceedingly rare. The concerns regarding needle track seeding have been specifically addressed by several authors,[21,26,27] who have found no cause for alarm because of its exceedingly low occurrence.

The technique of FNA we use is still essentially the same as that reported previously by us in 1981.[28] A 21-gauge needle is affixed to a 10-cc controlled syringe, retaining no air in the syringe barrel, and applying negative pressure by withdrawing the plunger. A minimum of two passes is made into the tumor. The needle is withdrawn and removed from the syringe, air is drawn into the cylinder, the needle is reapplied to the syringe, and a tiny droplet of specimen is applied to the glass slide to prepare a slide smear. The slides are placed immediately into a jar of absolute or 95% alcohol. Next, alcohol is withdrawn through the needle into the syringe and flushed a few times into another jar of absolute alcohol to prepare a cell block.

Imaging modalities

The introduction of high-resolution imaging in the form of computed tomography (CT) scans and magnetic resonance imaging (MRI) has revolutionized our ability to define the extent of various pathological processes throughout the body, and the salivary glands are no exception. Paradoxically, despite the level of technical advancement achieved, these modalities are not routinely used in the management of salivary gland tumors. Part of this is due to the fact that a histological diagnosis based on these images is still not possible given the current degree of sophistication. Additional imaging techniques that have been used in defining salivary gland pathology include ultrasound, sialography, and technetium scans.

Computed tomography

The ready availability and the cost of this imaging modality account for the popularity of CT scans if additional imaging studies are required by the clinician. While the ultimate choice of a CT scan or MRI may be dictated by nonclinical factors, the consensus is that CT scans are better in a patient with a history of inflammatory disorder while MRI is the modality of choice for palpable masses.[29,30] Specific clinical scenarios, as discussed below, may mandate the use of CT scans.

CT scans are particularly sensitive in the detection of calcium deposits in the salivary glands, a property which is useful in the diagnosis of elusive ductal calculi. This represents a marked advantage over MRI. Along the same lines, while extraglandular tumor spread is equally well visualized by both modalities, demonstration of subtle bony erosion or sclerosis requires the use of CT scans. Involvement of tumor into soft tissue is better visualized by MRI.

Cystic salivary lesions are another area where CT scans hold an advantage over MRI. The presence of a high water content in a majority of salivary gland tumors is presumed to be the cause of the inability of routine MRIs to distinguish between a cyst and a solid mass.

Artifacts from dental implants can have a negative impact on the quality of CT images. This can however be mitigated by special views. The facial nerve is not routinely imaged in CT scans and can represent a disadvantage when dealing with tumors with a predilection for perineural spread.

Magnetic resonance imaging

The distinction between benign and malignant tumors on MRI is predicated upon the difference in water content between the two types of tumor. The distinction however is not absolute. Som and Curtin[30] point out that high-grade malignancies tend to have low to intermediate signal intensities on all imaging sequences. Well-differentiated tumors, on the other hand, which include benign tumors and low-grade malignancies, tend to have a low T1 and high T2 signal intensity *(Table 14.2)*. This is explained by the fact that low-grade malignancies are generally well differentiated enough to produce secretory products, which therefore yield a higher net water content, reflected by a high T2 signal.

Contrast agents were developed to improve image resolution on MRI; among these, gadolinium-containing compounds are the most widely used. Gadolinium chelates were developed because of the high relaxivity of the gadolinium ion coupled with the relatively low toxicity of the complex with chelation of the metal ion.[31] Gadolinium therefore enhances lesion identification and characterization. Some authors have suggested that the routine use of gadolinium in MR studies of the salivary glands improves the quality of data obtained. The consensus, however, is that this adjunct is not necessary for the majority of cases.[30]

Kramer and Mafee[32] note that the intensity of the signal of the parotid gland is slightly less than that of subcutaneous fat,

and greater relative to muscle on T1-weighted, proton density-weighted, and T2-weighted images. Additionally the submandibular gland has a slightly lower signal intensity than the sublingual gland on proton density-weighted and T2-weighted sequences. This enables the distinction of the deep segment of the submandibular gland from the sublingual gland. These authors recommend conventional transverse T1-weighted and fast spin echo or short T1 inversion recovery T2-weighted techniques without gadolinium for tumors. Intravenous injection of paramagnetic contrast material, however, is extremely useful in evaluating perineural spread and cervical node involvement. MRI is particularly advantageous in delineating the margins of a lesion, thereby enabling clinicians to distinguish between multiple masses and lobulated solitary lesions. These differences in signal intensity as seen by MRI help to differentiate between the various neoplasms involving the salivary gland *(Table 14.2)*.

Ultrasound

Ultrasonography is most helpful in distinguishing solid from cystic lesions. Cystic lesions that are identified with ultrasound include simple lymphoepithelial cysts, cystic hygromas involving the salivary glands, ranulas, sialoceles and multiple lymphoepithelial cysts associated with human immunodeficiency virus (HIV). However the diagnostic capabilities of this modality are inferior to that of CT and MRI in solid masses. Color Doppler studies attempting to correlate pathology with flow patterns have likewise proven disappointing.

Technetium scan

The ability of salivary glands to concentrate technetium99m pertechnetate (Tc^{99m}) forms the basis of the use of this nuclear medicine technique in imaging salivary glands. The increased metabolic activity of the cells comprising Warthin's tumor produces the characteristic image of increased uptake. Oncocytomas are other lesions that may take up this tracer in excess of surrounding gland. Rarely, oncocytic rests in pleomorphic adenomas and oncocytic tumor metastases might also mimic this picture. Aside from Warthin's tumor, Tc^{99m} scans are not very useful in salivary gland imaging.

Sialography

Sialography is an invasive procedure which involves identification of the ductal opening of the gland to be studied, cannulation, injection of contrast material, and obtaining views in different planes. Sialograms or contrast delineation of the ductal structure of a salivary gland have very little application today in the face of near-perfect images produced by MRIs and CT scans.[33] Sialograms are useful in demonstrating ductal calculi and ductal disruptions secondary to trauma. Sialograms are said to be more sensitive than MRI in the diagnosis of Sjögren's syndrome in the early stages of the disease.[30] The sialographic appearance of Sjögren's syndrome is characterized by a uniformly distributed, punctate accumulation of contrast material throughout the gland, graphically described as a "leafless fruit-laden tree."[30]

Table 14.2 Distinction between benign and malignant tumors by magnetic resonance imaging

	T1	T2
Lymphoma	Low	High
Malignancy (high-grade)	Low	Low
Lipoma	Fat signal	Fat signal
Warthin's tumor	Intermediate	High
Pleomorphic adenomas	Low to intermediate	High
Hemangioma*	Intermediate	High

*Signal voids representing large-vessel phleboliths are characteristic. Venous malformations are best diagnosed by magnetic resonance imaging; true arteriovenous fistulae require an arteriogram for diagnosis.

Table 14.3 Salivary gland tumors		
Primary tumors		
Benign		
Epithelial	Pleomorphic adenoma (benign mixed tumor)	
	Monomorphic adenoma	
	Papillary cystadenoma lymphomatosum (Warthin's tumor)	
	Oncocytoma	
Nonepithelial	Hemangioma	
Malignant		
Epithelial	Mucoepidermoid carcinoma	
	Adenoid cystic carcinoma (cylindroma)	
	Acinic cell carcinoma	
	Malignant mixed tumor	
	Squamous cell carcinoma	
	Adenocarcinoma	
	Oncocytic carcinoma	
Nonepithelial	Lymphoma	
Metastatic tumors to salivary glands		
Melanoma		
Thyroid		
Kidney		
Breast		
Lung		
Colon		

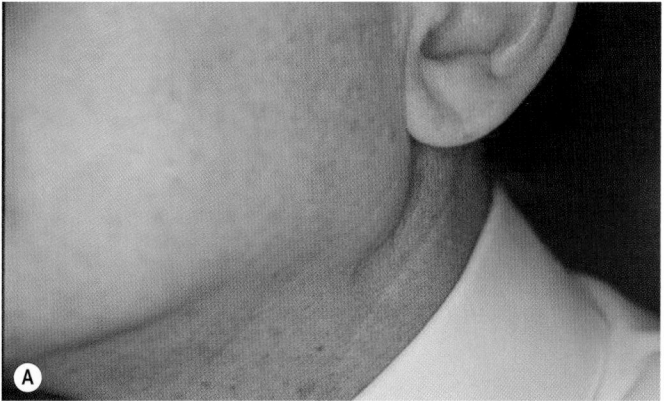
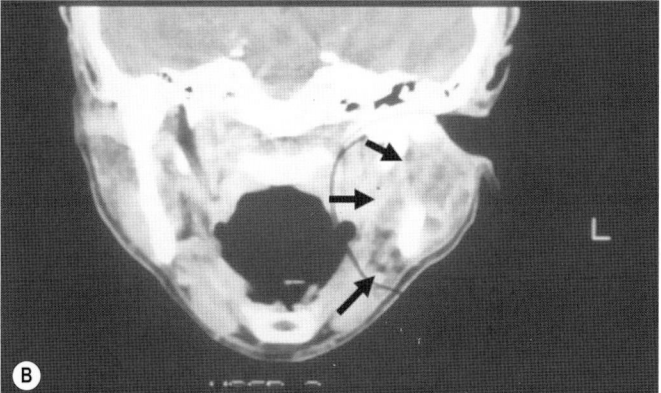
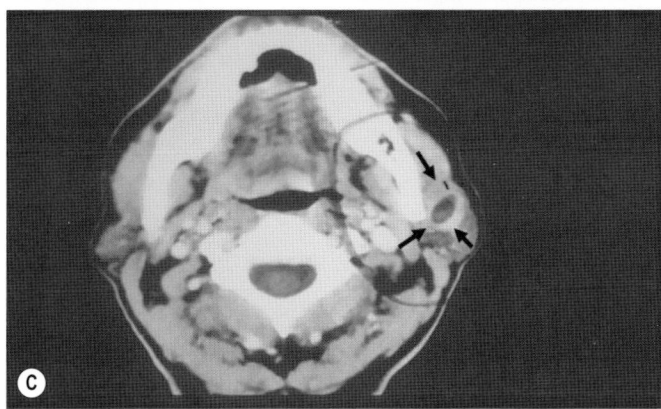

Fig. 14.6 (A) An abscess of the parotid gland is seen as a smooth mass at the angle of the jaw. The computed tomography scans **(B and C)** show a multiloculated collection.

Classification of tumors

The simplest way to classify salivary gland tumors is by their histologic cell types (epithelial or nonepithelial) and by their behavior patterns (benign or malignant) *(Table 14.3)*.

Nonneoplastic lesions

Sialadenosis

The salivary gland can enlarge for nutritional reasons not related to neoplastic cellular changes. These enlargements have been found associated with cirrhosis, malnutrition, or vitamin deficiency.

Sialadenitis

The gland can become enlarged due to inflammatory conditions. These can be due to trauma to the maxillofacial area, due to viruses (most commonly mumps or HIV),[34] or due to bacteria (most commonly *Staphylococcus aureus*) which can lead to abscess formation *(Fig. 14.6)*. Unusual causes of enlargement have been found to be related to sarcoidosis,[35,36] in which case, multiple salivary glands may be found to be enlarged.

Sialolithiasis

Stones in the ducts of the salivary glands *(Fig. 14.7)* are a common condition leading to a mass within the gland, or

enlargement of the gland secondary to obstruction of salivary flow. Most of these are found in the submandibular gland *(Fig. 14.8)*, and a lesser number are found in the parotid gland. Sometimes a sialogram may show no stones, but rather a stenosis from previous trauma that leads to obstructed or restricted flow *(Fig. 14.9)*.

Mucocele

These retention cysts of mucus production are most commonly found in the minor salivary glands. Frequently these are located in the lower lip, and they sometimes develop after trauma to the lip, laceration and suture repair, or secondary healing.

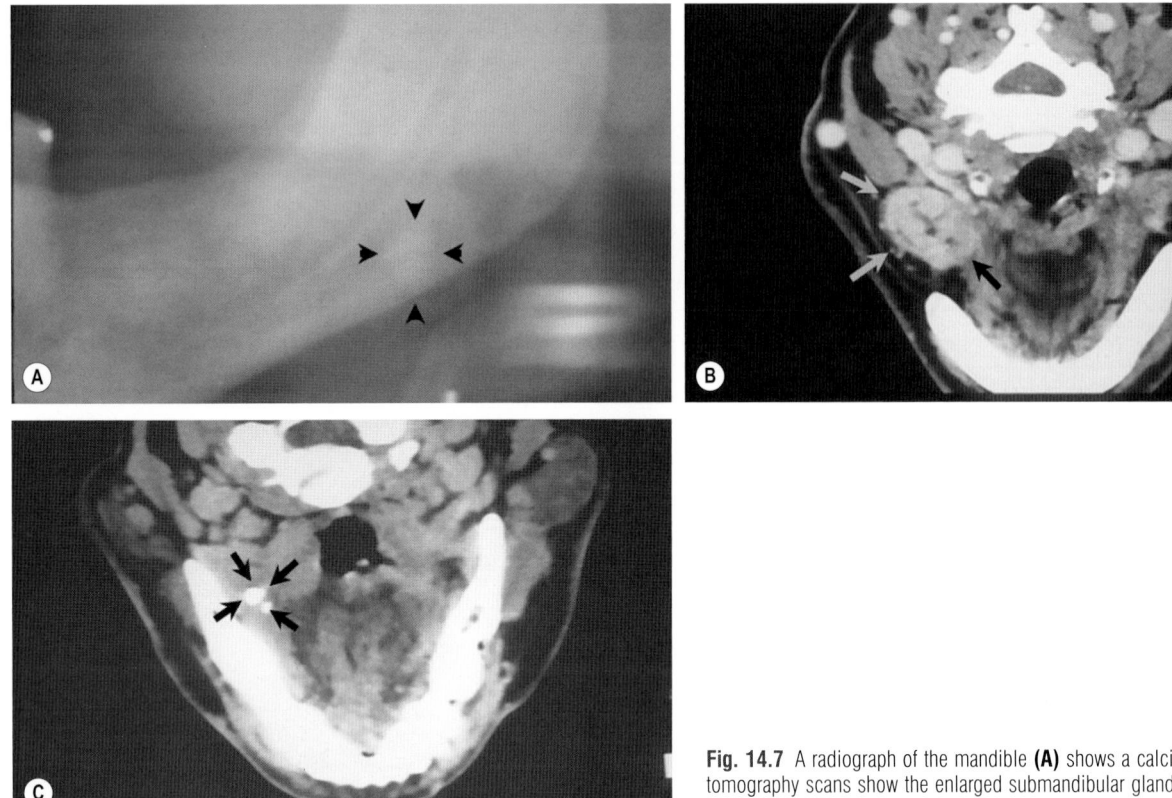

Fig. 14.7 A radiograph of the mandible **(A)** shows a calcified stone. The computed tomography scans show the enlarged submandibular gland **(B)** and the calcified stone **(C)**.

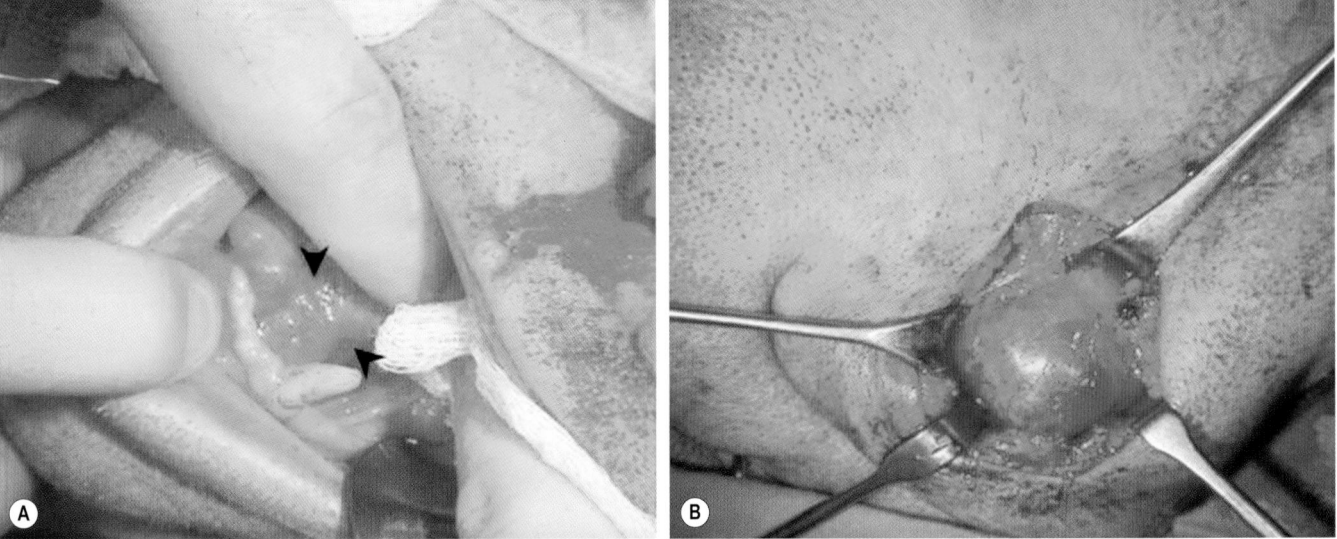

Fig. 14.8 An obstructed edematous Wharton's duct in the floor of the mouth **(A)** has led to an enlarged salivary cyst **(B)** within the submandibular gland.

Necrotizing sialometaplasia

This is an unusual and clinically disturbing lesion that has an uncertain cause. It may or may not be related to trauma to the oral mucosa, but is manifest as an enlarging, and often painless, ulceration.[37,38] They are more commonly found in the palatal mucosa *(Fig. 14.10)*, but can also be seen in the buccal mucosa or the lips.

Benign neoplastic lesions

Pleomorphic adenoma

Also known as the benign mixed tumor, pleomorphic adenoma is the most common tumor of the salivary glands. The tumor was originally believed to be "mixed" neoplastic cells derived from both duct epithelial cells and myoepithelial

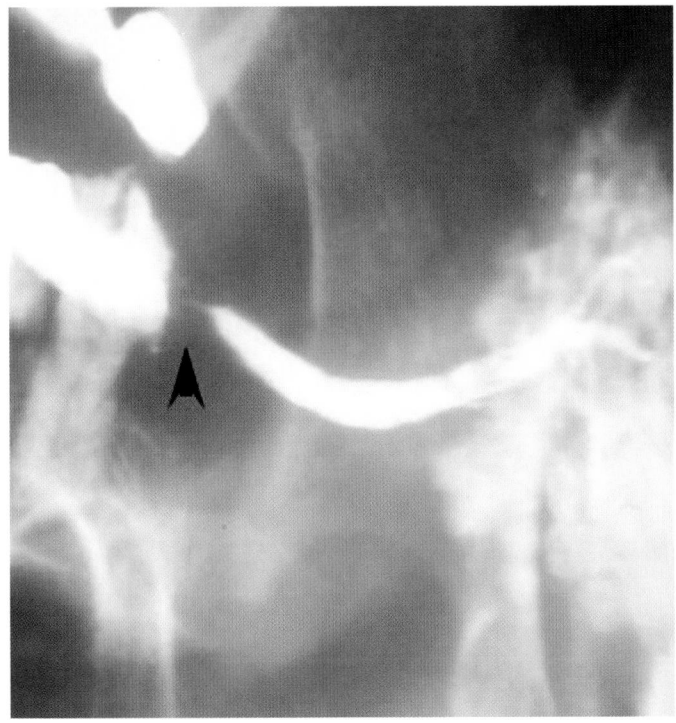

Fig. 14.9 An enlarged parotid gland was found to be due to a stenosis of the Stensen's duct when radiopaque dye is injected in a sialogram.

cells. However, these are now known to be neoplasms of purely the ectodermal cells.

They most commonly occur in the parotid gland (80–90% of cases), and appear as painless, "rubbery" firm, 1–2-cm masses in the deeper tissue. They are not attached to the overlying skin, and they do not cause any muscle dysfunction by pressure on the motor branches of the facial nerve. They can rarely be found bilaterally.[39]

Histologically, there is a distribution of mostly epithelial and stromal (mesenchymal) cells. These mesenchymal areas of the tumor may consist of chondroid or hyalinized stroma that have the appearance of hyaline cartilage on histologic examination.

Monomorphic adenoma

Although related to pleomorphic adenoma (benign mixed tumor), these tumors are usually manifest as single-cell variants of the benign mixed tumor. These tumors have been classified differently by a variety of authors, but the most widely used classification is that of Batsakis,[40] which describes the tumor to be derived from the duct cells. As such, they are either purely epithelial (basal cell adenoma) *(Fig. 14.11)*, or purely mesenchymal (myoepithelioma) tumors. Histologically, these tumors are found to grow by expansion against the salivary gland tissue and not by infiltration. Batsakis believes that, if left alone, these tumors would eventually develop into the pleomorphic variant of the adenoma.

Warthin's tumor (papillary cystadenoma lymphomatosum)

This benign tumor is the second most common tumor of parotid glands. It is found almost exclusively in the parotid

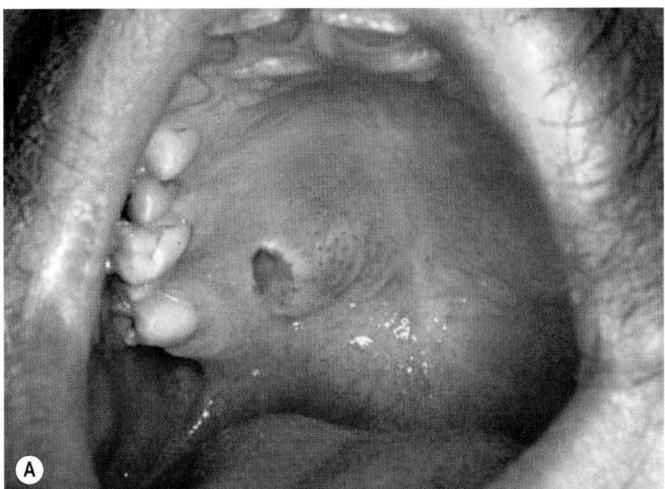
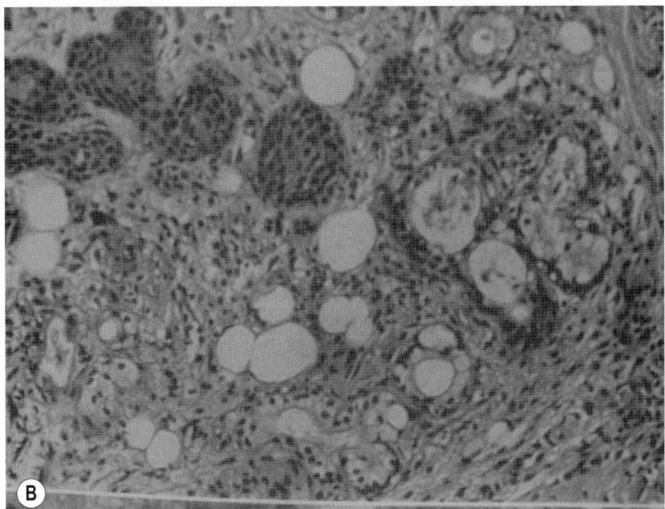
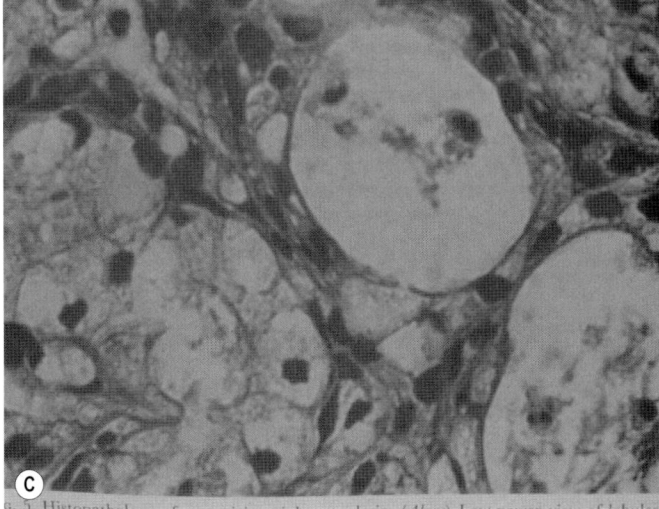

Fig. 14.10 (A) Necrotizing sialometaplasia presenting as an ulcer with sharp margins in the palate of a 56-year-old male. (B) Histologic examination of this lesion under low power shows liquefaction and necrosis of mucinous glands and marked inflammatory response. (C) High-power view shows destruction of gland, release of mucin, and acute inflammation. (Reproduced from Gahhos F, Enriquez RE, Bahn S, et al. Necrotizing sialometaplasia: a review of the literature and report of five cases. Plast Reconstr Surg. 1983;71:650, with permission.)

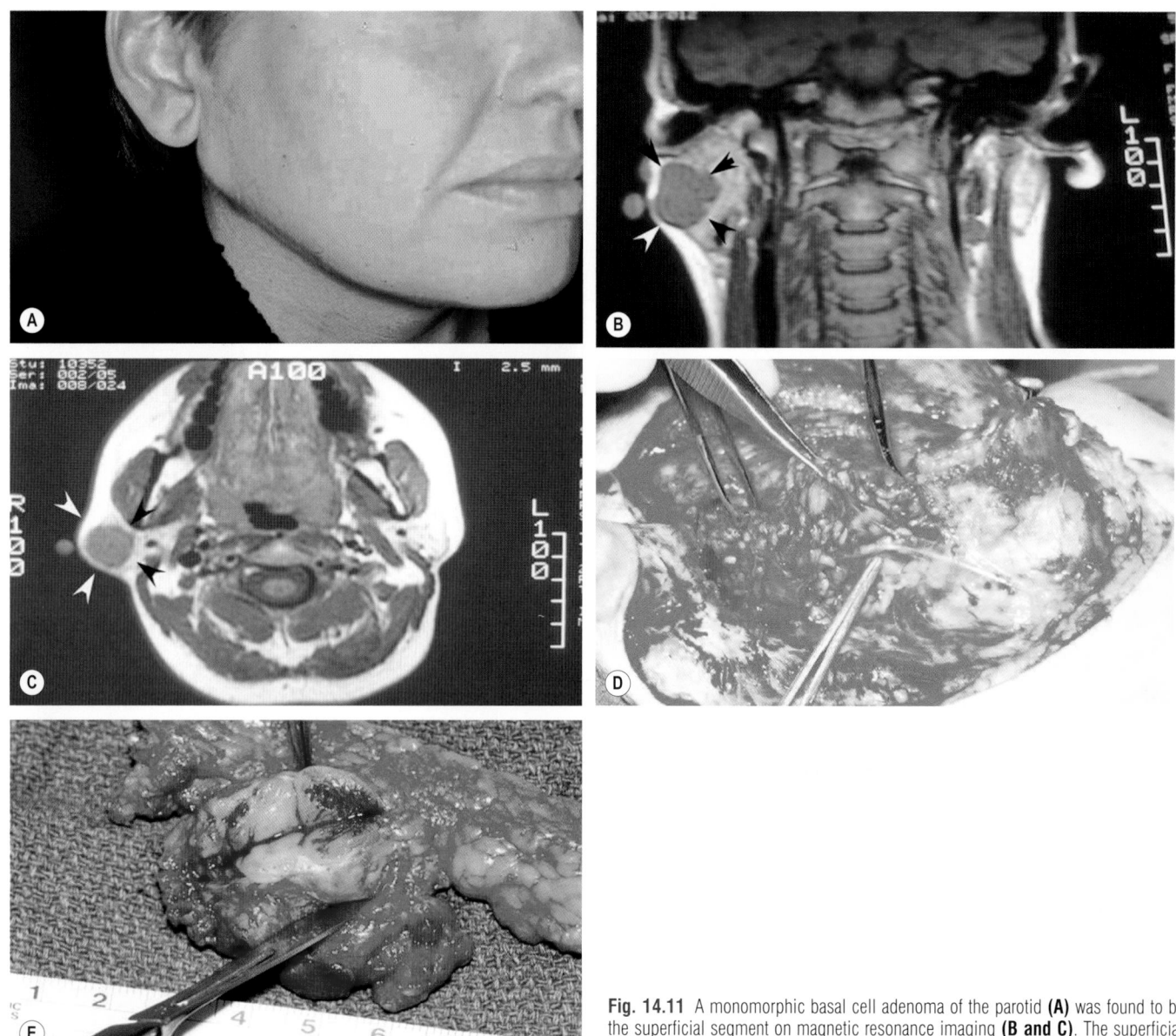

Fig. 14.11 A monomorphic basal cell adenoma of the parotid **(A)** was found to be in the superficial segment on magnetic resonance imaging **(B and C)**. The superficial parotidectomy **(D)** removed the tumor **(E)**.

gland, and is most commonly found in males between 50 and 60 years old.[41] It is clinically detected as a smooth mass, 3–4 cm in diameter, in the superficial segment of the gland *(Fig. 14.12)*, and may be found bilaterally in about 10% of patients.[42,43]

These tumors are derived from the proliferation of lymphoid tissues of periparotid or intraparotid lymph nodes. As such, they are believed to be proliferative tumors rather than neoplastic tumors. The diagnosis can be aided preoperatively by technetium scans, since the tumor consistently concentrates this isotope, and gives the appearance of a "hot gland."[44] A preoperative FNA biopsy may show the lymphoid tissue and confirm the diagnosis.

Oncocytoma

This is a benign neoplasm of the oncocytes, and represents less than 1% of all salivary gland tumors.[45] It is usually found in the parotid gland as an encapsulated lobular mass, often in elderly patients. It is believed by some to be a result of aging tissue in salivary glands rather than a true neoplastic development.

Hemangioma

These tumors are found mostly in the parotid glands, and 50% of these tumors are diagnosed in children.[46] In fact, they are the predominant tumor of parotid glands in children *(Fig. 14.13)*. The tumors are present at birth, and are usually identified within the first few months of life. The lesions are capillary, cavernous, or mixed vascular malformations. The capillary hemangiomas are the most common, and often grow rapidly for the first 6 months before undergoing spontaneous resolution over the next 5–6 years. The cavernous or mixed vascular malformations may continue to grow.

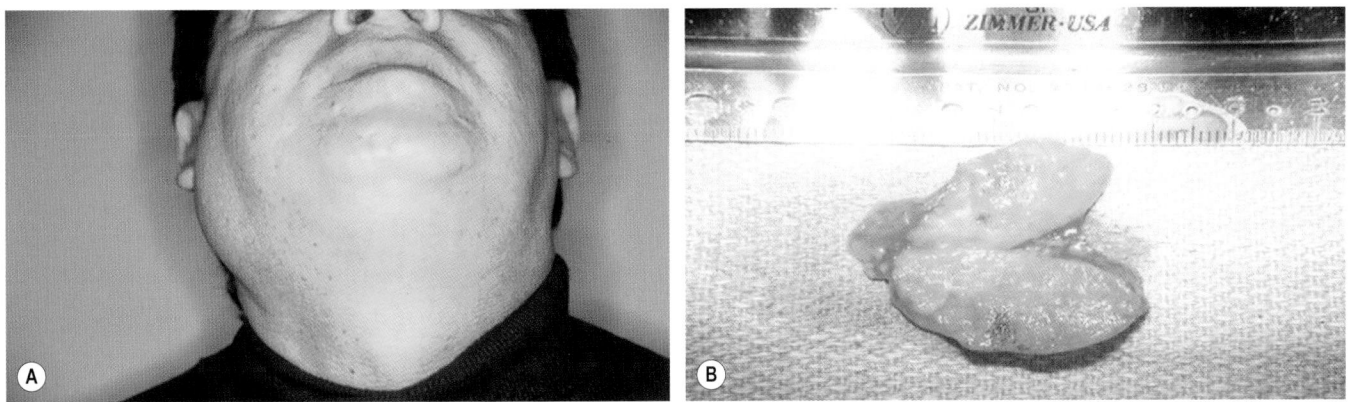

Fig. 14.12 A unilateral Warthin's tumor in a middle-aged male **(A)** was removed and shows the cystic lymphoid tissue on cut section of the tumor **(B)**.

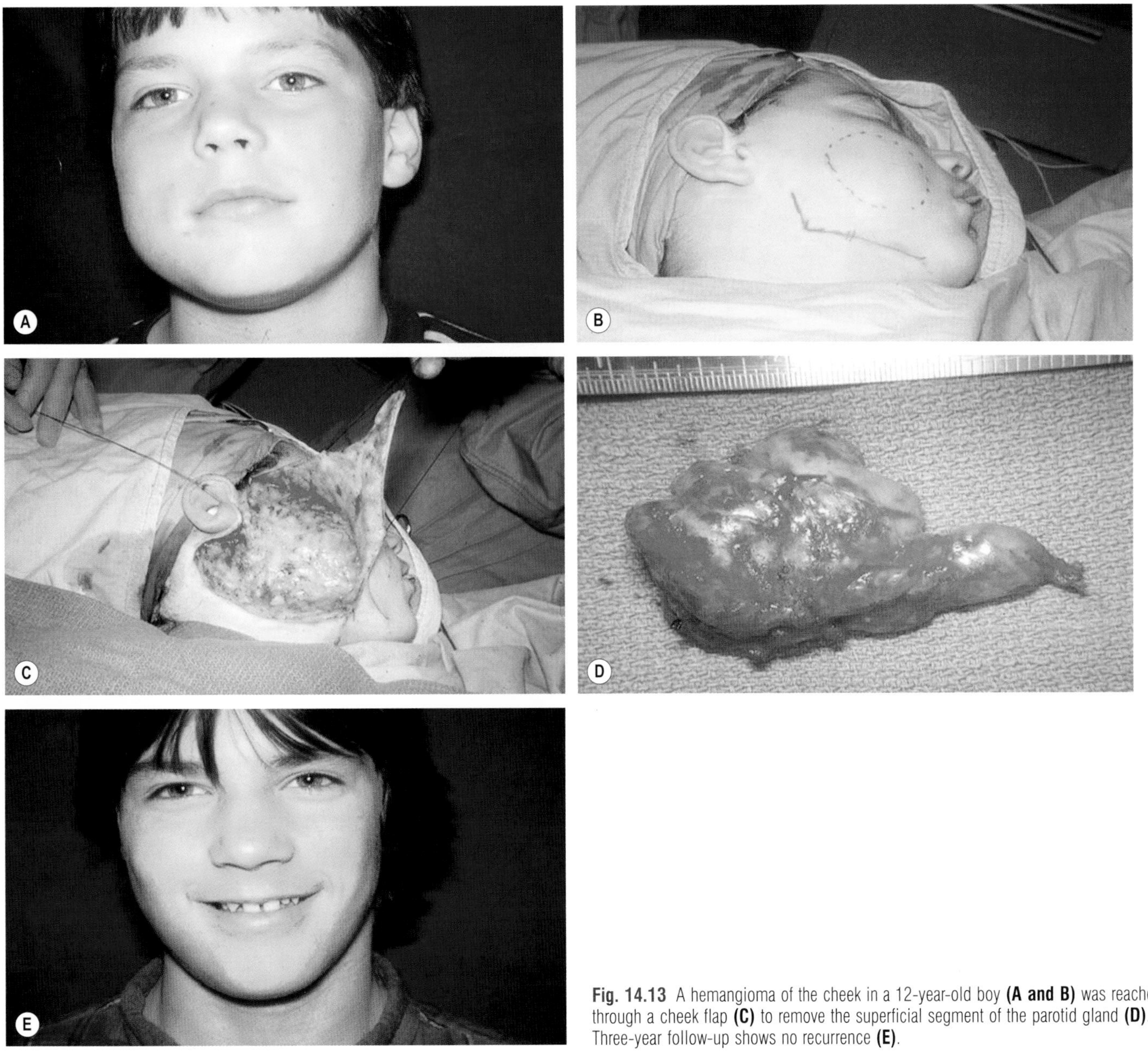

Fig. 14.13 A hemangioma of the cheek in a 12-year-old boy **(A and B)** was reached through a cheek flap **(C)** to remove the superficial segment of the parotid gland **(D)**. Three-year follow-up shows no recurrence **(E)**.

Table 14.4 Malignant tumors of parotid gland

Type	Percentage
Mucoepidermoid	24
Adenoid cystic	16
Acinic cell	15
Adenocarcinoma	13
Squamous cell	5
Undifferentiated	27

Table 14.5 Malignant tumors of submaxillary glands and sublingual glands

Type	Submandibular	Sublingual
Adenoid cystic	50%	45%
Mucoepidermoid	25%	40%
Adenocarcinoma	20%	
Malignant mixed	5%	

Malignant neoplastic lesions

Mucoepidermoid carcinoma

This tumor arises from the excretory ducts of the glands and represents the most common malignancy of salivary glands *(Tables 14.4 and 14.5)*. Mucoepidermoid carcinoma is the most common malignancy to occur in the parotid gland. Grossly, the tumor appears as a slow-growing, firm to hard mass within the salivary gland. If the tumor is neglected by the patient and it grows larger, there may be associated pain (from sensory nerve involvement) or ipsilateral weakness of certain facial muscles (due to tumor infiltration into branches of the facial nerve).

The tumors are characterized histologically by the presence of mucin-producing cells, squamous cells of the ducts or acini, and other cells with little differentiation and scant cytoplasm. They are classified as low-grade, intermediate-grade, or high-grade malignant lesions based on the histologic evaluation of the cell types predominating in the tumor.[47,48]

Adenoid cystic carcinoma (cylindroma)

These tumors are the second most common malignancy found in the parotid gland, and the most common among the submandibular and sublingual glands *(Tables 14.4 and 14.5)*. This tumor gets its name from its characteristic histologic pattern of cystic or cribriform arrangement that gives a "Swiss cheese" appearance *(Fig. 14.14)*. Clinically, the tumor appears as a firm 1–3-cm lesion that is fixed.

Acinic cell carcinoma

These are malignancies of the acinic cells of salivary glands, and are found overwhelmingly in the parotid gland. They are solid tumors that are 1–3 cm in diameter, but may also appear as cystic masses. The tumor can be multifocal, and 3% of these lesions are found bilaterally.[49]

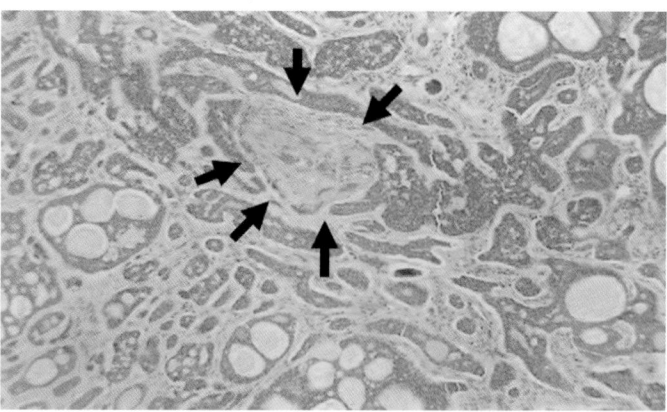

Fig. 14.14 Adenoid cystic carcinoma showing cystic and cribriform pattern typically scribed as "Swiss cheese." The center of this section shows the tumor cells invading nerve (arrows).

Adenocarcinoma

These tumors are classified by the very nature of being excluded from the above categories of glandular malignancies. As such, their true incidence is not known, but they probably represent about 3–5% of all salivary gland tumors.

Malignant mixed tumors

These tumors are most commonly malignant transformation from a benign pleomorphic adenoma. While it is believed that malignant cells may develop primarily with the basic pattern of a mixed tumor, the consensus remains that malignant mixed tumors and carcinomas arising in a pleomorphic adenoma are one and the same.

However, there is a difference between the recurrent benign mixed tumor, where the tumor is composed of well-circumscribed nodules growing in scar tissue and shows benign cytologic patterns, and the malignant mixed tumor, which is not circumscribed but shows invasion into adjacent tissue and nerves.[50]

Squamous cell carcinoma

These are very rare tumors of the salivary glands, and must be differentiated from squamous cell carcinomas metastatic to salivary glands, or underdiagnosed mucoepidermoid carcinoma. The true squamous cell carcinomas represent cancers arising from the salivary ducts themselves.

Oncocytic carcinoma

This is a malignant variant of the oncocytoma (itself representing only 1% of all salivary gland tumors), making this a very rare tumor.

Lymphoma

Clinically, these tumors represent the local manifestation of a systemic disease. When it involves salivary glands, it almost always involves the parotid gland, as this is the only salivary gland that contains lymph nodes or lymphoid tissue. These tumors are removed as an excisional biopsy of the lymph node *(Fig 14.15)*, and are evaluated histologically for diagnosis and classification of the type of lymphoma.

There is now an increasing incidence of acquired immunodeficiency syndrome (AIDS) diagnosed by the lymph node

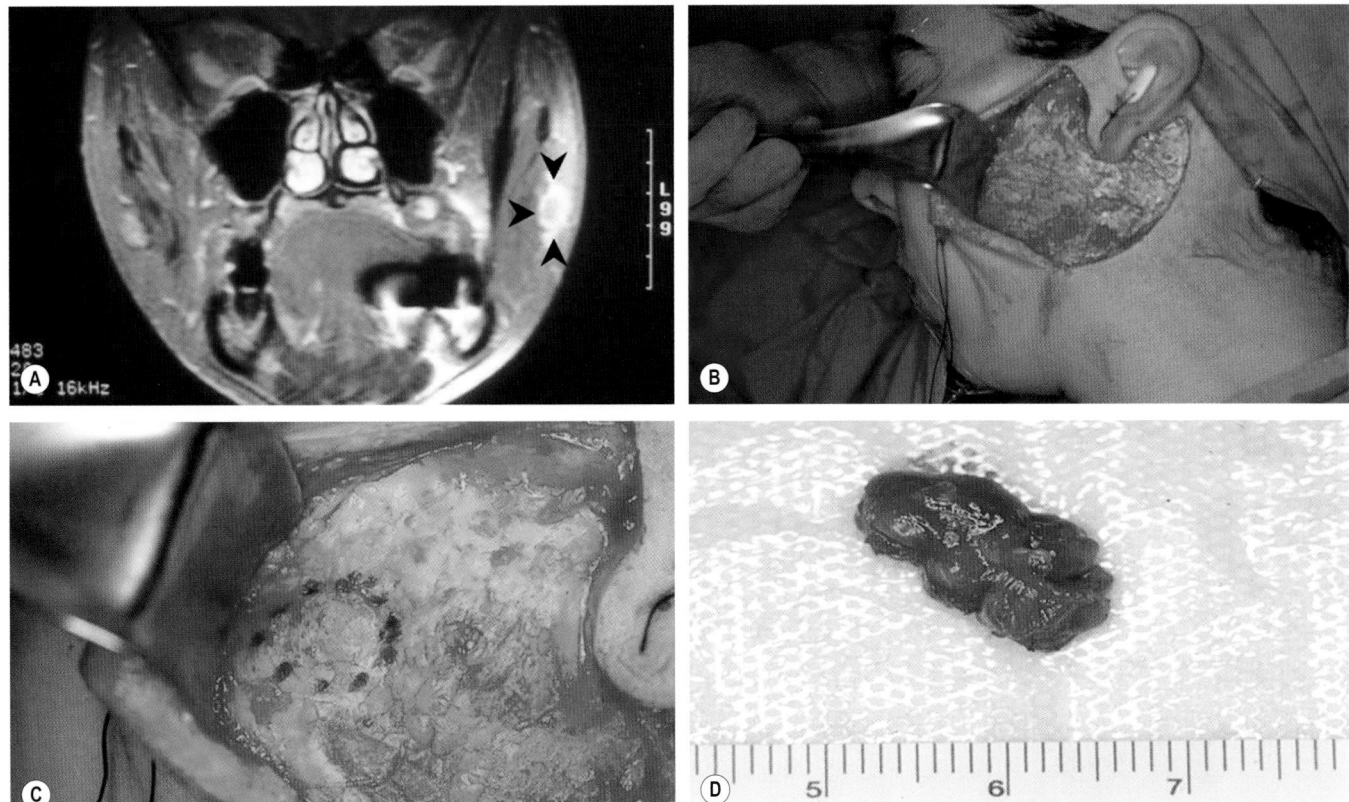

Fig. 14.15 Magnetic resonance imaging of the cheek identified a lymph node in the parotid gland **(A)**. A preoperative needle biopsy showed atypical lymphocytes. The mass was found in the superficial segment of the parotid **(B and C)**, was removed and found to be a lymph node **(D)** harboring a lymphoma.

manifestation of this viral disease.[34] Parotid gland swelling is often found in patients with HIV, and this manifestation can also be the initial presentation of the disease. Most commonly, the swelling is bilateral, painless and is a benign cystic lesion. The etiology has been postulated to be from compression due to intraparotid lymphadenopathy, and due to swelling as a result of the autoimmune phenomena.[51,52] Of note, this benign lesion has been found to be a reservoir of HIV-1.[53] In addition, patients with AIDS have been found to harbor Kaposi's sarcoma of the parotid gland.[54]

Metastatic tumors

Metastases to salivary glands account for 5–10% of salivary gland tumors. The parotid is the most common salivary gland to be involved with these metastases due to its rich lymphoid tissue. For that reason it is easy to understand that lymphatic metastases to the parotid gland most commonly arise from other malignancies in the head and neck area. A comprehensive series on metastasis to the parotid gland was performed by Conley and Arena in 1963.[55] Of the 81 cases of metastasis to the parotid, 46% were melanoma, 37% were squamous cell carcinoma, and 14% were from other malignancies. The most common in this small latter group was sarcomas, but also included cylindroma of the ear canal, and basal cell carcinoma.

Hematogenous spread to salivary glands can also be seen, and the parotid gland is again the most commonly involved.

While any cancer can spread to the parotid gland, the most common have been reported to be adenocarcinomas of the thyroid.

Treatment/surgical technique

Nonneoplastic lesions

Necrotizing sialometaplasia

Despite its disturbing appearance, necrotizing sialometaplasia is a self-limiting process that heals on its own; alternatively, it may be diagnosed by histologic examination after it is removed for not healing.

Benign neoplastic lesions

Pleomorphic adenoma

These lesions may be diagnosed preoperatively by cytologic examination of FNA biopsy. However, the diagnosis is usually made after the tumor mass is removed with surrounding normal gland by means of resection of the entire segment of the parotid gland superficial to the plane of the facial nerve *(Fig. 14.16)*. This procedure will usually result in a low incidence of recurrence (1%).[56] On occasion, the tumor is located in the deep segment of the parotid gland *(Fig. 14.17)*, requiring dissection of the facial nerve to protect the nerve, and subsequent removal of the deep tumor.

Recurrent pleomorphic adenomas are uncommon, but require careful management when they occur. They are best controlled by aggressive surgical removal and total parotidectomy when necessary, to achieve long-term control rates of better than 90%.[57] Postoperative radiation therapy has been shown to be effective in improving control rates in those patients at high risk for recurrence. Recurrences may also occasionally be manifest as a transformation to malignant mixed tumor.[58,59]

Monomorphic adenomas

Monomorphic adenomas exhibit benign behavior. If the tumor is removed surgically, recurrences are as acceptably low as that of the pleomorphic variant. Malignant transformations are believed to be rare.

Warthin's tumors

This entity can be surgically removed with a narrow margin of glandular tissue. Recurrences after resection are rare,[60] and may represent multicentric foci of lymphoid proliferation.[22] Alternatively, the tumor may be left alone, if the diagnosis is

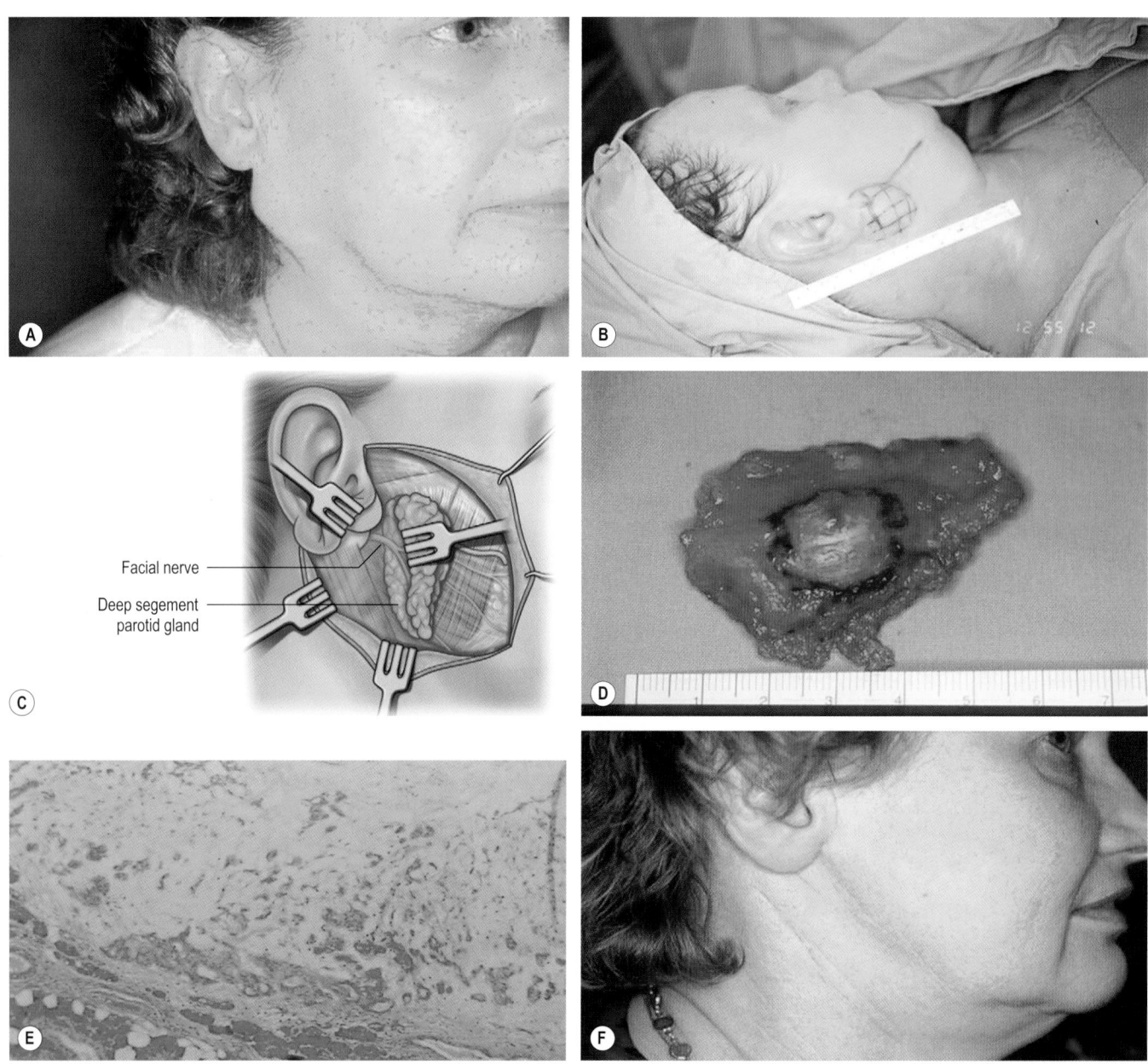

Fig. 14.16 A large pleomorphic adenoma **(A,B)** at the angle of the jaw was removed with the superficial segment of the parotid gland **(C)**. The horizontal plane of the dissection is along the branches of the facial nerve. The tumor is removed with the superficial segment of the gland **(D)**. Histologic examination **(E)** shows chondroid material (upper half). A shallowness is seen postoperatively at the site of the resected segment of the gland **(F)**.

Facial nerve
Deep segement parotid gland

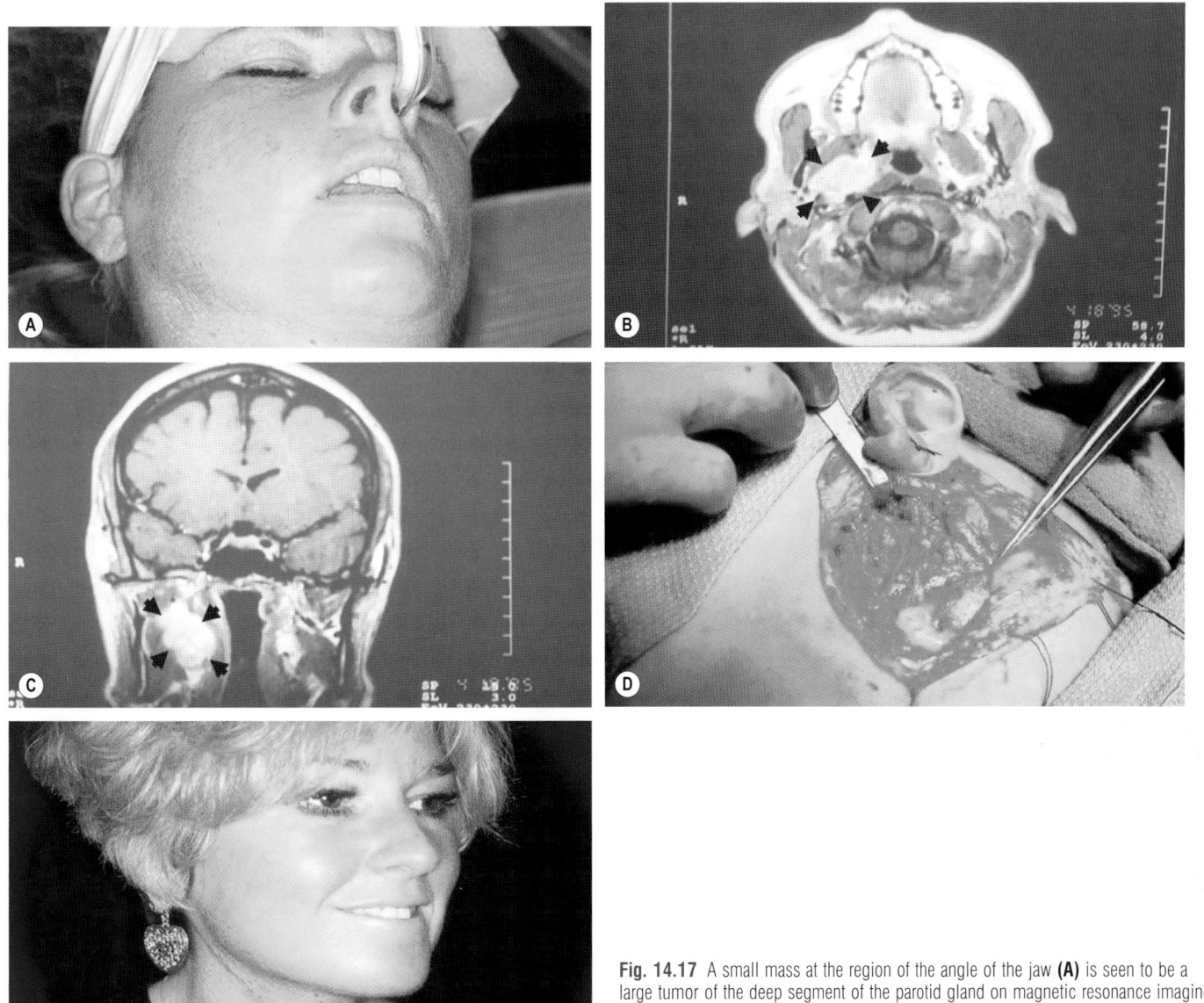

Fig. 14.17 A small mass at the region of the angle of the jaw **(A)** is seen to be a large tumor of the deep segment of the parotid gland on magnetic resonance imaging **(B and C)**. This required a dissection and retraction of the facial nerve to resect the tumor with the deep segment of the gland **(D)**. There is no hollow in the cheek postoperatively **(E)** because most of the superficial segment was retained.

confirmed preoperatively, and if the patient is willing to accept the facial appearance of fullness.

Oncocytoma

In managing oncocytoma, resection of the involved segment of the parotid gland is usually curative. Recurrences or malignant transformations are rare,[61] in which case resection with a good margin of normal tissue is required.

Hemangiomas

While capillary hemangiomas usually resolve spontaneously, cavernous or mixed vascular malformations may grow persistently. There is no indication for treatment with ionizing radiation, laser treatments, or freezing. When the tumor is expanding, a course of oral prednisone has been shown to be effective.[62] If regression is noted after 2 weeks, another week of treatment is indicated, followed by tapering of the dose. If

the growth continues despite treatment, early surgical removal is indicated to prevent physical occlusion of the external auditory canal.

Malignant neoplastic lesions

Mucoepidermoid carcinoma

The treatment of mucoepidermoid carcinoma should be guided by the grade of differentiation. The behavior of low-grade tumors can be similar to pleomorphic adenoma, and the incidence of occult microscopic metastases to regional nodes is less than 10%. Therefore, this variant of the tumor can be treated with superficial parotidectomy alone *(Figs 14.18 and 14.19)*, if the frozen section of the tumor reveals no tumor at the margins. If the permanent sections after the operation show evidence of tumor at the margins, postoperative radiation therapy would be indicated to decrease the chance of

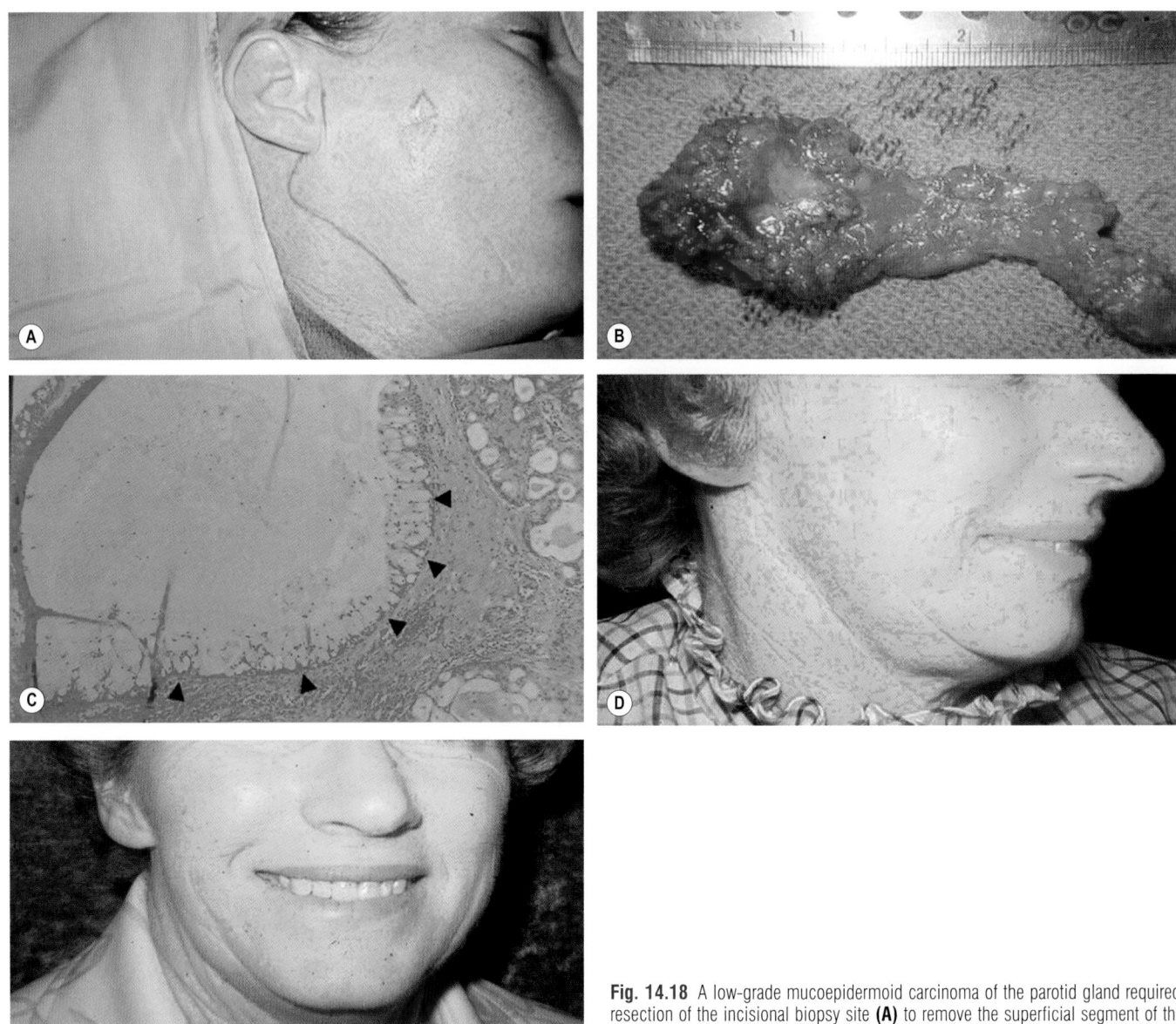

Fig. 14.18 A low-grade mucoepidermoid carcinoma of the parotid gland required resection of the incisional biopsy site **(A)** to remove the superficial segment of the parotid gland and tumor **(B)**. Histologic examination **(C)** shows well-differentiated cells (arrows) lining a mucin-producing gland. Six years after surgery **(D and E)**, there is no evidence of recurrence.

recurrence. These patients then need to be followed for evidence of future recurrence or cervical node involvement.

The intermediate-grade tumors have a more aggressive behavior with regard to local or regional involvement. In general, these tumors should be resected with preservation of the facial nerve if it is not involved with tumor. If a sample of the submandibular or jugulodigastric nodes shows any evidence of tumor, then a cervical lymph node dissection is indicated. Since the recurrence rate is reported to be 15–20%, postoperative radiation therapy to the tumor site and neck should be considered.

High-grade tumors are even more aggressive in their behavior. They have a greater tendency to metastasize to regional neck nodes (60%), and can infiltrate facial nerves (25%), leading to facial weakness. The treatment of these tumors requires a more aggressive approach with a total

parotidectomy and resection of any facial nerve branches that are involved with the tumor *(Fig. 14.20)*. Facial nerve grafting with a segment of the great auricular nerve may be indicated. Due to the high incidence of cervical node metastases *(Table 14.6)*, neck dissection is indicated for control. These patients should then be treated with a full course of postoperative radiation therapy to the site of the primary tumor and the neck.[63]

Adenoid cystic carcinoma

This entity is quite insidious and its surgical treatment requires aggressive resection of the gland to remove the tumor. Because of the affinity of the tumor for neural invasion both locally and at significant distances from the primary tumor, any nerves in the path of the tumor should be resected.[64] This may

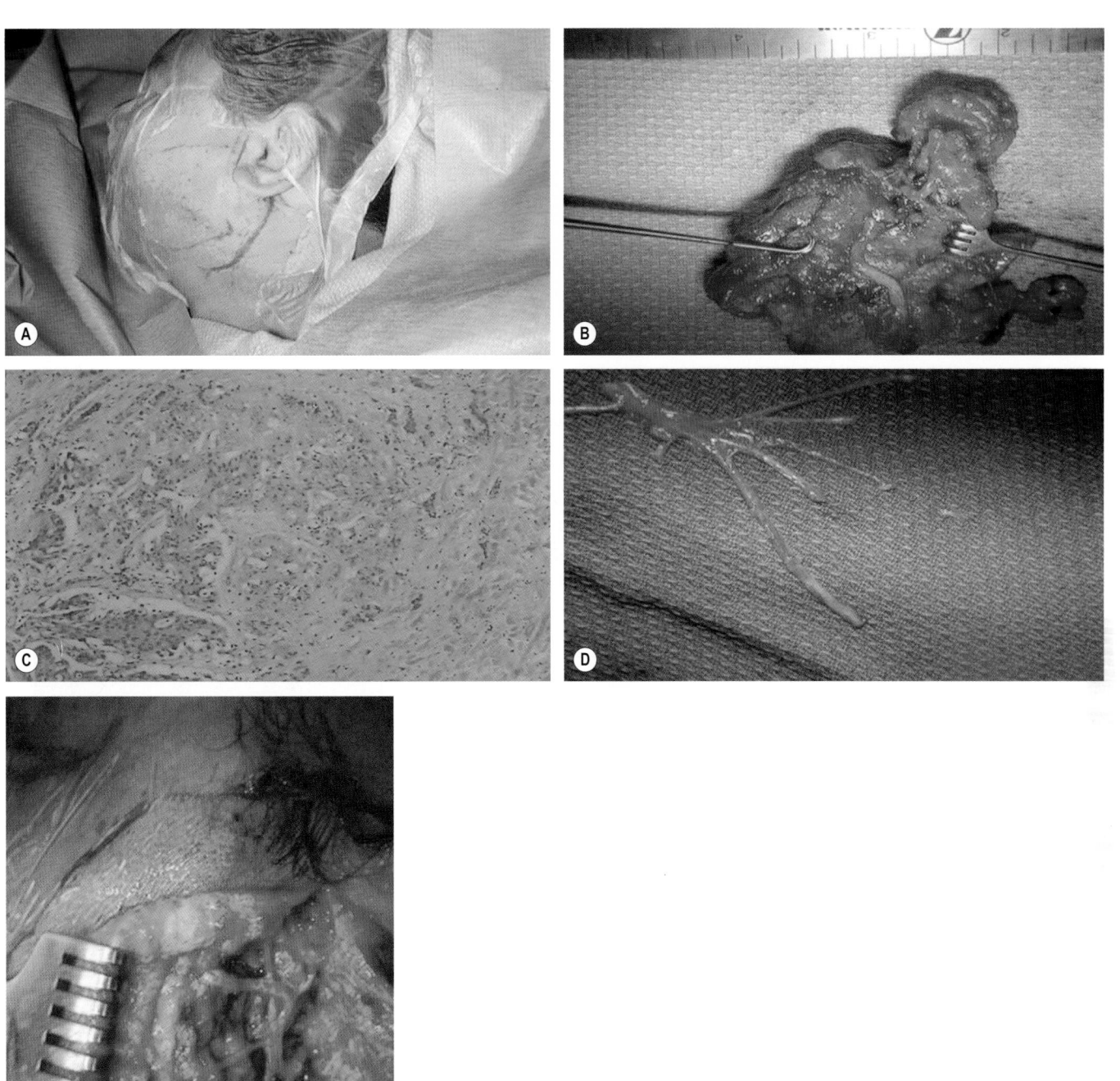

Fig. 14.19 A high-grade mucoepidermoid carcinoma of the parotid gland **(A)** necessitated total parotidectomy with resection of the facial nerve **(B)**. Histologic examination **(C)** shows poorly differentiated epidermal cells and no mucous glands. The great auricular nerve **(D)** was used to graft the facial nerve branches **(E)**.

require resection of the main trunk of the facial nerve, even into the temporal bone if it is involved. Otherwise, in these extensive cases, the recurrences would involve the skull base and cranial nerves as the tumor spreads into the central nervous system.

Adenoid cystic carcinomas are considered to be "radio-resistant" in that the recurrences cannot be "cured" with radiation therapy. However, radiation therapy as an adjuvant to surgery can suppress or slow down the growth rate.[65]

Therefore, this treatment modality has also been helpful in cases of unresectable recurrences.

Acinic cell carcinoma

Acinic cell carcinoma requires aggressive resection with total parotidectomy, resection of the facial nerve and repair with nerve grafts, and complete neck dissection if nodes are palpable. In patients with clinically negative nodes, elective lymphadenectomy may be considered in selected patients.

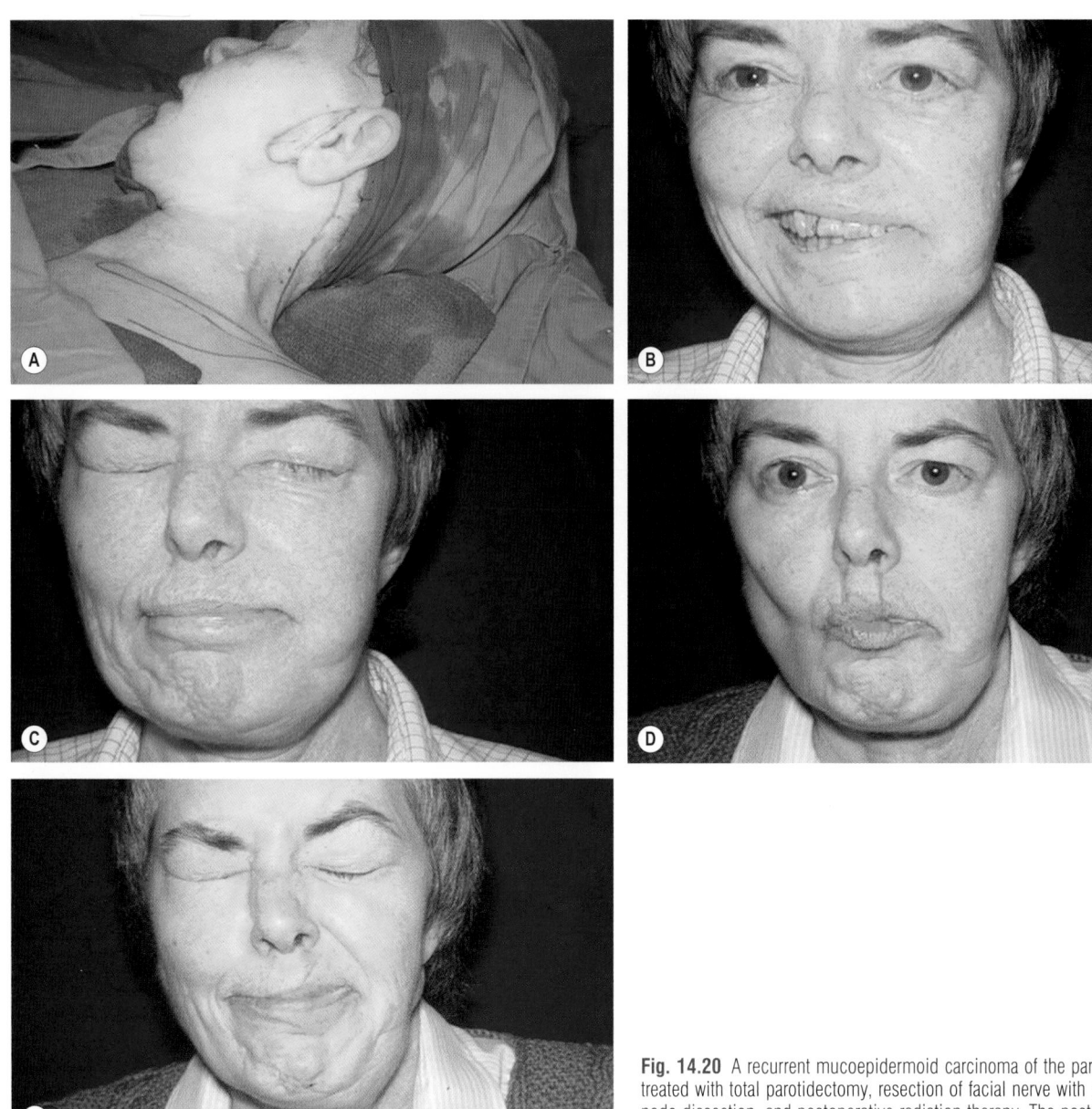

Fig. 14.20 A recurrent mucoepidermoid carcinoma of the parotid gland **(A)** was treated with total parotidectomy, resection of facial nerve with nerve graft, cervical node dissection, and postoperative radiation therapy. The postoperative left facial palsy **(B and C)** improved over the next 12 months **(D and E)**.

Table 14.6 Incidence of neck node metastases by tumor type

Type	Percentage
Squamous cell	70
Mucoepidermoid (high-grade)	60
Malignant mixed	30–50
Acinic cell	30
Adenocarcinoma	25
Adenoid cystic	10–15

Radiation therapy does not seem to be effective in controlling recurrences.

Adenocarcinomas

Adenocarcinomas located in the parotid gland are treated with wide resection *(Fig. 14.21)*, including sacrifice of the facial nerve, nerve grating, and cervical node dissection. Postoperative radiation therapy should be considered because of the frequent and rapid onset of recurrences.

Mixed malignant tumors

These lesions must be managed aggressively with total parotidectomy and resection of the facial nerve with nerve grafting. However, diagnosis of this tumor may be difficult with frozen section, for it may be initially interpreted as a pleomorphic adenoma, with the subsequent permanent

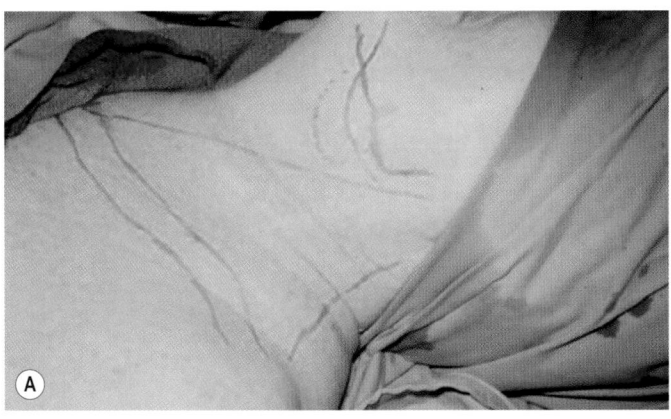 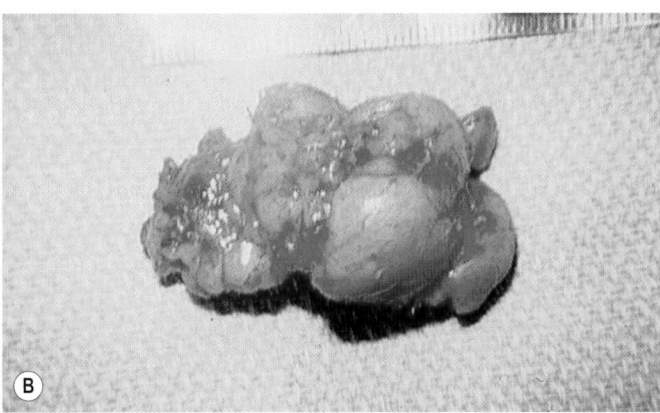

Fig. 14.21 Submandibular gland **(A)** was removed and found to be an adenocarcinoma **(B)**.

sections showing the features of malignant cells and aggressive invasion.

Oncocytic carcinoma

Oncocytic carcinoma should be treated with aggressive local resection, and cervical nodal dissection if lymph nodes are found to be involved.

Lymphoma

For lymphoma involving salivary glands, the treatment is nonsurgical (other than the excision of the nodal tissue for diagnosis) and is dictated by the histologic diagnosis of the node.

Outcomes, prognosis, and complications

Malignant neoplastic lesions

Mucoepidermoid carcinomas

Low-grade mucoepidermoid carcinomas have predominantly mucous cells and well-formed glandular cysts. Intermediate-grade lesions have a combination of the cell types (but cystic or glandular changes are infrequent), are locally invasive, and may metastasize. The 5-year cure rate of intermediate-grade mucoepidermoid carcinoma is reported to be as high as 90%. High-grade lesions have predominantly solid areas of squamous cells, with little or no glandular cysts or mucous cells. These tumors have a greater tendency to invade adjacent tissue, grow rapidly, and metastasize.

Adenoid cystic carcinomas

These lesions have a marked affinity for perineural invasion, leading to facial weakness and paralysis in 25–30% of patients.[66,67] Lymph node metastases are usually uncommon (10–15%); lymph node involvement is usually limited to the first echelon of nodes adjacent to the tumor.[67,68] These lesions behave in an unpredictable fashion, with some cases growing rapidly and leading to the patient's early demise, while others may exhibit very slow growth of pulmonary metastases lasting 20 years. Studies have reported 5-year survival rates of 75–80%, but the 10-year survival rates are 10–30% and the 15-year survival rates are 1–10%.

Acinic cell carcinomas

Acinic cell carcinomas have an aggressive biological behavior with finger-like extensions of growth into the adjacent tissues. Lymph node involvement is found in 30% of patients, and the tumor metastasizes commonly to lung, liver, and bones.

Adenocarcinomas

Adenocarcinomas appear as hard infiltrating masses that grow slowly. At the time of diagnosis, they are often associated with facial nerve involvement, cervical node metastases, or systemic organ metastases. The prognosis is poor, with 5-year survival reported at 25–50%.[69]

Mixed malignant tumors

These tumors have a poor prognosis, with 5-year survival rates reported to be about 40%.[70]

Squamous cell carcinomas

Squamous cell carcinomas have a high propensity for regional nodal spread.[71]

Frey syndrome

Postgustatory sweating (Frey syndrome) is caused by the interconnection of the cut parasympathetic nerve fibers of the surgically open and raw parotid gland to the cut sympathetic nerve fibers to the sweat glands of the overlying skin flap of the cheek. Since the sympathetic nerve fibers to the sweat glands are cholinergic fibers, when the patient eats food, the parasympathetic fibers of the gland stimulate the cholinergic fibers of the sweat gland to secrete. The patient then complains of sweating from the cheeks of the operative site when eating.

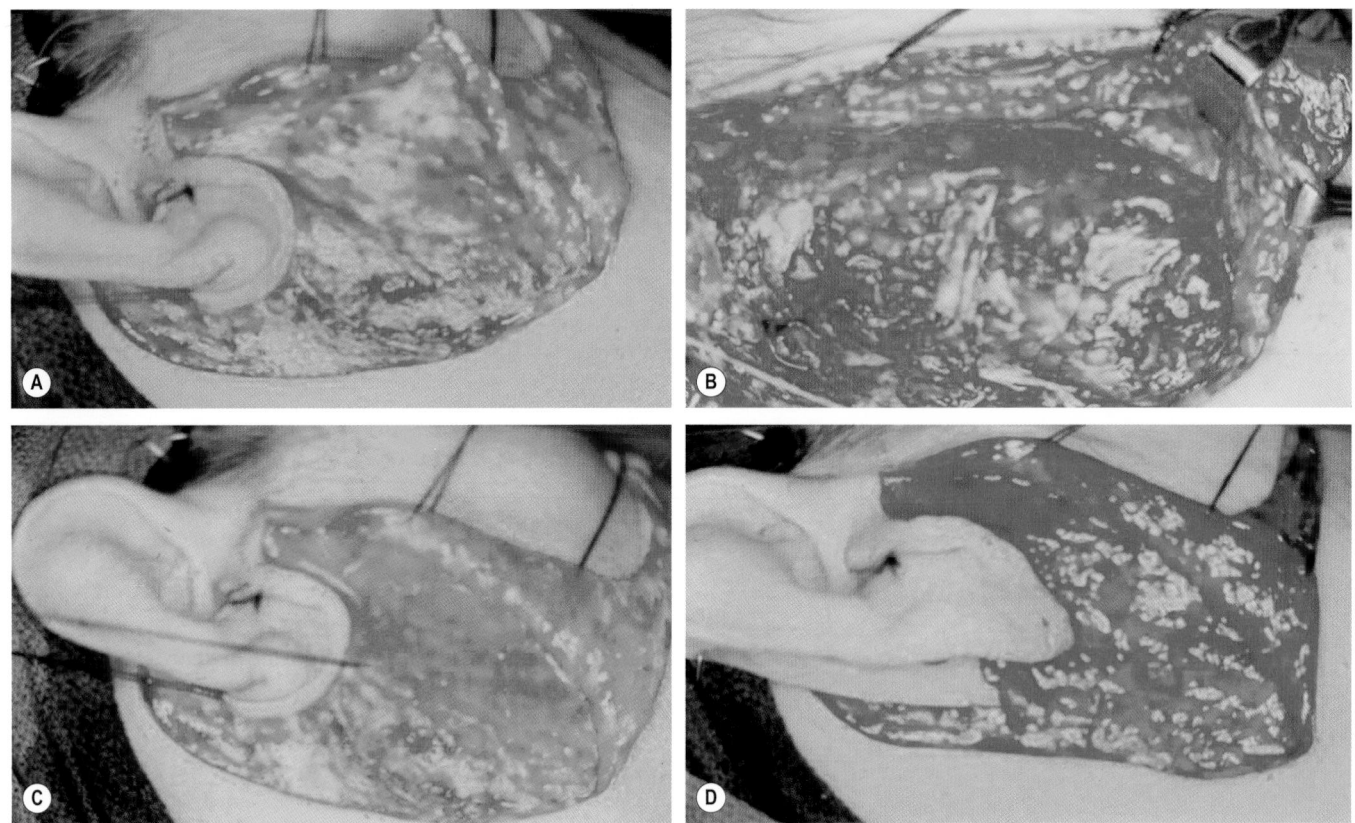

Fig. 14.22 After the cheek flap is elevated for a parotidectomy, the submuscular aponeurotic system is elevated **(A)** and preserved. Following completion of the parotidectomy **(B)**, the submuscular aponeurotic system is placed back over the exposed parotid resection **(C)** before the cheek flap is closed. If the peripheral edge of the submuscular aponeurotic system is preserved and rolled under, it can serve as soft tissue to fill in the hollow of the resected gland **(D)**.

This entity is often minimal and the incidence is reported in the literature to range from 7% to 50%[72–74] depending on the degree of symptoms necessary for diagnosis. Occasionally, there may be profuse sweating requiring intervention. In such cases, re-elevating the cheek flap will cut these fibers and scarring from the procedure may relieve the symptoms. It is best at these operations to place a sheet of fascia (fascia lata or temporalis fascia) in the intervening space.

Since 1978, our incidence of this syndrome has been reduced by elevating the SMAS that overlies the parotid gland *(Fig. 14.22A)* before performing the parotidectomy. The SMAS is then placed over the exposed remaining deeper segments of the parotid gland *(Fig. 22B–D)* to separate the parasympathetic nerves of the gland from the sympathetic nerves of the skin. In fact, folding over of the edges of SMAS can also help in filling the hollow of the resected superficial segment of the gland.

Access the complete references list online at **http://www.expertconsult.com**

11. Land C, Saku T, Hayashi Y, et al. Incidence of salivary gland tumors among atomic bomb survivors 1950–1987. Evaluation of radiation-related risk. *Radiat Res.* 1996; 146:28.

27. Qizilbash AH, Sianos J, Young JEM, et al. *Acta Cytol.* 1985;29:503.

38. Fowler CB, Brannon RB. Subacute necrotizing sialadenitis: report of seven cases and a review of the literature. *Oral Surg Oral Med Oral Path Oral Radiol Endod.* 2000;89:600.

41. Yoo GH, Eisele DW, Askin FB, et al. Warthin's tumor: a 40-year experience at the Johns Hopkins Hospital. *Laryngoscope.* 1994;104:799.

The authors report their experience with 132 cases of Warthin's tumor, and describe an increasing occurrence of this entity in women and African Americans. Nearly 90% of patients with Warthin's tumor were found to be smokers.

44. Higashi T, Murahashi H, Ikuta H, et al. Identification of Warthin's tumor with technetium-99m pertechnetate. *Clin Nucl Med.* 1987;12:796.

48. Goode RK, Auclair PL, Ellis GL. Mucoepidermoid carcinoma of the major salivary glands: clinical and histopathologic analysis of 234 cases with evaluation of grading criteria. *Cancer.* 1998;82:1217.

This study assessed the applicability of outcome predictors in minor salivary gland mucoepidermoid carcinoma to occurrences of this lesion in the major salivary glands. *Parotid gland tumors of a given histopathologic grade were found to have a better prognosis than similar tumors in the submandibular gland.*

55. Conley J, Arena S. Parotid gland as a focus of metastasis. *Arch Surg.* 1963;87:757.

    This is a widely cited primer on the anatomy, treatment, and prognosis of metastatic disease as it involves the parotid gland. The authors conclude that involvement of the parotid by any malignancy is associated with a grave outcome.

56. Laccourreye H, Laccourreye O, Cauchois R, et al. Total conservative parotidectomy for primary benign pleomorphic adenoma of the parotid gland: a 25-year experience with 229 patients. *Laryngoscope.* 1994; 104:1487.

    This series reports an extensive survival and complications analysis of patients presenting with primary benign pleomorphic adenoma of the parotid. Interestingly, surgeon experience, tumor spillage, and patient age/sex did not correlate with recurrence or facial nerve injury.

71. Spiro RH, Huvos AG, Strong EW. Malignant mixed tumor of salivary origin: a clinico-pathologic study of 146 cases. *Cancer.* 1977;39:388.

    Malignant mixed tumors were found to account for 6% of the salivary tumors examined over 30 years. The 15-year cure rate was 19%, with local recurrence being the most common cause of treatment failure.

15

Tumors of the facial skeleton: Fibrous dysplasia

You-Wei Cheong and Yu-Ray Chen

SYNOPSIS

- Craniofacial tumors comprise a wide variety of different tumor types at various locations in the craniofacial region. Management of craniofacial tumors in general is exemplified by the management of craniofacial fibrous dysplasia, discussed in this chapter.
- Craniofacial fibrous dysplasia is a benign fibro-osseous lesion in which normal craniofacial bone is replaced by fibro-osseous tissue.
- Fibrous dysplasia can present as monostotic or polyostotic, or associated with other conditions such as in McCune–Albright syndrome.
- Rapid enlargement and pain may indicate cystic degeneration or malignant transformation.
- Clinical assessment and computed tomography (CT) scan are performed as standard preoperative evaluation. Preoperative biopsy is performed in cases suspicious of malignancy.
- A multidisciplinary approach is required in the management of fibrous dysplasia, involving the craniofacial surgeon, neurosurgeon, ophthalmologist, and orthodontist.
- Indications for surgical intervention include aesthetic consideration, functional impairments, relieve of symptoms, and in situations where malignancy cannot be ruled out.
- Surgical intervention should not result in aesthetic and functional impairments greater than the original deficits.
- In the context of surgical approach, the craniofacial skeleton can be divided into four zones. Complete resection minimizes the possibility of recurrence. Shaving of the lesion is performed in selected cases.
- Fibrous dysplasia may present as a progressive and recurrent condition which requires long-term follow-up and treatment.

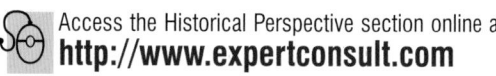

Access the Historical Perspective section online at
http://www.expertconsult.com

Introduction

Considering the complexity of the craniofacial anatomy, the topic of craniofacial tumors is both complex and broad.

Several important points have to be taken into consideration in the management of craniofacial tumors. These include proper assessment with accurate diagnosis, indepth understanding of the tumor pathology, indications and contraindications for surgical intervention, technical aspects of the various surgical options, availability of alternative treatments, and postoperative management of the patient. Operative planning must entail the extent of the resection, anticipation of the resulting defects, and the options available for reconstruction. In most cases, immediate reconstruction is warranted, as the defect often exposes vital structures or obliterates the containing walls of an anatomic space or cavity. Since various tissue and cellular types are located in the craniofacial region, a wide variety of tumor types occur in this location.

In this chapter, the focus is on craniofacial fibrous dysplasia. While by strict definition fibrous dysplasia is not considered a tumor, clinically it behaves like one. Therefore, by using it as a model, many of the principles applied in the management of fibrous dysplasia can be extended to other tumor types. Moreover operative techniques presented here can be applied as standard procedures for the resection and reconstruction of various other craniofacial tumors.

Basic science/disease process

Fibrous dysplasia is a benign bone lesion in which normal bone is replaced by fibro-osseous tissue. The lesion is reported to represent 5–7% of all benign bone tumors.[6] Fibrous dysplasia can present in a single bone (monostotic) or multiple bones (polyostotic), and also can be associated with other conditions such as in McCune–Albright syndrome.

The lesions of fibrous dysplasia develop during skeletal growth and have a variable natural evolution. Clinical presentation may occur at any age, with the majority of the lesions being detected by the age of 30 years. The lesions usually present at around 10 years of age and then progress throughout adolescence. At the initial stage, the lesions commonly present as painless swellings. The lesion may exhibit periods of dormancy intermixed with periods of growth. In many cases the progression of the disease stops after adolescence.

However there are cases where the lesions continue to progress after puberty.[7] The disease does not appear to have any gender predilection, except in McCune–Albright syndrome, which is more commonly found in females.[8]

Monostotic fibrous dysplasia is much more common than its polyostotic counterpart, accounting for as many as 80% of cases.[8] Although any bone in the body may be affected, the most frequently involved sites are the ribs, long bones, pelvis, jaws, and skull. Most of the lesions affecting the jaws are monostotic disease. On the other hand, skull involvement occurs in 27% of monostotic patients and up to 50% of polyostotic patients.[7] In the craniofacial region, fibrous dysplasia frequently involves, in descending order, the maxilla, mandible, frontal bones, sphenoidal bones, ethmoidal bones, parietal bones, temporal bones, and occipital bones.[2] Maxillary lesions may extend to include the zygoma, sphenoid bone, maxillary sinus, and floor of the orbit. In the mandible, the body area is the most frequently affected.

Multiple brownish skin pigmentations and endocrinopathies, such as precocious sexual development, hyperthyroidism, or hyperparathyroidism, indicate McCune–Albright syndrome. In McCune–Albright syndrome, the borders of the pigmented skin lesions are typically serrated or irregular, as opposed to the regular margins observed in the café-au-lait spots of patients affected with neurofibromatosis.[9] The association of soft-tissue myxoma, usually intramuscular, adjacent to lesions of fibrous dysplasia has been described in Mazabraud syndrome. The term "leontiasis ossea" describes a rare form of polyostotic fibrous dysplasia that involves the frontal and facial bones, resulting in marked deformities resembling a lion's face.[7] Another craniofacial entity, cherubism, is a hereditary fibro-osseous lesion, which symmetrically involves the mandible and maxilla. Although sometimes classified as a variant of fibrous dysplasia, cherubism is likely to be a form of giant cell reparative granuloma.[10]

Bone lesions found in fibrous dysplasia are characterized by woven ossified tissues, increased formation of bone matrix which does not mineralize normally, and extensive marrow fibrosis. Failure of bony maturation leaves a mass of immature isolated trabeculae enmeshed in dysplastic fibrous tissue that are turning over constantly but never quite completing the remodeling process.

Based on histological features, three main types of fibrous dysplasia can be identified: (1) Chinese writing type; (2) pagetoid type; and (3) hypercellular type.[2] Each type is differentiated on the basis of the amount, architecture, and cellularity of the bony tissue. The Chinese writing type is commonly found in the long bones and axial skeleton (rib, vertebrae). The bone trabeculae are thin and disconnected, with active osseous resorption by osteoclasts. Frequently resorption of the interior of bone trabeculae is observed (so-called dissecting resorption), similar to those observed in hyperparathyroidism. The osteogenic cells are star-shaped and numerous Sharpey fibers are present. The pagetoid type is commonly found in cases of fibrous dysplasia involving nongnathic craniofacial bones. The appearance is similar to osseous tissue found in Paget's disease, with dense and sclerotic trabecular tissue. The hypercellular type is characterized by the presence of discontinuous bone trabeculae distributed in an ordered and sometimes parallel fashion. Typically the sides of trabeculae are associated with multiple osteoblasts which are arranged in multiple layers. This type appears to

occur commonly in gnathic bones. Like the pagetoid variant, a significant amount of bone is present in the hypercellular type. It has been noted that fibrous dysplasia involving craniofacial bones produces radiologically hyperdense lesions compared to fibrous dysplasia in other sites.[11]

Many authors accept the premise that fibrous dysplasia represents a nonneoplastic, hamartomatous growth resulting from altered bone cell activity. Studies have shown that somatic mutation of the Gs-alpha gene occurs in osteoblastic cells derived from bone lesion in patients with fibrous dysplasia.[12] The mutation was first noted in patients with McCune–Albright syndrome but later was also identified in patients with isolated monostotic and polyostotic fibrous dysplasia. The mutation may induce abnormal osteoblastic cell proliferation or cell function in this disorder. Mutation in the Gs-alpha gene in osteoblastic cells leads to activation of adenylate cyclase, elevated cyclic adenosine monophosphate (cAMP) level and increased proliferation of abnormal osteoblastic cells, which results in overproduction of a disorganized collagenous matrix. Incidentally, it has been noted that an overactive cAMP signaling pathway also stimulates the growth of certain tissues such as gonads, thyroid, adrenal cortex, and melanocytes, leading to endocrinopathies and skin pigmentation, as noted in patients with McCune–Albright syndrome.[13] Yamamoto et al. noted that elevated level of cAMP in fibrous dysplasia lesions leads to increased level of interleukin-6 in patients affected by McCune–Albright syndrome. Increased interleukin-6 level in turn stimulates the activation of osteoclasts, leading to bone resorption, which is often observed in bone lesions of fibrous dysplasia.[14] This might explain why pamidronate, a bisphosphonate which inhibits osteoclast activity, can potentially produce an increase in the bony density in fibrous dysplasia and delay the spread of the lesions into surrounding bones.[15]

Malignant degeneration occurring within a fibrous dysplasia lesion is relatively uncommon. The malignant lesions usually develop in the third or fourth decade of life.[16] Malignancies can occur in both monostotic and polyostotic fibrous dysplasia, with frequency ranges from 0.5% (in monostotic) to 4% in McCune–Albright syndrome.[17,18] The most common histotypes are osteosarcoma, followed by fibrosarcoma, chondrosarcoma, and malignant fibrous histiocytoma.[19] The common symptoms of sarcomatous change are swelling and pain, usually developing rapidly. Radiographic imaging shows areas with poorly defined margins and osteolytic destruction. The lesions may extend through the bone cortex into the surrounding soft tissue. Periosteal reaction is usually not prominent. A coexisting aneurysmal bone cyst, or cystic degeneration of fibrous dysplasia, may clinically mimic a sarcomatous change. CT and magnetic resonance imaging (MRI) are useful in differentiating malignant lesions from the aforementioned benign cystic bone lesions. Biopsy is performed for histological diagnosis and grading.

The role of radiation in malignant transformation of fibrous dysplasia remains controversial. In a study of 28 cases of fibrous dysplasia with malignant transformation, 13 patients (46%) had received radiation therapy prior to the diagnosis of the malignant change. Generally, radiation is considered not effective in the management of fibrous dysplasia. Where is it possibile that radiation may actually induce sarcomatous change in fibrous dysplasia, it is not recommended in the management of fibrous dysplasia.[19,20] Malignancies arising from pre-existing fibrous dysplasia are typically aggressive. Urgent evaluation is needed if rapid swelling and pain occur in a pre-existing fibrous dysplasia lesion.[21,22] In treating malignant lesions of the jaws, Russ and Jesse state that surgical extirpation usually implies mandibulectomy or maxillectomy, depending on tumor location and extent.[23] The role of adjuvant radiation and chemotherapy remains debatable.[19,23] Despite aggressive treatment, local recurrence and distant metastasis are common.[16]

Diagnosis/patient presentation

The assessment of patients with craniofacial fibrous dysplasia involves history and clinical examination, radiological investigations, and tissue biopsy. For patients first presenting with fibrous dysplasia, important points to elicit in the history are the age at which symptoms first occurred, the timing and characteristics of pain, periods of rapid enlargement of the lesion, any previous treatment or procedures performed, and any symptoms suggestive of local effects, such as dystopia, diplopia, proptosis, blindness, nasal obstruction, sinusitis, hearing impairment, headache, tooth loss, and malocclusion. A rapidly enlarging lesion may indicate cystic degeneration or malignant transformation. Clinical examination is performed to assess the location and extent of the lesion, as well as the effects of local compression by the enlarging lesion.

All patients should undergo radiological imaging. Plain radiologic features of fibrous dysplasia are nonspecific and vary widely. The typical appearance is that of radiolucent lesions with a homogeneous ground-glass appearance and ill-defined margins. Occasionally the radiograph may reveal predominantly sclerotic lesions with or without accompanying lytic lesions. These nonspecific features make it difficult to differentiate fibrous dysplasia form other conditions such as ossifying osteoma and Paget's disease.[24,25]

At our center, CT scan of the craniofacial skeleton using 1-mm sections and three-dimensional reconstruction is routinely performed and is the investigation of choice. From the clinical findings and CT scan, the surgeon is able to obtain useful information regarding tumor size, location, any local invasion or compression. The CT appearance of fibrous dysplasia can be divided into three separate subtypes based on the proportion of ossified tissue and fibrous tissue within the lesion.[26] Pagetoid lesions have a mixture of radiodense and radiolucent areas of fibrosis. Sclerotic lesions are homogeneously dense in appearance. Cystic lesions contain one or more lucencies that are surrounded by a dense periphery.

MRI has been suggested some authors as a diagnostic tool for fibrous dysplasia.[27] Lesions have been described as areas with a decreased signal as well as sharply demarcated borders on both T1- and T2-weighted images.[28] However some authors have concerns regarding the potential of misdiagnosis with MRI.[29] The MRI features of fibrous dysplasia do not share the characteristics seen on plain radiography and CT. In fact, the MRI images of fibrous dysplasia often resemble that of tumors. This is particularly so when the lesions show intermediate signal intensities on T1-weighted images and high signal intensities on T2 images, and enhance brilliantly after injection of contrast material. The likelihood of correctly diagnosed fibrous dysplasia by MRI is high only when the signal intensities on both T1- and T2-weighted images are low despite the injection of contrast material.[30]

Bone scintigraphy may have some role in the diagnosis of fibrous dysplasia. The appearance of fibrous dysplasia on a bone scan is the result of increased tracer uptake in the diseased bone. Radionuclide scan has high sensitivity but low specificity, but it may be used for assessment of the extent of skeletal involvement in polyostotic disease.[31] Single-photon emission computed tomography (SPECT) has been reported to be sensitive in the detection of lesions that are not seen on CT.[32]

Histological samples can be obtained by an isolated incisional biopsy. Alternatively, tissue sample can be obtained at the time of surgical resection of the lesion itself. The caveat of the latter is that decision for a more radical resection cannot hinge on the result of the tissue biopsy. To avoid this scenario, it is recommended to do the biopsy as a separate procedure and wait for the result before the resection. In the scenario where the histologic sample is to be obtained during the operation, and if there are any doubts intraoperatively regarding the nature of the lesion, the resection part of the operation is deferred until final histological results are available. Although the histology of fibrous dysplasia is well established, cytological descriptions are rare. One group reported on fine-needle aspiration cytomorphology of fibrous dysplasia. The smears contained blood, occasional osteoclastic multinucleated giant cells, and frequent C-shaped fibrillary structures with dark central areas and lighter peripheries representing woven bone.[33] At present, the role of fine-needle aspiration cytology in fibrous dysplasia is still uncertain.

Biochemical markers such as serum alkaline phosphatase and urinary hydroxyproline are used occasionally to monitor disease progress and the response to the nonsurgical treatment.[24]

Patient selection

The mere presence of fibrous dysplasia of the craniofacial bones is not in itself an indication for intervention. Many small solitary lesions remain asymptomatic and static, requiring no treatment. Indications for surgical intervention in craniofacial fibrous dysplasia include aesthetic consideration, functional impairments, symptom relief, and in situations where malignancy cannot be ruled out. The most common indication for surgical intervention in fibrous dysplasia is a progressively enlarging bony lesion that causes visible and disfiguring deformity. This deformity may present as the disfiguring lesion itself, or as secondary telecanthus, dystopia, exophthalmos, or canting of the oral commissure. In most such cases, the objective of the operation is to restore a more aesthetically pleasing and symmetrical facial appearance. Operation is also indicated in the presence of functional impairments, for example, malocclusion and visual disturbance. Persistent pain is another indication for surgery. For cases where the diagnosis of the lesion is unclear and malignancy cannot be excluded, surgical intervention is also warranted.

Fibrous dysplasia of the anterior cranial base may compress the optic nerve and cause visual disturbance or even blindness. However controversy surrounds the management of fibrous dysplasia involving encasement of the optic canal, particularly in patients whose vision is normal. Lee *et al.* suggested that, while radiologic imaging showed that encasement of the optic canal causes narrowing of the canal, this alone does not result in visual loss.[34] Thus prophylactic decompression of the optic nerve is not indicated on the basis of the presence of encasement of the optic canal alone without visual symptoms, since the results of such imaging do not correlate with loss of vision. Moreover optic nerve decompression may associate with risks of failure of visual improvement after decompression or even blindness, even though the risks appear to be low in experienced hands.[35] In patients with optic canal encasement but without visual symptoms, regular observation with clinical examination and diagnostic imaging is more appropriate. Prophylactic decompression is not advised to be performed as a primary procedure, but as a procedure secondary to resection of the fibrous dysplasia lesion in the anterior skull base during the same operation. On the other hand, therapeutic decompression is advocated in patients with progressive deterioration of vision. For cases with sudden visual loss, it is recommended that decompression should be performed within 1 week of the onset of the symptom to maximize the chance of visual improvement.[35]

Some patients may present with a more acute clinical scenario. A previously diagnosed fibrous dysplasia may undergo cystic degeneration within the lesion. This usually manifests as pain and rapid enlargement of the lesion *(Fig. 15.1)*. Depending on its location, this may lead to disastrous complications, such as acute optic nerve compression with sudden deterioration of vision. Due to its rapidly progressing nature, cystic degeneration may clinically resemble malignant degeneration. While CT scan or MRI may aid in differentiating the two, sometimes revealing fluid level in the nonmalignant lesion, tissue biopsy may be needed to secure a more definite diagnosis. In cystic degeneration, total excision of the lesion is recommended.[24]

Contraindications for surgical intervention include: (1) the patient is not medically fit for general anesthesia and the surgical procedure; (2) the patient is not keen for operation; and (3) the surgical procedure is unlikely to meet the patient's expectations.

Treatment/surgical technique

Nonsurgical treatment

The aim of the treatment of fibrous dysplasia is to correct or prevent functional impairments, to improve symptoms, and to achieve aesthetic improvement. The mainstay of treatment for fibrous dysplasia remains surgical. However, some authors have proposed medical treatment as an adjunct to surgery. Bisphosphonates, for example, pamidronate, can alleviate pain and improve radiological appearance, presumably by inhibiting osteoclasts. Liens *et al.* reported that pamidronate 60 mg/day administered intravenously for 3 successive days had been given every 6 months for 18 months to nine patients. They noted that the treatment resulted in decreased intensity of bone pain, reduced bony resorption, and improved radiological features such as filling of lytic lesions.[36] Some authors recommend the use of vitamin D and calcium supplement, as

serum calcium is noted to be low in a subset of patients.[20] Steroids are currently used by some as a supportive therapy before and after surgical decompression of the optic nerve.[2] However medical treatment thus far has not proven to be effective in preventing the progress of the disease. As mentioned before, radiotherapy is not advisable in the management of fibrous dysplasia.

Preoperative considerations

Patients with craniofacial fibrous dysplasia are optimally treated through a multidisciplinary approach. Depending on the location of the lesion, referrals are made to appropriate disciplines for discussion and collaboration. Patients with upper craniofacial skeletal lesions are referred to a neuro-ophthalmologist. Formal ophthalmologic examination is performed. For this group of patients, if operation is contemplated, neurosurgical consultation is obtained. Such operations are performed jointly by the neurosurgeon and craniofacial surgeon. Orthodontic consultation is obtained for lesions involving the middle and lower face.

After elaborate consultations and discussion with the patient, a treatment plan is organized. While the overall treatment is multidisciplinary in nature, one particular physician must coordinate all the physicians involved and act as the principal caregiver to the patient, making sure that all goals and expectations are understood by all parties involved. At our center the role of principal caregiver is taken by the craniofacial surgeon.

Timing of operation

Timing of operation should be carefully considered and individualized for each patient. As a general rule, operation is delayed until after adolescence. This is to minimize recurrence and to intervene only after facial growth is complete. However there are situations in which early intervention is warranted. Operation in younger patients is performed in cases of cystic degeneration in which significant lesion expansion is associated with functional and aesthetic problems. For lesions which present a risk of optic compression, an earlier and more aggressive treatment approach is warranted. Lesions suspicious of undergoing malignant change should be investigated and treated promptly.

A patient may present to the craniofacial surgeon at any point in time during the course of the disease, frequently during early childhood. Because of variability in lesion growth rate, patient age (which affects school and job schedule), and degree of patient concern about the condition, there is often some leeway in the timing for operation. This largely depends on when the patient and family feel is the right time, with the surgeon offering guidance based on his/her knowledge and experience of the clinical behavior of the lesions. For nonmalignant lesions, we feel it is contraindicated to operate when the patient is not physically and psychologically ready. As one can see from the following examples, patients with craniofacial fibrous dysplasia will often be followed for a surgeon's entire career. To enhance the long-term partnership between the surgeon and the patient, it is important to remain somewhat flexible and acknowledge the patient's role and control in the management process.

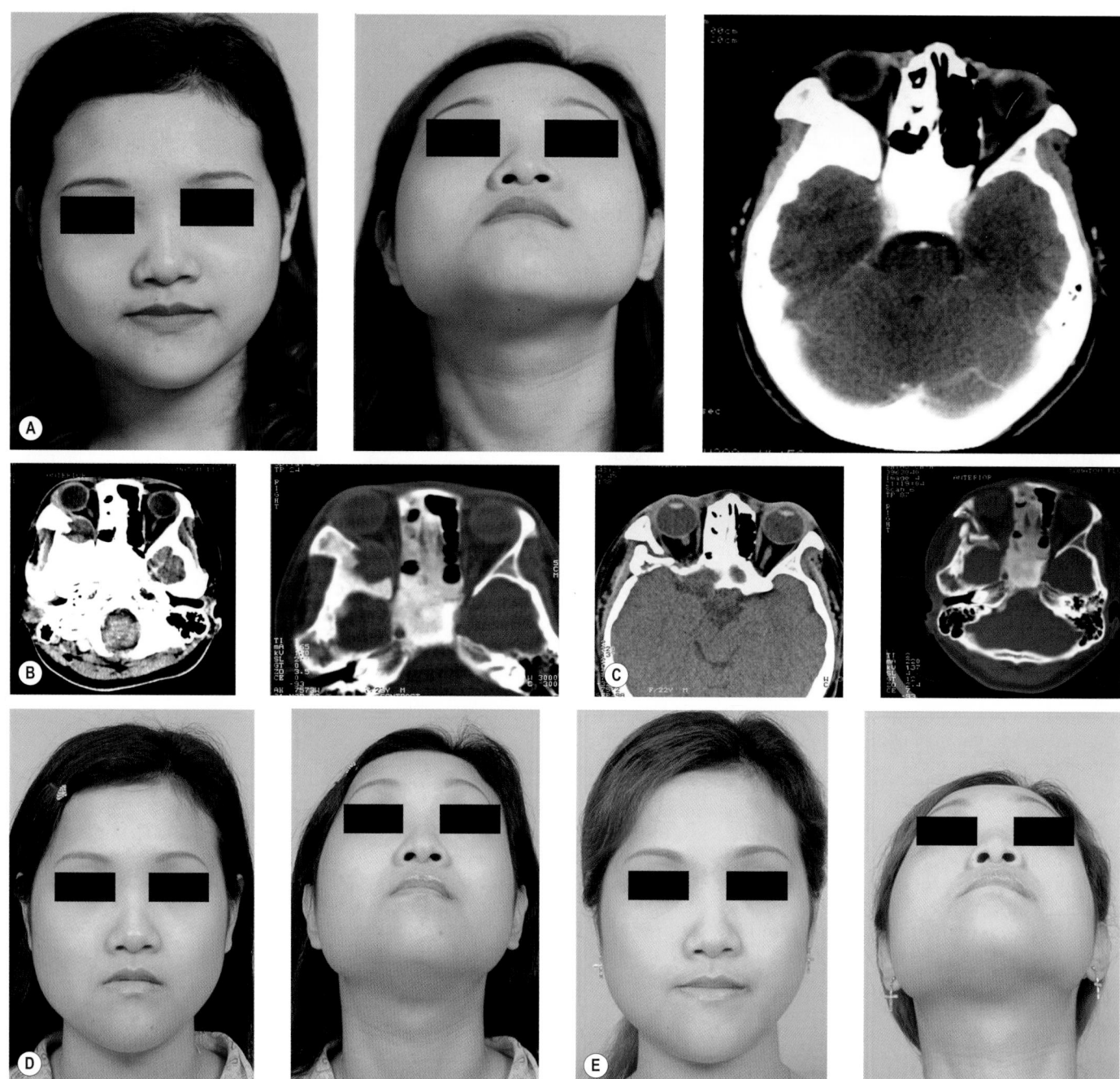

Fig. 15.1 Cystic degeneration of fibrous dysplasia associated with optic nerve compression. **(A1, A2)** A 22-year-old woman with fibrous dysplasia of the sphenoid, skull base, maxilla, zygoma, and mandible. **(A3)** At the time of initial computed tomography (CT) she has mild proptosis but no pain. **(B1, B2)** Eye pain developed 10 months later; repeated CT revealed a cystic mass of the right sphenoid ridge and sella within the lesion and compression of the right optic nerve. Transcranial excision of fibrous dysplasia, optic nerve decompression, and reconstruction of the lateral orbital wall and roof using split calvarial graft were performed. **(C1, C2)** CT was taken 6 months after the operation. **(D1, D2)** Three years following excision. **(E1, E2)** Seven years following the initial excision. In the interim, since the first operation, the patient underwent curettage of a cyst of the orbital floor and excision of fibrous dysplasia of the anterior maxilla. The floor and anterior maxilla were reconstructed with split-rib grafts. She also underwent curettage of a cystic mass of fibrous dysplasia of the mandible; this defect was reconstructed using bone graft from the inner cortex of the lower margin of the mandible. This case illustrates three points: **(1)** cystic degeneration of fibrous dysplasia; **(2)** optic nerve compression; and **(3)** need for close follow-up and re-resection when indicated. (Reproduced from Chen YR, Morris DE. Craniofacial tumours (fibrous dysplasia). In: Guyuron B, Eriksson E, Persing JA, eds *Plastic Surgery: Indications and Practice*. Philadelphia: Saunders Elsevier, 2009:437–454.)

The degree of deformity resulting from fibrous dysplasia is variable, as is a patient's perception of this. The surgeon must understand both his or her abilities and limitations in managing this condition. At some time points during the disease process, the surgeon may feel that the deformity, whether it is initial or residual, is of a minor degree such that he/she is not capable of achieving a level of improvement sufficient to meet the patient's expectations. In such cases, it is better to defer operation. Through serial examinations, photographic comparisons, and revisiting both surgeon's and patient's expectations, both will decide together when is the right time for operation or reoperation; this may be months to years later.

Surgical approach

Surgical approach is determined by tumor location. Any surgical procedure performed must not result in aesthetic and functional impairments worse than the original deformity. In the context of surgical approach, the craniofacial bones can be divided into four zones *(Fig. 15.2)*.[37] Zone 1 comprises the fronto-orbital, zygomatic, and upper maxillary regions, zone 2 the hair-bearing cranium, zone 3 the central cranial base, petrous mastoid, and pterygoid bones, and zone 4 the teeth-bearing bones, which are the maxillary alveolus and the mandible. These divisions are relevant in the surgical management of craniofacial fibrous dysplasia because they represent the logics applied in determining which surgical approach is to be used for a lesion in a particular location. Zone 1 is the most aesthetically apparent area in the whole craniofacial region. Complete resection of the lesion is advisable here to minimize the possibility of recurrence. Reconstruction is performed immediately, usually with bone grafts. Zone 2 is the cranium that is covered by hair-bearing scalp. Cosmesis is of less consequence in this area. Hence zone 2 lesions are generally treated with a more conservative surgical approach, for example, by shaving, which tends to restore a more normal bony contour. Zone 3 contains many important vascular structures as well as various cranial nerves. Surgical intervention in this area is avoided when possible. Lesions here are observed unless they develop symptoms such as visual disturbance secondary to optic nerve compression. In such a scenario, optic canal decompression is recommended. For lesions in zone 4, a more conservative approach is also preferred, at least at the initial stage. This is because resection of

teeth-bearing bones will result in the patient having to require dentures, which are less functional than the original dentition.

Craniofacial defects resulting from resection of fibrous dysplasia are reconstructed immediately using autogenous bone grafts. Traditionally, calvarium, rib, and iliac crest are the common donor sites. Many surgeons, including ourselves, prefer the use of calvarial bone graft, especially when the scalp has been elevated for exposure during the procedure. In addition to the reason of convenience where the calvarial bone is readily available, the resorption rate of calvarial bone graft is also noted to be low. In addition to the harvested bone grafts, segments of the resected specimen have also been used as graft material to reconstruct defects.

Zone 1

Operative approach

The eyes are protected by temporary tarsorrhaphy sutures. The head is positioned on a Mayfield head rest. The whole head is prepped to allow movement of the head during the operation for bone graft harvest and assessment for symmetry.

A bicoronal approach is used to gain adequate exposure of the lesion. At about 1.5 cm above the supraorbital rim, the dissection changes from subgaleal to subperiosteal plane. Dissection and soft-tissue elevation continue over the orbital roof, nasal dorsum, zygomatic arch, and anterior maxilla to obtain adequate exposure. Care should be taken to identify and preserve the lacrimal apparatus.

The planned osteotomy lines are marked. The osteotomies are designed to excise all abnormal-appearing bony lesions completely. For superficial lesions, these osteotomies are used to excise the actual bony lesions. For lesions situated deeper in the skull base, these same osteotomies may be used in the osteotomy and replacement approach. In this scenario, the osteotomized bone segment is removed to expose the deeper underlying lesion (for example, in the midline cranial base or nasal septum). After the lesion has been resected and removed, the osteotomized segment is replaced back into position.

The supraorbital osteotomy is used in the resection of lesions of the superior half of the orbit *(Figs 15.3A, 15.4)*. The neurosurgeon performs a frontal craniotomy and removes the bony plate to expose the frontal lobe. With gentle retraction of the frontal lobe and the placement of a malleable plate to protect the orbital contents, osteotomies are made through the supraorbital rim and orbital roof to remove the segment of bone containing the lesion. The osteotomies are made using a combination of burrs and saws. The orbitomaxillary osteotomy is used to resect lesions affecting the lateral orbital wall, maxilla, zygomatic body, and zygomatic arch. A frontotemporal craniotomy combined with osteotomies through the superolateral orbit and zygomatic arch, are made to facilitate the removal of the lesion *(Fig. 15.3B)*.

For lesions involving the inferior aspect of zone 1, the coronal flap alone may be insufficient for adequate exposure. In this case, a combination of coronal flap and Weber–Ferguson incision or degloving face incision along the buccal sulcus is employed *(Figs 15.5, 15.6)*. Osteotomies are performed through the glabella, orbit, nasal bones and maxilla above the level of the dental roots *(Fig. 15.3C)*. In this situation it is

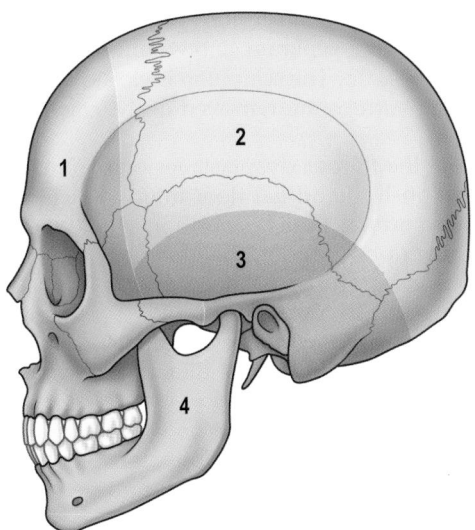

Fig. 15.2 Four zones of craniofacial dysplasia. (Redrawn from Chen YR, Morris DE. Craniofacial tumours (fibrous dysplasia). In: Guyuron B, Eriksson E, Persing JA, eds *Plastic Surgery: Indications and Practice.* Philadelphia: Saunders Elsevier, 2009:437–454.)

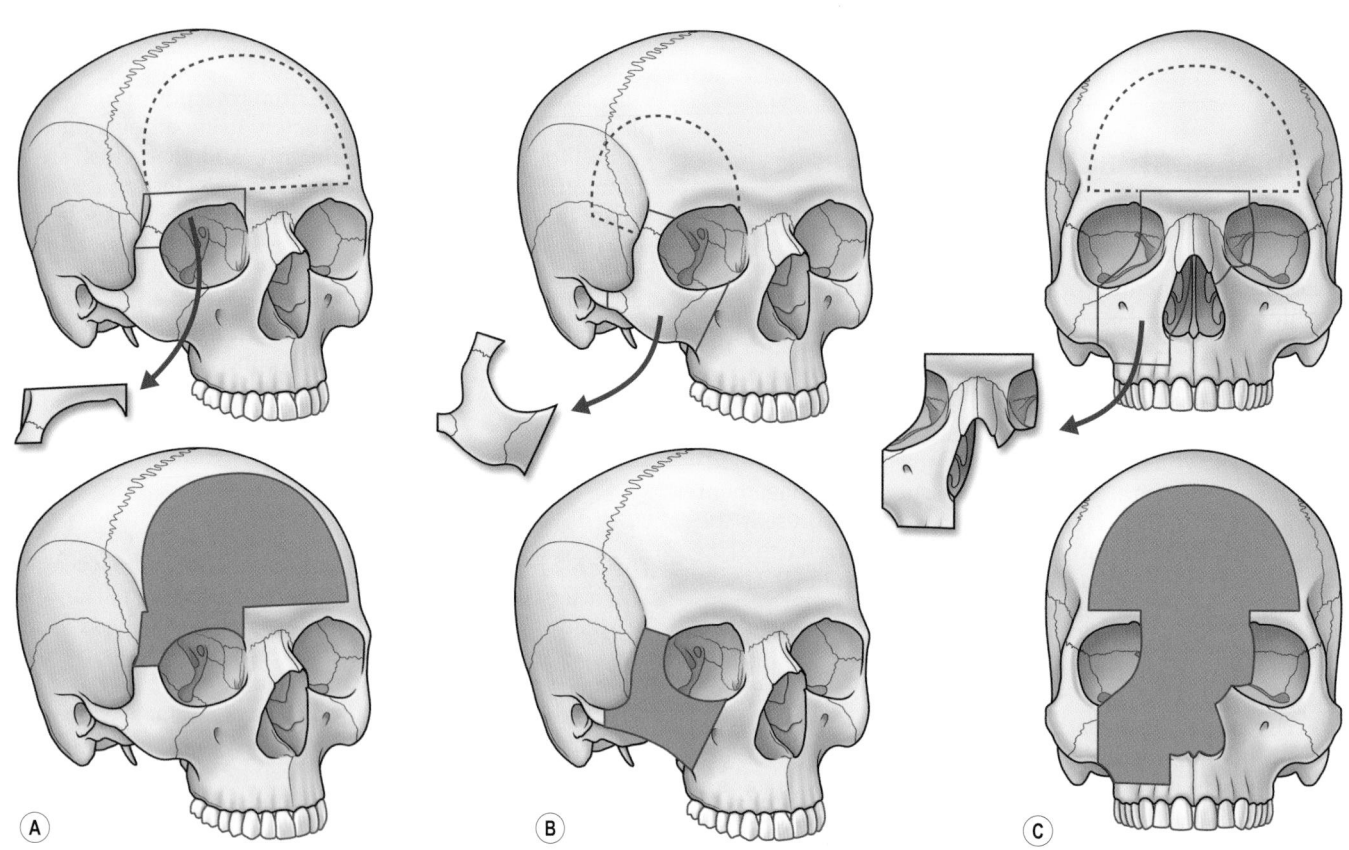

Fig. 15.3 Osteotomies used in resection of craniofacial fibrous dysplasia. **(A)** Supraorbital osteotomy. **(B)** Orbitomaxillary osteotomy. **(C)** Osteotomies through the glabella, orbit, nasal bones, and maxilla above the level of the dental roots. (Redrawn from Chen YR, Morris DE. Craniofacial tumours (fibrous dysplasia). In: Guyuron B, Eriksson E, Persing JA, eds *Plastic Surgery: Indications and Practice.* Philadelphia: Saunders Elsevier, 2009:437–454.)

particularly important to seal the extradural space from the nasopharynx, usually by using the galeal-frontalis flaps *(Fig. 15.7)*.

After the bone segment containing the lesion is removed, the defect is assessed and a construct designed for reconstruction. For defects involving the orbit, the goals of reconstruction are to restore symmetric skeletal form, symmetric orbital position and volume, normal anatomic compartmentalization, and to protect vital structures (i.e., globe and brain). We prefer to use split calvarial grafts assembled into a three-dimensional construct. Alternatively, a segment of titanium mesh can be plated to the construct to reconstruct one wall of the orbit.

Edges of the bone graft are burred to ensure a flush fit with no areas of prominence. Dural tenting sutures are placed to minimize dead space between the dura and the graft *(Fig. 15.8)*. To avoid palpable instrumentation or even a visible prominence, we prefer to use low-profile plates and screws in an area anterior to the hairline. In some cases the hardware is inset into a small groove burred on the graft and the adjacent native bone so that the plate and screws do not rise above the level of the graft and adjacent bone *(Fig. 15.9)*. In placing bone grafts, a step is burred along the native bone margin, into which the bone graft is inset *(Fig. 15.10)*. This is to provide additional support and increase the contact area between the graft and the adjacent native bone.

Hemostasis is secured and the wound is irrigated with saline, taking care to remove all bony debris. Any dural tears should be repaired with sutures. Two suction drains are placed (one anteriorly and one posteriorly) beneath the scalp flap, each exiting through a separate stab wound in the postauricular hair-bearing scalp. The scalp flap is closed in layers and the tarsorrhaphy sutures are removed at the conclusion of the operation.

Munro noted that the fibrous dysplasia lesion may reduce orbital volume and push the orbital floor inferiorly. He suggested that the new orbital roof be positioned at a height symmetrical with the opposite roof, the globe to be brought upwards through bone grafting the floor, and only enlarge orbital volume sufficiently to correct proptosis.[38] Canthoplasty is performed using clear nylon sutures. Canthal position is determined by comparison with that of the disease-free side.

Optic nerve decompression

The indications for optic nerve decompression have been mentioned. In cases where optic nerve decompression is required, exposure of the orbit is obtained as described above. The neurosurgeon proceeds with decompression of the optic canal under loupe or microscopic magnification. Microburrs are used to free the optic nerve completely from any bony impingement along its entire course within the optic cone *(Fig. 15.1)*.

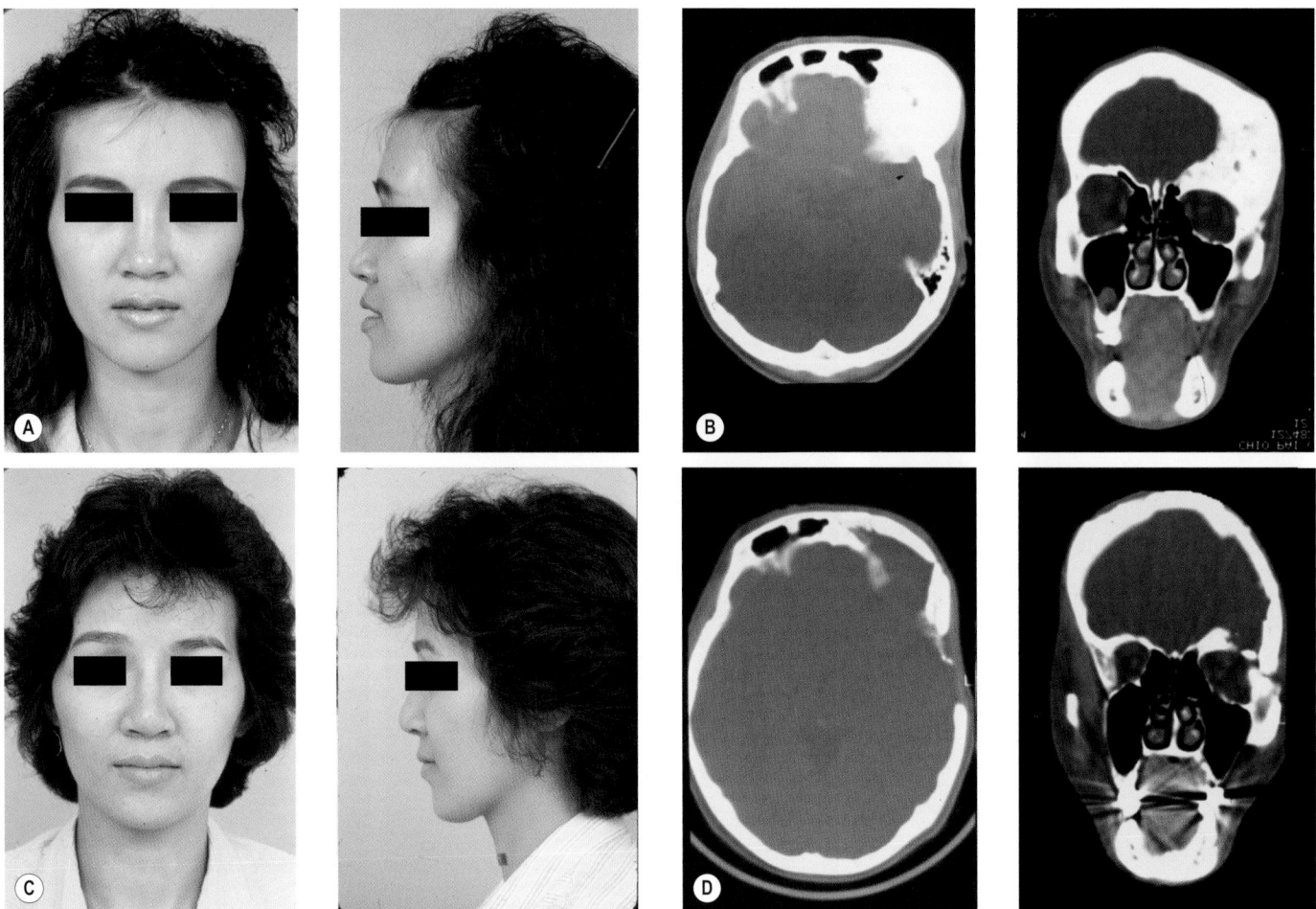

Fig. 15.4 **(A, B)** A 26-year-old patient presented with left fronto-orbital fibrous dysplasia in zone 1. **(C)** Three years after radical excision and primary calvarial bone graft reconstruction. **(D)** No recurrence on computed tomography follow-up. (Reproduced from Chen YR, Noordhoff MS. Treatment of craniomaxillofacial fibrous dysplasia: how early and how extensive? *Plast Reconstr Surg.* 1986:835–842.)

Zone 2

Operative approach

Zone 2 lesions are approached through a coronal incision as described above. For lesions posterior to the hairline, treatment is by shaving using burrs. The goal here is to restore anatomic form, contour, and symmetry. In these cases adequate bilateral exposure allows visual comparison and palpation for symmetry.

For more anterior lesions bordering on zone 1, a more aggressive approach is often taken, as this is a more visible location. A better cosmetic result can be achieved through excision, and the defect is immediately reconstructed with autogenous bone graft. Reconstruction with bone graft is much simpler in zone 2 compared to zone 1, as a single segment of bone graft is often sufficient.

Zone 3

This region contains major vessels and cranial nerves. Resection of fibrous dysplasia in this region is to be avoided whenever possible. The indication for operation in this region is for those lesions that cause functional deficits, for example, visual impairment. When indicated, optic nerve decompression is done with neurosurgical collaboration and may be done through a frontal craniotomy approach to the orbital roof. Alternatively a frontotemporal craniotomy or endoscopic nasal/transsphenoidal approach can be performed. The craniotomy approaches have been discussed in the zone 1 section.

Zone 4

Operative approach

For lesions in zone 4 (i.e., the maxilla and mandible), the goals of surgery are to re-establish a normal symmetrical three-dimensional skeletal form and to preserve a stable dental arch support. A more conservative approach such as shaving is preferred whenever possible. Radical resection might cause greater deformity or functional deficit than the lesion itself.

For fibrous dysplasia affecting the maxilla, the preferred approach is through an upper gingivobuccal incision. The soft tissues are elevated from the skeleton in the subperiosteal

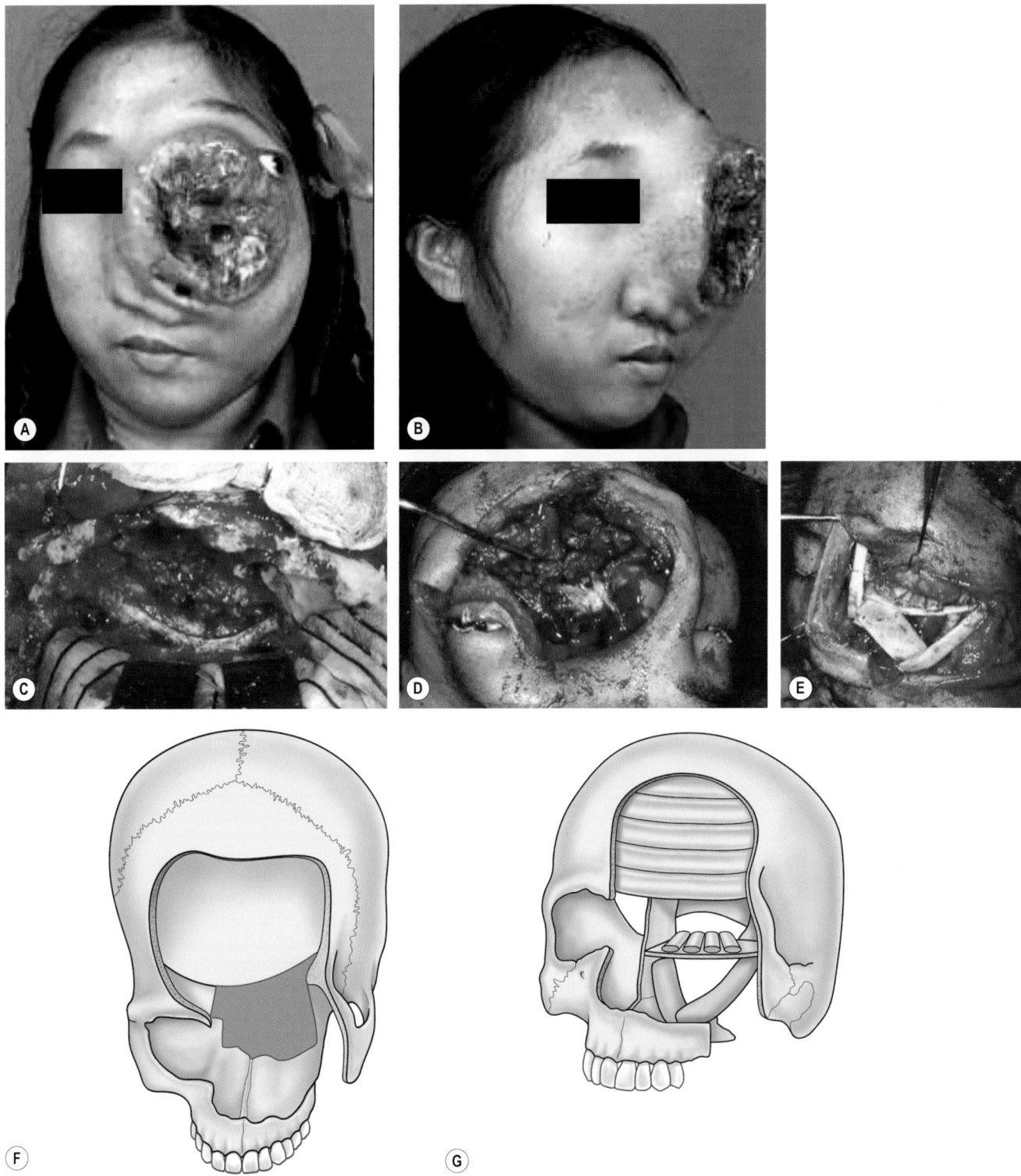

Fig. 15.5 A 20-year-old woman with a left fronto-orbital maxillary lesion. Overlying skin necrosis was secondary to the topical application of an herbal drug. **(A,B)** Biopsy revealed no malignancy. **(C)** Near-total excision with rib and iliac bone graft to reconstruct the left orbit, zygoma, and nasal bones. **(D)** The defect after resection. **(E)** Placement of bone grafts. **(F)** Anatomic configuration of the defect. **(G)** Configuration of the bone graft segments.

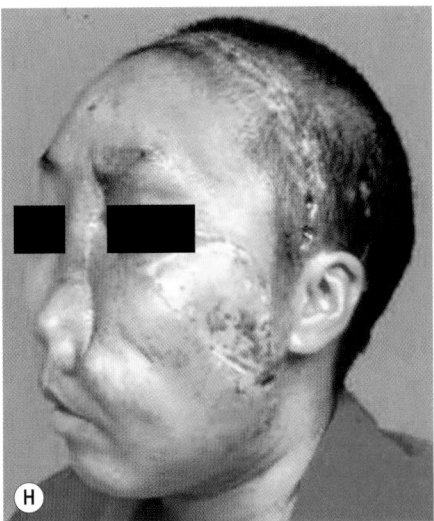
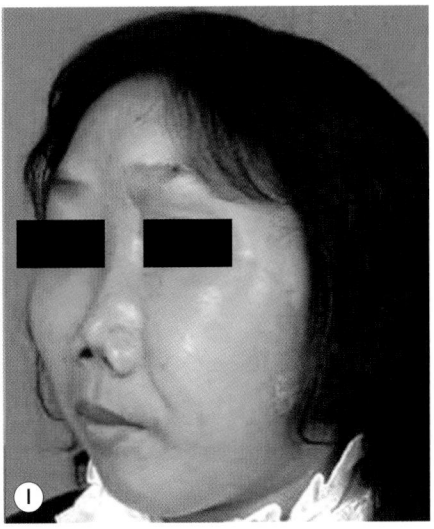
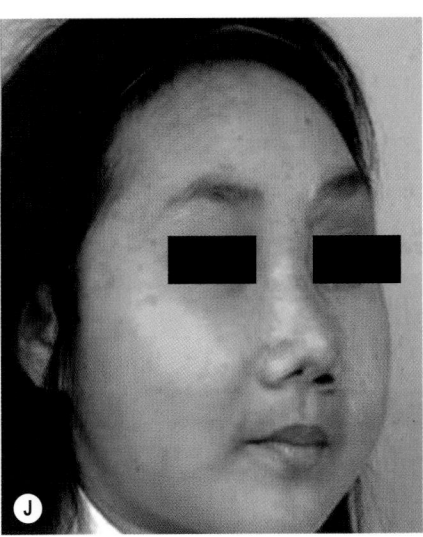

Fig. 15.5, cont'd **(H)** Lateral facial flap and full-thickness skin graft 1 month after initial resection. **(I)** Nineteen months following initial resection; patient had undergone two additional soft-tissue revisions. **(J)** Seven years after initial resection. In the interim, the patient underwent orthognathic surgery to shorten the midface. (Reproduced from Chen YR, Fairholm D. Fronto-orbito-sphenoidal fibrous dysplasia. *Ann Plast Surg.* 195;15:190–203.)

plane to expose the lesion widely. The extent of the lesion, or the portion that is causing deformity, is marked. Care should be exercised to avoid injuries to the infraorbital nerve and dental roots. With the assistant protecting the overlying soft tissues, the lesion is shaved with burrs. The wound is irrigated with copious amount of saline to remove bone particles, and closed with absorbable sutures.

In some cases, shaving may not be adequate. In this situation, the lesion is excised *(Figs 15.11, 15.12)*. We try to preserve the tooth-bearing portion of the maxilla. If the medial and/or lateral buttresses are sacrificed, these structures need to be reconstructed. The goals of reconstruction are to provide vertical support for the mid and lower facial skeleton and to restore a normal, symmetric contour and form. For immediate reconstruction, we prefer to use rib bone graft. This avoids exposing and potentially contaminating the dura while harvesting the calvarial graft in the same operation involving the oral cavity. The graft segments are placed to reconstruct the medial and lateral maxillary buttresses, vertically supporting the facial height. A step is burred along the periphery of the defect to facilitate inset of the grafts. This increases the area of contact between the graft and the adjacent native bone, and enhances stability of the inset graft *(Fig. 15.10)*. Additional graft segments are placed to reconstruct the remainder of bony defects. Reference is made to the contralateral side and to disease-free landmarks (e.g., infraorbital foramina, sides of the pyriform aperture) to achieve symmetry. The grafts are fixed with plates and screws. For lesions of the mandible, exposure is through a lower gingivobuccal incision. The lesions are marked and shaved. An attempt is made to preserve a symmetrical mandibular contour. With this approach, the mandibular arch remains in continuity. The level of the dental roots and mental foramina is marked to avoid injuries to these structures.

Despite a seemingly ideal reconstruction, some patients will require a subsequent orthognathic operation to correct a vertical height asymmetry or malocclusion *(Figs 15.5, 15.11)*. This may be secondary to bone graft resorption or to progressive fibrous dysplasia. In these cases the operation is planned carefully with the orthodontist. The goals of such an operation are to correct malocclusion and to level a canted occlusal plane. This usually involves an asymmetric LeFort 1 osteotomy in which the right and left sides are impacted or distracted to different degrees. Intraoperatively we find that the facebow combined with direct measurements is helpful in assessing symmetry.[39] For direct measurement, we expose both eyes and measure from the lower lid margin to the oral commissure, comparing both sides.

Postoperative care

Generally the patient is extubated in the operating room. If the operation involves craniotomy and exposure of the dura then the patient is admitted to the neurosurgical intensive care unit for neurological monitoring and a postoperative CT scan is done in the same evening or the next morning. Visual acuity is checked immediately postoperatively and serially while the patient is in the hospital. To reduce edema, the head of the bed is kept elevated to at least 30°. Cold packs are placed over the upper face beginning immediately postoperatively and continuing every hour for the next 24 hours.

For all patients intravenous antibiotics are continued for 2 days and changed to oral antibiotics to complete a 1-week course. If inserted, suction drains are left in place for 2–3 days. Patients are evaluated in clinic every 6 months to monitor tumor recurrence and potential late postoperative complications such as alopecia. The patient who undergoes optic nerve decompression requires repeated formal ophthalmologic assessment.

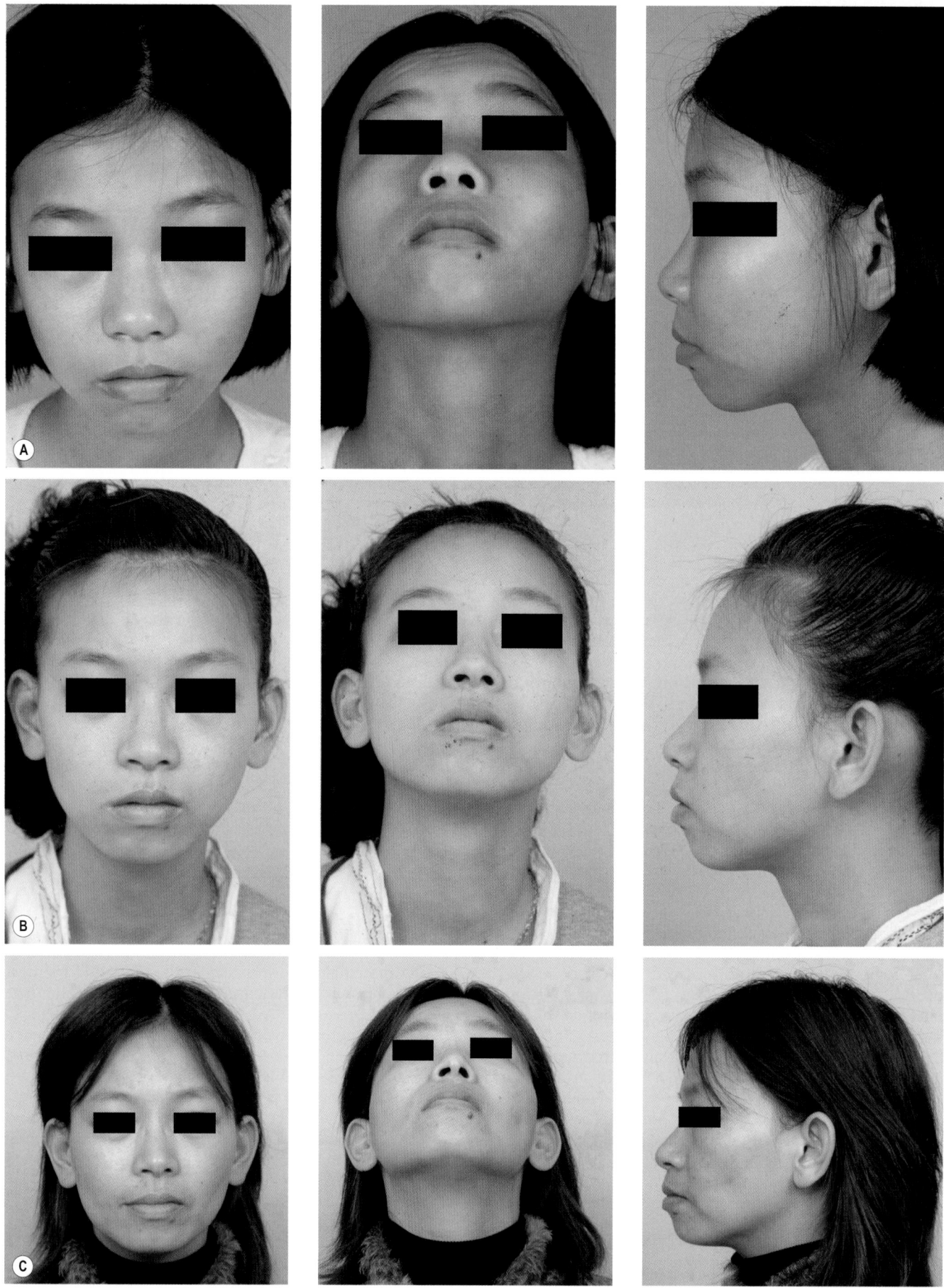

Fig. 15.6 (A) A 14-year-old patient presented with zone 1 fibrous dysplasia at the left zygomaticomaxillary region. Radical excision and rib graft reconstruction were performed through upper sulcus incision. **(B)** Five years after the operation. **(C)** Twenty-one years after operation. (Reproduced from Chen YR, Noordhoff MS. Treatment of craniomaxillofacial fibrous dysplasia: how early and how extensive? *Plast Reconstr Surg.* 1986:835–842.)

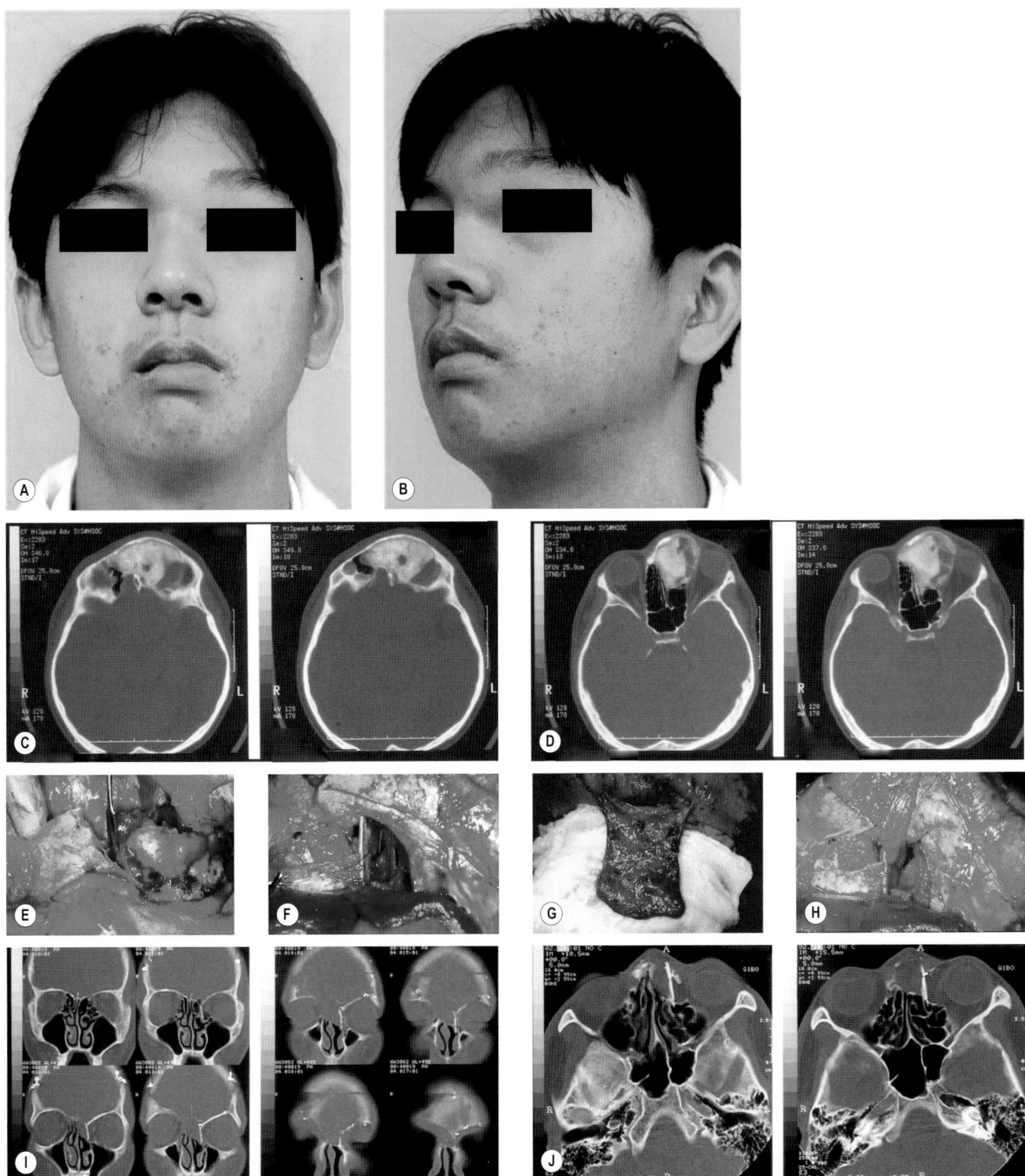

Fig. 15.7 A young male patient with osteoma of the fronto-naso-ethmoid region. **(A,B)** Photographs and **(C,D)** computed tomography (CT) scan at presentation. One month later he underwent radical excision of the ethmoid and nasal cavity. **(E)** Reconstruction was performed using galea-frontalis muscle flap and calvarial bone graft. **(F)** The defect after resection is shown. **(G)** The bone graft is seen supporting the left medial orbital wall. **(H)** The dissected galea-frontalis flap is inset overlying the bone graft. **(I,J)** CT 3 years after operation.

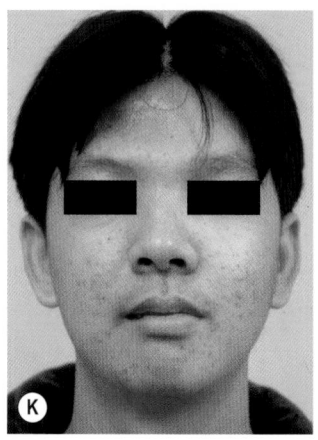
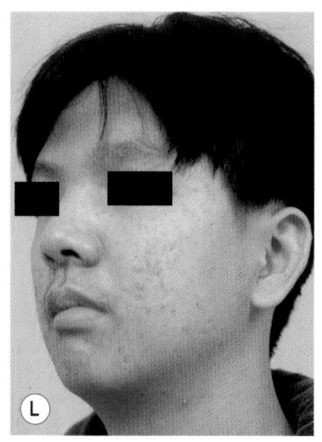
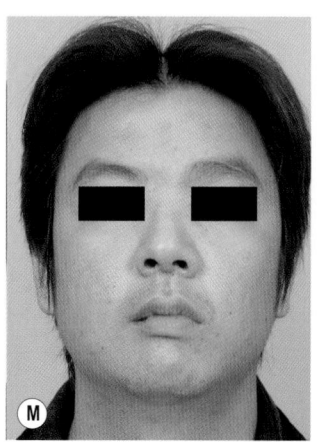
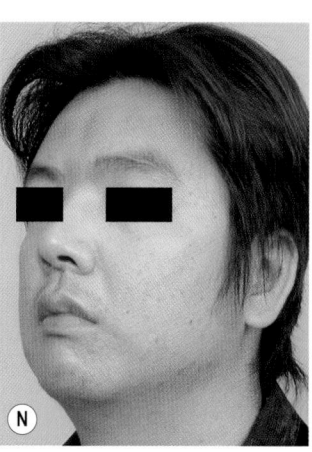

Fig. 15.7, cont'd (K,L) 1 year after operation and **(M,N)** 9 years after operation. (Reproduced from Chen YR, Morris DE. Craniofacial tumours (fibrous dysplasia). In: Guyuron B, Eriksson E, Persing JA. eds *Plastic Surgery: Indications and Practice.* Philadelphia: Saunders Elsevier, 2009:437–454.)

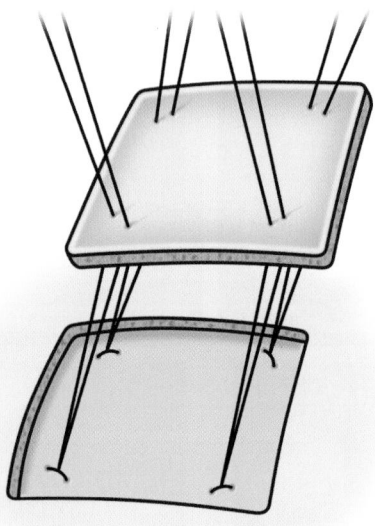

Fig. 15.8 Dural tenting sutures. Sutures are placed through the dura and tied; they are then passed through the holes drilled through the bone graft and retied.

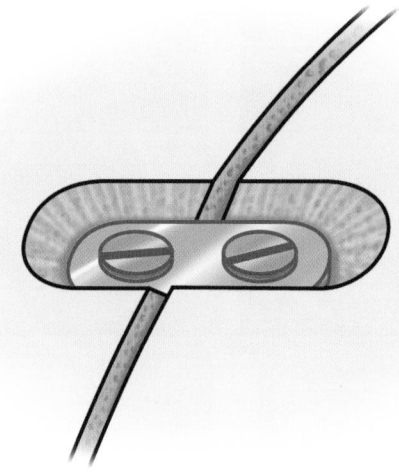

Fig. 15.9 Plates are inset into the bone to create a smooth contour. A groove is burred into the graft and the adjacent native bone just larger than the plate to allow inset.

Outcomes, prognosis, and complications

Potential complications

1. The superior sagittal sinus can be injured if an osteotomy is performed too close to the midline. If this occurs it is treated in collaboration with the neurosurgeon, by using Gelfoam packing, local pressure, and sutures.

2. Communication between the nasopharynx and the intracranial cavity can lead to epidural infection and meningitis. During reconstruction the nasopharynx and intracranial cavity must be separated by well-vascularized tissues. The galea-frontalis flap serves well for this purpose.

3. Errors in orbital reconstruction may result in improper globe positioning. This may lead to enophthalmos, telecanthus, or dystopia. There is a tendency for the globe to assume a more inferior position. To avoid this, additional strips of bone graft may be placed along the orbital floor for reinforcement.

4. Patients may complain of a palpable or even visible prominence of the plating beneath the skin. If there is

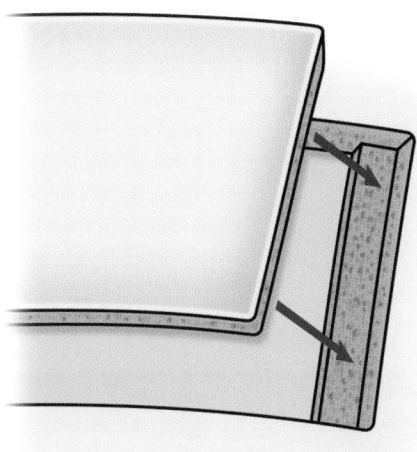

Fig. 15.10 A bony step is burred along the margin of the adjacent native bone to facilitate inset and support of the graft segment. Note the inner cortex ledge medially (arrows) that allows inset of the construct, and avoidance of a step-type defect.

no sign of infection, the patient is reassured and the hardware removed after bony union has occurred. This problem can be avoided by several means. When possible, place instrumentation posterior to the hairline, use low-profile plating, and use the minimal quantity required to achieve stability. In addition, the groove is burred into the graft and the adjacent native bone and the plate is inset into the groove to create a smooth contour.

5. Globe injury is best avoided by gentle anteroinferior traction of the scalp flap during exposure at and below the supraorbital rim.

6. Care should be taken to level the canthi at the end of the procedure. Visual comparison and measurements should be made to place the medial and lateral canthi at the same level compared to the contralateral side. In performing the canthopexy, a nonabsorbable suture is used to fix the canthal ligament to the periosteum.

7. If extensive dissection has been done to facilitate exposure of the bone, the patient may develop postoperative descent or "sagging" of the soft tissues. During reconstruction, sutures should be placed at sites of periosteal incision, to reattach and thereby resuspend the soft tissues.

8. Scalp alopecia is a complication to be avoided. We believe that wrapping the horseshoe portion of the head support with cotton bands helps to disburse the pressure between the head support and the scalp. Prepping and draping the entire head allow us periodically to lift and slightly rotate the head during the procedure, reducing prolonged pressure at any one location. The skin closure should be tension-free and any tension should be taken up by galeal sutures. After placing key sutures to mark the vertex, wound closure

is performed in a lateral to medial direction bilaterally. This allows slight advancement of the coronal flap from its bilateral inferior aspects towards the midline, thus reducing tension in the vertex region. Should alopecia occur, this is treated as a delayed secondary procedure, at least 6 months later. A small area of alopecia can be treated through excision and a local flap; a larger area may require tissue expansion.

9. For resection involving the maxillary alveolus and mandible, injuries to the dental roots and inferior alveolar nerve/mental nerve can be avoided by proper surgical planning and meticulous surgical technique. Minor injury to the nerve causes temporary hypoesthesia in the lower lip which usually will recover after few months. Severe nerve damage might lead to permanent sensory loss.

10. For resection involving the intraoral route, early complications include hematoma and intraoral wound dehiscence. These are largely preventable through adequate surgical technique. We prefer to close intraoral wounds in two layers. For the maxillary wound, several interrupted sutures are placed in the periosteal-muscular layers prior to mucosal closure. For the mandibular closure, the dissected periosteal edge is resuspended before the mucosa is closed. For cases involving orthognathic procedure, and for cases where there has been significant exposure of the mandibular angle, bilateral closed suction drains are placed. The tip is placed at the angle and the drain exits from the anterior aspect of the mucosal wound and is sutured around a tooth or to the orthodontics. These drains reduce edema and fluid accumulation within the dissected cavity. They are usually removed on postoperative day 1. Patients with a wound dehiscence are taken back to the operating room for irrigation and reclosure. Those with a palpable hematoma are also taken back to the operating room for evacuation and reclosure.

11. Infection of the intraoral wounds, if it occurs, usually presents subacutely from weeks to a few months after surgery. There may be a nidus such as a segment of free bone. Small, well-localized pus collections, or those that have spontaneously begun to drain intraorally, are treated in the clinic. Under local anesthetic, a portion of the wound overlying the fluctuance is opened. The wound is packed with single gauze. A more extensive collection warrants formal exploration, irrigation, and drainage in the operating room. For the patient with a recurring infection, formal exploration is recommended to remove any necrotic bone segment.

Secondary procedures

Patients may present with residual asymmetry from inadequate contouring during the initial procedure, or recurrent asymmetry secondary to progressive fibrous dysplasia. This possibility should be discussed with the patient preoperatively. The surgeon must decide whether reoperation is likely to improve the degree of deformity. It is advisable to wait at

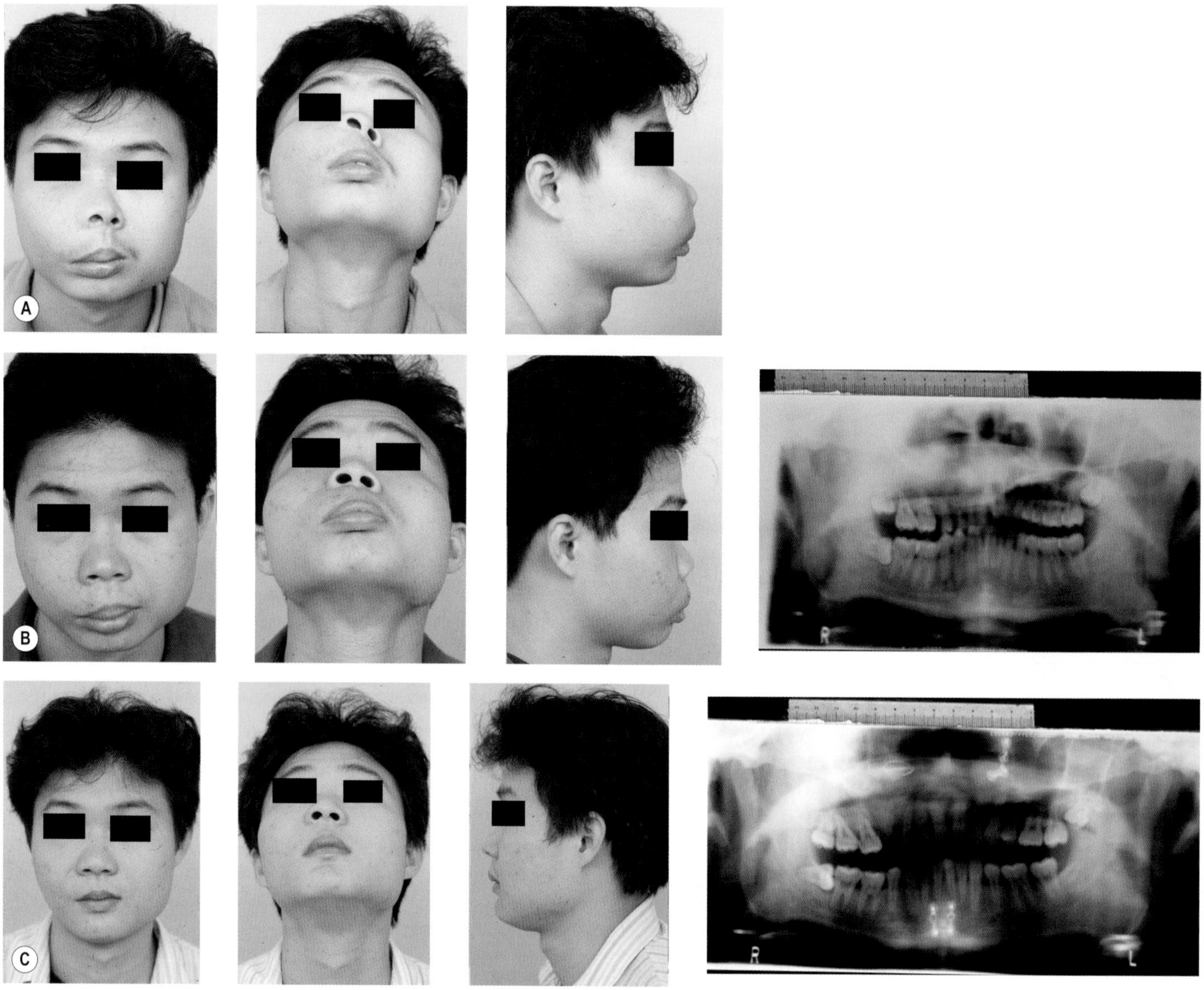

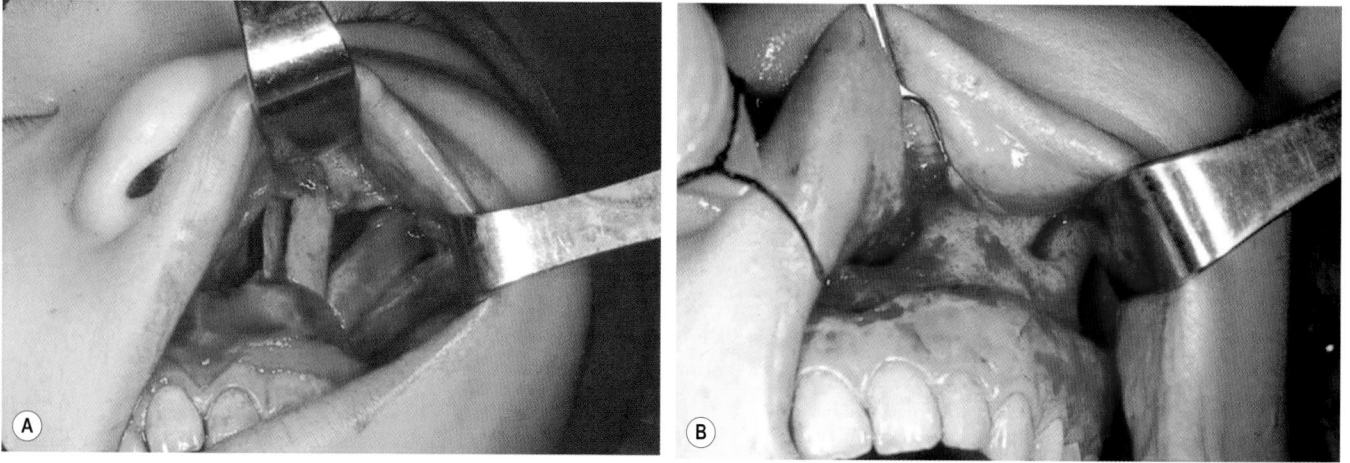

Fig. 15.11 **(A)** Right maxillary fibrous dysplasia in a 21-year-old patient. Resection with rib graft reconstruction was performed. **(B)** One year after the operation, malocclusion was noted at the anterior dentition **(B4)**. Wassmund and Kole anterior subapical osteotomies were performed to correct the malocclusion. **(C)** Two years after the resection. **(C4)** Panoramic view after Wassmund and Kole osteotomies.

Fig. 15.12 **(A)** Patient underwent resection and reconstruction using rib graft for a maxillary fibrous dysplasia lesion. **(B)** On re-exploration 3 years later for residual fibrous dysplasia, there is complete union between the native maxilla and rib grafts.

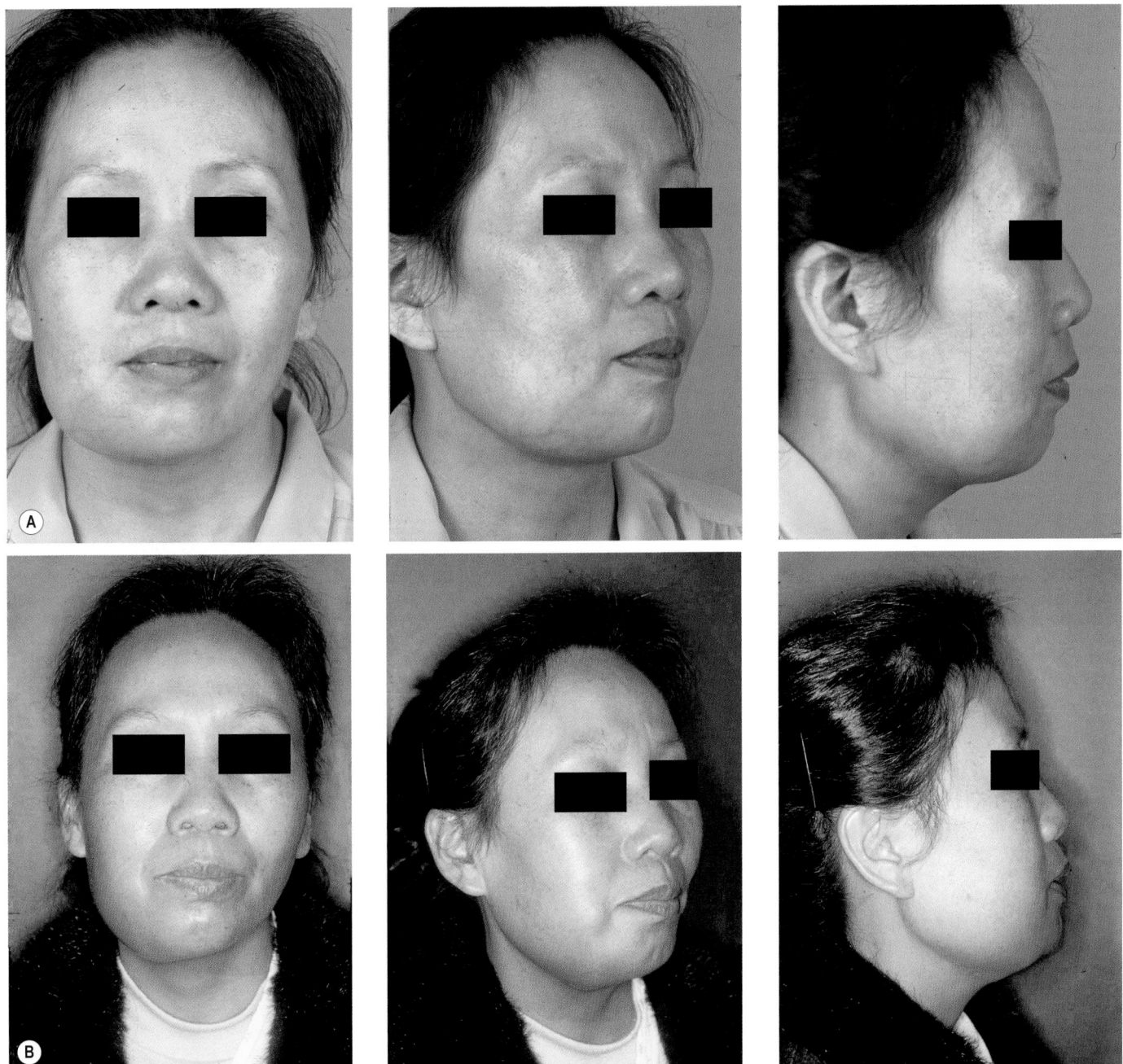

Fig. 15.13 (A) A 42-year-old patient diagnosed with right mandibular body fibrous dysplasia. Partial excision was performed. **(B)** The lesion recurred 5 years later. Right hemimandibulectomy was performed. Reconstruction was done with deep circumflex iliac artery osteocutaneous free flap.

least 6 months before any decision is made. This gives adequate time for edema to resolve so that a more accurate evaluation can be made.

Patients with zone 4 lesions may present months to years following the initial resection with an occlusal cant. This may be due to recurrent disease or graft resorption. Decision has to be made whether sufficient improvement can be achieved to justify reoperation. If so, the condition is evaluated with CT scan. Depending on the cause of the recurrent deformity, the treatment could be resection, additional bone grafting, or an orthognathic operation. Patients with a recurrent fibrous

dysplasia of the mandible can be treated with hemimandibulectomy and immediate reconstruction using a microvascular bone flap *(Fig. 15.13)*. In cases where reoperation is not warranted, the patient is counseled and it is prudent to wait.

Conclusion

Craniofacial fibrous dysplasia can cause significant functional and aesthetic deformities. At our center the principles and approaches in treating craniofacial fibrous dysplasia have

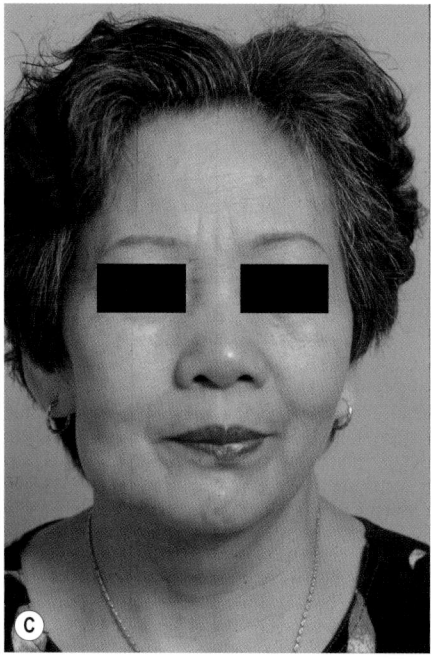
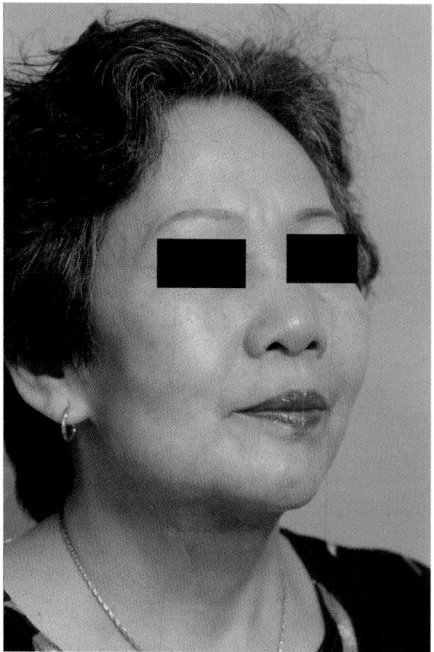
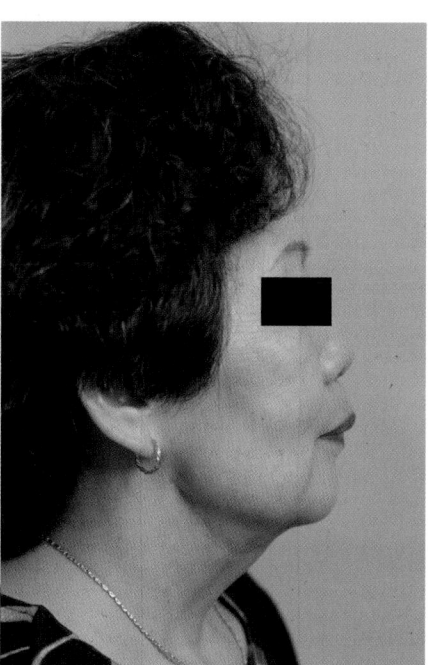

Fig. 15.13, cont'd (C) Appearance of the patient 10 years later.

evolved through the treatment of over 120 patients over the past two decades. Most of the patients have been followed up at Chang Gung Hospital by the senior author. A number of important points are to be highlighted here.

As these lesions are often located adjacent to important structures in the craniofacial region, management is best done through a multidisciplinary approach. The craniofacial surgeon coordinates inputs from various members in the multidisciplinary team and decides with the patient and family the decision for operation and the ideal timing. When operation is undertaken, effort is made to resect the lesion and reconstruct the defect at the same setting.

It is important to be sure of the diagnosis prior to planning a treatment approach. While this chapter focuses specifically on fibrous dysplasia, many of the operative principles discussed may serve as a model for treating other tumors occurring in the craniofacial skeleton. The surgeon however must consider the pathophysiology of the individual tumor at hand, and make appropriate adjustments regarding the extent and margins of resection, and the role of lymph node dissection, adjuvant or neoadjuvant therapy.

Due to the progressive and recurrent nature of fibrous dysplasia, patients with this disease are best served by a long-term caregiver who has become familiar with their individual disease and with their attitudes towards it.

Access the complete reference list online at **http://www.expertconsult.com**

2. Valentini V, Cassoni A, Marianetti TM, et al. Craniomaxillofacial fibrous dysplasia: conservative treatment or radical surgery? A retrospective study of 68 patients. *Plast Reconstr Surg*. 2009;123:653–660.
   An overview of craniofacial fibrous dysplasia. The article suggests that modern surgical technique allows an aggressive but definitive treatment with good aesthetic and functional results.

6. Dicaprio MR, Enneking WF. Fibrous Dysplasia. Pathophysiology, evaluation and treatment. *J Bone Joint Surg Am*. 2005;87:1848–1864.

7. Ozek C, Gundogan H, Bikay U, et al. Craniofacial fibrous dysplasia. *J Craniofac Surg*. 2002;13:382–389.

11. Riminucci M, Liu B, Corsi A, et al. The histopathology of fibrous dysplasia of bone in patients with activating mutations of the Gsα gene: site-specific patterns and recurrent histological hallmarks. *J Pathol*. 1999;187:249–258.
   The underlying pathogenesis of fibrous dysplasia involving the mutation of Gs alpha gene is discussed. Detailed descriptions are given regarding three different subtypes of fibrous dysplasia based on their histopathological characteristics, depending on the amount and structure of bone tissue within the bone lesion.

19. Ruggieri P, Sim FH, Bond JR, et al. Malignancies in fibrous dysplasia. *Cancer*. 1994;73:1411–1424.
   A retrospective study of 28 patients presented with malignant transformation occurring within fibrous dysplasia lesions. Clinical presentation, radiographic appearance, and microscopic features of the malignant lesions are discussed.

The controversial role of radiotherapy in the pathogenesis of these malignancies is also mentioned.

20. Kruse A, Pieles U, Riener MO, et al. Craniomaxillofacial fibrous dysplasia: A 10 year database 1996–2006. *Br J Oral Maxillofac Surg.* 2009;47:302–305

24. Chen YR, Chang CN, Tan YC. Craniofacial fibrous dysplasia: an update. *Chang Gung Med J.* 2006;29:543–548.

    Provides a comprehensive overview of craniofacial fibrous dysplasia, including the pathology, clinical features, diagnosis, and treatment.

26. Chen YR, Wong FH, Hsueh C, et al. Computed tomography characteristics of non-syndromic craniofacial fibrous dysplasia. *Chang Gung Med J.* 2002;25:1–8.

35. Tan YC, Yu CC, Chang CN, et al. Optic nerve compression in craniofacial fibrous dysplasia: the role and indications for decompression. *Plast Reconstr Surg.* 2007;120:19571962.

    Management of visual disturbance secondary to optic nerve compression is presented. The role of prophylactic and therapeutic optic nerve compression is discussed in detail.

37. Chen YR, Noordhoff MS. Treatment of craniomaxillofacial fibrous dysplasia: how early and how extensive? *Plast Reconstr Surg.* 1990;86:835–842.

16

Tumors of the lips, oral cavity, oropharynx, and mandible

John Joseph Coleman III and Anthony P. Tufaro

SYNOPSIS

- Cancer of the oral cavity and pharynx is thought to be caused by accumulated genetic alteration initiated by toxins from tobacco and promoted in the United States by alcohol intake.

- Tumors are staged according to the TNM system that considers anatomic subsite in the upper aerodigestive tract, size and adjacent extension for the primary tumor (T) number and laterality of cervical lymph nodes (N) and presence or absence of distant metastases (M).

- Surgery or radiotherapy are both effective in early stage tumors but surgery followed by postoperative adjuvant radiotherapy is preferable in Stage III or above tumors.

- The primary site and the cervical metastases or in some cases micrometastases are treated together as a composite resection or resection of the primary and neck dissection.

- Because of the anatomical complexity of the area, surgery and radiotherapy often interfere with the critical functions of respiration and alimentation. Resection and reconstruction should be designed to completely remove the cancer and preserve or restore as much function as possible.

- Extensive surgery with or without previous radiotherapy may result in difficult and dangerous complications such as osteoradionecrosis, fistula, carotid exposure and hemorrhage.

 Access the Historical Perspective section online at
http://www.expertconsult.com

Introduction

Cancer of the oral cavity and oral pharynx can create devastating damage to patients by interfering with the critical vegetative functions of respiration and alimentation and their corollary functions speech and swallowing. Patients in the United States and throughout the world who develop head and neck cancer often present with late stage disease which requires radical surgery and postoperative adjuvant radiotherapy increasing the risk of subsequent complications or deformity and dysfunction even if the therapy is successfully delivered. Moreover this patient population includes a high percentage of substance abusers since the known etiologies for this disease are carcinogens from tobacco and alcohol. A higher incidence of poverty, mental depression and malnutrition occur in these patients than in the general public adding further obstacle to their recovery and rehabilitation. Treatment must be tailored to these issues as well as to the fact that because of late stage presentation there is a high risk of tumor recurrence. These cancers usually recur within two years if they are not cured. Although there has not been a dramatic change in the mortality rate in the last 30 years, the efficient restoration to better function and appearance has been facilitated by the introduction of new reconstructive techniques particularly the widespread adoption of free tissue transfer.

The therapeutic approach to squamous cell carcinoma which makes up about 80% of cancers of the oral cavity and oropharynx comprises either surgery or radiotherapy for early stage disease (T_1, T_2) and surgery followed by postoperative adjuvant radiotherapy for later stage disease. The single stage surgery approach with synchronous extirpation and reconstruction followed by adjuvant radiotherapy has been accepted as the standard. Microsurgical techniques have allowed improved function and appearance by early reconstruction of the face, mandible and maxilla, oral cavity and pharynx. Although there has been some success with neoadjuvant or induction chemotherapy concurrent with or followed by radiotherapy, extirpative surgery and radiotherapy remain the standard of care. Cure rates are in the range of 70–90% for Stage I and II, 40–60% for Stage III and 30–50% for Stage IV.

Basic science

Head and neck cancer has long been considered a classic example of chemical carcinogenesis, most simply a two-part process where one carcinogen *initiates* the process and another promotes the subsequent growth of cancer. Tobacco is the initiating carcinogen most likely the polycyclic aromatic hydrocarbons such as benzopyrene which are produced in tobacco smoke. These are inhaled affecting the larynx and lung lining. They enter the blood stream and are secreted in the saliva where they can bathe the oral cavity and pharynx particularly in areas where saliva pools such as the floor of the mouth, the lateral tongue, the base of the tongue, the supraglottic larynx and the pyriform sinuses. These hydrocarbons affect the genetic material in the mucosal cells which are already in an inflammatory state because of the action of the promoting agent. In the Western world, the most common promoting agent is alcohol, as demonstrated by the high incidence of disease in patients who chronically use tobacco and alcohol. In South Asia which has a very high incidence of head and neck cancer *submucous fibrosis* appears to be the promoting factor with the tobacco and betel nut in *pan* an oral chew as the initiating factor. Other associations are with iron deficiency anemia in the Plummer–Vinson syndrome in Northern Europe and Vitamin A deficiency. Several occupational exposures have been considered promoting agents particularly nickel, radium, mustard gas, and wood dust.[32]

There has been a long recognized association between viral infection or colonization and head and neck cancer. Epstein–Barr virus infection is almost universal in patients with nasopharyngeal carcinoma. Recently, a strong epidemiologic association has been found between patients infected with human papilloma virus (HPV) and cancer of the tonsil and base of the tongue. It is theorized that the DNA from HPV type 16, 18, and 31 are highly active and may inactivate tumor suppressor genes resulting in tumor growth. Other genetics alterations have been frequently seen in head and neck cancer. Amplification of the oncogene cyclin has been reported. Mutation in the TP53 gene increases the risk of initial carcinogenesis and early recurrence and is seen more frequently in tobacco and alcohol use than in patients infected with the HPV suggesting different genetic pathways to a common neoplastic outcome.[33] Progression of head and neck cancers has been associated with amplification of the CDKN2A or p16 gene. Increased expression of the receptor for epithelial growth factor (EGFR) and certain EGFR mutations have been shown to predict poor prognosis and resistance to the tumor therapeutic cetuximab.

The final common pathway of the carcinogenic process in head and neck cancer appears to be decreased DNA repair capacity in the mucosal cells secondary to DNA repair gene polymorphisms. There are also disturbances in the cell cycle control systems that may be related to the accumulation of carcinogen metabolites.

The model of chemical carcinogenesis suggests that the entire mucosal field of the upper aerodigestive tract is at risk for development of cancer. Clinical and histologic evidence of this *field effect* is commonly seen in patients with head and neck cancer. The earliest or precancerous manifestation of this is *leukoplakia* or a white patch, a collection of hyperkeratotic hyperplastic cells with some mild dysplasia. *Erythroplakia* is a more aggressive change and may in fact harbor areas of invasive or *in situ* malignancy. This is an erythematous plaque, in which there is architectural disorganization of the mucosal cells and dysplasia with some nuclear alterations but no invasion of the basement membrane. *Carcinoma in situ* has frank

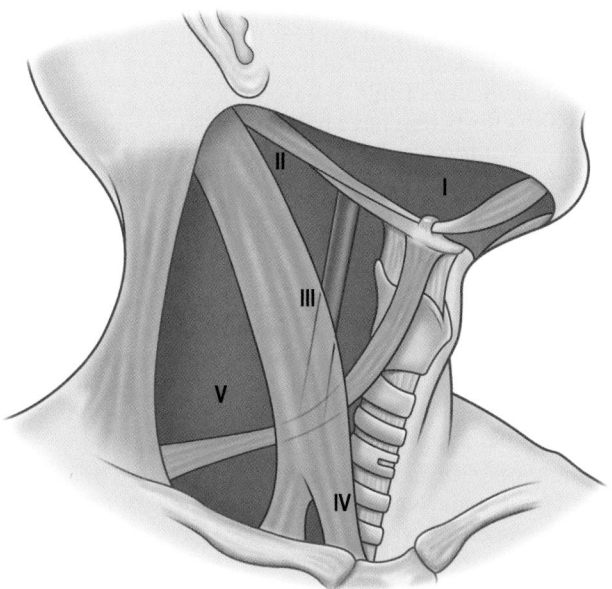

Fig. 16.1 Standardized description of lymph node anatomy.

malignant changes of the cells but confinement above the basement membrane. *Verrucous carcinoma* is a more indolent malignant change and frank *invasive carcinoma* invades into the underlying stroma. This field effect suggests that there might be a high incidence of synchronous primary cancers in the upper aerodigestive tract (5–7%) and a high incidence of secondary primary cancers a phenomenon that is seen clinically (20–30%). Although patients may have disseminated systemic carcinoma without cervical lymphadenopathy, the most common pathway of growth is locally, metastases to the regional lymph nodes and ultimately distant metastases *(Fig. 16.1)*.

Epidemiology

In the United States, head and neck cancer is a relatively uncommon disease making up about 3.2% of new cancers (c. 40 000/year) and 22% of cancer deaths (12 460).[32] The incidence is 270 cases per million US population as opposed to 520 million for colon cancer and 620 million for lung cancer. In the United States, if all the cancers of the head and neck are included, thyroid is the most common (29%), followed by larynx (15%), oropharyngeal mucosa (12%), and tongue (10%). The pathogenesis of thyroid cancer is completely different from that of mucosal carcinomas.[34] Most cancers of the upper aerodigestive tract arise from the respiratory epithelium and present as squamous cell carcinoma (80%), lip, tongue, tonsil, oropharynx, hypopharynx, larynx, and cervical esophagus. Adenocarcinoma is the second most common histology usually arising from the minor salivary glands in the area. Various types of sarcoma are less common.

Worldwide, particularly in developing countries, head and neck cancer is a bigger public health problem. It is estimated that there are 644 000 new cases and 300 000 deaths per year.[32] Including the world population, the most common site of presentation is the oral cavity. The countries with the highest *per capita* incidence of head and neck cancer are India followed by Australia, France, Brazil, and South Africa. In India, one-quarter of new cancers occur in the head and neck. In the US, the overall incidence of this disease is decreasing because of public health efforts that have been successful in diminishing tobacco use. Worldwide, however, the incidence and mortality is increasing and the 371 000 deaths from mouth and oropharyngeal cancer recorded in 2008 are projected to increase to 595 000 in 2030 because of the 40-year lag time related to tobacco effects in those countries more recently exposed to tobacco products such as in Africa and South-east Asia.[35] There has been a well established correlation between income and education and head and neck cancer, with an increased incidence in those patients suffering poverty and malnutrition.[36]

In the US, the male:female incidence ratio is three to one with a higher *per capita* incidence in blacks than whites, and an overall poorer survival in blacks. In Europe, 90% of patients affected are over 40 years of age and 50% are over 60. Worldwide, the ages are somewhat lower. In the developed world, there has been a rising incidence of disease in younger age groups, particularly related to HPV infection and probably its venereal transmission, since it is much more common in patients who have a family history of HPV infection or six or more sexual partners. This increase in head and neck cancers has paralleled a rapid rise in HPV infection in the developed world. These HPV associated tumors have a better survival rate than those related solely to tobacco and alcohol.[37]

As previously noted, the major risk factor is tobacco use which increases risk 5.25 times over nonsmokers in a dose-dependent relationship. Alcohol is both a co-factor and an independent risk factor with a two times greater incidence in nonsmoking consumers of alcohol. In a patient with a 40-pack/year history, who consumes five or more drinks/day, there is a 40 times increased risk of head and neck cancer.[38] Cessation of tobacco use alone or tobacco and alcohol use results in decreased risk approaching that of never having smoked or taken alcohol at 20 years.[39] Cessation also decreases the risk of metachronous upper aerodigestive tract tumors.

Patient presentation

Unfortunately, many patients with head and neck cancer present with advanced disease. The presenting symptom in 25% of patients with oral and oropharyngeal cancer and 50% of those with nasopharyngeal cancer is a mass in the neck representing regional metastases or at least Stage III disease. The site of the mass in the neck may predict the primary site of disease. Nodes in the submandibular or submental area (Level I) suggest primary cancer in the lip, anterior tongue or floor of the mouth; nodes in the jugulodigastric and upper jugular area (Level II) from the oral cavity, the oropharynx or nasopharynx; nodes in the mid-jugular area (Level III), oropharynx, hypopharynx or lateral tongue; nodes from the lower jugular area (Level IV), thyroid or visceral or breast primaries; and nodes in the posterior triangle (Level V), the scalp nasopharynx or parotid. A firm persistent cervical lymph node in a patient more than 40 years of age, particularly with a history of tobacco and alcohol use, should be considered head and neck cancer until proven otherwise.

Other symptoms at presentation are somewhat less specific but must be investigated, particularly if lasting longer than 3 weeks. These include sore throat, hoarseness, stridor and dysphagia. Unilateral ear pain may represent referred pain from lesions affecting structures innervated by the trigeminal or vagus nerves. History of smoking, alcohol use, previous infections or other diseases, previous malignancy and occupation are also important. Evidence of distant metastasis either dramatic on physical examination or more subtle by chemical or radiologic testing may be present. A careful and systematic examination of the upper aerodigestive tract must be performed by the use of direct inspection and palpation and use of laryngeal mirrors or a flexible nasolaryngoscope. Triple endoscopy (laryngoscopy, bronchoscopy, and esophagoscopy) to rule out synchronous malignancies was recommended in the past but is no longer considered cost-effective as a screening method. Signs of malignancy may include red or white patches on the mucosa, ulceration or mass on the tongue, tonsil, palate or elsewhere, poor dentition, or a loose tooth or teeth, edema of the tongue or other oral structures, nasal airway obstruction, proptosis or orbital mass, or unilateral ear effusion. Palpation may define a mass or elicit pain, suggesting ulceration or bony invasion. Examination of the neck and the rest of the body is critical in a targeted fashion to assess for regional or systemic metastases.

Further definition of the primary tumor site can be obtained by computerized tomography (CT) if bone is involved or magnetic resonance imaging (MRI) if the tumor is in soft tissue alone. Chest X-ray should be obtained in all patients because of the high incidence of primary and metachronous lesions. In later stage locoregional disease, particularly if there is a suspicion of distant metastases PET-CT scan may be useful although their sensitivity is greater than their specificity and several studies have shown no increase in accuracy of diagnosis when PET-CT is used to assess the neck.[40] The role of sentinel lymph node biopsy in evaluating the N0 neck has not been definitively determined. Clinically suspicious palpable masses in the neck should be evaluated by aspiration cytology which has a very high sensitivity and specificity. Nutritional parameters should be monitored as well as hemoglobin levels since many head and neck patients are malnourished, anemic and relatively dehydrated. If there is dysphagia or alimentary tract obstruction enteral feeding and rehydration should be undertaken prior to therapy although parenteral feeding has been shown to decrease survival. Because depression is 10 times more common in patients with head and neck than in the general public, a careful mental status examination and appropriate therapy should be undertaken prior to initiating major surgical or radiotherapeutic treatment.

Staging

Head and neck cancers like other solid tumors, are described for clinical purposes by staging. The American Joint Committee for Cancer (AJCC) and the Union Internationale Contre le Cancer (UICC) have established a method called TNM (tumor, nodal metastasis, metastases systemic), which characterizes the lesion in an anatomic fashion at the time of its clinical presentation *(Table 16.1)*. This system has been used relatively effectively to predict prognosis, determine treatment plans

Table 16.1 TNM clinical staging system for lip and oral cavity

T_x	Primary tumor cannot be assessed	N_x	Nodes cannot be assessed
T_0	No evidence primary tumor	N0	No evidence nodal metastasis
T_{is}	Carcinoma *in situ*		
T_1	≤2 cm in greatest dimension	N1	Single ipsilateral node <3 cm
T_2	2–4 cm	N2a	Single ipsilateral node 3–6 cm
		N2b	Multiple ipsilateral nodes 3–6 cm
		N2c	Bilateral or contralateral nodes <6 cm
		N3	Any lymph node >6 cm
T3	>4 cm		
$T4_a$	Lip: invasion of mandible, skin, floor of mouth, nerve OC: invasion of mandible, extrinsic tongue, maxilla, skin		
$T4_b$	Invasion of masticator space, skull base or carotid sheath		

Stage			
0	TisN0M0	IVA	T4aN012M0
I	T1N0M0		T123N2M0
II	T2N0M0	IVB	T4B any NM0
III	T3N0M0		T1–4A N3
	T123N1M0	IVC	any T any NM1

Modified from Patel SG, Shah JP. TNM staging of cancers of the head and neck: striving for uniformity among diversity. *CA Cancer J Clin.* 2005;55:242–258.[41]

Histologic variations, tumor thickness, such as the Breslow classification for melanoma and other parameters have been suggested as adjunct to the TNM system but have not been widely accepted. Present research is based on the concept that the head and neck cancer like all other cancers is the result of an accumulation of genetic alterations that results in clonal populations that exhibit independent growth mechanisms and outgrow the normal organ. This theory suggests that the addition of molecular markers of malignancy such as the abnormal expression of EGFR, Cyclin D1, HPV DNA, p53 gene and others be combined with TNM to better predict tumor behavior and prognosis and to help in selecting targeted therapies. Future research in this direction will determine the utility of these methods.[42]

Therapeutic choices

Decisions on types of therapy are made after appropriate work up and staging and are based to a great degree on site, size of the primary and involvement of adjacent structures. Because the head and neck is a compact area densely populated by critically important structures that greatly impact on appearance and function informed consent must be detailed and comprehensive. The main functions of the upper aerodigestive tract are respiration and alimentation and all therapies should attempt to eradicate the tumor while preserving as much of these functions as possible. Multiple quality-of-life (QOL) scales have been developed to quantify the problems created by head and neck tumors and the therapy that they require. Familiarity with these and their appropriate use will help the surgeon realistically counsel the patient.

The surgical oncologic principle of therapy is removal of the primary tumor with a margin of normal tissue surrounding it and removal from the neck preferably *en bloc*, any metastatic lymph nodes or draining nodes that have a high statistical probability of containing clinically occult metastases. The radiation oncologic principle is similar, lethal dose radiotherapy to the primary tumor and a lower dose to the surrounding area and sterilization of the draining cervical lymph nodes. For T1 and T2 tumors (those <4 cm in diameter), with no lymph node metastases surgery, resection of the primary site with or without neck dissection and radiation therapy of the primary site with or without the neck, give relatively equivalent disease free survival. When there are cervical nodal metastases, as in Stage III and IV disease, surgery followed by adjuvant radiotherapy is the most appropriate therapy. Radiation therapy is most frequently used for T1 or T2N0 cancers of the larynx and hypopharynx and nasopharynx and surgery more commonly used for T1 and T2N0 tumors of the oropharynx, oral cavity and paranasal sinuses. These choices are made to facilitate function since surgical resection of the larynx with subsequent esophageal or other nonlaryngeal speech creates a greater disturbance of function than radiation therapy. Surgical resection at the other sites may create little dysfunction and avoids the complications of radiotherapy such as xerostomia, progressive fibrosis, osteoradionecrosis and others.

The desire to preserve function and the discovery of chemotherapeutic combinations or targeted therapies that are more cytotoxic to head and neck cancers has lead to an increased

and to compare the effectiveness of various therapies. For the head and neck standard anatomic subsites have been determined, lips and oral cavity, pharynx, larynx, nasal cavity and paranasal sinuses, and thyroid gland. T-stage depends for the most part on size but also to some degree on adjacent structures affected. N-status depends on size, number and laterality of the cervical lymph nodes. M-status is self-evident.[41] The combination of characteristics describes the stage of the lesion. It is critical that the stage be accurately determined and recorded on presentation since it allows accurate translation of information and determination of prognosis and choice of therapy.

There has been much study oriented to improving the accuracy of staging systems in head and neck cancer. Anatomic staging provided by the TNM system may be inaccurate because of the difficulty in examining the head and neck with its complex anatomy, leading to underestimation of tumor size and the presence of lymph nodes particularly in the obese patient with a thick neck. Moreover, TNM staging does not address the variability of tumor biology and histology.

interest in organ preservation with induction chemotherapy and definitive radiotherapy. The success in laryngeal preservation demonstrated in the VA study and others has encouraged extension of this principle to other sites with mixed success in an attempt to avoid surgery altogether. Preradiotherapy or concurrent chemotherapy regimens have been used and a 62% organ salvage rate accomplished.[43] Salvage surgery (surgery for persistences and or recurrence) may be used if combined therapy is not successful. The use of chemotherapy as an adjuvant to radiotherapy in the postoperative setting has also been advocated but reports of it success are mixed.[44,45] The use of new reconstructive and extirpative techniques appears to have decreased the risks of complications for surgery performed after definitive radiotherapy and chemotherapy.[46]

Surgical access

Although significant progress has been made with endoscopic techniques and robotic mechanisms, adequate access and visualization remains critical to perform a satisfactory tumor resection. Access approaches are designed to expose the tightly packed structures held within the narrow confines of the upper aerodigestive tract while avoiding transection of important neurovascular structures to preserve sensation, motion or other special senses.

Lip splitting (labiotomy) incisions are usually planned as midline to allow the best symmetry and to avoid vascular embarrassment. Mandibulotomy should be midline or mesial to the egress of the mental nerve from the mandible to preserve sensation of the lip. If necessary, the mental nerve can be sacrificed and mandibulotomy performed on the vertical ramus above the entry of the inferior alveolar nerve to access the base of the tongue. Extension of the mandibulotomy can be along the floor of the mouth for exposure of the tonsil or retromolar trigone or midline through the tongue and palate to expose the nasopharynx, posterior pharynx or supraglottic larynx (Trotter approach). For access to the nose, paranasal sinuses and orbit, the incision in the superior alveolar sulcus (Caldwell–Luc) can expose the unilateral maxilla and be carried up to the infraorbital nerve or beyond. Extension of this approach across the midline and laterally along both sulci can be used to create a facial degloving incision to provide access to the total midface. When this incision is combined with a bilateral coronal incision it gives excellent access to the midface, orbits, skull base and sinuses. Unilateral exposure to the nose, sinuses, palate and orbit can be obtained by the Weber–Ferguson incision which extends from a midline upper lip splitting incision along the folds linking the juncture between the lip, cheek and nose, and extended above or below the eyelids or through the medial canthus depending on the structures that needs to be exposed *(Fig. 16.2)*.

Access to the oral cavity from the neck can be obtained through a retrosymphysial transverse incision entering the oral cavity from below and extending the incisions laterally until there is enough exposure to eviscerate the tongue without damaging the lingual nerve. Similarly more lateral pharyngotomy avoiding the hypoglossal and superior laryngeal nerves can provide limited exposure of the oropharynx, hypopharynx and larynx.

Oral cavity cancer

Lip

Evaluation and planning

Malignant lesions of the lip may include a diverse list of histopathologies, including minor salivary gland, neurogenic, and connective tissue; however, as is the case with all oral cavity sites, over 90% of all malignant lesions are squamous cell carcinoma (SCC). The discussions in this chapter will be limited to the diagnosis and management of squamous cell carcinoma.

The oral lip begins at the skin vermillion junction and is contiguous with the buccal mucosa and gingival sites. The etiologies most commonly associated with malignant lesions of the lip are tobacco use, solar exposure, and viral infections. Extension of disease from contiguous sites is also a common finding.

The lip represents the most common site of head and neck cancer, excluding cutaneous malignancies. The most common presentation is an ulcerated or exophytic lesion of the lower lip. Larger, infiltrative lesions may present with paresthesia secondary to mental nerve involvement *(Fig. 16.3)*.

The preoperative evaluation should include a complete exam of the head and neck. Second primary lesions or synchronous areas of dysplasia are not uncommon and should be addressed at the time of initial surgery. The clinical assessment of the primary tumor is of critical importance. Size and depth of invasion will guide the resection and subsequent reconstruction of the defect. All lesions that are either >T1, or exhibit invasion, >3–4 mm, or those that that present with paraesthesia should have imaging studies. Manual palpation alone may miss enlarged cervical nodes that contain metastatic disease. Furthermore, physical exam may be unreliable in the patient with a thick neck or scars from previous surgery. A contrast enhanced computed tomography study is usually readily available and can render information regarding metastasis and extension of disease. If this study is limited by dental artifact, an MRI will complement or replace the CT study and will be able to detect soft tissue disease, nodal involvement, perineural spread and bony invasion. In general PET imaging is not indicated as a routine study in the evaluation and management of malignant lesions of the lip.

Treatment

Surgical management is the primary treatment modality for malignant lesions of the lip. The use of definitive radiation therapy should be limited to those patients who cannot tolerate surgery. The use of radiation as definitive treatment carries the possibility of increased morbidity over surgery. The sequelae of trismus, xerostomia, dental caries and potential for osteoradionecrosis must be carefully considered prior to taking this course. The other significant aspect of this modality choice is that the use of adjuvant radiation will be limited or excluded from future treatment plans. While surgical excision and/or radiotherapy are regarded as equally effective, there are no large scale prospective trials to verify this.[47]

The prognosis for Stage I and II SCC of the lip is quite good. The 10-year recurrence free survival rates (RFS) are 94% and

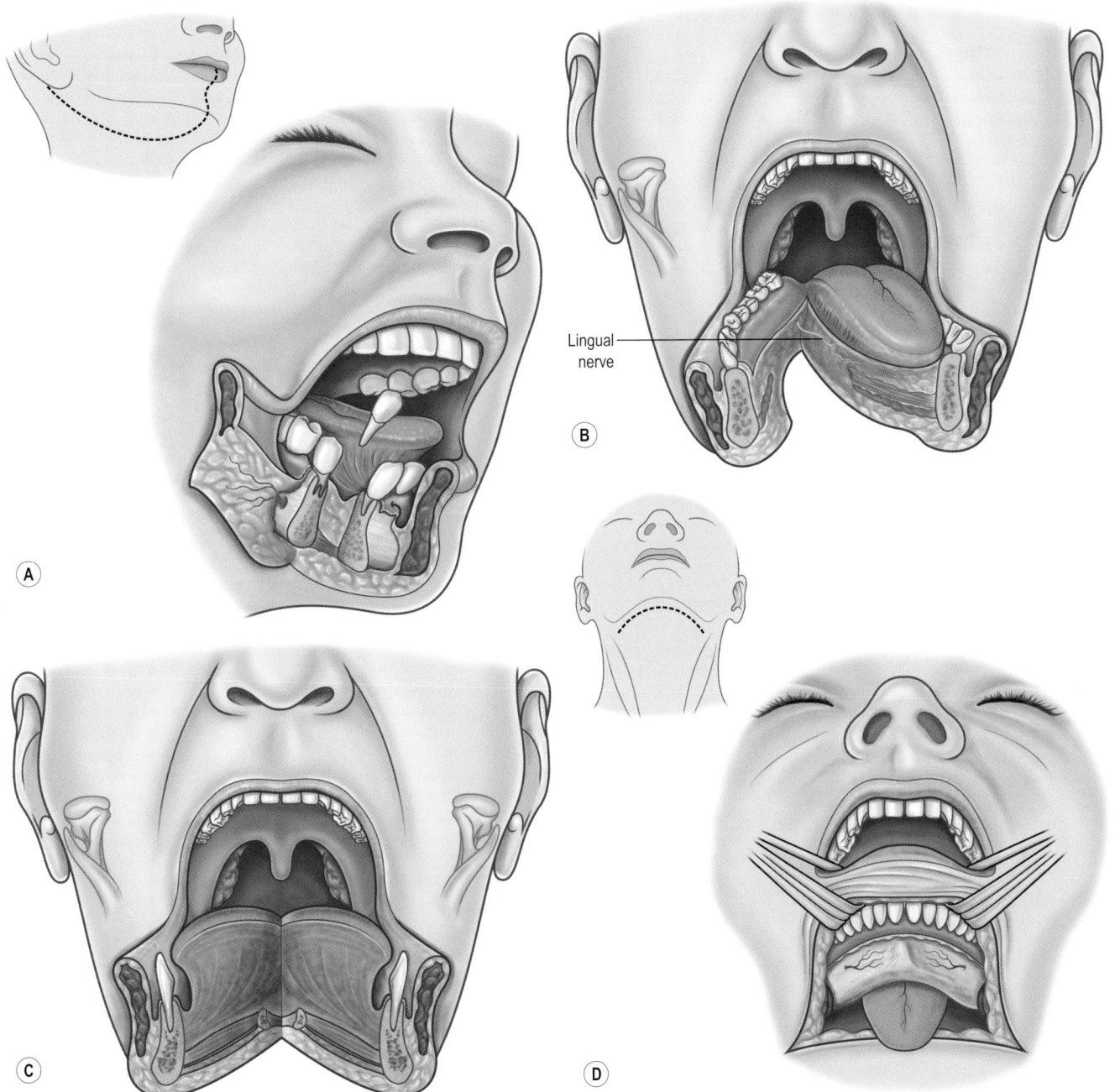

Fig. 16.2 Various methods of surgical access to tumors of the head and neck. **(A)** Midline labiotomy, paramedian mandibulotomy. **(B)** Midline labiomandibulotomy with paralingual extension. **(C)** Midline labiomandibuloglossotomy (Trotter). **(D)** Retrosymphysial approach.

27% for Stage I and II, respectively.[47] The initial tumor size will determine the final cosmetic and functional outcome. Lesions that require resection of the central portion of the lip that amount to less than ½ the lower lip can be closed with primary repair. A margin of at least 5 mm should be planned for smaller lesions. Locally advanced lesions, ≥T2, will need a margin of 1 cm. Smaller lesions can be resected as a wedge or full thickness "V" excision. The skin/vermillion junction at the margins of the resection should be marked so that it can be perfectly aligned at the time of reconstruction. A reconstructed vermillion that is off as little as 1–2 mm will be detectable. The apex of the wedge resection should not cross

adjacent anatomic structures such as the labiomental groove *(Fig 16.4)*. The resection can be planned as a "W" so that excision is maintained within aesthetic units. The resected tissue should be labeled prior to sending to pathology and the medial and lateral margins marked. Frozen section specimens should be taken from the patient's side of the resection for confirmation of adequacy of margin.

The reconstruction of the defect should begin with repair of the orbicularis oris. Once the muscle is repaired with absorbable suture, a few absorbable sutures can be placed in the mucosa. The skin/vermilion junction should be repaired with a permanent monofilament suture. A

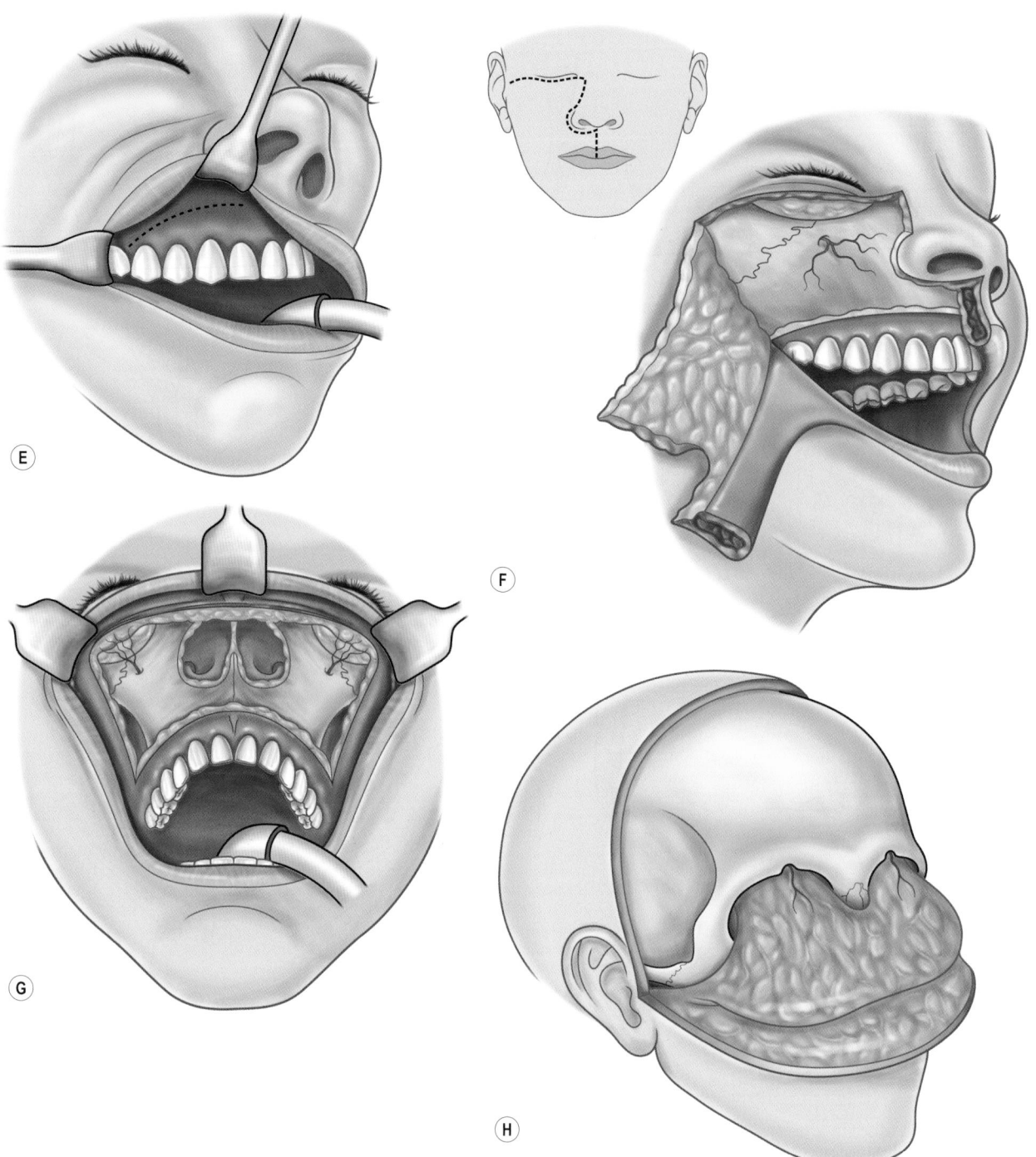

Fig. 16.2, cont'd **(E)** Buccoalveolar sulcus (Caldwell–Luc) approach. **(F)** Weber–Ferguson approach. **(G)** Midface degloving approach. **(H)** Bicoronal approach.

superficial scratch has been placed horizontally across the white roll at the point of resection; this ensures perfect realignment of this important landmark. Dermal and finally skin sutures are placed.

Lesions that approach the commissure are reconstructed with a full thickness pedicled flap from the upper lip. The reconstruction can be planned just slightly smaller than the resection. Once the specimen is removed and labeled the reconstruction flap is incised. An attempt should be made to preserve the superior labial artery. The medial skin incision

is made carefully through the skin and subcutaneous tissue. The apex of the flap is incised and the tissue rotated into position. It is important to maintain a 1 cm mucosal bridge on the oral side. Even if the artery is unable to be found the mucosal bridge will maintain the flap. Again a meticulous layered closure is mandated by repairing the muscle, mucosal surface, then vermillion is reapproximated and finally skin *(Fig. 16.5)*.

Resection of more than half of the upper or lower lip will require the use of adjacent tissues to reconstruct the defect.

Generally, the medial aspect of the cheek, particularly in older patients is the accepted donor site. Larger reconstructions, using Karapandzic or fan flaps, will cause significant microstoma, which is the primary limitation of these flaps. Free tissue transfers can incorporate a tendon for suspension of the soft tissue with improved function and aesthetics.

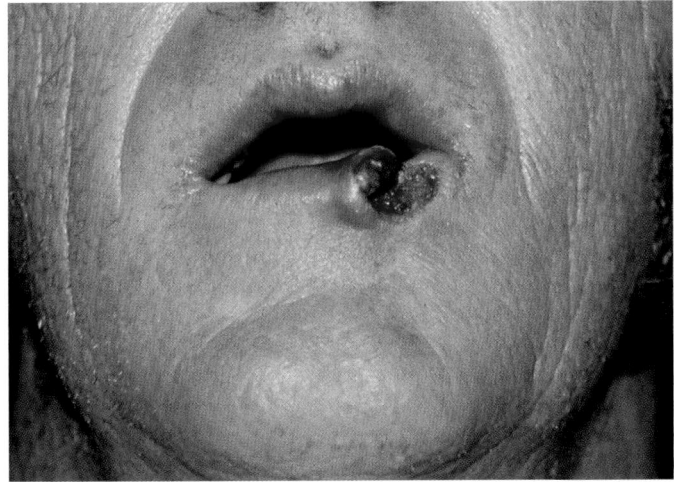

Fig. 16.3 Large infiltrating lip lesion causing paresthesia.

It is not uncommon for patients with a significant history of sun exposure to have a malignant lesion in conjunction with significant premalignant changes affecting the entire lower lip. In this case, the malignant and premalignant lesions should be addressed at the same operation. The full thickness excision can be combined with vermilionectomy. A mucosal advancement flap is mobilized from the buccal mucosa and sutured to the skin margin. The mucosa will initially crust over and should be kept moist with petroleum jelly.

Cervical metastasis

While the incidence of cervical metastasis is less common than that found with other oral sites, a small proportion of patients with lip primaries will present with or develop cervical metastatic disease. Only 2–12% of patients will present with positive nodes. While there is no conclusive evidence at this time, cancers originating in the upper lip and commissure appear to have the greatest risk of cervical metastasis.

The size of the primary and the histologic grade are two factors that play a role in metastasis. Tumors >2 cm have a 16–35% chance of developing lymph node metastases, while tumors <2 cm have a 4–7% chance of developing cervical disease.[48]

A comprehensive neck dissection is indicated for those patients who present with metastatic disease. If

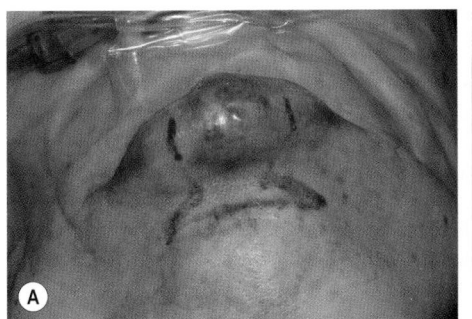
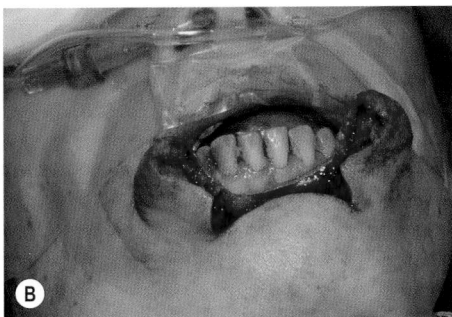
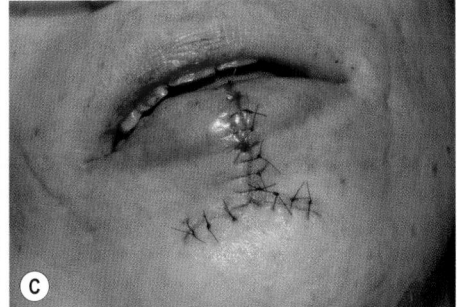

Fig. 16.4 (A) Lesion of central lower lip. **(B)** Resection defect. **(C)** Repair. Note alignment of vermillion margin.

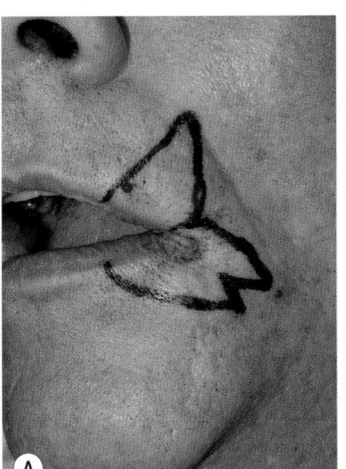
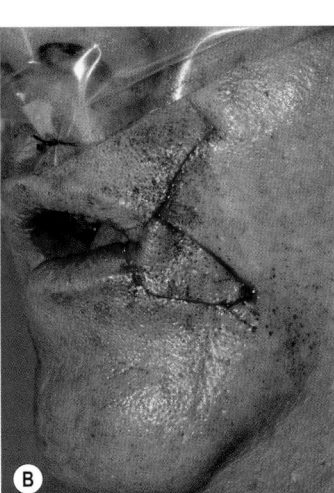
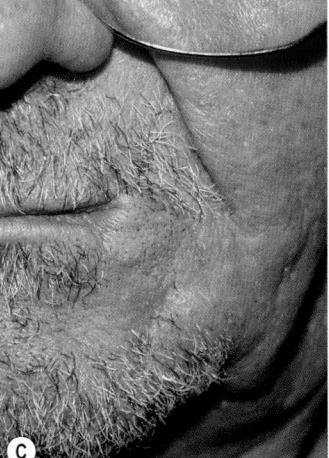
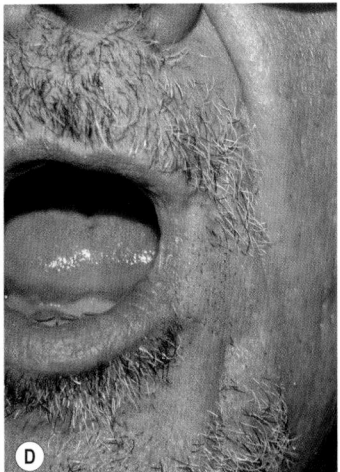

Fig. 16.5 (A) Recurrent squamous cell carcinoma at labial commissure. Resection designed as a "W" to maintain the resection within aesthetic units. **(B)** Flap from the upper lip transposed into defect. The "W" has been closed as a "V" and aesthetic units preserved. **(C)** Closed mouth view at 6 months postoperatively. **(D)** Functional view showing a mild amount of microstomia.

lymphadenopathy is detected in the parotid gland, it should be managed at the time of neck dissection.

Buccal mucosa

Evaluation and planning

SCC of the buccal mucosa is rare in the US and Western Europe. While it accounts for only 10% of all oral cavity carcinomas in the west, it is one of the most common cancers of Central and South Asia.[3] This is due to the habit of chewing tobacco mixed with lime and betel nut. Often it is difficult to find patients with disease whose site of origin is the buccal mucosa and not spread from a contiguous site. Patients with T1 or T2 tumors do not do well with a 5-year survival of 78% and 66%, respectively. Deeper invasion into muscle or Stensen's duct is associated with decreased survival.[49]

Treatment

Smaller tumors may be resected via a transoral technique. These excisions may be closed with primary closure or skin grafts. The need for a 1 cm margin will make primary closure very difficult. Larger lesions which extend onto the alveolar ridge of the mandible or maxilla will need to have the bone addressed, requiring either a marginal or segmental mandibulectomy or partial maxillectomy. Larger defects will be best addressed with fasciocutaneous free tissue transfer.

Management of the regional nodal bed has important implications on survival. In one study, the rate of occult nodal metastasis was at least 26%. Five-year survival rates for patients with and without positive neck nodes were 49% and 70%, respectively.[49] Elective selective neck dissection should be considered in N_0 patients with any tumor >T1. Adjuvant radiation therapy is included in the standard recommendations for patients with either: more than one positive lymph node, extracapsular extension, or close margins on final pathology. Positive margins are best addressed with re-excision.

One of the most significant problems in the management of this disease is the development of severe trismus. Even with the use of thin, supple fasciocutaneous flaps aggressive physical therapy must be instituted as soon after surgery as possible. Failure to do so will make it impossible for the patient to function normally.

Floor of mouth

Evaluation and planning

Primary tumors of the floor of mouth may be difficult to evaluate. The presence of dentition and close proximity to the mandible can make the extent of the tumor impossible to delineate without very careful physical examination. The tongue should be held with a gauze sponge and moved from side to side. The index finger of the opposite hand is used to retract soft tissue and palpate the lesion. A dental mirror is used to visualize the lingual surface of the alveolar ridge.

A large percentage, 43%, of patients present with Stage I or II disease. Five-year survival for Stages I through IV is 95%, 86%, 82%, and 52%, respectively.[50] There is a high risk of regional metastasis with occult lymph nodes found in 21% of patients with Stage I and 62% in patients with Stage II disease.[50]

Treatment

Smaller lesions can be resected via a transoral approach. The area can be left to heal by secondary intention or reconstructed with a split thickness skin graft. The lingual and hypoglossal nerves are at risk of injury when resecting floor of mouth lesions. The nerves are superficial and care must be taken to identify these structures and avoid injury.

Larger lesions will require better access. A mandibulotomy will allow excellent visualization of the entire lingual surface of the mandible, the floor of mouth, and contiguous areas of the ventral tongue. Marginal resections may be needed to obtain negative margins on the mandible. Larger lesions may also require a split thickness skin graft to avoid severe contracture seen with wounds left to heal by secondary intention. The best outcome for patients with larger defects is seen with reconstruction with a thin, supple fasciocutaneous flap, such as a radial forearm flap. This flap will offer protection to the underlying bone and avoid problems of wound breakdown and bone exposure, particularly in those cases of radiation failure or adjuvant radiation.

Patients with a carcinoma in the floor of the mouth are at a high risk of having metastatic regional disease. Some 30% of patients will present with positive nodes.[51] Smaller lesions (T1 and T2) that are not deeply infiltrated (1–2 mm) and are N0 can be managed with close observation following complete excision. Deeper lesions (>3 mm) can be treated with an elective supraomohyoid neck dissection. For lesions that cross the midline bilateral supraomohyoid neck dissections can be performed.

Patients with positive nodal disease are candidates for adjuvant radiotherapy, since locoregional recurrence remains a major source of treatment failure in these patients. The standard indications for adjuvant radiation are: more than 1 lymph node positive, extra nodal extension of disease, soft tissue disease, perineural/perivascular invasion, and close or microscopically positive margins.

Alveolar ridge lesions and retromolar trigone

Evaluation and planning

Only a small percentage of oral cavity malignancies are found on the alveolar ridge. They are usually found on the posterior aspect of the mandibular alveolar ridge. The retromolar trigone represents the small area of mucosal tissue overlying the mandibular third molar region and ascending ramus. It is continuous with buccal mucosa, maxillary and mandibular gingiva, tonsillar pillars, the soft palate, tongue, and pterygoid musculature.

Patients will often present with higher stage disease. The cervical metastasis rate has been reported to be 26% in a recent paper.[52] Because of the intimate approximation of the mucosa to bone, early involvement of the bone is not uncommon. Extension of the tumor into the masticator space is a poor prognostic indicator.

Management

Smaller lesions may be resected transorally and left to heal by secondary intention or closed with a skin graft or local flap. Unfortunately, most patients present with a higher stage disease.[52] Larger tumors will require some management of the mandible. Mandibulotomy may be required for adequate approach to the posterior oral cavity. Marginal mandibulectomy is indicated for tumors abutting the mandible or those with minimal cortical erosion. Tumors of the gingiva in the area of dentition exhibit early invasion as a function of tumor extending into cancellous bone via the dental socket and periodontal ligament (*Fig. 16.6*). In edentulous areas, the tumor extends through the gingiva into the alveolar process into the cancellous bone. Segmental mandibulectomy is indicated when there is extension of tumor into the cancellous bone.

Partial maxillectomy would be indicated for involvement of the maxillary alveolus. The defect can be closed with local flaps or dental appliances to obturate the defect (*Fig. 16.7*).

The overall 5-year survival rates for patients with squamous cell carcinoma of the alveolar ridge ranges from 50% to 65%. No significant survival difference has been observed between maxillary and mandibular lesions. The presence of cervical metastases markedly decreases survival. Backstrom *et al.* reviewed 125 patients with squamous cell carcinoma of the alveolar ridge and reported that the 5-year survival decreased from 41% to 7% in patients with cervical metastasis.[53] Adjuvant radiation therapy is indicated for close margins or microscopically positive margins, perineural, perivascular invasion, multiple positive nodes, or extracapsular spread.

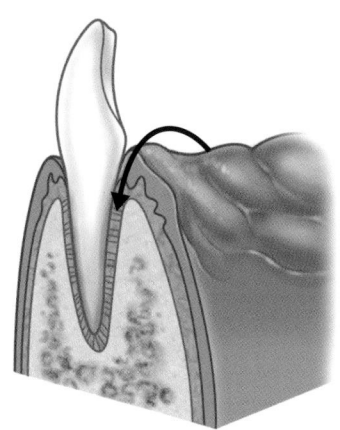

Fig. 16.6 Tumor progressing down the periodontal ligament into alveolar bone.

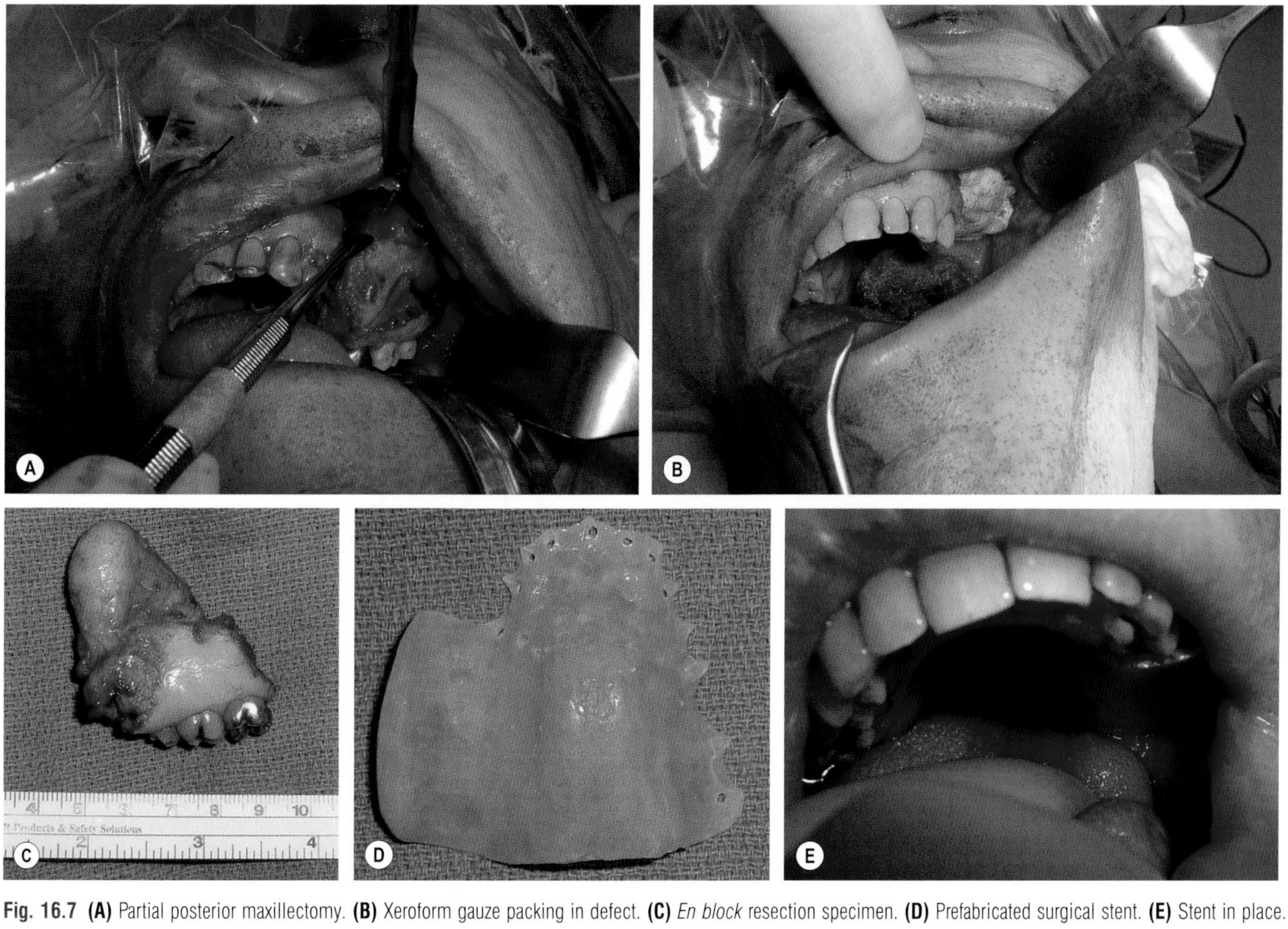

Fig. 16.7 (A) Partial posterior maxillectomy. **(B)** Xeroform gauze packing in defect. **(C)** *En block* resection specimen. **(D)** Prefabricated surgical stent. **(E)** Stent in place.

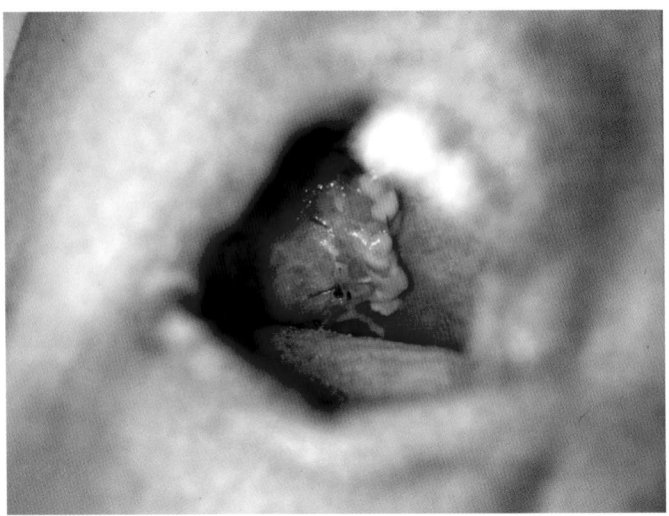

Fig. 16.8 Squamous cell carcinoma of the palate.

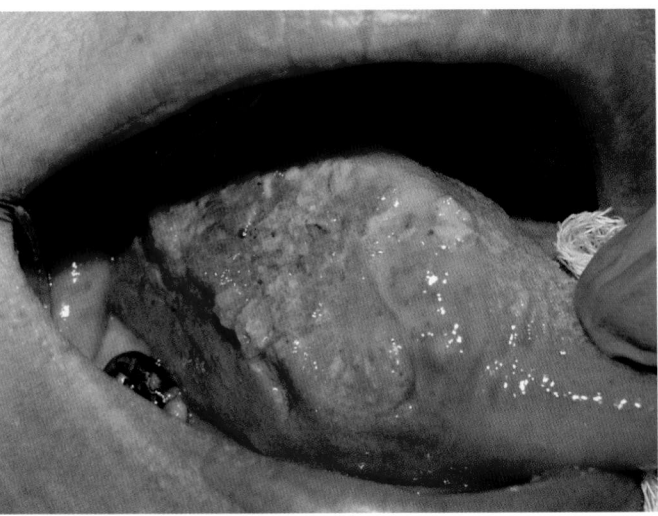

Fig. 16.9 Infiltrating squamous cell carcinoma of the tongue.

Hard palate

Evaluation and planning

Squamous cell carcinoma of the hard palate is a relatively rare disease in the United States. It is much more common in India and South Asia. It represents only 0.5% of all oral cancers in the United States, while in India, it represents about 40% of all oral cancers.[54]

Malignant tumors of the minor salivary glands of the hard palate are found to occur as frequently as squamous cell carcinoma.

The squamous cell carcinomas are usually well-differentiated which translates into a low occult cervical metastatic rate with only 10–25% of patients having clinically positive nodes. Level I and II nodes are the most commonly involved. The tumor is usually a painless mass of the hard palate. Larger tumors could invade the sinus or nasal cavity. A biopsy should be performed to rule out a salivary gland etiology *(Fig. 16.8)*.[55]

Management

Most smaller tumors can be resected periorally. The patient can have a stent fabricated prior to surgery. Following resection the palate can be covered with the stent and the defect can heal by secondary intention. Involvement of bone will require resection with adequate margins. The reconstructive options are a local flap and/or obturator/prosthesis. Larger invasive tumors will require maxillectomy with possible free tissue transfer and/or obturator/prosthesis.

Regional metastatic disease should be addressed with a neck dissection. Occult metastasis is not common. Adjuvant radiation therapy is indicated for patients with advanced disease, close margins, perineural/perivascular invasion or extranodal extension.

Evans and Shah state that the size of the primary tumor was a determining factor in survival. Patients with lesions >3 cm had a marked reduction in 5-year cure rates of 54% vs 16%.[56]

Oral tongue

Evaluation and planning

SCC of the tongue exceeds the total incidence of all other intraoral sites. The most common site of the primary tumor is the lateral border of the middle third of the oral tongue. Carcinoma of the anterior and middle third of the tongue is for the most part, either exophytic or ulcerative, while tumors of the posterior third of the tongue are often deeper, infiltrative extending into the intrinsic musculature of the tongue *(Fig. 16.9)*.

Tumors will often arise in areas of preexisting leukoplakia or erythroplasia. In areas of chronic glossitis, multiple independent synchronous foci of disease are possible. As the site of primary tumor moves posteriorly in the tongue, the histology will often change. Oral tongue lesions are often well to moderately differentiated while base of tongue carcinomas are usually less well-differentiated.

Regional metastasis of tongue carcinoma occurs more frequently than any other intraoral primary neoplasm. Middle third of tongue lesions metastasize more commonly than the anterior one third. Carcinoma of the base of the tongue has a very high incidence of metastases to both ipsilateral and bilateral cervical nodes.[57]

Patients with positive nodal disease need a definitive plan for management at the initial surgical intervention. The management of the nodal disease may be determined by the size and number of positive nodes. In most cases, definitive surgical therapy of the primary site and the cervical nodes, followed by adjuvant radiotherapy when appropriate is the best treatment paradigm. Adjuvant therapy is advised for patients with more than one positive node, extra capsular spread, a lymph node completely replaced by tumor, a large primary tumor or evidence of perineural/perivascular invasion. A patient who presents with a single positive node <2 cm may be managed with external beam radiation when a small primary tumor is being treated with radiation for definitive therapy. The use of external beam radiation as primary treatment will eliminate it as a treatment option subsequently in the case of local, regional failure.

The patient who presents with no clinical evidence of nodal disease (N0) may present a more complicated decision-making process. Factors that may help the surgeon make a comprehensive treatment plan take into account the potential risk of regional metastasis, the size of the primary tumor, the depth of tumor invasion, the grade of the tumor, and the location of the primary tumor. Patients with a short thick neck, which makes a clinical exam more difficult, or patients who may be unable to return on a frequent regular basis for follow up exams are factors that must also be considered by the surgeon when making the decision to observe or electively treat the N0 neck.

The risk of occult metastasis ranges from 20% to 40%.[58] Patients with tongue primaries have the highest risk of occult nodal disease, with a predictable pattern of metastases occurring from Level I through Level III.

If the decision is made to observe the N0 neck, that decision must be made with the knowledge that those patients who go on to develop regional disease will have lower rates of control.[59]

The most prudent course of treatment would dictate that those patients who have a 15–20% risk of occult nodal metastases undergo elective treatment of the levels most at risk. Spiro et al. found that tumor thickness of as little as a 2 mm depth correlated with an increased risk of nodal metastases.[60] With this knowledge, it is clear that even relatively small, invasive tumors present with a significant risk of regional disease.

The use of an elective supraomohyoid neck dissection, done in conjunction with the resection of the primary tumor, serves as an excellent diagnostic modality for staging as well as therapeutic modality.[61] This procedure carries with it little potential for morbidity. The management of malignant lesions of the tongue depends on the accurate staging of the primary site as well as the neck.

Radiation and surgery can show equivalent results for T1 and T2 disease. The 5-year disease free survival for both modalities is 80–90%. The use of radiation as the definitive modality of treatment may present significant problems in a population that has a 40% possibility of a second primary lesion.[62] The long-term complications of radiation are not trivial and include xerostomia, dental caries, potential for osteoradionecrosis, trismus, and many others. The most significant problem of definitive radiotherapy stems from the fact that the further use of radiation is eliminated from the treatment armamentarium for disease recurrence.

Management

The majority of patients are best managed with a resection of the primary tumor with at least 1 cm margins. The margins should be measured out and drawn on the tongue. Frozen sections should be sent on the patient tissue after the primary tumor has been resected. Positive margins need to be resected when possible.

T1 and T2 lesions of anterior and middle third of the tongue can be addressed with a wedge excision and layered closure. The tongue will be shortened and the tip will deviate to the resected side. The younger patient will rapidly adjust to the new size of the tongue and often will not require speech or swallowing therapy. Older patients may initially have difficulty with speech and eating and may benefit from speech and swallowing therapy.

Larger lesions which cross the midline are more problematic. Care must be taken to preserve at least one lingual artery and one lingual and hypoglossal nerve. An insensate and or immobile tongue is an almost insurmountable problem for rehabilitation. These problems will affect speech and swallowing, greatly impacting quality of life.

Larger posterior lesions will require a mandibulotomy for access. The defect created by the resection of larger lesions will require a skin graft or fasciocutaneous free tissue transfer for reconstruction. The use of a smaller thin radial forearm free flap will allow excellent range of motion. The reconstruction will be insensate and thus will make movement of the food bolus difficult. The patient may often require speech and swallowing therapy postoperatively.

Larger lesions and higher stages will require both surgery and adjuvant radiation for improved outcomes. The 5-year survival rates for Stage III and IV patients are 54% and 34%, respectively.[63]

Management of the mandible and maxilla

Marginal resection

Tumors that abut the lingual surface of the mandible will require a marginal resection. The uninvolved mandible will become the "deep" margin of resection. A marginal mandibular resection will leave the inferior border intact and reduce the functional deficit.

A marginal resection is contraindicated in cases of gross tumor invasion into bone, as identified on radiographs or clinical exam, tumor metastasis (i.e., renal cell, prostate) to bone, or evidence of invasion of the inferior alveolar canal and its contents, which may present as paraesthesia. Previous radiation to the mandible is also considered to be a contraindication to marginal resection. Marginal resections are very difficult in the edentulous mandible where residual bone stock is often atrophic. Patterns of bone resorption, with time, may leave the patient with a pencil thin mandible that is prone to fracture particularly if any bone is attempted to be resected. If a marginal resection is attempted in this setting, it may be prudent to "reinforce" the portion of the mandible left after resection with a reconstruction plate.

It is important to round all boney surfaces after the marginal resection. This will reduce the possibility of erosion and exposure (Fig. 16.10). The rounded bone edges will decrease stress and potential for fracture. This small step will improve the patient's ability to wear a prosthesis in the postoperative period. The defect created by the marginal resection can often be closed with the local tissue. The resection decreases the height of bone and mobilization of buccal soft tissue and the floor of mouth will often allow for primary closure. Closure in multiple layers will avoid breakdown of the wound and exposure of the resection margins. A radial forearm free tissue transfer is an excellent option for a more complicated reconstruction. The thin, soft nature of this flap allows it to drape over the bone and offer protection to the bone even in the face of adjuvant radiation.

Mandibulotomy

Tumors arising in the middle and extending into the posterior third of the tongue and floor of mouth, or lesions arising or

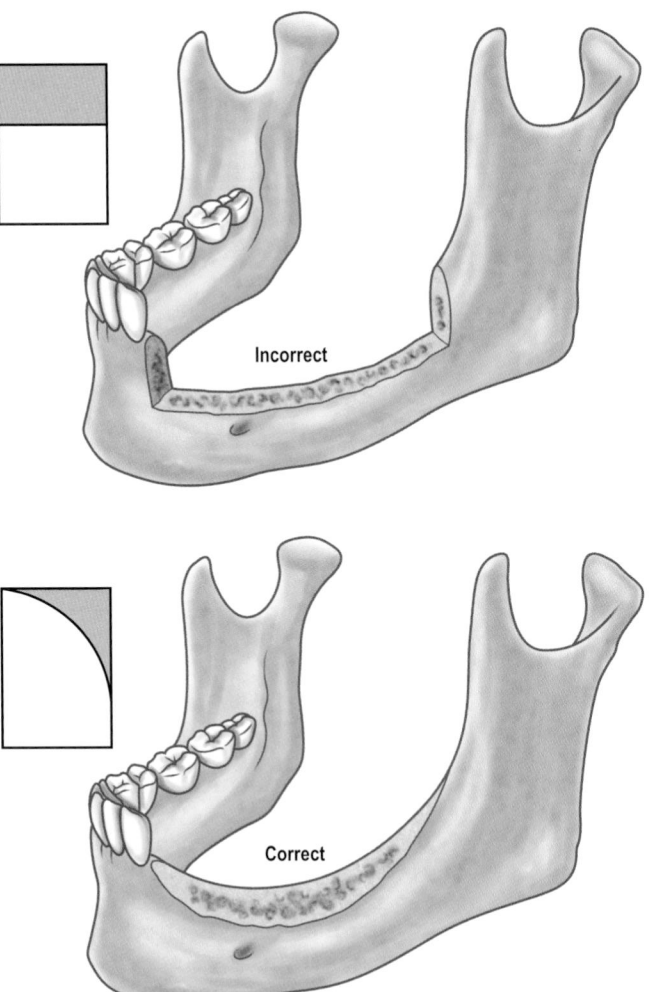

Fig. 16.10 Correct technique for marginal resection of the mandible.

extending into the oropharynx will need wider access for oncologic resection. The use of a mandibulotomy will allow wide and safe access to the posterior oral cavity back to the prevertebral space.

A panoramic radiograph of the mandible is obtained pre-operatively to plan proper placement of the osteotomy to avoid tooth roots and other anatomic and dental obstacles (bridgework, infected teeth, impacted teeth).

The osteotomy is planned just anterior to the mental nerve. This will allow for an easier osteotomy between the pre-molar roots and the canines where there is a natural divergence. This approach will preserve the inferior alveolar nerve and sensation to the lip and gingiva. If the mandibulotomy is placed in a more posterior position, the osteotomy will be in the direct portal of any radiation that may be needed in the postoperative period and the inferior alveolar nerve will be transected. Placement of the mandibulotomy in a more anterior position will usually require extraction of a tooth to facilitate the bone cut. If the tooth is not extracted, the roots of the anterior teeth are at high risk of injury and this situation raises the possibility of infection.

The mandibulotomy is carried out by dividing the lower lip and elevating a cheek flap. The mental nerve is identified

and a site selected for the osteotomy which is marked on the bone. A bone plate is fixed to the inferior border of the mandible with 2.0 mm screws placed in a bicortical fashion. The planned osteotomy should fall directly under the central hole of a 7-hole plate. This will allow for three screws on either side of the osteotomy. The holes are drilled and the screws placed. A smaller plate is now placed in the tension band position again with the central hole of a 5 or 7-hole plate over the osteotomy. These screws are placed in a monocortical fashion to avoid injury to the dental roots. The holes are drilled and the screws placed (*Figs 16.11A-D*).

The plates are now removed and held on the back table. The osteotomy is carried out with a sagittal saw. As the alveolar ridge is approached, the bone is scored and the final osteotomy is carried out with fine osteotomes. The mandible is now able to be opened and excellent access is given to the floor of mouth, posterior tongue and pharynx. Using cautery, the mucosa is carefully opened. As the mylohyoid muscle is divided, close attention must be paid to the hypoglossal and lingual nerves. They are found very superficially crossing from lateral to medial across the floor of the mouth. At the termination of the resection, the soft tissue is re-approximated with absorbable sutures. The muscles can be reapproximated with interrupted sutures in an effort to reconstruct the diaphragm of the floor of the mouth and ensure return to normal function. The bone plates are reapplied to the mandible in the predrilled holes. There should be a small bone gap to account for the thickness of the saw blade. Using this technique patients' occlusion will be unchanged from their presurgical occlusion (*Figs 16.11E-H*).

Management of the maxilla

Resection of the maxilla is indicated for the management of tumors arising on the gingiva, hard or soft palate or buccal sulcus. The maxillary ostectomy is indicated for tumors adherent to or invasive to the boney maxilla. Depending on the extent of invasion the maxillary resection may be as simple as an alveolectomy for small lesions progressing up through palatal fenestration, to partial/medial maxillectomy, on to complete maxillectomy (*Fig. 16.12*). For this discussion, we will limit the extent of resection to more localized tumors.

The surgical plan begins with axial and coronal CT imaging as well as a panoramic dental radiograph. Dental impressions preoperatively for the fabrication of stents are often important.

Small lesions are addressed with mucosal incisions down to bone with adequate margins. The bone is scored or sectioned with a cutting burr or saw. The final cuts are finished with fine osteotomes. The small defect can be dressed with petrolatum gauze and allowed to granulate in. The dressing is removed at 1 week and the area will mucosalize over. A dental stent or obturator will reduce discomfort and speed healing.

Large tumors will need to be addressed with an upper cheek flap, a Weber-Ferguson incision, for access. Attention to detail for placement of the skin incision is of great importance. The incision will be in the central gaze of all people the patient comes in contact with and the incision should be placed along the lines of esthetic units.

The cheek flap is elevated with adequate soft tissue margins. The infraorbital nerve is preserved if possible. The denuded portions of the cheek flap can be skin grafted. The maxillary

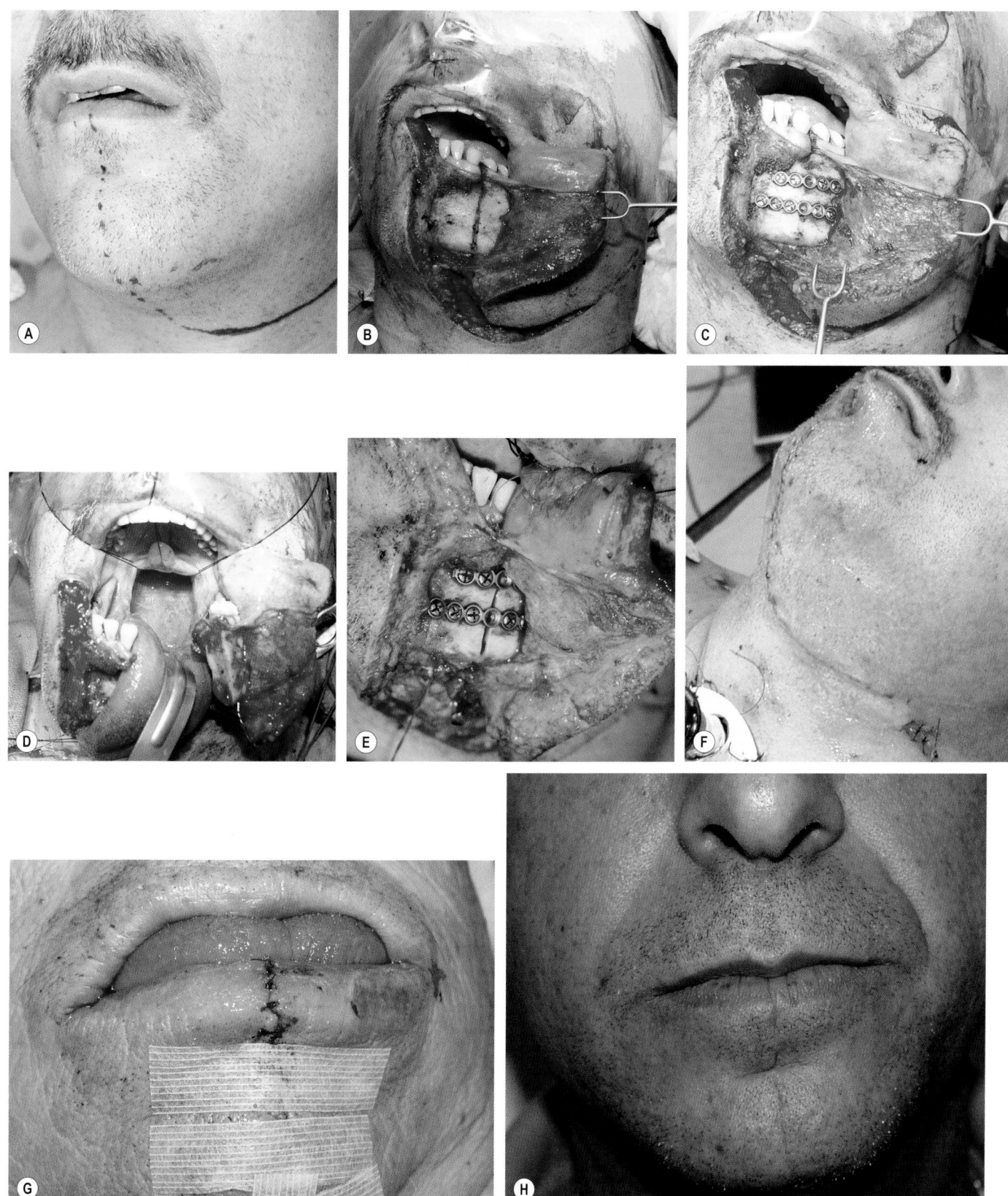

Fig. 16.11 **(A)** Mandibulotomy drawn out, splitting the lip in the midline. **(B)** Marking the position of the mandibulotomy just anterior to the mental nerve. **(C)** Two plates placed prior to completing the mandibulotomy. **(D)** Access possible with a mandibulotomy and floor of the mouth opened. **(E)** Bone plates placed with predrilled holes for proper position. Note the bone gap from the thickness of the saw blade. **(F)** Lateral neck closure. **(G)** Lip closure. Note alignment of vermillion. **(H)** Mandibulotomy 1 year postoperatively.

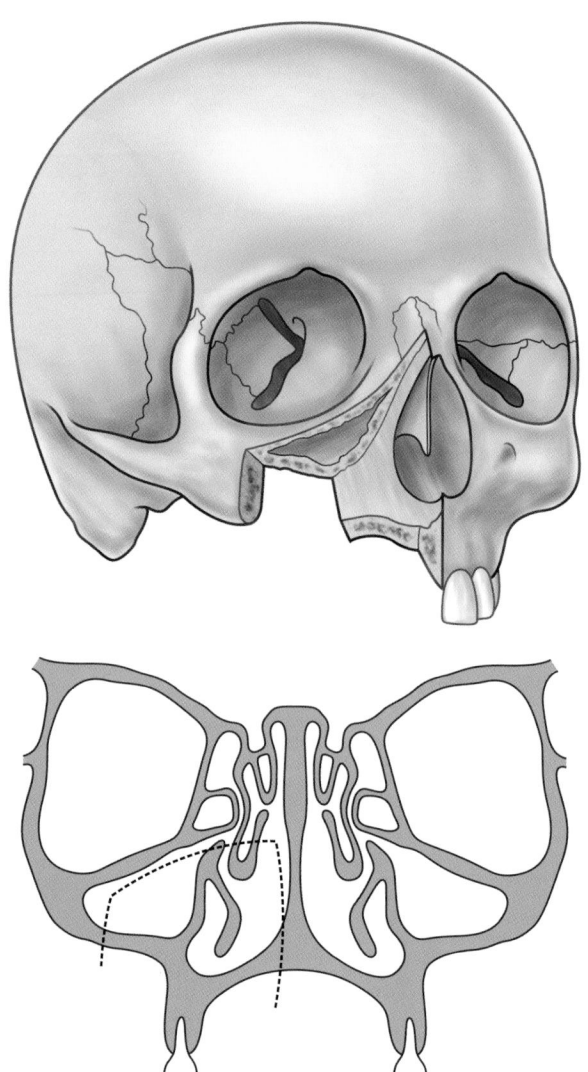

Fig. 16.12 Maxillectomy.

sinus can be covered with a skin graft if the mucosa is removed. The skin graft is sutured with chromic sutures and held in place with petrolatum gauze and a pre-fabricated stent is used to cover the defect and stabilize the packing. The stent and packing are removed at 1 week. The patient is instructed in daily irrigation and can obtain a final prosthesis in 2–4 months depending on healing *(Fig. 16.13)*.

Oropharynx

Oropharynx refers to tumors involving the soft palate, tonsils, base of tongue, posterior pharyngeal wall and vallecula. Malignant lesions of the oropharynx are uncommon and represent fewer than 1% of all malignancies. Smoking and alcohol exposure are the main etiologic factors. A recent troubling trend has been seen in young nonsmokers and nondrinkers who present with this disease. This trend appears to be related to HPV infection.

Oropharyngeal tumors tend to be more poorly-differentiated and have a higher propensity to exhibit early regional metastases, particularly base of tongue and tonsil lesions.[64]

Base of tongue

Base of tongue lesions account for 25–30% of all lingual squamous cell carcinomas. Because of the location, the deeply infiltrative nature of the tumor, most lesions are T2–T3 at presentation.[57] The majority of patients will present with clinically positive regional nodes at the time of initial diagnosis. Bilateral and contralateral nodal disease occurs in 20–30% of cases.[65]

Stage I and II cancers can be treated with either surgery or radiation as single modality therapy, with similar rates of local control and survival. The use of lasers and robotics to assist in access to base of tongue lesions and other difficult to approach areas will improve the willingness of surgeons and patients to accept surgery as the treatment of choice. At this time, definitive radiation therapy is the modality most commonly selected.

Due to the high rate of occult metastases, patients with N0 necks will require elective treatment. Some single therapy will be adequate. If radiation has been selected for management of the primary site, then the ipsilateral neck should be radiated. If surgery has been selected, then a supraomohyoid neck dissection is indicated. Treatment of both necks is indicated for midline lesions.

The 5-year disease specific survival and overall survival for base of tongue cancer are 65% and 45%, respectively for Stage I, and 54% and 62% for Stage II.[66] Cancer of the soft palate has a 5-year locoregional control, cause-specific survival and overall survival of 84%, 89%, and 52% for Stage I and 85%, 87%, and 61% for Stage II. The 5-year loco regional control, cause specific survival and overall survival rates of 92%, 100%, and 54% for Stage I and 88%, 86%, and 61% for Stage II tonsillar cancer. The management of advanced stage oropharyngeal cancers requires multidisciplinary multimodality therapy. The treatment paradigm has shifted toward chemoradiation protocols. Four acceptable options exist:

1. Surgery followed by adjuvant radiation
2. Definitive concurrent chemoradiation
3. Surgery followed by adjuvant chemoradiation
4. Induction chemotherapy followed by concurrent chemoradiation or sequential chemotherapy and radiation.

The use of nonsurgical organ preservation protocols for patients with advanced oropharyngeal cancers has evolved in an effort to decrease morbidity and improve quality of life. The selection of surgery followed by adjuvant radiation or concurrent chemoradiation is a decision that needs to be made based on the experience of the surgeon, the medical oncologist, and the radiation oncologist. The physical status of the patient and patient's wishes need to be factored into the equation. Concurrent chemoradiation has been compared to surgery plus adjuvant radiation in one randomized trial on advanced oropharyngeal cancers. There was no significant difference in 3-year disease-free survival between surgery plus adjuvant radiation and chemoradiation 50% vs 40% *(Fig. 16.14)*.[67]

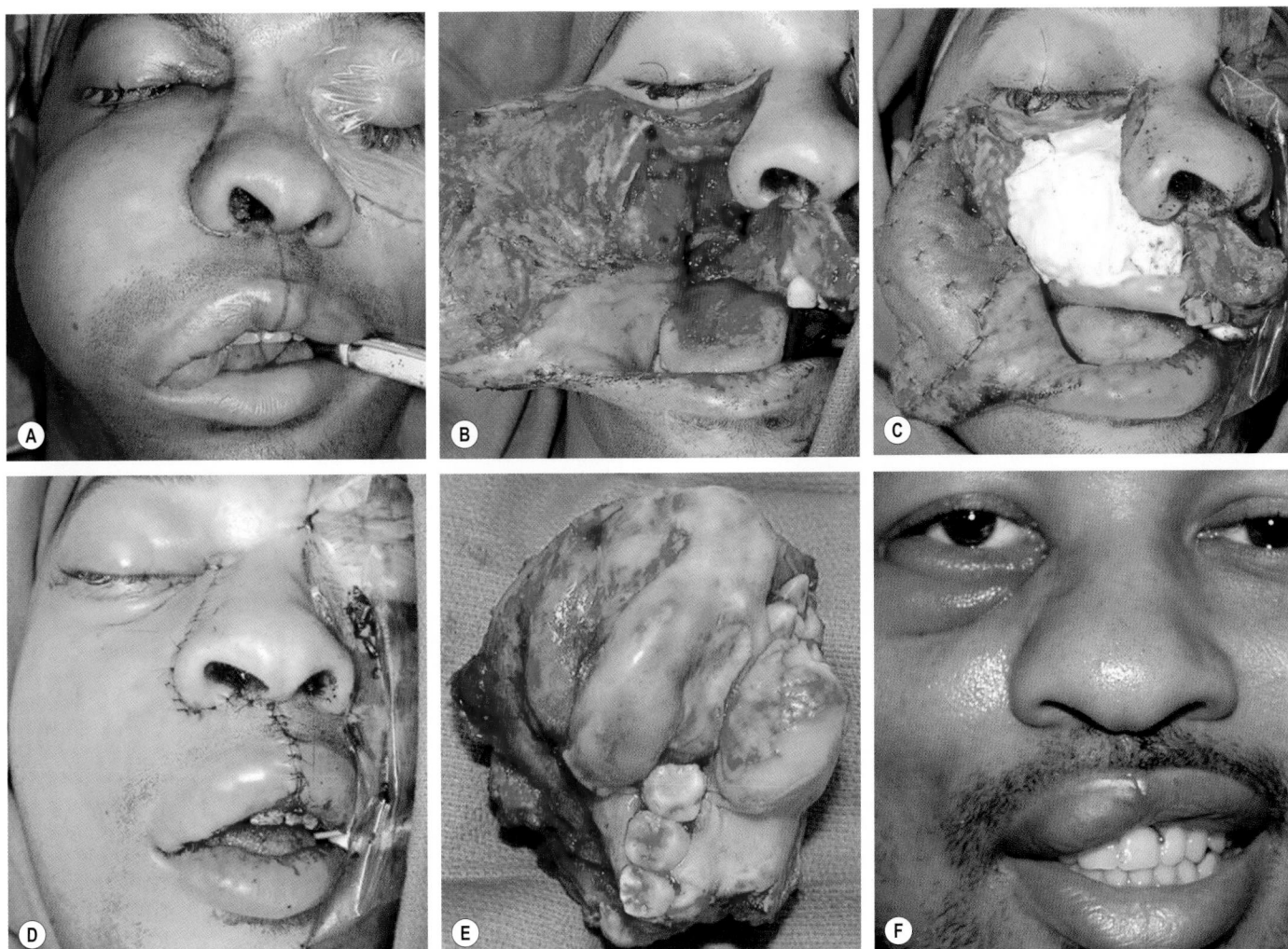

Fig. 16.13 (A) Maxillectomy incision marked out. **(B)** Completed maxillectomy. Including orbital floor. **(C)** A skin graft has been applied to the raw surface of the cheek. Xeroform packing is placed in the defect and a surgical stent is wired in place. **(D)** Immediate on table closure. **(E)** Large tumor growing over the occlusal surface of the dentition. **(F)** A 2-month postoperative photograph, with dental prosthesis in place.

Surgical approach

Neck dissection

The presence of nodal metastasis has a profound negative impact on patient survival, decreasing 5-year disease specific survival by 50%. The American Cancer Society states that over 40% of patients with oral cavity and pharyngeal squamous cell carcinomas present with regional metastasis at their initial examination. The risk of occult metastasis is relatively high for most primary oral cavity cancers and is directly related to the thickness of the primary tumor. Tumors of 2–5 mm in thickness have an occult metastatic rate of about 30%.

Levels I, II, and III are at the highest risk for occult metastasis from oral cavity primary tumors. The supraomohyoid neck dissection has been shown to be effective for the diagnostic staging and therapeutic management of the clinically N0 neck in patients at risk for occult metastasis. Approximately 30% of these patients will have positive nodal disease at pathologic evaluation.

In patients with clinical evidence of cervical nodal metastasis, a therapeutic neck dissection including Levels I–V is indicated *(Fig. 16.15)*. Most often, a therapeutic neck dissection for an oral cavity primary is a modified neck dissection, sparing the sternocleidomastoid muscle (SCM), the internal jugular vein, and the spinal accessory nerve.

Technique: supraomohyoid neck dissection

The incision is placed in a natural skin crease and extends from the mastoid area to the midline approaching the hyoid bone. The incision is two finger breaths below the angle of the mandible. The incision is carried through the platysma muscle, and superior and inferior subplatysmal flaps are raised. The greater auricular nerve and the marginal mandibular branch are identified and preserved. The marginal mandibular branch is found directly on the capsule of the submandibular gland and is elevated with either bipolar cautery or scissors. The nerve is retracted in a cephalad direction. Next, the fascia overlying the anterior border of the SCM is incised and the muscle freed of the investing fascia. The spinal accessory

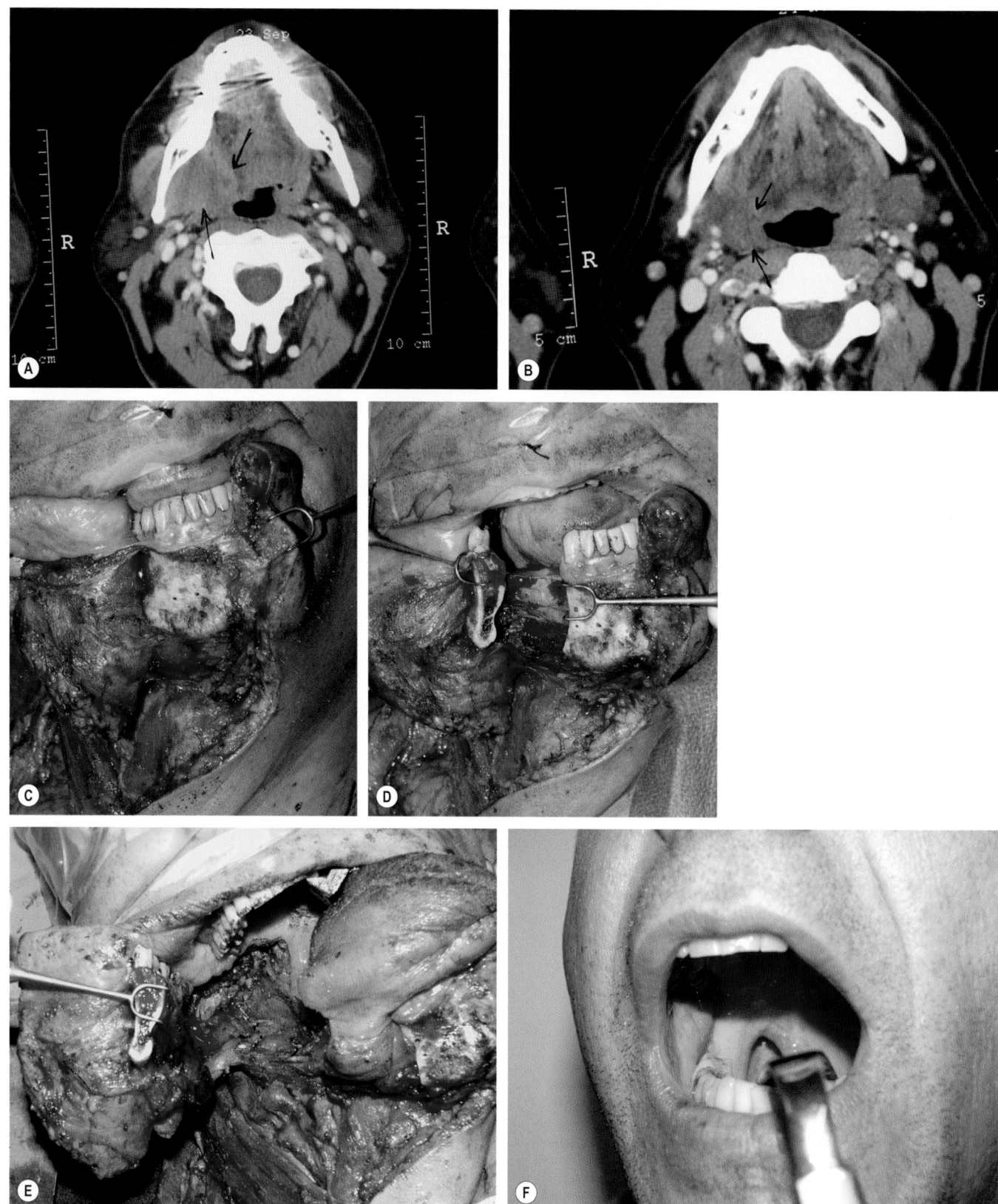

Fig. 16.14 **(A)** CT image of large oropharynx tumor. **(B)** CT image of oropharynx tumor after neo-adjuvant chemotherapy. **(C)** Lower cheek flap for mandibulotomy. **(D)** Mandibulotomy for approach to oropharynx. **(E)** Resection of oropharynx tumor. **(F)** Long-term outcome of radial forearm free flap for oropharynx tumor.

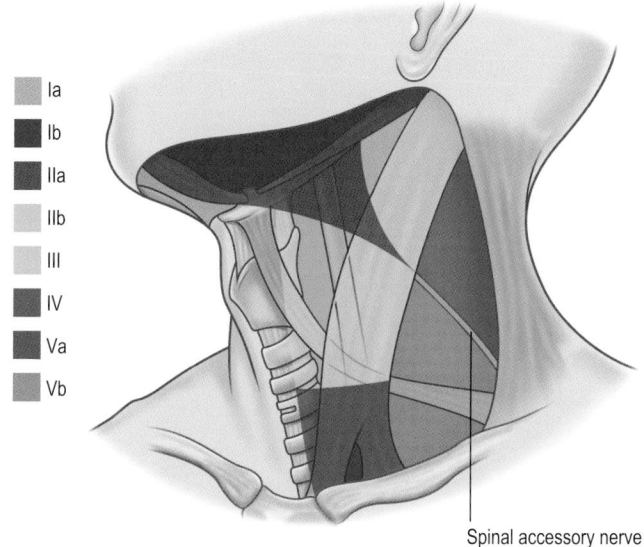

Fig. 16.15 Illustration of levels of cervical lymph nodes.

la
lb
lla
llb
lll
lV
Va
Vb

Spinal accessory nerve

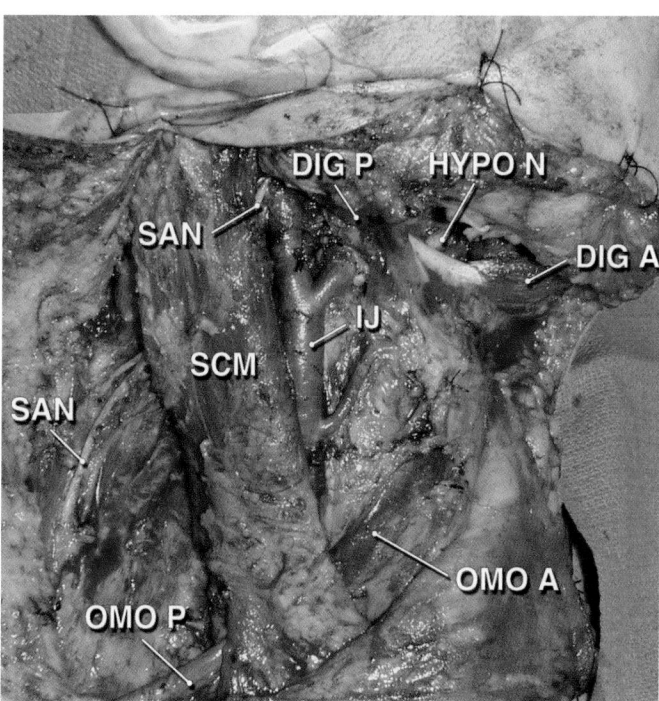

Fig. 16.16 Levels of cervical lymph nodes. SAN, spinal accessory nerve; SCM, sternocleidomastoid muscle; DIG P, digastric muscle posterior belly; DIG A, digastric muscle anterior belly; HYPO N, hypoglossal nerve; IJ, internal jugular vein; OMO A, omohyoid muscle anterior belly; OMO P, omohyoid muscle posterior belly.

nerve is identified as it passes deep to the posterior belly of the digastric muscle. The nerve is traced to the point it enters the SCM and is freed of its investing fascia using scissors or bipolar cautery. A Cushing nerve hook is used to retract the nerve. The fibrofatty node bearing tissue from Level IIB is passed deep to the nerve and the dissection proceeds down the internal jugular vein to the omohyoid muscle. The anterior belly of the omohyoid is followed to the hyoid bone. The electrocautery is used for this dissection. The fibrofatty tissue from the submental area is elevated using electrocautery. Care is taken to maintain good hemostasis in this area to avoid injury to the lingual and hypoglossal nerves. Cautery is used to dissect from anterior to posterior along the anterior belly of the digastric muscle. The dissection proceeds until the posterior edge of the mylohyoid muscle is identified. The mylohyoid is retracted in an anterior direction to expose the submandibular triangle. The gland is retracted posteriorly and the lingual nerve is identified in the cephalic portion of the submandibular triangle. Care is taken to identify the secretory-motor fibers going into the gland. They are clamped, divided and ligated. The hypoglossal nerve is identified as it crosses deep to the digastric tendon. The facial vein and artery are identified and divided. Wharton's duct will pass between the two nerves. The specimen is elevated posteriorly and the contents of Levels I, II, and III are delivered in continuity.

Technique: modified radical neck dissection

The upper transverse incision is the same as for the supraomohyoid dissection. A vertical incision is carried down to the midpoint of the clavicle in a lazy "S". This should be planned to lie over the sternocleidomastoid muscle. This will protect the deeper vascular structures if there is a dehiscence of the incision line, particularly if radiation may be used in the postoperative period *(Figs 16.16–16.18)*.

The operation begins in Level V. The posterior flap is elevated and care is taken to avoid injury to the spinal accessory nerve. It can be found by identifying the trapezius muscle and

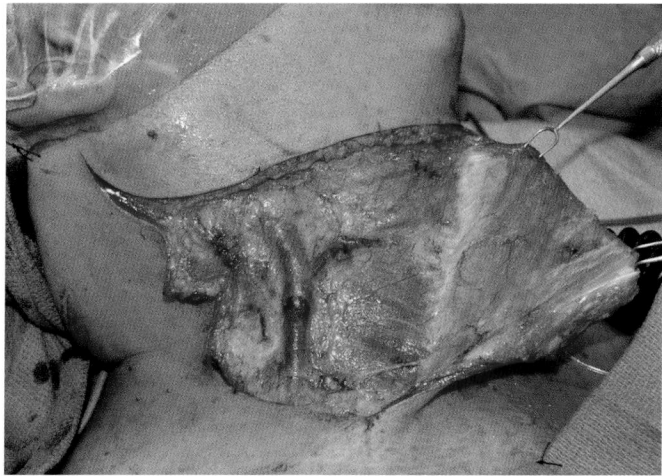

Fig. 16.17 Neck dissection. Subplatysmal flap dissection.

finding the nerve on the deep surface of the muscle where the nerve enters at the junction of the middle and distal thirds of the muscle. The spinal accessory nerve can also be identified exiting the posterior border of the SCM at Erb's point. This is found by tracing the great auricular nerve to the point where it exits from the posterior border of SCM and carefully spreading in the tissue just caudal to the great auricular nerve. The use of a nerve stimulator may be helpful for this portion of the dissection, particularly in patients with short thick necks. Of course, neck dissections are always done with the patient unparalyzed. Once the nerve is found and freed from investing tissue the dissection starts in the apex of the posterior

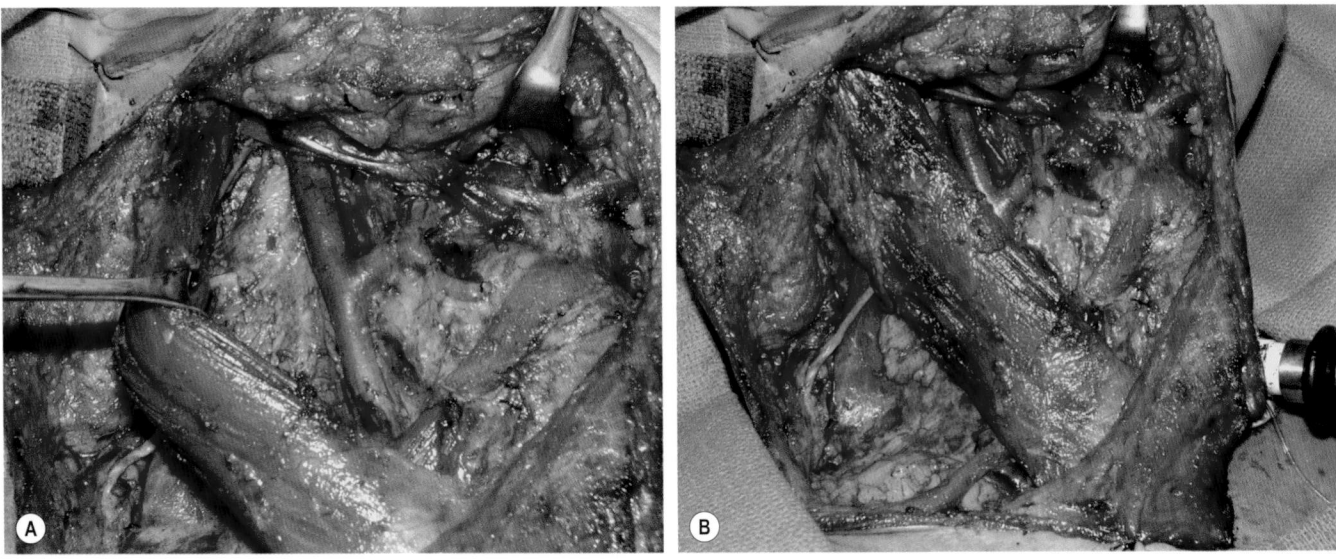

Fig. 16.18 (A) Neck dissection. Completed with SCM retracted to expose Levels I, II, III, IV. **(B)** Neck dissection. Completed exposing Level V.

triangle taking the fibrofatty node bearing tissue off of the deep muscles, the splenius capitis and levator scapulae. The dissection proceeds inferiorly and the specimen is passed under the spinal accessory nerve down to the clavicle. The specimen is elevated anteriorly and the posterior belly of the omohyoid is identified. This muscle will be freed and elevated so that the entire aspect of Level IV can be removed. The dissection should slow in this area to avoid injury to the brachial plexus, phrenic nerves and internal jugular vein. As the internal jugular vein is approached, at its confluence with the subclavian vein in the left neck, all tissue must be divided between clamps and ligated in an effort to avoid lymphatic leak or injury to the thoracic duct. The entire specimen is passed deep to the SCM and combined with the tissue from Levels I, II, and III. The dissection then proceeds as the supraomohyoid dissection. The flaps are closed over closed suction drains. The platysma muscle is closed with interrupted sutures. Deep dermal sutures of absorbable material are placed. Finally, the skin is closed with a subcuticular suture *(Fig. 16.18)*.

Major problems: avoidance and management

There are a broad range of complications associated with the surgical management of malignant lesions of the oral cavity and the oropharynx. They range from failure to effect an oncologic cure, to local wound breakdown and subsequent infection, salivary fistulae, and the whole spectrum of sequelae associated with neoadjuvant and adjuvant radiation therapy resulting in fibrosis of the soft tissues, trismus, all the way to injury to bone in the irradiated field. Due to the often difficult nature of achieving ideal and appropriate resection in the face of advanced or invasive disease, these complications are at times unavoidable; however, they may be minimized by careful planning, attention to detail, and adherence to the oncologic principles set forth in the previous sections.

Local recurrence

Return of tumor to the site of original resection is termed, local recurrence. Diagnosis is made by clinical evaluation, including radiologic investigation, of the site of primary disease or patient's complaints similar to the initial presentation of disease. The incidence of recurrence is the highest in the first 2–3 years post treatment. Local recurrence is likely due to incomplete initial resection with residual micro- or macroscopic disease present at the margin of extirpation. Adherence to the principle of achieving 1 cm margins in all planes is the most likely method to prevent local recurrence. Often, oral cancer is associated with a desmoplastic reaction in the surrounding tissues, making the margin of tumor spread indistinct and difficult to define clinically. When it is unclear whether appropriate margins have been achieved with wide excision, intraoperative frozen section with pathologic analysis should be undertaken in the plane which is in question. A 1 cm additional margin should be taken beyond the extent of pathologically positive frozen section. Management of local recurrence follows the same principles as primary resection with a goal of achievement of at least 1 cm margins. Often, resection of local recurrence is complicated by intervening radiation therapy creating concerns about appropriate wound healing underscoring the importance of adequate resection at the time of initial procedure. The management of local recurrence is a significant problem and should be addressed as soon as possible. The surveillance schedule for the first 2 years after initial management is directed at early diagnosis, with clinical examinations and imaging studies (CT, MRI, ultrasound).

Regional recurrence

Regional recurrence is defined as development of malignant spread of disease to the lymph nodes of the regional nodal basin after resection of the initial disease. This can be associated with local recurrence, but often, is not. Diagnosis of regional recurrence is made by clinical examination and imaging studies which are routinely performed in the postoperative period following resection. Avoidance of regional recurrence is best made by appropriate selection of patients for neck dissection at the time of initial operation. Suspicious lymph nodes should be biopsied preoperatively by fine-needle aspiration. Patients with biopsy proven nodal disease should receive a unilateral or bilateral neck dissection at the time of initial operation depending upon the distribution of nodal disease. Additionally, patients with primary tumors that have >2–3 mm invasion through the basement membrane should undergo a staging supraomohyoid neck dissection due to their propensity to have occult metastases. If the patient is found to have positive nodes in the supraomohyoid neck specimen, they are then candidates for adjuvant radiation for the involved neck.

Wound infection

Wound dehiscence can result in infections which are difficult to treat with antibiotics alone and may be complicated by the development of a salivary fistula. The most critical aspect in prevention of wound breakdown is meticulous attention to the suture line, which must be approximated completely, with apposition of tissue in a watertight fashion along the entire length of the incision. Meticulous closure in multiple layers, from the musculature of the floor of the mouth, to submucosa and oral mucosa, platysma muscle, dermal and epidermal layers, will help insure a watertight closure. Oral incision lines are constantly bathed in the salivary microbiologic milieu, which is conducive to infection of the underlying soft tissue and bone if the suture line is compromised in any way. Meticulous attention to the suture line is especially critical in patients after oncologic resection due to the impaired wound healing associated with subsequent radiation therapy after surgery. Additionally, appropriate perioperative antibiotics have been shown to diminish the likelihood of infection, but are not a substitute for appropriate closure. Broad spectrum antibiotics and debridement of infected tissue with packing and healing with secondary intention is the initial management of wound infection. Bony hardware in the region of wound, if stable may be left in place. If the hardware is mobile in the face of infection, it must be removed and further attempts at reconstruction deferred until the infection is managed. In the setting of intractable wounds, flap reconstruction is often required to facilitate the resolution of an infection.

Osteoradionecrosis

Radiation therapy is an important adjuvant to surgical resection for management of oral cancer, especially for local control of advanced disease, but it is not without its sequelae. Tissues surrounding the irradiated field are subject to devitalization, hypovascularity, and hypoxia. In the oral cavity, this can retard wound healing of the soft tissue and lead to devitalization and necrosis of the bone, also known as osteoradionecrosis (ORN). ORN and inevitable wound breakdown is highly associated with the development of infection. The incidence of ORN increases with more intense radiation exposure (>6000 Gray) and occurrence can either be spontaneous or associated with local trauma such as tooth extraction, biopsy, or surgery that stresses the regenerative capacity of the bone. The mandible is the bone most commonly affected by ORN after oral cancer resection. Proper attention to the details of mandibular resection will aid in the avoidance of problems. As discussed above, all bone cuts should be rounded to avoid sharp edges and osteotomies should be placed out of the direct line of radiation when possible. Soft tissue should be closed over the cut edges of bone. It is particularly helpful to have healthy muscle covering the bone. The incidence of ORN can be greatly diminished by thorough dental evaluation and extraction of infected or nonrestorable dentition in all patients with oral cancer who may conceivably receive radiation therapy. Extraction of diseased teeth should be carried out at least 3 weeks prior to radiation. All patients who receive radiation therapy should undergo prophylactic fluoride therapy daily for life to prevent radiation caries. Management of ORN involves hyperbaric oxygen and limited sequestrectomy only for early stage disease, with more advanced disease consisting of bone necrosis, soft-tissue defects, and cutaneous fistulas requiring radical debridement of nonviable and infected tissues. Reconstruction can be done using bone graft, but the hypoxic nature of the wound bed, especially in the setting of further irradiation, makes this an inadequate option for reconstruction. Free vascularized bone flaps are the optimal choice for reconstruction of ORN of the mandible requiring extensive debridement.[68]

Post-treatment surveillance

Surveillance in the postoperative period is a very important part of the care of the oncology patient. The purpose of this phase of care is to detect recurrence but the identification of second primary cancers is also an important aspect of close follow-up. The development of a second primary tumor is the most common cause of failure seen 36 months after initial treatment. A complete head and neck exam should be done on a regular basis. In the first post-treatment year, the exams should be done every 6–8 weeks. In the second year, exams are done every 8–10 weeks and every 10–12 weeks in the third year. Once the patient is out for 4 years, the surveillance exams are spaced out to twice per year. Patients who have survived 5 years advance to annual exams with a heightened suspicion for the identification of second primary tumors.

A complete history and examination are performed at every appointment. History should be directed at uncovering any changes in the patient's symptoms, including swallowing, pain, trismus, hoarseness, shortness of breath, or symptoms of aspiration. Patients who fail to regain lost weight or continue to experience weight loss should be carefully evaluated for recurrence.

There are limitations to physical exam brought about by body habitus and previous treatment. Radiation and surgery can give the soft tissues a "woody" indurated feeling making palpation of subtle changes difficult, even for the experienced examiner.

Computerized axial tomography and MRI are more sensitive for detection of local regional recurrence then physical exam alone. There should be attention to the fact that CT to the head and neck delivers a considerable amount of radiation to the area and its use as a routine surveillance modality should be limited. MRI is a very sensitive modality to detect soft tissue changes and does not deliver the radiation seen with CT. Ultrasonography is a very useful tool to identify suspicious areas that will require fine-needle aspiration.

The lung is the most common site for distant metastases in head and neck cancer. Head and neck cancer patients represent a group at high risk for lung cancer because of the site of their primary malignancy and their often seen smoking history. Because of these two factors, it is felt that chest CT is superior to chest X-ray for the detection of distant metastases, as well as second primary cancer.

PET scanning may have value in the head and neck cancer patient for the detection of local, regional recurrence, as well as distant metastases. It must be understood that PET scans done in the early postoperative period, within the first 3 months, may be misleading due to uptake secondary to ongoing postoperative and post-radiation inflammation. When using PET, it is most effective to obtain a PET/CT

which takes the physiologic data of PET and fuses it to the anatomic data of the CT.

It is probably not effective to use PET/CT as a routine surveillance screening tool.

Dental follow-up

Head and neck cancer patients need to get a dental exam and cleaning at least every 6 months. This group of patients is at high risk of local recurrence as well as second primary tumors. The dental exam can work as a screening tool for evaluation of mucosal changes. Radiation causes changes in salivary function, some of which will not return to normal. Thus, patients are at high risk of developing dental decay, and if left untreated can lead to devastating consequences. The dentist and dental hygienist should instruct the patient in oral care and the use of daily fluoride treatments.

 Access the complete references list online at **http://www.expertconsult.com**

22. Byers RM, El-Naggar AK, Lee YY, et al. Can we detect or predict the presence of occult nodal metastases in patients with squamous carcinoma of the oral tongue? *Head Neck*. 1998;20:138–144.

   A continuation of the work of this group at MD Anderson using a technique of careful orientation of the neck dissection specimen by the surgeon for the pathologist. They have calculated the risk of nodal metastasis in the N0 neck and demonstrated that the site of the primary tumor consistently predicts the site of lymph node metastases. Their data justifies the use of less than radical neck dissection in both the N0 and N+ neck. These anatomical studies are important since sentinel node biopsy has not been as specific and sensitive a diagnostic tool in the upper aerodigestive tract as it has been in the breast for breast cancer or on the skin for melanoma.

23. Coleman JJ. Complications in head and neck surgery. *Surg Clin N Am*. 1986;66:149–168.

24. Fletcher GH. Basic principles of the combination of irradiation and surgery. *Int J Radiat Oncol Biol Phys*. 1979;5:2091.

29. Ketcham A, Chretien P, Van Buren J, et al. The ethmoid sinuses: a reevaluation of surgical resection. *Am J Surg*. 1973;126:469–476.

   This is the landmark paper demonstrating the feasibility of intracranial–extracranial resection of tumors of the ethmoid sinuses. The authors present their series of resections showing a relatively low incidence of complications and mortality in patients with primary disease. This paper fostered the development of the craniofacial approach to skull base tumors, which was further enhanced by subsequent advances in reconstructive surgery. Of 56 patients with widely different histologies 54 underwent combined en bloc craniofacial resections Median survival was 8 years, with 49% 5-year survival and two hospital deaths, both after CSF leak. There were 32 major complications with CSF leak, representing five major and 12 minor complications. Putative advantages of this technique which have been further refined were: (1) accurate evaluation of the intracranial tumor extension; (2) protects the brain; (3) avoids cerebrospinal fistulization;

   (4) provides adequate hemostasis; (5) facilitates the en bloc tumor resection, and (6) selectively conserves the orbital contents.

32. Marur S, Forastiere A. Head and neck cancer: changing epidemiology diagnosis and treatment. *Mayo Clin Proc*. 2008;83:489–501.

   A detailed and comprehensive description of the epidemiology of squamous cell carcinoma of the head and neck, describing genetic, infectious chemical and other risk factors and highlighting the interactions of smoking, alcohol consumption and the mutation of tumor suppressor genes, as well as the infectious agents HPV and EBV. It also contains a well illustrated guide to disease presentation, diagnosis, and treatment although more heavily weighted toward chemoradiation rather than toward conventional therapies.

47. McCombe D, MacGill K, Ainslie J, et al. Squamous cell carcinoma of the lip: A retrospective review of the Peter MacCallum Cancer Institute experience 1979–1988. *Aust N Z J Surg*. 2000;70:358–361.

   In this retrospective series of 323 patients, the authors demonstrate many of the special characteristics of cancer of the lip, emphasizing its risk factors as smoking, chronic sun exposure, and advanced age. A subset of younger patients were found to have poorer prognosis than the overall group. Metachronous malignancy was found in 12.8% of the population and was best prevented by vermilionectomy at the time of excision of the index squamous cell carcinoma. Larger primary tumor size (T stage) and higher histologic tumor grade correlated with poorer prognosis. Local recurrence occurred in 3.3% of the T1 lesions and 6.5% of the T2; 2% of patients presented with clinically positive cervical lymphadenopathy and 4.3% of patients with N0 necks subsequently manifested metastatic disease to the neck. Recurrence-free survival was 92.5% and cause-specific survival 98% at 10 years. These authors felt that surgery and radiotherapy provide equivalent results and recommend that radiotherapy be employed when surgical extirpation would cause great disability or in the elderly patient.

48. Zitsch R, Park CW, Renner GT, et al. Outcome analysis for lip carcinoma. *Otolaryngol Head and Heck Surg.* 1995;113(5):589–596.

    This paper shows that SCCs of the upper lip and commissure have a poorer prognosis, grow more rapidly, ulcerate, and are more likely to metastasize.

50. Hicks WL, Loree TR, Garcia RI, et al. Squamous cell carcinoma of the floor of the mouth: a 20 year review. *Head and Neck.* 1997;19(5):400–405.

    It is shown in this paper that SCC of the floor of the mouth tends to be locally invasive. Surgery is the preferred treatment modality over radiation due to possible radiation injury to the mandible.

57. Ildstad ST, Bigelow ME, Remensnyder JP. Squamous cell carcinoma of the tongue. A comparison of the anterior two thirds of the tongue with its base. *Am J Surg.* 1983;146:456–461.

58. Vikram B, Strong EW, Shah JP, et al. Failure in the neck following multimodality treatment for advanced head and neck cancer. *Head and Neck.* 1984;6:724.

    This paper shows a decrease in failures in the neck when multimodality therapy is used. Irradiation must be started within 6 weeks after surgery.

60. Spiro RH, Huvos AG, Wong GY, et al. Predictive value of tumor thickness in squamous carcinoma confined to the tongue and the floor of the mouth. *Am J Surg.* 1986;152:345.

    This paper strongly suggests that measurement of tumor thickness may be a better way to select those oral cancer patients who are most likely to benefit elective treatment of the N0 neck.

61. Spiro JD, Spiro RH, Shah JP, et al. Critical assessment of supraomohyoid neck dissection. *Am J Surg.* 1988;156:286.

63. Franceschi D, Gupta R, Spiro RH, et al. Improved survival in the treatment of squamous cell carcinoma of the oral tongue. *Am J Surg.* 1994;166:451.

64. Jacobs CD, Goffinet DR, Fee Jr WE. Head and neck squamous cancers. *Curr Probl Cancer.* 1990;14(1):1–72.

67. Soo KC, Tan EH, Wee J, et al. Surgery and adjuvant radiotherapy vs concurrent chemoradiotherapy in stage III/IV nonmetastatic squamous cell head and neck cancer: a randomised comparison. *Br J Cancer.* 2005;93(3):279–286.

68. Jacobson AS, Buchbinder D, Hu K, et al. Paradigm shifts in the management of osteoradionecrosis of the mandible. *Oral Oncol.* 2010;46(11):795–801.

    This paper gives a thorough description of this complication of radiotherapy including its pathogenesis clinical and pathologic presentation and associated problems. It also presents a classification system, of osteoradionecrosis. Most important, however, it emphasizes the efficacy of microvascular tissue transfer as definitive early therapy and calls into question the previously widely accepted but rarely effective use of hyperbaric oxygen.

17

Carcinoma of the upper aerodigestive tract

Michael E. Kupferman, Justin M. Sacks, and Edward I. Chang

SYNOPSIS

▪ The incidence of head and neck cancer in the US is declining Head and neck squamous cell cancers (HNSCCs) as a group are the fifth most common malignancy among men worldwide.

▪ There is an association between some HNSCCs and human papillomavirus (HPV). Human papilloma virus-related HNSCC is reaching epidemic proportions in the US and will eclipse the incidence of cervical cancer over the forthcoming years.

▪ Cigarette smoking and chewing carcinogenic stimulants are a significant etiologic factor worldwide.

▪ Alcohol, too, is an important promoter of carcinogenesis and is a contributive factor in at least 75% of HNSCCs.

▪ Diagnosis is made by history, physical examination, and appropriate imaging.

▪ Any adult patient who presents with complaints of a neck mass should be considered a malignancy until proven otherwise.

▪ There is an emerging role for robotic surgery of the upper aerodigestive tracts in the management of HNSCC.

Introduction

The treatment of malignancies confined to the upper aerodigestive tract represents a formidable challenge. This challenge requires an intimate familiarity with anatomy, knowledge of the myriad of malignancies that afflict the region, and a multidisciplinary approach incorporating the efforts of medical and radiation oncologists, speech pathologists, and nutritionists, in addition to ablative and reconstructive surgeons. These coordinated groups optimize the treatment of these malignancies.

The upper aerodigestive tract includes the mouth, nose, paranasal sinuses, pharynx, larynx, trachea, and esophageal inlet. The goals of surgical management and reconstruction are not only to achieve complete resection, but also to consider postoperative function and aesthetics. A balance must be formed between obtaining adequate margins to limit the potential for recurrence and the avoidance of creating a defect that severely cripples or is unacceptable to the patient. The

ability to speak and swallow following treatment is of integral importance and has a tremendous impact on patient well-being and quality of life. Ultimately, the goal of therapies, including chemotherapy and radiation therapy, surgical extirpation, and reconstruction, is to maximize disease-free survival in conjunction with optimal function and quality of life.

Approximately 48000 new cases of head and neck cancer were projected to be diagnosed in the US, with over 11000 Americans succumbing to these malignancies in 2008.[1] Head and neck cancer, predominantly SCC, accounts for only 3% of all new cancer cases and only 2% of all cancer deaths in the US annually; however, these malignancies as a group are the fifth most common malignancy among men worldwide.[2] The overall incidence in the US appears to be decreasing in parallel with the increased awareness of the effects of cigarettes and smoking on the development of upper aerodigestive cancer; however, head and neck cancers continue to plague many parts of the world, especially where cigarette smoking and/or the chewing of carcinogenic stimulants is prevalent, and thus head and neck cancers will continue to be a major cause of cancer mortality worldwide.[2,3] A rising proportion of these cancers (particularly those found in the oropharynx) are attributable to oncogenic HPV[4,5] and the impact that the population-wide HPV vaccination will have on incidence rates has yet to be determined. This remains the most rapidly increasing segment of head and neck cancer incidence in the US today. Evidence is also suggestive that inherited factors and exposure to other environmental agents such as chromium, nickel, wood dust, industrial agents, and formaldehyde modulate risk and awareness will help refine prevention strategies in the future.[3,6,7]

This chapter aims to describe cancers of the upper aerodigestive tract in an anatomical fashion, but is not meant to be exhaustive. We will review the relevant anatomy, the American Joint Committee on Cancer staging criteria, and important treatment algorithms and considerations. Salivary gland tumors are addressed in a separate section (Chapter 14). It is the purpose of this chapter to summarize the surgical principles appropriate for all patients undergoing for carcinoma of the upper aerodigestive tract. Specific reconstructive modalities will be covered in subsequent chapters.

Incidence and prevalence

In the US, estimates for 2012 were for 26 740 new cases of oral cavity cancer, 13 510 new cases of pharyngeal cancer, and 12 360 new cases of laryngeal cancer.[4] While the US has noted an initial decrease in the incidence of head and neck malignancies, current studies have noted a recent increase in incidence.[5–8] In particular, while the median age at diagnosis for HNSCC is approximately 60 years, the incidence in patients younger than 45 years old appears to be increasing, presumably secondary to oncogenic strains of HPV.[9,10] Regarding cancer survivorship, approximately 350 000 individuals were living in the US with a history of head and neck cancer in November, 2007 (240 176 with a history of oral cavity/pharyngeal cancer and 93 096 with a history of laryngeal cancer). In 2008 in the US, 5390 deaths were predicted to be attributed to oral cavity cancer, 2200 to pharyngeal cancer, and 3670 to laryngeal cancer. However, head and neck cancer accounts for less than 2% of all cancer deaths in the US annually, and mortality rates appear to be decreasing.

Risk factors

Tobacco

The strength and consistency of the association between smoking and HNSCC have been demonstrated in numerous case-control and cohort studies with significant relative risks or odds ratios in the 3–12-fold range.[11–16] In addition, these follow-up studies have demonstrated a dose-dependent effect where higher pack years of smoking (packs per day × years of smoking) correlated with an increased risk while a longer duration since smoking cessation was associated with a decreased risk of developing a malignancy.[12,13,15,17] While there is a definitive relationship between tobacco use and upper aerodigestive SCC, the association with other mucosal malignancies such as nasopharyngeal and nasosinus carcinomas is less substantial.[18] The etiological relationship encompasses cigar and pipe smoking as well; however, the risk of second-hand smoke is less clear.[16,17,19,20] Regarding tobacco consumption and usage aside from smoking, there appears to be a strong correlation with the location of chewless tobacco or tobacco equivalents and the location of resultant malignancies. For example, such patients often develop SCC in dependent areas of the oral cavity such as the floor of mouth, larynx, and hypopharynx.[21] Similarly, in south central Asia where the use of such products is common, the gingivobuccal region is the most common site for HNSCC.[3,22] Furthermore, in South Central Asia "pano" (betel leaf, lime, catechu, and areca nut) is commonly chewed and is a strong risk factor independent of tobacco use for carcinoma of the oral cavity, one of the most common cancers in men and women in this region.[3,23,24]

Alcohol

Alcohol, too, is an important promoter of carcinogenesis and is a contributive factor in at least 75% of HNSCCs.[12,15,17] Furthermore, alcohol appears to have an effect on risk of HNSCC independent of tobacco smoking, but these effects are consistently significant only at the highest level of alcohol consumption.[6,12,15,16] While there is speculation as to the exact type of alcohol and the development of head and neck malignancies, it appears that the causative agent is the ethanol itself and the quantity consumed, regardless of the form in which it is consumed (i.e., beer, wine).[15,25] Nevertheless, it appears that the major clinical significance of alcohol consumption is that it potentiates the carcinogenic effect of tobacco at every level of tobacco use. However, this effect is most striking at the highest levels of exposure. The magnitude of this effect is at least additive, but may be synergistic in its carcinogenic effects.[12,15]

Infectious agents

Although it has been suggested that various infectious agents play a role in head and neck carcinomas, only EBV and HPV can be implicated as etiologic agents in head and neck carcinogenesis based on current scientific evidence. EBV appears to be associated with most nasopharyngeal carcinomas, and HPV (most commonly type 16 and 18) is associated with approximately 50% of oropharyngeal carcinomas.[5,6] HPV-related HNSCC appears to be a distinct biologic entity, with an excellent prognosis and exquisite chemo-radiosensititivty. HPV may also play a role in the etiology of SCC arising in the sinonasal tract.[26] While other infectious agents such as herpes simplex viruses and *Helicobacter pylori* have not been purported to be carcinogenic, no definitive evidence has been shown to support a causal relationship.[27–30] On the contrary, oropharyngeal cancer patients presenting without an extensive smoking history or tobacco exposures more commonly have HPV-16-associated tumors,[21] which may also suggest that there are synergistic interactions between the traditional oropharyngeal risk factors of tobacco and alcohol with HPV-16.[31] However, this is an area of continued research and investigation and brings into question whether the potential benefits of HPV-16 vaccination in preventing cervical cancer may extend to the prevention of upper aerodigestive malignancies as well.[10]

Laryngopharyngeal reflux

There is currently an active debate regarding the contribution of gastroesophageal reflux and consequent exposure of the upper aerodigestive tract to gastric contents and bacteria (i.e., *H. pylori*) in relation to the incidence of head and neck malignancies. Observational and anecdotal studies have long suggested that gastroesophageal reflux documented with 24-hour pH probe monitoring may be associated with laryngeal cancer.[32–37] Furthermore, a retrospective case-control study of 10 140 hospitalized patients and 12 061 outpatients with laryngeal and pharyngeal cancer and 40 561 hospitalized and 48 244 outpatient controls performed using US Department of Veterans Affairs databases demonstrated a significant increased risk of developing an upper aerodigestive cancer (laryngeal cancer).[38] However, a large Swedish cohort study of 66 965 patients with discharge diagnoses of heartburn, hiatal hernia, or esophagitis with a follow-up of 376 622 person-years concluded that there was no evidence of a causal association between gastroesophageal reflux and either laryngeal or pharyngeal cancer.[39]

Occupation/air pollution

Although occupational exposures probably play a minor role overall in the development of HNSCC, they are major risk factors for malignancies of the sinonasal region.[40–44] The most important exposures occur in the metalworking, refining, woodworking, and leather/textile industries.[40–43] Indoor air pollution is a significant problem in much of the developing world where indoor stoves using biomass or fossil fuels are the primary method of cooking and heating. Not only are these exposures likely risk factors for HNSCC, but they also contribute to the risk of paranasal sinus cancers and lung cancers, chronic pulmonary diseases, and childhood illnesses.

Anatomy

Oral cavity

The oral cavity is defined as starting at the vermilion border of the lips and extends posteriorly to include the buccal mucosa, anterior tongue, and floor of the mouth, hard palate, and upper and lower gingiva *(Fig. 17.1)*. The posterior border is defined by the circumvallate papillae of the tongue. Consequently, the mobile tongue occupies a major portion of the oral cavity and is contiguous with the floor of the mouth. The gingival mucosa overlying the mandibular and maxillary alveolar ridges adheres to the underlying periosteum. The hard palate forms the roof of the oral cavity and consists of mucosa overlying the palatine portion of the maxilla extending from the superior alveolar ridge to the junction with the soft palate, which lies in the oropharynx. Although the delineation between oral cavity and oropharynx might seem artificial, the distinction is important because of varying risk factors, natural history, individualized therapeutic approaches, and numerous functional considerations.

Pharynx

The pharynx is a musculomembranous tube suspended from the skull base to the level of the sixth cervical vertebra, supported by overlapping constrictor muscles (superior, middle, and inferior) and other muscles arising from the styloid process and skull base *(Fig. 17.2)*. This musculomembranous

conduit communicates with the oral cavity anteriorly, the nasopharynx superiorly, and the hypopharynx and larynx inferiorly. The nasopharynx is bounded by the skull base and represents the cranial-most segment of the pharynx and includes the soft palate, the adenoids, and superior portion of the pharyngeal walls, which contain the opening of the eustachian tubes.

The oropharynx begins at the circumvallate papillae of the tongue, and is bounded by the pharyngeal walls laterally, the

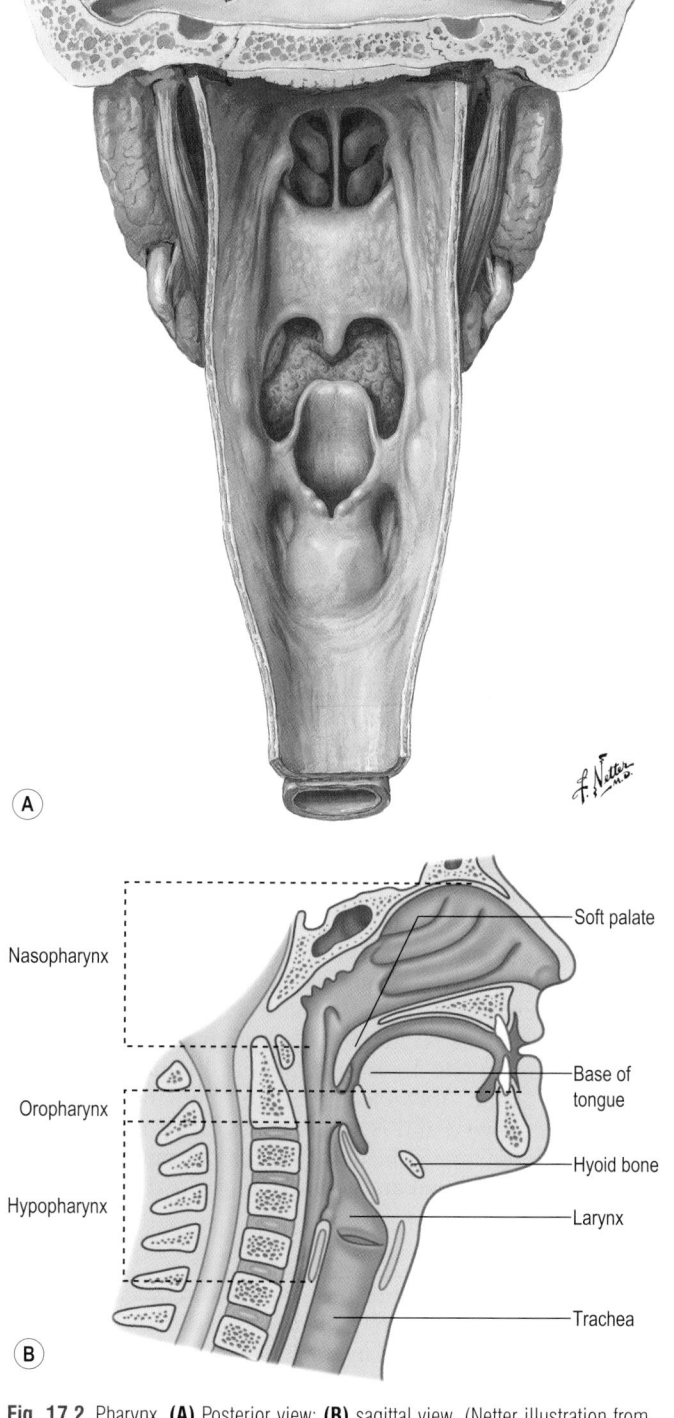

(A)

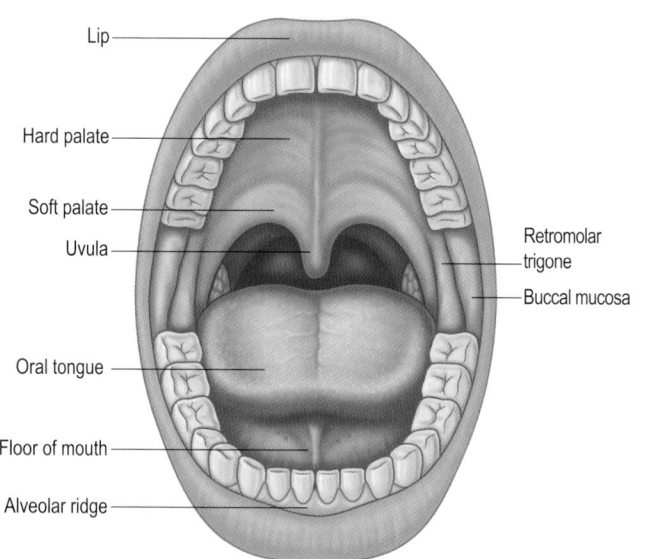

Lip
Hard palate
Soft palate
Uvula
Retromolar trigone
Buccal mucosa
Oral tongue
Floor of mouth
Alveolar ridge

Fig. 17.1 Anatomy of the oral cavity. (Reproduced from from Guyuron B, Erikkson E, Persing J, et al. Plastic surgery: indications and practice. Philadelphia, PA: Elsevier; 2008.)

Nasopharynx
Soft palate
Base of tongue
Oropharynx
Hyoid bone
Hypopharynx
Larynx
Trachea

(B)

Fig. 17.2 Pharynx. **(A)** Posterior view; **(B)** sagittal view. (Netter illustration from www.netterimages.com copyright Elsevier Inc. All rights reserved.)

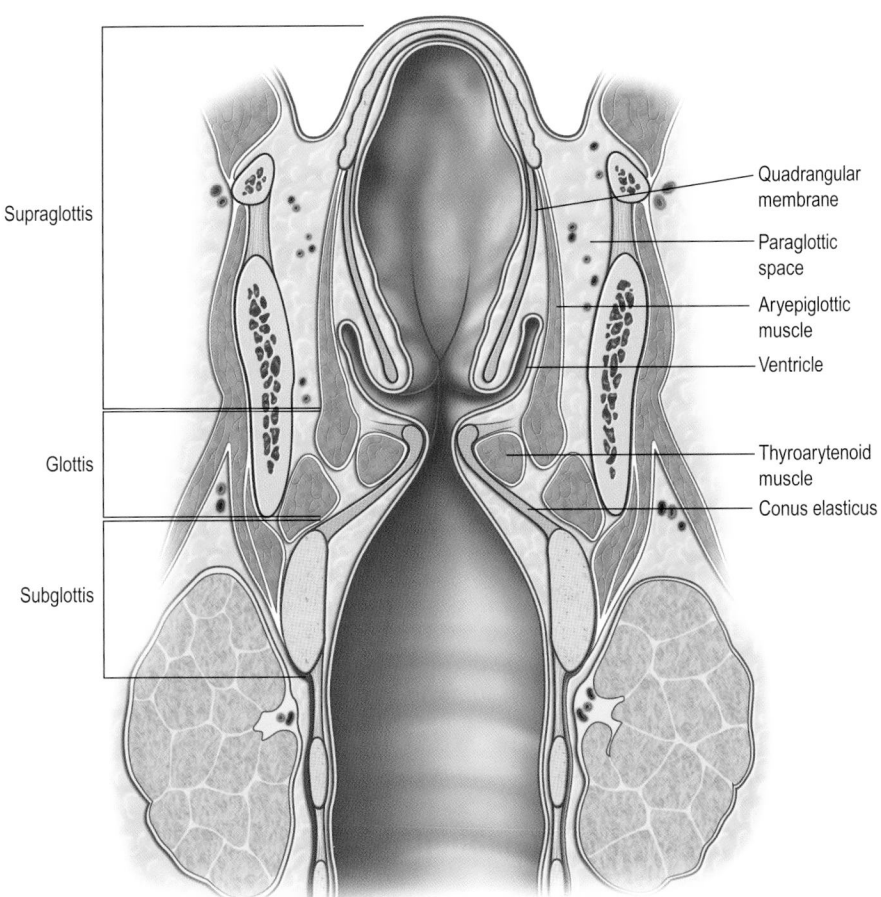

Supraglottis

Glottis

Subglottis

Quadrangular
membrane

Paraglottic
space

Aryepiglottic
muscle

Ventricle

Thyroarytenoid
muscle

Conus elasticus

Fig. 17.3 Coronal view of the larynx and its subsites.

soft palate superiorly, and the hyoid bone inferiorly. The oropharynx encompasses the tongue posterior to the circumvallate papillae, the base of tongue, valleculae, the uvula, tonsils, and the tonsillar pillars.

The oropharynx is divided into four sites of clinical importance: (1) the tonsillar area, which makes up the major portion of the lateral pharyngeal wall and blends with the tongue base, soft palate, and retromolar trigone; (2) the tongue base; (3) the soft palate; and (4) the posterior pharyngeal wall. Innervation of the pharynx is via the pharyngeal plexus, with contributions from the glossopharyngeal (cranial nerve IX: sensory) and vagus nerves (cranial nerve X: motor and sensory).

The hypopharynx is divided into three distinct regions: (1) the pyriform sinuses; (2) the posterior surface of the larynx (postcricoid area); and (3) the inferior, posterior, and lateral pharyngeal walls. The pyriform sinuses are paired mucosal pouches wrapped around the larynx, which funnel food around the larynx and into the esophagus. They are bounded superiorly by the pharyngoepiglottic folds and inferiorly by the cricoid cartilage. The sinuses come together at the esophageal introitus and cervical esophagus at the level of C6.

Larynx

The larynx consists of a mucosally covered cartilaginous framework (thyroid and cricoid cartilages) suspended from the hyoid bone above by the thyrohyoid membrane and attached below to the trachea *(Fig. 17.3)*. The opening to the larynx is continuous with the pharyngeal airway. Unlike the

rest of the pharynx, the mucosa of the larynx consists largely of columnar, ciliated, respiratory-type epithelium. Stratified squamous epithelium is found on the upper posterior epiglottis, aryepiglottic folds, and true vocal folds. It is important to note that, although there are lymphatics in the upper larynx, they are sparse in the true vocal folds, or glottis. The larynx is divided into three anatomic regions: the supraglottic larynx, the glottic larynx, and the subglottic larynx. The supraglottic larynx includes the epiglottis, aryepiglottic folds, and laryngeal surface of the arytenoids, false vocal cords, and ventricles. The glottic larynx is derived from the tracheobronchial anlage and consists of both true vocal cords and the mucosa of the anterior and posterior commissures. It extends from the lateral-most apex of the laryngeal ventricle to 1 cm below the free edge of the vocal folds toward the cricoid. It has few, if any, lymphatics. The subglottic larynx consists of the region bounded by the glottis above and the inferior border of the cricoid cartilage. Lymphatic supply to the subglottic larynx is extensive and bilateral. The infraglottic lymphatics drain to the cervical nodes through the cricothyroid membrane, while supraglottic lymphatics drain through the thyrohyoid membrane.

Nose and paranasal sinuses

The term "nose and paranasal sinuses" refers to the region of the upper aerodigestive tract that starts at the vestibule of the nose anteriorly, is covered by squamous epithelium, and extends posteriorly to the posterior choana, where the nasopharynx begins. The nasal cavity begins at the nostrils and ends at the nasal choanae, which communicate with the nasopharynx and include the vestibules, turbinates, septum, and choanae (Fig. 17.4). By definition, paranasal sinus malignancy does not include the nasopharynx unless by extension. It does include the paranasal sinuses, specifically, the maxillary, ethmoid, frontal, and sphenoid sinuses. Although the most common malignancy of the nose and paranasal sinuses is SCC, the nose and paranasal sinuses pose a particular set of problems that deserve separate consideration.

Neck

Anatomic considerations in the treatment of cancers of the head and neck must include a thorough understanding of the neural, vascular, and, especially, the lymphatic structures of the neck. Specifically, the digastric, omohyoid, sternocleidomastoid, and trapezius muscle all help contribute to organizing the neck into specific anatomical regions. These specific regions of the head and neck and the tumors that arise there have lymphatic drainage that have traditionally been thought of as being consistent and predictable. However, the use of sentinel lymph node biopsy in the management of HNSCCs would indicate that this may not be valid. Currently, the role of sentinel lymph node biopsy in the management of HNSCC is being evaluated.[45] There are six major groups of lymph nodes (paired bilaterally) in the head and neck,[46] although only levels I–V play a major role in aerodigestive tract HNSCC (Fig. 17.5).

Primary and secondary echelons of lymph node drainage have been defined for each major region of the head and neck mucosa. A standard rule of thumb is that the lymphatic drainage for any particular region is predicted by the arterial supply of that region. The lip, cheek, and anterior gingiva drain to submandibular and submental lymph node groups. In addition, the cheek and upper lip also drain to inferior parotid and facial nodes, while the posterior gingiva and palate drain to the internal jugular chain and lateral retropharyngeal groups. Lymphatic drainage for the tongue drains to the internal jugular, subdigastric, omohyoid, submandibular, and submental nodal groups. Midline lesions often drain bilaterally. The floor-of-mouth drainage is similar to that of the tongue. The upper portion of the pharynx drains directly to the upper cervical lymph nodes along the internal jugular chain. The oropharynx and tonsil drain through the parapharyngeal space to the midjugular region, particularly to the jugulodigastric nodes. Retropharyngeal nodes (nodes of Rouvière) and lateral pharyngeal nodes can also be involved and are always pathologic when clinically apparent. The regions of the hypopharynx and larynx drain primarily along the routes of their vascular supply to either the deep cervical nodes along the mid jugular (upper pharynx, larynx) or the deep nodes along the lower jugular and paratracheal region (lower pharynx, larynx) (Fig. 17.6).

For the purposes of local treatment, the various lymph node groups of the neck have been divided into levels. Level I includes the submental group of nodes (IA), located within the midline triangle bounded by the anterior bellies of the digastric muscles and the hyoid bone, and the submandibular group (IB), bounded by both bellies of the digastric muscle and the body of the mandible. Level II nodes consist of the upper jugular lymph nodes located in proximity to the upper third of the internal jugular vein and extending from the skull base to the level of the bifurcation of the carotid artery. The anterior and posterior boundaries are the lateral border of the sternohyoid muscle and the posterior border of the sternocleidomastoid muscle, respectively. Level II is further divided into those lymph nodes located anteroinferior to the vertical plane of the spinal accessory nerve (IIA) and those lymph nodes posterosuperior to the nerve (IIB). Level III nodes include those nodes located adjacent to the middle third of the internal jugular vein from the carotid bifurcation to the plane marked by the omohyoid muscle crossing over the jugular vein (the level of the cricoid cartilage). Anterior and posterior boundaries are the same as level II. Level IV nodes include the lower jugular group extending from omohyoid muscle above to the clavicle below. Level V nodes are those located in the posterior triangle in the region of the spinal accessory nerve and the transverse cervical artery. The anterior border of the trapezius muscle, the posterior border of the sternocleidomastoid muscle, and the clavicle below bound this level. This level, too, is further divided into Va and Vb nodes, with Va nodes being those nodes located above the plane along the inferior edge of the cricoid and including the chain of nodes superior to the spinal accessory nerve posterior to the sternocleidomastoid muscle. Level Vb nodes are below the cricoid plane, inferior to the spinal accessory nerve, and include the nodes along the transverse cervical artery and all of the supraclavicular fossa.

Patient evaluation

The initial evaluation of the patient with head and neck cancer of the upper aerodigestive tract requires knowledge of the risk factors, signs, symptoms, and physical findings associated with tumors of the various subsites within the head and neck. In addition to risk factors, the history of a patient with a potential head and neck cancer must focus on symptoms suggestive of that diagnosis. All patients should be asked about dysphagia (difficulty swallowing), odynophagia (pain on swallowing), weight loss, hoarseness, throat pain (especially if it is focal to a specific site or side), otalgia (ear pain), new cough, hemoptysis, and globus sensation (the sensation of something stuck in the throat). The patient should also be questioned about symptoms of gastroesophageal reflux, including heartburn, water brash (a bitter taste), and regurgitation. The majority of patients with pharyngeal tumors present with a unilateral neck mass, and the clinician should suspect a malignancy until proven otherwise. An early laryngeal cancer can present with hoarseness. Advanced laryngeal tumors may also cause dysphagia, odynophagia, or hemoptysis. Pharyngeal tumors may present with the same symptoms but more commonly present only with pain, persistent unilateral sore throat, or referred otalgia. However, the most common presenting sign in a patient with a pharyngeal cancer is a neck mass, indicating the presence of nodal metastasis. Otalgia can be caused by base of tongue, pharyngeal wall, and supraglottic tumors. The mechanism of this referred pain involves the vagus and glossopharyngeal nerves. The internal branch of the superior laryngeal nerve provides sensation to the supraglottic larynx and adjacent pharyngeal wall and base of tongue. Pain from these areas is referred to the ear through Arnold nerve, a branch of the vagus that innervates the external auditory canal. Tumors of the base of tongue and

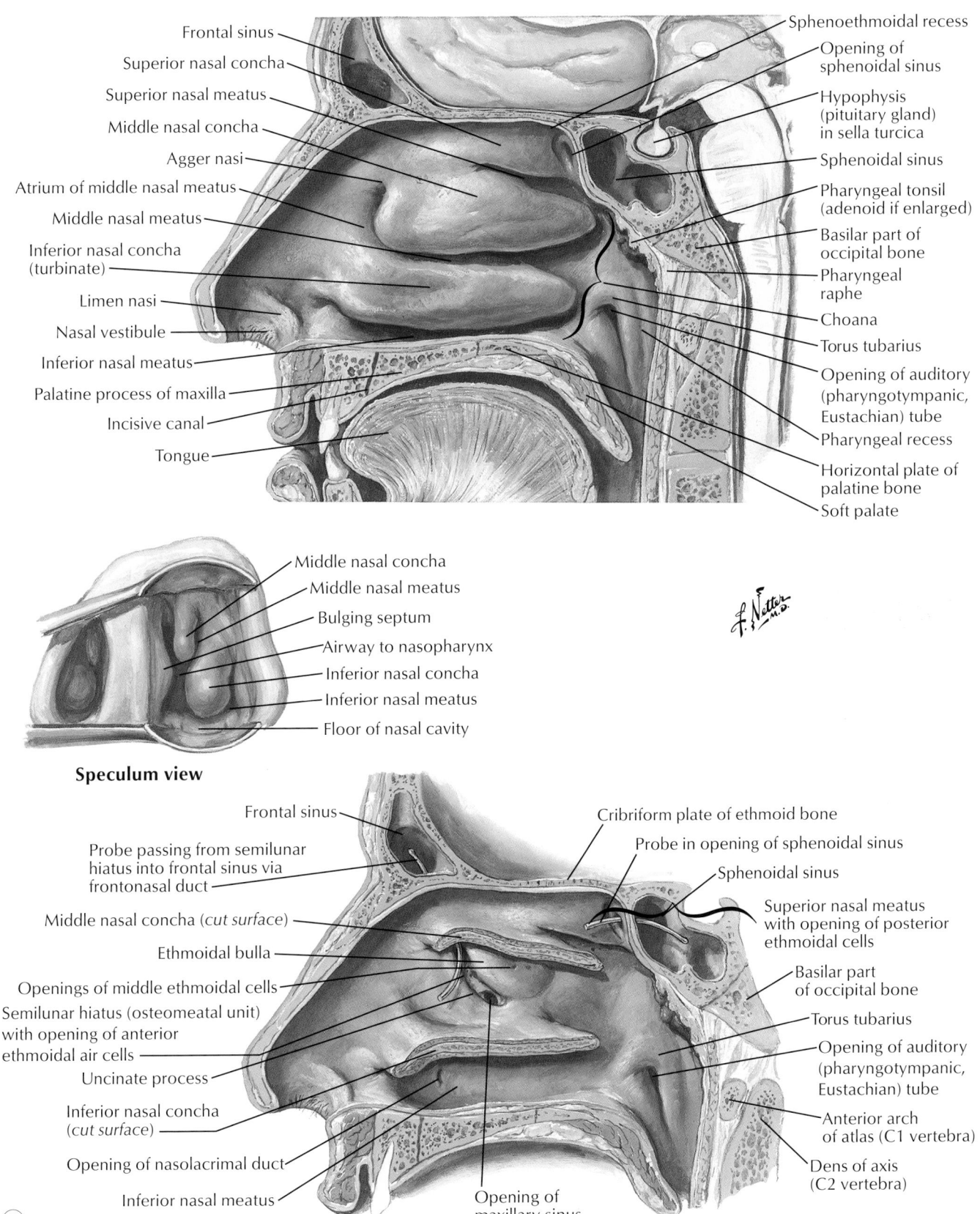

Fig. 17.4 Paranasal sinuses. **(A)** Sagittal section; **(B)** coronal and horizontal section. (Netter illustration from www.netterimages.com copyright Elsevier Inc. All rights reserved.)

Coronal section

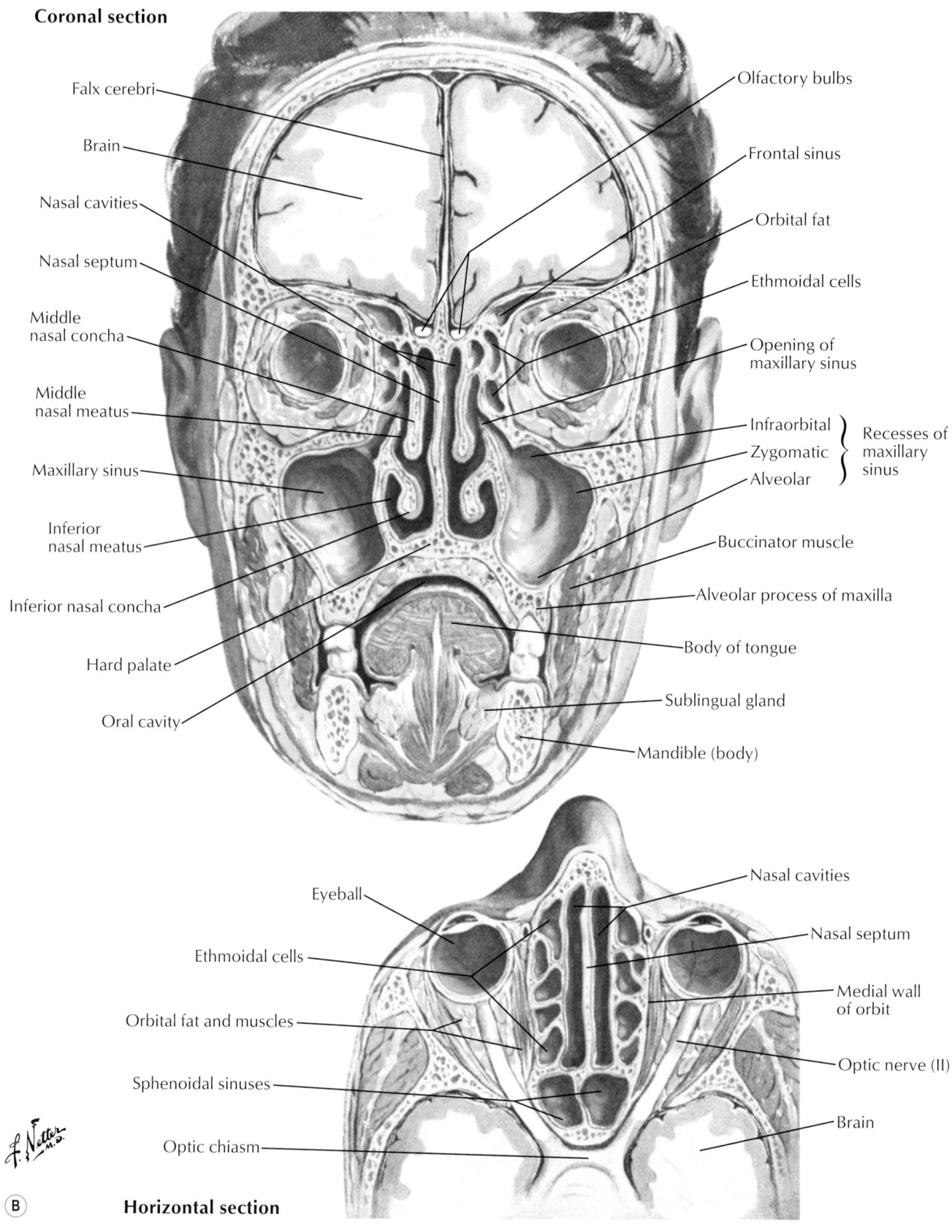

Falx cerebri

Brain

Nasal cavities

Nasal septum

Middle nasal concha

Middle nasal meatus

Maxillary sinus

Inferior nasal meatus

Inferior nasal concha

Hard palate

Oral cavity

Olfactory bulbs

Frontal sinus

Orbital fat

Ethmoidal cells

Opening of maxillary sinus

Infraorbital
Zygomatic } Recesses of maxillary sinus
Alveolar

Buccinator muscle

Alveolar process of maxilla

Body of tongue

Sublingual gland

Mandible (body)

Eyeball

Ethmoidal cells

Orbital fat and muscles

Sphenoidal sinuses

Optic chiasm

Nasal cavities

Nasal septum

Medial wall of orbit

Optic nerve (II)

Brain

(B)   **Horizontal section**

Fig. 17.4, cont'd

of the lips. Because of the accessibility of the oral cavity, and the morbidity of radiation-induced xerostomia, early tumors of this area (T1 and T2) are generally treated surgically. Locally advanced lesions (T3 and T4) are typically treated with combination therapy. While pre-malignant and small tumors of the lips can sometimes be treated with radiation or topical agents such as 5-fluorouracil or imiquimod, the standard treatment for lip cancers is surgery. Malignancies of the lip tend to be SCC while malignancies of the skin around the lip tend to be basal cell carcinomas. All lip cancers mandate assessment of the neck, but larger lip lesions warrant evaluation for possible selective neck dissection. Neck dissections are typically accomplished through an apron or visor-type incision and are often performed for advanced-stage lesions, although simultaneous neck and lip surgery may have implications for reconstructive options (*Fig. 17.7*). Synchronous neck dissections for lip cancers will impact reconstructive options, and the low incidence of occult cervical metastasis has led to a policy of neck observation for the majority of patients with lip cancers. Upper lip and commissure malignancies may drain to periparotid nodes, which require evaluation and possible superficial parotidectomy, in selected cases. Reconstruction of the lips will be discussed elsewhere (Chapter 10).

All tumors of the lip and oral cavity are staged using the tumor, node, and metastasis (TNM) classification (*Table 17.1* and *Fig. 17.8*). Postoperative irradiation is often indicated for oral cancers, which can pose challenges for reconstruction, dentition, and rehabilitation. The indications for adjuvant radiation in oral cancer include: close or positive margins, perineural invasion, multinodal metastasis, bony or soft-tissue invasion, and T3 or T4 tumors. While the lips comprise approximately 30% of cancers of the oral cavity, approximately 25–50% of oral cavity cancers occur in the mobile tongue. Because of the lack of anatomic barriers to spread, tongue cancer has a propensity for diffuse, infiltrative involvement, which is often difficult to gauge clinically. Curative resection, therefore, mandates an adequate cuff (generally 1 cm) around the lesion. T1 or T2 lesions are usually amenable to transverse wedge excision and subsequent direct closure or skin grafting. Large T2 lesions and larger lesions may require a paramedian mandibulotomy in order to obtain exposure for resection and reconstruction, which often requires free tissue transfer (*Fig. 17.9*). Floor-of-mouth cancers and cancers of the alveolar ridge comprise 30% of oral cavity malignancies and are intimately associated with the dentition and the mandible. If the cancer invades the bone, it may extend along the alveolar canal. Tumors of the retromolar trigone and buccal mucosa are often difficult to treat given their location and may require a mandibulectomy to gain appropriate access, exposure, and less common oncological control. Finally, tumors of the hard palate are uncommon and tend to originate from the minor salivary glands, which will be discussed later in this chapter. Depending on tumor size and location, resection may be performed perorally, through a transoral midface degloving approach, or through a Weber–Ferguson approach. Reconstruction of the hard palate (to maintain speech, feeding, and the separation of the oral cavity from the nasal cavity), nasal lining, and orbital floor may be required. Due to the high frequency of occult nodal metastasis, elective neck dissection is performed at the time of surgical resection. Clinical nodal disease mandates a therapeutic neck dissection.

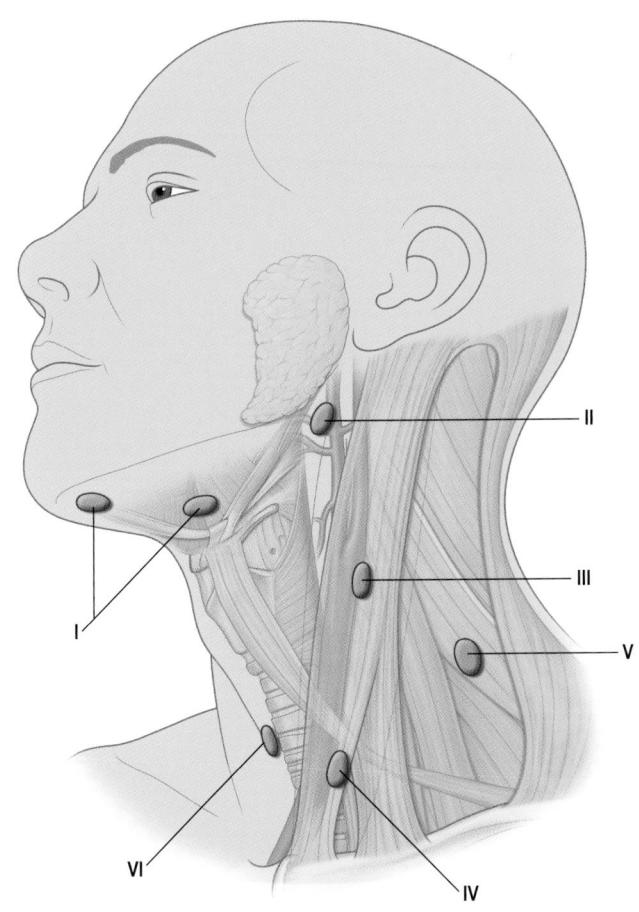

Fig. 17.5 Cervical lymphatic zones.

oropharyngeal wall may produce pain that travels in the glossopharyngeal nerve, which sends branches to the tympanic membrane and middle ear through Jacobson nerve, also allowing pain to be referred to the ear.

Patients may also present with symptoms of aural fullness, hearing loss, epistaxis, and unilateral or bilateral nasal obstruction, all of which can be attributed to a nasal cavity or nasopharyngeal tumor. If adults complain of unilateral hearing loss, otologic examination is mandatory to assess for a middle-ear effusion; if fluid is present, flexible nasopharyngoscopy is warranted to rule out a mass obstructing the eustachian tube orifice in the nasopharynx. Finally, any adult patient who presents with complaints of a neck mass should be considered a malignancy until proven otherwise.

Diagnosis and treatment

Oral cavity

The oral cavity begins at the lips and extends posteriorly to the circumvallate papillae and therefore is the area most accessible not only to direct examination, but also the area subjected to sun and ultraviolet exposure and resultant SCC

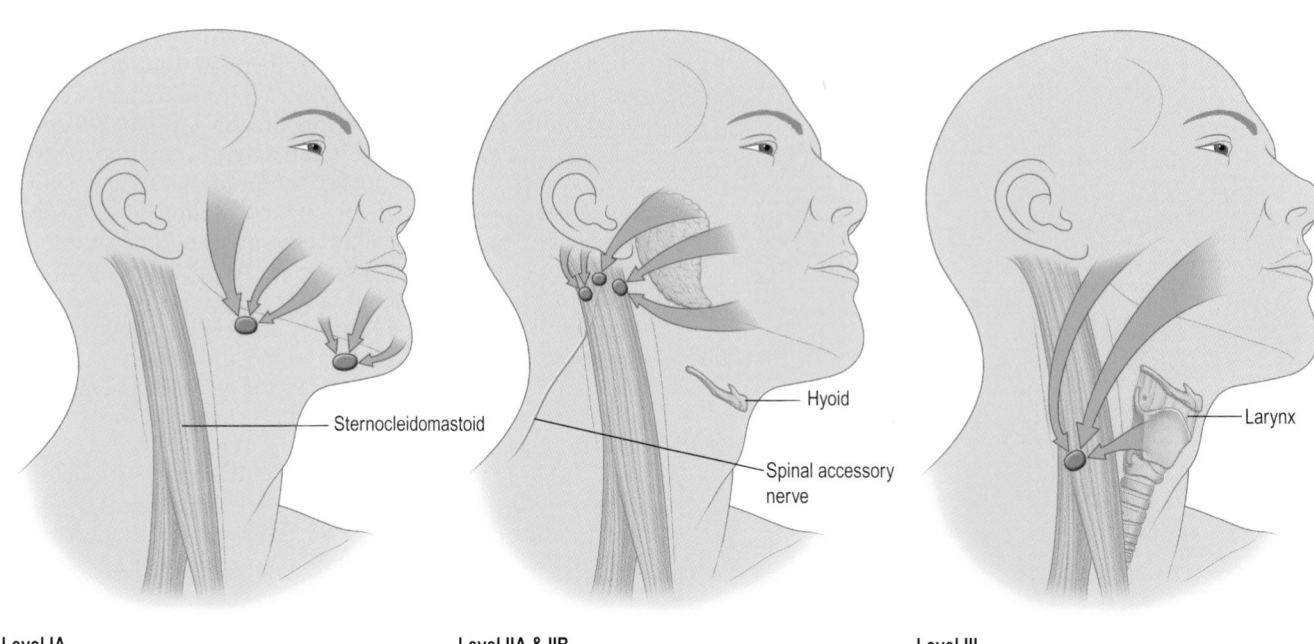

Level IA
- Floor of mouth, anterior oral tongue, anterior mandibular alveolar ridge, lower lip

Level IB
- Oral cavity, anterior nasal cavity, soft tissue of midface, submandibular gland

Level IIA & IIB
- oral cavity, nasal cavity, nasopharynx, oropharynx, hypopharynx, larynx, parotid gland (Greater risk of metastases from oral and larynx tumors to level IIA. Greater risk of metastases from oropharynx tumors to level IB)

Level III
- oral cavity, nasopharynx, oropharynx, hypopharynx, larynx

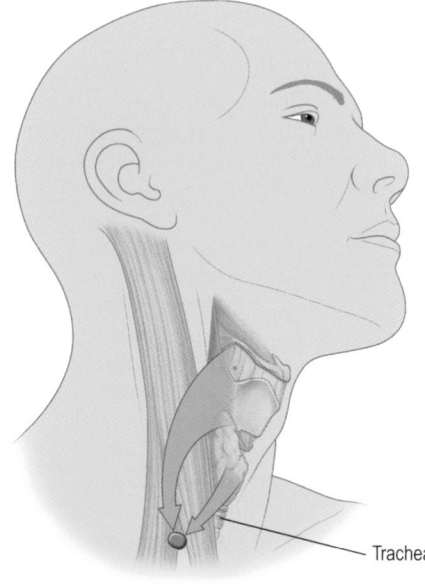
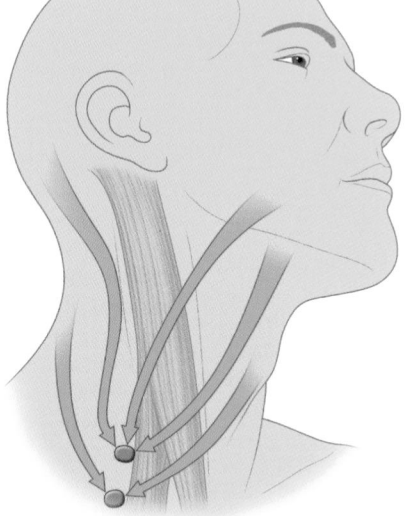
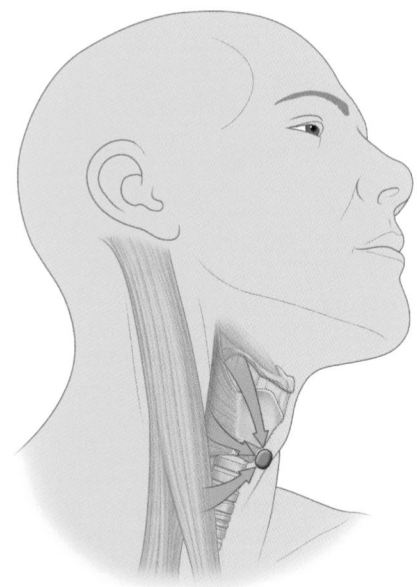

Level IV
- Hypopharynx, thyroid, cervical esophagus, larynx

Level VA & VB
- Nasopharynx, oropharynx, posterior scalp/neck skin

Level VI
- Thyroid gland and subglottic larynx, apex of piriform sinus, cervical esophagus

Fig. 17.6 Drainage pattern of head and neck lymph nodes.

Oropharynx

The oropharynx includes the base of tongue, faucial arches, tonsillar fossae, and posterior and lateral pharyngeal walls. The faucial arches include the anterior tonsillar pillars, soft palate, and uvula. The oropharynx extends superiorly to the plane of the soft palate and inferiorly to the plane of the hyoid bone. The anterior border is a ring formed by the circumvallate papillae of the tongue, the anterior tonsillar pillars laterally, and the border of the hard and soft palates superiorly. The clinical staging of oropharyngeal cancers depends primarily on tumor size and is similar to the staging of oral cavity

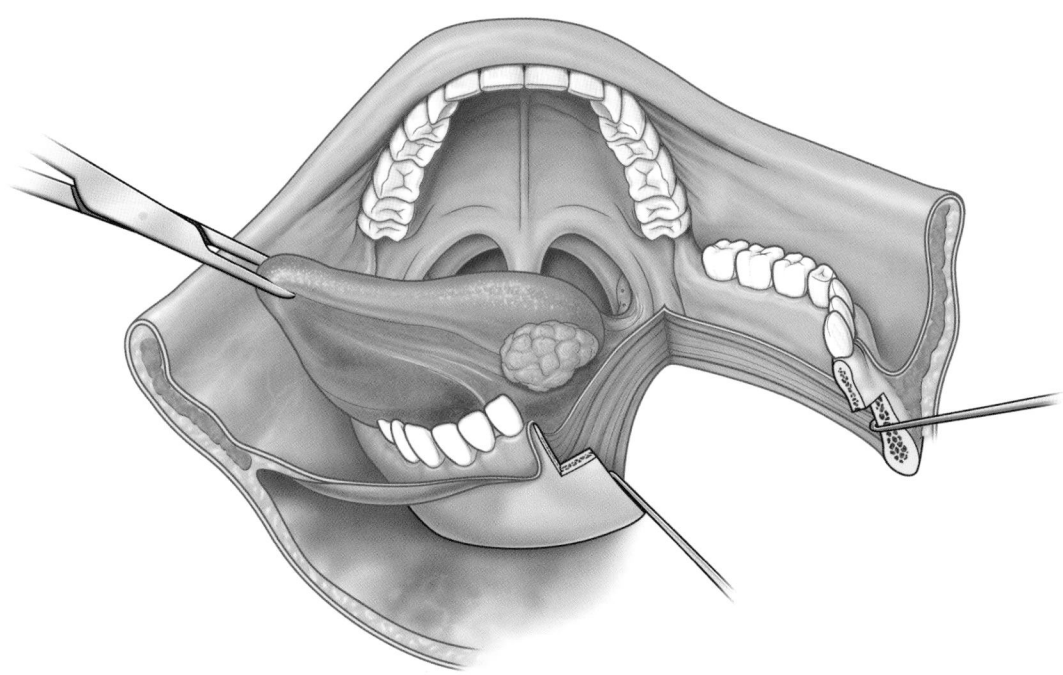

Fig. 17.7 Mandible-splitting approach for access to posterior tongue tumors. (Reproduced from from Guyuron B, Erikkson E, Persing J, et al. Plastic surgery: indications and practice. Philadelphia, PA: Elsevier; 2008.)

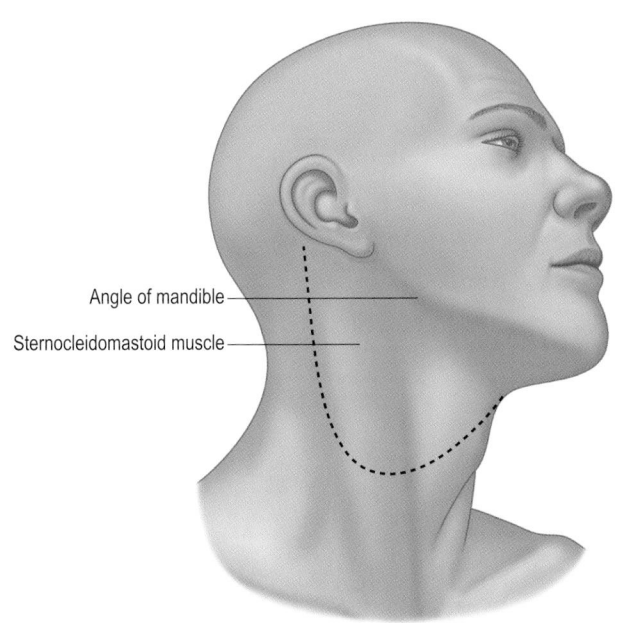

Angle of mandible

Sternocleidomastoid muscle

Fig. 17.8 Apron incision for access when performing neck dissections. (Reproduced from from Guyuron B, Erikkson E, Persing J, et al. Plastic surgery: indications and practice. Philadelphia, PA: Elsevier; 2008.)

cancers. Although tumors may arise from any site in the oropharynx, they arise most commonly from the palatine arch, which includes the tonsillar fossa and base of the tongue. Traditionally patients with oropharyngeal cancer are in their sixth and seventh decade of life with a significant history of tobacco use, although this demographic is changing with the rise of HPV-associated oropharyngeal cancers. The most common presenting symptom is a cervical mass of unknown etiology followed by chronic odynophagia (often unilateral) and referred otalgia. Change in voice, dysphagia, and trismus are late signs. Regional lymphatic metastases occur frequently and are related to the depth of tumor invasion and tumor size. Upper cervical nodes are generally first involved, but lower nodes can become clinically involved with skipping of the upper first-echelon nodes. Bilateral lymphatic metastases can occur, particularly with cancers of the soft palate, tongue base, and midline pharyngeal wall. The retropharyngeal lymph nodes are also common sites of metastasis and warrant evaluation when planning treatment.

Staging *(Table 17.2)*

The American Joint Committee on Cancer staging system for primary tumors of the oropharynx is as follows:

Tis Carcinoma *in situ*

T1 Tumor 2 cm or less in greatest dimension

T2 More than 2 cm but less than 4 cm

T3 Greater than 4 cm

T4 Invasion of bone, deep tongue muscles, skin.

Nodal staging

N0 No clinically detectable nodes

N1 Single ipsilateral node, less than or equal to 3 cm in diameter

N2a Single ipsilateral node, greater than 3 cm but less than 6 cm

N2b Multiple ipsilateral nodes, none greater than 6cm

N2c Bilateral or contralateral nodes, none greater than 6 cm

N3 One or more nodes greater than 6 cm present.

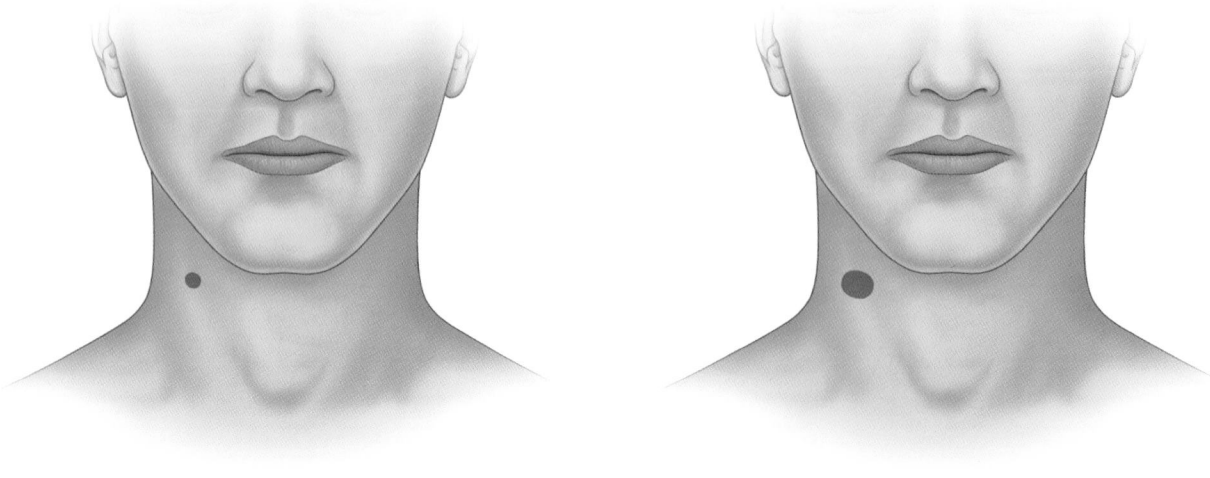

NI ≤3cm, single, ipsilateral   N2a >3≤6cm, single, ipsilateral

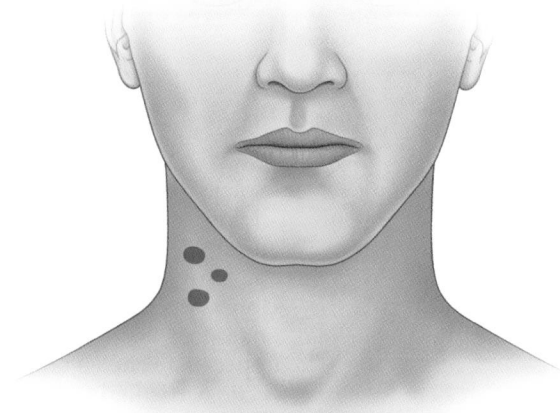

N2b ≤6cm, multiple, ipsilateral

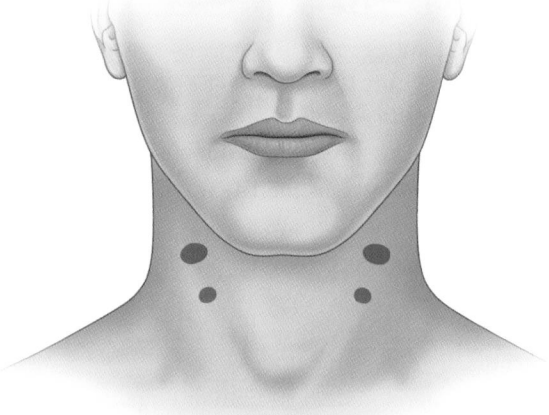

N2c ≤6cm, bilateral or contralateral

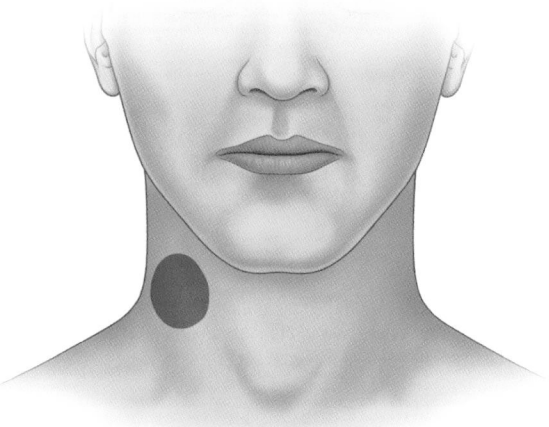

N3 >6cm

Fig. 17.9 Nodal (N) status determination.

The American Joint Committee on Cancer staging schema (TNM staging) is as follows and applies to all head and neck primaries:

Stage I T1 N0 M0

Stage II T2 N0 M0

Stage III T3 N0 M0 or T1, T2, or T3 N1 M0

Stage IV Any T4, N2 or N3, or M1 lesions.

Tonsil

The treatment of early tonsillar neoplasms (stages I and II) is usually radiation therapy as a single modality. Transoral wide local excision of small, superficial lesions may be locally effective, but does not address the high potential of occult lymph node metastasis, and thus a staging neck dissection should be performed if surgery is the primary treatment modality. While surgery and primary radiation offer comparable locoregional control for small tumors, many patients will require postoperative radiotherapy.[47] A role for transoral robotic surgery is emerging for selected tumors of the oropharynx, particularly the tonsillar region. Surgical management of advanced cancers requires extensive resections of the pharyngeal wall or mandible,[48,49] with free tissue transfer and postoperative radiotherapy. Patient function after intensive treatment is often poor, with a significant number dependent upon gastrostomy tube for nutrition and a tracheostomy for pulmonary toilet. Thus, a shift toward nonsurgical management with combined chemotherapy and radiotherapy approaches for tonsillar cancers has prevailed. However, radiation tends to have less short-term morbidity but significantly worse long-term morbidity, especially progressive radiation-induced fibrosis, which can cause wound-healing problems, long-term dysphagia, hoarseness, pain, or xerostomia that may also make future salvage operations and reconstructions more challenging. Stage III and IV tumors are most effectively treated with multimodality therapy, and some stage IV tumors are best treated with organ preservation protocols of chemotherapy and radiation. Surgery is often reserved for extensive disease and can result in severe deficits in speech and swallowing, as occur in the setting of a total glossectomy that may mandate a permanent feeding gastrostomy or tracheostomy.

The guiding principle for surgical resection is *en bloc* excision with adequate margins. As with most other head and neck sites, a mucosal and deep muscle margin of 1 cm is acceptable for the oropharynx; however, this may not be feasible when tumor is adjacent to structures such as the mandible, prevertebral fascia, skull base, or larynx. Small lesions of the tonsil may be amenable to transoral excision, but larger and more posterior lesions may require a lateral pharyngotomy, transhyoid (or suprahyoid) pharyngotomy, and mandible-splitting procedures with or without a median glossotomy to obtain adequate exposure. Mandibulectomy may also be used, but it causes functional and aesthetic morbidity, which is unwarranted if the mandible does not require excision for oncologic reasons. Most of these procedures require a temporary tracheotomy because of the potential for postoperative airway obstruction secondary to edema as well as to provide pulmonary toilet and to maintain control of the airway if postoperative bleeding occurs. Patients are decannulated once they can maintain their airway and pulmonary toilet.

Tongue base

Cancers of the base of the tongue pose a more difficult therapeutic problem than do tonsillar carcinomas. Most patients present with advanced disease due to the silent nature of these tumors, resulting in frequent regional metastases, greater treatment morbidity, and poor patient survival. Because of the functional deficits associated with gross total resection of even small tongue base cancers, most tumors are treated with definitive radiation with or without chemotherapy. However, advances in minimally invasive surgical approaches, particularly robotic surgery, have made surgical resection of these lesions more feasible. Owing to the rich network of lymphatics present in the base of the tongue, 75% of patients will present with stage III or IV disease. It is not uncommon for patients with small T1 or T2 tumors to develop multilevel, bilateral, or even contralateral metastases with lymph node involvement in 60% of patients. Overall 5-year survival rates range from 11% to 45%.[50,51] and 5-year survival rates decrease from over 60% for N0 patients to less than 30% for N1 patients.[50–53] Poor outcome is largely attributable to late diagnosis.[54] In retrospective analyses of various clinical trials, patients with HPV-positive tumors have a 75–80% 5-year survival after chemo-radiotherapeutic treatment. However, prospective studies that focus specifically on the HPV positive patients are necessary, as these patients may be more amenable to treatment de-intensification with minimally invasive surgery. Local recurrence is more frequent after radiation alone in most series,[50,53,55] and salvage rates for local failure are poor. Surgical management of early superficial primary tongue base tumors (T1) achieves results similar to those from radiation alone. In most cases, however, primary tumors are moderately advanced and require transcervical resection via mandibulotomy or lateral pharyngotomy approaches. Lateral pharyngotomy is used primarily to approach the lateral and posterior walls of the oropharynx and hypopharynx but can also be used for access to the base of tongue or supraglottic larynx. In general, large lesions require mandible-splitting procedures. Recently, the development of transoral robotic approaches has allowed for the resection of many of these tumors with less morbidity and with similar outcomes to the more aggressive open approaches.[56] Oropharyngeal lesions are aggressive and generally require selective or modified radical neck dissection, which is performed before the extirpation of the primary lesion. Due to the high rates of nodal metastases, patients should receive postoperative radiotherapy to the neck. Local tumor control rates are superior to those with radiation alone,[50,53] but regional control is poor if clinically positive nodes are present.

Elective neck dissection can serve an important role as a staging procedure, thereby providing a rationale for adjuvant radiation therapy. To date, no prospective randomized trial data are available that compare surgery alone with combined surgery with either pre- or postoperative radiation. Survival rates are significantly worse for patients with T4 and advanced nodal disease. Even with no laryngeal involvement, laryngectomy was traditionally performed with any total glossectomy to limit risks of aspiration postoperatively. Nonetheless, total glossectomy without laryngectomy has been effective in properly selected patients, but has been associated with severe deficits in quality of life due to impairments in speech, swallowing, and taste.

Soft palate and pharyngeal wall

Cancers of the soft palate and pharyngeal wall are less common than other oropharyngeal neoplasms. Soft-palate cancers can occur on the anterior surface of the palate and tend to be superficial. Posterior-wall lesions tend to be superficial with less tumor bulk than similarly staged lesions elsewhere in the oropharynx. Advanced lesions with deep invasion have ready access to the prevertebral fascia, infratemporal fossa, and skull base and can be associated with extensive submucosal spread with clinical skip areas. Such patients often present with skull base pain and neck stiffness. Radiation-based approaches as curative treatment are preferred in most cases, even for T3 primary tumors.[57] Resection of most soft-palate lesions is associated with severe functional disability. Small primary tumors with positive nodes can be effectively treated with definitive radiation to the primary tumor and neck. Neck dissections should be performed if disease in the neck persists at 6–8 weeks following the completion of external-beam therapy. Extensive pharyngeal wall cancers or palate cancers with extension to the tonsil and those cases with advanced regional metastases are usually treated with combined chemoradiotherapy approaches unless gross mandibular involvement is noted. Overall 5-year survival rates for soft-palate and faucial pillar cancers are 60–70% and range from 80–90% for T1 and T2 lesions to 30–60% for stages III and IV lesions.[58] Locoregional recurrence is the most frequent cause of failure.[59]

Hypopharynx

The hypopharynx comprises the piriform sinuses, postcricoid area, and posterior and lateral hypopharyngeal walls. The larynx lies anterior to the hypopharynx; the hypopharynx wraps around and behind the larynx. The hypopharynx represents one of the most lethal sites for SCC of the head and neck. The majority of patients note dysphagia as their primary complaint and occasionally otalgia which represents referred pain to the tympanic branch of cranial nerve IX.

Staging

T1 Confined to the site of origin

T2 Spread to an adjacent subsite or region without vocal cord fixation

T3 Fixation of the ipsilateral vocal cord

T4 Massive tumor with invasion of bone or the soft tissues of the neck.

Nodal staging

N0 No clinically detectable nodes

N1 Single ipsilateral node, less than or equal to 3 cm in diameter

N2a Single ipsilateral node, greater than 3 cm but less than 6 cm

N2b Multiple ipsilateral nodes, none greater than 6cm

N2c Bilateral or contralateral nodes, none greater than 6 cm

N3 One or more nodes greater than 6 cm present.

Lymph node metastases are clinically evident at time of diagnosis in 70–80% of patients[60–62] and are indicative of advanced disease. Bilateral and contralateral lymph node metastases occur in 10–20% of cases, particularly if tumors cross the midline of the hypopharynx. Primary tumor extension beyond the hypopharynx is common,[63,64] and the tumors have a propensity to spread submucosally to involve the oropharynx or esophagus. The majority (more than 75%) of hypopharyngeal cancers arise in the pyriform sinus, which tends to spread aggressively to neighboring structures such as the larynx, thyroid, and thyroid and cricoid cartilages. Because of the locale of hypopharyngeal cancers and their growth patterns and proximity to the larynx, surgical management often entails total laryngopharyngectomy.[65] Extension to the esophagus will necessitate a cervical esophagectomy. The remainder of hypopharyngeal malignancies is divided to 20% in the posterior pharyngeal wall, and approximately 5% in the postcricoid space.

Distant metastases at the time of diagnosis are rare; however, advanced hypopharyngeal cancers have the highest rate of distant metastases of upper aerodigestive cancers. Often surgical treatment requires a total laryngectomy, but radiation therapy, for early T1 and T2 and in combination with chemotherapy for T3 disease, has been investigated.[66] Retrospective analyses have consistently demonstrated that survival rates are lower and locoregional failure rates higher with radiation alone as compared with surgery or surgery and radiotherapy.[61,63,64,67–69] Small localized lesions of the pyriform sinus may be treated by radiation therapy alone or with partial laryngopharyngectomy, which typically results in a hemicircumferential defect of the hypopharynx, whereas total laryngopharyngectomy results in complete disruption of gastrointestinal continuity. Reconstructive options usually favor free tissue reconstruction with fasciocutaneous flaps for resurfacing of hemicircumferential defects and intestinal interposition flaps for complete defects. However, for patients with advanced disease, which is often the case, resection is followed by adjuvant radiation therapy. Resections may entail partial pharyngectomy, pharyngolaryngectomy, or total pharyngectomy combined with neck dissection and the associated difficulties in posttreatment function. Although free-flap reconstructions have improved results, there still remain the difficulties of lack of sensation and dysphagia.

Tumors arising in the lower hypopharynx or postcricoid mucosa often spread to involve the esophagus. Distal submucosal spread into the esophagus can be extensive and requires partial or total esophagectomy. Reconstruction with transposition of the stomach (gastric pull-up), jejunal free flap, or tubed fasciocutaneous free flap (either the anterolateral thigh or radial forearm flap) is currently recommended.[70–73] Treatment approaches with combined preoperative or postoperative radiation have dramatically improved the control of locoregional disease, but survival rates have not improved as substantially over those with surgery alone because of the increased rates of distant metastases. Postoperative radiation is currently preferred to preoperative radiation because of its lower local recurrence rates, fewer complications, and less difficulty in accurately assessing tumor margins.[61,67,68] The presence of lymph node metastases, extracapsular lymph node involvement, and direct extension of the primary tumor into the soft tissues of the neck are adverse prognostic factors and indications for postoperative chemoradiotherapy. Locoregional recurrence continues to account for the greatest number of deaths from disease.[74,75] Overall 5-year survival rates range from 10% to 30% for posterior pharyngeal wall cancers[76–80] and from 20% to 40% for pyriform sinus cancers.[60,61,63,67,69,75] Distant metastases are uncommon at the time of presentation, but may appear 2–5 years after primary therapy and seem to correlate with extent of regional lymph node involvement.[61,81] The rates of distant metastases range from 20% to 50%[61,75] and increase with the extent of lymph node disease.

Larynx

The larynx is divided into three subsites based on embryological development, which governs the vascular and lymphatic anatomy and therefore dictates differences in patterns of local spread, risks of lymphatic metastasis, and control rates. The anterior limit of the larynx includes the suprahyoid epiglottis, thyrohyoid membrane, and inner perichondrium of the thyroid cartilage, cricothyroid membrane, and anterior aspect of the cricoid cartilage. The pre-epiglottic space is important for staging supraglottic tumors; it extends from the thyrohyoid membrane anteriorly to the epiglottis posteriorly with the hyoepiglottic ligament superiorly. The glottis comprises the true vocal cords, anterior commissure, and posterior commissure. The superior limit of the glottis is the plane of the superior surface of the true vocal folds, which constitutes the floor of the laryngeal ventricles. The inferior limit is arbitrarily set as a plane 0.5 cm inferior to the vocal cords. The supraglottis extends from the tip of the epiglottis to the floor of the ventricles and includes the epiglottis, aryteno epiglottic folds, cuneiform and corniculate cartilages, arytenoids, false vocal cords, and pre-epiglottic space. The subglottis extends from the plane 1 cm below the vocal folds to the inferior edge of the cricoid cartilage. Below this is trachea, which is rarely the source of a primary tumor but is uncommonly involved by inferior spread of large laryngeal tumors.

The staging of supraglottic cancers is based on the subsite or region of the supraglottis involved in the cancer. Subsites include the false vocal cords, arytenoids, lingual and laryngeal surfaces of the epiglottis, and aryepiglottic folds. The epiglottis itself is also subdivided into the region extending above the plane of the hyoid and that below the hyoid. Suprahyoid epiglottic tumors tend to have a better prognosis than infrahyoid cancers, with the exception of those invading the aryepiglottic fold (marginal area) to involve the pyriform sinus. This, again, is due to the richer network of lymphatics in the infrahyoid portion of the epiglottis. Early cancers (T1 and T2) can involve one or more subsites but have normal vocal cord motion. Those cancers that cause fixation of the arytenoid or involve the postcricoid region, medial wall of the pyriform sinus, or pre-epiglottic space are staged T3. Those that extend beyond the larynx or invade thyroid cartilage are staged T4.

For supraglottic carcinomas, tumor staging is as follows:

T1 Confined to site of origin with normal vocal cord mobility

T2 Involving adjacent sites without cord fixation

T3 Limited to the larynx with spread to the hypopharynx (medial wall of the piriform sinus or postcricoid area) or pre-epiglottic space and/or vocal cord fixation

T4 Tumor extending beyond the larynx to involve the thyroid cartilage, soft tissues of the neck, or oropharynx (e.g., tongue base).

The staging of glottic carcinomas is also determined by functional and anatomic features. Cancers limited to the true vocal cords are T1 (T1a, one vocal cord involved; T1b, both vocal cords involved), and those with extension to an adjacent site or with impaired cord mobility are staged T2. Impaired vocal cord motion is due to muscular invasion and some element of paraglottic disease spread. Arytenoid fixation and vocal cord immobility upstage a lesion to a T3. Those tumors with cartilage involvement or extension outside the larynx are T4.

For glottic carcinomas, tumor staging is as follows:

T1 Confined to one or both vocal cords with normal mobility

T2 Supraglottic or subglottic extension and/or impaired vocal cord mobility

T3 Fixation of one or both vocal cords but confined to the larynx

T4 Tumor with thyroid cartilage invasion or extension beyond the larynx.

True subglottic cancers that are limited to the subglottic region (T1) or to the subglottis and true vocal cords (T2) are early cancers but, unfortunately, are diagnosed late because of a lack of symptoms. Fixation of the vocal cord (T3) and cartilage invasion or extension outside the larynx (T4) are associated with a worse prognosis.

For subglottic carcinoma, tumor staging is as follows:

T1 Confined to the subglottis

T2 Extending to the vocal cords, with normal or impaired mobility

T3 Confined to the larynx with cord fixation

T4 Massive tumor with cartilage invasion or extension beyond the larynx.

The true vocal cords present an effective boundary between supraglottic and subglottic lymphatic spread within the larynx. This anatomic barrier can be compromised by tumors involving the anterior or posterior commissures and with deeply invasive tumors that extend vertically across the true and false vocal cords (transglottic cancers). Normally, the inner perichondrium of the thyroid cartilage also presents an effective barrier to cancer spread. However, cancer involvement of the anterior commissure or transglottic extension is associated with invasion of the thyroid cartilage in 40–60% of cases.[82,83] Supraglottic cancers are usually more advanced than glottic cancers at the time of diagnosis because they do not generally produce early symptoms of hoarseness. Rather, the earliest symptoms of a supraglottic cancer are usually sore throat, dysphagia, referred otalgia, or the development of a neck mass representing regional metastasis. Airway compromise may be an early symptom with subglottic cancer.

Cancer of the glottic larynx is generally diagnosed at an earlier stage than are other head and neck sites, primarily owing to the early manifestation of symptoms, most commonly hoarseness. As a result, cure rates are generally higher than for other sites. Early supraglottic cancer is similarly treated with radiation, transoral endoscopic approaches, or open surgery. Radiation therapy is most effective in the treatment of smaller-volume, superficial lesions without cartilage destruction. Open surgery typically involves horizontal supraglottic laryngectomy and is an effective treatment of T1, T2, and select T3 tumors. Early subglottic laryngeal carcinoma is very rare, and is treated similarly to early-stage glottic and supraglottic tumors. Overall early laryngeal cancer (stages I and II) usually involves the glottis and represents 60% of laryngeal cancers. Early glottic tumors generally have a good prognosis with 90% 5-year patient survival for T1 lesions. Treatment options for T1 lesions include transoral laser resection or other partial laryngectomy procedures. Open vertical partial laryngectomy is generally reserved for T2 tumors, radiation failure, or limited local recurrences. Another operative option of interest is supracricoid subtotal laryngectomy. Conservation laryngeal procedures such as hemilaryngectomy and supraglottic laryngectomy, when they are feasible, will preserve speech and swallowing and avoid a permanent tracheostomy. Regardless, a multidisciplinary approach, with evaluation by a surgeon, medical oncologist, and radiotherapist with input from pathology, radiology, speech pathology, and dental prosthetics, is the standard of care for the complex patient with head and neck cancer. Further details of specific treatments are found within the subsite-specific sections.

The treatment of more advanced laryngeal cancers (T3 and T4) has historically included surgery with or without radiation therapy. Prospective randomized studies have shown convincingly that chemotherapy and radiation therapy (including surgical salvage) are equally effective in the long-term survival of patients with T3 laryngeal cancers as compared with surgery with or without radiation therapy. Approximately 60% of patients may preserve their larynx, and thus quality of life has significantly improved.[66,84] Speech communication profiles are clearly better in the group of patients randomized to the larynx preservation, but there was no determination of swallowing function.[85] Local control was poorer for patients with T4 lesions. Current standard of care argues that laryngeal preservation approaches or protocols be considered in treating such patients, with the corollary that patients with poor function at diagnosis will likely have poor laryngeal function after conservation treatment. Thus, a primary surgical approach should be strongly entertained for patients with significant aspiration based upon pretreatment swallowing studies. Many surgical procedures for laryngeal carcinoma involve the creation of a tracheal stoma. This area is sometimes at significant risk of tumor recurrence, which is most likely associated with paratracheal nodal metastases. For this reason, bilateral paratracheal dissections should be performed in T4 glottic cancers and radiation therapy provided postoperatively if metastases to this echelon of nodes are found pathologically. Once a stomal recurrence has developed, the prognosis is grave regardless of salvage treatment.

Supraglottic cancers

Important factors in selecting therapy for supraglottic cancers are tumor location, cord fixation, and pre-epiglottic extension. Tumors limited to the suprahyoid epiglottis are amenable to radiation with fields that encompass neck regions at risk of lymphatic metastases. Radiation is also effective for early lesions. Local control rates for patients with supraglottic tumors treated with radiation alone range from 68% to 94%, and survival rates are 50–89%. Small tumors of the suprahyoid epiglottis are amenable to endoscopic laser epiglottectomy. Lesions that involve the supraglottis anterior to the arytenoids may be treated with supraglottic laryngectomy *(Fig. 17.10)*. Involvement of both arytenoids and extension

inferiorly beyond the apex of the piriform sinus necessitate total laryngectomy because resection of both arytenoids would result in intractable aspiration. If the lesion extends superiorly and involves the pre-epiglottic space, vallecula, or tongue base, the involved regions will also need to be resected. If the supraglottis including a single arytenoid is involved, an extended supraglottic laryngectomy may be appropriate. All patients who undergo supraglottic laryngectomy will aspirate postoperatively, although this improves with time. If resection extends into the tongue base, aspiration will be worse. Tumors involving the aryepiglottic folds, pyriform sinuses, or infrahyoid epiglottis tend to be more aggressive, are deeply infiltrative, and frequently involve the pre-epiglottic space. Radiation alone is less effective than surgery, resulting in more frequent local recurrences that require surgical salvage. The addition of systemic concomitant chemotherapy will have a positive impact on the outcomes of patients with these tumors.

Pre-epiglottic extension of cancer carries a poor prognosis. However, such a situation can be managed effectively with horizontal supraglottic laryngectomy, which allows preservation of the voice but may still be subject to periodic aspiration. Paraglottic tumors are ominous and warrant thorough evaluation because the inferior limit of a supraglottic laryngectomy is through the most inferior aspect of the laryngeal ventricles, just above the true cords, and incomplete resection may result. The paraglottic space is the space bounded by the true and false vocal cords medially and the thyroid cartilage laterally. The thyroarytenoid muscles are within this space deep to the vocal ligament of the true cords. Deep to the ventricular folds, or false vocal cords, is paraglottic fat. Tumor involvement of the paraglottic space can impair vocal cord mobility through invasion of the thyroarytenoid muscle, vocal cord mucosa, or arytenoids.

The frequency of neck node metastases is at least 20% with T2 or greater tumors. Treatment of the clinically negative neck may be accomplished with surgery or radiation. Surgical approaches should include removal of bilateral primary nodal groups at risk of occult disease (levels II–IV). For T1 and T2 lesions, most authors demonstrate overall cure rates of 68–73%[63,86,87] with determinate 3-year survival rates of 80–85%[86–88] when elective neck dissection is included. While acceptable locoregional control can be achieved for supraglottic cancers, survival rates are adversely impacted due to the development of second primary tumors or intercurrent disease. Cure rates range from 73% to 75% for radiotherapy[89–92] and increase to 80–85% with the addition of surgical salvage.[93–95] Most recurrences are in the neck, and preservation of voice is successful in 65–70% of patients when salvage surgery is included.[93,96] Overall 5-year survival rates for supraglottic cancers range from 40% to 50%.[95,97] Local failures occur in approximately 10% of patients and regional failures in 15–20%. Rates of distant metastases range from 11% to 18%,[95,98,99] with rates approaching 30% in patients with stage IV disease.[100] Second primaries (20–25% of failures) are a major cause of death[91] and recurrent illness accounts for up to 20% of deaths.[99–101]

Glottic and subglottic cancers

Patients with glottic tumors often present with hoarseness while late symptoms include sore throat, dysphagia, hemoptysis, and odynophagia. Early lesions can be treated with radiation or surgery. Even relatively advanced lesions may be

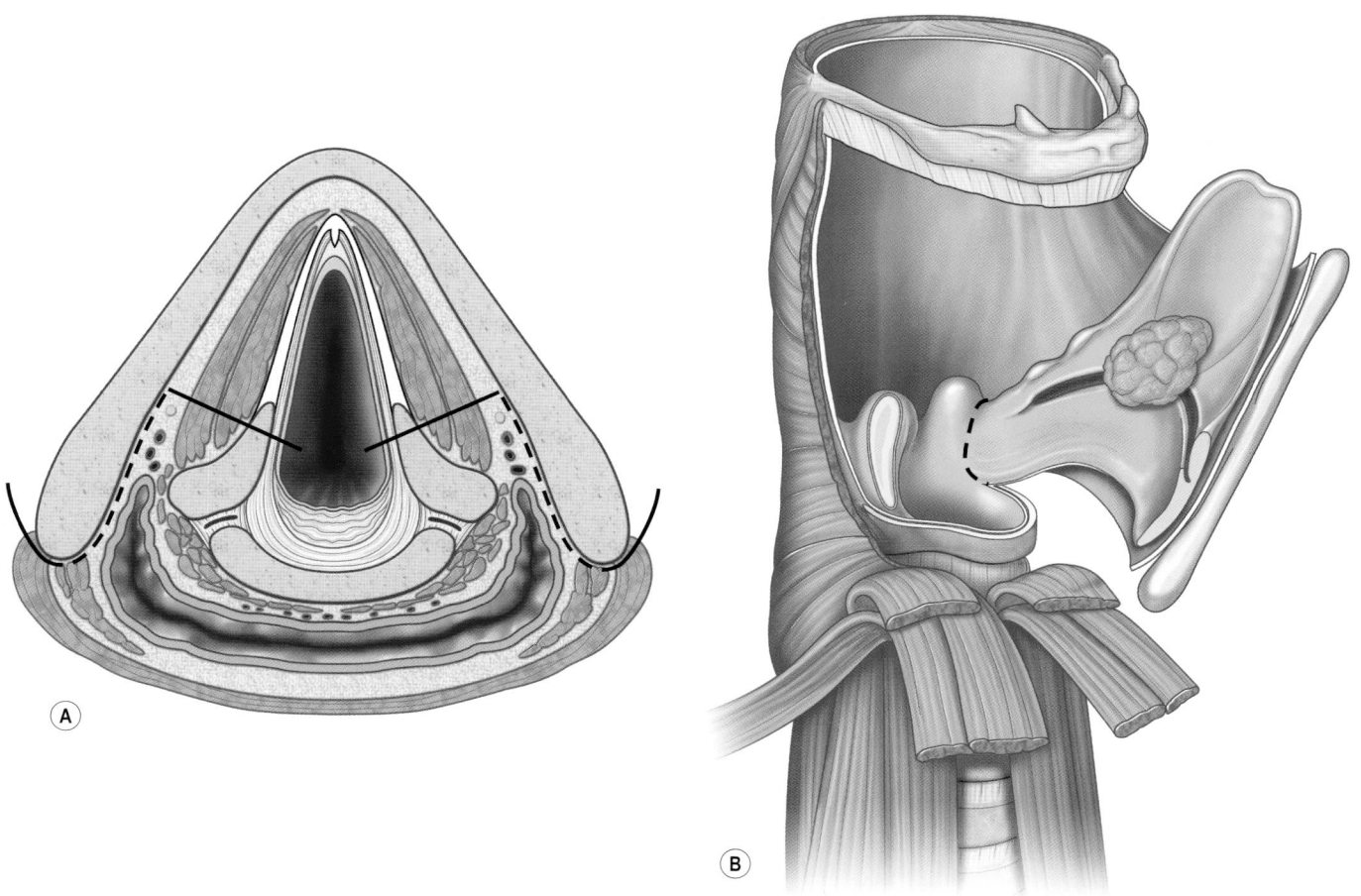

Fig. 17.10 Supracricoid laryngectomy shown from anterior oblique and sagittal views.

treated with surgery alone, depending on deep invasion and the status of the cervical lymphatics. The treatment of glottic cancer is greatly influenced by the secondary goal of voice preservation, and therefore the functional status of the vocal cords becomes the critical factor governing treatment. For small cancers (T1, T2) with mobile vocal cords, radiation therapy alone for cure achieves excellent local control rates; however, the actual quality of the voice is reduced following radiation (T1, 85–95%; T2, 65–75%), with overall survival rates similar to those for surgical resection.[102–105] Local recurrences after definitive radiation can often be salvaged with subsequent surgery and are more common in tumors involving the anterior commissure or the arytenoids. Recurrent glottic cancers after radiation are more frequent than with supraglottic cancers[106] and may require total laryngectomy for cure. Unfortunately, with a total laryngectomy, the ability to speak independently is sacrificed. A supracricoid laryngectomy is another primary or salvage treatment option of glottic carcinomas. Subglottic carcinomas are a rare variant of squamous carcinomas of the larynx possessing a high risk for paratracheal metastases, local recurrence, and death from disease.[107–109] Surgery is the preferred therapy, except in early superficial diseases of this site.[107–109] Although the stigma of laryngectomy remains, contemporary postoperative laryngeal rehabilitation offers quite acceptable functional

outcomes. The advent of tracheoesophageal punctures (TEPs), in conjunction with intense rehabilitation, has markedly improved the functional outcomes of laryngectomized patients. Laryngeal speech can be realized within 2 weeks after surgery. In the salvage surgical setting, TEP placement should be deferred for at least 3 months while the surgical site matures, particularly because early TEP placement may result in fistula formation and poor wound healing.

Survival figures in radiotherapy series are comparable to local control rates for surgery, reflecting the effectiveness of surgical salvage and the fact that few patients with early glottic cancer die of their disease. The 5-year survival rates for T1 lesions range from 85% to 95% with either primary surgery or radiation. Rates for T2 lesions are generally in the range of 75–85%, but these rates decrease by 10–15% (local control rates by 20–25%) when the mobility of the vocal cords is impaired[110] or when there is transglottic spread.[111] Lesions with impaired mobility owing to muscle invasion behave more like T3 cancers and have a poorer prognosis with radiotherapy alone.[101,102,112–114] Transglottic cancers and those with subglottic extension have higher rates of regional metastases and more often require total laryngectomy for cure **(Fig. 17.11)**. In selected patients with these more advanced lesions, extended supraglottic laryngectomy or supracricoid partial laryngectomy may effectively salvage the patient and avoid a

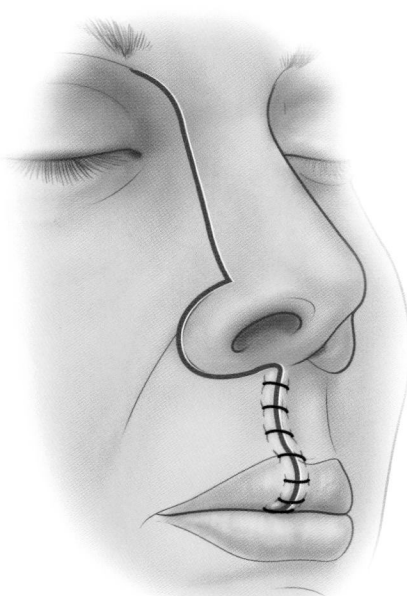

Fig. 17.11 Open lateral rhinotomy or Weber–Ferguson approach.

permanent stoma.[115,116] Voice quality is typically poor with these procedures, and permanent tracheostomy may be needed.

Management of advanced T3 glottic cancers has historically consisted of total laryngectomy with or without postoperative radiation therapy, although, in certain cases, T3 and T4 tumors treated with radiation alone can be effective in 70–80%,[117] and this is enhanced by the addition of systemic therapy with a platinum-based protocol. However, in patients with regional metastases, overall prognosis is poor and recurrence in the neck is a major problem when surgery alone is used. Consequently, elective modified or selective node dissections for staging purposes are recommended when surgery is performed for primary disease. Improved regional tumor control rates are achieved with the addition of adjuvant radiation therapy.[106] Surgery alone is curative in 50–80% of patients without nodal metastases,[91,113,118–120] but this decreases to less than 40% if metastases are present.[113,121,122]

Cancers that involve both the glottic and supraglottic regions (transglottic) are usually advanced and are associated with a high incidence (30–50%) of regional metastases.[111,123] Overall survival rates range from 50% to 55%,[112,121,124] with larynx preservation in 60–70% of these patients.[111,112,121]

Nose and paranasal sinuses

SCC of the nose and paranasal sinus is still the most common histology, but accounts for less than 50% of disease and overall represents a very small portion of malignancies of the upper aerodigestive tract. When taken as a whole, these malignancies account for only 0.2–0.8% of cancers diagnosed annually, or approximately 3% of cancers of the upper airway. The incidence is generally reported as 0.3–1 per 100 000 population.[125–127] These cancers tend to occur most commonly in the fifth decade of life and have been associated with tobacco use and environmental exposure to industrial agents, but they can occur at any age. Cancer of the nose and paranasal sinuses is rare in children except for some sarcomas, such as rhabdomyosarcoma.[128,129] The three most common malignant histologies of the paranasal sinuses are SCC, adenocarcinoma, and adenoid cystic carcinoma, but a number of other histologies are prevalent in this region, including sinonasal undifferentiated carcinoma (SNUC), neuroendocrine carcinoma, and esthesioneuroblastoma (often referred to as olfactory neuroblastoma).

Early symptoms usually include unilateral nasal airway obstruction, rhinorrhea, sinusitis, epistaxis, and, occasionally, dental problems such as dental pain, numbness, and loose teeth. Late symptoms include cranial nerve deficits, proptosis, facial pain and swelling, ulceration through the palate, and trismus, all of which are ominous signs and often reflect advanced disease. The critical component of early diagnosis is a low index of suspicion and a thorough endoscopic or fiberoptic examination of the entire nasal cavity to rule out benign disease such as nasal polyposis or uncomplicated acute or chronic sinusitis. Biopsy is indicated when a mass is found; however, these lesions can hemorrhage, especially neuroendocrine carcinoma, melanoma, and esthesioneuroblastoma, which have a propensity toward epistaxis. It is critical to consider minimizing exposure of uninvolved structures; therefore, biopsy only should be performed without Caldwell–Luc procedures, septoplasty, or entry into uninvolved sinuses. When evaluating the patient with a sinonasal mass, imaging plays an important part in not only the diagnosis and staging of these lesions, but also the surgical planning. Computed tomography and magnetic resonance imaging play complementary important roles in the evaluation of sinonasal neoplasms.[125,130] The staging of cancer of the paranasal sinuses is made radiographically.[126,128,131] Special note is made of "Ohngren's line," or the malignant plane. The plane is defined by an imaginary line drawn from the medial canthus to the ipsilateral angle of mandible and passes through the infraorbital foramen. Tumors above this line (suprastructure) are unfavorable, while those below (infrastructure) are considered favorable.

The most common sinonasal tumor is benign allergic nasal polyposis followed by inverting papilloma, which accounts for the majority of noninflammatory pathologies. It is generally felt that inverting papillomas arise from the squamous or schneiderian mucosa. Although inverting papillomas are benign, they can be very aggressive locally, causing destruction of vital structures, invasion of the orbit, diplopia, and significant deformities. Furthermore, these are associated with an approximately 15% incidence of malignancy. As a result of their aggressive nature and risk of malignancy, all inverting papillomas should be excised promptly and completely. Despite complete excision, these tumors can recur locally (9%) and degenerate into malignant disease. Surgical approaches include: (1) open transfacial; (2) midface degloving/sublabial; and (3) endoscopic. Surgical resections include: (1) medial maxillectomy; (2) infrastructure maxillectomy; (3) total maxillectomy with or without orbital exenteration; and (4) craniofacial resection. The open lateral rhinotomy incision lies along the side of the nose and extends from the medial canthus to the nasal ala, extending into the nasal vestibule and allows excellent visualization of the nasal cavity **(Fig. 17.11)**. The endoscopic approach is being increasingly used in the management of paranasal sinus cancers. This approach provides excellent visualization with angled telescopes, the ability to remove bone with high-speed drills and soft tissue with microdebriders, and can also be complemented by intraoperative surgical nagivation. However, this approach requires a high degree of comfort with the technology and experience with endoscopic techniques, as well as the ability to convert to an open approach when necessary. Some of the limitations include inability to repair large defects, access to the orbit, and the need for an experienced surgical assistant for a two-handed technique.

Traditionally, surgery with postoperative radiotherapy has been advocated for many of these tumors, with some exceptions. Although very effective for smaller tumors of select histologies, this approach provides poor control in advanced disease. This is because these tumors usually present with advanced disease involving the orbit, skull base, and soft tissues of the face. The shortcomings of traditional treatment have led to the incorporation of new approaches, including chemotherapy. Radiotherapy also plays a major role in the management of sinonasal malignancies. It is used both pre- and postoperatively and can be used in select cases as definitive therapy for small T1 and T2 lesions, especially those limited to the nasal vestibule and anterior nasal cavity.[132] Surgery with postoperative radiation therapy remains the standard of care for advanced sinonasal cavity tumors.

SNUC, neuroendocrine carcinoma, and esthesioneuroblastoma represent a spectrum of tumors with neuroendocrine differentiation that can be difficult to distinguish histologically. Immunohistochemistry is often necessary to diagnose these lesions accurately; they may also be confused with sinonasal melanoma, rhabdomyosarcoma, primitive neuroectodermal tumor, or lymphoma. SNUC is a rare but lethal cancer typically presenting as advanced disease in elderly patients. Traditional treatment has been surgery followed by postoperative radiation therapy, but this has provided poor long-term control. These tumors may be chemosensitive and a response to induction chemotherapy may identify patients for concomitant chemoradiotherapy as definitive treatment.[53,133–135] Surgical salvage after nonsurgical therapy has a uniformly dismal prognosis, but in light of the poor locoregional control achieved with traditional surgery and postoperative radiation therapy, most agree that study of concomitant chemoradiotherapy is warranted. Neuroendocrine carcinomas have also been traditionally treated with surgery and postoperative radiation therapy. However, the literature seems to suggest that they should be treated much like neuroendocrine carcinoma at other primary sites, such as small cell carcinoma of the lung.[136–138] Finally, esthesioneuroblastoma, or olfactory neuroblastoma, is a rare neoplasm of the sinonasal cavity, emanating from the olfactory neurofilaments at the cribriform plate. Invasion of the anterior cranial fossa occurs early in the disease process, and eventually involves the brain parenchyma.[128] Patients often present with nasal obstruction and epistaxis. Chemotherapy is reserved for patients with extensive intracranial or orbital disease that would otherwise require an extensive resection. In the induction setting, chemotherapy may be used for its cytoreductive properties, allowing complete surgical resection.[139] Surgical resection and post-operative radiation remain the standard of care.

Postoperative care

Postoperative care for the head and neck cancer patient undergoing treatment is specifically designed based on the type and location of the tumor removed. Following surgery, care is focused on airway management, wound care, and home care needs. Head and neck cancer patient patients are hemodynamically stable postoperatively, often encountering no adverse events. Patients undergoing small oral excisions and neck dissections can be transferred to a surgical floor and monitored by routine nursing care. For those patients undergoing more extensive resections requiring tracheotomy and major reconstruction, more acute and demanding attention is required. Dedicated units to observe for airway difficulties, pedicle or free flap viability, and hematoma formation are required. If these acute issues are controlled, then there is no requirement for prolonged intensive care unit admission.

Patients with head and neck cancer can have difficulty with oral secretions during the immediate postoperative period. Skilled nursing is essential to provide appropriate pulmonary hygiene. Safe and sterile suctioning provided at structured intervals and as needed to the oral cavity is critical to avoid airway obstruction. However, caution in these instances must be exercised if suture lines extend to the posterior oral cavity. Patient instruction is essential by nursing, mid-level providers, and the primary surgical team. Specifically, for patients undergoing total laryngectomy and receiving a tracheal stoma, this procedure requires meticulous cleaning every 6–8 hours and as needed to prevent the development of infection or airway obstruction. Patients also need to be educated that they may have increased nasal secretions due to anatomical changes following laryngectomy. A tracheostomy collar can supply humidified air and functions to moisturize this area, whose duties are normally maintained by the mouth and nose. Emergency equipment, including a bag valve mask and an extra laryngectomy tube, need to be at the patient's bedside at all times. In the event of a cardiac arrest, oxygen can be administered through the stoma via an adapter on the bag valve mask.

Meticulous wound care to the neck incision and stoma incisions is critical. Wounds should be cleaned with sterile saline and antimicrobial ointment applied to the incision site for the first 72 hours until epithelialization is complete. Closed suction drains placed into the neck under flaps evacuate blood and serous fluid from the surgical site. These drains are critical to preventing hematoma and seroma formation. Surgical incisions need to be examined routinely for signs of infection in the postoperative setting. If a patient undergoes laryngectomy with stoma creation, sterile gauze should be placed below the laryngectomy tube into order to prevent skin breakdown. Oral hygiene with normal saline or prescribed equivalent is essential to keep the oral cavity moist, free of contamination, and reduce odor.

Postoperative nutrition is essential for patients undergoing resection of tumors of the upper aerodigestive tract. In patients who are unable to swallow food on their own and who require prolonged enteral feeding, an open or percutaneous endoscopic gastrostomy (PEG) tube can be placed prior to surgery. In addition, nasogastric feeding tubes can be inserted at the time of surgery and converted to a PEG if the patient is unable to convert to oral feeds prior to discharge. A detailed nursing plan emphasizing early and intensive speech and swallowing therapy is essential for patients undergoing radical resections of the upper aerodigestive tract. For patients undergoing pharyngeal and esophageal reconstruction, it is imperative to coordinate care with the speech and swallowing specialist. Once the surgeon deems the reconstruction successful and the anastomosis healed, a barium swallow study can be performed to assess for function and for an anastomotic leak. If there is no evidence of fistula formation, the patient is advanced to an oral diet. If any question exists, the patient will remain on enteral feeds and a repeat swallowing study can be performed to rule out any leak. Patients undergoing less invasive procedures, which include oral resections and neck dissections without reconstruction, still need to be followed for speech and swallowing issues by skilled personnel. However, these patients can typically be followed as outpatients and discharged early from the hospital.

Outcomes, prognosis, and complications

The majority of deaths secondary to SCC of the upper aerodigestive tract occur during the first 5 years of diagnosis.[2] It is therefore imperative that these tumors be treated by a multidisciplinary team committed to providing extirpative expertise in addition to being able to provide adjuvant therapies such as chemotherapy and radiation. Surgical extirpation appropriately coordinated with nonsurgical modalities optimizes the successful treatment of these patients.

The stage of disease is correlated directly to the patient's prognosis. Survival for patients with stage I disease can exceed 80%. The development of nodal metastases reduces the survival of a patient with a small primary tumor by about half. Involvement of even a single lymph node is associated with a marked decline in survival. Locally advanced disease identified at the time of diagnosis, and including stages III and IV, results in a decrement in survival below 40%. Unfortunately, a significant majority of head and neck cancer patients will have stage III or IV disease at the time of diagnosis, and this is associated with an adverse outcome.

Even with aggressive primary treatment, the majority of the relapses that occur are confined to the head and the neck. Locoregional disease relapses account for a significant proportion of primary treatment failures. If distant disease does occur it is typically found in the lung. Overall prognosis for these patients with aerodigestive malignancies is typically related to the overall health status of the patient and stage of disease at the time of presentation.

Complications concerning the treatment of aerodigestive malignancies can be numerous. Specific problems related to nutritional status must be addressed both prior to and following surgery. Close coordination with nutritional support is critical in managing these patients appropriately. Maintaining adequate nutrition is paramount, as they can develop mucositis from both chemotherapy and radiation therapy, limiting the ability to tolerate an oral diet. The placement of a gastrostomy tube, either open or percutaneously, will help optimize caloric intake and improve hydration. Gastroesophageal reflux disease is a common finding in patients treated for SCC of the larynx and pharynx and must be treated with appropriate therapeutic interventions. Vigilance in attending to these patients postoperatively will help improve overall treatment outcomes.

Future directions and conclusions

Despite advances in multimodality regimens and surgical techniques, the survival of patients with upper aerodigestive malignancies who develop local regional recurrences and distant disease is poor. Lifestyle choices such as reducing the consumption of alcohol and eliminating or reducing smoking will help lead to prevention. The introduction of targeted molecular therapies has the potential to improve disease-free survival, with encouraging results demonstrated in selected early studies. An interdisciplinary team utilizing the appropriate resources best manages upper aerodigestive malignancies. Incorporating input from all involved clinicians and utilizing all available modalities is an approach that will prove to be successful in maximizing patient outcome and minimizing treatment-related morbidity for these malignancies.

Access the complete references list online at **http://www.expertconsult.com**

5. Chaturvedi AK, Engels EA, Anderson WF, et al. Incidence trends for human papillomavirus-related and -unrelated oral squamous cell carcinomas in the United States. *J Clin Oncol.* 2008;26:612.
   Investigates the impact of human papillomavirus (HPV) on the epidemiology of oral squamous cell carcinomas (OSCCs) in the US, and assesses differences in patient characteristics, incidence, and survival between potentially HPV-related and HPV-unrelated OSCC sites.

7. Carvalho AL, Nishimoto IN, Califano JA, et al. Trends in incidence and prognosis for head and neck cancer in the United States: a site-specific analysis of the SEER database. *Int J Cancer.* 2005;114:806–816
   Despite recent advances in the diagnosis and treatment of head and neck cancer, there has been little evidence of improvement in 5-year survival rates over the last few decades. To determine more accurate trends in site-specific outcomes as opposed to a more general overview of head and neck cancer patients, the authors analyzed the site-specific data collected in the Surveillance, Epidemiology, and End Results (SEER) Public Use Database 1973–1999. The site-specific analysis allows for a more accurate description of incidence, staging, treatment, and prognostic trends for head and neck cancer.

10. Sturgis EM, Cinciripini PM. Trends in head and neck cancer incidence in relation to smoking prevalence: an emerging epidemic of human papillomavirus-associated cancers? *Cancer.* 2007;110:1429–1435.
   The trends in head and neck cancer incidence and smoking prevalence are reviewed, discussing where such trends parallel

but also how and why they may not. In the US, public health efforts at tobacco control and education have successfully reduced the prevalence of cigarette smoking, resulting in a lower incidence of head and neck cancer. Vigilance at preventing tobacco use and encouraging cessation should continue, and expanded efforts should target particular ethnic and socioeconomic groups. However, an unfortunate stagnation has been observed in oropharyngeal cancer incidence and likely reflects a rising attribution of this disease to oncogenic human papillomavirus, in particular type 16 (HPV-16). For the foreseeable future, this trend in oropharyngeal cancer incidence may continue, but with time the effects of vaccination of the adolescent and young adult female population should result in a lower viral prevalence and hopefully a reduced incidence of oropharyngeal cancer. To hasten the reduction of HPV-16 prevalence in the population, widespread vaccination of adolescent and young adult males should also be considered.

45. Côté V, Kost K, Payne RJ, et al. Sentinel lymph node biopsy in squamous cell carcinoma of the head and neck: where we stand now, and where we are going. J Otolaryngol. 2007;36:344–349.

Evaluation of the existing literature on sentinel lymph node biopsy (SLNB) for early-stage oral and oropharyngeal head and neck squamous cell carcinoma (HNSCC) in clinically negative (N0) necks. Recent studies consistently showed high sensitivities > 93% for T1 and T2 HNSCC. SLNB has the potential to replace neck dissection in those patients. Data on T3 and T4 tumors were not as promising, although research is currently under way to determine the true metastasis detection rate. Appropriate technique is crucial for the complete detection of the sentinel nodes. For HNSCC sentinel lymphadenectomy, many studies have advocated the use of a colloid tracer and gamma probe detector, as well as the harvesting of a total of three nodes as a good standard technique.

46. Robbins KT, Shaha AR, Medina JE, et al. Committee for Neck Dissection Classification, American Head and Neck Society. Consensus statement on the classification and terminology of neck dissection. *Arch Otolaryngol Head Neck Surg.* 2008;134:536–538.

Standardization of terminology for neck dissection is important for communication among clinicians and researchers. New recommendations are made regarding the following: boundaries between levels I and II and between levels III/IV and VI; terminology of the superior mediastinal nodes; and the method of submitting surgical specimens for pathologic analysis.

18

Local flaps for facial coverage

Ian T. Jackson

SYNOPSIS

- Always consider the defect when panning a flap.
- Assess availability and laxity of local tissue.
- Rob Peter to pay Paul but only if Peter can afford it.
- Match the flap to the defect, not the defect to the flap.
- Keep your reconstruction as simple as possible.
- Good cosmesis is vital but function trumps cosmesis.
- Do not burn bridges.
- If unsure of how to proceed, for whatever reason, use a temporizing approach.

Introduction

As will be seen, nearly all the flaps described in this chapter are old flaps. The exceptions are the pre-fabricated flaps and the perforator flaps. This is because these old reconstructive techniques work well and continue to have a significant place in our armamentarium. The basic rule in facial flap surgery is not to choose the flap without consideration of the defect and careful examination of the characteristics of possible donor site positions, skin laxity and skin type. Most important, however, is the vascular supply of the area. It is this what will determine the feasibility, type and success of the reconstruction. In addition, it is advisable, if possible, to have several reconstructive options within the chosen donor site area. Above all, especially in resection of malignant neoplasms, the excision should not be designed to fit in with the chosen method of reconstruction. It is also important to keep in mind that complexity is frequently worse than simplicity. If reconstruction of the defect is beyond your reconstructive abilities, whether it be technique or knowledge, the use of a full-thickness skin graft is acceptable as long as the skin color and texture matches the local area. One should take into consideration that function in these cases is usually minimally or not at all impaired. In situations where there is concern as to the

pathology, a temporary dressing is applied until a definitive diagnosis becomes available. Once healing is complete a more satisfactory resection and a well-designed local flap reconstruction can be performed.

The basic rule in local flap surgery of the face is that you can rob Peter to pay Paul but only if Peter is sufficiently wealthy. On the face, cosmesis is of prime importance. There is a tendency not to consider tissue expansion in local flap surgery. The surgeon should think of using this technique when indicated, since it supplies the ideal skin cover and the amount of skin is usually plentiful. Also, there is only one surgical area. A variant of tissue expansion is used in many reconstructive efforts. When a wound is closed tightly or a flap which seems too small is used and yet the defect is closed, the biomechanical properties of creep and stress relaxation have been harnessed, and the skin elongates over time (*Table 18.1*). There is a limit to these mechanisms, and skin blood supply must also be considered. Familiarity with such techniques is essential in all flap procedures, and this knowledge is a "must" for all plastic surgeons, regardless of seniority.[1–3]

Flaps on the face have many designs and these are related to the area to be reconstructed and the size of the defect. It must not be forgotten, however, that there are only certain basic well-defined tissue manipulations; these are based on the concepts of advancement, transposition, and rotation. When required, these maneuvers can be improved upon by modifying the flap into an island. This, together with an extensive subcutaneous pedicle dissection, provides an extremely mobile flap. Contrary to some opinions, this mobilization will frequently produce better flap vascularization. This is probably related to freeing and altering of the subcutaneous tissues, thus reducing flap tension, also congestion of the flap can occur because of insufficient freeing of the flap base.

There are many challenges in facial reconstruction. The reasons for this are variations in color, texture, areas of hair-bearing skin, wrinkles, nerve supply, and function. In addition to these significant challenges, there are specific three-dimensional anatomic areas, including the nose, lips,

Table 18.1 Viscoelastic properties of the skin

Creep	When a sudden load is applied and kept constant, skin will stretch.
Stress relaxation	A constant load on the skin will cause lengthening. With time, the load required to maintain the lengthening decreases. This explains why white flaps will frequently become pink with time.

ears, eyelids, and eyebrows that require specific (and often difficult) reconstructive techniques in order to achieve optimal functional and aesthetic results.[2]

Another technique to consider, although it is not used much in the local flap area, is the musculocutaneous flap. Though originally conceived as a means of improving blood supply and making flaps more reliable, we now know that this is not necessary. However, muscle also adds bulk to a flap and there are situations where this is an asset.

Forehead and scalp

The characteristics of the forehead vary considerably with age and nationality. The smooth forehead of youth becomes the wrinkled forehead of seniority. The high, hair-free forehead of the Caucasian individual is different from the Indian or Arab forehead, which is small in all dimensions because of the anterior encroachment of hair; the former makes for much easier reconstruction than the latter. All foreheads have a limited amount of spare skin and, as a result, wide undermining and freeing are necessary to deal with many skin defects. Also, the forehead is surrounded by a frame with distinct outlines, mainly of hair that should not be disturbed, where possible (Table 18.1).

Rhomboid flap

This flap can be used, but as with all flaps, it is important to check if the tissue is available. In the forehead, vertical donor sites are preferred to horizontal sites, which may cause an upward shift of the eyebrows or downward repositioning the forehead hairline (Fig. 18.1).[3] Small rotation flaps or transposition flaps are also possibilities; however, these tend to "trapdoor" because of their round or oval design. In larger defects, a triple rhomboid may be used; this necessitates an excision of a hexagonal design (Fig. 18.2). Careful planning and assessment of the availability of loose skin in all three areas of flap harvest is essential.[3–5] In the temporal area, 3.5 cm flaps can be used, but this requires great care in order to prevent too great a shift of the hairline. This applies to reconstruction of any area on the nonhair-bearing scalp in proximity to the hairline edge (Fig. 18.3). Direct advancement flaps are possible but can only close smaller defects. Once again, the direction of hair growth must be considered. Island flaps are used only occasionally; they are frequently based on subcutaneous tissue rather than on definite blood vessels. This necessitates taking great care to maintain every subcutaneous strand possible and tension must be minimized.

Bilobed flaps can be used, but they tend to trapdoor or pincushion and are therefore obvious in any form of indirect lighting. Because of this, they are generally not recommended, though they do continue to be used and are sometimes the best way to reconstruct a given defect.[6,7] A small forehead with a lot of surrounding hair encroaching onto the forehead represents a considerable problem. Laser hair removal should be considered in such a patient. Large forehead reconstruction is treated by tissue expansion; this allows reconstruction by simple advancement or one of the expanded flaps described previously (Fig. 18.4).[8] Post-expansion size increases will decrease when the expander is removed and this must be taken into consideration when planning the reconstruction. Thus, a degree of over-expansion is strongly advised.

Eyebrow reconstruction

The eyebrow is complex and reconstruction is difficult, this is because hair grows in a fixed pattern that is not uniform and is difficult to reproduce exactly. A scalp island flap based on the temporal blood supply can be used, but the hair must be trimmed. The hair is often too dense and does not grow in the correct manner. In spite of this, the reconstructed eyebrow can be much appreciated by the patient, especially in the burned patient in whom both eyebrows are frequently involved. In such a patient, symmetry can be achieved. This, however, varies in degree. An alternative technique is micro-hair transplants with frequent trimming. These, unfortunately, rarely produce the unique anatomy and the density of the eyebrow hair. Eyebrow flaps must be designed with care to maintain the correct anatomic relationship (Fig. 18.5). Unfortunately, there may be a shortage of material available, and it may not be possible to have the eyebrow in the exactly desired anatomical position or size.

Nasal reconstruction

Many different flaps for nasal reconstruction have been described. In the bridgeline region, the glabella is the preferred donor site, and the variety of flaps can be the direct advancement type (Fig. 18.6), transposition (Fig. 18.7), bilobed (Fig. 18.8), rhomboid (Fig. 18.1), or island (Fig. 18.9). On the lateral aspect of the nose, bilobed (Fig. 18.8), rotation (Fig. 18.10), or transposition flaps (Fig. 18.11)[5–8] – all can provide excellent results. Fortunately, there is often more skin available in this area than expected.

To provide an acceptable nasal tip reconstruction, the bilobed flap is ideal, though, as already mentioned, it does have a tendency to trapdoor. The long advancement flap of Rintala,[9] which looks unreliable, usually works well but can cause some apprehension on the part of the surgeon and the patient due to skin color changes (Fig. 18.11). Another method is that of Schmidt,[10] in which the supraorbital area (i.e., just above the eyebrow) is tubed to a dimension that will reach to the nasal tip. Laterally, a nostril is made by dissecting a skin pocket and lining it with a skin graft and cartilage. The latter provides the required support and is placed if possible and if necessary. Remember – simple surgery if possible! Approximately 2–3 weeks after the initial reconstruction, this

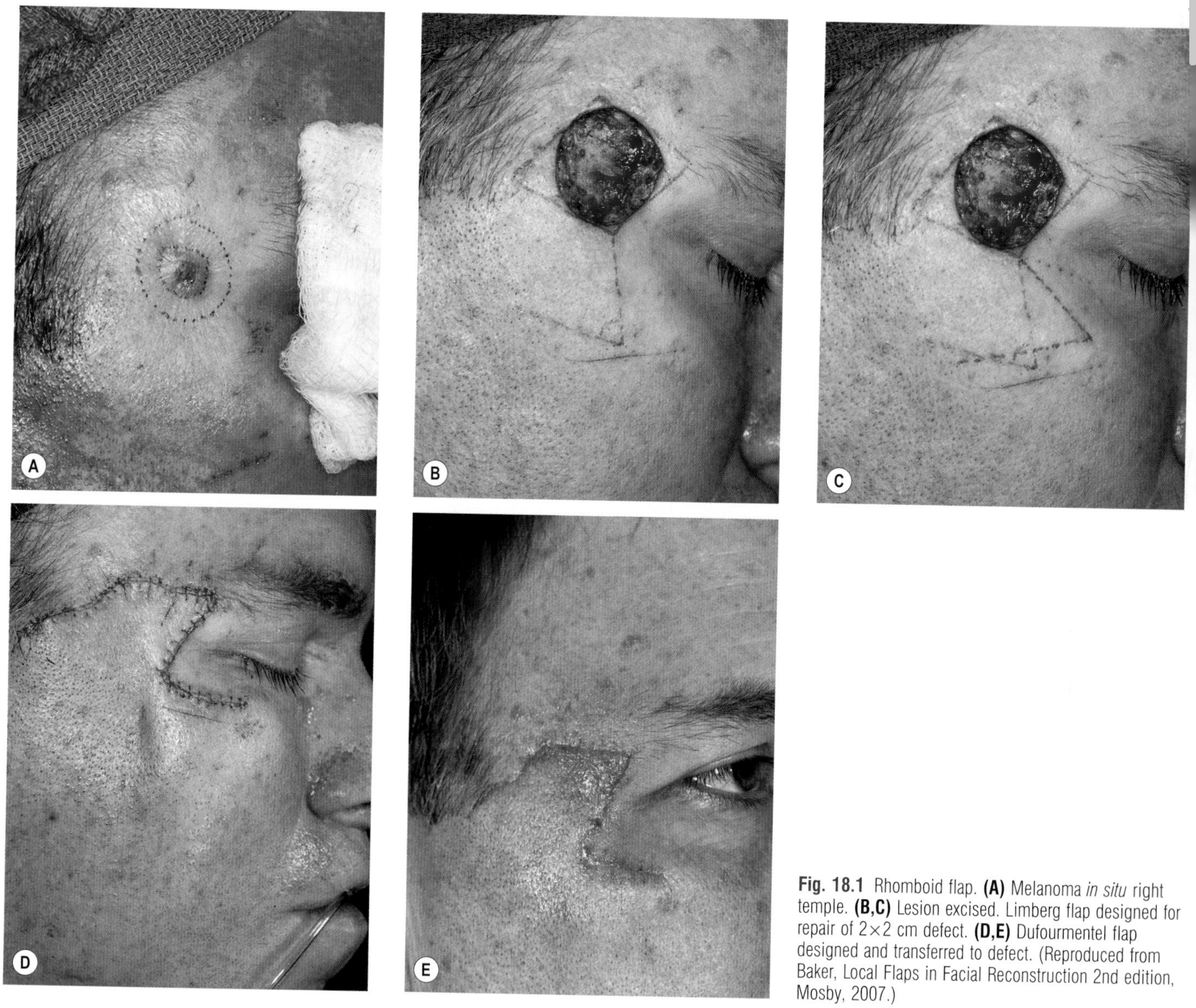

Fig. 18.1 Rhomboid flap. **(A)** Melanoma *in situ* right temple. **(B,C)** Lesion excised. Limberg flap designed for repair of 2×2 cm defect. **(D,E)** Dufourmentel flap designed and transferred to defect. (Reproduced from Baker, Local Flaps in Facial Reconstruction 2nd edition, Mosby, 2007.)

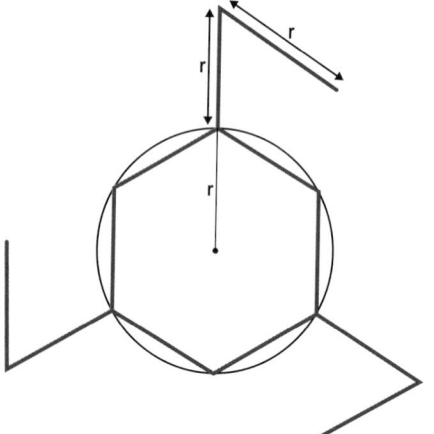

Fig. 18.2 Triple rhomboid flap. Circular cutaneous defect conceptualized as hexagon. Sides of hexagon are equal to radius (r) of circle. First side of flap created by direct extension equal in length to radius at alternative corners to prevent sharing of common sides. Second side of flap designed parallel to adjacent side of hexagon. (From Bray DA. Rhombic flaps. In: Baker SR, Swanson NA, eds. *Local flaps in facial reconstruction*. St Louis: Mosby; 1995:155, with permission.)

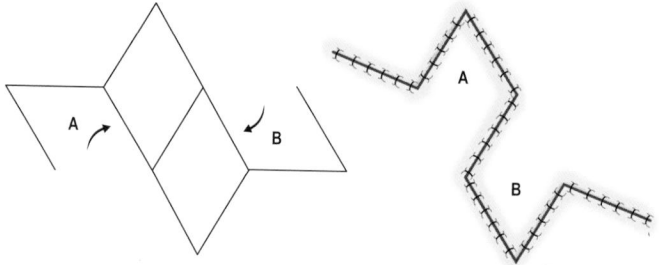

Fig. 18.3 Bilateral rhombic flaps designed for repair of large defect. Defect divided into two adjacent rhombuses **(A,B)** to assist with designing rhombic flaps.

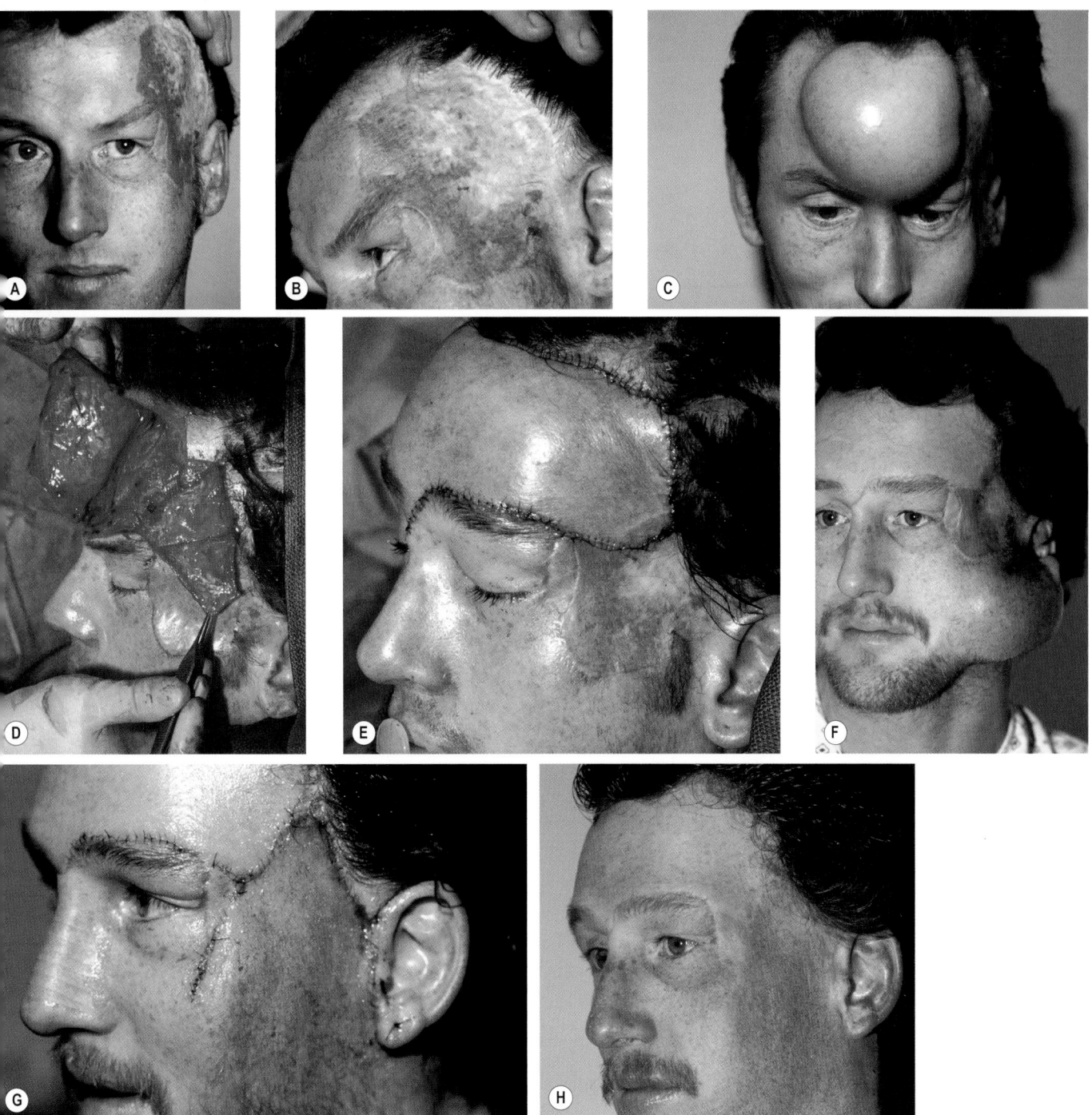

Fig. 18.4 Tissue expansion to achieve left defect closure. **(A,B)** Skin graft covering temple, anterior parietal scalp, and lateral cheek. **(C)** Expanded forehead skin. **(D)** following tissue expansion, expanded forehead skin used to cover defect created by partial resection of skin graft. **(E)** Expansion provided sufficient skin to cover temple. **(F)** Tissue expander beneath lateral cheek skin. **(G)** 6 days following removal of skin graft from cheek and reconstruction with expanded cheek advancement flap. **(H)** 6 months' postoperative. (Reproduced from Baker, Local Flaps in Facial Reconstruction 2nd edition, Mosby, 2007.)

composite is brought down to reconstruct the rim and the alar region *(Fig. 18.11)*. In the author's experience, this procedure is reliable and yields good results.

A composite graft from the ear is an excellent choice when the nostril is to be reconstructed. A cutout of the planned defect is made and transferred to the ear. A portion of the rim of a satisfactory size and shape is marked out. Using the markings, a full-thickness segment of the ear is removed. Lateral to or inferior to this, a long triangular full thickness of skin is taken in continuity with the posterior surface of the ear. Closure of the ear defect causes only a minor size reduction, which rarely seems to be a problem. The nose lesion is resected with lateral skin excess. The ear graft is then sutured in place with meticulous accuracy so that raw skin edges of the graft and ear oppose exactly, and the ear rim becomes the nostril rim. In this way, revascularization of the composite graft from

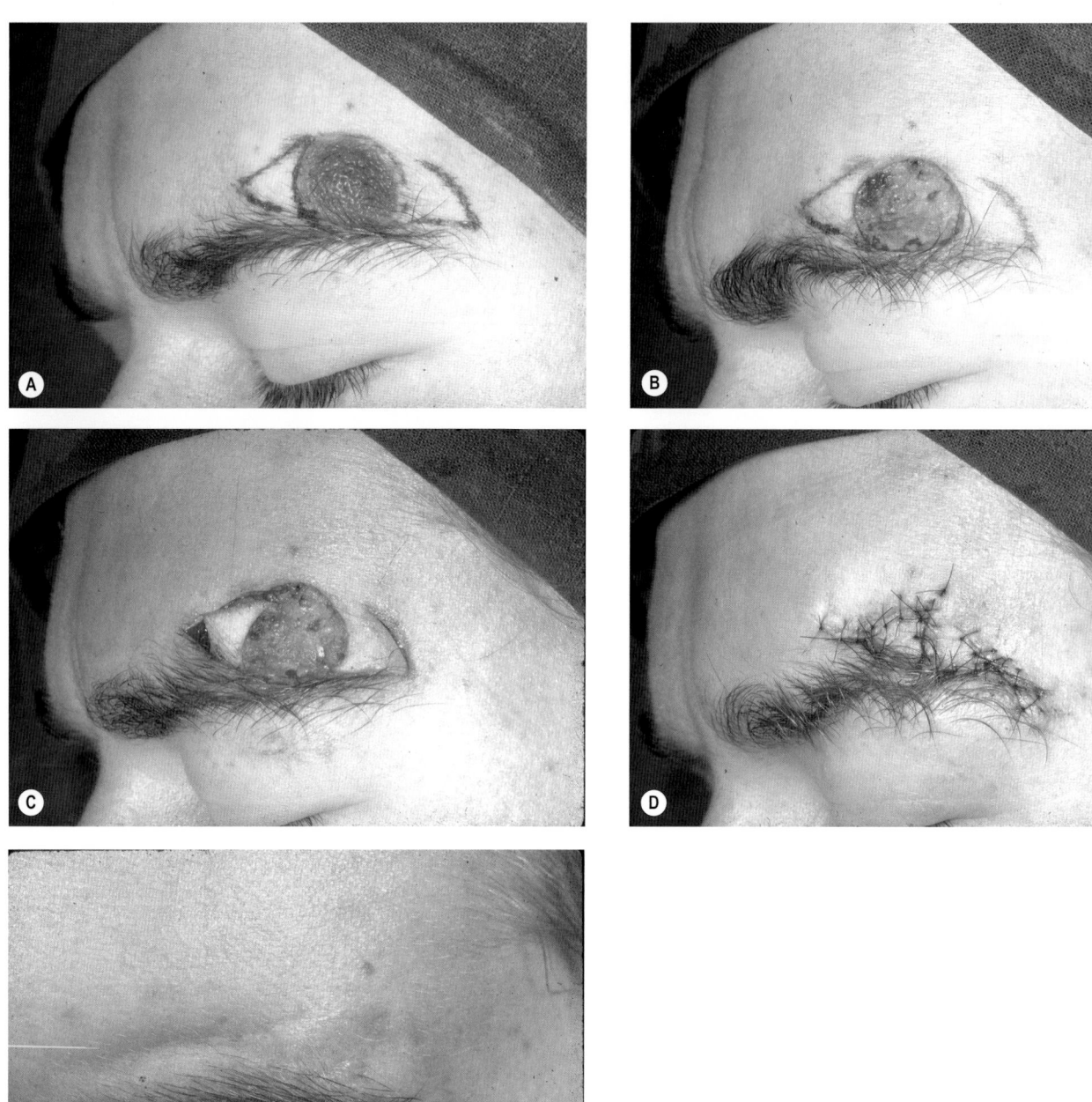

Fig. 18.5 Nevus of left supraorbital area involving eyebrow – hatchet flap reconstruction. **(A)** The planned excision has been drawn out together with bilateral hatchet flaps. **(B)** Nevus has been excised. It can be seen that the flap pedicles are superior for the lateral flap and inferior for the medial flap. **(C)** The flaps are elevated. **(D)** The flaps are transposed, and the secondary defect is closed. **(E)** Satisfactory end result with the eyebrow in a good position.

the full-thickness replacement area will occur with excellent results. The maximal dimensions of a composite graft are approximately 1 cm²; for defects greater than this, a composite flap of helical root is an excellent solution. A thin vertical forehead flap can also be used, but this must be based correctly (see below). When a more complex reconstruction is required (e.g., bilateral alar rims and columella), the total central forehead should be used. This area should be mapped and marked carefully to ensure that there is adequate tissue for the columella and alar rims. The flap is now elevated. The key to complete survival of the flap is the position of its base; this should be at

the medial canthal level or below. In this way, the vascular anastomosis on the side of the nose between the cheek and forehead vessels can provide a satisfactory flap to close the defect. With the base correctly positioned, the midline flap will comfortably reconstruct the nasal tip and the columella without tension and with absolute safety. The reason for poor results and failures is usually due to elevating the flap pedicle based on the brow area. Another problem is lack of understanding of the vascular anatomy (i.e., anastomosis between the facial and the forehead vascular systems in the superolateral area of the medial orbitolateral nasal area). The forehead

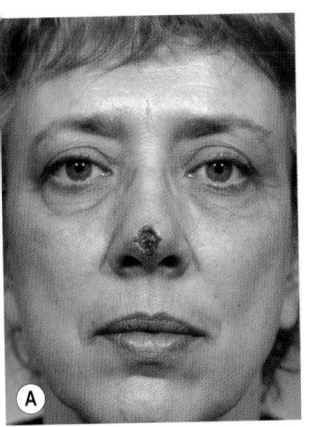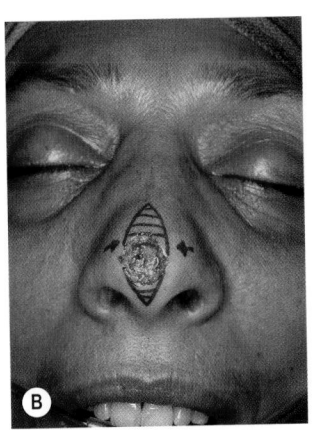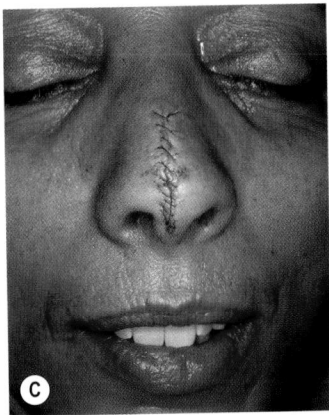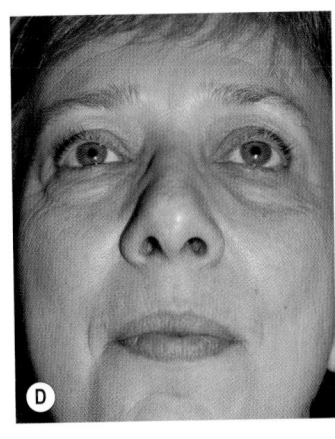

Fig. 18.6 Reconstruction of nasal defect with lateral advancement flaps. **(A)** 0.5×0.5 cm skin defect of nasal tip. **(B)** Primary wound closure planned. Anticipated standing cutaneous deformities (marked by horizontal lines). **(C)** Deformities excised and wound closed. **(D)** 1.5 years' postoperatively. (Reproduced from Baker, Local Flaps in Facial Reconstruction 2nd edition, Mosby, 2007.)

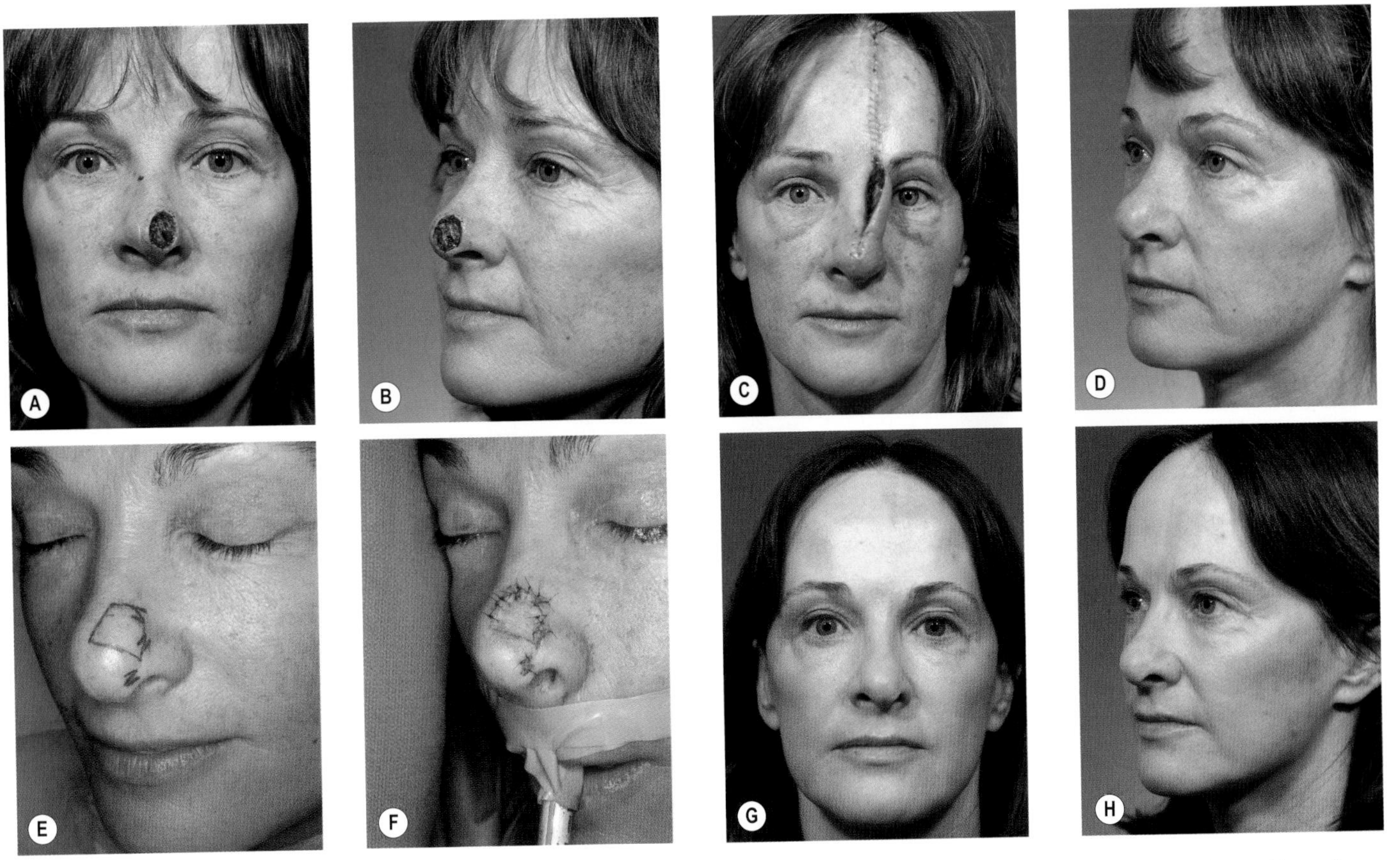

Fig. 18.7 Reconstruction of lateral nasal defect with forehead flap. **(A,B)** 1.5×1.5 cm skin defect of nasal tip. **(C)** Interpolated paramedian forehead flap used to repair defect. **(D)** 9 months' postoperative. Depressed scar surrounds lateral aspect of flap and mild trap-door deformity is present. **(E)** Nose marked for planned contouring procedure. Three Z-plasties positioned along depressed scar. **(F)** Flap thinned and Z-plasties performed. **(G,H)** 4 months following Z-plasties and full face carbon dioxide laser peel. (Reproduced from Baker, Local Flaps in Facial Reconstruction 2nd edition, Mosby, 2007.)

is closed directly, but if there is tension in the area just anterior to the hairline, it should be left to close spontaneously. The scar resulting from this rarely, if ever, requires any reconstruction The pedicle is divided at 2–3 weeks, depending on the inset, and the nasal tip is fashioned. Apart from thinning, it is unusual to require further adjustments *(Fig. 18.12)*. If there is any concern about vascularity, the flap base is delayed.

If a total nasal reconstruction is required, a larger amount of forehead skin is harvested in the transverse dimension, but again, the base should be positioned at or below the medial canthal ligament. The septal mucosa is used for lining. For closure of the midline forehead defect, the skin can frequently be mobilized extensively and advanced. If there is concern, a tissue expander can be inserted to expand the whole forehead.

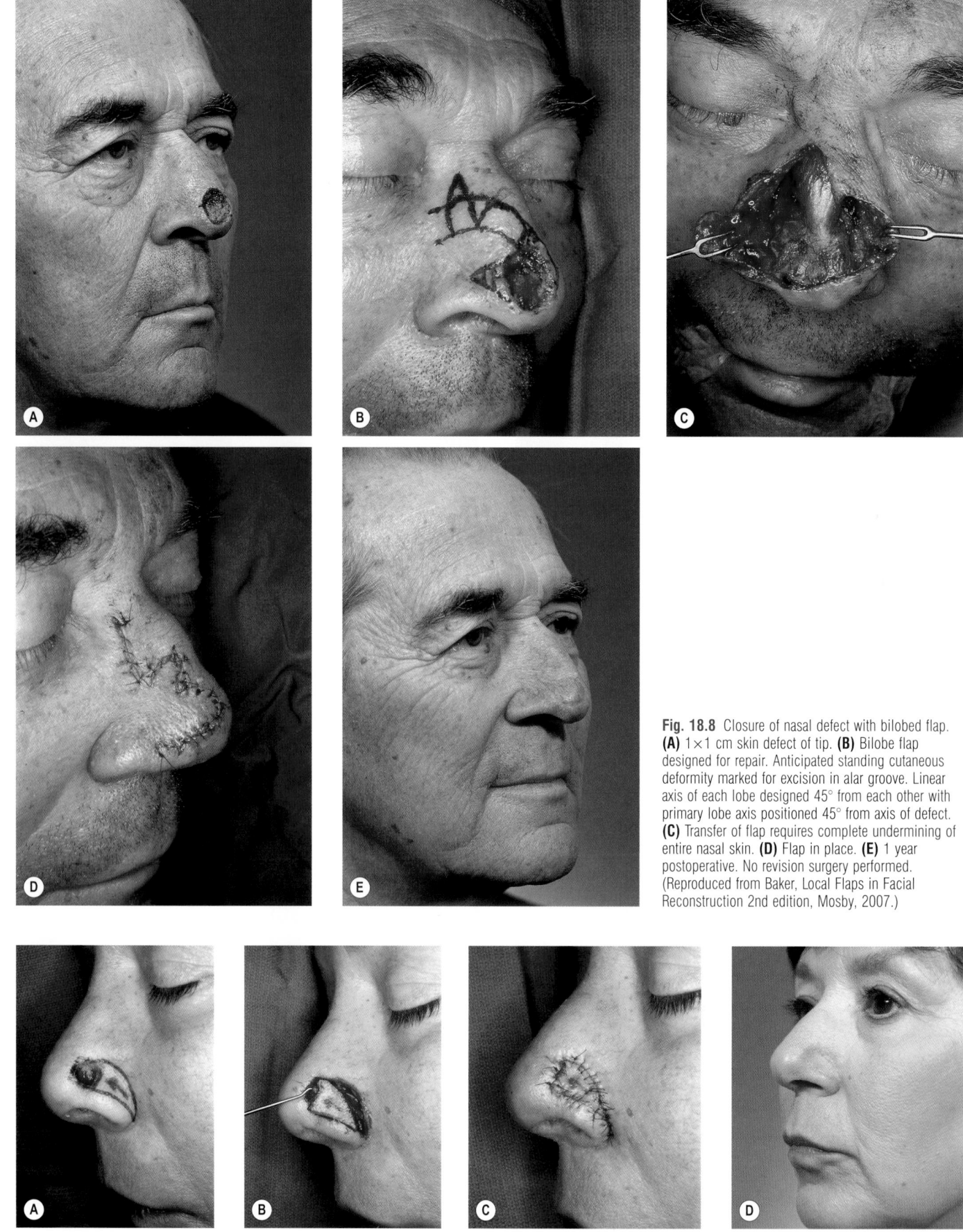

Fig. 18.8 Closure of nasal defect with bilobed flap. **(A)** 1×1 cm skin defect of tip. **(B)** Bilobe flap designed for repair. Anticipated standing cutaneous deformity marked for excision in alar groove. Linear axis of each lobe designed 45° from each other with primary lobe axis positioned 45° from axis of defect. **(C)** Transfer of flap requires complete undermining of entire nasal skin. **(D)** Flap in place. **(E)** 1 year postoperative. No revision surgery performed. (Reproduced from Baker, Local Flaps in Facial Reconstruction 2nd edition, Mosby, 2007.)

Fig. 18.9 (A) 0.8×0.7 cm skin defect of alar groove. V–Y island subcutaneous tissue pedicle advancement flap designed for repair. **(B)** Flap incised and advanced on nasalis muscle. **(C)** Flap in place. **(D)** 4 months' postoperative. (Reproduced from Baker, Local Flaps in Facial Reconstruction 2nd edition, Mosby, 2007.)

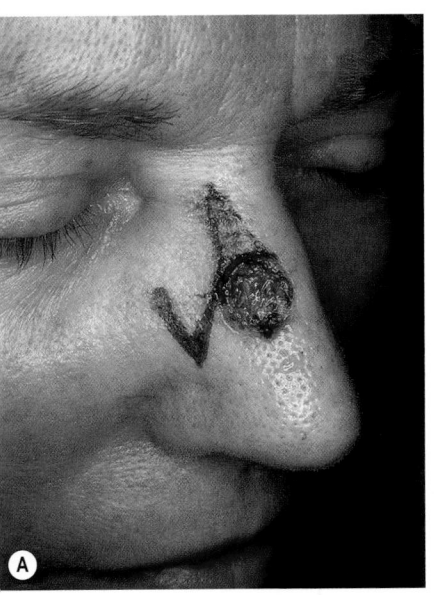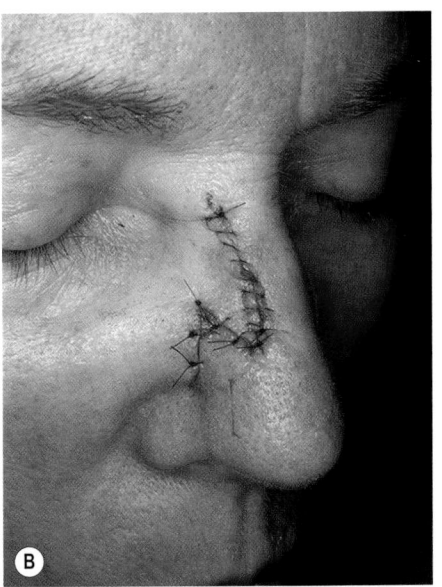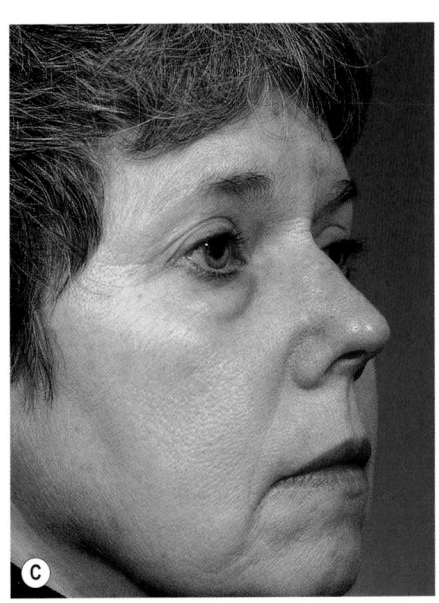

Fig. 18.10 (A) 1×0.8 cm skin defect of the dorsum. Transoperative flap designed for repair. Anticipated standing cutaneous deformity marked by horizontal lines. **(B)** Flap transposed. **(C)** 6 months postoperative. No revision surgery performed. (Reproduced from Baker, Local Flaps in Facial Reconstruction 2nd edition, Mosby, 2007.)

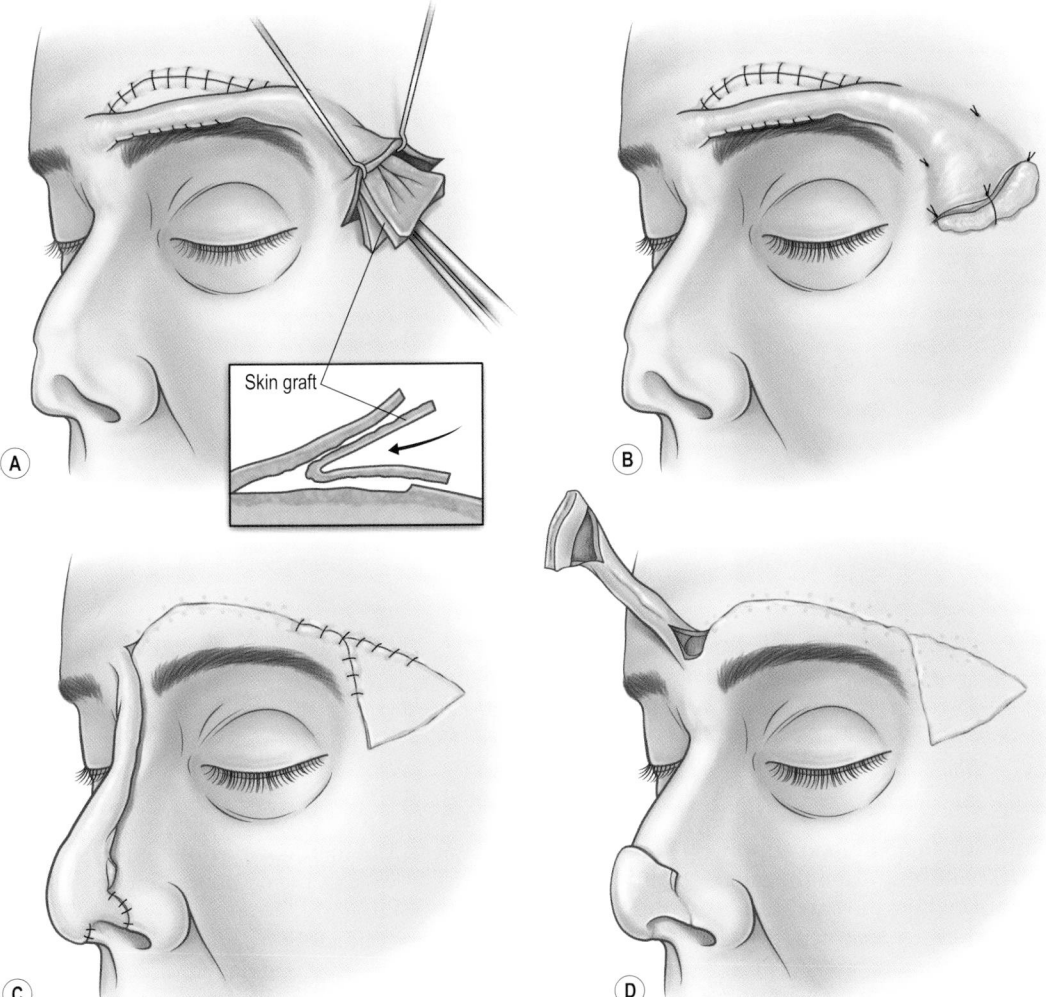

Skin graft

Fig. 18.11 Rintala dorsal nasal advancement flap to close nasal tip defect. **(A)** The basal cell carcinoma of the nasal tip is outlined, and the Rintala flap has been drawn out. The area of Burow's triangle resection is crosshatched on the forehead. **(B)** The excision is completed and the flap is elevated. **(C)** The flap is advanced after excision of the Burow triangles. The flap is pale, but this is due to epinephrine having been injected with the local anesthetic. **(D)** End result with slight scarring to the right of the nasal tip that settled uneventfully. (Reproduced from Baker, Local Flaps in Facial Reconstruction 2nd edition, Mosby, 2007.)

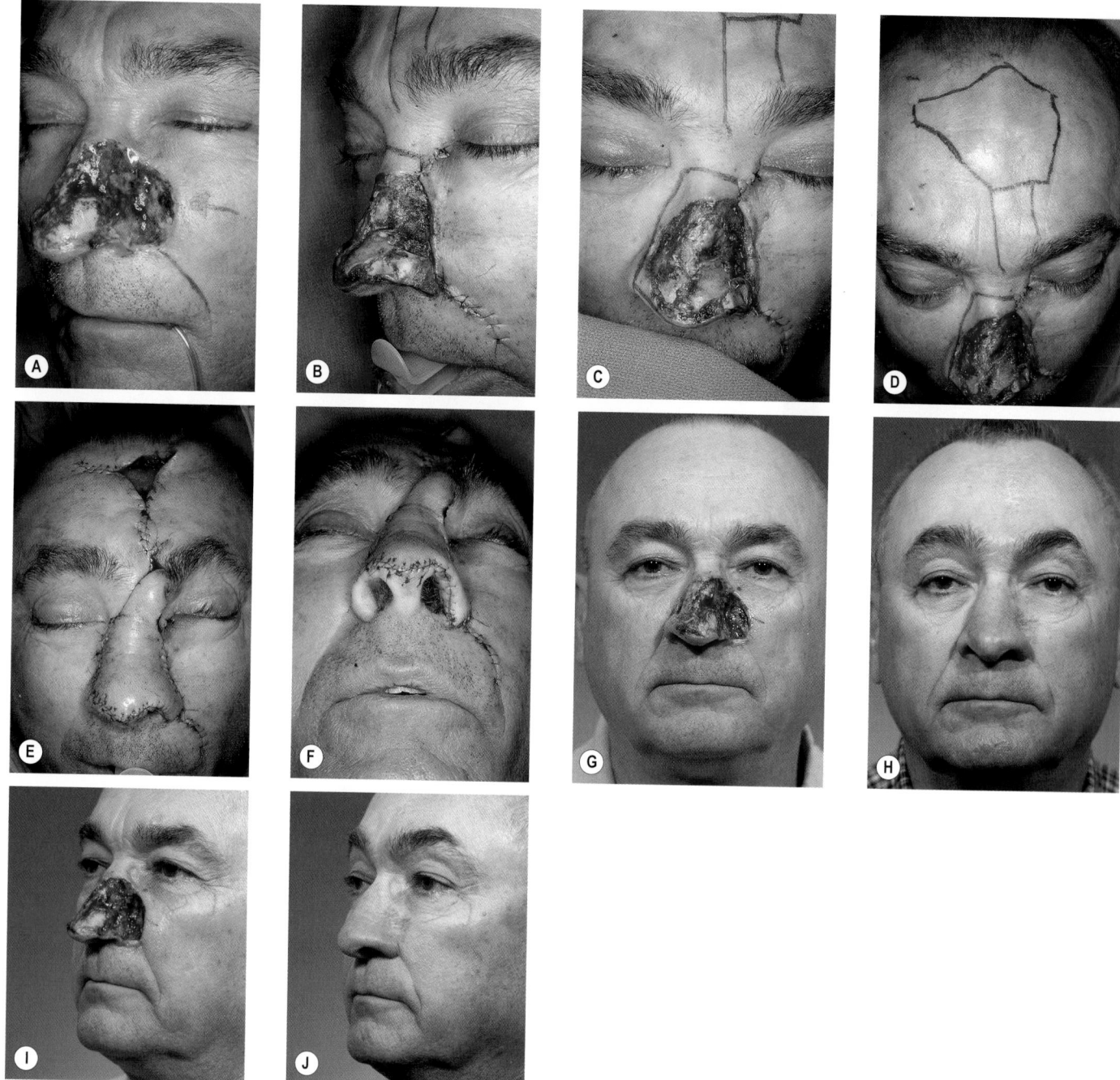

Fig. 18.12 Reconstruction of nasal tip and dorsum with forehead flap after resection of basal cell carcinoma. **(A)** 4×6 cm skin defect of dorsum, nasal tip, sidewall, and ala extending into cheek. Cheek advancement flap designed to repair cheek component of defect, **(B)** Cheek flap advanced to nasal facial sulcus. Auricular cartilage graft positioned for ala framework. **(C)** Remaining skin of dorsum and sidewall aesthetic units marked for excision. **(D)** Interpolated paramedian forehead flap design as covering flap. **(E,F)** Forehead flap transferred to nose. Portion of donor site left to heal by secondary incision. **(G–J)** Preoperative and 1 year, 4 months' postoperative. Contouring procedure performed. (Reproduced from Baker, Local Flaps in Facial Reconstruction 2nd edition, Mosby, 2007.)

This gives a large amount of skin with a good blood supply. If nasal support is needed, a cranial bone graft from the outer table of the skull is taken from an area where the curvature is similar to that required for the defect reconstruction, the shape can be chosen to some extent.[11] This may be done at the same time with secure screw stabilization of the bone graft in the forehead/nose junction. It may be safer to delay grafting to the time of flap division or to a third procedure. A less common method to reconstruct the tip of the nose is to use a

donor site from the neck, but there can be problems with color and texture of the neck skin and the contours, due to the softness of the subcutaneous tissue.

A long, transverse tube pedicle is raised transversely on the neck. After 2–3 weeks, one end is delayed, and this end is taken up 10 days later to reconstruct the tip. The flap is divided in 2–3 weeks and inset.

Noses may be prefabricated elsewhere (e.g., on the forearm using a radial flap) and subsequently transferred by microvascular techniques. Initially the results left a lot to e desired but with experience and technique refinement, he results are now much better and complications less roublesome.[12]

Eyelids

Partial lower lid defects

esions are frequently resected in a V fashion and the resultng defect can be carefully closed in layers. If this is not possible, the lower portion of the lateral canthal ligament is ivided through a small lateral canthal incision. This allows he lid to move medially, and closure can be obtained without ension. If there is too much tension, the incision and dissection are taken further laterally on the cheek. Closure is then btained without difficulty. The lateral incision is closed with Z-plasty in order to reduce any skin tension *(Fig. 18.13A–D)* *Fig. 18.13E–I)*.[13] ⊛ FIG **18.13E–I** APPEARS ONLINE ONLY

An extensive defect requires that a portion of nasal septum, vith mucosa attached on one side, be inserted with the mucosa toward the globe in order to form an internal lamella.[14] A portion of ear cartilage, with perichondrium in place of the mucosa, can also be used for support. Mucosalization of the inner surface occurs fairly rapidly. A cheek rotation flap of the required size then provides external cover *(Fig. 18.14)*. If the cheek skin is insufficient, prior expansion of the lateral cheek skin should be performed, or a narrow midline forehead flap can be used. The latter has the advantage of being a little more rigid. This, however, requires accurate sizing in all dimensions, also there will be a forehead scar. ⊛ FIG **18.14** APPEARS ONLINE ONLY

Partial upper lid defects

Reconstruction of the upper lid is a more difficult problem because the lid is vital for protection of the eye. It is best for the surgeon to sit at the head of the operating table and think of the upper lid as the lower lid and use the same techniques described for the lower lid modified to the required shape and size of the upper lid.

Any failure of reconstruction, particularly in the vertical dimension, may cause conjunctivitis and/or impaired vision. Without an adequate upper lid, the eye will be at risk for

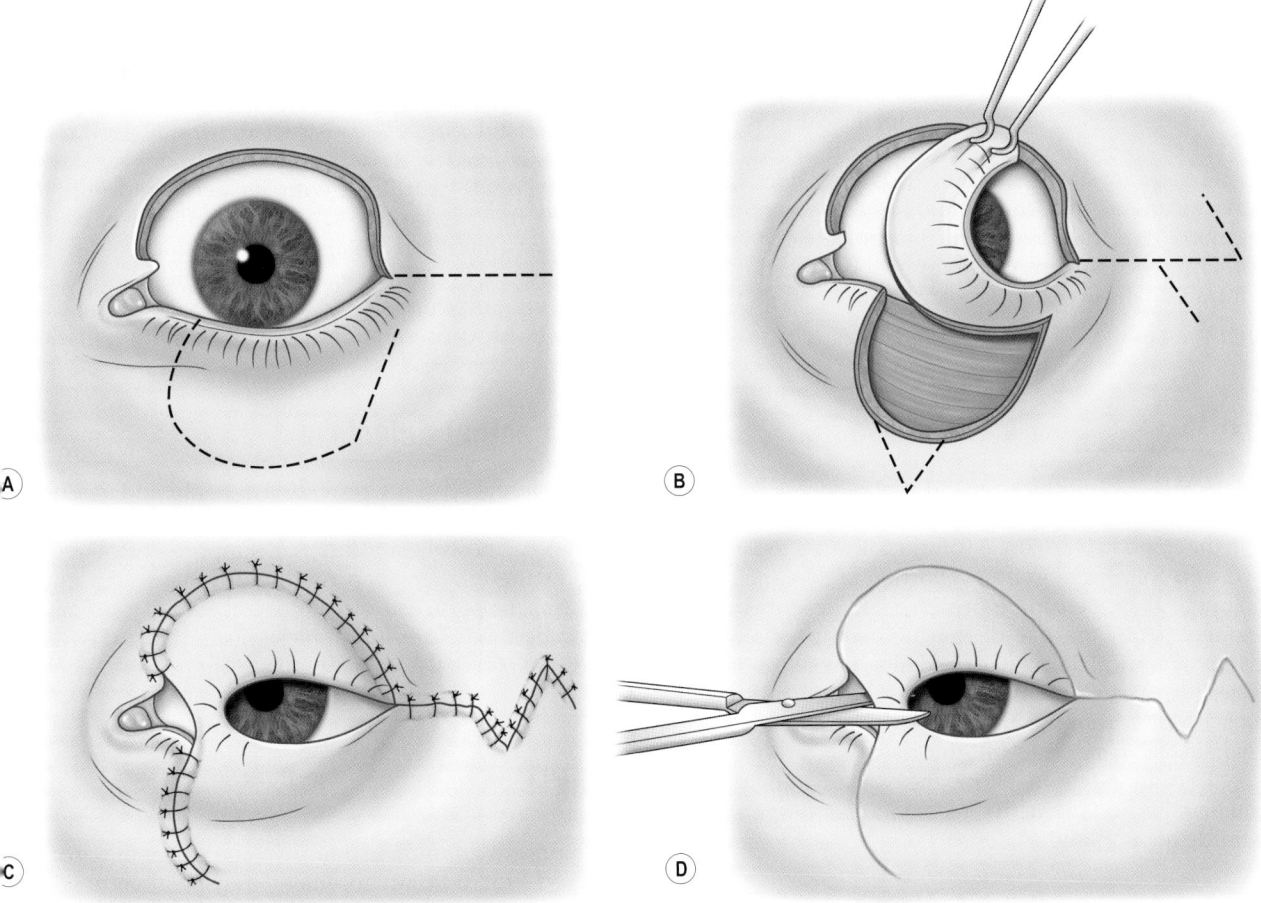

Fig. 18.13 Reconstruction of total upper eyelid defect with lower lid transposition. **(A–D)** Illustration of planned reconstruction of an upper eyelid defect with lower lid ransposition.

exposure, scarring, and loss of vision. Experience in eyelid surgery is essential.

Advancement flap

For a triangular defect in the upper lid (e.g., after tumor resection), an incision is made horizontally from the lateral canthus, followed by division of the superior limb of the lateral canthal ligament.[15] An incision is also made in the conjunctiva of the superior fornix. This alone will allow small defects to be easily closed. For the best result to be obtained laterally at the end of the horizontal skin incision, an unequal Z-plasty can be performed to deal with the dog-ear. As in the lower lid, accurate suturing and repositioning of the gray line, the lash line, and the rim conjunctival junction is essential *(Fig. 18.15)*. FIG **18.15** APPEARS ONLINE ONLY

Lid-switch flap (Abbé flap)

By using the same principles as the Abbé flap on the lip, a similar reconstruction can be used for defects of the upper lid *(Fig. 18.16)*.[16] There are marginal vessels in the lid, and a full-thickness V flap (the defect of which should close easily) can be taken from the lower lid, swung up, and sutured into the upper lid in layers. The lower lid defect closure requires the edges to come together directly without tension. If this does not occur, a small lateral canthal incision is made, and the inferior limb of the lateral canthal tendon is divided. If this is not sufficient, a long transverse incision from the canthus out to the temporal skin (incorporating a Z-plasty if necessary) will suffice to obtain tensionless closure. It is important that a preoperative examination of the mobility of the lower lid is carefully assessed. If necessary (e.g., in children), the conjunctiva is anesthetized with drops or rarely, general anesthesia. In adults, infraorbital nerve blocks can be used. FIG **18.16** APPEARS ONLINE ONLY

Free grafts

For larger defects, free, full-thickness lid replacements (composite grafts) have been employed. This is hazardous if it is performed in the standard fashion. A full-thickness lid replacement is used as a composite graft if a portion of conjunctiva and subconjunctival tissue can be preserved as described in the last segment. With the use of the methods previously described, a small vertical defect will need to be reconstructed. A full-thickness graft can be taken from the lower lid, and the conjunctiva is excised from the graft, leaving just enough for the full-thickness defect. The full-thickness skin portion remaining will be enough to allow the graft to survive; however, meticulous reconstructive technique is imperative. The lower lid defect is closed as described previously.

Large and total upper lid defects

For larger defects, the lower lid is used and the significant lower lid defect is reconstructed. A large full-thickness portion of lower lid is moved up on its marginal vascular pedicle. partial lower lid reconstruction is necessary. As the portion lower lid is turned up, the full thickness of the cheek advanced medially and grafted with nasal septum on its inne surface, as required *(Fig. 18.17)*.[15] FIG **18.17** APPEARS ONLINE ONLY

To reconstruct the upper lid, the whole lower lid is turne up. The lower lid reconstruction is based on an advancemer cheek flap lined with nasal septum, cartilage, and mucosa These pedicled lid reconstructions are left attached for 2– weeks, depending on the vascularity of the upturned flap Once the upper lid reconstruction is in position, small adjust ments are often necessary. Rearrangements are usuall required for the lateral canthus and occasionally to the edg of the lower lid or to provide adjustment of lower lid heigh With meticulous technique, a good cosmetic and functiona result can be obtained *(Fig. 18.13)*.[16] When a healthy eye present, a lid can be prefabricated on the forehead. A pock the size of the lid is designed and a mucosal graft is inserte When this reconstruction is complete, it is brought down o a vascular pedicle to replace the lid. The pedicle is divided 3 weeks. This protects the eye, but movement is minima unless there is some remaining orbicularis which can be use immediately or at a later date *(Fig. 18.18)*. FIG **18.18** APPEAR ONLINE ONLY

Total lower lid defects

These result from tumor resection, from trauma, or when th lower lid is used to reconstruct the upper lid *(Fig. 18.13* Reconstruction of the total lower lid is primarily performe for cosmesis.

The lower lid can be reconstructed with a cheek rotatio flap which is lined with oral mucosa or more satisfactoril using nasal septal cartilage with its perichondrium intac *(Fig. 18.18)*. In other instances, a forehead flap may be neces sary. This has the disadvantage of bulk, which can result i poor aesthetics. With time, however, the latter can b improved upon by debulking. With experience, there is n longer so much concern about ischemia resulting in skin o lid loss.

Medial canthal defects

Generally, forehead flaps provide a reliable and reasonabl good method of reconstruction. These flaps must be line with mucosa, however additional support is not require because of the inherent flap rigidity. It is very important t place a flap of sufficient size into the medial canthal are Failure to do this results in troublesome epiphora *(Figs 18.19 18.21)*. FIGS **18.19–21** APPEARS ONLINE ONLY

Cheek

Skin tumors are common in this area. The whole range of flap can be used – rotation, advancement, transposition, and islan type – with many variations required and usually availabl for each type of reconstruction.[17] Occasionally, for extremel large defects, a free flap may be required. (This is discusse in more detail in Chapter 10 of this volume).

Rotation

Because the cheek area is relatively large, rotation flaps may be designed in many sizes, depending on the position, shape and size of the defect to be reconstructed. When the area to be excised is triangulated, small flaps may simply be rotated around within a circle to close the defect. The design of rotation can be calculated by placing one end of a thread on the angle apex and the other at the edge of the defect. By rotating the outer end of the flap on the skin, the required circumference can be marked. In some instances, however, the flap edge may fall short. It is preferable to use the point to be closed as the length of the flap edge. By obtaining this measurement and rotating back to the donor area of the flap, adequate flap dimensions are achieved. Adjustments may be necessary along the line of the flap as the surgery progresses (*Figs 18.22, 18.23*).

Advancement

Advancement flaps can be used at any location on the cheek. As with the rotation flap, the advancement flap can be of any size. It is best to use natural lines, even if they diverge away from the defect, because this will still give a better and more natural cosmetic end result; by and large these areas provide flaps under less tension. The defect is outlined and resected, usually as a square, a circle or a rectangle. The flap is raised from one edge, dissection in a posterior direction provides sufficient skin and subcutaneous tissue to rotate and close the defect. Any excess skin at the anterior flap base is now resected. When an advancement flap is used to close a square defect, there are areas of excess skin related to the Burow's triangles, these are resected. Composite cheek and nose defects require composite reconstructions. The nose is resurfaced with a full-thickness skin graft, and an advancement

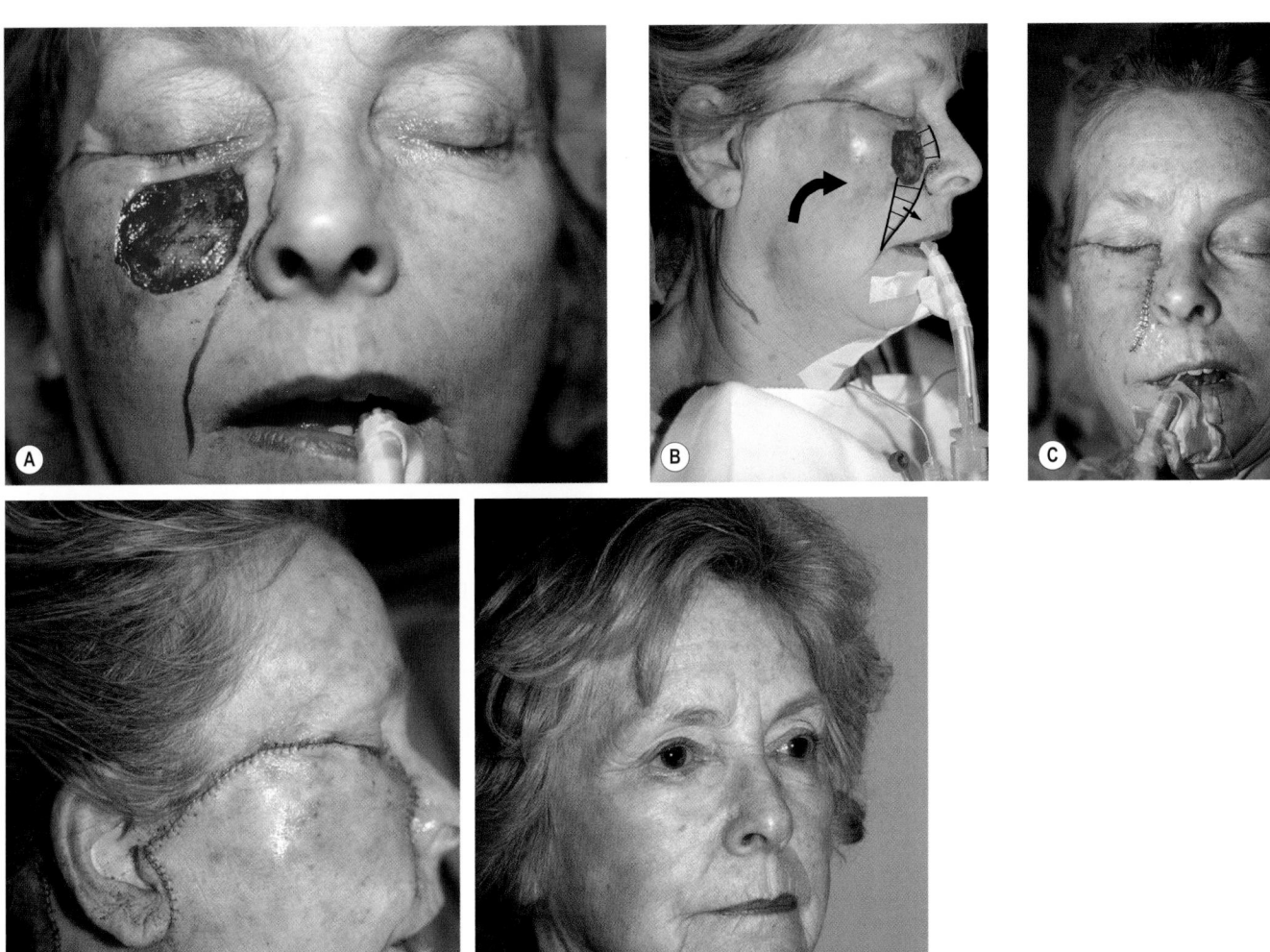

Fig. 18.22 Rotation cheek flap. **(A)** 4×3 cm medial cheek defect. Flap designed for repair. Incision for flap placed in subciliary line. Nasofacial sulcus and melolabial creases marked. Skin between defect and nasofacial sulcus and melolabial crease removed to position advancing border of flap in aesthetic boundary. **(B)** Incision for flap extended to preauricular crease and posterior auricular sulcus. Anticipated standing cutaneous deformity marked with horizontal lines on melolabial fold. **(C,D)** Flap in position. Note incision lines at level of lateral canthus. Medial border of flap positioned in nasofacial sulcus and melolabial crease. **(E)** Postoperative result with normal eyelid position and well-camouflaged scars. (Courtesy of Shaun R. Baker MD.)

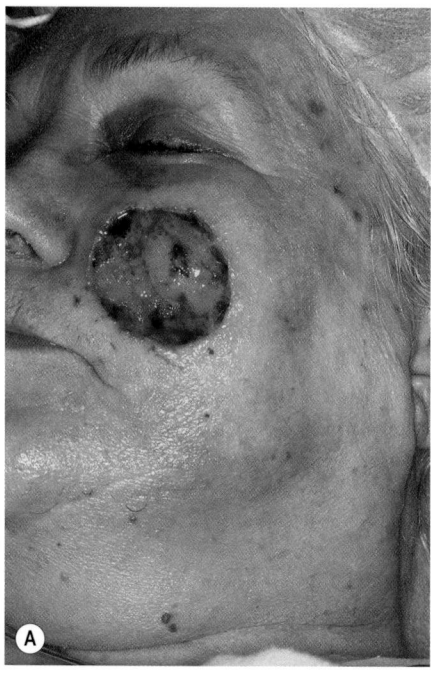
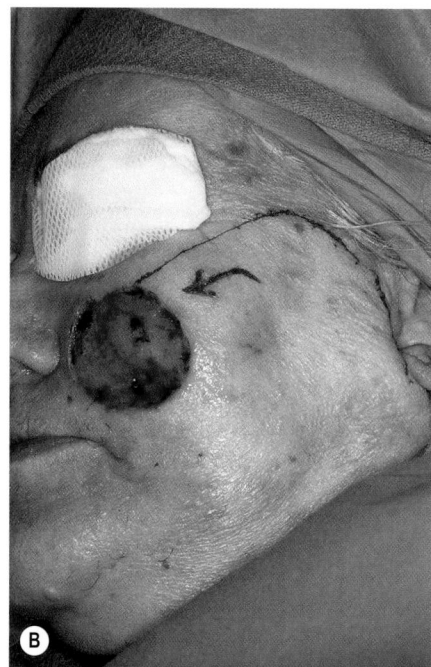
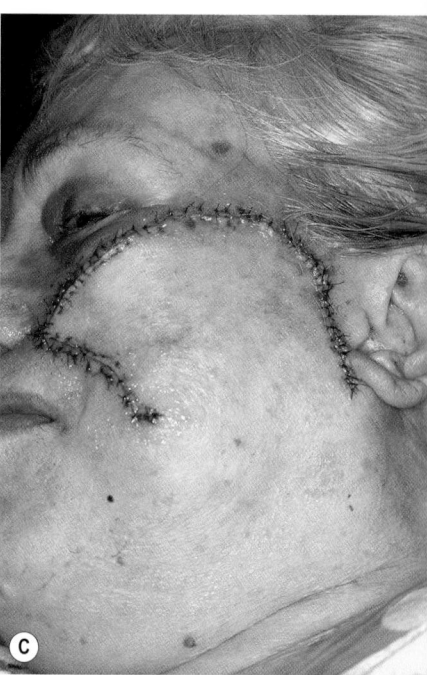

Fig. 18.23 Cheek rotation flap to close cheek defect. **(A)** 3×3 cm skin defect of medial cheek. **(B)** Rotation flap designed for repair. **(C)** Flap in place. Standing cutaneous deformity excised parallel to melolabial crease. (Courtesy of Shaun R. Baker MD.)

flap again with excision of Burow's triangles is used to reconstruct the cheek *(Fig. 18.24)*.

Transposition

A transposition flap is elevated from a nearby area and moved to close a defect while the base of the flap remains intact. Geometric flap planning is required. The rhomboid flap is an ideal example. The lesion is resected in a rhomboid design. Before this reconstruction, it is necessary to determine the location of excess skin by pinching the area between the thumb and index finger and determining the location of a 120° angle opposite this. The flap can then be taken from the area with the most available skin. The flap is rhomboid and should fit perfectly into the defect. As the flap is fitted into the defect, the donor site becomes significantly reduced. Because the design has corners, pincushioning rarely, if ever, occurs. The donor site can be closed directly *(Fig. 18.1)*. Any excess skin is resected.

Finger flap

The finger flap is similar to the rhomboid flap with removal of the corners, although it is usually longer and narrower *(Fig. 18.7)*. This flap is easy to design and use, but there tends to be shortening of the scar around its oval edge. The flap becomes elevated within the scar and forms a surface irregularity, referred to as an island or pincushion. Because the cosmetic result is not optimal, it is not advisable to use this flap for facial reconstruction.

Island flap

This technique can be used for advancement or transposition, but it must be employed with care because of the tendency to pincushion. It is similar to the flaps mentioned previously without the skin pedicle. The island flaps tend to be round or triangular; the triangular flap is less likely to pincushion. It is better to keep the dermis intact, but unfortunately, this is not always possible. The advantage of this variety of flap is that it is a one-stage procedure, and it is probably more flexible than the conventional flap. On the other hand, if care is not taken, these flaps can be devascularized more easily than standard pedicled flaps. This can occur by traction on or twisting of the pedicle or because of a tunnel that is too narrow and constricts the pedicle, compromising flap survival *(Fig. 18.9)*.

Large cheek defects

When large areas of the cheek require resection, it is possible to elevate the inferior skin of the cheek and neck.

This large amount of skin can be moved upward and medially, a combination of advancement and rotation. Such a flap will allow significant defects to be closed with the correct skin match and more importantly, it is tension-free. The scar can be hidden in the pre-auricular and pre-hairline area. The results from this technique can be excellent. It may be necessary to remove a lateral triangle of excess skin that results from the rotation *(Figs 18.23, 18.24)*. Care must also be taken when reconstructing defects in the male face. If possible,

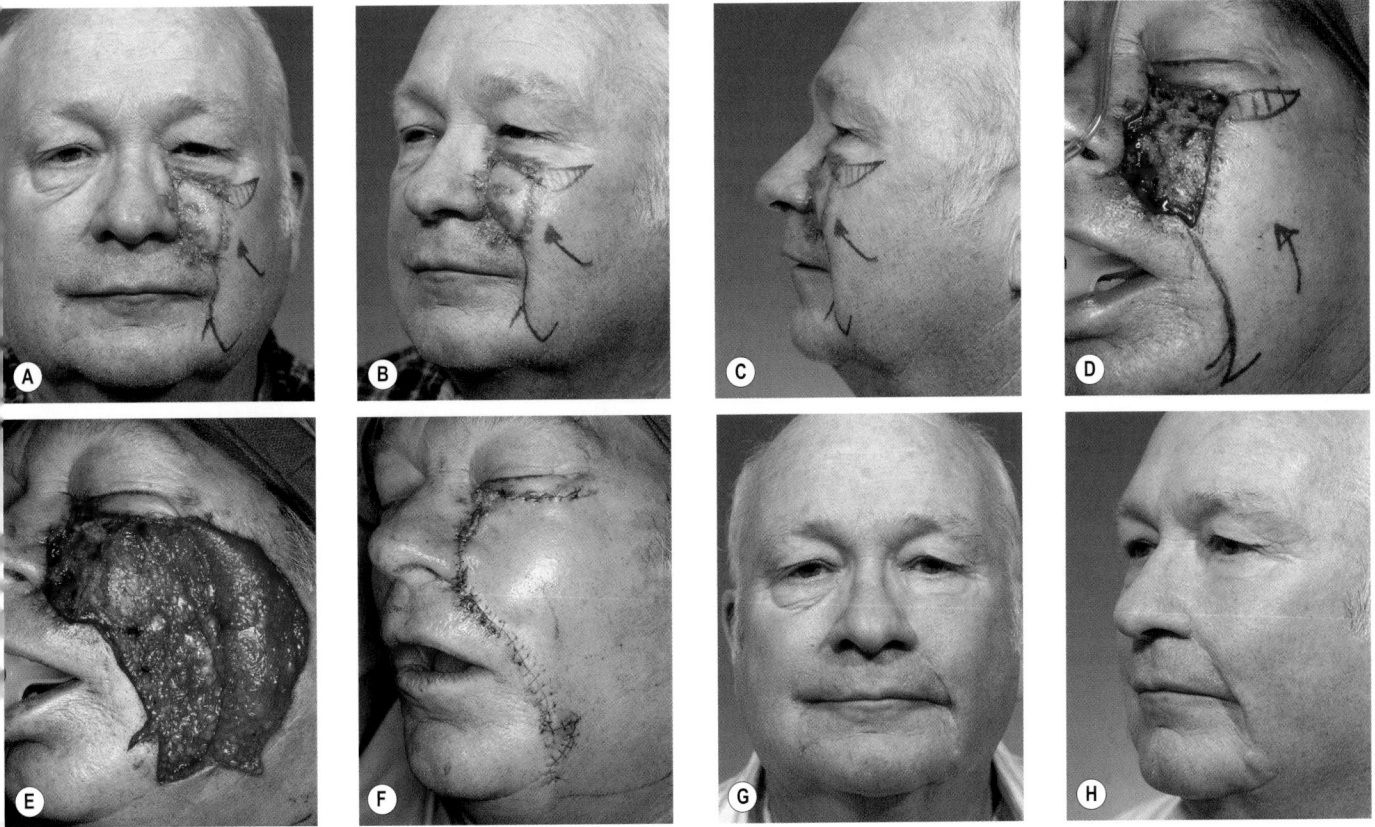

Fig. 18.24 (A–C) Melanoma *in situ* of medial cheek; 5×3 cm area marked for excision using square technique to ensure tumor-free margins. **(D–F)** Pivotal advancement flap designed for repair of defect following resection of lesion. Anticipated standing cutaneous deformity marked with vertical lines. Z-plasty designed at base of flap to eliminate need for equalizing Burow's triangle. **(G,H)** Melanoma excised, flap settled in position to give a good result. (Courtesy of Shaun R. Baker MD.)

hair-bearing skin should not be placed in the non hair bearing areas of the face.

Lips

The upper lip and lower lip must be considered individually because the methods used for reconstruction are not always applicable to both locations. (Further discussion on lip reconstruction can be found in Chapter 10 of this Volume.)

Upper lip

The Cupid's bow, the central mucosal excess, the position of the base of the nose, and the oral commissure are the areas to be considered in upper lip reconstruction. Any method that compromises the symmetry of these areas is not satisfactory. Unfortunately, when the defect is large, an optimal result may not be obtainable. (These techniques are discussed in more detail in Chapter 10 of this volume.)

Direct closure

Direct closure is used whenever possible, but care should be taken to realign the mucocutaneous margin and the white roll. In some instances, to prevent a notch on the free margin, a mucosal Z-plasty may be employed. This must be done with care. Dry (external) mucosa should be extraoral, and wet (internal) mucosa should be intraoral. If wet mucosa is exposed, it will be obvious because it is red and shiny and tends to crust when dry. The Cupid's bow is an important aesthetic area and should always be managed with great care. Its symmetry should not be compromised unless this is unavoidable. In full-thickness defects, accurate muscle reconstruction is mandatory to ensure symmetrical upper lip function.

Lateral and central defects can be closed directly, but judgment must be used. Any degree of asymmetry should be minimal. Orbicularis oris repair has previously been, to some extent, a neglected region. The muscle must be dissected out from the mucosa and the skin; the muscle topography is then examined and reconstructed with accuracy. Every measure should be taken to prevent examination and/or scanning. Magnification helps greatly and should always be used. In lip repair, there should be equal emphasis on aesthetics and function.

Larger defects

In the lateral and central areas of the upper lip, the perialar crescentic flap can be used (see Fig. 10.6). To allow the lip to advance without tension, a crescent of skin and deep subcutaneous tissue is removed from around the lateral area of the alar base by careful layered closure. It is important to construct the lower part of the crescent end at the alar base. This maintains the correct vertical height of the lip. In addition, the mucosa is incised transversely in the upper buccal sulcus. A fringe of mucosa should be left on the alveolus for accurate closure. This allows the whole lip segment to move medially, and large closure can be performed without tension. When there are large midline defects, these can sometimes be closed with bilateral perialar crescentic advancement flaps. The problem with this reconstruction is that it may result in a tight lip. In addition, the Cupid's bow may, more than likely, be compromised but this is unavoidable and further surgery may be required, as indicated.

Abbé flap

Traditionally, the Abbé flap was a full thickness V-shaped portion of the lower lip, which was taken up to expand the upper lip transversely.[18] Frequently, this was used to provide transverse release of the poorly repaired cleft lip. The labial vessels provide the blood supply. The upper lip is released by a vertical incision and the V-shaped defect of the upper lip is reconstructed using the Abbé flap. The lower lip vessel is then divided at 2–3 weeks. Although this gives nice release of the upper lip and provides bulk, there is a tendency to have a convexity bilaterally on either side of the flap and there tends also to be more movement in the lateral segments of the upper lip, with little or no movement of the flap.

In order to prevent these problems and to create a mobile upper lip which would give a more satisfactory result aesthetically and functionally, the author decided to change the design of the Abbé flap. The plan was to incise the flap anteriorly on the lower lip skin and posteriorly on the mucosa. On one side of the flap the incision is taken from the buccal sulcus over the lip mucosa and on to the skin. The lower lip muscles are dissected out leaving the mucosa and skin free of attachments. At this point, the muscles of the lower lip are intact and the mucosa and skin are sutured. In the upper lip, an incision is made and the orbicularis muscles are dissected out so that they can be freed and joined in the midline. This muscle dissection is extensive so that the muscles can be interdigitated in the midline. Care is taken not to disturb any nerves. This having been done, the lip dimensions are now satisfactory in terms of lip height and muscle bulk. The lower lip segment is now swung up into the upper lip defect and is sutured in position. Because of the very narrow pedicle, it is possible to have the flap placed in exactly the required position. This is almost like a full thickness graft of the skin and mucosa and therefore the division of the supplying vessel can be carried out in 2–5 days, although five is most frequent. This is significantly earlier than the conventional flap.[19] This flap is applicable to the cleft patient, particularly for the secondary bilateral cleft lip deformity.

At the second-stage procedure, it is necessary to rearrange the mucocutaneous junction with additional trimming of the flap. If the flap described above can be used, the lower lip muscle is left intact and the upper lip muscle is reconstructed. This results in good function of both lips in most cases.

Fan flaps

Fan flaps can be used for hemilip or total upper lip defects. These defects may be skin only or a full-thickness lip defect. Fan flaps can be standard or full thickness and are based on the perioral vasculature. The commissures are maintained and the flaps are rotated around them; thus, the anatomy of the mouth is maintained. However, fan flaps yield a much better result on the lower lip. This type of reconstruction has largely been overtaken by the perialar crescentic advancement flap.

Lower lip

In the lower lip, skin defects can be reconstructed with nasolabial flaps. These can be transferred as a two-stage procedure or in one stage, as island flaps. Pincushioning is a problem regardless of whether the flaps are round or square.

Full-thickness defects

In the lower lip, as opposed to the upper lip, larger defects can be closed directly because of the greater lip laxity. The closure should be performed in a careful, layered fashion in the following order: mucosa, muscle, and skin.

Karapandzic technique

By use of the Karapandzic technique, three-quarters of the lower lip can be reconstructed without difficulty (**Fig. 18.25**).[20] It has some resemblance to the perialar crescentic advancement flap, but it is a superior method. The reconstruction should replace the full thickness and depth of the lip. The skin is incised in a transverse direction to just beyond the nasolabial fold. Laterally, the vessels and nerves are dissected out and carefully preserved. The orbicularis muscle fibers are spread apart as far laterally as necessary. After this, it should be possible to move the leading edge to the midline or beyond, if necessary. It is best to use bilateral flaps and to perform a layered closure where they meet. In this way, a loose and symmetric lip is obtained, and the blood and nerve supply are maintained. Also, a properly functioning lip with a virtually normal anatomy is formed. The scars settle well and are acceptable from a cosmetic viewpoint.

Gillies fan flap

Until the Karapandzic procedure was published, the Gillies fan flap was considered to be the method of choice.[21] Full-thickness nasolabial flaps based on the labial vessels are swung around the commissure into the lower lip defect. These flaps can be unilateral or bilateral.

Comparison between Karapandzic and Gillies techniques

In the Karapandzic technique, the commissures are maintained and the width of the commissure is satisfactory. There is no need to supply lower lip mucosa. The flaps are neurotized and results in good lower lid function and sensation. In the Gillies reconstruction, the mouth is narrowed, and there is no mucosal cover of the flaps at the lip margin. Mucosal cover is supplied by advancing intraoral mucosa. Unfortunately, mucosa from this area is always red and shiny, and frequently has a tendency to crust when exposed to the air. The nerves are not kept intact, thus lip function and sensation are compromised. In spite of this, the function may be better than expected, especially in hemilip reconstruction.

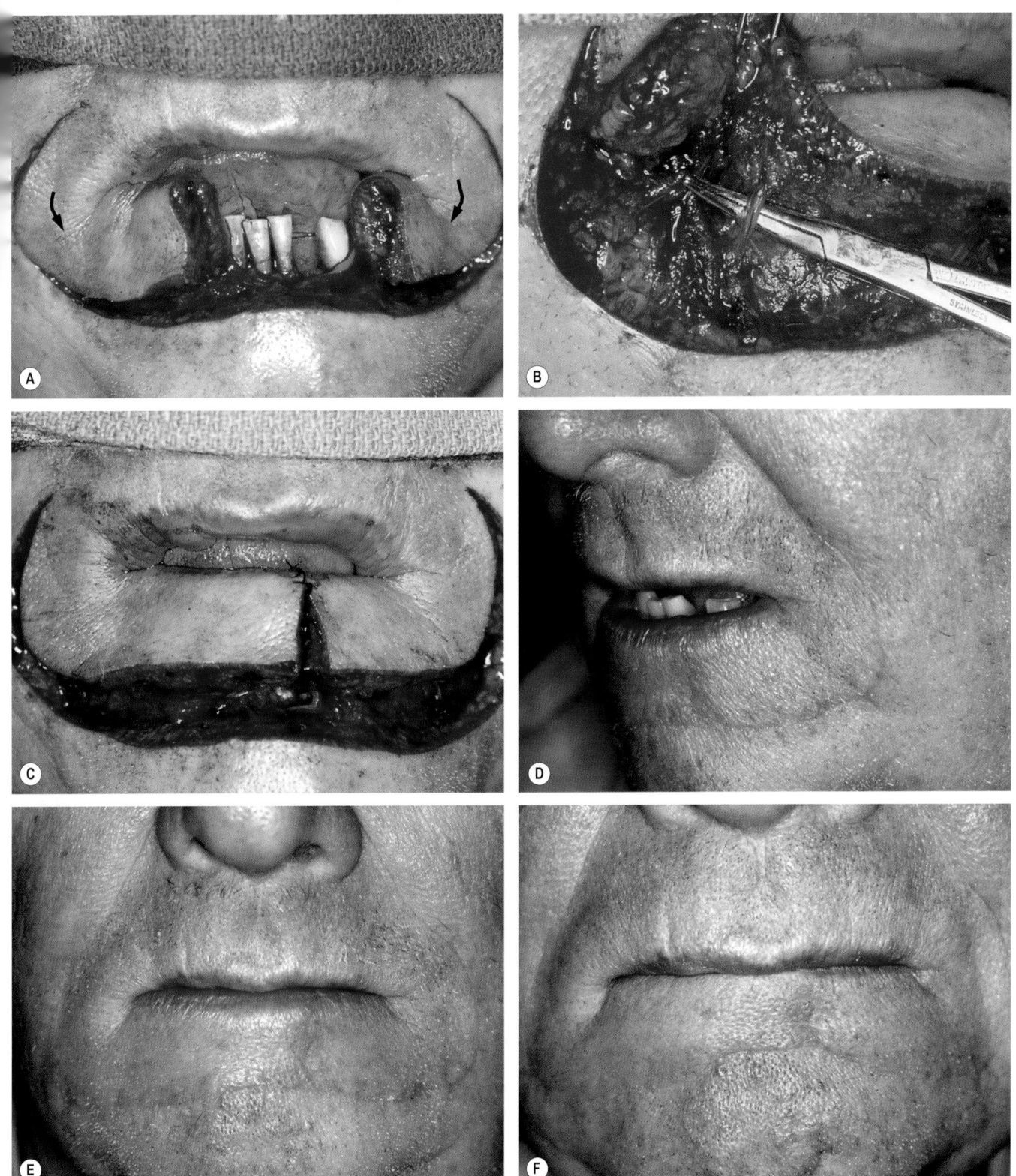

Fig. 18.25 Reconstruction of partial defect of lower lip with Karapandzic rotation–advancement flaps. **(A)** Full thickness defect of the lower lip. Bilateral Karapandzic flaps incised. **(B)** Demonstration of vessels preserved with "Karapandzic" technique of dissection. Compared to central lip, identification of peripheral margin of orbicularis muscle in the vicinity of commissures is more difficult. Releasing facial muscular attachments to orbicularis muscle may be performed lateral to actual peripheral margin of orbicularis muscle near commissures to insure consistency of thickness of muscular layer of flaps **(C)** Flaps approximated. **(D,E)** 6 months' postoperative. For proper lip height, flaps are designed with uniform width throughout length of flaps. For this reason, it is necessary to design flaps lateral to melolabial crease near commissure. **(F)** 1 year postoperative. Reconstructed lip has tightened, resulting from scar contraction. Such long-term changes are common. (From Renner G. Reconstruction of the lip. In: Baker SR, Swanson NA, eds. *Local flaps in facial reconstruction*. St. Louis: Mosby; 1995:368, with permission.)

Tongue flaps

Tongue flaps can be used to replace the lip red margin in reconstructions that do not supply the required amount of mucosa. Tongue flaps are also used in patients with advanced and extensive leukoplakial involvement of the lip mucosa. The traditional method is to use the dorsum of the tongue, but its color and surface irregularity make it aesthetically unsuitable as a lip mucosal substitute.

The undersurface of the tongue mucosa is smooth, may have good color, and can easily be transferred in a staged procedure *(Fig. 18.26)*. ⊛ FIG **18.26** APPEARS ONLINE ONLY

The flap is based anteriorly. It should be of a sufficient length and width. It is sutured into the lip defect. In 10 days, under local anesthesia, the flap is divided and inset. The tongue defect is closed directly. The mucosa tends to be a deeper shade of red and shinier than normal tongue mucosa. Crusting may occur and may require frequent application of petroleum jelly. Sensation is reduced as with any free transplant on the lip.

Total lower lip reconstruction

The Karapandzic technique can be used for total lower lip reconstruction, but the reconstructed lip is frequently too tight. The method of choice is bilateral fan flaps with resurfacing of the red lip with a flap from the undersurface of the tongue.[22] The Webster advancement technique, in which bilateral full-thickness horizontal advancement cheek flaps can be brought into place by excision of bilateral upper and lower vertical triangles at their bases, is another possibility. The mucosa is again supplied from the undersurface of the tongue. The scars in the nasolabial lines and around the chin heal well. The main problem is that the reconstructed lip is flat and tight and tends to trap-door. On occasion, two Abbé flaps from either side of the prolabial segment of the lip can be turned down to increase lip volume, but the end result is not particularly satisfactory from a cosmetic point of view. Function (e.g., drooling) may be improved to a variable degree. Not infrequently, free tissue transfer will be required to reconstruct a total lip defect. Discussion on this topic can be found in Chapter 10 of this Volume.

Commissure reconstruction

The commissure mucosa occasionally requires reconstruction. When analyzed, this can be divided into two rhomboids, one for each lip. Rhomboid flaps from the intraoral cheek area can resurface the defects without difficulty, and the donor sites can be closed directly. However, this is wet mucosa and is redder than the normal lip. Another method for larger defects (e.g., electrical burns) is to develop a large triangular mucosal island flap, advance its base to the commissure, and then use the considerable amount of tissue obtained as required. The donor site is closed directly. Later rearrangement of the mucosa is always required, but fortunately a sufficient supply is available after the procedure.

Finally, in some instances, lateral tongue flaps can be used to cover the upper and lower lip region at the commissure. These are divided after 10 days. These flaps are not widely used because anteriorly-based mucosal flaps have proved to be more satisfactory in terms of position and patient comfort.

Ear

The areas of the ear most often requiring excision and reconstruction are the rim and the conchal area. (Further material on ear reconstruction can be found in Chapter 7 in this Volume.)

Rim defects

It is frequently possible to excise a rim lesion and advance the rim by incising full thickness down to the lobule. There is no residual defect with this method *(Fig. 18.27)*. If there is concern about the viability of the tip of this flap or if the defect is larger, the posterior skin is dissected up and may be included into the rim. A larger flap with a large base has a better blood supply and is more likely to survive. It does not result in any ear deformity. In some instances, superior and inferior rim flaps will be used in conjunction with one another. Even larger defects are better reconstructed by postauricular flaps *(Fig. 18.28)*. The flap is elevated and sutured to the anterior edge

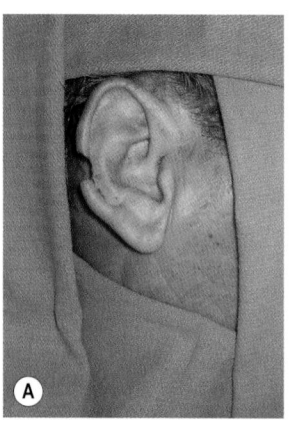 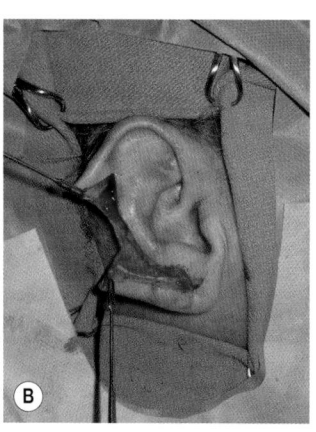 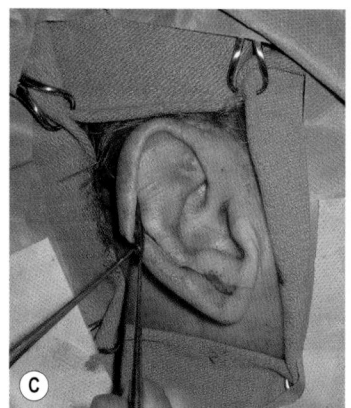 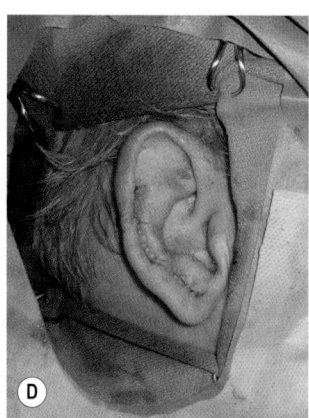

Fig. 18.27 (A) Helical defect following resection of a basal cell carcinoma. **(B)** Helical flaps are raised based on the posterior skin. **(C)** Flaps are dissected until advancement and closure without tension is possible. **(D)** Final appearance following closure. (Courtesy of Dr David Mathes.)

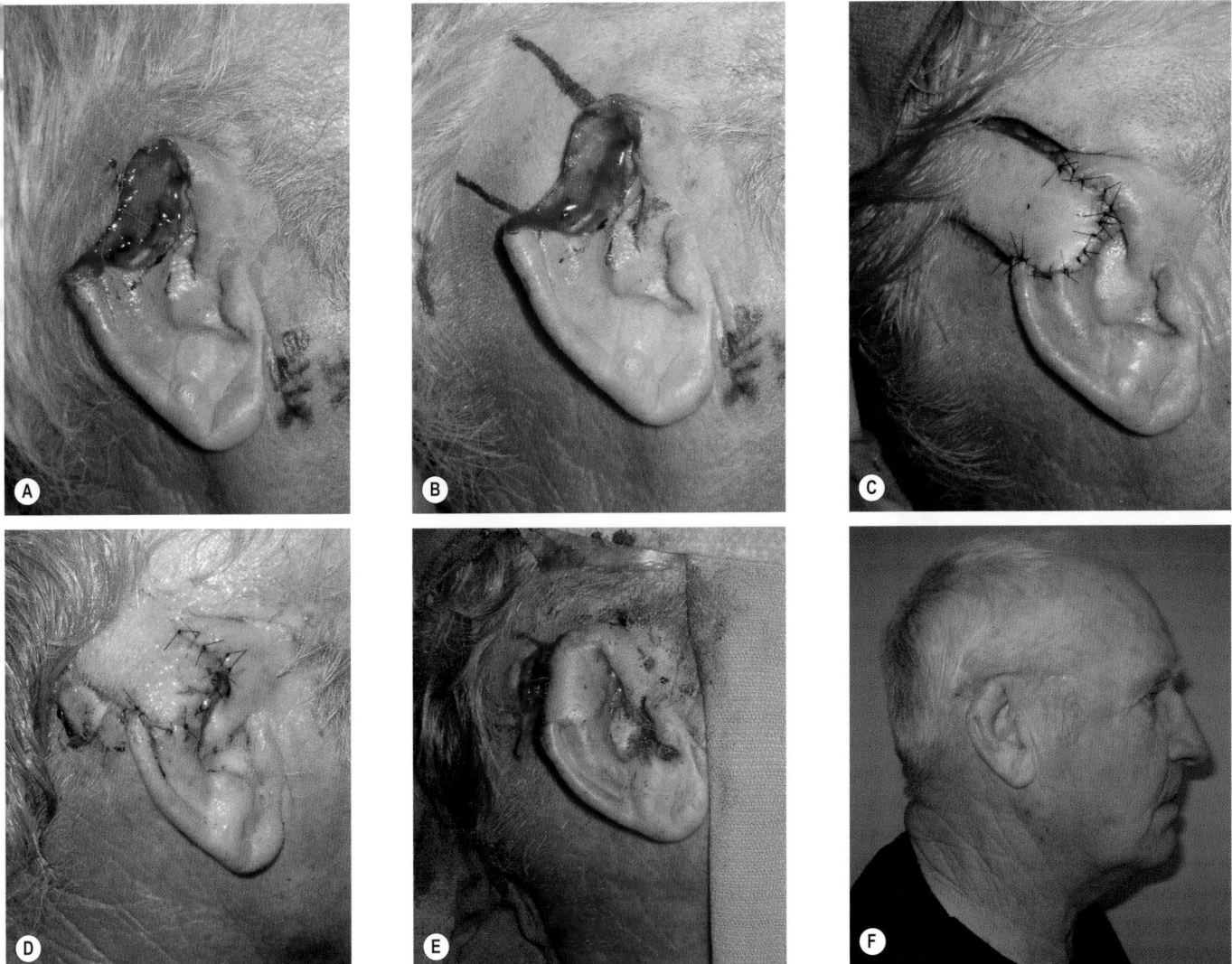

Fig. 18.28 **(A)** Defect of upper ear after resection of squamous cell carcinoma. **(B)** Post-auricular flap is designed, **(C)** raised and inset into defect. **(D)** Appearance prior to pedicle division and **(E)** following pedicle division. The intervening defect is skin grafted most easily with a post-auricular graft harvested more inferiorly than the defect and closed directly. **(F)** Late appearance. (Courtesy of Dr David Mathes.)

of the defect. After 3 weeks, a large flap is incised in the postauricular area, dissected up to provide laxity, and brought to the ear rim to provide more tissue. It is trimmed as necessary and sutured in place. Deep sutures can help in forming the shape as required. Further adjustments will most likely be necessary following on healing.

Anterior concha

If a lesion of significant size occurs in the anterior concha, resurfacing will be required. To achieve this, the lesion is resected together with the underlying conchal cartilage. The ear is then distracted forward, and a flap is designed with a central vertical pedicle based on the ear mastoid groove. The skin anterior and posterior to the groove is elevated, with some division of the subcutaneous hinge superiorly and inferiorly, it can be rotated into the ear defect. The posterior edge of the postauricular island is sutured to the posterior edge of

the defect, and the anterior edge of the island is sutured to the anterior edge of the defect. The posterior defect is closed directly. This will give an excellent result both on the anterior aspect of the concha and in the postauricular groove *(Fig. 18.29)*.[23]

In a large degloving of the ear, a temporal fascial flap is used to cover the defect. The flap is then covered with a full-thickness skin graft. This is a rare injury, but this technique can also be used in reconstruction of the congenitally absent ear. The end result is suboptimal because of the poor color of the skin graft. It may also have a shiny surface, especially if a split-thickness graft is used.

Skin expansion

Skin expansion for facial coverage is somewhat limited because it requires time for the expansion to be achieved. In

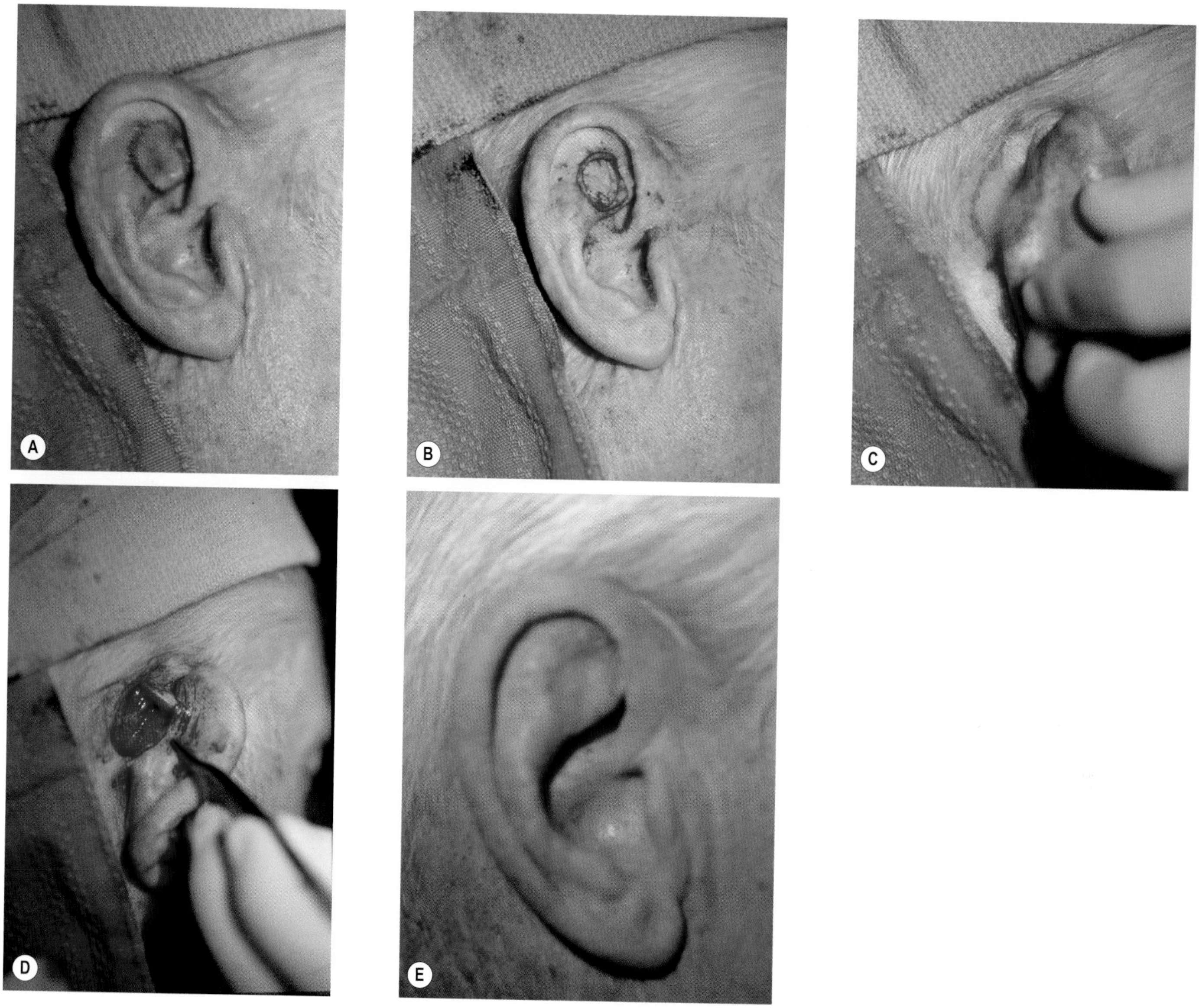

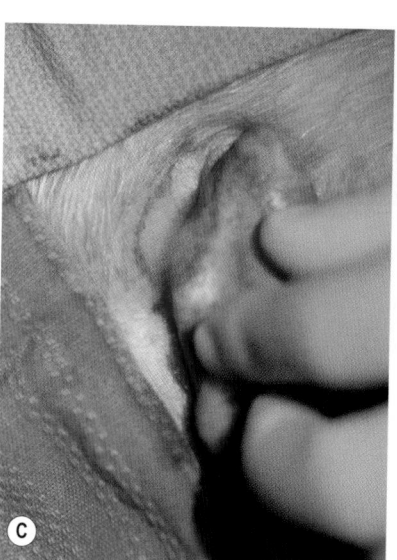

Fig. 18.29 **(A)** A 72-year-old man with a basal cell in the upper ear, marked for excision. **(B)** Defect includes anterior skin and underlying cartilage. **(C)** Post-auricular, superiorly based flap outlined. **(D)** Flap raised and tunneled into anterior defect. Small segment of flap is de-epithelialized and secondary defect is closed directly. **(E)** Final appearance of healed flap. (Courtesy of Dr Peter Neligan.)

some instances, immediate reconstruction may be required. In addition, the process of skin expansion is often uncomfortable and undesirable to the patient. However, if the time is available and only extra skin is required to reconstruct a defect, it is a good idea to gain some extra skin by this technique. The author favors expansion by use of external ports with inflation performed by the patient or relatives. This method leads to safe, efficient, and relatively comfortable expansion, particularly in children. This technique is especially useful when large amounts of skin are necessary *(Fig. 18.4).*[24]

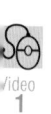

Perforator flaps in the face

Apart from the use of perforator free flaps for reconstruction of large defects in the head and neck, local perforator flaps have added to our choice of reconstructive options, particularly in the peri-oral region.[25] If one passes a Doppler probe along the course of the facial artery, one can appreciate crescendos of noise along the path of the artery. These represent perforators that supply the skin, arising in the facial artery and travelling vertically upward towards the skin. Flaps can be designed based on these perforators and used to reconstruct small defects. This technique is depicted in the video that accompanies this chapter. The perforator is identified, an exploratory incision is made along one side of the proposed flap in order to identify the perforator. A hand held Doppler is used to ascertain that the artery is open and that it remains open after rotation of the flap. This is the propeller principle, in which the flap is rotated through 180° on the perforator. This causes the perforator to twist. If the perforator is not adequately dissected, the surrounding soft tissue can cause constriction. Using the Doppler to check the artery provides a significant safety net.

Another newer flap that is extremely useful in reconstruction of the lower face and lips is the submental flap.[26] This flap is based on the submental branch of the facial artery that supplies perforators to the overlying skin. These perforators run alongside the anterior belly of the digastric muscle that can be harvested with the flap. This flap provides excellent color and texture match for the lower face, with the added advantage that the donor site is hidden under the chin where the patient cannot see it.

Conclusion

The use of facial tissue to close facial defects requires experience, artistry, and knowledge of skin biomechanics. The ability to close defects, large and small, and to produce cosmetically acceptable results is one of the great challenges of plastic surgery. It is important that plastic surgeons equip themselves with the knowledge and techniques required to meet this challenge and to provide patients with optimal functional and aesthetic results.

Bonus images for this chapter can be found online at http://www.expertconsult.com

Fig. 18.13 (E) Preoperative markings indicate the upper eyelid area to be resected. **(F)** The total upper eyelid is resected; the lower eyelid will be rotated up to reconstruct the upper eyelid with use of a medial pedicle. **(G)** The medial pedicle is divided, and the medial end of the lower lid is inset into the defect of the medial side of the upper lid. **(H,I)** A nasal septal chondromucosal graft is placed in position, and the cartilage is scored to make it bend as favorably as possible. A lateral cheek rotation flap is performed. Note the lateral Z-plasty to give as much medial movement as possible. This will give a good end result.

Fig. 18.14 Reconstruction of left lower eyelid with conchal-perichondrial graft and cheek advancement flap. This patient presented with a squamous cell carcinoma of the left lower eyelid with neck node involvement. **(A)** Skin operative plan drawn out. **(B)** After excision of lower eyelid and modified radical neck dissection with preservation of facial nerve. The lower eyelid is reconstructed with conchal cartilage with perichondrium facing toward the globe. **(C,D)** Advancement of cheek flap to reconstruct the lower eyelid. **(E)** Long-term result.

Fig. 18.15 Reconstruction of partial upper eyelid defect with advancement flap. **(A)** Basal cell carcinoma involving medial end of upper eyelid. **(B)** Operative plan of excision and rotation and advancement of the upper lid. **(C)** Excision of upper lid basal cell carcinoma. Note spoon to protect eye and the use of sharp pointed scissors to resect the lid. **(D)** Defect after excision of medial portion of the upper eyelid. **(E)** Lateral canthotomy performed superiorly. The lid is advanced with lateral Z-plasty in the temporal region. **(F)** End result.

Fig. 18.16 Coloboma of the upper eyelid – Abbé flap. **(A–C)** The defect can be seen, and the planned Abbé flap from the lower to the upper eyelid is outlined and shown in diagrammatic form. **(D)** The flap is in position. **(E)** The patient can close his eyelid satisfactorily.

Fig. 18.17 Reconstruction of upper and lower eyelid defect with a forehead flap after resection of medial canthal and upper and lower eyelid basal cell carcinoma. **(A)** Extent of the lesion can be seen. **(B)** The planned excision and the planned reconstruction with a forehead flap for the upper and lower lids and the medial canthal area. **(C)** Excision completed. Note large defect of upper and lower

eyelids, medial canthal area, and nasal area. **(D)** Reconstruction with a forehead flap. **(E)** Forehead flap sitting well in position. Reconstruction is performed by trimming of the forehead flap, harvesting of a chondromucosal flap from the septum, and elevating a cheek flap. **(F,G)** Cheek flap advanced and sutured into position. The eye has now been opened up. **(H,I)** Reconstruction complete. **(J)** Closure of lids. **(K)** Opening of lids.

Fig. 18.18 Total reconstruction of upper eyelid by a prefabricated composite forehead flap. **(A)** The preoperative appearance with no upper eyelid whatsoever. The lower eyelid is intact. **(B)** An upper eyelid is delayed vertically on the forehead with a bucket being designed under the forehead skin and subcutaneous tissue. **(C)** A mucosal graft is harvested, and holes are made in it to stretch it. **(D)** The mucosal graft is placed, mucosal side down, into the pocket in the center of the forehead with a small pack. Sutures are holding the mucosa in position. **(E)** Upper eyelid is released as much as possible. **(F)** Upper eyelid reconstruction being brought down to reconstruct the upper lid. Note the mucosa on the undersurface of the flap. **(G)** The lid is inset. **(H)** The lid reconstruction is complete and ready for levator muscle repositioning.

Fig. 18.19 Reconstruction of medial canthal area with island flap. **(A)** Basal cell carcinoma of the medial canthus. **(B)** Resection and proposed reconstruction outlined. **(C)** Island flap to reconstruct the medial canthal area together with transposition flap. **(D)** End result.

Fig. 18.20 Reconstruction of the medial canthal area and lid defects with forehead flaps. **(A)** Extensive basal cell carcinoma of left medial canthus. **(B)** Midline forehead flap elevated to reconstruct large post-resection defect of upper and lower lids, medial canthal area, and nose. **(C)** End result.

Fig. 18.21 Right forehead flap to medial canthus and lower lid defect. **(A)** Penetrating basal cell carcinoma. **(B)** Planned excision and tailored forehead flap. **(C)** Excision completed and flap in place. **(D)** End result.

Fig. 18.26 Resurfacing of the lower lip with a tongue flap. **(A)** Vascular malformation of the lower lip. **(B)** Tongue flap planned from undersurface of tongue. **(C)** Flap sutured to lip following resection of the malformation. **(D)** Result after 2 years.

Access the complete references list online at http://www.expertconsult.com

3. Jackson IT. *Local flaps in head and neck reconstruction*, 2nd ed. St. Louis: Quality Medical; 2007.

4. Limberg AA. The planning of local plastic operations on the body surface: theory and practice. In: Wolfe SA, (ed) trans. *Planirovanie mestnoplasticheskikh operatsiina poverkhnosti tela, 1906*. Lexington MA: Collamore Press; 1984.

7. McGregor JC, Soutar DS. A critical assessment of the bilobed flap. *Br J Plast Surg*. 1981;34:197–205.

13. McGregor IA. Eyelid reconstruction following subtotal resection of the upper or lower lid. *Br J Plast Surg*. 1973;26:346–354.

14. Mustardé JC. Eyelid repairs with costochondral grafts. *Plast Reconstr Surg*. 1962;30:267–272.

20. Karapandzic M. Reconstruction of lip defects by local arterial flaps. *Br J Plast Surg*. 1974;27:93–97.

In this classic paper, Dr Karapandzic describes the procedure which allows for preservation of the neurovascular bundles of the orbicularis oris in order to reconstruct defects of the lips. *This classic description focuses on reconstruction of lower lip defects.*

22. Jackson IT. Use of tongue flaps to resurface lip defects and close palatal fistulae in children. *Plast Reconstr Surg.* 1972;49:537–541.

This paper describes the technique of using an anterior tongue flap to reconstruct the vermillion, as well as more extensive lip defects. It also describes the use of the tongue flap for repair of palatal fistulae. In dentate patients, it is particularly important to ensure that precautions are taken to prevent the patient from biting the flap.

24. Keskin M, Kelly CP, Yavuzer R, et al. External filling ports in tissue expansion: confirming their safety and convenience. *Plast Reconstr Surg.* 2006;117(5):1543–1551.

25. Hofer SO, Posch NA, Smit X. The facial artery perforator flap for reconstruction of perioral defects. *Plast Reconstr Surg.* 2005;115(4):996–1003.

The concept of the facial artery perforator flap is discussed in a study of five clinical cases. The article concludes that this is a versatile flap due to a large arc of rotation and an aesthetically pleasing donor site. It is an ideal flap for one-stage reconstruction without secondary revisions.

26. Curran AJ, Neligan P, Gullane PJ. Submental artery island flap. *Laryngoscope.* 1997;107(11):1545–1549.

This paper describes the anatomy of the submental artery perforator flap. The artery is a branch of the facial artery. The perforators run alongside the anterior belly of digastric, which is harvested with the flap. Two cases are presented of lower face reconstruction using the submental flap.

19

Secondary facial reconstruction

Julian J. Pribaz and Rodney K. Chan

SYNOPSIS

- Secondary revision is an inevitable and indispensable part of facial reconstruction.
- An accurate diagnosis of the missing parts is as important in secondary reconstructions as during the primary reconstruction.
- A comprehensive reconstructive plan is needed from the start, including bailout strategies.

 Access the Historical Perspective section online at
http://www.expertconsult.com

Introduction

The goal of any reconstruction is to restore to normal, or as close to normal, form and function. This could only be completely achieved by replantation or in the future transplantation. All of our current reconstructive methods will always fall short of the ideal due to specific tissue characteristics. Hence the need for secondary, tertiary, or in fact multiple revisional procedures to achieve the best possible functional and aesthetic result. Indeed, the meaning of the word *plastic*, which is derived from the Greek *plastikos*, means to make or mold.

This chapter will address the principles and techniques utilized to enhance the final result of the initial primary reconstructive procedure. The sequence of reconstruction and timing in the application of these different techniques should be guided by basic principles. A well-thought-out reconstructive path is needed from the start so as not to "burn any bridges." Secondary facial reconstructions can be broadly separated into: (1) those that were part of the initial reconstructive plan; and (2) those that were unplanned and which may present to a different surgeon as a challenging case.

Basic science/disease process

Secondary facial reconstruction assumes a previous operative procedure, the cause of which in the head and neck may have a wide range of etiologies, from congenital malformations to various types of trauma, including burns, ballistic injuries, motor vehicle accidents, and animal bites. Tumors involving both bone and soft tissues, and infections may also have been the culprit. Each one of these etiologies has its own unique consequences.

Tissues may have been lost, displaced, or distorted. Both bone and soft tissues may have been involved. A common feature of all these etiologies is that along the way wounds were created and treated. These may have been simple and superficial but more likely, deep and complex. Healing may have been facilitated by primary or secondary closure, or involved a prior operative procedure utilizing tissue locally or afar. It should be remembered that there is renewed swelling and scarring at each interface, and that this occurs with each operative procedure, which in turn makes the outcome after each procedure somewhat unpredictable. It is usual and safe practice to allow the patient and the involved tissue to heal, the swelling to subside, and the scarring to mature before embarking on secondary and tertiary reoperative procedures.

Diagnosis/patient presentation

An accurate diagnosis of the deformity and an appraisal of the missing parts are essential. The deformity is compared with what is considered to be the "perceived normal." If the deficit is unilateral, the best guide is a comparison with the opposite side. With more extensive defects where both sides are involved, a consideration of baseline appearance as seen on an old photograph may serve as a guide to reconstruction. However, realistic goals must be set from the start as to what might be achievable with reconstruction.

An evaluation for secondary facial reconstruction begins with a thorough investigation into the history of the patient, in particular the operations and flaps that were previously utilized, paying close attention to the remaining donor vessels in the head and neck.[2] Next, an accurate diagnosis of the missing parts has to be made. While it is generally obvious what the missing parts are for a primary reconstruction that immediately follows extirpation, it is less obvious in secondary reconstructions where tissues have been pulled closed or healed secondarily. It takes an astute plastic surgeon to visualize what constitutes adequate contracture release and the resulting defect. This attention to making the correct comprehensive diagnosis is especially important when evaluating a patient whose primary reconstruction was performed elsewhere. Subsequent revisions are individualized and dictated by the area and underlying cause that required reconstruction. Therefore, a surgeon who specializes in secondary facial reconstructions needs to be well versed in all rungs of the reconstructive ladder, especially when many first-line options have already been utilized.

Patient selection

Facial defects and deformities should be evaluated in a systematic manner, starting from:

1. Overall magnitude and extent of the deformity and its anatomical location.
2. Displacement of major facial subunits; for example, the eyebrows, eyelids, nose, ear, and lips.
3. The extent of contour distortion.
4. Location and quality of the scarring that is present.
5. The color, texture, and quality of the skin.
6. The presence, absence, and distortion of specialized cutaneous features; for example, the hairline, sideburn, and beard area.
7. The quality of the subcutaneous tissues, volume and distribution.
8. The function or lack thereof of the underlying musculature.
9. The integrity or deformity of the underlying bony or cartilaginous support structures.
10. The status and quality of tissues lining the oral and nasal cavity.
11. The loss of other specialized components such as the lacrimal apparatus, teeth, and an adequate and mobile tongue.

The status of all these elements should first be appraised and a decision made regarding the best method of restoration.

In consideration of secondary reconstruction it is understood that a primary procedure has already been performed. The effectiveness of the first reconstruction has to be evaluated and sometimes it is necessary to advise the complete removal of an inadequate first reconstructive effort, to recreate the defect and start again from scratch. For complex reconstruction, it is ideal to have an expert evaluate the initial presenting problem and develop an appropriate and often-staged treatment plan. No complex facial defect or deformity can be expected to be adequately repaired in a single stage and thus if a staged repair is required, it is necessary to plan a correct sequence of procedures so to avoid "burning future bridges."

Treatment and surgical technique

Meticulous technique and planning should be emphasized at every step of a multistage facial reconstruction, as this makes subsequent operations more predictable. Planning and initial flap tailoring are critical first steps. Radiographs are useful to visualize the missing bony elements. We recommend the liberal use of preoperative and intraoperative models to simulate the missing soft tissues and/or bone in developing the plan.[3] This maneuver at the commencement of an operative procedure allows for tailored flaps to be designed at the most ideal donor site.

In general, the principles that are observed in secondary facial reconstructions are:

1. Restore to their normal location uninjured or partially injured anatomical features.
2. Repair scar contracture and if possible place the scars along the natural crease lines.
3. Restore the contour, which may involve debulking or augmenting soft facial parts with dermis fat grafts or autogenous fat grafting.[4,5]
4. Restoration of contour is more important than the presence of scars.
5. Replace "like with like," thus soft tissues should be replaced with soft tissues, and bony tissues with bone or bone substitutes.
6. Use local flap options with better color and texture match as advancement or transposition flaps to provide better cutaneous coverage of de-epithelialized, previously placed distant free flaps that may have been used.
7. Local specialized flaps, for example, hair-bearing flaps, to reconstruct specific subunits previously covered by large distant flaps are also used to help break up the scars and create an illusion of a more normal appearance.
8. If local flaps are not available to improve the color mismatch of distant flaps, consider the use of thin split-thickness skin grafts harvested from the scalp as overgrafts to resurface these areas after de-epithelialization of the existing flap.[6]
9. Carry out functional restoration of absent muscles of facial expression, especially for restitution of a smile and adequate closure of the eyelids and mouth. The options of free muscle transfer, with and without nerve grafts or local or regional muscle transfers of functioning muscle, can all be considered.
10. Restore adequate bony platform to repair bony contour deformities, or allow for dental rehabilitation with osseointegrated implants.
11. Carry out supplemental prosthetic reconstruction of nonreconstructible parts, for example, orbital and ear prostheses.

A few recurrent themes encountered in complex facial reconstructions are worthy of mention: (1) reconstruction of deficient intraoral and intranasal lining; (2) reconstruction of hair-bearing regions; as well as the use of (3) prefabrication and (4) prelamination as adjunctive techniques.

Intraoral and intranasal lining

Deficiency in intraoral and intranasal lining must be suspected in cases of internal or external perioral contractures, or when the lining is known to have been excised or irradiated.

Deficiency in intraoral lining can manifest as dry mouth, lack of facial movement, or lack of oral competence. Therefore, prior to commencement of any perioral reconstruction, intraoral scars must be fully released and the lining reconstructed. Otherwise, any attempts at external skin replacement will be suboptimal. Replacements of intraoral lining include skin grafts, regional flaps, and distant flaps. While skin graft might appear to be most appealing because of its availability and simplicity, we have not found it to be durable, especially in scarred or irradiated beds. Distant flaps such as anterolateral thigh flaps and radial forearm free flaps are certainly reliable methods of replacing lining. However, in cases of multiple prior operations, those flaps may have already been utilized or may be needed elsewhere. Furthermore donor vessels are usually scarce. The facial artery musculomucosal (FAMM) flap, a composite flap with mucosa and muscle taken from the lateral cheek, should be considered as an option. This is best done at the first operation when wide exposure and easy access to supple mucosa are available. When harvested with the overlying buccinator muscle, this is a robust flap that can cover widths of 2–2.5 cm. It can be based either superiorly (retrograde flow) or inferiorly (antegrade flow) to cover a variety of oronasal mucosal defects, including defects of the palate, alveolus, nasal septum, antrum, upper and lower lips, floor of the mouth, and soft palate *(Fig. 19.1)*.[7]

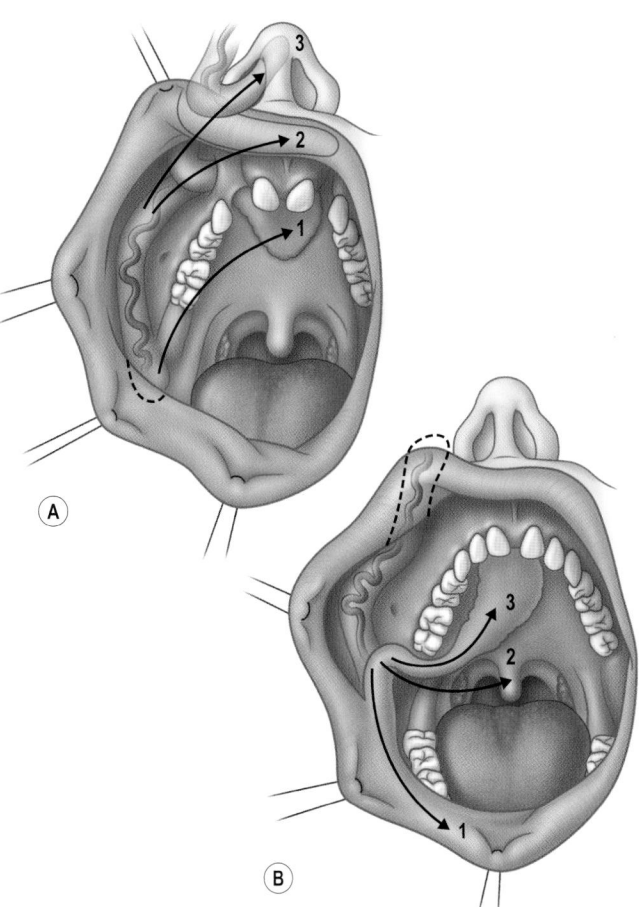

Fig. 19.1 (A) Superiorly based facial artery musculomucosal (FAMM) flap may be used for defects of the anterior palate, alveolus, maxillary antrum, nose, upper lip, and orbit. **(B)** Inferiorly based FAMM flap may be used for defects of the posterior palate, tonsillar fossa, alveolus, floor of mouth, and lower lip.[7]

With larger mucosal defects involving the floor of the mouth, the submental flap based on the submental branch of the facial artery is another useful regional option. Our experience indicates that this flap is generally very reliable with minimal donor site morbidity but should be used with caution if there was prior irradiation. Further it can be easily combined with the need for a neck dissection, though it is imperative to raise the flap and preserve its blood supply prior to commencement of the extirpative procedure.[8]

While vermilion is not strictly speaking intraoral lining, it is a specialized type of tissue that is impossible to reproduce. When vermilion is missing and cannot be borrowed from its neighboring areas, its appearance is much better matched with the use of nonkeratinized mucosa than the use of keratinized skin. In the early days of vermilion reconstruction, jejunal and gastric mucosa were attempted but were fraught with problems. The use of gastric mucosa in particular can be hypersecretory and its acidic contents ulcerogenic. FAMM flap, based superiorly for the upper lip and inferiorly for the lower lip, can give a good match for this specialized tissue.[9] Alternatively, the use of lingual mucosa or tattooing of keratinized skin can also be acceptable.

Hair-bearing flaps

Successful facial reconstructions, especially in males, need to recognize the pattern of hair growth particularly in the sideburn and beard areas in order to maintain symmetry. However, few sites are available as hair-bearing donors. The temporal scalp, frontal scalp, and the submental region can all give satisfactory results.[10] The frontal scalp can be transferred using the supratrochlear artery and the submental region can be transferred on the submental branch of the facial artery, though these areas may not be available. Temporal scalp skin contains an abundance of hair follicles and needs implantation of a heterotopic vessel as a first-stage reconstruction (see prefabrication, below).

Prefabrication

Prefabrication refers to the pretransfer implantation of a nonnative vascular pedicle into the tissue desired for reconstruction. It is used when the tissue desired for reconstruction cannot be practically transferred by alternate means. To optimize aesthetics in facial reconstruction, prefabrication is typically used to hand-pick thin tissues with cutaneous qualities most similar to the predisfigured part. The donor vessel can be any good length of vessel, including its surrounding fatty tissue.[11,12] The radial forearm fascial flap, the temporal parietal fascial flap, and the descending branch of the lateral femoral circumflex pedicles are all reliable donor vessels of good caliber. This is placed under the desired area of transfer and if needed can be placed over a tissue expander. This is an especially useful adjunct in cases of secondary facial reconstructions as first-line donor options are exhausted and new donor options need to be explored. This technique essentially creates a limitless number of donor sites.

Prelamination

Flap prelamination is a term first coined by Pribaz and Fine in 1994, referring to the pretransfer implantation of anything other than a vascular pedicle in the territory of an existing axial vascular bed.[13,14] In aesthetic facial reconstruction, prelamination is often used to assemble composite flaps that can be transferred as a unit that more closely approximates the predisfigured part.[11] Prelamination is a useful adjunct in both primary and secondary facial reconstructions of complex multifaceted defects.

Each of the selected cases of secondary facial reconstructions below demonstrates many of the basic dictums previously described. While secondary reconstructions can be broadly separated into two categories: (1) those that were part of the initial reconstructive plan; and (2) those that were unplanned and usually followed multiple other unsatisfactory reconstructions done elsewhere, it is on the second category that we want to focus. In the cases of secondary reconstructions that follow, we will first demonstrate our diagnosis of the missing elements and then the principles used to arrive at the reconstructive plan.

Case example 1

This patient is a 16-year-old girl with severe facial burns from hot-oil spill as a baby. She underwent initial reconstruction with staged tube pedicle flap from her groin for nose and chin reconstruction which unfortunately was totally inadequate (*Fig. 19.2*).

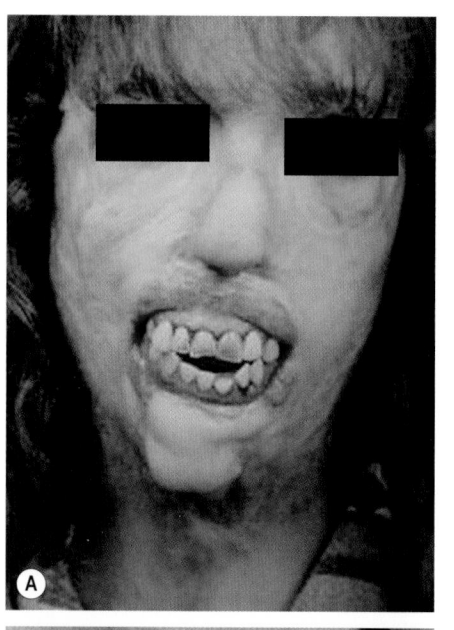
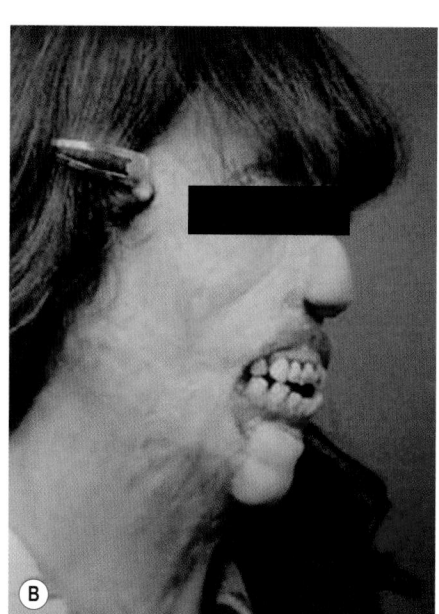
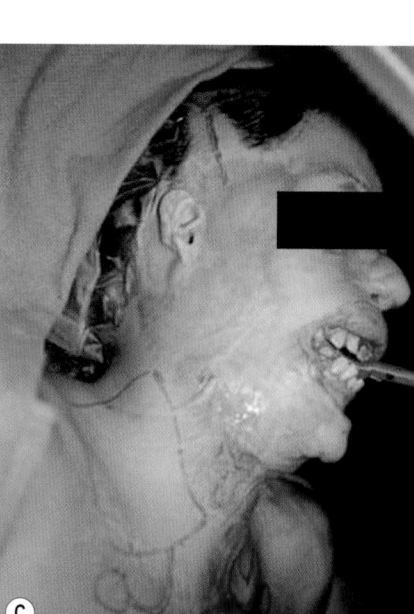
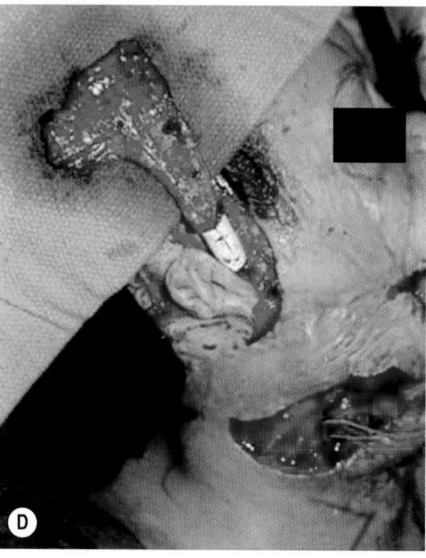
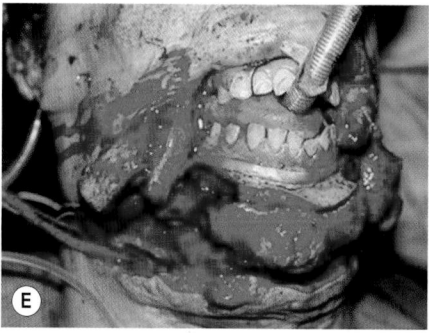
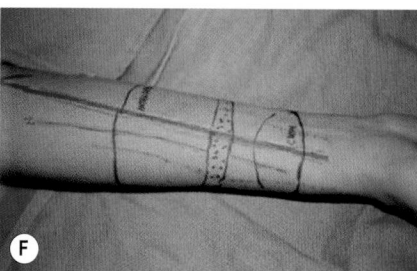

Fig. 19.2 A 16-year-old girl with severe facial burns from hot-oil spill as a baby. **(A, B)** Her initial reconstruction with staged tube pedicle flap from her groin for nose and chin reconstruction was unfortunately inadequate to give her oral competence and facial expression. **(C, D)** At the first stage, right neck skin is prefabricated using pedicled temporal parietal fascia flap over a tissue expander for upper lip reconstruction. **(E, F)** Lower lip and chin were reconstructed with free folded radial forearm flap and bilateral facial artery musculomucosal flaps.

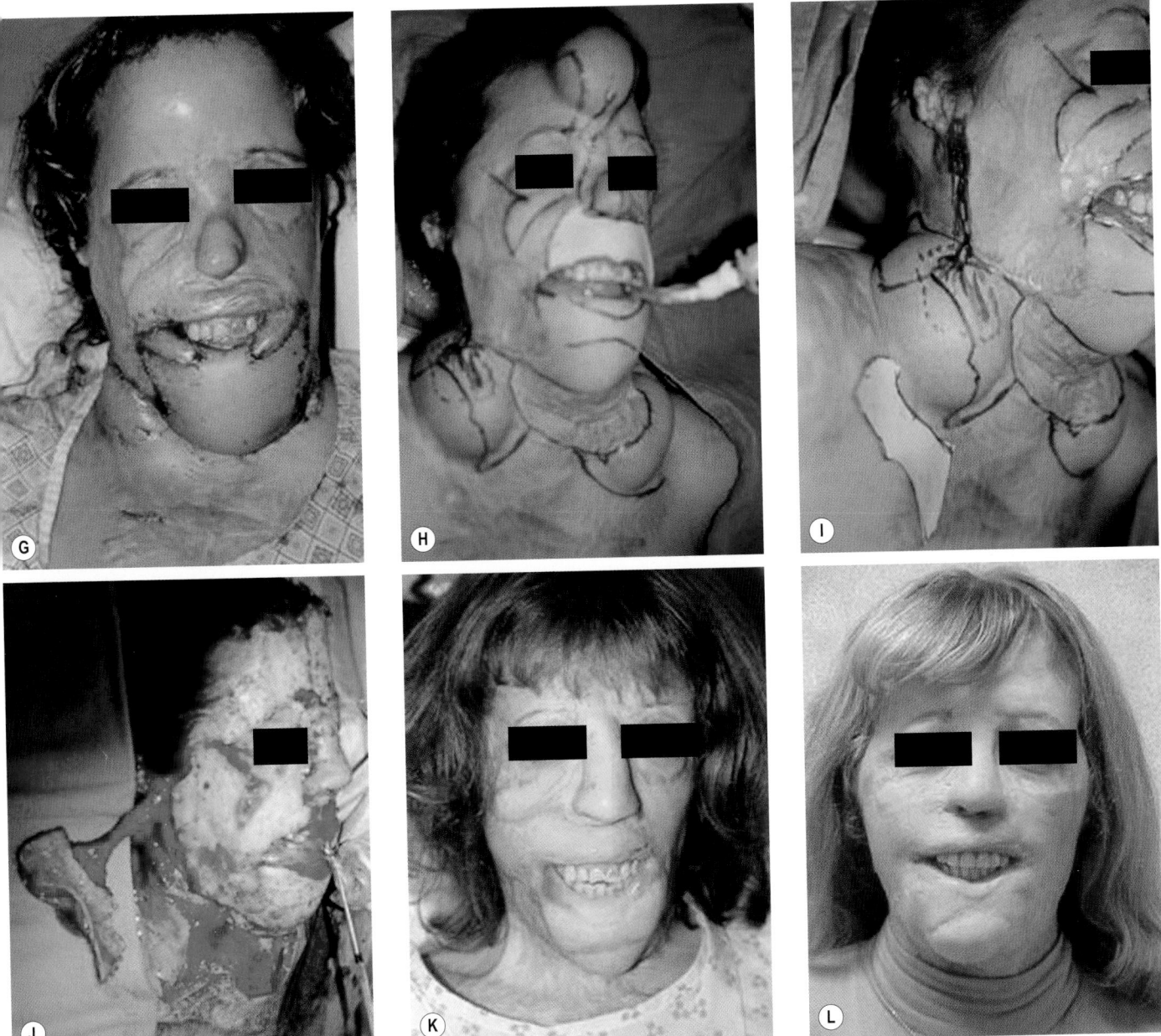

Fig. 19.2, cont'd **(G)** Her interim appearance with diminished lower incisor show is already evident. Tissue expander was placed under forehead flap for nasal reconstruction. At the second stage, her upper lip was reconstructed with the prefabricated expanded pedicle neck flap. **(H, I)** Template of the upper lip defect is seen and the course of the transposed pedicle outlined. **(J)** Her nose was reconstructed with the expanded forehead flap over lining flaps and cartilage grafts. **(K)** She was seen 3 months postoperatively with lower lip sagging. Dynamic temporalis muscle slings were designed to support her lower face and lips (not shown). **(L)** A satisfactory outcome is achieved 2 years following initial presentation. She has achieved oral competence and improved nasal aesthetics.[2]

Diagnosis

1. Full-thickness upper and lower lip loss and consequent lack of oral competence manifested as frequent oral caries and lack of facial expressions.

2. Nasal deformity with lack of tip projection and ill-defined facial-alar groove.

Reconstructive plan

Additional oral lining and external skin are needed to correct her upper and lower lip deficiencies. No local options are available. A radial forearm free flap is planned for lower lip reconstruction and a prefabricated neck flap is planned for upper lip reconstruction. Forehead flap and cartilage grafts will increase nasal projection and nasal skin quality. At the first stage, right neck skin was prefabricated using a pedicled temporal parietal fascia flap over a tissue expander for upper lip reconstruction. A tissue expander was also placed under forehead flap for nasal reconstruction. The lower lip and chin were reconstructed with free folded radial forearm flap. A three-dimensional template of the defect was made following contracture release which was then converted into a two-dimensional pattern before transposing on to the radial forearm.

She was seen immediately following lower lip free folded radial forearm flap and bilateral FAMM flap for vermilion reconstruction. At the second stage, her upper lip was reconstructed with the prefabricated expanded pedicle neck flap. Template of the upper lip defect is seen and the course of the transposed pedicle outlined. Her nose was reconstructed with a forehead flap over lining flaps and cartilage grafts. Sculpting of the supramental crease was also done at this time.

She was seen 3 months postoperatively with lower lip sagging. Bilateral dynamic temporalis muscle slings were designed to support her lower face and lips. She is seen immediately after her lower lip revision as well as sculpting of her nose. The mouth closes when the patient bites down. A satisfactory outcome is achieved 2 years following initial presentation. She has achieved oral competence and improved nasal aesthetics.[2]

This case illustrates multiple principles of secondary facial reconstruction:

1. Comprehensive diagnosis from the outset.
2. Use of templates for planning.
3. Prefabrication to bring in additional tissue, saving her from an additional free tissue transfer.

4. Use of FAMM flap for vermilion reconstruction.
5. Delayed use of forehead flap for resurfacing after previous distant flap.
6. Restoration of contour following free tissue transfer through debulking and placement of scars along natural creases.
7. Functional reconstruction of the lower lip with bilateral temporalis muscle flaps.

Case example 2

This patient is a 23-year-old female with a history of extensive burns and multiple facial skin grafts and releases who now desires better texture and uniformity (*Fig. 19.3*).

Diagnosis

The skin is irregular and noncompliant with no subcutaneous fat throughout her face and neck. She suffers from loss of normal nasal and facial contours from contractures of the face and nose.

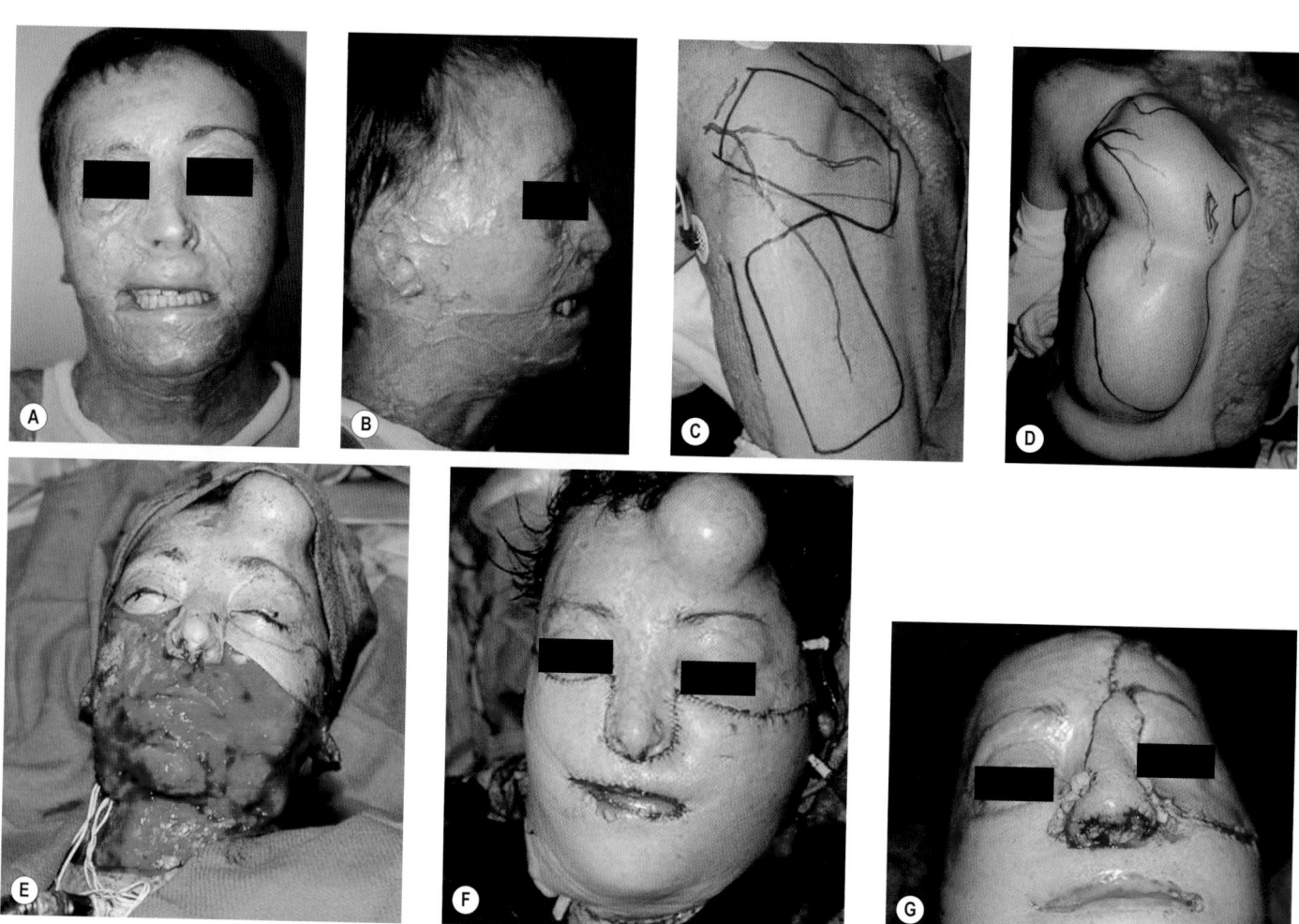

Fig. 19.3 A 23-year-old female with a history of extensive burns and multiple facial skin grafts and releases who now desires better texture and uniformity. **(A, B)** She suffers from loss of normal nasal and facial contours from contractures of the face and nose. **(C, D)** Facial resurfacing using an expanded free scapular/parascapular free flap was designed and outlined. **(E)** Following expansion, hypertrophic burn scar was excised from her face and neck. **(F)** She is seen immediately following free tissue transfer. **(G)** Expanded forehead flap was used for nasal resurfacing.

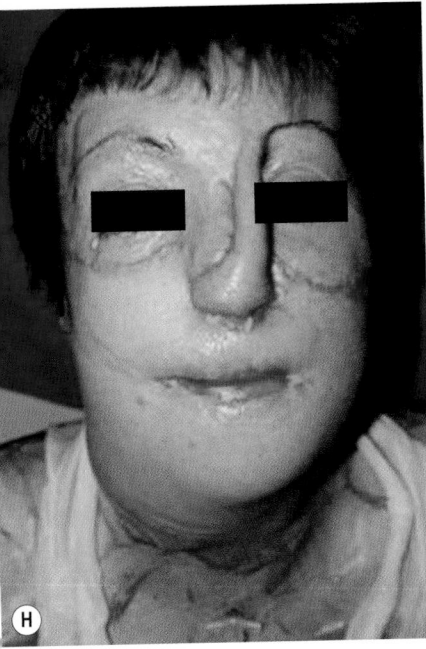 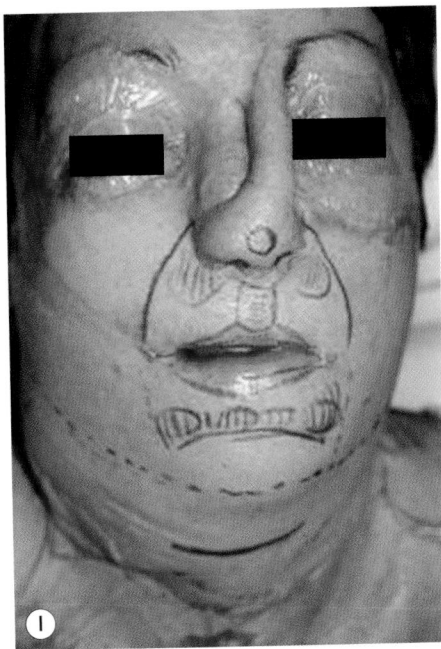 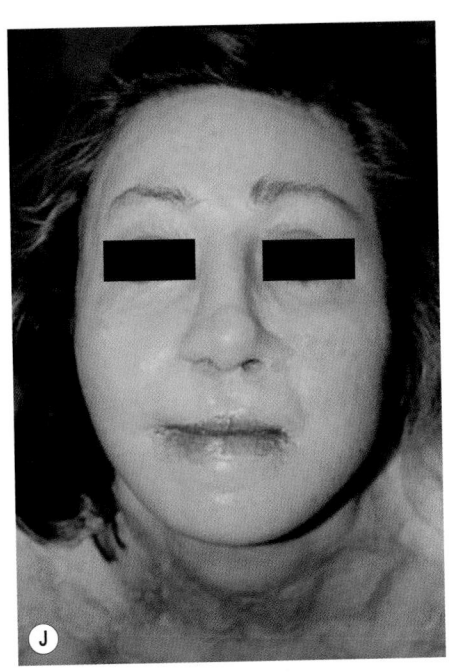

Fig. 19.3, cont'd (H) She is seen following healing of her free flap which still lacks normal facial and nasal contours. **(I)** Facial aesthetic units were recreated through debulking and placement of scars in lines of natural creases to recreate lines of the cheek, the philtrum, the upper lip, and chin. **(J)** Resurfacing of unstable skin has achieved a more uniform appearance of her face and neck.

Reconstructive plan

The intention was to carry out facial resurfacing using an expanded free scapular/parascapular free flap. She has few unburned donor sites large enough to resurface this area. Following expansion, hypertrophic burn scar was excised from her face and neck. Templating over the back was performed. She is seen immediately following free tissue transfer. Expanded forehead flap was used for nasal resurfacing. She is seen following healing of her free flap which still lacks normal facial and nasal contours. Facial aesthetic subunits were recreated through debulking and placement of scars in lines of natural creases to recreate separation between the cheek, the philtrum, the upper lip, and chin. Resurfacing of unstable skin has achieved a more uniform appearance of her face and neck. Attempts at further improving facial skin tone with laser resurfacing were partially successful and the patient is satisfied with her appearance with use of additional make-up.

This case illustrates multiple principles of secondary facial reconstruction:

1. Comprehensive diagnosis from the outset.
2. Use of templates for planning.
3. Delayed use of forehead flap for resurfacing.
4. Uniform resurfacing of the face and neck with expanded free flap.
5. Restoration of contour following free tissue transfer through debulking and placement of scars along natural creases.

Case example 3

The patient is a 17-year-old male (seen preinjury in *Fig. 19.4A*) following self-inflicted gunshot wound to the central one-third of his face with loss of bony support and left mandible. Reconstruction was first done elsewhere including open reduction, internal fixation of multiple bony fractures, rib grafts, and radial forearm free flap to separate the oro- and nasopharynx. Cantilever bone graft and forehead flap were performed for nasal reconstruction and subsequent Abbé flap for upper lip deficiency. The patient presented for secondary facial reconstruction 24 months after initial injury.

Diagnosis

1. Midface retrusion with lack of bony support.
2. Lack of nasal projection and ill-defined facial alar groove, deficient left alar.
3. Asymmetric lip with upper lip contracture and intraoral contracture.

Reconstructive plan

The intention was to carry out release of all intraoral contracture and reconstruct bony platform using free fibula flap. The contralateral facial artery is outlined in anticipation of extensive lining deficits. Midfibula osteotomy was performed to give support to both the maxilla and the mandible as a single free osteocutaneous flap. A large lining deficit is indeed seen following release. Both the fibular skin paddle as well as a superiorly based right FAMM flap can be seen during inset.

At a second stage, deficient left alar is reconstructed with free auricular flap of ascending helix and root of helix. Sixty-three months postinjury, after healing and edema subsided, a second forehead flap was done for nasal resurfacing. He is seen 8 years after the initial injury with symmetric lips lacking any external or internal oral contractures, improved midface, nasal projection, and nasal appearance.

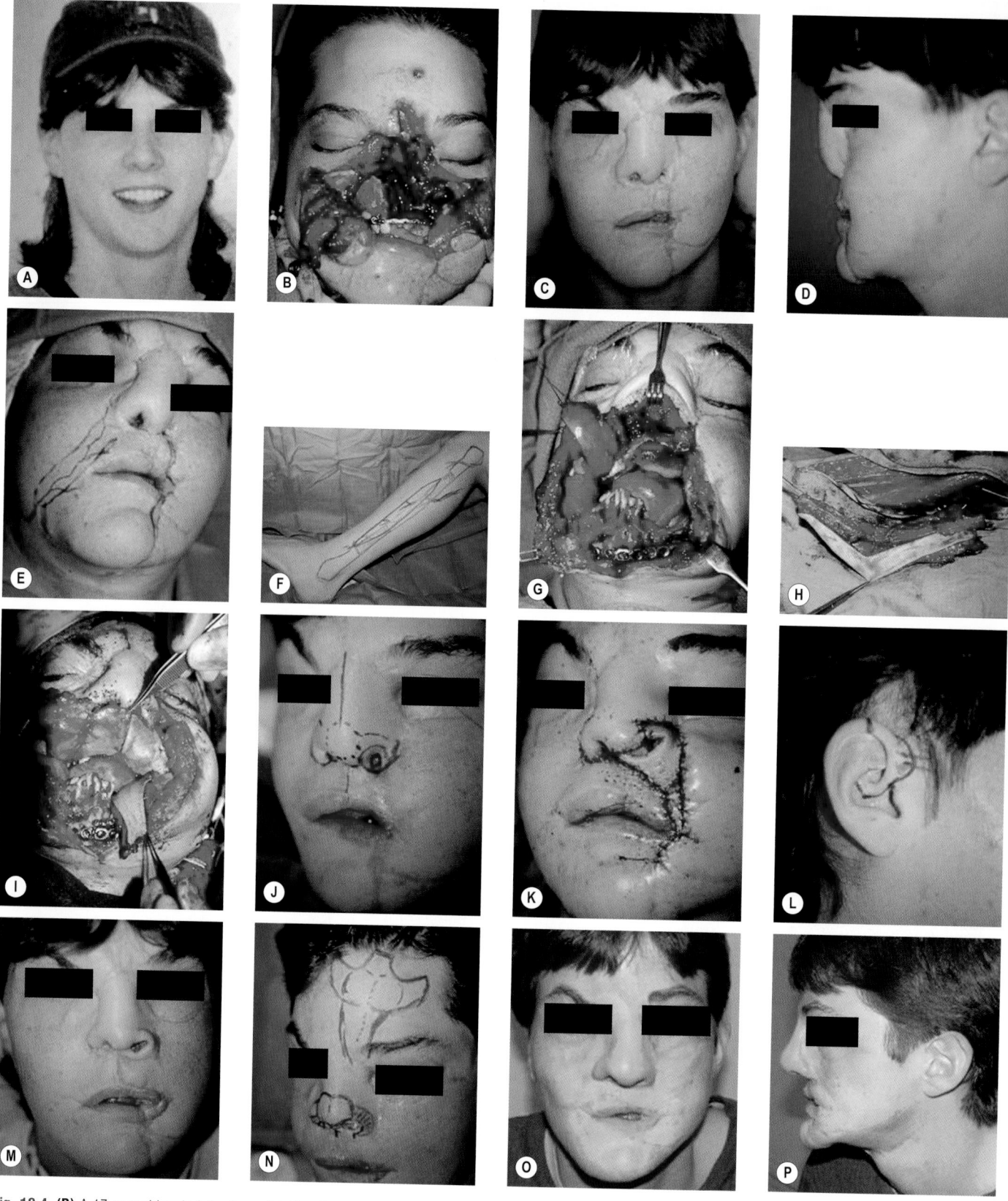

Fig. 19.4 **(B)** A 17-year-old male following self-inflicted gunshot wound to the central one-third of his face with loss of bony support and left mandible. **(A)** Preinjury appearance from an old photograph used as reference. Reconstruction first performed elsewhere included open reduction, internal fixation of multiple bony fractures, rib grafts, and radial forearm free flap to separate the oro- and nasopharynx. Cantilever bone graft and forehead flap were performed for nasal reconstruction and subsequent Abbé flap for upper lip deficiency. **(C, D)** The patient presented for secondary facial reconstruction 24 months after initial injury, lacking mid facial bony support, nasal projection, and asymmetric lip with upper lip and intraoral contractures. **(F)** Reconstructive plan included release of all intraoral contracture and reconstruction of bony platform using free fibula flap. **(E)** The contralateral facial artery is outlined in anticipation of extensive lining deficits. **(H)** Midfibula osteotomy was performed to give support to both the maxilla and the mandible. **(G)** A large lining deficit is indeed seen following release. **(I)** Both the fibular skin paddle as well as a superiorly based right facial artery musculomucosal flap are used for coverage. **(J–L)** At a second stage, deficient left alar is reconstructed with free auricular flap of ascending helix and root of helix. **(M, N)** Sixty-three months postinjury, after healing and edema subsided, a second forehead flap was done for nasal resurfacing. **(O, P)** He is seen 8 years after the initial injury with symmetric lips lacking any external or internal oral contractures, improved midface, nasal projection, and nasal appearance.

This case illustrates multiple principles of secondary facial reconstruction:

1. Comprehensive diagnosis from the outset, starting reconstruction from "scratch"
2. Adequate release of intraoral contracture a must, using FAMM flap and cutaneous portion of the free flap
3. Reconstruction of stable bony platform
4. Delayed use of second forehead flap for resurfacing.

Case example 4

A 39-year-old male presents with extensive left facial arteriovenous malformation (*Fig. 19.5*).

Diagnosis

He has a large deficit involving his cheek, upper and lower lip, intraoral lining, muscles of facial expression, and bony maxillary platform.

Reconstructive plan

This is a case of a planned multiple-stage reconstruction. He was primarily reconstructed using a tailored radial forearm folded flap, customized to defect with an alginate model. The folded portion was used for intraoral lining. Palmaris longus slings were used to suspend the lip and a contralateral FAMM flap was used for vermilion reconstruction. A planned delayed reconstruction of the maxillary platform was performed using a free fibula flap with osseointegrated implant for future dental rehabilitation. This was complicated by dehiscence of the radial forearm flap from the lateral alar with exposed plate. An extended forehead flap including a hair-bearing segment which was initially planned for mustache reconstruction was also able to cover the cheek defect. He was seen at 6 months postoperatively with excellent cheek projection and a symmetric mustache. At the time, he was still lacking all the facial mimetic muscles and thus had an asymmetric smile. A functional platysma-submental flap based on the submental branch of the facial artery and the cervical branch of the facial nerve was used for cheek reconstruction. One week later, muscle function was evident; 2 years later, he achieved a symmetric smile and symmetric hair growth.

This case illustrates many principles of secondary facial reconstruction:

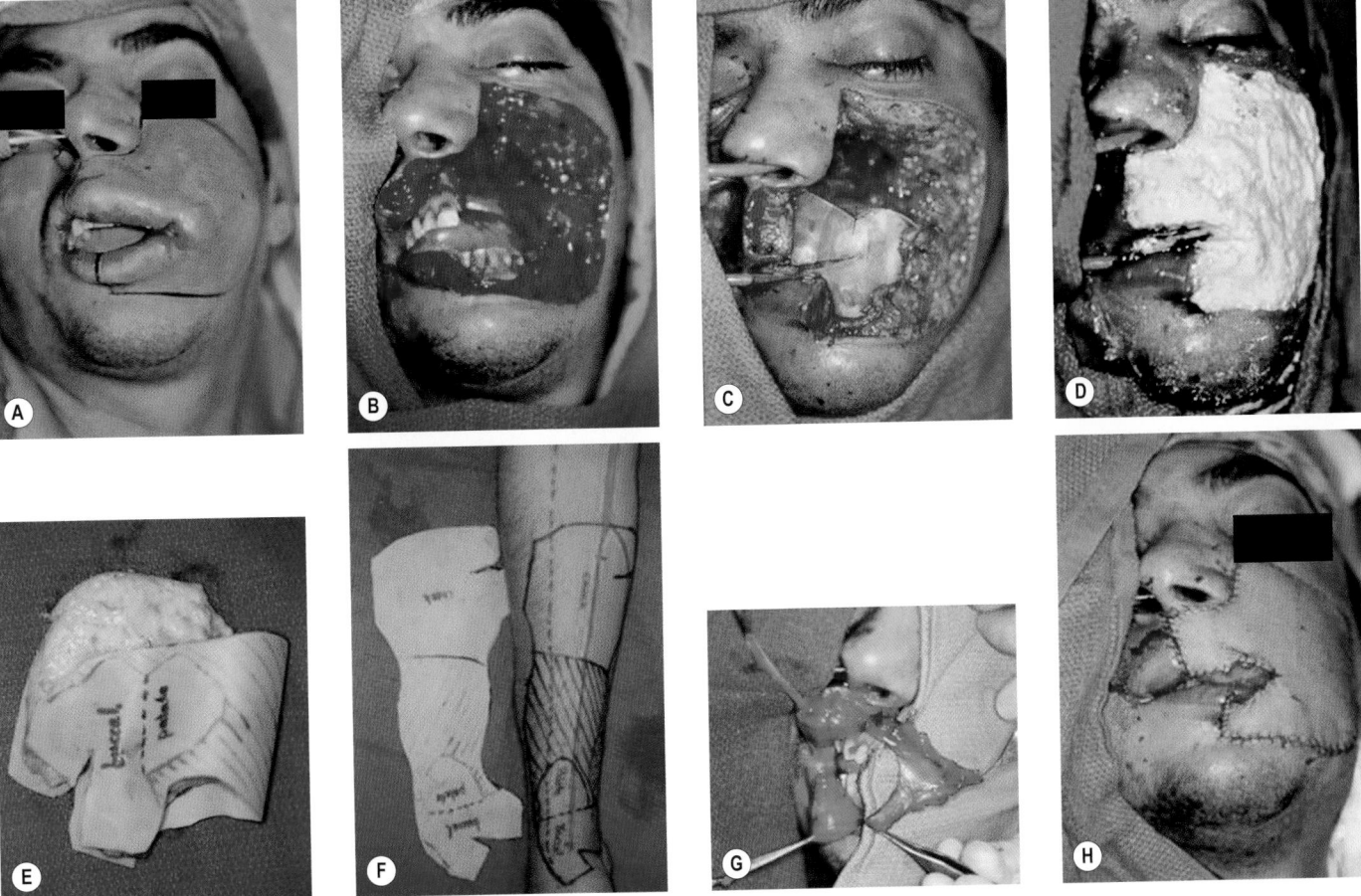

Fig. 19.5 (A) A 39-year-old male presents with extensive left facial arteriovenous malformation. **(B)** He has a large deficit involving his cheek, upper and lower lip, intraoral lining, muscles of facial expression, and bony maxillary platform. **(C, D)** He was primarily reconstructed using a tailored radial forearm folded flap, customized to the size, shape, and volume of the defect with an alginate model. **(E, F)** The folded portion was used for intraoral lining. **(G, H)** Palmaris longus slings were used to suspend the lip and a contralateral facial artery musculomucosal flap was used for vermilion reconstruction.

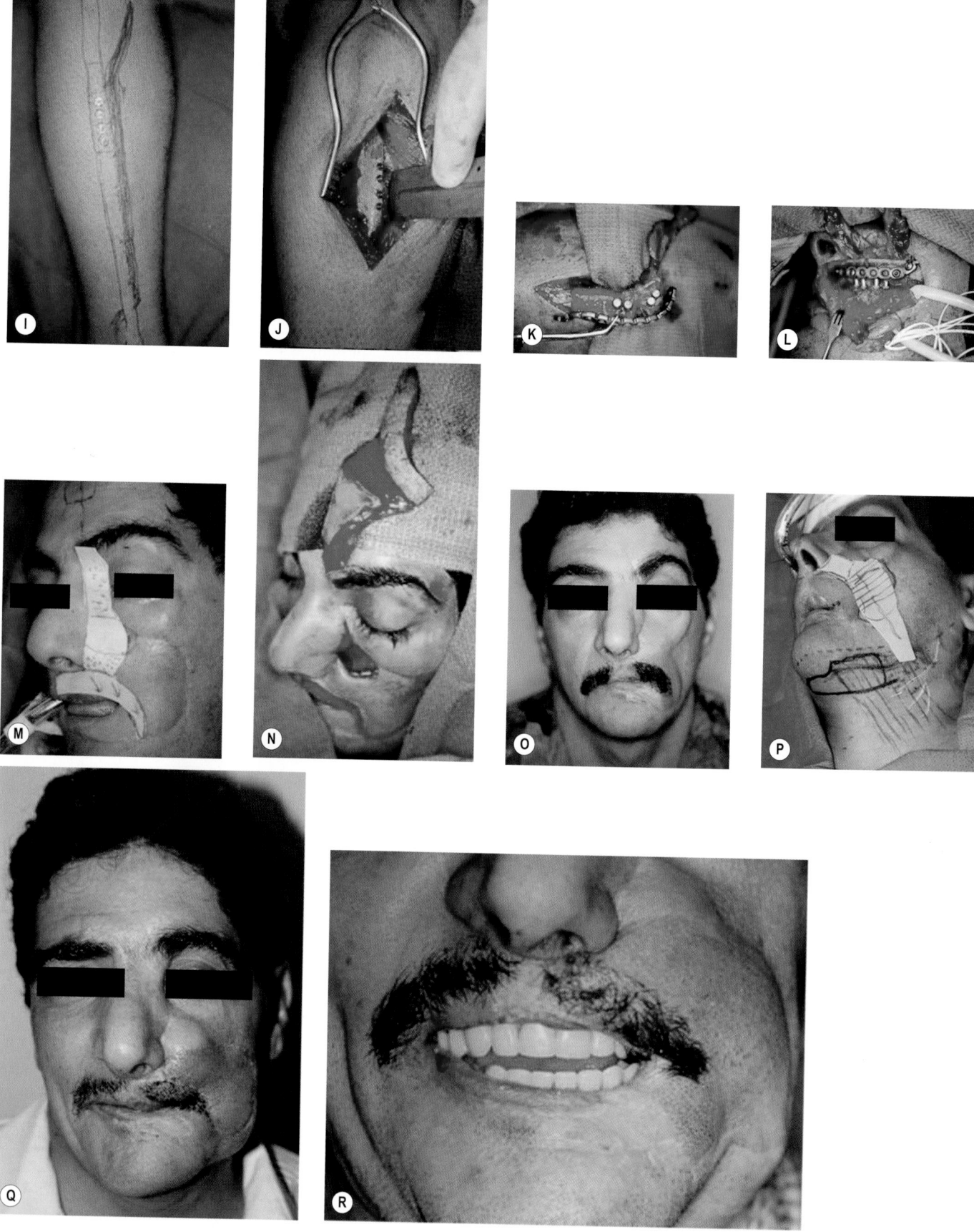

Fig. 19.5, cont'd **(I–L)** A planned delayed reconstruction of his maxillary platform was performed using a free fibula flap with osseointegrated implant for future dental rehabilitation. This was complicated by dehiscence of the radial forearm flap from the lateral alar with exposed plate. **(M, N)** An extended forehead flap, including a hair-bearing segment which was initially planned for mustache reconstruction, was also used to cover the cheek defect. **(O)** He was seen at 6 months postoperatively with excellent cheek project and symmetric mustache, though he still was missing all the facial mimetic muscles and had an asymmetric smile. **(P)** A functional platysma flap based on the submental branch of the facial artery and the cervical branch of the facial nerve was planned for cheek reconstruction. **(Q)** One week later, muscle twitching was evident. **(R)** Two years later, he achieved a symmetric smile and symmetric hair growth.

1. Comprehensive diagnosis from the outset.
2. Planning for a multiple-stage reconstruction from the start.
3. Use of alginate to model a three-dimensional volume loss and then converted to a two-dimensional defect on the donor site that can later be folded.
4. Use of FAMM flap for vermilion reconstruction.
5. Reconstruction of stable bony platform with dental implants in place.
6. Delayed use of forehead flap for resurfacing both the cheek and mustache reconstruction.
7. Use of local flaps secondarily to provide better color match and hair-bearing segments.

As evident from the patients presented, each case of secondary reconstruction is unique. While thinking "outside the box" is no doubt at times necessary, adherence to the basic principles demonstrated above will help guide the reconstruction.

Postoperative care

Postoperative care for each patient is unique and depends on the specific procedure performed. In the early postoperative period, this uniformly involves flap monitoring, perioperative antibiotics, and appropriate scar management. It is usual and safe practice to allow the patient and the involved tissue to heal, the swelling to subside, and the scar to mature before embarking on another tertiary procedure.

Outcomes, prognosis, and complications

Multiple operations are often required to achieve a finally acceptable outcome. This is discussed in detail with the patient from the start and the plan modified on an "as needed" basis. Realistic goals need to be communicated. Depending on the complexity of reconstruction, the number of secondary revisions necessary ranges from 2–3 for relatively simple defects to exceeding 20–30 for more complex defects. Once composite tissue allotransplantation becomes more widely available, patients with certain defects, especially those involving the central triangle of the face, should be pursued as transplant candidates. As such, local and regional flap options might actually become "lifeboats."

On assessing our own outcomes, it is of foremost importance as reconstructive surgeons to listen to our patients as they serve as our best teachers. Persistent complaints following reconstruction can be a hint as to what we can do better. To that end, we must strive to reintegrate the patient back to normalcy through our reconstructive means.

Complications are unfortunately a part of performing any complex reconstruction. Especially in areas of previous irradiation and severe scarring, blood supply is suboptimal and donor vessels are lacking. As Millard preached in his writings, each reconstructive plan must have a lifeboat, preferably even a lifesaver in a lifeboat.[15] For this reason, when first approaching a problem, the surgeon should go through the mental exercise of considering all the different options before deciding on the best one. The other options hence will serve as lifeboats when they become needed.

Access the complete reference list online at http://www.expertconsult.com

3. Pribaz JJ, Morris DJ, Mulliken JB. Three-dimensional folded free-flap reconstruction of complex facial defects using intraoperative modeling. *Plast Reconstr Surg.* 1994;93:285–293.
   Multifaceted free flaps are often needed in the reconstruction of complex facial defects. The article describes a simple technique to determine both the volume of tissue required and the localization of the various epithelial surfaces, thereby simplifying these complex reconstructions using an intraoperative alginate moulage.

7. Pribaz J, Stephens W, Crespo L, et al. A new intraoral flap: facial artery musculomucosal (FAMM) flap. *Plast Reconstr Surg.* 1992;90:421–429.
   First description of the FAMM flap by Pribaz et al. combining the principles of nasolabial and buccal mucosal flaps. The flap has proven to be reliable based either superiorly (retrograde flow) or inferiorly (antegrade flow) to reconstruct a wide variety of difficult oronasal mucosal defects, including defects of the palate, alveolus, nasal septum, antrum, upper and lower lips, floor of the mouth, and soft palate.

8. Taghinia AH, Movassaghi K, Wang AX, et al. Reconstruction of the upper aerodigestive tract with the submental artery flap. *Plast Reconstr Surg.* 2009;123:562–570.
   The article demonstrates the versatility of FAMM flaps specifically in lip and vermilion reconstruction. While lip and vermilion are specialized tissues that cannot be easily reproduced, FAMM flap has features similar to those of lip tissue that makes it an option when such losses are encountered. In this article, the anatomy, dissection, and clinical applications for the use of the FAMM flap in lip and vermilion reconstruction are discussed.

11. Mathy JA, Pribaz JJ. Prefabrication and prelamination applications in current aesthetic facial reconstruction. *Clin Plast Surg.* 2009;36:493–505.
   A review of prefabrication and prelamination techniques in facial reconstruction. Some of their unique abilities are presented, and their advantages, limitations, and technical pointers are provided. Relevant features and interdependencies among these procedures as they relate to aesthetic facial reconstruction are discussed.

13.   Pribaz JJ, Fine NA. Prelamination: defining the prefabricated flap – a case report and review. *Microsurgery*. 1994;15:618–623.

First paper to coin the term "prelamination" as modification of flaps prior to local or distant transfer were gaining wide acceptance. This article also clarifies the use of the term "prefabrication" which until then was used to describe all possible modifications. In this article, the term "prelamination" is used to refer to the implantation of tissue or other devices into a flap prior to transfer and suggests that prefabrication be restricted to the implantation of vascular pedicles.

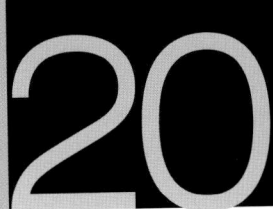

Facial transplant

Laurent Lantieri

SYNOPSIS

- Raising field with unanswered questions.
- High risk surgery.
- Necessity of lifelong treatment.
- Should be limited to patient with total destruction of orbicularis muscle.
- Indications are separated in two: Lower face transplant for destruction of orbicularis oris mostly indicated in ballistic traumas, full and upper face transplant indicated in destruction of orbicularis occuli mostly found in burned patients.
- Necessity of collaboration with many teams and strong logistic organization.

Introduction

Face transplant is a new rising field in plastic surgery, with only 20 transplants from November 2005 to February 2012.[1–9] However, six of those were realized in the year 2009, showing a great increase in their numbers. It is apparent that this will continue in the near future, but as in any innovative procedure, questions remain unanswered and only long-term follow-up will allow us to find those answers. Answers to the questions of risks–benefits balance; indications, and technical, immunological and ethical aspects are being progressively sought. Even if the number of face transplants is still small, the growing world expertise in composite tissue allotransplantation (CTA) is helping to answer some of these questions. CTA of various organs, such as the hands,[10] face,[1] bones,[11] joints,[12] abdominal wall,[13] represents over 100 patients today, with some of them having over 10 years of follow-up. CTA transplants are related to nonvital organs, mostly to restore function. The goal of the face transplant is to restore human appearance, which should not be limited to a static aspect but should also be a dynamic one. This dynamic transplant allows the restoration of communication capacity and social reintegration.[3]

Basic science

Immunosuppression

We easily forget that the first kidney transplant in France only survived 3 weeks,[14] as was the case for the first heart transplant[15] and the first liver transplant.[16] It is the understanding of Joseph Murray that the rejection was mostly due to an immunological phenomenon which led to intense research in immunology.[17] In 1972, Joseph Murray[18] explained his views on organ replacement and restoration of facial deformities, in his discourse to the Massachusetts Medical Society. Kidney transplantation was a developing field at that time, and face transplantation was not even a concept. Immunology was not then ready for CTA. In 1963, the first hand transplant was attempted and did not survive more than 3 weeks[19,20] because of lack of immunosuppressive therapy at the time. In the years after the first heart transplant, the mortality rate was such a concern that many teams abandoned the principle, even though the surgical technique was well established. Starting in 1976, cyclosporine[21] significantly improved the survival rate of patients by combining effective prevention of graft rejection and lack of hematologic toxicity. Other immunosuppressive agents introduced in recent years (tacrolimus,[22] mycophenolate mofetil,[23] monoclonal antibodies,[24,25] antilymphocyte serum[26]), have expanded the range of available therapeutic drugs in organ transplantation, allowing to cope with almost all situations of rejection. The standard immunosuppressive treatment of CTA is a scheme suitable for high immunological risk transplantation such as lung transplants.[27] It combines induction most of the time with antilymphocyte serum, which will cause lysis of effector cells responsible for acute cellular rejection, CD3+ T-lymphocytes, followed by maintenance therapy consisting of a three immunosuppressive drugs. Long after the first experimental work of Medawar,[28,29] the skin appeared to be the ultimate barrier requiring anti-rejection drug too toxic to be tolerated long term. Furthermore, the complexity of the human immune system and the presence of the immunocompetent element in transplanted tissue during CTA[30,31] could even be a threat by inducing graft-versus-host disease (GVHD) due to the presence of bone marrow and/or lymph nodes potentially involved in immune response. Since 1990, numerous studies were conducted in animals and in 1998, a team from Louisville showed that an immunosuppressive therapy combining Tacrolimus, Mycophenolate Mofetil and prednisone, could prevent the rejection of a complete transplanted limb, without major toxicity in a pre-clinical animal model (adult pig).[32] All this knowledge has led to relatively standardized protocols. Thus, the Lyon team, led by Dubernard[10,33] renewed the attempt to graft a hand, first unilateral then bilateral. If the unilateral graft eventually resulted in failure, this was due to the discontinuation of the patient, the first bilateral hand transplant was undoubtedly a success that has brought CTA to a clinical reality.[34]

We will focus here on the practical aspects of the treatment used in CTA. Today the standard treatment begins with an induction by injection of monoclonal or polyclonal antilymphocyte antibody. There is insufficient data so far between the choice of a monoclonal versus a polyclonal antilymphocyte antibody.[35] In practice *(Table 20.1)*, injection of antilymphocyte serum begins in the operating room just after the end anastomosis. The induction is then followed by a tri-therapy combining mycophenolate mofetil (MMF) and FK506 (tacrolimus) and steroids. The monitoring of this treatment requires accurate dosing in the days after surgery. Antilymphocyte serum needs a daily dosage of CD3+ T-lymphocytes. For tacrolimus, it is necessary to have a blood level of 10–15 ng per mL. For the Cellcept, repeated testing is performed to estimate the average concentration by using the area under curve (AUC) concept, which should be in the range of 40–50 ng/mL.

Other treatments are currently under study.[36] Apart from drugs, research protocols are directed towards tolerance induction. The concept was mostly developed by Starzl.[37–39] The principle is to prepare the donor or the graft so that the antigens of the transplanted organ are recognized as the antigens of the recipient. Many protocols exist in animals, but most involve a preparation by radiation which is not compatible with clinical practice. Recent approaches applicable in humans consist of a concomitant injection of hematopoietic stem cell from the donor. This bone marrow transplant can be a myeloablative protocol, i.e., removing the bone marrow recipient, which will change the immune system of the recipient and may cause a GVHD reaction. Thus, although particularly effective myeloablative approach is only used if there is a need for bone marrow associated to a solid organ transplant, as in the case in patients with myeloma with kidney failure, it is not applicable in the field of functional transplantation, as are CTAs. Nonmyeloablative protocols have been used in many animal models with success,[40,41] but we do not have conclusive results in humans. For some, the presence of bone marrow in the bones of the donor's hand is a true hematopoietic stem cell transplant and would explain the good results of these grafts. However, the comparison between the first three facial CTAs shows similar results in terms of immunosuppression with or without hematopoietic stem cells transplantation, as in the first transplant, or without, as in the two following. For others, the bone marrow transplant is only effective when transplanted with a vascularized bone which is the case in the hand and in transplants with mandible. This is not the case for the maxilla due to the relative paucity of bone marrow in the maxilla.

Some more subtle approaches seek a peripheral tolerance by treatment of blood cells trying to reduce the response of T-cells by causing antigen-presenting cells to a tolerogenic phenotype through apoptotic elements. This is the case of extracorporeal chemo-phototherapy (ECP),[42–44] where leukocyte cells are irradiated with UVA after leukapheresis and pretreated with psoralen. The principle of ECP is to induce apoptosis with UVA radiation after their presentation by psoralens. These leucocytes are immediately reinfused into the patient, where they undergo early apoptosis. Following apoptosis, the leucocytes are engulfed by macrophage or other antigen presenting cells such as immature cells in an anti-inflammatory environment. The anti-inflammatory pattern and the engulfment by immature cells without co-stimulatory molecules induces anergy by deleting effector T-cells that respond to the presented antigens. An increase in regulatory T-cells is also induced after ECP and may contribute to the allograft acceptance by the recipient. ECP has already been used for the great majority of solid organ transplantations to cure acute rejection episodes or in an attempt to prevent or cure chronic rejections.

For Starzl,[35–37] a pioneer of liver transplantation, tolerance should not be sought immediately, but should rather be a progressive approach through immunomodulation with rapid decline of anti-rejection treatment after the induction phase and adapted control of rejection. In light of his experience in transplantation of kidney and liver, he explained that in some cases, we may obtain a long-term safe treatment with low or no immunosuppression, by allowing the rejection to

Table 20.1 Induction protocol

MMF (CellCept)
  1 g preoperative
  2 g per day from day 1 to day 9 followed by 3 g per os
  Adaptation of doses of CellCept with mini-AUC
  Mini-AUC every week from d4: target AUC: 40–50 ng/mL
Tacrolimus (Prograf)
  0.2 mg/kg per day per os D1
  5 ng/mL until D7, 10–15 ng/mL during the first month
Thymoglobulin (TG)
  1.25 mg/kg: D0 to D10
  Perfusion on 10 h for the first perfusion (>4 h on next perfusion)
  Polaramine 2 amp IV and Prednisolone
  Monitoring with cell count of CD3
Prednisolone
  D0: 250 mg IV before TG (before surgery) and 250 mg in ICU
  D1: 250 mg before TG
  D2: 125 mg before TG
Prednisone
  D3: 60 mg before TG
  From D4 to D10: 30 mg before TG
  From D10 to D20: 20 mg/day then progressive diminution to obtain 10 mg/day at D30
Antiviral prophylaxis
  Valganciclovir 900 mg/day in case of CMV mismatch during 6 months
  Monitoring with CMV viremia

occur but by controlling it fast before the immune system is overwhelmed or the graft is damaged. The rejection will not only stimulate toxic T-cells but also regulatory cells. A long-term tissue chimerism should then occur even if never demonstrated in the transplanted patient. The results observed in our long-term follow-up in our team, are in favor of this hypothesis, as we have obtained a state of immunological stability, despite the strong decrease of immunosuppressive therapy.

Acute rejection is almost inevitable after the induction phase, when the rate of T-lymphocytes recovers at 3 weeks, but it is easily controlled by several boli of steroids. However, infection episodes can trigger other acute rejection episodes and need further specific treatment. Chronic rejection resulting in destruction of the graft, seen in all other transplants, has not been seen in a face transplant but is still a major threat. It seems however, that in the hand and face transplant patient with long-term follow-up, the grafts do not show any signs of degradation.

Face transplant only necessitates blood type compatibility. However, HLA matching can be a necessity in the case of patients who are sensitized, as seen in the burn patient who has received cadaver allograft, or after blood transfusion.[45] Each screened patient should have an anti-HLA serum test every 3 months during the preoperative period. HLA antibodies can appear also even in the absence of any recognized transplant, as certain viruses can mimic HLA antigens.[46] This explains the occasional apparition of these antibodies when very sensitive detection methods as Luminex[47] are used. In the case of a high level of positive HLA antibody, desensitization can be attempted but is often inefficient.[48] A virtual preoperative cross-match should be made and this has to be negative to allow transplantation, followed by postoperative real cross-match. If real cross-match is positive, then specific treatment by anti-CD20 monoclonal antibody and injection of immunoglobulin should be made to avoid humeral rejection.

Diagnosis and patient presentation

Patient selection

Contrary to hand transplants, indications for a face transplant seem somewhat difficult to determine. In the hand, we are looking at organ replacement in a patient with no hand, whereas in faces, there is a patient with no face and most of the patients can benefit from reconstruction using autologous tissue. However, there are elements in the face that cannot be reconstructed, which are the orbicularis muscle (orbicularis occuli and/or orbicularis oris). The indication should then be limited to this type of destruction. These are rarely isolated and can be seen in various etiologies, such as burns, ballistic traumas, animal bites and tumors. Many classifications have been published to try to score potential candidates. In our limited experience of five transplanted patients out of an initial 12 selected patients with a potential need of transplant, none of these classifications have been useful to determine the right indication. Indication for face transplant is a combination of three elements: the defect, the patient, and the transplantation team. Various traumas lead to a large variety of defects which are difficult to classify but that can be summarized in two types of transplant, depending on the kind of muscle destruction: *upper face transplant for orbicularis occuli and lower face transplant for orbicularis oris*. Full face transplant is a combination of both. The transplant can be limited to the lower face when the orbicularis oris is destroyed. This can be found in ballistic trauma where the mouth and the nose are destroyed and can be transplanted but the indication is related to the destruction of the mouth, not the nose. For the upper face, bilateral eyelid destruction, e.g., can be found in burn patient; the transplant is then justified and can be combined with other elements of the face like the ears and the nose. The indication is not limited to the anatomical aspect of the defect but should be estimated in combination with the immunological aspect and the psychological aspect, as even with the same defect some patients are not suitable for transplant due to immunological or psychological contraindications. In terms of immunology, some patients can be presensitized by either blood transfusion or a cadaveric skin graft. In the case of presensitization, an evaluation can be made for potential HLA compatible donors to estimate the possibility of having an organ in a reasonable time. If, for instance, the patient is presensitized to HLA A2, which is present in 50% of potential donors, only half of the potential donors will be suitable for this recipient. The enlistment has then to be carefully evaluated with the organ procurement organization and only done if the chances of transplant are real. The psychological evaluation of the patient is, of course, a key element to enlistment. Contraindications are mostly psychological instability, borderline personalities, addiction, and more generally, any psychiatric disorder that supposedly creates a doubt in the capacity of the patient to understand or to follow a lifelong treatment. The psychological and psychiatric evaluation takes time. During that process where the patients are hospitalized for evaluation, contact with different elements of the team are made. The nurses and assistant nurses have to be integrated into this process, as they are constantly confronted with the patient and can help to have a clear view of the adaptive capacity of the patient. Interestingly, it is probably the patients who have shown initially the best adaptive capacity, who have the best outcomes. An informed consent in such extreme surgery should be obtained with a clear understanding of the patient of the risks of the surgery but also that the transplantation implies a lifelong treatment. Ethical questions are raised for patients who are children, teenagers, and for emergency cases. Until more data are collected, it is for us to go early into this field with the simple question of free will. We advocate the use of time trade off (TTO) to evaluate the motivation of the patient. This consists of asking the patient how many years of life he will be ready to give to have perfect health. However, the TTO is only a tool. We have also been using quality-of-life scales, which are all adapted for disfigured patients evaluated for face transplant. If elements concerning the defect and concerning the patient (immunology and psychology) are not contraindicated, the third element is the transplantation team. All the members have to approve the case via several staff meetings. Rehearsals are mandatory to keep the spirit of teamwork and the instruments have to be regularly checked so that no logistic problem will appear during the procedure.

Surgical technique

While each recipient had particularities due to individual defects, common aspects of all the transplant harvests can be described. In all of our cases, the facial transplant is the first tissue harvested from a heart-beating brain-dead donor. Tracheotomy followed by alginate molding of the donor's face is done prior to any harvest, to allow reconstitution of the donor after harvesting. The harvest before cardiac arrest seems to be the most used technique. Contrarily to the hand or internal organ, the harvest of the face is a long procedure and the harvest on a nonbeating heart would lead to a very long warm ischemia. A long ischemia time could compromise the muscle function and could also change the immunologic impact due to the ischemia reperfusion injury, but improvement in organ preservation and surgical technique may prevent this in the future. Dissection on a beating heart donor helps to identify small vascular branches that could bleed if not correctly coagulated at the time of harvest. However, the restitution of the donor is fundamental and the molding should be done before any surgery. As the head and neck region is in the operative field; the anesthesiologists have then access to only the lower part of the donor. This disposition makes simultaneous removal of other organs impossible, even if all the transplant teams can, in theory, operate at the same time. The graft is washed with heparin-containing saline and transported in a standard icebox in preservation solution. Several organ preservation solutions have been used by different teams but none of them have been studied specifically for CTA. Once all the organs have been harvested and the resin mask, prepared during the operation, is fitted to the donor's face, the cadaver is returned to the family. We have tested several methods of reconstitution and the use of hard resin is the most efficient, as it can be done in a similar time as the harvest *(Figs 20.1–20.5)*.

Face transplant harvest

We recommend developing a reproducible and standardized technique.[49,50] The best technique is to harvest a full face transplant and to remove the unnecessary elements for the recipient. In this way, as all the elements are brought from the donor, the recipient team are confident as to what to remove on the recipient. Moreover, the reconstitution of the donor is easier. Basically, the drawing *(Fig. 20.6)* goes from the scalp as

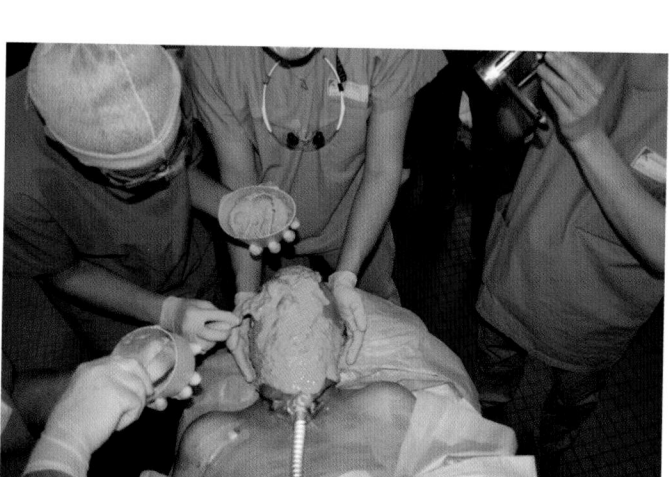
Fig. 20.1 Mold preparation.

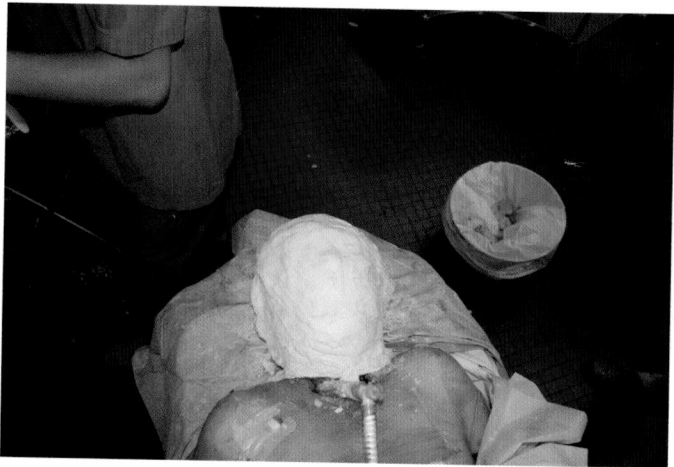
Fig. 20.2 Mold preparation 2.

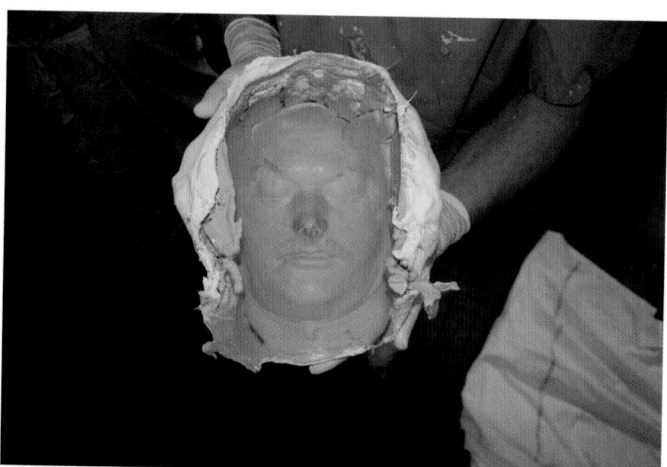
Fig. 20.3 Mold preparation 3.

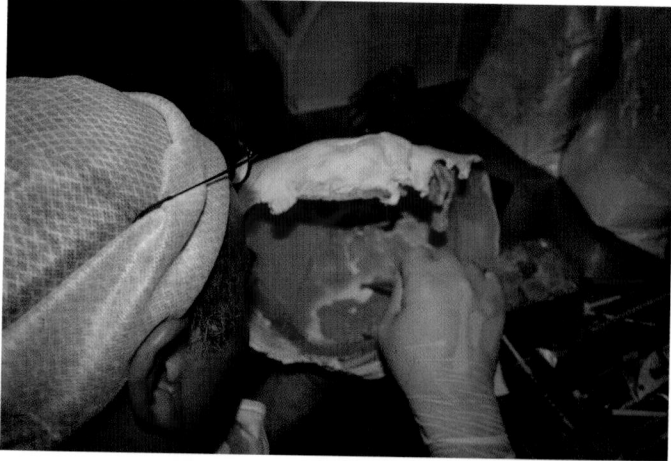
Fig. 20.4 Mask preparation.

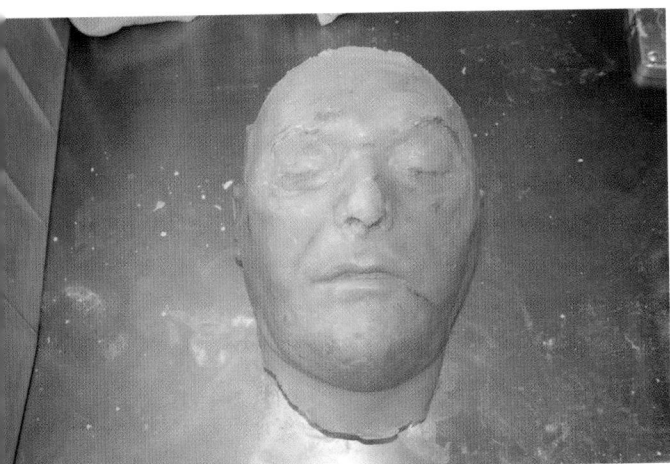

Fig. 20.5 Mask preparation 2.

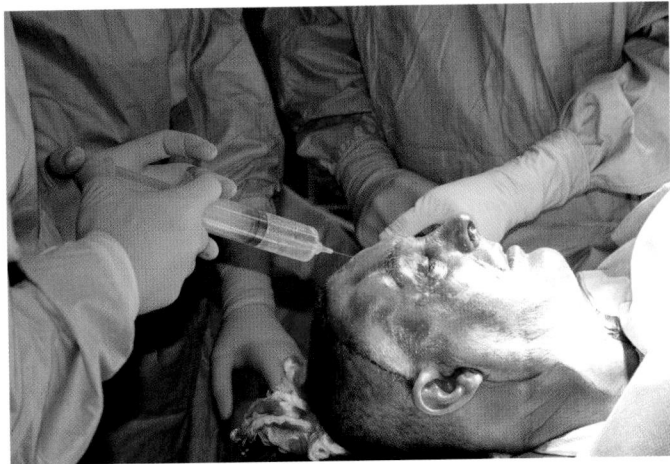

Fig. 20.6 Initial drawing and infiltration.

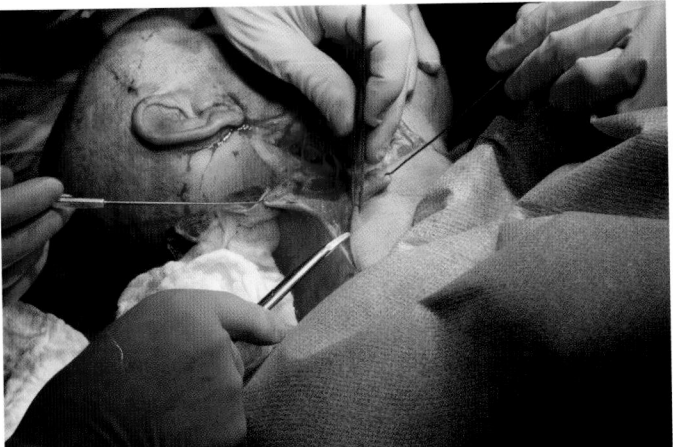

Fig. 20.7 External jugular dissection.

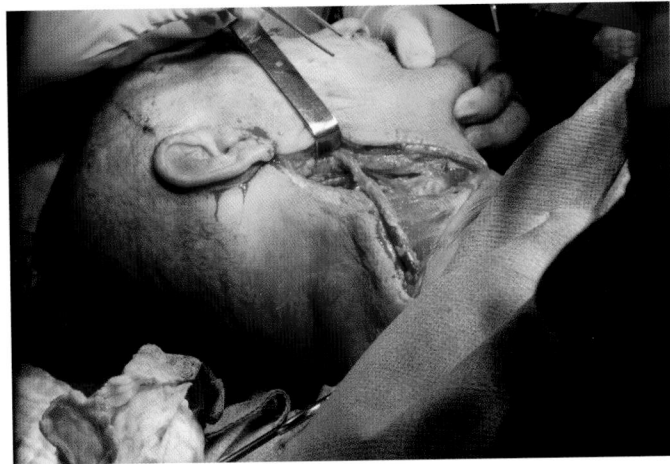

Fig. 20.8 External jugular dissection 2.

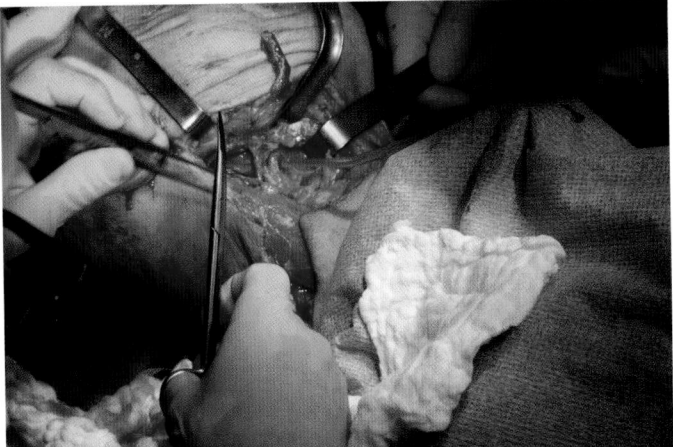

Fig. 20.9 Thyrolingofacial trunk and external carotid dissection.

a coronal incision; goes behind the ears and down to the neck, where a large skin flap has to be elevated and is only limited by the tracheotomy. The dissection starts in the neck with the approach of the external jugular vein on each side (Figs 20.7, 20.8). This vein has to be dissected as low as possible to allow

its use on the recipient. It is divided to have access to the deep vessels. The carotid artery and vein are isolated and followed upward. The thyrolingofacial trunk is then isolated (Figs 20.9–20.11). To have access to the different vascular branches, the hypoglossal nerve and the posterior part of the digastric muscle has to be divided (Fig. 20.12). This has to be done on both sides before proceeding to the next step. The facial nerve is approached through a parotidectomy access route. It is dissected until its bifurcation and transected at its exit from the stylomastoid foramen (Fig. 20.13). A 8-0 nylon is used to facilitate its location once on the recipient. To facilitate the approach, the external auricular conduit is transected. This way the facial nerve can be seen well and the maximum of nerve can be harvested. At that stage, several branches of the external carotid are still holding it back. The pharyngeal and lingual arteries have to be divided. One should take great care not to cut the facial artery at that stage, as it is running deep in the neck. The posterior auricular artery should be raised with the flap to allow scalp blood supply. For face transplant including the upper part and the scalp, the incision is sagittal and the flap is raised from posterior to anterior, followed by the forehead and including both ears (Figs 20.14, 20.15). The sagittal incision allows the harvest of the entire scalp. It is not

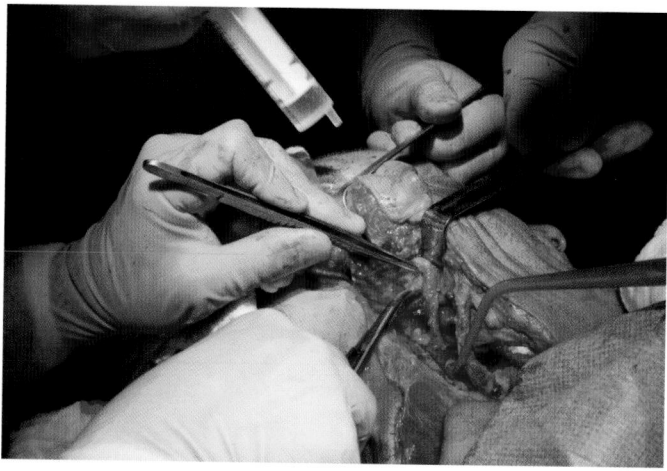

Fig. 20.10 Thyrolingofacial trunk and external carotid dissection 2.

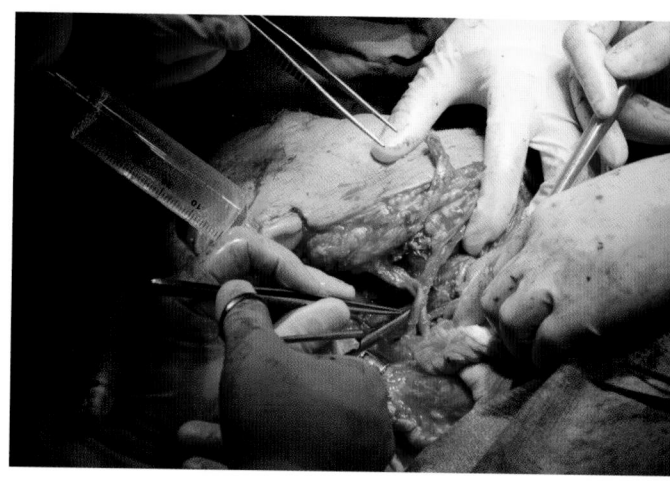

Fig. 20.11 Thyrolingofacial trunk and external carotid dissection 3.

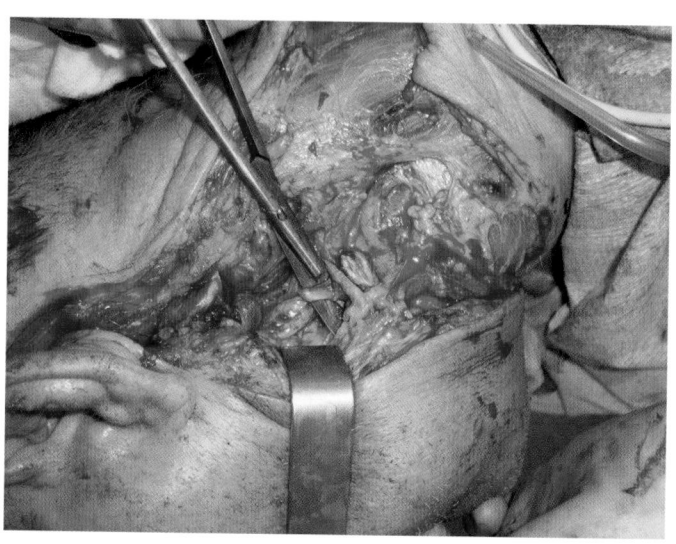

Fig. 20.12 Digastric division.

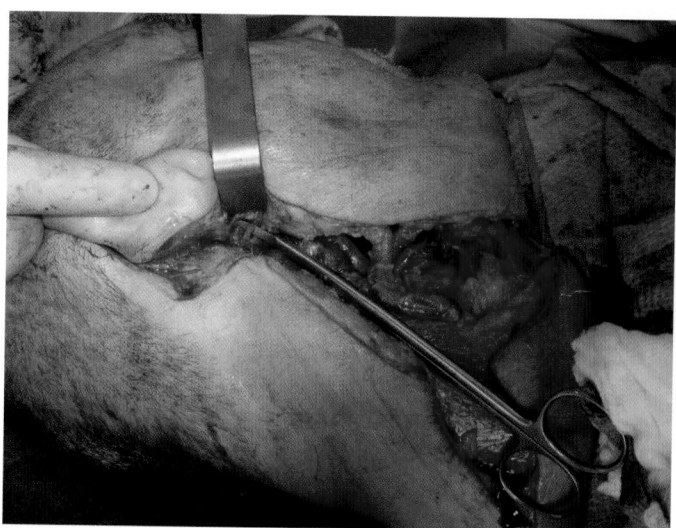

Fig. 20.13 Facial nerve.

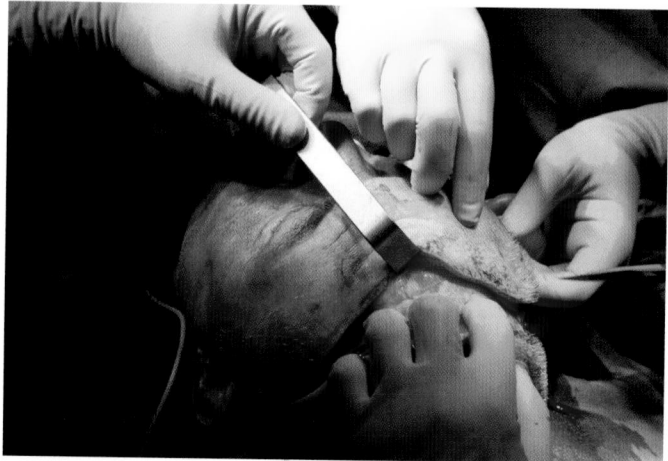

Fig. 20.14 Coronal approach.

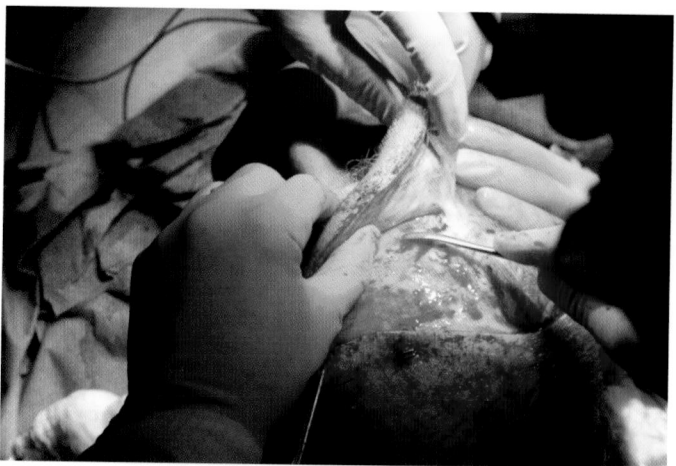

Fig. 20.15 Coronal approach 2.

necessary to harvest the occipital arteries. The dissection of these arteries is difficult and rarely reproducible, as they run very deep behind the sternocleidomastoid muscle. Our anatomical studies revealed that the superficial temporalis pedicle can perfuse at least 80% of the scalp and that the posterior auricular arteries are more important than occipital artery for scalp blood supply. The sagittal incision runs from the occipital area to the vertex. The scalp is dissected on a subperiosteal plane from backwards to forwards, as in a coronal approach. If the scalp is not necessary, a standard coronal approach is done. At that stage, the flap holds laterally by both maxillary arteries and vein just at the temporomandibular joint level. These vessels are ligated on both sides, which helps to have access to the orbital region *(Figs 20.16, 20.17)*. On the upper part of the flap, the dissection goes down to the levator muscle, which is divided after positioning a 3-0 nylon for easier repair *(Figs 20.18–20.21)*. The flap is then raised towards the front, following the masseter plane (beneath its aponeurosis) to the oral mucosa, along with the facial nerve, the parotid gland – including Stensen's duct, the superficial

portion, and part of the deep portion – the mental nerve, the orbicularis oris, and most of the smile muscles (including both the zygomaticus and levators). At the anterior edge of the masseter muscle, the dissection plane is subperiosteal at the level of the horizontal branch of the mandible and on the malar bone and the zygoma. The mental nerve is identified at its exit from the mental foramen and communicates with the oral cavity at the level of the cheek. The entire cheek mucosa is harvested along the parotid ostium. The buccal fat pad is left behind. On the dental part of the maxilla and mandible, the mucosa is cut at the gingival. The lateral canthus on each side is also divided after insertion of a 2-0 steel stitch, which will allow reinsertion *(Fig. 20.22)*. Infiltration will allow easy dissection of the eye conjunctiva which has to be incised at the border of the eyebulb. At that stage, the flaps holds medially only by the internal canthi. The lacrimal ducts are catheterized and the canthi are harvested with the nasal bone, by osteotomy. This osteotomy is wider than a rhinoplasty osteotomy to allow for the harvest of the medial canthi, the lacrimal duct, and bag. The infraorbital nerves are isolated on

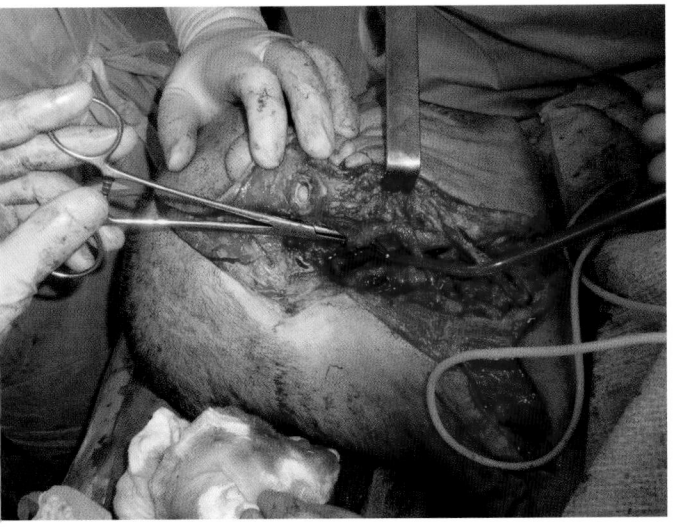

Fig. 20.16 Maxillary artery.

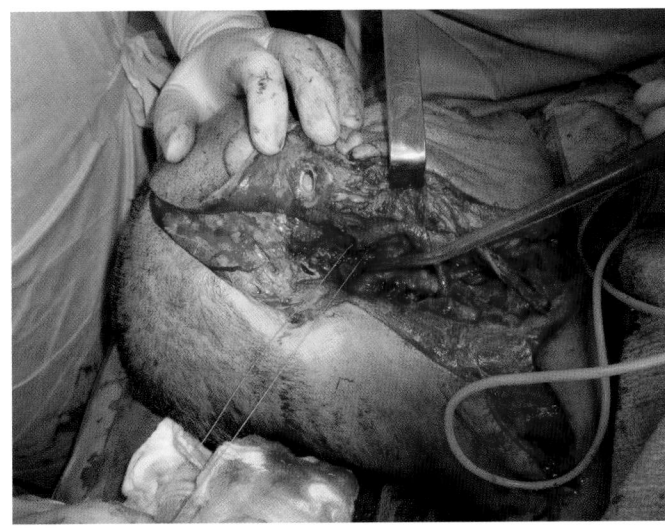

Fig. 20.17 Maxillary artery 2.

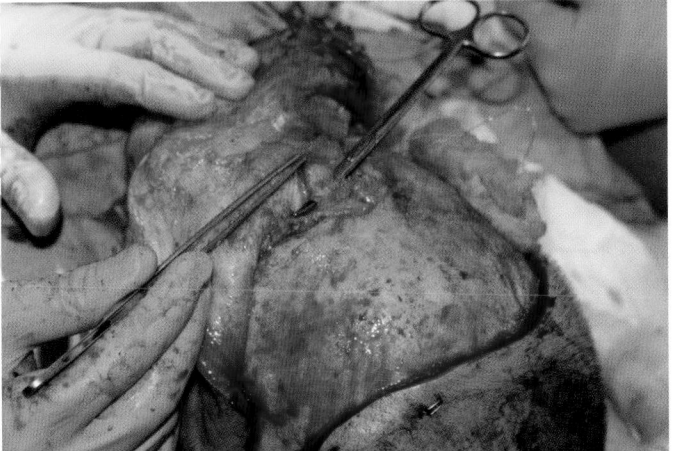

Fig. 20.18 Levator dissection.

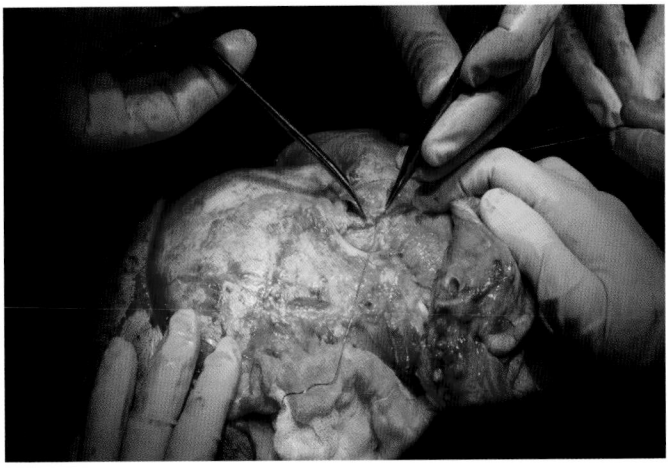

Fig. 20.19 Levator division.

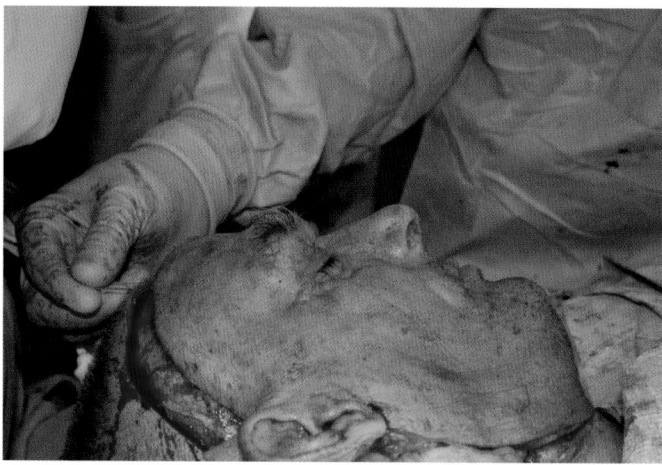

Fig. 20.20 Levator verification 1.

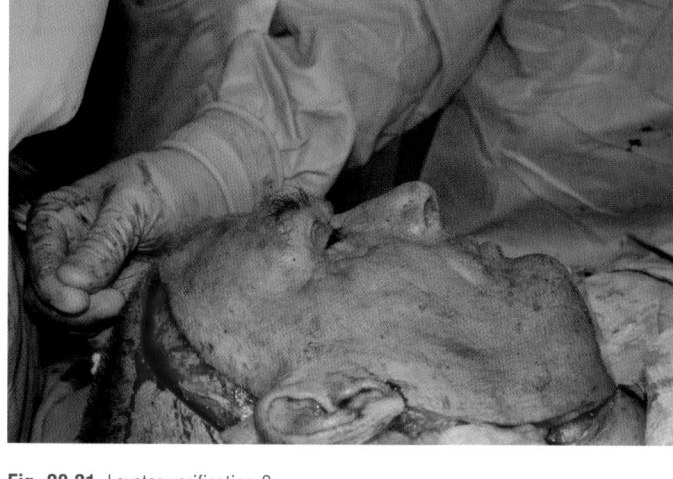

Fig. 20.21 Levator verification 2.

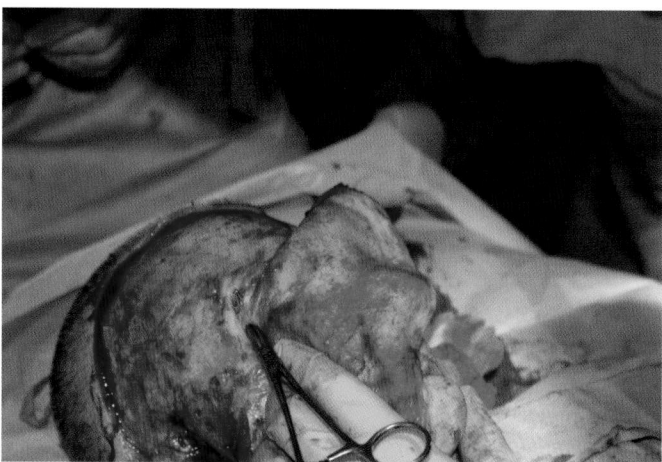

Fig. 20.22 External canthus dissection.

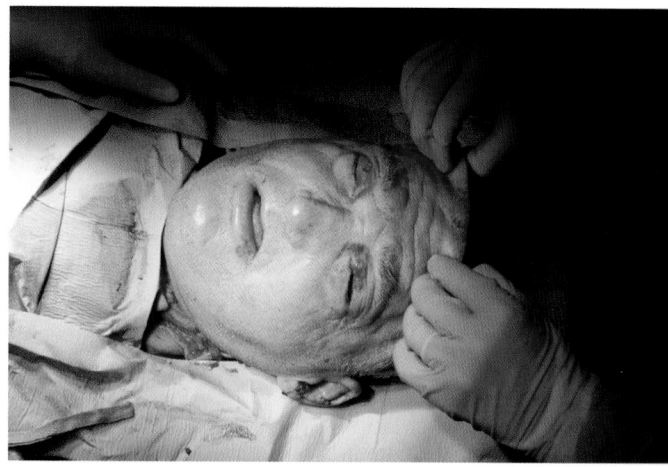

Fig. 20.23 Final dissection after medial osteotomy.

each side and transected at their foramen. The infraorbital nerve can be dissected on a longer route by a small osteotomy on the orbital margin. However, this is not relevant if the maxilla has to be transplanted at the same time as the rest of the face. In that case, the facial flap has to stay attached to the bone. This is also the case if the mandible is harvested, even if the main blood supply of the maxilla comes from the maxillary artery and the mandible from the dental artery. In practice, frank bleeding of the bone wedge can be seen once the transplant is revascularized showing that either periosteum vascularization or retrograde vascularization through the submental foramen is sufficient to vascularize the horizontal part of the mandible and. For the maxilla, the vascularization is probably due to the anastomosis between the facial artery and the maxillary artery through the infraorbital foramen. At that stage, the flap is almost completely liberated but remains attached in the submental region. The submaxillary gland is harvested with the facial artery which runs deep to it and the facial vein that runs superficially. As for any flap harvest, concentration has to be kept at maximum until the end, as the pedicle can be injured during the last moment. If so, it has to

be identified and repaired on the back table, before inset. At that stage, the transplant holds only by its blood supply: two external carotids and thyrolingofacial trunk *(Figs 20.23–20.29)*. The pedicle is divided. After harvest, the transplant is washed with heparinized saline followed by organ preservation solution and carried in a standard icebox *(Fig. 20.30)*. Before putting it in the icebox, an examination of the branches of the carotid artery is recommended, as the facial artery can easily be injured at the end of the dissection. The lacrimal duct catheters should also be secured *(Fig. 20.31)*. The cadaver is returned to the family with a painted resin mask prepared during the procedure, as explained previously (see Figs 20.4, 20.5). We recommend that people in charge of the facial reconstitution stay until the end of all harvested organs to allow the best possible restitution. In the case of lower face transplant, as for ballistic trauma, we advocate replacement of all of the lower part of the face as a cosmetic unit. The drawing of the flap begins in the glabella and follows the lateral limit of the nose and the infraorbital rim to the root of the helix *(Fig. 20.32)*. It then continues downward in the preauricular area to a location 5 cm below the mandibular angle, and

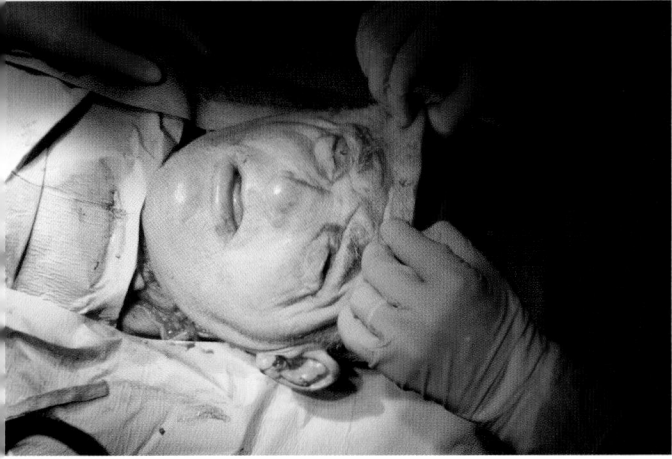

Fig. 20.24 Final dissection after medial osteotomy 2.

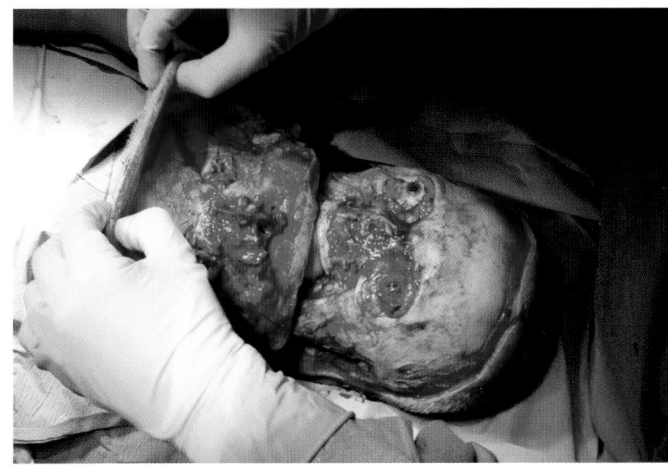

Fig. 20.25 Final dissection after medial osteotomy 3.

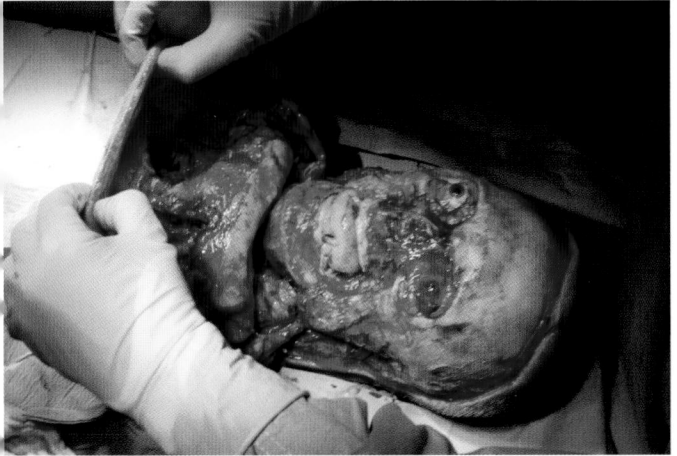

Fig. 20.26 Final dissection after medial osteotomy 4.

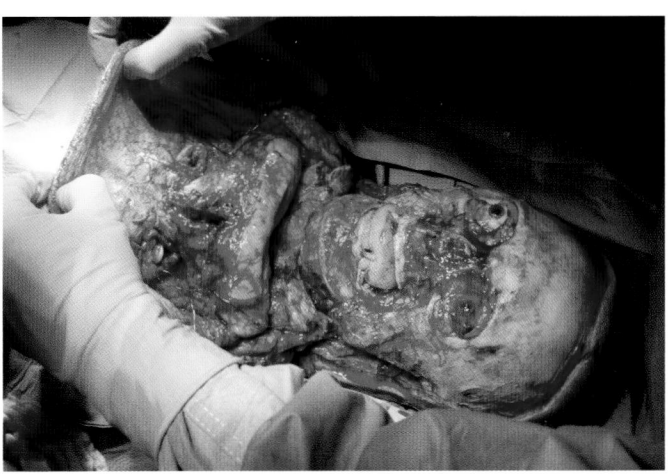

Fig. 20.27 Final dissection after medial osteotomy 5.

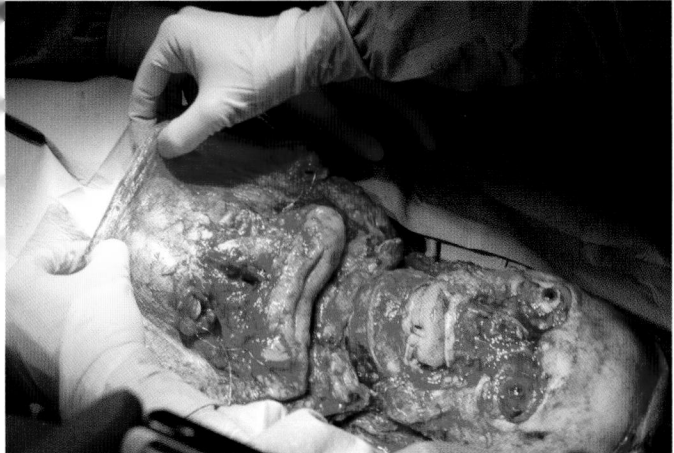

Fig. 20.28 Final dissection after medial osteotomy 6.

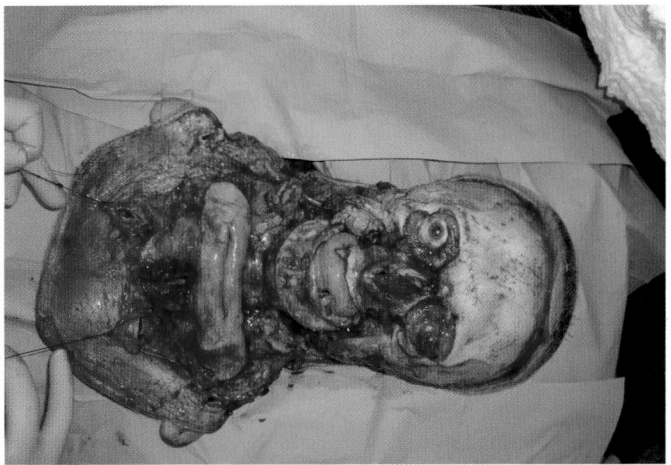

Fig. 20.29 Final dissection after medial osteotomy 7.

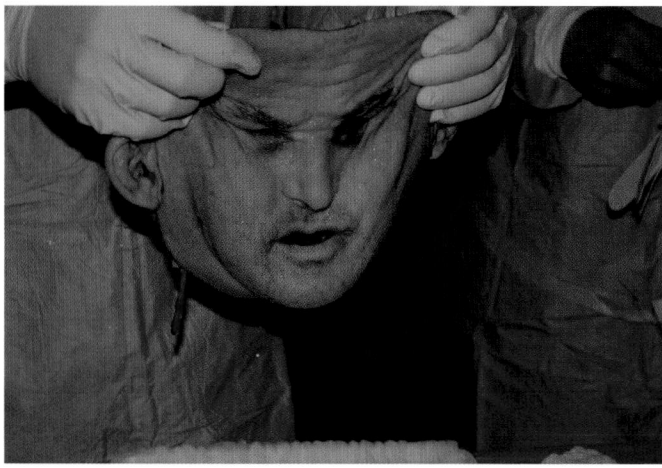

Fig. 20.30 Harvested transplant.

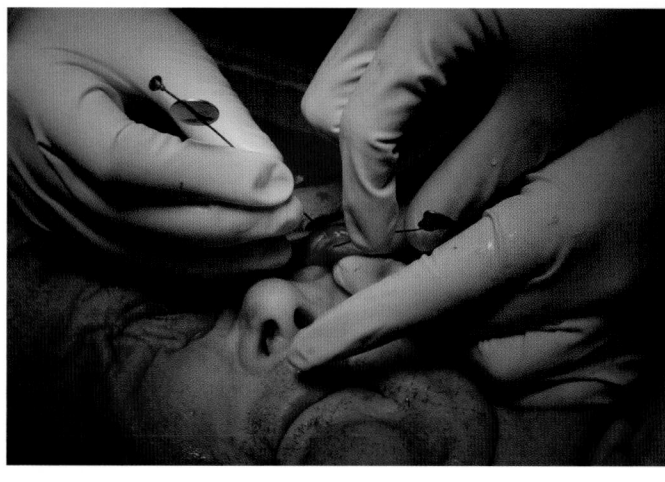

Fig. 20.31 Preparation of lacrimal ducts.

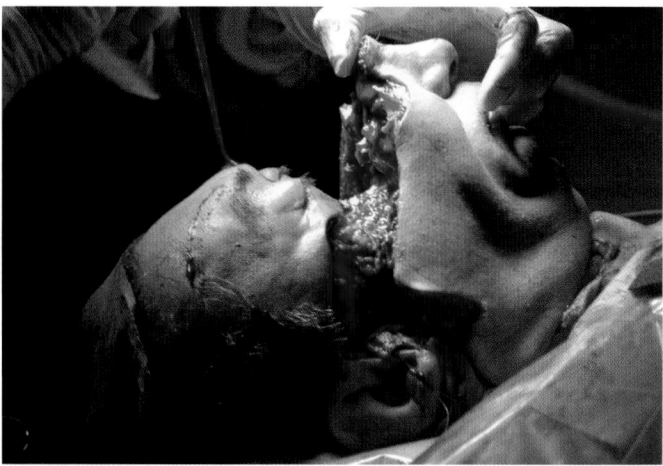

Fig. 20.32 Harvest of face transplant with maxilla and mandible.

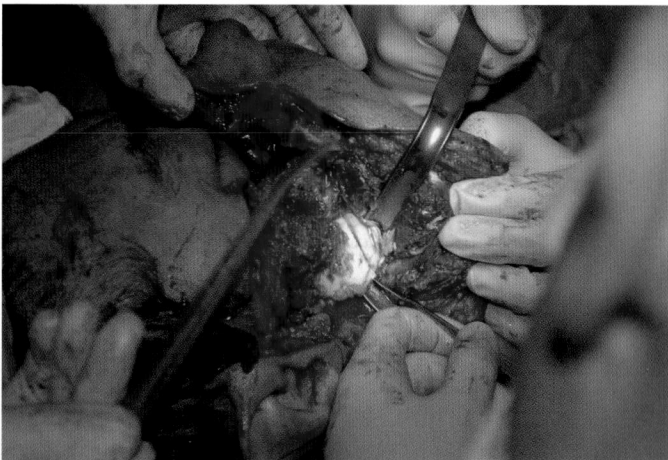

Fig. 20.33 Mandibular osteotomy.

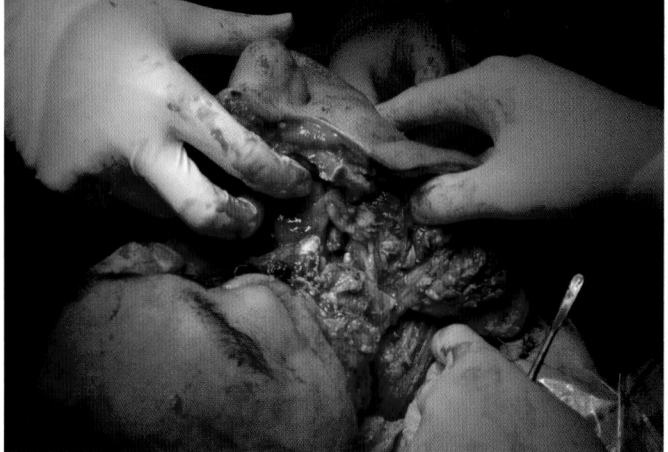

Fig. 20.34 Maxillary osteotomy.

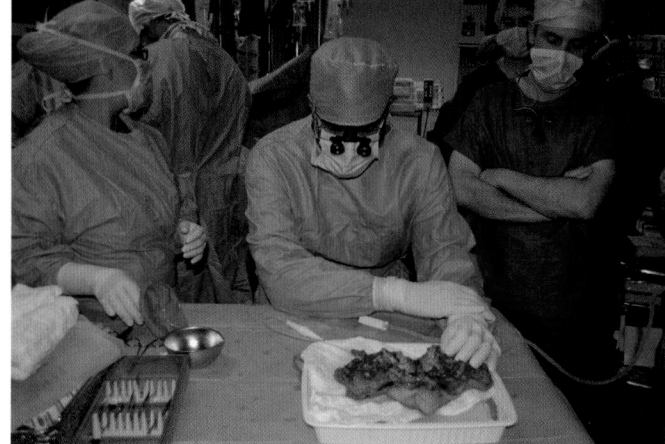

Fig. 20.36 Lower face transplant with mandible.

continues forward to join the opposite side in the anterior cervical area above the tracheotomy site. Osteotomy is carried out after vascular dissection. The maxilla and the mandible have to stay attached to the soft tissue to allow correct vascularization *(Figs 20.33–20.36)*. ⊕ FIG **20.35** APPEARS ONLINE ONLY

Recipient preparation

On the recipient, all scarred tissue should be debrided. As in conventional surgery, the respect of the cosmetic unit is a necessity to avoid a patchwork aspect but if this is true for the cutaneous aspect on the recipient where normal skin can be removed to allow cosmetic unit respect, it is obviously not true for the other elements *(Fig. 20.37)*. Any remaining muscle should be preserved as its function could be reactivated once liberated from scarred tissue. A superficial parotidectomy is realized on the recipient side, which allows the finding and distinguishing of upper and lower branches in the case of upper or lower transplant, and will allow suture without any tension. The arterial anastomosis are done as end end-to-end anastomosis on the external carotid artery and venous end-to-end anastomoses are performed on the thyrolingofacial trunks and on the external jugular when available *(Fig. 20.38)*. Thus, one should find two veins on each side, as the venous drainage seems to be mostly on the external jugular vessels. If no superficial vein is available as in the burn patient, the thyrolingofacial trunk can be anastomosed end-to-side on the external jugular, the final anastomosis being between the external jugular vein and the thyrolingofacial trunk, allowing full drainage with a long pedicle. After the first end-to-end anastomosis on the external carotid artery, the transplant is fully perfused, while the second anastomosis is performed after nervous repair going from one side to the other. The motor nerves (facial nerve) are always sutured but this can only be realized if the superficial parotidectomy has been correctly done. Individual suture to avoid dyskinesia is theoretically possible, however as explained above, the dissection of the facial nerve at a point of individualization of separate elements in the case of upper face transplant is not recommended, due to the risk of damaging the temporal vessels in the parotid gland. The sensory nerves (infraorbital and mental nerves) are sutured only when available. In the case of composite graft with bone this becomes impossible, as the nerves are included in the transplanted bones (see Figs 20.33, 20.34). The use of fibrin glue is helpful for nerve suture but also as a sealant to avoid postoperative hematoma. Bone fixation is performed when required with titanium plates and/or steel wire on the mandible and the maxilla. Bony fixation can be difficult due to discrepancies between the donor and the recipient, and it is necessary to take great care of this fixation which can necessitate several trimmings before correct fixation. In the case of mandibular transplant, the recipient remnant should be prepared carefully. Liberation of the masseter muscle may be necessary and section of the bony attachment of the temporal muscle tendon, as in an ankylosis. All sutures and fixation are done after unilateral venous and arterial anastomosis *(Fig. 20.39)*. The second side is done at the end. For the eyelid, if transplanted, the first step is to create a dacryocystorhinostomy by drilling a hole in the lateral wall of the nose *(Fig. 20.40)*. The lacrimal duct catheters are then passed into the nose *(Fig. 20.41)*. This operation should be done before suturing and fixing the bone. The nasal bone is then fixed with one screw which places the medial canthi *(Fig. 20.42)*. The lateral canthi are fixed with the previous steel wire *(Fig. 20.43)*. The end of the surgery is a simple skin closure *(Fig. 20.44)* *(Fig. 20.45)*. FIG **20.42, 20.43, 20.44** APPEAR ONLINE ONLY

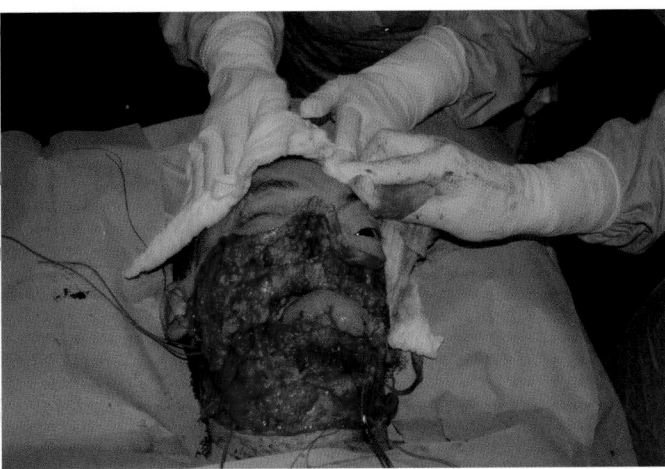

Fig. 20.37 Debridement of recipient for lower face transplant.

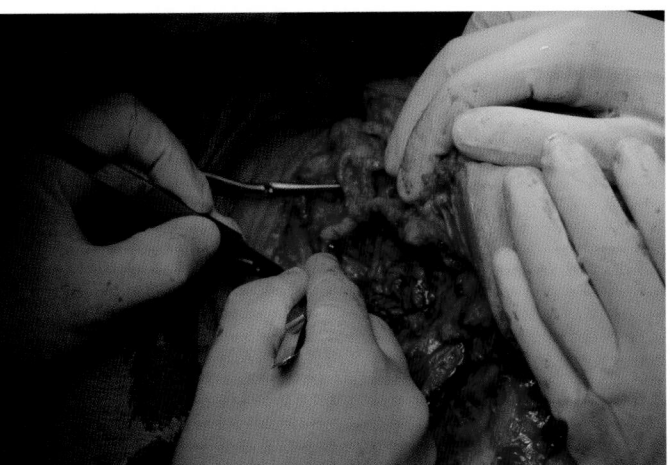

Fig. 20.38 Vascular anastomosis.

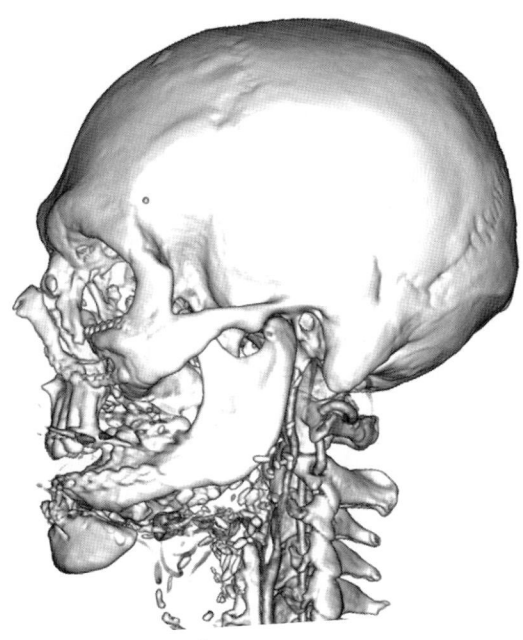

Fig. 20.39 Bone fixation.

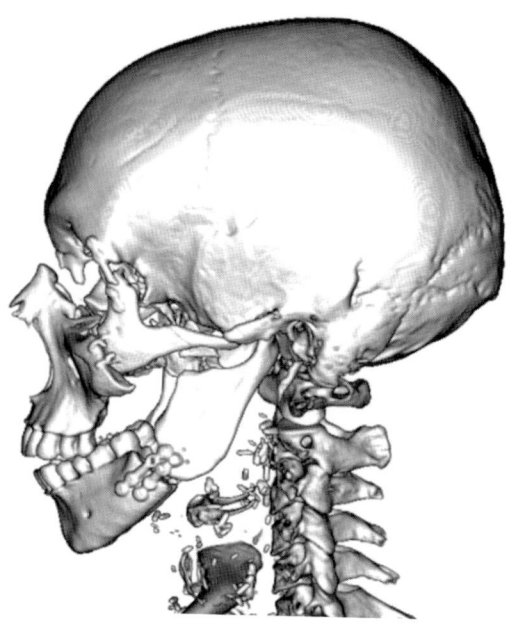

Fig. 20.40 Bone fixation 2.

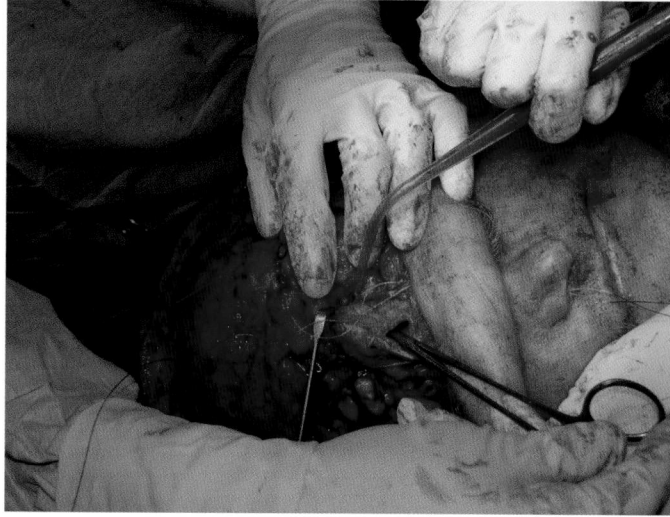

Fig. 20.41 Dacryocystorhinostomy.

Postoperative care

Infection prevention and treatment

Subsequent intercurrent infections can trigger rejection. This is particularly true in cytomegalovirus (CMV) infections.[51] Preventive treatment of these infections is possible in CMV-negative recipients, but we strongly recommend performing transplant in CMV-compatible status if possible. Prophylaxis for CMV infection consists of valganciclovir (900 mg/day for 6 months) if the donor and recipient statuses for CMV were: D+, R–. For the prevention of *Pneumocystis carinii* pneumonia, the patients receive trimethoprim-sulfamethoxazole (400 mg/day for 6 months). Our first recipient exhibited a prolonged valganciclovir-resistant viremia to CMV.[3] According to our CTA experience, viral infection (mostly related to CMV) appears to be more frequent compared with that in solid organ recipients: viral infection was reported in 34% of hand recipients,[52] and type 1 human herpes simplex virus has been reported after face CTA by several teams.[53] Infections appear to be an underestimated problem in the post-transplantation course of the immunocompromised recipients exposed to high-risk extended surgical procedures. Three of our four first recipients exhibited mild to severe bacterial infections in the early period, with dramatic consequences in one. As in solid organ transplant, such complications are related more to the surgical procedure than to an over-immunosuppression. In human hand transplants, the overall bacterial infection rate has been reported to be 11%.[46] According to our experience, we believe that postoperative bacterial infections are more frequent after facial CTA, and this should lead to specific prophylaxis and treatment for pre- and postoperative care. Preoperative bacterial mapping should be done as is postoperative regular bacterial counting. This is particularly true in transplantation for the burn patient who is often chronically infected with multiple resistant bacteria.

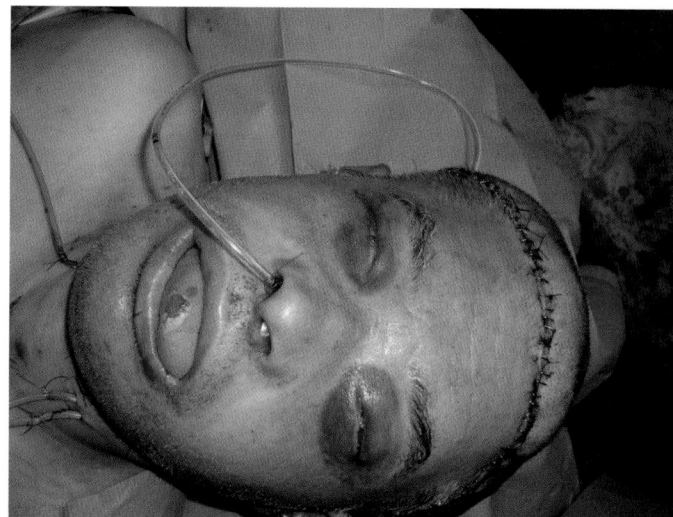

Fig. 20.45 Final closure.

Outcomes, prognosis, complications

Management of postoperative complications

As in any microsurgical procedure, thrombosis can occur leading to graft necrosis if not treated. To avoid such risk, the choice of large vessels is a necessity. However, in the multi-operated patient the recipient vessels can be in bad shape. The postoperative control of the artery by simple Doppler is possible. One should be aware that unilateral thrombosis can be very difficult do see clinically as the flap is totally perfused by one pedicle only. Any swelling, especially if asymmetrical, should be considered as a thrombosis and an echography and/or angioscanner should be done. Venous thrombosis can occur due to tension. Venous grafting is a possibility but can be replaced by re-routing the cephalic vein *(Figs 20.46, 20.47)*. The use of intravenous heparin is then necessary to avoid any new thrombosis. As the patient is in ICU for at least 2 weeks,

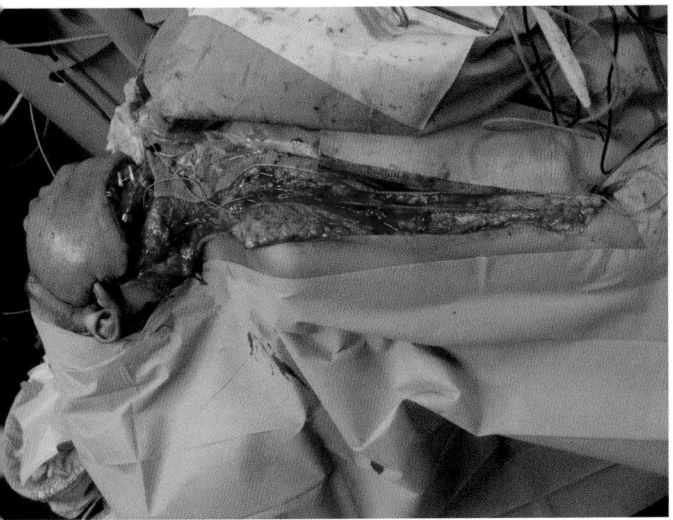

Fig. 20.46 Cephalic vein harvest.

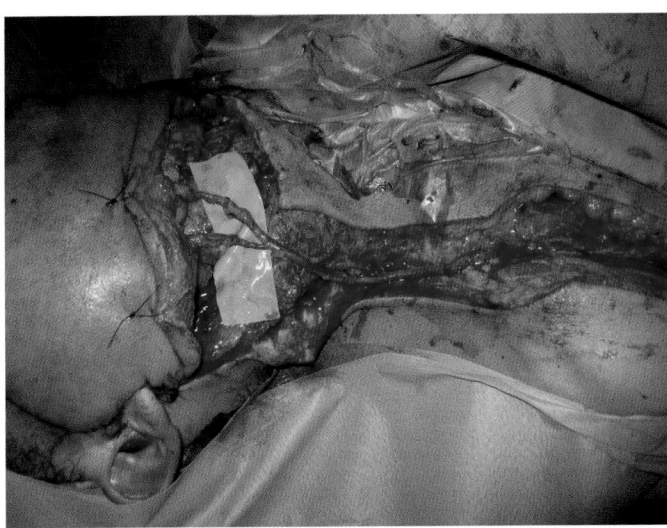

Fig. 20.47 Cephalic vein anastomosis.

all postoperative complications can be seen. Psychiatric problems can also be seen in postoperative period. These may not be different from those in any intensive surgery but confusion and agitation can be related to the use of steroids.

Follow-up

Transplantation has this particularity that long-term follow-up is a necessity. Any transplant requires monitoring. The advantage of CTAs is that they are visible and allow easy clinical monitoring. The rejection is characterized by inflammation followed by a macular erythematous rash preceding any necrosis. The onset of inflammation in the graft means biopsies must be performed in search of lymphocytic infiltration. Biopsies of the transplant should regularly be done to allow follow-up of potential rejection. The use of a histological classification, such as the Banff or Kanitakis[54,55] classification can be useful, but the clinical aspect is the key to estimating the presence or absence of rejection and to treat the patient. Biopsies should be made on different spots on the skin and the mucosa, as the rejection episode is generally not uniform. Beside histological and clinical follow-up, biological follow-up is a necessity, as in any transplant. Regular blood testing and clinical exam should follow for side-effects of the immunosuppressive treatment. Diabetes hypertension and chronic renal failure are the three major complications related to long-term immunosuppressive treatment. These blood tests are also a necessity to evaluate the compliance of the patient to the treatment. Physical therapy during the reinnervation process is important. Speech therapy helps the patient to improve and coordinates lip movement, which generally takes from 3–6 months. As of any transplanted patient, these patients have a higher risk of cancer, most of which are skin cancers that require a regular physical exam. Post-transplantation lymphoma disease also remains a major threat in these patients, as it has a high mortality rate if immunosuppression cannot stop immunosuppression, as seen in vital organs. This has never been seen in CTA so far, but will certainly be seen in the future as the number of transplanted patients increase.

Psychology

Some authors have argued that the psychological trauma resulting from the surgery would be so great that the procedure would cause more harm than good.[56,57] This was revealed to be absolutely false in our cases. We are not considering a patient with a normal face shifting from one face to another but rather a patient who is heavily disfigured with deep psychological scars. Thus, the surgery helps them to overcome the suffering psychological aspect. It is the stability of the patient during the process of evaluation which is the main argument to accept a patient on a program, and not the cause of disfigurement. A self-inflicted gunshot, for instance, is not a contraindication as far as the patient has to gain psychological stability. Borderline or bipolar personality can be contraindicating, as one should be sure that the patient will be able to take lifelong treatment. In the evaluation process, we are looking at the capacity of the patient to adapt to his disfigurement. The ideal candidate is paradoxically a patient who has good adaptation capacity and has managed to have some kind of social integration but at the same time expresses deep alteration of his quality of life. Before our first case, we thought that it would take a very long time for the patients to adapt to their new faces. We have since discovered that is not the case and that all patients have accepted their faces immediately, some of them describing the fact that they dream of themselves with their new face a couple of weeks after the transplant. Psychological support is however important as it is for patients sustaining any major surgery that necessitates intensive care and prolonged hospitalization.

Social reintegration

Social reintegration is the final goal of the surgery. It is correlated to the cosmetic and functional result. Cosmetic results necessitate respect of the cosmetic unit and correct nerve repair to restore facial animation. Even if a good cosmetic result can be achieved *(Figs 20.48–20.52)*, once surgery and immediate follow-up allows the patient to be discharged,

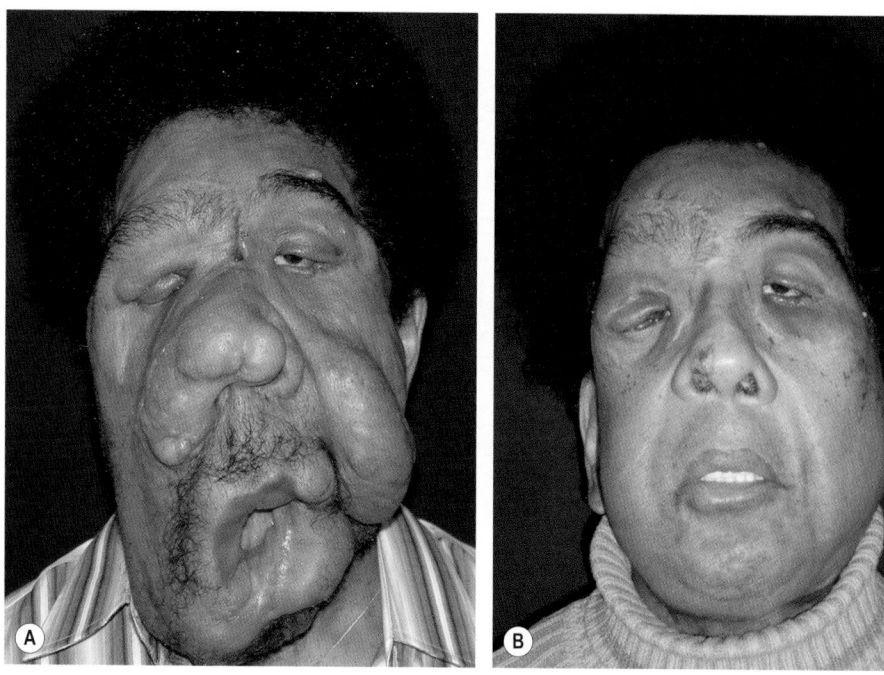

Fig. 20.48 Case 1: **(A)** Preoperative and **(B)** postoperative.

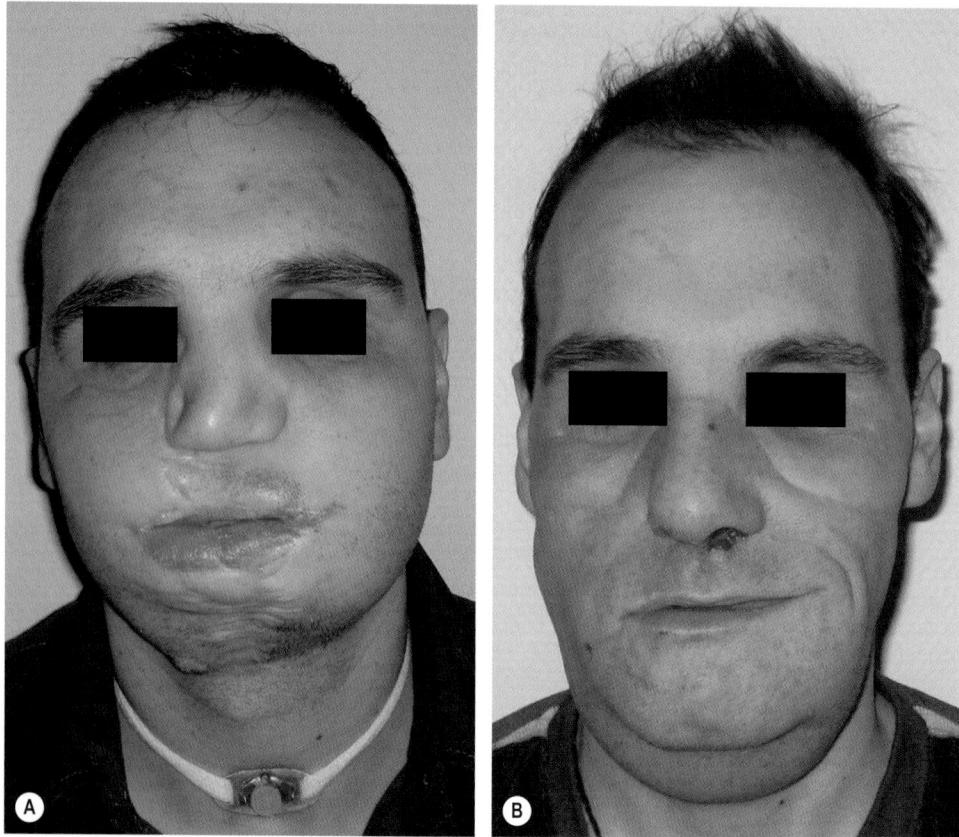

Fig. 20.49 Case 2: **(A)** Preoperative and **(B)** postoperative.

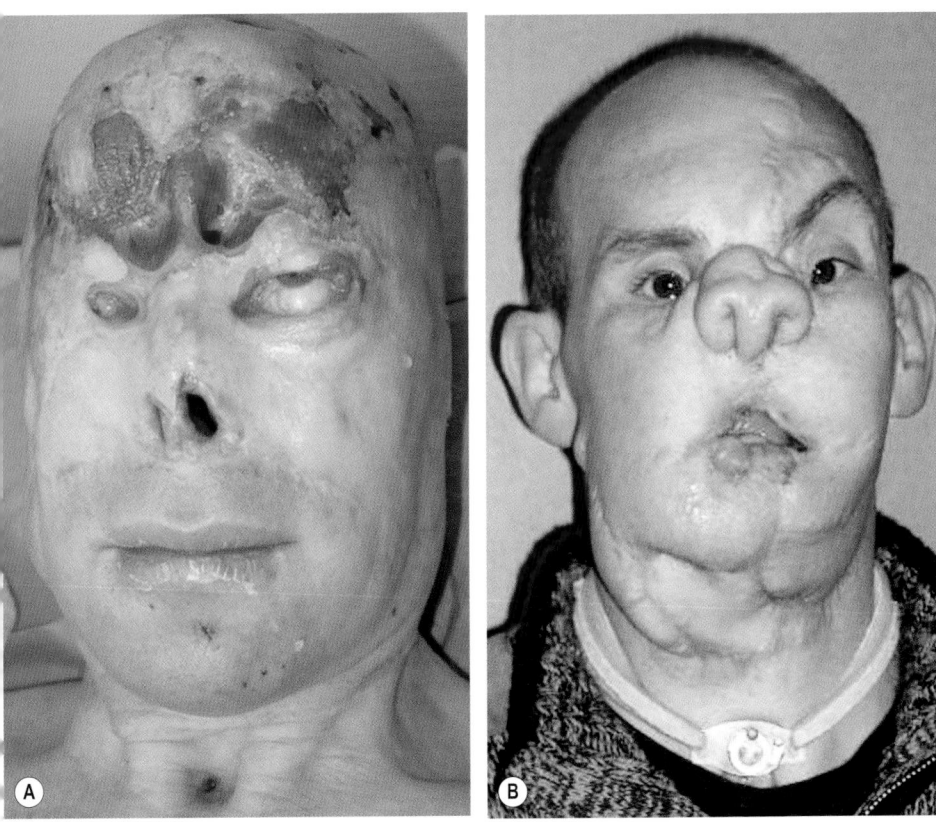

Fig. 20.50 Case 3: **(A)** Preoperative and **(B)** postoperative.

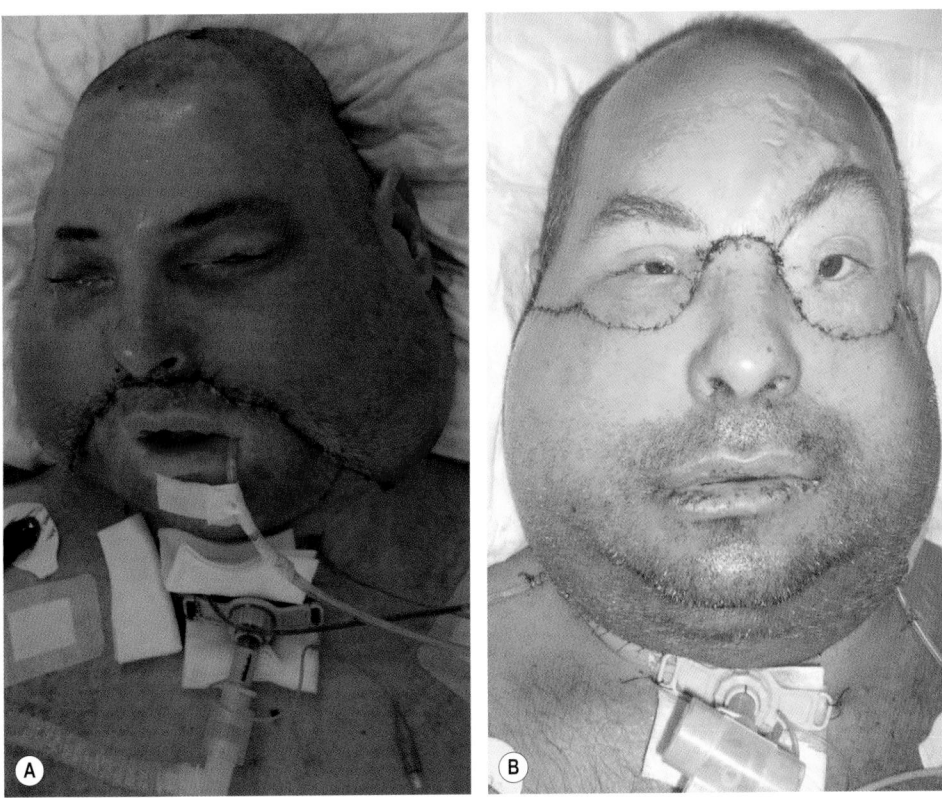

Fig. 20.51 Case 4: **(A)** Preoperative and **(B)** postoperative.

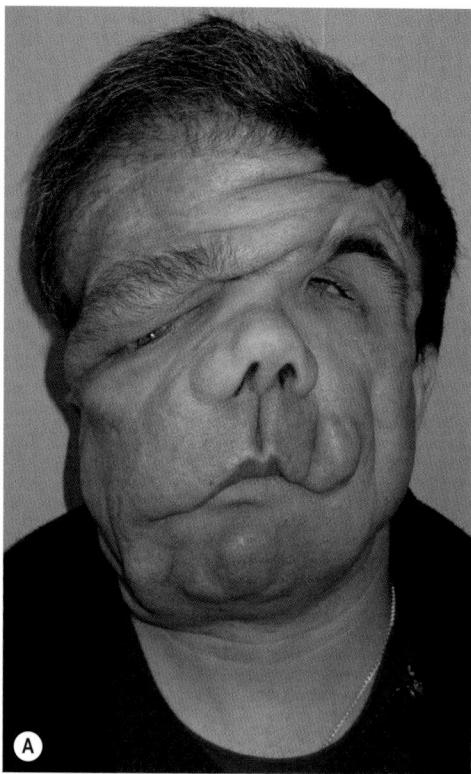 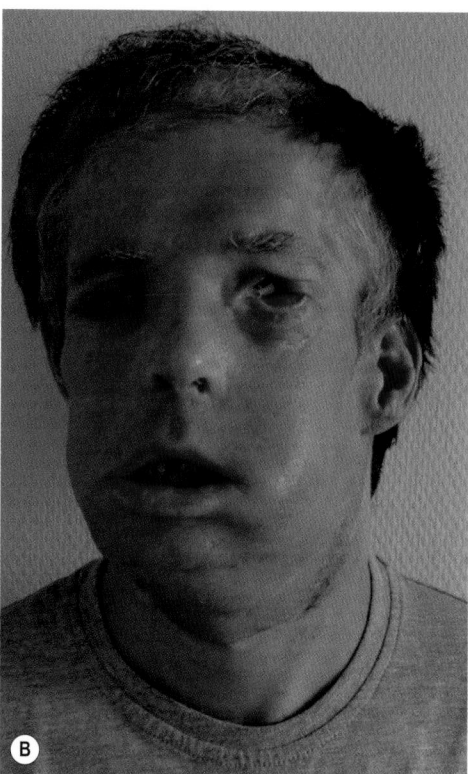

Fig. 20.52 Case 5: **(A)** Preoperative and **(B)** postoperative.

social workers should be involved to help the patient in his new life.

Revision surgery and secondary procedure

As in any reconstruction, a secondary procedure may be necessary. On the bony side, dental implants can be safely used as osteotomies if necessary. Scar revision, excision of skin and liposuction are also possible procedures. All these procedures should be done after evaluation of potential infection, local or general, as the patient is immunosuppressed. Vascular evaluation with CT angioscanner preoperatively is required as the anatomy is modified by the initial surgery. It is preferable to wait 6 months after transplant as any surgery can trigger a rejection episode. Injection of prednisolone immediately postoperative is useful to avoid rejection and treat potential swelling.

Access the Composite Tissue Allotransplantation Program section online at: **http://www.expertconsult.com**

Conclusion

We believe face transplants should reserved to a few centers where all the previously describe elements can be assured. I so, this new technology can bring a lot of relief for the patients who had previously no hope for any improvement. Quality of life improvement is one of the major goals of plastic surgery Face transplants, by giving back humanity to disfigured patients, brings this goal to the ultimate frontier. "It is of no use to give years to life if you don't give life to years".

 Bonus images for this chapter can be found online at **http://www.expertconsult.com**

Fig. 20.35 Lower face transplant.
Fig. 20.42 Nasal bone preparation.
Fig. 20.43 Lateral canthopexy.
Fig. 20.44 Final closure.

1. Dubernard JM, Lengele B, Morelon E, et al. Outcomes 18 months after the first human partial face transplantation. *N Engl J Med.* 2007;357: 2451–2460.

We performed the first human partial face allograft on November 27, 2005. Here we report outcomes up to 18 months after transplantation.

The postsurgical induction immunosuppression protocol included thymoglobulins combined with tacrolimus, mycophenolate mofetil, and prednisone. Donor hematopoietic stem cells were infused on postoperative days 4 and 11. Sequential biopsy specimens were taken from a sentinel skin graft, the facial skin, and the oral mucosa. Functional progress was assessed by tests of sensory and motor function performed monthly. Psychological support was provided before and after transplantation.

Sensitivity to light touch, as assessed with the use of static monofilaments, and sensitivity to heat and cold had returned to normal at 6 months after transplantation. Motor recovery was slower, and labial contact allowing complete mouth closure was achieved at 10 months. Psychological acceptance of the graft progressed as function improved. Rejection episodes occurred on days 18 and 214 after transplantation and were reversed. A decrease in inulin clearance led to a change in immunosuppressive regimen from tacrolimus to sirolimus at 14 months. Extracorporeal photochemotherapy was introduced at 10 months to prevent recurrence of rejection. There have been no subsequent rejection episodes. At 18 months, the patient is satisfied with the aesthetic result.

2. Guo S, Han Y, Zhang X, et al. Human facial allotransplantation: a 2-year follow-up study. *Lancet.* 2008;372:631–638.

The authors did a partial facial allotransplantation in 2006, and reports here the 2 year follow-up of the patient.

The recipient, a 30-year-old man from China, had his face severely injured by a bear in October, 2004. Allograft composite tissue transplantation was done in April, 2006, after careful systemic preparation. The surgery included anastomosis of the right mandibular artery and anterior facial vein, whole repair of total nose, upper lip, parotid gland, front wall of the maxillary sinus, part of the infraorbital wall, and zygomatic bone. Facial nerve anastomosis was done during the surgery. Quadruple immunomodulatory therapy was used, containing tacrolimus, mycophenolate mofetil, corticosteroids, and humanized IL-2 receptor monoclonal antibody. Follow-up included T lymphocyte subgroups in peripheral blood, pathological and immunohistochemical examinations, functional progress, and psychological support.

Composite tissue flap survived well. There were three acute rejection episodes at 3, 5, and 17 months after transplantation, but these were controlled by adjustment of the tacrolimus dose or the application of methylprednisolone pulse therapy. Hepatic and renal functions were normal, and there was no infection. The patient developed hyperglycemia on day 3 after transplantation, which was controlled by medication.

3. Lantieri L, Meningaud JP, Grimbert P, et al. Repair of the lower and middle parts of the face by composite tissue allotransplantation in a patient with massive plexiform neurofibroma: a 1-year follow-up study. *Lancet.* 2008;372:639–645.

4. Siemionow M, Papay F, Alam D, et al. First U.S. near-total human face transplantation-a paradigm shift for massive facial injuries. *Lancet.* 2009;374:203–209.

An innovative approach entailing a single surgical procedure of face allograft transplantation is a viable alternative and gives improved results.

On Dec 9, 2008, a 45-year-old woman with a history of severe midface trauma underwent near-total face transplantation in which 80% of her face was replaced with a tailored composite tissue allograft. We addressed issues of immunosuppressive therapy, psychological and ethical outcomes, and re-integration of the patient into society.

After the operation, the patient did well physically and psychologically, and tolerated immunosuppression without any major complication. Routine biopsy on day 47 after transplantation showed rejection of graft mucosa; however, a single bolus of corticosteroids reversed rejection. During the first 3 weeks after transplantation, the patient accepted her new face; 6 months after surgery, the functional outcome has been excellent. In contrast to her status before transplantation, the patient can now breathe through her nose, smell, taste, speak intelligibly, eat solid foods, and drink from a cup.

8. Eaton L. Spanish doctors carry out first transplantation of a full face. *BMJ.* 2010;340:c2303.

This was an article in the British Medical Journal and describes the first full face transplant. The operation was carried out at the end of March 2010 at Vall d'Hebron University Hospital in Barcelona.

Now Dr Barret, who has specialized in treating burns victims in the past and who has worked at the St Andrews Centre for Plastic Surgery and Burns in Chelmsford, Essex, believes that where someone has severe facial injuries it may be better to perform a full face transplantation than to try to patch them up with skin grafts.

The patient had lost the centre of his face—his nose, his mouth, the mandibles of the jaw, both cheekbones, his eyelids, and part of his soft tissue—in a "severe, high energy" accident. Dr Barret would not confirm reports that the injury was the result of a gunshot wound.

"He had sustained the injury in 2005 and had already had nine operations in another hospital in an attempt to restore his oral competence," he said.

In 2007 the team at the Barcelona hospital was alerted to the patient's plight and began to see whether the man, whose age is given as between 25 and 35, would be a suitable recipient of a face transplant. After psychological investigations doctors decided that he was a good candidate. Approval from the Madrid based National Organ Transplant Body was finally given in August 2009.

10. Dubernard JM, Owen E, Herzberg G, et al. Human hand allograft: report on the first 6 months. *Lancet.* 1999;353(9161):1315–1320.

18. Murray JE. Annual discourse – organ replacement, facial deformity, and plastic surgery. *N Engl J Med.* 1972;287(21):1069–1074.

    Plastic surgery, second only to obstetrics as the oldest surgical specialty, is tested most rigorously in the treatment of facial deformities. Through the centuries the mutilated nose cut off as punishment for murder, theft, or infidelity, the congenital cleft lip, and the face eaten by cancer or torn by trauma have forced the reconstructive surgeon to seek imaginative ways to restore both function and an aesthetically acceptable appearance.

28. Gibson T, Medawar PB. The fate of skin homografts in man. *J Anat.* 1943;77(Pt 4):299–310.4.

37. Starzl TE. Immunosuppressive therapy and tolerance of organ allografts. *N Engl J Med.* 2008;358(4):407–411.

49. Meningaud JP, Benjoar MD, Hivelin M, et al. The procurement of total human face graft for allotransplantation: A preclinical study and the first clinical case. *Plast Reconstr Surg.* 2010;15 June [Epub ahead of print].

21

Surgical management of migraine headaches

Bahman Guyuron and Ali Totonchi

SYNOPSIS

- Approximately 30 million Americans suffer from migraine headaches (MH) and lifetime prevalence is estimated to be 11–32%, including 18% of women and 6% of men.
- Poorly controlled or uncontrolled MH can be treated surgically.
- Before considering a patient for surgical management, he/she should be evaluated by a neurologist for diagnosis and medical management.
- In the surgical evaluation of patients with MH, the trigger site can be confirmed by botulinum toxin A (BTX-A) injection or nerve block. If the history or computed tomography (CT) scan findings are strongly indicative of a specific trigger site, this step can be bypassed.
- The four major trigger sites are: frontal, temporal, occipital, and nasal.
- In the frontal trigger site, the supraorbital and supratrochlear nerves are irritated while passing through the frowning muscles and this area is treated by resection of the glabellar muscle group (depressor supercilii, corrugator supercilii, and lateral portion of the procerus muscle) and replacement with fat graft.
- The temporal trigger site is treated by avulsion of the zygomaticotemporal branch of trigeminal nerve (ZTBTN) as it emerges from deep temporal fascia.
- The occipital trigger site is located in the posterior part of the neck where the greater occipital nerve is passing through the semispinalis capitis muscle and crosses over the occipital artery; treatment includes partial resection of the muscle, padding the nerve with a subcutaneous flap, and resection of the artery adjacent to the nerve.
- Rhinogenic trigger site is treated with septoplasty, elimination of contact points between the turbinate and the septum, reduction of enlarged turbinates, and decompression of concha bullosa or septa bullosa.

Introduction

Headaches are the seventh leading presenting complaint in ambulatory medical care in the US.[1] Nearly 30 million Americans suffer from MH and lifetime prevalence is estimated to be 11–32% across several countries. Eighteen percent of women and 6% of men are involved, and two-thirds of these patients do not benefit from over-the-counter medications. In women, MHs are more common than asthma (5%) and diabetes (6%) combined. MHs are ranked as number 19 among all diseases worldwide causing disability. Many of the available prophylactic medications harbor side-effects such as sedation, paresthesia, weight gain, cognitive impairment, and sexual dysfunction. The cost of migraine treatment and loss of time from work associated with MH impose a major economic burden on the patient and society, collectively exceeding $13 billion.[1-11]

Basic science/disease process

The diagnostic criteria of MH are shown in Box 21.1. There are two subtypes of migraine: migraine with aura and migraine without aura. Auras develop over 5–20 minutes, but last for less than 60 minutes, and are followed by a migraine. One out of three patients with MH experiences aura. MHs are usually frontotemporal, typically unilateral, and are characterized by recurrent attacks of pulsating, intense pain associated with nausea and photophobia. Traditional, nonsurgical treatment of MH can be nonpharmacologic or pharmacologic. Nonpharmacologic treatment of MH consists of avoidance of triggers, which commonly include caffeine, alcohol, or tobacco, and sometimes application of pressure, cold, or heat. Pharmacologic treatment can be further subdivided into acute analgesic, acute abortive, and prophylactic treatment. Acute analgesic treatment consists of pain control, acetaminophen, nonsteroidal anti-inflammatory drugs, analgesics, benzodiazepines, opioids, and barbiturates. The first-line acute abortive treatment is the use of triptans, although intravenous antiemetics and ergotamine can be used as well. Prophylactic treatment consists of beta-blockers, tricyclic antidepressants, and valproic acid.[12,13]

Box 21.1 Migraine headache diagnostic criteria

Migraine without aura

A. At least five attacks fulfilling criteria B–D

B. Headache attacks lasting 4–72 hours (untreated or unsuccessfully treated)

C. Headache has at least two of the following characteristics:
  a. Unilateral location
  b. Pulsating quality
  c. Moderate or severe pain intensity
  d. Aggravation by or causing avoidance of routine physical activity (e.g., walking or climbing stairs)

D. During headache at least one of the following:
  a. Nausea and/or vomiting
  b. Photophobia and phonophobia

E. Not attributed to another disorder

Migraine with aura

A. At least two attacks fulfilling criteria B–D

B. Aura consisting of at least one of the following, but no motor weakness:
  a. Fully reversible visual symptoms including positive features (e.g., flickering lights, spots, or lines) and/or negative features (i.e., loss of vision)
  b. Fully reversible sensory symptoms including positive features (i.e., pins and needles) and/or negative features (i.e., numbness)
  c. Fully reversible dysphasic speech disturbance

C. At least two of the following:
  a. Homonymous visual symptoms1 and/or unilateral sensory symptoms
  b. At least one aura symptom develops gradually over ≥5 minutes and/or different aura symptoms occur in succession over ≥5 minutes
  c. Each symptom lasts ≥5 and ≤60 minutes

D. Headache fulfilling criteria B–D for Migraine without aura begins during the aura or follows aura within 60 minutes

E. Not attributed to another disorder

(Adapted from International Headache Society website: http://i-h-s.org.)

Diagnosis/patient presentation

Preoperative history and considerations

Surgical treatment of a MH should only be considered after the diagnosis of MH is confirmed by a neurologist and more serious causes of headaches have been excluded. The proper surgical candidate is someone whose headaches are not controlled with traditional medical treatment and who has an acceptable surgical risk. Pregnant and nursing women are also typically excluded from surgical consideration. The constellation of symptoms leads the examiner to suspect the potential trigger site *(Table 21.1)*, which is further validated by physical examination.[28,32] The salient piece of information that helps to identify the trigger site is the site from which the pain starts. The patient is asked to complete a migraine form asking a number of critical questions. Keeping a monthly diary of MH prior to the surgery may provide more reliable information.

Hypertrophy of the corrugator supercilii muscle with vertical frown lines is a common finding and might be obvious in

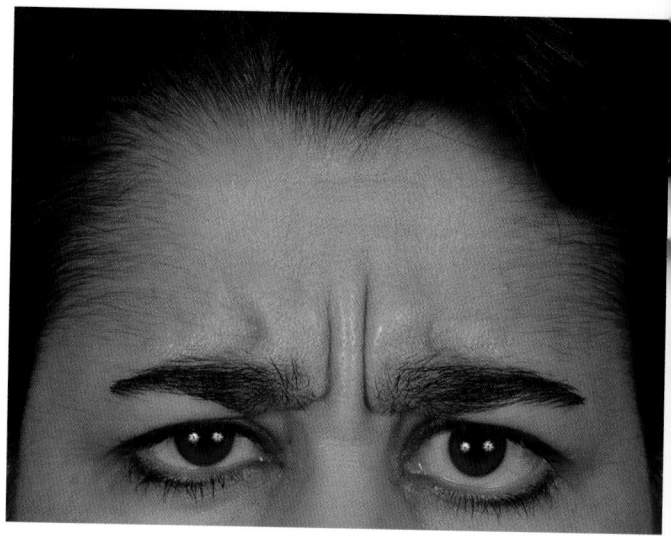

Fig. 21.1 Example of corrugator supercilii muscle hypertrophy.

patients with a frontal trigger site *(Fig. 21.1)*. The nasal exam includes a physical exam with or without endoscopic examination, which must be performed to detect septal deviation and turbinate hypertrophy with contact points between the septum and turbinates, concha bullosa and septa bullosa, and the findings are confirmed using a CT scan of the septum and sinuses *(Fig. 21.2)*.

Patient selection

Trigger sites

Currently, we have identified four common trigger sites: (1) frontal triggers, where glabellar muscles and possibly vessels compress the supratrochlear and supraorbital nerves and subsequent release of substance P and neurokines causes frontal headaches; (2) temporal triggers, where compression of ZTBTN by contraction of the temporalis muscle causes inflammation of the nerve and leads to temporal headaches; (3) occipital triggers, where the semispinalis capitis and occipital artery can compress the occipital nerve and cause occipital headaches; and (4) septonasal triggers, where intranasal structures compress the trigeminal end branches and cause paranasal and retrobulbar headaches.

There are several less common trigger sites, some of which are at intersections of nerves and arteries, such as the superficial temporal artery and the auriculotemporal nerve. The lesser occipital nerve and the third occipital nerve can also act as trigger sites.[26,27]

The role of botulinum toxin

BTX-A (Botox, Allergan, Irvine, CA) or abobotulinumtoxinA (Dysport, Medicis Aesthetics, Scottsdale, AZ) blocks the release of acetylcholine at the neuromuscular junction. A deadly neurotoxin produced by *Clostridium botulinum*, its clinical utility in MH has been gaining popularity over the last decade.[22,23]

Table 21.1 **The constellation of symptoms that aid in the diagnosis of migraine headache trigger sites**

	Frontal	Temporal	Rhinogenic	Occipital
Starting location of pain	Frontal area	Temple area	Behind the eye	At the point of exit of the greater occipital nerve from the semispinalis capitis muscle (3.5 cm caudal to the occipital tuberosity and 1.5 cm off the midline)
Time	Usually in the afternoon	Patient usually wakes up in the morning with pain	Patient commonly wakes up with pain in the morning or at night	Not specific
Exam, observation	Strong corrugator muscle activity causing deep frown lines on animation The points of emergence of the supraorbital and supratrochlear nerves from corrugator muscle or the foramen are tender to the touch Patients usually have eyelid ptosis on the affected side at the time of active pain Pressure on these sites may abort the headache during the initial stages Application of cold or warm compresses on these sites often reduces or stops the pain The pain is usually imploding in nature Stress-related	Sometimes associated with tenderness of the temporalis or masseteric muscle Clenching/grinding Rubbing or pressing the exit point of the zygomatico-temporal branch of the trigeminal nerve from the deep temporal fascia can stop the pain in the beginning Application of cold or warm compresses to this point may reduce or stop the pain The pain is characterized as imploding Stress-related	Commonly triggered by weather changes Rhinorrhea on the affected side Allergy-related Hormone-related, menstrual cycle-related The pain is usually described as exploding	Muscle tightness Heavy exercise-related Compression of this site can stop the pain in the early stage; at the later stage, this point is tender Application of cold or heat at this site may result in some improvement in the pain Stress-related
CT scan			Concha bullosa, septal deviation with contact between the turbinates and the septum, and septa bullosa	

CT, computed tomography.

BTX-A was first introduced over three decades ago as a treatment for strabismus,[33–36] and since has been used in many neuromuscular conditions, including oromandibular dystonia, laryngeal dystonia, cervical dystonia, writer's cramp, hemifacial spasm, and for aesthetic reasons.[37,38]

Since the original reports regarding the use of BTX-A for treatment of headache[19–21] and subsequent reports for its use in the determination of trigger sites,[23] the review of the neurology literature is contradictory in terms of success rate, possibly because these studies were not specific about the location of the injection.[39–42]

When BTX-A is used to identify trigger sites, the sites are injected systematically, starting with the most common and severe trigger site based on the patient's reported symptoms and physical examination. This is most often the corrugator supercilii muscle. First, 12.5 U BTX-A is injected with a long 30-gauge needle into the glabellar muscle sites. Patients then keep a headache diary, and refrain from taking prophylactic migraine medication unless contraindicated. Response to the injection over the subsequent 4 weeks will direct the next step. If the headache disappears completely, it means the injected site is likely to be the sole trigger site. If the headaches are improved but not eliminated, it means that the patient has additional trigger sites. If the patient does not respond to the injection, it means that the headaches are not likely to be triggered from the initial injection site (*Fig. 21.3*). Trigger sites are injected 1 month apart, up to a maximum of three injections. Those patients with trigger sites that observe at least 50% reduction in intensity or frequency of the headache from baseline are considered for surgical intervention.[28] Nerve blocks

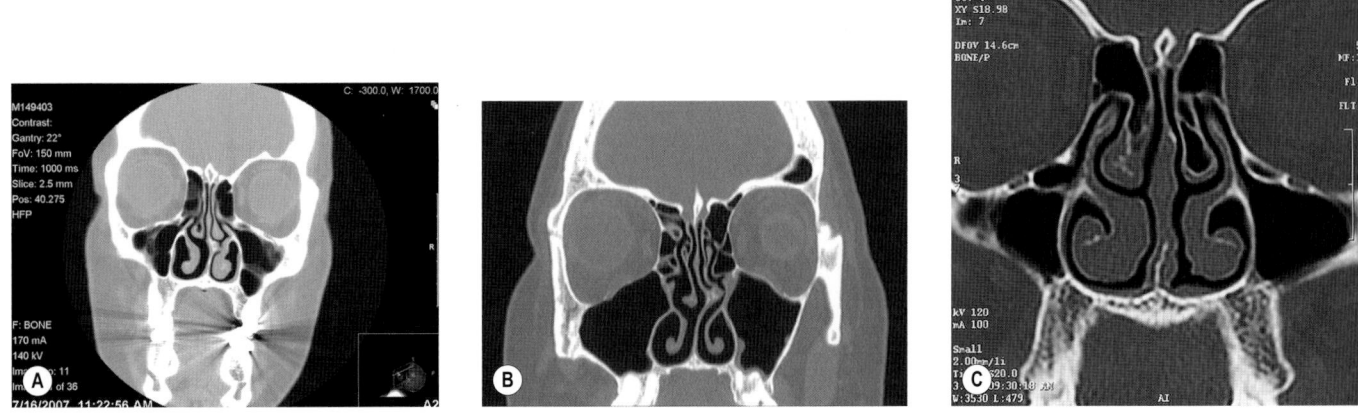

Fig. 21.2 (A) Combination of a large spur protruding into the left inferior turbinate, right middle turbinate concha bullosa, and extensive sinus disease. **(B)** Significant enough deviation of the septum to the left to touch the lateral wall of the nose and the left middle turbinate along with mild maxillary sinus disease. **(C)** Bilateral concha bullosa of the middle turbinates and Haller's cell.

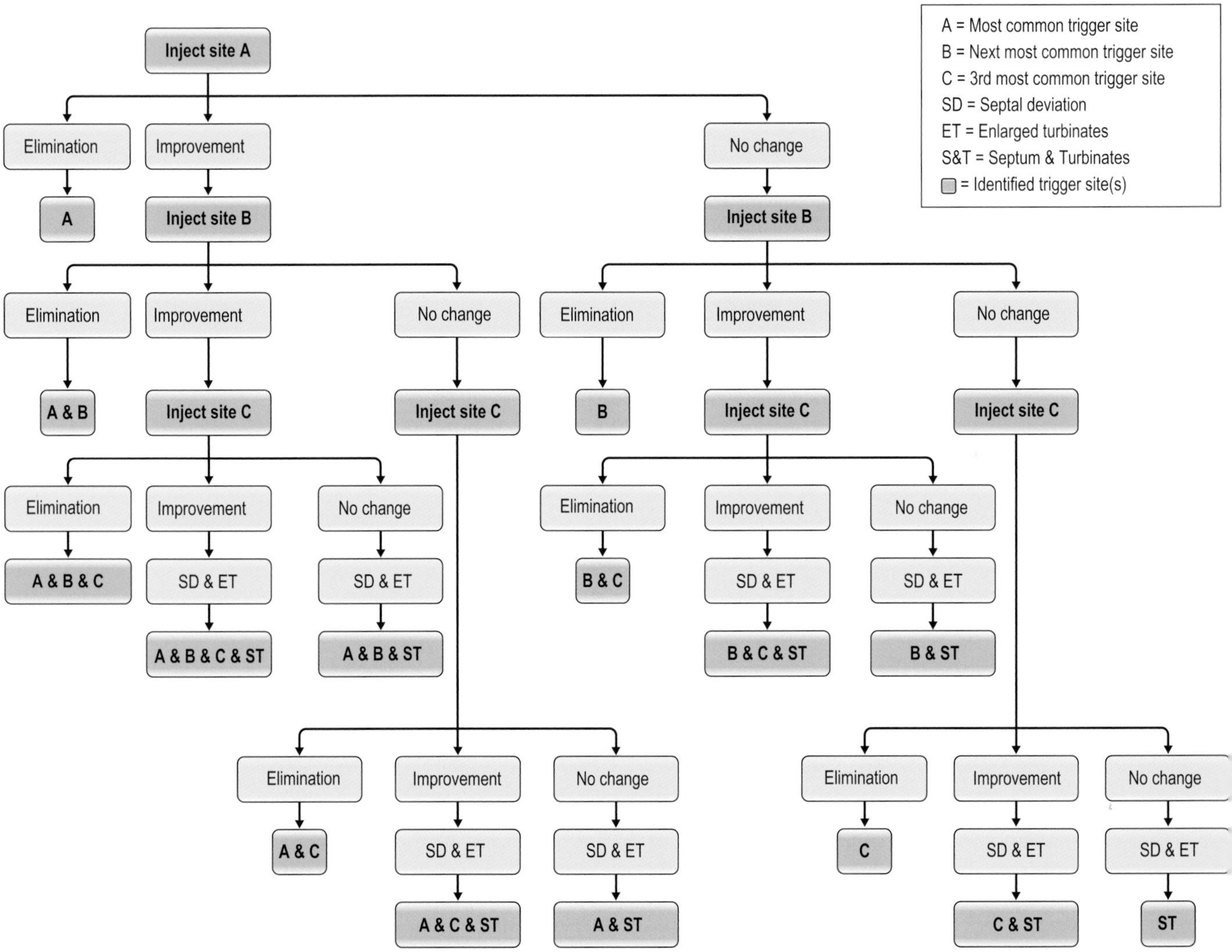

Fig. 21.3 Algorithm for diagnosis of migraine headache (MH) using botulinum toxin. Trigger sites are injected with 12.5 U botulinum toxin A with a 1-inch (2.5-cm) 30-gauge needle. Improvement is operationally defined as a 50% reduction in headache intensity or frequency from the baseline for 4 weeks. (Redrawn from Guyuron B, Kriegler JS, Davis J, *et al. Comprehensive surgical treatment of migraine headaches. Plast Reconstr Surg 2005;115:1–9.)

could be used similarly, but the timing of the injections is difficult since it has to be at the time of migraine episodes and the duration of effect is short.

The primary side-effect of BTX-A injected into the temporal area is atrophy of the temporal muscles and related hollowing of the temples and the reported hourglass deformity.[43] This disuse atrophy is temporary, and patients should be counseled appropriately. Eyelid ptosis is the second most common complication. Theoretically, strabismus might happen because of the high dose and deep injection in the temple or brow areas. Some patients have developed antibodies to BTX-A, rendering it relatively ineffective. This has been estimated to occur in over 7% of treated patients.[36,44] The use of non-A botulinum toxins for patients resistant to type A is currently being investigated.[36]

While BTX-A had a major role in the detection of the trigger sites and as the prognosticator during the initial phases of the development of this procedure, we currently do not use it routinely. A nerve block will serve a similar role if it is injected while the patient is in the early stages of the migraine cascade. The constellation of symptoms can serve as reliably as BTX-A in the detection of the trigger sites.

Treatment/surgical technique

Deactivation of frontal triggers

In the frontal trigger site, the supraorbital and supratrochlear nerves are passing through the glabellar muscles, including the corrugator supercilii, depressor supercilii, and procerus. The goal of surgery is to prevent compression of the nerves by the muscles, and complete resection is necessary for a favorable outcome.[19] The approach can be either transpalpebral[45,46] or endoscopic. The endoscopic approach is a better choice for those who suffer from MH triggered from both temporal and frontal sites.

Transpalpebral approach

Under intravenous sedation or general anesthesia, the face is prepped and draped. The upper tarsal crease is marked on each eyelid, with an incision length of approximately 1 inch (2.5 cm). Local anesthesia (0.5% lidocaine with 1: 100 000 epinephrine) is infiltrated into the eyelid. A skin incision is made with a 10c blade, and is extended through the orbicularis muscle. The plane between the orbicularis muscle and the septum is identified, and dissection is continued cephalad with a pair of baby Metzenbaum scissors. The depressor supercilii muscle comes into view first. The muscle is lighter in color than the corrugator supercilii and it is less friable. The muscle is then removed as thoroughly as possible. The corrugator supercilii muscle is identified next by its position over the supraorbital rim, as well as its darker color compared with the orbicularis oculi and depressor supercilii muscles. A small communicating vein is often seen between the supraorbital and supratrochlear vessels, deep to the muscle. The corrugator supercilii muscle is removed in a lateral to medial fashion using electrocautery as thoroughly as possible. Sometimes multitooth forceps serve effectively to remove the muscle completely around the nerve, while the supraorbital and supratrochlear nerves are preserved. Fat is harvested from the medial compartment of the upper eyelid and grafted to the site of the resected muscle. The fat graft serves three purposes: (1) it minimizes contour deformity resulting from a thorough muscle resection; (2) it protects the exposed nerve branches; and (3) it minimizes the recurrent function. The graft is sutured with 6-0 absorbable suture, and the skin incision is sutured with 6-0 plain catgut.[45,46]

Postoperatively, the patient is allowed to resume light activities on day 1, regular activities on day 7, and heavy exercise after 3 weeks. Patients usually sustain a reasonable amount of edema and ecchymosis which usually subside in 10–14 days.

Complications

The most common complication of this approach is persistent paresthesia of the forehead and frontoparietal scalp. Every patient experiences some anesthesia or paresthesia immediately after surgery. This includes the entire forehead and anterior scalp. This paresthesia nearly always resolves if the nerves have been preserved. There is a risk of asymmetry and dynamic imperfections as well, if the muscle is not removed thoroughly and evenly on both sides.

Endoscopic approach

After proper preparation of the face under sedation, the incision sites are marked. There are a total of five or six incisions, each one measuring 1–1.5 cm in length depending on the thickness of the scalp – one or two frontal incisions and two on either temple measuring 7 and 10 cm from the midline, all placed within the hair-bearing skin. For patients with a normal or short forehead, one midline incision is used while for patients with a longer or curved forehead, two midline incisions are utilized. Xylocaine containing 1:100 000 epinephrine is injected in the nonhair-bearing skin and Xylocaine containing 1:200 000 epinephrine is injected in the hair-bearing skin. The Endoscopic Access Device (EAD; Applied Medical Technology, Cleveland, OH) is used for hair control. The dissection is performed in the subperiosteal plane to the supraorbital rim and lateral orbital rim, and zygomatic arch. The procedure for ZTBTN resection is described below, and requires exposure of the zygomatic arch. For corrugator resection, attention is concentrated in the glabellar area. The supraorbital, supratrochlear nerve and corrugator muscle groups are exposed, and the periosteum is then released laterally, leaving the central portion intact over the mid glabellar area to prevent too much elevation of the medial eyebrows. The corrugator and depressor muscles are removed as thoroughly as possible along with medial fibers of the depressor supercilii muscle while the operating surgeon's nondominant finger is compressing the soft tissues against the grasper from the outside. Fat harvested from the temporal region is grafted to the corrugator site using the technique described by our group.[46,47] The junction of the zygomatic arch with the malar body is identified, a small rent in the deep temporal fascia is created cephalad to the arch, and the fat is harvested while the assistant is compressing on the buccal area.

Fascial sutures of 3–0 polydioxanone are placed for suspension of the temple area further laterally and cephalically to achieve some eyebrow lift if needed and displace the residual

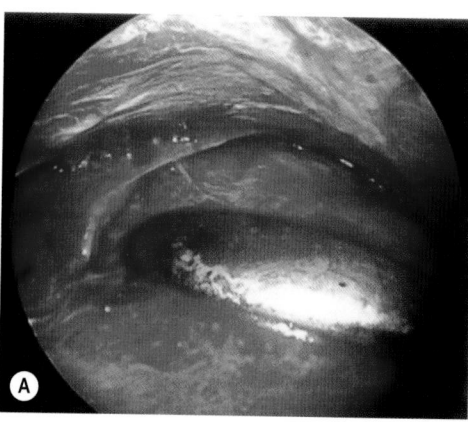
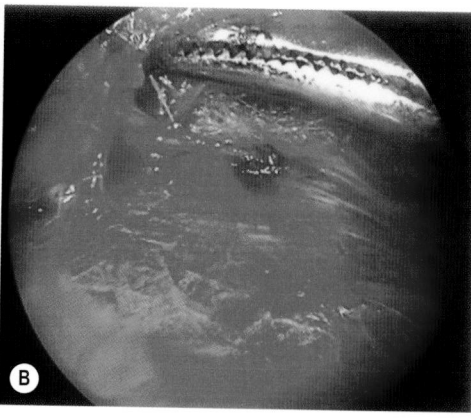

Fig. 21.4 Endoscopic view of the zygomaticotemporal branch of the trigeminal nerve. **(A)** The dissection is performed using a periosteal elevator. **(B)** The nerve can be seen superficial to the deep temporal fascia just under the grasping forceps.

distal ends of the nerve laterally. The suture suspends the superficial temporal fascia from the deep temporal fascia. A suction drain is placed in the incision and fixed with 5-0 plain catgut. Incisions are repaired with 5-0 polygalactin (Vicryl) and 5-0 plain catgut.[24] The endoscopic approach is used to provide access to both the temporal and frontal trigger sites, which are the two most common trigger sites.

Complications

Alopecia can occur at port sites, but is very unlikely. Every patient experiences complete anesthesia immediately after surgery; however, permanent paresthesia or anesthesia is unlikely. Inadequate resection of muscle may result in recurrence of the symptoms and dynamic irregularity of the forehead. Dimpling can occur on animation.[48] The temporal branch of the facial nerve is vulnerable to injury during the dissection.

Deactivation of temporal triggers

Temporal headaches are triggered primarily by contraction of the temporal muscle around the ZTBTN and probably compounded by the vessels irritating the nerves.

After appropriate preparation of the head and face, five or six 1–1.5-cm incisions are marked – two on each temple, usually 7 and 10 cm from the midline and one in the midline, only if the glabellar trigger site deactivation is intended. The forehead, temple, and malar regions are then injected with 1% lidocaine with 1:100 000 epinephrine. The hair-bearing scalp is injected with 0.5% lidocaine with 1:200 000 epinephrine. After the incisions are made with a no. 15 scalpel, they are deepened to the deep temporal fascia using the spreading effects of the baby Metzenbaum scissors. The dissection continues using an Obwegezer periosteal elevator and the EAD is inserted to allow the endoscope to be introduced. The periosteum is raised posteriorly and cephalically. Once dissection is completed on the right side, it is repeated on the left side.

A subperiosteal dissection is then carried out to the supraorbital rim, lateral orbital rim, zygomatic, and malar arches under endoscopic visualization. The dissection is continued immediately superficial to the deep temporal fascia until the ZTBTN is exposed *(Fig. 21.4)*. (It is absolutely crucial to the safety and success of this operation to avoid dissection too deep or too superficial to the deep temporal fascia; no fat should be left attached to the deep temporal fascia.) Grasping forceps or a long hemostat is used to dissect and avulse the nerve. It is important to avulse as much length of the nerve as possible to prevent re-coaptation. We usually remove a piece at least 2 cm long. Any bleeding vessels are coagulated and the proximal nerve end is allowed to retract into the temporalis muscle to reduce the risk of neuroma formation. The periosteum and arcus marginalis are released in the lateral orbital and supraorbital regions on patients older than 35 to facilitate rejuvenation.[24] The endoscopic devices are removed, and a single hook is placed on either side of the caudal portion of the incision. A 3-0 PDS suture is used to fix the superficial and intermediate temporal fascia to the deep temporal fascia laterally. A no. 10 TLS drain is placed, and the skin incisions are repaired with 5-0 poliglecaprone 25 (Monocryl) and 5-0 plain catgut interrupted stitches.

The drain is usually removed on postoperative day 2 and the patient is allowed to return to light activities the next day, to regular activities within 7 days, and to strenuous exercise within 3 weeks.

Complications

Every patient experiences transient anesthesia and paresthesia postoperatively. Fortunately, both of these are temporary. Permanent anesthesia and paresthesia are rare. Alopecia around the incisions can occur, and often is temporary. Patchy alopecia, perhaps related to the injection of epinephrine-containing local anesthetic, is a rare possibility. This type is also often temporary. Injury to the temporal branch of the facial nerve may rarely cause paralysis of the frontalis muscle. This complication is usually short-lasting as well. A neuroma, although a possibility after the avulsion of the nerve, has not been observed after this surgery.

Deactivation of occipital triggers

A 4-cm midline incision is designed in the hair-bearing caudal occipital region while the patient is seated. After induction of anesthesia, the patient is placed in a prone position with the shoulders raised by a gel roll and the neck stabilized. The area around the incision is shaved to a total width of approximately 3 cm. The incision site is then infiltrated with 1% lidocaine with 1:100 000 epinephrine *(Fig. 21.5A)*. The skin incision is made with a no. 10 scalpel and hemostasis is achieved with coagulation cautery. The incision is taken to the midline raphe *(Fig. 21.5B)*, and the trapezius fascia is incised

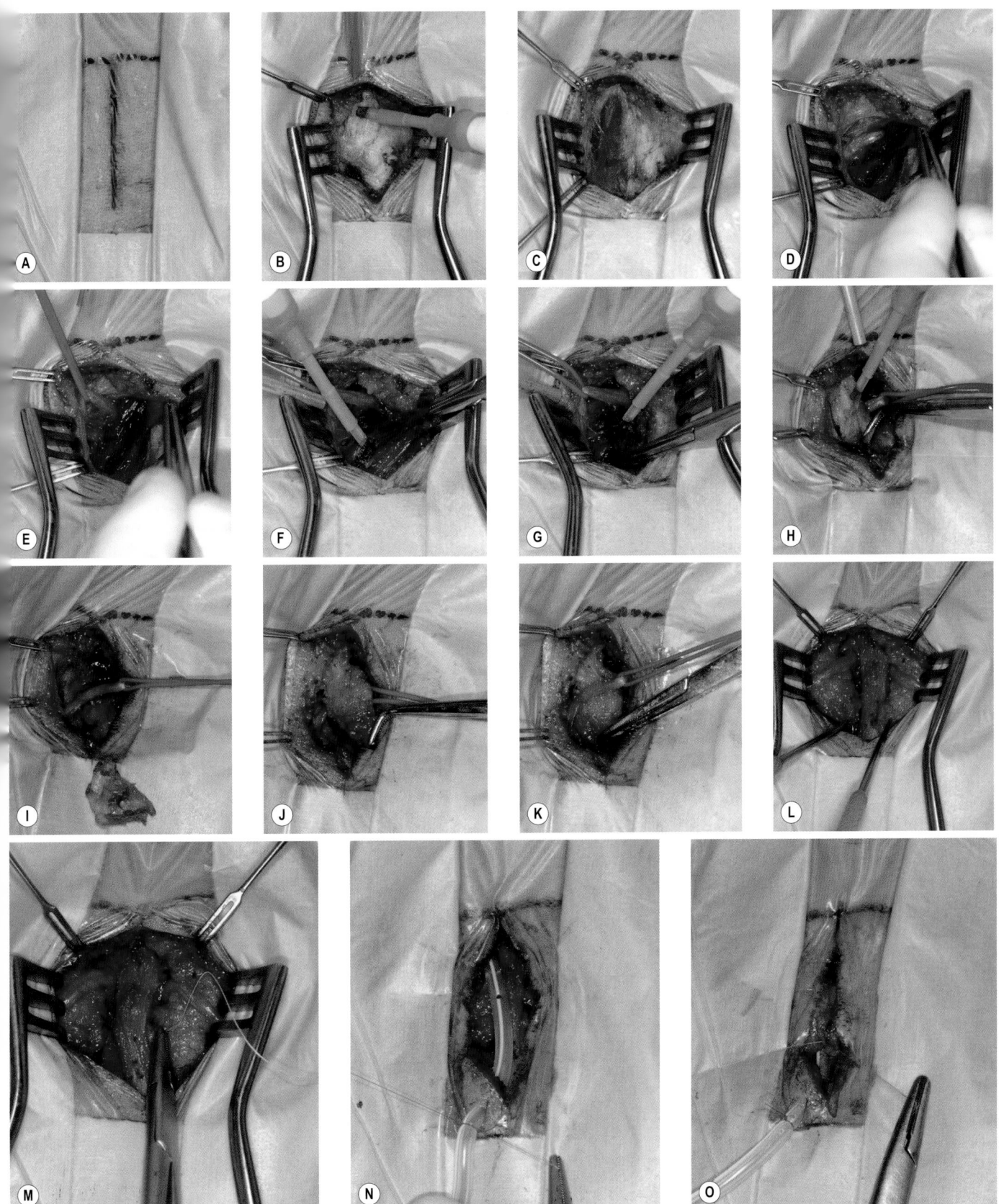

Fig. 21.5 Surgical technique for release of the occipital nerve for occipital migraines. **(A)** The 1.6-inch (4-cm) incision is designed in the caudal occipital region. **(B)** The incision is taken to the midline raphe and **(C)** the trapezius fascia is incised slightly away from the midline; the semispinalis muscle fibers can be identified by their vertical orientation. **(D)** Dissection continues subfascially and superficial to the muscle, and the trunk of the occipital nerve will be seen approximately 0.6 inch (1.5 cm) lateral to the midline and 1.2 inch (3 cm) caudal to the occipital protuberance. **(E–G)** A 1-inch (2.5-cm) length of muscle is dissected medial to the nerve, and transected. **(H–L)** A flap is designed to be placed under the nerve to protect it. **(M)** The flap is sutured to the midline raphe, and **(N)** a drain is placed. **(O)** The incision is closed in layers while attaching the subcutaneous flap to the midline raphe.

about 0.5 cm to the right of midline (*Fig. 21.5C*). The trapezius muscle, which rarely reaches the midline, has obliquely oriented fibers, and if encountered, it is divided and retracted laterally; the semispinalis capitus muscle fibers are identified by their vertical orientation and their location directly underneath the fascia. The semispinalis muscle is then further exposed following retraction of the trapezius fascia, and dissection is continued under the fascia. The trunk of the greater occipital nerve is easily located approximately 1.5 cm from the midline and 3 cm caudal to the occipital protuberance (*Fig. 21.5D*). Munion clamps are used to isolate the nerve. A vessel loop is placed around the nerve for retraction (*Fig. 21.5E*). A full-thickness, 1-inch (2.5-cm) length of muscle is dissected medial to the nerve, and is transected cephalically and caudally using cautery in the coagulation mode. The muscle resection is considered complete when no muscle fibers remain medial to the nerve (*Fig. 21.5F and 21.5G*). A small portion of the trapezius fascia and muscle immediately overlying the nerve is then removed (*Fig. 21.5H and 21.5I*). The nerve is traced laterally, ensuring no fascial bands remain superficial to the nerve, causing compression similar to carpal tunnel release. Occasionally, the nerve bifurcates within the muscle. In this case, it is necessary to remove muscle fibers between the two branches.

Dissection is continued laterally and superiorly along the direction of the nerve until the nerve reaches the subcutaneous adipose tissue. The occipital artery or its branches that are in contact with the nerve are cauterized using bipolar cautery. The third occipital nerve is avulsed, if visualized, and allowed to retract into the muscle. A 2 × 2-cm subcutaneously flap based caudally is elevated and passed under the nerve to isolate the nerve from muscle (*Fig. 21.5J and 21.5K*).

The procedure is repeated on the left side, if the patient is symptomatic, using an incision 0.5 cm from the midline. This leaves about 1 cm of the midline raphe intact. After completion of the procedure on the left side, the two subcutaneous flaps are sutured to the deepest portion of the midline raphe (*Fig. 21.5L and 21.5M*). A single drain is placed on the left side through a small stab wound and is passed to the right side under the midline raphe (*Fig. 21.5N*). 0.5 mL of the Kenalog 40-mg solution is injected in the perneurium and along the course of the nerve on each side. The wound is irrigated and repaired with 5-0 Monocryl to repair the subcutaneous tissue and to approximate the skin to midline raphe (*Fig. 21.5O*).

Complications

Infection or bleeding is rare after this procedure. Reattaching the skin to the midline raphe reduces the chance of seroma formation. Temporary anesthesia and paresthesia are expected. Permanent anesthesia and paresthesia are unlikely. Every patient experiences a slight depression in the removed muscle site.

Septonasal triggers

Septonasal triggers must be considered when injection of BTX-A in other trigger sites results in no change, improvement without resolution, or when the pain is mostly behind the eyes and commonly triggered by weather or hormonal changes, especially when the pain is daily and is worse in the morning. The main triggering factors are believed to be: (1)

deviated septum with a spur which is in contact with a turbinate; (2) concha bullosa; (3) septa bullosa; and (4) Haller cell. The main goal of surgery is to eliminate the contact point or decompress the concha or septa bullosa.

The face is prepped and draped after the induction of general anesthesia. The nose is packed with cocaine-soaked gauze and is infiltrated with 0.5% lidocaine with 1:200 000 epinephrine initially and 0.5% lidocaine containing 1:100 000 epinephrine after a few minutes. An L-shaped incision is made on the left side of the septum, and the mucoperiosteum is elevated. The opposite mucoperiosteum is accessed through an incision in the cartilage and elevated. If the patient has septa bullosa the posterior cephalic portion of the septal bone is removed enough to expose the sphenoid sinus. The deviated portion of the cartilaginous septum and bone is removed and a straight piece of cartilage is replaced. It is crucial to remove any existing spurs and eliminate any contact points between the turbinates and the septum. The mucoperiosteal flap is sutured back into place with 5-0 chromic running sutures. Doyle splints are placed and fixated with 4-0 Prolene sutures.

The Doyle stents are removed in 3–8 days. The patient may resume light activities on postoperative day 1 and heavy activities on postoperative day 7.

In some cases, the inferior turbinates are enlarged and require reduction. The inferior turbinates are infiltrated with 0.5% lidocaine containing 1:200 000 epinephrine, and 0.5% lidocaine containing 1:100 000 epinephrine after a few minutes. Turbinate scissors are used to resect the inferior turbinates conservatively. A partial infracture is performed and the area is cauterized. A patient who has concha bullosa or significant enlargement of the middle turbinates will require partial or complete resection of the middle turbinates. Using the sharp end of the septal elevator, the mucosa overlying the turbinate is incised and peeled off over the medial half of the turbinate. The medial wall of the concha bullosa is resected, raw margins are cauterized, and Doyle stents are inserted.

Complications

Temporary dryness of the nose occurs in 12% of our patients. At this time, we have not observed permanent dryness. Synechiae and sinus infection are rare. A small percentage of patients experience postoperative epistaxis, which, if significant enough, is treated with desmopressin without having to pack the nose.[49]

Conclusion

A patient who presents for surgical treatment for headaches should have a thorough headache evaluation. Trigger sites are then identified by the constellation of the presenting symptoms and, if practical, by systematically injecting 12.5 U BTX-A in frontal, temporal, and occipital trigger sites. For frontal trigger sites, corrugator muscle group resection is performed. For temporal trigger sites, the ZTBTN is avulsed. For occipital trigger sites, the semispinalis capitis muscle medial to the greater occipital nerve is resected. Septal and turbinate surgery is performed in patients who have evidence of septal deviation and enlarged turbinates, and whose clinical profile suggests septal and turbinate migraine triggers.

Access the complete references list online at **http://www.expertconsult.com**

9. Guyuron B, Varghai A, Michelow BJ, et al. Corrugator supercilii muscle resection and migraine headaches. *J Plast Reconstr Surg.* 2000;106:429–434; discussion 435–7.

   In this retrospective review, migraine headache status was assessed in patients undergoing forehead rejuvenation procedures involving resection of the corrugator supercilii. A strong correlation between corrugator removal and relief of migraine headaches was demonstrated.

14. Guyuron B, Tucker T, Davis J. Surgical treatment of migraine headaches. *Plast Reconstr Surg.* 2002;109:2183–2189.

   This is a prospective trial evaluating a surgical approach (corrugator resection, transection of the zygomaticotemporal branch of the trigeminal nerve, and temple soft-tissue repositioning) to managing migraine headaches. A significant improvement in symptomatology was demonstrated with surgery, and preoperative Botox injection was demonstrated to be useful in predicting this response.

15. Totonchi A, Pashmini N, Guyuron B. The zygomaticotemporal branch of the trigeminal nerve: an anatomical study. *Plast Reconstr Surg.* 2005;115:273–277.

16. Mosser SW, Guyuron B, Janis JE, et al. The anatomy of the greater occipital nerve: implications for the etiology of migraine headaches. *Plast Reconstr Surg.* 2004;113:693–697; discussion 698–700.

   It is theorized that trigger points along the greater occipital nerve may contribute to migraine headache symptomatology. This anatomic study assesses the course of the greater occipital nerve to enhance the efficacy of chemodenervation procedures.

27. Dash KS, Janis JE, Guyuron B. The lesser and third occipital nerves and migraine headaches. *Plast Reconstr Surg.* 2005;115:1752–1758; discussion 1759–1760.

28. Guyuron B, Kriegler JS, Davis J, et al. Comprehensive surgical treatment of migraine headaches. *Plast Reconstr Surg.* 2005;115:1–9.

   In this randomized prospective clinical trial, Botox injections were used to identify migraine headache trigger sites in diagnosed migraine sufferers. Site-specific surgical releases were shown to reduce migraine symptoms significantly compared to controls.

29. Guyuron B, Reed D, Kriegler JS, et al. A placebo-controlled surgical trial of the treatment of migraine headaches. *Plast Reconstr Surg.* 2009;124:461–468.

   This is a double-blind, sham surgery-controlled clinical trial that demonstrates the efficacy of trigger-point-specific surgical management of migraine headaches.

32. Guyuron B, Tucker T, Kriegler JS. Botulinum toxin A and migraine surgery. *J Plast Reconstr Surg.* 2003;112(Suppl):171S–173S; discussion 174S-176S.

PART 2

Pediatrics
Joseph E. Losee

22

Embryology of the craniofacial complex

Maryam Afshar, Samantha A. Brugmann, and Jill A. Helms

SYNOPSIS

- Analysis of human craniofacial development opens the door to understanding the basis for craniofacial dysmorphologies.
- Establishment of the craniocaudal and mediolateral axes is essential for proper craniofacial development.
- Neural crest cells are a multipotent, migratory mesenchymal population of cells that give rise to the majority of the facial skeleton.
- Facial clefting is a multifactorial disorder. Single mutations in multiple signaling pathways can result in facial clefting.
- Neurocranium is compromised of a cartilaginous and a membranous portion. Cartilaginous neurocranium is derived from embryonic mesoderm, while the membranous neurocranium is derived from cranial neural crest.
- Cranial sutures remain patent during infancy through an intricate balance between maintenance of undifferentiated cells and cells that have differentiated into osteoblasts.
- Derivatives of the five pharyngeal arches form parts of the human face and the neck.
- Three well known teratogens, retinoic acid, alcohol and cyclopamine, affect craniofacial development.

Introduction

Understanding normal development provides an essential framework for comprehending the basis for human craniofacial defects. Here, we take a "systems level" approach to describing the process of normal development and abnormal morphogenesis and, where applicable, provide information on the genetic or congenital basis for some common dysmorphologies. Our goal is to provide clinicians with an understanding of the relationship between the phenotypic presentation of a patient, the underlying gene mutations responsible for the defect, and how these gene mutations

adversely affect the behavior of cells that populate the craniofacial complex.

What is unique about craniofacial development?

Despite its remarkable topological complexity, one might legitimately wonder if craniofacial development is actually a relatively straightforward process. After all, craniofacial structures – like most organs and tissues in the body – arise from the growth and fusion of smaller embryological tissue blocks, whose initial organization is much simpler. Is there any reason to suspect that the factors controlling specification and morphogenesis in the craniofacial complex are different from those operating elsewhere in the body?

In fact, there are a number of unique features that clearly distinguish craniofacial development from the development of other tissues in the body. One of these unique features is the dual origin of craniofacial tissues: the skeletal scaffold and most of the connective tissues, including blood vessels, originate from a group of cells called the cranial neural crest, whereas the musculature and some parts of the skull originate from mesoderm. A second unique feature is the cadre of complex, reciprocal tissue–tissue interactions between the neuroectoderm, the mesenchyme, and facial ectoderm that drive normal development. A third novel feature is the elaborately choreographed morphogenetic movements – caused by both passive cell displacement and active cell migration – that define head development *(Fig. 22.1)*. An example of active cell migration is movement of cranial neural crest cells from the dorsal neural folds into the branchial arches and more ventral positions in the facial prominences *(Fig. 22.2)*. Any process that disrupts the rate, the timing, or the extent of these complex cellular behaviors can result in a craniofacial birth defect. In the following paragraphs, a brief overview of these early cellular movements, and the molecular pathways governing those movements, will be discussed.

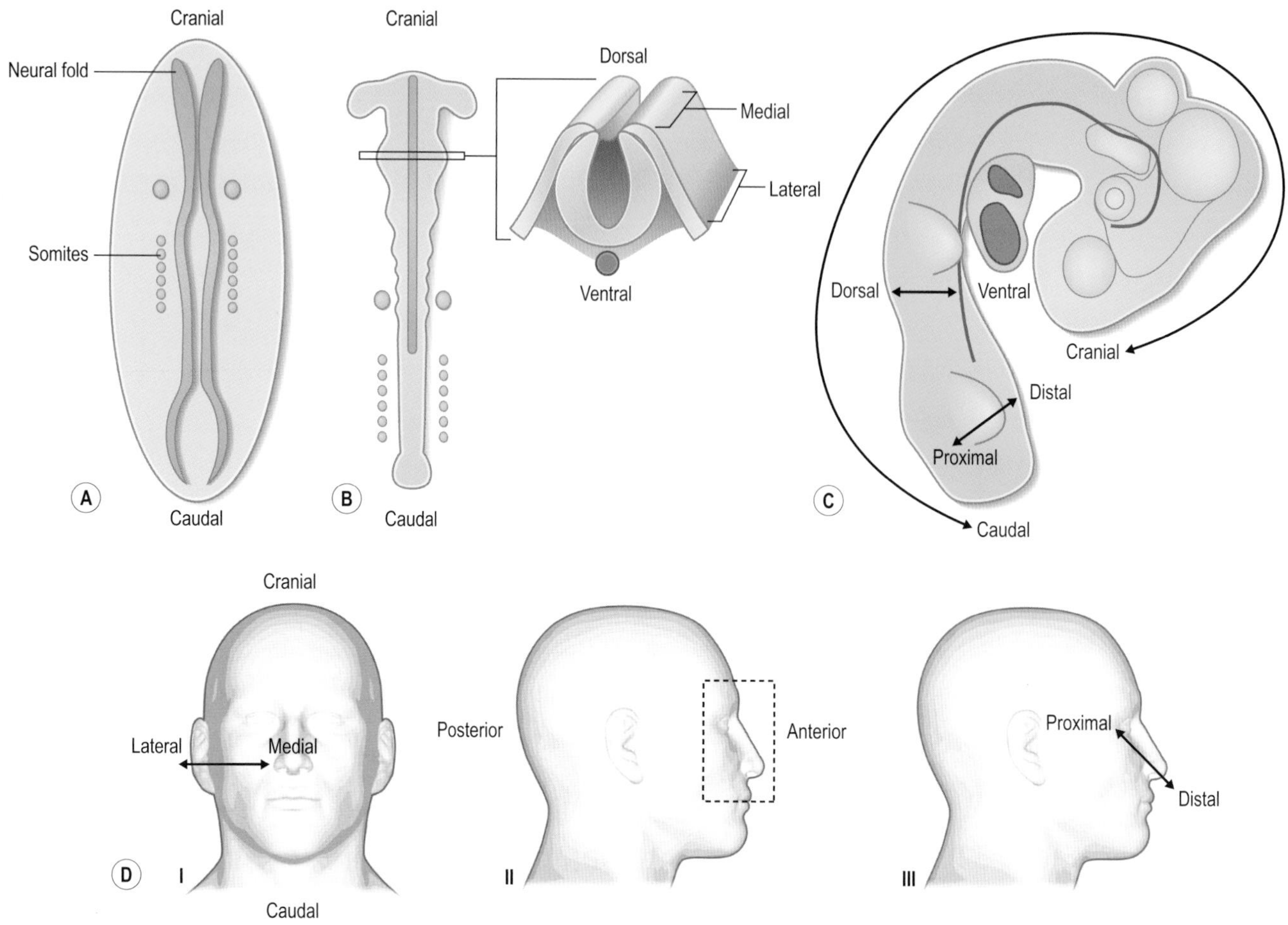

Fig. 22.1 Axes of embryo. **(A)** Dorsal view of human embryo during neurulation. **(B)** Frontal view of human embryo during neurulation. **(C)** Axes of human embryo after process of neurulation. **(D)** Illustration of human faces showing: **(I)** medial-lateral axes; **(II)** anterior-posterior and **(III)** proximal-distal axes.

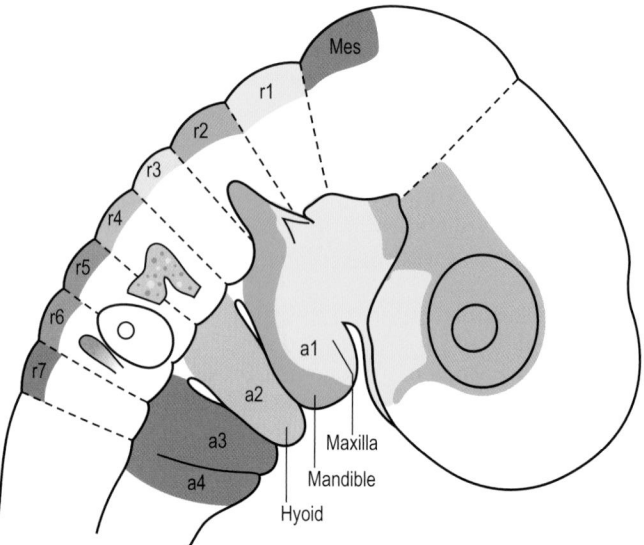

Fig. 22.2 Migration pattern of neural crest from rhombomeres to corresponding branchial arches. Rhombomeres are color-matched to branchial arches, indicating which rhombomere the neural crest cells in a particular arch or facial prominence comes from.

The initiation of craniofacial development

Gastrulation and the establishment of the craniocaudal and mediolateral axes

During the first week following fertilization of an ovum, the newly-formed zygote divides repeatedly into a solid mulberry-like cell mass known as the morula. As the morula traverses the fallopian tube and enters the uterus, cells continue to divide and the morula develops into a blastocyst. A blastocyst contains a fluid-filled cavity that separates cells into inner and outer layers, called the embryoblast and trophoblast, respectively. The trophoblast contributes to the formation of placental structures that support and nourish the developing embryo, while the embryoblast differentiates into the embryo itself. Implantation of the blastocyst into the uterine endometrium occurs during the 2nd week of development.

In the 3rd week of human development, the embryoblast grows, it divides into two, then three, layers. This process, called gastrulation, ultimately results in the formation of three primary germ layers (ectoderm, mesoderm, and endoderm)

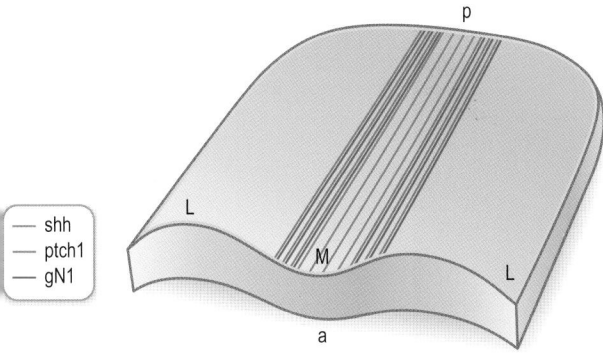

Fig. 22.3 Expression pattern of Sonic hedgehog (shh), patched (ptch) and Gli1 in the neural plate.

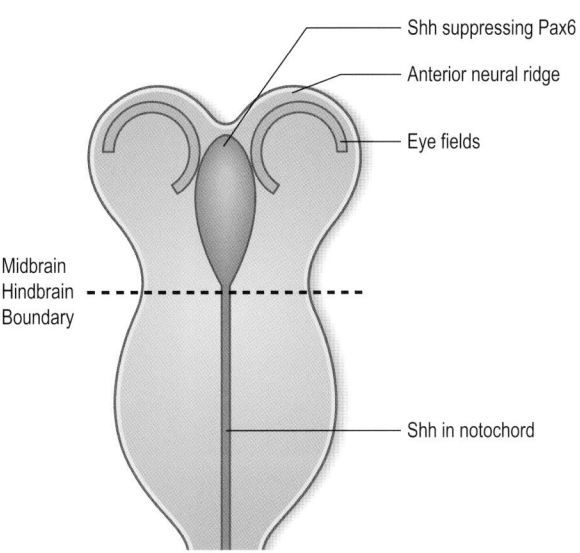

Fig. 22.4 Expression of Sonic hedgehog in the medial neural plate suppresses Pax6 expression and thus results in the development of two separate eye fields.

Even before this trilaminar disc of embryonic cells is established, however, it is apparent that the cranial (also known as rostral, or anterior) region of the embryo is distinct from the caudal (posterior) region *(Fig. 22.1)*. At the caudal end of the embryo, a group of cells known as the "primitive streak" emerges from the "primitive node." This epiblast-derived column of cells (chorda-mesoderm) progresses cranially via convergent extension movement until it reaches the prechordal plate, which is the site of the future mouth. The first cells to move anteriorly give rise to the pharyngeal endoderm and head mesenchyme.

By the end of the 4th and beginning of the 5th gestational week of human development, the craniocaudal (head to tail) axis is established. The mediolateral axis is also specified at this juncture, with "medial" denoting the midline of the embryo and "lateral" signifying the borders of the embryo *(Fig. 22.1)*. The molecular specification of the craniocaudal, mediolateral, and dorsoventral axis in vertebrates is obviously quite complex and is described in detail elsewhere.[1–3] For this review, we will limit our discussion to those molecular pathways that, when disrupted, produce the more common craniofacial malformations.

One of the earliest molecules that define the mediolateral axis is part of the "Hedgehog" family of secreted growth factors. Sonic hedgehog (shh), its receptor Patched (ptch), and at least one of its downstream targets, the transcription factor Gli1, are expressed in the medial region of the neural plate *(Fig. 22.3)*. In this midline domain, Shh signaling actively represses *Pax6*, a transcription factor that is required for the specification of the presumptive eye field in the anterior neural plate. Shh signaling normally represses *Pax6* expression in the midline of the presumptive eye field and in doing so, bifurcates into two, symmetrical regions *(Fig. 22.4)*. By this mechanism, a single eye field develops into two, separate eye fields. When Shh signaling is lost or disrupted at this stage of embryonic development, *Pax6* expression persists in the midline and as a consequence, only a single eye field is evident *(Fig. 22.5)*. Therefore, a loss of Hedgehog function at this early stage of development produces embryos with cyclopia (discussed below). This is a highly conserved pathway between various species and is present in all vertebrates *(Fig. 22.6)*. A single median eye is usually associated with an absence of the optic stalks, the optic chiasm, and the pituitary gland.[4] The

presence of a single eye is also accompanied by a proboscis, a medial tubular appendage lacking a nasal septum. ⊕ FIG 22.6 APPEARS ONLINE ONLY

Disruptions in mediolateral patterning produce severe HPE phenotypes

Cyclopia is the most severe manifestation of the malformation sequence known as "holoprosencephaly" (HPE). HPE is the most common structural malformation of the forebrain in humans, occurring in approximately 1:10–20000 live births.[5] In addition to cyclopia, HPE is associated with other craniofacial anomalies, including cebocephaly, ethmocephaly, and median cleft lip. Milder HPE phenotypes are known as microforms and they include microcephaly, microphthalmia, ocular hypotelorism, midfacial hypoplasia, and cleft lip with or without cleft palate.[6] In perhaps the mildest HPE phenotype, affected individuals exhibit only subtle midline abnormalities such as presence of a single upper central incisor.[6]

The etiology of HPE is as heterogeneous as its phenotypic presentation *(Table 22.1)*. Despite this, almost all of the gene mutations identified to date lead to a disruption in Hedgehog signaling.

Simultaneous with specification of the medial axis is patterning of the lateral regions of the anterior neural plate. Lateral plate patterning is regulated in large part, by members of the bone morphogenetic protein (BMP) family, which are expressed by cells located at the boundary between the neural and non-neural ectoderm *(Fig. 22.7)*. Signaling by BMP, plays an important role in the early stages of head formation and it is hypothesized that BMP activity promotes non-neural ectoderm while it inhibits neural ectoderm. This hypothesis is supported by mice with mutations in the extracellular antagonists that attenuate BMP, such as Chordin and Noggin, which display phenotypes remarkably analogous to human HPE sequence.[17]

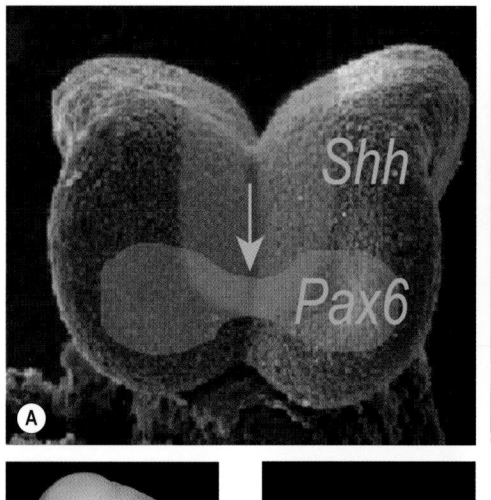
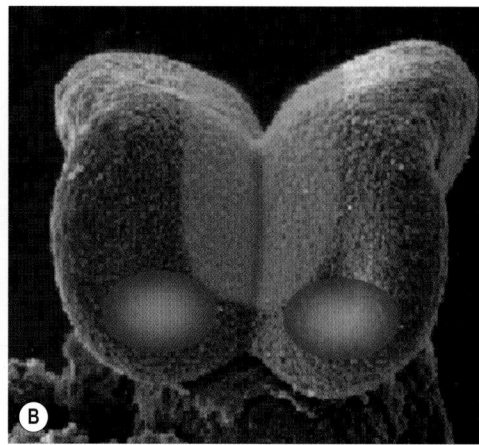
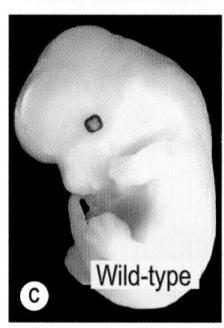
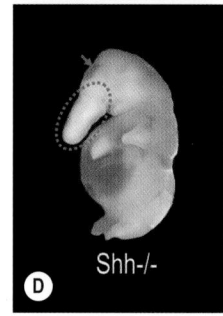

Fig. 22.5 (A) Shh expression (pink) in the medial neural plate with Pax-6 expression (green) in the dumbbell-shaped area which corresponds to the feature eye field. **(B)** Subdivision of Pax6 expression into two bilateral domains through expression of Shh. **(C)** Wild-type mouse embryo at embryonic stage 15.5. **(D)** Embryo exhibiting cyclopia (red arrow) with proboscis (dotted red circle) as a result of loss of Shh in the neural plate which has lead to persistence of a single Pax6 anterior midline.

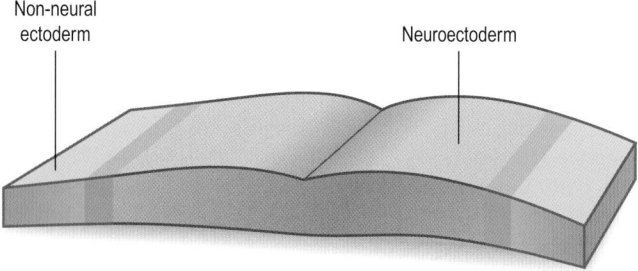

Fig. 22.7 BMP expression at the junction in between non-neural and neural ectoderm.

Table 22.1 Etiology of HPE genes

HPE causal genes	Initial report	Human	Mouse
Shh	Chiang et al. 1996[7] and Belloni et al. 1996[8]	X	X
Patched	Ming and Muenke 1998[9]	X	
Gli2	Roessler et al. 2003[10]	X	
Six3	Jeong et al. 2008[11] and Geng et al. 2008[12]	X	X
Zic2	Brown et al. 1998[13]	X	
TGIF	Gripp et al. 2000[14]	X	
Alcohol	Aoto et al. 2008[15]	X	X
Cyclopamine	Cordero et al. 2004[16]	X	X

Neurulation and the generation of the neural crest

During the process of neurulation, the neural plate "rolls up" to form the neural tube and in effect, this morphogenetic movement subdivides the ectoderm into two distinct tissues, the neural ectoderm, which will form the brain and spinal cord, and the non-neural (i.e., surface) ectoderm that will cover the embryo and later give rise to the epidermis *(Fig. 22.8)*.

In considering how the craniofacial tissues achieve their ultimate arrangement, it is helpful to remember that those regions of the neural plate that were once positioned in the center (medial region) eventually become positioned in the ventral part of the neural tube, and those regions that were lateral at the neural plate stage eventually become located dorsally in the neural tube *(Fig. 22.8)*. The reason that this repositioning is so important is that gene products, whose function it is to specify the midline of the neural plate, end-up having important roles in patterning the ventral neural tube. Likewise, molecules that regulate patterning in the lateral neural plate eventually have critical roles in dorsal neural tube specification. Two examples are Shh in the medial neural plate/ventral neural tube *(Fig. 22.3)* and BMPs in the lateral neural plate and dorsal neural tube *(Fig. 22.9)*.

Just prior to fusion of the neural folds, a population of cells emerges from the junction of the neural and non-neural ectoderm. This population of cells is known as the neural crest, and their role in head development is essential. In the head region, neural crest cells give rise to the majority of the neural, odontogenic, and skeletogenic tissues of the head, as well as melanocytes, some intrinsic eye muscles, pericytes, which

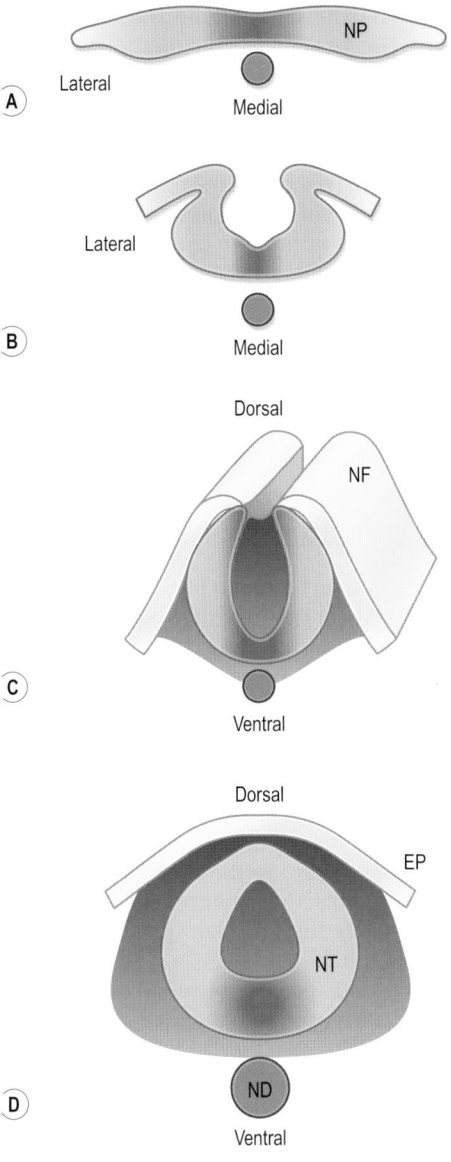

Fig. 22.8 Process of neurulation. **(A)** Neurulation starts with the formation of neural plate (NP). **(B)** Edges of the neural plate rise and form the neural folds **(C)**. **(D)** Neural folds (NF) meet in the midline to form the neural tube (NT) and the epidermis (EP). The notochord (ND) induces neural plate formation.

encase blood vessels in the head, and adipocytes In other parts of the body, neural crest cells yield neurons and glial cells of the entire peripheral nervous system and also endocrine cells.[18] The astounding amount of neural crest derivatives, coupled with their early embryonic appearance, have led some to refer to neural crest cells as the fourth germ layer.

Neural crest cells are derived from ectoderm, but through a carefully orchestrated process, they detach and acquire a mesenchymal (i.e., migratory) fate. This epithelial to mesenchymal transition (EMT) is a unique feature of normal neural crest cells, but is also seen in metastatic cells.[19] The highly invasive behavior of normal neural crest cells closely parallels cancerous cells that fail to respect tissue boundaries. As a consequence, considerable effort has gone into understanding the molecular regulation of neural crest cell formation.

Migration of the cranial neural crest into the facial prominences

In the head region, neural crest cell migration begins at the dorsal neural folds *(Fig. 22.10)*. Neural crest cells migrate from the dorsal neural tube into the prominences of the face; and, in avians, this migratory stream is divided into three components: those neural crest originating from rhombomere 2 migrate into the first arch; those arising from rhombomere 4 migrate into the second arch; and those neural crest cells from rhombomere 6 migrate into the third arch *(Fig. 22.2)*.[20] This migratory route appears to be largely the same in mammals and avians, and thus the majority of our detailed understanding of neural crest cell behavior has come from elegant experiments conducted using chick/quail chimeras by Nicole Le Douarin and colleagues.[21,22] Now, new imaging strategies can visualize, at the single cell level, the emigration of the cranial neural crest into the facial prominences, and these studies in large part, verify the earlier experiments.

Cranial neural crest mesenchymal cells migrate extensively throughout the embryo, most notably into the facial prominences. How do neural crest cells know which pathway to take, and where to end-up? New data indicate that this population of cells uses "cues" found on adjacent epithelial cells to direct their migration. This process is exemplified by the reciprocal signaling between cells expressing the Ephrins and

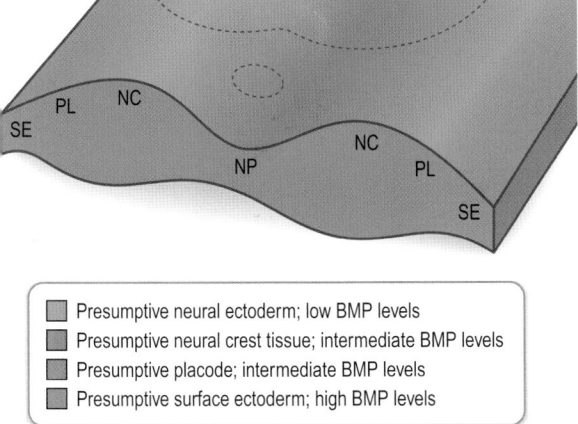

- ☐ Presumptive neural ectoderm; low BMP levels
- ☐ Presumptive neural crest tissue; intermediate BMP levels
- ☐ Presumptive placode; intermediate BMP levels
- ☐ Presumptive surface ectoderm; high BMP levels

Fig. 22.9 BMP expression in the neural plate.

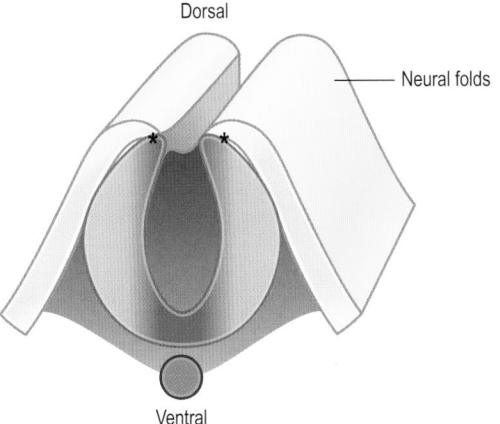

Fig. 22.10 Schematic drawing of dorsal neural folds (*), from where the neural crest cell arise.

cells expressing the Eph receptors, semaphorin III/collapsin I. Ephrins and Eph receptors are membrane bound proteins that function as a ligand-receptor pair.[23] Upon ligand-receptor binding, a molecular conduit for cross-talk is established between neural crest cells and adjacent tissues.[24,25] This was determined in part by experiments where truncated Ephrin receptors, which acted in a dominant negative fashion, were over-expressed in embryos. As a result of over-expression, neural crest cells failed to migrate appropriately, which indicated that Ephrin/Eph signaling was crucial for the proper migration of these cells. Subsequent experiments in avians indicate that Ephrin/Ephs act as bifunctional guidance cues, responsible for repelling some migrating neural crest cells and stimulating the migration of other cell types.[26] A more detailed understanding of Ephrin/Eph signaling will undoubtedly elucidate further how cranial neural crest migration is orchestrated during craniofacial development.

Establishment and fusion of the facial prominences

The basic morphology of the face is established between the 4th and 10th weeks of human development. The face is formed as a result of fusion of the midline frontonasal prominence, and three paired prominences, the maxillary, lateral nasal, and mandibular prominences (Fig. 22.11). Each of these prominences is filled with cranial neural crest cells that originated

at different positions along the neural tube (Fig. 22.2). The derivatives of each of the prominences will be discussed separately.

The frontonasal prominence

The frontonasal prominence gives rise to the forehead, midline of the nose, the philtrum, the middle portion of the upper lip, and the primary palate. Interruptions in frontonasal growth often result in a bilateral cleft lip, where the primary palate frequently "everts" (Fig. 22.12). In the mildest cases, clefts involving frontonasal prominence-derived structures may be limited to a notch in the vermillion border of the lip. In more severe cases, frontonasal clefts involve all of the tissues of the lip and these cases may most likely occur because of a failure of fusion between the frontonasal and maxillary prominences.

The lateral nasal prominences

The lateral nasal prominences give rise to the alae of the nose (Fig. 22.11). Clefts that involve the side of the nose often result from a failure in the fusion between the lateral nasal prominences and either the frontonasal or the maxillary processes (Fig. 22.13).

The maxillary prominences

The maxillary prominences give rise to the upper jaw and the sides of the face, the sides of the upper lip, and the secondary palate. The secondary palate separates the nasal passage from the pharynx, and this bony structure is derived from cranial neural crest cells that populate the maxillary prominences. In a stepwise manner, the palatal shelves extend vertically on either side of the tongue, and then subsequently rotate to a horizontal plane dorsal to the tongue, and fuse (Fig. 22.14). Initially, the palatal shelves are lined by an epithelium that, just prior to fusion, is partially sloughed off, leaving only the basal epithelial layer to cover the palatal shelves. This basal epithelial layer is known as the medial edge epithelium (MEE)

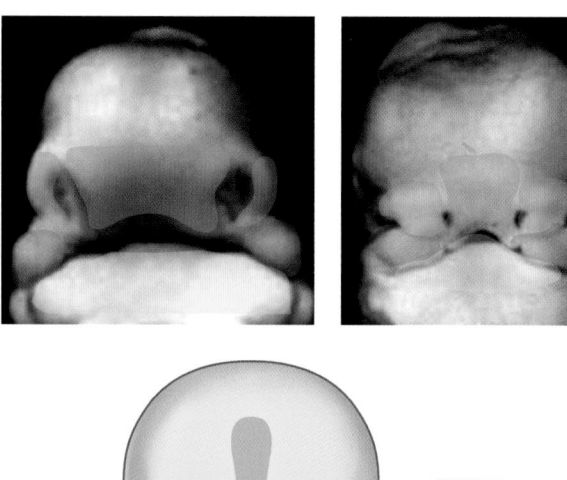

FNP
MXP
LNP
MNP

Fig. 22.11 Prominences of the vertebrate face. Frontonasal prominence (FNP), which contributes to the forehead, middle of the nose, philtrum and primary palate; maxillary prominence (MXP), which contributes to the sides of the face and lip and the secondary palate; lateral nasal prominence (LNP), which form the sides of the nose; and the mandibular prominence (MNP), which produce the lower jaw.

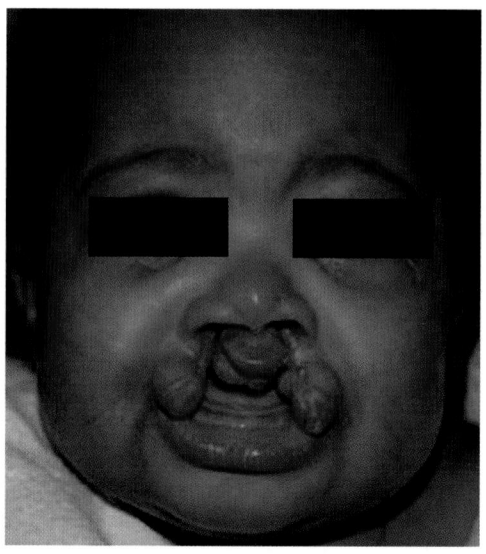

Fig. 22.12 Bilateral cleft palate with eversion of the primary palate.

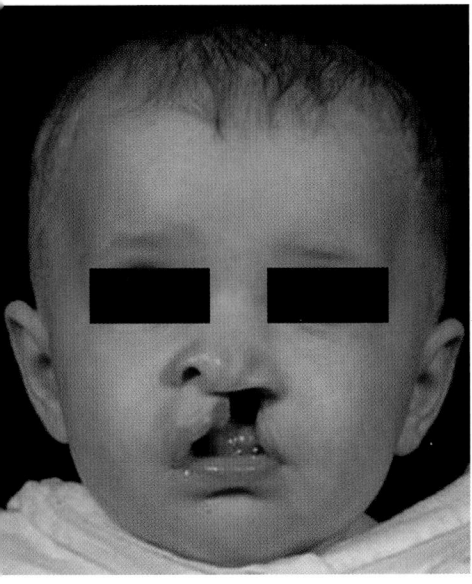

Fig. 22.13 Cleft involving the lateral nasal prominence.

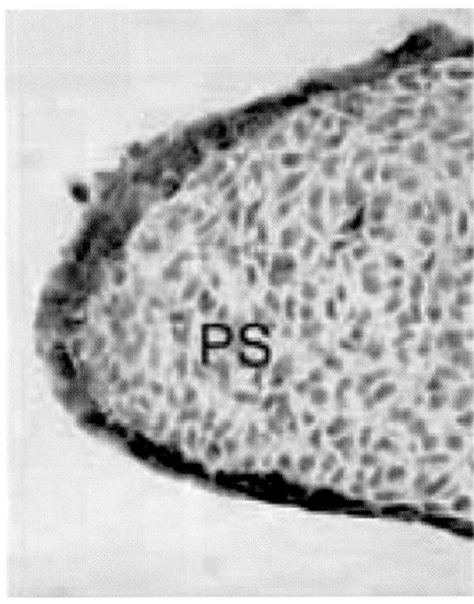

Fig. 22.16 TGFB3 expression, in the medial edge epithelium (black lining) of the mammalian palatal shelf (PS) (light blue).

and as the shelves grow towards the midline, the MEE of each shelf approximates and forms the midline epithelial seam (MES). The MES is then removed through the process of mesenchymal to epithelial transition (MET, the opposite of EMT), which leads to a confluence between the mesenchyme of the palatal shelves. Perturbations caused by genetic, mechanical, or teratogenic factors can occur at any of these steps, and frequently result in a cleft of secondary palate. Another type of secondary palatal clefting is palatal insufficiency, which is often caused by inadequate outgrowth of the maxillary prominences *(Fig. 22.15)*. ⊕ FIGS **22.14**, **22.15** APPEAR ONLINE ONLY

The mandibular prominences

The mandibular prominence forms the lower jaw and lip. Clefts of the lower jaw are very rare, presenting with a wide variety of phenotypes, ranging from a notch in the vermillion to a complete cleft of the lip involving the tongue, chin mandible and supporting structures of the neck and manubrium sterni.[27] The most extreme phenotype is associated with hypoplasia of the mandibular processes during the early embryonic period which will lead to the most severe cleft of the mandible while the most benign phenotype occurs later in embryonic development.[28]

In general, disruptions in the rate, the timing, or the extent of outgrowth of the facial prominences can all result in facial clefting. Remarkably, however, there appears to be some compensatory mechanisms that can overcome insufficient cell proliferation within a facial prominence and, through as-yet-unknown mechanisms, facial prominences can "repair" themselves *in utero*. In these rare cases (sometimes called "micro-clefts"), the result is a slight deformation in the vermillion border, with evidence of soft or hard tissue cleft. By understanding the mechanisms by which the body can repair these types of defects, we may gain insights into how a similar strategy could be employed to repair facial clefts *in utero*.

Advances in understanding the molecular causes of facial clefting

Using a combination of experimental approaches, researchers are discovering the specific signaling events and cellular processes that often go awry in cases of craniofacial clefting. This information is being used to develop more refined models of how craniofacial morphogenesis is normally regulated. These new data will undoubtedly form the basis for the treatment, and ultimately, the prevention of facial clefting.

Differentiation defects: the role of the TGF-β₃ in palatal fusion

TGF-β₃ is another member of the transforming growth factor beta superfamily and this gene is expressed by medial edge epithelial (MEE) cells just prior to the fusion of palatal shelves *(Fig. 22.16)*. *TGF-β₃* is essential for fusion between palatal shelves[29–31] since homozygous null *TGF-β₃* newborns exhibit a cleft secondary palate.[32] In the *TGF-β₃* null mutants the palatal shelves appear to approximate and adhere but the epithelial seam remains, and mesenchymal confluence does not occur. Further support for the role of *TGF-β₃* during palatal fusion comes from biochemical approaches. Antibodies that neutralize *TGF-β₃* prevent the fusion of the palatal shelves, supporting the finding that *TGF-β₃* is involved in the program regulating secondary palatal fusion.[33] Most data suggest that *TGF-β₃* plays a direct role in palatogenesis by mediating the breakdown of the epithelia that lie between the palatal shelves *(Fig. 22.17)*.

Inadequate growth of the facial prominences: defects in Wnt signaling and clefting

Mice carrying mutations in a member of the Wnt pathway exhibit clefting of the lip and palate.[34] In mice with mutation

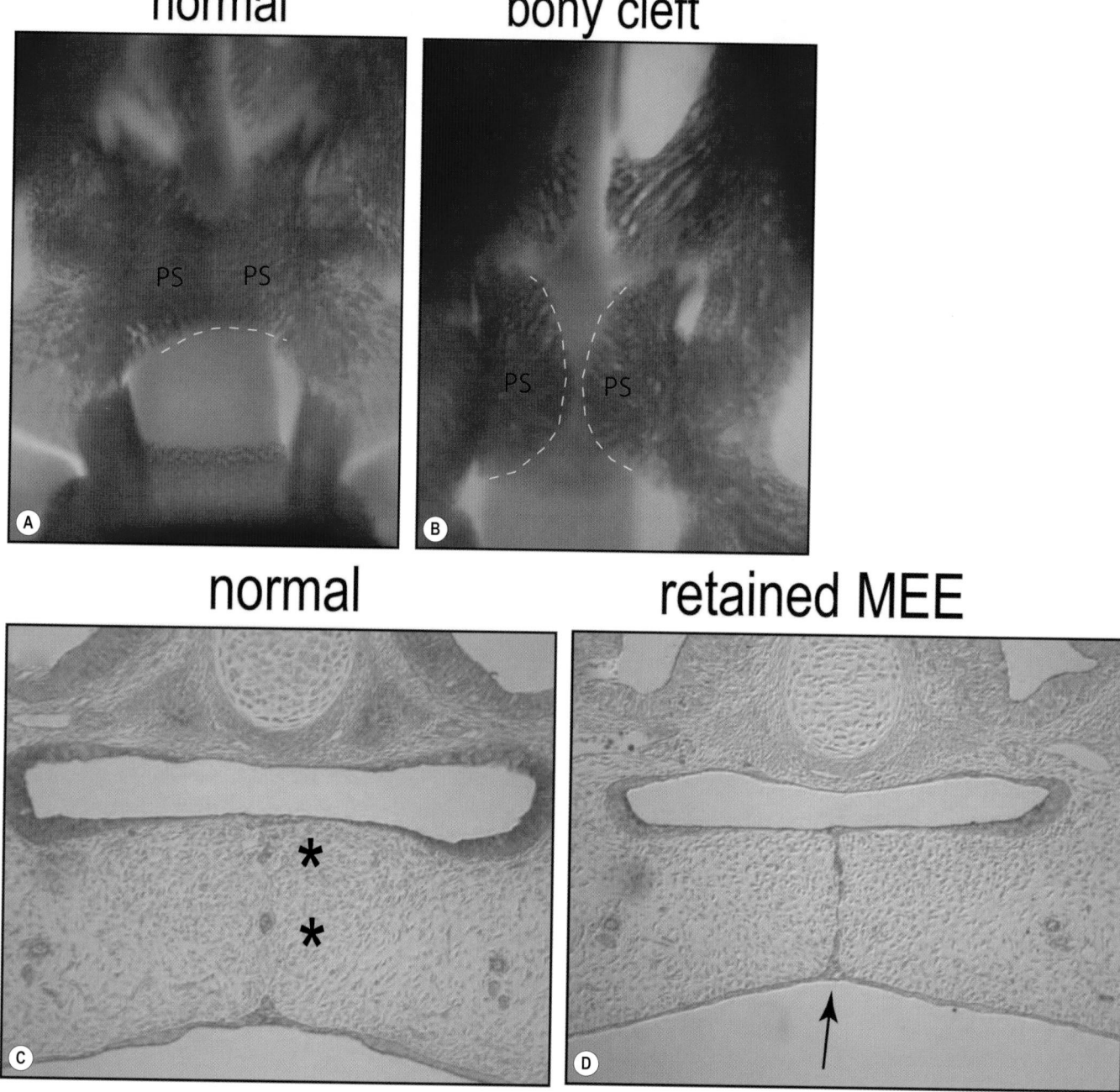

Fig. 22.17 Cleft palate in TGFB3 null mouse. **(A)** Transverse section through a developing wild type mouse (e14.5) palate demonstrating fusion in between the palatal shelves (PS). **(B)** Transverse section through the palate of a TGFB3 null t mouse (e14.5) demonstrating lack of fusion between the palatal shelves with formation of cleft of the secondary palate. **(C)** Transverse section through the palate of a developing wild type mouse (e 15.5) showing loss of medial edge epithelium of the palatal shelves. **(D)** Transverse section through the palate of a TGFB3 null mutant mouse (e15.5) with intact medial edge epithelium (MEE).

in Wnt9b, in particular, the basis for the clefting phenotype appears to be insufficient growth of the maxillary prominences.[35] Consequently, these prominences, from which the palatal shelves derive, fail to approximate and the result is palatal clefting.[36] Data from numerous laboratories, including our own, indicate that Wnt signaling plays a critical role in controlling cranial neural crest cell proliferation in the facial prominences.[37,38] When Wnt signaling is decreased, either by the removal of a ligand or by over-expression of a Wnt antagonist, the result is insufficient cell proliferation and facial clefting.

Mutation in FOXE1 associated with cleft lip and palate

FOXE1 (Forkhead box protein E1) is a member of a transcription factor family involved in embryonic pattern formation. Through positional cloning, candidate gene sequencing and developmental gene expression analysis, a strong correlation has been noted in between mutation in FOXE1 and occurrence of cleft lip and palate.[39] FOXE1 is expressed in the secondary palate epithelium of mice[40] and human embryos.[41] Furthermore, mice with a null mutation in FOXE1 have cleft palate and thyroid anomalies.[42] The FOXE1 gene is expressed at point of fusion between maxillary and the nasal processes, further supporting its role in palatogenesis.[39]

IRF genes and facial clefting

Another gene associated with facial clefting is the IRF6 (interferon regulatory factor) gene, which is part of a larger family of transcription factors that bind to specific DNA sequences and regulate gene expression. In mice, disruptions in Irf6 function results in clefting phenotypes.[43,44] In humans, mutations in IRF6 have been shown to cause Van Der Woude syndrome and popliteal pterygium syndrome, two clefting disorders.[45] There is also an increase risk of isolated cleft lip and palate in humans with variations in IRF6.[46,47] The occurrence of clefting in Irf6 mutant mice is hypothesized to be caused by defect in elevation of palatine shelves, secondary to inappropriate adhesions between the palatal shelves and oral epithelilum.[44]

Growth and ossification of the neurocranium

The neurocranium comprises that portion of the skull that protects the brain and functions as a protective bony case for this valuable organ. The neurocranium is further subdivided into two portions, the more ventral cartilaginous neurocranium (basicranium) and the dorsal membranous neurocranium, which form through two, distinct, processes.

The cartilaginous neurocranium

The basicranium forms the base of the skull and includes the sphenoid and ethmoid bones, the mastoid and petrous portions of the temporal bone, and the base of the occipital bone. Using experimental manipulations in chick embryos[22] and genetic fate-mapping approaches in mice,[48] the embryonic origins of the bones of the basicranium have been established. All skeletal elements that constitute the basicranium are derived from mesodermal cells that originate as part of the occipital somites and somitomeres.

Skeletal elements that comprise the basicranium form through endochondral ossification, where a cartilaginous template or anlage is first established and then is gradually replaced with a bony matrix through the process of vascular invasion. In addition, there are a number of skeletal elements associated with these mesoderm-derived bones that retain their cartilaginous fate, and they include the parachordal cartilage, the hypophyseal cartilages, and the ala orbitalis and temporalis (associated with the sphenoid bones), the trabeculae cranii (associated with the ethmoid bones), and the periotic capsule (associated with the temporal bones).

The membranous neurocranium

The membranous portion of the neurocranium forms the cranial vault, and is comprised of seven bones: the paired frontal, squamosal, and parietal bones, and the occipital bone. Unlike the basicranium, which is derived from embryonic mesoderm, the membranous neurocranium is derived from the cranial neural crest. There is some debate about the embryonic origins of the parietal bone, with some researchers claiming that this is a mesoderm-derived skeletal element[49] and others maintaining that it, along with the rest of the skull bones, have a cranial neural crest origin.[22]

The majority of the membranous neurocranium forms through the process of intramembranous ossification. Intramembranous ossification is distinguished from endochondral ossification because mesenchymal cells condense and directly differentiate into osteoblasts, without forming a cartilaginous intermediate. The occipital bone is a composite structure where the inferior portion forms via endochondral ossification and the superior portion forms via intramembranous ossification.

Histologically, the membranous neurocranium arises from skeletogenic mesenchyme located between the surface ectoderm and the underlying cerebral hemispheres. Bone formation is initiated when the neural crest-derived mesenchymal cells begin to secrete a collagenous matrix that mineralizes. This process begins separately in each of the bones, and expands radially until the bony (osteogenic) fronts nearly approximate one another. In humans, the primary cranial sutures include the frontal (between the frontal bones); the sagittal (between the parietal bones); the coronal (between the frontal and parietal bones), and the lambdoid (between the parietal and occipital bones) *(Fig. 22.18)*. Prior to suture fusion, 'soft spots' exists. These soft spots are clinically referred to as fontanelles. The most well known fontanelles are the anterior fontanel between the coronal, sagittal, and interfrontal suture, and the posterior fontanel, between the sagittal and lambdoid suture. While most of these sutures remain patent until the 3rd and 4th decade, the interfrontal suture undergoes physiologic fusion between the 6th and 8th months of life. The

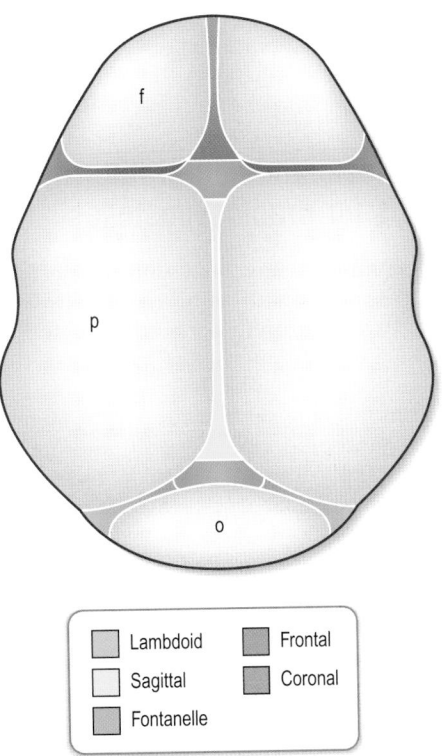

Lambdoid	Frontal
Sagittal	Coronal
Fontanelle	

Fig. 22.18 Cranial sutures.

osteogenic fronts of two opposing bones will eventually form the cranial suture complex, which is discussed in more detail in the following paragraphs.

Normal and pathological development of the sutures

Skull bones ossify during the fetal period and continue growing well into young adulthood. This growth is stimulated in large part by the expansion of the brain, and is achieved by the continuous differentiation of cells at the margins, or osteogenic fronts, of the individual bones. At the same time, this osteogenic differentiation is taking place, a subset of mesenchymal cells between the osteogenic fronts are maintained in an undifferentiated state. When the bones are nearly approximated, the regions of undifferentiated tissue become the sutures. Sutures remain open while the postnatal brain continues to grow, which leads to an interesting situation: cells in the middle of the suture complex must remain in an undifferentiated state, while adjacent cells differentiate into osteoblasts and add to the growing calvarial bone fronts. How these states of proliferation and differentiation are so precisely synchronized is the subject of much research.

A definitive answer to this question is still forthcoming but one thing is immediately obvious: destabilization of the delicate balance between cell proliferation and osteoblast differentiation is the basis for a number of pathological conditions in humans. The most common of these conditions is craniosynostosis (see below), which arises when mesenchymal cells in the suture region prematurely differentiate into osteoblasts and inadvertently fuse the cranial bones to one another. In other types of pathological conditions, such as cleidocranial dysplasia[50] or frontonasal dysplasias,[37] the skull bones fail to grow adequately. In these situations, the result is fibrous tissue covering the cerebral hemispheres without the benefit of ossification, clinically referred to as cranium occultum.

Balancing osteogenesis and cell proliferation: the molecular basis for craniosynostoses

Craniosynostosis is a common congenital defect affecting approximately 1 in 2000 to 2500 live births worldwide. Premature ossification disrupts growth perpendicular to the affected suture, which leads to compensatory growth of the skull in the parallel direction. Consequently, craniosynostosis results in a number of morphological and functional abnormalities including a dysmorphic cranial vault and facial asymmetry. A serious complication of craniosynostosis is increased intracranial pressure that can lead to blindness, deafness, and mental retardation.

There are over 100 craniosynostoses syndromes that have been described and attributed to specific mutations. Only a handful of these gene mutations have revealed a clear understanding of the molecular etiologies of isolated craniosynostoses; two of these mutations will be discussed here. First are patients with Saethre–Chotzen syndrome, who have mutations in the transcription factor *Twist*. Recent analyses indicate that mice with a single function copy of the Twist gene have craniosynostoses caused by inappropriate intermixing of neural crest-derived cells in the frontal bone with mesoderm-derived cells in the parietal bone.[51] Given the fact that humans with the same mutations exhibit nearly identical skeletal defects, it will undoubtedly prove interesting to determine how to circumvent this molecular defect to perhaps negate the effects of gene disruption on premature suture fusion. Mutations in the Wnt target gene, Axin2, are also associated with craniosynostoses, and in this case, in vitro data indicate that cells in which Wnt signaling is amplified have a tendency to differentiate prematurely into osteoblasts.[52] Axin2 homozygous mice have shorter snouts and premature fusion of the metopic suture, data that argue for a tight balance on the level of Wnt signaling for proper growth of the calvarial bones.

There have been significant advances in the management of craniosynostosis over the past four decades, but surgical intervention remains the only treatment to date. The surgical procedures typically involve strip craniectomies and cranial vault remodeling techniques to establish normal calvarial morphology. As our knowledge of the genetic and molecular factors dictating cranial suture fusion and maintenance of patency grows, we will undoubtedly develop new treatment strategies to treat the isolated forms of craniosynostosis.

Development of the viscerocranium

The bones of the facial skeleton comprise the viscerocranium. These bones are derived primarily from the cranial neural crest-derived mesenchyme of the first pharyngeal (branchial) arch. The cranial portion of the first arch gives rise to the maxillary prominences, which in turn develop into the maxilla, zygomatic bone, and the squamosal portion of the temporal bone. The caudal portion of the first arch gives rise to the mandibular prominences, which form the mandibular bone and the ossicles of the ear. Facial bones predominantly form via intramembranous ossification, with one notable difference: the mandible. Here, a cartilaginous anlage (Meckel's cartilage) forms a temporary structure that disappears in postnatal life. Its only remnant is the sphenomandibular ligament. Thus, despite the presence of a cartilaginous precursor, the mandible still forms through intramembranous ossification.

A number of disorders arise from the disruption of normal viscerocranial development. For example, hemifacial microsomia is a unilateral congenital hypoplasia of the craniofacial structures derived from the first and second arches, and is thought to occur due to trauma to the arches *in utero* between 30 and 45 days' gestation. Another craniofacial syndrome in which the viscerocranium is primarily affected, is Treacher Collins syndrome (also known as mandibulofacial dysostosis), an autosomal dominant disorder characterized by bilateral deficiencies in arch-derived structures. The genetic basis for Treacher Collins syndrome has been identified, and is due to perturbations in the nucleolar phosphoprotein, Treacle.[53]

Organization of the pharyngeal arches

In humans, the neck and parts of the face are derivatives of five distinct pharyngeal arches. The pharyngeal arches of human embryos initially resemble the gill arches of fish, except that the gill slits never become perforated. Instead, the external pharyngeal clefts between the arches remain separated from the apposed, internal pharyngeal pouches by thin pharyngeal membranes *(Fig. 22.19)*. Although the number of pharyngeal arches is somewhat variable among fish, five develop in human embryos corresponding to numbers 1, 2, 3, 4, and 6. Arch 5 either never forms in humans or forms as a short-lived rudiment and promptly regresses. Like so many other structures in the body, the pharyngeal arches form in craniocaudal succession: the first arch appears on day 22; the second and third arches appear sequentially on day 24; and the fourth and sixth arches appear sequentially on day 29.

Each arch gives rise to individual skeletal, visceral, arterial, muscular and nervous structures, and a summary of the derivatives of each arch is available in *Table 22.2*.

As the first pharyngeal arch (the mandibular arch), develops, it is remodeled to form a cranial maxillary swelling and a caudal mandibular swelling *(Fig. 22.20)*. These processes give rise to the upper and lower jaws, respectively. After the jaw evolves, the second-arch, (the hyoid arch) develops to serve as a bracing element to support them. This function is still detectable in humans. Derivatives of Reichert's cartilage, (second-arch cartilage) are shown in *Figure 22.21*. The third arch develops to form the lower rim of the hyoid bone as well

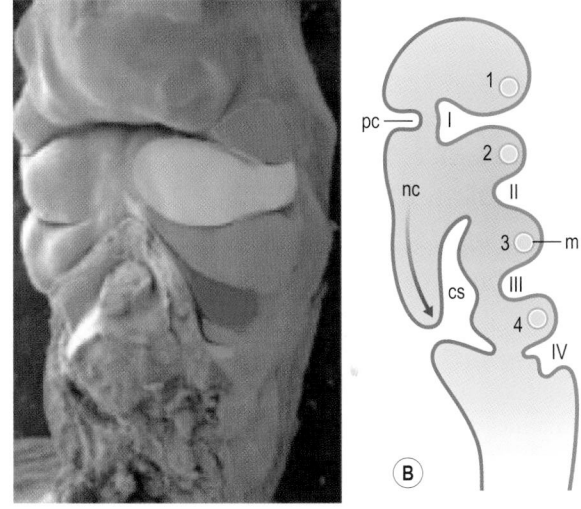

Fig. 22.19 Brachial arches. **(A)** Scanning electron image of pharyngeal arches. The arches are indicated by different colors. The first arch is divided into maxillary (1a, orange) and mandibular (1b, yellow) component. The second arch (2, green); third arch (3, purple); fourth arch (4, pink) and the residual sixth arch (6, blue). **(B)** The outgrowth of the pharyngeal clefts (pc) and pouches (white Roman numerals). The arches (1,2,3,4) are composed of a core of neural crest (nc, purple) and mesoderm (m, orange) surrounded by both surface ectoderm (blue) and pharyngeal endoderm (green).

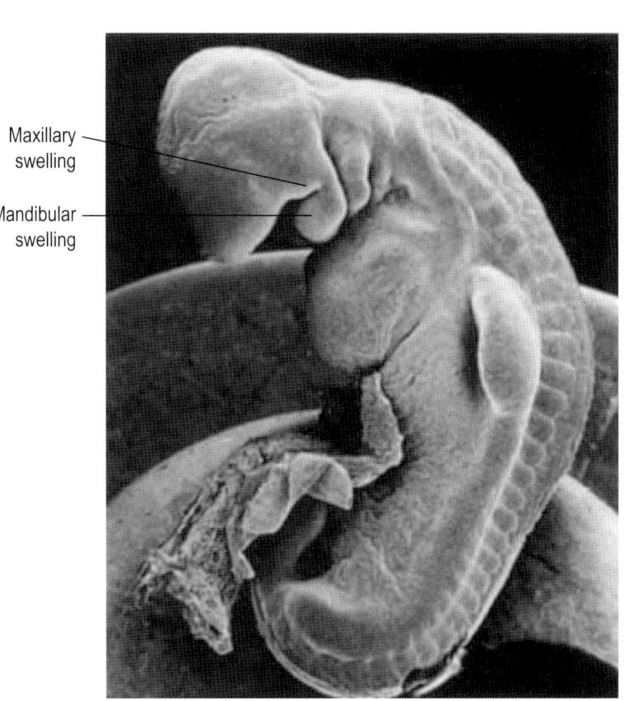

Fig. 22.20 Division of first branchial arch into the maxillary and mandibular prominences.

Table 22.2 Derivatives of the pharyngeal arches

Arch	Skeletal element	Musculature	Nerve	Artery
1st (mandibular and maxillary)	Incus, malleus, zygomatic, squamous. Part of the temporal, mandible and maxilla	Muscles of mastication	Trigeminal	Maxillary artery
2nd (hyoid)	Stapes, styloid process of temporal bone, stylohyoid ligament. Lesser horn and body of hyoid bone	Muscles of facial expression	Facial	Stapedial artery
3rd	Greater horns and lower body of hyoid	Muscles of the stylopharyngeus (throat)	Glossopharyngeal	Common carotid/internal carotid
4th and 6th	Cartilages of the larynx	Muscles of pharynx constriction, muscles of phonation, palatoglossus (tongue), muscles of upper esophagus	Vagus	Arch of aorta, right subclavian artery, original sprouts of pulmonary artery, ductus arteriosus, roots of pulmonary arteries

Modified from Moody SA, ed. Principles of Developmental Genetics. Burlington, MA: Academic Press; 2007, Ch. 30, Table 1).

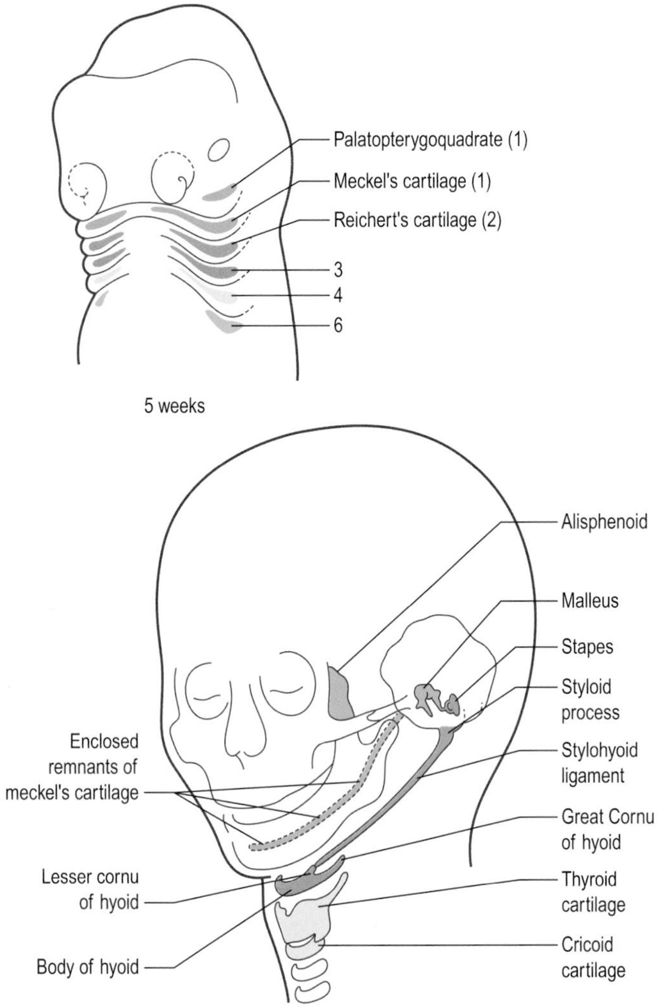

Fig. 22.21 Fate of pharyngeal arch cartilage.

as the root of the tongue, epiglottis and thyroid and inferior parathyroid *(Fig. 22.21)*. The fourth and sixth arches together give rise to the larynx; consisting of the thyroid cartilages, cuneiform, corniculate, arytenoid, and cricoid cartilages *(Fig. 22.21)*.

Disorders of arch development

After cleft lip and cleft palate, the most common group of facial malformations are defects caused by underdevelopment of the first and second arches, collectively known as craniofacial microsomia. Clinical manifestations of this condition include underdevelopment of external and middle ear, as well as underdevelopment of mandible, zygoma, maxilla, temporal bone, facial muscles, muscles of mastication, palatal muscles, tongue, and parotid gland. According to one theory, this malformation arises not from primary nonfusion of the maxillary and mandibular processes but, rather, from secondary ischemic necrosis caused by an expanding hematoma arising from the stapedial artery system. The stapedial artery provides the initial blood supply to this region of the maxillary and mandibular arches.[54]

The syndromes classified as mandibulofacial dysostoses closely resemble the above deformities but arise by very different mechanisms. In these disorders, underdevelopment of the lower face and mandible, and associated abnormalities of the palate and external ears result from mesenchyme deficits in the first and second pharyngeal arches.[55,56] This deficit has been explained as a result of defective migration or proliferation of neural crest cells or, alternatively, from excessive cell death.[53] One example of mandibulofacial dysostosis is DiGeorge syndrome, characterized by craniofacial defects, total or partial agenesis of the derivatives of the third and fourth pharyngeal pouches (the thymus and parathyroid glands), and cardiovascular anomalies. Although some cases of DiGeorge syndrome are associated with partial monosomy of chromosome 22, the syndrome also occurs among offspring of alcoholic women. Experiments have shown that acute administration of alcohol to animals during the period of third- to sixth-arch development can result in a spectrum of anomalies similar to DiGeorge syndrome.

Teratogens and their effects of craniofacial development

By studying the molecular and cellular bases by which teratogens exert their effects, we can gain a better understanding of the molecular and cellular regulation of normal development. While the abnormalities that arise following exposure to a specific teratogen may be diverse and highly variable, they are usually reproducible due to the fact that teratogens have distinct mechanisms of action and are selective with regard to their target cells, tissues, and organs. Numerous substances have been identified that have teratogenic effects during craniofacial development.[57] In particular, we will focus on three teratogens with well-known effects that disrupt the formation of the facial prominences.

Retinoids and retinoid-induced embryopathies

Clinical and experimental data generated over the past 60 years have clearly demonstrated that retinoic acid, a metabolite of vitamin A, can act as a powerful teratogen during embryogenesis. Both excesses and deficiencies of retinoic acid can lead to severe abnormalities in a variety of tissues.[58-60] The brain and the face in particular, appear to be especially sensitive to changes in the availability of retinoic acid during development.[58] Nervous system defects such as microphthalmia and holoprosencephaly, as well as facial anomalies such as midfacial hypoplasia and cleft lip/palate are all potential adverse outcomes following exposure to retinoic acid.

Retinoic acid, when delivered to the developing avian facial primordia, produces a wide range of morphological defects. Treatment with pharmacological doses of all-*trans*-retinoic acid at stage 20 gives rise to embryos in which the frontonasal mass is missing. At this same dosage and stage of delivery, the mandibular process remains unaffected. The prevailing data indicates that the craniofacial defects arise because teratogenic doses of retinoic acid disrupt the expression of *Shh* in the facial epithelium.[59] The insensitivity of the mandibular versus the frontonasal process to retinoid treatment is more difficult to understand. Retinoids may be differentially metabolized in the frontonasal as compared to the mandibular prominence, although this has not been demonstrated conclusively. One possibility is that the targets of retinoid action are not expressed in the mandibular prominence and therefore this tissue is relatively insensitive to high doses of retinoic acid.

Retinoid signaling has also been demonstrated to be critical for the development of the craniofacial tissues. The two classes of retinoid receptors in the head have distinct expression patterns in the neural epithelium, cranial nerves, sensory placodes, and neural crest cells. Blocking retinoid signaling produces a wide range of malformations in the neural tube and craniofacial region; for example, the hindbrain is open and the midbrain and forebrain are abnormally folded, the nasal capsule is missing, the optical axes are misaligned, and components of the otic capsule are reduced and aberrant. The secondary palate is clefted due to the fact that individual skeletal elements are either absent or severely malformed.

Alcohol effects

The effects of prenatal alcohol consumption leading to fetal alcohol syndrome (FAS) cause lifelong physical and mental impairment. Model systems to study FAS are uncovering the molecular and cellular mechanisms underlying these developmental impairments. The prevailing theory is that alcohol exerts its effects by interfering with retinoic acid (RA) synthesis and by causing increased RA degradation.[61] Other data indicate that ethanol exposure results in perturbations in Hedgehog signaling activity, with the consequence that Hedgehog target genes including *Ptch*, *Gli1*, *Gli2*, and *Gli3* are downregulated in the developing head. This causes neural crest cell death and craniofacial defects.[62]

Perturbations in cholesterol biosynthesis and metabolism

There is a striking overlap in the appearance of embryos exposed to teratogens such as cyclopamine and jervine, and those embryos whose cholesterol biosynthesis has been perturbed. An amazing amount of detective work went into discovering that the reason all of these animals have similar craniofacial defects is because they all negatively impinge on the Hedgehog signaling pathway. For example, the teratogenic effects of the plant *Veratrum californicum* have been well documented over the last 40 years because sheep which fed on this plant had offspring that were cyclopic. Over the intervening years, the active compounds in *Veratrum californicum* have been traced to cyclopamine and jervine.[63,64] When delivered to any pregnant animal, the result was offspring with cyclopia. It is now known that these molecules are steroidal alkaloids, which exert their teratogenic effect by perturbing cholesterol synthesis or transport.[65] Other drugs or gene mutations that perturb cholesterol biosynthesis or transport also cause cyclopia. For example, the loss of function of the megalin protein, a member of the low-density lipoprotein receptor family, produces craniofacial defects that resemble HPE.[66,67] Likewise patients with Smith–Lemli–Opitz syndrome, which is caused by a defect in a cholesterol biosynthetic enzyme, also exhibit mild forms of HPE.[4] These data show a clear link between teratogens such as cyclopamine, and perturbations in cholesterol. The link is that cholesterol is required for proper processing of the SHH protein, and it is now clear that cyclopamine directly affects this process by disrupting the function of the Hedgehog receptor, "Smoothened".[68]

Bonus images for this chapter can be found online at http://www.expertconsult.com

Fig. 22.6 Cyclopia in various species. **(A)** Unaffected chicken embryo. **(B)** Cyclopic chicken, with a single median eye (e, black arrow). **(C)** Lateral view of a wild-type, e15.5 mouse embryo. The eye (e, black arrow) and single telencephalic vesicle (*) are indicated. **(D)** e15.5 Shh null mouse embryo with cyclopia. The mutant lacks properly developed forebrain structures (*), and has the characteristic single medial eye (e, black arrow) and proboscis. **(E)** Unaffected kitten. **(F)** Cyclopic kitten.

Fig. 22.14 Coronal sections through a developing face demonstrating development of secondary palate. **(A)** Palatal Shelves from the maxillary process orient vertically on either side of the tongue. **(B)** Rotation of the shelves dorsal to the tongue. **(C)** Fusion of the medial edge epithelium (MEE) and formation of the midline epithelial seam.

Fig. 22.15 Schematic diagram of clefts secondary palate. **(A)** Diagram of ventral view of roof of the mouth showing the primary palate (blue) and secondary palate (orange). **(B)** Unaffected (nonclefted) palate. **(C)** Unilateral clefting of the secondary palate. **(D)** Bilateral clefting of the secondary palate. **(E)** Palatal insufficiency.

 Access the complete reference list online at **http://www.expertconsult.com**

8. Belloni E, Muenke M, Roessler E, et al. Identification of Sonic hedgehog as a candidate gene responsible for holoprosencephaly. *Nat Genet*. 1996;14(3):353–356.

    HPE represents one of the most variable and devastating craniofacial abnormalities. Through work done in this paper the prime genetic candidate for this disorder, Sonic Hedgehog (Shh), was identified. This discovery has led to extensive research on the Hedgehog family of secreted proteins and their role in early patterning of the neural plate and neural tube, and the range of human deformities associated with perturbations in this pathway.

11. Jeong Y, Leskow FC, El-Jaick K, et al. Regulation of a remote Shh forebrain enhancer by the Six3 homeoprotein. *Nat Genet*. 2008;40(11):1348–1353.

    Building off the knowledge of the role of Shh in HPE, authors of this paper used both genetic and biochemical experiments to investigate the mechanism of Shh regulation in the forebrain. Six3 mutations that cause HPE do so by failing to bind and activate the Shh forebrain enhancer. These data establish a link between Six3 and Shh regulation during normal forebrain development and in the pathogenesis of HPE.

12. Geng X, Speirs C, Lagutin O, et al. Haploinsufficiency of Six3 fails to activate Sonic hedgehog expression in the ventral forebrain and causes holoprosencephaly. *Dev Cell*. 2008;15(2):236–247.

16. Cordero D, Marcucio R, Hu D, et al. Temporal perturbations in sonic hedgehog signaling elicit the

spectrum of holoprosencephaly phenotypes. *J Clin Invest.* 2004;114(4):485–494.

Here, the authors demonstrate that the entire range of HPE phenotypes can be recapitulated by modulating the temporal activation of Shh in the brain first, and then within the face. These data establish a distinct role for Hedgehog signaling in facial morphogenesis, separate from its well known role in patterning the forebrain.

38. Brugmann SA, Goodnough LH, Gregorieff A, et al. Wnt signaling mediates regional specification in the vertebrate face. *Development.* 2007;134(18):3283–3295.

Wnt signaling is required for the generation of cranial neural crest cells; here, the authors show that Wnt signaling is also required for the proper growth and expansion of the facial prominences; specifically, Wnt signaling mediates the mediolateral axis of facial development and perturbations in this pathway are associated with hypertelorism and its related defects.

43. Rahimov F, Marazita ML, Visel A, et al. Disruption of an AP-2alpha binding site in an IRF6 enhancer is associated with cleft lip. *Nat Genet.* 2008;40(11): 1341–1347.

44. Ingraham CR, Kinoshita A, Kondo S, et al. Abnormal skin, limb and craniofacial morphogenesis in mice deficient for interferon regulatory factor 6 (Irf6). *Nat Genet.* 2006;38(11):1335–1340.

Mutations in IRF6 cause two orofacial clefting syndromes: Van der Woude and popliteal pterygium syndromes, and genetic variation in IRF6 confers risk for isolated cleft lip and palate. The authors used a transgenic murine model to demonstrate the role for IRF genes in oral epidermal development.

52. Liu B, Yu HM, Hsu W. Craniosynostosis caused by Axin2 deficiency is mediated through distinct functions of beta-catenin in proliferation and differentiation. *Dev Biol.* 2007;301(1):298–308.

53. Dixon J, Jones NC, Sandell LL, et al. Tcof1/Treacle is required for neural crest cell formation and proliferation deficiencies that cause craniofacial abnormalities. *Proc Natl Acad Sci U S A.* 2006;103(36): 13403–13408.

56. Calmont A, et al. Tbx1 controls cardiac neural crest cell migration during arch artery development by regulating Gbx2 expression in the pharyngeal ectoderm. *Development.* 2009;136(18):3173–3183.

23

Repair of unilateral cleft lip

Philip Kuo-Ting Chen, M. Samuel Noordhoff, and Alex Kane

SYNOPSIS

- Presurgical nasoalveolar molding.
- Modification of surgical techniques
  - Mohler's rotation incision
  - Mucosal flaps for nasal floor reconstruction, correction of mucosal deficiency in piriform area
  - Eliminate the perialar incision on advancement flap, limiting scars around the ala base and nostril floor
  - Mobilization of alar base
  - Nasal floor reconstruction with complete mucosal closure
  - Muscle release and reconstruction to simulate the philtral column
  - Anchoring of advancement flap to nasal septum for centralizing the Cupid's bow
  - Correction of central vermillion deficiency with triangular vermillion flap from lateral lip
  - Semiopen rhinoplasty with a reverse U incision on the cleft side and rim incision on the noncleft side
  - Atraumatic dissection to release the fibrofatty tissue from lower lateral cartilages
  - Advancement and fixation of the cleft side lower lateral cartilage to the noncleft side lower lateral cartilage and to the skin in an over-corrected position
  - Definition of the ala-facial groove with alar transfixion sutures.
- Postoperative maintenance of over-correction with silicone nasal conformer.

Introduction

Central and foremost, the multidisciplinary approach is essential to the satisfactory treatment of the cleft patients.[1] This includes surgeons, orthodontists, speech pathologists, pedodontists, prosthodontists, otolaryngologists, social workers, psychologists, as well as a photographer. In addition, the center's coordinator serves to coordinate all these specialties for the benefit of the patient as well as for gathering and recording vital information. All of these contribute to the care of cleft patients from infancy to adulthood. This is a time when lasting friendships and care contribute to the psychological, aesthetic, functional, and spiritual development of the person. The techniques presented here are based on the experience of the members of the Chang Gung Craniofacial Center over a period of 30 years in a Chinese population. They have also been tested in other racially diverse centers. The improved outcomes result from an integrated approach with presurgical management, surgical refinements and postsurgical maintenance.

Basic science/disease process

Prenatal diagnosis

Ultrasound examination for the diagnosis of prenatal anomalies and problems is common in many countries, and is helpful in the identification of serious fetal problems as well as cleft lip or palate. Prenatal diagnosis of cleft lip is usually made after 16–20 weeks' gestation. The detection rate has increased in recent years.[2-4] With the advancement of three-dimensional ultrasonography, visualization of the cleft lip has become more accurate.[5,6] The three-dimensional image is helpful for prenatal counseling because parents can visualize the face of the fetus clearly. It is important for the surgeon to take time and provide information regarding the treatment protocol and outcomes to the parents. In addition to professional counselors, cleft patients or their parents can personally explain how children with clefts can become normal functioning persons in society.

Genetics

The genetics of orofacial clefting are only partially understood; however, they are of great importance when counseling affected families. It is generally believed that isolated cleft palate is a genetic entity distinct from unilateral cleft lip with or without cleft palate.[7-9] This conclusion arises from both epidemiologic studies and the fact that embryologic events leading to cleft lip/palate and cleft palate occur at somewhat different times (3–7 weeks versus 5–12 weeks). It has long been assumed that both genetic and epigenetic factors play important roles in the etiology of clefts, and this is supported by the varying incidence of clefting with ethnicity, geographic location, and socioeconomic conditions.[10-12] Twin studies have clearly demonstrated a genetic basis for cleft lip/palate, with a 43% pairwise concordance rate in monozygotic twins versus a 5% concordance in dizygotic twins.[7,13,14]

The incidence of cleft lip/palate in white newborns is approximately 1 in 1000 (*Table 23.1*); isolated cleft palate occurs in about 0.5 in 1000. Annual reports in Taiwan indicate an incidence of 0.81–1.62 per 1000 for cleft lip with or without cleft palate and 0.47–0.66 per 1000 for isolated cleft palate.[10] While there are more than 250 syndromes associated with orofacial clefting,[11] most cases occur as an isolated abnormality; so-called nonsyndromic cleft lip/palate.[10] Given the incomplete understanding of the genetics of orofacial clefting and the imprecision in employing nonsyndromic versus syndromic nomenclature, estimates vary regarding the frequency of other malformations in children with clefts. In a large review of their center's experience, Rollnick and Pruzansky[16] identified other malformations in 35% of cleft lip/palate patients and 54% of cleft palate patients. Cleft lip/palate has an unequal gender distribution, favoring boys over girls, whereas this relationship is reversed in cleft palate only.[17] Cleft lip/palate affects the left side more often.[18,19]

Unaffected (i.e., noncleft) parents who have one child with cleft lip/palate have an estimated recurrence risk of 4%, which rises to 9% with two affected children. If one parent is affected, the risk of having a child with cleft lip/palate is also 4%, increasing to 17% if there is already both an affected parent and an affected child.[20] As the degree of familial relationship increases, recurrence risk decreases: first-, second-, and third-degree relatives have 4%, 0.7%, and 0.3% risk, respectively.[15] Recurrence risk increases with the severity of the cleft.[21]

The most appropriate genetic model for the inheritance pattern of nonsyndromic cleft lip/palate is a matter of considerable debate, and consensus has not been achieved. Classically, Fogh-Anderson proposed the idea that cleft lip/palate was transmitted by a gene of variable penetrance that could act dominantly or recessively, depending on the individual.[7,15] Multifactorial and multifactorial/threshold models have been widely advanced[22] and have predominated; others believe there is little evidence to support the concept

of transmission as a discontinuous threshold trait.[10] In the past decade, the prevailing method of genetic analysis of cleft lip/palate has been by allelic association, whereby "candidate" genes are selected on the basis of functional properties, expression pattern, chromosome location, or mouse homologues.[22] Numerous studies of this type have found significant association to the transforming growth factor-α (*TGFA*),[23] transforming growth factor-β3 (*TGFB3*),[24] retinoic acid receptor-α (*RARA*),[25] homeobox gene *MSX1*,[24] and *BCL3* proto-oncogene[26] loci. Although such studies are useful, their results must be interpreted with caution; it is not clear whether the ever-increasing implicated loci are truly representative of a large number of genes involved in the etiology of cleft lip/palate or whether this type of analysis has the ability to produce false-positive results.[15,22] The subtleties of the interplay between genes and environment in cleft lip/palate are yet to be uncovered, and new tools such as sophisticated linkage disequilibrium approaches may be needed to unravel these complexities.[15,22]

Classification of the clefts

Veau[27] suggested that all clefts be classified into four groups: group 1, cleft of the soft palate only; group 2, cleft of soft and hard palate; group 3, unilateral cleft of lip and palate; and group 4, bilateral cleft lip and palate. This simple classification has ignored the clefts of primary palate only and failed to separate the incomplete from the complete clefts of lip and palate.

Kernahan[28] reported the Y classification. The upper limbs represent right and left sides of the primary palate, that is, the lip, the alveolus, and the hard palate anterior to the incisive foramen. The lower limb represents the hard and soft palate posterior to the incisive foramen. The limitation of the Kernahan Y classification is that clefts of the secondary palate cannot be classified into right or left sides. The Y classification was modified (*Fig. 23.1*) into a better numeric system that allows a more accurate recording of all left or right clefts of the primary and secondary palate and is easily adapted to the computer.[29,30] In the modified Y classification, each right or left limb is assigned a number, 1–5 or 11–15, for the primary palate and 6–9 or 16–19, for the secondary palate, with 10 being a submucous cleft palate.

All clefts can also be recorded by letter codes. The first letter is the side of cleft (R, right; L, left), the second letter is the location of the cleft (P, primary palate; S, secondary palate posterior to incisive foramen), and the third letter represents the degree of cleft (C, complete; I, incomplete). This classification is simpler for communication and sorting compared with the modified Y, but is not as accurate. The letter coding is as follows: RPC, right primary complete; LPC, left primary complete; RPI, right primary incomplete; LPI, left primary incomplete; RSC, right secondary complete; LSC, left secondary complete; RSI, right secondary incomplete; and LSI, left secondary incomplete.

All clefts in the illustrations of patients in this chapter are classified according to the letter method and the modified Y numeric method. The numeric method is more accurate in recording partial clefts. Any combination of numbers can readily record the finer degrees of partial clefts. Examples of classification are shown in *Figures 23.2–23.5*.

Table 23.1 Incidence of cleft lip/palate in differing ethnic groups	
Ethnicity	Incidence per 1000 births
Amerindian	3.6
Japanese	2.1
Chinese	1.7
White	1.0
African-American	0.3

Data from Wyszynski DF, Beaty TH, Maestri NE. Genetics of nonsyndromic oral clefts revisited. Cleft Palate Craniofac J 1996; 33:406–417.[15] and Vieira AR, Orioli IM. Candidate genes for nonsyndromic cleft lip and palate. ASDC J Dent Child 2001; 68:229, 272–279.[12]

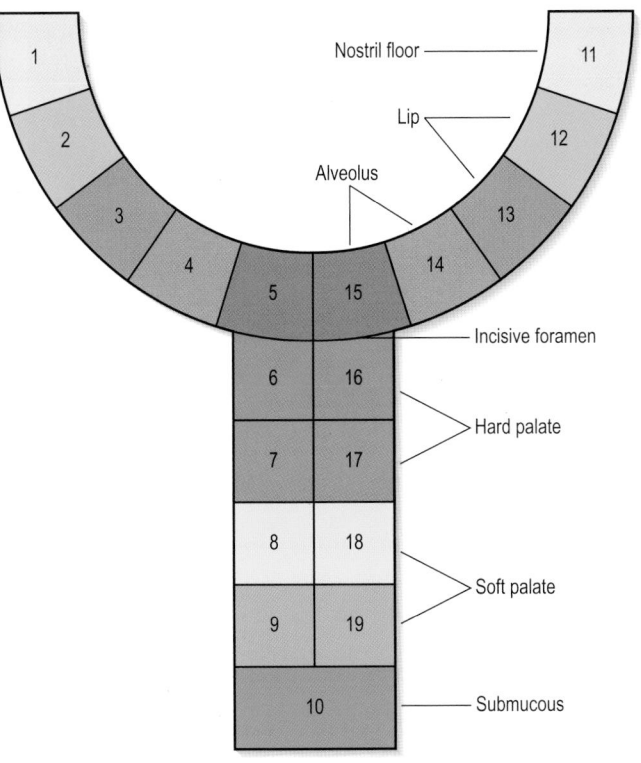

Fig. 23.1 A double Y uses numbers to classify clefts. Clefts of the primary palate anterior to the incisive foramen are numbered 1–5 and 11–15. Clefts of the secondary palate posterior to the incisive foramen are numbered 6–9 and 16–19. Any number combination is used to describe the type of cleft. (From Noordhoff MS, Huang CS, Wu J. Multidisciplinary management of cleft lip and palate in Taiwan. In: Bardach J, Morris HL, eds. Multidisciplinary Management of Cleft Lip and Palate. Philadelphia: WB Saunders; 1990:23.[29])

Diversity of the cleft pathology

Deficiencies of soft tissue, cartilage, and bone in cleft patients are difficult to evaluate accurately. There is an obvious difference in the availability of soft tissue among the following examples: (1) Left incomplete cleft of the primary palate (microform cleft lip, LPI, 13–14; *Fig. 23.2*); (2) Right incomplete cleft of the primary palate (incomplete cleft lip, RPI, 2–4; *Fig. 23.3*); (3) Left complete cleft of the primary and secondary palate (unilateral cleft lip and palate; LPC and LSC; 11–19; *Fig. 23.4*) and 4. Median facial dysplasia patient[31] *(Fig. 23.5)*. The surgeon can make an overall impression of cleft width, alar cartilage distortion, soft tissue deficiencies including the thickness and amount of orbicularis muscle, and underlying bony framework. Although impressions are useful, they cannot be quantitatively recorded.

Linear lip measurements of anthropometric marks provide a means of evaluating lip deficiencies. The quality and deficiency of the alar cartilage are impossible to evaluate accurately without a "cadaver-like" dissection. Deficiencies of bone can be recorded with three-dimensional computed tomographic scans, an accurate method of evaluating bone deficiencies but not practical in all patients. The computed tomographic scans *(Figs 23.2–23.5)* show a wide spectrum of bone deficiency that is present in the maxilla and alveolus. There is evident piriform deficiency in the occult cleft of *Figure 23.2*. There is a progressive deficiency of bone in the

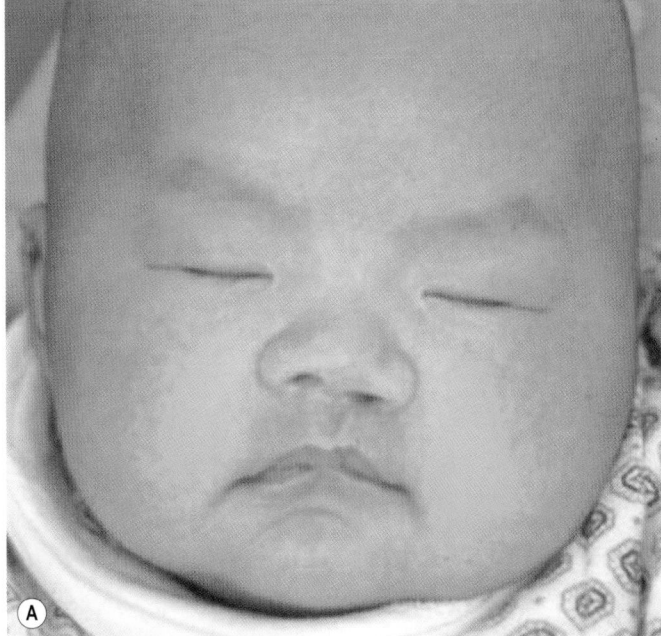

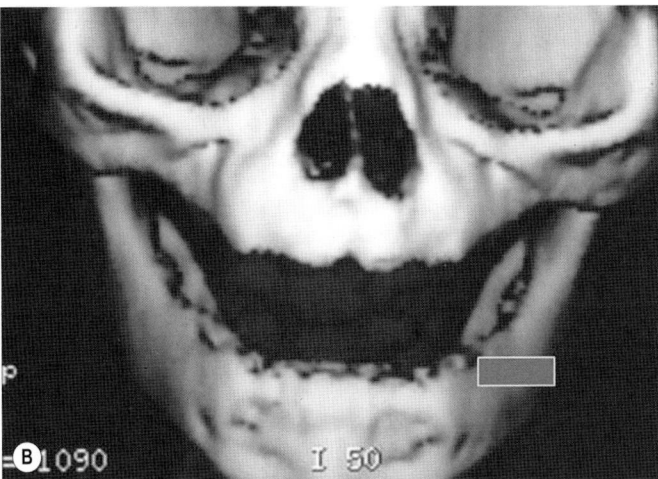

Fig. 23.2 A 1-month-old Chinese boy with a left occult cleft of the primary palate (left primary incomplete; LPI, 13–14). There is muscle separation and minimal elevation of the cleft-side Cupid's bow and a depressed left ala **(A)** due to deficient bone in the piriform area, as seen on the computed tomographic scan **(B)**.

piriform area and maxilla, as shown in Figures 23.3–23.5. These patients demonstrate a wide variety of bone, cartilage, and soft tissue deficiencies. This helps support the concept that all clefts are different, and the potential for normal growth probably varies considerably from patient to patient, in part because of these deficiencies.

Diagnosis/patient selection

Simple measurements with a caliper of important anthropometric points provide an inexpensive and accurate assessment of soft tissue deficiencies.[32] Measurements, on the basis of the anthropometric marks, are made at the time of surgery and recorded.

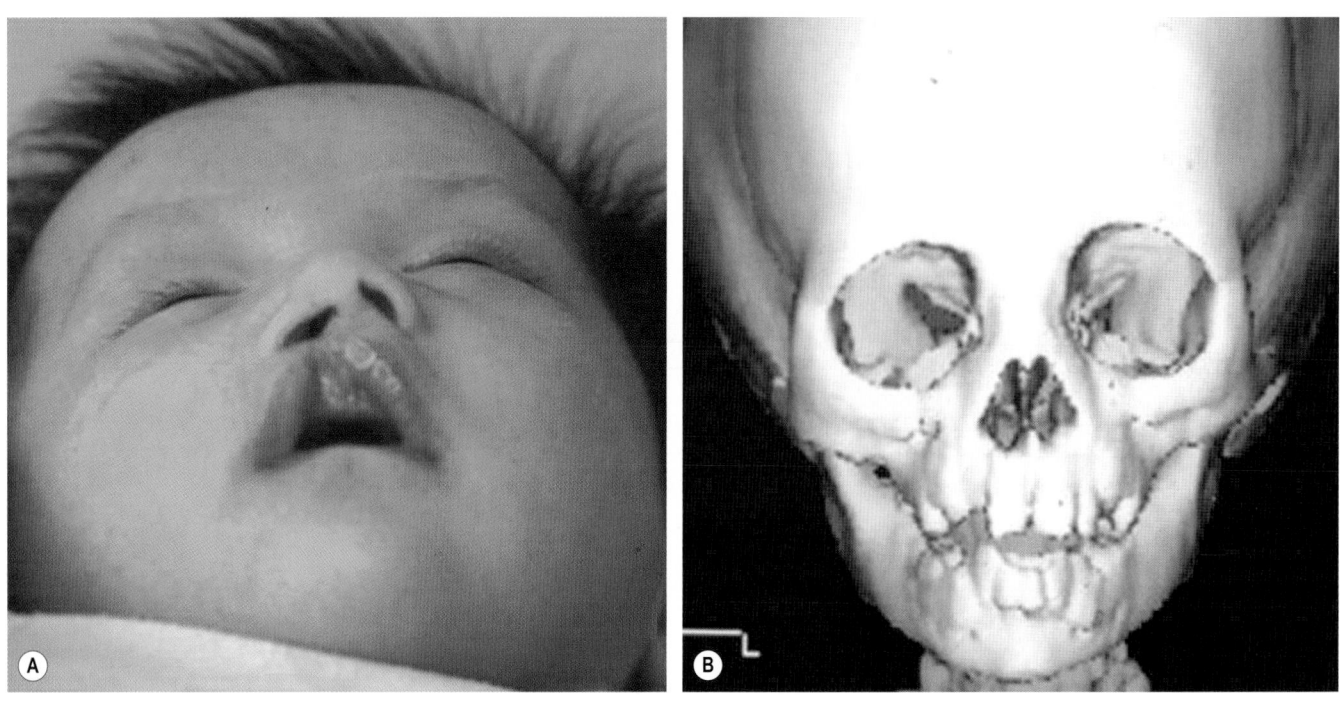

Fig. 23.3 A 2-month-old Chinese girl with a right incomplete cleft of the primary palate (right primary incomplete; RPI, 2–4). There is marked distortion and flattening of the right alar cartilage **(A)** The computed tomographic scan discloses deficient bone in the right maxilla and piriform area **(B)**.

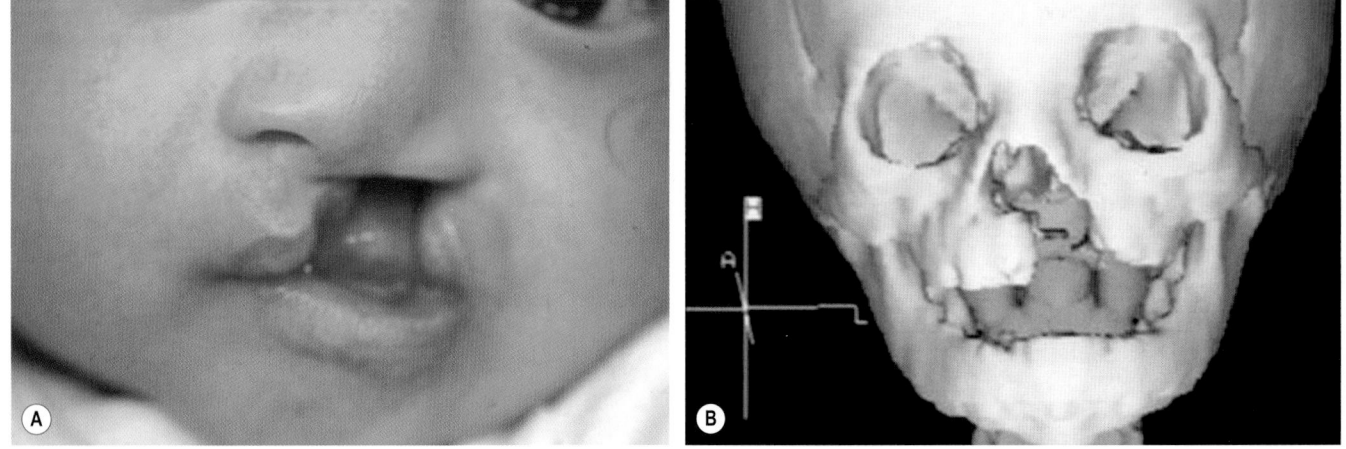

Fig. 23.4 Preoperative view at 1 month of a Chinese girl with a left complete cleft of the primary and secondary palate (left primary and left secondary complete; LPC, LSC, 11–19) **(A)**. The computed tomographic scan showed deficient bone in the cleft alveolus and piriform area **(B)**.

Lip measurements and markings

Cupids bow and vermillion

The points of the Cupid's bow (CPHR, IS, CPHL) are marked on the epidermis-vermillion junction line, the white skin roll (WSR), as identified by Millard.[33] The vermillion-mucosa junction line, the red line,[34] is also marked. This clearly defines the intervening vermillion and also helps identify the deficient vermillion beneath the cleft-side Cupid's bow. Other points marked are the base of the ala (SBAR, SBAL) and the commissure (CHR, CHL) *(Fig. 23.6)*.

The base of the cleft-side philtral column

The base of the cleft-side philtral column (CPHL') is a definite anatomic point but somehow difficult to identify. The red line always converges and meets the white skin roll medially. There is frequently a distinct point where the white skin roll changes directions and makes a slight curve about 3–4 mm before it meets the red line.[35,36] The base of the cleft-side philtral column is where the white skin roll changes direction and where the vermillion first becomes widest, usually 3–4 mm lateral to the converging point of red line and white skin roll. This is an important anatomic point for the cleft-side philtral

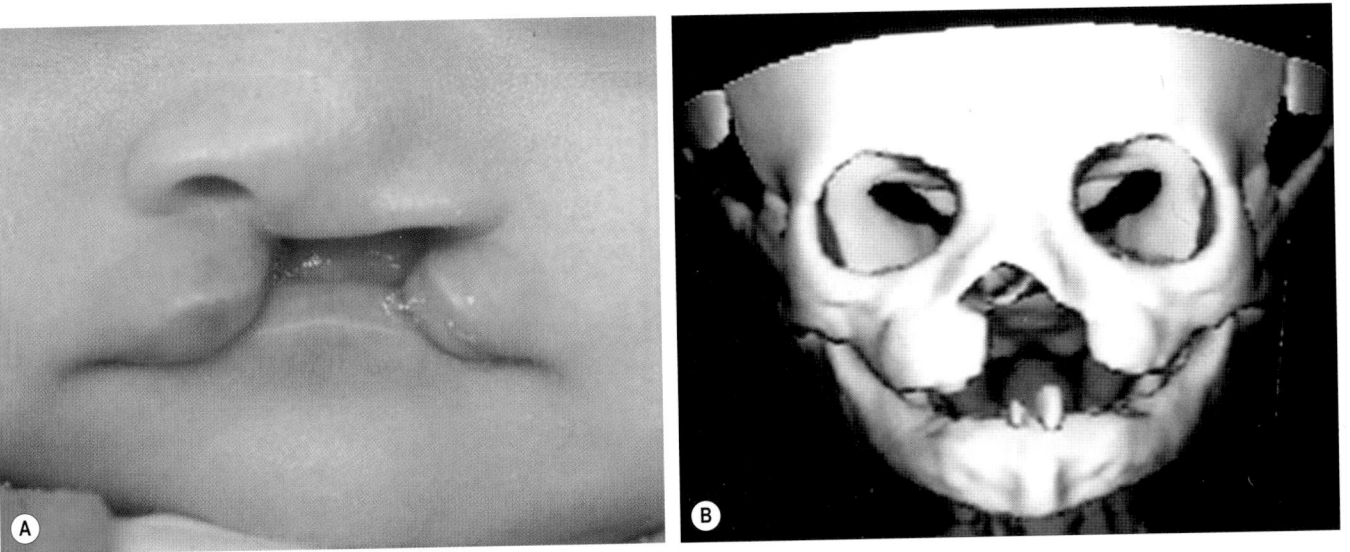

Fig. 23.5 A 1-month-old girl with left median facial dysplasia. There is wide cleft with indistinct Cupid's bow, deficient lip tissue and no lip frenum. The nose is severely depressed **(A)**. The computed tomographic scan showed severe deficient bone in the premaxilla, alveolus and piriform area **(B)**.

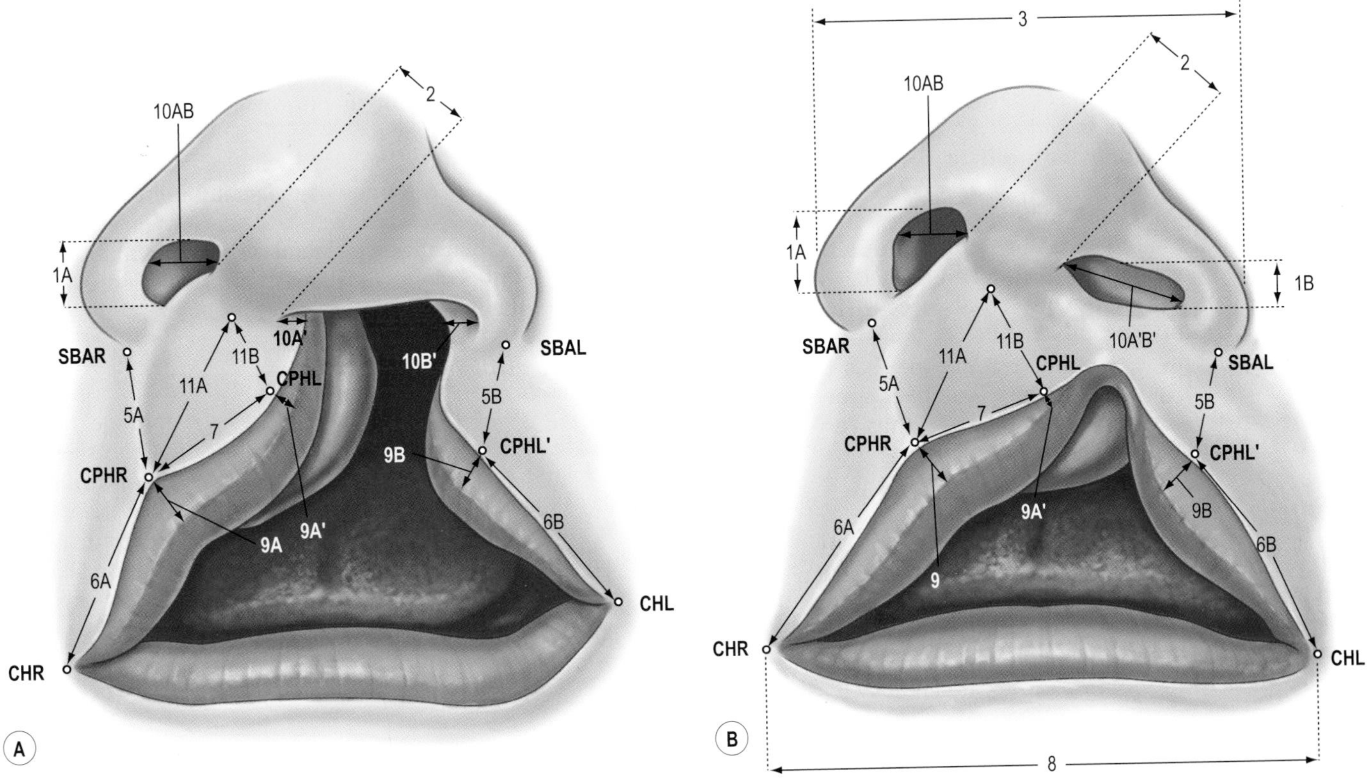

Fig. 23.6 (A) Unilateral complete cleft with anthropometric markings for measurements: CHR, CHL, commissure; right and left horizontal length; right and left vertical length; CPHR, noncleft-side philtral column; CPHL, cleft side Cupid's bow; CPHL', cleft-side philtral column; SBAR, SBAL, right and left base of ala. **(B)** Similar markings for the incomplete cleft lip. (From Noordhoff MS, Chen YR, Chen KT, et al. The surgical technique for the complete unilateral cleft lip-nasal deformity. Plast Reconstr Surg 1995; 2:167–174.[35])

column and should seldom be moved unless there is a severe discrepancy in horizontal or vertical measurements between the cleft side and noncleft side lips.

Evaluation of tissue deficiency or excess

Pool[36] noted areas of vital concern to the surgeon: the amount of tissue medial to the base of the ala and the vertical height of the lateral lip. In addition, the horizontal length of the lateral lip and the epidermal extension from the columella onto the premaxilla are important.

All other measurements for complete and incomplete clefts are recorded at the time of surgery for evaluation along with a record of the cleft deformity. The important measurements for the surgeon to evaluate are the vertical length (VR, VL) and the horizontal length (HR, HL).

Peaking of Cupid's bow

The discrepancy between the height from the central point of the base of columella to the two peaks of the Cupid's bow (CPHR and CPHL) is critical for leveling of the Cupid's bow. It was advocated that if the discrepancy is over 4 mm, it will be difficult to level the Cupid's bow with rotation-advancement technique.[33]

Lateral lip length and height

The short horizontal length on cleft side (HL) can be lengthened by moving point CPHL' medially, but this would shorten the vertical length (VL). Vertical length is more important aesthetically compared with the horizontal length. Therefore, vertical length is seldom sacrificed for horizontal length. The short vertical length can be increased by moving point CPHL' laterally, but this would result in an even shorter horizontal length that is already short. Extending the upper rotation-advancement incision around the ala can also increase the short vertical length. However, this results in an unacceptable perialar scar and should be avoided. It is stressed that point CPHL' is an anatomic point[34–36] similar to other anatomic points. It is not moved until all incisions, muscle dissection, and reconstruction are completed. The reason for this is that an increased vertical length of up to 4 mm can be achieved by adequate muscle dissection and redraping of the skin over the muscle, thus eliminating the need of perialar incisions or moving the point CPHL'.[35,37,38] In incomplete clefts, it is quite often to see a vertically long lateral lip. However, the measurements usually show the vertical height of the cleft side lip is similar to the noncleft side which means the cleft side lateral lip and the alar base are downward displaced. The vertically long lateral lip in incomplete clefts is just an illusion. Adequately mobilization of the cleft side alar base and lateral lip then advance the whole lateral complex superiorly and medially can always level the Cupid's bow thus vertical shortening of the lateral lip is seldom needed.

Columella and nasal floor skin

If the columella is narrow, a Mohler's rotation incision[39] would result in a very narrow columella base and should be avoided.[37] If there is deficient skin lateral to the base of the columella, use of C flap tissue to elongate the columella could result in a small nostril. In addition, it is advocated that increased vertical length of the advancement flap can be obtained by use of vestibular skin.[40] The disadvantage of vestibular skin is that it often includes hair follicles, which are unattractive. When there is deficient skin lateral to the base of the columella, the use of vestibular skin for increasing the length of the advancement flap would result in a small nostril. Careful evaluation of skin lateral to the columella and medial to the alar base is important to prevent a small nostril.

Deficient vermillion beneath the Cupid's bow

The vermillion beneath the cleft-side Cupid's bow is always deficient compared with the counterpart vermillion width on the noncleft side (Fig. 23.6).[35] Inadequate reconstruction of this deficient vermillion will result in free border deformities as seen in a straight-line vermillion closure.[34] The vermillion

medial to the base of the philtral column (point CPHL') fits into the deficient vermillion beneath the Cupid's bow.

Treatment/surgical technique

Overall cleft treatment plan in the Chang Gung Craniofacial Center

A genetic diagnosis and evaluation for other systemic conditions should be done at the time a prenatal diagnosis of the cleft is made. The newborn cleft baby should have a pediatric evaluation. Parents are counseled about feeding and given information for subsequent care and treatment. Presurgical nasoalveolar molding is started at 2 weeks or even earlier. It usually takes 3–4 months before the completion of the nasoalveolar molding (Fig. 23.7).[37]

The surgical approach

There are several different treatment plans leading to the surgical correction of the deformity (Fig. 23.8).[37] With effective presurgical nasoalveolar molding, a definitive cheiloplasty is done at the age of 3–5 months, when the alveolar gap is narrowed and nasal deformity is improved. Whenever presurgical orthopedics is not available or if the child is older than 3 months, a definitive cheiloplasty with nasal correction is done because presurgical orthopedics is usually not effective after 3 months. If there is a wide cleft (>12–15 mm) and an associated tissue deficiency, a nasolabial adhesion cheiloplasty is done at 3 months, followed by a definitive cheiloplasty at about 9 months.

Treatment after lip repair

A two-flap palatoplasty, with a Furlow technique for the soft palate, is done at 9–12 months. In most instances, a complete closure of all operative areas is attempted. Timing of alveolar bone grafting relates to the eruption of the central incisor and canine. It is determined by the orthodontist. This is usually at the age of 7–11 years. Speech evaluation starts at the age of 2.5 years. Early intervention for velopharyngeal

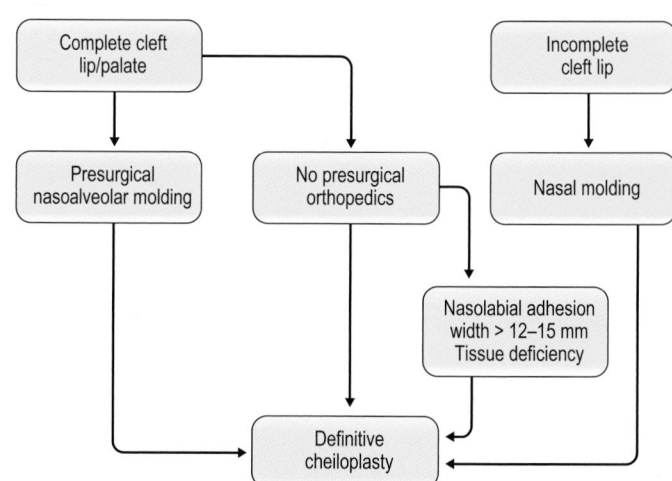

Fig. 23.7 Overall cleft treatment plan in the Chang Gung Craniofacial Center.

insufficiency is done as soon as possible on the basis of speech evaluation and nasopharyngoscopy. With continued improvement in the primary nasal reconstruction, secondary correction of nasal deformities can usually be delayed until facial growth is complete. However, if there is a significant nasal or

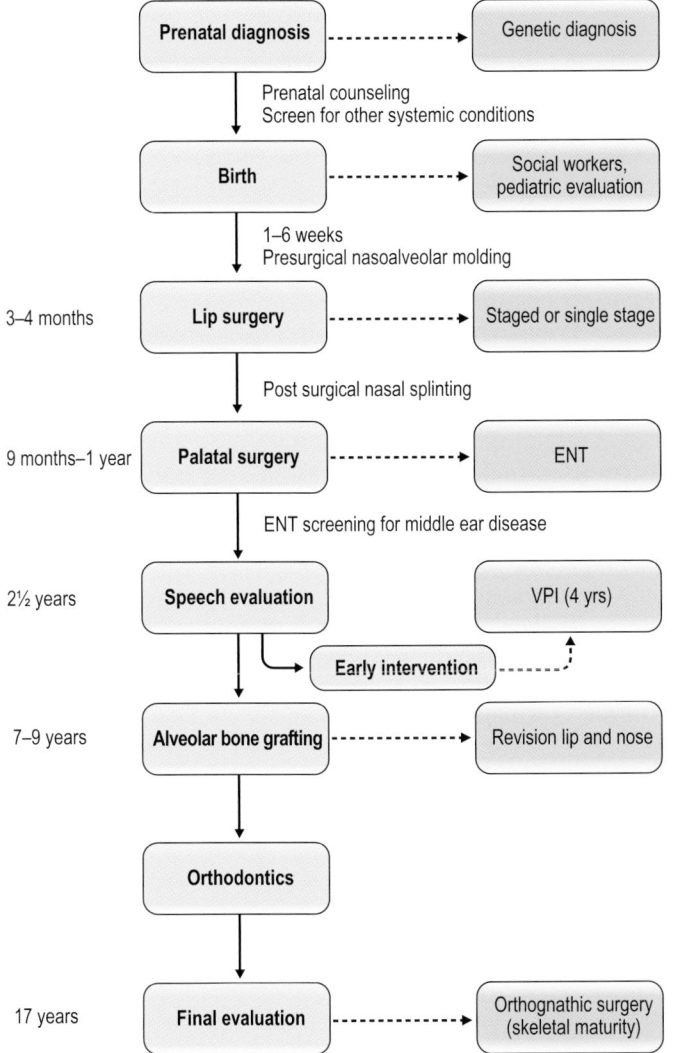

Fig. 23.8 Surgical algorithm for unilateral cleft lip repair in the Chang Gung Craniofacial Center.

lip deformity, or psychological reasons that warrant correction, secondary correction is done before the start of school. Orthodontic treatment during primary dentition is not done except for functional problems that can be corrected in a short time. Orthodontic treatment during mixed dentition is done to correct an anterior crossbite or align deviated incisors before alveolar bone grafting. Continuous orthodontic treatment in the mixed dentition is avoided. For most patients, a fixed orthodontic appliance is used to improve dental occlusion during permanent dentition. Orthognathic surgery is considered for maxillary hypoplasia associated with malocclusion at the time of skeletal maturity *(Fig. 23.7)*.[37]

Presurgical alveolar and nasoalveolar molding

There is a wide variation in the facilities and expertise for performing cleft surgery throughout the world. In many areas, the facilities, personnel, and finances are inadequate for comprehensive treatment. Therefore, presurgical care of the cleft infant may vary from nothing to a more complicated method such as nasoalveolar molding. However, some simple methods can be used to provide good care to the cleft child. It is important to begin the following techniques as soon after birth as possible, preferably within the first 2 weeks after birth.

Alveolar molding: external taping with or without dental plate

The external taping (nonsurgical lip adhesion) is the simplest technique for both presurgical molding of the maxillary halves and approximation of the alveolus. A strip of Micropore tape is placed across the cleft to approximate the upper lips. The objective of the tape is to simulate effects of an adhesion cheiloplasty and reposition the maxillary segments into proper alignment.[37,41] The external taping transfers the tension caused by the approximation of the cleft lip into an inward molding force on the premaxillary alveolus of the greater segment, gradually approximating the separated alveolus *(Fig. 23.9)*. A dental plate used in conjunction with the external taping keeps the tongue out of the cleft and prevents uncontrolled collapse of the dental arches. The central forces of the tongue pushing into the cleft and lateral muscle pull contribute to the cleft deformity *(Fig. 23.10)*. The dental plate is

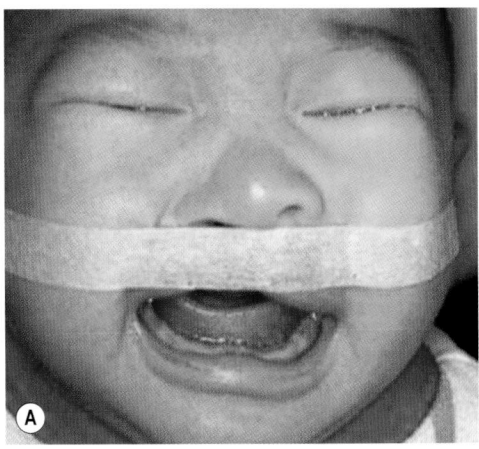

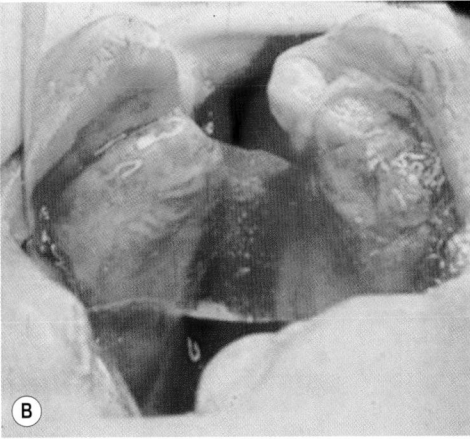

Fig. 23.9 Presurgical orthopedics with external tape and dental plate.
(A) Micropore tape across lip and cheek. **(B)** Dental plate in place to keep the tongue out of the cleft and to reposition the cleft maxilla and alveolus.

gradually ground out on its inner surface for controlled movement of the maxillary segments into their proper position.

Nasoalveolar molding

Liou's method

This method utilizes a molding bulb attached to a dental plate as an outrigger to mold the nose along with external taping

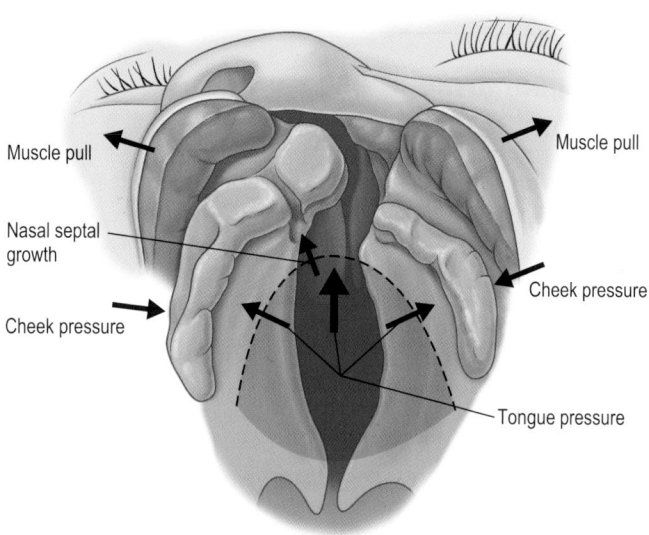

Muscle pull

Muscle pull

Nasal septal growth

Cheek pressure

Cheek pressure

Tongue pressure

Fig. 23.10 The forces that exert an influence on the cleft alveolus are the central tongue force, pushing the cleft laterally, and the tongue in the cleft alveolus, preventing approximation. Anteriorly, the muscle pulls laterally and the cheek pressure pushes posteriorly on the palate.

of the lip. The device is held to the palate with dental adhesives. The force from taping and counterforce from the molding bulb provide the combined force necessary to bring the alveolus into proper position. The nasal molding and alveolar molding are done at the same time, taking approximately 3 months.[37,42]

Overstretching of the nasal cartilage on the cleft side should be avoided. Nasal projection and the dental plate are modified or adjusted every 1–2 weeks until the arch and nose are properly positioned *(Fig. 23.11)*. A new molding device, with spring mechanism, is used at the Chang Gung Craniofacial Center in recent years. It can greatly lengthen the duration between each clinical visit from 1 week to 1 month, thus significantly reducing the burden of care for parents *(Fig. 23.12)*.

Grayson's method

Grayson[43,44] performs the nasal molding after alveolar approximation to avoid overstretching the nasal cartilage. The appliance consists of an acrylic or resin plate which fits over the maxillary dental arch (alveolar ridges), an acrylic retention arm or button, and a nasal stent. The nasal stent consists of a wire extending from the plate intranasally forming a kidney bean shape. This bilobed potion of the nasal stent is covered with soft acrylic. Alternatively, the nasal stent can be formed entirely from acrylic. Micropore tape applied to the lips and connected with orthodontic elastics hold the dental plate to the palate. Gradually adding soft resin on the inner surface of the buccal flange and grinding out the palatal surface of the dental plate approximates the alveolar shelves. The nasal projection is added and adjusted underneath the deformed cartilage. This technique should be started within the first 2 weeks after birth; careful monitoring is required every 1–2 weeks for a period of 3–6 months to complete it *(Fig. 23.13)*.

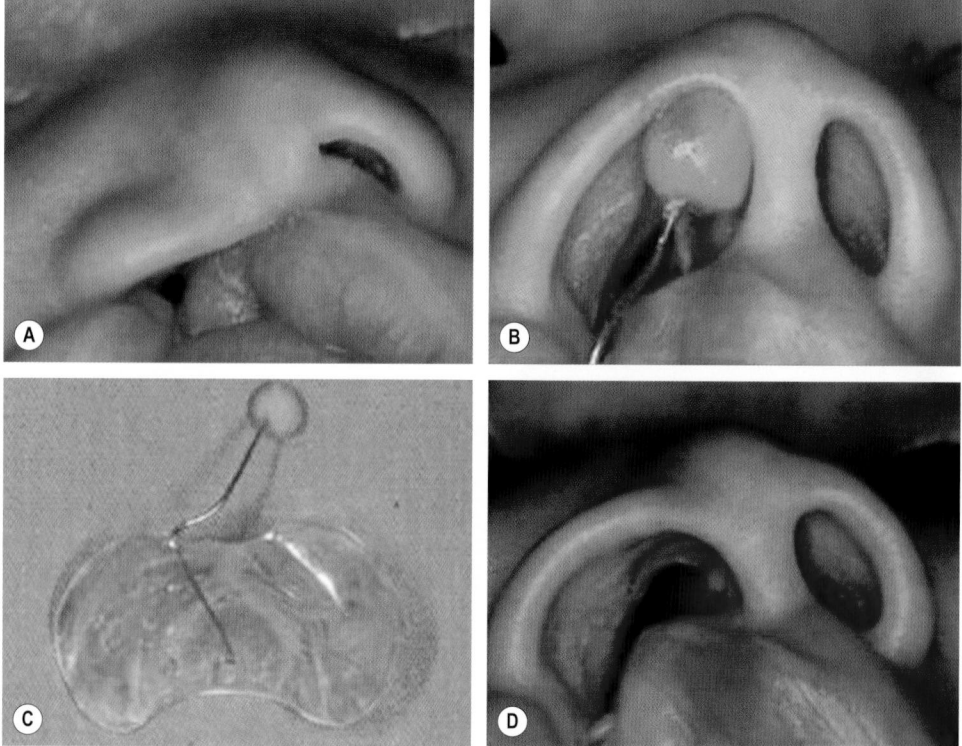

Fig. 23.11 Presurgical nasoalveolar molding, Liou's technique. Right complete cleft of primary and secondary palate (right primary and secondary complete; RPC, RSC, 1–9).
(A) Alveolus at 2 weeks before molding.
(B) During molding with dental plate and attached soft acrylic bulb in place at 1 month.
(C) The molding device and the dental plate.
(D) After molding at 3 months before operation.

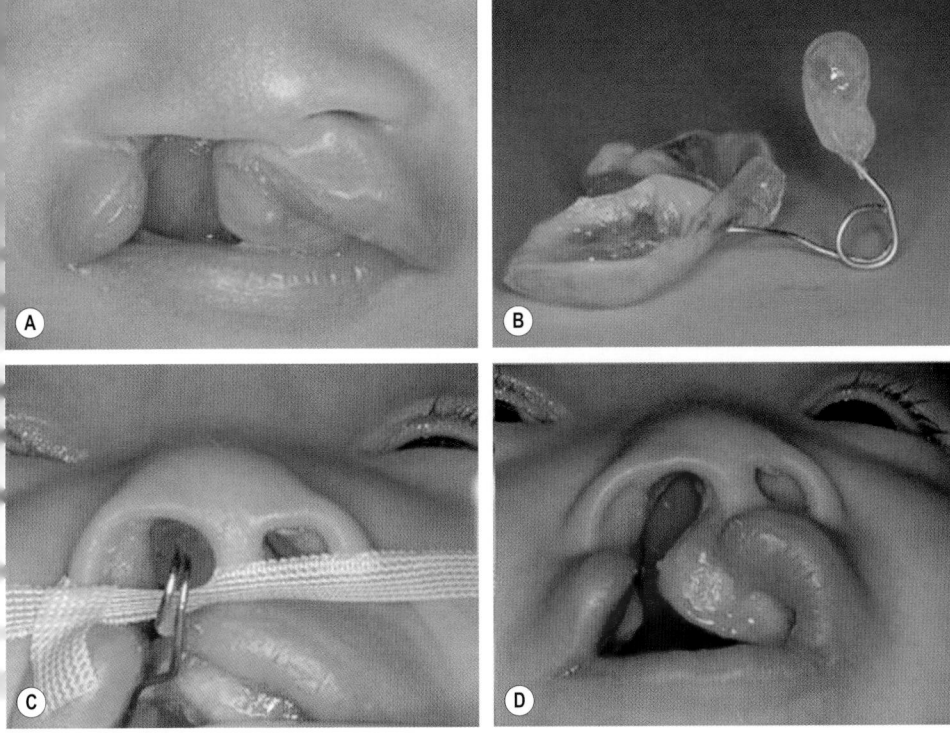

Fig. 23.12 New molding device by Liou's technique. Right complete cleft of primary and secondary palate (right primary and secondary complete; RPC, RSC, 1–9). **(A)** Initial visit at 2 weeks before molding. **(B)** The molding device with the spring mechanism and the dental plate. **(C)** During molding with dental plate and attached soft acrylic bulb in place at 2 month. **(D)** After molding at 3 months before operation.

Discussion of presurgical orthopedics

The primary objective of presurgical orthopedics is to correct the skeletal deformities of the cleft maxilla before surgery.[45–51] Keeping the tongue out of the cleft and replacing the pulling force from the separated lip muscle by tape traction across the lip accomplishes this purpose *(Fig. 23.9)*. Regardless of no improvement to facial growth,[52,53] presurgical orthopedics provides a better bony framework with a narrower cleft. Most surgeons, given a choice, would like a closely approximated cleft alveolus at the time of surgery.[54,55] It is also noted that there is a statistically significant increased narrowing of the cleft when the infant sleeps on the side compared with sleeping on the back.[56] Presurgical nasoalveolar molding can greatly improve the nasal shape before operation, thus facilitating nasal reconstruction.[43,44,57–59]

Surgical technique

Adhesion cheiloplasty: two-staged repair

The use of the adhesion cheiloplasty was first credited to Johanson.[60] The adhesion cheiloplasty is used as a routine part of the primary repair at some centers,[61–64] whereas it is used selectively at other centers.[35,65,66] A number of techniques are used. They vary from a simple type of lip adhesion[67,68] or a nasolabial adhesion,[62] to a more complex nasolabial adhesion used at the Chang Gung Craniofacial Center.[35,37] The incidence of dehiscence varies from 2–22%.[62,67,69] The incidence of nasolabial adhesion cheiloplasty decreased from 37% in 1986 to 1% in 1999 in the Chang Gung Craniofacial Center.[37] Factors contributing to a decreased incidence are more experienced cleft surgeons, improved presurgical orthopedics, and changing

the sleep position from the supine to the prone or side position, thus decreasing cleft width.[56]

The advantages and disadvantages of a two-stage nasolabial adhesion cheiloplasty

The advantages of a two-stage cheiloplasty are frequently stated to be narrowing of the cleft, decreased tension across the maxilla, easier correction of nasal deformity and development of more muscle or elongation of a short lip before definitive cheiloplasty.[70] If a preliminary nasolabial adhesion is warranted, it should produce better results with fewer secondary revisions and less disturbance of growth than a single-stage cheiloplasty.

In an evaluation of a two-stage procedure, Mulliken and Martinez-Perez[62] reported that 75% required nasal revision and 21% a revision of the lip. There are too many variables to determine whether an initial two-stage procedure or one-stage cheiloplasty gives a better result. In both instances, there will be a need for secondary procedures. This question relates to the surgeon's confidence in the ability to correct the problem, the timing of the procedure, and the desires of the patient or family.

Tension could possibly be decreased in a two-stage procedure, but even with an adhesion cheiloplasty, there is a muscular sling that causes increased tension, which molds the maxillary segments into position in a more gentle fashion.[71] There is no evidence to support the theory that a staged repair is better than a one-stage repair because of less tension.[72–77] Obtaining a better nostril with a two-stage procedure is also questioned.[62]

The biggest disadvantage of an adhesion cheiloplasty is the scarring. This makes dissection and mobilization of the tissues

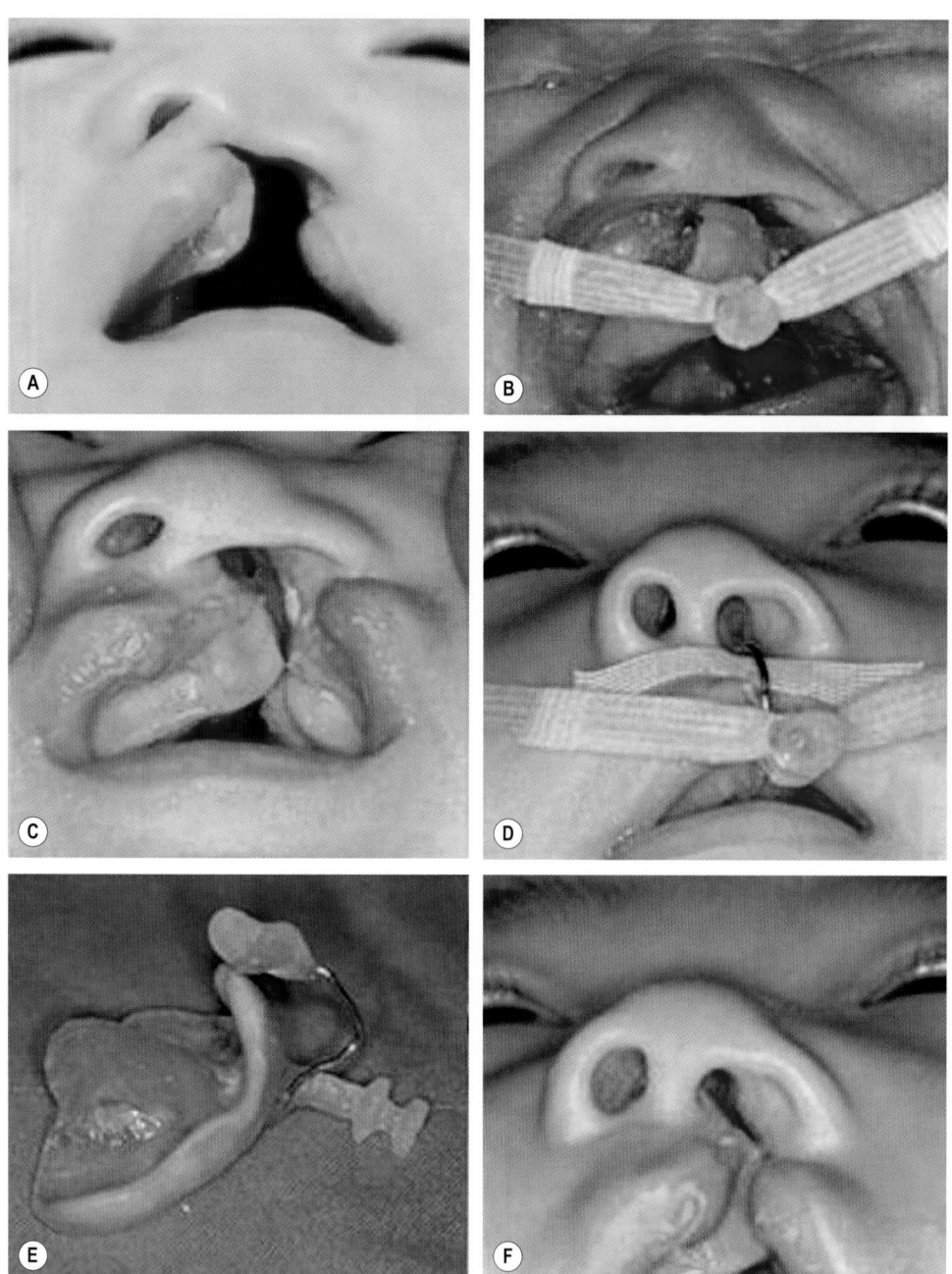

Fig. 23.13 Nasoalveolar molding, Grayson technique (left unilateral complete cleft of primary and secondary palate; LPC, LSC, 11–19). **(A)** Position of alveolus before nasoalveolar molding at 2 weeks. **(B)** During alveolar molding at 4 weeks. **(C)** Approximation of alveolus at 6 weeks. **(D)** Nasoalveolar molding. **(E)** The nasoalveolar molding device. **(F)** After nasoalveolar molding before surgery at 4 months.

more difficult than in a one-stage procedure. It is suggested that after lip adhesion, there is an increase in the vertical lip length and muscle volume, thus making the subsequent cheiloplasty easier and delivering a better result. A 10% increase in vertical height after nasolabial adhesions is reported, and this is an insufficient reason for advocating a preliminary adhesion cheiloplasty.[78]

Nasolabial adhesion cheiloplasty: surgical technique

An adhesion cheiloplasty is done in less than 1% of all clefts after the use of nasoalveolar molding in the Chang Gung Craniofacial Center. Current indications for a nasolabial adhesion cheiloplasty are: (1) An alveolar cleft >12–15 mm wide with an associated discrepancy of >5 mm in the vertical height between SBAR-CPHR and SBAL-CPHL'; (2) a complete cleft of the primary palate in which there is a prominent protruding premaxilla resulting in a long sagittal discrepancy between the premaxilla alveolus and maxilla.[37] Tissue deficiencies are more important than cleft width as a criterion in decision-making for a nasolabial adhesion cheiloplasty.

Markings

Standard markings and measurements for an adhesion cheiloplasty are similar to those of the complete unilateral clefts. However, vital landmarks CPHL and CPHL' and the vermillion medial to the base of the cleft-side philtral column (point CPHL') must not be violated *(Fig. 23.14)*.

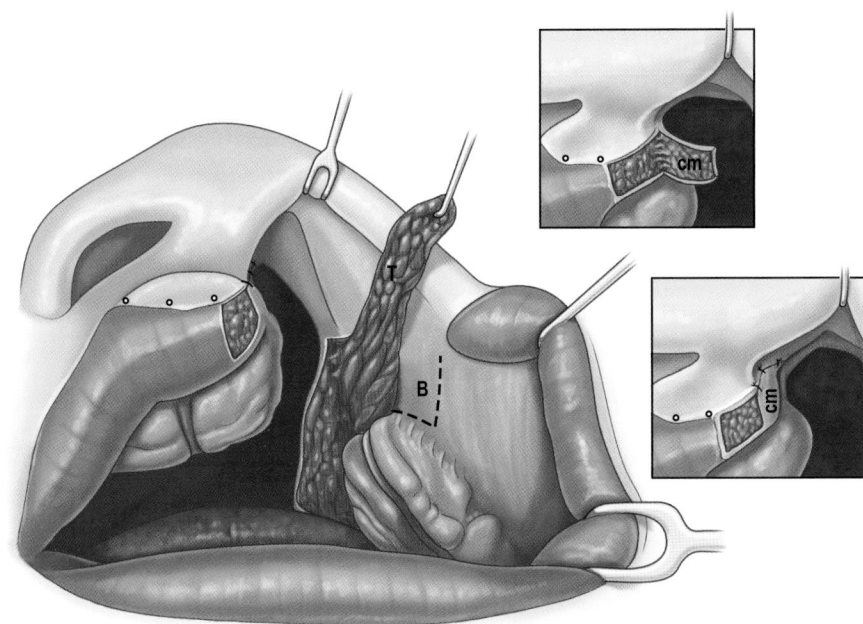

Fig. 23.14 Nasoalveolar adhesion. Insets: The incisions are on the skin border elevating a mucosal flap that is inserted along the skin columella-septal line behind the columella. The turbinate flap (T) is elevated, and the buccal mucosal flap (B) based on vestibular skin is marked for incision, varying the length according to the width of the cleft.

Elevation and insertion of C flap mucosa

An incision is made on the free edge of skin and mucosa on the noncleft side lip and extended posteriorly to the junction of columella skin and septal mucosa. All skin overlying the premaxilla is preserved. The mucosal C flap, based on the premaxilla, is incised and elevated. It is rotated and inserted behind the columella. This allows mobilization of the medial lip. There is no dissection of muscle *(Fig. 23.14)*.

Lateral lip incisions

The buccal mucosal flap and inferior turbinate (T) flap are elevated based on vestibular skin. The free edge of the lateral lip is opened, preserving the vermillion medial to CPHL' on the lateral lip. There is no muscle dissection. The fibrous attachments between the lower lateral cartilage (LLC) and piriform rim are released for mobilization of the alar base and LLC *(Fig. 23.15)*.

Mucosal flaps

With traction on a suspension suture through the dome of the upper lateral cartilage (ULC), the LLC is advanced and with its lateral crura sutured to the ULC. The T flap is rotated and sutured to the piriform rim. The buccal mucosal flap is folded on itself and sutured to the edge of the T flap *(Fig. 23.15)*.

Nostril floor closure

The leading edge of the folded buccal flap is advanced and sutured to the periosteum of the premaxilla. The buccal lip mucosa is advanced and sutured to the bridging mucosal flap and to the periosteum and mucosa of the premaxilla *(Fig. 23.16)*.

Muscle and skin closure

Several interrupted horizontal sutures are placed in the muscle, and the skin is closed. Of note, there is no dissection

between the nasal skin and the dome of the LLC, and no dissection over the maxilla.

Definitive cheiloplasty after adhesion

The adhesion cheiloplasty changes a complete cleft into an incomplete cleft. The definitive cheiloplasty can be performed around 6 months later after scar maturation. The technique described below is the technique used since the late 1990s in the Chang Gung Craniofacial Center. The rotation-advancement is more of a straight-line type of incision from the cleft side of the Cupid's bow to the base of the columella. The C flap is usually brought laterally, and the advancement flap is incised and advanced medially *(Fig. 23.17)*. As resurfacing of the piriform area with mucosal flaps was performed at the initial procedure, no dissection is needed over the maxilla. The LLC is released from the overlying skin through the base of the ala if necessary. Muscle repair, triangular flap augmentation of the deficient vermillion, skin closure, and nasal conformer placement is performed in sequence. An example of a two-stage cheiloplasty is shown in *Figure 23.18*.

Rotation advancement cheiloplasty for complete clefts

Video 1,2

The following principles are basic to the correction of the cleft deformity:

- Understanding of the embryologic development and anatomy
- Understanding of the nature of the deformity to be corrected
- Awareness of the different surgical procedures and their limitations
- Atraumatic surgical technique with delicate handling of tissues, sharp dissection, and careful hemostasis
- Limited dissection to avoid surgical trauma to adjacent tissues

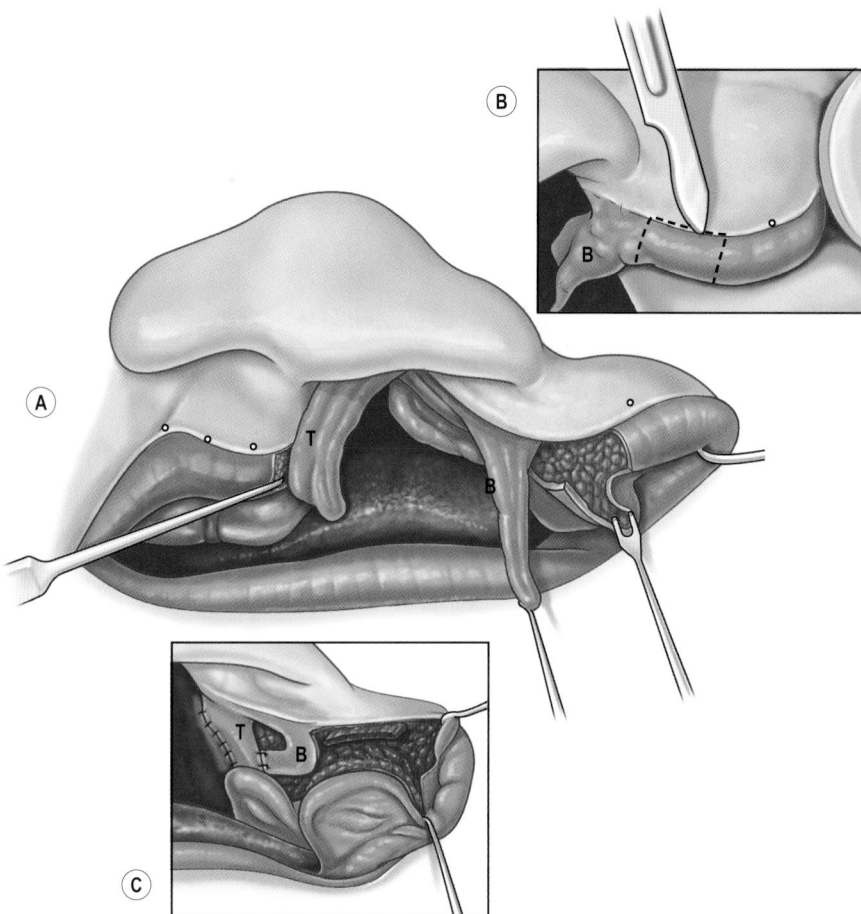

Fig. 23.15 Nasoalveolar adhesion. The turbinate (T) and buccal mucosal (B) flaps are elevated. Upper inset: The free edge of the lip is incised from the converging points of the red line and white skin roll to the base of the buccal flap, preserving the lateral lip vermillion and exposing the muscle. Lower inset: The turbinate flap (T) is rotated into the piriform area, and the free edge of the folded mucosal flap (B) is attached to the inferior edge of the turbinate flap.

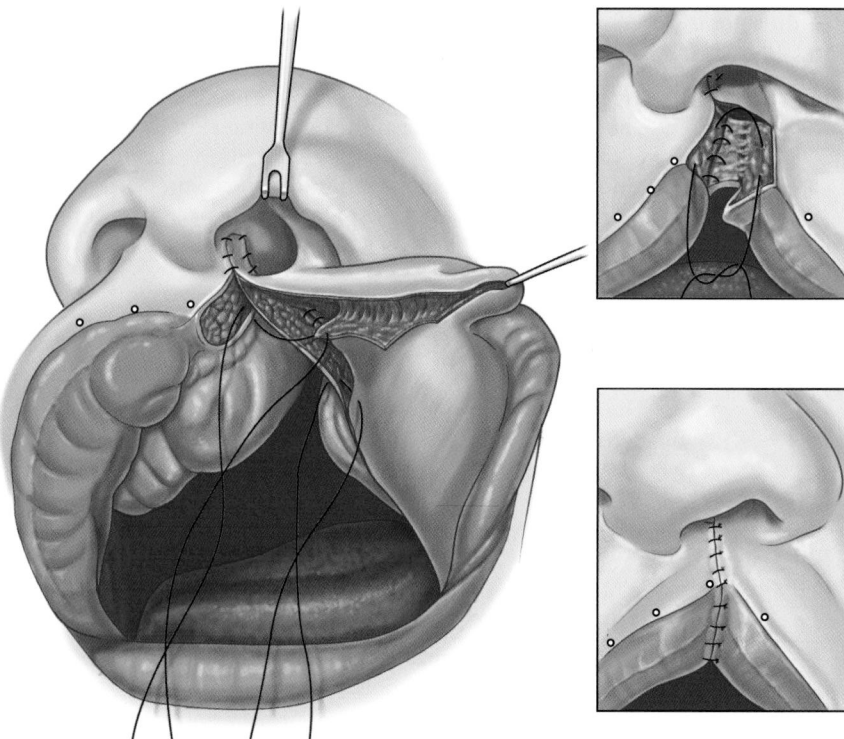

Fig. 23.16 Nasoalveolar adhesion. The leading edge of the folded mucosal flap is sutured to the periosteum of the premaxilla and the edge of the mucosal C flap. Insets: The posterior mucosa is closed, followed by several muscle sutures without muscle dissection, followed by skin closure.

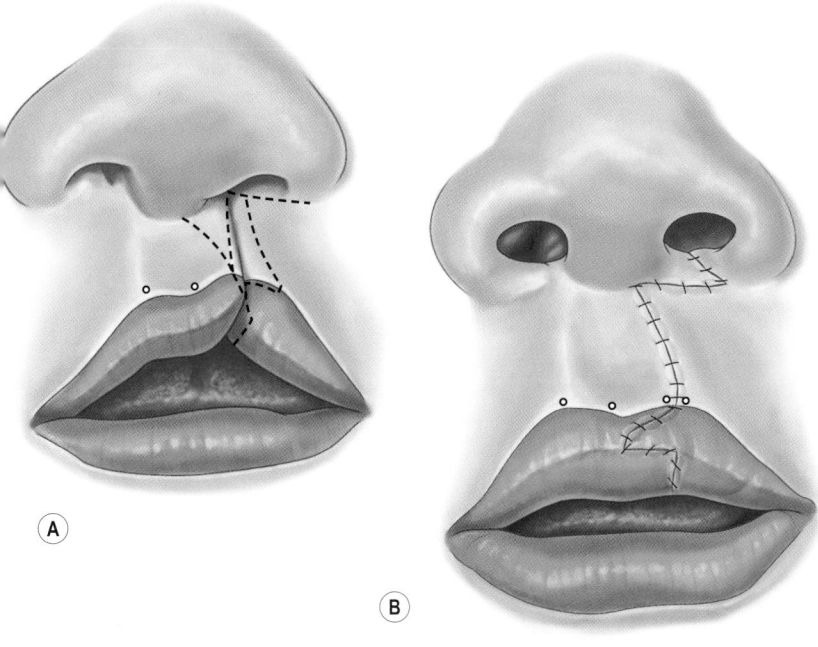

Fig. 23.17 Incision lines for the rotation-advancement flap. The two flaps are incised, and muscle is dissected for a distance of 2–4 mm. The two flaps are interdigitated with closure of mucosa, muscle, and skin. No dissection is necessary in the piriform or maxillary area. Release of the LLC is done through the base of the ala when indicated to achieve nostril symmetry.

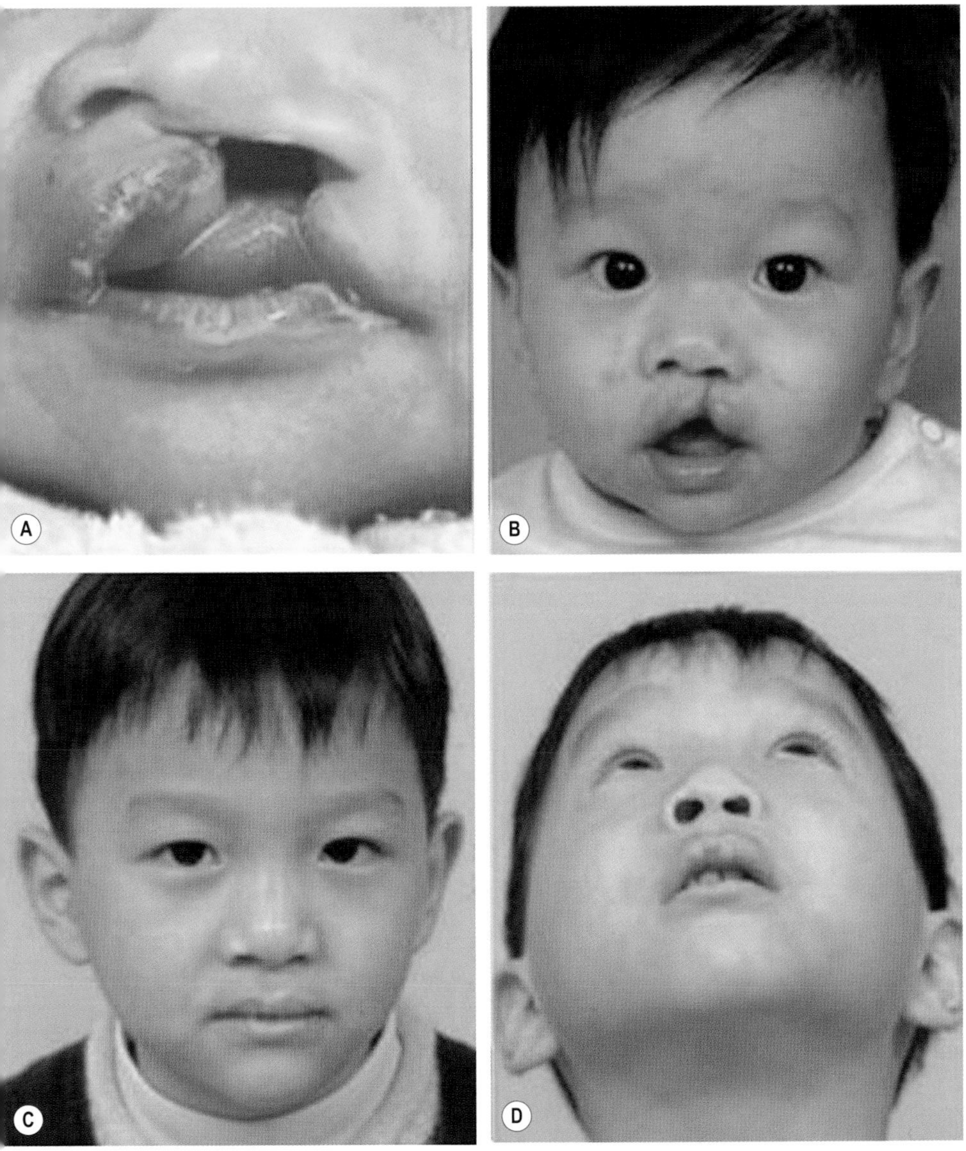

Fig. 23.18 (A) A 1-month-old Chinese boy with a left complete cleft of the primary and secondary palate (LPC, LSC, 11–19). Presurgical orthopedics was unsuccessful. The alveolar cleft was 10 mm wide, and there was associated vertical shortness of the lateral lip. **(B)** Postoperative view after a nasoalveolar adhesion cheiloplasty at 7 months. **(C,D)** Postoperative views at 5 years, when a definitive cheiloplasty was done.

- Knowledge of the healing process
- An alternative plan for complications or unexpected difficulties at the time of surgery as a lifeboat
- Understanding and awareness of the problems related to anesthesia, preoperative care, and postoperative care.

In addition to the basic principles that are applicable to any surgical procedure, some key concepts apply to the surgical technique in cleft repair. The key concepts of the surgical technique in the unilateral cheiloplasty are as follows:

- Mohler's rotation incision
- Mucosal flaps for nasal floor reconstruction, correction of mucosal deficiency in piriform area
- Eliminate the perialar incision on advancement flap, limiting scars around the ala base and nostril floor
- Mobilization of alar base
- Nasal floor reconstruction with complete mucosal closure
- Muscle release and reconstruction to simulate the philtral column
- Anchoring of advancement flap to nasal septum for centralizing the Cupid's bow
- Correction of central vermillion deficiency with triangular vermillion flap from lateral lip
- Semiopen rhinoplasty with a reverse U incision on the cleft side and rim incision on the noncleft side
- Atraumatic dissection to release the fibrofatty tissue from LLCs
- Advancement and fixation of the cleft side LLC to the noncleft side LLC and to the skin in an over-corrected position
- Definition of the alar-facial groove with alar transfixion sutures.

Medial incisions

The basic points for markings are shown in *Figure 23.6*. A Mohler's rotation incision line is marked as a curving line from CPHL going upward into the base of columella then turning back to the nasolabial junction of the noncleft side philtral column *(Fig. 23.19)*. The height of this rotation incision should be the same as the height of the noncleft side philtral column. The angle of the backcut is dependent on the width of columella. If the columella is wide, a wider angle can be made. The incision across the free border of the lip at CPHL should be at right angles to the axis of the white skin roll to facilitate subsequent lip closure. The muscle is freed from the skin in the subdermal plane for a distance of 2–3 mm *(Fig. 23.20, inset)*.

Adequate rotation

The muscle dissection on the noncleft side should reach the nasal floor of the noncleft side for adequate releasing of the abnormal muscle insertion to the columellar base *(Fig. 23.18)*.

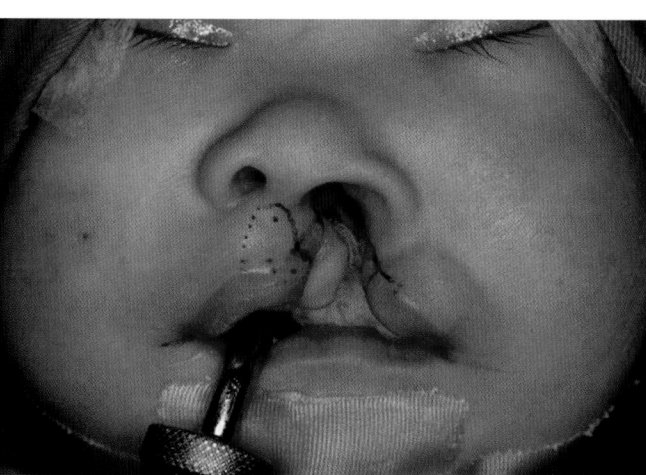

Fig. 23.19 Preoperative marking: CPHR, IS, CPHL, CPHL' and CHL as described in *Figure 23.6*. The C-flap (c) and C-flap mucosa (cm) are marked. The dotted line on the lip is the red line, which is the junction between vermillion and mucosa. Incision lines are shown on the lip extending from point CPHL lateral to the columella on the skin edge overlying the premaxilla extending superiorly along the junction line of columella skin and septal cartilage mucosa. The cleft-side base of the philtral column is also marked (CPHL'). The proposed incision lines are marked with the rotation incision in a Mohler's fashion. A small triangular white skin roll flap is designed above the CPHL'.

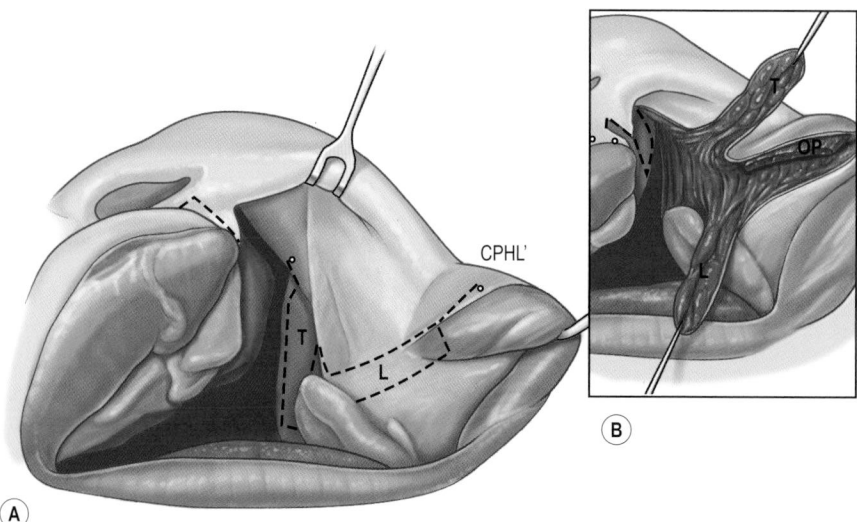

Fig. 23.20 The orbicularis peripheralis muscle (OP) is released in a subdermal plane. The abnormally inserted fibers of the nasalis, depressor septi, and levator muscles are released from the base of the ala. Inset (A): The muscle is freed from the skin in the subdermal plane for a distance of 2–3 mm.

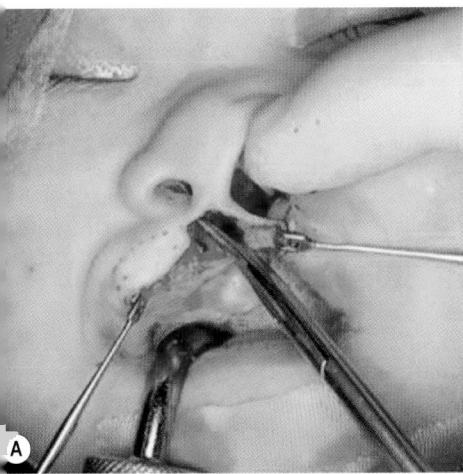
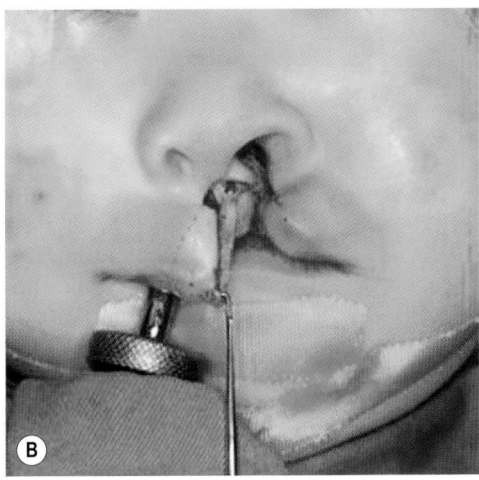

Fig. 23.21 (A) Traction on the free border of the lip helps to determine if the rotation is adequate. **(B)** The muscle dissection on the rotation flap should reach the nasal floor on noncleft side.

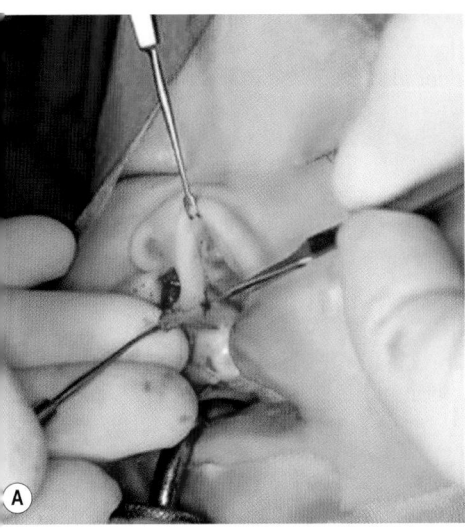
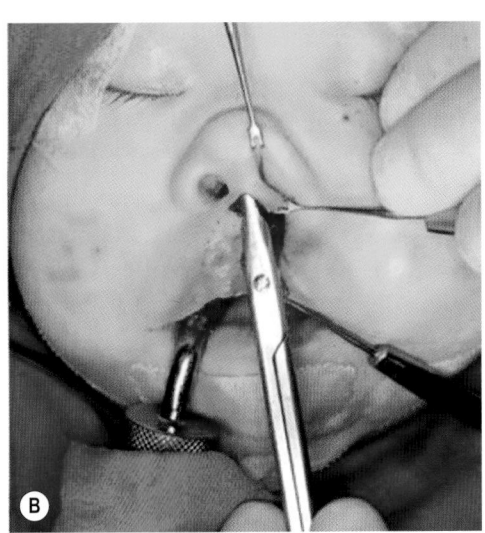

Fig. 23.22 (A) The incision line of the C-flap. **(B)** A blunt-tip scissors is used to release the foot plate of the medial crura of the cleft side lower lateral cartilage.

raction on the free border of the lip will determine if the otation is adequate, that is, both sides of the Cupid's ow at the same level *(Fig. 23.21)*. Even if the rotation is nadequate, extending the incision across the noncleft-side hiltral column should be avoided, as it will result in a verti-ally long lip. If the rotation fails to level the Cupid's bow, othing further is done until after muscle repositioning. A ack-cut, as advocated by Millard,[79] leaves a wide defect at he apex of the rotation incision. This defect is lower and vider than the defect after a Mohler's incision. It is better to e closed by a square-shape advancement flap. This area is lways the tightest and most difficult area of skin closure. herefore, to avoid a difficult, tight skin closure, a back-cut s avoided.

C-flap and footplate of medial crura

he C-flap incisions are made on a line that extends from oint CPHL along the junction of skin and mucosa to the most ateral point of the skin overlying the premaxilla. The incision n the premaxilla then turns superiorly at the junction of the olumellar skin and septal mucosa for a distance of 5 mm or

even longer *(Fig. 23.22)*. Blunt-tip tenotomy scissors are used to separate the medial crura of the cleft side lower lateral cartilage *(Fig. 23.22)*. This allows mobilization of the C-flap and repositioning of the downward displaced footplate of the medial crura of the cleft side lower lateral cartilage. The tip of the C-flap (point at CPHL) is rotated medially to fill in the defect on the columellar base after the Mohler's incision *(Fig. 23.23)*.

Lateral lip incisions

An L-flap[80] is marked based on the maxilla, extending on the free border of the lip to the point where the red line and white skin roll converge, preserving the vermillion on the lateral lip. The skin incision line on the free border of the lip starts from point CPHL'. A triangular shaped small WSR flap is designed *(Fig. 23.19)*. The width of the WSR flap is exactly the same as the width of WSR above the point CPHL'. The length of the WSR flap is only 1–2 mm. The incision line is then continued along the skin-mucosal junction on the piriform up to the inferior edge of the inferior turbinate then turning inward to include an inferior turbinate flap *(Fig. 23.23)*.

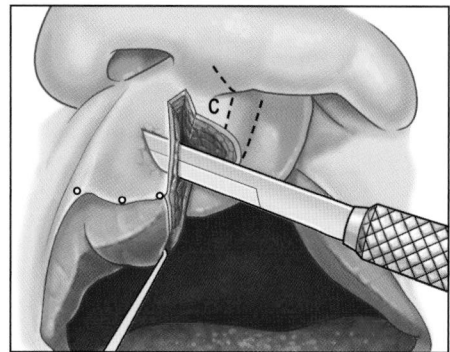

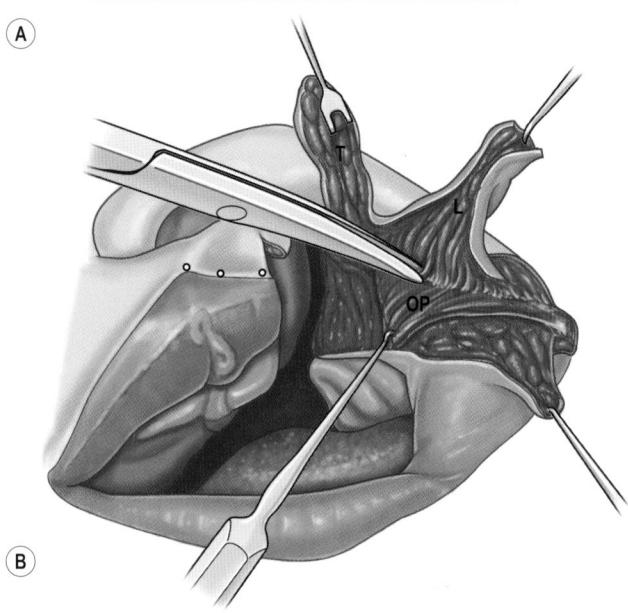

Fig. 23.23 (A) The tip of the C-flap adjacent to CPHL is rotated medially to fill the defect on columellar base after a Mohler's incision. Inset **(B)**: The completed dissection with an elevated turbinate (T) and mucosal flap (L) based on the maxilla. Markings for the mucosal flap L, based on maxilla and inferior turbinate flap T. The L-flap based on the maxilla extends to the converging red line and white skin roll, leaving the vermillion between this point and CPHL' available for reconstruction of the deficient vermillion beneath the cleft side of the Cupid's bow.

L-flap and inferior turbinate flap

The incision line on the inferior turbinate extends from the piriform rim inward on the upper and lower edges of the inferior turbinate for a distance of 1.5 cm, where a transverse cut is made. The inferior turbinate flap (T) is elevated in a retrograde fashion based on the vestibular skin. After elevation of the L and T flaps, the attachments of the LLC to the maxilla and ULC are released, allowing easy mobilization of the LLC and the lateral lip. Even in wide clefts, mobilization of the lip and cartilage is easily accomplished without an extensive dissection over the maxilla *(Fig. 23.23)*.

Orbicularis muscle dissection and alar base mobilization

The lateral lip mucosa is incised and dissected free for only 2 mm. Excessive dissection contributes to scarring and should be avoided. The orbicularis peripheralis muscle is bunched

up as a disorganized mass of fibers with numerous derma insertions.[81] By use of a blunt-nosed tenotomy scissors, th orbicularis peripheralis muscle is dissected along the edge c the dermis to a line extending from the base of the ala to th base of the philtral column CPHL'. The dissection is contir ued on a subdermal plane superiorly under and aroun the base of the ala. This releases the abnormal insertions c the paranasal muscles including the transverse portion of th nasalis muscle, the depressor septi, and the levator muscle of the upper lip and ala.[62,82,83] The Angular artery is used as landmark for the muscle dissection around the alar base. Th extent of dissection should be lateral to the vessel to assur most of the abnormal muscle insertions to the alar base ar released. Release of the muscle from the overlying skin an ala allows the tethered, bunched-up muscle to be stretchec effectively elongating the lateral lip. The skin will also stretc in a similar manner, gaining increased vertical heigh *(Fig. 23.20)*.

Elevation of orbicularis marginalis flap

The orbicularis marginalis (OM) flap is incised along the fre border of the lip to include the orbicularis marginalis muscle the vermillion medial to point CPHL', and the correspondin mucosa posteriorly. The OM flap is elevated to its base beneatl the philtral column (CPHL') in such a way that the volume c muscle at its base CPHL' is similar to the volume of muscl at the opposite point CPHR on the noncleft side of the lip. Th OM flap is cut squarely and not beveled *(Fig. 23.24)*.

Correction of piriform deficiency

The LLC is repositioned superiorly and fixed to the ULC witl interrupted polyglactin sutures *(Fig. 23.25)*. The T-flap base(on vestibular skin is rotated 90° to fill in the defect on pirifor rim. Its superior edge is sutured to the piriform edge. Th T-flap corrects mucosal deficiency and allows repositioning c the LLC and ala without restriction.

Nasal floor reconstruction and alar base repositioning

The L-flap is rotated medially behind the columella an(attached to the perichondrium of the previous incision behin(the columella. The inferior edge of the T-flap is sutured to th superior edge of the L-flap with interrupted 5–0 polyglactir sutures. The C-flap mucosa is rotated laterally and place(below the L-flap. It is attached to the maxilla and sutured t(the inferior edge of the L-flap. This gives good mucosal cover age of the nostril floor and lateral nostril wall without any raw surface or tension. The vestibular skin with attached al. is advanced over the mucosal bridge to the uppermost poin of the previous incision behind the columella. The upper fre(edge of the vestibular skin flap and bridging T and L flaps ar(closed with interrupted 5–0 polyglactin sutures. This gives good two-layer closure of the nostril floor and effectively cor rects the tissue deficiency in this area. The vestibular skin i advanced as far as necessary to achieve a slightly over corrected nostril width. This also advances and rotates the al inward into a position slightly over-corrected to the opposit side. Final positioning and closure of the nostril floor are don after muscle reconstruction *(Fig. 23.25)*.

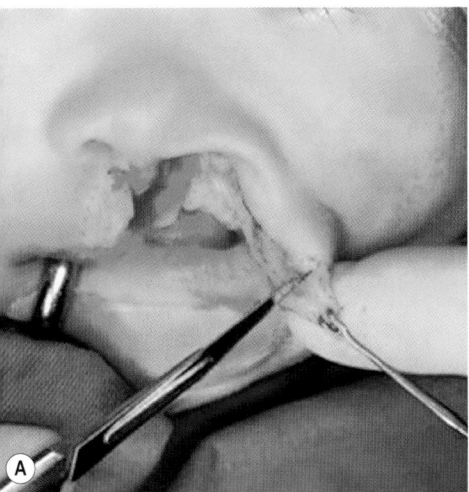 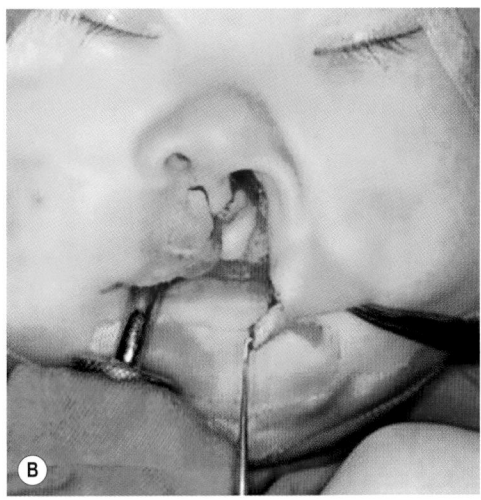

Fig. 23.24 (A,B) The incision along the skin edge from CPHL' to the base of the inferior turbinate and elevation of the OM flap on the lateral lip. The OM flap is elevated to its base beneath the philtral column (CPHL') in such a way that the volume of muscle at its base CPHL' is similar to the volume of muscle at the opposite point CPHR on the noncleft side of the lip.

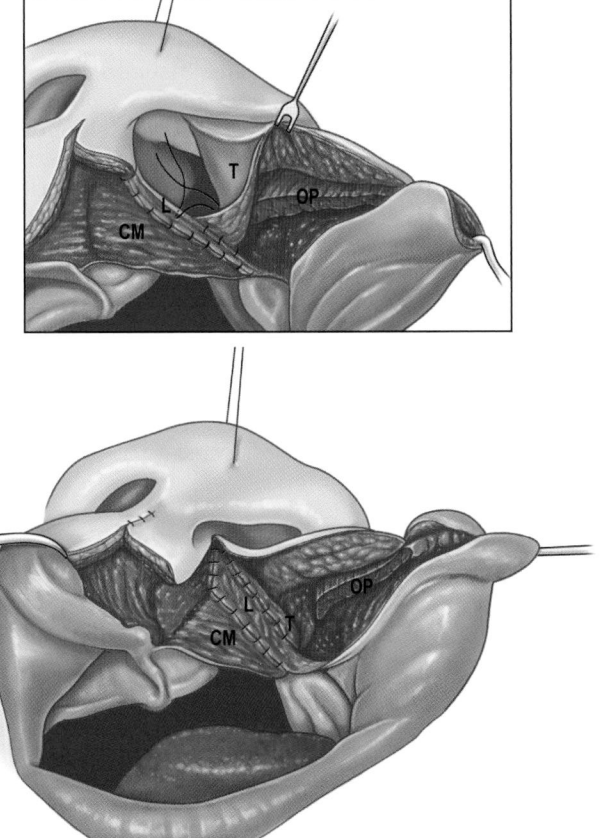

Fig. 23.25 (A) The LLC is freed from its fibrous attachments to the maxilla and ULC. There is no dissection over the maxilla. The LLC is elevated with a traction suture and fixed to the ULC in an elevated position. The turbinate flap (T) is rotated into the piriform area. The nostril floor is reconstructed with the L-flap behind the columella, and the CM flap mucosa is sutured lateral to the maxilla. **(B)** Completion of nostril floor reconstruction with advancement of the vestibular skin rotating the alar base inward. There is good mucosal closure with no open areas for secondary healing and scar contracture. OP, orbicularis peripheralis muscle.

Muscle reconstruction

The muscle is approximated with a 5–0 polydioxanone. A key suture is placed in the center of the muscle, opposite points CPHL and CPHL' and pulled downward to level the Cupid's bow. This is to assure the correct placement of each muscle suture. The first stitch is passed through the caudal edge of the nasal septum, catching the tip of the muscle (which is originally inserted above and lateral to the cleft side alar base) in the advancement flap in a mattress fashion and anchored to the septum. This anchoring suture helps to pull the lateral lip medially and centralize the Cupid's bow. The muscle sutures are placed in such a way that the lateral muscle is overlapping above the medial muscle to increase the muscle thickness and simulate a philtral column. The muscle in OM flap is also sutured in a mattress fashion to avoid any depression in this area after operation *(Fig. 23.26)*.

Philtral column reconstruction

To reconstruct the philtral column on the cleft side in unilateral clefts, several key steps are necessary. (1) *Skin incision line*: the Mohler's incision is more vertical and more lateral compared to the incision line of the traditional rotation-advancement technique. The final position of the suture line of the Mohler's incision is more similar to the position of the philtral column on the noncleft side. (2) *Muscle reconstruction*: the aforementioned muscle sutures place the muscle of the lateral lip above the muscle of the medial lip thus increasing the muscle thickness needed for a philtral column. (3) *Skin laxity*: besides the muscle thickness, loose skin is necessary to reconstruct a bulging philtral column. The mattress muscle sutures can horizontally approximate the muscle tighter than the skin. The "excessive" skin that appears after muscle reconstruction is preserved to provide enough laxity for the appearance of a philtral column.

Incisions for triangular vermillion flap

The vermillion flap is marked and incised on the OM flap, while the OM flap is held under tension. A No. 11 blade is laid on the incision line, drawing the knife across to ensure an accurate cut. After the vermillion flap is incised, an incision is made along or above the red line of the lip beneath the Cupid's bow opposite point CPHL, thus opening the lip for eventual insertion of the vermillion flap after muscle approximation. The width of the vermillion flap should correct the vermillion deficiency under the Cupid's bow. The tip of the vermillion flap should not cross the natural lip tubercle *(Fig. 23.27)*.

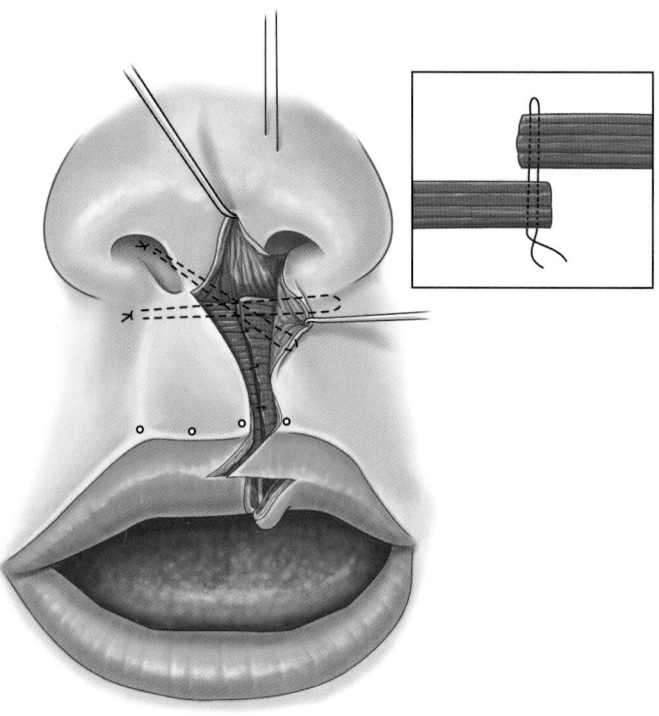

Fig. 23.26 Orbicularis peripheralis muscle closure (with septal anchoring suture). Inset: Overlapping the lateral muscle on the medial muscle for philtral column reconstruction.

Closure of the free border of the lip

Points CPHL and CPHL' are approximated with a fine 7–0 absorbable polyglactin suture. The excess mucosa opposite points CPHL and CPHL' on the free border of the lip is trimmed. The medial free border mucosa is also trimmed so the two edges fit together without excessive tissue. The vermillion triangular flap should fit into the medial opening beneath the Cupid's bow *(Fig. 23.28)*. Careful attention to excise excessive mucosa and muscle accurately is important. The most common error is to leave too much muscle or mucosa on the free border. Incisions on the vermillion are closed with continuous 7–0 polyglactin suture. The lateral lip buccal mucosa is trimmed and closed with interrupted fine absorbable sutures. The upper edge of the buccal mucosa is sutured to the C-flap mucosa that bridges the alveolar gap. This gives a complete mucosal closure without tension.

Incisions on nasal floor

The other tip of the C-flap (the most lateral point of skin overlying the premaxilla) is brought laterally. No lateral horizontal skin incision for the lateral advancement flap is made initially, as now the surgeon can better visualize how to make appropriate incisions that will eliminate incisions around the ala. Incisions around the ala are avoided and seldom needed. If the alar base and the peak of the Cupid's bow on the cleft side are still high, an incision is made inside the cleft side nasal floor (the direction shown in *Fig. 23.29*, left). This incision can vertically lengthen the lip and level the alar base and Cupid's bow. If the alar base is already leveled after muscle reconstruction, a nasal floor incision is made in the direction shown in *Figure 23.29* (right). Every attempt is made to preserve the nasal sill. The nasal sill is unique tissue very difficult to reconstruct in secondary deformities and should be carefully preserved in primary repairs. The nostril width on the cleft side is slightly over-corrected (narrower than the

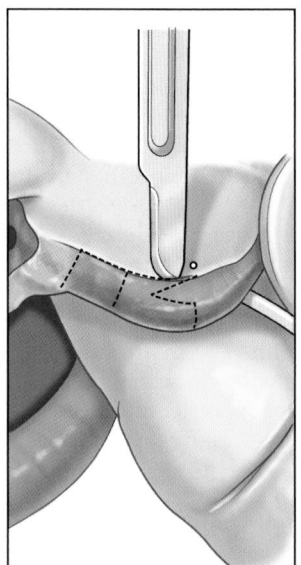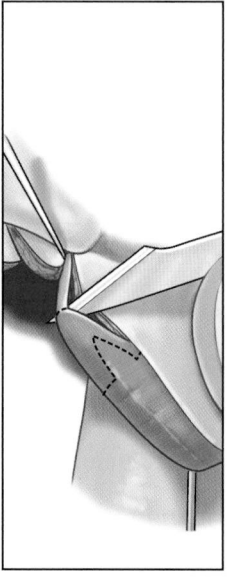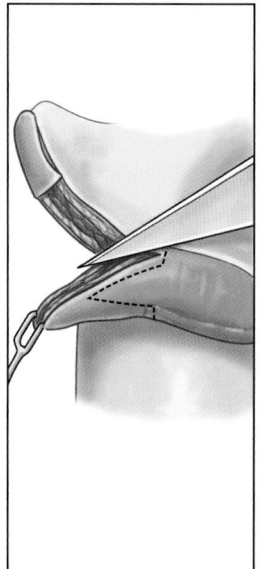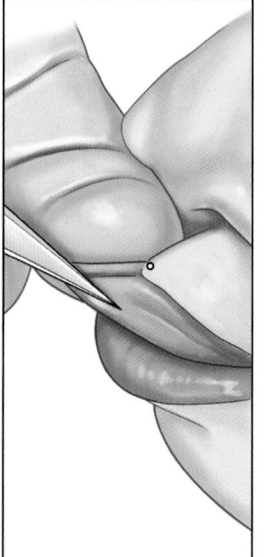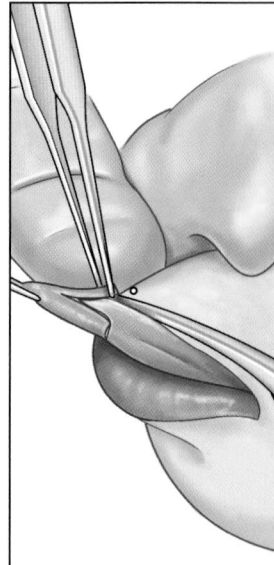

Fig. 23.27 The vermillion flap is marked and incised on the OM flap while the OM flap is held under tension. The width of the vermillion flap should correct the vermillion deficiency under the Cupid's bow. The tip of the vermillion flap should not cross the natural lip tubercle.

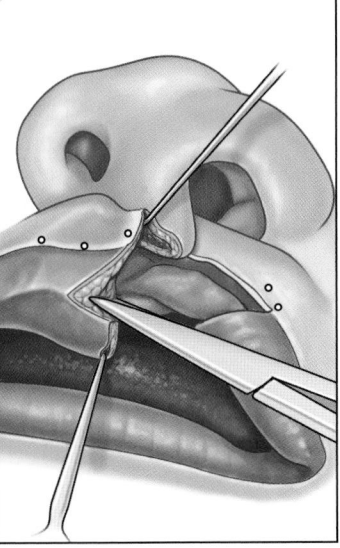
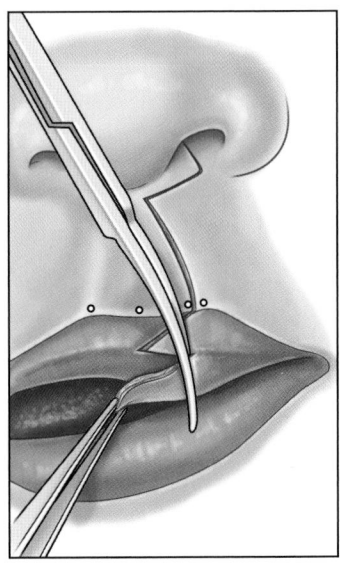
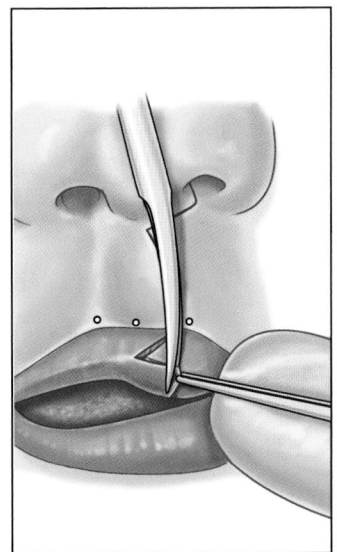
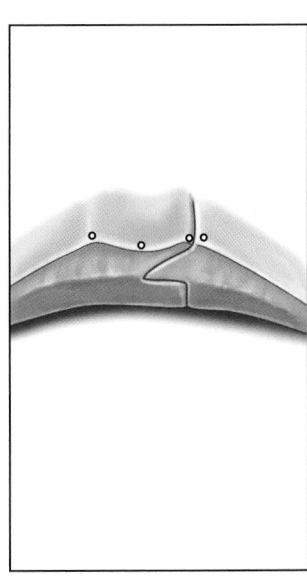

Fig. 23.28 Medially, the lip is opened on the red line beneath the Cupid's bow for insertion of the vermillion flap. The excessive tissue on both medial and lateral lips are carefully trimmed.

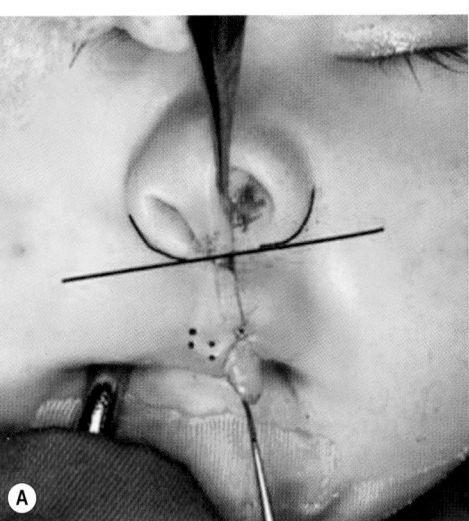
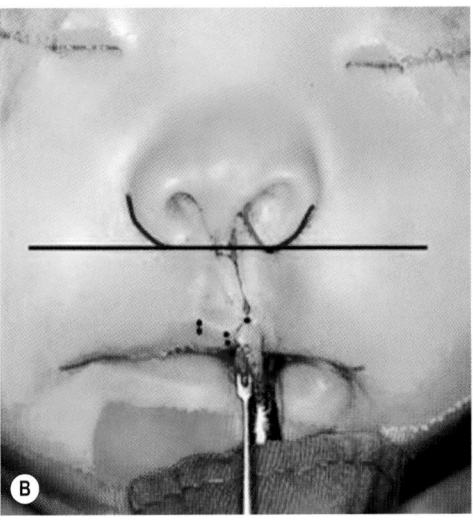

Fig. 23.29 (A) If the alar base and the peak of the Cupid's bow on the cleft side are still high, incision was made inside the cleft side nasal floor as the direction shown. This incision can vertically lengthen the lip and level the alar base and Cupid's bow. **(B)** If the alar base is already leveled after muscle reconstruction, incision is made as the direction shown to keep the alar base position.

noncleft side) as the authors' experience shows the cleft side nostril will widen with time after operation.

Final skin closure

The tip of the advancement flap is sutured to the most lateral point on the junction of the C-flap and the rotation flap. The suture line on the lateral part of the rotation flap thus mimics the philtral ridge. Excess skin on the nostril floor is excised as necessary with careful preservation of the nasal sill. The nasal floor is closed with 5–0 polyglactin sutures and lip skin is closed with 7–0 polyglactin sutures *(Fig. 23.30, left)*. The small triangular WSR flap on the lateral lip is directly approximated to the medial lip to reconstruct the bulging of the WSR. If the WSR on the medial lip is less prominent, a small horizontal incision can be made slightly above the point CPHL and the WSR flap from lateral lip can be inserted into medial lip for augmentation of the WSR above the CPHL.

Adequacy of rotation (small triangular flap)

It is important to make any necessary minor adjustments before finishing the operation. The cleft side Cupid's bow must be adequately rotated. If it is slightly elevated, a small hook is used to place the Cupid's bow under tension. A short transverse incision is made above the white skin roll to release the Cupid's bow into its proper position. An appropriately sized small triangular skin flap, 1–2 mm in width, is incised from the lateral lip and filled into the defect above the white skin roll. It is held with fine 7–0 polyglactin sutures *(Fig. 23.31)*. This small triangular skin flap is also helpful to improve the lip pout as it tightens the skin above the white skin roll.

Semi-open rhinoplasty

Previous long-term reports on primary nasal correction do not show any adverse effect on growth. Several techniques have

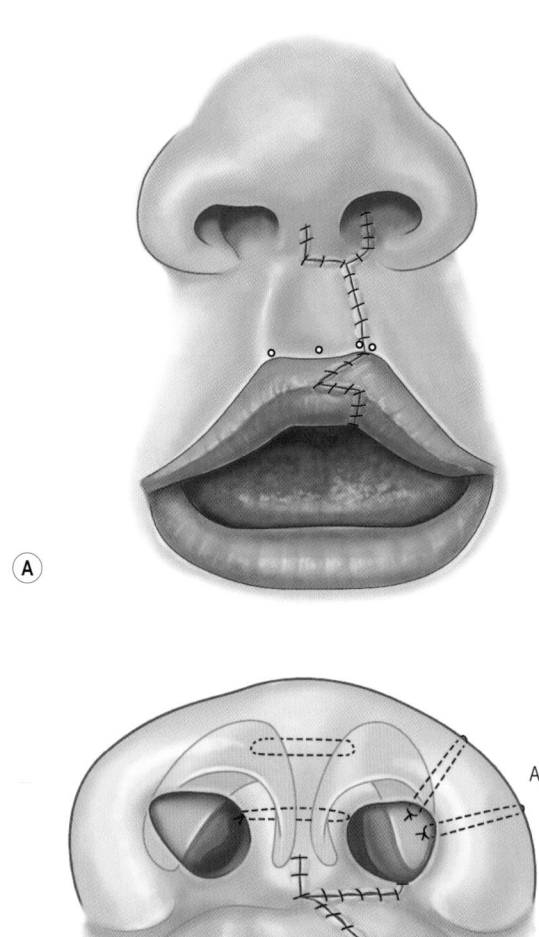

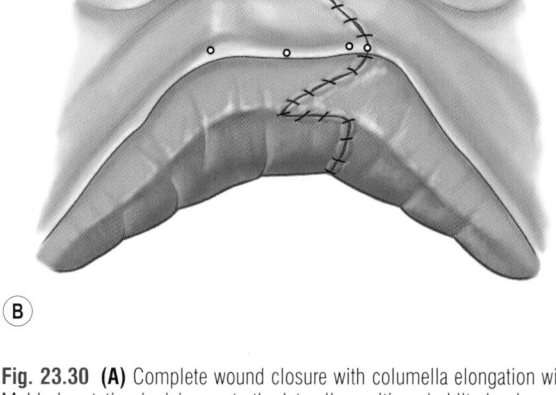

ATS

Fig. 23.30 (A) Complete wound closure with columella elongation with the Mohler's rotation incision; note the laterally positioned philtral column. **(B)** Alar transfixion sutures (ATS) of 5–0 absorbable monofilament are placed with traction on the LLC. One suture is placed in the vestibular skin. The remaining sutures catch the leading edge of the LLC, pass through the alar-facial groove and back near the rim of the ala, and are tied on the inner side. Notching of the skin disappears within 1–2 weeks.

been used in the Chang Gung Craniofacial Center for nasal reconstruction in unilateral clefts during the past 30 years.[34,35,37,84–86] The present technique is a semi-open rhinoplasty which, in the authors' experience, can achieve a clean and less traumatic dissection over the cartilaginous framework, better visualization, and better repositioning of the displaced cartilages. It can also preserve and even elongate the cleft side columella with careful tissue redistribution.

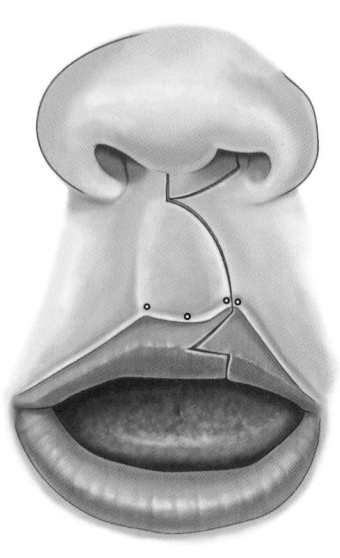

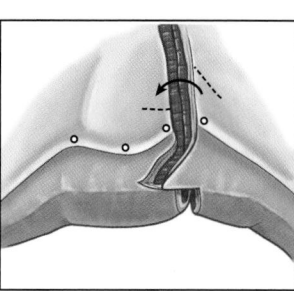

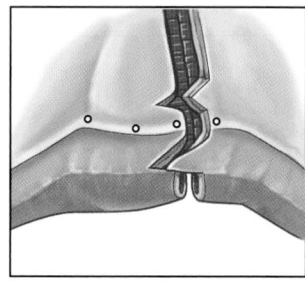

Fig. 23.31 The skin closure is depicted to show inadequate rotation and peaking of the Cupid's bow. A horizontal incision is made above CPHL on the cleft side of the Cupid's bow to rotate it down. An appropriately sized triangular flap from the lateral lip skin is inserted into this defect to correct the deformity.

Incision

A rim incision is marked on the noncleft side nostril and a reversed U incision[87] is marked on the cleft side. The reversed U incision is made about 1–2 mm higher than the alar rim on noncleft side *(Fig. 23.32A)*.

Release of fibrofatty tissue from LLCs

Incisions are made with No. 67 blade. The dissection is made above the LLCs with sharp scissors. The caudal edges of both LLCs are easily seen through these incisions, thus the dissection is less traumatic and avoids risk of iatrogenic injury to the cartilaginous framework *(Fig. 23.32B)*. The fibrofatty tissue on nasal tip is released from both LLCs *(Fig. 23.32B)*. The extent of dissection on the cleft side should be lateral to the groove on the caudal edge of the LLC to correct this groove.[88,89]

Repositioning of LLCs

The LLCs are approximated with 5–0 polydioxanone mattress sutures for medial rotation of the cleft side LLC *(Fig. 23.32C)*. The stitches are placed more laterally on the cleft side LLC for over-correction. Through-and-through sutures placed on the medial crura for further support to the LLCs *(Fig. 23.32C)*.

Trimming the excessive skin

After repositioning of the LLCs, there will always be some excessive skin on the upper part of the cleft side columella, below the reversed U incision. This excessive skin is responsible for the webbing of soft triangle in secondary cleft nasal deformities. This excessive skin is trimmed with a sharp scissor, and the wound is closed with 5–0 polyglactin sutures *(Fig. 23.32C)*.

Alar base position

The most important factor in achieving alar symmetry is releasing the abnormally attached paranasal muscles. In

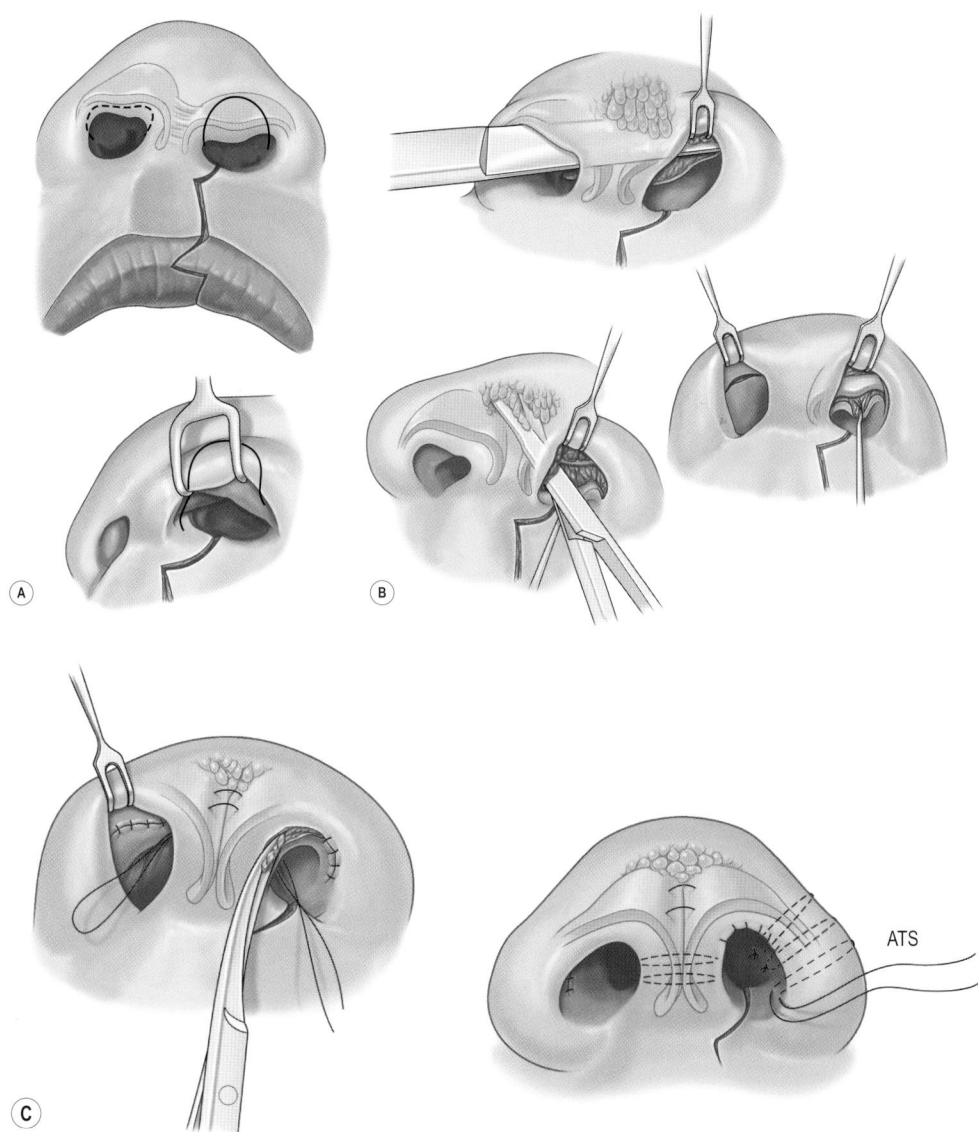

Fig. 23.32 **(A)** Semiopen rhinoplasty with a reversed U incision on the cleft side and a rim incision on the noncleft side. **(B)** Exposure of the caudal edge of the lower lateral cartilages (right upper). Release of the fibrofatty tissue from both LLCs with sharp dissection to avoid iatrogenic injury to the cartilages. The fibrofatty tissue should be completely released from the cartilages. **(C)** Careful trimming of the excessive skin after approximation of the LLCs (left). Additional sutures on medial crura and the alar transfixion sutures (ATS) (right).

reconstructing the nostril floor, the alar base is advanced farther to its proper width compared with the normal side. The alar-facial groove is further accentuated by the approximation of the lip musculature.

Creation of the alar-facial groove

Dissection between the skin and LLC releases the fibrous attachments between the skin and the LLC.[88] It also leaves a dead space under the skin. Mobilization of the alar base on cleft side will accentuate the vestibular webbing inside the cleft side nostril. Alar transfixion sutures help solve these problems and define the alar-facial groove. Two sutures are usually required. The lower suture is used to close the dead space and tack the vestibular webbing. The upper suture catches the leading edge of the LLC and helps to support the

LLC. Skin dimpling from the sutures disappears 2 weeks after surgery *(Fig. 23.32C, 23.30, right)*.

Examples of the results by the technique described are shown in *Figures 23.33–23.35*.

Adjustments at cheiloplasty

Making the necessary minor adjustments to achieve a satisfactory result is the enjoyment and challenge of cleft surgery. Every cleft is different and always needs minor adjustments.

Long vertical length of cleft side lip

A vertically long lateral lip is seldom encountered. It can be avoided by the septal anchoring suture used to suspend the lateral lip upward, and by trimming the excessive tissue on the nasal floor.

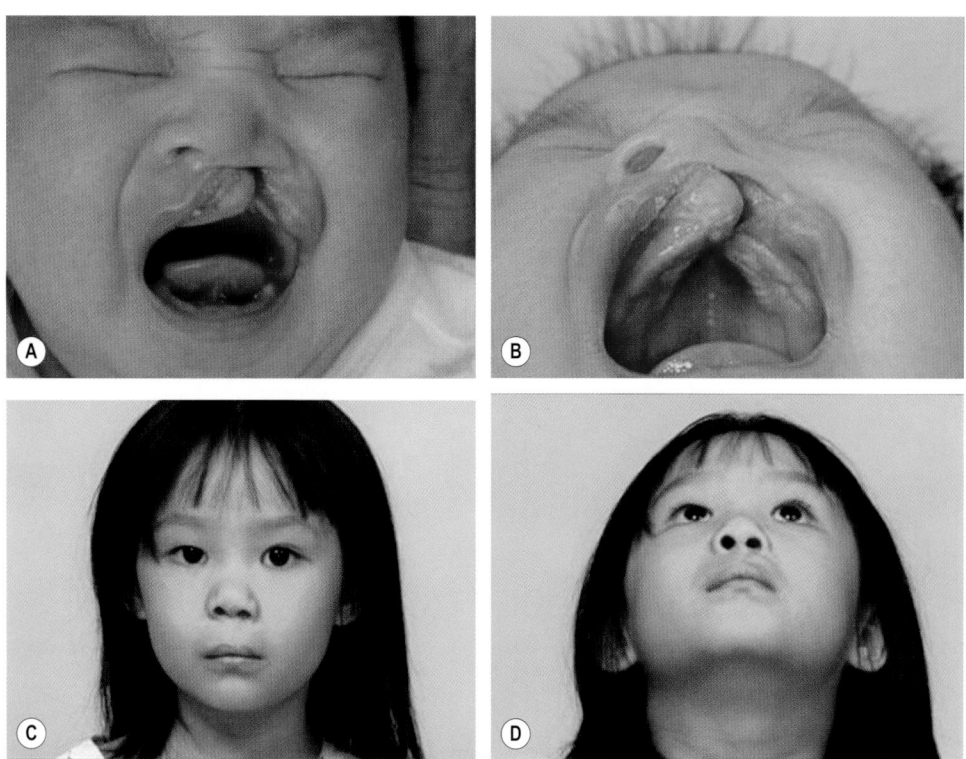

Fig. 23.33 (A,B) A 2-week-old girl with left complete cleft of primary palate (LPC, 11–15). **(C,D)** Postoperative views at the age of 6 years.

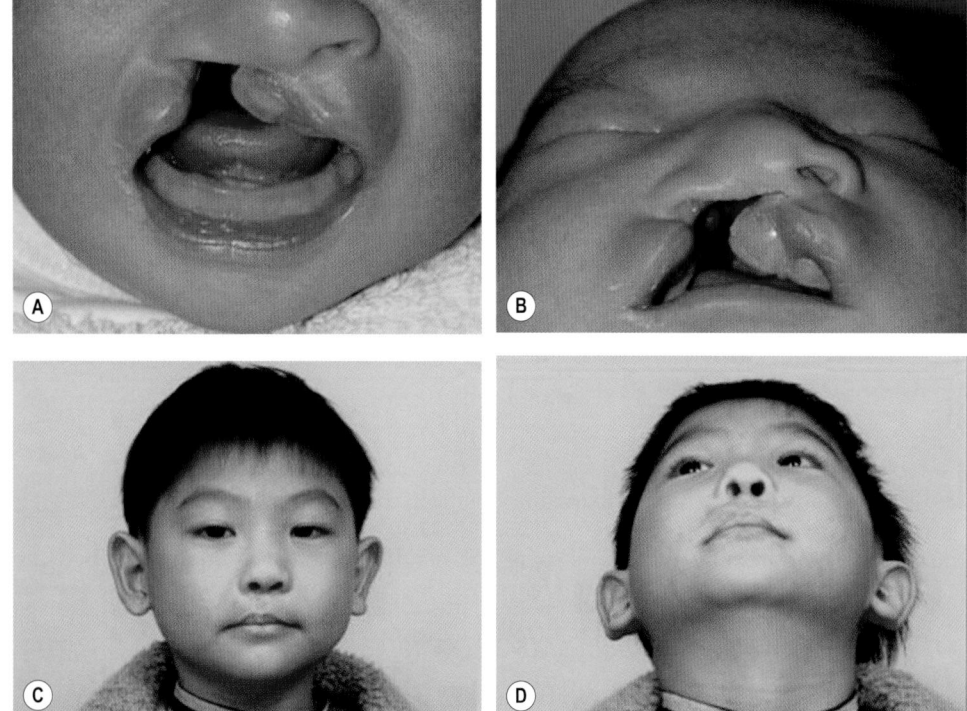

Fig. 23.34 (A,B) A 2-week-old boy with right complete cleft of primary and secondary palate (RPC, RSC, 1–9). **(C,D)** Postoperative views at the age of 5 years.

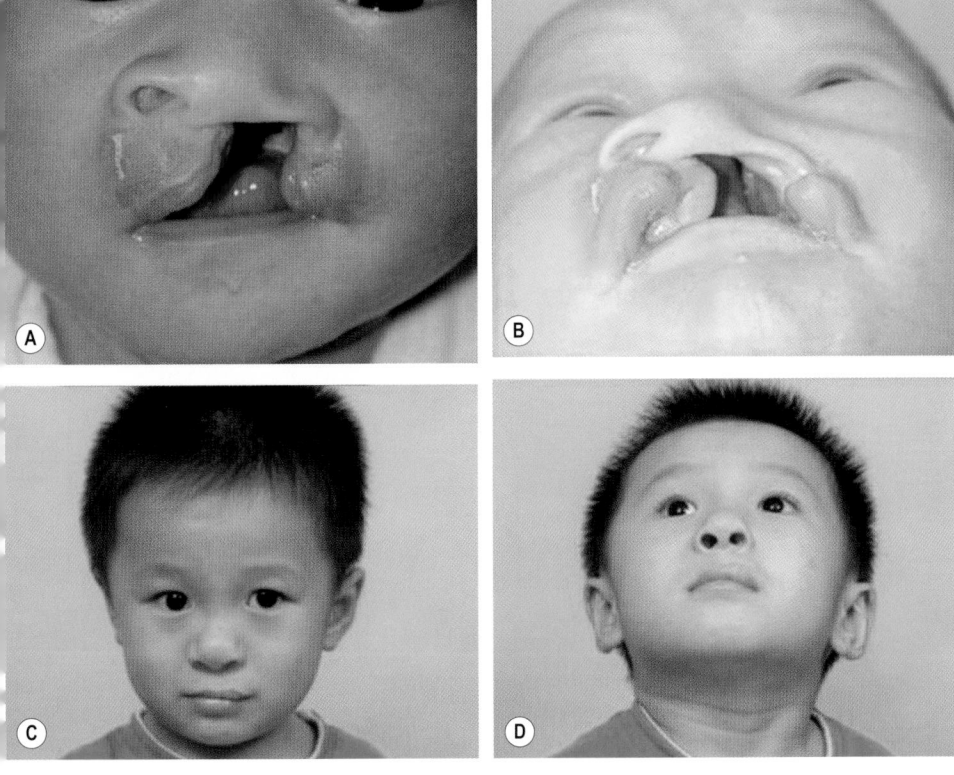

Fig. 23.35 (A,B) A 2-week-old boy with right complete cleft of primary and secondary palate (RPC, RSC, 1–9). **(C,D)** Postoperative views at the age of 4 years.

Short vertical length of cleft side lip

This is a common problem in most complete clefts. An adequate release and approximation of the orbicularis muscle will increase the vertical length by 3 to 4 mm. If the lip is still short, point CPHL' can be moved laterally 1 to 2 mm. Also, a small 1–2 mm triangular skin flap designed on the lateral lip can be inserted into the medial lip just above CPHL'. Last, a perialar incision can be made; however, this is done as a last resort.

Long horizontal length of cleft side lip

This is a relatively simple problem. Point CPHL' can be moved laterally as far as necessary to shorten the horizontal length.

Short horizontal length of cleft side lip

This problem is almost impossible to solve. After muscle dissection, release, and approximation, the horizontal length of the cleft-side lip will usually increase several millimeters. A horizontally short lip does not look bad compared with a vertically short lip with peaking of the Cupid's bow.

Long vertical height of noncleft side lip

Any vertical length over 12 mm on the noncleft side lip, e.g., on a 3-month old baby is excessively long and difficult to manage. To shorten this would entail excising a portion of a full-thickness segment of the lip, and that is seldom performed.

Free border of the lateral lip

If the lateral lip is too thin or deficient, the mucosa can be released, but this seldom corrects the problem. This is better corrected as a secondary procedure with use of temporoparietal fascia graft for lip augmentation.[90]

It is more often to see a bulging free border in incomplete clefts. The most accurate way to correct the excessiveness is to make incision along the red line, raise an inferiorly based mucosal flap with a thin layer of marginalis muscle, redrape the flap, and trim the excessive tissue *(Fig. 23.36)*.

Rotation advancement cheiloplasty for incomplete clefts

The incomplete cleft lip is sometimes surprisingly difficult to reconstruct. Also, the expectations for a good result are higher. It is a common mistake to underestimate the pathology and do less of a procedure in reconstruction. It is also a common mistake to have the impression that a vertically long lateral lip exists, and try to shorten the lip during the operation. Intraoperative measurements usually show the vertical height is similar between the two sides. The appearance of a vertically long lateral lip results from the downward displacement of the cleft side alar base. It is important to fully mobilize the alar base and reposition it cephalically, instead of vertically shortening the lateral lip.

Markings and incisions

The rotation incision and muscle dissection is made similar to complete clefts in a Mohler's fashion. The C-flap is raised similar to complete clefts. The incision on the advancement flap is made along the cleft edge. The WSR flap is also designed *(Fig. 23.37)*.

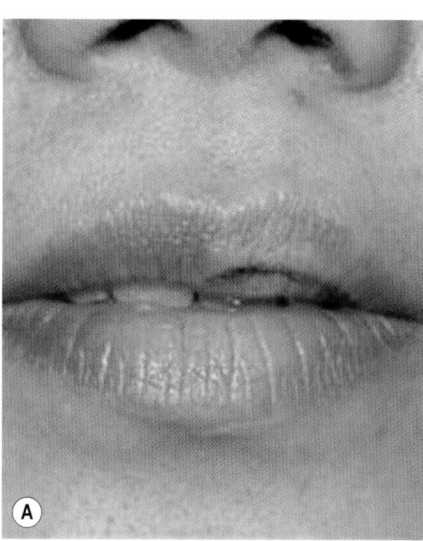
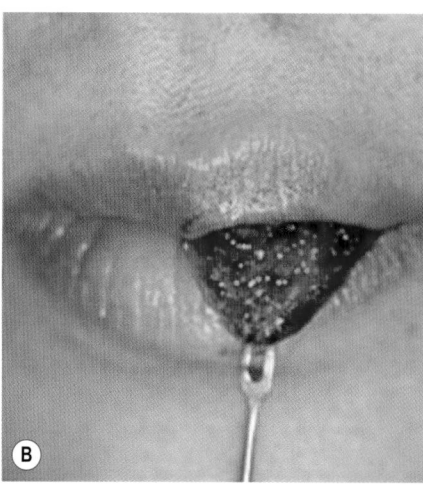
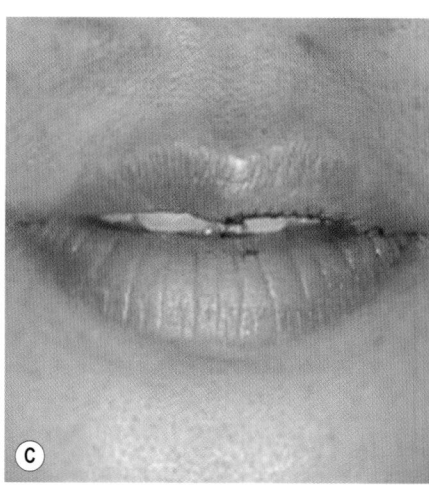

Fig. 23.36 The most accurate way to correct the excessiveness is to make incision along the extension of the red line from medial lip **(A)**, raising an inferiorly based mucosal flap with a thin layer of marginalis muscle **(B)**, re-draping the flap and trimming the excessive tissue **(C)**.

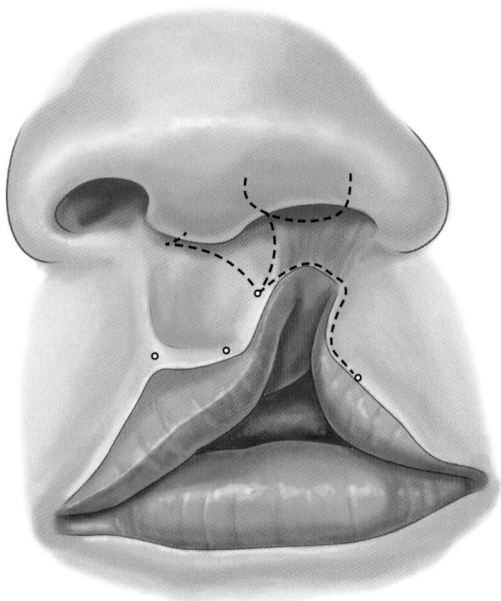

Fig. 23.37 Markings for incision lines in incomplete clefts with incision made along the free edge of the skin.

Nasal floor incision

A transverse incision is made inside the nasal floor at the junction of the skin and mucosa, leaving ample tissue on piriform area and premaxilla. A subperiosteal dissection is made from septum along the nasal floor to the piriform rim to raise the local tissue. The local flap will be used for correction of the nasal floor deficiency *(Fig. 23.38)*.

Dissection and release of muscle and elevation of OM flap

The technique and extent of muscle dissection is similar to complete clefts. Less muscle dissection tends to leave the abnormal muscle insertions to the alar base, which will cause the lateral and downward displacement of the alar base in secondary deformities. The OM flap is raised as in complete clefts.

Nasal floor reconstruction

The local tissue on the nasal septum and piriform area is turned over and sutured to each other, matching the height of the nasal floor on noncleft side nostril *(Fig. 23.39)*. The alar base is turned in, and the leading edge of the vestibular incision is sutured to the mucosa on the nasal floor as in complete clefts. Theoretically, placing Surgicel under the periosteum of the cleft side nasal floor could stimulate new bone formation, thus correcting the bony deficiency in this area. However, in a study performed by the authors, there was no benefit achieved in the overall aesthetic outcome.[91]

Muscle reconstruction

Muscle reconstruction is performed as in complete clefts, using an anchoring suture to the septum for centralizing Cupid's bow. Overlapping mattress muscle sutures are used to reconstruct the philtral column.

Nasal correction

Nasal correction is performed as in complete clefts with a rim incision on noncleft side nostril and reversed U incision on cleft side. The cartilage dissection, cartilage repositioning, alar transfixion sutures are the same. The cleft side nostril needs to be over-corrected (a taller and narrower nostril) as in complete clefts. An example of the result is shown in *Figure 23.40*.

Excessive free border

Although the "long lateral lip" is usually a false impression in incomplete clefts, it is not unusual to have some bulging on the free border of the cleft side lateral lip after leveling

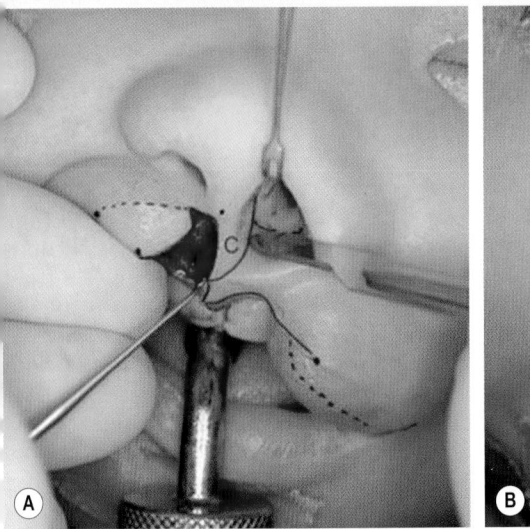
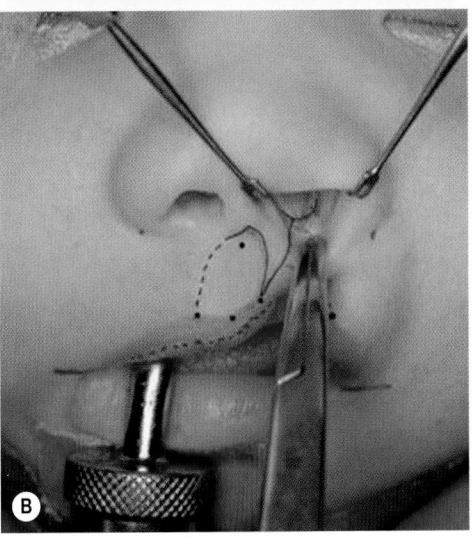

Fig. 23.38 The incision lines for C-flap and nasal floor: a transverse incision is made inside the nasal floor at the junction of skin and mucosa leaving ample tissue on piriform area and premaxilla.

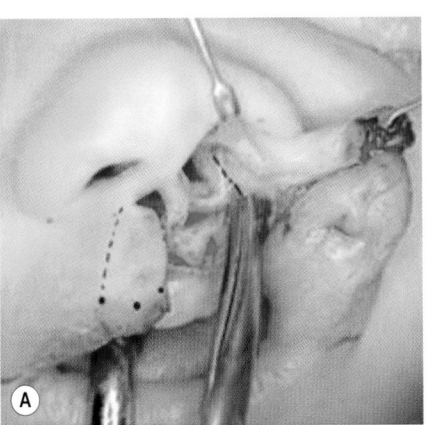
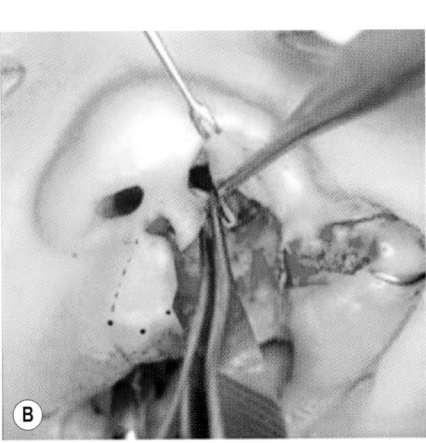
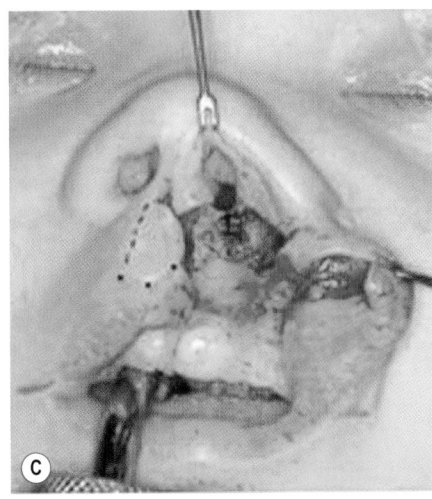

Fig. 23.39 The local tissue on nasal septum and piriform area (A) is turned over (B) and sutured with each other to match the height of the nasal floor on noncleft side nostril (C).

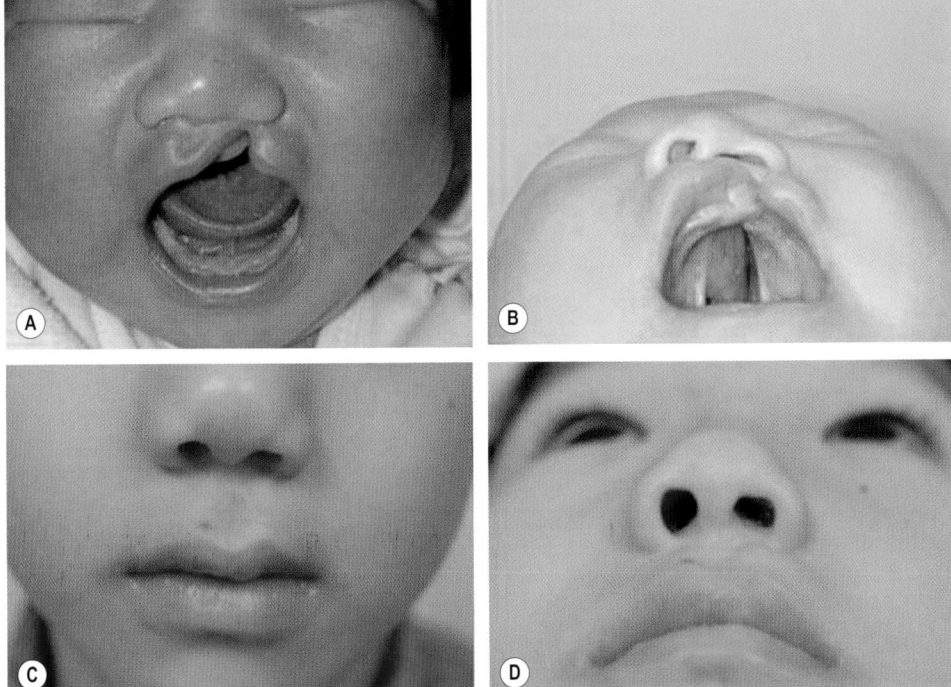

Fig. 23.40 (A,B) A 2-week-old boy with left incomplete cleft of primary and complete cleft of secondary palate (LPI, LSC, 12–19). (C,D) Postoperative views at the age of 7 years.

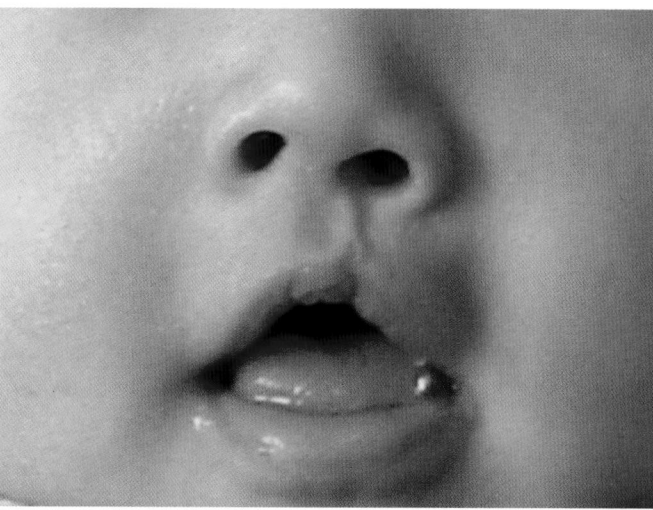

Fig. 23.41 A typical feature of a left occult cleft lip showing its characteristic pathologies.

Cupid's bow. If it is too prominent, the excessive free border can be trimmed using the technique shown in *Figure 23.36*.

Microform cleft lip

Pathology

The pathology presented in a microform cleft lip includes: nasal asymmetry, a philtral groove or striae parallel to the noncleft side philtral ridge, notching on free border of the lip, and disrupted white skin roll with high peaking of the Cupid's bow.[92] The orbicularis muscle ring is often disrupted or malaligned *(Fig. 23.41)*. Bony deficiency is often present as shown in *Figure 23.2*.

Discussion of different techniques

Surgical correction of microform cleft lip has received less attention in the literature because of its minor deformity. Efforts have been made to eliminate the external scar as with traditional rotation-advancement or straight-line closures. Cho[93] advocated orbicularis muscle interdigitation through an intraoral incision. Mulliken[92,94] suggested double uni-limb Z-plasties, muscle approximation and philtral ridge augmentation with a retro-auricular graft. The authors' preference is still a modified rotation advancement cheiloplasty similar to the technique used in incomplete cleft lips. It is felt that a rotation advancement cheiloplasty can better release the malaligned muscle, mobilize the displaced alar base, reconstruct the philtral column in both height and direction, and over-correct the cleft side nostril. It also allows for the excision of the groove or striae which is not parallel to the noncleft side philtral column. The repair almost always needs a triangular skin flap above the noncleft side Cupid's bow to correct the high peaking of the Cupid's bow. Although scaring is the major concern, scars are usually good if surgery is performed early (i.e., at 3 months) and parents follow instructions for postoperative scar care *(Fig. 23.42)*.

Postoperative care

Immediate postoperative care and monitoring is performed in the recovery room. The caregiver is allowed to enter the recovery room to hold the baby and is given instructions about maintaining the airway. A nurse specialist gives further instructions about the airway and subsequent care of the infant after return to ward. Instructions are given for clearing any mucus in the mouth or upper airway. A soft nipple with good flow is used with bottle-feeding. Feeding is started as soon as the baby desires. No arm restraints are used.

The wound is cleaned of any blood or mucus by a normal saline-soaked swab every 2–6 h. Antibiotic ointment is placed on the suture line after it is cleaned, keeping it from drying out or crusting. Normal saline sponges placed on the wound also seem to reduce pain and swelling. The infant and mother are discharged home the day after surgery and seen in the outpatient department in 5 days. At that time, skin sutures are removed under oral chloral hydrate sedation. The incision is treated with micropore tape and silicone sheeting *(Fig. 23.43)*. The patient is usually seen in another week and then periodically, to assure the parents are following the instructions. Massage of the lip scar is usually encouraged to hasten scar maturity.[37]

Postoperative maintenance of nasal shape

Postsurgical molding was first used in 1969 by Osada[95] and Skoog.[96] Friede[97] using an acrylic conformer, noted improvement in nasal contour. Matsuo[98,99] first reported presurgical molding in the unilateral incomplete cleft with a silicone conformer, and this was continued full time for 3 months postoperatively, and then at night for up to 12 months of age. The belief is that the deformed nasal cartilage is more easily molded while it is still plastic enough to be manipulated.

Subsequently, silicone nasal conformers have been used in many centers to support the LLC during the healing phase, and to prevent contracture and nasal stenosis.[35,37,100,101] Silicone nasal conformers have been used in the Chang Gung Center since the late 1980s.[102] The parents are instructed to use the conformers full-time for 6 months to 1 year if possible. The conformers need periodic adjustment to increase the height of the cleft side nostril, and maintain the nostril in an over-corrected position. The adjustments are made by adding silicone sheets (one millimeter in thickness) on top of the dome of the cleft side every 2–4 weeks *(Fig. 23.44)*. Success in nasal conformer use depends more upon the cooperation of the parents rather than the compliance of the patients.

Outcomes, prognosis and complications

Long-term results of lip morphology

A symmetrical balanced lip is the goal of cleft lip repair. A study was recently performed at the Chang Gung Craniofacial Center evaluating the long-term lip morphology in a group of 19 complete unilateral cleft lip patients operated on in 2002 with at least 4 years follow-up.[103] The surgical technique was

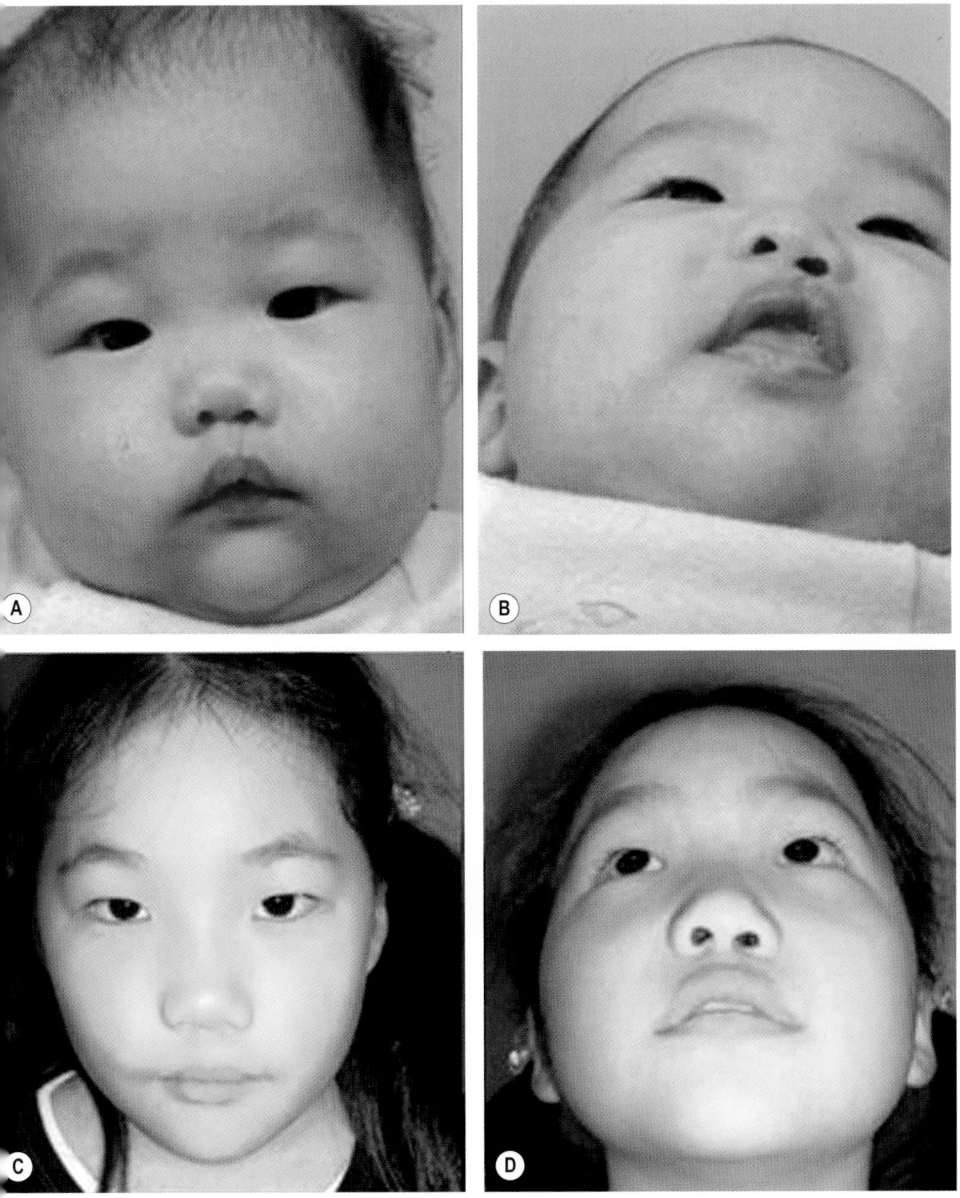

Fig. 23.42 (A,B) A 3-month-old girl with left occult cleft lip. **(C,D)** Postoperative views at the age of 7 years.

similar to the technique herein described, except for the septal anchoring muscle suture. There were statistically significant differences among the measurements in lip vertical height (VR, VL) and horizontal length (HR, HL), and in the measurements from the central columellar base to the points CPHR and CPHL, between initial intraoperative measurements and those at 3 months. However, the data at 4 years follow-up revealed that VR was significantly longer than VL; that HR was significantly longer than HL; and that the columella-CPHR was slightly shorter than columella-CPHL (however not significant). This demonstrated that Cupid's bow was deviated to the cleft side. Therefore, the authors now utilize a septal anchoring suture *(Fig. 23.45)*, to pull the cleft side lateral lip medially, thus helping to centralize the Cupid's bow.

Long-term result of nasal morphology

It is also important to know the outcomes of long-term nasal morphology following the integrated approach with

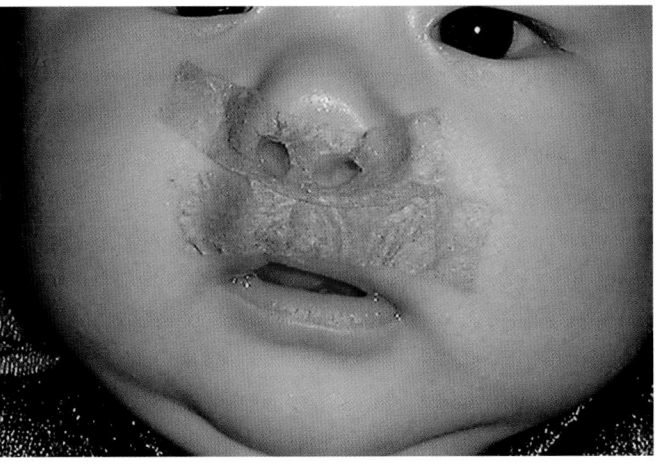

Fig. 23.43 Postoperative care with micropore tapes across the lip and silicone nasal conformer. The nasal conformer is held in nostril with tapes.

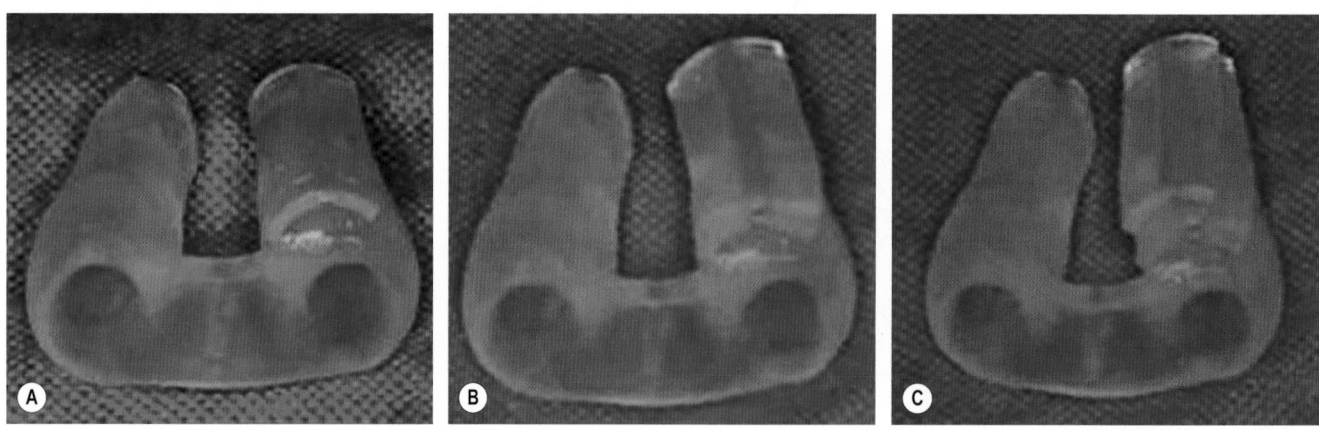

Fig. 23.44 The modification of the nasal conformer. Silicone sheets are added to the cleft side to increase the nostril height for maintenance of the nostril in over-corrected position.

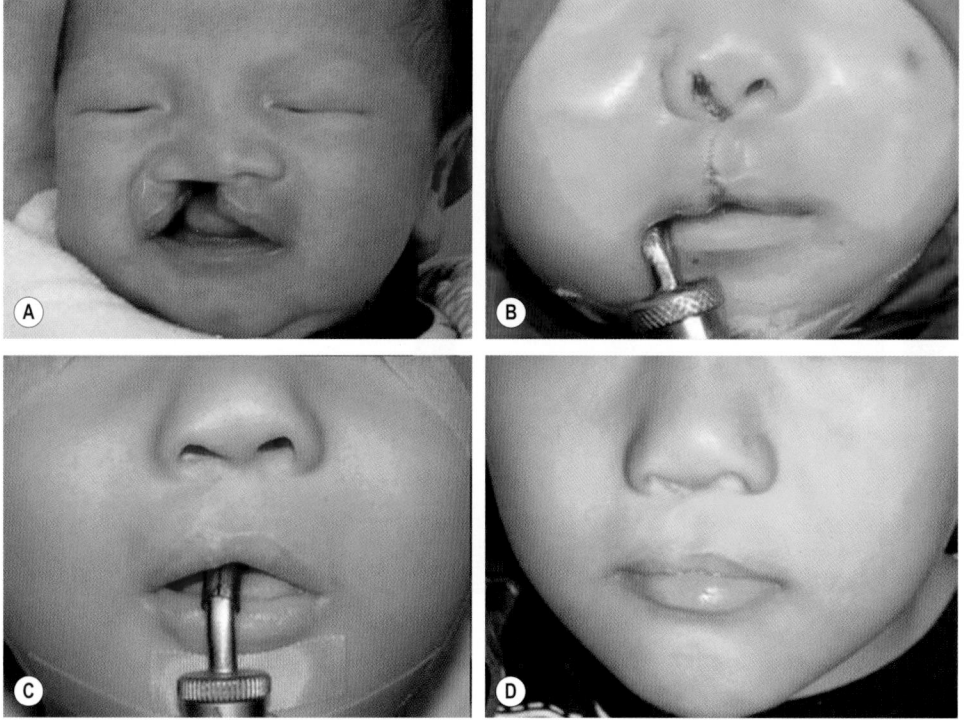

Fig. 23.45 Serial photographs of a boy with right complete cleft of primary and secondary palate. **(A)** 2 weeks old; **(B)** immediate after operation; **(C)** 1 year old before palate repair and **(D)** at the age of 5 years. The Cupid's bow though leveled, is deviated to the cleft side.

presurgical nasoalveolar molding, surgical refinement, and postsurgical maintenance. Two studies were conducted at the Chang Gung Craniofacial Center evaluating the long-term nasal morphology outcomes. The initial study evaluated nasal morphology in 25 patients operated on between 1997 and 1999. All patients underwent Liou's technique for nasoalveolar molding.[42] The surgical technique is similar to that described herein, except no cartilage dissection or repositioning was performed. Although the nasal shape was quite symmetrical immediately following surgery, at 3 years follow-up, there were significant differences among measurements of nostril height, columellar length and nostril width. The cleft side nostril height and columellar height were significantly

shorter than the noncleft side, and the cleft side nostril wa significantly wider *(Fig. 23.46)*. The recent study included group of patients who received the modified Grayson tech nique of nasoalveolar molding. The surgical techniqu included repositioning of the LLCs through bilateral rim inci sions. This study demonstrated better results when compare with the previous study; nonetheless, there was a simila trend in terms of relapse. Based on these observations, it is th authors' current practice to perform a reversed U incision o the cleft side, and to over-correct the cleft side nostril in it columellar height, nostril height and nostril width. As wel the cleft nostril needs to be maintained in the over-correcte position with postoperative modified silicone conformer use

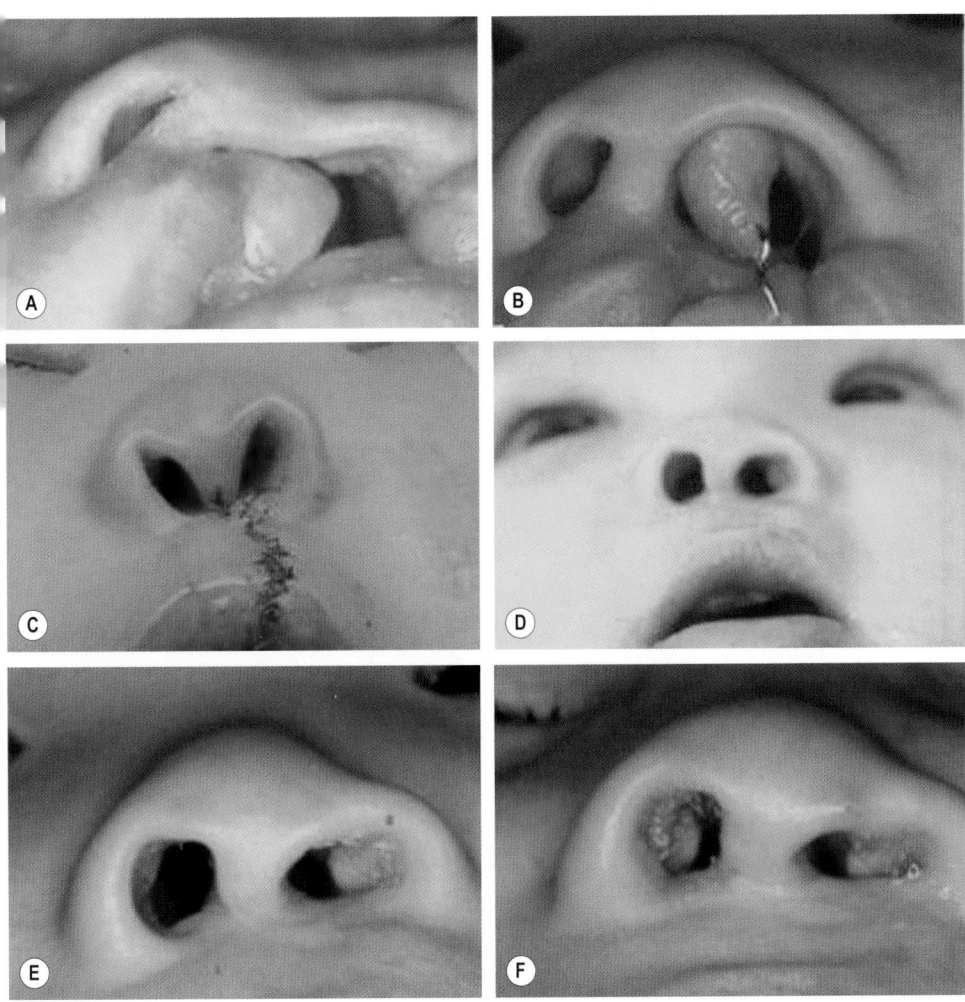

Fig. 23.46 Serial photographs of a girl with left complete cleft of primary and secondary palate. **(A)** 2 weeks old; **(B)** during nasoalveolar molding with Liou's method; **(C)** immediate after operation (without cartilage dissection and repositioning); **(D)** 1 year old before palate repair; **(E)** at the age of 1 year and half and **(F)** at the age of 3 years.

Satisfaction of patients

Patient and parental satisfaction is largely dependent upon psychosocial adaptation. A study performed in early 2000 at the Chang Gung Center evaluated the results in 77 patients receiving cleft lip repair in 1996. A total of 24% of patients required no revision of the nose or lip; 36% required a nasal correction; 10% a lip correction, and 28% required both a nasal and lip revision.[37] Approximately 60% of the patients requested lip or nose revision before school age. In recent years, with our integrated approach and improvement in outcomes, few patients now request revision before school age.

Complications

A total of 112 patients underwent unilateral cheiloplasty at the Chang Gung Craniofacial Center from January 2008 to November 2009. They were evaluated for postoperative complications. No instances of wound dehiscence were encountered. There was one minor separation of the nasal floor and two minor separations of the nasolabial junction that healed without problems. There were no wound infections except for five stitch abscesses (4.5%). Hypertrophic scarring was noted in 3% of the patients. There were no instances of postoperative bleeding.

Secondary procedures

Notching on Cupid's bow

It is not uncommon to have notching at the height of Cupid's bow on the cleft side. The similar appearance can have two different pathologies. The first scenario results from elevation of the point CPHL with correct position of the point CPHL' *(Fig. 23.47, left)*. Lowering CPHL can correct the deformity with a unilimb Z-plasty above the point CPHL. The white skin roll above CPHL should not be violated because of its unique nature.[104] The second scenario results from the downward displacement of CPHL' with CPHL in a correct position *(Fig. 23.47, right)*. A unilimb Z-plasty will result in an over-rotated Cupid's bow and should not be used. The technique to correct this deformity is described below.

Vertical discrepancy of the lateral lip

The vertically long lateral lip with CPHL' lower than CPHL is extremely difficult to correct and should be avoided in the primary cheiloplasty. It is corrected by complete opening of the lip, mobilizing the lateral lip, suspension of the lateral lip muscle to the nasal septum, and horizontal full thickness

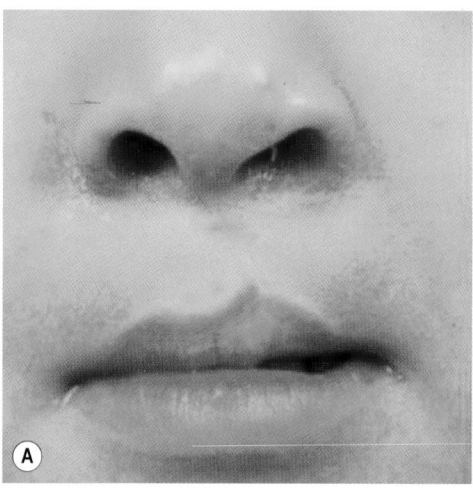
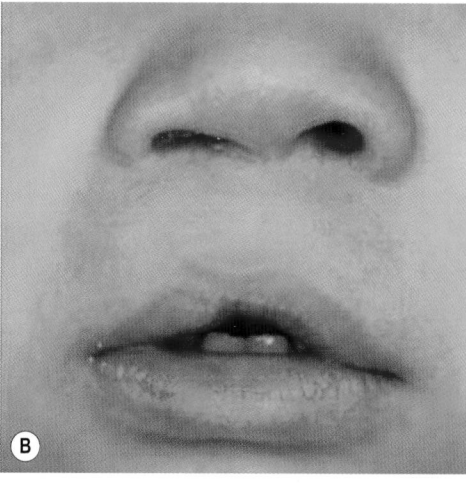

Fig. 23.47 Notching on Cupid's bow with different pathology: **(A)** the CPHL is elevated with CPHL' at good position. **(B)** CPHL at good position with CPHL' lower than its normal position.

shortening of the lip (skin, muscle, and mucosa). Over-rotation of the Cupid's bow is corrected in a similar fashion. The amount of nasal floor tissue that must be excised is usually beyond one's expectation. To elevate an over-rotated Cupid's bow of 1 mm usually requires more than 5 mm of tissue on nasal floor excision.

Secondary correction of a vertically short lateral lip, as measured from point SBAL and CPHL', also requires a complete opening of the lip. Greater rotation and advancement of the perialar skin and muscle from the cheek region to a position beneath the ala, is required for vertical lengthening of the lip.

Horizontal shortness of the lateral lip

Horizontal shortness of the lateral lip results from preoperative hypoplasia of the lip and in some instances, precludes a less optimal result. This pre-existing deformity is impossible to correct, and it is important to note at the time of surgery so the postoperative result can be thus evaluated.[105] The only possible solution is an Abbe flap, and this is rarely used.

Vermillion and free border problems

The free border of the lip consists of orbicularis marginalis muscle, which is covered with vermillion and mucosa.[85] Failure to reconstruct the vermillion adequately by a straight-line closure of the free border of the lip results in a characteristic deformity. The vermillion is deficient beneath the cleft side of Cupid's bow, and the red line is interrupted with a step-off appearance instead of the normal paralleling red line and white skin roll *(Fig. 23.48)*. Deformities of the free border of the lip are usually described as vermillion deformities in the literature without regard to whether the deformity consists of a vermillion deficiency, muscle separation, or excess or tight mucosa *(Fig. 23.49)*. With use of the triangular vermillion flap from the lateral lip, vermillion deficiencies are rare and seldom need correction.[34] Free border deformities that occur, despite placement of the vermillion flap, are usually not secondary to vermillion deficiency but due to muscle or mucosa problems.

A true vermillion deficiency is corrected by using the technique as described in primary repairs if the lateral lip is still

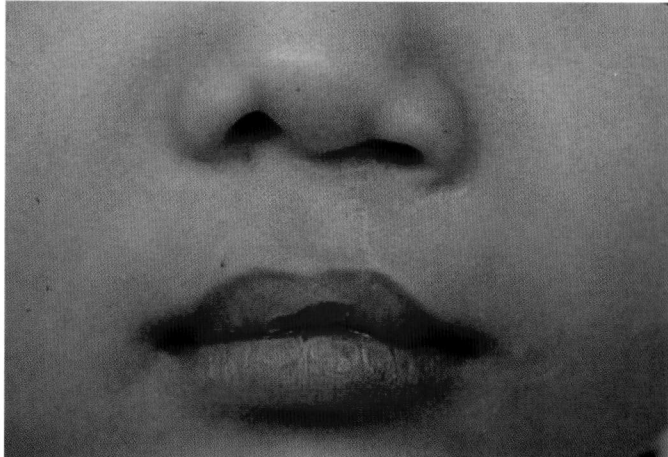

Fig. 23.48 Free border of the lip deformity with only vermillion deficiency; note the dry mucosa.

long enough. The point CPHL' is moved laterally according to the length of the deficient area. The vermillion medial to the new point CPHL' is designed as a triangular vermillion flap. It is advanced to replace the exposed mucosa under the point CPHL.

If the free border of the lip is thin without adequate orbicularis marginalis muscle, it can be augmented with temporoparietal fascia.[85] Any mucosal deficiency should be corrected at the same time with a local Z-plasty, VY-plasty or transposition flaps. Any excess mucosa or muscle can be accurately trimmed with the horizontal red line incision technique described above.

Wide nostril

It is the authors' current practice to over-correct the cleft side nostril *(Fig. 23.45)*. If the nostril is too narrow postoperatively, it can be improved by splinting with a silicone conformer. A wide nostril is corrected secondarily by a V-Y advancement of the alar base, fixing it to the nasal septum with a retention suture.

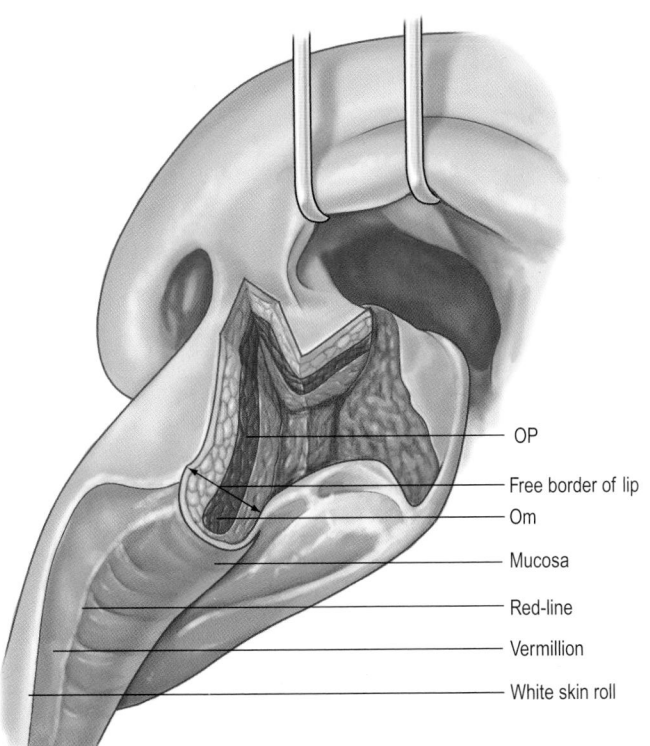

Fig. 23.49 The free border of the lip after incision. Note the orbicularis marginalis muscle covered by vermillion and mucosa and bordered by the white skin roll. The vermillion is deficient beneath the cleft-side Cupid's bow. Om, orbicularis marginalis muscle; OP, orbicularis peripheralis muscle.

OP
Free border of lip
Om
Mucosa
Red-line
Vermillion
White skin roll

Nostril hood at soft triangle

The hooding effect in the soft triangle of the cleft nostril is corrected by the reversed U incision, proper repositioning of the LLC, and careful trimming of any excessive skin in this area. The modified postoperative silicone conformer can maintain the nostril in its over-corrected position, and this helps to improve the deformity. As a secondary procedure, simple excision of the webbing usually is ineffective to correct the deformity. To adequately address the deformity, an open rhinoplasty with reversed U incision on the cleft side is necessary for adequate correction.

Inadequate correction of the LLC

At this time, it is impossible to obtain a satisfactory appearance of the nostril in all instances. This is likely due to cartilage deficiencies, fibrofatty tissue between the medial crura, and weakness of the alar cartilages. At the primary procedure, fibrofatty tissue should be dissected free from the cartilage and the LLCs approximated to each other with some over-correction. If the alar cartilage slumps after the initial surgery, it can be corrected with an open rhinoplasty and an additional cartilage graft at any age after 5 years.

Flared ala-facial groove

The flaring out of the alar base gives the nose an unattractive appearance. This is prevented at the time of surgery by

making sure that the alar base is medially advanced far enough. Also, adequate release of the abnormally inserted muscles around the alar base prevents the continuous pulling force causing the downward and lateral displacement of the alar base. Secondary correction of this deformity is much more difficult than correction of a wide nostril. It necessitates re-opening the lip, releasing the para-alar muscles adequately, rotating the ala inward, and a V-Y closure of the nostril floor. A retention suture placed between the nasal septum and alar base helps to maintain the new alar base position.

Vestibular webbing

Release of the alar base from the maxilla and rotating the ala medially will make the vestibular webbing inside the cleft side nostril more prominent. This can be corrected by alar transfixion sutures placed to tack the webbing. However, occasionally the webbing tends to recur postoperatively. Trimming of the webbing at initial surgery has been described and may give a better result compared to alar transfixion sutures. However, this excessive tissue might be useful to solve the lining deficiency in secondary rhinoplasty; and, in authors' opinion, should be preserved till secondary rhinoplasty.

Infrasill depression

A depression along the upper limb of the advancement flap can occur. This is rare with the technique described as it can be prevented by avoiding inappropriate excision of dermis on the free edge of the advancement flap. Good muscle approximation is also imperative. If correction is needed, it can be done by adequate muscle approximation, insertion of a dermal graft, or fat injection.

Secondary rhinoplasty

Correction of the nasal deformity in cleft lip patients is a challenging problem to every surgeon. The deformity is notorious for its resistance to surgical correction, because it involves all components of the nose: coverage, support, and lining. It is difficult to correct all these problems in a single operation.

In considering secondary nasal correction, a balanced skeletal base is the key factor for achieving a satisfactory result. Whenever possible, the hypoplastic maxilla with an asymmetric base for the nose must be corrected before a rhinoplasty is performed. This requires a combined evaluation and discussion between the orthodontist and the surgeon.

Alveolar bone grafting corrects the bony asymmetry between the alar bases. This surgery is done around the time of eruption of the permanent central incisor or canine tooth. In some instances, patients will refuse orthognathic surgery even in the presence of significant maxillary hypoplasia; in these situations, a corrective rhinoplasty still should be considered to improve facial features and the psychological impact.

An open tip rhinoplasty is used to correct the nasal deformity in most patients.[1] The procedure can provide undistorted exposure to the cartilaginous and bony framework. The pathologic deformities are addressed in a systematic approach and precise fashion by a combination of several rhinoplasty techniques. The following points are important to achieve a good correction:

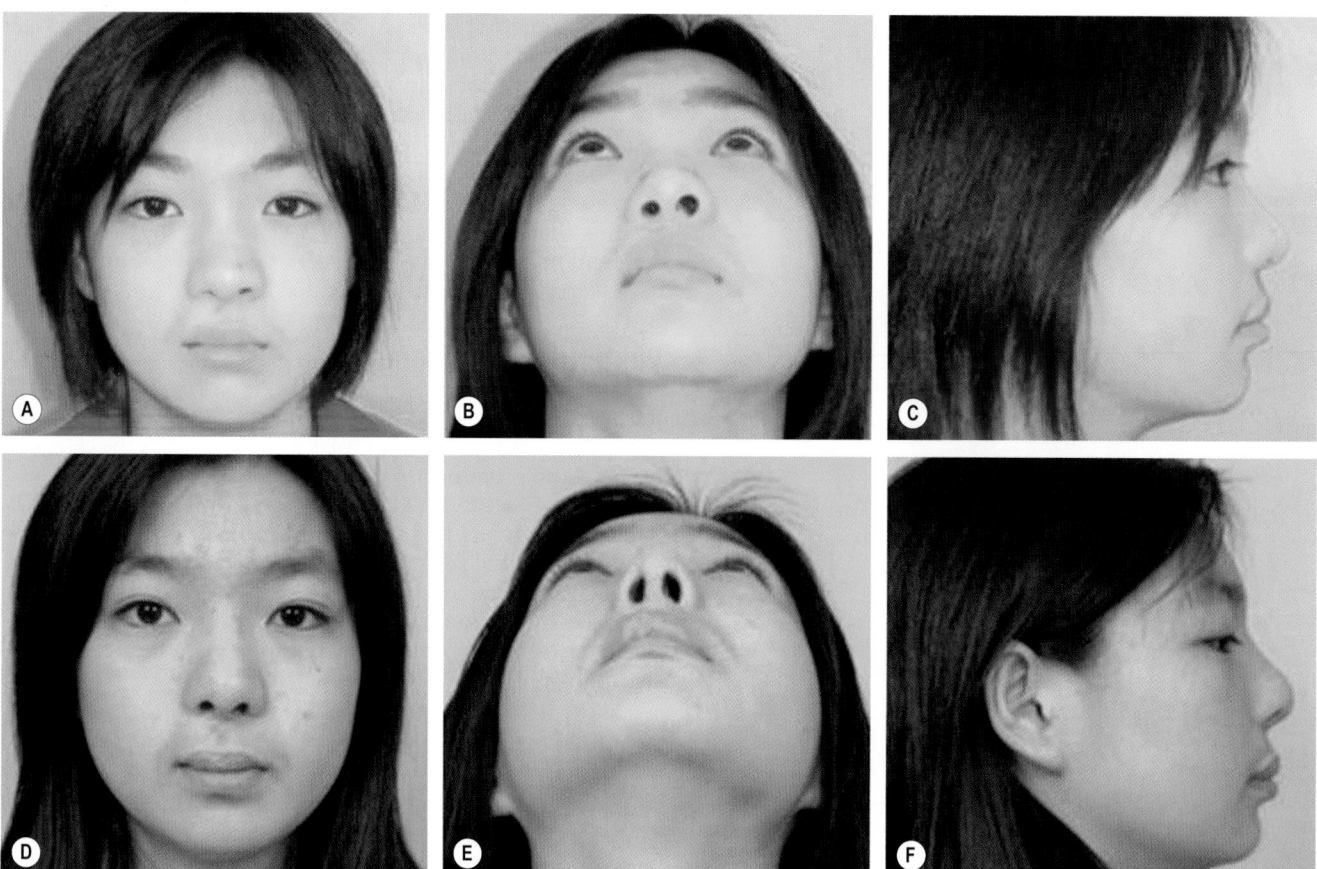

Fig. 23.50 An 18-year-old girl with right secondary cleft lip deformity. **(A)** The front, **(B)** worm's-eye view and **(C)** lateral views, before the revision. **(D,E,F)** same views after revision. The revision procedure included lip scar revision and philtral column augmentation. The nasal revision was an open rhinoplasty with insertion of a columellar strut, right alar rim cartilage graft and dorsal augmentation with diced cartilage graft.

- Symmetric dissection of covering skin
- Adequate release of any deficient mucosal lining with various techniques, including a Potter VY-plasty of the LLC, vestibular triangular flap, or an inferior turbinate flap
- Adequate mobilization of the deformed LLC with release of the interdomal ligaments, longitudinal fibers between the LLC and ULC, and lateral attachment to the piriform rim
- Use of a strong cartilaginous columellar strut
- Splinting the depressed alar rim with cartilage graft
- Correction of columellar deficiency and careful reshaping of the nostril hood
- Alar transfixion sutures
- Septal plasty when indicated.

At present, a satisfactory result is obtained in almost all cases *(Fig. 23.50)*.

Summary

The treatment of patients with cleft lip/palate continues to evolve, and it is hoped with better results in all areas:

functional, aesthetic, and psychological-spiritual. Current general concepts include the belief that passive movement of the maxillary arches is more physiologic than a rapid forced movement. Early presurgical nasoalveolar molding is a useful addition to the treatment of the cleft infant, achieving the benefits of close approximation of the maxillary segments, morphology easier for the surgeon to repair, and molding the nasal cartilages to better symmetry. However, the long-term outcomes of nasal molding are still lacking. The long-term effects of primary nasal cartilage surgery are positive; and, on this basis, the addition of nasal molding should not be detrimental. Not all caregivers may be unable to comply with such modern protocols because of a lack of personal resources, or the unavailable services such as in some developing countries. At the Chang Gung Craniofacial Center, protocol choices are provided to parents with explanations of the cost and time involved, making them a part of the decision process. Despite current protocols, no surgeon can always obtain satisfactory results; and, this likely is because of inherent growth problems, great variability of tissue deficiency, and the degree of parent and patient compliance.

29. Noordhoff MS, Huang CS, Wu J. Multidisciplinary management of cleft lip and palate in Taiwan. In: Bardach J, Morris HL, eds. *Multidisciplinary Management of Cleft Lip and Palate*. Philadelphia: WB Saunders; 1990:18–26.

33. Millard Jr DR, ed. The unilateral deformity. Cleft Craft: The Evolution of Its Surgery. Vol I. Boston: Little, Brown; 1976.

37. Noordhoff MS, Chen PKT. Unilateral cheiloplasty. In: Mathes ST, ed. Plastic Surgery. Vol 4. Philadelphia: WB Saunders; 2006.

39. Mohler L. Unilateral cleft lip repair. *Plast Reconstr Surg.* 1995;2:193–199.

This paper introduced a modification of the original rotation-advancement technique by changing the direction of the rotation incision to the "mirror-image of the noncleft side philtral column" that resulted in a more natural looking lip.

42. Liou EJ, Subramanian M, Chen PKT, et al. The progressive changes of nasal symmetry and growth after nasoalveolar molding: a three-year follow-up study. *Plast Reconstr Surg.* 2004;114(4):858–864.

This paper revealed that in patients with unilateral complete cleft lips, the nasal asymmetry was significantly improved after nasoalveolar molding and was further improved after primary cheiloplasty. However, after surgery, the nasal asymmetry significantly relapsed in the first year postoperatively and then remained stable and well afterward. The authors recommend (1) narrowing down the alveolar cleft as well as possible by nasoalveolar molding; (2) overcorrecting the nasal vertical dimension surgically; and (3) maintaining the surgical results using a nasal conformer.

44. Grayson BH, Garfinkle JS. Nasoalveolar molding and columellar elongation in preparation for primary repair of unilateral and bilateral cleft lip and palate. In: Losee JE, ed. *Comprehensive Cleft Care*. New York: McGraw Hill; 2009:701–720.

57. Barillas I, Dec W, Warren SM, et al. Nasoalveolar molding improves long-term nasal symmetry in complete unilateral cleft lip-cleft palate patients. *Plast Reconstr Surg.* 2009;123(3):1002–1006.

This paper demonstrated that the lower lateral and septal cartilages are more symmetric in patients with nasoalveolar molding compared with the surgery-alone patients. Furthermore, the improved symmetry can be maintained at 9 years of age.

62. Mulliken JB, Martinez-Perez D. The principle of rotation advancement for repair of unilateral complete cleft lip and nasal deformity: technical variations and analysis of results. *Plast Reconstr Surg.* 1999;104:1247–1260.

86. Salyer KE, Genecov E, Genecov D. Unilateral cleft lip-nose repair: A 33-year experience. *J Craniofac Surg.* 2003;14(4):549–558.

A 33-year experience in over 750 patients with a proven method of repair for primary unilateral cleft lip-nose is presented in this paper. Approximately 35% of them needed a minor revision in preschool age and most of them received an aesthetic rhinoplasty after growth was completed. This long term experience showed that with primary nasal reconstruction, self-esteem was enhanced in cleft patients.

102. Yeow VK, Chen PKT, Chen YR, et al. The use of nasal splints in the primary management of unilateral cleft nasal deformity. *Plast Reconstr Surg.* 1999;103(5):1347–1354.

This paper shows that postoperative nasal splinting in the primary management of the unilateral cleft nasal deformity serves to preserve and maintain the corrected position of the nose after primary lip and nasal correction, resulting in a significantly improved aesthetic result. The authors recommend that all patients undergoing primary correction of complete unilateral cleft deformity use the nasal retainer postoperatively for a period of at least 6 months.

24

Repair of bilateral cleft lip

John B. Mulliken

SYNOPSIS

- A child born with bilateral cleft lip should not have to suffer because of an ill-conceived and poorly executed primary repair. The operative principles for synchronous nasolabial repair are established:
  - Maintain symmetry
  - Secure primary muscular continuity
  - Design proper philtral size and shape
  - Construct median tubercle from lateral labial elements
  - Position/secure lower lateral cartilages and sculpt nasal tip and columella.

- The techniques based on these principles are within the repertoire of a well-trained surgeon whose practice is focused on children with cleft lip. Only the philtral columns and dimple seem just beyond the surgeon's craft.

- Preoperative dentofacial orthopedic manipulation of the premaxilla is necessary to permit synchronous closure of the primary palate. The surgeon must repair the bilateral cleft lip and correct the nasal deformity in three-dimensions based on knowledge of anticipated changes in the fourth-dimension. Modifications of the techniques used in repair of the most common complete form are needed for the less common bilateral variants, such as, binderoid, complete with intact secondary palate, symmetrical incomplete, and asymmetrical complete/incomplete.

- Outcomes can be assessed using preoperative and serial photography and documentation of revision-rates. Direct anthropometry is the "gold-standard" for quantification of the changing nasolabial features; however, it requires training and experience. Intraoperative anthropometry is used to record baseline dimensions and repeated as the child grows. Two-dimensional photogrammetry is applicable for certain linear and angular measurements if properly scaled. Computerized three-dimensional photogrammetry is a new methodology for quantifying nasolabial appearance. It is both accurate and reliable, and someday could be employed in intra- and inter-institutional comparative studies.

 Access the Historical Perspective section online at
http://www.expertconsult.com

Introduction

James Barrett Brown and his colleagues wrote that a bilateral cleft lip is twice as difficult to repair as a unilateral cleft and the results are only half as good.[1] Now, over one-half century later, many surgeons still seem resigned that the appearance of their patients after bilateral cleft lip repair cannot match those with repaired unilateral cleft lip. Too many infants born with bilateral cleft lip undergo old-fashioned, often multi-staged, procedures, and later have to endure sundry revisions throughout childhood and adolescence. Despite the surgeon's efforts, the stigmata of the repaired bilateral cleft lip and nose remain painfully obvious – even at a distance.

To the contrary, I have written that the appearance of a child with repaired bilateral cleft lip should be comparable to, and in many instances surpass, that of a repaired unilateral complete cleft lip.[2] This optimistic statement is based on two major advances in management of bilateral cleft lip over the past quarter century. First, is the recognition of the need for preoperative manipulation of the protuberant premaxilla. Second, is the acceptance of the principles and techniques of bilateral labial repair and especially the importance of synchronous correction of the nasal deformity.

Principles

Surgical principles, once established, usually endure, whereas surgical techniques continue to evolve. The following principles for repair of bilateral cleft lip were induced based on study of the literature and observations of residual deformities:[3]

1. *Maintain nasolabial symmetry*. Even the slightest differences between the two sides of the lip and nose will become more obvious with growth. Symmetry is the one

advantage a bilateral cleft lip has over its unilateral counterpart.

2. *Secure muscular continuity.* Construction of a complete oral ring permits normal labial function, eliminates the lateral bulges, and minimizes later distortion of the philtrum and interalar widening.

3. *Design the philtral flap of proper size and shape.* The philtrum rapidly elongates and widens, particularly at the columellar-labial junction.

4. *Construct the median tubercle using lateral* vermilion-mucosal elements. There is no white roll in the prolabium. Retained vermilion lacks normal coloration and fails to grow to full height.

5. *Position the slumped/splayed lower lateral cartilages and sculpt excess soft tissue in nasal tip and columella.* These maneuvers are necessary to establish normal nasal projection and columellar length/width.

Principles 1–4 needed definition, interpretation, and confirmation. Principle 5, primary correction of the nasal deformity, was a fundamental change in surgical strategy. The so-called "absent columella" is an illusion; nearby labial tissue need not be recruited to build it. "The columella is in the nose" became this surgeon's shibboleth. The columella can be exposed by anatomic positioning and fixation of the lower lateral cartilages and sculpting expanded skin in the soft triangles and upper columella.[4]

Third and fourth dimensions

Analogous to a sculptor working in marble, the surgeon must construct three-dimensional nasolabial features in flesh. Furthermore, unlike sculpture in stone, the repaired bilateral lip and nasal deformity changes with time – there will be normal growth, as well as abnormal alterations of the features. The nasolabial stigmata are attributable to the three-dimensional primary repair and the subsequent fourth-dimensional distortions.

Farkas and colleagues used direct anthropometry to document the normal patterns of nasolabial growth in Caucasians from age 1–18 years.[5] Fast-growing nasolabial features attain more than 75% of adult dimensions by age 5 years. For example, nasal height and width develop early, reaching a mean of 77% and 87% of adult size, respectively, by age 5 years. All labial landmarks grow rapidly, reaching approximately 90% of adult proportions by age 5 years. In contrast, tip protrusion and columellar length are slow-growing features; they attain a mean of only two-thirds of adult size by 5 years of age. These differences in nasolabial growth explain the well-recognized nasal stigmata and labial misproportions of a repaired bilateral cleft lip. The fast-growing features become overly long or too wide, i.e., interalar distance and philtral length and width. For example, in an early study of a small number of patients, it was determined that from time of initial closure to age 5 years, the philtrum had widened by a factor of 2.5 at the top and expanded two-fold between the peaks of Cupid's bow.[3] In contrast, nasal tip protrusion and columellar length remain abnormally short following conventional repair.

Applying *a posteriori* reasoning, the nasolabial features programmed for rapid growth in early childhood must be crafted on a small scale, whereas slow-growing features should be made slightly larger than the normal dimensions for an infant. Construction of the median tubercle is the exception to these guidelines. This normally fast-growing feature reaches 87% of adult height by age 5 years, but after bilateral cleft lip repair, the tubercle lags behind. Therefore, it must be fashioned to be as full as possible, anticipating insufficient growth.[2,6,7] There is also the unpredictable fourth-dimensional factor of central incisal show. Despite the surgeon's effort to craft a full median tubercle, augmentation may be necessary after eruption of the permanent central incisors and after the maxilla is in normal sagittal position.

Presentation

Bilateral cleft lip presents in three major anatomic forms: bilateral symmetrical complete (50%); bilateral symmetrical incomplete (25%), and bilateral asymmetrical (complete/incomplete) (25%).[45] The extent of the palatal cleft usually corresponds to the severity of the labial clefts. Bilateral complete cleft of the primary palate (lip and alveolus) is almost always associated with a bilateral complete cleft of the secondary palate. Bilateral symmetrical incomplete cleft lip is usually seen with minor or absent notching of the alveolar ridge with an intact secondary palate. There is more variation in palatal clefting in the asymmetrical bilateral forms: the palate can be either bilateral complete or unilateral complete on the major side.

Terminology for the contralateral bilateral asymmetric cleft lip requires further refinement. In general, the term "incomplete" cleft lip usually denotes that there is cutaneous continuity between the medial (nasomedial process) and the lateral (maxillary process). Incomplete cleft lip presents in a spectrum. At the severe end, there is a thin cutaneous band that some would argue constitutes a "complete" cleft lip. At the other end of the spectrum are the lesser-forms of incomplete cleft lip. Yuzuriha and Mulliken classified and defined these lesser-forms as *minor-form*, *microform*, and *mini-microform* as determined by the degree of disruption at the vermilion-cutaneous junction.[46]

Minor-form cleft lip extends 3–5 mm above the normal Cupid's bow peak, i.e., 50% or less of the normal cutaneous labial height. Other features are: deficient vermilion on medial side of the cleft; cutaneous groove and muscular depression; hypoplastic median tubercle; and minor nasal deformity.

Microform cleft lip is characterized by a notched vermilion-cutaneous junction in which the Cupid's bow peak is elevated less than 3 mm above normal. The other features are the same as in a minor-form, but they are less obvious. Nasal deformities include small depression of the sill, slightly slumped alar genu and 1–2 mm lateral displacement (and often under-rotation) of the alar base.

Mini-microform cleft lip is distinguished by a disruption of the white roll (vermilion-cutaneous junction) without elevation of the Cupid's bow peak. Usually there is a notch of the free mucosal margin. Muscular depression (particularly noticeable below the nostril sill) is variable as is the cleft nasal deformity.

This detailed subcategorization of the contralateral side in an asymmetrical bilateral cleft lip is important because the

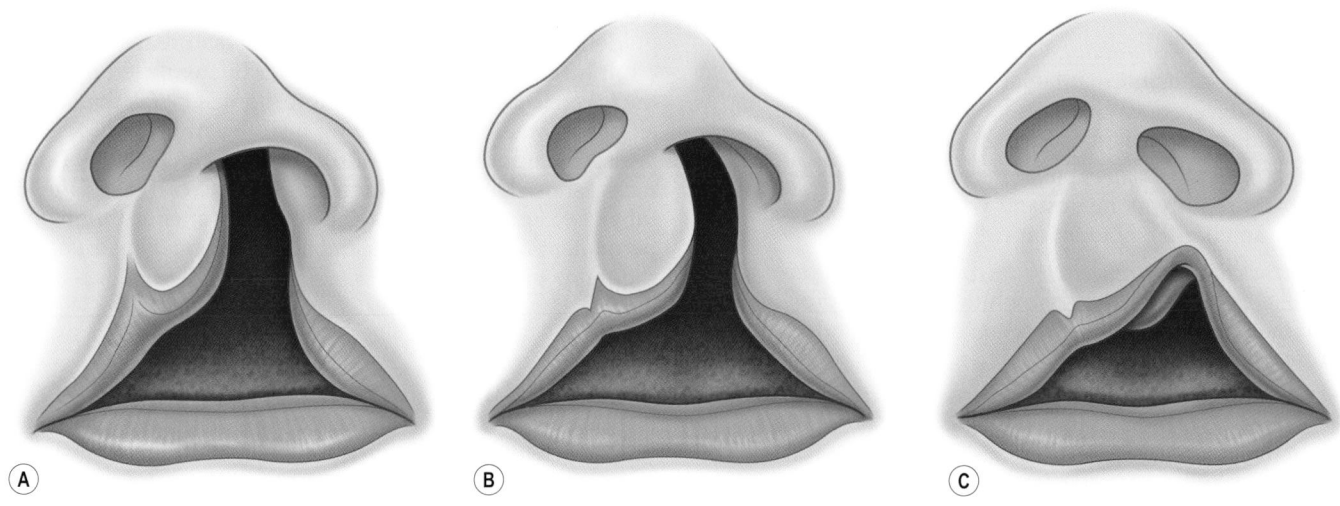

Fig. 24.1 Examples of asymmetrical bilateral cleft lip with a contralateral lesser form. **(A)** Left complete and right minor-form; **(B)** left complete and right microform; **(C)** left incomplete and right mini-microform.

extent of vermilion-cutaneous disjunction determines the operative strategy. Synchronous bilateral nasolabial repair is indicated for a contralateral incomplete cleft lip, including a minor-form. Correction of a contralateral microform or mini-microform is usually deferred until closure on the greater side. The type of contralateral (lesser-form) cleft lip not only guides the primary repair, it also foretells what revisions are likely to be necessary *(Fig. 24.1).*[45]

Video 1

Preoperative dentofacial orthopedics

Alignment of the three maxillary elements sets the skeletal stage for synchronous bilateral nasolabial repair. After retrusion and centralization of the premaxilla, the philtral flap can be designed in proper proportions, the nasal tip cartilages can be anatomically positioned, and the alveolar clefts can be closed, which stabilizes the maxillary arch and usually eliminates oronasal fistulas. Furthermore, premaxillary retropositioning minimizes the nasolabial distortions that occur during the rapid growth of early childhood.

There are two dentofacial orthopedic strategies: passive and active. A passive molding plate is retained by undercuts and maintains the transverse width of the maxillary segments. An external force is needed to retract the premaxilla, such as adhesive tape from cheek-to-cheek or an elastic band attached to a headcap. Bilateral labial adhesions have been tried since the mid-19th century; however, they often dehisce because of tension and the absence of prolabial muscle. Cutting and Grayson have popularized a more sophisticated version of a passive plate and taping called "nasoalveolar molding" (NAM).[44,47,48] Their plate produces differential pressure on the maxillary segments by selective reduction on the inner surfaces and addition of soft acrylic on the outer surfaces. After the alveolar gap is reduced to 5 mm, nasal molding begins. The nostrils are pushed upward by a bilobed acrylic nubbin on stainless steel prongs that are attached to the palatal plate.

A soft denture material is added across the nasolabial junction and a vertical tape is placed from prolabium-to-appliance to give a downward counterforce to the upward force applied to the nasal tips that stretch the columella. The premaxilla is gradually retracted by serial application of tape across the outrigger to the cheeks or to the labia. These tapes are changed daily by the parents. The apparatus must be adjusted weekly to modify the alveolar molding plate so as to narrow the maxillary segments. Although usually effective, NAM is labor-intensive and slow. There is no expansion of the maxillary elements with NAM; it is difficult to retract the premaxilla into alignment with the lesser segments. Unless there is adequate space in the arch, the premaxilla will abut the labial surface of the segments.

Complications with "NAM" include inflammation of the oral and nasal mucosa, blistering of the cheeks, trouble in feeding the infant, and difficulty in centralizing a badly torqued premaxilla. The skin of the columellar-labial junction can ulcerate if the horizontal prolabial band is too tight. There is also a potential risk that the molding plate could become dislodged and obstruct the airway; infants are obligatory nasal breathers until about age 3 months. A 5 mm diameter hole is placed in the center of the molding plate to minimize the possibility of this complication.[49]

The active-type dentofacial orthopedic device in current use is based on the protypic design by Georgiade and associates,[50] later refined and popularized by Millard and Latham.[51] The Latham appliance is constructed from a plaster cast of the upper jaw taken in the office. In the past, the appliance was fabricated in London, Ontario, Canada. A local, skilled prosthetist can also fabricate the custom-device. The appliance is pinned to the maxillary shelves with the infant under general anesthesia. An elastic chain on each side is connected to a transvomer wire that is looped under a roller in the posterior-superior section of the appliance and attached to cleats at the anterior edges of the maxillary plate. The parents turn the ratcheted screw daily to expand the anterior palatal segments. Visits are necessary at 1, 3, and 5 weeks to assure appropriate

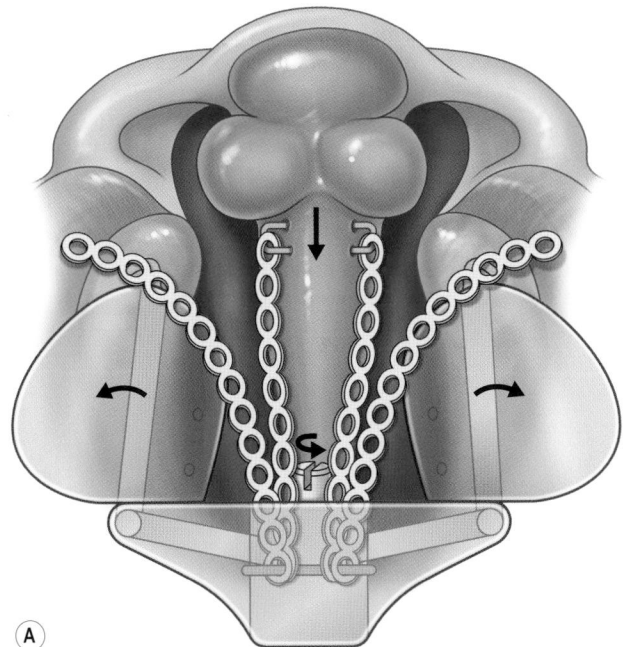

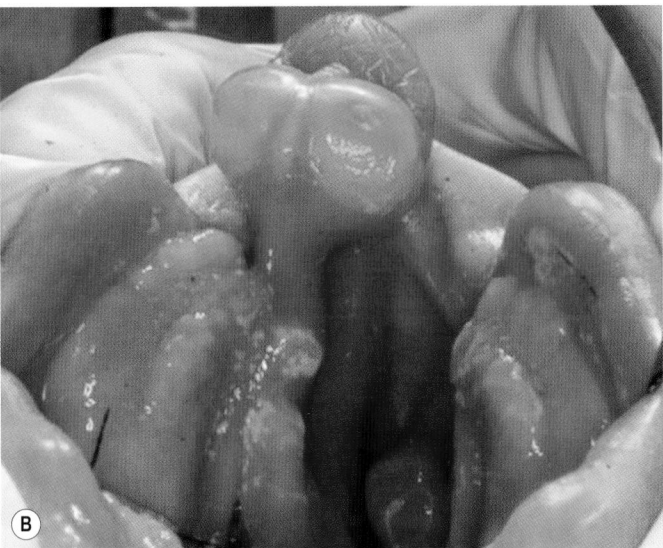

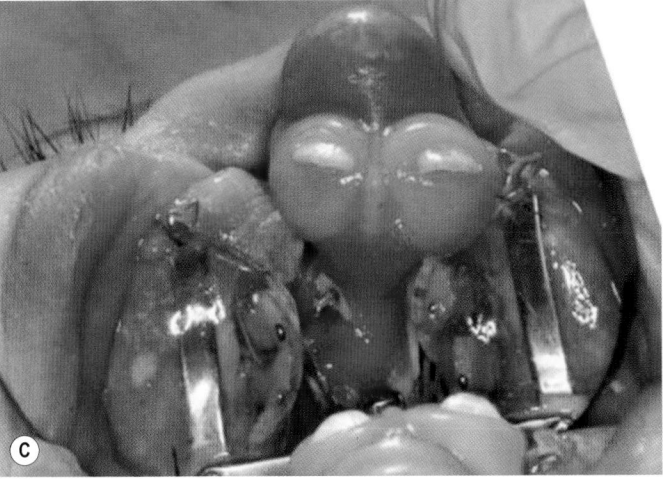

Fig. 24.2 (A) Latham appliance; **(B)** prior to insertion of device; **(C)** 6 weeks following dentofacial orthopedic manipulation.

fit and to adjust the bilateral elastic chains that retrocline the premaxilla. The process normally takes 6–8 weeks. The Latham appliance is effective in correcting premaxillary position in the sagittal plane; however the movement is more retroclination than retroposition. The appliance can also rectify premaxillary rotation, through differential traction, although there is little effect on vertical position *(Fig. 24.2)*.

The merits of passive versus active dentofacial orthopedics continue to be debated by proponents of each approach. Critics of active premaxillary orthopedics argue it causes midfacial retrusion.[52,53] Others have failed to document such an effect beyond that expected inhibition of vertical and forward maxillary growth in children with repaired bilateral cleft lip/palate and followed through the age of the mixed dentition.[54] There is also recent controversy about a possible deleterious effect of alveolar gingivoperiosteoplasty.

Traditional treatment protocols place undue emphasis on efforts to minimize inhibition of midfacial growth. Some degree of maxillary retrusion is an unavoidable consequence of closure of the cleft lip and cleft palate or both. The first priorities should be nasolabial appearance and speech. Midfacial retrusion is predictably corrected by maxillary advancement with the additional aesthetic benefits to nasal, labial, and malar projection.

Operative techniques

Video 1

The day of repair of a bilateral cleft lip and correction of the nasal deformity is the most important day in the child's life. It should be the first case in the morning, and probably the only operation for that day. The surgeon must work slowly and deliberately, taking as much time as necessary, without distractions, such as scheduled meetings, patients waiting in the office, and other obligations.

The technical details for repair of a bilateral complete cleft lip and nasal deformity are given below, followed by modifications used for the major anatomic variants of bilateral cleft lip. The reader will note that descriptions of the procedures do not follow the usual sequence of marking, dissection, and closure. Instead, the operative steps are portrayed as they proceed, which often requires turning attention from the lip to the nose, then back to the lip again, and ending with the final touches to the nose. Some leeway in the sequence of the operation is possible, but, in general this is not advisable, until considerable experience is gained in these procedures.

Bilateral cleft, complete cleft lip and palate

Markings

A sharpened tooth-pick is used for drawing and the ink is brilliant green dye (tincture) rather than methylene blue dye (aqueous). The anatomic points are designated using the standard anthropometric initialisms.[6] With the nostrils held upward with a double-ball retractor, the philtral flap is drawn first. Its dimensions are determined by the child's age at repair (usually 5–6 months), and less so by ethnicity. The length of the philtral flap (sn-ls) is set at 6–7 mm (normal male 11.4 ± 1.3 mm at 6–12 months); usually it is the same as the cutaneous prolabium. If the prolabial element is overly long, the philtral flap should be shortened appropriately. The width of the philtral flap is set at 2 mm at the columellar-labial junction (cphs-cphs) and 3.5–4 mm between the proposed Cupid's bow peaks (cphi-cphi) (normal male 6.7 ± 1.0 mm at 6–12 months). The sides of the philtral flap should be drawn slightly concave in anticipation of slight bowing with growth. Flanking flaps are drawn; these will be de-epithelialized and will come to lie beneath the lateral labial flaps in an effort to simulate philtral columns. These flanking flaps also add width and increase the vascularity of the philtral flap.

The proposed Cupid's bow peaks are carefully noted on the lateral labial elements and marked just atop the white roll above the vermilion-cutaneous junction. These points are situated so that there is some medial extension of white roll that will form the handle of the Cupid's bow and sufficient vermilion height to construct the median tubercle and raphe. Curvilinear lines are drawn at the juncture of the alar bases and lateral labial elements. Anthropometric dimensions are measured and recorded before proceeding. Lidocaine with epinephrine is injected into the nose and labial segments, and after the conventional 5–7 minute waiting time, the critical points, including the vermilion-mucosal junctions, are tattooed with tincture of brilliant green dye *(Fig. 24.3)*.

Labial dissection

First, all labial lines are lightly scored. The philtral flanking flaps are de-epithelialized, the extra prolabial skin is discarded, and the philtral flap is elevated (including subcutaneous tissue) up to the anterior nasal spine. The lateral white-roll-vermilion-mucosal flaps are incised; however, halt these incisions about 2–3 mm short of the tattooed lateral Cupid's bow peak-points. The lateral labial elements are disjoined from the alar bases, and the basilar flaps are freed from the piriform attachments by incision along the lower section of the vestibular cutaneo-mucosal junction.

The mucosal incisions are extended distal along the gingivolabial sulcus to the premolar region. With a double-hook on the muscular layer, the lateral labial elements are widely dissected off the maxillae in the supraperiosteal plane. The non-dominant ring finger is held on the infraorbital rim (to protect the globe) as the dissection is further extended over the malar eminence *(Fig. 24.4)*. Extensive release of the lateral labial segments is a critical maneuver so as to minimize tension at the muscular and cutaneous closure. The orbicularis oris bundles are dissected in the subdermal and submucosal plane for 1 cm, or a little further if necessary *(Fig. 24.5)*.

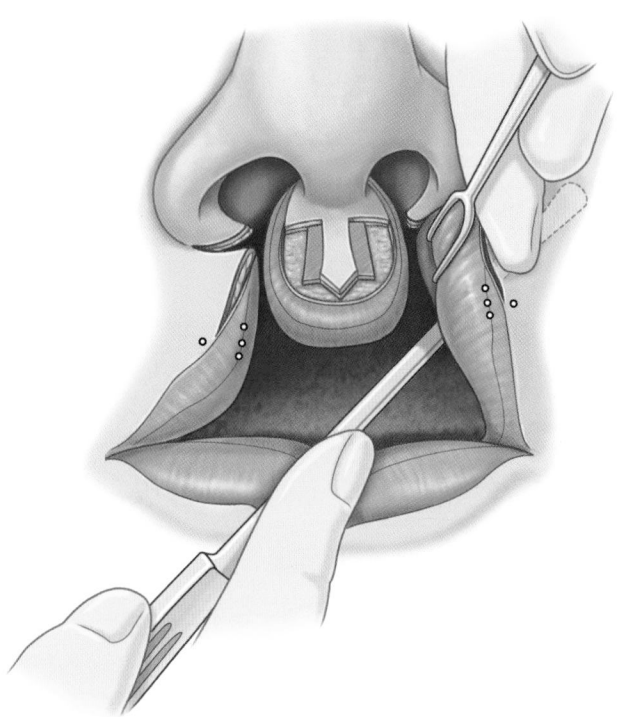

Fig. 24.4 Lateral labial elements dissected off maxilla in supraperiosteal plane, extending over the malar eminences.

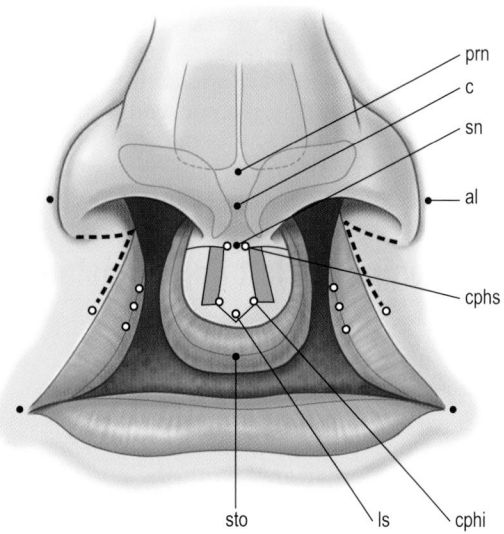

Fig. 24.3 Markings for synchronous repair of bilateral cleft lip and nasal deformity. Open circles denote tattooed dots. Anthropometric points: pronasale (prn); highest point of columella nasi (c); subnasale (sn); ala nasi (al); crista philtri superior (cphs); crista philtri inferior (cphi); labiale superius (ls); stomion (sto).

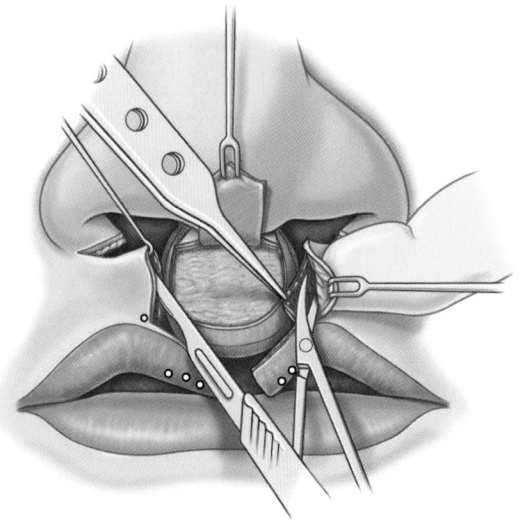

Fig. 24.5 Dissection of orbicularis oris muscle bundles in subdermal and submucosal planes.

Alveolar closure

The lateral nasal mucosal flaps are released from beneath the inferior turbinates, the medial nasal mucosal flaps are elevated from the premaxilla, and the nasal floors are closed. The premaxillary mucosal incisions are continued on each side and vertical incisions are made in the facing gingiva of the lesser segments. Often digital pressure on the pre-maxilla is necessary to permit the alveolar gingivoperiosteal closure.

The alar base flaps are advanced medially and the inner edge is sutured to the anterior edge of the constructed nasal floor. The thin strip of vermilion is trimmed off the premaxil-lary mucosa and the remaining mucosal flange is secured high to the premaxillary periosteum to construct the posterior side of the central gingivolabial sulcus *(Fig. 24.6)*.

Labial closure

Advancement of the lateral labial elements during closure of the sulci is critical. A back-cut is made at the distal end of the sulcal incision, and each sulcus is closed while the labial flap is being pulled mesially with a double hook. The advanced lateral labial mucosa forms the anterior wall of the central gingivolabial sulcus.

The orbicular bundles are apposed (end-to-end), inferiorly-to-superiorly, using simple polydioxanone sutures. Prior to completion of the muscular closure, a polydioxanone suture is placed on each side through the maxillary periosteum in the region of the origin of the depressor alae nasi and left untied. A polypropylene suture suspends the uppermost muscular elements to the periosteum of the anterior nasal spine *(Fig. 24.7A)*.

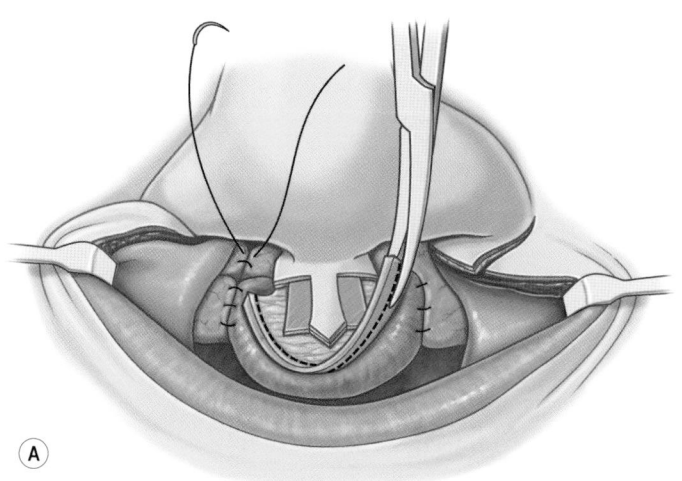
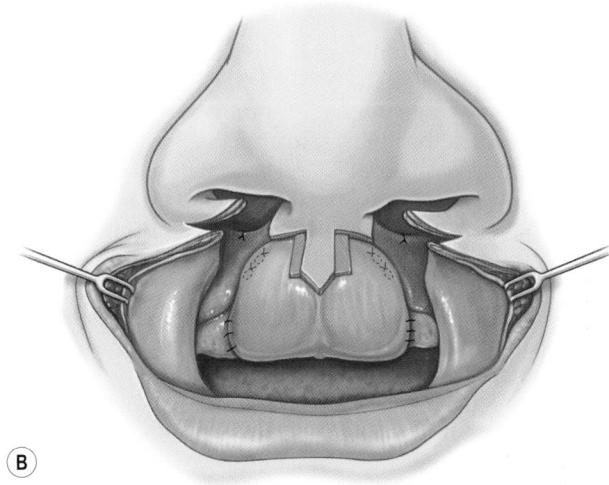

Fig. 24.6 (A) After completion of gingivoperiosteoplasty, redundant premaxillary vermilion is trimmed. **(B)** Remaining premaxillary mucosal flange sutured to periosteum forming posterior wall of anterior gingivolabial sulcus.

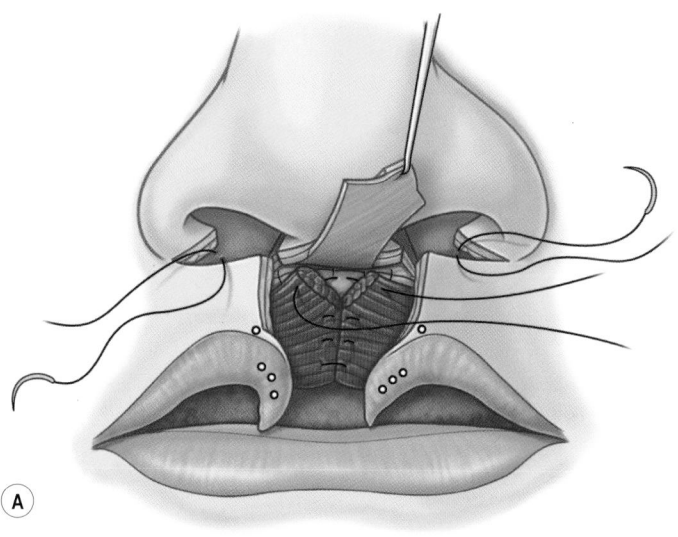
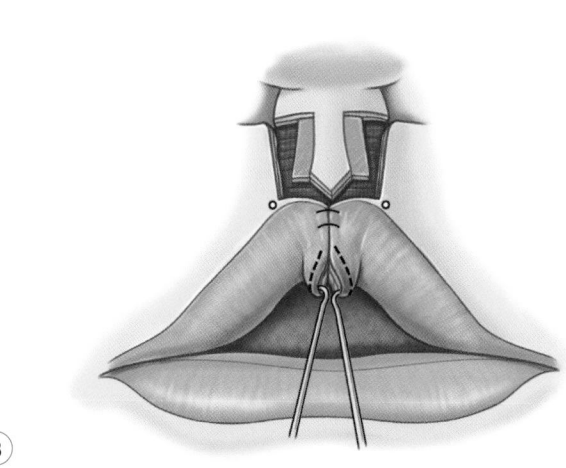

Fig. 24.7 (A) Apposition of orbicularis oris from inferior-to-superior; uppermost suture placed through periosteum of anterior nasal spine. **(B)** Lateral white-roll-vermilion-mucosal flaps trimmed to construct median tubercle and Cupid's bow.

Construction of the median tubercle begins with placement of a fine chromic suture, about 3 mm medial to the tattooed lateral Cupid's bow peak-point, joining the white-roll-mucosal flaps in the midline *(Fig. 24.7B)*. The excess vermilion-mucosa is successively trimmed from each flap, and the flaps are accurately aligned to form the median raphe. There is a natural inclination to save too much of the vermilion-mucosal flaps, resulting in a furrowed raphe. Attention is next focused on nasal repair before inset of the philtral flap.

Nasal dissection and positioning the lower lateral cartilages

The slumped/splayed lower lateral cartilages are visualized through bilateral rim incisions ("semi-open" approach). Fibrofatty tissue is dissected off the anterior surface of and between the cartilages; this is aided by elevation with a cotton-tipped applicator on the mucosal underside. Dissection is continued across the dorsal septum to expose the upper lateral cartilages *(Fig. 24.8)*.

With direct visualization, a horizontal mattress suture of 5–0 polydioxanone (P2 reverse cutting needle, Ethicon) is placed between the genua and left untied. Another mattress suture is inserted through each upper lateral cartilage and then through the ipsilateral lateral crus. Often it is possible to place a second suture to suspend the lateral crus to the upper lateral cartilage. Holding an intranasal cotton-tipped applicator, beneath the genu and tenting the nostril roof, facilitates the insertion and tying of these sutures *(Fig. 24.9)*.

The C-flap on each side of the columellar base is trimmed to 3–5 mm in length *(Fig. 24.10A)*. The alar bases are advanced medially, rotated endonasally, and sutured side-to-end to the C-flaps. Next, the tips of the alar base flaps are trimmed to complete closure of the sills. A "cinch suture" of polypropylene is placed through the dermis of each alar base, passing under the philtral flap, and tied to narrow the inter-alar dimension (al-al) to less than 25 mm (normal male 26 ± 1.4 mm at 6–12 months). The maxillary periosteal sutures, placed earlier, are brought above the muscular layer, inserted through the alar bases (superficial to the "cinch suture") and

tied. These sutures simulate the depressor alae nasi and also: (1) form the cymal shape of the sills; (2) prevent alar elevation with smiling; (3) minimize postoperative nasal widening *(Fig. 24.10B)*.

Final touches

Fashioning a philtral dimple seems just beyond the surgeon's skill, nevertheless, it is worth trying. One way to simulate this depression is to suture the dermis in the lower one-third of the philtral flap down to the orbicularis layer. The tip of the philtral flap is inset into the handle of Cupid's bow. The leading edge of the lateral labial flaps need not be trimmed before apposition to the philtral flap. A little extra lateral labial tissue helps to simulate the columns. There should be no tension at the philtral closure, which is done with fine,

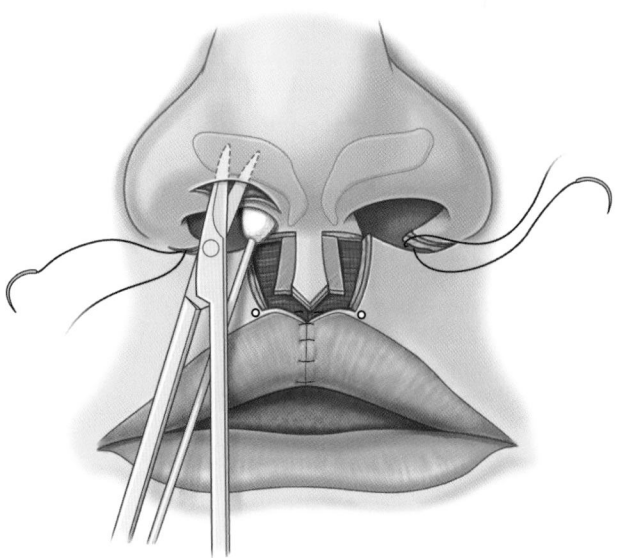

Fig. 24.8 Lower lateral cartilages exposed through rim incisions. Cotton-tipped applicator elevates nostril and helps display genua.

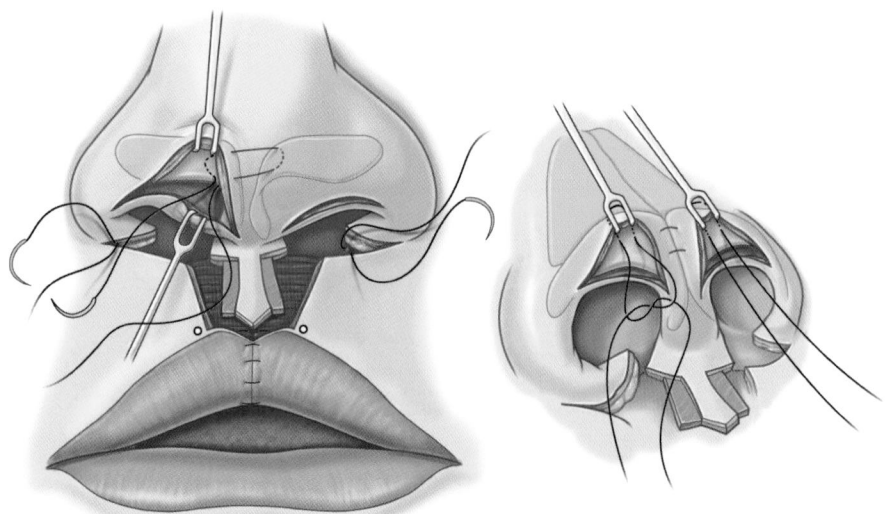

Fig. 24.9 Positioning dislocated and splayed lower lateral cartilages: **(A)** Apposition of genua with interdomal mattress suture; **(B)** suspension over ipsilateral upper lateral cartilage with inter-cartilaginous mattress suture.

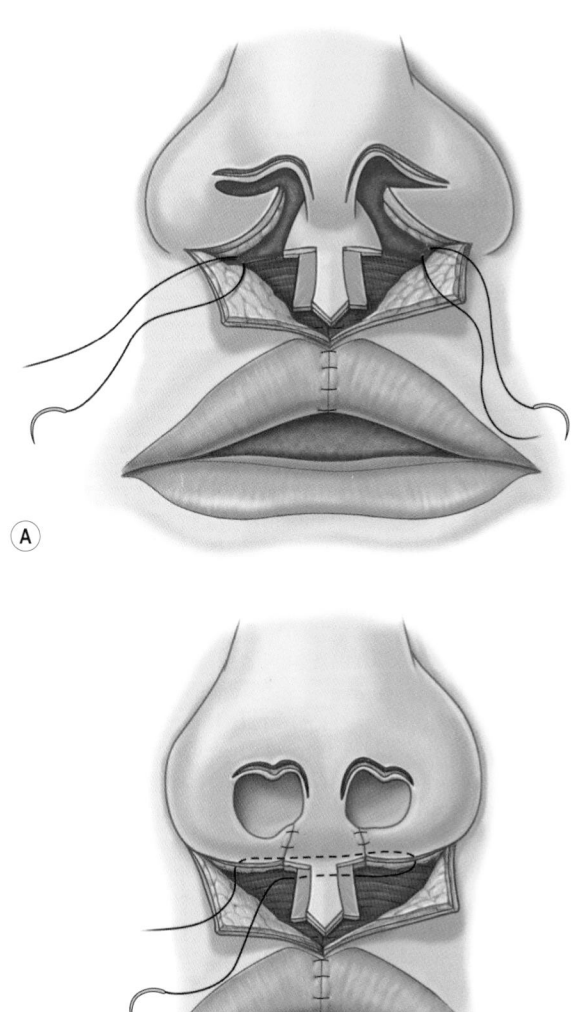

(A)

(B)

Fig. 24.10 (A) Columellar flaps shortened and alar bases trimmed. Note bilateral sutures in maxillary periosteum below alar bases – these sutures were inserted prior to completion of muscular closure. **(B)** Alar base flaps rotated endonasally and secured (side-to-end) to C-flaps. Interalar distance narrowed with cinch suture. Right maxillary periosteal suture to alar base has been tied – note cymal configuration (depression) of lateral sill.

interrupted dermal and percutaneous sutures. The cephalic margin of the labial flaps must be trimmed, corresponding to the position and cymal configuration of the sills *(Fig. 24.11)*. Closure of the labial flaps to the sills proceeds laterally-to-medially.

After anatomic positioning of the lower lateral cartilages, it is obvious that there is redundant domal skin in the soft triangles and in the upper columella. This extra skin is excised in a crescentic fashion from the leading edge of the rim incisions and extending inferiorly along each side of the columella *(Fig. 24.11)*. This resection narrows the nasal tip, defines and tapers the mid-columella, and elongates the nostrils.

Apposition of the genua also accentuates the extra lining (oblique webbing) in the lateral vestibules. Lenticular excision on the cutaneous side of the intercartilaginous junction flattens this lateral vestibular ridge *(Fig. 24.11, inset)*.

Immediately postoperative nasolabial anthropometry is documented and placed in the child's record *(Fig. 24.12)*.[6] The constructed columella (sn-c) is usually 5–6 mm, (normal male 4.7 ± 0.8 mm at 5 months). After the measurements, a strip of ¼ inch Xeroform® gauze is wrapped around a 19-gauge silicone tubing and a 1 cm segment is inserted into each nostril. These vented "stents" are removed after 48 h. Prolonged nostril splinting is difficult to maintain, likely to damage the sills, and probably unnecessary.

Postoperative care

A Logan bow is taped to the cheeks: (1) to protect the labial repair and (2) to hold an iced-saline sponge over the wound for 24 h postoperatively. The infant is discharged from hospital on the second postoperative day. The parents are instructed in suture-line care and how to keep the nostrils clean. Percutaneous sutures are removed 5–6 days postoperatively under general anesthesia using mask induction and insufflation. A ½ inch transverse Steri-Strip® (3M Health Care, St. Paul, Minnesota) is trimmed and placed over the labial scars; the tape is changed as needed for 6 weeks. Thereafter, the parents are instructed how to perform digital massage (with Pedi-Mederma®) for several months and counseled about the importance of application of sun-block ointment *(Fig. 24.13)*.

Technical modifications for bilateral variations

Late presentation of bilateral complete cleft lip/palate

Dentofacial orthopedics may not be available or practical in developing countries. Even in developed nations, a child with bilateral complete cleft lip/palate can present in late infancy, and, by that age, the premaxilla is rigid and preoperative manipulation is not possible. Rather than attempt labial closure over a protrusive premaxilla, consider ostectomy and set-back. There are two alternatives: (1) premaxillary set-back and nasolabial repair or (2) premaxillary set-back and palatoplasty. With careful attention to mucosal blood supply, premaxillary retropositioning can be safely done along with bilateral nasolabial closure. Another uncommon indication for the first alternative is partially successful dentofacial orthopedic preparation. *Caution:* Only a bilateral narrow isthmus of septal mucosa nourishes the premaxilla after the mucosal incisions and elevation necessary for alveolar gingivoperiosteoplasties and for resection of the premaxillary neck and inferior septal cartilage. The second alternative, premaxillary set-back, gingivoperiosteoplasties, and palatoplasty, is the safer procedure. It is recommended if the child is nearing age 1 year or older when speech is the first priority. Bilateral nasolabial repair on a solid maxillary foundation is scheduled later.

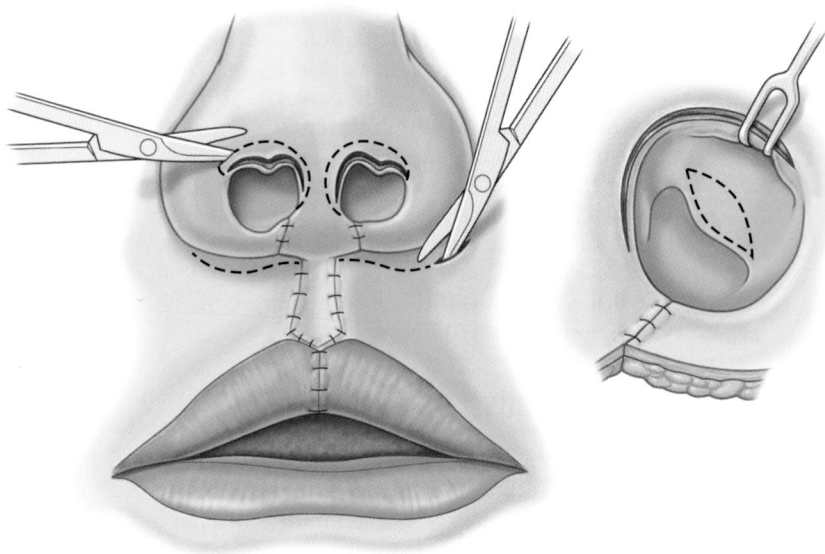

Fig. 24.11 Crescentic excision of expanded domal skin and lining extended into upper columella. Cyma-shaped resection of superior margin of lateral labial elements to fit curve of the alar base and sill. Lenticular excision of lateral vestibular web (inset).

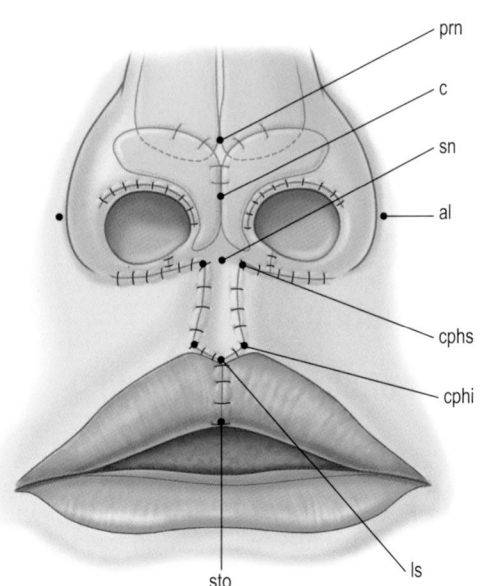

Fig. 24.12 Completed bilateral complete cleft lip/nasal repair. Pronasale (prn); highest point of columella nasi (c); subnasale (sn); ala nasi (al); crista philtri superior (cphs); crista philtri inferior (cphi); labiale superius (ls); stomion (sto).

Primary premaxillary retropositioning is likely to accentuate midfacial retrusion; however, nasolabial appearance and speech take precedence. The majority of children with bilateral complete cleft lip/palate will need maxillary advancement.

Binderoid bilateral complete cleft lip/palate

Nasal features in this rare bilateral variant include: orbital hypotelorism, hypoplastic bony/cartilaginous elements (including short septum and absent anterior nasal spine) and conical columella. Labial features are: hypoplastic prolabium/premaxilla (with a single incisor) and thin vermilion in the lateral labial segments.[55] The floppy premaxilla usually precludes an attempt at dentofacial orthopedic manipulation; furthermore, it is often unnecessary because the premaxilla is not procumbent.

Synchronous nasolabial repair is accomplished as described above, but there are some slight differences. Sometimes the premaxilla is so small that alveolar gingivoperiosteoplasties cannot be accomplished during labial closure. If necessary, a passive palatal plate can be used to maintain anterior maxillary width following nasolabial closure. The philtral flap need not be drawn overly-small in either height or width; it will expand very little with growth. The interalar dimension should be narrowed to slightly below age-matched normal because it will widen. Although the lower lateral cartilages are hypoplastic, usually they can be dissected, positioned and secured. The thin and tapered columella can be augmented when the child is older *(Fig. 24.14)*.

Secondary procedures are likely in a patient with the binderoid variant. These include dermal grafts to augment the median tubercle and to widen the narrow columellar base; cartilage grafts to the nasal tip, and a costochondral graft to build-up the nasal dorsum and project the tip, and maxillary advancement along with augmentation of the *fossae praenasale*.[55]

Bilateral complete cleft lip and intact secondary palate

Bilateral complete cleft lip/alveolus with intact secondary palate is another very rare form. The premaxilla is solid, thus obviating dentofacial orthopedics. If the premaxilla is not severely protrusive, it is usually possible to accomplish synchronous nasolabial repair and closure of the posterior premaxillary cleft. If this strategy is chosen, alveolar

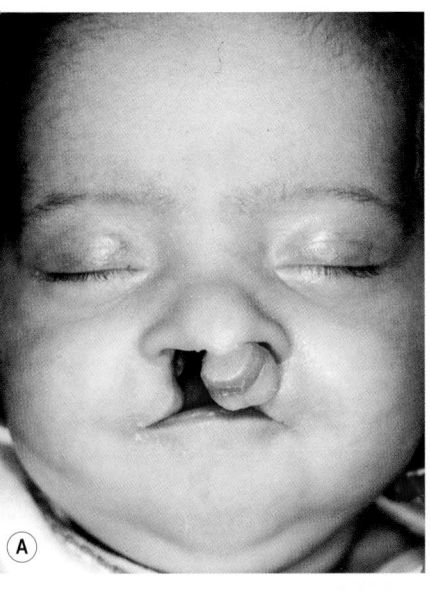
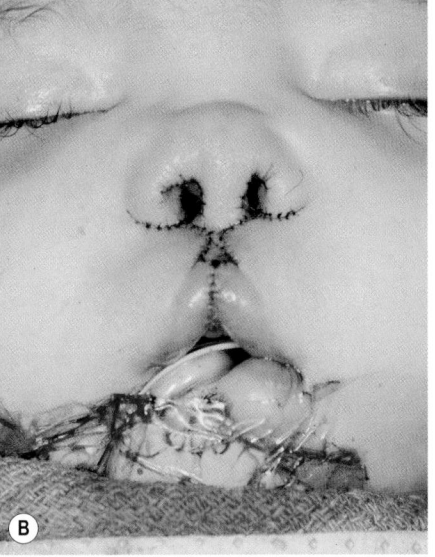

Immediate postoperative anthropometry documents under-corrected fast-growing features and over-corrected slow-growing features compared with normal values		
Intraoperative	Patient (7 months)	Normal (6–12 months)
n-sn	20.0[a]	26.9 ± 1.6
al-al	24.5	25.4 ± 1.5
sn-prn	10.5	9.7 ± 0.8
sn-c	6.0[a]	4.7 ± 0.8
cphs-cphs	1.5	NA
cphi-cphi	4.5[a]	6.5 ± 1.1
sn-ls	5.5[a]	10.7 ± 1.1
sn-sto	11.2[a]	16.0 ± 0.8
ls-sto	6.2	5.3 ± 1.4

Normal values expressed as norm ± SD. [a]Values outside SD. NA, not available.

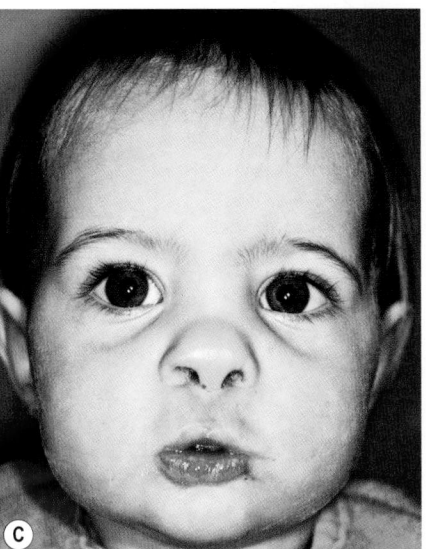
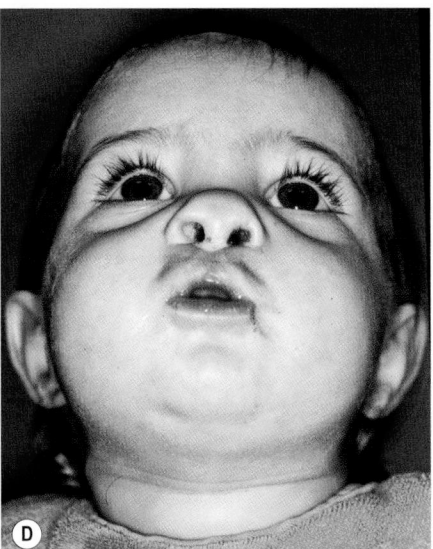
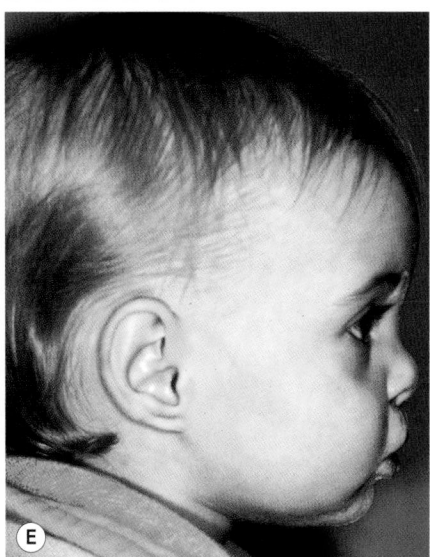

Fig. 24.13 (A) Bilateral complete cleft lip/palate. **(B)** Following synchronous nasolabial repair at 6 months. **(C,D,E)** At 4 months postoperative. Note columella/tip projection, hint of a philtral dimple, and normal columellar-labial angle.

gingivoperiosteoplasties should be delayed in order to preserve premaxillary blood supply. But, if the premaxilla is procumbent, consider a first-stage premaxillary ostectomy and set-back, along with closure of the alveolar clefts, and closure of the defect at the anterior edge of the hard palate. Bilateral nasolabial repair can be done safely at the second stage later in infancy. The alternative plan is premaxillary set-back, bilateral nasolabial repair and closure of the posterior premaxillary-palatal defect, leaving the facing edges of the alveolar clefts intact (to maintain blood supply to the premaxilla). The third strategy is premaxillary set-back, gingivoperiosteoplasties, nasolabial repair, and delayed closure of the premaxillary-palatal cleft (the latter is technically difficult). Midfacial retrusion is very unlikely following primary premaxillary set-back because the secondary palate is intact *(Fig. 24.15)*.

Bilateral incomplete cleft lip

One-quarter of all double labial clefts are incomplete and most are symmetrical.[45] Of all the bilateral variants, this is the most easily repaired. The design and execution are the same as for the bilateral complete form, including adjustments based on expected nasolabial changes with growth. There are two technical considerations that need to be underscored. The first relates to construction of the median tubercle. Usually, the tubercle should be formed using the lateral white-roll-vermilion-mucosal flaps. However, in the rare instance of a bilateral lesser-form (<50% of cutaneous labial height) and a prominent central white roll, the prolabial vermilion-mucosa may be utilized as the central segment. The next consideration is columellar length: measure sn-c. If columellar length is normal for the infant's age and the lower lateral cartilages are

Fig. 24.14 (A) Female infant with binderoid bilateral complete cleft lip/palate. **(B)** Floppy, diminutive premaxilla deviated to left centralized by Latham device. **(C)** After synchronous repair. Note thin vermilion in lateral labial elements. Midline tip incision is no longer used. **(D–F)** Appearance at age 5 years.

in nearly normal position, it may be unnecessary to position the cartilages and sculpt the tip. Nevertheless, interalar narrowing is always needed as this dimension is overly wide and will increase with growth. If the columella is short and the alar domes are splayed, the lower laterals should be apposed through the semi-open approach *(Fig. 24.16)*

Asymmetrical bilateral (complete/incomplete) cleft lip

Symmetry, the first principle of bilateral labial repair, should be foremost in mind when planning and executing closure of an asymmetrical variant. An algorithm for timing and techniques for repair of asymmetrical bilateral cleft lip is shown in *Figure 24.17*. If both greater and lesser side clefts are

incomplete or the lesser side is a minor-form, synchronous bilateral repair is indicated. However, if the greater side is incomplete and the contralateral side is microform or mini-microform, the incomplete side should be repaired first.

If the greater side is a complete cleft, it is initially managed by unilateral dentofacial orthopedics, followed by nasolabial adhesion and alveolar gingivoperiosteoplasty. Thus, the greater side is converted from a complete to an incomplete cleft. This levels the surgical field, and the options for the next stage become clear. If the contralateral (lesser side) cleft lip is a minor-form or a more severe incomplete, the second stage is simultaneous bilateral nasolabial repair. Keeping symmetry in mind, technical maneuvers on the complete side must be exaggerated because the distortions and tensions are greater than on the incomplete side. Even if the lower lateral cartilage is in near normal position on the incomplete side, use bilateral rim incisions and over-correct the cartilage on

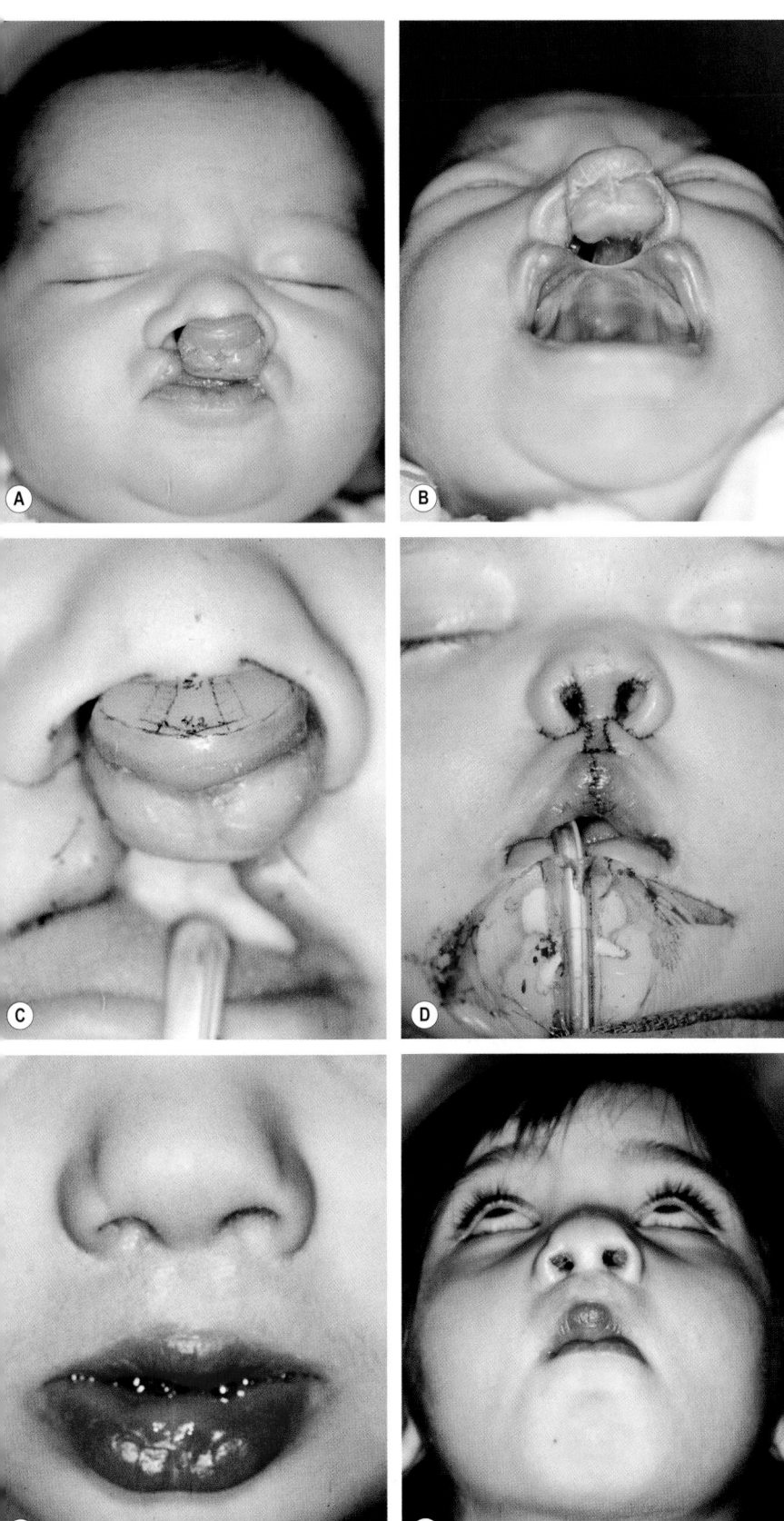

Intraoperative anthropometry. Slow-growing nasal protrusion and columella were crafted larger than normal but just within 1 SD

Intraoperative	Patient (6 months)	Normal (6–12 months)
n-sn	21.0[a]	26.9 ± 1.6
al-al	24.5	25.4 ± 1.5
sn-prn	10.5	9.7 ± 0.8
sn-c	5.0	4.7 ± 0.8
cphs-cphs	2.1	NA
cphi-cphi	4.5[a]	6.5 ± 1.1
sn-ls	5.5[a]	10.7 ± 1.1
sn-sto	13.0[a]	16.0 ± 0.8
ls-sto	7.0[a]	5.3 ± 1.4

Normal values expressed as norm ± SD. [a]Values outside SD. NA, not available.

Fig. 24.15 **(A)** Female infant with bilateral complete cleft lip/alveolus (van der Woude syndrome). **(B)** Intact secondary palate. **(C)** Markings for synchronous repair at age 6 months. **(D)** Following premaxillary set-back, alveolar gingivoperiosteoplasties and nasolabial repair. Palato-premaxillary defect closed and lower labial sinuses excised in second stage. **(E,F)** Appearance at age 2 years.

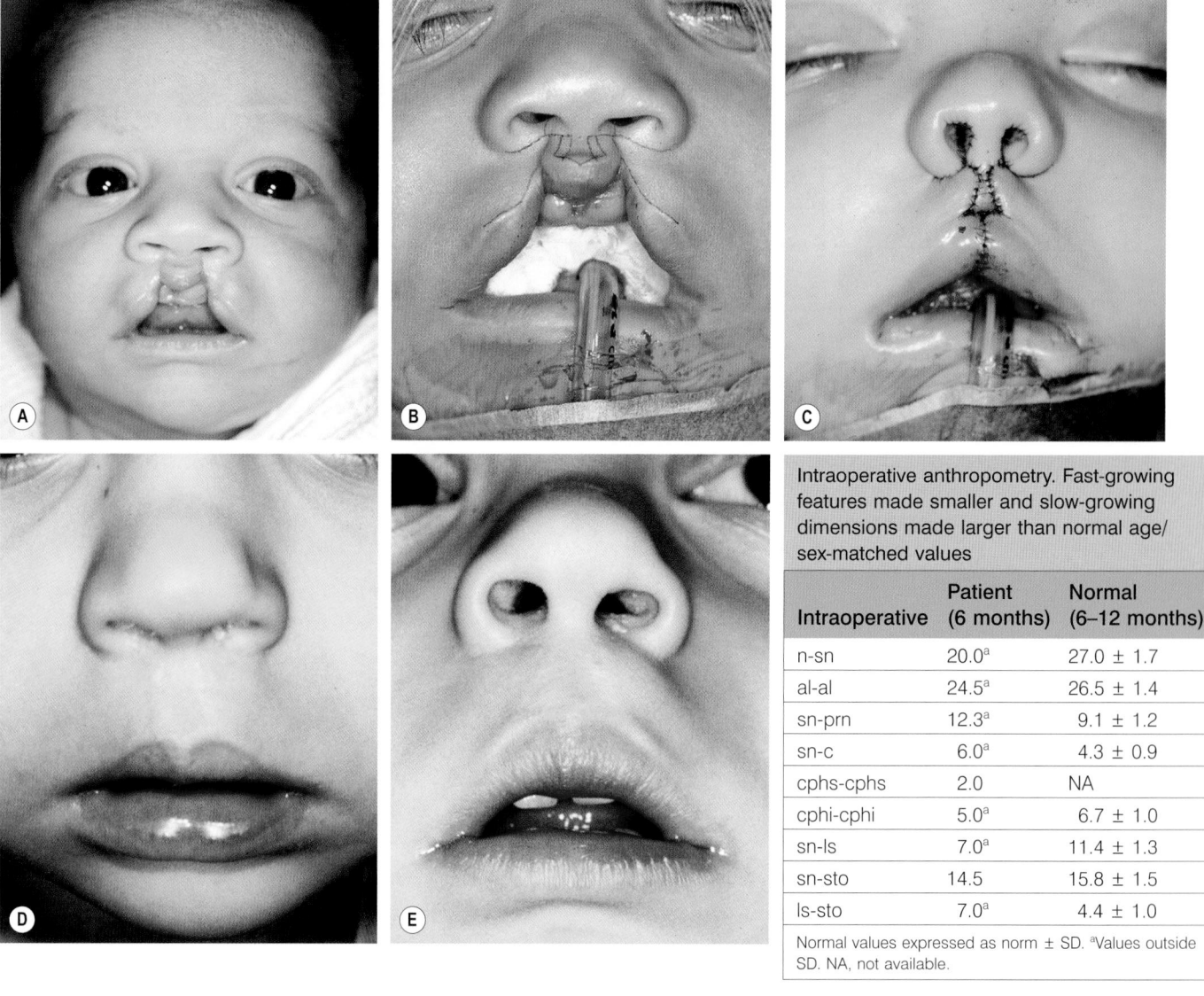

Intraoperative anthropometry. Fast-growing features made smaller and slow-growing dimensions made larger than normal age/sex-matched values		
Intraoperative	Patient (6 months)	Normal (6–12 months)
n-sn	20.0[a]	27.0 ± 1.7
al-al	24.5[a]	26.5 ± 1.4
sn-prn	12.3[a]	9.1 ± 1.2
sn-c	6.0[a]	4.3 ± 0.9
cphs-cphs	2.0	NA
cphi-cphi	5.0[a]	6.7 ± 1.0
sn-ls	7.0[a]	11.4 ± 1.3
sn-sto	14.5	15.8 ± 1.5
ls-sto	7.0[a]	4.4 ± 1.0

Normal values expressed as norm ± SD. [a]Values outside SD. NA, not available.

Fig. 24.16 (A) Bilateral symmetrical incomplete cleft lip. **(B)** Markings for synchronous closure at age 6 months. **(C)** Following nasolabial repair. **(D,E)** Appearance at age 1.5 years.

the complete side. There may be inequality of vermilion height at the junction forming the median raphe. This can be adjusted by a vermilion unilimb Z-plasty, usually with the triangular flap designed on the lesser side vermilion *(Fig. 24.18)*.

If the contralateral side is a microform cleft, it is best first to narrow the complete side by preoperative dentofacial orthopedics and repair it, either in one stage or two (after preliminary nasolabial adhesion), with alveolar gingivoperiosteoplasty. In so doing, observe the contralateral microform when designing the arc and position of the medial incision for rotation-advancement repair. Try to limit the incision at the columellar base and advancement of the lateral labial element so that the philtral suture-line will match the configuration of the contralateral microform. After the scar has remodeled, the contralateral microform is corrected using the double unilimb

z-plastic technique, including muscular apposition and dermal graft to augment the philtral ridge, and nasal correction.[56] Mirror-image symmetry is the goal with attention to philtral shape, Cupid's bow position, alar base placement and nostril axis.

If the lesser side cleft is mini-microform, often this can be corrected by vertical lenticular excision at the same time as repair on the greater side, although nothing is lost by waiting. Nasolabial asymmetries between the greater and lesser sides can best be judged when the child is older. Augmentation of the median tubercle is almost always necessary. If the Cupid's bow peak is too high on the repaired greater side, it is best to lower it (by unilimb Z-plasty) rather than adjust the mini-microform. Sometimes, a minor correction is needed to correct asymmetry of the nasal tip. Often a contralateral mini-microform does not need attention.[45]

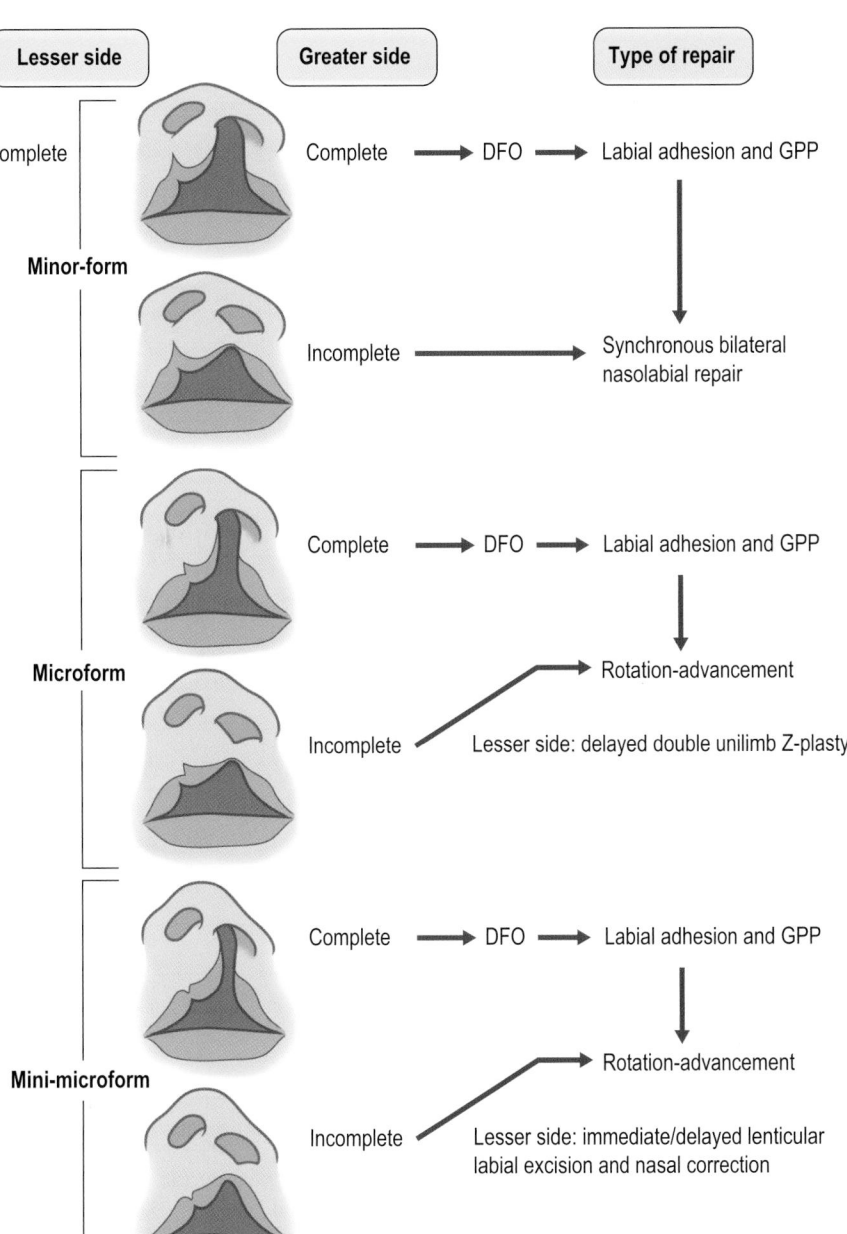

| Lesser side | Greater side | Type of repair |

Minor-form

Incomplete — Complete ⟶ DFO ⟶ Labial adhesion and GPP

Incomplete ⟶ Synchronous bilateral nasolabial repair

Microform

Complete ⟶ DFO ⟶ Labial adhesion and GPP

Rotation-advancement

Incomplete ⟶ Lesser side: delayed double unilimb Z-plasty

Mini-microform

Complete ⟶ DFO ⟶ Labial adhesion and GPP

Rotation-advancement

Incomplete ⟶ Lesser side: immediate/delayed lenticular labial excision and nasal correction

Fig. 24.17 Algorithm for correction of asymmetrical bilateral cleft lip (complete/incomplete) and contralateral incomplete or lesser-form cleft. DFO, dentofacial orthopedics; R-A, rotation-advancement; GPP, gingivoperiosteoplasty. (Modified from Yuzuriha S, Oh AK, Mulliken JB. Asymmetrical bilateral cleft lip: Complete or incomplete and contralateral lesser defect (minor-form, microform, or mini-microform). *Plast Reconstr Surg.* 2008;122:1494–1504.)

Outcomes

The surgeon's responsibility does not end with completion of nasolabial repair. There is an obligation to periodically assess the outcome of the procedure, and if possible, to continue to do so until skeletal growth is complete. Only by so doing, can the surgeon come to understand changes in the fourth dimension, learn from these observations, and apply this knowledge to succeeding infants with bilateral cleft lip.

Photography

Preoperative photographs are the basic minimum for documentation. They are unacceptable if taken when the child is on the operating table with the endotracheal tube in place. The surgeon must find the time and have the patience, to take preoperative frontal, submental and lateral views of the infant. Intraoperative photographs taken after cutaneous markings and immediately after the repair are also useful. The standard angle for the submental view should align the nasal tip on a line sighted half-way between the medial canthi and eyebrows. The submental photograph is essential for assessment of nasal configuration and symmetry. Photographs must be taken periodically during childhood, as well as before and after adolescent growth.

Standardized photographs can be used for panel-assessment of repaired bilateral cleft lip.[57] Although visual-perceptive analysis, using a predetermined rating scale, can be reliable, it is clumsy, time-consuming, and still subjective.

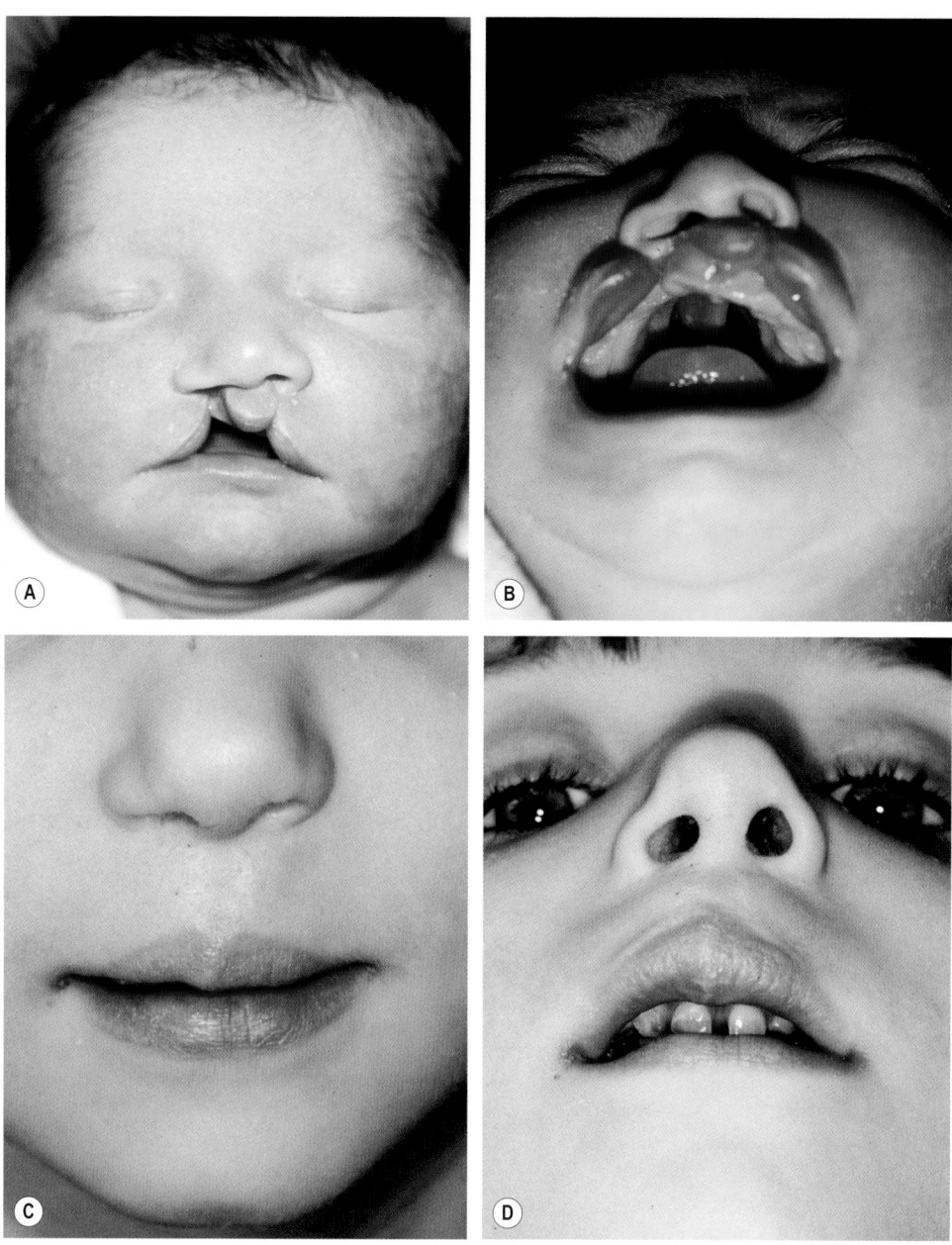

Fig. 24.18 **(A)** Asymmetrical bilateral cleft lip: right complete and left incomplete. **(B)** Bilateral complete cleft of secondary palate, submental view. **(C,D)** Age 6 years following first-stage right labial adhesion/gingivoperiosteoplasty and second-stage synchronous nasolabial repair.

Revision-rate

Most surgeons keep a mental tally of the kinds of revisions that are necessary after repair of a cleft lip. Documenting the types of secondary corrections guides the surgeon to make technical alterations during subsequent primary procedures. The surgeon's goal is to minimize the number of revisions. For a repaired bilateral deformity, the cutaneous lip should never need to be reopened; however, the nasal cartilages may require repositioning. The mucosal free margin often must be adjusted and, sometimes, nasal width has to be narrowed.

Symmetry is the one major advantage of a bilateral complete cleft lip as compared to a unilateral complete cleft lip. Any nasolabial asymmetry following closure and further distortions with growth will become increasingly obvious before the child attends school. These asymmetries remain relatively

unchanged during childhood; however, they often become magnified during adolescence. The age for kindergarten is a good time to assess the child for revision.

In a study of 50 consecutive nonsyndromic children (median age 5.4 years), the revision rate was 33% for those with bilateral complete cleft lip/palate as compared to 12% for those with bilateral complete cleft lip/alveolus and intact secondary palate.[58] The most common labial revision was resuspension of prolapsed anterior gingivolabial mucosa. This problem has since been minimized by trimming prolabial vermilion and securing the remaining mucosa to the premaxillary periosteum. Augmentation of a weak median tubercle with a dermal graft was also common; this was usually done at the time of alveolar bone grafting (age 9–11 years). Using the posterior iliac donor site, a thick dermal graft is easily taken, along with harvest of cancellous bone.[59]

The most frequent nasal distortion in this series was disproportionate widening of the inter-alar dimension; however, this rarely required correction during childhood. None of the children in this study required a secondary "columellar lengthening" or revision for an abnormally wide or long philtrum.

Given preoperative asymmetry, the revision-rate for asymmetrical bilateral cleft lip would be expected to differ slightly from that for the more common symmetrical complete forms. Indeed, our study showed the rate of nasolabial revision correlated with the degree of preoperative asymmetry between the greater and lesser sides. The lowest frequency of nasolabial revision was in the contralateral minor-form subgroup because symmetry is more likely achieved by synchronous bilateral correction. In contrast, the highest frequency of both nasal and labial revision (usually on the greater side) was in the contralateral mini-microform subgroup. This was predictable because the nearly normal configuration of a mini-microform makes it more difficult to attain primary symmetry. Conceptually, the complete/mini-microform type of bilateral cleft lip approaches the unilateral complete cleft lip deformity. In all of the contralateral lesser-forms, the most common labial deformity was a thin median tubercle, accentuated by a full mucosal free margin on the greater side. This deficiency of the tubercle can be explained by insufficient mesodermal contribution from the lesser side.

Reassessment of the frequency and types of nasolabial revisions must be undertaken after skeletal maturity. We analyzed the frequency of Le Fort I osteotomy and maxillary advancement in the major forms of bilateral cleft lip: 50% for bilateral incomplete or bilateral asymmetrical complete/incomplete and 75% for bilateral complete cleft lip/palate.[60] The high rate of maxillary advancement in our unit reflects our preference for operative correction for all patients with midfacial retrusion whatever the occlusal relationship. Le Fort I advancement is often combined with alloplastic onlay to the malar eminences to give a normal convex facial profile. Attempts to compensate for a small degree of maxillary retrusion at the dental level results in a relatively flat facial profile.

Revision-rate or need for secondary correction are essentially subjective criteria, i.e., the decision to proceed is determined by the surgeon's assessment and often made in agreement with the family and the older patient. Cephalometry has long been used by dental specialists to document skeletal growth in children with repaired cleft lip/palate. Similar quantitative methodology is needed to permit assessment of nasolabial appearance during childhood and adolescence.

Direct anthropometry

Farkas was the first to apply medical anthropometry to children with repaired bilateral cleft lip.[61] His reference book is invaluable.[62] It contains normative values for 28 nasal and 18 labial linear/angular measurements in a North American Caucasian population from birth (0–5 months and 6–12 months) and each year up to age 18. Direct anthropometry requires training, practice, and patience. The tools are a sliding Vernier caliper and a Castroviejo caliper. Locating the soft tissue landmarks and measuring nasolabial dimensions are usually easily accomplished in a child older than 5 years, but difficult-to-impossible in a younger child. Intraoperative anthropometry is used to assess severity of the deformity prior to the procedure and immediately after repair to record baseline nasolabial dimensions.[6] In an analysis of 46 consecutive repairs of bilateral complete cleft lip, intraoperative anthropometry confirmed the strategy of design in three dimensions in anticipation of the fourth dimension. All fast-growing nasolabial features were set smaller than age and sex-matched normal infants. The only exception was central vermilion-mucosal height (median tubercle) that purposely was made overly-full (on average 155% of normal). The slow-growing features, nasal protrusion and columellar height were also constructed longer than normal, 130% and 167%, respectively.

Direct anthropometry can be repeated as the child grows and compared to normal values based on sex and age. This was shown in a retrospective longitudinal analysis of 12 children with bilateral complete cleft lip who underwent repair with the same procedure as described herein.[4] Through age 4 years, nasal height and protrusion, as well as columellar length and width, were within 1 standard deviation of normal values. The interalar dimension was overly wide, about 1 standard deviation above normal. Nevertheless, the nose often did not appear wide because children with bilateral cleft lip tend to have minor orbital hypertelorbitism. The cutaneous lip was intentionally set short because this is less eye-catching than the typical long-lip appearance in these patients. Thus, total lip height was 1–2 standard deviations below normal, whereas, height of the median tubercle was 1 standard deviation above normal at 4 years. Fullness of the central red lip usually falls below normal in older children. Depending on the show of the permanent incisors, the median tubercle either is augmented or excess mucosa is trimmed. An example of a 8-year-old boy with repaired bilateral complete cleft lip/palate is shown in *Figure 24.19* with intraoperative and postoperative anthropometry.

Normative anthropometric measures are needed for the major ethnic groups. Farkas' book, in addition to Caucasian norms, includes data from Singapore for three age groups: 6 and 12 years (taken in school children) and 18 years (taken in army recruits and university students).[62] Indian anthropometry from infancy-to-adulthood is also available.[63] Kim and colleagues measured six nasolabial features in normal Korean children, age 5 years and younger, and compared the mean values to 30 children who had a modified "Mulliken repair" for three variants of bilateral cleft lip.[64] They found all nasolabial features were within 2 standard deviations of normal. Nasal tip protrusion and columellar length were below, whereas nasal width was slightly above, normal age-matched Korean noses.

Indirect anthropometry

Photogrammetry

Photogrammetry is the original type of indirect anthropometry. It eliminates any inaccuracies introduced in trying to measure the lip and nose in a frightened or fidgety child. However, measurements on two-dimensional photographs

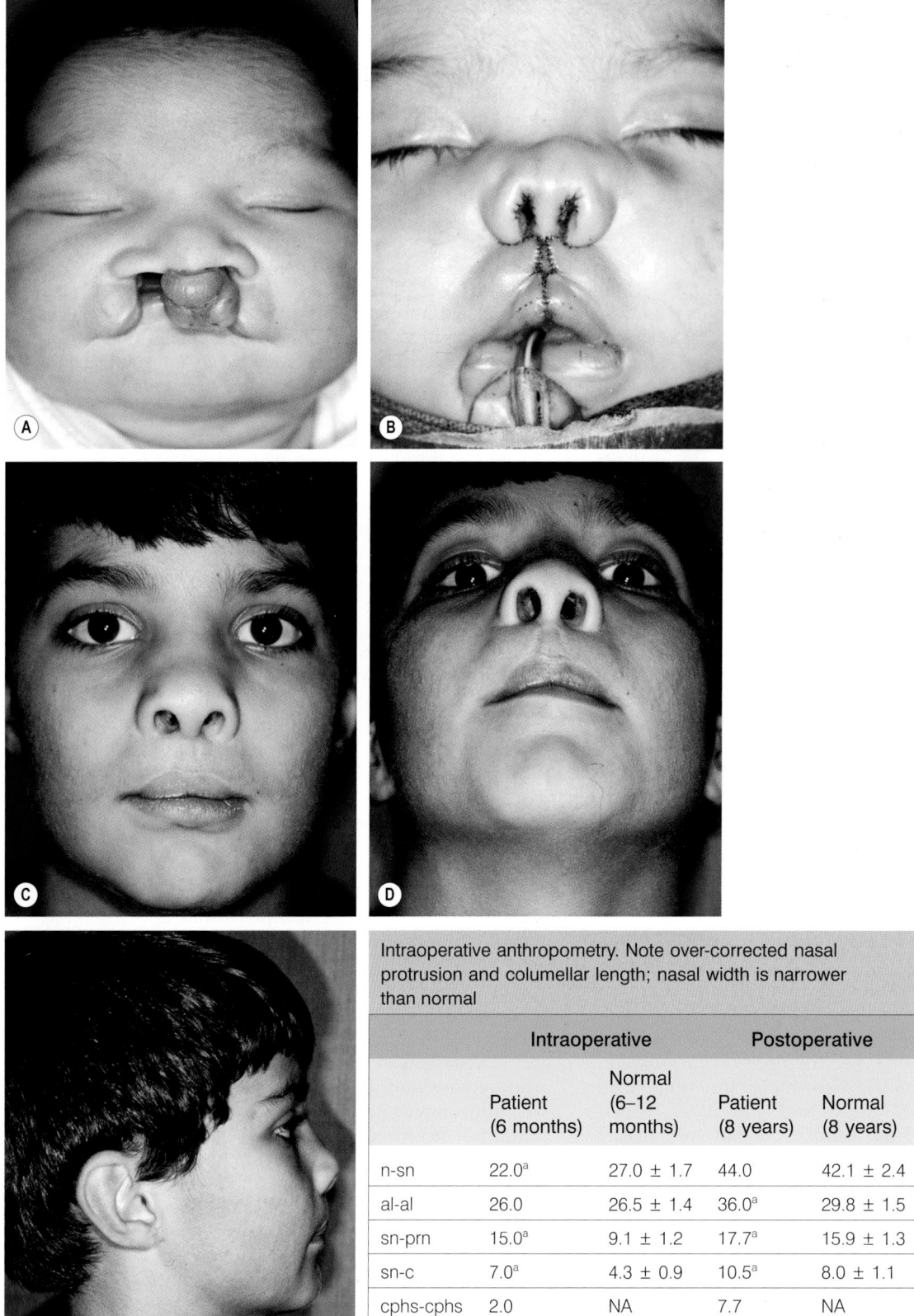

Intraoperative anthropometry. Note over-corrected nasal protrusion and columellar length; nasal width is narrower than normal

	Intraoperative		Postoperative	
	Patient (6 months)	Normal (6–12 months)	Patient (8 years)	Normal (8 years)
n-sn	22.0[a]	27.0 ± 1.7	44.0	42.1 ± 2.4
al-al	26.0	26.5 ± 1.4	36.0[a]	29.8 ± 1.5
sn-prn	15.0[a]	9.1 ± 1.2	17.7[a]	15.9 ± 1.3
sn-c	7.0[a]	4.3 ± 0.9	10.5[a]	8.0 ± 1.1
cphs-cphs	2.0	NA	7.7	NA
cphi-cphi	4.0[a]	6.7 ± 1.0	10.4[a]	8.8 ± 1.1
sn-ls	7.5[a]	11.4 ± 1.3	9.0[a]	14.0 ± 2.2
sn-sto	16.5	15.8 ± 1.5	16.0[a]	19.7 ± 1.8
ls-sto	7.0[a]	4.4 ± 1.0	7.8	8.0 ± 1.2

Normal values expressed as norm ± SD. [a]Values outside SD. NA, not available.

Fig. 24.19 (A) Bilateral complete cleft lip/palate. **(B)** Submental view following closure. **(C–E)** Appearance at age 8 years. Note nasal protrusion and columellar length are longer than normal; however nasal width and Cupid's bow width are above normal.

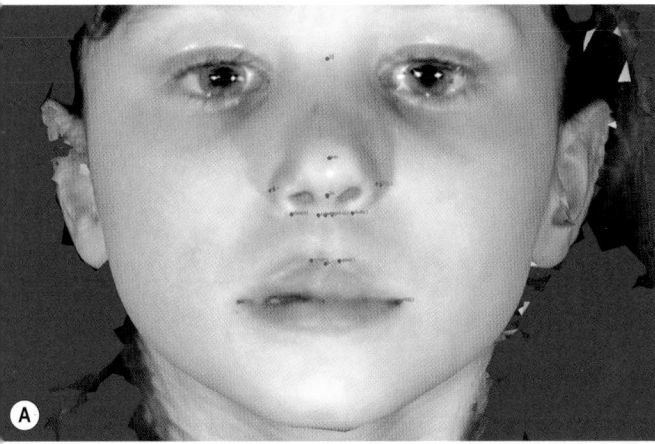

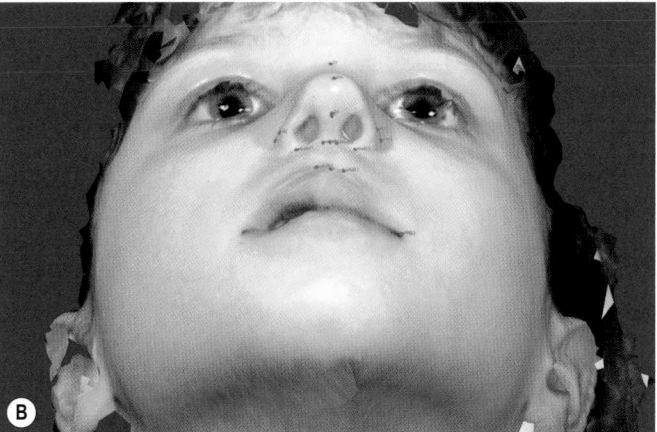

Intraoperative	Patient (6 months)	Normal (6–12 months)
n-sn	23.0[a]	26.9 ± 1.6
al-al	24.0[a]	25.4 ± 1.5
sn-prn	12.3[a]	9.7 ± 0.8
sn-c	6.0[a]	4.7 ± 0.8
cphs-cphs	2.0	NA
cphi-cphi	4.0[a]	6.5 ± 1.1
sn-ls	6.8[a]	10.7 ± 1.1
sn-sto	13.4[a]	16.0 ± 0.8
ls-sto	6.5	5.3 ± 1.4

Direct intraoperative anthropometric data on patient shown in Figure 24.18 (age 6 months).

Normal values expressed as norm ± SD. [a]Values outside SD. NA, not available.

Postoperative	Patient (6 years)	Normal (6 years)
n-sn	37.6	39.3 ± 2.7
al-al	26.5	27.5 ± 1.3
sn-prn	15.8[a]	14.5 ± 1.2
sn-c	L, 7.0; R, 6.4	7.5 ± 1.0
cphs-cphs	3.2	NA
cphi-cphi	6.7[a]	8.4 ± 1.3
sn-ls	11.5[a]	12.6 ± 1.3
sn-sto	20.3[a]	18.7 ± 1.7
ls-sto	9.7	8.0 ± 1.1

Indirect anthropometry (3D photogrammetry) at age 6 years (same patient as shown in Figure 24.18). Note changes in fast- and slow-growing features

Normal values expressed as norm ± SD. [a]Values outside SD. NA, not available.

Fig. 24.20 (A,B) Three-dimensional photogrammetry (Vectra® 3D imaging system): Anthropometric points located on frontal and submental images. (Same patient as in Figure 24.18.)

likely introduce errors due to magnification, variation in lightening, angulation, head position, and subject-to-camera distance. The magnification factor can be eliminated by including a standard metric in the photograph. Photogrammetry can only be used for linear measurements of certain nasolabial features, as well as for proportions and angles.[65] Examples of photogrammetric assessment in 15 patients with bilateral complete cleft lip, repaired by the operative techniques described herein, are found in a study by Kohout and colleagues.[66] The ratio of columellar length (sn-c) to nasal tip protrusion (sn-prn), the two slow-growing dimensions, was 0.47 ± 0.08, i.e., very close to the normal of 0.53 ± 0.02 at a mean age of 2 years. Changes in the columellar-labial angle were analyzed in a small cohort of children. This angle was obtuse in early childhood (128.5 ± 6.5°) (normal 102.5 ± 5.2°), but began narrowing after age 7 years and normalized by adolescence. Possible explanations for this change include either growth of the anterior-caudal septum, increasing obliquity of the lip, or increasing maxillary retrusion.

Liou and colleagues employed basilar photogrammetry to assess twenty-two young children with repaired bilateral complete cleft lip using the "NAM" protocol.[67] They determined that columellar length decreased in the 1st and 2nd years postoperatively, then started to increase in the 3rd year, but still lagged behind the normal length by 1.9 mm, whereas all other nasal dimensions increased significantly. Lee and co-workers also used photogrammetry to assess children who had undergone the NAM protocol and primary "retrograde" nasal correction.[68] They noted that columellar length was slightly less, but not statistically different, from a control group of children at an average age of 3 years.

Morovic and Cutting adapted some elements of primary nasal correction described herein and used photogrammetry with intermedial canthal distance as the scaling standard.[69] In 25 children, they calculated near normal columellar length and tip projection, but nasal width, columellar width, and nasolabial angles were significantly greater than the control values.

Stereophotogrammetry

Three-dimensional stereophotogrammetry is the most advanced way to quantitatively assess nasolabial appearance. Several systems are currently available: 3dMDface™ (3dMD,

Atlanta, GA) and Vectra® (Canfield Imaging Systems, Fairfield, NJ). The validity and reliability of these systems have been documented.[70,71] Synchronized high-resolution digital cameras capture images in milliseconds. Software algorithms merge the different overlapping images into a single three-dimensional image that can be viewed, turned in any direction, and analyzed on a computer. Standard anthropometric points are easily located after the image is appropriately maneuvered and the nasolabial dimensions are recorded *(Fig. 24.20)*. Furthermore, the digital images can be manipulated to calculate soft tissue projection and produce a numeric value for mirror-image symmetry of the nose or lip.

Conclusion

Every year, a cleft lip/palate team will treat only a few children born with a bilateral deformity or a variant. Every infant with this defect deserves a surgeon who has the requisite patience, precision, and passion to undertake the first operation. Indeed, the primary procedures are the major determinants of the child's appearance and ability to communicate. The surgeon also has the obligation to care for and assess these children well into adulthood – this requires singular commitment.

Access the complete reference list online at **http://www.expertconsult.com**

6.   Mulliken JB, Burvin R, Farkas LG. Repair of bilateral complete cleft lip: Intraoperative nasolabial anthropometry. *Plast Reconstr Surg.* 2001;107:307–314.

13.   Millard Jr DR. *Cleft Craft: The Evolution of Its Surgery.* Vol II. Boston: Little, Brown; 1977.

One definition of a "classic" is a great book that is often cited, but seldom read. In his conversational style of writing, Millard recounts the history of bilateral cleft lip repair as if he was an observer. The novice may find the organization of the book a little difficult to follow. Nevertheless, reading Millard's text is analogous to watching a master-surgeon in the operating room. The more experienced the visitor, the more gained by the experience.

44.   Cutting CB, Grayson BH, Brecht L, et al. Presurgical columellar elongation and primary retrograde nasal reconstruction in one-stage bilateral cleft lip and nose repair. *Plast Reconstr Surg.* 1998;101:630–639.

The article describes the prototype of a nasoalveolar molding appliance in preparation for synchronous nasolabial repair by Cutting's technique. The authors underscore that expansion of nasal lining is as important as stretching columellar skin. The principle of primary positioning the lower lateral cartilages is applied as described in this chapter; however, the technique differs.

45.   Yuzuriha S, Oh AK, Mulliken JB. Asymmetrical bilateral cleft lip: Complete or incomplete and contralateral lesser defect (minor-form, microform, or mini-microform). *Plast Reconstr Surg.* 2008;122:1494–1504.

This paper focuses on a subgroup of asymmetrical bilateral clefts that present with a lesser-form variant that is contralateral to a complete or incomplete cleft lip. The lesser-forms are defined based on extent of disruption at the vermilion-cutaneous junction: minor-form; microform, and mini-microform. These designations determine the methods of repair and correlate with frequency and types of revisions that are usually necessary.

55.   Mulliken JB, Burvin R, Padwa BL. Binderoid complete cleft lip/palate. *Plast Reconstr Surg.* 2003;111:1000–1010.

The authors define a rare subset of patients who have complete cleft lip/palate, nasolabiomaxillary underdevelopment, and orbital hypertelorism. One-half of the patients have a bilateral complete deformity, characterized by a diminutive single-toothed premaxilla. Necessary modifications in primary repair and in secondary correction of the hypoplastic soft tissue and skeletal elements are described.

57.   Lo L-J, Wong F-H, Mardini S, et al. Assessment of bilateral cleft lip nose deformity: A comparison of results as judged by cleft surgeons and laypersons. *Plast Reconstr Surg.* 2002;110:733–741.

58.   Mulliken JB, Wu JK, Padwa BL. Repair of bilateral cleft lip: Review, revisions, and reflections. *J Craniofac Surg.* 2003;14:609–620.

62.   Farkas LG, ed. *Anthropometry of the Head and Face.* 2nd edn. New York: Raven Press; 1994.

68.   Lee CT, Garfinkle JS, Warren SM, et al. Nasoalveolar molding improves appearance of children with bilateral cleft lip-cleft palate. *Plast Reconstr Surg.* 2008;122:1131–1137.

This study provides further proof of the principle of primary nasal correction. Photogrammetry was used to document columellar length in patients with bilateral cleft lip/palate who had nasal repair by the two-stage forked flap method versus primary nasal correction after nasoalveolar molding; both groups were compared to age-matched controls. Measurements to age 3 years showed nearly normal columellar length in the primary repair group without need for further nasal procedures, whereas secondary operations were recommended for all children who had forked flap columellar lengthening.

71.   Wong JY, Oh AK, Ohta E, et al. Validity and reliability of craniofacial anthropometric measurements of 3D digital photogrammetric images. *Cleft Palate Craniofac J.* 2008;45:232–239.

25

Cleft palate

William Y. Hoffman

SYNOPSIS

- Normal speech is the primary goal of cleft palate repair; minimizing effects of maxillary growth is also important but ultimately secondary.
- Cleft palate repair prior to 1 year of age (ideally 9–10 months) results in better speech outcomes than later repairs.
- The levator veli palatini muscle is longitudinally oriented in the cleft palate patient. Realignment of the muscle to a transverse and posterior position in the soft palate is the key to a successful functional result.
- Eustachian tube function is abnormal in cleft patients due to abnormal position of the tensor veli palatini muscle; this must be addressed in every cleft palate patient, usually with ventilating tubes.

Access the Historical Perspective section online at
http://www.expertconsult.com

Basic science

Embryology

The embryology of maxillary and palatal development is reviewed in detail in Chapter 21. In broad terms, the failure of fusion of the frontonasal and maxillary processes gives rise to the cleft of the primary palate, which includes the lip, alveolar process, and the hard palate anterior to the incisive foramen. This results in a cleft in the typical location between the premaxilla and the lateral maxilla, on either one or both sides. The lateral palatal shelves fuse later than the primary palate, around 7–8 weeks' gestation, as they rotate from vertical to horizontal orientation. This fusion proceeds from anterior to posterior, which helps to understand the spectrum of clefts of the secondary palate.

The levator palatini and other pharyngeal muscles are derived from the fourth branchial arch and are innervated by cranial nerve X (vagus). The sole exception to this is the tensor palatini muscle, which arises from the first branchial arch and is innervated by cranial nerve V (trigeminal).

Anatomy

Careful anatomic evaluation of each patient is of paramount importance in considering palatoplasty. Anatomic variability within the broad diagnosis of cleft palate will influence the timing and sequence of surgical repair as well as the type of repair. Optimal functional results depend directly on accurate analysis of the available structures and understanding of their long-term significance to function and facial growth (*Fig. 25.1*).

It is critical to understand the anatomy of the levator palatini muscle and the derangement of this anatomy that occurs in all clefts of the palate, including submucous cleft palate. Normally the levator muscle forms a transverse sling across the posterior half of the soft palate, and contraction causes the soft palate to move superiorly and posteriorly, contacting the posterior pharyngeal wall for velar closure, usually at the level of the adenoid pad. This action forms the characteristic "genu" seen on lateral views of the palate in motion.

In addition to being discontinuous across the cleft, the levator muscle runs more or less longitudinally along the cleft margin before it inserts aberrantly into the posterior border of the hard palate.[11–13] This results in ineffective contraction and inability to close the palate against the posterior pharyngeal wall. Air escape through the nose during speech produces a characteristic hypernasal quality. In addition, aberrant levator positioning as well as an abnormal fusion with the tendon of the tensor veli palatini muscle is thought to impair the function of the tensor muscle in assists with Eustachian tube function and is thought to be contributory to cleft otopathology.[14] A complete review of cleft otopathology is presented later in this chapter.

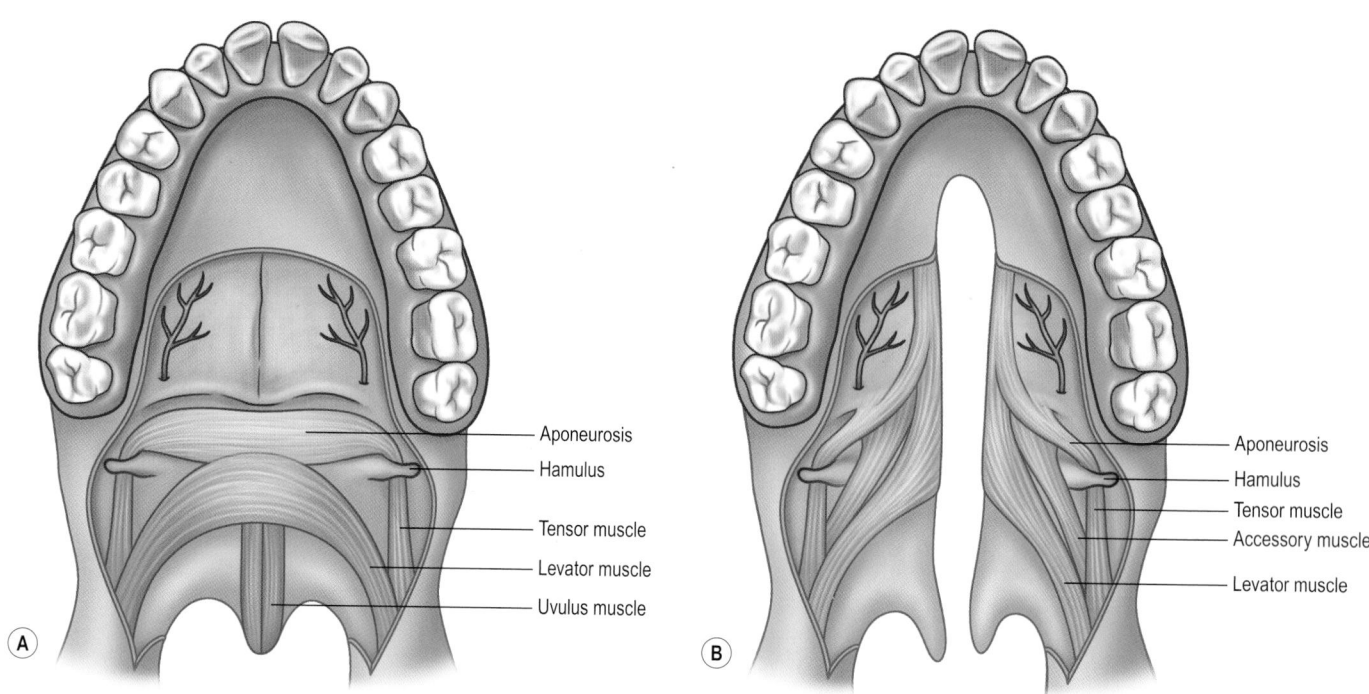

Fig. 25.1 **(A)** Normal anatomy: The levator veli palatini muscle can be seen forming a sling across the soft palate; the tensor veli palatini is shown coming around the hamulus to fuse with the levator. **(B)** Cleft palate: The muscles are seen running more or less parallel with the cleft margin.

Ear pathology

Alt was the first physician to note a correlation between ear disease and cleft palate in 1878.[15] Numerous studies have linked the presence of a cleft palate to abnormalities in Eustachian tube function. In multicenter studies, incidence of otitis media effusion has been found to be 96–100% in cleft patients, measured by both middle ear effusions on otoscopy and impedance testing and middle ear aspiration.[16,17] In the cleft palate, impairment of tubal dilation is thought to occur from complex misalignment of the paratubal musculature.[18,19] Both radiologic and manometric testing techniques have demonstrated abnormalities in active dilation of the eustachian tube.[20] In addition, intrinsic abnormalities of tubal cartilage framework rendering a Eustachian tube more collapsible have been noted. Although anatomic studies show that the levator veli palatini muscle does not directly actively open the Eustachian tube orifice, it is likely to have a secondary effect by influence on the tensor veli palatini and also with passive position of the orifice. The levator and tensor do share a common tendinous insertion near the hamulus and pulley position around the hamulus. In the cleft patient, the levator is connected solidly against the rigid posterior hard palate; the pulley effect around the hamulus cannot be activated and impairs opening of the tube. In addition, some theorize that constant bathing of the tube orifice with oropharyngeal refluxed material leads to inflammation and obstruction of drainage. Other studies have demonstrated adenoidal tissue at the level of the tubal dilator that could potentially contribute to mechanical obstruction.[21] Anatomic paratubal abnormalities and risk for serous otitis media and chronic audio-logic sequelae are present, regardless of cleft type, although Pierre Robin sequence has been postulated to be at even higher risk

for hearing loss because of potential for concomitant ossicular malformation.[22]

Chronic obstruction of drainage leads to serous otitis media, and long-standing effusion can result in hearing loss. Estimates are 20–30% incidence of pure tone hearing loss in cleft patients by audiography[23]; decreased hearing has been found in as many as half of cleft palate patients by other authors.[24] Untreated children with clefts and severe effusions may have total deafness. Whereas hearing loss is significant in any child, it may be even more so in a cleft patient in whom speech development may be abnormal.

It has long been suggested that closure of the palate reduces risk of permanent hearing loss. In retrospective studies, children who had undergone palatoplasty had significantly lower incidence of permanent hearing loss than did children with unrepaired cleft palates.[24] Although still controversial, palatoplasty is thought by most surgeons to reduce risk of chronic serous otitis media and hearing loss, although not by universal agreement. Nevertheless, serous otitis persists in most cleft patients for several years after palate repair, and myringotomy with placement of ventilating tubes remains the mainstay of treatment for this difficult problem.

Patient presentation

Cleft palate with cleft lip and alveolus

Although the primary palate and the secondary palate form at different stages of embryonic development, cleft palate is most commonly seen in combination with cleft lip. The alveolar portion of the cleft lies between the maxillary lateral incisor and canine tooth roots. This results in malposition of the maxillary lateral incisor and cuspid in both the deciduous and permanent dentition.[25,26] The maxillary lateral incisor on the cleft side is absent in 80–90% of cleft patients; when present, it may be smaller than the contralateral tooth or significantly dysmorphic[26–28] Absence of other teeth is not uncommon,[29] but it may be related to the surgery itself because adults who have not been operated on do not show the same patterns of hypodontia.[30] Asymmetry is common, resulting in alterations in first maxillary molar position.[31–33] In comparison to noncleft individuals, patients with unilateral cleft lip and palate have overall reduction in crown size[34] and delay of eruption of permanent dentition.[35] These findings support the theory of global dental growth potential disturbance associated with clefting. Interestingly, eruption of deciduous dentition is not significantly delayed.[36]

Unilateral complete cleft palate is characterized by direct communication between the entire length of the nasal passage and oropharynx. The nasal septum is deviated and buckled toward the cleft side. The absence of a portion of the inferior piriform aperture and the hypoplasia of the lateral nasal bony platform at the maxillary wall contribute to the cleft nasal deformity; the nasal base is depressed, the ala collapses, and the floor widens. The unilateral complete cleft is thus a full-thickness palatal defect of nasal mucosa, bony palate, velar musculature, and oral mucosa; all of these deficiencies must be addressed during the cleft palate repair or later at the time of alveolar cleft bone grafting.

In the bilateral complete cleft lip and palate, the premaxillary segment containing the central and lateral incisor tooth roots is discontinuous from the alveolar arch. The lateral segments often collapse inward and lingually, resulting in "locking out" of the premaxilla. Preoperative management with presurgical infant orthopedics (PSIO) may help prevent or treat lateral segment collapse and correct the anterior position of the premaxilla. If untreated, the anterior location of the premaxilla in this situation may result in anterior fistulas, which may in turn cause significant speech problems and nasal regurgitation of fluid. Later orthodontic treatment of the maxillary arch can align the segments before bone grafting.

Kernahan proposed a standardized reporting form to distinguish the variable presentations of cleft lip and palate, shown in *(Fig. 25.2)*.

Clefts of the secondary palate

Also called incomplete cleft palate, a cleft of the secondary palate may be variable, from an opening in the posterior soft palate to a cleft extending up to the incisive foramen. There is almost always a separation of the bony shelves of the hard palate, which is variable but may extend anteriorly to the incisive foramen. Most commonly, dentition is normal and symmetric.

Submucous cleft palate

Submucous cleft palate occurs when the palate has mucosal continuity but the underlying levator palatini muscle is discontinuous across the midline and longitudinally oriented, similar to the muscle anatomy in overt clefts of the palate. Calnan's classic triad of a midline clear zone (zona pellucida), a bifid uvula and a palpable notch in the posterior hard palate

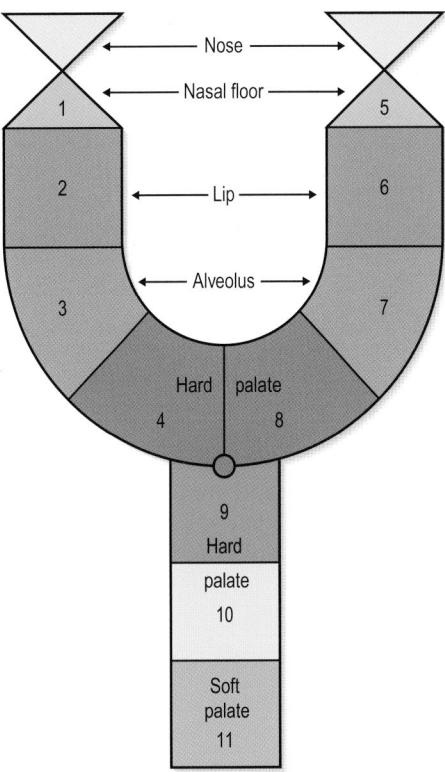

Fig. 25.2 Kernahan's classification of clefts allows for standardized reporting of the severity of both cleft lip and palate.

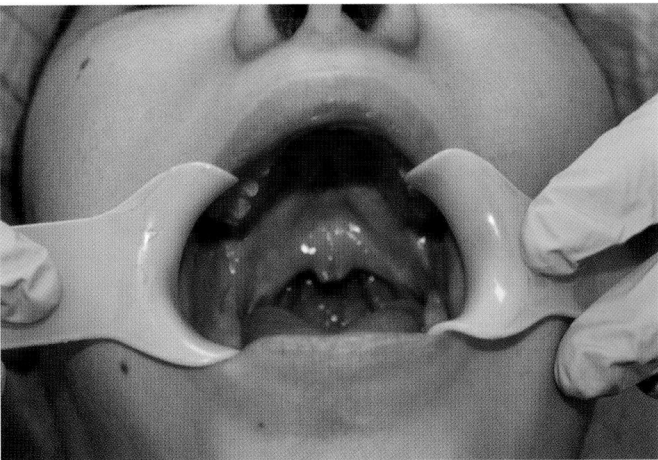

Fig. 25.3 Submucous cleft palate – note bifid uvula and thinning of central palate. On palpation there is a notch in the posterior hard palate rather than a posterior nasal spine.

is diagnostic of this condition. With contraction of velar musculature, a distinct midline muscle diastasis may be seen *(Fig. 25.3)*.

The significance of a submucous cleft may be difficult to assess clinically; the child with submucous cleft palate is often undiagnosed in infancy. In a study screening a large population of schoolchildren in Denver, the overall incidence of submucous cleft palate in the population was found to be 1 : 1200.[37] Another similar cohort study reported that 45–55% of patients with isolated submucous cleft palate were symptomatic with regard to speech, serous otitis media, or hearing loss.[38,39] In a large series of children with submucous cleft palate in Mexico, examination with fiberoptic nasendoscopy showed about one-third to have velopharyngeal insufficiency.[40] Other attempts to identify risk of speech problems with submucous cleft palate have been problematic because referrals to cleft palate clinics are usually based on the identification of speech issues rather than of the submucous cleft itself. Therefore, an infant identified with submucous cleft palate need not routinely undergo repair because a significant number of individuals with submucous cleft palate will not develop velopharyngeal insufficiency. Rather, these patients should be closely monitored with serial speech evaluations and audiometric surveillance.

Patients who present with velopharyngeal insufficiency and submucous cleft palate on examination require full evaluation, including speech evaluation and endoscopy.[41] Even in the absence of obvious findings on clinical examination, anatomic abnormalities are found in most patients (>90%) at the time of surgery[42,43]; thus, the so-called occult submucous cleft palate is simply one that is less obvious on clinical evaluation. There will still be rare patients, however, who have true palatopharyngeal disproportion and present with velopharyngeal insufficiency without any cleft, submucous or otherwise.

Corrective surgical technique for submucous cleft palate is focused on anatomic correction of the velar muscle diastasis. Although pharyngeal flaps and sphincter pharyngoplasty have been proposed as primary means of treatment,[40] most surgeons focus on repair of the abnormal levator muscle position.[44] The Furlow double opposing Z-plasty (see below) is an ideal procedure for these patients because there is no width discrepancy to be overcome.[45] This avoids the potential for nasal obstruction and sleep apnea in these patients if a pharyngeal flap is used.

Pierre Robin sequence

Pierre Robin described the triad of micrognathia, glossoptosis, and respiratory distress.[46] Of the children diagnosed with Pierre Robin sequence, 60–90% have cleft palate[47,48]; the palatal cleft is usually isolated to the velum and can be V shaped or, more typically, U-shaped.[49,50] In the past, this has been thought to be secondary to hyperflexion of the head in utero with resultant displacement of the tongue between the palatal shelves, preventing their fusion. More recently, extensive analysis of multiple syndromes associated with Pierre Robin sequence has delineated genetic associations, indicating that the etiology may not be such a simple mechanical event.[51–53] Infants with Pierre Robin sequence also have increased incidence of associated anomalies, particularly cardiac and renal problems.[54]

Newborns with Pierre Robin sequence may have severe respiratory and feeding difficulty because of the posterior displacement of the tongue. Initial treatment consists of placing the child prone and use of gastric lavage feeding tubes to push the tongue forward.[55] Nasal airways have been used for the same purpose with reported success rates of 80–90%.[56] If these conservative measures fail, surgical management of the airway may be required. A tongue-lip adhesion has been used as an alternative to tracheostomy and is generally effective.[57,58] More recently, mandibular distraction

osteogenesis has been used in neonates with success in averting tracheostomy, although long-term outcomes in regard to mandibular growth and dental development are not yet available.[59] In all cases, if management is focused on the upper airway, bronchoscopy should be performed to rule out any intrinsic subglottic problems (e.g., laryngomalacia) that might necessitate tracheotomy.

Palatoplasty in children with Pierre Robin sequence must be carefully timed with growth of the child, particularly the mandible. There is some controversy about "catch-up" growth of the mandible in children with Pierre Robin sequence; basically, there is good documentation of extra growth in the first year of life,[60,61] but growth is subsequently commensurate with that of normal children. Children with syndromes tend to have less growth than nonsyndromic cases. Late cephalometric evaluation has consistently shown that the children with Pierre Robin sequence have smaller mandibles than normal.[62] Closure of the palate narrows the effective area for respiration and can lead to respiratory distress. If the mandible attains reasonable size in the first year of life, palate repair can still be performed safely before 1 year of age. In the rare patient who has previously undergone tracheostomy, the palate should be repaired before decannulation. The risk of airway compromise after palatoplasty reaches 25%, with an emergent tracheostomy or reintubation rate of 11% at one institution.[63]

Syndromes

Multiple malformations or syndromes have been found frequently in cleft patients.[64] Cleft palate without associated cleft lip has been reported to be associated with a syndrome in as many as 50% of cases, while cleft lip and palate together have an incidence of syndromes of about 30%. Van der Woude syndrome is associated with a mutation in the interferon regulatory factor 6 (IRF6) gene that also causes popliteal pterygium syndrome; this is an autosomal dominant syndrome associated with lower lip sinus tracts ("lip pits"), and has variable penetrance including the full range of cleft lips as well as palates.

Children with cleft palate associated with an identified syndrome must be evaluated thoroughly and have individualized planning and timing of therapy. Infants with profound developmental delay and severely shortened life span projection should have surgical intervention delayed or should undergo palatoplasty under special circumstances only. In addition, syndromic children may have increased incidence of cardiac anomalies, requiring specific anesthetic and postoperative considerations. Repair of cleft palate in the hope that this will stimulate or allow a severely disabled child to speak gives unreasonable expectations and hope to parents; as noted before, it is critical to explain that palate repair may aid speech production but not speech development. Palate repair in severely disabled children can lead to altered airway status and obstructed upper airway in those with neuromuscular delay.

22q chromosomal deletion

Velocardiofacial syndrome, which is associated with a 22q chromosomal deletion, is detected by fluorescent immunohybridization (FISH). These children have a and the velocity of skeletal growth during puberty was blunted. However, duration of puberty and pubertal skeletal growth were prolonged an average of 1 year, resulting in final attained body height and radius length the same as those of control subjects.[69]

Numerous causes are thought to contribute to these differences in growth patterns. There are certainly feeding difficulties early in life before palate repair,[70] but it has also been suggested that intrinsic growth disturbances may be responsible for slow postnatal growth.[71] The increased frequency of ear and airway infections has been implicated in early growth retardation,[65] as have the multiple operative procedures that these children undergo.[70] Adding more confusion to the etiology is the fact that growth hormone levels may be diminished in cleft children. In summary, any growth disturbance is likely to be of multifactorial origin throughout infancy, childhood, and puberty. Fortunately, families can be counseled that most children attain norms of height, weight, and development.

Feeding and swallowing

The intact palate provides a barrier between the respiratory tract and the alimentary tract. To understand the difficulty cleft infants have with feeding, one must understand the normal role of the palate in sucking and swallowing. Oral intake is divided into two separate activities, generation of suction force (negative intraoral pressure) and swallowing. For negative intraoral pressure to be produced, the velum seals off the pharynx posteriorly; the lips close anteriorly, and negative pressure is produced by moving the tongue away from the palate and by opening the mandible. This effectively increases the intraoral volume within a closed system, resulting in generation of negative pressure. If the individual is unable to close the nasopharynx or to generate a seal of the lips, or if the palate is not intact at the point of contact with the tongue, negative pressure cannot be produced. This failure of velopharyngeal closure is the basis of difficulty with breast-feeding or normal bottle-feeding in the patient with cleft palate.

Suction on the nipple in a breast-feeding infant is thought to stabilize the nipple position while motion of the tongue against the nipple pushes fluid into the mouth. Ingestion through an artificial nipple is different; infants learn to manipulate the nipple and flow rates by closing the alveolus against the artificial nipple. Tongue motion is primarily used to transfer the bolus to the pharynx for swallowing. In the cleft infant, the communication between the oropharynx and nasopharynx prevents a seal of the tongue against the palate, and negative pressure cannot be generated. Suckling is therefore not productive, and breast-feeding is ineffective.

Most infants with clefts are unable to breast-feed. Infants with clefting limited to the posterior velum can often use posterior tongue position to generate a partial negative seal. The exception to this is the child with Pierre Robin sequence and isolated velar cleft, who can develop respiratory distress or ineffective suction from glossoptosis. Obviously, patients with isolated cleft lip and an intact palate should and do have little difficulty with breast-feeding.

Infants who are unable to breast-feed because of cleft palate have a number of options for feeding. Regimens and devices have evolved to nourish the infant, including specialty nipples

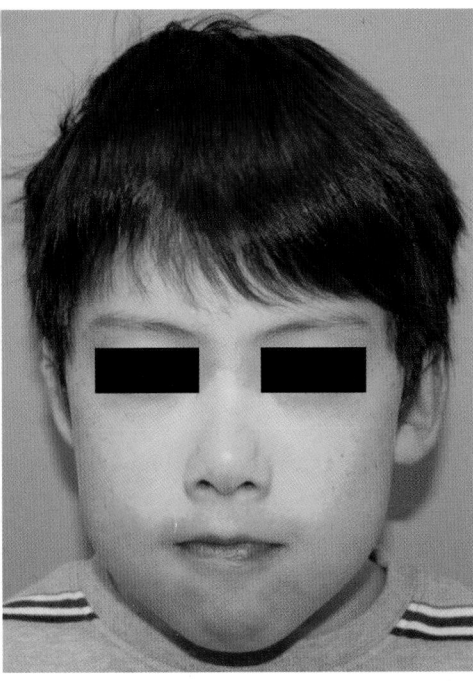

Fig. 25.4 Child with 22q. Note epicanthal folds, small nose.

characteristic "bird-like" facial appearance, soft palate dysfunction, developmental delay, and various cardiac conditions (*Fig. 25.4*). The same deletion gives rise to DiGeorge syndrome with associated B-cell and immune dysfunction; these children all need appropriate immunology referral and follow-up. The majority of these children does not have overt cleft palate and may not even have submucous clefts; usually the velar dysfunction is related to absence of movement of an otherwise normal soft palate. This may complicate decision-making, regarding surgery for speech in these patients.

Growth

At birth, the average weight is the same for cleft and unaffected newborns.[65,66] However, cleft infants have been shown to exhibit poor weight gain in early infancy. Studies observing infants with cleft lip and palate show initial growth retardation by the time they undergo surgical lip repair. When the same children reach the age for palatoplasty, they have significantly lagged on the growth curve. However, longitudinal studies show that after repair of the palate, average growth returns to normal compared with unaffected children by the age of 4 years. Stratification of risk within the longitudinal cohort shows pronounced growth retardation in associated syndromes and also in children with isolated clefts of the secondary palate.[67,68]

Children with orofacial clefting stabilize and continue normal growth to at least 6 years of age, with no statistically significant differences in height and weight when compared to unaffected children. In later childhood, however, average weight and height of children with cleft appear to diminish compared with those of control subjects. In a Danish study of skeletal maturity assessing both body height and radius length as an index of growth in male cleft patients, onset of puberty was found to be delayed on average by 6 months,

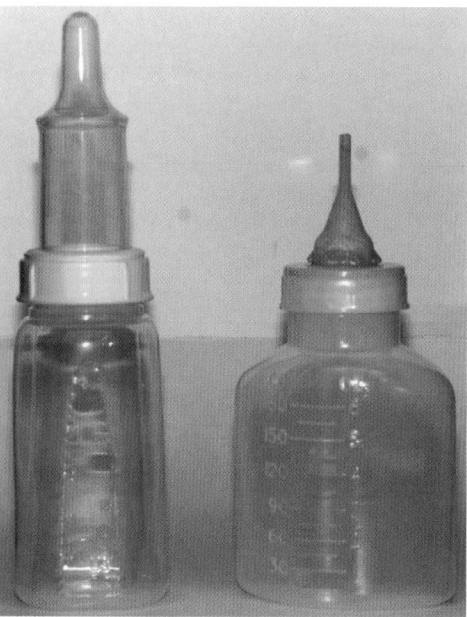

Fig. 25.5 Specialized bottles for cleft palate feeding. Left, Haberman feeder with reservoir in continuity with nipple. Right, Mead–Johnson feeder, which requires squeezing the bottle to improve flow of fluid.

such as lamb's nipples, crosscutting of standard nipples, and long soft nipples that place the liquid at the posterior tongue. Special flow bottles such as gravity flow and squeeze bottles allow the caregiver to carefully control the flow rate *(Fig. 25.5)*. The strategy of each technique is low resistance to flow, with controllable flow rate for optimal volume and minimal effort by the infant. All of these techniques are effective, and selection is generally by personal preference and the baby's acceptance of the method. Other key considerations are elevated head positioning during feeding and careful observation of feeding time and volume ingested.[72–75]

Swallowing involves a complex interaction of the tongue and pharynx. Coordinated swallowing is dependent on neuromuscular control and rhythmic coordinated contraction of the tongue and pharynx. Children with clefts generally do *not* have difficulty with swallowing and aspiration unless intrinsic neuromuscular abnormality of the tongue or pharynx is present. It is an error to ascribe aspiration simply to the presence of a cleft palate; indeed, aspiration with swallowing should stimulate an appropriate diagnostic evaluation, including thin barium swallow studies, bronchoscopy, and gastroscopy. Children may cough or sputter with reflux of the ingested material into the nose, particularly if volume or rate of feeding is excessive. During normal deglutition, the tongue moves the food bolus to the pharynx by complex interaction of tongue against palate. When the palate has an open cleft, food may reflux into the nasal passage. Nasal reflux is irritating to the nasal mucosa and can predispose to sinusitis and ulceration. In the older child, a persistent communication through a fistula in the palate may result in regurgitation of food through the nose, which is socially unacceptable.

Weight gain and skeletal growth confirm success of the feeding regimen. Once the palate is successfully closed surgically, special feeding methods are generally unnecessary.

Speech

The primary goal of palatoplasty is normal speech. Patients can grow and even thrive, despite feeding difficulties, but speech cannot be normalized if the palate is not repaired. The ability to partition the oropharynx and nasopharynx is crucial for normal speech production. The palate elevates during production of any sounds requiring positive pressure in the oropharynx; the levator palatini is primarily responsible for this movement *(Fig. 25.6)*.

Speech is a complex issue, and many factors may influence speech development in a child with a cleft palate. In addition to the importance of the palate itself, speech development may be influenced by motor or neurologic developmental delay (often seen in syndromes), by hearing, and by environmental stimuli. It is important to distinguish between speech production, which is primarily dependent on normal anatomic function, and speech development, which is influenced more by global developmental issues. Speech production also requires normal articulation, which in turn depends on tongue placement, lip competence, and dental position, all of which may be abnormal in cleft patients.[76]

If palate function is not corrected, velopharyngeal insufficiency results, with speech that is hypernasal, often with hoarse quality due to difficulty in directing airflow through the mouth. When complete closure cannot be anatomically or functionally obtained, compensatory mechanisms for sound production are learned. These are maladaptive patterns that interfere with global intelligibility and include glottal stops and pharyngeal fricatives. In addition, tongue placement for various phonemes is altered to achieve the most normal production of sounds. Eliminating these learned compensatory articulations is difficult, even with the best of speech and language therapy. Compensatory articulations may persist even in the face of a functional palate repair, especially in later repairs or secondary correction of velopharyngeal insufficiency.

Timing of palate repair

The normal palate serves several important functions, all related to functional separation of the oropharynx from the nasopharynx. Whereas the sine qua non for palate repair is normal speech, consideration of cleft palate surgery must balance developmental, dentofacial growth, and otologic issues as well.

Speech

The driving force for palatoplasty is the development of normal speech. Two crucial aspects of palatoplasty are important in optimal speech outcome: (1) surgical technique and (2) timing of palate repair. Victor Veau[11] first made the observation of a correlation between age at repair and speech outcome in 1931. He noted that children who had undergone repair before 12 months of age were much more likely to have normal speech than those with repair between 2 and 4 years of age. Children who underwent repair after 9 years of age had the worst speech outcome. The optimal time of palatoplasty still remains scientifically unproven. Confounding

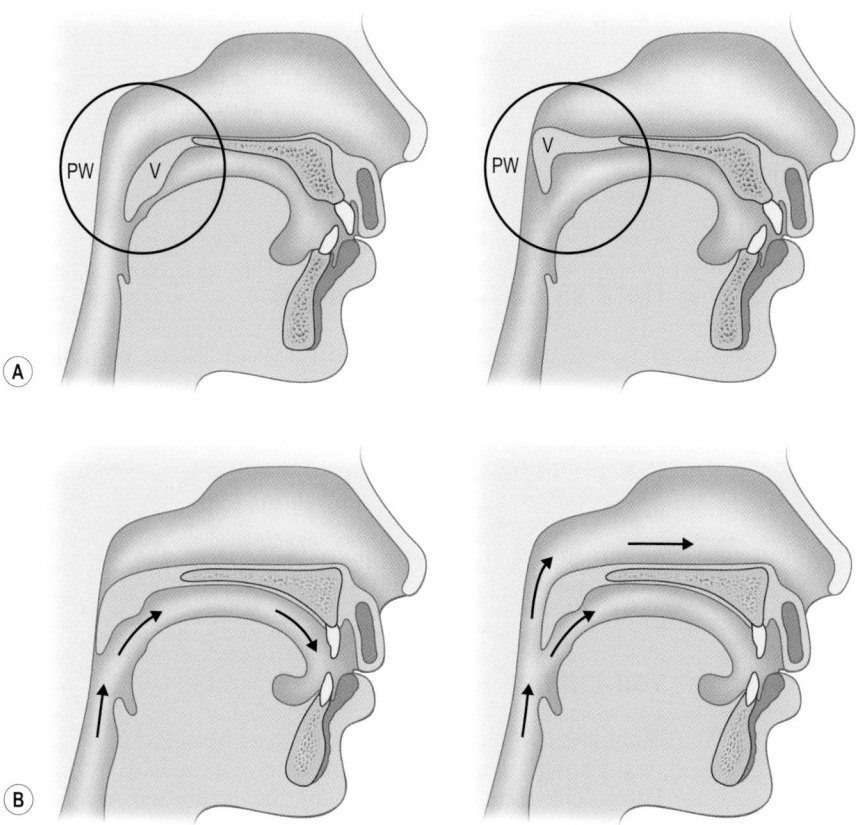

Fig. 25.6 (A) In the lateral cephalogram, the soft palate or velum ('V') is shown at rest (above left) and during speech, making contact with the posterior pharyngeal wall ('PW') (below right). **(B)** This line drawing shows the air flow during normal speech (left), with the velum making contact with the posterior pharynx to direct air out the mouth. If the velum is too short or movement is inadequate (right), air can escape through the nose during speech, creating velopharyngeal insufficiency (VPI).

variables of technique, surgeon's skill, lack of standardization of speech evaluations, and therapies preclude exact determination of optimal age at repair.[77]

Most would agree that the best speech results are correlated with closure of the palate near the time of the infant's beginning language acquisition, which for the normal-developing child is before 12 months of age.[78,79] Indeed, there is a body of evidence that phonologic development actually begins earlier, at 4–6 months of age.[80,81] Most studies of the timing of palatal repair have looked at secondary outcomes; increased compensatory articulations were shown in one study and increased need for pharyngeal flaps in another when the palate was repaired after 1 year of age. Although repairs before 1 year of age are now common, this is not a rigid chronologic milestone; rather, repair should be related to the child's speech development. Some studies have shown that if correction occurs even as late as 21 months, compensatory maladaptive patterns are infrequent. Despite the absence of hard evidence supporting earlier palate repairs, a growing body of opinion seems to support palate repair around 9–10 months of age for children with apparently normal development.[82,83] Very early repair of the palate (6 months or younger) has been proposed by some surgeons,[84–87] primarily as a means of improving feeding; however, long-term results are lacking for any large cohort of these patients. Prospective longitudinal assessment is currently in progress to attempt to better define the optimal timing of cleft repair.

Maxillary growth

Palatoplasty has been shown to detrimentally affect maxillary growth. Cephalometric analysis of adults with unrepaired cleft palate has shown normal maxillary dimensions and growth.[88,89] There is experimental evidence that the lip repair may restrict sagittal growth of the maxilla,[90,91] but in most patients, it seems that the palate repair is more significant. Many children with repaired cleft palate display typical findings of transverse maxillary deficiency requiring orthodontic widening of the maxilla once permanent teeth have erupted.

Transverse growth of the maxillary arch is narrowed in comparison with that in noncleft patients, resulting in typical malocclusion traits of crowding, lateral cross-bite, and open bite.[31,92–94] Whether the narrowed arch and maxillary growth inhibition result from surgical scarring[95,96] or intrinsic maxillary underdevelopment remains a matter of debate; most likely it is a combination of the two. There may be a sagittal growth deficiency as well; whereas 35–40% of children will develop an anterior crossbite, as many as 15–20% of children with cleft palate go on to require a Le Fort I maxillary advancement in some series. There is some evidence that the development of cross-bite and maxillary hypoplasia may be related to the severity of the original cleft.[97,98]

Although it might seem preferable to wait until a more advanced age for palate repair, given the growth effects on the maxilla, it is far more difficult to establish normal speech in older children after cleft repair than to correct occlusion with a combination of orthodontic treatment and orthognathic surgery.

Palate repair in the syndromic patient

Multiple malformations or syndromes have been found frequently in cleft patients.[64] Children with cleft palate associated with an identified syndrome must be evaluated thoroughly and have individualized planning and timing of therapy. Infants with profound developmental delay and severely shortened life span projection should have surgical intervention delayed or should undergo palatoplasty under special circumstances only. In addition, syndromic children may have increased incidence of cardiac anomalies, requiring specific anesthetic and postoperative considerations. Repair of cleft palate in the hope that this will stimulate or allow a severely disabled child to speak gives unreasonable expectations and hope to parents; as noted before, it is critical to explain that palate repair may aid speech production but not speech development. Palate repair in severely disabled children can lead to altered airway status and obstructed upper airway in those with neuromuscular delay.

Treatment/surgical technique

Technical considerations

A number of perioperative considerations must be addressed regardless of the type of repair used. The general health and the developmental status of the child play a role in the timing of the palate repair and are also important for anesthetic and surgical management. Audiology evaluation is routinely obtained preoperatively so that the otolaryngologist can place ventilating tubes in the tympanic membranes if indicated, saving the child an additional anesthetic.

The use of a RAE endotracheal tube facilitates placement of the Dingman gag without kinking the tube. The airway must be assessed constantly for problems; if lower central teeth are present, this can be a source of tube compression against the retractor. The Dingman gag, the most commonly used instrument for exposure, compresses the tongue and causes ischemia; if it is used for longer than 2 h, significant postoperative tongue swelling can occur. Lidocaine 0.5% and epinephrine 1 : 200 000 are infiltrated into the palate 7–10 min before incision; use of a 3-mL syringe makes the injection into the hard palate somewhat easier than with a larger syringe. A maximum of 1 mL/kg is used.

Palate repair is performed with the surgeon at the child's head, with use of a fiberoptic headlight or retractor. A rolled towel under the shoulders will extend the neck; it is important to assure that the child does not have any syndromes that predispose to cervical spine anomalies. The use of curved needle holders facilitates suture placement without obstruction of vision.

The most important aspect of surgical anatomy is the location of the greater palatine neurovascular bundle, which emerges through the greater palatine foramen through the lateral posterior hard palate. Incisions on each side are best made with the surgeon's contralateral hand to bevel the

incision away from the vascular pedicle. Circumferential freeing of the palatal attachments around the pedicle and gentle stretching of the pedicle out of the foramen are essential to obtain a tension-free closure of the oral flap.[99] In general, the goal is to obtain complete nasal and oral closure from front to back. In wide clefts, this may not be possible, particularly on the nasal surface. The most difficult area for closure, around the junction of the hard and soft palate, is the most common location for fistulas.

Hard vs soft palate closure

It is easier to understand cleft palate surgery by separating techniques used for the hard palate from those used for the soft palate. In general, all techniques use some form of mucoperiosteal flap for the hard palate closure; the soft palate repair emphasizes correction of the abnormal position of the levator palatini muscles. The location of the incision along the cleft margin can be varied to include more or less mucosa to be turned over for nasal lining. In the discussion below, the hard palate techniques are discussed first followed by soft palate closure.

von Langenbeck

Bernhard von Langenbeck introduced the use of mucoperiosteal flaps to close clefts of the secondary palate in the late 1800s. The initial description of the technique involved a simple approximation of the cleft margins with a relaxing incision that began posterior to the maxillary tuberosity and followed the posterior portion of the alveolar ridge. Some variation of the Langenbeck repair is still used commonly for clefts of the secondary palate. Intravelar veloplasty, or repair of the levator palatini muscle, as described below, is added today to reproduce the normal muscle sling (*Fig. 25.7*).

V-Y pushback (Veau–Wardill–Kilner)

George Dorrance (1877–1949) of Philadelphia realized that a distinct number of patients with cleft would develop velopharyngeal dysfunction caused by inability of the soft palate to touch the posterior pharyngeal wall.[100,101] In fact, he advocated muscle transposition but did so by fracturing the hamulus, which he believed would change the vector of muscle contraction and in combination with techniques of Langenbeck would lengthen the palate. He also advocated division of the major palatine neurovascular bundles to assist with the pushback. Thomas Kilner (1896–1964) was important in development of the V-Y palate repair along with Victor Veau and William E M Wardill (1893–1960). In addition, he pushed for palate repair at an earlier age, 12–18 months.[102]

The essence of the pushback repair is the central V incision on the hard palate that is then closed in a straight line, creating length on the oral side of the closure (*Fig. 25.8*). The initial description included osteotomy of the posterior hard palate at the greater palatine foramina to release the palatine vessels; circumferential dissection with release of the periosteum behind the vessels was subsequently advocated to stretch the vessels, which works as well with less risk of injury to this vital blood supply.[99,103] The nasal tissue is released and left open; some authors have proposed providing nasal lining

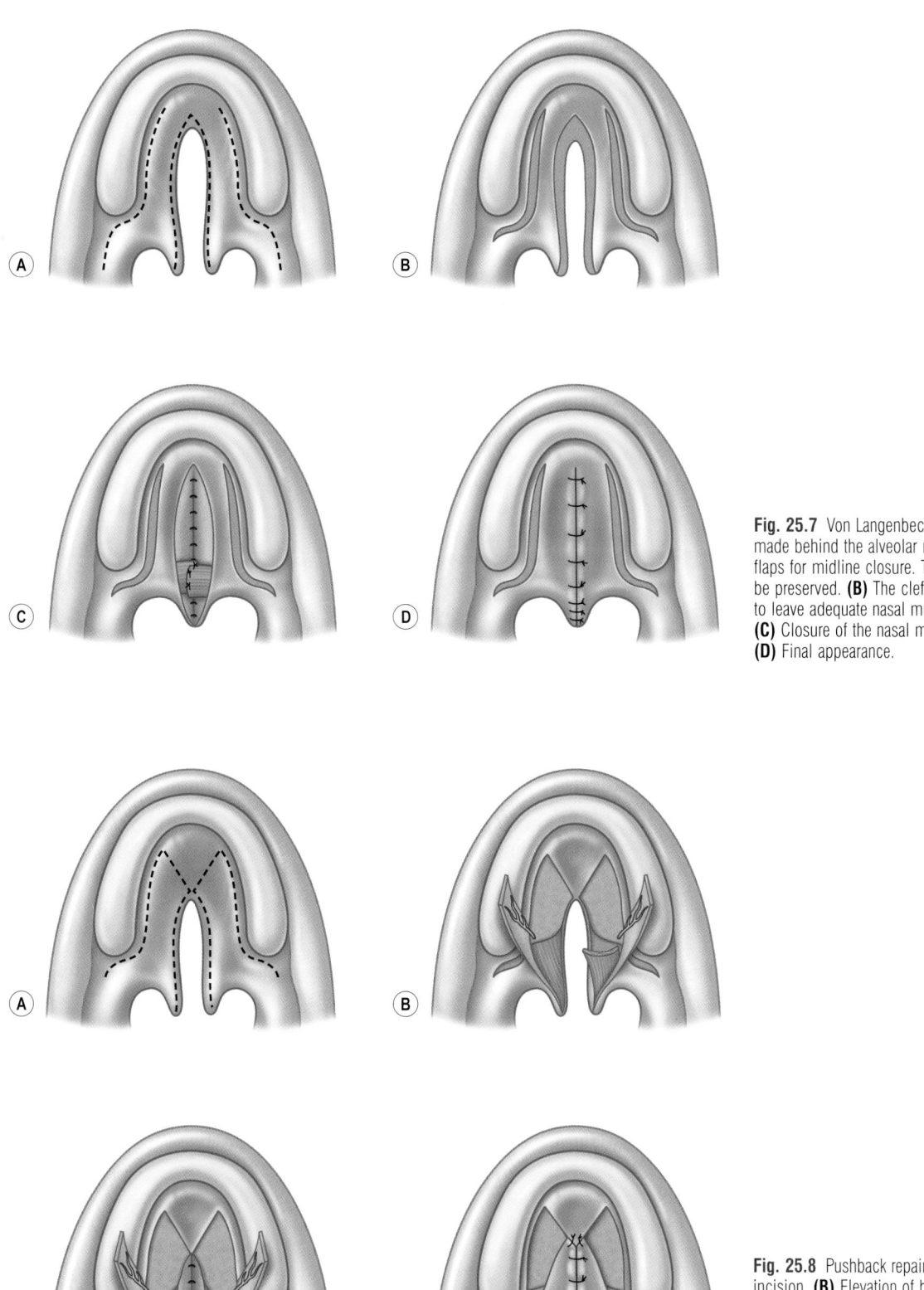

Fig. 25.7 Von Langenbeck repair. **(A)** Relaxing incisions are made behind the alveolar ridge, creating bilateral bipedicle flaps for midline closure. The greater palatine vessels must be preserved. **(B)** The cleft margins are incised in a manner to leave adequate nasal mucosa for complete closure. **(C)** Closure of the nasal mucosa and muscle repair. **(D)** Final appearance.

Fig. 25.8 Pushback repair. **(A)** Design of anterior "W" incision. **(B)** Elevation of bilateral mucoperiosteal flaps based on palatine vessels. The levator veli palatini muscles are freed from the posterior border of the hard palate. **(C)** The muscles are repaired across the midline of the soft palate. **(D)** The "Y" closure creates additional length but also leaves large raw areas bilaterally.

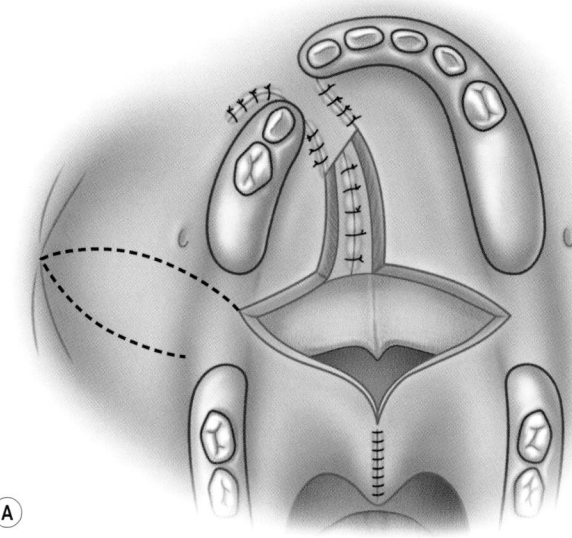

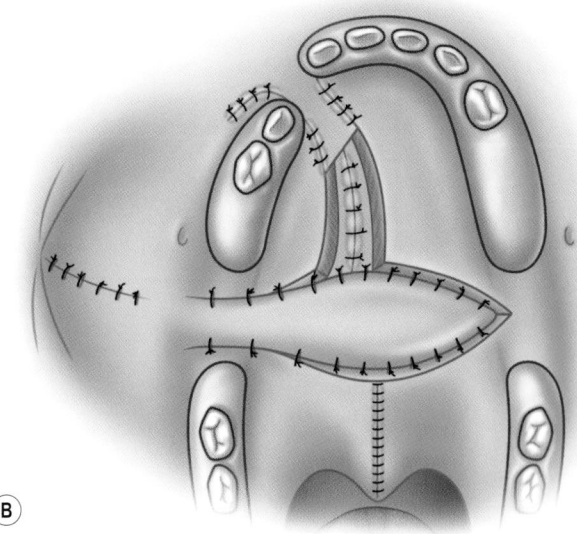

Fig. 25.9 (A) Buccal mucosal flap. Kaplan advocated use of this flap to elongate the nasal mucosa. **(B)** Flap transposed into the nasal surface. In some situations bilateral flaps can be used with the second flap lining the oral surface.

either with septal flaps,[104] or with buccal mucosa *(Fig. 25.9)*.[105] The soft palate is addressed with repair of the cleft margins and transverse closure of the levator muscle.

The pushback technique has the advantage of providing increased length for the palate and placing the levator muscle in a more favorable position. Large open areas are left anteriorly and on the nasal surface; as these close by contraction, a good deal of the length gain is lost. Additionally, the contraction of the oral mucosal defects results in loss of maxillary width anteriorly, a situation more difficult to correct than posterior maxillary narrowing. The arch may also be flattened anteriorly, a difficult problem for the orthodontist. The closure anteriorly in a complete cleft is a single layer of nasal mucosa only, which gives rise to a higher fistula rate in pushback repairs than in other techniques.[106]

Two-flap palatoplasty

Bardach and Salyer[107] originally described a technique of freeing mucoperiosteal flaps from the cleft margins only, arguing that the arch of the cleft would provide the length needed for central closure. This is certainly not a universal finding, and it is probably most applicable in relatively narrow clefts. The more extensive two-flap palatoplasty is a modification of the Langenbeck technique, extending the relaxing incisions along the alveolar margins to the edge of the cleft. This designs flaps entirely dependent on the circulation from the palatine vessels but also much more versatile in terms of their placement. In a complete unilateral cleft, the flap from the greater (medial) segment can be shifted across the cleft and closed directly behind the alveolar margin. This virtually eliminates fistulas in the anterior hard palate.[108]

The soft palate closure is accomplished with a straight-line closure in the typical two-flap technique. Intravelar veloplasty is an essential part of this closure *(Fig. 25.10)*.

Vomer flaps

There is confusion about the terminology applied to anterior closure of the nasal mucosa in complete cleft lip and palate. The original vomer flap is described as inferiorly based; an incision is made high on the septum, and the flap is reflected downward to provide a single-layer closure on the oral side. A number of European centers noted a high number of patients with maxillary retrusion, presumably from injury to the vomer-premaxillary suture, as well as a high fistula rate and changed to a two-layer anterior closure.[109–111]

Similar problems have not been found with superiorly based vomer flaps. This technique involves reflecting the mucosa from the septum near the cleft margin, dissecting only enough to close the nasal mucosa of the opposite side. In bilateral cleft palate, this requires a midline incision along the septum, and two flaps are reflected in each direction. This technique results in a two-layer closure of the hard palate mucosa, with low fistula rates and less effect on maxillary growth.[106]

Intravelar veloplasty

Although Victor Veau first advocated midline reapproximation of the levator palatini muscle, Braithwaite[112] was the first to perform more extensive muscle dissection for posterior repositioning and tension-free approximation. He emphasized careful dissection and freeing of the levator palatini from the posterior edge of the hard palate before approximation in the midline.

Cutting[113] has described a technique of veloplasty that includes division of the tensor palatini tendon and repositioning of the muscle at the hamulus. This method, known as radical levator transposition, requires an extensive dissection of the levator muscle, freeing it from both nasal and oral

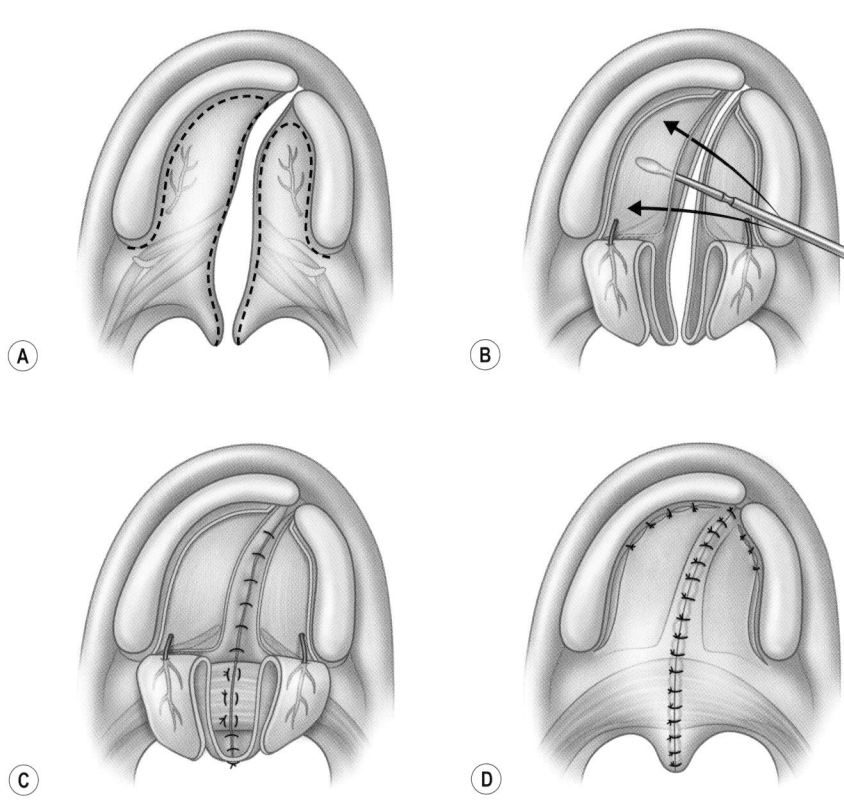

Fig. 25.10 Two flap palatoplasty. **(A)** The incisions are similar to the Langenbeck repair but meet the cleft margin just behind the alveolar ridge. **(B)** Mucoperiosteal flaps are developed on both sides with preservation of the greater palatine vessels. **(C)** The levator veli palatini muscle is freed from the posterior border of the hard palate and sutured across the midline. **(D)** Final closure. It is often possible to close much of the lateral incision and minimize raw areas.

mucosa *(Fig. 25.11)*. Although there is a reasonable thickness of oral mucosa, the adherence of the nasal mucosa to the muscle makes the dissection difficult on this side and at times results in perforation of the mucosa. Sommerlad described the use of the microscope for dissection of the muscle to reduce injury of the nasal mucosa. The tensor tendon is released just medial to the hamulus, and the levator muscle is overlapped to provide appropriate tension on the repair. This is presumably similar to the muscle overlap accomplished by Furlow's double opposing Z-plasty method. This technique has shown excellent speech outcomes in early evaluations. Both Cutting and Sommerlad[114] have proposed "re-repair" of the levator muscle when primary palatoplasty still results in velopharyngeal insufficiency.

Double opposing Z-plasty (Furlow)

Furlow[115] first described his technique for palate closure in the 1980s, adapting the Z-plasty principle to palatal closure. By alternating reversing Z-plasties of the nasal and oral flaps and keeping the levator palatini within the most posterior flaps, he reported initial early success in both speech outcomes and skeletal growth.

A Z-plasty is developed on both the oral and nasal surfaces of the soft palate but in opposite directions. For both of the Z-plasties, the central limb is the cleft margin, and the posteriorly based flap is designed to include the levator muscle. Furlow recommended that the posteriorly based oral flap be on the left side for a right-handed surgeon because the elevation of the muscle from the nasal mucosa is the most difficult part of the dissection *(Fig. 25.12)*.[116]

This technique addresses closure of the soft palate in a manner that provides complete nasal and oral closure as it re-establishes the levator sling. Because the nasal Z-plasty is placed more laterally a higher and presumably more functional sling is formed. The theoretical disadvantage of this technique is that it is nonanatomic in that it completely ignores the small longitudinal uvular muscle, but overall speech results have been comparable to or better than those with other techniques.[117,118]

Furlow described the use of relaxing incisions when necessary. The authors' preference is to combine a double opposing Z-plasty of the soft palate with a two-flap technique for the hard palate, resulting in a low fistula rate with good speech results. The chief problem may arise in very wide clefts, in which the distance to be traversed by the Z-plasty may be excessive. The anteriorly based oral flap can be joined to the relaxing incision to design an island flap based on the palatine vessels and giving considerably greater mobility, although this will shift the closure to the side of the posteriorly based flap. Another alternative is to extend the relaxing incision along the lateral border of the soft palate to allow oral closure and to use acellular dermal matrix for any nasal defects. A third alternative is to employ a straight-line closure in wide cases, reserving the Z-plasty as a secondary procedure if needed for speech.

Two-stage palate repair

The problem of maxillary growth after cleft palate repair has led some surgeons to advocate a two-stage approach to palatoplasty, with earlier repair of the soft palate only and later repair of the hard palate. The general protocol, originally

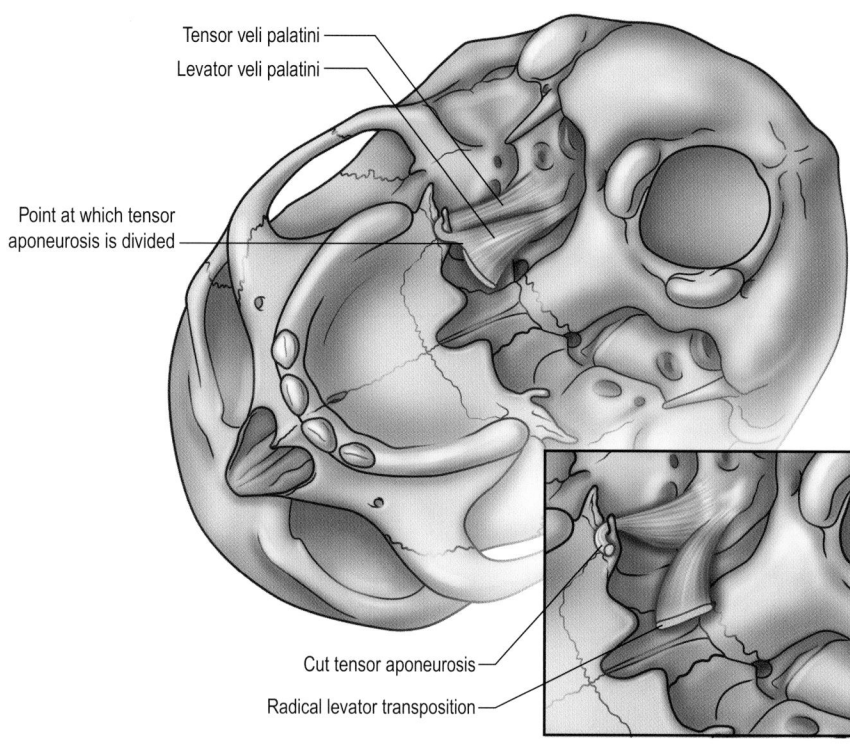

Tensor veli palatini

Levator veli palatini

Point at which tensor aponeurosis is divided

Cut tensor aponeurosis

Radical levator transposition

Fig. 25.11 Cutting's radical levator transposition; the levator veli palatini is freed completely from the posterior hard palate as well as from nasal and oral lining. The tensor tendon is cut medial to the hamulus to effect a complete release of the muscular sling.

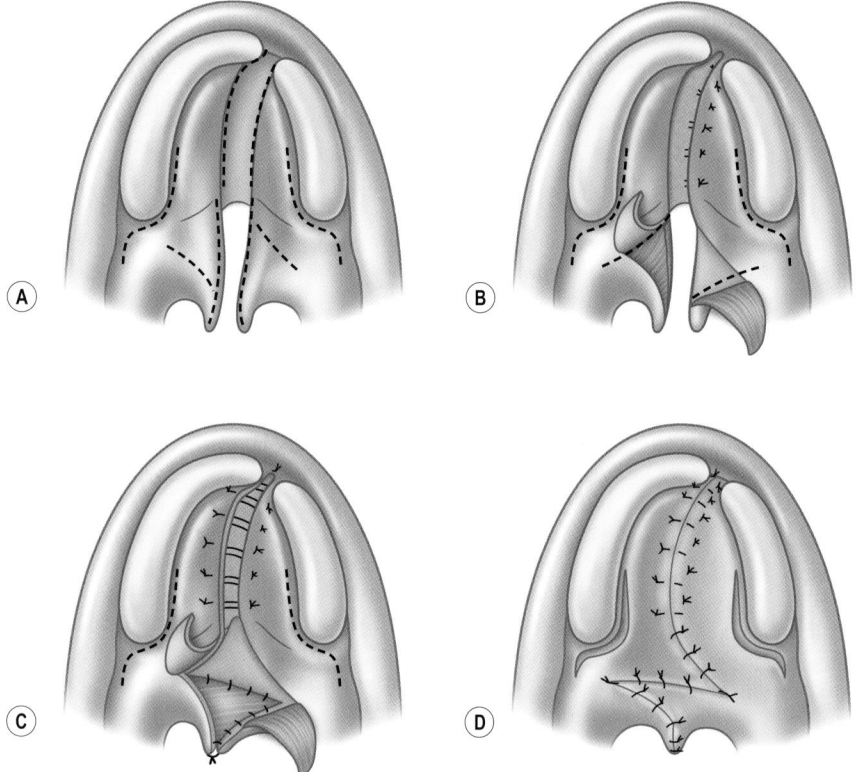

(A)

(B)

(C)

(D)

Fig. 25.12 Furlow double opposing Z-plasty. **(A)** The oral flap design is shown with the posteriorly based flap on the left side. If necessary the relaxing incisions can be continued up to the cleft margin behind the alveolus, similar to the two flap palatoplasty **(Fig. 25.9)** for the hard palate closure. **(B)** The left sided oral flap is raised with the levator muscle, the right sided flap above the muscle. The reverse pattern is planned for the oral side. A vomer flap is shown closing the nasal mucosa anteriorly. **(C)** The nasal flaps are transposed and the anterior oral mucosa closed. **(D)** The final appearance after transposition of the oral flaps.

introduced by Schweckendiek and Doz,[119] entailed repair of the soft palate at the same time as the cleft lip repair, around 4–6 months. The hard palate was obturated and repaired at about 4–5 years of age. Earlier ages have subsequently been proposed for hard palate repair, usually around 18–24 months.[120]

The rationale for this approach has been that the hard palate cleft narrows during the time between procedures, requiring less dissection and thus resulting in less maxillary growth disturbance. Although it is appealing on a theoretical basis, numerous studies have shown significantly poorer speech results from these two-stage procedures, with marginal if any salutary effect on the growth of the maxilla.[121–123] As noted before, good speech outcomes become more difficult to achieve with increasing age, whereas most maxillary growth problems can be addressed with orthodontic treatment and, if needed, surgical maxillary advancement.

Postoperative care

In the immediate postoperative period, breathing is the critical concern. The child with an open cleft palate has become accustomed to a larger than normal nasal airway which is virtually occluded after cleft palate repair, especially with the introduction of a small amount of blood or mucus in the nose. Postoperative hypoxemia is not uncommon, but generally resolves after 24–48 h.[124] The use of a traction suture in the tongue during the immediate period after extubation may avoid the need for utilizing any oral devices for maintaining the airway. Some centers use nasal trumpets routinely to improve ventilation. Monitoring with continuous pulse oximetry and minimizing narcotic use will help to avoid catastrophic problems. Acetaminophen 15 mg/kg alternating with ibuprofen 10 mg/kg will usually give adequate pain relief. Any patient who has had prolonged surgery (over 2 h) with the mouth gag in place should be observed for at least 48 h for tongue edema. Some surgeons routinely release the mouth gag at set intervals throughout the procedure, analogous to releasing the tourniquet during hand surgery.

Children with Pierre Robin sequence are a special group. These and any other children with syndromes that may affect breathing must be observed closely, even in an ICU setting, to be sure that there is no significant respiratory obstruction. Most Pierre Robin children stay additional time in the hospital for this reason.

Bleeding is not uncommon after palate repair. There are inevitably raw surfaces, which may ooze for 12–24 h. Bleeding can be reduced by surgery that takes less than 90–120 min because the epinephrine will still have some effect during emergence from anesthesia. Light pressure on the hard palate repair at the conclusion of the procedure will often control bleeding as well. The author has found that application of ice packs to the posterior neck is almost always effective in stopping postoperative bleeding in recovery or on the ward; this is a technique that has not been documented previously but has been used by experienced surgeons (Ousterhout, pers. comm. 1986).

Postoperative feeding is generally limited to liquids for 10–14 days, to prevent particulate matter lodging in the areas that are left open at the end of the procedure. Reducing or stopping intravenous fluids the morning after surgery causes some thirst, and almost all patients start to take adequate liquids under these circumstances. The parents must learn to time feeding 30 min or so after analgesic administration.

Arm splints may be used as well to prevent children from putting their fingers or more likely, foreign objects in the mouth.

Outcomes of cleft palate repair

Fistula

Fistula formation is one complication that has been studied in some detail. Fistulas may be a source of persistent nasal air loss even in the face of a functioning soft palate; they are also a source of nasal regurgitation of fluids. In one particularly extensive review of fistulas at a single institution, use of the Furlow repair was shown to markedly reduce fistulas relative to the V-Y pushback or von Langenbeck technique. The width of the cleft was the other factor in this multivariate analysis.[106] Late closure of fistulas may be difficult, especially in the hard palate, and the use of large mucoperiosteal flaps on the oral side is recommended to give the best outcome (*Fig. 25.13*).[125] If there is reason for delay of repair, a palatal plate may aid in obturating a fistula for speech purposes until surgical correction can be achieved.

Speech outcomes/VPI

Normal speech is the primary goal of cleft palate repair. Specifically this refers to the lack of velopharyngeal insufficiency and nasal air loss in speech. It can be difficult to interpret some studies, as it is common that "good" and "excellent" results are grouped together, or that the nasality is rated on a numerical scale. In general it is preferable to look at the presence or absence of nasality and ideally to use a binary outcome measure for analysis.

In the majority of studies in which some form of muscle repair is utilized, good speech results are obtained about 85–90% of the time. These results are in nonsyndromic cleft patients; syndromic patients will always have poorer results for a variety of reasons, but their good outcomes may be in the 50–60% range. It appears that width of cleft is related to outcome, as bilateral clefts often have worse speech outcomes, but there have been few studies looking at this in detail.

Some studies have examined the long-term stability of speech outcomes. In some patients nasality may develop in puberty or later, probably related to involution of the adenoid pad, but this is rare in our experience.

Maxillary growth

Normal maxillary growth is the secondary goal of palate repair. While some orthodontists might contest this, it is much more difficult to correct nasal speech after puberty than to perform a LeFort I maxillary advancement. It is clear that avoidance of large raw surfaces on the hard palate will improve maxillary growth long term, and that minimizing scar tissue will have a salutary effect as well. Fistula formation

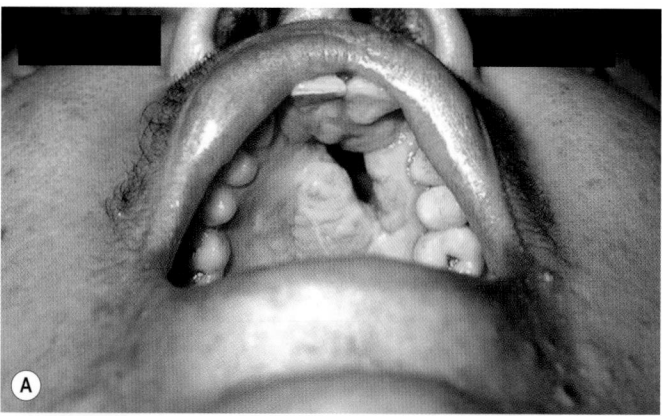

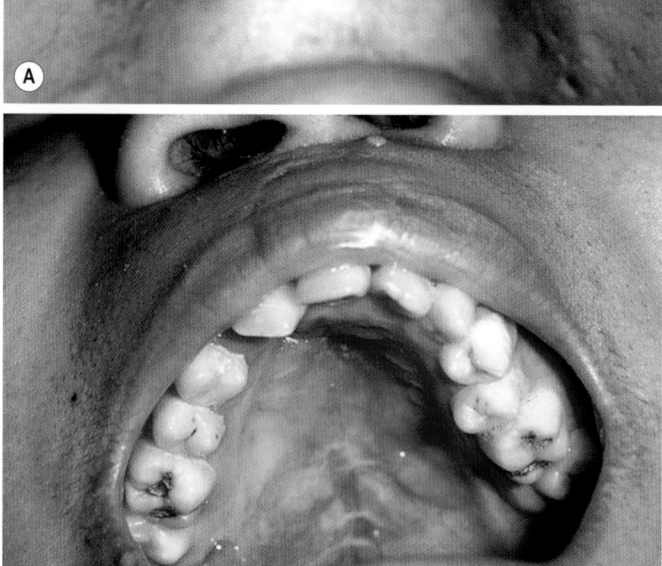

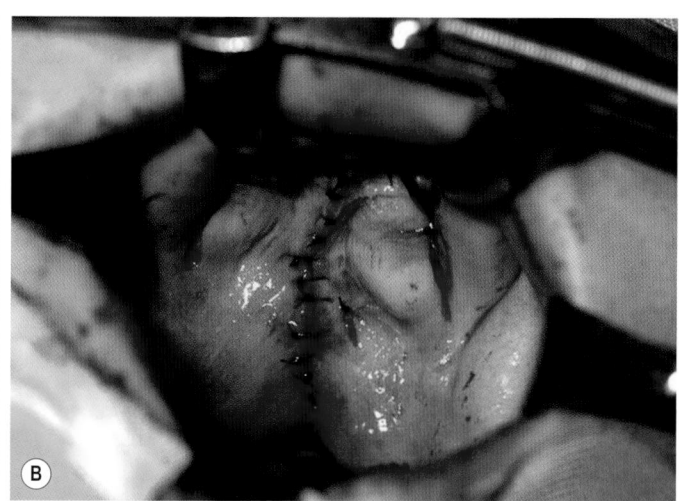

Fig. 25.13 (A) Fistula in hard palate. **(B)** Large mucoperiosteal flap for oral closure. **(C)** Repaired fistula.

requiring additional procedures will increase scar tissue and often decrease maxillary growth.

The need for maxillary advancement is highly variable, from 10–40% in nonsyndromic cleft patients. Because different centers have different surgeons as well as different protocols it is difficult to tease out the critical differences in practice that might account for these variations in outcome. Wider clefts and bilateral clefts have a higher rate of maxillary hypoplasia, possibly related to greater need for dissection at the time of palate repair.[126]

It is clear that syndromic patients have a higher rate of maxillary hypoplasia, which may well be genetically determined. In our review of van der Woude syndrome, the need for maxillary advancement was about 85% compared to less than 10% in a matched group of nonsyndromic unilateral cleft patients.

Conclusion

Cleft palate repair has undergone major changes in the past quarter century. Overall, results have improved as far as speech outcomes; this is probably due to the growth of centers for cleft care as well as to refinement of techniques. The team approach has decreased the number of operations needed to obtain better outcomes as the surgeon has gained knowledge from the other specialists involved in cleft care. The increased application of methods that incorporate reconstruction of the levator palatini muscle has produced much more predictable speech results. Current trends of earlier surgical intervention for cleft palate and presurgical alignment of the dental arches should result in still more predictable outcomes.

14. Huang MH, Lee ST, Rajendran K. A fresh cadaveric study of the paratubal muscles: implications for eustachian tube function in cleft palate. *Plast Reconstr Surg.* 1997;100:833–842.

Cadaveric dissections were performed to clarify possible ramifications of palatal clefting on eustachian tube function. Functional hypotheses are drawn from morphological findings.

43. Kaplan EN. The occult submucous cleft palate. *Cleft Palate J.* 1975;12:356–368.

45. Chen PK-T, Wu J, Hung KF, et al. Surgical correction of sub-mucous cleft palate with Furlow palatoplasty. *Plast Reconstr Surg.* 1996;97:1136–1146.

Sleep apnea is a recognized adverse outcome of pharyngeal flaps performed for velopharyngeal insufficiency (VPI). This report demonstrates that Furlow palatoplasty is a reliable alternative to pharyngeal flaps for the correction of VPI in the context of submucous cleft palate.

46. Robin P. Glossoptosis due to atresia and hypotrophy of the mandible. *Am J Dis Child.* 1934;48:541–547.

59. Denny AD, Talisman R, Hanson PR, et al. Mandibular distraction osteogenesis in very young patients to correct airway obstruction. *Plast Reconstr Surg.* 2001;108:302–311.

This clinical series correlates airway measurements before and after distraction with functional outcomes. The authors conclude that distraction improves tongue base position such that airway space is effectively increased.

91. Bardach J. The influence of cleft lip repair on facial growth. *Cleft Palate J.* 1990;27:76–78.

113. Cutting C, Rosenbaum J, Rovati L. The technique of muscle repair in the soft palate. *Operative Techniques Plast Surg.* 1995;2:215–222.

115. Furlow Jr LT. Cleft palate repair by double opposing Z-plasty. *Plast Reconstr Surg.* 1986;78:724.

Furlow describes his palatoplasty in the context of a 22-patient case series. Optimistic speech outcomes are reported.

120. Rohrich RJ, Byrd HS. Optimal timing of cleft palate closure. Speech, facial growth, and hearing considerations. *Clin Plast Surg.* 1990;17:27–36.

125. Emory Jr RE, Clay RP, Bite U, et al. Fistula formation and repair after palatal closure: an institutional perspective. *Plast Reconstr Surg.* 1997;99:1535–1538.

The authors report an 11.5% post-palatoplasty fistula rate. Local flaps are advocated to repair these lesions.

26

Alveolar clefts

Richard A. Hopper

SYNOPSIS

- Treatment of the alveolar cleft remains one of the most controversial topics in cleft care.
- Treatment protocols have varied in timing, technique, and selection of graft material.
- Currently the gold standard is secondary bone grafting with autogenous cancellous graft at the time of mixed dentition.
- Outcomes of proposed alternate treatments such as gingivoperiosteoplasty (GPP), primary bone grafting, and use of inductive proteins need to be compared to documented outcomes of this gold standard.
- Regardless of which technique is employed, coordination and communication between surgeon and orthodontist are essential for success.
- Failed or complex alveolar bone graft sites remain a considerable challenge. These recalcitrant alveolar clefts can benefit from recent applications of distraction osteogenesis techniques.

Access the Historical Perspective section online at
http://www.expertconsult.com

Introduction

- Compared to soft-tissue repair techniques, surgery on the bony alveolar defect in cleft lip and palate patients is relatively new.
- Early approaches including primary grafting in infancy fell into disfavor due to iatrogenic impairment of facial growth.
- Secondary bone grafting in mixed-dentition and primary GPP were introduced in the 1960s.
- Secondary bone grafting has become the gold standard for comparison of other techniques.
- Primary bone grafting and GPP remain controversial.

Practitioners in cleft care should understand the pros and cons of all options of alveolar cleft treatment regardless of their protocol of choice. Only in this way can the merits of new technologies and treatment protocols be fairly evaluated. The overriding goals of alveolar cleft treatment should be shared by all treatments and are listed in *Table 26.1*. The purpose of this chapter is to introduce the reader to the concepts of each treatment and to discuss the available literature regarding the success of each in achieving the treatment goals.

Basic science/disease process

Anatomy of the alveolar cleft

The alveolar cleft is more than a linear gap in the maxillary arch. With soft tissue removed the cleft is best visualized as a tornado, increasing in size from incisal to apical, becoming widest as it extends into the nasal cavity and distorts the surrounding anatomy *(Fig. 26.1)*. The soft-tissue distortion caused by this skeletal deficiency can be minimized by a correctly performed cleft lip repair, but not completely eradicated. In the patient with an untreated alveolar cleft, the alar base of the nose lacks the bony support of the noncleft side, and if release of the lateral nasal wall and reconstruction of the nasal component of the orbicularis oris muscle have not been achieved at the primary lip repair, the nasal base will remain attached to the hypoplastic piriform rim, with inferior and posterior malposition.

The fistula between oral and nasal cavities has three distinct boundaries. The nasolabial fistula is located at the apex of the cleft, high up in the labial sulcus, and consists of loose wet labial mucosa transitioning to nasal mucosa. The oronasal fistula extends from the incisive foramen to the alveolar process, and is a transition of attached palatal mucoperiosteum to nasal mucosa. At the corner of these two fistulas, at the alveolar process itself, attached alveolar gingiva is located, which is the only appropriate support lining of erupting teeth. Whichever technique is employed to close the soft tissues of

Table 26.1 Goals of treatment of the alveolar cleft

- Stable bone continuity of maxillary arch
- Separation of oral and nasal cavities
- Appropriate maxillary arch form and transverse width
- Stable environment for eruption of cleft-side canine
- Maintenance and bone support of all erupting teeth
- Keratinized gingival environment for erupted teeth
- Piriform bone support of nasal base
- Preserved anterior vestibule
- Uninhibited facial growth
- Minimized donor site morbidity

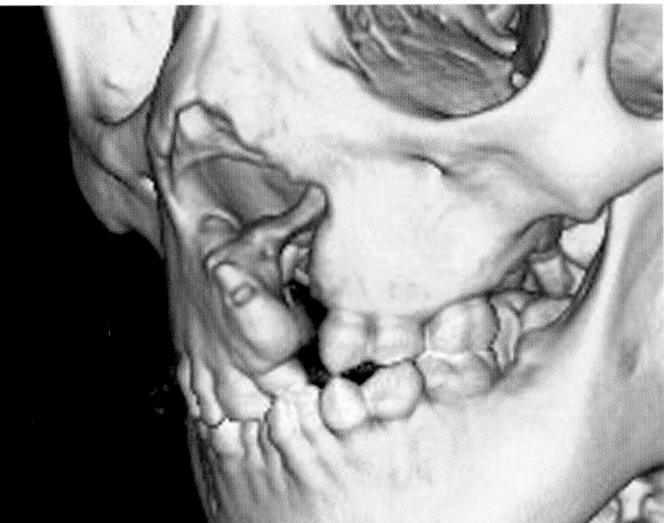

Fig. 26.1 Bony anatomy of an untreated unilateral cleft lip and palate in a 4-year-old. The lateral piriform rim is hypoplastic, increasing the width of the piriform opening on the cleft side, creating a tornado-shaped defect. The maxillary nasal crest is deviated away from the cleft, carrying the bony septum with it. The collapse of the ungrafted maxillary arch is apparent with a lingual crossbite of the lesser segment.

the nasolabial and oronasal fistulas, attached gingival tissue must be present at the anticipated site of eruption to ensure long-term support of the adult teeth.

Dental development

An alveolar cleft is associated with variable anomalies in dental development that must be taken into consideration with presurgical preparation, timing of surgery, surgical technique, and postsurgical orthodontic planning. Anomalies can include the number of teeth (missing teeth, supernumerary teeth), the location (mesial or distal to cleft), the shape (pegged or conical), the size (microdontic), the time of formation and/ or eruption, and crown and root malformations.[9,10]

A goal of successful alveolar cleft treatment is to provide a stable supporting environment for eruption of the permanent canine. The adjacent lateral incisor however must be taken into consideration prior to surgery with a coordinated surgical–orthodontic plan. The lateral incisor is often missing

in complete clefts; however, if present, it can be positioned either mesial or distal to the cleft. Although still debated, many consider that it is supernumerary when distal.[11]

It is important that the patient and family be informed before the bone graft procedure that in many cases a permanent lateral incisor is congenitally absent, will not erupt, or will be extracted as part of the treatment protocol.[12–15] The lateral incisor is extracted if it is needed to create space for the permanent canine to migrate and erupt through the newly grafted area. The orthodontist can then perform canine substitution of the lateral incisor if it was absent or not supernumerary.

Diagnosis/patient presentation

Gingivoperiosteoplasty

Prior to undergoing a GPP, the infant with a cleft must be evaluated by the practitioner coordinating the presurgical molding as well as the surgeon who will be performing the GPP. It must be emphasized that not all infants will be candidates for GPP due to individual variations of anatomy. Some infants with particularly wide unilateral clefts can be "mesenchymally deficient." Compressing and closing the alveolar cleft with molding and a GPP would unnaturally constrict the arch form. Isolated clefts of the primary palate are also difficult to predict if a GPP is possible. Due to the bony fusion of the secondary palate, the alveolar segments are more resistant to presurgical molding, and in some cases cannot be adequately aligned. Finally, in bilateral complete clefts, it is not always possible to align both sides of the premaxilla with the alveolar segments. In this case, one alveolar cleft can undergo a GPP to convert the arch form to a lesser and greater segment similar to a unilateral cleft. Assessment of parallel alveolar molding can be difficult, and benefits from a team presurgical evaluation *(Fig. 26.2.)* If the alveolar anatomy and presurgical molding outcome are favorable, a GPP can be offered to the family at the same time as the primary lip repair.

Primary bone grafting

Grafting at the time of primary dentition is practiced by relatively few centers, with the most published group being that of Rosenstein and Dado, who have used primary grafting as their approach to the alveolar cleft for over 20 years. Patient selection is based on the family's ability to undertake the staged surgical and orthodontic appliance protocol necessary to maintain arch relationship before and after grafting.[16]

Secondary bone grafting

As the patient is approaching the time of secondary bone graft, the craniofacial orthodontist and surgeon should discuss plans for timing of the graft, the fate of adjacent teeth, and the timing of arch expansion. Any dental morbidity such as poor hygiene or caries should be addressed by a pediatric dentist prior to the surgery. In some cases, primary teeth adjacent to the cleft should be extracted 3–6 weeks prior to grafting in order to ensure a viable mucosal seal of the oral surface of the

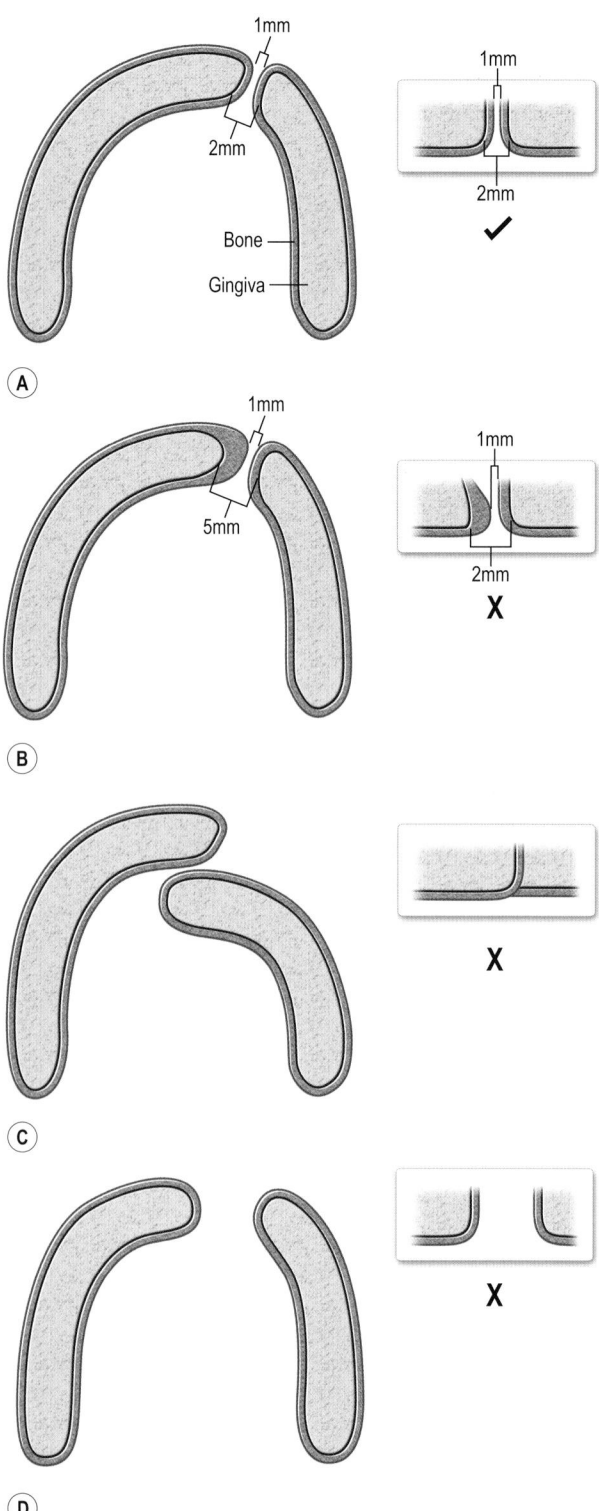

Fig. 26.2 **(A)** An appropriately molded unilateral alveolar cleft candidate for gingivoperiosteoplasty (GPP). There is parallel alignment of the alveolar cleft edges with a smooth arch form. **(B)** Gingival hypertrophy in the alveolar cleft is masking a bone gap that is too wide for a GPP. **(C)** A collapsed arch form not amenable to GPP. Although the edges are touching, the opposing bone segments within the cleft are not aligned for bone formation. **(D)** A mesenchymal-deficient arch form that should not undergo GPP. If this cleft was approximated with molding followed by a GPP that formed a bone fusion, it would unnaturally constrict the projection of the alveolar arch. Arch expansion with bone grafting of the alveolar gap is the indicated treatment.

grafted area. In most cases however, the teeth can be preserved until the time of grafting to maximize bone retention, avoid an additional procedure, and be extracted at the grafting surgery.

Arch expansion can be performed either before or after the graft surgery. Preoperative arch expansion allows the orthodontist to take full advantage of the mobility of the two or three ungrafted segments of the alveolus to achieve appropriate maxillary anterior and posterior arch width. When the graft is then placed and heals in the expanded cleft, the continuous maxillary arch form has an optimal relationship with the mandible. A collapsed overlapping alveolar cleft can also benefit from expansion, by increasing the access and visibility of the surgeon to the fistula at time of operation. The disadvantages of presurgical expansion however include overexpansion, such that the alveolar cleft becomes challenging to treat, due to simultaneous expansion of the oronasal fistula and resulting excessive tension on any soft-tissue repair. If an expander is in place at the time of surgery and obstructs the site, then replacement of the device with a custom acrylic retention splint at the time of surgery is indicated. Postoperative expansion should wait 6–8 weeks from the date of surgery, and conventional orthodontic movements should not be attempted before the cleft is grafted, but can start within 3 weeks of surgery.

Debate continues regarding the appropriate timing of a secondary bone grafting. The mixed-dentition phase is variable among patients, but typically falls between ages 6 and 11. Proponents of grafting early in mixed dentition believe that a stable healed graft prior to canine eruption results in a superior bone environment *(Fig. 26.3)*. El Deeb et al.[17] found that successful eruption of cuspids though the graft occurred when root formation of the canine adjacent to the cleft was one-fourth to one-half formed at the time of graft placement. Bergland et al.[18] found a higher proportion of graft failures and cases with lower interdental septa when grafting was done adjacent to fully erupted teeth compared to just before eruption. In comparison, Long et al. retrospectively performed detailed periapical radiograph analysis of bone formation and found no significant correlation between final graft success and the amount of canine crown eruption in the cleft at the time of grafting.[19]

Bone morphogenic protein

Recombinant human bone morphogenic protein-2 (rhBMP2) is a mitogen that has been demonstrated to stimulate osteoblastic activity and induce bone nodule formation in animals. It has been approved by the US Food and Drug Administration for clinical use in human spine fusion procedures, and has been shown to decrease nonunion, donor site morbidity, and operating time over autogenous grafting in this population.[20] More recent clinical applications have been on patients undergoing alveolar augmentation and implant placement[21] and early trials are now underway at individual centers for the treatment of alveolar clefts. The risk–benefit profile of rhBMP2 in these patients will remain unknown for the next decade. Patient selection should therefore be based on enrolment in an institutional review board-approved trial with appropriate consent and evaluation, including oversight by an independent data safety monitoring board.

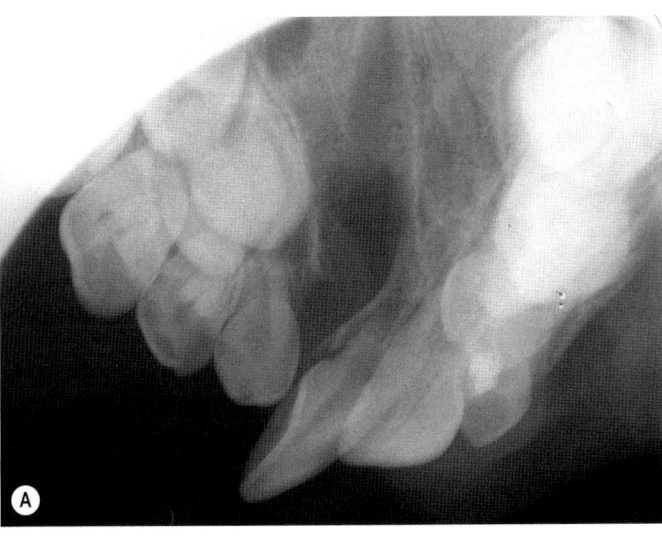 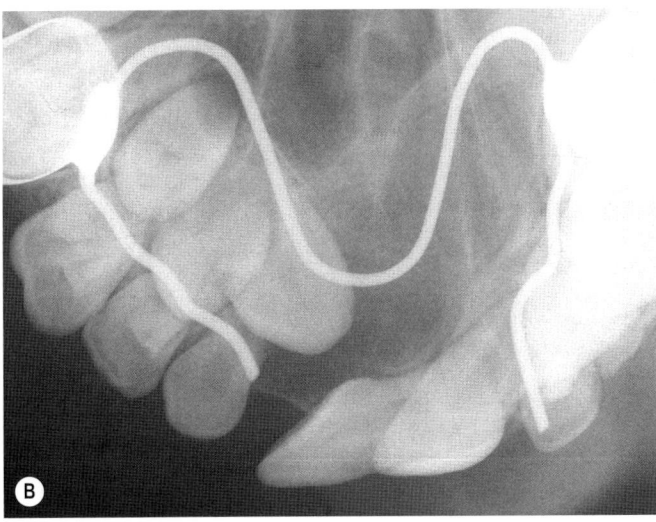

Fig. 26.3 (A) A unilateral alveolar cleft in mixed dentition ready for preoperative arch expansion and secondary bone grafting. The permanent canine is descending but is still covered with bone. The cleft extends from the alveolus up into the piriform cavity. **(B)** The same cleft after preoperative palate expansion and successful autogenous bone grafting. With the expansion and with orthodontic uprighting of the adjacent central incisor, there will be sufficient bone support and space for the erupting permanent canine.

Late bone grafting

Some centers have advocated delaying alveolar bone grafting in patients who are known to need a LeFort I osteotomy procedure at skeletal maturity in order to perform both simultaneously. This however has largely been abandoned in the presence of an erupting canine, since eruption into a bone graft is felt to provide better bone support and periodontal status.[12]

However, in any cleft center patients can present in permanent dentition without having had their alveolar cleft treated. In these cases, a combined segmental orthognathic and bone grafting procedure is required. Outcomes of these techniques however are not as favorable as grafting in mixed dentition followed by dental eruption into the graft and orthodontic movement.

Alveolar distraction

Successful primary or secondary treatment of the alveolar cleft should obviate the need for alveolar distraction in this patient population. Unfortunately there exist patients with "ungraftable" or "recalcitrant" alveolar clefts that have few options available to them other than undergoing transport distraction osteogenesis (TDO) of alveolar bone.[22] The typical patient who falls into this category has unhealthy, scarred gingiva, a large nasolabial and/or oronasal fistula, and a history of repeated unsuccessful bone grafts with infections and exposure. Another possible presentation is a previously grafted maxilla that has severe vertical deficiency along with scarred mucogingiva preventing additional graft augmentation. In both these cases, TDO is a useful tool to have in the cleft armamentarium.

In the wide "ungraftable" cleft patient *(Fig. 26.4)*, a tooth-bearing transport segment can be slowly moved into the gap, closing the fistula and converting the problem into a narrow cleft amenable to traditional secondary grafting. In the vertically deficient alveolus *(Fig. 26.5)*, a transport segment of

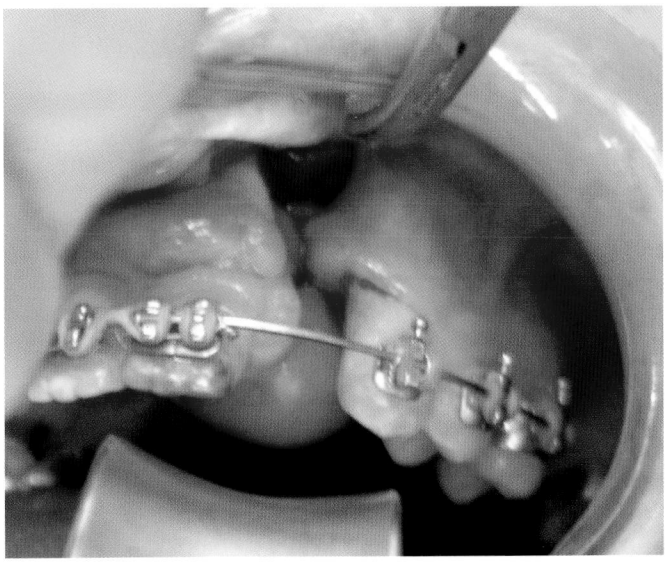

Fig. 26.4 A good candidate for interdental horizontal transport distraction. The patient had undergone three previous attempts at treatment of bilateral alveolar clefts, including transfer of a facial artery musculomucosal (FAMM) flap, seen hanging from the anterior palate. The patient has extensive scarring and a large tornado-shaped oronasal and nasolabial fistula. The recommended treatment was simultaneous closure of the nasal lining using the FAMM flap tissue with transport distraction of a three-tooth segment from the lesser segments, as shown in ***Figure 26.9***, followed by secondary bone grafting of the residual cleft.

superior maxillary bone, with or without prior bone augmentation, can be slowly lowered, leveling the alveolar ridge by gradually bringing the scarred attached gingival tissue along with the advancing bone front.

Factors that may have contributed to previous failed surgeries in patients with "recalcitrant" clefts must be carefully considered to avoid the plan for TDO suffering the same fate. Any dental caries or periapical disease must be addressed to minimize the infection risk during the period when the device is in place. Alcohol, smoking, and drug abuse must be ruled

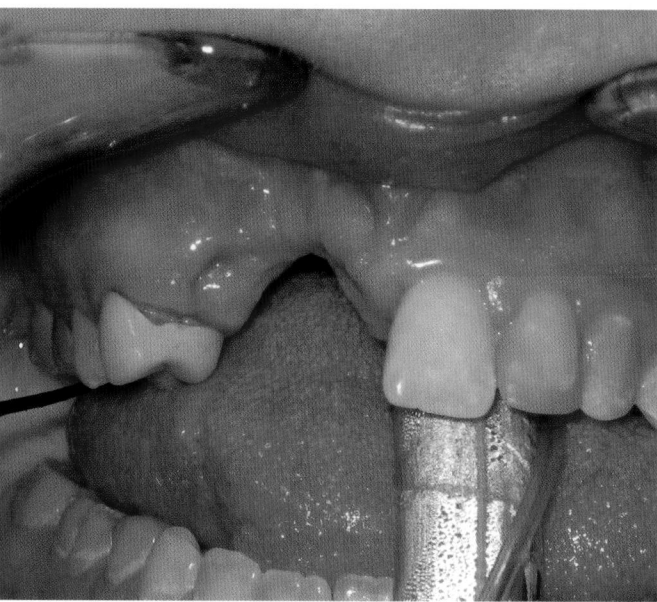

Fig. 26.5 A good candidate for vertical transport distraction. The patient had undergone six previous attempts of alveolar grafting with infection and graft loss. The result was vertical deficiency of the alveolus, loss of the adjacent three permanent teeth, and tight scarred gingival covering. The patient underwent stage cortical grafting and vertical transport distraction, as shown in *Figure 26.11*.

out, and the expectations on the patient must be discussed and documented. All current distraction devices require activation by the patient or caregiver and frequent follow-up during the period of activation. Therefore, a patient who is considered unreliable, noncompliant, or unable to return to clinic regularly is not a suitable candidate. TDO is currently reserved for patients past mixed dentition due to the risk to unerupted tooth follicles during the segmental osteotomies. Coordination with the patient's orthodontist or prosthodontist is essential in order to agree upon the desired goals of the procedure, and the endpoint of activation. Frequently the treatment plan may include arch expansion or tooth extraction, which should be performed prior to the TDO procedure. Written directions and a device-turning log should be carefully explained to the patient to avoid complications during activation. Perioperative chlorhexidine mouthwash should be used during activation with careful dental hygiene with a soft toothbrush.

Treatment/surgical technique

Gingivoperiosteoplasty

The GPP can be performed at any point of the primary cleft lip repair, but is easiest after all other dissection had been completed, and before repair of the lip elements. The "roof" of the GPP is the repair of the anterior palate (nasal floor) from the nasal sill back to the incisive foramen that is typically done with most modern cleft lip repairs. This is achieved by suturing the inferior edge of the reconstructed lateral nasal wall to a superiorly based mucoperiosteal vomer flap (nasal flap) *(Fig. 26.6)*. The incision along the vomer to create the leading edge of the vomer flap is at the level of the oral–nasal mucosa

demarcation. This demarcation is also visible on the opposing lateral nasal wall. The vomer flap vertical dissection is kept to the minimum needed to achieve closure of the nasal floor. After the mucosal incision, most of the vomer dissection can be achieved with an elevator, with the exception of the region of the premaxillary suture, which will require sharp dissection with a small blade. This nasal floor closure separates the nasal from the oral cavity back to the incisive foramen and provides the superior barrier of the guided tissue regeneration tunnel between the alveolar segments.

The "floor" of the GPP tunnel is created by elevating inferiorly based mucoperiosteal flaps from the oral edges of the alveolar cleft (oral flaps). These flaps are contained within the cleft itself, and extend from the labial surface of the alveolus back to the incisive foramen. They are typically 2–3 mm in vertical height, such that when they are inferiorly rotated, they meet across the oral boundary of the cleft and can be sutured together with everting resorbable 5-0 gut or Vicryl sutures.

The attached mucoperiosteum that remains within the alveolar cleft between the superior anteroposterior incision made to create the nasal closure flaps and the inferior one made to create the oral closure is the tissue used to close the anterior border of the GPP. The alveolar cleft can be visualized as a pyramid with the apex at the incisive foramen, where the superior and inferior vomer incisions converge. Anteriorly, these two incisions diverge, creating anteriorly based triangular flaps that are brought out from between the alveolar segments, pedicled anteriorly, and flipped across the cleft, closing the labial border of the GPP (labial flaps). In designing the GPP flaps, the incisions on one side of the cleft are shifted slightly superiorly, so that the labial flap covers the upper half of the labial border of the cleft, while on the contralateral side, the incisions are shifted inferiorly for the labial flap to cover the lower half. The superior edge of the upper labial flap is sutured to the lip mucosa, and the inferior edge of the lower labial flap is sutured to the anterior edge of the two oral flaps. In this fashion, a sealed guided tissue regeneration "chamber" is sealed nasally, orally, and labially by mucoperiosteal flaps, and contains two opposing bone surfaces on the mesial and distal walls. It is essential that this end goal is visualized throughout the GPP procedure to ensure that all soft-tissue interference is removed from the alveolar cleft during creation of the flaps, and that the flaps are positioned correctly to direct bone growth across the cleft.

Technical pitfalls of the GPP include elevation of the flaps in a submucosal instead of subperiosteal plane; inaccurate planning of flaps such that viability of the anteriorly based labial flaps is compromised; and trauma to the flaps from compressive handling with forceps. Frequently a deciduous tooth follicle is encountered during the flap dissection. Careful sharp dissection between the follicle and the periosteum is required to prevent disruption of dental eruption. If the flaps appear too thin or nonviable during the follicle dissection, the GPP should be aborted and the mucosa replaced.

Primary bone grafting

The protocols for primary bone grafting vary, but typically involve a staged approach of molding the maxillary arch segments in the first year of life followed by stabilization of the maxillary arch with an autogenous bone graft in infancy. In

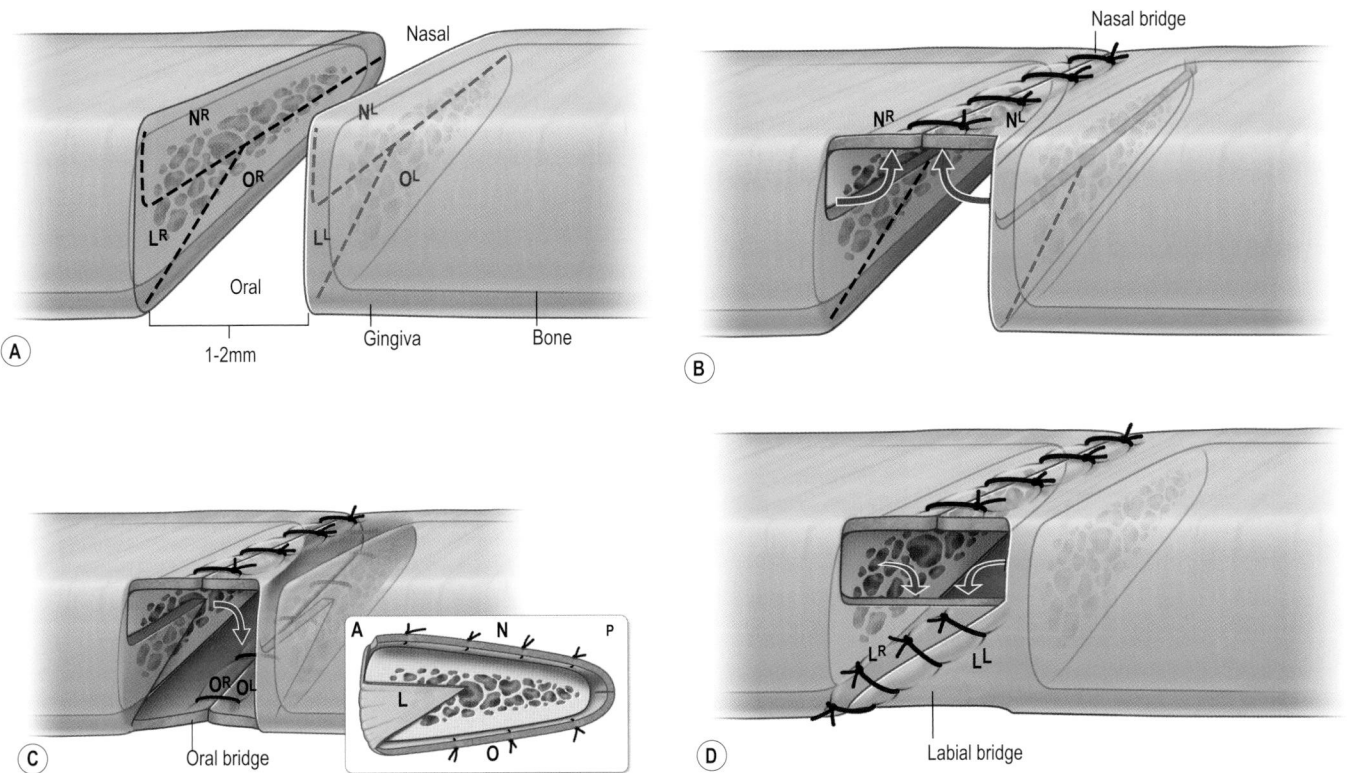

Fig. 26.6 Gingivoperiosteal flap design and elevation for the Millard-type gingivoperiosteoplasty. The dissection is limited to the tissues within the cleft. The flaps are named by the part of the periosteal tunnel they construct. See text for details. L^R, right labial flap; O^L, left oral flap; N^R, right nasal flap; A, anterior; P, posterior.

the protocol used by Rosenstein and Dado, a maxillary appliance is used prior to lip repair to align the alveolar segments.[16,23] Following a lip repair at 6–8 weeks of age, the appliance is modified to prevent posterior collapse of arch width while allowing the repaired lip musculature to mold and close the anterior cleft as a "butt joint." Once the cleft is molded to approximation, at around 4–6 months, the segments are stabilized with an autogenous split rib graft. The appliance is continued for 6–8 weeks postsurgery and the palate is closed at or before 1 year of age.

Secondary bone grafting

When performing a secondary bone grafting, the author uses chlorhexidine mouthwash and nasal antibiotic ointment in the days before surgery to decrease the bacterial load. The patient is positioned supine with a small support under the posterior iliac crest to facilitate the graft harvest. There should be two sterile fields to avoid contamination between the oral field and donor field.

The author follows a modification of the technique described by Abyholm et al.[24] *(Fig. 26.7)*. A superiorly based mucoperiosteal flap is raised off the lesser segment of the alveolus with a back-cut into the loose mucosa anterior to Stenson's duct. If the site immediately adjacent to the cleft has sufficient attached gingiva, this is included in the tip of the flap. If not, the attached gingiva of the one or two teeth distal to the cleft must be included in the flap, and when the flap is advanced, the papillae are shifted by one tooth width towards the cleft.

The lesser-segment flap is raised in a subperiosteal plane and then mobilized by performing a periosteal release across the undersurface of the flap, parallel to the occlusal surface, approximately 2.5 cm from the inferior edge. Since the periosteum contributes to the perfusion of the flap, the farther the release is performed from the edges of the flap, the better. This periosteal release is continued towards the cleft separating the labial mucosa from the cleft mucosa. For this release of labial mucosa, an angled blade is used to undermine the incision at the superior extent of the alveolar cleft labionasal fistula, taking care to cut up into the lip and not towards the nasal floor. This mobilizes the oral mucosa above the cleft along with the lesser-segment flap without violating the nasal cavity *(Fig. 26.7)*.

The opposing alveolar cleft mucosal surfaces are then cut from incisive foramen to labial surface of the alveolus, separating them into upper (nasal lining) and lower (oral lining) flaps. The upper mucoperisoteal nasal lining flaps are reflected out of the cleft and up into the piriform aperture and sutured to each other *(Fig. 26.7)* with a small curved needle repairing the labionasal fistula. If the space is too tight for a needle, the repair is done through the nose, passing a large needle from the nose into the cleft, through one of the lining flaps, and then passing it back from the cleft into the nose through the opposing lining flap and tying the knot inside the nostril. The lower oral lining flaps within the cleft are then reflected down into the mouth, such that they can be closed to each other with everting sutures to repair the oronasal fistula. If the cleft is too wide, then the anterior hard-palate tissue is raised as posteriorly based mucoperiosteal flaps pedicled on the greater

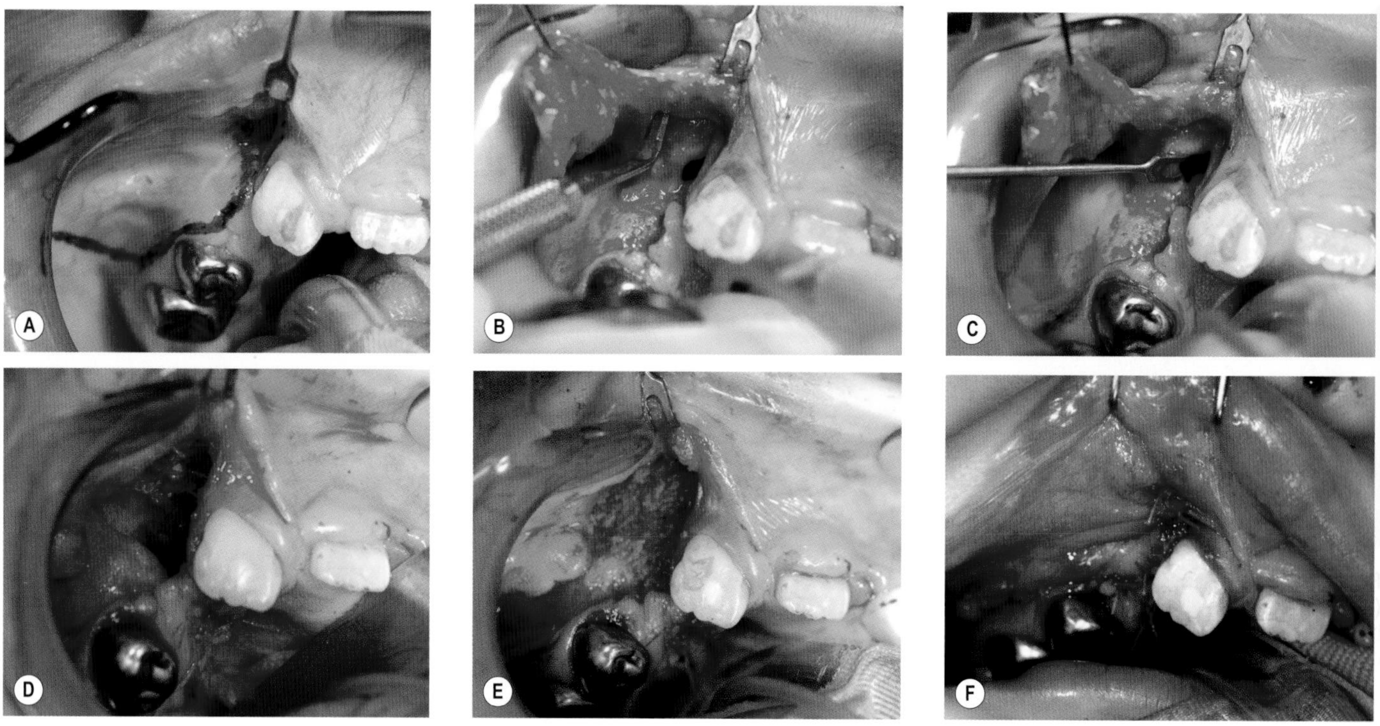

Fig. 26.7 Modified Abyholm technique for secondary bone grafting of a unilateral alveolar cleft. See text for details. **(A)** The superior-based lesser-segment flap for labial surface closure has been marked. The tip is covered with attached gingiva for transfer into the cleft. **(B)** The flap is raised off the lesser segment in a subperiosteal plane and cleft mucosa separated from the labial mucosa with an angled blade. **(C)** The opposing surfaces of mucosa within the cleft have been separated from alveolus to incisive foramen. The superior flaps (hook in place) are used to repair the nasal lining. **(D)** The two reflected superior mucosal flaps have been sutured together to close the nasal fistula and the two inferior flaps closed to repair the oral fistula. **(E)** Cancellous iliac crest bone graft has been packed within the cleft. **(F)** The lesser-segment mucoperiosteal flap is transposed across the labial surface of the graft without tension. The frenum was released secondarily.

palatine vessels, and sutured together to close the oral surface of the cleft without tension.

With closure of the oronasal fistula, the graft can now be harvested. Numerous donor sources of bone graft have been described,[25] but iliac crest cancellous bone graft is considered the gold standard *(Fig. 26.8)*. After the skin incision, the dissection proceeds directly down to the cartilage cap of the crest, without any muscle dissection or stripping. The cartilaginous crest is opened as an H-shaped incision to gain access to the underlying cancellous bone. The bone is harvested using a curette or gouge and stored in blood. If a cortical strut is planned to "reconstruct" the pyriform rim and provide a barrier between the graft and nasal lining, it is harvested from the inner table of the ilium. The graft donor site is then packed with gelfoam soaked with plain bupivicaine to minimize postoperative pain[26] and the cartilage tightly approximated prior to closing the skin.

If a cortical barrier strut is used, it is placed under the nasal lining repair, resting on the opposing edges of the piriform rim at the superior aspect of the cleft. The graft is then carefully packed into the prepared graft site, using a bone tamp to compress the pieces. If there is graft remaining after filling the cleft from incisive foramen to labial surface and from nasal lining to oral lining, the remaining bone is used to augment the deficient maxillary bone in the region of the cleft-side piriform rim. This onlay graft helps support the alar base of the nose, and can improve symmetry in the unilateral cleft nasal deformity. The lesser-segment mucoperiosteal buccal sulcus flap is then mesially advanced over the labial surface

of the graft and carefully secured with fine resorbable sutures to the mesial alveolus and oral palate. The most common site of dehiscence is at the junction of the lesser-segment flap and the oral lining repair, often at the edge of the central incisor crown. Meticulous atraumatic suture technique must be used in this area.

Postoperative care includes gentle oral hygiene with a soft manual toothbrush and antibiotic mouthwash. A mechanical soft diet is followed for 6 weeks. Radiographic preservation of the graft is assessed with a periapical film at 8–10 weeks. If a small portion of the graft site becomes exposed in the early postoperative course, it can often be salvaged with debridement of the exposed bone chip and antibiotic rinses. If the entire graft itself becomes contaminated or purulent, it must be removed, and the site allowed to heal before attempting a repeat graft.

For bilateral clefts, the same technique is used, but care must be taken to ensure that the U-shaped fistula behind the premaxilla is closed. If this has not been done adequately at the time of the palate repair, an angled blade is used to incise the posterior aspect of the premaxilla transversely, separating the mucosa into oral and nasal components. The nasal lining is repaired as in primary cases. The anterior hard-palate mucosa is then raised as unipedicled mucoperiosteal flaps and sutured to the oral mucosa of the posterior premaxilla. If the vascular supply of the premaxilla is tenuous, then the repair should be staged, doing each graft at different settings. As well, the repair can be staged with an initial soft-tissue oronasal fistula repair followed by standard bone grafting. A

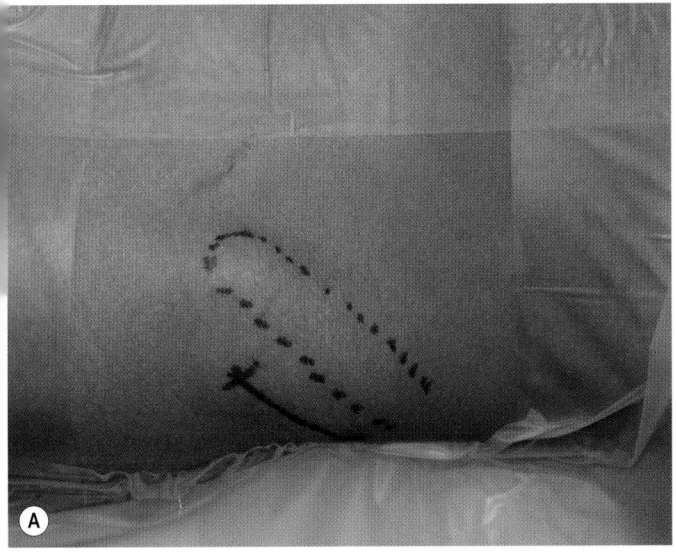
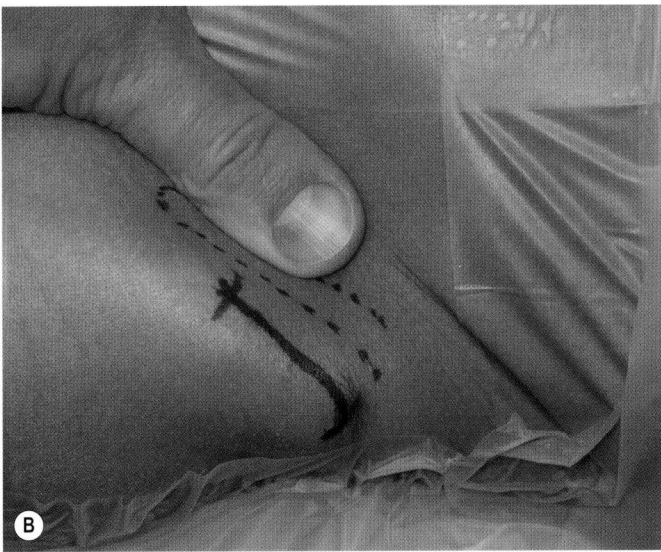

Fig. 26.8 Incision placement for harvesting iliac crest cancellous bone graft. **(A)** The anterior superior iliac spine and crest have been marked in dotted lines. **(B)** Upward traction is placed on the skin over the crest and the incision is marked along the iliac crest such that when the skin is released, the scar will lie off the crest and below the pant line. The incision should be 2 cm behind the anterior superior iliac crest to avoid iatrogenic damage to the lateral femoral cutaneous nerve. Excessive traction or transaction of the nerve will result in meralgia paresthetica.

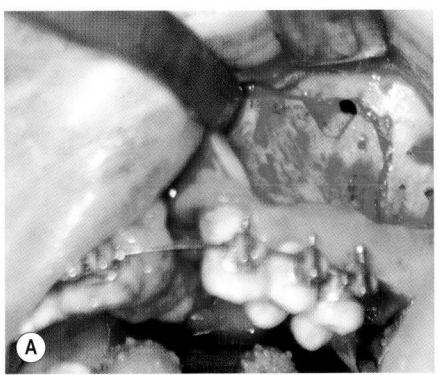
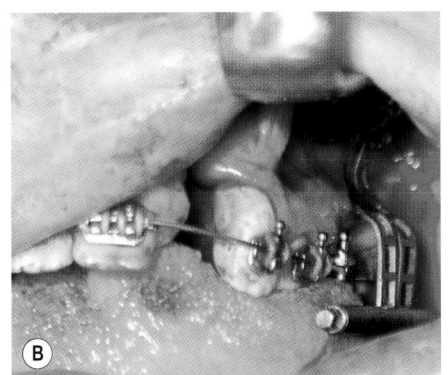
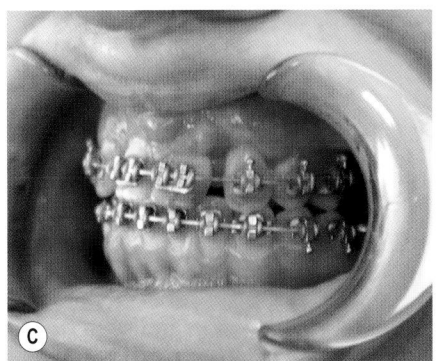

Fig. 26.9 The same patient shown in *Figure 26.4* undergoing horizontal alveolar transport distraction. See text for details. **(A)** An interdental osteotomy has been performed to create a three-tooth segment for transport. **(B)** The internal alveolar distraction device has been placed across the osteotomy. **(C)** Appearance postdistraction, consolidation, device removal, and secondary bone grafting. The patient is now ready for orthodontic alignment and dental restoration.

stabilization splint is essential for a bilateral cleft repair, or the mobility of the premaxilla postsurgery will prevent healing of the grafted clefts.

Occasionally at the time of bone grafting, unrestricted overgrowth at the premaxillary suture in patients with bilateral complete cleft lip and palate prevents the orthodontist from achieving the appropriate arch alignment needed for successful grafting. This can be seen in delayed or untreated clefts found in adopted children, when the lack of a repaired oral muscle sphincter did not mold the projecting premaxilla in early childhood. In these rare cases, premaxilla setback is required. This technique involves separating the premaxilla from the vomer and resecting a portion of the vomer and septum, allowing the entire premaxilla to be set back into alignment with the lesser segments.[27] This procedure carries the risk of necrosis of the premaxilla and loss of the anterior dentition, and should therefore only be performed when other options are not available.

Horizontal TDO of a tooth-bearing alveolar segment

This procedure is typically performed for a recalcitrant alveolar cleft with large oronasolabial fistula. The principle is to create a transport segment by separating an adjacent two- or three-tooth-bearing segment of the distal alveolus from the maxilla without damage to the tooth roots and without violation of the attached gingiva *(Fig. 26.9)*. The distraction device is then applied to the stable maxilla and the transport segment with an anterior/mesial vector, such that when the device is activated, the segment gradually closes the alveolar cleft until it is touching the premaxilla. At this point, the remaining cleft is amenable to standard grafting techniques. The device is then left in place and not activated during the 8–12-week consolidation period, during which the generate formed in the distraction gap distal to the transport segment gradually ossifies and stabilizes the transport segment. For large naso-orolabial fistulas, performing the nasal lining closure at the time of the device placement may be easier due to the improved visibility and access via the wide cleft. As the transport segment advances and the cleft and fistula are compressed, the repaired nasal lining will fold on itself and seal any remaining small holes, allowing the secondary grafting procedure to focus solely on closing the oral lining.

Activation of the device is initiated 5 days postoperation at 0.5–1 mm/day. Orthodontic guidance can be provided with brackets and an arch wire as long as the direction dictated by the orthodontic force is not competing with the distraction vector; otherwise, the device footplates and screws will be under strain. When performing simultaneous bilateral distraction for bilateral clefts, care must be taken to control protrusion of the ungrafted premaxilla as the transport segments contact it towards the end of activation (*Fig. 26.10*).

The device can be removed after 8–12 weeks of consolidation with simultaneous secondary grafting of the remaining approximated cleft.

Vertical alveolar TDO

Vertical alveolar TDO is useful for augmentation of a previously grafted cleft when the gingiva or previous surgeries have made augmentation with standard grafting techniques not possible (*Fig. 26.11*). Ten millimeters of vertical bone height below the maxillary sinus is the minimum required to perform an osteotomy and distraction without prior onlay grafting. If there is no or minimal bone below the maxilla, a cortical graft can be harvested as a separate procedure from the mandible angle, iliac crest, or outer calvarium and rigidly lag screwed as an onlay graft over the planned future osteotomy. The osteotomy and distraction can be performed 2–3 months later, transporting the increased bone volume from the incorporated onlay graft into the defect. The same activation and consolidation protocol for horizontal TDO is followed. During vertical distraction, however, the activation arm can often be covered with a custom temporary prosthesis created by the patient's prosthodontist.

Outcomes, prognosis, and complications

Gingivoperiosteoplasty

Long-term evaluation is just now becoming available of the Millard GPP protocol that used the Latham device to narrow the cleft such that a limited subperiosteal GPP could be performed. In evaluating their own patients, Millard *et al.*[28] found that a bony bridge formed in 63% of unilateral and 83% of

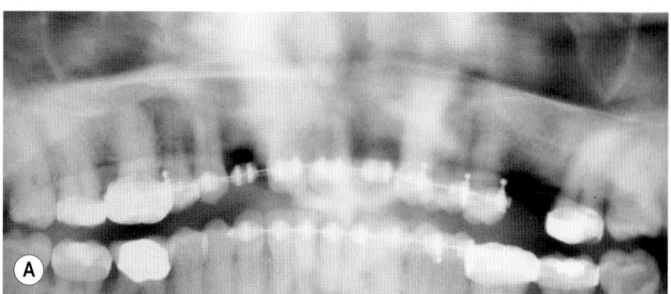

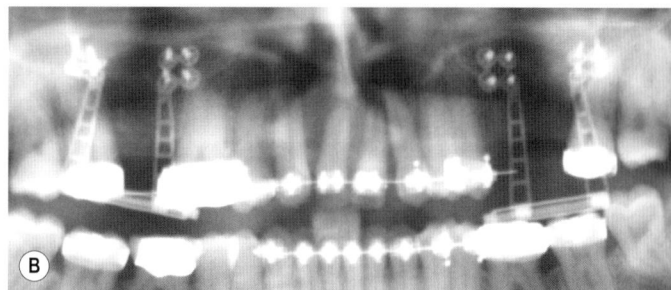

Fig. 26.10 Panorex radiograph of the bilateral transport distraction performed on the patient shown in *Figures 26.4 and 26.9*. **(A)** On the left side the patient had undergone a previous extraction, creating an ideal site for the interdental osteotomy. On the right side, the osteotomy is distal to the third tooth on the segment. **(B)** Postactivation, the canines are now adjacent to the central incisors and the alveolar clefts have been compressed. The distracted osteotomy contains generate tissue that will ossify during consolidation, effectively lengthening the maxillary arch.

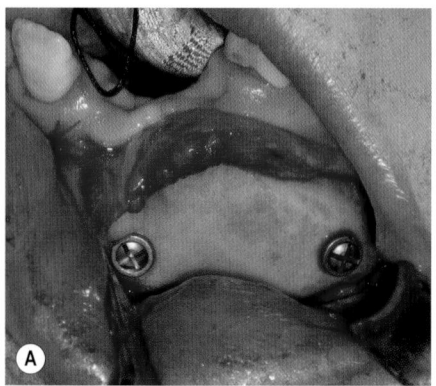
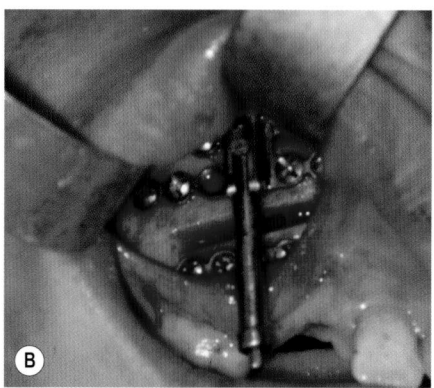
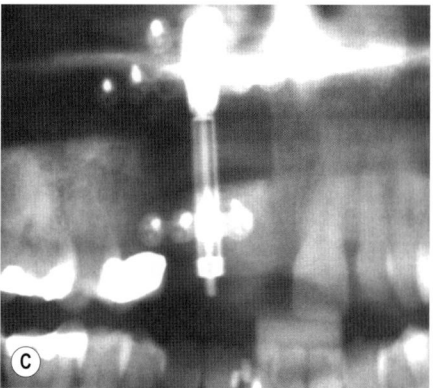

Fig. 26.11 The same patient shown in *Figure 26.5* undergoing vertical alveolar transport distraction. See text for details. **(A)** Since the vertical height of alveolus below the maxillary sinus was less than 10 mm, the site was augmented with an onlay autogenous split calvarial bone graft held in place with lag screws. **(B)** Three months later the lag screws are removed and a rectangular osteotomy is created within the consolidated graft. An internal vertical distractor has been placed across the osteotomy with a vector that will augment the vertical height of the alveolus and simultaneously lower the level of the gingival surface. **(C)** Radiograph of the device postactivation demonstrating alignment of the transport segment with the adjacent gum line. The generated tissue within the superior osteotomy site will consolidate over 2 months.

bilateral clefts and a very low percentage (3%) required secondary bone grafting. An increase in anterior crossbite was reported in patients treated with GPP, but they did not seem to require orthognathic surgery more frequently than did controls, though the follow-up was admittedly too short to tell definitively. Others, however, were less optimistic in their evaluations of these same patients. Henkel and Gundlach reported vertical growth disturbance of the maxilla in 42% of patients with unilateral and 40% of patients with bilateral clefts treated with Millard's technique.[29] Berkowitz et al.[30] analyzed the occlusion of these patients and found crossbites in 100% of patients treated with GPP, and he reported more difficulty in treating the crossbite deformity.[31,32] Matic and Power[31,32] retrospectively reviewed 65 unilateral and 43 bilateral clefts treated with Latham active molding and GPP. The clinical success rate compared to a historical group treated with secondary bone grafting was 41% for unilateral GPP and 58% for bilateral GPP, compared to 88% and 90% respectively for the secondary graft comparisons.

Grayson et al.[33] described the use of nasoalveolar molding (NAM) instead of the Latham device to narrow the cleft prior to GPP, with the theory that the more passive "guided molding" of NAM would be less detrimental on future facial growth and dental relationship. In retrospectively examining their cohort at mixed dentition, they reported bone formation in 80% of clefts with 73% not requiring secondary bone grafting.[34,35] In evaluating facial growth, they found no adverse effect on midface growth during mixed dentition, and on repeat analysis up to 18 years of age.[36,37] Continued prospective evaluation of the NAM and GPP protocol at other institutions will be required to determine if these results can be reproduced.

Primary bone grafting

On self-evaluation of this approach on 20 consecutive patients, Rosenstein et al.[23] reported no cephalometric evidence of impaired growth compared to a similar cohort who did not undergo primary grafting. Hathaway et al., at a separate center, retrospectively evaluated 17 patients who underwent primary grafting, and reported no difference in arch form compared to ungrafted clefts.[38] Ross evaluated cephalograms from 15 cleft centers and reported that grafting in infancy may have a negative effect on both vertical and horizontal midface growth, but it was not clear whether this was any greater than the effect of secondary bone grafting between the ages of 4 and 10 years.[39] The potential increased risk of exposing infants to an additional surgery and anesthesia in the first year of life must be weighed against the possible benefit of avoiding a secondary bone graft procedure in mixed dentition.[40]

Secondary bone grafting

Some of the most commonly used outcome measures for bone grafts are the Bergland scale[18] based on interdental height of bone, the bone height index,[41] based on the percentage of bone covering the roots of adjacent teeth, the Chelsea index,[42] measuring position and quality of bone, and the Kindelan bone-fill index[43] that is a four-point scale of percentage bone infill. All but the last require eruption of the permanent cuspid before they can be used. In addition to the variability of outcome measures, there is wide variation in the literature in timing of evaluation, as well as limitations inherent to plain film analysis such as rotation variability. Some have proposed cone beam computed tomography as a superior method of graft evaluation.[44,45]

In the context of these study limitations, the success rate of secondary alveolar bone grafting in the literature ranges from 70% to 80% in most studies,[41,43,46,47] to over 90% in a few reports.[48–51] Scottish cleft services reported a dramatic increase in graft success from 58%[52] to 76%[53] as a presumed result of a reorganization that decreased the number of surgeons performing bone grafts and establishment of nationally followed standard protocols.

Bone morphogenic protein

Isolated cleft centers have started trials for the use of rhBMP2 in the treatment of alveolar clefts in older patients given the increased failure rate of autogenous grafting in this population. A randomized trial of 21 skeletally mature patients with a unilateral cleft alveolar defect showed that patients treated with a collagen sponge soaked in rhBMP2 demonstrated improved bone healing and reduced donor morbidity and cost compared to those filled with autogenous iliac crest cancellous graft.[54] This group did not trial rhBMP2 in growing patients in mixed dentition due to their previous animal studies that demonstrated ectopic bone formation in 1%, as well as the high success rate of conventional autogenous grafting in this age group. Other centers have used rhBMP2 in place of autogenous grafting in growing children with evidence of bone formation,[55] but orthodontic outcomes are still pending. However, reported complications include ectopic bone formation, bone resorption or remodeling at the graft site, hematoma, neck swelling, and painful seroma. Other potential theoretical concerns include carcinogenicity and teratogenic effects.[56]

Late bone grafting

When an alveolar cleft is bone-grafted before eruption of the cuspid, there is greater than 80% chance of success, and the result provides adequate long-term periodontal support. With age this success rate drops sharply, approaching 50% at 25 years of age.[24,57] Grafting after eruption of permanent dentition also does not correct periodontal defects (i.e., inadequate periodontal ligament), even with subsequent orthodontic movement into the graft. The goal of grafting in adults is therefore no longer to provide support for erupted teeth, but rather to provide sufficient bone stock for prosthetic placement. In addition, the adult alveolar cleft is typically larger due to the poor health and loss of adjacent teeth. The technique of grafting an adult cleft involves rigid fixation of a corticocancellous graft with either resorbable or titanium fixation. Due to the slower incorporation of this graft architecture, an increased attention to the vascularity of the mucoperiosteal flaps and the nasal closure is essential. The cleft is also minimized by segmental maxillary osteotomies and advancement of the posterior segment into the cleft. In bilateral clefts, staging the surgery may be necessary. Implant placement should take place 3–4 months postgrafting to avoid loss of the graft.

Graft site augmentation

As with all bone, the alveolar graft requires mechanical stimulation to avoid resorption. Eruption of teeth into the graft and orthodontic movement of teeth can both provide this stimulation. In some cases where canine substitution is not performed, the bone graft placed to support the erupting canine may experience an "unstimulated" region adjacent to the central incisor due to the missing lateral incisor. In these cases, focal crestal resorption can occur and an alveolar augmentation procedure is required prior to implant placement at skeletal maturity.

Access the complete references list online at **http://www.expertconsult.com**

6.   Boyne PJ, Sands NR. Secondary bone grafting of residual alveolar and palatal clefts. *J Oral Surg*. 1972; 30:87–92.

   Landmark article largely recognized as initiating the popularity of secondary bone grafting. Boyne introduced the concept in the 1960s, advocating treatment towards the end of the first decade of life to minimize growth impairment while still supporting eruption of the adult dentition. Most of the described principles are still followed today.

12. Cassolato SF, Ross B, Daskalogiannakis J, et al. Treatment of dental anomalies in children with complete unilateral cleft lip and palate at SickKids hospital, Toronto. *Cleft Palate Craniofac J*. 2009;46: 166–172.

   Retrospective study of 116 children with complete unilateral cleft lip and palate treated since birth. The article quantifies dental anomalies in permanent dentition associated with complete unilateral cleft lip and palate and surveys treatment modalities used to address these problems.

16. Rosenstein S, Dado DV, Kernahan D, et al. The case for early bone grafting in cleft lip and palate: a second report. *Plast Reconstr Surg*. 1991;87:644–654; discussion 55–6.

17. El Deeb M, Messer LB, Lehnert MW, et al. Canine eruption into grafted bone in maxillary alveolar cleft defects. *Cleft Palate J*. 1982;19:9–16.

22. Liou EJ, Chen PK, Huang CS, et al. Interdental distraction osteogenesis and rapid orthodontic tooth movement: a novel approach to approximate a wide alveolar cleft or bony defect. *Plast Reconstr Surg*. 2000; 105:1262–1272.

   Detailed case based review of interdental transport distraction osteogenesis to treat wide alveolar clefts by the recognized expert.

24. Abyholm FE, Bergland O, Semb G. Secondary bone grafting of alveolar clefts. A surgical/orthodontic treatment enabling a non-prosthodontic rehabilitation in cleft lip and palate patients. *Scand J Plast Reconstr Surg*. 1981;15:127–140.

28. Millard DR, Latham R, Huifen X, et al. Cleft lip and palate treated by presurgical orthopedics, gingivoperiosteoplasty, and lip adhesion (POPLA) compared with previous lip adhesion method: a preliminary study of serial dental casts. *Plast Reconstr Surg*. 1999;103:1630–1644.

35. Sato Y, Grayson BH, Garfinkle JS, et al. Success rate of gingivoperiosteoplasty with and without secondary bone grafts compared with secondary alveolar bone grafts alone. *Plast Reconstr Surg*. 2008;121:1356–1367; discussion 68–9.

   Most recent retrospective evaluation by the NYU team of GPP outcomes with and without secondary bone grafting. They concluded that GPP alone or combined with secondary alveolar bone grafting results in superior bone levels when compared with conventional secondary alveolar bone grafting alone.

39. Ross RB. Treatment variables affecting facial growth in complete unilateral cleft lip and palate. *Cleft Palate J*. 1987;24:5–77.

53. McIntyre GT, Devlin MF. Secondary alveolar bone grafting (CLEFTSiS) 2000–2004. *Cleft Palate Craniofac J*. 2010;47:66–72.

   A good discussion article delineating some of the key components associated with quality and outcome of alveolar bone grafting. The authors relate the changes to the Scottish Regional Cleft Programme that increased graft success rate from 58% to 76%.

27

Orthodontics in cleft lip and palate management

Alvaro A. Figueroa and John W. Polley

SYNOPSIS

- Patients with oro-facial clefts are best treated through a team approach.
- Close collaboration between the orthodontist and surgeon is critical during the care of patients with oro-facial clefts.
- A developmental approach needs to be undertaken by orthodontists treating patients with oro-facial clefts.
- In infancy the orthodontist can support the surgeon with nasoalveolar molding and maxillary orthopedics.
- In the primary dentition stage the orthodontist can correct mild to moderate posterior and anterior crossbites.
- In the transitional dentition the orthodontist prepares the maxillary arch prior to bone grafting and premaxillary repositioning.
- In the full permanent dentition the orthodontists finalizes arch alignment and coordination.
- The orthodontists supports the surgeon during planning, preparation of appliances and follow up of patients requiring orthognathic surgery and/or distraction osteogenesis during adolescence.
- The orthodontist works closely with other specialists in pediatric dentistry, prosthodontics, oral and plastic surgery to rehabilitate the dental, oral and facial conditions of patients with oro-facial clefts.
- The application of new orthodontic diagnostic and treatment modalities to patients with oro-facial clefts is likely to improve treatment outcomes.

Introduction

The state of the art for the management of patients with oral facial clefts requires the use of a multidisciplinary approach as various structures, traditionally treated by several specialists, are involved. In the oral cavity, the cleft affects not only the soft and hard palate, but also the alveolus and dentition. The structural rehabilitation of these patients requires the surgical correction of the soft- and hard-tissue defects as well as the secondary effects of the cleft on maxillary development, dental support, and dental–occlusal alignment. The role of the orthodontist in cleft management is essential as the orthodontist assists the surgeon during all stages of reconstructive care: in the early stages, with presurgical nasal and maxillary orthopedics; during the transitional dentition stage, with alignment of the maxillary segments and dentition in preparation for secondary alveolar bone grafting; and during the permanent dentition and late adolescent years, by obtaining satisfactory dental and occlusal relationships and also to prepare the dentition for prosthetic rehabilitation and orthognathic surgery, if required. In addition, it has been the role of the orthodontist to monitor craniofacial growth and dental development, as well as the treatment effects on these patients through the use of roentgencephalometry.

With this approach, the management of the cleft patient has evolved dramatically in recent years. The reason for improved outcomes is based on refinements in primary and finishing surgical techniques, as well as timing and incorporation of other procedures such as presurgical orthopedics, orthodontics, and new prosthetic approaches utilizing resin-bonded prosthesis and/or osseointegrated implants.

It is our experience that patients treated within the context of the multidisciplinary approach can obtain excellent outcomes related to speech, ideal occlusion, satisfactory lip aesthetics, and skeletal balance *(Fig. 27.1)*. However, it is the secondary cleft nasal deformity that still gives the patient the "cleft stigmata." ⊛ FIG **27.1** APPEARS ONLINE ONLY

In recent years, new orthodontic and surgical treatment modalities have become available that may further improve outcomes in patients with orofacial clefts. In infancy, this includes the use of presurgical nasoalveolar molding techniques. In the mixed dentition, novel orthodontic–orthopedic approaches to correct maxillary hypoplasia are utilized; and, in the permanent dentition, the use of new appliances and dental materials to facilitate orthodontic treatment and the application of bone anchorage screws (BAS) to facilitate orthodontic tooth movement are employed. In addition, the use of distraction osteogenesis to improve the position of the maxilla in those cases with severe maxillary hypoplasia has become a well-accepted procedure. Finally the availability of new diagnostic techniques such as digital skull and dental models, three-dimensional (3D) photogrammetry, lower radiation computed tomography (CT) scans, cone beam CT (CBCT), and the development of 3D digital protocols to plan orthognathic surgery are now at the forefront of current orthodontic and surgical approaches. The efforts towards improvement of orthodontic and surgical treatment strategies developed for noncleft patients will benefit the challenging problems presented by cleft patients and are a welcome addition to the current treatment protocols.

In this chapter, some of the new orthodontic and surgical strategies that are of benefit to cleft patients will be presented. The reader is directed to previous publications that deal with the role of the orthodontist in the management of the cleft patient to complement the information presented in this chapter.[1–4]

Infancy

On many occasions, the surgeon is faced with an infant who has a severe cleft with marked distortions of not only the maxillary segments but also the cartilages of the nose. This situation can occur in both the unilateral and bilateral cleft lip and palate patient. Since 1995 we have introduced the use of nasoalveolar molding in the treatment protocol of those patients presenting with unilateral and bilateral clefts with premaxillary protrusion and hypoplastic columella with moderate to severe nasal distortions, following the general principles reported by Grayson and associates.[5–10] They utilize premaxillary and maxillary orthopedics with the additional purposes of not only aligning the maxillary and premaxillary segments, but also to reposition the nasal cartilages prior to lip repair.

Unilateral cleft lip

Evaluation of the cleft nose demonstrates the presence of severely distorted nasal cartilage with deviation of the nasal tip towards the noncleft side and severe angulation of the columella also to the noncleft side. In addition, we have observed that the soft tissues caudal to the lateral nasal cartilage may be hyperplastic and prominent. Repair of the lip under these conditions, even with surgical repositioning of the nasal cartilages, results in a suboptimal nasal morphology outcome, even though the lip repair is satisfactory. It is for this reason that we have now embarked on the process of orthopedic repositioning of the nasal cartilages, columella, nasal tip, and lateral wall of the vestibule in order to provide these patients with the best possible primary nasal reconstruction with minimally invasive surgical techniques. The procedure of presurgical infant nasal remodeling utilizing a modified intraoral plate was first described by Bennun and co-workers in Argentina.[11,12] Since then, it has been popularized in the US as nasoalveolar molding by Grayson et al.[5–10] The authors have used this technique since 1995 and have made some modifications.[13]

Our technique is as follows: the nasoalveolar molding plate is made utilizing a light cure orthodontic resin. A loop wire is incorporated to support the nasal conformer (nasal stent),

made of light cured acrylic, to reposition the nasal structures. The nasal stent is covered with soft acrylic to avoid irritation of the delicate tissues of the nasal mucosa. The palatal aspect of the plate is covered with soft-tissue liner in order to obtain perfect adaptation to the maxillary palatal shelves and undercuts created by the cleft (Figs 27.2 and 27.3). An exact fit of the plate is required for adequate retention, especially since we do not rely on external adhesive tape to maintain the plate in position. We utilize denture adhesive cream, after drying the plate and the oral mucosa prior to insertion. The parents are instructed to clean and replace the denture adhesive one to two times per day. Patients return on a weekly basis for adjustments to increase the length of the supporting wire and reshape the nasal stent. While the nasal molding is taking place, selectively grinding acrylic medial to the palatal shelves and adding acrylic lateral to the alveolar processes narrows the distance between the maxillary segments (Fig. 27.4). In addition, facial taping can be utilized to apply transverse pressure to the cleft segments and help with the cleft narrowing and nasal molding process (Fig. 27.5). FIGS 27.2–5 APPEAR ONLINE ONLY

The results expected from this technique include repositioning of the nasal tip towards the noncleft side with straightening of the columella and equalizing the height on the nasal domes as much as possible. In addition, the nasal stent is adjusted in such a way as to exert lateral pressure on the lateral nasal wall against the hyperplastic soft tissues caudal to the lateral nasal cartilage (Fig. 27.5). This results in a straighter nose with convex nasal cartilages and flattened hyperplastic lateral wall vestibular tissues.

At the time of surgery, the surgeon will repair the lip with medial repositioning of the base of the nose and narrowing of the nasal domes with tacking of the vestibular tissues to the lateral nasal wall. We believe that this combined effort will provide these patients with better noses that will require less extensive secondary revisions. The outcomes obtained with this technique are consistent and predictable and these variations of the molding technique have been incorporated with favorable results.

In cases that start with severe nasal distortion, we support the nasal molding with postsurgical nasal stents utilizing commercially available removable nasal stents.[13–15] The stent is usually kept in place using facial taping (Fig. 27.6) and is maintained for at least 2–3 months or for as long as the patient can deal with it comfortably. FIG 27.6 APPEARS ONLINE ONLY

Bilateral cleft lip

The patient with bilateral cleft lip and palate represents the most challenging condition for the reconstructive team. The premaxilla is extremely protrusive, the premaxilla and prolabium can be of variable size, the columella is deficient or almost nonexistent, the palatal clefts are wider than usual, and occasionally, the maxillary palatal shelves are collapsed. In addition, the nasal domes are wide apart and the tip projection is decreased (Fig. 27.7). It has been our experience that, in patients with bilateral cleft lip and palate, with a protrusive premaxilla, it becomes imperative that the premaxilla is repositioned into a more favorable relation with the maxillary segments in order to achieve definitive lip closure with minimal tension. If this is not done, a poor repair or failure with unfavorable consequences may occur. For this purpose, we have successfully utilized premaxillary orthopedics with an intraoral appliance that is retained with denture adhesive and has an elastic strap for premaxillary retraction.[16,17] This approach has allowed the surgeon to close the lip satisfactorily *(Figs 27.8 and 27.9)*. ⊕ FIGS 27.7–9 APPEAR ONLINE ONLY

In the bilateral cleft lip and palate patient the approach requires repositioning of the premaxilla prior to the nasal molding technique. For the last 20 years we have used a self-retaining intraoral plate[17] that has been modified from the original design.[16] This modification allows for easy adjustments and fewer frequent patient visits.

Grayson and coworkers[6–8,10] have utilized nasoalveolar molding for bilateral clefts. The appliance was intended to retract the premaxilla as well as molding the nasal cartilage and elongating the columella. Their plate design included retention through extraoral taping and elastics. We have modified the design utilizing our principles of a self-retained appliance[13,16,17] to avoid using facial taping to support the prosthesis. A light-cured resin plate is constructed to which orthodontic buttons or custom-formed wires are attached for retraction of the premaxilla with the elastomeric band. In addition the plate is relined with soft-tissue conditioner for close adaptation to the palatal tissues. After premaxillary retraction and repositioning are completed, the plate is modified by adding two wires that go into each nasal vestibule. The ends of the wires are bent in a loop and are covered with a light-cured acrylic covered with soft denture lining material (nasal stents). In addition, loops are bent about the level of the superior aspect of the prolabium for attachment of an elastomeric chain that has been covered with a soft-tissue denture liner. The purpose of the elastomeric chain across the prolabium is to hold it down, while the nasal prongs at the end of the wires are gradually elevated, lifting and medially repositioning the nasal domes and, at the same time, elongating the hypoplastic columella *(Fig. 27.8)*. The plate is used 24 hours a day, is removed daily for cleaning, and is held in position with the aid of a denture adhesive cream. In addition, the palatal aspect of the plate can be modified by adding material on the lateral aspects of the plate and removing acrylic on the medial aspects. This will allow for gentle and gradual repositioning of the maxillary segments, resulting in narrowing of the cleft. This technique has given the surgeon an improved situation for not only obtaining adequate lip repair but also providing a better situation for primary nasal reconstruction with remodeling of the nasal domes and nasal tip and elongation of the hypoplastic columella. The main advantage of this procedure is that it eliminates the need for secondary procedures for columella elongation in the early childhood years. All of the patients in whom this technique has been used have adjusted extremely well to the use of the appliance and the families have been extremely pleased with the results *(Fig. 28.9)*, as well as with the ease in which the orthopedic phase is carried out.

The described protocol has been well tolerated by patients and readily accepted by parents. This treatment protocol has been used for a few years and there are not enough long-term data to demonstrate the effects of the technique on the fully developed nasal structures. However, some patients are in the midteen years and the clinical impression at this time is that they will require less extensive nasal revision procedures at the completion of facial growth *(Fig. 27.10)*. ⊕ FIG 27.10 APPEARS ONLINE ONLY

Primary dentition

Orthodontic treatment at this stage is limited to the correction of certain posterior crossbites and anterior crossbites of mild to moderate degree.

Posterior crossbite

In the cleft patient, posterior crossbites are of both skeletal and dental origin. They are skeletal because the maxillary segments are usually collapsed after cleft palate surgery, especially in the canine region. In most instances, this change in arch form occurs prior to the eruption of the primary canines; therefore, at the time of eruption of these teeth, the maxillary cleft-side primary canine erupts medially to the lower one. In addition, this early relationship causes minor palatal displacement of the maxillary primary canine and labial displacement of the mandibular one.[3] This is an important observation, as this is the reason why cleft patients in the primary dentition rarely have occlusal or functional shifts. Patients in whom an occlusal shift is detected are those who are candidates for either selective tooth grinding or expansion procedures. Expansion can readily be accomplished but it should be noted that, after it is completed, unless a bone graft is placed, it has to be retained until the time of alveolar reconstruction with a bone graft. For this reason, we prefer to delay transverse expansion in the primary dentition until the patient is older and just prior to secondary alveolar bone-grafting procedures usually undertaken in the transitional dentition.

Anterior crossbite

Anterior crossbite of mild to moderate degree can be managed in the primary and transitional dentition stages utilizing elastic protraction forces delivered through a facial mask.[18–20] However, if it is noted that this crossbite is related to a moderate to severe skeletal maxillary hypoplasia, the patient is best managed with a surgical approach. If it is felt that the maxillary advancement is important at an early age due to its severity, it can be instituted by means of distraction osteogenesis.

Liou and Tsai[21] have introduced an intraoral technique for orthopedic advancement of the maxilla. They used a spring system with highly flexible wires to apply constant anterior pressure to the maxilla. Simultaneously they used a screw-type expander, which is regularly activated. After the screw reaches its limit, it is then turned backwards (contraction). This constant action results in activation of the circummaxillary suture complex and in this way maxillary protraction is obtained.[22] The technique has been applied to both cleft and noncleft patients with impressive outcomes and superior to conventional face mask therapy.[21]

Transitional dentition

This is the developmental stage in which a cleft patient, involving the alveolus, will receive the next surgical procedure after lip and secondary palate repair. In most instances, the dentition around the cleft presents severe malposition, limiting surgical access to the alveolar site *(Fig. 27.11)*. For this

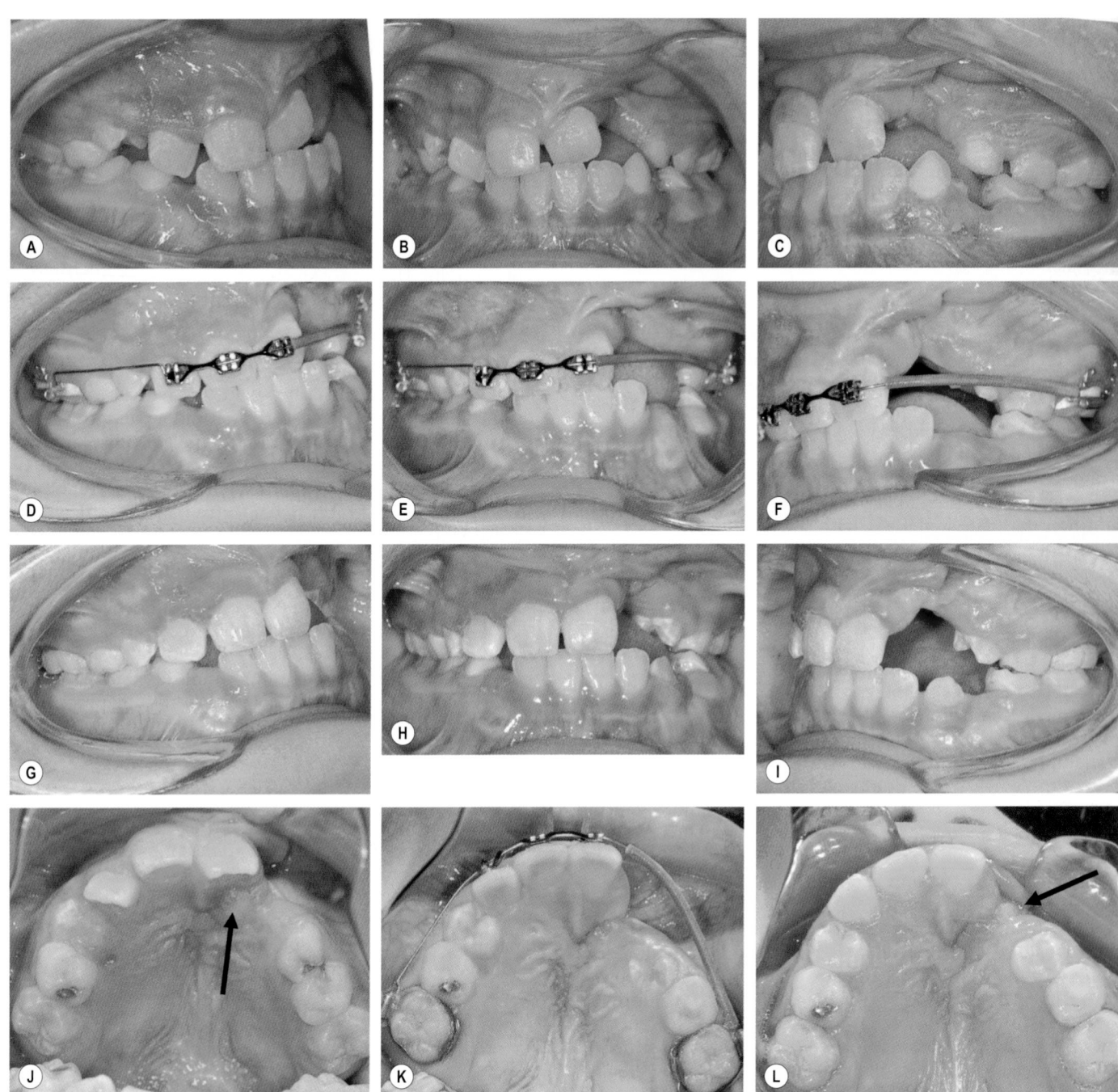

Fig. 27.11 (A–I) Patient with unilateral cleft lip and palate in the transitional dentition prior to orthodontic preparation for alveolar bone grafting (Top), after orthodontic treatment (center) and after bone graft (bottom). Note alignment of the dental arch with a simple segmental edgewise orthodontic appliance. **(J–L)** Occlusal views at similar stages, note missing lateral incisor and retained primary canine in the cleft area (arrow) (Left). This tooth was extracted prior to surgery. Note aligned arch prior to surgery (center). After surgery (right) the permanent canine erupted through the bone grafted area (arrow) (right).

purpose, the dentition adjacent to the cleft has to be reposi-tioned, preparing the cleft site for the secondary alveolar bone graft. Reconstruction of the cleft alveolus and anterior aspect of the maxilla is deferred until this stage, in an attempt to minimize the growth restriction resulting from surgical trauma and scarring.[23–25]

If it is determined that the patient requires orthodontic treatment for preparation of the surgical site, it should be initi-ated based on dental development of the permanent teeth to

be moved rather than chronological age.[3,13,26] It is known that cleft patients present with delay of dental development and eruption.[26,27] Orthodontic treatment should not be initiated until the near-complete root development of the incisors, on which orthodontic brackets will be placed *(Fig. 27.11M-O)*. Adherence to this guideline will result in minimal resorptive changes of the maxillary incisor roots. If the necessary treat-ment for secondary bone grafting of the maxilla is based on dental development rather than chronological age, a

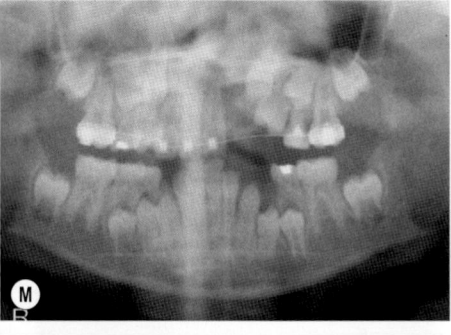
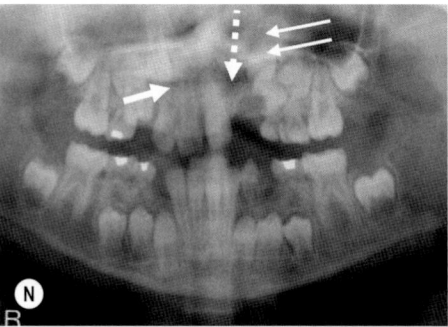
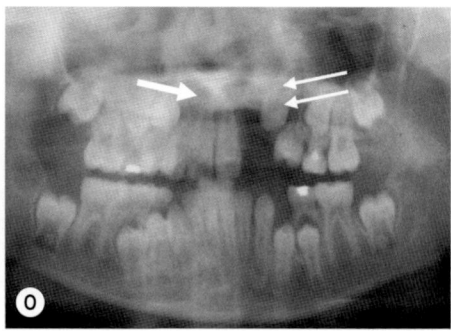

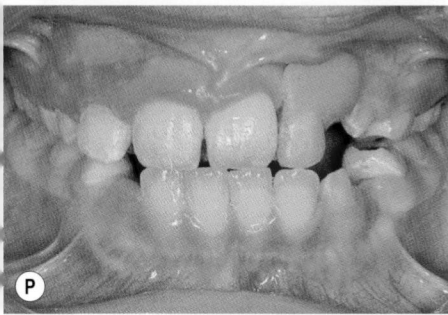

Fig. 27.11, cont'd (M–O) Panoramic radiographs at similar stages: note in the pretreatment radiographs (left, centre) complete apical root development of the maxillary incisors (single arrow), retained primary canine and missing lateral incisor (dotted arrow) and unerupted maxillary left canine (double arrows). After orthodontics and bone grafting (right) note intact maxillary incisor root apices (single arrow) and maxillary left canine erupting through the bone graft (double arrows). **(P)** After treatment an interim prosthesis was given to the patient replacing the missing lateral incisor (arrow).

safeguard for the adverse effects of surgery on growth is added. Our own studies[26] indicate that development and eruption of the cleft lateral incisor are markedly delayed when compared with a contralateral incisor *(Fig. 27.11M-O)*. This observation allows for placement of orthodontic appliances on the remaining incisors while the cleft lateral incisor has not yet erupted. When a viable cleft maxillary lateral incisor is present, this ensures its preservation and adequate bone support for eruption of both lateral incisor and canine after the bone graft.

When preparing the maxillary arch for a bone graft, it is necessary only to address the malposition of the incisors and the anterior collapse of the maxillary arch. The first stage is usually obtained through the use of a bonded edgewise appliance *(Fig. 27.11A-L)*. The use of new self-ligating brackets and highly flexible orthodontic arch wires permits slow and highly efficient tooth movement with minimal trauma and risk of root resorption. As the teeth slowly move, the surrounding thin alveolar bone remodels, maintaining adequate periodontal support even for those teeth adjacent to the cleft. The expansion of the arch can also be done with this appliance *(Fig. 27.12)*, but occasionally it has to be supported with a maxillary expander. The expander commonly used in our protocol is the quad helix expander *(Fig. 27.13)*. We rarely use a screw expander unless it is observed that the palatal tissues are severely scarred *(Fig. 27.14)*. Fortunately, with the use of more delicate surgical techniques, this latter situation is uncommon.

The expansion required for alveolar bone grafting should provide well-aligned maxillary segments with a minimal increase in the size of the alveolar gap. Wider alveolar gaps are difficult to close using local flaps.[28] In cases in which the clinician determines that the required expansion of the maxilla or repositioning of the premaxilla will create a wider gap between the maxillary segments, expansion and bone-grafting procedures are deferred until adolescence. At this time, the maxillary segments can be surgically mobilized and

approximated, allowing for closure with local flaps at the time of final orthognathic surgery.

After the maxillary segments and dentition are placed in their ideal positions, the patient is referred for secondary alveolar bone grafting.[29] Presurgical orthodontics in preparation for this reconstructive stage can be completed within a period of 6–12 months. Immediately prior to the bone graft, all appliances over the palate are removed and the labial aspects of the orthodontic wire are segmentalized for surgical access. In addition, supernumerary or primary teeth in the surgical site are extracted 8–12 weeks prior to surgery. This will provide the surgeon with intact gingival tissues for proper coverage of the bone graft.

The presence of alveolar bone is dependent on the presence of teeth. When the lateral incisor is present, with adequate crown and root anatomy and in favorable position, every attempt should be made to preserve it. If the lateral incisor erupts through the bone graft, suitable alveolar bone will be available in the alveolar ridge as well as for the erupting canine *(Fig. 27.15)*. If the permanent lateral incisor on the cleft side is missing or needs to be extracted due to its poor anatomy or position *(Fig. 27.11J-O)*, then the actively erupting canine could take its place and preserve the reconstructed alveolus.

Orthodontic treatment can be continued 8–12 weeks after bone graft surgery. As soon as appropriate maxillary arch and dental relations are achieved, the orthodontic appliances are removed and the patient is placed in retention until there is full permanent dentition. Teeth that were severely rotated prior to treatment need to be retained. Absent teeth can be temporarily replaced with a removable prosthetic appliance to improve aesthetics and limit the effects on speech production *(Fig. 27.11P)*.

Patients treated with the protocol outlined above complete the preparatory phase of orthodontic treatment in the preteen or early teen years. Patients are followed every 6 months to determine their craniofacial growth and dental development,

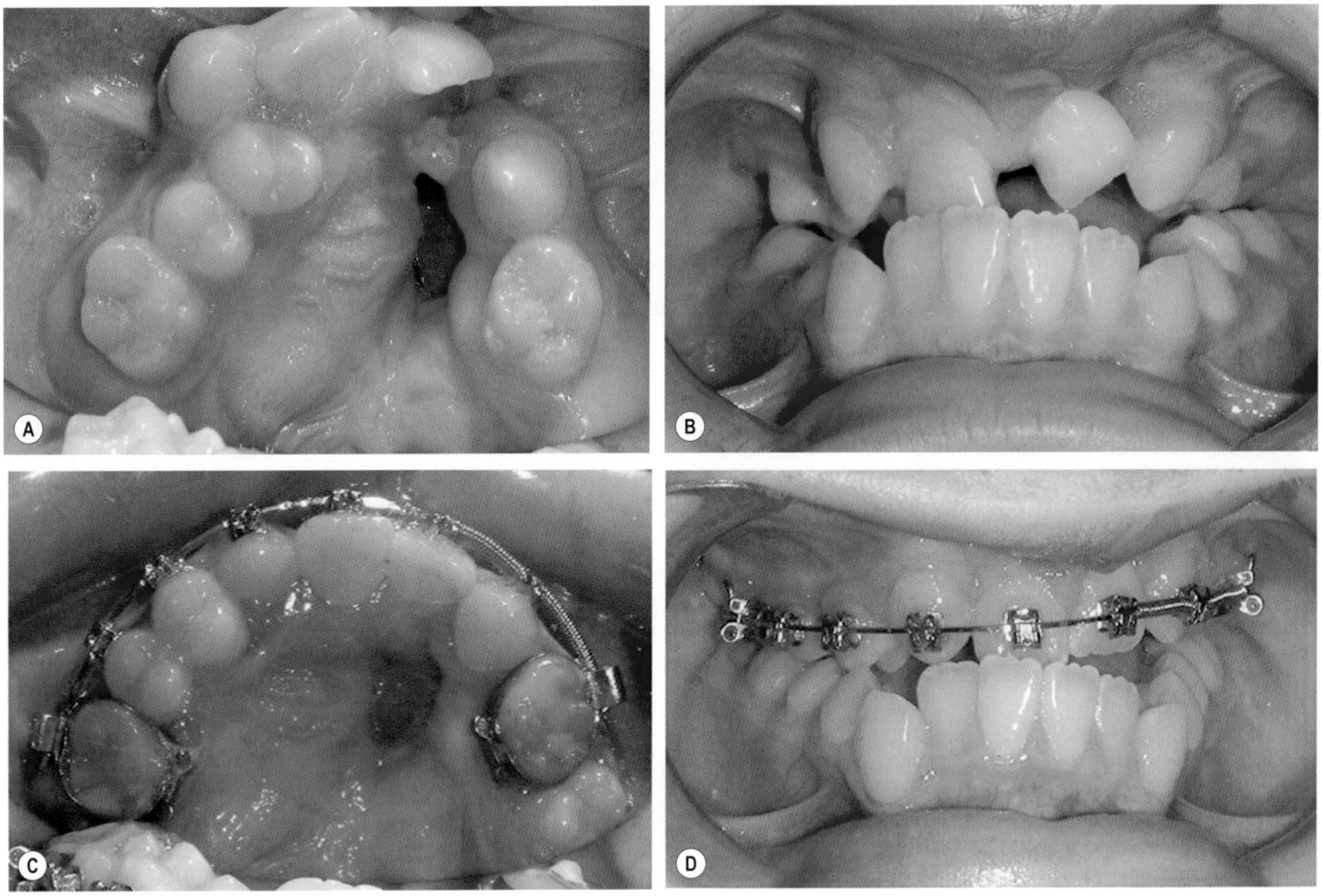

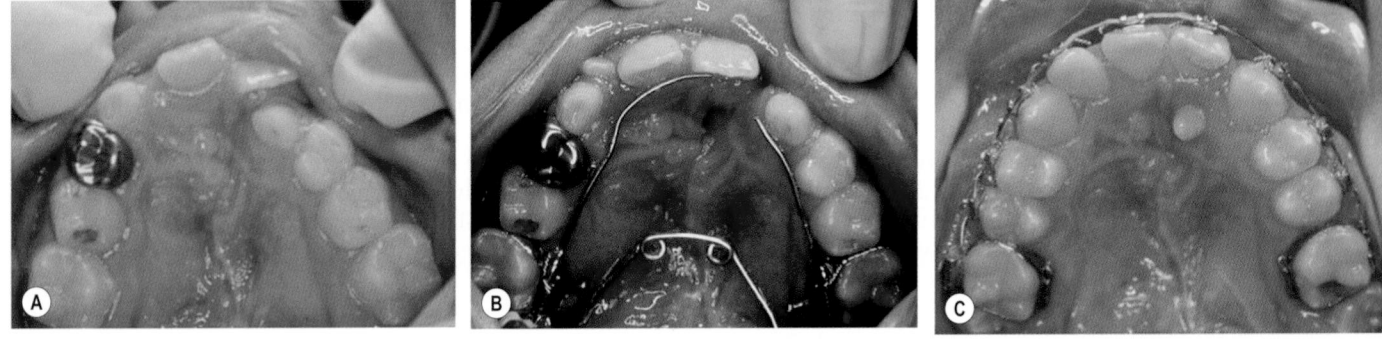

Fig. 27.12 (A–D) Maxillary arch expansion and dental alignment in a unilateral cleft lip and palate patient with severe scarring and collapse. Treatment was achieved in a slow fashion with the use of highly flexible wires and a self-ligating bracket.

Fig. 27.13 Patient with unilateral cleft lip and palate before orthodontic treatment in preparation for bone grafting **(A)**, during expansion with quad helix expander **(B)**, and after bone grafting with erupted cleft-side canine and peg cleft lateral incisor erupting palatal **(C)**. Note arch alignment after expansion and adequate arch form after expansion, bone grafting, and orthodontics.

especially eruption of the maxillary lateral incisor and canine on the cleft side. Occasionally, the maxillary canine is impacted and requires surgical exposure and orthodontic incorporation into the arch as the child is in the full permanent dentition. Impacted or severely malpositioned cleft-side maxillary lateral incisors are usually extracted *(Fig. 27.11J-L)*.

Finally, if it is determined that there is anteroposterior skeletal disharmony, the reconstructive team has to decide if it is

convenient to do the bone grafting in the transitional dentition or if it should be done in combination with future orthognathic surgical procedures. Patients in whom there is marked tissue deficiency, including maxillary hypoplasia and congenitally missing teeth, are likely candidates for postponement of the traditional approach for secondary alveolar bone grafting and will be treated later on in the permanent dentition in combination with orthognathic surgery. If it is

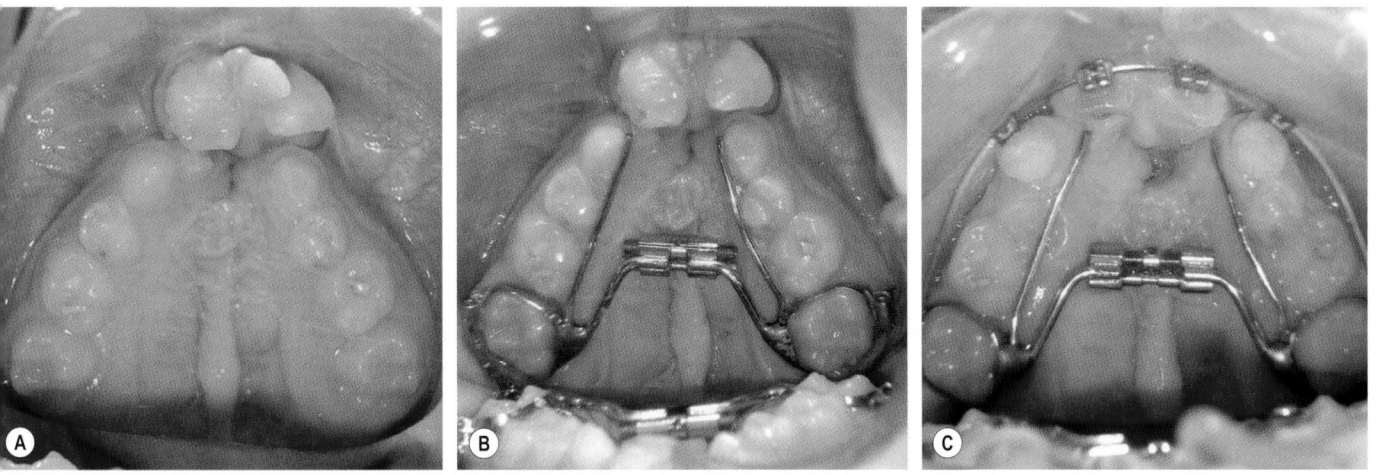

ig. 27.14 Intraoral views of a patient with bilateral cleft lip and palate with arch collapse **(A).** A rigid screw expander was used **(B).** After expansion **(C),** note improvement n arch form and opening of alveolar spaces in preparation for bone grafting.

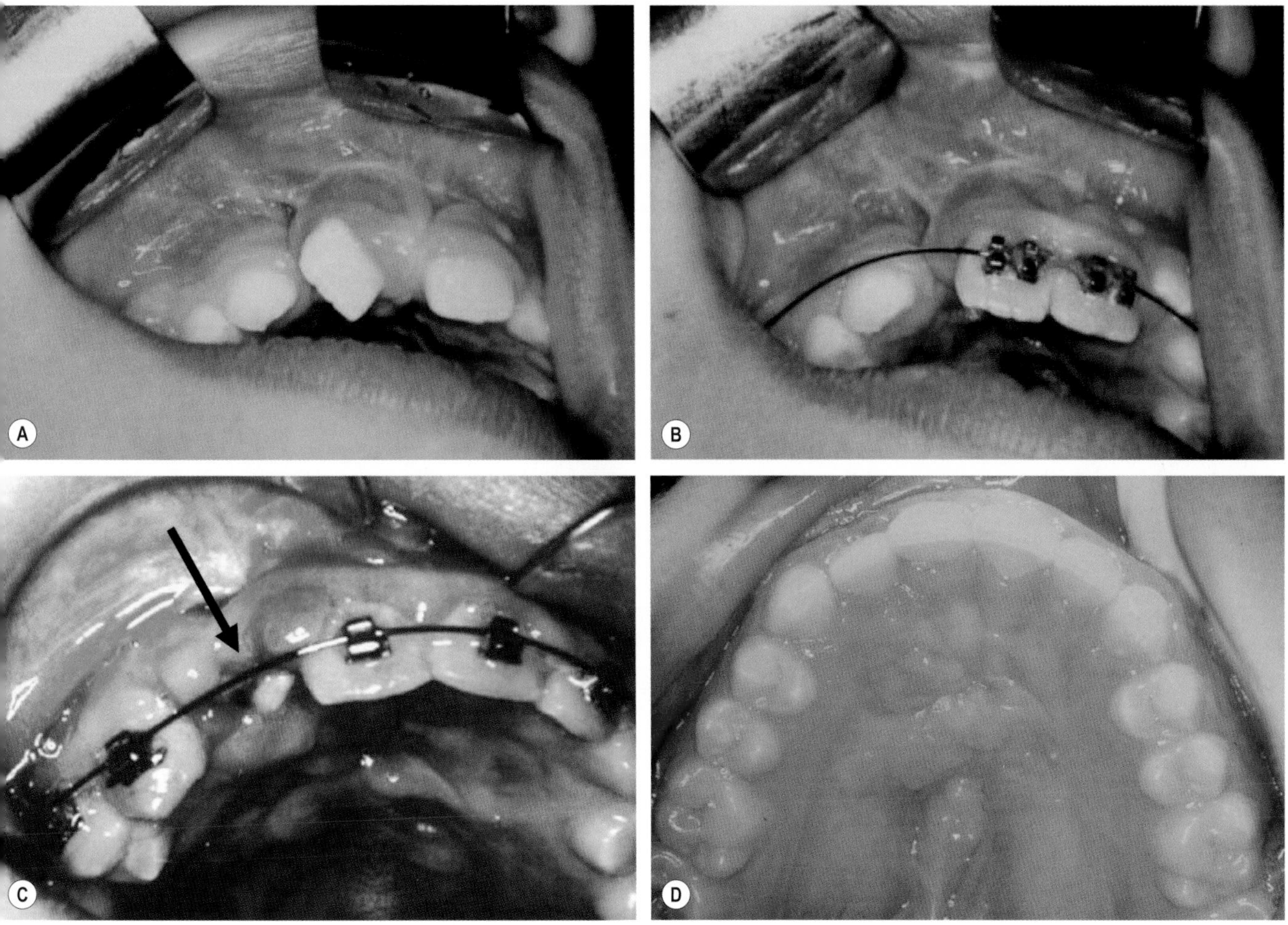

ig. 27.15 **(A–D)** Patient with right unilateral cleft lip and palate with permanent maxillary lateral incisor and canine present. After the bone graft the canine erupted with dequate gingival support. The lateral incisor erupted later on spontaneously (arrow) and was incorporated into the dental arch. At the completion of treatment the tooth was osmetically enlarged.

deemed important to preserve the dentition adjacent to the alveolar cleft, orthodontics are therefore indicated, even in the presence of a skeletal disharmony. The purpose of the orthodontic treatment is then to prepare the dentition for the alveolar bone graft and also to coordinate the maxillary arch to the mandibular arch for future orthognathic surgery that will be performed in the teen years. This approach minimizes the required orthodontic treatment prior to orthognathic surgery in the adolescent years.

Permanent dentition

At the time of an almost complete or complete permanent dentition, the orthodontist must perform definitive orthodontic treatment in the cleft patient. The goals are no different than those for noncleft patients but certain conditions must be kept in mind during treatment planning. These include: arch length requirements and need for dental extractions in cases of severe crowding; integrity of the dentition and supporting structures, especially for teeth adjacent to the alveolar cleft; unusual dental positions, such as impactions; dental transpositions; congenitally missing teeth or severely abnormal teeth that may need to be extracted requiring replacement either with a prosthesis or with orthodontic space closure, especially in the cleft region; maxillary and mandibular dental midlines and their relation to the facial midline; anterior/posterior, transverse, and vertical relationships of the maxilla and mandible to each other and to the face.[1-3,13]

The introduction of new flexible wires and self-ligating appliances permits physiologic forces allowing favorable soft-tissue and bone remodeling responses, especially on those severely malpositioned teeth adjacent to the cleft (Figs 27.12 and 27.16). Every attempt should be made to complete the case with class I cuspid and molar relationships with ideal overjet and overbite (Figs 27.1 and 27.17A). If the cleft lateral incisor is missing, the clinician must decide if this tooth needs to be replaced with a prosthesis or the space closed with orthodontics or with a combined surgical–orthodontic approach. Prosthetic replacement is usually reserved for those cases in which ideal class I cuspid relationships and overjet and overbite are present. In these cases, if the anatomy of the adjacent teeth to the dental gap is sound, a bonded prosthesis or an osseointegrated fixture can be utilized.[1-3,13,30,31]

In those cases with a missing lateral incisor, in which the maxillary canine has migrated forward and is erupting into the grafted alveolar ridge (Fig. 27.18), one must consider the replacement of the lateral incisor by the canine and moving all the posterior teeth forward. In a nonextraction case the cleft side will be finished with class II relations, but if lower bicuspids were extracted, the cleft-side occlusion should finish with class I relations (Fig. 27.1). In cases in which the outcome of the alveolar bone graft is not ideal, the clinician may want to move the canine forward into it to improve bone morphology rather than replacing the lateral incisor with an osseointegrated fixture or a prosthesis that might need additional bone grafting. In cases in which the canine has migrated forward into the lateral incisor position and ideal class I molar relations are present, the canine could be replaced with an osseointegrated implant (Fig. 27.17A and B). Other considerations that must be kept in mind to decide how to manage

the missing cleft-side maxillary incisor include the shape, size and color of the canine as well as the gingival contour in the area of the cleft.[3] If properly planned, both the prosthetic and orthodontic options to manage the missing cleft-side lateral incisor can provide outstanding results (Figs 27.1, 27.15, and 27.17A).

In situations in which the alveolar cleft is too wide for conventional bone grafting, the clinician may elect to shift the cleft-side posterior segment forward surgically and place the canine in the position of the missing lateral incisor. This assures not only closure of the alveolar defect, but also closure of the dental gap created by the missing cleft-side maxillary lateral incisor.[3,13,32] After bone grafting, it is not uncommon to find that the cleft-side maxillary canine has an unusual eruption path and is impacted. These teeth need to be managed surgically by exposing them so the orthodontist can incorporate them into the dental arch (Fig. 27.18A and B).

In some situations it is necessary to move teeth to close extraction spaces or reposition teeth within the arch to obtain better occlusal relations. In the past, intra-arch movements were difficult as the orthodontist depended on the adjacent teeth and patient cooperation using elastics or extraoral appliances for anchorage control. With the introduction of BAS also known in orthodontics as temporary anchorage devices the orthodontist's ability to achieve significant tooth movements has been enhanced.[33] BAS permit anteroposterior and vertical control of a single tooth or group of teeth during orthodontic treatment. The application of BAS is a simple office procedure. After completing the orthodontic treatment the BAS are simply removed without negative sequelae (Fig. 27.19).

Orthodontic management following the developmental approach outlined previously allows the clinician to take advantage of developmental and growth changes and permits the patient and family to recognize the need for distinct phases of orthodontic treatment which also allow for sufficient rest space between stages. This approach assures patient and family acceptance, compliance, and cooperation with the treatment protocol.

Orthognathic surgery and distraction procedures for the cleft patient

Skeletal and dental discrepancies between the maxilla and mandible are not uncommon in cleft patients. These discrepancies can be in the sagittal, transverse, and vertical planes. If the discrepancies are moderate to severe, they are best managed with a combined surgical/orthodontic approach. This approach results in substantial functional and aesthetic improvements in the cleft patient (Fig. 27.1).

It is generally accepted that patients with orofacial clefts have mandibles that are of normal size or slightly smaller.[3] For this reason, in most of the patients where the maxilla is extremely hypoplastic, the surgeon may want to do most of the sagittal correction with surgery just in the maxillary bone. In cases where there is skeletal open bite and marked mandibular deficiency or asymmetry, a two-jaw approach must be undertaken. The advantage of this surgical/orthodontic approach is that, with one operation, the reconstructive team can provide the patient with close to ideal occlusal relations with markedly improved function and aesthetics.

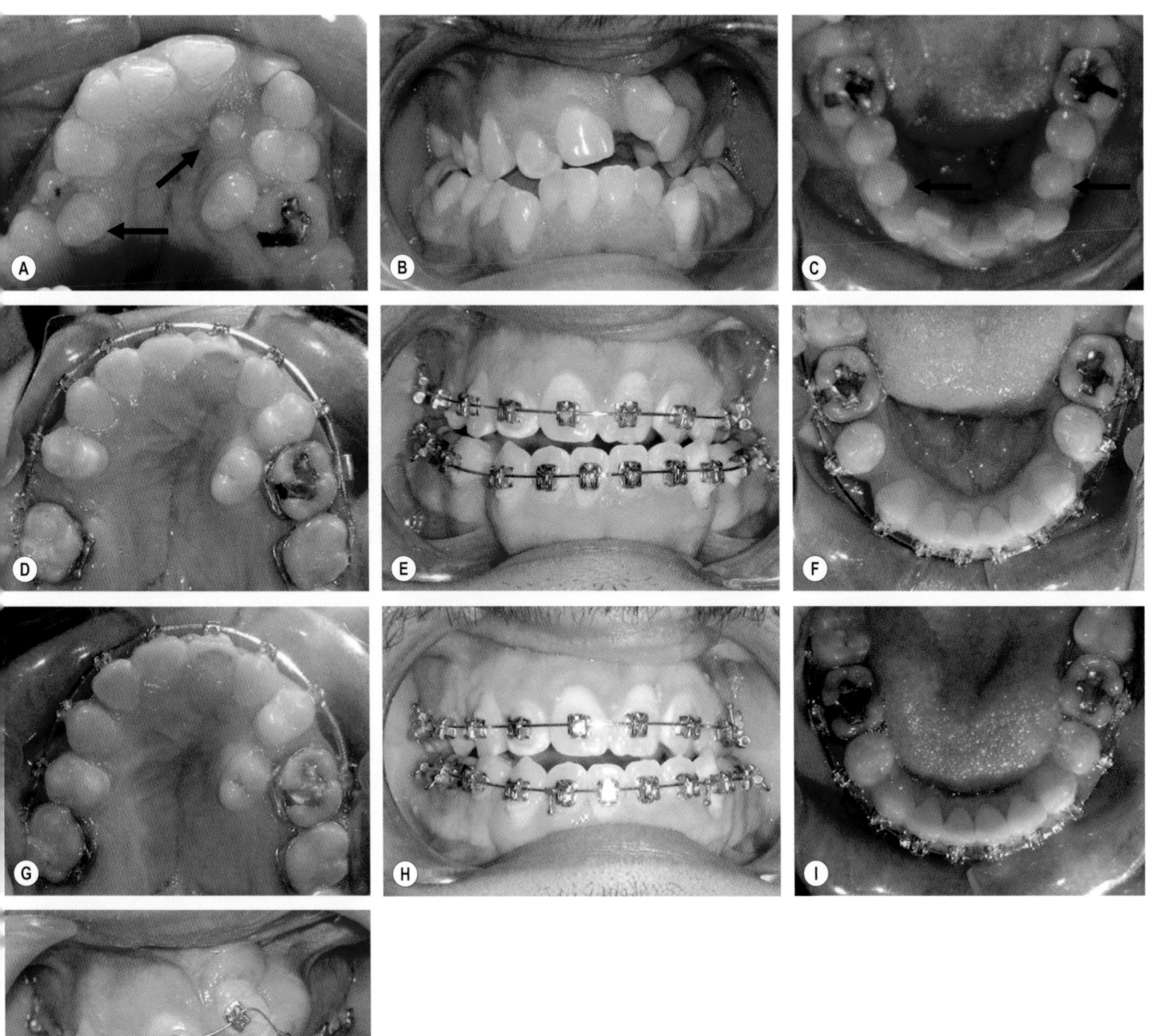

Fig. 27.16 Intraoral views of an adult patient with repaired unilateral cleft lip and palate. Before treatment **(A–C)**, note severely collapsed maxillary arch and crowding in both arches. A peg left maxillary incisor was present. Due to severe crowding dental extractions of teeth number 4, 7, 21, and 28 became necessary. Highly flexible wires and a self-ligating bracket system were used for treatment. Soon after leveling the gingival condition of the maxillary left central incisor was healthy **(D)**. After further alignment and space closure the gingival condition remained healthy. Space is being developed to incorporate number 13 into the arch **(E–I)**. Note initial high wire engagement **(J)**.

To assure success, close cooperation between the orthodontist and surgeon is required. It is the responsibility of the orthodontist to support the surgeon, so at the time of surgery, adequate occlusal relationships can be obtained. This, in turn, will add stability to the orthognathic procedure.

The planning for orthognathic surgery in the cleft patient is no different to that done for the patient with a noncleft dentofacial deformity. This includes a detailed clinical examination and collection of pertinent records prior to orthodontic treatment and again before surgery. All patients with palatal clefts who undergo maxillary advancement surgery are at risk

for velopharyngeal insufficiency, therefore, preoperative evaluation by the team speech and language pathologist is required before and after surgery to discuss potential risks and postoperative correction if necessary. After all the necessary records are obtained, the orthodontist will perform a cephalometric analysis and prediction surgical tracing to determine the required surgical movements. This can be done by hand tracing the X-rays or by using computerized imaging and cephalometric analysis. With the introduction of digital 3D software technology, based on CT scans and more recently CBCT, a new approach has been developed to assist surgeons

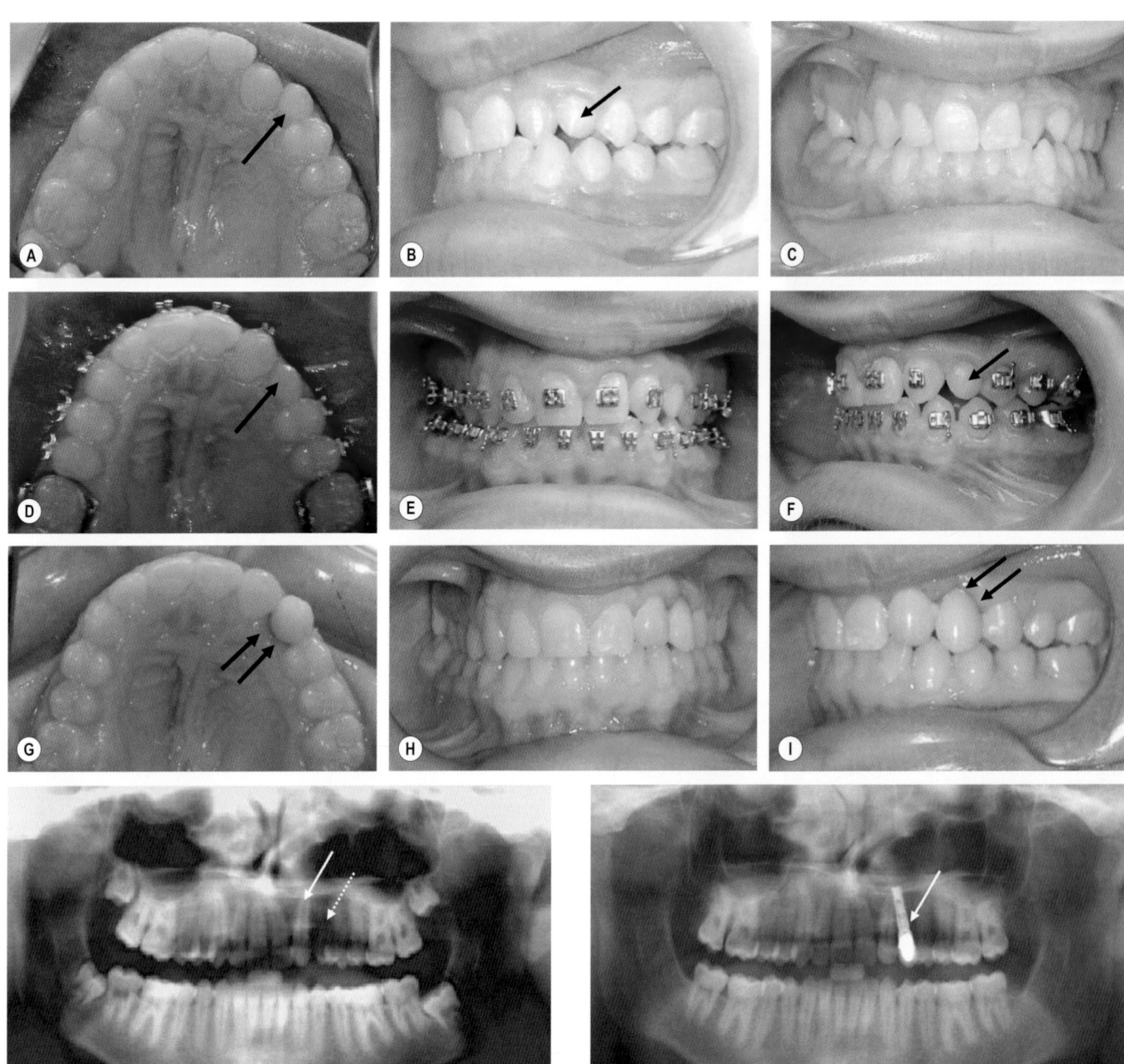

Fig. 27.17 (A–I) Intraoral views of a patient with left unilateral cleft lip and palate, who was missing the cleft-side maxillary lateral incisor, had the maxillary canine substituting the missing incisor and had a retained primary canine (single arrow). Since ideal posterior occlusion was present, it was decided not to close the space with orthodontics, but to replace the primary canine with an osseointegrated implant (double arrow). Note satisfactory occlusion and aesthetics after treatment. **(J, K)** Note in the pretreatment panoramic radiograph **(J)** the presence of the permanent maxillary left canine in the position of the missing lateral incisor (arrow), and the retained primary canine (dotted arrow). After treatment **(K)**, note replacement of the primary canine with an osseointegrated implant (arrow).

and orthodontists in the planning of craniomaxillofacial surgery.[35–39] This approach utilizes digital data from the scans, which in turn is managed by specialized software to create a 3D virtual model of the craniofacial skeleton. The desired surgical movements can be performed digitally. Based on the digital data, a physical model of the skull or the surgical splints can be constructed through stereolitography. This approach obviates the use of the traditional presurgical

planning that included use of a face bow and dental articulators to plan and do model surgery. Although the traditional approach has provided satisfactory outcomes, it can be inaccurate for complex movements and requires a sophisticated degree of proficiency acquired through experience. Delegation of this approach is not possible, and the surgeon and orthodontist need to spend significant laboratory time to plan surgery and prepare the needed surgical splints.

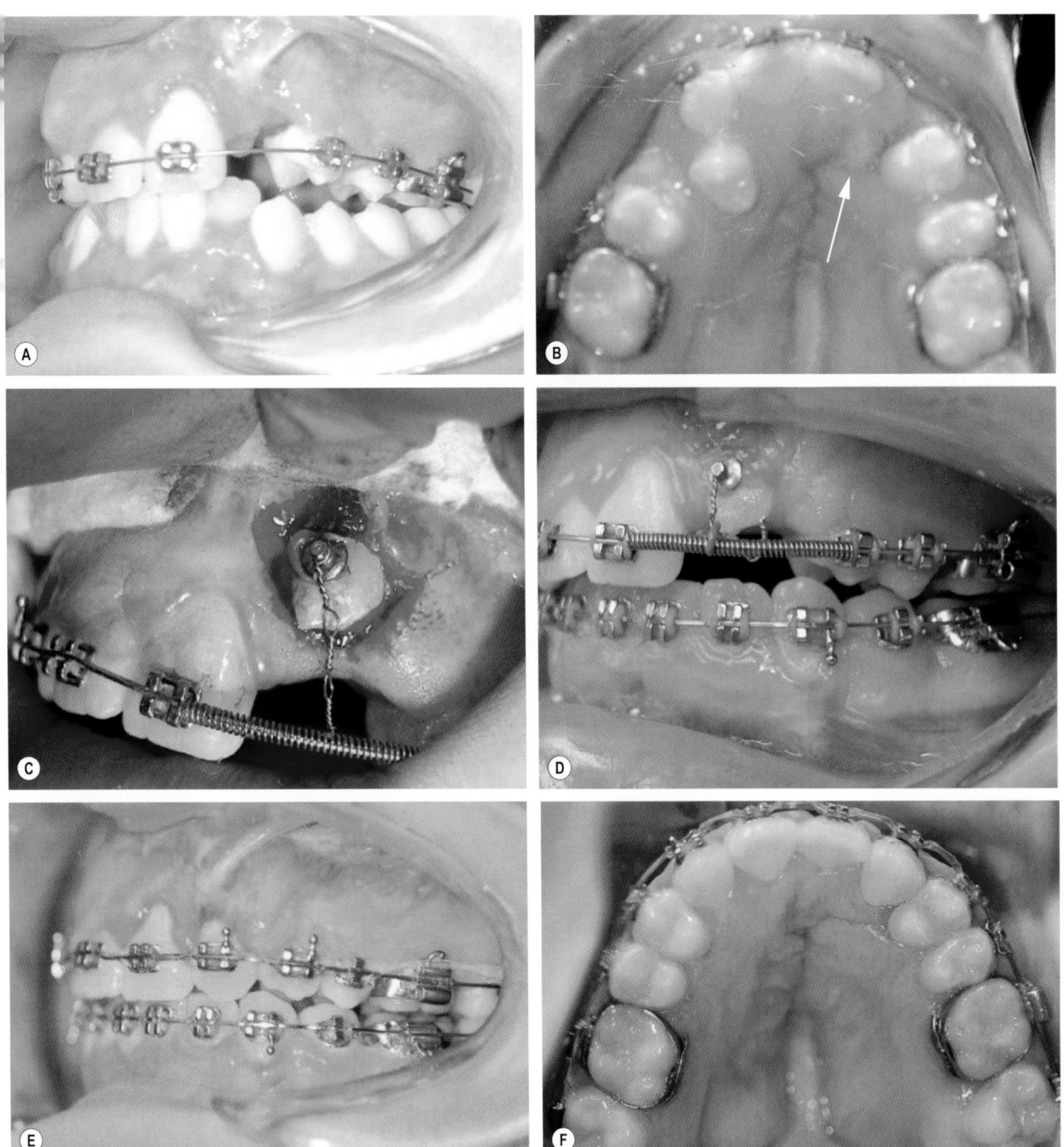

Fig. 27.18 **(A–F)** Intraoral views of a patient with left unilateral cleft lip and palate that was congenitally missing the right maxillary lateral incisor and the left one was peg-shaped (arrow). The peg incisor was extracted and the right maxillary canine was impacted and needed surgical exposure so it could be incorporated into the arch. Note satisfactory gingival and occlusal relations obtained after treatment. **(G, H)** Panoramic radiographs before **(G)** and after **(H)** treatment. Note high position of the left maxillary canine (arrow) and incorporation into the dental arch.

Significant research and technological developments have permitted accuracy of the new 3D methodology, especially the incorporation of accurate digital dental models from plaster casts into the maxillofacial model obtained through the CT and CBCT scans.[40–42] As 3D approaches become more familiar and accessible to clinicians, the planning *(Fig. 27.20)* and execution of complex maxillofacial surgery required by cleft patients should improve and predictable and successful outcomes should be routinely obtained. In addition the clinician should be able to delegate significant aspects of the

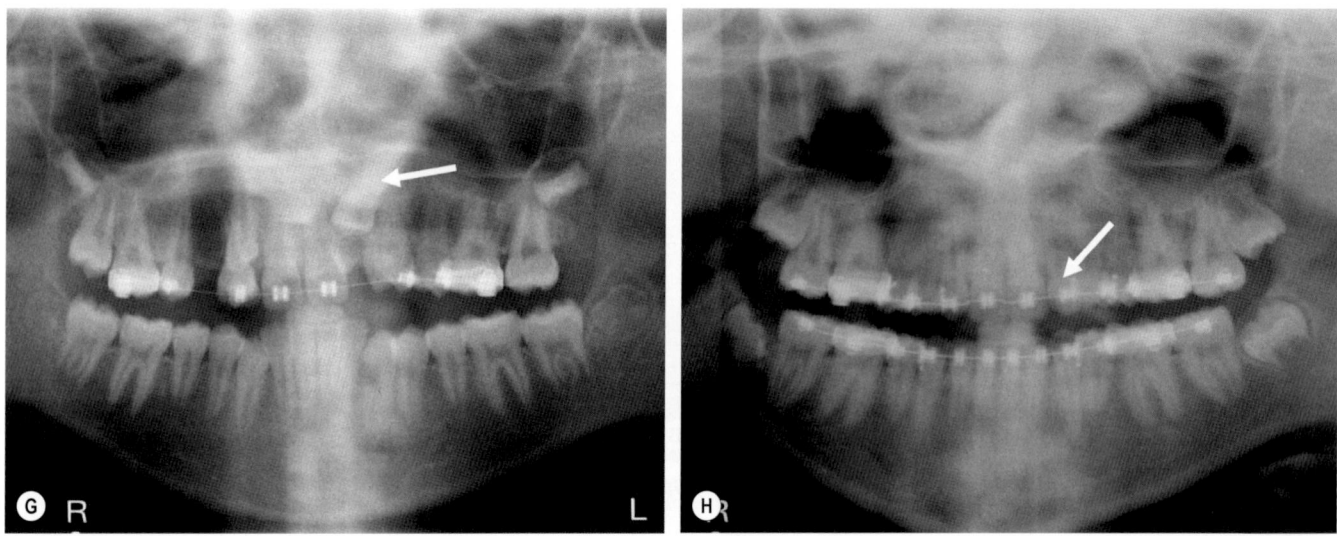

Fig. 27.18, cont'd

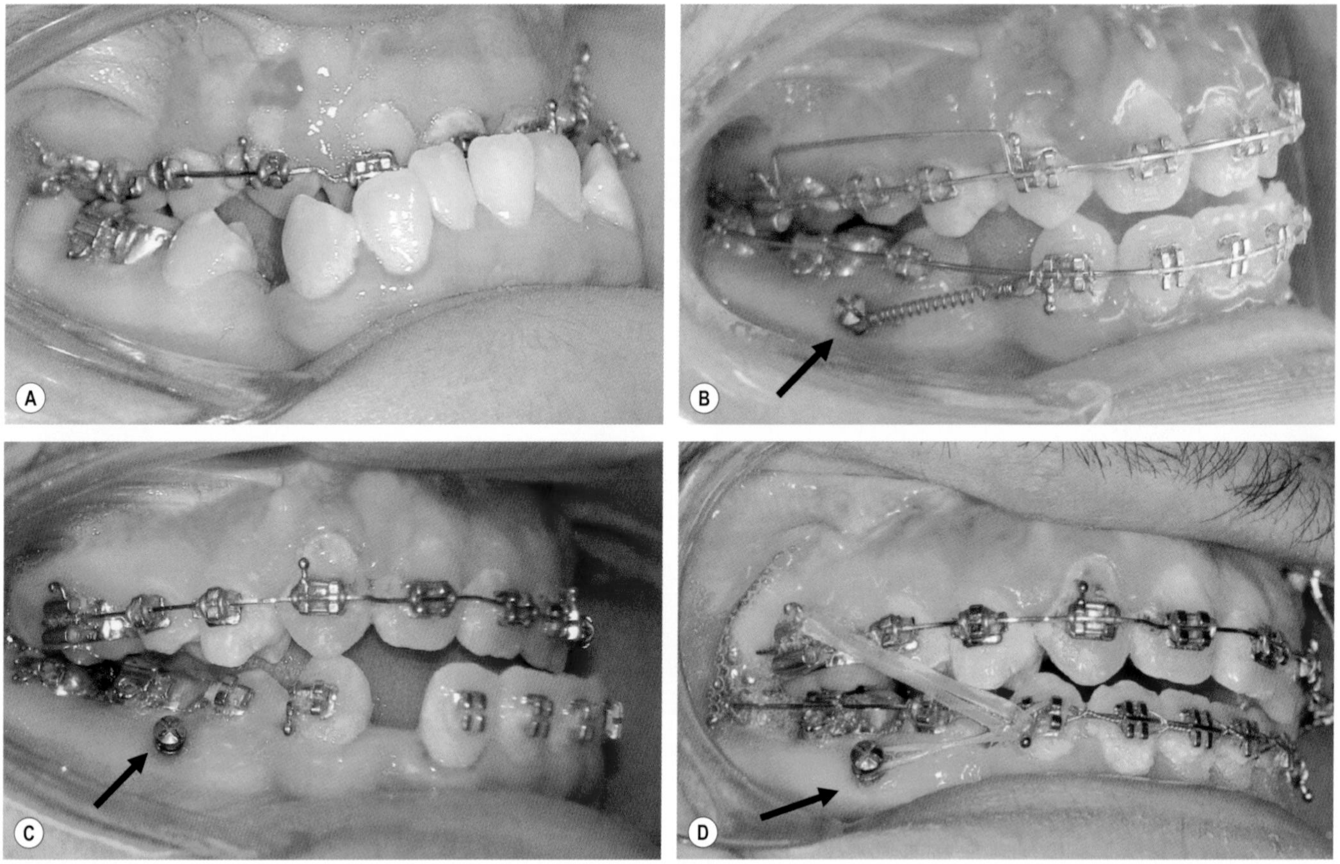

Fig. 27.19 (A–D) Intraoral views of a patient with unilateral right cleft lip and palate with anterior crossbite and severe maxillary and mandibular crowding. Maxillary lateral incisors and mandibular first bicuspids were extracted. After the maxillary arch was consolidated a anchorage screw (arrows) was used to assist with canine and incisor retraction. Note space closure and correction of the anterior crossbite.

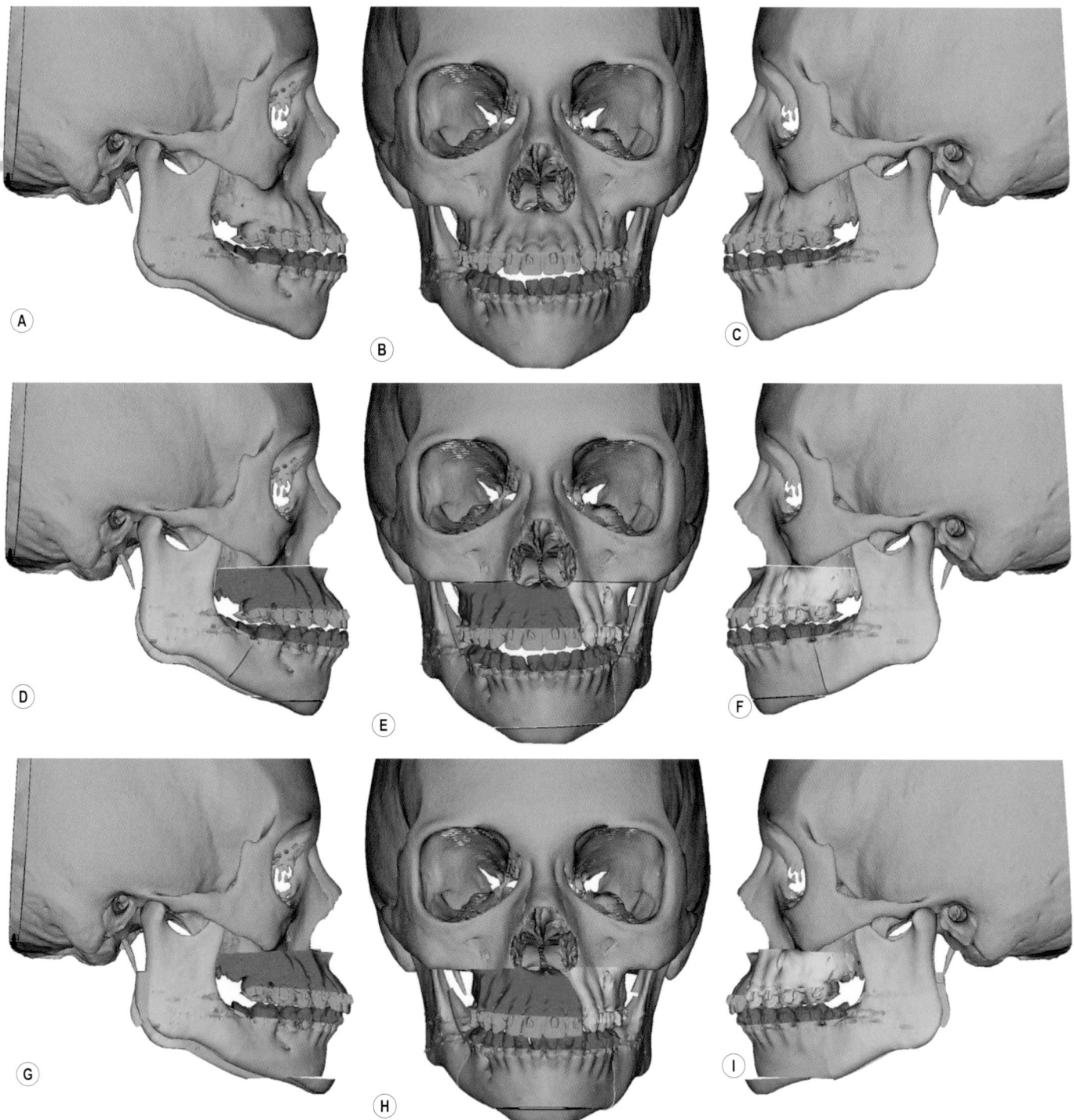

Fig. 27.20 Pretreatment **(A–C)** three-dimensional scans from a patient with maxillary deficiency and mandibular prognathism. Note: digital reproduction of the maxillary (green) and mandibular (blue) dentitions. A two-piece maxillary advancement (green-yellow) with mandibular setback (gray-light blue) and genioplasty (dark blue) were planned **(D–F).** The segments were repositioned and the dentofacial deformity and malocclusion were virtually corrected **(G–I).** From the digital models surgical splints and guides are manufactured, eliminating traditional dental model surgery. (Courtesy of Medical Modeling, Golden, Colorado.)

planning and splint fabrication procedures.[43,44] This approach gives the clinician a close approximation of the desired outcome, but he or she must be aware of the limited knowledge on soft-tissue responses (lip, nose, and velopharyngeal structures) relative to skeletal movement, especially in cleft patients. Additional research on 3D responses of the facial soft

tissues after maxillo/mandibular surgery is still needed. It is emphasized that it is the clinician and not the computer that will make the final treatment and surgical decisions. The 3D computerized technological advances allow the clinician diagnostic evaluation in all three planes of space, providing postsurgical evaluation that was not possible before. These include changes in airway volume after maxillary and mandibular surgery[45–47] and volumetric bone changes after alveolar bone grafting.[48,49]

Recently, however, there has been a resurgence of a "surgery first, orthodontics later" approach.[50,51] The desired approach, especially for the cleft patient, is opposite – "orthodontics first," followed by surgery and finishing orthodontics. Before surgery, the orthodontist must position all teeth within their supporting basal bones with the maxillary incisors in an ideal position relative to the palatal plane and the mandibular incisors in ideal axial inclination relative to the mandibular plane.

Both arches need to be properly coordinated to allow for ideal occlusal interdigitation at the time of surgery. In addition, the orthodontist must create interdental spaces to facilitate instrumentation, if interdental osteotomies are anticipated. The orthodontic appliance is used during the period of intermaxillary fixation and immediately after surgery for postsurgical elastic therapy *(Fig. 27.21)* and detailing of the occlusion. Close cooperation between the orthodontist and surgeon during the planning and initial orthodontic treatment stages should yield favorable occlusal, functional, and aesthetic outcomes *(Figs 27.1 and 27.21)*.

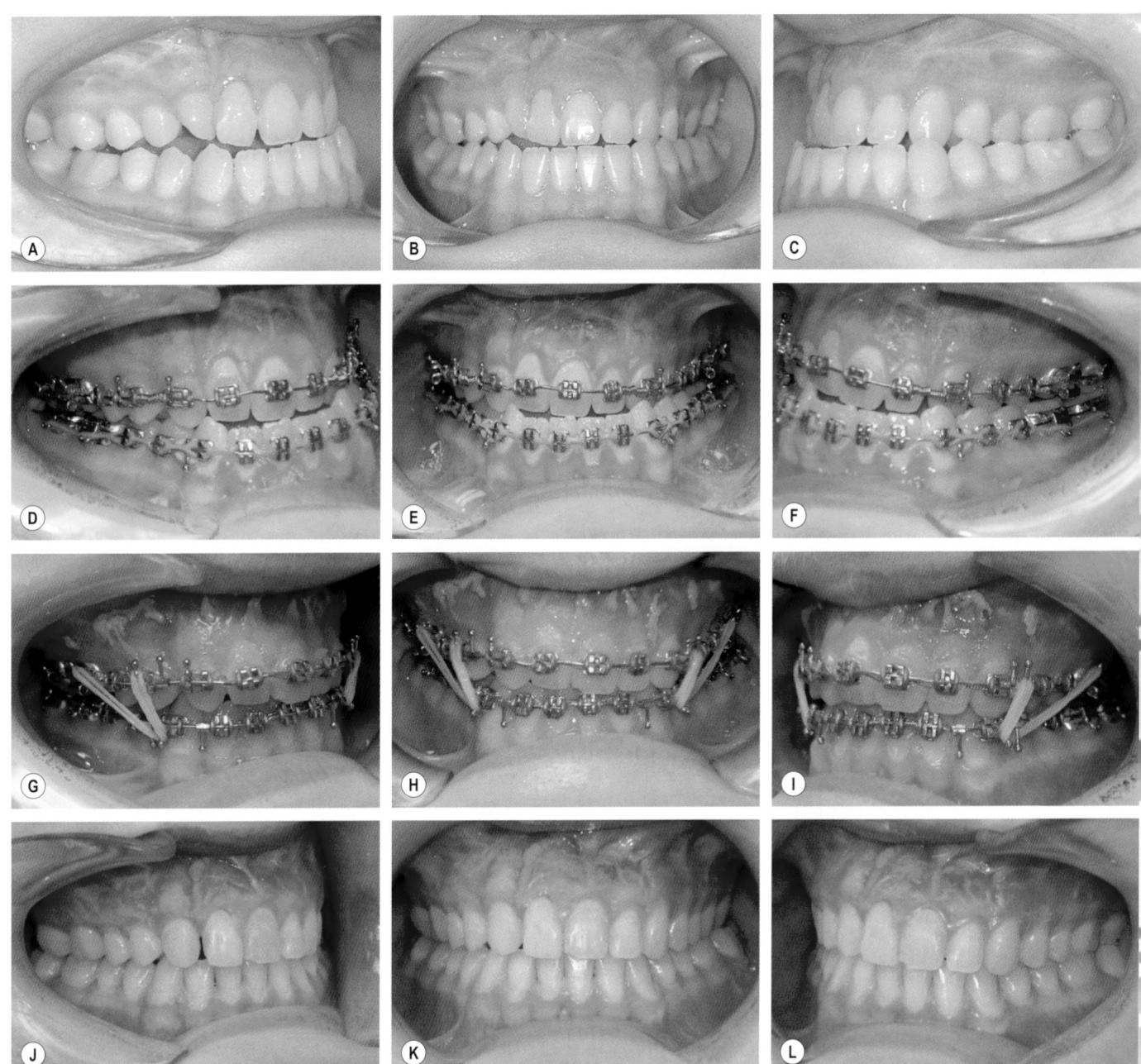

Fig. 27.21 Intraoral views of a patient with right unilateral cleft lip and palate with missing maxillary right lateral incisor and anterior crossbite **(A–C)**. After alveolar bone grafting and orthodontic alignment **(D–F)**, the patient underwent maxillary advancement with midline correction **(G–I)**. Note use of elastics to the orthodontic appliance for fixation and occlusal settling after surgery. After treatment, satisfactory occlusal relations were obtained. Note substitution of the missing right maxillary lateral incisor with the canine, with right class II molar relations and left class I molar and canine relations **(J–L)**.

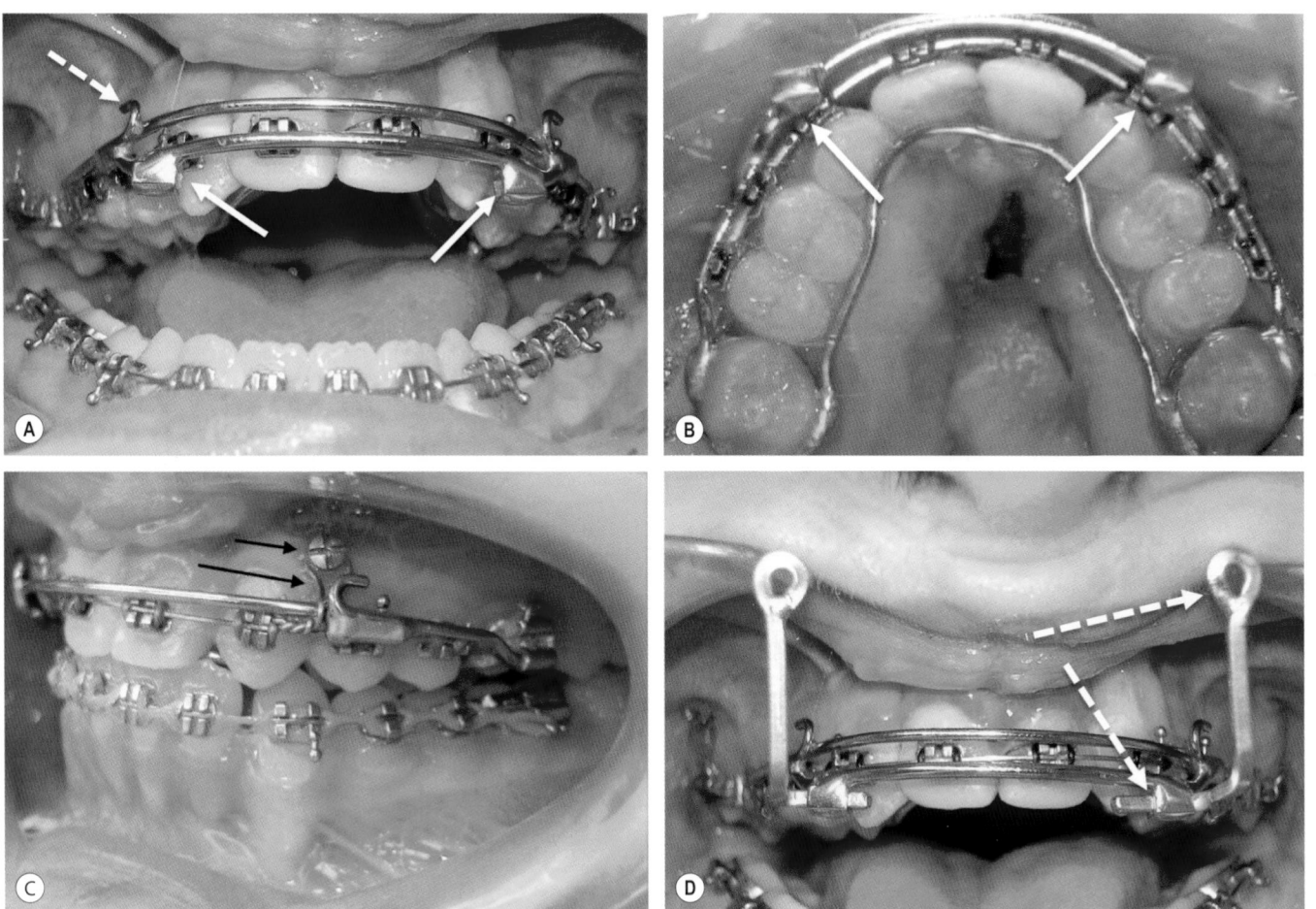

Fig. 27.22 Views of the intraoral splint with removable hooks used for maxillary and midface distraction with rigid external distraction. Note the square tubes (solid arrows) and retention face mask hooks (broken arrow) **(A)**. Occlusal view demonstrating labial and palatal bars soldered to the first molar bands and position of square tubes (arrows) **(B)**. At surgery, bone anchorage screws are placed and suspension wires are dropped to enhance anterior stability of the splint (arrows) **(C)**. Extraoral hooks with traction eyelets inserted through the square tubes of the splint (broken arrows) **(D)**.

In patients in whom the maxillary deficiency is severe and where there is substantial scarring or existing pharyngeal flaps, conventional orthognathic procedures are not reliable due to the inherent lack of stability and high relapse tendencies.[52,53] When performing conventional procedures in young patients with severe maxillary hypoplasia, one must wait until adolescence for surgical correction as these techniques rely on rigid fixation that requires substantial bone for placement of the hardware. Further, unerupted tooth buds might be injured during the application of rigid fixation plates. For young patients with severe maxillary deficiency, we have utilized distraction osteogenesis with a rigid external distraction (RED) device, and internal devices for patients with mild to moderate deficiencies. The technique of maxillary distraction utilizing a RED device has been previously described[54–58] and consists of five steps: (1) the fabrication of an intraoral splint that is used to deliver the distraction forces to the maxilla via the teeth; (2) a complete high Le Fort I osteotomy with septal and pterygomaxillary dysjunction; (3) the placement of a cranial halo with an external adjustable distraction screw system; (4) distraction; and (5) rigid and removable retention, as previously presented.

This technique has been applied to young children as well as adolescents and adults, with excellent functional and aesthetic results (*Figs 27.22 and 27.23*). The stability of the procedure has been remarkable and superior to that reported for conventional orthognathic surgical approaches.[56,58–61] The soft-tissue changes have also been superior to those reported when conventional orthognathic surgical techniques are used in cleft patients.[62,63] The velopharyngeal mechanism of these patients is minimally affected, especially for those patients having pharyngeal flaps who report improved articulation and resonance. Patients without pharyngeal flaps requiring major advancements can have postdistraction velopharyngeal incompetence requiring treatment with a pharyngeal flap or another type of pharyngoplasty.[64,65] To date, we have not seen negative effects on dental development, although, when performed in children under 6 years of age, we have noted on occasion rotation of a permanent second molar tooth bud as a result of increases in posterior arch length or surgical trauma.

Internal devices have been used in patients with less severe maxillary hypoplasia. The device used by the authors is a hybrid device (skeletal and dental anchorage) with the main advantage of not requiring a second operation for its removal.

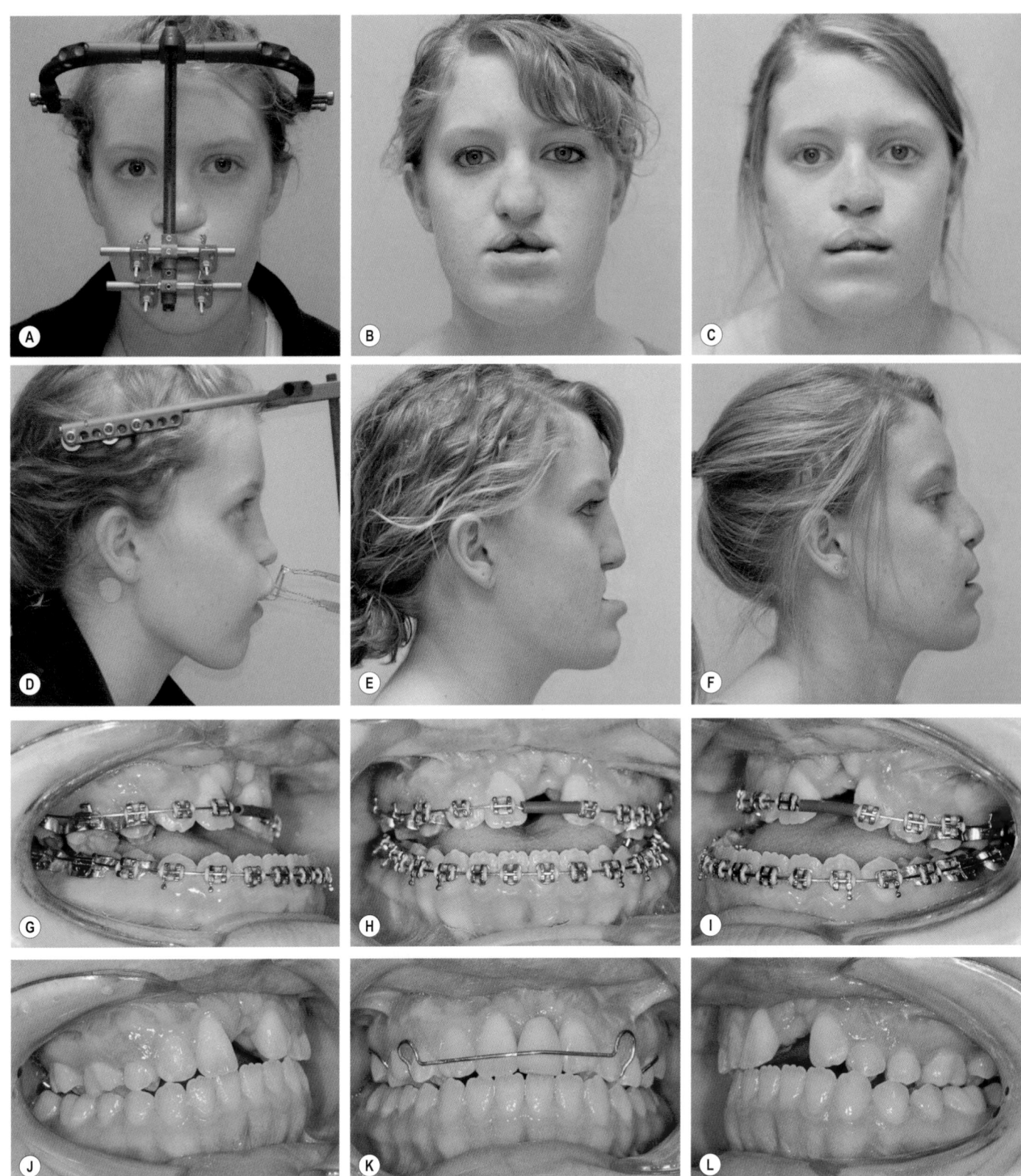

Fig. 27.23 (A–F) Facial photographs of a patient with bilateral cleft lip and palate with severe maxillary deficiency who underwent a high Le Fort I osteotomy and advancement with rigid external distraction **(A,D).** Before **(B,E)** and after **(C,F)** distraction frontal and profile views. Note dramatic facial balance improvement after treatment. Intraoral views before **(G–I)** and after **(J–L)** distraction. Note severe class III relations before treatment and restoration to a functional and aesthetic occlusion after treatment. Before treatment **(M)** note vertical and horizontal maxillary hypoplasia. After treatment **(N),** the amount of advancement is indicated by the horizontal arrow. The vertical arrows indicate the newly formed bone. Note absence of any fixation hardware, correction of preoperative open bite tendency, as well as anterior dental relations.

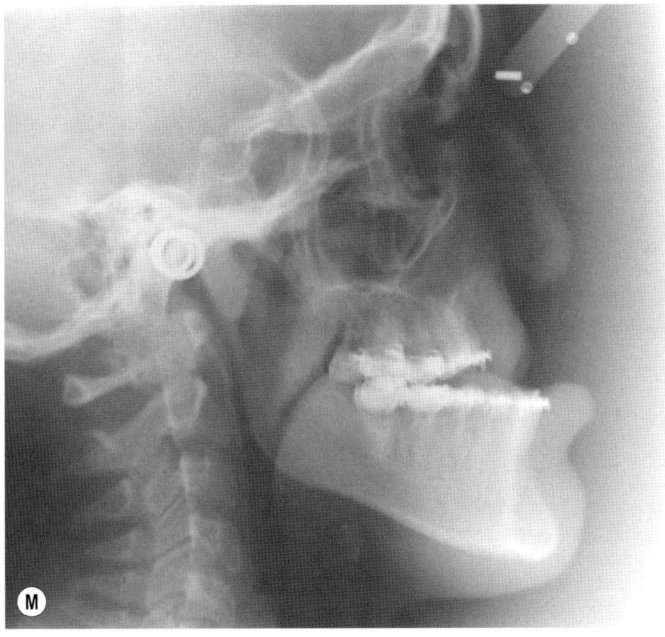
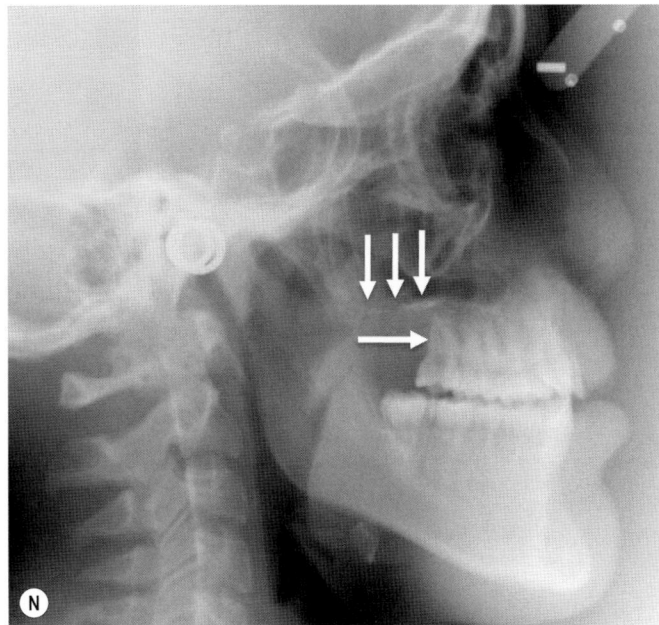

Fig. 27.23, cont'd

The device has been used successfully, with excellent functional and aesthetic outcomes[66] (*Figs 27.24–27.26*). 🔘 FIGS 27.24–26 APPEAR ONLINE ONLY

Maxillary distraction now offers a solution for the difficult cleft maxillary hypoplasia deformity. In addition, the technique has been expanded to other patients with syndromic conditions, such as Apert and Crouzon syndromes, and traumatic deformities.

Growth and orthodontic treatment

Since the orthodontist participates in the care of a cleft child from infancy into adulthood, it is imperative to recognize that abnormal facial growth will present an added challenge to the reconstructive team. It is understood that cleft patients do have different facial growth patterns than those seen in non-cleft individuals. However, cleft patients have significant growth potential. If this potential is not negatively affected by the reconstructive procedures required by the patient, it is likely that a favorable outcome will be obtained. Orthodontic treatment will be simplified if minimal growth disturbances affect the patient. Simplification and shortening of orthodontic treatment, which is usually the longest therapeutic intervention for many cleft patients, are desired as this will decrease the burden of care (e.g., patient, family, provider, public health system, society).

Cleft teams should strive to obtain optimal outcomes by critically assessing their protocols and incorporating proven strategies to manage their patients. It is accepted that surgery will likely create significant scarring in the infant maxilla, resulting in growth attenuation. Careful attention should be given to those protocols that minimize scarring in the anterior maxilla (i.e., delaying alveolar bone grafting and minimizing palatal scarring by avoiding damage to the maxillary body).[67,68] This, in turn, will result in less need for extended and complex orthodontic procedures.

Conclusion

The important contribution of the orthodontist to the comprehensive surgical orthodontic management of the cleft patient is illustrated. The role of the orthodontist is to support the surgeon with all aspects of craniofacial growth, dental development, occlusion, and treatment planning, so ideal outcomes can be obtained. With the addition of nasal alveolar molding as well as maxillary distraction osteogenesis, the traditional protocols for cleft management have been expanded. In addition, the incorporation of new technological advancements in orthodontics, such as highly flexible orthodontic arch wires, self-ligating orthodontic appliances, BAS, and accessibility to new 3D imaging technology, facilitates the required treatment interventions. It is hoped that these innovations will provide clinicians with new strategies for the difficult management of the cleft patient, and will provide the patient with outstanding outcomes. The treatment plan of the patient should be developed around the anatomical, functional, and developmental needs of the patient. Close cooperation between the surgeon and orthodontist is imperative for a successful outcome.

Bonus images for this chapter can be found online at **http://www.expertconsult.com**

Fig. 27.1 (A–I) Facial and **(J–R)** intraoral photographs; **(S–U)** panoramic and **(V–X)** lateral cephalometric radiographs of a patient with unilateral cleft lip and palate. The patient underwent lip and palate surgery in infancy. He had an alveolar bone graft in the transitional dentition. He had a diminutive tooth number 7 that was extracted and substituted with number 6. In late childhood, maxillary deficiency was noted and persisted until adolescence. He had orthodontic preparation of the dentition and underwent surgical maxillary advancement with rigid fixation. His treatment was successful, with satisfactory facial, occlusal, and skeletal outcomes.

Fig. 27.2 Dental cast **(A)** of an infant with unilateral cleft lip utilized to fabricate a palatal plate **(B)** to which a stainless-steel wire **(C)** is attached to fabricate the nasal stent required for molding the nasal structures.

Fig. 27.3 The wire to fabricate the nasal stent is left long **(A)**, measured relative to the height of the nose, and cut and bent, leaving an "adjustment loop" (lower arrow) and a terminal loop (upper arrow) to attach the nasal conformer part of the stent **(B)**. The end of the wire is covered by hard acrylic and lined with soft acrylic to fabricate the nasal stent (arrows) **(C)**. Patient without **(D)** and with **(E)** nasoalveolar molding plate in place.

Fig. 27.4 Facial photographs of a patient with unilateral cleft lip and palate before **(A)**, after nasoalveolar molding and before lip surgery, worm's-eye view **(B)** and frontal view **(C)**. Intraoral views before **(D)** and after **(E)** nasoalveolar molding. Note alveolar and palatal cleft narrowing and improved nasal form after nasoalveolar molding and prior to lip surgery. Frontal facial photograph after nasoalveolar molding and lip surgery **(F)**.

Fig. 27.5 Patient with unilateral cleft lip and palate undergoing nasoalveolar molding **(A)** and with facial taping **(B)**. Note rounding of the alar cartilage around the nasal stent.

Fig. 27.6 After nasoalveolar molding and lip surgery a nasal stent is inserted **(A)** and secured with tape **(B)**. Note base tapes adhering to the cheeks **(A)**, used to secure the nasal stent tape and to prevent skin irritation during frequent tape replacement.

Fig. 27.7 (A) Frontal, **(B)** profile, and **(C)** intraoral photographs of a patient with bilateral cleft lip and palate with protrusive and deviated premaxilla. She underwent premaxillary repositioning with an intraoral plate **(D)** with an anterior elastomeric chain **(E)**. **(F, G)** Frontal, **(H)** profile, and **(I)** intraoral photographs after premaxillary repositioning and prior to nasal molding. Note reduction of premaxillary asymmetry and protrusion as well as improved nasal form.

Fig. 27.8 After initial premaxillary repositioning, patient with bilateral cleft and palate undergoing nasal molding. Note two nasal stents added to the plate with an anterior elastomeric chain **(A, B)**. While the elastomeric chain is holding the premaxilla and prolabium down and back, the nasal stents elevate the nasal tip, repositioning the nasal domes towards the midline and elongating the columella **(C–E)**.

Fig. 27.9 Frontal, profile, and nasal photographs of a patient with bilateral cleft lip and palate who underwent presurgical nasoalveolar molding treatment and primary lip repair. Comparison of before **(A–C)** and after **(D–F)** nasoalveolar molding photographs illustrate reduction of premaxillary asymmetry and protrusion as well as improvement of nasal asymmetry. A satisfactory lip and nasal repair was obtained soon after lip surgery **(G–I)**. Four years after surgery **(J–L)**, the patient maintains excellent lip line, nose/lip relations, nasal symmetry, and projection.

Fig. 27.10 Long-term follow-up of a patient with unilateral cleft lip and palate treated with presurgical nasoalveolar molding, and only primary lip and palate repair and alveolar bone grafting. Close-up photos of the nose before **(A)** and after **(B)** nasoalveolar molding and feeding with the nasoalveolar molding prosthesis in place **(C)**. Facial photos before treatment **(D)**, postsurgery at 2 **(E)**, 9 **(F)** and 16 **(G)** years of age. Note satisfactory outcome with nice lip line and stable nasal symmetry.

Fig. 27.24 Intraoperative view **(A)** of the placement of a hybrid (bone–dental) internal maxillary distractor for Le Fort I maxillary advancement. Intraoral view **(B)** of the activating arm after incision closure. Note the horizontal arm of the distractor is wired through an intraoral metal splint (arrows). Cephalometric **(C)** and panoramic **(D)** radiographs demonstrating the buttress plates, adjustable and removable vertical stem, and horizontal distractor arm.

Fig. 27.25 After distraction and consolidation the device is removed in the office setting; the horizontal arms are unwired and removed from the vertical stems **(A, B)**. The vertical stem is unscrewed from the buttress plate and removed. The small vestibular wound is left to close spontaneously **(C, D)**.

Fig. 27.26 Before **(A–C)** and after **(D–E)** facial photographs of a patient with right unilateral cleft lip and palate and moderate maxillary hypoplasia who underwent Le Fort I maxillary advancement utilizing an internal adjustable and removable distraction device. Note improvement of facial convexity and lip/nose relations after treatment. Intraoral views before **(G–I)** and after **(J–L)** treatment. Note anterior crossbite and class III relations before treatment. The maxillary canines were used to replace the missing lateral incisors; she was completed with positive overjet and overbite and class II molar relations. Cephalometric and panoramic radiographs before **(M, O)** and after **(N, P)** treatment. Note moderate maxillary hypoplasia and concave profile before treatment as well as the still-erupting second maxillary molars. After treatment the maxilla was advanced, improving the skeletal and soft-tissue profile as well as anterior dental relations. Note continued eruption of maxillary second molars (horizontal arrows) and the buttress plates that remain after the distractor was removed (vertical arrows) after treatment.

Access the complete references list online at **http://www.expertconsult.com**

8. Grayson BH, Santiago PE, Brecht LE, et al. Presurgical nasoalveolar molding in infants with cleft lip and palate. *Cleft Palate Craniofac J.* 1999;36:486–498.

This article introduces the now-widespread concept of presurgical nasoalveolar molding. The authors conclude that nasoalveolar molding eliminates the need for surgical columella reconstruction.

52. Posnick JC, Dagys AP. Skeletal stability and relapse patterns after Le Fort I maxillary osteotomy fixed with miniplates: the unilateral cleft lip and palate deformity. *Plast Reconstr Surg.* 1994;94:924–932.

This study assesses relapse rates in 35 consecutive patients undergoing Le Fort I osteotomy with miniplate fixation and autogenous bone grafting. The authors found that miniplates do not prevent relapse in this population.

56. Polley JW, Figueroa AA. Rigid external distraction: its application in cleft maxillary deformities. *Plast Reconstr Surg.* 1998;102:1360–1372.

The authors present the use of rigid external distraction to correct maxillary hypoplasia in patients with facial clefts. Dramatic improvements in skeletal anatomy and soft-tissue deficiencies were observed.

58. Paresi Jr R, Felsten L, Shoukas J, et al. Maxillary distraction osteogenesis. In: Losee J, Kirschner, RE, eds. *Comprehensive cleft care*. New York: McGraw Hill; 2009:956–968.

This chapter offers a useful review of maxillary distraction in the context of orofacial clefting. Cephalometric evaluation is emphasized.

65. Guyette TW, Polley JW, Figueroa A, et al. Changes in speech following maxillary distraction osteogenesis. *Cleft Palate Craniofac J*. 2001;38:199–205.

Articulation and velopharyngeal function were assessed before and after maxillary distraction. Metrics included hyper/hyponasality, velopharyngeal passage dimensions, and articulation error.

28

Velopharyngeal dysfunction

Richard E. Kirschner and Adriane L. Baylis

SYNOPSIS

- Individuals with known or suspected velopharyngeal dysfunction (VPD) are best treated in the context of an interdisciplinary cleft/craniofacial team.

- Diagnosis of VPD requires obtaining a comprehensive patient history, perceptual speech evaluation, physical examination, and appropriate instrumental and imaging studies.

- Successful surgical management of VPD requires precision in diagnosis and individualization of treatment.

- VPD may be the result of velopharyngeal insufficiency, velopharyngeal incompetence, or velopharyngeal mislearning.

- Flexible fiberoptic nasopharyngoscopy should be completed as part of a standard preoperative evaluation to allow for direct visualization of the velopharyngeal mechanism during speech and surgical planning.

- Instrumental assessment of speech should always be interpreted in the context of the results of a comprehensive perceptual speech evaluation.

- Aerodynamic assessment of speech can provide the surgeon with information regarding velopharyngeal orifice size and timing to assist with treatment decision-making and judgment of surgical outcome.

- The primary goal of surgical management is to produce a competent velopharyngeal mechanism for speech while avoiding the complications of nasal airway obstruction.

Introduction

Normal speech is dependent upon the functional and structural integrity of the velopharynx, a complex and dynamic structure that serves to uncouple the oral and nasal cavities during sound production. Dysfunction of the velopharyngeal valve (referred to as VPD) may lead to hypernasality, nasal air emission, and compensatory articulation errors, all of which may impair speech intelligibility and lead to stigmatization. The goal of surgical intervention is to produce or restore velopharyngeal competence while avoiding the complications of

upper airway obstruction. Successful surgical management of VPD requires precision in diagnosis and individualization of treatment. Thus, optimization of surgical outcome is critically dependent upon a careful analysis of each patient's history, structural anatomy, and velopharyngeal dynamics – an analysis best performed with close collaboration between the surgeon, the speech pathologist, and the other members of the cleft/craniofacial team.

Anatomy and physiology of the velopharynx

Anatomy

The velopharyngeal port is defined anteriorly by the soft palate, or velum, laterally by the lateral pharyngeal walls, and posteriorly by the posterior pharyngeal wall. Closure of the velopharynx during speech is a voluntary action that is mediated by the motor cortex and that requires the coordinated action of the velopharyngeal musculature. The muscles of the soft palate include the levator veli palatini, the tensor veli palatini, the palatoglossus, the palatopharyngeus, and the musculus uvulae (Fig. 28.1). The levator takes its origin from the petrous portion of the temporal bone and from the medial aspect of the eustachian tube. Its fibers course anteriorly, inferiorly, and medially, inserting into the palatal aponeurosis and decussating with the levator fibers from the opposite side (Fig. 28.2). Contraction of the muscular sling formed by the paired levators is the primary mechanism for velar elevation and closure of the velopharyngeal port, although evidence suggests that the palatoglossus and palatopharyngeus muscles may act as antagonists to the levators to provide fine motor control of velar position during speech.[1,2] The musculus uvulae is a paired intrinsic muscle that likely contributes to velopharyngeal closure both by adding bulk to the dorsal surface of the velum and by contributing to velar stretch.[3–5] It is usually absent in patients with overt and submucosal clefts of the palate.[6]

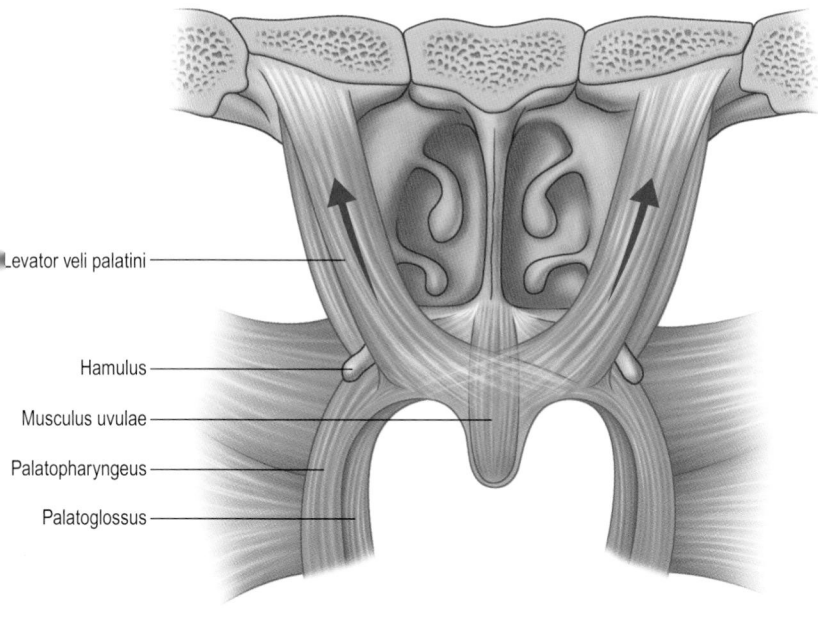

Levator veli palatini

Hamulus

Musculus uvulae

Palatopharyngeus

Palatoglossus

Fig. 28.1 Muscles of the velopharynx.

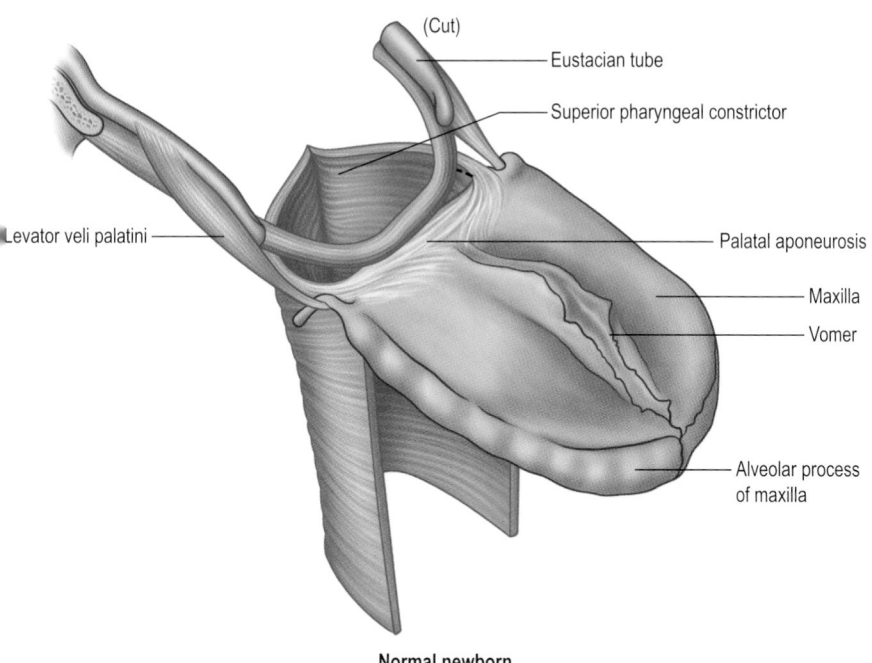

(Cut)

Eustacian tube

Superior pharyngeal constrictor

Levator veli palatini

Palatal aponeurosis

Maxilla

Vomer

Alveolar process of maxilla

Normal newborn

Fig. 28.2 Shematic of the levator veli palatini.

The superior pharyngeal constrictor is a broad, thin muscle that takes origin from the velum, the medial pterygoid, and the pterygomandibular raphe, inserting into the median pharyngeal raphe along with the constrictor muscle fibers from the opposite side. Contraction of the superior constrictor may contribute to velopharyngeal closure by effecting medial movement of the lateral walls and anterior movement of the posterior wall of the velopharynx.[7,8] The anatomy of the superior constrictor and its contribution to velopharyngeal closure, however, are highly variable.

With the exception of the tensor veli palatini, which is innervated by the third division of the trigeminal nerve (V_3), all of the muscles of the velopharynx receive motor innervation from the pharyngeal plexus, which is composed of fibers from the glossopharyngeal (IX), vagus (X), and accessory (XI) nerves.[9] Studies have suggested that the facial nerve (VII) may also play a minor role in velopharyngeal motor function.[10,11] It is important to note that, although the functional activity of the velopharyngeal valve (that is, uncoupling of the oropharynx and nasopharynx) during speech and swallowing may be similar, the neurological pathways for these activities are distinct. Velopharyngeal movements for speech are learned, voluntary activities that are controlled by the motor cortex, whereas similar movements for swallowing are primarily involuntary activities that originate from the brainstem.

Physiology

The velopharynx is a complex, three-dimensional valve which serves to uncouple the oropharynx and nasopharynx during speech and swallowing. This section will briefly discuss velopharyngeal function during speech.

It is widely accepted that the levator veli palatini is the muscle that is primarily responsible for velar motion and, hence, for velopharyngeal closure.[12] Fine motor control of velar position may also be governed by the palatoglossus and palatopharyngeus. As noted above, the paired musculus uvulae may play an important role in velar stretch and in filling the gap between the velum and the posterior pharynx during velopharyngeal closure. The relative contribution of the levator and of the superior pharyngeal constrictor to lateral pharyngeal wall movement has been the subject of some debate.

In normal individuals, the velum lifts posteriorly and superiorly during velopharyngeal closure. The normal point of contact with the posterior pharyngeal wall is located approximately three-quarters of the way back on the velum from the posterior nasal spine (*Fig. 28.3*). The site of velopharyngeal closure is usually at or just inferior to the palatal plane, but velar height, as well as the extent of velopharyngeal contact, varies systematically depending upon the phonetic context.[13–15]

The contribution of lateral pharyngeal wall movement to velopharyngeal closure varies amongst individuals with or without cleft palate and, as with velar movement, varies with the phonemic task. Maximal lateral pharyngeal wall displacement generally occurs at the level of velopharyngeal contact. Skolnick *et al.*[16] and Croft *et al.*[17] have described three basic patterns of velopharyngeal closure observed in normal subjects (*Fig. 28.4*): (1) coronal, in which closure is effected primarily by velar elevation; (2) circular (with or without Passavant's ridge), in which medial movement of the lateral pharyngeal walls contributes to velopharyngeal closure in near-equal proportion to the velum; and (3) sagittal, in which closure is effected primarily by medial movement of the lateral pharyngeal walls and the velum contacts the lateral walls rather than the posterior wall. Of these, the coronal pattern of closure is observed most commonly in both normal individuals and in patients with VPD.

In some individuals, a localized transverse ridge of tissue may be seen to form on the posterior pharyngeal wall during speech. This anterior movement of the posterior pharyngeal wall during velopharyngeal closure was first described by Passavant in 1863[18] and is therefore frequently referred to as "Passavant's ridge." Although some have written that its appearance is always indicative of pathologic velopharyngeal function, Croft *et al.*[17] have demonstrated that Passavant's ridge may play a role in velopharyngeal closure in both normal speakers and in those with VPD.

Electromyographic studies support the notion that normal velopharyngeal function requires the central coordination of velopharyngeal muscle activity with other articulatory movements.[19] Changes in velar position during sound production represent the end result of a complex interaction of several interrelated variables, including auditory and proprioceptive feedback. Moreover, for a single individual, there may be significant flexibility in the system of sound production such that there may be a limited but variable repertoire of velopharyngeal movements that may produce the same perceived sounds. Despite decades of speech science research, the precise neurophysiology of both normal and abnormal velopharyngeal function remains incompletely understood.

Basic science/disease process of velopharyngeal dysfunction

Velopharyngeal insufficiency

The first major diagnostic category of VPD is velopharyngeal insufficiency, a term used to denote an anatomic, or structural, defect responsible for inadequate closure of the velopharyngeal valve. Such defects may be congenital, as in cases of cleft palate or congenital velopharyngeal disproportion (i.e., a short soft palate relative to the depth of the pharynx) (*Fig. 28.5*), or they may be secondary to surgical procedures that alter velopharyngeal anatomy, as in cases of palatoplasty, tumor resection, or adenoidectomy. The most common congenital structural defects associated with VPD are cleft palate and submucosal cleft palate. The reported incidence of persistent VPD after cleft palate repair varies widely and is influenced by a large number of variables. In the absence of an oronasal fistula, however, VPD after palatoplasty is most commonly the result of impaired velar mobility, velopharyngeal disproportion, or a combination of both.

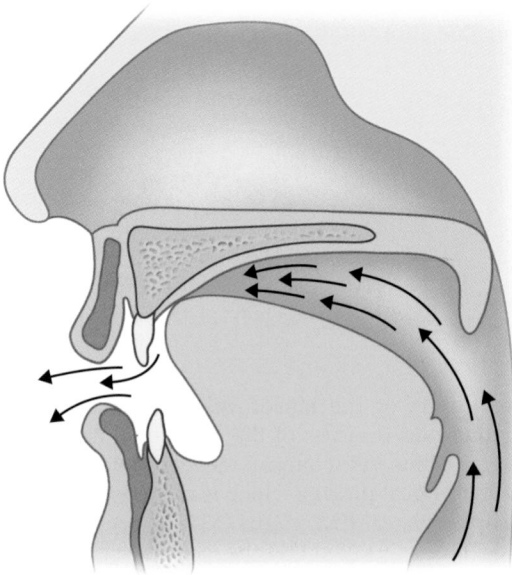

Fig. 28.3 Lateral view of normal velopharyngeal closure for speech during production of an oral pressure consonant.

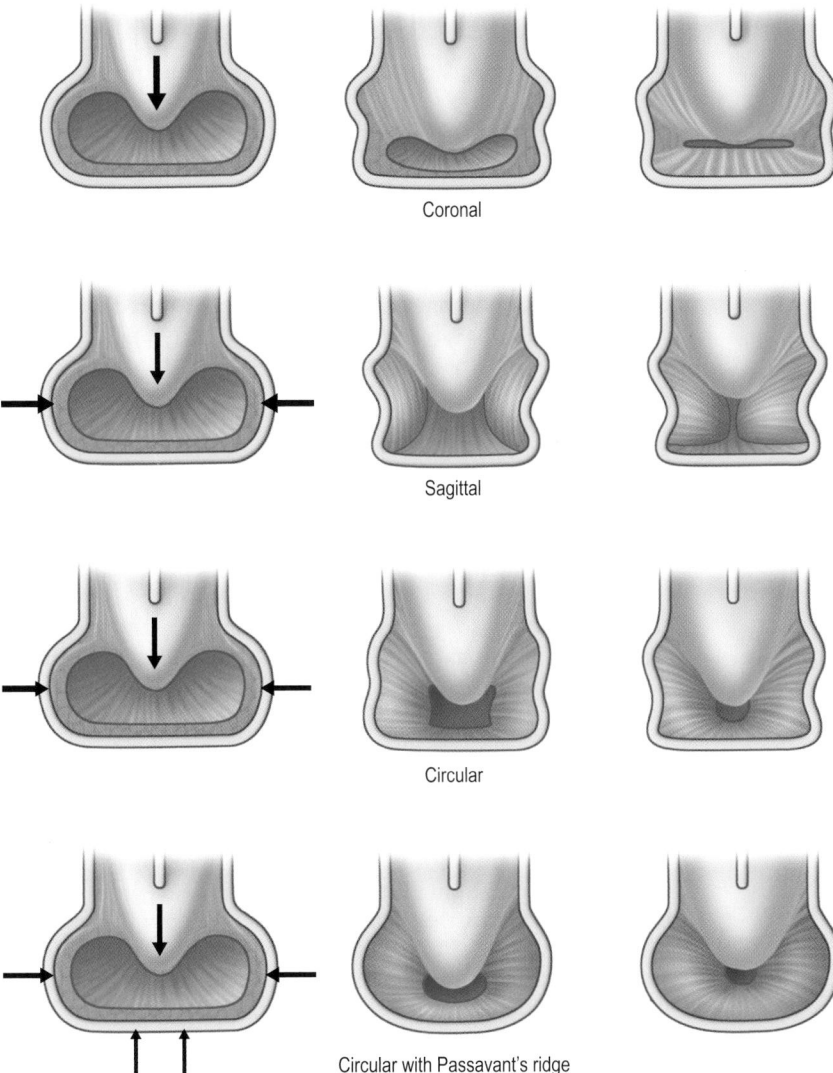

Coronal

Sagittal

Circular

Circular with Passavant's ridge

Fig. 28.4 Types of velopharyngeal closure patterns.

Since adequacy of velopharyngeal closure is largely a function of the ratio of pharyngeal depth to palatal length, patients with a proportionally short palate or deep pharynx may demonstrate incomplete velopharyngeal closure *(Fig. 28.5)*. Each of these conditions may be the result of either a congenital anomaly or an iatrogenic alteration in velopharyngeal architecture. Cicatricial changes following palatoplasty, for example, may lead to velopharyngeal insufficiency secondary to velar shortening. Congenital differences in skeletal architecture may also play a role in postpalatoplasty VPD. Patients with clefts have been demonstrated to have a broader nasopharynx than controls, likely the result of alterations in cranial base dimensions.[20–22] Osborne *et al.*[23] and Ross and Lindsay[24] have shown that a higher prevalence of upper cervical spine abnormalities in patients with clefts may result in increased pharyngeal depth. Likewise, platybasia, or flattening of the cranial base angle, may contribute to VPD by increasing pharyngeal depth, and thus the depth-to-length ratio. Ruotolo *et al.*[25] have shown that patients with 22q11.2 deletion syndrome, a condition associated with a high frequency of severe noncleft VPD, demonstrate several

predisposing skeletal and soft-tissue anomalies, including increased pharyngeal depth, platybasia, and cervical spine anomalies.

Velopharyngeal insufficiency may also be caused by postsurgical changes in velopharyngeal anatomy. In young children, velopharyngeal closure is most often velar-adenoidal. Removal of hyperplastic adenoids for the management of nasopharyngeal airway obstruction or chronic otitis media results in an acute increase in pharyngeal depth. In the majority of noncleft patients, the capacity for velar stretch allows the palate to accommodate for this change. In most cases, postadenoidectomy velopharyngeal insufficiency is transient, and resonance returns to normal within 6–12 months. VPD may persist, however, in a small number of patients, some of whom may have predisposing factors for VPD, including submucosal cleft palate, a short velum, a deep pharynx, or neuromuscular disorders. For patients with these conditions, the adenoids may play a critical role in velopharyngeal closure and even their normal involution may result in velopharyngeal insufficiency.[12] Careful assessment of velopharyngeal anatomy is therefore essential in all patients prior to

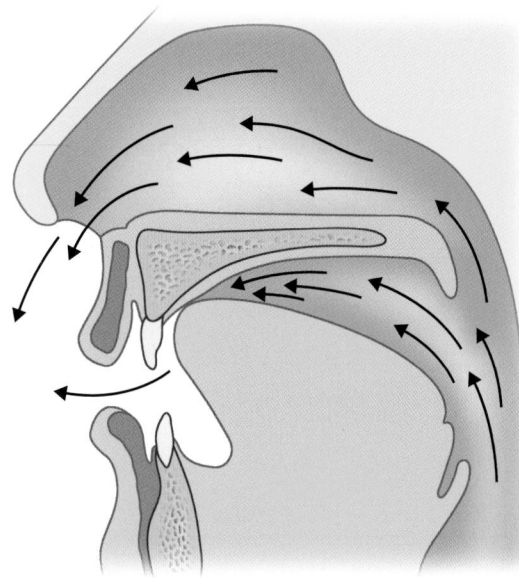

Fig. 28.5 Lateral view of inadequate velopharyngeal closure for speech due to a short soft palate (velopharyngeal insufficiency). The arrows represent the escape of air, pressure, and acoustic energy through the nasal cavity during speech.

adenoidectomy, and should be avoided if possible when anatomical factors that predispose to VPD are identified.

In some patients, irregularity of the surface contour of the adenoid pad may interfere with the ability of the velum to achieve complete velopharyngeal closure.[26] In others, enlarged tonsils may intrude between the velum and the posterior pharyngeal wall, resulting in incomplete closure.[27,28] In these cases, the first step in management should be a selective adenoidectomy or tonsillectomy, respectively, as such may be sufficient to solve the problem, obviating the need for any of the surgical procedures later described.

Velopharyngeal incompetence

The second major diagnostic category of VPD is velopharyngeal incompetence. This label is typically reserved for those cases of VPD known or suspected to be due to congenital or acquired neurological and/or neuromuscular causes such as cerebrovascular incidents, traumatic brain injury, brain tumor, abnormalities in muscle tone or function, and degenerative neuromuscular diseases. In velopharyngeal incompetence, there is typically no evidence of any underlying structural abnormality and palatal length is sufficient; however, the function of the velopharyngeal mechanism is suboptimal for speech production and/or swallowing. The speech sequelae of velopharyngeal incompetence are similar to that seen with velopharyngeal insufficiency, except that many of the individuals also demonstrate other features of dysarthria or other motor speech impairments (e.g., apraxia). Abnormal innervation of cranial nerves IX, X, or XI, or abnormalities in muscle tone/function may result in abnormal timing of palatal elevation which may also exacerbate the

perception of hypernasal speech, in excess of that predicted by velopharyngeal gap size alone. In addition, adults with velopharyngeal incompetence, depending on the etiology, frequently exhibit dysphagia and varying degrees of nasal regurgitation.

There are extensive possibilities for neurologic diagnoses that may be associated with congenital velopharyngeal incompetence including, but not limited to, cerebral palsy, myotonic dystrophy, muscular dystrophy, and congenital hypotonia. Asymmetrical velopharyngeal function, such as that typical of patients with hemifacial microsomia, is also a common cause of velopharyngeal incompetency. Acquired or "late" causes of velopharyngeal incompetence may include traumatic brain injury, cerebrovascular accident or brainstem stroke, and progressive diseases such as Parkinson's disease, amyotrophic lateral sclerosis, muscular dystrophies, multiple sclerosis, and other demyelinating diseases.[29-33]

Children and adults with motor speech disorders have also been shown to demonstrate velopharyngeal incompetence of varying degrees of severity. Apraxia of speech (also referred to as developmental apraxia of speech or childhood apraxia of speech, in children) is a neurologic condition resulting in difficulties with speech motor programming and control.[34] Apraxia may be characterized by inconsistent symptoms of VPD such as inconsistent nasalization of vowels or consonants and inconsistent nasal emission. In addition, many individuals with apraxia may exhibit a combination of both inconsistent hypernasality and hyponasality, providing additional evidence of the abnormal coordination of the palate during speech sound production. Younger children with apraxia may demonstrate some overlapping speech features often seen in children with congenital velopharyngeal incompetence of other causes. For example, children with a history of VPD may have a limited inventory of sounds and demonstrate difficulties learning to produce oral consonants in the first few years of life. These children may produce a pattern of compensatory articulation errors (i.e., glottal stop substitutions) or omit sounds completely. Children with apraxia have difficulty with generating the appropriate "motor program" (blueprint) for producing the sequence of motor movements to produce a sound, which is not typical of children with isolated VPD or clefting. The importance of obtaining a thorough speech pathology evaluation to diagnose these conditions differentially is critical for appropriate treatment decision-making.

Lastly, stress velopharyngeal incompetence is a special case of inadequate velopharyngeal closure for nonspeech behaviors. It is most commonly observed in wind musicians given the high pressure demands.[35,36] There may or may not be comorbid hypernasality or nasal emission in speech. In some cases, stress velopharyngeal incompetence may be an indicator of an underlying physical cause of velopharyngeal incompetence, which may have been masked, or very mild, in the past. In some cases, neurologic or structural causes of VPD (e.g., submucous cleft palate) are diagnosed following the presentation of stress velopharyngeal incompetence, further emphasizing the importance of a thorough clinical evaluation of all patients with any form of VPD.[37] Treatment for stress velopharyngeal incompetence may follow a similar course as that for speech disorders, although there have been reported cases of spontaneous recovery after a period of rest.

Velopharyngeal mislearning

The third, and lesser known, type of VPD involves velopharyngeal mislearning.[38] In this category, the velopharyngeal mechanism appears to be anatomically and physiologically capable of consistent and complete velopharyngeal closure for speech, despite the observation of inconsistent velopharyngeal closure for speech. In this type of VPD, the patient has mislearned how to produce certain speech sounds accurately. The most common example is that of phoneme-specific nasal emission, in which nasal airflow is produced as a complete substitution for an oral consonant, despite adequate velopharyngeal closure ability for other consonants.[39] Clinically, this will often be observed in a child with nasal emission heard on a selected set of sounds, most commonly S, Z, SH, or CH, but not on other sounds such as P, B, T, D, K, G. Another example of velopharyngeal mislearning is the case in which a child produces compensatory articulation errors (e.g., glottal stops) which may prevent or interfere with the achievement of adequate velopharyngeal closure for speech. The velopharyngeal movements during the production of these aberrant speech errors have been shown to be counterproductive (distal versus medial movement of the lateral pharyngeal walls) to the achievement of velopharyngeal closure for speech. A related example is that seen in children with congenital hearing loss with an inability to self-monitor their own speech production, resulting in nasalized speech errors with an otherwise physiologically intact velopharyngeal mechanism.

Velopharyngeal mislearning should be treated with behavioral speech therapy, not surgery. It is critical that a well-trained speech pathologist perform a thorough clinical evaluation to diagnose such conditions differentially in order to make the most appropriate treatment recommendations.

Combined types

In some cases, individuals with craniofacial anomalies and/or clefting may exhibit a combined disorder with evidence of both velopharyngeal insufficiency and velopharyngeal incompetency, resulting in a challenge for surgeons. Some patients with 22q11.2 deletion syndrome have been shown to demonstrate evidence of a combined type of VPD due to the combination of structural clefting disorders, increased pharyngeal depth, and hypotonia of the velopharynx.[40] Regardless of the type of VPD which is present, a complete and thorough physical exam, clinical speech evaluation, and any necessary instrumental or imaging studies should be completed to confirm the etiology and identify the most appropriate treatment plan.

Diagnosis/patient presentation

Patient history and physical exam

Individuals with known or suspected VPD are best treated in the context of an interdisciplinary cleft palate team. Regardless of age, the clinical examination typically includes a brief history and physical exam, perceptual speech evaluation, imaging and acoustic measures, and team discussion for treatment planning. The following information should be obtained during a patient interview when undergoing evaluation for VPD:

- Current patient/family concerns with speech
- Pregnancy history, complications, medication use, and any exposure to teratogens
- Birth and delivery history and complications
- Primary medical diagnoses (e.g., cleft palate, syndromes, cardiac defects, neuromuscular disease)
- History of any feeding or swallowing difficulties during infancy and any current swallowing concerns, including nasal regurgitation and difficulty with breastfeeding or bottlefeeding during infancy
- History of hearing loss or ear disease, including history of frequent ear infections or effusions
- History of snoring or symptoms of sleep apnea
- Surgical history, including prior tonsillectomy, adenoidectomy, and, if appropriate, cleft-related surgical history and timing
- History of any genetic testing and results
- Family history of cleft lip/palate, nasal speech, speech delay, or articulation/pronunciation difficulties; hearing loss, learning disabilities, and medical conditions
- Developmental history
- Speech therapy history.

Every patient, regardless of age, should undergo direct craniofacial and oral examination by the surgeon and speech pathologist with experience in clefting/craniofacial anomalies. The oral exam should be completed in an appropriate examination room and with appropriate lighting. Components of the examination should include an assessment of:

- Craniofacial symmetry
- Oral–facial movement and symmetry
- Dentition and occlusion
- Presence and location of any fistulae
- Presence of signs of submucous cleft palate, including bifid uvula, zona pellucida, and palpate for notch
- Soft palate length, symmetry, and degree of elevation and symmetry during phonation
- Tonsil size and symmetry.

The observations from the physical exam should be interpreted together with the clinical speech evaluation results. For example, if an exam reveals a submucous cleft palate but the patient has normal speech, surgical management would not be recommended. On the other hand, a normal oral exam with clinical speech findings suggestive of severe VPD does not negate the need for physical treatment. The findings from the oral examination may provide hints regarding the source or cause of VPD; however, imaging studies should be completed to confirm the etiology, size/shape, and consistency of the velopharyngeal gap, and to assess the surrounding anatomy of the upper airway.

Perceptual speech evaluation

Perceptual speech assessment is considered the gold standard in the diagnosis of speech disorders of persons with cleft palate and VPD.[41] Additional instrumental assessment and imaging are considered adjunct to the perceptual speech findings, which are the ultimate arbiter of a patient's need for treatment. Perceptual speech evaluation of this patient population should be completed by a speech pathologist with coursework, training, and continuing education in the area of cleft palate and craniofacial anomalies, whenever possible.

During the speech evaluation, the speech pathologist obtains the necessary clinical information regarding the presence and perceived severity of VPD, suspected etiology, and makes preliminary decisions regarding treatment recommendations to discuss with the team. In addition, the speech pathologist is making diagnostic decisions regarding the presence of comorbid conditions such as articulation disorders, voice disorders, and language difficulties. *Box 28.1* provides a list of common speech pathology terminology used for describing the speech characteristics associated with VPD.

BOX 28.1 Common speech pathology terminology

Intelligibility: perceived amount of speech (i.e., number of words) understood

Resonance: the perceptual balance of oral and nasal sound energy in speech. In speakers with velopharyngeal dysfunction, there is an abnormal escape of excessive nasal sound energy through the velopharyngeal port and into the nasal cavity, which is referred to as hypernasality

Hypernasality: perception of excessive nasal sound energy in speech, typically on vowels, glides (W, Y) and liquid sounds (L, R)

Hyponasality: perception of decreased nasal sound energy in speech, typically on nasal sounds M, N, and usually due to structural obstruction (e.g., enlarged adenoid pad, nasal congestion)

Mixed resonance: combination of both hypernasality and hyponasality perceived by a listener. Cul-de-sac resonance is sometimes considered a form of mixed resonance in which sound energy escapes to the anterior nasal cavity and becomes trapped by some form of nasal obstruction or constriction, such as a deviated septum

Nasal emission: abnormal escape of airflow through the nose during consonant production (can be audible or inaudible). When audible, may also be referred to as nasal turbulence

Compensatory articulation errors: a category of articulation errors typically observed in populations with cleft palate or velopharyngeal dysfunction, believed to result from an active strategy to regulate pressure and airflow for speech. Typically includes a pattern of producing sounds in a posterior place of the vocal tract such as the pharynx or larynx, where pressure and airflow can be "valved" prior to their escape to the level of the velopharynx or oral cavity

Glottal stop substitutions: the most common type of compensatory articulation errors seen in children with cleft palate or a history of velopharyngeal dysfunction, produced by adducting the vocal folds together and abruptly releasing the pressure beneath to create the sound of an oral pressure consonant. Often used as a replacement (substitution) for pressure consonants like P, B, T, D, K, G

Nasal substitutions: the active replacement of oral sounds P, B, T, D with nasal sounds M, N

Active nasal fricative: a learned articulatory behavior in which an oral sound (usually S, SH, CH) is replaced with a voiceless nasal sound (i.e., all airflow is emitted through the nose); this is sometimes accompanied by a nasal grimace

Weak pressure consonants: the perception of decreased pressure in oral consonants such as P, B, T, D, F, resulting from a fistula or velopharyngeal gap, causing these sounds to take on nasalization (e.g., the B sound is perceived as an M, the D is perceived as an N), even though the speaker is accurately attempting to produce the correct sound. Often co-occurs with nasal emission

Sibilant distortions: incorrect tongue placement resulting from faulty learning or malocclusion, resulting in imprecise production of sounds S and Z

The most common speech sequelae of VPD include reduced speech intelligibility; articulation disorders ranging from severe compensatory articulation disorders (e.g., pervasive use of glottal stop substitutions) to mild articulation errors and distortions secondary to malocclusion; reduced intraoral pressure of oral pressure consonants; audible nasal emission or nasal turbulence on oral pressure consonants; hypernasal resonance; possible hoarseness and decreased loudness.[41-43]

The components of a standard speech evaluation for the assessment of velopharyngeal closure for speech should include an assessment of intelligibility, resonance, voice, and articulation during a spontaneous speech sample, conversation, and/or picture description tasks.[44] A standard reading passage is suggested for use with adolescent and adult patients. Articulation skills should be assessed with standardized measures (i.e., a standardized articulation test), as well as word and sentence repetition tasks (standard lists available[44]). Oral-only or nasal-only stimuli (e.g., *Buy baby a bib, Pet the puppy, Mama made muffins*, etc.) are also used to assess resonance, nasal emission (audible and inaudible), and pressure for consonants. Special mirrors or listening tubes may also be utilized to evaluate the presence of inaudible nasal emission. The speech parameters are typically rated with five- or seven-point equal-appearing interval scales or other ratio-based scaling methods (e.g., visual analog scales).[41] In some centers, after the clinician rates each speech characteristic individually, a composite decision is made regarding the overall perceived adequacy of velopharyngeal closure for speech.

Audio or video recording of the speech examination should be completed whenever possible for clinical archiving, comparison pre–post treatment, assessment of speech outcome, and for potential research purposes. If clinical symptoms of VPD are present, additional diagnostic testing should follow. Standard speech evaluations for the cleft or VPD population should occur on at least an annual basis, and more frequently if there are changing needs (e.g., postsurgery, posttherapy). Speech evaluations after surgical management (e.g., pharyngeal flap) should occur at least 3–6 months postsurgery to allow for adequate time for healing, decrease in postoperative edema, and an initial period in which patients can "practice" speech with their newly modified speech mechanism.

Indirect measures of velopharyngeal closure for speech

When clinical speech evaluation suggests the presence of VPD, instrumental assessment of speech and velopharyngeal closure may be useful as an adjunct to perceptual judgments. Instrumental measures can provide confirmation of perceptual judgments and further evidence of the need for intervention, as well as allow for objective pre–post treatment measurements. The most popular clinical tools for indirect instrumental evaluation include acoustic assessment of nasality and aerodynamic testing.

Nasalance is an acoustic index of nasality which has been shown to correlate with perceptual judgments of resonance.[45] Nasalance can be measured using commercially available products such as the Nasometer (Kay Pentax) *(Fig. 28.6)*, Nasality Visualization System (Glottal Enterprises), Nasalview (Tiger DRS), and other similar systems. Nasalance is a ratio of the nasal sound energy divided by the sum of the oral plus nasal sound energy in the speech signal.[45] The patient wears a specialized headpiece with nasal and oral microphones that capture the speech signal while the patient reads or repeats a standardized speech sample *(Fig. 28.6)*. Automated analysis provides a nasalance score (expressed as a percentage), which is then interpreted against the perceptual speech observations. Nasalance can range from 0 to 100%; higher numbers represent a higher degree of nasality in speech. A variety of normative and "cutoff" scores have been suggested, which are dependent upon the type of speech stimuli used for the nasalance score calculation.[46–49] Surgeons and clinicians should exercise caution in reliance on nasalance scores, however, due to the variety of potential confounding variables that can artificially inflate or reduce nasalance scores. These include nasal turbulence, articulation errors, vocal hoarseness, mixed resonance, and equipment placement variations, which may reduce with the validity of this measure.[49–51] Nasalance should be considered a supplement to the perceptual speech evaluation, not a substitute for it.

Pioneered by Warren and colleagues,[52,53] pressure–flow testing was developed to obtain quantitative measurement of intraoral and nasal pressure and airflow, velopharyngeal orifice size, and velopharyngeal closure timing for speech. The schematic in *Figure 28.7* illustrates the type of instrumentation and set-up often utilized for aerodynamic assessment of velopharyngeal closure for speech. Custom-designed and commercially available aerodynamic systems, e.g., PERCI-SARS (Microtronics), offer both clinical and research applications for the assessment of velopharyngeal closure for speech. Warren and others[52–57] suggested the use of the word "hamper" as the speech stimulus for pressure–flow testing because of its /mp/ sound sequence which requires the velopharynx to open and close rapidly. An orifice of 10–20 mm^2 (or larger) during the /p/ sound of this stimulus has been shown to correlate highly with perceptual observations of hypernasality.[53] Some studies have suggested that even smaller gap sizes may be clinically significant, especially when variations in velopharyngeal timing are also present.[40,55–57] Pressure–flow testing provides quantitative data that are easy to interpret for diagnostic purposes. Some pressure–flow systems also offer the ability to use the information for biofeedback purposes for speech therapy. The disadvantages of pressure–flow testing include its cost and increased cooperation required for use with younger children.

Imaging

Imaging of the velopharynx is critical for making the most appropriate treatment decision. It is important for the surgeon to visualize the velopharyngeal mechanism *in vivo* during

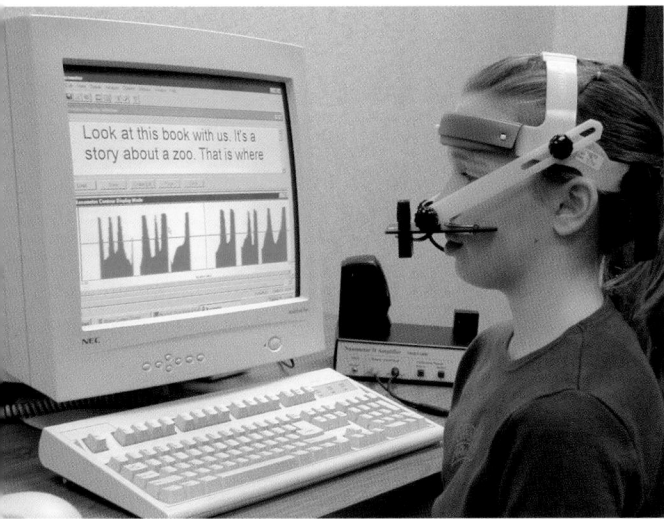

Fig. 28.6 Nasometer II. (Courtesy of Kay Pentax.)

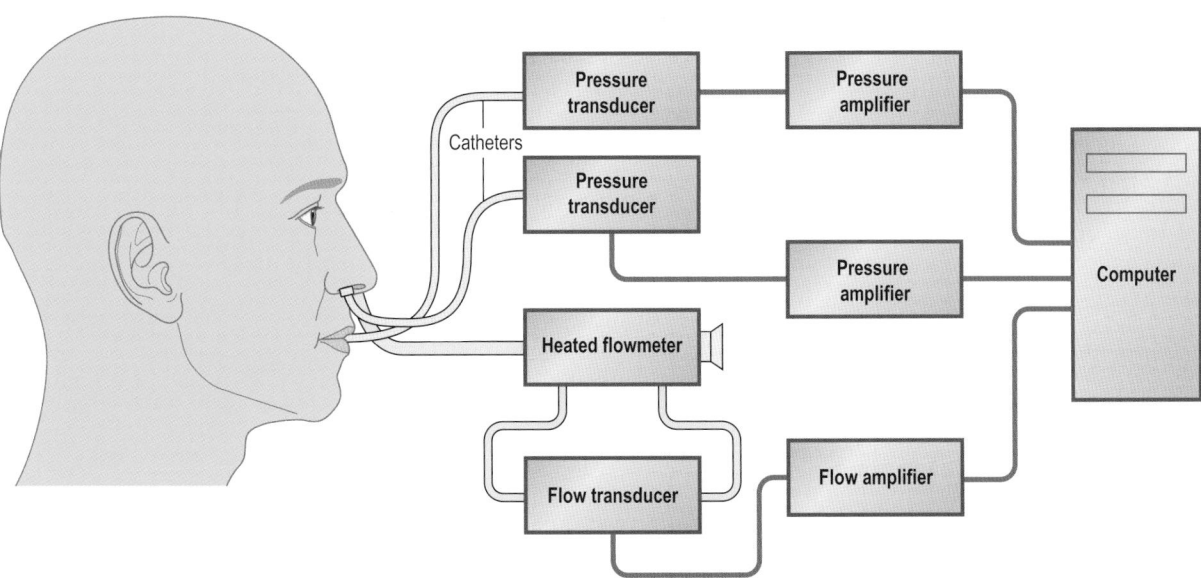

Fig. 28.7 Pressure–flow instrumentation for measuring intraoral pressure, nasal airflow, velopharyngeal orifice size, and velopharyngeal closure timing during speech.

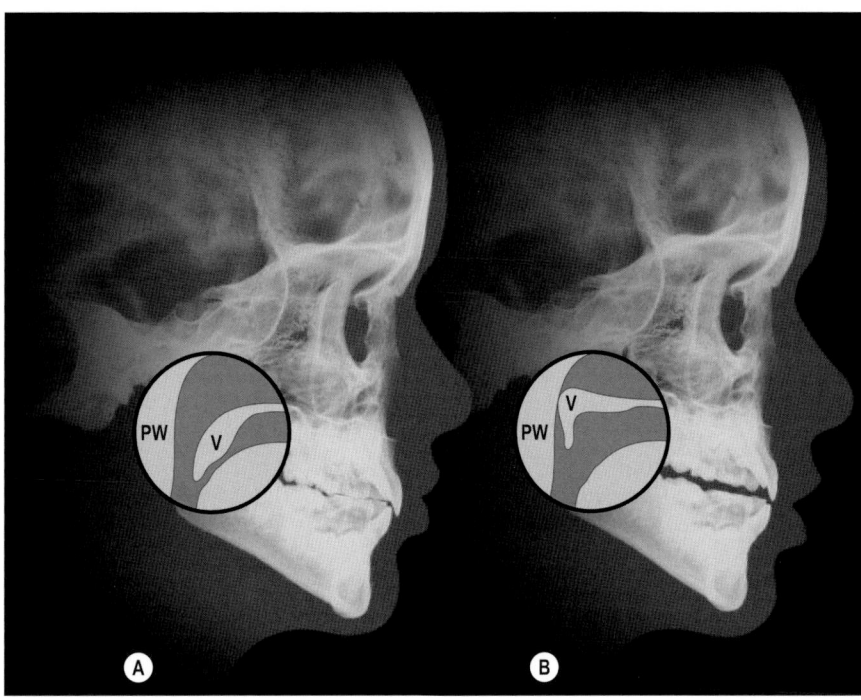

Fig. 28.8 Static lateral cephalometric radiographs of the velopharyngeal mechanism at rest compared with during oral speech. V, velum; PW, posterior pharyngeal wall.

speech in order to identify or confirm the etiology and extent of the problem, as well as to determine which type of surgical approach will best manage the speech problem. In addition, imaging is helpful for clarifying the status of the adjacent structures of the upper airway which could impact treatment planning, such as the size of the tonsils and adenoid pad. It is important that imaging be conducted with a trained speech pathologist in order to ensure that an appropriate speech sample is utilized so that diagnostic decisions are accurate. Imaging is best completed when a patient has the ability to produce at least some oral pressure consonants with accurate placement of the articulators and not just compensatory errors, in order to view the "best effort" of the velopharyngeal mechanism during speech.

Static radiographs

A basic lateral cephalometric radiograph obtained at rest (quiet breathing) and during sustained production of sounds, such as /u/ or /s/, is one of the oldest approaches to evaluate the velopharyngeal mechanism[58] *(Fig. 28.8)*. This type of image may be helpful for confirming palatal length and velar stretch, as well as tonsil and adenoid size; however there is no way of assessing connected speech and the dynamic function of the velopharyngeal mechanism.[59]

Video
1,2
Multiview videofluoroscopy

During multiview videofluoroscopy, a connected speech sample is recorded while motion fluoroscopy records the movement of the velopharyngeal mechanism from multiple angles. The benefit of this imaging approach is that it requires a lower degree of cooperation (as compared to nasopharyngoscopy) and also provides information regarding palatal length, pharyngeal depth, velopharyngeal gap size, and tonsil and adenoid size. Clinicians can examine the velopharyngeal

mechanism during connected speech (as compared to static images), which results in increased sensitivity to detect a smaller or inconsistent velopharyngeal gap; however, the radiation dose is higher than that of a traditional static radiograph. In this procedure, barium contrast is often instilled through the nose to help highlight the nasal surface of the velum and posterior pharyngeal wall, to aid in identification of the velopharyngeal gap. Multiple angles can be obtained, including lateral, frontal, base, and Towne's, with the lateral view as the most common.[60] Due to radiation exposure and the availability of other imaging options, videofluoroscopy for speech is becoming less common at many cleft centers.

Nasopharyngoscopy

Nasopharyngoscopy involves the passage of a flexible fiberoptic endoscope into the nasal cavity. Once the scope is positioned slightly above the velopharyngeal port, the view should allow for complete observation of all velopharyngeal structures during speech and swallowing, including anteriorly, the soft palate; posteriorly, the posterior pharyngeal wall or adenoid pad; and laterally, the lateral pharyngeal walls. Nasopharyngoscopy during speech is usually conducted by the surgeon, otolaryngologist, or a trained speech pathologist. Regardless, a speech pathologist should be present during the examination to model the correct speech stimuli for the patient to imitate during the procedure. Sufficient cooperation can be anticipated in most 4–5-year-olds, and even some mature 3-year-olds, when they have been shown to be capable of producing a sufficient speech sample. A topical anesthetic and decongestant and scope lubricant are often utilized for increased patient comfort and cooperation.

The scope should be inserted into the middle meatus of the nasal cavity whenever possible, as the inferior meatus may provide a view of the velopharyngeal port but is more prone

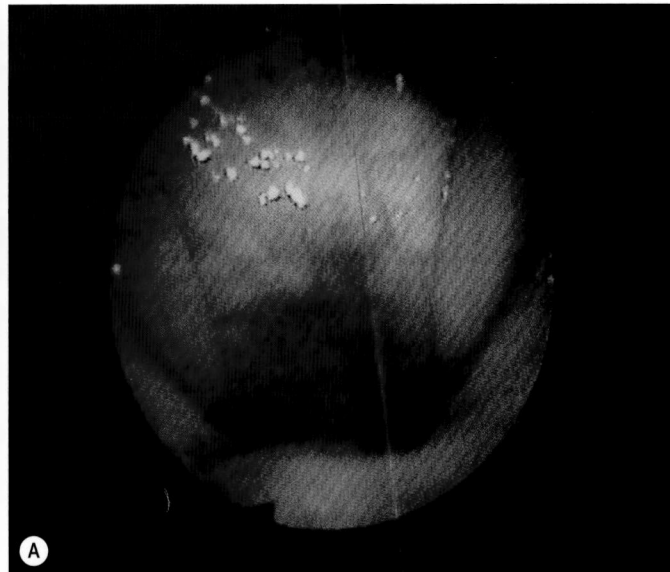

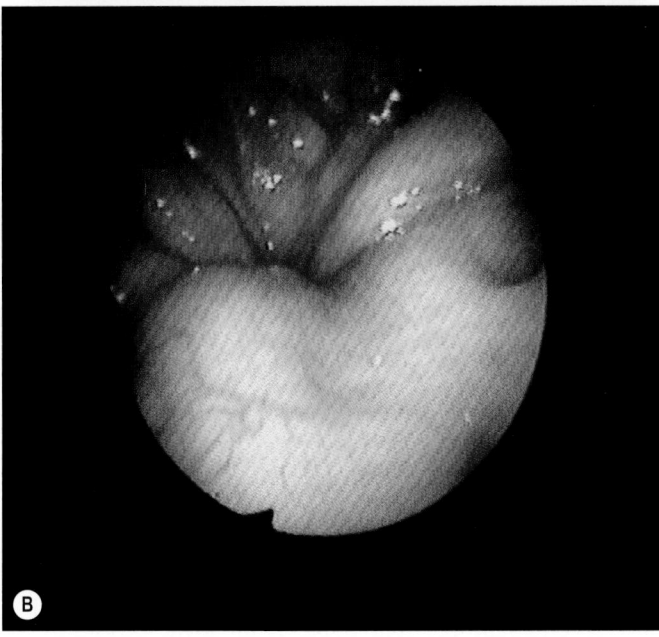

Fig. 28.9 Views of the velopharyngeal port during speech obtained by nasopharyngoscopy. **(A)** Inadequate velopharyngeal closure during speech resulting in a large central gap. **(B)** Complete closure of the velopharyngeal port during speech.

to artifact based on the viewing angle. The estimated size, shape, and consistency of the velopharyngeal gap can be viewed during speech and the type of velopharyngeal closure pattern can also be determined *(Fig. 28.9)*. Tonsil and adenoid size can be examined, as well as laryngeal structures, if needed. The benefit of nasopharyngoscopy is the direct view of the velopharyngeal mechanism from above the velopharyngeal port during speech, in color. Nasopharyngoscopy is also better for assessing small velopharyngeal gaps and asymmetrical velopharyngeal function, and velopharyngeal inadequacy persisting post-pharyngeal flap, and is the most direct assessment option for suspected occult submucous cleft palate. Another benefit of nasopharyngoscopy is that it may also be useful for slightly older children, adolescents, and

adults, who may benefit from biofeedback during speech therapy.

For multiview videofluoroscopy and nasopharyngoscopy, the speech sample should include words and phrases or sentences, which are carefully selected by the speech pathologist so that the patient's best attempts at velopharyngeal closure can be visualized during accurate articulation (and may also be contrasted with the least amount of velopharyngeal closure during nasal sounds or compensatory errors). Imaging exams should be audio- and video-recorded for later review whenever possible. Standard procedures for acquiring, rating, and interpreting videofluoroscopic and nasendoscopic images of the velopharynx during speech have previously been reported.[61]

Two other imaging methods, computed tomographic scans and magnetic resonance imaging (MRI), have been utilized for the assessment of velopharyngeal closure for speech, but primarily for research purposes. Dynamic MRI is still in the early stages of application for assessment of the velopharyngeal mechanism, with preliminary studies demonstrating the ability to capture the movement of the velopharyngeal mechanism during the phonation of vowels and consonants and limited speech tasks.[62–64]

Treatment/surgical techniques

The primary goal of surgical management is to produce a competent velopharyngeal mechanism while avoiding the complications of nasal airway obstruction, including hyponasality, obligate mouth-breathing, snoring, and obstructive sleep apnea. In all cases, surgical management should be individualized, taking into consideration each patient's velopharyngeal anatomy and function, as well as any comorbid conditions that may influence surgical outcome. All surgical procedures for the management of VPD seek to reduce the cross-sectional area of the velopharyngeal port and/or improve the dynamic function of the velopharyngeal valve. The procedures most commonly used for the management of VPD include Furlow double-opposing Z-palatoplasty, posterior pharyngeal flap, and sphincter pharyngoplasty. Posterior pharyngeal wall augmentation has been used less frequently.

Preoperative evaluation

In order to optimize surgical results while minimizing the likelihood of complications, all patients considered candidates for surgical management should undergo thorough preoperative evaluation. Individualization of surgical management is critical to optimizing surgical outcome. That is, differential management based upon specific anatomic and functional abnormalities allows for selection of the surgical technique most likely to achieve velopharyngeal competence in each patient.

The surgeon should elicit a thorough history, carefully assessing each patient for prior surgery on the palate, velopharynx, tonsils, and adenoids, as stated earlier in this chapter. The presence of associated syndromes and comorbid conditions should be noted, as should a prior history of upper-airway obstruction. Appropriate preoperative medical and anesthetic consultation should be obtained. Patients with a history of Pierre Robin sequence, loud snoring, or obstructive sleep apnea should undergo a careful preoperative evaluation of the airway, including polysomnography. In all such cases, stabilization of the upper airway should precede surgical management of VPD.

In addition to the perceptual speech evaluation, careful physical examination should be performed in all patients who may be candidates for surgical management of the velopharynx. Patients should be assessed for stigmata of syndromic diagnoses (e.g., 22q11.2 deletion syndrome) that may influence their management and outcome or those (i.e., Pierre Robin sequence) that may increase their risk for postoperative upper airway obstruction. Intraoral examination yields important information regarding oropharyngeal anatomy. Patients noted to have enlarged tonsils and/or adenoids should undergo tonsillectomy and adenoidectomy prior to posterior pharyngeal flap surgery in order to reduce their risk of postoperative upper airway obstruction. Examination of patients who have undergone prior tonsillectomy, however, may reveal scarring of the tonsillar pillars that may preclude sphincter pharyngoplasty. In patients who have undergone prior palatoplasty, the palate should be inspected carefully for velar dehiscence and oronasal fistulae. Patients with velar dehiscence should undergo re-repair of the palate prior to reassessment of velopharyngeal function and, if necessary, pharyngoplasty. Likewise, fistulae large enough to be of aerodynamic significance should be repaired and velopharyngeal function reassessed. Oropharyngeal examination may also provide useful information in those patients who present with persistent or recurrent velopharyngeal dysfunction after pharyngoplasty. For example, a pharyngeal flap appropriately positioned at the level of velar closure will be difficult to visualize on oral examination. The presence of a pharyngeal flap easily visible on the posterior pharyngeal wall below the palate should raise suspicion that the flap may be tethering the velum and impairing velopharyngeal closure.

In addition, preoperative imaging of the velopharynx is also essential to surgical planning. The diagnosis of VPD should be confirmed by nasendoscopy and/or multiview videofluoroscopy, as earlier described. The site, pattern, and symmetry of velopharyngeal closure should be noted, as should gap size, shape, and location. Imaging further allows the surgeon to assess orientation of the levator fibers, velar anatomy and function, and adenoid and tonsillar size and morphology. Markedly enlarged tonsils or irregularly shaped adenoids may impair velopharyngeal closure in some patients. Preoperative imaging allows the operator to assess the contribution of adenoid or tonsillar abnormalities to VPD, thereby avoiding misguided attempts at pharyngoplasty in patients for whom adenoidectomy or tonsillectomy is indicated as an initial procedure. Previous research has suggested that when a patient is observed to exhibit a short velum or decreased palatal elevation, but at least an average degree of medial movement of the lateral pharyngeal walls during speech, a pharyngeal flap procedure may be most likely to result in a better speech outcome. On the other hand, if a patient demonstrates average palatal length and elevation with minimal lateral pharyngeal wall contribution to velopharyngeal closure, a sphincter pharyngoplasty may be the more appropriate procedure. Surgeon experience, skill, and preference, as well as any potential concerns with airway obstruction in the patient's history, will also interact with imaging findings as part of the treatment decision-making process.

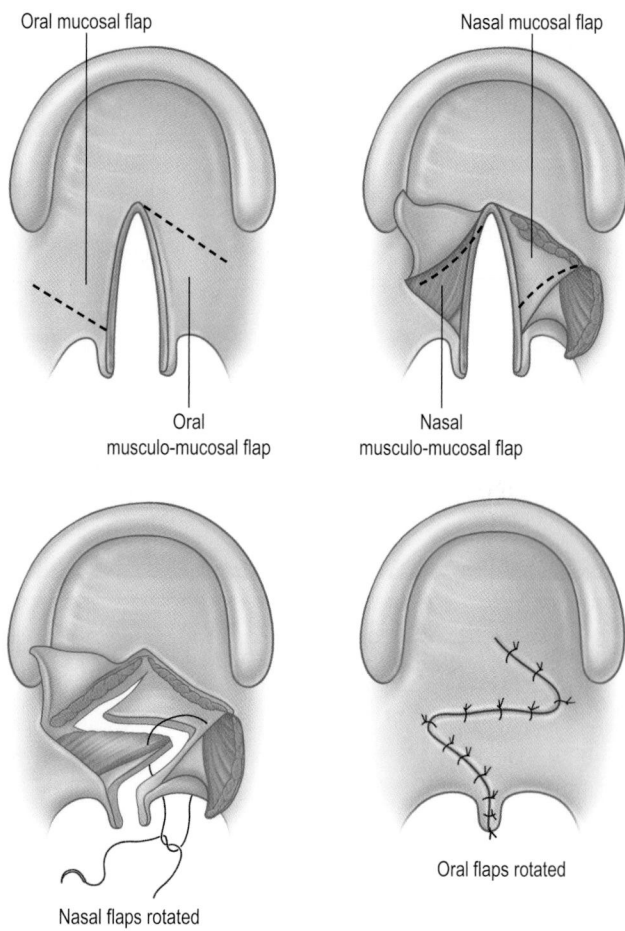

Fig. 28.10 Furlow palatoplasty.

Furlow double-opposing Z-palatoplasty (Fig. 28.10)

Although originally described for the primary repair of palatal clefts,[65] the Furlow double-opposing Z-palatoplasty incorporates several features that make it an ideal procedure in selected patients with VPD. Transposition of the posteriorly based myomucosal flaps reorients the levator muscles from the sagittal to the horizontal position, thereby reconstructing the levator sling. The Z-plasty design provides for palatal lengthening while avoiding velar shortening that may occur after straight-line closure. Thus, the Furlow Z-palatoplasty is well suited for the management of VPD in patients with an unrepaired submucosal cleft palate and in those who have undergone cleft palate repair without levator reconstruction. The technique is inappropriate, however, for patients in whom the levator muscle fibers are not sagittally oriented, as transposition of the myomucosal flaps would disrupt the anatomically normal or the previously reconstructed levator sling.

The design of the Furlow palatoplasty incorporates mirror-image Z-plasties on the oral and nasal aspects of the velum, such that the posteriorly based flaps contain both mucosa and the attached fibers of the levator veli palatini. In contrast, the anteriorly based flaps contain mucosa and submucosa alone. The Z-plasty design is determined by palatal anatomy, the incisions extending from the hamulus to the junction of the hard and soft palate at the cleft margin on one side and from the base of the uvula to the hamulus on the other. The posteriorly based flap is elevated in the nasal submucosal plane, thereby creating an oral myomucosal flap. Care must be taken to divide the levator fibers completely from the posterior edge of the hard palate in order to allow for complete posterior rotation of the flap and for horizontal repositioning of the levator. The contralateral flap is elevated in the oral submucosal plane, creating an anteriorly based mucosal flap.

The anteriorly based nasal mucosal flap is then developed by incising the nasal mucosa from the base of the uvula to a point just medial to the orifice of the eustachian tube. On the opposite side, the posteriorly based nasal myomucosal flap is incised along the posterior edge of the hard palate, again completely dividing the attachment of the levator to the bone. The nasal flaps are then transposed and sutured in place. Transposition of the oral flaps reconstructs the levator sling and completes the repair.

Several reports confirm the efficacy of the Furlow Z-palatoplasty in the management of VPD in selected patients with unrepaired submucosal cleft palate and with repaired overt clefts. In a series reported by Hudson et al.,[66] 85% of patients with VPD after primary palatoplasty demonstrated normal resonance after conversion to a Furlow Z-palatoplasty. Chen et al.[67] reported that the majority of patients with a velopharyngeal gap of less than 5 mm achieve velopharyngeal competence after Furlow repair, whereas the repair is far less successful when the gap size exceeds 10 mm. D'Antonio et al.[68] reported normal resonance after conversion to a Furlow Z-palatoplasty in six of eight patients with persistent VPD after cleft palate repair. All patients in their series demonstrated a central v-shaped notch in the posterior soft palate, good velar motion, and a "small" velopharyngeal gap.

High success rates for the management of VPD by Furlow palatoplasty have been reported in patients with submucosal cleft palate. As for previously repaired overt clefts, the likelihood of success in patients with submucosal clefts may be related primarily to gap size. Seagle et al.[69] reported that 83% of patients with VPD and submucosal cleft palate achieved velopharyngeal competence after Furlow repair, noting that successful outcomes are far more frequent in those patients in whom gap size measured less than 8 mm. Likewise, Chen et al.[70] reported that 97% of patients with submucosal clefts achieved velopharyngeal competence when gap size did not exceed 5 mm. Studies have confirmed that the Furlow Z-palatoplasty increases palatal length in most patients and have suggested that speech outcome after Furlow repair may be determined to a large extent by the degree of velar lengthening achieved,[68] an effect that is related primarily to the angles of the Z-plasty design. As noted above, however, the Z-plasty angles are determined not by any specific geometric design, but rather by the underlying palatal anatomy. As velar length decreases, the Z-plasty angles increase, thereby reducing the amount of velar lengthening effectively achieved following transposition of the flaps. Velopharyngeal competence after Furlow Z-palatoplasty, therefore, can be anticipated in the patient with a small velopharyngeal gap and good velar length but may be more difficult to achieve in patients with a large gap and short velum.

Complications after Furlow Z-palatoplasty include bleeding, oronasal fistula, and nasal airway obstruction. Fistula formation can be minimized by ensuring that the repair is completed with minimal tension. When necessary, lateral relaxing incisions should be employed in order to achieve a tension-free closure. Although mild obstructive apnea has been documented in patients following Furlow Z-palatoplasty, such has been noted to resolve in nearly all patients within 3 months of surgery.[71] When compared to patients who have undergone posterior pharyngeal flap surgery for the management of VPD, patients treated by Furlow repair demonstrate significantly lower incidence and severity of upper airway obstruction 6 months or more postoperatively.[72]

Posterior pharyngeal flap (Fig. 28.11)

The creation of midline flaps from the posterior pharyngeal wall represents the oldest surgical technique for the management of VPD. In 1865, Passavant published the first report describing the surgical management of VPD by adhesion of the soft palate to the posterior pharyngeal wall.[73] Schoenborn described the use of an inferiorly based pharyngeal flap in 1875 and of a superiorly based flap a decade later.[74,75] The superiorly based pharyngeal flap was described in the US by Padgett in 1930,[76] and by the middle of the 20th century, the procedure was widely employed as the standard surgical treatment for VPD.

The pharyngeal flap functions primarily as a central obturator of the velopharyngeal port. Closure of the lateral side ports during speech is dependent upon the medial movement of the lateral pharyngeal walls. Hence, this technique is optimally suited for patients with VPD that is characterized by the presence of a central gap and that is associated with good lateral pharyngeal wall motion. To be effective, the pharyngeal flap should be carefully placed at the level of attempted velopharyngeal closure as determined by preoperative imaging. Flaps that have been created too low or that have migrated inferiorly due to postoperative cicatricial changes may tether the velum and interfere with velopharyngeal closure. Patients with an asymmetrical velopharyngeal closure pattern should have flap design altered accordingly.

The width of the pharyngeal flap should be tailored to the functional and anatomic needs of each patient, again as determined by preoperative imaging. That is, patients with large gaps and those with relatively poor lateral pharyngeal wall motion may require a wider flap design in order to achieve velopharyngeal competence. Flap width is dependent not only upon the breadth of the flap itself, but also on the breadth of its inset on the posterior velum. Inset of the flap may be accomplished either by dividing the soft palate in the midline or by dissecting a submucosal pocket through a posterior transverse ("fishmouth") incision. The latter allows for somewhat greater flexibility in the design of flap width and lateral port dimensions.[77] Cicatricial change, or "tubing," of pharyngeal flaps may result in significant flap narrowing and, consequently, in deterioration of velopharyngeal function.[78] Pharyngeal flap narrowing can be minimized, however, by lining the raw surface of the flap with mucosal flaps of velar mucosa or by designing short, broad flaps. In all cases, the need to create wide flaps must be judiciously balanced against an associated increase in the risk of postoperative obstructive sleep apnea.

Careful surgical planning and individualization of flap design are essential to surgical success. Accurate interpretation of reported series is made difficult, however, by the use

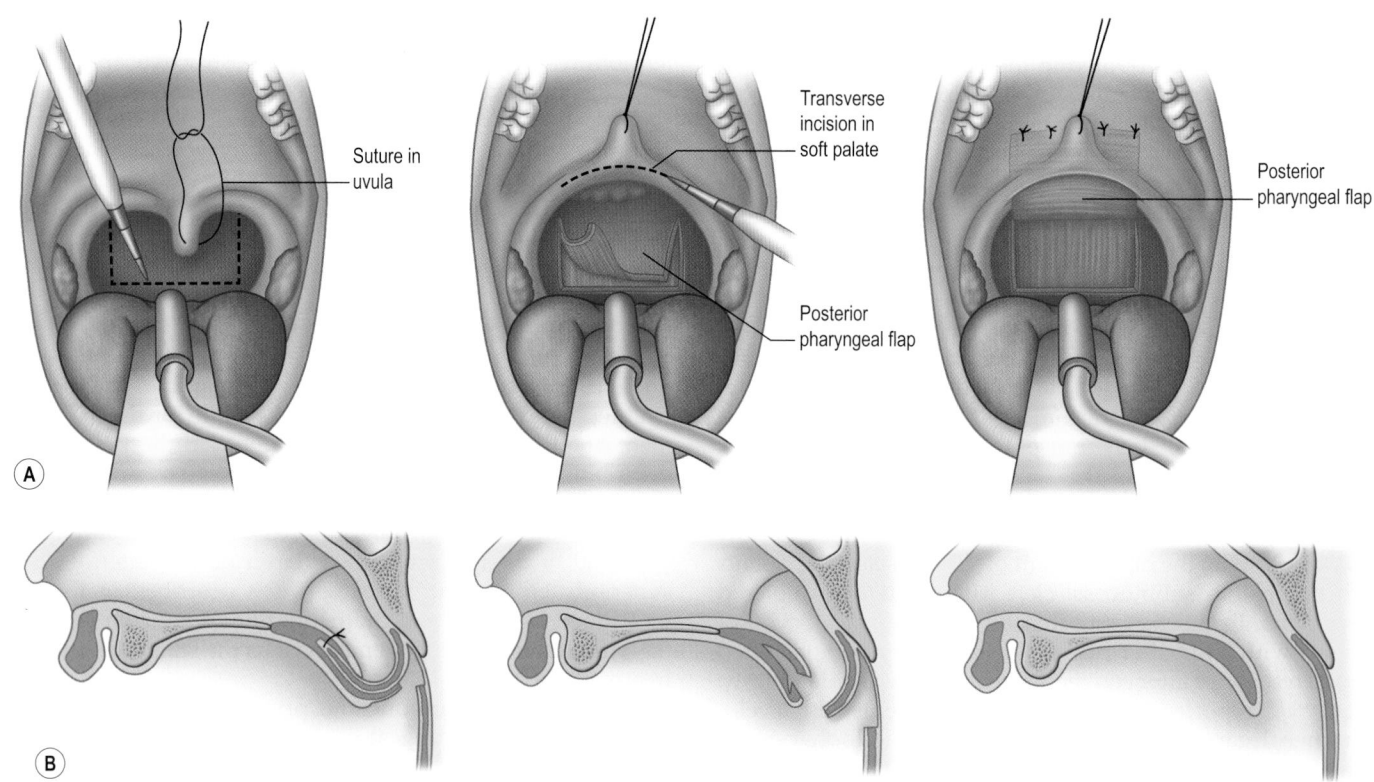

Fig. 28.11 (A, B) Posterior pharyngeal flap.

of different surgical techniques, heterogeneous patient populations, and nonstandardized, often unreliable measures of surgical outcome. Argamaso[77] reported that hypernasality was eliminated after pharyngeal flap surgery in 96% of 226 patients. Similarly, normal or borderline sufficient velopharyngeal function was achieved in 97% of 104 nonsyndromic patients described by Sullivan *et al.*[79] Cable *et al.*[80] reported stability in resonance scores over 14 years of follow-up after pharyngeal flap surgery, suggesting that surgical outcome after pharyngeal flap surgery is durable.

Several authors have expressed concerns regarding the negative impact of pharyngeal flap attachment on midfacial growth. Although several studies have yielded conflicting data, the majority of evidence from large series has failed to demonstrate that attachment of pharyngeal flaps has any significant long-term influence on maxillary development.[81]

Complications of pharyngeal flap surgery include bleeding, dehiscence, and nasal airway obstruction, including obstructive sleep apnea.[82] Rarely, deaths have been reported following the procedure, primarily related to airway compromise.[83] Fraulin *et al.*[84] reported that predictive factors for complications include the operator, associated medical conditions, concurrent surgical procedures, and an open flap donor site. Of all complications, upper airway compromise occurs most commonly. Nearly all patients experience transient nasal airway obstruction and perhaps mild obstructive apnea in the early postoperative period. The vast majority of patients demonstrate resolution of clinical and polysomnographic evidence of nocturnal upper airway obstruction within several months of surgery, as edema subsides. Wells *et al.*[85] documented clinical evidence of nocturnal upper airway

obstruction in 12 of 111 patients following pharyngeal flap surgery, three of whom required takedown of the flap. Nine of the 12 patients underwent polysomnographic evaluation, and this revealed obstructive apnea in only one patient. Thus, clinical evidence of postoperative nocturnal airway obstruction may not correlate with the presence of apnea. Syndromic patients and those with a history of Pierre Robin sequence may be at greater risk for airway compromise after pharyngeal flap surgery due to the presence of associated functional or anatomic airway abnormalities.[85,86] Similarly, patients with tonsillar enlargement may be at greater risk for postoperative upper airway obstruction and should therefore undergo tonsillectomy at or prior to the time of pharyngeal flap surgery.[87]

Postoperative monitoring of upper airway status, including continuous pulse oximetry, should be considered the standard of care for all patients following posterior pharyngeal flap surgery. For patients at high risk for postoperative airway obstruction, consideration should be given to the use of a nasopharyngeal airway, placed intraoperatively through one of the lateral ports, and to admission to the intensive care unit for overnight monitoring. Patients may be discharged from the hospital once they demonstrate adequate airway stability and oral fluid intake.

Sphincter pharyngoplasty *(Fig. 28.12)*

In 1950, Hynes[88] first described the technique of pharyngoplasty by transposition of musculomucosal flaps containing the salpingopharyngeus muscles. He later modified the technique to include the palatopharyngeus muscles, noting that success of the technique could be attributed to narrowing of

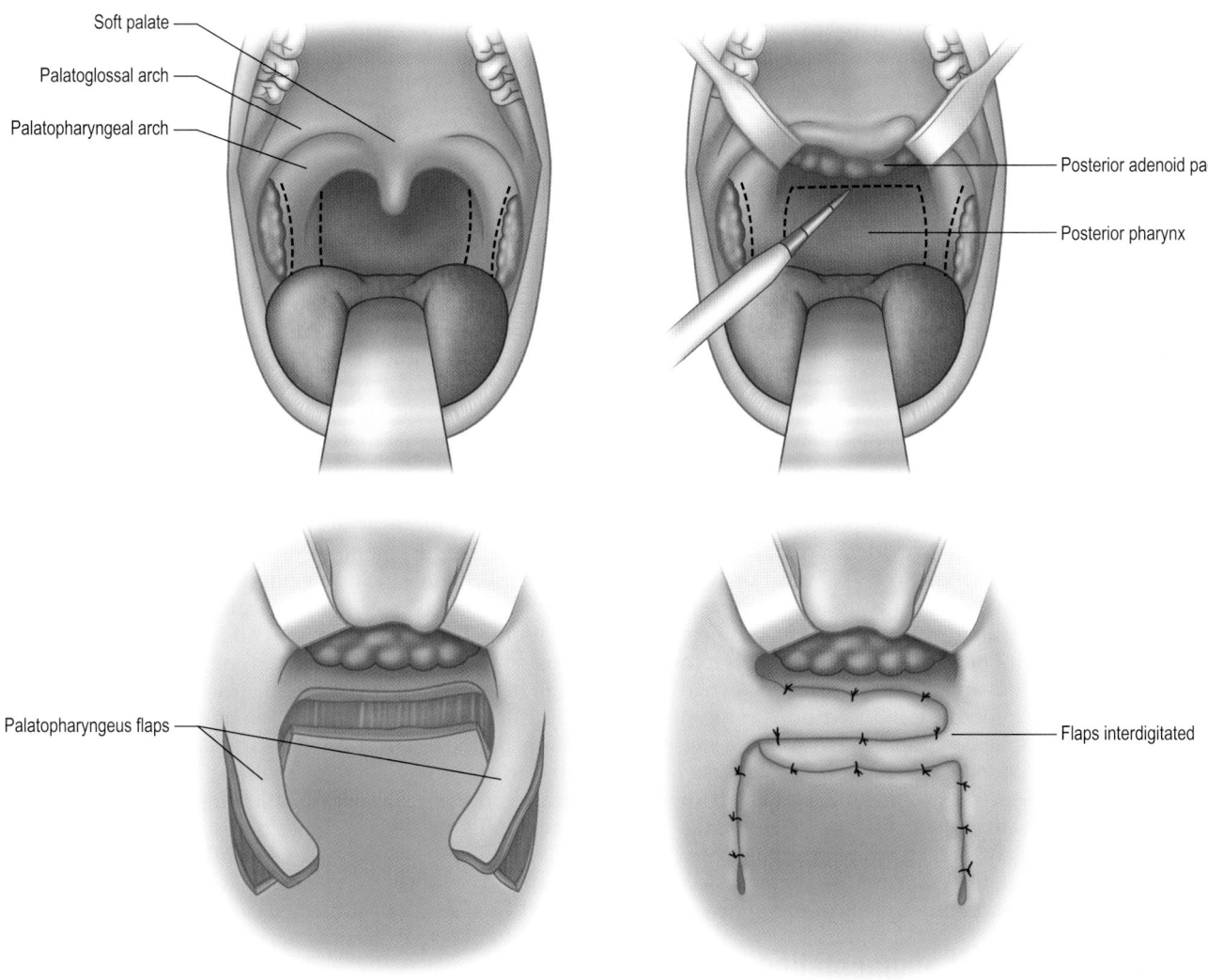

Fig. 28.12 Sphincter pharyngoplasty.

the velopharyngeal port and to augmentation of the posterior pharyngeal wall with bulky, "often contractile" flaps.[89,90] Orticochea[91] stressed the concept of creating a true "dynamic sphincter" in order to achieve velopharyngeal competence. He dissected bilateral palatopharyngeal myomucosal flaps and inset them into an inferiorly based mucosal flap on the posterior pharyngeal wall. Jackson and Silverton[92] later modified the procedure, eliminating the posterior pharyngeal flap, instead insetting the palatopharyngeal flaps into a transverse incision located higher on the posterior pharyngeal wall.

The surgical technique used most widely today represents a modification of the Hynes pharyngoplasty. Vertical incisions are made anterior to both posterior tonsillar pillars, and the palatopharyngeus muscles are exposed. The longitudinally oriented muscle fibers are carefully dissected from the posterolateral pharyngeal wall, so as to include the entire muscle in each of the flaps. Vertical incisions are then made posterior to the pillars, creating flaps that measure approximately 1 cm in width. On each side, the parallel incisions are joined by a transverse incision at the lowest aspect of the pillar, and the flaps are elevated. The flaps are then rotated medially and

inset into a transverse incision that connects the most superior aspect of the medial palatopharyngeal flap incisions.

Riski et al.[93] have stressed the importance of preoperative patient selection and of proper surgical planning for optimizing surgical outcome. Flap inset should be high on the posterior pharyngeal wall at the site of attempted velopharyngeal closure, as determined by preoperative imaging. Since a dynamic sphincter may be achieved in only a subset of patients,[94,95] anatomic factors, such as reduced port size and augmentation of the posterior pharyngeal wall, may be essential to achieving postoperative velopharyngeal competence. In a retrospective review of speech outcome in 48 patients who underwent sphincter pharyngoplasty, Shewmake et al.[96] reported that 85.4% achieved normal resonance. Riski et al.[97] reported that, of 139 patients who underwent sphincter pharyngoplasty, 78% demonstrated resolution of hypernasality and normal pressure–flow measurements. Most surgical failures were the result of the pharyngoplasty being placed too low on the posterior pharyngeal wall. Similarly, Witt et al.[98] noted that 16% of patients required pharyngoplasty revision, although the primary cause of failure was noted to be complete or partial flap dehiscence. In a series of 250 patients, Losken et al.[99] noted a revision rate of 12.8%, noting that persistent VPD after pharyngoplasty was more common in patients with 22q11.2 deletion syndrome. Failure was seen more often in patients with greater nasalance scores and velopharyngeal valve area on preoperative instrumental evaluation.

Several studies have compared speech outcome after posterior pharyngeal flap surgery and sphincter pharyngoplasty. Ysunza et al.[100] reported on 50 patients with cleft palate and residual VPD who were randomized to undergo one or the other procedure, finding no significant difference in the frequency of persistent VPD (12% and 16%, respectively) between the two groups. Similarly, Abyholm et al.[101] reported no significant difference in speech outcome 1 year following posterior pharyngeal flap or sphincter pharyngoplasty in a randomized multicenter trial.

Complications of sphincter pharyngoplasty are similar to those of posterior pharyngeal flap surgery and include bleeding, flap dehiscence, and upper airway obstruction. In a multicenter, prospective randomized trial of 97 patients, Abyholm et al.[101] noted that polysomnographic evidence of obstructive apnea 1 year after surgical management of VPD was rare, with no significant difference between patients undergoing posterior pharyngeal flap surgery and those undergoing sphincter pharyngoplasty. Saint Raymond et al.[102] examined polysomnograms of 17 patients before and after sphincter pharyngoplasty and found that the procedure induced no significant impairment in either the apnea–hypopnea index or the nocturnal oxygen saturation. Despite this, however, there was a notable reduction in slow-wave sleep and an increase in cortical microarousals postoperatively, suggesting that the reduction in nasopharyngeal airway diameter may increase airway resistance sufficiently enough to cause fragmentation of sleep architecture even in the absence of detectable sleep apnea.

Posterior pharyngeal wall augmentation

Augmentation pharyngoplasty, using both autologous tissues and alloplastic materials, has long been used by surgeons to reduce the size of the velopharyngeal orifice in patients with VPD. Long-term results have been variable and have depended upon both patient selection and the choice of augmentation material. Overall, the most durable results have been achieved in patients with good velar motion and relatively small velopharyngeal gap size.

In 1862, Passavant became the first to describe the use of local tissues to augment the posterior pharyngeal wall. In his initial description, he sutured the palatopharyngeal muscles together in the midline. In 1879, he described the use of a pedicled flap of posterior pharyngeal mucosa, rolled upon itself and inset across the posterior pharyngeal wall.[103] After disappointing results, the technique was abandoned. Hynes reported the use of myomucosal flaps containing the salpingopharyngeus (and later the palatopharyngeus) muscles nearly a century later.[88,89] In 1997, Witt et al. reported on the use of a rolled, superiorly based pharyngeal flap for posterior pharyngeal wall augmentation, noting no significant improvement in the speech of 14 patients treated.[104] In contrast, however, Gray et al.[105] reported good results using folded flaps in young patients with good velar motion.

In 1912, Hollweg and Perthes[106] described the use of autologous cartilage grafts inserted through a cervical incision. This procedure was later modified by others utilizing a transoral approach. Although many authors have reported some success with cartilage grafts placed into the posterior pharynx, the results and durability of these procedures have been variable. Denny et al.[107] reported elimination of hypernasality in 25% of 20 patients treated by retropharyngeal bone or cartilage grafts with lesser degrees of improvement seen in another 65%. Follow-up studies of the same cohort of patients, however, failed to document durability of the results achieved. The body of evidence suggests that some degree of graft migration and resorption after pharyngeal augmentation with cartilage appears inevitable. Recent reports have documented improvement in velopharyngeal function following injection of autologous fat into the posterior pharynx in selected patients,[108] although the application and effectiveness of this technique await greater experience and long-term follow-up.

The earliest attempts to augment the posterior pharyngeal wall by injection of exogenous material may have been those of Gersuny, who reported the use of petroleum jelly in 1900.[109] Although the technique achieved some success in improving patients' speech, the technique was associated with several serious complications, including blindness and death. In 1904, Eckstein[110] described injection of paraffin without untoward complications. Blocksma[111] reported augmentation pharyngoplasty using implantable blocks and injectable fluid Silastic. Although he noted improvement of speech in many patients, a high incidence of implant infection and extrusion led him to recommend the use of autologous implants as the preferred method for pharyngeal augmentation. Lewy published a single case report on the use of Teflon injection for the management of VPD in 1965.[112] Bluestone et al.[113] later reported success with Teflon injections in several patents, noting no instances of infection, extrusion, or foreign-body reaction. Smith and McCabe[114] documented complete elimination of hypernasality in 60% of 80 patients who underwent augmentation pharyngoplasty by Teflon injection. Furlow et al.[115] reported successful treatment of VPD by Teflon injection in 74% of 35 patients. Nevertheless, the risk of potentially serious complications has led the Food and Drug Administration to withdraw approval of its use for augmentation pharyngoplasty. Other exogenous materials that have been used to augment the posterior pharyngeal wall in patients with VPD include Proplast and calcium hydroxyapatite.

The majority of evidence suggests that posterior pharyngeal wall augmentation may be successfully used for the management of carefully selected patients with good velar motion and small-gap VPD. In order to be effective, augmentation should performed precisely at the level of attempted velar contact on the posterior pharyngeal wall as determined by preoperative imaging. To date, no single alloplastic material has been found to be uniformly safe, effective, and reliable, and single type of autologous graft has demonstrated consistent long-term stability. Therefore, augmentation pharyngoplasty should be considered only as a secondary option in carefully selected patients with VPD.

Nonsurgical treatment options

While surgery is the preferred treatment option for most cases of VPD, there may be patient-specific factors which cause nonsurgical options to be considered. Prosthetic or behavioral speech treatment may be appropriate for a select set of patients for whom surgery is not possible, not desired, or if the prognosis for surgical outcome is guarded.

Prosthetic treatment

Speech prostheses may be an appropriate treatment option for patients who have an unclear, guarded, or poor prognosis for improvement with surgery, such as: (1) when the diagnosis of VPD is unclear based on perceptual speech and/or imaging findings; (2) when the comorbid speech problems make it difficult to determine if surgical intervention will result in meaningful improvement in speech; and (3) when the patient has a known neuromuscular or degenerative condition that has been shown to result in suboptimal surgical outcomes. In addition, the patient may have known medical contraindications to having surgery or have cultural, religious, or other ethical conflicts with surgery. To be a good candidate for prosthetic management, the patient and family must demonstrate adequate compliance and dedication to completing the prosthetic treatment plan, which may require several visits, and be an appropriate dental candidate for fabrication of a speech prosthesis (i.e., demonstrate good dental hygiene).

The palatal lift and the speech bulb are the most commonly used speech prostheses[116] *(Fig. 28.13)*. A pediatric or general dentist, orthodontist, or prosthodontist may fabricate the device, usually with the input from the speech pathologist. A palatal lift is basically a standard orthodontic retainer with an extension posteriorly to "lift" up the soft palate. It is an appropriate treatment option for patients with a soft palate of sufficient length but lacks adequate movement during speech and/or swallowing, such as in cases of velopharyngeal incompetence. A speech bulb is more appropriate for patients with velopharyngeal insufficiency in which the palate is too short to contact the posterior pharyngeal wall. The speech bulb is similar to the palatal lift, with an addition of a "bulb" of acrylic material to fill in the remaining velopharyngeal gap during speech. Other types of obturators, without any posterior extension, may also be helpful for temporary or long-term obturation of palatal fistulae.

Behavioral speech therapy approaches

In selected patients with borderline or inconsistent VPD and/or velopharyngeal mislearning, at least a trial period of behavioral speech therapy may be helpful prior to proceeding with surgical management.[117,118] Speech therapy is always the most appropriate treatment for articulation errors, as surgery cannot change lip and tongue placement for the production of speech sounds. Speech therapy is also the most appropriate treatment for phoneme-specific nasal emission or phoneme-specific nasalization of sounds (velopharyngeal mislearning) as surgery cannot correct these articulation disorders.[119] There are also some behavioral speech therapy methods which may be effective for reducing mild or inconsistent hypernasality or nasal air emission, as well, especially when biofeedback is provided. If one considers the velum to be an articulator, just as the lips and tongue are, the idea of changing the "behavior" of the velum may be a reasonable goal. The patient must then be provided with the right tools and feedback, assuming that the underlying anatomy of the velopharyngeal mechanism otherwise appears intact. The ideal patient for such a treatment trial would have many of the following characteristics:

- Age 6–8 years or older.
- Intact cognitive skills.
- Intact motor skills.
- Adequate attention span and maturity.
- Normal hearing and vision.
- Good self-monitoring or speech self-correction skills.
- At least inconsistent velopharyngeal closure for speech.

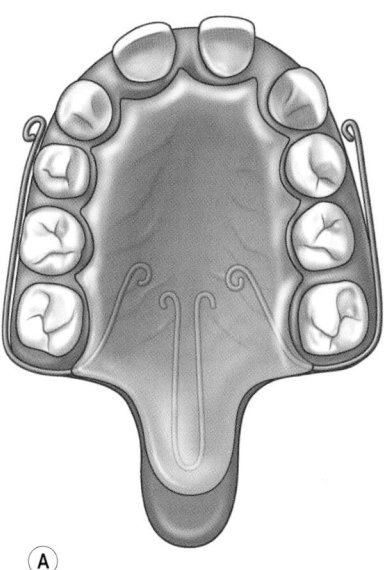
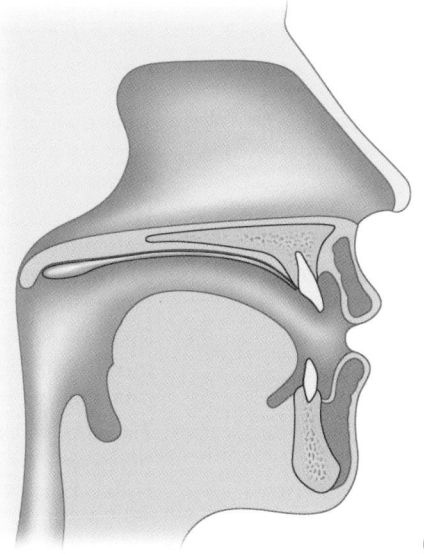
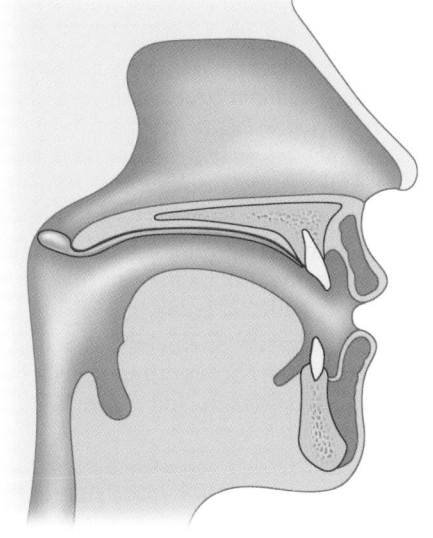

Fig. 28.13 (A) Schematic of a palatal lift (intraoral and lateral view). Note how the lift extends along the oral surface of the velum to lift it to the level of the palatal plane. The length of the palate is sufficient but, in cases of velopharyngeal incompetency, the function of the velopharyngeal mechanism is impaired. The palatal lift places the velum into position to provide adequate closure for speech and swallowing. **(B)** Speech bulb appliance assisting with velopharyngeal closure for speech. Note that the bulb fits up into the velopharyngeal orifice to obturate velopharyngeal port, as the length of the velum is insufficient to achieve closure independently.

- At least some accurate articulation skills already in the speech repertoire.
- Can demonstrates measurable change within the first few sessions of therapy.

Biofeedback is often a cornerstone of behavioral speech therapy to improve velopharyngeal closure for speech. Biofeedback may be provided through enhanced auditory, visual, or tactile–kinesthetic cues. Patients may benefit from technology that provides information during online speech production about oral pressure, nasal airflow, and nasalance. Nasopharyngoscopy is also a useful biofeedback tool as it allows for direct visualization of the velopharyngeal port and its movement during speech. It can be used for treating learned nasal emission and even glottal stop substitutions in selected patients.[120–122] Lastly, continuous positive airway pressure (CPAP) has been proposed as a treatment modality to improve velopharyngeal closure by "working" the muscles against artificially increased nasal resistance (nasal pressure) during speech for longer durations of time. The first round of CPAP clinical trials has yielded mixed speech outcome results.[123] In contrast, it should be stated that, although the velopharyngeal mechanism is a dynamic muscular system, "oral–motor exercises" of the lips, tongue, and palate have not been shown to be effective for improving long-term speech outcomes. Multiple studies have shown that palatal massage, electrical stimulation, swallowing exercises, blowing exercises, and blowing against resistance (i.e., horn/whistle programs), are not effective for improving speech.[124–126] Overall, significantly more research is needed to identify the most effective behavioral speech therapy approaches for improving velopharyngeal closure for speech.

Access the complete references list online at **http://www.expertconsult.com**

12. Peterson-Falzone SJ, Hardin-Jones MA, Karnell MP. Anatomy and physiology of the velopharyngeal system. In: Peterson-Falzone SJ, Hardin-Jones MA, Karnell MP, ed. *Cleft Palate Speech*. 3rd ed. St. Louis: Mosby; 2001:69–86.

17. Croft CB, Shprintzen RJ, Rakoff SJ. Patterns of velophrayngeal valving in normal and cleft palate subjects: a multi-view videofluoroscopic and nasendoscopic study. *Laryngoscope*. 1981;91:265–271.

    The authors studied 80 control subjects and 500 patients with velopharyngeal dysfunction using direct nasopharyngoscopy and multi-view videofluoroscopy. The incidence of the different patterns of velopharyngeal closure was found to be similar in frequency in both groups. The importance of these patterns is discussed in relation to the surgical management of patients with velopharyngeal dysfunction.

41. Kuehn DP, Moller KT. Speech and language issues in the cleft palate population: the state of the art. *Cleft Palate Craniofac J*. 2000;37:348–383.

    This summary paper covers all aspects of speech language assessment and treatment options relevant to cleft palate and velopharyngeal dysfunction. A review of the anatomy and physiology and instrumental assessment of the velopharyngeal mechanism is also provided.

42. Peterson-Falzone SJ, Hardin-Jones MA, Karnell MP. Diagnosing and managing communication disorders in cleft palate. In: *Cleft Palate Speech*. 4th ed. St. Louis: Mosby; 2010:221–247.

44. Henningsson G, Kuehn DP, Sell D, et al. Universal parameters for reporting speech outcomes in individuals with cleft palate. *Cleft Palate Craniofac J*. 2008;45:1–17.

    The Universal Parameters System (UPS) for rating speech in patients with cleft palate and velopharyngeal dysfunction is discussed. Examples of standard speech stimuli, a rating form, and various rating scales are included.

52. Warren DW, DuBois AB. A pressure-flow technique for measuring orifice area during continuous speech. *Cleft Palate J*. 1964;1:52–71.

61. Golding-Kushner KJ. Standardization for the reporting of nasopharyngoscopy and multiview videofluoroscopy: a report from an international working group. *Cleft Palate Craniofac J*. 1990;27:337–348.

    This manuscript describes a protocol for rating velopharyngeal structures and movement during speech using multiview videofluoroscopy and flexible nasopharyngoscopy. These standards were published as a result of an International Working Group meeting of experts in the field of clefting/velopharyngeal dysfunction and speech pathology.

67. Chen PK, Wu JT, Chen YR, et al. Correction of secondary velopharyngeal insufficiency in cleft palate patients with the Furlow palatoplasty. *Plast Reconstr Surg*. 1994;94:933–941.

    The results of this study demonstrate that a Furlow palatoplasty can satisfactorily correct velopharyngeal dysfunction in carefully selected patients. The most important factor is the size of the velopharyngeal gap. The majority of patients with a successful surgical outcome had a velopharyngeal gap less than 5 mm.

89. Hynes W. The results of pharyngoplasty by muscle transplantation in failed "cleft palate" cases, with special reference to the influence of the pharynx on voice production. *Ann R Coll Surg Engl*. 1953;13:17–35.

93. Riski JE, Serafin D, Riefkohl R, et al. A rationale for modifying the site of insertion of the Orticochea pharyngoplasty. *Plast Reconstr Surg*. 1984;73:882–894.

    The authors demonstrate the importance of insetting the sphincter pharyngoplasty at the site of attempted velopharyngeal closure. With this modification, successful outcomes were achieved in 93% of patients.

29

Secondary deformities of the cleft lip, nose, and palate

Evan M. Feldman, John C. Koshy, Larry H. Hollier Jr., and Samuel Stal

SYNOPSIS

- How did we get here? What led to this secondary deformity?
  - Spectrum of clefts: type and severity
  - Primary operative techniques
  - Technical expertise/experience
  - Growth
  - Timing of repair.
- Cut as you go.
- Prevention, prevention, prevention.

 Access the Historical Perspective section online at
http://www.expertconsult.com

Introduction

The etiology of secondary cleft deformities is multifactorial. The most influential factors leading to the development of a secondary deformity are the type and severity of the cleft, as well as the primary repair technique. Poor preoperative analysis and choice of technique will always lead to a secondary deformity. Matching the deformity to procedure takes a great deal of experience and flexibility by the surgeon. This experience and level of attention to detail can greatly affect results and the need for secondary correction. Tips and tricks learned by a single surgeon over a lifetime of performing cleft surgery can never truly be conveyed verbally or on paper. Lastly, because essentially all patients are operated on within the first year of life, the long period of dramatic growth and the resultant scar after the repair of the cleft structures both profoundly affect the end result. Delaying the definitive repair until a child has reached adolescence or adulthood may minimize the bony growth disturbance; however, early repair of the cleft deformity is mandatory for functional development and psychosocial benefit. Unrestrained growth of the cleft margins may result in even more severe secondary deformities, as the

repaired structures guide growth in an anatomic fashion. It is ideal to allow the facial structures to develop in a normal relationship to one another in the intended "functional matrix." Interestingly, this debate may become less important, as we learn more about whether these growth disturbances actually result from surgical insult or are simply sequelae of an intrinsic bony genetic defect. Correction of the unilateral cleft lip deformity was once thought to restrict the growth of the midface; however, based upon more recent animal studies, the hypoplasia may be secondary to an intrinsic growth deficit.[1–3]

Secondary procedures are, in many ways, more difficult than primary repairs. This is why preventing secondary deformities is of the utmost importance. Unlike the relatively uniform nature of the initial deformity, secondary problems are widely varied in both their appearance and etiology. Additionally, secondary procedures, by definition, involve previously operated on and heavily scarred tissue. Consequently, learning the techniques described in this chapter, while avoiding a "cookie-cutter" approach by intraoperatively tailoring the procedure to correct the defect uncovered after scar release, both allow the surgeon to express creativity and ultimately yields the best results. Even in the best of hands, the initial insult to the tissue can forever contribute to secondary deformities.

Basic science/disease process

Wound healing and growth

Secondary deformities occur for a number of reasons, including scarring, physical growth, and in some cases, technical error with the primary repair. Scarring affects individuals to varying degrees, and whether related to genetics or ethnic heritage, it can have profound results on aesthetic outcomes. The scar contraction can distort the fragile anatomic landmarks of the lip and nose, while excess scar tissue deposition can lead to unsightly irregularities in contour and color.

Additionally, physical growth is often referred to as the "fourth dimension" in cleft lip and palate surgery. The growth of the osseocartilaginous skeleton and soft tissues of the face is difficult to predict, and can very visibly affect outcomes. The original cleft lip surgery occurs months after birth with careful approximation and alignment of landmarks and facial structures in three dimensions; however, the human face undergoes rapid periods of growth from birth to 5 years of age and also during puberty, with final osseocartilaginous facial growth in normal children ending with the cessation of puberty. The subsequent changes in aesthetic outcomes that this "fourth dimension" will have are difficult to predict. Finally, technical error or poor technique selection can play a role in outcomes. Together, these factors allow secondary deformities of the cleft lip and palate to be the rule, and not the exception *(Figs 29.1, 29.2)*.

Diagnosis/patient presentation

Secondary deformity management is an integral part of treating the cleft lip and/or palate deformity. Patients with cleft lip and palate will undergo, on average, at least one nose and lip revision when followed into adolescence, with a significant number of individuals requiring multiple interventions.[4–6]

The reported incidence rates of palatal fistulas have varied greatly, with citations ranging from 0 to 76%; however, caution should be used when interpreting this data as definitions vary and asymptomatic fistulas are often excluded. Interestingly, over the past 5 years, reported palatal fistula rates have decreased. Using a variety of surgical techniques, authors report fistula rates between 0 and 12.9%, with 0–8.1% being symptomatic.[7–19]

Several studies have looked at the rates of fistula formation, and several strong factors have been identified. Studies have repeatedly demonstrated that surgeon experience is a major predictor of postoperative fistula rates.[7,20,21] Murthy *et al.* reviewed one surgeon's lifetime experience and noted that over 80% of his palatal fistulas occurred in the first 10 years of practice.[7] Additionally, Cohen *et al.* reported on three independently functioning surgeons: two had performed over 45 cleft palate repairs each and had fistula rates of 15% and 18%, while the third surgeon performed only 19 cleft palate repairs, and reported fistula rates of 63%.[21]

Studies have also demonstrated that the width of the initial palatal defect, the width of the palatal shelves, and ratio of the cleft width to the posterior arch width were significant predictors of palatal fistulas postoperatively.[21] Finally, other risk factors continue to be debated, including initial Veau classification of the defect, type of closure, age at repair, and gender.

Fistulas, regardless of size, represent a complex problem, as they are indicative of a significant scarring along a tense palatal closure. This is demonstrated by relatively high recurrence rates reported historically following fistula repair (25–100%)[11,21,22–31]; however, more recent data have demonstrated that fistula recurrence rates of 0–25%[7,11,23–25] are now being achieved.

Underlying each cleft lip and/or palate is a variable degree of skeletal deformity and hypoplasia. In a portion of these cases, the deficiency is mild and can be treated with orthodontics alone. On the other hand, for unilateral clefts, the reported incidence of orthognathic surgery varies between 26% and 48.5%, and for bilateral clefts is 24–76.5%.[21,26,27] The need ultimately varies based on threshold for performing orthognathic surgery.

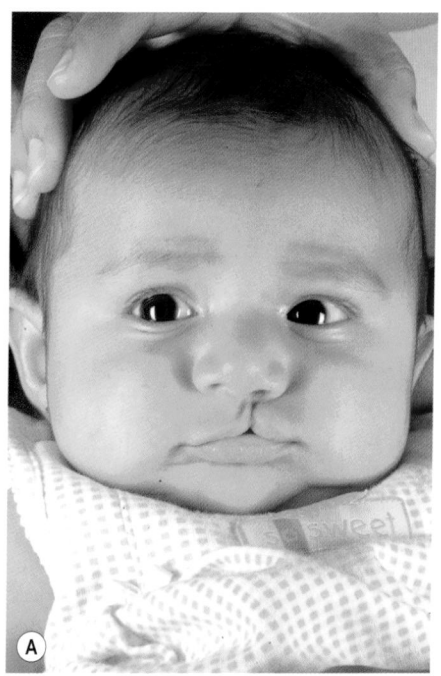 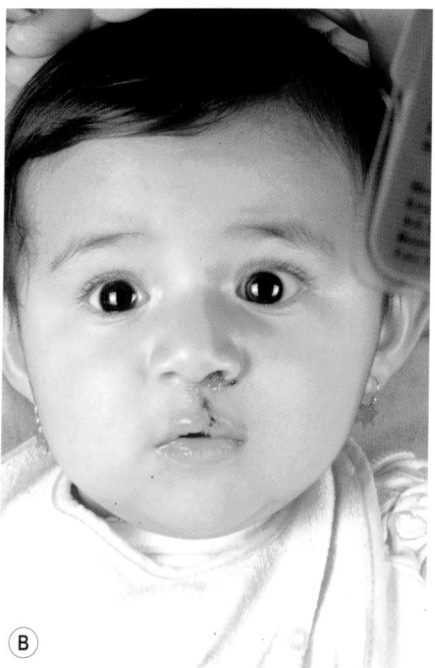 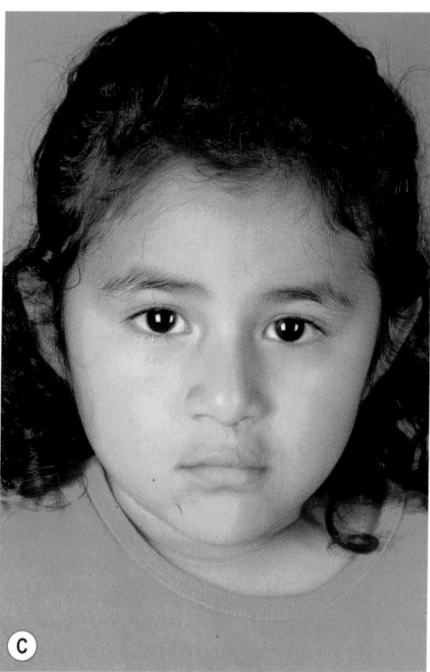

Fig. 29.1 (A–C) Even with perfect surgical technique, postoperative scarring and inflammation vary, resulting in a broad spectrum of secondary deformities.

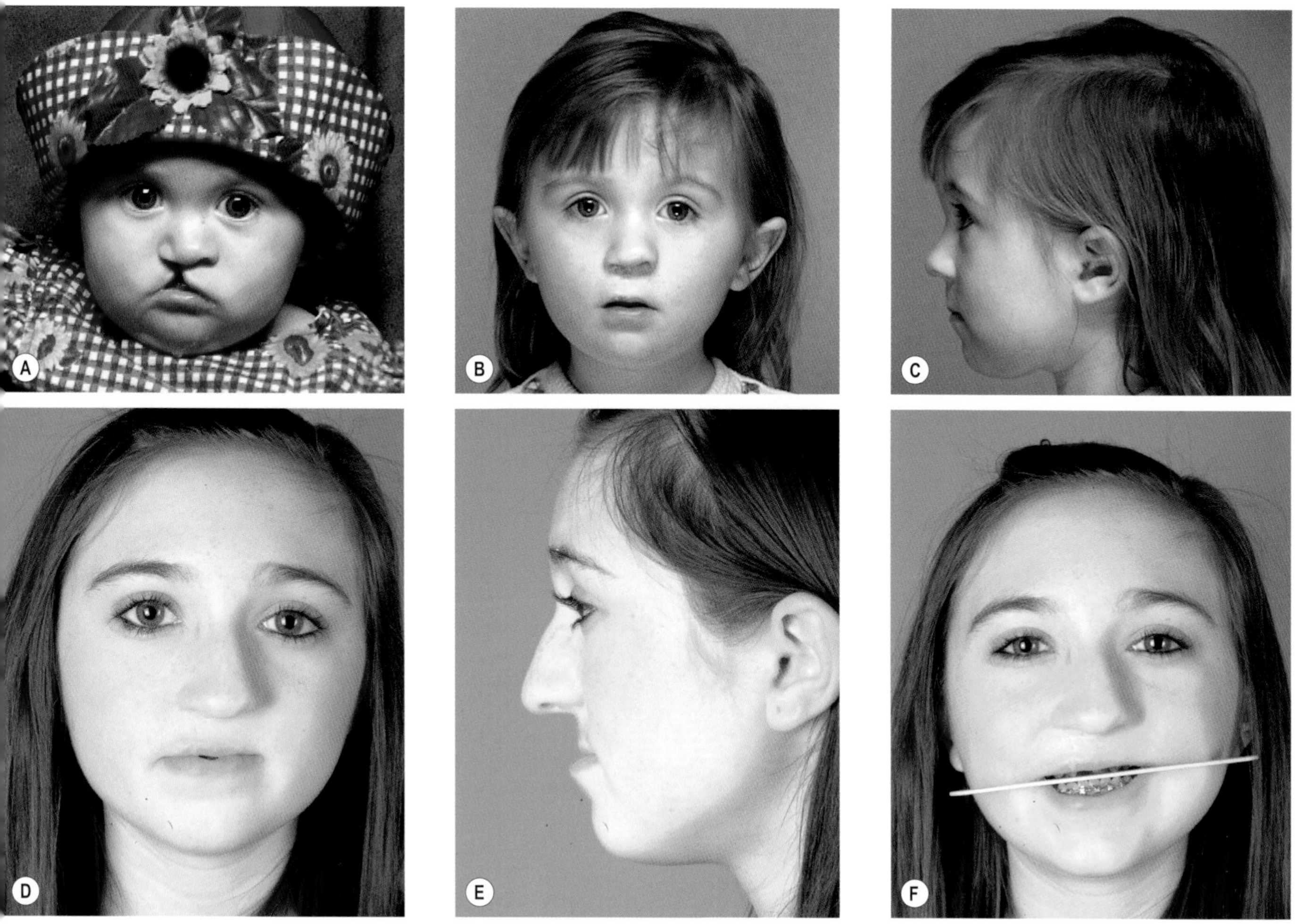

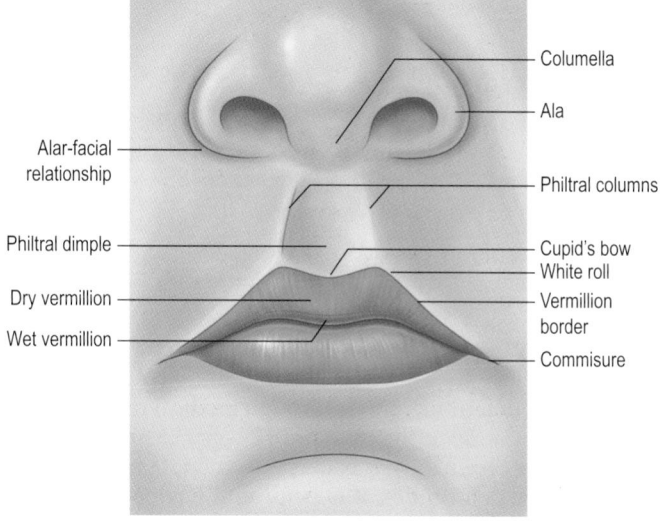

Fig. 29.2 (A–F) Beautiful early results can be drastically altered by abnormal and hypoplastic growth of the midface.

Cleft lip

Normal lip anatomy

The lips' surface can be divided into three portions: cutaneous, dry vermillion, and wet vermillion *(Fig. 29.3)*. Immediately underlying these superficial layers is a thin layer of connective tissue and fat, followed by a group of muscles which give the upper lip many of its structural and functional features *(Fig. 29.4)*. Other important aesthetic features include the contour and volume of the lips, provided by soft-tissue bulk and configuration.[28–31] Finally, the upper gingivobuccal sulcus plays an important role in the appearance and movement of the lip with animation.

Cleft lip anatomy

In the cleft lip, the anatomy is both disrupted and diminutive.[32] In general, the changes can be understood by dividing the discussion into the topics of: landmarks (philtral columns, white roll, cupid's bow), vermillion, and muscular continuity *(Fig. 29.5)*.

Fig. 29.3 Normal lip landmarks and features.

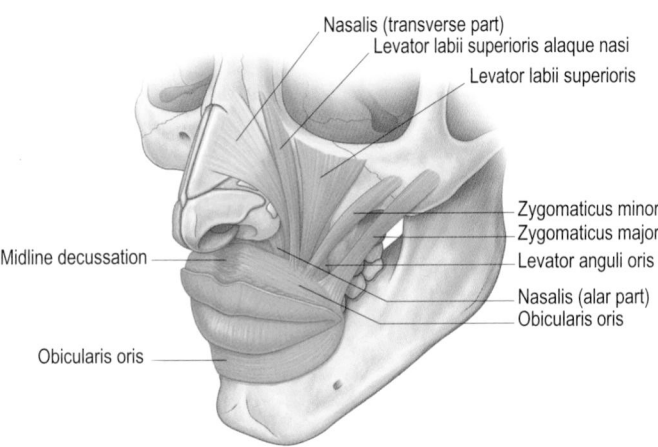

Nasalis (transverse part)
Levator labii superioris alaque nasi
Levator labii superioris
Zygomaticus minor
Zygomaticus major
Levator anguli oris
Nasalis (alar part)
Obicularis oris
Midline decussation
Obicularis oris

Fig. 29.4 The lip and nose are surrounded by a host of musculature that plays a role in its structure and function, and must be taken into consideration when correcting the cleft nose deformity.

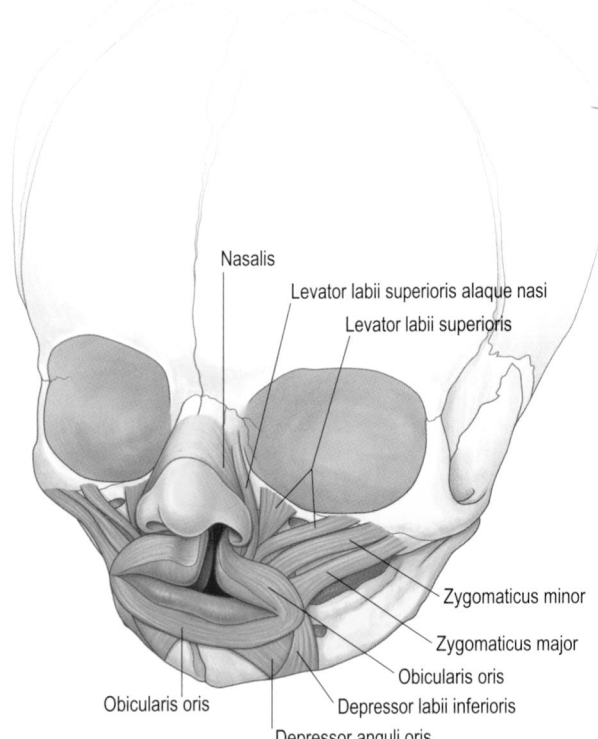

Nasalis
Levator labii superioris alaque nasi
Levator labii superioris
Zygomaticus minor
Zygomaticus major
Obicularis oris
Obicularis oris
Depressor labii inferioris
Depressor anguli oris

Fig. 29.5 Cleft anatomy and abnormal muscle insertions.

Evaluation

It is useful to determine, either through medical records and/or clinical assessment, the type of primary repair and if any secondary procedures have been performed. When evaluating secondary deformities, it is helpful to have a conceptual framework in place to evaluate the lip in a systematic matter. Objective methods have been described to evaluate secondary

deformities[33,34]; however, in day-to-day practice, these can be quite cumbersome. It helps, though, to take the essential elements from these to categorize deformities into five broad areas: scarring, lip, vermillion, muscle, and buccal sulcus.

Scarring should be evaluated for signs of immaturity (redness, firmness), contour changes, and for distortion of local structures. The degree and stage of scarring will dictate an early versus late intervention. Severe and worsening scarring may require an acute intervention (steroid injections), while stable or improving scars are best handled with close monitoring until full maturation.

Lip deformities include abnormal dimensions or landmark distortions of the philtral columns, cupid's bow, and lateral lip segments. The deformities include a short lip (philtral column on the cleft side is vertically shorter than the noncleft side), a long lip (philtral column on cleft side is vertically longer than the noncleft side), tight upper lip (decreased width between cupid's bow peaks and/or disparity in anteroposterior projection of the upper lip in relation to lower lip), wide upper lip (increased horizontal width between cupid's bow peaks), short lateral lip (cleft-side lateral lip segment is horizontally shorter than the lateral lip segment on the normal side), philtral column distortion, and cupid's bow distortion.

Vermillion deformities include thin or thick lip segments, vermillion mismatches (between the wet and dry vermillion), vermillion notching or border malalignment (between the white roll and vermillion), and the whistle deformity (median tubercle paucity resulting in nonapposition of upper and lower lip segments at rest). From a frontal view, the prominence and volume of the median tubercle should also be assessed. From a profile view, the lip should be evaluated for the break seen just above the white roll, as well as the anterior–posterior relationship between the upper and lower lip.

Deformities involving the muscle may result from inadequate muscle reapproximation during the primary repair or subsequent dehiscence. Orbicularis oris muscular dehiscence will present as bulging on either side of the lip repair with animation or a short and widened lip scar. However, since muscle reconstruction has become a standard part of the primary repair, the muscular deformities commonly seen now are more likely a result of inadequate disinsertion of the aberrant muscular attachments. Incomplete dissection of the aberrant attachments leads to more mild deformities, including tethering of the nasal ala, and a subtle relapse to the prior classic cleft appearance. While the orbicularis oris has always received great focus in cleft lip repair, the cleft lip and nose deformity involves a complex network of muscles in the oronasal region. Dissections performed by the authors have demonstrated that the lateral nasalis is also aberrantly inserted in the primary deformity and is often unaddressed during the primary repair. Additionally, the importance of creating a nasal floor and nostril sill during primary repair and subsequent secondary procedures cannot be overemphasized in achieving lasting results and preventing relapse of lateral and elevated alar position.

The buccal sulcus should be examined to determine how free the lip is from the maxilla. The deep aspect of the sulcus should extend up to the region of the columella–lip junction. If the lip is tethered, this can result from scar contracture or from a true paucity of tissue related to the initial deformity.

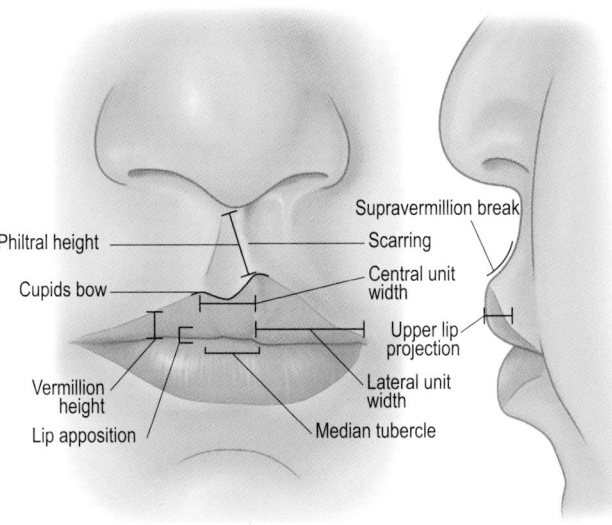

Fig. 29.6 Elements of analysis of secondary cleft lip deformities.

Labels in figure: Supravermillion break, Philtral height, Scarring, Cupids bow, Central unit width, Upper lip projection, Vermillion height, Lateral unit width, Lip apposition, Median tubercle

Any of the previously mentioned deformities can occur concomitantly, and as such, require the surgeon to prioritize treatment based on the importance and realistic potential benefit to the patient. The ultimate goal is a surgical plan that yields the best result, in the fewest number of operations (*Fig. 29.6*).

Patient selection

Timing

Proper intervention focuses on addressing functional impairments, as well as aesthetic deformities that could affect psychosocial development. To do the latter, one must have a solid understanding of how and when psychosocial factors affect outcomes, as well as the normal growth of the face. At about 6 years of age, the risk of teasing by peers increases substantially and may be a source of great distress for the cleft patient and the family. Consequently, all patients should be evaluated for secondary surgery at the age of 4 or 5 before the start of kindergarten. Decisions regarding timing are predicated on the severity of the problem relative to function and appearance, and balanced against both the emotional and physical maturity of the patient. As children progress into adolescence, they become more capable of expressing opinions about appearance, and their wishes should play an increasingly significant role in surgical decision-making.

Growth plays a role in outcomes, and studies have shown that roughly 87–93% of growth-related changes in labial landmarks occur by age 5.[35] Thereafter, certain growth-related changes are more predictable; however, scarring and other factors continue to affect long-term outcomes.

Scarring

While the corrected cleft lip deformity often looks its best at the first office visit, the process of scar maturation can result in significant color and contour abnormalities, distortion of adjacent mobile landmarks, and shortening of the lip dimensions. While these changes may necessitate a secondary correction, there are actions that can be taken during the healing process to minimize the severity of its sequelae. Parents should be advised to massage the scar with the lotion of their choice (vitamin E, cocoa butter, zinc, or Mederma), and utilize sun protection for at least 1 year to prevent persistent hyperpigmentation. These acute interventions are beneficial, not only for scar improvement, but also psychologically, as they involve the family in the care of the child. While silicone sheeting and hypoallergenic taping may be beneficial in the treatment of scars,[36] they may be difficult to maintain on the upper lip of a child and therefore yield varying results. Intralesional steroid injections may be started if there is evidence of hypertrophic or keloid scarring, or if the patient is at high risk for either of these. If the scar continues to be problematic after optimal conservative care, and a minimum of 12–18 months has been allowed for scar maturation, consideration should be given to a surgical revision.

Several surgical options exist for the treatment of secondary cleft lip scarring. The appropriate treatment selection should take into consideration the characteristics of the scar. Dermabrasion is a potential option for scars that are elevated. If scars are hypertrophic and have widened significantly, treatment with excision in the shape of a diamond or ellipse facilitates a straight-line closure. If the scar is depressed or overlies a philtral column a skin-only excision with a vest-over-pants closure (*Fig. 29.7*), or other bulking techniques (see philtral column distortion section, below) will be helpful.

Lip

Short lip

A vertically short lip can be caused by scar contraction, a primary deficiency of prolabial soft tissues, and/or inadequate primary rotation and advancement. A mild degree of shortening is not uncommon after repair because of scar contraction; however, this may improve over time. During the scar maturation process, patients can perform scar management, as discussed previously. If the deformity persists for more than 1 year or after the scar has matured, then consideration should be given to a surgical procedure.

The difference in lip height between normal and repaired sides is precisely measured to determine the amount of lengthening necessary. In patients with minor deformities (<2–3 mm), the shortness may be treated by a diamond-shaped scar excision or a unilimb Z-plasty to lengthen the philtrum; however, for lip shortening greater than 2–3 mm, these techniques may be insufficient. For this degree of lip shortening, one option is to perform a standard Z-plasty to lengthen the philtral column; however, it is important to remember that this technique places additional scars on the upper lip. For more significant degrees of shortening, or if additional scars from a Z-plasty are not preferable, the entire repair should be taken down and repeated (*Fig. 29.8*).

When a short philtral column persists due to underrotation of the flap, it is usually because of minimizing the backcut, and will always lead to vermillion notching and a vertically oriented, noncontinuous white roll. It is recommended to

Video 1

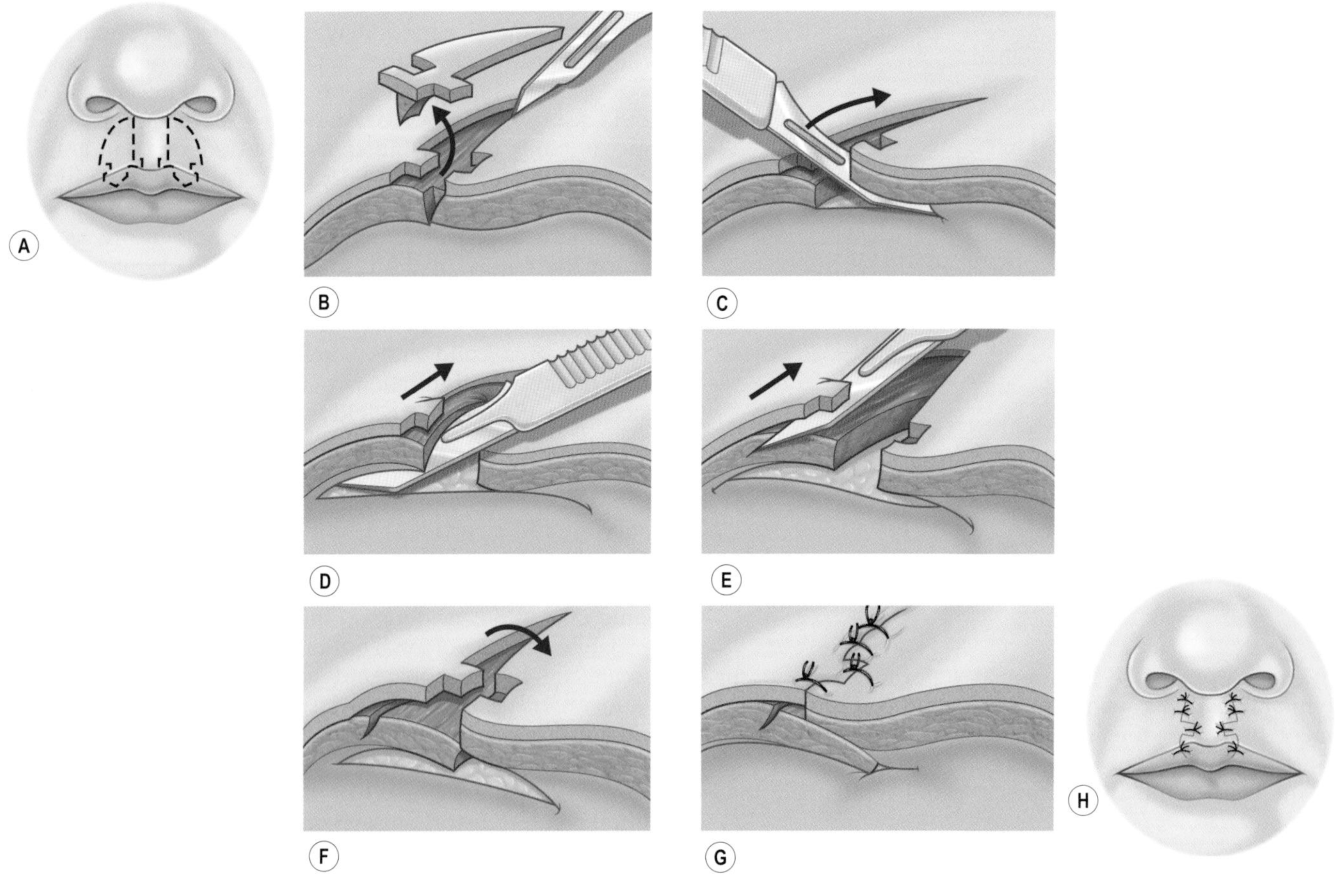

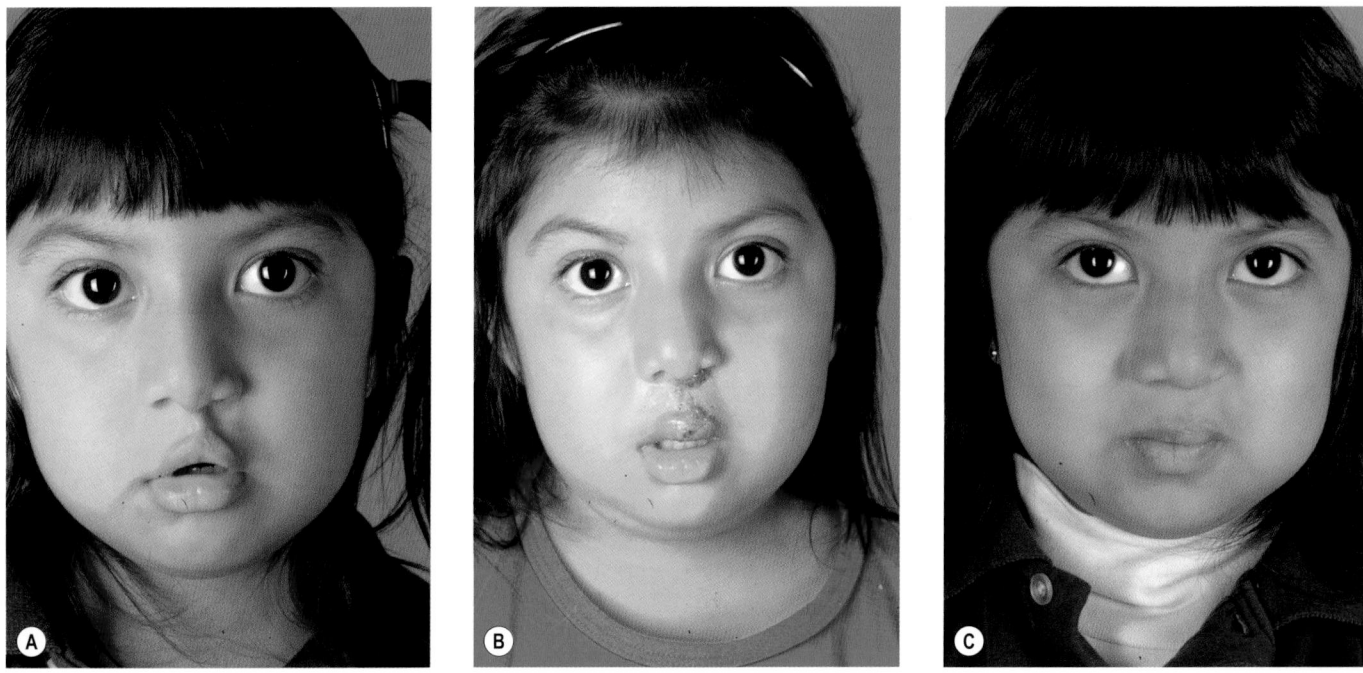

Fig. 29.7 (A–H) Illustration of the vest-over-pants closure, which buries de-epithelialized dermis underneath adjacent epidermis to add regional soft-tissue bulk.

Fig. 29.8 This patient demonstrates a short lip deformity, notched vermillion, and white roll discontinuity secondary to hypertrophic scarring. The patient subsequently underwent complete take-down of the repair, with repeat rotation advancement. **(A)** Preoperative photo; **(B)** 1-week postoperative photo; **(C)** 3–4-month postoperative photo.

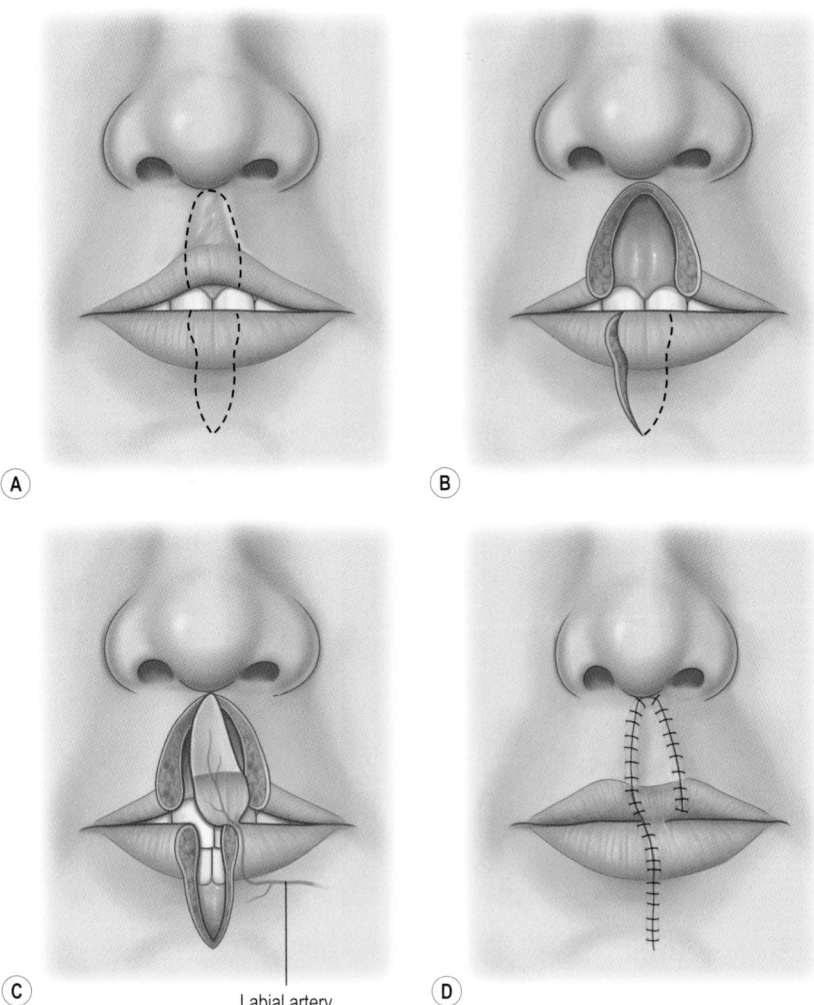

(A)   (B)   (C)   Labial artery   (D)

Fig. 29.9 (A–D) The Abbé flap allows for the transfer of full-thickness lower lip elements to the upper lip in cases of: (1) decreased upper lip anteroposterior projection; (2) excess scarring of the central aesthetic unit; and (3) significantly narrowed or shortened central aesthetic unit.

trade a slightly larger backcut/scar (even onto the columella and back down the normal philtral column) to obtain the necessary rotation.

Long lip

This deformity is rarely seen because of decreasing use of the Tennison repair; however, it can still occur for other reasons, such as overrotation of the medial lip segment. When addressing this deformity, it is tempting simply to excise lip tissue from beneath the alar base in an effort to "hitch up" the elongated cleft side. Experience has demonstrated that this does not yield acceptable results because of the underlying action of the orbicularis and gravity pulling down on the incision. Even suspension with permanent sutures fixed to bone is not always predictable. It is more preferable to take down the entire repair and excise tissue in all dimensions to correct the deformity.

Tight lip

Options for management of the horizontally tight lip deformity include fat injections to the upper lip and reduction of the lower lip through a wedge excision of inner lip tissue,

reducing lip bulk disparity. More significant deformities, however, are best treated with the Abbé flap.

The Abbé flap transfers full-thickness lip elements to the upper lip in a two-stage procedure by transfer of a lower lip segment based on the inferior labial vessels. The pedicled flap is then left in place for 2–3 weeks, before division and inset *(Fig. 29.9)*. While this flap is more commonly used with secondary bilateral cleft lip deformities, it can be used when there is: (1) decreased anteroposterior projection of the upper lip (particularly helpful in reducing the disparity in tissue volume between the upper and lower lip); (2) excess scarring of the central aesthetic unit; and (3) a significantly narrowed or shortened central aesthetic unit. Additionally, the flap provides a pseudodimple for the philtrum, a tuft of hair in males, and continuity of surface landmarks *(Fig. 29.10)*. This procedure, however, should not be the first choice, because of donor site morbidity, increased risk associated with two procedures, and patient discomfort associated with a 2–3-week period of flap delay between stages.

Wide lip

The horizontally wide lip can be caused by a number of factors. It is most frequently seen in bilateral clefts where the

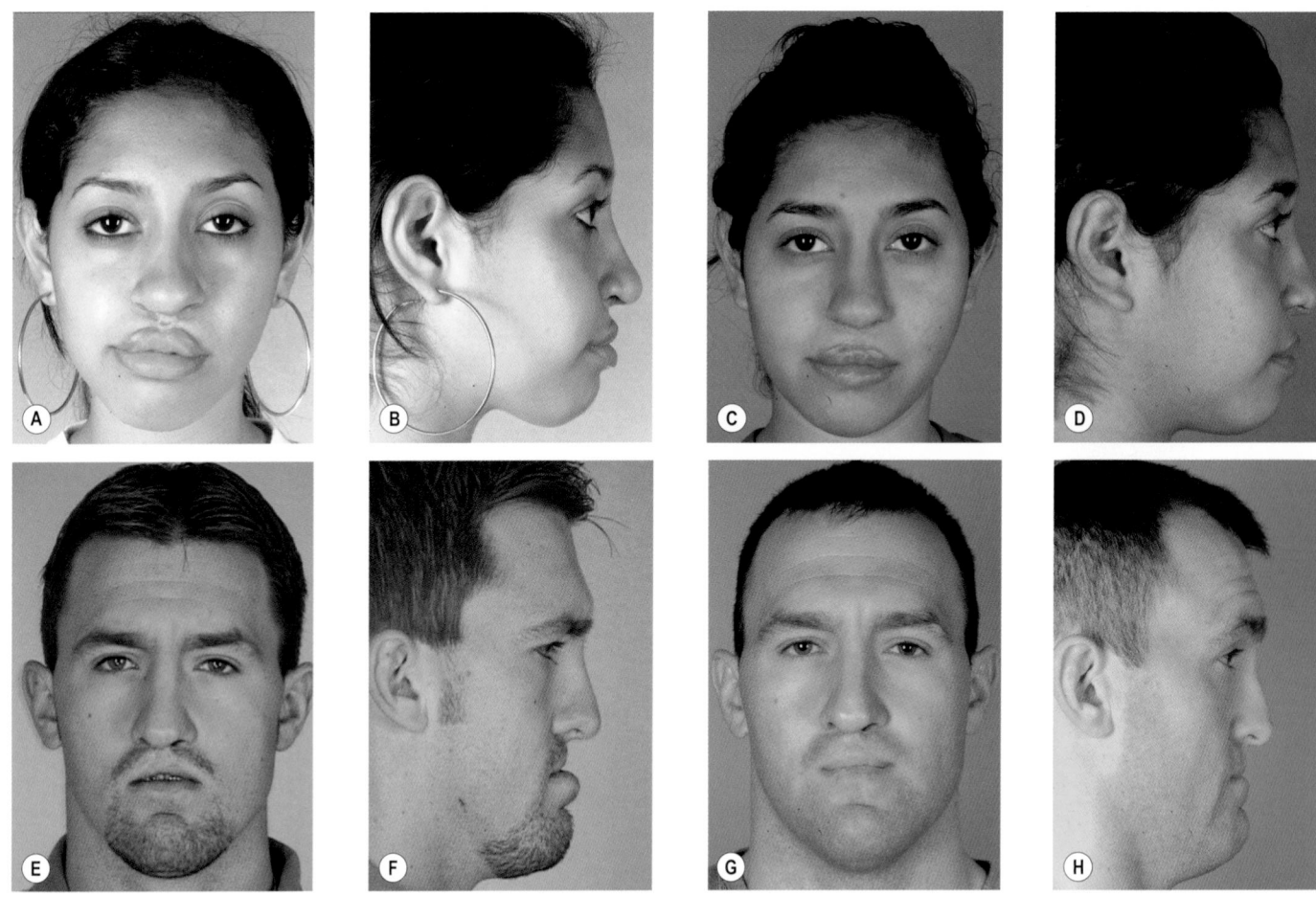

Fig. 29.10 A patient who was born with a bilateral cleft lip deformity **(A, B)** before and **(C, D)** 3 years after Abbé flap to correct a scarred and constricted philtrum and a tight lip. **(E, F)** A bilateral cleft lip patient with a short lip bilaterally accompanied by a paucity of central vermillion, and a tight upper lip. **(G, H)** Nine-year postoperative results post Abbé flap.

prolabial philtral segment was designed too wide at the time of initial operation. It can also be seen when persistent tension across the neophiltrum, secondary to a protruding maxilla or underlying orbicularis muscle function causes horizontal expansion of the prolabial soft tissue. The solution is excision of the excess philtral tissue, taking care to remember the tenets of lip surgery: meticulous approximation of the orbicularis oris and accurate approximation of philtral landmarks. Regardless of age at the time of the secondary procedures, the philtrum should be made smaller than the final desired size in anticipation of subsequent stretching.

Short lateral lip

A decrease in the horizontal width of the lateral upper lip segment is a common deformity, resulting from the need to achieve an optimal cupid's bow. This decrease in width of the lateral lip segment results after excision of its diminutive medial portion. Traditionally, the short lateral lip segment has been said to "stretch"; however, in our experience, this is not the case. Ultimately, though, intact central landmarks and good lip contour are more important than symmetry of the lateral lip segment.

Philtral column distortion

The philtral column can be affected by excessive scarring, short length, or a lack of prominence. In the case of excess scarring, the methods described in the section on scarring, above, can improve aesthetic outcomes. Shortened philtral columns can be addressed using methods described in the section on vermillion notching, below. Methods to recreate the philtral column, in general, involve either the addition or overlapping of soft tissue to add soft-tissue elevation. Fat grafts (free or dermal) have been used by some to augment the philtral column *(Fig. 29.11)*, and a "vest-over-pants" closure is an option to create the philtral column using local tissues. The latter method involves excision of the prior scar, with subsequent burial of the underlying dermis underneath the adjacent dermis to provide the bulk for the philtral column. Additional methods have been described, including using mattress sutures to reapproximate and evert the orbicularis, as well as vertical interdigitation of the orbicularis.[37]

Key principles of any procedures involving the region of the philtral columns include limited subcutaneous undermining, enough to allow a layered closure, and concomitantly releasing dermal orbicularis oris attachments that would

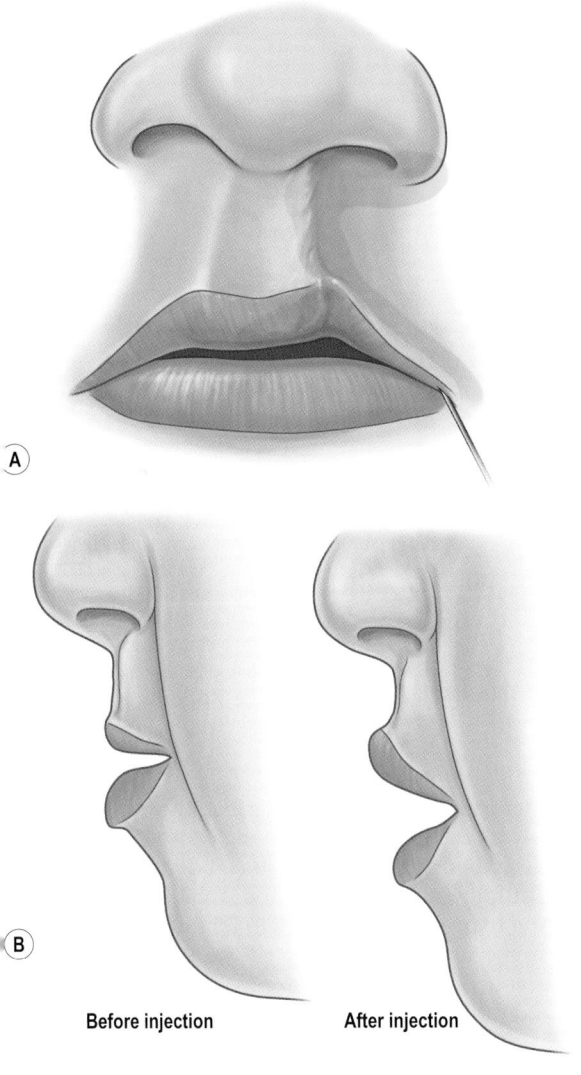

Before injection   **After injection**

Fig. 29.11 (A, B) These images demonstrate the concept behind free fat injections. Free fat is injected into a stab incision made near the oral commissure, and tunneled into the upper lip.

place additional tension on the wound. Care should be taken, however, to limit subcutaneous undermining to less than 5 mm, and not to cross the contralateral philtral column or central philtral dimple, thereby preventing landmark distortion and/or vascular compromise.

Cupid's bow distortion

Significant abnormalities of the cupid's bow in unilateral cleft lip deformities are usually the result of misalignment or notching, and can be corrected by local tissue rearrangement techniques, such as diamond excisions and Z-plasties. With more severe or complicated distortions, it may be necessary to take down the previous lip repair and to repeat rotation advancement. When there is a paucity of healthy and unscarred tissue for reconstruction, as seen after bilateral cleft lip repair, full-thickness lip elements can be acquired from the lower lip via the Abbé flap.

Vermillion

Thin lip

The goals for treating a thin lip deformity are to increase the amount of vermillion show, improve anteroposterior projection of the upper lip, and replace contour landmarks (the break point existing 3–4 mm above the upper lip vermillion and the prominent median tubercle). These goals are even more important in the female population, as increased vermillion show and volume are associated with increased attractiveness.[29,30] In cases of patients with adequate vermillion but a paucity of volume, fat grafting becomes an excellent option. This can be performed with either free fat injections or via a dermal fat graft.

Free fat grafting can be performed by harvesting adipose tissue from the lateral thigh or the periumbilical region, processing the fat, and subsequently injecting this into the upper lip via small stab incisions, just medial to the oral commissures *(Figs 29.11* and *29.12)*. In addition to increasing volume, there is much recent interest and reports of fat grafting improving the quality and color of overlying skin in scarred or radiated beds. While the procedure is simple in nature, it can become difficult if there is a significant amount of scar, making tunneling and multiple small-volume passes difficult. The authors have had more success fat grafting unscarred beds, as expanding the contracted, tight scar is quite challenging even with repeated injections.

Dermal fat grafts are composite grafts of dermis and subcutaneous fat that can be harvested and inserted *en bloc* via an intraoral incision into the upper lip. With the rapidly increasing success and interest in free fat grafting, the use of dermal fat grafts has dramatically decreased.

Bilateral clefts often have greater tissue deficiency than unilateral clefts, and subsequently have a greater risk of secondary deformity. Although local tissue rearrangement, as described before, may suffice for minor cases of vermillion deficiency, the deficiency in bilateral cleft lips is often more severe, requiring soft tissue that the adjacent areas cannot provide. These situations are best treated with an Abbé flap.

Video 2

Thick lip

A thick lip can be secondary to inadequate rotation advancement during the primary repair, excesses of tissue, or from inadequate depth of the gingivobuccal sulcus. If the thick lip results from a relative excess adjacent to an area of relative paucity, as is often seen with inadequate advancement rotation following the initial repair (festoons), the lateral lip element should be redistributed or readvanced to reduce the disparity. If the thick lip exists alone, then this can be treated with direct excision, via an incision on the inner aspect of the lip. Failure to create the gingivobuccal sulcus during primary repair can lead to inadequate suspension and a thick lip appearance, which can be corrected by recreation and deepening of the sulcus.

Video 3

Vermillion mismatch

The abnormal exposure and show of wet vermillion can be aesthetically and functionally displeasing, as the miscolored tissue is visibly apparent, and tends to become dry and

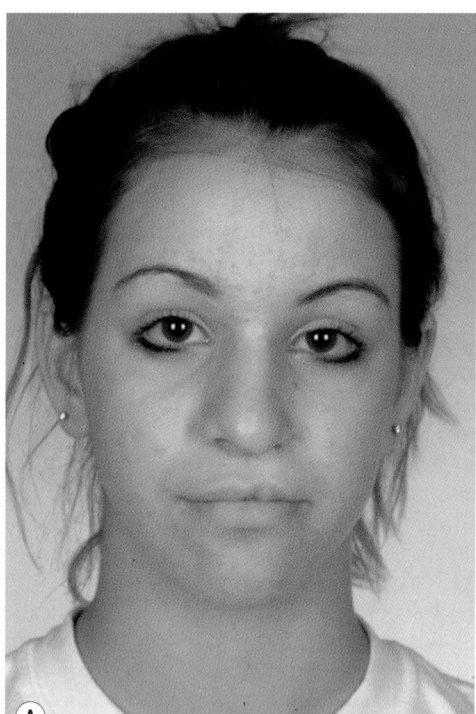

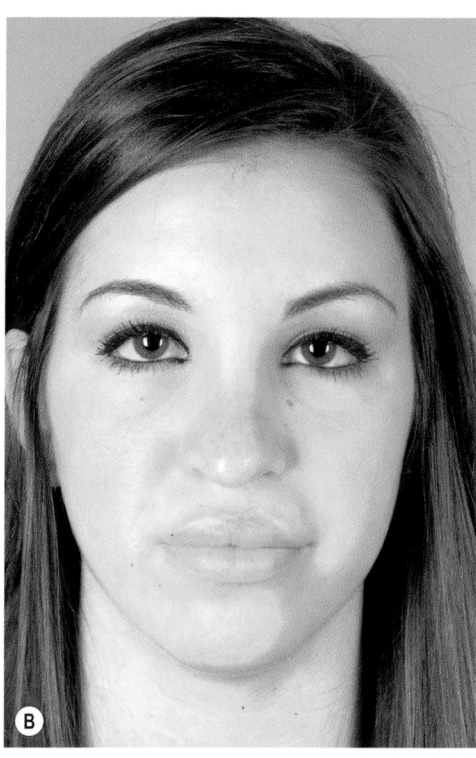

Fig. 29.12 (A, B) This patient has a preoperative paucity of vermillion centrally, as well as a thin lateral lip. After fat injections to the upper lip, the patient now has increased vermillion show and upper lip fullness. Fat grafting is a potent method to achieve these aesthetic outcomes, especially within the female population.

chapped very easily. If the color mismatch involves the median tubercle and adjacent structures, then excision of mucosa with subsequent medialization of adjacent, bilateral, undermined vermillion flaps can be used to close the defect, taking care to realign the wet–dry vermillion border. If the vermillion mismatch involves just the central tubercle and there is an adjacent lateral excess of vermillion, the wet and dry vermillion of the lateral elements can be used to recreate the central tubercle after it is excised.[38] Prevention, however, is the best treatment. Marking the wet–dry vermillion junction during primary repair, designing a triangle of dry vermillion on the lateral lip segment, and creating a half Z-plasty closure to supplement the medial lip segment deficient dry vermillion helps avoid the need for revision.

Vermillion notching/vermillion border malalignment

The etiology and treatment of vermillion notching or border malalignment are similar to the management of the short-lip/philtral deformity. Scar management, diamond excisions, Z-plasties, as well as local tissue rearrangement techniques (backcuts, M-plasties, V-Y advancements), should be used as necessary to correct any mild vermillion border malalignment. For more significant notching, the entire repair should be taken down and repeated.

Whistle deformity

The whistle deformity can occur secondary to scar contracture across the vermillion, failure to fill the central tubercle with lateral vermillion tissue, diastasis of the orbicularis muscle at the base of the nose (resulting in an upward pull on the central tissue), or a combination of these.[39] Many techniques to correct

the whistle deformity have been described, but the choice of repair should be based on the underlying cause. Methods that have been described include using local advancement flaps, fat grafting, autologous grafts, and the Abbé flap.

Local tissue rearrangement can help if a maldistribution of vermillion is the underlying cause. If the central deficiency occurs with concomitant lateral excess, then procedures to reposition and reorient the lateral tissue as advancement flaps should be undertaken.[40] Local options have classically involved V-Y advancements and Kapetansky's pendulum flaps. However, in the authors' opinion, this frequently results in a significant amount of scarring that can give the lip an unnatural feel and appearance with animation.

If there is not a disparity in vermillion bulk between the lip segments and adequate amounts of vermillion are present, this region may be augmented using free fat grafting.[41] Additionally, other fillers and autologous materials (palmaris longus grafts, temporoparietal fascial grafts, dermal fat grafts) have been used to augment the upper lip.

If the central tubercle vermillion bulk is deficient and there is no locally available tissue, consideration should be given to an Abbé flap – the workhorse for significant deformities. Lastly, the tongue flap can provide additional "nonlike" tissue to replace vermillion, and therefore is a last resort. With all interventions, care should be taken to place incisions that cross the wet–dry vermillion border as Z-plasties, W-plasties, or a lazy-S, to prevent future scar contracture. Ultimately, all possible causes of a whistle deformity must be addressed both to repair the deformity and to prevent its recurrence.

Orbicularis muscle deformities

Continuity of the orbicularis muscle is an important component in the appearance and function of the normal lip. Cleft lip defects involve a discontinuous orbicularis sphincter with the muscle aberrantly inserting into the cleft margins, columellar base, alar rim, and periosteum of the pyriform aperture. Failure to reconstruct the orbicularis adequately during the initial repair results in continued attachments to the alar base or columella, and this will cause worsening of the associated nasal deformity. After cleft lip repair, the muscle in continuity exerts pressure on the palatal shelves and premaxillary segment, bringing them together and directing them posteriorly. This provides an anatomic platform for the nose as well as support for the subcutaneous and dermal structures, preventing relapse or collapse into the bony cleft during scarring.

If the orbicularis is discontinuous, its repair must be incorporated into the secondary operation. This generally involves reopening the repair, dissecting the orbicularis from the overlying skin for several millimeters in the subdermal plane, and subsequent suture reapproximation. In the unilateral deformity, care should be taken not to dissect the orbicularis beyond the midportion of the philtrum, or the normal philtral dimple may be distorted. For optimal results, the surgeon must ensure that the orbicularis and nasalis musculature have been completely and widely taken down from the abnormal insertion points.

Buccal sulcus deformities

In general, deformities involving the superior gingivobuccal sulcus can be due to either an excess or deficit of tissue. If the problem is an excess of tissue, one can simply excise the excess and retack the mucosa to the nasal spine or the periosteum in the region of the columellar–lip junction. Deficiencies of the labial sulcus are most common after bilateral cleft lip repair and often reflect the underlying anatomy of the deformity rather than poor technique in the initial repair. Many techniques to bring in additional tissue to reconstruct the sulcus have been described, including local flaps, mucosal grafts, and split-thickness and full-thickness skin grafts. A common method uses a mucosal upper lip flap based inferiorly and extending into the upper lip. The prolabium is then dissected free off the premaxilla, and the flap is rotated into the columellar–lip junction region. Closure of the upper lip mucosa defect is then accomplished by approximating laterally based flaps of wet vermillion.[42] When the labial vermillion is insufficient, and other local rearrangement options are not possible, the best solution is a release of the sulcus and closure of the defect with grafting (*Fig. 29.13*). Buccal mucosa is the first choice for graft material, and a dental amalgam should be used as a stent to maximize graft take.

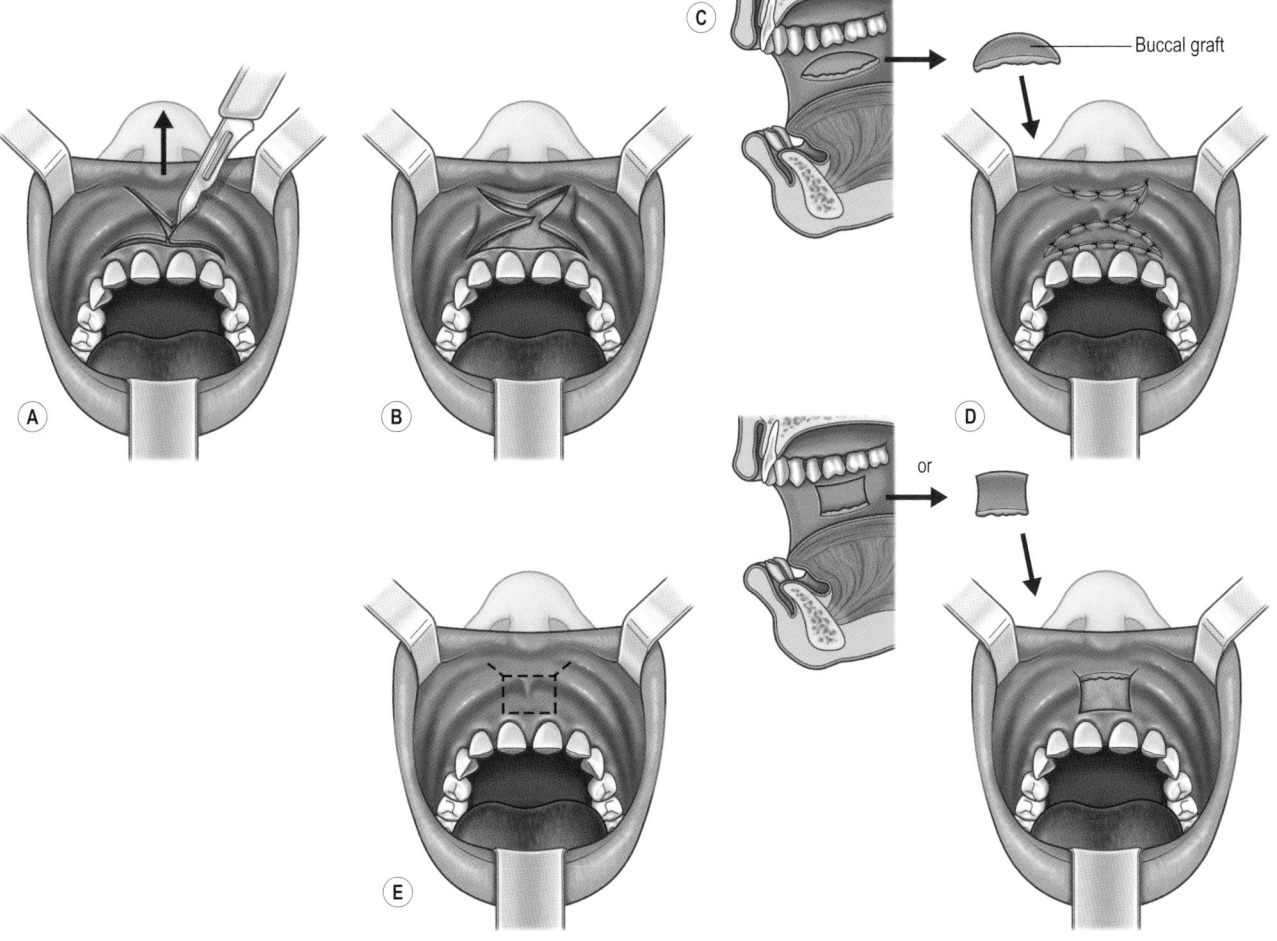

Fig. 29.13 (A–E) When there is a paucity of vermillion or gingival tissue for reconstruction of the superior buccal sulcus, recreation of the defect with grafts (buccal, split-thickness or full-thickness skin) is the next option.

Split-thickness and full-thickness skin grafts are distant options because of postoperative contraction and bulk, respectively.

Cleft palate

Evaluation

Palatal fistulas are significant complications seen after cleft palate repair. They vary in their clinical presentation, from asymptomatic to symptomatic (nasal air emission, hypernasal speech, and nasal regurgitation of fluid and food). Symptomatic fistulas are bothersome, as food within the fistula presents a hygiene problem as well as a potential source of infection. Semisolid foods tend to cause more problems than solids do. Interestingly, studies have not shown a significant association between the size of the fistula and clinical severity.[7,22]

Smith *et al.* introduced the Pittsburgh Classification Scheme[43] to categorize this complication based on anatomic location and recommended using a "+" sign to designate whether or not the fistula was symptomatic (*Table 29.1*). It is important to note that type VI and VII fistulas are a normal finding in certain clinical situations, and a type I fistula is of no perceivable clinical consequence.

Evaluation of secondary palatal deformities requires assessing both structure and function. Patients and/or families should be questioned regarding nasal regurgitation of food or liquid, a malodorous nasal smell, recurrent sinus infections, and hypernasal speech. The patient's palate should also be evaluated using a tongue blade and light source for complete exam of the hard and soft palates.

Patient selection

Timing

Symptomatic fistulas usually require surgical repair. If other procedures are planned, then asymptomatic fistulas can be addressed at that time.

Table 29.1 **The Pittsburgh fistula classification system**

Fistula type	Location
I	Uvula/bifid uvula
II	Soft palate
III	Soft–hard palate junction
IV	Hard palate
V	Incisive foramen
VI	Lingual-alveolar
VII	Labial-alveolar

In 2007, Smith et al. described a classification system for the standardized description of palatal fistulas, the Pittsburgh fistula classification system.[43] The "+" sign can be used to designate whether or not a fistula is symptomatic. It is important to note that fistula types VI and VII are a normal finding in certain clinical situations, type I fistulas are of no perceivable clinical consequence, and type V fistulas are for use with bilateral cleft lip and palates or Veau type IV clefts.

Treatment/surgical technique

The proper treatment of palatal fistulas requires an understanding of simple principles, and knowledge of the available treatment options, including local random flaps, local axial flaps, microvascular free tissue transfer, as well as the use of allograft.

Closure of the fistula should be performed in a two-layered fashion, forming a nasal and oral layer. These layers are usually formed by utilizing local random-pattern flaps from adjacent tissue. However, as the surrounding tissues are often scarred and tenuous, this can be difficult or may result in a repair that is prone to recurrence.

Nasal layer closure can be accomplished with turnover flaps from the mucosa lining the fistula. If this is inadequate, additional tissue can be retrieved from mucoperiosteal vomer flaps, or from mucosa off the posterior pharyngeal wall (for posterior fistulas). This last option is also valuable in individuals with underlying problems with velopharyngeal insufficiency, as this provides both a nasal layer and reduces the size of the velopharyngeal aperture.

Closure of the oral layer can be accomplished using local palatal mucoperiosteum; however, several key points are worth noting. First, flaps may be designed unilaterally or bilaterally, and may be elevated in either unipedicle or bipedicle fashion (based off the posterior greater palatine artery with or without the anterior incisive pedicle) (*Fig. 29.14*). Next, when closing the oral layer with local or adjacent tissue, it is critical to design these flaps to be much larger than the defect, as the scarred palatal mucosa is inelastic and often covers less of an area than it appears to when the flap is designed. As with all procedures, there should be minimal tension on these flaps at the time of closure. If there is a significant amount of tension on the repair, it may be helpful to osteotomize the greater palatine foramen to allow advancement of the neurovascular pedicle tethering the flap. Additionally, islandization of hemipalatal flaps can be performed to release additional tension.[1] Finally, one should avoid overlapping the nasal and oral layer suture lines, decreasing the chance that wound dehiscence will result in continuity between the oral and nasal cavity.

More recently, the use of biomaterials has been associated with a decrease in recurrence rates. Kirschner *et al.* used acellular dermis (Alloderm) to augment palatal fistula repair by sandwiching a thin sheet between the recreated nasal and oral mucosa layers (*Fig. 29.15*).[44] Losee *et al.* published their experiences with acellular dermal matrix and found that its use resulted in fistula recurrence rates of 10.9%, of which only one-third were symptomatic.[11] Despite these advances, there are still situations in which a tension-free repair is not possible with palatal tissue. In these situations, regional axial pattern flaps offer a viable option for the treatment of palatal fistulas.

There are three intraoral tissue options for palatal fistula closure: buccal mucosa, the tongue, and the posterior pharyngeal wall. The buccal mucosa and underlying soft tissue offer several options for donor tissue.[45] The buccal myomucosal flap raises mucosa with or without portions of the buccinator muscle and can be used for the reconstruction of either the nasal or oral layers. The flap is raised, leaving buccal fat pad, fascia and parotid duct undisturbed, and is then either rotated into the defect, or tunneled through the soft palate to reach the fistula site. Studies have shown that no major

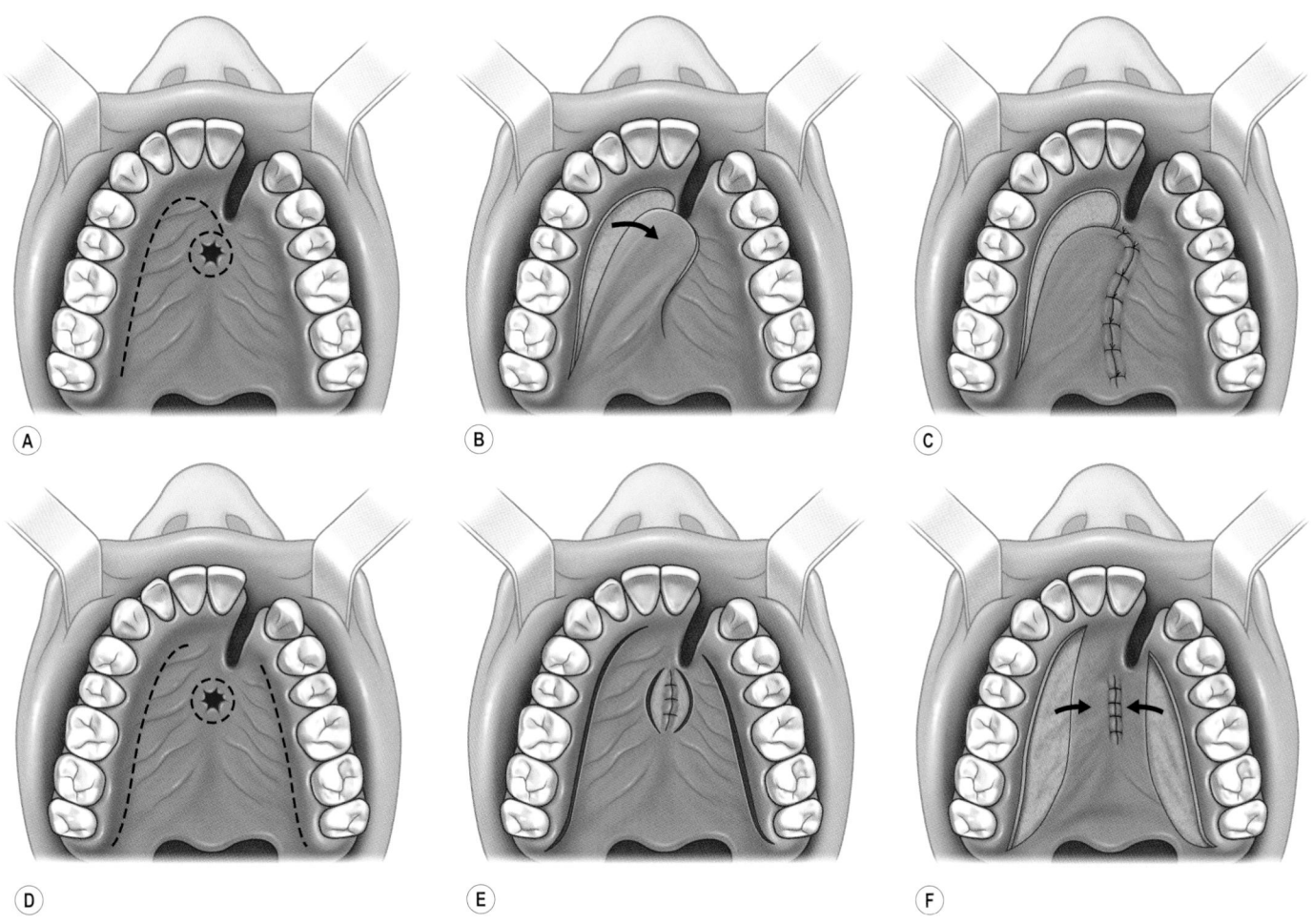

Fig. 29.14 (A–F) The first option for closure of palatal fistulas is local random-pattern tissue, which can be utilized in either a unipedicle or bipedicle fashion. It is important to note, however, that the majority of the peripheral hard palate is granulated mucosa after primary palatoplasty.

complications are shown in the cheek donor area.[46] The flap is limited because of its posteriorly based pedicle, having some difficulty reaching fistulas located in the far anterior portions of the palate.

The buccal tissue can also be harvested based on the facial artery. The facial artery myomucosal (FAMM) flap harvests mucosa, soft tissue, and a small amount of buccinator and orbicularis muscle *(Fig. 29.16)*. This axial flap can be based either superiorly (relying on retrograde flow) or inferiorly (relying on antegrade flow). The superiorly based flaps are primarily used to close defects involving the hard palate and alveolus, while inferiorly based flaps are used to close defects in the posterior hard palate, soft palate, and posterior portions of the alveolus. The flap is advantageous as its design prevents damage to the facial nerve and Stensen's duct. Additionally, because of its robust blood supply, the flap can be designed to be long (length-to-width ratio of 5:1), which subsequently allows the flap to be folded over on to itself and form a two-layered structure for palatal fistula closure. More recently, buccal soft tissues have been used in conjunction with the buccal fat pad to close palatal fistulas; however, long-term data are pending.[47]

For particularly recalcitrant defects, the tongue flap may be a consideration. The tongue has a rich submucous vascular plexus that allows the inclusion of healthy, well-vascularized tissue into the palatal defect. Initially, the flap was raised as a thick and bulky flap, but Assuncao later demonstrated that thin (5 mm at base, and 3 mm distally) flaps could be based anteriorly off the ranine arch, and via a two-stage procedure, could achieve a high rate of success[48] *(Fig. 29.17)*. This choice of reconstruction is suboptimal though in many ways, as the tongue must be tethered to the palate for 2–3 weeks, the texture and color are a poor match, and some data have demonstrated changes in articulation postoperatively.[49]

A more remote option includes the temporoparietal flap, axially based off the deep temporal artery, providing a thin flap with a reliable blood supply. Its use requires dissection of the temporalis, osteotomy of the zygoma, and placement of defect in the lateral maxilla allowing transfer into the defect.[50] The flap has been indicated by Van der Wal and Mulder[50] for large palatal defects in adult patients, as in children it may not be sufficiently developed for transposition. This treatment option is often not used for several reasons, including an extraoral scar, potential for temporal hollowing, osteotomy of the zygoma and maxilla, and possible facial nerve injury. Nonetheless, it remains useful for large, recurrent fistulas in adults after local options have been exhausted.

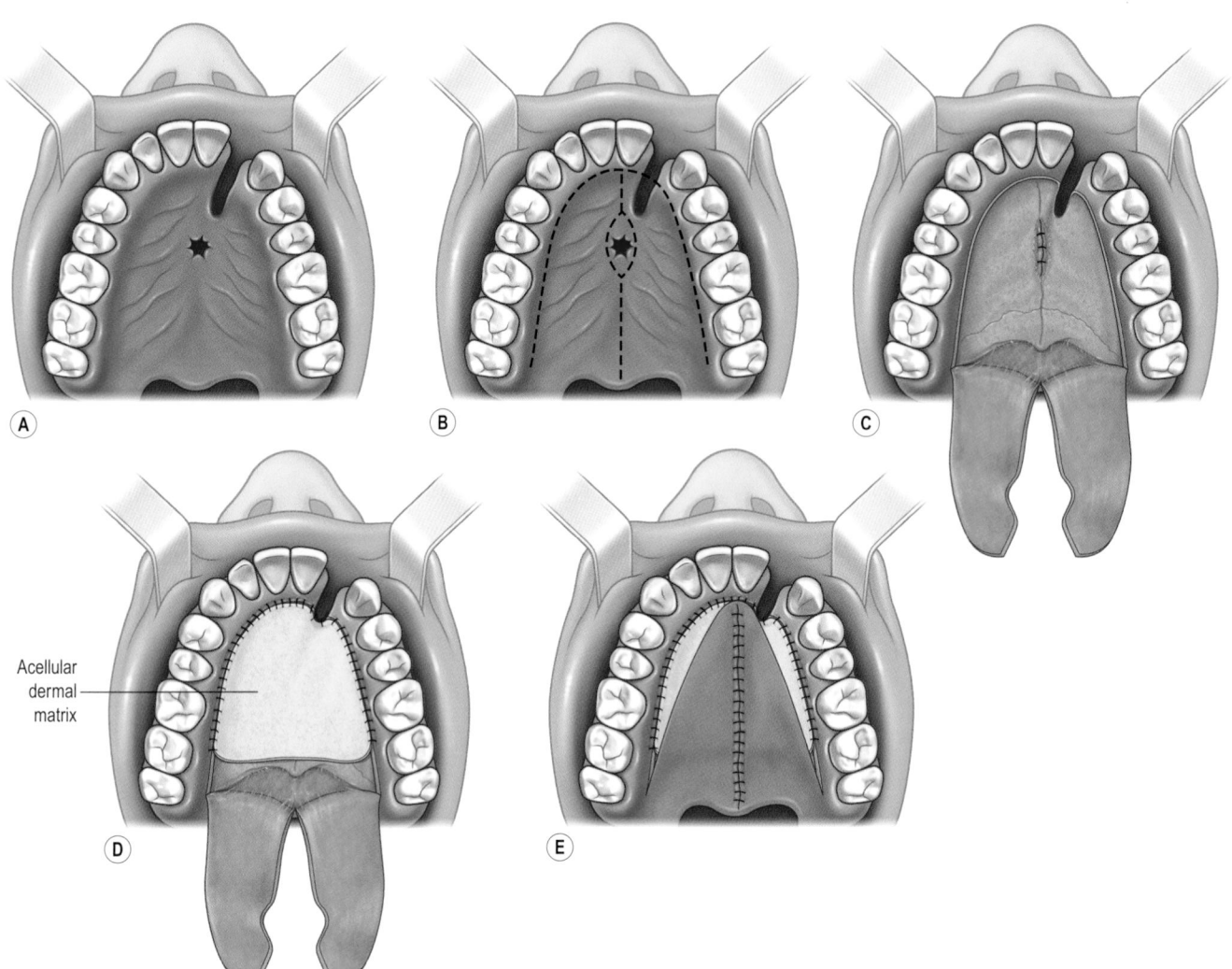

Fig. 29.15 (A–E) Placement of acellular dermal matrix provides a tool to achieve and bolster complete closure of the nasal lining.

Acellular dermal matrix

When local and regional flaps have failed, microvascular tissue transfer provides a final option for fistula closure, particularly for those with large, recalcitrant, anteriorly located fistulas in densely scarred palates. The radial forearm flap is the flap of choice because of its long and large-caliber pedicle, lack of tissue bulk, pliability, and potential to be folded over to provide both a nasal and oral layer.[51] Other options for free tissue transfer have been described, including first dorsal metatarsal artery dorsalis pedis flaps,[52] the osseous angular scapular flap,[52] and the lateral upper arm fasciocutaneous flap.[53] Reinert's group also described prelamination of a lateral upper arm fasciocutaneous flap via a two-stage procedure forming a bilayered flap, first embedding buccal mucosa and a silicone sheet beneath the flap weeks before harvest.[53,54]

Consideration must also be given in these cases to simple prosthetic obturation. Although creation of the obturator and ongoing care may be cumbersome, these prostheses can also incorporate teeth to disguise residual clefts within the alveolus.

In cases of alveolar bone graft failure leading to a persistent nasoalveolar fistula, bone grafting can be reattempted; and, if this fails, dento-osseous transport distraction osteogenesis can be performed.

Cleft nose

Normal anatomy

The nose can be viewed as a three-layered structure, including a cutaneous layer, an osseocartilaginous layer, and an inner layer of mucoperichondrium. The most significant layer, in terms of providing structural features, is the osseocartilaginous layer, which can be further divided into three regions: the upper, middle, and lower vault *(Table 29.2)*. Additionally, the nose has numerous muscles that involve the nasal base and lobules *(Fig. 29.4)*.

The tripod theory has been described to understand better the structural architecture of the nasal tip, base, and lobule. This theory describes the right and left lateral crura of the LLC as two legs of a tripod supporting the nasal tip, with the

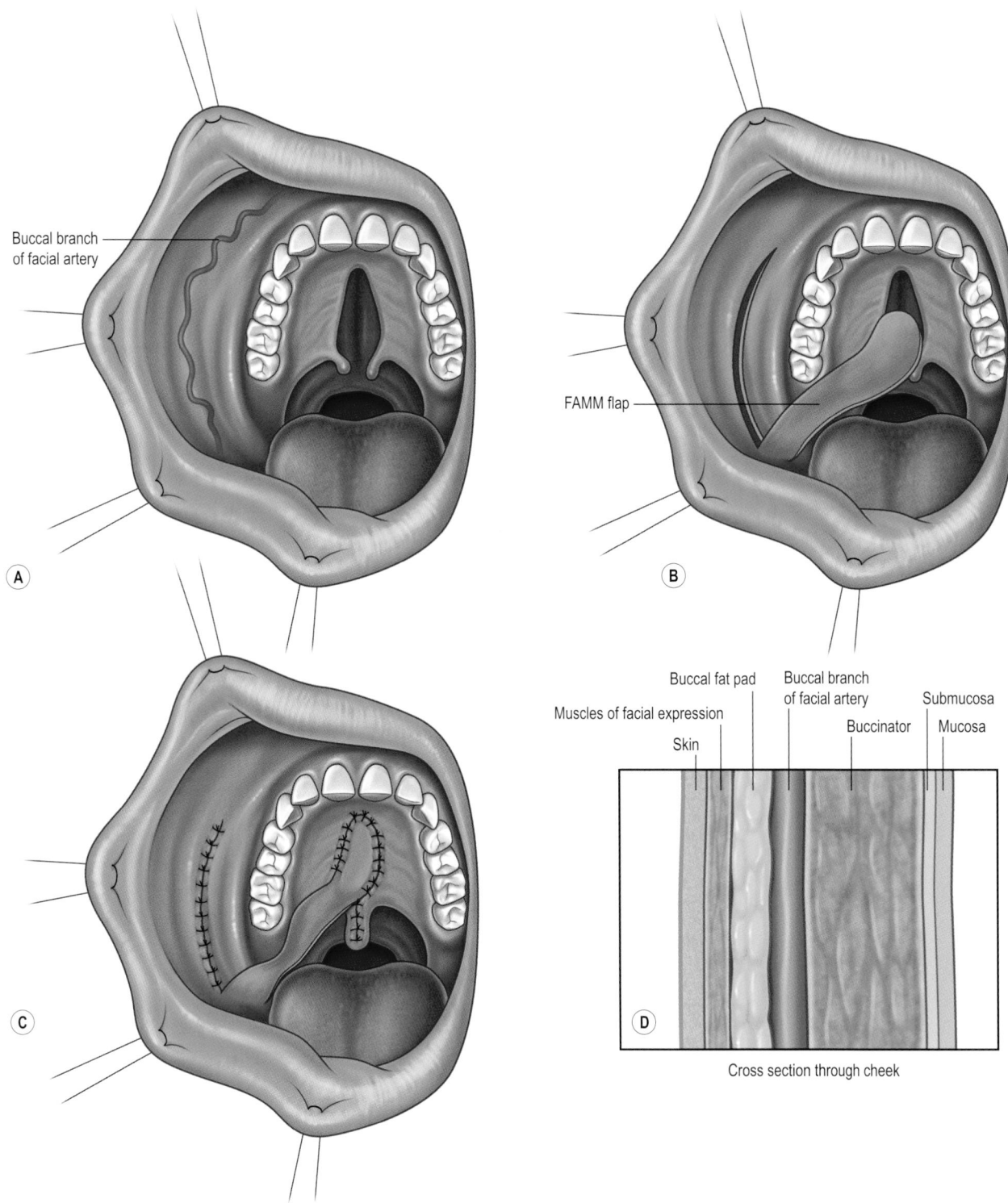

Buccal branch
of facial artery

FAMM flap

Buccal fat pad

Buccal branch
of facial artery

Muscles of facial expression

Buccinator

Submucosa

Mucosa

Skin

Cross section through cheek

Fig. 29.16 (A–D) Buccal tissue can be harvested via an axial pattern flap based off the facial artery. FAMM, facial artery myomucosal.

Table 29.2 **Classification of the osseocartilaginous skeleton of the nose**

Upper vault	Paired nasal bones Ascending/frontal processes of maxilla
Middle vault	Upper lateral cartilages
Lower vault	Lower lateral cartilages Medial crus Intermediate crus Lateral crus
Nasal septum	

adjoining medial crura functioning as the third leg. This simplistic view provides a general understanding of nasal tip dynamics, while in truth, the structural features of the nasal tip are provided by many structures *(Table 29.3)*.

Cleft nose anatomy

The anatomical nasal abnormalities with which unilateral and bilateral cleft lip patients present are somewhat similar although they differ in their laterality, extent of columellar and nasal tip involvement, and extent of deformity based on interventions already performed *(Figs 29.18–29.20)*. It is important to note that these abnormalities contribute to the nasal airflow obstruction commonly seen in cleft patients. Studies have shown that approximately 60% of patients have difficulty breathing through the nose[55] and have nasal airway

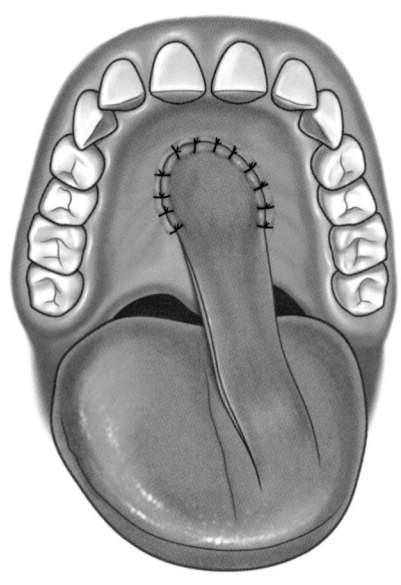

Fig. 29.17 The tongue offers another regional option for palatal fistula repair.

Table 29.3 **Structural features of the nasal tip**

Middle vault	Degree of apposition of the caudal medial crura and septum Overlap of ULC and LLC
Lower vault	Overlap of ULC and LLC Ligamentous connections between LLC and overlying skin Intermediate crus Lateral crus Interdomal ligamentous structures Accessory cartilages Piriform rim

ULC, upper lateral cartilage; LLC, lower lateral cartilage.
The tripod theory provides a simplistic understanding that the qualities of the nasal tip are provided by the medial crura/septum centrally, and the lateral crura from the sides. In truth, however, the nasal tip characteristics are provided by a number of structures.

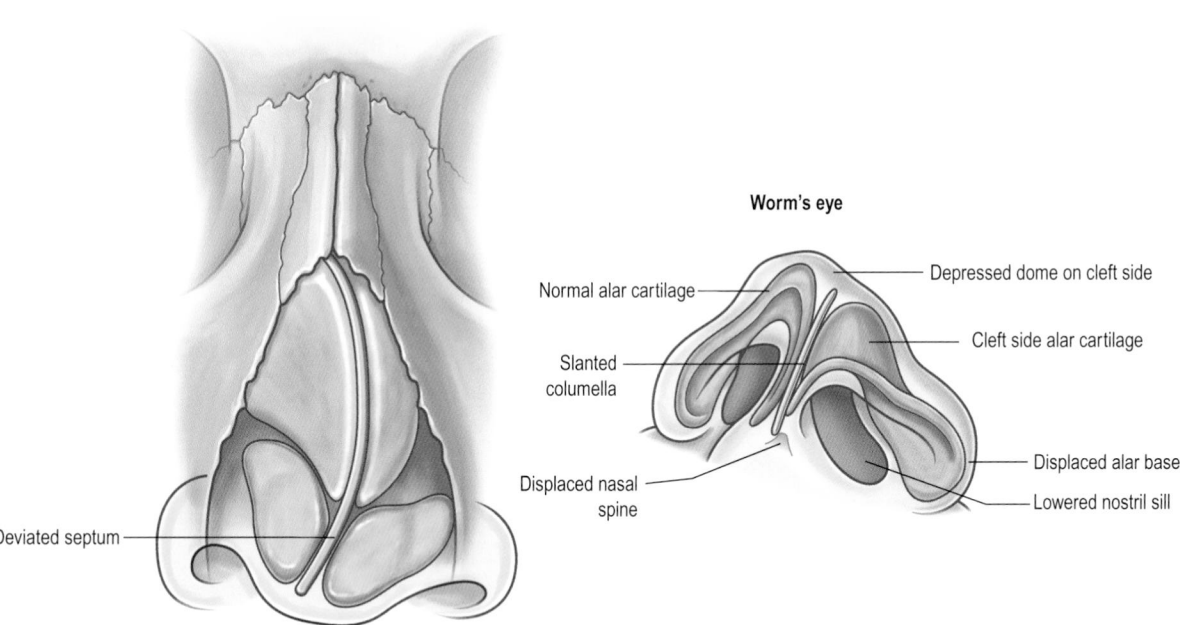

AP

Worm's eye

Normal alar cartilage

Slanted columella

Displaced nasal spine

Deviated septum

Depressed dome on cleft side

Cleft side alar cartilage

Displaced alar base

Lowered nostril sill

Fig. 29.18 The key aspects of the cleft nose deformity involve abnormalities of the osseocartilaginous skeleton. AP, anteroposterior.

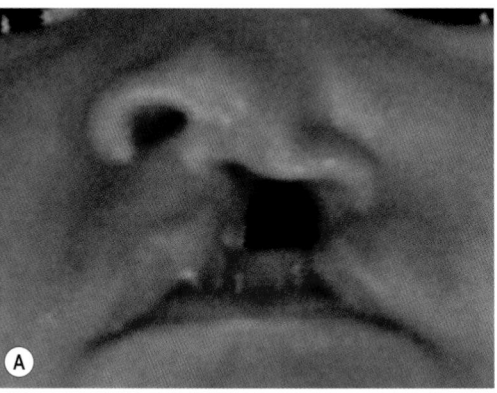
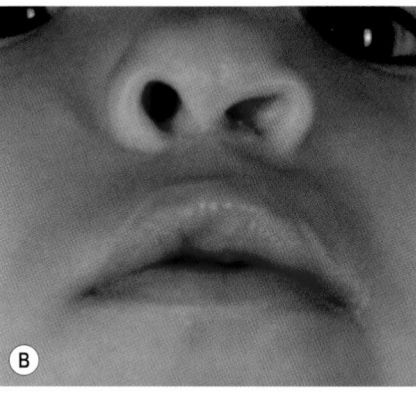
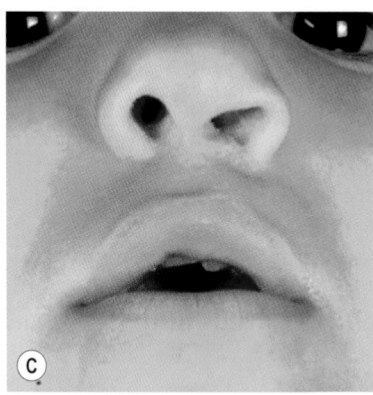

Fig. 29.19 (A–C) The classic cleft nose deformity as seen in *Figure 29.18* is not the same deformity seen secondarily by the plastic surgeon. Depending on the intervention performed, the initial severity of scarring, and subsequent growth, there may be a spectrum of secondary deformities.

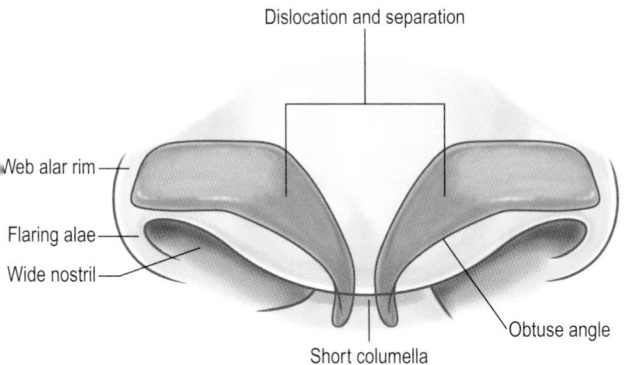

Fig. 29.20 The bilateral cleft nose deformity involves bilateral displacement and distortion of the osseocartilaginous skeleton of the nose. The shortened columella plays a prominent role in the bilateral deformity, and must be lengthened in subsequent procedures.

resistance 20–30% greater than normal.[55] Subsequently, the evaluation and treatment of secondary cleft nose deformities involve a proper assessment of both aesthetic and functional airway outcomes.

Evaluation

Recent advances in primary correction of the cleft nasal deformity have presented surgeons with the task of evaluating a spectrum of cleft nasal deformities. Patients who did not undergo primary nasal work always retained the key deformities and stigmata characteristic of the cleft nose. Patients with primary nasal correction have a spectrum of deformities based on the type and quality of repair performed in the first stage, as well as the degree of scarring and growth changes. However, in the authors' experience, patients who have undergone primary nasal correction always have a simpler definitive surgery with better results.

Evaluation of the secondary cleft nose deformity involves a proper history and physical exam. Patients need to be thoroughly questioned regarding the presence of nasal airway obstruction. Additionally, prior to any definitive nasal procedure, patients should be critically evaluated for underlying skeletal/midface hypoplasia. If maxillary or mandibular adjustment is necessary; this should be performed prior to rhinoplasty.

Physical examination of the nose can be complex; however, it helps to break it down into four areas: (1) frontal view; (2) profile view; (3) worm's eye/basilar view; and (4) internal view.[56] The nasal examination from the frontal view involves an outside-inside, top-down, medial-lateral approach. Initially, the nasal skin should be evaluated for thickness. Next, starting at the upper nasal vault, the nasal bones should be evaluated for symmetry and size. The middle vault should then be examined for vertical symmetry, upper lateral cartilage (ULC) collapse, and for internal valve incompetency (Cottle maneuver). Subsequently, the lower vault should be examined from a medial to lateral approach. The nasal tip should be analyzed for its morphology (bulbous, boxy, narrow, parenthesis), as well as for asymmetries. Next, the columella is examined for hemicolumellar height and width. The nasal ala is then examined for height, width, vertical position, position of the alar base, and the status of the nasal sill. Additionally, the pyriform rim and maxilla should be examined for hypoplasia.

From the profile view, five characteristics are examined. First, the depth of the radix is assessed. Second, the nasal dorsum is evaluated for the presence of a dorsal hump. Third, the nasal tip projection is evaluated. Fourth, the relationship between the columella and alar rim is examined for alar rim retraction. Fifth, the nasolabial angle is assessed.

From a worm's eye/basilar view, multiple features are assessed again to fully appreciate the three-dimensional nature of the nose and secondary deformities. First, the nasal tip position is evaluated. Next, the infratip lobule is assessed for size, shape, and symmetry. The columella is then checked for directionality and dimensions. The nostrils are assessed for their dimensions and symmetry, and the status of the nostril sill is also examined. Finally, the nasal alae are assessed for shape and symmetry.

On internal exam, the internal and external nasal valves are examined as sites for potential airflow disruption. The nasal septum is examined for the presence of deviation, spurs, and/or perforations. The inferior turbinates are subsequently evaluated for signs of hypertrophy, and finally, the nasal vestibule is examined for the presence of nasal synechiae.

This systematic approach represents one method of evaluating the cleft nose deformity where a treatment plan can be established[57]: (1) Is the pyriform rim/maxilla hypoplastic? (2) Is tip projection adequate? (3) Is projection of the bony dorsum deficient, normal, or overprojecting? (4) Is the position of the alar base adequate? (5) Are the shape and contour of the alar rim/lateral crus adequate? (6) Is the nasal airway obstructed? Further and more objective assessment can be performed with photographs, anthropometry, and nasometry.

Patient selection

Timing

The decision to operate on a patient with a secondary cleft nose deformity should be based on the severity of the deformity, the patient's and/or family's wishes, and the optimal timing for a procedure. The timing of secondary surgery on the cleft lip/nose deformity is subsequently based on the age of the patient, and the specific nature and aspects of the deformity. Revisionary procedures prior to entering preschool (age 4 or 5) are focused on reshaping, repositioning, and obtaining the optimal arc of rotation of the cleft-sided ala. In most situations, modification of the facial/nasal bones and septum should only be completed after the conclusion of nasal growth, to prevent disruption of growth centers. Cessation of growth has classically been thought to occur in the late teen years; however, there is firm anthropometric and cephalometric evidence demonstrating that the nose stops growing at the age of 11 or 12 years in females, and 13 or 14 years in males. If there is underlying midface hypoplasia requiring orthognathic surgery, the definitive rhinoplasty

should be delayed until this is completed. The final criterion is assuring that the patient is emotionally mature and capable of participating in the decision-making process preoperatively and in postoperative care.

Treatment/surgical technique

Efforts to correct the deformities associated with the secondary cleft nose are primarily focused on achieving: (1) nasal tip projection; (2) bony dorsum projection; (3) alar base position; (4) contour to the alar rim/lateral crus; (5) acute alar facial relationship; (6) an adequate nasolabial angle; and (7) nasal airway patency. Management of these goals requires decisions regarding access, technique, and supporting grafts *(Fig. 29.21)*.

Access

The two main options for access to the osseocartilaginous nasal skeleton include the closed or open approach, with each having its own pros and cons. The closed approach, which accesses the nasal structural components through an incision made within the nostril, provides minimally invasive access to the necessary nasal structures, allows accurate postoperative assessment of changes made, and provides natural pockets for the placement of grafts within the nose, all without causing the prolonged swelling seen with the open technique. While some surgeons argue that all procedures in rhinoplasty can be performed through a closed approach, the open approach has been used traditionally for more difficult and complicated procedures, especially when working on the nasal tip. The open approach uses a columellar incision to expose the nasal structures and provides superior

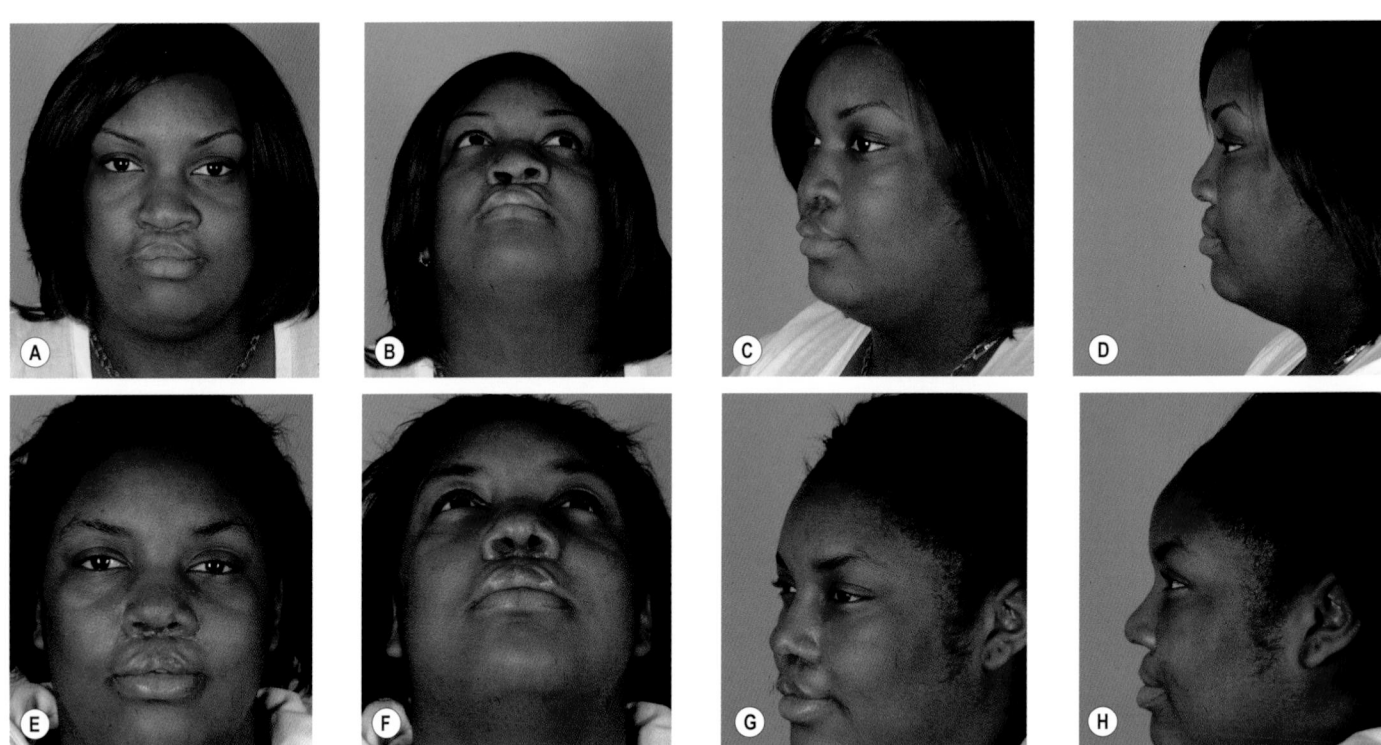

Fig. 29.21 (A–D) Preoperative pictures of a secondary bilateral cleft lip and nose deformity before undergoing definitive rhinoplasty. **(E–H)** One-week postoperative pictures demonstrating increased nasal tip projection, improved symmetry and width of the alar base, and corrected nostril orientation.

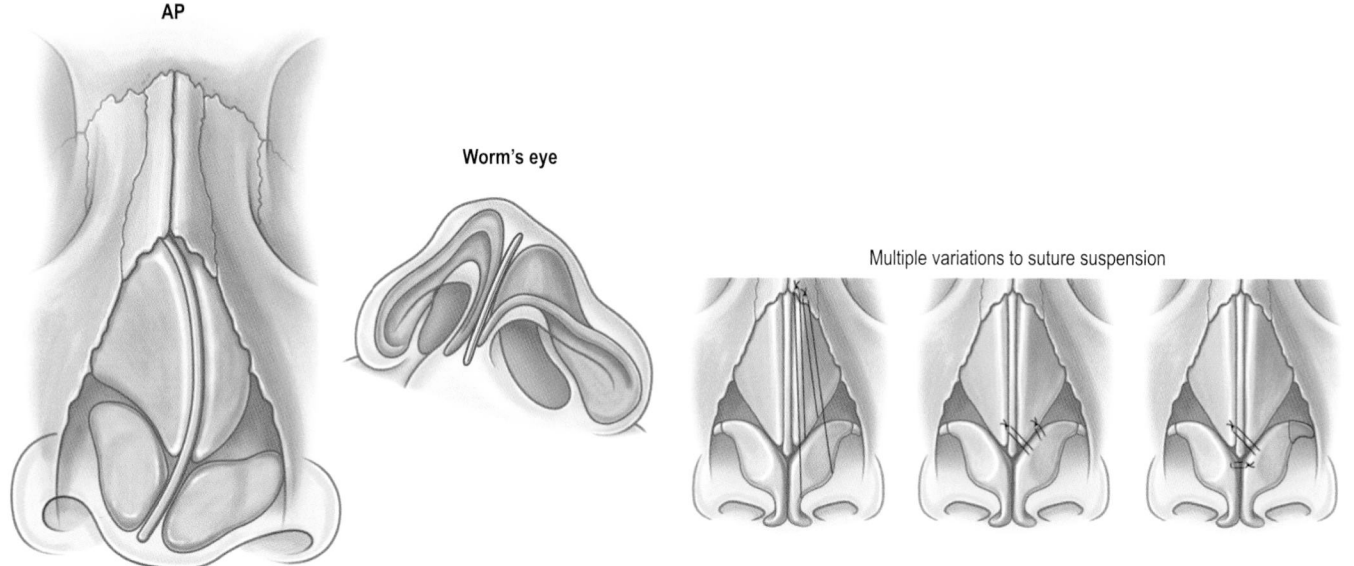

AP

Worm's eye

Multiple variations to suture suspension

Fig. 29.22 Suspension sutures apply force to reshape and reposition abnormal cartilaginous structures, utilizing appropriately placed and tensioned sutures, as demonstrated in these figures. AP, anteroposterior.

visualization and access; however, the external scar, loss of nasal tip support, interruption of columellar artery blood supply to the tip, and prolonged swelling are important downsides to this technique.

Technique

In the past, procedures to correct significant nasal tip depression, as seen with bilateral cleft-nasal deformity, focused on the skin and not the underlying structural support. Banked fork flaps, which use prolabial tissue to reconstruct the missing tissue, have been described and used in hopes of providing nasal tip projection. The procedure had its many downsides as it required a wide prolabium, resulted in significant secondary deformities,[58] and placed external scars along the upper lip. Subsequently, other methods were developed to address the nasal tip using similar principles under the same premise that the problem required more skin and soft-tissue recruitment.[59,60] The problem with these solutions, however, was that columellar lengthening, when performed without addressing the deformed cartilage, resulted in an abnormally long columella with significant secondary deformities. More recent techniques to recreate the columella have been performed in conjunction with structural modifications via a primary repair of the bilateral cleft lip/nose.

Outcomes have improved as techniques now address the underlying structural abnormalities in cleft nose deformities. The use of sutures to manipulate the cartilaginous and soft-tissue framework of the nose has revolutionized rhinoplasty. Suspension suture techniques have provided a way to manipulate the structural features of the nose in a less invasive fashion, reducing the need for excising and disturbing native tissues. Additionally, the acute effects of suspension techniques are reversible intraoperatively, compared to other methods which are mostly permanent.

The underlying principle is to manipulate mobile tissues by anchoring them to more immobile tissues using surgical

suture *(Fig. 29.22)*. Resuspension of the LLC involves the use of an infracartilaginous incision supplemented if necessary by medial dissection through the apex of existing lip incisions. The displaced ala is then completely freed from underlying structures, and a suture is placed through the desired point of the apex of the dome, and subsequently suspended to a superior position. Different authors have chosen different points for this "superior position," including to the contralateral ULC, tied over an external bolster, or to the contralateral LLC dome apex. The cleft-side LLC can be secured with a tapered needle on a polydioxanone suture to the dermis of the overlying skin envelope ("quilting sutures") by taking the stabilizing suture out through the skin and re-entering it through the same point, and tied intranasally *(Fig. 29.23)*. This may be facilitated by a small skin incision with a number 11 blade. Although this sometimes causes a small dimple of the overlying skin, this always resolves during the course of several weeks. Additionally, the technique maintains support for the repositioned skin envelope, and minimizes the problematic plica vestibularis. As well, these internal sutures obviate the need for external bolsters, which may cause scars on the nasal skin and upon their necessary early removal eliminate the established support.

The authors have recently developed a technique, the Stal–Feldman alar facial rotation excision, to address the alar base. This technique reshapes the nostril, eliminates excess ala, creates a full nostril sill, and narrows/transposes the alar base medially. These goals are accomplished while creating a more anatomic and acute alar facial relationship rather than the effacement commonly seen with Weir excision alone *(Fig. 29.24)*. This technique combines previously described alar–alar cinching sutures with a Weir excision when needed, and minimal sutures at the alar–cheek junction to avoid effacement. In unilateral deformities, the suture is passed across the base of the cleft side alar, across the nasal sill to the nasal spine, and back through the cleft-side alar base. In bilateral deformities, the suture is passed from alar base to alar base.

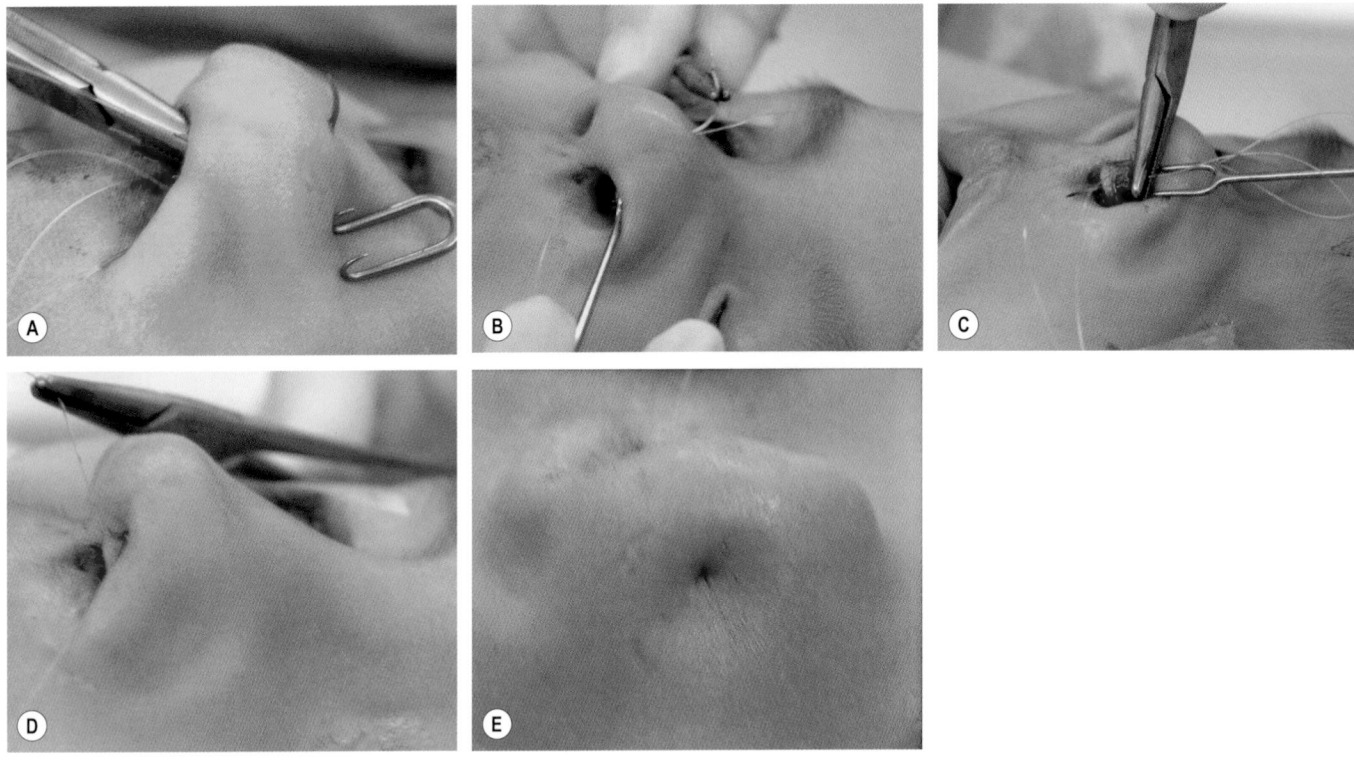

Fig. 29.23 (A–E) Quilting sutures function to suspend the lower lateral cartilage, reshape the nostril, and prevent alar lidding/plicae vestibularis by using the skin as an anchor point. Some skin dimpling can be seen postoperatively; however, this will resolve over time.

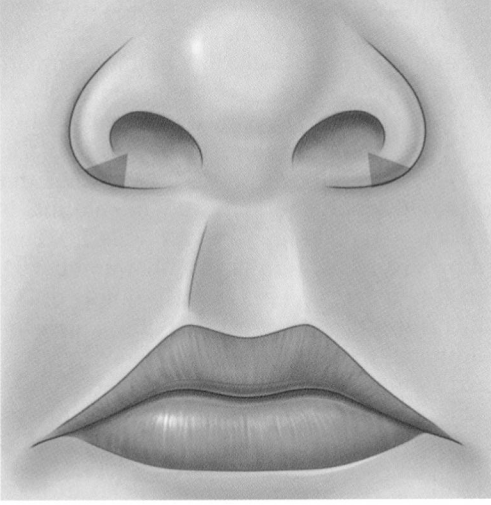

Mucosal-sparing

Fig. 29.24 The Weir excision is used to narrow the alar base.

This can be combined with a partial- or full-thickness wedge excision of skin and mucosa from the alar base or nostril sill depending on nostril size *(Fig. 29.25)*. For more severe cases of alar base displacement, release of the alar base from surrounding and deep structures, with subsequent repositioning, may be the best option.

Plastic surgeons[61,62] have developed approaches and techniques to modify the nasal tip. In general, these involve: (1) lateral crus resection/cephalic trim; (2) transdomal sutures;

(3) interdomal sutures *(Fig. 29.26)*; (4) lateral crural mattress sutures; and (5) columellar septal sutures.

Cephalic trim removes the attachments and overlap between the ULC and LLC, allowing independent movement and repositioning of the LLC. Transdomal sutures involve placing a mattress suture from the lateral portion of the alar dome or the lateral crus to the medial portion of the alar dome or medial crus. This reduces the distance between the lateral tip defining points, creating a narrower nasal tip. Next, interdomal sutures are passed between the middle crura in a mattress fashion, providing both symmetry and a reduction in interdomal width. Lateral crural sutures function to modify the curvature of the lateral crus, and are placed by passing a suture through the caudal aspect of the lateral crus, and then through a point laterally, approximately 4–6 mm away. This adjusts the convexity of the LLC and modifies the nostril flare. A columellar septal suture can then be used to adjust tip height, by suturing the medial crura together. Despite a surgeon's best efforts, suture modification of the tip may be inadequate to correct the deformity completely or provide enough support. Therefore, when suture modification is thought to be inadequate, one must consider additional support with cartilage grafts.

Supporting grafts

Columellar struts are particularly helpful in supporting the nasal tip, and are often used in combination with tip-modifying suture techniques. This graft is placed between the medial crura, and is often left free-floating *(Fig. 29.27)* to prevent constant motion against the nasal spine with lip movements. Alternatively, they can be fixed to the nasal

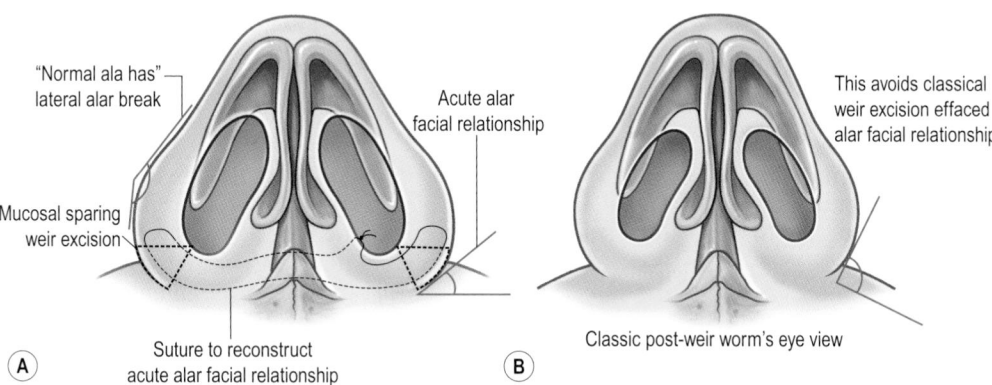

Fig. 29.25 (A, B) The Stal–Feldman alar facial rotation excision combines excision (partial or full-thickness lateral ala or nasal mucosa), if needed, with suturing techniques to reshape the nostril, narrow the alar base, maintain obtuse lateral alar break, and re-establish an acute alar facial relationship.

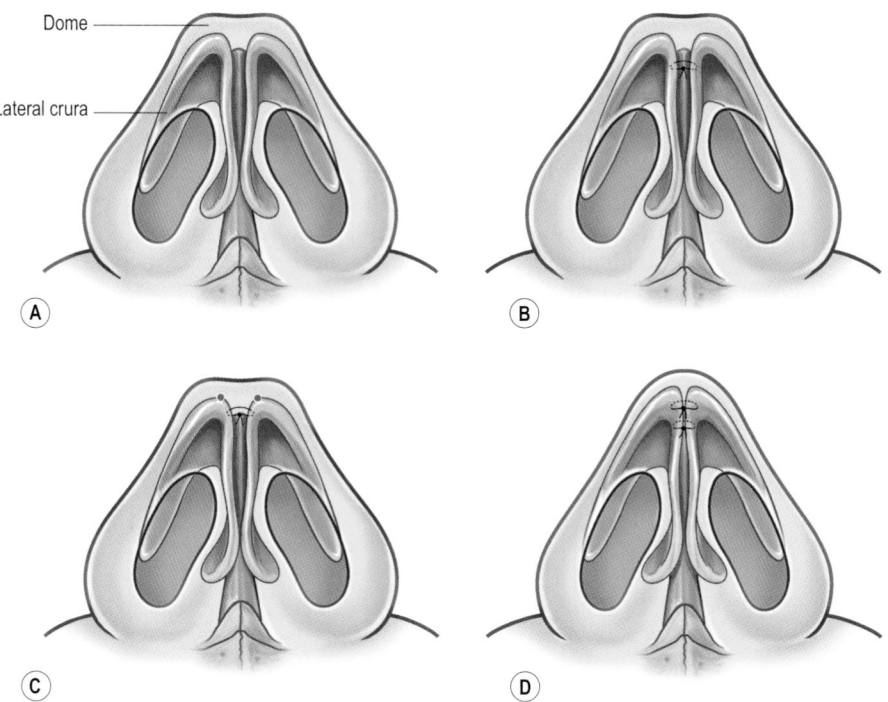

Fig. 29.26 (A–D) Sutures can also be used to reshape the nasal tip by modifying the relationship between the crus of the lower lateral cartilage between themselves or the contralateral lower lateral cartilage. These are used in conjunction with grafts to support the osseocartilaginous skeleton.

spine/premaxilla to give more support to the nasal tip; however, patients may complain of a stiff or fixed tip. Other grafts can be used to supplement and augment the cartilaginous skeleton of the nose, including spreader grafts, septal extension grafts, tip shield grafts, alar batten grafts, and dorsal onlay grafts.

Spreader grafts are placed between the dorsal septum and ULC. These grafts function to restore or maintain the internal nasal valve, straighten a deviated dorsal septum, improve the dorsal aesthetic lines, and reconstruct an open-roof deformity. The grafts are sutured to the septum, and may extend beyond the septal angle either to lengthen the nose or to increase tip projection.

Septal extension or extended spreader grafts function to control qualities of the nasal tip, including projection, support,

shape, rotation, and also create a supratip break. There are essentially three types of septal extension grafts. Types I and II supplement the nasal cartilaginous skeleton. Type I is similar to a dorsal spreader graft, except that it extends into the nasal tip between the medial crura. Type II grafts are paired batten grafts that extend diagonally into the nasal tip. Finally, type III grafts are attached directly to the anterior septal angle. Columellar struts or septal extension grafts can achieve 2–3 mm of additional tip projection when performed properly.

Additional grafts that can modify the appearance of the nasal tip include the tip graft and shield graft. The tip graft functions to camouflage tip irregularities, by placing graft tissue over the alar domes, and add to tip projection. The shield graft, popularized by Sheen, is placed over the caudal tip *(Fig. 29.28)*, not only modifying the appearance of the tip, but also augmenting the infratip lobule. In the authors' experience, shield grafts tend to have long-term problems with inadequacy and maintenance, and we subsequently prefer the use of onlay cartilage tip grafts.

Alar batten grafts are extra-anatomic support, placed in a pocket along the alar rim[15] *(Fig. 29.29)*. These grafts aid in opening the external nasal valve and also correct or prevent alar notching. Alar batten grafts should not be confused with lateral crural strut grafts. Crural strut grafts are placed underneath the LLC *(Fig. 29.29)*, while alar batten grafts are placed along the alar rim. Lateral crural struts structurally support the LLC, preventing collapse into the airway, giving the best opportunity to achieve LLC symmetry in a cleft nose.

Dorsal onlay grafts function to manipulate the appearance of the nasal dorsum by the application of cartilage (diced or intact) or other autogenous materials (Alloderm). Alloderm is used to smooth over minor contour deformities, while costal cartilage is used for significant augmentation of the nasal dorsum. Diced onlay grafts *(Fig. 29.30)* are used for moderate nasal dorsum deformities and have proven to be a safe, easy, and predictable manner to augment the nasal dorsum.[63]

Options for graft materials can be broken down into autologous, homografts (donated tissue from same species), and alloplastic. Autologous materials are generally preferred for their increased biocompatibility and low risk of infection and extrusion; however, they have associated donor site morbidity, a tendency to resorb, and in certain situations, come in finite amounts. In general, septal cartilage is thought to be the preferred source for grafts, as it provides a straight donor tissue that has a similar resilience to the native cartilaginous framework. Auricular cartilage and rib cartilage are additional options for donor sites, with costal cartilage being used in cases needing significant structural support.

Finally, bony osteotomies should be performed to address widened nasal bones and abnormal dorsal lines. They can

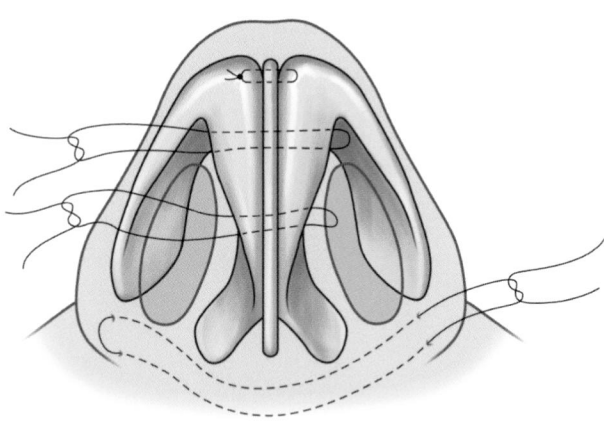

Fig. 29.27 Columellar struts involve the placement of a graft between the medial crus and suturing the structures together using mattress sutures. This improves nasal tip support and projection, columellar length, and nasolabial angle.

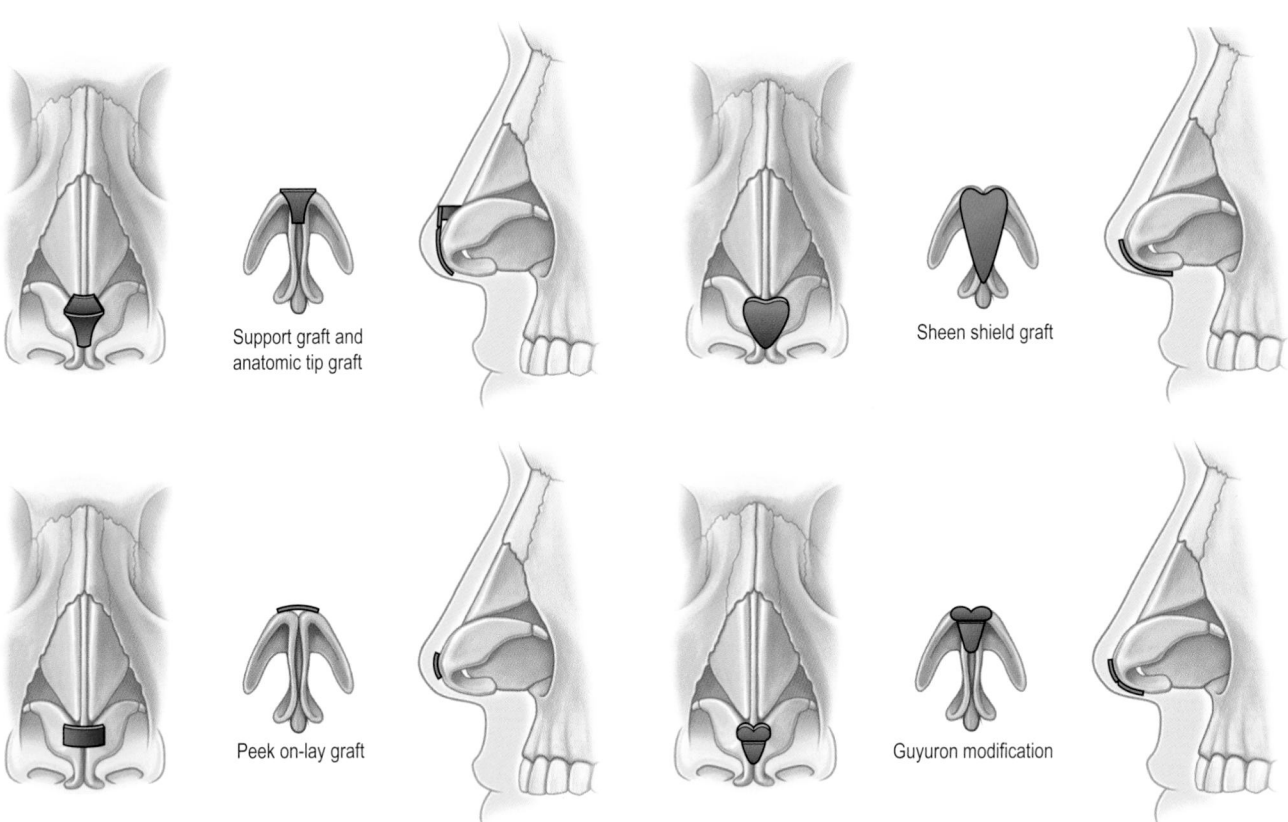

Support graft and anatomic tip graft

Sheen shield graft

Peek on-lay graft

Guyuron modification

Fig. 29.28 Shield grafts allow modification of the nasal tip and infratip lobule.

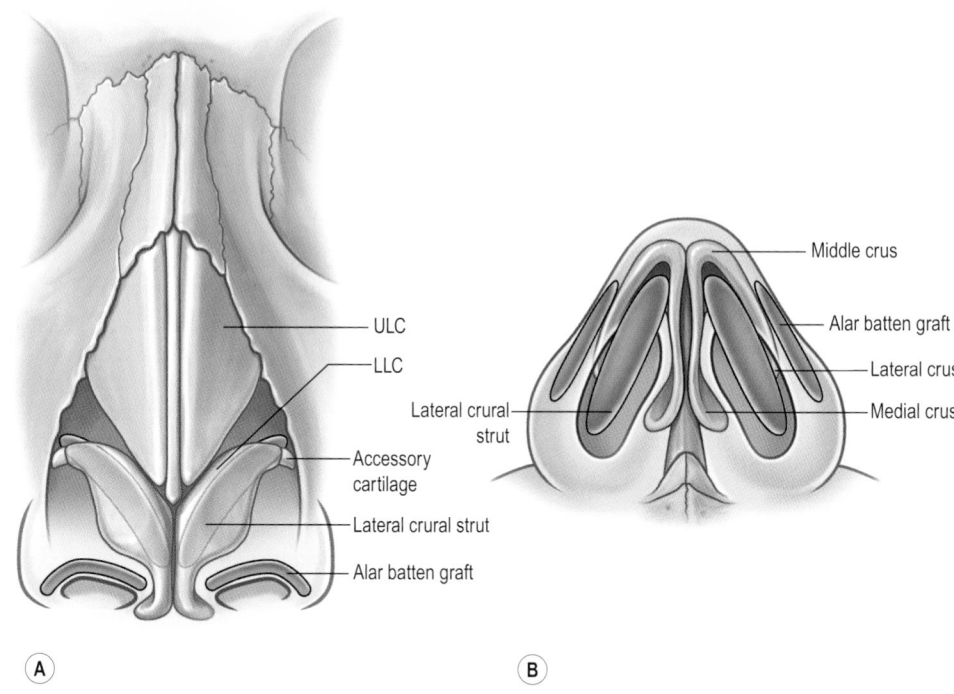

Fig. 29.29 (A, B) Alar batten grafts provide extra anatomical support to open the external nasal valve and prevent alar notching. Lateral crural strut grafts can alter the position, shape, or functional stability of the lower lateral cartilages. These supportive structures can be placed either uni- or bilaterally based on where support is needed. ULC, upper lateral cartilage; LLC, lower lateral cartilage.

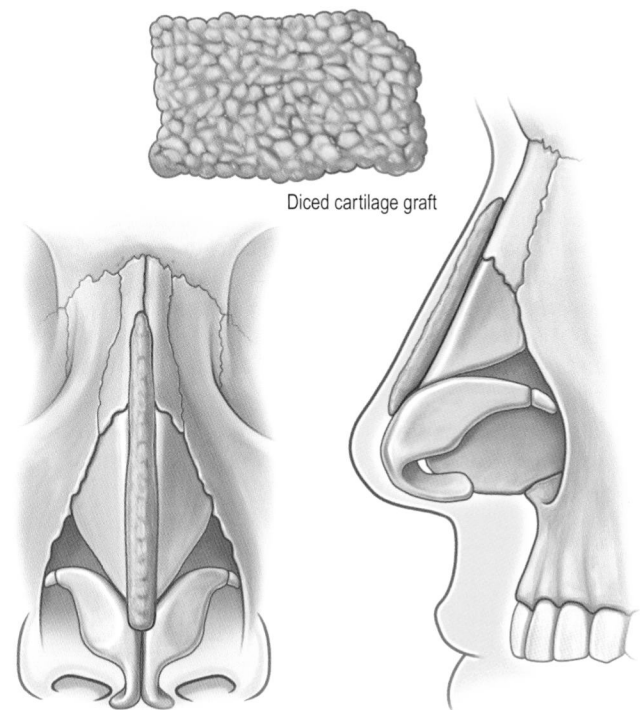

Fig. 29.30 (A, B) Diced cartilage can be used to augment the nasal dorsum and tip for mild to moderate deformities.

potentially improve both the aesthetics of the region and the functionality.

When "enough is enough"

The array of secondary deformities possible in patients with cleft lip and palate is formidable. When deciding on which deformities to treat operatively, one must determine their impact on the patient and the likelihood that a surgical procedure will substantially improve the problem. At some point in the operative sequence, further surgical intervention is unlikely to improve the patient's appearance or function significantly. Consequently, it is important to know when "enough is enough," that is, when the patient is unlikely to be helped by any further intervention.

Studies have demonstrated the potential for significant negative psychosocial impact of secondary deformities of the cleft lip and palate defect[64–66]; however, emphasis should not be taken away from the ability of these patients to function at a high level with both resilience and positive coping strategies.[67] Consequently, even though a vast array of techniques and procedures are available for modifying outcomes, surgery for secondary deformities should be reserved for those problems that are both bothersome to the patient and those which are likely to be improved by surgery. This can be a difficult reality for the plastic surgeon. As Marsh stated, the surgeon is at times more critical of the result than the patient is. Just as not every nasal dorsal hump needs to be removed, not every cleft lip nasal deformity needs to be revised. The enemy of good is better, particularly when better is unlikely.

Access the complete references list online at **http://www.expertconsult.com**

1. Weinzweig J, Panter KE, Seki J, et al. The fetal cleft palate: IV. Midfacial growth and bony palatal development following in utero and neonatal repair of the congenital caprine model. *Plast Reconstr Surg.* 2006;118:81–93.

4. Cohen SR, Corrigan M, Wilmot J, et al. Cumulative operative procedures in patients aged 14 years and older with unilateral or bilateral cleft lip and palate. *Plast Reconstr Surg.* 1995;96:267–271.

   In the 1990s, Cohen et al. set out to determine how extensive the role was that surgical procedures played in the lives of children with cleft lip and palate defects. This study looked at individuals from their institution who were over the age of 15, and reviewed the number and type of procedures that each individual had based on the original defect. They found that by the time individuals had reached the ages of 17 and 18, those with unilateral cleft lip and palate defects had on average ~6 operations, while those with bilateral cleft lip and palate defects had ~8 operations. On average, individuals in both groups had at least one lip and one nasal revision, with bilateral cleft lip and palate patients averaging two lip revision surgeries. While several of the procedures performed at that time are no longer necessary, and improved techniques have led to an overall reduction in the need for revisions, this article, among others, demonstrated that the management of a cleft lip and palate defect is an ongoing and extensive process.

11. Losee JE, Smith DM, Afifi AM, et al. A successful algorithm for limiting postoperative fistulae following palatal procedures in the patient with orofacial clefting. *Plast Reconstr Surg.* 2008;122:544–554.

21. Cohen SR, Kalinowski J, LaRossa D, et al. Cleft palate fistulas: A multivariate statistical analysis of prevalence, etiology, and surgical management. *Plast Reconstr Surg.* 1991;87:1041–1047.

   Cohen et al. performed a retrospective, multivariate analysis of patients who had been operated on for palatal fistula post cleft palate repair. They noted that fistulas occurred in a significant number of patients (23%), and noted that variables such as Veau classification, experience of the surgeon, and type of palatal closure affected the incidence rate of palatal fistulas. They also noted that factors such as age did not affect incidence rates. Other studies have been published that contest some of the conclusions drawn by this study, and many of the factors that influence palatal fistula incidence have been thoroughly debated. Nonetheless, it was clear that

there were some underlying causative factors that influence the risk of palatal fistulas, and once they occurred, they were a difficult problem to correct.

26. Daskalogiannakis J, Mehta M. The need for orthognathic surgery in patients with repaired complete unilateral and complete bilateral cleft lip and palate. *Cleft Palate Craniofac J.* 2009;46:498–502.

32. Mulliken JB, Pensler JM, Kozakewich HPW, et al. The anatomy of cupid's bow in normal and cleft lip. *Plast Reconstr Surg.* 1993;92:395–404.

   In the early 1990s, Mulliken et al. examined the gross and microscopic anatomy of the lip in normal individuals and those with cleft lips. The study reaffirmed and further characterized the anatomy of the normal lip, including the white roll, vermillion, and underlying orbicularis oris, but it also discussed the abnormalities underlying the cleft lip deformity. It was demonstrated that the dimunitive white roll found in cleft lips was associated with a hypoplasia of the pars marginalis, further demonstrating the role that dermal muscle insertions play in the landmarks of the upper lip. A great understanding of the underlying anatomy of the region has come to play a large role in the primary and secondary repair of the cleft lip deformity.

35. Farkas LG, Posnick JC, Hreczko TM, et al. Growth patterns of the nasolabial region: A morphometric study. *Cleft Palate Craniofac J.* 1992;29:318–323.

   Farkas et al. set out to determine the relationship between age and growth of the nasal and lip structures. They examined over 1500 North American Caucasian children and found that a majority of the lifetime growth of the upper lip occurred before the age of 5, while the majority of nasal growth after 1 year of age occurred between the ages of 5 and 18. Nasal growth was even more significantly delayed for nasal tip projection. The results of this study have played a major role in influencing the timing of interventions for cleft lip and palate cases, as well as influencing some of the technical details of the primary repair. However, it is important to take into consideration that underlying nasolabial growth in cleft lip and palate patients is abnormal, and the rules for growth in normal children do not necessarily apply to these patients.

61. Tebbetts JB. Shaping and positioning the nasal tip without structural disruption: A new, systematic approach. *Plast Reconstr Surg.* 1994;94:61–77.

30

Cleft and craniofacial orthognathic surgery

Jesse A. Goldstein and Steven B. Baker

SYNOPSIS

- Dentofacial deformities, in particular maxillary retrusion resulting in class III malocclusion, are typical of the cleft lip population. Of patients in this group, 25–30% have midface retrusion severe enough to require orthognathic surgery
- Orthognathic surgery should ideally be performed after facial growth is complete. If surgery is performed earlier, the likelihood is high that additional (though possibly less complicated) surgery may be required when the patient reaches skeletal maturity
- Treatment should favor expansive movements (anterior and inferior repositioning) to achieve class I occlusion rather than contractile movements (superior and posterior repositioning) in order to minimize premature aging.

Access the Historical Perspective section online at
http://www.expertconsult.com

Introduction

Orthognathic surgery is the term used to describe surgical movement of the tooth-bearing segments of the maxilla and mandible. Candidates for orthognathic surgery have dentofacial deformities that cannot be adequately treated with orthodontic therapy alone. Children with cleft lip and palate as well as certain craniofacial anomalies are especially prone to develop malocclusion. Indeed, where approximately 2.5% of the general population have occlusal discrepancies that warrant surgical correction, 25–30% of patients who undergo surgical correction of cleft lip and palate in infancy will have severe enough midface retrusion to require orthognathic surery.[1] Maxillary hypoplasia resulting in class III malocclusion is the typical deformity seen in patients with cleft and craniofacial deformities, but class II malocclusion, anterior open bites, occlusal cants and many other dentofacial deformities can also occur. Regardless of the etiology, patient examination and treatment-planning principles remain the same. The goal of orthognathic surgery, therefore, is to establish ideal dental occlusion with the jaws in a position that optimizes facial form and function.

Basic science

Growth and development

Timing of orthognathic surgery in the pediatric patient is key to good and predictable outcomes and is mediated by the development and maturation of the craniofacial skeleton. The foundation of maxillofacial growth relies on a complex interplay between genetic processes and micro- and macroenvironmental factors which must be understood to plan orthognathic procedures on patients with clefts and craniofacial disorders.

The osteogenesis of the maxillofacial skeleton occurs by way of two well-understood processes: intramembranous ossification and endochondral ossification. The cranial vault, upper face, midface, and a majority of the mandible arise from the former mechanism. Although there is a great amount of variability between individuals and genders, skeletal maturation generally progresses in a cranial-to-caudal direction with the cranial vault reaching close to adult size in early adolescence, followed closely by the upper face in the early teen years, the maxilla in the mid-teens, and the mandible in the late teen years *(Fig. 30.1)*.[3]

Dental eruption patterns proceed in a similar stepwise fashion, and the transition from mixed dentition (6–12 years of age) to permanent dentition (12–20 years of age) mirrors the maturation of the maxillofacial skeleton. Indeed, midface and lower face development is, in part, mediated by the budding deciduous and permanent dentition, providing regional signals to the alveolus and stimulating bony deposition. During this period, an alteration of tooth position can, in turn, alter the direction of growth of both the maxilla and mandible. Orthodontists take advantage of this active phase of development through their use of braces, palatal expanders, and various external devices to alter maxillary and

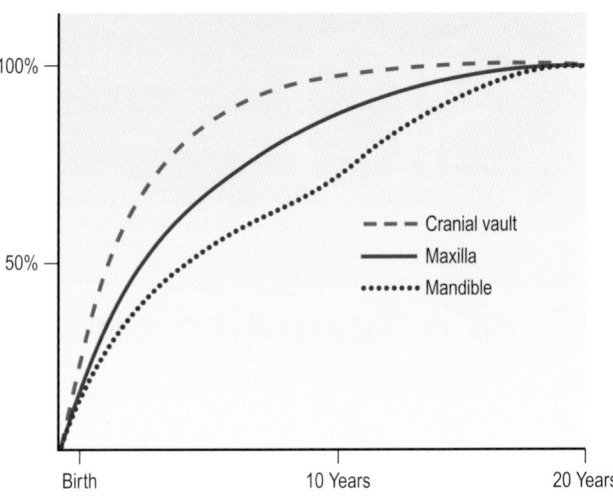

Fig. 30.1 Skeletal maturity of the cranial vault, the maxilla, and the mandible from infancy to skeletal maturity (scaled to 100% of adult size).

mandibular growth trajectories.[4] For this reason, surgical intervention is usually delayed until skeletal maturity is reached and orthopedic movements are no longer effective.

Diagnosis/patient preparation

Preoperative evaluation

The cleft and craniofacial team

The chance of a favorable surgical outcome is optimized if presurgical planning is performed in conjunction with a cleft/craniofacial team which includes plastic surgeons, otorhinolaryngologists, dentists, geneticists, orthodontists, and many others. Speech pathologists, for example, play an integral role in the evaluation of the velopharyngeal mechanism and the potential effects that maxillary advancement may have on speech nasality and articulation. A preoperative videonasoendoscopy has been shown to yield information that can aid in predicting postoperative hypernasality.

The orthodontist's role in the preoperative evaluation and management is critical. Prior to surgery, the potential surgical candidate requires a comprehensive workup that includes an analysis of the occlusal characteristics and the age of the facial skeleton, need for presurgical orthodontics, and possibly even palatal expansion. If orthognathic surgery is attempted before the facial skeleton reaches maturity, the need for revision surgery will be increased because of continued postoperative growth.

The history and physical examination

It is important to obtain a thorough medical, dental, and surgical history from every patient. Systemic diseases such as juvenile rheumatoid arthritis, diabetes, and scleroderma can affect treatment planning. With jaw asymmetries, a history of hyperplasia or hypoplasia from syndromic, traumatic, postsurgical or neoplastic etiologies affects treatment

considerations. Each patient should be questioned regarding symptoms of temporomandibular joint disease or myofascial pain syndrome. Motivation and realistic expectations are important for an optimal outcome. It is likewise important for patients to have a clear understanding of the procedure, recovery, and anticipated result. In younger patients, a family discussion in terms they can understand helps to alleviate preoperative anxiety. Orthognathic surgery is a major undertaking, and the patient and family must be appropriately motivated to undergo necessary preoperative and postoperative orthodontic treatment in addition to the surgery itself.

A complete physical exam should be performed on every patient prior to surgery. The frontal facial evaluation begins with the assessment of the vertical facial thirds (trichion to glabella, glabella to subnasale, and subnasale to menton) and the horizontal facial fifths (zygoma to lateral canthus, lateral to medial canthi, and intracanthal segment). The most important factor in assessing the vertical height of the maxilla is the degree of incisor showing while the patient's lips are in repose. Males should show at least 2–3 mm, whereas as much as 5–6 mm is considered attractive in females. If the patient shows the correct degree of incisor in repose, but shows excessive gingiva in full smile, the maxilla should not be impacted. It is more important to have correct incisor show in repose than in full smile. If lip incompetence or mentalis strain is present, it is usually an indicator of vertical maxillary excess.

The inferior orbital rims, malar eminence, and piriform areas are evaluated for the degree of projection. These regions often appear deficient in cleft patients, and maxillary advancement is therefore indicated; if they are prominent, posterior repositioning may be necessary. The alar base width should also be assessed prior to surgery since orthognathic surgery may alter this width which, in turn, may accentuate any asymmetries associated with a cleft nasal deformity. Asymmetries of the maxilla and mandible should be documented on physical examination, and the degree of deviation from the facial midline noted.

The profile evaluation focuses on the projection of the forehead, malar region, the maxilla and mandible, the nose, the chin, and the neck. An experienced clinician can usually determine whether the deformity is caused by the maxilla, the mandible, or both simply by looking at the patient. This assessment is made clinically and verified at the time of cephalometric analysis. The intraoral exam should begin with an assessment of oral hygiene and periodontal health. These factors are critical for successful orthodontic treatment and surgery. Any retained deciduous teeth or unerupted adult teeth are noted. The occlusal classification is determined, and the degrees of incisor overlap and overjet are quantified. The surgeon should assess the transverse dimension of the maxilla as prior cleft palate repair will often result in transverse growth restriction. If the mandibular third molars are present, they must be extracted 6 months prior to sagittal split osteotomy. Any missing teeth or periapical pathology should be noted, as should any signs or symptoms of temporomandibular joint dysfunction. These issues should be addressed prior to proceeding with orthognathic surgery. The term "dental compensation" is used to describe the tendency of teeth to tilt in a direction that minimizes dental malocclusion. For example, in a patient with an overbite (Angle class II malocclusion), lingual retroclination of the upper incisors and labial proclination of the lower incisors minimize the malocclusion

The opposite occurs in a patient who has dental compensation or an underbite (Angle class III malocclusion). Thus, dental compensation, which is often the result of orthodontic treatment, will mask the true degree of skeletal discrepancy. Precise analysis of the dental compensation is done on the lateral cephalometric radiographs.

If the patient desires surgical correction of the deformity, presurgical orthodondics will upright and decompensate the occlusion, thereby reversing the compensation that has occurred. This has the effect of exaggerating the malocclusion, but it also allows the surgeon to maximize skeletal movements. If the patient is ambivalent or not interested in surgery, mild cases of malocclusion may be treated by further dental compensation, which will camouflage the deformity and restore proper overjet and overbite. The importance of a commitment to surgery prior to orthodontics lies in the fact that dental movements for decompensation and compensation are in opposite directions, so this decision needs to be made prior to orthodontic therapy.[5]

Patient selection

Identifying the proper patient for orthognathic surgery is a key step to ensure satisfaction and successful outcomes. This includes amassing considerable data beyond a simple history and physical exam and should be coordinated with other members of the cleft/craniofacial team.

Cephalometric and dental evaluation

A cephalometric analysis and comparison to normative values can help the surgeon plan the degree of skeletal movement needed to achieve both an optimal occlusion and an optimal aesthetic result. A lateral cephalometric radiograph is performed under reproducible conditions so that serial images can be compared. This film is usually taken at the orthodontist's office using a cephalostat, an apparatus specifically designed for this purpose, and a head frame to maintain consistent head position. It is important to be certain the surgeon can visualize both the bony and soft-tissue features in order to facilitate tracing every landmark. Once the normal structures are traced, several planes and angles are determined (Fig. 30.2).

The sella–nasion–subspinale (SNA) and sell–nasion–supramentale (SNB) are the two most important angles in determining the positions of the maxilla and mandible relative to each other as well as the cranial base. These angles are determined by drawing lines from sella to nasion to A point or B point, respectively. By forming an angle with the sella and nasion, this position is referenced to the cranial base. A point provides information about the anteroposterior position of the maxilla. If the SNA angle is excessive, the maxilla exhibits an abnormal anterior position relative to the cranium. If SNA is less than normal, the maxilla is posteriorly positioned relative to the cranial base. The same principle applies to the mandible: B point is used to relate the mandibular position to the cranial base. The importance of the cranial base as a reference is that it allows the clinician to determine if one or both jaws contribute to a noted deformity. For example, a patient's class III malocclusion (underbite) could develop from several

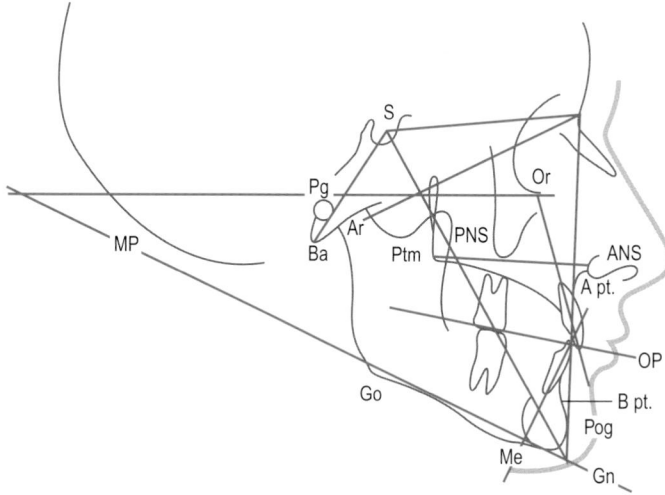

Fig. 30.2 The cephalometric radiograph is used to identify skeletal landmarks used in determining the lines and angles that reflect facial development. These measurements aid in determining the extent to which each jaw contributes to the dentofacial deformity. S, sella turcica, the midpoint of the sella turcica; N, nasion, the anterior point of the intersection between the nasal and frontal bones; **A**, "A point," the innermost point in the depth of the concavity of the maxillary alveolar process; **B**, "B point," the innermost point on the contour of the mandible between the incisor tooth and the bony chin; Ba, basale, the most inferior point of the skull base; Pg, pogonion, the most anterior point on the contour of the chin; Go, gonion, the most inferior and posterior point at the angle formed by the ramus and body of the mandible; Po, porion, the uppermost lateral point on the roof of the external auditory meatus; Or, orbitale, the lowest point on the inferior margin of the orbit; PNS, posterior nasal spine, the most posterior point on the maxilla; ANS, anterior nasal spine, the most anterior point on the maxilla; Gn, gnathion, the center of the inferior contour of the chin; Me, menton, the most inferior point on the mandibular symphysis; MP, mandibular plane, the line connecting the Go and the Gn; OP, occlusal plane.

different etiologies: a retrognathic maxilla and a normal mandible as is common in cleft patients, a normal maxilla and a prognathic mandible, a retrognathic mandible and a more severely retrognathic maxilla, or a prognathic maxilla and a more severely prognathic mandible. All of these conditions yield a class III malocclusion, yet each requires a different treatment approach. The surgeon can delineate the true etiology of the deformity by the fact that the maxilla and mandible can be independently related to a stable reference, the cranial base. Next, cephalometric tracings are performed.

Cephalometric tracings give the surgeon an idea of how skeletal movements will affect one another as well as the soft-tissue profile. They also allow the surgeon to determine the distances the bones will be moved to achieve the goals of specific procedure. Different tracing methods using acetate paper are used for isolated maxillary, isolated mandibular, or two-jaw surgeries. Much of the traditional hand cephalometric tracing, however. has given way to computer-aided cephalometric analysis which allows the surgeon to position the maxilla and mandible electronically on the cephalogram while recording the soft-tissue changes and measuring the degree of repositioning.

Complete dental records, including mounted dental casts, are needed to execute preoperative model surgery and fabricate surgical splints. Casts allow the surgeon to evaluate the occlusion both before and after articulation into proper positions. Analysis of new occlusion gives the clinician an idea of how intensive the presurgical orthodontic treatment plan will be. Casts also allow the clinician to distinguish between absolute and relative transverse maxillary deficiency. Absolute transverse maxillary deficiency presents as a posterior crossbite with the jaws in class I relationship. A relative maxillary transverse deficiency is commonly seen in a patient with a class III malocclusion. A posterior crossbite is observed in this type of patient, raising suspicions of inadequate maxillary width. However, as the maxilla is advanced or the mandible retruded, the crossbite is eliminated. Articulation of the casts into a class I occlusion allows the surgeon to distinguish easily between relative and absolute maxillary constriction.

Model surgery

Using the cephalometric tracings as a guide, the next step is to reproduce the maxillary and/or mandibular movements on articulated dental models. This allows for the fabrication of occlusal splints to be used intraoperatively to guide jaw repositioning in preparation for osteosynthesis. Model surgery begins by obtaining accurate casts of the patient's occlusion. If the surgeon does not have a dental laboratory, the orthodontist will obtain the casts. The success of the technical portion of orthognathic surgery correlates directly with the accuracy of the model surgery and splint fabrication.

Isolated mandibular surgery

It should be noted that if isolated mandibular surgery is being performed, the casts can be hand-articulated into the desired occlusion. The Galetti articulator is a useful tool that allows securing of casts with a screw mount. A universal joint allows the casts to be set in the desired relationship. Surgical splints can then be made from the articulator. If the maximum intercuspal position is the desired postoperative occlusion, a splint is unnecessary. The surgeon can osteotomize the mandible and secure it into its new position using the maximum intercuspal position as a guide to the new position. The surgeon should always verify the desired postoperative occlusion with the othrodontist prior to surgery.

Isolated maxillary and two-jaw surgery

A face bow is a device used to relate the maxillary model accurately to the cranium on an articulator. If a maxillary osteotomy is being performed, one set of models should be mounted on an articulator using the face bow. Two other sets of models are used in treatment planning. Next, an Erickson model block is used to measure the current position of the maxillary central incisors, cuspids, and the mesiobuccal cusp of the first molar. The face bow-mounted maxillary cast is placed on the model block. The maxillary model is then measured to the tenth of a millimeter vertically, anteroposteriorly, and end-on. By having numerical records in three dimensions, the surgeon can reproduce the maxillary cast's exact location, as well as determine a new location. Reference lines are circumferentially inscribed every 5 mm around the maxillary cast mounting. The distances the maxilla will move in an anteroposterior, lateral, and vertical direction have been determined from the previous cephalometric exam. These numbers are added or subtracted from the current values measured on the model block to determine the new

three-dimensional position of the maxillary cast. The occlusal portion of the maxillary cast is removed from its base using a saw. As much plaster is removed from the cast as is necessary to accommodate the new position of the maxilla. Once the model block verifies the maxilla is in its new position, the cast is secured with sticky wax or plaster to the mounting ring. Now it can be placed on the articulator. At this point, the surgeon has a mounting of the postoperative maxilla related to the preoperative mandible. An acrylic splint is made at this point. This splint is called the intermediate splint and is used in the operating room to index the new position of the maxilla to the preoperative position of the mandible. A second mounting with the casts in the occlusion desired by the orthodontist is used to make a final splint that represents the new position of the mandible to the repositioned maxilla. This is fabricated in a manner similar to the splint for isolated mandibular surgery. If the occlusion is good, intercuspal position can be used to position the mandible without the splint.

3D CT modeling

There are several computer-assisted design (CAD) programs that are now commercially available that can assist the surgeon with some or all of the preoperative patient preparation. A computed tomography (CT) scan is obtained with the patient wearing a bite jig that correlates natural head position to the three-dimensional (3D) CT image of the patient's face. Although conventional helical CT scans with fine cuts through the face are ideal, cone beam CT scans offer a comparable image quality with considerably less cost and radiation exposure (50 µSv compared to 2000 µSv). A cephalometric analysis can then be performed as well as simulated movements of the jaws and chin in any dimension. Once the osteotomy movements are verified by the surgeon, CAD/CAM technology is used to fabricate surgical splints for the patient. If necessary, 3D models of the patient can be made showing the exact proposed movement *(Fig. 30.3)*. Some systems can actually "wrap" a 2D digital image around the soft-tissue envelope of the 3D CT image, thus replicating a 3D image of the patient's face in color.

In these authors' experience, 3D CT modeling has demonstrated improved accuracy in diagnosis and treatment. The elimination of traditional model surgery saves the surgeon time in patient preparation. Finally, the 3D aspect of this treatment-planning approach enhances the surgeon's ability to predict how osteotomies may affect soft tissue of the face. These advantages facilitate the ability of the plastic surgeon to provide optimal care for these patients.

Developing a treatment plan

Once the data are obtained, the surgeon can determine which abnormalities the patient exhibits and the extent to which these features deviate from the norm. The treatment plan is the application of these data to provide the best aesthetic result while establishing a class I occlusion. The goal is not to "treat the numbers" in an attempt to normalize every patient. The appearance of the soft-tissue envelope surrounding the facial skeleton is the most crucial factor in determining the aesthetic success of orthognathic procedures, and the jaws

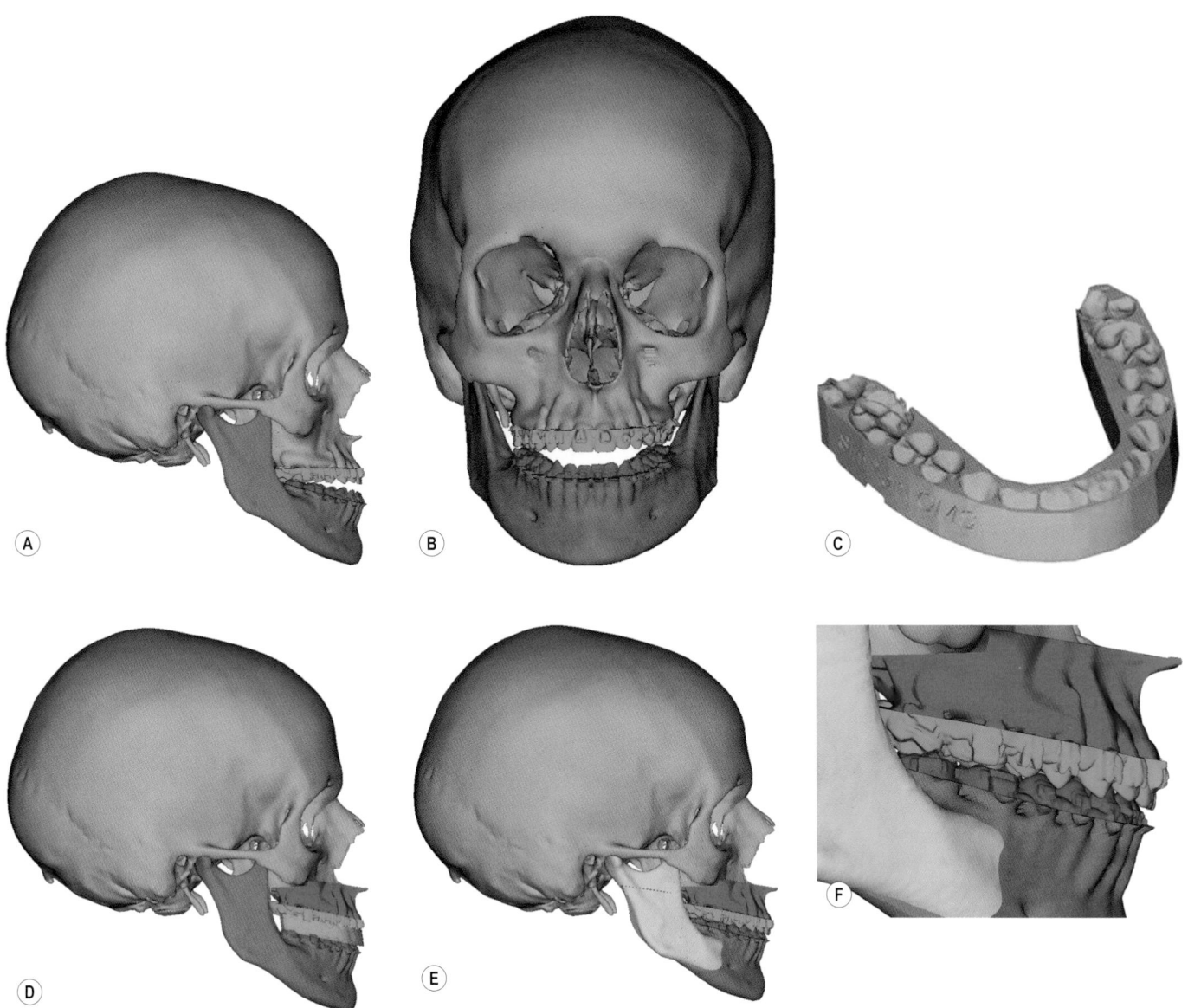

Fig. 30.3 Three-dimensional computed tomography reconstruction of patient with class III malocclusion and anterior open bite. **(A)** Lateral preoperative view. **(B)** Front preoperative view. **(C)** Three-dimensional representation of computer-designed intermediate splint which is fashioned for intraoperative use. **(D)** Lateral view after Le Fort I osteotomy has been simulated with intermediate splint in place. **(E)** Lateral postoperative view after Le Fort I and bilateral sagittal split osteotomies have been simulated with correction of class III malocclusion and anterior open bite. **(F)** Close-up view of predicted postoperative occlusion.

should be positioned so they provide optimal soft-tissue support.

Historically, skeletal movements that expanded the soft tissue of the face were less stable, so posterior and superior movements were preferred. Although these movements were more stable, they resulted in contraction of the facial skeleton with the associated soft-tissue features of premature aging. Since the introduction of rigid fixation systems, osteotomies that result in skeletal expansion have been achieved with a great degree of predictability. An attempt is made to develop a treatment plan that will expand or maintain the preoperative volume of the face. If a superior or posterior (contraction) movement of one of the jaws is planned, an attempt should be made to neutralize the skeletal contraction with an advancement or inferior movement of the other jaw or

the chin. It is important to avoid a net contraction of the facial skeleton as this may result in a prematurely aged appearance.

As skeletal expansion is increased, soft-tissue laxity is reduced and facial creases are softened. These effects increase the definition of the face, creating a more attractive appearance. It has been shown that skeletal expansion is aesthetically pleasing even if facial disproportion is necessary to achieve the expansion.[6] Women with successful careers as fashion models often exhibit slight degrees of facial disproportion and are considered beautiful. The aesthetic benefits the patient receives by expanding the facial envelope frequently justify the small degree of disproportion necessary to achieve them. Even in young adolescent patients who do not show signs of aging, one must not ignore these principles. A successful surgeon will incorporate these principles into the treatment plan of every patient so that, as the patient ages, the signs of aging will be minimized and a youthful appearance will be maintained as long as possible.

A class I occlusion can be achieved with the jaws in a variety of positions. The goal in treatment planning is to use the data from the patient's examination to predict the location of the jaws that will optimize the soft-tissue features of the face. By reducing the emphasis on "normal" values, and increasing the awareness of soft-tissue effects of skeletal movements, it is realized that skeletal disproportion often leads to a more favorable result.

Treatment/surgical technique

General principles and pertinent anatomy

Several principles have broad application to jaw surgery. Blood loss can be substantial in maxillofacial surgery and even small volumes can have significant clinical implications in the pediatric population. Standard techniques of head elevation, hypotensive anesthesia, blood donation, and the preoperative administration of erythropoietin are useful adjuncts to reduce blood loss, especially in the younger population. Before incisions are made, an antimicrobial rinse is helpful to minimize the intraoral bacterial count. A topical steroid is applied to the lips to reduce pain and swelling associated with prolonged retraction. Intravenous steroids may also be useful to reduce postoperative edema.

The occlusion desired may not be the same as maximum intercuspal position. The splint is useful in maintaining the occlusion in the desired location when it does not correspond to maximal intercuspal position. It is easy for the orthodontist to close a posterior open bite, but very difficult to close an anterior open bite with orthodontic treatment. At the end of the case it is important to have the anterior teeth and the canines in a class I relationship without an open bite.

Guiding elastics are useful postoperatively to control the bite. Class II elastics are placed in a vector to correct a class II relationship (maxillary lug is anterior to the mandibular lug). Class III elastics are applied to correct a class III discrepancy. With rigid fixation, the elastics will not correct malpositioned jaws. They serve only to help the patient adapt to the new occlusion. Minor malocclusions can be corrected with postoperative orthodontic treatment.

Certain skeletal movements are inherently more stable than others. Stable movements include mandibular advancement and superior positioning of the maxilla. Movements with intermediate stability include maxillary impaction combined with mandibular advancement, maxillary advancement combined with mandibular setback, and correction of mandibular asymmetry. The unstable movements include posterior positioning of the mandible and inferior positioning of the maxilla. The least stable movement is transverse expansion of the maxilla. Long-term relapse with rigid fixation has not been demonstrated to be clearly superior to nonrigid fixation in single-jaw surgery. However, in two-jaw surgery, rigid fixation results in less relapse. The judgment of the surgeon will dictate the extent to which the facial skeleton can be expanded without resulting in unacceptable relapse.

The maxilla is associated with the descending palatine artery, the infraorbital nerve, the tooth roots, and the internal maxillary artery. The internal maxillary artery runs about 25 mm from the pterygomaxillary junction, and the descending palatal artery descends into the posteromedial maxillary sinus. The infraorbital nerve exits the infraorbital foramen below the infraorbital rim along the mid pupillary line. The maxillary tooth roots extend within the maxilla in a superior direction. The canine has the longest root and is usually visible through the maxillary cortical bone.

The patient who presents with a cleft lip and/or palatal anomaly will have several anatomic differences when compared to an unaffected patient. The maxilla is typically deficient in both the anteroposterior and vertical dimensions. Because midface retrusion can be significant, it frequently appears that the mandible is prognathic, but it is rare that the mandible demonstrates a true prognathia. It is a relative prognathia secondary to the maxillary deficiency. Finally, because of lesser-segment collapse, the dental midline is often deviated toward the cleft side.

Despite having alveolar bone grafting performed, many cleft patients have deficient or missing bone in the region of the alveolus. Persistent palatal fistulas may be present as well. The lateral incisor is frequently missing in these patients and closure of this space must be taken into consideration at the time of treatment planning. If a large fistula is present in the alveolus, modifications of the Le Fort I procedure can be performed to facilitate a tension-free alveolar closure.

The important mandibular structures that may be injured with the mandibular osteotomy are the mental nerve, the inferior alveolar nerve, and the tooth apices. The third branch of the trigeminal nerve enters the mandibular foramen to become the inferior alveolar nerve. It runs below the tooth roots and exits at the level of the first and second premolars through the mental foramen. The region where it is most medial to the outer cortex is located near the external oblique ridge. This is where the vertical portion of the sagittal split osteotomy is made because it affords the largest margin of error.

Le Fort I osteotomy

The first step in any facial osteotomy is satisfactorily securing the nasal endotracheal tube; our preference is a nasal Ring–Adair–Elwin (RAE) endotracheal tube. The vertical position of the maxilla is recorded by measuring the distance between the medial canthus and the orthodontic arch wire. These vertical measurements are absolutely critical. The maxillary vestibule is injected with epinephrine prior to patient preparation. An incision is made with needle tip electrocautery 5 mm above the mucogingival junction from first molar to first molar. A periosteal elevator is then used to expose the maxilla around the piriform rim and infraorbital nerve. Obwegeser toe-in retractors are held by the assistant at the head of the operating table. As the dissection extends laterally, it is important to remain subperiosteal to avoid exposure of the buccal fat pad. A Woodson elevator is used to initiate reflection of the nasal mucosa, and a periosteal elevator is used to complete the dissection of the nasal floor and lateral nasal wall. A double-balled osteotome is used to release the septum from the maxilla and a uniballed osteotome is used to release the lateral nasal wall. The surgeon can insert a finger on

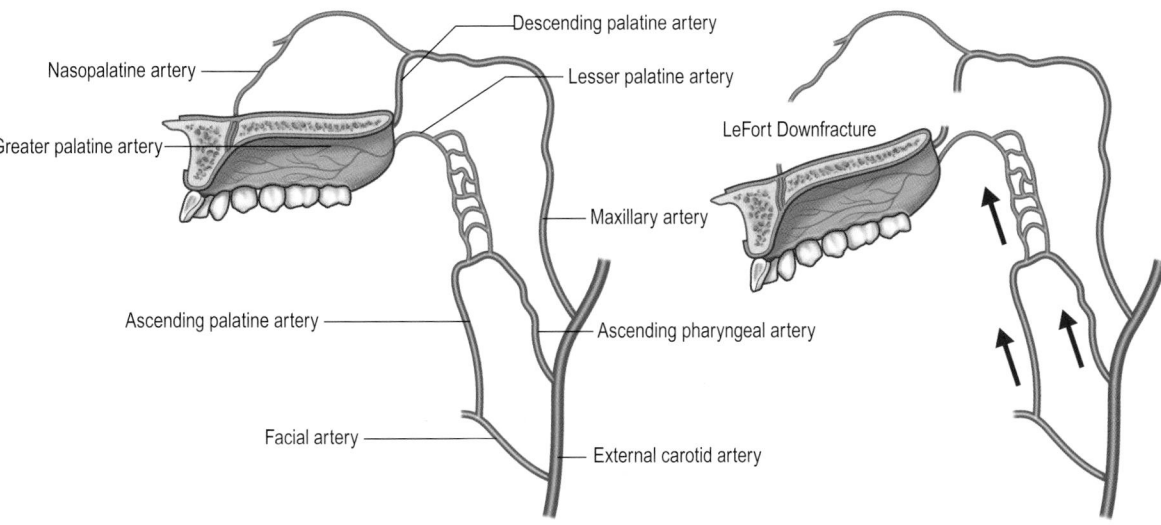

Fig. 30.4 Blood supply to maxilla before (left) and after (right) Le Fort I osteotomy and downfracture. After the nasopalatine and descending palatine arteries are transected, perfusion of the maxillary segment occurs via the lesser palatine artery.

the posterior palate to help feel when the cut is complete. A periosteal elevator is used to protect the nasal mucosa and then a reciprocating saw is used to make a transverse osteotomy from the piriform aperture laterally until the cut descends just posteriorly to the last maxillary molar and drops through the maxillary tuberosity. The cut should be made at least 5 mm above the tooth apices. This distance is determined from preoperative Panorex radiographs. If cuts are complete, the maxilla is downfractured with manual pressure.

An alternative is to use Rowe disimpaction forceps. These fit into the piriform aperture and on the palate to provide increased leverage for the downfracture. Pressure should be applied in a slow steady, controlled fashion, not in a series of quick movements. If the maxilla is not mobilized with relative ease, the cuts are likely not complete and should be re-evaluated. Once the downfracture is complete, a bone hook can be used by the assistant to hold the maxilla down while any remaining bony interferences are removed. The descending palatine arteries will be seen near the posteromedial maxillary sinus. These can be clipped prophylactically without compromising the blood supply to the maxilla *(Fig. 30.4)*. The splint is then used to place the maxilla in its proper position in occlusion with the mandible. Mandibulomaxillary fixation (MMF) is then applied with 26-gauge wires around the surgical lugs. The amount the maxilla will be impacted or elongated was determined in the treatment plan. This distance is added or subtracted from the medial canthal–incisor distance to determine the new vertical position of the maxilla. Four 2-mm plates, usually L-shaped, can be used to secure the maxilla. The MMF is released and occlusion verified prior to closure. If the alar base is wide, an alar cinch can be performed to normalize the width. Lip shortening may also result from closure. A V-Y closure at the central incisor can help alleviate this effect.

In patients who require increased cheek projection, a high Le Fort I osteotomy can be performed. This differs in that the transverse osteotomy is made as high as the infraorbital nerve will allow. If further cheek projection is necessary, bone grafts can be added. In the case of inferior or anterior positioning, gaps between the segments greater than 3 mm should be grafted with autogenous bone, cadaveric bone, or block hydroxyapetite. Finally, if simultaneous expansion of the maxilla is necessary, the maxilla can be split into two or more pieces to allow concurrent expansion.

Surgically assisted rapid palatal expansion

Correction of transverse maxillary constriction is common in patients with repaired cleft palates or those with craniofacial syndromes such as Apert's or Cruzon's syndrome. Such palatal constriction can be addressed in adolescence with non-surgical orthodontic appliances. As the sutures begin to close during late adolescence, relapse rates increase. A multiple Le Fort I osteotomy can be performed to provide simultaneous maxillary expansion, but the degree of relapse is high. In the young adult, the preferred procedure is the surgically assisted rapid palatal expansion (SARPE) procedure. The orthodontist places a palatal expander prior to the procedure. A Le Fort I osteotomy is performed to mobilize the maxilla completely from the upper face. A small osteotome is used to make a thin cut between the roots of the central incisors, and a midline split is completed to the posterior nasal spine. Separation is verified by activating the device. The maxilla is widened until the gingiva blanches and then is relaxed several turns to avoid ischemia. The SARPE offers the best stability for maxillary expansion in the young adult and older patient. Transverse deficiencies of the mandible can be corrected with a similar technique, that of distraction osteogenesis (DO).

Bilateral sagittal split osteotomy

The endotracheal tube placement and epinephrine injection are carried out in a similar fashion to the Le Fort I osteotomy.

The mucosal incision is made with electrocautery about 10 mm from the lateral aspect of the molars and extends from the mid-ramus to the region of the second molar. If insufficient tissue is left on the dental side of the incision, closure is more difficult. A periosteal elevator is used to expose the lateral mandible and the anterior coronoid process in a subperiosteal plane. As the coronoid process is exposed, placement of a notched coronoid retractor may facilitate the dissection. A curved Kocher forcep with a chain can be clamped to the coronoid process and the chain secured to the drapes. To optimize blood supply, subperiosteal dissection is limited to those areas required to complete the osteotomy. A J-stripper is used to release the inferior border of the mandible from the attachments of the pterygomasseteric sling. The eternal oblique ridge and inferior border of the mandible should be exposed. The medial aspect of the ramus is also dissected subperiosteally. The mandibular nerve should be identified. A Seldin elevator is inserted medial to the ramus and protecting the nerve. A Lindemann side-cutting burr is used to make a cut on the medial ramus that is parallel to the occlusal plane and extends about two-thirds of the distance to the posterior ramus.

The osteotomy proceeds from medial to lateral until the burr is in the cancellous portion of the ramus. Mandibular body retractors are then placed and a fissure burr or a reciprocating saw is used to make an osteotomy from the mid-ramus down along the external oblique ridge, gently curving to the inferior border of the mandible. The cuts are verified with an osteotome, and then large osteotomes are inserted and rotated to separate the segments gently. The tooth-baring segment is referred to as the distal segment, and the condylar portion as the proximal segment.

The inferior alveolar nerve should be identified and found in the distal segment. If part of the nerve is located within the proximal segment, it should be gently released with a small curette. After both osteotomies are complete, the distal segment is placed into occlusion and secured by tightening 26-gauge wire loops around the surgical lugs. If a surgical splint is necessary to establish a required occlusion, it is placed between the teeth before MMF wiring. The proximal segments are then gently rotated to ensure they are seated within the glenoid fossa. When each condyle is comfortably seated within the fossa, it is rotated to align the inferior borders of the two segments and secured into position with a clamp. Three lag screws are placed at the superior border of the overlapping segments on each side of the mandible. To ensure that the transbuccal trocar will be placed properly, a hemostat is placed at the proposed screw location and pointed toward the cheek. A small stab incision is made in the skin, and the trocar is placed through the tissue bluntly until the tip enters the oral incision. The trocar is then exchanged for a drill guide, and the 2.0-mm and 1.5-mm drills are used in the lag sequence to make three holes through the overlapping portion of the proximal and distal segments. The screw lengths are measured and the screws inserted. The MMF is released, and the mandible is gently opened and closed to verify the occlusion. If a malocclusion is noted, the most likely etiology is that one or both condyles were not seated properly during application of fixation. The screws should be removed and replaced until the correct occlusion is established. The wounds are irrigated and closed with interrupted 4-0 chromic sutures.

Intraoral vertical ramus osteotomy

A second technique for correcting mandibular prognathism or asymmetry is the intraoral vertical ramus osteotomy. The incision is the same as described above. A subperiosteal dissection is performed from the lateral ramus and a LeVasseur Merrill retractor is used to hold this tissue laterally. An oscillating saw is then used to make a vertical cut from the sigmoid notch to the inferior border of the mandible. The osteotomy must be made posterior to the mandibular foramen on the medial side. The antilingula is a useful landmark, and is found as an elevation on the lateral mandible, indicating the approximate location of the mandibular foramen. After both sides of the mandible are complete, the distal segment is moved into occlusion, making sure that the proximal segments remain lateral to the distal segments posteriorly. Because rigid fixation is difficult to apply, a single wire, or no fixation at all, is used, and the patient remains in MMF for 6 weeks. This osteotomy can be done from an external approach but this incision results in a scar on the neck.

Two-jaw surgery

Moving the maxilla and the mandible in one procedure requires osteotomizing both jaws and precisely securing them into position as determined by the treatment plan. If proper treatment planning, model surgery, and splint fabrication are performed, each jaw should be able to be placed into its desired position with precision. The mandibular bony cuts are started first but terminated prior to osteotomy completion. The maxillary osteotomy is made, and the maxilla is placed into its new position using the intermediate splint. The splint is used to wire the teeth into MMF, allowing for indexing the new position of the maxilla to the preoperative (uncorrected) position of the mandible. With the condyles gently seated, the maxillomandibular complex is rotated so that the maxillary incisal edge is at the correct vertical height. The maxilla is plated into position, the MMF is released, and the intermediate splint removed. Next the mandibular osteotomies are completed, and the distal segment of the mandible is placed into the desired occlusion using the final splint. If the teeth are in good occlusion without the splint, the final splint may not be necessary to establish the desired occlusal relationship. Wire loops secure the occlusal relationship and the rigid fixation is completed as previously described.

Genioplasty

Including a genioplasty in the treatment plan can be a powerful adjunct to mandibular movements, either by offsetting soft-tissue collapse secondary to posterior mandibular repositioning or by augmenting anterior mandibular movement. When performed asymmetrically, a genioplasty may also correct for minor mandibular asymmetries.

After adequate local anesthetic infiltration, the mucosa is incised from canine to canine with needle tip electrocautery 5 mm below the mucogingival junction. The mentalis is transected, being sure to leave enough muscle cuff to allow for reapproximation during closure. Failure to do so can result in a ptotic soft-tissue envelope, or "witch's chin" deformity. Next, the dissection is carried out in a subperiosteal fashion identifying and protecting the mental nerves bilaterally. Using

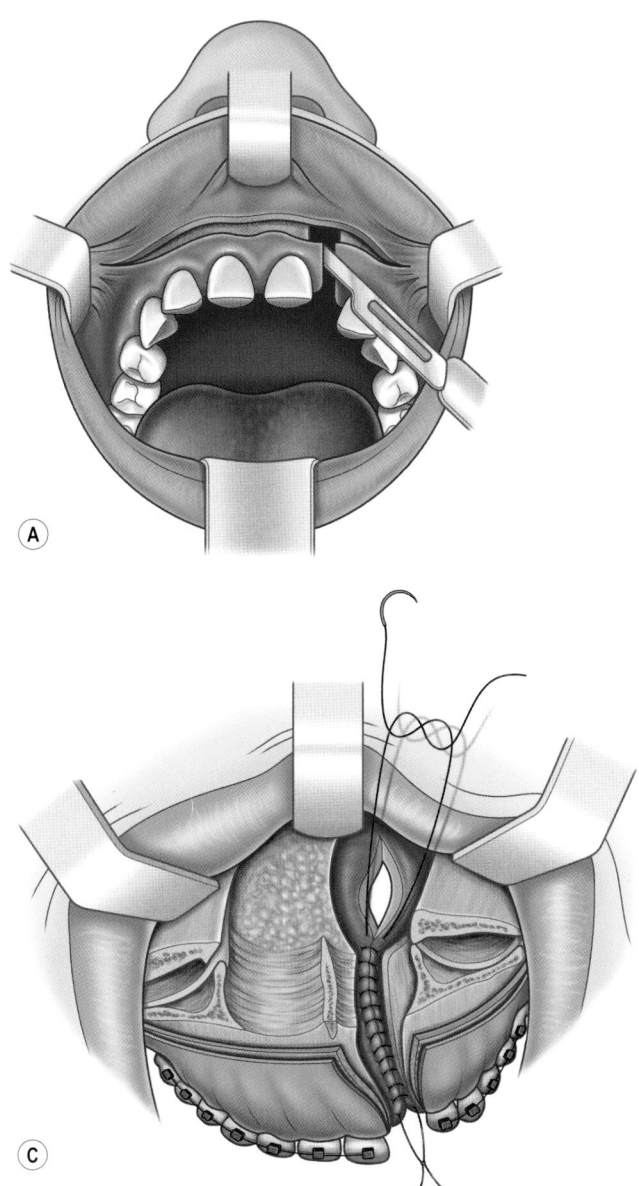

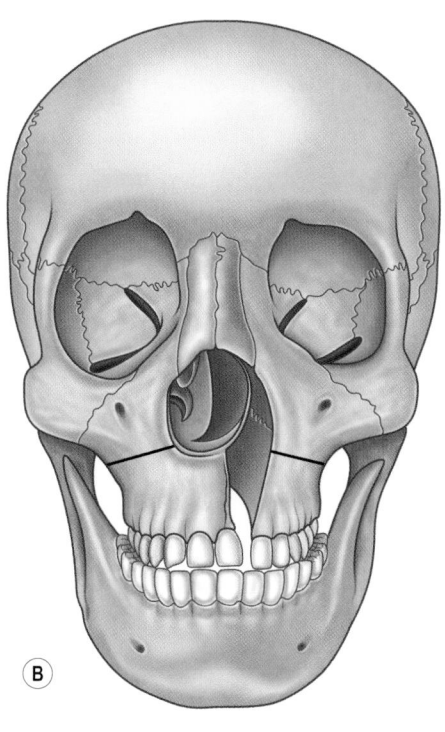

Fig. 30.5 (A) For patients with a unilateral cleft lip, the incision is made similar to a standard Le Fort I osteotomy, except an alveolar dissection is used if supplemental bone grafting or fistula closure is necessary. **(B)** The Le Fort osteotomy allows compression of the maxillary segments if necessary to close a pre-existing fistula. **(C)** Fistula repairs are easier after compression of the segments and exposure of nasal and palatal tissue.

a reciprocating saw, the mandibular midline is gently marked to aid in centric fixation. The transverse osteotomy is made approximately 3 mm below the mental foramina in order to protect the intraosseus course of the mental nerves and the canine tooth roots. The trajectory of the osteotomy can be varied depending on the type of correction required. The mobilized segment is then fixed into the desired position with plates and screws, using the midline mark as a guide. The mentalis is then repaired and the mucosa closed.

Cleft surgery

Orthognathic surgery in cleft lip/palate patients is done similar to noncleft patients with the exception of several important modifications that are necessary to maintain blood supply and assist in fistula closure.

In a unilateral cleft lip patient, the standard maxillary incision can be made with little jeopardy to the premaxillary

blood supply *(Fig. 30.5)*. Each side of the cleft has an incision made similar to that of the alveolar bone graft incision. This allows for a two-layer closure of the palatal and nasal mucosa. If supplemental bone grafting needs to be done at this time, harvested bone can be placed into the alveolar gap after fixation has been applied. If a wide fistula is present, the surgeon can compress the maxillary segments to reduce the size of the alveolar space. This ensures the soft-tissue closure is under minimal tension and the chance of fistula closure is optimized. The canine may now be adjacent to the central incisor, but the restorative dentist can fabricate a prosthetic crown for the canine to make it look like a lateral incisor.

In the bilateral cleft patient, care must be taken not to make the vestibular incision across the premaxilla. The premaxillary blood supply originates from the vomer and the buccal mucosa. Since the vomer will be split, the majority of blood flow to the premaxilla must course from the premaxillary buccal mucosa. A circumvestibular incision that violates this

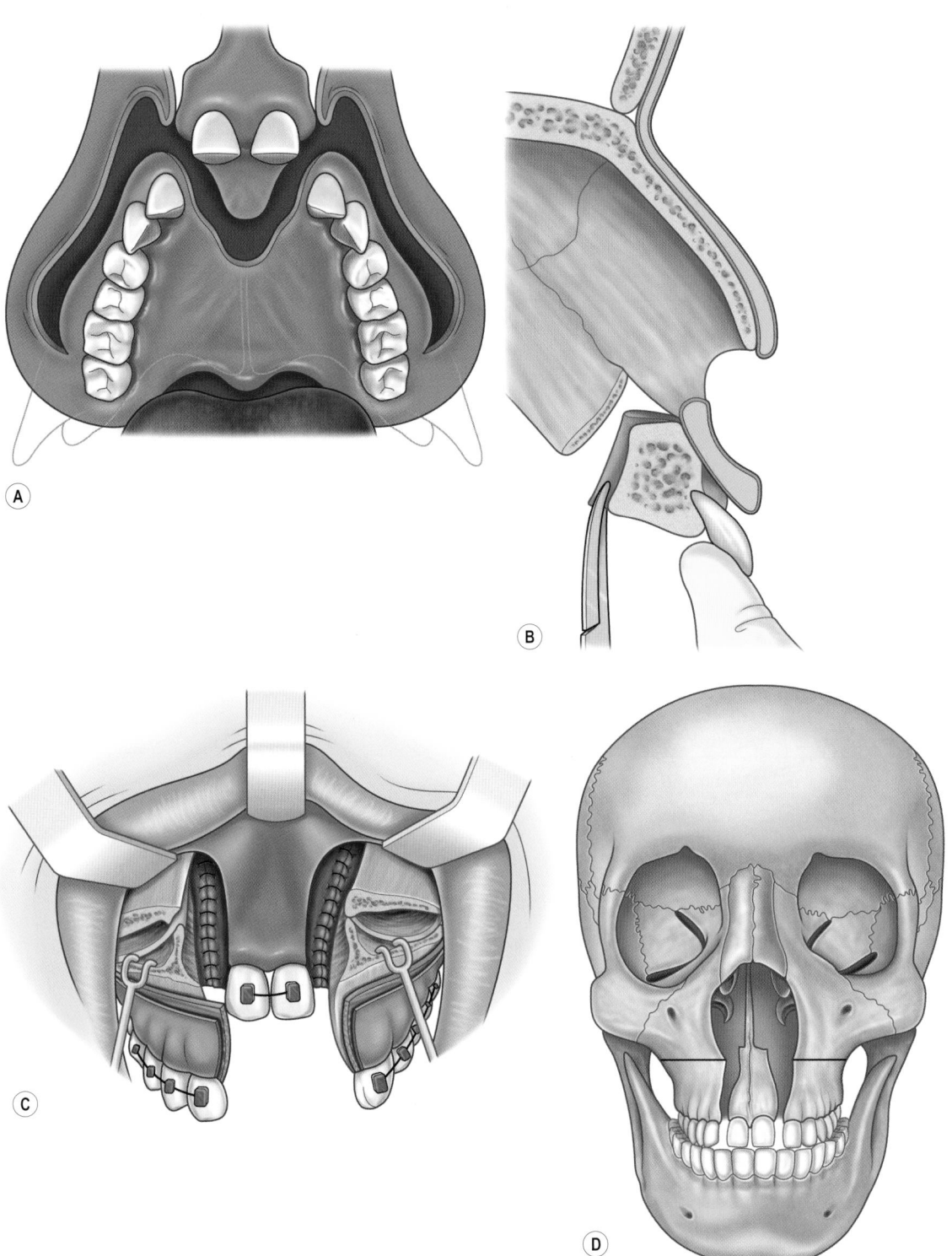

Fig. 30.6 **(A)** For patients with a bilateral cleft, care is taken to avoid incisions across the premaxilla. **(B)** The premaxillary osteotomy is completed from a posterior approach. **(C)** Fistula repairs or supplemental bone grafting can be done at this time. **(D)** Compression of the maxillary segments can be performed if wide fistulas are present.

mucosa will severely jeopardize the blood supply of the premaxillary segment *(Fig. 30.6)*. To minimize the risk of complications, the incision is stopped just lateral to the alveolar cleft on each side. One minimizes reflection of the mucosa from the premaxilla in order to preserve the blood supply. The osteotomy of the premaxillary segment is made from a posterior approach just anterior to the incisive foramen. This allows mobilization of the segment without violation of the buccal mucosa. Similar to the unilateral cleft maxilla, residual fistulae and inadequate alveolar bone may be present. If either is identified, it can be corrected by a two-layer mucosal closure and bone grafting into the alveolar defect. If large gaps are present that may jeopardize fistula closure, the segments can be compressed at the alveolar gaps to reduce tension of the repair. Postoperative orthodontics and prosthetic restorations of the teeth can correct almost any postoperative dental aesthetic irregularities.

Once the incision is made, the mucosa is reflected in a subperiosteal plane to expose the piriform aperture, the zygomatic buttress, and the posterolateral maxilla. A reciprocating saw is used to make a high Le Fort I osteotomy in most cases. A high Le Fort I osteotomy is cut horizontally in a lateral direct line from the piriform aperture to the zygomatic buttress. One takes this line as high as possible while staying at least 5 mm below the inferior orbital foramen. A vertical cut is now made from the lateral edge of the horizontal cut and taken to an area about 5 mm above the tooth root apices. The lateral nasal walls are cut with a uniball osteotome and mallet. The vomer and septum can be reached through the lateral maxillary osteotomies so the mucosa remains preserved. The pterygomaxillary junction can be separated with a 10-mm curved osteotome or the maxillary tuberosity can be cut posterior to the last molar in the arch. The latter choice makes downfracture easier and results in fewer complications. Downfracture is now completed with either digital pressure or application of the Rowe disimpaction forceps. If a wide alveolar fistula is present, the greater and lesser segments can be compressed at the alveolus. The occlusion that would result from segment compression would be evaluated on the dental casts during preoperative model surgery. Any deficiency of alveolar bone can be corrected with supplemental bone grafts after application of fixation, and fistulas can be corrected as well.

The surgical splint is then placed to orient the new position of the maxilla to the mandible. Wire loops (26-gauge) are used to place the patient in maxillomandibular fixation. It is extremely important to make sure the condyles are seated as the maxillomandibular complex is rotated to its new vertical dimension. Generally, cleft patients have vertical maxillary deficiency in addition to the sagittal deficiency. This requires the maxilla to be positioned inferiorly to its new position. If vertical lengthening greater than 5 mm is required, bone grafts are placed between the osteotomy segments to reduce relapse. Rigid fixation is now used to secure the maxilla into its new position. If any instability remains across the maxillary segments, a small plate can be placed across the segments to reduce mobility and maintain the bone graft. Because the osteotomized cleft maxilla results in a multisegment maxilla, the surgical splints are wired in place for 6–8 weeks in order to allow for bone healing.

Distraction osteogenesis

DO is a useful technique to gain large advancements reliably with relatively low rates of relapse. This technique takes advantage of osteoinductive properties of tension and stress across the osteotomy to expand the mandibular or maxillary segment rapidly while allowing the soft tissue to relax over time. Without the need for anatomic reduction or rigid fixation at the time of surgery, DO is often technically easier and faster than traditional orthognathic surgery. Moreover, various methods of distraction allow for precise control in several different vectors to position the osteotomized segment

accurately in space with relation to the cranial base and other dentofacial landmarks.

Basic approaches to commonly encountered problems

The following paragraphs outline basic treatment approaches to commonly encountered dentofacial deformities commonly seen in orthognathic patients.

Skeletal class II malocclusion

Conditions such as Treacher–Collins syndrome, Sickler syndrome, and Pierre Robin sequence are often associated with class II malocclusion, which is almost always caused by mandibular retrognathia and is almost always best treated by mandibular advancement *(Fig. 30.7)*. The mandible is small, and forward positioning is an expansile movement that enhances facial form. If the maxilla is also slightly deficient or in a normal position, one may consider a bimaxillary advancement to enhance further facial soft-tissue definition, especially in more mature patients. If the malocclusion is minimal and there is little pre-existing dental compensation, one may choose to have the orthodontist intentionally compensate the dentition to correct the occlusion and avoid surgery. In contrast, if the malocclusion appears minimal but there is dental compensation, the skeletal discrepancy will be more significant after the orthodontist decompensates the dentition, and the patient may be a good surgical candidate.

Skeletal class III malocclusion

A class III malocclusion may be treated by advancing the maxilla, posteriorly positioning the mandible, or by combining these procedures. It is important to consider the contributions of the mandible and the chin separately as each may require different treatments to achieve aesthetic goals. If some posterior positioning of the mandible is necessary, one may advance the maxilla to counteract the skeletal contraction produced from posteriorly positioning the mandible. Additionally, the patient may benefit from an advancement genioplasty, counteracting any skeletal contraction occurring from a mandibular setback. As in the class II patient, a minor malocclusion with minimal dental compensation may be corrected with orthodontic treatment alone. In contrast, a minor malocclusion with dental compensation may become a significant malocclusion after dental decompensation, and the patient will be a good surgical candidate.

Maxillary constriction

Patients can present with a maxilla that is narrow in a transverse dimension. Maxillary constriction may occur as an isolated finding or as one of multiple abnormalities. Up to about 15 years of age, the orthodontist can usually expand the maxilla nonsurgically with a palatal expander. If orthopedic expansion cannot be done, a SARPE can be performed. If the maxilla requires movement in other dimensions, a two-piece (or multipiece) Le Fort I osteotomy can be performed to place the maxilla in its new position while simultaneously achieving transverse expansion *(Fig. 30.8)*.

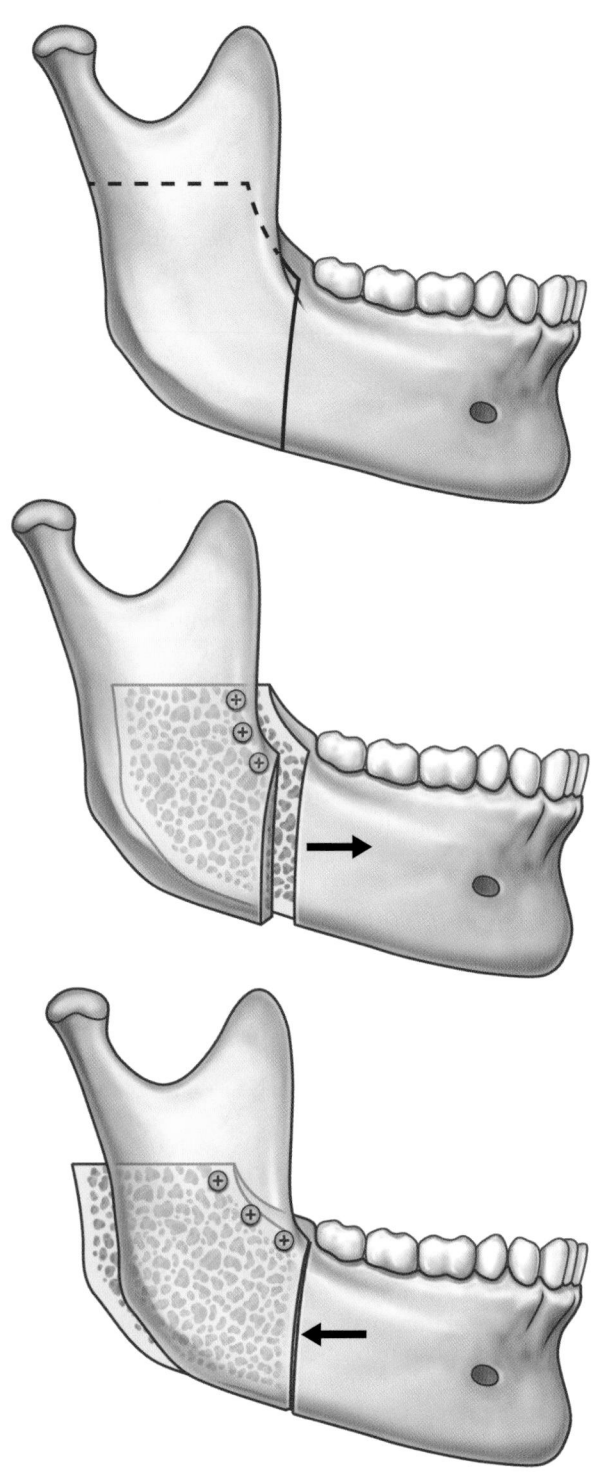

Fig. 30.7 Mandibular sagittal split osteotomies demonstrating mandibular advancement and mandibular setback.

Apertognathia

An anterior open bite is caused by a premature contact of the posterior molars and is commonly seen in patients with syndromic craniosynostoses such as Apert or Crouzon syndromes. The recommended treatment is a posterior impaction

of the maxilla. By reducing the vertical height of the posterior maxilla, the mandible can come into occlusion with the remaining mandibular teeth. Posterior maxillary impaction does not necessarily result in incisor impaction; the posterior maxilla is simply rotated clockwise and upward using the incisal tip as the axis of rotation. Therefore, incisor show should not be affected. If a change in incisor show is also desired, the posterior impaction is performed, and then the whole maxilla can be inferiorly positioned or impacted to its new position *(Fig. 30.9)*.

Vertical maxillary excess

Vertical maxillary excess is typically associated with lip incompetence, mentalis strain, and an excessive degree of gingival show (long-face syndrome). The treatment approach is to impact the maxilla to achieve the proper incisor show with the lips in repose. Impaction, however, may result in skeletal contraction, so the surgeon must consider anterior repositioning of the jaws to neutralize the associated adverse soft-tissue effects. As the maxilla is impacted, the mandible rotates counterclockwise (with respect to a rightward-facing patient) to maintain occlusion. This rotation results in anterior positioning of the chin and is called mandibular autorotation. The opposite occurs if the maxilla is moved in an inferior direction. In this case, the chin point rotates in a clockwise direction, resulting in posterior positioning of the chin point. It is important to note these effects on the cephalometric tracing during treatment planning because a genioplasty may be required to re-establish proper chin position.

Short lower face

A short lower face is marked by insufficient incisor show and/or a short distance between subnasale and pogonion. Treatment is aimed at establishing a proper degree of incisor show. The facial skeleton should be expanded to the degree that provides optimal soft-tissue aesthetics. As the maxilla is inferiorly positioned, resulting clockwise mandibular rotation leads to a posterior positioning of the chin. The surgeon needs to assess the new chin position preoperatively on the cephalometric prediction tracing to determine if an advancement genioplasty will be necessary to counter the effects of mandibular clockwise rotation.

Postoperative care

Postoperative care of patients undergoing orthognathic surgery is paramount to a successful surgical outcome and a satisfied patient and family. Close adherence to an oral hygiene regimen, including regular tooth brushing and chlorhexidine mouth rinses, will minimize the risk of postoperative infection, as will a short course of antibiotics targeted toward common mouth flora. Additionally, steps taken to reduce swelling, including ice, head elevation, and anti-inflammatory medication such as Solu-Medrol, will greatly improve patient comfort. A soft diet for at least the first 3 weeks postoperatively will help reduce the risk of malunion or hardware failure. As well, guiding elastics are usually employed for the first 2–3 weeks.

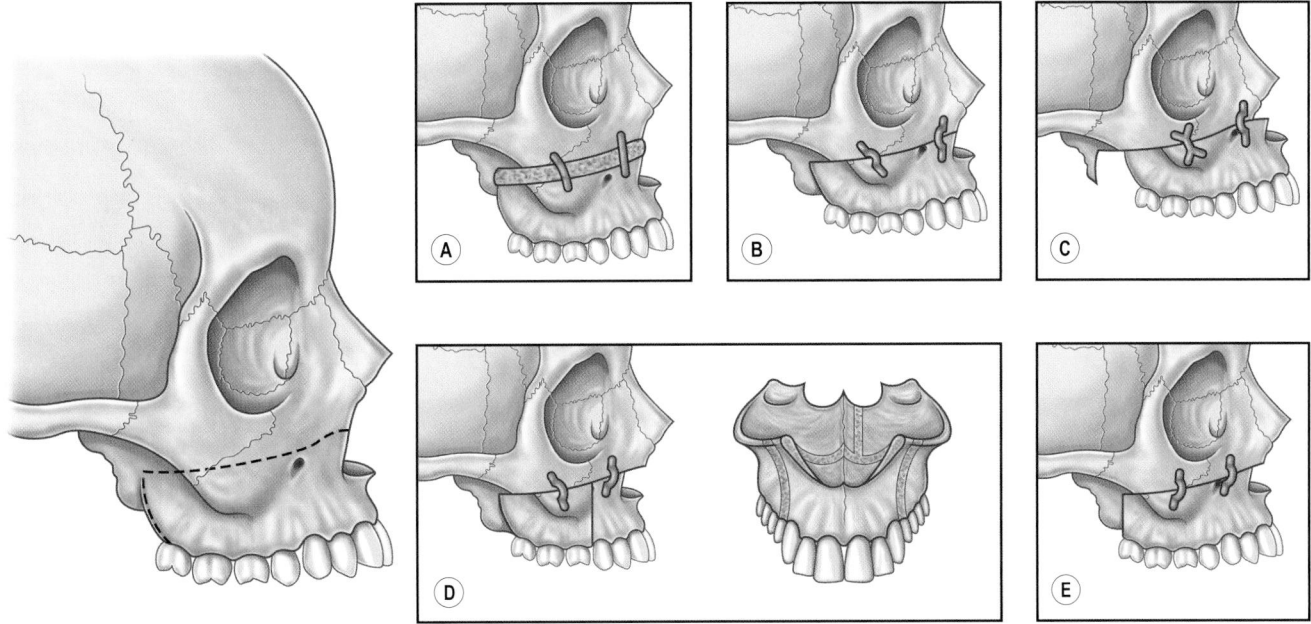

Fig. 30.8 (A–E) Le Fort I osteotomies demonstrating maxillary advancement, impaction, setback, and multipiece Le Fort.

Outcomes, prognosis, and complications

Accurate assessment of orthognathic surgical outcomes is essential to maintaining safe practices, maximizing patient satisfaction, and effectively evaluating an ever-changing field. Indeed, this importance is echoed in the ways investigators have analyzed postoperative results. These range from measurement tools such as three-dimensional CT scanning and volumetric analyses (used to evaluate postoperative changes in bony and soft tissues immediately and over time) to questionnaires assessing patient-reported satisfaction scales and quality of life. While there is currently no universally accepted tool to demonstrate patient outcomes after orthognathic surgery accurately and reliably, with reasoned and reasonable expectations on the part of the patient, family, and surgeon alike, orthognathic surgery can result in high levels of satisfaction from both a functional and aesthetic level.

Of particular importance to the cleft and craniofacial population is the effect of orthognathic surgery on speech. It is generally accepted that the etiology of velopharyngeal insufficiency (VPI) in the cleft patient is due to the malalignment or shortening of the palatal musculature, as well as growth, development, and/or surgical sequelae that can lead to abnormal structural relationships. Given the intricate attachment of the muscular apparatus of the velum to the maxilla, it follows that movement of the maxilla can change the preoperative velopharyngeal function.

Janulewicz *et al.* performed a retrospective study of the change in velopharyngeal function of 54 cleft lip and palate patients who underwent maxillary advancement with or without a mandibular setback procedure over a 21-year period.[7] As summarized in *Table 30.1*, their study shows a

Table 30.1 Comparison of preoperative and postoperative speech variables

Total number of patients: 54	Pre-op evaluation % (n)	Post-op evaluation % (n)
VP function: competent	42% (23)	18% (10)
VP function: borderline competent	36% (20)	40% (22)
VP function: borderline incompetent	9% (5)	22% (12)
VP function: complete VPI	13% (7)	20% (11)
Normal nasality	40% (22)	40% (22)
Mild hypernasality	18% (10)	29% (16)
Moderate hypernasality	4% (2)	15% (8)
Severe hypernasality	4% (2)	2% (1)
Hyponasality	33% (18)	15% (8)
Reduced sibilant IOAPs	26% (14)	35% (19)
Reduced fricative IOAPs	16% (9)	26% (14)
Reduced plosive IOAPs	6% (3)	22% (12)
Anterior dentition errors	64% (35)	47% (26)
Mean speech score	2.46	4.24

VP, velopharyngeal; VPI, velopharyngeal incompetence; IOAP, intraoral air pressure.
(Reproduced from Janulewicz J, Costello BJ, Buckley MJ, et al. The effects of Le Fort I osteotomies on velopharyngeal and speech functions in cleft patients. *J Oral Maxillofac Surg.* 2004;62:308–314.)

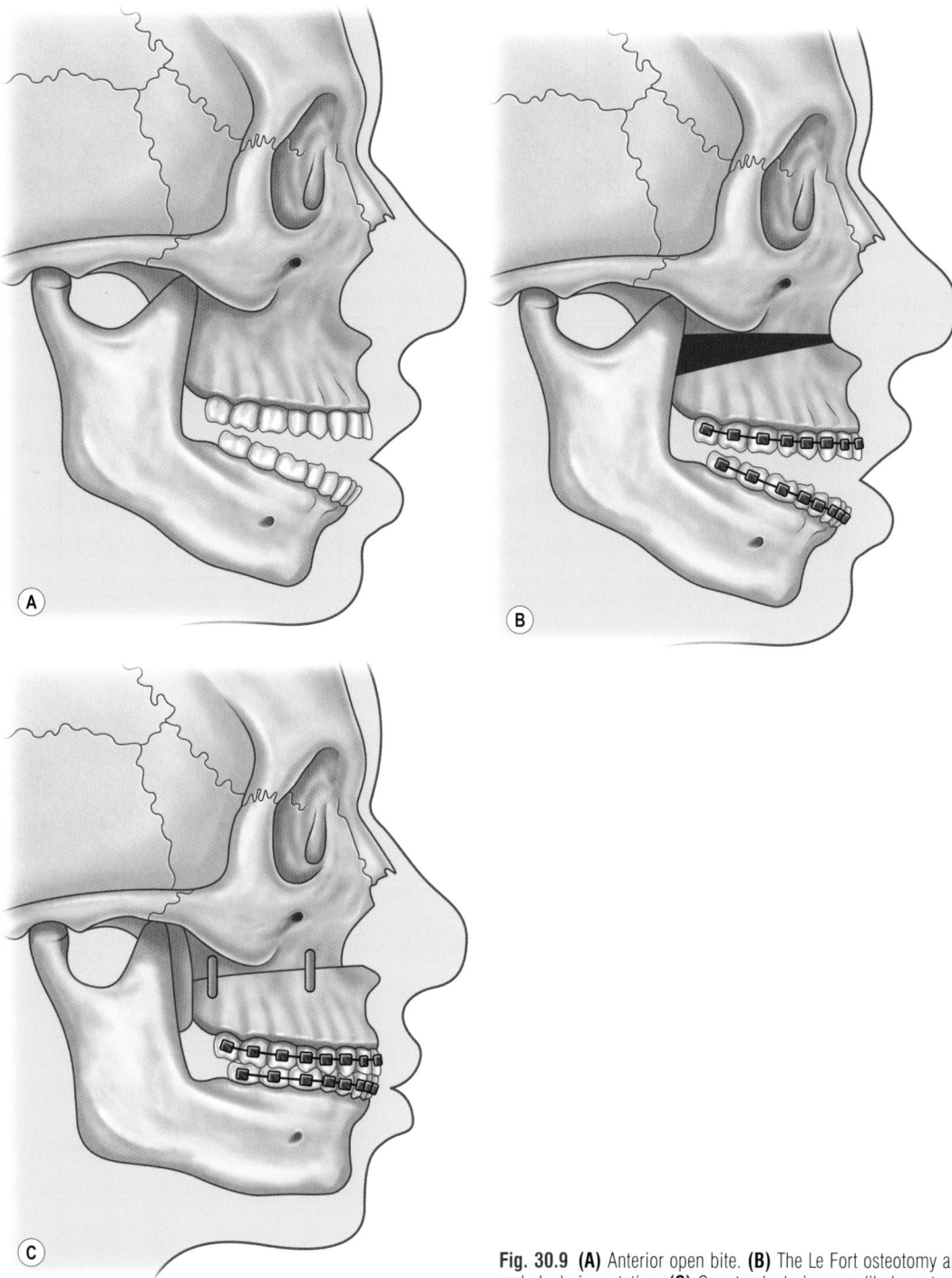

Fig. 30.9 (A) Anterior open bite. **(B)** The Le Fort osteotomy allows posterior impaction of the maxilla and clockwise rotation. **(C)** Counterclockwise mandibular autorotation closes the anterior open bite.

decline in competent velopharyngeal function (from 42% to 18%), an increase in both borderline incompetence (from 9% to 22%) and complete VPI (from 13% to 20%). The authors also noted that the quality of speech declined, as evidenced by the increase in overall objective speech score from 2.46 to 4.24 (the higher the score, the worse the speech). In contrast, the authors noted that articulation defects improved, although the improvement did not achieve statistical significance. Preoperatively 84% (46 patients) had at least one articulation defect as compared to 73% (40 patients) postoperatively.

Other published studies have shown similar results or no change in VPI function following jaw surgery. In their study, Phillips et al.[8] showed that the extent of anteroposterior movement of the maxilla is unrelated to velopharyngeal deterioration and is not a useful predictor. In their study of 26 cleft patients (16 unilateral complete and 9 bilateral complete cleft lips and palates), Phillips et al. demonstrated that all patients with perceived hypernasal speech preoperatively had hypernasality after advancement. Furthermore, 9 of 12 patients who had preoperative nasopharyngoscopy showing borderline or inadequate VP closure developed postoperative VPI. Based on these results, Phillips *et al.* conclude that preoperative assessment can predict postoperative speech and velopharyngeal function.

In summary, it appears that, while a positive effect on articulation might be achieved by orthognathic surgery, it might be at the expense of velopharyngeal function. Further prospective, controlled studies would be helpful in elucidating the relationships between maxillary advancement and speech.

Posnick and Tompson[9] performed a retrospective study evaluating relapse in cleft patients who had undergone orthognathic surgery between 1987 and 1990. They found that there was no significant difference in outcome between patients who had maxillary surgery alone and those who had operations on both jaws. Furthermore, the outcome did not vary significantly with the type of autogenous bone graft used or the segmentalization of the osteotomy. All 35 patients included in the study underwent a modified Le Fort I maxillary osteotomy with varied degrees of horizontal advancement, transverse arch widening, and vertical change. Eleven of the 35 patients also required mandibular surgery, consisting of sagittal split osteotomies. In 13 of 35 patients a pharyngoplasty was in place at the time of maxillary Le Fort I osteotomy. The results of the study are summarized in *Table 30.2*.

The mean horizontal advancement achieved for the group was 6.9 mm; 5.3 mm was maintained 1 year later (mean relapse 1.6 mm). In 11 of the 35 patients the relapse was less than 1.0 mm. For the 13 patients who had a pharyngoplasty at the time of the Le Fort I osteotomy, the mean horizontal advancement was 8.2 mm immediately after the operation and 6.5 mm 1 year later. Stability of the vertical displacement was also evaluated. No maxillary vertical change was necessary in 12 of 35 patients. The mean vertical displacement of the maxilla in patients who underwent vertical displacement was 2.1 mm; 1.7 mm was maintained 1 year later. The authors concluded that neither horizontal nor vertical relapse was related to the extent of movement. The overjet from the cephalometric radiographs at the 1-year postoperative interval was maintained in all patients, whereas a positive overbite was maintained in only 30 of 35 patients (85%).

Other investigators have found a correlation between relapse and the degree of advancement. To identify factors associated with relapse after orthognathic surgery in the cleft lip/palate patient, Hirano and Suzuki[10] performed a retrospective study on 58 cleft patients who underwent orthognathic surgery over a 10-year period. From their study, they identified the following factors related to relapse:

1. Horizontal advancement: In their series the mean horizontal relapse was 24.1% of the mean advancement. There was significant correlation between extent relapse and advancement. The authors report that complete surgical mobilization of the maxilla is important in preventing relapse.

2. Vertical displacement (inferior positioning): In their study the mean inferior vertical elongation was 3.0 mm with a relapse of 2.1 mm. Based on their study, the authors recommend a 2-mm overcorrection in inferior positioning of the maxilla.

3. Rotation, clockwise or counterclockwise: The authors report that most of their surgical rotation was lost and relapse was seen in both clockwise and counterclockwise rotations. They suggest overcorrection to mitigate the effects of relapse.

4. Type of cleft: Orthognathic surgery in a bilateral cleft patient was more likely to result in relapse, according to their study. They attribute the increase in likelihood of relapse to increased scarring of palatal tissues and multiple missing teeth.

5. Previous alveolar bone grafting: Although studies have reported the value of alveolar bone grafting in establishing stability of advancement and minimizing relapse, the study by Hirano and Suzuki[10] found no association between alveolar bone graft and the rate of relapse in unilateral cleft lip and palate patients.

6. Number of missing teeth: The study by Hirano and Suzuki[10] also found no correlation between the number of missing teeth and relapse although the authors stress that multiple missing teeth can compromise the stability of the occlusion.

7. Type of orthognathic surgery: There was no difference in the relapse rate between patients undergoing maxillary surgery alone and those who underwent two-jaw surgery.

While both relapse and worsening VPI can occur with the movements performed in orthognathic surgery, they are a result of primary deficiencies in the soft tissue due to prior scar formation as well as the underlying deformity and thus are under only limited surgeon control. There are several complications, however, on which the surgeon can have a direct effect.

Improper positioning of the jaws is noted by malocclusion or an obvious unaesthetic result. Special care must be taken to ensure proper condyle positioning during fixation of the mandibular osteotomy. If malocclusion results from improper condyle position during fixation, it must be removed and reapplied. The same is true for improper indexing of the splint. For this reason, it is wise to verify splint fit prior to surgery. Meticulous treatment planning prior to surgery minimizes splint-related problems.

Measures to reduce the chance of an unfavorable mandibular split should always be employed. Removal of mandibular

Table 30.2 Patients with unilateral cleft lip and palate undergoing Le Fort I osteotomy with miniplate fixation: mean horizontal/vertical displacement and relapse

Time after surgery	Effective horizontal mean advancement (mm)	Effective vertical mean change (mm)
1 week	6.9 ± 2.6	2.1 ± 2.4
6–8 weeks	6.3 ± 2.6	1.9 ± 2.1
1 year	5.3 ± 2.7	1.7 ± 2.0

(Reproduced from Posnick JC, et al. Cleft-orthognathic surgery: the unilateral cleft lip and palate deformity. In: Craniofacial and maxillofacial surgery in children and young adults, Vol. 2, chapter 34. WB Saunders, 2001.)

third molars 6 months prior to the osteotomy allows time for sockets to heal, decreasing the chance of a bad split. If the segments do not appear to be easily separating, the surgeon should verify that the osteotomies are complete. Excessive force that could increase the chance of an uncontrolled mandibular split should be avoided. If an unfavorable split occurs, the segments can be plated to re-establish normal anatomy, and the proximal and distal segments can then be secured into the desired position with rigid fixation.

Bleeding may occur from any area, but most commonly from the descending palatine artery in the maxilla. This can be stopped with packing or by placing a hemoclip on the artery. Bone wax is useful for bleeding bony edges.

Nerve damage is rare, but can occur. The nerves associated with these procedures are the infraorbital, inferior alveolar, and mental nerve. If a transaction is witnessed, coaptation with 7-0 suture nylon suture is recommended. The patient should be informed that there is approximately a 70% chance of some paresthesia immediately after surgery, but permanent changes are seen in only 25% of patients.

The incidence of nonunion or malunion is rare after surgery. If a malunion occurs, the jaw may need to be osteotomized again to move it into proper position. A nonunion requires secondary bone grafting to establish osseous continuity.

Secondary procedures

The need for secondary procedures in orthognathic surgery is uncommon, especially when careful patient selection and preoperative evaluation are employed. However, orthognathic surgery rarely can completely resolve the preoperative dentofacial deformity. Indeed, maxillary and mandibular movements, in addition to altering occlusal relationships and skeletal proportions, may highlight features previously de-emphasized by malocclusion. In such cases, procedures such as rhinoplasty, fat grafting, or malar augmentation may help restore facial harmony.

It is important to realize that underlying issues related to the primary cleft or craniofacial disorder may not be fully addressed with orthognathic surgery. For example, patients with repaired clefts who undergo orthognathic surgery to address a class III malocclusion may still need surgeries to complete their dental rehabilitation. Bone grafting and vestibuloplasty may be as necessary after orthognathic surgery as before.[11] Likewise, in the setting of persistent edentulous spaces, osseointegrated implants which are resistant to orthopedic movements should be utilized only after jaw surgery and postoperative orthodontics have determined final tooth positions.

References

1. DeLuke DM, Marchand A, Robles EC, et al. Facial growth and the need for orthognathic surgery after cleft palate repair: literature review and report of 28 cases. *J Oral Maxillofac Surg*. 1997;55:694–697; discussion 7–8.

2. Obwegeser H. Surgery of the maxilla for the correction of prognathism. *SSO Schweiz Monatsschr Zahnheilkd*. 1965;75:365–374.

3. Enlow EH. Craniofacial growth and development: normal and deviant patterns. In: Posnick JC, ed. *Craniofacial and maxillofacial surgery in children and young adults*. Philadelphia: W B Saunders; 2000:22–35.

   In this comprehensive chapter, the author provides a detailed account of the development of the craniofacial skeleton, under both normal conditions and in disease states. It highlights the temporal relationship between growth of the cranial skeleton and the facial skeleton as well as the differences among genders and in specific conditions craniofacial abnormalities.

4. Mao JJ, Wang X, Kopher RA. Biomechanics of craniofacial sutures: orthopedic implications. *Angle Orthod*. 2003;73:128–135.

5. Tompach PC, Wheeler JJ, Fridrich KL. Orthodontic considerations in orthognathic surgery. *Int J Adult Orthodon Orthognath Surg*. 1995;10:97.

6. Selber JC, Rosen HM. Aesthetics of facial skeletal surgery. *Clin Plast Surg*. 2007;34:437–445.

   This article highlights the changing paradigm in orthognathic treatment planning from one based on pure cephalometric analysis to one encompassing an evaluation of the aesthetic facial soft-tissue proportions.

7. Janulewicz J, Costello BJ, Buckley MJ, et al. The effects of Le Fort I osteotomies on velopharyngeal and speech functions in cleft patients. *J Oral Maxillofac Surg*. 2004;62:308–314.

8. Phillips JH, Klaiman P, Delorey R, et al. Predictors of velopharyngeal insufficiency in cleft palate orthognathic surgery. *Plast Reconstr Surg*. 2005;115:681–686.

   This article is a retrospective examination of 26 patients who underwent orthognathic advancement. Assessments of speech and velopharyngeal function before and after orthognathic surgery and the role of nasopharyngoscopy are detailed.

9. Posnick JC, Tompson B. Cleft-orthognathic surgery: complications and long-term results. *Plast Reconstr Surg*. 1995;96:255–266.

   This article is a retrospective evaluation of 116 patients with cleft palate who underwent orthognathic surgery to correct malocclusion. The authors report a mean follow-up of 40 months and describe common complications and outcomes.

10. Hirano A, Suzuki H. Factors related to relapse after Le Fort I maxillary advancement osteotomy in patients with cleft lip and palate. *Cleft Palate Craniofac J*. 2001;38:1–10.

    This article is a retrospective study of 58 patients (42 unilateral cleft and 16 bilateral cleft) who underwent orthognathic surgery to correct maxillary hypoplasia. The authors report a mean follow-up period of 2.5 years. Based on cephalometric and statistical analyses, the authors elucidate factors related to relapse after Le Fort I maxillary advancement.

11. Baker S, Goldstein JA, Seiboth L, Weinzweig J. Posttraumatic maxillomandibular reconstruction: a treatment algorithm for the partially edentulous patient. *J Craniofac Surg*. 2010;21:217–221.

31

Pediatric facial fractures

Joseph E. Losee and Darren M. Smith

SYNOPSIS

- Traumas that would likely produce fractures in adults often do not in children due to intrinsic anatomical factors.
- In addition to the unique anatomy of the pediatric patient, future growth and development must be accounted for when addressing these injuries.
- A growing appreciation of the pediatric craniofacial skeleton's resilience and the utility of late orthodontics is making practitioners more comfortable with conservative strategies.
- In deciding between operative and conservative management of pediatric facial fractures, the practitioner is essentially weighing the risk of growth disturbance against the benefit of precise reduction and rigid fixation.
- Craniofacial development, along with the resilience of the pediatric skull and supporting structures, often facilitates a less invasive approach to managing these complex injuries.

 Access the Historical Perspective section online at
http://www.expertconsult.com

Introduction

Facial fractures are relatively uncommon in children. Traumas that would likely produce fractures in adults often do not in children due to intrinsic anatomical factors such as larger fat pads, decreased pneumatization of sinuses, increased skeletal flexibility secondary to more malleable bone stock, and compliant sutures. Parental supervision also prevents many would-be fractures.[1] The same structural characteristics of the pediatric craniofacial skeleton that thwart fracture are responsible for the unique injury patterns that are observed when bony injury does occur. Pediatric facial fracture evaluation begins with the ABCs of trauma and proceeds through clinical and radiographic assessment, culminating in conservative or operative management. In addition to the unique anatomy of

the pediatric patient, future growth and development must be accounted for when addressing these injuries. A conservative approach is advised whenever feasible, and long-term follow-up is mandatory to ensure adequate outcomes and inform future practice. The objective of this chapter is to provide the reader with an understanding of the anatomical and growth-related factors that make pediatric craniofacial fracture repair a unique entity, and to offer a discussion of specific treatment modalities in this context.

Basic science/disease process

Incidence

Pediatric facial fractures comprise less than 15% of all facial fractures and increase in frequency with age.[4,5] One review found 54% of fractures to occur in the skull, one-third in the upper and middle thirds of the face, and the remainder in the lower third.[6] In the authors' cohort, orbital fractures were the most common across all age groups.[7] Pediatric orbital fractures represent anywhere from 3% to 45% of facial fractures.[8–11] Midface fractures are uncommon (10.4% of facial fractures in the authors' series), likely secondary to the protection of the midface by the prominent forehead and mandible in children, in addition to the robust anatomy of this region.[12] Zygomaticomaxillary complex (ZMC) fractures are the most common of the rare midface fractures.[1] Nasal fractures comprise up to 50% of pediatric facial fractures.[8,13] Nasal and maxillary fractures were the most common osseous injury among infants in the US National Trauma Databank, while mandible fractures supplanted these in older teenagers, with mandible fractures being the overall most common facial fracture.[5] Mandible fractures are often cited as the most common pediatric facial fracture, accounting for 20–50% of all pediatric facial fractures.[8,11,14,15] The prominence of this structure explains these findings. Of mandible fractures in the authors' series (n = 179), condylar head and subcondylar fractures were most common (48%).[16] Anatomical distribution varies with age;

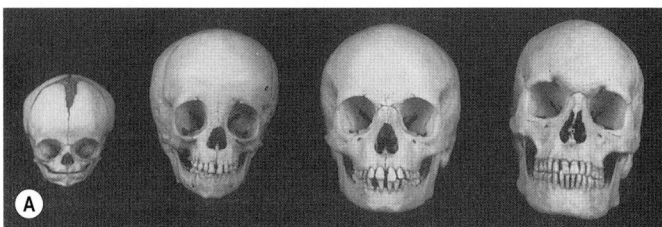 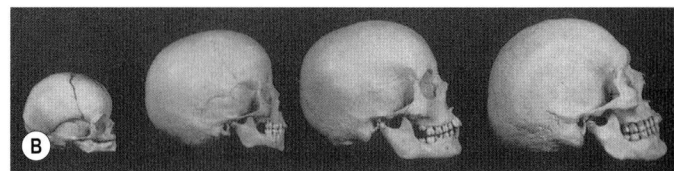

Fig. 31.1 **(A)** Frontal view and **(B)** side view of the growing craniofacial skeleton. Note the decreasing cranial-to-facial ratio and increasing facial prominence. (Reproduced from Mathes S, Hentz V. Plastic surgery, 2nd ed. Philadelphia, PA: Elsevier; 2006.)

condylar fracture incidence decreases, while body and angle fractures increase.[17]

Demographics

In the authors' series,[7] there was a 69%:31% male-to-female ratio. A total of 62.6% of patients were admitted to hospital, and 18.6% to an intensive care unit. In all, 35.9% of facial fractures underwent operative management. Half (48%) of fractures were sustained by patients 12–18 years of age; 6–11-year-olds accounted for 32% of fractures and children under 5 years of age contributed 20% of fractures.[7] Similar patterns have been observed by other authors.[1,4,5,18] Per the US National Trauma Databank, motor vehicle collision (MVC), assault, and falls were the most common cause of facial fracture across all age groups.[5] In the context of MVC, unrestrained children were significantly more likely to sustain facial fractures: 65–70% of children involved in all-terrain vehicle or bicycle accidents were not wearing helmets.[5] In the authors' series, the cause of injury varied by age: violence, assault, and MVC were the most common causes of injury in 12–18-year-olds, while activities of daily living caused the most fractures in 0–5-year-olds. Orbital fractures were the most common fracture type across all age groups. Naso-orbital ethmoid (NOE) fractures were the least common.[7]

Associated injuries

Facial fractures are high-energy injuries, and as such are heavily associated with other injuries. The authors conducted a unique review of all patients with *International Statistical Classification of Diseases 9* (ICD-9) codes indicative of facial fracture presenting to the emergency department of their center (*n* = 782). Children were included regardless of whether they were treated operatively or conservatively, or as inpatients, outpatients, by plastic surgery, or by any of the other services handling facial traumas.[7] The goal was to improve patient capture and remove selection bias that may otherwise have been present due to admission status, treating specialty, or need for operative intervention. In this series, excluding soft-tissue injuries, brain trauma was the injury most commonly associated with facial fractures across all age groups. A total of 55% of patients with facial fractures had associated injuries: 81% of these were considered "serious" and included cardiovascular, cervical spine, or intra-abdominal trauma. Some 47% had neurological injuries (60% of these were concussions), and 3% had ophthalmologic injuries, including blindness. In all, 1.4% died as a result of their injuries.

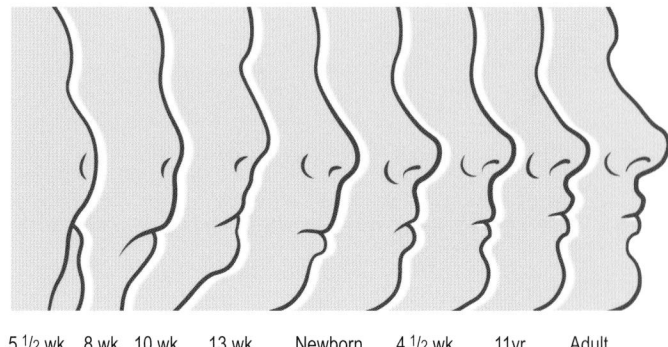

5 1/2 wk   8 wk   10 wk   13 wk   Newborn   4 1/2 wk   11yr   Adult

Fig. 31.2 Schematic of growing face, in profile. Note decreased protection of face afforded by cranium, and increasing prominence (and exposure to injury) of mandible.

Growth and development

Craniofacial development is the culmination of a complex and incompletely understood interaction between intracellular processes, intercellular signaling, and environmental influences. Cranial-to-facial ratio decreases with maturity from 8:1 at birth to 2:1 in adulthood[19] *(Figs 31.1 and 31.2)*. The cranium grows secondary to the brain, which triples in size during the first year of life.[19–22] This is a continuous process that is 25% complete at birth, 75% complete at 2 years, and 95% complete by 10 years. Facial growth is sporadic: it is 40% complete at 3 months, 70% at 4 years, 80% by 5 years, pauses until puberty, and resumes until 17 years of age.[19] The upper face grows secondary to brain and ocular development; midfacial growth follows the development of the nasal capsule and dentition. Orbital growth is complete by 6–8 years and nasal growth is largely complete by 12–14 years. The palate and maxilla achieve two-thirds adult size by 6 years.[23] At birth, the mandible is formed by two bones joined by cartilage at the symphysis, ossifying within the first year of life. The majority of permanent teeth erupt by 12 years of age. The gonial angle becomes increasingly acute, the ramus and body enlarge, and the distance between the dentition and the inferior mandibular border increases. Cortical bone replaces tooth buds as the primary component of mandibular volume. The inferior alveolar nerve is displaced superiorly to rest midway from the superior and inferior mandibular borders. The mental foramen migrates to rest ultimately beneath the first or second permanent premolar.[24]

The decreased bone mineral content of the infant skull yields increased tolerance to force without fracture; fractures

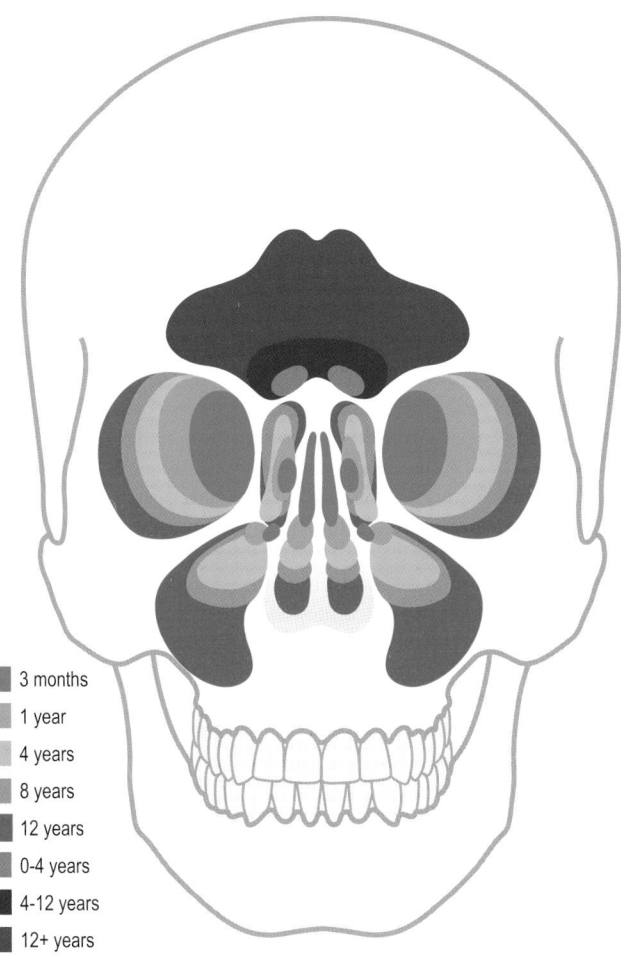

3 months

1 year

4 years

8 years

12 years

0-4 years

4-12 years

12+ years

Fig. 31.3 Pneumatization of the sinuses. Fracture patterns evolve with sinus development.

that do occur are more likely to be incomplete "greensticks." In addition to mineralization, sinus pneumatization and dental eruption are responsible for the evolving craniofacial load-bearing capacity and subsequent fracture patterns *(Figs 31.3 and 31.4)*. The maxillary sinus is aerated at 12 years of age; the frontal sinus is not aerated until adulthood. Oblique craniofacial fractures precede the Le Fort patterns seen in adulthood as an incompletely pneumatized frontal sinus transmits energy directly from the site of impact to the supraorbital foramen and then to the orbit and zygoma. In one large study, Le Fort fractures were only seen in patients greater than 10 years of age.[18] Forehead fractures in children may develop into growing skull fractures (documented in 0.6–2% of pediatric skull fractures).[25] These lesions develop secondary to brain pulsations transmitting through occult dural disruptions and driving a growing bony diastasis. Another consequence of the underdeveloped frontal sinus is an increased incidence of isolated orbital roof "blow-in" fractures.[26] Blindness also occurs with increased frequency due to the direct transmission of force to the orbit.[26] Trapdoor fractures are more common secondary to greater bony elasticity.[27] Children tend to have fractures without enophthalmos or vertical orbital dystopia (VOD), likely secondary to more robust supporting structures existing in this population. Enophthalmos and VOD require composite injury to bone, ligaments, and periosteum allowing for an increase in intraorbital volume *(Fig. 31.5)*.

Isolated midface fractures are rare in children as this region is shielded by the prominent forehead and mandible.[28] Palatal splits are more common secondary to incomplete ossification of the hard palate. These injuries represent significant potential for growth disturbances secondary to the presence of growth centers in the maxilla and nasal capsule and because the midface is retruded relative to the cranium at this age.[8,29,30] Incomplete zygomaticofrontal (ZF) suture union leads to fracture dislocations characterized by inferior displacement of the zygoma and orbital floor, further contributing to oblique fracture patterns.[23] Oblique fracture patterns are also encouraged

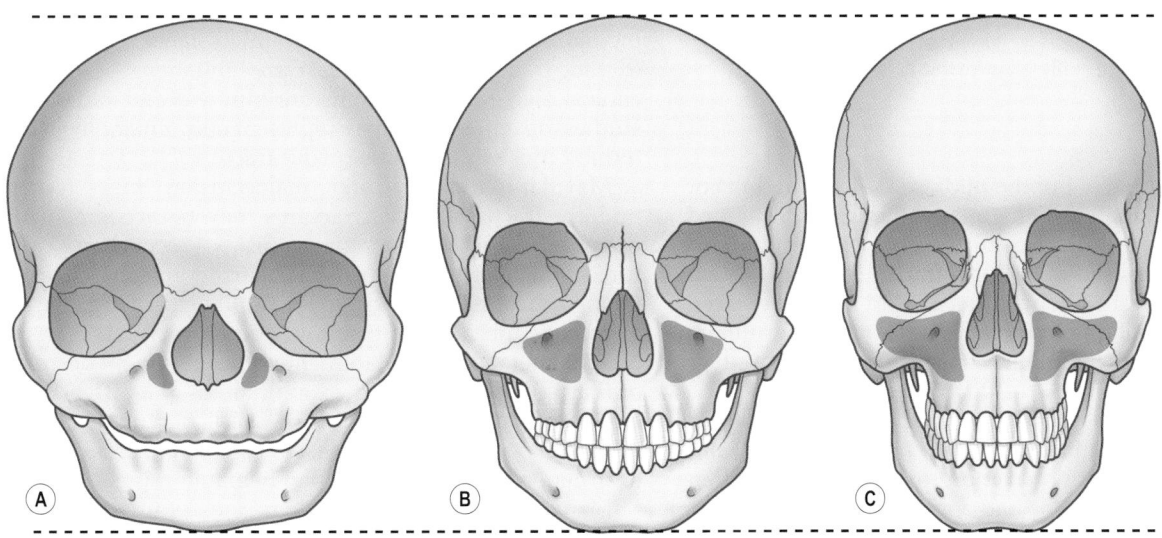

Fig. 31.4 (A–C) Development of the maxillary sinuses. The maxillary sinus plays an important role in determining how traumatic force will be transmitted through the midface.

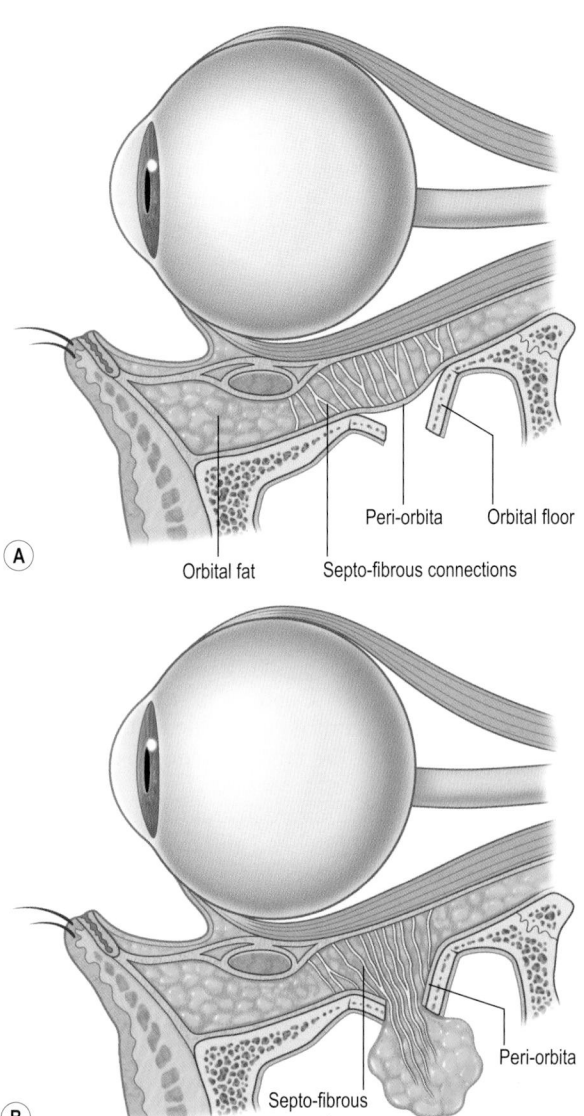

Fig. 31.5 Sagittal section of the orbit. **(A)** Orbital floor fracture with preserved orbital volume secondary to intact periorbita. **(B)** In contrast, the herniation of orbital contents secondary to disrupted periorbita in association with a floor fracture. It is the injury depicted in **(B)** that is required for enophthalmos or vertical orbital dystopia.

by the underdevelopment of the midface skeleton and major buttress systems. Until 10 years of age, the underdeveloped maxillary sinus transmits force to the alveolus, resulting in alveolar fractures instead of Le Fort I fractures. Le Fort IIs are replaced by unilateral NOE fractures. Le Fort IIIs are replaced by multifragment oblique craniofacial fractures.[18] The authors have consistently seen oblique fracture patterns in their patients *(Figs 31.6–31.8)*.[31]

The less mineralized, more compliant pediatric mandible is more resistant to comminuted fractures. Condylar head and subcondylar fractures are seen more frequently in children due to incomplete ossification and a relatively weak condylar neck *(Figs 31.9 and 31.10)*. While certain regions of the mandible are classically highlighted as growth centers (e.g., condyles and lingual tuberosity), condylectomy and differential masticatory strain studies point to a more diffuse,

dynamic process by which morphological change proceeds via coordinated bone deposition and resorption.[24] Heightened awareness of potential growth disturbance and temporomandibular joint (TMJ) ankylosis is, however, justified in the setting of condylar fractures given an incomplete understanding of these injuries' implications.

Diagnosis and presentation

The importance of a consistent approach to craniofacial trauma cannot be overemphasized. The first step in treating acute craniofacial injuries is ensuring that the trauma ABCs have been completely addressed. The craniofacial surgeon's most direct interaction with this process will likely be in assuring a secure airway in cases where anatomy has been severely distorted. While infants are obligate nasal breathers, their nasal airway is relatively narrow and thus easily obstructed.[32] Meticulous hemostasis must be achieved given a child's relatively decreased blood volume and ability to mask significant losses with normotension prior to rapid decompensation.[32,33] Hypothermia is also more likely to be problematic given a child's increased surface area-to-volume ratio.[32]

A systematic physical exam is performed. Eyelid hematoma, hearing loss, hemotympanum, and cranial nerve (CN) palsy may herald skull base fractures. Exophthalmos and inferior globe displacement may represent a supraorbital or roof fracture. Ptosis may be present secondary to levator paralysis. Orbital trauma will likely be accompanied by periorbital echymosis and subconjunctival hematoma. Extraocular muscle restriction may cause diplopia *(Figs 31.11 and 31.12)*. Forced duction is required to rule out muscle entrapment in obtunded patients. Superior orbital fissure syndrome (internal and external ophthalmoplegia (CN II, IV, VI paralysis), proptosis, and CN V paresthesia) and orbital apex syndrome (superior orbital fissure syndrome with blindness secondary to CN II involvement) must be emergently addressed *(Fig. 31.13)*. In nasal-orbital-ethmoid fractures, a bowstring test (palpation of the bony medial canthal attachment on lateral distraction of the lower eyelid) will assess the integrity of the medial canthal tendon. Intraorbital distance is assessed to exclude traumatic telecanthus. Gaze limitations – even if other clinical signs and symptoms are minimal and radiographic studies are equivocal – may represent entrapment in an entity termed the "white-eyed blowout fracture."[34]

Maxillary mobility and malocclusion may represent midface fractures. ZMC fractures may be accompanied by upper buccal sulcus hematoma, epistaxis secondary to a fractured maxillary sinus, a preauricular depression, cheek flattening, or lateral canthal dystopia. Impingement of a depressed zygomatic arch on the coronoid process may yield trismus. Medial lateral wall displacement with subsequent decrease in orbital volume may yield exophthalmos *(Fig. 31.14)*. Nasal deviation, compressibility of the nasal dorsum, and septal hematoma must be appreciated on exam. Nasal airway obstruction may represent septal hematoma.

Many pediatric patients are in mixed dentition; aside from wear facets, preinjury dental records are the surgeon's only ally in establishing preoperative occlusion. Occlusive splints can be fabricated based on these materials. Signs and symptoms consistent with mandible fracture include malocclusion,

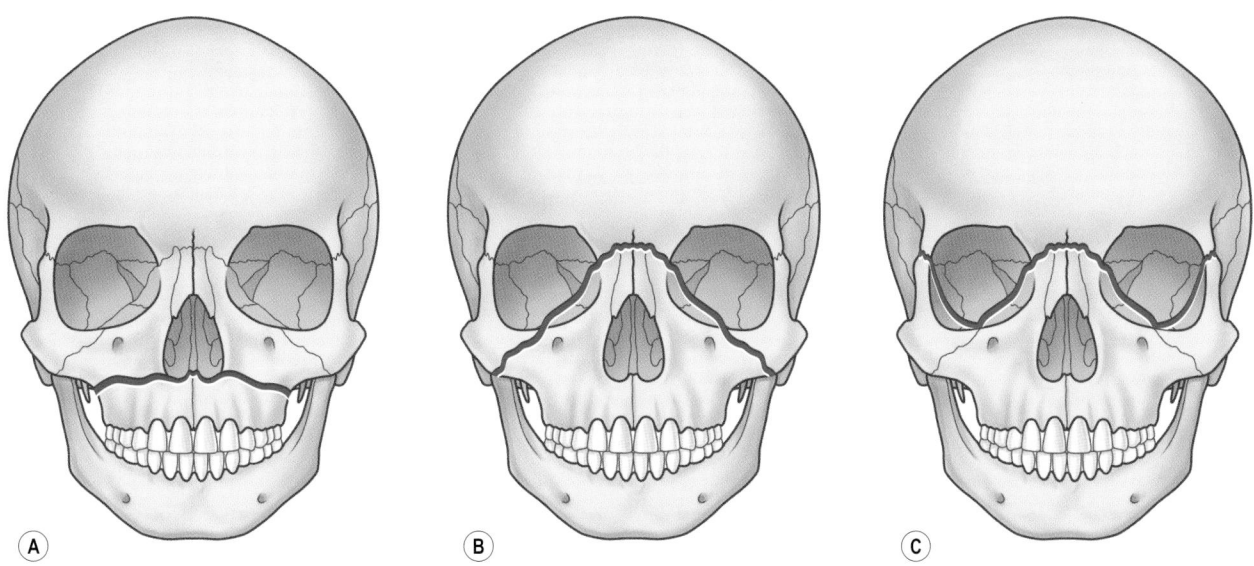

Fig. 31.6 These are the classic Le Fort fracture patterns described in adult craniofacial fractures: **(A)** Le Fort I; **(B)** Le Fort II; **(C)** Le Fort III. Children exhibit distinct fracture patterns, as described in the text and demonstrated in *Figures 31.7 and 31.8*.

drooling, trismus, decreased maximal incisive opening, discomfort on mandibular excursion against symphyseal pressure, and dental step-off. The TMJ can be evaluated by palpating the external auditory canal while ranging the jaw. Certain patterns of malocclusion are associated with specific fractures. Anterior open bite often results from bilateral condylar fractures secondary to loss of mandibular height and premature posterior contact. Unilateral posterior condylar fracture may result in contralateral posterior open bite. Mandible fractures must trigger suspicion for cervical spine fractures given the proximity and high-energy nature of these injuries.

Patient selection

In deciding between operative and conservative management of pediatric facial fractures, the practitioner is essentially weighing the risk of growth disturbance against the benefit of precise reduction and rigid fixation. Below is a fracture-specific discussion of anatomical and developmental factors to aid the practitioner in making informed decisions on a fracture-by-fracture basis. While some favor delaying intervention until swelling resolves, others note the pediatric craniofacial skeleton's resilience: loose fragments may adhere within 3–4 days of injury.[23] Converse advocated prompt repair in the 1960s.[35] The authors maintain that if the decision is made to operate, this should be done early so long as the degree of swelling is not prohibitive.

Indications for operative management of cranial base and skull fractures include significant displacement, cerebrospinal fluid (CSF) leak persisting despite conservative measures, intracranial hematoma, deformed facial contour, frontal-lobe contusion with mass effect, and growing skull fracture.

In adults, there are fairly straightforward criteria for operative management of orbital fractures (fracture area greater than 1 cm^2 or if over 50% of an orbital wall is involved).[36–40] Other indications include superior orbital fissure syndrome and frontal-temporal-orbital fractures resulting in exophthalmos. Operative indications in children are less clear; it is likely that enophthalmos and VOD are less likely in children secondary to more robust orbital periosteum and supporting ligaments *(Fig. 31.5)*. Stronger supporting structures may render open reduction, internal fixation (ORIF) less necessary in these fractures. The authors analyzed operative necessity in the context of a three-group orbital fracture classification system ($n = 81$): type 1, pure orbital fractures (limited to the orbit without extension to adjacent bones); type 2, craniofacial fractures (oblique fractures extending from the skull into the orbital roof and face); type 3, orbital fractures contributing to described patterns (impure blowout, ZMC, NOE) *(Table 31.1)*.[41] Type 1 fractures were nonoperative (88%) unless there was evidence of acute enophthalmos, VOD, or muscle entrapment on forced duction. Type 2 fractures were managed conservatively and tracked with serial scans until an absolute operative indication was encountered (17% were ultimately operative). Type 3 fractures were more likely (72%) to require operative intervention. Overall, 23 (28.3%) orbits were managed operatively.[41] Success with this conservative strategy is evidenced by a low rate of adverse outcomes.

Conservative management is indicated for minimally displaced and greenstick midface fractures, especially in younger children. Displaced and unstable fractures require ORIF. Nasal fractures warrant immediate intervention if a septal hematoma is evident. While closed reduction is often inadequate secondary to insufficient release of tension on the septum, cartilages, and bony pyramid, aggressive open treatment in children has significant potential to affect facial growth adversely. Therefore a closed reduction is usually offered to children with definitive open management delayed until skeletal maturity.

Dentoalveolar fractures are usually nonoperative, while displaced mandibular fractures require operative

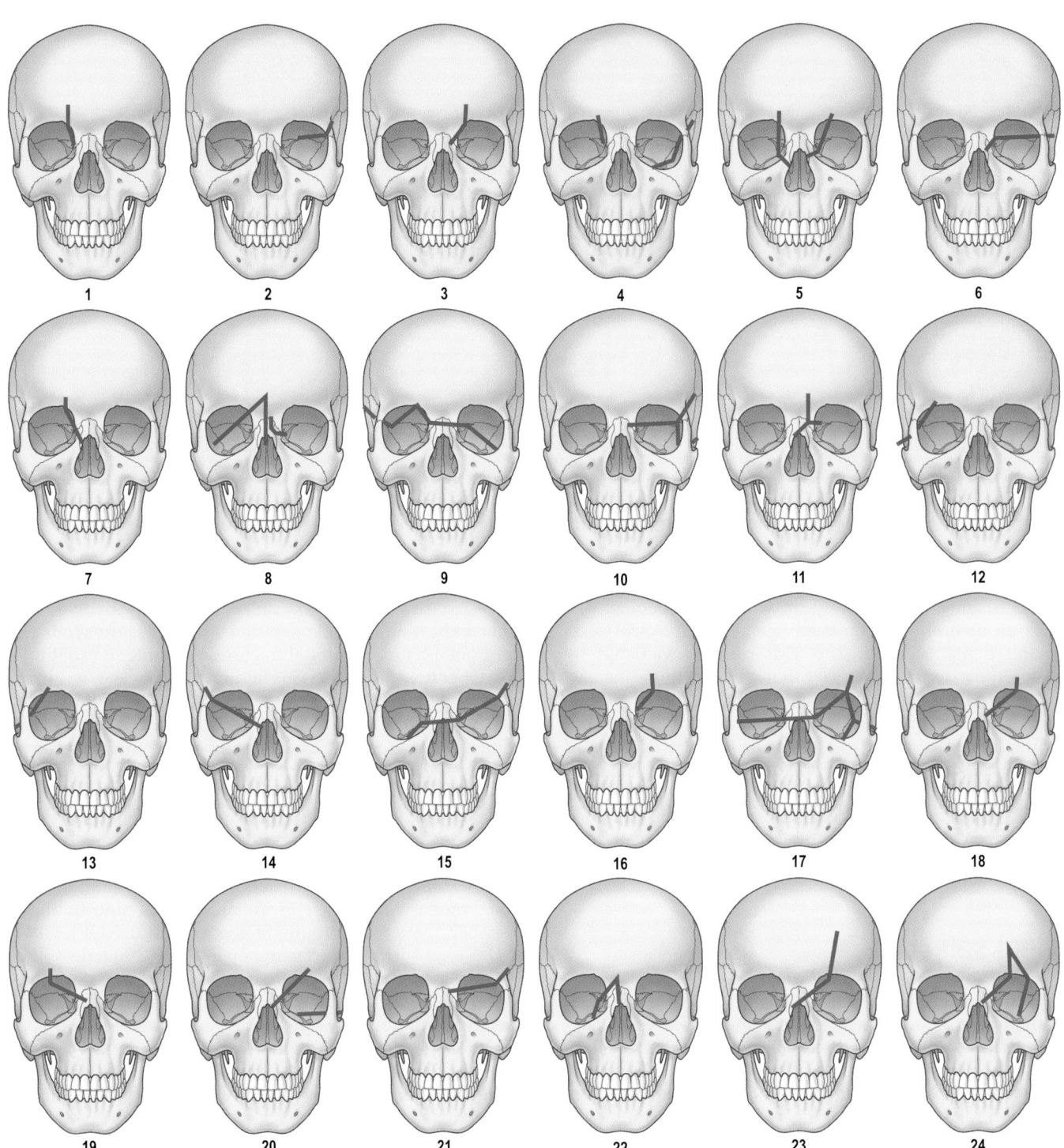

Fig. 31.7 Schematic examples of the oblique craniofacial fracture patterns encountered in children.

management. Conservative management is warranted if these fractures are isolated, minimally displaced, and occlusion is preserved.[17] Assuming preserved occlusion, the operative indications for condylar fractures are more controversial. The pediatric condyles ("vascular bony sponges"[42]) are regarded as growth centers, sensitive to disruptions of blood supply and morphology with resultant susceptibility to ankylosis and altered mandibular development. Intracapsular injuries should be managed conservatively to minimize growth

disturbance and TMJ ankylosis; the pediatric mandible has the potential to undergo restitutional remodeling (condylar head regeneration). Some argue for a more aggressive approach to dislocated condylar neck fractures in older children since the condyles are less likely to regenerate in children greater than 7 years of age, and may require eventual osteotomy and cartilage grafting for TMJ function and normalization of occlusion.[43,44] In the case of bilateral neck fractures in the older patient, ORIF of one side is reasonable, with a short

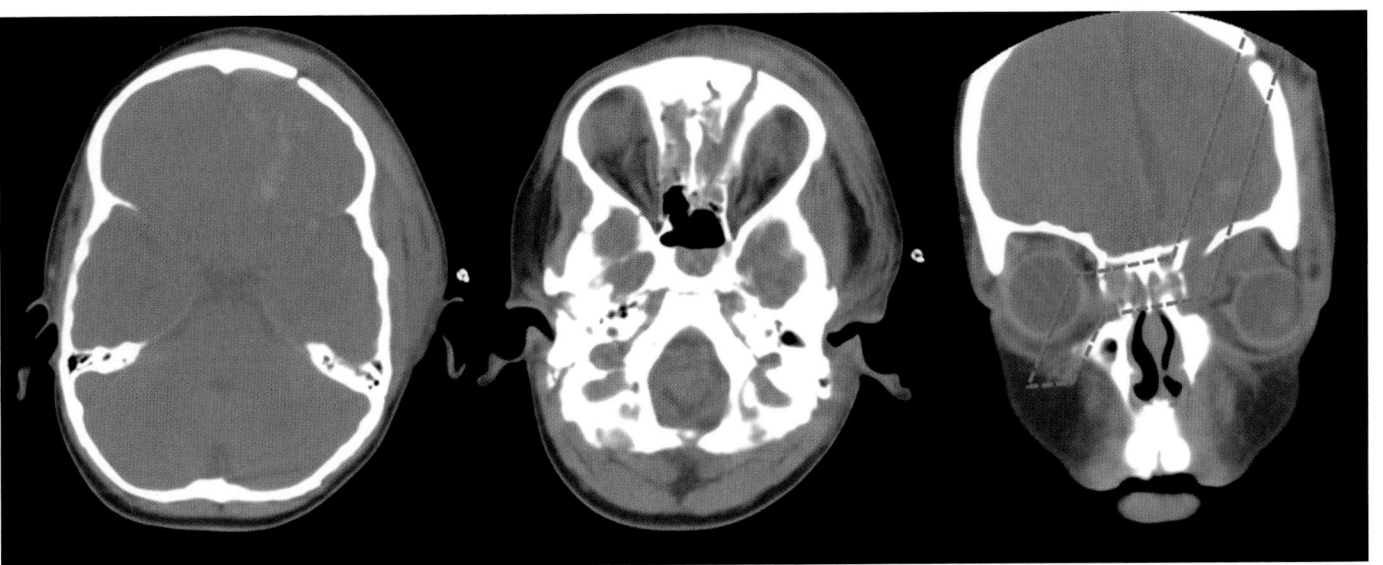

Fig. 31.8 Computed tomography (CT) scans in the axial plane demonstrate an oblique fracture at the level of the cranium (left) and cranial base (center). Right, the CT scan represents a sagittal reconstruction of the same patient, with the course of the oblique fracture outlined in red.

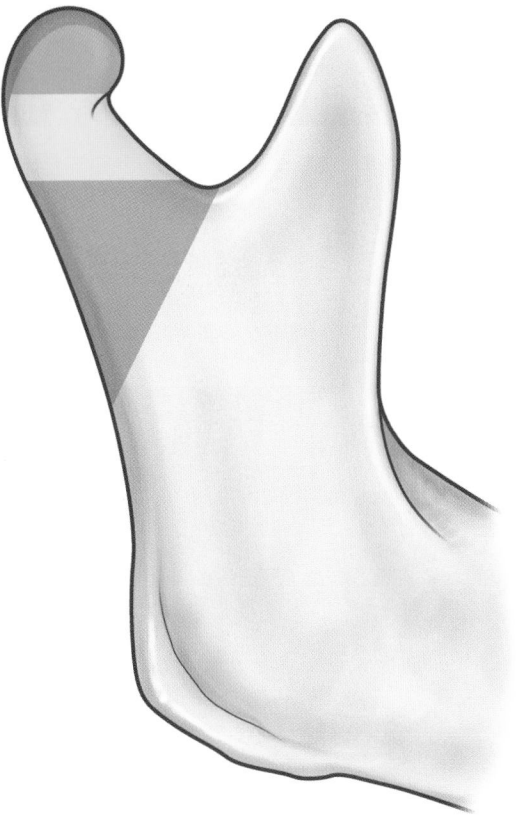

Fig. 31.9 Anatomical vocabulary pertaining to the mandibular condyle. The condylar head is green (except its articular surface, which is blue), the condylar neck is yellow, and the subcondylar region is orange. Vague terminology in reference to these structures often causes confusion in the clinic and in the literature.

Table 31.1 The authors' orbital fracture classification system	
Type 1	**Pure orbital fractures**
1a	Floor fractures
1b	Medial wall fractures
1c	Roof fractures
1d	Lateral wall fractures
1e	Combined floor and medial wall fractures
Type 2	**Craniofacial fractures**
2a	Growing skull fractures
Type 3	**Orbital fractures associated with common fracture patterns**
3a	Fractures of the floor and inferior orbital rim
3b	Zygomaticomaxillary fractures
3c	Naso-orbitoethmoid fractures
3d	Other fracture patterns

course of intermaxillary fixation. Other indications for open management include a foreign body in the TMJ, failure to normalize occlusion with closed management, and a condyle displaced into the middle cranial fossa. Every effort should be made to avoid open management for intracapsular fractures, high condylar neck fractures, coronoid fractures, and any fracture in which there are no barriers to motion and baseline occlusion is preserved.[17] A condylar head fracture in the presence of another mandible fracture is an indication for ORIF of the other fracture to allow for early TMJ motion. Of the 96 consecutive patients in the authors' series, 53% underwent operative management.[16] Each child undergoing surgery had a 64.7% chance of an adverse outcome as compared to 45% in children receiving conservative therapy. However, none of the adverse outcomes recorded (i.e., limited

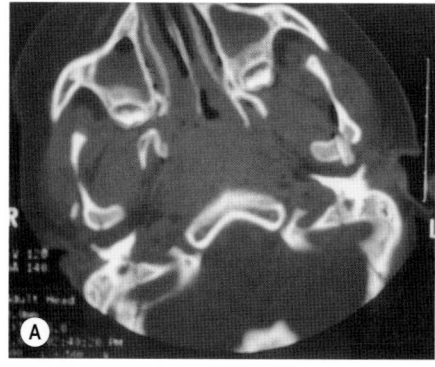
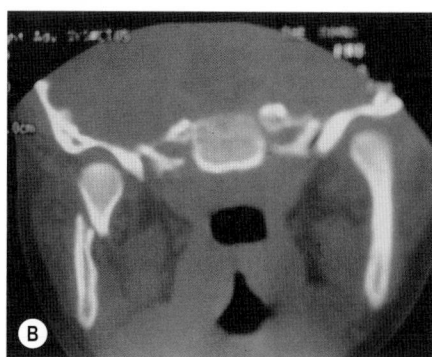
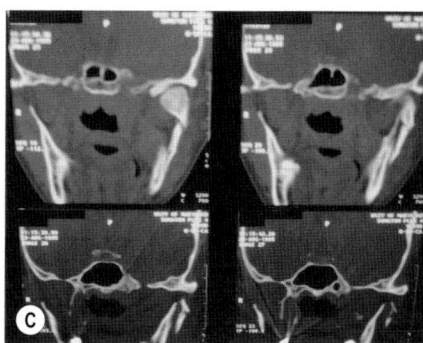

Fig. 31.10 (A) Axial computed tomography scan demonstrating condylar head fractures. **(B)** Coronal view of a condylar neck fracture; **(C)** serial coronal views of a subcondylar fracture. (Reproduced from Mathes S, Hentz V. Plastic surgery, 2nd ed. Philadelphia, PA: Elsevier; 2006.)

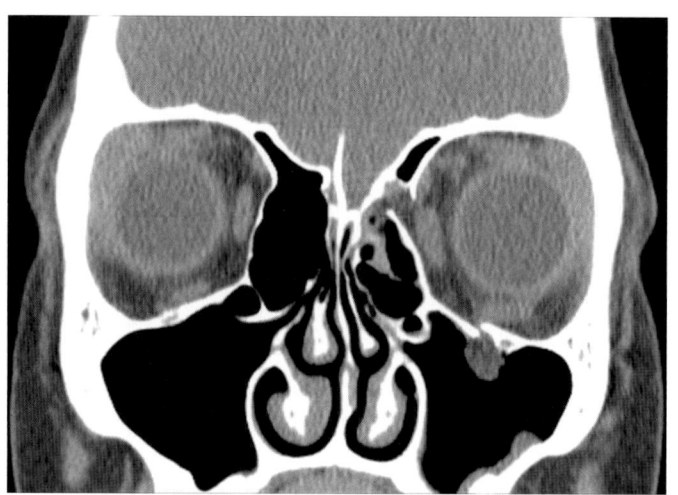

Fig. 31.11 Coronal computed tomography scan demonstrating an orbital floor fracture with an entrapped inferior rectus muscle on the patient's left side.

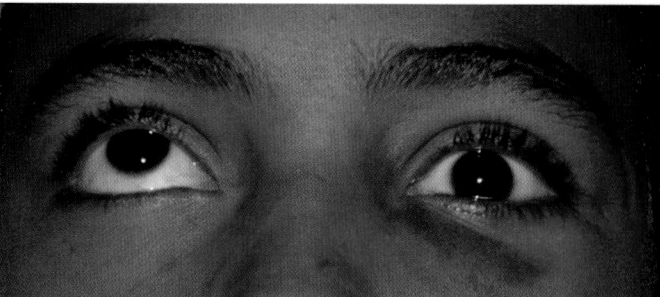

Fig. 31.12 Patient with an entrapped left inferior rectus. He is being instructed to "look up," but is unable to do so with his left eye due to the entrapped inferior rectus.

TMJ opening, persistent pain) was of functional significance.

Treatment/surgical technique

General principles

Certain principles may be applied to the management of all pediatric craniofacial fractures. The younger the patient, the higher the threshold for operative intervention. While it is critical to visualize fracture lines adequately, periosteal stripping should be minimized as, in accordance with Moss and Salentijn's "functional matrix" principle, stripping may adversely affect growth and development.[45] Growth disturbances are felt by some to be minimized by using absorbable plating systems in skeletally immature patients.

Cranial base/frontal skull fractures

Goals of cranial base and skull fracture repair include protection of the neurocapsule, dural reconstruction and control of

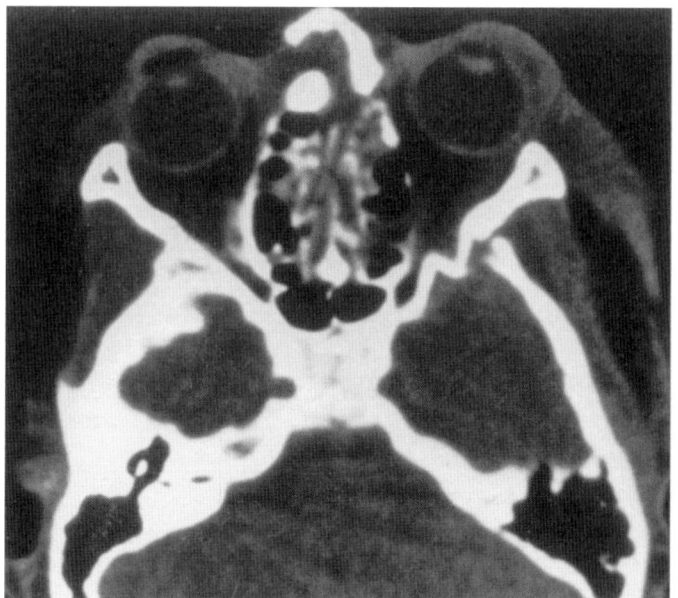

Fig. 31.13 Superior orbital fissure (SOF) syndrome may well result from the injury demonstrated in this axial computed tomography scan, in which a left frontal-temporal-orbital fracture has collapsed the SOF. (Reproduced from Mathes S, Hentz V. Plastic surgery, 2nd ed. Philadelphia, PA: Elsevier; 2006.)

CSF leaks, prevention of infection, and aesthetic restoration of craniofacial contour. A functioning sinus capable of adequate drainage through growth and development must be achieved. A coronal incision allows for craniotomy and ORIF *(Figs 31.15–31.17)*. After exposing fractures with subperiosteal dissection, fracture fragments must be removed to inspect the underlying dura. Epidural hematomas are evacuated and dural lacerations are repaired by the pediatric neurosurgical team. The bone fragments are then replaced and fixated. Caution must be exercised in manipulating frontal-temporal orbital fractures given the proximity to the middle meningeal artery. For patients mature enough to have a frontal sinus, Rodriguez *et al.* present a useful algorithm of approach.[46] If the nasofrontal duct is obstructed, obliteration or cranialization is indicated *(Fig. 31.18)*. Advantages of cranialization over obliteration include wide exposure of the injured area and single-stage elimination of the sinus as a potential focus

of infection. If the duct is traumatized but still patent, nondisplaced anterior and posterior table fractures can be carefully followed. Severely displaced anterior table fractures can be reconstructed. If the frontal sinus is preserved, serial CTs must be followed to ensure proper sinus development and adequate drainage, and the nasofrontal ducts may be stented via an endonasal approach. The presence of a CSF leak directs management decisions regarding frontal sinus fractures.[47] Leaks are observed for 4–7 days of bed rest and possible lumbar drain, and cranialization performed if the leak persists. If the leak stops, and the nasofrontal duct is unobstructed, the sinus may be preserved. In the case of an auto-corrected leak with an obstructed duct, anterior table ORIF is accompanied by "partial obliteration" (use of fracture fragments to obliterate only the nasofrontal duct and the base of the frontal sinus) following complete removal of sinus mucosa.

Bone loss is a difficult problem, especially in children too old (over 2 years) to heal large calvarial defects spontaneously, yet in whom split calvarial grafts are unavailable due to an underdeveloped diploic space (under approximately 9 years).[48,49] Significant donor site morbidity (infection, pain, hemorrhage, and nerve injury) in up to 8% of patients,[50] as well as low tissue yield, limits the usefulness of autogenous bone grafts. Bone substitutes are limited by a lack of biocompatibility and susceptibility to infection.[51] In patients with favorable wound conditions, the authors favor a bilaminate construct composed of intra- and extracranially placed bioresorbable mesh with interposed demineralized bone matrix mixed with bone dust and chips.[52] The authors are optimistic that a potential future role exists for protein therapy in pediatric craniofacial reconstruction.[53,54]

Orbital fractures

The goals of orbital fracture treatment include the restoration of globe position and the correction of diplopia. If ORIF is necessary, the transconjunctival approach to the orbit is preferred secondary to good cosmesis and a lower risk of ectropion. If lateral exposure is necessary, a subciliary or mid-lid incision avoids the lateral cantholysis that would be necessary with a transconjunctival incision. If medial exposure is necessary, a transcaruncular approach with/without a coronal incision is performed. A gingival buccal sulcus incision can be added if necessary. Herniated tissues are reduced from the fracture, the fracture is cleared of debris, and stable foundations for fixation and grafting are identified. When reduction is achieved, the residual defect is repaired with resorbable

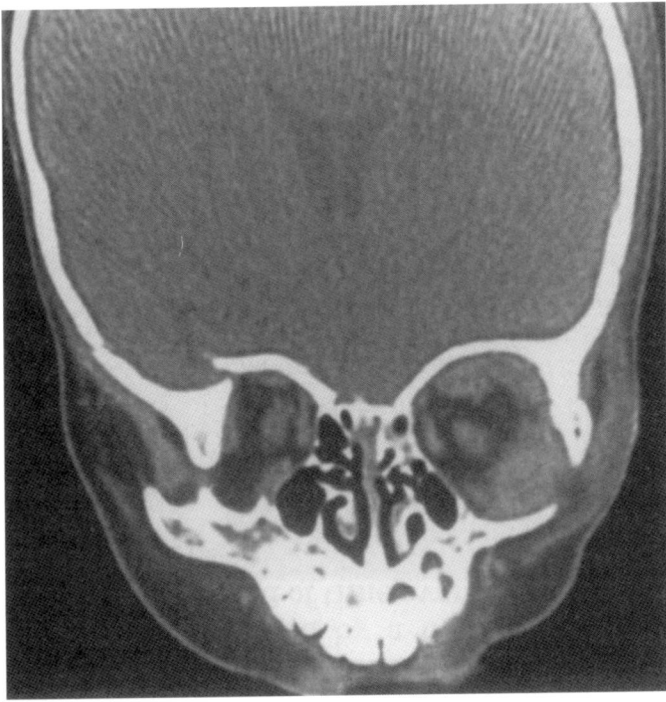

Fig. 31.14 Coronal computed tomography scan demonstrating a right frontal-temporal-orbital fracture. The lateral orbital wall is compressed medially, decreasing orbital volume and resulting in exophthalmos. (Reproduced from Mathes S, Hentz V. Plastic surgery, 2nd ed. Philadelphia, PA: Elsevier; 2006.)

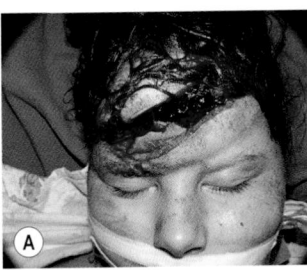
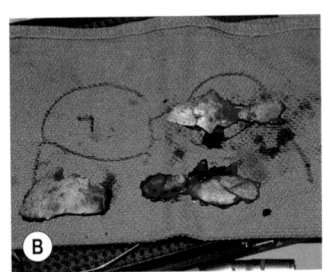
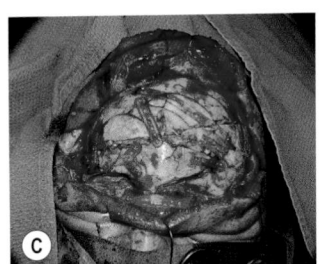
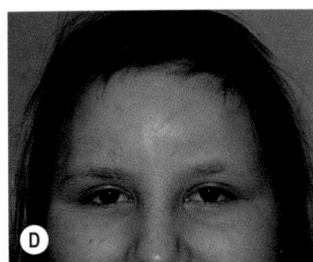

Fig. 31.15 **(A)** Frontal bone fracture after a motor vehicle collision. The bone fragments are mapped out as shown in **(B)** before they are reconstructed with absorbable plates, as in **(C)**. **(D)** The 6-month follow-up result. (Reproduced from Guyuron B, Erikkson E, Persing J, et al. Plastic surgery: indications and practice. Philadelphia, PA: Elsevier; 2008.)

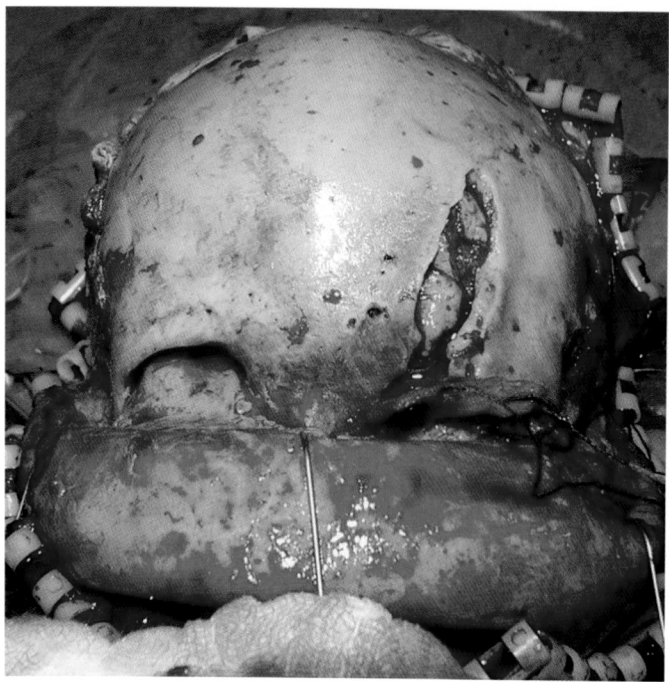

Fig. 31.16 Fracture of frontal bone.

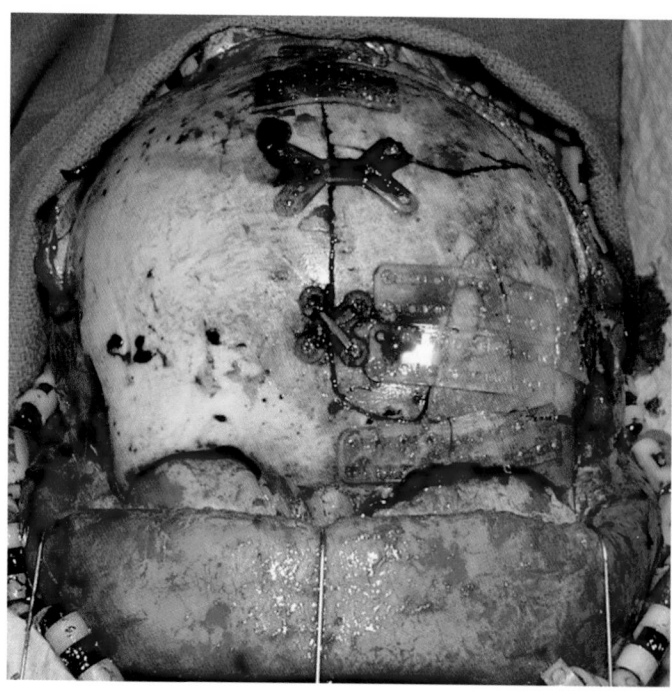

Fig. 31.17 The fracture shown in **Figure 31.16** has been reconstructed according to the method depicted in **Figure 31.15**.

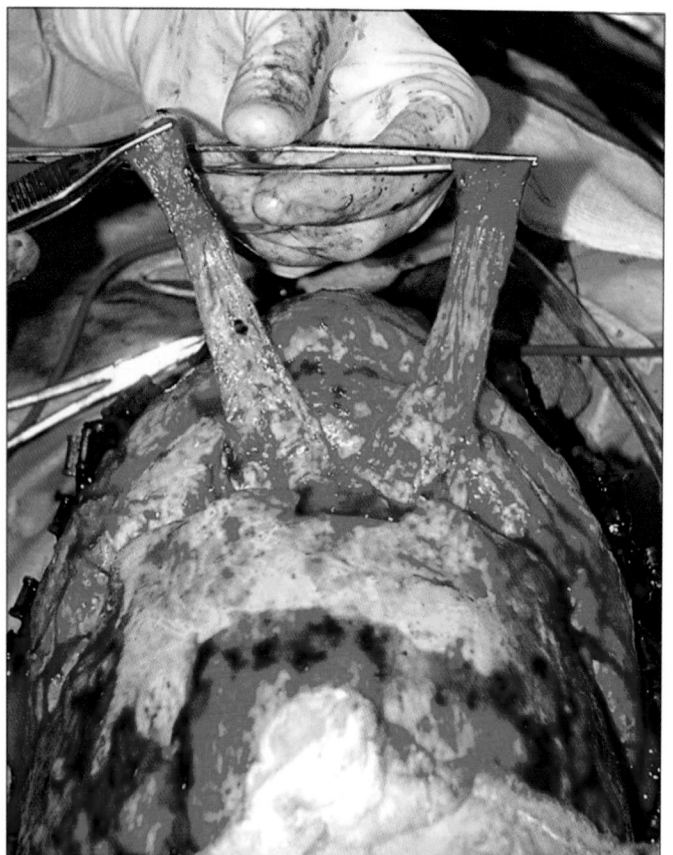

Fig. 31.18 Galeal flaps pedicled at the level of the brow have been raised to line the reconstructed anterior cranial base. A maneuver such as this is required to ensure that a barrier is in place to protect the intracranial contents from "the outside world." (Reproduced from Guyuron B, Erikkson E, Persing J, et al. Plastic surgery: indications and practice. Philadelphia, PA: Elsevier; 2008.)

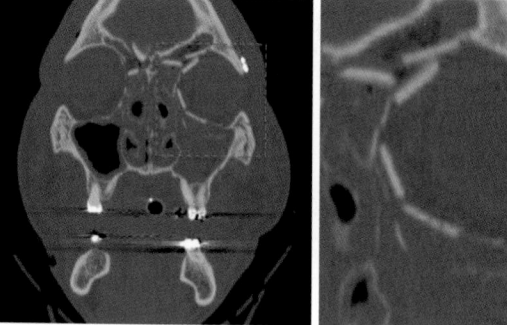

Fig. 31.19 Coronal computed tomography scan demonstrating orbital reconstruction with split calvarial grafts (the image on the right is a magnified view of the area outlined in red in the image on the left).

mesh or split calvarial graft *(Fig. 31.19)*. Care must be taken to resuspend midface soft tissues.

Maxillary and midface fractures

Minimally displaced maxillary fractures in young children may be managed conservatively with a soft diet. Palatal split fractures may require ORIF or may be splinted with mandibulomaxillary fixation (MMF). Incompletely developed dentition renders arch bars difficult to apply, often requiring creative strategies such as circummandibular wiring and piriform suspension wiring *(Figs 31.20 and 31.21)*. Depending upon the patient's age, shorter courses of MMF are acceptable: some authors advocate fixation for 1 week or less,[1] followed by dental elastics in the very young. When ORIF is necessary, the operator must avoid injuring developing tooth buds when plating the facial buttresses.

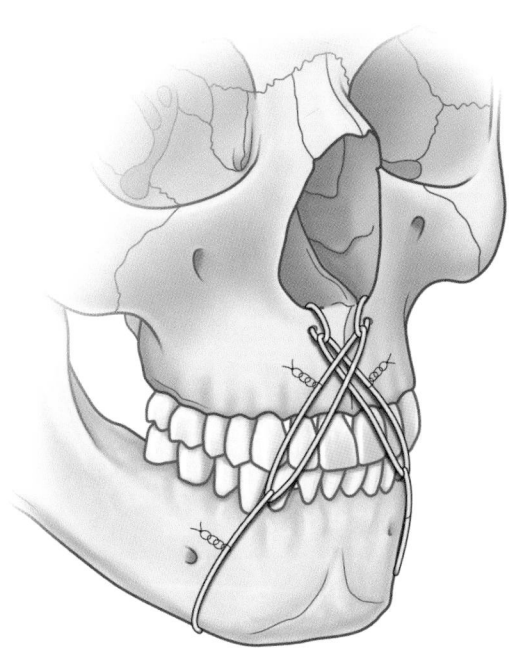

Fig. 31.20 Creative mandibulomaxillary fixation strategies are often required in children.

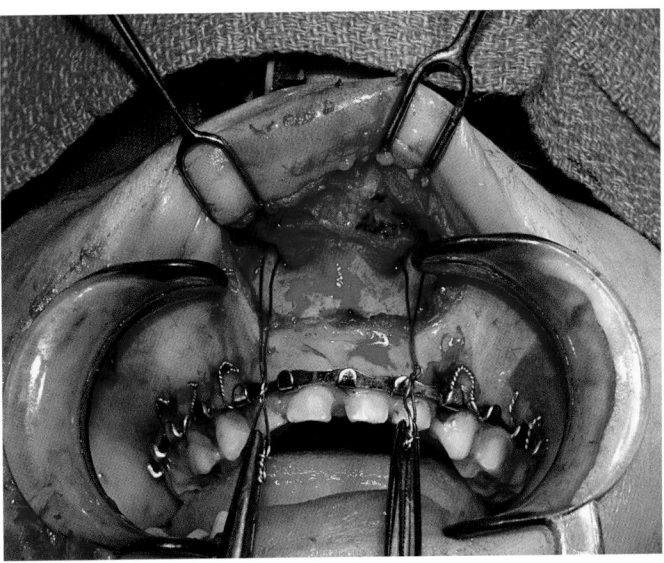

Fig. 31.21 Drop piriform wires being placed for mandibulomaxillary fixation in a pediatric patient. (Reproduced from Guyuron B, Erikkson E, Persing J, et al. Plastic surgery: indications and practice. Philadelphia, PA: Elsevier; 2008.)

Zygomaticomaxillary complex fractures

Operative goals in ZMC fracture management include resolution of orbital injury (VOD, enophthalmos), correction of malocclusion, and the restoration of appearance (malar flattening). The zygoma is aesthetically responsible for the malar eminence, and an inferiorly displaced zygoma may displace the lateral canthus with it by way of the tendon's attachment to Whitnall's tubercle. Access to the ZF suture may be gained through a subciliary incision, a subconjunctival approach with lateral cantholysis, or the lateral portion of an upper lid blepharoplasty incision. Additional exposure is obtained with an upper buccal sulcus incision. Some authors have reported that medially impacted large fragment fractures may be addressed through an upper gingival buccal sulcus incision alone with exposure of the anterior face of the zygoma, fracture reduction, and confirmation of orbital floor continuity with endoscopy via the maxillary sinus.[23] It is generally accepted that adequate reduction at the lateral wall of the orbit or the greater wing of the sphenoid is essential to proper reconstruction; reduction must also be achieved at the lateral orbital rim / ZF suture, inferior orbital rim, and the zygomaticomaxillary (ZM) buttress. Fixation is then performed sequentially at the ZF suture, the inferior orbital rim, and the ZM buttress. The operator must ensure that orbital volume and morphology are not altered by the initial injury or the reduction, and floor reconstruction may be required in the procedure.[26]

Nasal and naso-orbital ethmoid fractures

Nondisplaced or minimally displaced fractures may be externally splinted. In the case of a displaced fracture, due to the significant potential for growth disturbance with aggressive open management of nasal injuries in children, many favor

Table 31.2 Age-specific norms for interorbital distance	
Age	**Normal interorbital distance**
Newborn	10–15 mm
2-year-old	20 mm
12-year-old	25 mm
Adult	35 mm
IOD = dacryon to dacryon or IOD = medial intercanthal distance (MICD): 4–6 mm.	

acute closed reduction and external fixation whenever feasible. An elevator or knife handle may be passed endonasally to outfracture depressed nasal bones and maxillary frontal process fragments. Conversely, infracture may be achieved with digital repositioning. The septum may be relocated with Asch forceps. When necessary, fractures are splinted internally and externally. Septal hematomas must be managed early with an incision through the mucoperiostium. If bilateral septal incisions are made, overlap must be avoided as septal perforation may result. Dead space may be eliminated with septal quilting sutures or internal splints to compress the mucopericondrium to the septal cartilage.

NOE fractures are characterized by posterior and lateral displacement of the nasal bones and medial orbital rims, with fractures of the medial orbital walls and ethmoids. A free medial orbital rim segment containing the insertion of the medial canthus (the "central fragment") *(Fig. 31.22)* results in traumatic telecanthus. Even if not immediately apparent, telecanthus may develop 7–10 days after trauma. Intercanthal distance must be restored to age-specific norms *(Table 31.2)* by reduction of the medial orbital rims. If necessary, the medial canthal tendons are reattached with transnasal wires passing superior and posterior to the posterior lacrimal crest. A cantilever bone graft is employed to restore the nasal dorsal

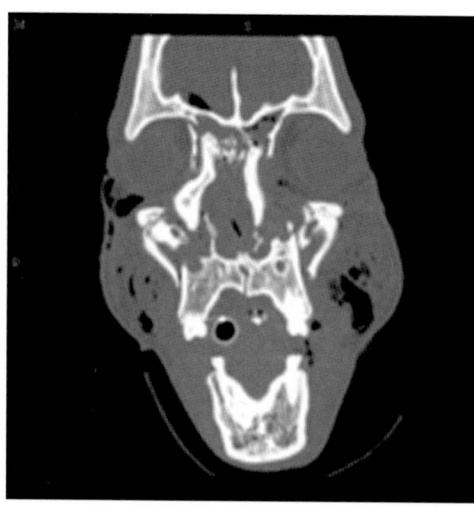

Fig. 31.22 Coronal computed tomography scan demonstrating bilateral naso-orbital ethmoid fractures with their requisite "central fragments."

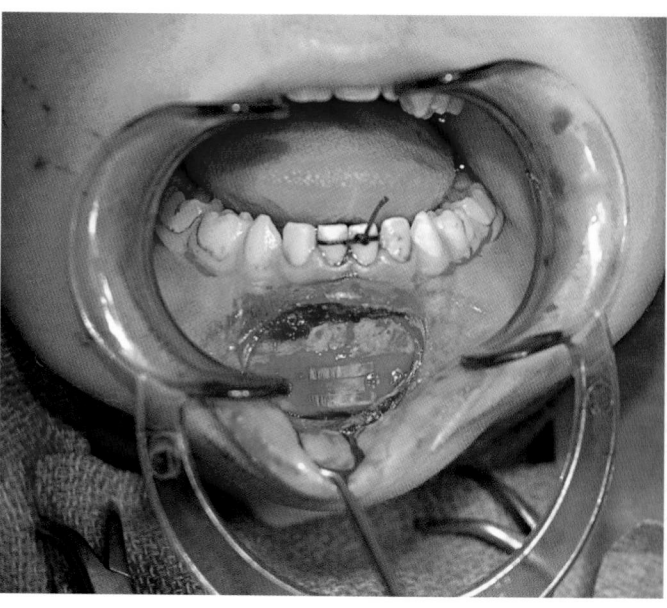

Fig. 31.23 Circumdental suture functions as a bridle wire in combination with an inferiorly placed monocortical adsorbable plate for a symphyseal fracture in a child. (Reproduced from Guyuron B, Erikkson E, Persing J, et al. Plastic surgery: indications and practice. Philadelphia, PA: Elsevier; 2008.)

height. Complicated NOE fractures are exposed by coronal, inferior orbital rim, and gingival buccal sulcus incisions. A high index of suspicion must be maintained for fractures extending to the anterior skull base.

Mandible fractures

Goals in the management of mandible fractures include the restoration of normal occlusion and the achievement of bony union while minimizing potential growth disturbance and injury to developing tooth follicles. Dentoalveolar fractures can often be managed conservatively with occlusive splinting, arch bars, or bonded wires in combination with soft diet, good oral hygiene, and mandible rest. Nondisplaced or minimally displaced mandibular fractures with normal occlusion in young children may be treated with immobilization with a "jaw bra" and/or cervical collar and liquid diet. Minor malocclusions after fracture healing can be managed with orthodontics. If necessary, MMF may require creativity in children *(Figs 31.20 and 31.21)*.

Condylar head fractures are treated with a short course of rest followed by physical therapy (such as gum chewing). Unilateral condylar neck fractures are often adequately managed with closed reduction, arch bars, and contralateral elastics. Bilateral condylar neck fractures with a loss of posterior height and resultant anterior open bite may require a more aggressive approach. In younger children, these fractures can be managed with closed reduction and external fixation (MMF for 2–3 weeks); adolescents may require formal ORIF.

Whenever possible, existing lacerations and an intraoral approach should be utilized in pediatric mandible fractures requiring open management. Given the immature mandible's ability to remodel under masticatory forces, as well as its amenability to orthodontic manipulation, it is wise to accept imperfect reduction and occlusion in order to preserve developing tooth follicles.

If bony fixation is necessary in young patients, monocortical screws should be utilized and hardware should be placed at the inferior mandibular border to avoid injury to developing tooth buds. Alternatively, interosseous wiring of the

mandibular border and a dental bridle wire may be adequate in combination with a short course of MMF *(Fig. 31.23)*. Transosseous wiring and bicortical screws may be considered after 11 years of age (or as early as 8 years of age for symphyseal fractures).[17]

Postoperative care

In the postoperative period, appropriate rest and supervision are paramount in preventing undue stress to operative repairs. Steroids may be given after extensive manipulation of the orbital contents. The surgeon should maintain a low threshold for aggressive evaluation (i.e., CT scan, ophthomologic evaluation, etc.) after orbital surgery in the presence of unexpected pain, regardless of visual acuity. For nasal fractures, if intranasal splinting is used, it may be discontinued after 1 week, and external splints should remain in place for 2 weeks. Antibiotic prophylaxis is used if internal splints are employed. Mandible fractures warrant a period of jaw rest. If conservatively managed, stabilization can be enhanced with a cervical collar, jaw bra, or ACE wrap. Depending upon patient age, some argue that metallic fixation used for ORIF should be removed once adequate healing has occurred to minimize growth effects.

Outcomes, prognosis, and complications

General principles

Outcomes and complications in pediatric facial fractures are understudied. A broad range of complication rates in the

Table 31.3 Authors' classification system for adverse outcomes in pediatric facial fractures

Classification	Definition	Example
Type 1	Intrinsic to fracture	Loss of permanent tooth with mandible fracture
Type 2	Secondary to intervention	Marginal mandibular nerve injury during open reduction, internal fixation of mandibular fracture
Type 3	Subsequent to growth and development	Asymmetric mandibular growth after condylar fracture

literature (2.6–21.6%) implies vague documentation of these injuries.[18,55,56] Photographic, radiographic, and functional documentation over time is essential in developing literature to inform our ongoing treatment of these potentially life-altering injuries. Meaningful outcomes analysis in this field is dependent on improved standardization of data collection.[57] To this end, the authors have introduced a classification system to facilitate the clear characterization and discussion of adverse outcomes in these injuries.[58] Type 1 complications are intrinsic to the fracture itself (i.e., blindness following orbital fracture, tooth loss following mandibular fracture). Type 2 complications are directly secondary to an intervention: conservative or surgical management (i.e., ectropion following subciliary incision, enophthalmos following orbital fracture repair). Type 3 complications are subsequent to growth and development with potential contributions of the fracture itself and subsequent treatment *(Table 31.3)*.

Infection, nonunion, and malunion are rare in comparison to adults secondary to increased osteogenesis, less frequent indications for open reduction, and a lower frequency of severely displaced fractures in children.[13] To the contrary, disturbances in growth and development secondary to facial trauma and its management are a common concern. Growth disturbance secondary to facial trauma is, however, an incompletely understood phenomenon. The contribution of hardware to growth retardation is not clear. In one study, the authors report 6 of 96 children with facial fractures undergoing ORIF to have experienced delayed or restricted growth. As they state, however, it is impossible to separate the developmental effects of fixation from other intrinsic and extrinsic factors.[59] Mustoe *et al.* concluded that closed reduction of nasal fractures is not deleterious for growth[60]; invasive rhinoplasty is similarly benign according to Ortiz-Monasterio and Olmedo.[61] Other authors express significant concern for subsequent growth effects.[62,63] Complete resection of the septum, as in hypertelorism correction, is well documented to have devastating effects on the growth and development of the midface.[64] Metallic cranial hardware may pose a direct hazard to growing children as it may translocate intracranially secondary to cranial bone deposition *(Figs 31.24 and 31.25)*.

Cranial base/skull fractures

These injuries may be complicated by CSF leak, meningitis, sinusitis, mucoceles, mucopyoceles, or brain abscesses. CSF leaks usually resolve spontaneously within 1 week; if the leak persists, a 5–7-day lumbar drain trial should precede operative intervention.[65,66] A cranial base fracture with an occult dural disruption may lead to a "growing skull fracture" secondary to cerebral pulsations enlarging even innocent-appearing cranial base fractures. Growing skull

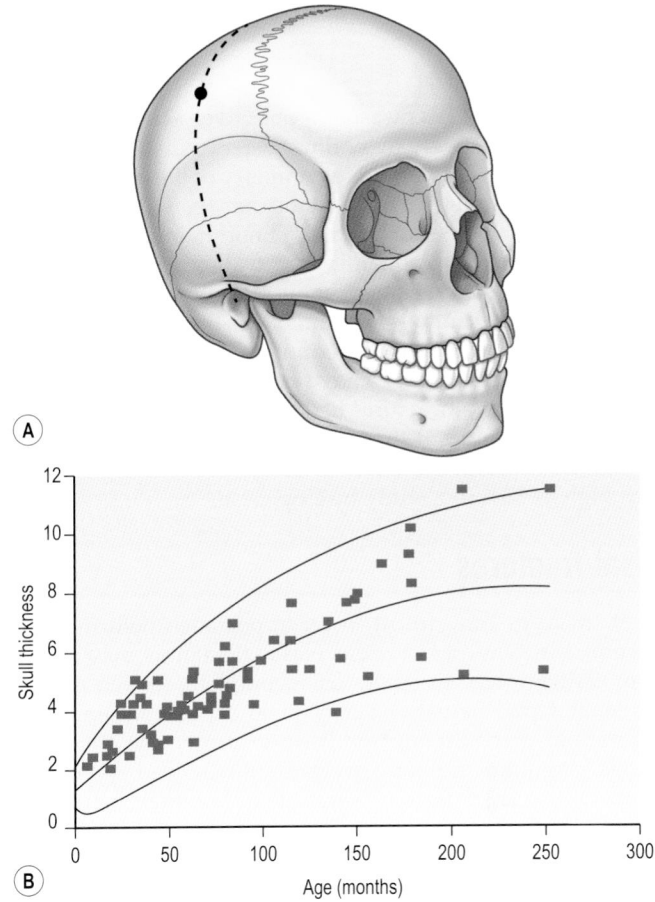

Fig. 31.24 **(A, B)** The skull increases in thickness with craniofacial development in a relationship reported by Pensler and McCarthy. (Redrawn from Pensler J, McCarthy JG. The calvarial donor site: an anatomic study in cadavers. *Plast Reconstr Surg.* 1985;75:648.)

fractures complicate 0.03–1% of skull fractures, and usually occur in patients younger than 3 years of age.[67,68] Missed growing skull fractures may lead to gliosis, lateral ventricular dilation, cerebral herniation, pulsatile exophthalmos, and VOD.[25] In the authors' series, 40% of patients with skull fractures exhibited an adverse outcome: type 1: 5%, type 2: 20%, and type 3: 35%, including growing skull fractures, CSF leaks, enophthalmos, VOD, ptosis, amblyopia, and exophthalmos.

Orbital fractures

The most worrisome adverse outcomes of orbital reconstruction include persistent diplopia and enophthalmos.

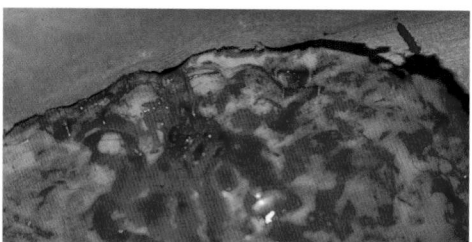

Fig. 31.25 Endocranial surface of a calvarial bone flap demonstrating transcranial migration of metallic hardware in a pediatric patient. (Reproduced from Guyuron B, Erikkson E, Persing J, et al. Plastic surgery: indications and practice. Philadelphia, PA: Elsevier; 2008.)

Enophthalmos can be measured objectively by exophthalmometry or subjectively by noting posterior displacement of the globe on worm's-eye view, asymmetry of the upper eyelid creases, and asymmetry in the distance between ciliary margin and superior and inferior limbus.[41] Enopthalmos can sometimes be corrected by orbital floor or wall bone grafting, but may require osteotomies and bony relocation and possibly lateral or medial canthal adjustment. In the authors' series, 10.7% of isolated orbital fractures suffered adverse outcomes: type 1: 3.6%, type 2: 3.6%, and type 3: 3.6%. Three patients with isolated orbital fractures had enopthalmos, all less than the clinically significant threshold of 2 mm. Persistent diplopia did not occur in the authors' series, but was reported to be as high as 36% in a study by Cope *et al.*[41,69]

Nasal fractures

Nasal fractures may result in an appearance deformity or functional airway obstruction. Nasal deviation may result from cartilaginous warping or incomplete reduction. An untreated septal hematoma may yield septal thickening or perforation, and ultimate saddle-nose deformity. Excessive callous formation and bony overgrowth may lead to a dorsal hump. One study reports a 5% rate of late lacrimal obstruction after ORIF of NOE fractures. This is managed with dacrocystorhinostomy.[70] In the authors' series, 21.7% of nasal fractures exhibited adverse outcomes (type 1: 8.7% and type 3: 17.4%) consisting of persistent nasal deformity or airway obstruction.[71] Secondary corrective surgery should be delayed until after skeletal maturity unless clinically significant nasal airway obstruction is present.

Zygomaticomaxillary complex fractures, maxillary and midface fractures

Adverse outcomes following ZMC fracture repair include persistent V2 hypothesia, enophthalmos, VOD, facial widening, malar flattening, canthal deformity, and ectropion secondary to lower lid approaches. Maxillary fractures may result in nasolacrimal obstruction or malocclusion. Zygomatic-coronoid ankylosis may occur after severe zygomatic fracture.[23]

Mandible fractures

Mandible fractures may be complicated by growth disturbances or functional impairment such as malocclusion,

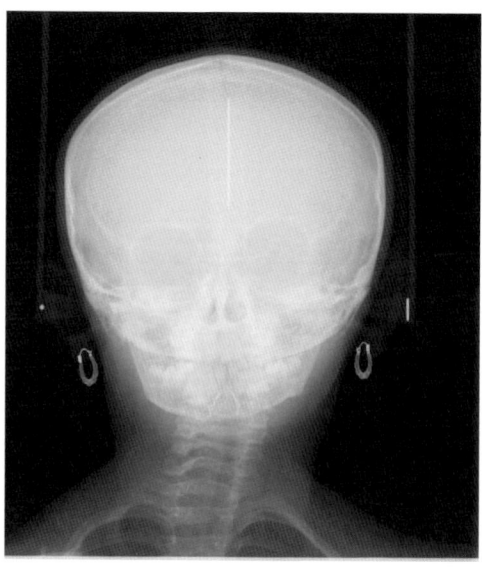

Fig. 31.26 Cephalogram of a patient 2 years after a left mandibular body fracture. The left mandibular ramus, angle, and body demonstrate decreased growth relative to the contralateral side.

trismus, or TMJ ankylosis. Marginal mandibular nerve injury may result from surgery. In the authors' series of 179 mandible fractures in 96 patients, type 1 outcomes were seen in 20.0% of operative patients and in 0% of conservatively managed patients ($P = 0.05$), type 2 outcomes were seen in 13.3% of operative patients and in no conservatively managed patients ($P = 0.115$), and type 3 outcomes were seen in 66.7% of operative patients and in 45.0% of conservatively managed patients ($P = 0.402$).[16] In another reported series, patients were at most risk for growth disturbances and facial asymmetry if they sustained mandibular fractures between 4 and 7 years of age and least likely to have growth sequelae if they were injured prior to 4 years of age (children greater than 11 years of age experienced an intermediate rate of growth disturbance) *(Fig. 31.26)*. The authors of this series explain this age distribution by positing that children in the youngest group have better condylar blood flow, allowing for regeneration and avoidance of growth disturbances; moreover, they note that the majority of mandibular growth spurts occur at either end of their 4–7-year-old age group.[72]

Secondary procedures

Imola et al. provide a useful overview of secondary procedures that may be required in managing craniofacial fractures.[73] Soft-tissue deformity and the evolution of a scarred soft-tissue envelope are the single greatest barriers to optimal outcomes. Poorly reduced fractures may require osteotomy and repeat ORIF. Traumatic telecanthus may require transnasal fixation; if the medial canthus must be reinserted, it is essential to ensure sufficiently superior and posterior positioning. Dorsal nasal deficiency may exacerbate the appearance of telecanthus, and this may also be surgically addressed. Mandibular growth disturbances may necessitate advancement genioplasty or distraction. Secondary correction of enophthalmos requires anterior globe repositioning, reduction of the orbital contents, and osteotomy and repositioning of skeletal components. VOD may require four-wall osteotomies for optimal results.[73] Diplopia is most likely to occur secondary to extraocular muscle dysfunction as opposed to globe malposition; the inferior rectus and superior oblique are the muscles most commonly involved. Growing skull fractures require dural repair and cranioplasty. Hardware removal may be indicated to minimize growth disturbances, avoid risks associated with transcranial migration, or if the hardware is causing discomfort or aesthetic concern.

Conclusions

The craniofacial skeleton undergoes a dramatic structural and topographical metamorphosis as it matures from the infant to the adult state. The neonatal skull is profoundly different from its adult counterpart, and therefore responds to traumatic forces with unique injury patterns. Specific functional and aesthetic criteria must be met in reconstructing the various regions of the pediatric craniofacial skeleton. These objectives must be achieved with strategies that properly balance respect for future growth. Craniofacial development, along with the resilience of the pediatric skull and supporting structures, often facilitates a less invasive approach to managing these complex injuries.

Access the complete references list online at **http://www.expertconsult.com**

17. Smartt Jr JM, Low DW, Bartlett SP. The pediatric mandible: ii. management of traumatic injury or fracture. *Plast Reconstr Surg*. 2005;116:28e–41e.

18. Ferreira PC, Amarante JM, Silva PN, et al. Retrospective study of 1251 maxillofacial fractures in children and adolescents. *Plast Reconstr Surg*. 2005;115:1500–1508.

    This large series describes more than 900 pediatric facial fracture patients. Demographics and associated injuries were assessed.

24. Smartt Jr JM, Low DW, Bartlett SP. The pediatric mandible: I. A primer on growth and development. *Plast Reconstr Surg*. 2005;116:14e–23e.

    This is an excellent review of the literature pertaining to human mandible development. It sets the stage for the companion article, "The pediatric mandible: II. Management of traumatic injury or fracture," also cited here.

25. Havlik RJ, Sutton LN, Bartlett SP. Growing skull fractures and their craniofacial equivalents. *J Craniofac Surg*. 1995;6:103–110; discussion 111–102.

41. Losee J, Afifi A, Jiang S, et al. Pediatric orbital fractures: classification, management, and early follow-up. *Plast Reconstr Surg*. 2008;122:886–897, 2008.

46. Rodriguez ED, Stanwix MG, Nam AJ, et al. Twenty-six-year experience treating frontal sinus fractures: a novel algorithm based on anatomical fracture pattern and failure of conventional techniques. *Plast Reconstr Surg*. 2008;122:1850–1866.

    Frontal sinus fractures often represent difficult management decisions. Here, an extensive clinical experience is distilled into a practical, clearly presented algorithm.

53. Smith DM, Afifi AM, Cooper GM, et al. Bmp-2-based repair of large-scale calvarial defects in an experimental model: regenerative surgery in cranioplasty. *J Craniofac Surg*. 2008;19:1315–1322.

    BMP-2 is shown to address subtotal cranial defects effectively in a rabbit model. Clinical implications are discussed.

54. Smith DM, Cooper GM, Mooney MP, et al. Bone morphogenetic protein 2 therapy for craniofacial surgery. *J Craniofac Surg*. 2008;19:1244–1259.

    This review presents an introduction to BMP-2 for craniofacial surgeons. Topics range from molecular mechanisms to clinical concerns.

58. Losee J, Chao M. Complications in pediatric facial fractures. *Cranial Maxillofac Trauma Reconstr*. 2009;2:103–112.

72. Demianczuk AN, Verchere C, Phillips JH. The effect on facial growth of pediatric mandibular fractures. *J Craniofac Surg*. 1999;10:323–328.

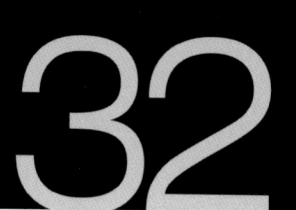

Orbital hypertelorism

Eric Arnaud, Daniel Marchac, Federico Di Rocco, and Dominique Renier

SYNOPSIS

- Hypertelorism is not a disease in itself; it is just a symptom which may belong to various conditions.

- It is mainly present in facial clefts but may accompany faciocraniosynostosis, where craniosynostosis has to be corrected independantly before 1 year of age.

- Surgical treatment of hypertelorism can be undertaken after age 4 and preferably before age 8 (at completion of cerebral growth and before frontal sinus growth).

- The technique of correction depends upon the degree of interorbital distance and on the occlusion.

- According to the degree of interorbital distance, the technique is based on a two-, three- or four-wall mobilization, through a subcranial or a transcranial approach.

- If the occlusion is normal, the osteotomy is a box-shift type; if the occlusion is angulated, a facial bipartition osteotomy and medialization of the two hemifaces are performed.

- Rhinoplasty is best performed at the end of growth: it represents one of the most important morphological improvements of the whole therapeutic sequence.

- Minor additive procedures contribute to the completion of the result: epicanthus correction, medial and lateral canthopexy, and fat grafting in the temporal region.

- Intellectual development in patients with facial clefts is usually good.

 Access the Historical Perspective section online at
http://www.expertconsult.com

Introduction

Craniofacial malformations are disorders that affect both the cranium and the face. In faciocraniosynostoses, the facial mal-development is associated with craniosynostosis (premature fusion of one or several sutures). In facial clefts, the major anomaly affects the face, and is occasionally associated with

a cranial problem. Hypertelorism is not a disease in itself; rather, it is a symptom or associated finding which accompanies some craniofacial conditions. Hypertelorism is defined by the abnormal increase in the interorbital distance (between the bony orbits). The abnormality may be symmetrical or asymmetrical.

In embryonic development, the development of the face occurs early, between the fourth and eighth weeks of gestation. When one observes that the midportion of the face develops immediately anterior to the forebrain, it is obvious that there is a close relationship between the face and the brain. Lateral to this midline prominence, paired elements appear: the nasal placodes and the maxillary processes. These structures merge in the midline whilst the frontonasal prominence is displaced in a cephalic direction. This prominence narrows to form the bridge and roo t of the nose. The developing eyes present as optic vesicles "outpouching" from the brain, and are initially positioned far laterally. The optic vesicles move closer together as the frontonasal prominence narrows. Simultaneously, the tip of the nose is derived from the paired medial elements, as the paired maxillary and mandibular processes fuse to form the lower part of the face. Clefts of the midline craniofacial structure occur when this delicate sequence of events is disrupted.

Basic science and disease process

If the frontonasal prominence remains in its embryonic position, the optic placodes cannot migrate toward the midline, and this results in orbital hypertelorism, often associated with various anomalies of the forehead and nose. It had been said that "the face predicts the brain," and the importance of the centrofacial anomaly appears to parallel the forebrain defect.[1] Conversely, interrupted development of the medial prominence may lead to an absence of midline structures with excessive narrowing, such as cyclopia or ethmocephaly. Hypertelorism alone is a mild degree of this sequence at the orbital level.

The associated maxillary anomalies seen with hypertelorism consist mainly of insufficient anterior growth in the upper maxilla, resulting in maxillary retrusion. Since the face is physiologically underdeveloped in infancy, facial anomalies may be more apparent later in childhood when facial growth is completed.

There is little known of the genetics of craniofacial malformations, likely due to the limited number of cases. As major facial clefts are rare, most of our knowledge of the pathogenesis of these malformations is based on studies of the formation of cleft lip and palate. Nevertheless, the role of heredity is obvious in the more frequent clefts of the lip, palate, and the lateral aspects of the orbit.

Radiation, infection, and maternal metabolic imbalances, which can be involved in cleft lip, have not been reported to be responsible for craniofacial malformations. Drugs and chemicals such as tretinoin, thalidomide, corticosteroids, and even aspirin are known to be responsible for malformations; and, while facial development occurs early in pregnancy,[2] mothers may ingest various drugs while unaware of being pregnant. Causal environmental and hereditary factors probably play varying epigenetic roles in the formation of particular malformations.

Various systems of classification have been proposed for craniofacial clefts; two of them are of special value when assessing craniofacial anomalies. These are the "median facial clefts" and the Tessier classification, an orbitocentric cleft classification.

Diagnosis of hypertelorism and patient presentation in facial clefts

Median facial clefts

Median facial clefts can be divided into two categories: those presenting with a deficiency of tissue and missing parts, and those without lack of tissue but presenting with a widening malformation.

Midline tissue deficiency malformations are almost always linked with a forebrain deficiency. The term "arhinencephaly" has been used, but holoprosencephaly, a name proposed by De Myer et al.,[1] better reflects the lack of median tissues. On the basis of this brain–facial linkage, and including some concepts of Cohen and associates, the holoprosencephalic malformations present with hypotelorism, as opposed to hypertelorism.[3]

In contrast with the previous group, near-normal to excess tissue midline disorders do not have a high correlation between the facial anomalies and the underlying brain. The deformities can range from a notch in the upper lip and a widened nose to the most severe form of midline cleft. The term "frontonasal dysplasia," suggested by Sedano et al. for this group of anomalies,[4] is used widely, especially amongst geneticists. Frontonasal dysplasia and holoprosencephaly are therefore at opposite ends in this system of classification of midline anomalies.

This classification does not take into account all the asymmetrical and paramedian anomalies. For easier definition and treatment implications, the authors use the Tessier classification, which is based on surgical experience.

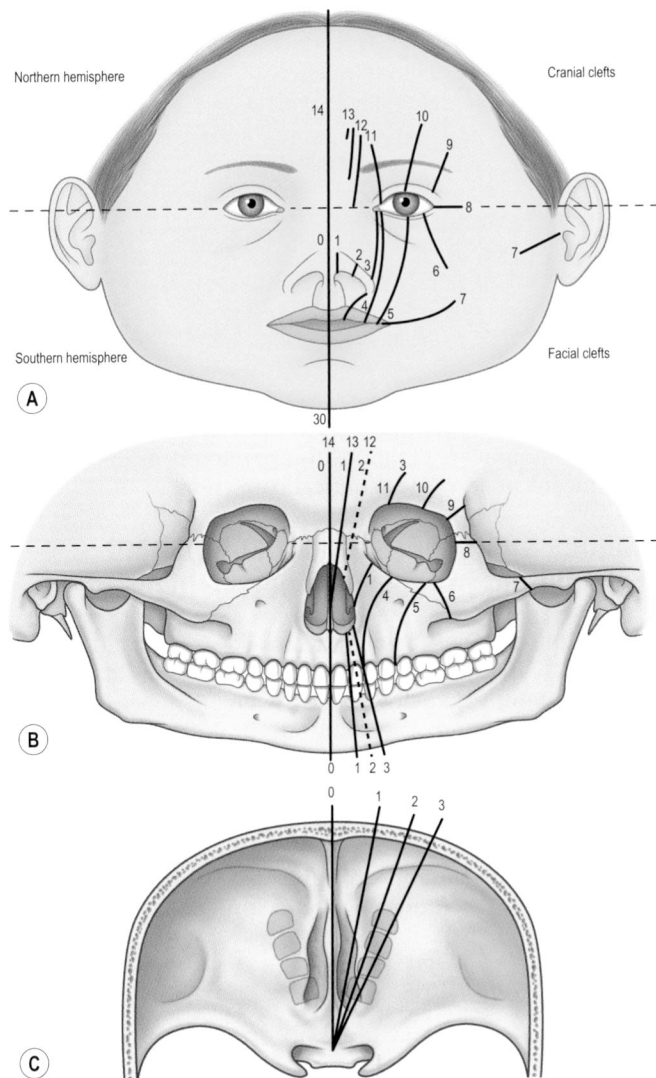

Fig. 32.1 (A–C) Tessier classification.

Tessier classification of facial clefts

In the Tessier classification,[5] the orbit is the reference landmark, common to both the cranium and the face. The clefts, numbered from 0 to 14, rotate around the orbit and follow constant lines through the skeleton and soft tissues *(Fig. 32.1)*. Clefts can be mostly cranial if they run upward from the eyelid (7–14) or mostly facial if they run downward from the palpebral fissure (0–6). They are craniofacial if the upper and lower pathways are connected.

The following combinations can be clinically observed: 0 and 14, 1 and 13, 2 and 12, 3 and 11, and 4 and 10. This concept of additive facial and cranial clefts equaling 14 is helpful when examining the patient and often allows identification of malformation along its entire length, above and below the orbit. The severity of the cleft is highly variable and can range from a slight soft-tissue indentation to a complete open cleft. The soft-tissue and skeletal clefts are, on the whole, superimposable. However, a detailed description of the soft-tissue defect, in relation to the skeletal cleft, is more reliable, because the skeletal landmarks are more consistent. The Tessier classification defines the 0–14 cleft as a midline widening, present in frontonasal dysplasia.

Unilateral and bilateral forms of clefting are found in various combinations, mainly asymmetrical when bilateral. Three-dimensional computed tomography has greatly facilitated diagnosis, whilst magnetic resonance imaging explores the brain, looking for an associated malformation. Stereolithographic models, constructed from computed tomography images, are also available, and may be useful for diagnosis and surgical planning as these malformations are uncommon and rarely identical.

Some isolated facial clefts, such as those affecting the lateral aspect of the face in Treacher–Collins syndrome (bilateral 6, 7, and 8 clefts), do not present any surgical interest for the neurosurgeon. The central and paramedial clefts affecting the face and cranium are of neurosurgical interest, as the cranium is the means of access for surgical correction.

Diagnosis of hypertelorism and patient presentation in faciocraniosynostosis

Hypertelorism is not the main feature of faciocraniosynostosis, and is variable in its presentation.[6] When mild, it is frequently left untreated; however, when more noticeable, it can be addressed through a separate surgical step. Depending on the dental occlusion, and particularly the horizontal position of the upper maxillary arch, the treatment of hypertelorism will vary between an orbital shift and a facial bipartition. The timing of treatment is variable according to the pathology; however, in the authors' experience, skull expansion for craniosynostosis treatment should precede hypertelorism correction.[7,8]

Crouzon's syndrome

Described by Crouzon in 1912,[9] this syndrome involves only the face and cranium and is not associated with other anomalies elsewhere on the limbs or trunk. The fundamental dysmorphology is an underdeveloped midface presenting with exorbitism secondary to insufficient depth of the orbits, hypoplasia of the malar bones, and a class III malocclusion. Hypertelorism may be present but is usually mild. The nose is short. Brachycephaly is usually present; however, scaphocephaly, plagiocephaly, or even a cloverleaf skull may be present. With an extended classification, the association of facial retrusion and craniosynostosis might be named as a related Crouzon's anomaly. Commonly, the diagnosis of Crouzon's syndrome is difficult to make during the first year of life, even if brachycephaly is obvious. It is often difficult to know whether the midface will be affected, even on radiological examination. Midface retrusion and exorbitism appear later in life. In some cases, however, the diagnosis is evident at birth.

Severe maxillary retrusion may produce airway obstruction with mandatory mouth breathing. There is a great variability of expression, and both severe and mild forms can be observed in the same family.

The strategy of treatment of faciocraniosynostosis is either two-staged[10–12] (fronto-orbital first, then facial advancement later) or a frontofacial monobloc advancement,[13–15] preferably with distraction.[16] Whenever present, the hypertelorism might be corrected around 4–5 years of age, usually with an orbital

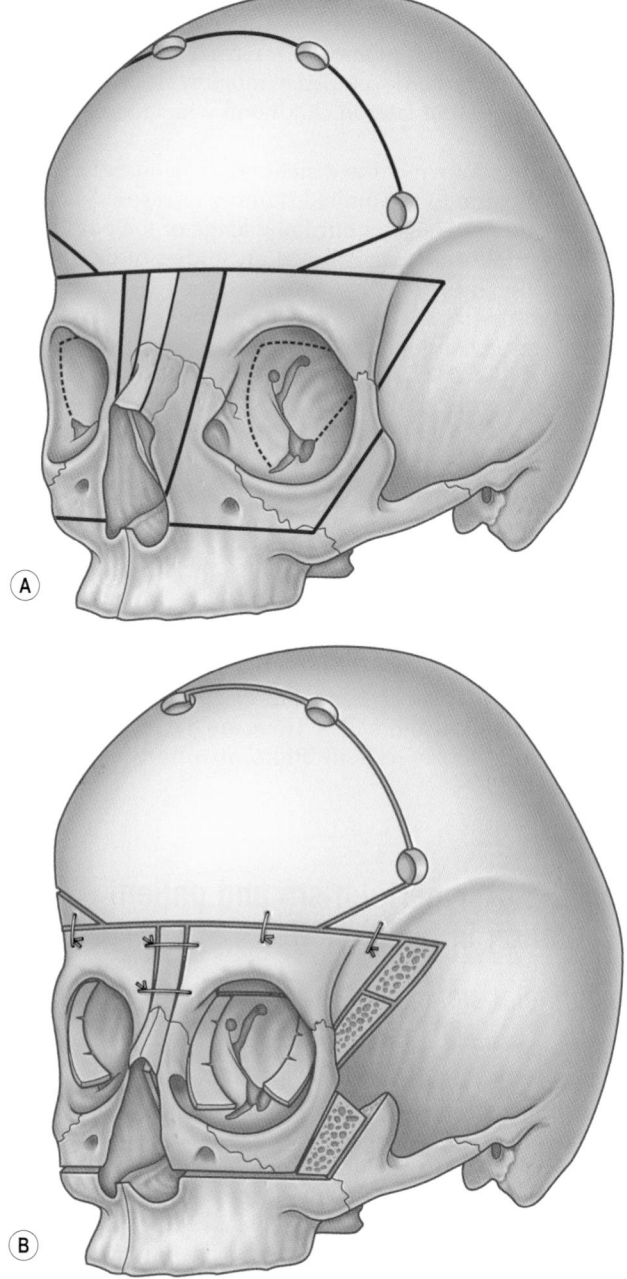

(A)

(B)

Fig. 32.2 Box-shift mobilization of orbits. **(A)** Before mobilization of the orbits; **(B)** after mobilization of the orbits.

shift *(Fig. 32.2)*, because in Crouzon's disease, the maxillary arch is normal (at least in the horizontal dimension).

Pfeiffer's syndrome

Described by Pfeiffer in 1964, this syndromic entity is an association of faciocraniosynostosis and anomalies of the hands and feet. The brachycephaly induced by bicoronal synostosis is often asymmetrical and is associated with midface retrusion secondary to maxillary hypoplasia. Hypertelorism is often present in this syndrome. The thumbs and great toes are broad with a varus deviation, and may be associated with soft-tissue syndactylies, the latter being difficult to diagnose early in life. Some severe forms exist, with marked perinatal frontofacial retrusion resulting in visual and respiratory problems. This condition is sometimes associated with a cloverleaf skull.

The strategy of treatment is similar to that for Crouzon's, but Pfeiffer's syndrome is often more severe than Crouzon's, with a higher tendency to relapse after surgical advancement.

Apert's syndrome (acrocephalosyndactyly)

First described by Apert in 1906,[17] this syndrome is easy to recognize because of the associated syndactylies of the hands and feet. The severity of syndactyly is scored according to Cohen and Kreiborg.[18] Type 1 is syndactyly of the central three digits, type 2 is syndactyly of digits 2–5, and type 3 is syndactyly of all five digits.

The craniofacial involvement is always marked at birth, in contrast with that in Crouzon's, with brachycephaly (sometimes asymmetrical) associated with facial retrusion. Both coronal sutures are fused, although some rare cases present with unilateral coronal synostosis or without any synostoses (4 cases without synostoses in our series). The hypertelorism and the anterior open bite add to the distinction from Crouzon's disease. In fact, the maxillary alveolar arch is higher than the posterior part of the palate. Another main difference with Crouzon's is the frequent sagittal dehiscence of the sutural system with the forehead frequently remaining wide open during the first year of life; this contributes to the abnormally wide forehead and face in this syndrome. Associated abnormalities of the central nervous system are more frequent than in other syndromic craniosynostoses. The exception is Chiari-like malformations, which are common in Crouzon's, but, due to premature fusions of the lambdoid sutures, are uncommon in Apert's.[19] Because of these patients' divergent frontal plane, bipartition procedures are more adapted to correct Apert's-associated hypertelorism. Nevertheless, skull expansion (either anterior or posterior) is performed first, usually before 1 year of age to address the craniosynostotic skull.

Craniofrontonasal dysplasia

In the group of craniofacial dysplasias (see discussion of median facial clefts with frontonasal dysplasia, below), some cases present with a bicoronal craniosynostosis, including a subgroup called craniofrontonasal dysplasia. There is a brachycephaly, often marked, associated with the facial anomalies of frontonasal dysplasia, which include hypertelorism, broad nasal bridge, and bifid nose; soft-tissue syndactyly may also be present.

Craniofrontonasal dysplasia is far more common in females than in males, consistent with its X-linked inheritance. In the authors' series, 36% of cases were familial, and 91% of patients were females.

Patient selection

Orbital shift or bipartition?

The choice between orbital shift and bipartition is mainly linked to a series of factors:

- The maxillary arch: if the maxillary arch is narrow and inverted with the incisors being higher than the molars, bipartition is the operation of choice because it widens the maxilla and improves the angle of the upper dentition. On the other hand, if the maxillary arch and occlusion are normal, it is preferable to avoid an interpterygomaxillary disjunction.
- The axis of the orbits: if the axis is normal, a horizontal mobilization is satisfactory; if the orbits are laterally and downwardly oblique, bipartition is required.
- The nasal fossae: if they are narrow, bipartition and medialization of the upper face improve the airways by enlarging the lower part of the face.
- Extent of the hypertelorism: bipartition is the operation of choice in the most severe cases, whereas orbital shift is indicated for more limited displacements.
- The bipartition procedure can also be used to get access to a lesion of the cranial base. Some midline clefts are associated with an encephalocele of the ethmoidosphenoidal area. After midline splitting, easy access to the encephalocele can be obtained.

Treatment/surgical technique

Surgical principles in facial clefts

Tessier's breakthrough collaboration between plastic and neurological surgery allowed him to conceptually minimize the surgical border existing between the face and the skull and dramatically enhance the surgical treatment of upper facial clefts.[20] Tessier demonstrated that the frontocranial route was a good approach to access the nose and orbits and that frontocranial problems can be treated simultaneously with facial problems. The fear of contamination from the facial cavities was so great among neurosurgeons in 1967 that, for their first case, Tessier and his neurosurgical colleague, Guyot, placed a dermal skin graft on the dura of the anterior cranial fossa after it had been elevated, voluntarily sacrificing both the olfactory nerves. A few months later, they performed the combined craniofacial approach. By 1970, a one-stage procedure to address the orbits from superior and inferior approaches was considered safe, and the olfactory nerves could be preserved (Converse).[21] Preliminary disinfection of the nasal cavities, dissection of the mucosal domes and their immediate repair if opened, preservation or perfect repair of dura, changing of instruments if passing through the facial cavities, and perioperative antibiotic therapy were preventive measures that helped to avoid infection, osteitis, and meningitis.

There are two ways to mobilize the orbits when correcting orbital hypertelorism. The treatment planning varies according to the severity of the hypertelorism, the maxillary structure, and the age of the patient. An orbital shift can simply be performed in cases of normal or subnormal dental occlusion. In cases of restricted transverse maxillary structures, mobilization of both hemifaces (necessitating a facial bipartition) can be performed to correct the hypertelorism and the arched palate at the same time.

The classic approach described by Tessier et al. in 1967[20] consisted, after removal of the enlarged medial portion, of an en bloc mobilization of the orbits medially, the lower

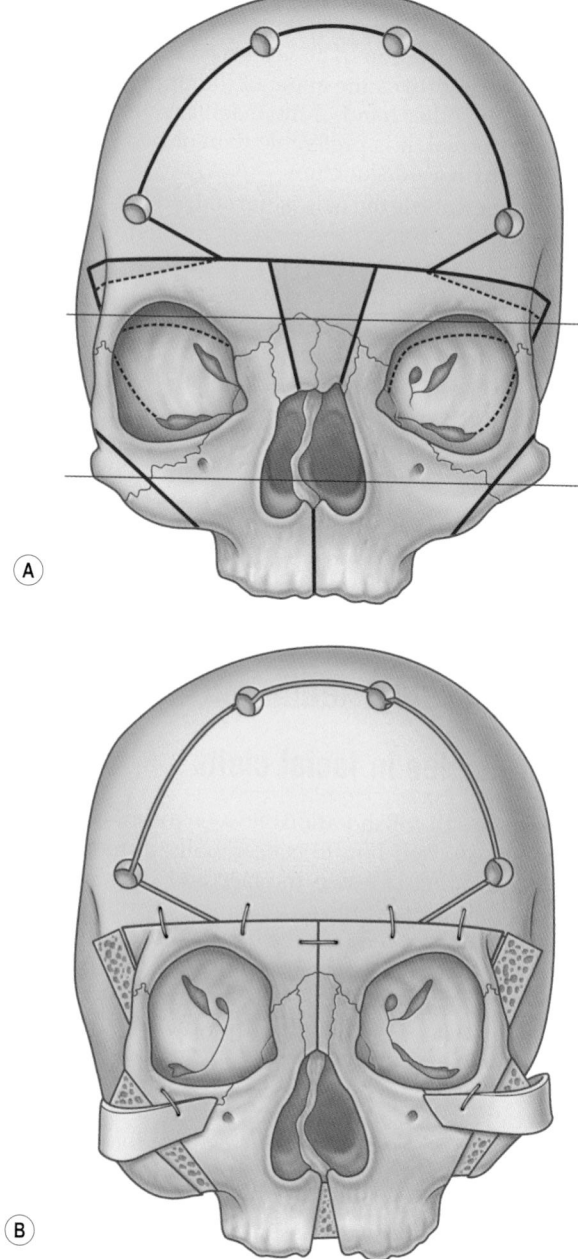

Fig. 32.3 Medialization of the two hemifaces after bipartition. **(A)** Before medialization; **(B)** after medialization.

horizontal cuts being situated below the infraorbital rim, through the malar bone and the maxilla. In Tessier's protocol, especially in adult patients, a supraorbital bar is kept in place in order to ensure stability of the mobilized orbits.[22]

Bipartition, proposed by van der Meulen[23,24] and developed by Tessier,[25,26] represents a mobilization of the two hemifaces *(Fig. 32.3)*. Instead of cutting below the orbits, the surgeon makes the osteotomies through the zygomatic arch, the pterygomaxillary junction and medially through the palate. The medial resection must have a "V" shape because there will be an element of rotation, along with a narrowing on the midline. The rotation allows for widening of the maxillary arch and

the nasal fossae and also for changing the axis of the orbits, which have a lateral slant.

Surgical techniques in facial clefts

Principles

The two main aims of surgery for this condition are to bring the orbits closer together and to create a nose of normal appearance. The basic anatomical anomaly is an increase in both the interorbital distance and the nasal bones whilst the glabellar region is much wider than normal. The enlarged portion of the midline structures is removed and, after mobilization of the orbits, the nasal skeleton is adjusted with the help of a bone graft if more dorsal projection is needed *(Fig. 32.4)*.

This combined approach allows the surgeon to move the orbits and repair bony anomalies of the fronto-orbitonasal complex. Orbital displacement is key to the treatment of major craniofacial clefts. The orbit can be moved on a horizontal, vertical, anterior, or posterior axis to correct all anomalies. Reconstruction of a missing orbital roof or part of the forehead, canthopexies, and correction of soft-tissue problems can be performed simultaneously.

Not all hypertelorisms are symmetrical, and asymmetrical cases are more complex to correct. The cranial base is also asymmetrical and so the different distortions must be carefully evaluated by computed tomography three-dimensional reconstructions. Sometimes both orbits have to be moved in different directions.[26,27]

The age at operation is important. If there is a cranial cleft, it is better to wait for the median frontal defect to ossify before surgery is scheduled. The neurosurgical approach is by means of a frontal bone flap. Its lower part depends on the variable elevation of the orbital rim, often including elevation of one side and transverse displacement on the opposite side.

Soft-tissue anomalies, such as skin excess, may be treated initially by sagittal resection or can be postponed as this tissue may contract over time. Another reason to delay midline skin resection is that dorsal nasal bone grafting, which is almost mandatory to achieve adequate nasal correction, requires some degree of skin excess.

In minor cases, a limited procedure with one- to three-wall mobilization may suffice.

Infrafrontal correction of hypertelorism

In the least significant hypertelorisms (less than 35 mm interorbital distance), a single medial wall mobilization can be undertaken. This procedure can be performed through a limited subciliary incision, but the authors prefer a coronal approach unless medial skin excess makes a nasal incision mandatory. The thin bone of the medial wall of the orbit can be easily in-fractured *(Fig. 32.5)*.

In selected cases presenting with mild symmetrical hypertelorism (35–40 mm), large frontal sinuses, and a high pituitary sella, the supraorbital rim and roof of the orbits can be left in place with mobilization of the other three walls.[20,28–31] However, this method is less effective for the correction of the orbital distance than the box-shift osteotomy. This subcranial approach can be used in a horizontal shift or a bipartition whenever the cribriform plate is high enough. Raveh and

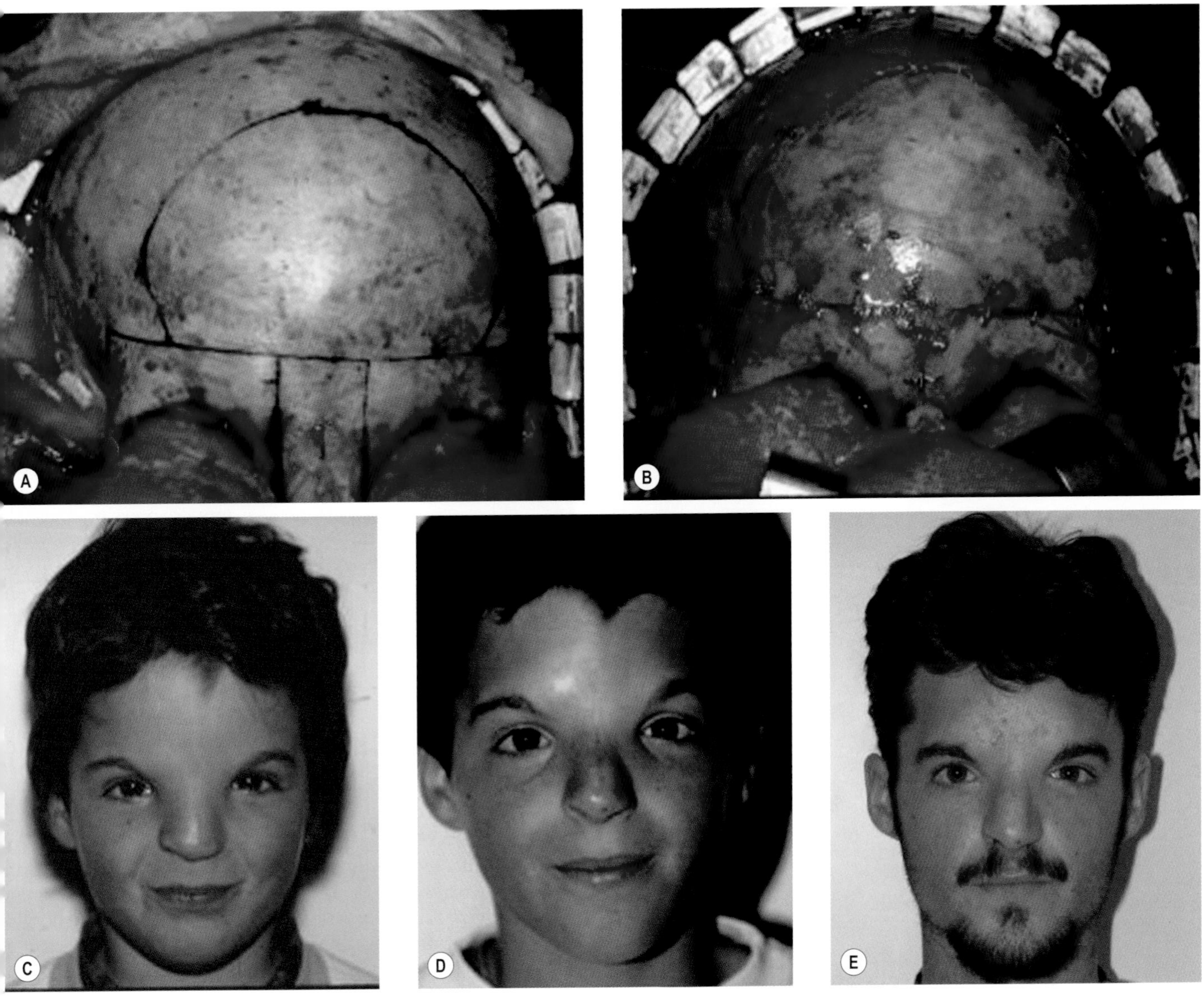

Fig. 32.4 Box-shift osteotomy for midline cleft. (A) Before osteotomy: note both lateral spurs, avoiding the need for supraorbital bar. (B) After medial shift. (C) Age 5 years, before treatment. (D) Age 6 years, after operation. (E) Age 21 years.

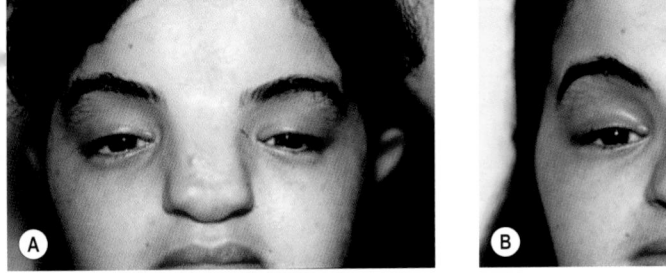
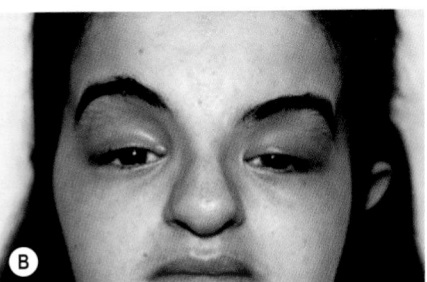
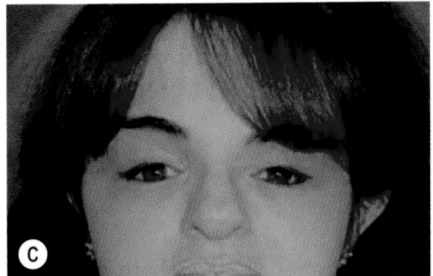

Fig. 32.5 Three-wall medialization osteotomy (horizontal shift). (A) Before treatment at age 7 years. (B) After operation. (C) At age 21 years.

Vuillemin[32] used this inferior intracranial approach, cutting the orbital roof and the ethmoidal cells from below, without a frontal craniectomy. They claimed to have good control of the dura and a shorter recovery period due to less aggressive surgery.

The periorbital regions are widely dissected through a coronal approach and subciliary incisions. The osteotomies are performed posteriorly enough to keep a wide bony platform that will push the globe medially. Medially, the nasal mucosa is dissected from under the nasal bones through a

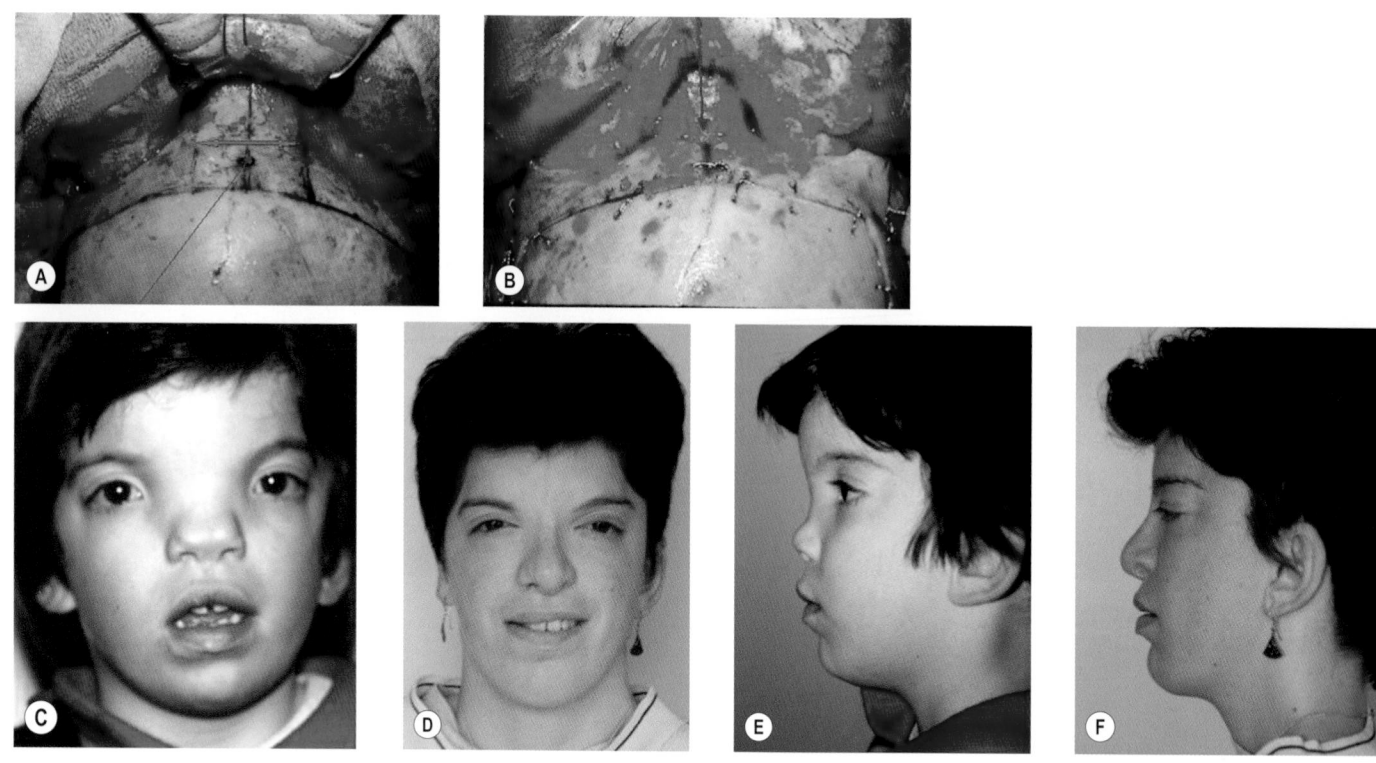

Fig. 32.6 Box-shift osteotomy for midline cleft. **(A)** Before osteotomy: note maximum width of bony resection. **(B)** After medial shift. **(C)** Front view at age 4 years before treatment. **(D)** Front view at age 25 years. **(E)** Lateral view at age 4 years before treatment. **(F)** Lateral view at age 25 years.

retrograde approach. A trephine hole can be created from above to improve access for the interorbital resection, allowing the nasal bones to be lifted and affording control of the superior medial wall segments. Should a dural tear occur, a frontal flap can be elevated for intracranial repair. The rest of the osteotomies are performed as in the intracranial approach. The mobilization must be carefully performed because the three-wall bony orbit is fragile. Stabilization is performed medially with stainless-steel wires. Repositioning of the nasal bones and control of the canthi are performed last before closure.

Box-shift osteotomies (symmetrical orbital hypertelorism)

When the interorbital distance is greater than 40 mm (*Fig. 32.6*), the neurosurgical approach is critical because it allows access to the orbital roof and the central ethmoidosphenoidal area. Only in rare circumstances, and in older patients, is it possible to move the lower three-quarters of the orbits and remove the excess width of the central nose below the cribriform plate while leaving the roof of the orbits intact. This extracranial approach is only possible if the cribriform plate is very high and the deformity is minimal.

Like most craniofacial teams, the authors prefer to use the frontal approach to have a clear view of the anterior cranial fossa; this also facilitates dura repair if necessary. In hypertelorism, anomalies of the midline often exist and good exposure is essential for dural control. Of note, duplication of the crista galli apophysis is not uncommon.

Frontal craniectomy

Frontal craniectomy allows access to the orbital roofs and medial structures. The design of the frontal craniectomy must be carefully planned by the craniofacial surgeon. The lower limit is of importance. Some surgeons, following Tessier's technique, prefer to keep a bridge of bone intact at the lower part of the forehead between the frontal flap and the mobilized orbits to maintain stability. If this is to be performed, the supraorbital rim to be preserved is about 1 cm in height; the preserved frontal bridge also measures 1 cm, and the lower limit of the frontal craniotomy must be at least 2 cm above the orbits. Many craniofacial surgeons, including the authors, do not preserve this horizontal band; the lower limit of the craniectomy with this approach is 1 cm above the orbits. This approach facilitates access to the anterior cranial fossa. An anteroposterior landmark and a stable point of fixation are fundamental. For these reasons, the authors preserve a low lateral spur of frontal bone, with the frontal craniotomy flap taking an upward angle at about the middle of the orbits (*Fig. 32.2*).

The frontal flap must be elevated with care as anomalies are frequently encountered (e.g., a very deep groove for the longitudinal sinus or a thick, or even bifid, crista galli). After the frontal flap has been elevated, careful dissection of the dura from the orbital roofs and from the edge of the greater wing of the sphenoid bone and the adjacent part of the temporal fossa is performed. The central region around the cribriform plate is the most challenging portion of the dissection. If the cribriform plate is normal or only moderately altered, the resection necessary to decrease the distance between the orbits is performed in the ethmoidal cells on either side of the cribriform plate. Sometimes, the cribriform plate is highly abnormal with the olfactory grooves widely separated and running close to the medial walls of the orbits. In these cases, sacrifice of the olfactory nerves is unavoidable during a large medial resection.

Meticulous repair of the dura is mandatory after resection of the olfactory nerves. A periosteal patch is often useful to reinforce the closure. The central resection is performed by the craniofacial surgeon who has previously dissected the nasal mucosal domes by proceeding cephalad from below the nasal bones. The paranasal osteotomies are performed vertically at a slightly divergent angle. The transverse posterior osteotomy is then performed. It is usually made in front of the crista galli if the olfactory nerves are intact. In the most severe cases, this osteotomy is performed posteriorly, removing most of the ethmoid bone. The medial resection is lifted *en bloc* and the nasal mucosal domes are exposed. If they are not intact, immediate suturing of the nasal mucosa is performed.

Osteotomies of the orbit

Next, the osteotomies are performed through the orbital roof, lateral orbital wall, and posteromedial wall. The lower osteotomies vary according to whether orbital shift or bipartition is being performed. The orbits are then brought together and contact is established in the midline. All the interposing elements, such as an enlarged superior nasal septum or residual posterior ethmoidal cells, must be removed. The dura must be carefully protected during these maneuvers. After the orbits are rigidly fixated in the midline by wires or miniplates, the neurosurgical portion of the procedure is almost complete. Dural integrity and hemostasis are ensured in the anterior and temporal cranial fossae, and the frontal bone flap is secured back in place.

Bone grafts from the cranial vault are needed to close the gaps in the orbital walls and often to build up the nasal dorsum. Sometimes, in adolescents and adults, it is possible to split the frontal bone flap and use the posterior aspect for bone grafts. More often, it is necessary to take bone grafts from the cranial vault. Specifically, a thick, straight 5-cm segment is necessary for nasal reconstruction. It is convenient to take these bony pieces posterior to the frontal flap. In the authors' practice, bone dust from the burr holes and small residual bony fragments are mixed with fibrin glue and used to occlude the vault defects after the graft removal.

The optic nerve is not straight; it has laxity that allows it to follow the displacement of the eyeball. Even a significant displacement is well tolerated by the optic nerves. To permit a good medial displacement of the eyeball, it is essential that the medial wall of the orbit is also displaced towards the midline. If the osteotomy is too anterior, there will be a step effect, limiting the displacement of the ocular globes.

A secondary rhinoplasty will most likely be necessary to achieve an optimized aesthetic result.

Bipartition with intracranial approach (large symmetrical hypertelorism with arched palate)

This technique varies slightly from the box-shift, but many surgical steps are identical. Differences are as follows *(Fig. 32.3)*:

- V-shape resection of bone at the nose
- absence of osteotomy in the maxilla at the lower limit of the orbit
- osteotomy at the pterygomaxillary junction
- the medialization part of the upper face creates an opening at the palatal level *(Fig. 32.7)*.

Asymmetrical cases

Asymmetrical cases are more difficult to correct than symmetrical ones. Sometimes each orbit must be moved in different directions whilst on other occasions only one of the orbits is involved in the planned displacement. The cranial base is also asymmetrical; the various distortions must be carefully evaluated by computed tomography with three-dimensional reconstructions. Paramedian clefts create a situation in which the affected orbit is displaced laterally and inferiorly to a variable degree. A defect in the frontal bone is often associated. The orbit may be reduced in size (anophtalmia or microphtalmia). Various anomalies of the maxillary and nasal portion of the face may also be associated.

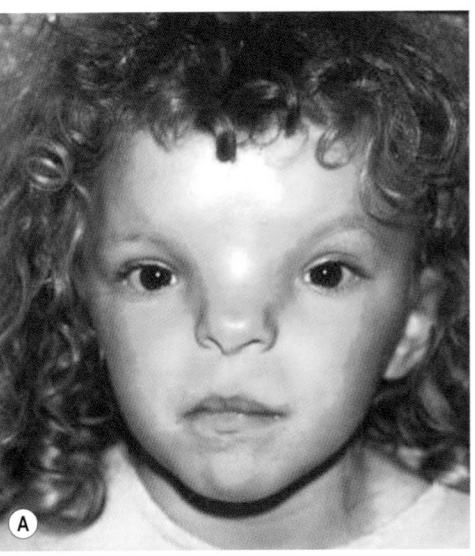
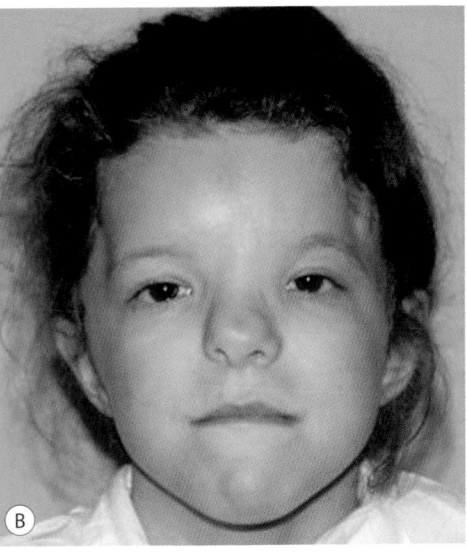

Fig. 32.7 Hypertelorism correction by bipartition for a frontocranial dysplasia. **(A)** Before treatment at age 4.5 years. **(B)** After treatment (observe temporal hollowness, to be corrected secondarily).

After the anomaly has been evaluated and classified according to the Tessier system (see previous discussion), a plan of treatment is devised. The correction must be planned from top to bottom; that is, the frontal and orbital regions must be reconstructed first. In most cases, a bilateral asymmetrical correction is required. The neurosurgical approach is by means of a frontal bone flap, its lower limit being carefully planned because of the variable reconstructions of the supraorbital rim, often including elevation on one side. Transverse movement only is performed on the affected side. In the paramedian clefts, the ethmoidal region is asymmetrical and dural elevation should be performed with care. After the orbits are properly positioned, the frontal bone flap is adjusted and wired into place.

Sometimes only one orbit is displaced, usually inferiorly, with one globe inferior to the other; this condition is defined as orbital dystopia. In these situations, displacement of the entire orbit *en bloc* is the solution. Partial maneuvers such as elevation of the roof and placement of bone grafts on the floor usually produce disappointing results. This *en bloc* displacement of the orbit requires a frontal flap to gain access to the roof. This frontal flap can be unilateral and corresponds to the width of the orbital osteotomy. The frontal segment removed to permit elevation of the supraorbital rim is utilized as a bone graft placed below the orbit to maintain the elevation and fill the resultant bony gap.

In some cases of asymmetrical clefting, an asymmetrical bipartition has been used.

Timing and indications for surgery in faciocraniosynostosis

Without early treatment, intracranial hypertension can lead to optic atrophy and visual loss in craniosynostosis. This is observed mainly in Crouzon's syndrome and in oxycephalies. In the series of Hôpital Necker Enfants-Malades, papilledema was observed in 35% and optic atrophy in 10% of Crouzon's cases. In the other syndromes, papilledema was observed in only 4–5% and no optic atrophy was observed.[19] Because of these risks, and as previously mentioned, strategic management of faciocraniosynostosis usually demands at least a two-stage procedure[7,8,11,12] followed by later refinements. The skull is operated upon first and the face secondarily. Apert's

syndrome is definitely the most difficult to treat, and might require the largest number of additional procedures.

Orbits

In Necker's experience, the surgical treatment of the associated hypertelorism is delayed until after the frontal advancement and after 4 years of age.[7,8] This strategy provides a thick enough skull bone to perform stable fixation after mobilization of the osteotomized segments. The choice between the orbital shift and the facial bipartition depends on a series of factors:

- The maxillary arch: if the maxillary arch and occlusion are normal, it seems preferable to avoid an interpterygomaxillary disjunction, and box-shift osteotomies are sufficient; this is the case in Crouzon's and Apert's. Conversely, if the maxillary arch is narrow and inverted, the incisors being higher than the molars, bipartition is the operation of choice because it widens the maxilla and improves the angle of the upper dentition.
- The axis of the orbits: if the axis is normal, a horizontal mobilization is satisfactory. If they are laterally and downwardly oblique, bipartition corrects these anomalies.
- The nasal fossae: if they are narrow, bipartition improves the airways, especially if a narrowing in the upper part of the face is associated with a widening of the maxillary arch.

These last three criteria are all present in Apert's, and therefore bipartition is the procedure of choice for these patients. The bipartition can be performed with a facial Le Fort III advancement as a combined second step, sometimes by means of osteodistraction. In cases of a Le Fort III osteotomy combined with bipartition and distraction, we would use the combination of internal and external distraction devices *(Fig. 32.8)*.

Face

Le Fort classically described three types of maxillary disjunction depending on the transversal level of the facial fractures. Since the surgical facial advancements approximately reproduce these fracture lines on the face, Tessier gave the names of Le Fort I, II, and III to the facial osteotomies. Although Gillies was the first to perform a facial advancement in the

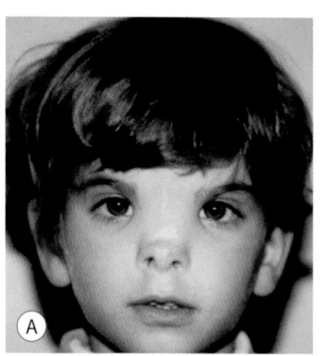
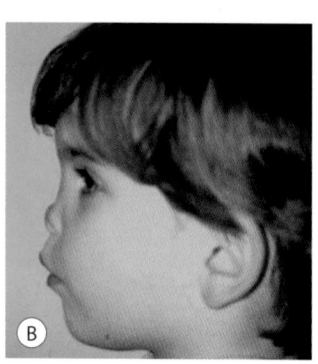
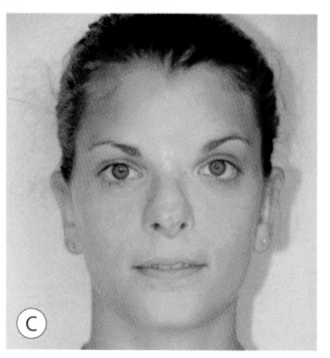
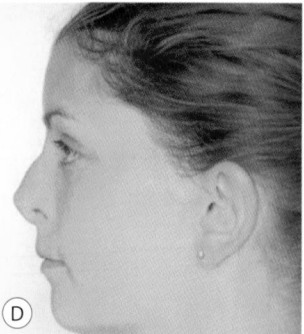

Fig. 32.8 Box-shift osteotomy for midline cleft. **(A)** Before osteotomy: front view at age 4 years. **(B)** Before osteotomy: lateral view at age 4 years. **(C)** Front view at age 23 years after augmentation rhinoplasty (observe good quality of midline nasal scar for skin excess). **(D)** Lateral view at age 23 years after augmentation rhinoplasty (nasal revision to be performed for hump removal).

late 1940s,[33] Tessier[10] really developed the Le Fort III type of advancement, his lines of osteotomies being deeper than those of Gillies, located behind the lacrimal apparatus. The facial advancement is usually of the Le Fort III type.

Patients who have previously undergone forehead advancement normally have facial retrusion to a variable degree. As a rule, we prefer to delay the facial advancement until there is permanent dentition and a stable occlusive relationship can be achieved. When the deformity is moderate, there is no difficulty in convincing the patient and the family to wait. In patients with more severe deformity, the social and psychological pressure is high, as well as the demands of the family and often the child. In most severe cases, difficulties in chewing and breathing as well as significant inferior exorbitism are also present. In these situations, after a warning that another operation (usually a Le Fort I) will be necessary after permanent dentition is in place, we perform a facial advancement.

In Apert's, the advancement will be combined with a facial bipartition, as mentioned earlier. This procedure is performed before final dentition has erupted; therefore no attempt to correct the open bite is made.

Surgical technique of hypertelorism correction in faciocraniosynostosis

Because faciocraniosynostoses are essentially characterized by backward displacement of the forehead and midface, both having to be moved forward, this condition can be treated by advancing the forehead and the face either separately or simultaneously, possibly in combination with the correction of the hypertelorbitism. The classical management includes an initial anterior skull remodeling and, later, a facial advancement as a second step, as detailed previously. In cases where early frontofacial advancement is performed, the hypertelorism is corrected secondarily.[7,8]

Hypertelorism correction by bipartition in combination with Le Fort III osteotomy (Figs 32.9 and 32.10)

The combination of hypertelorism and maxillary anomalies makes the facial bipartition the logical operation in treating Apert's syndrome. This may be combined with a distraction if indicated.

Coronal approach

The scalp is incised after subcutaneous infiltration with epinephrine solution; the incision follows the scar of the previous skull expansion if present. Exposure of the calvarial vault in the subgaleal or supraperiosteal plane might be complicated by scar tissue and bony dehiscence. Complete dissection of the periorbita is conducted in the subperiosteal plane. Exposure of the root of the nose, as well as the lateral walls of the orbits and the zygomatic arches, is performed after undermining both temporalis muscles.

Subcranial osteotomies

The lower three-quarters of the orbits, the nose, the malar bones, and the upper maxilla, are to be mobilized. Bony cuts are performed with a reciprocating saw in a bilateral manner. The lateral cut of the orbit is usually started at the frontozygomatic junction, then continued on to the floor of the orbit to reach the sphenomaxillary fissure. Care must be taken to avoid cutting through the lower orbital rim with an anteriorly based osteotomy so as not to fracture the inferior orbital wall in a shallow, distorted orbit. The zygomatic arch is easily transected. The root of the nose is horizontally sectioned while a 3-mm cranial buttress is maintained. A medial V-shaped resection is then performed; the osteotomy is extended downward to the medial wall of each orbit, taking care to be posterior enough to avoid disruption of the medial canthus. Finally, a bilateral pterygomaxillary disjunction is made from above through the pterygoid fossa, with a finger inside the mouth to control the position of the chisel.

An epinephrine solution is also infiltrated under the palatal mucosa. A medial bony cut might be necessary through a small mucosal opening behind the incisors. This will allow for rotation of the two hemipalates. At this point the two hemifaces are free enough to be mobilized independently. A combined movement of upper medialization and inferior lateralization allows the rotation of both hemifaces to correct the hypertelorism and the down-slanting of the eyelids.

Osteosynthesis and grafts

Osteosynthesis with metallic wires or miniplates is necessary in the orbital region at the lateral junction of the orbital wall and at the zygomatic arch in order to maintain the advancement. Bone grafts, usually taken from the outer table of the parietal calvaria, are mandatory at the root of the nose and in the upper part of the lateral orbital walls. The grafts at the frontozygomatic junction are triangular, whereas two quadrangular grafts, like two parts of the roof of a house, are required at the root of the nose. Bone grafts might be useful to fill the gaps at the lateral orbital walls to prevent enophthalmos if a significant advancement is performed at the Le Fort III level.

An archbar is anchored on the teeth with metallic wires to maintain stability at the maxillary level.

Closure of the scalp is conducted in the usual manner after the temporal muscles have been transposed anteriorly to fill the temporal defect created by the medialization of the lateral walls of the orbits.

If distractors are used for a combined advancement, a few technique modifications would be employed:

- The nose and lateral aspects of the frontozygomatic regions would be grafted but not rigidly fixated.
- In case of external distraction, the pulling wires would preferably be at the pyriform apertures (*Fig. 32.9*).
- In case of internal distracters, a transfacial pin would be useful for fixation of both hemifaces (*Fig. 32.10*). Internal distracters may be left as consolidators for a longer period of time (3–4 months).

Postoperative care

Like all major transcranial craniofacial procedures, postoperative care depends on the procedure itself and its implications

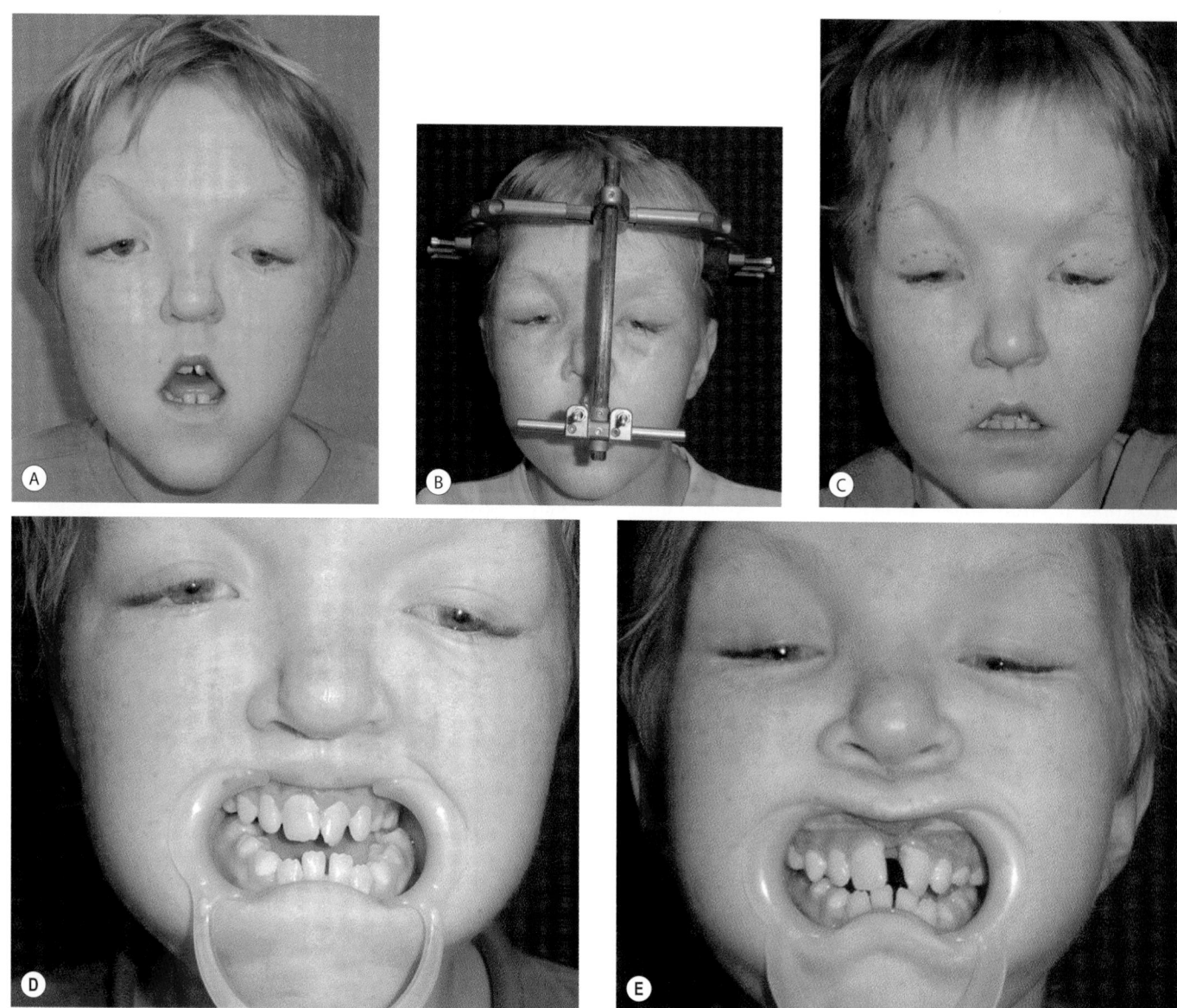

Fig. 32.9 Le Fort III with bipartition and external distraction in an Apert patient aged 11 years (observe gap between incisors) before orthodontic treatment. **(A)** Front view before surgery. **(B)** Front view with external distractor in place. **(C)** Front view after surgery (observe normalization of eyelid cants). **(D)** Occlusion before surgery. **(E).** Occlusion after surgery.

for systemic homeostasis. Close monitoring is best achieved in a specialized pediatric intensive care unit for at least the first 24 hours. It is not uncommon in our experience that the degree of postoperative airway edema may dictate a prolonged intubation extending up to 3 or 4 days. After such a delay, it is likely that the acute phase of the initial swelling, sometimes impressive after 48 hours at the eyelid level but also in the airway, has nearly, if not completely, resolved. A conservative approach to the airway may avoid unwanted reintubation after an early extubation. This is a significant risk after bilateral hemifacial medialization, even if this procedure enlarges the airway at the base of the nose.

Postoperative bleeding secondary to the various osteotomy lines must be carefully monitored, especially in the context of pre- and intraoperative blood loss and possible resultant

coagulopathy. Prophylactic antibiotic therapy is usually not extended beyond 48 hours according to guidelines for an invasive craniofacial procedure with exposed contaminated spaces (ethmoidal sinus, frontal sinus if present).

The prophylactic preoperative tarsorrhaphy is left in place until after successful extubation. The tarsorrhaphy will protect the cornea from ulcer formation and reduce potentially severe chemosis (conjunctival edema). When a box-shift osteotomy has been performed, the subciliary stiches are best removed at day 3 and replaced by Steri-Strips. Sutures from a midline excess skin excision are removed at day 5 like any other facial closure, unless a subcuticular intradermal running suture has been placed.

Prevention of complications remains a key issue in the postoperative period.

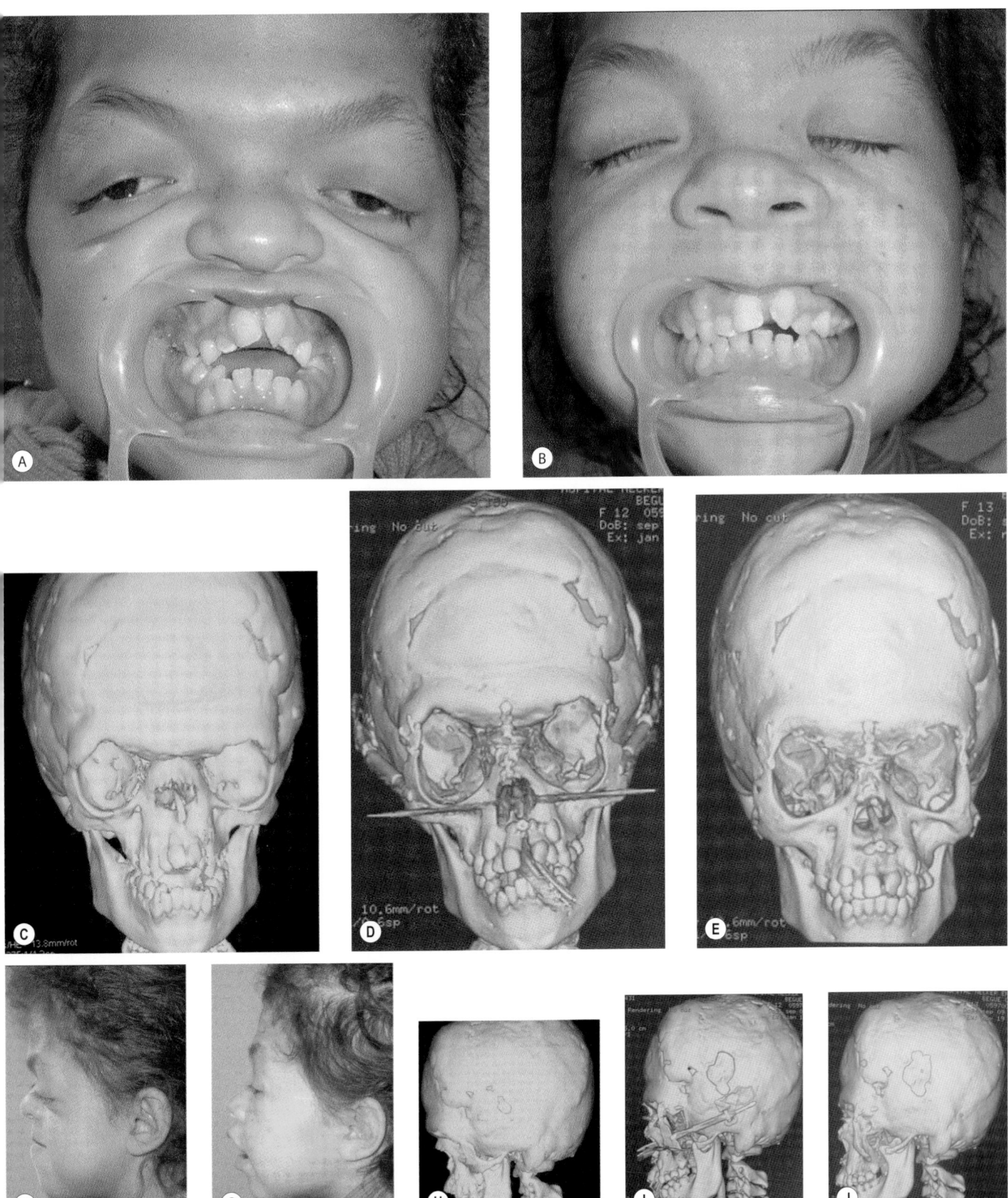

Fig. 32.10 Le Fort III with bipartition and internal distraction (observe transfacial pin during distraction period), and modification of angulation of the maxillary arch. **(A)** Front view before; **(B)** front view after procedure. **(C)** Computed tomography (CT) scan before Le Fort III (observe retrusion of the midface). **(D)** CT scan during distraction with transfacial pin. **(E)** CT scan after distraction and removal of distractors. **(F)** Lateral view before advancement. **(G)** Lateral view after advancement. **(H)** Lateral CT scan before advancement. **(I)** Lateral CT scan during distraction with internal devices. **(J)** Lateral CT scan after distraction.

Outcomes, prognosis, and complications

Possible complications may be separated into acute and delayed occurrences. As previously mentioned, acute complications must be vigilantly prevented during the initial postoperative period:

- Excessive bleeding, mainly related to a coagulopathy induced by important preoperative transfusion, is a risk.
- Cerebrospinal fluid leakage through the nose is not uncommon and may require lumbar drainage if persistent after 3 days of lumbar punctures. Rhinorrhea represents a risk of meningitis and can be avoided by careful dissection in the retroglabellar region.
- Infection linked to an insufficient cranialization of the frontal sinus (if a frontal sinus was present at the time of surgery to require cranialization). This may be best prevented by operating early after the age of 4 years, when the frontal sinus has usually not yet developed. Infection may arise anywhere from a few days to a few months postoperatively.
- Ophthalmological complications such as keratitis or chemosis are best prevented by the initial tarsorrhaphy. Blindness represents an exceptionally rare but dramatic complication, and all patients should be warned accordingly. The possibility of a postoperative strabismus is more common, and care should be taken to sufficiently medialize the medial orbital walls posterior to the osteotomies so as to avoid a step-off that may impinge on the medial rectus muscles. Failure to carry the medialization far enough posteriorly may also contribute to an insufficient medialization of the globes despite a satisfactory medialization of the bony orbits.
- In the long term the most important complication is an insufficient correction. This is most likely to occur not by relapse, but by soft-tissue relaxation, especially at the medial canthi. To this extent the medial canthus fixation tends to be disappointing and frequently necessitates a secondary correction (*Fig. 32.11*). The secondary rhinoplasty greatly contributes to the aesthetic outcome, but must be delayed until adulthood.
- Temporal hollowing is not uncommon, especially if the hypertelorism correction is the second major procedure after a cranioplasty or after a bipartition, which tends to deepen the temporal fossa.

Secondary procedures

Soft-tissue problems are more complex to treat than bony irregularities.

Some craniofacial malformations involve only the skeleton, e.g., mild symmetrical orbital hypertelorism, orbital dystopia, frontal or malar asymmetries, and malposition. Correction can be achieved through hidden approaches, such as bicoronal or vestibular incisions, or through palpebral infraciliary approaches, all of which leave almost invisible scars.

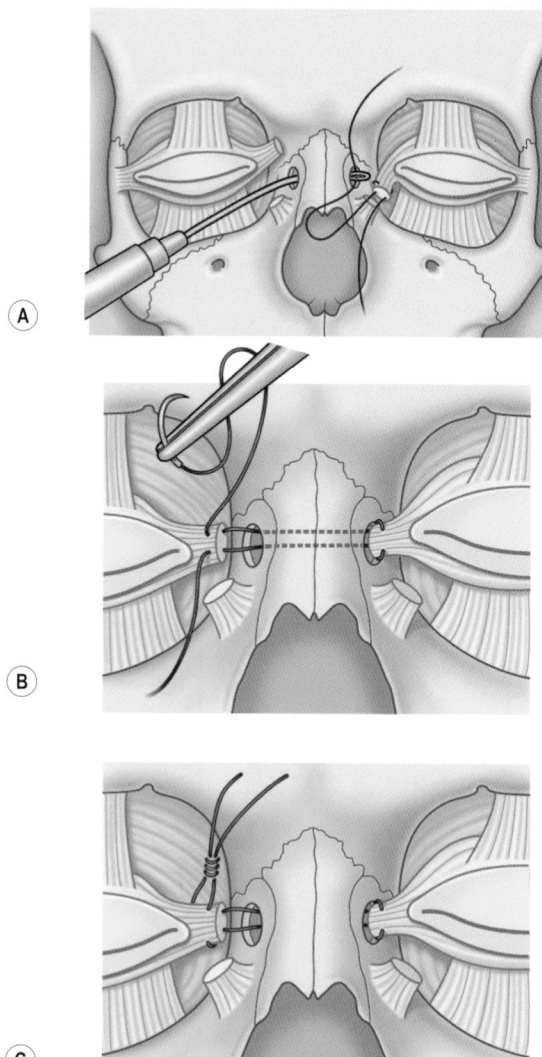

Fig. 32.11 (A–C) Secondary correction of medial canthus disinsertion.

Temporal hollowness can be addressed by fat grafting according to the Coleman technique. Repeated treatments may be necessary.

Excess skin can be adjusted and will retract. After correction of moderate hypertelorism, the excess skin of the glabellar region and dorsum of the nose retracts with the help of good undermining and a bone graft to lift the dorsum of the nose. Possible future soft-tissue correction must be considered in the initial treatment plan such that skeletal access is achieved without sacrificing potential cutaneous flap options. For example, if a frontal skin flap is planned, the design of the coronal incision may have to be altered to avoid violating the future pedicle.

It is usually much easier to reconstruct the skeleton than to correct soft-tissue deficiencies. All the resources of plastic surgery can rarely achieve a perfect contour with minimal scars. The authors briefly consider the primary soft-tissue problems encountered in major congenital craniofacial malformations at the end of this chapter.

Regardless, the final rhinoplasty will be the most important element of the definitive aesthetics result.

Refinements in hypertelorism correction (in clefts or craniosynostotic patients)

Irregularities are frequent in the frontal region, the nose, and the temporal fossae. Refinements may be performed early or delayed until the completion of craniofacial growth, after 15 years of age. Techniques to obtain a satisfactory contour have classically included bone remodeling, bone grafting, and the onlay of biomaterials. More recently, fat grafting as described by Coleman has proven useful to correct minor anomalies such as temporal hollowing.

Soft-tissue refinements are aesthetically relevant for the final result and may be divided into several subcategories, as follows.

Canthus correction

During the surgical correction of hypertelorism, it is preferable to maintain the bony attachment of the medial canthus. In so doing, one avoids the need for medial canthus reattachment, which is always possible but is sometimes unreliable in the long term. Even when the medial canthal ligament is preserved, if the medial bony resection is 2 cm, the postoperative intercanthal distance may be reduced by only 1 cm, demonstrating 50% efficacy at the soft-tissue level. It might be necessary to reinsert the medial canthal ligaments under increased tension (with a transnasal technique: *Fig. 32.11*) and correct an epicanthal fold (easily achieved with Y-V plasty or a Del Campo technique (asymmetric Z-plasty).[34]

The lateral canthus is less well defined and it is easily repositioned with a lateral suspension, if necessary, at the end of the craniofacial procedure. If this correction proves insufficient in the long term, a lateral canthopexy may be performed secondarily through a small lateral incision.

Scalp and eyebrows

Hairline distortion is frequently observed in craniofacial clefts and reflects the continuity of the cleft at the scalp level. Hair growing down on to the forehead can be removed. Unwanted hair can be incorporated into a frontal skin resection that facilitates exposure, or excision may be achieved secondarily. Eyebrows can be clefted or displaced. Differential repositioning of the forehead and scalp can correct eyebrow displacement, usually by lowering the high side.

Nose

In symmetrical hypertelorism presenting with an excess of skin at the level of the nasal dorsum, it is advisable to avoid the easy solution of midline skin excision. Some of these median scars do very well with time and become hardly visible, but others stretch, become pigmented, and are very prominent. It is therefore better to count on skin retraction, as previously discussed.

If there is a cleft affecting the nose, it should be corrected at the time of the craniofacial procedure to utilize the relative excess soft tissue obtained by the undermining performed around the nose. A cleft can be closed by reapproximation of tissues with plasties at the alar margins, but if there is a tissue deficiency, various nasal flaps should be considered. The excess skin existing on the upper part of the nose can be transferred to the lower part.

In some cases, the nose is very distorted and the shortage of skin is obvious from the start. The frontal area is the best zone from which to obtain the missing skin. On other occasions, correction of the hypertelorism creates an excess of soft tissue at the level of the forehead that can be used as a frontal flap. Sometimes, a preliminary frontal skin expansion may be necessary to provide the required soft tissue. The potential need for nasal reconstruction should be carefully considered early in the planning process as the usually preferred coronal approach may require modification if soft-tissue recruitment becomes necessary in this context.

Eyelids and orbits

Clefts of the eyelids primarily involve the lower eyelid and are addressed during the midface reconstruction, as are oculonasal clefts. The craniofacial clefts discussed in this chapter may also result in pathology of the orbits.

If there is anophthalmia or microphthalmia, the bony orbit does not develop to its normal size. The preferred treatment is a progressive enlargement of the conjunctiva,[35,36] but conformers are very difficult to place; intraorbital expanders are much more efficient and can produce an almost normal growth of the orbit with a prosthesis fitted afterwards. Nevertheless, this orbital expansion is difficult to execute and requires very close follow-up. If orbital expansion fails or is not attempted, a micro-orbit must be faced. This orbit should first be placed in proper position, vertically and horizontally, in relation to the other orbit. It can then be surgically enlarged by expanding the whole circumference. Access to the orbital roof is obtained with a localized frontal craniotomy, as for an orbital dystopia. The secondary soft-tissue work of creating a good cavity capable of retaining an ocular prosthesis, and building up the short, retracted eyelids with auricular composite grafts, is often more difficult and time-consuming than the skeletal work.

Oculomotor disorders

Numerous conditions in craniofacial surgery may present with oculomotor disorders, especially when hypertelorism is apparent. The rule is to perform the bony work first and secondarily to address any oculomotor disorders that are present. Further discussion of the treatment of oculomotor disorders is beyond the scope of this chapter.

Recurrences of hypertelorism

In our experience, hypertelorism recurrences are not frequent if the repair has been performed after 4 years of age, at the completion of skull growth. This recurrence rate would be different if the hypertelorism were corrected earlier; for instance, at 1 year of age the brain is still undergoing significant growth which might counteract medialization of the orbits. An exceptional circumstance of orbital hypertelorism relapse has been encountered with an interorbital encephalocele which had recurred because of ventriculoperitoneal shunt dysfunction. The encephalocele acted as an interorbital expander that progressively enlarged the tissues between the orbital cavities.

Conversely, the inherent lack of growth in faciocraniosynostosis may produce relative relapse of any associated maxillary retrusion, but this finding does not require further revision.

Careful analysis with three-dimnensional computed tomography helps tremendously in planning for precise bony work.[37] Nevertheless, minor primary undercorrection of hypertelorism is more frequent than actual recurrence, despite satisfactory bony work. This finding underscores the importance of soft-tissue refinements, especially with regard to nasal correction, which will eventually determine the success of the clinical outcome. In older patients, nasal deformity may not only be the presenting chief complaint; it might also be the final and most important step of the surgical correction.[38,39]

Craniofacial surgery is teamwork

It is obvious from the congenital craniofacial malformations discussed in this chapter that the only possible approach to these patients is via a craniofacial team. Once the team members have examined the patient, and with the invaluable help of modern imaging, a plan of treatment is drawn up by the plastic surgeon and the neurosurgeon to incorporate all the morphological and functional aspects of the correction. These operations are too complex to be performed without significant previous experience with the problems involved. Such experience can only be obtained if these operations are performed in a limited number of specialized centers.

Access the complete references list online at **http://www.expertconsult.com**

5. Tessier P. Anatomical classification of facial, craniofacial and laterofacial clefts. *J Maxillofac Surg*. 1976;4:69.

7. Marchac D, Renier D, Broumand S. Timing of treatment for craniosynostosis : a 20 year experience. *Br J Plast Surg*. 1994;47:211–222.

   The authors report their extensive experience in this 983-patient series. With early diagnosis, brachycephalies are corrected between 2 and 4 months of life; other craniosynostoses are addressed in the second half of the first year of life.

9. Crouzon O. Dysostose craniofaciale héréditaire. *Bull Soc Med Hôp Paris*. 1912;33:D:-15.

10. Tessier P. Osteotomies totales de la face: Syndrome de Crouzon, syndrome d'Apert, oxycephalies, scaphocephalies, turricephalies. *Ann Chir Plast*. 1967; 12:273.

13. Ortiz-Monasterio F, Fuente del Campo A, Carillo A. Advancement of the orbits and the midface in one piece, combined with frontal repositioning for the correction of Crouzon's deformities. *Plast Reconstr Surg*. 1978;6:507.

   The authors advocate composite advancement of the orbits and midface in addition to frontal advancement for the management of Crouzon's syndrome. They caution that, while they are optimistic, their data do not have sufficient follow-up to demonstrate the longevity of their results.

16. Arnaud E, Marchac D, Renier D. Reduction of morbidity of frontofacial advancement in children with distraction. *Plast Reconstr Surg*. 2007;120:1009–1026.

   This is a prospective analysis of 36 patients undergoing monobloc distraction for faciocraniosynostosis. The authors assessed their outcomes and concluded that their use of internal distraction reduced the risks inherent to monobloc advancement.

17. Apert E. De l'acrocephalosyndactylie. *Bull Soc Med Hop Paris*. 1906;23:1310.

19. Renier D, Sainte-Rose C, Marchac D, et al. Intracranial pressure in craniostenosis. *J Neurosurg*. 1982;57: 370–377.

   Pre- and postoperative intracranial pressure (ICP) measurements were taken in 23 craniosynostosis patients. Elevated ICP normalized after surgery. A correlation was noted between elevated ICP and lower cognitive testing.

21. Converse JM, Ransohoff J, Matthew E, et al. Ocular hypertelorism and pseudohypertelorism. Advances in surgical treatment. *Plast Reconstr Surg*. 1970;45:1.

   This review begins with a discussion of the definition of hypertelorism and associated diagnoses. A detailed survey of corrective procedures follows.

22. Tessier P. Experience in the treatment of orbital hypertelorism. *Plast Reconstr Surg*. 1974;53:4.

33

Craniofacial clefts

James P. Bradley and Henry K. Kawamoto Jr.

SYNOPSIS

- Congenital craniofacial clefts are abnormal disfigurements of the face and cranium occurring in a variety of patterns and varying degrees of severity
- Craniofacial clefts are thought to occur spontaneously, except for syndromes with clefting combinations numbers 6, 7, and 8), like Treacher–Collins syndrome or hemifacial microsomia
- If normal embryologic neuroectoderm migration and penetration do not occur, the epithelium breaks down to form a facial cleft. The severity of the cleft is proportional to the failure of penetration by the neuroectoderm
- Tessier's numeric classification from number 0 to number 14 (facial clefts = numbers 0–8 and cranial clefts = numbers 9–14) offers a descriptive, easy-to-understand system for rare craniofacial clefts and is treatment-oriented
- Median craniofacial dysplasias consist of hypoplastic (tissue deficiency), dysraphia (normal tissue but clefted), and hyperplastic (tissue excess) malformations
- During infancy (3–12 months), functional problems, soft-tissue clefts, and midline cranial defects (e.g., encephaloceles) may be corrected
- In older children (6–9 years), midface and orbital reconstruction with bone grafting or a facial bipartition may be performed
- At skeletal maturity orthognathic and final soft-tissue corrective procedures may be performed.

Introduction

Congenital craniofacial clefts are abnormal disfigurements of the face and cranium with deficiencies, excesses, or even a normal (but separated) amount of tissue occurring along linear regions.[1-4] Of all congenital facial anomalies, craniofacial clefts are among the most disfiguring. They may be seen in a variety of patterns and varying degrees of severity. Although at first glance they appear to defy definable patterns, most craniofacial clefts occur along predictable embryologic lines.[5] Craniofacial clefts may be either unilateral or bilateral and one cleft type can manifest on one side of the face, while a different type is present on the other side.

Classifications of craniofacial clefts

Craniofacial malformations are rare, and have multiple variations and a spectrum of severity. For diagnostic and treatment purposes, the use of similar terminology describing embryologic maldevelopment, genetic etiology, or anatomic landmarks is beneficial. Organization of the seemingly heterogeneous clefting malformations is necessary for both morphogenetic understanding and knowledge of surgical anatomy for treatment. Therefore, orderly systems of classification have been described.[1-4]

The American Association of Cleft Palate Rehabilitaion (AACPR) separated craniofacial clefts into four categories based on pathologic location: (1) mandibular process clefts; (2) naso-ocular clefts; (3) oro-ocular clefts; and (4) oroaural clefts.[6] First, mandibular process clefts group malformations of the mandible and lower lip. Second, naso-ocular clefts include malformations located between the nasal ala and the medial canthus. Third, oro-ocular clefts consist of clefting anomalies connecting the oral cavity to the orbit between the medial and lateral canthus. Fourth, oroaural clefts describe anomalies involving the region from the oral commissure to the auricular tragus. Subsequent to the AACPR classification, Boo-Chai made modifications based on surface anatomic landmarks, including skeletal components.[7] The oro-ocular clefts were subdivided into two types, the oromedial canthus and orolateral canthus, with the infraorbital foramen as a reference point.

The Karfik classification has an embryologic and morphologic basis and is divided into five groups: (1) group A: rhinencephalic malformations; (2) group B: anomalies of the first and second branchial arch; (3) group C: orbitopalpebral malformations; (4) group D: craniocephalic malformations (e.g., Apert and Crouzon syndrome); and (5) group E: atypical deformities from congenital tumors, atrophy, hypertrophy, and true oblique clefts which cannot be related to any embryologic fusion line.[8] Group A, the rhinencephalic malformations, was further divided into two subtypes: group A1, axial malformations derived from frontonasal promenince, and group A2, paraxial malformations adjacent to the nasal region. Group B, anomalies of the first and second branchial arch, was also further divided into two subtypes: group B1, composed of the lateral otocephalic malformations (craniofacial microsomia, Treacher–Collins syndrome, Pierre Robin sequence, and auricular malformations) and group B2, including the mandibular midline malformations.

The Van der Meulen classification used the term "dysplasia" since some of the malformations did not represent true clefts.[9] The defects were labeled by the name of the developmental area (facial processes and bones) that is involved. The malformations are believed to occur before or during the fusion of the facial processes, but before the start of ossification (*Fig. 33.1*).

Median craniofacial clefts require special consideration because of variation in malformations and deformations. With tissue agenesis and holoprosencephaly at one end (the hypoplasias), and frontonasal hyperplasia and excessive tissue (the hyperplasias) at the other end, median anomalies with normal tissue volume occupy the middle portion of the spectrum.[10] Noordhoff *et al.* limited the term "holoprosencephaly" to cases of alobar brain and preferred the term "dysplasia"rather than "dysgenesis."[11] Thus, for clarification, median craniofacial dysplasias have been organized and divided into:

I: median craniofacial hypoplasia (tissue deficiency or agenesis)

II: median craniofacial dysraphia (normal tissue volume but clefted)

III: median craniofacial hyperplasia (tissue excess or duplication).

Under each division further subclassification is used to describe the specific anomalies of the number 0–14 clefts (*Table 33.1*).

I: Median craniofacial hypoplasia (tissue deficiency and/or agenesis)

A. Holoprosencephalic spectrum (alobar brain)

1. Cyclopia: described as a single eye in a single orbit. Arrhinia exists with proboscis often located above the single orbit. Microcephaly is also a component.

2. Ethmocephaly: severe hypotelorism exists but the orbits are separate anatomically. Again, arrhinia is present; however, the proboscis is located in between the orbits.

3. Cebocephaly: moderate to severe hypotelorism is noted. There is a proboscis-like rudimentary nose in a more typical nasal position.

4. Primary palate agenesis: the primary palate, including the premaxillary segment and associated midline structures, is absent or severely deficient. Hypotelorism is seen.

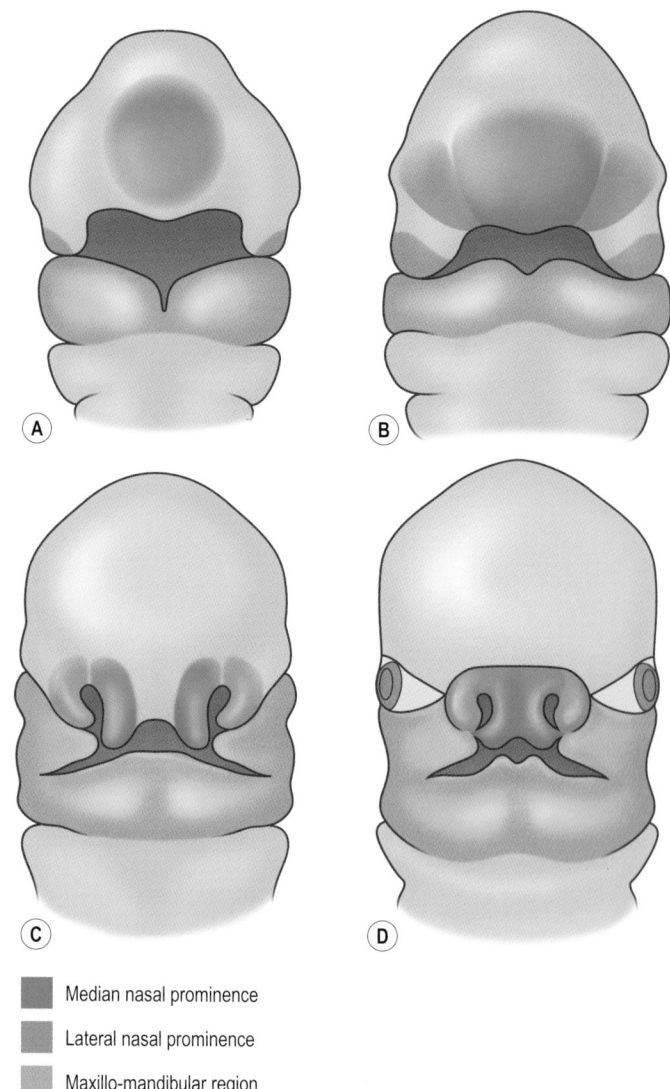

Median nasal prominence

Lateral nasal prominence

Maxillo-mandibular region

Fig. 33.1 Embryology of the face. Illustration depicting facial development at: **(A)** 27 days; **(B)** 33 days; **(C)** 39 days; and **(D)** 46 days with migration of median nasal prominence, lateral nasal prominence, and maxillomandibular region.

B. Median cerebrofacial hypoplasia (lobar brain)

In this condition, midline facial hypoplasia and midline cerebral malformations exist. Unilateral or bilateral cleft lip and palate may be present.

C. Median facial hypoplasia

Midline facial hypoplasia exists without gross cerebral involvement. Unilateral or bilateral cleft lip and palate may again be present.

D. Microforms of median facial hypoplasia

Microform variants of median facial hypoplasia may occur when there are mild deficiencies from maldevelopment of the median facial structures. Unilateral or bilateral cleft lip and palate can also be found. This group also includes:

1. Binder syndrome or anomaly (maxillonasal dysplasia) patients have characteristic flat nasomaxillary facial

Table 33.1 Classification of median craniofacial dysplasia

Subclassification	Description
I. Median craniofacial hypoplasia	**Tissue deficiency**
A. Holoproencephalic spectrum (alobar brain)	Single holistic brain with midline facial hypoplasia or agenesis *(Fig. 33.1)*. Four subclassifications: cyclopia, ethmocephaly, cebocephaly, primary palate agenesis
1. Cyclopia	1. Single eye in a single orbit, arrhinia with proboscis often located above the single orbit and microcephaly *(Fig. 33.2)*
2. Ethmocephaly	2. Severe hypotelorism but separate orbits. Arrhinia with proboscis located between the orbits *(Fig. 33.3)*
3. Cebocephaly	3. Severe hypotelorism. Proboscis-like rudimentary nose *(Fig. 33.4)*
4. Primary palate agenesis	4. Premaxillary segment missing or hypoplastic *(Fig. 33.5)*
B. Median cerebrofacial hypoplasia (lobar brain)	Separate lobes to brain but with midline cerebral malformation; midline facial hypoplasia *(Fig. 33.6)*
C. Median facial hypoplasia	Midline facial hypoplasia without gross cerebral involvement *(Fig. 33.7)*
D. Microforms of median facial hypoplasia	1. Binder anomaly (maxillonasal dysplasia) *(Fig. 33.8)* 2. Central maxillary incisor anomaly *(Fig. 33.9)* 3. Absent upper lip frenulum *(Fig. 33.10)*
II. Median craniofacial dysraphia	**Normal tissue volume but clefted**
A. True median cleft	Isolated cleft of the upper lip or abnormal split between the median globular process. It can be an incomplete *(Fig. 33.11)* or complete form *(Fig. 33.12)*
B. Anterior encephalocele	Cystic malformation in which central nervous structures are abnormally displaced or herniated through a defect in the cranium *(Figs 33.3 and 33.14)*
III. Median craniofacial hyperplasia	Tissue excess or duplication. All forms of excess tissue starting from just thickened or duplicated nasal septum to the more severe forms of frontonasal dysplasia *(Figs 33.15 and 33.16)*

region with deficient or absent nasal spine and a negative overjet from class III anterior incisor relationship.

2. Abnormalities of the maxillary central incisors: three variants of this include:
   (a) absent central maxillary incisors
   (b) single maxillary central incisor
   (c) hypoplastic central maxillary incisors.
3. Absence of upper lip frenulum

II: Median craniofacial dysraphia

Median craniofacial dysraphia describes a midline anomaly that has normal tissue volume but clefting or an abnormal separation of midline structures is present. Within the spectrum of median craniofacial dysplasia there is a group of malformations which have normal tissue volume but have abnormally split (true median cleft lip) or displaced (encephalocele). This group is better placed as median tissue defects midway between hypoplasia and hyperplasia.

A. True median cleft

A true median cleft may manifest as an isolated cleft of the upper lip, "0 cleft," not associated with either hypoplasia or hyperplasia. Alternatively, a true median cleft may have tissue deficiency or agenesis, e.g., absent nasal septum. A true

median cleft may also occur with tissue excess, e.g., duplicated nasal septum. With median craniofacial dysraphia a true median cleft has separated but there is a normal tissue amount. The upper lip deformity is a true median cleft lip with a split between the median globular processes. This is opposed to a "false" median cleft with agenesis of the globular processes. With the true median cleft the separation passes between the central incisors. The cleft may continue posteriorly as a cleft of the primary and/or secondary palate. When the cleft encroaches into the interorbital region, orbital hypertelorism may be seen.

B. Anterior encephaloceles

An encephalocele is a cystic congenital malformation in which central nervous system structures have herniated through a defect in the cranium in communication with cerebrospinal fluid pathways. They occur between normally developed zones, where a weakness permits brain to escape. The mass further pushes fields apart.

Anterior encephaloceles are divided into frontoethmoidal and basal groups. In frontoethmoidal encephaloceles, the defect occurs at the junction of the frontal and ethmoidal bones (the foramen cecum).[12] Nasoethmoidal encephalocele is considered a Tessier number 14 cleft or frontonasal dysraphia in Mazzola's morphological classification. Basal encephaloceles are associated with a defect at or behind the crista galli and, in some cases, they may protrude through a defect in the sphenoid bone and are called transsphenoidal encephalocele.[13]

III: Median craniofacial hyperplasia (tissue excess or duplication)

This spectrum of anomalies includes all forms of excess tissue starting from just thickened or duplicated nasal septum towards the more severe forms of frontonasal dysplasia.

"Frontonasal dysplasia" was the most widely known of these types of hyperplasias.[14] Objections are raised about the terminology of this condition. Typically, the term "dysplasia" refers to the whole spectrum of abnormal tissue development starting from tissue agenesis and hypoplasia all the way to the other extreme of hyperplasia and excess tissue.

The basic defect of median craniofacial hyperplasia is not known. Embryologically, if the nasal capsule fails to develop properly, the primitive brain vesicle fills the space normally occupied by the capsule, thus producing anterior cranium bifidum occultum and leading to morphokinetic arrest in the positioning of the eyes and nostrils, which tend to maintain their relative fetal positions.[15,16] Experiments have shown that a reduction in the number of migrating neural crest cells results in these multiple defects.[17,18]

Other nasal findings may range from a notched broad nasal tip to completely divided nostrils with hypoplasia and even absence of the prolabium and maxilla with a median cleft lip. In addition, variable notching of the ala is described. Occasionally associated abnormalities include accessory nasal tags, low-set ears, conductive hearing loss, mild to severe retardation, basal encephalocele, and agenesis of the corpus callosum. Importantly, a high incidence of ocular abnormalities is described. More distant anomalies include tetralogy of Fallot, absence of the tibia, and others. When hypertelorism is severe or when extracephalic anomalies occur, mental deficiency appears to be more likely and more severe.[14,15,17]

The Tessier classification of craniofacial clefts was described in 1976.[1] This classification has proven to be the most complete and has withstood the test of time. This insightful classification was based on the extensive personal experience by Tessier in the anatomy laboratory, in the operating room, and from his embryologic knowledge. The terminology is uniform and the characterizations of specific features are detailed. It is also reproducible by clinicians evaluating craniofacial clefts. In addition, the classification links the clinical observations with underlying skeletal deformity documented by preoperative three-dimensional (3D) computed tomography (CT) scan imaging and confirmed during surgery. Correlation of the clinical appearance with the surgical anatomic findings improves the clinical utility of this system for the craniofacial surgeon. Distinctive features such as Tessier craniofacial clefts are described below.

Epidemiology and etiologic factors

The true incidence of craniofacial clefts is unknown because of their rarity and because of the difficulty in recognizing sometimes subtle physical findings in mild malformations. However, the incidence of craniofacial clefts has been estimated at 1.4–4.9 per 100 000 live births.[1–3] The incidence of rare craniofacial clefts compared to common cleft lip and palate malformations may range from 9.5 to 34 per 1000.[3]

Most rare craniofacial clefts occur sporadically. However, the role of heredity in the causation of rare craniofacial clefts seems to occur in Treacher–Collins syndrome and in some familial cases of Goldenhar syndrome. A dominant gene defect (TCOF-1) causes Treacher–Collins syndrome.[19] Although penetrance is somewhat variable, the malformation is very consistent. In a TCOF-1 gene knock-out animal model, regional massive cell death affected crest cell mesenchymal migration and resulted in zygomatic abnormalities. Constriction limb deformities (amniotic band syndrome) have also been associated with rare facial clefting. Coady *et al.* found a statistically significant association between craniofacial clefts and limb ring constrictions.[20]

Based on animal and human clinical studies, many environmental factors have also been shown to cause facial clefts. These investigations produced four major categories: (1) radiation[21,22]; (2) infection[23,24]; (3) maternal metabolic imbalances[25]; and (4) drugs and chemicals.[26] A considerable number of drugs and chemicals have teratogenic potential but few have been shown to cause craniofacial malformations in humans. Some medications, including those containing retinoic acid, are being looked at as a cause of facial malformations.[27]

Although the teratogenic potential of drugs and their effect on facial development are known, the critical phase of embryologic differentiation and development occurs when a mother may be unknowingly pregnant. Teratologists are confronted with the problem of multiple factors acting on numerous pathways and have no simple answer that universally explains the formation of a particular cleft.

Embryologic craniofacial development

The understanding of normal morphogenesis occurring in the embryo and fetus allows the clinician to describe and classify craniofacial clefts of infants and adults. Likewise, the study of rare craniofacial clefts lends clues to facial and neuroembryology. A traditional summary of normal facial development and newer understanding of genetically determined development zones of the face based on neuroembryology is outlined below.

The three primary germ layers, ectoderm, mesoderm, and endoderm, are the basis for tissue and organ formation.[28] In the third week of gestation, the primitive tissues of the trilaminar embryo give rise to notochordal and prechordal mesoderm. Simultaneously, the rostral ectoderm differentiates to form highly specialized neural crest cells, which are responsible for the ultimate development of the brain and midline facial structures.[29] The ectoderm forms a neural plate with bilateral folds which conjoin into a neural tube. During closure of the neural tube, neural crest cells (mesenchyme) migrate into underlying tissue, forming pluripotential stem cells. The embryonic prominences of the face are formed by the migration of these neural crest cells. A segmental pattern of ventral migration of neural crest, termed rhombomeres, provides the precursors of cartilage, bone, muscle, and connective tissue of the face and head.

Any defect in the quantity and quality of this migrating ectomesenchyme is manifest as a craniofacial malformation from severe holoprosencephaly to minor clinical stigmata of craniofacial clefts like dimples or skin tags.[30] Another cause for arrested development causing dysplasias and dystopias (the abnormal formation and location of structures) is abnormal development or involution of embryologic arteries.[31]

Starting at the fourth week of gestation, the face assumes a recognizable form.[32] Between 4 and 8 weeks of gestation the crown–rump length increases from approximately 3.5 mm to 28 mm. The double-layer stomodeal membrane creates the opening for the primitive mouth. An overhanging frontonasal prominence represents the superior border of the stomodeum.[2] Five prominences (the frontonasal and paired maxillary and mandibular) formed by neural crest migration surround the stomodeum (Fig. 33.1). The frontonasal prominence is formed by neural crest cells migrating ventrally from the mesencephalic region and contributes to the frontal and nasal bones. The maxillary and mandibular prominences are formed by more caudally located migrating neural crest cells that encounter pharyngeal endoderm in their ventral migration around the aortic arches.

Optic vesicles appear from lateral envaginations of the diencephalons and induce lens placodes in ectoderm and neural crest migration to form the sclera. Defective optic vesicle formation results in microphthalmos, or anophthalmos. The movement of this optic tissue from lateral to medial results from the narrowing frontonasal prominence and expansion of the lateral face. Inadequate transition of the eyes produces hypertelorism and overmigration produces hypotelorism or even median cyclopia.[33]

During the sixth week, the medial nasal processes enlarge and coalesce in the midline. The nasal placodes arise from ectodermal tissue inferolateral to the frontonasal prominence and cephalad to the stomodeum. Nasal placodes invaginate into the face to form nasal pits and elevations at the margins produce a horseshoe-shaped median and lateral nasal prominences. The caudal extensions of the medial nasal processes, the globular processes, are united with the developing maxillary processes to form the upper lip. The medial nasal process gives rise to the nasal tip, the columella, the philtrum, and the premaxilla. The nasal alae are derived from the lateral nasal processes. The frontonasal process contributes the bridge and the root of the nose.

The posterior aspect of each nasal pit is separated from the oral cavity by an oronasal membrane. Failure of this membrane to disintegrate normally leads to choanal atresia.[34] The paired median nasal processes merge with the frontonasal prominence to form the majority of the frontal process. These structures gradually enlarge and superiorly displace the frontonasal prominence. During the sixth week, the two median nasal processes coalesce in the midline and their most caudal limbs, the premaxillary prominence, expand above the stomodeum. The nasal tip, philtrum, columella, cartilaginous septum, and primary palate are derived from these paired median elements. Cephalad to the medial nasal process, the frontonasal process persists to form the nasal dorsum and root. Elevation of the lateral nasal prominence creates the nasal alae. Defects during this development may be midline and produce arrhinia or a bifid nose.

The maxillary processes are paired mesodermal masses that lie cephalad to the mandibular arch and ventral to the optic neuroectoderm. These triangular masses enlarge, separate from the mandibular arch, and then migrate ventrally. The maxillary process ultimately coalesces with the mesoderm of

the globular processes to form the upper lip. The cheek, maxilla, zygoma, and secondary palate are also derived from the maxillary processes. Between the maxillary prominence and lateral nasal prominence a depression exists with a solid rod of epithelial cells.[35] The ends of this rod form a connection from the nasal pit to the conjunctival sac (nasolacrimal duct). With inadequate neural crest cell migration a fissure within the line of this duct may persist as an oblique facial cleft.

The stomodeal aperture is reduced by migrating mesenchyme fusing the maxillary and mandibular prominences to form the oral commissures. Inadequate neural crest cells result in macrostomia while excessive tissue produces microstomia or macrostomia. The mandibular prominence lies between the stomodeum and the first branchial groove, which delineates the caudal limits of the face. The paired free ends of the mandibular arch enlarge and converge ventrally during the sixth week. The lower lip and mandible are developed from this arch. Paired lateral pharyngeal elevations of the arch unite to form the anterior portion of the tongue.

The external and middle ear are also formed during the sixth week of gestation. The tragus and the crus of the helix are derived from three hillocks at the caudal border of the first branchial arch. The malleus and incus of the middle ear are also formed by the first branchial arch. The remainder of the external ear is formed from three hillocks on the cephalic border of the second branchial arch. The stapes of the middle ear is also formed by the second branchial arch.

During a short 4-week period, there is a coordination of cell migration, cellular interaction, and apoptosis. Failure of this intricate program will result in clefts that will usually fall along predictable embryonic lines.

Failure of fusion

Two theories exist that describe how embryologic failure or errors result in craniofacial cleft malformations. First, the "fusion failure" theory suggests that clefts are created when fusion of facial processes fail.[36] Second, the "failure of mesodermal penetration" theory implicates the lack of mesoderm and neuroectoderm migration and penetration into the bilaminar ectodermal sheets as the cause of craniofacial clefts.[37] Although most of the current knowledge is based on animal cleft lip and palate studies, rare craniofacial clefts may be produced by similar mechanisms.

The "failure of fusion" theory, proposed by Dursy in 1869 and His in 1892, purported that the free edges of the facial processes unite in the central region of the face.[35] As various processes fuse, the face gradually forms. When epithelial contact is established between opposing facial processes, mesodermal penetration completes the fusion. Dursy suggested that the upper lip is created when finger-like advancing ends of the maxillary process and the paired global process unite. He asserted that disruption of this sequence results in craniofacial cleft anomalies.

Proponents of the mesodermal penetration theory believed that the finger-like ends of the facial processes do not exist. Warbrick[38] and Stark et al. and Ehrmann[39] suggest that the central facial processes are composed of bilamellar sheets of ectoderm. This bilamellar membrane is bordered by epithelial seams, which delineate the principal processes. During development, the mesenchymal tissue migrates and penetrates this double-layered ectoderm, called the "epithelial wall." Caudal to the stomodeum, the lower face is formed by the branchial arches. The arches consist of a thin sheet of mesoderm, which lie between the ectodermal and endodermal layers. The neural crest cells of neuroectodermal origin, which arise from the dorsolateral surface of the neural tube, migrate under the ectoderm and supplement the mesoderm of the frontonasal process and branchial arches.[40] Most of the craniofacial skeleton is believed to be formed by these neural crest cells. If neuroectoderm migration and penetration do not occur, the epithelium breaks down to form a facial cleft. The severity of the cleft is proportional to the failure of penetration by the neuroectoderm. Unfortunately, the precise nature of the proposed mechanisms in the formation of rare craniofacial clefts is not known. Nevertheless, the concepts of fusion and mesodermal penetration provide an understanding of the problems of the rare craniofacial cleft.

Neuromeric theory

Newer understanding of neuroembryology suggests that a direct relationship exists between the development of the nervous system and those structures to which its contents are dedicated. The neural tube is conceived as a series of developmental zones within the central nervous system.[41,42] Six prosomeres provide a cartesian system to organize the tracts and nuclei of the prosencephalon (forebrain). The mesencephalon (midbrain) and rhomboencephalon (hindbrain) are subdivided into two mesomeres and 12 rhombomeres respectively. Each of these neuromeres is defined by a unique overlap of several genetic coding zones along the axis of the embryo. In the hindbrain and caudally to the coccyx these neuromeric units are defined by the Homeobox series of genes (Hox genes). In the forebrain, a more complex series of genes is used, such as Sonic hedgehog (Shh), Wingless (Wnt), and Engrailed (En).

The unique "barcode" for each neuromeric zone is shared with all cells exiting from a particular level to form the mesoderm and endoderm of the embryo. For example, the Hox gene which codes for the rhombomeres 2 and 3 (which make up the first pharyngeal arch-PA1) is shared with the mesoderm that makes up those arches. This same Hox gene is also shared with the neural crest cells which subsequently move into the mesodermal "zones" of PA1. The migrating neural crest cells then provide the instructions for differentiation into the appropriate facial tissues. Thus, all the bones and soft tissues of the face can be thought of as genetically determined "fields" with defined cellular content and a fixed position in space. With the folding of the embryo, these fields are placed into their correct topologic positions and a three-dimensional form results.

This system permits the "mapping" of the face into developmental zones with distinct spatial origins in their precursor tissue units. The midline mesoderm of the nasal and ocular fields is of different origin, innervation, and blood supply from all surrounding mesodermal elements. When all the developmental zones are accounted for, the occurrence of craniofacial clefts is nothing more than an orderly progression of deficiency states in the precursor fields, resulting in varying degrees of absence of soft-tissue functional matrix or underlying bone. The anatomic and clinical observations of Tessier and his classification system are exactly compatible with this map. Variations include: (1) clefts number 2 and 3 fall within

the same zone (cleft number 3 being more posterior) and (2) clefts number 4 and 5 represent varying degrees of involvement in the same zone of the maxilla. Tessier's classification system has been widely adopted by surgeons and other clinicians and has stood the test of time. However, geneticists and embryologists have been slow to embrace his numeric organization of craniofacial clefts because it could not previously be understood by existing theories of embryologic developmental. The consistency of these newer neuroembryologic theories with Tessier's classification of craniofacial clefts reinforces the importance of Tessier's descriptions. With progression of the neuromeric theory, the value of Tessier's organization of rare craniofacial clefts should become apparent to embryologists and geneticists.

Patient selection

Distinctive features of Tessier craniofacial clefts

Tessier developed a classification for rare craniofacial clefts based on his anatomical and operative observations and experiences (*Fig. 33.2A*). The clefts are numbered from 0 to 14, follow well-defined zones of the face and orbit, and correlate with embryologic developmental maps (*Fig. 33.2B*). The numbered clefts relate soft-tissue clinical features to underlying bony involvement verified by operative findings and more recently preoperative 3D CT assessments.

The eyelids and orbits define the horizontal axis dividing the face into upper and lower hemispheres. Tessier used these landmarks, because the orbit belongs to both the cranium and the face. Thus, the orbit separates the numbered cranial clefts from the facial clefts. In addition, the following combinations of numeric clefts are often clinically observed: 0 and 14, 1 and 13, 2 and 12, 3 and 11, 4 and 10, 5 and 9, and 6 and 8. Clefts 5–9 are considered lateral clefts, because they pass lateral to the infraorbital foramen. Tessier cleft number 7 is the most lateral craniofacial cleft.

The clinical expression of the craniofacial cleft is highly variable. Tessier reported that the soft-tissue and skeletal components were seldom affected to the same extent. Skeletal landmarks are more constant and reliable than the soft-tissue landmarks. Typically, facial clefts located medial to the infraorbital foramen had greater soft-tissue involvement than clefts found lateral to the foramen. By contrast, facial clefts located lateral to the infraorbital foramen had greater bony disruption than clefts found medial to the foramen. Finally, bilateral forms of the clefts are found in varying combinations, often creating an asymmetric malformation.

The craniofacial clefts, as described below, use the Tessier classification to relate soft-tissue features to underlying skeletal involvement. The severity of involvement of regional structures influences the therapeutic strategy. The order of description below consists of facial clefts from medial to lateral followed by cranial clefts from lateral to medial.

Number 0 cleft

The number 0 cleft has been called median craniofacial dysraphia, centrofacial microsomia, frontonasal dysplasia,

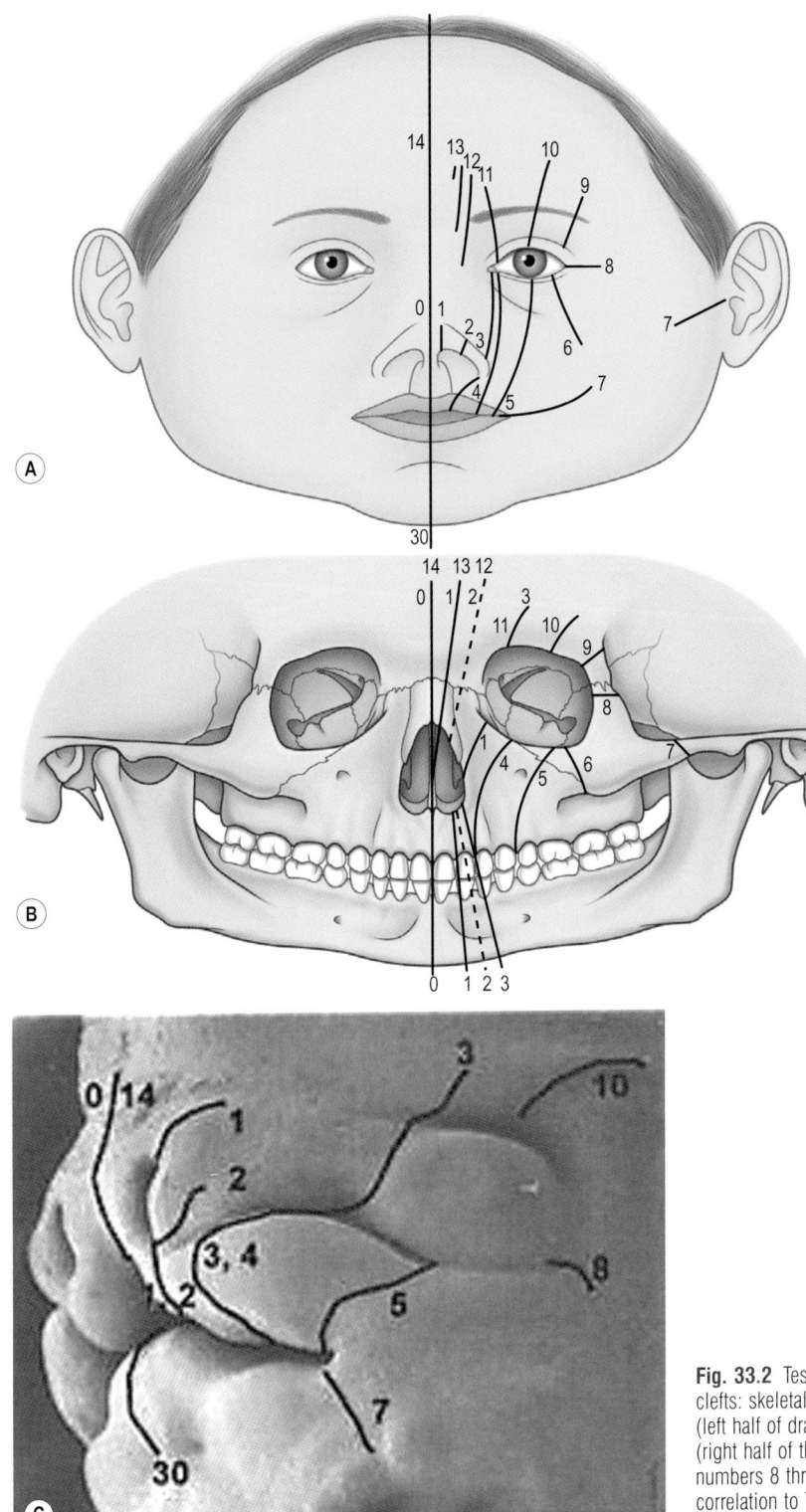

Fig. 33.2 Tessier classification of craniofacial clefts. **(A, B)** Illustration of Tessier clefts: skeletal locations of numeric clefts are depicted on the right side of the face (left half of drawing). Soft-tissue landmarks are outlined on the left side of the face (right half of the drawing). Facial clefts are numbers 0 through 7 and cranial clefts are numbers 8 through 14. Mandibular midline facial cleft is number 30. **(C)** Embryology correlation to Tessier facial clefts: Tessier-numbered craniofacial clefts are shown correlating with growth center junctions in this 45-day-old fetus.

median cleft face syndrome, or holoprosencephaly; but, for accuracy, it is the facial manifestation or lower half of "median craniofacial dysplasia," as described above.[43,44] Patients with this midline facial cleft may have a cranial extension or a number 14 cleft. As mentioned above, the number 0 Tessier craniofacial clefts are unique in that there may be a deficiency, normal, or excess tissue. With tissue agenesis and holoprosencephaly at one end (the hypoplasias), and frontonasal hyperplasia and excessive tissue (the hyperplasias) at the other end, median anomalies with normal tissue volume occupy the middle portion of the spectrum.

Median craniofacial hypoplasia (deficiency of midline structures)

A deficiency may manifest as hypoplasia or agenesis in which portions of midline facial structures are missing *(Fig. 33.3)*. This developmental arrest may range from the mildest form of hypoplasia of the nasomaxillary region and hypotelorism to a severe form of cyclopia, ethmocephaly, or cebocephaly. The subcategories *(Table 33.1)* demonstrate that the severity of facial anomalies correlate well with the severity of brain abnormality and mental retardation. A CT scan of the brain can differentiate between alobar and lobar brain anomalies and clarify the spectrum of holoprosencephalic patients. Clinically it may be important to distinguish among patients with poor brain differentiation who may die in infancy from those with a better prognosis.

Soft-tissue deficiencies

Soft-tissue deficencies with Tessier 0 clefts include the upper lip and nose. Agenesis or hypoplasia may result in a false median cleft lip and absence of philtral columns. When a wide central cleft exists, it typically extends the length of the upper lip and up into the nasal floor *(Fig. 33.3A, B)*. With nasal anomalies, the columella may be narrowed or totally absent. The nasal tip may be depressed from lack of septal support. The septum may often be vestigial with no caudal attachment to the palate. Dental abnormalities may include absent central maxillary incisors, single maxillary central incisor, and/or hypoplastic central maxillary incisors.

Skeletal deficiencies

Skeletal deficiencies range from separation between the upper central canines to absence of the premaxilla and a cleft of the

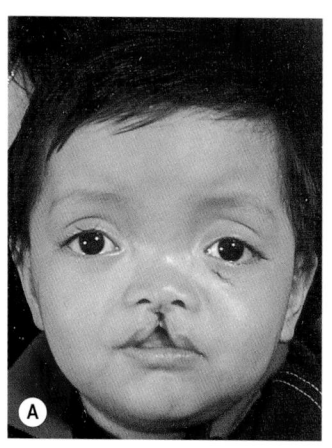
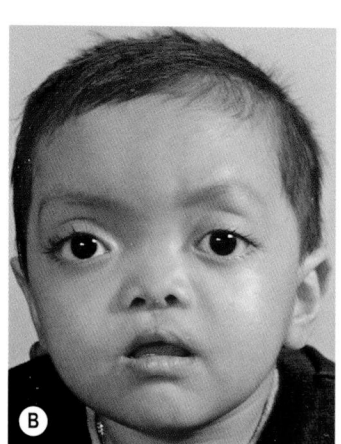
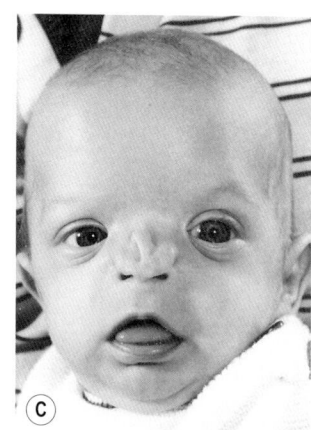
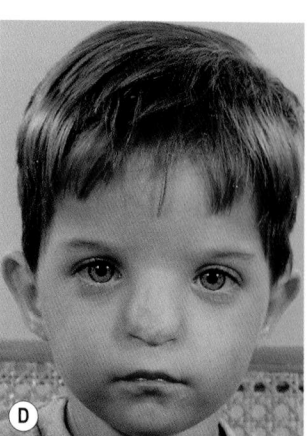

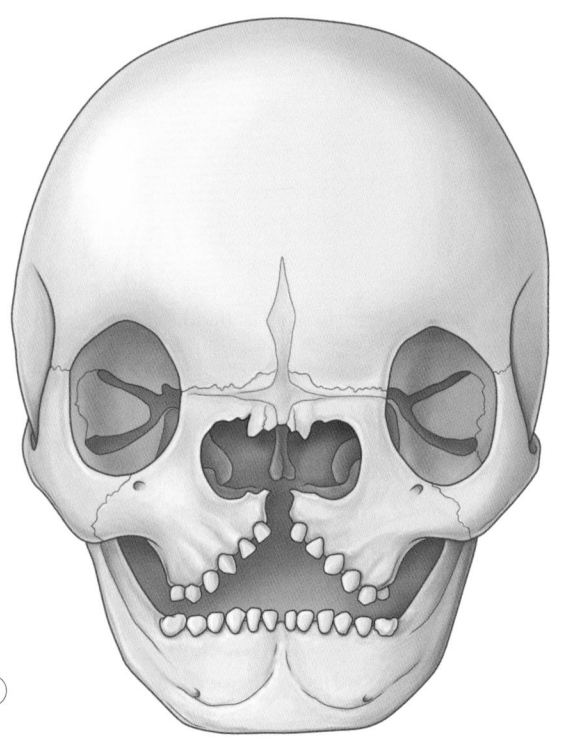

Fig. 33.3 Number 0 cleft. **(A,B)** Patient with a true median cleft lip palate, cleft palate, hypertelorbitism and sphenoethmoidal encephalocele (not seen). **(A)** Preoperative view. **(B)** Postoperative view after median cleft lip repair. **(C,D)** Patient with excessive midline tissue manifested by bifid nose and an accessory band of skin on the nasal dorsum. **(C)** Preoperative view. **(D)** Postoperative view after initial nasal surgery. **(E)** Illustration of skeletal involvement demonstrates separation between the central incisors, widening of the nasal region, and orbital hypertelorism.

secondary palate *(Fig. 33.3C)*. Nasal deficiency may include partial or total absence of the septal cartilage and even nasal bones. The bone defect may extend cephalad into the area of the ethmoid sinuses and result in hypotelorism or cyclopia. Nasomaxillary deficiencies like these may be seen in Binder syndrome.

Median craniofacial dysraphia (normal tissue volume but clefted)

These Tessier 0 clefts placed between the hypoplasias and hyperplasias have normal tissue volume but are abnormally split (true median cleft lip) or displaced (encephalocele).

Soft-tissue involvement

When an isolated cleft of the upper lip is not associated with tissue deficiency (e.g., absent nasal septum) or tissue excess (e.g., duplicated septum) it is considered a "true" median cleft lip. With a true median cleft lip there is a split between the median globular processes, whereas with a false median cleft lip an agenesis of the globular processes may occur. An encephalocele is a cystic congenital malformation in which central nervous system structures herniate through a defect in the cranium in communication with cerebrospinal fluid pathways.[45] They occur between normally developed zones, where a weakness permits the brain to escape the cranial space. The mass may further push the developmental fields apart.[42]

Skeletal involvement

When the true median cleft passes between the central incisors, the cleft can continue posteriorly as a midline cleft palate. When the cleft encroaches into the interorbital region, hypertelorbitism may occur. Anterior encephaloceles are divided into basal and frontoethmoidal groups. In frontoethmoidal encephaloceles, the defect occurs at the junction of the frontal and ethmoidal bones (the foramen cecum).[12] Basal encephaloceles are associated with a defect at or behind the crista galli and, in some cases, they may protrude through a defect in the sphenoid bone.

Median craniofacial hyperplasia (excess of midline tissue)

This spectrum of midline anomalies includes all forms of excess tissue starting from just thickened or duplicated nasal septum *(Fig. 33.3B)* towards the more severe forms of frontonasal dysplasia.

Soft-tissue midline excess

Soft-tissue midline excess tissue may be manifested in the lip with broad philtral columns or a duplication of the labial frenulum. The nose may be bifid with a broad columella and mid dorsal furrow. The alar and upper lateral cartilages may be displaced laterally.

Skeletal excess

Skeletal excess in a widened number 0 facial cleft can be seen as a diastema between the upper central incisors. A duplicate nasal spine may exist. A characteristic keel-shaped maxillary alveolus is seen. Anterior teeth are angled toward the midline creating an anterior open bite. Central midface height is shortened. The cartilaginous and bone nasal septum is thickened or duplicated. The nasal bones and nasal process of the maxilla are broad, flattened, and displaced laterally from the midline. Ethmoidal and sphenoidal sinuses may be enlarged, contributing to symmetrical widening of the anterior cranial fossa and hypertelorism. The cribriform plate is low and the breadth of the crista galli is exaggerated. The body of the sphenoid is broadened with displacement of the pterygoid plates away from the midline.

Number 1 cleft

This paramedian facial cleft was first delineated by Tessier.[1] Van der Meulen *et al.* nominated this cleft as a type 3 nasoschizis nasal dysplasia.[9] The number 1 facial cleft continues cranially as a number 13 cleft.

Soft-tissue involvement

The number 1 cleft, similar to the common cleft lip, passes through the cupid's bow and then the alar cartilage dome. Notching in the area of the soft triangle of the nose is a distinct feature *(Fig. 33.4A)*. The columella may be short and broad. The nasal tip and nasal septum deviate away from the cleft. Soft-tissue furrows or wrinkles may be present on the nasal dorsum if the cleft extends in a cephalic direction. The cleft is evident medially to a malpositioned medial canthus and telecanthus may result. With a cranial extension as a number 13 cleft, vertical dystopia is present.

Skeletal involvement

A keel-shaped maxilla exists with the anterior incisors facing toward the cleft creating an anterior open bite. An alveolar cleft is rare but would pass between the central and lateral incisors. This paramedian cleft separates the nasal floor at the pyriform aperture just lateral to the nasal spine *(Fig. 33.4B)*. The cleft may extend posteriorly as a complete cleft of the hard and soft palate. Extension of the cleft in a cephalad direction is through the junction of the nasal bone and the frontal process of the maxilla. The nasal bones are displaced and flattened. Ethmoidal expansion leads to hypertelorism. Also, there is asymmetry of the greater and lesser sphenoid wings, the pterygoid plates, and anterior cranial fossa.

Number 2 cleft

Soft-tissue involvement

This other paramedian facial cleft also may begin in the region of the common cleft lip. However, the nasal deformity is in the middle third of the alar rim and distinguishes the number 2 cleft *(Fig. 33.5)*. In the number 2 cleft, the ala is hypoplastic whereas, in the number 1 cleft, the ala is merely notched at the dome; and, in the number 3 cleft, the alar base is displaced. The lateral aspect of the nose is flattened and the dorsum is broad. The eyelid is not involved; the cleft passes medially to the palpebral fissure. Although the medial canthus is displaced, the lacrimal duct is usually not involved. If the cleft

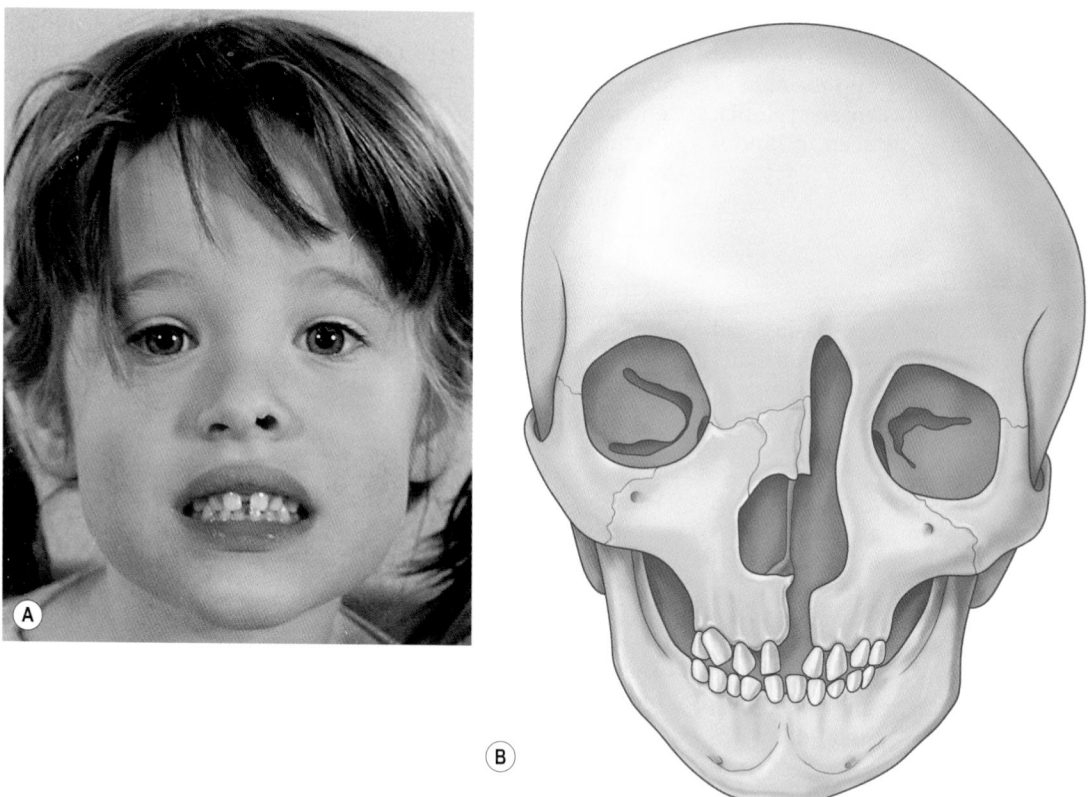

Fig. 33.4 Number 1 cleft. **(A)** Patient with notched left alar dome and orbital dystopia. **(B)** Skeletal involvement is through the piriform aperture just lateral to the nasal spine and septum. The orbit is displaced laterally.

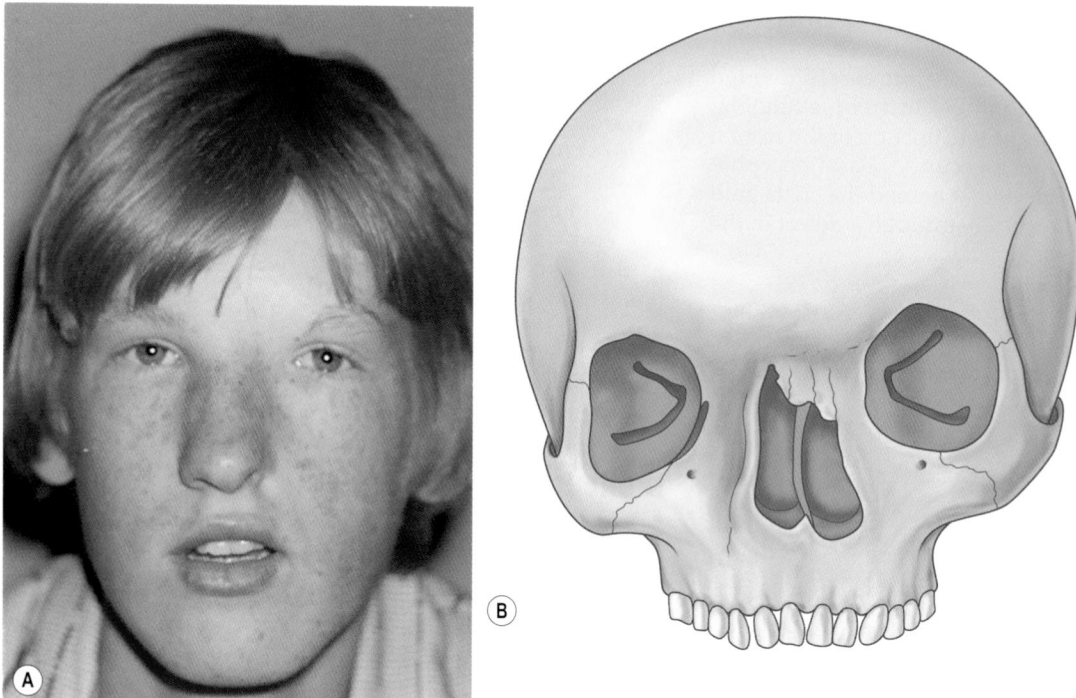

Fig. 33.5 Number 2 cleft. **(A)** Patient with hypoplasia of the middle third of the right nostril rim causing the appearance of alar base retraction. The lateral nose is flattened. The medial border of the eyebrow is also distorted as evidence of a number 12 cranial cleft. There is also orbital dystopia and displacement of the right medial canthus. **(B)** Skeletal involvement shows deformity of the piriform aperture and nasal bone.

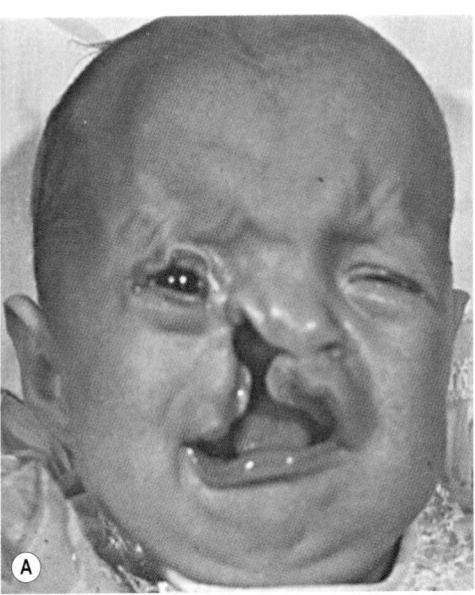

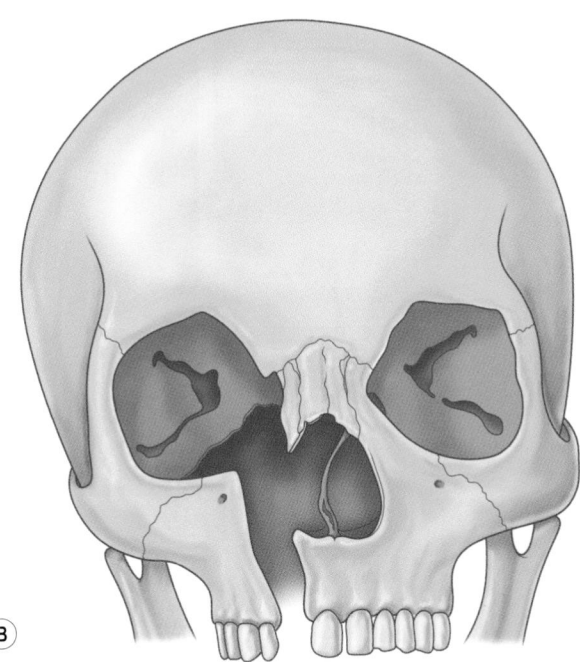

Fig. 33.6 Number 3 cleft. **(A)** Patient with complete form has a right cleft lip and palate and severe shortening of tissues between the right alar base and medial canthus. The right nasal ala is displaced superiorly, the medial canthus is displaced inferiorly, and the nasolacrimal system is disrupted. **(B)** Skeletal involvement is between the lateral incisor and the canine extending up through the lacrimal groove. The cleft creates a direct communication among the orbital, maxillary sinus, nasal, and oral cavities.

continues in a cephalad direction as a cranial number 12 cleft, then distortion of the medial brow is noted.

Skeletal involvement

The number 2 cleft begins between the lateral incisor and the canine. It extends into the pyriform aperture, lateral to the septum and medial to the maxillary sinus. A hard- and soft-palate cleft may occur. The nasal septum may be deviated away from the cleft. The cleft distorts the nasal bones as it passes between the nasal bones and the frontal process of the maxilla. Ethmoidal sinus involvement may result in orbital hypertelorism. Asymmetry of the greater and lesser sphenoid wings and anterior cranial base is present.

Number 3 cleft

The number 3 cleft is the most common of the Tessier craniofacial clefts. Morian reported the first case and later classified this as a Morian type I cleft.[46] It is also referred to as a Tessier oronaso-ocular cleft. The cephalad continuation of the cleft is a number 11 cleft. In contrast to a common cleft lip and palate, a number 3 cleft has the following: (1) an equal distribution between males and females; and (2) an occurrence of one-third on the right, one-third on the left, and one-third bilateral. When bilateral clefting occurs, a number 4 or 5 facial cleft may be seen contralateral to the number 3 cleft.

Soft-tissue involvement

The number 3 cleft begins similar to a number 1 and 2 cleft, passing through the philtral column and floor of the nose. Deficiency of tissue between the alar base and lower eyelid

results in a shortened nose on the affected side. The cleft passes between the medial canthus and the inferior lacrimal punctum (*Fig. 33.6A*). The lacrimal system, particularly the lower canaliculus, is disrupted. Blockage of the nasolacrimal duct and recurrent infections of the lacrimal sac are common. The inferior punctum is displaced downward and drainage may occur directly on to the cheek instead of into the nasal cavity.

The medial canthus is inferiorly displaced and may be hypoplastic. Colobomas of the lower eyelid are medial to the inferior punctum. In mild forms, colobomas may be the only obvious evidence of this cleft. In mild cases it is important to check a CT scan for bony involvement and maintain an index of suspicion for disruption of the lacrimal system. Involvement of the globe is rare but microphthalmia may occur. Typically, the eye is malpositioned inferiorly and laterally. Injury to the eye, including corneal erosions, ocular perforation, and loss of vision may result from desiccation unless globe is protected.

Skeletal involvement

Osseous characteristics of this facial cleft include involvement of the orbit and direct communication of the oral, nasal, and orbital cavities (*Fig. 33.6B*). The cleft begins between the lateral incisor and the canine. In contrast to the number 1 and 2 facial clefts, the anterior maxillary arch is flat in the number 3 cleft. The number 3 cleft disrupts the frontal process of the maxilla and then terminates in the lacrimal groove. In the severest form the cleft is bilateral and skeletal disruption is significant. With bilateral cases the contralateral facial cleft may be a number 4 or 5 cleft. There may be narrowing of the ethmoid and sphenoid sinuses. Both the orbital floor and anterior cranial base are displaced inferiorly.

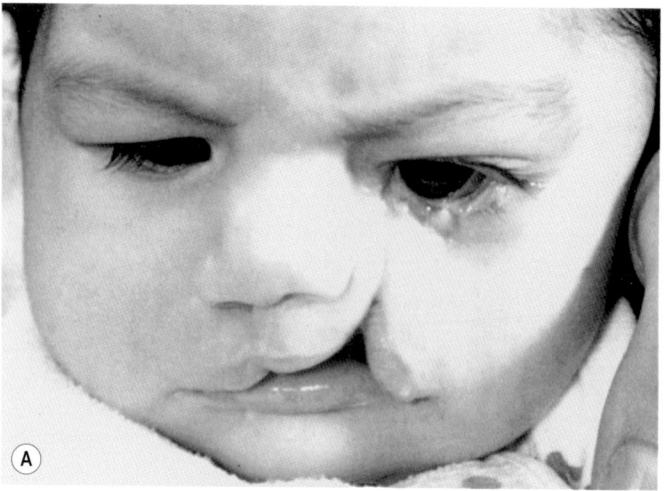

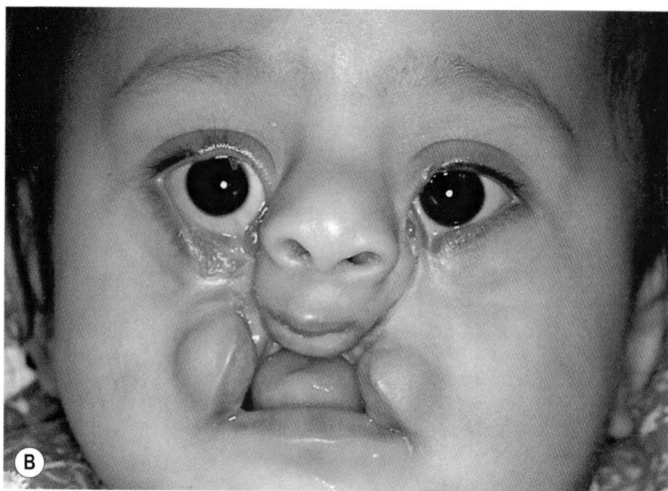

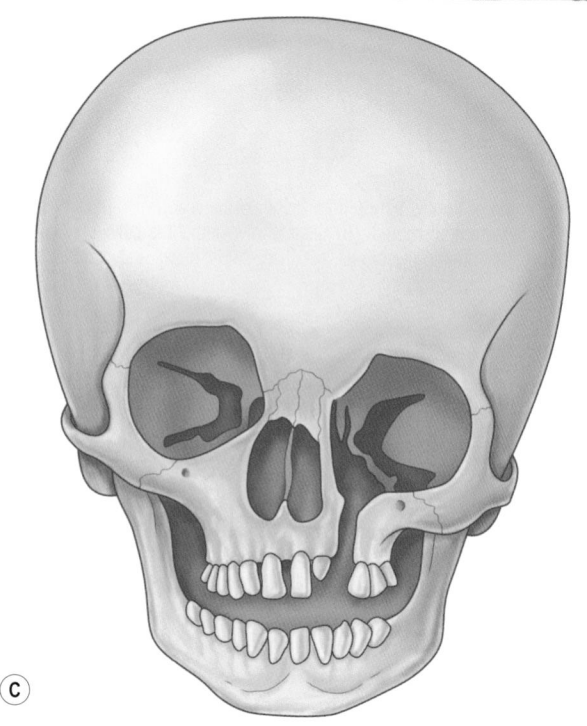

Fig. 33.7 Number 4 cleft. **(A)** Patient with left-side cleft that begins lateral to cupid's bow and terminates in the lower eyelid medial to the punctum. **(B)** Bilateral clefting of the upper lip lateral to cupid's bow and malar extension to the lower eyelids with asymmetric involvement. **(C)** Skeletal involvement begins between the lateral incisor and canine and extends through the maxilla between the infraorbital foramen and the piriform aperture. The orbit, maxillary sinus, and oral cavities communicate.

Number 4 cleft

The number 4 cleft occurs lateral to the nose and other median facial structures. The cleft has been called meloschisis (separation of cheek). Dick reported the first case in the English literature and von Kulmus may have recorded the initial description in Latin in 1732.[47] The cleft has also been classified or referred to as oro-ocular (AACPR), orofacial cleft,[1] and medial maxillary dysplasia.[1,48] The cranial continuation of the cleft is the number 10 cleft. For unilateral number 4 facial clefts it is estimated that a distribution exists for right to left side of 2 to 1.3 and a distribution exists for male to female of 2.5 to 1. In contrast, bilateral cases occur in equal numbers of males and females. Bilateral cases are associated with contralateral craniofacial clefts numbers 3, 5, and 7.

Soft-tissue involvement

As opposed to numbers 1, 2, and 3 facial clefts, the number 4 cleft begins lateral to cupid's bow and the philtral column and medial to the oral commissure *(Fig. 33.7A)*. The orbicularis oris muscle is located in the lateral lip element with no muscle centrally. The cleft passes lateral to the nasal ala. Although the ala is not involved and the nose is intact, it is displaced superiorly. Bilateral involvement pulls the nose upward *(Fig. 33.7B)*. The cleft extends through the cheek and into the lower eyelid lateral to the inferior punctum. The lower eyelid and lashes may extend directly into the lateral aspect of the cleft. The medial canthus and nasolacrimal system are normal. Globe is typically normal but microphthalmia and anophthalmos may be seen.

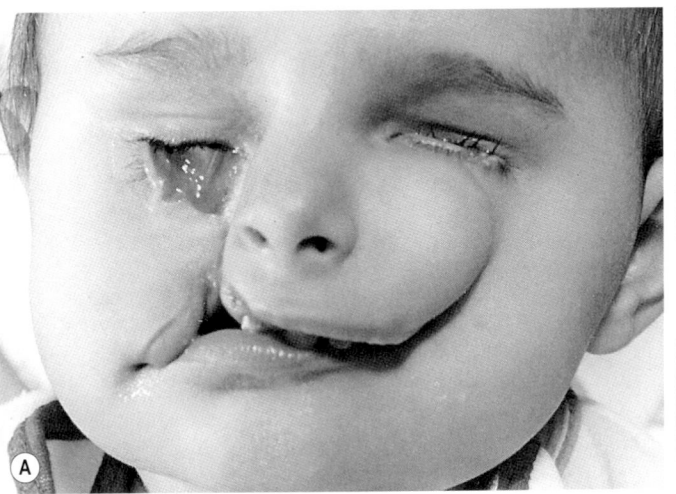

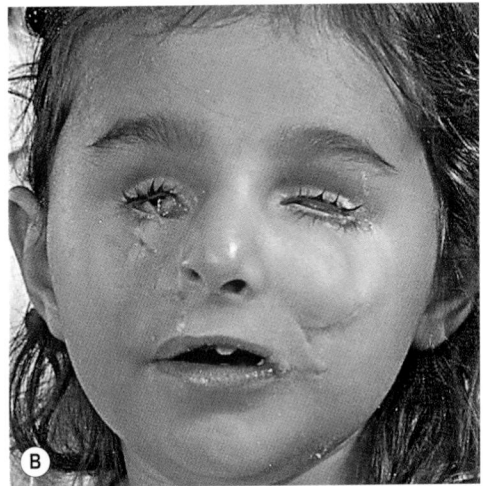

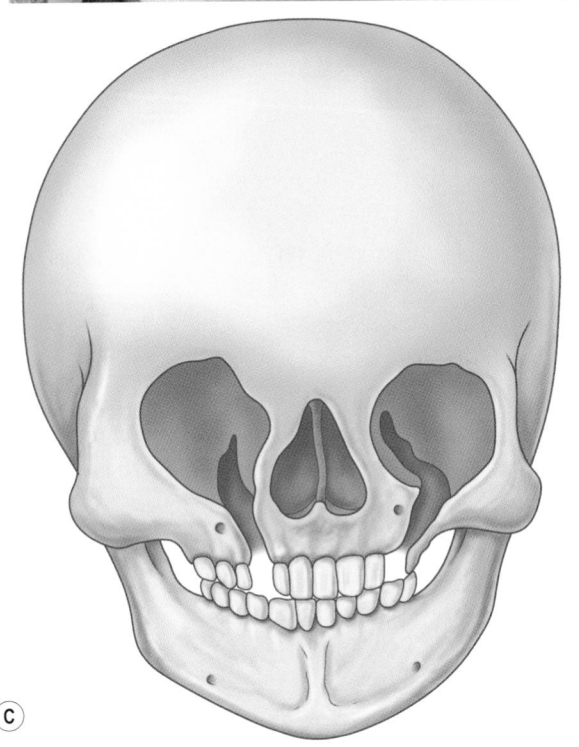

Fig. 33.8 Number 4 cleft (right) and number 5 cleft (left). **(A)** This patient demonstrates bilateral facial clefts with a number 4 cleft that begins lateral to cupid's bow and extends up to the medial third of the lower eyelid while the number 5 cleft begins just medial to the oral commissure and extends up the lateral cheek to the middle of the eyelid. **(B)** Postoperative view of same patient after repair of bilateral clefts. **(C)** Skeletal involvement in the number 4 cleft begins between the lateral incisor and canine and passes medial to the infraorbital foramen. In the number 5 cleft, the cleft begins at the premolars and extends lateral to the infraorbital foramen.

Skeletal involvement

Skeletal involvement is usually less extensive than the number 3 cleft. The alveolar cleft begins between the lateral incisor and the canine *(Fig. 33.7C)*. The cleft extends lateral to the pyriform aperture to involve the maxillary sinus. The medial wall of the maxillary sinus is intact. A confluence exists between the oral cavity, maxillary sinus, and orbital cavity but not the nasal cavity. The cleft then passes medial to the infraorbital foramen. This landmark defines the boundary between the medial number 4 facial cleft and lateral number 5 facial cleft. The number 4 cleft terminates at the medial aspect of the inferior orbital rim. With an absent medial orbital floor and rim, the globe may prolapse inferiorly. In bilateral cases the medial midface and premaxilla are protrusive. The sphenoid body is asymmetric and pterygoid plates are displaced but the anterior cranial base is unaffected.

Number 5 cleft

This facial cleft is the rarest of the oblique facial clefts. It has been called the oculofacial cleft II, Morian III cleft, a lateral maxillary dysplasia, or an oro-ocular type II cleft (AACPR classification).[1,49] The cephalad progression of the number 5 cleft is the number 9 cleft. One-fourth of cases are unilateral, one-fourth of cases are bilateral, and one-half of cases are combined with another facial cleft.

Soft-tissue involvement

The number 5 facial cleft begins just medial to the oral commissure and coursed along the cheek lateral to the nasal ala *(Fig. 33.8A, B)*. The cleft terminates in the lateral half of the lower eyelid. Although the globe is typically normal, microphthalmia may occur.

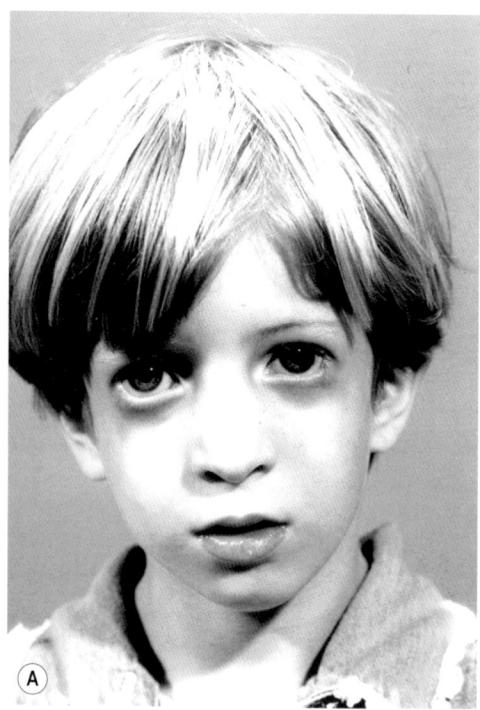

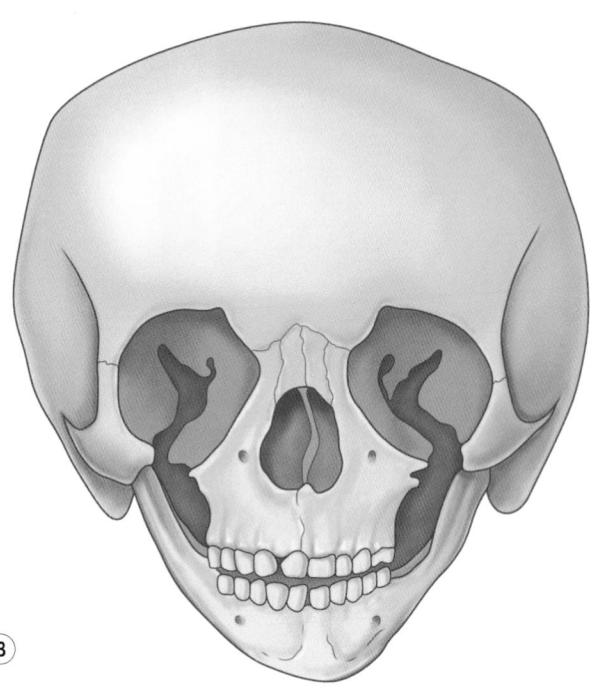

Fig. 33.9 Number 6 cleft. **(A)** Patient with an incomplete form of Treacher–Collins syndrome shows bilateral linear malar hypoplasia. **(B)** Skeletal involvement occurs in the region of the zygomatic-maxillary suture. The zygoma is hypoplastic.

Skeletal involvement

The alveolar cleft begins lateral to the canine in the region of the premolars. In contrast to the number 4 cleft, the number 5 cleft then courses lateral to the infraorbital foramen and terminates in the lateral aspect of the orbital rim and floor *(Fig. 33.8A, C)*. The cleft is separated from the inferior orbital fissure. The maxillary sinus may be hypoplastic. Prolapse of orbital contents through the lateral orbital floor defect into the maxillary sinus causes vertical orbital dystopia. The lateral orbital wall may be thickened and the greater sphenoid wing abnormal. The cranial base is normal.

Number 6 cleft

This zygomaticmaxillary cleft represents an incomplete form of Treacher–Collins syndrome. It was nominated a maxillozygomatic dysplasia by Van der Meulen *et al.*[49] Similar and often more severe cleft facial features are seen in Nager syndrome. Nager syndrome patients also may have radial club deformities of the upper extremities.

Soft-tissue involvement

The cleft is often identified as a vertical furrow, due to hypoplastic soft tissue, from the oral commissure to the lateral lower eyelid *(Fig. 33.9A)*. This line of hypoplasia runs through the zygomatic eminence along an imaginary line from the angle of the mandible to the lateral palpebral fissure. The lateral palpebral fissure is pulled downward. The lateral canthus is displaced inferiorly. This may create an appearance of a severe lower lid ectropion and an antimongoloid slant. Colobomas appear in the lateral lower eyelid and mark the cephalic end of the cleft.

Skeletal involvement

The number 6 facial cleft is along the zygomatic-maxillary suture separating the maxilla and zygoma *(Fig. 33.9B)*. There is no alveolar cleft but a short posterior maxilla may result in an occlusal tilt. Choanal atresia is common. The cleft enters the orbit at the lateral third of the orbital rim and floor. It connects to the inferior orbital fissure. The zygoma is hypoplastic with an intact zygomatic arch. There is narrowing of the anterior cranial fossa. The sphenoid is normal.

Number 7 cleft

This temporozygomatic facial cleft is the most common craniofacial cleft. Other descriptive terms of this cleft include: craniofacial microsomia, hemifacial microsomia, otomandibular dysostosis, first and second branchial arch syndrome, auriculobranchiogenic dysplasia, hemignathia and microtia syndrome, oroaural cleft (AACPR), a group B1 lateral otocephalic branchigenic deformity, and zygotemporal dysplasia.[49–52] Goldenhar syndrome (oculo-auriculo-vertebral spectrum) is an autosomal-dominant more severe form additionally with epibulbar dermoids and vertebral anomalies.[53] The number 7 cleft is also seen in Treacher–Collins syndrome. The incidence is approximately 1 in 5600 births. There is a slight (3:2) male predominance and bilateral involvement.

Soft-tissue involvement

The cleft begins at the oral commissure and runs to the preauricular hairline. The intensity of expression varies from a mild broadening of the oral commissure with a preauricular skin tag to a complete fissure extending toward the microtic ear

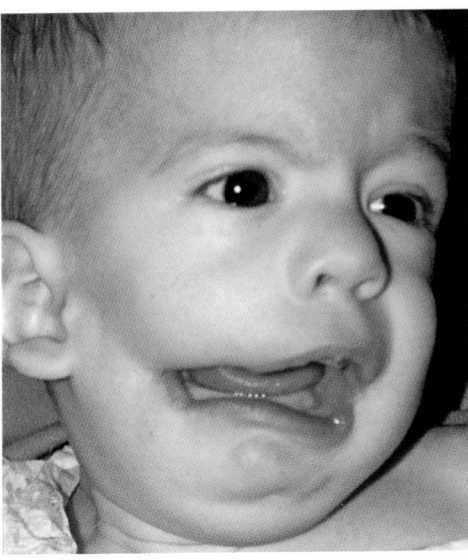

Fig. 33.10 Number 7 cleft. Patient with a complete fissure of the right oral commissure which extends toward the external ear, resulting in macrosomia. (Courtesy of D Horowitz.)

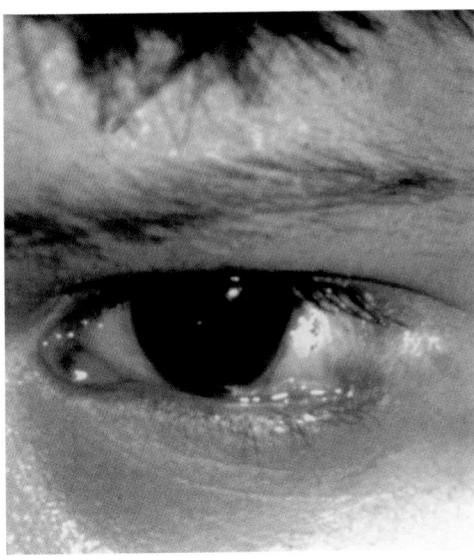

Fig. 33.11 Number 8 cleft. In this patient's left eye the lateral commissure of the palpebral fissue is obliterated by a dermatocele. This cleft separates the facial and cranial clefts.

(Fig. 33.10). Typically the cleft does not extend beyond the anterior border of the masseter. However, the ipsilateral tongue, soft palate, and muscles of mastication (cranial nerve V) may be underdeveloped. The parotid gland and parotid duct may be absent. Facial nerve weakness (cranial nerve VII) may be present. External ear deformities range from preauricular skin tags to complete absence. External ear and middle-ear abnormalities have been documented by Longacre et al.,[52] Grabb,[55] and Converse et al.[54] Preauricular hair is usually absent in patients with craniofaical microsomia. Patients with Treacher–Collins often have preauricular hair from the temporal region pointing to the oral commissure. The ipsilateral soft palate and tongue are often hypoplastic.

Skeletal involvement

Osseous anomalies in a number 7 cleft include a wide range. The skeletal cleft passes through the pterygomaxillary junction. Tessier believed that the cleft is centered in the region of the zygomaticotemporal suture. The posterior maxilla and mandibular ramus are hypoplastic in the vertical dimension, creating an occlusal plane that is canted cephalad on the affected side. The coronoid process and condyle are also often hypoplastic and asymmetric, contributing to a posterior open bite on the affected side. The zygomatic body is severely malformed, hypoplastic, and displaced. In the most severe form, the zygomatic arch is disrupted and is represented by a small stump. The malpositioned lateral canthus is caused by a hypoplastic zygoma that results in the inferiorly displaced superolateral angle of the orbit. Occasionally severely deforming number 7 clefts can cause true orbital dystopia. The abnormal anterior zygomatic arch continues posteriorly as a normal zygomatic process of the temporal bone. The cranial base is asymmetric and tilts causing an abnormally positioned glenoid fossa. The anatomy of the sphenoid is abnormal and there can be a rudimentary medial and lateral pterygoid plate.

Number 8 cleft

This frontozygomatic cleft located at the lateral canthus is the equator of the Tessier craniofacial time zones *(Fig. 33.11)*. It is the temporal continuation of the orolateral canthus cleft (AACPR), the commissural clefts of the ophthalmo-orbital disorders, and zygofrontal dysplasia.[48] The number 8 cleft divides the facial clefts from the cranial clefts. The number 8 cleft rarely occurs alone but is usually associated with other craniofacial clefts. It appears to be the cranial extension of the number 6 cleft. The bilateral occurrence of the combination of numbers 6, 7, and 8 craniofacial clefts is unique. Tessier believed that this pattern of clefts best describes the Treacher–Collins syndrome *(Fig. 33.12)*. Infants with Goldenhar's syndrome will typically have more soft-tissue involvement, while those with Treacher–Collins syndrome tend to have more severe bony abnormalities.

Soft-tissue involvement

The number 8 cleft extends from the lateral canthus to the temporal region. A dermatocele may occupy the coloboma of the lateral commissure. Occasionally hair markers can be seen along a line between the temporal area and the lateral canthus. The soft-tissue malformation presents as a true lateral commissure coloboma (dermatocele) with absence of the lateral canthus. Abnormalities of the globe, in the form of epibulbar dermoids, are also often present, especially in Goldenhar's syndrome.

Skeletal involvement

The bony component of the cleft occurs at the frontozygomatic suture. Tessier noted a notch in this region in patients with Goldenhar syndrome (combination number 6, 7, and 8 clefts). In the complete form of Treacher–Collins syndrome (combination number 6, 7, and 8 clefts) the zygoma may be hypoplastic or absent and the lateral orbital wall missing *(Fig.*

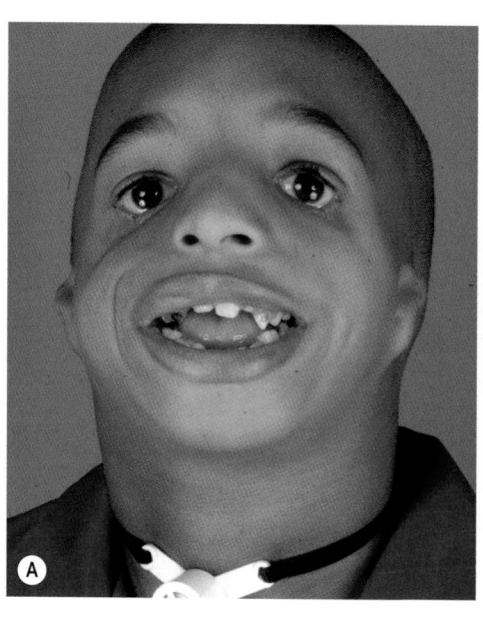
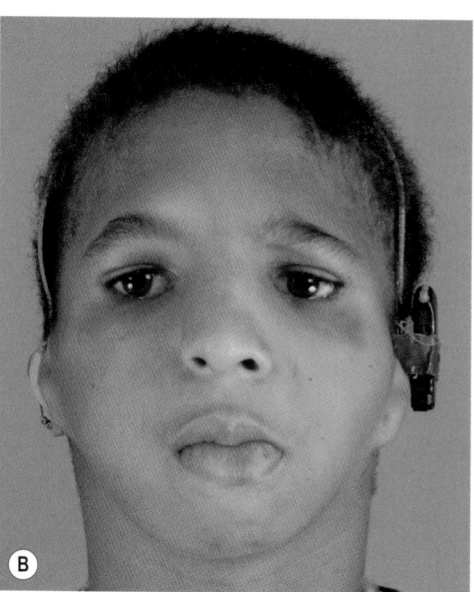
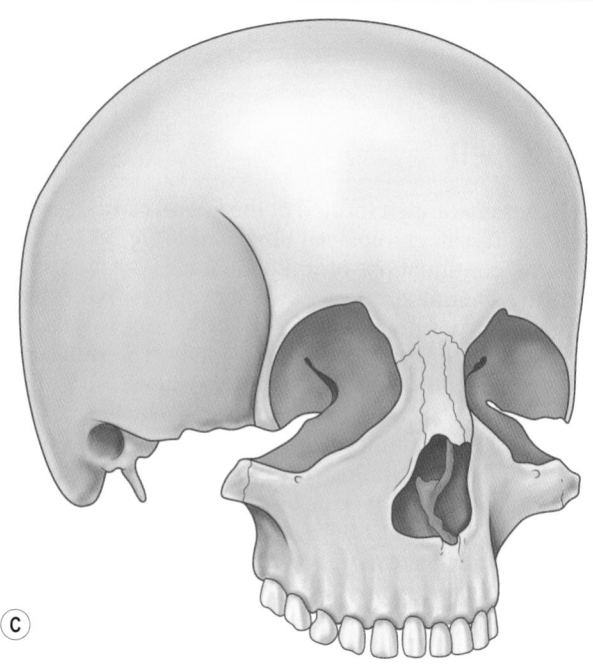

Fig. 33.12 Combination number 6, 7, and 8 cleft. **(A)** Patient with Treacher–Collins syndrome demonstrates malar hypoplasia, antimongoloid slant to palpebral fissure, and a retruded chin. **(B)** Postoperative image after malar reconstruction with cranial bone grafts, eyelid reconstruction with lid switch flaps, and mandibular distraction to remove the tracheostomy. Subsequently the patient underwent bilateral total ear reconstruction. **(C)** Skeletal involvement in the complete form includes absence of the zygoma, lateral orbital wall (greater wing of sphenoid provides remaining portion of the lateral wall), and lateral orbital floor.

33.12C). Thus, the lateral palpebral fissure's only support is the greater wing of the sphenoid and downward slanting occurs. With this defect there is soft-tissue continuity of the orbit and temporal fossa.

Number 9 cleft

This upper lateral orbit cleft is the rarest of the craniofacial clefts. The number 9 cleft begins the medial movement through the cranial clefts. This defect was nominated frontosphenoid dysplasia by Van der Meulen.[48] It is the cranial extension of the number 5 facial cleft.

Soft-tissue involvement

The number 9 cleft is manifested by abnormalities of the lateral third of the upper eyelid and eyebrow. The lateral

canthus is also distorted. In the severe form, microphthalmia is present *(Fig. 33.13)*. The superolateral bony deficiency of the orbits allows for a lateral displacement of the globes. The cleft then extends cephalad into the temporoparietal hair-bearing scalp. The temporal hairline is anteriorly displaced and a temporal hair projection is often seen in the number 9 cleft. Furthermore, a cranial nerve VII palsy in the forehead and upper eyelid is common.

Skeletal involvement

The bony defect of the number 9 cranial cleft extends through the superolateral aspect of the orbit. Distortion of the upper part of the greater wing of the sphenoid, the squamosal portion of the temporal bone and surrounding parietal bones may be present. This hypoplasia of the greater wing of the sphenoid results in a posterolateral rotation of the lateral

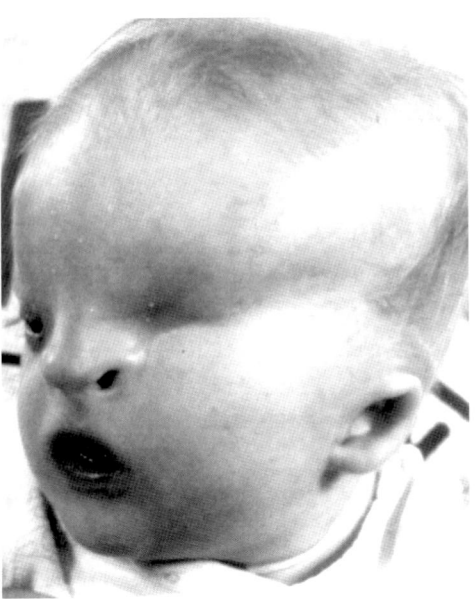

Fig. 33.13 Number 9 cleft. Patient with left-side rare number 9 cleft through the superolateral orbital roof with micophthalmia.

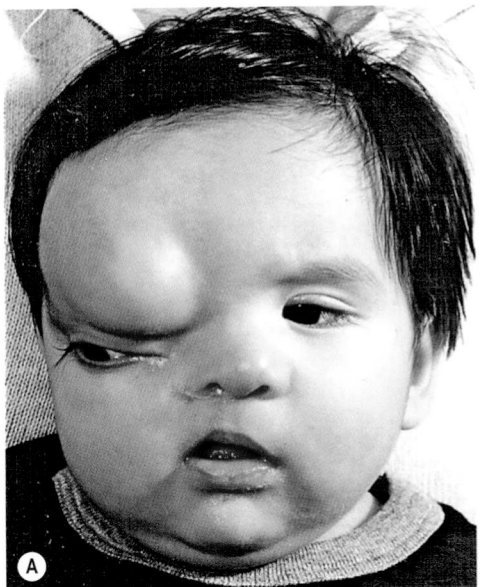

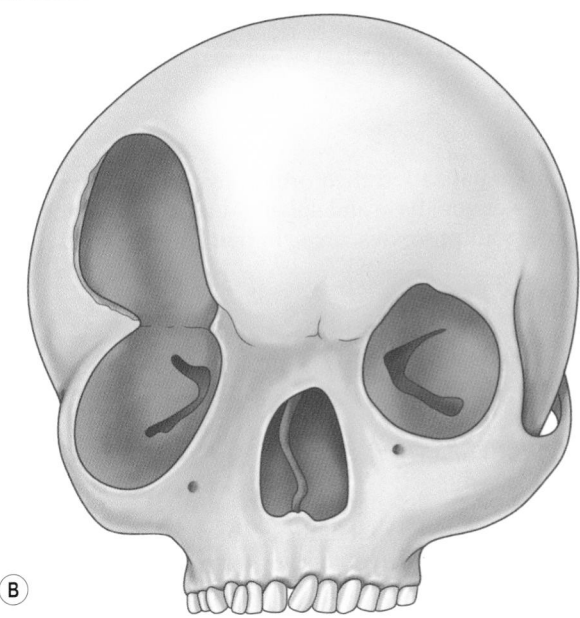

Fig. 33.14 Number 10 cleft. **(A)** Patient with fronto-orbital encephalocele in the mid right forehead. This fills the void from the cleft defect in the center of the left superior orbital rim. The right globe is displaced downward. **(B)** Skeletal defect and asymmetric hypertelorism are demonstrated on the right.

orbital wall. The pterygoid plates may be hypoplastic. There may be a reduction in the anteroposterior dimension of the anterior cranial fossa.

Number 10 cleft

This upper central orbital cleft has also been classified as a frontal dysplasia group.[48.] The number 10 cleft is the cranial extension of a number 4 cleft.

Soft-tissue involvement

The number 10 cleft begins at the middle third of the upper eyelid and eyebrow. The lateral eyebrow may angulate temporally. The palpebral fissure may be elongated with an amblyopic eye displaced inferolaterally *(Fig. 33.14A)*. The entire upper eyelid may be absent in severe forms (ablepharia). Colobomas and other ocular anomalies may be present. Frontal hair projection may connect the temporoparietal region to the lateral brow.

Skeletal involvement

The bony component of the number 10 cranial cleft occurs in the middle of the supraorbital rim just lateral to the superior orbital foramen *(Fig. 33.14B)*. Often an encephalocele occupies the defect through the frontal bone and a prominent bulge is observed in the forehead. The orbit may be deformed with a lateroinferior rotation. Orbital hypertelorism may result in severe cases. The anterior cranial base may also be distorted.

Number 11 cleft

This upper medial orbital cleft is the cranial extension of the number 3 cleft. Van der Muelen *et al.* included this malformation in their frontal dysplasia group.[48]

Soft-tissue involvement

The medial third of the upper eyelid may show involvement with a coloboma. The upper eyebrow may have a disruption evident which extends up to the frontal hairline *(Fig. 33.15)*. A tongue-like projection at the medial third of the frontal hairline may also be identified.

Skeletal involvement

The number 11 cleft may be seen as a cleft in the medial third of the supraorbital rim if it passes lateral to the ethmoid bone. If the cleft passes through the ethmoid air cells to produce

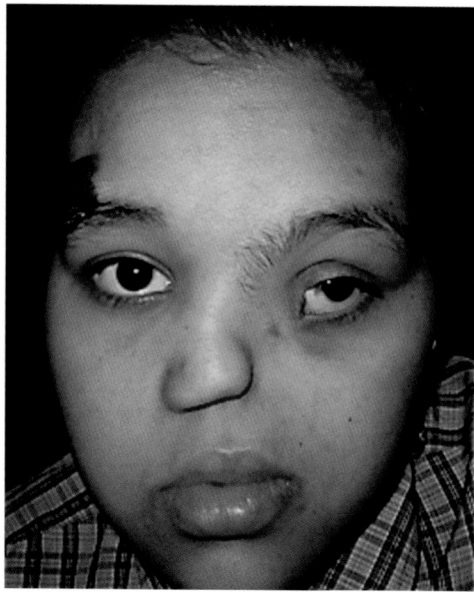

Fig. 33.15 Number 11 cleft. Patient with coloboma in medial third of left upper eyelid extending through the medial third of the eyebrow.

extensive pneumatization then orbital hypertelorism is seen clinically. The cranial base and sphenoid architecture, including the pterygoid processes, are symmetric and normal.

Number 12 cleft

The number 12 cleft is the cranial extension of the number 2 cleft.

Soft-tissue involvement

The soft-tissue cleft lies medial to the medial canthus and colobomas extend to the root of the eyebrow. There is a lateral displacement of the medial canthus with an aplasia of the medial end of the eyebrow. There are no eyelid clefts. The forehead skin is normal with a short downward projection of the paramedian frontal hairline *(Fig. 33.16A)*.

Skeletal involvement

The number 12 cleft passes through the flattened, frontal process of the maxilla *(Fig. 33.16B)*. It then travels superiorly, increasing the transverse dimension of the ethmoid air cells, producing orbital hypertelorism and telecanthus. The frontal and sphenoid sinuses are also pneumatized and enlarged. The remainder of the sphenoid and frontal bones are normal. The frontonasal angle is obtuse. The cleft is located lateral to the olfactory groove, thus the cribriform plate is normal in width. Encephaloceles have not been observed with this cleft. The anterior and middle cranial fossae are widened on the cleft side, but otherwise normal.[57]

Number 13 cleft

The number 13 cleft is the cranial extension of the paramedian, facial number 1 cleft *(Fig. 33.17)*.

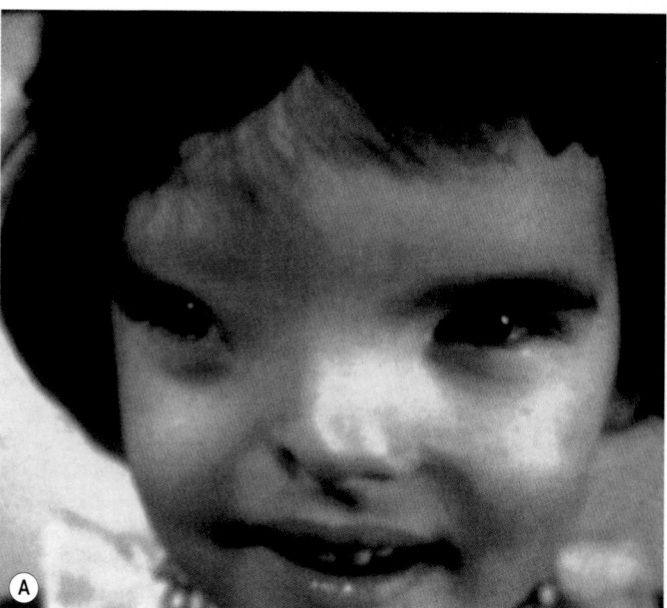

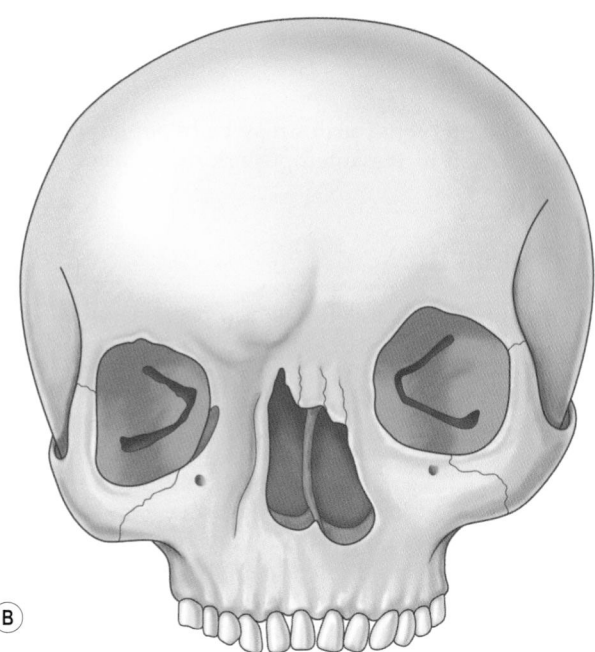

Fig. 33.16 Number 12 cleft. **(A)** Patient with right cleft has orbital hypertelorism and a disturbance of the left medial eyebrow. **(B)** Skeletal involvement of right-side clefting through the frontal process of the maxilla displacing the orbit laterally and hypertelorism results.

Soft-tissue involvement

There is typically a paramedian frontal encephalocele, which is located between the nasal bone and the frontal process of the maxilla. The soft-tissue cleft is medial to intact eyelids and eyebrows. The medial end of the eyebrow, however, can be displaced inferiorly. A V-shaped frontal hair projection can also be seen.

Skeletal involvement

Changes in the cribriform plate are the hallmark of a number 13 cleft. The paramedian bony cleft traverses the frontal bone,

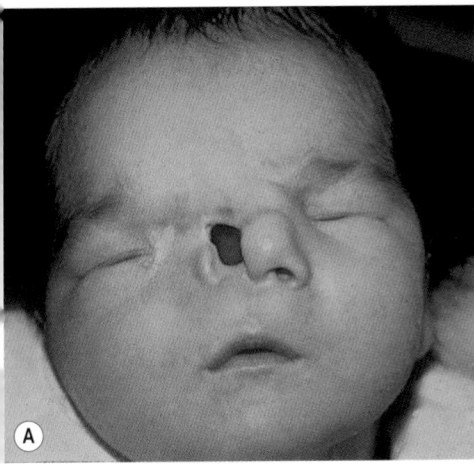

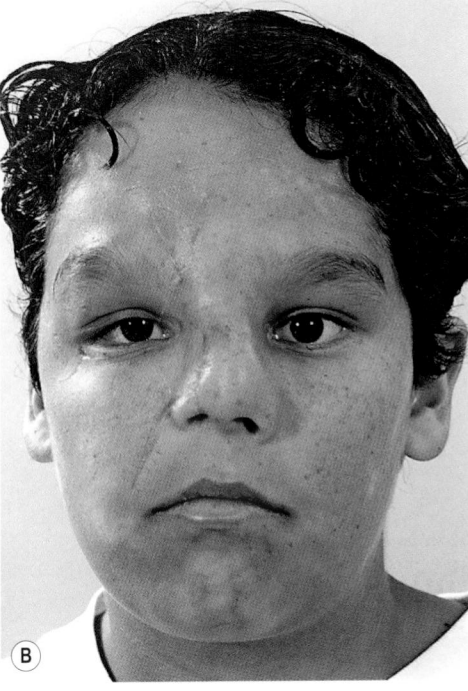

Fig. 33.17 Number 13 cleft. **(A)** Patient with a right cleft which begins cleft through the right alar dome (number 1 cleft) and extends to the frontal bone to cause right-sided telorbitism. **(B)** Postoperative image after corrective facial bipartition and nasal reconstruction with forehead flap.

then courses along the olfactory groove. There is widening of the olfactory groove, the cribriform plate, and the ethmoid sinus, which results in hypertelorism. A paramedian frontal encephalocele can cause the cribriform plate to be displaced inferiorly, leading to orbital dystopia. Unilateral and bilateral forms of the number 13 cleft exist, similar to most of the other craniofacial clefts. When the cleft is bilateral, some of the most extreme cases of hypertelorism can be seen.[2]

Number 14 cleft

The number 14 cleft occurs in the midline forehead and cranium as an extension of number 0 clefts. As in the number 0 clefts or median craniofacial dysraphia, described above, there may be a tissue deficiency, tissue excess, or normal amount of tissue but clefted in some way.

Soft-tissue involvement

Similar to its facial counterpart, the number 14 cleft can be produced as an agenesis or an overabundance of tissue. When agenesis occurs, orbital hypotelorism is generally seen. Included in this group of craniofacial malformations are the holoprosencephalic disorders, which include cyclopia, ethmocephaly, and cebocephaly *(Fig. 33.18A)*. The cranium is typically microcephalic and there is hypotelorism. A complete absence of midline cranial base structures can occur, causing the orbits to coalesce. Malformations of the forebrain are usually proportional to the degree of facial abnormality. An extensively involved number 14 cleft can severely handicap the newborn and life expectancy is usually limited from hours to months.

At the other end of the spectrum, hypertelorism is associated with the number 14 cleft *(Fig. 33.18B)*. The terms frontonasal and frontonasoethmoid dysplasia were used by Van der Meulen to categorize this group.[48] Lateral displacement of the orbits can be produced by midline masses such as a frontonasal encephalocele or a midline frontal encephalocele *(Fig. 33.18C, D)*. Cohen *et al.* thought that the basic fault in embryologic development lies in the malformation of the nasal capsule and the developing forebrain remains in a low position.[56] A morphokinetic arrest of the normal medial movement of the eyes occurs and the orbits remain in their widespread fetal position. Flattening of the glabella and extreme lateral displacement of the inner canthi are also seen. The periorbita, including the eyelids and eyebrows, are otherwise normal. A long midline projection of the frontal hairline marks the superior extent of the soft-tissue features of this midline cranial cleft.

Skeletal involvement

The frontal encephalocele herniates through a medial frontal defect. The caudal aspect of the frontal bone is flattened, giving the glabellar region a flattened and indistinct position. No pneumatization of the frontal sinus is evident; however, the sphenoid sinus is extensively pneumatized. The crista galli and the perpendicular plate of the ethmoid are bifid and there is an increased distance between the olfactory grooves *(Fig. 33.18E)*. When the crista galli is severely enlarged, preservation of the olfactory nerve is often not possible during the surgical correction of hypertelorism. The crista galli and ethmoids are widened and caudally displaced. Consequently, the cribriform plate, which is normally located 5–10 mm below the level of the orbital roof, can be caudally displaced up to 20 mm.[58] The greater and lesser wings of the sphenoid are rotated and result in a relative shortening of the middle cranial fossa. The anterior cranial fossa is upslanting, causing a harlequin eye deformity on plain radiographs.

Number 30 cleft

The median cleft of the lower jaw was first described by Couronne. These median clefts of the lower lip and mandible are caudal extensions of the number 14 cranial cleft and number 0 facial cleft *(Fig. 33.19)*. The number 30 clefts include: mandibular process clefts, midline branchiogenic syndrome, and intermandibular dysplasia.

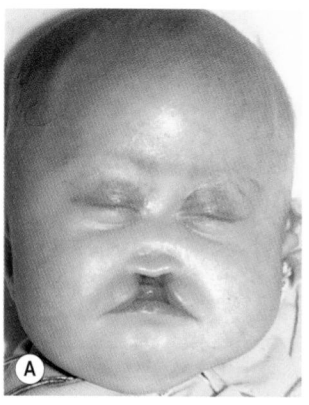 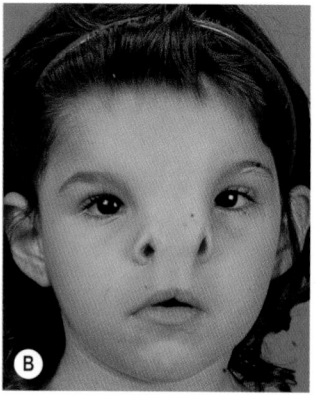 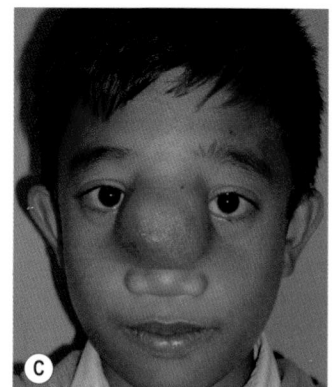 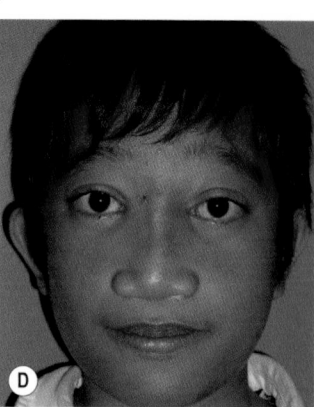

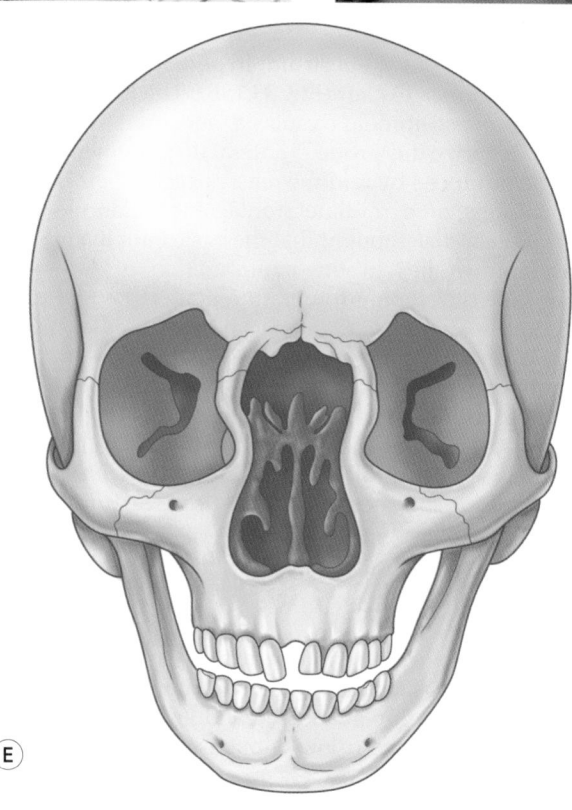

Fig. 33.18 Number 14 cleft. **(A)** Patient with number 14 cleft, holoproencephaly, a form of median craniofacial hypoplasia (tissue deficiency). **(B)** Patient with number 14 cleft, frontonasoethmoidal encephalocele, a form of median craniofacial dysraphia (normal tissue but clefted). **(C)** Patient with number 14 cleft, craniofrontonasal dysplasia, a form of median craniofacial hyperplasia (excess tissue). **(D)** Postoperative image after corrective encephalocele repair, medial orbit repositioning, and nasal bone grafting. **(E)** Skeletal involvement shows displacement of the frontal process of the maxilla, the nasal bones, and medial orbital walls laterally. This large defect is often occupied by an encephalocele.

Soft-tissue involvement

Soft-tissue involvement of this midline cleft may be as mild as a vermillion notch in the lower lip. However, often the entire lower lip and chin may be involved. The anterior tongue may be bifid and attached to the split mandible by a dense fibrous band. Ankyloglossia and total absence of the tongue have been reported with midline mandibular clefts. The anterior neck strap muscles are often atrophic and replaced by dense fibrous bands which may restrict chin flexion.

Skeletal involvement

Skeletal involvement is typically a cleft between the central incisors extending into the mandibular symphysis. This anomaly is thought to be caused by failure of fusion of the first branchial arch. However, associated neck anomalies are felt to be caused by failure of fusion of other lower branchial arches. The hyoid bone at times is absent and the thyroid cartilages may fail to form completely.

Summary

The clinical expression of craniofacial clefts is highly variable and ranges from a mild, barely noticeable *forme fruste* (microform) to a disfiguring, complete defect of skeletal and soft tissue. Tessier's description of craniofacial clefts based on bony and soft-tissue landmarks provides a classification which can be validated by neuroembryology. Craniofacial clefts, far from being considered oddities, will allow plastic surgeons in the future to refine and understand the developmental architecture of the face.

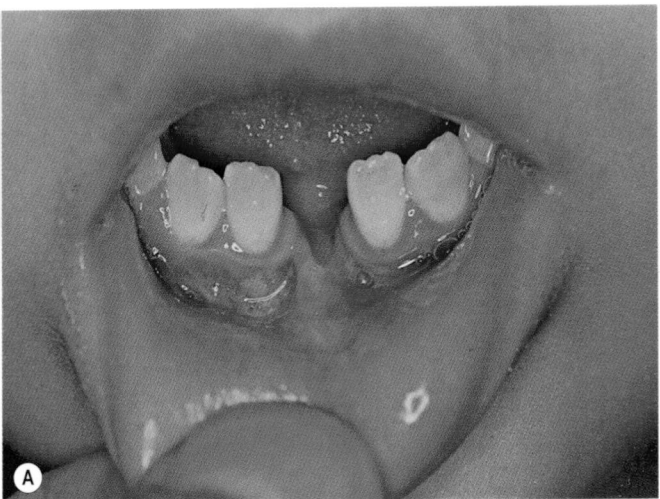

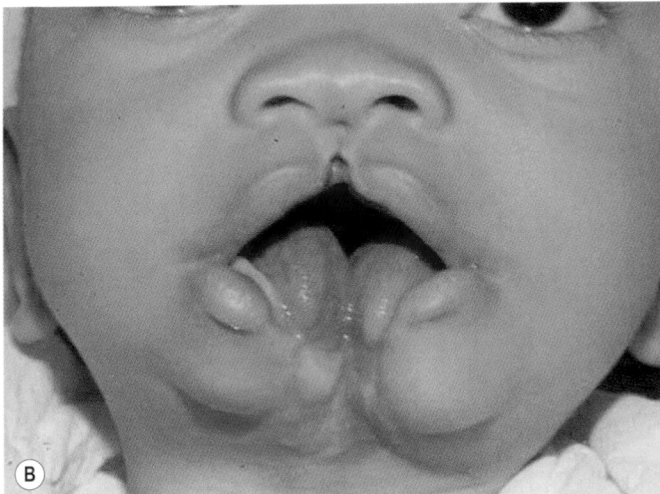

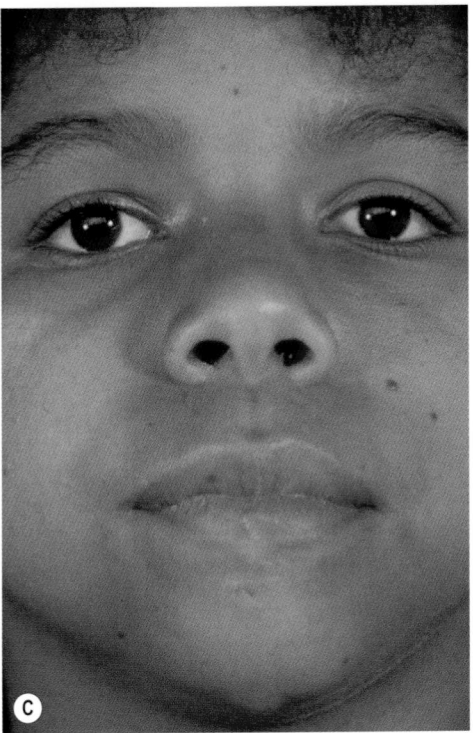

Fig. 33.19 Number 30 cleft. **(A)** Close-up intraoral view of patient with number 30 cleft showed dental separation of central incisors and bony cleft. **(B)** Preoperative view of patient with number 30 cleft with a deep tongue groove and fusion to the clefted mandible. (Courtesy of Cassio Raposo du Amaral, MD.) **(C)** Postoperative view of same patient with number 30 midline mandibular cleft after skeletal and soft-tissue repair. (Courtesy of Cassio Raposo du Amaral, MD.)

Treatment

Treatment of craniofacial clefts

Standardized treatment plans are not always possible because of the variety of craniofacial clefts and levels of severity. However, guiding principles are helpful in determining the proper timing and stages for corrective surgery.[2–4] If there are functional problems, like ocular exposure, or airway problems, or if the malformation is severe, then surgery should be performed early. If the malformation is mild, surgery should be delayed. During infancy (3–12 months), soft-tissue clefts and midline cranial defects (e.g., encephaloceles) may be corrected. Midface and orbital reconstruction with bone grafting may be performed in older children (6–9 years). Orthognathic

procedures are delayed until skeletal maturity (14 years or greater).

Surgical techniques used for correction of craniofacial clefts depend upon the anatomic regions that are involved. For timing and general corrective protocols, the deformities may be grouped into: (1) midline and paramedian clefts (numbers 0–14, numbers 1–13, 2–12, or other combinations); (2) oronaso-ocular clefts (numbers 3–11, 4–10, 5–9); and (3) lateral clefts including constellation of numbers 6, 7, and 8 clefts like Treacher–Collins syndrome of craniofacial microsomia.

First, for midline clefts, proper diagnosis into median craniofacial hypoplasia (tissue deficiency), median craniofacial dysplasia (normal tissue volume but separated), or median craniofacial hyperplasia (tissue excess) is helpful for proper treatment planning. Midline clefts may have symmetrical deformities like bifidity of the nasal cartilages or

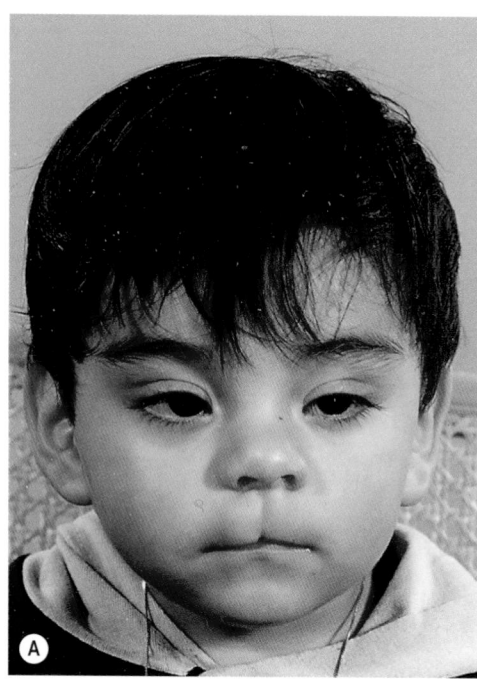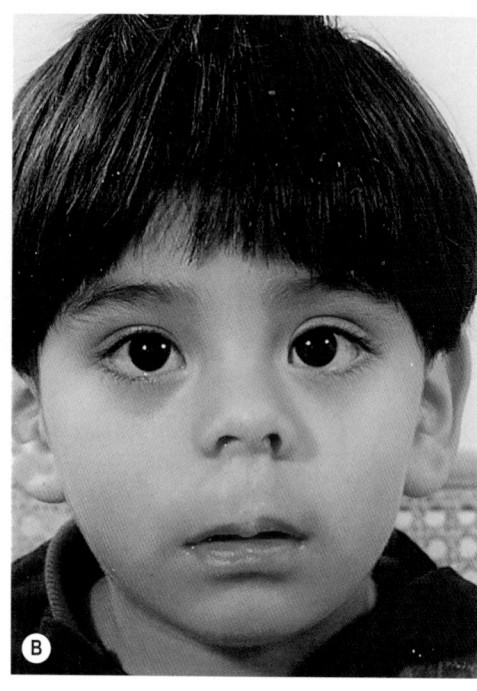

Fig. 33.20 Number 0 cleft correction. **(A)** Preoperative frontal view of patient with midline incomplete cleft lip. **(B)** Postoperative frontal view of patient after intraoral repair of orbicularis oris muscle without cutaneous scar.

symmetrical hypertelorbitism, while paramedian clefts manifest asymmetry with unilateral nasal notching or horizontal and vertical orbital dystopia. For the upper lip, correction of cleft defects involves aligning the white roll and vermillion, and restoring muscular continuity as in a common cleft lip repair. Microform variations may be corrected with intraoral muscle repair, Z-plasty of the white roll, and no cutaneous scar *(Fig. 33.20)*. For lateral clefts, lip reconstruction is performed with a rotation-advancement repair.

For the nose, a median cleft correction may be done in early childhood with a primary rhinoplasty used to unify bifid nasal cartilages after excision of intervening fibrofatty tissue. For paramedian defects, the nose is reconstructed with cartilage grafts or composite skin-cartilage grafts, particularly for asymmetries and soft triangle notching. Alar retraction may be corrected with local rotation flaps or Z-plasty flaps. Secondary nasal reconstruction may be performed with a septoplasty or even cantilevered cranial bone grafts. Correction of duplication of the nasal septum should be reserved until the end of nasal growth.

For orbital dystopia, correction with an orbital box osteotomy has been described for these deformities; however, a facial bipartition allows for more versatility, especially in patients with mixed dentition when occlusal correction is not paramount. A facial bipartition requires bilateral monobloc osteotomies: in the anterior zygomatic arch, lateral orbital wall, orbital roof, medial orbital wall, orbital floor, pterygomaxillary buttresses, and septum (during the midface downfracture). Anterior encephalocele reduction and cranial base bone graft may be necessary before midline fixation *(Fig. 33.21)*.[59] For these large anterior encephaloceles, subsequent cleft palate repair may require a pharyngeal flap for nasal lining. With paramedian (numbers 1–13, 2–12) clefts, vertical adjustment of a facial bipartition segment may be necessary to correct vertical, as well as horizontal, orbital dystopia *(Fig. 33.22)*. For these procedures, the misaligned occlusal plane is

usually temporary and correctable. Subsequent medial canthoplasty may also be necessary.

Second, for oro-naso-ocular clefts (numbers 3–11, 4–10, 5–9), the original descriptions for correction of the soft-tissue component of these clefts involved the use of Z-plasty flaps. These flaps were designed to lengthen the foreshortened distance between the medial canthus and nasal alar base on the affected side. Presently, flaps are designed to respect aesthetic units by leaving scars along aesthetic lines.[57] For repair, complete dissection of the cleft is necessary. Small orbital floor bone graft or bone graft matrix may be used to fill the cleft defect and separate the orbit from the maxillary sinus. A banner flap from along the median nasal sidewall may be rotated into a subciliary incision beneath the affected lower eyelid and a transnasal medial canthopexy may be performed. Oro-naso-ocular clefts may also present with large encephaloceles from cranial defects *(Fig. 33.23)*. In these cases a staged approach in infancy may be appropriate for optimal correction. Of note, for the lateral lip cleft repair (numbers 4 and 5 clefts), the intervening tissue between the philtral column and lateral cleft should be excised.

The third treatment group, the lateral craniofacial clefts (numbers 6, 7, and 8) include the constellation of clefts like Treacher–Collins syndrome and craniofacial microsomia. For the oral commissure (as in cleft number 7), macrostomia may affect feeding, saliva control, and speech acquisition and should be addressed at an early age. The oral commissure should be corrected for symmetry and fall approximately below the medial canthal vertical line. Orbicularis oris muscle fibers should be reoriented and interlaced at the neo-oral commissure, and the cleft should be closed in a straight line. The medial aspect may be closed with a small Z-plasty so that the vertical limb is along the nasolabial fold. For the lower lip (as in cleft number 30), a vertical excision with bilateral extensions (not crossing the labiomental fold) with a layered closure is performed.[60]

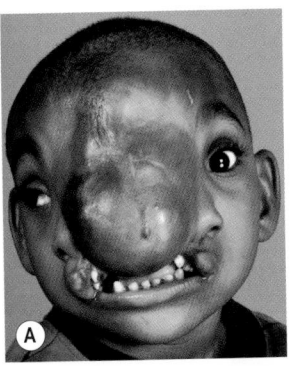
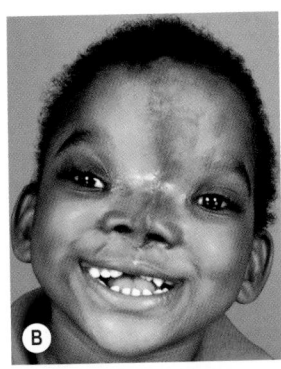
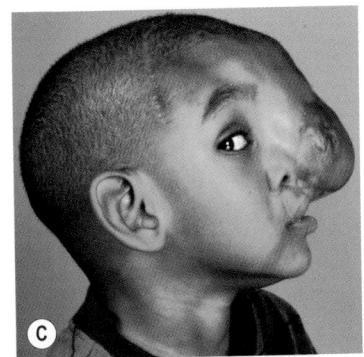
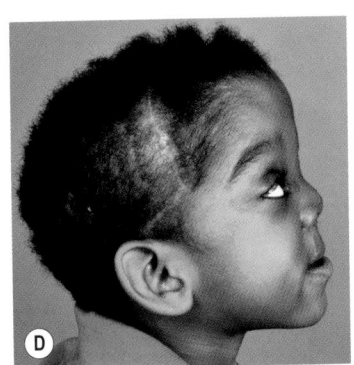

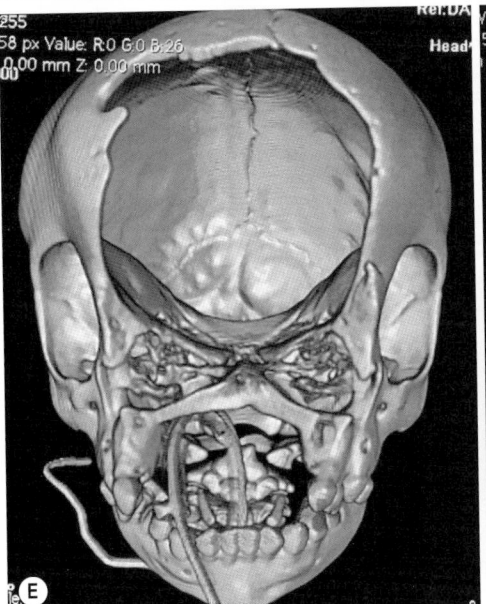
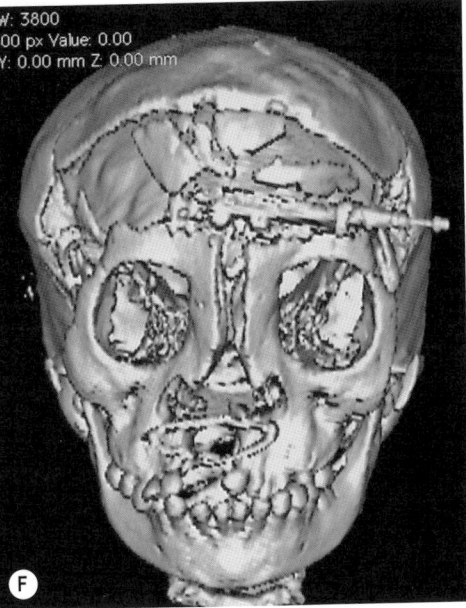

Fig. 33.21 Number 0, 14 cleft correction. **(A,B)** Frontal views of patient with Tessier numbers 0–14 craniofacial cleft. **(A)** Preoperative image demonstrating large midline frontonasal encephalocele. **(B)** Postoperative image after gradual orbital contraction procedure and median cleft lip and nose repair. **(C,D)** Lateral views of patient with Tessier numbers 0–14 craniofacial cleft. **(C)** Preoperative image demonstrating the anterior displacement of the encephalocele with functional problems of independent ocular movement and drooling. **(D)** Postoperative image after corrective procedures. Functional improvements in ocular, oral competence, and speech were noted. **(E)** Preoperative three-dimensional computed tomography scan with large central osseous defect and 81-mm interdacryon distance. **(F)** Postoperative image after orbital contraction with midline device in place.

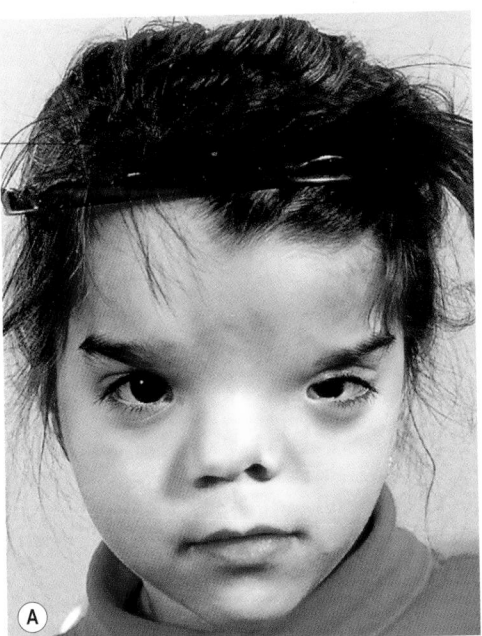
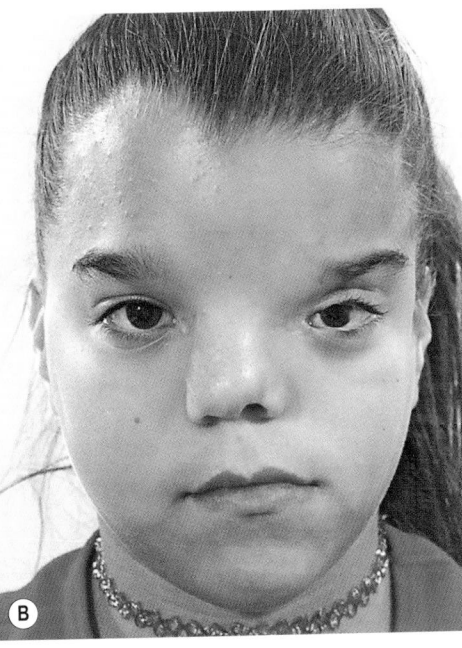

Fig. 33.22 Number 2, 12 cleft correction. **(A)** Preoperative view shows left nasal alar cephalad malposition, orbital dystopia, and hairline malformation. **(B)** Postoperative view after facial bipartition and medial canthoplasty. Future nasal correction will be needed.

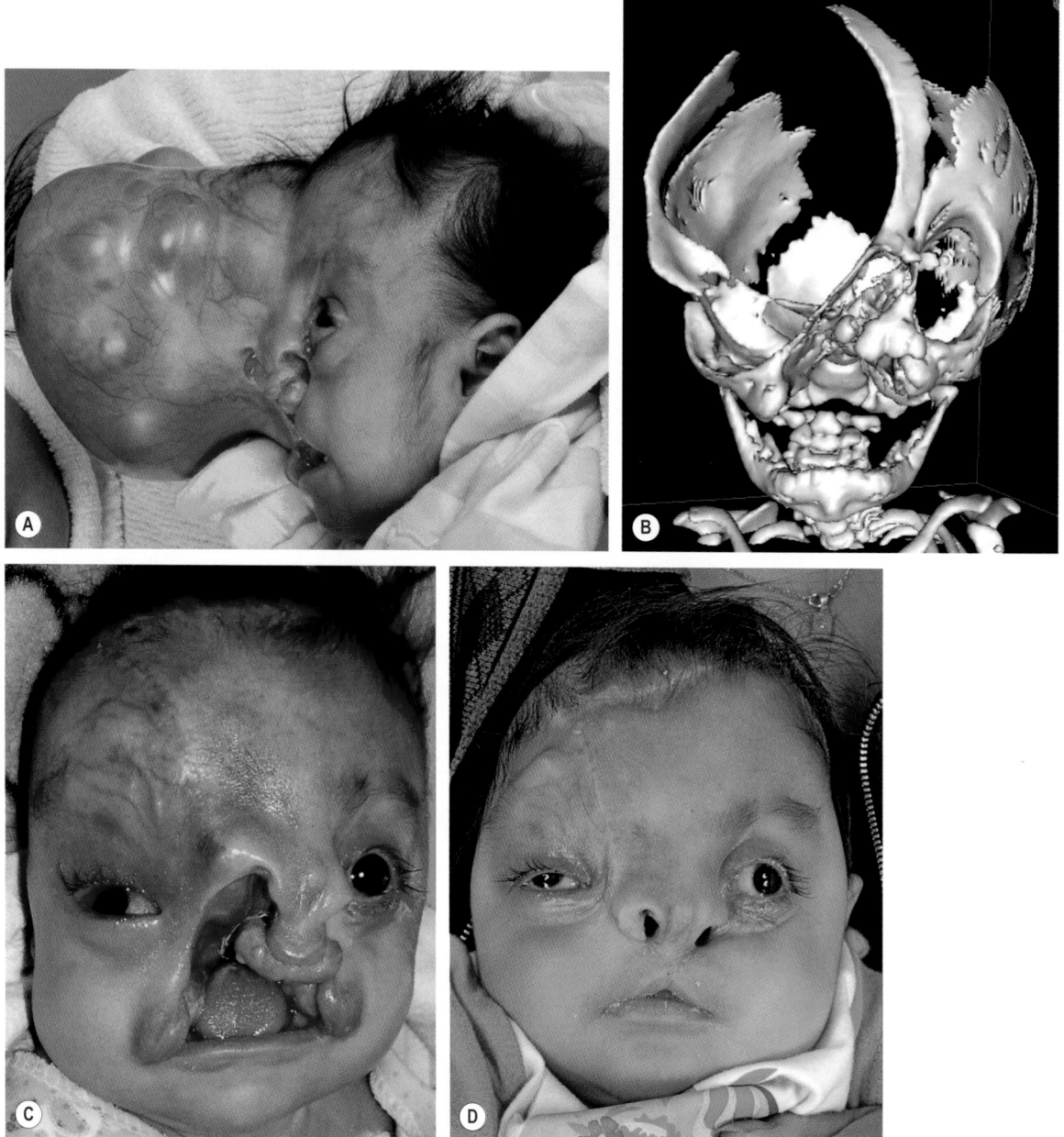

Fig. 33.23 Number 3, 10 cleft correction. **(A)** Preoperative left lateral image demonstrated a large right frontoencephalocele. A right-side numbers 3 and 10 and a left-side number 3 craniofacial cleft were present. **(B)** Computed tomography scan revealed significant bony defect of the right fronto-orbital region, encephalocele cyst, and bony deformity. **(C)** After the first procedure of encephalocele repair and right fronto-orbital reconstruction, the patient showed improvement but still had orbital and facial cleft deformities. **(D)** Postoperative frontal images after bilateral cleft lip repair and right nasoforehead rotation and medial canthal repositioning. Future reconstructive procedures will be necessary.

For mandibular reconstruction (as in cleft combinations 6, 7 and 8 in both craniofacial microsomia and Treacher–Collins syndrome), costochondral grafts may be used for severe deformities, and distraction osteogenesis for moderate deformities in mid-childhood (6–8 years).[61] For mild maxillary deformities resulting in an occlusal cant, correction can wait until adulthood with a Le Fort I osteotomy with or without a concomitant mandibular procedure.

Surgical correction of the periorbital region is necessary in many craniofacial clefts. For the eye, urgent intervention is necessary if the eye is exposed and at risk of corneal ulceration. However, early reconstructive procedures for globe protection must be balanced to allow enough eye opening to prevent deprivation amblyopia. For the eyelid, "lid switch" transposition flaps are used for skin/muscle deficiencies. Palatal grafts may be used for lower lid conjunctival lining. The orbit may be reconstructed with cranial bone grafting to restore orbital continuity and correct dystopia. Accurate repositioning of the medial canthus may be performed with transnasal wiring. Lateral canthopexies are sometimes needed to achieve symmetry. Correction of number 8 (lateral eye) clefts are performed with Z-plasty flaps. For the lacrimal apparatus, disruption of the canalicular system may be corrected with Silastic stents or formal dacryocystorhinostomy.

Outcomes and complications

Proper timing and technique of staged corrective procedures will minimize perioperative complications and long-term sequelae. If early functional problems like globe exposure are not addressed, then corneal ulceration and blindness may result. Likewise, speech problems may develop, as in more common cleft lip and palate deformities. Complications may occur for specific soft- or hard-tissue correction because of the difficult nature of these procedures.

Summary

Craniofacial clefts are highly variable and range from mild (barely noticeable) *forme fruste* (microform), to disfiguring, complete defects of the skeletal and soft tissue. Tessier's description of craniofacial clefts based on bony and soft-tissue landmarks provides a classification which has been validated by neurometric theory of neuroembryology. For corrective surgery, guiding principles are helpful in determining the proper timing and stages, like addressing functional problems (ocular exposure, airway problems) early. General corrective protocols may be grouped into: (1) midline and paramedian clefts (numbers 0–14, 1–13, 2–12); (2) oro-naso-ocular clefts (numbers 3–11, 4–10, 5–9); and (3) lateral clefts (numbers 6, 7, 8; like Treacher–Collins syndrome of craniofacial microsomia).

Access the complete references list online at **http://www.expertconsult.com**

1. Tessier P. Anatomical classification of facial, cranio-facial and latero-facial clefts. *J. Maxillofac. Surg.* 1976;4:69.

   Tessier introduces his now ubiquitous classification scheme for craniofacial clefts in this account. Cleft position is described in reference to the orbit.

2. Kawamoto Jr HK. The kaleidoscopic world of rare craniofacial clefts: order out of chaos (Tessier classification). *Clin. Plast. Surg.* 1976;3:529.

3. Kawamoto Jr HK. Rare craniofacial clefts. In: McCarthy JG, ed. *Plastic surgery*. Philadelphia: Saunders; 1990:2922–2973.

4. Bradley JP, Kawamoto HK. Rare craniofacial clefts. In: Grabb WC, Smith JW, eds. *Plastic surgery*. Philadelphia: Saunders; 1990:2922–2973.

5. Carstens MH. Functional matrix repair: A common strategy for unilateral and bilateral clefts. *J. Craniofac. Surg.* 2000;11:437–469.

9. Van der Meulen JC, Mazzola R, Vermey-Keers C, et al. A morphogenetic classification of craniofacial malformations. *Plast. Reconstr. Surg.* 1983;71:560.

   The authors describe a new classification scheme for craniofacial clefts. Pathogenesis and cerebral involvement are emphasized.

10. Allam K, Wan D, Kawamoto HK, et al. The spectrum of median craniofacial dysplasia. *Plast. Reconstr. Surg.* 2011;127:812–821.

    Midline craniofacial malformations are further defined from an embryological perspective. The authors separate these entities into hypoplasias (tissue deficiency), dysraphias (normal amount of tissue, but clefted), and hyperplasias (tissue excess).

11. Noordhoff SM, Huang CS, Lo LJ. Median facial dysplasia in unilateral and bilateral cleft lip and palate: a subgroup of median cerebrofacial malformations. *Plast Reconstr Surg.* 1993;91:996–1005.

    A group of patients characterized by midface anomalies without cerebral involvement is identified. Topics ranging from anatomical considerations to growth potential are addressed.

57. Longaker MT, Lipshutz GS, Kawamoto Jr HK. Reconstruction of Tessier number 4 clefts revisited. *Plast. Reconstr. Surg.* 1997;99:1501.

58. Tessier P. Orbital hypertelorism. 1. Successive surgical attempts, material and methods, causes and mechanisms. *Scand. J. Plast. Reconstr. Surg.* 1972;6:135.

    Orbital hypertelorism is described. An extensive case series informs observations on diagnosis and management.

34

Nonsyndromic craniosynostosis

Derek M. Steinbacher and Scott P. Bartlett

SYNOPSIS

- Craniosynostosis is the pathologic fusion of one or more cranial vault sutures, usually resulting in an abnormal head shape. Nonsyndromic craniosynostosis occurs in a sporadic, nonfamilial fashion, in the absence of an associated genetic syndrome.

- The fused cranial suture results create a cranial deformity, with areas of restricted growth and compensatory bossing, as well as the potential for functional and organic issues (increased intracranial pressure (ICP) being the most significant).

- Diagnosis entails a clinical examination and computed tomography (CT) corroboration. The optimal timing of treatment is during infancy, between 6 and 9 months.

- Conventional open techniques and new modalities (including springs and distraction osteogenesis) can be entertained.

- The choice of operation depends on the specific suture fused and the degree of dysmorphology. In general, the technical surgical goals entail: releasing the area of sutural fusion, repositioning the bone in an anatomic but overcorrected location, eliminating secondary compensatory changes, filling in osteotomy gaps with bone dust slurry, and closing the soft tissue relatively tension-free.

- The physiologic goal is to mitigate functional problems (e.g., intracranial hypertension and developmental delay, optic disc atrophy, and strabismus).

- Complications can be divided into early or late events.

- Secondary revisions may be necessary involving either the soft tissue, bone, or both.

- On rare occasions, the complete intracranial procedure must be repeated. However, major morbidity and mortality are exceedingly uncommon in the modern approach and management of craniosynostosis.

 Access the Historical Perspective section online at
http://www.expertconsult.com

Introduction

Craniosynostosis is the pathologic fusion of one or more cranial vault sutures, usually resulting in an abnormal head

shape. Nonsyndromic craniosynostosis refers to an isolated entity, without an associated genetic syndrome, occurring in approximately 1 in 1800 to 1 in 2500 births. Typically in nonsyndromic forms only one suture is involved, termed simple craniosynostosis, though occasionally two or more sutures may be affected (complex craniosynostosis). The type of synostosis is denoted based on the suture fused, with sagittal being the most common and lambdoid the least. There is recent evidence that the distribution of metopic and unicoronal synostosis (UCS) is changing, with a relative increase in metopic craniosynostosis.[1,2] Midline synostoses (sagittal and metopic) appear more apt to occur among twins.[3] Gender predilection demonstrates male preference for sagittal synostosis (4:1), while females are slightly more prone to unilateral coronal synostosis (3:2).[4] A complex, multifactorial set of etiologic factors is at work in nonsyndromic craniosynostosis given the differences in population incidence, proportion of family cases, male-to-female distribution, and phenotypic severity among and between types of sutural synostosis.[5]

Basic science/disease process

Nonsyndromic craniosynostosis most frequently occurs in a sporadic and nonfamilial fashion. The mechanistic cause and biochemical changes at the suture appear to stem from a variety of genetic and environmental factors. The genetic influence, however, is poorly understood. Ephrin-A4 (EFNA4) is, as yet, the only identified gene proposed to play a role in nonsyndromic craniosynostosis.[26] Autosomal-dominant familial inheritance, in the absence of a known identifiable gene, is reported to account for approximately 8–14% of nonsyndromic synostoses.[5,27]

About 2% of sagittal synostosis cases are familial.[28] Coronal synostosis demonstrates an 8–10% positive family history.[5] Bicoronal synostosis is more apt to be inherited than UCS.[27] Older paternal age may contribute more to coronal than sagittal synostosis. Metopic synostosis is thought to be familial in up to 10% of cases.[29,30] Seemingly nonsyndromic coronal and metopic synostosis can be associated with a subtle presentation of phenotypic features in Muenke and Saethre–Chotzen syndromes. FGFR3 and TWIST gene mutations should be tested in cases of craniosynostosis with suspected familial inheritance.[26,31] Lambdoid synostosis occurs so infrequently that it is difficult to quantify the incidence of heritable cases. There have been a few case reports denoting lambdoidal synostosis within families.[32–34]

Environmental effects on suture biology are also suggested to promote synostosis. Antenatal head compression, from multiple gestation, large infant size, abnormal intrauterine lie, or uterine abnormalities, has been reported in association with nonsyndromic craniosynostosis. Graham and Smith describe two cases of metopic synostosis and one case of coronal synostosis secondary to bicornuate uterine morphology, cephalic compression in the pelvis from a triplet gestation, and a constricted *in utero* lie after early descent, respectively.[35] Higginbottom *et al.* recounted three cases of craniosynostosis also resulting from external force to the head, one each from breech position, amniotic band, and a morphologic abnormality of the uterus.[36] Twin studies demonstrate an increase in craniosynostosis, providing further evidence that gestational constraint contributes to premature sutural fusion in all twin types, while monozygotic twins may have the additional influence of genetic factors.[5]

The concept of intrauterine constraint is borne out in experimental models. Animal studies demonstrate that intrauterine constraint results in 88% suture fusion, with FGFR2 and transforming growth factor-β (TGF-β) expression being enhanced in the fused sutures.[37–39] In addition to TGF-β, other growth factors shown to upregulate from head constraint, possibly influencing sutural stenosis, include: BMP-4, Noggin, and Indian hedgehog.[38,40,41] However, restriction of sutural expansion in lambs by rigid plating across the coronal sutures 8 weeks antepartum demonstrated persistently patent sutures, by CT scan and histologically, despite the phenotypic appearance of bicoronal synostosis.[42]

A host of other nongenetic risk factors have been reported in association with nonsyndromic craniosynostosis. Maternal smoking, white maternal race, advanced maternal age, gestation at high altitude, use of nitrosatable drugs (e.g., nitrofurantoin), paternal occupation (e.g., agriculture, forestry), fertility treatments, endocrine abnormalities (e.g., hyperthyroidism), and warfarin ingestion during gestation have all been linked to craniosynostosis.[43–48]

Regardless of the genetic and environmental influences, it is theorized that fusion of the suture occurs as either a primary or secondary event. Ossification of the suture as the principal cause was first suggested by Virchow, and others have since agreed.[16,17,49–52] An increased number of osteoblasts at the affected suture results in calvarial ossification and subsequent suture fusion.[49,50,52–55] This concept intimates that any change in cranial base length, brain volume, cerebrospinal fluid (CSF) volume, and ICP are secondary to the primary event at the suture (sutural fusion).

The fusion of the suture as a secondary issue to either cranial base underdevelopment or diminished brain growth has also been proposed. Gunther, in 1931, first suggested that delayed growth of the cranial base was the first step leading to sutural fusion.[56] Moss furthered this theory, stating that the skull base abnormality promoted tight dural attachments adjacent to the vault sutures.[57] He postulated that suture fusion results when these dural connections tether the osseous plates and prevent the stretch at the cranial sutures prompted by normal brain growth.[58,59] This implies that diminished cranial base length is the primary problem resulting in secondary sutural fusion, and possible changes to the brain and CSF volume.

Lack of intrinsic brain growth potential has also been suggested to cause early fusion of cranial sutures.[59] Diminished brain growth subjacent to the suture, hence less stimulus and stretch on the vault sutures, may portend sutural fusion. Marsh *et al.* compared a series of infants with nonsyndromic coronal synostosis to normal control infants on CT scan, demonstrating dysmorphic brain features in the former group.[60]

Fellows-Mayle and colleagues tested the three theories of sutural fusion in a rabbit model using the Path analysis.[61] The primary suture fusion model was found to describe best the causal nature of both early- and delayed-onset craniosynostosis. In any event, once the suture ossifies early, a downstream series of events is initiated with aesthetic, growth-related, and functional consequences.

The events that succeed the fused cranial suture relate to restriction of brain expansion in the area subjacent to the stenosis. Skull expansion is restricted in vectors perpendicular to the fused suture and, with forces directed elsewhere, compensatory bulges develop, usually parallel to the fused suture.[16,17] Delshaw *et al.* outlined four concepts describing the changes in cranial vault expansion that occur as a result of diminished growth at the fused suture.[62,63]

1. "Cranial vault bones that are prematurely fused act as a single bone plate with decreased growth potential.

2. Abnormal asymmetrical bone deposition occurs at perimeter sutures with increased bone deposition directed away from the bone plate.

3. Perimeter sutures adjacent to prematurely fused suture compensate in growth more than perimeter sutures distant to sutural stenosis.

4. A nonperimeter suture that is contiguous to the premature fused suture undergoes enhanced symmetrical bone deposition along both edges."

These events and compensations lead to an abnormal head shape as well as the potential for functional and organic issues. For instance, diminished orbital size results in exorbitism, globe prominence, and resultant corneal abrasion or irritation. Changed orbital dimensions can also result in differential extraocular muscle excursion between sides. This can portend strabismus and/or visual problems. Similarly, with one coronal suture affected, the heightened orbital distance results in a more superior location of the lid margin and levator apparatus, occasionally resulting in lagophthalmos, and worsening corneal exposure. In cases when both coronal sutures are fused, hypertelorism may be present, rarely affecting binocular vision.

More significantly, the fusion of cranial sutures is associated with increased ICP. The risk with a single suture synostosis is less than with multiple sutures (14% versus 47%), but a valid risk nonetheless in all cases.[64] Recent reports demonstrate that, even in mild cases of nonsyndromic synostosis, a significant proportion exhibit intracranial hypertension (defined as >17 mmHg) on lumbar puncture.[65] Increased ICP occurs because the compartment (cranial vault) is too tight for its contents (brain). Additionally, there may be a discrepancy between CSF production and egress. The pressure on the brain portends neurologic sequelae, including headaches, nausea, vomiting, visual problems, and motor, behavioral, and intellectual delay.

Diagnosis/patient presentation

Parents or pediatricians notice an abnormal forehead or head shape at or shortly following birth. The child is then frequently referred to a craniofacial surgeon or a neurosurgeon. Occasionally, the pediatrician may confuse true craniosynostosis with deformational change and advocate a conservative, observational approach. This results in diagnostic delay. The verification of true synostosis can also be delayed when the synostosis is mild (incomplete) and the head shape is not markedly abnormal, or in cases with later, symmetric, postnatal sutural fusion. History may reveal a multiple gestation or abnormal intrauterine lie. Family history should be elicited and referral to genetics made where appropriate. Headaches, visual disturbances, lethargy, and vomiting are signs of increased cranial pressure and may be difficult to elicit in infants. Intracranial hypertension can also manifest as papilledema on fundoscopic exam or by decreased red color saturation. The opthamologic exam should also note eye muscle function, as stramismus or opthalmoplegia can occur from bony changes to the orbits in craniosynostosis.

Physical examination is the cornerstone in the diagnosis of craniosynostosis. Symmetric brain enlargement is inhibited by the fused sutures and compensatory cranial bulges occur where sutures are patent. The cranium takes on a characteristic shape depending on the suture(s) involved *(Fig. 34.1)*. Palpation and sometimes even visual inspection can reveal the presence of ridging at fused suture lines. Head circumference and cephalic index are adjunctive measurements that may support the diagnosis *(Table 34.1)*. However, visual inspection and palpation remain the most effective means of confirming the diagnosis. Fusion of multiple sutures should raise greater concern for a genetic or familial cause and for intracranial hypertension.

True craniosynostosis must be differentiated from positional plagiocephaly. A comprehensive discussion of deformational plagiocephaly is outside the scope of this chapter, but we will address important distinguishing features from synostotic plagiocephaly *(Table 34.2)*. Deformational occipital flatness has risen dramatically following the "back to sleep" campaign advocated by the American Academy of Pediatrics.[66] Infants with positional plagiocephaly usually have a history of sleeping supine with the head consistently turned toward one side.[67] Torticollis frequently occurs with positional plagiocephaly. The shortened sternocleidomastoid muscle favors ipsilateral head turning, or conversely, the ipsilaterally flattened occiput leads to the torticollis secondarily.[68]

When clinical suspicion strongly supports the diagnosis, a three-dimensional (3D) CT scan is a necessary adjunct to document the presence and extent of synostosis. A high-resolution scan will readily illustrate the fused suture and allow analysis from several angles. The CT scan also allows for assessment of ventricular size, defects of the corpus callosum, and presence of brainstem abnormalities. Importantly, radiologic signs of increased ICP can be witnessed. The characteristic "thumbprinting" or "copper-beaten" patterns, when evident on 3D scan or the scout film, suggest raised cranial pressure *(Fig. 34.2)*. Similarly, 2D cuts can show loss of gyral folding and

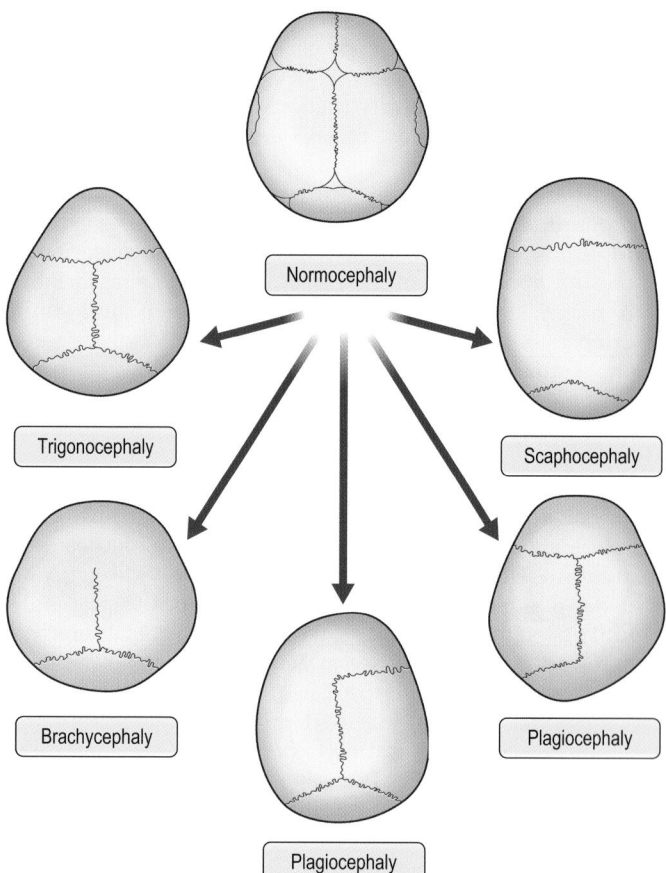

Fig. 34.1 Characteristic skull shape depending on sutural involvement in craniosynostosis.

Table 34.1 Cephalic index (CI), based on maximal cranial length and maximal cranial width: $CI = Wd/L \times 100$, where Wd is the maximal cranial width and L is the maximal cranial length

Cephalic index	Suggested diagnosis
<71	Hyperdolichocephalic
71–76	Dolichocephalic/scaphocephalic (as with sagittal)
76–81	Mesocephalic
81–81.5	Brachycephalic (as with bicoronal)
>85.5	Hyperbrachycephalic

(Reproduced from Bennaceur S, Petavy-Blanc AS, Chauve J, et al. Human cephalic morphology. Anthropometry. In: Laffont A, Durieuz F, eds, *Encyclopédie médicochirurgicale*. Elsevier; 2005:85–103).

blunted cisternae along the endocranial surface, consistent with the brain trying to expand against an immobile, restrictive cranial vault. The CT scan also may aid in surgical planning and serves as a baseline study to compare against postoperative changes.

Sagittal synostosis develops following fusion of the midline, sagittal suture *(Table 34.3)*. This results in a "boat-shaped" head (i.e., scaphocephaly) with an expanded anteroposterior dimension and a narrowed bitemporal distance. Cephalic index is consistent with dolichocephaly (<76). A sagittal ridge

Table 34.2 Differentiating synostotic from deformational plagiocephaly

	Flat forehead	Flat occiput	
	Unicoronal synostosis (UCS)	Unilateral lambdoid synostosis	Deformational plagiocephaly
Primary feature	Ipsilateral forehead retrusion	Ipsilateral occipital flatness	Ipsilateral occipital flatness
Compensatory changes	Contralateral forehead may be bossed	Ipsilateral mastoid bulge (canted skull base)	Ipsilateral forehead may be bossed
	No change in occiput	Ipsilateral forehead, no change or recessed	Contralateral forehead may be retruded
Ipsilateral ear position	Anterior and superior	Varied Posterior and inferior	Varied Anterior
Periorbital region	Ipsilateral Wide palpebral fissure Higher retruded supraorbital rim, brow Harlequin on X-ray	Usually unaffected in anatomic head position	Usually unaffected May have contralateral retrusion of fronto-orbital zygomatic region
Nasal radix	Deviated towards affected side	Midline in anatomic head position	Midline
Head shape from above	Ipsilateral forehead retrusion	Trapezoid	Parallelogram
Incidence	Rare	Very rare	Common

Table 34.3 Scaphocephaly

Suture fused	Features
Sagittal	Elongated anteroposterior head Frontal and occipital prominence Biparietal narrowness

may be appreciated on palpation. Fusion of the anterior sagittal suture contributes to significant frontal bossing. Similarly, an occipital bulge results from involvement of the posterior sagittal suture. Varying degrees of frontal or occipital prominence can occur depending on the extent and location of synostosis along the sagittal suture.

Plagiocephaly is a general term denoting an asymmetric coronal plane of the cranium. The twisted head shape is the result of unilateral coronal synostosis, unilateral lambdoid synostosis, or positional molding *(Table 34.2)*. Some object to the term "plagiocephaly" as anatomically imprecise. Referral by the affected suture is the preferred terminology, but the general phenotypic descriptor "plagiocephaly" is still often encountered.

UCS is termed "anterior plagiocephaly" *(Table 34.4)*. UCS demonstrates a flattened ipsilateral forehead and supraorbital rim, a raised eyebrow, and a widened palpebral opening on the affected side. The lateral orbital rim and ipsilateral temporal area also appear deficient. The root of the nose deviates toward the affected suture. The ear may be displaced anterior and superior on the side of coronal fusion. The contralateral forehead is often bossed, which is a compensatory change. The occipital region is usually unaffected and symmetric, which, along with the pathognomonic orbital changes, differentiates UCS from other causes of plagiocephaly. Facial asymmetry can occur, particularly if the UCS is left unchecked. When present, the chin deviates to the unaffected side secondary to changed position of the glenoid fossa.[63,69] The affected orbit is vertically taller and narrower than the contralateral side on frontal 3D CT. Intraorbitally, the ipsilateral steep superior orbital fissure and sphenoid wing is known as the harlequin deformity. Patency of the frontosphenoidal suture should also be investigated on CT scan as the disease process can continue to this terminal extension of the coronal suture. In rare cases, frontosphenoidal synostosis alone can result in morphology that mimics UCS.[70]

Bicoronal synostosis is symmetric, does not cause plagiocephaly, and is more likely to be either familial nonsyndromic or associated with a syndrome *(Table 34.5)*. Fusion of both coronal sutures results in brachycephaly (flat head), marked by increased biparietal diameter, and decreased anteroposterior diameter leading to a blunted forehead and supraorbital ridge. In certain cases, there can be a compensatory increase in parietal height causing turribrachycephaly (tall flat head).

Unilateral lambdoidal synostosis is a very rare cause of plagiocephaly ("posterior plagiocephaly") *(Table 34.6)*. It is characterized by a cant of the posterior skull base with occipital flatness on the affected side and an ipsilateral inferiorly displaced mastoid bulge. In some cases there is secondary

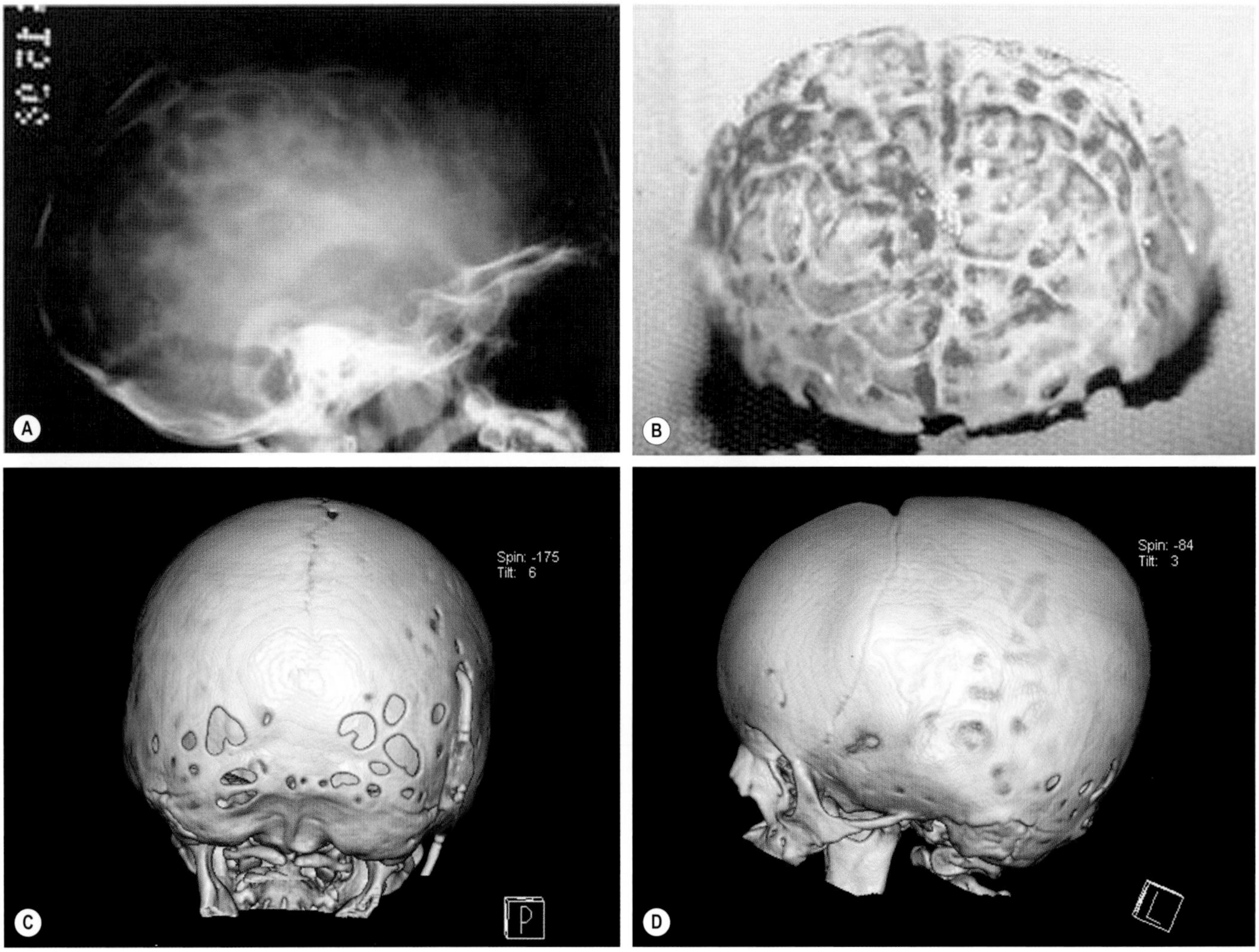

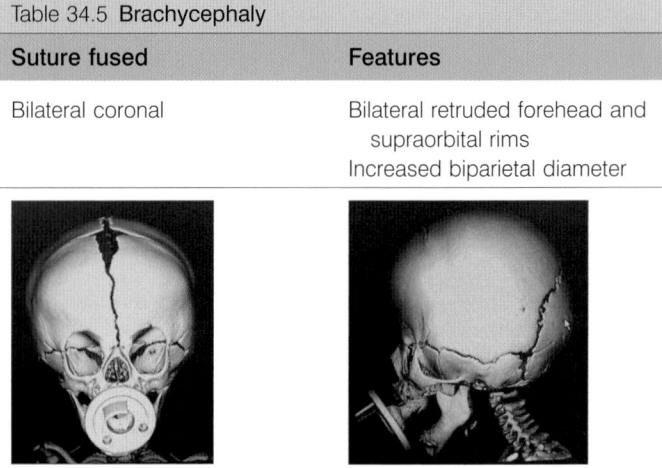

Fig. 34.2 Radiologic signs of increased cranial pressure – "thumbprinting." (Reproduced from Weinzweig J, Baker SB, Whitaker LA, et al. Delayed cranial vault reconstruction for sagittal synostosis in older children: an algorithm for tailoring the reconstructive approach to the craniofacial deformity. *Plast Reconstr Surg*. 2002;110:397–408.)

Table 34.4 Anterior plagiocephaly

Suture fused	Features
Unilateral coronal 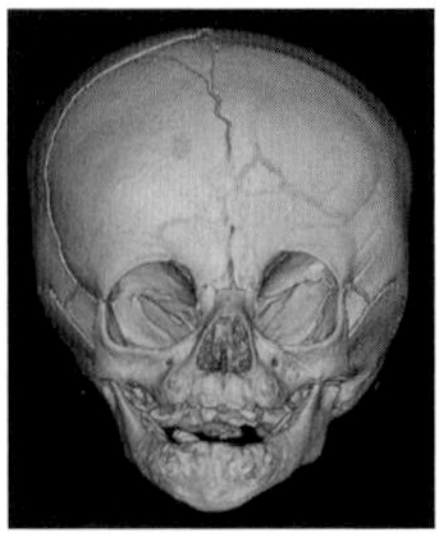	Ipsilateral Retruded forehead and supraorbital rim Raised eyebrow Widened palpebral fissure Radix deviates to affected ear anterior and superior Contralateral forehead bossed 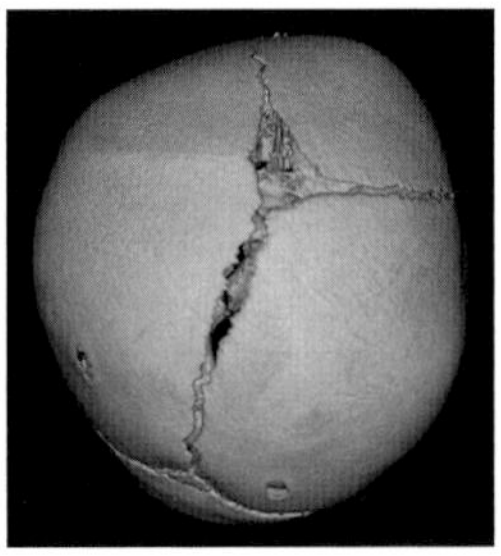

Table 34.5 Brachycephaly

Suture fused	Features
Bilateral coronal	Bilateral retruded forehead and supraorbital rims Increased biparietal diameter

Table 34.6 Posterior plagiocephaly

Suture fused	Features
Unilateral lambdoid	Ipsilateral occipital flatness Ipsilateral mastoid bulge Ear inferior

Table 34.7 Trigonocephaly

Suture fused	Features
Metopic	Keel-shaped forehead Bitemporal narrowing Hypotelorism

contralateral forehead prominence, providing an overall trapezoid head shape when viewed from above.[71] Clinically, the ipsilateral ear position is inferior, but quite varied in terms of anteroposterior placement. However, CT scan always shows the affected ear is closer to the anterior nasal spine.[72–74] CT also demonstrates deviation of the posterior cranial fossa toward the affected lambdoid suture, with a symmetric anterior fossa.

Trigonocephaly refers to the triangular-shaped head that occurs with early fusion of the metopic suture *(Table 34.7)*. The metopic suture ordinarily closes at 8 months of life.[75] The spectrum of severity can range from a metopic ridge alone to significant ridging with marked trigonocephaly. The features of metopic synostosis include a keel-shaped forehead, bitemporal narrowing, parietal expansion, supraorbital and lateral orbital retrusion, and hypotelorism. Metopic synostosis is most apt to be associated with midline brain aberrations and one report suggests a higher than usual concomitant presentation of Chiari I malformation.[76]

Patient selection

Infants with a confirmed diagnosis of craniosynostosis should be evaluated by a multidisciplinary team. Genetics input is essential to rule out an associated syndrome, especially in cases of bicoronal synostosis. Additionally, laboratory testing for TWIST and FGFR3 gene mutations may be warranted in familial instances of single-suture synostoses or in those cases with suggestive phenotypic features. The neurosurgeon is an intraoperative participant in the care of these patients and preoperatively evaluates the status of the brain parenchyma and associated abnormalities (e.g., hydrocephalus, Chiari malformation). A neuro-ophthalmologist examines the optic disc for papilledema, and can investigate red color saturation and visual evoked potentials, as well as ophthalmoplegia and strabismus. Other critical craniofacial team members include the psychologist and audiologist.

The decision to operate depends on appearance and functional concerns. Cases of mild deformity with partial fusion, without clinical evidence of intracranial hypertension or developmental delays, can be managed by observation. More significant dysmorphology, especially with the suggestion of increased brain pressure, should be treated operatively. The treatment goals in craniosynostosis are: (1) release the fused sutures to allow for brain growth and development; (2) normalize the head and forehead shape; and (3) mitigate functional issues (e.g., intracranial hypertension and developmental delay, optic disc atrophy, and strabismus).

The parents should be given a realistic appraisal of the benefits of surgery from both an appearance and functional vantage point. Parents should be counseled that a tendency toward recurrence of the synostotic morphology may occur, secondary to diminished growth in the region, and, as a result, the child's deformity will be operatively overcorrected. Additionally, secondary deformities (e.g., temporal hollowing), also from lack of growth, may pose an aesthetic concern to the child several years postoperatively, requiring secondary extracranial intervention. Rarely, repeat intracranial procedures may be required.

The principal functional concerns relate to ICP elevation which can lead to neurologic impairment (e.g., developmental delay, visual loss). Treatment of the synostotic cranium is intended to avoid such potential brain malfunction related to increased ICP.[77] This raises the question of the utility of preoperative ICP monitoring. In cases where the parents are committed to surgical correction of the child and/or in the presence of papilledema or other suggestive symptoms or signs of intracranial hypertension, subjecting the infant to formal ICP monitoring is not warranted. However, when parents are uncertain if they wish to pursue operative treatment, despite moderate to severe dysmorphology, and when clinical or radiologic (e.g., "copper-beaten" or "thumbprinting" on 3D CT) indicators of intracranial hypertension are lacking, ICP monitoring could be considered. If ICP is shown to be elevated on lumbar puncture or intracranial monitoring in such children, this provides impetus to proceed with operative correction. It is clear that the presence of papilledema represents only a fraction of the cases of true intracranial hypertension.[78,79] However, the invasiveness of ICP testing should be weighed against its utility in operative decision making. Realistic expectations with regard to correction or prevention of developmental delay should be articulated to the parents, as such a result obviously cannot be guaranteed.

The optimal timing of treatment is during infancy, between 6 and 9 months.[49,77,80] This is to harness the force of the rapidly growing brain, allowing brain expansion to influence the newly unrestricted calvarial plates. Additionally, the cranial bone in this age group remains malleable and easy to mold and shape, and bony defects, created during calvarial repositioning, are more apt to reossify completely. The infant is also more prepared to endure the anesthetic risk and the hematopoietic nadir has passed by 6 months. Additionally, intervention during this time may result in normalization of the cranial base.[52,81] Delay in surgery after 1 year of life is not advocated as it may result in further progression of the dysmporhology, possible secondary compensatory aberrations (including asymmetry of the facial skeleton), and development of neuropsychiatric problems.[82] However, some have claimed that surgical delay until after 12 months may carry the benefit of reduced need for secondary revision.[83] Proponents of endoscopic techniques prefer intervention even earlier than 6 months, to take further advantage of brain doubling size.

Treatment/surgical technique

Preparation

Cranial vault remodeling procedures are best performed in a pediatric hospital or surgical suite with a pediatric intensive care unit (ICU) and a pediatric anesthesia team. An anesthesia team comfortable with the pediatric airway and hemodynamic function is critical. Traditionally the chief cause of mortality with cranial vault remodeling was related to blood loss. This has lessened with appropriate recognition and maneuvers by both the surgical and anesthesia teams. The rare, but present, risk of air embolism is assessed by cardiopulmonary status and end-tidal CO_2 recordings. Invasive hemodynamic monitoring (arterial line) is required and typically central venous access is obtained prior to initiating the procedure. Cross-matched blood and fresh frozen plasma should be available in the room at the start of the case.

The anesthesia team should diligently follow hemodynamic parameters and hemoglobin levels throughout the case, with low threshold for transfusion. Systemic administration of antifibrinolytics (e.g., aprotinin or aminocaproic acid) may be beneficial in reducing blood loss and is an ongoing study at our center.[84–86] Blood loss is a continual process occurring from the expansive surface area created by the scalp flap, calvarial plates, and dura. In rare instances, acute significant blood loss can occur and, when present, is most frequently related to dural sinus tears in the setting of repeat operation with osseous-dural adhesions. Placement of so-called blocking stitches (running interlocking 2-0 Prolene) on either side of the planned coronal incision and injection of vasoconstrictors (e.g., epinephrine–kenalog mixture) along the incision and planned area of dissection help minimize bleeding from the scalp flap. Blocking sutures are preferred to Rainey clips for the possible reduced incidence of alopecia.[87] Similarly, needle point electrocautery is ill advised along the incision because of damage to follicles leaving a wider, hairless scar.[88] However, electrocautery is utilized in those cases where epinephrine is contraindicated (e.g., long QT syndrome). Supraperiosteal dissection along the cranium and subperiosteal dissection

intraorbitally also diminish blood loss. Vigilant hemostatic control of oozing surfaces by use of bone wax, electrocautery, and bipolar, as indicated, should also be performed.

The child is typically positioned supine for abnormalities involving the frontal region. Occipital dysmorphology is better approached from a prone position. A modified prone position ("sphinx") may be required for simultaneous anterior and posterior cranial vault remodeling. The authors prefer a staged approach in such cases if possible, to minimize blood loss, and to give more complete access to a single anatomic site (and therefore a more complete correction), rather than a somewhat limited access to two anatomic areas.

A coronal incision is required for most cranial vault remodeling procedures. The incision should be placed from ear to ear, overlying the vertex, and attention paid to potential future procedures or presence of existing incisions (e.g., ventricular shunt). The design can be a straight line or zigzag. The scar is most noticeable in the temporal region and a zigzag pattern is preferred at least in this location, and is often continued along the entire length of incision.[89] The knife blade should be beveled anteriorly to preserve viable hair follicles, allowing growth through the scar (i.e., trichophytic closure). If an endoscopic approach is pursued, this typically requires two shorter incisions, one posterior and anterior.[90] Occasionally an upper-eyelid incision is needed in endoscopic techniques to address the orbital rim position.[91]

The choice of operation depends on the specific suture fused and the degree of dysmorphology. In general, the technical surgical goals entail: releasing the area of sutural fusion, repositioning the bone in an anatomic but overcorrected location, eliminating secondary compensatory changes, filling in osteotomy gaps with bone dust slurry, and closing the soft tissue relatively tension-free. Open cranial vault remodeling provides necessary access and freedom to accomplish these goals. Comprehensive, open techniques are preferred to treat craniosynostosis with increasing severity of the deformity. The limited approaches (e.g., endoscopic or linear craniectomy) may be applicable for milder skull deformities, certainly not involving more than a single suture, in younger patients (<3–6 months).[4] These limited or endoscopic approaches do not reposition hypoplastic bony segments, but rather rely on the expanding brain, alone or coupled with helmet therapy, to correct the skull deformity.[90] The frontal region must be addressed in metopic and coronal synostoses and most effectively done in a full-access manner.

Stabilization of repositioned bone segments is best performed with sutures, wires, or resorbable plates and screws. The objective is to create a stable construct but not to restrict brain growth and subsequent skull expansion. Titanium or metallic plates are not utilized in infants undergoing cranial remodeling for fear of transcranial migration with subsequent growth.[92–96] Free-floating forehead techniques have been attempted in the past, but, without stability, a permanent deformity may result.[97] Obviously, limited or endoscopic techniques do not utilize fixation, as they involve strip suturectomies and/or barrel staves only.

Sagittal synostosis

There are many options for treating sagittal suture fusion. In the neonatal period, when the anteroposterior deformity may be mild, a simple strip craniectomy (sagittal synostectomy),

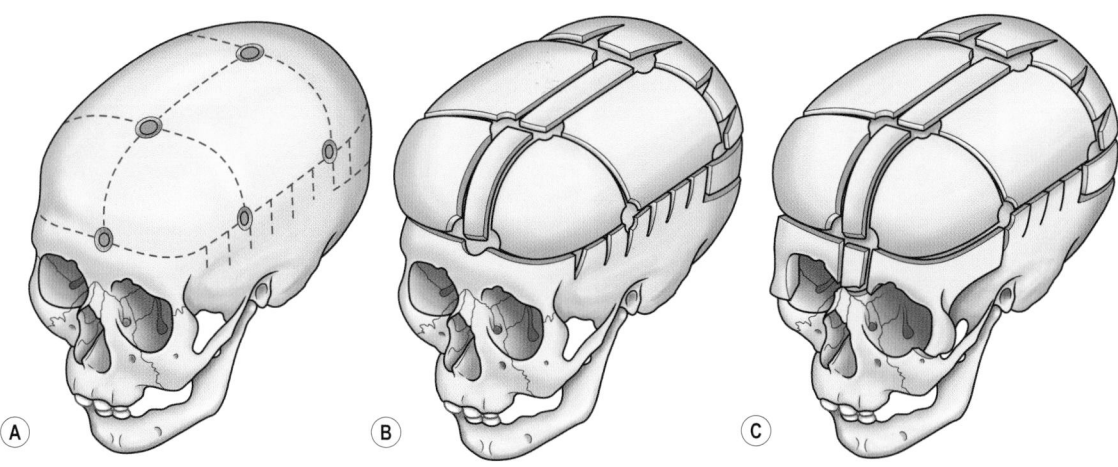

Fig. 34.3 (A–C) Total vault expansion for sagittal synostosis. (Reproduced from Weinzweig J, Baker SB, Whitaker LA, et al. Delayed cranial vault reconstruction for sagittal synostosis in older children: an algorithm for tailoring the reconstructive approach to the craniofacial deformity. *Plast Reconstr Surg*. 2002;110:397–408.)

or variation thereof, may be performed. This can be done by either an open or an endoscopic approach. The space created between parietal bones at the vertex may allow the head shape to normalize with brain growth (the fronto-occipital distance shortens and the biparietal distance expands).[63] However, a semblance of frontal bossing or occipital prominence can persist over time. Additionally, the medial border of the parietal bones, at the site of the suturectomy, can refuse with recurrence and progression of scaphocephaly noted. This is not an attractive surgical option for infants older than 6 months because: (1) it does not adequately correct the scaphocephaly; and (2) permanent osseous defects can result along the vertex.

The endoscopic approach for treatment of craniosynostosis was introduced by Jimenez and Barone.[90] The original cohort included 4 infants all under 3 months of age, with a follow-up period for approximately 1 year. The technique described includes a strip craniectomy with lateral barrel staves. A crucial component of this approach is use of the molding helmet postoperatively. Early results were successful gauging by aesthetic criteria. Additional practitioners have reported on using endoscopic access for treatment of sagittal synostosis, with various modifications.[98] It has been demonstrated that, in infants younger than 3–6 months of age, treatment of sagittal synostosis by suturectomy and parasagittal osteotomies can be effective.

If the dysmorphology is more significant, but still minimal frontal prominence, the "pi" procedure can be performed. The pi procedure was first described in 1978 by Jane *et al.* and produces immediate correction of the fronto-occipital length and biparietal width.[99] Technically, it involves two parallel parasagittal ostectomies of the two parietal bones, connected with a transverse ostectomy, located behind the coronal suture and extending to the temporal region (resembling the Greek symbol for pi). The dura is dissected free from the endocranial surface of the frontal bone and the remaining fused sagittal suture, to prevent buckling when reapproximating new bone edges. Displacing the frontal bone posteriorly results in bulging of the brain laterally. These two movements are key to improving the morphology of scaphocephaly. Though probably not more effective than strip craniectomy during the

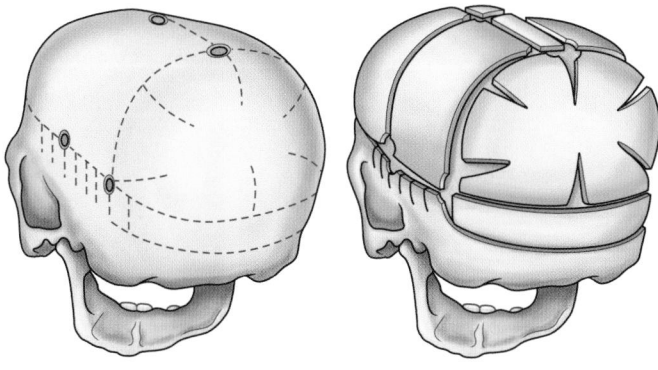

Fig. 34.4 Occipital repositioning as part of total vault remodeling in sagittal synostosis. (Reproduced from Weinzweig J, Baker SB, Whitaker LA, et al. Delayed cranial vault reconstruction for sagittal synostosis in older children: an algorithm for tailoring the reconstructive approach to the craniofacial deformity. *Plast Reconstr Surg*. 2002;110:397–408.)

neonatal period, the pi procedure offers the advantage of immediate aesthetic correction of head shape and improved efficacy in older infants (e.g., 8 months).

Moderate to severe scaphocephaly is best corrected by total cranial vault reconstruction, as the more limited techniques described will not adequately correct the dysmorphology[100–102] *(Fig. 34.3)*. This is best done between 6 and 9 months and entails excision of the frontal, parietal, and occipital bone plates, which are molded, reshaped, and repositioned *(Fig. 34.4)*. The occipital region is advanced forward and the frontal prominence retropositioned *(Fig. 34.5)*. When performed in children older than 2 years, few, if any, calvarial defects are left because they are less apt to reossify.[102]

Unicoronal synostosis

The primary treatment goal in UCS involves alleviating the fronto-orbital asymmetry. This entails advancing the supraorbital and lateral orbital rims, reducing the height of the ipsilateral orbit, advancing the ipsilateral frontal bar, and

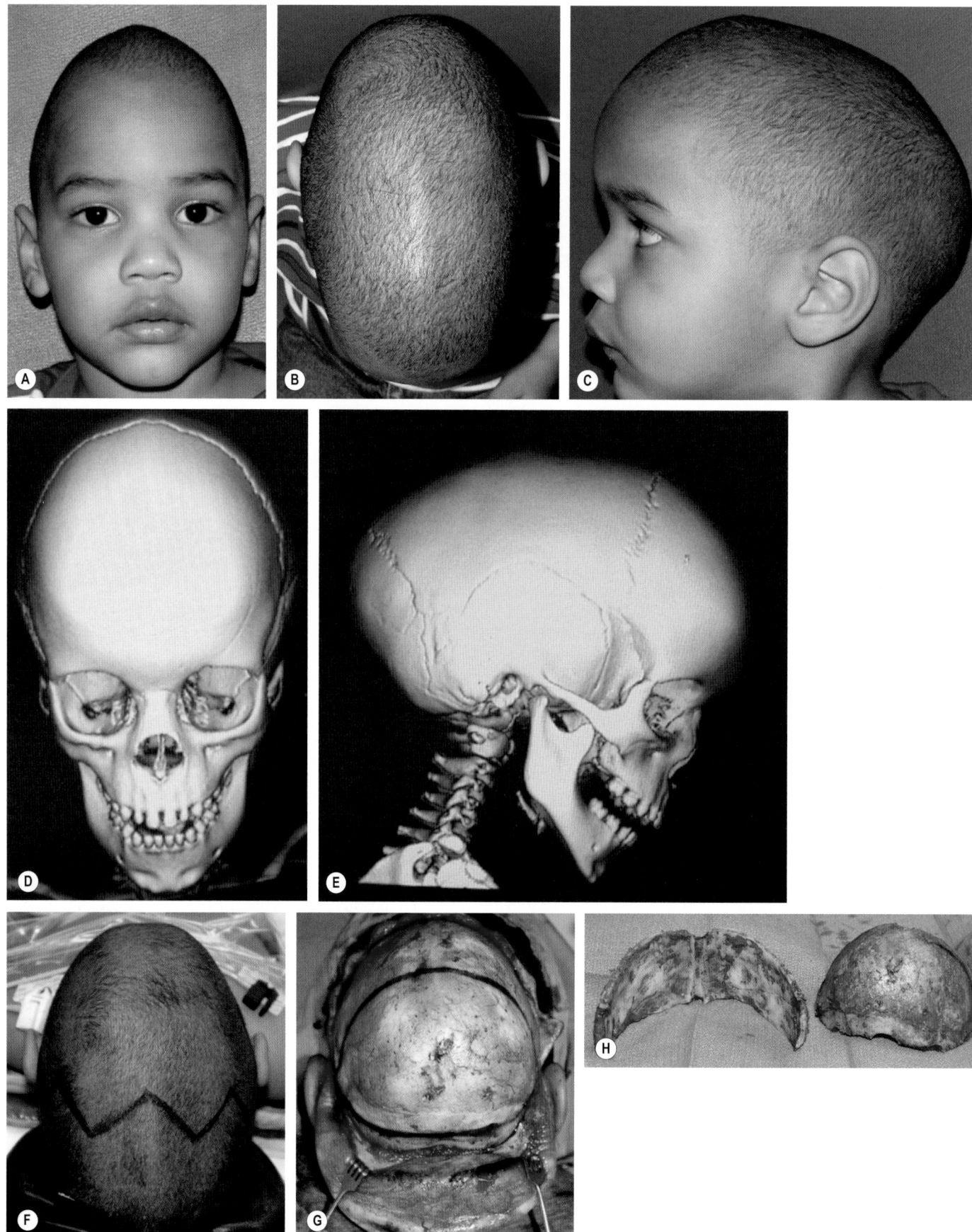

Fig. 34.5 Treatment of sagittal synostosis. **(A–C)** Preoperative photographs. **(D, E)** Preoperative computed tomography (CT) scans. **(F–J)** Intraoperative posterior vault reshaping. **(K–O)** Intraoperative frontoparietal reshaping. **(P–R)** Postoperative CT scans. **(S–U)** Postoperative head shapes.

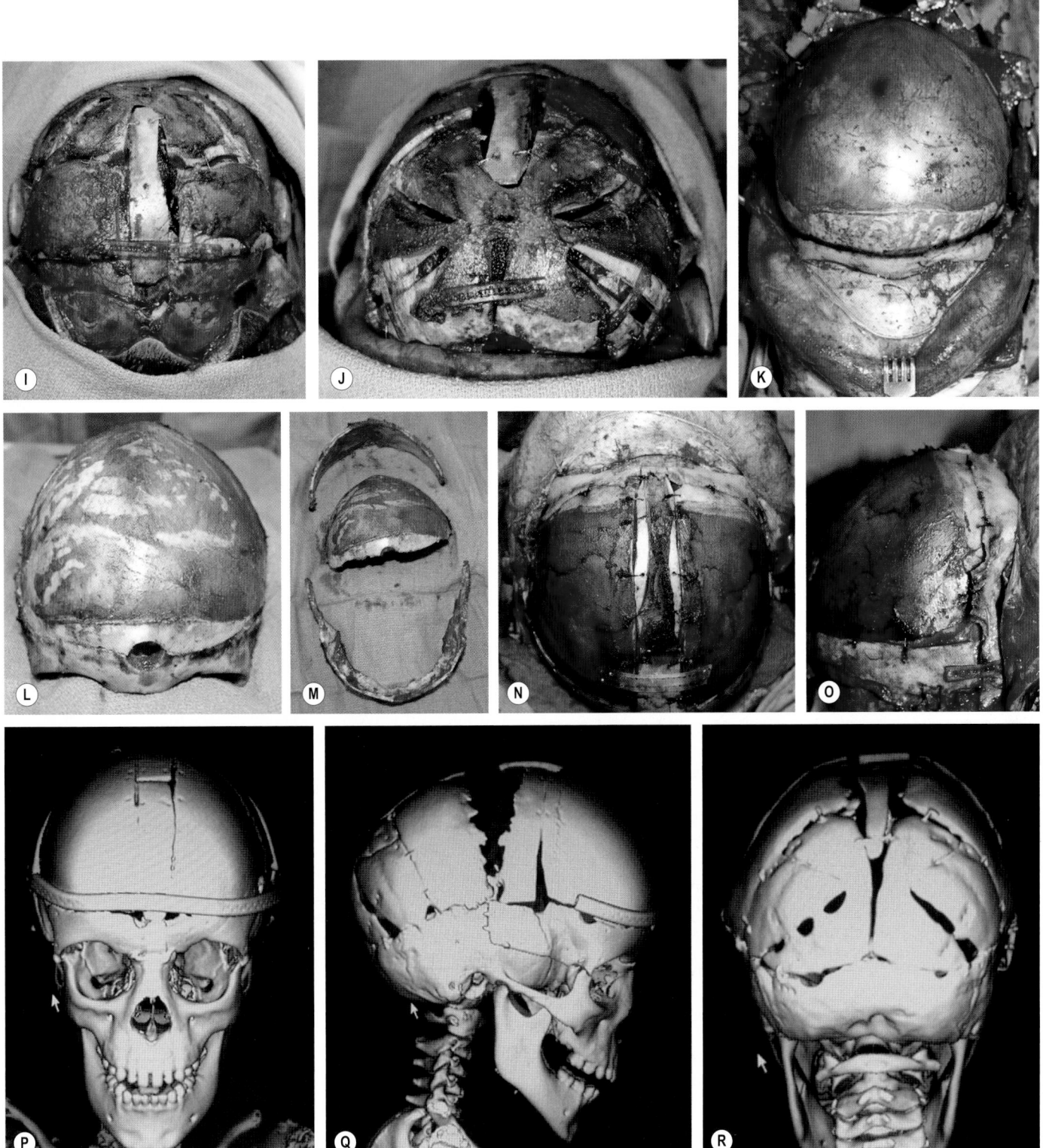

Fig. 34.5, cont'd

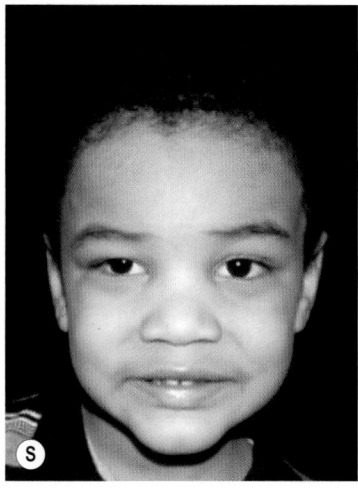
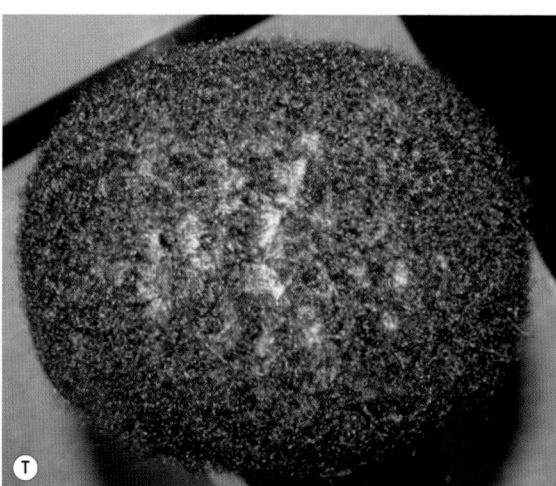
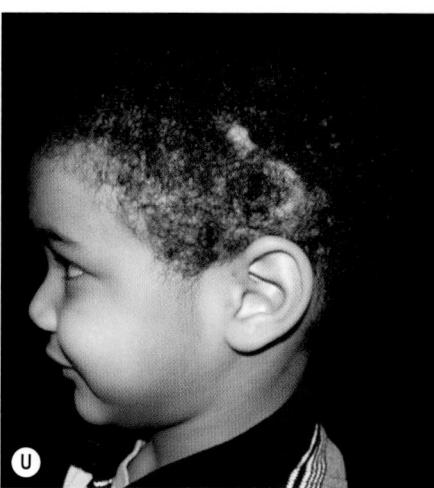

Fig. 34.5, cont'd

diminishing the contralateral compensatory forehead bulge, if present. These are complex movements not readily amenable to simple conservative techniques. However, treatment in early infancy by suturectomy followed by helmet therapy has been proposed.[103–105] Jimenez and Barone[104] reported on 50 patients, mean age 3.5 months, who underwent an endoscopic unicoronal synostectomy followed by approximately 12 months of postoperative molding. The authors conclude that this technique proved effective in 43% of cases. No mention is made regarding additional treatments required in those cases that were not effective.[104] Other attempts at limited craniectomies through small incisions have been reported.[106] The advantages of less blood loss, shorter operative time, and earlier discharge from the hospital are laudable goals, but this should be weighed against providing the most complete and durable correction of the dysmorphology. Further study is warranted for endoscopic, limited approaches to the coronal suture. As of now these techniques are not effective in all cases of UCS, and certainly should not be entertained in infants older than 6 months.

The most effective and comprehensive approach to correct the complex craniofacial changes associated with UCS, particularly in older infants and those with more significant dysmorphology, is forehead reshaping and fronto-orbital advancement. A bifrontal or unifrontal advancement may be performed, depending on the severity of the deformity.[107] A bilateral craniotomy is typically necessary coupled with advancement of the ipsilateral or bilateral supraorbital band *(Fig. 34.6)*. The objective of the fronto-orbital advancement is to position the supraorbital rim 12–13 mm anterior to the cornea. An 8–15-mm magnitude of bandeau advancement is usually required on the affected side. There are several techniques and modifications attributed to the fronto-orbital advancement, depending on the correction sought and the severity of the deformity.[108–111] Simultaneous to repositioning the orbital rim, the ipsilateral forehead is advanced, the orbital height may be reduced, and the contralateral forehead is recessed or contoured as necessary *(Fig. 34.7)*. One described technique involves discarding the abnormal supraorbital bar and replacing it with reshaped frontal bone from the contralateral side.[112] We prefer unilateral or differential bilateral frontal bandeau advancement with

reshaping of the contralateral forehead compensations. A canthopexy may be performed to lower the affected side lateral canthus if an upward slant is present. Some advocate including the nasal bones in continuity with the frontal bar and uprighting the nasal radix deviation by closing wedge osteotomy.[113] Others feel the nasal root deviance corrects by adolescence with the lack of continued "pull" toward the fused suture.[114]

Bicoronal synostosis

Correcting bilateral forehead and supraorbital rim width and retrusion (brachycephaly) is necessary to normalize frontofacial balance and to afford orbital protection. An early approach to this was the floating forehead, where no fixation was performed and subsequent brain growth was intended to expand the forehead anteriorly.[115] This has fallen out of favor, giving way to techniques that precisely position the bone segments and employ fixation for a stable construct. Current techniques involve a bifrontal craniotomy and creation of a bilateral frontal bandeau *(Fig. 34.6)*. The anterior dimension is advanced, creating greater forehead prominence, and the supraorbital rim is positioned 2–3 mm ahead of the corneal zenith. The width is narrowed by creating a midline endocranial flexion or a median ostectomy of the repositioned frontal bones. In bicoronal synostosis the height of the skull may also be increased (turribrachycephaly). This can be addressed by barrel staves and greenstick fracture of the posterior parietal bones or occipital plates.

Metopic synostosis

The primary objective in surgically correcting metopic synostosis involves anterior cranial vault expansion, thereby alleviating the bitemporal constriction and triangular head appearance.[63] The intent is to round the forehead shape and also to improve hypotelorism. An endoscopic strip craniectomy procedure has been reported as an attempted treatment. This technique may have some utility in young infants, but, as with UCS, it is not effective in all patients and not appropriate for older infants. In their same series with UCS, Jimenez

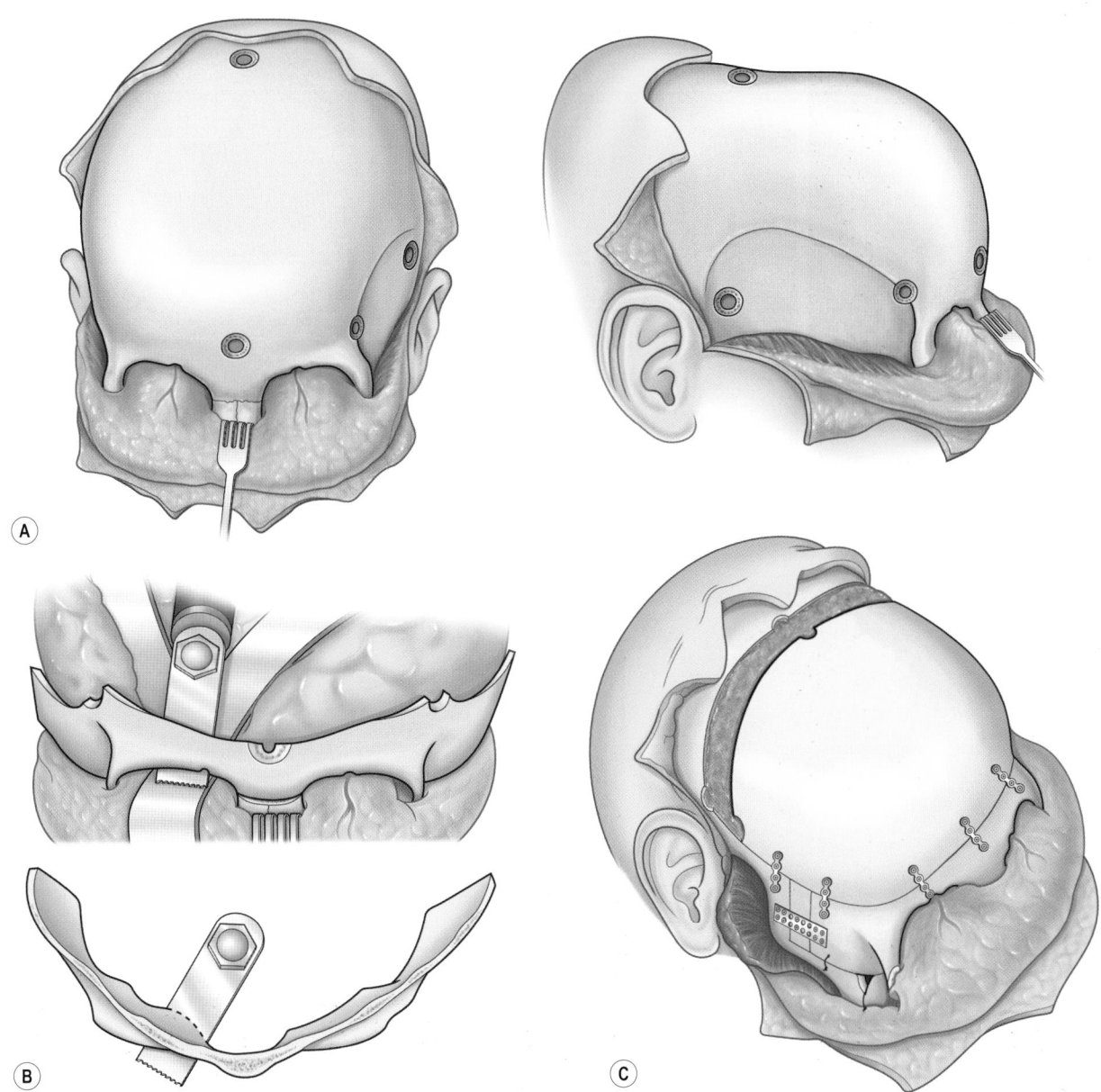

Fig. 34.6 Fronto-orbital advancement. **(A)** Exposure, craniotomy, and frontal bandeau lines. **(B)** Creating the bandeau. **(C)** Completed fronto-orbital advancement. (Redrawn from an illustration by Dr. David Low.)

and Barone reported on 50 infants with metopic synostosis treated in this fashion, also shown to be 43% effective.[104]

Several more comprehensive techniques have been described in an attempt to correct the morphologic sequelae seen in metopic synostosis.[97,115–121] Selber *et al.* reviewed the refinement in technical approach to fronto-orbital reconstruction in metopic infants over a 30-year period. The current iteration entails splitting the fronto-orbital bar in the midline and interposing a bone segment to increase the bitemporal and interorbital distance *(Figs 34.8 and 34.9)*. The new construct exhibits a more obtuse endocranial angle, witnessed by advancement and expansion of the lateral rims and temporal region. This bandeau is then held in place by sutures at the zygomaticofrontal region and temporally with resorbable plates. An intervening bone graft is often utilized at the temporal gap created from the advancement of the fronto-orbital

construct. The goal is to overcorrect the hypoplastic bone segments, especially the temporal and lateral orbital regions, which are most prone to regress toward the original deformity (secondary to impaired growth potential).

Lambdoid synostosis

Lambdoid synostosis is rare and the literature on surgical treatment has previously been clouded by the diagnostic confusion with positional plagiocephaly. Endoscopic strip craniectomies and molding therapy have been advocated by some in young infants, with evaluation at long-term follow-up still ongoing.[122] In cases of limited occipital flattening, an open broad synostectomy with barrel staves and outfracture of the ipsilateral occipital bone may be successful. The corrected occipital area requires a minimum of semirigid fixation, as the

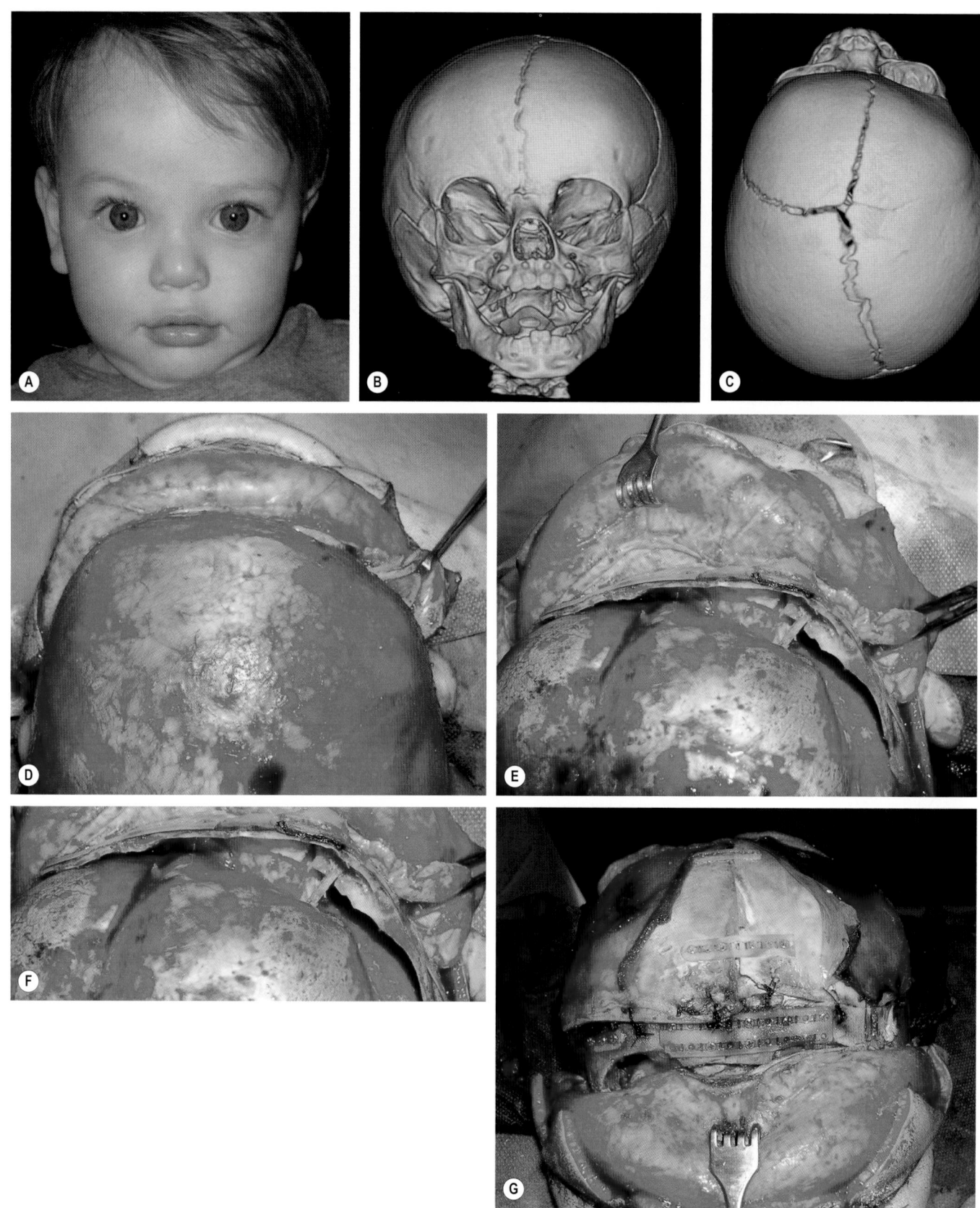

Fig. 34.7 Treatment of right unicoronal synostosis. **(A)** Preoperative frontal photograph. **(B, C)** Preoperative computed tomography (CT) scans. **(D)** Intraoperative: craniotomy and hemi-bandeau. **(E, F)** Intraoperative: bandeau positioning and overcorrection. **(G)** Intraoperative: fixation with resorbable plates.

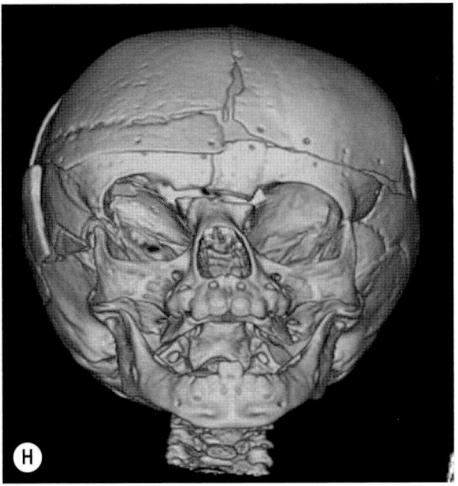

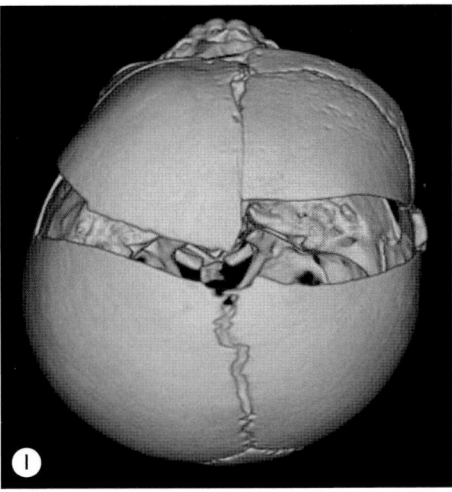

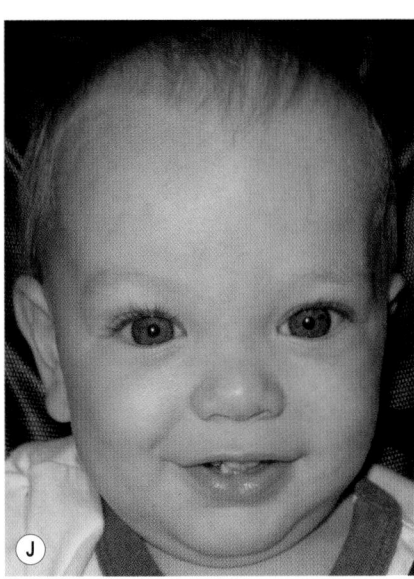

Fig. 34.7, cont'd (H, I) Postoperative CT. (J) Postoperative photographs.

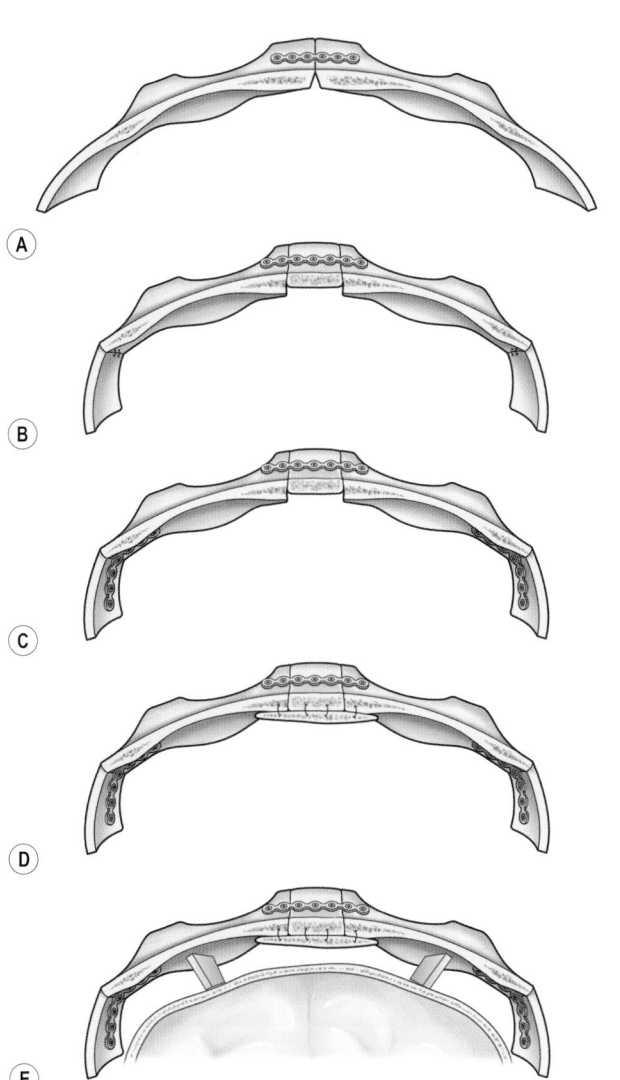

Fig. 34.8 (A–E) Variations of the frontal bandeau in metopic synostosis.

child will have the tendency to lie supine, resulting in relapse or restitution of the original defect in the presence of an unstable construct. Older infants and children with more severe dysmorphology require treatment by skull vault remodeling. We recommend a switch cranioplasty with occipital bar advancement.[123] The posterior vault bone flap is hemisected, and each half is transposed to the opposite side and rotated 90–180° to achieve best fit. These are fixed anteriorly with resorbable plates and bone gaps are filled with graft fragments or a bone dust–fibrin mixture *(Fig. 34.10)*.

Springs

A relatively new adjunct used in the treatment of single suture synostosis entails slow active bone movement aided by springs.[124] The concept is similar to gradual distraction but is not immediately controllable and the forces imparted are unequal along the length of the spring arm. This was first shown to be experimentally effective in rabbits by Persing *et al.*[125] This technique was popularized in clinical practice by Lauritzen *et al.*, where spring-assisted expansion was first utilized in a turricephalic infant and in a child with Apert syndrome.[124] Lauritzen *et al.* have since reported the utility of springs in over 100 clinical cases involving sagittal, metopic, biroconal, and multisuture synostoses[126] *(Fig. 34.11)*. Important treatment parameters include using this technique in children younger than 6 months (3 months or sooner is preferable), and recognizing that the amount of bony transposition imparted by the spring is typically 6 cm or less.[127] As the closed spring is permitted to open, a force of 7–10 N is created, but this can vary depending on the type of spring.[127] Experimental models have demonstrated increased bony thickness adjacent to the springs and that growth vector modification may occur in perimeter sutures.[128,129] Concerns for transmigration or erosion of the spring arm through the bone have been substantiated in animal models, but this occurs simultaneously with the bone plate movement and may have little clinical consequence.[127]

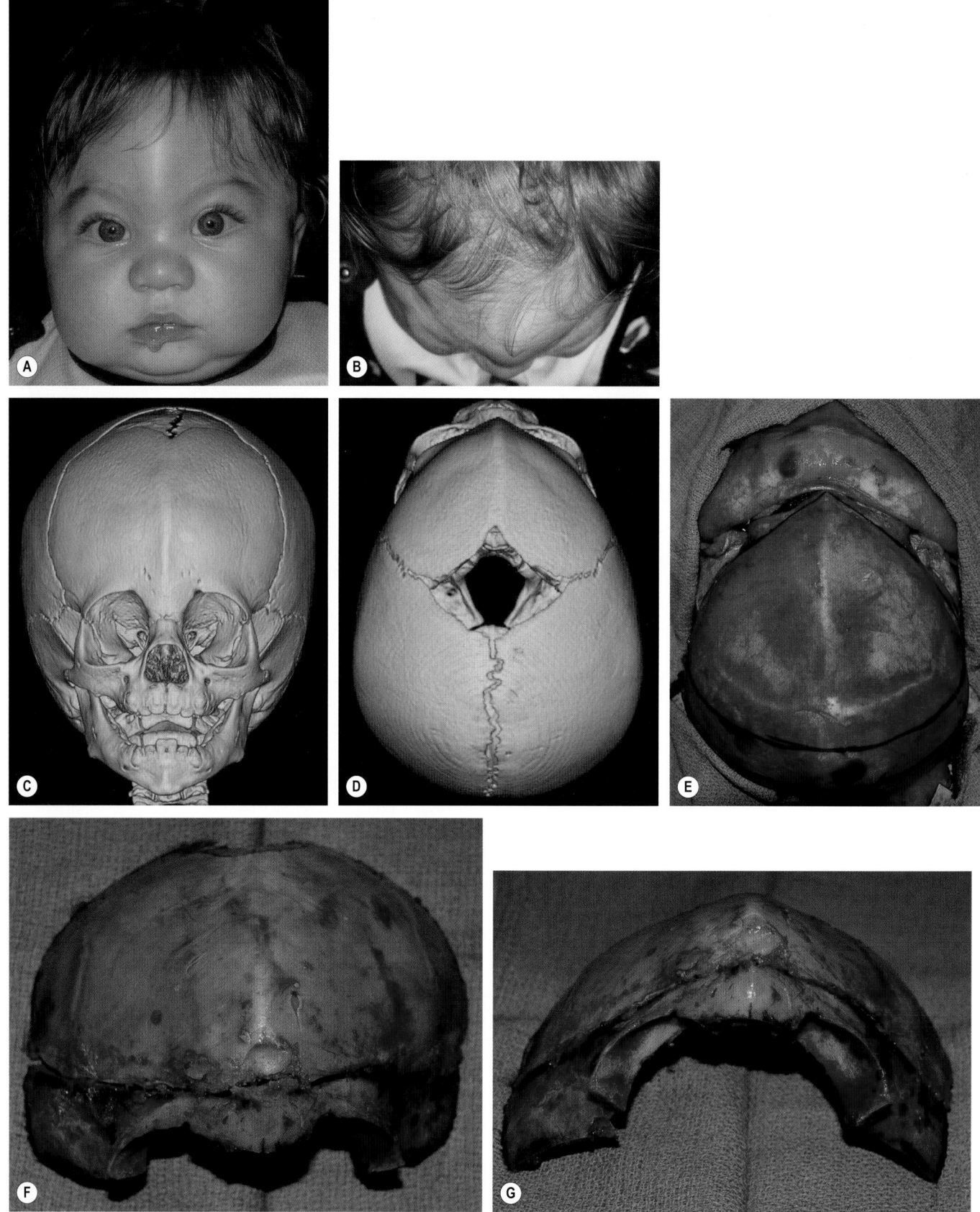

Fig. 34.9 Treatment of metopic synostosis. **(A, B)** Preoperative photographs. **(C, D)** Preoperative computed tomography (CT) scans. **(E–G)** Intraoperative.

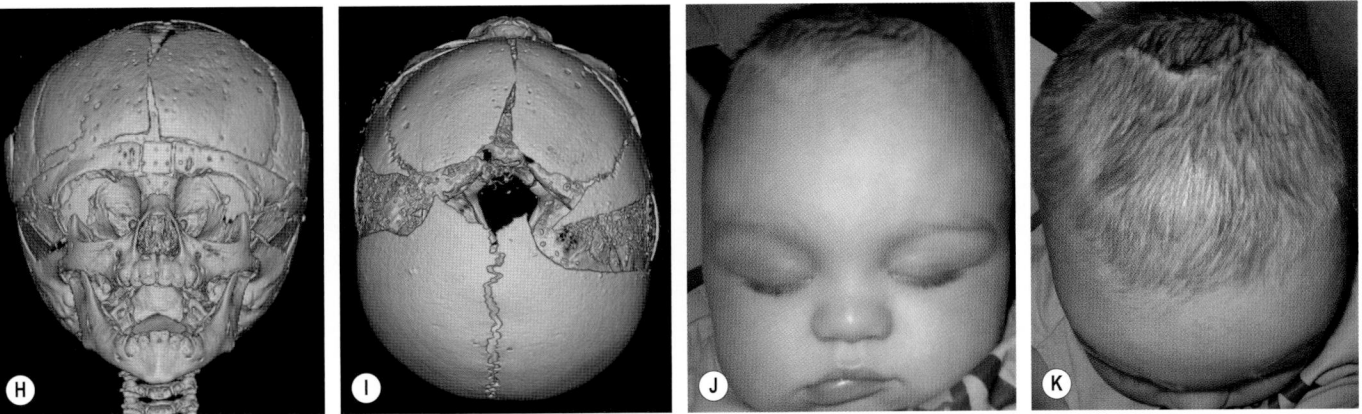

Fig. 34.9, cont'd (H, I) Postoperative CT scans. **(J, K)** Postoperative photographs.

The spring device is most widely reported for treatment of sagittal synostosis.[126,130] The concept of the strip craniectomy allowing brain growth to remodel the vault shape is furthered by imparting the active gradual force of the closed spring. Intuitively, the spring force required in a younger infant is less, compared with an older infant with thicker bone.[130] Both a single and paired springs have been reported as effective when placed along the sagittal suture. Biparietal widening is promoted, and, as mentioned, is more effective in younger infants, but does not readily address any significant antero-posterior elongation. The lazy-S sagittal incision provides easy access, but is not ideal if anterior or posterior vault reshaping is required at a later time.[126,130] Maltese et al. suggest springs are useful in the treatment of metopic synostosis as well. They note that hypotelorism can be corrected and have made the modification of outfracturing the frontotemporal segments to address bitemporal constriction (this element is not effectively changed by placement of a spring along the metopic suture).[131] Cases of bicoronal synostosis and multisutural synostosis have been reported and shown to be effective in selected cases.[126]

A few minor complications have been noted, most often related to spring dislodgment. Modifications in spring foot-plate design have been implemented to help reduce this issue. Additionally, springs should be placed such that, if they do dislodge, they do not end up intraorbitally or intracranially. Reasons cited for reluctance of spring techniques include unpredictability, or lack of control, and requirement for a second operation to remove the spring. Advantages over complete vault remodeling include diminished operative morbidity (less significant dissection and bone manipulation) and minimal immediate tension on the soft-tissue closure. Clearly, for older children, asymmetric stenoses, and cases of more severe dysmorphology, spring expansion techniques are of limited utility.

Distraction

Distraction osteogenesis is another technique to reposition cranial vault bones gradually while encouraging intervening bone fill between segments. Its use and benefits for simultaneous movement of the midface and frontal region (monobloc) have been championed for well over a decade.[132] The applicability for treatment of single-suture synostoses is a logical foray. Barone et al. demonstrated the effectiveness of distraction in the rabbit cranial vault, experimentally, and commented on the dense bone regenerated between distracted edges.[133] Hirabayashi et al. first reported the clinical use of distraction for fronto-orbital advancement in an infant with brachycephaly.[134] A multitude of examples have since been reported, including for single suture involvement, multi-suture synostosis, and both syndromic and nonsyndromic children.[135–139] The published cases have principally involved the treatment of fronto-orbital deformities and biparietal narrowness. Posterior (occipital) distraction is an area undergoing current investigation.[140] To date, reported cases of vault remodeling utilizing distraction have not objectively evaluated the aesthetic outcome. One author stated subjectively that "good cosmetic results were achieved" when distraction was used for a single case of bicoronal synostosis.[134] Another report, comparing conventional remodeling with distraction, claimed "more satisfactory skull shaping control" was achieved when the distraction technique was employed.[135] However, improvement of appearance is not even mentioned in the majority of reports.[137–139] Rather, the major focus in the literature has been on the feasibility, technical specifics, stability, magnitude of advancement, and complications.

In contradistinction to the spring modality, distraction is best reserved for children at least 6 months of age. Younger infants have poorer-quality bone with less reliable screw retention. Additionally, the thin caliber of the bone can result in screws penetrating intracranially. As children get older the bone thickness and quality improve. As a result, it is not surprising that the effectiveness of distraction has been demonstrated in school-aged children with various cranial vault abnormalities.[138]

The types of distractor used are typically those fabricated for the mandibular skeleton and adapted to fit the cranial skeleton. It is reported that internal distractors are better tolerated by patients, whereas external devices are easier to place by the surgeon.[141] However, most major centers have altogether abandoned use of external distractors for any application, as internal-buried distractors are less bulky, more readily tolerated by the patient, less prone to hardware site infections, and do not create pin tract scars. The number of distractors required for effective vault movement is an area of debate.

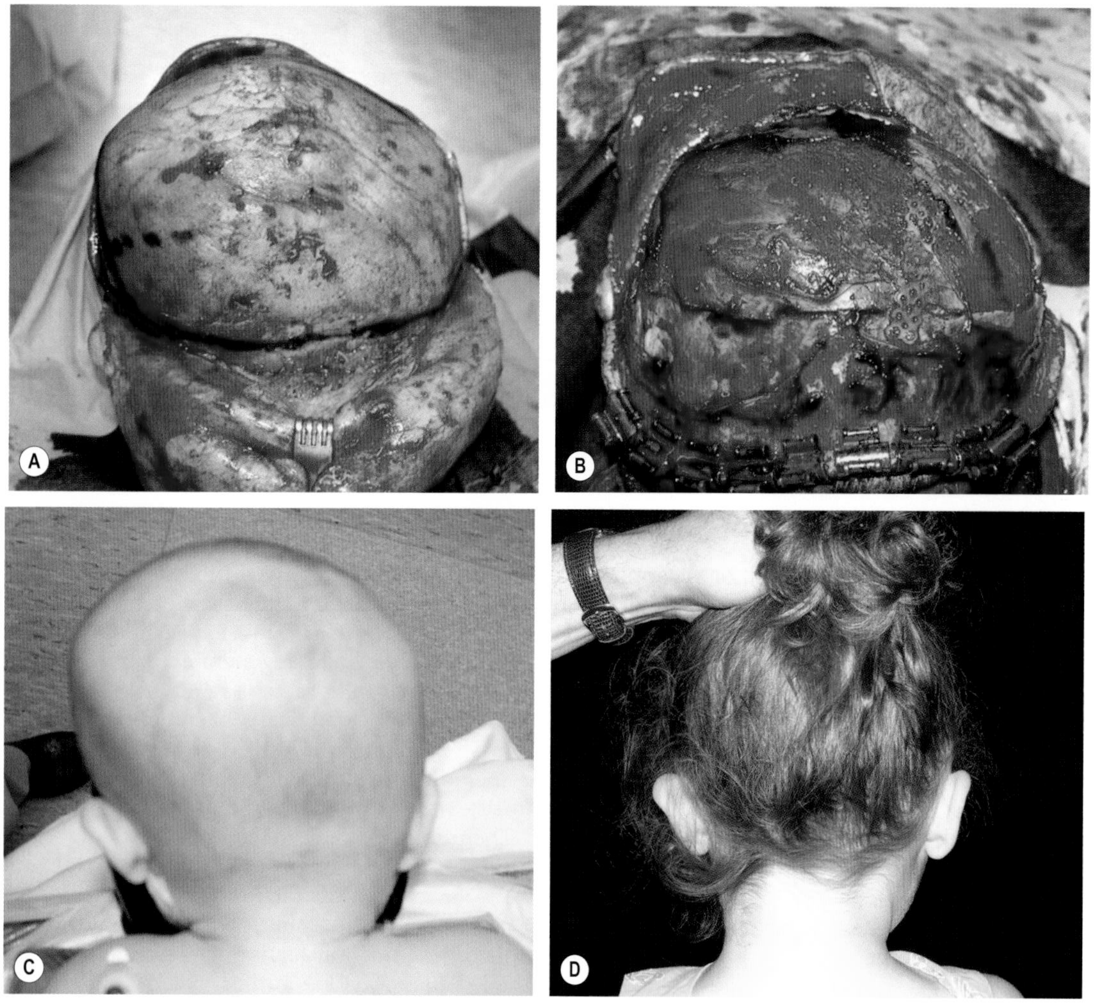

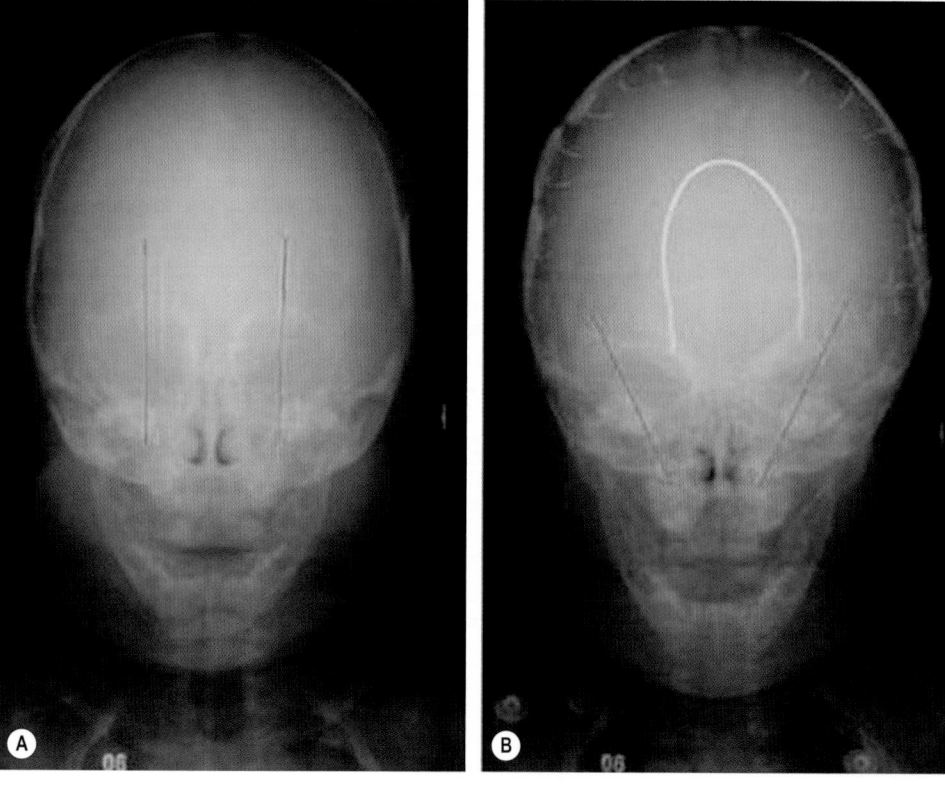

Fig. 34.10 Treatment of lambdoid synostosis. **(A, B)** Switch cranioplasty and occipital bar advancement. **(C, D)** Before and after head shape, from posterior.

Fig. 34.11 (A, B) Springs in craniosynostosis, attempting to widen the fronto-orbital region. (Reproduced from Lauritzen CG, Davis C, Ivarsson A, et al. The evolving role of springs in craniofacial surgery: the first 100 clinical cases. *Plast Reconstr Surg*. 2008;121:545–554.)

Advocates for multiple devices (three or four) cite greater control and strength provided (less chance of device failure).[142–144] Those in favor of fewer devices (one or two) prefer the relative simplicity and theoretically reduced chance for overlapping or colliding vectors.[145–147] Additionally, placement of fewer distractors correlates with less blood loss, and reduces the chance of inflammation and device malfunction. Obviously in multiple suture synostoses, multiple sets of distractors are required. One case of combined sagittal and lambdoid synostosis was addressed with two pairs of distractors (e.g., two devices each on the sagittal and lambdoid areas) for biparietal widening and occipital expansion, respectively.[138]

The surgical technique entails similar osteotomies as used in conventional approaches, but limited dural dissection is performed. The dura is left adherent to the endocranial surface so that it is expanded along with the vault bones. When using distraction, the osteotomies must be placed precisely so that the parallel bone edges do not collide during the trajectory of advancement *(Fig. 34.12)*. Similarly, the distraction devices must be positioned such that vector imparted does not result in bony interferences. Preoperative planning and simulation may aid in the appropriate placement of both osteotomies and devices.

Reported cranial vault distraction protocols usually entail a latency of 3–5 days, an activation rate of 1 mm/day, and a consolidation period that equals twice the duration of active distraction. As with any application of distraction osteogenesis, there exists a balance between too rapid a rate of activation (resulting in poor bony regenerate) and too slow a rate (resulting in premature consolidation). In addition to limiting further expansion, premature ossification can contribute to device breakage.[139] One group reports adjusting the rate of distraction according to a 3D CT scan obtained at 10 mm of distraction.[139] If this interval scan demonstrates very dense regenerate, the distraction rate is increased. Conversely, if the intervening tissue is inadequate, the distraction rate is slowed. Instead of CT radiation, there may be a role for ultrasound in evaluating the regenerate for this purpose.[148]

Distraction conveys advantages related to operative morbidity, stability, and durability. Compared to conventional remodeling procedures, typical perioperative benefits using distraction include shorter operative time, diminished blood loss, and a shorter hospital stay (unless the child is activated in the hospital, in which case hospital stay is longer). Distraction also has the advantage of mitigating extradural dead space, achieving a greater magnitude of advancement, and promoting soft-tissue acclimatization. Additionally, the dural and periosteal blood supplies are maintained, the need for bone grafts are obviated, and there is possibly less chance for relapse.

Disadvantages of cranial vault distraction include the inability to reshape gross contour abnormalities (e.g., correction of flattened/hypoplastic areas or compensatory bulges). For instance, the supraorbital rim and frontal slope can be advanced as one unit, but the relationship between the two areas is not readily altered. Instead of direct manipulation of bone segments, there is reliance on secondary molding from the brain. Additional downsides to vault distraction include a longer time period necessary to achieve final results, the requirement of patient compliance and parental involvement, the need for a second stage to remove the devices, and minor complications associated with the device.

Complications occur in approximately 30% of patients, although they are typically minor.[139] Reported problems have included skin infection (related to device prominence or distraction arm exposure), device dislodgement or deformation, and, occasionally, device breakage.[139] Skin inflammation or infection is usually managed conservatively, using local measures and cleansing. Device dislodgment is minimized by securing the distractor with multiple screws per footplate in

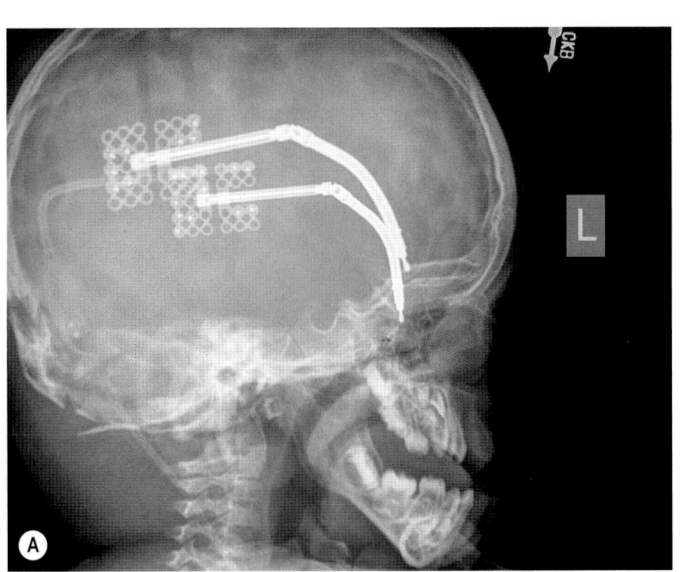
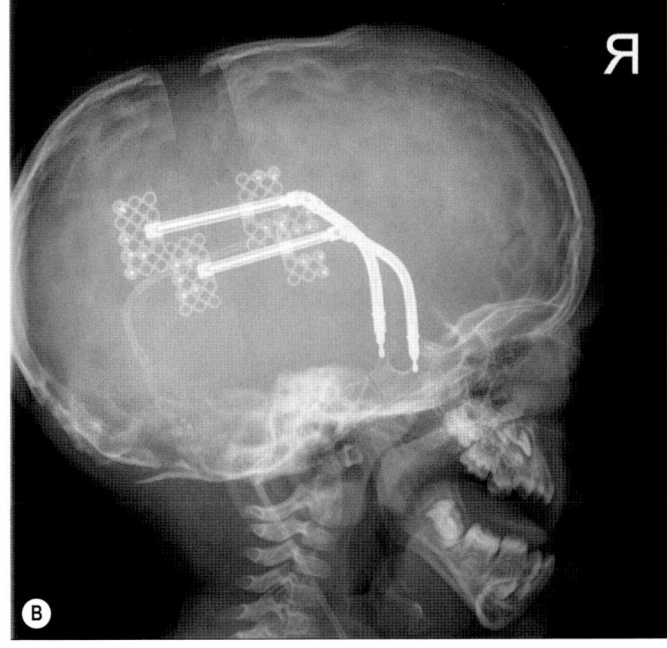

Fig. 34.12 (A, B) Cranial vault expansion using distraction osteogenesis.

high-quality bone. Proper positioning of the osteotomies and devices, aided by preoperative planning and intraoperative attention, also minimizes device failure and improper trajectory. Steps to avoid device breakage include use of a stronger-caliber device (i.e., at least 2-0 thickness), placing multiple distractors (for load sharing), extensive scalp dissection or galeal scoring, and preventing early consolidation (by maintianing a quick activation pace).

Clearly, distraction osteogenesis has utility for treatment of craniosynostosis. Despite several limitations to its application, additional study, refinement in technique, and outcomes assessment will allow distraction to become an increasingly accepted modality in the management of vault abnormalities. However, for significant dysmorphology involving the anterior vault and orbital region, conventional open treatment methods remain the standard of care.

Postoperative care

Cases of major cranial vault reconstruction should be admitted to the ICU postoperatively. Hemodynamic function and neurologic/visual status are monitored. Blood products are given as needed for hemodynamic instability or blood loss anemia. Intravenous normal saline is infused for fluid replacement and maintenance. Perioperative antibiotics are administered for 72 hours. Serum electroytes are followed and an age-appropriate diet is instituted. The craniofacial dressing is removed on the second postoperative day. Output from the subgaleal drain is monitored, emptied, and recorded regularly. Typically the drain is removed on the third postoperative day, regardless of output quantity, so long as the drainage caliber is serosangineous. In this instance the scalp flap is usually adherent to the calvarium and removal of the drain does not result in subcutaneous fluid accumulation. In cases where the drainage is clear, and/or known dural tears or CSF leaks are present, a trial of clamping or removing the Jackson Pratt (JP) drain from suction, alternating with restoration of suction, can be pursued. This prevents continual active suction of CSF and encourages the dural defect to close. Our center has developed a worksheet, based on averages of consecutive cranial vault remodeling patients, that denotes a range of expected JP drain outputs, hemoglobin values, and other variables, stratified by patient age.[149] This is useful for parents, ICU nurses, and ICU physicians alike in the early management of these children.

Parents are advised that, although not usually present immediately postoperatively, significant periorbital edema will ensue, peaking on the second or third postoperative day, in infants who have undergone frontal reconstruction. Children who have undergone posterior reconstruction, and were positioned prone, are likely to have significant periorbital edema immediately postoperatively from prolonged positional dependence. Measures to minimize postoperative edema include gentle dissection along anatomical planes, intraoperative local injection of steroid periorbitally, and systemic administration of corticosteroids.[150–152] Our practice is to obtain a postoperative 3D CT scan once the JP drain is removed. This is to analyze the position of the manipulated bone segments and hardware in the reconstruction, and to serve as a baseline postoperative study. The child is typically discharged from the hospital on the third or fourth postoperative day. The first follow-up visit takes place at 3–4 weeks, with subsequent visits typically at 12 weeks, 6 months, 1 year, and annually or biennially thereafter.

Outcomes, prognosis, and complications

Early complications following vault remodeling are rare. Potential postoperative infectious sequelae include wound infection, meningitis, osteomyelitis, and line infection. Wound infection and dehiscence occur in less than 1% of cases.[153–155] This is principally due to the robust blood supply of the craniofacial region, with a possible contribution from perioperative antibiotics and 100% oxygen administration.[156,157] Meningitis is also infrequent. When this does occur it is typically in the setting of a persistent CSF leak. Closure of the leak is encouraged by relieving active drainage suction (JP clamping trial) or, when necessary, a lumbar drain. Inflammation surrounding a dural opening actually may assist in occluding the CSF egress. In addition to halting the CSF leak, treatment of meningitis includes appropriate antibiotic therapy.

Osteomyelitis of repositioned bone plates is a rare, but potentially devastating, complication associated with cranial vault remodeling.[155] Infection is more apt to occur in older children where sinus boundaries are crossed. If recognized early, limited debridement and administration of both parenteral and local (e.g., catheter irrigation) antibitotics can eradicate the infection and encourage bone healing. In more widespread or lately realized situations, more significant debridement and ostectomy may be required, leaving spans of unprotected dura. This frequently necessitates long-term antimicrobial therapy and staged reconstruction of the calvarial vault.

Line infections are another potential rare cause of infection. Central lines are most often held responsible. The subclavian line has the least incidence of infection, while the jugular location has a higher rate because of the piston effect occuring with neck movement. Groin lines should be altogether avoided because of intertriginous contamination and a higher likelihood of infection. Rarely a bacteremia can develop and lines should be removed and cultured. Echocardiogram may be necessary to exonerate the presence of infective endocardial vegetations.[153]

Postoperative fever is usually not infectious in origin. Postsurgical stress and inflammatory mediators can impart a febrile response. Additionally, blood contacting the meninges, the breakdown of blood products, and transfusion reactions can also be responsible for pyrexia.

Coagulopathy may result following large-volume blood transfusion. Increases in bloody JP output and other clinical signs of bleeding should be monitored. Changes in mental status should prompt an emergent CT scan to investigate for intraparencyhmal hemorrhage. Coagulation laboratories should be closely monitored with a low threshold for clotting factor and platelet replacement if necessary.

Intraparecyhmal hemorrhage may also predispose the patient to seizure activity that may require pharmacologic antiseizure prevention. Bleeding within the posterior cranial

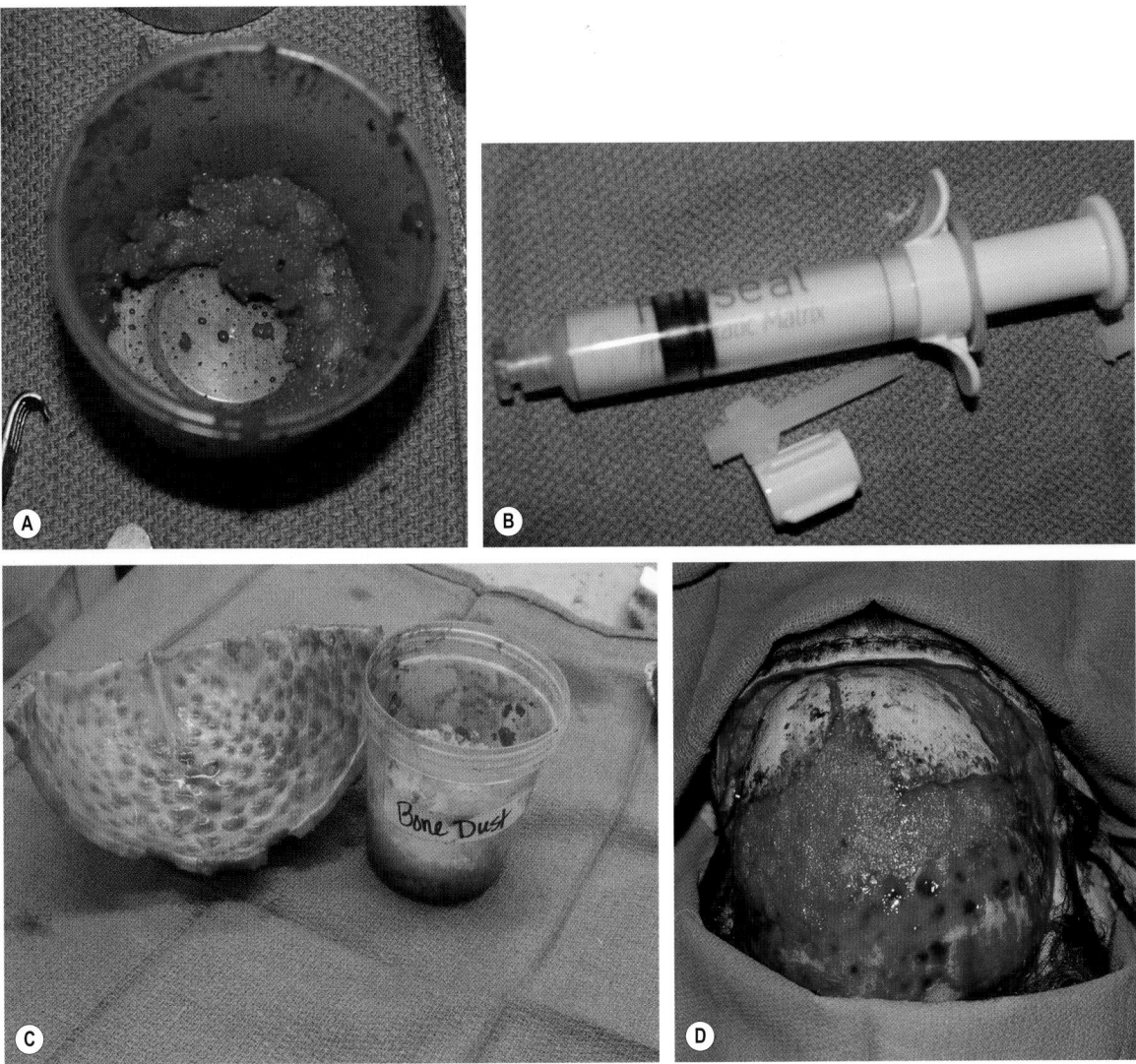

Fig. 34.13 (A–D) Example of bone particulate mixed with fibrin glue to fill craniotomy advancement gaps.

fossa, particularly in patients with pre-existing brainstem malformations, is especially worrisome and has the potential for dire consequences. Rare reports of optic nerve injury or infarction can lead to blindness following cranial vault reconstruction. One reported case indicated a delayed presentation, after discharge from the hospital, thought to be an ischemic bilateral optic nerve injury predisposed by prolonged prone position and blood loss.[158]

During the years and months following cranial vault remodeling, morphologic changes, relating to growth and durability of the bony construct, may ensue. The most frequent are bony gaps or contour irregularities, from incomplete ossification between advanced calvarial segments, and secondary deformities pursuant to growth disturbances and a recapitulation toward the original dysmorphology.

Gaps between repositioned bone segments typically regenerate bone, when created during infancy. The osteogenic dural surface promotes rapid reossification in this age group. Occasionally, large defects, especially when present in older children, may persist permanently. If these gaps are small and not visibly noticeable, no intervention is required and they

can be observed.[159] No restriction relating to gym class or sports is required, though some have advocated protective helmets for the theoretic risk of penetrating injury to the brain.[153] If the defects are very large or are esthetically bothersome, split calvarial bone or particulate bone may be used to fill the defects. Most practitioners currently pro forma fill bone gaps or stepoffs with bone particulate at the time of the initial vault remodeling. The bone is harvested from the endocranial surface of the craniotomy bone and mixed with fibrin glue *(Fig. 34.13)*.

The Whitaker classification describes surgical outcome in reference to the extent of secondary or repeat procedures required[160]. This is divided into four categories and evaluated at earliest 1–2 years from the initial procedure *(Table 34.8)*. The classification is stratified based on increasing need for revision: I, excellent result, no revisions necessary; II, satisfactory result, soft-tissue revision indicated; III, marginal result, bony irregularities present, requiring contouring with bone grafts or alloplast/osteobiologicals; IV, unacceptable result, repeat craniotomy and/or fronto-orbital reshaping necessary.[160] Fewer than 30% of single-suture nonsyndromic

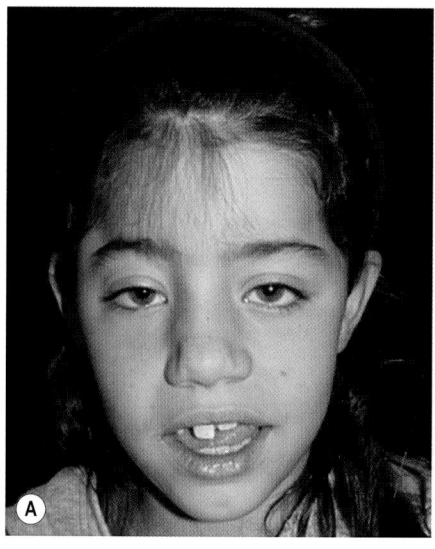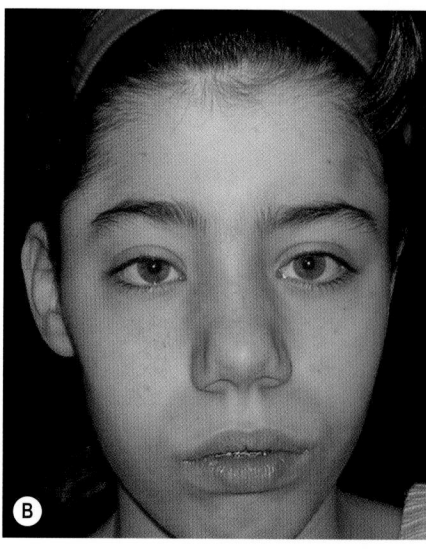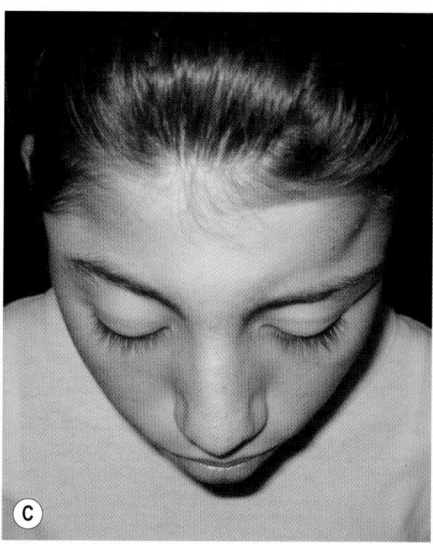

Fig. 34.14 (A–C) Temporal hollowing occurring during the years following right unicoronal synostosis correction by fronto-orbital advancement.

Table 34.8	Whitaker classification for surgical revision
I	Excellent result, no revisions necessary
II	Satisfactory result, soft-tissue revision indicated
III	Marginal result, bony irregularities present, requiring contouring with bone grafts or alloplast/osteobiologicals
IV	Unacceptable result, repeat craniotomy and/or fronto-orbital reshaping necessary

(Reproduced from Whitaker LA, Bartlett SP, Schut L, et al. Craniosynostosis: an analysis of the timing, treatment, and complications in 164 consecutive patients. *Plast Reconstr Surg.* 1987;80:195.)

reconstructions typically benefit from secondary revisions during the years following the primary surgery (Whitaker II–IV). Most reports put the value of reoperation at well below 10%, but with increasing scrutiny, subtle asymmetries and contour irregularities exist in many patients who do not elect to undergo a revisional procedure.[161–164] The vast majority of nonsyndromic children are categorized postoperatively as Whitaker II–III. The need for secondary surgery depends on the type and severity of the original synostosis, the age of operation, and the technique used.[135] The highest rate of reoperation in nonsyndromic children is reported with bicoronal synostosis.[63] Evidence is mounting that many of these previously described "nonsyndromic" children actually carry a genetic abnormality underlying their condition. Among single-suture synostoses, total vault remodeling of sagittal fusion has been reported as most apt to require reoperation (6%).[163] Others feel that asymmetric deformities involving an unbalanced cranial base and orbital inequalities are more difficult to normalize primarily and therefore more prone to requiring secondary adjustments, compared with symmetric abnormalities.[135] The deviation of skull base may underlie incomplete resolution of facial asymmetry following treatment for UCS (e.g., radix and chin point deviations) *(Fig. 34.14)*. Correction of metopic synostosis, though

symmetric, frequently has the penchant toward return of orbital rim retrusion and temporal narrowing. As a function of age, reoperation was required more often in infants treated sooner than 6 months compared to 6–12 months,[165] though, interestingly, other reports show no effect of age on need for revision.[166,167] In terms of timing for reoperation, in the rare case that a complete repeat operation is required (Whitaker IV), the optimal timing is between age 3 and 5. The majority of the brain growth is completed by age 3 and interpersonal childhood interactions occur around age 5.[135] Despite similar surgical techniques in syndromic children, the pendulum swings toward Whitaker III–IV, with presence of more marked postoperative deficiencies.

Soft-tissue problems that develop typically relate to brow and canthal position, or scar thickness and quality. Hollowness in the temporal region is of bony origin, but certain practitioners may advocate augmenting the temporal soft tissue using autologous fat grafting as camouflage. Contour irregularities are ubiquitous and may be secondary to inadequately reossified bone gaps, overlapped bony edges, or hardware. The necessity to shape these is typically an aesthetic decision and can be accomplished by a combination of rotary burr reduction of bulges and augmentation of depressions. This is usually pursued after the age of 7. The most concerning development after cranial vault remodeling is failure to correct the primary deformity adequately, or tendency toward restitution of the original dysmorphology. It is clear that deficient growth of the repositioned, hypoplastic bone segments is responsible for the recapitulation of the deformity ("recurrence") and the presence of secondary deformities (e.g., temporal hollowness)[135,168] *(Fig. 34.14)*.

Even single-suture synostoses have tendency to recur toward original head shape.[135,162] Fearon *et al.* demonstrated that growth following single-suture synostosis correction falls off with time.[162] This effect was witnessed in all types of single-suture synostosis (metopic, coronal, sagittal, and lambdoid), when surgically corrected children were evaluated over an average 8-year follow-up period.[135] Growth impairment appeared greatest in vectors perpendicular to the fused suture, implying the effect of the primary process and/or incomplete surgical normalization. This suggests that simply surgically normalizing the head shape is insufficient treatment. The vault-remodeling procedure should overcorrect the hypoplastic areas and overcontour locations of future expected deficiencies in an attempt to compensate for the differential growth that will occur. The authors felt, though not corroborated statistically, that the growth disturbance was proportional to the original severity of the deformity. Also, it appeared that growth was poorer in children treated at an earlier age. As previously mentioned, timing of treatment should balance the possible need for reoperation, potential magnitude of growth disturbance, and workability of bone, with the likelihood of persistent bony gaps, the durability of the construct, and attempted avoidance of neuropsychiatric issues.[135]

In addition to morphologic outcome and propensity toward recurrence of the abnormal head shape, the effect on functional issues imparted by craniosynostosis correction should be addressed. Strabismus, often present in UCS, does not appear to improve following fronto-orbital advancement and reconstruction. Parents are counseled that eye patching or extraocular muscle surgery may be required at some point postoperatively, as determined by the ophthalmologist, and that the craniosynostosis correction is not intended to improve ocular motility.[169] The effect of vault reshaping on intracranial hypertension is an area sparking significant interest. Inagaki *et al.* reported on a population of children with mild craniosynostosis who underwent ICP measurements before and after surgical correction. They found that the relatively high proportion of children with preoperative increase in ICP (>17 mmHg) experienced normalization of pressure following treatment.[65] This is important for two reasons: (1) even morphologically mild cases of synostosis demonstrate ICP elevation; and (2) vault expansion relieves the elevated pressure (theoretically mitigating the ill effects produced by prolonged intracranial hypertension). This is indirectly demonstrated on the evidence that release of fused futures has a positive effect on brain metabolism.[170] There is also clinical evidence that cranial expansion in craniosynostosis will impart benefit against the known negative neurologic sequelae accompanying increased ICP (e.g., neurocognitive delay), compared to individuals who are left untreated.

Intellectual capacity and neuropsychiatric development can be impaired in patients with longer-standing, uncorrected craniosynostosis.[171] Intelligence quotient is shown to be diminished in children older than 1 year with uncorrected synostosis compared to children who undergo cranial vault remodeling earlier than age 1.[172,173] A review of children with metopic synostosis demonstrated behavioral and developmental problems that interestingly did not correlate with the severity of head abnormality.[174] Sagittal synostosis, once thought only to pose an aesthetic problem, has been shown by sophisticated neuropsychologic testing to result in learning disability when not surgically addressed.[175] Behavioral indicators for intracranial hypertension can be assessed in late-presenting older children with craniosynostosis. A history of developmental delay, irritability, headaches, and vomiting suggests a pressure component in these children, and favors surgical expansion for symptomatic relief. A recent review of children presenting older than 2 years old demonstrated improvement of neurologic symptoms (e.g., headaches, nausea) and presumed correction of intracranial

hypertension by cranial vault-remodeling procedures in this subset.[176]

Secondary procedures

Secondary procedures can be divided into those for soft tissue or bony deformities. Frequent soft-tissue modifications include: scar revision, canthopexy, brow lift, fat grafting, and oculoplastic procedures (strabismus surgery, ptosis repair). Hard-tissue interventions may include: bone grafting defects, autologous or alloplastic augmentation of contour deficiencies, hardware removal, or, rarely, repeat intracranial vault reshaping.

Scar revision can be performed at any time by exicision, either as a singular procedure, or frequently whenever the coronal incision is reopened to address deeper bony contour irregularities. A wide, hairless scar can be noticeable and bothersome, especially when hair is worn short or is thin in caliber. Closure under tension, from a significant osseous advancement, and genetic propensity contribute to thick unaesthetic scars. Attempts to avoid unsightly scars on initial closure include a trichophytic closure, and limited use of both electrocautery and compressive scalp clips, though despite our best efforts, scarring remains unpredictable.

There are several techniques to perform canthopexy for differential angulation of the lateral canthal position (most typically seen in UCS).[177] This may be performed at the time of the initial fronto-orbital reshaping, but it is controversial as to whether a canthopexy is always necessary. As a delayed procedure, the canthopexy technique could involve osseous wiring, deep and superior to the zygomaticofrontal suture,[178] or various suture approaches involving the lateral canthal tendon or lateral palpebral commissure and periosteum of the internal lateral orbital rim.[179]

Asymmetric brow position may be addressed as a secondary procedure. The practitioner should recognize that underlying bone inequalities may contribute to the differential brow position (relatively raised or lowered). For instance, supraorbital ridge retrusion and flattening of the forehead may position the brow higher (akin to the original deformity in UCS). In these instances, bony augmentation of the supraorbital region will aid in properly positioning the brow. Soft-tissue brow-lifting procedures are numerous in the aesthetic literature. Common effective procedures include rotation of the coronal flap away from the side of desired lift and bone fixation and suture techniques.[180,181] A combination of addressing the underlying bony support and soft-tissue brow pexy techniques should be employed to correct brow position effectively.

Fat-grafting techniques can serve to camouflage hollow areas or depressions. Most commonly, temporal concavities can be observed following fronto-orbital advancement procedures as a result of bony deficiency[168] *(Fig. 34.14)*. Though not addressing the tissue type responsible for the problem, fat grafting is a less invasive technique to provide bulk and improve contour in these areas.[182] The principal issue relates to its unpredictability, in terms of how much resorbs. Patients may require several repeat rounds of fat injections. Depression of medial epicanthal folds may be witnessed following trigonocephaly correction. This can be alleviated using an onlay bone graft to the depressed nasal radix (effectively tenting up the medial soft tissue). Strabismus surgery and ptosis repair are outside the scope of this chapter, but may be necessary and typically performed by the ophthalmologist member of the craniofacial team.

Full-thickness bony gaps may be addressed by a variety of materials. Autologous bone grafting is preferable, by way of particulate bone or larger-segment cranial bone grafting, depending on the size of the defect. BMP and growth factors may be added to particulate bone, or possibly used alone. Ridges or irregularities can be smoothed by rotary burr, rasp, or ostectomy; and hardware can be removed (e.g., wires or nonresorbing plates) when they contribute to sharp spots or edges. Rarely, prominent wires can begin to thin overlying skin or predispose to pressure ulcers. Areas of prominence juxtaposed with concavities are addressed by a combination of reducing the bulges and augmenting the depressions. Bone grafting and alloplastic augmentation (e.g., hydroxyappatite bone paste, calcium phosphate cement, methylmethacrylate, porous polyethylene, or peak implants) are techniques to impart larger area contour changes as a secondary cranioplasty procedure. These techniques exhibit varying degrees of effectiveness and are largely dependent on surgeon preference and experience with the specific material.[159]

Access the complete references list online at **http://www.expertconsult.com**

16. Persing JA, Jane JA, Shaffrey M. Virchow and the pathogenesis of craniosynostosis: a translation of his original work. *Plast Reconstr Surg.* 1989;83:738–742.

22. Shillito Jr J, Matson DD. Craniosynostosis: a review of 519 surgical patients. *Pediatrics.* 1968;41:829–853.

64. Renier D, Sainte-Rose C, Marchac D. et al. Intracranial pressure in craniosynostosis. *J Neurosurg.* 1982;57:370–377.

   The authors assessed pre- and postoperative intracranial pressure (ICP) in 92 cases of craniosynostosis. Preoperatively elevated ICP normalized over several weeks after surgery. ICP was inversely correlated with intelligence.

80. Persing JA, Babler WF, Winn HR, et al. Age as a critical factor in the success of surgical correction of craniosynostosis. *J Neurosurg.* 1981;54:601.

   Coronal sutures were artificially immobilized to simulate craniosynostosis in a rabbit model, and surgical release was performed at various time points. Cranial growth was most improved with earlier suture release.

93. Persing JA, Posnick J, Magge S, et al. Cranial plate and screw fixation in infancy: an assessment of risk. *J Craniofac Surg.* 1996;7:267–270.

99. Jane JA, Edgerton MT, Futrell JW, et al. Immediate correction of sagittal synostosis. *J Neurosurg.* 1978;49:705–710.

   The authors described a series of 22 sagittal sysnostosis corrections. They noted that refusion of the sagittal suture did not occur, despite the fact that no specific measures to prevent this occurrence were undertaken.

107. Bartlett SP, Whitaker LA, Marchac D. The operative treatment of isolated craniofacial dysostosis (plagiocephaly): A comparison of the unilateral and bilateral techniques. *Plast Reconstr Surg.* 1990;85:677.

   This is a retrospective review of isolated plagiocephaly repairs. The authors conclude that excellent outcomes can be achieved with both unilateral and bilateral approaches, and that special consideration should be given to assuring adequate correction in the temporal region to maximize positive outcomes.

118. Havlik RJ, Azurin DJ, Bartlett SP, et al. Analysis and treatment of severe trigonocephaly. *Plast Reconstr Surg.* 1999;103:381.

119. Whitaker LA, Bartlett SP, Schut L, et al. Craniosynostosis: an analysis of the timing, treatment, and complications in 164 consecutive patients. *Plast Reconstr Surg.* 1987;80:195.

   Outcomes in craniofacial procedures performed in patients stratified by age were compared. The authors conclude that craniofacial procedures may best be delayed until after 7 years of age, but cranial surgery may best be performed earlier in life.

153. Fearon J, Ruotolo R, Kolar J. Single suture craniosynostoses: Surgical outcomes and Long-term growth. *Plast Reconstr Surg.* 2009;123:635–642.

35

Syndromic craniosynostosis

Jeffrey A. Fearon

SYNOPSIS

- Syndromic craniosynostoses have coexisting anomalies aside from fused cranial sutures.
- Treatment paradigms are best applied according to patient phenotype, and not genotype.
- The avoidance of neurocognitive delays requires a focus on the prevention of both sleep apnea and chronic elevations in intracranial pressure.
- The management of the syndromic craniosynostoses should be relegated to dedicated craniofacial teams, comprised of experienced subspecialists.

 Access the Historical Perspective section online at
http://www.expertconsult.com

Introduction

Craniosynostosis, or any anomalous fusion of cranial sutures, may affect either a single suture, or multiple sutures. In general, most infants presenting with a single sutural synostosis will not have a syndrome, while those with multiple sutural craniosynostoses will probably have one. However, syndromes have been described in association with only a single sutural synostosis, and various patterns of multiple sutural fusions (often referred to as the "complex craniosynostoses") may occur without comprising a true syndrome. By definition, all syndromic craniosynostoses have additional anomalies that occur in embryologically distinct areas apart from the skull. The syndromic craniosynostoses are relatively uncommon, and of all the anomalies treated by craniofacial surgeons, they can present some of the greatest treatment challenges. The optimal care of patients with these unusual syndromes is best relegated to experienced craniofacial teams, comprised of multiple subspecialists. These teams are able to maximize outcomes and also allow for the coordination of care, which can reduce the total number of operative procedures affected children must endure.

Basic science/disease process

As the field of craniofacial genetics has matured, a more complete picture of the molecular basis for the syndromic synostoses is emerging. Today, over 150 different craniosynostosis syndromes have been described.[14] The majority of syndromic craniosynostoses are the result of an FGFR-related mutations, which are primarily autosomal-dominant.[15] In addition to the more commonly encountered Apert, Crouzon, and Pfeiffer syndromes, other FGFR-related craniosynostosis syndromes include: Muenke, Crouzon with acanthosis nigricans, Jackson–Weiss, and Beare–Stevenson (Table 35.1). Among the non-FGFR mutations are: Boston-type craniosynostosis (MSX2), the Philadelphia type, and Saethre–Chotzen (TWIST 1). All the FGFR-associated craniosynostoses are gain-of-function mutations, and while MSXS is also a gain-of-function mutation, the TWIST mutation represents a loss of function.[16] Notably, the TWIST mutation has been reported to occur in association with an increased incidence of breast and renal cancers; however, a subsequently published multicenter Australian study has failed to support these earlier findings.[17–19]

The majority of infants born with one of the syndromic craniosynostoses will present with bilateral coronal craniosynostosis, either in isolation or associated with other sutural synostoses. In addition, there may be variable effects on the development of the midface, as well as the hands and feet. It has been noted that some genes expressed in craniofacial development are also expressed in limb development.[20,21] Among the most commonly encountered syndromic craniosynostoses is Crouzon syndrome, which is notable for the presence of phenotypically normal hands and feet. Pfeiffer syndrome is recognizable by the presence of enlarged thumbs and halluces, and Apert syndrome may be easily identified by the associated complex syndactylies of the hands and feet. With a fairly recent explosion of research in molecular genetics, many surgeons were hopeful that gene testing would finally provide specific and accurate diagnoses for each of the phenotypically unique craniofacial syndromes. Thus far, this has proven not to be the case. Not only can the same mutation cause different syndromes, but different mutations may be associated with the same syndrome.[22,23] For example, identical mutations have been noted in individuals with Crouzon syndrome, Pfeiffer syndrome, and Jackson–Weiss syndrome, suggesting that unlinked modifier genes, or epigenic factors, play an important role in determining the final phenotype.[24,25] Apert syndrome has been shown to result from at least two separate amino acid missense substitutions: Ser252Trp or Pro253Arg. The former has been reported to occur slightly more commonly (over 60% of cases) and is associated with a less severe form of syndactyly, but with an increased frequency for cleft palates.[26] Moreover, within syndromes there can be significant phenotypic variability. For example, Pfeiffer syndrome has been phenotypically subclassified into three separate types: type I is described as the "classic Pfeiffer" and represents a milder presentation; type II is notable for a cloverleaf (or Kleeblattschädel) skull deformity; and type III is reserved for the most severely affected children. In spite of these differences, no specific genetic mutations have been noted to correlate with each of these described phenotypes.[27]

Diagnosis/patient presentation

Most physicians begin their evaluation of an infant with an abnormal skull shape by ordering a radiological study, such as a computed tomography scan, in order to ascertain the specific diagnosis. However, these studies are most often unnecessary, as the diagnosis of syndromic craniosynostoses can usually be made solely on the basis of a careful physical examination.[28] Having an appreciation for how the skull is affected by sutural fusion (with growth inhibition occurring perpendicular to fused sutures and compensatory growth occurring in the remaining open sutures) enables the astute examiner to diagnose correctly which sutures are fused. Further differentiation between syndromes can be made by examination of the fingers and toes. *Table 35.2* lists some of the more commonly presenting syndromes, along with some identifying phenotypic characteristics.

Even more important than attempting to establish which specific syndrome a child might have is first to determine if there are any potentially acute impediments to life, such as an airway obstruction or feeding impairment (e.g., inadequate intake, reflux, aspiration). Concerns for potentially detrimental raised intracranial pressure, albeit extremely important, usually take a secondary role in this initial evaluation, because of the low likelihood for issues in the first few months of life. This is because in infancy, the remaining open sutures are usually effective in compensating for those that are fused. Nevertheless, in formulating a lifelong treatment strategy for any child with syndromic craniosynostosis, the author believes that there are two primary areas worthy of focus that have the potential to prevent neurocognitive loss, and maximize development: (1) avoiding prolonged periods of hypoxia; and (2)

Table 35.1 FGFR-related craniosynostoses

Syndrome	Percentage caused by FGFR1 mutations	Percentage caused by FGFR2 mutations	Percentage caused by FGFR 3 mutations
Muenke			100%
Crouzon		100%	
Crouzon with acanthosis nigricans			100%
Jackson–Weiss		100%	
Apert		100%	
Pfeiffer type I	5%	95%	
Pfeiffer type II		100%	
Pfeiffer type III		100%	
Beare–Stevenson		<100%	
FGFR2 isolated coronal synostosis		100%	

(Adapted from Robin NH, Falk MJ, Haldeman-Englert CR. FGFR-related craniosynostosis syndromes. Gene Reviews. Available online at: www.genetests.org.)

Table 35.2 Clinical findings in selected FGFR-related syndromic craniosynostoses

Syndrome	Skull shape	Midface	Hands and feet
Apert	Moderate to severe brachycephaly with occasional severe turribrachycephaly	Moderate hypoplasia	Pansyndactylies of hands and feet (thumbs can be free, and partial syndactylies of small fingers and toes may occur)
Crouzon	Brachycephaly	Mild to moderate hypoplasia	Generally unaffected
Muenke	Unilateral or bilateral brachycephaly	Mild to none	Variable carpal and tarsal fusions
Pfeiffer type I	Brachycephaly	Moderate	Broad thumbs and halluces. Variable limited syndactyly
Pfeiffer type II	Cloverleaf skull deformity with pansynostoses	Moderate	Broad thumbs and halluces. Variable limited syndactyly
Pfeiffer type III	Pansynostoses with marked turricephaly	Moderate to severe	Broad thumbs and halluces. Variable limited syndactyly

avoiding prolonged periods of raised intracranial pressure. The initial management of any child born with one of the syndromic craniosynostoses typically involves more medical management, rather than surgical. As the affected infant moves farther along the severity continuum, the likelihood for airway compromise increases, as does the potential for feeding issues. Any suspicion for airway compromise should be further evaluated with polysomnography.

In early infancy, central sleep apnea (typically associated with an acquired Chiari I malformation, which results in brainstem compression) is less commonly identified as the cause for impaired ventilation, and obstructive sleep apnea is far more likely. The etiology for any observed obstructive sleep apnea may be multifactorial, but is most often directly related to mid facial hypoplasia. This hypoplasia elevates the palate, which correspondingly reduces the size of the nasal airway. This resultant diminished nasal airway is different from a true choanal atresia, which is caused by a congenital persistence of tissues separating the nose form the mouth. The reduced nasal aperture associated with syndromic craniosynostosis is best left untreated because of the dismal success rates that have been observed following any early surgical intervention.[29] Other causes for airway obstruction include: tracheomalacia, tracheal stenosis (especially with type II Pfeiffer syndrome), and gastroesophageal reflux (antireflux medication should be considered for all syndromic infants).[30] Feeding issues are commonly seen in conjunction with airway obstruction, and associated neuromuscular immaturity may result in silent aspiration; therefore, feeding evaluations are often useful. When obstructive sleep apnea is identified, more conservative treatments include use of continuous positive airway pressure masks and tonsillectomies. Some surgeons have reported performing frontofacial advancements in infancy; however, there is currently no evidence to support these early interventions, and such treatments may be considered as falling outside the current mainstream of care.[31,32] On the other hand, temporary tracheostomies have been attributed to lowering mortality rates for the more severe patterns of syndromic craniosynostosis, and should be considered in all infants and younger children who have failed the more conservative therapies.[30] Typically, the incidence for airway compromise can be expected to increase with age, as the mid facial hypoplasia becomes more progressive.

In addition to airway management, the second critical area of focus for any child with syndromic craniosynostosis is the avoidance of raised intracranial pressure. As with airway issues, the potential for raised intracranial pressure increases over time. Unfortunately, the clinical determination of elevated intracranial pressure is an extremely challenging endeavor. There have been no published studies evaluating either the specificity or sensitivity of any of the often-cited clinical signs for raised intracranial pressure. Currently, it is unknown exactly how high, or for how long intracranial pressure needs to be elevated before there are irreversible adverse effects on cognitive function. Nevertheless, some attempts to determine the presence of potentially elevated intracranial pressure must be made. There are studies using direct measurement techniques, which suggest that when more than one suture is fused (even when there is a normal skull volume), intracranial pressure is more likely to be elevated.[33–35] Given the invasive nature of obtaining direct intracranial pressure measurements, it is not reasonable to perform serial testing for elevations in intracranial pressure in every child with syndromic craniosynostosis. Instead, secondary assessments for intracranial pressure are used, such as: the physical assessment of fontanels or other skull defects (to assess dural tension), serial head circumference measurements (to look for changes along the growth curves), fundoscopic examinations (to assess for papilledema), reversed visual evoked potentials, and magnetic resonance imaging scanning (to monitor for decreasing ventricular size, enlargement of the optic nerves, or progressive tonsillar herniation).[35–40] Some believe that chronic elevations in intracranial pressure may result in observable changes in the skull radiographs, such as imprinting ("copper-beaten," and/or thinning of the bone); however, there are no supportive studies to confirm this relationship, nor does this finding appear to correlate with intelligence.[41] Although it may seem intuitive that progressive skull malformations might correlate with increased intracranial pressure and developmental issues, this relationship has thus far not been supported by retrospective single sutural synostosis studies.[42,43]

In addition to the need for evaluating a child for potential airway compromise and raised intracranial pressure, additional anomalies must be considered. The association between cerebellar tonsillar herniation and syndromic craniosynostosis was first described over 30 years ago; since that time, studies have shown that these Chiari malformations are an acquired defect, and are likely exacerbated by ventriculoperitoneal shunting.[44–46] Chiari malformations have been observed to occur infrequently in Apert syndrome, often in Crouzon syndrome, and almost always in the more severe presentations for Pfeiffer syndrome.[30,37,47] It is important to screen all children for this condition with routine magnetic resonance imaging, because, when symptomatic, Chiari malformations may lead to central sleep apnea, disordered swallowing, syringomyelia, or even potentially fatal central sleep apnea. In addition to Chiari malformations, children need to be followed for the potential development for hydrocephalus, which is often not diagnosed until after a skull expansion procedure has been performed.

Another important concern in children born with syndromic craniosynostosis is exposure-related visual loss. As a result of altered orbital growth, severe proptosis may occur, resulting in impaired lid coverage and corneal scarring. Some infants with syndromic craniosynostosis (primarily with Apert syndrome) may also have submucous, or complete clefts of the secondary palate. There is also a higher incidence of cardiac anomalies among the syndromic craniosynostoses, particularly atrial and ventricular septal defects.[48] Malrotation of the gut appears to be more common in Pfeiffer syndrome, and should be radiologically evaluated with an upper gastrointestinal series with a small-bowel followthrough, when indicated.[30]

Patient selection

Identification of the ideal time to operate on a child, and determining which operation should be performed, cannot be decided on a syndrome-by-syndrome basis. Instead, it is better to consider the child's phenotypic presentation. In this regard, it is useful to recognize that the syndromic synostoses actually represent a continuum of birth defects. At one end of this syndromic craniosynostosis spectrum would be the isolated bilateral coronal craniosynostoses (without any associated mid facial hypoplasia, and only minimally impaired cranial growth), and at the other end would be the severely constricted Kleeblattschädel skull deformities and complete pansynostoses (with extremely deficient mid facial growth, and associated severe airway anomalies) *(Fig. 35.1)*. Appreciating where each child falls on this continuum allows surgeons to apply treatment algorithms specific to the problems encountered.

The timing for the initial surgical intervention for any of the craniosynostoses has not been specifically studied. The two goals for treating the affected skull of any child with syndromic craniosynostosis are to normalize appearance, and to prevent sustained elevations in intracranial pressure (sufficient to impact cognition). Implicit among these goals is to accomplish them as safely, and with as few procedures, as possible. Studies examining long-term calvarial growth following single sutural corrections have shown that growth is not normal postoperatively.[49,50] Considering the rapid growth of the brain in infancy, delaying surgical intervention has the benefit of achieving a better longer-term result. This is partly because early surgical intervention must contend with the reduced mechanical rigidity of the thin infant skull that impairs the ability to achieve any significant enlargement of the calvaria. Moreover, earlier surgical intervention has the disadvantage of the rapidly growing brain quickly occupying any achievable increase in intracranial volume. Conversely, delaying surgery might potentially result in a preventable visual or developmental loss.[36,38] Studies measuring intracranial pressure in children with craniosynostosis suggest that elevated pressure is more likely when multiple sutures are fused, that elevated pressures may inversely correlate with mental function, and that surgery can successfully reduce intracranial pressure.[33–35] However, more important than treating raised intracranial pressure is the prevention of avoidable developmental delays; this particular parameter is something that is much harder to measure. Some studies have suggested that earlier surgery (under 1 year of age) is associated with higher IQ scores.[51,52] Nevertheless, these retrospective studies may have been influenced by selection biases (i.e., well-educated parents may be more likely to bring their child to a physician earlier for treatment).

Given the absence of well-designed studies, surgeons must currently use their best judgment in determining how long it is safe to delay surgical enlargement of the skull. The number of fused sutures, the presence of widely patent decompressing sutures, and the degree of the presenting skull deformity are all factors that may influence the timing for skull decompression procedures. If concerns for intracranial pressure elevations are low, it is likely that the older the child is at the time of surgery, the better the long-term result.

Treatment/surgical technique

Of all the congenital craniofacial anomalies, treatment of the syndromic craniosynostoses can present some of the greatest challenges. Although the vast majority of published literature has been retrospective and anecdotal, much has nevertheless been learned from observation. The aforementioned goals of treatment, which are to normalize both function and appearance, need to be accomplished as safely and with as few operations as possible. The management of the syndromic craniosynostoses requires a team of dedicated specialists, and is ideally reserved for those centers that have both a focused interest in these complex problems and sufficient expertise to provide safe and efficient care. Underscoring the challenges of treating the more severe syndromic craniosynostoses are the significant mortality rates that have been described within this particular subpopulation (reportedly as high as 66–85%).[53,54] The timing for skull surgery, and the selection of the best operative procedure, varies with the child's phenotype. At the milder end of the syndromic craniosynostosis

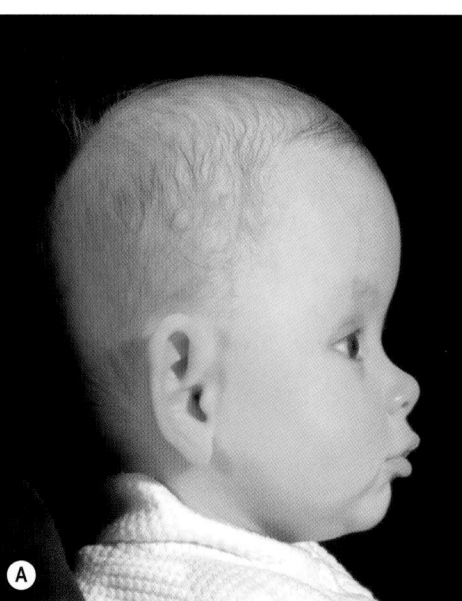

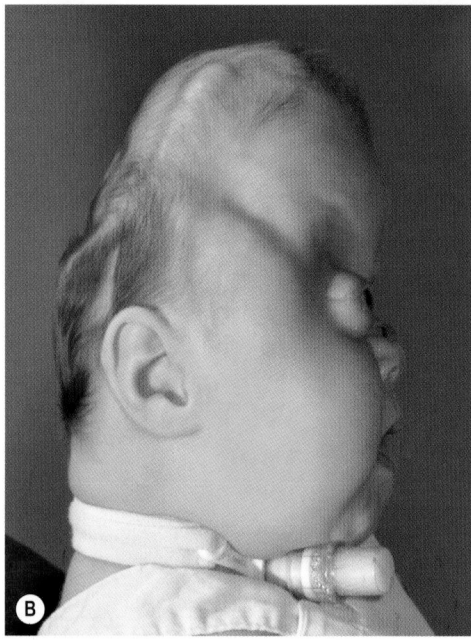

Fig. 35.1 The syndromic craniosynostosis spectrum can vary from isolated bicoronal synostosis as seen in Muenke craniosynostosis **(A)** to the pansynostoses that may be seen in association with Pfeiffer syndrome **(B)**.

spectrum, presenting with a more moderate degree of brachycephaly (especially when there is a split metopic or sagittal suture that offers some degree of decompression), the author will delay surgery until the open bony defects have closed, or the dura begins to become tense. As the degree of skull deformity progresses along the severity continuum, progressive turricephaly will be seen. If allowed to progress beyond a moderate stage, an increased skull height can be exceedingly difficult to correct later, therefore making significant turricephaly a relative indication for earlier surgical intervention.

The surgical procedure for any child falling along the mild to moderate end of the syndromic craniosynostosis spectrum consists of enlargement of the anterior fossa. The goal of surgery is to increase intracranial volume by bringing the supraorbital bandeau as far forward as possible, while simultaneously lowering any anterior turricephaly. Surgery performed in children under 9 months of age is more challenging because of the inherent weakness of the thin, relatively immature skull; as a result, any small degree of advancement obtained at this early age will be quickly eradicated by the rapidly growing brain (clinically evident by the rapid reappearance of brachycephaly). Perhaps it is for this reason that some surgeons have advocated beginning with a posterior decompression.[55,56]

However, there are also a number of compelling reasons that argue against early posterior skull surgery in children with syndromic synostosis. To begin with, acquired Chiari malformations, although relatively uncommon for Apert syndrome, have been reported to occur in 70% of children with Crouzon syndrome and up to 100% of children with the more severe Pfeiffer presentations.[30,37,47] Given these incidences, there is a high likelihood that a low posterior fossa enlargement, with decompression of the foramen magnum, will be necessary. However, early decompressions of the foramen magnum (performed under a year of age) typically offer only transient benefits because of subsequent bony regrowth. Therefore, it can be argued that it is better to hold posterior skull enlargement in abeyance, pending the development of a symptomatic Chiari. Additionally, it is well recognized that, following anterior remodeling procedures, the frontal bone can develop subsequent irregularities with growth. If the posterior parietal and upper occipital region has been surgically preserved, this unaltered smooth bone can be exchanged for the irregular frontal bone at skeletal maturity, bringing the benefit of a lifelong aesthetically pleasing forehead. However, if the posterior skull was surgically altered in infancy, this later correction will not be possible. Therefore, it is the author's opinion that, for the majority of children with syndromic craniosynostosis, it is probably best to begin with an anterior cranial vault remodeling procedure, at some point over a year of age.

There are multiple techniques that can be used to enlarge the frontal fossa, and most utilize some form of a supraorbital bandeau, or vertical bar, of varying lengths. Once cut, the bandeau can be advanced into the desired location, and the frontal bone is reattached. The exact positioning of the bandeau is critical, for as the bandeau goes, so goes the rest of the reconstruction. Some surgeons prefer to use a horizontally short bandeau, which extends laterally only as far as the lateral orbital rim (*Fig. 35.2*).[7,51,57] This particular bandeau design lacks any inherent stability; therefore, very rigid

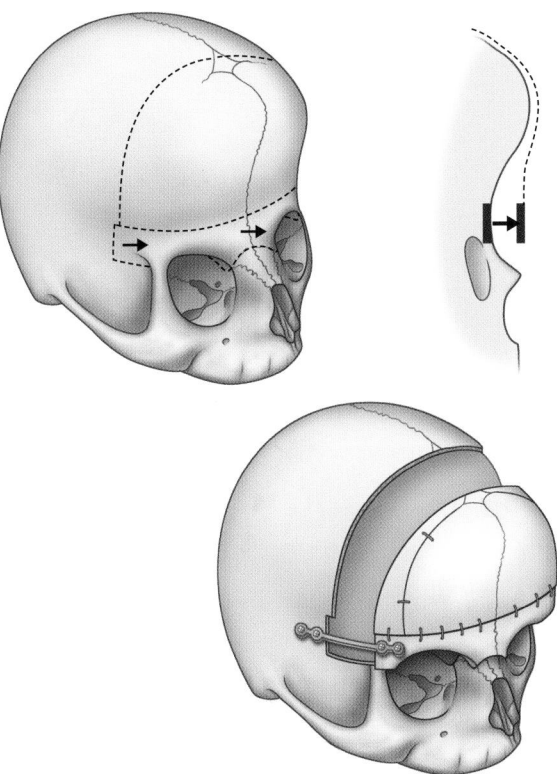

Fig. 35.2 Enlargement of the anterior fossa may be performed utilizing a horizontally short bandeau. This technique requires use of a plating system in order to provide lateral stability. However, significant advancements with this osteotomy design may result in an increase in temporal hollowing.

osseous fixation is required in order to stabilize the advancement. For this reason, most surgeons prefer a longer horizontal bandeau design with a tenon-type tongue-in-groove joint that extends posteriorly across the temporal bone, providing inherent stability (*Fig. 35.3*).[58–60] However, when the deformity resulting from coronal synostosis is analyzed, it turns out that the ideal vector for bandeau advancement is not the simple forward horizontal movement that is often described.[61] Instead, the bandeau needs to be moved in both a forward and inferior direction, in order to obtain an ideal anatomically overcorrected repositioning. There are numerous possible bandeau osteotomies which can be employed three-dimensionally to overcorrect the observed displacement precisely.[62] For example, for isolated bilateral coronal craniosynostosis (with elevation and recession of the supraorbits, but with a normal forehead width), a stair-step osteotomy can be used to advance and stabilize the bandeau (*Fig. 35.4*). For those cases in which the forehead (and temporal region) has developed a compensatory excess width, custom osteotomies can be used to narrow the bandeau while simultaneously advancing and lowering the supraorbits (*Fig. 35.5*). The frontal bone can also be removed without designing a true bandeau (and also without cutting into the frontal sinuses, avoiding contamination of the surgical field), and then this bone is either repositioned or replaced with another bone flap in both a more forward and inferior position via temporal insets (*Fig. 35.6*). As previously noted, the longer that surgery can be delayed, the more stable the bone, the greater the

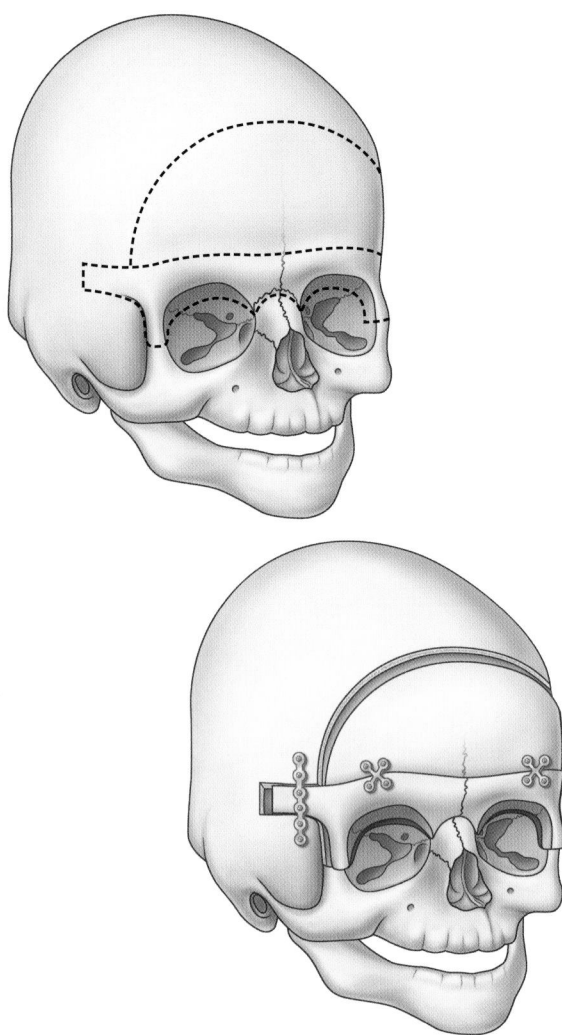

Fig. 35.3 Use of a longer bandeau design, with a tenon-type tongue-in-groove joint, provides inherent stability, and may offer a smoother transition into the temporal region. A potential problem with this particular osteotomy design is that it does not inferiorly reposition the supraorbit, which is always necessary with coronal synostosis.

achievable advancement, and the longer the correction will last before needing to be repeated. Nevertheless, all timing considerations must also take into account the goal of preventing any potentially irreversible developmental delays from prolonged raised intracranial pressure. Given the need to balance the concerns for intracranial pressure and desire to reduce the total number of operations, the author prefers to delay cranial remodeling, for those patients falling along the milder end of the syndromic craniosynostosis spectrum, until about 15 months of age.

Treatment of the more severely affected infants with syndromic craniosynostosis often requires a more aggressive approach. Faced with a child with pancraniosynostosis, elevated intracranial pressure will quickly ensue, and surgeons need to be prepared to perform earlier decompressions, often as soon as the infant can safely tolerate this significant procedure (12–16 weeks of age). Severely affected skull configurations are notable for pronounced turricephaly, that may or may not be associated with varying degrees of a cloverleaf deformity. For these pansynostoses, the author prefers to perform an isolated midvault decompression for a number of reasons. To begin with, no attempt should be made to address the aesthetically important forehead with an early decompression (the thin bone makes any significant frontal advancement impossible, and early surgery only makes subsequent frontal advancements extremely challenging). Similarly, the low posterior skull should not be expanded at this early time, not only because the thin bone will not permit adequate expansion, but also because a later Chiari decompression will likely be required. Finally, as a result of the associated skull base compression, venous hypertension will ensue, resulting in enlargement of transosseous veins, which are most prominent in the low central occipital region (*Fig. 35.7*). These dilated veins should ideally be preserved, as ligation has been cited as the cause of a postoperative mortality.[63] The exception to perform early posterior decompressions is for those infants who are noted to have a severe Chiari malformation and have already required placement of a ventriculoperitoneal shunt. This combination may indicate the need for very early decompression of the foramen magnum, because shunt failures in this particular subgroup can be devastating.

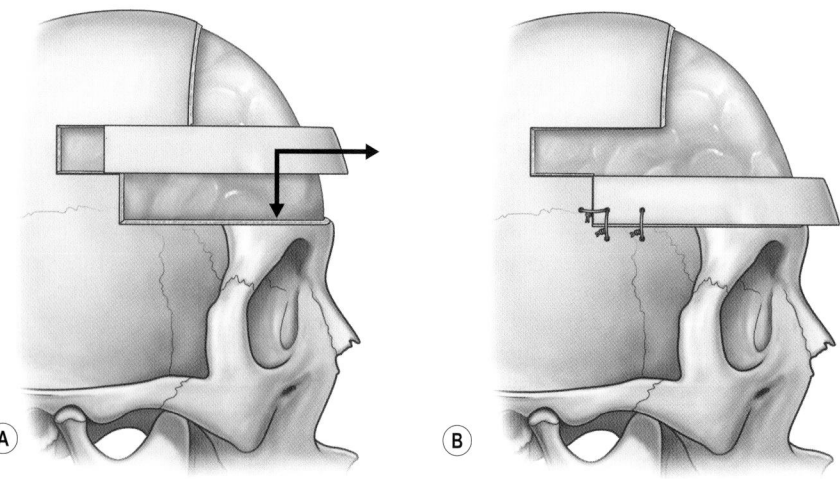

(A) (B)

Fig. 35.4 (A, B) A stair-step osteotomy can be used to advance and stabilize the bandeau. This design permits both a forward advancement and a simultaneous inferior repositioning of the bandeau.

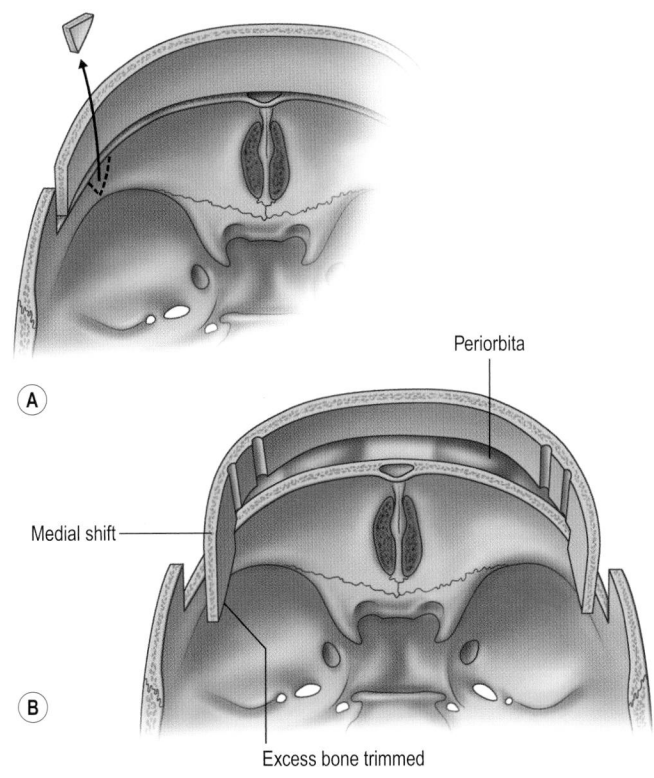

(A)

Periorbita

Medial shift

(B)

Excess bone trimmed

Fig. 35.5 (A, B) When there is an anomalous increase in frontotemporal width, skull base osteotomies can be performed: these are designed to narrow the bandeau while simultaneously advancing and lowering the supraorbits.

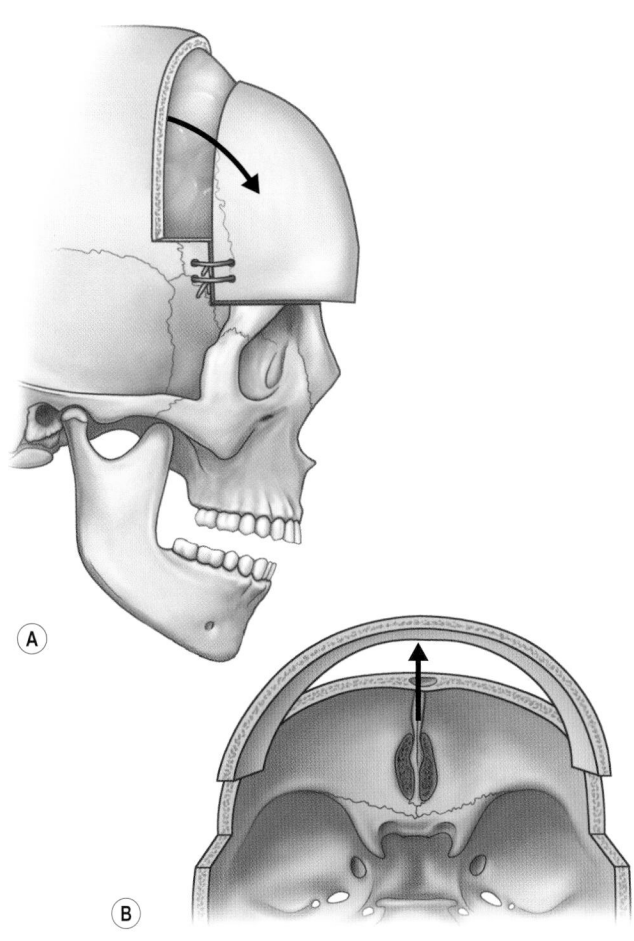

(A)

(B)

Fig. 35.6 (A) As an alternative to using a standard bandeau, a low frontal osteotomy can be performed to remove almost the entire frontal bone. **(B)** This bone segment is then repositioned (or rotated 180°) and inset in a more anterior and inferior position. This particular design permits preservation of frontal sinus (avoiding potential contamination), and is particularly useful when the lower bandeau is of poor quality.

The midvault decompression procedure requires removal and replacement of the parietal bones, with a special focus on those areas of abnormal compression *(Fig. 35.8)*. This procedure can be demanding as keels of bone are often encountered, which extend deeply into the sulci of the brain *(Fig. 35.9)*. The performance of any procedure at this early stage of growth means that a subsequent cranial vault enlargement will almost certainly be needed before the child has reached 18 months of age, or earlier. Careful monitoring for clinical signs for elevated pressure, and the development of an acquired Chiari malformation, needs to be performed. Recently, some authors have advocated performing posterior skull distractions in infancy.[64] The current downsides to this technique appear to include: the requirement for two operative procedures (one to place the device and the other to remove it), the likelihood for higher complication rates (from mechanical problems), and the fact that the use of distraction devices has not been shown to offer any advantages over decompressive procedures. In addition, because of the relative softness on bone in infancy, early distraction often creates an undesirable skull configuration, with an accentuated prominence noted at the device–bone interface. Hopefully, comparative studies will be performed in the future that may further elucidate the indications, if any, for calvarial distraction. Finally, all anterior cranial vault advancements performed in early childhood should be accompanied by the placement of absorbable suture temporary tarsorraphies, in order to prevent postoperative chemosis, which in children with significant proptosis may result in blindness.[30]

The second major area of treatment for patients with syndromic craniosynostosis is the compromised airway that can result from the associated mid facial hypoplasia. Patients who present with mid facial deficiencies need to be followed both clinically and with serial polysomnography. The determination of the ideal time for surgical advancement of the midface is based on two indications. The first is the development of obstructive sleep apnea, which is not amenable to any less invasive correction (i.e., medication, tonsillectomy, and use of a continuous positive airway pressure mask at night). Although some authors have reported mid facial advancement in infancy, these early advancements are at best only transiently helpful and, pending supportive studies, this early intervention cannot currently be recommended.[31,32,65] Therefore, for younger children presenting with refractory obstructive sleep apnea, the author favors placement of a temporary tracheostomy until the patient is over 5 years of age, at which time a mid facial advancement can be safely and effectively performed.

The second indication for a mid facial advancement is based on the child's psychosocial development. Typically,

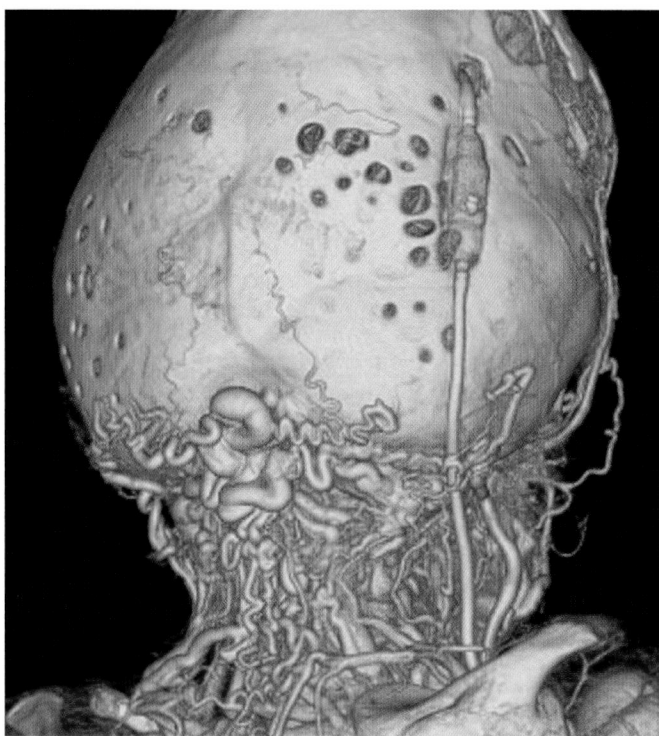

Fig. 35.7 Low, posteriorly draining enlarged transcranial veins are commonly seen with the more severe phenotypic presentations of Apert and Pfeiffer syndrome. Ideally, these vessels should be preserved in order to avoid potentially life-threatening brain edema.

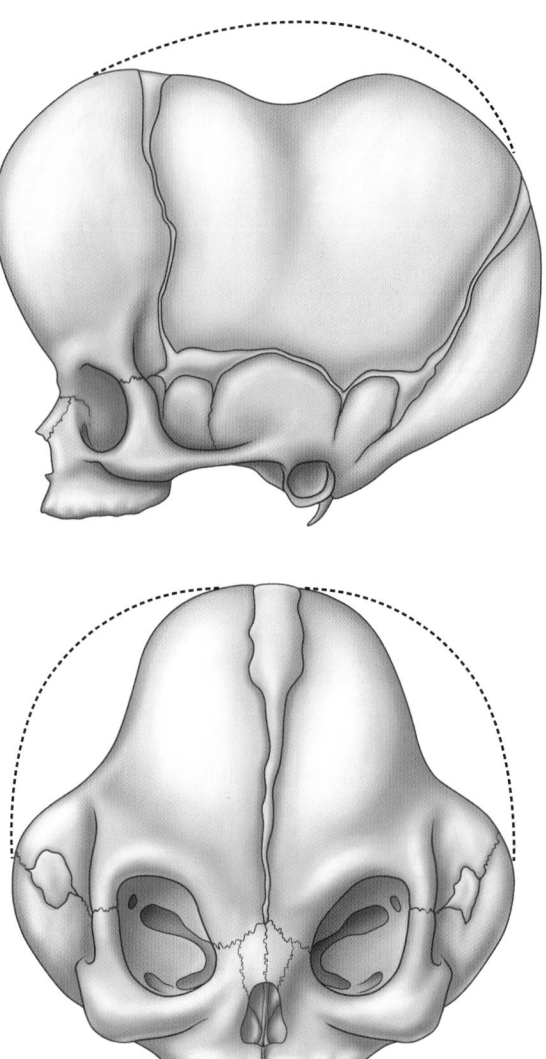

Fig. 35.8 A midvault cranioplasty can effectively decompress infants affected with pansynostosis. This procedure entails careful removal and replacement of the abnormally indented parietal bones.

issues associated with appearance will present later in childhood, and vary with numerous social factors. Children's parents are best suited to ascertain when teasing is beginning to have an effect on their child. Although a number of different osteotomy patterns have been described for advancing the hypoplastic midface, they can all be placed into one of two basic groups: (1) those requiring intracranial exposure; and (2) those that do not. Of the intracranial advancements, the most commonly used technique is the frontofacial advancement (also known as "the monobloc"), first described by Ortiz-Monasterio *et al. (Fig. 35.10)*.[66] This procedure has the advantage of simultaneously advancing the midface, and enlarging the anterior cranial fossa, potentially saving the child an additional operative procedure.

Another intracranial mid facial advancement is the facial bipartition *(Fig. 35.11)*.[67–70] Although initially described for the treatment of hypertelorism, the bipartition can also be used to advance the midface, while simultaneously reducing intraorbital distance, and theoretically sagittally bending the midface in a more aesthetically pleasing way. The subcranial mid facial advancement is achieved utilizing a Le Fort III osteotomy pattern *(Fig. 35.12)*. In skeletally mature patients with permanent dentition, the Le Fort III osteotomy can be combined with a Le Fort I osteotomy, which permits simultaneous vertical lengthening of the midface *(Fig. 35.13)*. While many surgeons chose to correct mid facial hypoplasia utilizing a monobloc procedure, at the current time most surgeons prefer the subcranial Le Fort III. The popularity of the Le Fort III may be for a number of reasons, including: the indications for enlarging the anterior cranial fossa and advancing the

midface rarely correspond temporally; the midface usually requires a differential advancement (typically, two to three times the amount of advancement needed for the forehead); and the reported complication rates for frontofacial advancements are much higher than with the subcranial procedures (because of the necessary breach of the anterior floor of the frontal fossa, exposing the intracranial space to the nasal sinuses).[71]

The greatest challenges facing any type of mid facial advancement are in actually obtaining the required advancement, and being able to achieve the necessary stabilization. These challenges, especially in the younger growing child, lead a number of craniofacial surgeons to turn to utilization of distraction techniques. Currently, two types of distraction techniques are being used: (1) laterally based semiburied distraction devices; and (2) centrally based external halo devices *(Figs 35.14 and 35.15)*.[31,72–77] Of these two techniques, the centrally based halo distraction offers the advantages of providing a better correction of the central "dish face" deformity, allowing manipulation of the distraction vector postoperatively, and having a lower complication rate (this technique has been reportedly used to salvage semiburied device failures).[75,78] For many reasons, advancement of the midface in skeletally immature children needs to focus on positioning the malar eminences in an overcorrected position, and should not in any way attempt to normalize occlusal relationships. To begin with, the maxilla typically shows no forward growth following mid facial advancement, while the mandible will continue to grow postoperatively.[79–82] In addition, correction of the vertical maxillary hypoplasia needs to wait until the eruption of secondary dentition is complete, at which time either an isolated Le Fort I or a Le Fort III with a Le Fort I can be performed in order to accomplish the required vertical facial lengthening.[75]

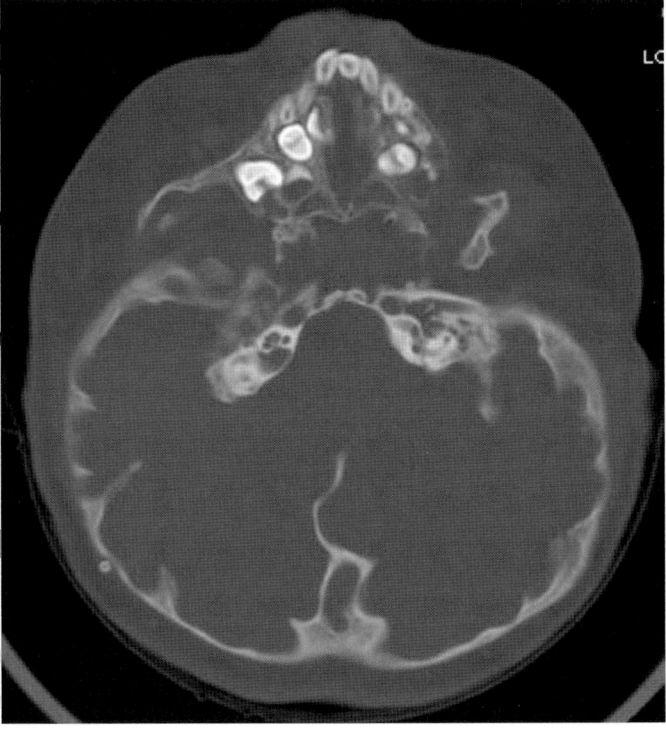

Fig. 35.9 Posterior keels of bone, which extend deep into dural invaginations, can be expected in patients with pansynostoses, particularly Pfeiffer syndrome.

Postoperative care

Both cranial remodeling procedures and mid facial advancements are often associated with moderate to massive amounts of blood loss, and may be further complicated by challenging airways.[83–85] As a result, the postoperative care of patients with syndromic craniosynostosis requires comprehensive pediatric anesthetic and intensive care management. The ability to minimize blood loss, and resultant volume shifts, can substantially contribute to a smoother postoperative recovery. With increased surgical experience, operative times are typically reduced. Moreover, techniques such as preoperative erythropoietin administration, intraoperative blood recycling, the judicious use of bone wax, and the use of meticulous electrocautery may all help to minimize the need for perioperative blood transfusions.[86,87] Postoperatively, "third-space" volume shifts occur secondary to changes in capillary permeability, leading to the accumulation of fluid in both the intracranial advanced epidural "dead space" and subgaleal space. Hemoglobin levels will generally fall over the first few postoperative days, prior to reaching equilibrium 3–4 days later. As the estimated blood loss approaches a majority of the patient's calculated total blood volume, it is important to monitor for potential dilutional coagulopathies. Disturbances in acid–base balance can also be expected from intraoperative

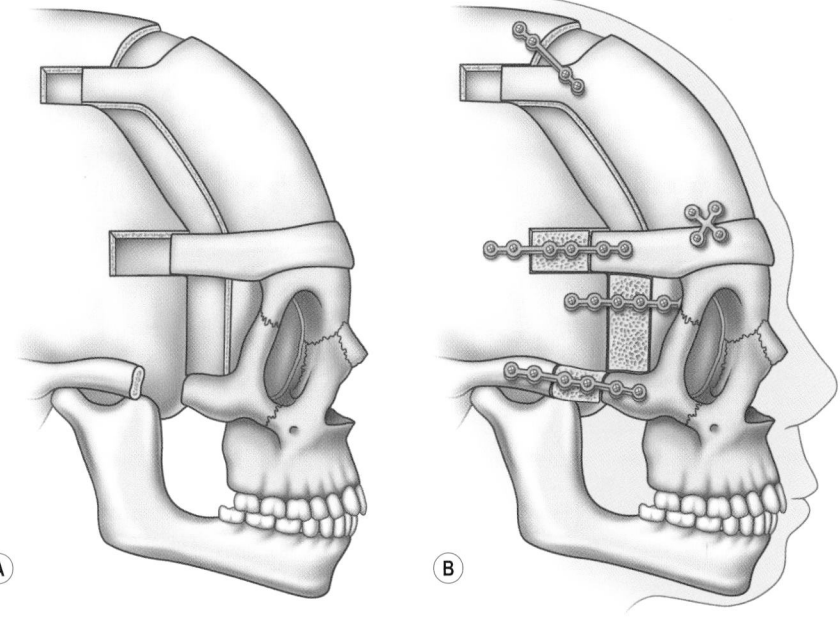

(A)　　　(B)

Fig. 35.10 (A) The monobloc frontofacial advancement simultaneously enlarges the anterior cranial fossa and advances the midface. **(B)** However this procedure does result in a connection between the sinuses and the intracranial cavity, necessitating placement of some biologic barrier (i.e., pericranial flap) to separate these two spaces, or use of distraction techniques.

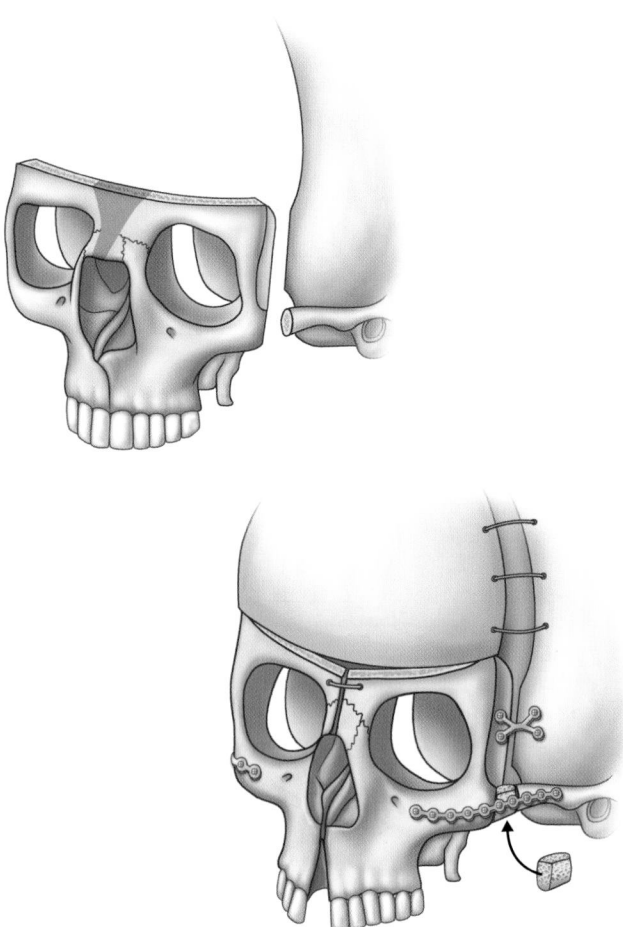

Fig. 35.11 The facial bipartition splits the midface through a combined intracranial and extracranial exposure. This permits simultaneous mid facial advancement, reduction in the intraorbital distance, and sagittal bending of the face. This procedure also results in a connection between the sinuses and the intracranial cavity, necessitating placement of some biologic barrier (i.e., pericranial flap) to isolate these two spaces.

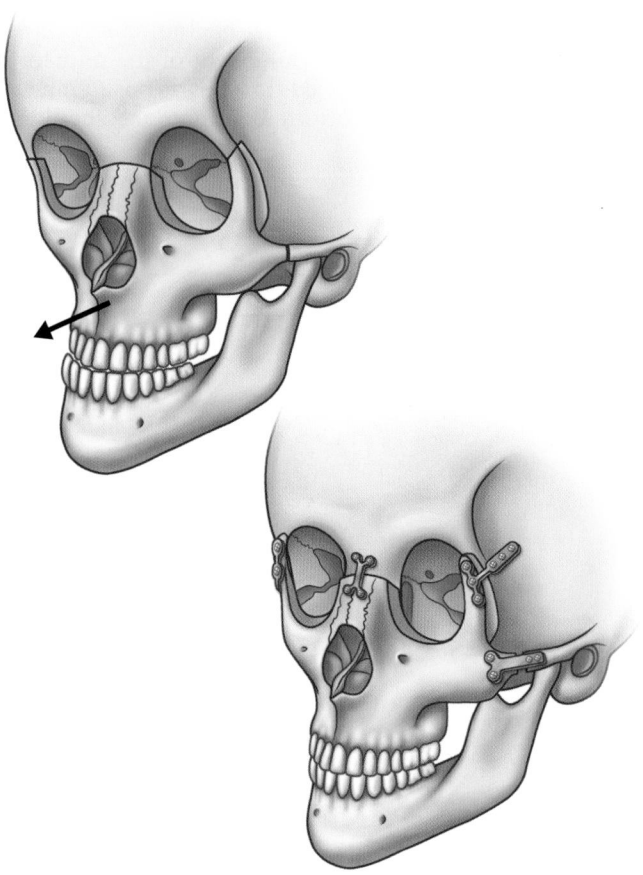

Fig. 35.12 The traditional Le Fort III osteotomy is a subcranial procedure that advances the midface as a single segment. Lateral orbital z-plasties help to stabilize the advancement.

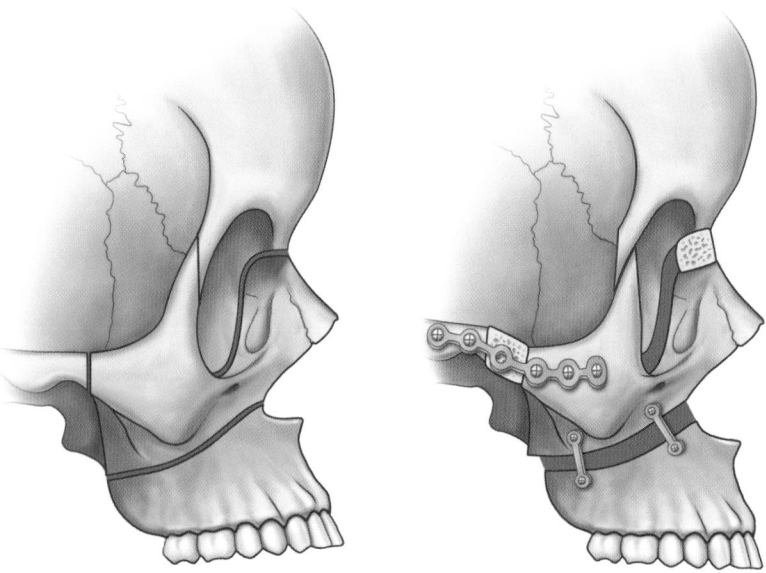

Fig. 35.13 The Le Fort III with a Le Fort I is a two-piece mid facial advancement that permits vertical facial lengthening and idealization of the dental occlusion, while independently repositioning the malar eminences.+

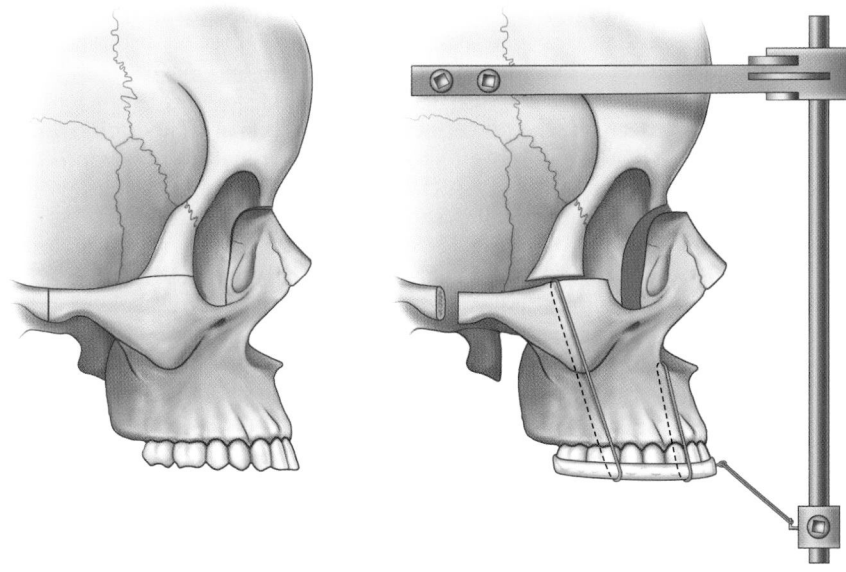

Fig. 35.14 The halo distraction Le Fort III utilizes low lateral orbital straight-line osteotomies, and offers the potential for significantly greater maxillary advancements. This technique permits vector changes postoperatively, during the advancement phase.

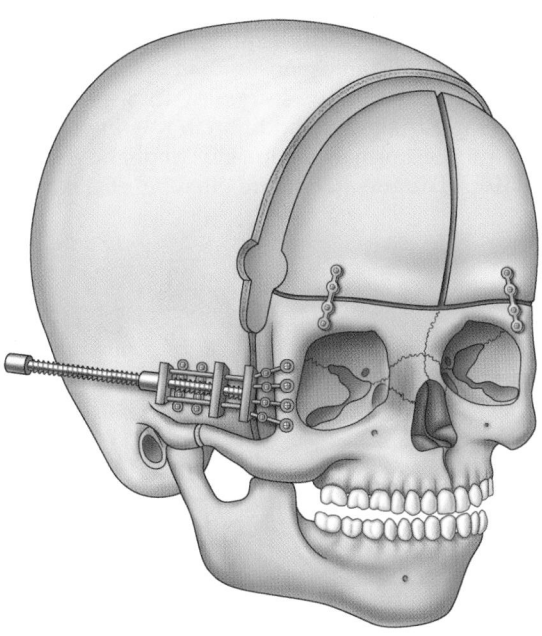

Fig. 35.15 Semiburied lateral facial distraction devices can be used to advance either a subcranial Le Fort III osteotomy, or a monobloc (pictured). These devices do not permit vector changes during distraction, and may exacerbate a central "dish face" deformity.

hypoperfusion-associated anaerobic metabolism (resulting in lactic acid production), which can be exacerbated by hypoventilation immediately following extubation (especially with subsequent narcotic administration). Some pediatric intensivists will choose to treat this postoperative acidosis with sodium bicarbonate, which may result in secondary hypokalemia (from the intracellular transport of potassium).[88] Other intensive care specialists argue that it is better to allow this early acidosis to correct on its own without intervention, as the perioperative hypoventilation abates and normal ventilation permits the loss of carbon dioxide.

It is also important to follow the patient's overall mental status closely, in order to monitor for the potential development of a subcranial hematoma, or for the syndrome of inappropriate antidiuretic hormone (which, when identified, is best initially treated with a restriction in free water intake).[89,90] For those children undergoing mid facial advancements, airway monitoring is critically important, and protocols for managing airway compromise need to be established, and readily implemented when necessary.

Outcomes, prognosis, and complications

Measuring treatment outcomes in syndromic craniosynostosis is a challenging endeavor, given that the goals of surgery (the prevention of developmental delays and the normalization of appearance) result in outcomes that are exceedingly difficult to quantify. Few studies have examined the need for secondary procedures following primary craniosynostosis corrections, and these have reported reoperative rates between 2 and 13%.[50,59,91,92] Only one study has focused on reoperative rates in the syndromic synsotoses, and this study cited a reoperative rate of 37%, with an average 6-year follow-up.[93] Unfortunately, none of these studies evaluate reoperative rates at skeletal maturity, and most do not even define the criteria used to decide the need for a secondary procedure. A number of factors can potentially influence the need for secondary cranial vault remodeling procedures: the age of the initial operation (with earlier surgery resulting in more total procedures), the degree of growth inhibition (which is partially syndrome-related), the success of the procedure, and the criteria used to determine the need for a secondary procedure. There are no long-term assessments of cognitive function; however, some studies suggest a correlation between early surgery and higher IQ scores (although these retrospective study cannot show causation).[51,94]

Outcomes have been evaluated following Le Fort III halo distraction, and these studies have documented postoperative skeletal stability without relapse; although following distraction, no further forward growth of the maxilla has been noted.[79,82] While some studies have measured improvements in airway diameter following Le Fort III distraction, only one has assessed changes in postoperative ventilation (measured by pre- and postoperative polysomnography), and this study confirmed improvements in airway exchange.[79,95,96] While few studies have tried to assess treatment outcomes, complication rates have been more extensively examined. Infection rates following cranial vault remodeling procedures have been reported to be between 2.5% and 6.5%, with secondary procedures and longer operative times cited as potential risk factors.[97–99] A number of retrospective studies have examined mortality rates following intracranial procedures. These reports suggest an experience-related decline in mortality rates, with incidences falling from 2.2% to 0.1%.[100–105]

Secondary procedures

Aside from the two major craniofacial procedures (cranial vault remodeling and mid facial advancement) that are typically required for treatment of the syndromic craniosynostoses, a number of adjunctive procedures have been described: some that are often beneficial, and others that are probably unnecessary. Although a few authors have reported the need for intracranial hypertelorism corrections in patients with syndromic synostosis, this author believes that these procedures are almost never useful.[106,107] This is because, in most instances,

the increased intraorbital distance actually falls within the mild to mild-to-moderate range of telorbitism, which does not satisfy the usual requirements for directed orbital translation.[108] In addition, with appropriate mid facial advancement, the nasal dorsum can be brought forward sufficiently to decrease the perception of any significant hypertelorism.

All children affected with Apert syndrome require treatment for their associated syndactylies, and numerous techniques for digital separation have been reported.[109,110] The author prefers a two-staged approach to separate all 10 fingers and toes; however, this comprehensive treatment paradigm requires a dedicated team approach.[111] As the skeletal growth approaches completion, digital osteotomies are usually necessary to correct the clinodactyly that may occur.

With the completion of facial growth, if malar projection is relatively normal, an isolated Le Fort I is typically required both to maximize occlusal relationships, and to lengthen the midface vertically. Following this orthognathic procedure, additional malar augmentation can be realized by the use of allogenic implants (which in some cases may mitigate the need for a repeat Le Fort III). Some surgeons are currently exploring the use of "structural fat grafting"; however, there are not yet any compelling long-term data evaluating permanency.

Lastly, a rhinoplasty is typically required for most children affected with syndromic craniosynostosis, in order to correct the "beak deformity" that occurs secondary to displacement of the lower lateral cartilages. In addition to rotating the alar cartilages into a more normal relationship, cephalic rotation of the tip and dorsal augmentation are often beneficial.

Access the complete references list online at **http://www.expertconsult.com**

2. Goodrich JT, Tutino M. An annotated history of craniofacial surgery and intentional cranial deformation. *Neurosurg Clin North Am.* 2001;12:45–68, viii.

7. Marchac D. Radical forehead remodeling for craniostenosis. *Plast Reconstr Surg.* 1978;61:823–835.
   This classic article marks the progression from treating craniosynostosis with strip craniectomies to a true remodeling procedure. It was also one of the earliest to depict a frontal bandeau.

11. Gillies H, Harrison SH. Operative correction by osteotomy of recessed malar maxillary compound in a case of oxycephaly. *Br J Plast Surg.* 1950;3:123–127.
    This is the first description of a Le Fort III-type osteotomy for advancing the midface. Although his osteotomy lines did not actually follow the "true" Le Fort III pattern, this report is the first to attempt to advance the "whole face and palate."

13. Tessier P. The definitive plastic surgical treatment of the severe facial deformities of craniofacial dysostosis. Crouzon's and Apert's diseases. *Plast Reconstr Surg.* 1971;48:419–442.
    It is likely that patients presenting with Apert and Crouzon syndrome were the real catalyst that spurred Tessier to develop techniques upon which the foundations of craniofacial surgery were built. This article describes some of Tessier's early forays into treating these rare anomalies.

30. Fearon JA, Rhodes J. Pfeiffer syndrome: a treatment evaluation. *Plast Reconstr Surg.* 2009;123:1560–1569.
    This article is one of the first to describe the comprehensive care of patients with Pfeiffer syndrome, and details a more updated approach to treating the syndromic craniosynostosis.

34. Renier D, Sainte-Rose C, Marchac D, et al. Intracranial pressure in craniostenosis. *J Neurosurg.* 1982;57:370–377.

66. Ortiz-Monasterio F, del Campo AF, Carrillo A. Advancement of the orbits and the midface in one piece, combined with frontal repositioning, for the correction of Crouzon's deformities. *Plast Reconstr Surg.* 1978;61:507–516.
    This paper is the earliest description of a combined "orbitofacial advancement," which was later to become known as the monobloc advancement.

79. Fearon JA. Halo distraction of the Le Fort III in syndromic craniosynostosis: a long-term assessment. *Plast Reconstr Surg.* 2005;115:1524–1536.

93. McCarthy JG, Glasberg SB, Cutting CB, et al. Twenty-year experience with early surgery for craniosynostosis: II. The craniofacial synostosis syndromes and pansynostosis – results and unsolved problems. *Plast Reconstr Surg.* 1995;96:284–295; discussion 96–8.

105. Whitaker LA, Munro IR, Salyer KE, et al. Combined report of problems and complications in 793 craniofacial operations. *Plast Reconstr Surg.* 1979;64:198–203.

36

Craniofacial microsomia

Joseph G. McCarthy, Barry H. Grayson, Richard A. Hopper, and Oren M. Tepper

SYNOPSIS

- Patients with craniofacial microsomia (CFM) require the care of a skilled multidisciplinary clinical team.
- Phenotypic features of CFM are highly variable. While the three structures most commonly affected include the auricle, mandible, and maxilla, abnormal development can occur in any of the derivatives of the first or second branchial arches.
- During the evaluation of CFM, it is essential to assess for retroglossal airspace narrowing and obstructive sleep apnea via endoscopy and sleep studies, particularly in bilateral cases.
- Distraction osteogenesis (DO) of the mandible should be considered in neonates and infants with CFM who exhibit severe respiratory compromise and who may otherwise require a tracheostomy.
- Vectors of mandible distraction (vertical, oblique, or horizontal) should be planned according to treatment goals.
- In cases of severe mandibular hypoplasia, staged procedures with grafting (nonvascularized or vascularized bone) should be performed, often followed by DO.
- If two-jaw surgery is to be performed for CFM, a two-splint (intermediate splint) technique is used and the technique is usually deferred until skeletal maturity has been achieved.
- Orthodontic monitoring is important throughout the years of growth and development. Interventions are especially important during and after the distraction process to prevent undesired movements (i.e., anterior open bite, lateral shift) and in the period surrounding two-jaw surgery.

 Access the Historical Perspective section online at
http://www.expertconsult.com

Basic science/disease process

Incidence

The reported incidence of CFM ranges from 1 in 3500 to 1 in 26 550 live births, with a commonly quoted incidence of 1 in 5600 live births. When one considers the presence of congenital ear tags and mild unilateral mandibular hypoplasia, the incidence is obviously much higher. It is the second most common craniofacial anomaly after cleft lip and palate.

Grabb reported a male predominance, with a male-to-female ratio of 63 : 39, and Rollnick reported a similar ratio of 191 : 103. The clinical series of Horgan *et al.* reported an equal sex ratio of 59 males to 62 females.

Etiopathogenesis

The underlying cause or etiopathogenesis of CFM remains a subject of debate. The prevailing theory was that CFM was a sporadic event, possibly precipitated by exposure to teratogens. Other studies have instead suggested a fundamental role for genetic transmission in some patients. The etiology of CFM is probably heterogeneous among individuals, with variable contributions from extrinsic and intrinsic factors. Support for a teratogenic etiology of CFM is based largely on animal studies. Poswillo exposed mouse embryos to triazine by maternal administration of the drug, causing CFM-like phenotypes *(Fig. 36.1)*. Focal hematomas arising from disruption of the stapedial artery were also observed. Although a "stapedial artery hemorrhage etiology" is attractive because the vessel is a second branchial arch derivative, a causative association between the bleeding and the deformities has not been made. The hemorrhages occurred 14 days after administration of the teratogen, and there was no clear temporal relationship between the hemorrhage appearance and the associated phenotypic deformity. When mice are exposed to triazine later in development (10 days of gestation), all animals developed deformities; however, only a third showed evidence of a hematoma. The authors concluded that triazine has a direct teratogenic effect and the stapedial artery findings were simply a side-effect. In contrast to those described by Poswillo, these animals demonstrated more evidence of bilateral deformities and inner-ear anomalies. Intermittent occlusion of the internal carotid system of fetal sheep late in gestation has been shown to result in deformities similar in

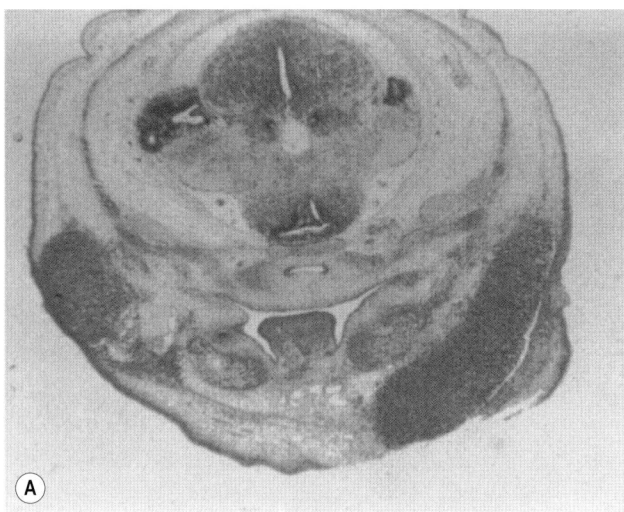
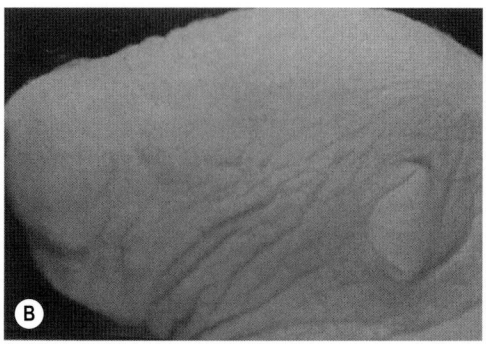
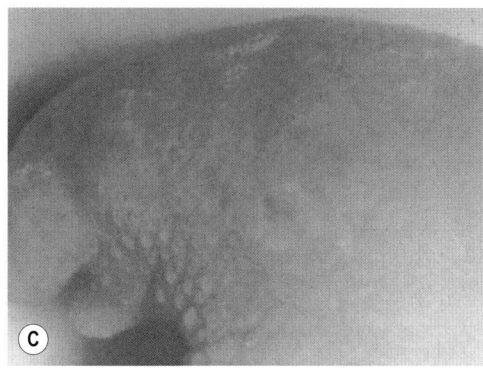

Fig. 36.1 Mouse phenocopy of craniofacial microsomia induced by the administration of triazine. **(A)** Histologic section of the head showing bilateral hematomas. The smaller one is in the ear region (right), and the large one encompasses the ramus and angle of the mandible (left). **(B)** Upper panel, normal ear–jaw relationship at full term in the normal animal. Lower panel, the diminutive helix and abnormal mandible in the unilateral craniofacial microsomia phenocopy. (Reproduced from Poswillo D. The pathogenesis of the Treacher–Collins syndrome [mandibulofacial dysostosis]. *Br J Oral Surg*. 1975;13;1.)

appearance to CFM. The vascular disruption hypothesis, therefore, cannot be excluded.

Rats exposed to etretinate, a retinoic acid derivative, show deformities comparable to the first and second branchial arch syndromes. This finding is consistent with the finding that neural crest cells express large amounts of retinoic acid-binding proteins. Furthermore, when retinoic acid is administered early in development, it interferes with cell migration. When administered later in gestation, however, retinoic acid kills ganglionic placodal cells, resulting in a deformity similar to mandibulofacial dysostosis (Treacher–Collins).

Human case studies also support a teratogen-based etiology for CFM. Thalidomide and ethanol administration during pregnancy and gestational diabetes are exogenous other factors that have been implicated.

Support of a genetic etiology of CFM has come from both animal and human studies. A transgenic mouse model for CFM with an insertional deletion on mouse chromosome 10 has been described with an autosomal-dominant mode of transmission and 25% penetration. The affected animals display low-set ears, unilateral microtia, and jaw asymmetry, without evidence of middle-ear abnormality. Second branchial arch hematomas were also observed in the embryos.

Human genetics studies have documented a positive family history in 9.4% of 32 probands, 21% of 57 probands, 26% of 88 probands, and 44% of 82 probands. Kaye *et al*. performed segregation analysis on 74 families of probands with CFM and rejected the hypothesis that genetic transmission is not a causative factor. The evidence favored autosomal-dominant inheritance; however, recessive and polygenic models were not distinguishable. Despite the suggestion of autosomal-dominant transmission, they found only a 2–3% overall recurrence rate in first-degree relatives. This figure compares to the 10% recurrence risk in first- and second-degree relatives reported by the same group in an earlier study of 294 individuals with CFM. Graham *et al*. described a family with a strong autosomal-dominant transmission of Goldenhar-like phenotype with linkage to a mutation at locus 8q13.

The high variability and low penetrance of CFM may be explained in terms of genetic transmission by a number of theories. Compensation of defective genes by adjacent normal genes has been described in a cleft palate mouse model, and it may explain the variability of CFM. Another mechanism may be "maternal rescue," a mechanism by which transplacental transfer of a normal maternal gene product may compensate for an abnormal fetal gene. The low penetrance of CFM may be explained by differential expression of maternal and paternal DNA sequences (genomic imprinting) or by only a limited number of cells possessing the abnormal gene (mosaicism).

Studies on the incidence and expression of craniofacial anomalies in twins have provided insight into the etiology of CFM. Mulliken's group described 10 twin pairs with CFM. Only one of the pairs, who were monozygotic, was concordant for the anomaly. Other twin studies have noted a high level of discordance of CFM among monozygotic twins. Even among concordant monozygotic twins, the anomaly can be mirror image. One theory to explain the discordant findings is that vascular insufficiency of the first and second branchial arch occurs in monozygotic twins with a shared placenta (monochorionic) and unequal circulation. Arguing against this is the observation that discordance is not limited to monochorionic twins but is also observed in dichorionic pairs. Monozygotic discordance would appear to refute the teratogen theory of CFM; however, monozygotic twins have been reported to respond to *in utero* teratogens in a discordant manner.

In summary, the exact etiology of CFM is not known. It is likely to involve a number of factors ranging from abnormal genes with various intrinsic modifiers to extrinsic insults such as teratogens or vascular events. It is also probable that, as in patients with cleft palate, the population of patients with CFM is a heterogeneous group. Some individuals with the phenotype may be part of a family with a dominant abnormal gene expression, in which case the recurrence risk would approach 50%. In other individuals with a purely environmental etiology, recurrence would be negligible. The empirically stated recurrence rate of 2–3% for CFM should be recognized as a group summary and placed in context when an individual or family with this phenotype is counseled.

Embryology

The ear serves as a frame of reference in this syndrome because of its developmental relationship with the jaw. A brief review of the phylogeny and ontogeny of the auricle and hearing apparatus is helpful in understanding the embryogenesis of the malformation in the patient with CFM.

The two principal divisions of the organ of hearing are derived from different embryonic anlagen. The sensory organ in the inner ear is derived from the ectodermal otocyst; the sound-conducting apparatus in the external and middle ear comes from the gill structures.

The membranous labyrinth has its beginning in the 3½-week-old human embryo as a thickening of the ectoderm in the side of the head – the otic placode. This area is enfolded to become the otic pit and is subsequently pinched off to become the otocyst. By means of a series of folds, the otocyst differentiates in the 3-month-old fetus into the endolymphatic duct and sac, the semicircular endolymphatic ducts, the utricle, the saccule, and the organ of Corti. By the fifth month of fetal life, the sensory end organ of the ear attains adult form and size as the cartilaginous otic capsule ossifies.

It is speculated that the aquatic ancestors of humans swam in seas not yet as salty as today's oceans and that endolymph, entrapped by the enfolding otocyst, closely resembles in chemical composition the dilute salt water of the primeval sea. Our ancient aquatic forebears did not require any special mechanism to transmit sound to the inner ear. As in today's fish, sound was readily transmitted from the sea through the skin to the fluid of the inner ear.

When these ancestors struggled out of the seas on to dry land, a new problem appeared. A mechanical device was needed to convert air vibrations of large amplitude and small force into fluid vibrations of small amplitude and large force. The gill structures, no longer needed for breathing, became converted into such a mechanism. The first branchial groove became the external auditory meatus and canal; the first pharyngeal pouch became the eustachian tube and middle ear. Instead of the branchial groove and pharyngeal pouch

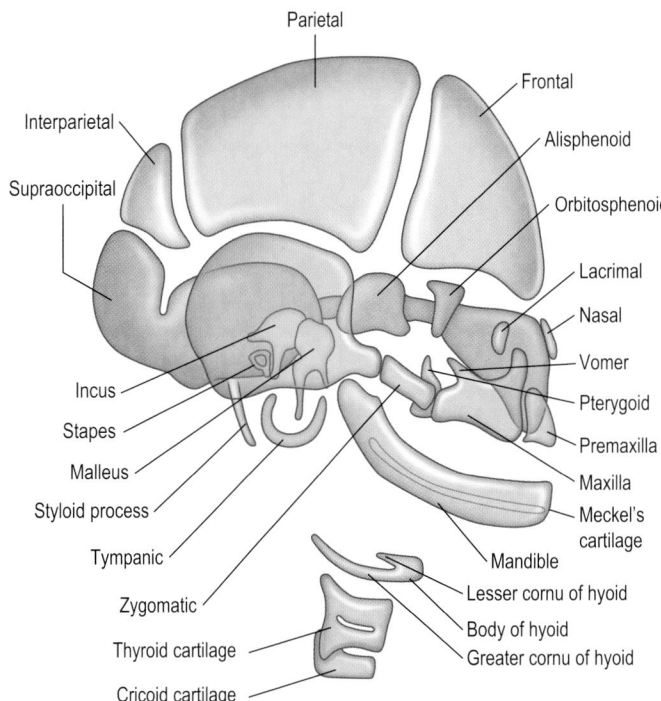

Fig. 36.2 Schematic drawing: the visceral arch cartilages appear in green; the cranial base cartilages appear in purple. The remaining skeletal elements are the intramembranous bones of the face and cranial vault (blue). (Adapted from Hamilton WJ, Mossman H. Human embryology, 4th ed. Cambridge, England: W. Heffer; 1972.)

connecting to become a gill cleft, a thin intervening layer of tissue remained to form the tympanic membrane.

The mandible, incus, and malleus develop from the cartilage of the first branchial arch (Meckel cartilage) *(Fig. 36.2)*. The stapes (with the exception of the footplate, which originates from the otic capsule), styloid process, and hyoid bone develop from the cartilage of the second branchial arch (Reichert cartilage). The large area of the tympanic membrane, connected by the lever system of the ossicular chain to the small area of the oval window, provides the ear with an effective mechanism to overcome the sound barrier between air and water.

By the third fetal month, the external auricle has been formed from the first and second branchial arches on either side of the first branchial groove, which is the primary shallow, funnel-shaped external auditory meatus *(Fig. 36.3)*. From the inner end of the primary meatus, a solid cord of ectodermal cells extends farther inward, with a bulb-like enlargement adjacent to the middle ear. It is not until the seventh fetal month that the cord canalizes, beginning medially to form the tympanic membrane and extending laterally to join with the primary meatus to form the completed external auditory meatus. The external and middle ears, although capable of transmitting sound to the inner ear, are not yet of adult form and size.

In the seventh fetal month, pneumatization of the temporal bone begins. At birth, the eustachian tube inflates; the fetal mesoderm tissue in the middle ear and antrum continues to resorb until the epithelium lies close to the periosteum, and pneumatization of the temporal bone proceeds.

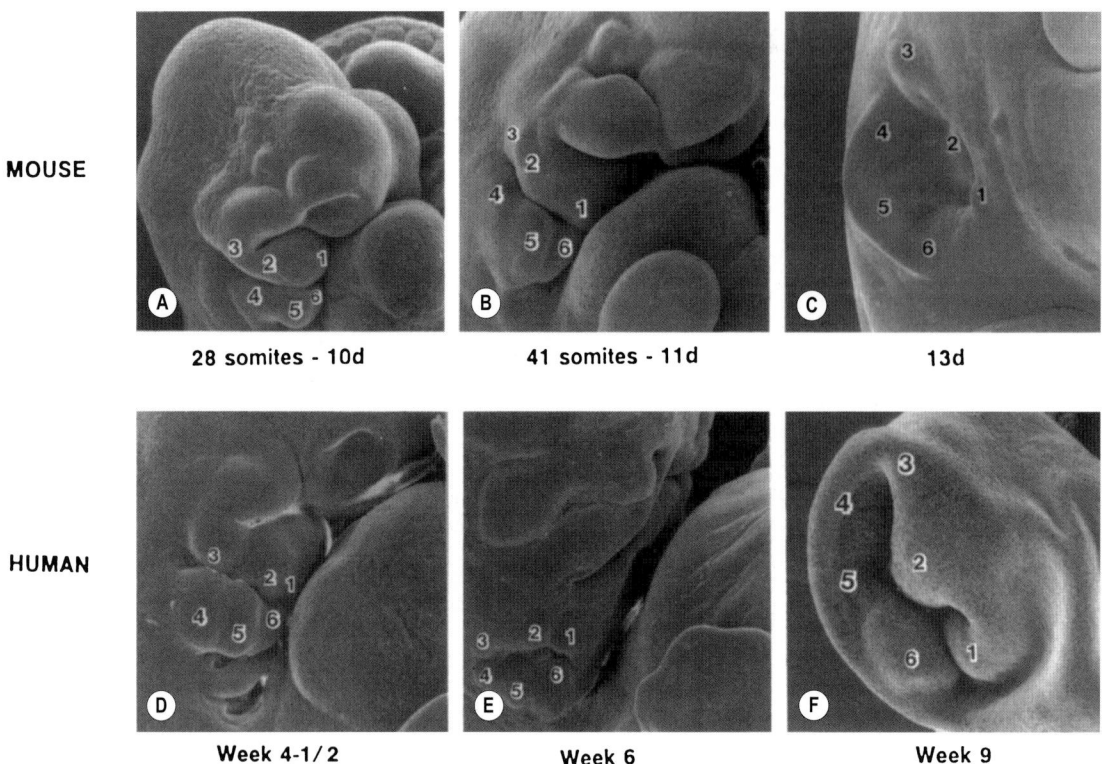

MOUSE

28 somites - 10d   41 somites - 11d   13d

HUMAN

Week 4-1/2   Week 6   Week 9

Fig. 36.3 Comparison of external ear development in the mouse (upper panel), on which most experimental studies have been conducted, and the human (lower panel). The various growth centers (auricular hillocks, which are six in number) are virtually the same in the two species. (Reproduced from Jarvis BL, Sulik KK, Johnston MC. Congenital malformations of the external, middle, and inner ear produced by isotretinoin exposure in fetal mouse embryos. *Otol Head Neck Surg.* 1990;102;391–401.)

The external auditory meatus, entirely cartilaginous at birth (except for the narrow incomplete ring of the tympanic bone), deepens by growth of the tympanic bone to form the adult osseous meatus. Except for pneumatization of the petrous apex, which may continue into adult life, the external and middle ears finally attain adult form and size in late childhood (in contrast to the inner ear, which becomes adult in fetal life). It is generally accepted that the first branchial arch furnishes the anterior part of the auricle; the second arch provides the structures of the remaining external ear.

The maxilla, palatine bone, and zygoma develop from the maxillary process of the first branchial arch, whereas the mandible forms from the mandibular process. Meckel cartilage, the primary jaw of lower vertebrates, represents the temporary skeleton of the first pharyngeal arch; the two symmetric cartilaginous bars describe a parabolic arch that serves as a model and guide in the early morphogenesis of the mandible.

Three main regions of Meckel cartilage should be considered: (1) the distal portion, which becomes incorporated into the anterior part of the body of the mandible; (2) a middle portion, which gives rise to the sphenomandibular ligament and contributes to the mylohyoid groove of the mandible; and (3) the proximal or intratympanic portion, which differentiates into the malleus, the incus, and the anterior malleolar ligament.

Pathology

A fundamental characteristic of the syndrome is the variable manifestation of the pathologic findings.

The deformity in CFM usually has the three major features of auricular, mandibular, and maxillary hypoplasia. The hypoplasia, however, can also involve adjacent anatomic structures: the zygoma, the pterygoid processes of the sphenoid bone, the temporal bone (the middle ear; the mastoid process is small and acellular), the frontal bone, the facial nerve, the muscles of mastication, the parotid, the cutaneous and subcutaneous tissues, the tongue, the soft palate, the pharynx and the floor of the nose.

Whereas the jaw and ear deformities are the most conspicuous in the majority of patients, the first and second branchial arches and the structures derived from them are intimately interlinked with the chondrocranium and membranous bones of the skull; associated deformities of the temporal bone and other cranial bones are inevitable. In extreme forms of the dysplasia, widespread craniofacial involvement is evident *(Fig. 36.4)*. As Pruzansky stated, maldevelopment in one area may trigger a "domino effect," with involvement of the entire craniofacial skeleton including microphthalmos, orbital dystopia, and orbitofacial clefts.

Skeletal tissue

The most conspicuous deformity of unilateral CFM is the hypoplasia of the mandible on the affected side. The ramus is hypoplastic or even absent, and the body of the mandible curves upward to join the vertically reduced ramus. The chin is deviated to the affected side. On the "normal" or "less affected" side, the body of the mandible is also characterized by abnormalities in the skeletal and soft-tissue anatomy. The

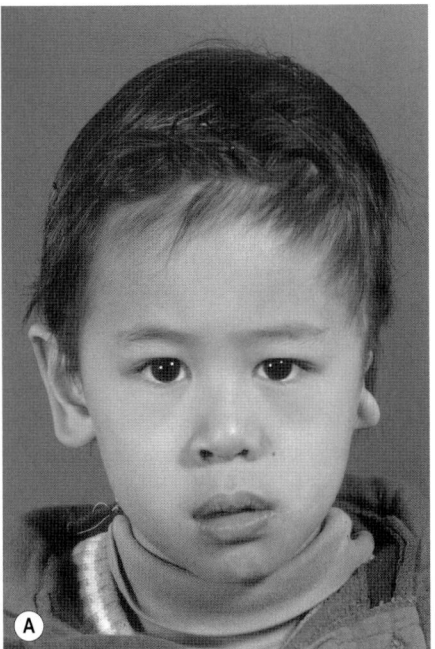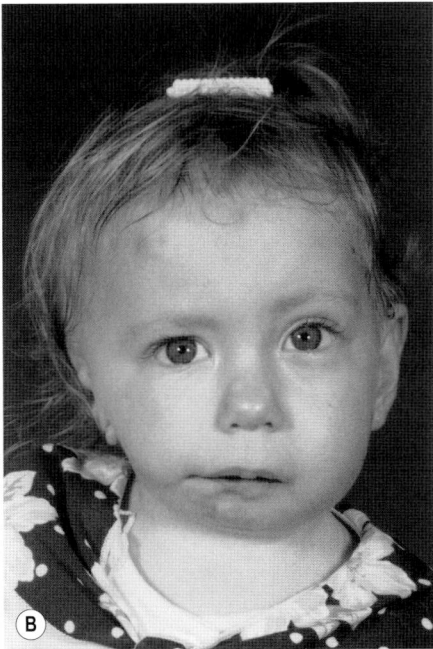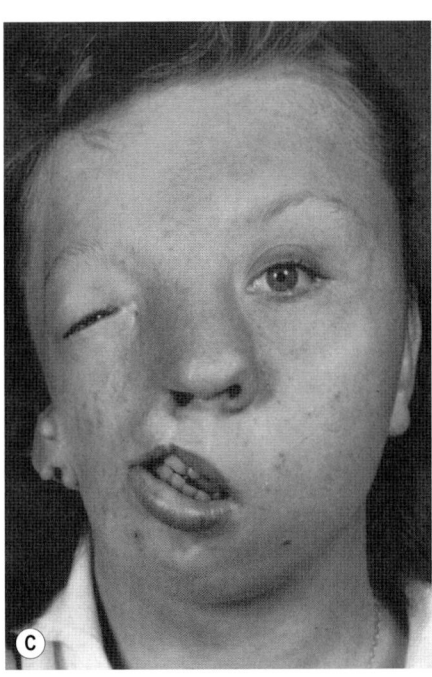

Fig. 36.4 Variable clinical manifestations of unilateral craniofacial microsomia. **(A)** Mild example characterized by microtia, canting of the oral commissure and alar base plane, deficiency of the affected cheek soft tissues, and deviation of the chin to the affected side. **(B)** Moderate example. Note the microtia, deficient cheek soft tissue, macrostomia, canting of the oral commissure, and retruded and deviated chin. **(C)** Severe example with microtia, microphthalmos, retrusion of the brow, occlusal cant, elevation of the oral commissure, and deviation of the chin.

body of the "normal" mandible shows an increased horizontal dimension and an increase in the gonial angle. The increase in length of soft- and hard-tissue structures on the less affected side may represent compensatory growth, secondary to the growth deficiency on the affected side.

Ramus and condyle malformations vary from minimal hypoplasia or blunting of the condyle to its complete absence in association with hypoplasia or agenesis of the ramus *(Fig. 36.5)*. In all patients, condylar anomalies can be demonstrated, and this finding may be pathognomonic of the syndrome. As a consequence, the spatial relationships of the malformed or deficient skeletal parts, as well as the associated neuromuscular components, become of paramount importance in the diagnosis and planning of treatment.

The posterior wall of the glenoid fossa is partially formed by the tympanic portion of the temporal bone, which provides the bony portion of the external auditory canal in the normally developed ear. When there is hypoplasia of the temporal bone, the posterior wall of the glenoid fossa cannot be identified. The infratemporal surface is flat, and the hypoplastic ramus is often hinged on this flat surface at a point anterior to the contralateral "unaffected" temporomandibular joint.

Mandibular growth deficiency usually is closely related to the degree of hypoplasia of the condyle. In more severe conditions there is considerable disparity in condylar growth between the affected and contralateral sides. The cant of the occlusal plane (higher on the affected side) is caused by the short, hypoplastic ramus and by hypoplasia of the ipsilateral maxillary dentoalveolar process *(Fig. 36.6)*. The floor of the maxillary sinus and of the nose on the affected side is canted at a higher level. In some patients, the base of the skull is elevated on an inclined plane similar to the inclined occlusal plane. Anteroposterior and superoinferior dentoalveolar and

skeletal dimensions are reduced on the affected side. Crowded dentition, with a characteristic tilt of the anterior maxillary and mandibular occlusal planes upward on the affected side, is often noted.

Craniofacial bones other than the mandible or maxilla can be involved, especially the tympanic and mastoid portions of the temporal bone; the petrous portion usually is remarkably spared. The styloid process is frequently smaller on the affected side. The mastoid process can have a flattened appearance, and there can be partial or complete lack of pneumatization of the mastoid air cells *(Fig. 36.7)*.

The zygoma can be underdeveloped in all its dimensions, with flattening of the malar eminence. A decrease in the span of the zygomatic arch results in a decrease in the length of the lateral canthal–tragal line on the affected side.

Disparities in the vertical axis of the orbit can be seen, with or without evidence of microphthalmos *(Fig. 36.8)*. Often in this situation, there is flattening of the ipsilateral frontal bone – an appearance of plagiocephaly without radiographic evidence of coronal synostosis.

Nonskeletal (soft) tissue

The relationship between the soft tissue and skeletal dysmorphology of CFM is not fully understood. One theory is that they are independent manifestations of the same genetic or environmental event. Another possibility is that one is primarily involved, whereas the other is only a secondary event.

The "functional matrix" theory of Moss attributes the overall growth and development of the head to the development of the soft-tissue matrix and functional spaces. The matrix is composed of cells, tissues, organs, and air volumes

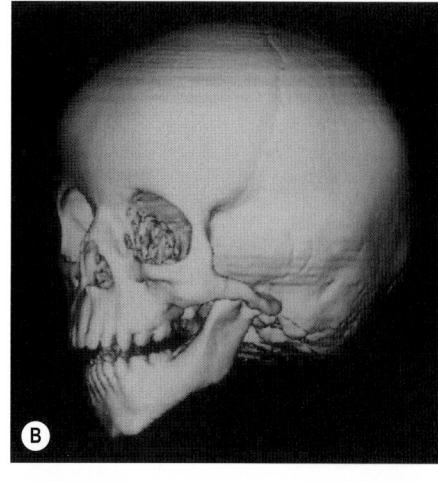
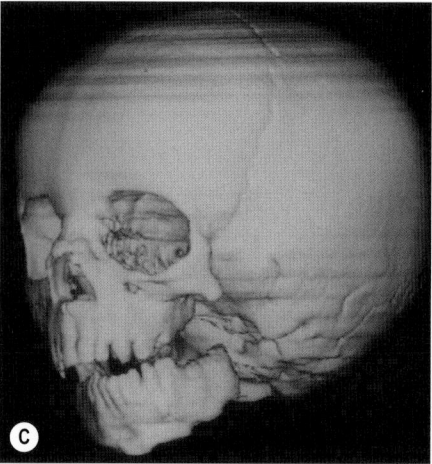
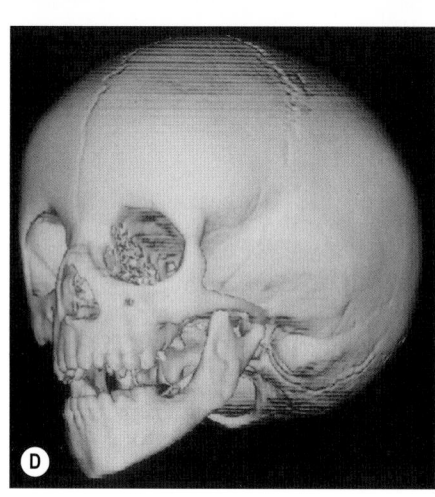
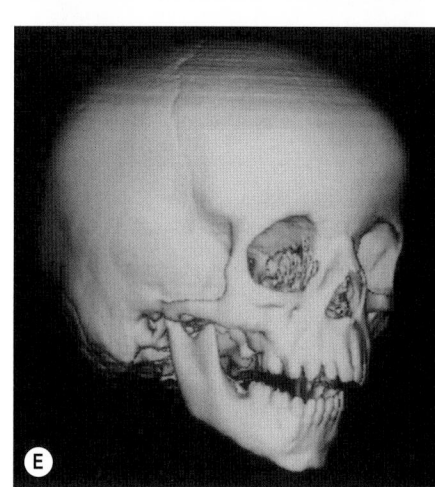
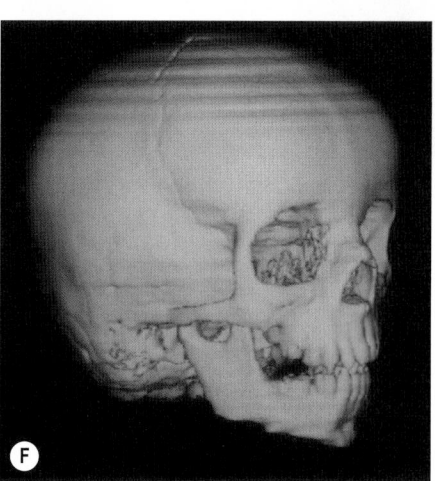

Fig. 36.5 Three-dimensional computed tomography scans of three unilateral craniofacial microsomia cases demonstrating increasing severity as viewed from left to right. The affected side of each case is on the top panel, with the corresponding normal or contralateral side on the lower panel. The three cases correspond to the Pruzansky classification of mandibular deformity described later in the chapter: class I (left), class II (center), class III (right).

that serve a functional role. The associated "hard" tissues, such as bone and cartilage, serve to protect and support the functional matrix. Their morphology is solely determined by the functional matrix. As summarized by Moss, "bones do not grow, they are grown." This theory has been supported by animal research examining the effect of transposition of muscles of mastication on bone morphology. Investigation of the effect of soft tissue on bone shape in humans with unilateral CFM has been limited to computed tomographic (CT) analysis. Results of these studies do suggest that changes in the muscles of mastication can elicit a postnatal change in bone morphology but that the opposite – bone changes affecting muscle – does not take place *(Fig. 36.9)*. It can be speculated that, if the functional matrix theory is validated, future treatment of CFM may be limited to early manipulation of the soft-tissue matrix to elicit a secondary effect on the associated bone.

Muscles of mastication

Muscle function, especially that of the lateral pterygoid muscle, is impaired in many patients with CFM. The right

muscle is responsible for the lateral movement of the mandible to the left side, whereas the left muscle controls movement to the right. Both sides act synergistically in executing protrusive opening movements. In patients with CFM, a severe limitation of protrusive and lateral movements secondary to hypoplasia of the lateral pterygoid muscle is observed.

The impact of this factor is apparent both on the developing musculature and on the morphology of the attached bone. An alteration in mandibular movements (opening, lateral, and protrusive) comparable with the degree of mandibular deficiency is often noted.

When the patient opens the mouth, the deviation toward the affected side is produced not only by the skeletal asymmetry but also by the minimal or absent contribution of the ipsilateral medial and lateral pterygoid muscles in countering the opposing actions of the muscles on the unaffected side. The condyle on the less affected side is displaced abnormally downward and laterally when the mandible is depressed, almost to the point of dislocating the condyle from the glenoid fossa. No discernible condylar movement can be elicited on the affected side during opening and protrusive movements of the mandible. Thus, in testing for lateral pterygoid muscle weakness, one finds an inability to shift the jaw laterally

Congenital hearing loss may be due to a malformed inner ear, hypoplasia of the cochlear nerve and brainstem auditory nuclei, or hypoplasia and impaired function of cranial nerves IX through XII.

Nervous system

A wide variety of cerebral anomalies exist in CFM and may include ipsilateral cerebral hypoplasia, hypoplasia of the corpus callosum, hydrocephalus of the communicating type and obstructive type, intracranial lipoma, and hypoplasia and impression of the brainstem and cerebellum. Other associated abnormalities include cognitive delay, epilepsy, and encephalographic findings suggestive of epilepsy.

Cranial nerve abnormalities are frequent in CFM and can range from arhinencephaly of the bilateral type and unilateral type to unilateral agenesis and hypoplasia of the optic nerve with secondary changes in the lateral geniculate body and visual cortex, congenital ophthalmoplegia and Duane retraction syndrome, hypoplasia of the trochlear and abducens nuclei and nerves, congenital trigeminal anesthesia, and aplasia of the trigeminal nerve and motor and sensory nucleus.

The most common cranial nerve anomaly is facial paralysis secondary to agenesis of the facial nerve in the temporal bone or hypoplasia of the intracranial portion of the facial nerve and facial nucleus in the brainstem. Any cranial nerve can be clinically involved in patients with CFM, and it is likely that hypoplasia or agenesis of a portion of the entire cranial nerve trunk and corresponding brainstem nuclei represents the pathoanatomic substrate of the clinical dysfunction. In the clinical setting the most common finding is dysfunction of the marginal mandibular nerve on the affected side.

Skin and subcutaneous tissue

The deficiency of soft tissues on the affected side in CFM is evident from the reduced distance between the mastoid process and the oral commissure or lateral canthus of the eye. The skin and subcutaneous tissue show varying degrees of hypoplasia, particularly in the parotid-masseteric and auriculomastoid areas. Hypoplasia or aplasia of the parotid gland can place the branches of the facial nerve in a superficial and surgically vulnerable position.

In the series of patients described by Grabb, 10% had malformations of the eyes and eyelids or palate. Transverse facial clefting, ranging from macrostomia to a full-thickness defect of the cheek, can be present (*Fig. 36.11*). The clefts probably result from a failure of the maxillary and mandibular processes to fuse. In embryonic development, the lateral commissure of the oral fissure is initially situated at the point of bifurcation of the maxillary and mandibular processes. With fusion of these and development of the muscles of mastication, the original broad mouth is reduced in size. In addition, the parotid glands, originally located near the embryonic oral commissure, grow laterally toward the developing ear, but the parotid duct papillae remain in their more medial position.

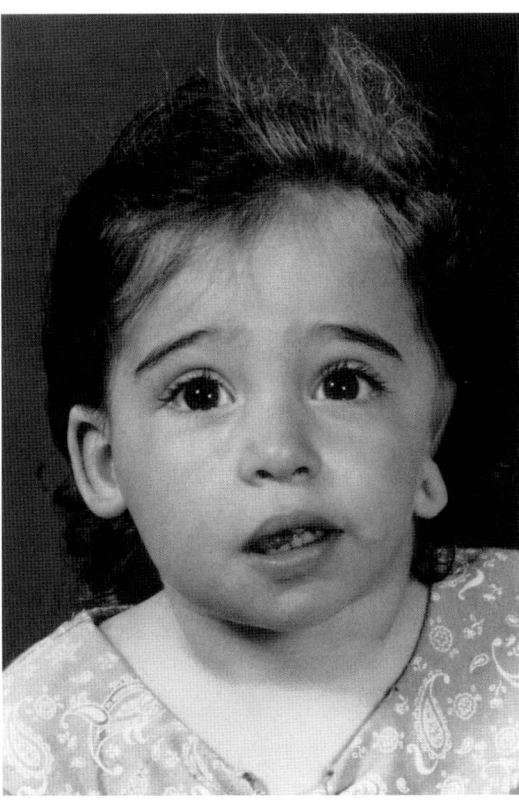

Fig. 36.6 Patient with left-sided craniofacial microsomia demonstrating the characteristic occlusal and nasal cant upward on the affected side along with associated cheek hypoplasia and ear anomaly.

toward the unaffected side and to deviate the midline of the chin toward the affected side during opening and during forceful protrusion.

In many cases, the coronoid process is absent, and there is reduction in the size of the temporalis muscle. The associated masseter and medial pterygoid muscles are also grossly deficient.

Ear

Auricular malformations are a usual manifestation of the syndrome. Meurman proposed a classification of the auricular anomalies based on the studies of Marx (1926): grade I, distinctly smaller malformed auricles with most of the characteristic components; grade II, vertical remnant of cartilage and skin with a small anterior hook and complete atresia of the canal; and grade III, an almost entirely absent auricle except for a small remnant, such as a deformed lobule (*Fig. 36.10*).

In a comprehensive study, Caldarelli *et al.*, using air and bone conduction audiometry and temporal bone tomography, evaluated 57 patients with CFM. It was observed that the degree of Meurman auricular deformity does not correlate exactly with hearing function. The type of hearing loss, although usually assumed to be conductive in origin, can be determined only by audiometry. Tomography, not auricular morphology, is the only indicator of middle-ear structure. The unaffected ear may also harbor abnormalities in structure and function and should be evaluated.

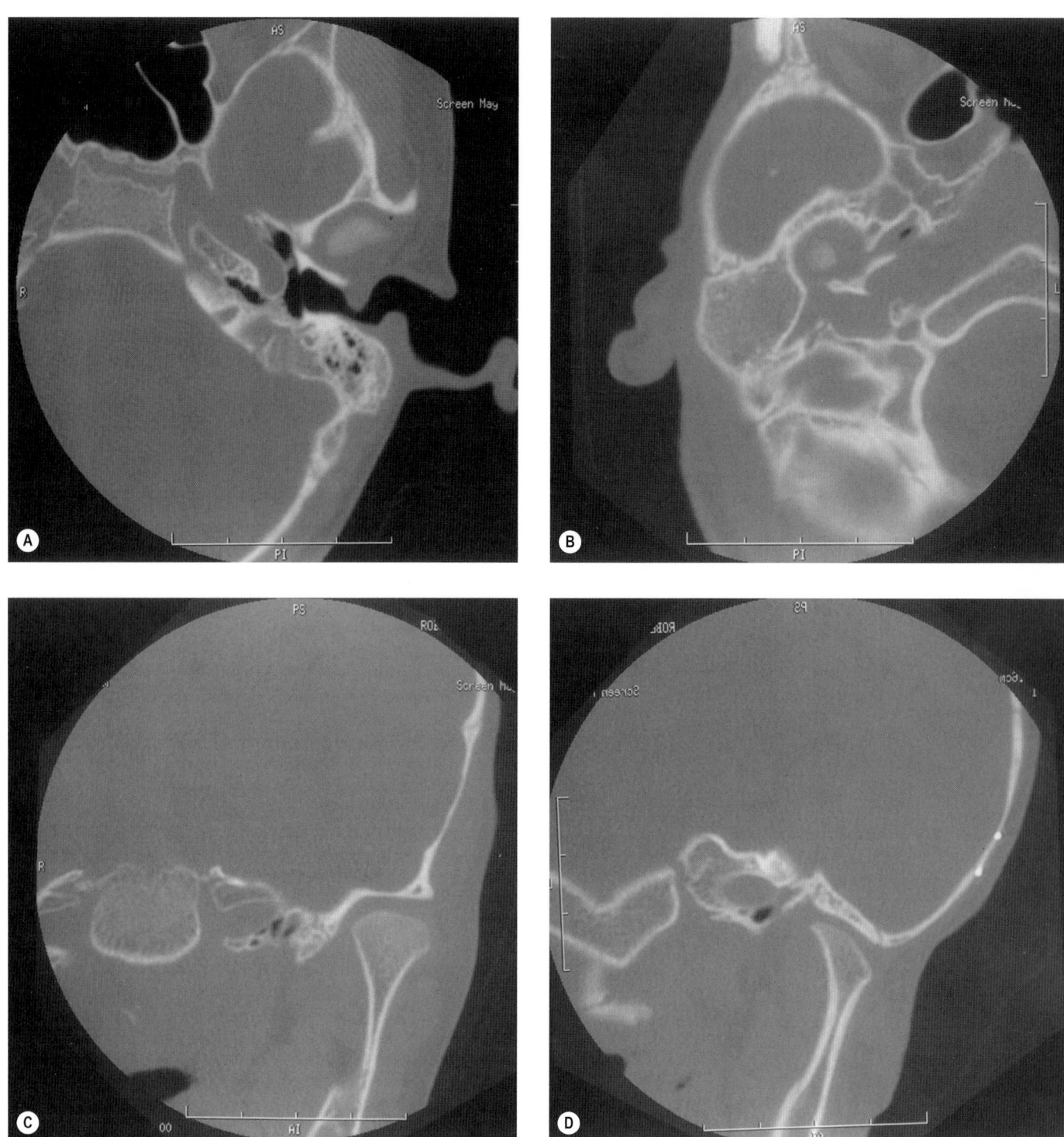

Fig. 36.7 Computed tomography scan images of condylar and temporal abnormalities in unilateral craniofacial microsomia compared with the contralateral side. Upper panel, axial cuts through the temporal bone at the level of the condylar head. Upper left, on the less affected side, normal lateral location of the glenoid fossa and pneumatization of the mastoid bone are visualized. Upper right, on the affected side, the glenoid fossa and condylar head are medially displaced, and there is an absence of air cells in the mastoid bone. Lower panel, coronal cuts through the condylar and temporal bone. Lower left, on the less affected side, there is normal condylar morphology with level articulation with the temporal bone. Lower right, on the affected side, the condylar head is dysmorphic and articulates with the temporal bone at an angle.

Extracraniofacial anatomy

Horgan *et al*. reviewed 121 cases of CFM and reported that 67 patients (55%) had at least one extracraniofacial (vertebral, cardiac, genitourinary) anomaly, with some having up to seven malformations. They also identified a relationship between the presence of these malformations and the severity of the craniofacial bone and soft-tissue involvement. The spectrum and incidence of associated malformations are listed in *Table 36.1*.

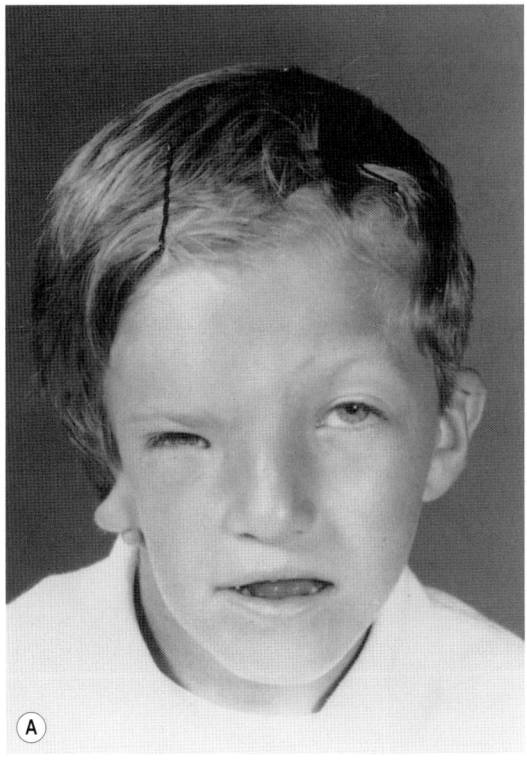 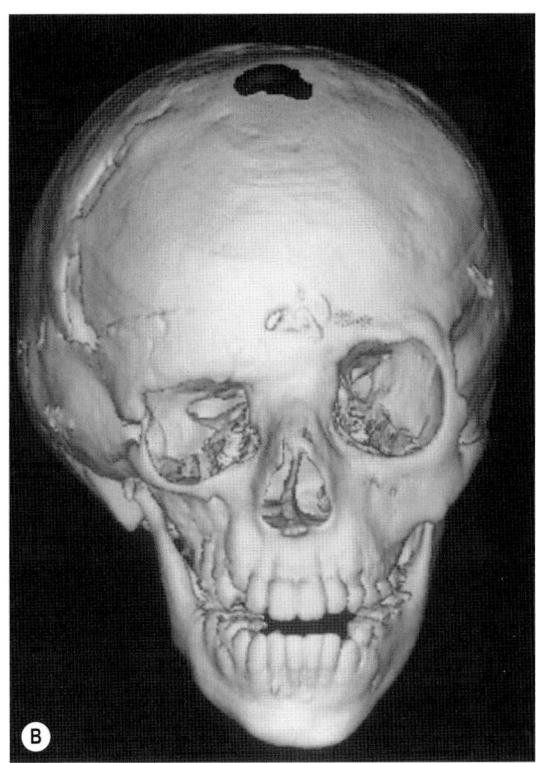

Fig. 36.8 **(A)** Craniofacial microsomia with orbital and frontal bone involvement (right side). There is vertical orbital dystopia. **(B)** The congenital fronto-orbital asymmetry persists even after cranial vault remodeling.

Table 36.1 **The spectrum and incidence of associated extracranial malformations**

	Principal anomalies	**Associated anomalies**	
Mandibular	Mandibular hypoplasia (89–100%) Malformed glenoid fossa (24–27%)	Craniofacial Velopharyngeal insufficiency (35–55%)	General Vertebral/rib defects (16–60%) Cervical spine anomalies (24–42%)
Ear	Microtia (66–99%) Preauricular tags (34–61%) Conductive hearing loss (50–66%) Middle-ear (ossicle) defects	Palatal deviation (39–50%) Orbital dystopia (15–43%) Ocular motility disorders (19–22%) Epibulbar dermoids (4–35%) Cranial base anomalies (9–30%)	Scoliosis (11–26%) Cardiac anomalies (4–33%) Pigmentation changes (13–14%) Extremity defects (3–21%)
Midfacial	Maxillary hypoplasia Zygomatic hypoplasia Occlusal canting	Cleft lip and/or palate (15–22%) Eyelid defects (12–25%) Hypodontia/dental hypoplasia (8–25%)	Central nervous system defects (5–18%) Genitourinary defects (4–15%) Pulmonary anomalies (1–15%)
Soft tissue	Masticatory muscles Hypoplasia (85–95%) Macrostomia (17–62%) Seventh-nerve palsy (10–45%)	Lacrimal drainage abnormalities (11–14%) Frontal plagiocephaly (10–12%) Sensorineural hearing loss (6–16%) Preauricular sinus (6–9%) Parotid gland hypoplasia Other cranial nerve defects (e.g., V, IX, XII)	Gastrointestinal defects (2–12%)

The prevalence rates were summarized from 19 reports in the literature from 1983 to 1996. Studies based on selected samples were omitted to minimize selection bias. It was recognized by the authors that the prevalence rate may be falsely elevated because the reporting tertiary centers may have a referral bias of more severely affected patients.
(Adapted from Cousley RR, Calvert ML. Current concepts in the understanding and management of hemifacial microsomia. *Br J Plast Surg*. 1997;50:536–551.)

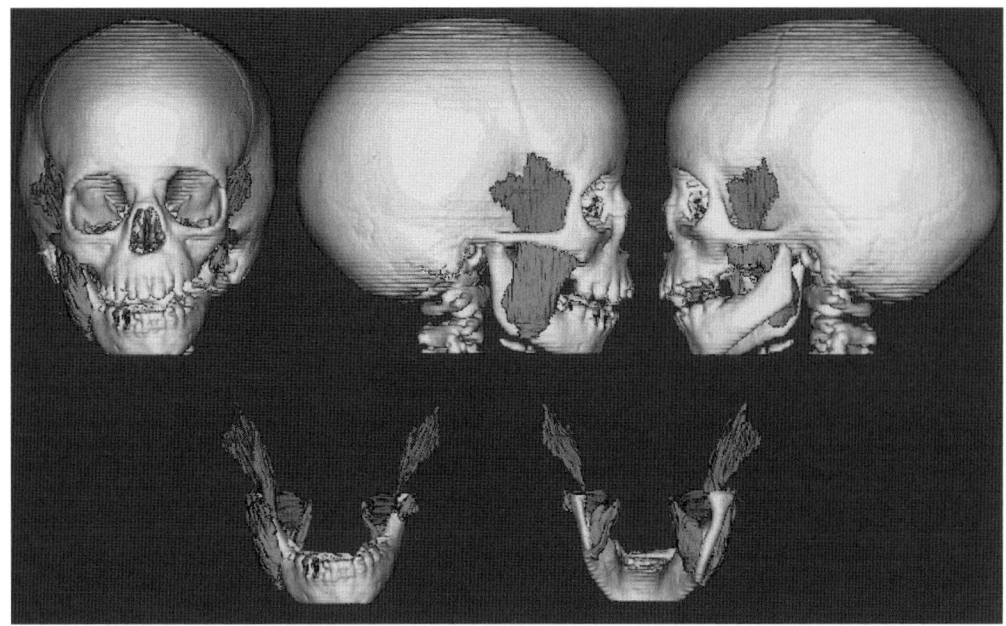

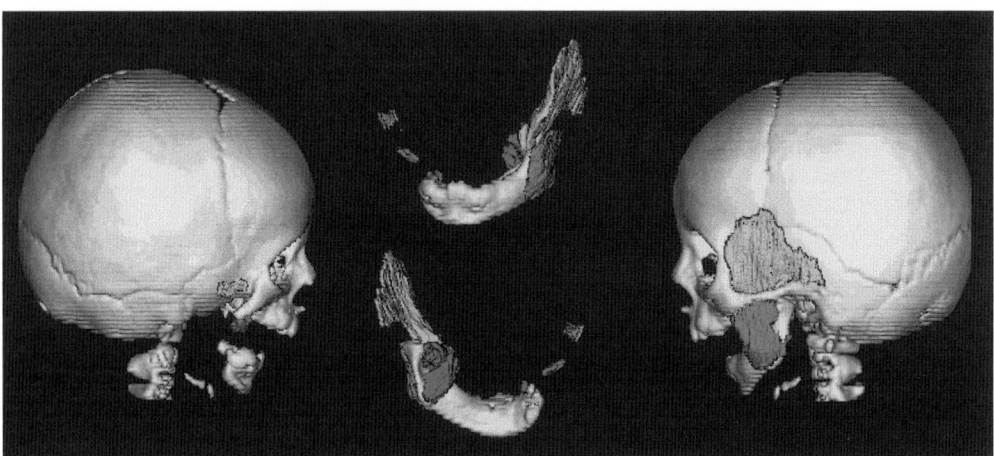

Fig. 36.9 Top panel, computed tomography (CT) images of a child with unilateral (left) craniofacial microsomia and grade I Pruzansky mandible. The images show composites of the osseous surface and segmented masticatory musculature derived from CT data. Bottom panel, images of a child with unilateral (right) craniofacial microsomia and grade III Pruzansky mandible. CT images show composites of the osseous surface and segmented masticatory musculature derived from CT data. (Courtesy of Drs. Alex Kane and Jeffrey Marsh, Washington University, St. Louis.)

Natural history

There are two schools of thought concerning the natural history or behavior of CFM (without any therapeutic intervention). One asserts that the severity of skeletal deformity is not progressive, with growth of the affected side paralleling that of the unaffected or less affected side. The other school of thought is that CFM is a progressive anomaly, with inhibited growth on the affected side resulting in increasing facial asymmetry with age. The natural history of the soft-tissue changes in CFM is not known since they are more difficult to document and quantitate.

Rune *et al.* examined the facial growth of 11 patients with unoperated unilateral CFM by use of metallic implants and roentgen stereophotogrammetry. They reported a mild increase in occlusal cant in 5 patients and stable or improving occlusal cant in the remaining 6. The authors concluded that asymmetry of the jaw does not increase with time; however,

only 1 patient in their study group had reached skeletal maturity at the time of the study. Polley *et al.* retrospectively examined longitudinal posteroanterior cephalograms of 26 patients with unoperated unilateral CFM. The patients were divided into three groups on the basis of Pruzansky mandibular grading. Both vertical and horizontal asymmetries were analyzed by a combination of angular and linear measurements. They reported that growth on the affected side paralleled that on the unaffected side, regardless of the grade of severity or side that was affected.

Kearns *et al.* interpreted the significant changes in gonial height difference and in intergonial angle, as reported in the Polley paper, to indicate a progressive vertical asymmetry that is correlated with the severity of mandibular deformity. This reinterpretation was consistent with their findings when they retrospectively examined 67 patients with unoperated unilateral CFM by horizontal angular analysis of posteroanterior cephalograms. They divided the patients into two groups

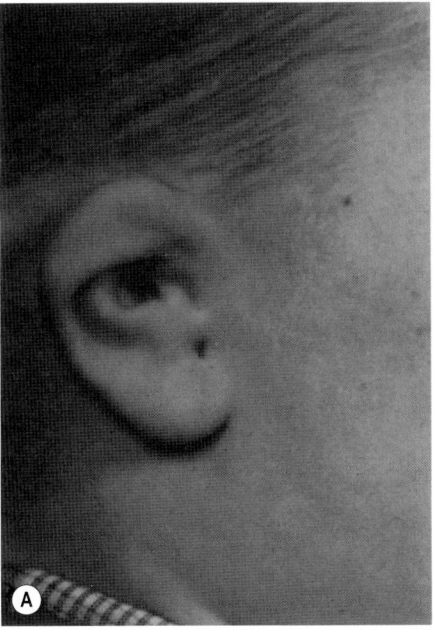 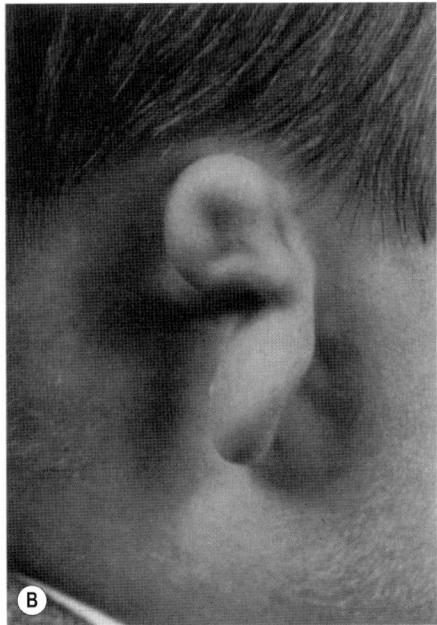 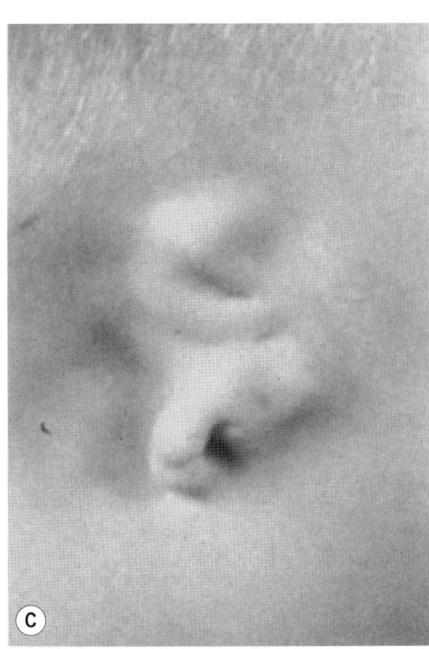

Fig. 36.10 Example of three grades of auricular anomalies in the Meurman classification. **(A)** Grade I: small malformed ear with most components present. **(B)** Grade II: vertical remnant of skin and cartilage. There is atresia of the external auditory meatus. **(C)** Grade III: the auricle is almost entirely absent except for a misplaced lobule and diminutive skin and cartilage remnants.

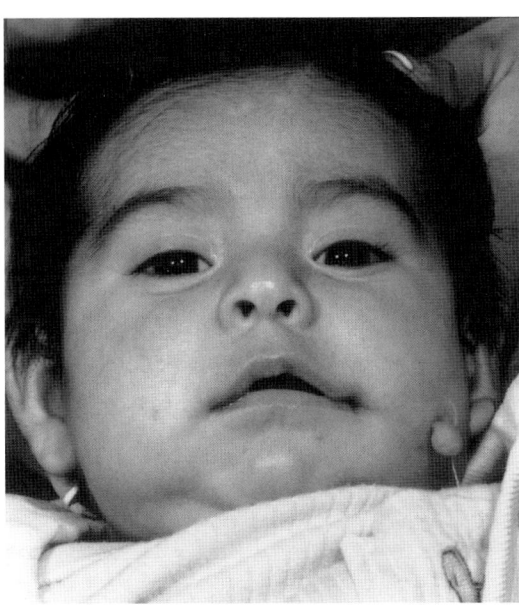

Fig. 36.11 Transverse facial cleft in a patient with left unilateral craniofacial microsomia. The soft-tissue cleft is manifest by the left macrostomia. The soft-tissue deficiency extends towards the tragal region.

based on the Pruzansky classification; they found no significant changes in group I but significant changes in all measurements in group II.

If the true natural history of CFM is progression, early surgical intervention may be indicated in an attempt to minimize the deformity. If, instead, CFM remains relatively stable, one could argue that surgery can be deferred to minimize the need for revisionary procedures, provided that there is neither a significant functional (respiratory, masticatory) or dysmorphic problem. The topic is again discussed later in the section on growth studies.

Diagnosis/patient presentation

Differential diagnosis

The differential diagnosis of facial asymmetry includes temporomandibular joint ankylosis, Romberg syndrome, postirradiation deformity, condylar hyperplasia, and hemifacial hypertrophy. Treacher–Collins syndrome or severe orbitofacial clefts can also be confused with bilateral CFM; however, the deformed ramal and condylar findings so characteristic of CFM are not present. Postnatal trauma or infection that affects the condylar cartilage can result in decreased mandibular growth, with a secondary effect on the growth of the surrounding ipsilateral craniofacial skeleton. Unlike the postnatal deformities, CFM is characterized by deficient soft-tissue and external ear malformations on the affected side as well as more widespread involvement of the skeleton, including the temporal bone, mastoid, and skull base. Minimal diagnostic criteria for CFM have been suggested by Cousley and Calvert as (1) ipsilateral mandibular and ear defects or (2) asymmetric mandibular or ear defects in association with either (a) two or more indirectly associated anomalies or (b) a positive family history of CFM. Indirectly associated anomalies were defined as those "not normally related either in terms of developmental fields or function."

It is difficult to determine the true ratio of unilateral to bilateral CFM. Patients diagnosed with unilateral involvement often have subtle abnormalities of the ear, mandible, or orbit on the contralateral side. Grabb reported 12 bilateral cases in his series of 102 (12%), Meurman reported 8 in 74 (11%), and Converse reported 15 in a series of 280 (5%). In contrast, in a review of 294 oculoauriculovertebral patients, 98 (33%) had some form of bilateral involvement, and the ear involvement was symmetric in 34 of these. Mulliken reported 34 cases (28%) with bilateral involvement among 121 cases

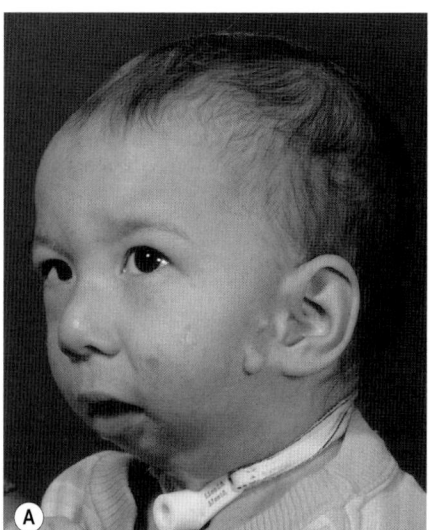
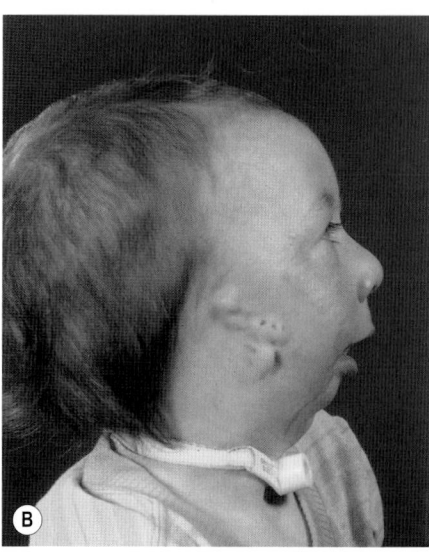
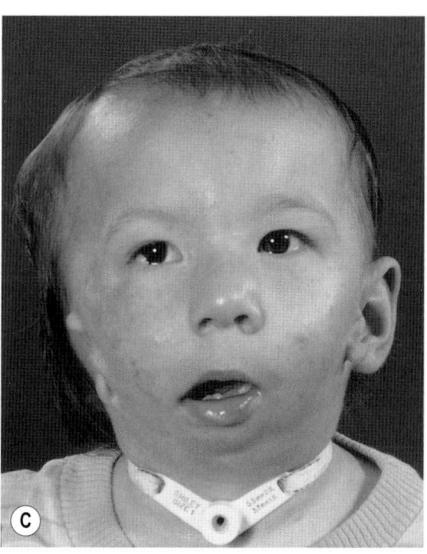

Fig. 36.12 Patient with bilateral craniofacial microsomia of the Goldenhar variant. The right side of the face is more severely affected with a Meurman III ear deformity, epibulbar dermoid, cheek soft-tissue deficiency, and micrognathia. The left side of the face is less affected; however, a mandibular abnormality is evident along with a pretragal cartilaginous remnant and skin tag. Severe micrognathia and respiratory obstruction usually indicate bilateral involvement.

of CFM. The higher ratio of bilateral involvement in more recent reviews may be due to an increased appreciation/documentation of subtle contralateral soft-tissue anomalies (macrostomia, cheek hypoplasia, preauricular skin tags) by the examining physician *(Fig. 36.12)*.

Classification systems

Multiple classification systems have been described for CFM, thus rendering comparison of different clinical experiences confusing. An ideal classification system would be one that describes accurately all anatomic components of CFM and the associated severity to facilitate communication among health professionals, to allow comparison of clinical experiences, and to formulate classification-based comprehensive treatment protocols. No classification system has yet achieved this ideal.

Pruzansky reported a grading system of progressive mandibular deficiency: grade I, minimal hypoplasia of the mandible; grade II, functioning but deformed temporomandibular joint with anteriorly and medially displaced condyle; or grade III, absence of the ramus and glenoid fossa. This classification was later modified by Kaban, Padwa, and Mulliken *(Fig. 36.13 and Table 36.2)*. With this system and a modification of the three-grade auricular malformation classification of Meurman, Pruzansky divided his patients into nine groups. In a later report, his group continued to support this classification scheme but recognized the limitation of describing the variable CFM population solely on the basis of jaw and ear malformations. The variability of anatomic involvement in CFM had been recognized by Converse 10 years earlier, when he and his colleagues appreciated the involvement of the soft tissue and muscles of mastication. In their division of 15 bilateral CFM patients into four groups, the first three groups were based on ear and mandible findings, whereas the fourth included facial soft tissue and bone involvement.

The comprehensive phenotypic classification system, described by Tenconi and Hall and based on 67 patients with CFM, was one of the first to incorporate the ocular and extracranial findings in CFM, such as ocular dermoids,

Table 36.2 Pruzansky classification of mandibular deformity with Kaban, Padwa, and Mulliken modification

Type	Description
I	All mandibular and temporomandibular joint components are present and normal in shape but hypoplastic to a variable degree
IIa	The mandibular ramus, condyle, and temporomandibular joint are present but hypoplastic and abnormal in shape
IIb	The mandibular ramus is hypoplastic and markedly abnormal in form and location, being medial and anterior. There is no articulation with the temporal bone
III	The mandibular ramus, condyle, and temporomandibular joint are absent. The lateral pterygoid muscle and temporalis, if present, are not attached to the mandibular remnant

(Adapted from Kaban LB, Padwa BL, Mulliken JB. Surgical correction of mandibular hypoplasia in hemifacial microsomia: the case for treatment in early childhood. *J Oral Maxillofac Surg.* 1998;56:628–638.)

microphthalmos, limb deficiencies, and vertebral, heart, or renal abnormalities. Type I was unilateral, divided into classic, microphthalmic, bilateral asymmetric, and complex types; type II was unilateral with limb deficiency type; type III was unilateral of the frontonasal type and type IV was unilateral, Goldenhar type, divided into type A (unilateral) and type B (bilateral).

Munro and Lauritzen described a five-part surgical-anatomic classification scheme divided according to the skeletal deformity but oriented toward treatment considerations. The classification is determined by whether the skeleton is complete (type I) or incomplete (types II–V), whether the occlusal plane is level (type Ia) or tilted (types Ib–V), and whether the orbit is involved (types IV and V). The classification forms the basis of a treatment plan for the skeletal abnormalities of the face *(Fig. 36.14)*.

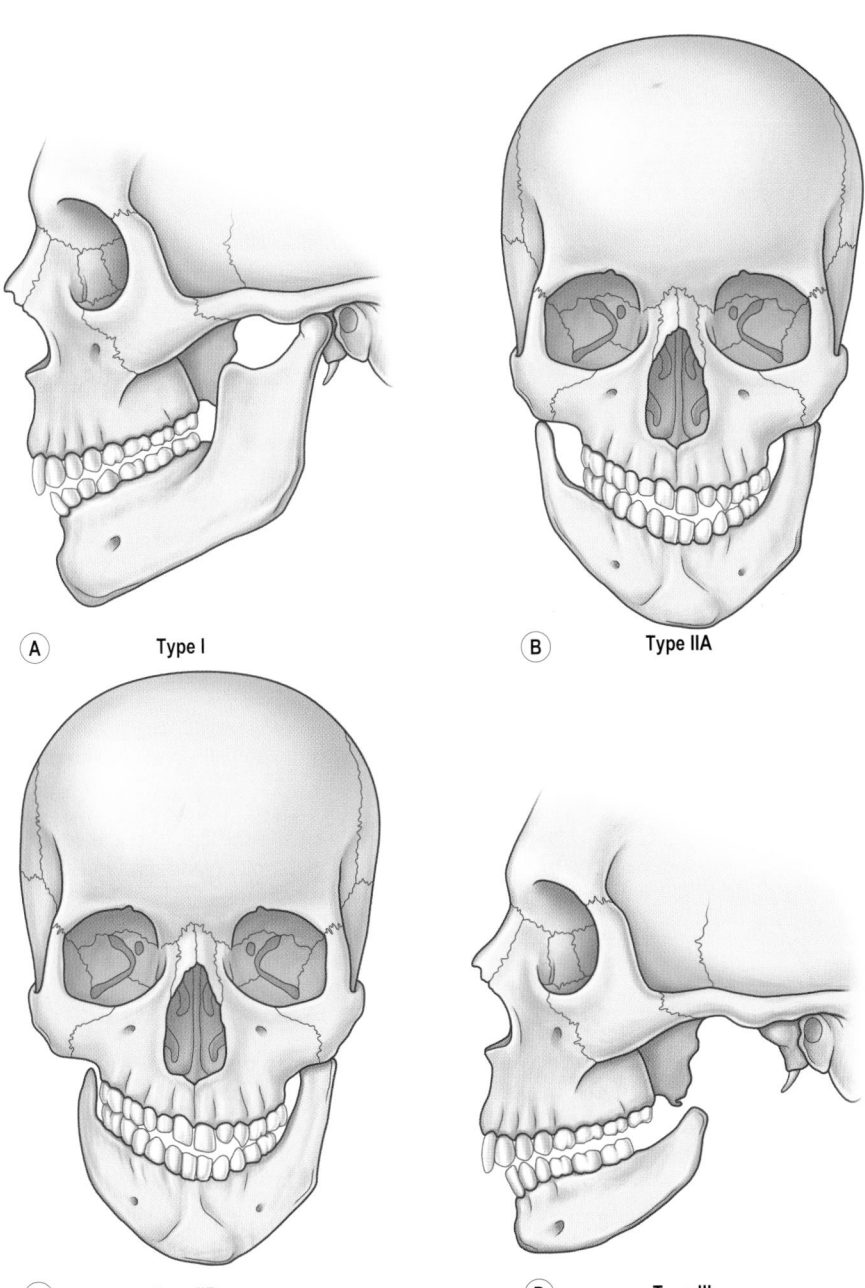

Fig. 36.13 Pruzansky classification of the mandibular deformity, as modified by Kaban *et al.* **(A)** Type I: the mandibular deficiency is only mild. **(B)** Type IIA: the condyle and ramus are small, but the condyle and glenoid fossa are anatomically oriented. However, a flattened condyle can be hinged on a flat, often hypoplastic infratemporal surface. The coronoid process may be absent. **(C)** Type IIB: this is similar to type IIA except that the vertical or superoinferior plane of the condyle ramus is medially displaced. There is not a functioning glenoid fossa. **(D)** Type III: there is absence of the ramus, condyle, and coronoid process.

David *et al.* devised an alphanumeric (SAT) coding classification in the spirit of the TMN classification system of malignant tumors *(Table 36.3)*. The SAT classification system grades skeletal (S), auricle (A), and soft tissue (T) anomalies on an increasing numeric scale of severity. S_1, S_2, and S_3 skeletal deformities are similar to the three grades of mandibular hypoplasia described by Pruzansky, with S_4 and S_5 representing mandible changes with orbital involvement. A_0 describes a normal ear, and A_1, A_2, and A_3 are increasing degrees of malformation. T_1, T_2, and T_3 are mild, moderate, and major soft-tissue defects, respectively.

The OMENS classification of CFM, described by Vento, LaBrie, and Mulliken, also uses alphanumeric codes to classify patients according to the severity of malformation of different anatomic components *(Table 36.4)*. Similar to the SAT classification, it grades ear anomalies (E in OMENS, A in SAT) in four grades from 0 to 3 and soft-tissue defects (S in OMENS, and T in SAT) in three grades. Unlike in the SAT classification, however, the skeletal component is broken down into four orbital (O) and four mandibular (M) grades of deformity. The mandibular grading system includes the subdivision of Pruzansky type II into IIa and IIb, as first proposed by Kaban and associates. Facial nerve involvement is also addressed as the N in OMENS. Both SAT and OMENS systems can be used to describe separately each side in a patient with bilateral CFM.

Photography

Baseline photography should be obtained using standardized lighting and head positioning with lips at rest. Standardized records should include full face, submental vertex, bird's eye, lateral, oblique smile, and occlusal views. Functional facial nerve views are also requisite.

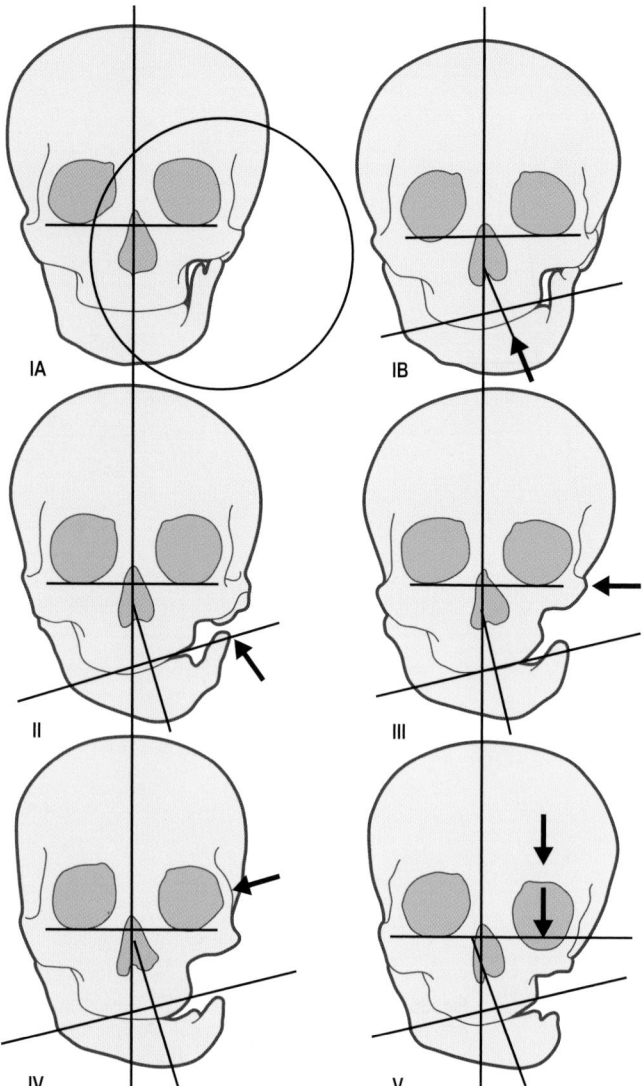

Fig. 36.14 Classification of unilateral craniofacial microsomia based on the pathologic skeletal anatomy (after Munro and Lauritzen). In the upper panel, the circle designates the usual site of skeletal involvement. The midsagittal, midincisor, orbital, and occlusal planes are illustrated. See text for details.

The development of three-dimensional camera systems provides a helpful tool for quantitatively documenting the deformity and recording volumetric and contour changes following surgical interventions; it is also an important component of the preoperative planning process.

Cephalometrics

Despite the popularity of CT and cone beam imaging in imaging the craniofacial skeleton, cephalograms remain essential in serial examination of the facial bones, as follow-up after orthognathic jaw surgery, during the activation phase of DO, and in determining and documenting changes of the facial skeleton.

In the standard cephalometric technique, the ear rods of the cephalostat are inserted in the external auditory meatus, and the patient's head is placed in the Frankfort horizontal or natural head position. The patient with CFM usually has one

Table 36.3 SAT classification

Skeletal	
S_1	Small mandible with normal shape
S_2	Condyle, ramus, and sigmoid notch identifiable but grossly distorted; mandible strikingly different in size and shape from normal
S_3	Mandible severely malformed and strikingly different in size and shape from normal
$S_4 S_3$	Mandible plus orbital involvement with gross posterior recession of lateral and inferior orbital rims
$S_5 S_4$	Defects plus orbital dystopia and frequently hypoplasia and asymmetric neurocranium with a flat temporal fossa
Auricle	
A_0	Normal
A_1	Small, malformed auricle retaining characteristic features
A_2	Rudimentary auricle with hook at cranial end corresponding to the helix
A_3	Malformed lobule with rest of pinna absent
Soft tissue	
T_1	Minimal contour defect with no cranial nerve involvement
T_2	Moderate defect
T_3	Major defect with obvious facial scoliosis, possible severe hypoplasia of cranial nerves, parotid gland, and muscles of mastication; eye involvement; cleft of face or lips

(Adapted from David DJ, Mahatumarat C, Cooter RD. Hemifacial microsomia: a multisystem classification. *Plast Reconstr Surg*. 1987;80:525–535.)

ear positioned inferior and anterior to the other. If the malpositioned ear is used in this technique, the head is incorrectly oriented to the X-ray beam and the film. The technician should project an imaginary line from the normal ear, perpendicular to the midsagittal plane and passing to the opposite side of the head. The x–y coordinates of this point, in millimeters, should be recorded directly on the cephalogram for future reference. Clinical determination of the midsagittal plane can be made by tipping the head down and observing the gross shape of the calvaria from above.

The classic lateral cephalogram provides information on maxillomandibular relationship, as well as the deviation of the bone and soft-tissue profile from documented norms. The posteroanterior and basilar cephalograms are equally important in assessing patients with CFM in that they allow documentation of the facial midline and the degree of facial asymmetry in three dimensions (*Fig. 36.15*).

Grayson *et al.* described the technique of multiplane cephalometry. With lateral, coronal, and basilar radiographs, skeletal landmarks can be identified in three coronal and three axial planes and used to construct an estimation of the midline for each plane. These midlines are compared with the midsagittal plane, which is determined by relatively stable bilateral structures such as the occipital condyles, the center of the foramen magnum, and the medial axis of the spheno-occipital synchondrosis. By use of this technique, a phenomenon termed warping can be observed within the skeleton of the

Table 36.4 OMENS classification

Orbit	
O_0	Normal orbit size and position
O_1	Abnormal size
O_2	Abnormal position
O_3	Abnormal size and position
Mandible	
M_0	Normal mandible
M_1	Mandible and glenoid fossa are small ("minimandible")
M_2	Mandibular ramus short and abnormally shaped
M_{2A}	Glenoid in acceptable position
M_{2B}	Temporomandibular joint medially displaced
M_3	Complete absence of ramus, glenoid fossa, and temporomandibular joint
Ear	
E_0	Normal
E_1	Mild hypoplasia and cupping
E_2	Absence of external auditory canal
E_3	Malpositioned lobule with absent auricle
Nerve	
N_0	No facial nerve involvement
N_1	Upper facial nerve involvement
N_2	Lower facial nerve involvement
N_3	All branches affected
Soft tissue	
S_0	No soft-tissue deformity
S_1	Minimal (mild) tissue deformity
S_2	Moderate tissue deformity (between the two extremes)
S_3	Major (severe) subcutaneous and muscular deficiency

(Adapted from Vento AR, LaBrie RA, Mulliken JB. The OMENS classification of hemifacial microsomia. *Cleft Palate Craniofac J.* 1991;28:68–76, discussion 77.)

patient with CFM. The midline constructs deviate progressively laterally as one passes anteriorly from the skull base to the piriform rim in the coronal plane and inferiorly from the orbits to the mandible in the axial plane.

Computed tomography

CT, including cone beam imaging, has become a fundamental diagnostic and evaluation tool for all patients with CFM. Unlike cephalography, CT can image both bone and soft tissue, and it does not have the problem of superimposition of skeletal landmarks. Axial and coronal cuts provide detailed information on the bone and soft-tissue asymmetry and the severity of malformation throughout the entire craniofacial skeleton. For the young patient who cannot be evaluated with conventional cephalographic imaging because of lack of cooperation, a CT or cone beam scan, performed under sedation or general anesthesia, has provided information for early treatment planning *(Fig. 36.16)*.

Because data derived from the CT scan are computer-based, programs can be written to present the information in any number of formats, including three-dimensional CT and multiplanar reformation. Three-dimensional presentation of CT images provides a visual summary of the underlying skeleton, which can be viewed and analyzed at any angle. Another useful manipulation of CT data is multiplanar reformation (CT/MPR), or DentaScan, which processes axial CT scan information to obtain true cross-sectional images and panoramic views of the mandible and maxilla similar to a Panorex *(Fig. 36.16)*. This is invaluable in imaging tooth follicles in relation to available bone stock in the immature patient who is too young for conventional dental imaging and in whom mandibular distraction is planned.

Cone beam CT scan technology allows detailed imaging of the maxillomandibular complex at reduced cost, radiation exposure, and time as compared to conventional helical CT scans.

Endoscopy

In patients with respiratory insufficiency or sleep apnea, endoscopy is indicated to document the site of obstruction. In bilateral CFM, and occasionally in unilateral CFM, there can be life-threatening retroglossal narrowing secondary to mandibular deficiency. Moreover, endoscopy can also rule out other sites of obstruction along the respiratory tract.

Sleep studies

In patients with obstructive sleep apnea, sleep studies (polysomnography) can define the degree of the respiratory dysfunction and are invaluable, along with interpretation of the clinical symptoms and endoscopic findings, in determining whether surgical intervention, i.e., mandibular distraction, is indicated.

Patient selection

The evolution or development of surgical/orthodontic techniques for the correction of the skeletal and soft-tissue defects of the patient with CFM mirrors the history of plastic surgery: bone grafts, osteotomies, DO, dermis-fat grafts, local flaps, microvascular free flaps, and autogenous fat injections. It is the treatment challenge posed by the patient, usually a severe asymmetric deformity, often accompanied by a functional deficit, and the need to integrate a multidisciplinary treatment team that have attracted the plastic surgeon.

The surgical reconstructive requirements of the patient with CFM vary from patient to patient and are dependent on the individual anatomic and functional deficiencies. The skeletal reconstructive efforts have traditionally been directed at correction of the mandibular deficiency, usually involving the ramus and body, as well as the condyle and temporomandibular joint. Along with mandibular hypoplasia, there is invariably an associated pathologic process involving the maxilla and zygoma. The associated occlusal problems, especially in the unilateral type, include upward canting of the occlusal

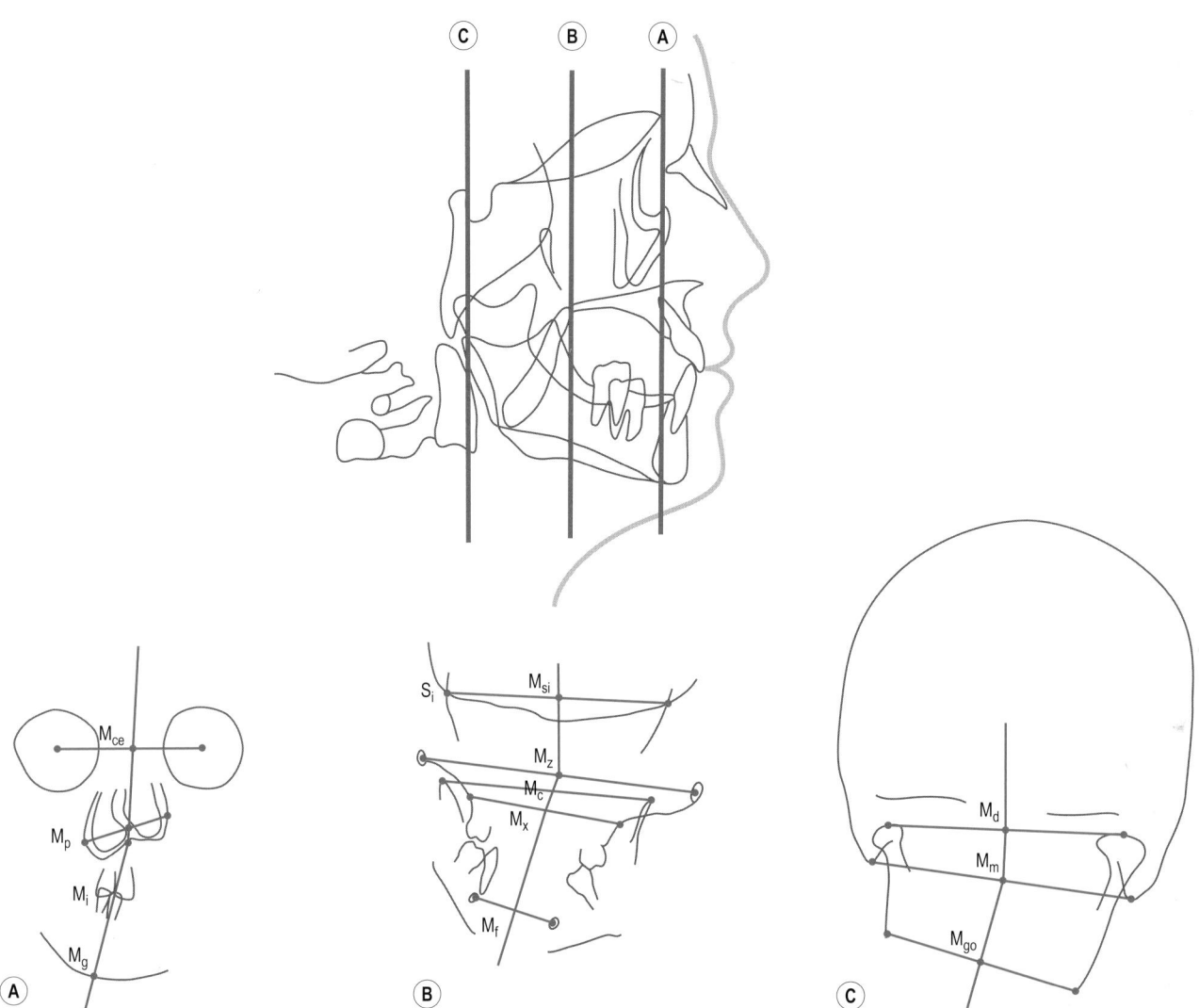

Fig. 36.15 Top, the three vertical planes of the face. Separate tracings are made on the same radiograph, corresponding to structures derived from the lateral view in or near the three planes indicated. Bottom, **(A)** straight lines connecting M_{ce}, M_p, M_i, and M_g result in a segmented construct whose angles express asymmetry of structure in this facial plane. **(B)** Midline construct of the B plane. **(C)** Midline construct of the C plane. (Reproduced from Grayson B, McCarthy JG, Bookstein F. Analysis of craniofacial asymmetry by multiplane cephalometry. *Am J Orthod.* 1983;84;217.)

plane, skeletal crossbite, and shifting of the dental midline. In a small percentage of patients, the fronto-orbital area can be deficient. Along with the skeletal deficits there is usually soft-tissue hypoplasia of varying degree. In summary, the clinician is usually dealing with a composite skeletal and soft-tissue deformity – "bone carpentry" alone is often insufficient in the global treatment of the patient with craniofacial microsomia.

Other variables that must be considered are the functional needs (respiratory, otologic, masticatory, speech, and psychosocial) of the patient and the role of subsequent growth and development of the affected and neighboring anatomic parts. The clinician must first consider the functional requirements, especially sleep apnea and other types of respiratory deficiency associated with micrognathia and glossoptosis. With severe respiratory insufficiency, it had been traditional to treat the child with a tracheostomy but mandibular distraction can often obviate the need for tracheostomy, if it is confirmed there is single-level obstruction. Such individuals invariably

have feeding problems, and a gastrostomy may also be indicated. A child will occasionally have poor function of the palpebral sphincter, and treatment may be required to protect the cornea. In children with bilateral craniofacial microsomia, the hearing deficits are so severe that speech development is impeded and hearing devices may be required. Cervical vertebral abnormality can be associated with a Chiari malformation and other central nervous system anomalies have also been reported.

The timing of surgical intervention has been the subject of a long-running controversy. The school advocating osteotomies only in the adult or adolescent patient has included Poswillo, who thought that such surgery in the growing child would interfere with the functional matrix and impede subsequent craniofacial growth and development. Using a similar argument, Obwegeser also advocated deferring jaw surgery until skeletal and dental maturity had been reached. He popularized reconstruction of the temporomandibular joint and

The development of distraction techniques by McCarthy and colleagues at New York University represented a true paradigm shift in the treatment of patients with either unilateral or bilateral craniofacial microsomia. The techniques are simpler and associated with less morbidity, especially infection; they obviate the need for intermaxillary fixation, autogenous bone graft harvesting, or blood transfusion. Advocates of mandibular distraction recommend the technique in infancy if there is clinical evidence of sleep apnea and in children with severe dysmorphism. Early mandibular reconstruction with distraction, however, does not preclude subsequent mandibular surgical procedures, depending on mandibular growth and development.

Soft-tissue hypoplasia is a prominent feature of craniofacial microsomia, especially in the cheeks (parotid-masseteric) and auriculomastoid areas. The results of nonvascularized dermis-fat grafts are unpredictable, including a residual contour irregularity or even loss of the entire graft. Vascularized flap transfers are preferred because of long-term survival and the ability to deliver large volumes of fat. This concept was first established by the insertion of a tube flap in the preauricular area and the use of a de-epithelialized pedicle flap. These flap techniques have been superseded, however, by the introduction of de-epithelialized microvascular free flaps of dermis and fat. Restoration of soft-tissue contour with microvascular transfers of omentum has fallen out of favor because of the requisite need for a laparotomy and a secondary procedure to resuspend the omentum. In recent years the technique of serial autogenous fat injections, as advocated by Coleman, has gained considerable popularity as an alternative method of augmenting the deficient soft tissue.

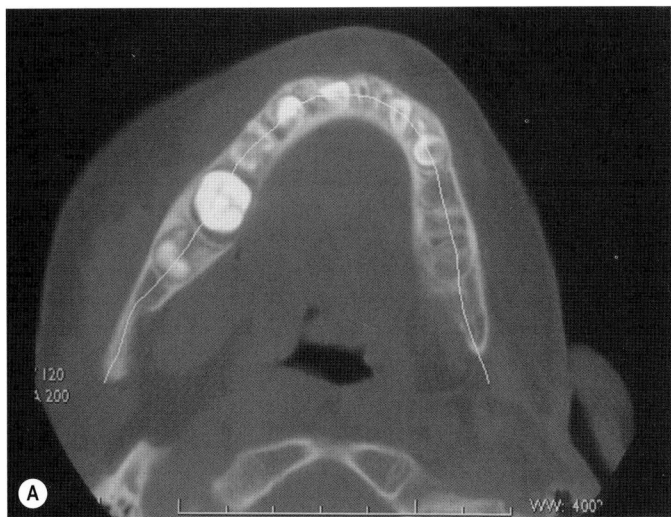

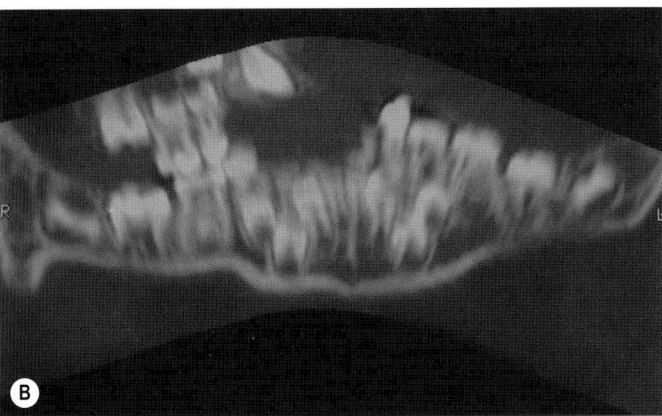

Fig. 36.16 Computed tomography multiplanar reformation (CT/MPR) or DentaScan imaging of a unilateral craniofacial microsomia mandible with primary dentition. The tooth follicles of the secondary dentition can be visualized to aid in planning osteotomies and pin placement. Upper, axial CT scan through mandibular occlusion. Lower, reformatted DentaScan. Note the tooth follicles crowding in the rami.

zygomatic arch with rib grafts, as well as the rotation of the lower half of the craniofacial skeleton inferiorly and medially by the combination of a Le Fort I osteotomy, bilateral sagittal split osteotomy of the mandibular rami, and three-dimensional genioplasty.

Advocates of osteotomies in children included Dingman and Grabb, who recommended a metatarsal bone graft reconstruction of the affected mandibular ramus. Converse and Rushton described a 12-year-old with unilateral CFM who also underwent a horizontal osteotomy of the ramus with insertion of an iliac bone graft in the resulting defect; a bite block was constructed to open the occlusion on the affected side. Delaire recommended elongation of the affected ramus between the ages of 4 and 6 years by an inverted-L osteotomy with insertion of rib grafts in the horizontal component of the resulting defect. Converse *et al.* advocated a two-stage procedure during the period of mixed dentition to correct the maxillomandibular asymmetry. Other proponents of childhood osteotomies and bone grafts included Murray *et al.* and Munro and Lauritzen, who also reported subsequent elongation and growth of the rib-grafted mandibular segment.

Treatment/surgical technique

Tracheostomy or gastrostomy

In the neonatal period, tracheostomy can be a lifesaving maneuver in patients with severe respiratory distress, but the need for this treatment modality has been lessened in recent years with the introduction of mandibular distraction. Some newborns who require perinatal endotracheal intubation can successfully tolerate extubation several days later. If extubation is not possible, distraction or tracheostomy must be considered.

For infants with severe eating problems, a gastrostomy is indicated to improve the nutritional status of the child and to provide the calories essential for growth and development. The nutritional problem is often aggravated by the increased energy requirements associated with respiratory insufficiency and is often corrected by mandibular distraction.

Commissuroplasty

Commissuroplasty or closure of the lateral facial cleft is indicated in patients with a macrostomia or a true lateral facial cleft. Vermilion and oral mucosal flaps are designed after the site of the projected oral commissure is determined *(Fig. 36.17)*. The flaps are approximated and sutured with resorbable sutures. The orbicularis muscle stumps are skeletonized and closed in a vest-over-pants fashion with resorbable

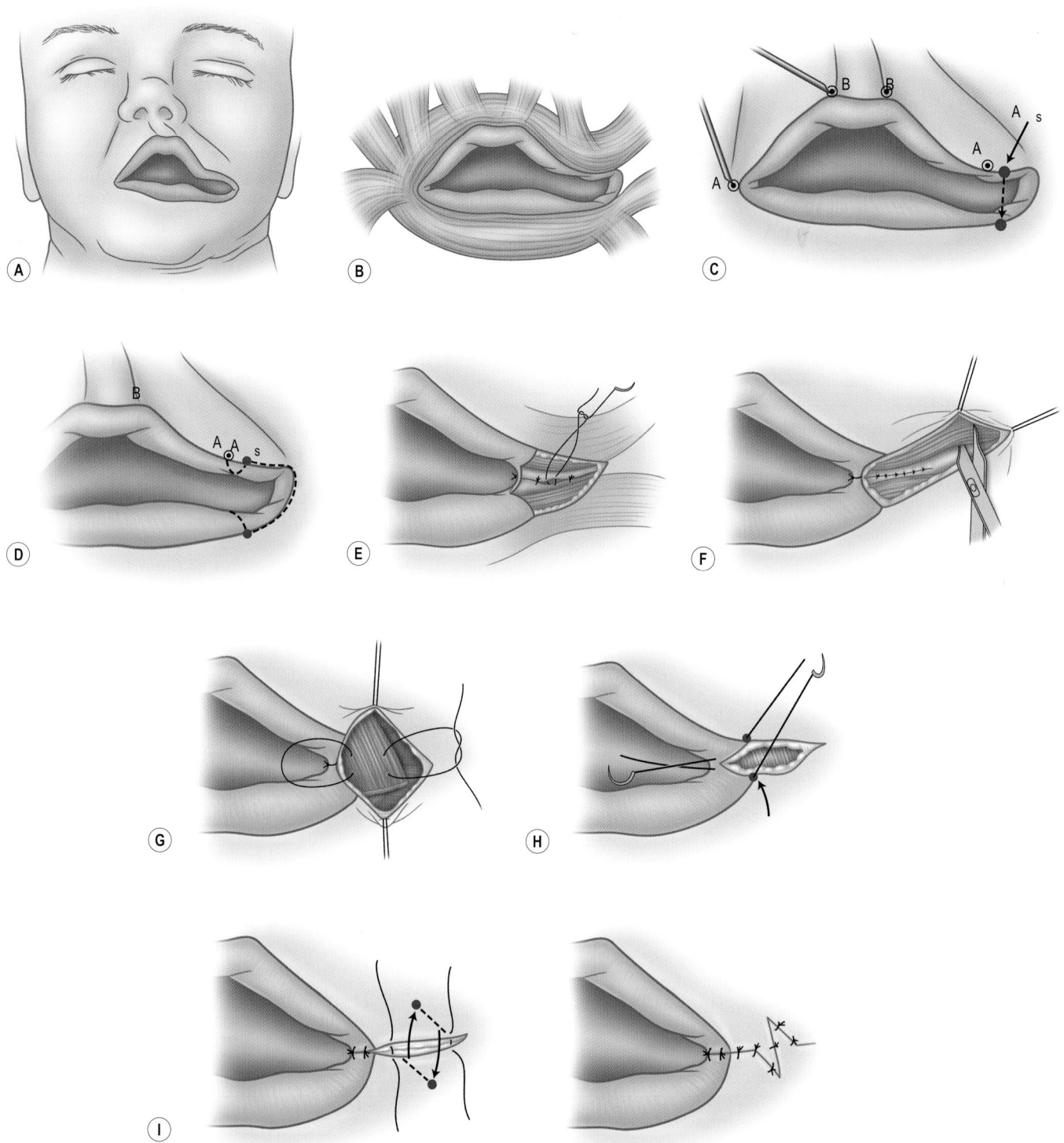

Fig. 36.17 Correction of lateral facial cleft (McCarthy technique). **(A)** Preoperative appearance, left-sided lateral facial cleft. **(B)** Disruption of the orbicularis sphincter at the commissure. **(C)** Markings are made on the white line with ink: A, oral commissure on unaffected side. B, philtral column on unaffected side. B', philtral column on affected side. A', proposed oral commissure (distance = AB). A's is made more lateral (overcorrected) because of the expected postoperative contraction. A dot is placed opposite on the lower lip. **(D)** Proposed vermilion turnover flap (outlined by the interrupted line). **(E)** Closure of the oral mucosa. **(F)** The upper and lower orbicularis muscle bundles are skeletonized and divided. **(G)** Vest-over-pants closure of upper and lower divided ends of orbicularis muscle bundles. **(H)** A simple suture is placed at the white lines at A's (see **C**). **(I)** Proposed Z-plasty closure. The resulting central limb must lie in the direction of the nasolabial fold.

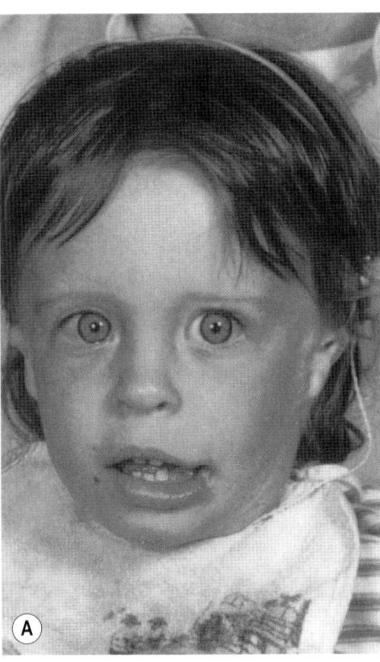
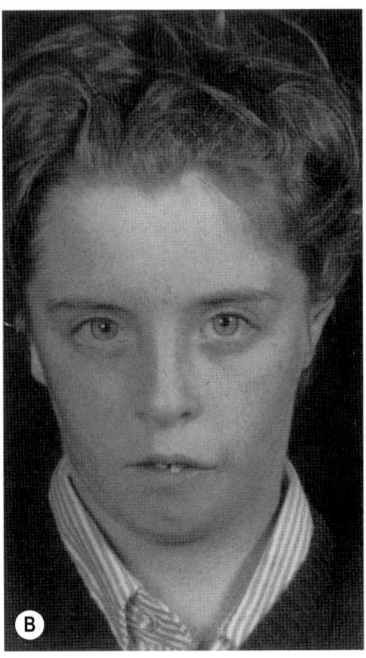

Fig. 36.18 A 2-year-old boy with left-sided lateral facial cleft (macrostomia) and bilateral microtia. **(A)** Preoperative appearance. **(B)** After correction by the technique illustrated in Figure 36.17.

sutures. The cutaneous closure is incorporated in a Z-plasty designed to simulate the nasolabial fold. Closure is accomplished with nylon sutures *(Fig. 36.18)*.

Mandibular distraction

Mandibular distraction can be employed at any age from the neonate to the adult. The technique involves an osteotomy on one or both sides of the mandible with the application of either an extraoral *(Fig. 36.19)* or intraoral/semiburied *(Fig. 36.20)* distraction device. The semiburied device is reserved for those patients with an adequate bone stock in the ramus and body of the mandible (type I or IIA, B). It is especially helpful when a vertical vector (see *Fig. 36.23*, below) is indicated. After a latency period of approximately 5 days, the device can be activated at the rate of 1 mm/day. In children younger than 3 years, it is appropriate to employ a rate of 1.5 mm/day to avoid premature consolidation. In the neonate, for whom intubation is critical, the latency period can be reduced to 1 or 2 days and the activation rate accelerated to 2 mm/day to reduce the length of endotracheal intubation.

In patients with unilateral craniofacial microsomia, activation of the distraction device is continued until there is leveling or overcorrection of the occlusal plane, inferior displacement of the ipsilateral oral commissure, and movement of the chin point to or beyond the midline *(Fig. 36.21)*. Such parameters should be overcorrected in the growing child. In the younger patient with bilateral mandibular deficiency, the technique is employed bilaterally, and activation is continued until the mandibular anterior teeth are either edge to edge with, or anterior to, the maxillary anterior teeth. The technique is applicable in patients of all ages with either unilateral or bilateral *(Fig. 36.22)* craniofacial microsomia. Of note, for those patients requiring distraction for improvement of airway, an additional criterion to consider for ending distraction activation is evidence of improved retroglossal airspace on lateral cephalogram or endoscopy.

In preoperative planning, CT scans (axial and three-dimensional) are essential in defining the skeletal pathologic process and determining whether there is adequate bone stock for the osteotomy and device pin placement. A curved reformat of the CT data yields a DentaScan that is helpful in documenting the position of unerupted tooth follicles. In the extremely hypoplastic ramus with dental crowding, preliminary removal of tooth follicles may be necessary.

The vectors of distraction are important and are determined by the placement of the pins and distraction device in relation to the maxillary occlusal plane *(Fig. 36.23)*. In the patient with unilateral craniofacial microsomia, the surgical goal is to increase the vertical or superoinferior dimension of the ramus (vertical vector). In bilateral distraction, surgeons should consider the vector of distraction and how this relates to the clinical goal. In order to correlate distraction vector with mandibular movement, our group recently studied this question in 15 patients and found that a horizontal vector produces substantial downward vertical movement, while a vertical vector results in greater horizontal projection of the mandible. While this may seem counterintuitive, this can be better understood if one considers the three-dimensional effects of distraction lengthening. With vertical vector distraction, posterior facial height increases, thus enabling counterclockwise rotation of the mandible and increased projection of the chin point as the symphyseal plane uprights. On the other hand, horizontal vector distraction does not create a posterior open bite that would allow for counterclockwise autorotation. As a result, horizontal distraction tends to maintain an existing steep maxillary occlusal plane and thus move the pogonion in a downward vertical direction. An oblique vector represents an intermediate orientation.

With the introduction of multiplanar distraction devices and the development of the concept of molding of the regenerate by maxillomandibular elastic band/wire therapy (see section on management of the occlusion: the role of the orthodontist later in this chapter), the clinician has the capability of achieving closure of an anterior open bite.

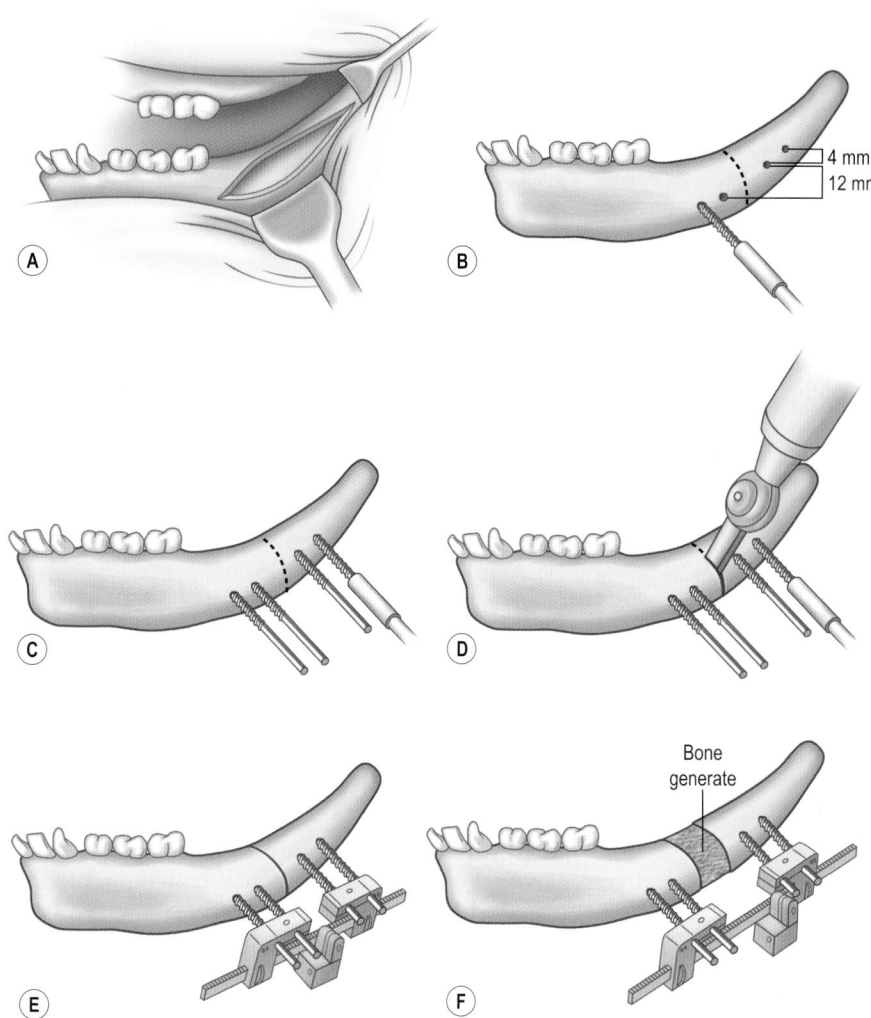

Fig. 36.19 Technique of extraoral distraction. **(A)** Intraoral incision (can also use transcutaneous submandibular incisions). **(B)** Line of osteotomy and sites of insertion of self-drilling pins. **(C)** Partial osteotomy and insertion of fourth pin. **(D)** Completion of osteotomy. **(E)** The device has been attached. **(F)** Generation of bone after activation of the device.

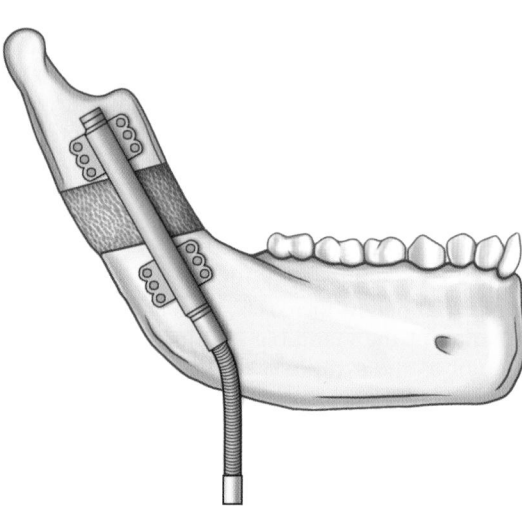

Fig. 36.20 Schematic drawing of an internal/semiburied mandibular distraction device. The device is shown in the consolidation phase after completing activation.

With the accumulation of clinical experience, it has been demonstrated that mandibular distraction can be repeated (secondary distraction), that previously inserted rib or iliac grafts of adequate volume can also be distracted, and that the temporomandibular joint can be reconstructed by the technique of transport distraction *(Fig. 36.24)*. In transport distraction, a reverse L-shaped osteotomy is made in the ramal segment. A distraction device is placed across the osteotomy, and the leading edge of the transport segment is driven in the direction of the pseudoglenoid fossa. The leading edge of the transport segment develops a fibrous cartilage surface that simulates the articular surface of the condyle.

Maxillomandibular distraction is also possible by performing a concomitant Le Fort I osteotomy (incomplete) at the time of the mandibular osteotomy (see *Fig. 36.9*). The patient is placed in intermaxillary fixation, and as mandibular distraction proceeds, the maxillary segment is moved in an inferior and anterior direction. Thus, the occlusal cant is corrected, the oral commissure is lowered, and the chin is moved to the midline.

The technique is especially indicated in the older child in whom spontaneous or orthodontically guided descent of the maxillary dentoalveolus into the posterior open bite resulting from unilateral mandibular distraction is not possible (see section on management of the occlusion: the role of the

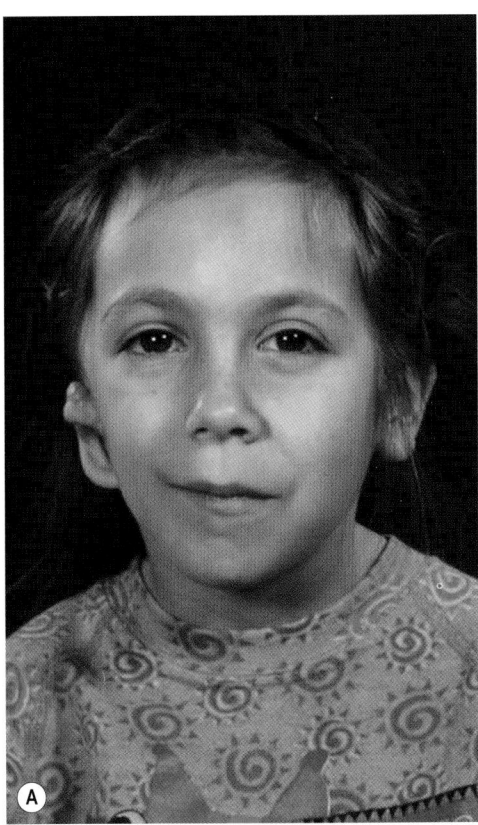
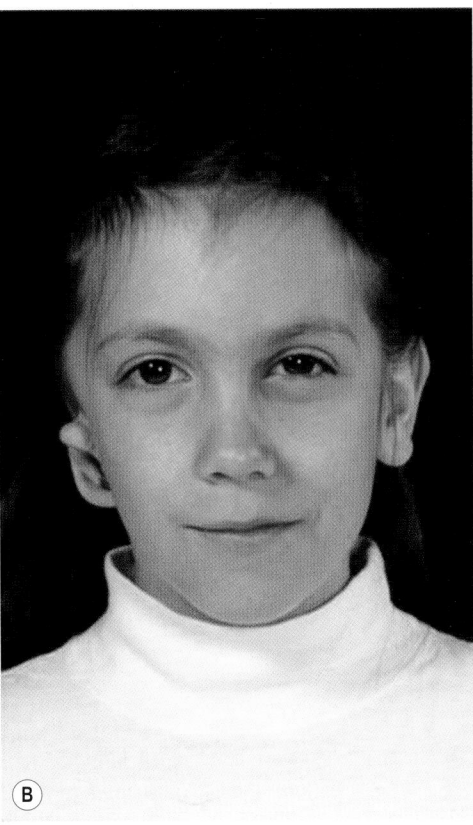

Fig. 36.21 Example of a patient with moderate craniofacial microsomia who underwent unilateral distraction of the right mandible. **(A)** Note the characteristic features of chin point deviation and an occlusal cant to the affected side. **(B)** Postoperative result demonstrating the improved chin point position and soft-tissue contour.

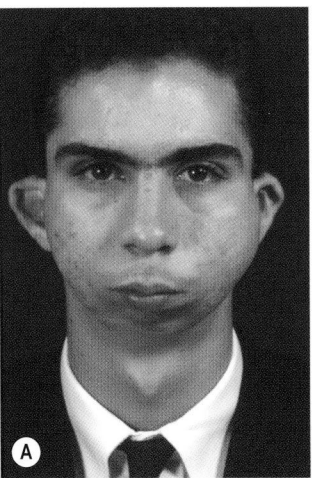
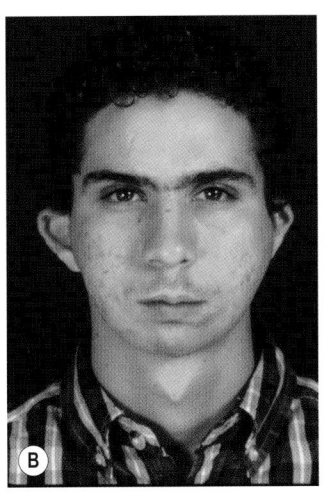
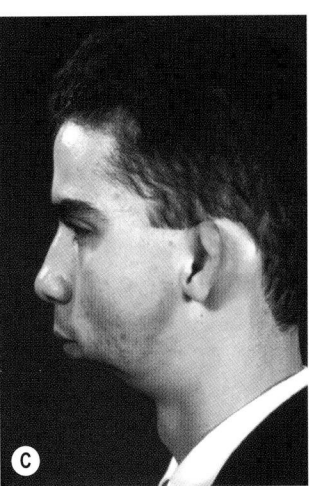
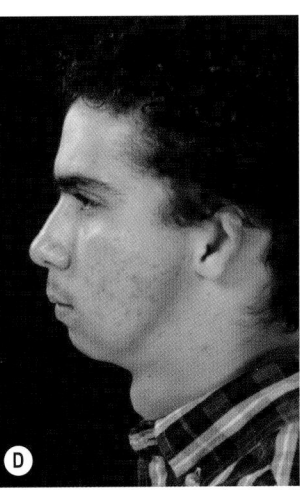

Fig. 36.22 A clinical example of a patient with severe bilateral craniofacial microsomia. Preoperative frontal **(A)** and lateral views **(C)** demonstrate a severely retrognathic appearance with minimal definition of his chin. Postoperative views **(B, D)** following bilateral distraction.

orthodontist later in this chapter). The Le Fort I corticotomy can also be performed on the younger patient without fear of injury to the unerupted maxillary teeth.

Bone grafts

Rib or iliac bone grafting has been the traditional method of reconstructing the type III mandibular skeletal defect (absence of the ramus and condyle) *(Fig. 36.25)*. Through a coronal incision, complemented by a submandibular Risdon incision,

the mandibular remnant is exposed in a subperiostal plane. The projected location of the glenoid fossa is determined through the coronal incision. If the zygomatic arch is missing, this becomes part of the bone graft reconstruction. The cartilaginous end of the iliac crest or two-tier rib graft is placed in a groove of the reconstructed zygomatic arch, and the cartilaginouos portion, simulating a condyle, prevents ankylosis. Rigid skeletal fixation is achieved at the mandibular remnant, and the patient is placed in intermaxillary fixation, which is removed at approximately 8 weeks. Subsequent growth of the

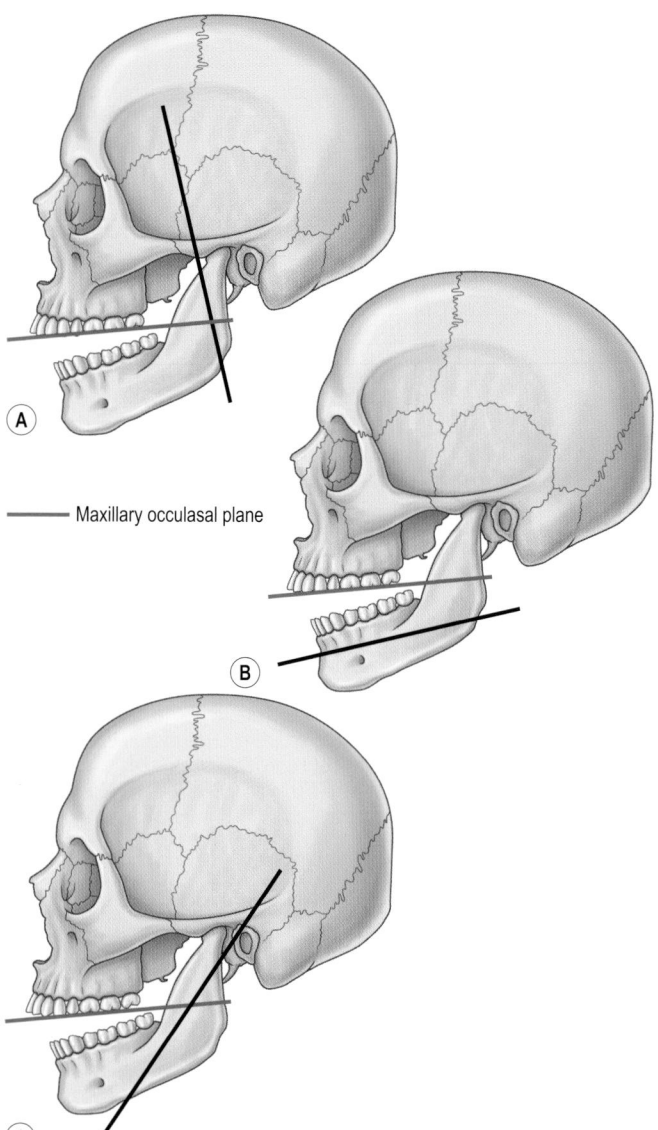

Maxillary occulasal plane

Fig. 36.23 Vectors of distraction. **(A)** The vertical vector is 90° to the maxillary occlusal plane and is indicated for the patient with deficiency localized to the mandibular ramus. **(B)** The horizontal vector is relatively parallel to the maxillary occlusal plane and is indicated for deficiency of the mandibular body. **(C)** The oblique vector is between the vertical and the horizontal vectors and is indicated for correction of combined mandibular ramus body deficiency.

mandible is unpredictable, but the patients can undergo distraction of the bone graft-reconstructed mandibular site at a later date *(Fig. 36.26)*.

An alternative technique is the reconstruction of the missing ramus/condyle with a microvascular fibula free flap with or without a skin "paddle" to correct the soft-tissue deficiency.

Maxillomandibular orthognathic surgery

In the skeletally mature patient, traditional maxillomandibular orthognathic surgery is indicated. The mandibular osteotomies include the bilateral sagittal split of the ramus and the vertical or oblique osteotomy of the ramus. Obwegeser combined the Le Fort I maxillary osteotomy with bilateral sagittal split of the mandibular ramus and genioplasty *(Fig. 36.27)* to ensure leveling of the occlusal plane and establishment of the optimal occlusal relationships. The Le Fort I osteotomy is repositioned, according to preoperative plans, and rigid skeletal fixation is achieved with plates and screws. The sagittal split and vertical or oblique osteotomies allow repositioning of the tooth-bearing mandibular segments. Fixation, especially in the sagittal split procedure, is achieved with lag screws or plates. Genioplasty, usually in three planes, completes the procedure *(Fig. 36.28)*.

Careful planning is essential. The occlusal cant observed in unilateral CFM results from a reduction in the vertical dimension of the maxilla and mandible on the affected side. Some patients may also show, superimposed on this growth abnormality, facial findings characteristic of the long-face or short-face syndrome, as manifested by excessive or deficient maxillary gingival exposure at rest or on smiling. The objectives of surgery are to correct the occlusal cant while at the same time optimizing the lip–incisor relationship.

There are three potential movements of the Le Fort I segment for correction of the defect *(Fig. 36.29)*. In the first example, the left side is affected but the skeletal and soft-tissue relationship is normal on this side. In this example, when the patient smiles, an excessive amount of teeth and gingivae shows on the less affected (right) side. The Le Fort I segment is illustrated as elevated or impacted on the right side only, correcting the cant of the occlusal plane. In the second example, the left side is affected and the maxilla is vertically deficient on this side. The patient, on smiling, shows a normal amount of gingivae and dental structures on the less

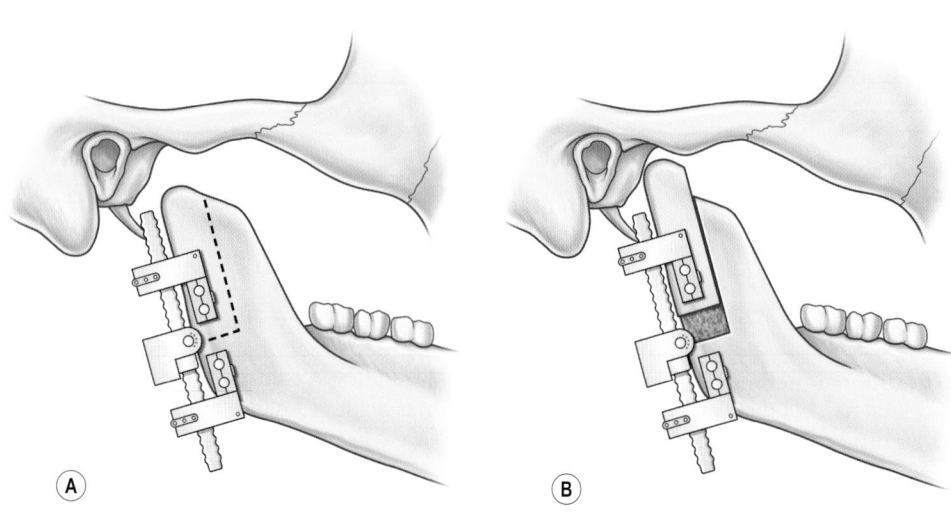

Fig. 36.24 Technique of transport distraction. **(A)** L-shaped osteotomy (interrupted lines) and application of the distraction device. **(B)** With activation of the device, bone is generated in the ramus, and a condyle (with a fibrocartilage cap) is advanced into a pseudoglenoid fossa.

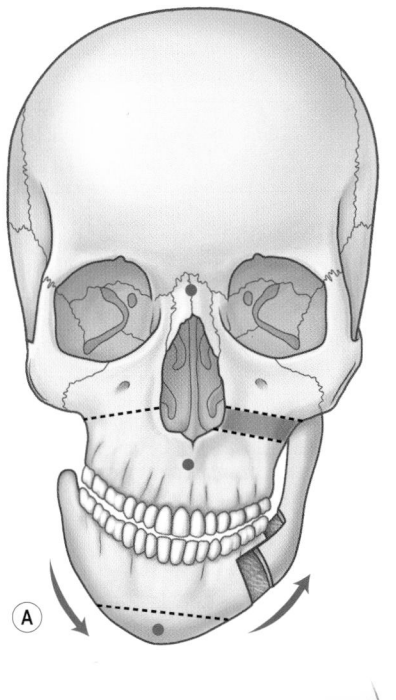
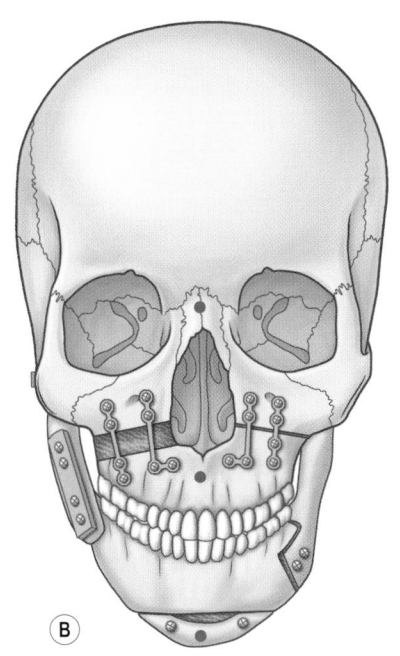

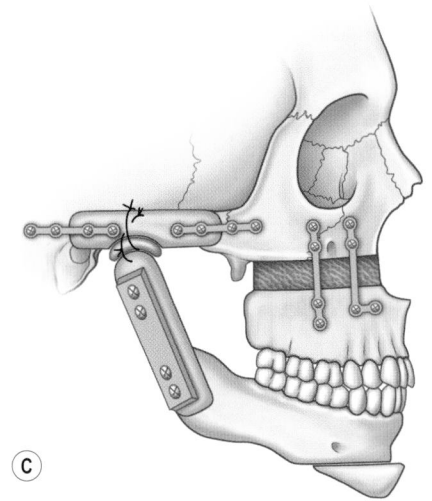
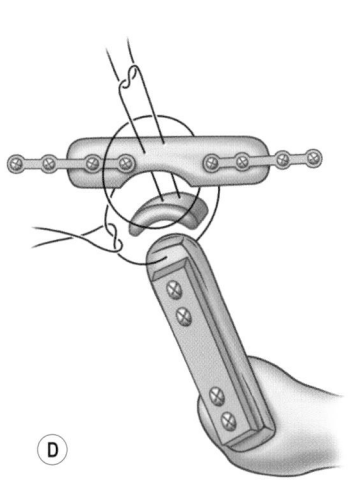

Fig. 36.25 Technique of bone graft reconstruction of the mandibular ramus, condyle, and glenoid fossa in unilateral craniofacial microsomia. **(A)** The dots designate the asymmetry of the craniofacial midline, and the arrows show the projected movement of the mandible. Note the Le Fort I line of osteotomy and the area of osteotomy on the unaffected side of the maxilla. In the mandible, the genioplasty and sagittal split osteotomies are illustrated. **(B)** After osteotomy and movement of the maxillary and mandibular segments and double-tier bone graft reconstruction of the ramus, condyle, and glenoid fossa. A bone graft has been placed in the maxillary defect. Rigid skeletal fixation has been established across the Le Fort I, sagittal split, and genioplasty osteotomies. **(C and D)** Lateral views illustrating the details of the ramus, condyle, and glenoid fossa (bone graft) reconstruction. Note that the cartilage cap is interposed between the bone grafts, reconstructing the ramus, condyle, and glenoid fossa (undersurface of the zygomatic arch). A resorbable suture approximates these.

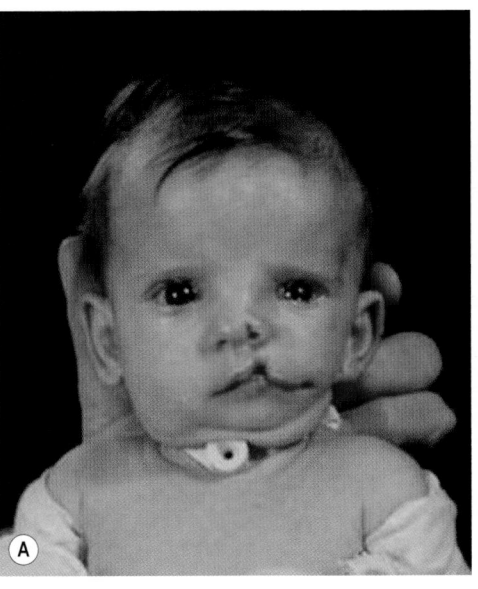
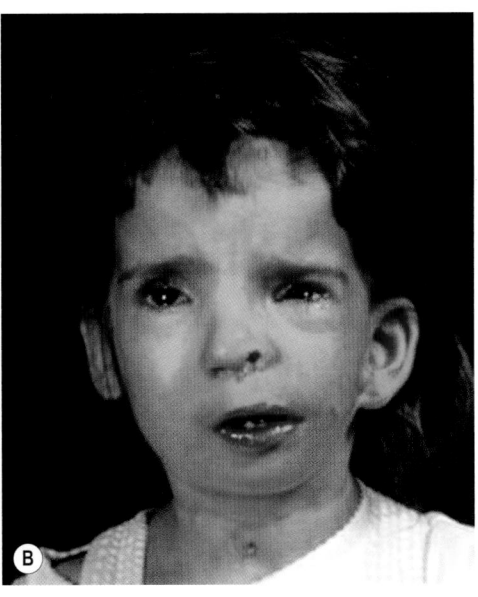

Fig. 36.26 (A) An example of a patient with left-sided craniofacial microsomia and significant clefting is shown. This patient presented with a Pruzansky III mandible, and underwent bone graft reconstruction of her left mandibular ramus. **(B)** Subsequent distraction of her bone graft was then performed with improvement in symmetry.

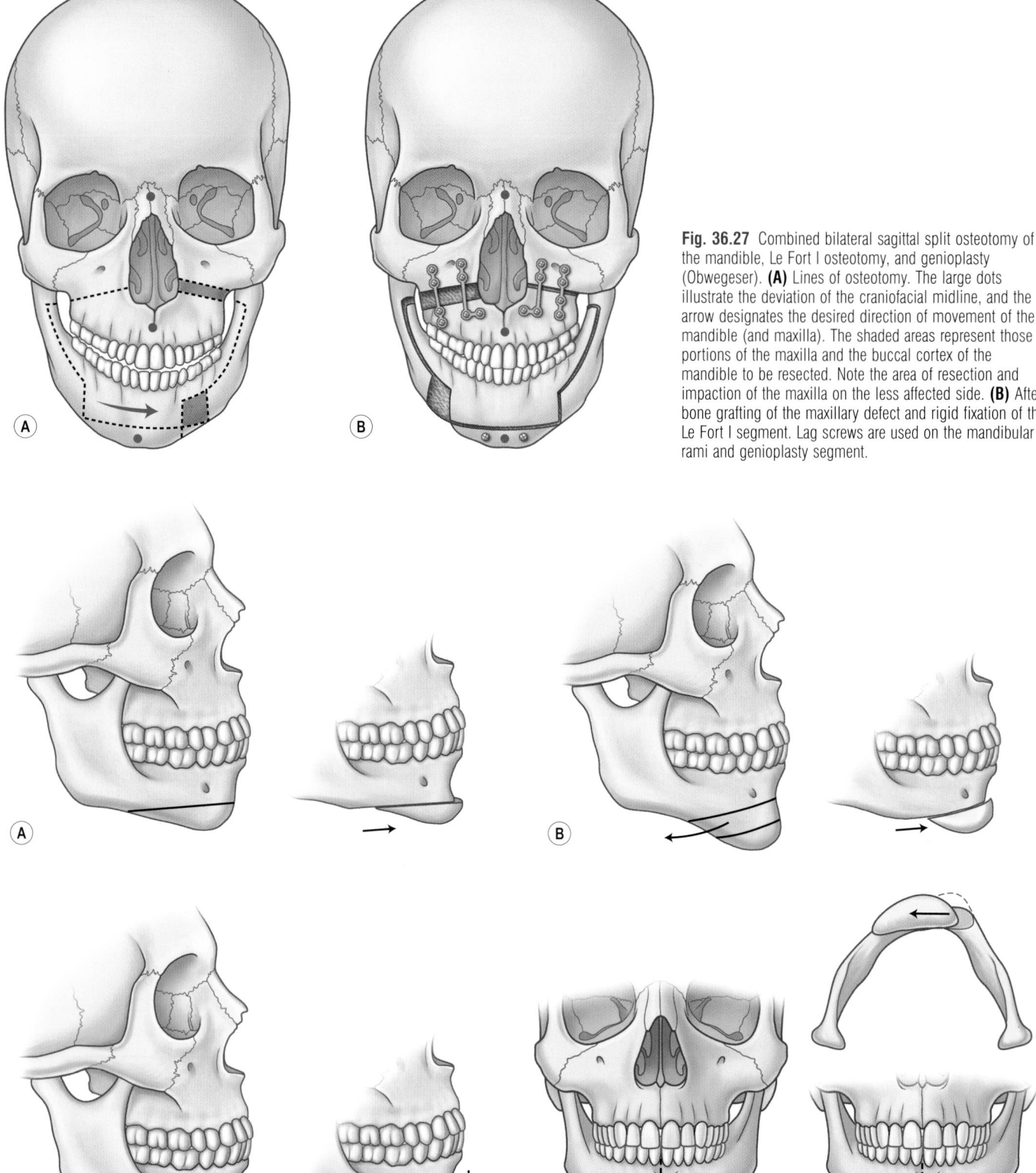

Fig. 36.27 Combined bilateral sagittal split osteotomy of the mandible, Le Fort I osteotomy, and genioplasty (Obwegeser). **(A)** Lines of osteotomy. The large dots illustrate the deviation of the craniofacial midline, and the arrow designates the desired direction of movement of the mandible (and maxilla). The shaded areas represent those portions of the maxilla and the buccal cortex of the mandible to be resected. Note the area of resection and impaction of the maxilla on the less affected side. **(B)** After bone grafting of the maxillary defect and rigid fixation of the Le Fort I segment. Lag screws are used on the mandibular rami and genioplasty segment.

Fig. 36.28 Location and orientation of the advanced genioplasty segment. **(A)** In advancement in the *z*-axis, the osteotomy is placed well below the mental foramina to avoid injury to the inferior alveolar nerve. The angulation of the osteotomy allows forward advancement of the chin without any vertical changes. **(B)** Simultaneous advancement and vertical reduction of the chin. Note that two parallel osteotomies are performed with an intervening osteotomy. **(C)** Simultaneous advancement and vertical elongation of the chin. The interposition material typically employed is blocks of porous hydroxyapatite. **(D)** Lateral shifting of the symphyseal segment in the *x*-axis to restore lower face symmetry.

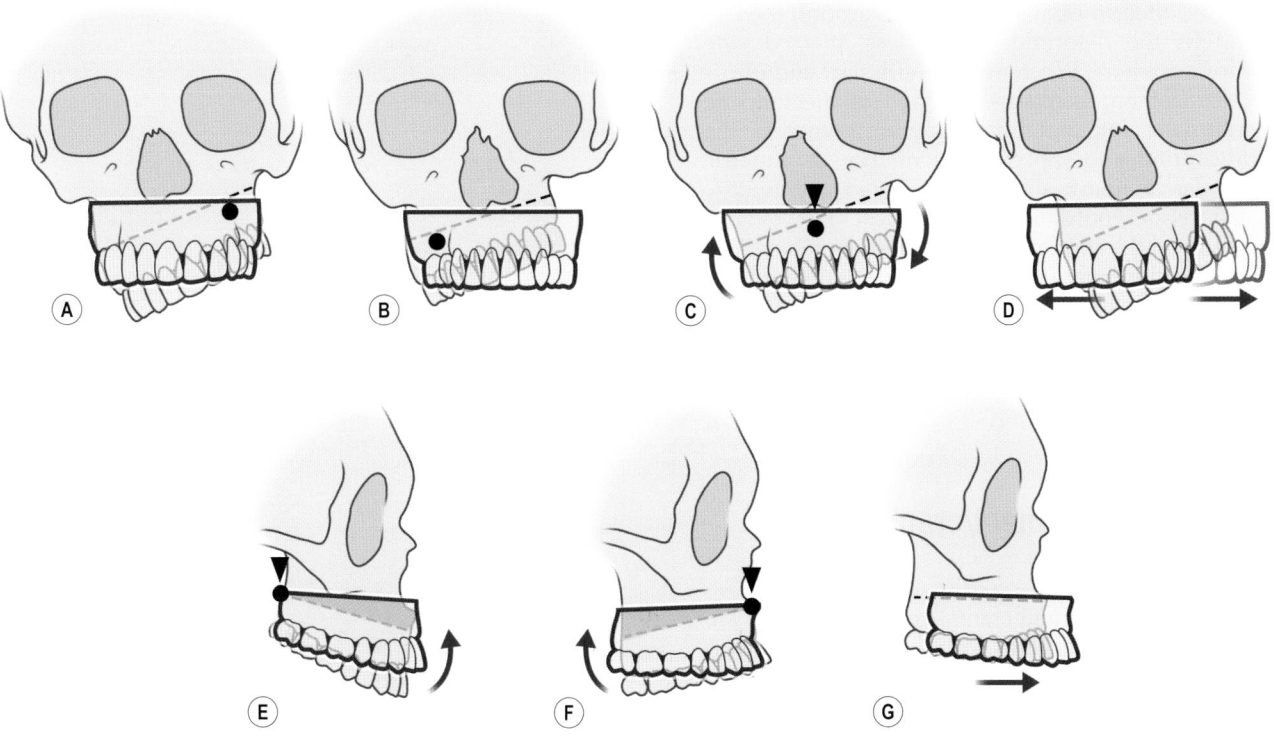

Fig. 36.29 Correction of the occlusal cant. **(A–C)** Vertical changes with the Le Fort I segment (large dot = pivot point); dotted lines represent the preoperative position and bold lines represent the postoperative position of the Le Fort I segment. Arrows designate direction of skeletal movement. **(D)** Horizontal changes with the Le Fort I segment. **(E and F)** Anterior and posterior impaction of the Le Fort I segment in a superior direction. **(G)** Anterior advancement. Rigid skeletal fixation is not illustrated.

affected (right) side and a deficient amount of these structures on the affected (left) side. For the skeletal and soft-tissue relationship to be improved on the affected side, the Le Fort I segment is displaced inferiorly on the left side only. Note that the center of rotation is on the right as the occlusal plane is leveled. In the third example, the patient's left side is affected and the teeth appear slightly above the drape of the lips. The right side shows an excessive amount of gingiva on smiling. Correction of the occlusal cant is achieved by rotating the Le Fort I segment around a point at the midline (i.e., impaction on the right, lowering on the left). It should be emphasized that the skeletal deformity may also require other types of correction by movement of the Le Fort I segment to the left or right in the horizontal dimension. On evaluation of the lateral cephalogram, correction of the deformity may require that the segment be rotated superiorly or inferiorly either anteriorly or posteriorly in combination with advancement or setback of the osteotomized segment.

Two-splint technique

In the correction of the skeletal asymmetry in unilateral CFM when simultaneous surgery of both jaws is planned, two interocclusal splints are employed. The first or intermediate splint is used to establish the position of the osteotomized maxillary segment by referencing it to this splint that is wired to the nonosteotomized mandible. The mandible and splinted maxillary segment are rotated around the condyles and mobilized superiorly, ensuring accurate condylar "seating." The maxilla is fixed into position with plates and screws. The intermediate splint is removed, and a second or definitive splint is wired to

the maxillary dentition. The mandibular osteotomies are completed, after which the mandible is guided into its planned position as it is wired into the definitive splint. Rigid fixation of the mandibular segments is then established.

The two-splint procedure functions only when both condyles and rami are of normal shape and size – usually not the case in unilateral craniofacial microsomia. The unequal ramal heights and condylar pathologic anatomy result in an asymmetric path of closure for the affected mandible. The mandibular body follows a path of opening and closing that is oblique rather than parallel to the craniofacial midsagittal plane. This complex three-dimensional motion cannot be accurately reproduced on conventional dental articulators. Thus, the intermediate splint does not accurately position the Le Fort I segment when the mandible is rotated upward toward the maxilla. Establishing the position of the Le Fort I segment is therefore dependent on calculations of the planned change derived from the results of mock surgery on articulated study models, mock surgery on the cephalograms, and three-dimensional cephalometric or CT images.

Unilateral versus bilateral ramus osteotomies to reposition the mandible

The mandible and maxilla in unilateral CFM demonstrate a true bilateral deformity. The primary deformity, by virtue of its effect on altering jaw position and function, induces compensatory shape and size changes on the unaffected or "less affected" side. This is seen as a bowing-out and elongation of the mandibular body and ramus on the less affected side. When the mandible is repositioned only by osteotomizing or bone grafting the affected ramus and rotation around the less affected condyle, the deformity of the less affected side becomes more apparent. When the mandibular midline is centered in this fashion, the contour of the less affected side appears abnormally full and thrust laterally, whereas the affected side continues to appear deficient. The asymmetric bony mandibular anatomy and the associated asymmetric overlying soft tissue contribute to this effect. However, a ramal osteotomy on the contralateral side permits repositioning of the mandibular body in a manner that reduces, rather than emphasizes, the asymmetry. The optimally repositioned mandible results in minimal lateral displacement of the less affected mandibular body while maximal inferior and lateral displacement of the affected side is obtained. Soft-tissue augmentation of the cheek on the affected side is often required to achieve more symmetric craniofacial contour.

Fronto-orbital advancement/cranial vault remodeling

Fronto-orbital advancement and cranial vault remodeling are occasionally indicated in the child with retrusion of the ipsilateral supraorbital rim and frontal bone. A combined craniofacial route is required to provide surgical access to the frontal bone, orbits, and nasal radix. After an anterior craniotomy, a fronto-orbital advancement is performed. The frontal bone (forehead) can be reconstructed by remodeling the native frontal bone or replacing it with a harvested cranial bone graft.

Autogenous fat injections

Autogenous fat, harvested from the abdominal wall, flanks, or buttocks and injected into the deficient facial soft tissues, has become an effective treatment modality in serially improving craniofacial contour. Serial injections or treatments are required and successful graft incorporation cannot be predicted due to variable early resorption. It should also be noted that fat injections also improve the quality of the overlying skin (dermal thickness and cutaneous contour) after they are revascularized.

Microvascular free flap

The microvascular free flap has become the surgical workhorse in augmenting the severely deficient soft tissue of the cheek and preauricular and neck regions *(Fig. 36.30)*. The preferred donor site is the parascapular area, and different components of the flap can be used to restore the contour of the temporal, cheek, and upper lip regions. It is wise to defer the free flap until the underlying skeletal deficiencies have been corrected. Soft-tissue restoration with a microvascular free flap can camouflage any underlying postsurgical skeletal irregularities *(Fig. 36.31)*. However, secondary recontouring procedures are often indicated.

Although autogenous dermis-fat grafts have been recommended, long-term survival is less predictable, and there can be residual contour irregularities from resorption and scarring of the graft. They have largely been replaced by autogeneous fat grafting techniques.

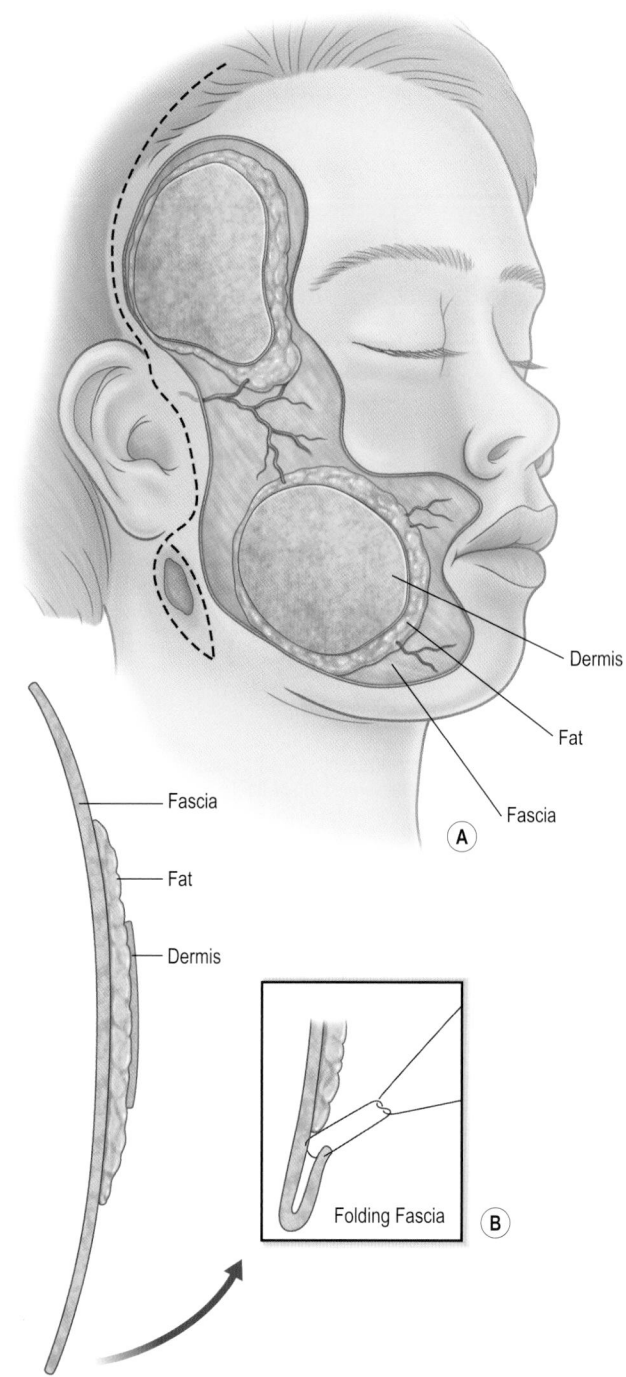

Fig. 36.30 (A) Schematic drawing showing lines of incision and soft-tissue deficits that are reconstructed by use of a composite de-epithelialized dermis, fat, and fascial flap. **(B)** Cross-sectional line drawing showing how folding of the fascia into multiple layers enables reconstruction of variable layers of subtle soft tissue. (Reproduced from Siebert JW, Longaker MT. Microsurgical correction of facial asymmetry in hemifacial microsomia. *Operative Techniques Plast Reconstr Surg*. 1994;1:94.)

Auricular reconstruction

Auricular reconstruction is required in patients with microtia. The multistaged reconstruction is usually deferred until the child is at least 8 years of age (see Chapter 7).

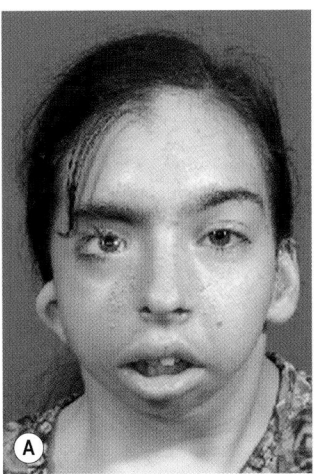 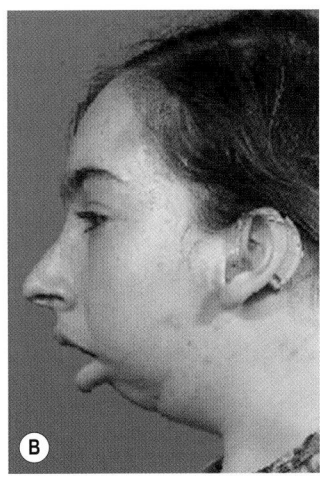 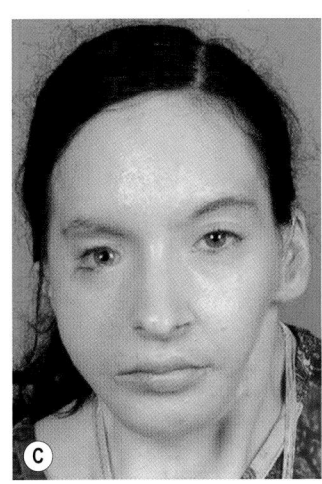 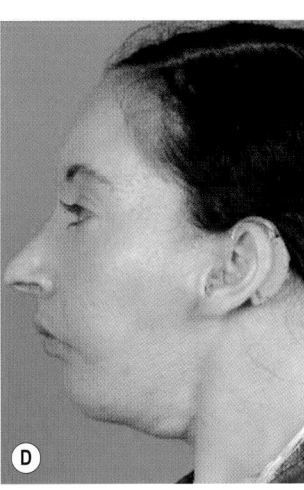

Fig. 36.31 Patient with right-sided craniofacial microsomia who required reconstruction of her mandible with composite bone and overlying soft tissue **(A, B).** An osteocutaneous parascapular free flap was subsequently performed to provide soft tissue as well as additional bone stock after bilateral sagittal split osteotomies, LeFort I, and genioplasty **(C, D).** Performed with Dr. John Siebert.

Management of the occlusion: the role of the orthodontist

Early intervention

Because the deciduous dentition is often used in the early interceptive orthodontic and surgical phases of care, the patient is referred for a pedodontic oral health evaluation between the ages of 12 and 18 months. This is intended to provide the parents with guidelines for their child's dental care and to begin preparing the child behaviorally to cooperate with oral examination and treatment.

The objectives of orthodontic treatment, in the deciduous dentition, are aimed at preventing or intercepting the development of severe malocclusion and enhancing skeletal growth. A typical example is to provide adequate space for the eruption of the adult dentition by expansion and enlargement of the maxillary arch. In the mandibular dental arch, prevention of space loss due to premature shedding of a deciduous tooth may be achieved with a lingual arch space maintainer. On occasion, a mandibular first or second molar tooth bud may be present lying in the path of the anticipated distraction osteotomy or in the site of a planned bone graft. In some circumstances, the orthodontist may presurgically use orthodontic forces to erupt the tooth and to guide it out of the surgical site, sparing its early demise.

A review of the orthodontic literature shows that attempts have been made to use functional orthodontic appliance therapy to correct "mild" mandibular asymmetry in patients with craniofacial microsomia. The orthodontic literature is replete with papers debating the ability of functional appliance therapy to improve mandibular growth in children found among the "normal" population. It is doubtful that children born with mandibular anomalies of moderate to severe deficiency will achieve lasting benefit, if any, from functional appliance therapies. The authors are of the opinion that functional appliance therapy in this population causes undesirable dentoalveolar compensations; therefore in instances of significant functional deficit (airway, swallowing, psychosocial) we favor early mandibular DO or bone graft reconstruction.

Predistraction orthodontic management

As in the preparation of a patient for orthognathic surgery, predistraction orthodontics may include removal of dental compensations, coordination of dental arch widths, and correction of occlusal plane disharmony and crowding. After these objectives are achieved with fixed orthodontic appliances, passive rectangular arch wires and surgical hooks are placed for the use of intermaxillary guiding elastics during the active stage of distraction. Before consolidation of the newly formed bone (generate), it is possible to mold the generate with intermaxillary elastics and to adjust the vector of distraction to achieve the planned occlusion. In the young child, an occlusal splint might be required at the end of device activation to maintain the leveled mandibular occlusal plane while interocclusal space is maintained for the postdistraction correction of the maxillary occlusal plane. The postdistraction-activation splint also serves to reduce or negate the effect of the masseter muscle contraction and compression of the newly formed generate.

Orthodontic management during active distraction

The vectors of distraction may be further modified by the use of intermaxillary elastics during the activation phase. After a bone generate is formed by activation of the distraction device, up to the first few weeks of consolidation, intermaxillary elastics can alter the skeletal and dental relationships. Intermaxillary elastics may be worn in class II, class III, vertical, or transverse directions during the activation phase. Anterior vertical intermaxillary elastics may be helpful in reducing an anterior open bite and may be employed transversely to correct or to prevent lateral shifting of the mandible *(Fig. 36.32).* In some patients for whom an open bite has been closed, intermaxillary elastics may be worn during the consolidation period for skeletal and dental retention.

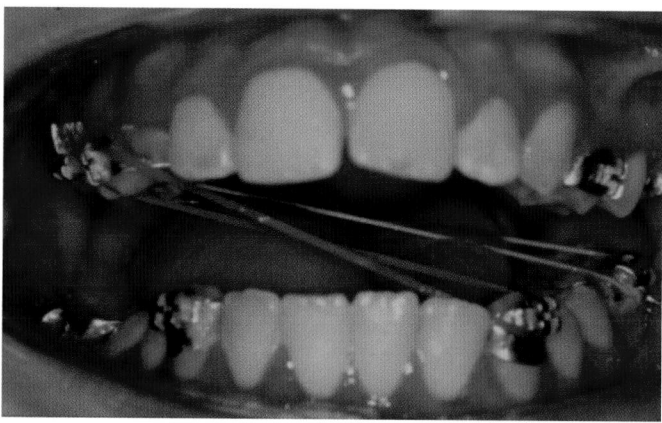

Fig. 36.32 Translingual elastics preventing laterognathism during activation of a unilateral distraction device.

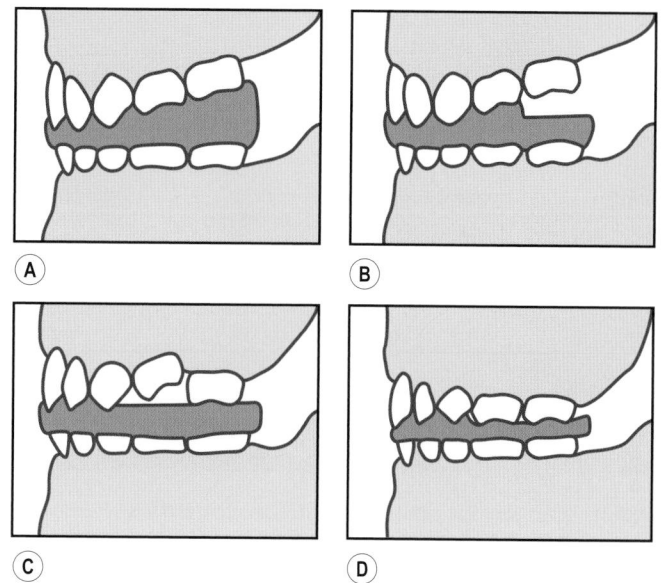

Fig. 36.33 Management of posterior open bite after unilateral mandibular distraction. **(A)** Postdistraction open bite with occlusal bite plate. **(B)** Serial reduction of bite plate occlusal to the posterior maxillary molar. **(C)** Eruption of the posterior maxillary molar to the bite plate followed by progressive anterior reduction of the bite plate. **(D)** After occlusal eruption of the maxillary dentition to the reduced surface of the bite plate.

The progress of distraction is monitored by documenting changes in the relationships of the maxillary and mandibular dentition and changes in the orientation of the occlusal plane, oral commissure, and position of the chin. In general, and especially in the growing child, activation of the device continues until the deformity is overcorrected (e.g., anterior crossbite in a bilateral patient and lowering of the commissure and occlusal plane on the affected side below that of the contralateral side in the unilateral patient). The amount of overcorrection is influenced by the amount of expected postdistraction growth remaining in the craniofacial skeleton. A young child with much growth ahead would be overcorrected more than a child who is approaching completion of growth. With the expectation that postdistraction growth will be "syndromic" and inadequate to keep up with the "normal side," there is a need for overcorrection of the ramus in the very young child.

Postdistraction orthodontic management

In unilateral distraction cases, the orthodontist is often confronted with a treatment-induced posterior open bite on the distracted side and crossbite on the contralateral side. The open bite may be managed with gradual adjustment of a bite plate *(Fig. 36.33)*. The crossbite resulting from mandibular shift across the midsagittal plane may be corrected by a combination of transpalatal arches, lingual arches, intermaxillary cross elastics, and palatal expansion devices.

The posterior open bite that is often observed after unilateral distraction results from vertical lengthening of the ramus and consequent lowering of the mandibular occlusal plane on the affected side. It is important to prevent relapse of the mandibular occlusal plane correction resulting from uncontrolled occlusal overeruption of the mandibular teeth and alveolus. The posterior open bite plate is adjusted gradually to achieve eruption of the maxillary teeth and dentoalveolar process down to the level of the mandibular occlusal plane. During several months, the posterior superior surface of the appliance is serially reduced under pairs of maxillary teeth to allow their gradual eruption and inferior descent. The ability of the maxillary dentoalveolus to hypererupt is lost in later years.

After vertical unilateral distraction of the mandibular ramus, the mandibular body shifts toward the contralateral side, often resulting in posterior crossbites. The crossbite on the distracted side shows the maxillary teeth buccal to the mandibular teeth. On the contralateral side, the maxillary teeth are palatal to the mandibular teeth (palatal crossbite). The palate may be expanded to correct the crossbite with a classic palatal expansion device. Maxillary palatal expansion typically occurs bilaterally: as the palatal crossbite is corrected, the buccal crossbite may be accentuated. To prevent this, intermaxillary cross elastics may be worn on the side of the buccal crossbite. The lower molars may be supported by a lingual arch to minimize the tendency for the cross elastic to tip the lower molars out toward the buccal aspect while the maxillary molars are tipped to the palatal aspect and into improved occlusal relationship with the lower dental arch.

Treatment algorithm

Neonatal period and infancy

In the evaluation of the newborn or infant, the surgeon must assess the respiratory function of the child. With a severe mandibular deficiency and associated glossoptosis, the nasal and oral pharyngeal spaces are severely constricted. A pediatric otolaryngologist is invaluable in documenting the respiratory status of the patient by physical and endoscopic examination. Pulse oximetry and sleep studies (polysomnography) complement the evaluation.

Endotracheal intubation is occasionally indicated after delivery. If it appears that the need for endotracheal intubation will be prolonged, tracheostomy has traditionally been the technique employed. With the development of mandibular distraction, it has been demonstrated that distraction of the mandible can obviate the need for a tracheostomy. Whichever modality is selected, the clinician must ensure that, by one method or another, the airway must be secured.

Infants with sleep apnea often have associated feeding problems. Gavage feeding can be provided initially, but if the feeding problem continues, gastrostomy should be considered to ensure adequate calorie intake for the child. The nutritional requirements of the infant are accentuated by the energy demands associated with respiratory distress. Feeding problems are usually relieved when the sleep apnea has been corrected.

Fronto-orbital advancement and cranial vault remodeling may also be indicated in a small percentage of patients with a fronto-orbital deformity. Such surgery should be delayed until the child is at least 12 months of age.

A few patients may also require repair of an associated cleft of the lip, alveolus, hard or soft palate, and this should be repaired at the appropriate age. It is also the optimal time to repair a macrostomia or lateral facial cleft.

Removal of ear tags or cartilaginous remnants in the cheeks is always satisfying for the parents, and this can also be done in the first year.

Early childhood

During the period of early childhood (18 months through 3 years), mandibular reconstruction can be undertaken in the child with respiratory insufficiency or a moderate or severe example of skeletal deficiency.

For the child with a type III mandible (absent ramus and condyle), autogenous rib or iliac bone grafting of the hypoplastic mandible should be undertaken. As mentioned previously, such bone (neomandible) is amenable to a distraction procedure at a later stage provided there is adequate bone volume. Treatment would result in an improved airway and facial appearance. It would also facilitate orthodontic work in establishing a functional occlusion.

For the patient with a type IIA or IIB deformity, mandible distraction could be undertaken especially if there is associated respiratory insufficiency or significant facial dysmorphism that could impair psychosocial development. In the unilateral case, activation of the distraction device should continue until the occlusal plane and affected oral commissure are lowered below the unaffected side and sufficient anterior thrust of the mandible and chin is achieved to improve the retroglossal airway and facial appearance.

Soft-tissue augmentation is not undertaken at this stage. In like fashion, the child is not a suitable candidate for orthodontic therapy or auricular reconstruction.

Childhood

Childhood is defined as the period from 4 through 13 years when there is active craniofacial growth and development. For much of this time, the child is in the period of mixed dentition. Primary mandibular distraction could be undertaken during this period if there is a respiratory deficiency or evidence of a significant dysmorphism, as

characterized by occlusal cant, disparity of the oral commissure, and chin asymmetry and retrusion.

Experience has shown that in the patient undergoing mandibular distraction before 3 years of age there is usually a spontaneous descent of the associated maxillary dentoalveolus with mandibular distraction. Beyond that age, there are two choices for managing the cant of the maxillary occlusal plane. In the first program, mandibular distraction can be accomplished and an orthodontic bite block constructed at the time of device removal to fill the resulting posterior void between the maxillary and mandibular dentition. During the subsequent year, the orthodontist can gradually reduce the bite block to allow serial descent of the maxillary dentoalveolus. In the alternative method, combined maxillomandibular distraction is performed with a combined Le Fort I corticotomy, sparing the unerupted maxillary dentition, and mandibular osteotomy with distraction device application. With activation of the device and intermaxillary fixation, there is associated distraction of the maxilla with leveling of the occlusal plane.

It is during the childhood years that auricular reconstruction is undertaken and microvascular free-flap or serial fat injection augmentation of the cheek soft tissues can be considered.

Orthodontic therapy can be instituted as early as 4 years of age, depending on the level of the patient's cooperation. The following treatment options must be considered by the orthodontist:

1. early intervention by a pediatric dentist to prepare the teeth for any orthodontic therapy
2. early orthodontic intervention:
   • maxillary arch expansion to provide space for the adult dentition
   • mandibular lingual arch space maintenance
   • forced eruption of a molar tooth bud out of the proposed path of the mandibular osteotomy to prevent extraction of a molar
3. distraction stabilization appliance for unilateral ramal vertical lengthening
4. bite block therapy for controlled dentoalveolar elongation of the ipsilateral maxillary posterior segment.

Adolescence and adulthood

Adolescence/adulthood is defined as that period when craniofacial growth and development are completed, usually at a minimum of 16 years for girls and 17 years for boys. Treatment planning at this stage does not have to take into consideration the important variable of subsequent growth and development. The role of the orthodontist involves preoperative planning as well as presurgical and postsurgical orthodontic therapy.

Orthognathic surgery plays a role at this point because in a single surgical maneuver the craniofacial skeletal structure can be restored and optimal occlusion achieved as part of a combined orthodontic and surgical rehabilitation program. The surgical procedure described by Obwegeser (Le Fort I osteotomy, bilateral sagittal split osteotomy of the mandible, and genioplasty) has proved to be the therapeutic workhorse in this clinical situation.

In recent years, with the development of refined distraction devices and techniques, the role of maxillomandibular distraction in the mature patient can be considered. For example, a Le Fort I osteotomy can be performed with three-dimensional repositioning of the maxilla and rigid skeletal fixation. Intraoral mandibular distraction can then be performed, and the mandible and its occlusion can be "docked" into the repositioned maxilla. The distraction technique also improves soft-tissue contour and is associated with a lower rate of relapse. The development of the concept of molding of the generate by a combination of multiplanar distraction devices and skeletally anchored intermaxillary elastics ensures the achievement of optimal occlusion and skeletal structure.

Genioplasty alone is the only skeletal reconstruction required in patients with a mild deformity characterized only by chin retrusion and asymmetry. A three-dimensional genioplasty can provide anterior advancement of the chin and three-dimensional repositioning to correct asymmetry.

Any soft-tissue deficiencies must also be addressed with a variety of techniques such as fat injections or microvascular free flaps.

Growth studies

Mandibular growth in unilateral craniofacial microsomia: a controversy

Polley and colleagues described the skeletal growth from early childhood to maturity of patients with unilateral CFM who did not undergo surgery. They reported that mandibular asymmetry is not progressive in nature. The authors of this chapter also agree that the "mandibular asymmetry is not progressive in nature"; however, a controversy exists around describing the ramal growth rates that are responsible for maintaining a constant ratio of size difference between the left and right mandibular rami during the years of mandibular growth. Polley et al. stated that "growth of the affected side in these patients parallels that of the nonaffected side." The authors take the contrary position that growth of the affected side occurs at a rate that is less than that of the unaffected side, a finding that in itself is responsible for the gradual return to asymmetry after early unilateral mandibular distraction in growing children with unilateral craniofacial microsomia. Close examination of the data published by Polley et al. shows that the ratio of affected ramus length to unaffected ramus length remains the same over time because of, rather than in spite of, different rates of growth on each side of the mandible.

In a longitudinal study of 12 patients with unilateral CFM who underwent correction of the mandibular deformity by DO (average age 4.8 years at the time of procedure), clinical and cephalometric examinations were performed for a follow-up period of 9 years. In the period of observation after distraction, the 12 mandibles showed cephalometric and clinical evidence of growth. The nondistracted rami grew at a greater rate than the distracted rami. A reduction of the distracted ramal length, averaging 3.46 mm, occurred in the first year following surgery (*Fig. 36.34*).

Thereafter, the distracted rami grew at a rate of 0.77 mm/ year while the unaffected rami grew at a rate of 1.3 mm/year.

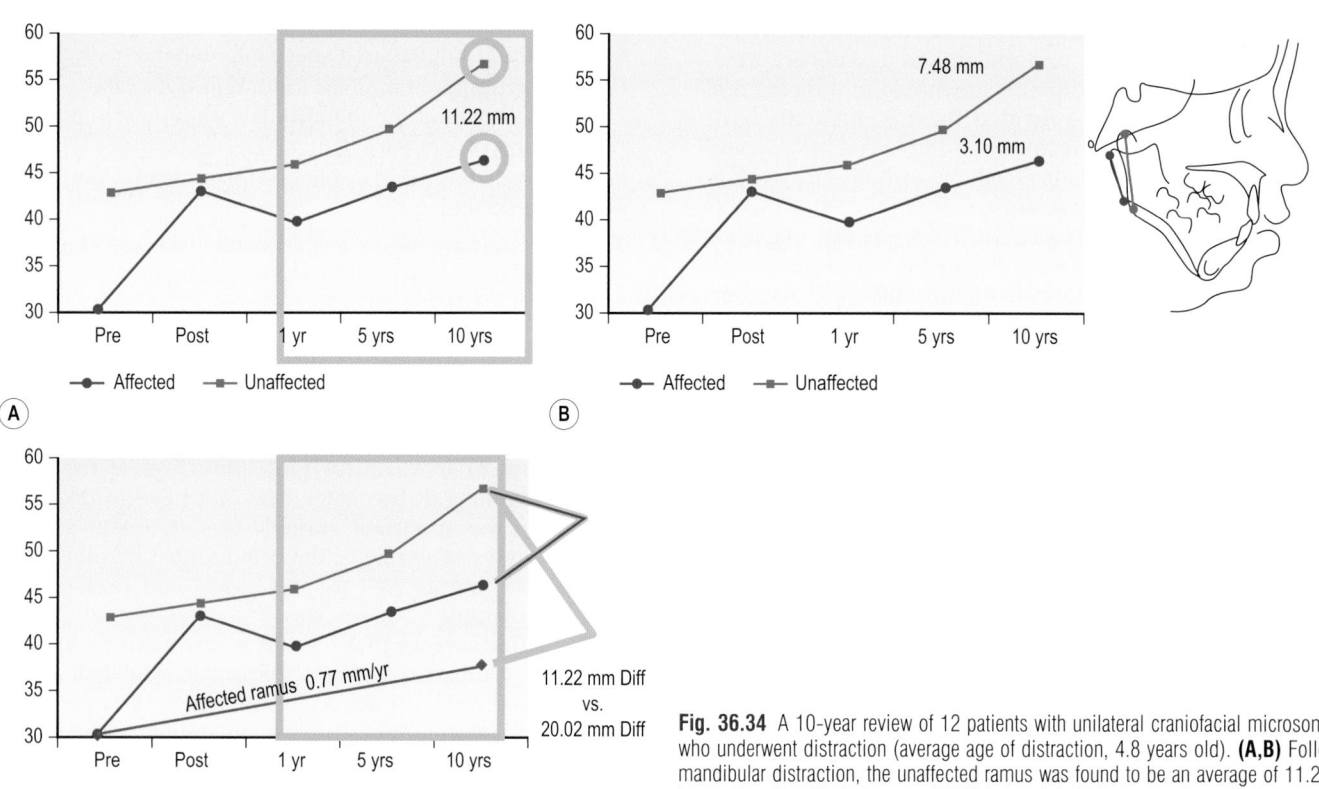

Fig. 36.34 A 10-year review of 12 patients with unilateral craniofacial microsomia who underwent distraction (average age of distraction, 4.8 years old). **(A,B)** Following mandibular distraction, the unaffected ramus was found to be an average of 11.22 mm longer than the affected ramus. **(C)** This translated into a rate of growth that was significantly greater in the unaffected ramus (1.3 mm/year) versus the affected side (0.7 mm/year).

Thus, over a period of 9 years following mandibular distraction, the affected rami increased in size by 6.93 mm while the unaffected rami increased in size by 11.73 mm. At the conclusion of the 9-year follow-up, the unaffected ramus was on average 11.22 mm longer than the affected ramus *(Fig. 36.34)*.

Thus, 10 years following distraction facial asymmetry reappears; however, it is probably not as severe as if distraction were not performed. In the interval the patient has improved craniofacial form and occlusal relationships.

References

1. Grayson BH, McCormick S, Santiago PE, et al. Vector of device placement and trajectory of mandibular distraction. *J Craniofac Surg.* 1997;8:473.

2. Shetye PR, Grayson BH, Mackool RJ, et al. Long-term stability and growth following unilateral mandibular distraction in growing children with craniofacial microsomia. *Plast Reconstr Surg.* 2006;118:985.

3. Hollier LH, Kim JH, Grayson B, et al. Mandibular growth after distraction in patients under 48 months of age. *Plast Reconstr Surg.* 1999;103:1361–1370.

4. McCarthy JG, Katzen JT, Hopper R, et al. The first decade of mandibular distraction: lessons we have learned. *Plast Reconstr Surg.* 2002;110;1704–1713.

5. Dec W, Peltomaki T, Warren SM, et al. The importance of vector selection in preoperative planning of unilateral mandibular distraction. *Plast Reconstr Surg.* 2008;121:2084.

6. Vendittelli BL, Dec W, Warren SM, et al. The importance of vector selection in preoperative planning of bilateral mandibular bilateral distraction. *Plast Reconstr Surg.* 2008;122:1144.

   This study relates the vector of distraction with the rotation/ movement of the mandible. Pre- and postoperative cephalograms of 15 patients undergoing bilateral distraction were reviewed and demonstrated that a horizontal vector resulted in vertical translation of the mandible, whereas a vertical vector resulted in greater horizontal movement of the symphysis and counterclockwise rotation.

7. Kaban LB, Moses MH, Mulliken JB. Surgical correction of hemifacial microsomia in the growing child. *Plast Reconstr Surg.* 1988;82;9.

   This study is the first to demonstrate the benefits of surgical intervention during childhood for patients with craniofacial microsomia. Twenty patients were reviewed and were divided into those undergoing lengthening with interposition bone graft (n = 10) and those having total reconstruction of the ramus. All patients demonstrated reduction in secondary deformity.

8. Obwegeser HL. Correction of the skeletal anomalies of otomandibular dystosis. *J Maxillofac Surg.* 1974;2;73.

   Landmark paper in which Obwegeser reports his approach to older patients with craniofacial microsomia (then commonly termed "otomandibular dystosis"). Cases are presented ranging from mild bone hypoplasia to patients requiring total reconstruction of the glenoid, temporal bone, zygoma, and lateral orbit.

9. Mccarthy JG, Schreiber JS, Karp NS, et al. Lengthening of the human mandible by gradual distraction. *Plast Reconstruct Surg.* 1992;89;1.

   First study to demonstrate the successful use of distraction osteogenesis of the craniofacial skeleton in humans. Gradual lengthening of the mandible via distraction is reported in four patients.

10. Siebert JW, Longaker MT. Microsurgical correction of facial asymmetry in hemifacial microsomia. *Operative Techniques Plast Reconstr Surg.* 1994;1;93.

    Microsurgical techniques have become an important adjunct to the treatment of craniofacial microsomia in providing soft tissue, as well as bone if needed. Siebert and colleagues report their experience with free-flap reconstruction for soft-tissue deficiency in patients with craniofacial microsomia.

37

Hemifacial atrophy

Peter J. Taub, Lester Silver, and Kathryn S. Torok

SYNOPSIS

- Pathogenesis of progressive hemifacial atrophy may be a lymphocytic neurovasculitis or a variant of localized scleroderma.
- When selecting appropriate patients for treatment, several factors are important, including the age of the patient and the nature and the complexity of the deformity (i.e., tissue types affected).
- In most patients, the disease is at first progressive but then is noted to abate on its own.
- Patients with cutaneous features treated with immunosuppression in combination with methotrexate have been found to have cessation of disease progression and reversal/improvement of disease damage.
- Surgical treatment options offer the largest amount of tissue with excellent safety and should be used in conjunction with fillers to provide the best possible outcome.

 Access the Historical Perspective section online at
http://www.expertconsult.com

Introduction

The condition of progressive hemifacial atrophy (PHA) has no definite pathogenesis, although there have been multiple suggestions for its etiology. Most recently, Pensler et al.[1] called this a lymphocytic neurovasculitis involving chronic cell-mediated vascular injury with incomplete endothelial regeneration, associated with the trigeminal nerve. Historically, it has been thought that congenital hemifacial atrophy may be a type of localized scleroderma, especially when it is noted in the forehead as the "en coup de sabre" (ECDS) or saber mark. Whether these two are different entities or whether this is the same disorder in a different form (i.e., localized scleroderma) is still not clear in the literature. In more recent years, Rogers[2] reviewed 772 cases of PHA and there was a further definitive review in 1983 by Lewkonia and Lowry.[3] The disorder has been shown to occur with other body asymmetries and has been described with a host of neurological features. Many neurology articles point out that, although less common, bony deformities can be present along with the soft-tissue defect. Bilateral cases have been reported but are unusual.

Patient selection and treatment

When selecting appropriate patients and options for treatment, several factors need to be considered. These include:

- The age of the patient
- The nature and complexity of the deformity (i.e., which tissue types are affected)
- The presence of associated disorders and conditions
- The patient's understanding of the problem and the options for treatment.

Of importance in patient selection is the timing of the surgery. It has been generally assumed that reconstructive surgery is best performed after the disease has "burned itself out" and this could involve a delay up to 2 years following what looks like the end of progression. However, the literature also suggests that earlier treatment with vascularized tissue, such as a free flap, is possible and that doing so may stop further tissue wasting (i.e., it may interrupt the progression of the disease). However, at this time, the more accepted opinion is to wait until the disease has run its course. Most importantly, the treatment of this disorder is determined by the patient's individual deformity, ranging from mild to moderate to severe. In the mild deformity, injectable materials have a place as well as the use of fat injections. Other materials can be used for this purpose as well (i.e., fat, fascia, dermis, acellular dermis). These materials can be used in more severe deformities, often as an adjunct to surgery. However, in more severe deformities the tendency is to use free tissue transfers. In all deformities, combinations of buried materials, injected materials, and free flap transfers in some combination all have a role to play.

The original free tissue transfers, as muscle and/or myocutaneous flaps, although generally satisfactory, were found to be slightly bulky. Free omental transfer has the downside of requiring an abdominal exploration and is somewhat harder to fix in place in the facial area. Consequently, free fasciocutaneous flaps have become the present choice, and several have been described (groin, anterolateral thigh, and superficial inferior epigastric flaps), with consideration given to the needs of the deformity. However, the most common free tissue transfers now used are based on the circumflex scapular pedicle that allows bulk and pliability as well as better fixation. This can be taken in various combinations, including bone if needed.

Etiopathogenesis

The exact etiology of PHA is not well understood, but is felt to have a strong autoimmune and neurogenic component. Certain histologic findings have supported a combination of the two, which may be best described as a "lymphocytic neurovasculitis."[5]

Autoimmune process

PHA is likely a variant of the autoimmune disease localized scleroderma, specifically the subtype of linear scleroderma that affects the face, termed ECDS. Many times it is hard to differentiate these two entities as ECDS often leads to atrophy of subcutaneous tissue and facial bones causing hemifacial atrophy later in the disease course. Besides the clinical appearance, other etiologic, histologic, and clinical manifestations are similar between PHA and ECDS, which lends support to the theory of different spectra of the same disease. Both share similar characteristics, including age of onset, female preponderance, neurological involvement, lymphocytic infiltrate on biopsy, and a clinical course of evolution for several years followed by stabilization. Positive autoantibodies, such as antinuclear antibody, which are found in ECDS, have also been demonstrated in "classic" PHA (hemifacial atrophy without sclerodermatous skin changes).[20–22]

Histologic findings

The histological findings in PHA and ECDS are similar, though there are a few differences. Idiopathic PHA usually is without significant cutaneous involvement, as compared to ECDS, where cutaneous findings of hyperpigmented and/or sclerotic linear markings are expected. However, skin biopsies performed in patients with idiopathic PHA with no apparent cutaneous findings have demonstrated a cellular infiltrate similar to localized scleroderma. A perivascular infiltrate of mononuclear cells, mostly lymphocytes and monocytes, has been demonstrated in the dermis,[23] with a particular focus surrounding the dermal neurovascular bundles, termed "lymphocytic neurovasculitis" by Mulliken and colleagues.[1] Under electron microscopy, degenerative alterations of the vascular endothelia were also documented. These findings suggest an autoimmune disease process, similar to that of localized scleroderma.

There are a few histologic differences noted between ECDS/localized scleroderma and PHA. Although the dermal collagen fibrils appear more closely packed in patients with PHA,[5] they are not as homogenized and fragmented as seen in ECDS. The elastic fibers are preserved and dermal appendages (hair follicles and sebaceous glands) are hypoplastic in PHA compared to the destruction of elastic fibers and atrophy of dermal appendages seen in ECDS/localized scleroderma.[24,25]

Neurogenic process

Several clinical manifestations support a neurogenic origin of PHA. The distribution of facial atrophy typically follows a dermatome of the trigeminal nerve, being unilateral in 95% of cases and only rarely crossing the midline. Pensler et al.[1] reported the initial distribution of atrophy among the divisions of the trigeminal nerve in 41 patients with PHA to be 35% in V_1, 45% in V_2, and 20% in V_3, with eventual progression of disease to involve 65% in V_1, 80% in V_2, and 50% in V_3.[5] Neuritis of the trigeminal nerve is suggested by several patients experiencing episodes of pain in the involved area prior to the onset of tissue atrophy.[26] An internet survey of 205 PHA patients by Stone reported that 46% of responders experienced facial pain.[27] The dermal lymphocytic infiltrate centered around neurovascular bundles in the dermis on histology also supports a neurologic target.[5] Though most patients with PHA do not experience facial sensory, sympathetic, or parasympathetic dysfunction, some do experience peripheral facial nerve palsy, ocular motor palsy, and optic neuritis.[28,29]

Another theory involving the nervous system is the hyperactivity of the sympathetic nervous system, specifically inflammation of the superior cervical ganglion, causing features of PHA. Experimental animal studies support this hypothesis. Resende et al. ablated the superior cervical ganglion of rabbits, cats, and dogs and observed clinical features consistent with PHA within 30 days, such as localized alopecia, keratitis, enophthalmos, and hemifacial atrophy with slight bone atrophy.[30] Moss et al. also observed similar findings in an experimental rat model after unilateral cervical sympathectomy.[31]

Clinical, radiological, and cerebrospinal fluid (CSF) laboratory findings of patients with PHA highly support that the disease affects the central nervous system (CNS), likely in an autoimmune fashion. The clinical manifestations of CNS involvement are found in approximately 8–20% of patients with PHA (the same as that found in ECDS).[23] These are usually expressed as seizures, chronic headaches, and/or optic neuritis; and less commonly as neuropsychiatric disorders, deterioration of intelligence, and/or ischemic stroke. When brain imaging is performed in symptomatic patients, abnormalities such as atrophy and calcinosis are common, with up to 63% of 49 patients evaluated by Kister et al. having multiple or diffuse brain lesions on magnetic resonance imaging (MRI).[28] Lumbar puncture analysis of CSF reveals findings consistent with an inflammatory process with the presence of oligoclonal bands and elevated IgG levels.[30] Further evidence supporting inflammation of the CNS includes histologic findings of brain biopsies of PHA patients, which demonstrate the same changes as seen in the ECDS form of localized scleroderma: chronic perivascular lymphocytic inflammation with some vessels showing intimal thickening and hyalinization.[33]

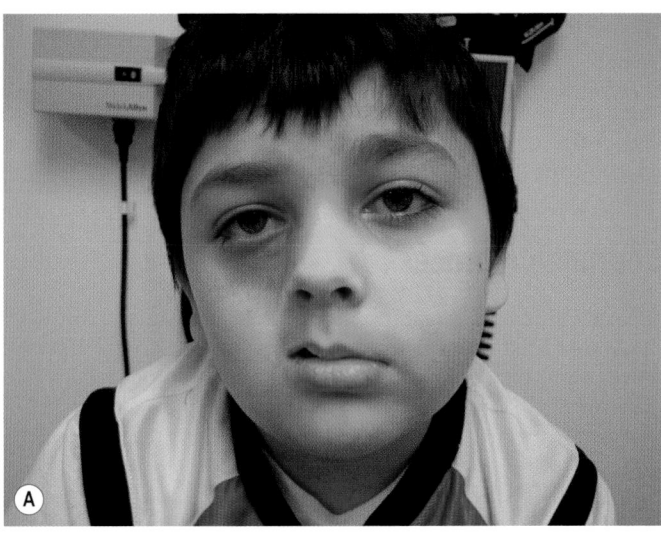
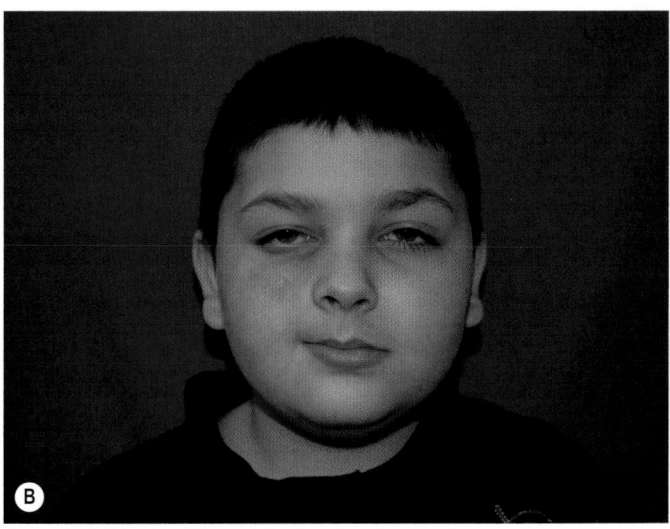

Fig. 37.1 **(A)** An 8-year-old boy with right hemifacial atrophy demonstrating absence of the medial lower eyelashes and a hyperpigmented lesion of the cheek with associated subcutaneous atrophy. **(B)** The patient three months postoperative, after two treatments with autologous structural fat grafting.

Infection hypothesis

As in most autoimmune diseases, infectious agents have been postulated as an etiologic agent in PHA. The development of clinical disease manifestations has been noted to follow viral or bacterial infections. The most notorious suspect for both PHA and ECDS was *Borrelia burgdorferi*[34,35]; however, further studies have not substantiated this finding.[36,37] The viral infections indicated, such as Epstein–Barr virus, correlate with the typical exposure to these infectious agents in the first and second decades of life, and are more likely coincidental rather than etiologic factors.

Trauma

The role of trauma inducing PHA is quite controversial; however, in several patients a specific history of trauma to the affected area is elucidated, especially following tooth injury or extraction.[38,39] In a self-report survey of 205 patients with PHA 12% reported injuries they thought could be directly related to their disease onset.[27] There have not been any standardized epidemiological studies to verify this hypothesis.

Epidemiology

The incidence of PHA is not well defined but is tightly associated with that of the ECDS subtype of localized scleroderma, since many reviews reporting and summarizing these diseases are combined together.[23,27,40,41] The incidence of localized scleroderma is approximately 3 per 100 000 people and the prevalence is 50 per 100 000 people. Of those with localized scleroderma, approximately 40% have the linear subtype, and only 30% of these affect the face and/or scalp, termed ECDS.[42] Therefore, an estimated incidence of 5 per 1 000 000 people and prevalence of 8 per 100 000 people is calculated for PHA. There is no racial predilection of PHA. There is a slight female predominance, with most studies having female-to-male ratios

between 2.2:1 and 3:1.[23,27] The median age of onset for most studies is 10 years old with a general range of 5–15 years of age,[23,27,41] which is consistent with ECDS.[42,43] Most cases of PHA are sporadic; however a few familial cases have been reported.[44]

Clinical manifestations

The initial clinical manifestations include both cutaneous findings and subcutaneous atrophy. A survey of initial symptoms reported by 49 patients with PHA demonstrates 37% having hyperpigmentation or darkening of the skin, 22% having a hypopigmented spot or streak of skin, 6% with alopecia of the scalp, medial eyebrow or eyelashes, and 24% noticed an "indentation" signifying subcutaneous atrophy *(Fig. 37.1)*.[45] The subcutaneous atrophy typically evolves first on the cheek or temple and later extends to the brow, angle of mouth, and/or neck.[46] Later in the disease course, atrophy or growth arrest of the underlying bone and cartilage can occur, causing further facial deformity. Facial muscles may become atrophic, but they tend to maintain their normal function. The disease typically progresses slowly over several years (2–10 years) and then tends to enter a stable phase.[38,46]

Cutaneous and subcutaneous involvement

Pigmentary changes in the cutaneous tissue are a common finding in PHA. The hyperpigmentation is often described as a "bluish" discoloration and is commonly mistakenly for a bruise that does not heal *(Fig. 37.2)*. This is thought to reflect increased vascularity during the active or inflammatory phase of the disease.[47] At times, the initial blue, violaceous, or erythematous phase is short and goes unnoticed, leaving behind a brown discoloration and/or areas of hypopigmentation. These discolorations are typically distributed in a dermatomal distribution along the trigeminal nerve.[5] If the skin lesion becomes fibrotic (thickened skin) or atrophic and forms a well-demarcated linear depression (groove) in a

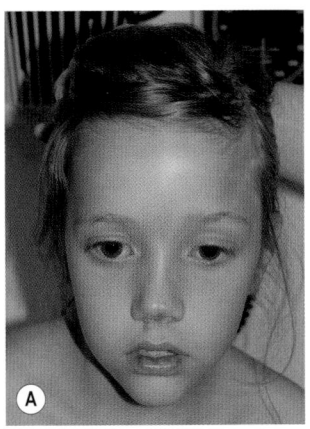
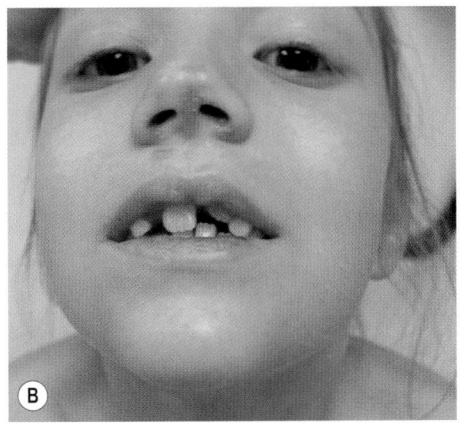
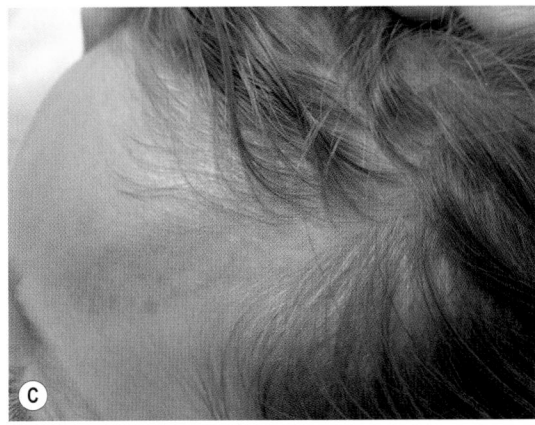

Fig. 37.2 A 7-year-old girl with active "en coup de sabre," demonstrating an erythematous lesion on **(A)** the nose, **(B)** philtrum, and **(C)** left forehead.

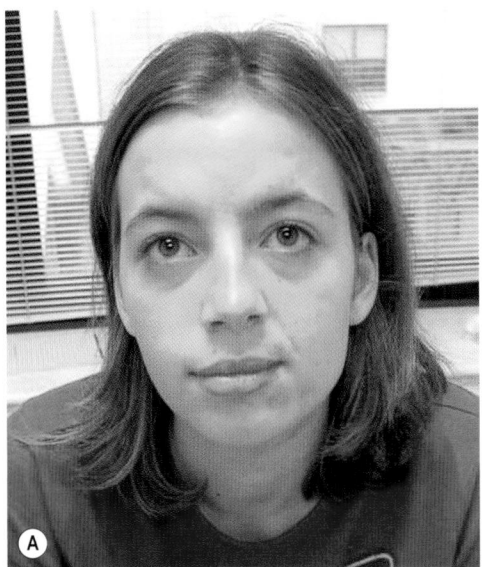
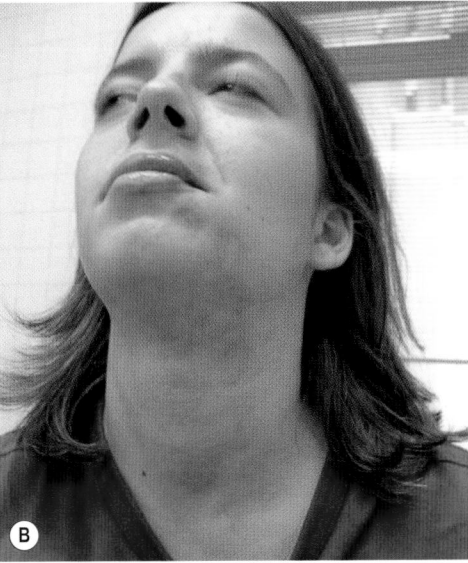

Fig. 37.3 (A) An 18-year-old female with long-standing "en coup de sabre" for 5 years leading to left progressive hemifacial atrophy. **(B)** Other associations include the plaque morphea lesions of the neck.

frontoparietal or hemifacial distribution, it is considered to be ECDS morphea or linear scleroderma of the head.[48]

For many patients with ECDS after skin and subcutaneous induration and atrophy, the deeper tissues become involved, leading to the development of hemifacial atrophy. Therefore, the end result of ECDS appears the same as PHA without sclerodermatous changes *(Fig. 37.3)*.

Cutaneous disease damage parameters include discoloration, both hyperpigmentation and hypopigmentation, dermal atrophy (signified by shiny skin and visible veins), subcutaneous atrophy (described as a flattening or concavity of the subcutaneous tissue), and skin thickening/fibrosis at the center of the lesion.[49] Several skin appendages reside in the dermis, including sweat glands and hair follicles; therefore, alopecia of the scalp, eyebrow, and eyelashes is not uncommon.[50] The severity of disease damage, in regard to subcutaneous atrophy, when evaluated by Pensler *et al.*[1] using multivariate analysis in a group of 42 patients with PHA, was found not to be significantly influenced by trigeminal nerve distribution, side of face, age of onset, or extent (surface area) of the disease process.[5]

Musculoskeletal involvement

The facial musculature undergoes atrophy and thinning, mostly affecting masseteric muscles, tongue, and palatal muscles, though function is usually preserved. The degree of skeletal hypoplasia is dependent upon the age of onset, with those younger than 10 at onset having the highest risk.[26] It is hypothesized that the facial skeleton does not undergo atrophy, as the subcutaneous tissue, but likely fails to develop (hypoplastic) during this period of bony growth, possibly due to the adjacent inflammatory and atrophic process of the overlying skin and subcutaneous tissue. The maxilla and mandible are most often involved, with both sagittal and vertical undergrowth, causing appearance and dental abnormalities. Since hypoplasia of either maxilla and/or mandible is unilateral, profound tilting of the occlusal plane develops. Although enophthalmos is common when PHA involves the V_1 distribution, the radiographic measurements of the skeletal orbit are normal, and the enophthalmos is more related to the atrophy of the periorbital subcutaneous tissues rather than skeletal hypoplasia.[5]

Central nervous system involvement

CNS manifestations occur in approximately 8–21% of patients with PHA and include seizures, hemiparesis, migraine headaches, neuropsychiatric disturbances, ischemic stroke, and intellectual deterioration.[23,27,28,41,43] These same manifestations and frequency of CNS involvement are reported in association with ECDS. Most patients have CNS symptoms years after the onset of cutaneous or subcutaneous findings, with a mean of 4.3 years, though a minority (approximately 16%) will have neurologic symptoms preceding cutaneous/subcutaneous involvement.[28]

The most common CNS manifestation is localization-related seizures. In a literature review by Kister *et al.* of a cohort of 54 patients with PHA and/or ECDS who experienced neurologic symptoms, 73% experienced epilepsy and, in 33% of these, seizures were described as being refractory to medications.[28] In comparison to other autoimmune disorders of the CNS, such as multiple sclerosis (MS), the brain lesions of PHA (and ECDS) appear to be more epileptogenic.[51] In comparison to MS, focal CNS neurological symptoms were uncommon in PHA, with 11% of patients upon presentation, and 35% of patients overall, reported to have deficits (excluding facial palsy). The literature review of 54 cases by Kister *et al.*[28] reported neuropsychiatric symptoms in 15% of cases, and headaches in 35%. Stone's internet survey of 205 patients with PHA demonstrated that 46% of the patients reported anxiety, 10% reported depression, and 52% reported migraine headaches.[27]

In those experiencing neurological symptoms, brain imaging is often abnormal. In Kister's review, 49 of the 54 patients with PHA had an MRI performed: 90% revealed an abnormality. In each patient at least one T2 hyperintensity was observed, mainly in the subcortical white matter, followed by corpus callosum, deep gray nuclei, and brainstem.[28] Other abnormalities detected on MRI are intraparenchymal calcifications and brain atrophy. Blaszczyk *et al.* reported an association between calcifications and focal epilepsy.[41] Brain atrophy has been observed and varies from being very focal and related to adjacent subcutaneous atrophy to more widespread, involving an entire cerebral hemisphere; however, as with cutaneous disease, the atrophy "respects" the midline and typically does not cross over to the opposite hemisphere.[28] There is not a direct correlation between the degree of severity of skin and subcutaneous involvement and brain lesions, and several patients with PHA are neurologically asymptomatic in spite of visible brain lesions.[52] The percentage of patients with PHA or ECDS who are neurologically asymptomatic with brain lesions is unknown given the small cohort studies, which do not routinely image all patients with these conditions.

In Kister's cohort of 54 patients, 20 had a magnetic resonance angiography or cerebral angiogram performed, eight (40%) of which had vascular abnormalities consistent with vasculitis. Of these cases, biopsy-proven low-grade cerebral vasculitis was observed in three cases.[28] Brain biopsies of other select cases have found brain parenchymal inflammation with a perivascular lymphocytic cuffing.[53] Sclerosis, fibrosis, and gliosis of brain parenchyma, meninges, and vasculature have also been reported.[54] CSF findings in PHA/ECDS also support an inflammatory process by demonstrating oligoclonal bands and elevated IgG levels.[32]

Ocular involvement

A variety of ocular abnormalities have been associated with PHA, including alterations of the adnexal structures, anterior or posterior segments of the eye, and the optic nerve. The frequency of involvement is unknown; however, a large portion of those in Kister's study and those in Stone's internet survey report eye findings, 29% and 46% respectively, with uveitis, optic neuritis, and globe retraction being the most common.[27] Significant enophthalmos, principally due to soft-tissue atrophy, is demonstrated in the majority of patients with facial atrophy in the first trigeminal nerve distribution.[5] Ocular muscle paralysis, ptosis, Horner syndrome, heterochromia iridis, and dilated fixed pupil have been reported. Inflammatory conditions of the eye have also been demonstrated, including uveitis (anterior and posterior), episcleritis, keratitis, choroiditis, and papilledema.[55,56] A careful ophthalmologic examination using a slit lamp is recommended in patients with PHA and/or ECDS to assess for an inflammatory-fibrotic process, which may be arrested by immunosuppressive therapy.

Oral involvement

The tongue and upper lip of the affected side of the face are often markedly atrophic. The maxilla and mandible may be underdeveloped (hypoplastic), resulting in malocclusion and altered dentition. Often, there is a unilateral posterior crossbite as a result of jaw hypoplasia, and an abnormally skewed high-arched palate may also be observed (*Fig. 37.4*). Radiographically, the teeth may have atrophic roots causing delayed tooth eruption and crowding, but affected teeth are normal and vital clinically.[57] Thirty-five percent of the 201 PHA patients surveyed by Stone complained of difficulty

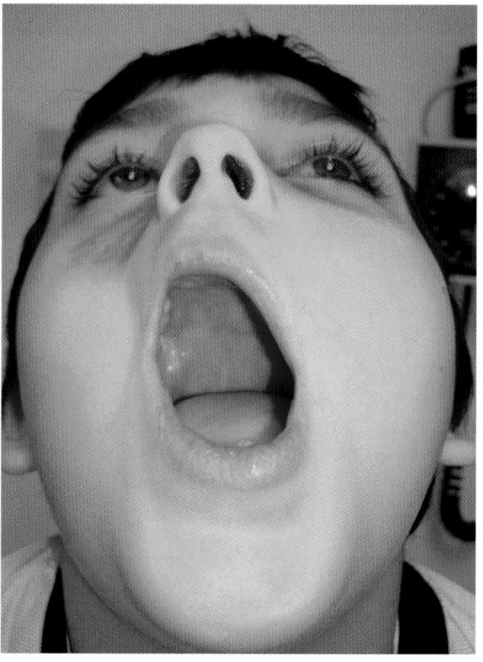

Fig. 37.4 This 8-year-old boy has progressive hemifacial atrophy and an associated high-arched palate with associated malocclusion.

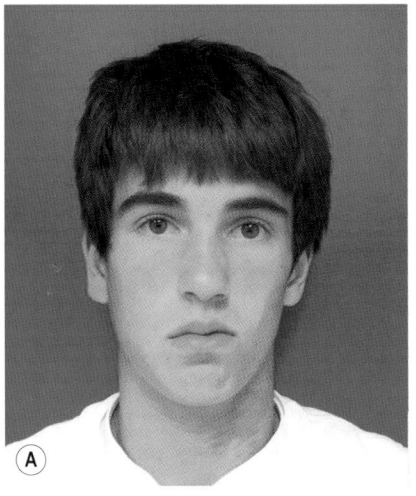
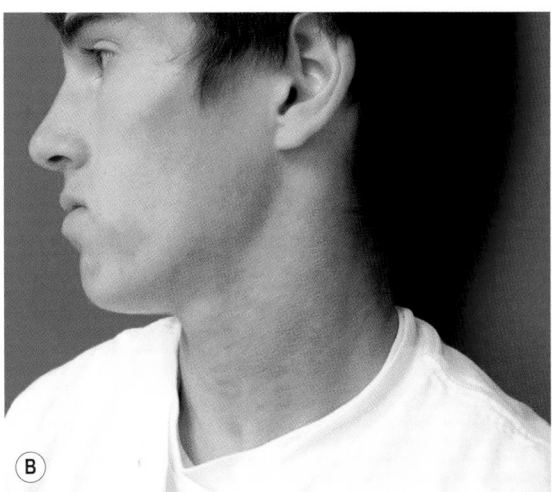
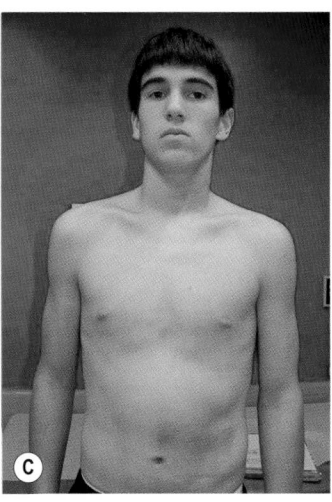

Fig. 37.5 A 13-year-old boy with progressive hemifacial atrophy **(A)** involving the left face with coexistent generalized plaque morphea of **(B)** neck and **(C)** abdomen.

opening or closing the jaw or jaw pain.[27] Early dental referral is helpful in realigning dentition with orthodontic equipment for better functional and cosmetic outcome.

Laboratory findings and prognostic indicators

A review of the literature and case series demonstrates that initial laboratory testing of inflammatory markers for disease activity assessment is of limited use, with only approximately 10% of the patients having an elevated white blood cell or eosinophil count, and 20% having an elevated sedimentation rate.[52,58] Autoantibodies, on the other hand are quite common, with antinuclear antibody positivity in 40–50% of cases, demonstrating nucleolar, speckled, and homogeneous staining patterns.[52,59,60] Specific antibodies to extractable nuclear antigens have also been found, including anti-single-stranded DNA (ss-DNA), antihistone, anti-double-stranded DNA, anti-centromere, and anti-Scl-70 antibodies. Although these antibodies reflect autoimmune disease as an etiologic agent for PHA, they are not specifically associated with active or inactive disease. However, two of the antibodies, ss-DNA and antihistone antibody, have been correlated with disease severity and progressive disease features, such as larger surface area of the lesion and continued spreading of the lesion in those with ECDS/PHA.[60]

A clinical prognostic indicator of disease severity regarding skeletal involvement is young age of onset. Pensler *et al.*[1] found that age under 10 years was a significant risk factor for profound skeletal dysplasia.

Differential diagnosis

The main two entities included in the differential diagnosis of PHA are congenital hemifacial atrophy and the ECDS subtype of localized scleroderma. Congenital hemifacial atrophy is present at birth and includes diminution in the size of teeth on the involved side, as does PHA, but it is not progressive

like PHA. In contrast, ECDS is difficult to distinguish from PHA, and there are many who argue they are variants of the same disease rather than two distinct entities, as noted earlier. As ECDS resolves from an active stage, atrophy of the skin, subcutaneous tissue, and bone is morphologically identical to that of the atrophy seen in PHA. Some would categorize ECDS that results in hemifacial atrophy as a subtype of PHA. A few possible differentiating features that are more distinct to ECDS compared to "classic" PHA are scalp and forehead involvement, and induration of the skin and subcutaneous tissues during the acute phase. However, this is not clear as histologic evidence supports a similar lymphocytic infiltration in both entities, as well as shared neurological and ophthalmologic features. There is considerable overlap between the two entities, with 30–40% of patients being classified as having coexistent ECDS and PHA.[23,28] In addition, there are several patients with PHA in association with different subtypes of localized scleroderma affecting other parts of the body besides scalp and face, such as deep, generalized and plaque morphea *(Fig. 37.5)*.[61]

Other forms of lipoatrophy are usually not localized to the face, such as lipodystrophy from congenital diseases such as progeria, Dunnigan syndrome, and Kobberling syndrome. Other identified causes of widespread lipoatrophy are endocrine disorders, such as hyperthyroidism and diabetes, other autoimmune diseases, such as systemic sclerosis and dermatomyositis, and drug-induced atrophy, the most notorious being the protease inhibitors for the treatment of human immunodeficiency virus. Other craniofacial conditions present with bone hypoplasia (i.e., hemifacial microsomia); however, these syndromes are associated with clinical features distinct from PHA.

Treatment/surgical technique

Role of immunosuppression

Patients with PHA having any cutaneous features of localized scleroderma (erythema/purple hue, induration, dyspigmentation, or thickness/fibrosis) or the appearance of a

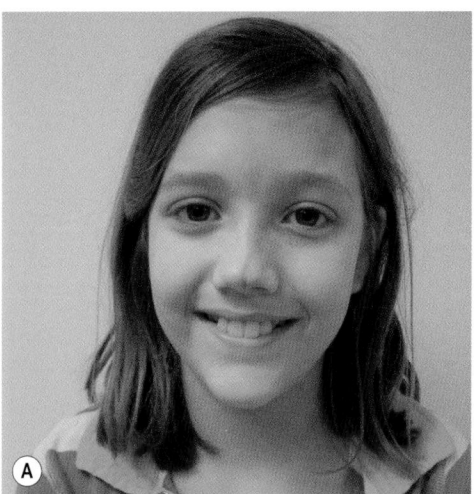 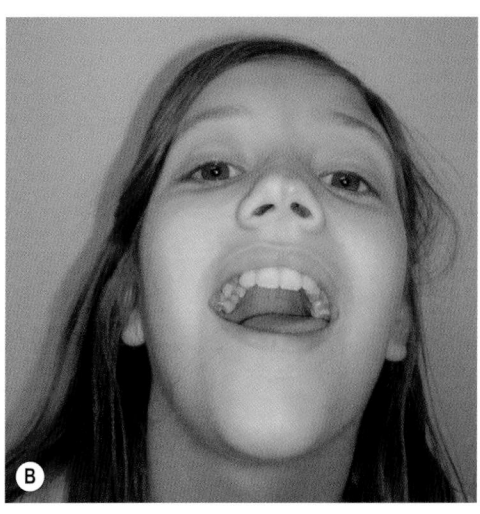

Fig. 37.6 (A, B) The 7-year-old girl pictured in *Figure 37.2*, 3 years after initial immunosuppressive therapy with prednisone and methotrexate and continued low-dose therapy.

demarcated line, as in ECDS, should be considered candidates for immunosuppressive therapy. Patients with these features treated with immunosuppression, typically corticosteroids in combination with a disease-modifying agent such as methotrexate, have been found to have cessation of disease progression and reversal/improvement of disease damage *(Fig. 37.6)*. For example, hyperpigmented skin becomes lighter, sclerotic skin softens, subcutaneous atrophy is less noticeable with some "filling in" of fat, hair growth is observed in areas of alopecia, and tongue atrophy is less dramatic.[62–65] Many PHA patients with neurological manifestations, such as seizures and optic neuritis, have shown benefit from immunosuppressive therapy, and some of these manifestations have flared after weaning off therapy.[66] After a period of 3–5 years on immunosuppressive therapy with an improved or stable clinical examination, immunosuppression is weaned off as the disease is felt to have "burned out" at that point. After an observation period of stable disease off medications, typically 1 year, then it is felt to be "safe" for reconstruction.

Nonsurgical intervention

The use of nonsurgical alloplastic filling agents is advantageous for facial contour reconstruction on account of their absence of a donor site and their abundant supply. These however are counterbalanced by their increased susceptibility to local tissue responses, including capsule formation, seroma development, infection, and extrusion as well as their material cost. Examples include silicone gel, hydroxyapatite beads, and hyaluronic acid. As well, use of these agents in the immature patient must be given special consideration.

Grafting of autogenous material, such as fat, is advantageous because fat may be easily harvested from the patient from one or more sites with almost no donor site morbidity and no functional loss. In the exceptionally thin patient, subcutaneous fat might be difficult to identify. There is no possibility of rejection, only atrophy of some portion of the grafted tissue. A dermal fat graft may be similarly used; the de-epithelialized graft is harvested as one unit with the hope that "take" will be improved.

Surgical intervention

The surgical treatment options currently offer the largest amount of tissue with excellent safety. They should be used in conjunction with fillers to provide the best possible outcome.[67] Local, pedicled flaps have been described to reconstruct deficits and deformities in the head and neck. However, their lack of adequate bulk has limited their role in cases of extensive soft-tissue deficit *(Fig. 37.7)*. Soft tissue, based on the superficial temporal pedicle, is the most obvious choice and may be rotated inferiorly to fill more superficial depressions. Attempts to augment the bulk of the flap using a free dermis–fat graft sandwiched between the folded superficial temporal fascia have been described.[68]

Numerous free flaps have been used to correct the facial contour deformities in patients with PHA, including muscle, fat, and often a combination of tissue types, offering benefits over any single type alone.

Smaller deficits may be reconstructed with smaller muscle or fascial flaps, such as the gracilis and radial forearm adipofascial flap, respectively *(Figs 37.8, 37.9)*.[69] Conversely, the deep inferior epigastric perforator can provide more soft-tissue bulk. In the heavier patient, the omentum provides an adequate source of fat for soft-tissue volume.[70–72] It may be supplied by either the right or left gastroepiploic arteries, and harvest requires entering the abdomen, by either traditional or laparoscopic means. The omentum lacks internal structure and often leads to soft-tissue descent with time. Other choices include the superficial inferior epigastric flap,[73,74] the transverse rectus abdominis muscle flap,[75] and the deltopectoral flap.[76,77]

Song *et al.* were the first to report the harvest and application of the anterolateral thigh adipofascial flap in 1984 *(Fig. 37.10)*.[78] Advantages include the ability to harvest the flap in the supine position away from the area of inset, the large, reliable skin flap available, its proximity to muscles that may be incorporated for bulk, and its relatively long vascular pedicle. The donor site defect may be closed directly in the absence of sufficient tension or covered with a skin graft. Disadvantages include the variability of the skin perforators and the potentially tedious dissection of the pedicle if it courses within the muscle for an extended length.[79]

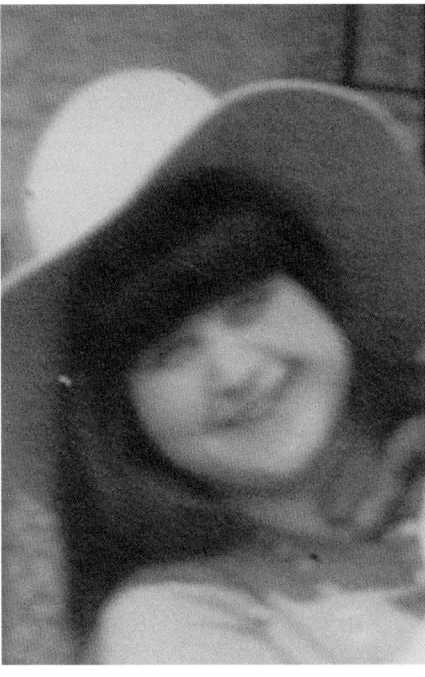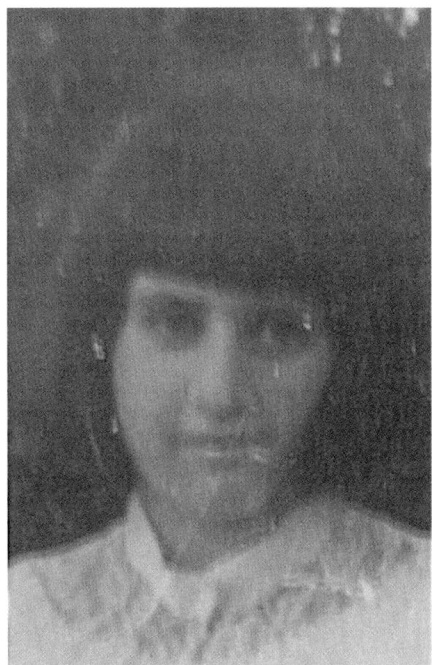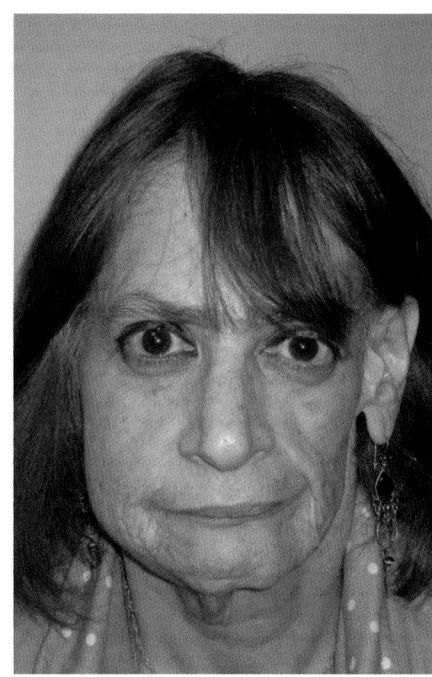

Fig. 37.7 A 59-year-old woman diagnosed with progressive hemifacial atrophy and treated with a tubed pedicle flap from the abdomen to the wrist and eventually to the face, where it was inset via a parotid incision.

If bone augmentation is required, a vascularized costo-chondral graft taken with a latissimus dorsi musculocutaneous flap has been described.[80]

Scapular and parascapular flap

The scapular and parascapular adipofascial flap based on the circumflex scapular pedicle are the most useful flaps for restoring facial volume.[81–84] Advantages include its relatively straightforward harvest, posterior-torso donor scar, and minimal functional deficit. The disadvantage is positioning the patient in either a prone or lateral decubitus to harvest. The authors prefer the lateral decubitus position so the patient does not need to be turned during the case. However, less than adequate exposure of the contralateral face for comparison is achieved.

The technique of soft-tissue augmentation of the face begins with marking the patient for either a local, pedicled flap or a distant, free flap *(Fig. 37.11A)*. This should be done prior to positioning the patient in the operating room. A transparency of the defect can then be created using X-ray film *(Fig. 37.11B)*. Once anesthetized, the patient is carefully positioned either in a true lateral decubitus position or supine with the ipsilateral shoulder turned to expose the posterior torso if a scapular or parascapular flap is to be used. The apex of the skin paddle is centered over the triangular space bounded by the teres minor, teres major, and long head of triceps. The vessel within the triangular space is checked with the Doppler. The axillary artery gives off the subscapular artery, which in turn gives rise to the circumflex scapular artery about 1–4 cm from its origin. Occasionally, the circumflex scapular artery can arise directly off the axillary artery. The circumflex scapular artery usually travels with paired

venae comitantes and the subscapular artery travels with a single vein. The circumflex scapular artery enters the posterior torso via the triangular space and gives off a transverse cutaneous scapular branch and a vertical parascapular branch. The latter supplies the parascapular flap. The transparency made from the defect can then be used to maximize soft-tissue harvest *(Fig. 37.11C)*.

The incisions at the donor and recipient sites are injected with lidocaine and epinephrine. Lubrication is placed in the eyes and a temporary tarsorrhaphy can be used to protect the corneas. The face is prepped with dilute Betadine solution to prevent keratitis.

The procedure begins with creation of the subcutaneous pocket on the face. The extent of the dissection must extend beyond the borders of the atrophy to allow for adequate contouring. Suitable recipient vessels are identified for the anastomosis. At the conclusion of this portion of the dissection, careful hemostasis is achieved with a bipolar electrocautery and counted sponges are left beneath the dissected skin envelope.

The flap is then harvested from the posterior torso, without having to turn the patient significantly. The trapezius and infraspinatus muscles should be identified early in the dissection since they serve as important landmarks for flap dissection, which should proceed from medial to lateral and inferior to superior. Flap elevation is best performed in the looser areolar tissue just above the muscular fascia. If flap elevation proceeds deep to the fascia, the dissection can become confusing as to where the pedicle exits the triangular space.

The flap can be completely de-epithelialized and buried or left with a thin cutaneous paddle, incorporated into the closure and available for postoperative flap monitoring

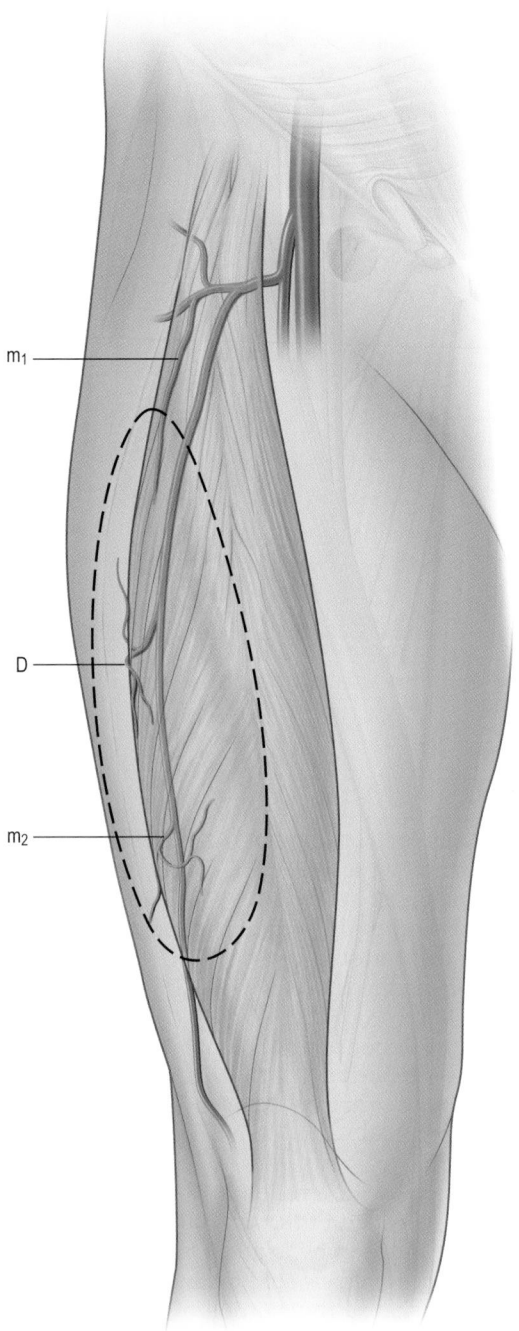

Fig. 37.8 The anatomy of the anterolateral thigh flap. D, septocutaneous perforators of the descending branch of the circumflex femoral artery; m₁, musculocutaneous perforators of the transverse branch of the lateral circumflex femoral artery; m₂, musculocutaneous perforators of the descending branch of the lateral circumflex femoral artery.

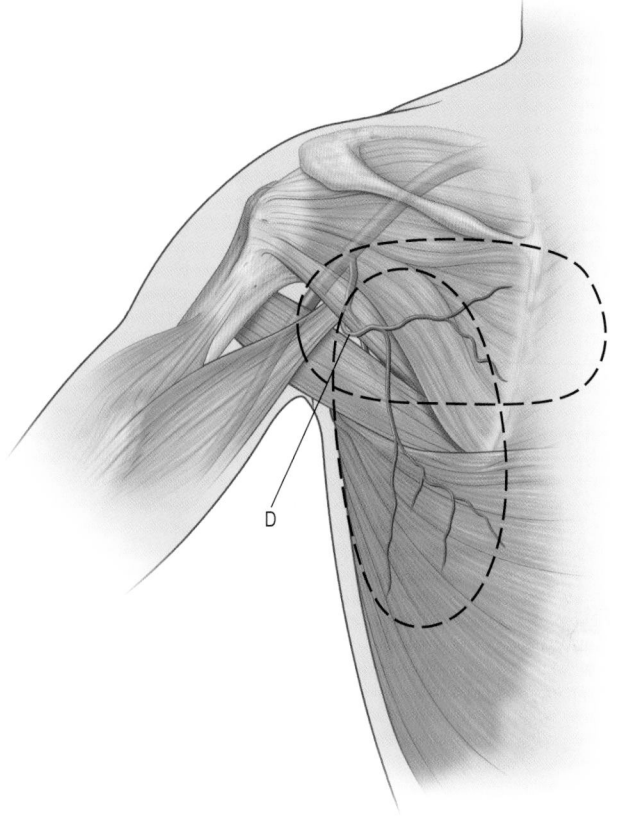

Fig. 37.9 The anatomy of the parascapular flap. D, circumflex scapular artery.

(Fig. 37.11D). The terminal flap ends should be contoured and fixed to the skin with overlying bolsters. Several points of fixation are required. At each point, a narrow roll of Vaseline gauze is fabricated as a tie-over bolster. Fixation involves passing a smooth nylon or Prolene suture completely through one side of the Vaseline gauze bolsters. It is then passed through the skin and into the pocket for the flap. A mattress suture is used to grab the flap and the suture is passed back into the pocket and out of the skin in proximity to the entrance point. It then passes through the other end of the bolster and is left long while each of the remaining sutures is placed. When all are completed, each is tied down, making sure the flap is passed into each of the pockets that have been dissected out *(Fig. 37.11E)*.

A single small drain is left in the face and a second larger drain is left in the donor site. The former is removed prior to discharge if the output is sufficiently small. The latter is left in longer because of its tendency to continue to drain serous fluid. The wounds are closed in layers and the face dressed with bacitracin to avoid pressure over the flap.

Even in the absence of a skin paddle, an audible Doppler signal through the skin should be recorded every hour for the first day and then every 2 hours for the second day. Patients are kept NPO for the first night and then gradually advanced to clears and a regular diet.

Outcomes, prognosis, and complications

The outcomes from soft-tissue augmentation are usually quite good, with symmetry the ultimate goal. Reconstructive success is predicated more on identifying the tissue types involved with precise location of the deficit and choosing an

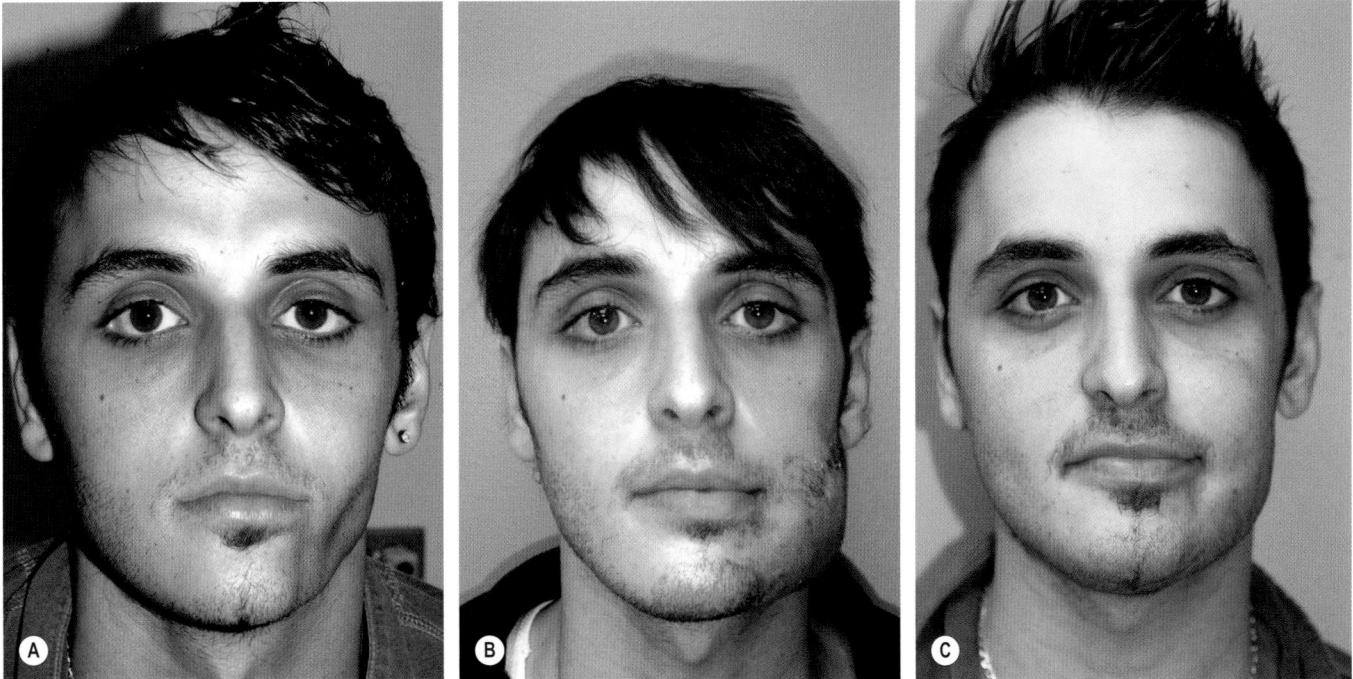

Fig. 37.10 (A) Preoperative photograph of a 20-year-old male with localized progressive hemifacial microsomia affecting primarily the left lower face. **(B)** Postoperative photograph following harvest and inset of a free gracilis flap. **(C)** Postoperative photograph following revision of the free gracilis flap by debulking.

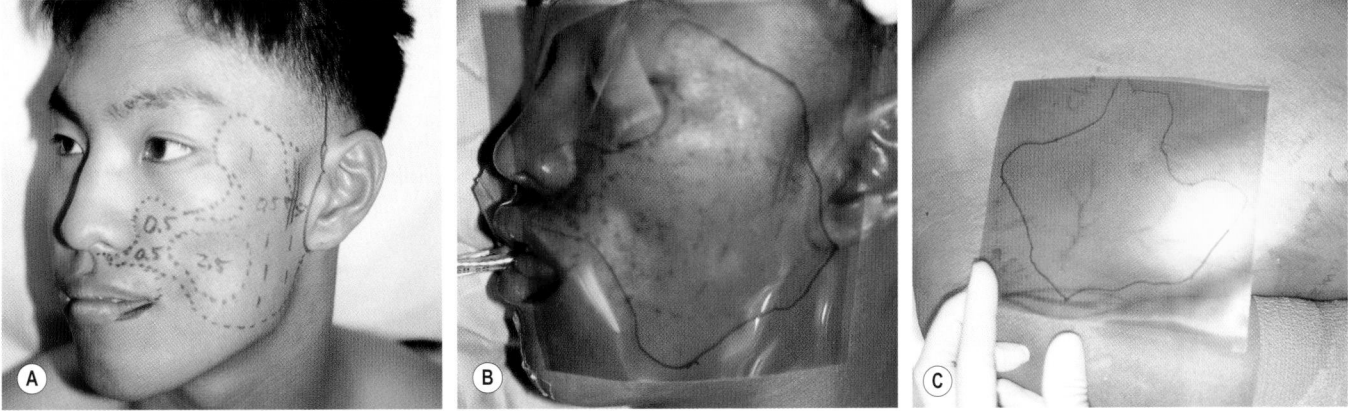

Fig. 37.11 (A) Preoperative photograph of a 25-year-old male with more diffuse progressive hemifacial microsomia. **(B)** Intraoperative photograph demonstrating the use of X-ray film to map the extent of involvement and soft-tissue requirement. **(C)** Intraoperative photograph demonstrating transfer of the template to the posterior torso prior to harvest of a parascapular free flap.

appropriate intervention strategy. Incorporating multiple options is reasonable and often preferable.

Secondary procedures

Once inset, revision should be part of every treatment protocol. It would be exceedingly unusual for the exact amount of tissue to be harvested and placed at the initial procedure. Edema progresses during surgery and blurs the boundaries between normal and deficient tissue.

The first revision is not planned sooner than 6 months following flap placement, allowing edema to resolve and secondary blood supply from the surrounding tissues to develop. Some patients may benefit from waiting even longer if continued changes in the face are noted. Debulking the flap may be achieved with either direct excision or suction lipectomy or a combination of the two.

The existing incisions are usually sufficient for access to the flap. At 6 months, it is unlikely that interruption of the pedicle would lead to compromise of the flap. However, the location of the vascular pedicle should be known so it may be avoided and bleeding minimized. Again, bolsters may be

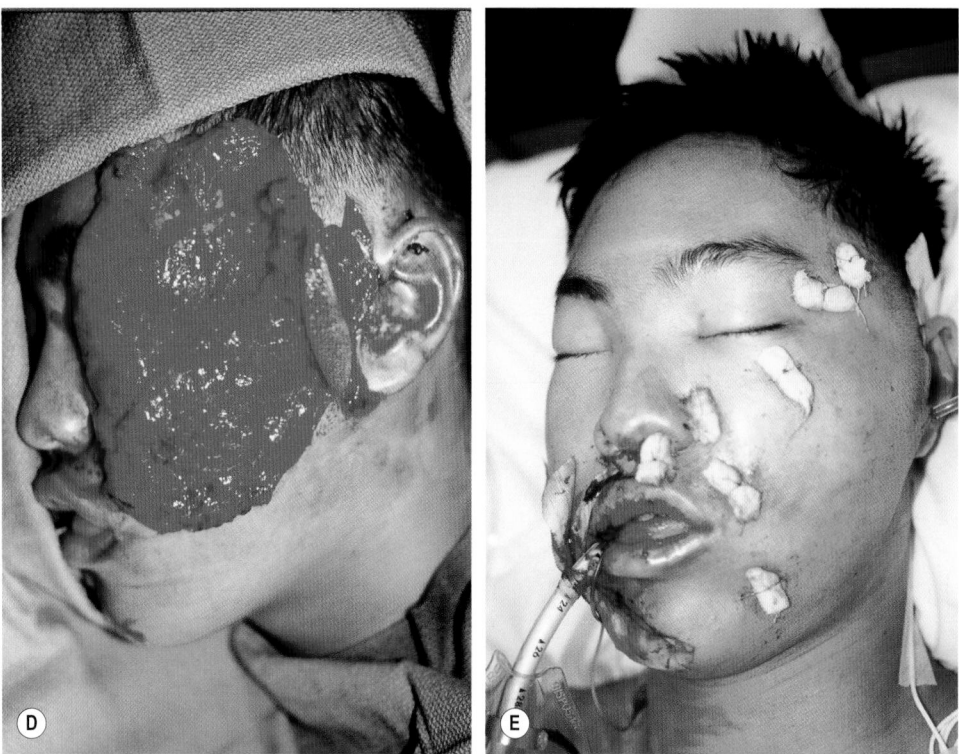

Fig. 37.11, cont'd **(D)** Intraoperative photograph of the flap positioned over the ipsilateral face prior to inset. Note the thin, vertical skin paddle left over the proximal portion of the flap that is used to monitor the viability of the flap postoperatively. **(E)** Intraoperative photograph following inset of the free parascapular flap. Note the use of Vaseline gauze tie-over bolsters to hold the distal margins of the flap in their respective subcutaneous pockets.

used to fix underlying soft tissue into place. Further refinements of the flap are certainly plausible to address persistent concerns.

Debulking of the flap is usually one component of the revision along with further addition of soft tissue to areas that remain deficient. In the latter instance, flap tissue from contiguous areas may be rotated from overly bulky areas to regions with persistent lack of volume. Similarly, additional autogenous fat or alloplastic filler may be used for smaller areas of need.

Access the complete references list online at **http://www.expertconsult.com**

1. Pensler JM, Murphy GF, Mulliken JB. Clinical and ultrastructural studies of Romberg's hemifacial atrophy. *Plast Reconstr Surg*. 1990;85:669–674; discussion 675–676.

    The article documents both the clinical features and the accompanying sonographic findings seen with hemifacial atrophy.

23. Tollefson MM, Witman PM. En coup de sabre morphea and Parry–Romberg syndrome: a retrospective review of 54 patients. *J Am Acad Dermatol*. 2007;56:257–263.

    This well-cited article points out the cutaneous and subcutaneous manifestation of hemifacial atrophy.

27. Stone J. Parry–Romberg syndrome: a global survey of 205 patients using the Internet. *Neurology*. 2003;61: 674–676.

    The article highlights the various clinical features seen with hemifacial microsomia.

64. Uziel Y, Feldman BM, Krafchik BR, et al. Methotrexate and corticosteroid therapy for pediatric localized scleroderma. *J Pediatr*. 2000;136:91–95.

    The article identifies methotrexate as a nonsurgical disease-modifying treatment for localized scleroderma, which has similar features to hemifacial microsomia.

81. Longaker MT, Siebert JW. Microvascular free flap correction of severe hemifacial atrophy. *Plast Reconstr Surg*. 1995;96:800–809.

    This article covers the important means of treating hemifacial atrophy, namely microvascular free tissue transfer.

38

Pierre Robin sequence

Christopher G. Zochowski and Arun K. Gosain

SYNOPSIS

- Pierre Robin sequence (PRS) is not a syndrome.
- PRS is a clinical triad consisting of glossoptosis, retrognathia, airway compromise, and possibly clefting of the secondary palate.
- PRS can be an isolated entity or found in the clinical setting of a syndromic child.
- The spectrum of symptoms is vast and an efficient multidisciplinary workup is necessary.
- This workup must begin with an evaluation of the airway.
- The respiratory distress can be managed for many children with PRS and a base-of-tongue airway obstruction with prone positioning and supplemental oxygen.
- If the respiratory distress is not corrected, then airway stenting may be of benefit.
- If this measure fails then many surgical measures are described. There is controversy over which surgical route is best.
- Nutritional support is paramount if this patient population is to thrive. Depending on the patient, specialized bottles, nipples, feeding positions, and feeding tubes may be utilized.
- This craniofacial patient must be followed chronically by many specialties as many systems may be involved.

Historical perspective

To devise future treatments of a clinical entity, one must understand the history of it. The earliest account of a presentation of PRS dates back to 1822 by St. Hilaire, followed by Fairbain in 1846. Later in the 19th century, attempts were made to subclassify the clinical entity by Taruffi into those with "hypomicrognatus" and those with "hypoagnathus." These descriptions demonstrate that as early as the 19th century clinicians understood that a major component of this entity was the mandible. There was a misunderstanding, however, that the mandible was small in size, as compared to the current understanding of a retropositioned mandible. In 1891 Lanneloague and Monard described 4 cases that were significant as 2 of the patients had clefting of the palate. In 1902 Shukowsky presented a case of a hypoplastic mandible causing respiratory distress.

Despite earlier descriptions, the condition bears the name of the French stomatologist Dr. Pierre Robin. Dr. Robin lived from 1867 to 1949 and was a professor in the French School of Stomatology as well as editor of the periodical *Stomatologie*. His main contribution to the body of knowledge regarding PRS was the dissemination of it. Beginning in 1923 he wrote 17 articles on the problems of "glossoptosis" and is credited with introducing the term. He highlighted the severity of the potential respiratory complications and the difficulty these children have with feeding and weight gain. Robin felt that the more severe cases were quite dire and wrote, "I have never seen a child live more than 16–18 months who presented with hypoplasia such as the lower maxilla was pushed more than 1 cm behind the upper." To combat the airway compromise Robin preferred a "monobloc" appliance to keep the mandible forward to restore the normal mandibulomaxillary relationship. Unfortunately, Robin drew many extraneous associations to this cohort and overestimated the incidence of the clinical entity at 3 out of 5 live births (*Fig. 38.1*).

In 1902, Shukowsky performed the first tongue lip adhesion (TLA) by simply suturing the tongue to the lip but the description was not published until 1911. This was successful in 1 patient, but another patient died of asphyxia when the suture pulled through the tongue. The use of TLA was not widely accepted during these initial descriptions. There followed a period of four decades when the treatments for respiratory distress in this cohort consisted of external traction devices placed on the mandible. One such device consisted of a pediatric back brace with a halo from which traction was applied. This was maintained for 4 weeks and was usually successful in alleviating the airway compromise. This modality, however, led to a significant amount of temporomandibular joint ankylosis. Then, in the 1940s, Douglas published a refined technique of TLA and a resurgence in the technique occurred.[1]

PRS has evolved in name since the early descriptions as the understanding of the etiopathogenesis has advanced. Initially,

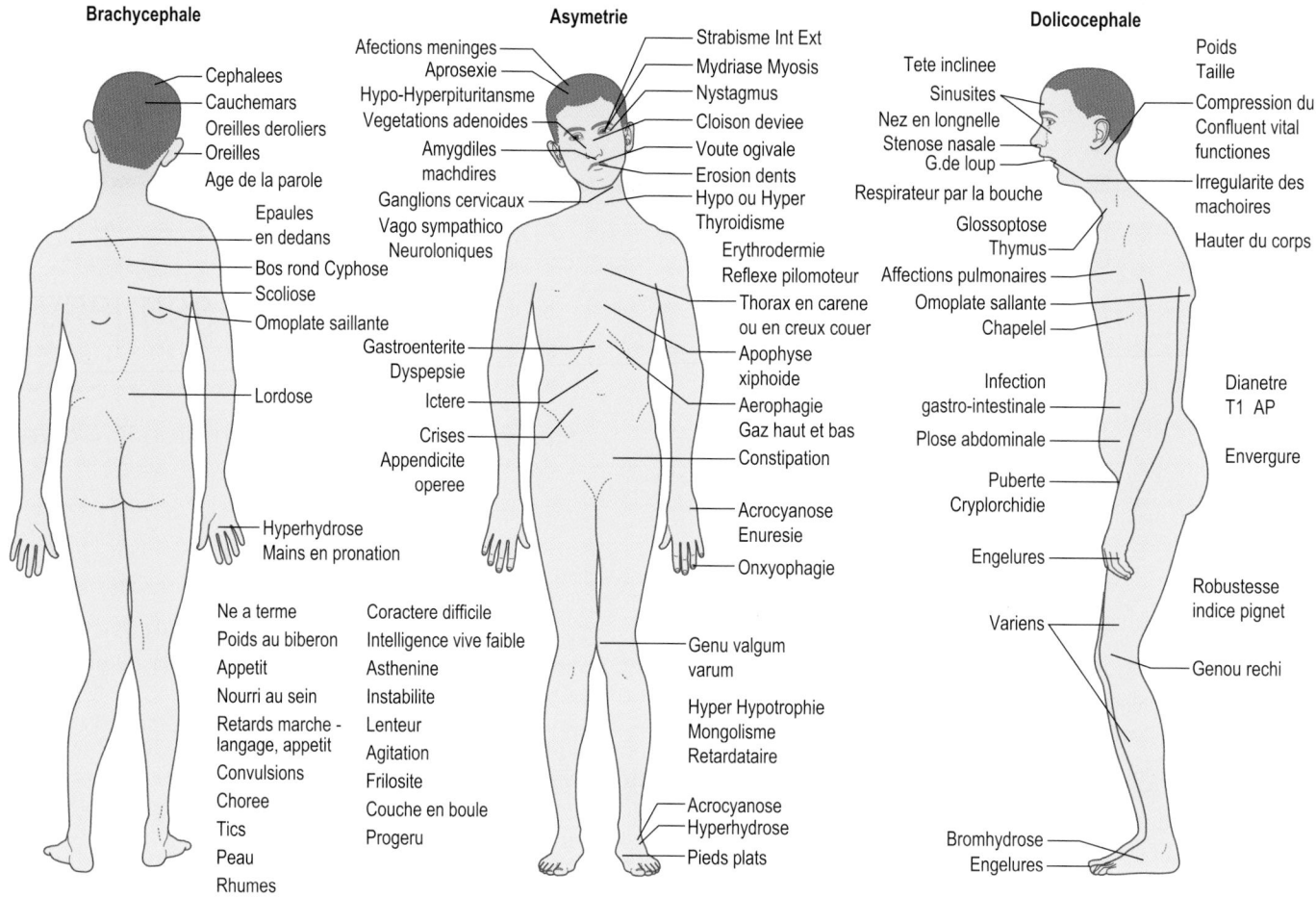

Fig. 38.1 Dr. Robin postulated many clinical associations with glossoptosis.

the clinical constellation was termed "Pierre Robin syndrome." In 1976 Gorlin, Pinborg, and Cohen created the term "Pierre Robin anomalad," noting that this entity was not a syndrome.[2] The term "anomalad" was used to describe an etiologically nonspecific complex that could occur with various syndromes of known or unknown origin or in isolation. Some authors began to use the phrase "Robin complex" but this was shortly replaced by "Pierre Robin sequence" (PRS) or "Robin sequence" by Pashayan and Lewis in 1984.[3] Purists feel that eponyms should not include first names and prefer "Robin sequence."

In the last three decades, with advances in distraction osteogenesis, new debate has arisen. Many new techniques have been described and many series published. These all strive for the same goal of relieving the obstruction of the tongue base. The debate over which surgical technique is best will likely continue as new technologies arise.

Basic science/disease process

PRS is a clinical triad consisting of glossoptosis, retrognathia, airway obstruction, and possibly clefting of the secondary palate. The term "glossoptosis" refers to a posteriorly displaced tongue that obstructs the airway and does not refer to

an enlarged tongue. The cleft palate is not obligatory for the diagnosis and can exist as either a U- or V-shaped cleft and is present in approximately 50% of cases *(Fig. 38.2)*. PRS can be an isolated entity or found in the clinical setting of a syndromic child.

The incidence of PRS varies widely with estimates ranging between 1 in 5000 live births to 1 in 50 000 live births. Most accept the number to be closer to 1 in 8500 live births. A total of 4.5% of infants born in a high-volume delivery hospital will require neonatal intensive care unit (NICU) admission for respiratory distress, and 1% of this group will have PRS.

There is no difference in incidence between boys and girls except in the X-linked form. The X-linked form is characterized by cardiac malformations and club feet in addition to the classic findings.

Estimates of mortality have improved as both the understanding of and treatment options for PRS have evolved. As stated above, Robin painted a bleak picture for any child with PRS. In 1946 Douglas reported greater than 50% mortality with conservative treatment.[1] The major cause of mortality was felt to be secondary to aspiration. Current ranges of mortality for patients with PRS are between 2.1% and 30%. In 1994, Caouette-Laberge *et al.*[4] stratified mortality after subclassification into three groups. For those with adequate respiration in prone positioning and the ability to be bottle-fed, the mortality was found to be 1.8%. For those with adequate

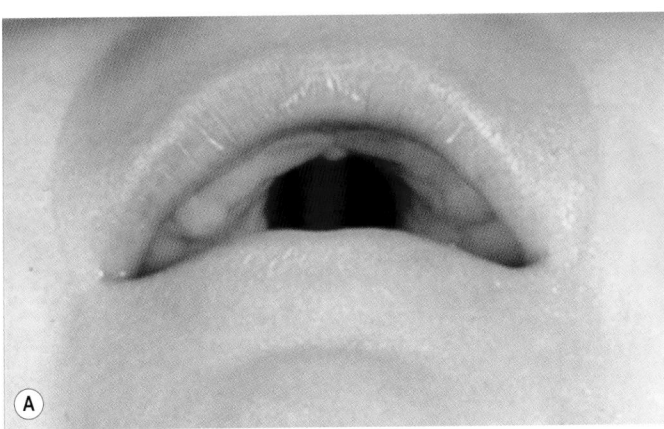
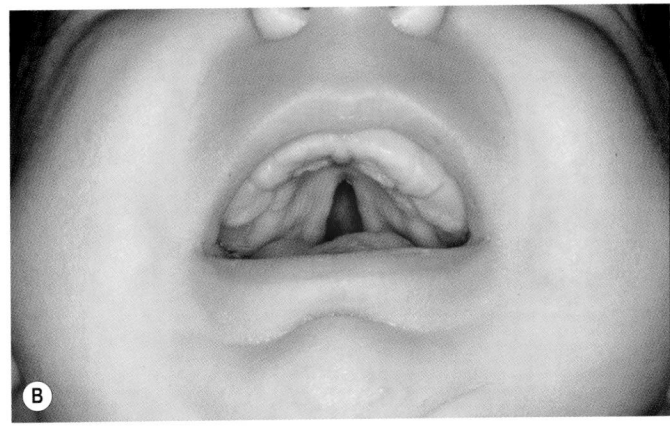

Fig. 38.2 **(A)** This child with Pierre Robin sequence demonstrates the classic U-shaped cleft palate. **(B)** The cleft palate in Pierre Robin sequence may also take the form of a V.

respiration in prone positioning but the requirement of gavage feeds, the mortality was 10%. For those with respiratory distress necessitating endotracheal intubation and gavage feeds the mortality was 41%.

The etiology of PRS is still unclear. As the clinical entity is considered a sequence, there can be many postulated causes. Before any etiological considerations, a clear understanding of the difference between a syndrome and clinical sequence is important. A syndrome refers to a group of signs and symptoms that vary in degree of expression but ultimately result from a single pathological insult. A sequence describes a spectrum of anomalies that may be instigated by varying disease processes but ultimately converge in the same phenotypic findings. This differentiation is germane as a cohort of patients with PRS will be syndromic, like those with Stickler syndrome. The converse does not hold true as not all patients with Stickler syndrome have the phenotypic findings of PRS *(Fig. 38.3)*. Approximately 80% of patients with PRS are nonsyndromic.

Shprintzen[5] hypothesized that the etiology is multifactorial. The mandible may be programmed to be retrognathic if the child has an associated syndrome such as Treacher–Collins, Nager, or Stickler syndrome. This was termed a "malformational" cause. The retrognathic mandible can be from a "deformational" cause such as intrauterine growth constriction. The growth constriction can be caused by a multigravid pregnancy, oligohydramnios, or a uterine anomaly. This could place the child's chin in a flexed position into the chest and restrict growth.

Chiriac and colleagues[6] postulated three theories regarding the etiology of PRS. In the "mechanical theory," the inciting event is mandibular hypoplasia that occurs in the 7th to 11th week of gestational life from various etiologies. The effect is a tongue that rides high in the oral cavity and interferes with the movement of the lateral palatine processes as they progress from a vertical to horizontal orientation *(Fig. 38.4)*. Experimental animal models have mimicked this theory by inducing intrauterine constriction, inducing the triad of findings consistent with PRS. Some feel these events lead to a U-shaped palatal cleft in PRS due to the blockage by the tongue; however others feel that the cleft can be either U- or V-shaped. In the "neurological maturation theory," a neuromuscular delay occurs in the musculature to the tongue,

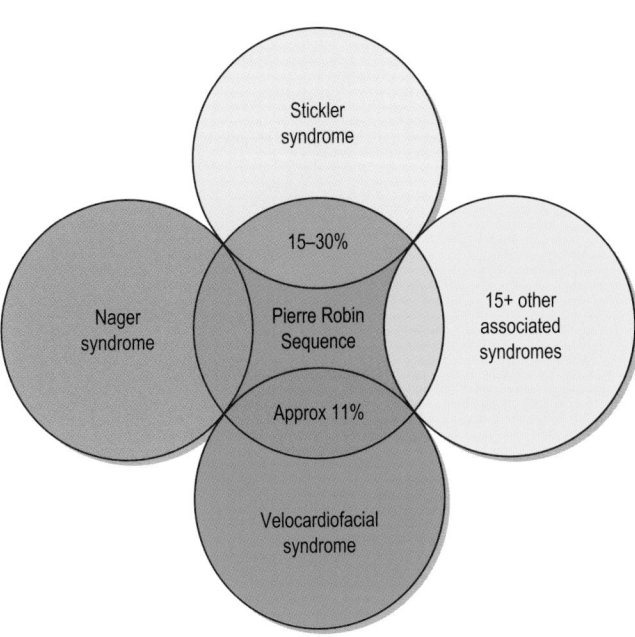

Fig. 38.3 There are many syndromes associated with Pierre Robin sequence; however it can be found in isolation as well.

pharyngeal pillars, and palate. The delay has been noted on electromyogram to the respective sites of these patients. In the "rhombencephalic dysneuralation theory," motor and regulatory organization of the rhombencephalus is related to a major complication in development.

Cohen[7] also described several distinct mechanisms of etiopathogenesis: malformation, deformation, and connective tissue dysplasia. The final mechanism demonstrates a link between diseases of "connective tissue dysplasia" and PRS. An example of this is PRS and Stickler syndrome. Many authors agree upon the influence of intrauterine exposure to teratogens in the formation of PRS. Possible teratogens include alcohol, trimethadione, and hydantoin.

Due to the multiple syndromes associated with PRS and the still unknown etiopathogenesis, analysis of inheritance can be difficult. Cohen in 1978[8] reported up to 18 associated syndromes with PRS. This list includes: Stickler syndrome,

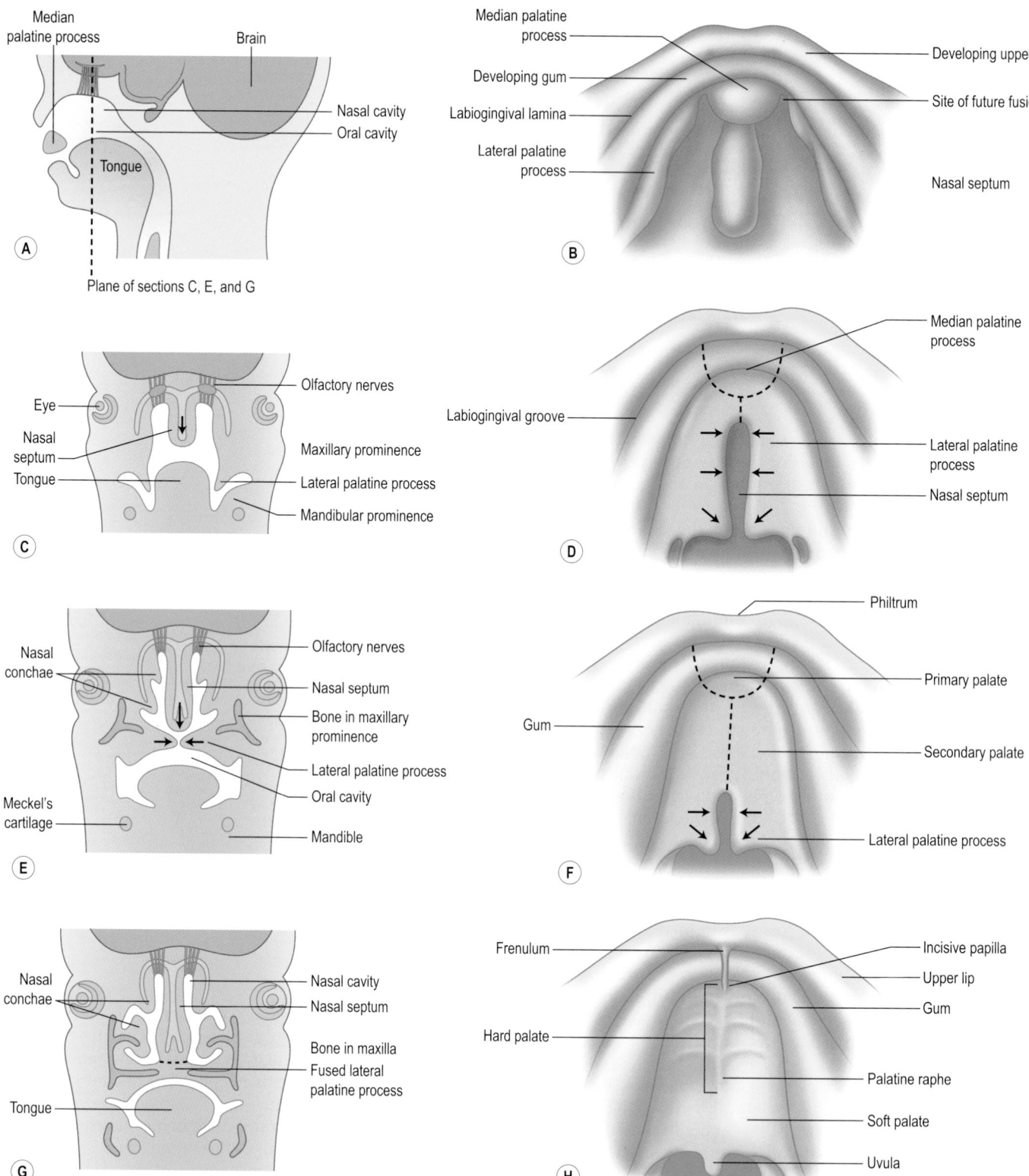

Fig. 38.4 (A–H) The embryology of the tongue and palate is important for understanding the cleft palate in Pierre Robin sequence. The retropositioned tongue blocks the movement of the lateral palatine processes from a vertical to horizontal position.

velocardiofacial syndrome, Moebius syndrome, del6q, Marshall syndrome, Treacher–Collins syndrome, Catel–Mancke syndrome, Kabuki syndrome, Nager syndrome, fetal alcohol syndrome, Weissenbacher–Zweymuller syndrome, popliteal pterygium, CHARGE association, Andersen–Tawil syndrome, collagen XI gene sequence, and achondrogenesis type II. The list of recognized associations can be quite extensive *(Table 38.1)*.

Review of the literature of PRS demonstrates relevance in loci 2q24.1-33.3, 4q32-qter, 17q21-24.3, SOX9 gene on 17q24.3-q25.1, GAD67 on 2q31, PVRL1 on 11q23-q24, KCNJ2 mRNA, TCOF1, GAD67, COL2A1, COL9A1, COL11A1, and COL11A2.[9] The roles of these genes are still not fully understood. They can have a causative role, make the condition more likely, be significant in the associated syndrome, or be coincidental to another process.

The most frequently associated syndrome with PRS is Stickler syndrome. This is thought to be caused by a mutation in the COL2A1 (12q13) gene, COL9A1, COL11A1 (1p21) or COL11A2 (6p21), which affects type 2 and sometimes type 11 collagen. Stickler syndrome can be characterized by midline clefting, a flat midface, a hypoplastic mandible, a flat nasal bridge, a long philtrum, epicanthal folds, prominent eyes, retinal detachments, cataracts, joint hypermobility, and sensorineural hearing loss. Molecular genetic testing for COL2A1, COL9A1, COL11A1, and COL11A2 is available in clinical laboratories, but is most often a clinical diagnosis.

Another associated syndrome is Shprintzen syndrome or velocardiofacial syndrome. The etiopathogenesis is felt to be secondary to a deletion in 22q11. Characteristics are a cleft palate, retrognathic mandible, long upper lip and philtrum, an elongated face, almond-shaped eyes, a wide nose, small ears, conductive hearing loss, slender digits, hypoparathyroidism, immune dysfunction, and learning disabilities. The cardiothoracic anomalies include pulmonary atresia, ventricular septal defects, and hypoplastic pulmonary arteries. Approximately 15% of patients have PRS, and 35% have cleft palate. Conversely, velocardiofacial syndrome is found in up to 11% of patients with PRS.

Nager syndrome, or acrofacial dysostosis, demonstrates autosomal-recessive or autosomal-dominant inheritance. The craniofacial features are similar to mandibulofacial dysostosis. These patients have hypoplasia or agenesis of the thumbs, radius, and of one or more metacarpals. A cleft palate is present. Lower eyelid colobomas may be present, and the child may be short in stature. The mandibular hypoplasia can be severe and there is not a clinical growth "catch-up" period as in children with isolated PRS.

In twin studies, a higher incidence of twinning was noted with PRS (9%) versus the general population (1%). Family members of a child with PRS have a 13–27% incidence of cleft lip or palate.

In a study of 47 children with isolated Robin sequence, Carrol et al.[10] reported 9 cases with a positive family history and a distribution of familial cases compatible with autosomal-dominant inheritance of reduced penetrance and variable expressivity. It is unclear, however, if many of the investigations were careful to exclude those with syndromic PRS. This is especially true in those cases of PRS associated with Stickler syndrome that may not manifest ocular and skeletal anomalies until later in childhood. In another study assessing children with isolated PRS, there was a family

Table 38.1 There are many recognized syndromes associated with Pierre Robin sequence. The postulated genetic locus is shown for several syndromes

Abruzzo–Erickson syndrome

Achondrogenesis type II: 12q13.11-q13.2, COL2A1

ADAM sequence (anionic deformity, adhesions, mutilations)

Amniotic band disruption

Andersen–Tawil: 17q23.1-q24.2, KCNJ2 gene

Beckwith–Wiedemann syndrome: locus 11p15.5, 11p15.5, 11p15.5, 5q35. p57, H19, LIT1

Bruce–Winship syndrome

Campomelic syndrome

Carey–Fineman–Ziter

Catel–Mancke syndrome

Cerebrocostomandibular syndrome

CHARGE association

Chitayat syndrome

Collagen XI gene sequence

Congenital myotonic dystrophy

Del (4q) syndrome

Del (6q) syndrome

Diastrophic dysplasia

Distal arthrogryposis–Robin sequence

Donlan syndrome

Dup (11q) syndrome

Femoral dysgenesis–unusual facies syndrome

Fetal alcohol syndrome

Froster contracture–torticollis syndrome

Kabuki syndrome

Larsen syndrome: 3p14.3, mutations in FLNB (Filamin B) gene

Marshall syndrome: COL11A1

Martsolf syndrome: 1q41 gene encoding protein RAB3GAP2

Miller–Dieker syndrome: 17p13.3

Möbius syndrome: 13q12.2-q13

Nager syndrome: 9q32

PARC syndrome (poikilodermia, alopecia, retrognathism, cleft palate)

Persistent left superior vena cava syndrome

Popliteal pterygium syndrome

Postaxial acrofacial dysostosis (Miller syndrome)

Radiohumeral synostosis

Richieri–Costa syndrome

Robin–oligodactyly syndrome

Sanderson–Fraser syndrome

Spondyloepiphyseal dysplasia congenital: 12q13.11-q13.2, COL2A1

Stickler syndrome: 12q13.11-q13.2, COL2A1, COL9A1, COL11A1, COL11A2

Stoll syndrome

Toriello–Carey syndrome

Treacher–Collins syndrome: mutation in the "treacle" gene (TCOF1), locus 5q32-q33.1

Velocardiofacial syndrome: microdeletion at the q11.2 band of chromosome 22

Weissenbacher–Zweymuller syndrome (otospondylomegaepiphyseal dysplasia) (type II Stickler or "nonocular Stickler syndrome"): gene COL11A2 locus 6p21.3

history of cleft lip or cleft lip and palate in 27.7%. No relatives had a history of PRS; however it is a possibility that the manifestations were present, not acknowledged at a young age, and outgrown in time in the family members.

Diagnosis/patient presentation

The presentation of PRS can be quite varied along the spectrum of severity. To recall, the triad of retrognathia, glossoptosis, and airway obstruction is required for the diagnosis of PRS. A cleft of the secondary palate may be present as well and has been described in up to 50% of patients. This may involve the soft palate only, or the soft and hard palate. In addition, some have described an indicative U-shaped cleft with PRS, but a V-shaped cleft can exist as well.

The respiratory disturbances are just as varied and may be profound at birth, requiring emergent intubation, or mild, and only noted during perturbing settings. In severe cases, periodic desaturations may occur, retractions may be visible, stridor may be audible, or hypoxia and hypoxemic neurological injury can result. These children can progress to develop cor pulmonale. By definition, the child with PRS must have an obstruction localized to the level of the base of the tongue. Additional levels of airway involvement can exist, and 10–15% of infants with PRS have been found to have laryngomalacia. The overall incidence of tracheomalacia in the general population is difficult to determine. Data from the Sophia Children's Hospital in Rotterdam suggest an incidence of 1 in 2100 newborns.[11]

Infants with PRS may also have cardiac anomalies. Congenital heart defects are associated with PRS in 14% of cases.[12,13] As mentioned previously, those with syndromic PRS may have cardiac findings specific to the named syndrome, as in velocardiofacial syndrome, persistent left superior vena cava syndrome, and Andersen–Tawil syndrome.

Infants with PRS may also present with feeding difficulties and failure to thrive. Poor feeding, long feeding times, hypoxia during feeding, gagging, vomiting, aspiration, frequent pneumonia, and gastroesophageal reflux disease are possible. The failure to thrive in this cohort has dual causality from both the poor intake and from the increased metabolic demand from laboring to breath and prolonged feeding times.

The diagnosis of PRS can be made on clinical exam postnatally; however, with the evolution of better ultrasound techniques, the suspicion may arise prenatally if severe retrognathia and a cleft palate are visualized. The early prenatal diagnosis may lead to the recommendation for delivery in a tertiary care facility. In this setting the child would benefit from a coordinated effort by perinatologists, neonatologists, specialized nutritionists, speech pathologists, and surgical subspecialists.

Patient selection

As stated previously, the best setting for a child with suspicion of PRS is in a tertiary care institution with a multidisciplinary pediatric team. This team should include a pediatric pulmonologist, speech therapist, nutritionist, anesthesiologist, otolaryngologist, and craniofacial surgeon.

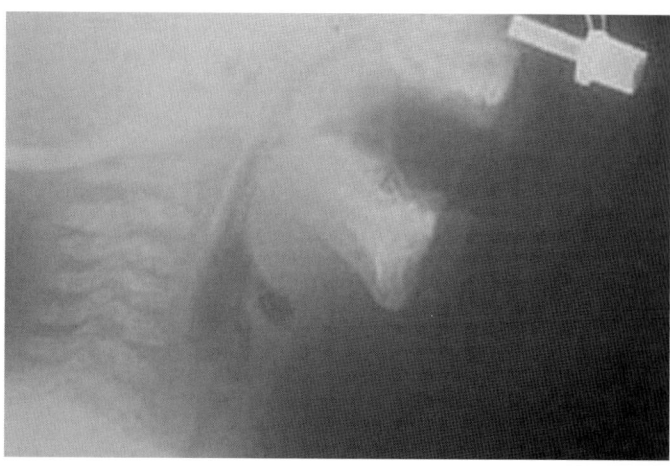

Fig. 38.5 A lateral radiograph demonstrating a nasopharyngeal tube bypassing the base-of-tongue obstruction.

The first interaction with the patient may occur in the delivery suite. As respiratory distress may be lethal, the airway is of paramount importance. For the child suspected of having PRS, resuscitation according to the American Academy of Pediatrics Neonatal Resuscitation Program begins with prone positioning and supplemental oxygen. If this fails then a laryngeal mask airway (LMA) or nasopharyngeal airway can be attempted *(Fig. 38.5)*. If this modality fails, then endotracheal intubation may be necessary and can be aided with a fiberoptic laryngoscope. Due to the retrognathic mandible and glossoptosis, there have been many descriptions of specialized ways to insert the endotracheal tube, but these are in the controlled environment of an operating room. All the prior steps are contingent on the neonate's cardiopulmonary status, the skill of the physician managing the airway, and the availability of proper equipment. If all else fails in the acute setting, an emergent tracheotomy may be warranted. If a child is diagnosed with multiple congenital anomalies prenatally, an EXIT (*ex utero* intrapartum treatment) procedure may be a viable option. In this scenario, the airway can be secured while the child is still receiving placental circulation.

The interaction with the PRS child does not necessarily begin in the delivery suite. The child may have lesser symptoms, as in isolated PRS. Once clinical suspicion of PRS is recognized, a stepwise workup should ensue. The workup should be centered on the significant effects experienced by the PRS patient: the presence of desaturations and feeding difficulties. One must also be mindful of any failed measures previously attempted for the patient. The workup should utilize methods that are readily accessible and begin with least invasive modality.

A thorough history should be obtained that includes the mother's history and the prenatal course. Other pathologies and scenarios may be at work and one should not only focus on the overt anatomical findings. Key points to elucidate from the history are maternal alcohol or drug consumption, infections during pregnancy, prenatal care and screening, and a family history of syndromes.

The pathognomonic mandible must be assessed. A metric is needed for growth and progress of the diminutive mandible. This can be simply obtained by using a wooden end of a

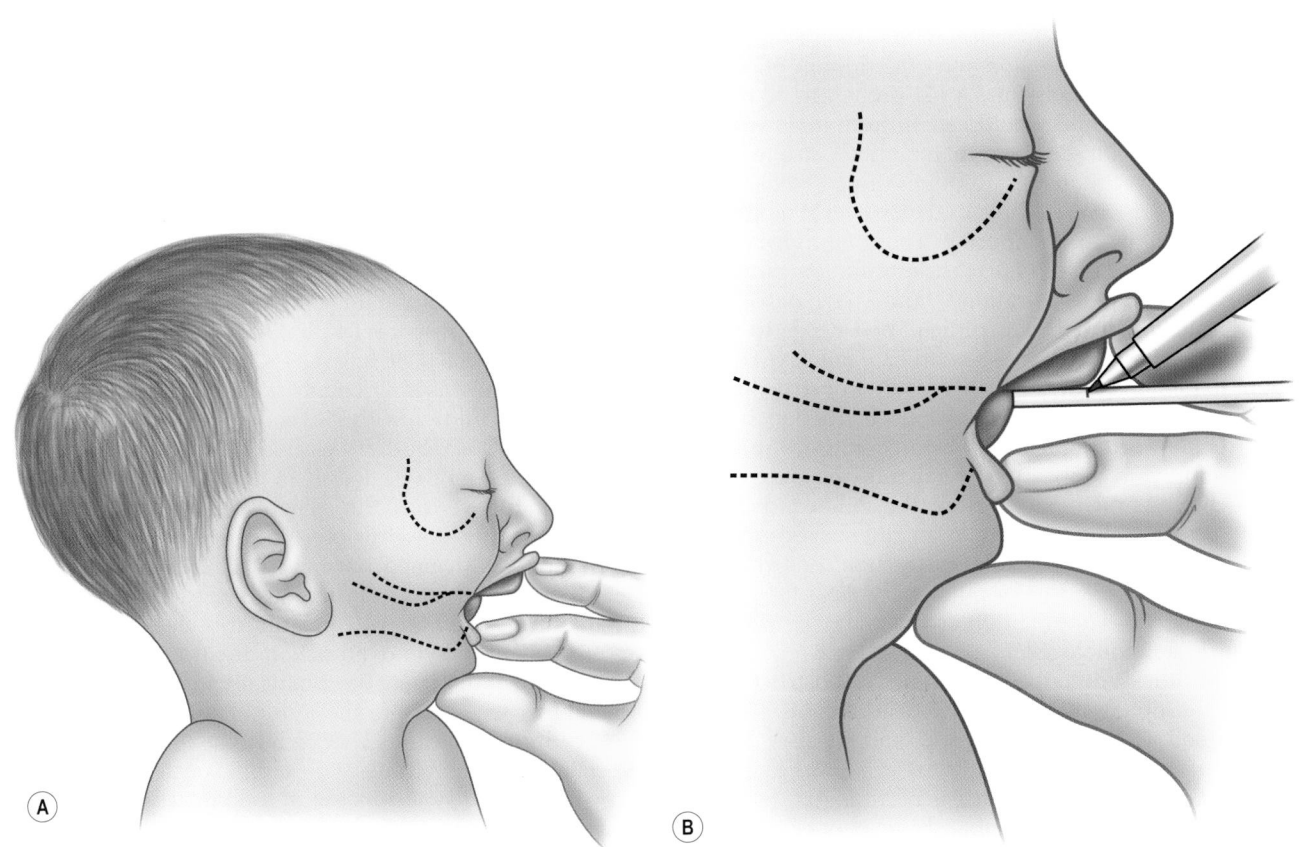

Fig. 38.6 (A) The objective measurement of the mandibular–maxillary discrepancy should be standardized with the child in the upright position with the mandible gently supported without translating it out of position. **(B)** The mandibular maxillary discrepancy is then measured by marking the distance from the most anterior aspect of the mandibular alveolus to the most anterior aspect of the maxillary alveolus on a cotton-tipped applicator. This is then measured with a ruler.

cotton-tipped applicator to measure the maxillary–mandibular discrepancy (MMD).[14,15] The stick is pressed against the anterior aspect of the gingiva of the mandibular alveolus and a mark is made at the anterior aspect of the maxillary alveolus *(Fig. 38.6)*. This value can be variable if not done systematically. As the mandible has a tendency to fall posteriorly in the supine position, the MMD should be obtained with the child upright. The MMD should not act as an absolute for selecting a treatment modality for the child with PRS. Some authors have stated that an MMD of 8–10 mm is an indication for surgical treatment. Robin himself[16] stated that no infant lived past 18 months of age when the MMD was greater than 10 mm. Surgical indications should arise from the overall clinical picture and endoscopic assessment.

The respiratory assessment is paramount in selecting the proper treatment when PRS is clinically suspected. For the clinical entity to exist there must be a respiratory obstruction, and the clinician must evaluate for desaturations. These desaturations can happen at any time, from birth to the point at which the native growth of the mandible helps the base of the tongue clear the airway or the oropharyngeal musculature gains the control required to keep the airway patent. Some feel that the obstructive events in newborns with PRS increase in frequency in the initial 4 weeks of life. Therefore, a false sense of security should not occur after a brief evaluation. In a series by Gosain and Nacamuli,[17] 18 patients presented in

the first week of life and 3 patients presented between 12 and 33 months of age. The respiratory assessment should include continuous pulse oximetry in different scenarios, such as when the child is awake, sleeping, and feeding. The monitoring time required for the sleeping group should be a minimum of 12 hours for neonates and a regular period of sleep for children. The criteria for desaturations are defined as having any single oxygen saturation value less than 80% at any time or if oxygen saturation values are less than 90% for 5% or more of the monitored time. Based on this assessment, the children are placed into two groups: those with desaturations and those without. If a child is found to have no desaturations during sleep but is clinically still suspicious, a formal sleep study is obtained. If the sleep study is positive then the child is placed in the positive desaturation group. For those without desaturations, a screening for feeding difficulties is undertaken.

The feeding assessment begins by plotting the child on a growth chart to determine the starting point and successive trend in weight. In a child with PRS, a downward trend in weight can be seen without treatment. The child can also be assessed by visual observation of feeding. This should be with continuous pulse oximetry to assess for desaturations. Children with PRS usually have prolonged feeding times that are consistently greater than 30 minutes per bottle. These children may also gag and cough during feeds or even become hypoxic. In addition, it has been suggested that up to 87% of infants with PRS have gastroesophageal reflux. The PRS child is already predisposed to aspiration and the addition of significant reflux only compounds this. A pH probe can be utilized to determine if the child would benefit from treatment.

Those children with a diminutive mandible and with feeding difficulties but without desaturations during feeds are treated with nasogastric tube feeding, oral pharyngeal motion studies, and close follow-up monitoring. Those with desaturations while feeding are placed into the desaturation group.

All children who have desaturations should have nasoendoscopy and bronchoscopy. This is difficult and needs to be done in the NICU with equipment to reintubate quickly. This is paramount to demonstrate the proper level of obstruction. There are three main subdivisions: no visible obstruction, infraglottic obstruction, or tongue base obstruction. Care must be taken not simply to stop after visualizing the base-of-tongue obstruction. As mentioned before, the child can have a double lesion. If the nasendoscopy in a child suspected of having PRS demonstrates no visible obstruction, one must suspect a central nervous system or pulmonary disorder. It is appropriate to obtain the consultation of a pediatric neurologist and pediatric pulmonologist.

Sher and colleagues[18] described four types of obstruction seen via flexible nasopharyngoscopy in 53 children with PRS. Type 1 is described as "true glossoptosis," and consists of a tongue that contacts the posterior pharynx at a level below the soft palate *(Fig. 38.7)*. Type 2 consists of a tongue that is displaced posteriorly as in type 1 but at the level of or above the soft palate, such that the palate becomes sandwiched between the tongue and posterior pharyngeal wall in the upper oropharynx *(Fig. 38.8)*. Type 3 consists of an obstruction caused by a medial collapse of the lateral pharyngeal walls *(Fig. 38.9)*. Type 4 consists of the pharynx collapsing or constricting as a sphincter *(Fig. 38.10)*. In the analysis by Sher et al.,[18] 59% were classified as type 1, 21% were type 2, 10% were type 3, and 10% were type 4. As stated earlier, 10–15% will also present with laryngomalacia, and the clinician must recognize this. Occasionally the craniofacial surgeon will be consulted after intubation or tracheostomy. These patients will still require endoscopic evaluation.

The child suspected of having PRS must be assessed for hearing difficulties as this cohort is at higher risk. In one analysis, 83% of children with PRS had some degree of hearing loss versus 60% of children with a cleft palate only. The hearing loss was more profound in children with PRS, and typically conductive in nature. There was also an increased incidence of middle-ear effusions, but the middle- and inner-ear anatomy was deemed normal in all. If a palatal cleft is present there will exist an anomalous insertion of the tensor veli palatini and levator veli palatini muscles. This predisposes eustachian tube to dysfunction. In addition, the orifice of the eustachian tube may be chronically inflamed from continuous reflux secondary to the cleft palate. If the child with PRS is syndromic, the associated syndrome may carry with it the specific otologic findings. An example of this is PRS associated with Stickler syndrome, with a significant incidence of sensorineural hearing loss.

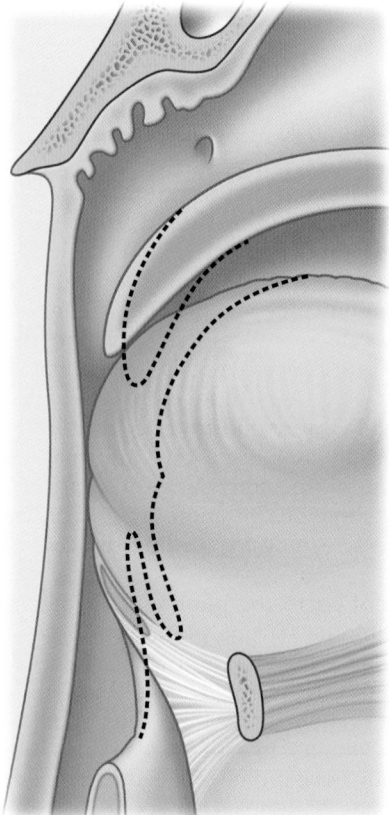
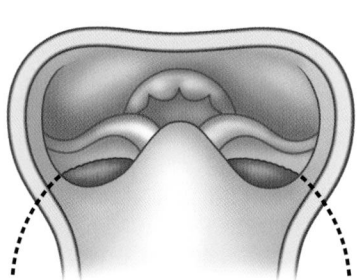
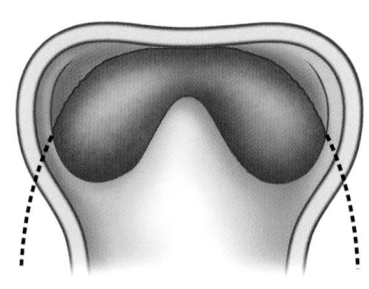

Fig. 38.7 Description of the types of obstruction seen endoscopically in children with Pierre Robin sequence. Type 1 obstruction is described as "true glossoptosis," and consists of a tongue that contacts the posterior pharynx at a level below the soft palate. (Reproduced from Sher AE, Sphrintzen RJ, Thorpy MJ. Endoscopic observations of obstructive sleep apnea in children with anomalous upper airways: predictive and therapeutic value. Int J Pediatr Otorhinolaryngol 1986; 11:135.)

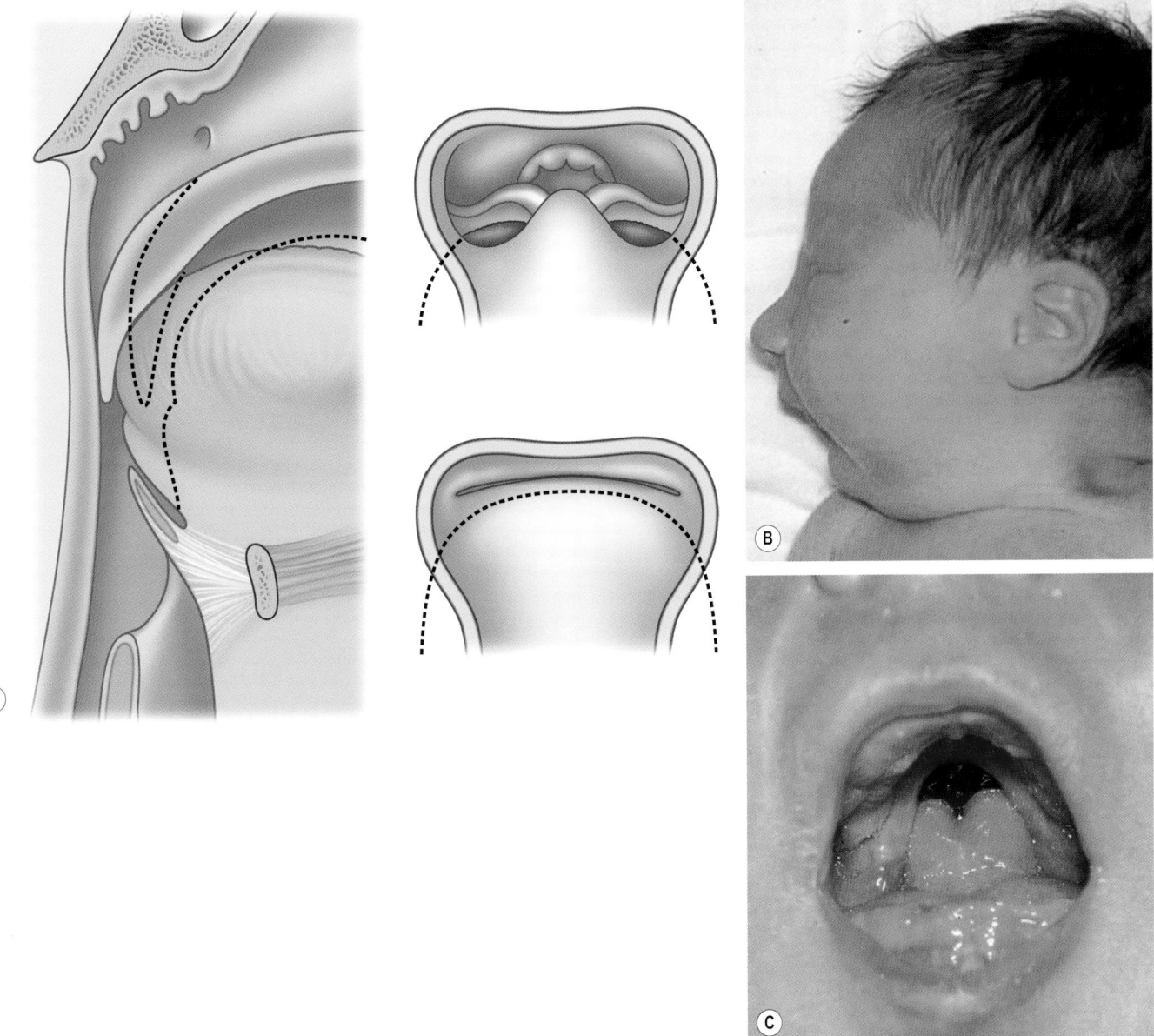

Fig. 38.8 **(A)** Type 2 obstruction consists of a tongue that is displaced posteriorly as in type 1 but at the level of or above the soft palate, such that the palate becomes sandwiched between the tongue and posterior pharyngeal wall in the upper oropharynx. **(B, C)** This child demonstrates a cleft palate with the tongue displaced cranially above the palate.

Treatment

The treatment chosen must take into account the entire spectrum of causality in PRS. As in the diagnostic workup of these patients, one must begin with the least invasive, most appropriate modality first. The treatment of the airway obstruction, if present, takes precedence. There are two main categories for airway management: nonsurgical and surgical.

To begin a discussion of the treatment of the airway obstruction, the underlying mechanism must be understood. Robin[19] described the mechanism as a tongue that is displaced posteriorly due to the retrognathic mandible. Others have similarly described the tongue base acting as a "ball valve" draping over the glottis *(Fig. 38.11)*. The muscular coordination of the

oropharynx also plays a role in the obstruction, highlighting the multifactorial mechanism of obstruction in PRS. The neuromuscular impairment may predispose the airway to collapse. Inadequate functioning of the genioglossus was described by Delorme et al.[20] In this description, the genioglossus is shortened and rotates the tongue posteriorly. Delorme and colleagues went on to postulate that this causes the retropositioned mandible, and not the converse. This theory is not widely accepted and demonstrates the complexity and lack of consensus of the possible etiology.

Another point of contention is the role that a cleft palate plays in degree of symptoms in PRS. Some feel that this anatomic finding will exacerbate the upper airway obstruction. Hotz and Gnoinski[21] theorized that the tongue may become impacted in the palatal cleft, perpetuating the posterior

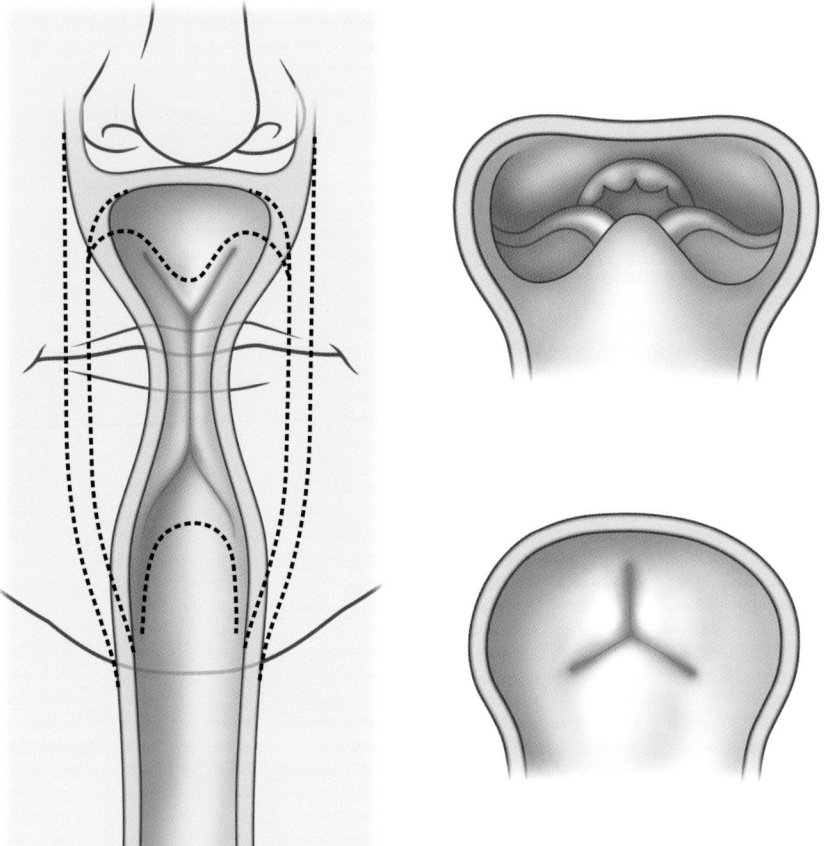

Fig. 38.9 Type 3 obstruction consists of an obstruction caused by a medial collapse of the lateral pharyngeal walls.

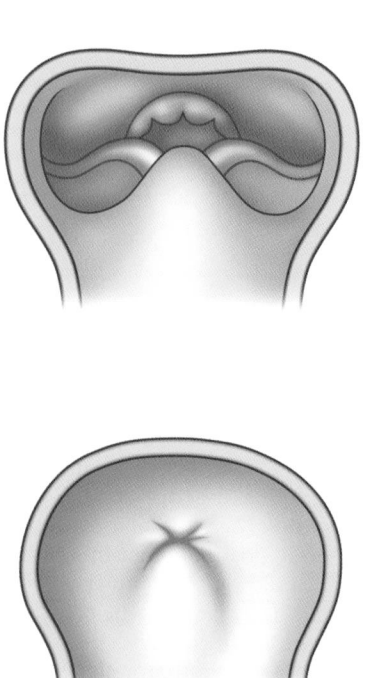

Fig. 38.10 Type 4 obstruction consists of the pharynx collapsing or constricting as a sphincter.

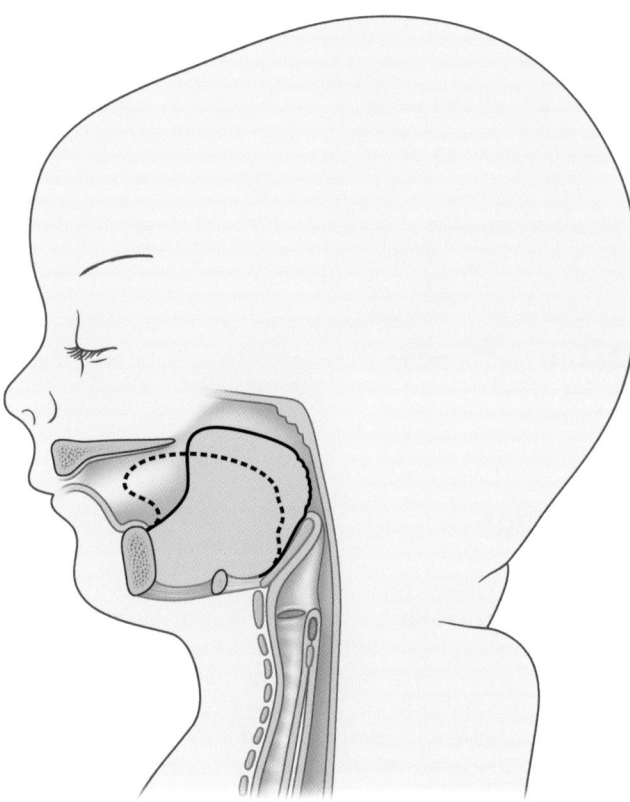

Fig. 38.11 The tongue displaces posteriorly and can act as a ball valve. The dashed line demonstrates the normal position of the tongue. The solid line depicts the possible position of the tongue in Pierre Robin sequence.

positioning of the tongue and upper airway obstruction. Others assert that the cleft may be beneficial and act as an oronasal passage for air.

Nonsurgical airway management

The algorithm for the acute management of the airway in this cohort was described earlier. Cardiopulmonary monitoring is an absolute during this critical time. If desaturations are present in a child with a diminutive mandible, prone positioning should be attempted. The benefit of this maneuver was described by Robin in 1934[22] and radiographically confirmed by Sjolin in 1950.[23] This acts to displace the chin and tongue base forward. Cogswell and Easton[24] showed that the least resistance to airflow for children with PRS is in the prone position. This maneuver can be bolstered by providing the child with supplemental oxygen. If effective, the prone position must be maintained 24 hours a day, even during feeding, baths, and diaper changes *(Fig. 38.12)*.

If prone positioning fails, then a 3-mm nasopharyngeal airway should be placed. Some authors recommend placement to a depth of 8 cm or until the resolution of the obstruction occurs. A recent series demonstrated excellent success in 20 neonates with PRS managed with prone positioning and placement of a nasopharyngeal airway.[25,26] In this report, the nasopharyngeal stent remained indwelling for an average of 44 days and the children remained in hospital during this time. In another report, the median hospital stay was 10 days with the aid of home healthcare services. In this series the average time to removal of the nasopharyngeal airway was 105 days. With proper training, the parents can care for the nasopharyngeal airway without the assistance of a home nurse.

If nasopharyngeal stenting is not successful, then nasal continuous positive airway pressure can be undertaken. An LMA may be attempted. If this fails, then an endotracheal tube can be inserted through the LMA. In the moment of the airway compromise, some instruments may not be readily accessible or timely; therefore some steps may be skipped and the child may need immediate endotracheal intubation.

All of the aforementioned measures depend on the severity of the obstruction and the neuromuscular control of the neonate. Some children on the lower end of the spectrum do well with prone positioning or other nonsurgical measures and are ultimately managed at home with the aid of a home pulse oximeter. Those children on the more severe end of the spectrum, such as many with an associated syndrome, will require some form of life-saving surgical intervention.

Surgical airway management

Surgical management of the airway in children with PRS may be required in the acute setting. A tracheostomy may be unavoidable in certain circumstances, as in the child with PRS with an infraglottic obstruction, or if other surgical methods were employed and the child is still failing to thrive.

The placement of a tracheostomy is not a procedure without morbidity. The management of the tracheostomy site is very labor-intensive and costly for parents and healthcare providers. The neonatal tracheostomy tube is prone to mucus plugging and malposition due to the small size of the neonatal airway and the smaller diameter of the internal lumen of the tube. Some children with PRS may require the tracheostomy for 2–4 years before decannulation. During this time, significant granulation tissue formation and stenosis can occur. It has been suggested that long-term speech, behavior, and developmental problems are associated with pediatric tracheostomy. There have also been implications of moderate to severe intellectual impairment associated with pediatric tracheostomy.

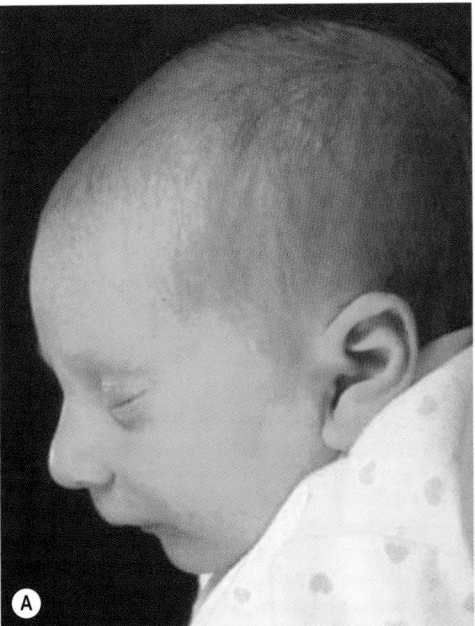
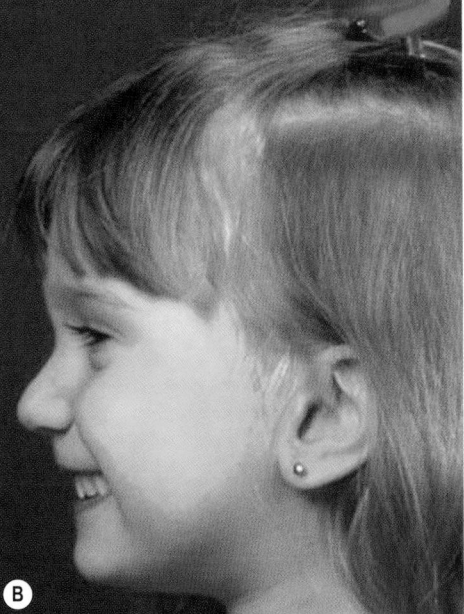

Fig. 38.12 A female with isolated Pierre Robin sequence treated with prone positioning alone at 1 week old versus 3 years old. This demonstrates the ability of the mandibular growth to "catch up" in nonsyndromic cases.

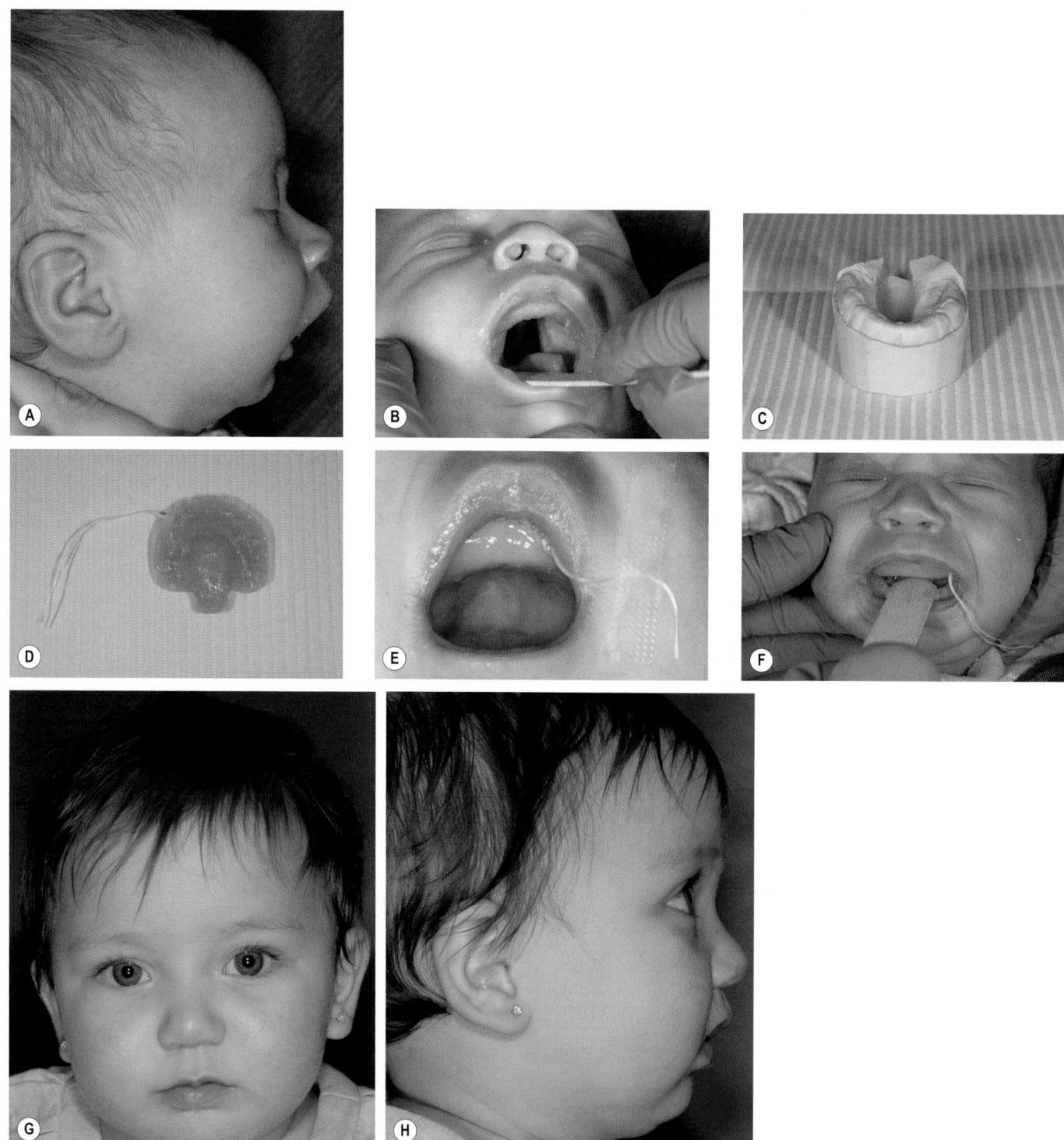

Fig. 38.13 (A) A 3-month-old female with isolated Pierre Robin sequence with respiratory desaturations. On initial exam she had a mandibular maxillary discrepancy of 4 mm. **(B)** The patient had a cleft palate. **(C, D)** A mold was made and a dental plate was fashioned. **(E, F)** The plate fits comfortably and is held in place with dental adhesive. **(G, H)** The patient at 6 months of age with a mandibular–maxillary discrepancy of zero. She was not requiring supplemental oxygen and was feeding well.

During the workup of the child suspected to have PRS, nasendoscopy may reveal tongue base obstruction. In addition to the airway manipulations described earlier, some centers have found success with the use of a palatal plate. A pediatric dentist can fashion this acrylic plate from an impression of the maxilla, and it can be affixed to the palate with denture paste. The plate acts to push the base of the tongue anteriorly *(Fig. 38.13)*. Anteriorly placed knobs can stimulate the tongue similar to the effect from manual massage. The plate is not used as a traction device. In a recent report, a dental plate was used successfully in 122 neonates (91%) diagnosed with PRS and was unsuccessful in only 12 (9%). Of the

12, 9 underwent glossopexy successfully, 4 were intubated, and 1 child received a tracheostomy.

Many procedures have been described over the years for PRS, but all share a similar theme of moving the base of tongue anteriorly relative to the mandible. This can be accomplished with soft-tissue or skeletal techniques.

Soft-tissue techniques

A TLA can aid in the resolution of the airway obstruction. Originally described by Shukowsky in 1911,[27] the tongue was simply sutured to the lower lip. The concept was popularized by Douglas in 1946.[1] In Douglas' technique, a rectangular area is denuded under the tongue, along the floor of the mouth, on the alveolus, and on to the lower lip. The tongue is then brought forward, and the raw surfaces are coapted. A mattress tension suture passes from the dorsum of the tongue to the chin. This technique was modified by Routledge in 1960,[28] and more recently modified by Argamaso.[29] TLA remains a mainstay of treatment. The procedure is comprised of elevating a proximally based rectangular mucosal flap from the ventral surface of the tongue and a complementary superiorly based mucosal flap from the labial surface of the lower lip (*Figs 38.14–38.17*). The flaps are approximately 1 × 1.5 cm in size. Care is taken to protect Wharton's ducts. If a short or tight lingual frenum is present, a frenulotomy or a frenectomy can be beneficial. In the modification described by Argamaso,[29] the genioglossus muscle is detached from the mandible with a small periosteal elevator. The tongue-based flap is sutured to the lower side of the opposing defect in the mucosa of the lower lip. The exposed tongue musculature is then sutured to the exposed orbicularis oris and anterior soft tissues through a small incision caudal to the mandibular symphysis.

Additionally, a larger suture is passed in a circummandibular fashion into the muscular substance of the tongue. Several authors have described using various methods to accomplish this, including Keith needles or an awl. The sutures are then usually tied over a button. A nasopharyngeal tube should be placed and left indwelling for 2–3 days. Feeds should be administered by a nasogastric tube to prevent sucking while healing. These children should remain in an intensive care setting during the postoperative period as they are extubated in a guarded manner and to ensure that the airway remains adequate afterwards.

The timing of the takedown of a TLA cannot be overstressed. Some authors recommended repair of the cleft palate, if present, at the same time as the TLA takedown. This methodology can lead to a later than necessary TLA takedown and oromotor retardation. In addition, a combined cleft palate repair and TLA takedown may produce substantial airway edema and respiratory compromise. Conservative guidelines include evaluation of the child at 1 month of age to assure the TLA was successful. Afterwards, evaluations should be every 2 months until the adhesion is taken down. The evaluation focuses on tongue motion, which is quite infantile and possibly dormant early in life. As the child matures the tongue will exhibit rhythmic muscular movements. A good clinical indicator of tongue maturity is active motion in response to touch. The decision to take down the TLA does not hinge solely upon this, but also upon the MMD and overall clinical picture. A MMD of less than 3 mm is usually a good prognostic indicator that the TLA can be taken down safely. Using these guidelines, most are able to be reversed by 6–7 months of age. Elective palate repair is performed separately at the routine time interval, which is at age 11–12 months at our institution. To take down the TLA, the two mucosal flaps are incised and the intervening tissue between these flaps is

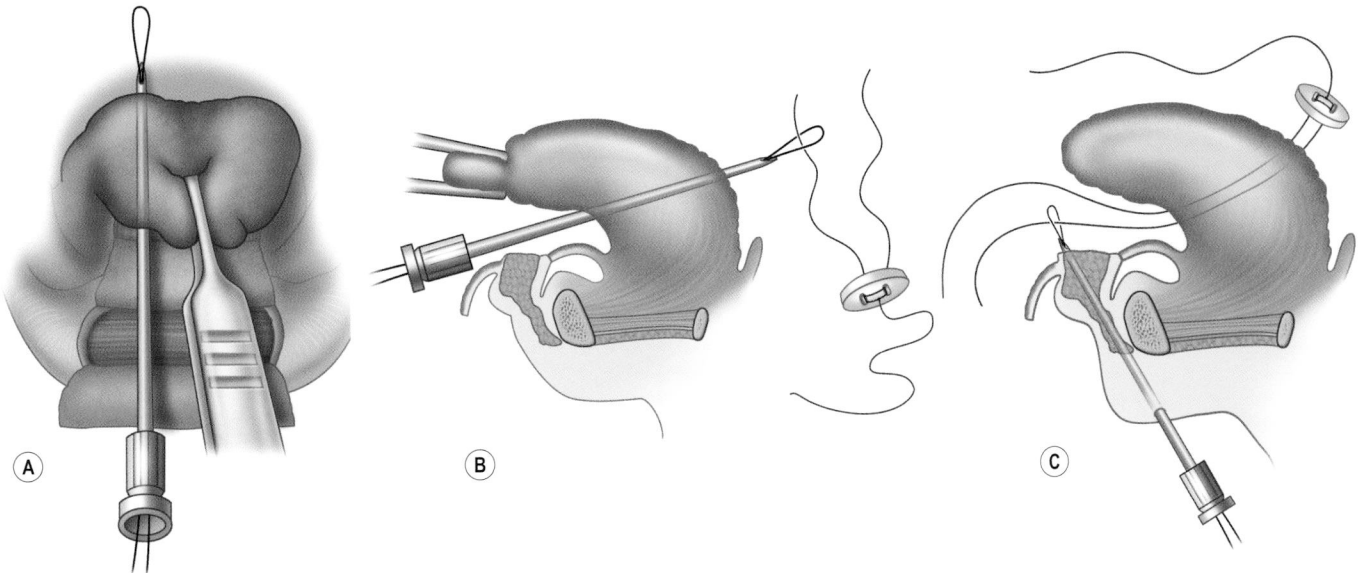

Fig. 38.14 (A–C) In a tongue lip adhesion a posteriorly based flap is elevated from the tongue and a corresponding mucosal flap is elevated from the labial surface of the lower lip. Care is taken not to injure Wharton's ducts. The tongue-based flap is inset to the caudal margin of the defect created by the elevation of the lip-based flap. A nonresorbable suture is then passed through the tongue and brought through the raw surface created by the flap elevation. The suture is then passed through the raw surface created by the labial flap, taking care to catch orbicularis oris. The suture is then brought out through the submental area by passing anterior to the mandible. The labially based flap is then inset into the tongue defect.

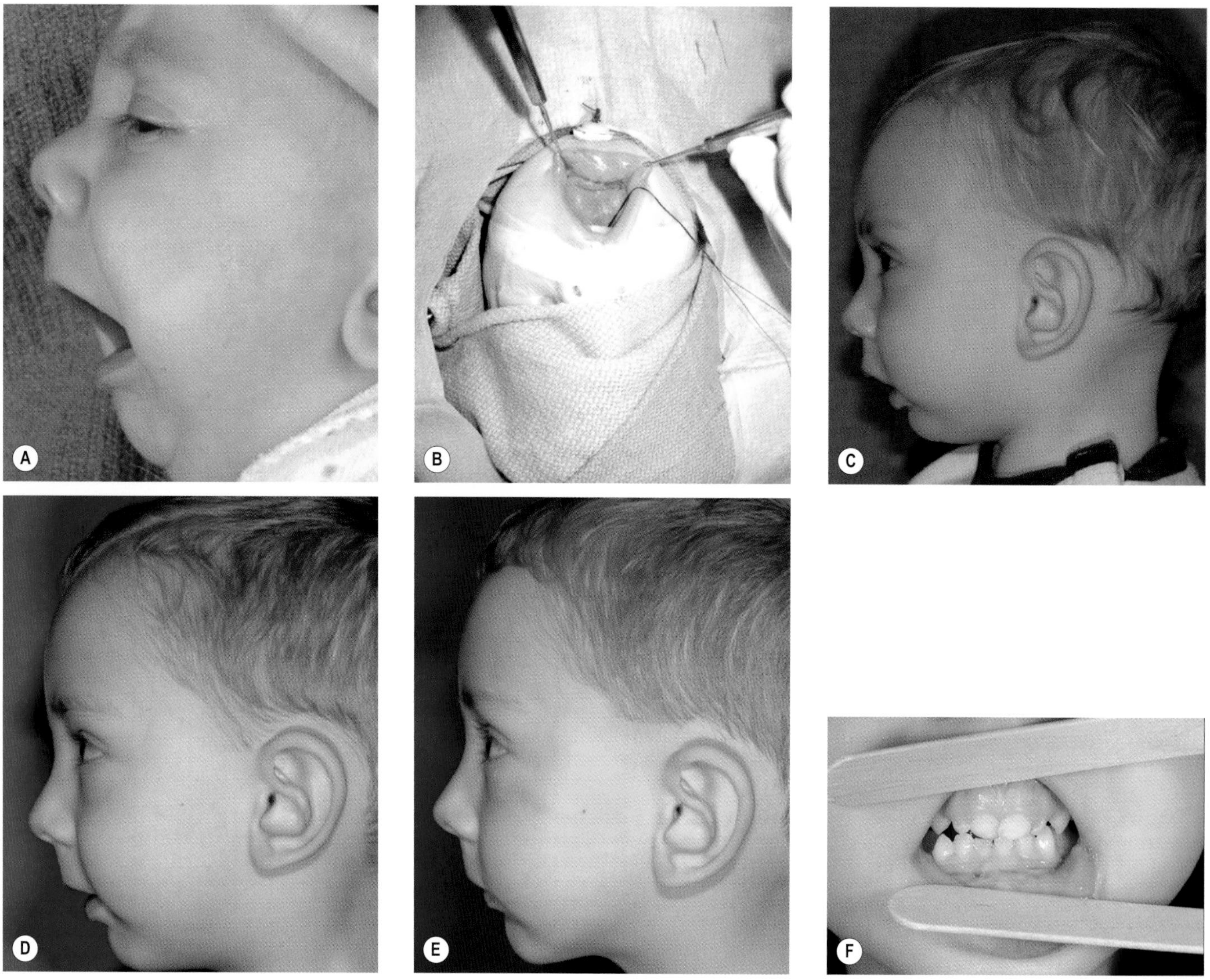

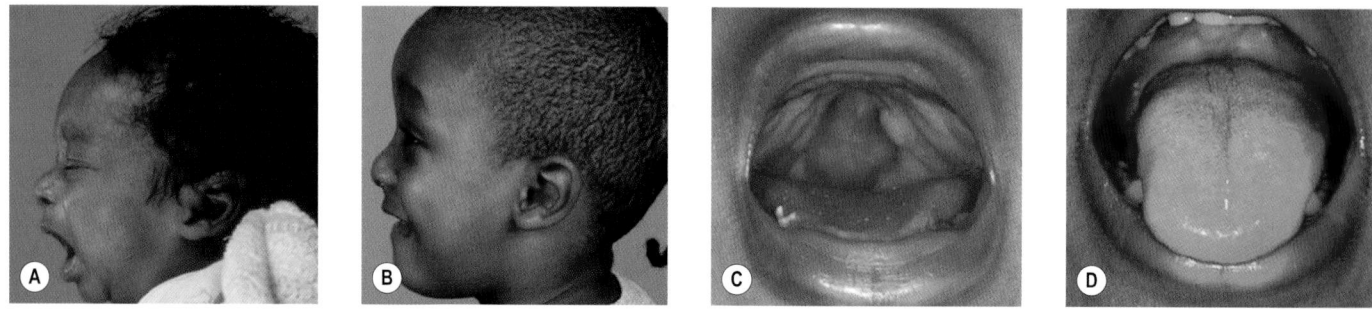

Fig. 38.15 (A) A child with Pierre Robin sequence. **(B)** The child was treated with a tongue lip adhesion. **(C–F)** The patient did well throughout childhood and demonstrated good mandibular growth over time.

Fig. 38.16 (A–D) Another child treated successfully for airway compromise and feeding difficulties with tongue lip adhesion alone.

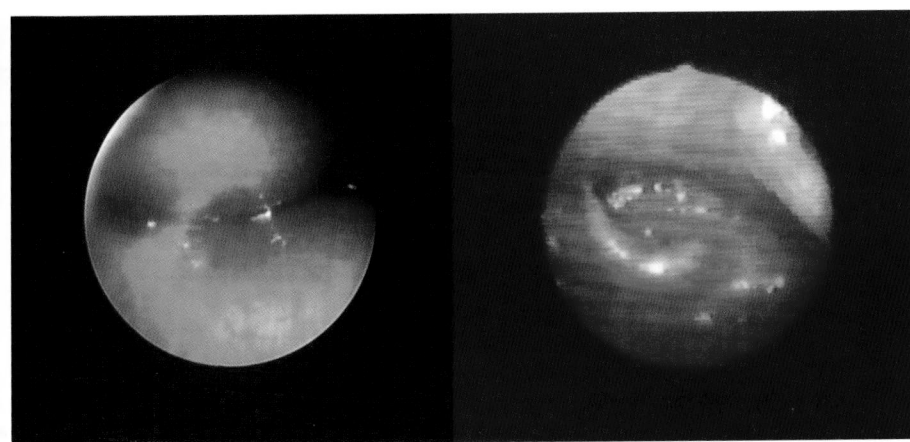

Fig. 38.17 Left, The same patient as in *Figure 38.16* demonstrating glossoptosis on nasendoscopy. Right, the airway is cleared 3 days after tongue lip adhesion.

divided by electrocautery. The flaps are then closed such that no raw surfaces remain that may result in synechiae. Using this protocol, the authors have not had any residual tongue dysmorphia or impairment in tongue motility.

Rogers et al.[30] reported a success rate of 80% of 24 neonates with PRS treated with TLA. Huang and colleagues[31] reported a 70% success rate with TLA, with success defined as weight gain, extubation, or prevention of tracheotomy. In a series by Schaefer and colleagues,[17] 10 of 21 neonates with PRS were treated with prone positioning alone, 7 were treated successfully with TLA in 9 attempts, 2 required tracheostomy, and 3 underwent mandibular distraction.

Critics of TLA state that the sutures easily cut through the friable tissues of the tongue, adhesion rarely occurs, detrimental scarring of the tongue forms, airway obstruction persists, and the possible injury to Wharton's ducts is significant. Denny challenged the use of TLA in favor of distraction osteogenesis. In his series of 11 patients with PRS, only 2 were successfully treated with TLA alone. Five patients required secondary surgical intervention for recurrent airway obstruction within 4 months.[32] The authors suggest that TLA should be considered as a temporizing management option.

Kirschner et al.[33] sought to answer the criticisms of TLA in a series of 33 patients with PRS, of which 29 were treated with TLA. The rate of dehiscence was observed to be 17.2%. This occurred exclusively when the procedure was comprised of mucosal adhesion alone with no muscle incorporation. In addition, 5 of the 6 patients who ultimately required a tracheostomy were syndromic patients. This highlights the importance of subgroup analysis in PRS.

Some feel that speech development can be affected due to the tongue being affixed anteriorly during this critical time. LeBlanc and Golding-Kushner[34] examined this and found that children who underwent TLA had minimal long-term effects on speech development. Glossopexy seemed to affect only early speech production by delaying sound production. Once the TLA is taken down, patients "catch up" by accelerated development. The morphologic changes seen in the TLA cohort, such as thick lower lip mucosa, a blunted lingual apex, and lingual deviation on protrusion, were noted to be temporary. The TLA cohort was equal to patients with cleft palate and their syndrome-matched counterparts in the maintenance of articulatory integrity, and their development of speech sound production at 18 months.

Overall, some series suggest a higher failure rate with TLA for PRS. This appears to be surgeon-dependent and technical. Several measures that can improve results are creating an adequate labial mucosal cuff, and ensuring adequate tongue muscle to lip muscle coaptation.

Other soft-tissue procedures have been described other than TLA. Oecononopoulas[35] described the use of a heavy silk suture through the base of the tongue that is affixed to the cartilaginous portion of the mandible about 1 cm lateral to the midline. Hadley and Johnson[36] also devised a technique where the pull focused on the tongue base. In this description, a towel clamp is used to pull the tongue by the tip, and a nasopharyngeal tube is moved in and out of position to test for adequate airway clearance. Then, a 0.062-inch (0.2-cm) or 0.045-inch (0.1-cm) Kirschner wire is driven from one angle of the mandible, through the tongue base, and out through the contralateral angle, taking care to stay anterior to the endotracheal tube and avoiding injury to the inferior alveolar nerve and tooth buds (Fig. 38.18). In some descriptions, a silk traction suture was used in place of a towel clamp and remained in place even after extubation as a precaution.

Lewis et al.[37] described a tensor fascia latae sling in 1968. In this technique, a long strip of tensor fascia latae, approximately 0.5–0.75 cm wide, is harvested. A 1-cm submental incision is made and dissection courses to the inferior border of the mandible. A fascial carrier is placed via the incision through the floor of the mouth. The tongue is held in an anterior position and the fascial carrier is brought out of the tongue laterally at the junction of the middle and posterior thirds. The fascial graft is placed into the eye of the fascial carrier and withdrawn through the submental incision. The remaining intraoral fascial graft is pulled transversely through the substance of the tongue to the contralateral side. It is then withdrawn through the tongue, floor of the mouth, and the submental incision (Fig. 38.19). Care must be taken not to place this too posteriorly in the tongue as the anterior tongue can drape posteriorly and cause a second obstruction. Proper tension can be set and the anterior caudal ends of the fascia are anchored to the periosteum of the symphysis. The proponents of this technique cite the ease and speed of the procedure. This technique does not require secondary procedures to "take down" the sling. The obvious shortcoming of this technique is the donor site morbidity.

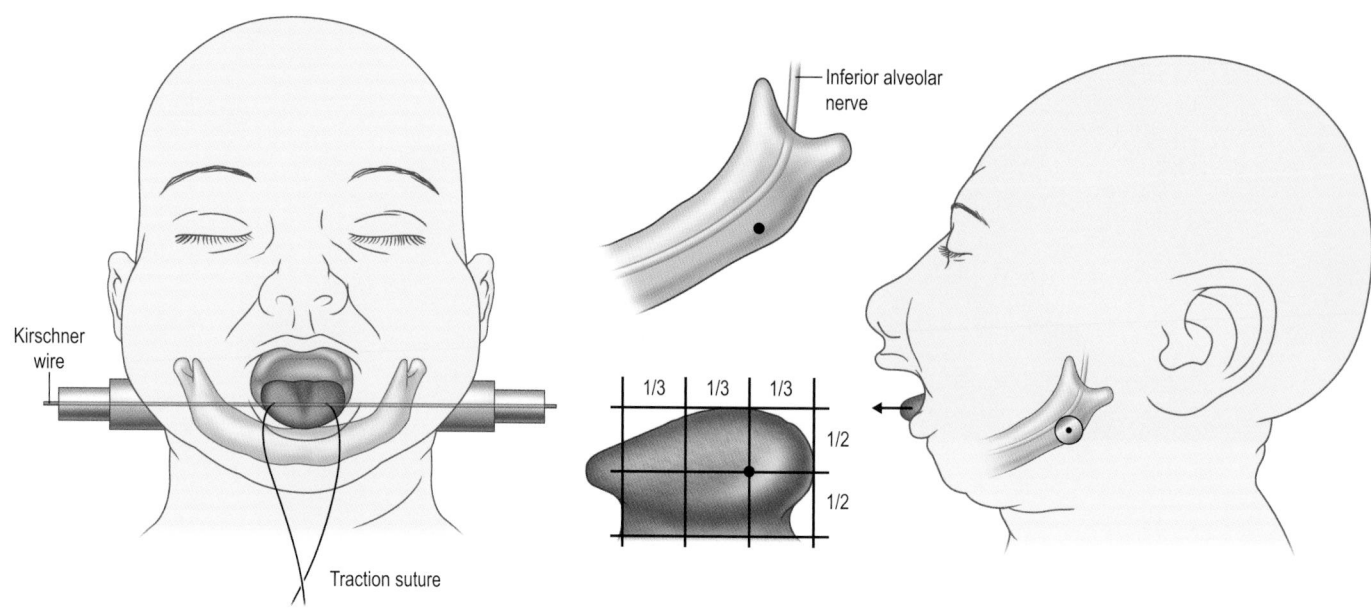

Fig. 38.18 Hadley and Johnson[36] described a technique in which a Kirschner wire is passed from mandibular angle to mandibular angle with the tongue under tension.

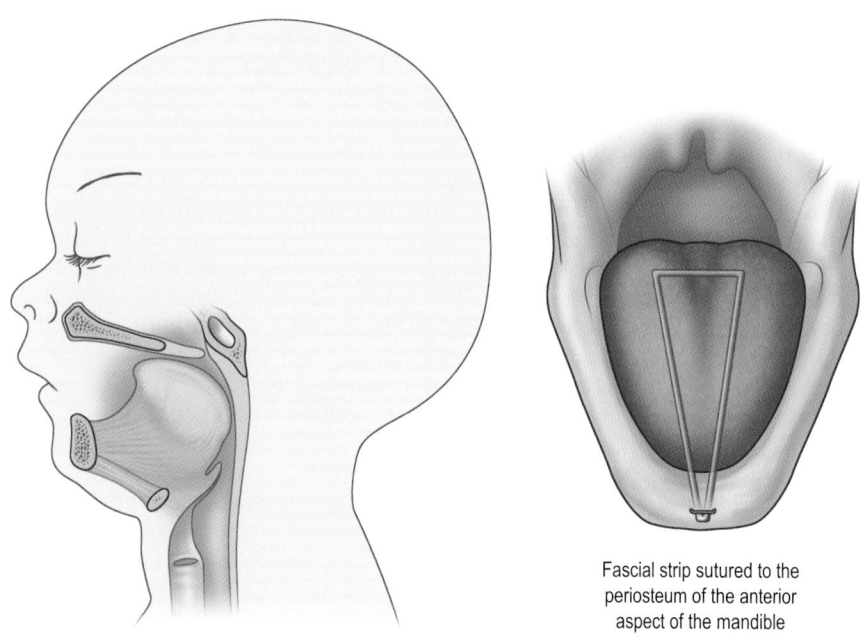

Fascial strip sutured to the periosteum of the anterior aspect of the mandible

Fig. 38.19 The tensor fascia latae has been described as a sling. In this technique, the tensor fascia latae graft is looped around the base of the tongue posteriorly and anchored to the mandible anteriorly.

Bergoin and colleagues[38] describe a procedure termed "Hyomandibulopexie." In this technique the ventral anterior surface of the tongue and mandible is anchored to the hyoid bone with 3-0 braided nylon sutures. This technique was rarely used as it was felt to interfere with potential mandibular growth and made intubating the child difficult.

Lapidot and Ben-Hur[39] felt that the TLA described by Douglas[1] restricts free movement of the mobile segments of the tongue and that this may hinder growth of the mandible. Instead, in their description, 18-gauge steel wire is placed into the most posterior midline portion of the tongue base. The steel wire is then directed anterior and caudally to arise below the hyoid bone *(Fig. 38.20)*. The opposite end of the wire is tunneled submucosally to the foramen cecum and then directed inferiorly to emerge at the superior aspect of the hyoid.

In other techniques, the vector of pull on the tongue is altered. In the Duhamel procedure,[40] heavy nylon suture is passed across the most posterior aspect of the body of the tongue, exits laterally through the cheeks or oral commissures, and then tied over buttons.

Delorme and colleagues[20] felt that the musculature of the floor of the mouth is under increased tension, causing the tongue to protrude cranially and posteriorly, and a full

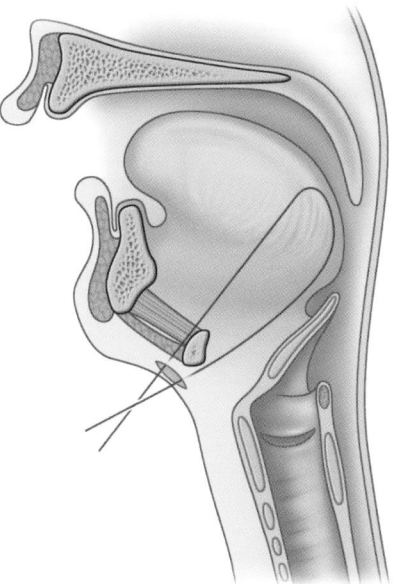 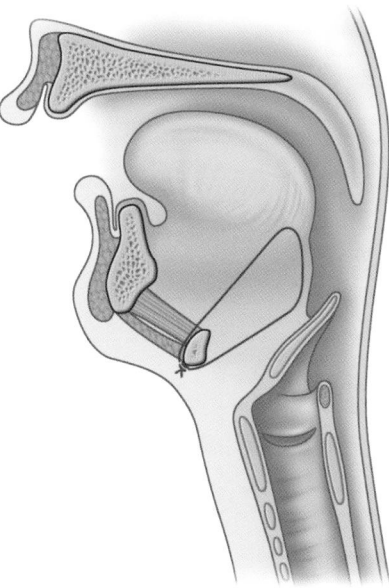

Fig. 38.20 The technique described by Lapidot and Ben-Hur[51] uses an 18-gauge steel wire that is placed into the most posterior midline portion of the tongue base. The steel wire is then directed anterior and caudally to arise below the hyoid bone. The opposite end of the wire is tunneled submucosally to the foramen cecum and then directed inferiorly to emerge at the superior aspect of the hyoid.

soft-tissue release from the anterior mandible is required to relieve the airway obstruction *(Figs. 38.21 and 38.22)*. Through a 2-cm submental incision the periosteum is incised at the lower border of the mandibular symphysis. Then the wide periosteal release of the floor of mouth musculature is done from the medial border of the mandible as far posteriorly as the angles of the mandible. This includes release of the origins of the genioglossus, geniohyoid, and mylohyoid muscles. The child remains intubated for 1–2 weeks. Caouette-Laberge and colleagues used this technique successfully in 11 of 12 patients.[4] Breugem and colleagues[41] treated 14 patients with subperiosteal release. Seven patients were treated successfully and avoided tracheostomy. Of the 7 requiring tracheostomy, only 1 was nonsyndromic. Dudiewicz *et al.*[42] felt that success with this technique could be obtained by combining the subperiosteal release with closure of the cleft palate. It was felt that a properly repaired cleft palate provides a barrier against the posterior displacement of the tongue.

Overall, all of the soft-tissue techniques strive toward the same goal: to pull the base of the tongue forward relative to the mandible. We feel that this is most logically carried out in our hands by pulling the tongue longitudinally toward the lip as in a TLA.

Skeletal techniques

Procedures in this category can further be divided into those that apply traction on the mandible versus those that distract the mandible. Traction applied to mandible as a treatment for PRS is of historical note. One major drawback of this technique is that the circummandibular wires at the parasymphysis can cut through the thin bone in neonates. One method affixes an acrylic plate to the mandible by circummandibular wires and the tension is distributed evenly, preventing cut-through *(Fig. 38.23)*. The weight needed to clear the airway obstruction has been noted to be 50–200 grams. The traction

is released for feeds after 1–2 weeks. Then the traction device utilizes decreasing amounts of weight and may remain in place for up to 5 weeks. This is all done under constant cardiopulmonary monitoring.

With the advent of distraction osteogenesis, the armamentarium of the craniofacial surgeon was expanded for many purposes. In 1927 Rosenthal[43] performed the first mandibular osteodistraction procedure using an intraoral tooth-borne appliance. The work of Ilizarov with the long bones advanced the body of knowledge exponentially. In 1972, Cosman and Crikelair[44] reported 3 cases of respiratory difficulty associated with retrognathia that responded to mandibular advancement. In 1989, McCarthy[45,46] clinically applied the technique of extraoral osteodistraction on 4 children. In 1997 Guerrero et al.[47] were the first to report the results of intraoral mandibular distraction for widening of transverse deficiencies in 11 patients. In 1994, McCarthy developed a miniaturized bone-borne uniguide mandibular distractor. In 1994 Havlik and Bartlett,[48] and later Haug and colleagues[49] reported on the treatment of severe micrognathia using extraoral distraction devices. Many reports followed on the application of intraoral appliances *(Fig. 38.24)*.

The mechanism of action of clearing the airway with mandibular distraction in PRS is similar to that described previously. The tongue base moves anteriorly by its attachments to the distracted mandible, pulling the tongue out of the hypopharynx *(Fig. 38.25)*. The aperture of the airway is increased in an anteroposterior dimension. After approximately 8 mm of distraction, the tongue posture visibly changes on a daily basis. This change in tongue posture to a normal horizontal position on the floor of the mouth is a clinical indicator for the timing of extubation.

Selection of mandibular distraction to address tongue base position in infants with PRS entails three fundamental decisions: (1) What portion of the mandible is to be lengthened? (2) What vector of distraction is to be used? (3) What type of device is to be used? In answer to the first two questions,

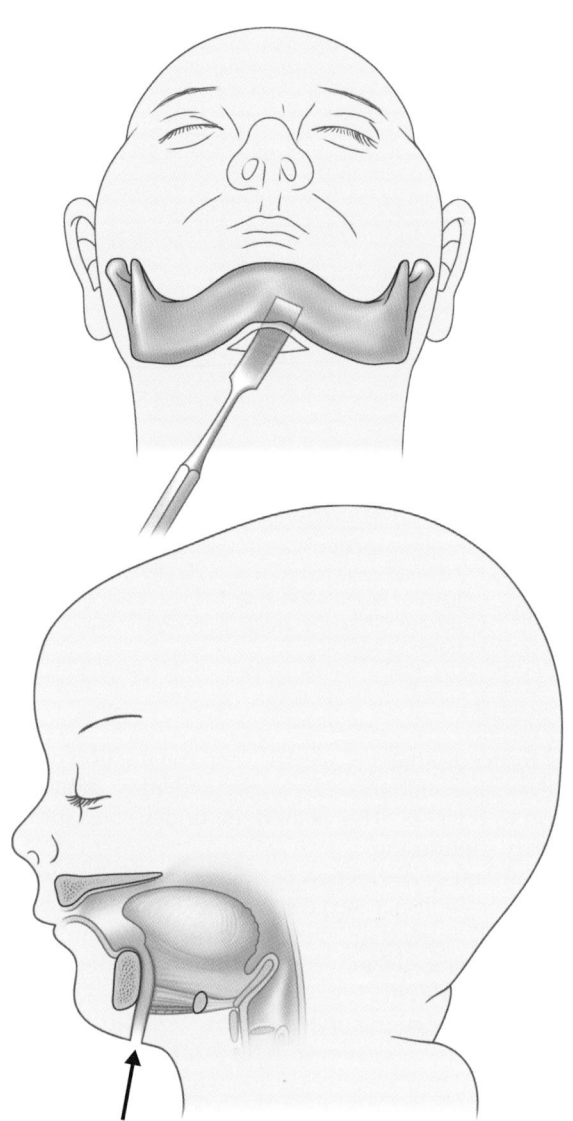

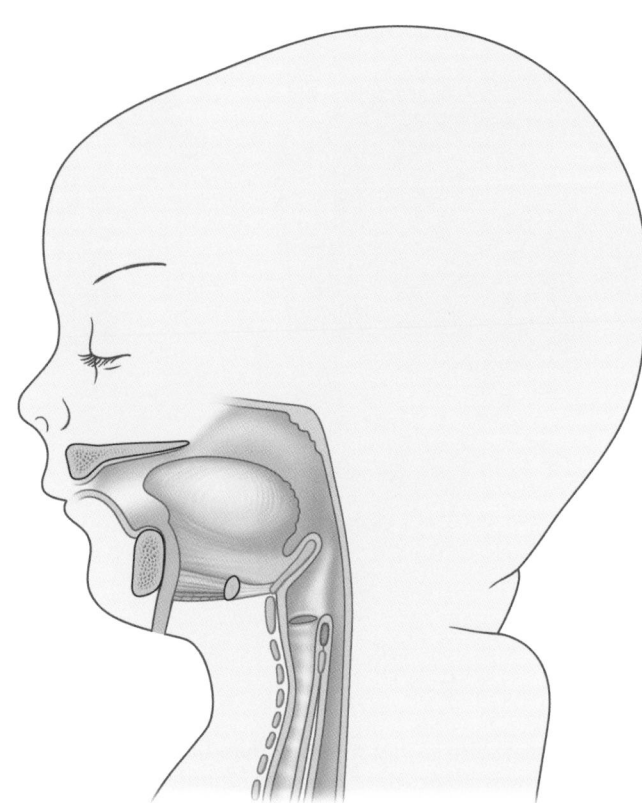

Fig. 38.22 The wide periosteal release is done as far posteriorly as the angles of the mandible. This includes release of the origins of the genioglossus, geniohyoid, and mylohyoid muscles.

Fig. 38.21 In the procedure described by Delorme and colleagues,[20] a subperiosteal release of the floor of the mouth musculature is done through a 2-cm submental incision.

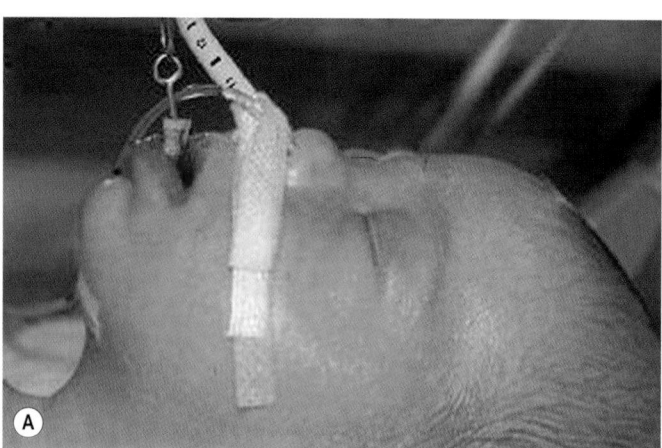

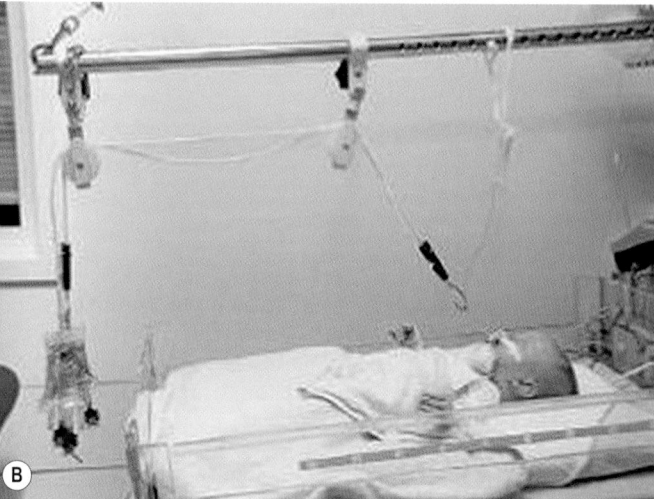

Fig. 38.23 (A, B) A demonstration of using traction on the mandible to relieve the airway obstruction. In this technique, an acrylic plate is fixed to the mandible and traction is applied to the plate.

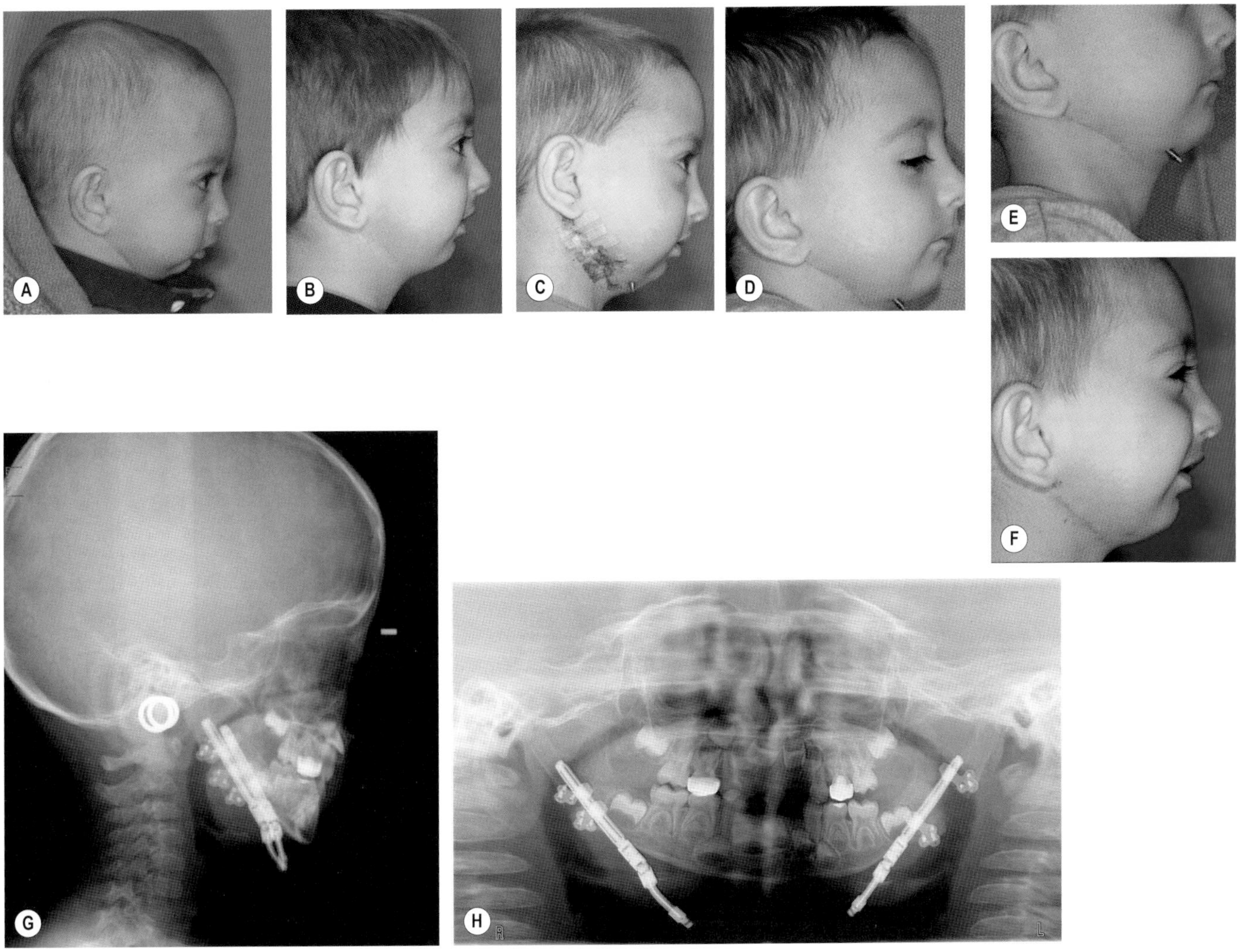

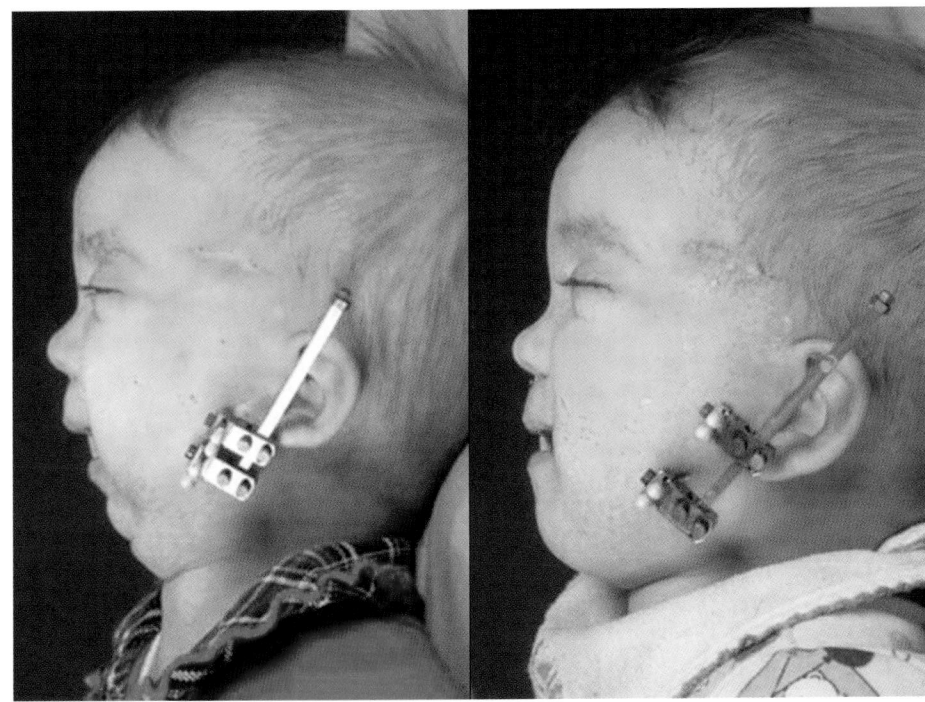

Fig. 38.24 A child with Pierre Robin sequence treated with mandibular distraction osteogenesis via an intraoral distractor.

Fig. 38.25 A child with Pierre Robin sequence treated with mandibular distraction osteogenesis via an external distractor. The mandibular–maxillary discrepancy was dramatically improved.

infants with PRS invariably have a short mandibular ramus. Therefore, our preference is to lengthen the ramus rather than the body of the mandible. However, this can be technically challenging in a very diminutive mandible. While it is technically easier to lengthen the body of the mandible, one must realize that the body of the mandible is a "tooth bank" and not only is one likely to eliminate or injure tooth roots at the site of osteotomy and/or device fixation, but there will inevitably be a gap in the permanent dentition where distraction took place. We therefore advocate osteotomy in the ramus of the mandible above the occlusal plane so as to minimize risk to the inferior alveolar nerve. Selection of vector of distraction will depend on the patient's presentation. However, neonates with PRS who require distraction to open the airway present during the first month of life, and orthodontic assessment cannot be made. Therefore, one must use basic principles more than orthodontic assessment in selecting the vector of distraction. A rough guide to distraction vector when lengthening the ramus is to remain parallel to the posterior border of the ramus. This usually produces a distraction vector approximately 60° from the occlusal plane, providing components both to lengthen the ramus and to advance the chin point forwards. Autorotation of the mandible secondary to ramus lengthening will also bring the chin point forward. In answer to the third question, what type of device is to be used? one may choose between external and internal distraction devices. If one chooses an external distraction device, the osteotomy may be created through an intraoral or an extraoral incision. If one chooses an intraoral approach, local anesthetic containing adrenaline is injected over the oblique line and the buccal surface of the mandible. A lateral vestibular incision is made on both sides. Subperiosteal dissection is done to expose the gonial angles and the posterior mandibular body. Selection of pinhole sites is very important as this dictates the vector of distraction. Before placing the percutaneous pins, the skin is bunched or pulled cephalically for better cosmesis of the final scars.

The neonatal mandibular bone is brittle and narrow, thus precision is important. The unerupted tooth follicles should also be avoided. The pins should be tested and ensured to be in good bone stock. It is prudent to place the pins and temporarily affix the distractor before completing the corticotomies so as to return the mandible to its original reduction following completion of corticotomies. Circular vertical corticotomies are made just anterior to the ascending ramus. The corticotomy can be made with a mechanical saw at the buccal cortex, superior border, and inferior border of the mandible. Following corticotomy, an osteotome is used as a lever to insure that the proximal and distal segments are independently mobile, therefore insuring that the osteotomy is complete. Fixation of the distraction device can now be completed to stabilize the mandible. Note that if the distractor was completely fixed prior to this point, one could not insure completion of the osteotomy, which could predispose to premature consolidation and/or device failure during distraction. The intraoral incision is then closed with resorbable sutures. The ability to distract must be checked while in the operating room and then the device is returned to the starting position. One must take note of the starting MMD.

Distraction is usually initiated after a latency period of 3 days, and the rate of distraction is 1.5–2 mm in children under 1 year of age. Note that, at the age when PRS patients undergo distraction, the distraction parameters are accelerated over those used in older patients to prevent premature consolidation. The child recovers in the intensive care unit. The MMD is recorded to ensure effective distraction. The pins are cleaned with peroxide, and antibiotic ointment is applied twice daily. Distraction continues until the desired MMD is obtained and the base-of-tongue obstruction is clinically cleared. The consolidation phase varies at different centers, but we recommend a consolidation period of 8 weeks.

If an extraoral incision is used, the incision is made at the site of pin placement. The platysma is then divided and care must be taken not to injure the marginal mandibular nerve. One should use a nerve stimulator and avoid the use of local anesthetic so as to maintain motor nerve function. The pterygomasseteric sling is incised and the masseter is stripped, and the buccal cortex of the mandible is exposed. The pin placements and corticotomies are done in a similar fashion to that previously described, and device fixation should follow mobilization of the mandible.

Internal devices may also be used for distraction. While there are many ways to approach device placement, we prefer to use an intraoral approach to the mandibular ramus, similar to that described for placement of the external device. It is important to note that vector of distraction is fixed once the device is fixed, and therefore positioning of the intraoral device is critical to the final outcome. Even if one places the osteotomy above the occlusal plane, fixation of the distal portion of the device will inevitably be in the region of tooth roots, and monocortical screws are recommended. We make two stab incisions through the skin corresponding to the region of proximal and distal segment fixation. These stab incisions are used to pass the screwdriver, using self-drilling and self-tapping monocortical screws (3.5-mm length) for device fixation. Although the device is positioned prior to completing the osteotomy, it must be removed to insure completion of the osteotomy prior to final fixation. Our preference is to bring the activation unit out through a submandibular stab wound for ease of access during the distraction process, although many surgeons bring the activation out through an intraoral incision and keep the device within the mouth. Advantages of internal distraction over external devices include one-to-one bone lengthening with device activation, whereas external devices may torque at the pin level and not achieve one-to-one distraction. The internal device is also less prone to device dislodgement due to trauma, and there are no stretched scars in the skin that are inherent when using external distraction pins. Disadvantages of internal devices include the need for wider exposure for device placement, fixed distraction vector at the time of device placement as opposed to multidimensional external units, and the need for a second operation for device removal. At this time, there are no good resorbable fixation units by which internal devices could be fastened to the mandible, although many groups are currently working on this technology. Once these resorbable fixation devices are available, it will obviate the need for a second operation, since the distraction devices will simply be pulled away from their resorbable fixation units once the consolidation process is complete.

Proponents of mandibular distraction osteogenesis feel that the need for a tracheostomy can be avoided, airway obstruction caused by the tongue base can be relieved, scars are cosmetically acceptable, and the mandible can be redistracted if needed.[50]

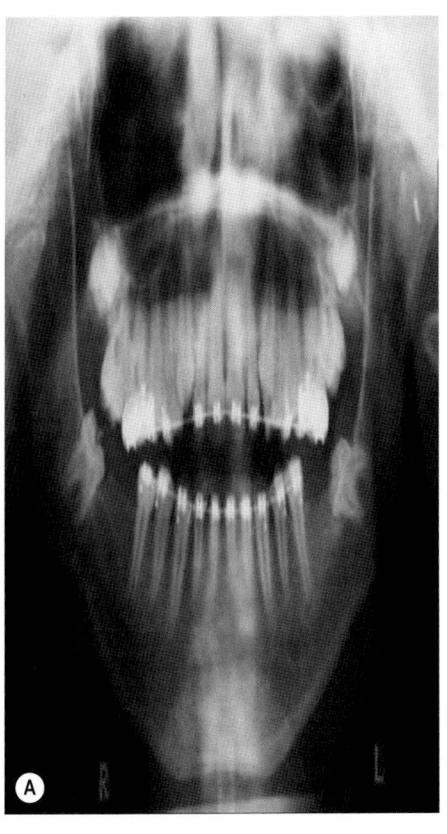

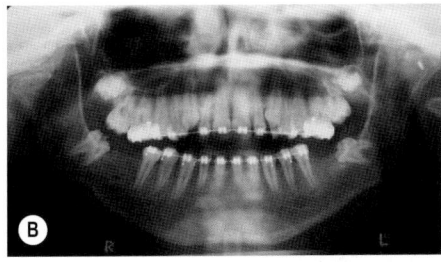

Fig. 38.26 (A, B) Abnormally positioned second molars 8 years after second mandibular distraction osteogenesis.

The potential shortcomings of this technique are related to a significant risk of complications and the gradual improvement in the airway. Depending on the protocol, distraction usually progresses at a rate of 0.5–2 mm a day. The child may still require prolonged intubation or a tracheostomy during this time. A recent analysis of the literature[51A] demonstrated an overall complication rate of 20.5–35.6% for mandibular distraction osteogenesis for varied indications *(Figs 38.26 and 38.27)*. Relapse was significant in 64.8% of cases. Other significant complications were injuries to the tooth roots in 22.5%, hypertrophic scarring in 15.6%, nerve injury in 11.4%, infection in 9.5%, inappropriate vector of distraction in 8.8%, device failure in 7.9%, fusion error in 2.4%, and temporomandibular injury in 0.7%. Another shortcoming is that a second procedure is required for removal of the appliance and there exists the possible need to redistract later in life. The procedure itself requires the periosteum to be stripped and an osteotomy to be made, and this can theoretically restrict growth. The ability to distract is also contingent on the age of the child and size of the mandible. Distraction is not offered for neonates younger than 39 gestational weeks, as the mandible may not be physically able to maintain the fixation of the device.

There is an ongoing debate over whether to choose distraction of the mandible over other surgical methods such as TLA. Some authors feel that distraction should be a last resort and less invasive measures be attempted first. This is done with the expectation that the growth of the mandible will experience a "catch-up phase" of growth. The literature is replete with evidence for and against this postulate. The natural history of mandibular growth is defined by the associated syndrome. The syndromic child may not experience the same rate of mandibular growth.[52] If the child continues to

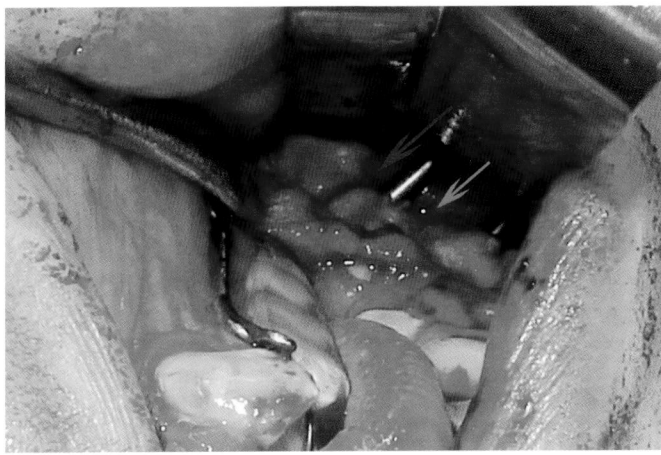

Fig. 38.27 Intraoperative view demonstrating the two distal pins of the distraction device remaining in bone. A fracture has resulted between these pins (small arrow) distal to the site of premature fusion of the initial osteotomy site (large arrow).

demonstrate airway difficulties after 6–7 months of age, then the mandibular growth was inadequate to clear the tongue base sufficiently and distraction may be warranted. In this setting, endoscopy should be repeated to ensure that there are no other sites of airway obstruction that were not evident earlier in life.

Some feel that mandibular distraction should be performed earlier in the algorithm for PRS and replace TLA. Dauria and Marsh[53] proposed such an approach. Denny and Kalantarian[50] completed this task successfully in a series of 5 consecutive neonates with PRS with bilateral mandibular distraction

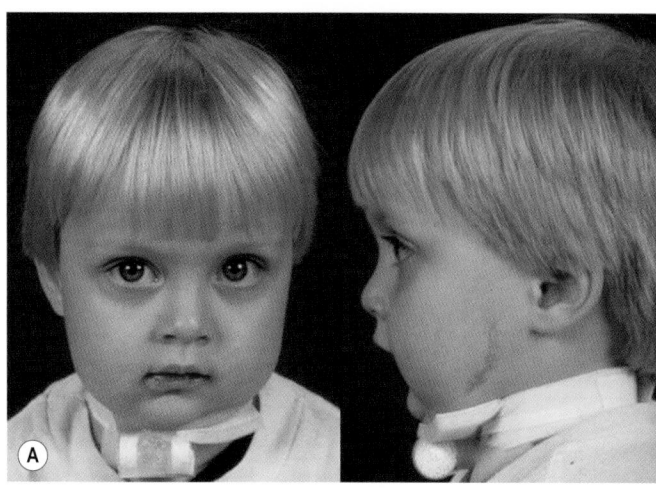
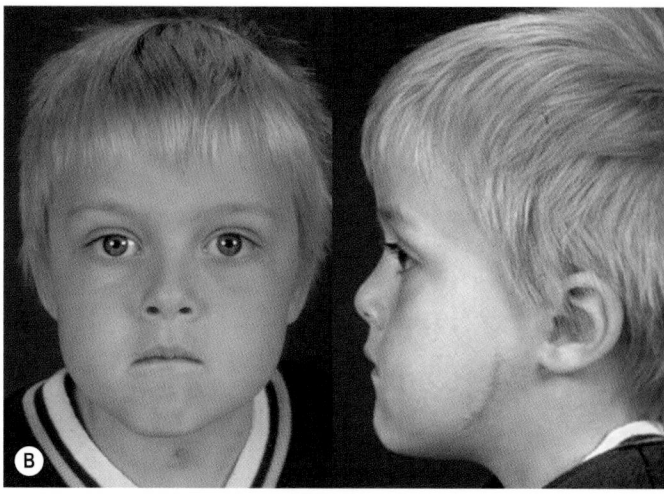

Fig. 38.28 (A) A 3-year-old boy with Pierre Robin sequence with persistent tracheostomy following one attempt at mandibular distraction. **(B)** Successful decannulation after second mandibular distraction and tracheal reconstruction.

osteogenesis. All avoided tracheostomy, had complete elimination of respiratory symptoms, and were extubated before completion of the active distraction process. All 5 patients remained extubated without airway support.

A recent series by Sati and colleagues[54] retrospectively assessed 15 isolated PRS patients treated with TLA from 1994 to 2004 and 24 treated with mandibular distraction osteogenesis from 2004 to 2009. Comparison of distraction osteogenesis with TLA demonstrated no difference in age at the time of surgery, age at palatal closure, or length of ICU stay. The distraction osteogenesis group was extubated sooner postoperatively. There were no postprocedure tracheostomies in the distraction osteogenesis group, compared to 4 in the TLA group. There were 12 complications in the TLA group, compared to 4 in the distraction osteogenesis group. It is unclear what criteria were used in determining the time for extubation. If this was the main parameter by which these cases were assessed, the clinicians could have had a bias to extubate later in patients with TLA. This is of particular relevance since the two groups were done at different time periods, and using subjective assessments of when to extubate could have varied and been based on the clinician's confidence in the intervention.

One must keep in mind that distraction progresses at a set rate, and some cases may require a tracheostomy despite distraction *(Fig. 38.28)*. The proposition of distraction as an earlier option is more attractive as the technology improves. There has been a progression from pin-retained external devices to internal distractors. However, the use of internal distractors in this young cohort is difficult as there is not enough room subperiosteally to accommodate the device. Recently, the potential for resorbable mandibular distraction devices has created new excitement. This would theoretically limit the procedure burden on the child to one and limit the potential complications from general anesthetic. At the present time multiple companies are working towards a clinically useful internal distractor. Currently, none has proven reliable for clinical use due to the anchor being weak.

In summary, both methods of soft-tissue and skeletal procedures can successfully clear the airway obstruction. It is the responsibility of the treating physician to ensure that the source of the obstruction is solely localized at the base of the tongue. After the proper workup is completed, the technique chosen follows surgeon preference. As stated above, for isolated base-of-tongue obstruction in a neonate with isolated PRS that has failed nonsurgical measures, we prefer to attempt a TLA. If the respiratory distress is not alleviated, then mandibular distraction osteogenesis is warranted. If the child has an associated syndrome, then we prefer mandibular distraction osteogenesis over TLA, such as in a child with Nager syndrome and PRS *(Fig. 38.29)*.

Treatment of the nutritional deficit

One cannot forget to treat the feeding difficulties in PRS, as a malnourished child will have difficulty thriving regardless of technique employed. The neonate has minimal skills for coordination of the aerodigestive structures beyond that provided at a reflex level. In PRS, the retrognathia may prevent anteriorization of the tongue and sufficient latching. Some feel that the child is unable to generate sufficient negative pressure due to the cleft palate, but feeding difficulties exist in those without a cleft palate.

In addition to the anatomic and oromotor reasons for poor feeding, these children experience behavioral conditioning as well. Feeding can be a noxious experience, with gagging, choking, and vomiting. This negative reinforcement may need to be addressed by a behavioral psychologist and nutritionist working in conjunction.

Maintenance of an open airway while trying to feed uses a great deal of calories, contributing to the overall deficit in the Pierre Robin patient. Relieving the airway obstruction will allow the child to overcome feeding difficulties and gain weight.

There are many described measures that can be attempted to aid in feeding. Manual support of the mandible during feeding can improve the quality of the seal and function of the labial sphincter. This can also help to relieve the base-of-tongue obstruction. Another technique is to move the nipple

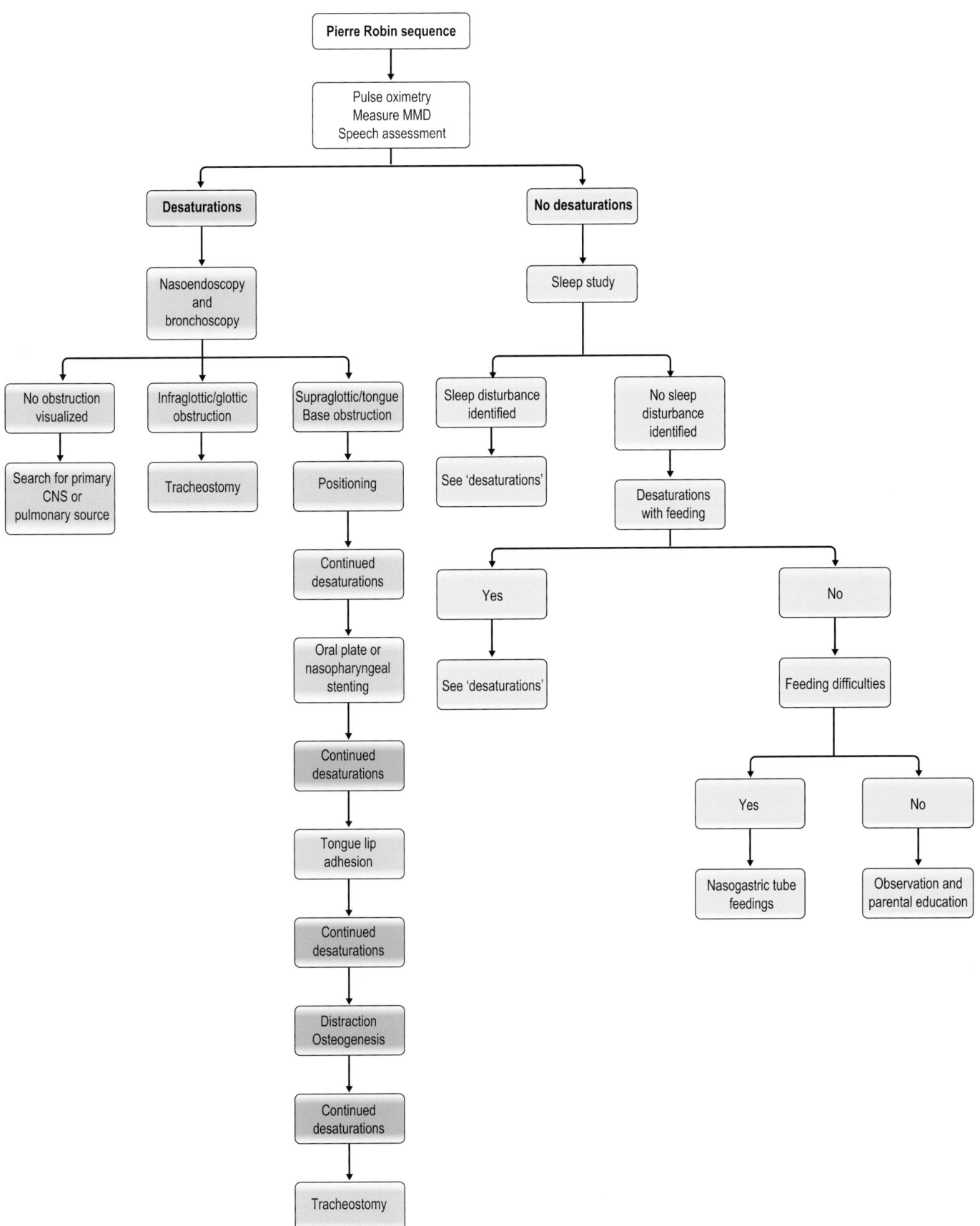

Fig. 38.29 Overall algorithm for assessment and treatment for a child suspected of having Pierre Robin sequence. MMD, maxillary–mandibular discrepancy; CNS, central nervous system.

or bottle in a rhythmic fashion to stimulate better sucking. Benefit has also been seen in placing the nipple on to the substance of the tongue.

Breastfeeding is often difficult and requires considerable effort and modification of technique. As a result, many of these neonates are bottle-fed with specialized bottles and nipples. The principle of specialized bottle-feeding is to allow a steady stream of milk, usually by a modified nipple that prevents negative-pressure build-up, and a soft bottle for the parent to regulate the outflow. These nipples are usually softer and longer than traditional nipples. The nipple is long enough to allow contact with the tongue, but not long enough to promote gagging. The nipple may need to be inserted completely, therefore a nipple with a narrow base is desirable. A larger opening can be fashioned in the nipple, but this must be done with caution so as not to cause aspiration.

If the neonate is unable to take oral feeds with specialized nipples and bottles, then nasogastric or orogastric feeds should be administered. In a study assessing 9 patients with PRS, all patients required an initial period of support with nasogastric tube feeding, and 67% also required total parenteral nutrition supplementation at some point. One must be mindful that the use of a feeding tube may increase the risk for the development of gastroesophageal reflux.

Another study assessed the long-term need for supplemental nutrition based on subgroup analysis of neonates with isolated PRS, syndromic PRS, and those with unique anomalies with PRS. Tube feeds were needed in 53%, 67%, and 83% respectively. In the isolated group, feeding supplementation was usually needed for 0–3 months and for 4–18 months in the syndromic group. A successful diet was observed in approximately 90% of these two groups at 3 years. Of note, even 42% of those treated with prone positioning demonstrated feeding difficulties. This highlights the importance of specialized feeding methods even in the "milder" cases.

The typical neonate with PRS should be fed 150–165 mL/kg per day of 20 kcal/oz formula or breast milk which equates to 100–110 cal/kg per day. Optimal weight gain should be 20–30 g/day. If this weight gain is not observed, then the supplementation should be increased. If the child tolerates breastfeeding or is bottle-fed breast milk, it should be fortified with powdered term formula or medium-chain triglyceride oil instead of human milk fortifier, as the phosphorus contained may promote neonatal tetany.

Treatment of otologic conditions

Placement of myringotomy tubes has been shown to be effective in preventing recurrent bouts of otitis media and may restore normal levels of hearing. These children should be followed closely by a pediatric otolaryngologist. The treatment plan may be tailored to the associated syndrome if not isolated PRS.

Secondary procedures

As 50% of these children will have an associated cleft palate, addressing the timing is an important consideration. Descriptions of palate repair at the time of TLA takedown have been described, and the authors' preference against this was previously discussed. There are reports of emergent tracheostomy when this combined approach has been performed.[55] At our institution, the cleft palate repair is performed at the routine time interval, which is at 11–12 months of age.

As with other children with cleft palates, the nurturing of speech is important. Later procedures to correct velopharyngeal insufficiency may be required. It has been shown that children with PRS may have a higher risk of airway compromise after pharyngeal flap procedures.

Access the complete references list online at **http://www.expertconsult.com**

1. Douglas B. The treatment of micrognathia associated with obstruction by a plastic procedure. *Plast Reconstr Surg.* 1946;1:300.

2. Cohen MM. The Robin anomalad – its specificity and associated syndromes. *J Oral Surg.* 1976;34:587.

   This work is significant as it highlights the evolving understanding of Pierre Robin sequence and the syndromes associated with it. PRS is one of the more well-known eponyms by name, but few in the medical world understand the etiopathogenesis. This paper highlights that the clinical entity is not a syndrome, and can be found in isolation or in a syndromic child. Many associations are pooled in this work.

5. Shprintzen RJ. The implications of the diagnosis of Robin sequence. *Cleft Palate Craniofac J.* 1992;29:205.

   This is a comprehensive review article that does well to organize the contemporary knowledge of that time. This paper illustrates the debate of "mandibular catch-up" that was beginning at that time after the inception of mandibular distraction osteogenesis.

9. Jakobsen LP, Knudsen MA, Lespinasse J, et al. The genetic basis of the Pierre Robin sequence. *Cleft Palate Craniofac J.* 2006;43:155–159.

   Most articles on Pierre Robin sequence will merely mention the genetic basis in a paragraph, but this more recent work attempts to discuss the topic comprehensively. As previously discussed, there are many syndromes associated with PRS, and this work discusses the associated genes for each and inheritance patterns. This paper is important as it discusses this topic from a different perspective, that of a geneticist.

14. Schaefer RB, Gosain AK. Airway management in patients with isolated Pierre Robin sequence during the first year of life. *J Craniofac Surg.* 2003;14:462–467.

15. Schaefer RB, Stadler 3rd JA, Gosain AK. To distract or not to distract: an algorithm for airway management in isolated Pierre Robin sequence. *Plast Reconstr Surg.* 2004;113:1113–1125.

   This paper delineates a comprehensive treatment pathway that provides a safe methodology for treating the child with Pierre Robin sequence. Many issues are discussed that treat the global issues, such as airway issues, glossoptosis, and feeding these patients. The article discussed the difference in treatment options due to differences in severity seen between the isolated and syndromic subsets of PRS. Tongue lip adhesion demonstrated favorable results in this work in the isolated PRS group.

16. Robin P. Glossoptosis due to atresia and hypotrophy of mandible. *Am J Dis Child* 1934;48:541–547.

33. Kirschner RE, Low DW, Randall P, et al. Surgical airway management in Pierre Robin sequence: is there a role for tongue-lip adhesion? *Cleft Palate- Craniofac J.* 2003;4:13–18.

50. Denny AD, Kalantarian B. Mandibular distraction in neonates: a strategy to avoid tracheostomy. *Plast Reconstr Surg.* 2003;109:3.

    Denny and Kalantarian demonstrate the efficacy of mandibular distraction osteogenesis in their work. The surgical tool is very powerful in relieving the airway obstruction. The use of tongue lip adhesion is less stressed. This highlights that the surgical modality used may ultimately be what works best for that surgeon in addition to patient factors.

52. Rogers G, Lim AA, Mulliken JB, et al. Effect of a syndromic diagnosis on mandibular size and sagittal position in Robin sequence. *J Oral Maxillofac Surg.* 2009;67:2323–2331.

55. Antony AK, Sloan GM. Airway obstruction following palatoplasty: analysis of 247 consecutive operations. *Cleft Palate Craniofac J.* 2002;39:145–148.

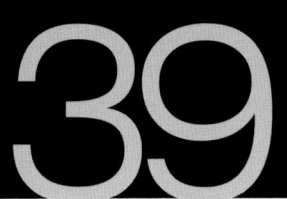

Treacher–Collins syndrome

Fernando Molina

SYNOPSIS

- Treacher–Collins syndrome is a congenital craniofacial malformation that involves the bone and soft tissues of the middle and lower facial thirds. Specifically, the orbits, zygomaticomaxillary complex, and mandible are affected.
- Coloboma of the lower eyelids, inferior obliquity of the palpebral fissures, lateral canthal dystopia, and notching of the upper eyebrows and eyelids are characteristic.
- Surgical reconstruction should include techniques to repair both soft-tissue and skeletal deformities.
- Parietal bone grafts are used to augment the malar eminence. Bilateral distraction osteogenesis corrects hypoplasia of the mandibular ramus and body with simultaneous improvement of respiratory and digestive function.
- Colobomas and macrostomia are repaired prior to bony reconstruction, and microtia is treated between 9 and 10 years of age.

 Access the Historical Perspective section online at
http://www.expertconsult.com

Introduction

The abnormal development of the first and second branchial arches results in bilateral Tessier clefts 6, 7, and 8 with the concomitant stigmata of Treacher–Collins syndrome. While Treacher–Collins syndrome occurs as an autosomal-dominant disorder in 1 per 50000 live births, 60% of cases arise as sporadic mutations. The syndrome is most successfully treated in staged procedures addressing bone and soft tissues.

Airway management is the primary concern when treating infants born with Treacher–Collins syndrome. The narrow pharynx and short mandible may cause obstructive sleep apnea and subsequent neonatal death. Early mandibular distraction may avoid the need for tracheostomy in severely affected neonates.

The malar region may be reconstructed with free calvarial bone grafts. Bilateral mandibular distraction, with distraction vectors carefully planned to improve the length of the ascending ramus, will correct micrognathia and anterior open bite. Orthodontic maneuvers will allow for growth of the posterior vertical dimension of the maxilla.

Colobomas and macrostomia are repaired prior to bony reconstruction. Microtia is usually corrected at approximately 9–10 years of age.

Basic science/disease process

Treacher–Collins syndrome, or mandibulofacial dysostosis, is a complex congenital craniofacial malformation that most strikingly involves the middle and lower thirds of the face, affecting both bony structures and soft tissues. It is transmitted by an autosomal-dominant gene of variable penetrance and phenotypic expressivity. The severity of the disease increases in successive generations.[7,8] Fifty percent of the cases reported in the literature do not have a documented family history, and thus an influence of exogenous factors on expressivity of the mutation may be inferred. Advanced paternal age is considered a risk factor. These genetic anomalies cause bilateral defects in structures derived from the first and second branchial arches.

Diagnosis/patient presentation

Patients with mandibulofacial dysostosis may present with all or most of the following features (*Box 39.1*): an inferior obliquity and shortening of the palpebral fissures, coloboma of the lower eyelids, dystopia of the lateral canthi, absence of eyelashes, and notching of the eyebrows and upper eyelids. The craniofacial skeleton is also involved: the malar bone is hypoplastic or absent, along with the zygomatic arch. The maxilla is narrow and underprojected with a high and narrow palate.

Box 39.1 Characteristic clinical features of Treacher–Collins syndrome

Eyelids

Antimongoloid obliquity of palpebral fissures

Coloboma of lower eyelids

Dystopia of lateral canthi

Shortening of palpebral fissure

Absence of eyelashes

Notching of eyebrows and upper eyelids

Orbits

Inferior portion of lateral wall is often absent

Inferior migration of superolateral portion of frontal bone

Malar bone

Hypoplastic or absent

Absence of zygomatic arch

Maxilla

Narrow and underprojected

High and narrow palate

Mandible

Hypoplastic

Vertical occlusal plane

Class III malocclusion with anterior open bite

Long and retruded chin

Nose

Protruded with a broad base

Flattened frontonasal angle

Narrow pharynx

Others

Microtia and ear deformities

Absence of external auditory canal

Abnormalities of middle ear

Macrostomia

Possible velopharyngeal insufficiency

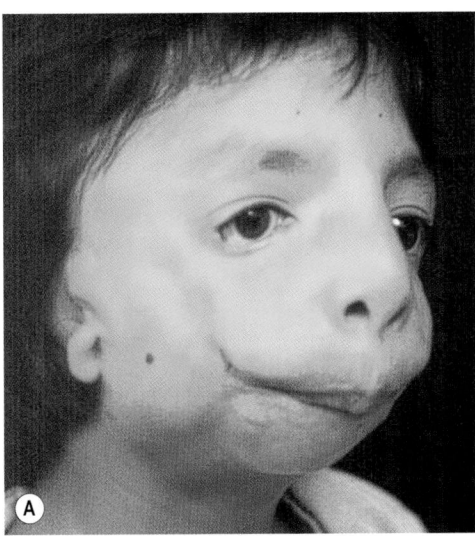
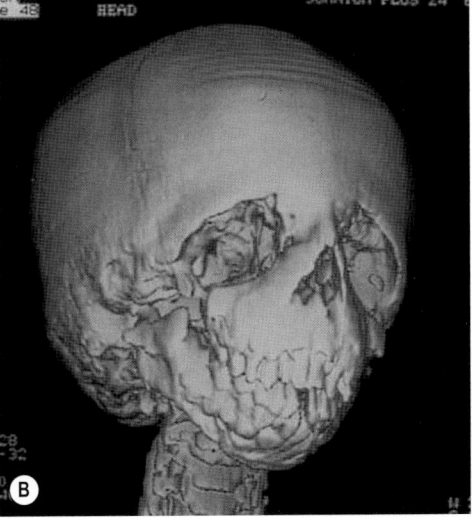

Fig. 39.1 (A) A 7-year-old boy with Treacher–Collins syndrome presenting with severe coloboma of the lower eyelids, hypoplastic maxilla, underprojected and narrow maxilla. There is bilateral microtia and macrostomia. The mandible shows severe hypoplasia, including at the menton. **(B)** Three-dimensional computed tomography scan, showing the absence of the zygoma and malar bone and the lack of the inferolateral orbital floor. The mandible has a very short ascending ramus and the posterior aspect of the maxilla is also very short vertically.

The mandible is hypoplastic with a severe shortening of the ascending ramus; the condyle is severely affected as well. The chin is long and retruded; the mandibular body is short and typically features an exaggerated antegonial notch. Micrognathia of different degrees is also observed, with an anterior open bite. The nose is protruded and broad with a flattened frontonasal angle. Other clinical features include ear deformities or microtia, absence of the external auditory canal, anomalies of the middle ear, and macrostomia[9] *(Fig. 39.1)*.

Radiographically, the Waters and posterior–anterior views, as well as frontal tomograms, show hypoplasia of the malar bones and partial or complete absence of the zygomatic arches. The shape of the orbits is abnormal secondary to the partial or total absence of the lateral wall and floor of the orbits.[10]

The lateral cephalogram demonstrates normal upper anterior face height with a reduced posterior face height, resulting in a vertical occlusal plane and shortening of the choanae. The sphenoethmoid angle is more acute and the angle between the anterior cranial base and the palatal plane is more obtuse. Mandibular retrognathism is present, with shortening of the ramus and the body of the mandible. The chin is long and retruded.[11]

The absence of the zygomatic bone is responsible for the absence of the lateral orbital rim and for the poor definition of the inferior orbital rim. For the same reason, there is no clear separation between the orbital cavity, the temporal fossa, and the infratemporal fossa. The zygomatic arches are hypoplastic or absent, and the aponeurosis of the hypoplastic temporal muscle is in direct continuity with the aponeurosis of the masseter muscle.[12]

According to Tessier's classification, the zygomatic bone is absent because of the confluence of clefts 6, 7, and 8. The number 6 cleft is situated between the maxilla and the zygomatic bone, opening the infraorbital fissure. The number 7 cleft is a temporozygomatic cleft accounting for the malformations of the ears and the macrostomia. The number 8 cleft

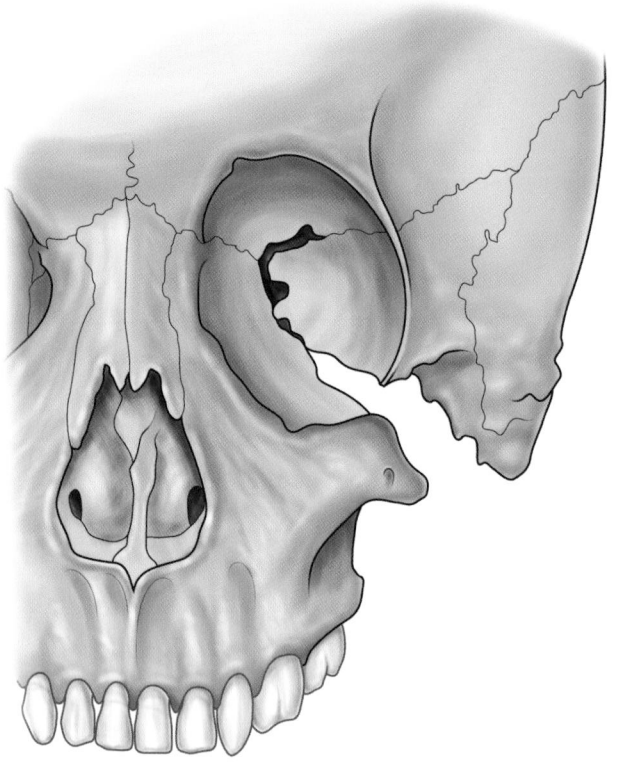

Fig. 39.2 According to Tessier, the confluence of craniofacial clefts 6, 7, and 8 produces the hypoplasia or absence of bony structures, including the zygoma, orbit, maxilla, and ascending ramus of the mandible.

involves the frontozygomatic suture[6] *(Fig. 39.2)*. There exists a wide spectrum of phenotypic expressivity, and some clinical features are present in a less evident fashion. Likewise, there are asymmetric cases resulting from different penetrance of the deformity on each side of the face.

Computed tomographic scans with three-dimensional reconstruction show the affected bone structures in detail.

Patient selection

A careful physical exam is required to ensure an adequate functional assessment of the retropharyngeal space. Significant micrognathia can produce respiratory distress, and some patients require a tracheostomy or mandibular distraction at a very early age. It is also important to assess hearing and speech. Dental impressions must be obtained to plan mandibular or maxillomandibular procedures in older patients.

Treatment and surgical technique

Treatment is aimed at correcting the colobomas, reconstructing the malar bones and zygomatic arches, establishing an adequate maxillomandibular relationship with functional occlusion, harmonizing thze profile by improving the proportional relationship between the different regions of the face, and correcting the auricular malformations and macrostomia.

Surgical intervention is divided into four stages. The first stage includes the correction of functional emergencies when present. Respiratory distress is addressed with mandibular distraction or tracheostomy very early in life. Corneal exposure is addressed with eyelid reconstruction. The second stage of reconstruction consists of zygomaticomaxillary reconstruction with cranial bone grafts.[13,14] Generally, these procedures are performed between 2 and 4 years of age. The third stage of reconstruction, mandibular distraction, is performed between 3 and 6 years of age. The goal is bilateral elongation of the ascending ramus and closure of the anterior open bite.[15,16] The fourth stage is distraction osteogenesis of the reconstructed zygomaticomaxillary complexes and lateral orbits. This distraction should be performed when zygomaticomaxillary growth is observed to be the limiting factor in global craniofacial growth. This stage is frequently performed between 5 and 8 years of age.

Colobomas

Colobomas usually occur in the lower eyelid and are full-thickness defects. Reconstruction should therefore include all eyelid components. The most popular procedure consists of a myocutaneous flap from the superior eyelid rotated down to cover the defect in the inferior eyelid. Essentially, a Z-plasty is designed along the borders of the coloboma *(Fig. 39.3)*, the defect is defined in the inferior eyelid, and the superior eyelid flap is raised and rotated into the inferior defect. A release of the orbital septum is mandatory to correct the position of the lateral canthus. A tarsoconjunctival reconstruction is seldom required.

Zygoma

Zygomaticomaxillary reconstruction has undoubtedly received most of the attention from experts on this topic. Various alloplastic and autologous materials, including silicone, dermis-fat grafts, cartilage grafts, and many others, have been used with varying degrees of success for this reconstruction. Many believe that calvarial bone grafts are the best option for the reconstruction of the zygomatic arch and malar bone. Some characteristic challenges of this procedure include: the large amount of bone required, bone grafts must be adapted to the contour of the defect, the new bone structure must achieve the necessary projection, and secondary bone resorption must be avoided.[13,14,17–19]

The parietal bone is the author's preferred donor site. A paper template is made including the malar bone, zygomatic arch, and the lateral aspect of the orbit. The template is used to design bilateral bone grafts, each as a single unit, from both parietal regions. The curvature of the donor region will be used to achieve natural contour and projection of the new zygomaticomaxillary structure. The left parietal region is used to reconstruct the right side of the face and vice versa *(Fig. 39.4)*. The free bone grafts are fixed to the subjacent bone structure at the orbit and the maxilla with 3–4 screws, 16 mm in length. This is usually sufficient for stable immobilization. The new zygomatic arch should reach laterally to the bone ridge at the external auditory canal. In addition to the rigid fixation, the posterior surface of the graft should have good contact with the masseter muscle and the rest of the local soft tissues such that bony resorption is minimized *(Fig. 39.5)*. In

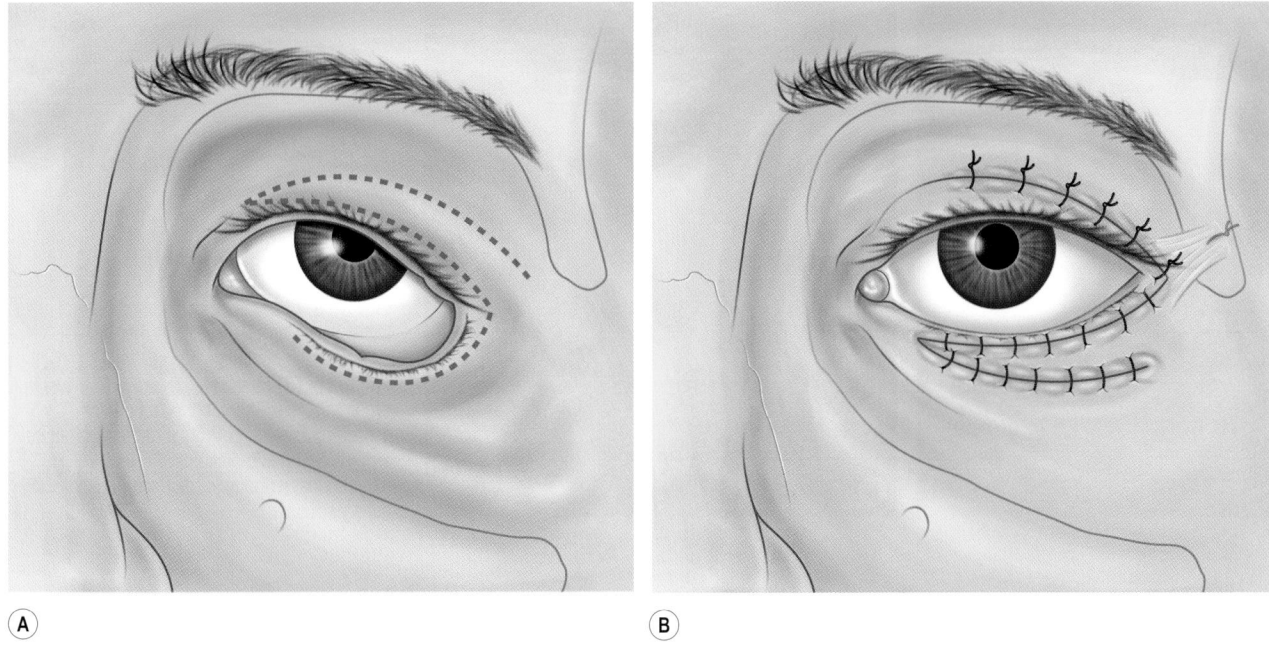

Fig. 39.3 (A) Procedure for coloboma correction. Planning for a simultaneous rotation upper eyelid myocutaneous flap is outlined. **(B)** The result after the flap rotation, including the lateral canthopexy. The ligament has been reattached 4–5 mm superior to its original insertion.

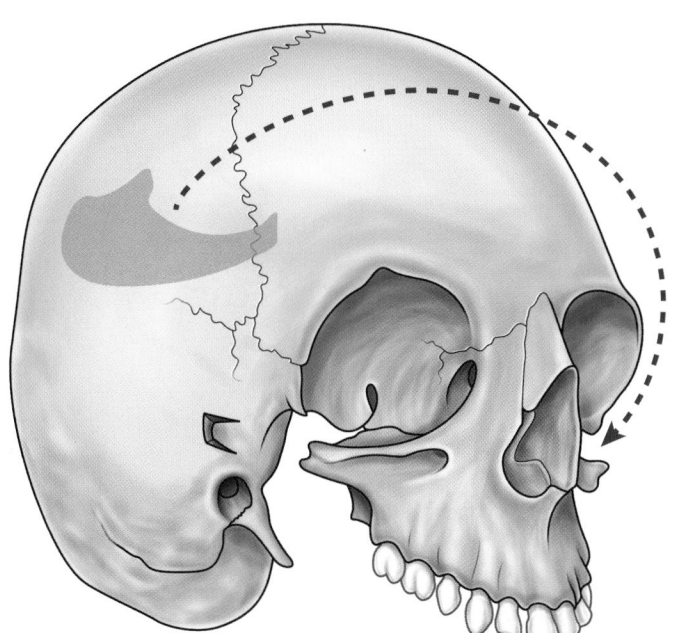

Fig. 39.4 Using a template, a bicortical parietal bone graft is harvested. The right graft will be transferred to the left zygomaticomaxillary region. The natural curvature of the bone will produce an excellent projection of the reconstructed region.

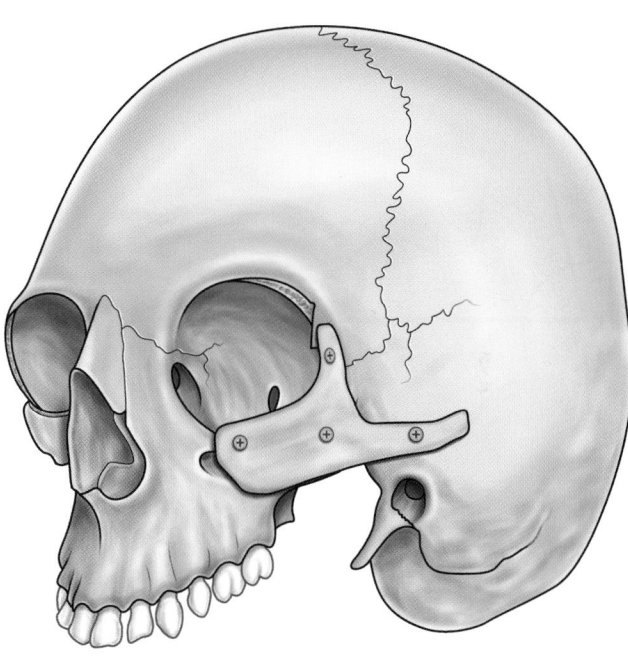

Fig. 39.5 The free parietal bone graft is fixed with 3–4 screws to the deeper bone structures. The bone graft should be adapted to the contour of the receiving bone to reduce bone resorption.

addition, a subperiosteal suspension of the cheek soft tissues is performed with 3–4 monofilament sutures attached to the temporalis. If necessary, the lateral canthus is resuspended at this time.

With these techniques, a natural appearance is restored to the zygomaticomaxillary region with good contour and excellent projection. The subperiosteal suspension of overlying soft tissues adds volume to the region and

redraping of the periorbital skin produces an aesthetic result *(Fig. 39.6)*.

In the past, composite temporoparietal flaps had been widely used; however the muscle is always hypoplastic and its rotation produced secondary depression at the external temporal fossa.[14,18,19] This procedure also sacrificed precise shaping of the osteomuscular flap to preserve vascularity. Even so, with this technique, only 60% of the muscle's contact

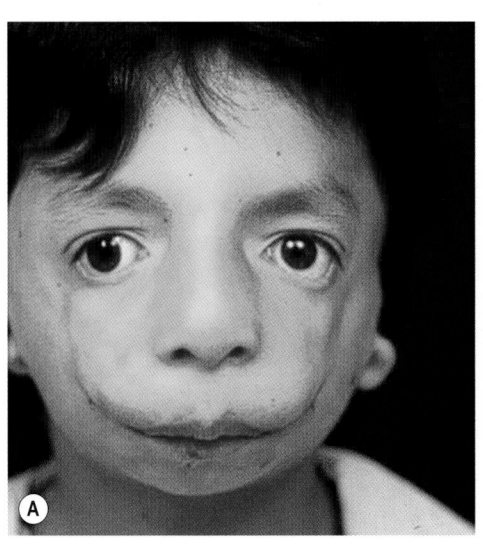
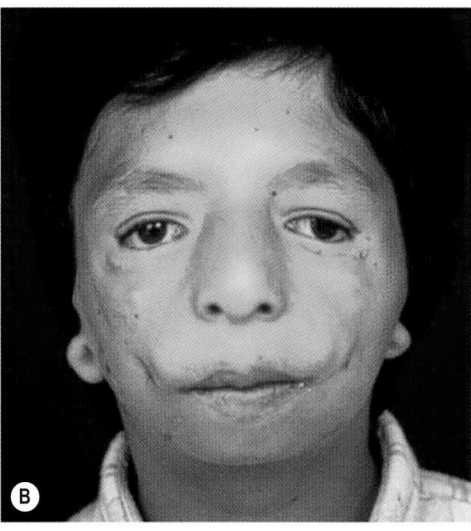

Fig. 39.6 (A) Preoperative frontal view of a 7-year-old boy presenting with all the characteristic features of severe Treacher–Collins syndrome. **(B)** Postoperative result after bilateral zygomaticomaxillary reconstruction and coloboma correction. Notice the new structure at the bizygomatic distance. Bilateral bidirectional mandibular distraction has also been performed.

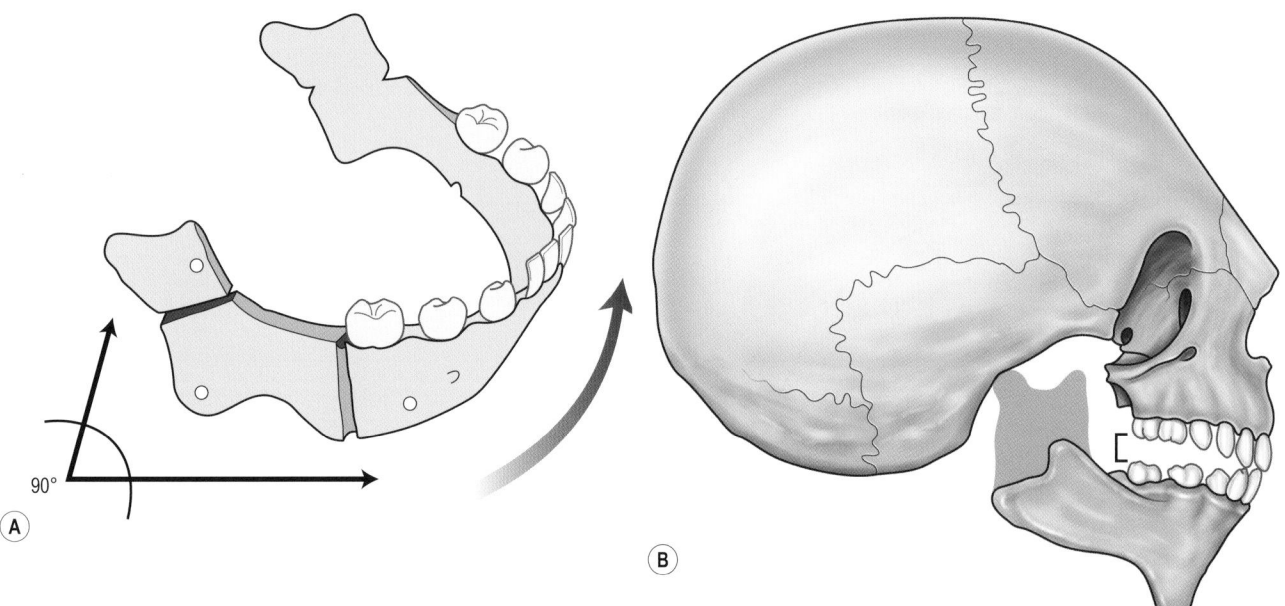

Fig. 39.7 (A) The diagram shows the corticotomies performed at each side of the mandible. Notice the position of pin insertion at the ascending ramus, the angle, and the mandibular body. Also note the relationship that should be obtained between the vertical and horizontal distraction vectors. **(B)** Once elongation of the ascending ramus has been obtained, an important posterior open bite will be produced. The use of bite blocks is gradually diminished to allow for the vertical growth of the posterior maxilla.

with underlying bone can be maintained. This does not represent a considerable blood supply if we consider that 80% of the blood supply of cranial bones comes from the dura mater and only 20% is derived from the periosteum.[10]

Mandible

Micrognathia in Treacher–Collins presents a unique problem in which the mandibular anatomy is hypoplastic in all dimensions. Moreover, patients suffer from chronic respiratory and digestive problems. The deformity is usually bilateral, affecting mainly the ramus and the body, both in form and volume. For these patients, a bidirectional, bilateral solution is required.

In these cases two corticotomies are performed: a vertically oriented one in the mandibular body and a horizontally oriented one in the ascending ramus. Three pins are used: a central one at the mandibular angle, a second in the mandibular body, and a third in the central aspect of the ascending ramus. One bidirectional distraction device is used on each side, each with two distraction rods to allow independent, precise elongation of each segment. The central pin acts as a fixed pivot point for distraction of the ramus and body *(Fig. 39.7)*.

Elongation of the ascending ramus produces an important posterior open bite. At the body, the lengthening is minimal: just enough to overcorrect the molar relationship and to close the classic anterior open bite of the deformity. Precisely planned distraction vectors are critical to obtaining the proper degree of mandibular elongation and resultant occlusal changes. The relationship between the vertical (ramus) and the horizontal (body) vectors has to be less than 90°. These vectors will produce an exaggerated counterclockwise mandibular rotation closing the open bite and creating an open bite between the retromolar region and the posterior aspect of the maxilla. Posterior bite blocks are placed and gradually reduced in the vertical dimension to control growth of the posterior maxilla, closing the open bite by increasing the posterior maxillary vertical dimension.

Most of these patients present with a typical facial convexity with deficient soft tissue of the lower third of the face and neck, absence of definition in the submental angle, and shortened suprahyoid muscles. Patients with the most severe phenotype are frequently tracheostomy-dependent, and the ability to open their mouth is minimal or nonexistent. With bone distraction, all tissues from skeleton to skin are simultaneously elongated without the inconvenience of bone grafts or tissue expansion. In contrast, after conventional osteotomies and bone grafts, the contracted muscles and overlying

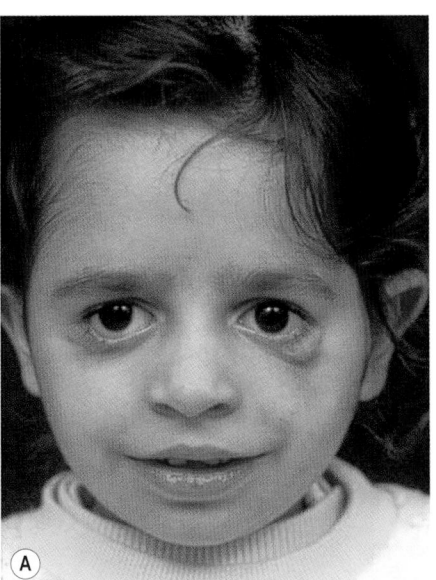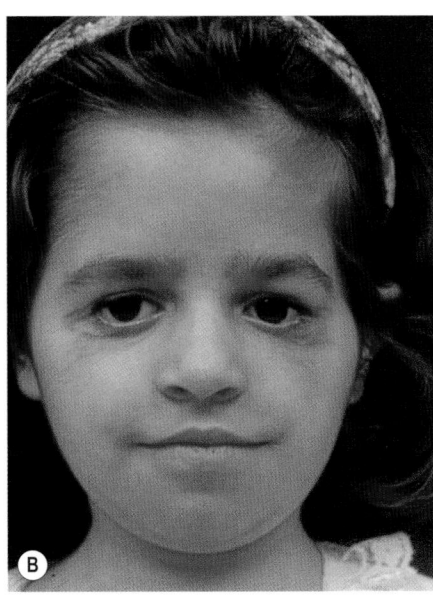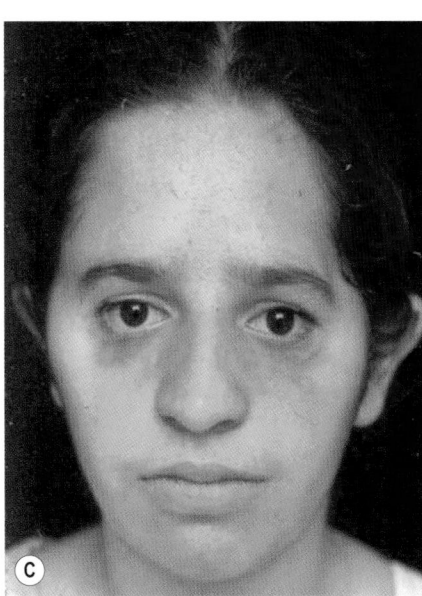

Fig. 39.8 (A) Preoperative view of a 3-year-old girl with Treacher–Collins syndrome. Coloboma correction has already been performed. **(B)** Postoperative view at 5 years old. The bilateral bidirectional mandibular distraction has reconstructed the inferior portion of the face. The rotation of the mandible has closed the anterior open bite. **(C)** Postoperative view at 11 years old. The maxilla and the mandible show a nearly normal relationship. The grafted zygomaticomaxillary region, however, demonstrates delayed growth. At this time the patient is ready for zygomaticomaxillary distraction and fat injection.

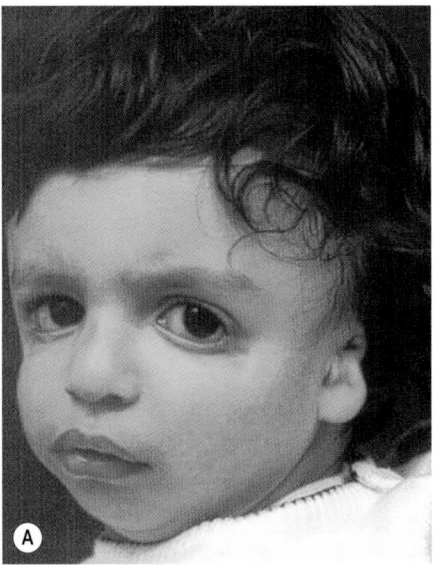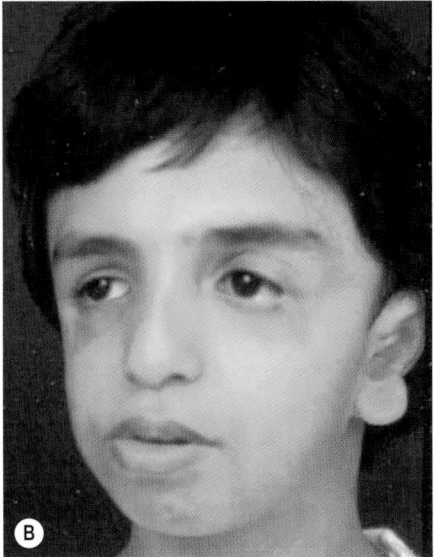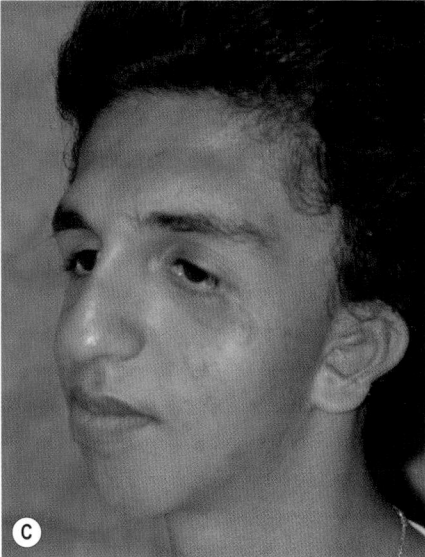

Fig. 39.9 (A) Preoperative view of a 2-year-old boy with classic Treacher–Collins syndrome. **(B)** At 7 years old, after coloboma correction, zygomaticomaxillary bone grafting, mandibular distraction, and ear reconstruction. **(C)** At 16 years old: after distraction, new bone formation has produced excellent zygomaticomaxillary volume. Two sessions of fat injection have obtained excellent facial contour and definition.

soft-tissue envelope act as a counterforce to the bony advancement, often causing bony relapse and necessitating multiple procedures to achieve optimal aesthetic results. Tissue expansion increases the amount of skin, but other soft tissues such as muscles, vessels, and nerves remain unchanged.

The overall functional and aesthetic results with bidirectional mandibular distraction are satisfying *(Fig. 39.8)*. The neck takes on a more normal shape with a well-defined submental angle, the muscles and soft tissues of the floor of the mouth are elongated, as are the masticatory muscles, and

the chin takes on a more prominent position. These anatomical changes reconstruct the inferior third of the face, lending improved proportionality to the entire face. Once a more normal size and shape of the mandible have been achieved, these patients are able to open their mouths to receive orthodontic and dental treatment. Additionally, we have noted improvements in deglutition and respiration. Often, those patients with tracheostomies can be decannulated, and those with feeding tubes are routinely converted to oral feeding.

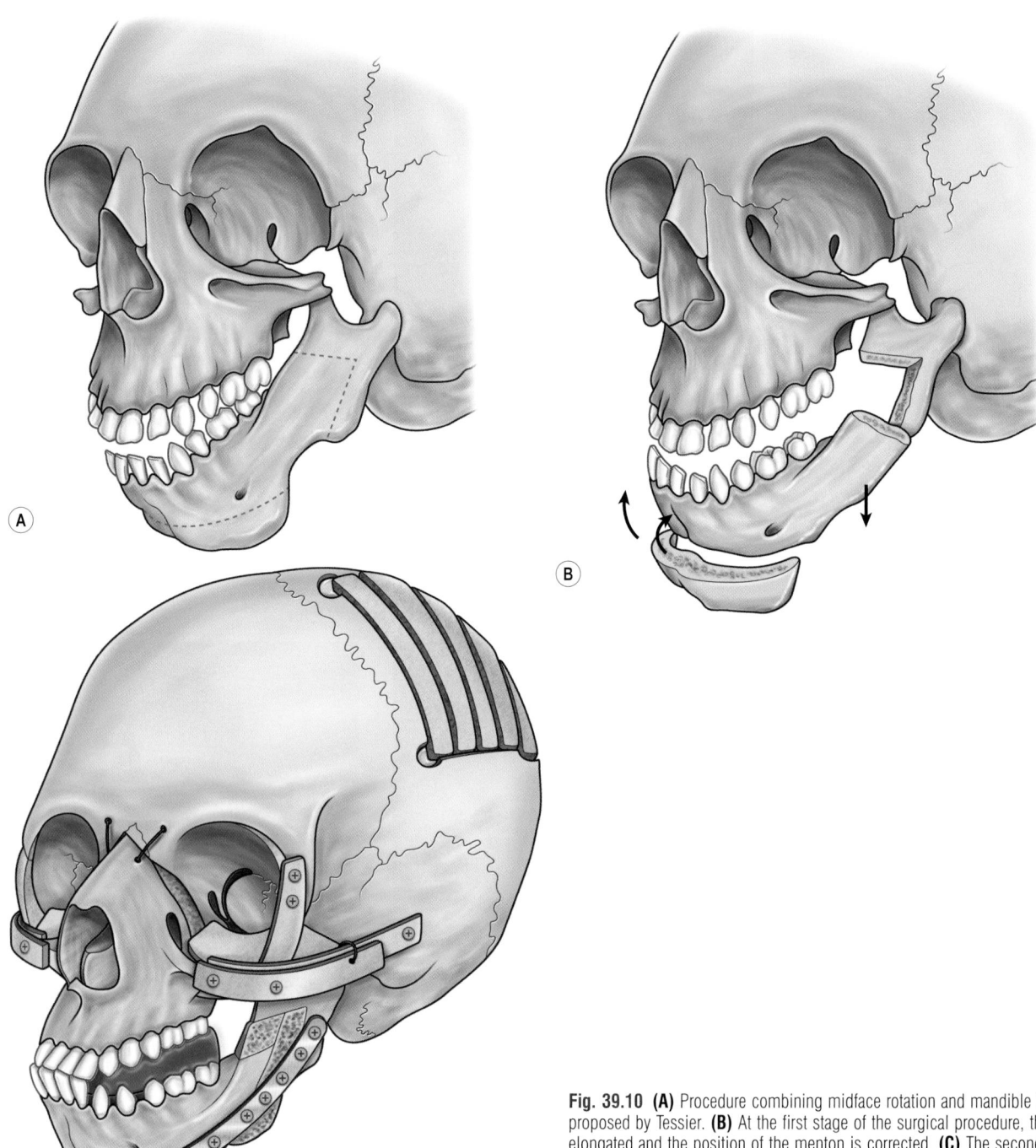

Fig. 39.10 **(A)** Procedure combining midface rotation and mandible lengthening as proposed by Tessier. **(B)** At the first stage of the surgical procedure, the mandible is elongated and the position of the menton is corrected. **(C)** The second stage of the procedure includes the midface osteotomy, adapting the occlusion to the new dimension of the mandible. Additional calvarial bone grafts can be added to the orbit and zygoma.

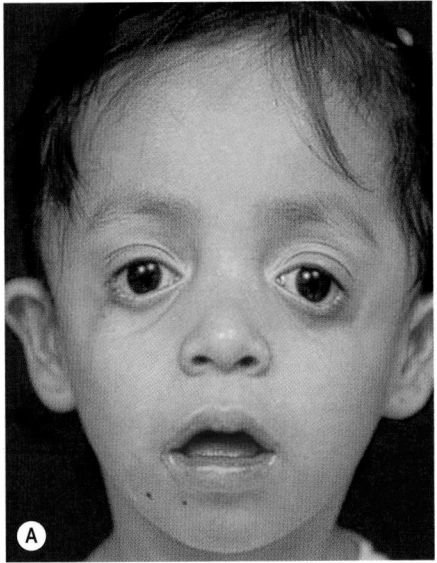 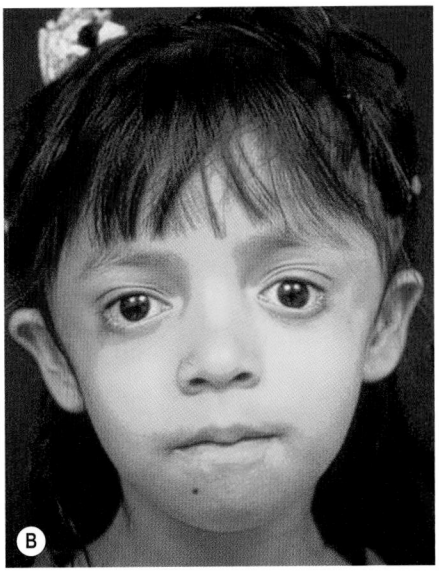 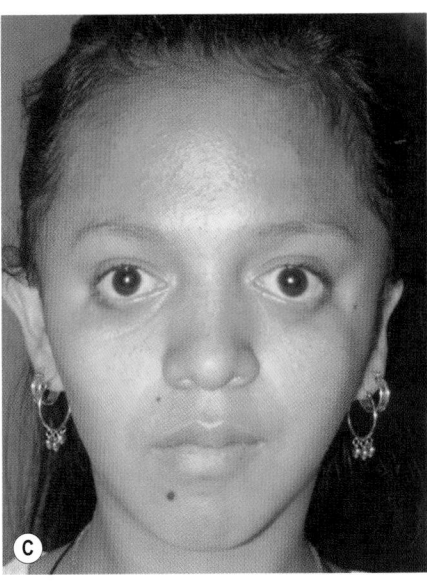

Fig. 39.11 (A) Preoperative fontal view of a 3-year-old girl. Severe colobomas, hypoplastic zygomaticomaxillary region, micrognathia, and anterior open bite are present. **(B)** At 5 years old, after zygomaticomaxillary bone grafting and bilateral bidirectional mandibular distraction. Notice the new bone structure at the bizygmatic areas and the inferior third of the face. **(C)** Postoperative view at 17 years old; volume has been added to the malar eminences after distraction osteogenesis of the bone grafts. Final refinements of the facial contour have been obtained after fat injection.

Distraction of zygomaticomaxillary region

At 7–10 years of age, the grafted zygomaticomaxillary complexes are distracted. The orbitomalar-zygomatic region can be accessed via a coronal approach. An osteotomy is designed to include the zygomatic arch, the posterior aspect of the malar bone, the inferior third of the lateral orbital wall, and the inferior orbital rim medially to the infraorbital foramen. A buried distraction device is fixed to the parietal bone, and its tip is anchored to the posterior aspect of the malar eminence. After 5 days of latency, activation of the device begins at a rate of 1 mm/day. New bone formation is observed and a well-defined malar structure is the result *(Fig. 39.9)*.

Orthognathic procedures

For selected adult patients, classical osteotomies with a combination of midface rotation and mandibular lengthening are still utilized.[20] With a Le Fort III osteotomy, the midface is rotated and placed in proper relationship to the mandible using the frontonasal angle as a fulcrum *(Fig. 39.10)*. As a result, the maxilla has a more pronounced anterior projection. As well, it approximates a more appropriate horizontal plane, allowing greater lengthening of the mandible, both vertically and sagittally. Unfortunately, the tight soft-tissue envelope sometimes restricts bony repositioning and can be a significant cause of relapse.

Postoperative care

Orthodontic manipulation is absolutely necessary to obtain good final functional occlusion. The use of orthodontic elastics during the consolidation period allows for "callus" manipulation, properly positioning the mandible in relation to the maxilla. Intraoral myofunctional devices, such as the Fränkel III style, are used in the long term to maintain the bone structures and teeth in an excellent relationship.

Secondary procedures

To define the final contour of the cheeks, zygomatic region, and gonial angle, fat grafting is becoming a very important adjunctive technique. In our experience, fat grafting is indicated after 15 years of age as a final refinement of the soft-tissue contour and volume *(Fig. 39.11)*. Fat is harvested from the abdomen, prepared for injection, and grafted with 2-mm cannulas. Fat is deposited in fine layers beginning supraperiosteally and proceeding superficially to an intramuscular plane, and concluding with small quantities delivered to the subcutaneous plane. In each cheek 15–20 cc of fat is inserted.

 Access the complete references list online at **http://www.expertconsult.com**

1. Gorlin RJ, Cohen MM, Levin LS. *Syndromes of the head and neck*. 3rd ed. New York: Oxford University Press; 1990.

3. Treacher Collins E. Case with symmetric congenital notches in the outer part of each lid and defective development of the malar bones. *Trans Ophthalmol Soc UK*. 1900;20:109.

4. Franceschetti A, Zwahlen P. Un Syndrome nouveau: La dysostose mandibulo-faciale. *Bull Schweiz Akad Med Wiss*. 1994;1:60.

6. Tessier P. Vertical and oblique facial clefts (orbitofacial fissures). In: Mustarde JC, ed. *Plastic surgery in infancy and childhood*. Philadelphia: WB Saunders; 1971:94.

10. Fuente del Campo A, Martínez Elizondo L, Arnaut E. Treacher–Collins syndrome (mandibulofacial dysostosis). *Clin Plast Surg*. 1994;21:613–623.

    The authors present their technique to normalize facial proportions in Treacher–Collins syndrome.

11. Garner L. Cephalometric analysis of Berry–Treacher–Collins syndrome. *Oral Surg Oral Med Oral Pathol*. 1967;23:320.

12. Marsh JL, Celin SE, Vannier MW, et al. The skeletal anatomy of mandibulofacial dysostosis (Treacher–Collins syndrome). *Plast Reconstr Surg*. 1986;78:460.

    This paper is an observational study of 3D craniofacial CT scans of patients with Treacher–Collins syndrome. The authors find that the zygomatic process of the temporal bone is the most frequently aplastic component of these patients' craniofacial skeletons.

14. McCarthy JG, Zide BM. The spectrum of calvarial bone grafting: introduction of the vascularized calvarial bone flap. *Plast Reconstr Surg*. 1984;73:687.

    The authors describe traditional methods of bone grafting. A vascularized calvarial flap (based on the temporal vessels) is then presented; it is noted that vascularized bone flaps are ideal for devitalized recipient sites, such as may be encountered in midface reconstruction for Treacher–Collins syndrome.

15. Molina F, Ortiz Monasterio F. Extended indications for mandibular distraction: unilateral, bilateral and bidirectional. *International Craniofacial Congress*. 1993;5:79.

16. Molina F, Ortiz Monasterio F. Mandibular elongation and remodeling by distraction: A farewell to major osteotomies. *Plast. Reconstr. Surg*. 1995;96(4):825–842.

    The authors discuss a novel corticotomy-based method for mandibular distraction. Improved facial symmetry was noted in their cohort, with no observed relapse.

19. Van der Meulen JCH, Hauben DJ, Vaandrager JM, et al. The use of a temporal osteoparietal flap for the reconstruction of malar hypoplasia in Treacher–Collins syndrome. *Plast Reconstr Surg*. 1984;74:687.

    The temporalis muscle provides an axial vascular supply to the temporal periosteal bone flap described in this paper. The osseous component of the flap may seed further bone growth when this flap is used for malar reconstruction in patients with Treacher–Collins syndrome.

20. Tessier P, Tulasne JF. Treacher–Collins syndrome. Combined rotation of the midfacial segment and mandibular lengthening. In: Marchac D, ed. *Craniofacial surgery*. Berlin: Springer-Verlag; 1987:369.

40

Congenital melanocytic nevi

Bruce S. Bauer and Neta Adler

SYNOPSIS

■ Congenital melanocytic nevi (CMN) are composed of clusters of nevomelanocytes that are generally present at birth but occasionally arise as late as several years. These lesions arise from melanocytic stem cells that migrate from the neural crest to the embryonic dermis and upward into the epidermis. They may also migrate into the leptomeninges.

■ Although the bulk of these lesions are small and benign, some cover large portions of the body or can be in conspicuous locations, and may create an aesthetically displeasing appearance, resulting in psychological issues. Furthermore, their potential for malignant degeneration causes anxiety for the parent, primary care physician, and surgeon alike.

■ Small pigmented nevi are present in 1 in 100 births, large nevi are present in only 1 in 20000 births, and the giant lesions are even less common. As a result, most surgeons have little experience with them and little opportunity to develop a rational protocol for their treatment.

■ The goal of this chapter is to review the pathophysiology and natural history of CMN, summarize the risk of malignant degeneration, and provide a rational approach to treatment.

 Access the Historical Perspective section online at **http://www.expertconsult.com**

Introduction

- CMN consist of clusters of nevomelanocytes that develop *in utero*. Although many congenital nevi are visible at birth, some are "tardive," probably because they are too small to be detected at birth or do not have sufficient melanin.[1,2]
- CMN are one of the risk factors for eventual development of cutaneous and extracutaneous melanoma, with larger nevi having greater risk. Based on that, CMN are usually classified according to their estimated largest diameter in

adulthood. Small nevi are up to 1.5 cm, medium are 1.5–19.9 cm and large nevi are those with estimated diameter of more than 20 cm. Giant nevi are 50 cm or larger. Giant nevi are usually accompanied by multiple smaller satellite nevi.

- Congenital nevi present in approximately 1% of births,[3] large CMN occur in approximately 1:20000 births,[4] and giant lesions (>50 cm) are even less common.[5]
- While most surgeons are familiar with treating the small and intermediate-size nevi, it is difficult to gain enough experience when approaching more extensive lesions.
- Many strategies have been tried for removal and reconstruction of large and giant nevi. When direct excision and primary closure are not a possibility then tissue expansion is the "workhorse" treatment modality for many medium to large nevi. Facial nevi that cross multiple aesthetic units as well as involving the periorbital area may require expansion in combination with full-thickness skin graft (expanded or nonexpanded). Finally, some unique cases may benefit from a free flap and tissue expansion as an adjunct procedure to close the donor site.

Basic science/disease process

The etiology of CMN remains unclear. The development of CMN is determined *in utero* between the fifth and 24th weeks of gestation. One of the theories of melanocyte differentiation is that, as the neural tube develops during early embryogenesis, melanoblasts migrate from the neural crest along the leptomeninges to the embryonic dermis.[6] From the embryonic dermis, the progenitor melanocytic cells migrate into the epidermis, where they differentiate into dendritic melanocytes.

Dysregulated migration, proliferation, and differentiation of melanocytes in the skin and leptomeninges are implicated in the pathogenesis of CMN and neurocutaneous melanosis (NCM).[8,9]

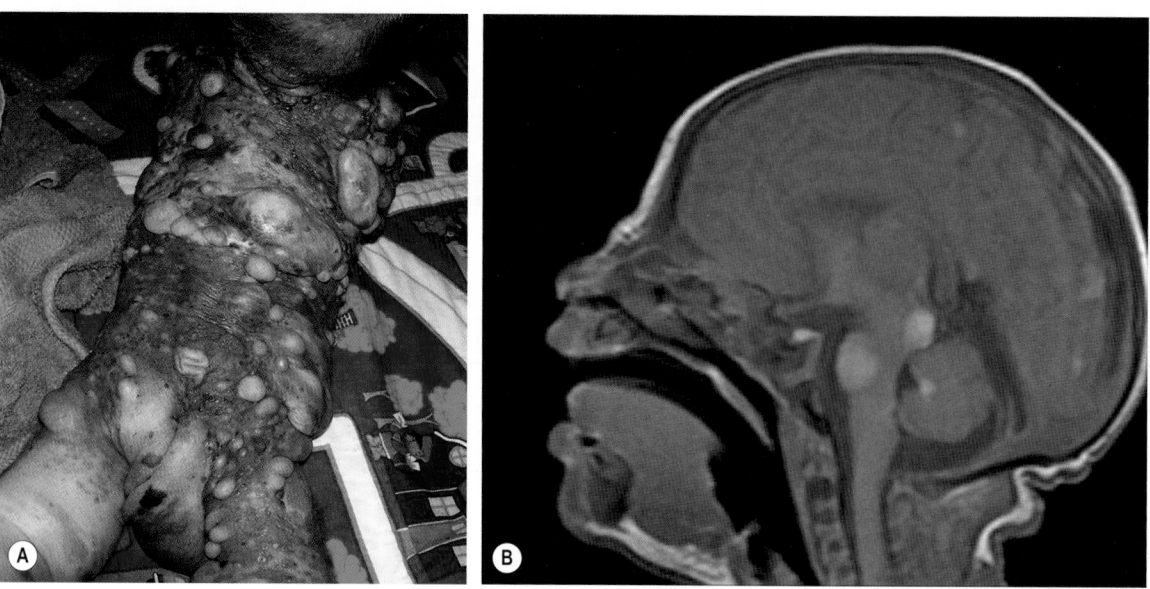

Fig. 40.1 (A) This child with near-total body nevus shows marked variation in nevus thickness, color, and surface architecture. Multiple areas of thick, neural nevus are present. **(B)** A T1-weighted image on magnetic resonance imaging demonstrates several lesions typical of neurocutaneous melanosis.

Several molecular signaling pathways have been associated with the pathogenesis of CMN. Melanocyte development appears partially under the control of c-met and c-kit proto-oncogenes, which encode met and kit proteins, respectively. Hepatocyte growth factor (HGF), also known as scatter factor (SF), is a multifunctional regulator of epithelial cells expressing the tyrosine kinase receptor encoded by c-met. Overexpression of HGF/SF, which is a ligand for the met protein receptor, is implicated in perturbations of melanocyte proliferation, differentiation, survival, and migration.[10] Transgenic mice overexpressing HGF/SF are born with cutaneous and leptomeningeal melanocytosis.[11] HGF/SF also functions in regulating the migration and differentiation of premyogenic cells during embryogenesis.[11] It has been shown that overexpression of this signaling molecule in mice may lead to rhabdomyosarcoma,[12] a tumor that on rare occasions also arises in patients with large CMN.[13,14] Furthermore, studies with met null mice suggest that met plays a role in NCM, because met knockout mice do not develop NCM.[12] Overexpression of HGF/SF and/or met, and sustained activation of met, could explain the mechanism of cutaneous and leptomeningeal melanoma and rhabdomyosarcoma development in individuals with CMN. C-kit, a proto-oncogene that encodes the kit tyrosine kinase receptor for the ligand known as SCF, also plays a role in melanocyte development. In tissue cell culture, c-kit-expressing neural crest cells give rise to clones containing only melanocytes.[15] Proliferative nodules, consisting of aggregates of epithelioid or spindled immature benign melanocytes in the dermis of CMN, highly express c-kit.[16] Moreover, kit can activate N-RAS, which is an oncogene that is mutated in some cases of nodular melanoma.[17] N-RAS mutations have also been reported in CMN,[18] suggesting a possible genetic link between CMN and melanoma.

The exact risk for development of melanoma in CMN is not clear. While the relative risk for the incidence of melanoma in patients with large CMN compared to a control group is reported to be high, between 52 and 1046,[19,20] the absolute risk is estimated between 1.25% and 10%.[20,21] Patients with small and medium-sized CMN have a lower risk of melanoma, with a reported relative risk of 9.545 and an absolute risk between 0 and 4.9%.[20,22] Also, many of the articles discussing the issue of relative risk of melanoma do not differentiate between cutaneous and extracutaneous melanoma and the presence of NCM may be the greater risk factor in subsequent risk of malignancy.

NCM is characterized by an excess deposition of melanocytes along the leptomeninges *(Fig. 40.1)*. It can occur in both patients with large CMN and those with multiple small or medium-sized CMN. Patients with large CMN located on the posterior axis are thought to have greater risk for NCM but, on a multivariate analysis, the only risk factor for NCM in patients with large congenital nevi is having multiple satellite nevi: more than 20 satellites had a 5.1-fold increased risk for NCM compared with patients with fewer satellites.[23] The true incidence is not known, but symptomatic NCM may affect 6–11% of patients with large CMN. Symptomatic NCM has a poor prognosis. Symptoms frequently present in early childhood. Neurologic symptoms can manifest themselves as seizures, developmental delay, hydrocephalus, and delayed motor development.

Rarely, other tumors, such as rhabdomyosarcoma and liposarcoma, are associated with CMN.

Diagnosis/patient presentation

Small to medium-sized CMN usually present as round to oval homogeneous pigmented lesions, light to dark brown in color, with sharply demarcated borders, mamillated surface, and hypertrichosis. However, larger CMN, in particular, may show asymmetry, irregular borders, multicolored pigment pattern, rugous texture, and a nodular surface. In addition, large CMN are often associated with many smaller satellite nevi. As the child grows, especially at puberty, the CMN may change color, becoming lighter or darker, developing hair, becoming more heterogeneous or more homogeneous. CMN may spontaneously regress and some patients may develop vitiligo. Nodular proliferation may be present from birth or develop at a later age. CMN are usually asymptomatic; however, patients with larger lesions may present with pruritus, xerosis, skin fragility, erosions, or ulcerations and decreased ability to sweat from the involved skin *(Fig. 40.2)*.

A review of dermoscopy patterns in congenital nevi found that most nevi demonstrate a reticular, globular, or reticuloglobular pattern. The findings varied with age and the anatomic location of the nevus, with the globular pattern found more often in younger children and the reticular pattern found in patients aged 12 years or older.[24]

Because of the increased risk of melanoma associated with congenital nevi, attempts have been made to distinguish congenital nevi from acquired nevi on the basis of histology. Distinguishing histologic features include: (1) involvement by nevus cells of deep dermal appendages and neurovascular structures (including hair follicles, sebaceous glands, arrector pili muscles, and within walls of blood vessels); (2) extension of nevus cells to deep dermis and subcutaneous fat; (3) infiltration of nevus cells between collagen bundles; and (4) a nevus cell-poor subepidermal zone.[25–27] In contrast to congenital nevi, acquired nevi are usually composed of nevus cells that are limited to the papillary and upper reticular dermis and do not involve the appendages.

In cases associated with a high index of suspicion for the presence of NCM, magnetic resonance imaging of the central nervous system is a useful diagnostic tool *(Fig. 40.1B)*.

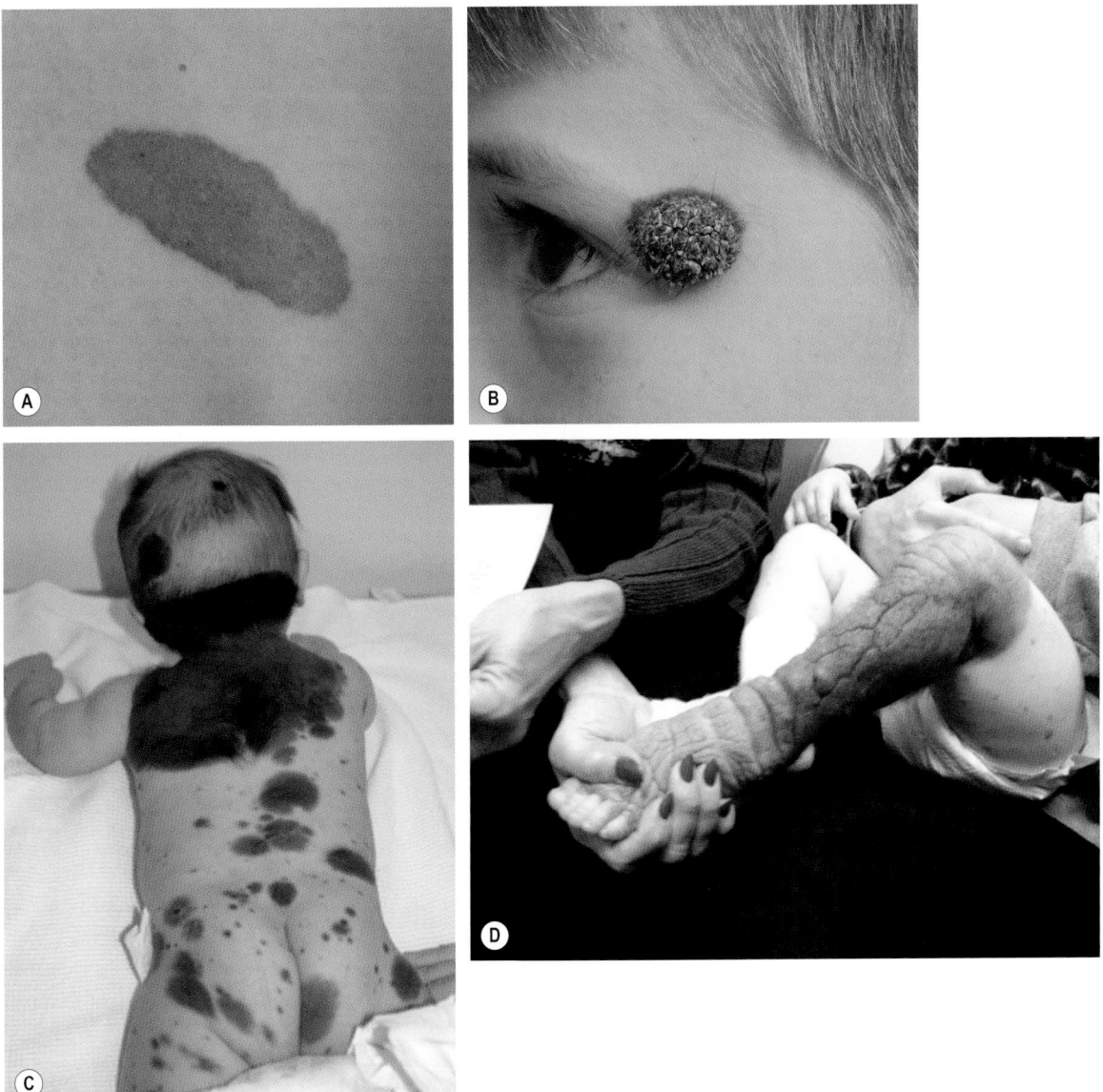

Fig. 40.2 Nevi present with widely variable appearance and size. **(A, B)** Small and medium nevi may be flat with uniform color and border, or thick and verrucous. **(C)** They may present as large nevi with multiple small and medium satellite nevi, or **(D)** on the lower extremity they may become thick, cerebriform-like, and associated with severe pruritus and chronic breakdown.

Patient selection

The treatment of large and giant nevi is controversial. Although the risk of malignant transformation in congenital pigmented nevi is well established,[28–32] many feel that the risk of developing melanoma is too low to warrant the unsightly scars or grafts that may follow treatment. There is no evidence in the literature that demonstrates decrease in occurrence of melanoma after excision of large congenital melanocytic lesion. Furthermore, these patients have an increased risk of extracutaneous melanoma.[32,33] Others feel that, in the presence of NCM, the greatest risk lies within the central nervous system, so the excision of the cutaneous lesion can only have limited benefits. However, the appearance of these lesions clearly produces a stigma with significant psychological implications. The challenge for the surgeon involved in treating these often complex lesions is to develop treatment modalities that not only accomplish the excision of all or most of the nevus but also lead to an optimal aesthetic and functional outcome.

Although the lifetime risk of malignant melanoma for small and medium congenital pigmented nevi is reported to be 0–4.9%,[34] the risk of melanoma is nearly nil prior to puberty for small nevi,[35,36] and so one may comfortably wait until the child is old enough to excise the lesion under local anesthesia. If the lesion is located in an area where the excision and reconstruction may not likely be accomplished under local anesthesia or where there may be the possibility of a better final scar with earlier excision, then early excision under general anesthesia may be warranted. Certainly, many nevi positioned in prominent parts of the face may present as a significant source of peer ridicule starting quite early in the school years and delaying the excision in an effort to avoid a general anesthetic is not in the child's best interest.

The authors advocate treatment of large and giant nevi by 6 months of age in most cases. Although many of the tissue expansion procedures used in the treatment of large nevi can be applied to older children and adults, the intolerance for repeated procedures and the decreased elasticity of the skin may make the excision of extensive lesions impractical in older patients. Also, for larger nevi the greatest risk for malignancy is in the first few years.[37,38]

Treatment/surgical technique

Many strategies have been tried for the removal and reconstruction of large and giant nevi. Serial excision can often debulk these massive lesions but rarely remove them completely. Excision and split-thickness skin graft have generally poor functional and aesthetic outcomes. Dermabrasion, curettage, chemical peel, and laser treatment all have problems with recurrence since these modalities only eliminate the superficial portion of the nevus while the cells of congenital pigmented nevi can usually be found as deep as the subcutaneous fat and sometimes even in deeper structures.[29] This group of "partial-thickness" excision, while potentially reducing the overall number of nevus cells and lightening the degree of pigmentation, is commonly associated with later bleedthrough of the deep nevus cells, but may be manifest as both abnormal skin coloration and hypertrichosis *(Fig. 40.3)*.

There is also difficulty following the lesions for malignant transformation because of the scarring. The long-term effects of laser treatment on the remaining nevus cells remain to be determined.

Juvenile skin, although elastic, does not have the laxity of an adult skin and local flaps used in adults are often difficult in children. When direct excision and primary closure are not a possibility then tissue expansion is the "workhorse" treatment modality for many medium to large nevi. Facial nevi that cross multiple aesthetic units, as well as involving the periorbital area, may require expansion in combination with full-thickness skin graft (expanded or nonexpanded). Finally, some unique cases may benefit from a free flap and tissue expansion as an adjunct procedure to close the donor site.

Partial-thickness excision

Partial-thickness excision of large and giant nevi has taken the form of early dermabrasion, curettage, laser, or more recently, excision, leaving the underlying subcutaneous fat in place, to minimize contour deformities and covering this with a dermal collagen substructure and very thin split-thickness skin graft or even culture skin. These latter approaches have been particularly applied to the extremities where techniques such as expansion are not as readily applied. The potential downside of each of these approaches is that, while the surface nevus population may be reduced, the deeper nevus cells will frequently "bleed through" over time, leaving an even more significant deformity at an age when complete excision may no longer be an option. Circumferential grafting of the extremities with these approaches can still also result in significant late functional disturbance.

Serial excision

Serial excision is the excision of a lesion in more than one stage. The inherent viscoelastic properties of skin are used, allowing the skin to stretch over time. These techniques enable wound closure to be accomplished with a shorter scar than if the original lesion was elliptically excised in a single stage and to reorient the scar closer to the relaxed skin lines. This technique can be applied to small or medium nevi, depending on the location of the nevus and the laxity of the local skin *(Fig. 40.4)*. However, with each stage of the serial excision there is some recoil and serial excision alone, near sensitive areas like the lower eyelid and oral commissure, may create tissue shortage and long-term distortion of structures that would not arise if tissue expansion had been applied rather than serial excision alone.

Excision with skin graft reconstruction

As noted above, the depth of the congenital nevus requires excision to the fascial level if one is to limit the risk of leaving nevus behind, either to "bleed through" later, or to undergo degeneration with potentially late identification. However skin grafts do have some role in the treatment of congenital nevi.

On the face (periorbital region and ear) expanded and nonexpanded full-thickness skin grafts provide good match in both color and thickness for the recipient area. Likewise,

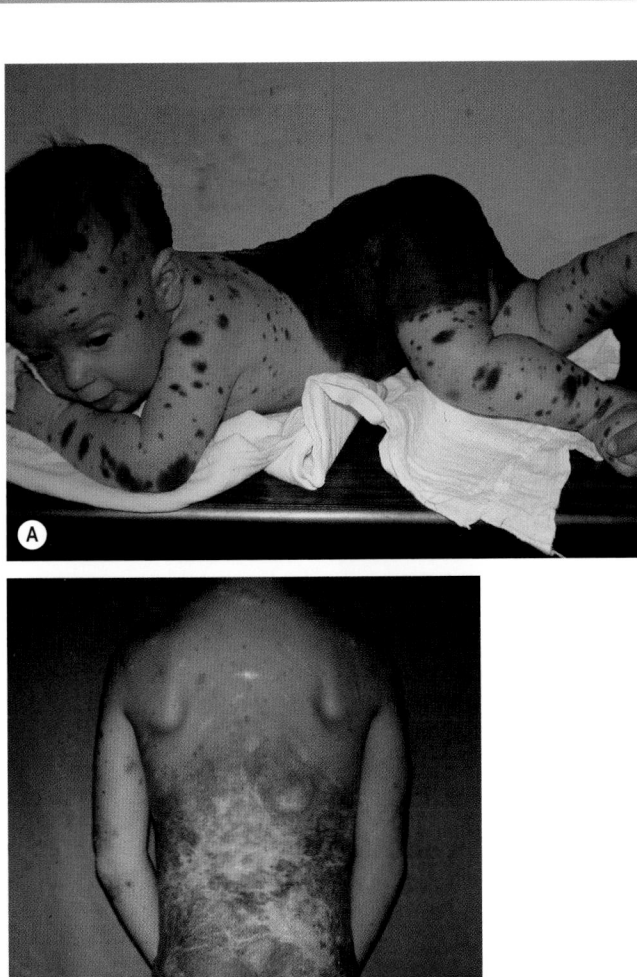

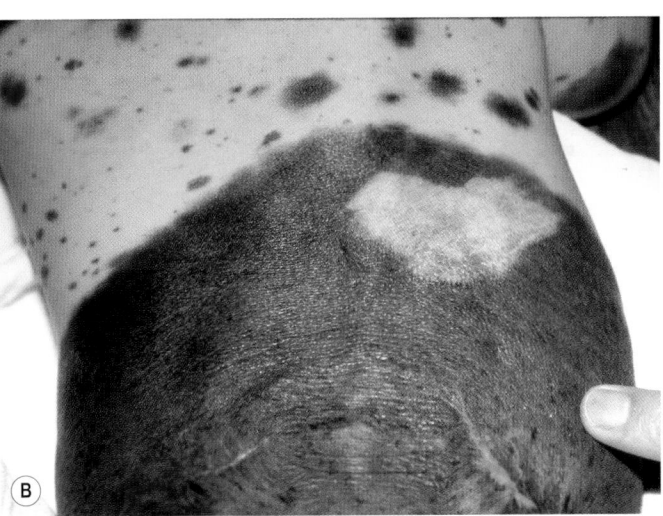

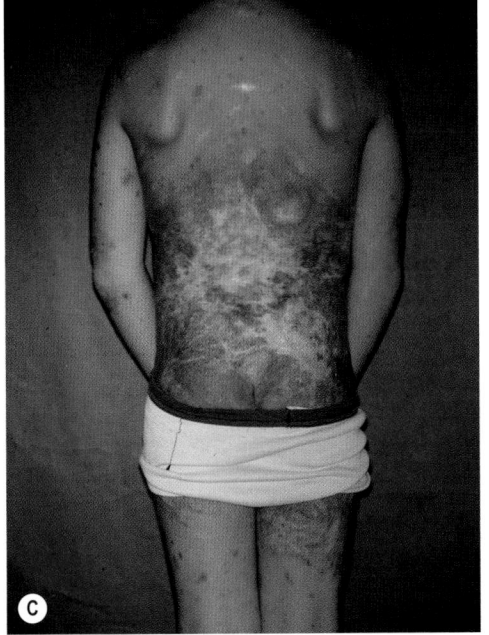

Fig. 40.3 **(A)** This infant has a giant nevus and multiple satellite nevi. **(B)** The light area within the nevus was dermabraded in the neonatal period. **(C)** At 7 years of age, despite partial-thickness excision with a dermatome at 3 months of age, nevus cells are present throughout the back and even in the initially dermabraded area, despite its continued lighter appearance.

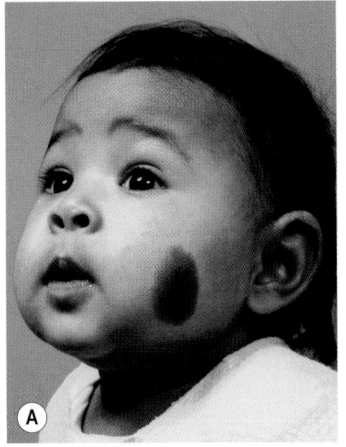
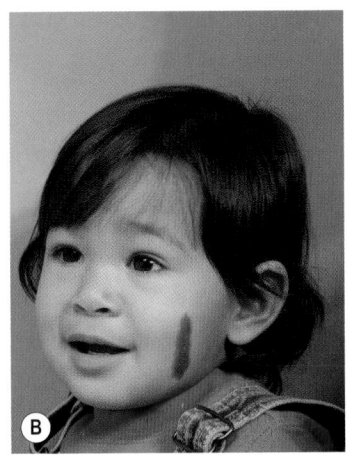
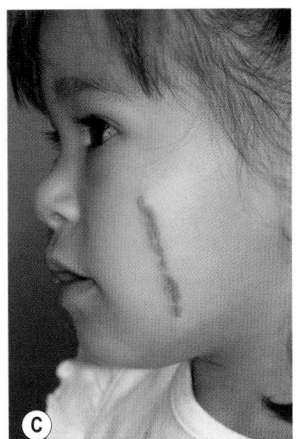
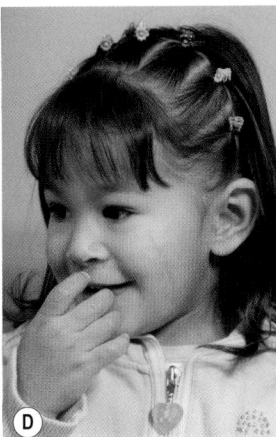

Fig. 40.4 A medium-sized nevus of the cheek is excised in three surgeries with the benefit of reducing the length of the final scar as well as avoiding potential distortion of the surrounding facial structures. **(A)** Preoperatively; **(B)** 6 months after first-stage excision; **(C)** 6 months after second-stage excision; and (D) 4 months after the third and final stage.

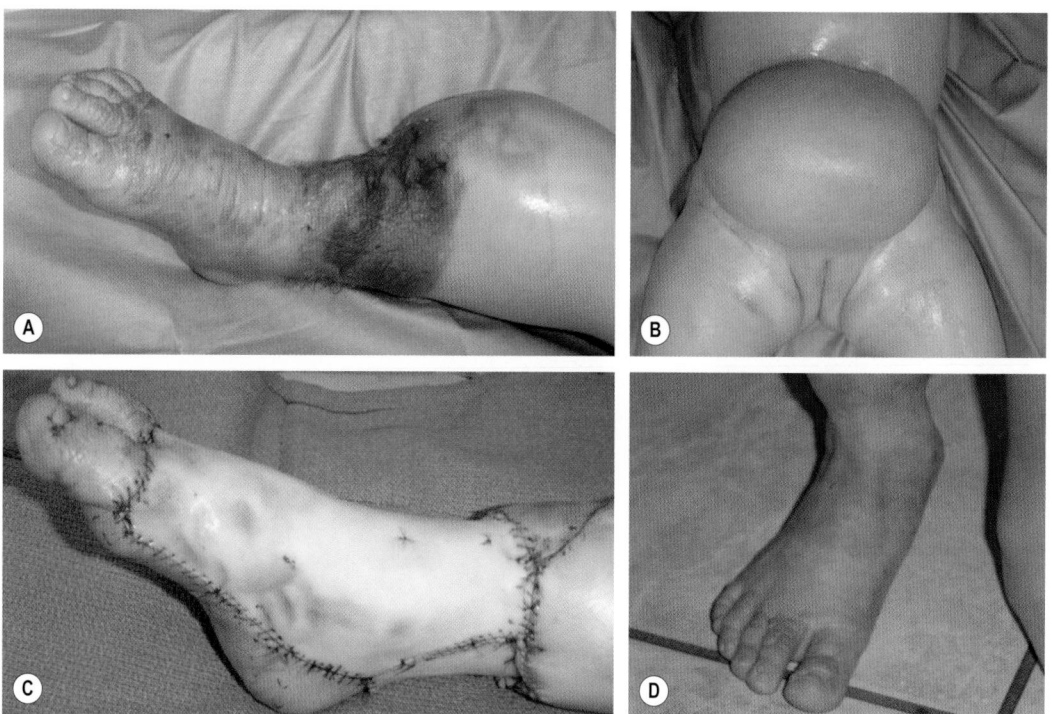

Fig. 40.5 An expanded full-thickness skin graft provides both good functional and aesthetic reconstruction on the dorsum of the foot and lower quarter to one-third of the leg. **(A, B)** In this patient expansion was carried out both regionally and at the graft donor site in the lower abdomen and bilateral groin. **(C)** At completion of grafting with the expanded full-thickness skin graft and advancement of the expanded adjacent skin flap to minimize the step-off between flap and graft. **(D)** The result at 1 year postgrafting.

expanded full-thickness skin grafts are an excellent choice for coverage on the dorsum of the hand and foot (and distal third of the leg) *(Fig. 40.5)*. However, if the excision is being carried to the fascial level, the contour deformity produced following excision and skin graft to the extremities and trunk can be significant, and result in both aesthetic and functional defects later in life.

Use of split-thickness skin grafting on the trunk, even when done with nonmeshed medium-thickness grafts, can still result in considerable late deformity with potential associated functional defects where the graft skin does not keep up with surrounding growth. The one area of the trunk that can be grafted without significant late contour deformity is the back because of the relatively uniform flat surface. Significant contour deformities develop later where the grafting is carried on to the flanks and anterior trunk (particularly in heavier individuals where the border between grafted and nongrafted skin can create quite dramatic deformities) *(Fig. 40.6)*. Skin grafting of the back can however provide a means of excising a large segment of the nevus, in an area of potentially greater risk of degeneration, and enhance the dermatologist's ability to map and follow the remaining lesion.

Tissue expansion

Several types of tissue expanders exist based on shape, size, and type of filling valve. The shape that the authors most commonly use in treatment of congenital nevi is rectangular. Expander volumes have a wide range and vary according to the anatomic site. Saline is delivered in a controlled fashion via the valve port which is located at some distance from the expander, overlying firm tissue. While integrated ports have been used by some surgeons, we use remote ports in all cases with none externalized despite the fact that the parents typically do the expander injections. Since the skin overlying the port can be readily anesthetized with a topical anesthetic, we see no benefit in externalizing the ports.

Consideration for the incisions, expander placement, and flap movement in relation to the defect and postoperative scars requires preoperative planning and discussion with the patient and family. In regard to donor site, one must match color, texture, and contour of the recipient site to maximize the aesthetic and functional outcome. The donor site tissue must be free of infection, or have stable scars, to minimize the risk of expander failure or extrusion. Careful selection of expander size is also imperative in areas with thin donor skin, in order to avoid expander folds or prominence which can create areas of excessive pressure and skin compromise. In the majority of the cases, the expanders are placed through an incision within the border of the lesion. In cases where the expansion has been used repeatedly and scars are present both at the border of the remaining nevus and at junctions of prior flaps, the new expanders should be placed through those scars that are least likely to be stressed by the weight or pull of the new expander (i.e., away from the most dependent points). In other cases, like unstable scar, vascular tumor, and craniofacial deformities, the incisions are planned outside the border of defect or on occasion at a distant site. A pocket is dissected to allow placement of the expander with placement of the port in a separate pocket over a region with firm skeletal support for ease of outpatient filling. Partial fill of the expander

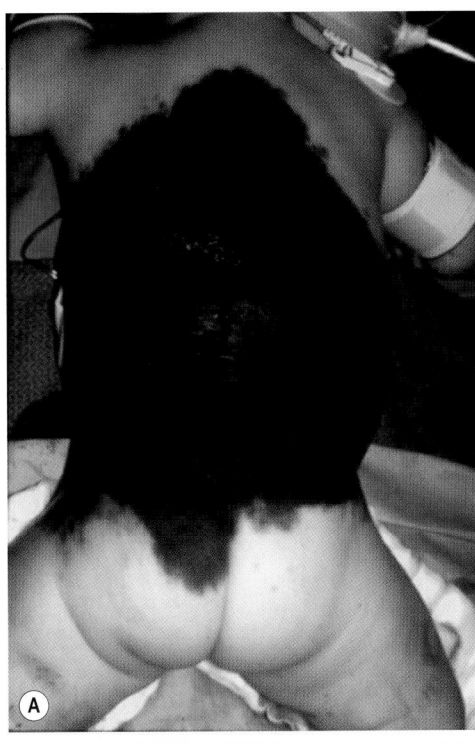

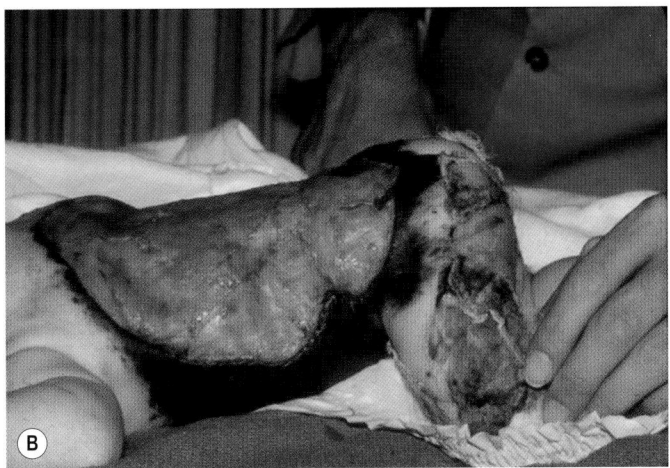

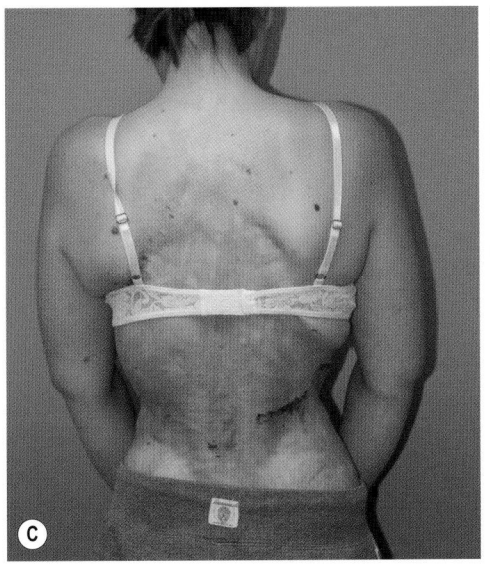

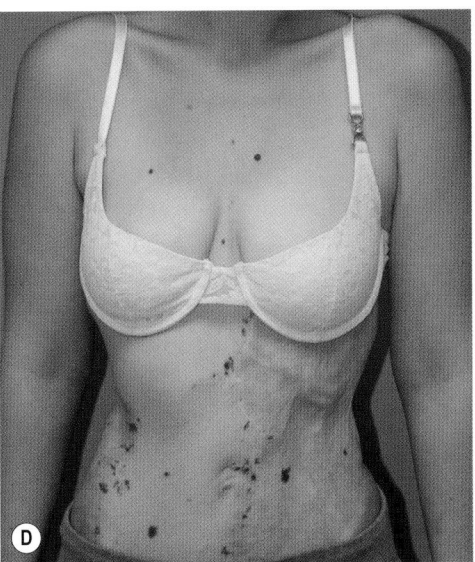

Fig. 40.6 (A) This case, treated early in our giant nevus experience, had the unusual feature of fixation of the nevus to the deep tissues of the back and invasion of the underlying latissimus muscle, requiring a deeper-plane excision. **(B)** One week postexcision the nonmeshed split-thickness skin graft was healing well. **(C, D)** A significant contour deformity is seen 22 years later, after excision of the remaining nevus only to fascial level.

(10–20% of the listed volume) ensures the expander is properly positioned without surface folds that can cause pressure against the skin flap to be expanded. Closed suction drains are placed for a few days (3–10 days) to control the potential dead space from wide undermining.

Serial injections are started 7–10 days postinsertion provided the skin flaps are in excellent condition and continue on a weekly basis for about 10–12 weeks. Most pediatric patients go on a home expansion protocol with injections performed by the parents under the direction of our nursing staff and surgeons.

If another set of expanders is needed to excise the lesion fully (serial expansion) we usually wait 4–6 months between them.

A broad-spectrum antibiotic is started upon surgery and is continued until the drains are removed. By maintaining a low threshold for placing the expander patient back on antibiotic in the presence of suspected beginning of infection, most infections can be controlled before potential loss of the expander.

The design of an expanded flap is of major importance. While the early dogma of tissue expansion emphasized designing advancement flaps only, experience over more than two decades has demonstrated that expanded transposition and rotation flaps may frequently be preferable. It provides greater versatility in flap design and range.[39,40] The high vascularity of expanded flaps, gained by the process of expansion, makes this design safe. In the expanded transposition flap, the base of the flap is also expanded, which allows advancement of the base of the flap in addition to the transposition of the tissues and thus provides greater coverage than advancement only.

Regional consideration in pediatric tissue expansion

The optimal choice of treatment still varies by body region, and we will discuss the most pertinent issues and considerations necessary for successful tissue expansion in each body region.

Scalp

The expander is placed in a pocket dissected subgaleal but staying above the periosteum. Flaps are designed taking into consideration the orientation of the major scalp vessels (superficial temporal, postauricular, occipital vessels and contribution from supraorbital vessels). Port placement in the preauricular area is favored when an expander does not encroach on the area because of the ease of palpation, limited risk to the overlying skin, and low risk of migration. The expanders used in scalp reconstruction are usually of 250, 350, or 500 cc volume (although 70 cc expanders may be used for medium-sized nevi). Large and giant nevi might require serial expansion with a larger expander placed after each stage to distribute expansile forces evenly over the hair follicles. As previous studies have shown, tissue expansion itself does not induce proliferation of hair follicles but can more than double the size of the scalp without visible decrease in hair density.[41] Despite former thoughts that expansion may affect cranial vault morphology, it usually self-corrects within 3–4 months.[42,43]

The use of expanded transposition flaps versus simple advancement flap design has greatly reduced the number of serial expansion required and has resulted in improved reconstruction of hair direction and hairline *(Fig. 40.7)*.

Face and neck

Large and giant nevi of the face are the most visible of these lesions and also represent the area where unsightly scarring is most readily visible; consequently, the planning and execution of the reconstructive plan must be very detailed.

To achieve an optimal aesthetic and functional result in the facial and cervical regions, one must adhere to the subunit principle. This dictates incision placement so the final result has the scar hidden in a natural crease (e.g., nasolabial fold). Undue tension on facial structures (brow, eyelid, mouth) can cause disfigurement such as brow asymmetry or ptosis, anterior hairline asymmetry, lower lid and oral drooping, especially when using cervical skin flaps cephalad to the cervicomandibular angle.

Neale and associates report 10% lower eyelid ectropion rate and >10% lower lip deformity in this context.[44] Judicious flap design and the use of expanded transposition and rotation flaps, as well as the use of multiple expanders and overexpansion, are recommended to minimize these complications.

For forehead lesions, in general one should always use the largest expander possible under the uninvolved forehead skin, occasionally even carrying the expander under the lesion. It is important to avoid elevation of either the ipsilateral or contralateral brow since it can only be returned to the preoperative position with the interposition of additional nonhair-bearing forehead skin. Expansion of the deficient area alone will not reliably lower the brow once a skin deficiency exists.[45] Overreaching with the expanded flap both risks flap compromise and increases the risk of brow and hairline distortion. Accepting the need for repeat forehead expansion to complete the forehead reconstruction may also limit the length of the scar above the brow on the uninvolved side.

For periorbital reconstruction, expanded full-thickness skin grafts can also achieve better functional and aesthetic results than split-thickness skin grafts. Pre-expansion of a donor site will allow a single, large full-thickness skin graft to be harvested for reconstruction of the eyelids,[46] canthus, and the region between eyelid and brow, without the multiple "seams" that follow the use of multiple smaller grafts. The supraclavicular area is the ideal donor site for grafts to be placed on the face because of excellent color and texture match. Part of the expansion provides for the graft tissue, with the remainder used for primary closure of the donor site. Donor site expansion also allows harvest of free flaps from distant sites to cover complete cheek or forehead aesthetic units when regional tissue is not available. Where previously we carried the single graft on to the nasal dorsum when the nevus involved the periorbital area and nose, we now use flaps from expanded forehead for that coverage (often combined with excision of nevus of the forehead) *(Fig. 40.8)*.

The eyebrow may be reconstructed at the same time as the eyelid, treated after the adjacent forehead or eyelid nevus is excised, or left unresected as an important aesthetic landmark *(Fig. 40.8C)*. When the eyebrow is heavily involved with the nevus, it is our current practice to leave a small portion of the nevus unexcised, to mimic the normal eyebrow. If the nevus is darkly pigmented in a fair-skinned child, the residual lesion may be lightened through laser treatment at a later time. The long-term effectiveness of this approach has not yet been established though. The residual brow nevus is closely followed, and if changes occur either in surface character or color, leading to concerns about potential degeneration, the involved brow is excised and reconstructed. A reconstructive option includes an island flap of temporal scalp based on a branch of superficial temporal artery. If the temporal scalp is minimally involved with nevus and there is a plan for simultaneous expansion of the temporal scalp, the island flap can be planned from the area of maximally expanded flap, with the effect that the hair density is lessened in expansion, and the resultant reconstructed brow will likewise not be too dense. However, for patients where the temporal scalp is involved with nevus, reconstruction with micrografts or strip grafts may become necessary. These are decisions that may not be possible to make until the late teens or adult years.

Trunk

The most common location of giant nevi was found to be over the posterior trunk, often extending anteriorly in a dermatome distribution.

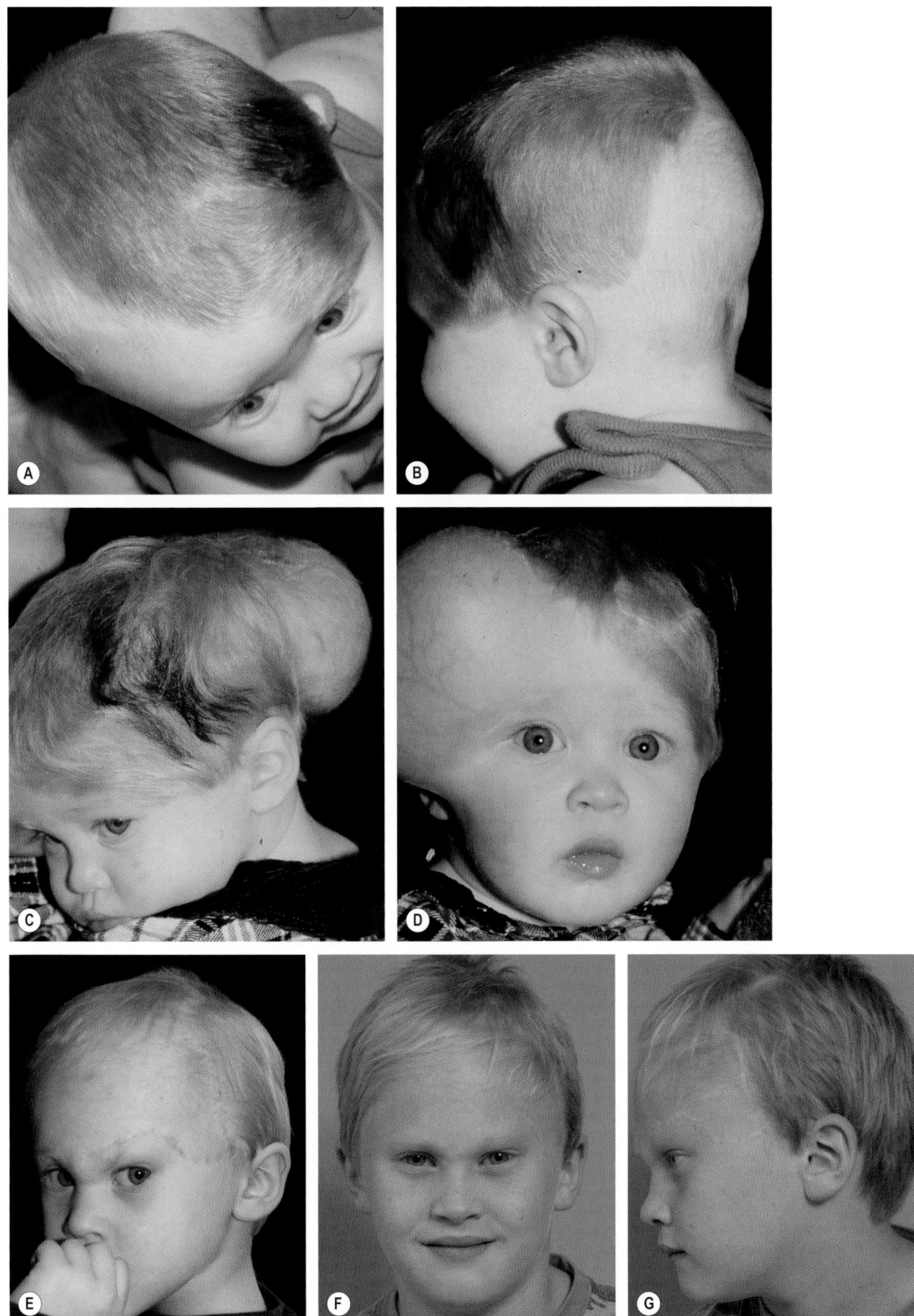

Fig. 40.7 (A, B) This infant was born with a large nevus of nearly half the scalp and left lateral forehead. **(C, D)** Expanders were placed posterior to the nevus and beneath the normal forehead and adjacent scalp at 6 months of age. **(E)** The appearance of the reconstructed scalp and forehead at 2 years of age and 1 year postexcision of the remaining scalp nevus requiring a second expansion. Forehead width, hairline, and hair direction are well oriented. Some residual excess skin is present in the glabellar area. **(F, G)** Six years following completion of the expansion and minor revision of the scars along the brow, the patient has excellent symmetry and a natural hairline and direction of hair growth.

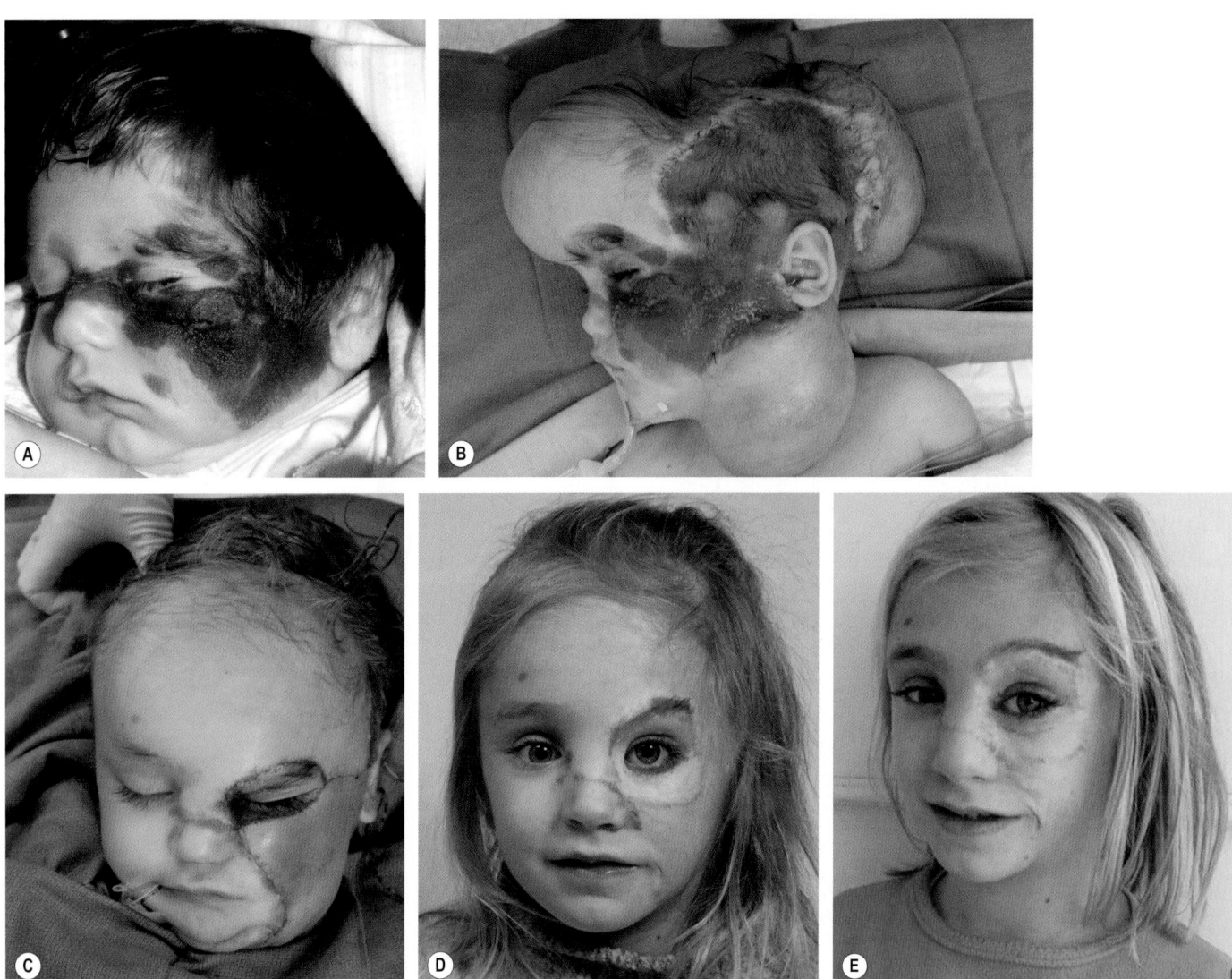

Fig. 40.8 (A) This infant was born with a thick mamillated hairy nevus with deeply pigmented areas centrally and light pigmentation along the borders which gradually darkened. **(B)** Three expanders are shown in place and, with hair trimmed, the full extent of the nevus is visible. **(C)** Nevus of the forehead, cheek, nose, and scalp is excised following well-planned expander placement. The eyelid and brow were not addressed at this point. **(D)** Three years postexpansion, prior to further excision of the nevus of the eyelid, revision of graft and scar of brow and canthal region. The upper and lower eyelids were grafted with a single-piece expanded full-thickness skin graft from the supraclavicular are. **(E)** At 7 years of age, the eye and brow symmetry is good and the patient is ready for minor revision with both surgery and laser.

Tissue expansion can be very effective on the anterior trunk, provided that the lesion is confined to either the lower abdomen or central abdomen and that there is sufficient uninvolved skin above, or above and below the nevus to expand. Expansion must be avoided in or around the area of the breast bud in females and lesions of the breast should be left until after breast development. Flaps below the chest can be designed as transposition or rotation flaps rather than direct downward advancement to avoid pulling down the areola–nipple complex.

Alternatively, expanded flaps can be advanced transversely across the abdomen, reinsetting the umbilicus in the same manner as in a standard abdominoplasty *(Fig. 40.9)*.

The use of expanded transposition flaps has enabled excision of nevi of the upper back/neck and back/buttock/perineal region, where previously it was thought that only skin grafting was possible. Tissue expanders in the 500–750 cc range are used most commonly in infants and young children. Serial expansion with careful planning has made possible the excision of progressively larger nevi of the back and buttocks, with excellent outcomes. Subsequent expansions, as a child gets older, are carried out using expanders in the 250–500 cc size for shoulders and upper back and 1000–1200 cc size for the lower back/buttocks *(Figs 40.10 and 40.11)*.

In patients with giant nevi involving the entire or near-entire back, flanks, and abdomen, and with markedly variegated nevus architecture or color, one may decide to excise the greater part of the nevus of the back alone, and cover this with split-thickness (nonmeshed) skin grafts *(Fig. 40.6)*. Some literature suggests that this is the area at greatest risk of degeneration, and when color, texture, or character of the nevus makes follow-up difficult, excision may be warranted to "simplify" follow-up. We recognize that split-thickness

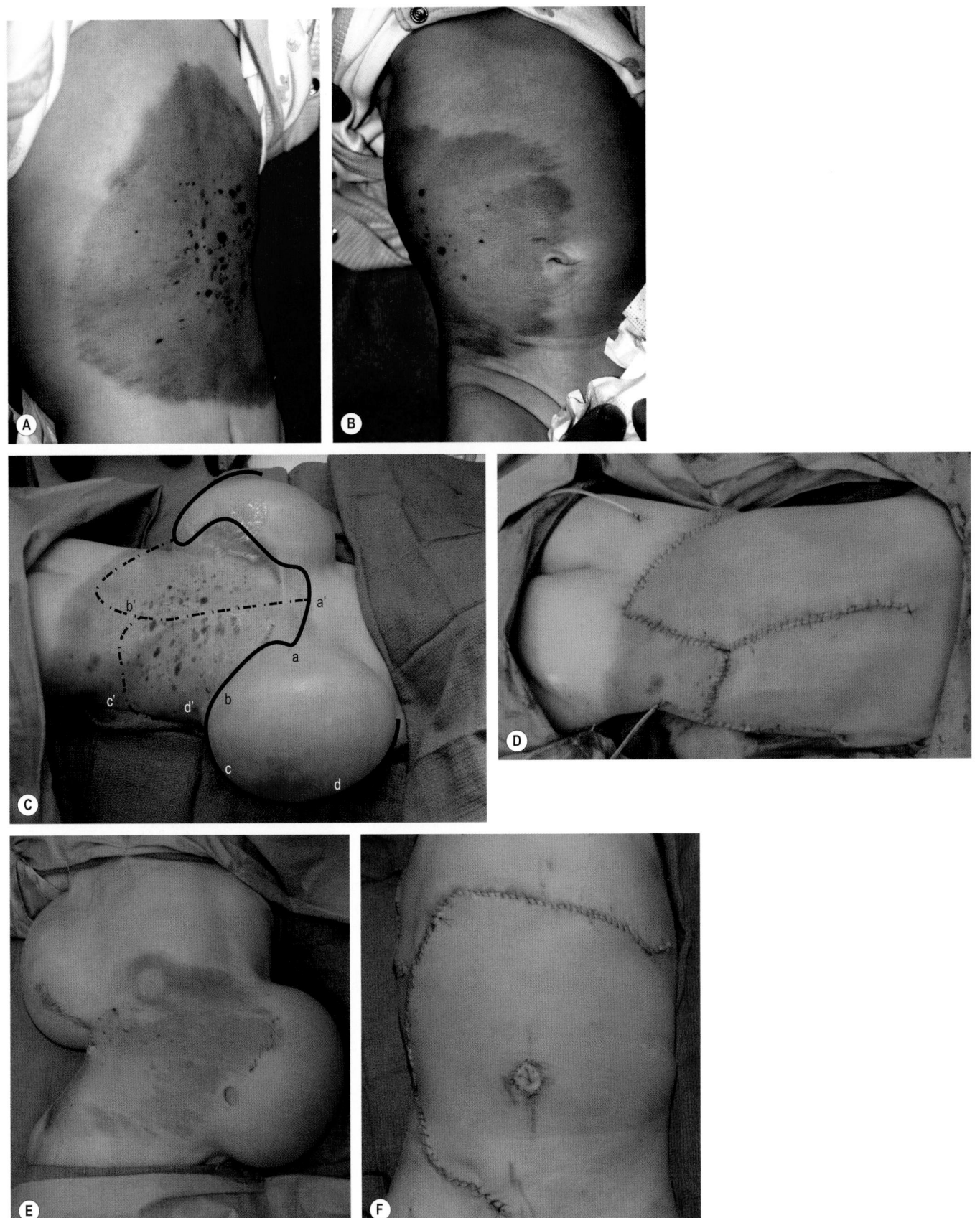

Fig. 40.9 (A, B) This large nevus covers the greater part of the back and wraps around to the right half of the lower chest and abdomen. **(C, D)** At completion of the first expansion of the back the flaps are transposed to cover most of the back. The flaps are designed with a superomedial base and a back cut across the lateral part of the flap (point c to d). This design allows a greater coverage of normal tissue due to the advancement of the base of the flap (point d to d'). **(E)** The second set of expanders is placed beneath one of the previously expanded back flaps and beneath the uninvolved left abdominal skin. **(F)** The expanded flaps, anterior and posterior, join on the right flank as the abdominal flap is advanced transversely across the abdomen and the umbilicus is delivered through the flap.

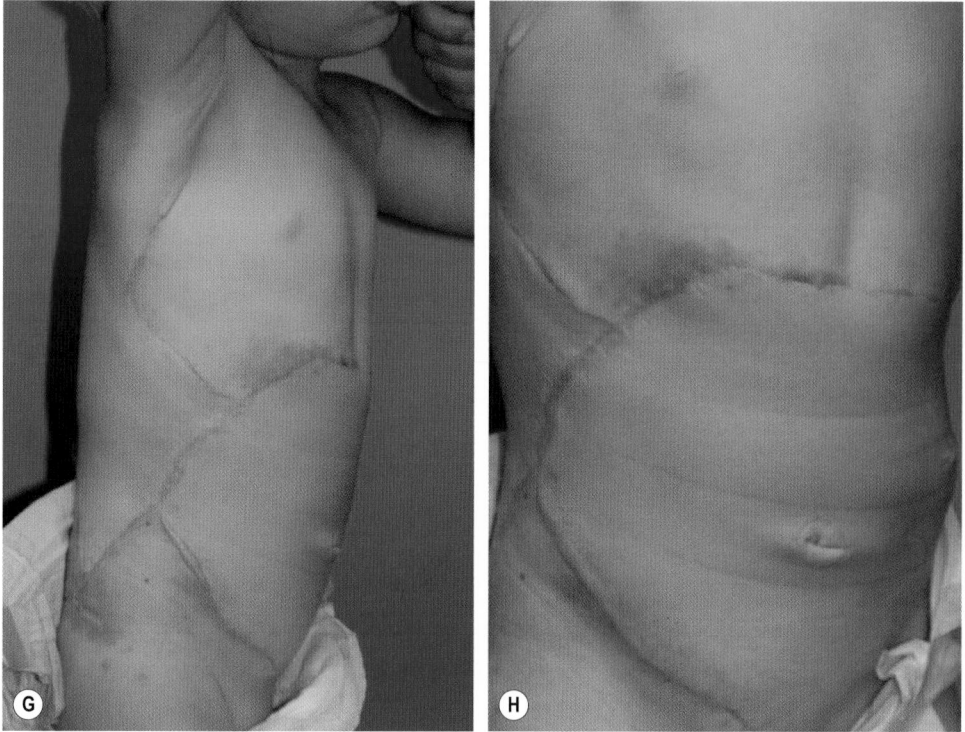

Fig. 40.9, cont'd (G, H) Anterior and lateral views 2 months postoperatively show only small areas of remaining nevus that can be excised from the upper abdomen without further expansion and without risk of downward pull on the right breast.

skin grafts elsewhere on the trunk and extremities may be associated with significant deformity and potential functional disturbance during growth, so we recommend against grafting elsewhere. The back is the only area where split-thickness skin grafting may provide a reasonable aesthetic result as long as the graft is not meshed.

Extremities

Tissue expansion of the extremities has been viewed classically as of limited value and is associated with a higher risk of complications.[47,48]

The geometry of the extremity, as well as the limited flexibility of the skin (particularly in the lower extremity), makes regional expansion of limited use. Expanded flaps can be moved effectively in a circumferential direction, but move poorly in an axial direction. However, attempts to move a limited amount of skin to reconstruct the defect when the nevus is more than a third of the circumference of the extremity can result in significant constriction of the extremity, particularly in the upper arm *(Figs 40.12–40.14)*.

In the past decade, the authors have begun to find a way around these limitations.[49] Large expanded transposition flaps from the scapular region are used to cover the upper arm and shoulder. For circumferential nevi from the mid humeral level to the wrist, expansion of the flank creates a large pedicled flap through which the forearm can be placed during vascularization of the flap from the recipient bed. After 3 weeks the pedicle is divided. Expanded full-thickness skin grafts have been used effectively for the

dorsum of the hand, with excellent aesthetic outcome *(Fig. 40.12)*.

Although pedicled flaps are not readily available for coverage of more extensive lesions of the arm, thigh, or leg, the authors have had success with expanded free flaps from the abdomen and scapular region. Alternatively, when the patient is seen in early infancy, an expanded pedicle flap from the posterior thigh/buttock to the leg from knee to ankle affords the same benefits as an expanded pedicle flap from the abdomen/flank to the upper extremity *(Fig. 40.14)*. These procedures have been used only in very carefully selected cases, and the optimum timing of these complex reconstructive procedures is still under consideration.

Satellite nevi

Satellite nevi may appear anywhere over the course of the first few years of life, and their number seems to correlate directly with the likelihood of NCM.[23] They may vary in size from small to medium lesions *(Figs 40.2, 40.3, and 40.11)*. To date, no case of melanoma has been reported arising in a satellite nevus.[50] With this in mind, it is generally agreed that the primary reason for excision of satellite nevi is an aesthetic one. A significant benefit may also result from excising multiple satellite nevi on the face before the child enters his or her school years. In addition, some of the larger satellites on the extremities may be excised in infancy and early childhood (simultaneously with other procedures on the major lesion) by relatively simple serial excision techniques; if left to later childhood and adolescence, the reduced flexibility of the sur-

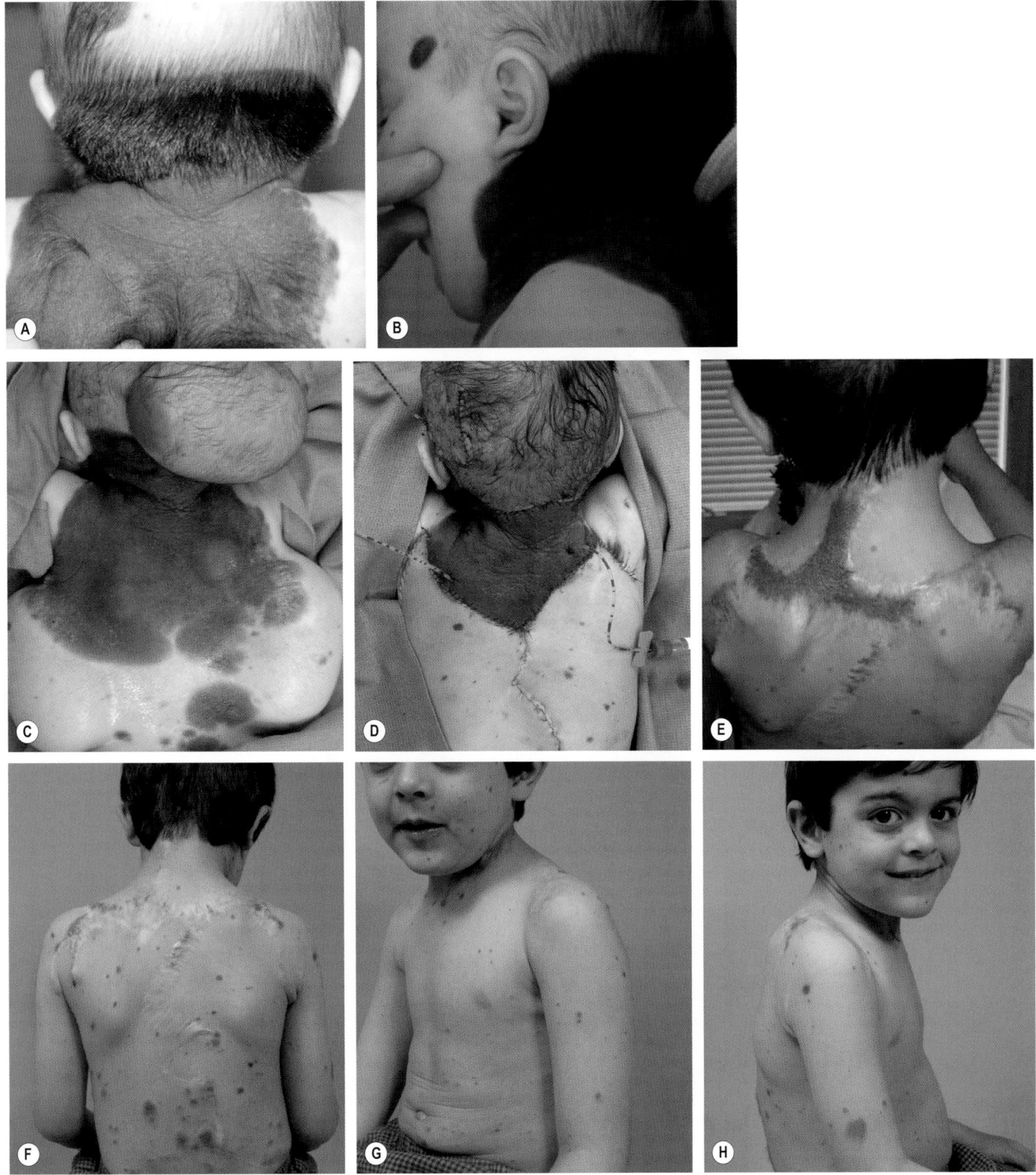

Fig. 40.10 (A, B) This patient, shown fully in *Figure 40.2C*, showed thick, deeply pigmented nevus over the occiput, neck, and upper back with multiple satellite nevi on the remaining trunk, extremities, and face. **(C, D)** The first expanders were placed in the occiput above the nevus and bilateral back/flanks below the nevus. This allowed excision of scalp nevus and the lower portion of the back nevus and brought normal back skin to join normal shoulder skin lateral to the remaining neck/shoulder nevus. **(E)** At 3 years of age the expanded flaps have been advanced further toward the midline of the posterior neck prior to final excision. **(F–H)** As in other patients with some uninvolved skin in the anterior shoulders, he was able to undergo serial expansion of the shoulder flaps to complete the shoulder, neck, and upper back nevus excision. Although some of the satellites remain and scars have widened in the upper back, the shoulder, neck, and upper arm contour is normal and the scars are positioned so as to avoid any inhibition of growth or function.

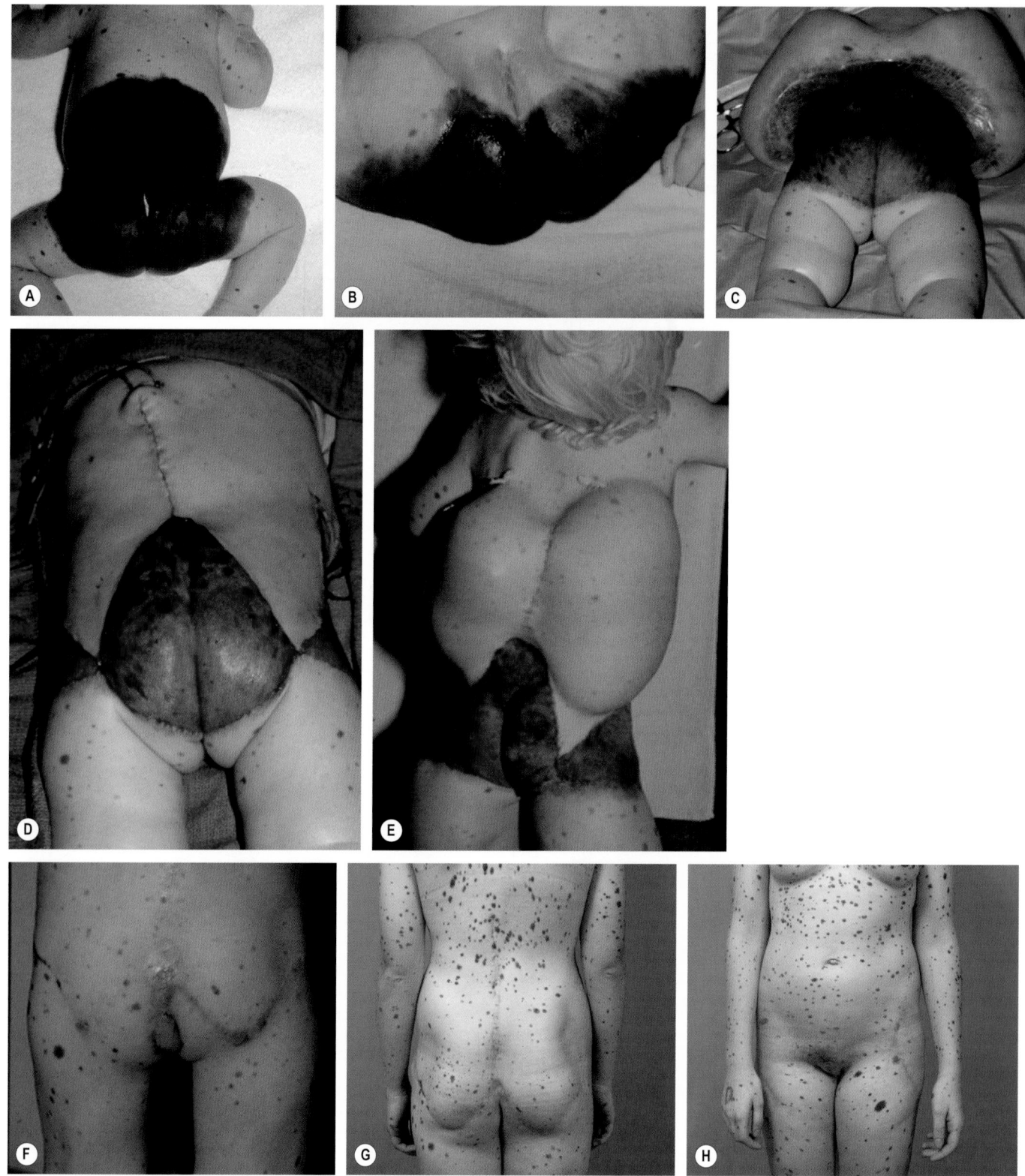

Fig. 40.11 (A, B) This infant was born with a large nevus of the lower half of the back, buttocks, perineum, and upper thigh. **(C, D)** Expanded transposition flaps create the length and flap orientation to allow. **(E, F)** repeat expansion and coverage of the remaining buttocks, perineum, and perianal areas. **(G, H)** The patient is seen 13 years later with no additional scar revisions. While she has extensive involvement with small satellite nevi, the scars from the excision and reconstruction were clearly positioned to avoid significant contour deformities and growth disturbance.

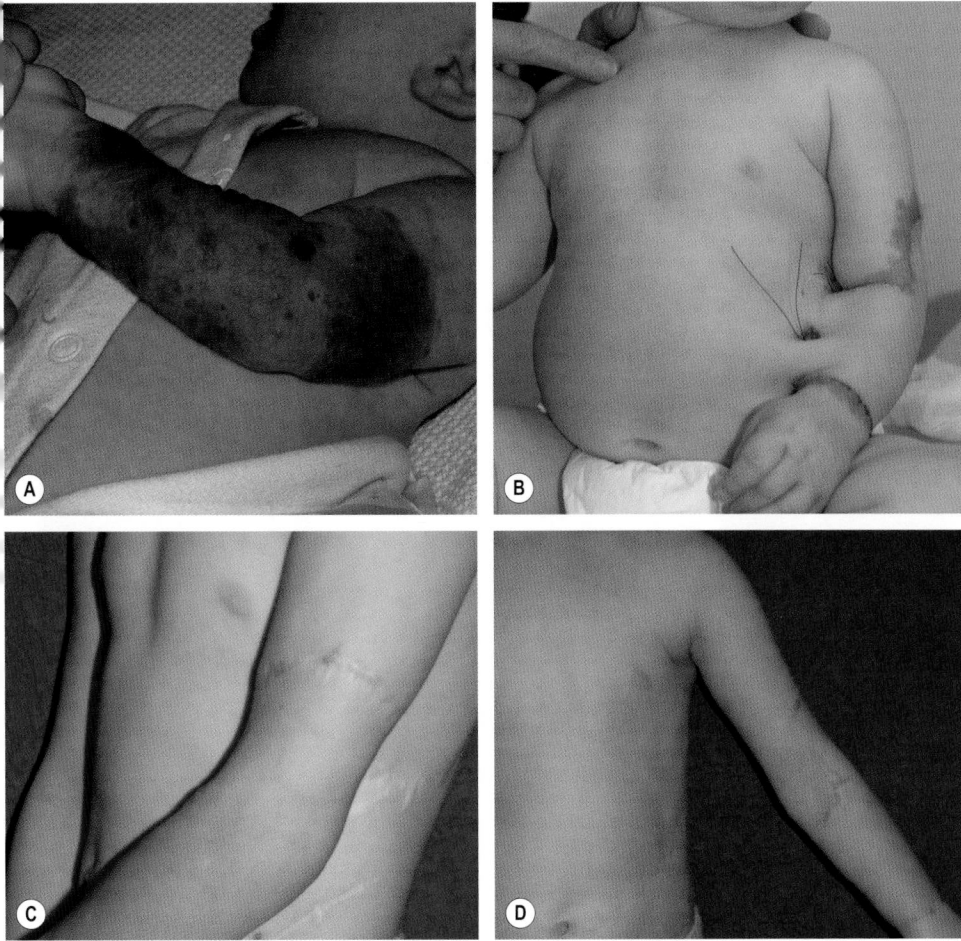

Fig. 40.12 (A, B) This child with circumferential nevus of the arm was treated with an expanded pedicle flap from the abdomen and flank. Following 3 months' expansion the expander is removed, the nevus excised, and the arm passed into a tunnel of expanded skin which is secured around the arm with large bolster sutures. The pedicle is divided at 3 weeks, then additional excision of a narrow strip of remaining nevus both proximal and distal to the flap allows finetuning of the scars. **(C, D)** The patient is shown 3 years after division of the flap with excellent contour of the arm, and an aesthetically acceptable donor site.

rounding tissues may no longer allow excision without expansion or grafting.

Postoperative care

Parents are often more comfortable having their child observed for the first night postoperatively. The patients may be monitored for pain or hematoma formation. The dressing is changed daily for several days (antibiotic ointment on suture line with Xeroform gauze above and soft padding). The drains are usually removed 3–10 days postoperatively, depending on the amount of discharge. Serial injections are started 7–10 days after insertion, provided the skin flaps are in excellent condition. After one or two postoperative visits and a teaching session, most patients start home expansion directed by the parents or guardians. Parents are provided with a printed card to record the schedule and amount of saline injected throughout the expansion process. They are encouraged to take digital photos and record the process and keep us well informed.[51] A local anesthetic cream can be put on the skin above the port prior to the injection to minimize pain. The expansion should be performed until the skin is tense but not extremely painful to the patient or of any compromise to the skin.

Outcomes, prognosis, and complications

Beyond site-specific complications of tissue expansion mentioned earlier, major complications may involve infection, expander exposure, and flap ischemia. Traditionally, it has been taught that early postoperative infection should be managed with expander removal and antibiotics; however, early detection of infection and maintaining a low threshold for antibiotic use may avoid expander loss. Small extrusions of the expander when the surrounding wound is stable may allow for some additional expansion and expander salvage. Minor complications include pain during expansion (which is transient), seroma, "dog ears" at donor site, and widening of scars.[51,52]

Given the relative scarcity of large and giant nevi, it has been difficult for many surgeons to accumulate large enough

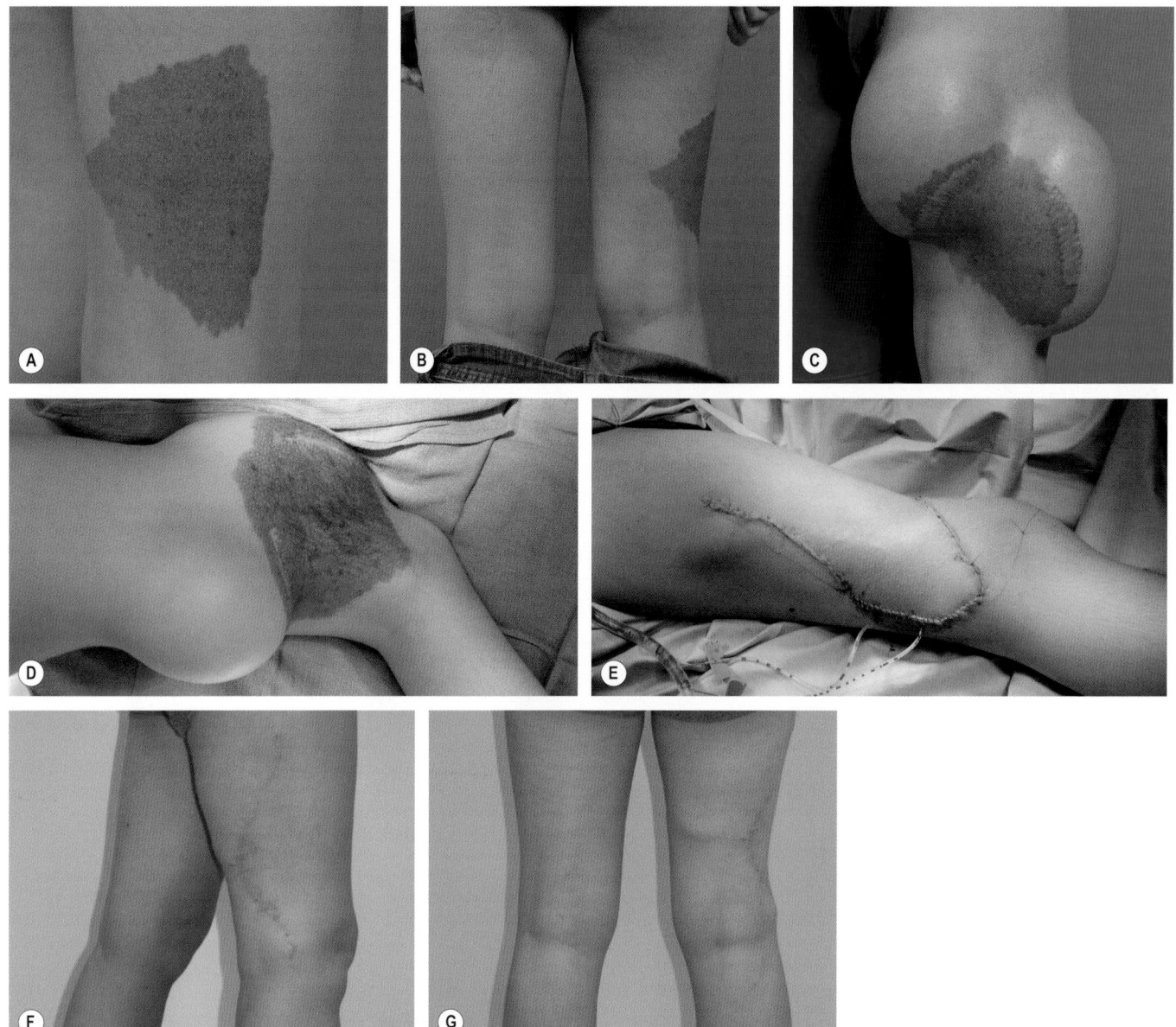

Fig. 40.13 (A, B) This young teen presented with a large nevus of the anterolateral thigh. **(C)** The appearance after 13 weeks of expansion. **(D, E)** The greater part of the nevus is excised (leaving only a small strip of nevus at its posterior border) and the flap transposed, releasing the flap just above the knee so as to place the scar in the least visible position and minimize risk of a significant contour deformity that would arise with direct advancement of the flap. **(F, G)** The final result is shown at 3 years following excision of the final segment of the nevus, with excellent contour and the scar positioned to avoid later functional disturbance.

numbers of cases to draw conclusions regarding the effectiveness of varied surgical options with respect to risk reduction of degeneration and/or functional and aesthetic outcomes. Since 1988, the authors have closely followed the efficacy of early treatment of large and giant nevi in different body regions with a series of now over 300 patients. Long-term follow-up, and the repetition of patterns of involvement in each affected area, has given us a unique opportunity to compare varied approaches of excision as well as the need for secondary surgical procedures, either to improve the aesthetic outcome or to deal with late functional problems. We have continued to modify the treatment protocol to improve outcomes, and to minimize the need for secondary surgery.

In regions that do not lend themselves readily to tissue expansion, early in our experience, efforts were directed at excising the nevus and skin-grafting the defect. It became clear after relatively short follow-up that when lesions were excised to a depth assuring complete or near-total removal, split-thickness skin graft reconstruction resulted in poor aesthetic outcomes, and, when carried circumferentially around the trunk or extremities, later growth of the child resulted in a worsening contour defect with potential growth disturbance. In an effort to improve aesthetic outcomes, and provide reconstructions having a greater chance of keeping up with growth, large full-thickness grafts were harvested from expanded donor sites. The relative size constraints of full-thickness grafts were virtually eliminated. However, when

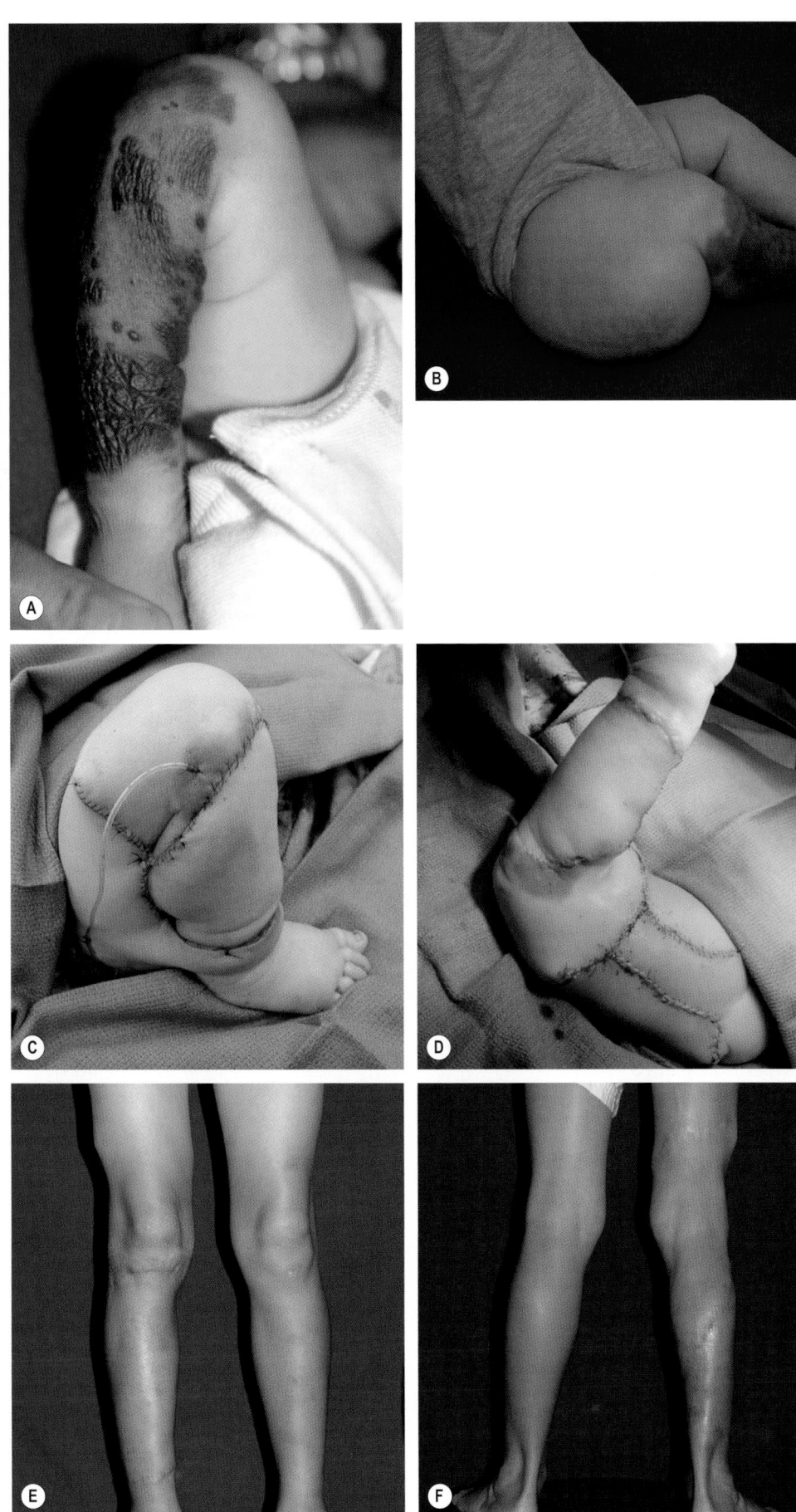

Fig. 40.14 (A) The flexibility of the infant's leg is used to advantage for the excision of this circumferential nevus extending from knee to just above the ankle. **(B)** The posterior thigh was expanded starting at 4 months of age. **(C)** At 7 months of age the greater part of the nevus was excised and the defect reconstructed with an expanded pedicled flap from the posterior thigh, held in place by slipping the foot beneath a "bucket handle" of skin which lay between the initial incision used to place the expander, and the proximal border of the flap. **(D)** The pedicle was divided after 3 weeks and the "bucket handle" bipedicle flap converted to a unipedicle flap and used for partial coverage of the donor defect on the posterior thigh. **(E, F)** The excellent contour of both the leg and proximal thigh is evident on the two views of the patient 6.5 years following the excision and flap reconstruction.

following these patients into the teen years, despite relatively normal skin surface appearance and growth, contour deformities were great enough to suggest limiting even full-thickness skin grafting to the dorsum of hand or foot, and the periorbital area. In the extremities these late deformities were avoided with the selective use of expanded pedicle flaps, as well as the use of free tissue transfer with subsequent expansion of the transferred tissue to increase its coverage.

Recognizing the increasing difficulty of tissue expansion with age, some of these procedures are only effective if done when the patient is young. While not totally ruling out any procedures (other than the expanded pedicle flap from posterior thigh to lower leg) for reconstruction in older children/adults, one must accept that, at present, many patients with giant nevi extending from waist to knee are best monitored, rather than subjected to unsightly scars and possible functional disturbance. Free tissue transfer, either with or without prior expansion, allows for the harvest of larger flaps with improved ease of donor site closure, and may provide a means of correcting some late deformities secondary to either complications of earlier treatment, or poor choice of the initial treatment option.

Access the complete references list online at **http://www.expertconsult.com**

9. Kovalyshyn I, Braun R, Marghoob A. Congenital melanocytic naevi. *Australas J Dermatol*. 2009;50:231–240.

   A comprehensive review about congenital melanocytic nevi, including pathogenesis, natural history, and complications.

20. Zaal LH, Mooi WJ, Klip H, et al. Risk of malignant transformation of congenital melanocytic nevi: a retrospective nationwide study from The Netherlands. *Plast Reconstr Surg*. 2005;116:1902–1909.

    Retrospective study of national database of patients with large and giant congenital nevi from the Netherlands. The authors compared melanoma rates between patients with giant nevi and the general population over a 10-year period and revealed an increased rate of melanoma in patients with giant congenital melanocytic nevi when compared with the general population.

33. Bittencourt FV, Marghoob AA, Kopf AW, et al. Large congenital melanocytic nevi and the risk for development of malignant melanoma and neurocutaneous melanocytosis. *Pediatrics*. 2000;106:736–741.

36. Rhodes AR, Melski JW. Small congenital nevocellular nevi and the risk of cutaneous melanoma. *J Pediatr*. 1982;100:219–224.

39. Bauer BS, Margulis A. The expanded transposition flap: shifting paradigms based on experience gained from two decades of pediatric tissue expansion. *Plast Reconstr Surg*. 2004;114:98–106.

   This paper demonstrates the advantages of transposition flaps used in tissue expansion when compared with advancement flaps.

45. Bauer BS, Few JW, Chavez CD, et al. The role of tissue expansion in the management of large congenital pigmented nevi of the forehead in the pediatric patient.

   This paper suggests guidelines for treatment of forehead and scalp congenital nevi with an emphasis on preserving or reconstructing the landmarks of hairline, hair direction, and brow position.

46. Bauer BS, Vicari FA, Richard ME, et al. Expanded full-thickness skin grafts in children: case selection, planning, and management. *Plast Reconstr Surg*. 1993;92:59–69.

47. Pandya AN, Vadodaria S, Coleman DJ. Tissue expansion in the limbs: a comparative analysis of limb and non-limb sites. *Br J Plast Surg*. 2002;55:302–306.

49. Margulis A, Bauer BS, Fine NA. Large and giant congenital pigmented nevi of the upper extremity: an algorithm to surgical management. *Ann Plast Surg*. 2004;521:158–167.

52. Manders EK, Schenden MJ, Furrey JA, et al. Soft-tissue expansion: concepts and complications. *Plast Reconstr Surg*. 1984;74:493–507.

   Review of the early concepts of how and why expansion works and discuss potential complications with avoidance techniques.

41

Pediatric chest and trunk defects

Lawrence J. Gottlieb, Russell R. Reid, and Justine C. Lee

SYNOPSIS

- Pediatric trunk defects require multidisciplinary comprehensive care in order to maximize patient safety and successful outcome.
- Reconstructive surgery for the pediatric patient requires consideration for the paucity of tissue available in a small body habitus, the necessity for growth, and the tenuous physiology that may accompany children afflicted with congenital defects.
- Closure of ventral body wall defects may pose significant challenges to the neonatal circulation whereas closure of dorsal body wall defects must address exposed neural elements.

Introduction

Patients with severe congenital trunk defects are frequently diagnosed during prenatal ultrasonography sessions or at birth and require the coordination of multiple disciplines, including reconstructive plastic surgery. Reconstructive surgery for the pediatric patient requires consideration for the paucity of tissue available in a small body habitus, the necessity for growth, and the tenuous physiology that may accompany children afflicted with congenital defects. Body wall defects have the potential risk of exposing vital structures and subsequent infection. Closure of ventral body wall defects may pose significant challenges to the neonatal circulation whereas closure of dorsal body wall defects must address exposed neural elements.

Embryology

Development of the body wall begins at the fourth week of gestation when the mesoderm organizes into the paraxial, intermediate, and lateral plate layers. The paraxial mesoderm, adjacent to the neural tube, differentiates into the skeletal support and surrounding soft tissue that characterize the dorsal body wall and encase the central nervous system.

Intermediate mesoderm forms the urogenital structures. Lateral plate mesoderm differentiates into both the soft-tissue and skeletal components of the ventral body wall. The lateral plate mesoderm, with ectoderm covering, folds and fuses at the end of the fourth week of gestation.[1,2] Congenital ventral body wall defects result from the lack of lateral plate fusion.

Thoracic wall defects

Pectus excavatum

Pectus excavatum, also known as funnel chest, is the most common congenital anterior thoracic wall deformity, occurring in 1 in 300 live births. It is characterized by a depression of the sternum as well as costal cartilage displacement. Males outnumber females 3:1 and patients are predominantly Caucasian. Pectus excavatum is usually identified within the first year of life, although more subtle variations are frequently not noticed until teenage years.

Pectus deformities often carry a familial component; however the etiology remains unclear. Mendelian patterns of inheritance are not identified and no definitive genetic mutations have been found, although associations with Marfan's syndrome, Poland's syndrome, scoliosis, clubfoot, and syndactyly are known. All of the current evidence points to either genetic mutations with incomplete penetrance or multifactorial causes.

Clinical presentation and evaluation

Patients with pectus excavatum exhibit a depressed sternum that is frequently greater on the right with sternal retraction on inspiration.[3,4] Both the body of the sternum and the costal cartilages at the sternocostal junction have posterior angulation (Fig. 41.1). Rounded sloping shoulders, mild dorsal kyphosis, and a protuberant abdomen are associated findings but may be related to postural changes that patients exhibit secondary to a conscious or subconscious attempt to hide their deformity.

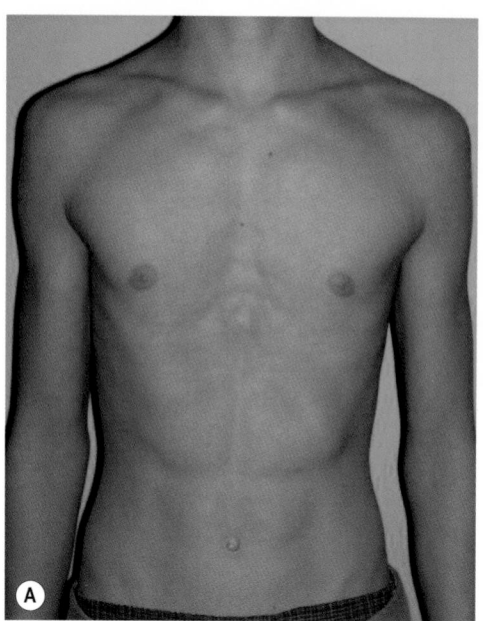
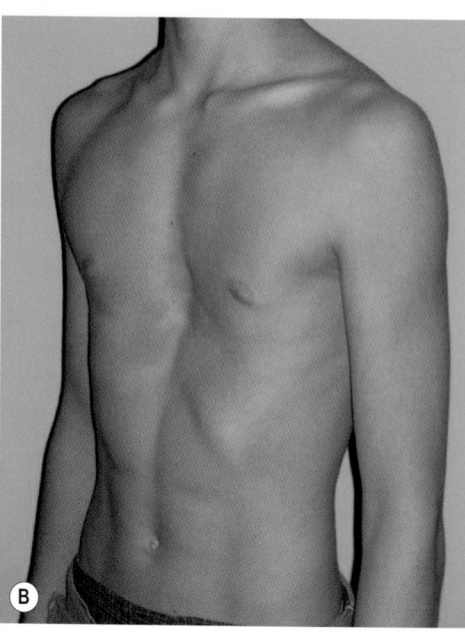

Fig. 41.1 Pectus excavatum is the most common congenital anterior thoracic wall defect and is characterized by a depression deformity in the sternum and costal cartilage displacement. A male predominance exists. **(A)** Anterior view of patient with pectus excavatum. **(B)** Oblique view of patient. Note the decrease in anterior–posterior distance between the sternum and the vertebral column.

Proper identification of the extent of structural irregularity, physiologic limitations, and psychological responses to the deformity are crucial in treatment decision-making. Basic workup should include chest radiographs, pulmonary function tests, electrocardiogram, and chest computed tomography (CT) scan *(Fig. 41.2)*. Haller and others stratified anatomic severity of pectus excavatum by defining the pectus severity index (PSI) using measurements obtained from CT scans.[5,6] The PSI is calculated by dividing the internal transverse thoracic width by the smallest anterior–posterior distance between the vertebrae and the most depressed portion of the chest wall. Normal values range between 2.5 and 3.25. Operative intervention usually occurs with PSI values greater than 4.8.[7]

Surgical indications

Most patients are asymptomatic and seek elective intervention for the correction of contour deformities, especially when the features become more prominent during the pubertal growth spurt. Although cardiopulmonary compromise is controversial, anatomically severe versions of pectus excavatum are thought to benefit from surgical intervention.[8,9] Kelly suggests that surgery is indicated when two or more of the following occur: a severe, symptomatic deformity; progression of deformity; paradoxical respiratory chest wall motion; CT scan with a PSI greater than 3.25; cardiac or pulmonary compression or pathology; significant body image disturbance; or failed repairs.[10] Surgical correction is considered safe in children older than 7 years of age; however, timing has been a subject of controversy.

Treatment

Some patients with mild deformities can be satisfactorily treated with physical therapy to improve their posture and increase the bulk of their pectoralis muscles. Surgical correction of pectus excavatum can be categorized into contour camouflage and contour repair procedures. Camouflage of the

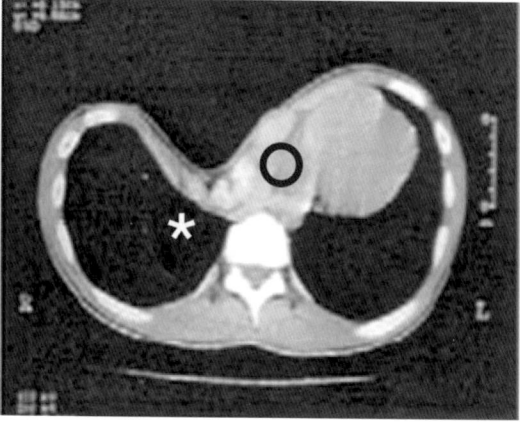

Fig. 41.2 Pectus excavatum deformity on computed tomography (CT) scan. CT scan of pectus excavatum deformities illustrates both the severity of sternal depression as well as the morphology of the depression and its effects on the involved organs. The pectus severity index (PSI) utilized CT scans to stratify deformities by dividing the internal thoracic width by the smallest anterior–posterior distance. Operative intervention is usually performed if the PSI is greater than 4.8.

contour deformities has been successfully accomplished with autologous tissue or custom prosthetics. The disadvantage of autologous tissue is the donor site scar and potential morbidity. Flaps containing muscle should not be relied on for volume correction only unless innervated and able to contract, as the muscle will invariably atrophy if not innervated and contracting. The most common contour camouflage technique is placement of customized silicone implants[11–14] *(Fig. 41.3)*. Satisfactory results are obtained with silicone implants with few short-term complications other than seroma formation. Additional problems with prosthetics are displacement and visualization of edges, especially in thin patients. Autologous reconstruction has been used as an alternative to prosthetics in selected patients.[15–18] Recently, Sinna *et al.* described a combination of approaches covering a custom implant with

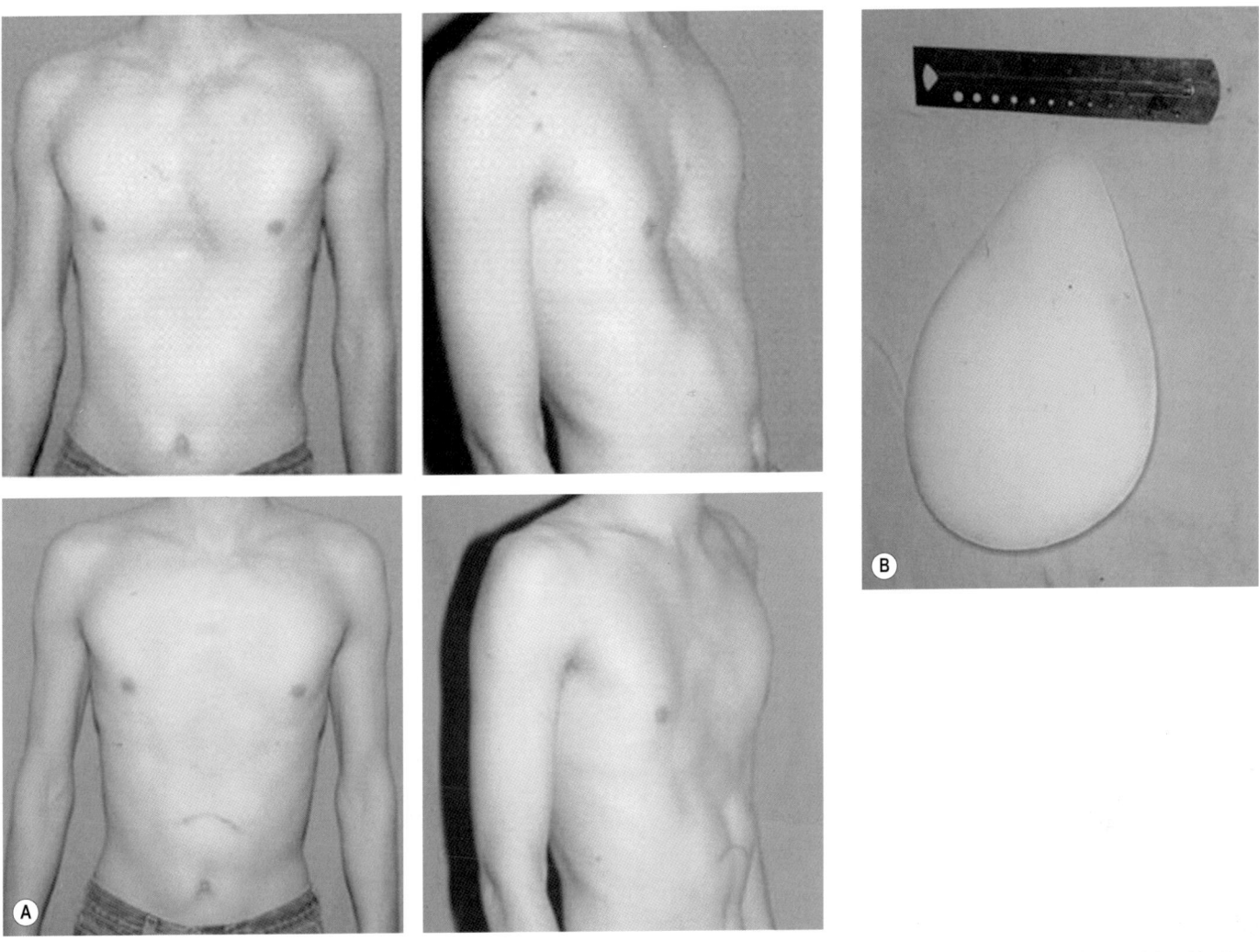

Fig. 41.3 Contour camouflage using silicone implants in pectus excavatum. Customized silicone implants are a common method of camouflaging contour deformities in pectus excavatum. **(A)** Preoperative **(i, ii)** and postoperative **(iii, iv)** photographs following implant insertion. A transverse epigastric incision was used for insertion. **(B)** Custom silicone implant.

bilateral de-epithelialized thoracodorsal artery perforator flaps.[19] Injection of autologous fat or prosthetic soft-tissue fillers has also been described.[20,21]

Whereas contour camouflage techniques are most appropriate for patients with mild deformities, patients with moderate to severe deformities are better suited for contour repair techniques. Ravitch described an open repair technique of elevating bilateral pectoralis muscle flaps with resection of abnormal costal cartilages followed by transverse osteotomy of the sternum and fixation in a corrected position[4] *(Fig. 41.4)*. Since his report, the Ravitch procedure has been modified in many ways: from preserving the perichondrium to minimal cartilage resection and varying technique to support the sternum.[22,23] Haller and colleagues describe supporting the elevated sternum by overlapping the sternal ends of the costal cartilages over the costal ends in a tripod fixation.[24,25] Almost all open techniques utilize a transverse inframammary crease or a short chevron incision, except for older patients or Marfan patients where a vertical midline incision is usually used. Bilateral pectoralis major and upper rectus abdominis muscles are disinserted from the sternum and ribs bilaterally and raised to expose the costal cartilages. With or without sacrifice of the perichondrium, the costal cartilages are resected to a greater or lesser degree. Since Ravitch's initial experience, it has become clear that the most medial and most lateral portions of the costal cartilages should be preserved in young children to minimize secondary growth disturbances. The sternal angulation is corrected with a transverse wedge osteotomy that is done at the level of the third or fourth intercostal space corresponding to the upper edge of the sternal depression. The osteotomy can then be secured with sutures, wire, or rigid fixation plates.[26,27] The xiphoid process is detached from the sternum and allowed to retract down.

Horizontal sternal fixation techniques are not universally used but are considered by many to be important for sternal support. Many surgeons have supported the sternum with a metallic strut developed by Adkins and Blades.[28] Fonkalsrud and colleagues report on a modified open technique with minimal cartilage resection and use of the Adkins strut in 450 patients.[29] Most of these patients had retrosternal placement but more recently they have converted to a suprasternal strut to facilitate removal (at 6 months) and minimize the need to

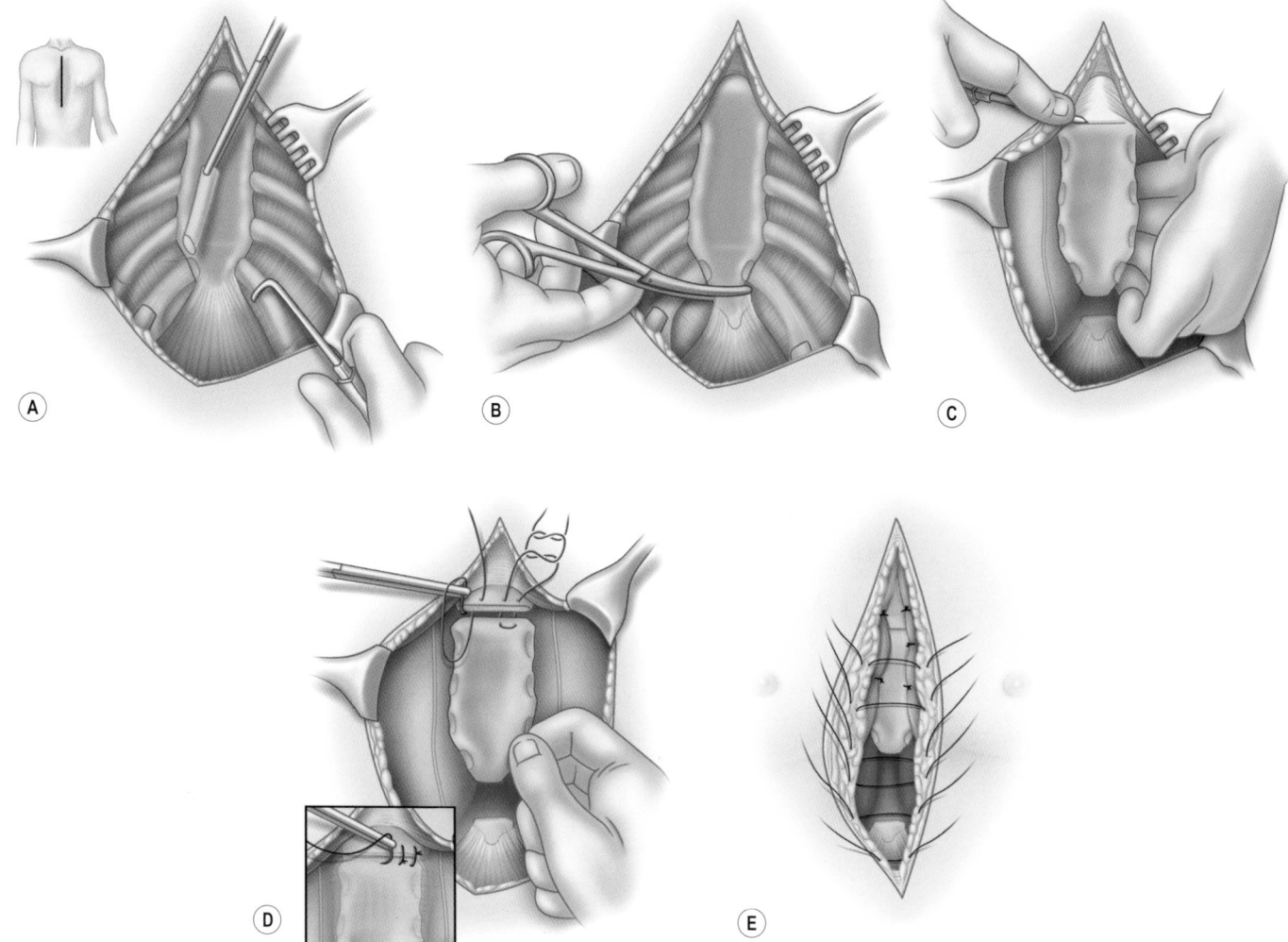

Fig. 41.4 Ravitch repair. In 1949, Ravitch described his classic approach to pectus excavatum repair. **(A)** Starting with a midline incision, the pectoralis muscles are incised and elevated to expose the sternum and the sternocostal junction. **(B)** The lowest two costal cartilages are resected with perichondrium and the xiphoid is osteotomized to begin mobilization of the sternum. **(C)** Five costal cartilages are divided bilaterally and a single cortex osteotomy is made superiorly. **(D)** The inferior sternum is reapproximated at a corrected position and secured with braided silk mattress sutures. **(E)** The pectoralis muscles are reapproximated midline and the skin incision is closed. (Reproduced from Ravitch MM. The operative treatment of pectus excavatum. *Ann Surg.* 1949;129:429–444.)

enter the pleural cavity. Hayashi and Maruyama describe the use of a vascularized rib strut based on the anterior intercostal branch of the internal mammary artery instead of a metallic strut.[30] Robicsek *et al.* have extensive experience reporting on over 600 patients treated with a retrosternal Marlex mesh "hammock" technique with excellent long-term results.[31] Recently, bioabsorbable mesh placed for retrosternal support in the Robicsek technique has been reported and found to be associated with decreased inflammatory reaction, decreased postoperative pain, and elimination of the risk of retrosternal metal support device dislodgment.[32]

A radical method to repair contour deformities of the sternum uses a sternal turnover bone graft.[33] This technique has been met with problems of sternal avascular necrosis due to the interruption of blood supply. Vascularized sternal turnover bone flaps with microvascular anastomoses of the internal mammary vessels were later developed to prevent such complications and have been successful in several reports.[34–36]

With the development and advances in thoracoscopy, minimally invasive repair of pectus excavatum (MIRPE) has emerged as a viable option.[37,38] MIRPE, also called the Nuss procedure, involves a thoracoscopic exposure of the sternum and the placement of a bent bar *(Fig. 41.5)*. Unlike the Ravitch and modified Ravitch procedures, skeletal resection is avoided and the operative time is significantly shorter. However, complications such as bar dislocation, bar extrusion, and costal erosion have been reported.[39] In addition, a second procedure to remove the bar is required. Absorbable transsternal bars have been used in the Nuss procedure but they are associated with higher breakage rates.[40]

The immediate complications of pectus excavatum contour repair are rare beyond pneumothorax and wound infection. Especially in the Ravitch procedure without rigid fixation, recurrence can occur as a late complication. Secondary thoracic deformity is a serious late complication that has been observed in patients who undergo correction at an early age. Thought to be due to the interruption of growth centers and

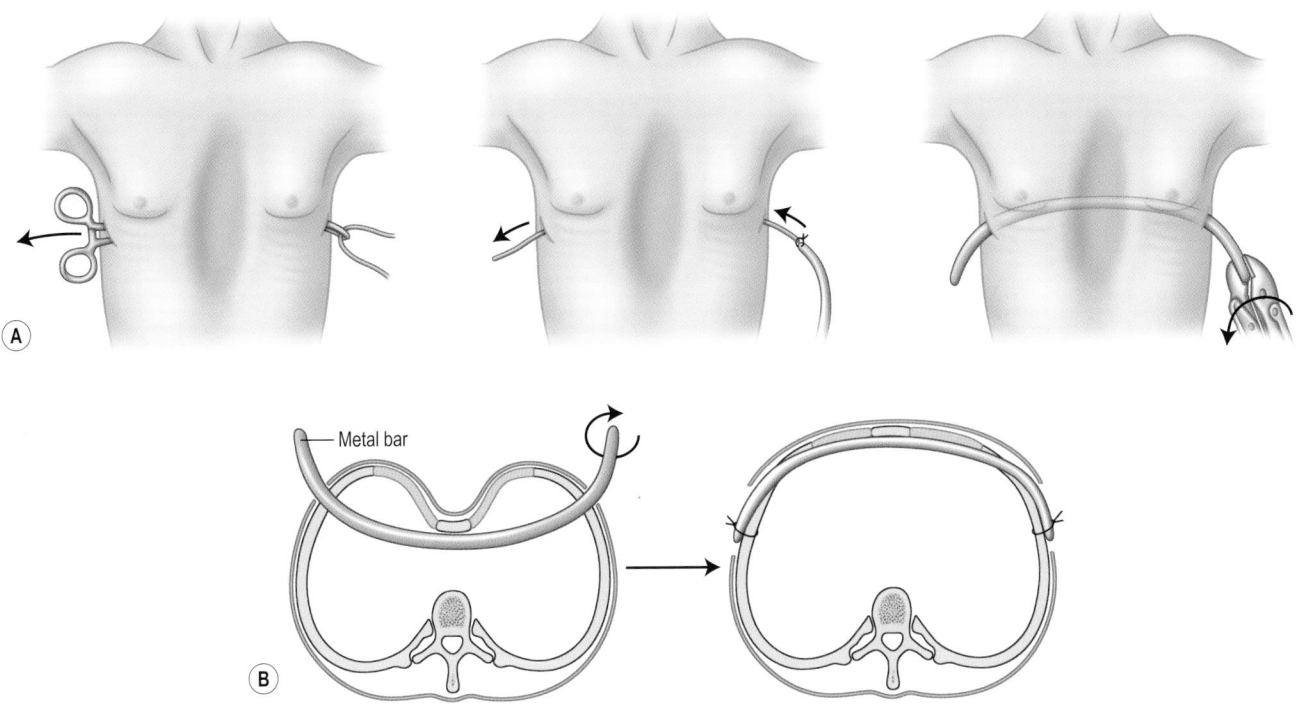

Fig. 41.5 The Nuss repair, also known as the minimally invasive repair of pectus excavatum (MIRPE), is a thoracoscopic method of contour repair using a bent bar. **(A)** A Kelly clamp is advanced across the mediastinum underneath the sternum (left panel). The clamp guides the placement of a bent bar into the substernal space (middle and right panels). **(B)** For the insertion, the bar follows the concave curvature of the deformed thorax (left). Once in place, the bar is rotated 180° on its axis such that it forces the sternum anteriorly into a convex formation (right). (Reproduced from Nuss D, Kelly RE Jr, Croitoru DP, et al. A 10 yr review of minimally invasive technique for the correction of pectus excavatum. *J Pediatr Surg*. 1998;33:545.)

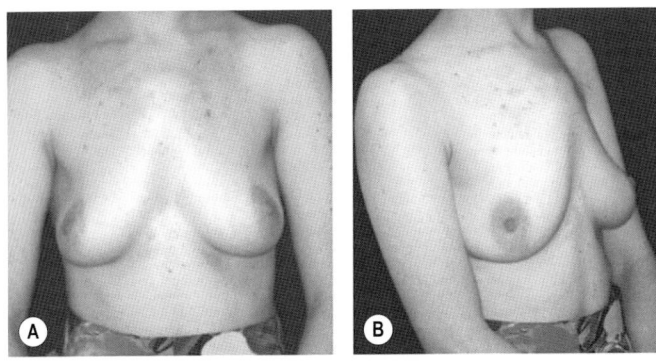

Fig. 41.6 Pectus carinatum is an anterior protrusion thoracic deformity that is the reverse of pectus excavatum but is generally considered to be in the same spectrum of deformities. Shown here are anterior (left) and oblique (right) photographs of a 28-year-old woman with pectus carinatum.

intrathoracic scar formation, the patients develop narrowed thoraces and severe pulmonary impairment. Haller *et al.* coined this phenomenon as acquired Jeune's syndrome.[41]

Pectus carinatum

Pectus carinatum, although less common in presentation compared to pectus excavatum, is considered to be in the same spectrum of deformities. It is characterized as a protrusion deformity of the anterior thoracic wall *(Fig. 41.6)*. Similar to pectus excavatum, pectus carinatum does not have a defined etiology. The incidence is between 1 in 10 000 and 1 in 1000 live births and is six times more common in males.

Clinical presentation and surgical indications

Three types of anterior thoracic protrusion deformities have been described in the pectus carinatum spectrum.[42] The chondrogladiolar type is the most common version and is characterized by anterior displacement of the body of the sternum with costal cartilage concavity. Asymmetric mixed deformities can also occur with displacement of the costal cartilages on one side with normal positioning of the sternum. Prominence of the chondromanubrial junction with a depressed sternum represents the third and least common type. Unlike pectus excavatum, younger patients do not have cardiopulmonary compromise and tend to display subtle findings on clinical exam. Patients tend to be diagnosed at a later age and seek surgical correction for their contour irregularities. Pectus carinatum can also be an acquired defect secondary to pectus excavatum repair.[43]

Treatment

Skin incisions for pectus carinatum reconstruction are usually transverse inframammary fold incisions. Classically, the pectoralis and rectus muscles are elevated to expose the costal cartilages and the sternum. For the chondrogladiolar deformity, subperichondrial resection of the costal cartilages is combined with a single or double osteotomy to return the sternum

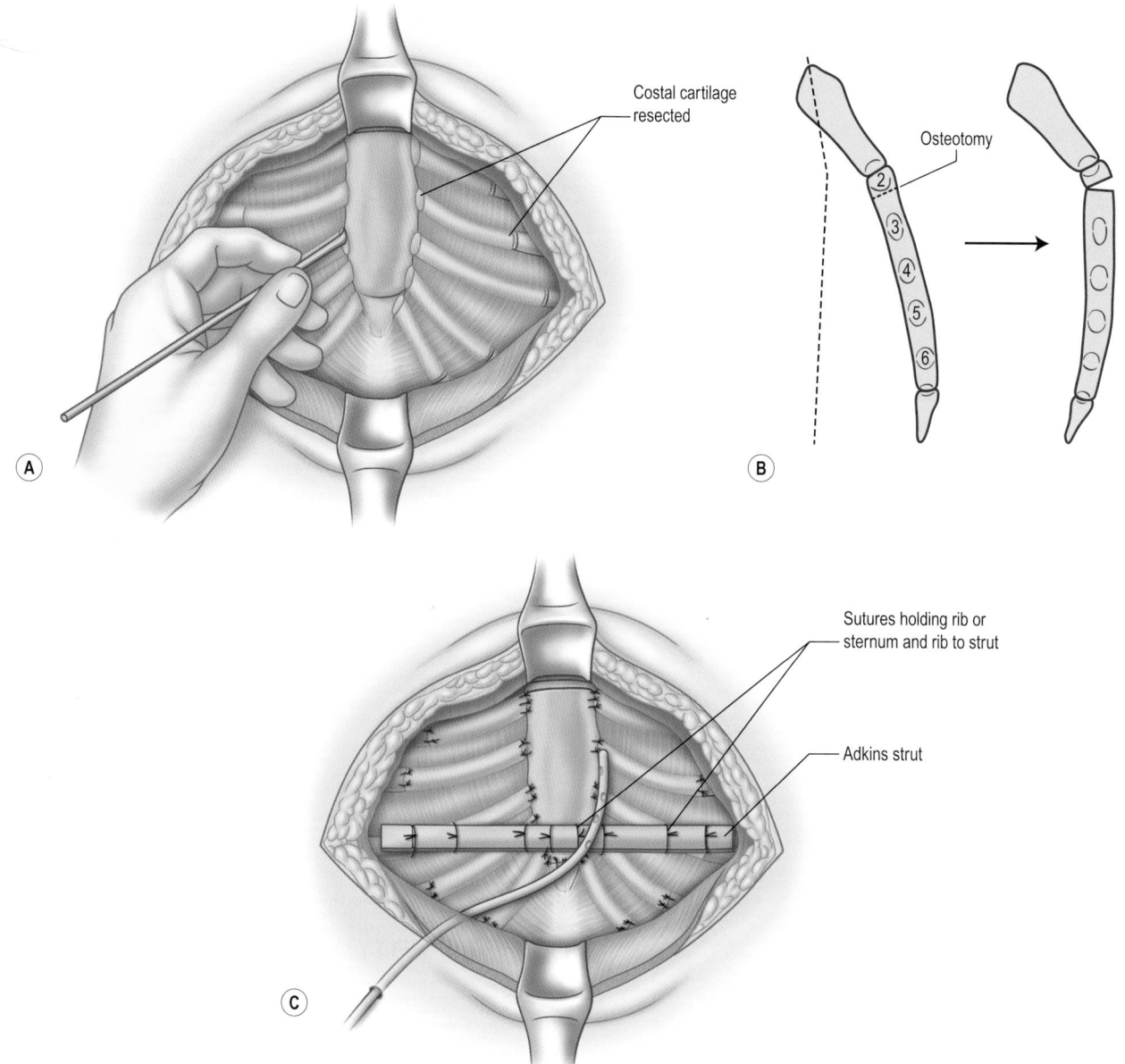

Fig. 41.7 For the modified Ravitch approach for pectus carinatum repair, a chevron incision is made inferior to the nipples and the pectoralis and rectus muscles are reflected to expose the sternum and costal cartilages. **(A)** A section of costal cartilage is resected with perichondrium. **(B)** Following costal cartilage resection, the anterior table of the sternum is osteotomized to reposition the sternum. Shown here are lateral diagrams of the osteotomy. **(C)** An Adkins strut with a normal anterior thoracic contour is then wired to ribs laterally. The repositioned sternum and medial costal cartilages are sutured to the strut. (Modified from Fonkalsrud EW, Anselmo DM. Less extensive technique for repair of pectus carinatum. *J Am Coll Surg* 2004;198:898 and Shamberger RC, Welch KH. Surgical correction of pectus carinatum. *J Pediatr Surg.* 1987;22:48–53.)

to the correct alignment[42] *(Fig. 41.7)*. For the asymmetric deformities, sternal positioning is corrected after costal cartilage resection with a wedge osteotomy. Recent refinements in this procedure include a method in which costal cartilages are resected through splitting the muscle along its fibers rather than elevating the entire muscle.[44] Nonsurgical means of correction using orthotics have been described in small case series with subjective improvement of carinatum.[45] However, the results do not have long-term follow-up and it is not clear that young patients can tolerate wearing a brace for extended periods of time.

Jeune's syndrome

Asphyxiating thoracic dystrophy, Jeune's syndrome, is a rare familial autosomal-recessive osteochondrodystrophy characterized by a narrow, immobile thorax and a protuberant abdomen[46] *(Fig. 41.8)*. Though the early descriptions were in neonates who succumbed to respiratory insufficiency, subsequent reports have demonstrated that Jeune's syndrome has a variable expression and may result in viability.[47] In patients who have less severe versions of Jeune's syndrome, renal failure occurs in adulthood.

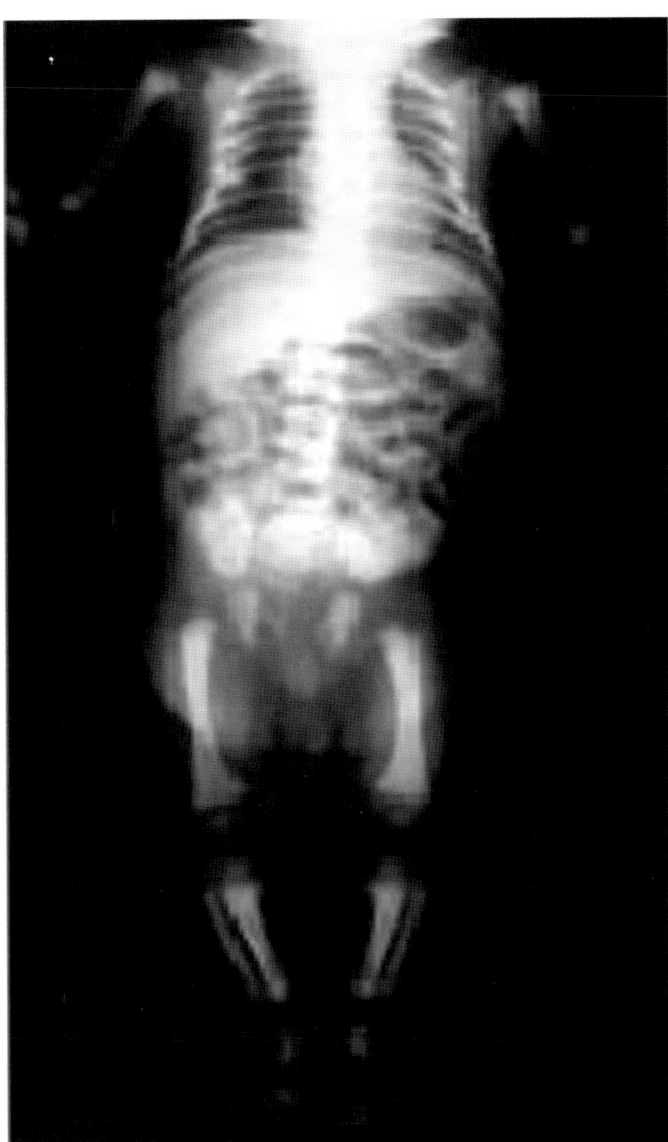

Fig. 41.8 Radiograph of a 3-month-old infant with Jeune's syndrome, asphyxiating thoracic dystrophy. Note the horizontal orientation of the ribs, the characteristic "bell-shaped" thorax, shorter lower limbs, and pelvic abnormalities. (Reproduced from Morgan NV, Bacchelli C, Gissen P, et al. A locus for asphyxiating thoracic dystrophy, ATD, maps to chromosome 15q13. *J Med Genet.* 2003;40:431–435.)

Clinical presentation and surgical indications

Jeune's syndrome can be variably expressed.[48] The neonate with severe Jeune's syndrome is generally described as having a narrow, bell-shaped thorax that is narrowed in both the transverse and sagittal dimensions with mild brachydactyly. The ribs are short, wide, and barely reach the anterior axillary line. Histologic examination of the costochondral junction reveals disordered endochondral ossification. These patients have severe restrictive lung disease and frequently require mechanical ventilation. In contrast, patients who have a moderate expression of Jeune's syndrome tend to have a narrow thorax without respiratory compromise, severe brachydactyly, and renal failure at a later age. These patients are usually identified upon presentation for renal transplantation or renal

replacement therapy. Finally, the mildest form of Jeune's syndrome may be manifested with only polydactyly and severe brachydactyly. Surgical correction is indicated in those patients undergoing respiratory compromise.

Treatment

Operative intervention in Jeune's syndrome is focused on expansion of the thoracic cavity. Two methods have emerged as successful options: median sternotomy and lateral thoracic expansion thoracoplasty. The median sternotomy technique usually requires addition of bone graft, stainless steel struts, or prosthetic spacers.[49–52] Alternatively, Davis and colleagues described a lateral thoracic expansion technique *(Fig. 41.9)*. In this procedure, ribs 4 through 9 are differentially transected, separated from periosteum, and different ribs are secured together in an expanded fashion with titanium plates.[53–55] The authors noted excellent results in patients over 1 year of age and new bone formation with this method. Waldhausen and colleagues report success with a technique using a vertical expandable prosthetic titanium rib thoracoplasty for the treatment of children with thoracic insufficiency syndrome. Two patients in their series had Jeune's syndrome.[56]

Ectopia cordis

Ectopia cordis represents a spectrum of four rare congenital deformities uniformly characterized by a midline sternal defect. The incidence of ectopia cordis is 0.8 per 100 000 live births and can vary from asymptomatic benign clefts to severe conditions with high mortality rates. Many cases can be diagnosed by prenatal ultrasound *(Fig. 41.10)*.

Clinical presentation and surgical indications

Multiple investigators have provided anatomic classifications of ectopia cordis. Cervical ectopia cordis is the most severe version with superior displacement of the heart and craniofacial deformities. Thoracic ectopia cordis describes the classic extrathoracic heart without soft tissue or bony covering. Thoracoabdominal ectopia cordis is a combination of both thoracic wall and abdominal wall defects *(Fig. 41.11)*. These defects are associated with Cantrell's pentalogy, which includes a midline supraumbilical defect, low sternal defect, anterior diaphragmatic defect, pericardial defect, and intracardiac anomalies.[57] Finally, bifid sternum is a relatively benign finding with a cleft upper sternum that rarely causes significant physiologic disturbance *(Fig. 41.12)*. Surgical correction is necessary in thoracic, thoracoabdominal, and cervical ectopia cordis with the initial goal of coverage of the heart followed by ultimately returning the heart to the thoracic cavity when patients have developed sufficient reserve. Coordinated multidisciplinary care involving obstetricians, neonatologists, critical care anesthesiologists, cardiothoracic surgeons, and plastic surgeons is critical to reduce mortality in these high-risk neonates.

Treatment

Thoracic and thoracoabdominal ectopia cordis repair is most successful when performed in a staged manner. The first step

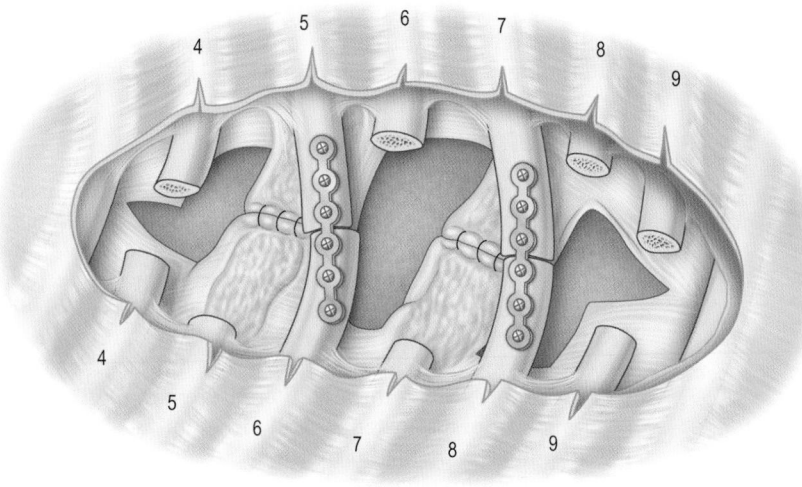

Fig. 41.9 Jeune's syndrome repair. The lateral thoracic expansion technique as described by Davis involves transection of ribs 5 through 9 and rigid fixation of alternate ribs. The thoracic cavity is expanded by increasing the amount of space between ribs. (Reproduced from Davis JT, Heistein JB, Castile RG, et al. Lateral thoracic expansion for Jeune's syndrome: midterm results. *Ann Thorac Surg.* 2001;72:872.)

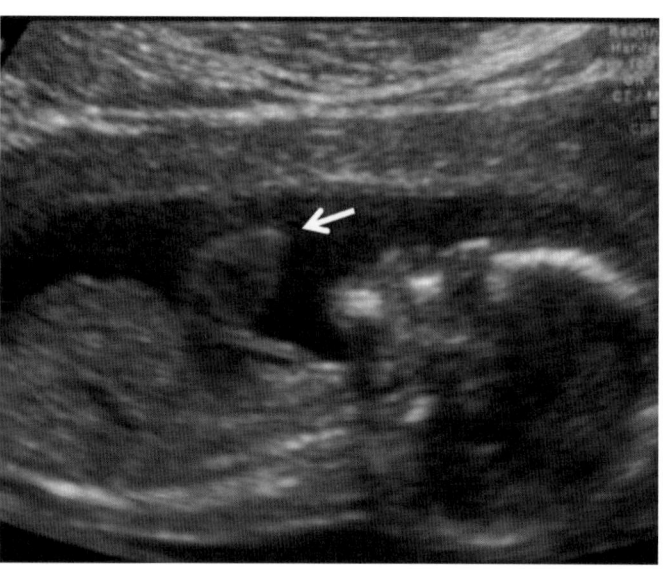

Fig. 41.10 Prenatal ultrasound diagnosis of ectopia cordis. Prenatal ultrasound of 32-week-old fetus demonstrating extrathoracic heart (arrow).

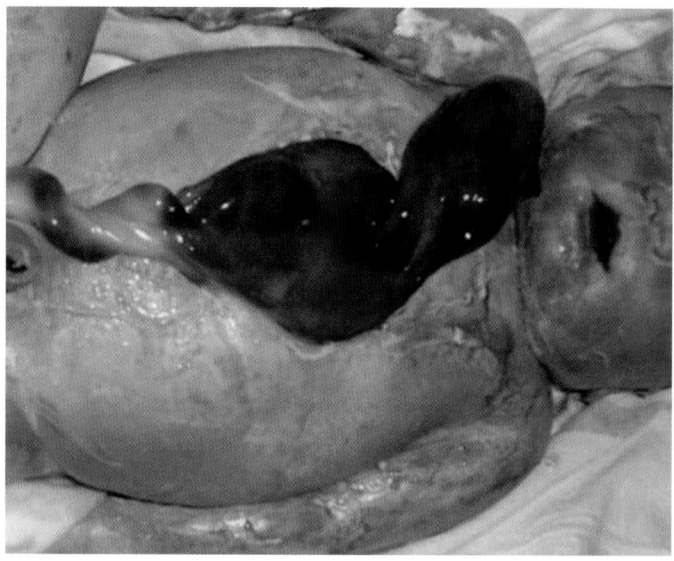

Fig. 41.11 Thoracoabdominal ectopia cordis. Same patient as **Figure 41.10** with ectopia cordis, midline supraumbilical defect, and low sternal defect.

is performed within the first several hours of life and involves coverage of the exposed heart with bilateral pectoral skin flaps, split-thickness skin grafts, or synthetic or biologic mesh. There should be no attempt at returning the heart to the thoracic cavity at this point due to the cardiopulmonary compromise that will occur with compression.[58] At several months to 2 years of age, the patient receives chest wall reconstruction and repositioning of the heart. Chest wall reconstruction can take the form of musculocutaneous flaps over autologous rib grafts as well as alloplastic custom-made struts.[59,60] Hochberg and colleagues[59] described a method of elevating the pectoral and rectus muscles as a unit and transposing bipedicled musculocutaneous flaps medially with relaxing incisions laterally. The resulting donor sites were skin-grafted on the lateral aspects of the patient. Outcomes for cervical, thoracic, and

thoracoabdominal ectopia cordis are poor. Most patients do not survive beyond the perioperative period.

Sternal clefts without an exposed heart are significantly less complicated. Surgical repair is usually performed within the first month of life. Bilateral pectoralis major muscle advancement flaps over rib grafts have yielded good cosmetic results.[61] Rigid fixation with titanium plates also has been reported.[62]

Poland's syndrome

Poland's syndrome is a rare disorder that is characterized by the unilateral absence of the sternal head of the pectoralis major muscle, breast hypoplasia or aplasia, absent or deformed ribs, axillary alopecia, and ipsilateral upper extremity shortening and brachysyndactyly.[63,64] Poland's syndrome has been reported to have an incidence around 1 to 30 000 live births, with males outnumbering females.[65] The etiology is unknown. One suggested mechanism for Poland's syndrome is subclavian artery insufficiency occurring around the sixth week of gestation with the right side affected twice as often as the left.

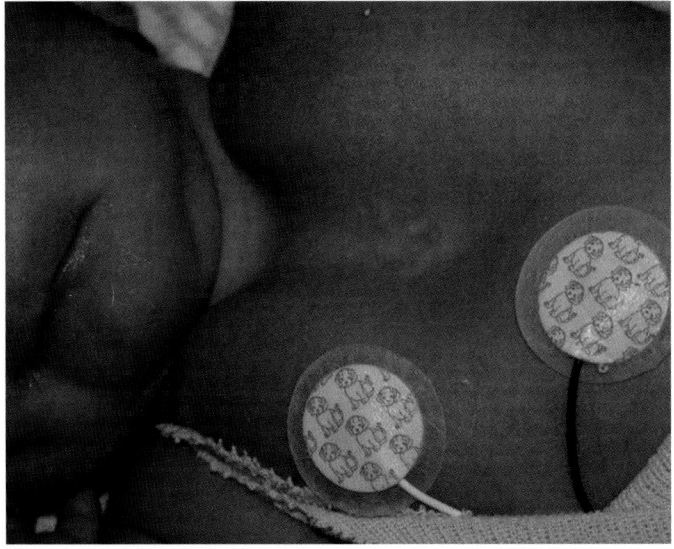

Fig. 41.12 Bifid sternum is a benign condition in the spectrum of ectopia cordis defects. Similar to more severe forms, a failure of sternum fusion is evident. However, the thoracic contents are positioned anatomically and there are no associated physiologic abnormalities.

Alternatively, unilateral developmental failure of the lateral plate mesoderm has also been proposed.

Clinical presentation and surgical indications

Pediatric patients with Poland's syndrome are heterogeneous. The pathognomonic feature is the absence of the sternal head of the pectoralis major muscle with anterior axillary fold deficiency *(Fig. 41.13)*. Varying degrees of chest wall and hand involvement may occur *(Fig. 41.14)*. In rare severe circumstances, depression deformities can occur with attenuation of ribs 2–5 with absence of anterior cartilage leading to paradoxical motion of the chest wall or lung herniation Some patients have a carinate deformity on the contralateral side. In one-third of patients, the breast is affected and can range from hypoplasia to complete absence. The latissimus dorsi muscle may be attenuated. Diagnosis of Poland's syndrome is possible by prenatal ultrasound but is usually best evaluated with postnatal physical exam.

Basic workup for Poland's syndrome begins with the postnatal physical exam. The trunk and upper extremities need to be examined in entirety with comparison to the contralateral side. The presence of the pectoralis major, serratus anterior, and latissimus dorsi should be confirmed by palpation. A standard chest radiograph is necessary to visualize the ribs. Computed tomography or magnetic resonance imaging with contrast may be helpful for surgical planning. The primary surgical indication for repair at a young age is ribcage aplasia,[66] resulting in cardiopulmonary compromise. At later ages, surgery is usually performed for concerns of contour abnormalities in both males and females.

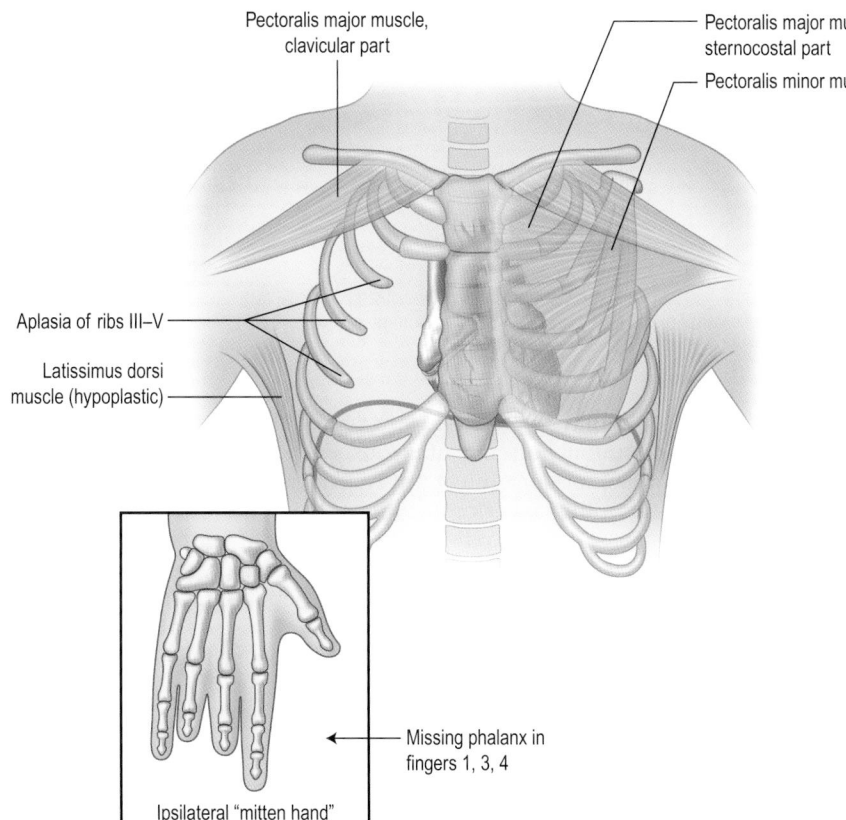

Pectoralis major muscle, clavicular part

Pectoralis major muscle, sternocostal part

Pectoralis minor muscle

Aplasia of ribs III–V

Latissimus dorsi muscle (hypoplastic)

Missing phalanx in fingers 1, 3, 4

Ipsilateral "mitten hand"

Fig. 41.13 Poland's syndrome is characterized by a unilateral absence of the sternal head of the pectoralis major muscle, breast hypoplasia or aplasia, absent or deformed ribs, axillary alopecia, and ipsilateral upper-extremity shortening and brachysyndactyly. (Reproduced from Fokin AA, Robicsek F. Poland syndrome revisited. *Ann Thorac Surg.* 2002:74:2218.)

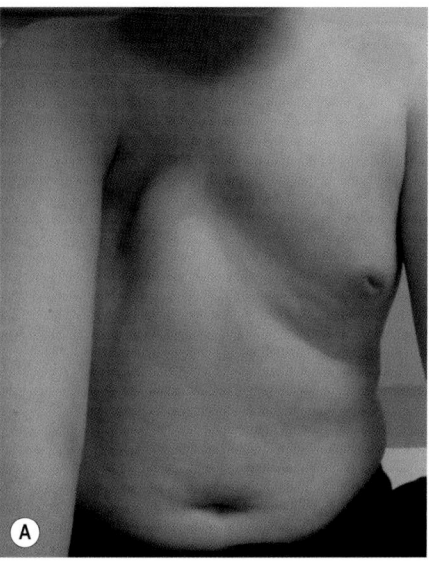 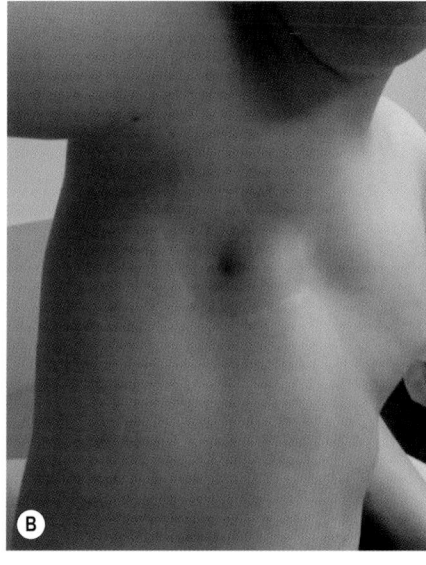 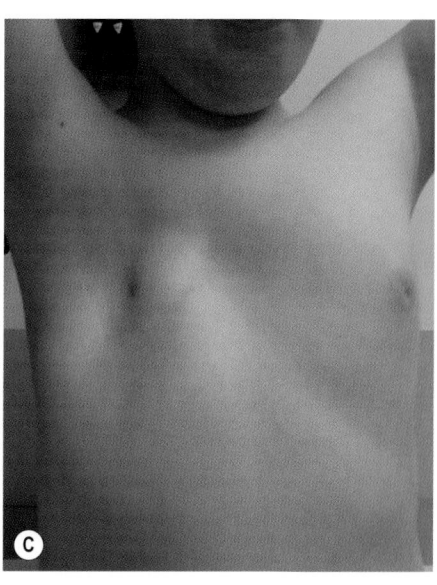

Fig. 41.14 Poland's syndrome is a rare disease with a male predominance. **(A)** A young boy with right-sided Poland's syndrome. **(B, C)** Note the presence of a hypoplastic nipple and the absence of the sternal head of the pectoralis major.

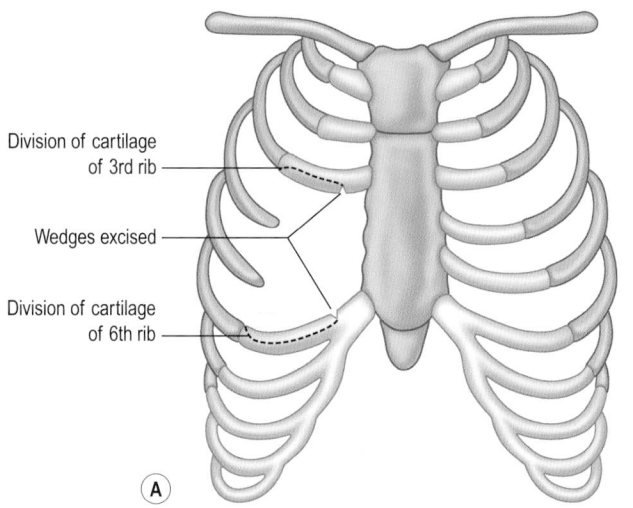 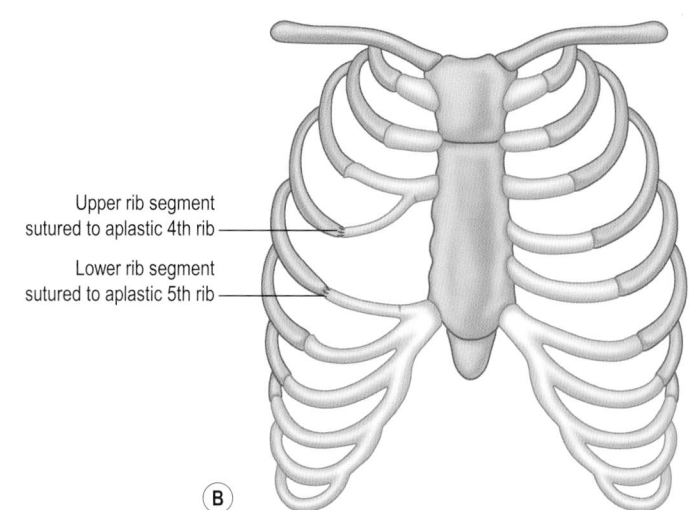

Fig. 41.15 (A, B) Split-rib graft repair for Poland's syndrome. Skeletal support in Poland's syndrome can be achieved by excising the existing superior and inferior costal cartilages, splitting the cartilages, and refixation to the abnormal ribs. (Reproduced from Fokin AA, Robicsek F. Poland syndrome revisited. *Ann Thorac Surg.* 2002:74:2218.)

Treatment

A heterogeneous spectrum of reconstructive options exists for correction of Poland syndrome. Mild forms of Poland's syndrome generally have a strictly soft-tissue deficiency. Similar to adult breast reconstruction, both silicone prostheses as well as autologous tissue reconstruction have been described. Custom prosthetic implants for chest wall deformities have a high incidence of displacement, erosion, discomfort, and edge visibility, especially in thin individuals.[67] Multiple groups have provided evidence that pedicled latissimus dorsi flaps with or without silicone implants can be accomplished with excellent results, improving chest wall contour in a staged fashion (56). Some groups have modified this method with the use of minimally invasive endoscopy to elevate the latissimus.[68,69] Free tissue transfer such as the transverse rectus abdominis musculocutaneous, deep inferior epigastric perforator, superior gluteal artery perforator (SGAP), and antero-lateral thigh perforator flaps have been used for breast reconstruction and soft-tissue camouflage/fill of contour defects.[70,71] Contralateral latissimus dorsi microneurovascular transfer has been described for functional replacement of the missing pectoralis muscle as well as reconstructing a more normal appearance to the anterior axillary fold when the ipsilateral latissimus dorsi muscle is attenuated or otherwise unusable.[72]

In more severe presentations of Poland's syndrome, bony support for chest wall reconstruction has traditionally been accomplished with autologous split-rib grafts *(Fig. 41.15)* or Marlex mesh *(Fig. 41.16)*.[73,74] Both techniques have met success;

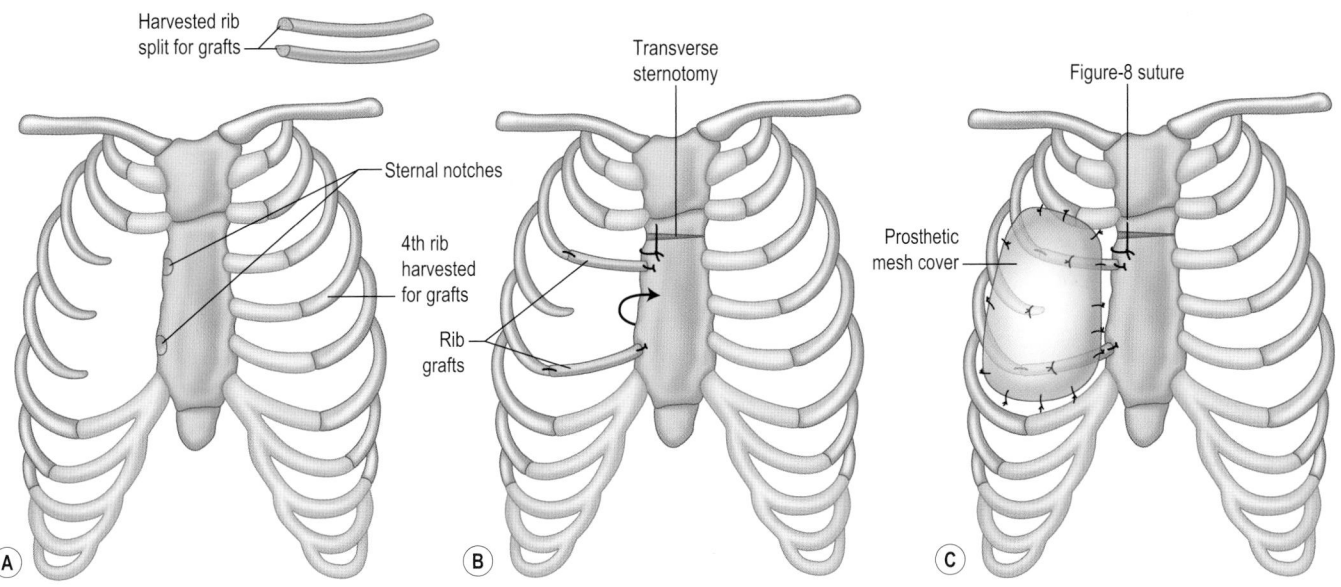

Fig. 41.16 (A–C) Mesh usage in Poland's syndrome repair. In additional to autologous split-rib grafts, Marlex mesh placed above the rib grafts serves to correct the skeletal contour deformity. However, the appearance of the thorax after either rib grafts alone or Marlex mesh over rib grafts is flattened. The contour deformity also requires addition of soft tissue or prostheses over the bony reconstruction. (Reproduced from Fokin AA, Robicsek F. Poland syndrome revisited. *Ann Thorac Surg*. 2002:74:2218.)

however, Marlex mesh placement tends to result in a flattened appearance and, therefore, tends to be performed in conjunction with latissimus dorsi flaps. Alternatively mesh prostheses with rib graft, molded silicone prostheses, as well as cryopreserved costal cartilage have been described with varying success.[13,75,76] Symmetry of the carinate deformity on the contralateral side may subsequently be corrected with a sternal osteotomy and rotation.

Abdominal wall defects

Omphalocele and gastroschisis

Omphalocele and gastroschisis are congenital abdominal wall defects occurring in 1 in 4000–7000 live births and 1 in 10 000 live births, respectively.[77] Omphaloceles have a tendency to be larger in size than gastroschisis and involve the herniation of bowel, liver, and other organs into the umbilical cord with amniotic sac covering. Gastroschisis differs from omphalocele in that the umbilical cord is intact and evisceration of the bowel occurs through a defect in the abdominal wall without amniotic sac covering. Males and females are equally affected. The genetic causes of omphalocele and gastoschisis are unknown but the two are thought to be different entities.

Clinical presentation and surgical indications

The abdominal wall defect in both omphalocele and gastroschisis ranges from 4 to 7 cm in diameter. Giant omphaloceles are defined as omphaloceles with a diameter greater than 5 cm.[78] Patients with omphalocele frequently have concurrent genetic disorders such as chromosomal abnormalities, Beckwith–Wiedemann syndrome, ectopia cordis, and OEIS (omphalocele, exstrophy of bladder, imperforate anus, and

spinal defect) sequence *(Fig. 41.17)*.[79] In contrast, an estimation of approximately 14% of gastroschisis is associated with unrelated genetic defects.[80]

Treatment

Reconstructive methods for omphalocele and gastroschisis are directly related to the size of the ventral abdominal wall defect and the magnitude of the intraabdominal "loss of domain" (LOD). Small defects can be closed primarily or with minimal undermining of surrounding soft tissues. Giant omphaloceles usually cannot be closed primarily due to lack of tissue or severe physiologic consequences from decreased venous return due to LOD. In gastroschisis, the lack of amniotic sac covering results in the exposure of a large surface area, therefore adequate fluid resuscitation along with early physiologic coverage is crucial to survival of the neonate. Complications from the defect or subsequent closure include pneumonia, bowel obstruction, ileus, sepsis, and necrotizing enterocolitis.

Nonsurgical treatment of large omphaloceles has been accomplished with sclerosing agents such as 0.25% Mercurochrome or 0.5% silver nitrate until surrounding tissues are sufficiently expanded for definitive closure. However, healing by secondary intent in omphaloceles runs the risk of infection and is therefore not an ideal solution.

Surgical closure techniques are frequently staged or delayed. In 1948, the first description of omphalocele closure with staged skin flaps was reported.[81] Although the closure was successful, the disadvantage of using skin alone was the resultant large ventral hernia. A more definitive closure would necessitate the reapproximation of fascia or the interposition of a synthetic or alloplastic material.

Reapproximation of fascia in large abdominal wall defects requires expansion of abdominal wall. Silastic silo placement is a widely used method simultaneously to "push" the

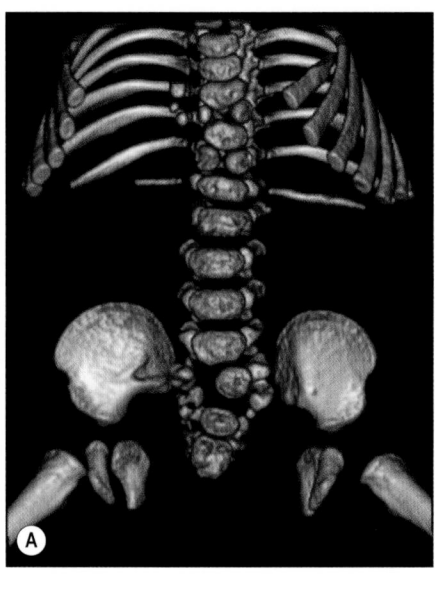
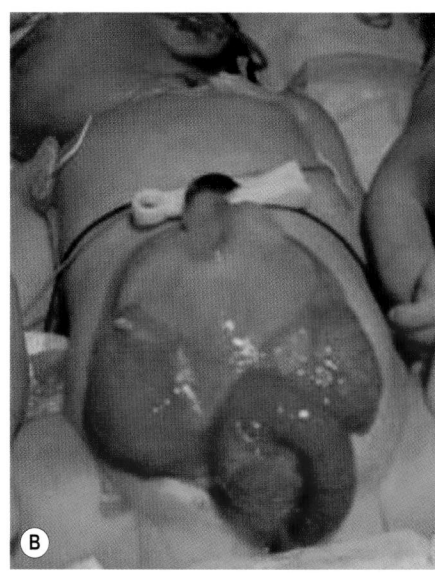
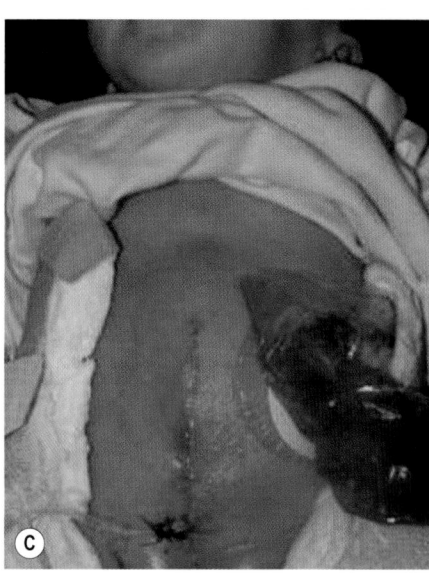

Fig. 41.17 (A) Three-dimensional reconstruction of computed tomography scan of neonate with omphalocele, exstrophy of bladder, imperforate anus, and spinal defect (OEIS). Note the wide pelvic separation of pubic symphysis and spinal defects. **(B)** Preoperative view of same neonate with OEIS demonstrating extensive abdominal wall defect. **(C)** Postoperative photograph of patient a few weeks after multistaged omphalocele repair, genitourinary reconstruction, abdominal closure, and orthopedic correction of pelvis.

abdominal contents back into the abdominal cavity, which then stretches the abdominal wall allowing for slow reversal of LOD and subsequent closure. Under sterile conditions, a silo is placed over the abdominal viscera with its edges secured to the fascial opening. The silo is slowly tightened postoperatively (allowing the abdominal cavity to accommodate to the increased volume slowly) until all of the viscera returns to the abdominal cavity. Silo rupture from the fascial edge due to the tension from reduction is a known complication. In the event of silo rupture, salvage by negative-pressure wound therapy directly on bowel contents has been described in a small case series as a bridge to definitive closure.[82] Intraperitoneal tissue expansion is an alternative method of abdominal wall expansion to treat LOD. In two reports, intraperitoneal tissue expansion was performed with an intrapelvic expander over the course of 3–5 weeks.[83,84] Both groups reported successful closure with low complication rates. Finally, the component separation technique has also been described in giant omphalocele closure. In 10 children with giant omphaloceles and a median age of 6.5 months, component separation was performed by incising the external oblique aponeurosis.[85] Unlike the previous techniques, closure was performed after a period of nonoperative therapy until complete re-epithelialization of the omphalocele. Complications in 3 patients included central line sepsis, midline skin necrosis, and hematoma.

Fascial substitution can be accomplished using prosthetic or bioprosthetic materials. The early reports of prosthetic implantation included a Teflon sheet attached to the peritoneum and a Marlex sheet to the anterior rectus sheath as a secondary procedure.[86] Bioprosthetic materials such as pericardial patches[87] and Alloderm have also been described in case reports.[88] Secondary procedures after abdominal closure are frequently required. In omphalocele patients, umbilicoplasty is performed either in an immediate or delayed fashion.[89,90] Bladder and cloacal exstrophy is often associated with omphalocele. Reconstruction of the urogenital system is addressed in another chapter in this text (vol. III, Chapter 44).

Posterior defects

Embryology

The neurectoderm begins as a single sheet of cells. At 4 weeks of gestation, the same time the body wall develops from the lateral plate mesoderm, neural plates emerge and migrate towards each other to form the neural tube.[91] Fusion occurs in an anterior to posterior direction and in a cephalad to caudad manner. Failure of anterior closure results in diastematomyelia and anterior meningocele. Failure of posterior closure results in the spina bifida spectrum.[92]

Spina bifida

Spina bifida is classified into three major groups. Spina bifida aperta is an open myelocele with no covering over the neural elements. Neurologic loss is present at birth. Spina bifida cystica encompasses meningoceles, meningomyeloceles, and syringomyeloceles. Meningoceles account for 14% of neural tube defects and usually occur in the lumbar spine. Meningoceles are defined by the herniation of meninges without cord elements. Meningomyeloceles occur at the conus medullaris and are characterized by a herniation of the meninges with spinal cord through the vertebrae. Meningomyelocele is the most common neural tube defect, accounting for 85% of all neural tube defects with a worldwide prevalence of 0.17–6.39 per 1000 live births.[93] It is frequently associated with motor and sensory deficits. Syringomyeloceles refer to a meningocele with a dilated central canal. Spina bifida occulta is the most benign neural tube defect with minimal clinical significance. Patients frequently present with dermal sinuses, a posterior hair patch, or lipoma but do not usually have neurologic symptoms.

Clinical presentation and evaluation

Patients with spina bifida cystica are frequently diagnosed with prenatal ultrasound and upon birth. Exposed cord in spina bifida cystica has a thin membranous meninges sac and needs to be prevented from desiccation with moist dressings to preserve neurologic function.

Evaluation of the neonate should begin with consultation by the neurosurgeon and the reconstructive surgeon for coverage of cord elements. Frequently, neural tube defects are accompanied by other defects such as limb deformities and neuropathic bladder requiring consultations to orthopedics and urology, respectively.

Surgical indications

Prior to the 1960s, meningomyelocele patients bore a mortality rate of approximately 65–75% within the first 6 months of life with rare survival to 6 years of age.[94,95] Since that time, early closure has been recognized to be essential to prevention of infection and is now considered standard of care. Successful closure within 24–48 hours of life has resulted in survival to approximately 85% at 3 months, 60–70% at 1 year, and 40–50% at 3 years.[96] Despite advances, patients continue to suffer from significant morbidity due to coexisting conditions such as hydrocephalus and tethered cord. On the other hand, meningoceles with adequate skin coverage can be deferred until 3 months of age. Bony defects in spina bifida are generally not addressed.

Treatment

As mentioned above, early physiologic closure of exposed spinal elements is essential. The primary goals are to protect cord elements, avoid infection and seal any cerebrospinal fluid leak. Soft-tissue closure over the dural repair, whether with muscle, skin grafts, or skin flaps, is important to maintain the integrity of the dural repair.

Historically, primary skin closure of meningomyeloceles accounted for approximately 75% of all repairs.[97] The remaining 25% of large meningomyelocele defects required other means of reconstruction *(Table 41.1)*. Sizable defects up to 20 cm² have been accomplished with modest skin undermining. De Brito Henriques *et al.* described obtaining primary closure in 15 of 16 patients with defects up to 64 cm² using acute intraoperative tissue expansion with an intermittent skin traction technique.[98] The disadvantage in this approach was the increase in operative time necessary to perform the intraoperative slow traction technique.

Variations of random-pattern skin flaps and fasciocutaneous flaps have been described by a number of investigators to prevent the skin edge necrosis common to primary closure. Adjacent tissue rearrangements, including rotation, transposition, advancement, Z-plasty, and Limberg flaps, have all been described using dermal vascular supply. Cruz and colleagues described a creative double Z rhomboid skin flap in which margins of skin were excised in the form of a rhombus with adjacent angles of 60° and 120°. Two sets of 60° equilateral

Z-plasty flaps were drawn on opposite sides of the defect by extending incisions from the 120° angles and transposed into the defect.[99] Despite the success of this report, local tissue rearrangements relying on random-pattern blood supply are generally not reliable for large defects. The amount of skin and subcutaneous tissue required for coverage is usually not well perfused without defined perforator or axial vascular supply, thus resulting in frequent wound breakdown.

Although random-pattern skin flaps are usually not reliable for large defects, the development of such flaps contributed to the design of geometric-pattern fasciocutaneous, musculocutaneous, and perforator-based flaps providing a more reliable tension-free skin closure technique *(Figs 41.18 and 41.19)*.

Doppler confirmation of perforators in the base of these flaps has been helpful in intraoperative planning. Three vascular perforator territories were identified by Iacobucci *et al.* during the description of bilateral superior and inferior fasciocutaneous transposition flaps.[100] Superolaterally, parascapular and scapular fascial branches of the circumflex scapular artery represent the dominant blood supply to the superior transposition flap. The vascular pattern of the middle third of the area originates from muscular perforators and lateral cutaneous branches of the costal groove segment of the lower intercostal arteries. The inferior flap receives contributions from the superficial circumflex iliac artery perforators. Permutations of this flap include the fasciocutaneous Z advancement rotation flap and a bilateral rotational transposition flap with curvilinear incisions.[101,102] Both of these flaps are robust flaps based on the preservation of the thoracolumbar fascia and the perforating vessels. The curvilinear advancement rotation flap has the added advantage of moving skin incisions such that they do not overlie the dural repair incision line.

One of the most common fasciocutaneous transposition techniques utilizes V-Y advancement from the flanks. Several modifications of this technique have been reported such as placing the apical extensions of the V incisions such that they are supplied by paraspinous perforators, preserving skin bridges at the superior and inferior aspects of the bilateral flaps,[103–105] and the design of crescentic-shaped flaps in our practice.

Several other fasciocutaneous flap designs reported in smaller numbers of studies include the large bilobed transposition, the rhomboid perforator, and the unequal Z-plasty.[106–109] Both the bilobed and the rhomboid flaps are elevated in the classical manner with careful attention to the incorporation of perforating vessels. Mutaf's unequal Z-plasty, however, has unique geometric criteria.[110] The advantage of this flap design is that, after transposition, the skin incisions are not overlying the dural repair but the excision of skin in the conversion to a triangular defect and the rather complicated design limit its utility.

The unilateral island SGAP flap was described by Duffy *et al.* for smaller defects averaging 4.8 × 6.8 cm².[111] Despite preservation of the perforator pedicle with a cuff of muscle, flaps in this were commonly plagued with venous congestion.

Though bony reconstruction is not thought to be required for meningomyelocele repairs, Mustarde proposed an innovative method of reconstructing a bony spinal canal under turnover paraspinal muscle flaps *(Fig. 41.20)*.[112] Following closure of the dura, the paraspinal muscles are incised and transverse

Table 41.1 Meningomyelocele repairs

Type	Method	Number of patients	Timing	Defect size (average or range)	Complications	Reference
Skin flap, muscle flap, skin graft	Skin flaps, reverse and advancement latissimus, STSG	Total: 74 Skin flap (37) Lateral flap (5) STSG (32)	Acute	Primary: 22.7 cm² STSG: 37.3 cm²	Primary: 41% flap necrosis, 13.5% CSF leak, 10.8% sepsis, 2.7% death STSG: 6.3% partial graft loss, 6.3% CSF leak, 3.1% sepsis, no deaths	122
Skin flap	Double Z rhomboid	10	Acute	4–23 cm²	Partial flap necrosis in 1 patient, CSF leak in 1 patient	99
Fasciocutaneous	Modified bipedicled VY	11	Acute	7–40 cm²	None	106
Fasciocutaneous	Bilateral rotation advancement	5	Acute	30–80 cm²	None	103
Fasciocutaneous	Bilateral rotation advancement	9	5 acute, 4 delayed	24–48 cm²	Skin necrosis in 1 patient	102
Fasciocutaneous	Triangular unequal Z-plasty	5	Acute and delayed	54–102 cm²	Hematoma in 1 patient	110
Fasciocutaneous	Bilobed	20	Acute	38.4 cm²	Partial flap loss with CSF leak in 1 patient	107
Fasciocutaneous	Bilobed	5	Acute	12.25–36 cm²	None	108
Fasciocutaneous	Z advancement rotation, bilateral	11	10 acute, 1 delayed	45–114 cm²	None	101
Fasciocutaneous	Rhomboid	1	Acute	42 cm²	None	109
Fasciocutaneous	Modified Limberg flap	4	Acute	16–68 cm²	Wound breakdown in 1 patient	129
Fasciocutaneous	Bipedicled flap	12	Acute	6–7 cm (width)	None	130
Musculocutaneous	Reverse latissimus island, unilateral	12	7 acute, 5 salvage	Unknown	2 patients with minor wound breakdown at medial aspect of donor site	92
Musculocutaneous	Latissimus transposition, STSG to secondary defect	2	Delayed	Unknown	None	131
Musculocutaneous	Proximally based latissimus island, bilateral	20	Delayed	6 ± 1.2 cm²	None	114
Musculocutaneous	Unilateral and bilateral latissimus (bipedicled, proximal, and reverse flow)	23	Acute	35–74.16 cm²	Wound dehiscence in 2 patients, distal flap necrosis in 2 patients	132

Table 41.1 Meningomyelocele repairs—cont'd

Type	Method	Number of patients	Timing	Defect size (average or range)	Complications	Reference
Musculocutaneous	Rhomboid latissimus transposition	30	Acute	Maximum 60 cm²	Unknown	133
Muscle and Musculocutaneous	Latissimus, gluteus with STSG	8	Acute	97.9 cm²	CSF leak until VP shunting in all cases	134
Musculocutaneous	Latissimus, VY advancement	1	Acute	117 cm²	None	135
Muscle	Reverse latissimus, unilateral with STSG over muscle	1	Acute primary repair, salvage	Unknown	None on salvage	115
Musculocutaneous	SGAP	6	Acute	32.64 cm²	Venous congestion common, epidermolysis in 1 patient	111
Musculocutaneous	Bilateral latissimus with gluteal fascia, relaxing incisions	19	Most acute, some delayed	20–50 cm²	None	118
Musculocutaneous	Latissimus and/or trapezius	82	Acute	Unknown	None	120
Musculocutaneous	Bilateral interconnected latissimus and gluteus maximus	9	Acute	42–80 cm²	None	121
Osteomusculocutaneous	Paraspinous muscle/bifid spine turnover ± STSG	Unknown	Acute	Unknown	Unknown	112
Osteomusculocutaneous	Latissimus, trapezius	6	Acute and salvage	Unknown	None	117

STSG, split-thickness skin graft; SGAP, superior gluteal artery perforator; CSF, cerebrospinal fluid; VP, ventriculoperitoneal.

processes are osteotomized. The paraspinal muscles are brought together in the midline and covered with a split-thickness skin graft.

Mustarde's paraspinous muscle advancement and turnover flaps have been found to be useful to others in providing a well-vascularized layer above the closed neuroplacode.[113] Skin closure can then be performed by skin graft, direct closure, or a variety of flaps. The particular advantage of paraspinous muscle flap closure is that it protects the dural repair should there be any overlying skin breakdown.

Muscle and musculocutaneous flaps frequently involve usage of the latissimus dorsi muscle. Unilateral proximally based latissimus flaps are most useful for higher lesions whereas reverse and island flaps can reach low lumbosacral defects.[92,114,115] However, many of these defects require bilateral muscle flaps,[116] as recognized first by Desprez et al.[117] The

authors documented 6 children, ranging from neonates to 2 years of age, with large meningomyeloceles that were closed with bilateral bipedicled advancement of the latissimus dorsi and trapezius muscles through lateral skin incisions. The muscles were transected laterally and advanced medially. Bifid spinous processes were osteotomized similar to Mustarde's technique of reconstructing the spinal canal. The lateral incisions were closed with V-Y advancement flaps. Moore and colleagues modified this technique with relaxing incisions along the lateral border of the latissimus in the posterior axillary line.[118] Dissection is carried out under the latissimus muscle with elevation of the thoracolumbar fascia in continuity with the superficial gluteal fascia. Intercostal and lumbosacral perforators are divided medially. The paraspinous fascia is incorporated to provide additional strength to the deep layer of the closure. While the authors reported no

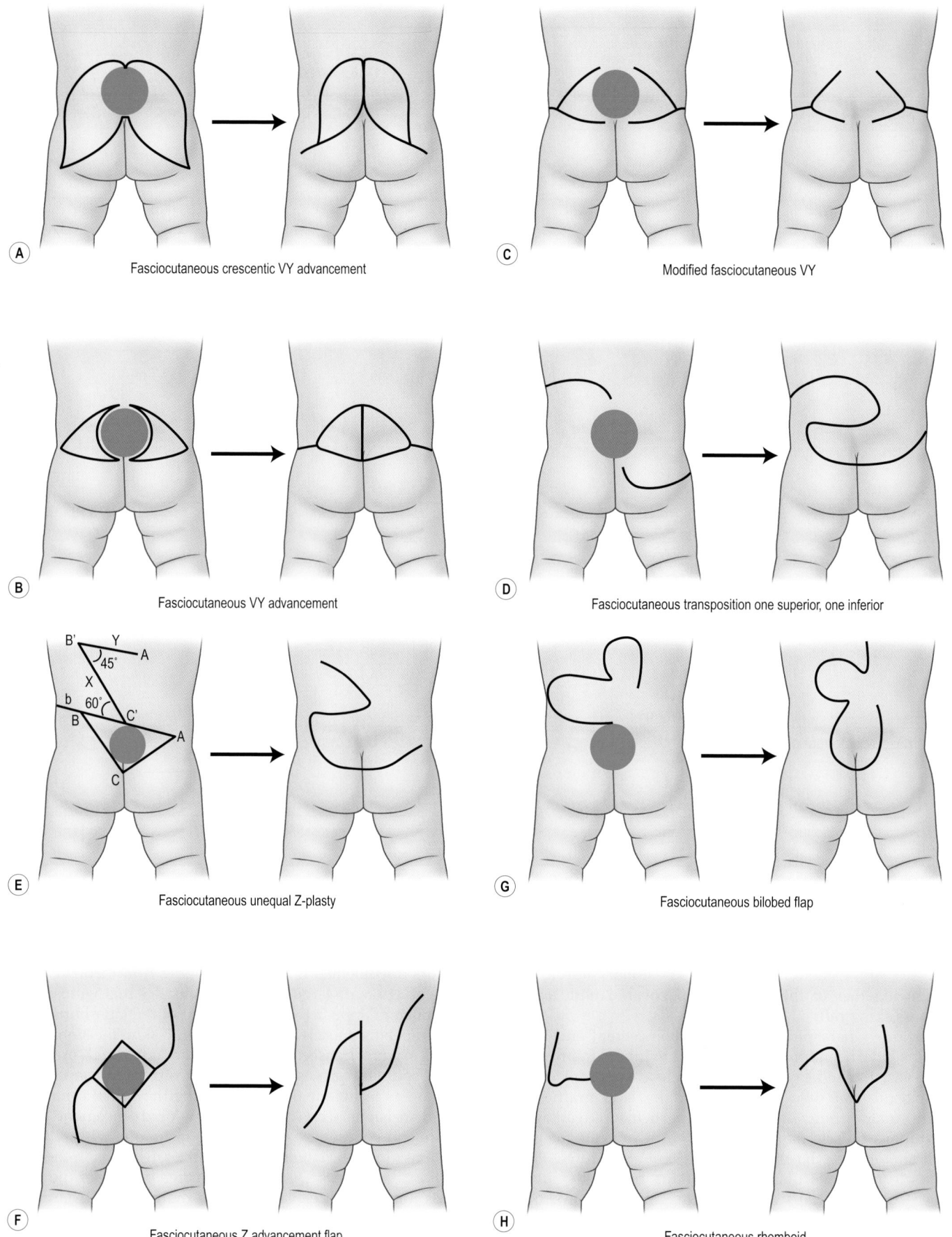

Fig. 41.18 Fasciocutaneous flaps in meningomyelocele repair. **(A)** Bilateral crescentic V-Y advancement. **(B)** Classic bilateral V-Y advancement. **(C)** Modified bipedicle V-Y advancement. **(D)** Superior and inferior rotational transposition. **(E)** Unequal Z-plasty. **(F)** Z advancement. **(G)** Bilobed transposition. **(H)** Rhomboid transposition.

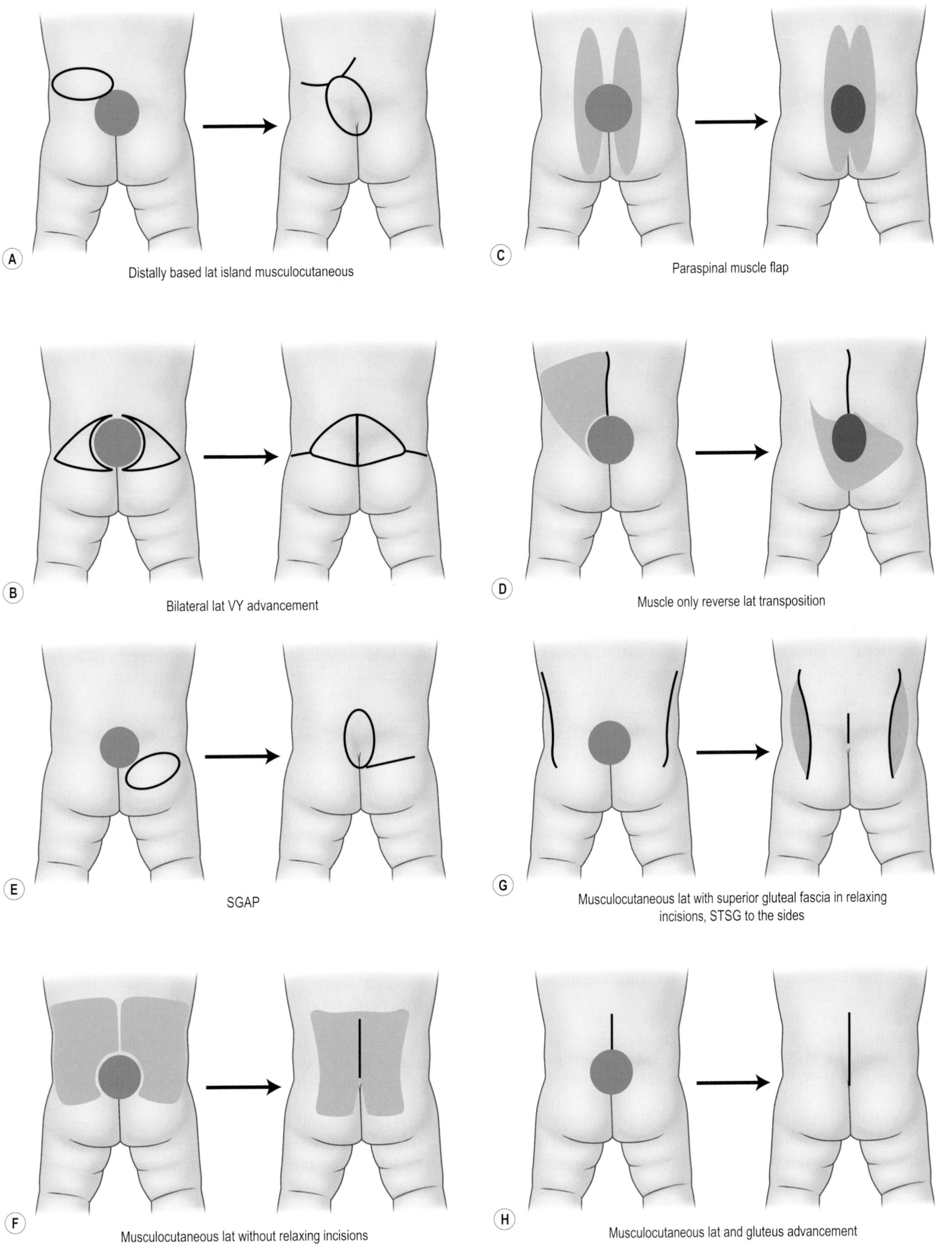
A
Distally based lat island musculocutaneous
C
Paraspinal muscle flap
B
Bilateral lat VY advancement
D
Muscle only reverse lat transposition
E
SGAP
G
Musculocutaneous lat with superior gluteal fascia in relaxing incisions, STSG to the sides
F
Musculocutaneous lat without relaxing incisions
H
Musculocutaneous lat and gluteus advancement

Fig. 41.19 Muscle and musculocutaneous flaps in meningomyelocele repair. **(A)** Distally based latissimus musculocutaneous advancement. **(B)** Bilateral latissimus V-Y musculocutaneous advancement. **(C)** Paraspinous muscle advancement or turnover. **(D)** Distally based latissimus turnover muscle flap with split-thickness skin graft coverage over flap. **(E)** Superior gluteal artery perforator (SGAP) interposition. **(F)** Bilateral latissimus musculocutaneous advancement. **(G)** Bilateral latissimus musculocutaneous advancement with lateral relaxing incisions covered with split-thickness skin grafts (STSG). **(H)** Bilateral latissimus and gluteus maximus interconnected musculocutaneous advancement.

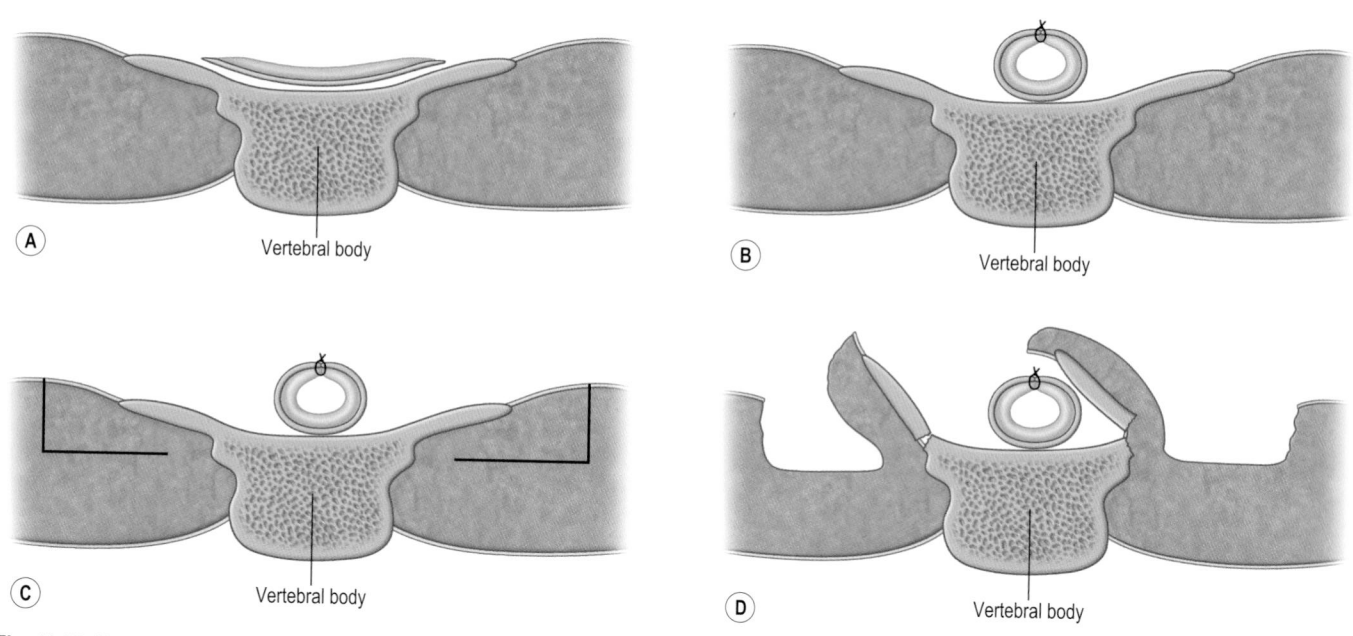

Fig. 41.20 (A–D) Mustarde osteomuscular flaps for spinal canal reconstruction. In 1968, Mustarde proposed the usage of bifid spinal processes in the reconstruction of the spinal canal. He argued that the skin cover alone was insufficient as a means of protecting the spinal cord. Following dural closure, the paraspinal muscles are incised laterally. The spinal processes are osteotomized and the paraspinal muscle flaps with the associated spinal processes are combined into turnover flaps. (Reproduced from Mustarde JC. Reconstruction of the spinal canal in severe spina bifida. *Plast Reconstr Surg.* 1968;42:109–114.)

complications from this series, the maximum defect they closed was 50 cm². The need for skin grafts in the relaxing incisions added scarring to the patient, making this technique less desirable. In contrast, McCraw *et al.* reported 82 patients who received a similar bilateral latissimus dorsi and trapezius musculocutaneous advancement flap without the need for relaxing incisions.[119,120]

A more extensive version of the bilateral latissimus musculocutaneous advancement was proposed by Ramirez and colleagues.[121] In 9 neonates with large thoracolumbar meningomyeloceles, the authors elevated the thoracolumbar fascia over the paraspinous muscles to the lateral border of the latissimus with perforator obliteration. The gluteus maximus is then deoriginated from the iliac crest and sacrum and dissected free from the gluteus medius. The entire unit, comprised of latissimus dorsi connected to gluteus maximus, is then advanced bilaterally without relaxing incisions and closed in the midline.

Skin grafting over dural closures was popularized by Luce and Walsh.[122] The authors retrospectively reviewed their experience of 74 neonates that included management by primary closure (*n* = 37), latissimus muscle flaps (*n* = 5), and split-thickness skin grafts (*n* = 32). The population of patients treated with wide skin flap undermining displayed significant wound-healing complications resulting in higher rates of cerebrospinal fluid leak, sepsis, and death. Despite success with latissimus flaps, the concern for blood loss led these authors to prefer closure with split-thickness skin grafts (either temporary xenograft or immediate autologous skin grafts). They noted that conversion to grafting decreased all immediate complications seen with primary closure and did not cause large-volume blood loss. Skin grafting, therefore, offers a simple way to obtain rapid coverage of dural repairs; however,

it lacks adequate soft tissue to protect the repair from trauma. In long-term follow-up, lumbosacral skin grafts did not have an increase in skin ulceration but thoracolumbar and thoracic patients covered with split-thickness skin grafts not only had an increased incidence of skin ulceration but also had an increased incidence of developing a gibbus deformity when compared to primary skin closure techniques.[123] The etiology of the gibbus deformity and the association with skin graft reconstruction of thoracolumbar and thoracic meningomyeloceles are not clear. Considering the results of this long-term follow-up study, skin grafts should only be used in the thoracolumbar and thoracic regions as a temporizing measure for immediate neonatal closure. Mustoe *et al.* reported the use of tissue expansion and delayed primary closure in older children who had poor-quality skin coverage over their spinal defects.[124]

Authors' preferred method

Meningomyeloceles display heterogeneity, therefore necessitating the need for a varied armamentarium of reconstructive options individualized to each patient, with the goal of providing reliable closure using well-vascularized tissue without tension *(Fig. 41.21)*. While many of the studies mentioned above refer to measurements, the size of the defect is less important then the relative amount of the uninvolved surrounding back skin *(Fig. 41.22)*.

Our primary goals are to protect cord elements, avoid infection, and seal any cerebrospinal fluid leak. With that, surgery within the first 24 hours of life is routine, performed by a multidisciplinary team of neurosurgeons and plastic surgeons. After closure of the spinal placode by the neurosurgeon *(Fig. 41.23)*, the plastic surgery team provides a

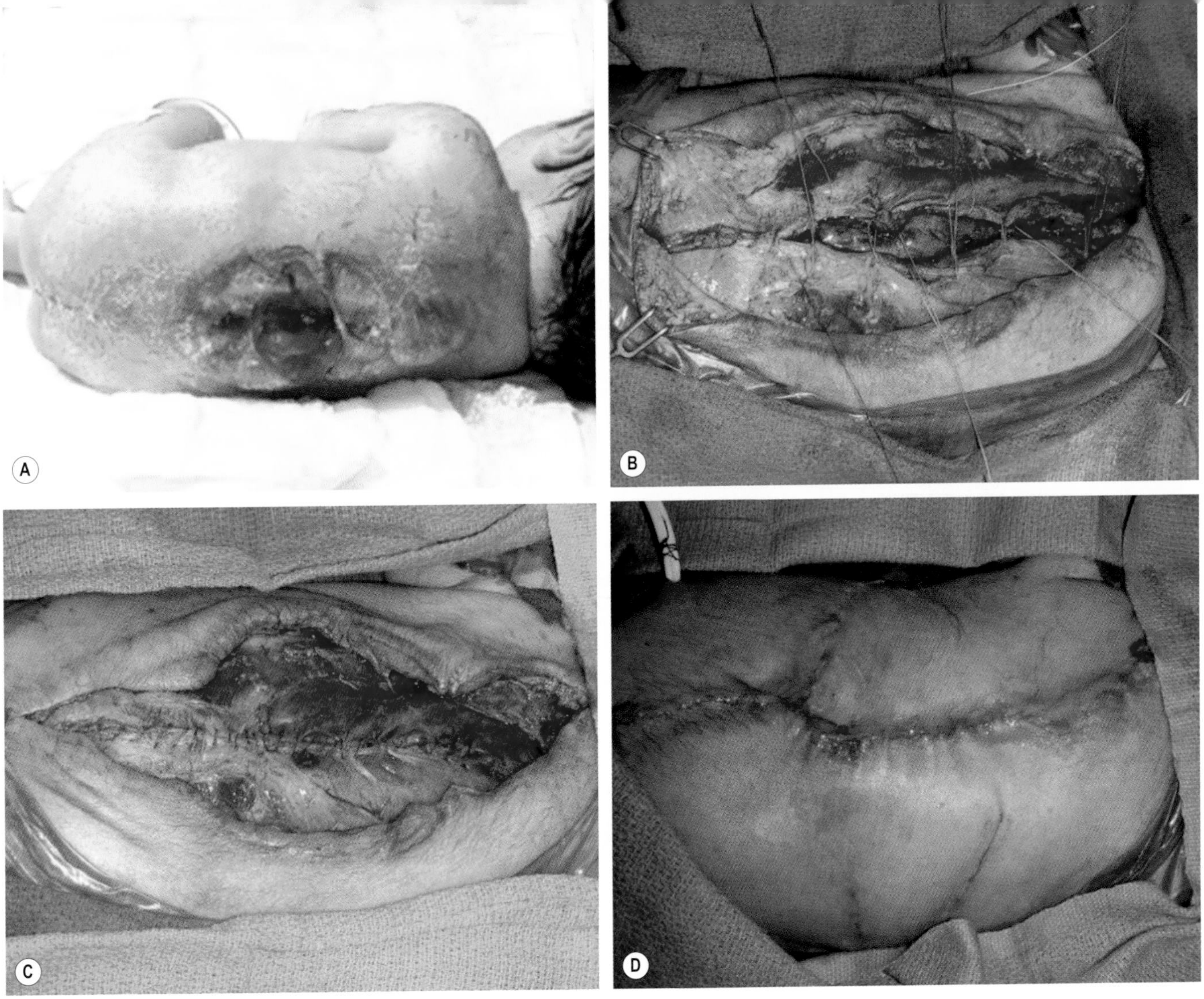

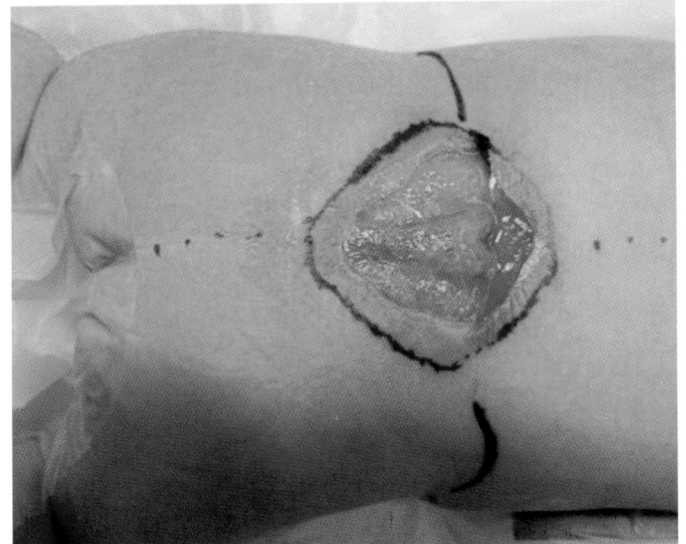
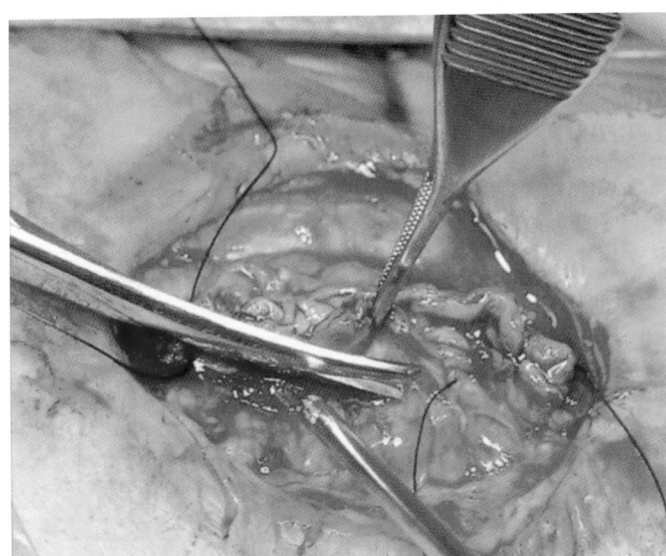

Fig. 41.21 Thoracolumbar meningomyelocoele involving most of the back. **(A)** Note the fine membrane covering most of the defect. **(B, C)** After neural tube repair and reinforcement with paraspinous muscles, gluteus, latissimus, and trapezius muscles advanced to midline with minimal undermining. **(D)** V-Y relaxing incision through skin and subcutaneous tissue to allow for tension-free midline closure.

Fig. 41.22 Lumbosacral meningomyelocele. There is clearly not enough skin lateral to the defect to allow for primary closure without tension. Location of iliac crests is marked, as is the midline (dotted line) and edge of compromised skin.

Fig. 41.23 Meningomyelocele. Neurosurgeons preparing to close the neural elements prior to any soft-tissue closure.

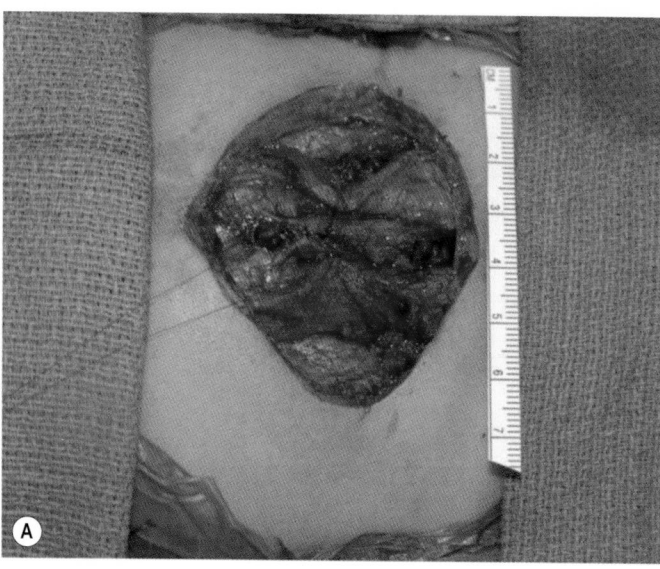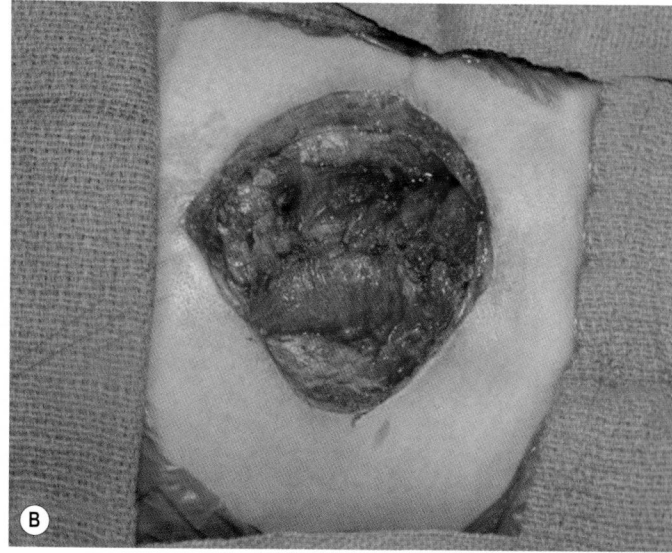

Fig. 41.24 Paraspinal muscle flaps. **(A)** Lateral edges of paraspinous muscles are incised and being advanced to ward midline. **(B)** Paraspinous muscle flap closure completed, providing a well-vascularized layer to protect the spinal closure beneath it.

multilayer, tension-free, well-vascularized definitive closure. The first layer above the neural closure is paraspinous turn-over flaps to help seal and protect the neural repair *(Fig. 41.24)*. Perforator-based crescent-shaped V-Y advancement/rotation flaps are then performed to provide well-vascularized tissue. This flap is designed so that the tail of the Y is oriented to where there is most skin laxity laterally. Its goal is to minimize skin tension in the midline. With a paucity of skin lateral to the defect, the crescent design of the V-Y allows for recruitment of tissue from the lateral buttock and thigh area. Flaps used to close lumbar sacral defects are based on gluteal perforators advancing and rotating the skin from inferior lateral to midline *(Fig. 41.25)*. Flaps used to close thoracolumbar defects are usually based on the paraspinal or latissimus perforators rotating the skin (with or without muscle) from superior lateral to midline, similar to the case report described by Sarifakioglu *et al.*[116]

Sacrococcygeal teratoma

Sacrococcygeal teratomas are the most common congenital tumors in the posterior trunk, with an incidence of 1 in 40 000 live births with a female predominance.[125] Teratomas are thought to originate from embryonic cell material derived from totipotent cells, thus organ parts are frequently found with elements or various different tissue types. Sacrococcygeal teratomas uniformly can undergo malignant transformation with increasing age and are therefore usually removed shortly after birth. When the tumors are excised during the neonatal period, the patients tend to recover well with rare incidence of malignancy and recurrence. Malignant tumors require adjuvant chemotherapy.

Clinical presentation and surgical indications

Patients are usually identified at birth with a midline round, cystic, or solid mass attached at the sacrum or coccyx.

Teratomas grow in the posterior and inferior direction with stretching of the muscles surrounding the tumor. Large tumors may cause difficulty in delivery. There is occasional intra-abdominal extension.

Treatment

Resection is usually performed shortly after birth when the neonate is deemed medically stable to undergo surgery. The resulting defect usually can be closed primarily with local tissue rearrangement. One case report of a giant sacrococcygeal teratoma resection with a resulting skin defect has required advancement of gluteal musculocutaneous flaps for closure.[126]

Other posterior malformations

Dermal sinus and postanal pits are congenital back lesions that rarely require extensive reconstruction.[127] Dermal sinuses are found in the midline back, between the occiput and the sacrum, and sometimes associated with an angioma. Infection of the sinus tract can result in recurrent meningitis.

Postanal pits occur over the coccyx and appear to track similar to pilonidal cysts. Asymptomatic pits pose no danger and can be observed. When infected, postanal pit resection usually only requires primary closure.

Neonates with tethered cord frequently present with a tuft of hair or an angiomatous lesion at the site of tethering. Neurosurgical repair is important for the prevention of future neurologic dysfunction. Skin is virtually always primarily closed.

Diastematomyelia presents similarly to tethered cord.[128] The spinal cord is divided with a median septum and patients tend to have focal neurologic deficits. Prognosis is excellent for such patients and primary closure is routine.

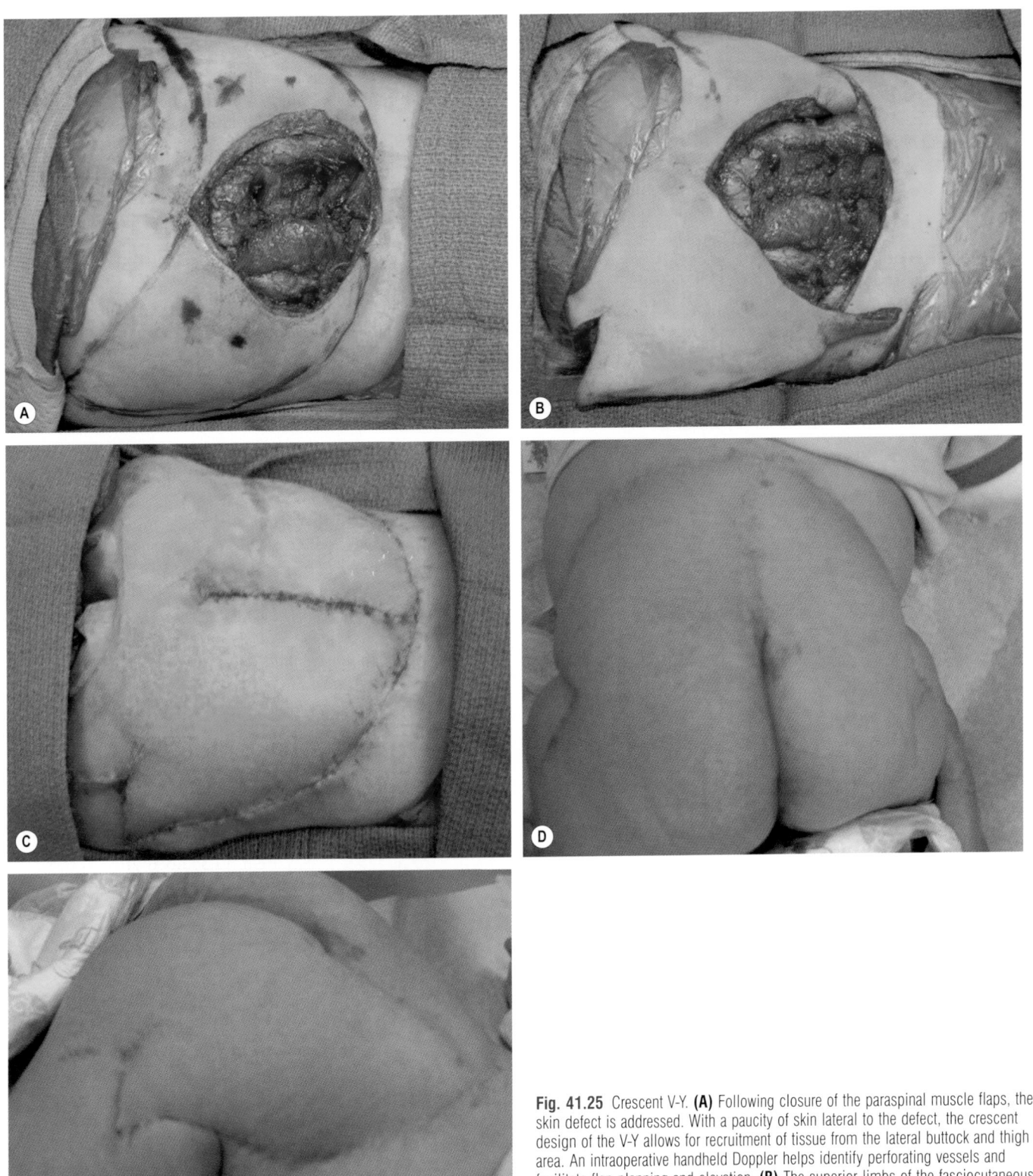

Fig. 41.25 Crescent V-Y. **(A)** Following closure of the paraspinal muscle flaps, the skin defect is addressed. With a paucity of skin lateral to the defect, the crescent design of the V-Y allows for recruitment of tissue from the lateral buttock and thigh area. An intraoperative handheld Doppler helps identify perforating vessels and facilitate flap planning and elevation. **(B)** The superior limbs of the fasciocutaneous crescent V-Y advancement flaps with V-Y back-cuts are incised and the flap is isolated on its main perforators. The inferior limbs are only completed (to islandize a true V-Y flap) if needed to release tension. **(C)** Skin closure accomplished without tension in the midline. V-Y back-cut converted to a Z to facilitate insetting of the lateral tip of the flap. **(D, E)** Incisions at 3 months postoperatively.

Access the complete references list online at **http://www.expertconsult.com**

3. Ravitch MM. The operative treatment of pectus excavatum. *Ann Surg.* 1949;129:429.

Ravitch presents the anatomical basis and physiological consequences of pectus excavatum in this classic paper. The indications for surgery are discussed at length and largely the same as current indications. Excellent diagrams of his procedure as well as case studies are shown.

6. Haller Jr JA, Kramer SS, Lietman SA. Use of CT scans in selection of patients for pectus excavatum surgery: a preliminary report. *J Pediatr Surg.* 1987;22:904–906.

37. Nuss D, Kelly Jr RE, Croitoru DP, et al. A 10-year review of a minimally invasive technique for the correction of pectus excavatum. *J Pediatr Surg.* 1998;33:545–552.

42. Shamberger RC, Welch KJ. Surgical correction of pectus carinatum. *J Pediatr Surg.* 1987;22:48–53.

The authors present their extensive experience on pectus carinatum correction. They discuss the evolution of their procedure and compare their study to other major series.

53. Davis JT, Heistein JB, Castile RG, et al. Lateral thoracic expansion for Jeune's syndrome: midterm results. *Ann Thorac Surg.* 2001;72:872–877; discussion 8.

59. Hochberg J, Ardenghy MF, Gustafson RA, et al. Repair of thoracoabdominal ectopia cordis with myocutaneous flaps and intraoperative tissue expansion. *Plast Reconstr Surg.* 1995;95:148–151.

73. Haller Jr JA, Colombani PM, Miller D, et al. Early reconstruction of Poland's syndrome using autologous rib grafts combined with a latissimus muscle flap. *J Pediatr Surg.* 1984;19:423–429.

Prior to this work, Poland's syndrome was corrected with a method of skeletal support along with synthetic mesh. This novel work introduces the usage of autologous tissue coverage over rib grafts and represents an important collaboration between pediatric and plastic surgery.

77. Weber TR, Au-Fliegner M, Downard CD, et al. Abdominal wall defects. *Curr Opin Pediatr.* 2002;14:491–497.

A comprehensive review of abdominal wall defects including anatomy, embryology, etiology, management, and advances in research is presented.

95. Laurence KM. Effect of early surgery for spina bifida cystica on survival and quality of life. *Lancet.* 1974;1:301–304.

122. Luce EA, Walsh J. Wound closure of the myelomeningocoele defect. *Plast Reconstr Surg.* 1985;75:389–393.

The authors' extensive experience with meningomyelocele reconstruction is reported. They discuss the complications encountered with wide undermining of skin flaps and the progression to muscle flaps and skin grafts.

42

Pediatric tumors

Sahil Kapur and Michael L. Bentz

SYNOPSIS

- Pediatric tumors are highly varied in origin, pathophysiology, and clinical presentation.
- These tumors can be highly malignant or benign masses with complex presentations and can be grouped and treated based on their growth characteristics and local complications.
- Pediatric masses can also be embryological tissue remnants or have their origin due to errors along the pathways of embryological development.
- These masses can commonly present as acute or chronic reactions to infections, leading to lymphadenopathy.

Introduction

Pediatric tumors are highly varied in origin, pathophysiology, and clinical presentation and therefore have different modes of treatment associated with them. This chapter presents tumors that are benign masses but have complex presentations, such as the neurofibromatosis group of tumors that have multiple systemic signs but can be grouped and treated based on their local craniofacial/ophthalmologic complications. Another spectrum of tumors, the juvenile aggressive fibromatosis group, are masses that originate from myofibroblastic tissue and can exhibit a highly aggressive growth pattern. Pediatric masses can also have their origin due to errors along the pathways of embryological development. Tumors such as dermoids present in a continuum of dermoids to encephaloceles. Fusion errors in development can lead to branchial arch pathology, and the presence of embryologic tissue remnants can lead to thyroglossal duct cysts. Pediatric tumors can also be highly malignant, such as the soft-tissue sarcoma group of tumors, including rhabdomyosarcomas, or can be benign masses that have potential for malignant transformation, such as pilomatrixomas. Finally, masses can be present as acute or chronic reactions to infections leading to lymphadenopathy.

This chapter attempts to present a spectrum of pathology which varies from chromosomal errors causing aggressively growing lesions, errors during embryogenesis leading to maldevelopment of tissue structures or remnant tissue, malignant transformation of various tissue types, and the effect of infectious pathology on normal tissue.

Neurofibromatosis

Synopsis

- Neurofibromatoses are a group of inherited disorders with established diagnostic criteria based on symptoms of presentation.
- Craniofacial presentation of this disease is classified based on surgical treatment options available.

Introduction

Neurofibromatoses are a set of inherited disorders comprising neurofibromatosis-1 (NF-1), NF-2, and schwannomatosis. All of these lead to the formation of benign nerve sheath tumors.[1]

Basic science/disease process

NF-1 is an autosomal-dominant disorder with complete penetrance and variable expression. Chromosome 17 is involved. The incidence is 1/3000, and the average age of children at the time of presentation is 7 years.[1–3]

NF-2 is a completely different entity from NF-1. It is much rarer, occurring with an incidence of 1/25000. It is associated with a gene mutation on chromosome 22 and is characterized by bilateral vestibular schwannomas and juvenile subcapsular lens opacity. Schwannomatosis, on the other hand, is even rarer, with an incidence of 1/40000. It is characterized by subcutaneous, peripheral nerve, and spinal schwannomas without vestibular schwannomas and ophthalmologic features of NF-2.

The discussion below pertains mainly to the treatment of various clinical features of NF-1.

Café-au-lait spots

Diagnosis/patient presentation

Café-au-lait spots are characterized as cutaneous, hyperpigmented lesions, typically 20–30 mm in diameter. They contain keratinocytes with increased macromelanosomes. Greater than six lesions are found in 90–99% of cases.[4,5]

Treatment/surgical technique

Surgery is rarely recommended. Laser treatment can be considered for cosmetic improvement.[6,7]

Lisch nodules

Diagnosis/patient presentation

Lisch nodules are dome-shaped, melanocytic hamartomas found on the surface of the iris.[4,5] They appear around age 10, and are present in nearly all people with NF-1 by age 20.

Treatment/surgical technique

No treatment is required.

Optic nerve gliomas

Diagnosis/patient presentation

Optic nerve gliomas are the most common central nervous system tumors in NF-1 patients. They occur in 15% of cases and are histologically identified as low-grade pilocytic astrocytomas.[4,5,8] They are relatively indolent and sometimes asymptomatic. If symptomatic, they can cause proptosis, squint, abnormal color vision, visual field loss, pupillary abnormalities, and hypothalamic dysfunction.[7]

Treatment/surgical technique

Treatment involves vincristine and cisplatinum.[9] Surgery is necessary if proptosis is present, and if there is a need to debulk extensive chiasmal gliomas.

Glomus tumors

Diagnosis/patient presentation

Glomus tumors are usually solitary lesions, but occur in multiples in individuals with NF-1. They present under fingernails with symptoms of cold sensitivity and increased localized tenderness.[10]

Treatment/surgical technique

Treatment is local excision.

Craniofacial manifestation

Diagnosis/patient presentation

In the craniofacial region, the orbitotemporal area is most commonly involved. Orbitotemporal neurofibromatosis-associated skeletal malformations and deformities include[11–17]:

- sphenoid wing hypoplasia, which leads to expansion of the middle cranial fossa into the posterior orbit and causes proptosis
- remodeling and/or decalcification of the posterior orbit
- supraorbital tumors, which cause defects of the orbital roof and lead to a downward and outward displacement of the globe
- thinning of the lateral and inferior orbital rims
- depression of the orbital floor and elevation of the orbital roof and supraorbital rim, which increases orbital volume
- dysplasia and downward dislocation of the zygoma
- progressive plexiform neurofibromatosis of the temporal area, which leads to continued enlargement of the eyelids, excessive mechanical ptosis, pulsating proptosis, eye pain, and epiphora.

Treatment/surgical technique

Treatment is based on Jackson's classification[11,14]:

- Article I. Class 1: significant soft-tissue involvement with minimal bone involvement and normal vision
  - Treatment involves debulking of the soft-tissue component of the tumor through an anterior, lateral, or anterolateral orbitotomy. If blepharoptosis is present, levator resection is performed.[16] In cases where only a partial resection is carried out, a technique of netting the remaining tissue using Teflon mesh has been proposed[18] *(Fig. 42.1)*.
- Article II. Class 2: soft-tissue and bone involvement with normal vision
  - Treatment involves an intracranial approach for tumor debulking and posterior orbital wall reconstruction.[16] After the tumor is debulked, the herniated temporal lobe is reduced and bone grafts, obtained from splitting the contralateral frontal bone, are used to reconstruct the posterior and superior orbital walls. Orbital volume is increased with osteotomies and the globe is elevated by raising the canthal ligaments and building the floor. A two-stage approach has been suggested in which the intracranial portion of tumor debulking and orbital reconstruction is completed in stage 1. A second-stage procedure is performed in which subcutaneous debulking, eyelid, face, and orbital reconstruction is completed[19] *(Fig. 42.2)*.
- Article III. Class 3: soft-tissue and bone involvement with blindness or an absent globe
  - Treatment involves debulking the tumor with exenteration. An orbital approach is used to reduce the herniated temporal lobe into the middle cranial fossa. The bony defect is covered with a split-rib/bone graft. The orbital volume is reduced and its position is adjusted with osteotomies and bone grafts. Finally, an orbital prosthesis is fitted.

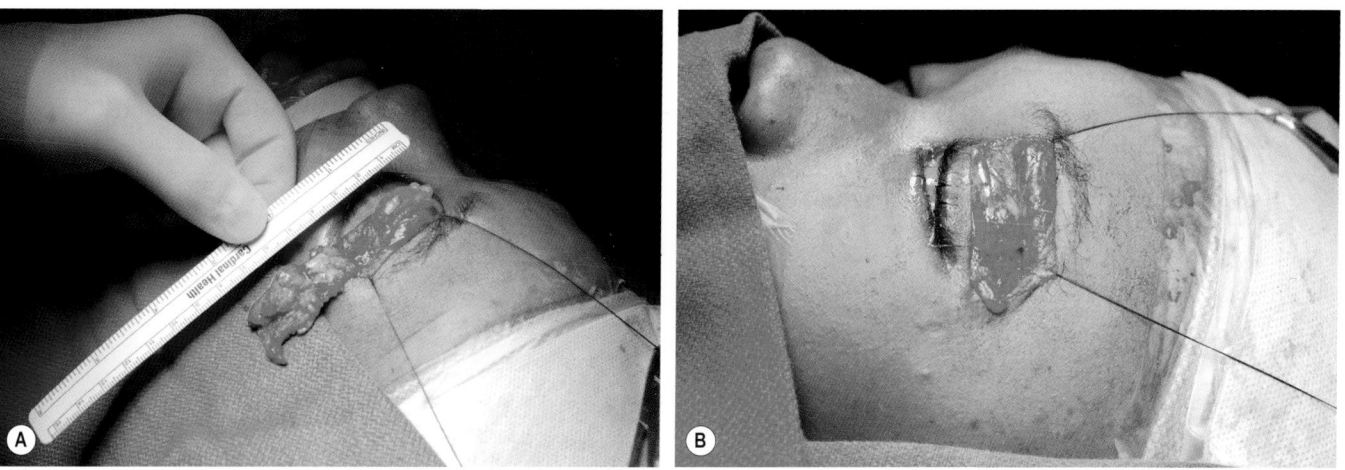

Fig. 42.1 (A, B) Anterior orbitotomy with debulking of left orbitotemporal neurofibromatosis. (Courtesy of Dr. Delora L. Mount.)

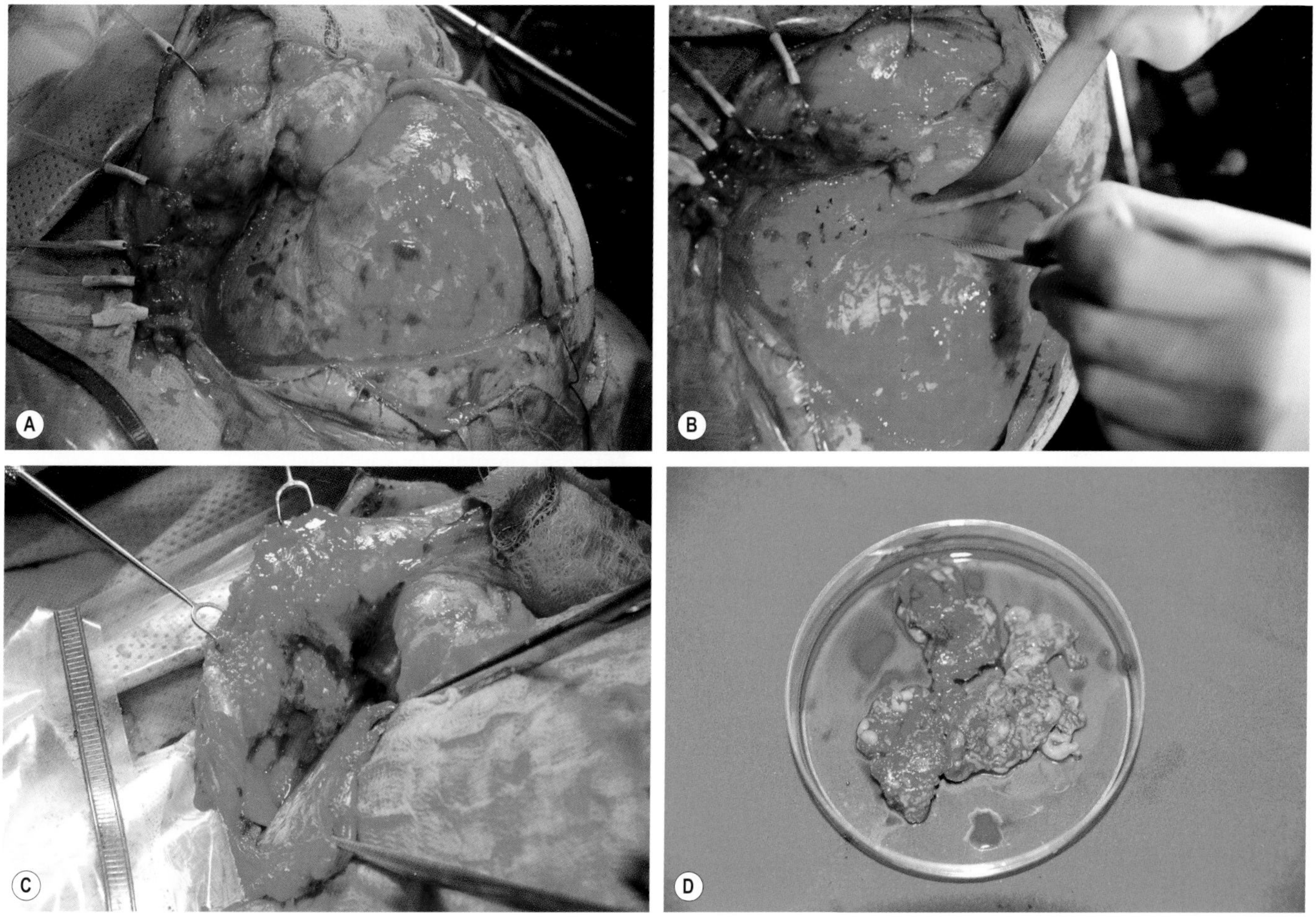

Fig. 42.2 (A) Stealth-guided left frontal craniotomy, orbital osteotomy, orbital roof/anterior clinoid resection, extradural orbitofrontal tumor dissection, and periorbital cranial reconstruction for craniofacial neurofibromatosis. **(B)** Stealth-guided left frontal craniotomy, orbital osteotomy, orbital roof/anterior clinoid resection, extradural orbitofrontal tumor dissection, and periorbital cranial reconstruction for craniofacial neurofibromatosis. **(C)** Stealth-guided left frontal craniotomy, orbital osteotomy, orbital roof/anterior clinoid resection, extradural orbitofrontal tumor dissection, and periorbital cranial reconstruction for craniofacial neurofibromatosis. **(D)** Specimen: neurofibroma lesion. (Courtesy of Dr. Delora L. Mount.)

Neurofibromas

Diagnosis/patient presentation

Nerve sheath tumors arise between the dorsal root ganglion and terminal nerve branches.[4,5,20] They are composed of Schwann cells, fibroblasts, mast cells, and perineural cells.[7,20,21] Localized cutaneous neurofibromas are the most common nerve sheath tumors. They present as multiple slow-growing, pedunculated lesions that progressively increase in prominence.[7] These lesions can be surgically excised for symptomatic benefit. This, however, may lead to hypertrophic scarring. The benefits of carbon dioxide laser treatment have not been clearly established. Diffuse cutaneous neurofibromas present as a plaque-like thickening of the dermis and subcutaneous tissue, and are most frequently found in the head and neck region. These are nondestructive, soft, compressible lesions that grow along the fibrous septa in children and young adults. Removal of these subcutaneous lesions may lead to neurological deficits in the region of the concerned nerve. Localized intraneural fibromas are the second most frequent type of neurofibroma, and represent fusiform enlargement of peripheral nerves. These are the most common neurofibromas of the upper extremity, and account for 85% of cases.[22] Spinal and cranial nerves may also be involved. Massive soft-tissue neurofibromas (elephantiasis neurofibromatosa) lead to distortion of the face and require complete excision.[23] Plexiform neurofibromas are composed of nerve sheath cells proliferating along the length of the nerve and are associated with hypertrophy of the overlying soft tissue, hyperpigmentation, and hypertrichosis of the overlying skin. Plexiform neurofibromas occur in 16–40% of patients with NF. These lesions involve the trunk (43–44%), extremities (15–38%), and head and neck (18–42%).[20] They are congenital in origin and become evident by 2 years of age. Plexiform neurofibromas are locally destructive lesions that grow during periods of hormonal change, and may involve multiple nerve branches and plexi.[24]

Treatment/surgical technique

Preoperative contrast-enhanced computed tomography (CT), magnetic resonance imaging (MRI), angiography, and embolization have been recommended.[20,21,22,25] The highly vascular nature of these lesions makes surgical removal complicated.[24] Multiple nonsurgical management options, such as farnesyl transferase inhibitors, antiangiogenesis drugs, and fibroblast inhibitors, are being explored.[26] Tumors resected in children below the age of 10 years recur in 60% of cases, while those resected above the age of 10 years recur in 30% of cases.[27]

Malignant degeneration of peripheral nerve sheath tumors

Diagnosis/patient presentation

There is an 8–13% lifetime risk for these tumors to undergo malignant degeneration. This occurs predominantly between the ages of 20 and 35.[4,7] Medium and large nerves of the thigh, buttock, brachial plexus, and paraspinous areas are involved. Signs of malignant degeneration include increased pain, new neurological deficits, sphincter disturbance, rapid increase in the size of the neurofibroma, or change in texture.[28] Fluorodeoxyglucose positron emission tomography helps with the quantification of glucose metabolism in the cells, and can help distinguish between benign and malignant lesions.[29,30]

Treatment/surgical technique

Prompt surgical intervention is necessary, which consists of debulking and nerve grafting. Complete removal with tumor-free margins is necessary. Adjuvant radiotherapy for tumors larger than 5 cm, high-grade lesions, or incompletely excised tumors is recommended.[7,28]

Malignant schwannomas (neurofibrosarcomas)

Diagnosis/patient presentation

Neurofibrosarcomas can involve either the cervical vagus nerve or the sympathetic chain and present as parapharyngeal masses, with paresthesia, pain, and muscle weakness.[31] They may also be of parotid origin. Children with NF-1 are at increased risk for developing these lesions.[32]

Treatment/surgical technique

Surgery is the primary treatment modality. Adjuvant chemotherapy and radiation may be indicated. Local recurrence and lung metastases are common.[33]

Juvenile aggressive fibromatosis

Synopsis

- Fibroblastic or myofibroblastic neoplasms are locally aggressive lesions.
- Different presentations include:
  - fibromatosis colli
  - congenital solitary or generalized fibromatosis
  - infantile digital fibroma
  - gingival fibromatosis
  - juvenile nasopharyngeal angiofibroma.

Basic science/disease process

Fibroblastic or myofibroblastic neoplasms are locally aggressive lesions. The average age of onset is the third decade of life. These tumors, however, may also occur during the first month of life. About 5% of cases are found in the hand.[34]

Fibromatosis colli

Diagnosis/patient presentation

Fibromatosis colli presents as solitary tumors of the sternocleidomastoid muscles (SCM) and are the most common cause of neonatal torticollis. The tumors are first seen between 3 and 4 weeks of age. They develop in the lower portion of the SCM and may involve both sternal and clavicular heads of the muscle. The diagnosis is made through fine-needle aspiration that yields fibroblasts, degenerative atrophic skeletal muscle cells, and numerous giant muscle cells. Natural regression of the tumor is seen during the first 6 months of life. Torticollis is associated with fibromatosis colli in 23–33% of patients and may continue after treatment in 17% of patients because of progressive fibrous replacement of the muscle tissue.[35]

Treatment/surgical technique

Surgery involves releasing both heads of the SCM through a limited transverse incision. The clavicular head is readvanced and attached to the sternal head to lengthen the muscle and preserve the anatomic landmarks of the sternal column. Surgery is performed on patients in whom torticollis persists for 1 year.[36]

Congenital fibromatosis

Diagnosis/patient presentation

Congenital fibromatosis can present in a solitary or generalized form. Solitary lesions can be seen as well-demarcated, firm, palpable masses (<3 mm) in skin, subcutaneous tissue, and muscle or as hyperlucent masses in bone. These lesions are usually present at birth, but additional lesions may develop later.

Treatment/surgical technique

Treatment is surgical resection. The rate of recurrence is about 32%.[37]

Infantile digital fibroma

Diagnosis/patient presentation

These generally appear as single or multiple gelatinous or firm nodules on fingers or toes. They are rare and are seen in both males and females. They are generally harmless but are removed because of the discomfort they cause by rubbing on footwear. The diagnosis can be confirmed with a skin biopsy that shows spindle-shaped cells and collagen fibers in the dermis. A radiograph is usually taken to determine the extent of the lesion (Fig. 42.3).

Treatment/surgical technique

Surgical procedure is relatively simple and calls for shaving off the lump. Recurrence rate after surgery is high.

Outcomes, prognosis, and complications

A conservative approach can also be undertaken because many fibromas can resorb and disappear by themselves over 2–3 years.

Gingival fibroma

Diagnosis/patient presentation

Gingival fibromas are common lesions of the oral cavity caused by chronic irritation that leads to connective tissue

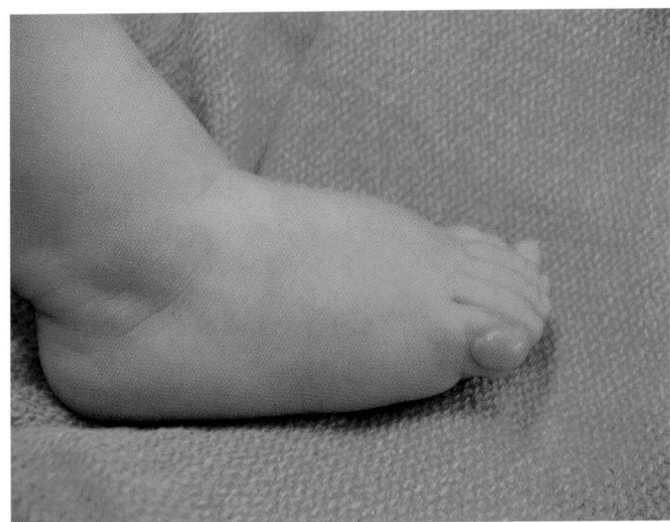

Fig. 42.3 Infantile digital fibroma. (Courtesy of Dr. Michael L. Bentz.)

hyperplasia. They occur on any oral mucosal surface, including the tongue, palate, cheek, and lip. The lesions are pale, smooth and firm, with sessile or pedunculated bases, and are usually less than 1 cm in diameter.

Treatment/surgical technique

Treatment is surgical excision. Recurrence is rare if the source of irritation is removed.

Juvenile nasopharyngeal angiofibroma

Diagnosis/patient presentation

Juvenile nasopharyngeal angiofibromas are benign, locally aggressive, vascular lesions, typically found in adolescent males between the ages of 10 and 17. They originate in the posterolateral nasopharynx, near the sphenopalatine foramen, and present with nasal obstruction and epistaxis. About 66% of patients present with local disease and 20% have intracranial invasion. CT scans show widening of the pterygopalatine fossa and the pterygomaxillary fissure. MRI is used to delineate the soft-tissue invasion, while angiography helps determine the vascular supply. Given the highly vascular nature of these tumors, biopsy should not be attempted.

Treatment/surgical technique

Treatment involves embolization followed by surgery. A transpalatal, transfacial, midface degloving approach or Le Fort I osteotomy approach can be used. An anterior subcranial approach is used for transcranial lesions.[38–40]

Outcomes, prognosis, and complications

The recurrence rate is 73%, but can be as high as 90% with positive margins. Recurrence usually occurs within 3 months of excision.[34]

Dermoids

Synopsis

- They are present from birth and consist of both ectoderm and endoderm.
- Dermoids commonly arise in the head and neck. They can grow large to compress adjacent structures.
- Different types include: nasal dermoids, intradural dermoids, extraangular dermoids, and dermoid cysts of the neck.

Introduction

Dermoids are present from birth, and form due to embryonic inclusion of germ cells between fusing tissue layers. They commonly arise in the head and neck.

Nasal dermoids

Basic science/disease process

Between the third and eighth week of embryogenesis, when the neural groove deepens to form the neural tube, incomplete sequestration of the neuroectoderm from the somatic ectoderm leads to a persistent connection of the foramen cecum with the fonticulus nasofrontalis, and the foramen cecum with the prenasal space. These connections cause the formation of nasal dermoids, dermal sinuses, gliomas, and encephaloceles.[41] Nasal dermoids can be present at any point between the glabella and the base of the columella. Intracranial extension can exist via the tract through the nasal septum and foramen cecum, or through the widened frontonasal suture (fonticulus nasofrontalis) and foramen cecum. In these cases, the presence of the dermoid between the leaves of falx and a bifid crista galli are noted *(Fig. 42.4)*.

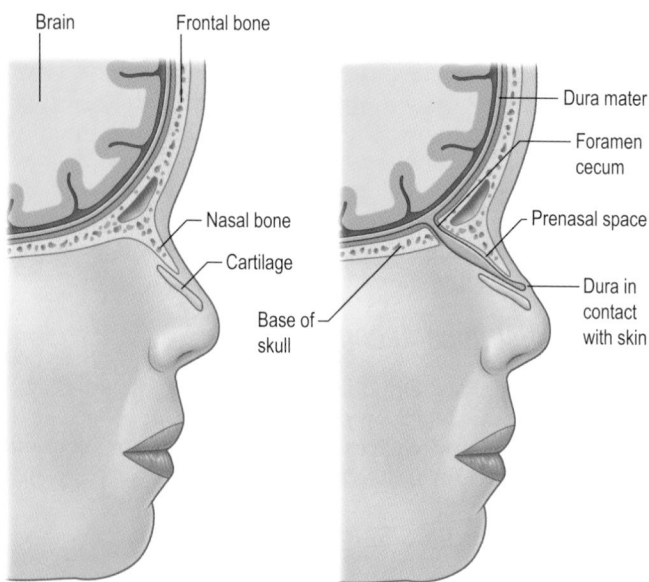

Fig. 42.4 Dermoid embryology.

Diagnosis/patient presentation

Dermoids present as firm, cystic lesions, or infected persistent abscesses. They expand slowly and cause destruction of the nasal bones and widening of the nasal ridge. MRI can help differentiate between normal anatomic variants of the anterior cranial base versus the intracranial extension of dermal sinus tracts. CT scans can help delineate the bony anatomy of the nose and the cranial base, and help in operative planning with the use of three-dimensional reconstruction.[42,43]

Treatment/surgical technique

Dermoid cysts or sinuses that are present at the columella usually extend to the nasal spine. Resection involves a circumscribed removal of the sinus tract. If a cyst is associated with it, it is dissected through the labial sulcus. Sinuses and cysts that are present from the radix to the nasal tip, but are without intracranial extension, are excised in combination with an open rhinoplasty approach. This approach has been reported to have improved exposure of the osteotomies, the upper lateral cartilages, and the septum[44] *(Fig. 42.5)*. A closed

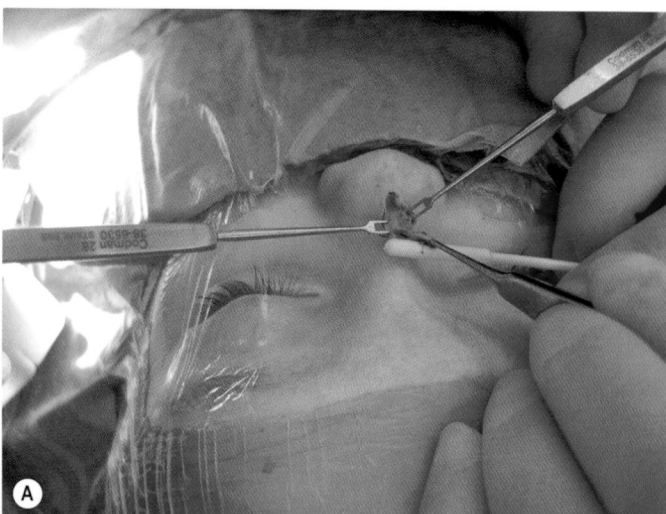

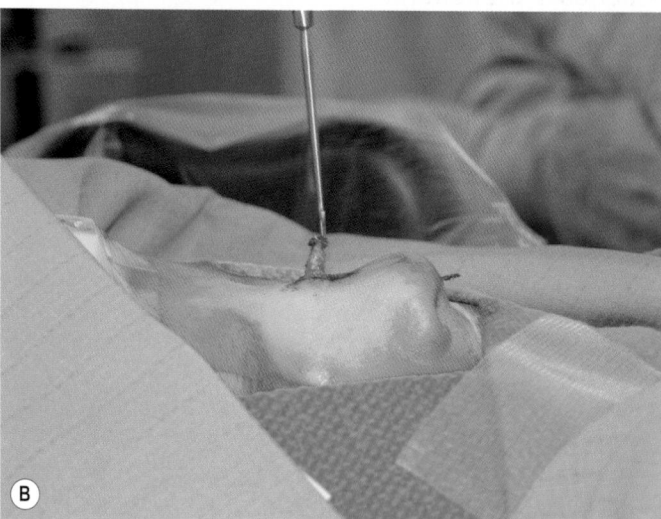

Fig. 42.5 (A, B) Excision of nasal dermoid without intracranial extension. (Courtesy of Dr. Diane G. Heatley.)

rhinoplasty technique has been proposed for the excision of superficial distal nasal-tip dermoids. Since most nasal dermoid cysts are confined to the superficial nasal area, this technique can prove to be beneficial.[45] For lesions with suspected/confirmed intracranial extension, failure to excise the tract completely can lead to abscess formation, meningitis, or osteomyelitis.[46,47] Multiple approaches have been proposed.[48-61] The traditional approach calls for combining an intracranial procedure such as a bifrontal craniotomy, with an extracranial procedure, such as a transverse, vertical, inverted U, lateral rhinotomy, or rhinoplasty to address the entire sinus tract.[48,49]

A second approach, described as the "keystone" technique, involves a bifrontal craniotomy superior to the supraorbital rims, two paramedian sagittal osteotomies extending down the length of the nasal bones, followed by outfracturing of the keystone component. This technique allows complete exposure of the sinus tract and enhanced exposure of the anterior cranial base.[53] A similar subcranial transglabellar approach involves horizontal osteotomies above the suprarorbital rims and at the level of the nasal bones, and vertical osteotomies at the supraorbital rims to expose the intracranial portion of the dermoid. This technique allows one to approach the lesion from one direction, thereby maintaining a single field. It is also attributed to require decreased frontal-lobe retraction and therefore has a lower risk of contusions, cerebral edema, and long-term neurological defects.[55] The osteotomy size is smaller than the traditional frontal craniotomy approach, which reduces the risk of dural tears or cerebrospinal fluid leaks[58] (*Fig. 42.6*).

Outcomes, prognosis, and complications

The recurrence rate of nasal dermoids after surgical excision is 12%.[61] A meta-analysis showed that the rate of complications with the traditional craniofacial approach was 30% while the subcranial approach reduced the complication rate to 16%.[57] Complications included tension pneumocephalus, cerebrospinal fluid leakage, subdural hematoma, longer operative times, and longer intensive care unit stays.[58,59]

Secondary procedures

Immediate reconstruction is preferred and may involve the use of conchal or costal cartilage grafts, as well as bone grafts for reconstruction of the cartilaginous skeleton of the nose. Reconstruction of "keystone" skull base defects can be carried out with bone grafts taken from the parietal bone of the skull. The origin of the frontal sinus may be disturbed, and the resulting defect, if not in continuity with the sinus, can occasionally be corrected using hydroxyapatite cement.

Intradural dermoids and dermal sinus tracts

Basic science/disease process

The incomplete sequestration of neuroectoderm and somatic ectoderm during embryogenesis can lead to persistent dermal sinus tracts from the occiput to the sacrum.[62,63] About 1% of these tracts are found in the cervical spine, 10% in the thoracic spine, 41% in the lumbar spine, and 35% in the lumbosacral spine.[64] These sinus tracts are cephalically oriented, lined with

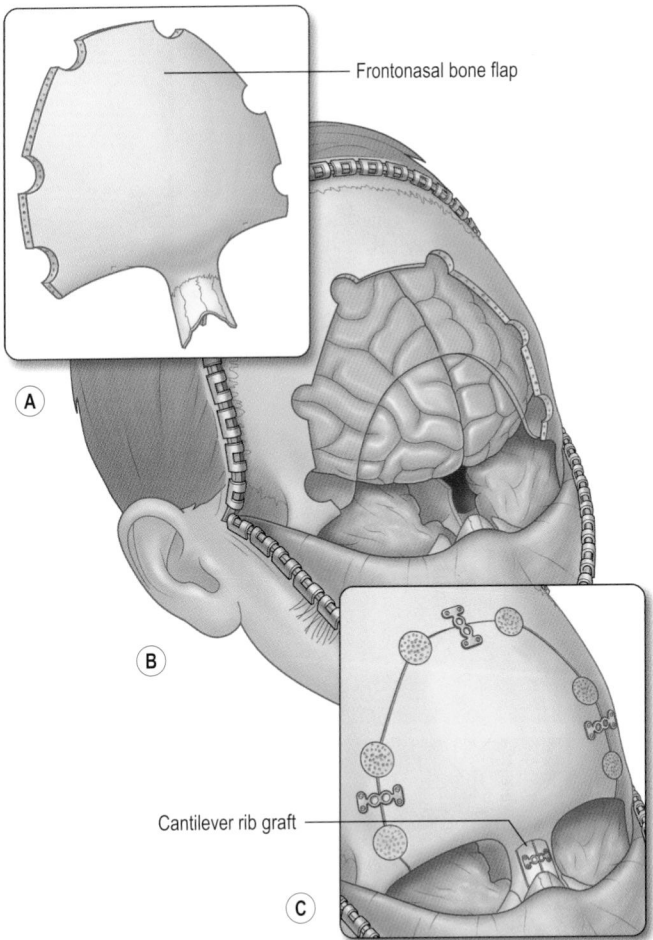

Fig. 42.6 Subcranial approach to intracranial dermoids. **(A)** Frontonasal bone fragment. **(B)** Subcranial approach with simultaneous access to the frontal lobe, the anterior skull base, and the nasal cavity. **(C)** Reconstruction with replacement of the frontonasal bone fragment, cantilever rib grafts to the nasal dorsum, and orbital floor reconstruction with split calvarial bone graft.

stratified epithelium, and may lead to the vertebral column, ending as intradural dermoid cysts.[62]

Diagnosis/patient presentation

Dermal sinus tracts can present as hypertrichosis, skin tags, abnormal pigmentation, subcutaneous lipomas, or angiomata.[65,66] The presence of these tracts can also lead to recurrent bacterial meningitis. Additionally, traction on the spinal cord can occur and can lead to symptoms of motor weakness, autonomic irritation, or sphincter dysfunction. MRI is the imaging tool of choice, and helps with the evaluation of other associated pathologies such as inclusion tumors, dermoids, epidermoids, teratomas,[67-74] split cord malformations[75,76] and tethered cords[77] (*Fig. 42.7*).

Treatment/surgical technique

Surgical excision involves tracing the tract through the subcutaneous tissue, lumbosacral fascia, and bony defect. If the dura is involved, laminectomy is necessary to open the dura and

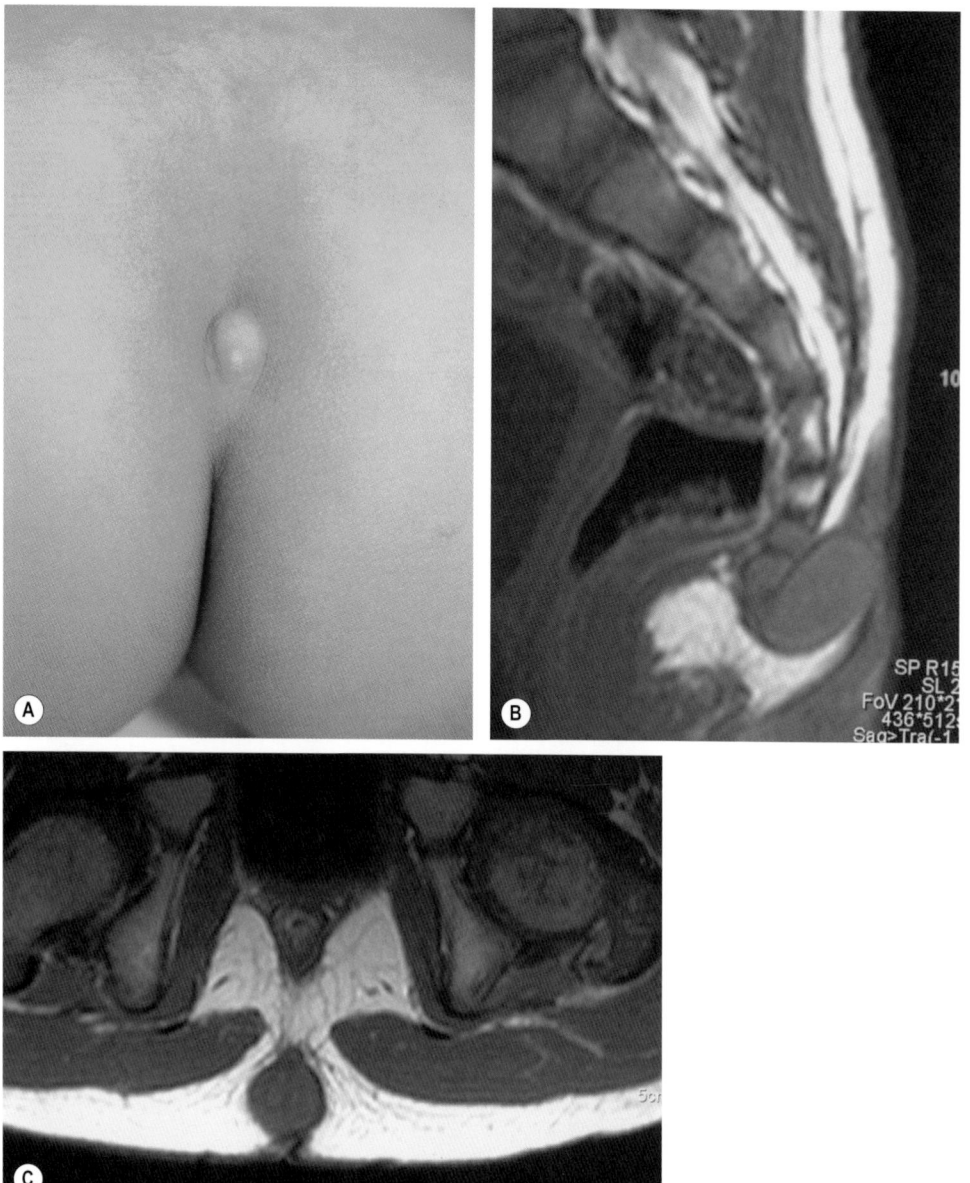

Fig. 42.7 (A) External manifestation of intradural dermoid. **(B, C)** Magnetic resonance imaging showing intradural dermoid. (Courtesy of Dr. Dennis P. Lund.)

explore the intradural space. Laminectomy may be required to inspect the intradural extension within the subarachnoid space. Intramedullary dermoids located at the conus are usually associated with cephalic extension. Occasionally, there is an associated thickened tethered cord, which requires sectioning of the filum.[77] The presence of adhesions at the site of previous resection and associated progressive neurologic deficits require re-exploration and lysis of adhesions.[78,79]

External angular dermoids

Basic science/disease process

External angular dermoids are usually fixed to the orbital rim periosteum and the frontozygomatic suture, with very rare intraosseus extension. Intraosseus extension presents as

intraosseus cysts that can very rarely erode intracranially.[80] External angular dermoids usually lie along the trajectory of the Tessier number 10 cleft. They may also be present more medially at the brow and supraorbital region. If they approach the frontonasal junction, they need to be evaluated as frontonasal dermoids.

Diagnosis/patient presentation

External angular dermoids are slow-growing and rarely exceed 4 cm in size. Size varies based on sweat gland activity.[80]

Treatment/surgical technique

Most lesions are excised through an incision in the lateral portion of the upper lid. Dermoids are generally found underneath the orbicularis muscle. If the dermoid is large with extension temporally, a hairline incision can be made to gain access. Endoscopic-assisted excision is discouraged laterally because it has been associated with injury to the facial nerve.

Dermoid cysts of the neck

Basic science/disease process

In contrast to dermoids of the head, which are found in different fusion planes, these present as subcutaneous masses. About 28% of them are dermal in origin. They are located in the midline of the neck and are composed of ectodermal tissue, sebaceous glands, and hair.[81–83] The epidermoid cyst is the most common dermoid cyst.[83]

Diagnosis/patient presentation

In newborns, these can present as masses in the floor of the mouth, with extension to the midline of the neck.[84]

Branchial cleft anomalies

Synopsis

- Each branchial arch, pouch, and groove complex forms a particular area of the head and neck.
- The first and second branchial cleft anomalies comprise 98% of all such anomalies. The third and fourth branchial cleft anomalies form the other 2%. Definitive treatment involves surgical excision.

Introduction

Fusion of branchial arches takes place between the third and sixth weeks of gestation. Failure of fusion of these arches leads to branchial cleft anomalies, which present as cysts, internal sinuses, external sinuses, fistulas, or combinations of the above. A branchial anomaly is present inferior to all the embryonic derivatives of its associated arch, and superior to all the embryonic derivatives of the next arch.[85] Cysts are the most common and are lined by squamous or columnar epithelium. Cysts and the masses associated with them are usually found in the anterior cervical triangle near lymph tissue.[86] Internal sinuses present with infection and halitosis. External sinuses present as openings in the middle to lower neck in the anterior cervical triangle or by the external ear.

Second branchial cleft anomaly (90%)

Basic science/disease process

A complete second branchial cleft begins near the sternal origin of the SCM, passes along the anterior border of the SCM lateral to the hypoglossal and glossopharyngeal nerves, and ends at the tonsillar fossa, superior to the hypoglossal and glossopharyngeal nerves *(Fig. 42.8)*.

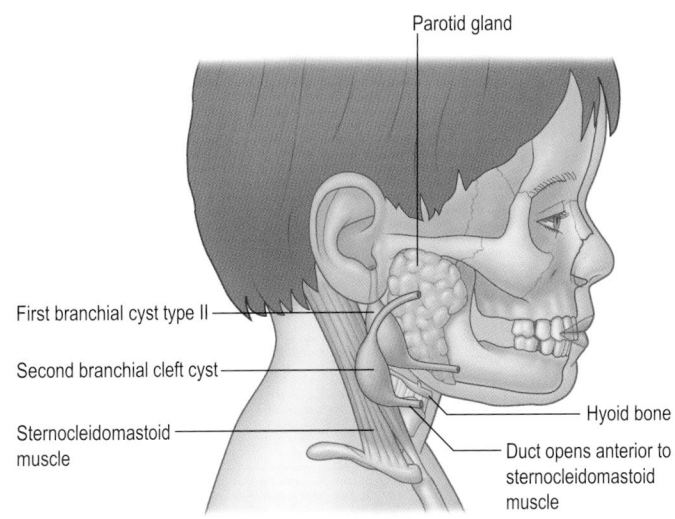

Fig. 42.8 Branchial cleft.

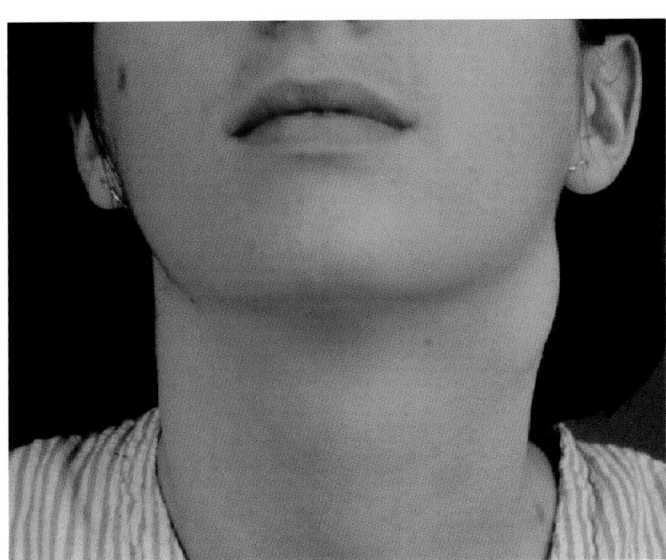

Fig. 42.9 Second branchial cleft cyst. (Courtesy of Dr. Diane G. Heatley.)

Diagnosis/patient presentation

Cystic masses are more common. Sinuses and fistulas may be present along the superior two-thirds of the tract.[87] The tract may be a blind sinus, or may extend all the way up to the tonsillar fossa, leading to chronic salivary drainage problems. These lesions also present as recurrent deep neck infections, and CT scans are helpful in recognizing them[88] *(Fig. 42.9)*.

Treatment/surgical technique

Fistulous tracts can be identified by injecting methylene blue or radiopaque material into the tract followed by a CT scan.[89] This step can be avoided since the tract may easily be followed during the excision. While dissecting out the tract, care is taken to preserve the hypoglossal and glossophargyneal nerves, and the internal and external carotid arteries. If the

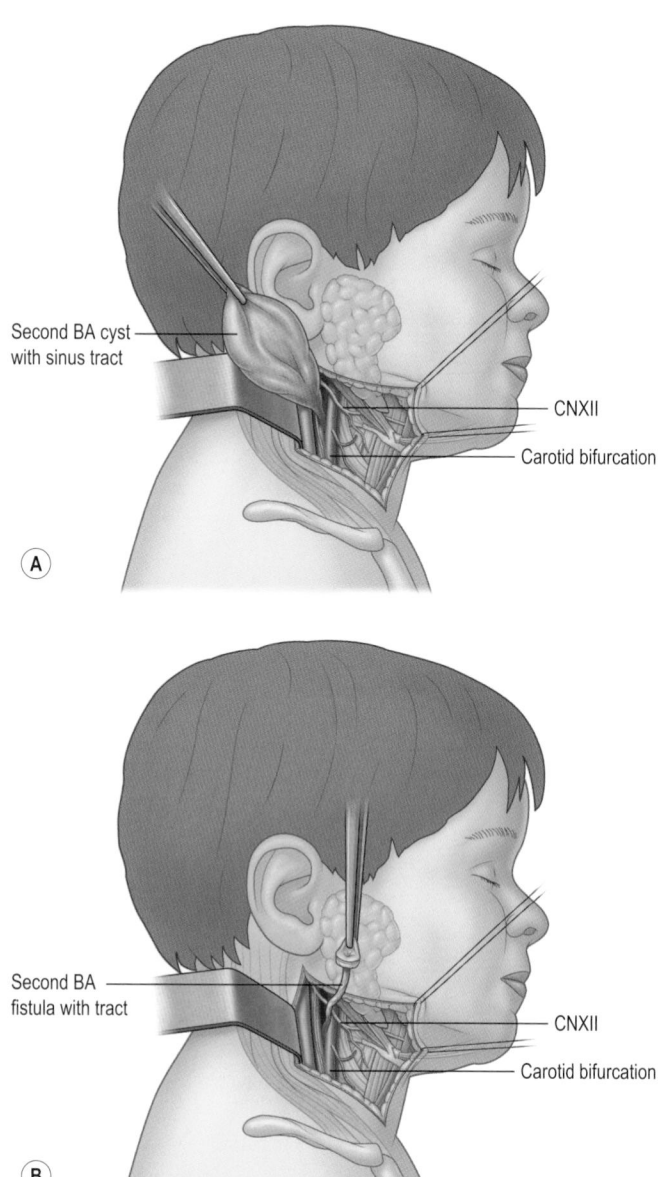

Fig. 42.10 **(A, B)** Excision of second branchial cleft cyst.

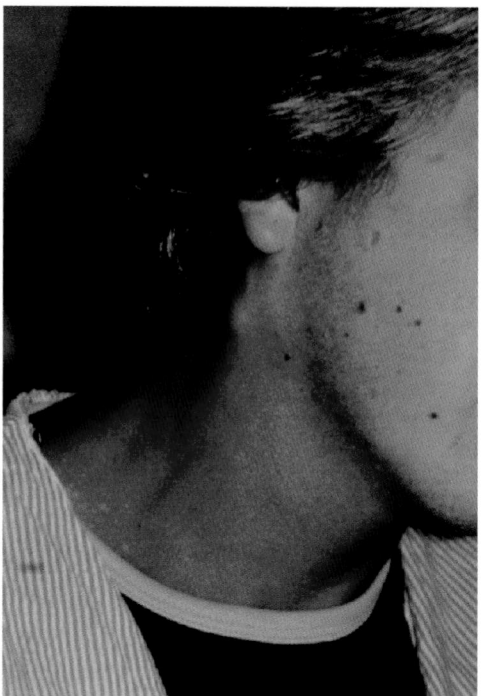

Fig. 42.11 First branchial cleft cyst. (Courtesy of Dr. Diane G. Heatley.)

tract extends into the base of the tonsillar fossa, the tonsil may need to be resected *(Fig. 42.10)*.

First branchial cleft anomaly (8%)

Basic science/disease process

Normal fusion of the first branchial arch presents as the external auditory meatus.

A complete nonfusion of the first arch leaves a cleft extending from the external auditory canal traveling along and under the border of the mandible up to the midline.

Diagnosis/patient presentation

About 66% of the associated lesions are cysts. These usually present as masses in the parotid region along with pits or depressions near the external auditory meatus.[90] Sinuses and fistulas are less common. These tracts may pass through the parotid gland and their excision may jeopardize facial nerve branches. Fistulas can be traced from the junction of the ear and cartilaginous canal to the overlying skin *(Fig. 42.11)*.

Fistulas present as two types:

1. The type 1 anomaly is a duplication of the membranous external meatal canal and is composed of ectodermal elements. The tract begins medial, anteroinferior, or posterior to the pinna and conchal cartilages. It then runs parallel to the external canal and has a blind end in the middle tympanic region.

2. The type 2 anomaly is a duplication of the membranous ear canal and the auricle and therefore contains both ectodermal and mesodermal structures. The tract begins with an opening in the anterior neck, superior to the hyoid bone and anterior to the SCM. It extends superiorly through subcutaneous tissue, pierces the substance of the parotid gland, and then passes superficial, deep, or in between two branches of the facial nerve.[91,92]

Treatment/surgical technique

Incision and drainage of infected cysts may be necessary before definitive surgery. The sinus/fistulous tracts extend into the parotid gland and their excision may jeapordize the facial nerve.[87,92,93] Complete excision consists of a superficial parotidectomy with facial nerve dissection.

Third branchial cleft anomaly

The third branchial cleft anomaly presents with a tract that has an opening along the anterior border of the SCM and extends deep to the carotid artery, toward or through the thyrohyoid membrane. It originates at the base/cranial end of the pyriform sinus and then passes above the superior laryngeal nerve.[94]

Fourth branchial cleft anomaly

The fourth branchial cleft anomaly begins at the apex of the pyriform sinus and passes through the cricothyroid membrane beneath the superior laryngeal nerves. It then travels inferiorly in the tracheoesophageal groove, posterior to the thyroid gland and into the thorax. The tract then loops around the arch of the aorta on the left and the subclavian artery on the right and courses superiorly, posterior to the common carotid artery. It finally makes another loop around the hypoglossal nerve and terminates at the medial border of the SCM. The descending portion of the tract has the highest likelihood of being infected. Patients present with respiratory distress, mediastinal abscesses, and suppurative thyroiditis.[95,96]

Outcomes, prognosis, and complications

Recurrence rates are increased when there is a history of multiple preoperative infections associated with the anomaly, and when there is no epithelial tissue found in the specimen.[85]

Thryoglossal duct cysts

Synopsis

- A persistent embryological remnant of the descending thryoglossal duct gives rise to a cyst.
- This clinically presents in the first two decades of life.
- Treatment involves excision using the Sistrunk technique.

Introduction

Thyroglossal duct cysts are the most common tumors of the anterior cervical region, which are usually located in the midline at or below the level of the hyoid. They are persistent embryological remnants of the descending thyroglossal duct.

Basic science/disease process

During the third week of gestation, thyroid gland development begins at the foramen cecum, at the junction of the tongue and pharynx. As the thyroid anlage begins to descend, the fusion of the second branchial arch causes the gland to move more anteriorly. The thyroglossal duct passes superficially, through or just deep to the hyoid bone. The duct tissue differentiates into thyroid gland and the midportion of the duct disintegrates. If this middle area persists, then it can differentiate to give rise to columnar, ciliated, or squamous epithelium, thereby forming a cyst. These cysts are found anterior and inferior to the hyoid bone and present during the first or second decades of life.

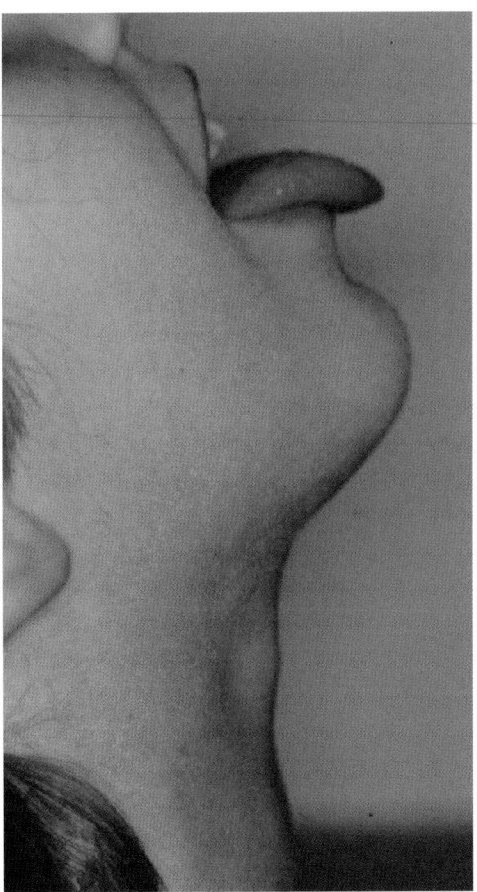

Fig. 42.12 Movement of thyroglossal duct cyst with tongue protrusion. (Courtesy of Dr. Diane G. Heatley.)

Diagnosis/patient presentation/ patient selection

Thyroglossal duct cysts are tethered to the hyoid bone and therefore move with swallowing and tongue protrusion *(Fig. 42.12)*. They are usually painless masses unless they become infected. If the cysts are infected or rupture, thyroglossal duct sinus tracts can form. These sinus tracts then drain clear or cloudy mucus.[87,97,98]

Treatment/surgical technique

Treatment involves surgical excision using the Sistrunk technique. A curvilinear incision is made over the cyst followed by excision of the full duct up to the foramen cecum along with the central 1 cm of the hyoid bone.[99] Thyroid scans should be done to ensure that the tissue is not functioning ectopic thyroid gland. Hormonal evaluation, CT, or ultrasound scans may also be performed.[97,100]

Outcomes, prognosis, and complications

Recurrence is possible if lingual thyroid tissue is left behind. In this case, treatment may involve a transoral excision of tongue tissue around the foramen cecum. The Sistrunk technique reduced the recurrence rate from 20–49% to less than 5%.[101]

Pilomatrixoma

Synopsis

- These are ectodermal in origin and arise from the outer root sheath cells of the hair follicle.
- These tumors usually occur in the head and neck region of children.
- Treatment is surgical excision, with radiation therapy for malignant lesions.

Introduction and history

In 1880, this lesion was first described by Malherbe and Chenantais, who thought this arose from sebaceous glands and called them calcifying epitheliomas of Malherbe.[102]

In 1961, Forbes and Helwig[103] proposed this to be a benign lesion and gave it the name, pilomatrixoma.

Basic science/disease process

Pilomatrixomas originate from the outer root sheath cells of the hair follicle in the lower dermis and form a connective tissue capsule. Histologically, these tumors are seen as noninvasive islands of basaloid cells with hyperchromatic nuclei and no nucleoli. The other major component of the tumor consists of cells that show a central unstained area, representing the shadow of a lost nucleus, called ghost cells. These tumors are well demarcated and are completely or partially surrounded by fibrosis or an inflammatory reaction.[104] Malignant transformation has not been reported in children but it has in adults. In adults, pilomatrical carcinoma behaves similarly to basal cell carcinoma and has similar metastatic potential.[105] Pilomatrical carcinomas show invasive nests of tumor cells with irregular borders, large vesicular nuclei, prominent nucleoli, multiple mitotic figures, and focal necrosis.

Diagnosis/patient presentation

The average age at presentation is 7 years with a peak between ages 8 and 13 years.[106–108] These tumors commonly occur in regions of fine vellus hair growth in children, such as the cheeks and periorbital area[106] *(Fig. 42.13)*. Female preponderance of the tumor and a history of regional trauma in 9% of patients have been reported.[104,107] The frequency of having multiple tumors is about 2–3%, although rates as high as 10% have also been reported.[105] Multiple tumors are noted in patients with Gardner's syndrome, Steinert's disease, myotonic dystrophy, and sarcoidosis.[107,109–111] When the skin is tented and the tumor is palpated below it, one can feel multiple nodules.[112] The freely mobile characteristic of the mass rules out dermoid cyst and its nodular nature helps rule out epidermal cysts. Fine-needle aspiration determines cytology; the presence of ghost cells, basaloid cells, and calcium deposits, and helps solidify the diagnosis.[113] Ultrasound is cheap,

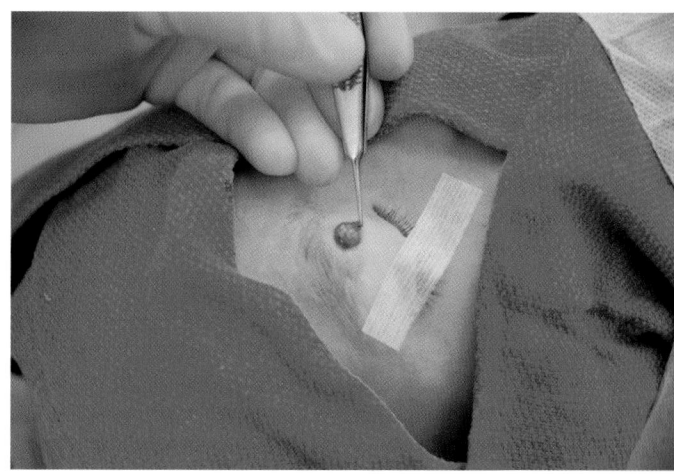

Fig. 42.13 Excision of pilomatrixoma. (Courtesy of Dr. Delora L. Mount.)

effective, and helps determine the relationship of the tumor with the parotid gland.[114]

Treatment/surgical technique

Treatment for the malignant lesion is wide local excision. Reconstruction is deferred for 1 year, while observing for recurrence. Radiation may help for locoregional control.[105]

Benign lesions are completely excised. When the tumor adheres to the skin, overlying skin is resected. Surgery is generally curative and recurrence is rare.[115] Treatment with incision and curettage has been reported for large tumors in cosmetically significant areas.

Postoperative care

Malignant lesions have a high likelihood of recurrence, thus patients need to be observed for recurrence.

Outcomes, prognosis, and complications

The rate of recurrence of benign lesions is very low and patients have an excellent prognosis. Metastatic spread occurs in 6% of patients with malignant lesions.[108] Metastatic lesions are usually found in the lungs, but have also been reported in the lymph nodes, liver, pleura, kidney, and heart.[116]

Soft-tissue sarcomas

Rhabdomycosarcoma

Synopsis

- This is a malignant tumor of mesenchymal origin.
- In the head and neck the most common presentations are in the orbit, nasopharynx, paranasal sinuses, and middle ear.
- Three histological types include embryonal, alveolar, and pleomorphic rhabdomyosarcoma.

Introduction

Rhabdomyosarcoma is the most common of the pediatric soft-tissue sarcomas. It is the third most common solid, extracranial, pediatric tumor (after Wilms tumor and neuroblastoma) and is diagnosed in about 250 patients annually.

Basic science/disease process

Rhabdomyosarcomas generally originate from mesenchymal cells committed to becoming skeletal muscle cells. They have, however, also been found to arise from viscera such as the prostate, gallbladder, and urinary bladder. The tumors resemble different stages of prenatal muscle formation. There are three histological types: embryonal, alveolar, and pleomorphic. The embryonal type is more common in infants and young children; the alveolar type is more common in adolescents and young adults; and the pleomorphic type is generally found in older adults. Rhabdomyosarcomas are found to be present in multiple syndromes such as Li–Fraumeni, Beckwidth–Wiedemann, and a subset in Gorlin syndrome.

Diagnosis/patient presentation

Patients most commonly present with lesions in the head and neck, genitourinary tract, and extremities.[117] In the head and neck, the most common presentations involve the orbit (20–40%), nasopharynx, paranasal sinuses, and the middle ear.[118] Embryonal tumors are found in 80–85% of cases, alveolar tumors in 10–15%, and pleomorphic tumors in 5% of cases. Embryonal rhabdomyosarcomas occur between birth and age 15. The median age at presentation for rhabdomyosarcomas is 5 years.[119] These tumors tend to present as fungating masses in the conjunctiva and vagina or as obstructive masses in the genitourinary tract and biliary system. They cause proptosis and diplopia when they involve the orbit and neurological manifestations when they involve nerve roots in the paraspinal region. Rhabdomycosarcomas of the temporal bone present with hearing loss, otalgia, and otorrhea *(Fig. 42.14)*. CT scans of the head and skull base and lumbar puncture are used to evaluate for extension of the disease into the skull, meninges, and brain.

Treatment/surgical technique/postop care

Treatment depends on the stage. Primary modalities are multidrug chemotherapy and external-beam radiation therapy. If complete remission is not obtained, adjuvant radiation therapy and surgery are carried out. Surgical involvement (staging and treatment) is mutilating and leads to functional loss as a result. Primary excision should be attempted only if complete excision can be accomplished without functional or cosmetic consequences.

Outcomes, prognosis, and complications

Patients undergoing the primary treatment modality have a 74% 5-year survival rate, while 33% have recurrent metastatic disease that is fatal. Metastases occur through blood or lymphatic channels to lymph nodes, lungs, bones, or brain.[120]

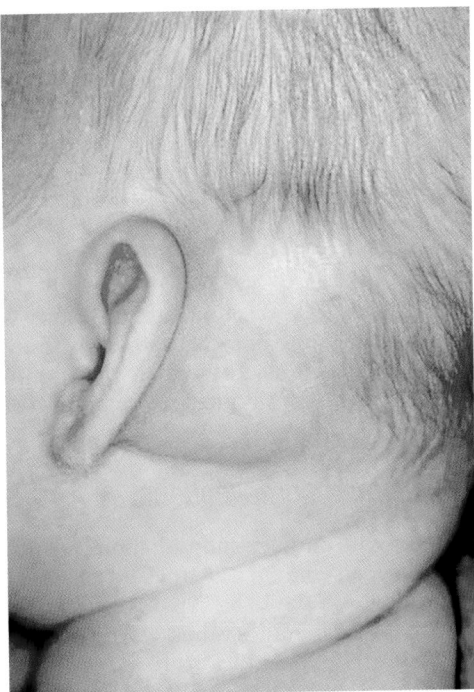

Fig. 42.14 Rhabdomyosarcoma. (Courtesy of Dr. Diane G. Heatley.)

Secondary procedures

Secondary excision may be considered after chemotherapy, based on the judgment of the surgeon. If the tumor still remains unresectable, then radiotherapy is employed.

Synovial soft-tissue sarcoma

Synopsis

- These sarcomas arise form synovioblastic differentiation of pluripotent mesenchymal stem cells.

Introduction

Synovial soft-tissue sarcomas are the most common soft-tissue sarcoma of the hands and feet, and represent 8–10% of all malignant somatic soft-tissue neoplasms.

Basic science/disease process

These sarcomas arise from synovioblastic differentiation of pluripotent mesenchymal stem cells. Histological studies show a biphasic pattern of pseudoepithelial cells and spindle cells with a fibrosarcomatous appearance.[121]

Diagnosis/patient presentation

Synovial soft-tissue sarcomas present as solitary, well-circumscribed lesions in the upper or lower extremities (80%). They are para-articular, never arise within the joint, and are not associated with normal synovial tissue. Nonextremity sites include the trunk (8%), retroperitoneum/abdomen (7%), and head and neck (5%).[122] Common locations in the neck include parapharyngeal/retropharyngeal spaces, larynx, pharynx, tongue, and tonsils.[123] The most common symptom is a painless mass that has existed for several weeks to years. These lesions may also present as chronic contractures, acute arthritis, bursitis, or as tumors following trauma. Up to 30% of synovial soft-tissue sarcomas have calcifications on radiographs. MRI is the imaging modality of choice and it shows the tumors to be sharply marginated and largely cystic.

Treatment/surgical technique

The treatment of choice is surgical excision, with pre- or postoperative radiation therapy. Adjuvant chemotherapy may improve local control if the tumor size is greater than 5 cm. The goal of surgery is to obtain tumor-free margins of 1–3 cm.[124–127]

Outcomes, prognosis, and complications

The overall survival rates with surgery and radiation therapy are shown to be 76% at 5 years and 57% at 10 years. Disease-free survival rates have been shown to be 59% at 5 years and 52% at 10 years. The rate of local failure is below 20% but the rate of metastatic spread at 10 years has been shown to be 44%. Tumors greater than 5 cm in size have worse survival rates.[127] Complications at 5 years are 7%, and at 10 years are 9%. These include fractures, fibrosis, soft-tissue necrosis, neuropathy, and edema. Most common sites of metastases are lung (74–81%), lymph nodes (12–23%), and bone (10–20%).[128]

Alveolar soft-part sarcoma

Synopsis

- This is a rare tumor that occurs primarily in skeletal muscles or musculofascial planes of extremities.

Introduction

Alveolar soft-part sarcoma is a rare neoplasm of unknown etiology or histogenesis but poor prognosis.

Basic science/disease process

Alveolar soft-part sarcomas account for 1% of all soft-tissue sarcomas. They occur primarily in skeletal muscles or musculofascial planes of extremities, and in the head and neck region in children.

Diagnosis/patient presentation

Children, adolescents, and young adults between the ages of 15 and 35 years are more likely to carry this diagnosis. The tumor has a predilection for females and usually presents as a soft, painless, slow-growing mass. Most patients have metastases at the time of diagnosis.

Treatment/surgical technique

Wide local excision is the mainstay of treatment. Metastatic spread occurs to lungs, bone, central nervous system, and liver.

Outcomes, prognosis, and complications

Survival has been reported as 82% at 2 years, 59% at 5 years, and 47% at 10 years.[129–131] Alveolar soft-part sarcomas can recur more than 10 years after primary resection.

Lymphadenopathy

Synopsis

- Acute bacterial lymphadenitis presents with mild fever, tender, indurated, and erythematous lymph nodes or systemic toxicity.
- Chronic regional lymphadenopathy is observed in diseases such as cat-scratch disease.
- Cervical tuberculous adenitis (scrofula) begins with a pulmonary infection that spreads to the lymph nodes.

Introduction

About 30% of lymph nodes are found in the head and neck region.[132] Posterior auricular and occipital lymph nodes drain the posterior scalp and the superficial portion of the postero-superior neck.[133] Preauricular and infraorbital nodes drain the temporal scalp, lateral eyelids, conjunctiva, and cheek. These nodes are connected to the parotid lymph nodes in the lateral parotid gland. Submandibular and submental nodes drain the teeth, gum, tongue, and buccal mucosa. The deep cervical lymph node chain runs along the internal jugular vein, deep to the SCM. Its superior portion drains the tongue and the posterior pharynx. Its inferior portion drains the larynx, trachea, thyroid, and esophagus. Superficial cervical nodes lie superficial to the SCM. The anterior chain of nodes runs along the internal jugular vein, while the posterior chain is present in the posterior triangle. These nodes receive drainage from the superficial tissues of the neck, mastoid process, posterior auricular nodes, and the nasopharynx. The tonsillar nodes drain the palatine tonsils.

Bacterial lymphadenitis

Basic science/disease process

Bacterial lymphadenitis usually occurs in children less than age 4, and is preceded by an upper respiratory tract infection or pharyngitis. It can present with mild fever, tender, indurated, and erythematous lymph nodes or systemic toxicity. Submandibular nodes are affected in half of the patients. Upper cervical nodes are affected in 25% of patients. The most common causative organisms in children under the age of 3 include: *Staphylococcus aureus* and *Streptococcus agalactiae* (group G streptococcus). Sepsis is most likely in this age group. In children over the age of 3, *Staphylococcus aureus* and *Streptococcus pyogenes* (group A streptococcus) are the most common organisms. Bacterial lymphadenitis can also be caused by *Escherichia coli* and anaerobes in the setting of periodontal disease.

Diagnosis/patient presentation

Staphylococcus aureus adenitis is most likely to cause an abscess. About 30% of acutely infected lymph nodes suppurate in 2 weeks.[134,135] Group A streptococcus adenitis causes bilateral jugulodigastric node enlargement, fever, severe sore throat, frontal headache, abdominal pain, toxic appearance, and exudative tonsillitis. It may also present with minimal systemic symptoms and nontender adenopathy.

Treatment/surgical technique

Treatment of acute lymphadenitis involves incision and drainage. This prevents migration of the disease into the chest and abdomen via fascial planes.

Chronic regional lymphadenopathy

Basic science/disease process

Cat-scratch disease is the most common cause of chronic regional lymphadenopathy affecting the head and neck region in children and young adults.[136–139] Up to 50% of cases involve head and neck nodes. The bacterial organisms involved are *Bartonella henselae* and *Afipia felis*, which are transmitted via a cat scratch or bite.[140]

Diagnosis/patient presentation

The clinical course of this disease begins with the formation of a red papule at 3–12 days at the site of inoculation. The papule progresses to a vesicle, then to a pustule, which develops an eschar and then resolves. This is followed by lymphadenopathy a week later. About 85% of patients develop a deep enlarged lymph node at the site of inoculation. Proximal lymph nodes may be skipped, with distal nodes developing lymphadenopathy.[141,142] The disease is self-limiting, but may lead to complications in 5–13% of cases.

Treatment/surgical technique

Antibiotic therapy is used for highly symptomatic patients. Surgical excision of enlarged lymph nodes is advocated if the nodes become fluctuant.[139]

Outcomes, prognosis, and complications

Complications include encephalopathy, erythema nodosum, thrombocytopenic purpura, Parinaud's oculoglandular syndrome, and hepatitis.[139,143] If the patient is immunocompromised, then lymphadenopathy may progress to bacillary angiomatosis, which is characterized by disseminated disease and cutaneous nodular lesions.

Cervical tuberculous adenitis (scrofula)

Basic science/disease process

Cervical tuberculous adenitis is caused by inhaled mycobacteria, which lead to a pulmonary infection. The infection eventually spreads to regional lymph nodes via lymph vessels or distal lymph nodes via blood vessels.[144]

Diagnosis/patient presentation

Scrofula typically presents in children under the age of 6 as painless enlarging masses. Lower anterior and posterior cervical lymph nodes are involved bilaterally. Tonsillar and submandibular lymph nodes may also be involved. Symptoms include fever, weight loss, night sweats, and decreased appetite. Lymph nodes will occasionally develop suppurative changes and produce draining sinuses. Generalized lymphadenopathy can develop from miliary spread of the disease. The diagnosis is made using erythrocyte sedimentation rate (ESR), tuberculin skin tests, chest radiographs, and fine-needle aspiration.[145]

Treatment/surgical technique

Surgical excision is recommended to prevent the formation of chronic draining fistulas, especially if open wounds are present. If the tuberculin skin test is positive, cultures are sent and four-drug therapy, consisting of rifampin, isoniazid, pyrazinamide, and ethambutol, is started. The course of treatment is 6 months. Treatment may be tapered to two-drug therapy based on culture results.

Atypical nontuberculous mycobacteria

Basic science/disease process

Mycobacterium scrofulaceum and *M. avium-intercellulare* are the most common atypical nontuberculous mycobacteria responsible for this lymphadenopathy. Both organisms are commonly found in the south-eastern US. The site of entry is the mouth, followed by spread to regional lymph nodes.

Diagnosis/patient presentation

Patients present with unilateral lymphadenopathy mainly involving submandibular nodes. Nodes are initially painless and mobile but eventually become inflamed, fixed, and suppurative *(Fig. 42.15)*. Infection spreads locally to

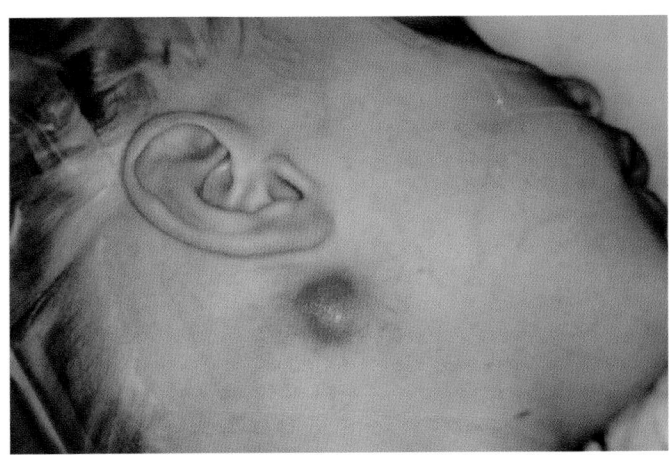

Fig. 42.15 Atypical mycobacterial abscess. (Courtesy of Dr. Dennis P. Lund.)

subcutaneous surrounding tissues leading to chronically draining sinus tracts. The age of presentation is between 1 and 5 years, and patients usually do not have systemic symptoms. They have a normal ESR, chest radiograph, and white cell count. Definitive diagnosis is made through culture.[146]

Treatment/surgical technique

Definitive treatment involves surgical excision with or without medical therapy. These organisms are more resistant to antituberculosis drugs. If there exists a suspicion for an atypical mycobacterial infection, the treatment consists of a combination of clarithromycin, ethambutol, rifampin, and ciprofloxacin while awaiting results.[147]

Access the complete references list online at http://www.expertconsult.com

11. Jackson IT, Carbonnel A, Portparic Z, et al. Orbitotemporal neurofibromatosis: classification and treatment. *Plast Reconstr Surg.* 1993;92:1–11.

This article divides the clinical presentation of orbitotemporal neurofibromatosis into three groups, based on orbital and soft-tissue involvement, and the state of the eye. The treatment methods differ based on the severity of presentation and therefore this classification helps guide the treatments used. The article presents 24 patients who are followed for a maximum of 12 years.

28. Ferner RE, Gutmann DH. International consensus statement on malignant peripheral nerve sheath tumours in neurofibromatosis 1. *Cancer Res.* 2002;62:1573–1577.

41. Sessions RB. Nasal dermal sinuses: new concepts and explanations. *Laryngoscope.* 1982;92:1–28.

This is a classic paper that describes, evaluates, and unifies the various existing theories describing the etiology of dermoids. The paper shows how dermoids and encephaloceles are a continuum in the manifestation of congenital anterior cranial base defects. The diagrams in the paper clearly illustrate the surgical anatomy of these defects.

50. Hanikeri M, Waterhouse N, Kirkpatrick N, et al. The management of midline transcranial nasal dermiod sinus cysts. *Br J Plast Surg.* 2005;58:1043–1050.

57. Kellman RM, Marentette L. The transglabellar/subcranial approach to the anterior skull base: a review of 72 cases. *Arch Otolaryngol Head Neck Surg.* 2001;127:687–690.

This paper describes the transglabellar/subcranial approach to the anterior skull base in patients who have dermoids with intracranial extension. Through a retrospective analysis

of 72 cases in two academic medical centers it analyses parameters such as average operating room time, complication rates, and length of ICU stay and compares them to results published for traditional craniofacial approaches.

85. Schroeder JW, Mohyuddin N, Maddalozzo J. Branchial anomalies in the pediatric population. *Otolaryngol Head Neck Surg.* 2007;137, 289–295.

This paper reviews the presentation, evaluation, and treatment of branchial anomalies. It accomplishes this task through a retrospective study involving 97 pediatric patients with branchial anomalies who were treated over a 10-year period. The associated complications and the rates of recurrence after treatment are also discussed.

99. Sistrunk WE. The surgical treatment of cysts of the thyroglossal tract. *Ann Surg.* 1920;71:121–122.

110. McCulloch TA, Singh S, Cotton DWK. Pilomatrix carcinoma and multiple pilomatrixomas. *Br J Dermatol.* 1996;134:368–371.

115. Prousmanesh A, Reinisch JF, Gonzalez-Gomez I, et al. Pilomatrixoma: a review of 346 cases. *Plast Reconstr Surg.* 2003;112: 1784–1789.

This article examines the cause, clinical and histological presentation, management, and treatment outcomes of pilomatrixoma. A retrospective review of patient records spanning a period of 11 years is conducted, during which 346 pilomatrixomas were excised from 336 patients at Children's Hospital in Los Angeles. The study concludes that the treatment of choice is surgical excision and that the rate of recurrence is low.

116. Aslan G, Erdogan B, Aköz T, et al. Multiple occurrence of pilomatrixoma. *Plast Reconstr Surg.* 1996;98:510–533.

43

Conjoined twins

Oksana Jackson, David W. Low, and Don LaRossa

SYNOPSIS

- Conjoined twins are one of the most uncommon congenital anomalies, with an incidence between one in 50 000 and one in 100 000 births
- Conjoined twins are classified by dorsal or ventral site of fusion and anatomic region of fusion
- Separation of conjoined twins requires a multidisciplinary team approach
- Understanding the shared anatomy through preoperative imaging studies and investigations is critical to successful separation
- Careful planning and insertion of tissue expanders is almost always necessary to accomplish wound closure
- Intensive care monitoring and support, nutritional supplementation, and pressure-reducing strategies are essential for successful separation.

 Access the Historical Perspective section online at **http://www.expertconsult.com**

Basic science/disease process

Incidence

Conjoined twins are one of the most uncommon congenital anomalies. The typical form of monozygotic twinning occurs in 4 per 1000 live births, and dizygotic fraternal twinning in approximately 10–15 per 1000. Twin births therefore occur in about 1 in 90 live births.[12] The incidence of conjoined twins has been estimated at between one in 50 000 and one in 100 000 pregnancies. Spencer has reported that 1% are stillborn, and 40–60% die shortly after birth, so the true incidence is closer to 1:200 000 live births.[5,13] Recent reports of prenatally diagnosed conjoined twins indicate that more than a fourth of cases die *in utero* and one-half die immediately after birth, leaving only 20% potential survivors who are candidates for separation.[14] In all reports, females predominate over males by approximately three to one. However, in reports of stillborn conjoined twin pairs, males predominate over females.[5,10,15–17]

Classification

A number of classification systems exist and each categorizes conjoined twins by their most prominent site of union together with the suffix "pagus," a Greek word meaning "that which is fixed." The most commonly used system, both clinically and historically in the literature, was adapted from that proposed by Potter and Craig, and simplified to include the five most common forms of conjoined twinning, listed here in order of decreasing frequency: thoracopagus, omphalopagus, pygopagus, ischiopagus, and craniopagus.[18] These five types are summarized below and illustrated in *(Fig. 43.4)*. Additionally, the number of shared anatomic structures can be described with the prefixes "di-," "tri-," and "tetra-," combined with the involved parts, "prospus" (face), "brachius" (upper extremity), and "pus" (lower extremity). For example, ischiopagus twins may have three (tripus) or four (tetrapus) legs.

The thoracopagus type is the most common, occurring in 74% of cases. Infants with this form of twinning face each other, have major junctions between the chest and abdomen, and may have conjoined livers, hearts, and upper gastrointestinal structures *(Fig. 43.5; case 6, below)*. Separation may be limited by the degree of cardiac involvement. Conjoined six-chamber hearts are common in thoracopagus twins and have never been separated successfully; only a single successful case of separation of twins with conjoined atria has been reported.[19] Advances in prenatal diagnosis and the development of fetal surgery have improved perinatal survival in cases where separation is deemed appropriate. For example, the EXIT procedure (*ex utero* intrapartum treatment) has been recently used at the Children's Hospital of Philadelphia in the separation of thoracopagus twins. In this case, one twin had a normal heart that perfused a co-twin with a rudimentary heart, and EXIT allowed prompt control of the airway and

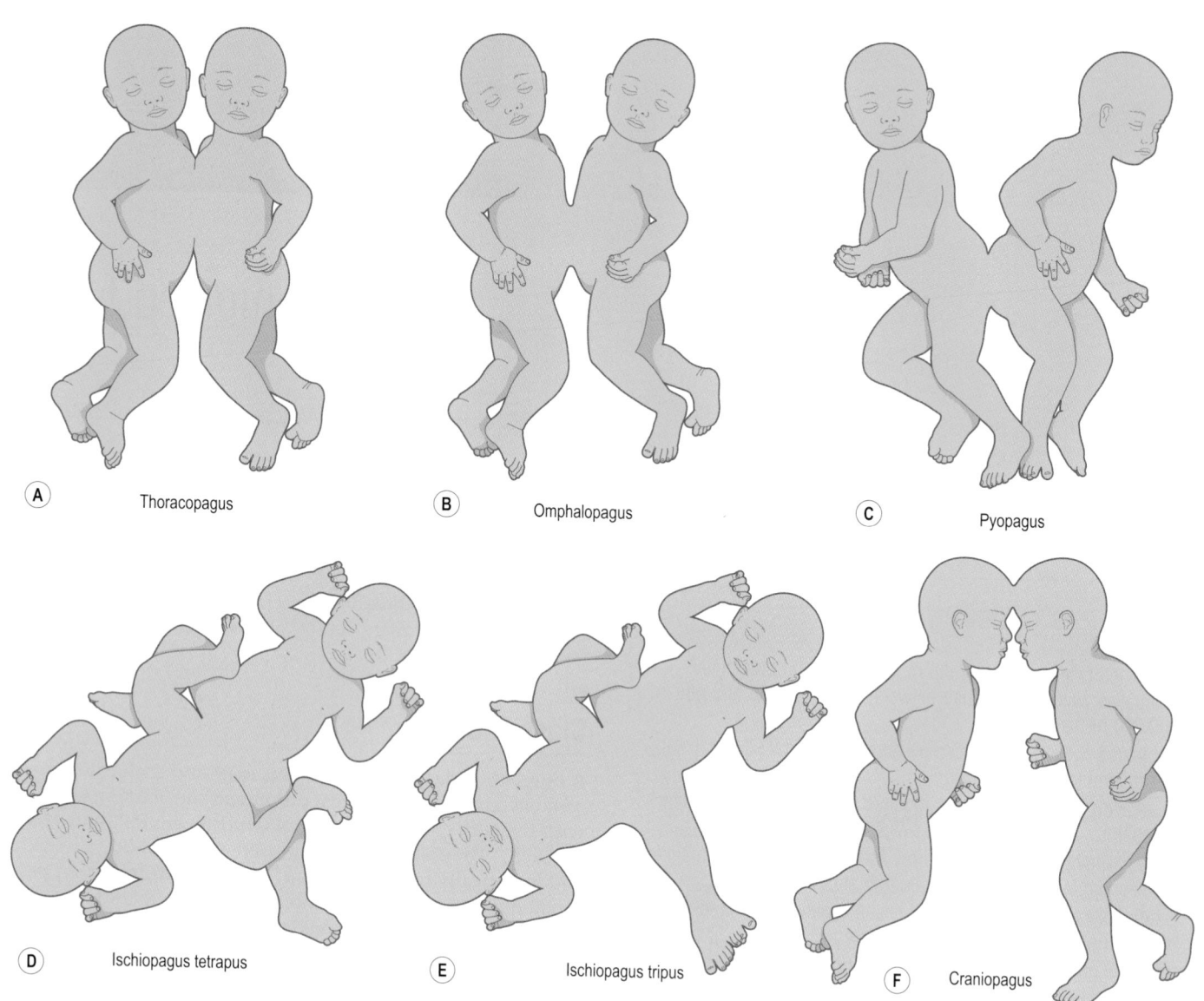

A   Thoracopagus   B   Omphalopagus   C   Pyopagus

D   Ischiopagus tetrapus   E   Ischiopagus tripus   F   Craniopagus

Fig. 43.4 Clinical classification of conjoined twins: thoracopagus, omphalopagus, pygopagus, ischiopagus (both tetrapus and tripus forms illustrated), and craniopagus.

circulation prior to clamping the umbilical cord, leading to survival of the normal co-twin.[14]

In omphalopagus twins, there is fusion in the abdominal area with variable connections of the liver, biliary tree, and gastrointestinal tracts. In isolated omphalopagus forms, there is no cardiac connection (case 8, below).

Pygopagus twins are joined at the level of the sacrum and commonly face away from each other. There is usually a shared spinal cord, and the perineal structures and rectum also may be fused. Pygopagus twins represent about 17% of conjoined twins.[12]

In the ischiopagus type, the junction is at the pelvic level with sharing of the genitourinary structures, rectum, and liver *(Fig. 43.5)* (cases 5 and 7, below). These twins may each have a single normal leg and a common fused leg, referred to as a tripus, or four legs may be present. The tripus, when present, usually has dual neural and vascular supply and preoperative determination of perfusion is important in planning separation. Often, the tripus is sacrificed and the soft tissue used for

closure of each twin, leaving each with a single leg. In a unique case, Zuker *et al.* reported successful transplantation of an entire extremity from a dying twin to her sister, thus leaving the surviving one with two functional legs.[20]

The least common and perhaps the most difficult to separate is the craniopagus type because the cranial union often involves a variety of neural and vascular connections.[12,21,22] Craniopagus twins represent 2–6% of conjoined twins and occur with an incidence of one in 2.5 million births.[9] They can share scalp, calvarium, dural sinuses, and surfaces of the brain, but the face, foramen magnum, and spine remain separate. Even when the cerebral cortices are contiguous, craniopagus twins do not share neuronal pathways, as demonstrated by completely independent behavior and by electroencephalogram studies. Facial and skull asymmetry can occur, as well as other intracranial and extracranial abnormalities. The site of fusion can vary significantly, and rotation about this site of union can produce a variety of anatomic orientations.[3,8,21,23] A number of authors have classified craniopagus twins by the

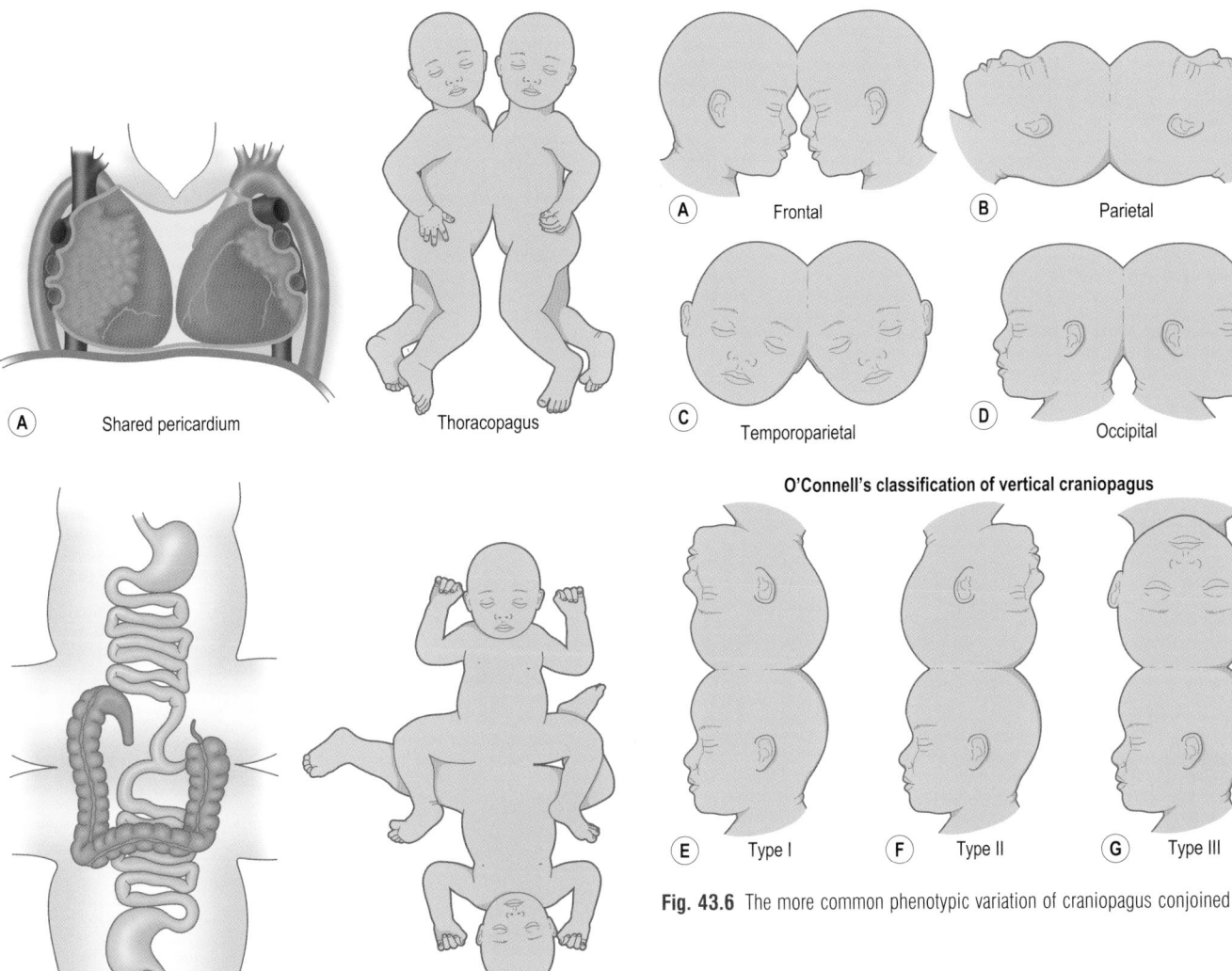

Fig. 43.6 The more common phenotypic variation of craniopagus conjoined twins.

Fig. 43.5 Within each type of union, the anatomy of conjoined twins can be quite variable. The anatomic features on the left of the illustration describe the anatomy of the twins depicted on the right. These are examples of two common types, amenable to surgical separation. **(A)** Thoracopagus twins with separate hearts but a shared pericardium. **(B)** Tetrapus ischiopagus twins with shared intestine from distal ileum and single colon, rectum, and anus.

site, degree of fusion, or alignment of the twins.[24,25] The more common phenotypic variations described in case reports in the literature are illustrated in *(Fig. 43.6)*.

An alternative classification system was proposed by Spencer, based on the analysis of embryologic data and the teratology of over 1200 cases. She divided conjoined twins into dorsal and ventral forms of union, joined in one of eight anatomic sites *(Fig. 43.7)*. This classification system specifically defines and restricts the anatomy of fusion between the different types of conjoined twinning, thus attempting to standardize the nomenclature for purposes of predicting separability, surgical planning, and outcomes after surgery, as well as for consistent documentation for research purposes.[26] In Spencer's embryologic classification system, ventral unions

are oriented ventrally or ventrolaterally, and the union always includes the umbilicus, whereas dorsal unions are united dorsally or dorsolaterally and do not include the thoracic or abdominal viscera or the umbilicus. Ventral unions are further subdivided into rostral, caudal, or lateral. These eight types with their definitions and restrictions are listed below.[26]

Ventral

Rostral

1. Cephalopagus: fused from the top of the head to the umbilicus.
2. Thoracopagus: united from the upper thorax to the umbilicus and always involving the heart.
3. Omphalopagus: joined primarily in the area of the umbilicus and never including the heart.

Caudal

4. Ischiopagus: united from umbilicus through pelvis and sharing external genitalia and anus.

Lateral

5. Parapagus: sharing a conjoined pelvis with one symphysis pubis and one or two sacrums *(Fig. 43.7A)*

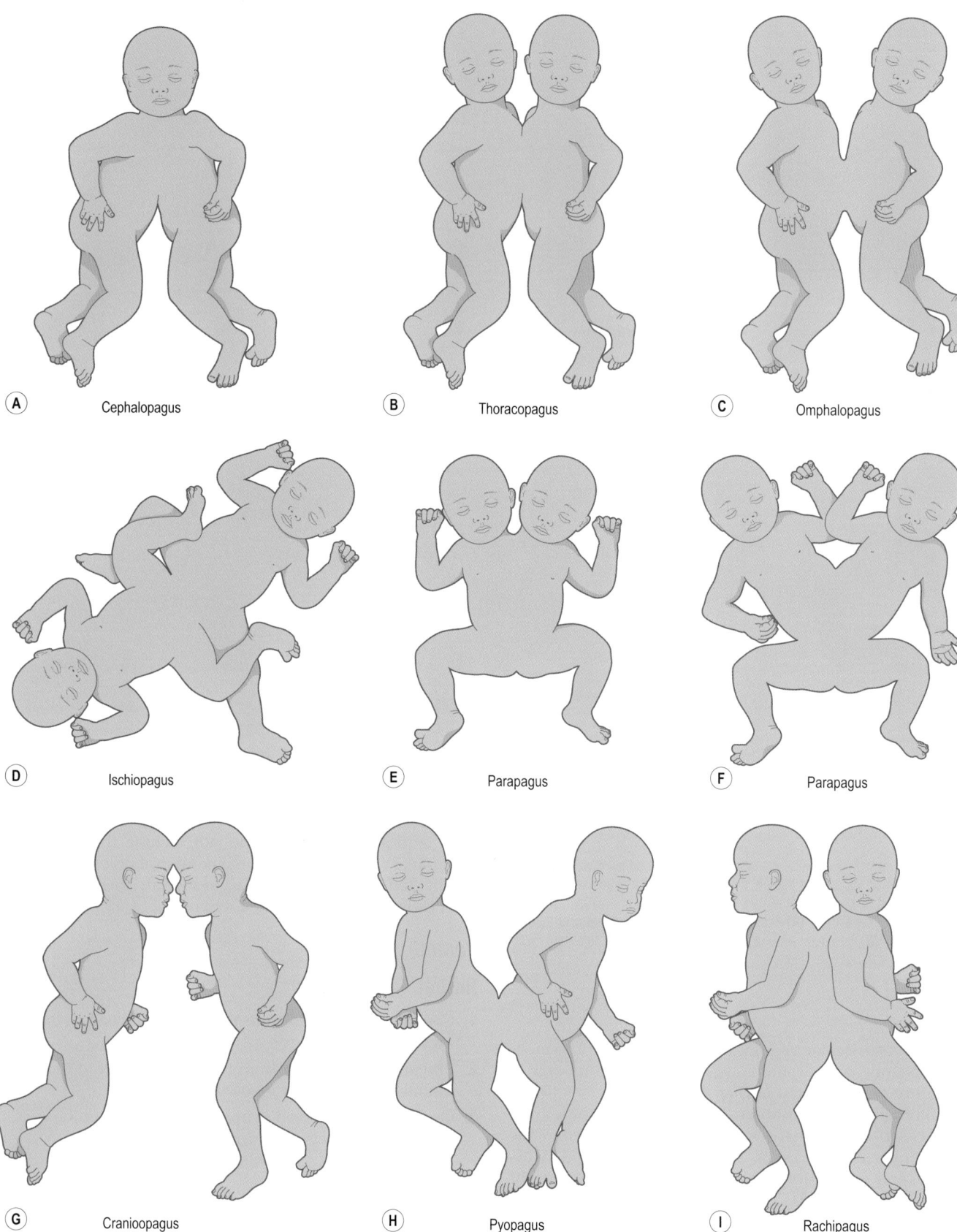

A Cephalopagus

B Thoracopagus

C Omphalopagus

D Ischiopagus

E Parapagus

F Parapagus

G Cranioopagus

H Pyopagus

I Rachipagus

Fig. 43.7 (A) The eight types of conjoined twins, as classified by Rowena Spencer[26] based on the theoretical site of union and divided into ventral and dorsal forms of junction.

anlage of the heart, the diaphragm, the oropharyngeal and cloacal membranes, the neural tube, and the periphery of the embryonic discs, each site corresponding to specific types of conjoined twinning. The unions are always homologous, meaning the fusion occurs head to head, tail to tail, front to front, back to back, or side by side but never head to tail or front to back. Spencer's "spherical theory" proposes that conjoined twins united dorsally "float" in a shared amniotic cavity, and those united ventrally "float" on the sphere of a shared yolk sac. In both cases, they can be oriented from rostral to caudal, depending on the relative temporal–spatial relationship of the embryonic discs during fusion[28] *(Fig. 43.8)*.

Diagnosis/patient presentation

Prenatal evaluation

The diagnosis of conjoined twins can be made as early as the 12th week of gestation on prenatal ultrasound. First-trimester or early second-trimester ultrasound findings suggestive of conjoined twins include a fixed position of the twin bodies on serial examinations, lack of a separating membrane between the twins, and inability to separate the fetal bodies and skin contours.[29,30] Once the diagnosis is suspected, evaluation should continue with serial ultrasounds, magnetic resonance imaging (MRI), and echocardiography to define better the extent of the union and the anatomy of the shared organs, to determine the presence of any associated abnormalities, and to monitor the pregnancy for complications[14] *(Fig. 43.9)*.

Careful cardiac evaluation is essential given the high incidence of thoracopagus types. Both ultrafast fetal MRI with three-dimensional reconstruction and echocardiography are useful in determining the cardiac structure and function. Prenatal echocardiography may be superior to postnatal scans because the amniotic fluid provides a good buffer for scanning, and positioning of the transducer may be difficult postnatally against the small pericardial window. Delineation of the conjoined cardiac anatomy has been achieved as early as the 20th week of gestation, although third-trimester studies are most reliable; even those may underestimate the severity of disease when compared with autopsy studies.[12,14,29] Echocardiography can also be utilized while on placental support during the EXIT procedure, as was reported by MacKenzie *et al.* at the Children's Hospital of Philadelphia and proved critical in delineating the relationship of the great vessels in preparation for immediate separation.[14]

The presence of other anomalies, even in organ systems not related to the conjoining, may affect survival and need to be ascertained prenatally as well. Observed anomalies include congenital diaphragmatic hernia, abdominal wall defects, neural tube defects, club foot, imperforate anus, esophageal atresia, and cystic hygroma.[14] Serial scans also are necessary to monitor the pregnancy for the unique complications that are known to occur in multifetal gestations such as twin–twin transfusion syndrome, co-twin demise, and oligohydramnios-polyhydramnios sequence, as well as for the effects of cross-circulation on the pregnancy such as polyhydramnios and hydrops. Polyhydramnios is noted in 50% of cases of conjoined twin gestations and may require treatment during pregnancy to prevent complications such as preterm labor.[12,31]

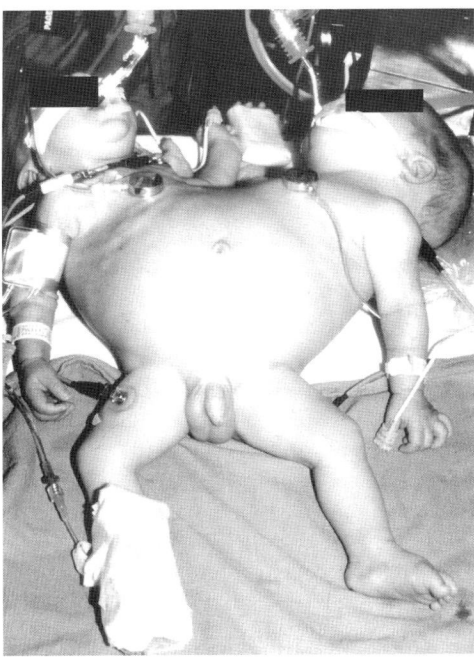

Fig. 43.7, cont'd (B) Parapagus conjoined twins with a single pelvis.

Dorsal

6. Craniopagus: united on any portion on the skull except the face or foramen magnum, and the trunks are never united.
7. Pygopagus: sharing sacrococcygeal and perineal regions, and sometimes the spinal cord.
8. Rachiopagus: fused dorsally above the sacrum, and exceedingly rare.

Asymmetrical forms of conjoined twinning often occur, resulting in a smaller and larger twin; these are termed "parasitic" followed by their closest classification. When one twin is significantly smaller and less well developed, it is often malnourished and has other physiologic problems which can complicate potential separation. On some occasions, the smaller twin may die and much of the deceased twin may be absorbed. Conjoined twins whose union and anatomy are intermediate between different types are termed "atypical conjoined twins."[26]

Etiology

Two theories have been proposed to explain the embryology resulting in conjoined twins. The classic theory of incomplete fission, described by Zimmerman,[27] proposes that there is incomplete separation of the embryonic discs of twins arising from a uniovular gestation between 13 and 16 days after fertilization. More recently, Spencer[28] proposed an alternative theory of secondary fusion of two originally separate monovular embryonic discs. This theory postulates that, during the third or fourth week of development, previously separate embryonic discs reunite either dorsally or ventrally at specific sites where the surface ectoderm is either absent or normally programmed to fuse or break down. These sites include the

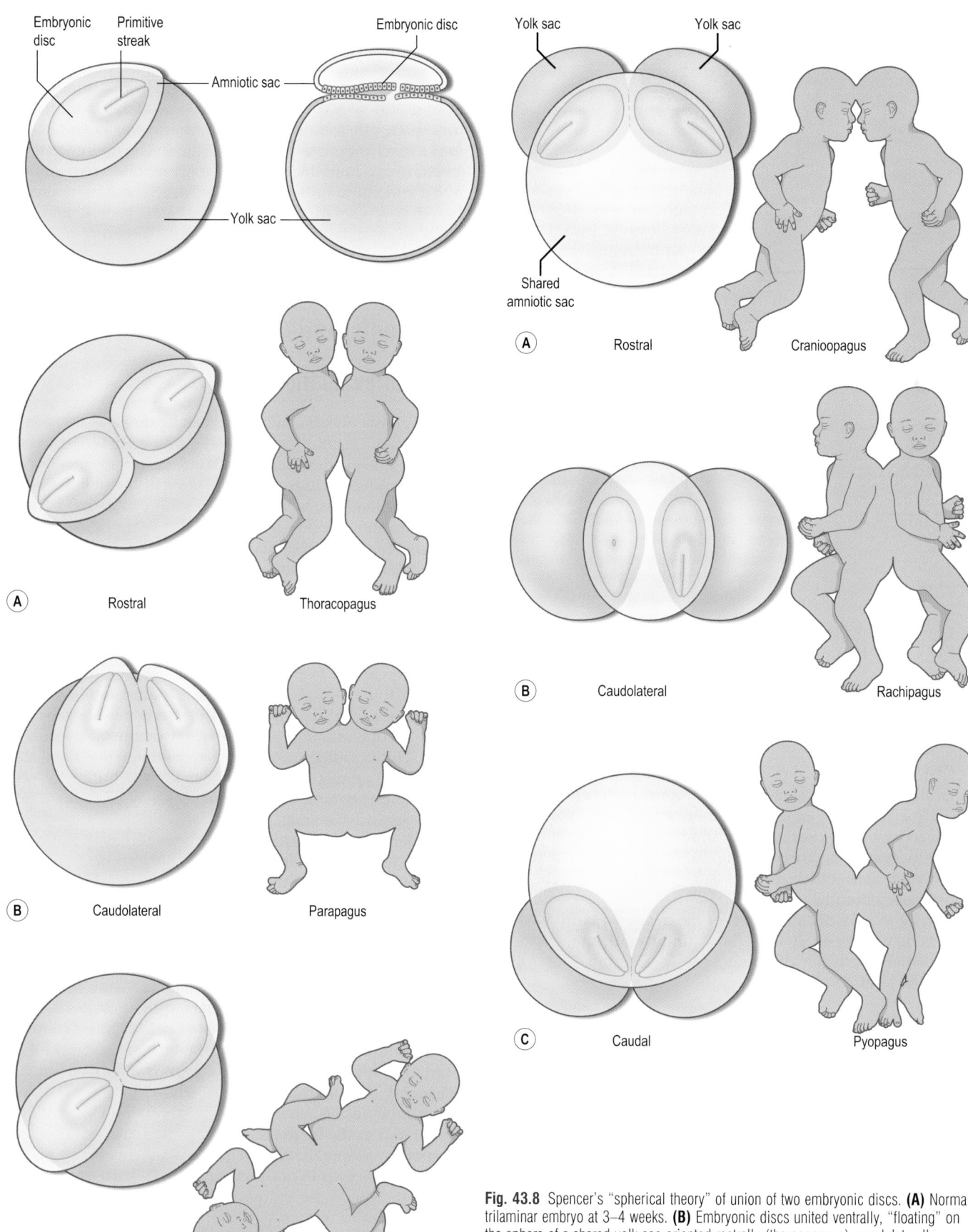

Fig. 43.8 Spencer's "spherical theory" of union of two embryonic discs. **(A)** Normal trilaminar embryo at 3–4 weeks. **(B)** Embryonic discs united ventrally, "floating" on the sphere of a shared yolk sac oriented rostrally (thoracopagus), caudolaterally (parapagus), and caudally (ischiopagus). **(C)** Embryonic discs united dorsally, "floating" in a shared amniotic cavity oriented rostrally (craniopagus), middorsally (rachipagus), and caudally (pygopagus).

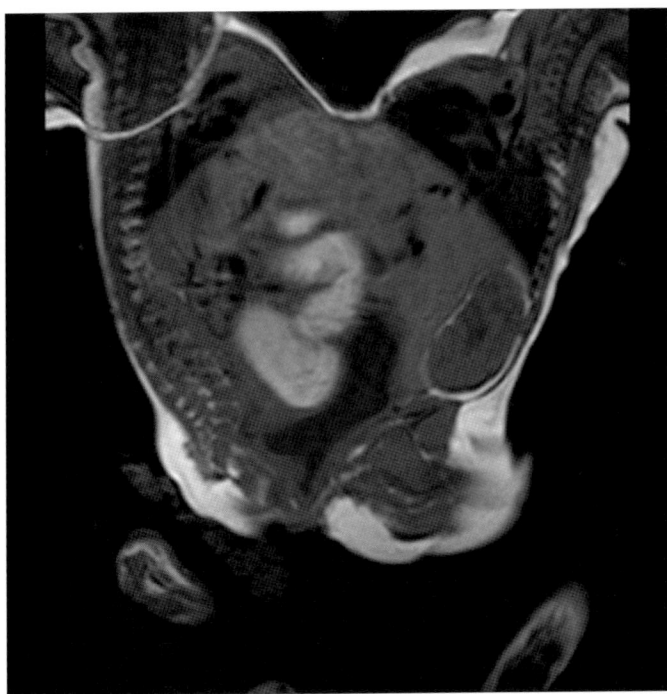

Fig. 43.9 Prenatal magnetic resonance imaging of ischiopagus twins with conjoined livers and colon and a cloacal malformation (case 7).

Ethical, religious, and moral issues surrounding conjoined twin pregnancies and separation are complex. Accurate prenatal diagnosis and early determination of the extent and severity of the twin union enable determination of the feasibility of separation and prediction of postnatal outcomes. This is critical in early counseling of families so that the options of termination versus near-term cesarean delivery can be discussed. Elective termination is recommended in cases where there is cerebral or cardiac fusion, and parents may also elect termination when the anticipated severity of deformity and quality of life following separation is unacceptable.[12] Early assessment also provides time for parental adjustment and predelivery planning; the involvement of psychologists, social workers, and ethicists may beneficial in this decision-making and counseling process.

Treatment/surgical technique

Obstetric management

Near-term cesarean delivery at 36–38 weeks of gestation after confirming lung maturity and delivery at or near a pediatric surgical center is the recommended obstetric management. Although a number of vaginal deliveries have been reported in the literature, cesarean section is preferred for the safest management of the fetuses and the mother. Cesarean section also provides the opportunity for utilizing the EXIT procedure for the management of twins expected to have rapid cardiac deterioration.

Twins who survive delivery fall into three groups, determined predominantly by their cardiac anatomy: those who die shortly after birth, those who survive to planned separation, and those who require emergent separation after birth. Those who do not require emergent separation have a survival rate of 80–90% in most series. Emergent separation is required when one twin is dead or dying and threatening the survival of the other twin, or when a life-threatening and correctable congenital anomaly is present in one or both twins such as intestinal atresia, malrotation, ruptured omphalocele, or anorectal agenesis. Survival in this situation falls to 30–50%. The obvious advantages of delayed separation include diminished risks of anesthesia, ability to confirm the anatomy and evaluate for other congenital anatomies, and the ability to ensure adequate wound coverage with preseparation tissue expansion.[12,14,15,32]

Preoperative planning

Elective separation may take place as early as 2–4 months after delivery. Maintenance in an intensive care setting during this time allows for close monitoring and stabilization of the infants, and nutritional supplementation as necessary to optimize growth and development preoperatively. Detailed postnatal investigations continue to confirm the conjoined anatomy and other possible congenital anomalies. Computed tomography scanning in addition to MRI may provide useful information about shared organs as well as skeletal anatomy, while MRI is preferred for delineating vascular anatomy; gastrointestinal contrast studies and angiography also may be utilized but have been less helpful.[3,10]

Assembly of a multidisciplinary team of various surgical subspecialists, neonatologists, anesthesiologists, and nurses, as well as the development of a comprehensive surgical and perioperative management plan, is critical to the success of twin separation. Two distinct anesthesia and surgery teams should be assembled, and the anesthetic management plan and operative steps in separation should be predetermined and reviewed. Both schematic diagrams as well as three-dimensional models may be useful in planning separation.[3,33] Logistic details, including patient positioning, placement of lines and monitors, and operative room set-up and instrumentation, should not be overlooked.

Essential preoperative planning also includes proposed management of the soft tissues at the time of separation. If the shared anatomy allows for separation and survival of both twins, then wound closure becomes a critical issue. Assessment of the anticipated soft-tissue deficiency will determine the need for preseparation tissue expansion to accomplish stable wound closure. Without adequate skin coverage, the child is at risk for exposure of important viscera, frank evisceration, and sepsis. If the closure is too tight, embarrassment of cardiac and pulmonary function can occur, which can be fatal. Additional support materials may be necessary when large defects of the body walls, particularly the chest, abdomen, and pelvic floor, are created after separation. The plastic surgeon, therefore, is an essential member of the surgical team attempting twin separation.

Delineation of the vascular skin territories is important in planning the line of separation between co-twins, especially in cases of ischiopagus tripus where the common leg is to be sacrificed and the soft tissue divided for reconstruction and closure of both twins. Although magnetic resonance angiography and angiographic studies can illustrate large-vessel anatomy and extremity perfusion, they are inadequate at assessing the precise vascular territories of the skin at the level of the pelvis and along the extremity. Fluorescein previously has been used to evaluate perfusion and viability of skin flaps, ischemic extremities, injured bowel, and burn wounds.[34–38] The traditional fluorescein test uses qualitative visual assessment of tissue fluorescein delivery by inspection under ultraviolet light. A quantitative technique of intravenous fluorescein mapping employing a fiberoptic perfusion fluorometer was reported by Ross et al.[39] as helpful in defining the vascular territories and the line of separation between a pair of complicated ischiopagus twins at the Children's Hospital of Philadelphia in 1984[39,40] *(Fig. 43.10).*

Role of the plastic surgeon

The separation of conjoined twins challenges the plastic surgeon to provide sufficient soft tissue to cover a significant area of intrinsic deficiency. Twin separation is analogous to separation of a simple or complex syndactyly, a congenital anomaly well known to plastic surgeons. As in the separation of syndactyly, insufficient tissue is present for resurfacing the conjoined interface so that skin grafts are generally needed, except in the simplest types. Likewise, the soft-tissue deficit in conjoined twins is twice the surface area of the canal joining the twins.[41] A variety of methods for providing soft-tissue coverage have been reported in the literature and include the use of skin grafts and skin substitute products, local skin flaps, pneumoperitoneum, and tissue expansion.

Skin grafting represents the least useful primary method of coverage in these patients. Skin grafting can be used only in the smallest of defects and requires an intact body wall for a bed. Only under the most extreme circumstances would a skin graft primarily be applied to abdominal viscera, although skin grafting is often used secondarily to treat wound-healing complications, not uncommon after twin separation. Today, various skin substitute products are available and can be used to cover deficient areas of skin and also to reconstruct fascial defects.[42–44] As in traditional abdominal wall and chest wall reconstruction, both synthetic and biologic materials can be utilized, although biologics are much preferred in the pediatric population and where soft-tissue coverage may be precarious. Dermal replacement materials and other biologic meshes are favorable because they are quickly revascularized and promote ingrowth of new tissue; thus they are compatible with growth and are easily managed if exposure occurs.[45–47] Random-pattern or arterialized flaps of skin or skin and muscle can be used for coverage of small defects. Few case reports from the literature describe their use for coverage other than utilization of the third leg with fillet and sacrifice of the tripus. Indeed, many of the successful ischiopagus tripus separations have used the third leg for soft-tissue coverage.

Pneumoperitoneum has been reported by several surgical groups in the past. Mestel et al. utilized pneumoperitoneum in an ischiopagus tripus twin pair. They injected 500–1500 cc of air every 3 days and were able to increase the abdominal circumference by 12 cm. At separation, there was insufficient skin and the tripus was sacrificed to achieve a successful closure.[48] Yokomori et al. used pneumoperitoneum in conjunction with tissue expanders in an ischiopagus tripus twin

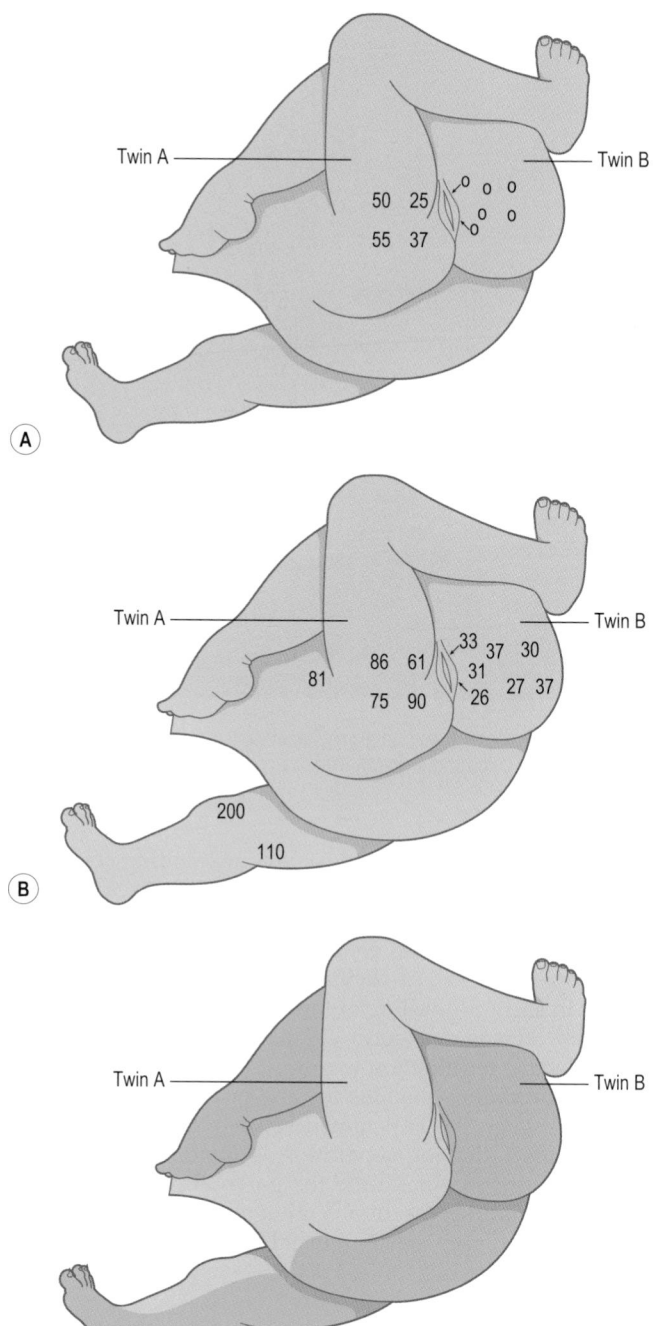

Fig. 43.10 (A–C) Technique of dermofluorometry demonstrating differential skin perfusion of the pelvis and lower extremities in a case of ischiopagus tripus twins. (Reproduced from Ross AJ 3rd, O'Neill JA, Jr., Silverman DG, et al. A new technique for evaluating cutaneous vascularity in complicated conjoined twins. *J Pediatr Surg.* 1985;20:743–746.)

pair, but again the tripus was sacrificed for successful coverage at the time of separation.[49] Wen-Sung Hung and co-workers also utilized pneumoperitoneum in an ischiopagus tripus with twice-weekly injection of 500–1500 cc of air. The circumference was increased by 19 cm, but again, the third leg was sacrificed for closure.[50] Although infection was felt to be a potential risk of pneumoperitoneum, it was not encountered by any of the investigators. In all three cases, however, an insufficient amount of soft tissue was generated to achieve successful closure without sacrifice of the third shared leg.

Tissue expansion represents a great advance in the ability to provide adequate soft-tissue coverage for the separation of conjoined twins. Although Neumann first introduced the concept in 1957, it was not until 1976 that tissue expansion became popular, with the introduction of the Radovan expander.[51,52] Since then, tissue expansion has been used widely by plastic surgeons for a variety of conditions where additional skin is needed. The first report of the successful use of tissue expansion for the separation of conjoined twins was by Zuker and his co-workers in 1986 for the successful separation of an ischiopagus conjoined twin pair. Five subcutaneous and two intraperitoneal expanders were used. One twin was closed successfully, but in the second, Marlex mesh reinforcement of the abdominal wall and split-thickness skin grafting were needed to complete the closure.[53] Numerous reports have followed, utilizing tissue expansion in both the intraperitoneal and subcutaneous positions.[41,53-55]

We advocate subcutaneous tissue expansion with placement of the maximum number of tissue expanders possible in all areas surrounding the canal separating the infants. They should be placed on the extremities in tripus cases as well, to facilitate harvest of adequate skin and subcutaneous tissue flaps without sacrifice of the lower extremities. Smooth-walled overtextured tissue expanders should be used for two reasons. In infants, the subcutaneous tissue layer is thin. Tissue expanders with a hard backing produce sharp edges which can gradually erode through the skin at the margin of the expander. In addition, capsule formation is reduced with a textured implant surface, and thus, further thinning of the skin can occur. Distant ports rather than integral ports are also preferred for the same reason. The thin skin overlying the tissue expander is subject to breakdown from repeated injections during the expansion process, thus increasing the risk of expander exposure with integral ports.

Clinical experience

The following eight cases of conjoined twin separation review our experience with the separation of conjoined twins at the Children's Hospital of Philadelphia between 1980 and 2007. These examples highlight the lessons we have learned and present principles in surgical technique and patient management that may be helpful to future teams attempting conjoined twin separation.

Case 1:

thoracopagus and ischiopagus twins (1980)

Separation of this male thoracopagus and ischiopagus twin pair (*Fig. 43.11*) was performed at 2.3 years of age and represented the first use of tissue expanders in our series (1980). One large circular 1000-cc Radovan expander was inserted beneath their shared abdominal skin through an incision in the xiphoid region and the umbilicus was released from its attachment to the abdominal wall. Despite the extra skin generated, it was inadequate and resulted in a tight closure on the smaller twin, resulting in cardiopulmonary insufficiency and death. His skin was harvested and was frozen for eventual use for coverage of

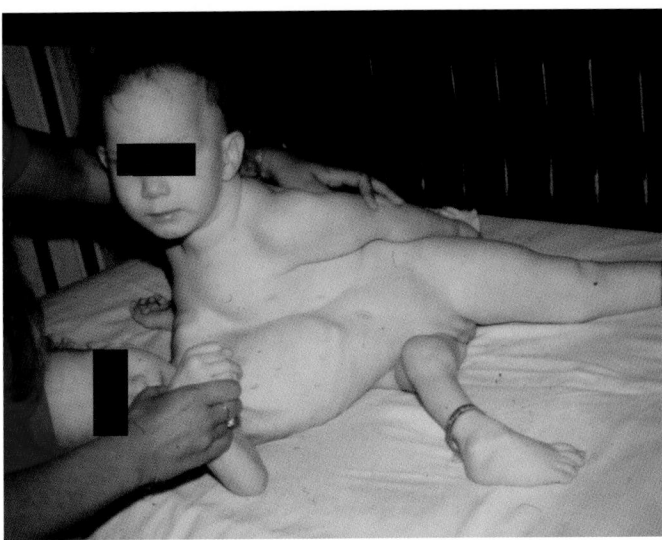

Fig. 43.11 Thoracopagus and ischiopagus twins prior to separation. Tissue expanders were used for the first time at the Children's Hospital of Philadelphia in 1980 to generate additional skin prior to separation.

open wounds on the surviving twin. The skin grafts were frozen in liquid nitrogen after sequential passage through increasing concentrations of glycerol in saline, as described by Lehr and co-workers.[56] Closure of the surviving twin was achieved using the capsule along with the expanded skin. Granulation tissue developed on the capsular surface over ensuing days and was successfully grafted with skin that had been harvested from the deceased twin.

Case 2:

ischiopagus twins (1984)

This ischiopagus tripus conjoined twin pair were joined from the sternum to the pelvis with a shared liver, terminal ileum, and colon. Each twin had a separate normal lower extremity and a shared extremity. Fluorescein studies were used in this case and proved quite helpful in assessing the territories of skin perfusion and determining the lines of separation. Preoperative studies demonstrated a clear line of separation along the pelvis and extremity with the blood supply to the extremity predominantly coming from twin A. The twins were separated along this line and the extremity was given to twin A. A pedicled flap from the shared thigh based on the lower abdomen of twin B was used to complete the cutaneous closure of twin B. Injection of fluorescein was performed again intraoperatively to assess the viability of this pedicled flap prior to closure and any nonviable tissue was trimmed. Because the knee joint of the shared extremity was not stable, the knee was disarticulated and the distal flap of skin and muscle used to complete the closure of twin A (*Fig. 43.10*).

Case 3:

omphalopagus and ischiopagus twins (1988)

This omphalopagus and ischiopagus twin pair had a less complex connection between the infants from xiphoid to pelvis. They were treated with a single 1000-cc Radovan expander beneath the shared abdominal skin. The expander was introduced through a single incision in the xiphoid region with release of the umbilicus. Expansion was initiated in the hospital but was completed on an outpatient basis. A successful surgical separation with complete skin coverage was achieved without difficulty at 14.5 months of age without the need for skin grafts.

Case 4:

ischiopagus twins (1992)

In this ischiopagus twin pair, additional expanders were used because of the soft-tissue inadequacy experienced in the first twin pair separation. At 3 months of age, a 700-cc round Radovan expander was used to expand the conjoined abdominal region and two smaller 250-cc rectangular expanders were used on the back, all with remote ports. Four days postoperatively, some skin necrosis was evident in the upper abdomen and the twins were taken back to the operating room. The area of necrosis was excised and the single abdominal tissue expander was replaced with two smaller 250-cc expanders. The patients were initially treated on a regular bed mattress with frequent, regular rotation from the abdomen to the back. Despite this, chronic pressure on their backs caused a threatened exposure of the posterior expanders. Transfer to a Clinitron bed improved the situation to some degree but the skin continued to thin over the posterior expanders. This prompted earlier surgical separation, which was performed at 5 months of age. The expanded abdominal skin was converted into bi-pedicled flaps to achieve closure and the remaining defects were grafted with autogenous split-thickness skin grafts. Once again, despite the use of additional expanders, there was insufficient soft tissue for complete wound coverage with the expanded skin. Further expansion would have been desirable.

Case 5:

ischiopagus tripus twins (1993)

This ischiopagus tripus twin pair was treated at 3.5 years of age using multiple rectangular tissue expanders. Two expanders were placed on the shared lower extremity, one on the anterior aspect and the other on the posterior aspect of the upper thigh, another was inserted on the back, and two more were placed in the abdominal region *(Fig. 43.12)*. They were expanded over a period of 3 months with a total of 6 liters of saline. During the expansion process, there was threatened erosion of the skin from the firm backing on the rectangular abdominal expander, and it was replaced with a smooth-walled expander. The twins were treated in a Clinitron bed for the entire expansion period, thus eliminating the problems with skin breakdown on the back. However, continuous movement of the legs caused chronic abrasion of the expanded skin overlying the tissue expander in the tripus against the expanded abdominal skin, and therefore, the legs were immobilized in a cast. Separation was successful with sufficient soft tissue to cover both twins without sacrifice of the tripus.

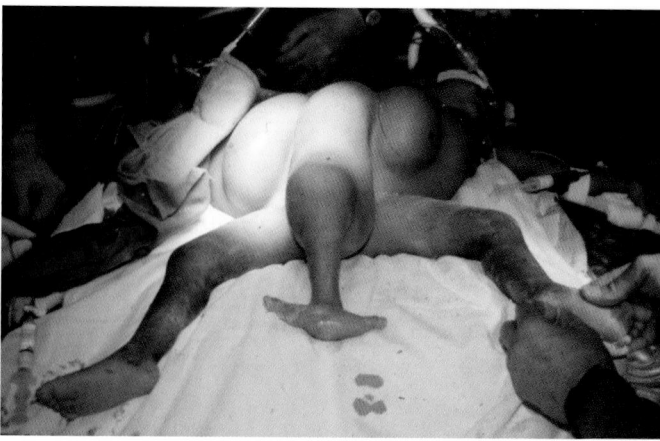

Fig. 43.12 Ischiopagus tripus twins – the abnormal tripus extremity is clearly demonstrated.

Case 6:

thoracopagus and omphalopagus twins (1999)

This thoracopagus and omphalopagus twin pair was separated at 6 months of age. They were joined from the level of the manubrium to the umbilicus with a shared liver, diaphragm, and chest cavity, although their hearts were not joined *(Fig. 43.13)*. At 3 months of age, three rectangular-shaped 500-cc remote port tissue expanders were placed, one superior to the area of union in the thoracic area, and the other two at the inferior lateral aspect of the junction in the lower abdomen. These were filled over the next 3 months and produced ample expanded skin. At the time of separation, Gore-Tex® patches were used by the general surgeons to close the chest cavities in both twins; there was sufficient soft tissue for uneventful and stable closure over these prostheses.

Case 7:

ischiopagus twins (2001)

This ischiopagus twin pair was separated at 7 months of age. They had joined livers, a shared colon, and both had a cloacal malformation requiring a shared colostomy shortly after birth. Four expanders originally were placed in the thoracic and abdominal regions at 3 months of age *(Fig. 43.14A)*. The patients were taken back to the operating room twice during the expansion process because of expander complications. The thoracic expander was removed due to some overlying skin necrosis and one of the lateral abdominal expanders was removed due to threatened exposure and a seroma. One month later two additional expanders were placed in the thoracic and abdominal regions since a greater soft-tissue requirement was anticipated. Expansion was resumed uneventfully, and separation was performed 3 months later. Vicryl mesh was used in closure of the abdominal wall due to contamination from the colostomy during the procedure with a plan for more definitive abdominal wall reconstruction in the future.

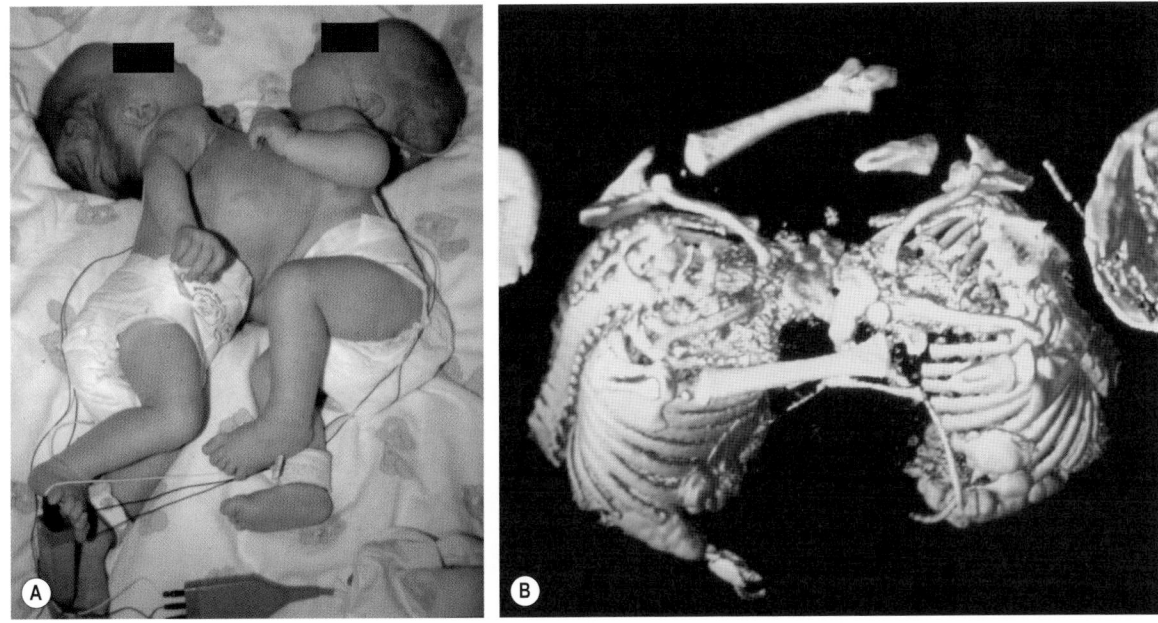

Fig. 43.13 (A) Thoracopagus and omphalopagus twins. **(B)** Three-dimensional computed tomography scan was helpful in demonstrating shared skeletal structures.

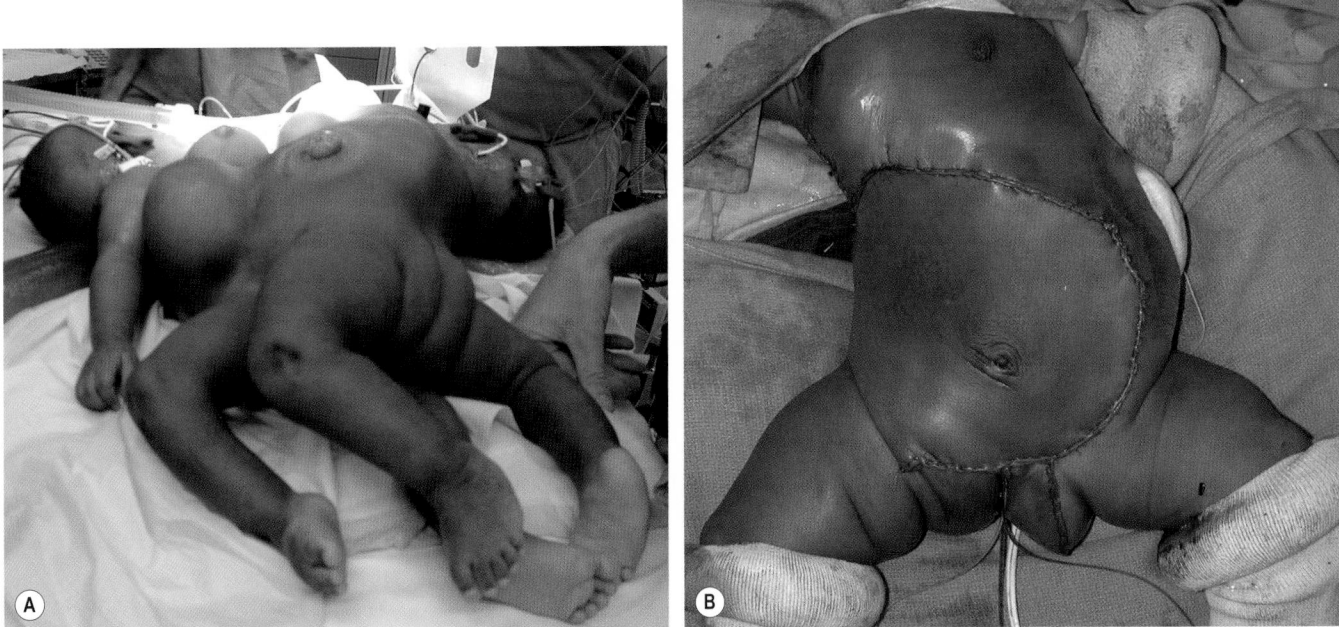

Fig. 43.14 (A) Ischiopagus twins with shared liver and colon, with tissue expanders in place. The shared colostomy is visible. **(B)** Twin A with complete skin closure of abdominal wall.

Local advancement and rotation flaps of the expanded thoracic and abdominal skin were used and complete coverage of the abdominal defect was obtained in one twin. In the second twin, a small lateral defect remained after rotation of the abdominal skin flap; vacuum-assisted closure therapy hastened wound healing, and the defect was eventually covered with an autologous skin graft *(Fig. 43.14B)*.

Case 8:

omphalopagus twins (2007)

This pair shared a portion of liver and duodenum. Four expanders were placed in subcutaneous pockets, but one developed a leak during the expansion process. Acellular dermal matrix was used to compensate for insufficient skin coverage over the central abdomen *(Fig. 43.15)*.

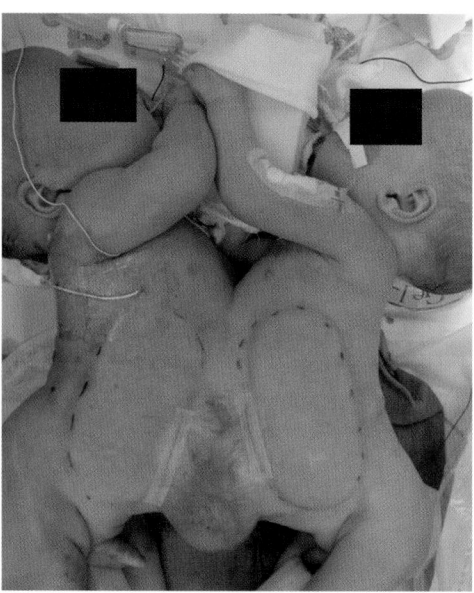

Fig. 43.15 Omphalopagus twins with newly placed expanders. The injection ports are dorsally located. Two additional expanders were placed on the contralateral side.

Postoperative care

Supportive care in an intensive care unit setting with meticulous monitoring is essential for postoperative stabilization of the separated infants. Elective paralysis and ventilation for 24–48 hours are preferable during the immediate postoperative period for fluid and electrolyte replacement and cardiac stabilization. Perioperative antibiotics and strict infectious precautions also are recommended to avoid sepsis.

Perioperative pressure reduction strategies are critical for successful management of the soft tissues. A Clinitron bed is recommended during tissue expansion to optimize soft-tissue viability and prevent pressure-related ulcerations in dependent areas or over the expanders. This should be continued during the early postoperative period of immobilization to augment postoperative wound healing, especially when flaps and grafts have been utilized in closure. Adjunctive techniques such as frequent turning, supportive gel padding, and immobilization of the extremities when necessary to prevent traumatic ulcerations, also should be employed.

Continued nutritional support is equally critical. More often than not, one of the infants is smaller and less well nourished. The stress of prolonged treatment and repeated operations compounds this problem, placing the infants at greater risk for wound-healing and infectious complications. In this situation, the use of supplemental parenteral or enteral feedings is beneficial, and should be considered in most cases.

Outcomes, prognosis, and complications

Wound-healing complications are common postoperatively. Postoperative vacuum-assisted closure therapy can be useful in managing wound dehiscence or flap losses, and secondary skin grafting and surgical revision are frequently necessary to manage soft-tissue wounds and unacceptable scarring.

The overall success of conjoined twin separation depends on the experience and preparedness of the treating team and the resources available at the pediatric specialty center. Recent advances in imaging techniques for prenatal diagnosis, pre- and postoperative critical care management, and anesthetic care have improved outcomes and survival rates in general. Comprehensive long-term care by a multispecialty team is critical in the management of these patients from prenatal diagnosis to postoperative follow-up to address their complex issues. Follow-up at the same institution is recommended due to the anatomic complexity of these patients, and it also allows for determination of long-term outcomes.

Access the complete references list online at **http://www.expertconsult.com**

1. Bates AW. Conjoined twins in the 16th century. *Twin Res.* 2002;5:521–528.

3. Redett R, Zucker RM. Conjoined twins. In: Bentz M, Bauer BS, Zucker RM, eds. *Principles and practice of pediatric plastic surgery.* St. Louis: Quality Medical Publishing; 2008:185–212.
   A well-rounded account of perioperative and operative considerations relating to the separation of conjoined twins is presented.

5. Spitz L. Surgery for conjoined twins. *Ann R Coll Surg Engl.* 2003;85:230–235.

6. Spitz L, Kiely EM. Conjoined twins. *JAMA.* 2003;289: 1307–1310.
   The authors begin with an account of conjoined twin reports in history. A review of classification, diagnosis, and management follows.

10. Spitz L. Conjoined twins. *Br J Surg.* 1996;83:1028–1030.
    This brief reports offers the author's perspective from an experience of 10 sets of conjoined twins over a decade. Special mention is made of the potential for heavy intraoperative blood loss and the fragility of these patients after separation.

12. O'Neill Jr JA. Conjoined twins. In: Grosfeld JL, O'Neill Jr JA, Fonkalsrud EW, et al, eds. *Pediatric surgery.* Philadelphia: Mosby; 2006,
    This chapter is a review of topics ranging from prenatal diagnosis to ethical considerations related to conjoined twins. Particularly useful is the authors' systems-based approach to surgical technique.

14. Mackenzie TC, Crombleholme TM, Johnson MP, et al. The natural history of prenatally diagnosed conjoined twins. *J Pediatr Surg.* 2002;37:303–309.

21. Walker M, Browd SR. Craniopagus twins: embryology, classification, surgical anatomy, and separation. *Childs Nerv Syst*. 2004;20:554–566.

28. Spencer R. Theoretical and analytical embryology of conjoined twins: part I: embryogenesis. *Clin Anat*. 2000;13:36–53.

This review spans over 1200 cases of conjoined twins. Observations drawn from these cases form the basis for a discussion of the embryology leading to this pathology.

41. Zubowicz VN, Ricketts R. Use of skin expansion in separation of conjoined twins. *Ann Plast Surg*. 1988;20: 272–276.

44

Reconstruction of urogenital defects: Congenital

Mohan S. Gundeti and Michael C. Large

SYNOPSIS

- Reconstruction of cloacal or urogenital sinus abnormalities is complex, often requiring multiple surgical disciplines and multiple stages.
- Hypospadias is common, perhaps increasing in incidence, and may be managed through multiple surgical approaches.
- Penoscrotal transposition and chordee commonly accompany hypospadias and may be treated concomitantly.

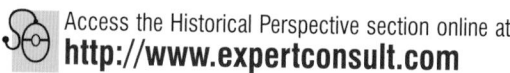

Access the Historical Perspective section online at
http://www.expertconsult.com

Introduction

The reconstructive techniques for congenital urogenital defects are broad-ranging, and the indications for intervention vary from emergent to elective. Herein the authors will discuss the normal development of the urogenital tract, followed by a discussion of some common female and male disorders and their surgical repairs. Cloacal and urogenital sinus disorders, as well as variant presentations that may include clitoromegaly, exstrophy, and/or epispadias, will be addressed first. What follows will concentrate on the spectrum of hypospadias disorders and some representative surgical techniques.

In general, reconstructive techniques for urologic disorders have satisfactory outcomes, but the importance of proper surgical timing and patient selection may not be understated. Vaginal agenesis is associated with Mayer–Rokitansky–Kuster–Hauser syndrome, wherein the proximal two-thirds of the vagina is absent. A mesonephric duct abnormality has been proposed as the etiology, with diagnosis often occurring in the workup of primary amenorrhea. Potential problems after vaginoplasty may include graft foreshortening, injury to

adjacent urinary structures, and problems secondary to prolonged postoperative immobilization.

Bladder exstrophy tends to occur in nulliparous, young females' offspring, with a recurrence risk of 1:275 and a risk of 1:70 in progeny. Patients have a low-set umbilicus and wide pubic diastasis. The pubic bone is shortened by 30%, with external rotation of the posterior pelvis. The clitoris or penis is short and bifid, and the urinary sphincter mechanism is underdeveloped. Nearly all patients have radiographic evidence of vesicoureteral reflux, and the incidence of inguinal hernias is increased. Treatment is discussed primarily in Volume 4, Chapter 13.

Cloacal exstrophy occurs when the anterior rectal and bladder walls do not develop. Prenatal ultrasound may illustrate an anterior infraumbilical cystic mass with separated pubic rami, rocker-bottom feet, and meningomyelocele. The newborn will have an exstrophied, shortened cecum that separates two exstrophied hemibladders. The ileum is prolapsed, the testes undescended, and the penis or clitoris small and bifid. The cloacal membrane is thought to have been persistent or overgrown, preventing mesenchymal ingrowth and thereby resulting in fusion of the genital ridges caudal to the membrane. Similar to bladder exstrophy, the posterior pelvis is externally rotated, the pubis is shortened, and pubic diastasis may be severe. Other associated abnormalities include spina bifida, lower limb deformities, uterine and vaginal duplication or agenesis, upper urinary tract anomalies, and gastrointestinal disorders, including short-gut syndrome.

Hypospadias occurs when the development of the urethral spongiosum and prepuce halts, resulting in a meatal location proximal to that of the distal glans. A hypospadic meatus is often accompanied by penile chordee as the normal embryological correction of curvature is likewise arrested. The severity of hypospadias is dictated by meatal location, ranging from perineal to glanular (*Figs 44.1, 44.2*). The more severe the hypospadias, the more likely it is accompanied by chordee and penoscrotal transposition (*Figs 44.3 and 44.4*).

Basic science/disease process

Development

The cloaca appears during the second gestational week, with the urorectal septum forming during week 4 *(Fig. 44.5)*. The urorectal septum fuses with the cloacal membrane by week 7. Defects of the cloacal membrane may result in bladder or cloacal exstrophy and epispadias. The mullerian ducts fuse to become the uterovaginal canal. Distally, the urogenital sinus forms the vestibule and the intervening sinovaginal bulbs canalize to form the distal vaginal canal. Paramesonephric abnormalities are frequently associated with ipsilateral renal anomalies, partly based upon their proximity during development. Anomalies of agenesis and fusion may occur. When the urogenital sinus fails to develop into the distal vagina, atresia results; agenesis occurs when the proximal third of the vagina fails to develop in a 46XX phenotypic female. Transverse septa arise from failure of fusion or canalization of the urogenital sinus and mullerian ducts. Meyer–Rokitansky–Kusler–Hauser syndrome consists of mullerian aplasia, often accompanied by renal and cervicothoracic dysplasias. ⊛ FIG **44.5** APPEARS ONLINE ONLY

Between weeks 7 and 8 of gestation, the male gonads differentiate secondary to the transcription of the *SRY* gene, thereby producing testosterone. The distance between anus and genitalia increases, the phallus elongates, the genital folds fuse, the preputial folds form and fuse dorsally, and during the 11th gestational week, the urethral folds fuse ventrally. If the genital folds fail to fuse, as in hypospadias, the preputial folds also fail to fuse ventrally, resulting in excessive dorsal

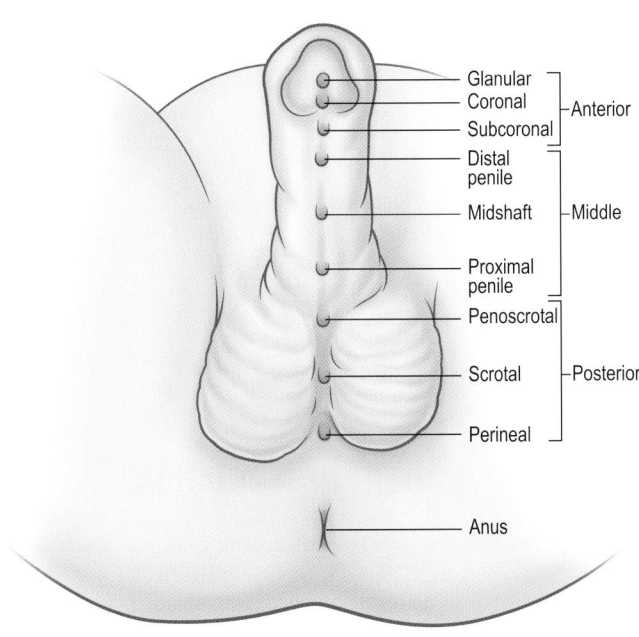

Fig. 44.1 Spectrum of hypospadias. (Reproduced from Wein: Campbell-Walsh Urology, 9th ed. © 2007 Saunders.)

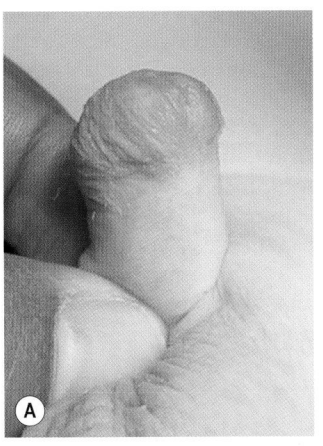 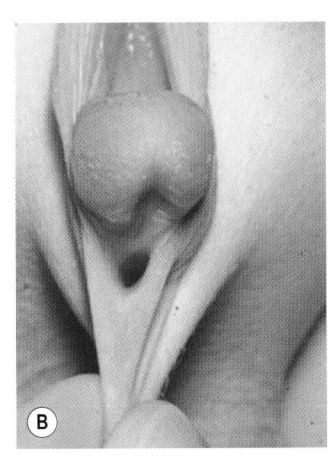 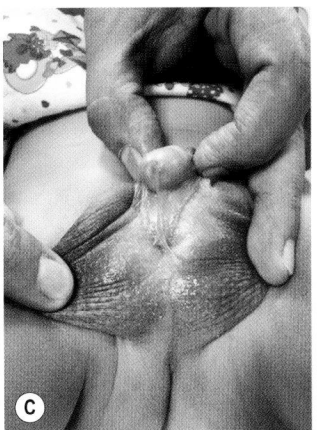 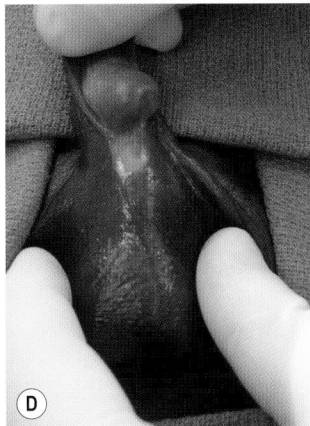

Fig. 44.2 **(A)** Glanular, **(B)** coronal, **(C)** penoscrotal, and **(D)** perineal hypospadias.

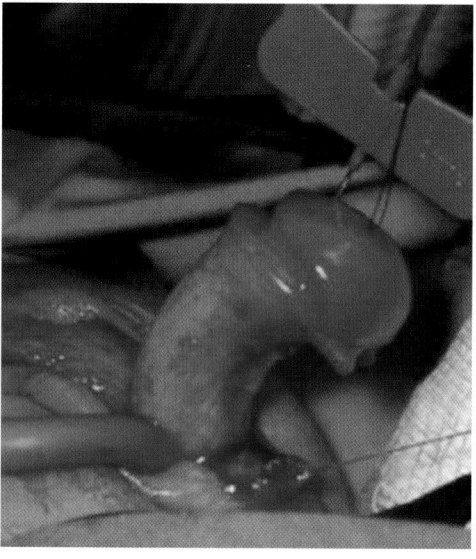

Fig. 44.3 Intraoperative depiction of chordee.

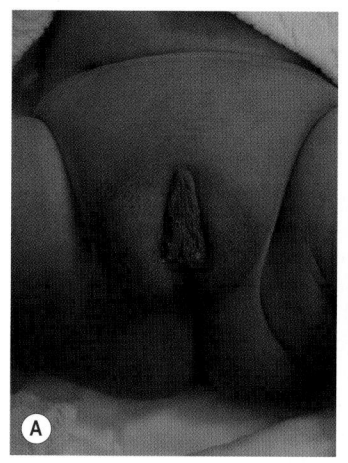
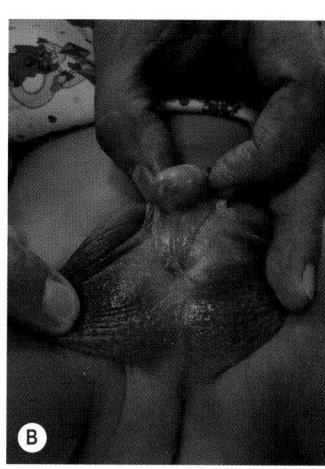

Fig. 44.4 (A, B) Penoscrotal transposition.

preputial tissue. By week 16, the glandular urethra forms. The glandular portion of the urethra is lined by squamous epithelium which likely also arises from urogenital sinus origin, but then undergoes differentiation.[14] Histologically, the hypospadic urethral plate contains sinusoids of urethral spongiosum and no scar tissue. The innervation of the hypospadic penis is like that of the normal penis: the pedendal nerve gives off the dorsal nerve which travels as two bundles on either side of 12 o'clock.

Epidemiology/incidence

The incidence of vaginal agenesis is 1:5000 female births, congenital adrenal hyperplasia 1:5000–15000, bladder exstrophy 1:30000 with male-to-female ratio 3:1, and cloacal exstrophy 1:800000, with male-to-female ratio 2:1. The incidence of hypospadias is roughly 1:300 male births, an increase from 2:1000 male births in 1970. There is nearly a ninefold increase in hypospadias in monozygotic twins.

Etiology

Urogenital sinus abnormalities may be isolated or associated with congenital adrenal hyperplasia, most often due to 21-hydroxylase deficiency. Overdevelopment of the cloacal membrane preventing medial migration of mesenchyme with subsequent membrane rupture underlies current models of the exstrophy–epispadias complex. Cloacal exstrophy is associated with cardiovascular, central nervous system, respiratory, gastrointestinal, and musculoskeletal abnormalities. Most cases are sporadic, with unbalanced translocations being hypothesized as causative in select cases. Neurologic and spinal defects may be related to dorsal mesenchymal

disruption or underlying tendency for separation of the spinal cord from vertebrae in the presence of a cloacal exstrophy. Regarding hypospadias, a polygenic, multifactorial etiology is most likely. Some cases may be caused by testosterone, dihydrotestosterone, or androgen receptor deficiencies, but these are found in only 5% of cases. Theories of chordee include incomplete development of the urethral plate, abnormal urethral meatal mesenchyme, and disproportional corporal growth.

Diagnosis/patient presentation

The workup of a newborn with ambiguous genitalia should involve multiple disciplinary teams and critical associations such as congenital adrenal hyperplasia should be ruled out. Fluid and electrolyte balance and blood pressure control should be maintained. Examination should note any suprapubic mass or ascites, sacral dimples, genitalia curvature and size, palpability of gonads, location of anus and perineal orifices, and pigmentation. Karyotype and adrenal biochemical studies should be undertaken, with prompt replacement of cortisol and fludrocortisone in cases of congenital adrenal hyperplasia. *In utero* exposure to androgenic substances should be investigated, as should a family history of infantile death. Radiographic and endoscopic evaluations of the genitalia and urinary tract are indicated, including abdominal X-ray and ultrasound, genitography, echocardiography, lumbar magnetic resonance imaging, and cystoscopy with vaginoscopy. Exstrophy is often diagnosed *in utero*, and neonatal intensive care is mandatory. Older patients with isolated vaginal atresia or transverse vaginal septa may present with amenorrhea or a distended upper vagina.

Hypospadias is frequently diagnosed at birth on physical examination, although later diagnoses are not uncommon. Patients with impalpable gonads and hypospadias have a disorder of sexual differentiation until proven otherwise, and karyotype is indicated.

Patient selection

For the patient with vaginal agenesis, the techniques and timing remain controversial. It is apparent that the majority of patients undergoing vaginoplasty as infants require additional vaginal surgery. When vaginal defects are associated with clitoromegaly, as in congenital adrenal hyperplasia, the surgeon has two fundamental options: perform an uncomplicated clitoroplasty with deferred vaginoplasty or a complex clitorovaginoplasty with deferred minor introitus repair in postpuberty.

Patients presenting with the exstrophy–epispadias complex are managed with a staged procedure.[15] Bladder and abdominal closures with bilateral osteotomy are performed in the newborn period. Epispadias repair occurs 6–12 months later, and bladder neck reconstruction with ureteral reimplantation in another 4–5 years if indicated.

Patient selection is most pertinent to hypospadias repair. The meatal location, glans volume, penile length, presence of penoscrotal transposition and/or chordee, and width and depth of the urethral plate all weigh in the surgeon's selection of technique. In general, distal hypospadias may be treated by tubularized incised plate (TIP) procedure with meatoplasty and glanuloplasty (MAGPI) techniques, while proximal hypospadias are frequently treated by two-staged graft or onlay island flap repairs.

The optimal timing for hypospadias repair is 6 months of age in a full-term male. Ninety-two percent of pediatric urologists perform a TIP procedure for distal hypospadias .[13] Proximal hypospadias without curvature is repaired by TIP or onlay island flap by equal proportions of urologists, while proximal hypospadias with severe chordee is most often repaired by a staged repair.[16] Intramuscular testosterone injections of 25 mg/dose or 2 mg/kg/dose may be administered up to three times prior to repair in an attempt to improve penile vascularity and tissue robustness, thereby facilitating subsequent surgery.

Treatment/surgical technique

Vaginal reconstruction

Vaginal agenesis

Reconstruction may involve grafts of the skin, intestine, or buccal mucosa. In the Abbé–McIndoe procedure, a Y incision is made on the median raphe between urethra and anus. A Foley catheter facilitates dissection posterior to the urethra. The neovaginal walls are formed by partial-thickness skin grafts harvested from the hip and buttock. Partial-thickness grafts are best in the adult population, while full-thickness grafts may be utilized in adolescents. The exact dimensions of the neovagina must be tailored to the individual, with a young adult having depth of 10–14 cm. The skin grafts are sutured to one another with epidermal surface positioned to line the interior of the vagina. These grafts may be molded around a Heyer–Schulte vaginal stent which is then seated and inflated into position to facilitate take. The Y incision flaps are approximated to the graft edges, and the labia majora are sutured to each other to prevent distal migration of the stent. The patient remains on bedrest for at least 5 days and constipating medication is administered. After this, the labia are separated, the stent deflated and the graft examined. Upon discharge, the patient is taught how to remove, wash, and replace the stent daily. A stent or dilator is encouraged for a minimum of 6 months to minimize retraction, and intercourse is appropriate after 3 months. Vulvobulbocavernosus, gracilis, or rectus myocutaneous flaps are frequently utilized for vaginal reconstruction in the adult population following radical pelvic surgery.

The use of bowel results in mucus production which may require daily douching and result in odor or ulcerations.[17] While bowel preparation has historically been advised, the authors have found it to be unnecessary.[18,19] A Pfannenstiel incision is appropriate, although a midline incision may also be employed. A 10-cm segment of mobile sigmoid or ileum may be taken out of continuity and anastomosed directly to the skin dimple *(Fig. 44.6)*. While some surgeons detubularize and subsequently fold the bowel to form the neovagina, the authors find this unnecessary and perform a simple proximal-limb closure with 2-0 absorbable suture. The distal aspect of the bowel limb is anastomosed in recessed fashion to skin flaps or the rudimentary vagina is cases of proximal atresia. The bowel anastomosis may be hand-sewn or stapled.

Within bowel constructs, stenosis occurs more often with ileum than with colon.[20] The type of bowel utilized depends upon surgeon preference and patient anatomy (e.g., cloacal exstrophy will require ileal vaginoplasty). Some advocate the usage of sigmoid colon as the proximity of its mesentery allows for free passage into the low pelvis.[21] Vaginal reconstruction is cautioned in patients with cervical agenesis as severe ascending bacterial infections have resulted in some patients.

Lastly, buccal mucosal vaginoplasty has been reported with success at 6–18-month follow-up.[3,22] The buccal mucosa grafts may be quilted, and after development of the neovaginal space, single or multiple grafts are utilized to line the cavity. A stent or mold is placed following suturing of the graft to the vaginal bed. Others advocate usage of minced 0.5 mm^2 micromucosal grafts derived mechanically from bilateral buccal grafts.[23] These micromucosal grafts are spread on to five gelatin strips, each $2.5 \times 6 \text{ cm}^2$, to line the anterior, posterior, apical, and lateral walls with a 5-mm interpatch distance. Likewise, a silicone vaginal stent with drainage holes and luminal packing is placed to maintain counterpressure. Regardless of technique, the surgeon must place tantamount importance on patient compliance as disuse or failure to dilate may result in atrophy. It is our practice that vaginoplasty is best performed once the patient is considering sexual activity or of appropriate age for performing periodic manual dilations.

Hints and tips

- Mineral oil may be injected to facilitate separation of the vaginal stent from graft following an Abbé–McIndoe procedure
- The proximal extent of the bowel vaginoplasty limb may be sutured to the sacrum or paraspinous ligaments to minimize potential prolapse[21]
- For buccal mucosal repairs, each cheek may yield a graft of approximately 3×7 cm. The graft should be harvested from inside the vermillion border extending posterior, inferior to Stensen's duct

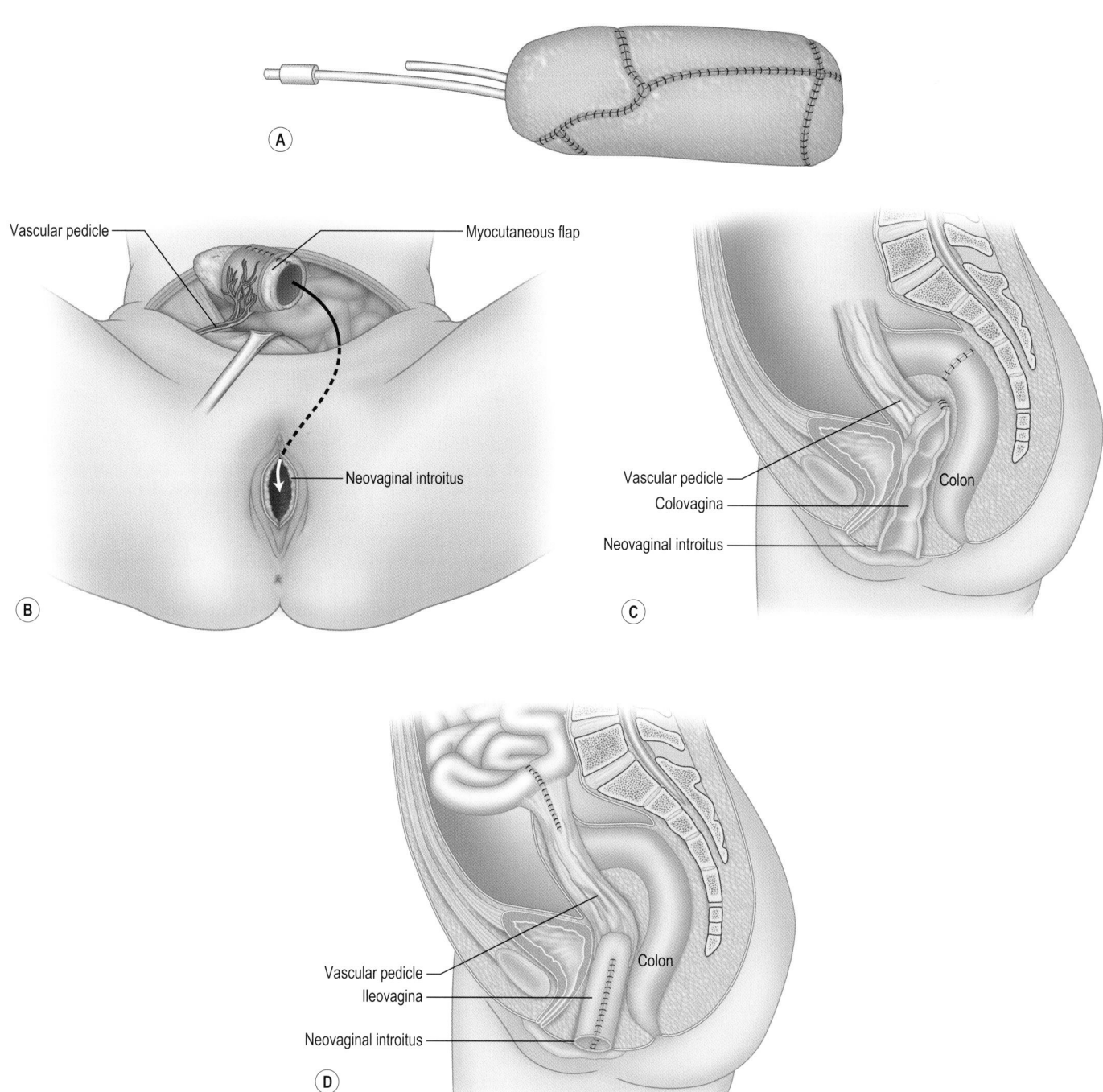

Fig. 44.6 (A, B) Myocutaneous flap vaginoplasty. Schematic depiction of bowel vaginoplasty: **(C)** colovaginoplasty and **(D)** ileovaginoplasty.

Urogenital sinus and clitoromegaly

Abnormalities of the urogenital sinus may be divided into low or high confluence defects. A confluence of the urogenital sinus distal to the urinary sphincter is considered low; those proximal are high. Repair may involve reduction clitoroplasty, development of labial folds, and construction of a capacious vagina. Prone positioning is preferred, at least initially, for advanced repairs.

Lower confluences may be repaired by cut-back vaginoplasty for simple labial adhesions, flap vaginoplasty, or vaginal pull-through. In a flap vaginoplasty, a posterior perineal flap is fashioned anterior to the rectum *(Fig. 44.7)*. The posterior urogenital sinus wall is incised and subsequently sutured to either side of the interposing posterior skin flap. The anterior vaginal wall remains intact.

For some low and all high confluence sinuses, complete separation of the urethra from vagina, or total urogenital mobilization, may be indicated with subsequent pull-through vaginoplasty. The authors prefer the technique described by Rink and Adams in which the anal sphincter remains intact while still permitting adequate operative exposure.[24] The

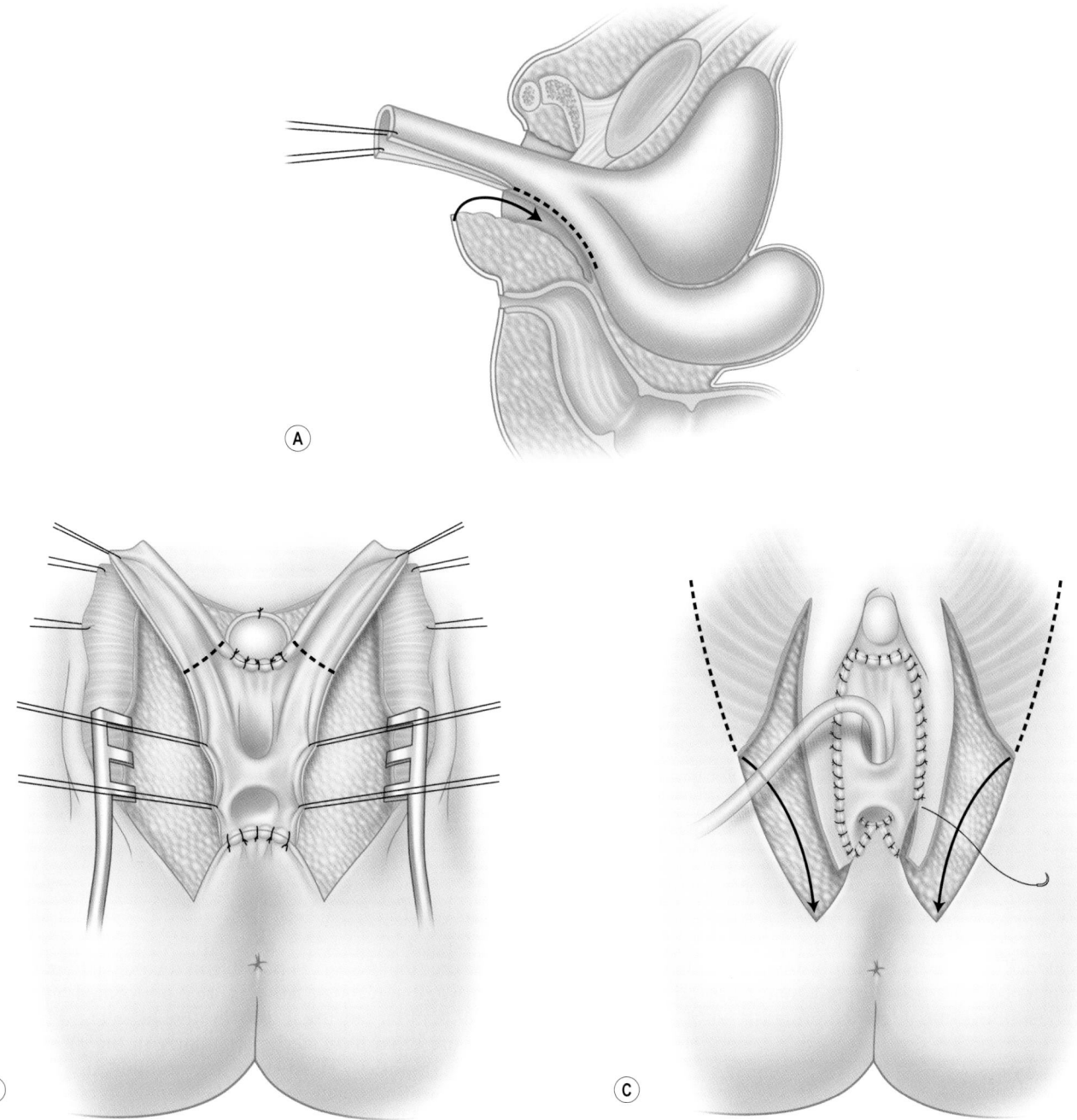

Fig. 44.7 (A–C) Urogenital sinus repair. (Reproduced from Rink RC, Cain MP. Urogenital mobilization for urogenital sinus repair. *Br J Urol Int*. 2008;102:1182–1197.)

patient is initially supine for the creation of a posterior U-shaped incision, as above, but then placed prone after mobilization of the posterior flap with or without clitoral reduction. Traction sutures allow for increasingly proximal dissection around the sinus, and the posterior sinus is again split at midline until the urethral confluence is visualized. The anterior vaginal wall is further dissected free from the urethra, with Rink and Adams designating this as the most challenging but most critical step of the operation. Preputial flaps may be needed to bridge between the distalmost extent of the mobilized vagina and the perineal skin. The labia minora are constructed from phallic skin.

With regard to clitoroplasty, the glans clitoris, the tunics, and the neurovascular bundles are preserved while excess erectile tissue may be debulked laterally.[25] A U-flap is created anterior from the perineum to each lateral ventral aspect of the phallus *(Fig. 44.8)*. A single incision connects the two flaps along the perineal raphe. The phallus is then degloved, leaving the ventral strip intact. Buck's fascia is incised, and the cavernosa are separated from the tunics and

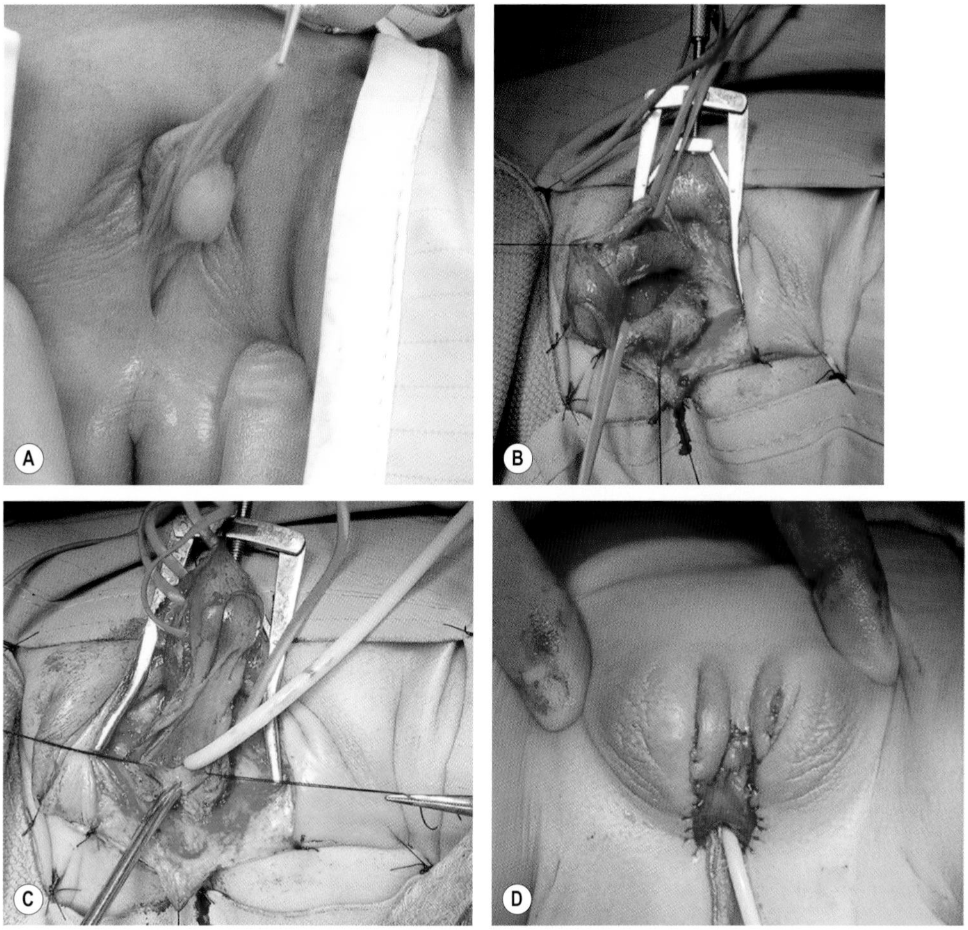

Fig. 44.8 (A–D) Corresponding intraoperative sequence of urogenital sinus repair with feminizing genitoplasty.

suture-ligated. The glans is then approximated to the ends of the foreshortened cavernosa. They connect posterior to the urethra. The authors often defer clitoroplasty until puberty.

Hints and tips

• Endoscopic elucidation of the confluence is critical in planning urogenital sinus repair *(Fig. 44.9)*
• A Fogarty balloon may help with intraoperative vaginal manipulation
• Identification and preservation of the neurovascular bundles are critical for successful clitoroplasty ⊛ FIG **44.9** APPEARS ONLINE ONLY

Cloacal exstrophy

With cloacal exstrophy, repair is most frequently staged. Initially, omphalocele closure with terminal colostomy and bladder plate approximation is performed *(Figs 44.10 and 44.11)*. The second stage consists of mobilization and closure of the bladder halves with midline fixation of the bladder and posterior urethra as deep as possible in the pelvis *(Fig. 44.12)*. Phallic or vaginal reconstruction is often performed only after successful bladder closure. Postoperative bowel and bladder regimens are often indicated, particularly in the presence of spinal abnormalities. Third-stage repair often involves the creation of continent catheterizable channels to bladder and bowel. ⊛ FIGS **44.10, 11B-H** APPEAR ONLINE ONLY

Bladder exstrophy

Plastic film is utilized to keep the bladder mucosa moist between birth and repair. In the neonatal period, bladder and abdominal closure is performed similar to that for second-stage cloacal exstrophy repair and is combined with osteotomies *(Fig. 44.12)*. Epispadias repair and reflux procedures are staged. For a more complete description, please see Volume 4, Chapter 13.

Female epispadias

Female epispadias ranges in severity from simply a patulous meatus to a complete dorsal separation of urethra and urinary sphincter *(Fig. 44.13)*. The clitoris may be bifid, the mons shallow, and the labia minora underdeveloped. Repair often involves tapering of the urethra with excision of dorsal redundancy and subsequent genitoplasty *(Fig. 44.14)*. The urethra is reconstructed over a catheter, and the mons tissue is utilized as a second layer for closure. In the Ransley–Gundeti modification, the dorsal redundant tissue is excised, the posterior urethral plate tubularized, and the anterior urogenital diaphragm reconstructed; however, additional sutures are placed to anchor the distal urethra to the reconstructed urogenital

diaphragm *(Fig. 44.14)*. This modification is thought to recreate more readily the physiologic anterior angulation of the distal female urethra. ⊗ FIG **44.14** APPEARS ONLINE ONLY

Urethral reconstruction for hypospadias with or without chordee and penoscrotal transposition

The goal of hypospadias repair is to allow for standing urination and normal ejaculatory function, while providing a slit-like terminal meatus. The technique should be simplistic with readily reproducible results. The prepuce may or may not be reconstructed depending upon cultural and patient expectations. Scrotoplasty may be performed for significant penoscrotal transposition *(Fig. 44.15)*. Baskin and Ebbers delineate five steps apparent in all hypospadias repairs: orthoplasty (straightening of the penis), urethroplasty, meato- and glanuloplasty, scrotoplasty, and epithelial coverage.[26] Herein the authors will highlight some of the more common repair techniques.

Meatoplasty and glanuloplasty

The MAGPI repair is best suited for the individual with a distal or anterior hypospadias. Oftentimes these patients are able to void with a straight stream, but the repair is requested for social, cultural, or parental concerns. The initial incision is circumferential, 5 mm proximal to the glans, and degloving is performed, allowing for orthoplasty *(Fig. 44.16)*. Any bridge within the urethral plate is incised and then repaired in Heineke–Mikulicz fashion so that the distal glanular groove and the more proximal hypospadic meatus are in continuity. A stay stitch allows for distal advancement of the meatus, and the glans edges are subsequently trimmed and approximated in two-layer fashion.

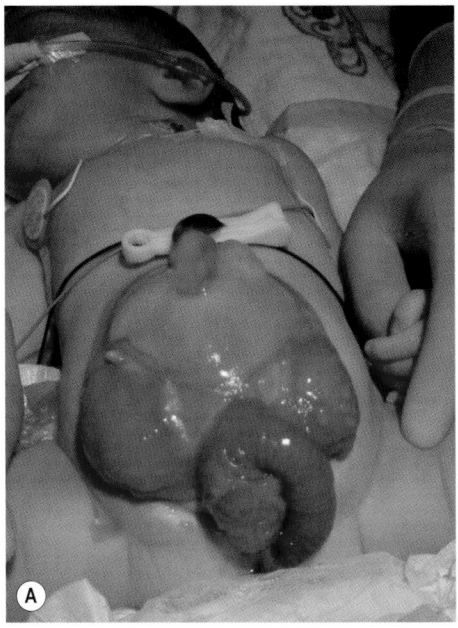

Fig. 44.11 Cloacal exstrophy repair for *Figure 44.10*.

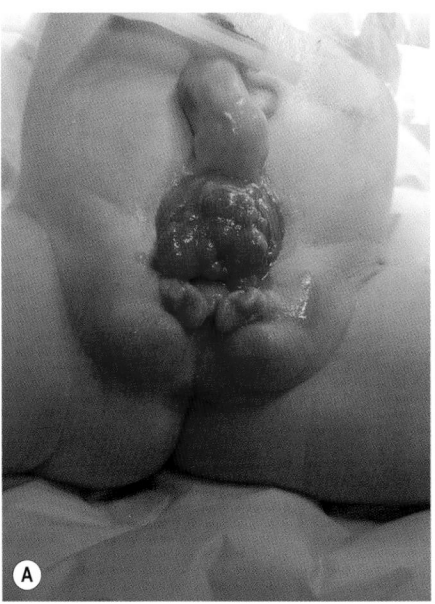

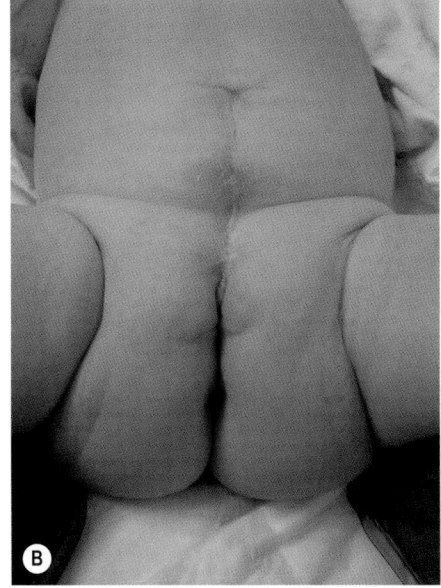

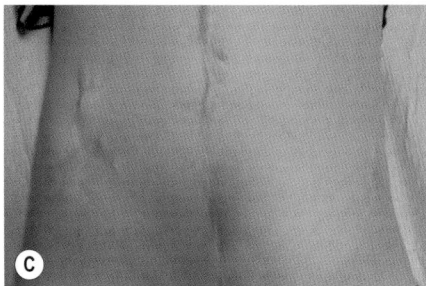

Fig. 44.12 (A, B) Female bladder exstrophy repair. **(C)** Final late appearance.

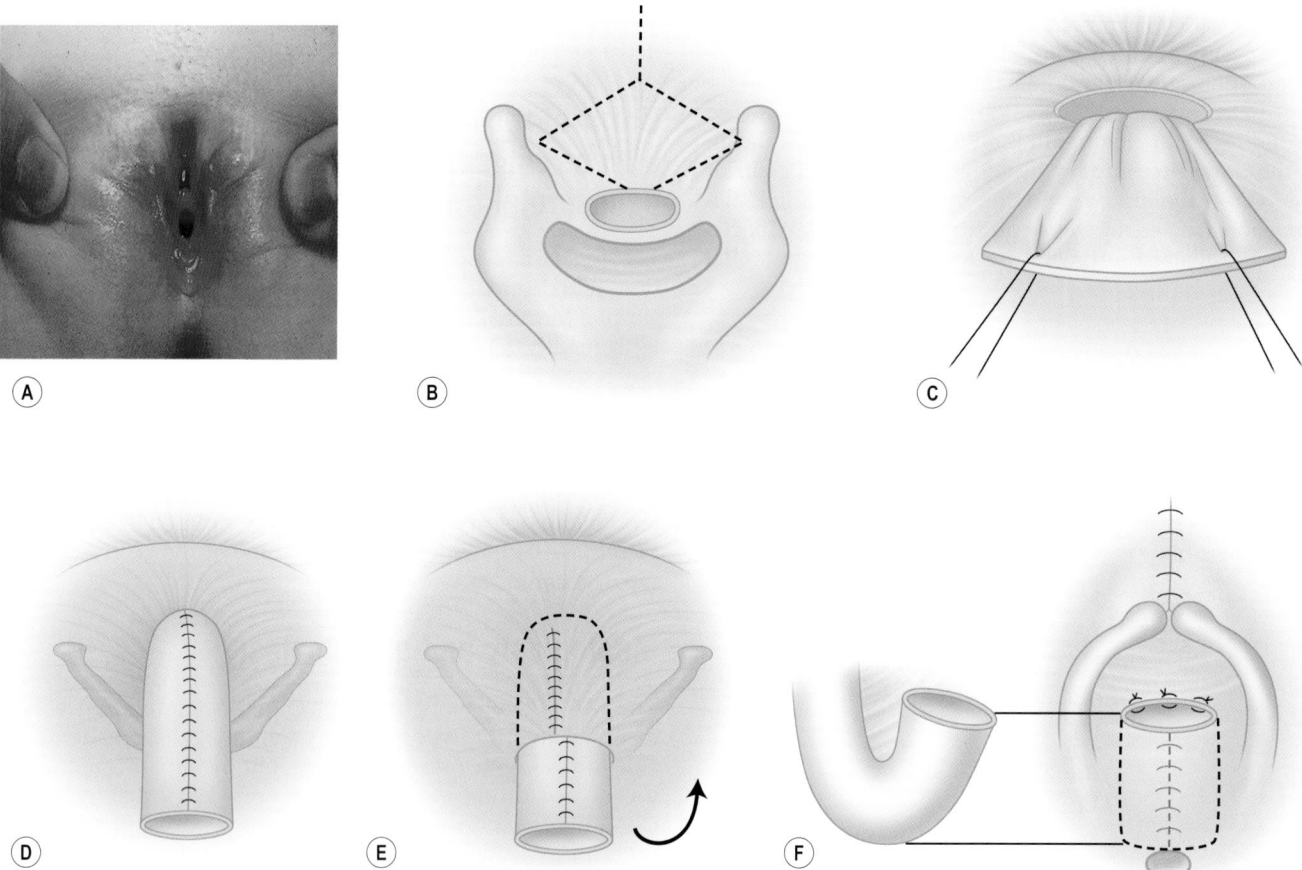

Fig. 44.13 **(A)** Ransley–Gundeti technique of female epispadias repair. **(B)** Female episadias: triangulated area of excess diamond-shaped skin. **(C)** Urethral plate mobilization. **(D)** Neourethra formation. **(E)** Pelvic floor tissue approximation over the neourethra. **(F)** Completed female episadias urethral reconstruction, showing the urethral angulation technique.

Tubularized incised plate repair

Easily reproducible, the TIP repair is our initial choice for patients with distal hypospadias. The urethral plate is measured in width, and diluted epinephrine may be injected prior to incision. A vertical incision is made alongside each edge of the urethral plate, and a crossing incision connects the two at the proximal extent of the meatus. The depth of the lateral incisions is based upon the glans volume and plate size; the crossing incision should be exceptionally thin, serving simply to disconnect the ventral penile skin from the underlying urethra while avoiding entrance into the urethral lumen (*Fig. 44.17*). Similar to the MAGPI repair, a circumferential incision extends each side from the crossing incision, approximately 5 mm from the coronal margin. The penis is degloved, chordee is assessed, and orthoplasty is performed if indicated. The midline of the plate is then incised utilizing an ultrafine-tipped ophthalmologic knife, and the plate is tubularized around a 5 French feeding tube which serves as a urethral stent. Glans flaps are created laterally. A second layer of dartos tissue or spongiosal tissue is rotated to cover the urethral suture line. The glans is reapproximated in two layers, and the shaft is closed at midline to complete the repair. In the case

of a very shallow urethral groove or small glans, a free graft may be interposed between the posterior TIP defect, thereby allowing for larger ultimate circumference[27].

Hints and tips

- A glans traction suture helps with intraoperative manipulation of the penis
- Placement of a penile tourniquet aids in visualization and may be periodically released during repair
- Minimization of tissue handling and creation of tension-free anastomoses optimize tissue health
- Bipolar electrocautery forceps are preferable to monopolar forceps for hemostasis
- 2.5× or greater loupes or the surgical microscope may improve tissue manipulation

Onlay island flap repair

Onlay island flap repair is commonly employed for midshaft hypospadias defects, although distal applications also exist.[28]

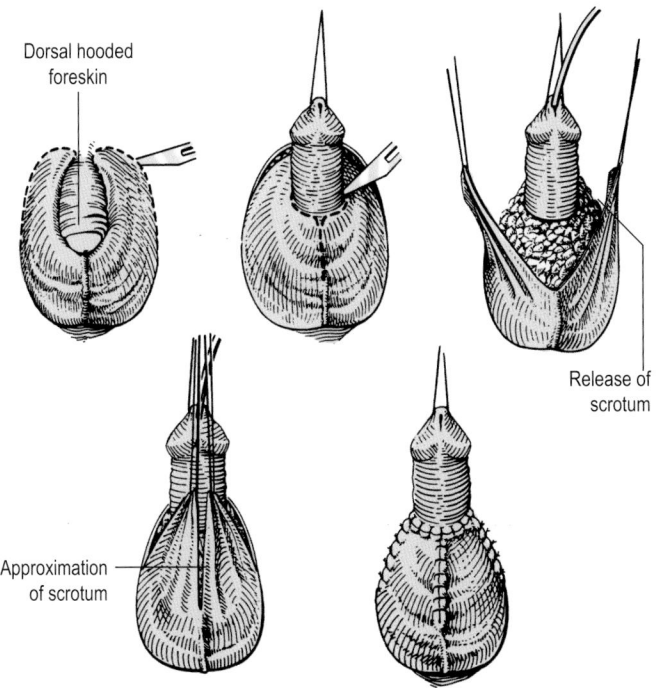

Dorsal hooded foreskin

Release of scrotum

Approximation of scrotum

Fig. 44.15 Penoscrotal transposition correction. (Reproduced from Wein: Campbell-Walsh Urology, 9th ed. © 2007 Saunders.)

chosen approach to orthoplasty will follow. After complete degloving of the penis, less than 10% of patients with hypospadias require penile straightening.[29] A Gittes test is performed, during which a penile tourniquet is tightened, and a small-gauge butterfly needle is placed through the glans directly into one of the corpora cavernosa. Sterile saline is slowly injected into the corpus until an erection is achieved, and any chordee is elucidated. As anatomic studies have shown a paucity or absence of neural structures at the 12 o'clock position of the penile shaft, the authors repair all instances of chordee by simple midline plication and no longer perform historical, more elaborate techniques[26].

Hints and tips

- Glans-to-glans approximation is critical in preventing meatal regression after meatoplasty and glanuloplasty (MAGPI) repair
- After degloving and orthoplasty of the penis, an initially distal hypospadias may now appear proximal and require a more extensive repair. Likewise, in a patient with poor distal urethral tissue, proximal dissection to healthy spongiosum may convert a distal hypospadic meatus to a proximal defect
- Submucosal injection of the buccal mucosa with lidocaine with 0.5% epinephrine facilitates harvest prior to defatting

---

Two stay stitches are placed at corners of the prepuce *(Fig. 44.18)*. Similar to a TIP repair, U-shaped and circumferential subcoronal incisions are performed. Degloving and orthoplasty follow, after which the distance from meatus to distal glans tip is measured. A rectangular preputial onlay graft is harvested and rotated to the ventrum along its pedicle. A second layer of vascularized inner preputial tissue may be utilized for coverage before glans approximation and closure.

Two-stage repair

For proximal hypospadias, a two-stage repair often affords the greatest chance for long-term success, albeit with the limitation of multiple surgeries separated by 6 months or more. A subcoronal circumferential incision is made as well as a longitudinal incision from glans tip to hypospadic meatus *(Figs 44.19-44.21)*. Once healthy urethral plate is identified, the remaining distal plate is excised. The glans is split longitudinally, and the resulting urethral defect measured. If of sufficient size, the prepuce may be utilized as either a pedicled flap or free graft. If insufficient, a free graft of buccal mucosa is performed with a 1:1 ratio of graft to site sizing. The buccal tissue has an extensively vascularized lamina propria, so long-term shrinkage is minimal. Second-stage repair is performed by tubularization of the graft with second-layer coverage before final epithelial approximation *(Fig. 44.20)*.

Orthoplasty

While discussion of chordee repair is contained elsewhere (Volume 4, Chapter 13), a brief description of the authors'

Postoperative care

Graft vaginoplasty is commonly followed by a minimum of 5 days' bedrest. A spica cast is often placed to ensure adequate perineal immobilization. Vaginal dilation may be started as soon as 3 weeks postoperatively, although others have recommended keeping a vaginal stent in place for the first 3 months with daily vaginal douching.[19,27] Routine home dilation of sigmoid and ileal vaginoplasties may be performed if, upon sexual activity, the caliber is inadequate.[16,18] For cloacal exstrophy, ureteral stents are typically removed 2 weeks postoperatively, and suprapubic tube clamping is performed at 4 weeks with measurement of postvoid urinary residual volumes. A common follow-up imaging schedule may involve renal ultrasound prior to suprapubic tube removal and then every 3 months with urine culture for 1 year.

Bladder and cloacal exstrophy repairs involve placement of a lower extremity spica cast and external fixator for 6 weeks. Urinary catheters remain for 6–8 weeks, and an evaluation under anesthesia is performed 3 months postoperatively. Periodic ultrasound examination of the kidneys is indicated, as well as a continence evaluation at 4–5 years of age. Epispadias repair may be followed by annual renal ultrasound. Noninvasive assessments of voiding and continence are done postoperatively, and bladder neck reconstruction may be indicated if incontinence is bothersome or severe.

Hypospadias repair is primarily an outpatient procedure. Pain control is ameliorated by a preoperative caudal nerve block. A soft 5 French feeding tube is utilized to stent the urethra. A dressing consisting of three supportive Duoderm strips followed by a Tegaderm wrap serves to keep the penis elevated, thereby minimizing swelling (video).

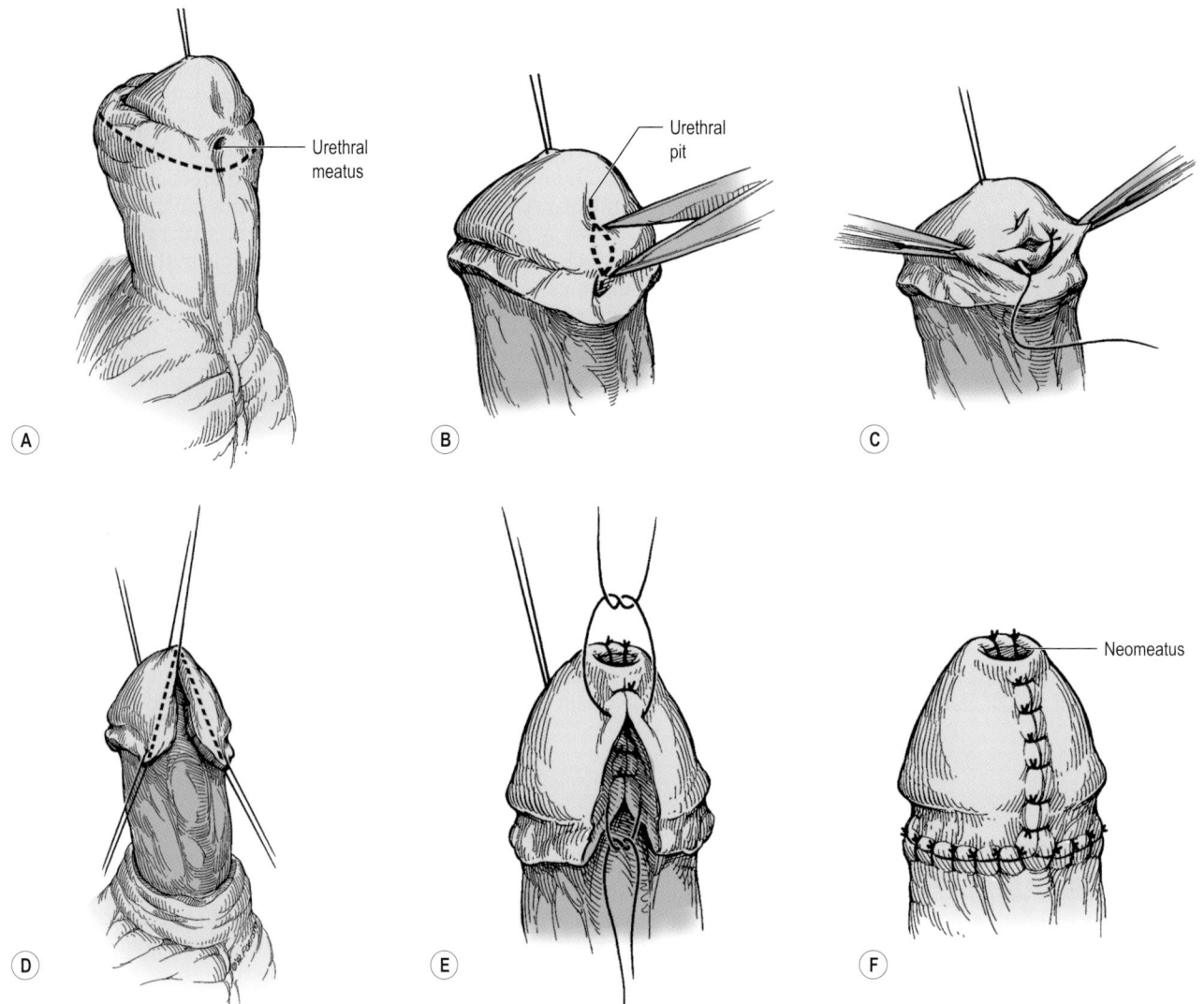

Fig. 44.16 (A–F) Meatoplasty and glanuloplasty (MAGPI) for distal hypospadias defects. (Reprinted from Duckett JW: Hypospadias. In Walsh PC, Retik AB, Vaughan ED Jr, Wein AJ [eds]: Campbell's Urology, 7th ed. Philadelphia, WB Saunders, 1998.)

Outcomes, prognosis, and complications

Evidence-based prospective studies are lacking, and most conclusions are based upon large retrospective series. Regarding vaginal replacement, the intestinal neovagina appears to have a lower incidence of stenosis than the McIndoe skin neovagina.[20] Neither age nor pelvic geometry (android versus gynecoid) appears to affect outcomes for sigmoid vaginoplasty, with satisfactory cosmetic results being noted in all 23 patients reviewed.[19] Diversion colitis is unique to sigmoid constructs. If vaginal stenosis occurs and serial dilations are unsuccessful, secondary procedures are best performed after puberty. Patients with high imperforate anus may undergo vaginoplasty derived from their mucus fistula, thereby avoiding the need for a bowel anastomosis.[21] As for cloacal surgery, the presence of a perineal raphe, an anal dimple, normal reflexes, and normal spine and magnetic resonance imaging serve as positive predictors of postoperative fecal continence.[30]

The mantra of the first chance being the best chance is certainly true for hypospadias repair. While successful outcomes are the norm, those who have poor surgical outcomes are at risk for scarring and abnormal-appearing genitalia, difficulty urinating, and long-term sexual and relationship difficulties. Bleeding and hematoma formation are the most common complications. A second layer of coverage is the single best measure for preventing urethrocutaneous fistula formation. Less common complications include meatal stenosis, infection, urethral diverticula and stricture, balanitis xerotica obliterans, and repair breakdown.

With regard to the MAGPI repair, Duckett and Snyder have described 1000 patients with fistulae in 0.5%, meatal retraction in 0.06%, and chordee in 0.1% at mean follow-up of 2 months.[31]

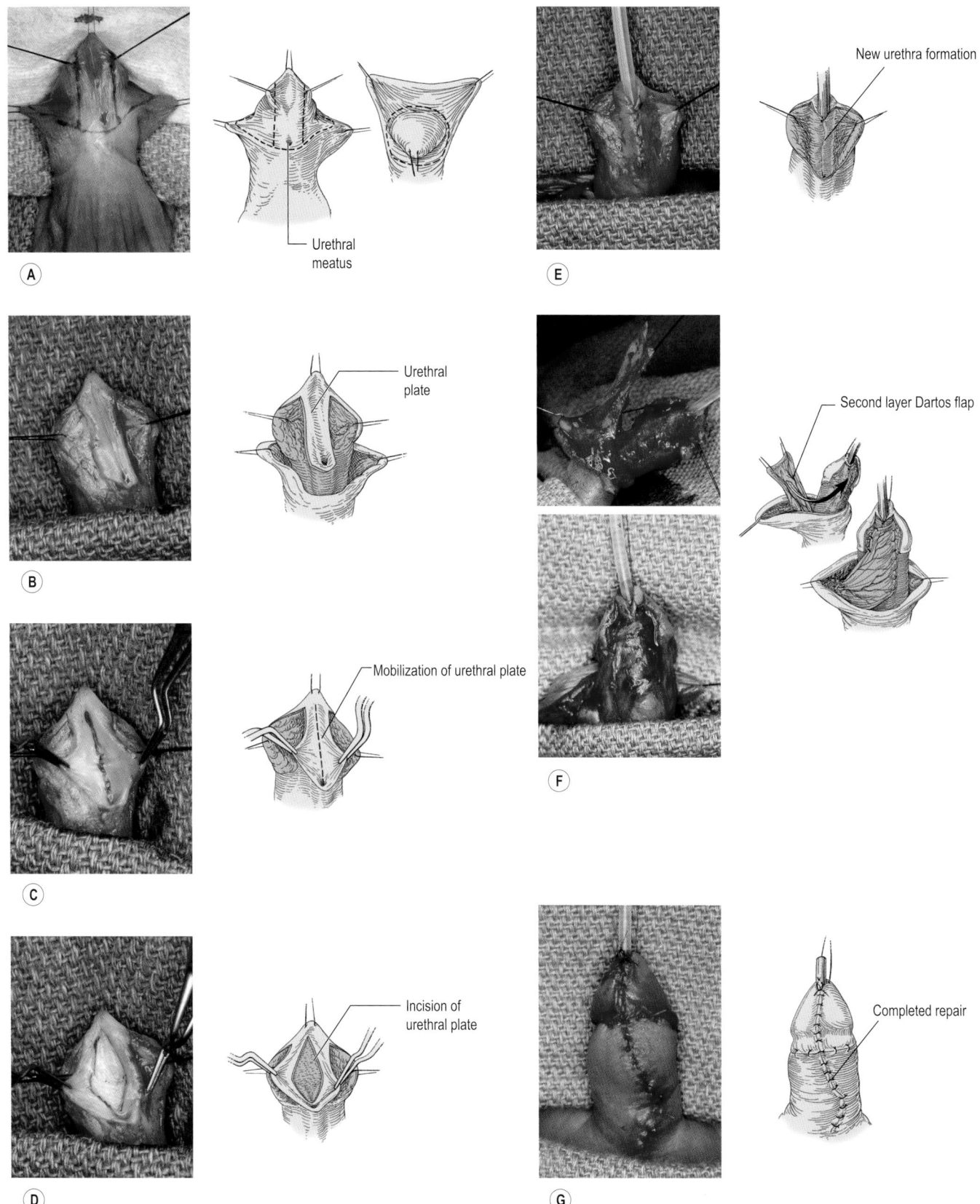

Fig. 44.17 (A–G) Tubularized incised plate (TIP) repair for hypospadias defects. (Reprinted from Retik AB, Borer JG: Primary and reoperative hypospadias repair with the Snodgrass technique. World J Urol 1998;16:186.)

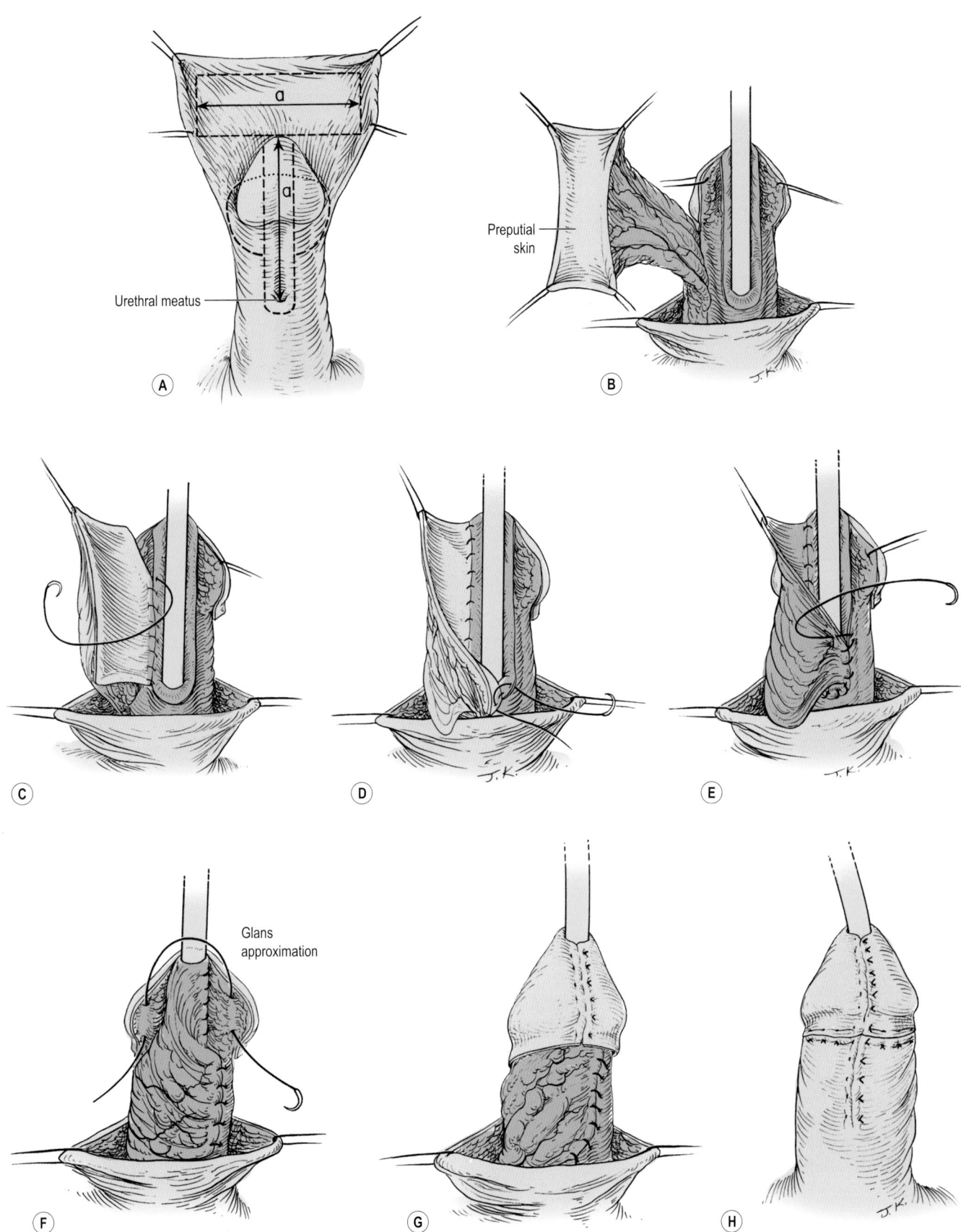

Fig. 44.18 (A–H) Onlay island flap repair for hypospadias defects. (Reprinted from Atala A, Retik AB: Hypospadias. In Libertino JA [ed]: Reconstructive Urologic Surgery, 3rd ed. St. Louis, Mosby–Year Book, 1998.)

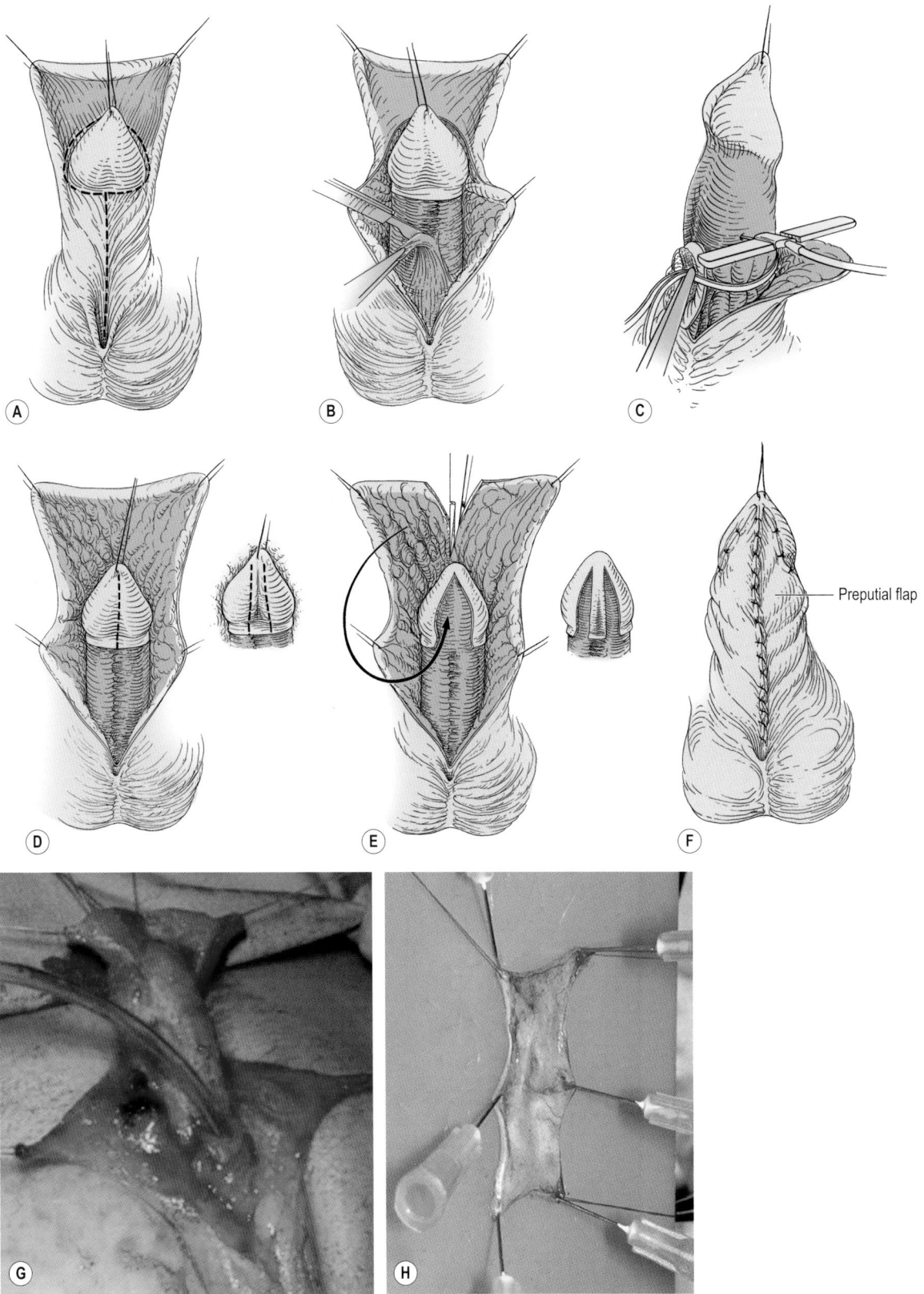

Fig. 44.19 (A–F) First stage of two-stage hypospadias repair with preputial flap - vascularized. **(G,H)** The authors' technique for free preputial/buccal graft for first stage hypospadias repair. (Reprinted from Retik AB, Borer JG: Primary and reoperative hypospadias repair with the Snodgrass technique. World J Urol 1998;16:186.)

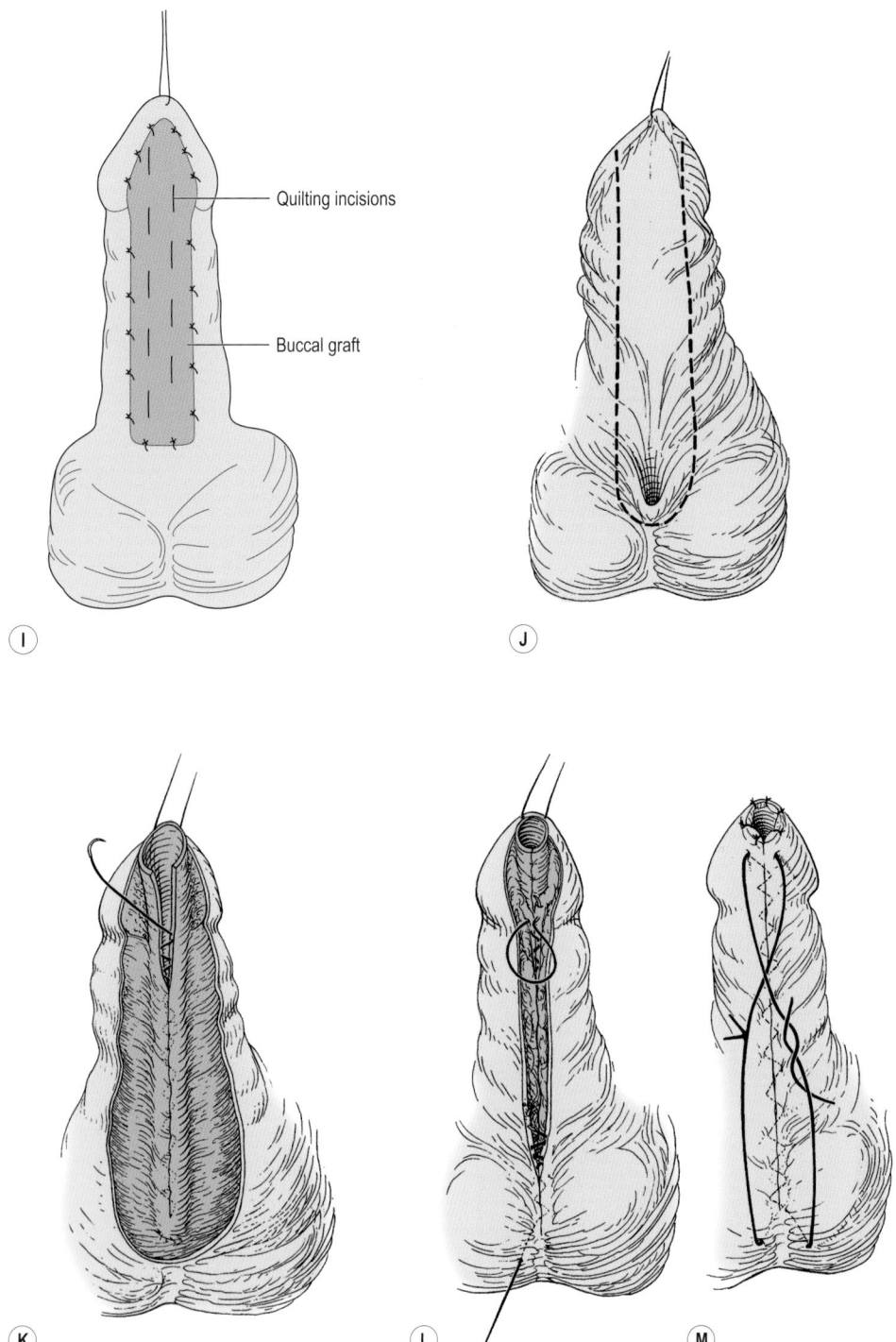

Quilting incisions

Buccal graft

I

J

K

L

M

Fig. 44.19, cont'd (I–M) Second-stage hypospadias repair of two stage repair.

These results have failed to be reproduced, with other groups noting at 2 years nearly 15% had complete meatal regression.[32] Data for the TIP repair are evolving. A multicenter review of over 2000 patients suggested a complication rate of 9%.[33] Fistulae occur in 5%, meatal stenosis in 2%, and glans dehiscence in 5%.[34]

A large series of onlay island flap repairs shows a 6% urethrocutaneous fistula and 9% reoperation rate.[35] In a review of 600 patients with two-stage repair, the majority preputial, a first-stage revision was required in 4%, and second-stage fistulae occurred in 6%, although the use of a dartos flap for second-layer closure may serve to limit this rate further.[36] Unfortunately, data regarding long-term cosmesis, urinary function, and sexual function remain quite limited.

Secondary procedures

Secondary procedures for urogenital repairs are common and often planned. Stenosis following vaginoplasty is often treated by serial dilation, either postoperatively or deferred until puberty. Genitoplasty and clitoroplasty often require revision at puberty. Regarding hypospadias, distal or midshaft hypospadias repairs should be single-staged and definitive. When complications such as urethrocutaneous fistulae do occur, primary repair, while attempted by some, is cautioned. Our experience has echoed that of Bracka, where two-stage buccal mucosa repair has yielded good results for those with previous failed hypospadias repair.[36]

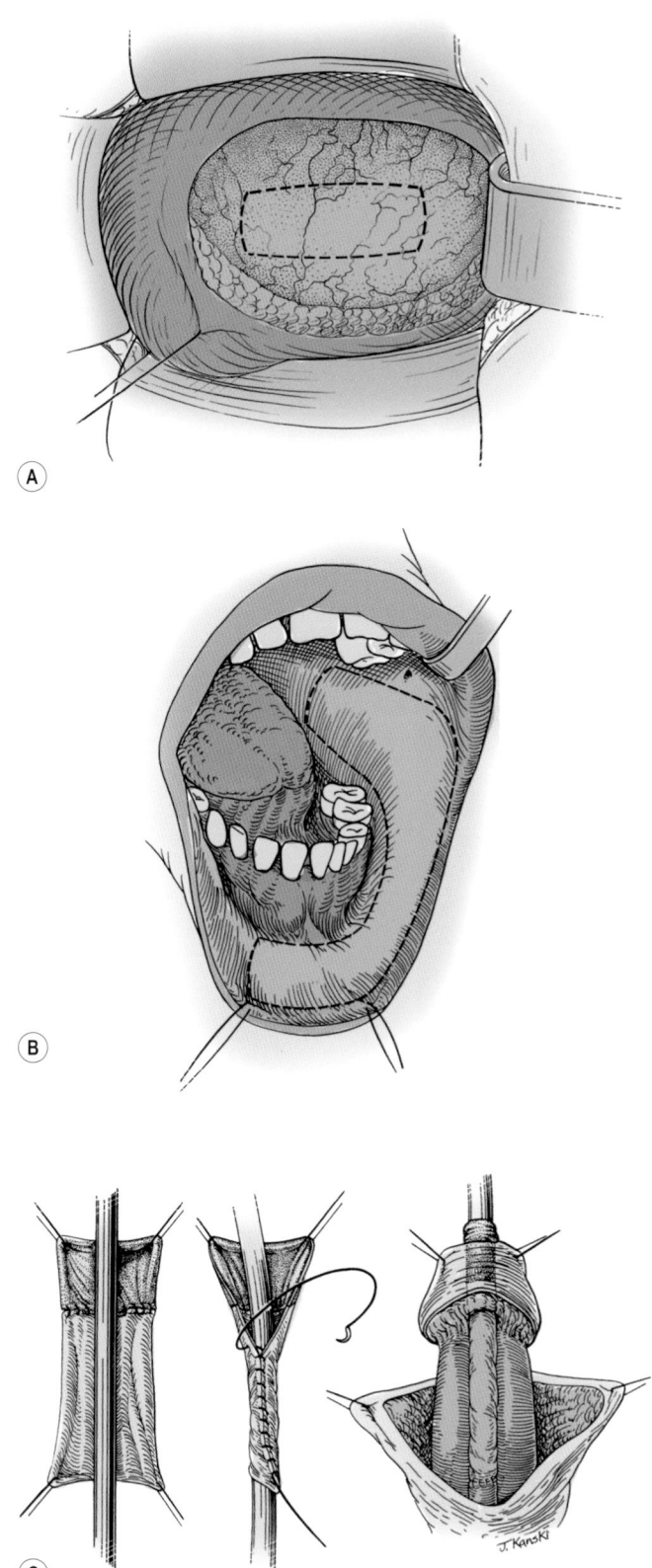

Fig. 44.20 (A, B) Harvesting the buccal mucosal graft. **(C)** Tubularization of the buccal mucosal graft.

Bonus images for this chapter can be found online at
http://www.expertconsult.com

Fig. 44.5 Development of the urogenital tract. (Modified from Larsen WJ: Human Embryology. New York, Churchill Livingstone, 1997.)
Fig. 44.9 Endoscopic view within common channel of urogenital sinus demonstrating urethral (ventral) and vaginal (dorsal) orifices.
Fig. 44.10 (A–D) Cloacal exstrophy repair. (Reproduced from Wein: Campbell-Walsh Urology, 9th ed. ©2007 Saunders.)
Fig. 44.11 (B–D) Corresponding intraoperative images of cloacal exstrophy repair for *Figure 44.10*. **(E–G)** Second stage cloacal exstrophy repair. **(H)** The final appearance late life.
Fig. 44.14 (A–K) Schematic of female epispadias repair. (Reproduced from Wein: Campbell-Walsh Urology, 9th ed. ©2007 Saunders.)

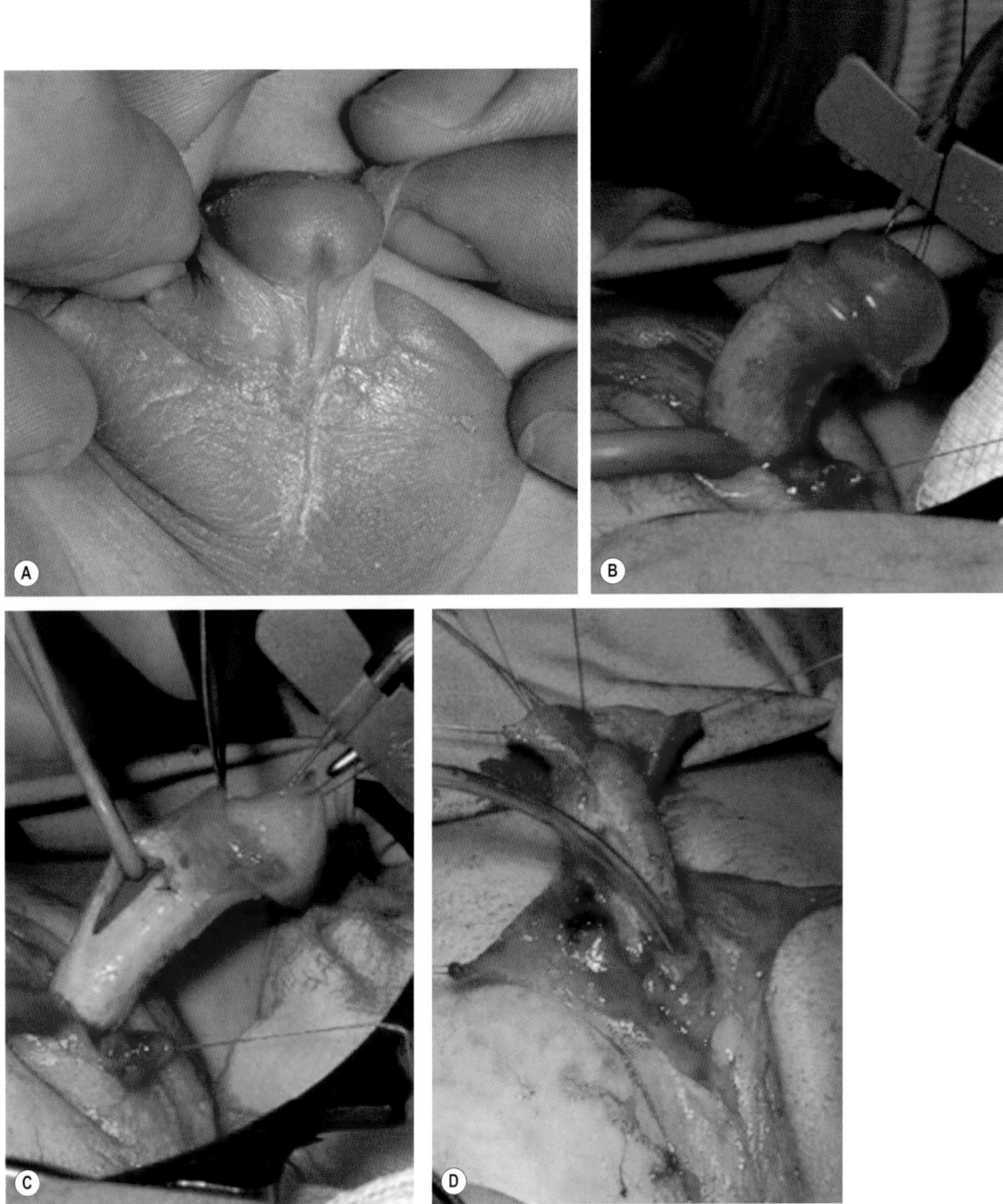

Fig. 44.21 Two-stage hypospadias repair depicting dorsal plication for chordee correction. **(A)** Perineal hypospadias; **(B)** chordee; **(C, D)** correction of chordee;

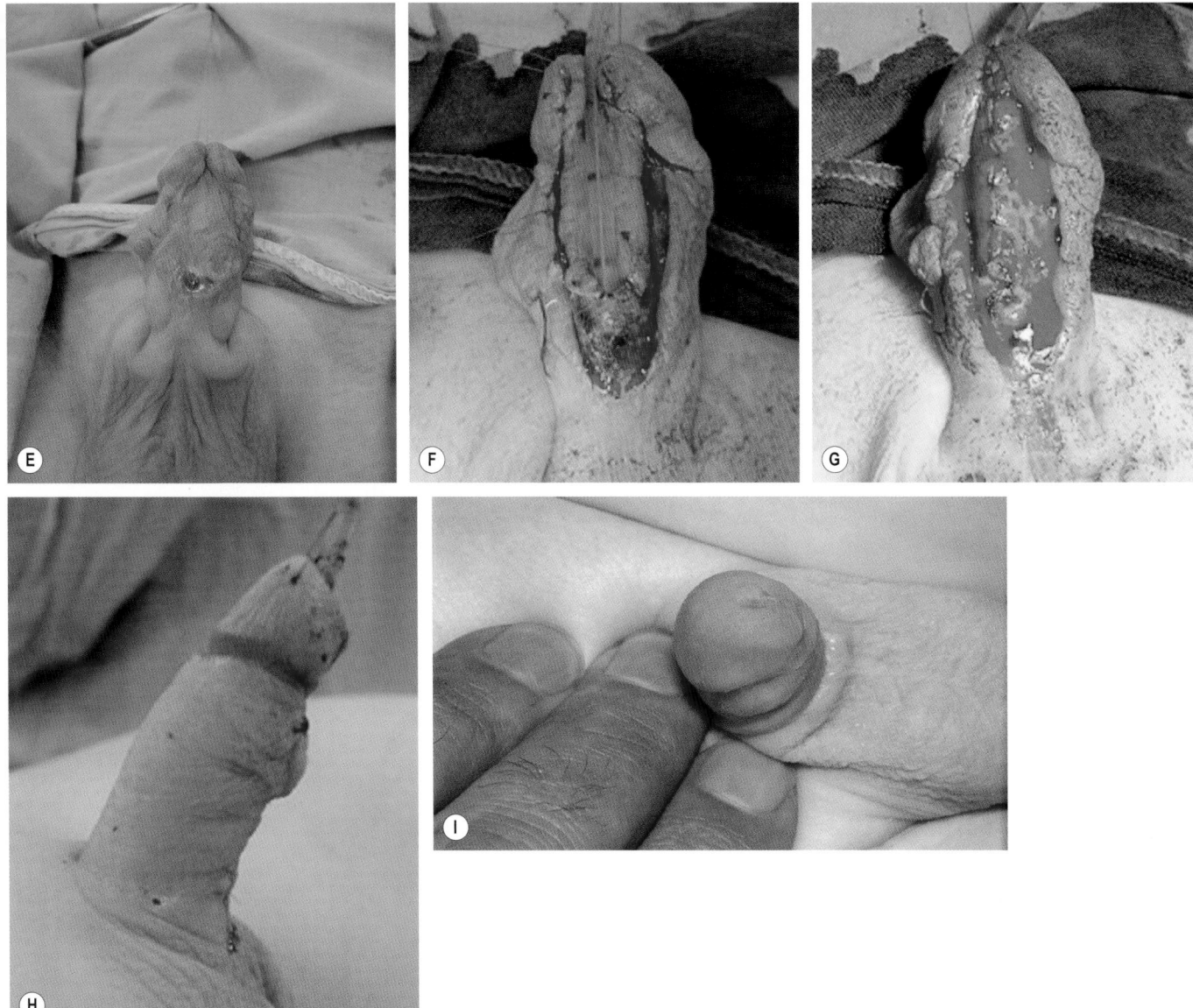

Fig. 44.21, cont'd **(E)** completed first stage repair six months postoperative; **(F–H)** Second stage hypospadias repair depicting free preputial and delayed tubularization. **(I)** the final appearance one year after the second stage repair.

Access the complete references list online at **http://www.expertconsult.com**

16. Cook A, Khoury AE, Neville C, et al. A multicenter evaluation of technical preferences for primary hypospadias repair. *J Urol.* 2005;174:2354.

18. Gundeti MS, Godbole PP, Wilcox DR. Is bowel preparation required before cystoplasty in children? *J Urol.* 2006;176:1574.

19. Rajimwale A, Furness III PD, Brant WO, et al. Vaginal construction using sigmoid colon in children and young adults. *Br J Urol Int.* 2004;94:115.

    A large retrospective review of the surgeons' experience with sigmoid vaginoplasty, comparing pre- and postpubertal patient outcomes.

20. Hensle TW, Dean GE. Vaginal replacement in children. *J Urol.* 1992;148:677.

24. Rink RC, Adams MC. Feminizing genitoplasty: state of the art. *World J Urol.* 1998;16:212.

    A review of the Indiana University surgical approach to disorders of sexual differentiation.

25. Baskin LS, Erol A, Li YW, et al. Anatomical studies of the human clitoris. *J Urol.* 1999;162:1015.

26. Baskin LS, Ebbers MB. Hypospadias: anatomy, etiology, and technique. *J Pediatr Surg.* 2006;41:463.

    A comprehensive review of hypospadias, highlighting recent advancements in surgical technique.

28. Elder JS, Duckett JW, Snyder HM. Onlay island flap in the repair of mid and distal penile hypospadias without chordee. *J Urol.* 1987;138:376.

34. Snodgrass W, Koyle M, Manzoni G, et al. Tubularized incised plate hypospadias repair: results of a multicenter experience. *J Urol.* 1996;156:839.

    Results of 148 patients undergoing TIP repair at six centers are reported.

36. Bracka A. Hypospadias repair: the two stage alternative. *Br J Urol.* 1995;7:31.

    A single surgeon's experience of 600+ two-stage hypospadias repairs.

*Note: **Boldface** roman numerals indicate volume. Page numbers followed by f refer to figures; page numbers followed by t refer to tables; page numbers followed by b refer to boxes.*

A

Aase syndrome, **VI**:573t
Abbé flap
  lip reconstruction, **III**:259–265, 261f–262f, 454
  partial upper lid defects, **III**:450
  secondary cleft deformities, **III**:637, 637f–638f
abdomen
  abdominal viscera flap classification, **I**:521, 521t
  abdominal wall reconstruction, **IV**:279–296
    background information, **IV**:279–280
    complications
      adhesions, **IV**:294
      pain management, **IV**:294–295
      recurrences, **IV**:294
      secondary hernias, **IV**:294
      seromas, **IV**:294
      wound breakdown, **IV**:294
    disease process, **IV**:280, 281f
    flap classifications, **I**:553t, 555f
    muscle/musculocutaneous flaps, **I**:553–554
    outcome assessments, **IV**:293
    patient presentation and diagnosis, **IV**:280–282
    patient selection, **IV**:282–283
    postoperative care and follow-up
      abdominal binders, **IV**:293
      analgesia, **IV**:293
      antibiotic therapy, **IV**:292–293
      drain management, **IV**:293
      limited physical activity, **IV**:293
      muscle relaxation, **IV**:293
      nutritional support, **IV**:292
      postoperative management, **IV**:291–292
    prognosis, **IV**:293–294
    reconstructive zones, **I**:553f
    research summary, **IV**:295
    secondary procedures, **IV**:295
    surgical technique and treatment
      abdominal wall transplantation, **IV**:290
      adjunctive techniques, **IV**:291, 292f
      autologous tissue repair, **IV**:289
      bioburden reduction, **IV**:283–284
      component separation method, **IV**:284–289, 285f–289f
      fascia lata grafts, **IV**:289, 290f
      negative-pressure wound therapy, **IV**:284
      parastomal hernia repair, **IV**:290
      primary suture technique, **IV**:284
      tissue expansion, **IV**:289–290, 291f

abdomen *(Continued)*
      abdominal wall transplantation, **IV**:290
    anatomical characteristics
      blood supply, **II**:533–534, 533f
      embryology, **II**:530–534
      fascial layers, **II**:531–533
      general characteristics, **IV**:227–230, 227f, **V**:412, 413f
      lymphatic system, **II**:533
      musculature, **II**:531–533, 532f, **IV**:228–229, 229f, **V**:412, 413f
      nerves, **II**:534, 534f, **IV**:230, **V**:412, 413f
      schematic diagram, **II**:531f
      skin, **II**:531–533
      umbilicus, **II**:531
      vascular anatomy, **II**:533–534, 533f, **IV**:229–230, 229f, **V**:412, 413f
    congenital melanocytic nevi (CMN), **III**:844–848, 847f–848f
    liposuctions, **II**:521–522
    lower bodylift/belt lipectomy surgery, **II**:568–598
      anatomical considerations, **II**:568–569, 569f
      complications
        deep vein thrombosis (DVT), **II**:593–594
        dehiscence, **II**:591
        general discussion, **II**:589–595
        infections, **II**:592
        psychological difficulties, **II**:594–595
        pulmonary embolisms, **II**:593–594
        seromas, **II**:590
        tissue necrosis, **II**:592–593, 595f
        wound separation, **II**:590–591
      disease process
        massive weight loss patients, **II**:569, 570f
        normal weight patients group, **II**:570, 572f–573f
        20–30 pounds overweight group, **II**:569, 571f
      general discussion, **II**:568
      markings
        horizontal mons pubis marking, **II**:581–582, 583f
        inferior back marking, **II**:584, 584f
        lateral mons to anterior superior iliac spine (ASIS) marking, **II**:582, 583f
        posterior vertical midline marking, **II**:583–584, 584f
        superior back marking, **II**:584–585, 584f
        superior horizontal abdominal marking, **II**:582–583, 583f
      surgical guidelines, **II**:580–585

abdomen *(Continued)*
      vertical alignment marking, **II**:585
      vertical midline marking, **II**:581
    outcome assessments
      characteristics, **II**:588–595
      group I patients, **II**:589f–590f
      group II patients, **II**:591f–592f
      group III patients, **II**:593f–594f
    patient presentation and diagnosis
      back roll presentations, **II**:571, 578f
      body mass index (BMI), **II**:570, 574f
      buttocks variations, **II**:577f
      commonalities, **II**:570–571
      fat deposition pattern, **II**:570, 574f–575f
      hanging panniculi, **II**:576f
      skin/fat envelope, **II**:570, 574f–575f
    patient selection
      belt lipectomy/central bodylift, **II**:572–574, 574b
      general discussion, **II**:571–580
      lower bodylift type II (Lockwood technique), **II**:571–572, 573b, 579f
      preoperative assessment, **II**:577–580
      selection criteria, **II**:574–576, 577b
    postoperative care and follow-up, **II**:588, 588b
    secondary procedures, **II**:595
    surgical procedures
      anesthesia, **II**:585–588
      dissection techniques, **II**:587f
      goals, **II**:580, 580b
      markings, **II**:580–585, 583f–584f
      positioning, **II**:587f
      positioning sequence, **II**:585
      suturing techniques, **II**:585–588, 586f
    surgical technique and treatment
      belt lipectomy, **II**:580–585
      circumferential excisional procedures, **II**:580–585, 580f–582f
      excisional tension, **II**:580–585, 580f–582f
    upper bodylift considerations, **II**:595, 596f–597f
    zones of adherence, **II**:568–569, 569f
  pediatric abdominal wall defects
    omphalocele and gastroschisis
      characteristics, **III**:865–866
      clinical presentation and evaluation, **III**:865, 866f
      surgical indicators, **III**:865
      treatment strategies, **III**:865–866
  photographic guidelines, **I**:110, 115f–116f
  progressive hemifacial atrophy (PHA), **III**:797f
  robotic surgery, **I**:863

abdominal aortic aneurysms (AAA) repair,
    I:843
abdominoplasty, II:530–558
    abdominal contouring
        giant pannus, II:640–643, 643f–644f
        hidden penis, II:640, 643f
        major weight loss (MWL) patient, II:639b
        mons correction, II:640, 641f–642f
        operative planning and technique,
            II:639–640
        patient evaluation, II:639
        surgical variations, II:640–643, 640f–641f
    abdominal wall defects, II:535
    aesthetic procedures
        abdominoplasty with umbilical
            transection
            characteristics, II:541
            indicators, II:542
            markings, II:542
            operative technique, II:542, 543f–544f
            outcome assessments, II:542, 544f
            patient selection, II:542
            postoperative care and follow-up, II:542
            preoperative procedures, II:542
        circumferential abdominoplasty, II:551
        documentation, II:539
        fleur-de-lis type abdominoplasty
            abdominal contouring, II:640–643,
                640f–641f
            characteristics, II:548–549
            indicators, II:549
            markings, II:549–550, 550f
            operative technique, II:550
            outcome assessments, II:550–551, 551f
            patient selection, II:549
            postoperative care and follow-up,
                II:550
            preoperative procedures, II:550
        high-lateral-tension (HLT)
            abdominoplasty
            characteristics, II:547
            indicators, II:547
            markings, II:547, 549f
            operative technique, II:548
            outcome assessments, II:548, 549f
            patient selection, II:547
            postoperative care and follow-up,
                II:548
            preoperative procedures, II:547–548
        major weight loss (MWL) patient, II:551
        markings, II:537, 538f
        mini/short scar abdominoplasty
            anesthesia, II:540
            characteristics, II:539
            indicators, II:539–540
            markings, II:540, 540f
            operative technique, II:540–541
            outcome assessments, II:541, 542f
            patient selection, II:539–540
            postoperative care and follow-up,
                II:541
            preoperative procedures, II:540
        pre/intra/postoperative management,
            II:537–538
        reverse abdominoplasty
            characteristics, II:551–552
            indicators, II:552
            markings, II:552–553, 553f

abdominoplasty (Continued)
    Scarpa's fascia preservation
        characteristics, II:551
        indicators, II:551
        operative technique, II:551
        outcome assessments, II:551, 552f–553f
    scar-position measurements, II:537
    standard abdominoplasty
        characteristics, II:542–545
        indicators, II:545
        markings, II:545
        operative technique, II:545–546,
            546f–547f
        outcome assessments, II:546–547, 548f
        patient selection, II:545
        postoperative care and follow-up,
            II:546
        preoperative procedures, II:545
    surgical technique and results, II:539, 540t
    tissue pinching, II:537, 538f
    vertical abdominoplasty, II:553
    wound closure, II:538–539, 539f
    anatomical considerations
        blood supply, II:533–534, 533f
        embryology, II:530–534
        fascial layers, II:531–533
        lymphatic system, II:533
        musculature, II:531–533, 532f
        nerves, II:534, 534f
        schematic diagram, II:531f
        skin, II:531–533
        umbilicus, II:531
        vascular anatomy, II:533–534, 533f
    atypical scars, II:554–555, 556f
    background information, II:559
    circumferential abdominoplasty, II:551
    complications, II:557–558
    contraindications, II:558
    deformity classifications, II:535, 535f
    externus belt, II:554, 556f
    goals, II:530
    incidence, II:530
    infiltration, I:143, 144f
    major weight loss (MWL) patient, II:551
    mons pubis management, II:557, 557f
    pathology, II:535
    patient selection
        informed consent, II:537
        patient history, II:536
        patient preoperative instructions, II:537
        photographic documentation, II:536–537
        physical examination, II:536, 536f
        preoperative markings, II:537
    umbilicoplasty, II:553–554, 554f–555f
abductor digiti minimi (ADM) tendon,
    VI:758
abductor hallucis, III:295t
abductor pollicis brevis (APB) muscle, VI:212
abductor pollicis longus (APL) muscle, VI:51,
    211, 211f
ablative laser treatments, IV:454, 454t, 484
abrasions, I:241, III:29, 30f, 43
Abruzzo–Erickson syndrome, III:807t
absent thumb, VI:546t
absorptive powders, pastes, and fibers, I:289t
acanthomas, I:720
accessory auricles, I:732–733, 733f
accidental radiation exposure, I:673–674

acellular dermal matrix (ADM)
    chest wall reconstruction, IV:239, 240f
    lower extremity reconstructive surgery,
        IV:128–129, 130f
    omentum reconstruction, V:474–476, 477f
    palatal fistula repair, III:642, 644f
    revisionary breast surgery
        basic principles, V:68–69
        capsular contracture, V:52–53, 52f,
            336–340
        clinical signs, V:79t
        comparison studies, V:70t
        complications, V:78–79, 79t
        omentum reconstruction, V:474–476, 477f
        patient presentation and diagnosis, V:71
        patient selection, V:71, 72t
        preoperative/postoperative Baker
            classifications, V:79, 79t
        prognosis and outcomes, V:78–79
        surgical technique and treatment
            augmentation versus augmentation
                mastopexy, V:79t
            capsular contracture, V:77–78, 77f, 79t
            implant stabilization, V:75–76, 75f–76f
            lamellar separation, V:73–75, 73f
            lower pole coverage, V:73–75, 73f–76f
            placement indicators, V:71–78, 72f, 73b
            tissue thickeners, V:76–77
    skin grafts, I:342, IV:480, 482–484
    surgical innovation, I:851–852, 851f
acetone, IV:395
achondrogenesis, III:805–807, 807t
Acinetobacter, IV:513–514
acinic cell carcinoma
    characteristics, III:370
    classifications, III:365t
    incidence, III:376t
    outcomes and complicatons, III:377
    parotid gland, III:370t
    surgical technique and treatment,
        III:375–376
acne, II:19–20, 77
acne scars, I:311–312, II:69, 75f
acquired and congenital defects, I:44
acquired cicatricial alopecia, III:111t
acquired cranial and facial bone deformities,
    III:226–242
    access incisions
        coronal incisions, III:226–227, 227f
        intraoral incisions, III:227
        lower eyelid incisions, III:227
    background and general characteristics,
        III:226
    bone grafts
        donor site considerations, III:227,
            228f–229f
        soft-tissue cover, III:227
    complications, III:242
    postoperative care and follow-up,
        III:240–242
    prognosis and outcomes, III:242
    secondary procedures, III:242
    surgical technique and treatment
        chin implants, III:240, 240f–241f
        irradiated orbit, III:235–238
        mandibular fractures, III:238–240, 239f
        mandibular reconstruction, III:240
        maxillary buttresses, III:236–238

acquired cranial and facial bone deformities
    (Continued)
    maxillary reconstructiion, III:238–240,
        238f
    posttraumatic enophthalmos, III:234–235,
        237f
    specific defects
        cranium, III:228, 230f–231f
        nasoethmoid area, III:232, 234f
        nose, III:228–229, 231f–233f
        orbitozygomatic region, III:232–234,
            235f–236f
acquired facial paralysis, III:284
acquired pigment cell nevus, I:724, 724f
acquired vaginal defects, IV:326–335
    anatomical characteristics, IV:326, 327f
    complications, IV:334
    etiology, IV:326
    patient presentation and diagnosis,
        IV:326–327, 327f
    patient selection, IV:327–328
    postoperative care and follow-up
        immediate postoperative period, IV:333
        long-term recovery, IV:333–334
    prognosis and outcomes, IV:334
    surgical technique and treatment
        basic principles, IV:328–333
        flap reconstruction
            bilateral gracilis flaps, IV:331–333,
                332f–333f
            flap reconstruction options, IV:327t
            modified Singapore fasciocutaneous
                flap, IV:328, 329f
            pedicled rectus myocutaneous flap,
                IV:328–329, 330f–331f
            reconstruction algorithm, IV:328f
        goals, IV:328–333, 328b
acral lentiginous melanoma, I:752–753, 754f
acrocephalosyndactyly, III:689
    See also Apert syndrome
acrochordon, I:730, 730f
acrosyndactyly, VI:540f
actin, VI:349
actinic keratosis, I:736, 736f, VI:316–317, 317f
ActiveFX™ laser, II:71t, 73
active immunotherapy, I:205–206, 206f
activin, I:270t, 274
acute rejection, I:819
acute ulnar collateral ligament (UCL) tear,
    VI:155, 155f
acute wounds, I:241–242, 241f
ADAM sequence (anionic deformity,
    adhesions, mutilations), III:807t
ADAMTS (a disintegrin and
    metalloproteinase with thrombospondin
    motifs) family, VI:412–413
AdatoSil 5000, II:47–48, 47t
    See also soft-tissue fillers
adductor brevis muscle, IV:15t–16t, 18f, 19t,
    20f–22f
adductor longus muscle, IV:15t–16t, 18f, 19t,
    20f–22f
adductor magnus muscle, IV:15t–16t, 18f, 19t,
    20f–22f
adductor pollicis (ADP) muscle, VI:52, 212
adenine, I:177–182, 177f
adenocarcinoma
    characteristics, III:370
    classifications, III:365t
    incidence, III:376t

adenocarcinoma (Continued)
    outcomes and complicatons, III:377, 377f
    parotid gland, III:370t
    submandibular gland, III:370t
    surgical technique and treatment, III:376
adenoid cystic carcinoma (cylindroma)
    characteristics, III:370, 370f
    classifications, III:365t, 370t
    incidence, III:376t
    outcomes and complicatons, III:377
    surgical technique and treatment,
        III:374–375
adenosine monophosphate (AMP), I:575f,
    821–822
adenosine triphosphate (ATP), I:256f, 258, 575,
    575f–576f, IV:195–196, VI:228–229
adenoviruses, I:186–187, 188t
adhesion cheiloplasty
    advantages/disadvantages, III:525–526
    two-stage palate repair, III:525
adhesions, III:8–10, IV:294
adhesives and glues
    characteristics, I:792b
    cyanoacrylates, I:793
    fibrin tissue adhesives, I:793
    platelet gels, I:793
    research background, I:792–793
adipose-derived stem/stromal cells (ASCs)
    cell surface receptors, I:219–220, 219f–220f
    characteristics, I:217–218, 217f
    delivery methods, I:220
    fat grafting, I:345–346, II:327–328
    harvesting methods, I:218–219, 218f
    induced pluripotent stem cells, I:236
    in vitro differentiation protocols
        adipogenic differentiation, I:221, 222f
        chondrogenic differentiation, I:221
        osteogenic differentiation, I:220–221, 221f
    in vivo model
        clinical correlates, I:223
        future trends, I:223, 224f–225f
        nude athymic mouse 4-mm calvarial
            defect, I:221–223, 222f
    mouse versus human ASCs, I:219
    regenerative qualities, V:583–584
    tissue engineering, I:369–371
adipose tissue engineering, I:387f, 389–390,
    389f
adolescents
    aesthetic surgery, I:45–46, 45t
    gender identity disorder, IV:341
adoptive immunotherapy, I:204–205, 205f
Adson test, VI:65, 66f
adult brachial plexus injury
    characteristics, VI:790t
    electrodiagnostic studies, VI:797–798
    etiology, VI:793
    evaluation examinations, VI:794f–795f,
        795–796, 796t
    general discussion, VI:793
    infraclavicular brachial plexus injury,
        VI:802–803
    level 1 injury
        characteristics, VI:798–802
        functioning free muscle transplantation
            (FFMT), VI:801–802
        nerve transfer, VI:799–800
        pedicled muscle transfer, VI:800–801
        reconstructive strategies, VI:800
    level 2 injury, VI:802

adult brachial plexus injury (Continued)
    level 3 injury, VI:802
    level 4 injury, VI:802–803
    motor examination, VI:794f–795f, 795–796,
        796t
    nerve transfer
        basic procedure, VI:799–800
        closed-target nerve transfer, VI:799
        end-to-side neurorrhaphy nerve transfer,
            VI:799–800
        extraplexus nerve transfer, VI:799
        functioning free muscle transplantation
            (FFMT), VI:801–802
        intraplexus nerve transfer, VI:799
        pedicled muscle transfer, VI:800–801
        proximal nerve transfer versus distal
            nerve transfer, VI:799r
        recommended induction exercises,
            VI:800t
        reconstructive strategies, VI:800
    outcome assessments, VI:805
    palliative reconstruction procedures, VI:805
    patient history, VI:793–794
    postoperative care and rehabilitation, VI:805
    pre- and retroclavicular injury, VI:802
    preoperative assessment and diagnosis,
        VI:794–795
    reconstructive strategies
        elbows, VI:800, 801t
        fingers, VI:800, 801t, 802f, 803t
        shoulder, VI:800, 801t
    research summary, VI:805, 815
    sensory examination
        basic procedure, VI:796
        British Medical Research Council (BMRC)
            Scale/Chuang modification, VI:796t
        Horner's syndrome, VI:796
        plain X-ray and imaging studies, VI:796
        Tinel's sign, VI:796
    surgical technique and treatment
        characteristics, VI:798–805
        Chuang's angle, VI:804–805, 804f
        exploration techniques, VI:803–805, 804f
        functioning free muscle transplantation
            (FFMT), VI:801–802
        infraclavicular brachial plexus injury,
            VI:802–803
        infraclavicular dissection, VI:804–805,
            804f
        level 1 injury, VI:798–802
        level 2 injury, VI:802
        level 3 injury, VI:802
        level 4 injury, VI:802–803
        pedicled muscle transfer, VI:800–801
        pre- and retroclavicular injury, VI:802
        supraclavicular dissection, VI:803–804,
            804f
    vascular injury, VI:798
advancement flap
    cheek reconstruction, III:271–272, 272f,
        451–452, 453f
    classifications, I:513f
    partial upper lid defects, III:450
adverse drug interactions, I:145
advertising ethics, I:59–60, 59f–60f
Aegineta, Paulus, IV:393, V:153–159
Aeromonas hydrophila, VI:241–242
aesthetic facial surgery
    patient safety, I:131–132
    psychological aspects, I:39

aesthetic practice liabilities, I:100–101
aesthetic prostheses, VI:870, 871f
aesthetic surgery
   adolescent aesthetic surgery, I:45–46, 45t
   aesthetic nasal reconstruction, III:134–186
      defect classification
         adversely located defects, III:139–140
         composite defects, III:140
         deep defects, III:140
         large defects, III:140
         small defects, III:139
         superficial defects, III:139
      disease process, III:134–135
      false planning assumptions
         donor site considerations, III:135
         extra tissue transfer, III:135
         flap design, III:135
         scars, III:135
         single flap approach, III:136
         supportive frameworks, III:135–136
         tissue expansion, III:135
         tissue preservation, III:135
      forehead donor site
         expansion considerations, III:158–159
         expansion delay, III:159–160
         expansion technique, III:159–160
         harvesting guidelines, III:160
         primary closure, III:155
         scars within the forehead territory,
            III:156–157
         surgical delay procedures, III:157–158
      intranasal lining flaps
         applications, III:166t
         basic procedure, III:164f–166f
         detailed characteristics, III:163–166
         isolated unilateral mid-vault lining
            loss, III:166–167
         operative technique, III:166–170,
            167f–169f
      local flaps
         bilobed flap, III:143–145, 144f–145f,
            446f
         dorsal nasal flap, III:143, 144f–145f
         forehead flaps, III:148–155, 149f
         one-stage nasolabial flap, III:145–146
         single-lobe transposition flap, III:143,
            144f–145f
         surgical guidelines, III:142–146
         three stage full-thickness forehead flap,
            III:151–152, 152f
         three stage full-thickness forehead flap
            (stage 1), III:152–153, 153f–159f
         three stage full-thickness forehead flap
            (stage 2), III:153–155
         three stage full-thickness forehead flap
            (stage 3), III:155, 155t
         two-stage forehead flap, III:148,
            150f–151f
         two-stage forehead flap (stage 1),
            III:148–151
         two-stage forehead flap (stage 2),
            III:151, 151t
         two-stage nasolabial flap, III:146–148,
            146f–147f
         two-stage nasolabial flap (stage 1),
            III:146
         two-stage nasolabial flap (stage 2),
            III:146–148

aesthetic surgery (Continued)
      nasal contour and support restoration
         basic principles, III:160–179
         composite grafts, III:161
         design guidelines, III:160, 160t
         facial artery myomucosal (FAMM) flap,
            III:163
         free flap nasal reconstruction,
            III:173–174
         graft fixation, III:161
         hard-tissue support replacement,
            III:160
         harvesting guidelines, III:161
         hingeover lining flaps, III:162
         inadequate platforms, III:174
         intranasal lining flaps, III:163–166,
            164f–166f, 166t
         lining restoration, III:161
         material selection, III:160–161
         microvascular transfer, III:173
         modified folded forehead flap,
            III:170–172, 170f–171f
         nasal lining restoration, III:174–179
         nasolabial flap, III:163
         prelaminated flap technique, III:162
         residual lining advancement,
            III:161–162
         second forehead flap, III:163
         second lining flaps, III:162–163
         skin graft linings, III:172–173
         soft-tissue support and contouring,
            III:161
         timing considerations, III:160
      nasal cover restoration
         adversely located defects, III:146–148
         deep defects, III:146–148
         healing by secondary intention,
            III:140–141
         large defects, III:146–148
         local flaps, III:142–146
         primary repair procedures, III:141
         skin grafts, III:141–142
         small/superficial defects, III:140–141
      nasal lining restoration
         Burget–Walton approach, III:175f
         Menick–Salibian approach, III:176f
         mid-vault defects, III:174
         operation 1, III:174–177
         operation 2, III:177
         operation 3, III:177–178
         operation 4, III:178
         operation 5, III:178–179
         subtotal and total nasal defects, III:174,
            175f–181f
      outcomes and complicatons, III:179–181
      patient presentation and diagnosis,
         III:135
      regional unit repair
         basic principles, III:138–139
         contralateral normal, III:138
         donor site considerations, III:138
         exact dimensions and outline, III:138
         exact foil templates, III:138
         old scars, III:139
         preliminary operationa, III:139
         stable platforms, III:139
         subcutaneous framework restoration,
            III:139

aesthetic surgery (Continued)
         subunit principle, III:138
         surgical staging, III:139
         tissue transfer, III:138–139
         wound healing, III:138–139
      secondary procedures
         do-over revisions, III:184
         major revisions, III:184
         minor revisions, III:181–184
         secondary revisions, III:181–184,
            182f–184f
      skin grafts
         basic principles, III:141–142
         full-thickness forehead skin graft,
            III:141, 142f
         operative technique, III:141–142
         preauricular and postauricular skin
            grafts, III:141
      surgical goals, III:134
      surgical planning and preparation
         central facial units, III:136–137, 137f
         defect classification, III:139–140
         false planning assumptions, III:135–136
         modern approach, III:136, 136t, 137f
         peripheral facial units, III:136, 137f
         regional unit repair principles,
            III:138–139
         traditional approach, III:135
      surgical technique and treatment
         challenges, III:140–179
         forehead donor site, III:155–160
         nasal contour and support restoration,
            III:160–179
         nasal cover restoration, III:140–155
         zones of nasal skin quality, III:140
   beauty doctors, I:26–27, 28f
   female genital aesthetic surgery, II:655–677
      aesthetic ideals, II:669
      labia majora reduction, II:673–674,
         674f–676f
      labia minora reduction
         characteristics, II:669–673
         outcomes and complicatons, II:672–673,
            672f–673f
         surgical technique, II:670–672,
            671f–672f
      lipodystrophy, II:674–676, 675f–677f
      mons correction, II:640, 641f–642f
      mons pubis descent, II:674–676,
         675f–677f
      post-bariatric surgery reconstruction,
         II:640, 641f–642f
      research summary, II:677
      self-esteem issues, II:655, 669
      vulvar anatomy, II:669
   male genital aesthetic surgery, II:655–677
      enhancement procedures, II:655
      flaccid versus erect penis measurements,
         II:655–656
      hidden penis
         characteristics, II:665–668, 665f–666f
         outcome assessments, II:668
         post-bariatric surgery reconstruction,
            II:640, 643f
         surgical technique, II:667–668,
            667f–669f
      patient selection and examination, II:656
      penile anatomy, II:656

aesthetic surgery (Continued)
  penile enlargement reconstruction
    dermal fat graft and Alloderm removal,
      II:661–662, 661f
    fat removal, II:660–661
    outcomes and complicatons, II:662
    postoperative care and follow-up, II:662
    reconstructive issues, II:660–662
    VY advancement flap reversal, II:658f,
      660, 661f
  penile girth enhancement
    allograft dermal matrix grafts, II:660
    challenges, II:659–660
    dermal and dermal fat grafts,
      II:659–660
    fat injections, II:658f–659f, 659
  penile lengthening
    basic procedure, II:656–658, 657f–658f
    outcome assessments, II:657–658, 659f
    VY advancement flap, II:656–658,
      657f–658f
  penoscrotal web, II:662, 663f
  research summary, II:677
  scrotal enlargement, II:662, 664f
  self-esteem issues, II:655
origins, I:25–26
patient safety, I:131–132
postwar aesthetic surgery, I:28
psychological aspects, I:39
rhinoplasty, I:26f
Affirm™ laser, II:71t, 72
Afipia felis, III:891
Agee endoscopic carpal tunnel release
  (ECTR), VI:509
agency law, I:98
aging process
  classic aging characteristics, II:184–193, 185f
  eyes, II:116, 116f
  fat grafting, II:328, 329f
  neck, II:313–315
  skin, II:15
  soft-tissue fillers, II:44–45
Agrimonia pilosa, V:33t–35t
air embolism, IV:433t
air-fluidized (AF) beds, IV:364–366, 364f
air pollution, III:421–422
airway management, I:132
alar base surgery, II:177
Albucasis (Abu-l-Qasim), I:14–15
alcohol, IV:395
alcohol consumption, III:421, 515
aldehydes, IV:395
alemtuzumab, I:821, 825–826
alfentanil, IV:427
alginate, I:289t
alkaline phosphatase (ALP), I:428, 432t, 434f,
  IV:104
Allen's test, VI:40b, 52–53, 60
allergic reactions to anesthesia, I:146
allergic rhinitis, II:454, 458
Allium sativum, V:33t–35t
AlloDerm
  Asian rhinoplasty, II:175
  breast augmentation, V:52f, 69–71, 70t
  burn wound treatment, IV:415, 415t
  dermal graft and repair, I:340–342
  lower extremity reconstructive surgery,
    IV:128–129, 130f
  nipple-areola complex reconstruction,
    V:515–516

AlloDerm (Continued)
  penile girth enhancement, II:660
  soft-tissue fillers, II:45t, 46
allogeneic bone grafts
  advantages, I:459–460
  allograft bone incorporation, I:460
  bone graft formulations, I:460
  disease transmission risk, I:459
  immunogenicity, I:460
  processing and preservation techniques,
    I:459
Allograft, IV:128–129
allografts
  bone, I:830, IV:174–175, 180–181, 180f
  cartilage, I:831
  characteristics, IV:412t–414t
  definition, I:815
  nerve repair and grafting, I:473–474, 473t,
    475f, 831
  penile girth enhancement, II:660
  skin grafts, I:325t, 829
AlloMax, V:69, 70t
aloesin, II:24
aloe vera, II:22
alopecia, II:206, VI:646
alpha hydroxy acids (AHAs)
  characteristics, II:18–19
  facial skin resurfacing, II:66–67
  glycolic acid, II:19
  lactic acid, II:18–19
aluminum (Al) alloys, I:786–787
alveolar clefts, III:584–594
  anatomical characteristics, III:584–585, 585f
  background information, III:584
  complications, III:592–594
  dental development, III:585
  goals, III:584, 585t
  patient presentation and diagnosis
    alveolar distraction, III:587–588, 587f–588f
    bone morphogenetic proteins (BMPs),
      III:586
    cleft palate with cleft lip and alveolus,
      III:570–571, 571f
    gingivoperiosteoplasty (GPP), III:585, 586f
    late bone grafts, III:587
    primary bone grafts, III:585
    secondary bone grafts, III:585–586, 587f
  prognosis and outcomes
    bone morphogenetic proteins (BMPs),
      III:593
    gingivoperiosteoplasty (GPP), III:592–593
    graft site augmentation, III:594
    late bone grafts, III:593
    primary bone grafts, III:593
    secondary bone grafts, III:593
  surgical technique
    gingivoperiosteoplasty (GPP), III:588,
      589f
    horizontal alveolar transport distraction,
      III:591–592, 591f–592f
    primary bone grafts, III:588–589
    secondary bone grafts, III:589–591,
      590f–591f
    vertical alveolar transport distraction,
      III:592, 592f
alveolar ridge
  anatomical characteristics, III:422f
  cancer management
    preoperative assessment, III:406
    treatment strategies, III:406–407, 407f, 427

alveolar soft-part sarcoma
  characteristics, III:890
  complications, III:890
  disease process, III:890
  patient presentation and diagnosis, III:890
  prognosis and outcomes, III:890
  surgical technique and treatment, III:890
Amalian, II:47t
Amazing Gel, II:48t
  See also soft-tissue fillers
ambiguous genitalia, IV:336–338
amelanotic melanoma, I:753, 755f
amelia See congenital transverse arrest
American Academy of Orthopaedic Surgeons
  clinical practice guidelines for the treat-
    ment of carpal tunnel syndrome, VI:507t
American Association for Hand Surgery
  (AAHS), VI:xlvii
American Association of Oral and Plastic
  Surgeons, I:24
American Board of Plastic Surgery, VI:xliv
American Joint Committee on Cancer (AJCC)
  Staging Manual, I:750–761, III:400–401,
    IV:105, 105t, V:286–287
American Recovery and Reinvestment Act
  (2009), I:85
American Society for Aesthetic Plastic Surgery
  (ASAPS), I:57–58, II:2–3
American Society of Anesthesiologists (ASA)
  risk classification system, I:125, 125t–126t
American Society of Gene and Cell Therapy,
  I:192
American Society of Plastic Surgeons (ASPS)
  Code of Ethics, I:57–58
  historical background, I:24
amitriptyline, IV:427
amniocentesis, I:199
amniotic band disruption, III:807t
ampicillin, II:21t
amputations
  acute wounds, I:241
  burn reconstruction, IV:451–453
  Chopart amputation, IV:208
  cold injury/frostbite, IV:458–459, 459f
  decision-making process, IV:65–66, 86
  diabetic foot ulcers, IV:194–195
  Dupuytren's disease, VI:361
  ear reconstruction, III:209, 212, 213f–214f
  fingers, I:766–768, 769f
  foot reconstruction
    diabetic foot ulcers, IV:194–195
    hindfoot amputations, IV:216–217
    midfoot amputations, IV:208
    transmetatarsal amputation, IV:207
  Lisfranc amputation, IV:208
  lower extremity reconstructive surgery,
    IV:83, 132–133
  mangled upper extremities, VI:256
  psychosocial aspects, VI:246–247
  replantation and revascularization surgery,
    VI:228–249
    complications, VI:248–249
    general discussion, VI:228
    ischemia–reperfusion pathophysiology,
      VI:228–229
    outcome assessments, VI:247–248, 247t
    patient presentation and diagnosis
      patient selection indications and
        contraindications, VI:230–231,
        230t–231t

amputations (*Continued*)
  replantation centers, **VI**:229–230, 229t, 230f
  transportation considerations, **VI**:229, 229f
  postoperative care and follow-up
    anticoagulant agents, **VI**:244–245
    postoperative monitoring, **VI**:245–246, 246b, 246t
    postoperative therapy, **VI**:246
    psychosocial aspects, **VI**:246–247
  secondary procedures, **VI**:248f, 249
  surgical technique and treatment
    artery repair, **VI**:233–234, 234f
    bone fixation, **VI**:232–233, 232b, 232f
    distal amputations, **VI**:241–242, 241f
    ectopic replantation, **VI**:243, 244f
    multiple digit replantations, **VI**:237–238, 237f–240f
    nerve repair and grafting, **VI**:235
    operative sequence, **VI**:231–232, 231f
    pediatric replantation, **VI**:244
    proximal amputations, **VI**:238–241, 238f–240f
    ring avulsion injuries, **VI**:242, 242b, 242t, 243f
    single-digit amputation, **VI**:241f
    skin closure, **VI**:235
    tendon graft and repair, **VI**:233, 233b
    thumb replantation, **VI**:235–237, 236f–237f
    vein repair, **VI**:234–235, 235f
  sarcoma-related reconstruction, **IV**:110
  surgical innovation, **I**:5
  traumatic ear injuries
    complete amputation, **III**:42
    partial amputation with a narrow pedicle, **III**:42
    partial amputation with a wide pedicle, **III**:41f, 42
  traumatic nose injuries, **III**:44
  upper extremity amputees, **VI**:870–880
    aesthetic prostheses, **VI**:870, 871f
    body-powered prostheses, **VI**:870–871
    control mechanisms, **VI**:870–871
    general characteristics, **VI**:870
    prosthetics–composite tissue allotransplantation (CTA) comparisons, **VI**:879–880
    residual limb surgery
      neuroma management, **VI**:876
      soft-tissue improvement, **VI**:875–876, 875f–876f
      targeted muscle reinnervation (TMR), **VI**:871, 876–879
    surgery–prosthesis considerations
      elbow disarticulation/long trans-humeral amputation, **VI**:874–875
      finger amputation, **VI**:872, 872f
      general discussion, **VI**:872–875
      partial hand, **VI**:872, 873f
      shoulder disarticulation/proximal transhumeral amputation, **VI**:875
      wrist disarticulation/transradial amputation, **VI**:873–874, 873f–874f
    targeted muscle reinnervation (TMR)
      characteristics, **VI**:876–879
      myoelectric prostheses, **VI**:871

amputations (*Continued*)
    shoulder disarticulation level, **VI**:877–879, 878f–879f, 879t
    transhumeral level, **VI**:876–877, 876f–877f
    transradial level, **VI**:879
anaerobic bacteria, **I**:249–250
anaplastic large cell lymphoma (ALCL), **V**:37
ancient Egypt, **I**:11–12
Andersen–Tawil syndrome, **III**:805–807, 807t
André–Thomas sign, **VI**:58–59
androgen antagonists, **IV**:341t
anesthesia
  abdominal wall reconstruction, **IV**:283
  American Society of Anesthesiologists (ASA) risk classification system, **I**:125, 125t–126t
  buttock augmentation, **II**:609
  carpal tunnel syndrome surgery, **VI**:507–509, 507b, 508f
  closed rhinoplasty, **II**:427–435
  cosmetic surgery, **II**:9
  eutectic mixture of local anesthetics (EMLA), **III**:26
  facial skeletal augmentation, **II**:342
  facial soft-tissue injuries
    auricular nerve, **III**:27
    cheeks, **III**:27, 27f–28f
    chin, **III**:27, 28f
    ears, **III**:27–29, 29f
    Erb's point, **III**:27
    facial field block, **III**:26–29
    forehead, **III**:26, 27f
    general discussion, **III**:26–29
    glabella, **III**:26, 27f
    jaw, **III**:27
    local infiltration, **III**:26
    lower eyelid area, **III**:27, 27f–28f
    lower lip, **III**:27, 28f
    neck, **III**:27
    nose, **III**:27, 27f–28f
    scalp, **III**:26, 27f
    teeth, **III**:27, 27f–28f
    topical anesthetics, **III**:26
    upper eyelid area, **III**:26, 27f
    upper lip, **III**:27, 27f–28f
  flexor tendon injuries, **VI**:207
  hair transplantation, **II**:503–504
  infraorbital nerve anesthesia, **III**:57
  lateral SMASectomy, **II**:233
  liposuctions, **II**:514–515
  local anesthesia, **I**:137–149
    absorption, **I**:147
    action variability, **I**:146–147
    carbonated anesthesia, **I**:140, 140f, 148
    comparative pharmacology, **VI**:96t
    complications
      adverse drug interactions, **I**:145
      allergic reactions, **I**:146
      bradycardia, **I**:145
      cardiovascular toxicity, **I**:146
      central nervous system toxicity, **I**:146
      hypertension, **I**:145
      hypotension, **I**:145
      nausea and vomiting, **I**:145
      respiration, **I**:144–145
      reversal effects, **I**:145

anesthesia (*Continued*)
      tachycardia, **I**:145
      toxicity diagnosis and treatment, **I**:146, 146b
    epinephrine, **I**:139, 140f, 147–148
    general discussion, **I**:137
    infiltration
      abdominoplasties, **I**:143, 144f
      breast augmentation, **I**:142–143, 143f
      breast reduction, **I**:141–142, 141f–142f
      characteristics, **I**:140–144
      facelifts, **I**:140, 141f
      liposuctions, **I**:143–144, 144f
    patient selection, **I**:137–138
    pharmacokinetics, **VI**:94
    pharmacology, **VI**:94–96
    pre-emptive effects, **I**:148–149
    premedication, **I**:138
    research summary, **I**:149
    secondary rhinoplasty, **II**:468
    sedation choice, **I**:138
    sedation drugs, **I**:138–139
    selection guidelines, **VI**:95–96, 95t
      anesthetic drugs, **I**:139
      carbonated anesthesia, **I**:140, 140f
      characteristics, **I**:139–140
      vasoconstricting agents, **I**:139–140
    toxicity, **I**:147–148, **VI**:94–95, 101–102
    vasoconstrictive effects, **I**:147
    vasoconstrictors, **VI**:95
  lower bodylift/belt lipectomy surgery, **II**:585–588
  microvascular free-flap surgery, **I**:611
  mini/short scar abdominoplasty, **II**:540
  open rhinoplasty, **II**:389–390
  regional anesthesia techniques
    axillary block, **VI**:99–100, 101f
    Bier block, **VI**:97
    characteristics, **VI**:96–100
    digital blockade, **VI**:96–97
    infraclavicular block, **VI**:99, 100f
    interscalene block, **VI**:97, 98f
    intravenous regional anesthesia, **VI**:97
    supraclavicular block, **VI**:97–99, 99f
    wrist block, **VI**:97
  secondary rhinoplasty, **II**:468
  upper extremity surgery, **VI**:92–105
    anatomical characteristics
      axillary sheath, **VI**:92–94
      brachial plexus, **VI**:92–94, 93f
      microneuroanatomy, **VI**:94
      nerve innervation, **VI**:93f
      perineurial environment, **VI**:92–94
      sonoanatomy, **VI**:94
    complications
      characteristics, **VI**:100–102
      evaluation and management, **VI**:101
      infections, **VI**:102
      local anesthetic toxicity, **VI**:94–95, 101–102
      peripheral nerve injury, **VI**:100
      vascular injury, **VI**:102
    goals, **VI**:92
    local anesthesia
      comparative pharmacology, **VI**:96t
      pharmacokinetics, **VI**:94
      pharmacology, **VI**:94–96
      selection guidelines, **VI**:95–96, 95t

Note: **Boldface** *roman numerals indicate volume. Page numbers followed by f refer to figures; page numbers followed by t refer to tables; page numbers followed by b refer to boxes.*

anesthesia (Continued)
    toxicity, VI:94–95, 101–102
    vasoconstrictors, VI:95
    outcome assessments
        anesthetic types, VI:102–103
        clinical outcomes, VI:102
        operating room cost and efficiency, VI:103
        patient satisfaction, VI:102
    perioperative pain management
        chronic postoperative pain, VI:104, 104t
        general discussion, VI:103–104
        peripheral catheters, VI:103
        preemptive analgesia, VI:103–104
        risk factors, VI:104t
    regional anesthesia techniques
        axillary block, VI:99–100, 101f
        Bier block, VI:97
        characteristics, VI:96–100
        digital blockade, VI:96–97
        infraclavicular block, VI:99, 100f
        interscalene block, VI:97, 98f
        intravenous regional anesthesia, VI:97
        supraclavicular block, VI:97–99, 99f
        wrist block, VI:97
    special cases
        cardiac patients, VI:103
        pediatric patients, VI:103
    vertical scar reduction mammaplasty, V:182
    See also patient safety
aneuploidy, I:185
aneurysmal bone cysts, VI:328–329, 328f
aneurysms, I:677t, VI:324, 325f, 474, 479–481, 481f
Angelman syndrome, I:183
angiogenesis
    pedical flap viability augmentation, I:580
    skin wound healing, I:271
    tissue expansion effects, I:624
    tissue-specific stem cells, I:230, 231f
    trunk, IV:220
    wound healing, I:250–252, 251f, 260
angiography
    cutaneous and soft-tissue tumors, I:710
    hand ischemia, VI:472, 472f
angiokeratoma, VI:668t
angioleiomyoma, I:731–732
angioma cavernosum, I:676–678
angioma racemosum, I:676–678
angioma simplex, I:676–678
angiosarcomas, I:671, 741–742, 741f
angiosome
    arterial perforators, I:482, 483f
    characteristics, I:480–482
    computed tomography angiography, I:483f
    cutaneous arteries, I:482f
    vessel networks, I:483f
angular artery, IV:222f, 223
animal bites, VI:343
animal-skin nevus, I:724, 725f
animation, I:865, 867t
ankle brachial pressure index (ABPI), I:279–281
ankles
    anatomical characteristics
        fascial system
            characteristics, IV:52–56
            extensor retinacula, IV:52, 52t, 54f
            flexor retinaculum, IV:52–54, 52t, 54f
            peroneal retinaculum, IV:54, 54f, 54t

ankles (Continued)
    functional role, IV:50–61
    innervation, IV:60f, 61
    skeletal structure, IV:50, 52f
    vascular supply
        dorsalis pedis, IV:59, 60f
        peroneal artery, IV:47f, 59–61, 61f–62f
        posterior tibial artery, IV:47f, 59
    burn reconstruction, IV:443t, 444, 509
    liposuctions, II:525
ankylosing spondylitis, VI:406–408
annular pulleys, VI:29–32, 30f, 179–182, 180f
anorexia nervosa, I:49–50, 49b
anterior circumflex humeral artery, IV:225–227, 226f
anterior intercostal artery perforator (AICAP) flap, V:308, 488
anterior interosseous nerve (AIN) syndrome
    characteristics, VI:510–511
    nonsurgical management, VI:511
    surgical technique and treatment, VI:511, 512f–513f
anterior plagiocephaly, III:729, 730f, 730t
anterior segmental ostectomy, II:178, 181–182
anterior superior iliac spine (ASIS), VI:264–266
anterolateral thigh flap
    foot reconstruction, IV:211
    lower extremity reconstructive surgery, IV:68–69, 69f, 75, 75f–76f, 81f, 88f
    male genital reconstructive surgery, IV:304–310, 306f, 311f
    mangled upper extremities, VI:274–275, 275f–276f
    oral cavity and mouth reconstruction, III:321–322
    perineal reconstruction, IV:388–389, 390f–391f
    phalloplasty, IV:311f, 323, 324f–325f
    pharyngoesophageal reconstruction
        flap design and harvesting, III:339–341, 340f–342f
        flap inset guidelines, III:342–347, 343f–348f
        frozen neck, III:352–353
        isolated cervical esophageal defects, III:354
        oral diet, III:356t
        postlaryngectomy pharyngocutaneous fistulas, III:353–354, 353f–354f
        selection guidelines, III:338–339
    scalp and forehead reconstruction, III:130
    tongue reconstruction, III:309t–310t
anterolateral thigh perforator flap, IV:145, 145f–146f
anthropometrics
    background information, II:354–365, 355f
    bilateral cleft lip surgery
        direct anthropometric measurements, III:565, 566f
        indirect anthropometric measurements
            photogrammetry, III:565–567
            stereophotogrammetry, III:567–568, 567f
    chin, II:360, 361f
    eyes, II:358, 358f
    facial beauty ideals, II:177
    forehead, II:356–358, 357f–358f
    lips, II:360, 360f
    neoclassical canons, II:356b

anthropometrics (Continued)
    nose, II:358–359, 359f
    soft tissue facial analysis, II:355–356, 356b, 356f–357f, 356t
    unilateral cleft lip
        general discussion, III:519–522
        lip measurements and markings
            base of the cleft-side philtral column (CPHL'), III:520–521, 521f
            columella, III:522
            Cupid's bow, III:520, 521f
            Cupid's bow peaking, III:522
            lateral lip length and height, III:522
            nasal floor skin, III:522
            tissue deficiency/excess evaluation, III:521
            vermillion, III:520, 521f
            vermillion deficiency, III:522
antibiotics, II:21t, III:82, IV:85, 196–197, 217, 292–293, VI:333
anticoagulant agents, I:582, IV:85, VI:244–245
anti-IL-2, I:821t, 825
anti-inflammatories, II:21t
antilymphocyte globulin, I:821t, 824
antimicrobial dressings, I:289t
antioxidants
    coenzyme Q10, II:27
    dry skin care, II:18
    general discussion, II:27–28
    grape seed extract, II:27
    green tea, II:27–28
    lycopene, II:28
    resveratrol, II:27
    sensitive skin care, II:23–24
    vitamin C, II:27
    vitamin E, II:27
antiproliferative agents
    azathioprine, I:821–823, 822t, 833t
    mycophenolate mofetil, I:822–823, 822t, 833t
antiseptics, IV:367
antithrombin, I:243f
antithymocyte globulin, I:821t, 824
apertognathia, III:666, 668f
Apert syndrome
    complications, VI:614
    epidemiology, VI:610
    outcome assessments, VI:614
    pathogenesis, VI:610
    patient presentation and diagnosis, III:689, VI:610, 611f, 611t, 613f, 644–645, 645f, 682
    patient selection, VI:612
    postoperative care and follow-up, VI:614
    secondary procedures, VI:614
    surgical innovation, III:226
    surgical technique and treatment
        basic procedure, VI:612–614
        finger separation, VI:612
        metacarpal synostosis, VI:614
        preferred treatments, VI:611f, 612t–613t, 613f
        thumb and first web separation, VI:612–614
    syndromic craniosynostosis, I:197, 197f, 197t, III:749–750, 750t
    thumb hypoplasia, VI:573t
apical ectodermal ridge (AER), VI:526–530, 529f–530f
apical segmental setback ostectomy (ASO), II:179

aplasia cutis congenita (ACC), **III:**110–111, 111f
Apligraf, **I:**337, 794t, 795, **IV:**128–129, 415t, 522
apnea–hypopnea index (AHI), **III:**96, 102–103
apocrine cystadenoma, **I:**722–723, 723f
apocrine glands, **I:**322
apocrine nevus, **I:**723
apoptosis, **I:**661–662
Apple, **I:**79
Applied Physics Laboratory (APL), **I:**860–861
apraxia, **III:**618
Aquamid, **II:**48t
　See also soft-tissue fillers
Arabian surgery, **I:**14–15
Arbeitsgemeinschaft für Osteosynthesefragen (AO) principles, **VI:**106, 107t
arbutin, **II:**24–25
arcuate line, **IV:**227–230, 227f
areola reconstruction, **V:**516–518, 517b, 517f–518f
　See also nipple-areola complex
Argiform, **II:**48t
　See also soft-tissue fillers
argon lasers, **III:**30
arms
　liposuctions, **II:**521
　nerve compression syndromes, **VI:**510, 510f
　post-bariatric surgery reconstruction, **II:**652
　upper limb contouring, **II:**617–633, **V:**558–581
　　causal factors, **II:**617, 618f–620f
　　complications, **II:**629–631, 629t
　　demand increases, **II:**617, **V:**558–564
　　outcomes and complicatons, **V:**563–564
　　pathophysiology, **V:**558–559
　　patient presentation and diagnosis, **II:**617–620, **V:**559–564
　　patient selection
　　　arm surface anatomy, **II:**624f
　　　laboratory work-up, **II:**623
　　　physical examination, **II:**620–624, 621f–622f
　　　plan formulation, **II:**622–623
　　　preoperative assessment, **II:**623
　　　sagittal view of arm anatomy, **II:**625f
　　　selection guidelines, **V:**559–560
　　　thromboembolic disease prophylaxis, **II:**623–624
　　Pittsburgh Rating Scale, **V:**559–560, 559t
　　post-bariatric surgery reconstruction, **II:**652
　　postoperative care and follow-up, **II:**629, **V:**562–563
　　prognosis and outcomes, **II:**629–631, 630f–632f
　　secondary procedures, **II:**632–633, 632f
　　surgical technique
　　　basic procedure, **V:**560–562, 561f–563f
　　　marking, **II:**624–626, 627f
　　　operative procedures, **II:**626–629, 627f–629f
　　　surface anatomy, **II:**624, 624f–626f
　　　surgical tips, **V:**562b
Arnica montana, **V:**33t–35t
Arnold's nerve, **III:**27–29, 29f
arrow flap, **V:**503t, 507, 507f
ArteFill (Artecoll), **II:**47–48, 47t, 49t
　See also soft-tissue fillers

Arteplast, **II:**48t
　See also soft-tissue fillers
arterial malformation (AM), **I:**677t, **VI:**668t
arterial puncture, **IV:**433t
arterial territories, **I:**482–484, 484f
arterial ulcers, **I:**253–254
arteriovenous fistula and arteriovenous malformation (AVM), **I:**735, 736f, **IV:**433t
arteriovenous hemangioma, **I:**678t
arteriovenous malformation (AVM)
　causal factors, **VI:**684–690
　classification systems, **I:**676–677, 677t, **VI:**668t
　clinical manifestations, **I:**698–699
　diagnostic work-up, **VI:**670t
　pathogenesis, **I:**696–698, **VI:**685–686
　patient presentation and diagnosis, **VI:**669, 670f, 686–687, 686f–688f
　Schobinger clinical staging system, **VI:**686t
　Schobinger staging system, **I:**698–699, 699t
　surgical technique and treatment, **VI:**669–672, 671t, 687–690, 689f
　terminology, **I:**678t
　treatment strategies
　　embolization, **I:**700
　　intervention guidelines, **I:**699–700
　　resection, **I:**689f, 700
artery repair, **VI:**233–234, 234f
ArteSense, **II:**48t
　See also soft-tissue fillers
articularis genu muscle, **IV:**15t–16t, 18f, 19t, 20f–22f
ascorbic acid, **I:**282, **II:**18, 27
Asian facial cosmetic surgery, **II:**163–183
　beauty ideals, **II:**163–164
　blepharoplasty
　　anatomical considerations, **II:**164–165, 165f–166f
　　eyelid characteristics, **II:**164
　　outcomes and complicatons, **II:**170–172
　　postoperative care and follow-up, **II:**170
　　preoperative assessment, **II:**166–167, 166f–167f
　　surgical technique and treatment
　　　incisional methods, **II:**168, 169f
　　　lateral canthoplasty, **II:**170, 171f–172f
　　　medial epicanthoplasty, **II:**169, 170f–171f
　　　nonincisional methods, **II:**167–168, 167f–168f
　　　partial incisional methods, **II:**168, 168f
　　　subclinical ptosis repair, **II:**169
　facial bone surgery
　　beauty ideals, **II:**177
　　facial contouring surgery
　　　malar reduction surgery, **II:**180–181, 180f
　　　mandible angle ostectomy, **II:**179, 179f–180f
　　　narrowing genioplasty, **II:**181, 181f
　　historical background
　　　anterior segmental ostectomy, **II:**178
　　　malar reduction, **II:**177–178
　　　mandible angle reduction, **II:**178
　　　orthognathic surgery, **II:**178
　　malar reduction surgery
　　　bicoronal approach, **II:**181
　　　intraoral infracture technique with incomplete osteotomy, **II:**181

Asian facial cosmetic surgery (Continued)
　　　intraoral L-shaped ostectomy, **II:**181
　　　surgical technique, **II:**180–181, 180f
　　orthognathic surgery
　　　bimaxillary protrusion, **II:**181–182
　　　jaw rotation, **II:**181, 182f–183f
　　outcomes and complicatons
　　　mandible angle reduction, **II:**182
　　　zygoma reduction, **II:**182
　　patient presentation and diagnosis
　　　chin, **II:**178–179
　　　dentoalveolar protrusion, **II:**179
　　　facial profiles, **II:**179
　　　mandible angle, **II:**178
　　　zygoma, **II:**178
　　surgical technique and treatment
　　　anterior segmental ostectomy, **II:**181–182
　　　facial contouring, **II:**179–181
　　　orthognathic surgery, **II:**181–182
　rhinoplasty
　　contracted nose
　　　dermal fat graft, **II:**176
　　　derotation grafts, **II:**176, 176f
　　　rib cartilage graft, **II:**176
　　　septal extension grafts, **II:**176
　　　surgical technique and treatment, **II:**173–176
　　general discussion, **II:**172–173
　　historical background, **II:**173
　　low profile nasal dorsum augmentation
　　　implant materials, **II:**173–174
　　　one-piece augmentation rhinoplasty, **II:**174
　　　preoperative view, **II:**174f
　　　two-piece augmentation rhinoplasty, **II:**174, 174f
　　nasal skeleton, **II:**172–173
　　outcomes and complicatons
　　　capsular contractures, **II:**177
　　　implant deviation, **II:**176
　　　implant exposure, **II:**176
　　　implant infection, **II:**176
　　patient presentation and diagnosis
　　　blunt nasal tip, **II:**173
　　　broad nasal dorsum, **II:**173
　　　general discussion, **II:**173
　　　short/contracted nose, **II:**173
　　　underprojected nasal tip, **II:**173
　　secondary procedures
　　　alar base surgery, **II:**177
　　　forehead augmentation, **II:**174f, 177
　　　genioplasty, **II:**177
　　　paranasal augmentation, **II:**177
　　soft tissue profile, **II:**172–173
　　surgical technique and treatment
　　　bulbous nose, **II:**175, 176f
　　　contracted nose, **II:**173–176
　　　low profile nasal dorsum augmentation, **II:**173–174, 174f
　　　septal extension grafts, **II:**175–176, 175f
　　　short nose, **II:**175–176, 475–476, 478f–479f
　　　underprojected nasal tip, **II:**174–175
　　underprojected nasal tip
　　　alloplastic materials, **II:**175
　　　cartilage grafts, **II:**175
　　　general discussion, **II:**174–175

Note: **Boldface** roman numerals indicate volume. Page numbers followed by f refer to figures; page numbers followed by t refer to tables; page numbers followed by b refer to boxes.

Asian facial cosmetic surgery (Continued)
onlay cartilaginous grafts, II:175
septal extension grafts, II:175, 175f
aspirin, I:582, 615–617, II:21t, VI:244–245
assets, I:67–68, 71f
asymmetrical bilateral cleft lip, III:560–562, 563f–564f
asymmetric tuberous breast deformity
Case III (asymmetric tuberous breast deformity)
patient presentation and diagnosis, V:533
preoperative assessment, V:533
surgical procedures, V:533
Case IV (Type II tuberous breast)
operative sequence, V:533–534
patient presentation and diagnosis, V:534f–535f
postoperative result, V:534
preoperative assessment, V:533
Case VI (Type III flap), V:534–537
Case V (severe bilateral mammary hypoplasia and tuberous deformity)
patient presentation and diagnosis, V:534, 536f
post-lipostructure result, V:534
general considerations, V:532
patient presentation and diagnosis, V:533–534
ataxia telangectasia mutated (ATM) gene, I:662
atheroma, I:719, 720f
Atléan BTCP, II:48t
See also soft-tissue fillers
atresia, I:677t
atrophic rhinitis, II:454, 458
atypical (dysplastic) nevus, I:745–746, 747f
atypical (dysplastic) nevus syndrome, I:746–747
atypical mole, I:724
atypical nontuberculous mycobacteria
disease process, III:891
patient presentation and diagnosis, III:891–892, 891f
surgical technique and treatment, III:892
augmentation mammaplasty, V:13–38
adolescent aesthetic surgery, I:45t, II:5f
autologous fat grafts, V:591–595, 593f–595f
background information, V:13
breast reconstruction considerations, V:380
diagnostic imaging, V:270–271, 271f
endoscopic approaches, V:81–96
background and general characteristics
general discussion, V:81–82
illumination and imaging technology, V:82
latissimus dorsi (LD) flap, V:82–83
optical cavities, V:81–82
support systems, V:82
endoscopic augmentation mammaplasty
breast anatomy, V:83
outcomes and complicatons, V:87–88, 88f
patient presentation and diagnosis, V:83
patient selection, V:83–84
postoperative care and follow-up, V:87–88
surgical technique and treatment, V:84–87, 84f–87f
fat grafting, I:342–346, 346f–347f

augmentation mammaplasty (Continued)
gender identity disorder surgery, IV:348–350
iatrogenic disorders, V:97–118
background information, V:97
breast implants
implant malposition, V:112–116
saline implants, V:13–14, 110, 110f
silicone gel implants, I:789–790, 790f, V:14–15, 102–109
sponges, V:101–102, 102f
steroid atrophy, V:110, 110f
implant malposition
double-bubble deformity, V:116, 116f
inadequate muscle release, V:113, 114f
plane of insertion, V:112–113, 113f
submusculofascial plane, V:114–115, 114f
symmastia, V:115–116, 116f
transaxillary dissection, V:115, 115f
injection materials
background information, V:97–101
liquid silicone injections, V:98–100, 99f–100f
paraffin injections, V:97–98, 98f
polyacrylamide hydrogel injections, V:100–101, 100f–101f
post-pregnancy secondary ptosis, V:117, 117f
ptosis, V:116–117, 117f
saline implants
autoinflation, V:111–112, 112f
capsular calcification, V:110, 110f
deflation, V:110–111, 111f
ripples and folds, V:111, 111f
silicone gel implants
capsular calcification, V:107–109, 108f–109f
capsular contracture, V:106–107, 106f–107f
characteristics, I:789–790, 790f
closed capsulotomy, V:107, 107f–108f
developmental background, V:14–15
double-bubble deformity, V:116, 116f
first generation implants, V:14–15, 103f
fourth and fifth generation implants, V:15
hematomas, V:104–105, 104f–105f
historical background, I:789–790, V:102–109
implant disruption, V:103–104, 103f
implant malposition, V:112–113, 113f
infections, V:105–106, 105f–106f
second generation implants, V:14–15, 104f
third generation implants, V:14–15, 104f
infiltration, I:142–143, 143f
informed consent, V:17–19
mastopexy
basic procedure, V:139–143
operative technique, V:142–143
preoperative/postoperative comparisons, V:143f
surgical tips, V:142b
measurement and analysis, V:16–17, 19f, 25f
operative planning
implant selection
filling material, V:24–25
implant shape, V:25–27, 28f–29f

augmentation mammaplasty (Continued)
implant size determination, V:25, 25f
implant surface texture, V:25, 26f–27f
incision length and placement, V:19–20
inframammary incision, V:19, 27–30
periareolar incision, V:19, 30–31
pocket position
subfascial position, V:21f
subpectoral position, V:22f–24f, 28f–29f
surgical guidelines, V:20–27, 20f
surgical technique and treatment
inframammary incision, V:27–30
periareolar incision, V:30–31
preoperative markings, V:27–32
surgical guidelines, V:27b, 30b
transaxillary incision, V:31
transumbilical incision, V:32
transaxillary incision, V:19, 31
transumbilical incision, V:19–20, 32
patient presentation and diagnosis
hard tissue asymmetry, V:17f–18f
ideal breast structure, V:16f
patient history and examination, V:15–16
soft tissue asymmetry, V:18f
patient safety, I:132
patient selection, V:16–17
perioperative complications
delayed complications
implant rupture and deflation, V:37, 79t
periprosthetic capsular contracture, V:36–37
hematomas, V:32–37, 79t
medication and herbal supplement avoidance list, V:33t–35t
Mondor's disease, V:35–36
nipple sensitivity, V:32–37
seromas, V:32–37, 79t
wound infections, V:35, 79t
postoperative care and follow-up, V:32
psychological aspects, I:40–41
revisionary surgery, V:39–80
acellular dermal matrix (ADM)
basic principles, V:68–69
capsular contracture, V:52–53, 52f
clinical signs, V:79t
comparison studies, V:70t
complications, V:78–79, 79t
patient presentation and diagnosis, V:71
patient selection, V:71, 72t
preoperative/postoperative Baker classifications, V:79, 79t
prognosis and outcomes, V:78–79
surgical technique and treatment, V:71–78
background and challenges, V:39–40
biological responses, V:40
body responses
encapsulation processes, V:71
published research, V:69–71
regeneration processes, V:69
resorption processes, V:69
capsular contracture
acellular dermal matrix (ADM), V:52–53, 52f, 336–340
Baker classifications, V:36t, 46–53, 362, 362t
blood supply, V:49f
capsulectomy, V:47, 48f–49f
capsulotomies, V:47

augmentation mammaplasty (Continued)
  etiology, V:46t
  mastopexy, V:47, 48f
  neo subpectoral pocket conversion,
    V:50–52, 51f
  nipple-areola complex, V:49f
  subgландular to subpectoral
    conversion, V:50, 50f–51f
  surgical options, V:47t
  causal factors, V:67–68, 68b
  clinical signs, V:79t
  implant malposition
    characteristics, V:53, 53f–54f
    etiology, V:53–55, 54f
    treatment strategies, V:55–58, 55t,
      56f–57f
  outcomes and complicatons, V:65–66, 66t,
    78–79, 79t, 263–264
  patient presentation and diagnosis
    acellular dermal matrix (ADM), V:71
    classifications, V:41–42, 42f
    indicators, V:42–44
    patient history, V:40–44, 41t
    physical examination, V:40
  patient selection, V:42–44, 71, 72t
  postoperative care and follow-up, V:65,
    262–263
  preoperative/postoperative Baker
    classifications, V:79, 79t
  prognosis and outcomes, V:78–79
  published research, V:69–71
  secondary procedures, V:37
  surgical technique and treatment
    augmentation versus augmentation
      mastopexy, V:79t
    breast asymmetry, V:61–63, 62f–63f
    capsular contracture, V:46–53, 49f,
      77–78, 77f, 79t, 264
    implant failure, V:58–59
    implant malposition, V:53, 53f–54f, 79t
    implant pocket options, V:44–65, 44t,
      45f
    implant stabilization, V:75–76, 75f–76f
    lamellar separation, V:73–75, 73f
    lower pole coverage, V:73–75, 73f–76f
    placement indicators, V:71–78, 72f,
      73b
    preoperative assessment, V:44–65
    rippling/implant edge palpability,
      V:59–61, 61f
    size changes, V:64–65
    soft tissue changes, V:63–64, 64f
    surgical tips, V:44b
    tissue thickeners, V:76–77
  tissue changes, V:68–69
secondary procedures, V:37
silicone chemistry, V:14
surgical technique and treatment
  inframammary incision, V:27–30
  periareolar incision, V:30–31
  preoperative markings, V:27–32
  surgical guidelines, V:27b, 30b
  transaxillary incision, V:31
  transumbilical incision, V:32
augmentation pharyngoplasty, III:628
auras, III:491–492
auricular cartilage, I:398–404, 413–419
auricular nerve, III:27

auricular reconstruction, III:187–225
  acquired deformities (loss of auricular
    tissue)
    amputated ears, III:209, 212, 213f–214f
    cartilage replantation, III:210, 212
    composite graft, III:210, 210f
    dermabraded amputated auricle
      replantation, III:211, 211f
    microsurgical ear replantation, III:212
    skin coverage considerations, III:207–212,
      209f
    tissue attached by a narrow pedicle,
      III:209, 210f
  acquired partial defects, III:217
  anatomical considerations, III:187, 188f
  associated deformities, III:190, 191b, 191t
  bilateral microtia, III:204
  classifications, III:189, 190b, 190f
  constricted ears, II:489–490, III:204,
    205f–206f
  craniofacial osteointegration, I:800–802,
    800t, 801f
  cryptotia, II:490, III:204, 206f–207f
  deformities with loss of auricular tissue
    auricular skin loss, III:214
    full-thickness defects, III:214
    prosthetics, III:217
    skin coverage considerations, III:215–217
    trauma-acquired defects, III:214–215, 216f
  deformities without loss of auricular tissue
    cauliflower ear, III:212, 215f
    contour irregularities, III:212
    external auditory canal stenosis, III:212,
      215f
    otohematoma, III:212, 215f
  etiology
    developmental factors, III:189, 190f
    hereditary factors, III:189
    incidence, III:189
  general discussion, III:187
  microtia
    bilateral microtia, III:204
    clinical characteristics, III:190–191, 190f
    patient selection, III:191–192
    surgical technique and treatment
      preoperative assessment, III:192
      rib cartilage graft, III:194, 195f
      surgical planning and preparation,
        III:192–194
      surgical staging, III:192
  middle-ear surgery, III:187–189
  prominent ear
    antihelical fold restoration, III:206–207
    conchal alteration, III:206
    lateral cartilage surface alteration, III:207
    medial cartilage surface alteration, III:207
    pathology, III:204–206, 208f
    treatment strategies, III:206
  regional defects
    acquired earlobe deformities, II:492,
      III:220–221, 223f
    helical rim, III:218–219, 219f
    lower-third auricular defects, III:220,
      222f
    middle-third auricular defects, III:220,
      221f
    upper-third auricular defects, III:219–220
  secondary reconstruction, III:202–204

auricular reconstruction (Continued)
  structural support
    composite grafts, III:218, 219f
    contralateral conchal cartilage, III:217
    ipsilateral conchal cartilage, III:217–218,
      218f
  surgical technique and treatment
    acquired partial defects, III:217
    conchal definition, III:197–198, 199f–200f
    first stage
      adult patient framework modifications,
        III:195, 196f
      framework fabrication, III:194
      framework implantation, III:195–196
      postoperative activities, III:197
      rib cartilage graft, III:194, 195f
    hairline management, III:201–202, 203f
    lobule rotation, III:197, 198f
    Nagata technique, III:202
    posterior auricular region detachment,
      III:198–200, 201f
    preoperative assessment, III:192
    residual tissue utilization, III:217
    secondary reconstruction, III:202–204
    surgical planning and preparation,
      III:192–194, 194f
    surgical staging, III:192, 192f–193f
    technique variations, III:202
    tragal construction, III:197–198, 199f–200f
  tumors
    benign tumors, III:221
    malignant tumors, III:221–222
autografts
  bone, I:829–830
  cartilage, I:830–831
  definition, I:815
  nerve grafts, I:831, VI:707, 708f, 708t
  skin grafts, I:325t, 828–829
autologous fat grafts See fat grafting
autologous fillers, II:45b, 46
autologous nerve grafts, I:472–474
autologous vein grafts, I:472–473
automobile accidents, III:49, IV:63
autosomal inheritance, I:182–183, 182f
avascular necrosis, II:371f, 372
Avena sativa, II:18
Avicenna, VI:xliii–xliv
avulsions
  acute wounds, I:241
  facial soft-tissue injuries, III:31–32, 33f
  mangled upper extremities, VI:256, 256f
  nerve injuries, I:466t, 467–468, 468f, VI:792,
    792f–793f
  traumatic nose injuries, III:43–44, 44f
axial pattern flap, I:515, 515f
axillary artery, IV:225–227, 226f
axillary block, VI:99–100, 101f
axillary contouring, V:558–581
  demand increases, V:558–564
  outcomes and complicatons, V:563–564
  pathophysiology, V:558–559
  patient presentation and diagnosis,
    V:559–564
  patient selection, V:559–560
  Pittsburgh Rating Scale, V:559–560, 559t
  postoperative care and follow-up, V:562–563
  surgical technique and treatment, V:560–
    562, 561f–563f, 562b

axillary contractures, **IV**:445, 448f–449f, 507, 507f
axillary lymphadenectomy, **I**:771–777, 775f
axonotmesis, **I**:464–465, 465t, **VI**:698–700, 699t, 793
azathioprine, **I**:821–822, 822t, 833t
azelaic acid, **II**:21t
Azficel-T, **II**:46

B
baby oil, **IV**:395
babysitter technique, **III**:291–292, 291f–292f
bacillus Calmette-Guérin (BCG), **I**:205–206, 206f
bacitracin, **IV**:410
back
    anatomical characteristics
        general characteristics, **IV**:220–223, 221f
        musculature, **IV**:221–223, 222f, 224f
        vascular anatomy, **IV**:222f, 223, 224f
    back roll presentations, **II**:571, 578f
    body contouring
        back rolls, **V**:570–573
        outcomes and complicatons, **V**:573
        pathophysiology, **V**:570–571
        patient presentation and diagnosis, **V**:571
        patient selection, **V**:571–572
        postoperative care and follow-up, **V**:573
        surgical planning, **V**:571–572
        surgical technique and treatment, **V**:572, 573f
        surgical tips, **V**:572b
        transverse excisional upper bodylift, **V**:570f, 572
    soft-tissue reconstruction, **IV**:256–278
        flap closure
            adjacent tissue transfers, **IV**:268
            basic principles, **IV**:259–260
            erector spinae muscle flaps, **IV**:260–262, 260f–267f
            external oblique flaps, **IV**:268–269
            latissimus muscle/myocutaneous flap, **IV**:262–263, 268f–270f, 272f–273f
            pedicled omental flap, **IV**:267–268
            perforator flaps, **IV**:268
            spine closure, **IV**:260–269
            superior gluteal artery flap, **IV**:264–265, 277f
            trapezius muscle flap, **IV**:263–264, 274f–276f
        free flap coverage
            bone grafts, **IV**:271
            soft tissue flaps, **IV**:270
        historical background, **IV**:256
        patient presentation and diagnosis
            midline back wounds, **IV**:256–257
            nonmidline back wounds, **IV**:257
        postoperative care and follow-up, **IV**:277
        regional flap selection
            cervical spine area, **IV**:271
            lumbar area, **IV**:272
            lumbosacral region, **IV**:272–273
            thoracic area, **IV**:271–272
        special clinical situations
            cerebrospinal fluid leaks, **IV**:276–277
            chronic hardware exposures, **IV**:275
            esophageal fistula, **IV**:275
            lipomas of the spine, **IV**:275–276
            prophylactic closure of back incisions, **IV**:274

back (Continued)
            pseudomeningocele repair, **IV**:276–277
            tethered cord surgery, **IV**:275–276
        treatment strategies
            flap closure, **IV**:259–274
            free flap coverage, **IV**:270–271
            lateral back wounds, **IV**:273–274
            local wound care, **IV**:257, 257f–258f
            operative debridement, **IV**:258–259, 259f–260f
            regional flap selection, **IV**:271–273
            tissue expansion, **IV**:269–270
            vascularized bone reconstruction, **IV**:271
bacterial lymphadenitis
    disease process, **III**:890
    patient presentation and diagnosis, **III**:891
    surgical technique and treatment, **III**:891
baical skullcap root, **V**:33t–35t
Baker classification of contracture, **V**:36t, 46–53, 46t, 79t, 362, 362t
bak foong pill, **V**:33t–35t
balance sheets, **I**:67–68, 71f
baldness
    male-pattern baldness, **I**:633–635
    types and patterns, **II**:497–498
Baller–Gerold syndrome, **VI**:573t
Banff grading scale, **VI**:849t, 850f
Bannayan-Riley-Ruvalcaba (BRR) syndrome, **VI**:669, 690
    See also PTEN (phosphatase and tensin homologue)-associated vascular anomaly (PTEN-AVA)
Bardet–Biedl syndrome, **VI**:617t
bariatric surgery
    abdominal wall reconstruction, **IV**:282
    advantages, **II**:635–636, 636t
    post-bariatric surgery reconstruction, **II**:634–654
    abdominal contouring
        giant pannus, **II**:640–643, 643f–644f
        hidden penis, **II**:640, 643f
        major weight loss (MWL) patient, **II**:639b
        mons correction, **II**:640, 641f–642f
        operative planning and technique, **II**:639–640
        patient evaluation, **II**:639
        surgical variations, **II**:640–643, 640f–641f
    arm contouring
        demand increases, **V**:558–564
        outcomes and complicatons, **V**:563–564
        pathophysiology, **V**:558–559
        patient presentation and diagnosis, **V**:559–564
        patient selection, **V**:559–560
        Pittsburgh Rating Scale, **V**:559–560, 559t
        postoperative care and follow-up, **V**:562–563
        surgical technique and treatment, **V**:560–562, 561f–563f, 562b
    back contouring
        back rolls, **V**:570–573
        outcomes and complicatons, **V**:573
        pathophysiology, **V**:570–571
        patient presentation and diagnosis, **V**:571
        patient selection, **V**:571–572
        postoperative care and follow-up, **V**:573

bariatric surgery (Continued)
        surgical planning, **V**:571–572
        surgical technique and treatment, **V**:572, 573f
        surgical tips, **V**:572b
        transverse excisional upper bodylift, **V**:570f, 572
    body contouring centers of excellence, **II**:653
    complications, **II**:653
    gynecomastia
        excision of gynecomastia with nipple repositioning, **V**:575–579, 578f–580f
        outcomes and complicatons, **V**:579
        pathophysiology, **V**:573–574
        patient presentation and diagnosis, **V**:574
        patient selection, **V**:574–575, 575t
        postoperative care and follow-up, **V**:578
        pseudogynecomastia, **V**:575t, 576f–577f
        surgical markings, **V**:575–576, 576f–577f
        surgical technique and treatment, **V**:576–578, 578f–580f
        surgical tips, **V**:578b
    lower bodylift (LBL)/buttock contouring
        major weight loss (MWL) patient, **II**:644b
        markings, **II**:645, 646f–647f, 649f
        operative technique, **II**:645, 647f–649f
        patient evaluation, **II**:644–645
        patient selection, **II**:645
        postoperative care and follow-up, **II**:645
    male chest contouring
        excision of gynecomastia with nipple repositioning, **V**:575–579, 578f–580f
        outcomes and complicatons, **V**:579
        pathophysiology, **V**:573–574
        patient presentation and diagnosis, **V**:574
        patient selection, **V**:574–575, 575t
        postoperative care and follow-up, **V**:578
        pseudogynecomastia, **V**:575t, 576f–577f
        surgical markings, **V**:575–576, 576f–577f
        surgical technique and treatment, **V**:576–578, 578f–580f
        surgical tips, **V**:578b
    mastopexy
        breast reshaping, **V**:564–570
        dermal suspension, **V**:566–570, 568f
        outcomes and complicatons, **V**:567–570
        pathophysiology, **V**:564, 564b
        patient presentation and diagnosis, **V**:564–565
        patient selection, **V**:565–566
        postoperative care and follow-up, **V**:567
        surgical goals, **V**:565b
        surgical planning, **V**:565–566, 566t, 569f–570f
        surgical tips, **V**:567b
        total parenchymal reshaping mastopexy, **V**:566–570
    patient presentation and diagnosis
        patient history, **II**:636–637
        physical examination, **II**:637
        preoperative assessment, **II**:637
        preoperative counseling and education, **II**:637–638

bariatic surgery *(Continued)*
    patient selection
        body contouring, **II**:638, 638t
        body mass index (BMI), **II**:638–639
        intraoperative procedures, **II**:638–639, 638t
        patient safety, **II**:638–639, 638t
        psychological considerations, **II**:638
    secondary procedures, **II**:653
    staging and combination procedures, **II**:653
    surgical technique
        abdominal contouring, **II**:639–643
        arms, **II**:652
        breast, **II**:652
        lower bodylift (LBL)/buttock contouring, **II**:644–645
        male chest, **II**:652
        trunk, **II**:652
        upper extremities, **II**:652
        vertical thigh-lift, **II**:645–652
    total parenchymal reshaping mastopexy
        surgical markings, **V**:566
        surgical technique and treatment, **V**:566–567, 568f
    vertical thigh-lift
        complications, **II**:652
        major weight loss (MWL) patient, **II**:648b
        markings, **II**:649–652, 650f
        operative technique, **II**:651f–652f, 652
        patient evaluation, **II**:645–648
        patient selection, **II**:648–649
        postoperative care and follow-up, **II**:652
Baronio, Giuseppe, **I**:20
Barr body, **I**:181
bar surfactants
    characteristics, **II**:16
    combination bars, **II**:16
    superfatted soaps, **II**:16
    synthetic detergent bars, **II**:16
    transparent soaps, **II**:16
Bartonella henselae, **III**:891
basal cell carcinoma
    characteristics, **I**:737, 737f, **III**:117–118, 118f, **VI**:317, 317f
    dermoscopic analysis, **I**:709, 709f
    histological classification, **I**:738b
    surgical margins, **I**:717
    tumor colors, **I**:709
basiliximab, **I**:821t
Baumann skin-typing system (BSTS), **II**:14–15, 14t, 19t
Baumeister lymphatic vessel reconstruction technique, **IV**:95–96, 96f
Bayh-Dole Act (1980), **I**:847
Bayne and Klug classification of radial longitudinal deficiency, **VI**:558, 558t, 559f
Bayne classification of ulnar longitudinal deficiency, **VI**:567, 568f, 568t
Bean syndrome, **VI**:668t
Beare–Stevenson syndrome, **I**:197, 197f, 197t, **III**:749–750, 750t
Beautical, **II**:48t
    See also soft-tissue fillers
beauty doctors, **I**:26–27, 28f
Beautygel, **II**:47t

Becker's melanosis/Becker's pigmented hairy nevus, **I**:725
Beckwith–Wiedemann syndrome, **III**:807t
bed sores, **I**:279
bell flap, **V**:508, 508f, 508t
Bell, Sir Charles, –**VI**:2
belt lipectomy, **II**:568–598
    anatomical considerations, **II**:568–569, 569f
    complications
        deep vein thrombosis (DVT), **II**:593–594
        dehiscence, **II**:591
        general discussion, **II**:589–595
        infections, **II**:592
        psychological difficulties, **II**:594–595
        pulmonary embolisms, **II**:593–594
        seromas, **II**:590
        tissue necrosis, **II**:592–593, 595f
        wound separation, **II**:590–591
    disease process
        massive weight loss patients, **II**:569, 570f
        normal weight patients group, **II**:570, 572f–573f
        20–30 pounds overweight group, **II**:569, 571f
    general discussion, **II**:568
    major weight loss (MWL) patient, **II**:644b
    markings, **II**:645, 646f–647f, 649f
    operative technique, **II**:645, 647f–649f
    outcome assessments
        characteristics, **II**:588–595
        group I patients, **II**:589f–590f
        group II patients, **II**:591f–592f
        group III patients, **II**:593f–594f
    patient evaluation, **II**:644–645
    patient presentation and diagnosis
        back roll presentations, **II**:571, 578f
        body mass index (BMI), **II**:570, 574f
        buttocks variations, **II**:577f
        commonalities, **II**:570–571
        fat deposition pattern, **II**:570, 574f–575f
        hanging panniculi, **II**:576f
        skin/fat envelope, **II**:570, 574f–575f
    patient selection, **II**:645
        belt lipectomy/central bodylift, **II**:572–574, 574b
        general discussion, **II**:571–580
        preoperative assessment, **II**:577–580
        selection criteria, **II**:574–576, 577b
    postoperative care and follow-up, **II**:588, 588b, 645
    secondary procedures, **II**:595
    surgical technique and treatment
        circumferential excisional procedures, **II**:580–585, 580f–582f
        excisional tension, **II**:580–585, 580f–582f
        markings
            horizontal mons pubis marking, **II**:581–582, 583f
            inferior back marking, **II**:584, 584f
            lateral mons to anterior superior iliac spine (ASIS) marking, **II**:582, 583f
            posterior vertical midline marking, **II**:583–584, 584f
            superior back marking, **II**:584–585, 584f
            superior horizontal abdominal marking, **II**:582–583, 583f
            surgical guidelines, **II**:580–585

belt lipectomy *(Continued)*
        vertical alignment marking, **II**:585
        vertical midline marking, **II**:581
    surgical procedures
        anesthesia, **II**:585–588
        dissection techniques, **II**:587f
        goals, **II**:580, 580b
        markings, **II**:580–585, 583f–584f
        positioning, **II**:587f
        positioning sequence, **II**:585
        suturing techniques, **II**:585–588, 586f
    upper bodylift considerations, **II**:595, 596f–597f
    zones of adherence, **II**:568–569, 569f
Benelli mastopexy technique
    basic procedure, **V**:127–132
    surgical technique
        areola fixation, **V**:131f
        basic procedure, **V**:128–132
        dissection techniques, **V**:128f
        flap attachment, **V**:129f–130f
        flap types, **V**:129f
        gland plication invagination, **V**:131f
        markings, **V**:128f
        round block suture, **V**:131f
        U stitches, **V**:131f
benign cutaneous and soft-tissue tumors
    benign appendage-origin tumors
        apocrine cystadenoma, **I**:722–723, 723f
        chondroid syringoma, **I**:723, 723f
        nevus sebaceous, **I**:721, 721f
        pilomatricoma, **I**:721–722, 721f
        steatocystoma multiplex, **I**:723, 724f
        syringoma, **I**:722, **III**:117, 117f
        trichilemmal cyst, **I**:722, 722f
    benign epithelial-origin tumors
        dermoid cyst, **I**:720, 721f
        epidermal nevus, **I**:718, 718f
        epidermoid cyst, **I**:719, 720f
        keratoacanthoma, **I**:719, 719f, **VI**:315–316, 316f
        milia, **I**:719–720
        seborrheic keratosis, **I**:719, 719f, **VI**:316
    benign mesenchymal-origin tumors
        accessory auricles, **I**:732–733, 733f
        acrochordon, **I**:730, 730f
        arteriovenous fistula and arteriovenous malformation (AVM), **I**:735, 736f
        capillary malformation
            hemangioma simplex, **I**:734, 734f–735f
            strawberry hemangioma, **I**:734–735, 735f
        cavernous hemangioma, **I**:735, 735f
        dermatofibroma, **I**:729, 729f, **VI**:316, 316f
        fibroma pendulum, **I**:730, 730f
        glomus tumors, **I**:734
        granulomas, **I**:733–734, 733f–734f
        hypertrophic scars, **I**:730, 731f
        juvenile xanthogranuloma, **I**:729–730, 729f–730f
        keloid scars, **I**:730, 730f
        leiomyoma, **I**:731–732
        lipoma, **I**:731, 731f–733f
        lymphatic malformation, **I**:736
        mucous cyst of the oral mucosa, **I**:736, 736f
        osteochondrogenic tumors, **I**:732, 733f
        rhabdomyoma, **I**:732
        soft fibroma, **I**:730

*Note: **Boldface** roman numerals indicate volume. Page numbers followed by f refer to figures; page numbers followed by t refer to tables; page numbers followed by b refer to boxes.*

benign cutaneous and soft-tissue tumors
    (Continued)
    venous malformation, I:735, 735f
    xanthoma, I:729, 729f
benign neural crest-origin tumors
    Becker's melanosis, I:725
    blue nevus, I:727
    Mongolian spot, I:726–727, 728f
    neurofibroma, I:728, 728f, VI:320, 320f
    neuromas, I:727
    nevus of Ito, I:726, 727f
    nevus of Ota, I:725–726, 726f
    nevus spilus, I:725, 726f
    pigment cell nevus
        acquired pigment cell nevus, I:724, 724f
        characteristics, I:723–725
        congenital pigment cell nevus, I:724,
            725f
        dysplastic nevus, I:724, III:113–114, 114f
        juvenile melanoma, I:724–725, 726f
        lentigo simplex, I:723–724, 724f
    schwannoma, I:727, 728f, VI:320, 320f
benign masseteric hypertrophy (BMH), III:17
benign pigmented nevus, VI:315, 315f
Bennett's fracture, VI:157, 157f
benzodiazepine, IV:427
benzopyrene, III:398–399
Bernard-Burow cheek advancement,
    III:265–268
Bernoulli's principle, II:452–453
β-catenin signaling, I:428–429
beta-blockers, II:21t
beta hydroxy acid (BHA), II:19
biceps femoris muscle, IV:15t–16t, 18f, 19t,
    20f–22f, 35f
biceps femoris muscle flap, IV:139–140
Bichat's fat pad, II:270–272, 271f–272f
Bier block, VI:97
biglycan (BGN), I:432, 432t
bilateral cleft lip, III:550–568
    bilateral variation modifications
        asymmetrical bilateral cleft lip, III:560–
            562, 563f–564f
        bilateral complete cleft lip and intact
            secondary palate, III:558–559, 561f
        bilateral incomplete cleft lip, III:559–560,
            562f
        binderoid bilateral complete cleft lip/
            palate, III:558, 560f
        late presentation, III:557–558
    challenges, III:550–551
    characteristics, III:508f
    multidimensional nasolabial features,
        III:551
    orthodontic treatment
        distraction procedures, III:602–611,
            609f–611f
        growth considerations, III:611
        infants, III:596–597
        orthognathic surgery, III:602–611, 607f
        permanent dentition, III:602–611
        transitional dentition, III:597–602, 601f
    outcome assessments
        direct anthropometric measurements,
            III:565, 566f
        general discussion, III:563–568
        indirect anthropometric measurements
            photogrammetry, III:565–567
            stereophotogrammetry, III:567–568,
                567f

bilateral cleft lip (Continued)
        photographic documentation, III:563
        revision rates, III:564–565
    patient presentation, III:551–552, 552f
    preoperative dentofacial orthopedics,
        III:552–553, 553f
    research summary, III:568
    surgical principles, III:550–551
    surgical technique
        alveolar closure, III:555, 555f
        labial closure, III:555–556, 555f
        labial dissection, III:554, 554f
        lower lateral cartilage positioning, III:556,
            556f–557f
        markings, III:553–554, 554f
        nasal dissection, III:556, 556f–557f
        philtral dimple, III:556–557, 558f
        postoperative care and follow-up, III:557,
            559f
        timing considerations, III:553–557
bilateral facial paralysis, III:284
bilateral microtia, III:204
bilateral pedicle TRAM flap, V:393–410
    background and general characteristics,
        V:393–394
    circulatory zones, V:395f
    outcomes and complicatons, V:407–410
    patient selection, V:395–396
    postoperative care and follow-up, V:406
    secondary procedures, V:410
    surgical technique and treatment
        external and internal oblique
            components, V:404f
        fascial and muscle strips, V:400f, 403f
        fascial closure, V:405f
        inferomedial dissection, V:402f
        lateral muscle dissection, V:401f
        markings, V:397f, 400f
        medial dissection, V:402f
        medial suprafascial dissection, V:399f
        muscle and fascial pedicle control,
            V:402f
        pedicle arrangement, V:403f–404f
        pedicle length, V:403f
        preoperative assessment, V:396
        Prolene mesh, V:405f
        shaping guidelines, V:405–406, 406f–409f
        surgical procedures, V:396–405,
            397b–399b
        tunnel positions, V:398f
    vascular anatomy, V:394–395, 394f
bilateral sagittal split osteotomy, III:661–662
biliopancreatic diversion (BPD), II:636, 636t
bilobed flap, III:143–145, 144f–145f, 446f
bimaxillary protrusion, II:181–182
binderoid bilateral complete cleft lip/palate,
    III:558, 560f
Bio-Alcamid, II:48t
    See also soft-tissue fillers
Biobrane®, IV:412t–414t
biodegradable polymers, I:791–792
BioDigital Systems, I:866–867, 867f–868f
bioengineering
    bioengineered skin substitutes, I:793–795
    engineered skin replacements, I:289t, 290
    nerve repair and grafting, I:476
    skin grafts, I:337–338
biofilms, I:250
Bioformacryl, II:48t
    See also soft-tissue fillers

Bioinblue, II:48t
    See also soft-tissue fillers
Biologic, II:49t
    See also soft-tissue fillers
biological debridement, IV:366–367
biological wound dressings, IV:410–415,
    412t–414t
biologic brachytherapy, I:6
biologic fillers, II:45t, 46–47, 47t, 49t
biomaterial-based implants, I:786–797
    bioprosthetic mesh, I:795–796, 795b
    bovine fetal dermis, I:796
    bovine pericardium, I:796
    future trends, I:796–797
    human acellular dermal matrix (HADM),
        I:796
    porcine acellular dermal matrix (PADM),
        I:796
    small intestinal mucosa, I:796
biomaterial scaffolds
    stem cell delivery, I:233–234, 233f
    tissue repair, reconstruction, and
        regeneration, I:187–189, 189f
biomedical burden, I:212–213, 213f
Bioplastique, II:48t
    See also soft-tissue fillers
bioprosthetic mesh, I:795–796, 795b
biopsies
    core needle biopsy, IV:106, V:272–273,
        272f–273f
    epidermolysis bullosa, IV:520, 521f
    excisional biopsies, IV:106–107
    excisional biopsy, I:273
    fine-needle aspiration (FNA), IV:106, V:272
    hand tumors, VI:313
    image-guided core biopsy, V:271–272, 272f
    incisional biopsies, IV:107
    Jamshidi core needle bone biopsy, IV:358–
        360, 361f
    melanoma detection, I:764
    reoperative biopsies, IV:107–108
    sarcomas
        core needle biopsy, IV:106
        excisional biopsies, IV:106–107
        incisional biopsies, IV:107
        reoperative biopsies, IV:107–108
    scalp and forehead disorders, III:120
    stereotactic biopsy, V:271–272, 272f
    ultrasound guidance biopsy, V:271–272,
        272f–273f
bipedicle flap delay, I:513f
BIRADS (Breast Imaging Reporting and Data
    System) classification, V:268, 268t
bis(2-chloroethyl)nitrosourea (BCNU),
    I:779–781
bite wounds
    animal bites, VI:343
    characteristics, VI:343–344
    clenched-fist injuries, VI:343, 344f
    human bites, VI:343–344
B-K mole syndrome, I:747
bladder
    exstrophy and epispadias
        male genital reconstructive surgery,
            IV:301–303, 302f–303f
        surgical technique and treatment
            bladder exstrophy, III:912–913, 913f
            female epispadias repair, III:912–913,
                914f
    tissue engineering, I:394–395

bladder *(Continued)*
    urogenital defect reconstruction,
            III:906–924
        embryology, **III:**907–908
        epidemiology, **III:**908
        etiology, **III:**908
        outcomes and complicatons, **III:**916–921
        patient presentation and diagnosis,
            III:908–909
        patient selection, **III:**909
        postoperative care and follow-up, **III:**915
        secondary procedures, **III:**921
        surgical technique and treatment
            bladder exstrophy, **III:**912–913, 913f
            female epispadias repair, **III:**912–913,
                914f
Blair–Brown grafts, **I:**325–326
Blair, Vilray, **I:**23–24, 27, **VI:**xlv–xlvi
blastocyst, **III:**504–505
bleach, **IV:**461–463
bleomycin, **I:**309–310, 692–693
blepharitis, **IV:**521
blepharoplasty, **II:**108–137
    Asian blepharoplasty
        anatomical considerations, **II:**164–165,
                165f–166f
        eyelid characteristics, **II:**164
        outcomes and complicatons, **II:**170–172
        postoperative care and follow-up, **II:**170
        preoperative assessment, **II:**166–167,
                166f–167f
        surgical technique and treatment
            incisional methods, **II:**168, 169f
            lateral canthoplasty, **II:**170, 171f–172f
            medial epicanthoplasty, **II:**169,
                170f–171f
            nonincisional methods, **II:**167–168,
                167f–168f
            partial incisional methods, **II:**168, 168f
            subclinical ptosis repair, **II:**169
    complications, **II:**135–136
        impacts, **II:**138–139
        major complications, **II:**140t
        minor complications, **II:**139t
        pre-existing conditions, **II:**141t
    corneal protection, **II:**140, 142f
    facelift techniques, **II:**203
    goals, **II:**108, 109b
    patient presentation and diagnosis
        evaluation examinations, **II:**116, 117f
        ocular examination
            external examination, **II:**118, 119f
            extraocular muscles, **II:**120
            globe, **II:**120
            malar eminence, **II:**119f, 120
            orbits, **II:**120
            pupils, **II:**120
            tear film, **II:**119f, 120–121
            tear troughs, **II:**120, 120f
            visual acuity, **II:**118, 119f
        photographic documentation, **II:**121,
                121b
        physical examination
            medical and ophthalmic history,
                II:116–121, 117b
            ocular examination, **II:**118–121
        unintentional eye appearance deception,
                II:121

blepharoplasty *(Continued)*
    patient selection
        anatomic-directed therapy
            eyelid ptosis/retraction, **II:**121–122
            globe position, **II:**122
            lower eyelid tonicity, **II:**121
            malar prominence, **II:**122
            optimal brow positioning, **II:**122, 123f
            tear trough deformities, **II:**122, 123f
            upper eyelid position, **II:**121
        preoperative assessment, **II:**121, 121b
    periorbital anatomy
        blood supply, **II:**112, 114f
        eyelids, **II:**111, 111f
        facial nerve, **II:**112–115, 115f
        forehead, **II:**110–111, 110f–111f
        general discussion, **II:**108–115
        lateral retinaculum, **II:**109, 109f–110f
        lower eyelid area, **II:**112
        medial orbital vault, **II:**110, 110f
        orbital anatomy, **II:**108–109, 109f
        retaining ligaments, **II:**112, 114f
        sensory nerves, **II:**112–115, 114f
        septal extension, **II:**112, 114f
        temporal region, **II:**110–111, 110f
        trigeminal nerve, **II:**112–115
        upper eyelid area, **II:**111–112, 113f
    postoperative care and follow-up,
                II:134–135
    secondary blepharoplasty, **II:**138–162
        corneal protection, **II:**140, 142f
        eyelid zones, **II:**140, 141f
        lower eyelid area
            anatomical analysis, **II:**148–151, 148f,
                151f
            canthoplasty techniques, **II:**151–160,
                155f–156f, 155t
            chemosis, **II:**162, 162f
            complications, **II:**160–162
            dermal orbicular pennant lateral
                canthoplasty (DOPLC), **II:**156,
                158f–159f
            distraction test, **II:**150, 153f
            ectropion, **II:**150–151, 154f
            excessive fat resection, **II:**160–162, 161f
            eyelid malposition, **II:**148–151, 152f
            inadequate fat resection, **II:**160–162, 161f
            inferior retinacular lateral
                canthoplasty/canthopexy (IRLC),
                II:156–157, 160f
            lateral bone-to-canthus relationship,
                II:149–150, 152f
            lower lid eversion, **II:**150–151, 154f
            medial canthus-to-lateral canthus
                relationship, **II:**150, 153f
            midface elevation and fixation, **II:**157,
                161f
            midlamellar cicatricial retraction,
                II:150f
            patient evaluation, **II:**148–151, 149t
            persistent malar bags, **II:**161f, 162
            snap test, **II:**150, 153f
            surgical procedures, **II:**151–160, 155t
            tarsal strip lateral canthoplasty,
                II:155–156, 156f–157f
        upper eyelid area
            Fasanella–Servat operation, **II:**146f
            Herring's law, **II:**145, 147f

blepharoplasty *(Continued)*
        patient evaluation, **II:**142–145, 142t,
                143f–144f
            ptosis, **II:**143–145, 144f–146f
            retraction, **II:**145, 147f
    special cases
        male blepharoplasty, **II:**137
        people of color, **II:**137
    subperiosteal facelift
        lower eyelid area, **II:**270–273, 270f
        upper eyelid area, **II:**268–270, 269f
    surgical technique and treatment
        aesthetic enhancement, **II:**123
        blepharoptosis
            basic principles, **II:**124–127
            surgical technique, **II:**126–127, 127f
        canthopexy, **II:**131–133, 133f–134f
        lower eyelid surgery
            basic principles, **II:**127–131
            burn wound treatment, **IV:**486–488,
                488f
            orbicularis suspension, **II:**130–131
            orbital fat excision, **II:**128–130
            transconjunctival blepharoplasty, **II:**128,
                129f–131f
            transcutaneous blepharoplasty, **II:**128
        midfacelift, **II:**132–133, 135f–136f
        upper eyelid surgery
            anchor/invagination blepharoplasty,
                II:124, 126f
            burn wound treatment, **IV:**486, 487f
            general discussion, **II:**123–124
            orbital fat excision, **II:**124, 126f
            simple skin blepharoplasty, **II:**124, 125f
    youthful and beautiful eyes characteristics,
                II:115–116, 115f
blindness, **III:**56, 74
Blix curve, **VI:**28f
blog defamation law, **I:**98–99
blood group antigens, **I:**816
blood stem cells, **I:**261–264, 261f
blood vessels
    skin grafts, **I:**321
    tissue engineering, **I:**392
    tissue-specific stem cells, **I:**230, 231f, 232
blue nevus, **I:**727, 744f, 745
blue-ocean strategy, **I:**66
blue rubber bleb syndrome (BRBS), **I:**695,
                VI:668t, 682–684
B lymphocytes, **I:**817
Bockenheimer lesions, **I:**695, **VI:**668, 668t
body contouring
    abdominal contouring
        giant pannus, **II:**640–643, 643f–644f
        hidden penis, **II:**640, 643f
        major weight loss (MWL) patient, **II:**639b
        mons correction, **II:**640, 641f–642f
        operative planning and technique,
                II:639–640
        patient evaluation, **II:**639
        surgical variations, **II:**640–643, 640f–641f
    centers of excellence, **II:**653
    major weight loss (MWL) patient,
                V:558–581
    arms
        demand increases, **V:**558–564
        outcomes and complicatons, **V:**563–564
        pathophysiology, **V:**558–559

*Note: **Boldface** roman numerals indicate volume. Page numbers followed by f refer to figures; page numbers followed by t refer to tables; page numbers followed by b refer to boxes.*

body contouring (Continued)
    patient presentation and diagnosis,
      V:559–564
    patient selection, V:559–560
    Pittsburgh Rating Scale, V:559–560, 559t
    postoperative care and follow-up,
      V:562–563
    surgical technique and treatment,
      V:560–562, 561f–563f, 562b
  back
    back rolls, V:570–573
    outcomes and complicatons, V:573
    pathophysiology, V:570–571
    patient presentation and diagnosis,
      V:571
    patient selection, V:571–572
    postoperative care and follow-up, V:573
    surgical planning, V:571–572
    surgical technique and treatment,
      V:572, 573f
    surgical tips, V:572b
    transverse excisional upper bodylift,
      V:570f, 572
  gynecomastia/male chest contouring
    excision of gynecomastia with nipple
      repositioning, V:575–579, 578f–580f
    outcomes and complicatons, V:579
    pathophysiology, V:573–574
    patient presentation and diagnosis,
      V:574
    patient selection, V:574–575, 575t
    postoperative care and follow-up,
      V:578
    pseudogynecomastia, V:575t, 576f–577f
    surgical markings, V:575–576, 576f–577f
    surgical technique and treatment,
      V:576–578, 578f–580f
    surgical tips, V:578b
  mastopexy
    breast reshaping, V:564–570
    dermal suspension, V:566–570, 568f
    outcomes and complicatons, V:567–570
    pathophysiology, V:564, 564b
    patient presentation and diagnosis,
      V:564–565
    patient selection, V:565–566
    postoperative care and follow-up,
      V:567
    surgical goals, V:565b
    surgical planning, V:565–566, 566t,
      569f–570f
    surgical tips, V:567b
    total parenchymal reshaping
      mastopexy, V:566–570
  secondary procedures, V:579
  total parenchymal reshaping mastopexy
    surgical markings, V:566
    surgical technique and treatment,
      V:566–567, 568f
  patient safety, II:638–639, 638t
  psychological considerations, II:638
body dysmorphic disorder (BDD), I:50–51,
  50b, II:7–8, 447–448
body image
  definition, I:30–31
  developmental stages
    adolescence, I:31
    early childhood, I:31
    older adults, I:31
    school-age children, I:31

body image (Continued)
  emotional response and behavior, I:31
  plastic surgery effects, I:31–32
body mass index (BMI)
  bariatric surgery, IV:282
  major weight loss (MWL) patient, II:570,
    574f
  obesity, II:634–635, 635t, 638–639
  upper limb contouring, II:617
body-powered prostheses, VI:870–871
bone
  acquired cranial and facial bone
    deformities, III:226–242
    access incisions
      coronal incisions, III:226–227, 227f
      intraoral incisions, III:227
      lower eyelid incisions, III:227
    background and general characteristics,
      III:226
    bone grafts
      donor site considerations, III:227,
        228f–229f
      soft-tissue cover, III:227
    complications, III:242
    postoperative care and follow-up,
      III:240–242
    prognosis and outcomes, III:242
    secondary procedures, III:242
    surgical technique and treatment
      chin implants, III:240, 240f–241f
      cranium, III:228, 230f–231f
      irradiated orbit, III:235–238
      mandibular fractures, III:238–240, 239f
      mandibular reconstruction, III:240
      maxillary buttresses, III:236–238
      maxillary reconstructiion, III:238–240,
        238f
      nasoethmoid area, III:232, 234f
      nose, III:228–229, 231f–233f
      orbitozygomatic region, III:232–234,
        235f–236f
      posttraumatic enophthalmos, III:234–
        235, 237f
  allografts, I:830, IV:174–175, 180–181, 180f
  alveolar clefts, III:584–594
    anatomical characteristics, III:584–585,
      585f
    background information, III:584
    complications, III:592–594
    dental development, III:585
    goals, III:584, 585t
    patient presentation and diagnosis
      alveolar distraction, III:587–588,
        587f–588f
      bone morphogenetic proteins (BMPs),
        III:586
      gingivoperiosteoplasty (GPP), III:585,
        586f
      late bone grafts, III:587
      primary bone grafts, III:585
      secondary bone grafts, III:585–586, 587f
    prognosis and outcomes
      bone morphogenetic proteins (BMPs),
        III:593
      gingivoperiosteoplasty (GPP),
        III:592–593
      graft site augmentation, III:594
      late bone grafts, III:593
      primary bone grafts, III:593
      secondary bone grafts, III:593

bone (Continued)
  surgical technique
    gingivoperiosteoplasty (GPP), III:588,
      589f
    horizontal alveolar transport
      distraction, III:591–592, 591f–592f
    primary bone grafts, III:588–589
    secondary bone grafts, III:589–591,
      590f–591f
    vertical alveolar transport distraction,
      III:592, 592f
  Asian facial bone surgery
    beauty ideals, II:177
    facial contouring surgery
      malar reduction surgery, II:180–181,
        180f
      mandible angle ostectomy, II:179,
        179f–180f
      narrowing genioplasty, II:181, 181f
    historical background
      anterior segmental ostectomy, II:178
      malar reduction, II:177–178
      mandible angle reduction, II:178
      orthognathic surgery, II:178
    malar reduction surgery
      bicoronal approach, II:181
      intraoral infracture technique with
        incomplete osteotomy, II:181
      intraoral L-shaped ostectomy, II:181
      surgical technique, II:180–181, 180f
    orthognathic surgery
      bimaxillary protrusion, II:181–182
      jaw rotation, II:181, 182f–183f
    outcomes and complicatons
      mandible angle reduction, II:182
      zygoma reduction, II:182
    patient presentation and diagnosis
      chin, II:178–179
      dentoalveolar protrusion, II:179
      facial profiles, II:179
      mandible angle, II:178
      zygoma, II:178
    surgical technique and treatment
      anterior segmental ostectomy,
        II:181–182
      facial contouring, II:179–181
      orthognathic surgery, II:181–182
  autografts, I:829–830
  bone homeostasis and turnover
    basic principles, I:432–438
    bone regeneration
      angiogenesis, I:443t–444t
      bone morphogenetic proteins (BMPs),
        I:434–436, 435t, 443t–444t
      fibroblast growth factor (FGF), I:435t,
        437–438, 441–442, 443t–444t
      mesenchymal stem cells (MSCs),
        I:425–434, 434f
      molecular mechanisms, I:434–438,
        435t
      platelet-derived growth factor (PDGF),
        I:435t, 438, 443t–444t
      transforming growth factor-β (TGF-β)
        superfamily, I:435t, 436–437,
        443t–444t
      vascular endothelial growth factor
        (VEGF), I:435t, 438, 443t–444t
    mechanotransduction, I:433
    Wolff's law, I:433
  burn reconstruction, IV:446, 450f

bone (Continued)
  cellular composition
    extracellular matrix (ECM), **I:**431–432, 432t
    osteoblasts
      characteristics and functional role, **I:**427t, 428
      major signaling pathways, **I:**428–429
      transcriptional regulation, **I:**429
    osteoclasts
      characteristics and functional role, **I:**427t, 430–431
      differentiation mechanisms, **I:**431
    osteocytes
      characteristics, **I:**427t, 429
      functional role, **I:**427t, 429–430
      histology, **I:**429
      mechanotransduction, **I:**433
  chemical composition
    inorganic phase, **I:**427
    organic phase, **I:**427
  giant cell tumors of the bone, **VI:**329, 329f
  microanatomy
    cortical versus cancellous bone, **I:**425–426, 426f
    formation processes, **I:**425–432
    haversian system, **I:**426, 426f
    osteon, **I:**426, 426f
  osteosarcoma, **I:**741, 741f, **VI:**329, 655, 656f
  repair and grafting, **I:**425–463
  skeletal reconstruction, **IV:**174–188
    allogeneic bone grafts
      advantages, **I:**459–460
      allograft bone incorporation, **I:**460
      bone graft formulations, **I:**460
      disease transmission risk, **I:**459
      immunogenicity, **I:**460
      processing and preservation techniques, **I:**459
    bone grafts, **I:**425–463
      acquired cranial and facial bone deformities, **III:**227, 228f–229f
      age factors, **I:**444
      allogeneic bone grafts, **I:**459–460
      allografts, **IV:**174–175
      back soft-tissue reconstruction, **IV:**271
      blood supply, **I:**441–442, 442f
      bone graft healing and graft survival, **I:**448–449
      bone morphogenetic proteins (BMPs), **IV:**174–175, 186–187
      bone remodeling, **I:**444–448
      bone substitutes, **I:**460
      bone transfers, **I:**448
      calvarium harvests, **I:**454–455, 454f
      constriction band syndrome, **VI:**642
      cortical versus cancellous bone grafts, **I:**449
      craniofacial microsomia (CFM), **III:**781–782, 783f
      donor site considerations, **III:**227, 228f–229f
      fibula harvests, **I:**452
      fracture fixation, **I:**442
      fracture healing, **I:**438–444
      greater trochanter harvests, **I:**452
      harvesting methods, **I:**449–455
      ilium harvests, **I:**449–452, 450f–451f

bone (Continued)
      Le Fort III osteotomy–bipartition correction technique, **III:**695
      olecranon harvests, **I:**452
      orbital fractures, **III:**55
      primary bone repair, **I:**439, 439f–440f
      rib harvests, **I:**452–454, 453f
      secondary (callus) bone repair, **I:**439–441, 439f, 441f
      soft-tissue cover, **III:**227
      surgical technique and treatment, **IV:**176–177
      tibia harvests, **I:**452, 452f
      vascularized bone flaps, **IV:**175, 175f
      xenogeneic bone grafts, **I:**460
    bone remodeling
      age factors, **I:**448
      blood supply, **I:**448
      distraction osteogenesis, **I:**446–447, 447f
      influencing factors, **I:**447–448
      ossoeintegration, **I:**445
      osteoconduction, **I:**445
      osteoinduction, **I:**444–445
      patient factors, **I:**448
      radiation therapy (RT), **I:**448
    bone transfers
      allogeneic bone grafts, **I:**459–460
      basic principles, **I:**459
      bone graft healing and graft survival, **I:**448–449
      bone substitutes, **I:**460
      cement pastes, **I:**460–462
      clinical considerations, **I:**449
      cortical versus cancellous bone grafts, **I:**449
      fibula harvests, **I:**452
      greater trochanter harvests, **I:**452
      harvesting methods, **I:**449–455
      ilium harvests, **I:**449–452, 450f–451f
      indicators, **I:**448
      olecranon harvests, **I:**452
      prefabricated polymers, **I:**462
      rib harvests, **I:**452–454, 453f
      tibia harvests, **I:**452, 452f
      vascularized bone flaps, **I:**455–459
      xenogeneic bone grafts, **I:**460
    cement pastes
      BoneSource, **I:**461
      calcium phosphate (CaP), **I:**460–461
      Norian SRS/CRS, **I:**461
      osteoactive materials, **I:**461–462
    distraction osteogenesis
      basic principles, **I:**446–447
      histology, **I:**446–447, 447f
    facial injuries, **III:**49–88
      causal factors, **III:**49
      initial assessment, **III:**49–51
    foot reconstruction, **IV:**196
    lower extremity reconstructive surgery, **IV:**83, 83f
    patient presentation and diagnosis, **IV:**175–176
    postoperative care and follow-up
      adjunct therapy, **IV:**186–187
      postoperative aesthetic conditions, **IV:**187–188
      postoperative monitoring, **IV:**186

bone (Continued)
    prefabricated polymers
      Medpor, **I:**462
      methylmethacrylate, **I:**462
    research summary, **IV:**188
    sarcoma-related reconstruction, **IV:**111–112, 111f
    skeletal defects, **IV:**174
    surgical technique and treatment
      allograft reconstruction, **IV:**180–181, 180f
      bone grafts, **IV:**176–177
      distraction osteogenesis, **IV:**179–180, 179f
      Ilizarov technique, **IV:**179–180, 179f
      periosteal and osteoperiosteal grafts, **IV:**178–179
      reconstruction methods, **IV:**176
      upper extremities, **IV:**181–185
      vascularized bone transfer, **IV:**177–178, 177f–178f
      vascularized epiphyseal reconstruction, **IV:**185–186, 186f–187f
    vascularized bone flaps
      advantages, **I:**455–459
      vacularized calvarium, **I:**457–459, 458f
      vacularized fibula, **I:**455, 457f
      vascularized iliac transfer, **I:**455, 456f
      vascularized rib, **I:**456–457
      vascularized scapula, **I:**455–456, 458f
    stiff hand
      extension contracture, **VI:**451–452, 451f
      flexion contracture, **VI:**450
    tissue expansion effects, **I:**623–624
Bone Anchored Hearing Aide (BAHA), **I:**799–800, 800f
bone distraction, **I:**6–7
bone marrow-derived mesenchymal stem cells (BMSC)
  clinical correlates, **I:**228
  current research and applications, **I:**224–226
  definitions, **I:**223–224
  gene therapy, **I:**190
  in vitro tissue harvest and differentiation protocols, **I:**226
  in vivo models, **I:**226–228
  tendon substitutes/engineered tendons, **I:**352–353
  wound healing, **I:**262, 262f
bone morphogenetic proteins (BMPs)
  alveolar clefts, **III:**586, 593
  bone grafts, **IV:**174–175, 186–187
  bone homeostasis and turnover
    bone regeneration, **I:**434–436, 435t, 443t–444t
    functional role, **I:**435–436
  bone tissue engineering, **I:**393
  craniofacial development
    lateral plate patterning, **III:**505, 506f
    neural crest generation, **III:**506–508, 507f
  current research and applications, **I:**225f
  gene regulation, **I:**180–181
  hand plate development, **VI:**530
  osteoblasts, **I:**428
  potential applications, **I:**213–214
  skin wound healing, **I:**274

*Note: **Boldface** roman numerals indicate volume. Page numbers followed by f refer to figures; page numbers followed by t refer to tables; page numbers followed by b refer to boxes.*

bone regeneration
　　bone marrow-derived mesenchymal stem
　　　　cells (BMSC), I:227
　　tissue-specific stem cells, I:230, 230f, 232
bone sarcoma
　　characteristics, IV:101–102
　　epidemiology, IV:103
　　imaging methods, IV:104, 104f
　　Muskuloskeletal Tumor Society staging
　　　　system, IV:105t
　　outcome assessments, IV:115–116
　　patient presentation and diagnosis,
　　　　IV:103–104, 104f
　　patient selection, IV:104
　　pediatric tumors, VI:655, 656f
　　preservation options
　　　　complex approaches, IV:112
　　　　general discussion, IV:110–112
　　　　neuromuscular units, IV:111
　　　　skeletal reconstruction, IV:111–112, 111f
　　　　vascular surgery, IV:112
　　recurrence management, IV:116–125
　　surgical resection techniques
　　　　amputation indicators, IV:110
　　　　biopsies
　　　　　　core needle biopsy, IV:106
　　　　　　excisional biopsies, IV:106–107
　　　　　　fine-needle aspiration (FNA), IV:106
　　　　　　incisional biopsies, IV:107
　　　　　　reoperative biopsies, IV:107–108
　　　　lymph node dissection, IV:110
　　　　nerve involvement, IV:109
　　　　osseous involvement, IV:109
　　　　primary osseous sarcomas, IV:109
　　　　specimen handling, IV:109
　　　　surgical revisions, IV:107–108, 108t
　　　　vascular involvement, IV:108
　　　　wound closure, IV:109
　　treatment strategies
　　　　chemotherapy, IV:106
　　　　radiation therapy (RT), IV:106
　　　　surgical goals, IV:104–105
　　　　surgical planning, IV:105
　　　　surgical treatment, IV:105–106
　　tumor growth and metastasis, IV:103
bone scans, VI:312
bone sialoprotein (BSP), I:428, 431–432, 432t
BoneSource, I:461
bone tissue engineering, I:392–393
borderline personality disorder, I:36
Borges, Albert F., I:316
Borrelia burgdorferi, III:794
Boston-type craniosynostosis, I:197t,
　　III:749–750
botulinum toxin (BTX), VI:495
botulinum toxin type-A (BoNT-A), II:30–43
　　background information, II:30
　　facial muscles, II:34f
　　migraine headaches, III:492–495, 494f
　　patient selection, II:33
　　pharmacology/pharmacokinetics
　　　　action mechanisms, II:31
　　　　adverse effects, II:32
　　　　BoNT-A commercial sources, II:31
　　　　contraindications, II:32
　　　　patient presentation and diagnosis,
　　　　　　II:31–32
　　　　recommended dosage, II:32–33
　　postoperative care and follow-up, II:42
　　potential adverse reactions, II:42

botulinum toxin type-A (BoNT-A) (Continued)
　　prognosis and outcomes, II:42
　　rejuvenation guidelines, II:30b
　　secondary procedures, II:42
　　treatment technique
　　　　brow elevation, II:37
　　　　crow's feet, II:34–37
　　　　depressor anguli oris, II:41
　　　　forehead, II:34
　　　　general discussion, II:33–42
　　　　glabella, II:33–34, 35f–36f
　　　　hyperhidrosis, II:42
　　　　lower eyelid area, II:34–37
　　　　mentalis, II:39f–40f, 41
　　　　nasolabial folds, II:37–38, 38f
　　　　neck, II:37, 38f
　　　　perioral lines, II:39–41, 39f–40f
　　　　surgical complication repair, II:41
botulinum toxin type-B (BoNT-B), II:31
Bouchard's nodes, VI:417–425
boutonnière deformity
　　characteristics, VI:223–224, 223f
　　preoperative assessment, VI:223–224
　　secondary reconstruction, VI:224, 224f
　　tenotomy, VI:224, 224f
Bouvier maneuver, VI:58–59, 764–765, 764f
bovine collagen See soft-tissue fillers
bovine fetal dermis, I:796
bovine pericardium, I:796
Bowen's disease, I:736–737
boxcar scars, II:69
Boyes superficialis transfer, VI:748t, 750–752,
　　752f
brachial plexus
　　adult brachial plexus injury
　　　　characteristics, VI:790t
　　　　electrodiagnostic studies, VI:797–798
　　　　etiology, VI:793
　　　　evaluation examinations, VI:794f–795f,
　　　　　　795–796, 796t
　　　　general discussion, VI:793
　　　　infraclavicular brachial plexus injury,
　　　　　　VI:802–803
　　　　level 1 injury
　　　　　　characteristics, VI:798–802
　　　　　　functioning free muscle transplantation
　　　　　　　　(FFMT), VI:801–802
　　　　　　nerve transfer, VI:799–800
　　　　　　pedicled muscle transfer, VI:800–801
　　　　　　reconstructive strategies, VI:800
　　　　level 2 injury, VI:802
　　　　level 3 injury, VI:802
　　　　level 4 injury, VI:802–803
　　　　motor examination, VI:794f–795f,
　　　　　　795–796, 796t
　　　　nerve transfer
　　　　　　basic procedure, VI:799–800
　　　　　　closed-target nerve transfer, VI:799
　　　　　　end-to-side neurorrhaphy nerve
　　　　　　　　transfer, VI:799–800
　　　　　　extraplexus nerve transfer, VI:799
　　　　　　functioning free muscle transplantation
　　　　　　　　(FFMT), VI:801–802
　　　　　　intraplexus nerve transfer, VI:799
　　　　　　pedicled muscle transfer, VI:800–801
　　　　　　proximal nerve transfer versus distal
　　　　　　　　nerve transfer, VI:799t
　　　　　　recommended induction exercises,
　　　　　　　　VI:800t
　　　　　　reconstructive strategies, VI:800

brachial plexus (Continued)
　　　　outcome assessments, VI:805
　　　　palliative reconstruction procedures,
　　　　　　VI:805
　　　　patient history, VI:793–794
　　　　postoperative care and rehabilitation,
　　　　　　VI:805
　　　　pre- and retroclavicular injury, VI:802
　　　　preoperative assessment and diagnosis,
　　　　　　VI:794–795
　　　　reconstructive strategies
　　　　　　elbows, VI:800, 801t
　　　　　　fingers, VI:800, 801t, 802f, 803t
　　　　　　shoulder, VI:800, 801t
　　　　research summary, VI:805, 815
　　　　sensory examination
　　　　　　basic procedure, VI:796
　　　　　　British Medical Research Council
　　　　　　　　(BMRC) Scale/Chuang
　　　　　　　　modification, VI:796t
　　　　　　Horner's syndrome, VI:796
　　　　　　plain X-ray and imaging studies,
　　　　　　　　VI:796
　　　　　　Tinel's sign, VI:796
　　　　surgical technique and treatment
　　　　　　characteristics, VI:798–805
　　　　　　Chuang's angle, VI:804–805, 804f
　　　　　　exploration techniques, VI:803–805,
　　　　　　　　804f
　　　　　　functioning free muscle transplantation
　　　　　　　　(FFMT), VI:801–802
　　　　　　infraclavicular brachial plexus injury,
　　　　　　　　VI:802–803
　　　　　　infraclavicular dissection, VI:804–805,
　　　　　　　　804f
　　　　　　level 1 injury, VI:798–802
　　　　　　level 2 injury, VI:802
　　　　　　level 3 injury, VI:802
　　　　　　level 4 injury, VI:802–803
　　　　　　pedicled muscle transfer, VI:800–801
　　　　　　pre- and retroclavicular injury, VI:802
　　　　　　supraclavicular dissection, VI:803–804,
　　　　　　　　804f
　　　　vascular injury, VI:798
　　anatomical characteristics, VI:92–94, 93f
　　disputed anatomy, VI:790, 791f
　　gross anatomy, VI:789, 791f
　　microanatomy, VI:790–791
brachial plexus injuries, VI:789–816
　　adult brachial plexus injury
　　　　British Medical Research Council
　　　　　　(BMRC) Scale, VI:795–796, 796t
　　　　characteristics, VI:790t
　　　　Chuang modification, VI:796t
　　　　electrodiagnostic studies, VI:797–798
　　　　etiology, VI:793
　　　　evaluation examinations, VI:794f–795f,
　　　　　　795–796, 796t
　　　　general discussion, VI:793
　　　　Horner's syndrome, VI:796
　　　　motor examination, VI:794f–795f,
　　　　　　795–796, 796t
　　　　outcome assessments, VI:805
　　　　palliative reconstruction procedures,
　　　　　　VI:805
　　　　patient history, VI:793–794
　　　　plain X-ray and imaging studies,
　　　　　　VI:796, 797f–798f
　　　　postoperative care and rehabilitation,
　　　　　　VI:805

brachial plexus (Continued)
　preoperative assessment and diagnosis, VI:794–795
　research summary, VI:805, 815
　sensory examination, VI:796, 796t
　surgical technique and treatment, VI:798–805
　Tinel's sign, VI:796
　vascular injury, VI:798
avulsion injuries, VI:792f–793f
classifications, VI:791t
degree of nerve injuriy, VI:793
general discussion, VI:789
infant obstetric brachial plexus palsy
　background information, VI:806–812
　clinical examination, VI:806–808, 808f–809f
　clinical presentation, VI:806, 807f
　imaging methods, VI:809f
　injury type incidence, VI:810t
　intraoperative findings, VI:810t
　nerve graft results, VI:811–812, 812f–813f
　outcome assessments, VI:811, 812t
　postoperative care and follow-up, VI:810–811, 811f
　preoperative preparations, VI:808
　reconstructive strategies, VI:810, 810t
　rupture–avulsion injuries, VI:810, 810t–811t
　rupture injuries, VI:810, 810t
　surgical technique and treatment, VI:808–809
　surgical timing, VI:808
level of injury, VI:791f, 791t, 792
obstetric brachial plexus palsy
　characteristics, VI:805–806, 805b
　infant obstetric brachial plexus palsy, VI:806–812
　injury type incidence, VI:810t
　intraoperative findings, VI:810t
　nerve graft results, VI:811–812, 812f–813f
　outcome assessments, VI:811, 812t
　postoperative care and follow-up, VI:810–811, 811f
　research summary, VI:815
　rupture–avulsion injuries, VI:810, 810t–811t
　rupture injuries, VI:810, 810t
　sequelae obstetric brachial plexus palsy, VI:812–815
pathophysiology, VI:793
pediatric brachial plexus injury
　characteristics, VI:790t, 805–806, 805b
　infant obstetric brachial plexus palsy, VI:806–812
　injury type incidence, VI:810t
　intraoperative findings, VI:810t
　nerve graft results, VI:811–812, 812f–813f
　outcome assessments, VI:811, 812t
　postoperative care and follow-up, VI:810–811, 811f
　research summary, VI:815
　rupture–avulsion injuries, VI:810, 810t–811t
　rupture injuries, VI:810, 810t

brachial plexus (Continued)
　sequelae obstetric brachial plexus palsy, VI:812–815
research summary, VI:815
rupture injuries, VI:792f
sequelae obstetric brachial plexus palsy
　characteristics, VI:812–815
　elbow deformity reconstruction, VI:815
　examination chart, VI:814t
　forearm and hand deformity reconstruction, VI:815
　shoulder deformity reconstruction, VI:813–815
microvascular thrombosis prevention, VI:245
nerve origins, VI:696f
obstetric brachial plexus palsy
　characteristics, VI:790t, 805, 805b
　infant obstetric brachial plexus palsy
　　background information, VI:806–812
　　clinical examination, VI:806–808, 808f–809f
　　clinical presentation, VI:806, 807f
　　imaging methods, VI:809f
　　injury type incidence, VI:810t
　　intraoperative findings, VI:810t
　　nerve graft results, VI:811–812, 812f–813f
　　outcome assessments, VI:811, 812t
　　postoperative care and follow-up, VI:810–811, 811f
　　preoperative preparations, VI:808
　　reconstructive strategies, VI:810, 810t
　　rupture–avulsion injuries, VI:810, 810t–811t
　　rupture injuries, VI:810, 810t
　　surgical technique and treatment, VI:808–809
　　surgical timing, VI:808
　injury type incidence, VI:810t
　intraoperative findings, VI:810t
　nerve graft results, VI:811–812, 812f–813f
　outcome assessments, VI:811, 812t
　postoperative care and follow-up, VI:810–811, 811f
　research summary, VI:815
　rupture–avulsion injuries, VI:810, 810t–811t
　rupture injuries, VI:810, 810t
　sequelae obstetric brachial plexus palsy
　　characteristics, VI:812–815
　　elbow deformity reconstruction, VI:815
　　examination chart, VI:814t
　　forearm and hand deformity reconstruction, VI:815
　　shoulder deformity reconstruction, VI:813–815
brachioplasty, II:617–633, V:558–581
causal factors, II:617, 618f–620f
complications, II:629–631, 629t, V:563–564
demand increases, II:617, V:558–564
pathophysiology, V:558–559
patient presentation and diagnosis, II:617–620, V:559–564
patient selection
　arm surface anatomy, II:624f
　laboratory work-up, II:623
　marking, II:624–626, 627f

brachioplasty (Continued)
　operative procedures, II:626–629, 627f–629f
　physical examination, II:620–624, 621f–622f
　Pittsburgh Rating Scale, V:559–560
　plan formulation, II:622–623
　preoperative assessment, II:623
　sagittal view of arm anatomy, II:625f
　surface anatomy, II:624, 624f–626f
　thromboembolic disease prophylaxis, II:623–624
Pittsburgh Rating Scale, V:559–560, 559t
postoperative care and follow-up, II:629, V:562–563
prognosis and outcomes, II:629–631, 630f–632f, V:563–564
secondary procedures, II:632–633, 632f
surgical technique and treatment, V:560–562, 561f–563f, 562b
brachycephaly, III:729, 730f, 730t
brachydactyly
　brachymesophalangy, VI:637f, 639–640
　brachymetacarpia, VI:638f, 640, 640f
　causal factors, VI:637
　clinical manifestations, VI:635–641, 636f–638f
　clinodactyly
　　characteristics, VI:630, 636, 638f, 640
　　outcomes and complicatons, VI:632
　　pathogenesis, VI:630
　　patient presentation and diagnosis, VI:630–631, 631f
　　patient selection, VI:631
　　postoperative care and follow-up, VI:632
　　radiographic imaging, VI:637f
　　secondary procedures, VI:632
　　surgical technique and treatment, VI:546t, 631–632, 631f, 640
　Kirner's deformity, VI:639f
　Mohr–Wriedt syndrome, VI:636, 638f, 646
　polydactyly
　　characteristics, VI:639f
　　classification systems, VI:535–537, 535f–536f
　symbrachydactyly
　　classification systems, VI:537, 537f–538f
　　patient presentation and diagnosis, VI:549–550, 550f, 609f, 640–641, 640f–641f, 645f
　　surgical technique and treatment, VI:546t
　syndactyly
　　characteristics, VI:635f, 639f
　　classification systems, VI:535–537, 535f, 537f, 605f
　　epidemiology, VI:604
　　outcomes and complicatons, VI:608–609, 609f
　　pathogenesis, VI:604
　　patient presentation and diagnosis, VI:564–565, 604, 606f
　　patient selection, VI:604–605
　　postoperative care and follow-up, VI:608
　　secondary procedures, VI:609
　　surgical technique and treatment
　　　basic procedure, VI:605–608, 605b, 608b
　　　complete and complex syndactyly, VI:608

Note: **Boldface** roman numerals indicate volume. Page numbers followed by f refer to figures; page numbers followed by t refer to tables; page numbers followed by b refer to boxes.

brachydactyly (Continued)
    fingertip separation, **VI:**608
    incomplete syndactyly, **VI:**608
    lateral soft tissue defects, **VI:**606–607,
        608f
    timing considerations, **VI:**546t
    web creation, **VI:**606, 607f
    treatment strategies, **VI:**637–639
    See also Apert syndrome
brachymesophalangy, **VI:**637f, 639–640
brachymetacarpia, **VI:**638f, 640, 640f
brachytherapy, **I:**656–657
Braden scale for predicting pressure sore risk,
    IV:362t–363t
bradycardia, **I:**145
bradykinin, **I:**268–269
brain-derived neutrophic factor (BDNF), **I:**232
Branca family, **I:**16–18
branchial cleft anomalies
    characteristics, **III:**885, 885f
    first branchial cleft anomaly
        disease process, **III:**886
        patient presentation and diagnosis,
            III:886, 886f
        surgical technique and treatment, **III:**886
    fourth branchial cleft anomaly, **III:**887
    second branchial cleft anomaly
        disease process, **III:**885, 885f
        patient presentation and diagnosis,
            III:885, 885f
        surgical technique and treatment,
            III:885–886, 886f
    third branchial cleft anomaly, **III:**886–887
Brand EE4T transfer, **VI:**766–767, 766f
Brand EF4T transfer, **VI:**767, 767f–768f
Brand–Moberg modification, **VI:**827–830,
    828f–829f
Brava bra, **I:**7, **V:**601, 601f
BRCA mutations, **V:**266–267, 453, 454f
breakeven analysis, **I:**73f
Breakthrough Series model, **I:**170
breast augmentation, **V:**13–38
    adolescent aesthetic surgery, **I:**45t, **II:**5f
    autologous fat grafts, **V:**591–595, 593f–595f
    background information, **V:**13
    botulinum toxin type-A (BoNT-A), **II:**41
    breast reconstruction considerations, **V:**380
    diagnostic imaging, **V:**270–271, 271f
    endoscopic approaches, **V:**81–96
        background and general characteristics
            general discussion, **V:**81–82
            illumination and imaging technology,
                V:82
            latissimus dorsi (LD) flap, **V:**82–83
            optical cavities, **V:**81–82
            support systems, **V:**82
        endoscopic augmentation mammaplasty
            breast anatomy, **V:**83
            outcomes and complicatons, **V:**87–88,
                88f
            patient presentation and diagnosis,
                V:83
            patient selection, **V:**83–84
            postoperative care and follow-up,
                V:87–88
            surgical technique and treatment,
                V:84–87, 84f–87f
    fat grafting, **I:**342–346, 346f–347f
    gender identity disorder surgery,
        IV:348–350

breast augmentation (Continued)
    iatrogenic disorders, **V:**97–118
        background information, **V:**97
        breast implants
            implant malposition, **V:**112–116
            saline implants, **V:**13–14, 110, 110f
            silicone gel implants, **I:**789–790, 790f,
                V:14–15, 102–109
            sponges, **V:**101–102, 102f
            steroid atrophy, **V:**110, 110f
        implant malposition
            double-bubble deformity, **V:**116, 116f
            inadequate muscle release, **V:**113, 114f
            plane of insertion, **V:**112–113, 113f
            submusculofascial plane, **V:**114–115,
                114f
            symmastia, **V:**115–116, 116f
            transaxillary dissection, **V:**115, 115f
        injection materials
            background information, **V:**97–101
            liquid silicone injections, **V:**98–100,
                99f–100f
            paraffin injections, **V:**97–98, 98f
            polyacrylamide hydrogel injections,
                V:100–101, 100f–101f
        post-pregnancy secondary ptosis, **V:**117,
            117f
        ptosis, **V:**116–117, 117f
        saline implants
            autoinflation, **V:**111–112, 112f
            capsular calcification, **V:**110, 110f
            deflation, **V:**110–111, 111f
            ripples and folds, **V:**111, 111f
        silicone gel implants
            capsular calcification, **V:**107–109,
                108f–109f
            capsular contracture, **V:**106–107,
                106f–107f
            characteristics, **I:**789–790, 790f
            closed capsulotomy, **V:**107, 107f–108f
            developmental background, **V:**14–15
            double-bubble deformity, **V:**116, 116f
            first generation implants, **V:**14–15, 103f
            fourth and fifth generation implants,
                V:15
            hematomas, **V:**104–105, 104f–105f
            historical background, **I:**789–790,
                V:102–109
            implant disruption, **V:**103–104, 103f
            implant malposition, **V:**112–113, 113f
            infections, **V:**105–106, 105f–106f
            second generation implants, **V:**14–15,
                104f
            third generation implants, **V:**14–15,
                104f
    infiltration, **I:**142–143, 143f
    informed consent, **V:**17–19
    mastopexy
        basic procedure, **V:**139–143
        operative technique, **V:**142–143
        preoperative/postoperative comparisons,
            V:143f
        surgical tips, **V:**142b
    measurement and analysis, **V:**16–17, 19f, 25f
    operative planning
        implant selection
            filling material, **V:**24–25
            implant shape, **V:**25–27, 28f–29f
            implant size determination, **V:**25, 25f
            implant surface texture, **V:**25, 26f–27f

breast augmentation (Continued)
    incision length and placement, **V:**19–20
    inframammary incision, **V:**19, 27–30
    periareolar incision, **V:**19, 30–31
    pocket position
        subfascial position, **V:**21f
        subpectoral position, **V:**22f–24f, 28f–29f
        surgical guidelines, **V:**20–27, 20f
    surgical technique and treatment
        inframammary incision, **V:**27–30
        periareolar incision, **V:**30–31
        preoperative markings, **V:**27–32
        surgical guidelines, **V:**27b, 30b
        transaxillary incision, **V:**31
        transumbilical incision, **V:**32
        transaxillary incision, **V:**19, 31
        transumbilical incision, **V:**19–20, 32
    patient presentation and diagnosis
        hard tissue asymmetry, **V:**17f–18f
        ideal breast structure, **V:**16f
        patient history and examination, **V:**15–16
        soft tissue asymmetry, **V:**18f
    patient safety, **I:**132
    patient selection, **V:**16–17
    perioperative complications
        delayed complications
            implant rupture and deflation, **V:**37, 79t
            periprosthetic capsular contracture,
                V:36–37
        hematomas, **V:**32–37, 79t
        medication and herbal supplement
            avoidance list, **V:**33t–35t
        Mondor's disease, **V:**35–36
        nipple sensitivity, **V:**32–37
        seromas, **V:**32–37, 79t
        wound infections, **V:**35, 79t
    postoperative care and follow-up, **V:**32
    psychological aspects, **I:**40–41
    revisionary surgery, **V:**39–80
        acellular dermal matrix (ADM)
            basic principles, **V:**68–69
            capsular contracture, **V:**52–53, 52f
            clinical signs, **V:**79t
            comparison studies, **V:**70t
            complications, **V:**78–79, 79t
            patient presentation and diagnosis,
                V:71
            patient selection, **V:**71, 72t
            preoperative/postoperative Baker
                classifications, **V:**79, 79t
            prognosis and outcomes, **V:**78–79
            surgical technique and treatment,
                V:71–78
        background and challenges, **V:**39–40
        biological responses, **V:**40
        body responses
            encapsulation processes, **V:**71
            published research, **V:**69–71
            regeneration processes, **V:**69
            resorption processes, **V:**69
        capsular contracture
            acellular dermal matrix (ADM),
                V:52–53, 52f, 336–340
            Baker classifications, **V:**36t, 46–53, 362,
                362t
            blood supply, **V:**49f
            capsulectomy, **V:**47, 48f–49f
            capsulotomies, **V:**47
            etiology, **V:**46t
            mastopexy, **V:**47, 48f

breast augmentation *(Continued)*
    neo subpectoral pocket conversion,
      V:50–52, 51f
    nipple-areola complex, **V:**49f
    subglandular to subpectoral
      conversion, **V:**50, 50f–51f
    surgical options, **V:**47t
  causal factors, **V:**67–68, 68b
  clinical signs, **V:**79t
  implant malposition
    characteristics, **V:**53, 53f–54f
    etiology, **V:**53–55, 54f
    treatment strategies, **V:**55–58, 55t,
      56f–57f
  outcomes and complicatons, **V:**65–66, 66t,
    78–79, 79t, 263–264
  patient presentation and diagnosis
    acellular dermal matrix (ADM), **V:**71
    classifications, **V:**41–42, 42f
    indicators, **V:**42–44
    patient history, **V:**40–44, 41t
    physical examination, **V:**40
  patient selection, **V:**42–44, 71, 72t
  postoperative care and follow-up, **V:**65,
    262–263
  preoperative/postoperative Baker
    classifications, **V:**79, 79t
  prognosis and outcomes, **V:**78–79
  published research, **V:**69–71
  secondary procedures, **V:**37
  surgical technique and treatment
    augmentation versus augmentation
      mastopexy, **V:**79t
    breast asymmetry, **V:**61–63, 62f–63f
    capsular contracture, **V:**46–53, 49f,
      77–78, 77f, 79t, 264
    implant failure, **V:**58–59
    implant malposition, **V:**53, 53f–54f, 79t
    implant pocket options, **V:**44–65, 44t,
      45f
    implant stabilization, **V:**75–76, 75f–76f
    lamellar separation, **V:**73–75, 73f
    lower pole coverage, **V:**73–75, 73f–76f
    placement indicators, **V:**71–78, 72f, 73b
    preoperative assessment, **V:**44–65
    rippling/implant edge palpability,
      V:59–61, 61f
    size changes, **V:**64–65
    soft tissue changes, **V:**63–64, 64f
    surgical tips, **V:**44b
    tissue thickeners, **V:**76–77
  tissue changes, **V:**68–69
  secondary procedures, **V:**37
  silicone chemistry, **V:**14
  surgical technique and treatment
    inframammary incision, **V:**27–30
    periareolar incision, **V:**30–31
    preoperative markings, **V:**27–32
    surgical guidelines, **V:**27b, 30b
    transaxillary incision, **V:**31
    transumbilical incision, **V:**32
breast cancer, **V:**266–295
  diagnosis
    BIRADS (Breast Imaging Reporting and
      Data System) classification, **V:**268,
      268t
    clinical breast examination, **V:**267–268
    general discussion, **V:**267–271

breast cancer *(Continued)*
  histologic methods
    characteristics, **V:**271–273
    core needle biopsy, **V:**272–273,
      272f–273f
    excisional biopsy, **V:**273
    fine-needle aspiration (FNA), **V:**272
    image-guided core biopsy, **V:**271–272,
      272f
    stereotactic biopsy, **V:**271–272, 272f
    ultrasound guidance biopsy, **V:**271–272,
      272f–273f
  imaging methods
    breast implants, **V:**270–271, 271f
    magnetic resonance imaging (MRI),
      V:268–270, 270f
    mammography, **V:**268, 269f
    ultrasonography, **V:**268, 269f
  epidemiology, **V:**266
  inflammatory breast cancer, **V:**275f
  locally advanced breast cancer, **V:**275f
  outcomes and complicatons, **V:**286–287,
    286f–287f
  pathogenesis, **V:**266–267
  patient selection, **V:**273–274, 274f
  postmastectomy breast reconstruction
    basic principles, **I:**640–647
    chest wall irradiated areas, **I:**645–647
    delayed reconstruction, **V:**291–292,
      291f–292f, 358, 359f
    expander device, **I:**642–643, **V:**292f
    immediate postmastectomy breast
      reconstruction
      acellular allogenic dermal matrix
        (ADM), **I:**644–645, 644f
      basic procedure, **V:**287–291
      breast implants, **V:**353
      deep inferior epigastric perforator
        (DIEP) flaps, **V:**288f
      expander-implant insertion, **V:**353–354,
        354f
      latissimus dorsi (LD) flap, **V:**288,
        289f–290f
      muscle coverage, **I:**643–645
      prosthesis insertion, **V:**356–358
      radiation therapy (RT), **V:**290
      second-stage surgery, **V:**356, 357f
      skin reducing mastectomy, **V:**354–356,
        355f
      submuscular position, **I:**643–644
      subpectoral (dual-plane) position, **I:**644
      transverse rectus abdominis
        myocutaneous (TRAM) flaps,
        V:288f
    prosthesis insertion
      basic procedure, **V:**356–358
      capsulectomy, **V:**357f
      contralateral adjustments, **V:**356–358
      inframammary fold reconstruction,
        V:357f
      large breast augmentation, **V:**358
      medium breast augmentation,
        V:357–358
      small breast augmentation, **V:**356–357
    secondary breast reconstruction, **I:**645,
      646f
    secondary procedures, **V:**292–294, 293f
    skin reducing mastectomy, **V:**354–356, 355f

breast cancer *(Continued)*
  radiation treatment
    breast conservation, **I:**665
    chemotherapy sequencing, **I:**668
    nodal draining area irradiation, **I:**665–666
    postmastectomy radiation (PMRT), **I:**665
    radiotherapy techniques, **I:**666–668,
      666f–667f
    research background, **I:**664–668
  secondary procedures, **V:**292–294, 293f
  surgical technique and treatment
    breast-conserving therapy (BCT)
      algorithmic approach, **V:**279f–280f
      basic principles, **V:**274–280
      oncoplastic surgery, **V:**277–280,
        278f–280f
      surgical technique, **V:**276–277,
        276f–277f
    mastectomies
      characteristics, **I:**202, 203f, **V:**280–286
      extended radical mastectomy, **V:**281f
      modified radical mastectomy, **V:**285,
        285f
      nipple-sparing mastectomy, **V:**282–284,
        284f–285f
      nodal evaluation, **V:**286, 286f
      prophylactic mastectomy, **V:**284
      skin-sparing mastectomy, **V:**282,
        283f–284f, 288f
      total mastectomy, **V:**281–282, 281f
    treatment and reconstruction, **I:**43
breast-conserving therapy (BCT), **V:**482–498
  basic principles, **V:**482–483
  breast cancer surgery
    algorithmic approach, **V:**279f–280f
    basic principles, **V:**274–280
    oncoplastic surgery, **V:**277–280, 278f–280f
    surgical technique, **V:**276–277, 276f–277f
  complications, **V:**495
  endoscopic approaches, **V:**82–83
  flap classification and vascular anatomy
    anterior intercostal artery perforator
      (AICAP) flap, **V:**308, 488
    dorsal intercostal artery perforator
      (DICAP) flap, **V:**488
    intercostal artery perforator (ICAP) flap,
      V:486f–488f, 487–488
    lateral intercostal artery perforator
      (LICAP) flap, **V:**487f–488f, 488
    lateral thoracodorsal flap (LTDF),
      V:306–308
    latissimus dorsi (LD) flap, **V:**306–308,
      309f, 311f, 485–489, 486f
    pedicled flaps, **V:**489, 492f
    serratus anterior artery perforator (SAAP)
      flap, **V:**486f–488f, 488–489
    superior epigastric artery perforator
      (SEAP) flap, **V:**308, 486f, 489
    thoracodorsal artery perforator (TDAP)
      flap, **V:**308, 486–487, 486f–488f
  flap design
    flap choice, **V:**489, 490f–492f
    markings, **V:**490f–492f, 492–493, 494f–495f
    preoperative perforator mapping,
      V:489–492, 490f–492f, 494f–495f
    surgical technique, **V:**490f–492f, 493,
      494f–495f
  general discussion, **V:**482

Note: **Boldface** *roman numerals indicate volume. Page numbers followed by f refer to figures; page numbers followed by t refer to tables; page numbers followed by b refer to boxes.*

breast-conserving therapy (BCT) *(Continued)*
  oncoplastic approach, **V:**296–313
    algorithmic approach, **V:**279f–280f
    basic principles, **V:**277–280
    benefits, **V:**312
    contour deformities, **V:**278f
    definition, **V:**296
    lumpectomy deformities, **V:**278f
    margin status and management, **V:**298
    outcomes and complicatons, **V:**310–312
    Paget's disease of the nipple, **V:**278f
    postoperative care and follow-up, **V:**310
    preoperative assessment, **V:**297–298, 297b
    secondary procedures, **V:**310–312, 312t
    surgical planning, **V:**301–312
    timing considerations, **V:**297–298,
      299f–300f
  patient presentation and diagnosis
    batwing mastopexy, **V:**308f
    decision-making process, **V:**483–485, 485f
    donut type mastopexy, **V:**308f
    inferior pedicle mastopexy, **V:**305f, 307f
    lateral quadrantectomy type defect,
      V:303f
    latissimus dorsi (LD) flap, **V:**306–308,
      309f, 311f
    margin status and management, **V:**298
    oncologic safety, **V:**310
    patient selection, **V:**483
    preoperative assessment, **V:**297–298, 297b
    superior pedicle mastopexy, **V:**304f
    timing considerations, **V:**297–298,
      299f–300f, 484–485
    volume displacement reconstruction,
      V:302–306, 304f–305f, 483–484
    volume replacement reconstruction,
      V:306–310, 309f, 483–484
  postoperative care and follow-up,
    V:493–495
  prognosis and outcomes, **V:**495
  secondary procedures, **V:**495–497, 496f–497f
  surgical technique and treatment
    basic procedure, **V:**485
    batwing mastopexy, **V:**308f
    breast cancer
      algorithmic approach, **V:**279f–280f
      basic principles, **V:**274–280
      oncoplastic surgery, **V:**277–280,
        278f–280f
      surgical technique, **V:**276–277,
        276f–277f
    donut type mastopexy, **V:**308f
    inferior pedicle mastopexy, **V:**305f, 307f
    lateral quadrantectomy type defect,
      V:303f
    latissimus dorsi (LD) flap, **V:**82–83,
      306–308, 309f, 311f
    oncologic safety, **V:**310
    oncoplastic resection, **V:**301, 311f
    outcomes and complicatons, **V:**310–312
    postoperative care and follow-up, **V:**310
    secondary procedures, **V:**310–312, 312t
    superior pedicle mastopexy, **V:**304f
    treatment algorithms, **V:**301–310, 301f,
      302t, 303f
    volume displacement reconstruction,
      V:302–306, 304f–305f
    volume replacement reconstruction,
      V:306–310, 309f, 483–484
  tumor-to-breast ratio, **V:**296–297, 297f

breast implants, **V:**336–369
  applications, **V:**336
  diagnostic imaging, **V:**270–271, 271f
  evolutionary development
    dimensions, **V:**352–353
    filling material, **V:**352–353, 352f
    shape, **V:**352, 352f
    shell, **V:**352
  expander-implants
    adjustable, permanent expander-implants,
      V:366–367
    average operative time, **V:**364t
    basic procedure, **V:**338–340
    breast envelope preservation, **V:**367–368
    capsular contracture, **V:**362, 362t–364t
    cellulitis, **V:**359, 360f
    clinical studies, **V:**362, 363t
    complication frequency, **V:**363–365, 364t
    complications, **V:**359
    delayed reconstruction, **V:**342f, 358, 359f
    erythema, **V:**359
    evaluation studies, **V:**365
    expander failure or malfunction,
      V:360–361, 360f–361f, 364t
    fat injections, **V:**365, 368
    flap-based reconstruction, **V:**367
    hematomas, **V:**359, 359f, 364t
    implant malposition, **V:**363t
    implant removal, **V:**363t
    implant rupture and deflation, **V:**361–362,
      363t
    infections, **V:**361–363, 363t–364t
    insertion procedures, **V:**353–354
    outcome assessments, **V:**363–365
    persistent serous drainage, **V:**359–360
    postoperative care and follow-up,
      V:358–359
    preoperative/postoperative comparisons,
      V:340f–341f
    secondary procedures
      cosmetic revision surgery, **V:**365, 366f
      fat injections, **V:**365, 368
      nipple reconstruction, **V:**365–366
    skin necrosis, **V:**360, 360f, 363t
    wrinkle formation, **V:**363t
  implant malposition
    clinical signs, **V:**79t
    double-bubble deformity, **V:**116, 116f
    inadequate muscle release, **V:**113, 114f
    incidence, **V:**79t
    plane of insertion, **V:**112–113, 113f
    submusculofascial plane, **V:**114–115,
      114f
    symmastia, **V:**115–116, 116f
    transaxillary dissection, **V:**115, 115f
  implant selection
    filling material, **V:**24–25
    implant shape, **V:**25–27, 28f–29f
    implant size determination, **V:**25, 25f
    implant surface texture, **V:**25, 26f–27f
  outcomes and complicatons
    capsular contracture, **V:**264, 336–340, 362,
      362t–364t
    cellulitis, **V:**359, 360f
    clinical studies, **V:**362, 363t
    erythema, **V:**359
    expander failure or malfunction,
      V:360–361, 360f–361f
    hematomas, **V:**359, 359f
    infections, **V:**361–363

breast implants *(Continued)*
    persistent serous drainage, **V:**359–360
    skin necrosis, **V:**360, 360f
  patient presentation and diagnosis
    exclusion criteria, **V:**345–346, 347f
    inclusion criteria
      contralateral adjustments, **V:**346
      large breast reconstruction, **V:**346, 350f
      medium breast reconstruction, **V:**346,
        349f
      small breast reconstruction, **V:**346, 348f
  perioperative complications
    delayed complications
      implant rupture and deflation, **V:**37, 79t
      periprosthetic capsular contracture,
        V:36–37
    hematomas, **V:**32–37, 79t
    medication and herbal supplement
      avoidance list, **V:**33t–35t
    Mondor's disease, **V:**35–36
    nipple sensitivity, **V:**32–37
    seromas, **V:**32–37, 79t
    wound infections, **V:**35, 79t
  postoperative care and follow-up, **V:**32,
    358–359
  reconstructive paradigms
    contralateral adjustments, **V:**343f
    cosmetic breast reconstruction,
      V:344f–345f
    indications and contraindications, **V:**343f
    mastectomy techniques, **V:**343f
    radiation therapy (RT), **V:**347f
    surgical strategy, **V:**340–344
  saline implants
    autoinflation, **V:**111–112, 112f
    capsular calcification, **V:**110, 110f
    decision guidelines, **V:**24–25
    deflation, **V:**110–111, 111f
    developmental background, **V:**13–14
    ripples and folds, **V:**111, 111f
  scientific research, **V:**336–340
  secondary procedures, **V:**37
  silicone gel implants
    capsular calcification, **V:**107–109,
      108f–109f
    capsular contracture, **V:**106–107,
      106f–107f
    characteristics, **I:**789–790, 790f
    closed capsulotomy, **V:**107, 107f–108f
    decision guidelines, **V:**24–25
    developmental background, **V:**14–15
    double-bubble deformity, **V:**116, 116f
    first generation implants, **V:**14–15, 103f
    fourth and fifth generation implants, **V:**15
    hematomas, **V:**104–105, 104f–105f
    historical background, **I:**789–790,
      V:102–109
    implant disruption, **V:**103–104, 103f
    implant malposition, **V:**112–113, 113f
    infections, **V:**105–106, 105f–106f
    second generation implants, **V:**14–15, 104f
    third generation implants, **V:**14–15, 104f
  sponges, **V:**101–102, 102f
  steroid atrophy, **V:**110, 110f
  surgical technique and treatment
    delayed reconstruction, **V:**358, 359f
    expander-implant insertion, **V:**353–354,
      354f
    immediate postmastectomy breast
      reconstruction, **V:**353

breast implants (Continued)
  inframammary incision, **V:**27–30
  periareolar incision, **V:**30–31
  preoperative markings, **V:**27–32
  preoperative project, **V:**346–352, 350f–351f
  prosthesis insertion
    basic procedure, **V:**356–358
    capsulectomy, **V:**357f
    contralateral adjustments, **V:**356–358
    inframammary fold reconstruction, **V:**357f
    large breast augmentation, **V:**358
    medium breast augmentation, **V:**357–358
    small breast augmentation, **V:**356–357
  second-stage surgery, **V:**356, 357f
  skin reducing mastectomy, **V:**354–356, 355f
  surgical guidelines, **V:**27b, 30b
  tissue preservation, **V:**353–358
  transaxillary incision, **V:**31
  transumbilical incision, **V:**32
BREAST-Q, **I:**162–164, 171
breast reconstruction
  anatomical and physiological considerations, **V:**412
  autogenous breast reconstruction, **V:**457–471
    background information, **V:**457–458
    reconstruction population, **V:**458–470
  autologous fat grafts, **V:**582–604
    adipose-derived stem/stromal cells (ASCs), **V:**583–584
    applications, **V:**582–583
    contour deformities
      patient selection, **V:**584–595
      post-flap reconstruction, **V:**584t, 586, 587f–588f
      post-implant reconstruction, **V:**584–586, 584t, 585f
      radiation-caused deformities, **V:**584t, 586, 588f–589f
    harvesting considerations, **V:**583–584
    outcomes and complicatons
      graft survival, **V:**602
      infections, **V:**602
      liponecrotic cysts, **V:**602
      mammographic abnormalities, **V:**602
      neoplasia, **V:**602–603
      persistent swelling, **V:**602
    patient presentation and diagnosis, **V:**584
    patient selection
      congenital deformities, **V:**584t, 591, 591f
      contour deformities, **V:**584–595
      indicators, **V:**584t
      lumpectomy deformities, **V:**584t, 586–590, 590f
      primary breast augmentation, **V:**591–595, 593f–595f
      total breast reconstruction, **V:**595
    postoperative care and follow-up, **V:**601, 601b
    radiation deformities, **V:**583–584
    research summary, **V:**604
    secondary procedures, **V:**603–604, 603f
    surgical technique and treatment
      basic procedure, **V:**595–601
      Brava bra, **V:**601, 601f

breast reconstruction (Continued)
      cannulas, **V:**596f, 598f, 599–601, 600f
      centrifuges, **V:**598f, 600f
      Coleman method, **V:**598, 598f
      contour deformities, **V:**596f
      Cytori™ fat harvest system, **V:**598–599, 600f
      fat harvesting and processing, **V:**597–598, 597f
      injection techniques, **V:**599–601, 600f
      LipiVage™ fat harvest system, **V:**598–599, 599f
      Lipokit™ fat harvest system, **V:**598–599, 600f
      Luer-to-Luer connector, **V:**598, 598f
      markings, **V:**596f
      strainers/straining methods, **V:**598–599
      V-shaped dissectors, **V:**597f
  autologous reconstruction, **V:**411–412
  breast anatomy, **V:**1–12
    anatomical relationships, **V:**6f
    blood supply, **V:**6–8, 7f–8f
    Cooper's ligaments, **V:**3–5
    development stages, **V:**2–3, 2f–4f
    general discussion, **V:**1
    ideal breast structure, **V:**1–2, 2f, 16f
    lymphatic system, **V:**8, 9f
    milk lines, **V:**2–3, 2f
    musculature
      external oblique, **V:**10f, 11
      intercostal dissection, **V:**10f
      internal oblique, **V:**10f
      pectoralis major, **V:**9–11, 10f
      pectoralis minor, **V:**10f
      rectus abdominis, **V:**10f, 11
      serratus anterior, **V:**10–11, 10f
    nipple areola complex, **V:**5, 10f
    parenchyma, **V:**3–5, 6f
    ptosis, **V:**3–5, 5f, 10f
    research summary, **V:**11
    schematic diagram, **V:**4f
    sensory innervation, **V:**9
    skeletal support, **V:**5–6
    structure, **V:**4f
    surgical indications, **V:**11
  deep femoral artery perforator (DFAP) flap, **V:**464–467, 468f–469f
  deep inferior epigastric perforator (DIEP) flaps
    imaging methods, **V:**326
    immediate postmastectomy breast reconstruction, **V:**288f
  disease process, **V:**458
  endoscopic approaches, **V:**81–96
    background and general characteristics
      general discussion, **V:**81–82
      illumination and imaging technology, **V:**82
      latissimus dorsi (LD) flap, **V:**82–83
      optical cavities, **V:**81–82
      support systems, **V:**82
    breast anatomy, **V:**88
    outcomes and complicatons, **V:**93–96
    patient presentation and diagnosis, **V:**88–89
    patient selection, **V:**89
    postoperative care and follow-up, **V:**93

breast reconstruction (Continued)
    surgical technique and treatment
      basic procedure, **V:**89–93
      completed dissection, **V:**93f
      dissector instrumentation, **V:**91f
      hemostasis, **V:**94f
      instrumentation, **V:**90f
      laparotomy pad, **V:**91f
      markings, **V:**89f
      scissor dissection, **V:**92f–93f
      wetting solutions, **V:**90f
  fat grafting, **I:**342–346, 346f–347f
  hypoplastic breast
    basic principles, **I:**647–648
    immature breast, **I:**648
    Poland syndrome, **I:**648, 649f
    tuberous breast, **I:**647
  imaging methods, **V:**326–335
    color Doppler imaging, **V:**328
    future trends, **V:**331–335
    hand-held Doppler ultrasound, **V:**327–328
    magnetic resonance imaging (MRI), **V:**328–329, 329f
    multidetector-row computed tomography (MDCT)
      basic principles, **V:**328–329
      deep inferior epigastric perforator (DIEP) flaps, **V:**326, 327f–328f
      radiological protocol, **V:**329, 330f, 332f–334f
    radiological protocol
      lympho-magnetic resonance imaging (MRI), **V:**334f
      multidetector-row computed tomography (MDCT), **V:**329, 330f, 332f–334f
      noncontrast magnetic resonance imaging (MRI), **V:**329, 334f
      perforator selection guidelines, **V:**330–331, 330f, 332f–333f
    research summary, **V:**331–335
  inferior gluteal artery perforator (IGAP) flap
    advantages, **V:**459–464
    anatomical characteristics, **V:**461–463
    complications, **V:**464
    patient selection, **V:**460–461
    postoperative care, **V:**464
    surgical technique, **V:**463–464, 464b, 467f–468f
  latissimus dorsi (LD) flap, **V:**370–392
    anatomical characteristics, **V:**370–372, 371f
    contraindications, **V:**381
    general discussion, **V:**370
    outcomes and complicatons
      donor site morbidity, **V:**390
      flap necrosis, **V:**390
      follow-up consultations, **V:**389–390
      partial breast reconstruction, **V:**306–308, 309f, 311f, 485–489, 486f
    patient presentation and diagnosis, **V:**372
    patient selection and indicators, **V:**372–374, 373f–375f
    postoperative care and follow-up, **V:**389
    research summary, **V:**390

breast reconstruction (Continued)
  secondary procedures
    secondary thoracodorsal nerve ligation,
      V:389
    timing considerations, V:389
    tissue expansion, V:389
  specific indicators
    augmentation mammaplasty, V:380
    large ptotic breasts, V:380–381
    partial mastectomy defects, V:380
    patient selection, V:374–376, 375f
    post-mastectomy defects, V:380
    prophylactic mastectomy, V:381
    radiation therapy (RT) history,
      V:376–378, 376f–379f
    thin or unreliable skin flaps, V:380, 380f
    transverse rectus abdominis
      myocutaneous (TRAM) flap
      candidates, V:374–376, 375f
  surgical technique
    basic procedure, V:381–387
    deep fat attachment, V:384f
    design guidelines, V:383f–384f
    elevation and transposition, V:385f
    flap shape, V:387f
    patient positioning, V:384f
    skin island placement, V:382f–383f, 386f
    surgical variants, V:387–389, 388f
  lumbar artery perforator (LAP) flap,
    V:467–470, 470b, 470f
  major weight loss (MWL) patient
    breast reshaping, V:564–570
    dermal suspension, V:566–570, 568f
    outcomes and complicatons, V:567–570
    pathophysiology, V:564, 564b
    patient presentation and diagnosis,
      V:564–565
    patient selection, V:565–566
    postoperative care and follow-up, V:567
    surgical goals, V:565b
    surgical planning, V:565–566, 566t,
      569f–570f
    surgical tips, V:567b
    total parenchymal reshaping mastopexy
      surgical markings, V:566
      surgical technique and treatment,
        V:566–567, 568f
  mastectomies, V:411–412
  muscle/musculocutaneous flaps, I:546–549,
    548f–549f
  nipple-areola complex
    characteristics, V:500f
    flap designs adjacent to scars
      double-opposing tab flap, V:511t,
        512–513, 512f–513f
      general discussion, V:511–513
      S-flap, V:511–512, 511f, 511t
      spiral flap, V:513, 513f
    flaps with autologous graft augmentation
      cartilage grafts, V:514, 514f
      fat grafts, V:514–515, 514f
    inferior pedicle breast reduction, V:168f,
      171f–172f
    mastectomy planning, V:419, 419f
    mastopexy
      inverted-T technique, V:146–147
      major weight loss (MWL) patient,
        V:566–570
      outcomes and complicatons, V:148–150
      periareolar techniques, V:126–133

breast reconstruction (Continued)
    postoperative care and follow-up,
      V:147–148
    vertical/short scar techniques,
      V:133–146
  post-mastectomy reconstructiion,
    V:430–432, 432f–433f
  pull-out/purse-string flap techniques
    bell flap, V:508, 508f, 508t
    double opposing peri-areolar/
      purse-string flap, V:508–510, 508t,
      509f–510f
    general discussion, V:507–510
    top-hat flap, V:510, 510f
  reconstruction process
    areola deformities, V:248–249, 250f
    areola hypopigmentation, V:249–251
    areola reconstruction, V:516–518, 517b,
      517f–518f
    asymmetries, V:251
    autologous fat grafts, V:407–410,
      514–515, 514f
    batwing mastopexy, V:308f
    complications, V:245, 519, 519b
    composite nipple graft, V:500–502,
      501f–502f
    donut type mastopexy, V:308f
    flap designs adjacent to scars,
      V:511–513
    flaps with allograft augmentation,
      V:515–516, 516f
    flaps with alloplastic augmentation,
      V:515
    flaps with autologous graft
      augmentation, V:514–515
    flap techniques, V:501t
    general discussion, V:499
    inferior pedicle mastopexy, V:307f
    latissimus dorsi (LD) flap, V:309f
    mastopexy revision, V:254–261,
      258f–263f
    nipple areola ischemia, V:247–248,
      248f–249f
    nipple loss, V:148, 243t, 253–254, 255f
    nipple malposition, V:149, 243t, 252,
      252f–253f
    nipple retraction, V:252
    omentum reconstruction, V:476f–477f,
      480
    outcome assessments, V:519
    patient presentation and diagnosis,
      V:499–500, 500f
    patient selection, V:500
    postmastectomy breast reconstruction,
      V:292–294, 293f
    postoperative care and follow-up,
      V:518, 518f
    pull-out/purse-string flap techniques,
      V:507–510
    secondary/revisional procedures, V:519
    surgical technique and treatment,
      V:500–516
    symmetry, V:480
    traditional flaps, V:502–507
  traditional flaps
    arrow flap, V:503t, 507, 507f
    C–V flap, V:503t, 506–507, 506f, 514–515
    general discussion, V:502–507
    skate flap, V:502–504, 503f–505f, 503t
    star flap, V:503t, 504–506, 505f

breast reconstruction (Continued)
  omentum reconstruction, V:472–481
    basic principles, V:472–473
    complications, V:480–481
    patient selection, V:473
    postoperative care and follow-up, V:480
    prognosis and outcomes, V:480–481
    secondary procedures, V:481
    skin preservation, V:472
    surgical technique and treatment
      acellular dermal matrix (ADM),
        V:474–476, 477f
      bilateral reconstruction, V:476–477,
        478f–480f
      epigastric region closure, V:477–480
      implants, V:474–476, 476f
      laparoscopic harvesting, V:473,
        473f–474f
      lipofilling, V:476
      nipple-areola complex reconstruction,
        V:480
      pectoralis major muscle, V:474–476
      prostheses, V:474, 475f, 479f
      reconstruction process, V:473–474, 474f
  partial breast reconstruction, V:482–498
    basic principles, V:482–483
    breast-conserving therapy (BCT),
      V:277–280, 482
    complications, V:495
    flap classification and vascular anatomy
      anterior intercostal artery perforator
        (AICAP) flap, V:308, 488
      dorsal intercostal artery perforator
        (DICAP) flap, V:488
      intercostal artery perforator (ICAP)
        flap, V:486f–488f, 487–488
      lateral intercostal artery perforator
        (LICAP) flap, V:487f–488f, 488
      lateral thoracodorsal flap (LTDF),
        V:306–308
      latissimus dorsi (LD) flap, V:82–83,
        306–308, 309f, 311f, 485–489, 486f
      pedicled flaps, V:489, 492f
      serratus anterior artery perforator
        (SAAP) flap, V:486f–488f, 488–489
      superior epigastric artery perforator
        (SEAP) flap, V:308, 486f, 489
      thoracodorsal artery perforator (TDAP)
        flap, V:308, 486–487, 486f–488f
    flap design
      flap choice, V:489, 490f–492f
      markings, V:490f–492f, 492–493,
        494f–495f
      preoperative perforator mapping,
        V:489–492, 490f–492f, 494f–495f
      surgical technique, V:490f–492f, 493,
        494f–495f
    oncoplastic approach, V:296–313
      algorithmic approach, V:279f–280f
      basic principles, V:277–280
      benefits, V:312
      contour deformities, V:278f
      definition, V:296
      lumpectomy deformities, V:278f
      margin status and management, V:298
      outcomes and complicatons, V:310–312
      Paget's disease of the nipple, V:278f
      postoperative care and follow-up, V:310
      preoperative assessment, V:297–298,
        297b

breast reconstruction (Continued)
    secondary procedures, V:310–312, 312t
    surgical planning, V:301–312
    timing considerations, V:297–298, 299f–300f
  patient presentation and diagnosis
    batwing mastopexy, V:308f
    decision-making process, V:483–485, 485f
    donut type mastopexy, V:308f
    inferior pedicle mastopexy, V:305f, 307f
    lateral quadrantectomy type defect, V:303f
    latissimus dorsi (LD) flap, V:82–83, 306–308, 309f, 311f
    margin status and management, V:298
    oncologic safety, V:310
    patient selection, V:483
    preoperative assessment, V:297–298, 297b
    superior pedicle mastopexy, V:304f
    timing considerations, V:297–298, 299f–300f, 484–485
    volume displacement reconstruction, V:302–306, 304f–305f, 483–484
    volume replacement reconstruction, V:306–310, 309f, 483–484
  postoperative care and follow-up, V:493–495
  prognosis and outcomes, V:495
  secondary procedures, V:495–497, 496f–497f
  surgical technique and treatment
    basic procedure, V:485
    batwing mastopexy, V:308f
    donut type mastopexy, V:308f
    inferior pedicle mastopexy, V:305f, 307f
    lateral quadrantectomy type defect, V:303f
    latissimus dorsi (LD) flap, V:306–308, 309f, 311f
    oncologic safety, V:310
    oncoplastic resection, V:301, 311f
    outcomes and complicatons, V:310–312
    postoperative care and follow-up, V:310
    secondary procedures, V:310–312, 312t
    superior pedicle mastopexy, V:304f
    treatment algorithms, V:301–310, 301f, 302t, 303f
    volume displacement reconstruction, V:302–306, 304f–305f
    volume replacement reconstruction, V:306–310, 309f, 483–484
  tumor-to-breast ratio, V:296–297, 297f
  patient presentation and diagnosis
    deep femoral artery perforator (DFAP) flap, V:464–467, 468f–469f
    lumbar artery perforator (LAP) flap, V:467–470, 470b, 470f
    reconstruction population, V:458–470
    transverse upper gracilis free flap (TUG)
      anatomical characteristics, V:458–459, 460f
      complications, V:459
      patient selection, V:458
      postoperative image, V:460f
      surgical technique and treatment, V:459, 459b, 461f–462f

breast reconstruction (Continued)
  perforator surgery
    background and general characteristics, V:435–436
    deep inferior epigastric perforator (DIEP) flaps
      anatomical characteristics, V:327f, 436–439, 437f–438f
      imaging methods, V:326, 327f–329f
      immediate postmastectomy breast reconstruction, V:287–291, 288f
      outcomes and complicatons, V:452
      patient presentation and diagnosis, V:439–440
      patient selection, V:440–441
      postoperative care and follow-up, V:451–452
      preoperative assessment, V:439–440
      secondary procedures, V:453
      surgical technique, V:442–451
    future trends, V:331–335
    ideal perforator vessel, V:327, 327f–329f
    patient presentation and diagnosis
      computed tomography (CT) imaging, V:440, 441f–442f
      preoperative assessment, V:439–440
      ultrasound evaluation, V:440
    perforator selection guidelines, V:330–331, 330f, 332f–333f
    recipient vessels, V:439, 439f
    research summary, V:331–335
  post-bariatric surgery reconstruction, II:652
  postmastectomy breast reconstruction
    basic principles, I:640–647
    chest wall irradiated areas, I:645–647
    complications
      clinical studies, V:362, 363t
      expander failure or malfunction, V:360f–361f
      infections, V:361–363
      skin necrosis, V:360f
    delayed reconstruction, V:291–292, 291f–292f, 358, 359f
    expander device, I:642–643, V:292f
    expander-implants
      adjustable, permanent expander-implants, V:366–367
      average operative time, V:364t
      basic procedure, V:338–340
      breast envelope preservation, V:367–368
      capsular contracture, V:362, 362t–364t
      cellulitis, V:359, 360f
      clinical studies, V:362, 363t
      complication frequency, V:363–365, 364t
      complications, V:359
      cosmetic revision surgery, V:365, 366f
      delayed reconstruction, V:342f, 358, 359f
      erythema, V:359
      evaluation studies, V:365
      expander failure or malfunction, V:360f–361f, 364t
      fat injections, V:365, 368
      flap-based reconstruction, V:367
      hematomas, V:359, 359f, 364t
      implant malposition, V:363t
      implant removal, V:363t

breast reconstruction (Continued)
    implant rupture and deflation, V:361–362, 363t
    infections, V:361–363, 363t–364t
    insertion procedures, V:353–354
    nipple reconstruction, V:365–366
    outcome assessments, V:363–365
    persistent serous drainage, V:359–360
    postoperative care and follow-up, V:358–359
    preoperative/postoperative comparisons, V:340f–341f
    secondary procedures, V:365–366
    skin necrosis, V:360, 360f, 363t
    wrinkle formation, V:363t
  immediate postmastectomy breast reconstruction
    acellular allogenic dermal matrix (ADM), I:644–645, 644f
    basic procedure, V:287–291
    breast implants, V:353
    deep inferior epigastric perforator (DIEP) flaps, V:288f
    expander-implant insertion, V:353–354, 354f
    latissimus dorsi (LD) flap, V:288, 289f–290f
    muscle coverage, I:643–645
    prosthesis insertion, V:356–358
    radiation therapy (RT), V:290
    second-stage surgery, V:356, 357f
    skin reducing mastectomy, V:354–356, 355f
    submuscular position, I:643–644
    subpectoral (dual-plane) position, I:644
    transverse rectus abdominis myocutaneous (TRAM) flaps, V:288f
  outcomes and complicatons
    cellulitis, V:359, 360f
    erythema, V:359
    expander failure or malfunction, V:360–361
    hematomas, V:359, 359f
    persistent serous drainage, V:359–360
    skin necrosis, V:360
  patient presentation and diagnosis
    exclusion criteria, V:345–346, 347f
    inclusion criteria, V:346
    large breast reconstruction, V:346, 350f
    medium breast reconstruction, V:346, 349f
    small breast reconstruction, V:346, 348f
  postoperative care and follow-up, V:358–359
  prosthesis insertion
    basic procedure, V:356–358
    capsulectomy, V:357f
    contralateral adjustments, V:356–358
    inframammary fold reconstruction, V:357f
    large breast augmentation, V:358
    medium breast augmentation, V:357–358
    small breast augmentation, V:356–357
  reconstructive paradigms
    contralateral adjustments, V:343f
    cosmetic breast reconstruction, V:344f–345f

breast reconstruction (*Continued*)
  indications and contraindications,
    V:343f
  mastectomy techniques, **V:**343f
  radiation therapy (RT), **V:**347f
  surgical strategy, **V:**340–344
  secondary breast reconstruction, **I:**645,
    646f
  skin reducing mastectomy, **V:**354–356,
    355f
  surgical technique and treatment
    delayed reconstruction, **V:**358, 359f
    expander-implant insertion, **V:**353–354,
      354f
    immediate postmastectomy breast
      reconstruction, **V:**353
    prosthesis insertion, **V:**356–358
    second-stage surgery, **V:**356, 357f
    skin reducing mastectomy, **V:**354–356,
      355f
    tissue preservation, **V:**353–358
  reconstructive burn surgery, **IV:**506
  secondary procedures, **V:**292–294, 293f,
    470–471
  superior gluteal artery perforator (SGAP)
    flap
    advantages, **V:**459–464
    anatomical characteristics, **V:**461–463
    complications, **V:**464
    patient selection, **V:**460–461
    postoperative care, **V:**464
    surgical technique, **V:**463–464, 464b,
      465f–467f
  tissue expansion
    basic principles, **I:**640–647
    chest wall irradiated areas, **I:**645–647
    expander device, **I:**642–643, **V:**292f
    immediate postmastectomy breast
      reconstruction
      acellular allogenic dermal matrix
        (ADM), **I:**644–645, 644f
      muscle coverage, **I:**643–645
      submuscular position, **I:**643–644
      subpectoral (dual-plane) position, **I:**644
    secondary breast reconstruction, **I:**645,
      646f
  total breast reconstruction, **V:**595
  transverse rectus abdominis myocutaneous
    (TRAM) flaps
    autogenous breast reconstruction,
      V:457–458
    basic procedure, **I:**546–549, 549f
    bilateral pedicle TRAM flap, **V:**393–410
      background and general characteristics,
        V:393–394
      circulatory zones, **V:**395f
      external and internal oblique
        components, **V:**404f
      fascial and muscle strips, **V:**400f, 403f
      fascial closure, **V:**405f
      inferomedial dissection, **V:**402f
      lateral muscle dissection, **V:**401f
      markings, **V:**397f, 400f
      medial dissection, **V:**402f
      medial suprafascial dissection, **V:**399f
      muscle and fascial pedicle control,
        V:402f
      outcomes and complicatons, **V:**407–410
      patient selection, **V:**395–396
      pedicle arrangement, **V:**403f–404f

breast reconstruction (*Continued*)
      pedicle length, **V:**403f
      postoperative care and follow-up,
        V:406
      preoperative assessment, **V:**396
      Prolene mesh, **V:**405f
      secondary procedures, **V:**410
      shaping guidelines, **V:**405–406,
        406f–409f
      surgical procedures, **V:**396–405,
        397b–399b
      tunnel positions, **V:**398f
      vascular anatomy, **V:**394–395, 394f
    free TRAM flap, **V:**411–434
      abdominal closure, **V:**426–428, 429f
      anatomical and physiological
        considerations, **V:**412
      complications, **V:**430, 431f
      delayed versus immediate
        reconstruction, **V:**414
      flap dissection, **V:**419–422, 420f–421f,
        423f
      flap inset guidelines, **V:**426, 427f–428f
      general discussion, **V:**411
      mastectomy planning, **V:**419, 419f
      nipple-areola complex reconstruction,
        V:430–432, 432f–433f
      patient presentation and diagnosis,
        V:414–416
      patient selection, **V:**416–418
      pedicled versus free TRAM, **V:**414–415
      postoperative care and follow-up,
        V:428–429
      procedure selection, **V:**417–418
      radiation therapy (RT), **V:**415–416
      recipient vessels, **V:**422–426, 424f–425f
      research summary, **V:**432
      risk factors, **V:**416–417
      surgical technique and treatment,
        V:418–428
      timing considerations, **V:**414
    patient selection, **V:**374–376
    schematic diagram, **I:**548f
    surgical manipulation, **I:**578
  transverse upper gracilis free flap (TUG)
    anatomical characteristics, **V:**458–459,
      460f
    complications, **V:**459
    patient selection, **V:**458
    postoperative image, **V:**460f
    surgical technique and treatment, **V:**459,
      459b, 461f–462f
breast reduction, **V:**152–164
  adolescent aesthetic surgery, **I:**45t
  Biesenberger technique, **V:**154, 155f
  central mound technique, **V:**156–159, 160f
  complications, **V:**243t
  evaluation examinations, **V:**162–163
  evidence-based medicine and health service
    research, **I:**160–161, 161f
  historical background, **V:**153–159
  inferior pedicle breast reduction, **V:**165–176
    background and general characteristics,
      V:154–156, 165–166
    case studies, **V:**172–175, 173f–174f
    complications, **V:**175
    inferior pedicle technique with Wise-
      pattern skin excision, **V:**156, 159f,
      161f
    patient selection, **V:**166

breast reduction (*Continued*)
    planning and marking guidelines
      asymmetrical cases, **V:**168, 168f
      equilateral triangle marking, **V:**166–167,
        167f
      inframammary fold, **V:**167
      preoperative markings, **V:**166, 167f
      symmetry assessments, **V:**168
      transverse incisions markings, **V:**167
    research summary, **V:**175
    surgical technique and treatment
      apical suture, **V:**171f
      basic procedure, **V:**168–172
      de-epithelialization, **V:**169f
      flap thickness evaluation, **V:**170f
      inferior pedicle with inverted-T skin
        closure, **V:**159f, 161f
      medial and lateral triangle excision,
        V:170f
      nipple-areola complex, **V:**168f,
        171f–172f
      postoperative results, **V:**172f
      preoperative/postoperative
        comparisons, **V:**173f
      symmetry evaluation, **V:**172f
  infiltration, **I:**141–142, 141f–142f
  L short-scar mammaplasty, **V:**206–215
    background and general characteristics,
      V:206–207
    complications, **V:**213
    patient selection, **V:**206–207
    planning and marking guidelines, **V:**207,
      208f–209f
    reduction results, **V:**210f–214f
    research summary, **V:**214–215
    surgical technique, **V:**207–210, 209f
  mammary hypertrophy, **V:**152–153, 161–162,
    240f–241f
  McKissock vertical bipedicled
    dermoglandular flap with Wise-pattern
    skin excision, **V:**156, 157f–158f
  McKissock vertical dermoglandular flap
    with Wise-pattern skin excision, **V:**156,
    159f
  Passot technique, **V:**154, 154f
  patient presentation and diagnosis,
    V:162–163
  psychological aspects, **I:**41–42
  revisionary surgery, **V:**242–265
    incidence, **V:**242
    outcomes and complicatons, **V:**245
    pathophysiology, **V:**244
    patient history, **V:**242–244
    patient presentation and diagnosis, **V:**244
    postoperative care and follow-up,
      V:244–245, 262
    preoperative assessment, **V:**244
    research summary, **V:**264
    surgical re-intervention
      areola deformities, **V:**248–249, 250f
      areola hypopigmentation, **V:**249–251
      asymmetries, **V:**251
      contour abnormalities, **V:**247
      fat necrosis, **V:**251
      flap necrosis, **V:**246
      hematomas, **V:**245–246, 246f
      mastopexy revision, **V:**254–261,
        258f–263f
      nipple areola ischemia, **V:**247–248,
        248f–249f

breast reduction (Continued)
nipple loss, **V:**148, 243t, 253–254, 255f
nipple malposition, **V:**149, 243t, 252–253, 252f–253f
nipple retraction, **V:**252
postoperative care and follow-up, **V:**246
re-do breast reduction, **V:**254, 256f
scars, **V:**246–247
wound excision and re-closure, **V:**246–247
Schwarzmann technique, **V:**154, 155f
sculpted pillar vertical reduction mammaplasty, **V:**228–241
background and general characteristics, **V:**228
complications, **V:**236–239, 239f–241f
patient selection, **V:**228–229
planning and marking guidelines, **V:**229, 229f–230f
research summary, **V:**239
surgical technique
basic procedure, **V:**229–236
large breast reduction, **V:**236, 238f
moderate breast reduction, **V:**236, 237f
small breast reduction, **V:**235, 236f
wound closure, **V:**231–235, 232f–235f
short scar periareolar inferior pedicle reduction (SPAIR) mammaplasty, **V:**194–205
background and general characteristics, **V:**159, 194–195
complications
areolar spreading, **V:**204
fat necrosis, **V:**203–204
general discussion, **V:**203–205
hypertrophy recurrence, **V:**204–205
polytetrafluoroethylene (PTFE) infection/exposure, **V:**204
shape distortion, **V:**204
patient selection, **V:**195–196
planning and marking guidelines, **V:**196, 197f–198f
reduction results
large breast reduction, **V:**202–203, 203f
modest breast reduction, **V:**202, 203f
small breast reduction, **V:**201–203, 202f
research summary, **V:**205
surgical technique, **V:**196–201, 200f–201f
Strombeck horizontal bipedicle technique, **V:**156, 156f
superomedial pedicle with Wise-pattern skin closure, **V:**156–159, 161f
vertical scar reduction mammaplasty, **V:**177–193
comparison studies, **V:**178t
complications
frequency, **V:**189–192, 191t
scar healing, **V:**190, 191f
under-resection, **V:**192
wound dehiscence, **V:**191
Hall-Findlay technique, **V:**159, 178t
historical background, **V:**177–180
Lassus technique, **V:**156–159, 177–180, 178t
Lejour technique, **V:**159, 178t
Lista technique, **V:**178t
medial pedicle breast reductions, **V:**189, 190f
nipple-areola complex, **V:**179f

breast reduction (Continued)
patient selection
patient characteristics, **V:**180–181
symptoms, **V:**180
planning and marking guidelines
perioperative care, **V:**181
skin marking, **V:**181–182, 181f, 183f
postoperative care and follow-up, **V:**188
research summary, **V:**192
superior pedicle breast reductions, **V:**188–189, 189f
surgical technique and treatment
anesthesia, **V:**182
breast shaping, **V:**186–187, 187f
de-epithelialization, **V:**184, 184f
dressings and wound care, **V:**188
infiltration, **V:**182–184
liposuction, **V:**185
patient positioning, **V:**182
pedicle selection, **V:**182, 184f
surgical excision, **V:**184–185, 185f–186f
wound closure, **V:**187–188, 187f–188f
breasts
anatomical characteristics, **V:**1–12
anatomical relationships, **V:**6f
blood supply, **V:**6–8, 7f–8f
Cooper's ligaments, **IV:**224, **V:**3–5, 120–121, 120f
development stages, **V:**2–3, 2f–4f
general discussion, **V:**1
ideal breast structure, **V:**1–2, 2f, 16f
lymphatic system, **V:**8, 9f
milk lines, **V:**2–3, 2f
musculature
external oblique, **V:**10f, 11
intercostal dissection, **V:**10f
internal oblique, **V:**10f
pectoralis major, **IV:**225f, **V:**9–11, 10f
pectoralis minor, **IV:**225f, **V:**10f
rectus abdominis, **V:**10f, 11
serratus anterior, **IV:**224–225, **V:**10–11, 10f
nipple areola complex, **V:**5, 10f
parenchyma, **V:**3–5, 6f
ptosis, **V:**3–5, 5f, 10f, 121f
research summary, **V:**11
schematic diagram, **V:**4f, 120f
sensory innervation, **V:**9
skeletal support, **V:**5–6
structure, **V:**4f
surgical indications, **V:**11
vascular anatomy, **IV:**225–227, 226f
breast ptosis
background information, **V:**119–120
pathophysiology
basic principles, **V:**120–121
breast anatomy, **V:**120f
breast base anomaly classifications, **V:**123f
breast development, **V:**123f
classifications, **V:**122f
Cooper's ligaments, **V:**120–121, 120f
procedural guidelines, **V:**122t
Regnault classification, **V:**121, 121f
von Heimburg's tuberous breast classification, **V:**121, 124t
ptosis types, **V:**122f
Regnault classification, **V:**121f

breasts (Continued)
lymphatic system, **V:**8, 9f
nontuberous congenital breast asymmetry
bilateral but different surgical procedure, **V:**537–538
bilateral but similar surgical procedure, **V:**537–538
case studies
Case VII (volume asymmetry), **V:**538, 539f
Case VIII (volume asymmetry), **V:**538, 540f
Case IX (severe hypoplasia), **V:**538–541, 542f–543f
Case X (severe asymmetry), **V:**544
dermal apron, **V:**544, 545f
general considerations, **V:**537–538, 537b
monolateral operation, **V:**537
photographic guidelines, **I:**110, 113f–114f
surgical indications, **V:**11
tuberous breast deformity, **V:**521–547
asymmetric tuberous breast deformity
Case III (asymmetric tuberous breast deformity), **V:**533
Case IV (Type II tuberous breast), **V:**533–534, 534f–535f
Case VI (Type III flap), **V:**534–537
Case V (severe bilateral mammary hypoplasia and tuberous deformity), **V:**534, 536f
general considerations, **V:**532
autologous fat grafts, **V:**591
background information, **V:**521–522
case studies
asymmetric tuberous breast deformity, **V:**533–537, 534f–536f
Case I (bilateral symmetric tuberous breast), **V:**523f–524f, 531
Case III (asymmetric tuberous breast deformity), **V:**533
Case II (severe tuberous breast deformity), **V:**524f–526f, 531–532
Case IV (Type II tuberous breast), **V:**533–534, 534f–535f
Case VI (Type III flap), **V:**534–537
Case V (severe bilateral mammary hypoplasia and tuberous deformity), **V:**534, 536f
glandular flap Type III, **V:**534–537
severe tuberous breast deformity, **V:**524f–526f, 531–532
classifications
background information, **V:**526–529
Type I tuberous breast, **V:**523f–526f, 526
Type II tuberous breast, **V:**526–527, 527f–528f, 529b
Type III tuberous breast, **V:**529, 529b
glandular correction flaps
characteristics, **V:**529–531
glandular flap Type I, **V:**530
glandular flap Type II, **V:**530
glandular flap Type III, **V:**530
glandular flap Type IV, **V:**530–531
pathogenesis, **V:**522
patient presentation and diagnosis
diagnosis, **V:**522–529, 523b
evaluation examinations, **V:**526–529

breasts *(Continued)*
 postoperative care and follow-up,
  V:544–545
 surgical technique and treatment
  case studies, V:531–532
  general considerations, V:529, 529b
  glandular correction flaps, V:529–531
  intraoperative sequence, V:532
  suturing techniques, V:544–545
 terminology, V:521–522
Breslow classification of melanoma, I:753–756,
 756f
Bricker, Eugene M, VI:xlvi–xlvii
bridge plating, VI:113, 115f
British Medical Research Council (BMRC)
 Scale, VI:716, 716t, 795–796, 796t
bromelain, V:33t–35t
bronchopleural fistula
 outcome assessments, IV:252
 pathogenesis, IV:252
 schematic diagram, IV:254f
 surgical technique and treatment, IV:252
Brophy, Truman, I:23–24
browlift surgery
 basic principles, II:203
 botulinum toxin type-A (BoNT-A), II:37, 41
 complications, II:105–106, 105f–106f
 patient presentation and diagnosis
  aesthetics, II:98f–100f, 99–100
  forehead aging, II:98–99, 98f–99f
 postoperative care and follow-up, II:105
 prognosis and outcomes, II:105–106
 secondary procedures, II:106, 106f
 surgical technique
  anterior hairline approach, II:101–102, 102f
  direct suprabrow approach, II:104
  endoscopic approach, II:102–103, 103f
  general discussion, II:100–105
  lateral brow approach, II:103–104, 104f
  open coronal approach, II:100–101, 101f
  subperiosteal facelift, II:274, 274f
  suture suspension browplexy, II:105
  temple approach, II:103, 103f
  transpalpebral approach, II:103, 104f
  transpalpebral browplexy, II:104–105
Brown, James Barrett, VI:xlv–xlvi
brown recluse spider bite, VI:336
Bruce–Winship syndrome, III:807t
Brummer "winch" operation, VI:825f
buccal fat pad, III:10–11, 309t
buccal mucosa
 anatomical characteristics, III:308, 422f
 cancer management
  complications
   acute complications, III:333
   chronic complications, III:333–334
  decision-making process
   basic procedure, III:311–313
   immediate postoperative appearance,
    III:314f
   myocutaneous perforator flap, III:313f
   patient follow-up, III:312f–314f
   radial forearm flap, III:311f
   squamous cell carcinomas (SCCs),
    III:311f–313f
   ulnar forearm flap, III:312f
 diagnosis and treatment, III:427
 preoperative assessment, III:406
 soft tissue flaps, III:309t
 surgical technique and treatment, III:406

buccal mucosa *(Continued)*
 cleft palate surgery, III:576–578, 578f
 male genital reconstructive surgery, IV:307,
  309f
buccal space, II:84–85
buccal sulcus deformities, III:641–642, 641f
Buck's fascia, II:656, 661–662, 661f, IV:299f
Buerger's disease, VI:474
bulb (hair follicle), I:321, 322f
bulbous nose, II:175, 176f
bulimia nervosa, I:49–50, 49b
Buncke, Harry J, VI:xlvii
Bunnell ring finger flexor digitorum
 superficialis transfer, VI:755–756,
 755f–757f, 761t
Bunnell, Sterling, –VI:2
Bunnell test, VI:53–54, 53f
bupivacaine, I:139, 140f, 147–148
 comparative pharmacology, VI:96t
 patient safety, I:129–130
 selection guidelines, VI:95–96, 95t
 toxicity, VI:95
Burget–Walton surgical approach, III:175f
Burian, Frantisek, I:23
buried penis *See* hidden penis
Burke, Jack, I:368
Burkhalter extensor indicis proprius transfer,
 VI:754–755, 754f–755f
burns
 burn reconstruction, IV:500–510
  extremity burn reconstruction, IV:435–455
  facial burn wound treatment, IV:468–499
   acute facial burns, IV:470–473
   complications, IV:497
   damage assessments, IV:468–473, 469f
   depth of burn determination, IV:470
   epidemiology, IV:468
   nonsurgical management, IV:473
   outcome assessments, IV:497–498
   postoperative care and follow-up,
    IV:497
   secondary procedures, IV:498–499
   surgical management, IV:473–484
  general discussion, IV:500
  hypertrophic scars, IV:501, 501f–502f
  outcome assessments, IV:509
  postoperative care and follow-up, IV:509
  research summary, IV:509
  surgical technique
   axillary contractures, IV:507, 507f
   breast reconstruction, IV:506
   cheeks, IV:490–491, 506
   ears, IV:473, 491–492, 496f, 498–499,
    505–506
   elbows, IV:507
   eyebrows, IV:504–505
   eyelids, IV:470–473, 485–488, 486f–487f,
    498–499, 504–505, 504f
   facial burn deformities, IV:504–506
   fascial flaps, IV:503
   fingers, IV:508, 508f
   hands, IV:507–509, 508f
   lips, IV:505
   local flaps, IV:502–503, 503f
   lower extremities, IV:509
   muscle flaps, IV:503
   nail deformities, IV:509
   neck, IV:506
   nose, IV:473, 488–489, 498–499, 505
   perineum, IV:506–507

burns *(Continued)*
  scalp, III:119–120, 120f, IV:492–493,
   498–499, 504, 504f
  scar release, IV:501–502, 502f
  skin grafts, IV:502
  skin substitutes, IV:502
  tissue expansion, IV:503
  web space contractures, IV:508
  wound closure, IV:502–503
  wrists, IV:508, 508f
 timing considerations, IV:500–501
 wound contraction, IV:501
 burn wound treatment, IV:393–434
  acute management, IV:393
  assessment strategies
   body surface area calculations,
    IV:402f
   burn size estimation, IV:402f
   patient presentation and diagnosis,
    IV:402–408, 403t
   Wallace's rule of nines, IV:402f
  burn types
   chemical burns, IV:396
   electrical burns, IV:396–397, 396f, 396t
   nonaccidental burns, IV:397
   thermal burns, IV:394–396
  compartment syndrome
   decompressive laparotomy, IV:431f
   detailed characteristics, IV:428–431
   early escharotomy, IV:430f
   escharotomy incisions, IV:429f–430f
   escharotomy lines, IV:428f
   extensive escharotomies, IV:431f
   full thickness burn escharotomies,
    IV:429f
   hand escharotomies, IV:429f
   periocular escharotomies, IV:430f
   zigzag escharotomies, IV:430f
  complications
   adrenal insufficiency, IV:428
   compartment syndrome, IV:428–431
   deep vein thrombosis (DVT), IV:431
   gastrointestinal (GI) complications,
    IV:431
   heparin-induced thrombocytopenia,
    IV:432
   heterotopic ossification, IV:431–432
   hypertrophic scars, IV:434
   hypothermia, IV:434
   infections, IV:427–428, 428f, 432–434
   inflammatory response, IV:432
   neutropenia, IV:432
   peripheral and central-line insertion,
    IV:433–434, 433t
   potential complications, IV:428b
   secondary sclerosing cholangitis (SSC),
    IV:434
   skin graft loss, IV:427
  epidemiology, IV:393–397
  historical background, IV:393
  initial evaluation and treatment
   airway management, IV:401f
   associated injuries, IV:400f
   burn history, IV:401b
   burn unit referrals, IV:400b
   guidelines, IV:399–402
   inhalation injury indicators, IV:401b
   major burns, IV:400b
   nonaccidental burn or scald indicators,
    IV:401b

burns (Continued)
   moderate to severe burns
      conservative versus surgical therapy,
         IV:416
      cultured epithelial autografts (CEA),
         IV:420f
      debridement, **IV:**417f
      full-thickness skin graft, **IV:**420f
      healed lower limb donor sites, **IV:**419f
      inflated scrotal tissue, **IV:**418f
      initial treament strategies, **IV:**408–421
      local pivot flaps, **IV:**420f
      monitoring strategies, **IV:**410
      pneumatic tourniquets, **IV:**417f
      radial forearm flap, **IV:**421f
      reconstruction techniques, **IV:**420–421,
         421b
      resuscitation formulae, **IV:**409, 409t
      skin substitutes, **IV:**418f
      split-thickness skin graft, **IV:**417f–419f
      staples, **IV:**419f
      surgical equipment, **IV:**416f
      surgical technique and treatment,
         IV:416–420
      tissue expansion, **IV:**418f
      topical ointments, **IV:**410
      wound dressings, **IV:**410–416
   nutritional therapy
      amino acids, **IV:**425
      anabolic steroids, **IV:**423–425
      β-blockers, **IV:**425
      catabolism-induced complications,
         IV:421–425, 421t, 422b
      endocrine and glucose monitoring,
         IV:423
      enteral nutrition/parenteral nutrition,
         IV:423, 423f
      hepatic protein monitoring, **IV:**423
      importance, **IV:**421–425
      metabolic rate versus burn size,
         IV:421t
      nutrition formulae, **IV:**423, 424t
      stress response, **IV:**422b
   pain control
      miscellaneous drugs, **IV:**427
      opioid analgesics, **IV:**427
      simple analgesics, **IV:**427
   pathophysiology
      burn shock, **IV:**398
      hypovolemia and fluid extravasation,
         IV:399
      local response, **IV:**398
      mediators, **IV:**399
      skin characteristics, **IV:**397–402
      systemic response, **IV:**398
   patient presentation and diagnosis
      assessment strategies, **IV:**402–408
      burned genitalia, **IV:**407, 407f
      carboxyhemoglobinemia, **IV:**408t
      deep partial thickness burns, **IV:**403t,
         405–406
      epidermal burns, **IV:**403t, 404, 404f
      full thickness injuries, **IV:**403t, 406–407,
         406f–407f
      inhalation injuries, **IV:**407–408, 408t
      intubation indicators, **IV:**408b
      management protocols, **IV:**405f
      reconstruction priorities, **IV:**404b

burns (Continued)
      superficial partial thickness burns,
         IV:403t, 404–405, 406f
      typical findings, **IV:**403t
   rehabilitation
      basic principles, **IV:**425–434
      complications, **IV:**427–434
      occupational therapy treatments/
         physiotherapy, **IV:**425b
      pain control, **IV:**426–427, 427b
      patient positioning, **IV:**426f
      pressure garments, **IV:**426f
      pressure management, **IV:**426f
   risk factors, **IV:**394
   stress response
      emergent phase, **IV:**422
      fluid shift phase, **IV:**422
      hypermetabolic phase, **IV:**422
      metabolic abnormalities, **IV:**422b
      resolution phase, **IV:**422
      systemic response, **IV:**422b
   surgical goals, **IV:**393
   thermal burns
      contact burns, **IV:**394–395, 395f
      flash and flame burns, **IV:**394
      scalds, **IV:**394, 394f
      tar, **IV:**395–396
   wound dressings
      biological wound dressings, **IV:**410–
         415, 412t–414t
      characteristics, **IV:**410–416, 411b
      physiological wound dressings,
         IV:415–416
chemical injury, **IV:**396, 460–464
electrical burns
   burn wound treatment, **IV:**396–397
   electric current effects, **IV:**396t
   patient presentation, **IV:**396f
   reconstructive surgeries, **IV:**435–436
   scalp and forehead, **III:**119–120, 120f
extremity burn reconstruction, **IV:**435–455
   acute phase surgery
      joint reconstruction, **IV:**441–442,
         442f–443f, 445f
      skin grafts, **IV:**441
      skin substitutes, **IV:**441
   axillary contractures, **IV:**507, 507f
   burn-related accidents, **IV:**435
   complications
      axillary contractures, **IV:**445, 448f–449f
      bone exposure, **IV:**446, 450f
      elbow contractures, **IV:**445–446
      heterotopic ossification, **IV:**446
      scar retraction, **IV:**444–445
      skeletal-muscle complications, **IV:**446
      unstable healing, **IV:**444
   elbows, **IV:**507
   electrical burns, **IV:**435–436
   fingers, **IV:**508, 508f
   hands, **IV:**507–509, 508f
   nail deformities, **IV:**509
   patient presentation and diagnosis
      compartment syndrome, **IV:**437–439,
         437f–440f
      emergency surgical procedures,
         IV:437b
      escharotomy incisions, **IV:**429f–430f,
         437–439, 437f–440f

burns (Continued)
      escharotomy lines, **IV:**428f
      extensive escharotomies, **IV:**431f
      fluid infusion and edema, **IV:**436–437
      full thickness burn escharotomies,
         IV:429f
      hand escharotomies, **IV:**429f
      preoperative assessment, **IV:**436–440
      related trauma, **IV:**439–440
      zigzag escharotomies, **IV:**430f
   patient selection, **IV:**440
   postoperative care and follow-up
      active mobilization, **IV:**444
      ankles, **IV:**444
      compression garments, **IV:**447f
      elbows, **IV:**443
      hips/flanks, **IV:**443–444
      joint position, **IV:**443t
      knees, **IV:**444
      passive mobilization, **IV:**444
      patient positioning, **IV:**443
      physio-kinesitherapy tasks, **IV:**447f
      shoulder, **IV:**443
      treatment strategies, **IV:**442–444
      wrists, **IV:**443
   prognosis and outcomes, **IV:**444–446
   secondary procedures
      amputations, **IV:**451–453
      fasciocutaneous flaps, **IV:**449–450
      free flaps, **IV:**450
      general characteristics, **IV:**446–454
      laser treatments, **IV:**454, 454t
      lipofilling, **IV:**453–454
      myocutaneous flaps, **IV:**449–450
      nerve repair and grafting, **IV:**450–451
      rotation flaps, **IV:**448–449, 453f–454f
      skin expansion, **IV:**450
      skin grafts, **IV:**447–448
      skin substitutes, **IV:**448
      tendon retraction, **IV:**451
      Z-plasty technique, **III:**269f, **IV:**447,
         451f–454f
   surgical technique and treatment
      acute phase surgery, **IV:**441
      characteristics, **IV:**440–442
   web space contractures, **IV:**508
   wrists, **IV:**508, 508f
facial burn wound treatment, **IV:**468–499
   acute facial burns
      ears, **IV:**473
      eyes/eyelids, **IV:**470–473
      mouth, **IV:**473
      nose, **IV:**473
      treatment strategies, **IV:**470–473,
         471f–472f
   complications, **IV:**497
   damage process
      acute facial burns, **IV:**470–473
      damage assessments, **IV:**468–473,
         469f
      depth of burn determination,
         IV:470
   epidemiology, **IV:**468
   flaps
      basic principles, **IV:**480–481
      indicators, **IV:**480b
      trapeze-plasties, **IV:**481
      Z-plasty, technique, **IV:**481, 481f

Note: **Boldface** *roman numerals indicate volume. Page numbers followed by f refer to figures; page numbers followed by t refer to tables; page numbers followed by b refer to boxes.*

burns (*Continued*)
  inadequate donor-site skin
    dermal substitutes, **IV:**480, 482–484
    general discussion, **IV:**482–484
    tissue expansion, **IV:**482, 483f
  nonoperative facial reconstructive adjunct
      techniques
    corrective cosmetics, **IV:**485
    fat transplantation, **IV:**485
    hair transplantation, **IV:**485
    laser therapy, **IV:**484, 484f
    prosthetics, **IV:**485
    steroid treatments, **IV:**485
  nonsurgical management, **IV:**473
  outcome assessments, **IV:**497–498
  postoperative care and follow-up, **IV:**497
  secondary procedures, **IV:**498–499
  skin grafts
    advantages, **IV:**474
    basic principles, **IV:**479
    composite grafts, **IV:**480
    full-thickness skin graft, **IV:**479–480
    skin substitutes, **IV:**480, 482–484
    split-thickness skin graft, **IV:**479
  specific areas
    cheeks, **IV:**490–491, 506
    commissure, **IV:**473, 489–490, 495f
    ears, **IV:**473, 491–492, 496f, 498–499,
        505–506
    eyebrows, **IV:**485, 498–499
    eyelids, **IV:**470–473, 485–488, 486f–487f,
        498–499, 504–505, 504f
    forehead, **IV:**485, 498–499
    lower eyelids, **IV:**486–488, 488f
    lower lip and chin, **IV:**489, 492f–494f,
        498–499
    medial canthus scars, **IV:**488
    neck, **IV:**493–494, 498–499, 506
    nose, **IV:**473, 488–489, 498–499, 505
    scalp, **III:**119–120, 120f, **IV:**492–493,
        498–499, 504, 504f
    severe cervical burn scars and
        contractures, **IV:**494
    upper eyelids, **IV:**486, 487f
    upper lip, **IV:**489, 490f–491f, 498–499
  specific surgical techniques
    scar replacement with local skin,
        IV:478, 478f
    serial excision, **IV:**478
    W-plasty technique, **IV:**478–479, 478f
  surgical management
    algorithmic approach, **IV:**475–477,
        476f–477f
    basic principles, **IV:**474–475
    flaps, **IV:**480–481
    inadequate donor-site skin, **IV:**482–484
    skin grafts, **IV:**479–480
    specific techniques, **IV:**478–479
    surgical techniques, **IV:**473
    total wound healing/scar maturation,
        IV:474–475, 474f
  total wound healing/scar maturation
    aesthetic units, **IV:**474, 475f
    ancillary techniques, **IV:**475, 475b, 476f
    diagnosis, **IV:**474
    functional restoration, **IV:**474, 475f
    local flaps, **IV:**474
    reconstruction planning, **IV:**474
    skin grafts, **IV:**474
    skin-matching considerations, **IV:**475

burns (*Continued*)
      surgical goals, **IV:**475
      timing considerations, **IV:**474–475, 474f
  nonaccidental burns, **IV:**397
  psychological considerations, **I:**42–43
  scalp and forehead, **III:**119–120, 120f
  thermal burns
    contact burns, **IV:**394–395, 395f
    flash and flame burns, **IV:**394
    scalds, **IV:**394, 394f
    tar, **IV:**395–396
  tissue expansion, **I:**629, 638f, **IV:**497
Burow's triangles, **I:**304, **III:**34–36, 37f,
    265–268
Burton classification, **VI:**432, 432t
Burton–Pelligrini procedure, **VI:**437–439, 438f
business plans, **I:**80–82, 81f
business principles, **I:**64–91
  accounting
    balance sheets, **I:**67–68, 71f
    breakeven analysis, **I:**73f
    cash flow summary, **I:**68, 72f
    financial ratios
      characteristics, **I:**68–69
      efficiency ratios, **I:**69
      leverage ratios, **I:**69
      liquidity ratios, **I:**69
      profitability ratios, **I:**69
    generally accepted accounting principles
        (GAAP), **I:**67–69
    income statements, **I:**67, 70f
  economics, **I:**73–74
  entrepreneurship, **I:**80–82, 81f
  ethics, **I:**87–88, 88b
  finance
    discounted cash flow, **I:**72–73
    goals, **I:**69–73
    net present value, **I:**72–73
    opportunity cost, **I:**71–72
    return on investment, **I:**73
    time value of money, **I:**70–71
  healthcare–industrial complex, **I:**64–65
  human resource management, **I:**83–84
  innovation, **I:**78–80
  leadership, **I:**88–90, 89f
  legal and regulatory considerations
    American Recovery and Reinvestment
        Act (2009), **I:**85
    business ownership categories, **I:**84–86
    Dodd–Frank Wall Street Reform and
        Consumer Protection Act (2010), **I:**86
    Patient Protection and Affordable Care
        Act (2010), **I:**86
    Sarbanes–Oxley Act (SOX, 2002), **I:**85
  marketing strategy, **I:**75–76, 75f
  negotiation, **I:**86–87
  operations/operational effectiveness,
      I:76–78
  Six Sigma program case study, **I:**78b
  strategic principles, **I:**65–67, 66f
  supply-and-demand theory, **I:**73–74
  sustainable enterprise, **I:**82–83
butter, **IV:**395
buttocks
  aesthetic analysis
    basic principles, **II:**600–602, 600f
    ethnic ideals, **II:**603f–604f, 603t
    lateral mid-buttock/hip contour, **II:**601,
        601f
    lateral view aesthetics, **II:**602, 602f–603f

buttocks (*Continued*)
    lower inner gluteal fold/leg junction,
        II:601, 601f
    upper inner gluteal/sacral junction,
        II:600–601, 601f
    V-zone, **II:**600–601, 601f
  anatomical characteristics
    fascial system, **IV:**5
    innervation, **IV:**5–8, 7f
    musculature, **IV:**5, 5t
    skeletal structure, **IV:**2–5, 3f–4f
    vascular supply, **IV:**5, 7f
  buttock augmentation, **II:**599–616
    advantages/disadvantages, **II:**605t
    complications
      capsular contracture, **II:**614
      chronic pain, **II:**615
      hematologic and metabolic
          disturbances, **II:**614
      hyperpigmentation/skin discoloration,
          II:615
      implant exposure, **II:**614
      implant malposition, **II:**615, 615f
      implant rotation, **II:**615
      infections, **II:**613–614
      micro fat grafting (MFG), **II:**613–614
      neuropraxia, **II:**614–615
      seromas, **II:**614
      skin ulceration, **II:**615
      wound dehiscence, **II:**614, 614f
    ethnic ideals, **II:**603f–604f, 603t
    general characteristics, **II:**599
    implant placement and selection
      general discussion, **II:**599
      implant shape selection, **II:**607
      implant size determination, **II:**607–608,
          608f
      implant size selection, **II:**608
      intramuscular implant surgical
          technique, **I:**806–808
      intramuscular plane, **II:**606–607
      lateral view, **II:**608
      muscle height to width ratio, **II:**607,
          608f
      placement and selection, **II:**605–608
      sciatic nerve, **II:**607f
      subcutaneous plane, **II:**606, 606f
      subfascial plane, **II:**607, 607f
      submuscular plane, **II:**606, 607f
    intramuscular implant surgical technique
      anesthesia, **II:**609
      drains, **II:**610
      expanders, **II:**610
      implant placement/closure, **II:**610–611
      incision design/selection, **II:**609–611,
          610f
      markings, **II:**609
      muscle dissection, **II:**610
      positioning, **II:**609
      preoperative preparations, **II:**609
      sizers/implant size, **II:**610
      skin flap dissection, **II:**610
    micro fat grafting (MFG)
      complications, **II:**613–614
      general discussion, **II:**599
      postoperative care and follow-up,
          II:612
      pre-surgical markings, **II:**608–609
      surgical technique, **II:**609
    patient presentation and diagnosis, **II:**603

buttocks *(Continued)*
  patient selection
    aesthetic goals, **II**:605, 605t
    body frame determination, **II**:604
    guidelines, **II**:604–605
    potential candidates, **II**:604–605
  postoperative care and follow-up
    implant-based augmentation, **II**:613
    micro fat grafting (MFG), **II**:612
    patient activity, **II**:612–613
  prognosis and outcomes, **II**:613–615
  secondary procedures
    additional augmentation, **II**:616
    general discussion, **II**:615–616
    liposuction, **II**:616
    scar revision, **II**:616
  subfascial implant surgical technique
    markings, **II**:611, 611f
    surgical technique, **II**:611–612,
      611f–613f
  volume redistribution, **II**:603, 604f
congenital melanocytic nevi (CMN),
  III:844–848, 850f
fat deposition pattern, **II**:577f
gluteal aesthetic ideals, **II**:599–600, 600f, 603f
gluteus maximus muscle
  breast reconstruction, **V**:292
  characteristics, **I**:516f, **IV**:5
  clinical applications, **I**:523f–524f
  gluteal aesthetic ideals, **II**:600, 600f
  perineal reconstruction, **I**:557
  pressure sores, **I**:562–565, 566f–568f
gluteus medius muscle, **IV**:5
gluteus minimus muscle, **IV**:5
liposuctions, **II**:523, 524f
photographic guidelines, **I**:110, 115f–116f
post-bariatric surgery reconstruction
  major weight loss (MWL) patient, **II**:644b
  markings, **II**:645, 646f–647f, 649f
  operative technique, **II**:645, 647f–649f
  patient evaluation, **II**:644–645
  patient selection, **II**:645
  postoperative care and follow-up, **II**:645
topographical anatomy, **II**:600, 600f
buttresses, midface
  See midface buttress fractures
Butyrospermum parkii, **II**:18
Byzantine Empire, **I**:14

C
cadaver dissection, **I**:15f
cadaveric skin, **IV**:410–415
café-au-lait spots
  characteristics, **I**:725, 726f
  patient presentation and diagnosis, **III**:878
  surgical technique and treatment, **III**:878
calcifying epithelioma, **I**:721–722, 721f
calcineurin inhibitors, **I**:822t, 823
calcium (Ca)
  calcium alginate, **I**:289t
  calcium hydroxyapatite, **II**:47t
  calcium phosphate (CaP), **I**:445, 460–461
  calcium phosphates, **I**:792
  intracellular Ca²⁺ overload, **I**:576–577, 576f
  tricalcium phosphate, **II**:48t.
  see also soft-tissue fillers
Caldwell–Luc technique, **III**:402, 403f–404f,
  436

calvarium harvests, **I**:454–455, 454f
Camellia sinensis, **II**:27–28
cameras, **I**:117–119
Camitz palmaris longus transfer, **VI**:756–758,
  757f–759f, 761t
Campbell hand injury severity scale (HISS),
  VI:247
Camper, Petrus, **I**:18
Camper's fascia, **II**:656, **IV**:227–230, 227f
campomelic syndrome, **III**:807t
camptodactyly
  characteristics, **VI**:628
  epidemiology, **VI**:628
  outcomes and complicatons, **VI**:630
  patient presentation and diagnosis,
    VI:628–629
  patient selection, **VI**:629
  postoperative care and follow-up, **VI**:630
  secondary procedures, **VI**:630
  surgical technique and treatment, **VI**:546t,
    629–630, 629f–630f
Canadian Institutes for Health Research
  (CIHR), **I**:168–169
cancellous bone grafting, **I**:449
cancellous (trabecular) bone, **I**:426
cancer management
  background information, **I**:201
  cancer treatments
    biologics, **I**:206
    chemotherapy, **I**:204
    historical background, **I**:201–207
    immunotherapy, **I**:204–206, 205f–206f
    ionizing radiation, **I**:202–204
    neoadjuvant therapy, **I**:201–207
    photodynamic therapy, **I**:206–207
    surgery, **I**:202, 203f
  head and neck cancer
    cervical lymph nodes, **III**:415f
    complications
      dental follow-ups, **III**:418
      general discussion, **III**:416–418
      local recurrence, **III**:416
      osteoradionecrosis (ORN), **III**:417
      post-treatment surveillance, **III**:417–418
      regional recurrence, **III**:416–417
      wound infections, **III**:417
    epidemiology, **III**:399–400
    lymph node anatomy, **III**:399f
    medical challenges, **III**:398
    neck dissection
      basic procedure, **III**:413–416, 427, 429f
      modified radical neck dissection,
        III:414f–416f, 415–416
      supraomohyoid neck dissection,
        III:413–415
    nodal status determination, **III**:429–431,
      430f
    oral cavity/mouth/tongue/mandibular
      reconstruction, **III**:307–335
      acute complications, **III**:333
      challenges, **III**:307–308
      chronic complications, **III**:333–334
      decision-making process, **III**:311–313
      defect factors, **III**:310–311, 310t
      disease process, **III**:308
      flap options, **III**:310t
      free tissue transfer, **III**:311
      local/regional flaps, **III**:309t, 311

cancer management *(Continued)*
      patient factors, **III**:308–310, 310t
      patient presentation and diagnosis,
        III:308
      patient selection, **III**:308–316
      postoperative care and follow-up,
        III:332–333
      prognosis and outcomes, **III**:333–334
      secondary procedures, **III**:334
      skin grafts, **III**:311
      soft tissue flaps, **III**:309t
      surgical technique, **III**:316–332
    pathogenesis, **III**:398–399
    patient presentation and diagnosis, **III**:400
    psychological aspects, **I**:43–44
    radiation treatment, **I**:668–669
    risk factors
      alcohol, **III**:421
      gastroesophageal reflux, **III**:421
      infectious agents, **III**:421
      pollution exposure, **III**:421–422
      tobacco, **III**:421
    surgical access, **III**:402, 403f–404f
    therapeutic choices, **III**:401–402
    TNM clinical classification system,
      III:308, 400–401, 401t
    upper aerodigestive tract, **III**:420–439
      anatomical considerations, **III**:422–424
      diagnosis and treatment, **III**:427–437
      epidemiology, **III**:420
      future trends, **III**:438
      incidence, **III**:421–427
      outcomes and complicatons, **III**:438
      patient evaluation, **III**:424–427
      postoperative care and follow-up,
        III:437–438
      prevalence, **III**:421–427
      risk factors, **III**:421–422
  management approaches, **I**:208–210
  pathobiology
    critical mass, **I**:207
    tumor classifications, **I**:208
    tumor margins, **I**:207–208
  penile cancer, **IV**:313, 314f
  research summary, **I**:210
  See also breast cancer; tumors
Candida albicans, **VI**:337
Canterbury Tales (Chaucer), **V**:119–120
canthopexy, **II**:131–133, 133f–134f
Capanna technique, **IV**:180
capillary-arteriovenous malformation
  (CAVM), **I**:677t
capillary hemangioma, **I**:678t
capillary-lymphatic arteriovenous
  malformation (CLAVM), **I**:677t
capillary-lymphatic malformation (CLM),
  I:677t
capillary-lymphatic-overgrowthvascular-
  epidermal nevus (CLOVE)
  See CLOVES syndrome
capillary-lymphatic-venous malformation
  (CLVM), **I**:677t
capillary malformation-arteriovenous
  malformation (CM-AVM)
  classification systems, **I**:677t
  pathogenesis, **I**:692f, 696–698, 700, **VI**:691
  patient presentation and diagnosis, **VI**:691
  surgical technique and treatment, **VI**:691

capillary malformations (CM)
    classification systems, **I:**676–677, 677t, **VI:**668t
    clinical manifestations, **I:**688–689
    diagnostic work-up, **VI:**670t
    hemangioma simplex, **I:**734, 734f–735f
    pathogenesis, **I:**688, **VI:**675
    patient presentation and diagnosis, **VI:**669, 670f, 675, 677f
    strawberry hemangioma, **I:**678t, 734–735, 735f
    surgical technique and treatment, **VI:**669–672, 671t
    terminology, **I:**678t
    treatment strategies, **I:**679f, 689–690
capillary malformation venous malformation (CMVM), **VI:**668t, 682–684
capillary-venous malformation (CVM), **I:**677t
capsaicin, **V:**33t–35t
capsular calcification
    saline implants, **V:**110, 110f
    silicone gel implants, **V:**107–109, 108f–109f
capsular contracture
    Asian rhinoplasty, **II:**177
    breast augmentation, **V:**36–37, 263–264
    breast implants, **V:**336–340, 362, 362t–364t
    buttock augmentation, **II:**614
    classification systems, **V:**36t
    closed capsulotomy, **V:**107, 107f–108f
    revisionary breast surgery
        acellular dermal matrix (ADM), **V:**52–53, 52f
        Baker classifications, **V:**46–53, 362, 362t
        blood supply, **V:**49f
        capsulectomy, **V:**47, 48f–49f
        capsulotomies, **V:**47
        clinical studies, **V:**363t
        etiology, **V:**46t
        mastopexy, **V:**47, 48f
        neo subpectoral pocket conversion, **V:**50–52, 51f
        nipple-areola complex, **V:**49f
        subglandular to subpectoral conversion, **V:**50, 50f–51f
        surgical options, **V:**47t
        surgical technique and treatment, **V:**46–53, 49f, 77–78, 77f, 79t
    silicone gel implants, **V:**106–107, 106f–107f
capsulectomy, **V:**47, 48f–49f
capsulotomies, **V:**47, 107, 107f–108f
carbonated anesthesia, **I:**140, 140f, 148
carbon (C) alloys, **I:**786–787
carbon dioxide resurfacing lasers, **II:**21t, 461–462, **IV:**484
carboxyhemoglobinemia, **IV:**407–408, 408t
cardiovascular disease, **I:**226–228
cardiovascular toxicity, **I:**146
Carey–Fineman–Ziter syndrome, **III:**807t
carpal fractures
    epidemiology, **VI:**161, 162f
    magnetic resonance imaging (MRI), **VI:**85
carpal tunnel syndrome
    American Academy of Orthopaedic Surgeons clinical practice guidelines for the treatment of carpal tunnel syndrome, **VI:**507t
    anatomical considerations, **VI:**505, 506f
    basic procedure, **VI:**401–402, 401f
    etiology, **VI:**505
    nonsurgical management, **VI:**507

carpal tunnel syndrome (*Continued*)
    outcomes and complicatons, **VI:**401, 509–510, 509b
    patient presentation and diagnosis, **VI:**364–365, 505–507, 507b
    patient selection, **VI:**507
    post-nerve injury/surgery rehabilitation, **VI:**856–857
    postoperative care and follow-up, **VI:**401
    prevalence, **VI:**505–510
    secondary procedures, **VI:**401–402
    surgical technique and treatment
        Agee endoscopic carpal tunnel release (ECTR), **VI:**509
        anesthesia, **VI:**507–509, 507b, 508f
        Chow technique, **VI:**509
        endoscopic carpal tunnel release (ECTR), **VI:**509
        open carpal tunnel release (OCTR), **VI:**507–509
        palmaris brevis/thenar muscle preservation, **VI:**509f
    surgical tips, **VI:**402b
Carpenter syndrome, **VI:**573t
carpometacarpal (CMC) joints
    carpometacarpal (CMC) arthroscopy
        basic principles, **VI:**434–439
        Burton–Pelligrini procedure, **VI:**437–439, 438f
        dorsal wedge extension osteotomy, **VI:**435
        Eaton–Littler procedure, **VI:**435–437, 436f
        simple trapeziectomy, **VI:**437
        stage II-IV surgical procedures, **VI:**437
        trapeziectomy with ligament reconstruction and/or tendon interposition, **VI:**437–439, 438f–439f
        volar ligament reconstruction, **VI:**435–437
        Weilby suspensionplasty, **VI:**438, 439f
    fractures and joint injuries, **VI:**138–139, 153, 153f
    tetraplegic restoration
        IC group 4 and 5 patients, **VI:**834–838
        stable thumb CMC joints
            extensor phase, **VI:**838
            flexor phase, **VI:**838
            treatment strategies, **VI:**834–838
        unstable CMC joints
            extensor phase, **VI:**837
            flexor phase, **VI:**837
            postoperative care and follow-up, **VI:**837–838
            treatment strategies, **VI:**837
Carpue, Joseph Constantine, **I:**18–19, 19f
Carrol-Girard Screw, **III:**65
Carroll tests, **I:**835–837, **VI:**848
cartilage
    allografts, **I:**831
    Asian rhinoplasty, **II:**175
    autografts, **I:**830–831
    autologous fillers, **II:**46
    bone marrow-derived mesenchymal stem cells (BMSC), **I:**227–228
    characteristics, **I:**397–398, 398f
    chondrosarcoma, **I:**741, **VI:**329
    histologic studies, **I:**398f
    nasal anatomy
        anatomical characteristics, **II:**450–452
        characteristics, **II:**382–386

cartilage (*Continued*)
        external nasal valve, **II:**384f, 452f, 455
        internal nasal valve, **II:**384f, 452f, 455
        lower lateral cartilages, **II:**384f
        nasal ligaments, **II:**382f
        nasal vaults, **II:**382f, 384f
        schematic diagram, **II:**383f
        septum, **II:**384f–385f, 451f
        stabilization, **II:**385f
    repair and grafting, **I:**397–424
        autologous cartilage grafts
            auricular cartilage graft, **I:**398–404, 399f–405f
            general discussion, **I:**398–408
            nasal cartilage graft, **I:**404–407, 405f–407f
            nipple-areola complex reconstruction, **V:**514, 514f
            rib cartilage graft, **I:**407–408, 408f–411f
        autologous perichondrial grafts, **I:**408–413, 412f
        ear reconstruction, **III:**210, 212
        secondary rhinoplasty, **II:**470, 470f–471f
        tissue engineering
            auricular cartilage, **I:**413–419
            basic principles, **I:**413
            endonasal rhinoplasty, **I:**393–394, 394f
            facial contouring, **I:**419–421
            future trends, **I:**423–424
            in vitro cartilage engineering, **I:**423–424
            joint cartilage repair and reconstruction, **I:**421–423
            research background, **I:**413
            rhinoplasty, **I:**419–421
            stem cell-based cartilage engineering, **I:**423
            three-dimensional (3D) structural control, **I:**424
    xenografts, **I:**831
case studies
    evidence-based medicine and health service research
        case-control studies, **I:**155–156, 156f
        case series/case reports, **I:**156
    human resource management, **I:**84b
    innovation, **I:**80b
    Six Sigma program, **I:**78b
cash flow summary, **I:**68, 72f
cat bites, **VI:**343
CATCH 22, **I:**194–195
Catel–Mancke syndrome, **III:**805–807, 807t
Cat-eye syndrome, **VI:**573t
cationic liposomes, **I:**186, 187f, 188t
cat-scratch disease, **III:**891
cauliflower ear, **III:**212, 215f
cavernous hemangioma, **I:**678t, 735, 735f
CD4/CD8 T lymphocytes, **I:**47–48, 818–819, 827–828
CD25 T lymphocytes, **I:**827–828
cell adhesion molecules (CAMs), **I:**819–820
cell-assisted lipotransfer (CAL), **I:**345–346, 345f–347f
cell death, **I:**661–662
cellulite, **II:**509, 524–525
cellulitis, **II:**411, **V:**359, 360f, **VI:**336
Celsus, Aulus Cornelius, **I:**13–14, 14f
cement pastes
    BoneSource, **I:**461
    calcium phosphate (CaP), **I:**460–461
    Medpor, **I:**462

cement pastes (Continued)
  methylmethacrylate, **I**:462
  Norian SRS/CRS, **I**:461
  osteoactive materials, **I**:461–462
Center for Devices and Radiological Health
    (CDRH), **I**:847–849
central longitudinal deficiency, **VI**:546t
central nervous system
  local anesthesia effects, **I**:146
  progressive hemifacial atrophy (PHA),
    III:796
central polydactyly
  patient presentation and diagnosis, **VI**:618
  surgical technique and treatment, **VI**:546t,
    622, 622f
central ray deficiency
  associated syndromes, **VI**:565t
  characteristics, **VI**:563–564, 563b, 564f
  classification systems, **VI**:565t
  outcomes and complicatons, **VI**:566–567
  pathogenesis, **VI**:564
  patient presentation and diagnosis,
    VI:564–565, 564f
  patient selection, **VI**:565
  postoperative care and follow-up, **VI**:566
  secondary procedures, **VI**:567
  surgical technique and treatment, **VI**:565,
    565f–566f
cephalic trim, **II**:397, 398f
cephalic vein harvest, **III**:484–485, 485f
cephalometrics
  basic principles, **II**:360–363
  bone landmarks, **II**:363f
  craniofacial microsomia (CFM), **III**:774–775,
    776f
  facial profile classifications, **II**:361f
  malocclusions, **II**:362f
  maxillary and mandibular dental arches,
    II:362f
  orthodontic considerations, **II**:363–364
  software programs, **II**:363f
  temporomandibular joint (TMJ), **II**:364–365,
    364f
cephalopagus twins, **III**:896f–897f
ceramics, **I**:375, 792
cerebral cavernous malformation (CCM),
    I:677t, 693–694
cerebral palsy *See* spastic hand
cerebrocostomandibular syndrome, **III**:807t
cervical lymphadenectomy, **I**:771, 773f–774f
cervical lymph nodes, **III**:415f, 424, 427f
cervical myelography, **VI**:796
cervical spine injuries, **IV**:355–356, **VI**:817
cervical tuberculous adenitis (scrofula)
  disease process, **III**:891
  patient presentation and diagnosis, **III**:891
  surgical technique and treatment, **III**:891
cesium (Cs), **I**:656
chamomile, **II**:22
Champy technique, **III**:80–81, 80f
Chang Gung Craniofacial Center cleft
    treatment plan
  orthodontic treatment, **III**:522–523
  patient presentation and diagnosis,
    III:522–523, 522f
  surgical approach, **III**:522, 523f
Charcot deformities, **IV**:195
CHARGE association, **III**:805–807, 807t

charged couple devices (CCDs), **I**:117–119
charlatan doctors, **I**:27
Chase, Robert A, **II**:108–109
Chaucer, Geoffrey, **V**:119–120
Chauliac, Guy of, **I**:15
check rein ligaments, **VI**:13b, 456f
cheekbones, **II**:178
cheeks
  anesthesia, **III**:27, 27f–28f
  cheek flaps, **I**:22–23, 23f
  facial paralysis, **III**:291
  high SMAS technique, **II**:257–258
  melanoma excisions, **I**:766, 767f
  reconstructive surgeries, **III**:254–277
    burn wound treatment, **IV**:490–491, 506
    composite defects, **III**:274, 275f
    facial nerve, **III**:274
    importance, **III**:254–255
    local flaps
      anterolateral thigh flap, **III**:274
      cheek rotation advancement flap,
        III:271–272, 272f, 451, 451f–452f
      finger flap, **III**:452
      free tissue transfer, **III**:272
      island flap, **III**:452
      large cheek defects, **III**:452–453
      radial forearm flap, **III**:274
      scapular and parascapular flaps,
        III:273, 275f
      selection guidelines, **III**:271–274
      soft tissue cheek reconstruction,
        III:272–273
      submental artery flap, **III**:272,
        273f–274f
      transposition flap, **III**:452
    operative technique
      advancement flap, **III**:451–452, 453f
      basic principles, **III**:271
      finger flap, **III**:452
      island flap, **III**:452
      large cheek defects, **III**:452–453
      local flaps, **III**:271–274
      rotation flaps, **III**:451, 451f–452f
      transposition flap, **III**:452
    reconstructive burn surgery, **IV**:490–491,
      506
    research summary, **III**:274–276
    surgical guidelines, **III**:254
  traumatic injuries
    evaluation examinations, **III**:25, 25f
    facial nerve injury, **III**:45
    parotid duct repair, **III**:45, 45f
    surgical technique and treatment,
      III:44–45
chemical burns, **IV**:396
chemical carcinogenesis, **III**:398–399
chemical injury
  chemical burns, **IV**:396
  upper extremities, **IV**:456–467
    characteristics, **IV**:460–464
    complications, **IV**:464
    corrosive agents
      characteristics, **IV**:461
      patient presentation and diagnosis,
        IV:462
      phenol, **IV**:461–463
      secondary surgical treatment, **IV**:463
      white phosphorus, **IV**:461–463

chemical injury (Continued)
  desiccants
    characteristics, **IV**:461
    patient presentation and diagnosis,
      IV:462
    secondary surgical treatment, **IV**:463
    sulfuric acid, **IV**:461–463
  disease process
    classifications, **IV**:460–461
    corrosive agents, **IV**:461
    desiccants, **IV**:461
    oxidizing agents, **IV**:460–461
    pathophysiology, **IV**:460
    protoplasmic poisons, **IV**:461
    reducing agents, **IV**:461
    vesicants, **IV**:461
  oxidizing agents
    characteristics, **IV**:460–461
    chromic acid, **IV**:460–461, 463
    patient presentation and diagnosis,
      IV:461–462
    secondary surgical treatment, **IV**:463
    sodium hypochlorite, **IV**:461–463
  patient presentation and diagnosis
    characteristics, **IV**:461–462
    corrosive agents, **IV**:462
    desiccants, **IV**:462
    oxidizing agents, **IV**:461–462
    protoplasmic poisons, **IV**:462
    reducing agents, **IV**:462
    vesicants, **IV**:462
  patient selection, **IV**:462
  postoperative care and follow-up,
    IV:464
  prognosis and outcomes, **IV**:464
  protoplasmic poisons
    characteristics, **IV**:461
    formic acid, **IV**:461–463
    hydrofluoric acid, **IV**:461–462, 464
    patient presentation and diagnosis,
      IV:462
    secondary surgical treatment,
      IV:463–464
  reducing agents
    characteristics, **IV**:461
    hydrochloric acid, **IV**:461–463
    patient presentation and diagnosis,
      IV:462
    secondary surgical treatment, **IV**:463
  research summary, **IV**:456
  secondary procedures, **IV**:464
  secondary surgical treatment
    characteristics, **IV**:463–464
    corrosive agents, **IV**:463
    desiccants, **IV**:463
    oxidizing agents, **IV**:463
    protoplasmic poisons, **IV**:463–464
    reducing agents, **IV**:463
    vesicants, **IV**:463
  surgical technique and treatment
    primary treatment, **IV**:462–463
    secondary treatment, **IV**:463–464
  vesicants
    characteristics, **IV**:461
    mustard gas, **IV**:461–463
    patient presentation and diagnosis,
      IV:462
    secondary surgical treatment, **IV**:463

chemical peeling methods
  characteristics, II:62
  patient selection and treatment, II:66–67
  wound healing biology
    characteristics, II:62–63
    inflammatory response, II:62
    proliferation phase, II:62
    remodeling phase, II:63
chemokines
  inflammatory mediators, I:819–820
  skin wound healing, I:275
  wound healing, I:244–245
chemotherapy
  breast cancer, I:668
  cutaneous and soft-tissue tumors, I:717–718
  sarcomas, IV:106
Cheng's defect classification, III:317t–318t
Chen scale, VI:247, 247t
chest
  anatomical characteristics
    general characteristics, IV:223–227, 225f
    musculature, IV:224–225
    vascular anatomy, IV:225–227, 226f
  male chest
    body contouring
      excision of gynecomastia with nipple
        repositioning, V:575–579, 578f–580f
      outcomes and complicatons, V:579
      pathophysiology, V:573–574
      patient presentation and diagnosis,
        V:574
      patient selection, V:574–575, 575t
      postoperative care and follow-up,
        V:578
      pseudogynecomastia, V:575t, 576f–577f
      surgical markings, V:575–576, 576f–577f
      surgical technique and treatment,
        V:576–578, 578f–580f
      surgical tips, V:578b
    post-bariatric surgery reconstruction,
      II:652
  pediatric chest and trunk defects,
    III:855–876
    abdominal wall defects, III:865–866
    congenital defects, III:855
    ectopia cordis
      characteristics, III:861–862, 862f
      clinical presentation and evaluation,
        III:861, 862f–863f
      surgical indicators, III:861
      treatment strategies, III:861–862
    embryology, III:855
    Jeune's syndrome
      characteristics, III:860–861, 861f
      clinical presentation and evaluation,
        III:861
      surgical indicators, III:861
      treatment strategies, III:861, 862f
    omphalocele and gastroschisis
      characteristics, III:865–866
      clinical presentation and evaluation,
        III:865, 866f
      surgical indicators, III:865
      treatment strategies, III:865–866
    pectus carinatum
      characteristics, III:859–860, 859f
      clinical presentation and evaluation,
        III:859
      surgical indicators, III:859
      treatment strategies, III:859–860, 860f

chest (Continued)
    pectus excavatum
      characteristics, III:855–859
      clinical presentation and evaluation,
        III:855–856, 856f
      minimally invasive repair of pectus
        excavatum (MIRPE), III:858, 859f
      Ravitch repair, III:857, 858f
      surgical indicators, III:856
      treatment strategies, III:856–859,
        857f–858f
    Poland syndrome
      characteristics, III:862–865
      clinical presentation and evaluation,
        III:863, 863f–864f
      surgical indicators, III:863
      treatment strategies, III:864–865,
        864f–865f
    posterior defects
      dermal sinuses, III:874
      diastematomyelia, III:874
      embryology, III:866
      postanal pits, III:874
      sacrococcygeal teratoma, III:874
      spina bifida, III:866–874
    sacrococcygeal teratoma
      characteristics, III:874
      clinical presentation and evaluation,
        III:874
      surgical indicators, III:874
      treatment strategies, III:874
    spina bifida
      characteristics, III:866–874
      clinical presentation and evaluation,
        III:867
      meningomyeloceles, III:868t–869t,
        872–874, 873f
      paraspinal flap method, III:872–874,
        873f–875f
      surgical indicators, III:867
      treatment strategies, III:867–872,
        868t–869t, 870f–872f
    thoracic wall defects
      ectopia cordis, III:861–862
      Jeune's syndrome, III:860–861
      pectus carinatum, III:859–860
      pectus excavatum, III:855–859
      Poland syndrome, III:862–865
  photographic guidelines, I:110, 113f–114f
  post-bariatric surgery reconstruction, II:652
  reconstructive surgeries, IV:239–255
    bronchopleural fistula
      outcome assessments, IV:252
      pathogenesis, IV:252
      schematic diagram, IV:254f
      surgical technique and treatment, IV:252
    chest wall osteomyelitis
      outcome assessments, IV:252
      pathogenesis, IV:252
      surgical technique and treatment,
        IV:252
    chest wall sections, IV:240t
    chest wall tumors
      outcome assessments, IV:249
      pathogenesis, IV:247
      patient presentation and diagnosis,
        IV:247, 247f
      patient selection, IV:247
      surgical technique and treatment,
        IV:248f, 249

chest (Continued)
    empyema
      outcome assessments, IV:252
      pathogenesis, IV:252
      surgical technique and treatment,
        IV:252
      treatment strategies, IV:253f
    flaps
      latissimus dorsi (LD) flap, I:552–553,
        IV:241, 243f–244f
      muscle/musculocutaneous flaps,
        I:552–553
      omentum, IV:245, 246f–247f
      pectoralis major muscle, IV:241,
        241f–242f
      rectus abdominis, I:552–553, IV:244–
        245, 245f
      serratus anterior muscles, I:552, IV:244,
        244f
    mediastinitis/sternal wounds
      outcome assessments, IV:251
      pathogenesis, IV:249
      patient presentation and diagnosis,
        IV:249
      surgical technique and treatment,
        IV:249–251, 250f–252f
      wound classifications, IV:249t
    muscle-sparing thoracotomy, IV:239, 240f
    osteoradionecrosis (ORN)
      pathogenesis, IV:252–253, 254f
      surgical technique and treatment,
        IV:253
    patient selection, IV:247
    secondary procedures, IV:255
    skeletal support, IV:239, 240f
    traumatic chest wall deformities
      occurrence, IV:253
      outcome assessments, IV:255
      patient presentation and diagnosis,
        IV:253
      patient selection, IV:253–255
      surgical technique and treatment,
        IV:253–255, 255f
  robotic surgery, I:863
Chiari malformations, III:751
CHILD (congenital hemidysplasia with
  ichthyosiform erythroderma and limb
  defects) syndrome, VI:573t
children
  amputations, VI:230–231, 230t–231t, 244
  chest and trunk defects, III:855–876
    abdominal wall defects, III:865–866
    congenital defects, III:855
    ectopia cordis
      characteristics, III:861–862, 862f
      clinical presentation and evaluation,
        III:861, 862f–863f
      surgical indicators, III:861
      treatment strategies, III:861–862
    embryology, III:855
    Jeune's syndrome
      characteristics, III:860–861, 861f
      clinical presentation and evaluation,
        III:861
      surgical indicators, III:861
      treatment strategies, III:861, 862f
    omphalocele and gastroschisis
      characteristics, III:865–866
      clinical presentation and evaluation,
        III:865, 866f

children (Continued)
  surgical indicators, III:865
  treatment strategies, III:865–866
pectus carinatum
  characteristics, III:859–860, 859f
  clinical presentation and evaluation,
    III:859
  surgical indicators, III:859
  treatment strategies, III:859–860, 860f
pectus excavatum
  characteristics, III:855–859
  clinical presentation and evaluation,
    III:855–856, 856f
  minimally invasive repair of pectus
    excavatum (MIRPE), III:858, 859f
  Ravitch repair, III:857, 858f
  surgical indicators, III:856
  treatment strategies, III:856–859,
    857f–858f
Poland syndrome
  characteristics, III:862–865
  clinical presentation and evaluation,
    III:863, 863f–864f
  surgical indicators, III:863
  treatment strategies, III:864–865,
    864f–865f
posterior defects
  dermal sinuses, III:874
  diastematomyelia, III:874
  embryology, III:866
  postanal pits, III:874
  sacrococcygeal teratoma, III:874
  spina bifida, III:866–874
sacrococcygeal teratoma
  characteristics, III:874
  clinical presentation and evaluation,
    III:874
  surgical indicators, III:874
  treatment strategies, III:874
spina bifida
  characteristics, III:866–874
  clinical presentation and evaluation,
    III:867
  meningomyeloceles, III:868t–869t,
    872–874, 873f
  paraspinal flap method, III:872–874,
    873f–875f
  surgical indicators, III:867
  treatment strategies, III:867–872,
    868t–869t, 870f–872f
thoracic wall defects
  ectopia cordis, III:861–862
  Jeune's syndrome, III:860–861
  pectus carinatum, III:859–860
  pectus excavatum, III:855–859
  Poland syndrome, III:862–865
childhood plastic surgeries
  acquired and congenital defects, I:44
  adolescent aesthetic surgery, I:45–46, 45t
  craniofacial deformities, I:44–45
  tissue expansion, I:629
congenital melanocytic nevi (CMN), III:844
epiphyseal growth plate, VI:651–666
  anatomical characteristics, VI:651–652,
    652f
  epiphyseal transfer
    harvesting methods, VI:660–664
    indicators, VI:659–660

children (Continued)
    proximal humerus reconstruction,
      VI:659–660, 659f–660f
    vascular supply, VI:660, 661f
  growth plate closure, VI:652–654
  outcomes and complicatons, VI:664–665,
    665f
  patient presentation and diagnosis
    trauma injuries, VI:654–655
    tumors, VI:655–656
  patient selection, VI:656, 656f
  physeal arrest
    bar resection, VI:657–658, 657f–658f
    corrective osteotomies, VI:658–659
    epiphysiodesis, VI:657
    lengthening or shortening treatments,
      VI:658–659
    observational studies, VI:657
    partial physeal arrest completion,
      VI:657
    physeal distraction, VI:657
  postoperative care and follow-up
    donor sites, VI:664
    recipient sites, VI:664
  proximal fibular epiphysis harvesting
    anterior tibial pedicle exposure, VI:661,
      662f
    basic procedure, VI:660–664
    biceps femoris tendon, VI:662, 663f
    distal osteotomy, VI:662
    interosseous membrane dissection,
      VI:662, 663f
    peroneal nerve dissection, VI:661–662,
      662f
    proximal tibiofibular joint capsulotomy,
      VI:662, 663f
    skin incision, VI:661, 661f
    vascular pedicle dissection, VI:662–664,
      664f
  puberty-related skeletal assessments,
    VI:652–654, 653f
  secondary procedures
    donor sites, VI:665
    recipient sites, VI:665
  surgical technique and treatment
    epiphyseal transfer, VI:659–664
    physeal arrest, VI:656–659
  trauma injuries
    fracture classifications, VI:654–655,
      654f–655f
    fracture treatment, V:410
    incidence and distribution, VI:654
  tumors
    bone sarcoma, VI:655, 656f
    congenital chondrodysplasia,
      VI:655–656
  vascular anatomy, VI:652
flexor tendon injuries, VI:196–197
pediatric brachial plexus injury
  characteristics, VI:790t, 805–806, 805b
  infant obstetric brachial plexus palsy
    background information, VI:806–812
    clinical examination, VI:806–808,
      808f–809f
    clinical presentation, VI:806, 807f
    imaging methods, VI:809f
    injury type incidence, VI:810t
    intraoperative findings, VI:810t

children (Continued)
    nerve graft results, VI:811–812,
      812f–813f
    outcome assessments, VI:811, 812t
    postoperative care and follow-up,
      VI:810–811, 811f
    preoperative preparations, VI:808
    reconstructive strategies, VI:810, 810t
    rupture–avulsion injuries, VI:810,
      810t–811t
    rupture injuries, VI:810, 810t
    surgical technique and treatment,
      VI:808–809
    surgical timing, VI:808
  injury type incidence, VI:810t
  intraoperative findings, VI:810t
  nerve graft results, VI:811–812, 812f–813f
  outcome assessments, VI:811, 812t
  postoperative care and follow-up,
    VI:810–811, 811f
  research summary, VI:815
  rupture–avulsion injuries, VI:810,
    810t–811t
  rupture injuries, VI:810, 810t
  sequelae obstetric brachial plexus palsy
    characteristics, VI:812–815
    elbow deformity reconstruction, VI:815
    examination chart, VI:814t
    forearm and hand deformity
      reconstruction, VI:815
    shoulder deformity reconstruction,
      VI:813–815
pediatric facial fractures, III:671–685
  associated injuries, III:672
  background information, III:671
  demographics, III:672
  growth and development factors
    basic principles, III:672–674
    condylar head fractures, III:678f
    cranial-to-facial ratio, III:672f
    Le Fort fracture patterns, III:675f
    mandibular condyle, III:677f
    oblique craniofacial fracture patterns,
      III:676f–677f
    orbital region, III:674f
    sinus development, III:673f
  incidence, III:671–672
  orbital fracture classification system,
    III:677t
  orbital fractures, III:54, 54f
  outcomes and complicatons
    adverse outcome classifications, III:683t
    basic principles, III:682–683
    cranial base/skull fractures, III:683
    mandible fractures, III:684, 684f
    maxillary and midface fractures,
      III:684
    metallic cranial hardware, III:683f–684f
    nasal fractures, III:684
    orbital fractures, III:683–684
    zygomaticomaxillary complex
      fractures, III:684
  patient presentation and diagnosis,
    III:674–675, 678f–679f
  patient selection, III:675–678
  postoperative care and follow-up, III:682
  research summary, III:685
  secondary procedures, III:684–685

children (Continued)
surgical technique and treatment
basic procedure, III:678
cranial base/frontal skull fractures, III:678–679, 679f–680f
mandible fractures, III:681f–682f, 682
maxillary and midface fractures, III:680, 681f
nasal and naso-orbital ethmoid fractures, III:681–682, 681t, 682f
orbital fractures, III:679–680, 680f
zygomaticomaxillary complex fractures, III:681
pediatric hand fractures, VI:139, 158, 158f
pediatric hand radiographs, VI:71–72, 72f–73f
pediatric plastic surgeries
acquired and congenital defects, I:44
adolescent aesthetic surgery, I:45–46, 45t
craniofacial deformities, I:44–45
tissue expansion, I:629
pediatric tumors, III:877–892
background and general characteristics, III:877
branchial cleft anomalies
characteristics, III:885, 885f
first branchial cleft anomaly, III:886
fourth branchial cleft anomaly, III:887
second branchial cleft anomaly, III:885–886, 885f
third branchial cleft anomaly, III:886–887
dermoids
dermal sinus tracts, III:883–884
external angular dermoids, III:884–885
general characteristics, III:882
intradural dermoids, III:883–884
nasal dermoids, III:882–883, 882f
neck cysts, III:885
epiphyseal growth plate
bone sarcoma, VI:655, 656f
congenital chondrodysplasia, VI:655–656
lymphadenopathy
atypical nontuberculous mycobacteria, III:891–892
bacterial lymphadenitis, III:890–891
cervical tuberculous adenitis (scrofula), III:891
characteristics, III:890
chronic regional lymphadenopathy, III:891
neurofibromatoses
café-au-lait spots, III:878
congenital fibromatosis, III:881
craniofacial manifestation, III:878, 879f
definition, III:877
disease process, III:877–878
fibromatosis colli, III:880–881
general discussion, III:877
gingival fibroma, III:881
glomus tumors, III:878
infantile digital fibroma, III:881, 881f
juvenile aggressive fibromatosis, III:880
juvenile nasopharyngeal angiofibroma, III:881
Lisch nodules, III:878
neurofibromas, III:880
neurofibrosarcomas, III:880
optic nerve gliomas, III:878

children (Continued)
peripheral nerve sheath malignancies, III:880
pilomatrixoma
characteristics, III:888
complications, III:888
disease process, III:888
patient presentation and diagnosis, III:888, 888f
postoperative care and follow-up, III:888
prognosis and outcomes, III:888
surgical technique and treatment, III:888
soft-tissue sarcomas
alveolar soft-part sarcoma, III:890
rhabdomycosarcoma, III:888–889
synovial soft-tissue sarcoma, III:889–890
thryoglossal duct cysts
characteristics, III:887
complications, III:887–888
disease process, III:887
patient presentation and diagnosis, III:887, 887f
prognosis and outcomes, III:887–888
surgical technique and treatment, III:887
trigger thumb
etiology, VI:648
general discussion, VI:648–649
timing considerations, VI:546t
treatment strategies, VI:648–649
upper extremities
epiphyseal growth plate, VI:651–666
anatomical characteristics, VI:651–652, 652f
growth plate closure, VI:652–654
patient presentation and diagnosis, VI:654–656
patient selection, VI:656, 656f
puberty-related skeletal assessments, VI:652–654, 653f
surgical technique and treatment, VI:656–664
vascular anatomy, VI:652
physical examinations, VI:67
surgical technique and treatment
anesthesia, VI:103
epiphyseal growth plate, VI:651–666
chimeric flaps, I:612, 612f
chin
anesthesia, III:27, 28f
anthropometric analysis, II:360, 361f
Asian facial bone surgery, II:178–179
burn wound treatment, IV:489, 492f–494f, 498–499
chin augmentation
adolescent aesthetic surgery, I:45t
botulinum toxin type-A (BoNT-A), II:41
characteristics, II:346, 349f–350f
implant augmentation versus sliding genioplasty, II:348
surgical technique, II:347–348, 350f–351f
chin implants, III:240, 240f–241f
Treacher Collins syndrome, III:828–830
Chinese agrimony, V:33t–35t
Chinese peony, V:33t–35t
Chinese writing-type fibrous dysplasia, III:381
Chitayat syndrome, III:807t

chitosan, I:376f
chlorine (Cl)
hydrochloric acid, IV:461–463
sodium hypochlorite, IV:461–463
chloroprocaine, VI:96t
cholesterol biosynthesis and metabolism, III:515
chondrodysplasia, VI:655–656
chondroid syringoma, I:723, 723f
chondroitin, V:33t–35t
chondrosarcoma, I:741, IV:103, 247, 248f, VI:329
Chopart amputation, IV:208
Chordin, III:505
chorionic villus sampling (CVS), I:199
Chow technique, VI:509
chromatin, I:181–182, 181f
chromium (Cr)
chromic acid, IV:460–461, 463
cobalt-chromium alloys, I:787
metal alloy compositions, I:786–787
chronic nerve compression
numerical grading scale
median nerve, IV:154t
peripheral nerves, IV:154t
tibial nerve, IV:155t
ulnar nerve, IV:155t
outcomes and complicatons, IV:172–173, 172t
pathogenesis, IV:153–155
patient presentation and diagnosis, IV:157
patient selection, IV:158
postoperative care and follow-up, IV:170–172, 172f
Pressure-Specified Sensory Device (PSSD), IV:154, 158f
research background, IV:151–152
surgical technique and treatment
basic procedure, IV:164–170
medial ankle tunnel release, IV:167f
peroneal nerves, IV:168f–170f
surgical tips, IV:164b, 166b
tarsal tunnel, IV:167f
tibial nerve, IV:171f
tarsal tunnel decompression, IV:172t
chronic regional lymphadenopathy
complications, III:891
disease process, III:891
patient presentation and diagnosis, III:891
prognosis and outcomes, III:891
chronic rejection, I:819
chronic ulnar collateral ligament (UCL) tear, VI:155–156, 156f
chronic wounds
arterial ulcers, I:253–254
definition, I:253–256
diabetic ulcers, I:254–255, 254f
foot injuries, IV:196
pressure ulcers, I:255–256
treatment strategies, I:287
venous ulcers, I:253
wound infection, I:249–250
Chuang modification, VI:796t
chylothorax, IV:433t
cicatrices See scars
cicatricial alopecia, III:109–110, 111t
circumferential abdominoplasty, II:551
circumferential dermatolipectomy
anatomical considerations, II:568–569, 569f
characteristics, II:551

circumferential dermatolipectomy (Continued)
  complications
    deep vein thrombosis (DVT), II:593–594
    dehiscence, II:591
    general discussion, II:589–595
    infections, II:592
    psychological difficulties, II:594–595
    pulmonary embolisms, II:593–594
    seromas, II:590
    tissue necrosis, II:592–593, 595f
    wound separation, II:590–591
  disease process
    massive weight loss patients, II:569, 570f
    normal weight patients group, II:570, 572f–573f
    20–30 pounds overweight group, II:569, 571f
  general discussion, II:568
  outcome assessments
    characteristics, II:588–595
    group I patients, II:589f–590f
    group II patients, II:591f–592f
    group III patients, II:593f–594f
  patient presentation and diagnosis
    back roll presentations, II:571, 578f
    body mass index (BMI), II:570, 574f
    buttocks variations, II:577f
    commonalities, II:570–571
    fat deposition pattern, II:570, 574f–575f
    hanging panniculi, II:576f
    skin/fat envelope, II:570, 574f–575f
  patient selection
    belt lipectomy/central bodylift, II:572–574, 574b
    general discussion, II:571–580
    lower bodylift type II (Lockwood technique), II:571–572, 573b, 579f
    preoperative assessment, II:577–580
    selection criteria, II:574–576, 577b
  postoperative care and follow-up, II:588, 588b
  secondary procedures, II:595
  surgical technique and treatment
    belt lipectomy
      anesthesia, II:585–588
      dissection techniques, II:587f
      goals, II:580, 580b
      markings, II:580–585, 583f–584f
      positioning, II:587f
      positioning sequence, II:585
      suturing techniques, II:585–588, 586f
      excisional tension, II:580–585, 580f–582f
      surgical rationale, II:580–585
    upper bodylift considerations, II:595, 596f–597f
  zones of adherence, II:568–569, 569f
circumflex iliac osteocutaneous flap, III:322, 323f
circumflex scapular and thoracodorsal pedicles, I:530f
circumflex scapular artery, IV:222f, 223
cisplatin, I:779–781
citalopram, I:51
Claoué, Charles, I:24
Clark classification of melanoma, I:753–756, 756f
Clark's nevus, I:724
clavicle, IV:185

clawing of the fingers
  Bouvier maneuver, VI:764–765, 764f
  Brand EE4T transfer, VI:766–767, 766f
  Brand EF4T transfer, VI:767, 767f–768f
  donor muscle-tendon selection, VI:764–765, 765f
  Fritschi PF4T transfer, VI:767–768
  Littler modification, VI:764–765
  modified Stiles–Bunnell technique, VI:764–766, 765f
  pulley insertions, VI:764–765, 764f–765f
  static procedures, VI:763–764, 763f–764f
cleansers
  bar surfactants
    characteristics, II:16
    combination bars, II:16
    superfatted soaps, II:16
    synthetic detergent bars, II:16
    transparent soaps, II:16
  characteristics, II:16
  liquid surfactants, II:16
cleft lip surgery
  bilateral cleft lip, III:550–568
    bilateral variation modifications
      asymmetrical bilateral cleft lip, III:560–562, 563f–564f
      bilateral complete cleft lip and intact secondary palate, III:558–559, 561f
      bilateral incomplete cleft lip, III:559–560, 562f
      binderoid bilateral complete cleft lip/palate, III:558, 560f
      late presentation, III:557–558
    challenges, III:550–551
    multidimensional nasolabial features, III:551
    orthodontic treatment
      distraction procedures, III:602–611, 609f–611f
      growth considerations, III:611
      infants, III:596–597
      orthognathic surgery, III:602–611, 607f
      permanent dentition, III:602–611
      transitional dentition, III:597–602, 601f
    outcome assessments
      direct anthropometric measurements, III:565, 566f
      general discussion, III:563–568
      indirect anthropometric measurements, III:565–568
      photogrammetry, III:565–567
      photographic documentation, III:563
      revision rates, III:564–565
      stereophotogrammetry, III:567–568, 567f
    patient presentation, III:551–552, 552f
    preoperative dentofacial orthopedics, III:552–553, 553f
    research summary, III:568
    surgical principles, III:550–551
    surgical technique
      alveolar closure, III:555, 555f
      labial closure, III:555–556, 555f
      labial dissection, III:554, 554f
      lower lateral cartilage positioning, III:556, 556f–557f
      markings, III:553–554, 554f
      nasal dissection, III:556, 556f–557f

cleft lip surgery (Continued)
      philtral dimple, III:556–557, 558f
      postoperative care and follow-up, III:557, 559f
      timing considerations, III:553–557
  closed rhinoplasty, II:442
  Le Fort I osteotomy, III:663–665, 663f, 669t
  nineteenth century, I:19–20
  orthodontic treatment, III:595–613
    bilateral cleft lip
      distraction procedures, III:602–611, 609f–611f
      growth considerations, III:611
      infants, III:596–597
      orthognathic surgery, III:602–611, 607f
      permanent dentition, III:602–611
      transitional dentition, III:597–602, 601f
    distraction procedures, III:602–611, 609f–611f
    growth considerations, III:611
    infants
      bilateral cleft lip, III:596–597
      treatment strategies, III:596–597
      unilateral cleft lip, III:596
    management goals, III:595–596
    orthognathic surgery, III:602–611, 607f–608f
    permanent dentition, III:602–611, 603f–606f
    primary dentition
      anterior crossbite, III:597
      posterior crossbite, III:597
    research summary, III:611
    transitional dentition, III:597–602, 598f–601f
    unilateral cleft lip
      Chang Gung Craniofacial Center treatment plan, III:522–523
      distraction procedures, III:602–611, 609f
      growth considerations, III:611
      infants, III:596
      orthognathic surgery, III:602–611, 607f–608f
      permanent dentition, III:602–611, 603f–606f
      transitional dentition, III:597–602, 598f–601f
  orthognathic surgery, III:663–665, 663f–664f
  patient presentation and diagnosis, III:570–571, 571f
  Renaissance, I:15–16, 16f
  secondary cleft deformities, III:631–654
    cleft lip
      cleft lip anatomy, III:633, 634f
      evaluation examinations, III:634–635, 635f
      normal lip anatomy, III:633, 633f–634f
      patient selection, III:635
      scarring considerations, III:635, 636f
      timing considerations, III:635
    etiology, III:631
    lips
      Cupid's bow, III:639
      long lip, III:637
      philtral column reconstruction, III:638–639, 639f
      short lateral lip, III:638
      short lip, III:635–637, 636f

cleft lip surgery (Continued)
  tight lip, III:637, 637f–638f
  wide lip, III:637–638
  patient presentation and diagnosis,
      III:632
  vermillion
    buccal sulcus deformities, III:641–642,
        641f
    orbicularis muscle deformities,
        III:640–641
    thick lip, III:639
    thin lip, III:639, 640f
    vermillion mismatch, III:639–640
    vermillion notching/vermillion border
        malalignment, III:640
    whistle deformity, III:640
  wound healing and growth, III:631–632,
      632f–633f
training simulators, I:867, 867f
unilateral cleft lip, III:517–549
  adjustment surgeries
    free border of the lateral lip, III:539,
        540f
    general discussion, III:537–539
    long horizontal length of cleft side lip,
        III:539
    long vertical height of cleft side lip,
        III:539
    long vertical length of cleft side lip,
        III:537
    short horizontal length of cleft side lip,
        III:539
    short vertical length of cleft side lip,
        III:539
  Chang Gung Craniofacial Center
      treatment plan
    orthodontic treatment, III:522–523
    patient presentation and diagnosis,
        III:522–523, 522f
    surgical approach, III:522, 523f
  characteristics, III:519f–521f
  classification systems, III:518–519, 519f
  complications, III:545
  general discussion, III:517
  genetic considerations, III:517–518, 518t
  incidence, III:517–518, 518t
  microform cleft lip
    pathology, III:542, 542f
    surgical correction techniques, III:542,
        543f
  nasoalveolar molding
    Grayson's method, III:524, 526f
    Liou's method, III:524, 524f–525f
  nasolabial adhesion cheiloplasty
    advantages/disadvantages, III:525–526
    C flap mucosa elevation and insertion,
        III:527, 527f
    lateral lip incisions, III:527, 528f
    markings, III:526, 527f
    mucosal flaps, III:527, 528f
    muscle and skin closure, III:527
    nostril floor closure, III:527, 528f
    post-adhesion definitive cheiloplasty,
        III:527, 529f
    surgical technique, III:526–527
    two-stage palate repair, III:525
  orthodontic treatment
    Chang Gung Craniofacial Center
        treatment plan, III:522–523
    distraction procedures, III:602–611, 609f

cleft lip surgery (Continued)
    growth considerations, III:611
    infants, III:596
    orthognathic surgery, III:602–611,
        607f–608f
    permanent dentition, III:602–611,
        603f–606f
    transitional dentition, III:597–602,
        598f–601f
  outcome assessments
    long-term lip morphology, III:542–543,
        544f
    long-term nasal morphology, III:543–
        544, 545f
    patient and parental satisfaction, III:545
  pathological diversity, III:519, 519f–521f
  patient presentation and diagnosis
    anthropometrics, III:519–522
    lip measurements and markings,
        III:520–522, 521f
    prenatal diagnosis, III:517
  research summary, III:548
  rotation advancement cheiloplasty
      (complete clefts)
    adequate rotation, III:530–531, 531f,
        535, 536f
    alar base mobilization, III:532
    alar base repositioning, III:532, 533f
    basic principles, III:527–539
    C flap incisions, III:531, 531f–532f
    final skin closure, III:535, 536f
    free border of the lip closure, III:534,
        535f
    inferior turbinate flap, III:532, 532f
    lateral lip incisions, III:530f, 531, 532f
    medial incisions, III:530, 530f
    muscle reconstruction, III:533, 534f
    nasal floor incisions, III:534–535, 535f
    nasal floor reconstruction, III:532, 533f
    orbicularis marginalis flap elevation,
        III:532, 533f
    orbicularis muscle dissection, III:532
    philtral column reconstruction, III:533
    piriform deficiency correction, III:532,
        533f
    preoperative markings, III:530f
    semi-open rhinoplasty, III:535–537
    triangular vermillion flap incisions,
        III:533–534, 534f
  rotation advancement cheiloplasty
      (incomplete clefts)
    basic principles, III:539–542
    excessive skin trimming, III:540–542
    markings and incisions, III:539, 540f
    muscle dissection and release, III:540
    muscle reconstruction, III:540
    nasal correction, III:540, 541f
    nasal floor incisions, III:540, 541f
    nasal floor reconstruction, III:540, 541f
    orbicularis marginalis flap elevation,
        III:540
  secondary procedures
    Cupid's bow, III:545, 546f
    flared ala-facial groove, III:547
    free border repair, III:546, 546f–547f
    horizontal shortness of the lateral lip,
        III:546
    infrasill depression, III:547
    lower lateral cartilage correction,
        III:547

cleft lip surgery (Continued)
    secondary rhinoplasty, III:547–548, 548f
    soft triangle of nostril hood, III:547
    vermillion repair, III:546
    vertical discrepancy of the lateral lip,
        III:545–546
    vestibular webbing, III:547
    wide nostril repair, III:546
  semi-open rhinoplasty
    alar base positioning, III:536–537
    alar-facial groove creation, III:537,
        538f–539f
    background information, III:535–537
    excessive skin trimming, III:536, 537f
    fibrofatty tissue release, III:536, 537f
    incisions, III:536, 537f
    lower lateral cartilage repositioning,
        III:536, 537f
  surgical technique and treatment
    adhesion cheiloplasty, III:525
    adjustment surgeries, III:537–539
    alveolar molding, III:523–524,
        523f–524f
    Chang Gung Craniofacial Center
        treatment plan, III:522–523
    microform cleft lip, III:542
    nasoalveolar molding, III:524
    nasolabial adhesion cheiloplasty,
        III:526–527
    postoperative care and follow-up,
        III:542, 543f
    postoperative management of nasal
        shape, III:542, 544f
    presurgical orthopedics, III:523f, 525
    rotation advancement cheiloplasty
        (complete clefts), III:527–539
    rotation advancement cheiloplasty
        (incomplete clefts), III:539–542
cleft palate surgery, III:569–583
  nineteenth century, I:19–20
  orthodontic treatment, III:595–613
    distraction procedures, III:602–611,
        609f–611f
    growth considerations, III:611
    infants, III:596–597
    management goals, III:595–596
    orthognathic surgery, III:602–611,
        607f–608f
    permanent dentition, III:602–611,
        603f–606f
    primary dentition
      anterior crossbite, III:597
      posterior crossbite, III:597
    research summary, III:611
    transitional dentition, III:597–602,
        598f–601f
  palatal development
    anatomical characteristics, III:569, 570f
    ear pathology, III:570
    embryology, III:569
  patient presentation and diagnosis
    cleft palate with cleft lip and alveolus,
        III:570–571, 571f
    feeding and swallowing difficulties,
        III:573–574, 574f
    growth factors, III:573
    incomplete cleft palate, III:571
    multiple syndromes, III:572
    Pierre Robin sequence, III:572
    secondary palate clefts, III:571

cleft palate surgery (Continued)
　　speech development, III:574, 575f
　　submucous cleft palate, III:571–572, 571f
　　22q chromosomal deletion, III:572–573, 573f
　Pierre Robin sequence (PRS), III:804–808, 805f
　postoperative care and follow-up, III:581
　prognosis and outcomes
　　fistula formation, III:581, 582f
　　maxillary growth, III:581–582
　　speech outcomes, III:581
　research summary, III:582
　secondary cleft deformities, III:631–654
　　cleft palate
　　　evaluation examinations, III:642
　　　palatal fistulas, III:642, 643f
　　　patient selection, III:642
　　　Pittsburgh fistula classification system, III:642, 642t
　　　surgical technique and treatment, III:642–644, 643f–646f
　　　timing considerations, III:642
　　etiology, III:631
　　patient presentation and diagnosis, III:632
　　wound healing and growth, III:631–632, 632f–633f
　surgical technique and treatment
　　Furlow double-opposing z-palatoplasty, III:579, 580f
　　hard versus soft palate closure, III:576
　　intravelar veloplasty, III:578–579, 580f
　　Langenbeck repair technique, III:576, 577f
　　technical perioperative considerations, III:576
　　timing considerations
　　　general discussion, III:574–576
　　　maxillary growth, III:575–576
　　　multiple syndromes, III:576
　　　speech development, III:574–575
　　two-flap palatoplasty, III:578, 579f
　　two-stage palate repair, III:579–581
　　Vomer flaps, III:578
　　V-Y palate repair (Veau–Wardill–Kilner), III:576–578, 577f–578f
clefts
　alveolar clefts, III:584–594
　　anatomical characteristics, III:584–585, 585f
　　background information, III:584
　　complications, III:592–594
　　dental development, III:585
　　goals, III:584, 585t
　　patient presentation and diagnosis
　　　alveolar distraction, III:587–588, 587f–588f
　　　bone morphogenetic proteins (BMPs), III:586
　　　cleft palate with cleft lip and alveolus, III:570–571, 571f
　　　gingivoperiosteoplasty (GPP), III:585, 586f
　　　late bone grafts, III:587
　　　primary bone grafts, III:585
　　　secondary bone grafts, III:585–586, 587f

clefts (Continued)
　　prognosis and outcomes
　　　bone morphogenetic proteins (BMPs), III:593
　　　gingivoperiosteoplasty (GPP), III:592–593
　　　graft site augmentation, III:594
　　　late bone grafts, III:593
　　　primary bone grafts, III:593
　　　secondary bone grafts, III:593
　　surgical technique
　　　gingivoperiosteoplasty (GPP), III:588, 589f
　　　horizontal alveolar transport distraction, III:591–592, 591f–592f
　　　primary bone grafts, III:588–589
　　　secondary bone grafts, III:589–591, 590f–591f
　　　vertical alveolar transport distraction, III:592, 592f
　classification systems, III:518–519, 519f
　cleft hands, VI:535f, 540f, 564, 565t
　cleft palate
　　feeding and swallowing difficulties, III:573–574, 574f
　　growth factors, III:573
　　incomplete cleft palate, III:571
　　multiple syndromes, III:572
　　palatal development
　　　anatomical characteristics, III:569, 570f
　　　ear pathology, III:570
　　　embryology, III:569
　　Pierre Robin sequence, III:572
　　secondary palate clefts, III:571
　　speech development, III:574, 575f
　　submucous cleft palate, III:571–572, 571f
　　22q chromosomal deletion, III:572–573, 573f
　craniofacial clefts, III:701–725
　　characteristics, III:701
　　classifications
　　　classification systems, III:701–704, 703t
　　　median craniofacial dysraphia, III:703–704, 703t
　　　median craniofacial hyperplasia (tissue excess or duplication), III:703t, 704
　　　median craniofacial hypoplasia (tissue deficiency or agenesis), III:702–703, 703t
　　clinical expression, III:720
　　differential defects, III:509, 509f–510f
　　embryology, III:686, 702f
　　epidemiology, III:704–706
　　etiology
　　　embryologic craniofacial development, III:702f, 704–705
　　　failure of fusion theory, III:705–706
　　　neuromeric theory, III:706
　　FOXE1 (Forkhead box protein E1) mutation, III:510–511
　　general discussion, III:509–511
　　inadequate growth, III:509–510
　　IRF6 (interferon regulatory factor) gene, III:511
　　median craniofacial dysraphia
　　　anterior encephaloceles, III:703–704
　　　characteristics, III:703–704
　　　number 0 cleft, III:709

clefts (Continued)
　　　skeletal involvement, III:709
　　　soft-tissue involvement, III:709
　　　true median cleft, III:703
　　median craniofacial hypoplasia (tissue deficiency or agenesis)
　　　holoprosencephalic spectrum (alobar brain), III:702
　　　median cerebrofacial hypoplasia (lobar brain), III:702
　　　median facial hypoplasia, III:702
　　　microform variants, III:702–703
　　　number 0 cleft, III:703t, 708–709, 708f
　　　skeletal deficiencies, III:708–709, 708f
　　　skeletal excess, III:709
　　　soft-tissue deficiencies, III:708, 708f
　　　soft-tissue midline excess, III:709
　　number 0 cleft
　　　characteristics, III:706–709
　　　median craniofacial dysraphia, III:709
　　　median craniofacial hyperplasia (tissue excess or duplication), III:709
　　　median craniofacial hypoplasia, III:703t, 708, 708f
　　　treatment strategies, III:722f–723f
　　number 1 cleft
　　　characteristics, III:709
　　　skeletal involvement, III:709, 710f
　　　soft-tissue involvement, III:709, 710f
　　number 2 cleft
　　　skeletal involvement, III:711
　　　soft-tissue involvement, III:709–711, 710f
　　　treatment strategies, III:723f
　　number 3 cleft
　　　characteristics, III:711
　　　skeletal involvement, III:711, 711f
　　　soft-tissue involvement, III:711, 711f
　　　treatment strategies, III:724f
　　number 4 cleft
　　　characteristics, III:712–713
　　　skeletal involvement, III:712f, 713
　　　soft-tissue involvement, III:712, 712f
　　number 5 cleft
　　　characteristics, III:713–714
　　　skeletal involvement, III:713f, 714
　　　soft-tissue involvement, III:713, 713f
　　number 6 cleft
　　　characteristics, III:714
　　　skeletal involvement, III:714, 714f
　　　soft-tissue involvement, III:714, 714f
　　number 7 cleft
　　　characteristics, III:714–715
　　　skeletal involvement, III:715, 715f
　　　soft-tissue involvement, III:714–715, 715f
　　number 8 cleft
　　　characteristics, III:715–716, 715f–716f
　　　skeletal involvement, III:715–716, 716f
　　　soft-tissue involvement, III:715
　　number 9 cleft
　　　characteristics, III:716–717
　　　skeletal involvement, III:716–717
　　　soft-tissue involvement, III:716, 717f
　　number 10 cleft
　　　characteristics, III:717
　　　skeletal involvement, III:717
　　　soft-tissue involvement, III:717, 717f

Note: **Boldface** roman numerals indicate volume. Page numbers followed by f refer to figures; page numbers followed by t refer to tables; page numbers followed by b refer to boxes.

clefts (Continued)
    number 11 cleft
        characteristics, III:717–718
        skeletal involvement, III:717–718
        soft-tissue involvement, III:717, 718f
    number 12 cleft
        characteristics, III:718
        skeletal involvement, III:718, 718f
        soft-tissue involvement, III:718, 718f
    number 13 cleft
        characteristics, III:718–719, 719f
        skeletal involvement, III:718–719
        soft-tissue involvement, III:718
    number 14 cleft
        characteristics, III:719
        skeletal involvement, III:719, 720f
        soft-tissue involvement, III:719, 720f
    number 30 cleft
        characteristics, III:719–720, 721f
        skeletal involvement, III:720
        soft-tissue involvement, III:720
    orbital hypertelorism, III:686–700
        Apert syndrome, III:689
        craniofrontonasal dysplasia, III:689
        Crouzon syndrome, III:688, 688f
        embryology, III:686
        faciocraniosynostosis, III:688–689
        median facial clefts, III:687
        oculomotor disorders, III:699
        outcomes and complicatons, III:698
        pathogenesis, III:686–689
        patient presentation and diagnosis,
           III:687–688
        patient selection, III:689
        Pfeiffer syndrome, III:688–689
        postoperative care and follow-up,
           III:695–696
        recurrences, III:699–700
        secondary procedures, III:698–700,
           698f
        surgical technique and treatment,
           III:689–695
        Tessier cleft classification system,
           III:687–688, 687f
    outcomes and complicatons, III:725
    patient selection
        number 0 cleft, III:706–709
        number 1 cleft, III:709
        number 2 cleft, III:709–711
        number 3 cleft, III:711
        number 4 cleft, III:712–713
        number 5 cleft, III:713–714
        number 6 cleft, III:714
        number 7 cleft, III:714–715
        number 8 cleft, III:715–716
        number 9 cleft, III:716–717
        number 10 cleft, III:717
        number 11 cleft, III:717–718
        number 12 cleft, III:718
        number 13 cleft, III:718–719
        number 14 cleft, III:719
        number 30 cleft, III:719–720
        Tessier cleft classification system,
           III:687–688, 687f, 706, 707f
    research summary, III:725
    transforming growth factor-β (TGF-β)
        superfamily, III:509, 509f–510f
    treatment strategies
        basic procedure, III:721–725
        number 0 cleft, III:722f–723f

clefts (Continued)
        number 2 cleft, III:723f
        number 3 cleft, III:724f
    Wingless (Wnt) signaling defects,
        III:509–510
craniofacial microsomia (CFM), III:767, 771f
lateral nasal prominences, III:508, 509f
nonsyndromic cleft lip and palate, I:193–194
orofacial clefts, I:193
orthognathic surgery, III:655–670
secondary cleft deformities, III:631–654
    cleft lip
        cleft lip anatomy, III:633, 634f
        evaluation examinations, III:634–635,
           635f
        normal lip anatomy, III:633, 633f–634f
        patient selection, III:635
        scarring considerations, III:635, 636f
        timing considerations, III:635
    cleft nose
        cleft nose anatomy, III:646–647,
           646f–647f
        decision-making process, III:653
        evaluation examinations, III:647–648
        normal anatomy, III:644–646, 646t
        patient selection, III:648
        surgical technique and treatment,
           III:648–653
        timing considerations, III:648
    cleft palate
        evaluation examinations, III:642
        palatal fistulas, III:642, 643f
        patient selection, III:642
        Pittsburgh fistula classification system,
           III:642, 642t
        surgical technique and treatment,
           III:642–644, 643f–646f
        timing considerations, III:642
    etiology, III:631
    lips
        Cupid's bow, III:639
        long lip, III:637
        philtral column reconstruction,
           III:638–639, 639f
        short lateral lip, III:638
        short lip, III:635–637, 636f
        tight lip, III:637, 637f–638f
        wide lip, III:637–638
    patient presentation and diagnosis,
        III:632
    vermillion
        buccal sulcus deformities, III:641–642,
           641f
        orbicularis muscle deformities,
           III:640–641
        thick lip, III:639
        thin lip, III:639, 640f
        vermillion mismatch, III:639–640
        vermillion notching/vermillion border
           malalignment, III:640
        whistle deformity, III:640
        wound healing and growth, III:631–632,
           632f–633f
syndromic cleft lip and palate, I:194–195
velopharyngeal insufficiency (VPI),
    III:667–670, 667t
    See also cleft lip surgery; cleft palate
        surgery; hypertelorism
Cleland's ligaments, VI:5, 7f, 347, 348f, 350f
clenched-fist injuries, VI:343, 344f

Cleopatra's needle, V:99
clindamycin, II:21t
Clinical Queries, I:151
clinical target volumes (CTV), I:663
clinodactyly
    characteristics, VI:630, 636, 638f, 640
    outcomes and complicatons, VI:632
    pathogenesis, VI:630
    patient presentation and diagnosis,
        VI:630–631, 631f
    patient selection, VI:631
    postoperative care and follow-up, VI:632
    radiographic imaging, VI:637f
    secondary procedures, VI:632
    surgical technique and treatment, VI:546t,
        631–632, 631f, 640
    See also brachydactyly
cloacal exstrophy repair
    embryology, III:907–908
    epidemiology, III:908
    etiology, III:908
    outcomes and complicatons, III:916–921
    patient presentation and diagnosis,
        III:908–909
    patient selection, III:909
    postoperative care and follow-up, III:915
    secondary procedures, III:921
    surgical technique and treatment, III:912,
        913f
clomipramine, I:51
clonidine, II:21t, IV:427
closed capsulotomy, V:107, 107f–108f
closed rhinoplasty, II:413–449
    augmentation phase
        columellar grafts, II:436
        dorsum and radix, II:436
        graft donor sites
           alloplastic materials, II:439–440
           calvarial bone, II:439
           conchal cartilage, II:439
           costal cartilage, II:439
           general discussion, II:439–440
           maxillary augmentation, II:440
        graft selection, II:436–437
        lateral wall grafts, II:436
        spreader grafts, II:436
        tip grafts, II:436–437, 437f–438f
    complications
        circulatory complications, II:445
        general discussion, II:444–446
        graft problems, II:444–445
        hematomas, II:446
        hemorrhage, II:445
        iatrogenic airway obstruction, II:444
        infections, II:445–446
        lacrimal duct injury, II:446
        red nose, II:446
        rhinitis, II:445
        septal collapse, II:446
        septal perforation, II:445
        skeletal problems, II:444
        soft-tissue problems, II:444
    dissatisfied patients
        body dysmorphic disorder (BDD),
           II:447–448
        primary versus secondary candidates,
           II:446–447
        prior versus current surgeon, II:447
        reoperations, II:448
        surgeon–patient relationship, II:446–448

closed rhinoplasty (Continued)
dressings, II:439
nasal aesthetics
potential complications and revisions, II:424
preoperative photographs, II:423
surgical goals, II:423–424
surgical guidelines, II:423–424
open rhinoplasty-caused deformities, II:448–449, 449f
patient selection
false planning assumptions, II:421–422
patient interview, II:422
preoperative assessment
evaluation examinations, II:422–423
external nose, II:423
septum, II:423
turbinates, II:423
valves, II:423
primary versus secondary candidates, II:422
postoperative care and follow-up, II:439–441
secondary rhinoplasty, II:448–449
septal graft specimen, II:436–437
surgical planning
decision-making process, II:427
endonasal rhinoplasty, II:425
general discussion, II:424–427
nasal base size–bridge height balance, II:425, 426f
skin thickness and distribution, II:424, 424f
teach-yourself concept, II:427
tip lobular contour, II:424–425, 425f
surgical technique and treatment
general discussion, II:427–435
routine order
alar cartilage resection, II:433–434
anesthesia, II:427–435
dorsal resection, II:428, 428f–433f
intracartilaginous incisions, II:428, 428f
nasal spine-caudal septum resection, II:433
septoplasty, II:434–435
skeletonization, II:427–428
spreader graft tunnels, II:434–435, 435f
upper lateral cartilage resection, II:434
turbinectomy
alar wedge resection, II:435–436
characteristics, II:435–436
graft placement, II:435–436
osteotomy
basic procedure, II:435
goals, II:435
wound closure, II:435–436
variants
cleft lip nasal deformity, II:442
donor site-depleted patient, II:443
ethnic rhinoplasty, II:441–442
male rhinoplasty, II:441
nasal deviation, II:441, 442f
older adults, II:442–443
rhinophyma, II:443, 443f
closed-target nerve transfer, VI:799
closed wounds, I:285–286, 286t
Clostridium botulinum, II:31, III:492–495
Clostridium perfringens, IV:196–197, 312–313

CLOVES syndrome
classification systems, VI:668, 668t
pathogenesis, I:698f, 705, VI:691
patient presentation and diagnosis, VI:688f, 692
surgical technique and treatment, VI:692
coagulase-negative staphylococci, I:249–250
cobalt (Co)
cobalt-chromium alloys, I:787
metal alloy compositions, I:786–787
cocaine, III:26–29
Cochrane Database of Systematic Reviews, I:152–153
Code of Ethics, I:57–58
Coelst, Maurice, I:24, 24f
coenzyme Q10, II:18, 27
coffeeberry, II:18
Coffin–Siris syndrome, VI:573t
Cohen syndrome, VI:573t
Coilingel, II:47t
cold injury/frostbite
upper extremities, IV:456–467
classifications, IV:456–460
complications, IV:459–460
disease process
freezing phase, IV:457
pathophysiology, IV:456–457
rewarming phase, IV:457
nonsurgical interventions
adjunctive therapy, IV:458
field management, IV:458
rapid rewarming, IV:458
splinting, IV:458
patient presentation and diagnosis
clinical assessment, IV:457
physical examination, IV:457–458
radiographic imaging, IV:457–458
patient selection, IV:458
postoperative care and follow-up, IV:459
prognosis and outcomes, IV:459–460
research summary, IV:456
secondary procedures
hyperbaric oxygen therapy, IV:460
sympathectomy, IV:460
thrombolytics, IV:460
surgical technique and treatment
amputations, IV:458–459, 459f
length salvage, IV:459
nonsurgical interventions, IV:458
cold intolerance
peripheral nerve injuries, VI:717–718
replantation and revascularization surgery, VI:248–249
Coleman method, II:332–335, 336f, V:598, 598f
collagenases, I:269–271, VI:353–354, 354f–355f
collagens, I:243f, 270–271, 289t, 320, 431–432, 432t, VI:348–349
collagen XI gene sequence, III:805–807, 807t
collateral ligaments
hands and wrists, VI:13f
hand stability assessment, VI:49–50, 49f–50f
knee skeletal structure, IV:32f
stiff hand, VI:449, 451, 454, 454f
Colles fascia
anatomical characteristics, IV:298–299
female perineum, IV:230–235, 233f
male perineum, IV:235, 236f–237f

colloidal oatmeal, II:23
colobomas, III:829f, 830, 831f, 833f, 835f
color Doppler imaging
basic principles, V:328
color duplex Doppler imaging, I:501
cutaneous and soft-tissue tumors, I:709–710
vascular anatomical research, I:501
columellar scars, II:481–482, 482f
columellar strut graft, II:397–398, 398f
combination bars, II:16
combined polydactyly, VI:616, 617t
combined vascular malformations
classification systems, I:677t, VI:668t
diagnostic work-up, VI:670t
patient presentation and diagnosis, VI:670f
surgical technique and treatment, VI:669–672, 671t
comedogenesis, II:20
commissure, III:287f, 456, IV:489–490, 495f
commissuroplasty, III:777–779, 778f–779f, IV:505
common determinant (CD) cells, I:818–819, 827–828
common warts, VI:314–315, 315f
compartment syndrome
burn wound treatment
decompressive laparotomy, IV:431f
detailed characteristics, IV:428–431
early escharotomies, IV:430f
escharotomy incisions, IV:429f–430f
escharotomy lines, IV:428f
extensive escharotomies, IV:431f
full thickness burn escharotomies, IV:429f
hand escharotomies, IV:429f
periocular escharotomies, IV:430f
zigzag escharotomies, IV:430f
lower extremities
burn reconstruction, IV:437–439, 437f–440f
lower leg, IV:37
trauma injuries, IV:84–85
upper extremities, IV:437–439, 439f–440f
competition models, I:66, 66f
complementary metal oxide semiconductor (CMOS) sensors, I:117–119
complement cascade, I:817
complex lacerations, III:31, 32f
complex regional pain syndrome (CRPS), VI:486–502
background and general characteristics, VI:486–487, 487f, 488t
nerve compression syndromes, VI:497t, 498f, 503–525
pathophysiology, VI:487–490, 488f–489f
patient presentation and diagnosis
adjunctive diagnostic measures, VI:492–493
clinical diagnosis, VI:488t, 491–493, 491f–492f
epidemiology, VI:490
patient characteristics, VI:490–491
precipitating events, VI:490
peripheral nerve injuries, VI:717
postoperative care and follow-up, VI:497
prognosis and outcomes, VI:497–499
research summary, VI:501
secondary procedures, VI:499–501

*Note: **Boldface** roman numerals indicate volume. Page numbers followed by f refer to figures; page numbers followed by t refer to tables; page numbers followed by b refer to boxes.*

complex regional pain syndrome (CRPS) (*Continued*)
  treatment strategies
    basic principles, **VI**:493–495, 493f
    drug therapy, **VI**:494
    emerging treatments
      botulinum toxin (BTX), **VI**:495
      intravenous ketamine infusion therapy, **VI**:494–495
    interventional therapies, **VI**:494
    invasive pain management therapies, **VI**:495
    peripheral nerve surgery
      joint denervation surgery, **VI**:497t
      nerve compression syndromes, **VI**:497t, 498f
      patient selection, **VI**:495, 496f
      perioperative pain management, **VI**:495–497
      surgical technique, **VI**:489f, 497, 498f–500f
    physical therapy and rehabilitation, **VI**:493
    psychological support, **VI**:493–494
    spinal cord stimulation, **VI**:495
component dorsal hump reduction, **II**:391–392, 391f
composite nipple graft, **V**:500–502, 501f–502f
composite tissue allotransplantation (CTA)
  face transplants, **III**:473–490
    background information, **III**:473
    cephalic vein harvest, **III**:484–485, 485f
    complications, **III**:484–485
    face transplant harvest
      basic procedure, **III**:476–482
      coronal approach, **III**:478f
      digastric division, **III**:478f
      external canthus dissection, **III**:480f
      external jugular dissection, **III**:477f
      facial nerve, **III**:478f
      final dissection after medial osteotomy, **III**:480f–481f
      harvested transplant, **III**:482f
      initial drawing and infiltration, **III**:477f
      lacrimal duct preparation, **III**:482f
      levator dissection and division, **III**:479f
      levator verification, **III**:480f
      lower face transplant, **III**:482f
      mandibular osteotomy, **III**:482f
      maxillary artery, **III**:479f
      maxillary osteotomy, **III**:482f
      thyrolingofacial trunk and external carotid dissection, **III**:477f–478f
    immunosuppression, **III**:473–475, 474t
    patient selection, **III**:475
    postoperative care and follow-up
      follow-up consultations, **III**:485
      infection prevention and treatment, **III**:484
      psychological support, **III**:485
      social reintegration, **III**:485–488, 486f–488f
    prognosis and outcomes, **III**:484–488
    recipient preparation
      basic procedure, **III**:482–483
      bone fixation, **III**:483f–484f
      dacryocystorhinostomy, **III**:484f
      final closure, **III**:484f
      lower face debridement, **III**:483f
      vascular anastomosis, **III**:483f

composite tissue allotransplantation (CTA) (*Continued*)
    research summary, **III**:488
    revision surgeries, **III**:488
    secondary procedures, **III**:488
    surgical technique
      basic procedure, **III**:476–483
      face transplant harvest, **III**:476–482
      mask preparation, **III**:476f–477f
      mold preparation, **III**:476f
      recipient preparation, **III**:482–483
  microvascular surgery, **I**:620
  prosthetics–composite tissue allotransplantation (CTA) comparisons, **VI**:879–880
  surgical innovation, **I**:2–3
  tissue transplantation challenges, **I**:815, 831–834, 837–839
  upper extremity surgery, **VI**:843–854
    challenges, **VI**:852
    complications, **VI**:850–851
    donor and recipient selection, **VI**:845–846, 846t
    emerging insights
      chronic rejection, **VI**:852–853, 853t
      cortical plasticity, **VI**:852
      future trends, **VI**:854
      immunomodulatory strategies, **VI**:853–854
      neural integration, **VI**:852
      tolerance approaches, **VI**:853–854
    epidemiology, **VI**:843–844
    evolutionary development
      chronology, **VI**:845
      experimental background, **VI**:844–845
      immunology, **VI**:844
    procedural aspects
      donor limb procurement, **VI**:846–847, 847f
      recipient surgery, **VI**:847, 848f
    prognosis and outcomes, **VI**:850–851
    program establishment and implementation, **VI**:845
    prosthetics–composite tissue allotransplantation (CTA) comparisons, **VI**:879–880
    protocol-related considerations
      immunomonitoring, **VI**:850
      maintenance immunosuppression, **VI**:847, 849f, 853–854
      rehabilitation and functional assessment, **I**:835–837, **VI**:848, 849f
      rejection assessments, **VI**:849–850, 849f–851f, 849t
    upper extremity transplantation versus replantation, **VI**:851–852
composite tissue grafts, **I**:365f, 366
compound motor action potential (CMAP), **VI**:504
compound muscle action potentials (CMAPs), **VI**:797–798
compound nevi, **I**:744, 744f
computed tomography (CT)
  angiosome studies, **I**:480–482, 483f
  brachial plexus injuries, **VI**:796
  computed tomography angiography
    hand ischemia, **VI**:472, 473f
    perforator flaps, **IV**:69f–70f, 73f
    vascular anatomical research, **I**:501, 502f

computed tomography (CT) (*Continued*)
    vascular imaging, **VI**:89–90
    vascular injury, **IV**:67–68
  craniofacial fibrous dysplasia, **III**:382
  craniofacial microsomia (CFM), **III**:775, 777f
  cutaneous and soft-tissue tumors, **I**:710
  deep inferior epigastric perforator (DIEP) flaps, **V**:440, 441f–442f
  epiphyseal growth plate, **VI**:656
  facial injuries
    frontal bone and sinus fractures, **III**:51
    injury assessment, **III**:51
    midface buttresses, **III**:71
    nasoethmoidal orbital fractures, **III**:61
    orbital fractures, **III**:54
  facial soft-tissue injuries, **III**:26
  fracture assessment, **VI**:107
  functional role, **I**:868–869, 869f
  hand and wrist evaluations
    advantages/disadvantages, **VI**:78–82, 81t
    bony tumors, **VI**:81–82
    fractures and dislocations, **VI**:78–79, 81f
    soft-tissue masses, **VI**:313
    tumors, **VI**:313
  head and neck cancer detection, **III**:400, 417–418
  melanoma detection, **I**:762–764, 762f
  multidetector-row computed tomography (MDCT)
    basic principles, **V**:328–329
    deep inferior epigastric perforator (DIEP) flaps, **V**:326, 327f–328f
    radiological protocol, **V**:329, 330f, 332f–334f
  nasal disease and obstructions, **II**:457f
  pectus excavatum, **III**:856, 856f
  salivary gland tumors, **III**:363–364
  sarcoma detection, **IV**:103–104
  scalp and forehead reconstruction, **III**:120
  single-photon emission computed tomography (SPECT), **III**:382
  temporomandibular joint (TMJ) dysfunction, **III**:92
  three-dimensional (3D) computed tomography (CT), **I**:662–664, **III**:658, 659f
  vascular anatomical research, **I**:501, 502f
  vascular anomalies, **VI**:669
  velopharyngeal dysfunction (VPD), **III**:623
  wrist injuries, **VI**:166–169
computer-based simulation
  basic principles, **I**:865
  functional role
    surgical planning simulators, **I**:868–869, 869f
    training simulators, **I**:865–868, 866f–868f, 867t
  future trends, **I**:869–870
  implementation, **I**:865
  physical–behavioral–genomics model, **I**:869–870, 869f
  use rationale, **I**:865
concept of beauty, **II**:1–2
condylar fractures
  facial injuries, **III**:83, 83f
  temporomandibular joint (TMJ) dysfunction, **III**:90–91
congenital alopecia, **VI**:646
congenital chondrodysplasia, **VI**:655–656
congenital cicatricial alopecia, **III**:111t

congenital defects
  Apert syndrome
    characteristics, **VI:**610, 644–645, 645f
    complications, **VI:**614
    epidemiology, **VI:**610
    outcome assessments, **VI:**614
    pathogenesis, **VI:**610
    patient presentation and diagnosis, **VI:**611f, 611t, 613f, 682
    patient selection, **VI:**612
    postoperative care and follow-up, **VI:**614
    secondary procedures, **VI:**614
    surgical technique and treatment
      basic procedure, **VI:**612–614
      finger separation, **VI:**612
      metacarpal synostosis, **VI:**614
      preferred treatments, **VI:**611f, 612t–613t, 613f
      thumb and first web separation, **VI:**612–614
  brachydactyly
    brachymesophalangy, **VI:**637f, 639–640
    brachymetacarpia, **VI:**638f, 640, 640f
    causal factors, **VI:**637
    clinical manifestations, **VI:**635–641, 636f–638f
    clinodactyly
      characteristics, **VI:**630, 636, 638f, 640
      outcomes and complicatons, **VI:**632
      pathogenesis, **VI:**630
      patient presentation and diagnosis, **VI:**630–631, 631f
      patient selection, **VI:**631
      postoperative care and follow-up, **VI:**632
      radiographic imaging, **VI:**637f
      secondary procedures, **VI:**632
      surgical technique and treatment, **VI:**546t, 631–632, 631f, 640
    Kirner's deformity, **VI:**639f
    Mohr–Wriedt syndrome, **VI:**636, 638f, 646
    polydactyly
      characteristics, **VI:**639f
      classification systems, **VI:**535–537, 535f–536f
    symbrachydactyly
      classification systems, **VI:**537, 537f–538f
      patient presentation and diagnosis, **VI:**549–550, 550f, 609f, 640–641, 640f–641f, 645f
      surgical technique and treatment, **VI:**546t
    syndactyly
      characteristics, **VI:**635f, 639f
      classification systems, **VI:**535–537, 535f, 537f, 605f
      epidemiology, **VI:**604
      outcomes and complicatons, **VI:**608–609, 609f
      pathogenesis, **VI:**604
      patient presentation and diagnosis, **VI:**564–565, 604, 606f
      patient selection, **VI:**604–605
      postoperative care and follow-up, **VI:**608
      secondary procedures, **VI:**609
      surgical technique and treatment, **VI:**546t, 605–608, 605b, 608b
    treatment strategies, **VI:**637–639

congenital defects *(Continued)*
  breast reconstruction, **V:**584t, 591, 591f
  childhood plastic surgeries, **I:**44
  congenital alopecia, **VI:**646
  constriction band syndrome
    bone grafts, **VI:**642
    clinical manifestations, **VI:**641–642, 642f
    surgical treatment, **VI:**546t, 641–642, 642f–643f
    toe-to-hand transplantations, **VI:**642, 643f
  craniofacial clefts, **III:**701–725
    characteristics, **III:**701
    classifications
      classification systems, **III:**701–704, 703t
      median craniofacial dysraphia, **III:**703–704, 703t
      median craniofacial hyperplasia (tissue excess or duplication), **III:**703t, 704
      median craniofacial hypoplasia (tissue deficiency or agenesis), **III:**702–703, 703t
    clinical expression, **III:**720
    differential defects, **III:**509, 509f–510f
    embryology, **III:**686, 702f
    epidemiology, **III:**704–706
    etiology
      embryologic craniofacial development, **III:**702f, 704–705
      failure of fusion theory, **III:**705–706
      neuromeric theory, **III:**706
    FOXE1 (Forkhead box protein E1) mutation, **III:**510–511
    general discussion, **III:**509–511
    inadequate growth, **III:**509–510
    IRF6 (interferon regulatory factor) gene, **III:**511
    median craniofacial dysraphia
      anterior encephaloceles, **III:**703–704
      characteristics, **III:**703–704
      number 0 cleft, **III:**709
      skeletal involvement, **III:**709
      soft-tissue involvement, **III:**709
      true median cleft, **III:**703
    median craniofacial hypoplasia (tissue deficiency or agenesis)
      holoprosencephalic spectrum (alobar brain), **III:**702
      median cerebrofacial hypoplasia (lobar brain), **III:**702
      median facial hypoplasia, **III:**702
      microform variants, **III:**702–703
      number 0 cleft, **III:**703t, 708–709, 708f
      skeletal deficiencies, **III:**708–709, 708f
      skeletal excess, **III:**709
      soft-tissue deficiencies, **III:**708, 708f
      soft-tissue midline excess, **III:**709
    number 0 cleft
      characteristics, **III:**706–709
      median craniofacial dysraphia, **III:**709
      median craniofacial hyperplasia (tissue excess or duplication), **III:**709
      median craniofacial hypoplasia, **III:**703t, 708, 708f
      treatment strategies, **III:**722f–723f
    number 1 cleft
      characteristics, **III:**709
      skeletal involvement, **III:**709, 710f
      soft-tissue involvement, **III:**709, 710f

congenital defects *(Continued)*
  number 2 cleft
    skeletal involvement, **III:**711
    soft-tissue involvement, **III:**709–711, 710f
    treatment strategies, **III:**723f
  number 3 cleft
    characteristics, **III:**711
    skeletal involvement, **III:**711, 711f
    soft-tissue involvement, **III:**711, 711f
    treatment strategies, **III:**724f
  number 4 cleft
    characteristics, **III:**712–713
    skeletal involvement, **III:**712f, 713
    soft-tissue involvement, **III:**712, 712f
  number 5 cleft
    characteristics, **III:**713–714
    skeletal involvement, **III:**713f, 714
    soft-tissue involvement, **III:**713, 713f
  number 6 cleft
    characteristics, **III:**714
    skeletal involvement, **III:**714, 714f
    soft-tissue involvement, **III:**714, 714f
  number 7 cleft
    characteristics, **III:**714–715
    skeletal involvement, **III:**715, 715f
    soft-tissue involvement, **III:**714–715, 715f
  number 8 cleft
    characteristics, **III:**715–716, 715f–716f
    skeletal involvement, **III:**715–716, 716f
    soft-tissue involvement, **III:**715
  number 9 cleft
    characteristics, **III:**716–717
    skeletal involvement, **III:**716–717
    soft-tissue involvement, **III:**716, 717f
  number 10 cleft
    characteristics, **III:**717
    skeletal involvement, **III:**717
    soft-tissue involvement, **III:**717, 717f
  number 11 cleft
    characteristics, **III:**717–718
    skeletal involvement, **III:**717–718
    soft-tissue involvement, **III:**717, 718f
  number 12 cleft
    characteristics, **III:**718
    skeletal involvement, **III:**718, 718f
    soft-tissue involvement, **III:**718, 718f
  number 13 cleft
    characteristics, **III:**718–719, 719f
    skeletal involvement, **III:**718–719
    soft-tissue involvement, **III:**718
  number 14 cleft
    characteristics, **III:**719
    skeletal involvement, **III:**719, 720f
    soft-tissue involvement, **III:**719, 720f
  number 30 cleft
    characteristics, **III:**719–720, 721f
    skeletal involvement, **III:**720
    soft-tissue involvement, **III:**720
  orbital hypertelorism, **III:**686–700
    Apert syndrome, **III:**689
    craniofrontonasal dysplasia, **III:**689
    Crouzon syndrome, **III:**688, 688f
    embryology, **III:**686
    faciocraniosynostosis, **III:**688–689
    median facial clefts, **III:**687
    oculomotor disorders, **III:**699

*Note: **Boldface** roman numerals indicate volume. Page numbers followed by f refer to figures; page numbers followed by t refer to tables; page numbers followed by b refer to boxes.*

congenital defects (Continued)
outcomes and complicatons, III:698
pathogenesis, III:686–689
patient presentation and diagnosis, III:687–688
patient selection, III:689
Pfeiffer syndrome, III:688–689
postoperative care and follow-up, III:695–696
recurrences, III:699–700
secondary procedures, III:698–700, 698f
surgical technique and treatment, III:689–695
Tessier cleft classification system, III:687–688, 687f
outcomes and complicatons, III:725
patient selection
number 0 cleft, III:706–709
number 1 cleft, III:709
number 2 cleft, III:709–711
number 3 cleft, III:711
number 4 cleft, III:712–713
number 5 cleft, III:713–714
number 6 cleft, III:714
number 7 cleft, III:714–715
number 8 cleft, III:715–716
number 9 cleft, III:716–717
number 10 cleft, III:717
number 11 cleft, III:717–718
number 12 cleft, III:718
number 13 cleft, III:718–719
number 14 cleft, III:719
number 30 cleft, III:719–720
Tessier cleft classification system, III:687–688, 687f, 706, 707f
research summary, III:725
transforming growth factor-β (TGF-β) superfamily, III:509, 509f–510f
treatment strategies
basic procedure, III:721–725
number 0 cleft, III:722f–723f
number 2 cleft, III:723f
number 3 cleft, III:724f
Wingless (Wnt) signaling defects, III:509–510
Freeman–Sheldon syndrome, VI:646, 646f
general discussion, VI:634
generalized skeletal abnormalities, VI:642–644
genetically-caused disease
characteristics, I:192–198
craniosynostosis, I:195–196
nomenclature, I:192–193
nonsyndromic cleft lip and palate, I:193–194
orofacial clefts, I:193
syndromic cleft lip and palate, I:194–195
syndromic craniosynostosis, I:196–198, 197t
Haas syndrome, VI:645–646, 646f
hands, VI:526–571, 634–650
Apert syndrome, VI:644–645, 645f
brachydactyly
brachymesophalangy, VI:637f, 639–640
brachymetacarpia, VI:638f, 640, 640f
causal factors, VI:637
clinical manifestations, VI:635–641, 636f–638f
clinodactyly, VI:636, 637f–638f, 640

congenital defects (Continued)
Kirner's deformity, VI:639f
Mohr–Wriedt syndrome, VI:636, 638f, 646
polydactyly, VI:639f
symbrachydactyly, VI:640–641, 640f–641f, 645f
syndactyly, VI:635f, 639f
treatment strategies, VI:637–639
camptodactyly
characteristics, VI:628
epidemiology, VI:628
outcomes and complicatons, VI:630
pathogenesis, VI:628
patient presentation and diagnosis, VI:628–629
patient selection, VI:629
postoperative care and follow-up, VI:630
secondary procedures, VI:630
surgical technique and treatment, VI:546t, 629–630, 629f–630f
central ray deficiency
associated syndromes, VI:565t
characteristics, VI:563–564, 563b, 564f
classification systems, VI:565t
outcomes and complicatons, VI:566–567
pathogenesis, VI:564
patient presentation and diagnosis, VI:564–565, 564f
patient selection, VI:565
postoperative care and follow-up, VI:566
secondary procedures, VI:567
surgical technique and treatment, VI:565, 565f–566f
child and family assessments
diagnostic imaging, VI:543–544
hand control development, VI:541t, 542–543, 542f
ossification timing/growth plate closure, VI:543f
patient and family history, VI:541–542
physical examination, VI:541t, 542–543, 542f–543f
support systems, VI:539–544
surgical congenital hand clinic, VI:541
weight-bearing development, VI:543f
classification systems, VI:526–527
congenital alopecia, VI:646
congenital longitudinal arrest, VI:555–556
congenital transverse arrest
assessment strategies, VI:548, 549f
general considerations, VI:548b
outcomes and complicatons, VI:553–555
pathogenesis, VI:548–549
patient presentation and diagnosis, VI:549–550, 549f–550f
patient selection, VI:550–553
postoperative care and follow-up, VI:550–553
secondary procedures, VI:555
surgical technique and treatment, VI:550–553
constriction band syndrome
bone grafts, VI:642
clinical manifestations, VI:641–642, 642f

congenital defects (Continued)
surgical treatment, VI:641–642, 642f–643f
toe-to-hand transplantations, VI:642, 643f
development anomalies
background information, VI:534–535
classification systems, VI:534–535
modified classification of congenital anomalies of the hand and upper limb, VI:537–539, 538f–541f, 538t
Swanson/IFSSH classification, VI:535–537
symbrachydactyly, VI:537, 537f–538f, 546t
syndactyly, VI:535–537, 535f, 537f
terminology, VI:534–535
diagnosis, VI:544
embryology, VI:526–534
Freeman–Sheldon syndrome, VI:646, 646f
general discussion, VI:634
generalized skeletal abnormalities, VI:642–644
Haas syndrome, VI:645–646, 646f
limb development
embryology, VI:526–534
hand development timing, VI:527t
molecular controls, VI:527–530, 529f–530f
upper limb morphogenesis, VI:527, 527t, 528f–529f
macrodactyly
clinical manifestations, VI:634–635, 635f
Hong Kong survey, VI:635t
proteus syndrome, VI:635
surgical technique and treatment, VI:636f
Madelung's deformity, VI:646–647, 647f
Mohr–Wriedt syndrome, VI:646
multiple exotoses, VI:642–644, 644f
phocomelia
characteristics, VI:556, 556b
outcomes and complicatons, VI:557
pathogenesis, VI:556
patient presentation and diagnosis, VI:556, 556f
patient selection, VI:556
postoperative care and follow-up, VI:557
secondary procedures, VI:557
surgical technique and treatment, VI:556–557
Pierre–Robin syndrome, VI:646, 646f
Poland syndrome, VI:644–647, 644f
polydactyly
associated syndromes, VI:617t
central polydactyly, VI:546t, 618
characteristics, VI:616
classification systems, VI:535–537, 535f–536f
epidemiology, VI:616
genetic considerations, VI:616–617
outcomes and complicatons, VI:622–623, 623f, 623t
pathogenesis, VI:616–617
patient selection, VI:618
postaxial polydactyly, VI:546t
potassium titanium oxide phosphate (KTP) lasers, VI:622

congenital defects *(Continued)*
  radial polydactyly, **VI:**564–565, 617–618, 617f, 617t
  secondary procedures, **VI:**623
  surgical technique and treatment, **VI:**619–622
  ulnar polydactyly, **VI:**617t, 618
  radial hypoplasia/aplasia
    characteristics, **VI:**557, 557b
    classification systems, **VI:**558t, 559f
    outcomes and complicatons, **VI:**563
    pathogenesis, **VI:**557–558
    patient presentation and diagnosis, **VI:**558–560, 558f–559f
    patient selection, **VI:**560
    postoperative care and follow-up, **VI:**563
    secondary procedures, **VI:**563
    surgical technique and treatment, **VI:**560–563, 560f–562f
    timing considerations, **VI:**546t, 547f
  research summary, **VI:**647–648
  surgical indicators
    appearance, **VI:**544–545, 545f
    functionality, **VI:**544, 545f
    timing considerations, **VI:**545–547, 546f–547f, 546t
  terminology, **VI:**527
  thumb hypoplasia, **VI:**572–602
    abductor digiti quinti minimi muscle (ADQM) transfer, **VI:**587–588, 589f
    associated conditions, **VI:**573–574, 573t
    characteristics, **VI:**572
    classification systems, **VI:**574, 574f
    clinical presentation, **VI:**574–583
    deficient first web space, **VI:**586–587
    etiology, **VI:**573
    Fanconi anemia (FA), **VI:**573t, 574
    flexor digitorum superficialis (FDS) transfer, **VI:**588–590
    four-flap Z-plasty, **VI:**585f, 586–587
    Holt–Oram syndrome, **VI:**573t, 574
    inadequate index finger, **VI:**599–600
    incidence, **VI:**572–573
    interphalangeal (IP) joint motion, **VI:**590
    metacarpophalangeal joint instability, **VI:**587, 588f
    outcomes and complicatons, **VI:**597–599
    patient presentation and diagnosis, **VI:**574–583
    patient selection, **VI:**583–584
    pollex abductus, **VI:**578f, 590
    pollicization technique, **VI:**590–594, 591f–593f
    poor/absent palmar abduction (opposition), **VI:**587–590
    postoperative care and follow-up, **VI:**597
    secondary procedures, **VI:**599–600
    surgical technique and treatment, **VI:**586–594
    tendon graft stabilization, **VI:**587
    thrombocytopenia absent radius (TAR) syndrome, **VI:**573t, 574
    timing considerations, **VI:**546t, 583–584, 583f

congenital defects *(Continued)*
  Type I (mild hypoplasia), **VI:**574–575, 575f, 584, 585f, 597
  Type II (moderate hypoplasia), **VI:**575–577, 576f, 578f, 584, 597
  Type III (severe hypoplasia), **VI:**577, 579f–580f, 584, 587, 588f, 597
  Type IV (floating thumb), **VI:**577, 581f, 586
  Type V (aplasia), **VI:**577, 582f, 586
  Type VI (cleft hand), **VI:**579–580, 594–595, 598
  Type VI (symbrachydactyly thumb), **VI:**580–581, 595, 598
  Type VII (constriction ring syndrome), **VI:**581, 595–596, 599
  Type VIII (five-fingered hand), **VI:**581–582, 596, 599
  Type IX (radial polydactyly), **VI:**582–583, 596, 599
  Type X (syndromic short skeletal thumb ray), **VI:**583, 596–597, 599
  VACTERL association, **VI:**573t, 574
  tissue development/differentiation
    general discussion, **VI:**530–534
    innervation, **VI:**534, 534f
    myogenesis, **VI:**532–534, 533f
    skeletogenesis, **VI:**531–532, 532f
    vasculogenesis, **VI:**530–531, 531f
  trigger thumb
    etiology, **VI:**648
    general discussion, **VI:**648–649
    treatment strategies, **VI:**648–649
  ulnar hypoplasia/aplasia
    associated syndromes, **VI:**567t
    characteristics, **VI:**567
    classification systems, **VI:**567, 568f, 568t–569t
    incidence, **VI:**567–570
    outcomes and complicatons, **VI:**570
    pathogenesis, **VI:**567
    patient presentation and diagnosis, **VI:**567–569, 567f–569f
    patient selection, **VI:**569
    postoperative care and follow-up, **VI:**570
    secondary procedures, **VI:**570
    surgical technique and treatment, **VI:**569–570, 570f
  macrodactyly
    classification systems, **VI:**541f
    clinical manifestations, **VI:**634–635, 635f
    Hong Kong survey, **VI:**635t
    proteus syndrome, **VI:**635
    surgical technique and treatment, **VI:**636f
  Madelung's deformity, **VI:**646–647, 647f
  male genital reconstructive surgery
    disorders of sex development (DSD), **IV:**303–304
    exstrophy and epispadias, **IV:**301–303, 302f–303f
    hidden penis, **IV:**304, 304f–305f
    severe penile insufficiency, **IV:**304–306, 306f
  Mohr–Wriedt syndrome, **VI:**646
  multiple exotoses, **VI:**642–644, 644f

congenital defects *(Continued)*
  nontuberous congenital breast asymmetry
    bilateral but different surgical procedure, **V:**537–538
    bilateral but similar surgical procedure, **V:**537–538
    case studies
      Case VII (volume asymmetry), **V:**538, 539f
      Case VIII (volume asymmetry), **V:**538, 540f
      Case IX (severe hypoplasia), **V:**538–541, 542f–543f
      Case X (severe asymmetry), **V:**544
    dermal apron, **V:**544, 545f
    general considerations, **V:**537–538, 537b
    monolateral operation, **V:**537
  Pierre–Robin syndrome, **VI:**646, 646f
  research summary, **VI:**647–648
  thumb hypoplasia, **VI:**572–602
    associated conditions, **VI:**573t
    Fanconi anemia (FA), **VI:**573t, 574
    general discussion, **VI:**573–574
    Holt–Oram syndrome, **VI:**573t, 574
    thrombocytopenia absent radius (TAR) syndrome, **VI:**573t, 574
    VACTERL association, **VI:**573t, 574
  characteristics, **VI:**572
  classification systems, **VI:**574, 574f
  clinical presentation
    general characteristics, **VI:**574–583
    Type I (mild hypoplasia), **VI:**574–575, 575f
    Type II (moderate hypoplasia), **VI:**575–577, 576f, 578f
    Type III (severe hypoplasia), **VI:**577, 579f–580f
    Type IV (floating thumb), **VI:**577, 581f
    Type V (aplasia), **VI:**577, 582f
    Type VI (cleft hand), **VI:**579–580
    Type VI (symbrachydactyly thumb), **VI:**580–581
    Type VII (constriction ring syndrome), **VI:**581
    Type VIII (five-fingered hand), **VI:**581–582
    Type IX (radial polydactyly), **VI:**582–583
    Type X (syndromic short skeletal thumb ray), **VI:**583
  etiology, **VI:**573
  inadequate index finger, **VI:**599–600
  incidence, **VI:**572–573
  outcomes and complicatons
    Type I (mild hypoplasia), **VI:**597
    Type II (moderate hypoplasia), **VI:**597
    Type III (severe hypoplasia), **VI:**597
    Type VI (cleft hand), **VI:**598
    Type VI (symbrachydactyly thumb), **VI:**598
    Type VII (constriction ring syndrome), **VI:**599
    Type VIII (five-fingered hand), **VI:**599
    Type IX (radial polydactyly), **VI:**599
    Type X (syndromic short skeletal thumb ray), **VI:**599
  patient presentation and diagnosis, **VI:**574–583

congenital defects (Continued)
patient selection, VI:583
pollicization technique
basic principles, VI:590
dissection and exposure, VI:590
general discussion, VI:590–594
incisions, VI:590, 592f–593f
operative technique, VI:591f–593f
outcomes and complicatons, VI:598
skeletal shortening, VI:594
skin closure and web construction,
VI:594
tendon and intrinsic muscle
rebalancing, VI:594
postoperative care and follow-up, VI:597
secondary procedures, VI:599–600
surgical technique and treatment
abductor digiti quinti minimi muscle
(ADQM) transfer, VI:587–588,
589f
deficient first web space, VI:586–587
flexor digitorum superficialis (FDS)
transfer, VI:588–590
four-flap Z-plasty, VI:585f, 586–587
interphalangeal (IP) joint motion,
VI:590
metacarpophalangeal joint instability,
VI:587, 588f
pollex abductus, VI:578f, 590
pollicization technique, VI:590–594,
591f–593f
poor/absent palmar abduction
(opposition), VI:587–590
tendon graft stabilization, VI:587
Type III (severe hypoplasia), VI:587,
588f
Type VI (cleft hand), VI:594–595
Type VI (symbrachydactyly thumb),
VI:595
Type VII (constriction ring syndrome),
VI:595–596
Type VIII (five-fingered hand), VI:596
Type IX (radial polydactyly), VI:596
Type X (syndromic short skeletal
thumb ray), VI:596–597
timing considerations, VI:546t, 583–584,
583f
treatment strategies
Type I (mild hypoplasia), VI:584, 585f
Type II (moderate hypoplasia), VI:584
Type III (severe hypoplasia), VI:584
Type IV (floating thumb), VI:586
Type V (aplasia), VI:586
trigger thumb
etiology, VI:648
general discussion, VI:648–649
timing considerations, VI:546t
treatment strategies, VI:648–649
tuberous breast deformity, V:521–547
asymmetric tuberous breast deformity
Case III (asymmetric tuberous breast
deformity), V:533
Case IV (Type II tuberous breast),
V:533–534, 534f–535f
Case VI (Type III flap), V:534–537
Case V (severe bilateral mammary
hypoplasia and tuberous
deformity), V:534, 536f
general considerations, V:532
autologous fat grafts, V:591

congenital defects (Continued)
background information, V:521–522
case studies
asymmetric tuberous breast deformity,
V:533–537, 534f–536f
Case I (bilateral symmetric tuberous
breast), V:523f–524f, 531
Case III (asymmetric tuberous breast
deformity), V:533
Case II (severe tuberous breast
deformity), V:524f–526f, 531–532
Case IV (Type II tuberous breast),
V:533–534, 534f–535f
Case VI (Type III flap), V:534–537
Case V (severe bilateral mammary
hypoplasia and tuberous
deformity), V:534, 536f
glandular flap Type III, V:534–537
severe tuberous breast deformity,
V:524f–526f, 531–532
classifications
background information, V:526–529
Type I tuberous breast, V:523f–526f,
526
Type II tuberous breast, V:526–527,
527f–528f, 529b
Type III tuberous breast, V:529, 529b
glandular correction flaps
characteristics, V:529–531
glandular flap Type I, V:530
glandular flap Type II, V:530
glandular flap Type III, V:530
glandular flap Type IV, V:530–531
pathogenesis, V:522
patient presentation and diagnosis
diagnosis, V:522–529, 523b
evaluation examinations, V:526–529
postoperative care and follow-up,
V:544–545
surgical technique and treatment
case studies, V:531–532
general considerations, V:529, 529b
glandular correction flaps, V:529–531
intraoperative sequence, V:532
suturing techniques, V:544–545
terminology, V:521–522
urogenital defect reconstruction, III:906–924
defect occurrence, III:906
embryology, III:907–908
epidemiology, III:908
etiology, III:908
outcomes and complicatons, III:916–921
patient presentation and diagnosis,
III:908–909
patient selection, III:909
postoperative care and follow-up,
III:915
secondary procedures, III:921
surgical technique and treatment
bladder exstrophy, III:912–913, 913f
female epispadias repair, III:912–913,
914f
meatoplasty and glanuloplasty,
III:913–915, 914b, 916f
tubularized incised plate (TIP) repair,
III:914, 917f
urethral reconstruction, III:913, 915f
vaginal reconstruction, III:909–912
See also hypertelorism; Poland
syndrome

congenital dermal melanocytosis, I:726–727
congenital facial paralysis, III:284
congenital fibromatosis
patient presentation and diagnosis, III:881
surgical technique and treatment, III:881
congenital hemangioma (CH)
classification systems, I:677t, VI:668t
clinical manifestations, I:687
pathogenesis, VI:673–674
patient presentation and diagnosis, VI:674,
676f
surgical technique and treatment, VI:674
treatment strategies, I:687
congenital lipomatosis overgrowth, vascular
malformations, epidermal nevi, and
scoliosis syndrome See CLOVES
syndrome
congenital longitudinal arrest, VI:555–556
congenital melanocytic nevi (CMN),
III:837–854
epidemiology, III:837
etiology, III:837–838
neurocutaneous melanosis (NCM),
III:837–838, 838f
pathogenesis, III:837–838
patient presentation and diagnosis,
III:838–839, 839f
patient selection, III:840
surgical technique and treatment
excision with skin graft reconstruction,
III:840–842, 842f–843f
extremities, III:848, 849f–853f
face and neck, III:844, 846f
partial-thickness excision, III:840
pediatric tissue expansion, III:844
satellite nevi, III:848–851, 849f
scalp, III:844, 845f
serial excision, III:840, 841f
tissue expansion, III:842–844
treatment strategies, III:840–851, 841f
trunk, III:844–848, 847f–850f
congenital myotonic dystrophy, III:807t
congenital nevi, I:745, 745f–746f
congenital nevomelanocytic nevus (CNN),
III:112–113, 114f
congenital pigment cell nevus, I:724, 725f
congenital transverse arrest
assessment strategies, VI:548, 549f
general considerations, VI:548b
outcomes and complicatons
distraction augmentation manoplasty,
VI:554, 554f
foot donor site, VI:554–555
free nonvascularized phalangeal transfer,
VI:553–554
free phalangeal transfer, VI:554–555
free toe transfer, VI:555, 555f
prosthetics, VI:553
secondary procedures, VI:555
pathogenesis, VI:548–549
patient presentation and diagnosis,
VI:549–550, 549f–550f
patient selection, VI:550–553
postoperative care and follow-up,
VI:550–553
surgical technique and treatment
carpal level, VI:551
forearm level, VI:550–551
metacarpal level, VI:551–553, 551f–553f
transhumeral level, VI:550

conjoined twins, **III**:893–905
  classification systems, **III**:893–897, 894f–897f
  dorsal unions, **III**:897
  etiology, **III**:897, 898f
  incidence, **III**:893
  outcomes and complicatons, **III**:904
  postoperative care and follow-up, **III**:904
  prenatal evaluation, **III**:897–899, 899f
  surgical technique and treatment
    clinical case studies
      ischiopagus tripus twins, **III**:902b, 902f
      ischiopagus twins, **III**:901b–903b, 903f
      omphalopagus and ischiopagus twins,
        III:901b–902b
      omphalopagus twins, **III**:903b, 904f
      thoracopagus and ischiopagus twins,
        III:901b, 901f
      thoracopagus and omphalopagus
        twins, **III**:902b, 903f
    obstetric management, **III**:899
    plastic surgery role, **III**:900–901
    preoperative planning, **III**:899–900, 900f
  ventral unions
    caudal unions, **III**:895, 898f
    lateral unions, **III**:895, 898f
    rostral unions, **III**:895, 898f
connective tissue growth factor (CTGF),
  I:270t, 284
constricted ears, **II**:489–490, **III**:204, 205f–206f
constriction band syndrome
  bone grafts, **VI**:642
  clinical manifestations, **VI**:641–642, 642f
  surgical treatment, **VI**:546t, 641–642,
    642f–643f
  toe-to-hand transplantations, **VI**:642, 643f
contact burns, **IV**:394–395, 395f
continuous positive airway pressure (CPAP),
  I:127, **III**:96, 102–103
Contour Threads, **II**:319
contracted nose
  dermal fat graft, **II**:176
  derotation grafts, **II**:176, 176f
  rib cartilage graft, **II**:176
  septal extension grafts, **II**:176
  surgical technique and treatment, **II**:173–176
contract law, **I**:97
cooperatives, **I**:85
Cooper, Samuel, **IV**:393
Cooper's ligaments, **IV**:224, **V**:3–5, 120–121,
  120f–121f, 522
copper (Cu)
  deficiency disorders, **I**:282
  glycyl-L-histidyl-L-lysine-Cu^{2+} (GHK-Cu),
    II:18
Cordyceps sinensis, **II**:23
core needle biopsy, **IV**:106, **V**:272–273,
  272f–273f
corneal protection, **II**:140, 142f
Cornelia de Lange syndrome, **VI**:567t
cornification, **I**:320
cornified nail bed
  characteristics, **VI**:124
  surgical technique and treatment, **VI**:124
corporations, **I**:85
corrective cosmetics, **IV**:485
corrugators, **II**:110–111, 110f, **III**:15
Corset (Feldman) platysmaplasty, **II**:320f
Cortesi, GB, **I**:18

cortical bone, **I**:425–426, 426f, 449
corticosteroids
  infantile hemangioma (IH)
    intralesional corticosteroids, **I**:682
    systemic corticosteroids, **I**:682–684
    topical corticosteroids, **I**:682
  rheumatoid arthritis, **VI**:372–373, 380b
  secondary rhinoplasty, **II**:481
  sensitive skin, **II**:21
  transplantation immunology, **I**:821, 822t
cosmetic surgery, **II**:1–12
  age distribution, **II**:3t
  Asian facial cosmetic surgery, **II**:163–183
    beauty ideals, **II**:163–164
    blepharoplasty
      anatomical considerations, **II**:164–165,
        165f–166f
      eyelid characteristics, **II**:164
      incisional methods, **II**:168, 169f
      lateral canthoplasty, **II**:170, 171f–172f
      medial epicanthoplasty, **II**:169,
        170f–171f
      nonincisional methods, **II**:167–168,
        167f–168f
      outcomes and complicatons, **II**:170–172
      partial incisional methods, **II**:168, 168f
      postoperative care and follow-up,
        II:170
      preoperative assessment, **II**:166–167,
        166f–167f
      subclinical ptosis repair, **II**:169
      surgical technique and treatment,
        II:167–170
    facial bone surgery
      anterior segmental ostectomy, **II**:178,
        181–182
      beauty ideals, **II**:177
      facial contouring, **II**:179–181
      historical background, **II**:177–178
      malar reduction, **II**:177–178
      mandible angle reduction, **II**:178, 182
      orthognathic surgery, **II**:178, 181–182
      outcomes and complicatons, **II**:182
      patient presentation and diagnosis,
        II:178–179
      surgical technique and treatment,
        II:179–182
      zygoma reduction, **II**:182
    facial contouring surgery
      malar reduction surgery, **II**:180–181,
        180f
      mandible angle ostectomy, **II**:179,
        179f–180f
      narrowing genioplasty, **II**:181, 181f
    malar reduction surgery
      bicoronal approach, **II**:181
      intraoral infracture technique with
        incomplete osteotomy, **II**:181
      intraoral L-shaped ostectomy, **II**:181
      surgical technique, **II**:180–181, 180f
    orthognathic surgery
      bimaxillary protrusion, **II**:181–182
      jaw rotation, **II**:181, 182f–183f
    rhinoplasty
      alar base surgery, **II**:177
      blunt nasal tip, **II**:173
      broad nasal dorsum, **II**:173
      bulbous nose, **II**:175, 176f

cosmetic surgery (*Continued*)
    capsular contractures, **II**:177
    contracted nose, **II**:173–176
    forehead augmentation, **II**:174f, 177
    general discussion, **II**:172–173
    genioplasty, **II**:177
    historical background, **II**:173
    implant deviation, **II**:176
    implant exposure, **II**:176
    implant infection, **II**:176
    low profile nasal dorsum
      augmentation, **II**:173–174, 174f
    nasal skeleton, **II**:172–173
    outcomes and complicatons, **II**:176–177
    paranasal augmentation, **II**:177
    patient presentation and diagnosis,
      II:173
    secondary procedures, **II**:177
    septal extension grafts, **II**:175–176, 175f
    short/contracted nose, **II**:173
    short nose, **II**:175–176, 475–476,
      478f–479f
    soft tissue profile, **II**:172–173
    surgical technique and treatment,
      II:173–176
    underprojected nasal tip, **II**:173–175
  endoscopic approaches, **V**:81–96
    background and general characteristics
      general discussion, **V**:81–82
      illumination and imaging technology,
        V:82
      latissimus dorsi (LD) flap, **V**:82–83
      optical cavities, **V**:81–82
      support systems, **V**:82
    endoscopic augmentation mammaplasty
      breast anatomy, **V**:83
      outcomes and complicatons, **V**:87–88,
        88f
      patient presentation and diagnosis, **V**:83
      patient selection, **V**:83–84
      postoperative care and follow-up,
        V:87–88
      surgical technique and treatment,
        V:84–87, 84f–87f
  gender distribution, **II**:3t
  historical background, **I**:27
  patient management
    friends and family as patients, **II**:5–6
    ideal patient, **II**:3–4
    initial consultation
      first contact, **II**:6
      nurse's assessment, **II**:6
      patient coordinator, **II**:7
      photographic consent, **II**:6–7
      post-consultation follow-up letter, **II**:7
      preoperative consent, **II**:9
      presurgery anesthesia evaluation form,
        II:9
      surgeon's assessment, **II**:6
    patient acceptance
      financial expectations, **II**:8–9
      informed consent, **II**:8
      surgical expectations, **II**:8
    patient motivation, **II**:3–4
    patient rejection
      guidelines, **II**:7–8, 7f
      timing, **II**:7–8
      wording, **II**:8

*Note: **Boldface** roman numerals indicate volume. Page numbers followed by f refer to figures; page numbers followed by t refer to tables; page numbers followed by b refer to boxes.*

cosmetic surgery (Continued)
    postoperative care and follow-up
        discharge guidelines, II:9–10
        follow-up consultations, II:9–10
    research summary, II:11
    second and subsequent consultations,
        II:7
    special patient groups
        male cosmetic surgery patient, II:4, 4f
        young cosmetic surgery patient, II:4–5,
            4f–5f
    unhappy patients
        colleague's patient, II:10–11
        communication skills, II:10–11
    postoperative care and follow-up
        discharge guidelines, II:9–10
        follow-up consultations, II:9–10
    procedure increases, II:2f
    research summary, II:11
    societal interest
        concept of beauty, II:1–2
        societal acceptance, II:2–3
        surgeon advertising, II:3
    top five surgical procedures, II:2f
    unsatisfactory results
        characteristics, II:10
        happy patients, II:10
        patient management
            colleague's patient, II:10–11
            communication skills, II:10–11
        unhappy patient and surgeon, II:10
        unhappy patient/happy surgeon, II:10
CosmoDerm/CosmoPlast, II:45t, 47, 49t
    See also soft-tissue fillers
costal cartilage, II:396, 397f, 439
cost–benefit analysis (CBA), I:167
cost-effectiveness analysis (CEA), I:167
costoclavicular compression test, VI:65, 66f
cost–utility analysis (CUA), I:167
counter-transference, I:34
Cowdan syndrome, VI:669, 690
cranio-carpo-tarsal dystrophy, VI:646, 646f
craniofacial deformities, I:44–45, III:655
craniofacial development, III:503–516
    craniofacial clefts
        differential defects, III:509, 509f–510f
        FOXE1 (Forkhead box protein E1)
            mutation, III:510–511
        general discussion, III:509–511
        inadequate growth, III:509–510
        IRF6 (interferon regulatory factor) gene,
            III:511
        transforming growth factor-β (TGF-β)
            superfamily, III:509, 509f–510f
        Wingless (Wnt) signaling defects,
            III:509–510
    craniosynostoses, III:512
    facial prominence establishment and
        fusion
        characteristics, III:508–509, 508f
        frontonasal prominence, III:508, 508f
        lateral nasal prominences, III:508, 509f
        mandibular prominences, III:509
        maxillary prominences, III:508–509
    general discussion, III:503
    initiation stage
        bone morphogenetic proteins (BMPs),
            III:505, 506f
        craniocaudal and mediolateral axes,
            III:504–505

craniofacial development (Continued)
    cyclopia, III:505
    disruptions and malformations, III:505,
        506t
    gastrulation, III:504–505
    holoprosencephaly (HPE), III:505, 506t
    Sonic hedgehog (Shh) expression, III:505,
        505f–506f, 506t
    neurocranium growth and ossification
        cartilaginous neurocranium, III:511
        characteristics, III:511–512
        cranial sutures, III:511f
        membranous neurocranium, III:511–512,
            511f
    neurulation
        Ephrin/Eph signaling, III:507–508
        neural crest generation, III:506–508, 507f
        neural crest migration pattern, III:504f,
            507–508, 507f
    pharyngeal arches
        characteristics, III:512–515, 513f–514f,
            513t
        developmental disorders, III:514
    suture development, III:512
    teratogens
        cholesterol biosynthesis and metabolism,
            III:515
        developmental effects, III:514–515
        prenatal alcohol consumption, III:515
        retinoids and retinoid-induced
            embryopathies, III:514–515
    unique features
        embryo axes, III:504f
        general discussion, III:503
        neural crest migration pattern, III:504f
    viscerocranium development, III:512
craniofacial fibrous dysplasia, III:380–397
    assessment and diagnosis considerations,
        III:380
    complications, III:392–393
    disease process, III:380–382
    pathogenesis, III:380–382
    patient presentation and diagnosis, III:382
    patient selection, III:382–383, 384f
    postoperative care and follow-up, III:389
    research summary, III:395–396
    secondary procedures, III:393–395,
        395f–396f
    surgical technique and treatment
        nonsurgical treatments, III:383
        operation timing, III:383–385
        preoperative assessment, III:383
        surgical approach
            optic nerve decompression, III:384f,
                386
            zonal procedure, III:385–389, 385f
            zone 1, III:385–386, 386f–393f
            zone 2, III:387
            zone 3, III:387
            zone 4, III:387–389, 394f
craniofacial microsomia (CFM), III:761–791
    disease process
        associated syndromes, III:769t
        auricular malformation, III:767, 771f
        embryology, III:763–764, 763f–764f
        etiopathogenesis, III:761–763, 762f
        extracraniofacial anatomy, III:768
        muscle function, III:766–767
        natural growth behavior, III:770–771
        nervous system anomalies, III:767

craniofacial microsomia (CFM) (Continued)
        nonskeletal (soft) tissue, III:765–766, 770f
        pathology, III:764, 765f
        skeletal tissue, III:764–765, 766f–769f
        skin and subcutaneous tissue, III:767,
            771f
    incidence, III:761
    mandibular growth studies, III:790–791,
        790f
    patient presentation and diagnosis
        cephalometrics, III:774–775, 776f
        classification systems, III:772–773, 772t,
            773f–774f, 774t–775t
        computed tomography (CT), III:775, 777f
        differential diagnosis, III:771–772, 772f
        endoscopic approaches, III:775
        photographic documentation, III:773–774
        sleep studies, III:775
    patient selection, III:775–777
    surgical technique and treatment
        auricular reconstruction, III:786
        autogenous fat injections, III:786
        bone grafts, III:781–782, 783f
        commissuroplasty, III:777–779, 778f–779f
        fronto-orbital advancement/cranial vault
            remodeling, III:786
        gastrostomy, III:777
        mandibular distraction, III:779–781,
            780f–782f
        maxillomandibular orthognathic surgery,
            III:784f
        Le Fort I osteotomy, III:782–786,
            784f–785f
        two-splint technique, III:785
        unilateral versus bilateral ramus
            osteotomies, III:785–786
    microvascular free flap, III:786, 786f–787f
    occlusion management
        early intervention, III:787
        orthodontic management during active
            distraction, III:787–788, 788f
        postdistraction orthodontic
            management, III:788, 788f
        predistraction orthodontic
            management, III:787
    tracheostomy, III:777
    treatment algorithms
        adolescence and adulthood, III:789–790
        childhood, III:789
        early childhood, III:789
        neonatal period and infancy, III:788–789
craniofacial surgery
    acquired cranial and facial bone
        deformities, III:228, 230f–231f
    craniofacial clefts, III:701–725
        characteristics, III:701
        classifications
            classification systems, III:701–704, 703t
            median craniofacial dysraphia,
                III:703–704, 703t
            median craniofacial hyperplasia (tissue
                excess or duplication), III:703t,
                704
            median craniofacial hypoplasia (tissue
                deficiency or agenesis), III:702–703,
                703t
        clinical expression, III:720
        differential defects, III:509, 509f–510f
        embryology, III:686, 702f
        epidemiology, III:704–706

craniofacial surgery (Continued)
 etiology
  embryologic craniofacial development,
   III:702f, 704–705
  failure of fusion theory, **III:**705–706
  neuromeric theory, **III:**706
 FOXE1 (Forkhead box protein E1)
  mutation, **III:**510–511
 general discussion, **III:**509–511
 inadequate growth, **III:**509–510
 IRF6 (interferon regulatory factor) gene,
  III:511
 median craniofacial dysraphia
  anterior encephaloceles, **III:**703–704
  characteristics, **III:**703–704
  number 0 cleft, **III:**709
  skeletal involvement, **III:**709
  soft-tissue involvement, **III:**709
  true median cleft, **III:**703
 median craniofacial hypoplasia (tissue
  deficiency or agenesis)
  holoprosencephalic spectrum (alobar
   brain), **III:**702
  median cerebrofacial hypoplasia (lobar
   brain), **III:**702
  median facial hypoplasia, **III:**702
  microform variants, **III:**702–703
  number 0 cleft, **III:**703t, 708–709, 708f
  skeletal deficiencies, **III:**708–709, 708f
  skeletal excess, **III:**709
  soft-tissue deficiencies, **III:**708, 708f
  soft-tissue midline excess, **III:**709
 number 0 cleft
  characteristics, **III:**706–709
  median craniofacial dysraphia,
   III:709
  median craniofacial hyperplasia
   (tissue excess or duplication),
   III:709
  median craniofacial hypoplasia,
   III:703t, 708, 708f
  treatment strategies, **III:**722f–723f
 number 1 cleft
  characteristics, **III:**709
  skeletal involvement, **III:**709, 710f
  soft-tissue involvement, **III:**709, 710f
 number 2 cleft
  skeletal involvement, **III:**711
  soft-tissue involvement, **III:**709–711,
   710f
  treatment strategies, **III:**723f
 number 3 cleft
  characteristics, **III:**711
  skeletal involvement, **III:**711, 711f
  soft-tissue involvement, **III:**711, 711f
  treatment strategies, **III:**724f
 number 4 cleft
  characteristics, **III:**712–713
  skeletal involvement, **III:**712f, 713
  soft-tissue involvement, **III:**712, 712f
 number 5 cleft
  characteristics, **III:**713–714
  skeletal involvement, **III:**713f, 714
  soft-tissue involvement, **III:**713, 713f
 number 6 cleft
  characteristics, **III:**714
  skeletal involvement, **III:**714, 714f
  soft-tissue involvement, **III:**714, 714f

craniofacial surgery (Continued)
 number 7 cleft
  characteristics, **III:**714–715
  skeletal involvement, **III:**715, 715f
  soft-tissue involvement, **III:**714–715,
   715f
 number 8 cleft
  characteristics, **III:**715–716, 715f–716f
  skeletal involvement, **III:**715–716, 716f
  soft-tissue involvement, **III:**715
 number 9 cleft
  characteristics, **III:**716–717
  skeletal involvement, **III:**716–717
  soft-tissue involvement, **III:**716, 717f
 number 10 cleft
  characteristics, **III:**717
  skeletal involvement, **III:**717
  soft-tissue involvement, **III:**717, 717f
 number 11 cleft
  characteristics, **III:**717–718
  skeletal involvement, **III:**717–718
  soft-tissue involvement, **III:**717, 718f
 number 12 cleft
  characteristics, **III:**718
  skeletal involvement, **III:**718, 718f
  soft-tissue involvement, **III:**718, 718f
 number 13 cleft
  characteristics, **III:**718–719, 719f
  skeletal involvement, **III:**718–719
  soft-tissue involvement, **III:**718
 number 14 cleft
  characteristics, **III:**719
  skeletal involvement, **III:**719, 720f
  soft-tissue involvement, **III:**719, 720f
 number 30 cleft
  characteristics, **III:**719–720, 721f
  skeletal involvement, **III:**720
  soft-tissue involvement, **III:**720
 orbital hypertelorism, **III:**686–700
  Apert syndrome, **III:**689
  craniofrontonasal dysplasia, **III:**689
  Crouzon syndrome, **III:**688, 688f
  embryology, **III:**686
  faciocraniosynostosis, **III:**688–689
  median facial clefts, **III:**687
  oculomotor disorders, **III:**699
  outcomes and complicatons, **III:**698
  pathogenesis, **III:**686–689
  patient presentation and diagnosis,
   III:687–688
  patient selection, **III:**689
  Pfeiffer syndrome, **III:**688–689
  postoperative care and follow-up,
   III:695–696
  recurrences, **III:**699–700
  secondary procedures, **III:**698–700, 698f
  surgical technique and treatment,
   III:689–695
  Tessier cleft classification system,
   III:687–688, 687f
 outcomes and complicatons, **III:**725
 patient selection
  number 0 cleft, **III:**706–709
  number 1 cleft, **III:**709
  number 2 cleft, **III:**709–711
  number 3 cleft, **III:**711
  number 4 cleft, **III:**712–713
  number 5 cleft, **III:**713–714

craniofacial surgery (Continued)
  number 6 cleft, **III:**714
  number 7 cleft, **III:**714–715
  number 8 cleft, **III:**715–716
  number 9 cleft, **III:**716–717
  number 10 cleft, **III:**717
  number 11 cleft, **III:**717–718
  number 12 cleft, **III:**718
  number 13 cleft, **III:**718–719
  number 14 cleft, **III:**719
  number 30 cleft, **III:**719–720
  Tessier cleft classification system,
   III:687–688, 687f, 706, 707f
 research summary, **III:**725
 transforming growth factor-β (TGF-β)
  superfamily, **III:**509, 509f–510f
 treatment strategies
  basic procedure, **III:**721–725
  number 0 cleft, **III:**722f–723f
  number 2 cleft, **III:**723f
  number 3 cleft, **III:**724f
 Wingless (Wnt) signaling defects,
  III:509–510
facial injuries, **III:**49–88
 causal factors, **III:**49
 condylar and subcondylar fractures,
  III:83, 83f
 edentulous mandible fractures, **III:**83–84,
  84f
 facial transplantation, **III:**131
 frontal bone and sinus fractures
  clinical examination, **III:**51
  complications, **III:**53
  computed tomography (CT), **III:**51
  injury patterns, **III:**51
  nasofrontal duct, **III:**51, 52f
  surgical technique and treatment,
   III:52–53, 52f
 gunshot wounds
  delayed versus immediate
   reconstruction, **III:**85
  immediate and high velocity gunshot
   wounds, **III:**86–87
  low velocity gunshot wounds, **III:**85–87
  treatment strategies, **III:**86–87, 86f
 initial assessment
  blunt trauma craniofacial injuries,
   III:50–51
  clinical examination, **III:**50–51
  computed tomography (CT), **III:**51
  general discussion, **III:**49–51
  timing considerations, **III:**49–50
 lower facial fractures, **III:**75
 mandibular fractures
  antibiotics, **III:**82
  characteristics, **III:**75
  Class I fractures, **III:**77–78
  Class II fractures, **III:**78
  Class III fractures, **III:**78–80
  classification systems, **III:**76–77
  clinical examination, **III:**76
  comminuted fractures, **III:**78, 79f
  complications, **III:**82–83
  dental wiring and fixation techniques,
   III:75–76
  diagnosis, **III:**76
  displacement direction and extent,
   III:77

*Note: **Boldface** roman numerals indicate volume. Page numbers followed by f refer to figures; page numbers followed by t refer to tables; page numbers followed by b refer to boxes.*

craniofacial surgery (Continued)
  edentulous mandible fractures,
    III:83–84, 84f
  fracture line direction and angulation,
    III:77, 77f
  internal fixation devices, III:80–83
  intraoral approach, III:79
  muscle function considerations,
    III:76
  open reduction treatment, III:78–79
  reduction and fixation principles,
    III:78, 78f
  surgical indicators, III:79–80
  teeth, III:77
  temporomandibular joint, III:76–77
  third molar extraction, III:81, 81f
  treatment strategies, III:77
  midfacial fractures
    complications, III:74
    Le Fort classification of facial fractures,
      III:71–75, 72f
    midface buttresses, III:70–71, 70f
    nasal fractures, III:57–59, 58f
    nasoethmoidal orbital fractures,
      III:60–61
    postoperative care and follow-up,
      III:74
    zygoma, III:63–65
  orbital fractures
    blow-out fractures (children), III:54,
      54f
    blow-out fractures (floor of the orbit),
      III:54
    characteristics, III:53–57
    complications, III:56–57
    computed tomography (CT), III:54
    infraorbital nerve anesthesia, III:57
    operative technique, III:55
    orbital apex syndrome, III:57
    physical examination, III:53–54, 54f
    postoperative care and follow-up,
      III:56
    schematic diagram, III:53f
    superior orbital fissure syndrome,
      III:57
    surgical anatomy, III:53
    surgical technique and treatment,
      III:54–55
    timing considerations, III:55
    treatment indicators, III:54
  panfacial fractures
    complications, III:84–85, 85f
    definition, III:84–85
    postoperative care and follow-up,
      III:85
    surgical sequence, III:84
    treatment strategies, III:84
  upper facial fractures
    frontal bone and sinus injury patterns,
      III:51
    orbital fractures, III:53–57
  orthognathic surgery, III:655–670
    complications, III:667–670
    growth and development factors,
      III:655–656, 656f
    model surgery
      basic procedure, III:658
      isolated mandibular surgery, III:658
      isolated maxillary and two-jaw surgery,
        III:658

craniofacial surgery (Continued)
  patient presentation and diagnosis
    cleft/craniofacial team, III:656
    patient history and examination,
      III:656–657
    preoperative assessment, III:656–657
  patient selection
    cephalometric and dental evaluation,
      III:657–658, 657f
    general discussion, III:657–660
    model surgery, III:658
    three-dimensional (3D) computed
      tomography (CT) models, III:658,
      659f
    treatment planning process, III:658–660
  postoperative care and follow-up, III:666
  prognosis and outcomes, III:667–670,
    667t
  secondary procedures, III:670
  surgical technique and treatment
    apertognathia, III:666, 668f
    basic procedure, III:660
    bilateral sagittal split osteotomy,
      III:661–662
    cleft lip surgery, III:663–665, 663f–664f
    distraction osteogenesis, III:665
    genioplasty, III:662–663
    intraoral vertical ramus osteotomy,
      III:662
    Le Fort I osteotomy, III:610f–611f,
      660–661, 661f, 663f, 667f–668f, 669t
    maxillary constriction, III:665, 667f
    short lower face, III:666
    skeletal anatomy, III:660
    skeletal class II malocclusions, III:665,
      666f
    skeletal class III malocclusions, III:665
    surgically assisted rapid palatal
      expansion (SARPE) procedure,
      III:661
    two-jaw surgery, III:662
    vertical maxillary excess, III:666
    velopharyngeal insufficiency (VPI),
      III:667–670, 667t
  pediatric facial fractures, III:671–685
    associated injuries, III:672
    background information, III:671
    demographics, III:672
    growth and development factors
      basic principles, III:672–674
      condylar head fractures, III:678f
      cranial-to-facial ratio, III:672f
      Le Fort fracture patterns, III:675f
      mandibular condyle, III:677f
      oblique craniofacial fracture patterns,
        III:676f–677f
      orbital region, III:674f
      sinus development, III:673f
    incidence, III:671–672
    orbital fracture classification system,
      III:677t
    outcomes and complicatons
      adverse outcome classifications, III:683t
      basic principles, III:682–683
      cranial base/skull fractures, III:683
      mandible fractures, III:684, 684f
      maxillary and midface fractures,
        III:684
      metallic cranial hardware, III:683f–684f
      nasal fractures, III:684

craniofacial surgery (Continued)
  orbital fractures, III:683–684
  zygomaticomaxillary complex
    fractures, III:684
  patient presentation and diagnosis,
    III:674–675, 678f–679f
  patient selection, III:675–678
  postoperative care and follow-up, III:682
  research summary, III:685
  secondary procedures, III:684–685
  surgical technique and treatment
    basic procedure, III:678
    cranial base/frontal skull fractures,
      III:678–679, 679f–680f
    mandible fractures, III:681f–682f, 682
    maxillary and midface fractures,
      III:680, 681f
    nasal and naso-orbital ethmoid
      fractures, III:681–682, 681t, 682f
    orbital fractures, III:679–680, 680f
    zygomaticomaxillary complex
      fractures, III:681
  robotic surgery, I:862–863
  surgical innovation, I:8
  See also hypertelorism
craniofrontonasal dysplasia, III:689
craniopagus twins, III:893–897, 894f, 896f–898f
craniosynostosis
  characteristics, I:195–196, III:749
  faciocraniosynostosis
    Apert syndrome, III:689
    characteristics, III:688–689
    craniofrontonasal dysplasia, III:689
    Crouzon syndrome, III:688, 688f
    general discussion, III:686
    Pfeiffer syndrome, III:688–689
    surgical indicators and timing
      face, III:694–695
      general discussion, III:694–695
      orbits, III:694, 694f
      surgical technique, III:695
  molecular bases, III:512
  nonsyndromic craniosynostosis, III:726–748
    definition, III:726
    pathogenesis, III:726–728
    patient presentation and diagnosis
      anterior plagiocephaly, III:729, 730f,
        730t
      brachycephaly, III:729, 730f, 730t
      cephalic index (CI), III:728t
      characteristics, III:728–731
      plagiocephaly, III:729, 729t
      posterior plagiocephaly, III:729–731,
        731f, 731t
      scaphocephaly, III:728–729, 729f, 729t
      skull shape, III:728f
      synostotic versus deformational
        plagiocephaly, III:729t
      thumbprinting patterns, III:728, 730f
      trigonocephaly, III:731, 731f, 731t
    patient selection, III:731–732
  syndromic craniosynostosis, III:749–760
    characteristics, I:196–198, 197t, III:749
    complications, III:759–760
    disease characteristics, III:749–750, 750t
    fibroblast growth factor receptor
      (FGFR)-related mutations, III:749–
      750, 750t
    patient presentation and diagnosis,
      III:750–751, 750t

craniosynostosis (Continued)
  patient selection, III:751–752, 752f
  postoperative care and follow-up,
     III:757–759
  prognosis and outcomes, III:759–760
  secondary procedures, III:760
  surgical technique and treatment
     anterior fossa enlargement, III:753f
     bandeau design, III:754f
     basic techniques, III:752–757
     facial bipartition, III:758f
     Le Fort III osteotomy, III:758f–759f
     low frontal osteotomy, III:755f
     low posteriorly draining enlarged
        transcranial veins, III:756f
     midvault cranioplasty, III:756f
     monobloc frontofacial advancement
        procedure, III:757f
     posterior keels of bone, III:757f
     skull base osteotomies, III:755f
     stair-step osteotomy, III:754f
Cremaster muscle, IV:235, 236f–237f
CREST syndrome, VI:409
"crossed fingers" sign, VI:58–59
cross finger flaps, VI:130–131, 133f
Crouzon syndrome
  characteristics, I:197, 197f, 197t, III:749–750,
     750t
  patient presentation and diagnosis, III:688,
     688f
  surgical innovation, III:226
crow's feet, II:34–37
cruciate pulleys, VI:29–32, 30f, 179–182,
     180f
crush/compression injuries, I:466–467, 466t,
     VI:256, 256f, 261f
cryotherapy, I:308–309, 718
cryptotia, II:490, III:204, 206f–207f
crystalline arthropathy, VI:407t, 409–410
cubital tunnel syndrome
  anatomical considerations, VI:513–514
  clinical signs, VI:514t
  hand therapy, VI:857
  outcomes and complicatons, VI:513b,
     515–516
  patient presentation and diagnosis, VI:514
  patient selection, VI:514
  surgical technique and treatment
     endoscopic decompression, VI:515
     intramuscular transposition, VI:515
     medial epicondylectomy technique,
        VI:515, 516f
     simple decompression, VI:514–515
     subcutaneous transposition, VI:515
     submuscular transposition, VI:515
cultured epithelial autografts (CEA),
     I:336–337, 337f, IV:411, 420f
curcumin, II:24
cutaneomucosal venous malformation
     (CMVM), I:677t, 693–694
cutaneous and soft-tissue tumors, I:707–742
  benign cutaneous and soft-tissue tumors
     benign appendage-origin tumors
        apocrine cystadenoma, I:722–723, 723f
        chondroid syringoma, I:723, 723f
        nevus sebaceous, I:721, 721f
        pilomatricoma, I:721–722, 721f
        steatocystoma multiplex, I:723, 724f

cutaneous and soft-tissue tumors (Continued)
        syringoma, I:722, III:117, 117f
        trichilemmal cyst, I:722, 722f
     benign epithelial-origin tumors
        dermoid cyst, I:720, 721f
        epidermal nevus, I:718, 718f
        epidermoid cyst, I:719, 720f
        keratoacanthoma, I:719, 719f, VI:315–
           316, 316f
        milia, I:719–720
        seborrheic keratosis, I:719, 719f, VI:316
     benign mesenchymal-origin tumors
        accessory auricles, I:732–733, 733f
        acrochordon, I:730, 730f
        arteriovenous fistula and arteriovenous
           malformation (AVM), I:735, 736f
        capillary malformation, I:734–735
        cavernous hemangioma, I:735, 735f
        dermatofibroma, I:729, 729f, VI:316, 316f
        fibroma pendulum, I:730, 730f
        glomus tumors, I:734
        granulomas, I:733–734, 733f–734f
        hemangioma simplex, I:734, 734f–735f
        hypertrophic scars, I:730, 731f
        juvenile xanthogranuloma, I:729–730,
           729f–730f
        keloid scars, I:730, 730f
        leiomyoma, I:731–732
        lipoma, I:731, 731f–733f
        lymphatic malformation, I:736
        mucous cyst of the oral mucosa, I:736,
           736f
        osteochondrogenic tumors, I:732, 733f
        rhabdomyoma, I:732
        soft fibroma, I:730
        strawberry hemangioma, I:734–735,
           735f
        venous malformation, I:735, 735f
        xanthoma, I:729, 729f
     benign neural crest-origin tumors
        acquired pigment cell nevus, I:724, 724f
        Becker's melanosis, I:725
        blue nevus, I:727
        congenital pigment cell nevus, I:724,
           725f
        dysplastic nevus, I:724, III:113–114, 114f
        juvenile melanoma, I:724–725, 726f
        lentigo simplex, I:723–724, 724f
        Mongolian spot, I:726–727, 728f
        neurofibroma, I:728, 728f, VI:320, 320f
        neuromas, I:727
        nevus of Ito, I:726, 727f
        nevus of Ota, I:725–726, 726f
        nevus spilus, I:725, 726f
        pigment cell nevus, I:723–725
        schwannoma, I:727, 728f, VI:320, 320f
  malignant cutaneous and soft-tissue tumors
     basal cell carcinoma
        characteristics, I:737, 737f, III:117–118,
           118f, VI:317, 317f
        dermoscopic analysis, I:709, 709f
        histological classification, I:738b
        surgical margins, I:717
        tumor colors, I:709
     malignant appendage-origin tumors
        extramammary Paget's disease, I:739,
           739f
        Merkel cell carcinoma, I:716t, 739, 739f

cutaneous and soft-tissue tumors (Continued)
        sebaceous carcinoma, I:738, 738f
        sweat gland carcinoma, I:738
        trichilemmal carcinoma, I:738, 738f
     malignant epithelial-origin tumors
        actinic keratosis, I:736, 736f, VI:316–
           317, 317f
        Bowen's disease, I:736–737
        squamous cell carcinomas (SCCs),
           I:737, 737f, III:118–119, 118f,
           VI:317, 317f
     malignant mesenchymal-origin tumors
        angiosarcomas, I:741–742, 741f
        chondrosarcoma, I:741, VI:329
        dermatofibrosarcoma protuberans
           (DFSP), I:739, 739f
        Kaposi's sarcoma, I:742
        leiomyosarcoma, I:740, 740f
        liposarcoma, I:740, 740f
        malignant fibrous histiocytoma (MFH),
           I:739–740, 740f, VI:321, 322f
        osteosarcoma, I:741, 741f, VI:329
        rhabdomyosarcoma, I:741
  patient presentation and diagnosis, I:710
     angiography, I:710
     clinical staging system, I:711, 716t
     computed tomography (CT), I:710
     dermoscopic analysis, I:709, 709b, 709f
     Doppler imaging, I:709–710
     inspection and palpation, I:707–709
     magnetic resonance imaging (MRI), I:710
     pathogenic diagnosis, I:710–711
     positron emission tomography (PET),
        I:710
     scintigraphy, I:710
     TNM clinical classification system/pTNM
        pathologic classification system,
        I:711, 712f–714f, 715b, 750–761, 752t
     tumor colors, I:709b
     ultrasound imaging, I:709–710
     X-ray analysis, I:710
  treatment strategies
     chemotherapy, I:717–718
     cryotherapy, I:718
     electrocoagulation therapy, I:718
     immunotherapy, I:718
     laser treatments, I:718
     lymph node dissection
        axillary lymph node dissection,
           I:714–715
        inguinal lymph node dissection, I:715
     radiation therapy (RT), I:717
     reconstructive surgeries, I:717
     sclerotherapy, I:718
     wide excision, I:711–712, 717b
cutaneous horns, VI:314, 314f
cutaneous myxoma, I:736
cutaneous paddle inserts, IV:388f
cutaneous sarcoidosis, III:115–116, 116f
cutaneous squamous cell carcinoma (cSCC),
     III:118–119, 118f
  See also squamous cell carcinomas (SCCs)
cutis marmorata telangiectatica congenita
     (CMTC), I:677t, 690
C–V flap, V:503t, 506–507, 506f, 514–515
cyanoacrylates, I:793
cyclic adenosine monophosphate (cAMP),
     I:626f, III:381

Note: **Boldface** *roman numerals indicate volume. Page numbers followed by f refer to figures; page numbers followed by t refer to tables; page numbers followed by b refer to boxes.*

cyclooxygenase-2 (COX-2), I:433
cyclooxygenase inhibitors, II:21–22
cyclosporine, I:822t, 823, 833t
Cymetra, II:45t, 46–47
cysteine, I:269–271
cystic hygroma, I:678t
cytokines
    Dupuytren's disease, VI:349
    inflammatory mediators, I:819–820
    macrophages, I:816
    mesenchymal stem cells (MSCs), I:225–226
    osteoarthritis, VI:412–413
    radiation therapy (RT), I:662
    scars, I:309–310
    skin aging, II:15
    skin wound healing, I:270t, 275
    wound healing, I:244–245
cytosine, I:177–182, 177f
cytotoxic T-lymphocyte-associated antigen (CTLA-4), I:783

D
dacarbazine (DTIC), I:778–781
daclizumab, I:821t
Dakin solution, IV:410
Daniel's defect classification, III:317t
danshen, V:33t–35t
Darrach procedure, VI:382–384
Dartigues, Louis, I:24
Dartmouth Atlas Project, V:315–316, 316f
Dartos fascia, IV:235, 236f–237f, 298–299, 299f
da Vinci, Leonardo, VI:xliii–xliv
da Vinci system
    advantages/disadvantages, I:856
    craniofacial surgery, I:862
    design features, I:855–856, 856f
    FDA approval, I:855–857
    training simulators, I:865–868
DEAE Sephadex, II:48t
    See also soft-tissue fillers
debridement
    burn wound treatment, IV:416–420, 417f
    facial soft-tissue injuries, III:29
    foot injuries, IV:198–199, 200f
    mutilated/mangled hands, VI:251, 251f
    pressure sores, IV:366–368, 368f
    tar burns, IV:395–396
dedifferentiation processes, I:261–264, 261f
deep circumflex iliac artery, IV:229–230, 229f
deep circumflex iliac artery composite flap, I:529f
deep external pudendal artery, IV:232–235, 234f, 238f
deep femoral artery perforator (DFAP) flap, V:464–467, 468f–469f
DeepFX™ laser, II:71t, 73
deep inferior epigastric artery (DIEA), IV:229–230, 229f
deep inferior epigastric perforator (DIEP) flaps, V:435–456
    anatomical characteristics, V:327f, 436–439, 437f–438f
    breast reconstruction
        background and general characteristics, V:435–436
        delayed reconstruction, V:291f
        immediate postmastectomy breast reconstruction, V:287–291, 288f
        outcomes and complicatons, V:452

deep inferior epigastric perforator (DIEP) flaps (Continued)
    patient presentation and diagnosis
        computed tomography (CT) imaging, V:440, 441f–442f
        preoperative assessment, V:439–440
        ultrasound evaluation, V:440
    patient selection, V:440–441
    postoperative care and follow-up, V:451–452
    recipient vessels, V:439, 439f
    secondary procedures
        BRCA-2 mutation, V:453, 454f
        mammary hypertrophy, V:453, 455f
        nipple-areola complex, V:453, 453f
    shaping guidelines
        breast conus, V:448f, 449–451, 450f
        breast envelope, V:449f, 451
        breast footprint, V:447–449, 448f
        general discussion, V:447–451
        nipple-areola complex, V:449f
    surgical technique
        closure, V:447
        golden rules, V:447b
        intramuscular dissection, V:444f–445f, 446
        operative procedures, V:443–447
        preoperative markings, V:442–443, 444f–445f
        shaping guidelines, V:447–451
        submuscular dissection, V:444f–445f, 446–447
        suprafascial dissection, V:443–446, 444f–445f
        umbilicus creation, V:447
    imaging methods, V:326, 327f–329f
deep palmar arch, VI:469
deep peroneal nerve, IV:48t
deep space infections, VI:338–339, 338f
deep vein thrombosis (DVT)
    abdominal wall reconstruction, IV:283
    abdominoplasty, II:591
    brachioplasty, II:629t
    burn wound complications, IV:431
    facelifts, II:194
    liposuctions, II:525–527
    lower bodylift/belt lipectomy surgery, II:585–588, 593–594
    post-bariatric surgery reconstruction, II:638–639
Defense Advanced Research Projects Agency (DARPA), I:860–861
deformation, I:192
dehiscence
    abdominoplasty, II:557–558
    buttock augmentation, II:614, 614f
    lower bodylift/belt lipectomy surgery, II:591
    reduction mammaplasty, V:191
    scalp and forehead reconstruction, III:131–132
DEKA Research and Development, I:860–861
del (4q) syndrome/del (6q) syndrome, III:807t
DeLange dwarfism, VI:565t
de Lange syndrome, VI:565t, 567t, 573t
Delpech, Jacques Mathieu, I:19
deltopectoral flaps, III:274f, 309t, 318–319, 319f
deltopectoral triangle, IV:223–227
Demodex folliculorum, II:20–21

dendritic cells, I:818
denial, I:32, 37–38
dental occlusal views, I:110
dentoalveolar protrusion, II:179
dentofacial deformities
    characteristics, III:655
    orthognathic surgery
        complications, III:667–670
        growth and development factors, III:655–656, 656f
        model surgery
            basic procedure, III:658
            isolated mandibular surgery, III:658
            isolated maxillary and two-jaw surgery, III:658
        patient presentation and diagnosis
            cleft/craniofacial team, III:656
            patient history and examination, III:656–657
            preoperative assessment, III:656–657
        patient selection
            cephalometric and dental evaluation, III:657–658, 657f
            general discussion, III:657–660
            model surgery, III:658
            three-dimensional (3D) computed tomography (CT) models, III:658, 659f
            treatment planning process, III:658–660
        postoperative care and follow-up, III:666
        prognosis and outcomes, III:667–670, 667t
        secondary procedures, III:670
        surgical technique and treatment
            apertognathia, III:666, 668f
            basic procedure, III:660
            bilateral sagittal split osteotomy, III:661–662
            cleft lip surgery, III:663–665, 663f–664f
            distraction osteogenesis, III:665
            genioplasty, III:662–663
            intraoral vertical ramus osteotomy, III:662
            Le Fort I osteotomy, III:610f–611f, 660–661, 661f, 663f, 667f–668f, 669t
            maxillary constriction, III:665, 667f
            short lower face, III:666
            skeletal anatomy, III:660
            skeletal class II malocclusions, III:665, 666f
            skeletal class III malocclusions, III:665
            surgically assisted rapid palatal expansion (SARPE) procedure, III:661
            two-jaw surgery, III:662
            vertical maxillary excess, III:666
            velopharyngeal insufficiency (VPI), III:667–670, 667t
deoxyguanosine triphosphate (dGTP), I:822–823
deoxyribonucleic acid (DNA)
    characteristics, I:177–182, 177f
    epigenetic mechanisms, I:181–182, 181f
    gene expression, I:179–180
    gene regulation, I:180–181, 180f
    genomic DNA organization, I:178–179, 178f
dependent clingers, I:37
dependent personality, I:35
depositions and narratives, I:93
depressive disorders, I:47–48, 48b
depressor anguli oris, II:41, III:282, 282f

depressor supercilii, III:15–16
de Quervain's tendonitis, VI:364–367, 366f
dermabrasion, II:21t
Dermagraft, I:338, 794t, 795
dermal apron, V:544, 545f
dermal graft and repair *See* skin grafts
DermaLive/DermaDeep, II:48t
    See also soft-tissue fillers
Dermalogen, II:45t, 46–47
dermal orbicular pennant lateral canthoplasty
    (DOPLC), II:156, 158f–159f
dermal papilla, I:321, 322f
dermal sinuses, III:874
dermal substitutes
    Apligraf, I:337, 794t, 795
    bioengineered skin substitutes, I:793–795
    burn reconstruction, IV:441, 448, 502
    burn wound treatment, IV:411b, 412t–415t
    commercial product comparisons, I:794t
    Dermagraft, I:338, 794t, 795
    Epicel, I:794t, 795
    epidermolysis bullosa, IV:522, 523f–524f
    facial burn wound treatment, IV:480,
        482–484
    Integra, I:794, 794t, IV:448
    lower extremity reconstructive surgery,
        IV:128–129, 130f
    skin grafts, I:335–336, 335t, 336f
    skin wound healing, I:289t
dermal vascularization, I:321
Dermamatrix, V:69–71, 70t
dermatofibroma, I:729, 729f, VI:316, 316f
dermatofibrosarcoma protuberans (DFSP),
    I:739, 739f
dermatologic exfoliative disorders, IV:511–517
    See also skin
dermis, I:320, 322f, II:44–45, IV:397–402
dermoid cyst, I:720, 721f
dermoids
    dermal sinus tracts, III:883–884
    external angular dermoids
        disease process, III:884
        patient presentation and diagnosis,
            III:884
        surgical technique and treatment,
            III:884–885
    general characteristics, III:882
    intradural dermoids
        disease process, III:883
        patient presentation and diagnosis,
            III:883, 884f
        surgical technique and treatment,
            III:883–884
    nasal dermoids
        complications, III:883
        disease process, III:882, 882f
        patient presentation and diagnosis,
            III:882
        prognosis and outcomes, III:883
        secondary procedures, III:883
        surgical technique and treatment,
            III:882–883, 882f–883f
    neck cysts
        disease process, III:885
        patient presentation and diagnosis,
            III:885
Desert hedgehog gene, I:428–429
desmoid tumor, I:736

desmoplastic melanoma, I:753, 755f
De-Solv-It, IV:395
deviated nose with dorsal hump
    outcome assessments, II:407
    surgical goals, II:406
    surgical plan, II:407
    systematic analysis, II:405–406, 406f
deviated septum
    nasal disease and obstructions, II:454–455,
        454f–456f
    surgical technique and treatment
        characteristics, II:458–461
        complications, II:463
        C-shaped anteroposterior deviation,
            II:459, 460f
        C-shaped cephalocaudal deviation, II:459,
            460f
        localized deviation, II:461
        open rhinoplasty, II:392–393
        postoperative care and follow-up,
            II:462–463
        prognosis and outcomes, II:463, 463f–464f
        secondary procedures, II:463
        septal tilt, II:459, 459f
        S-shaped anteroposterior deviation,
            II:459, 460f
        S-shaped cephalocaudal deviation, II:459,
            460f
devil's claw, V:33t–35t
dextran, I:582, 615–617, VI:244–245
diabetes
    bone marrow-derived mesenchymal stem
        cells (BMSC), I:227
    diabetic ulcers, I:254–255, 254f, 281,
        IV:194–195
    foot reconstruction
        diabetic ulcers, IV:194–195
        hemorheologic abnormalities, IV:194f,
            195–196
        neuropathic changes, IV:195
    lower extremity reconstructive surgery,
        IV:134, 134f–135f
diacylglycerol (DAG), I:626f
diagnostic tools, II:354–372, VI:68–91
    anthropometrics
        background information, II:354–365, 355f
        chin, II:360, 361f
        eyes, II:358, 358f
        facial beauty ideals, II:177
        forehead, II:356–358, 357f–358f
        lips, II:360, 360f
        neoclassical canons, II:356b
        nose, II:358–359, 359f
        soft tissue facial analysis, II:355–356,
            356b, 356f–357f, 356t
    congenital hand deformities, VI:543–544
    general discussion, II:354, VI:68
    hand tumors, VI:312–313, 313f
    nerve repair and grafting, VI:725
    orthognathic surgical procedures
        blood supply, II:366f
        cephalometrics
            basic principles, II:360–363
            bone landmarks, II:363f
            facial profile classifications, II:361f
            malocclusions, II:362f
            maxillary and mandibular dental
                arches, II:362f

diagnostic tools *(Continued)*
        orthodontic considerations, II:363–364
        software programs, II:363f
        temporomandibular joint (TMJ),
            II:364–365, 364f
    complications
        avascular necrosis, II:371f, 372
        dental and periodontal complications,
            II:371
        hemorrhage, II:371
        neurosensory loss, II:371
        unfavorable aesthetic outcomes, II:371
    genioplasty, II:367–368, 368f
    mandibular osteotomies, II:366–367, 367f
    maxillary osteotomy, II:368–370, 369b,
        369f–370f
    postoperative care and follow-up,
        II:370–371
    surgical technique, II:365–366
    vascular networks, II:366f
    radionuclide imaging, VI:90
    vascular imaging techniques, VI:89–90, 90f
    wrist injuries, VI:166–169
    See also computed tomography (CT);
        magnetic resonance imaging (MRI);
        radiographic imaging
diapedesis, I:245, 246f
diastematomyelia, III:874
diastrophic dysplasia, III:807t, VI:573t
diet and exercise, II:635, 636t
dietary supplements, V:33t–35t
differentiation processes, I:261–264, 261f
difficult patients
    dependent clingers, I:37
    entitled demanders, I:38
    hateful patients, I:36–37
    manipulative help-rejecting complainers,
        I:38–39
    self-destructive deniers, I:37–38
DiGeorge syndrome, III:514
digital Allen's test, VI:60
digital arteries, VI:469
digital cameras, I:117–119
digital fascia, VI:347, 348f
digital joints, I:421–423
digital single lens reflex (dSLR) cameras,
    I:117–119
digital subtraction angiography (DSA),
    VI:89–90
dihydrotestosterone (DHT), II:497–498
dimethyl sulfoxide (DMSO), IV:466
diplopia, III:56
dipyradimole, I:617
Disabilities of the Arm, Shoulder and Hand
    (DASH) Outcome Measure, I:835, VI:247,
    848, 856
discoid lupus erythematosus (DLE), III:115,
    115f
discounted cash flow, I:72–73
disease-modifying antirheumatic drugs
    (DMARDs), VI:372–373, 380b
disorders of sex development (DSD),
    IV:303–304, 336–338, 337t
disruption, I:192–193
disruptive technology, I:843–844, 844f
dissatisfied patients, I:52, 53b
distal amputations, VI:241–242, 241f
distal arthrogryposis–Robin sequence, III:807t

distal humerus malrotation measurement, **VI:**63, 64f
distal interphalangeal (DIP) joint
  distal interphalangeal (DIP) arthrodesis
    fixation techniques
      axial compression screw, **VI:**415–416, 416f
      characteristics, **VI:**414–416
      interosseous wiring, **VI:**415
      K-wire fixation, **VI:**415
      tension band wire technique, **VI:**415
    indicators, **VI:**414
  distal interphalangeal (DIP) fusion
    biomechanical effects, **VI:**414
    complications
      infections, **VI:**417
      nonunion occurrences, **VI:**417
    distal interphalangeal (DIP) arthrodesis
      fixation techniques, **VI:**414–416
      indicators, **VI:**414
    distal interphalangeal (DIP) arthroplasty, **VI:**417
    mucous cysts, **VI:**417
  Dupuytren's disease, **VI:**350–353
  fractures and joint injuries, **VI:**138–139, 141–142, 142f
  osteoarthritis
    biomechanical effects, **VI:**414
    diagnosis, **VI:**414, 415f
    distal interphalangeal (DIP) arthrodesis
      fixation techniques, **VI:**414–416
      indicators, **VI:**414
    surgical indicators, **VI:**414
  replantation and revascularization surgery, **VI:**241–242, 241f
distally based flaps, **I:**531, 531t
distal phalanx fractures
  nail ridges, **VI:**121
  patient presentation and diagnosis, **VI:**120
  reconstructive surgeries, **VI:**120–121
  surgical technique and treatment, **VI:**120
distal radioulnar joint (DRUJ)
  magnetic resonance imaging (MRI), **VI:**86–88
  radiographic imaging, **VI:**75f, 374f
  rheumatoid arthritis
    basic principles, **VI:**374–376
    distal ulna resection (Darrach procedure)
      basic procedure, **VI:**382–384
      chevron incision, **VI:**382f
      outcomes and complicatons, **VI:**383–384
      postoperative care and follow-up, **VI:**383
      pronator quadratus release, **VI:**383f
      radiographic imaging, **VI:**384f
      secondary procedures, **VI:**384
      surgical tips, **VI:**384b
      ulnar head exposure, **VI:**382f
      ulnar head removal, **VI:**383f
      ulnar stump stabilization, **VI:**384f
    radiographic imaging, **VI:**374f
    stability assessment, **VI:**54–55, 56f
distortion, **I:**33
distraction osteogenesis
  basic principles, **I:**446–447
  histology, **I:**446–447, 447f
  orthognathic surgery, **III:**665
  skeletal reconstruction, **IV:**179–180, 179f

DMAIC model (define, measure, analyze, improve, control) of process improvement, **I:**77–78
Dodd–Frank Wall Street Reform and Consumer Protection Act (2010), **I:**86
dog bites, **VI:**343
Domagk, Gerhard, **VI:**xliii–xliv
Donlan syndrome, **III:**807t
Doppler imaging, **I:**500–501, 709–710, **IV:**193, 194f, 470
Dorrance, George, **III:**576–578
dorsal artery of the clitoris, **IV:**232–235, 234f
dorsal intercostal artery perforator (DICAP) flap, **V:**488
dorsalis pedis, **IV:**59, 60f
dorsal metacarpal artery flaps, **VI:**134, 135f
dorsal nasal flap, **III:**143, 144f–145f
dorsal scapular artery, **IV:**222f, 223
Doryphorus, **II:**355f
double-bubble deformity, **V:**116, 116f
double opposing peri-areolar/purse-string flap, **V:**508–510, 508t, 509f–510f
double-opposing tab flap, **V:**511t, 512–513, 512f–513f
double-opposing Z-plasty, **VI:**288f
doxycycline, **I:**692–693, **II:**21t
dressings, wound, **I:**287–288, 289t, **IV:**410–416
drooling, **III:**76
Drucker, Peter, **I:**79, 88–89
dry skin
  basic skin care formulations
    antioxidants, **II:**18
    characteristics, **II:**16–18
    cleansers
      bar surfactants, **II:**16
      characteristics, **II:**16
      liquid surfactants, **II:**16
    moisturizers
      characteristics, **II:**16–18
      emollients, **II:**18
      humectants, **II:**17–18
      occlusives, **II:**17
  causal factors, **II:**15–19
  clinical signs, **II:**16
  hydroxy acids
    alpha hydroxy acids (AHAs)
      characteristics, **II:**18–19
      glycolic acid, **II:**19
      lactic acid, **II:**18–19
      patient selection and treatment, **II:**66–67
    beta hydroxy acid (BHA), **II:**19
Duchenne's sign, **VI:**58–59, 514t
dug out neck deformity, **II:**294, 295f
Duoderm®, **IV:**412t–414t
dup (11q) syndrome, **III:**807t
Dupuytren, Guillaume, **IV:**393
Dupuytren's disease, **VI:**346–362
  arterial insufficiency, **VI:**360b
  clinical manifestations
    digital fascia, **VI:**347, 348f
    first webspace, **VI:**347–348, 348f
    Garrod's nodules, **VI:**352f
    general characteristics, **VI:**351–353
    general discussion, **VI:**346–348
    nodule formation, **VI:**351f
    palmar and palomodigital disease, **VI:**352f
    palmar fascia, **VI:**347, 347f
    plantar fibromatosis, **VI:**352, 352f

Dupuytren's disease (*Continued*)
  complications, **VI:**359–360, 360b
  definition, **VI:**346–348
  digital anatomy, **VI:**349t, 350f–351f
  disease process, **VI:**349–351, 349t, 351f
  epidemiology, **VI:**346
  pathogenesis, **VI:**348–349
  patient presentation and diagnosis
    clinical manifestations, **VI:**351f–352f
    differential diagnoses, **VI:**353
    patient history, **VI:**351–353
    physical examination, **VI:**351–353
  patient selection, **VI:**353
  postoperative care and follow-up, **VI:**359
  prognosis and outcomes, **VI:**359–360
  research summary, **VI:**361
  secondary procedures
    amputation, **VI:**361
    indicators, **VI:**360–361
    proximal interphalangeal (PIP) arthrodesis, **VI:**361
    skeletal traction, **VI:**361
    total volar tenoarthrolysis, **VI:**361
    wedge osteotomy, **VI:**361
  treatment strategies
    general discussion, **VI:**353–359
    injection treatments, **VI:**353–354, 354f–355f
    modality therapy, **VI:**353
    surgical treatment
      check rein release technique, **VI:**358, 358f
      dermatofasciectomy, **VI:**355t, 359
      local fasciectomy, **VI:**355t, 356
      open fasciotomy, **VI:**355t, 356
      percutaneous (needle) aponeurotomy, **VI:**354–355, 355b, 355t, 356f
      radical fasciectomy, **VI:**355t, 358–359
      regional fasciectomy, **VI:**355t, 356–358, 357f–358f, 358b
      surgical options, **VI:**354–359, 355t
Duran–Houser method, **VI:**198–199, 198f
Durkan's median nerve compression test, **VI:**505–507
dye lasers, **I:**718
Dyggve–Melchior–Clausen syndrome, **VI:**573t
dynamic tenodesis effect, **VI:**55–56
dysplasia, **I:**193
dysplastic nevus, **I:**724, **III:**113–114, 114f
dysrhythmias, **IV:**433t

E
EARLi flap *See* latissimus dorsi (LD) flap
earlobe keloids, **III:**220, 223f
ears
  anatomical characteristics, **III:**19, 107f, 187, 188f
  anesthesia, **III:**27–29, 29f
  auricular cartilage graft, **I:**398–404, 399f–405f
  autologous cartilage harvesting, **II:**395–396, 396f
  burn wound treatment, **IV:**473, 498–499
  craniofacial microsomia (CFM), **III:**761–791
    disease process
      associated syndromes, **III:**769t
      auricular malformation, **III:**767, 771f
      embryology, **III:**763–764, 763f–764f
      etiopathogenesis, **III:**761–763, 762f
      extracraniofacial anatomy, **III:**768

ears (Continued)
    muscle function, III:766–767
    natural growth behavior, III:770–771
    nervous system anomalies, III:767
    nonskeletal (soft) tissue, III:765–766,
        770f
    pathology, III:764, 765f
    skeletal tissue, III:764–765, 766f–769f
    skin and subcutaneous tissue, III:767,
        771f
    incidence, III:761
    mandibular growth studies, III:790–791,
        790f
    occlusion management
        early intervention, III:787
        orthodontic management during active
            distraction, III:787–788, 788f
        postdistraction orthodontic
            management, III:788, 788f
        predistraction orthodontic
            management, III:787
    patient presentation and diagnosis
        cephalometrics, III:774–775, 776f
        classification systems, III:772–773, 772t,
            773f–774f, 774t–775t
        computed tomography (CT), III:775,
            777f
        differential diagnosis, III:771–772, 772f
        endoscopic approaches, III:775
        photographic documentation,
            III:773–774
        sleep studies, III:775
    patient selection, III:775–777
    surgical technique and treatment
        auricular reconstruction, III:786
        autogenous fat injections, III:786
        bone grafts, III:781–782, 783f
        commissuroplasty, III:777–779,
            778f–779f
        fronto-orbital advancement/cranial
            vault remodeling, III:786
        gastrostomy, III:777
        mandibular distraction, III:779–781,
            780f–782f
        maxillomandibular orthognathic
            surgery, III:782–786, 784f–785f
        microvascular free flap, III:786,
            786f–787f
        occlusion management, III:787–788
        tracheostomy, III:777
    treatment algorithms
        adolescence and adulthood, III:789–790
        childhood, III:789
        early childhood, III:789
        neonatal period and infancy,
            III:788–789
    embryology, III:187–189
    osteointegrated ear reconstruction,
        I:800–802, 800t, 801f
    otoplasty, II:485–493
        adolescent aesthetic surgery, I:45t
        complications, II:492–493
        definition, II:485
        ear deformities, II:485
        patient dissatisfaction, II:493
        patient presentation and diagnosis
            anatomical structure, II:486f
            asymmetry, II:486

ears (Continued)
        lower third area, II:486
        main components, II:486f
        middle third area, II:486
        overall size and shape, II:485
        upper third area, II:485
    patient selection, II:486
    postoperative care and follow-up, II:492
    prognosis and outcomes, II:492–493
    secondary procedures, II:493
    surgical technique and treatment
        aging, elongated ear lobes, II:491
        anatomic considerations, II:487–492
        constricted ears, II:489–490, III:204,
            205f–206f
        cryptotia, II:490, III:204, 206f–207f
        earlobe deformities, II:290–293, 292f,
            492, III:220–221, 223f
        earring-related complications, II:491
        large ears, II:488–489
        near-ear facelift deformities, II:491–492
        normal-sized prominent ears,
            II:487–488
        prominent ear, III:204–207, 208f
        retroauricular deformities, II:492
        scars, II:492
        Stahl's ear deformity, II:490–491,
            490f–491f
        tragal deformities, II:290, 291f, 492
    palatal development, III:570
    photographic guidelines, I:110
    reconstructive surgeries, III:187–225
        acquired deformities (loss of auricular
            tissue)
            amputated ears, III:209, 212, 213f–214f
            cartilage replantation, III:210, 212
            composite graft, III:210, 210f
            dermabraded amputated auricle
                replantation, III:211, 211f
            microsurgical ear replantation, III:212
            skin coverage considerations, III:207–
                212, 209f
            tissue attached by a narrow pedicle,
                III:209, 210f
        acquired partial defects, III:217
        anatomical considerations, III:187, 188f
        associated deformities, III:190, 191b, 191t
        bilateral microtia, III:204
        burn wound treatment, IV:473, 491–492,
            496f, 498–499, 505–506
        classifications, III:189, 190b, 190f
        constricted ears, II:489–490, III:204,
            205f–206f
        craniofacial osteointegration, I:800–802,
            800t, 801f
        cryptotia, II:490, III:204, 206f–207f
        deformities with loss of auricular tissue
            auricular skin loss, III:214
            full-thickness defects, III:214
            prosthetics, III:217
            skin coverage considerations,
                III:215–217
            trauma-acquired defects, III:214–215,
                216f
        deformities without loss of auricular
            tissue
            cauliflower ear, III:212, 215f
            contour irregularities, III:212

ears (Continued)
        external auditory canal stenosis,
            III:212, 215f
        otohematoma, III:212, 215f
    etiology
        developmental factors, III:189, 190f
        hereditary factors, III:189
        incidence, III:189
    first stage
        adult patient framework modifications,
            III:195, 196f
        framework fabrication, III:194
        framework implantation, III:195–196
        postoperative activities, III:197
        rib cartilage graft, III:194, 195f
    general discussion, III:187
    local flaps
        anterior concha, III:457, 458f
        rim defects, III:456–457, 456f–457f
    microtia
        bilateral microtia, III:204
        clinical characteristics, III:190–191, 190f
        patient selection, III:191–192
        preoperative assessment, III:192
        rib cartilage graft, III:194, 195f
        surgical technique and treatment,
            III:192–194
    middle-ear surgery, III:187–189
    prominent ear
        antihelical fold restoration, III:206–207
        conchal alteration, III:206
        lateral cartilage surface alteration,
            III:207
        medial cartilage surface alteration,
            III:207
        pathology, III:204–206, 208f
        treatment strategies, III:206
    regional defects
        acquired earlobe deformities, II:492,
            III:220–221, 223f
        helical rim, III:218–219, 219f
        lower-third auricular defects, III:220,
            222f
        middle-third auricular defects, III:220,
            221f
        upper-third auricular defects,
            III:219–220
    secondary reconstruction, III:202–204
    structural support
        composite grafts, III:218, 219f
        contralateral conchal cartilage, III:217
        ipsilateral conchal cartilage, III:217–
            218, 218f
    surgical technique and treatment
        acquired partial defects, III:217
        conchal definition, III:197–198,
            199f–200f
        first stage, III:194–197
        hairline management, III:201–202, 203f
        lobule rotation, III:197, 198f
        Nagata technique, III:202
        posterior auricular region detachment,
            III:198–200, 201f
        preoperative assessment, III:192
        residual tissue utilization, III:217
        secondary reconstruction, III:202–204
        surgical planning and preparation,
            III:192–194, 194f

ears (Continued)
surgical staging, III:192, 192f–193f
technique variations, III:202
tragal construction, III:197–198, 199f–200f
tumors
benign tumors, III:221
malignant tumors, III:221–222
robotic surgery, I:862–863
tissue expansion, I:637–638
traumatic injuries
anatomical considerations, III:40
auditory canal stenosis, III:41–42
causal factors, III:39–42
complete amputation, III:42
evaluation examinations, III:25, 25f, 40
hematomas, III:40–41, 41f
lacerations, III:41, 41f
partial amputation with a narrow pedicle, III:42
partial amputation with a wide pedicle, III:41f, 42
Treacher Collins syndrome, III:828–830
tumors
benign tumors, III:221
malignant tumors, III:221–222
eating disorders, I:49–50
Eaton classification, VI:432, 432t, 433f
Eaton–Littler procedure, VI:435–437, 436f
ecchymosis, II:526
eccrine glands, I:322
eccrine nevus, I:723
ectasia, I:677t
ectodermal dysplasia, I:195
ectopia cordis
characteristics, III:861–862, 862f
clinical presentation and evaluation, III:861, 862f–863f
surgical indicators, III:861
treatment strategies, III:861–862
ectopic replantation, VI:243, 244f
ectrodactyly–ectodermal dysplasia–cleft syndrome (EEC) syndrome, VI:565t, 573t
edema
extremity burn reconstruction, IV:436–437
liposuctions, II:526
lymphedema, I:672
melanoma treatment, I:781t
periareolar surgical technique with mesh support, V:226
rhinoplasty complications, II:411
skin wound healing, I:288
edentulous mandible fractures, III:83–84, 84f
efficiency ratios, I:69
Egypt See ancient Egypt
Eichoff test, VI:56
eicosapentaenoic acid, V:33t–35t
18q-syndrome, VI:573t
Eikenella corrodens, VI:334, 344
elastic cartilage, I:397, 398f
elastins, I:320
elastolytic scars, II:69
elbows
adult brachial plexus injury reconstructive strategies, VI:800, 801t
burn reconstruction, IV:443, 443t, 445–446, 507
elbow disarticulation/long transhumeral amputation, VI:874–875
free-functioning muscle transfer, VI:787

elbows (Continued)
joint denervation surgery, VI:497t
nerve compression syndromes, VI:510, 510f
physical examination
bony landmarks, VI:61, 62f
distal humerus malrotation measurement, VI:63, 64f
joint instability, VI:61–63, 63f
lateral ligament complex
accessory collateral ligament, VI:61, 62f
annular ligament, VI:61, 62f
lateral ulnar collateral ligament, VI:61, 62f
radial collateral ligament, VI:61, 62f
medial collateral ligament complex, VI:61, 62f
pivot shift test maneuver, VI:63, 64f
posterolateral rotatory instability (PLRI), VI:63
puberty-related skeletal assessments, VI:653, 653f
sequelae obstetric brachial plexus palsy, VI:813–815
spastic hand surgery, VI:460, 461f
tetraplegic restoration
biceps to triceps transfer
advantages/disadvantages, VI:821–822
postoperative care and follow-up, VI:822, 822f
surgical technique, VI:821–822, 821f
deltoid to triceps transfer
postoperative care and follow-up, VI:825
surgical technique, VI:822–824, 822b, 823f–824f
hygiene considerations, VI:821f
importance, VI:820–825
elective lymph node dissection (ELND), I:756–761
electrical burns
burn wound treatment, IV:396–397
electric current effects, IV:396t
patient presentation, IV:396f
reconstructive surgeries, IV:435–436
scalp and forehead, III:119–120, 120f
electric arc, IV:435–436
electrocoagulation therapy, I:718
electromyography, VI:504–505, 700–701
electronic medical records
data collection integration, I:170–172
'meaningful use' concept, I:171
patient-reported outcomes (PRO) research, I:171–172
privacy laws, I:121
electron therapy, I:655–656
electroporation, I:186, 188t
Electrostatic Detection Apparatus (ESDA) test, I:95–96
Elevess, II:45t, 47, 49t
See also soft-tissue fillers
ellagic acid, II:25
Ely, Edward, I:25–28
emblicanin, II:25
embolic therapy, I:684
embolisms, IV:433t
embryoblast, III:504–505
embryology
abdominoplasty, II:530–534
craniofacial clefts, III:686, 702f
craniofacial development, III:504–505, 504f

embryology (Continued)
craniofacial microsomia (CFM), III:763–764, 763f–764f
ears, III:187–189
genital embryology
genetic sex, IV:297
gonadal sex, IV:297–298
phenotypic sex, IV:298, 298f
hands, VI:468
lower extremities, IV:1, 2f
nail/nail bed, VI:117
palatal development, III:569
pediatric chest and trunk defects, III:855
Pierre Robin sequence (PRS), III:805, 806f
tissue engineering, I:368–369
trunk, IV:220
urogenital defect reconstruction, III:907–908
See also limb development (embryology)
embryonic stem cells (ESCs), I:213f, 260–261, 369–371
emollients
characteristics, II:18
oatmeal, II:18
shea butter, II:18
empyema
outcome assessments, IV:252
pathogenesis, IV:252
surgical technique and treatment, IV:252
treatment strategies, IV:253f
enabling technology, I:843
enchondromas, VI:85, 327, 327f
en coup de sabre (ECDS), III:114–115, 115f, 792, 795f
endocanthion, II:356t
endochondral ossification, I:440
endonasal rhinoplasty, II:425
endoscopic carpal tunnel release (ECTR), VI:509
endothelial cells, I:270t, 678–680
endothelial progenitor cells (EPC), I:190–191, 230, 369–371
endothelin-1 (ET-1), I:573–574, 574f, 580–581
endothelium-derived contracting factors (EDCFs), I:573–574, 574f
endothelium-derived relaxing factors (EDRFs), I:573–574, 574f
end-to-side neurorrhaphy nerve transfer, VI:799–800
Engrailed (En) gene, III:706
Enneking's classification system of musculoskeletal sarcomas, VI:329–330, 330t
enophthalmos, III:56
Enterococcus faecalis, I:249–250
entitled demanders, I:38
entonox, IV:427
entrepreneurship, I:80–82, 81f
enzymatic debridement, IV:366–367
Ephrin/Eph signaling, III:507–508
epicanthal fold, II:164–165
Epicel®, I:794t, 795, IV:415t
epidermal growth factor (EGF), I:189–190, 270t, 275, 625f
epidermal inclusion cysts, VI:314, 314f
epidermal nevus, I:718, 718f
epidermal stem cells, I:262–263, 262f, 296
epidermis, I:319–320, 322f, II:44–45, IV:397–402
epidermoid cyst, I:719, 720f, III:116–117, 116f

epidermolysis bullosa, **IV:**511–525
  general discussion, **IV:**511
  mitten hand deformity, **IV:**523f–524f
  outcomes and complicatons, **IV:**522
  pathogenesis, **IV:**517–518, 518t
  patient presentation and diagnosis
    biopsies, **IV:**520, 521f
    blistering, **IV:**518f–520f, 519–520
    characteristics, **IV:**518–520, 518f–519f
    hyperkeratosis, **IV:**519f
    squamous cell carcinoma, **IV:**520f
    syndactyly, **IV:**519f
  patient selection, **IV:**521
  postoperative care and follow-up, **IV:**522
  surgical technique and treatment
    skin substitutes, **IV:**522, 523f–524f
    surgical care, **IV:**521–522
    wound care, **IV:**521–522
epigenetic mechanisms, **I:**181–182, 181f
epinephrine
  facial soft-tissue injuries, **III:**26–29
  infiltrating wetting solutions, **II:**516t, 517
  patient safety, **I:**129–130
  selection guidelines, **I:**139, 140f, **VI:**95–96, 95t
  toxicity, **I:**148, **VI:**94–95
  vasoconstrictive effects, **I:**147
epistaxis, **II:**410–411
epithelioid sarcoma, **I:**742, **VI:**321, 323f
eponychial deformities
  characteristics, **VI:**125
  surgical technique and treatment, **VI:**125, 125f
Epstein–Barr virus, **III:**399, 421
Epworth Sleepiness Scale (ESS), **III:**96–97
erbium-doped yttrium aluminum garnet (YAG) lasers, **III:**30
Erb's palsy, **VI:**806, 807f
Erb's point, **III:**27
Erlich, Paul, **VI:**xliii–xliv
erythema, **I:**652, **II:**77, **V:**359
erythema multiforme, **IV:**512–514, 512t
  See also toxic epidermal necrolysis (TEN)
erythromycin, **II:**21t
Escherichia coli, **III:**890
esophageal fistula, **IV:**275
esophagus
  anatomical characteristics, **III:**337, 337f
  reconstructive surgeries, **III:**336–359
    anatomical considerations, **III:**337, 337f–338f
    anterolateral thigh flap
      flap design and harvesting, **III:**339–341, 340f–342f
      flap inset guidelines, **III:**342–347, 343f–348f
      frozen neck, **III:**352–353
      isolated cervical esophageal defects, **III:**354
      oral diet, **III:**356t
      postlaryngectomy pharyngocutaneous fistulas, **III:**353–354, 353f–354f
      selection guidelines, **III:**338–339
    complications
      anastomotic strictures, **III:**357–358, 357f
      neck wound infection, **III:**358
      pharyngocutaneous fistula, **III:**357

esophagus *(Continued)*
      defect types, **III:**337t
      guidelines, **III:**336
      jejunal flap
        flap harvesting, **III:**349–350, 349f–350f
        flap inset guidelines, **III:**350, 350f
        oral diet, **III:**356t
      outcome assessments, **III:**356–357
      patient selection, **III:**337–339
      postoperative care and follow-up
        general postoperative care, **III:**354–355
        oral diet, **III:**355–356, 355f, 356t
        voice rehabilitation, **III:**356, 356f
      preoperative assessment
        donor site evaluation, **III:**338
        flap selection, **III:**338–339, 339f, 339t
        medical evaluation, **III:**337–338
        radiotherapy and surgery history, **III:**338
      radial forearm flap
        flap design, **III:**347, 348f
        flap harvesting, **III:**347–349, 348f–349f
        oral diet, **III:**356t
      secondary procedures
        flap debulking, **III:**358
        tracheal stomaplasty, **III:**358, 358f
      surgical technique and treatment
        anterolateral thigh flap, **III:**339–347
        frozen neck, **III:**352–353
        isolated cervical esophageal defects, **III:**354
        jejunal flap, **III:**349–350
        postlaryngectomy pharyngocutaneous fistulas, **III:**353–354, 353f–354f
        radial forearm flap, **III:**347–349
        recipient vessel selection, **III:**351–352, 351f–352f, 351t
        transverse cervical vessels, **III:**351–352, 351f–352f
essential oils, **II:**17
Esser, Johannes, **I:**22–23, 24f
Esthelis/Fortelis/Belotero, **II:**47t
esthesioneuroblastoma, **III:**436–437
Esthirase, **II:**47t
Estlander flap, **III:**259, 263f, 276f
17β-estradiol, **IV:**341t
estrogen, **IV:**341t
estrogen receptor (ER), **V:**266–267
ethanol, **I:**692–693, 696
ether, **IV:**395
ethics, **I:**55–63
  advertising, **I:**59–60, 59f–60f
  business principles, **I:**87–88, 88b
  ethics complaints, **I:**57t
  expert witness testimony, **I:**62, 92–93
  friends and family as patients, **II:**5–6
  gene therapy, **I:**191–192
  MBA oath, **I:**88b
  monetary relationships, **I:**61–62
  moral decisions and consequences, **I:**55
  operating rooms, **I:**61
  outpatient relationships, **I:**60–61
  patient–surgeon relationship, **I:**58–59
  professional associations, **I:**57–58
  providers and third-party payers, **I:**61–62
  research summary, **I:**62
  tissue engineering, **I:**388
ethnic rhinoplasty, **II:**441–442

eutectic mixture of local anesthetics (EMLA), **I:**682, **III:**26
evidence-based medicine and health service research, **I:**150–175
  comparative effectiveness analysis
    challenges
      economic study types, **I:**167
      limitations, **I:**167–168
      perspectives, **I:**166
      research summary, **I:**168
      study designs, **I:**167
    key concepts, **I:**166
    national research priority, **I:**166
  future trends
    electronic medical records
      data collection integration, **I:**170–172
      'meaningful use' concept, **I:**171
      patient-reported outcomes (PRO) research, **I:**171–172
    knowledge translation
      background information, **I:**168–169
      implementation barriers, **I:**169
      Knowledge To Action model, **I:**169, 169f
    learning collaboratives, **I:**170
    multicenter clinical trials network, **I:**168
  large-database analysis
    data sources
      administrative claims data, **I:**159
      clinical registries, **I:**158–159, 158t
      epidemiology, **I:**160
      large cohort studies, **I:**160
      plastic surgery applications, **I:**160–161, 161f
    population-based research
      effectiveness versus efficiency, **I:**156–157, 157f
      mortality rates, **I:**157f
      sample size effects, **I:**157–158, 157t
    usage guidelines
      administrative claims data, **I:**159–161
      small-area variations, **I:**159
      volume–outcome analysis, **I:**159–160, 160t
  medical practice variations, **V:**316–317
  outcome usefulness
    healthcare quality, **I:**172–174
    patient decision aids, **I:**174
    performance measures, **I:**172–173
    public reporting, **I:**173–174
  patient-reported outcomes (PRO) research
    electronic medical records, **I:**171–172
    measure development guidelines, **I:**162–164, 163f
    modern psychometric methods, **I:**164
    preference-based measures
      key concepts, **I:**164–165
      quality-adjusted life years (QALYs), **I:**164–165
      utilities and values, **I:**164–165, 165f
    questionnaires, **I:**161–162
    reliability and validity measures, **I:**162, 162f
    terminology and definitions, **I:**161–162
  research summary, **I:**174–175
  sources
    existing literature evaluations, **I:**150–151, 151f
    general discussion, **I:**150–153

evidence-based medicine and health service
  research *(Continued)*
    literature search strategies
      Clinical Queries, I:151
      general discussion, I:151
      PICO approach, I:151
      PubMed, I:151
    meta-analysis, I:151–152, 152f
    systematic reviews, I:152–153
  study designs
    case-control studies, I:155–156, 156f
    case series/case reports, I:156
    characteristics, I:153–156
    cohort studies, I:155, 155f–156f
    experimental studies
      large multicenter trials, I:154–155
      patient preference trials, I:154
      randomized controlled clinical trials,
        I:153–154, 154t
    levels of evidence, I:153t
    observational studies, I:155
Evolution, II:48t
  See also soft-tissue fillers
Ewing's sarcoma, IV:103
excisional biopsies, IV:106–107
excisional biopsy, V:273
excisional wounds, I:286–287
expanded polytetrafluoroethylene (ePTFE),
  I:790
expert witness testimony, I:62, 92–93
express warranty, I:94–95
extensor carpi radialis brevis (ECRB) tendon,
  III:295t, VI:51, 211, 211f, 825–826
extensor carpi radialis longus (ECRL) tendon,
  VI:51, 211, 211f
extensor carpi ulnaris (ECU) synergy test,
  VI:55, 57f
extensor carpi ulnaris (ECU) tendon, VI:52,
  211, 211f
extensor digiti minimi (EDM) tendon, VI:51,
  211, 211f
extensor digitorum brevis muscle flap, IV:59f,
  205–206, 206f
extensor digitorum communis (EDC) tendon,
  VI:51, 211, 211f
extensor digitorum longus (EDL), IV:35f–36f
extensor hallucis longus (EHL), IV:35f–36f
extensor indicis propius (EIP) tendon, VI:211,
  211f
extensor indicis proprius (EIP) tendon, VI:51
extensor pollicis brevis (EPB) muscle, VI:51,
  211, 211f
extensor pollicis longus (EPL) tendon
  extensor tendon injuries, VI:211, 211f, 213f
  hand anatomy, VI:51
  tetraplegic restoration
    key pinch restoration, VI:826–827, 827f,
      831f
    wrist extension, VI:825f
extensor retinacula, IV:52, 52t, 54f
extensor tendon injuries, VI:210–227
  anatomical characteristics
    extrinsic muscles, VI:211, 211f
    functional anatomy
      extrinsic muscles, VI:213
      intrinsic muscles, VI:212–213
      joint extension mechanisms, VI:213
      linked chains, VI:212, 212f
    general discussion, VI:211–212
    intrinsic muscles, VI:211–212, 212f

extensor tendon injuries *(Continued)*
  complications, VI:221
  hand therapy, VI:862–865, 865f
  outcome assessments, VI:221
  patient presentation and diagnosis, VI:213,
    213f–214f
  patient selection, VI:213–214, 214b
  postoperative care and follow-up, VI:220–
    221, 221f
  research summary, VI:227
  secondary procedures
    boutonnière deformity
      characteristics, VI:223–224, 223f
      preoperative assessment, VI:223–224
      secondary reconstruction, VI:224, 224f
      tenotomy, VI:224, 224f
    challenges, VI:221b
    delayed sagittal band reconstruction,
      VI:225, 225b, 225f
    hanging fingertip, VI:221–222, 222f
    missing tendons, VI:225
    soft-tissue management/staged
      reconstruction, VI:226–227, 226f–227f
    swan-neck deformity, VI:222–223,
      222f–223f
    tendon transfers versus tendon grafts,
      VI:225
  surgical technique and treatment
    suturing techniques, VI:214, 214f, 215b
    zone I
      chronic injuries, VI:216
      mallet finger, VI:214–216, 215f–217f
      open injuries, VI:216
    zone II, VI:217, 217f
    zone III
      characteristics, VI:217–218
      closed injuries, VI:217, 218f
      open lacerations, VI:218, 218f
    zone IV, VI:218–219
    zone V
      human bites, VI:219, 219f
      partial lacerations, VI:219
      sagittal band, VI:219
    zone VI, VI:219
    zone VII, VI:219–220
    zone VIII, VI:220
    zone IX, VI:220
  treatment challenges, VI:210
extensor tendon ruptures
  basic procedure, VI:404–406, 405f–408f
  outcomes and complicatons, VI:405–406
  postoperative care and follow-up, VI:405
  surgical tips, VI:406b
external angular dermoids
  disease process, III:884
  patient presentation and diagnosis, III:884
  surgical technique and treatment,
    III:884–885
external anterior scrotal artery, IV:235, 238f
external auditory canal stenosis, III:212, 215f
external oblique muscle
  abdominal wall reconstruction, I:553t, 554
  anatomical characteristics, IV:228–229, 229f
  back wounds, IV:268–269
external posterior scrotal artery, IV:235, 238f
externus belt, II:554, 556f
extracellular matrix (ECM)
  bone composition, I:431–432, 432t
  extra cellular matrix–growth factor
    interactions, I:275

extracellular matrix (ECM) *(Continued)*
  regenerative medicine, I:368
  scar biology and formation, I:300
  skin wound healing, I:269–271, 271f, 278
  wound healing, I:242, 250–252, 251f
extracellular polymeric substances (EPS), I:250
extramammary Paget's disease, I:739, 739f
extraplexus nerve transfer, VI:799
extraskeletal Ewing's sarcoma, I:742
extravasation injury
  upper extremities, IV:456–467
    causal factors, IV:464–467
    complications, IV:466–467, 467f
    disease process
      characteristics, IV:464–465
      cytotoxic agents, IV:464–465
      osmotically active agents, IV:464
      vasoconstrictive agents, IV:464
    patient presentation and diagnosis,
      IV:465, 465f
    patient selection, IV:465
    postoperative care and follow-up, IV:466
    prognosis and outcomes, IV:466–467
    research summary, IV:456
    secondary procedures, IV:467
    surgical technique and treatment
      cytotoxic agents, IV:466
      osmotically active agents, IV:466
      treatment strategies, IV:465–466
      vasoconstrictive agents, IV:466
extremities expansion, I:650
extrinsic tightness test, VI:54
eyebrows
  anthropometric analysis, II:356–358, 358f
  browlift surgery
    basic principles, II:203
    botulinum toxin type-A (BoNT-A), II:37,
      41
    complications, II:105–106, 105f–106f
    patient presentation and diagnosis
      aesthetics, II:98f–100f, 99–100
      forehead aging, II:98–99, 98f–99f
    patient selection, II:100
    postoperative care and follow-up, II:105
    prognosis and outcomes, II:105–106
    secondary procedures, II:106, 106f
    surgical technique
      anterior hairline approach, II:101–102,
        102f
      direct suprabrow approach, II:104
      endoscopic approach, II:102–103, 103f
      general discussion, II:100–105
      lateral brow approach, II:103–104,
        104f
      open coronal approach, II:100–101,
        101f
      subperiosteal facelift, II:274, 274f
      suture suspension browplexy, II:105
      temple approach, II:103, 103f
      transpalpebral approach, II:103, 104f
      transpalpebral browplexy, II:104–105
  burn wound treatment, IV:485, 498–499
  congenital melanocytic nevi (CMN), III:844,
    846f
  facial paralysis, III:286, 286t, 287f
  hypertelorism correction, III:699
  optimal brow positioning, II:122, 123f
  reconstructive burn surgery, IV:504–505
  reconstructive surgeries, III:441, 444f
  soft-tissue fillers, II:51

eyebrows (Continued)
surgical technique and treatment
basic procedure, **III**:34–38
Burow's triangles, **III**:37f
local brow advancement flaps, **III**:36–38, 37f
local flaps, **III**:441, 444f
local grafts, **III**:38
eyeglobe, **II**:120, 122, **III**:252–253, 252t
eyelids
anatomical characteristics, **II**:111, 111f, 164–165, 165f, **III**:19, 20f
Asian blepharoplasty
anatomical considerations, **II**:164–165, 165f–166f
eyelid characteristics, **II**:164
outcomes and complicatons, **II**:170–172
postoperative care and follow-up, **II**:170
preoperative assessment, **II**:166–167, 166f–167f
surgical technique and treatment
incisional methods, **II**:168, 169f
lateral canthoplasty, **II**:170, 171f–172f
medial epicanthoplasty, **II**:169, 170f–171f
nonincisional methods, **II**:167–168, 167f–168f
partial incisional methods, **II**:168, 168f
subclinical ptosis repair, **II**:169
burn wound treatment, **IV**:470–473, 485–488, 486f–488f, 498–499, 504–505, 504f
colobomas, **III**:829f, 830, 831f, 833f, 835f
corneal protection, **II**:140, 142f
cutaneous and soft-tissue tumors
clinical staging system, **I**:716t
TNM clinical classification system/pTNM pathologic classification system, **I**:715b
ethnic differences, **II**:113f
eyelid ptosis/retraction, **II**:121–122
eyelid repair
botulinum toxin type-A (BoNT-A), **II**:34–37
burn wound treatment, **IV**:470–473, 485–488, 486f–488f, 504–505, 504f
facelift techniques, **II**:203
fat grafting, **II**:332f
high SMAS technique, **II**:257–258
nineteenth century, **I**:20, 21f
subperiosteal facelift
lower eyelid area, **II**:270–273, 270f
upper eyelid area, **II**:268–270, 269f
eyelid skin deficiencies/eyelid malposition, **II**:308
eyelid zones, **II**:140, 141f
hypertelorism correction, **III**:699
lid lamellae, **III**:57
lower eyelid area
access incisions, **III**:227
anatomical characteristics, **II**:112
anesthesia, **III**:27, 27f–28f
facial paralysis, **III**:287–289, 287f, 290f
lower eyelid surgery
basic principles, **II**:127–131
burn wound treatment, **IV**:486–488, 488f
large defects, **III**:450

eyelids (Continued)
orbicularis suspension, **II**:130–131
orbital fat excision, **II**:128–130
partial lower lid defects, **III**:449
total lower lid defects, **III**:450
transconjunctival blepharoplasty, **II**:128, 129f–131f
transcutaneous blepharoplasty, **II**:128
lower eyelid tonicity, **II**:121
secondary blepharoplasty
anatomical analysis, **II**:148–151, 148f, 151f
canthoplasty techniques, **II**:151–160, 155f–156f, 155t
chemosis, **II**:162, 162f
complications, **II**:160–162
dermal orbicular pennant lateral canthoplasty (DOPLC), **II**:156, 158f–159f
distraction test, **II**:150, 153f
ectropion, **II**:150–151, 154f
excessive fat resection, **II**:160–162, 161f
eyelid malposition, **II**:148–151, 152f
inadequate fat resection, **II**:160–162, 161f
inferior retinacular lateral canthoplasty/canthopexy (IRLC), **II**:156–157, 160f
lateral bone-to-canthus relationship, **II**:149–150, 152f
lower lid eversion, **II**:150–151, 154f
medial canthus-to-lateral canthus relationship, **II**:150, 153f
midface elevation and fixation, **II**:157, 161f
midlamellar cicatricial retraction, **II**:150f
patient evaluation, **II**:148–151, 149t
persistent malar bags, **II**:161f, 162
snap test, **II**:150, 153f
surgical procedures, **II**:151–160, 155t
tarsal strip lateral canthoplasty, **II**:155–156, 156f–157f
subperiosteal facelift, **II**:270–273, 270f
vertical shortening, **III**:57
medial canthal defects, **III**:450, **IV**:488
reconstructive burn surgery, **IV**:470–473, 485–488, 486f–487f, 498–499, 504–505, 504f
secondary facelifts, **II**:308
soft-tissue injuries, **III**:38–39, 38f–40f
Treacher Collins syndrome, **III**:828–830
upper eyelid area
anatomical characteristics, **II**:111–112, 113f
anatomic-directed therapy, **II**:121
anesthesia, **III**:26, 27f
epicanthal fold, **II**:164–165
facial paralysis, **III**:287–289, 287f–289f
partial upper lid defects
Abbé flap, **III**:450
advancement flap, **III**:450
decision-making process, **III**:449–450
full-thickness skin graft, **III**:450
lower lid transposition, **III**:449f
ptosis, **III**:57
secondary blepharoplasty
Fasanella–Servat operation, **II**:146f
Herring's law, **II**:145, 147f

eyelids (Continued)
patient evaluation, **II**:142–145, 142t, 143f–144f
ptosis, **II**:143–145, 144f–146f
retraction, **II**:145, 147f
subperiosteal facelift, **II**:268–270, 269f
upper eyelid surgery
anchor/invagination blepharoplasty, **II**:124, 126f
burn wound treatment, **IV**:486, 487f
general discussion, **II**:123–124
orbital fat excision, **II**:124, 126f
simple skin blepharoplasty, **II**:124, 125f
total upper lid defects, **III**:450
eyes
aging process, **II**:116, 116f
anthropometric analysis, **II**:358, 358f
burn wound treatment, **IV**:470–473
corneal protection, **II**:140, 142f
nasoethmoidal orbital fractures
characteristics, **III**:60–61
classification systems, **III**:61–63, 62f
clinical examination, **III**:60–61, 61f
complications, **III**:63
computed tomography (CT), **III**:61
surgical pathology
causal factors, **III**:60
interorbital space, **III**:60
traumatic orbital hypertelorism, **III**:60
traumatic telecanthus, **III**:60
treatment strategies
basic procedure, **III**:61–63
canthal reattachment, **III**:63
central fragment considerations, **III**:63
lacrimal system injury, **III**:63
orbital fractures
characteristics, **III**:53–57
complications
blindness, **III**:56
diplopia, **III**:56
enophthalmos, **III**:56
implant migration or hemorrhage, **III**:56
lid lamellae, **III**:57
ocular globe injuries, **III**:56
retrobulbar hematoma, **III**:56
upper eyelid ptosis, **III**:57
vertical shortening of the lower eyelid, **III**:57
computed tomography (CT), **III**:54
infraorbital nerve anesthesia, **III**:57
nasoethmoidal orbital fractures
causal factors, **III**:60
characteristics, **III**:60–61
classification systems, **III**:61–63, 62f
clinical examination, **III**:60–61, 61f
complications, **III**:63
computed tomography (CT), **III**:61
interorbital space, **III**:60
lacrimal system injury, **III**:63
traumatic orbital hypertelorism, **III**:60
traumatic telecanthus, **III**:60
treatment strategies, **III**:61–63
orbital apex syndrome, **III**:57
physical examination, **III**:53–54, 54f
postoperative care and follow-up, **III**:56
schematic diagram, **III**:53f
superior orbital fissure syndrome, **III**:57

Note: **Boldface** *roman numerals indicate volume. Page numbers followed by f refer to figures; page numbers followed by t refer to tables; page numbers followed by b refer to boxes.*

eyes (Continued)
surgical anatomy, III:53
surgical technique and treatment
basic procedure, III:55–56
bone grafts, III:55
cutaneous exposures, III:55
endoscopic approaches, III:55
forced duction test, III:55, 55f
goals, III:54–55
inorganic implants, III:56
orbital floor restoration, III:55, 56f
timing considerations, III:55
treatment indicators
blow-out fractures (children), III:54, 54f
blow-out fractures (floor of the orbit),
III:54
guidelines, III:54
osseointegrated orbital reconstruction,
I:802–803, 802b, 803f
periorbital anatomy
blood supply, II:112, 114f
eyelids, II:111, 111f
facial nerve, II:112–115, 115f
forehead, II:110–111, 110f–111f
general discussion, II:108–115
lateral retinaculum, II:109, 109f–110f
lower eyelid area, II:112
medial orbital vault, II:110, 110f
orbital anatomy, II:108–109, 109f
retaining ligaments, II:112, 114f
sensory nerves, II:112–115, 114f
septal extension, II:112, 114f
temporal region, II:110–111, 110f
trigeminal nerve, II:112–115
upper eyelid area, II:111–112, 113f
photographic guidelines, I:107–108, 109f
progressive hemifacial atrophy (PHA),
III:796
toxic epidernal necrolysis (TEN), IV:516
trauma evaluations, III:25
Treacher Collins syndrome, III:828–830
youthful and beautiful eyes characteristics,
II:115–116, 115f

F
Facebook, I:98–99
facelifts
basic principles, II:184–207
anatomy and patient presentation
bony skeleton, II:192, 192f–193f
classic aging characteristics, II:184–193,
185f
deep fascia, II:191–192
facial fat, II:186–188, 187f–188f, 239
facial muscles, II:189, 190f
facial shape changes, II:188–189, 188f
malar fat pad, II:186–188, 186f–188f
nerve anatomy, II:192–193
ptosis, II:185f, 186–188
retaining ligaments, II:189–191, 191f,
239
skin, II:185–186, 185f
superficial musculoaponeurotic system
(SMAS), II:189
volume loss/volume gain, II:185f,
186–188, 239–240
ancillary techniques
blepharoplasty, II:203
browlift surgery, II:203
lip procedures, II:204–205, 204f

facelifts (Continued)
midfacelift, II:204
volume augmentation, II:203–204
volume removal, II:203
general discussion, II:184
nerve anatomy
facial nerve, II:192–193, 194f
sensory nerves, II:193, 195f–196f
patient selection, II:193–195
research summary, II:206
surgical complications
alopecia, II:206
hematomas, II:205, 205f
infections, II:206, 206f
motor nerve injury, II:205–206
sensory nerve injury, II:205
skin loss, II:206
unsatisfactory scars, II:206
surgical conditions, II:196
surgical technique
ancillary techniques, II:203–205
deep tissue surgery, II:200
dressings, II:205
facelift incisions, II:197–200, 198f–201f
neck surgery, II:202–203, 203f
postoperative care and follow-up,
II:205
repositioning approaches, II:196–205
skin flap mobilization and closure,
II:200–202, 202f
subcutaneous facelifts, II:197, 200f–201f
beauty doctors, I:27, 28f
deep tissue surgery, II:208–215
basic principles, II:200
facial aging, II:208
research summary, II:212
subcutaneous facelifts
loop sutures, II:209–210, 210f, 223–231
MACS (minimal access cranial
suspension) lift, II:209–210, 210f,
216–217, 217t, 223–231
skin-only facelifts, II:208–210, 209f
SMAS plication, II:209, 210f, 224–225
subperiosteal facelift, II:212, 214f
supra-platysmal plane facelift
basic principles, II:210–212, 211f
deep plane facelift, II:211, 213f
dual plane facelift, II:211–212, 214f
SMAS ectomy, II:210–211, 212f
extended SMAS technique, II:238–256
aesthetic analysis and treatment
challenges, II:239–240
facial fat descent, II:239
volume loss/volume gain, II:239–240,
240f–241f
zygomaticus major muscle, II:240,
241f
anatomical considerations, II:239
background information, II:238
facial asymmetry, II:249–251, 251f–252f
facial shape evaluations
bizygomatic diameter, II:242, 242f
facial length, II:242, 243f
facial width, II:242, 242f
general discussion, II:242
malar region convexity versus
submalar region concavity, II:242,
243f–244f
malar volume, II:242, 242f
relative vertical heights, II:242, 243f

facelifts (Continued)
neck correction procedures
incisions, II:254–255
platysma muscle release, II:252–255,
253f–254f
SMAS fixation versus platysmaplasty,
II:254, 255f
radial expansion
aesthetic advantages, II:244, 245f–246f
characteristics, II:241–244
dual plane facelift, II:244
facial shape and contour, II:242
mandibular ramus height/mandibular
body length, II:243
research summary, II:255
retaining ligaments, II:239
SMAS fixation, II:251–252, 253f
surgical technique
basic principles, II:244–247, 247f
SMAS elevation, II:245–246, 248f–249f
SMAS fixation, II:246–247, 249f,
251–252, 253f
surgical variations
general discussion, II:248–249
release, II:248–249, 250f
facial skin resurfacing, II:76f
fat grafting, II:330–332, 330f–332f
high SMAS technique, II:257–265
ancillary procedures, II:262–263, 264f
complications, II:265
development process, II:259–260,
259f–260f
patient consultation, II:257–258
postoperative care and follow-up,
II:263–265
superficial subcutaneous fatty mass,
II:258, 258f
surgical planning, II:260
surgical technique, II:260–262, 261f–263f
zygomaticus major muscle, II:259f
infiltration, I:140, 141f
lateral SMASectomy, II:232–237
advantages, II:233
operative procedures
anesthesia, II:233
neck and jowl defatting, II:234, 316
open submental incision, II:234, 235f
platysmaplasty, II:234, 235f–237f
platysma resection, II:234–235, 235f
skin closure, II:236–237, 236f–237f
skin flap elevation, II:233–234
SMAS plication, II:235–236, 236f
temporal and earlobe dog-ears,
II:236–237
temporal hairline incisions, II:233, 234f
vectors and contouring, II:235–236, 236f
MACS (minimal access cranial suspension)
lift, II:223–231
background information, II:223
inappropriate skin shifts, II:300–301
patient expectations, II:226–227
patient selection
evaluation examinations, II:225–226
facial skeletal structure and asymmetry,
II:226
facial volume, II:226
forehead rejuvenation, II:226
glabellar rhytides, II:226
jowls, II:226
medical history, II:226

facelifts (Continued)
neck, II:226
ocular region, II:226
previous surgeries, II:226
skin characteristics, II:226
platysma-SMAS plication (PSP), II:216–217, 217t
research summary, II:231
subcutaneous facelifts, II:209–210, 210f
surgical foundation
basic principles, II:224–225, 224f
extended MACS procedure, II:225f
facial nerves, II:226f
microimbrication, II:225f
short scar incision, II:225f, 228f
surgical strategy
anchor points, II:227, 228f
basic guidelines, II:227–231
cheek sutures, II:228
malar sutures, II:228–229
neck sutures, II:227–228, 228f, 316
skin advancement and resection, II:229–231, 229f–231f
skin incision and undermining, II:227
surgical sequence, II:227
near-ear facelift deformities
classifications, II:491–492
earlobe deformities, II:290–293, 292f, 492
retroauricular deformities, II:492
scars, II:492
tragal deformities, II:290, 291f, 492
patient safety, I:131–132
patient selection
eyelid repair, II:332f
facial atrophy, II:332f
fat grafting, II:330–332, 330f–331f
lips, II:331f
platysma-SMAS plication (PSP), II:216–222
advantages/disadvantages, II:219–221
background information, II:216–217
comparison studies, II:217t
neck-related procedures, II:219t, 220–221, 316
outcome assessments
assessment results, II:218–219, 219t
complications, II:219
neck-related procedures, II:219t
preoperative–postoperative comparisons, II:221f–222f
ProForma assessment, II:217–218, 218t
synchronous procedures, II:219t
research summary, II:221
surgical technique, II:217, 217f–218f, 220f, 234, 235f
psychological aspects, I:39
secondary facelifts, II:277–312
patient considerations, II:308–309
planning considerations, II:311
secondary deformities
general discussion, II:278
secondary aging deformities, II:278, 278f
secondary surgical deformities, II:278–308
secondary surgical deformities
characteristics, II:278–308
cross-hatched scars, II:288–290, 290f
drapery lines, II:303f
earlobe deformities, II:290–293, 292f

facelifts (Continued)
eyelid skin deficiencies/eyelid malposition, II:308
facial atrophy, II:306–308, 307f
fat injections, II:306–308, 307f
hairline displacement and disruption, II:279–282, 279f–283f
hair loss, II:282–284, 283f–284f
inappropriate skin shifts, II:300–301, 301f–302f
inappropriate SMAS shifts/SMAS injury, II:304, 304f
large digastric muscles, II:296–297, 297f
laser resurfacing, II:308
over-excision of buccal fat, II:294, 295f
over-excision of subcutaneous fat, II:293–294, 293f–294f
over-excision of subplatysmal fat, II:294, 295f
poorly situated scars, II:284–288, 285f–289f
prominent submandibular glands, II:294–296, 296f
residual jowl, II:300, 300f
residual platysma bands, II:297–299, 298f
skin deficiencies, II:301–303
skin slough, II:303
smile block, II:304–305, 304f
temporal face compression, II:301
tightness and wrinkling, II:301–303, 302f–303f
tragal deformities, II:290, 291f, 492
unaesthetic facial implants, II:305
uncorrected and under-corrected mid-face deformities, II:299–300, 299f–300f
un-rejuvenated forehead, II:305–306, 306f
un-rejuvenated peri-oral region, II:306
wide scars, II:288, 289f
technical considerations, II:309
subcutaneous facelifts
basic principles, II:197, 200f–201f
high SMAS technique, II:257–258, 258f
loop sutures, II:209–210, 210f, 223–231
MACS (minimal access cranial suspension) lift, II:209–210, 210f, 216–217, 217t, 223–231
skin-only facelifts, II:208–210, 209f
SMAS ectomy
basic principles, II:224–225
supra-platysmal plane facelift, II:210–211, 212f
SMAS plication, II:209, 210f, 224–225
subperiosteal facelift, II:266–276
advantages, II:266–267, 267f–268f
background information, II:266
deep tissue surgery, II:212, 214f
dissection approaches, II:266–267, 267f–268f
functional role, II:275
surgical results, II:274f–275f, 275
surgical technique
browlift surgery, II:274, 274f
fat grafting, II:273
forehead and upper eyelid area, II:268–270, 269f

facelifts (Continued)
lower face and neck, II:273–275, 274f
midface and lower eyelid area, II:270–273, 270f–273f
patient consultation, II:267–275
rejuvenation enhancement methods, II:273
superficial musculoaponeurotic system (SMAS)
basic principles, II:189
extended SMAS technique, II:238–256
aesthetic analysis and treatment, II:239–240
anatomical considerations, II:239
background information, II:238
facial asymmetry, II:249–251, 251f–252f
facial shape evaluations, II:242
neck correction procedures, II:252–255, 253f–254f
radial expansion, II:241–244
research summary, II:255
retaining ligaments, II:239
SMAS fixation, II:251–252, 253f
surgical technique, II:244–247
surgical variations, II:248–249
facial aging
dissection planes, II:89–91, 90f
suture placement, II:91
facial skin resurfacing, II:76f
high SMAS technique, II:257–265
ancillary procedures, II:262–263, 264f
complications, II:265
development process, II:259–260, 259f–260f
patient consultation, II:257–258
postoperative care and follow-up, II:263–265
superficial subcutaneous fatty mass, II:258, 258f
surgical planning, II:260
surgical technique, II:260–262, 261f–263f
zygomaticus major muscle, II:259f
lateral SMASectomy, II:232–237
advantages, II:233
operative procedures, II:233–237
platysma-SMAS plication (PSP), II:216–222
background information, II:216–217
comparison studies, II:217t
outcome assessments, II:217–219
surgical technique, II:217, 217f–218f, 234, 235f
secondary facelifts
inappropriate skin shifts, II:300–301, 301f–302f
inappropriate SMAS shifts/SMAS injury, II:304, 304f
over-excision of buccal fat, II:294, 295f
over-excision of subcutaneous fat, II:293–294, 293f–294f
over-excision of subplatysmal fat, II:294, 295f
residual jowl, II:300, 300f
residual platysma bands, II:297–299, 298f
smile block, II:304–305, 304f
temporal face compression, II:301

*Note: **Boldface** roman numerals indicate volume. Page numbers followed by f refer to figures; page numbers followed by t refer to tables; page numbers followed by b refer to boxes.*

facelifts (Continued)
    uncorrected and under-corrected
        mid-face deformities, II:299–300,
        299f–300f
    SMAS ectomy
        background information, II:232–233
        basic principles, II:224–225
        supra-platysmal plane facelift,
        II:210–211, 212f
    SMAS plication, II:209, 210f, 224–225,
        235–236, 236f
face transplants, III:473–490
    background information, III:473
    cephalic vein harvest, III:484–485, 485f
    complications, III:484–485
    follow-up consultations, III:485
    immunosuppression, III:473–475, 474t
    infection prevention and treatment, III:484
    patient selection, III:475
    postoperative care and follow-up, III:484
    prognosis and outcomes, III:484–488
    psychological support, III:485
    research summary, III:488
    revision surgeries, III:488
    secondary procedures, III:488
    social reintegration
        postoperative case, III:486f–487f
        preoperative case, III:486f–488f
        surgical goals, III:485–488
    surgical technique
        basic procedure, III:476–483
        face transplant harvest
            basic procedure, III:476–482
            coronal approach, III:478f
            digastric division, III:478f
            external canthus dissection, III:480f
            external jugular dissection, III:477f
            facial nerve, III:478f
            final dissection after medial osteotomy,
                III:480f–481f
            harvested transplant, III:482f
            initial drawing and infiltration, III:477f
            lacrimal duct preparation, III:482f
            levator dissection and division, III:479f
            levator verification, III:480f
            lower face transplant, III:482f
            mandibular osteotomy, III:482f
            maxillary artery, III:479f
            maxillary osteotomy, III:482f
            thyrolingofacial trunk and external
                carotid dissection, III:477f–478f
        mask preparation, III:476f–477f
        mold preparation, III:476f
        recipient preparation
            basic procedure, III:482–483
            bone fixation, III:483f–484f
            dacryocystorhinostomy, III:484f
            final closure, III:484f
            lower face debridement, III:483f
            vascular anastomosis, III:483f
facial aging
    anatomical characteristics, II:78–92
        aging changes
            general discussion, II:86
            muscle aging, II:86
            skin, II:86
            subcutaneous tissue, II:86
        cavity anatomy, II:82–83, 82f
        facial nerve branches, II:85–86, 85f
        facial regions, II:79f

facial aging (Continued)
        facial spaces
            bone changes, II:87, 87f–88f
            buccal space, II:84–85
            characteristics, II:83–85
            premasseter space, II:84, 84f, 90f
            prezygomatic space, II:84, 84f, 90f
            retaining ligaments, II:87
            upper temporal space, II:83–85, 83f, 90f
        five-layer construct
            deep fascia, II:79f–80f, 82
            general discussion, II:79–82
            musculo-aponeurotic layer, II:79f–80f,
                81
            platysma auricular fascia (PAF),
                II:81–82, 81f
            retaining ligaments, II:79f–80f
            skin, II:79–80, 79f–80f
            subcutaneous tissue, II:79f–81f, 80–81
            topographical anatomy, II:81–82, 81f
        regional changes
            forehead, II:88
            lower face, II:89
            mid-cheek, II:88–89, 89f
            temple, II:88
        soft tissue layers, II:78
    correction considerations
        dissection planes, II:89–91, 90f
        suture placement, II:91
    deep tissue surgery, II:208
    research summary, II:91
facial analysis, II:177, 355–356, 356b, 356f–
    357f, 356t
facial artery musculomucosal (FAMM) flap,
    III:163, 309t, 462–463, 463f, 643, 645f
facial atrophy, II:306–308, 307f, 328, 329f, 332f,
    334f
facial attractiveness, II:1–2
facial burn wound treatment, IV:468–499
    acute facial burns
        ears, IV:473
        eyes/eyelids, IV:470–473
        mouth, IV:473
        nose, IV:473
        treatment strategies, IV:470–473,
            471f–472f
    complications, IV:497
    damage process
        acute facial burns, IV:470–473
        damage assessments, IV:468–473, 469f
        depth of burn determination, IV:470
    epidemiology, IV:468
    nonoperative facial reconstructive adjunct
        techniques
        corrective cosmetics, IV:485
        fat transplantation, IV:485
        hair transplantation, IV:485
        laser therapy, IV:484, 484f
        prosthetics, IV:485
        steroid treatments, IV:485
    nonsurgical management, IV:473
    outcome assessments, IV:497–498
    postoperative care and follow-up, IV:497
    secondary procedures, IV:498–499
    specific areas
        cheeks, IV:490–491, 506
        commissure, IV:473, 489–490, 495f
        ears, IV:473, 491–492, 496f, 498–499,
            505–506
        eyebrows, IV:485, 498–499

facial burn wound treatment (Continued)
        eyelids, IV:470–473, 485–488, 486f–487f,
            498–499, 504–505, 504f
        forehead, IV:485, 498–499
        lower eyelids, IV:486–488, 488f
        lower lip and chin, IV:489, 492f–494f,
            498–499
        medial canthus scars, IV:488
        neck, IV:493–494, 498–499, 506
        nose, IV:473, 488–489, 498–499, 505
        scalp, III:119–120, 120f, IV:492–493,
            498–499, 504, 504f
        severe cervical burn scars and
            contractures, IV:494
        upper eyelids, IV:486, 487f
        upper lip, IV:489, 490f–491f, 498–499
    surgical management
        algorithmic approach, IV:475–477,
            476f–477f
        basic principles, IV:474–475
        flaps
            basic principles, IV:480–481
            indicators, IV:480b
            trapeze-plasties, IV:481
            Z-plasty technique, IV:481, 481f
        inadequate donor-site skin
            dermal substitutes, IV:480, 482–484
            general discussion, IV:482–484
            tissue expansion, IV:482, 483f
        skin grafts
            advantages, IV:474
            basic principles, IV:479
            composite grafts, IV:480
            full-thickness skin graft, IV:479–480
            skin substitutes, IV:480, 482–484
            split-thickness skin graft, IV:479
        specific techniques
            scar replacement with local skin,
                IV:478, 478f
            serial excision, IV:478
            W-plasty technique, IV:478–479, 478f
        surgical techniques, IV:473
        total wound healing/scar maturation
            aesthetic units, IV:474, 475f
            ancillary techniques, IV:475, 475b, 476f
            diagnosis, IV:474
            functional restoration, IV:474, 475f
            local flaps, IV:474
            reconstruction planning, IV:474
            skin grafts, IV:474
            skin-matching considerations, IV:475
            surgical goals, IV:475
            timing considerations, IV:474–475,
             474f
Facial Cripples, I:21
facial fat, II:186–188, 187f–188f, 239
facial feminization, IV:348–350
facial fractures, III:49–88
    causal factors, III:49
    condylar and subcondylar fractures, III:83,
        83f
    edentulous mandible fractures, III:83–84,
        84f
    gunshot wounds
        delayed versus immediate reconstruction,
            III:85
        immediate and high velocity gunshot
            wounds, III:86–87
        low velocity gunshot wounds, III:85–87
        treatment strategies, III:86–87, 86f

facial fractures (Continued)
  initial assessment
    blunt trauma craniofacial injuries, III:50–51
    clinical examination, III:50–51
    computed tomography (CT), III:51
    general discussion, III:49–51
    timing considerations, III:49–50
  lower facial fractures
    mandibular fractures
      antibiotics, III:82
      characteristics, III:75
      Class I fractures, III:77–78
      Class II fractures, III:78
      Class III fractures, III:78–80
      classification systems, III:76–77
      clinical examination, III:76
      comminuted fractures, III:78, 79f
      complications, III:82–83
      dental wiring and fixation techniques, III:75–76
      diagnosis, III:76
      displacement direction and extent, III:77
      edentulous mandible fractures, III:83–84, 84f
      fracture line direction and angulation, III:77, 77f
      internal fixation devices, III:80–83
      intraoral approach, III:79
      muscle function considerations, III:76
      open reduction treatment, III:78–79
      reduction and fixation principles, III:78, 78f
      surgical indicators, III:79–80
      teeth, III:77
      temporomandibular joint, III:76–77
      third molar extraction, III:81, 81f
      treatment strategies, III:77
  midfacial fractures
    complications
      airway management, III:74
      bleeding, III:74
      blindness, III:74
      cerebral spinal rhinorrhea or otorrhea, III:74
      infections, III:74
      late complications, III:74–75
      malocclusion, III:74–75
      malunion occurrences, III:74
      nasolacrimal duct injury, III:75
      nonunion occurrences, III:74
    Le Fort classification of facial fractures
      background information, III:71–75
      goals, III:71
      Le Fort I level fractures/transverse (Guerin) fractures, III:71, 72f, 73
      Le Fort II level fractures/pyramidal fractures, III:72f–73f, 73–74
      Le Fort III level fractures/craniofacial dysjunction, III:72f–73f, 73–74
    midface buttresses
      alveolar fractures, III:71
      characteristics, III:70–71, 70f
      clinical examination, III:70–71
      computed tomography (CT), III:71
      treatment strategies, III:71

facial fractures (Continued)
  nasal fractures
    closed reduction treatment, III:59–60
    complications, III:60
    K-wire support, III:59
    nasal septum fractures and dislocations, III:58–59, 58f
    open reduction treatment, III:59
    soft tissue contracture, III:59–60, 59f
    types and locations, III:57, 58f
  nasoethmoidal orbital fractures
    causal factors, III:60
    characteristics, III:60–61
    classification systems, III:61–63, 62f
    clinical examination, III:60–61, 61f
    complications, III:63
    computed tomography (CT), III:61
    interorbital space, III:60
    lacrimal system injury, III:63
    traumatic orbital hypertelorism, III:60
    traumatic telecanthus, III:60
    treatment strategies, III:61–63
  postoperative care and follow-up, III:74
  zygoma
    anterior treatment approach, III:65–66
    buttress articulations and alignment, III:66–67
    characteristics, III:63–65
    classification systems, III:65–67
    closed reduction treatment, III:66
    complications, III:69
    compound comminuted fractures, III:69–70
    diagnosis, III:64–65
    high energy fractures, III:67–68, 68f
    posterior approach (coronal incisions), III:66
    reduction methods, III:67
    surgical pathology, III:64–65
  panfacial fractures
    complications, III:84–85, 85f
    definition, III:84–85
    postoperative care and follow-up, III:85
    surgical sequence, III:84
    treatment strategies, III:84
  pediatric facial fractures, III:671–685
    associated injuries, III:672
    background information, III:671
    demographics, III:672
    growth and development factors
      basic principles, III:672–674
      condylar head fractures, III:678f
      cranial-to-facial ratio, III:672f
      Le Fort fracture patterns, III:675f
      mandibular condyle, III:677f
      oblique craniofacial fracture patterns, III:676f–677f
      orbital region, III:674f
      sinus development, III:673f
    incidence, III:671–672
    orbital fracture classification system, III:677t
    orbital fractures, III:54, 54f
    outcomes and complicatons
      adverse outcome classifications, III:683t
      basic principles, III:682–683
      cranial base/skull fractures, III:683
      mandible fractures, III:684, 684f

facial fractures (Continued)
      maxillary and midface fractures, III:684
      metallic cranial hardware, III:683f–684f
      nasal fractures, III:684
      orbital fractures, III:683–684
      zygomaticomaxillary complex fractures, III:684
    patient presentation and diagnosis, III:674–675, 678f–679f
    patient selection, III:675–678
    postoperative care and follow-up, III:682
    research summary, III:685
    secondary procedures, III:684–685
    surgical technique and treatment
      basic procedure, III:678
      cranial base/frontal skull fractures, III:678–679, 679f–680f
      mandible fractures, III:681f–682f, 682
      maxillary and midface fractures, III:680, 681f
      nasal and naso-orbital ethmoid fractures, III:681–682, 681t, 682f
      orbital fractures, III:679–680, 680f
      zygomaticomaxillary complex fractures, III:681
  upper facial fractures
    frontal bone and sinus fractures
      clinical examination, III:51
      complications, III:53
      computed tomography (CT), III:51
      injury patterns, III:51
      nasofrontal duct, III:51, 52f
      surgical technique and treatment, III:52–53, 52f
    orbital fractures
      blow-out fractures (children), III:54, 54f
      blow-out fractures (floor of the orbit), III:54
      characteristics, III:53–57
      complications, III:56–57
      computed tomography (CT), III:54
      infraorbital nerve anesthesia, III:57
      operative technique, III:55
      orbital apex syndrome, III:57
      physical examination, III:53–54, 54f
      postoperative care and follow-up, III:56
      schematic diagram, III:53f
      superior orbital fissure syndrome, III:57
      surgical anatomy, III:53
      surgical technique and treatment, III:54–55
      timing considerations, III:55
      treatment indicators, III:54
facial injury surgery, III:49–88
  causal factors, III:49
  condylar and subcondylar fractures, III:83, 83f
  edentulous mandible fractures, III:83–84, 84f
  facial transplantation, III:131
  gunshot wounds
    delayed versus immediate reconstruction, III:85
    immediate and high velocity gunshot wounds, III:86–87
    low velocity gunshot wounds, III:85–87
    treatment strategies, III:86–87, 86f

*Note: **Boldface** roman numerals indicate volume. Page numbers followed by f refer to figures; page numbers followed by t refer to tables; page numbers followed by b refer to boxes.*

facial injury surgery (Continued)
  initial assessment
    blunt trauma craniofacial injuries, III:50–51
    clinical examination, III:50–51
    computed tomography (CT), III:51
    general discussion, III:49–51
    timing considerations, III:49–50
  lower facial fractures
    mandibular fractures
      antibiotics, III:82
      characteristics, III:75
      Class I fractures, III:77–78
      Class II fractures, III:78
      Class III fractures, III:78–80
      classification systems, III:76–77
      clinical examination, III:76
      comminuted fractures, III:78, 79f
      complications, III:82–83
      dental wiring and fixation techniques, III:75–76
      diagnosis, III:76
      displacement direction and extent, III:77
      edentulous mandible fractures, III:83–84, 84f
      fracture line direction and angulation, III:77, 77f
      internal fixation devices, III:80–83
      intraoral approach, III:79
      muscle function considerations, III:76
      open reduction treatment, III:78–79
      reduction and fixation principles, III:78, 78f
      surgical indicators, III:79–80
      teeth, III:77
      temporomandibular joint, III:76–77
      third molar extraction, III:81, 81f
      treatment strategies, III:77
  midfacial fractures
    complications
      airway management, III:74
      bleeding, III:74
      blindness, III:74
      cerebral spinal rhinorrhea or otorrhea, III:74
      infections, III:74
      late complications, III:74–75
      malocclusion, III:74–75
      malunion occurrences, III:74
      nasolacrimal duct injury, III:75
      nonunion occurrences, III:74
    Le Fort classification of facial fractures
      background information, III:71–75
      goals, III:71
      Le Fort I level fractures/transverse (Guerin) fractures, III:71, 72f, 73
      Le Fort II level fractures/pyramidal fractures, III:72f–73f, 73–74
      Le Fort III level fractures/craniofacial dysjunction, III:72f–73f, 73–74
    midface buttresses
      alveolar fractures, III:71
      characteristics, III:70–71, 70f
      clinical examination, III:70–71
      computed tomography (CT), III:71
      treatment strategies, III:71
    nasal fractures
      closed reduction treatment, III:59–60
      complications, III:60

facial injury surgery (Continued)
      K-wire support, III:59
      nasal septum fractures and dislocations, III:58–59, 58f
      open reduction treatment, III:59
      soft tissue contracture, III:59–60, 59f
      types and locations, III:57, 58f
    nasoethmoidal orbital fractures
      causal factors, III:60
      characteristics, III:60–61
      classification systems, III:61–63, 62f
      clinical examination, III:60–61, 61f
      complications, III:63
      computed tomography (CT), III:61
      interorbital space, III:60
      lacrimal system injury, III:63
      traumatic orbital hypertelorism, III:60
      traumatic telecanthus, III:60
      treatment strategies, III:61–63
    postoperative care and follow-up, III:74
    zygoma
      anterior treatment approach, III:65–66
      buttress articulations and alignment, III:66–67
      characteristics, III:63–65
      classification systems, III:65–67
      closed reduction treatment, III:66
      complications, III:69
      compound comminuted fractures, III:69–70
      diagnosis, III:64–65
      high energy fractures, III:67–68, 68f
      posterior approach (coronal incisions), III:66
      reduction methods, III:67
      surgical pathology, III:64–65
  panfacial fractures
    complications, III:84–85, 85f
    definition, III:84–85
    postoperative care and follow-up, III:85
    surgical sequence, III:84
    treatment strategies, III:84
  upper facial fractures
    frontal bone and sinus fractures
      clinical examination, III:51
      complications, III:53
      computed tomography (CT), III:51
      injury patterns, III:51
      nasofrontal duct, III:51, 52f
      surgical technique and treatment, III:52–53, 52f
    orbital fractures
      blow-out fractures (children), III:54, 54f
      blow-out fractures (floor of the orbit), III:54
      characteristics, III:53–57
      complications, III:56–57
      computed tomography (CT), III:54
      infraorbital nerve anesthesia, III:57
      operative technique, III:55
      orbital apex syndrome, III:57
      physical examination, III:53–54, 54f
      postoperative care and follow-up, III:56
      schematic diagram, III:53f
      superior orbital fissure syndrome, III:57
      surgical anatomy, III:53
      surgical technique and treatment, III:54–55
      timing considerations, III:55
      treatment indicators, III:54

facial ligaments
  aging process, II:87
  anatomical characteristics, II:79f–80f, 189–191, 191f
  extended SMAS technique, II:239
  periorbital ligaments, III:9f
  retaining ligaments, II:112, 114f, III:8–10, 10f–11f
facial lipoatrophy, II:54–55, 330
facial muscles, II:34f, 189, 190f, III:280–282, 281f
facial mutilations, I:20–23, 22f
facial nerve
  anatomical characteristics
    buccal branch, III:12f, 13
    cervical branch, III:12f, 13–14
    deep fascia, III:6
    frontal/temporal branch, III:12–13, 12f
    general characteristics, III:11–14, 278–280
    marginal mandibular nerve, III:12f, 13
    periorbital area, II:112–115, 115f
    scalp and forehead, III:107–108, 108f
    schematic diagram, III:9f, 12f, 279f, 295f
    sensory nerve connections, III:14
    zygomatic branch, III:12f, 13
  botulinum toxin type-A (BoNT-A), II:41
  facelifts, II:192–193, 194f, 226f
  facial nerve branches, II:85–86, 85f, III:108f
  reconstructive surgeries, III:274
  salivary glands, III:362f
  traumatic injuries, III:45
facial nevi, III:844, 846f
facial paralysis, III:278–306
  anatomical considerations
    facial musculature, III:280–282, 281f
    facial nerve, III:278–280, 279f, 295f
    upper lip, III:280–281, 282f, 282t
  classifications, III:284, 285t
  definition, III:278
  functional considerations, III:304–305, 305f
  historical background, III:278
  Möbius syndrome, III:284, 297–298, 300f, 305f
  outcomes and complicatons, III:303–304
  patient presentation and diagnosis, III:282–284, 283f
  patient selection, III:284–285
  postoperative care and follow-up, III:303, 303t
  research summary, III:305–306
  secondary procedures, III:304
  treatment strategies
    cross-facial nerve graft, III:293–295, 293f–295f
    microneurovascular muscle transplantation
      basic procedure, III:292–297
      gracilis muscle transplantation, III:295–297, 295t, 296f–298f
      operative technique, III:292–293, 295t
      smile analysis, III:292, 293f
      two-stage microneurovascular transplantation, III:293–295, 295t
    muscle transplantation in the absence of seventh-nerve input, III:297–298, 299f–300f
    nerve transfers, III:291–292, 291f–292f
    nonsurgical management, III:285–286, 286t
    planning strategies, III:285

facial paralysis (Continued)
  regional muscle transfer, III:298–300, 301f
  soft-tissue rebalancing
    characteristics, III:302
    lower lip, III:302, 303f
  static slings, III:300–302, 301f
  surgical management
    cheeks, III:291
    decision-making process, III:286–291, 286t
    eyebrows, III:286, 286t, 287f
    lips, III:287f, 291
    lower eyelid area, III:287f, 289–291, 290f
    nasal airways, III:287f, 291
    upper eyelid area, III:287–289, 287f–289f
  two-stage microneurovascular trans-plantation, III:293–295, 293f–295f
facialplasty
  See facelifts
facial reconstruction, I:798–813
  beauty doctors, I:27, 28f
  craniofacial osteointegration
    advantages, I:799, 799b
    ancillary autogenous procedures, I:810, 810b, 811f
    disadvantages, I:799b
    future trends, I:812–813
    historical background, I:798
    implant considerations
      bone bed, I:805
      bone preparation, I:805, 805f
      implant load, I:805
      implant materials, I:804
      implant–tissue interface, I:804–805
    indicators and applications
      Bone Anchored Hearing Aide (BAHA), I:799–800, 800f
      ear reconstruction, I:800–802, 800t, 801f
      reconstruction applications, I:799–804
    maintenance regimen, I:809, 810f
    midfacial reconstruction, I:803–804, 804f
    osseointegrated nasal reconstruction, I:802, 802b, 802f–803f
    osseointegrated orbital reconstruction, I:802–803, 802b, 803f
    prognosis and outcomes
      general discussion, I:810–812
      individual implant success rates, I:810–811
      prosthetic success, I:812
      skin response, I:812, 812f
    prosthetic construction, I:808–809, 809f–810f
    surgical technique, I:806–808, 807f–808f
    treatment planning process, I:805–806
  local flaps, III:440–460
    basic principles, III:440–441
    cheeks
      advancement flap, III:451–452, 453f
      finger flap, III:452
      island flap, III:452
      large cheek defects, III:452–453
      rotation flaps, III:451, 451f–452f
      transposition flap, III:452
    ears
      anterior concha, III:457, 458f
      rim defects, III:456–457, 456f–457f

facial reconstruction (Continued)
  eyebrow reconstruction, III:441, 444f
  eyelids
    large defects, III:450
    medial canthal defects, III:450
    partial lower lid defects, III:449
    partial upper lid defects, III:449–450
    total lower lid defects, III:450
    total upper lid defects, III:450
  facial burn wound treatment, IV:474
  lips
    commissure reconstruction, III:456
    lower lip, III:454–456
    upper lip, III:453–454
  nasal reconstruction
    basic procedure, III:441–449
    bilobed flap, III:143–145, 144f–145f, 446f
    dorsal nasal flap, III:143, 144f–145f
    forehead flaps, III:148–155, 149f
    interpolated paramedian forehead flap, III:445f, 448f
    lateral advancement flaps, III:445f
    one-stage nasolabial flap, III:145–146
    Rintala dorsal nasal advancement flap, III:447f
    three stage full-thickness forehead flap, III:151–152, 152f
    three stage full-thickness forehead flap (stage 1), III:152–153, 153f–159f
    three stage full-thickness forehead flap (stage 2), III:153–155
    three stage full-thickness forehead flap (stage 3), III:155, 155t
    transoperative flap, III:447f
    two-stage forehead flap, III:148, 150f–151f
    two-stage forehead flap (stage 1), III:148–151
    two-stage forehead flap (stage 2), III:151, 151t
    two-stage nasolabial flap, III:146–148, 146f–147f
    two-stage nasolabial flap (stage 1), III:146
    two-stage nasolabial flap (stage 2), III:146–148
    V-Y advancement flap, III:446f
  partial upper lid defects
    Abbé flap, III:450
    advancement flap, III:450
    decision-making process, III:449–450
    full-thickness skin graft, III:450
    lower lid transposition, III:449f
  perforator flaps, III:458–459
  research summary, III:459
  scalp and forehead, III:123–127, 124f, 126f, 441, 442f–443f
  skin expansion, III:457–458
  skin viscoelasticity, III:441t
  reconstructive burn surgery
    challenges, IV:504–506
    cheeks, IV:490–491, 506
    ears, IV:473, 491–492, 496f, 498–499, 505–506
    eyebrows, IV:504–505
    eyelids, IV:470–473, 485–488, 486f–487f, 498–499, 504–505, 504f

facial reconstruction (Continued)
  lips, IV:505
  neck, IV:506
  nose, IV:473, 488–489, 498–499, 505
  Renaissance, I:17f
  rhomboid flap, III:441, 442f–443f
  secondary facial reconstruction, III:461–472
    case study 1
      diagnosis, III:465
      patient description, III:464b–466b, 464f–465f
      reconstructive plan, III:465–466
    case study 2
      diagnosis, III:466
      patient description, III:466b–467b, 466f–467f
      reconstructive plan, III:467
    case study 3
      diagnosis, III:467
      patient description, III:467b–469b, 468f
      reconstructive plan, III:467–469
    case study 4
      diagnosis, III:469
      patient description, III:469b–471b, 469f–470f
      reconstructive plan, III:469–471
    complications, III:471
    etiology, III:461
    goals, III:461
    patient presentation and diagnosis, III:461–462
    patient selection, III:462
    postoperative care and follow-up, III:471
    prognosis and outcomes, III:471
    surgical technique and treatment
      flap prelamination, III:464–471
      hair-bearing flaps, III:463
      intraoral and intranasal lining, III:462–463, 463f
      planning guidelines, III:462–471
      prefabricated flaps, III:463
  soft-tissue injuries, III:23–48
    anesthesia
      auricular nerve, III:27
      cheeks, III:27, 27f–28f
      chin, III:27, 28f
      ears, III:27–29, 29f
      Erb's point, III:27
      facial field block, III:26–29
      forehead, III:26, 27f
      general discussion, III:26–29
      glabella, III:26, 27f
      jaw, III:27
      local infiltration, III:26
      lower eyelid area, III:27, 27f–28f
      lower lip, III:27, 28f
      neck, III:27
      nose, III:27, 27f–28f
      scalp, III:26, 27f
      teeth, III:27, 27f–28f
      topical anesthetics, III:26
      upper eyelid area, III:26, 27f
      upper lip, III:27, 27f–28f
    diagnostic studies
      computed tomography (CT), III:26
      general discussion, III:26
      X-ray analysis, III:26
    etiology, III:23–24, 24f

facial reconstruction (Continued)
  general discussion, III:23
  patient presentation and diagnosis
    diagnostic studies, III:26
    evaluation examinations, III:24
    general discussion, III:24–26
    head and neck evaluations, III:24–25
    provider consultations, III:26
  provider consultations
    dentists, III:26
    ophthalmologists, III:26
  research summary, III:46
  skin considerations, III:23–24
  surgical technique and treatment
    abrasions, III:29, 30f
    anesthesia, III:26–29
    avulsions, III:31–32, 33f
    cheeks, III:44–45
    complex lacerations, III:31, 32f
    ears, III:39–42
    eyebrows, III:34–38, 37f
    eyelids, III:38–39, 38f–40f
    irrigation and debridement, III:29
    lips, III:46, 47f–48f
    neck, III:46
    nose, III:42–44
    oral cavity and mouth, III:45–46
    scalp, III:33–34, 33f, 35f–37f
    secondary intention healing, III:32–33
    simple lacerations, III:30, 31f
    traumatic tatoo, III:29–30, 30f
  systematic head and neck evaluations
    airway evaluation, III:25
    basic procedure, III:24–25
    cheek examination, III:25, 25f
    ear examination, III:25, 25f, 40
    eye examination, III:25
    nose examination, III:25
    oral cavity and mouth examination,
      III:25
  twentieth century, I:20–23, 22f–23f
facial skeletal augmentation, II:339–353
  complications, II:352
  craniofacial deformities, II:339
  general discussion, II:339
  patient presentation and diagnosis
    characteristics, II:339–340
    facial anthropometries, II:340
    neoclassical canons, II:340, 356b
    physical examination, II:340
    radiology assessments, II:340
  patient selection
    general discussion, II:340–342
    orthognathic surgery
      adjunct therapy, II:340, 341f
      alternatives, II:340, 341f
      rejuvenation therapy, II:340–342, 341f
      skeletal enhancement, II:340
      skeletal versus soft-tissue augmentation,
        II:342
  postoperative care and follow-up, II:351–352
  prognosis and outcomes, II:352
  secondary procedures, II:352
  surgical technique and treatment
    anesthesia, II:342
    chin augmentation
      characteristics, II:346, 349f–350f
      implant augmentation versus sliding
        genioplasty, II:348
      surgical technique, II:347–348, 350f–351f

facial skeletal augmentation (Continued)
  implants/implant materials
    guidelines, II:342
    hematoma prevention, II:343
    immobilization, II:343
    mandible implants, II:346–351
    midface implants, II:343–346
    polyethylene, II:343
    positioning, II:343
    shape considerations, II:343
    silicone, II:342
  incisions, II:342
  infraorbital rim
    Jelks and Jelks categorized globe–
      orbital rim relationships, II:343–
      344, 344f
    surgical technique, II:344, 345f
  malar region
    characteristics, II:345
    surgical technique, II:345–346, 348f–349f
  mandible implants
    chin augmentation, II:346
    general discussion, II:346–351
    ramus, angle, and body considerations,
      II:348, 351, 351f–352f
  midface implants
    general discussion, II:343–346
    infraorbital rim, II:343–344, 344f
    malar region, II:345
    pyriform aperture, II:344
  pyriform aperture
    characteristics, II:344, 346f
    surgical technique, II:344–345,
      346f–347f
facial skin resurfacing, II:60–77
  chemical peeling methods
    characteristics, II:62
    patient selection and treatment, II:66–67
    wound healing biology
      characteristics, II:62–63
      inflammatory response, II:62
      proliferation phase, II:62
      remodeling phase, II:63
  complications
    acne, II:77
    characteristics, II:76
    infections, II:77
    milia, II:77
    pigmentary changes, II:77
    prolonged erythema, II:77
    scarring, II:77
  fractional photothermolysis, II:61, 61f, 65,
    65f
  laser–tissue interactions
    laser properties, II:63–64
    molecular bases, II:63–64
  nonablative facial skin rejuvenation (NSR),
    II:64–65
  patient presentation and diagnosis, II:65–66
  patient selection and treatment
    acne scars, II:75f
    chemical peeling methods, II:66–67
    complications, II:76
    deeper heating long pulse skin tightening
      procedures, II:70, 71f
    facelifts, II:76f
    fractional photothermolysis, II:70–74, 71t
    laser treatments, II:67–70, 68f
    perioral lines, II:74–76, 74f–75f
    photodynamic therapy, II:69–70, 70f

facial skin resurfacing (Continued)
  postoperative care and follow-up, II:76
  selective photothermolysis (SPT)
    characteristics, II:64
    reaction types
      biostimulation, II:64
      photochemical reactions, II:64
      photothermal reactions, II:64
      surface cooling, II:64
  treatment strategies
    chemical peeling methods, II:62, 66–67
    fractional photothermolysis, II:61, 61f,
      70–74, 71t
    laser treatments, II:60–62
facial soft-tissue injuries, III:23–48
  etiology, III:23–24, 24f
  general discussion, III:23
  patient presentation and diagnosis
    diagnostic studies
      computed tomography (CT), III:26
      general discussion, III:26
      X-ray analysis, III:26
    evaluation examinations
      diagnostic studies, III:26
      head and neck evaluations, III:24–25
      immediate life-threatening injuries, III:24
      provider consultations, III:26
    general discussion, III:24–26
    provider consultations
      dentists, III:26
      ophthalmologists, III:26
    systematic head and neck evaluations
      airway evaluation, III:25
      basic procedure, III:24–25
      cheek examination, III:25, 25f
      ear examination, III:25, 25f, 40
      eye examination, III:25
      nose examination, III:25
      oral cavity and mouth examination,
        III:25
  research summary, III:46
  skin considerations, III:23–24
  surgical technique and treatment
    abrasions, III:29, 30f
    anesthesia
      auricular nerve, III:27
      cheeks, III:27, 27f–28f
      chin, III:27, 28f
      ears, III:27–29, 29f
      Erb's point, III:27
      facial field block, III:26–29
      forehead, III:26, 27f
      general discussion, III:26–29
      glabella, III:26, 27f
      jaw, III:27
      local infiltration, III:26
      lower eyelid area, III:27, 27f–28f
      lower lip, III:27, 28f
      neck, III:27
      nose, III:27, 27f–28f
      scalp, III:26, 27f
      teeth, III:27, 27f–28f
      topical anesthetics, III:26
      upper eyelid area, III:26, 27f
      upper lip, III:27, 27f–28f
    avulsions, III:31–32, 33f
    cheeks
      basic procedure, III:44–45
      facial nerve injury, III:45
      parotid duct repair, III:45, 45f

facial soft-tissue injuries (Continued)
  complex lacerations, **III:**31, 32f
  ears
    anatomical considerations, **III:**40
    auditory canal stenosis, **III:**41–42
    causal factors, **III:**39–42
    complete amputation, **III:**42
    hematomas, **III:**40–41, 41f
    lacerations, **III:**41, 41f
    partial amputation with a narrow
      pedicle, **III:**42
    partial amputation with a wide pedicle,
      III:41f, 42
  eyebrows
    basic procedure, **III:**34–38
    Burow's triangles, **III:**37f
    local brow advancement flaps,
      III:36–38, 37f
    local grafts, **III:**38
  eyelids, **III:**38–39, 38f–40f
  irrigation and debridement, **III:**29
  neck, **III:**46
  nose
    abrasions, **III:**43
    amputations, **III:**44
    avulsions, **III:**43–44, 44f
    basic procedure, **III:**42–44
    lacerations, **III:**43
  oral cavity and mouth
    basic procedure, **III:**45–46
    lips, **III:**46, 47f–48f
    oral mucosa repair, **III:**46
    tongue, **III:**46
  scalp, **III:**33–34, 33f, 35f–37f
  secondary intention healing, **III:**32–33
  simple lacerations, **III:**30, 31f
  traumatic tatoo, **III:**29–30, 30f
facio-auriculo-vertebral spectrum, **VI:**573t
faciocraniosynostosis
  Apert syndrome, **III:**689
  characteristics, **III:**688–689
  craniofrontonasal dysplasia, **III:**689
  Crouzon syndrome, **III:**688, 688f
  general discussion, **III:**686
  Pfeiffer syndrome, **III:**688–689
  surgical indicators and timing
    face, **III:**694–695
    general discussion, **III:**694–695
    orbits, **III:**694, 694f
  surgical technique, **III:**695
Fallopio, Gabriele, **I:**18
familial atypical mole and melanoma
  syndrome (FAMMM), **III:**113–114, 114f
familial cutaneous and mucosal venous
  malformation, **VI:**668t
Fanconi anemia, **VI:**617t
Fanconi anemia (FA), **VI:**573t, 574
fan flaps, **III:**454
Farkas, Leslie, **II:**355
Fasanella–Servat operation, **II:**144–145, 146f
fascia lata grafts, **IV:**289, 290f
fascial flaps
  lower extremity reconstructive surgery,
    IV:75
  Mathes–Nahai Classification, **I:**517–519,
    518f
  reconstructive burn surgery, **IV:**503
  tissue expansion, **I:**630

fascial graft and repair
  clinical application, **I:**348, 349f–350f
  definition, **I:**348–350
  future trends, **I:**348–350
  surgical technique, **I:**348
Fascian, **II:**45t, 46
fasciocutaneous flaps
  advantages/disadvantages, **I:**539
  arc of rotation, **I:**539–540
  extremity burn reconstruction, **IV:**449–450
  lower extremity reconstructive surgery
    anterolateral thigh perforator flap, **IV:**145,
      145f–146f
    characteristics, **IV:**143–147
    foot reconstruction, **IV:**211–214, 215f–216f
    groin/superficial circumflex iliac
      perforator flap, **IV:**143, 143f–144f
    lateral thigh/profunda femoris perforator
      flap, **IV:**144–145, 144f
    medial thigh septocutaneous flap,
      IV:143–144, 144f
    sural flap, **IV:**146, 146f
    thoracodorsal artery perforator, **IV:**147,
      147f
    trauma injuries, **IV:**81, 81f–82f
  male genital reconstructive surgery,
    IV:307–310
  mangled upper extremities, **VI:**254–255,
    266–275
  Mathes–Nahai Classification, **I:**517–519, 518f
  oral cavity and mouth reconstruction,
    III:319–322
  scalp and forehead reconstruction, **III:**130
  selection guidelines, **I:**542
  spina bifida, **III:**867–872, 868t–869t,
    870f–871f
  type A fasciocutaneous flaps, **I:**518, 519t,
    520f
  type B fasciocutaneous flaps, **I:**518, 519t,
    520f
  type C fasciocutaneous flaps, **I:**519, 519t,
    520f
  vascular anatomical research, **I:**504
  vascularized bone flaps, **I:**526f
fat embolism syndrome (FES), **IV:**84
fat grafting, **II:**327–338
  adipose-derived stem/stromal cells (ASCs),
    I:345–347, 345f–347f, **II:**327–328
  aging process, **II:**328, 329f
  Asian rhinoplasty, **II:**176
  autologous fillers, **II:**46
  breast reconstruction, **V:**582–604
    adipose-derived stem/stromal cells
      (ASCs), **V:**583–584
    applications, **V:**582–583
    autologous fat grafts, **V:**407–410, 514–515
    contour deformities
      patient selection, **V:**584–595
      post-flap reconstruction, **V:**584t, 586,
        587f–588f
      post-implant reconstruction, **V:**584–586,
        584t, 585f
      radiation-caused deformities, **V:**584t,
        586, 588f–589f
    harvesting considerations, **V:**583–584
    outcomes and complicatons
      graft survival, **V:**602
      infections, **V:**602

fat grafting (Continued)
      liponecrotic cysts, **V:**602
      mammographic abnormalities, **V:**602
      neoplasia, **V:**602–603
      persistent swelling, **V:**602
    patient presentation and diagnosis, **V:**584
    patient selection
      congenital deformities, **V:**584t, 591,
        591f
      contour deformities, **V:**584–595
      indicators, **V:**584t
      lumpectomy deformities, **V:**584t,
        586–590, 590f
      primary breast augmentation,
        V:591–595, 593f–595f
      total breast reconstruction, **V:**595
    postoperative care and follow-up, **V:**601,
      601b
    radiation deformities, **V:**583–584
    research summary, **V:**604
    secondary procedures, **V:**603–604, 603f
    surgical technique and treatment
      basic procedure, **V:**595–601
      Brava bra, **V:**601, 601f
      cannulas, **V:**596f, 598f, 599–601, 600f
      centrifuges, **V:**598f, 600f
      Coleman method, **V:**598, 598f
      contour deformities, **V:**596f
      Cytori™ fat harvest system, **V:**598–599,
        600f
      fat harvesting and processing,
        V:597–598, 597f
      injection techniques, **V:**599–601, 600f
      LipiVage™ fat harvest system,
        V:598–599, 599f
      Lipokit™ fat harvest system, **V:**598–
        599, 600f
      Luer-to-Luer connector, **V:**598, 598f
      markings, **V:**596f
      strainers/straining methods, **V:**598–599
      V-shaped dissectors, **V:**597f
  clinical application, **I:**342–346, 344f–347f
  complications, **II:**337–338, 338f
  contraindications, **II:**330–332
  definition, **I:**342–347
  future trends, **I:**346–347, 348f
  liposuctions, **II:**332, 333f
  nipple-areola complex reconstruction,
    V:407–410, 514–515, 514f
  patient presentation and diagnosis,
    II:328–330
  patient selection
    evaluation examinations, **II:**330–332
    eyelid repair, **II:**332f
    facelifts, **II:**330f–331f
    facial atrophy, **II:**332f, 334f
    hands, **II:**332, 333f
    liposuctions, **II:**333f
    lips, **II:**331f
  penile girth enhancement, **II:**659–660
  postoperative care and follow-up,
    II:335–337
  prognosis and outcomes, **II:**337–338
  secondary procedures, **II:**338
  soft-tissue fillers, **II:**55f
  subperiosteal facelift, **II:**273
  surgical innovation, **I:**7
  surgical technique

fat grafting (Continued)
    Coleman method, II:332–335, 336f, V:598, 598f
    harvesting methods, I:342f–343f, II:334, 334f–335f, V:597–598, 597f
    placement methods, II:335, 336f–337f
    refinement methods, II:334–335, 335f–336f
    viability studies, II:327
fat necrosis
    abdominoplasty, II:557–558
    bilateral pedicle TRAM flap reconstruction, V:407–410
    breast reduction, V:251
    periareolar surgical technique with mesh support, V:226, 226t
    sculpted pillar vertical reduction mammaplasty, V:238, 239f
    short scar periareolar inferior pedicle reduction (SPAIR) mammaplasty, V:203–204
    vertical scar reduction mammaplasty, V:191t
fat transplantation, IV:485
fat tumors See lipoma
FDA-approved biological fillers, II:45t
FDA-approved synthetic fillers, II:47t
fecal incontinence, IV:363–364
Federal False Claims Act, I:96
fee splitting, I:61–62
feet
    anatomical characteristics
        cutaneous innervation, IV:46f, 51f, 61
        extensor digitorum brevis muscle flap, IV:59f
        fascial system
            characteristics, IV:52–56
            extensor retinacula, IV:52, 52t, 54f
            fascial compartments, IV:54–56, 56f–57f, 56t
            flexor retinaculum, IV:52–54, 52t, 54f
            peroneal retinaculum, IV:54, 54f, 54t
            plantar fascia, IV:54, 55f
        functional role, IV:50–61
        innervation, IV:46f, 51f, 60f
        motor nerves, IV:61
        musculature, IV:42f, 44f, 56–58, 56f–57f, 56t, 58t, 59f
        skeletal structure, IV:50, 53f
        vascular supply
            dorsalis pedis, IV:59, 60f
            peroneal artery, IV:47f, 59–61, 61f–62f
            posterior tibial artery, IV:47f, 59
    burn reconstruction, IV:509
    cutaneous innervations, I:255f
    diabetic ulcers, I:254–255, 254f
    melanoma excisions, I:767–768, 771f
    Mohr–Wriedt syndrome, VI:636, 638f
    muscle/musculocutaneous flaps, I:560–562, 562f–563f
    photographic guidelines, I:114
    reconstructive surgeries, IV:189–219
        anatomic location-based reconstruction
            ankle and foot dorsum, IV:205–207, 206f
            anterolateral thigh flap, IV:211
            extensor digitorum brevis muscle flap, IV:205–206, 206f
            fasciocutaneous flaps, IV:211–214, 215f–216f
            gracilis muscle, IV:211
            heel pad flaps, IV:209

feet (Continued)
            hindfoot amputations, IV:216–217
            intrinsic muscle flaps, IV:209, 210f
            lateral arm flap, IV:211, 213f
            lateral supramalleolar flap, IV:206–207
            medial plantar artery flap, IV:209
            microvascular free flap, IV:211–216
            midfoot amputations, IV:208
            neurovascular island flap, IV:207–208
            parascapular flap, IV:211, 212f
            pedicle flaps, IV:205–217
            plantar forefoot, IV:207
            plantar hindfoot, IV:208–216, 210f, 212f–216f
            plantar midfoot, IV:208
            radial forearm flap, IV:211, 214f
            rectus abdominis, IV:211
            serratus anterior muscles, IV:211
            suprafascial flaps, IV:208
            sural artery flap, IV:209–211
            toe fillet flap, IV:207
            transmetatarsal amputation, IV:207
            V-Y plantar flap, IV:207
        disease process
            angiosomes, IV:189–190
            compartment pressure measurement, IV:190
            gait analysis, IV:190–191, 191f–192f
        outcome assessments, IV:217–218
        patient presentation and diagnosis
            antibiotic therapy, IV:196–197
            bone assessment, IV:196
            Charcot deformities, IV:195
            chronic wounds, IV:196
            clinical evaluations, IV:191–192
            connective tissue disorders, IV:192
            diabetic foot ulcers, IV:194–195
            hemorheologic abnormalities, IV:194f, 195–196
            infection identification, IV:196–197
            ischemia, IV:193, 194f
            neuropathic changes, IV:195
            venous stasis ulcers, IV:192–193
        patient selection
            decision-making process, IV:197
            limb function, IV:197
        postoperative care and follow-up, IV:217
        research summary, IV:218
        soft tissue reconstruction
            angiosomes, IV:201
            closure techniques, IV:201–205, 202f–205f
        surgical technique and treatment
            anatomic location-based reconstruction, IV:205–217
            soft tissue reconstruction, IV:201–205
        trauma effects, IV:189
        treatment strategies
            debridement, IV:198–199, 200f
            external fixation, IV:199–201
            trauma and crush injuries, IV:198, 198f
            wound management, IV:199
    tissue expansion, I:650
    toe-to-hand transplantations, VI:280–281, 280f, 295–296, 296f, 555, 555f, 642, 643f
felon, VI:337–338, 337f
female genital aesthetic surgery, II:655–677
    aesthetic ideals, II:669
    labia majora reduction, II:673–674, 674f–676f

female genital aesthetic surgery (Continued)
    labia minora reduction
        characteristics, II:669–673
        outcomes and complicatons, II:672–673, 672f–673f
        surgical technique, II:670–672, 671f–672f
    lipodystrophy, II:674–676, 675f–677f
    mons correction, II:640, 641f–642f
    mons pubis descent, II:674–676, 675f–677f
    post-bariatric surgery reconstruction, II:640, 641f–642f
    research summary, II:677
    self-esteem issues, II:655, 669
    vulvar anatomy, II:669
female perineum
    characteristics, IV:230–235
    cross-section diagram, IV:231f
    schematic diagram, IV:232f–233f
    urogenital triangle, IV:233f
    vascular anatomy, IV:232–235, 234f
female-to-male transsexual surgery
    female-to-male chest surgery, IV:349–350
    metaidoioplasty, IV:315–318, 317f, 346
    pars fixa of the urethra creation, IV:314–315, 316f–317f
    phalloplasty
        anterolateral thigh flap, IV:311f, 323, 324f–325f
        basic procedure, IV:318–323
        fibula flap, IV:323
        perforator flaps, IV:323
        radial forearm flap
            aesthetic phallus, IV:319, 320f
            donor site considerations, IV:321, 321f
            general discussion, IV:318–323
            minimal morbidity, IV:321
            normal scrotum, IV:321, 322f
            one-stage procedure, IV:319
            operative technique, IV:318, 319f–320f, 324f–325f
            research summary, IV:322–323
            sexual intercourse, IV:321–322, 322f
            surgical goals, IV:318–322
            tactile and erogenous sensation, IV:319–321
            voiding while standing, IV:321
        vaginectomy, IV:314–315, 315f
femoral dysgenesis–unusual facies syndrome, III:807t
femoral-fibular-ulnar deficiency syndrome, VI:567t
femur, IV:10f, 183
fenfluramine, II:635
fentanyl, IV:427
fetal alcohol syndrome (FAS), III:515, 805–807, 807t
fetal aminopterin effects, VI:573t
fetal valporate effects, VI:573t
feverfew, II:21t, 22, V:33t–35t
Fgf gene expression, VI:527–530, 529f
fibrin, I:243f, 244, 793
fibrinogen, I:243f, 244
fibroblast growth factor (FGF)
    adipose-derived stem/stromal cells (ASCs), I:219
    bone regeneration, I:435t, 437–438, 441–442, 443t–444t
    Dupuytren's disease, VI:349
    fat grafting, I:345

fibroblast growth factor (FGF) (Continued)
  fibroblast growth factor receptor (FGFR)-
    related mutations, III:749–750, 750t
  gene regulation, I:180–181, 180f
  pedical flap viability augmentation,
    I:580–582
  skin wound healing, I:270t, 274–275
  tissue engineering, I:381, 381f
  wound healing, I:234, 244
fibroblasts
  aging process, II:44–45
  induced pluripotent stem cells, I:237
  scars, I:264–265
  skin wound healing, I:268f, 269–271, 270t,
    271f, II:63
fibrocartilage, I:397, 398f
fibroma pendulum, I:730, 730f
fibromatosis colli
  patient presentation and diagnosis,
    III:880–881
  surgical technique and treatment, III:881
fibronectin, I:243f, 244, 270–271, VI:348–349
fibrosarcoma, IV:103
fibrous dysplasia, III:380–397
  assessment and diagnosis considerations,
    III:380
  complications, III:392–393
  disease process, III:380–382
  pathogenesis, III:380–382
  patient presentation and diagnosis, III:382
  patient selection, III:382–383, 384f
  postoperative care and follow-up, III:389
  research summary, III:395–396
  secondary procedures, III:393–395,
    395f–396f
  surgical technique and treatment
    nonsurgical treatments, III:383
    operation timing, III:383–385
    preoperative assessment, III:383
    surgical approach
      optic nerve decompression, III:384f,
        386
      zonal procedure, III:385–389, 385f
      zone 1, III:385–386, 386f–393f
      zone 2, III:387
      zone 3, III:387
      zone 4, III:387–389, 394f
fibrous histiocytoma, I:729
fibroxanthoma, I:736
fibula
  fibula flap, IV:323
  fibula harvests, I:452
  fibular nerve, IV:51f
  schematic diagram, IV:34f
fibula osteoseptocutaneous flap, III:323, 324t
Filatov, Vladimir, I:21–22
films, I:289t
finance
  discounted cash flow, I:72–73
  goals, I:69–73
  net present value, I:72–73
  opportunity cost, I:71–72
  return on investment, I:73
  time value of money, I:70–71
financial ratios
  characteristics, I:68–69
  efficiency ratios, I:69
  leverage ratios, I:69

financial ratios (Continued)
  liquidity ratios, I:69
  profitability ratios, I:69
Fine Lines, II:49t
  See also soft-tissue fillers
fine-needle aspiration (FNA), III:363, 363f,
    IV:106, V:272
finger flap, III:452
fingers
  adult brachial plexus injury reconstructive
    strategies, VI:800, 801t, 802f, 803t
  anatomical characteristics, VI:14f
  arterial system, VI:468–469
  boutonnière deformity
    characteristics, VI:223–224, 223f
    preoperative assessment, VI:223–224
    secondary reconstruction, VI:224, 224f
    tenotomy, VI:224, 224f
  burn reconstruction, IV:508, 508f
  clawing of the fingers
    Bouvier maneuver, VI:764–765, 764f
    Brand EE4T transfer, VI:766–767, 766f
    Brand EF4T transfer, VI:767, 767f–768f
    donor muscle-tendon selection, VI:764–
      765, 765f
    Fritschi PF4T transfer, VI:767–768
    Littler modification, VI:764–765
    modified Stiles–Bunnell technique,
      VI:764–766, 765f
    pulley insertions, VI:764–765, 764f–765f
    static procedures, VI:763–764, 763f–764f
  finger amputation, VI:872, 872f
  finger extension restoration, VI:774–775
  finger flexion restoration, VI:775f, 776
  fractures and joint injuries
    treatment strategies
      carpometacarpal (CMC) joints, VI:153,
        153f
      distal interphalangeal (DIP) joint,
        VI:141–142, 142f
      external fixation, VI:144, 145f
      hemi-hamate replacement arthroplasty
        (HHRA), VI:144–147, 146f–147f,
        147b
      internal fixation, VI:141–153
      metacarpal fractures, VI:150–153, 867
      metacarpal head fractures, VI:151
      metacarpal neck fractures, VI:151–152,
        151f
      metacarpal shaft fractures, VI:152, 152f
      metacarpophalangeal (MCP) joint,
        VI:150, 150f
      middle phalanx base articular fractures,
        VI:143–148, 143f
      middle phalanx shaft fractures, VI:142
      multiple metacarpal fractures, VI:152
      phalangeal fractures and dislocations,
        VI:141
      proximal interphalangeal (PIP) joint,
        VI:142–143, 143f, 144b
      proximal phalanx head fractures,
        VI:147
      proximal phalanx shaft and base
        fractures, VI:148, 149f
      surgical options, VI:141–153
      unicondylar fractures, VI:147–148, 148f
  free-functioning muscle transfer, VI:785–787
  hanging fingertip, VI:221–222, 222f

fingers (Continued)
  index finger abduction, VI:770–771, 771f
  intrinsic muscles, VI:211–212, 212f
  mallet finger
    aluminum splint, VI:216f
    lateral view, VI:215f–216f
    posteroanterior view, VI:215f–216f
    postoperative doorstop, VI:217f
    stack splint, VI:216f
    surgical procedures, VI:214–216
  melanoma excisions, I:766–768, 768f–769f
  Neviaser accessory abductor pollicis longus
    and free tendon graft, VI:771, 771f
  osteoarthritis, VI:414
  rheumatoid arthritis
    basic principles, VI:376–379
    boutonnière deformity
      basic procedure, VI:379f, 396–398, 399f
      outcomes and complicatons, VI:398
      patient presentation and diagnosis,
        VI:378f, 380f
      postoperative care and follow-up,
        VI:398
      surgical tips, VI:398b
      thumb deformities, VI:399–400, 400f
    flexion and volar subluxation, VI:377f
    metacarpophalangeal (MCP) arthrodesis
      basic procedure, VI:395
      outcomes and complicatons, VI:395
      postoperative care and follow-up,
        VI:395
    metacarpophalangeal (MCP) arthroplasty
      basic procedure, VI:392–394, 392f, 394f
      entrance point, VI:392f
      final implant position, VI:394f
      osteotomy, VI:393f
      postoperative care and follow-up,
        VI:393–394
      PyroCarbon implants, VI:392f
    metacarpophalangeal (MCP)
      synovectomy and soft tissue
      reconstruction
      basic procedure, VI:390–391, 390f–391f
      outcomes and complicatons, VI:391,
        391f
      postoperative care and follow-up,
        VI:391
      secondary procedures, VI:391
      surgical tips, VI:395b
    operative procedures
      boutonnière deformity, VI:396–398
      metacarpophalangeal (MCP)
        arthrodesis, VI:395
      metacarpophalangeal (MCP)
        arthroplasty, VI:392–394
      metacarpophalangeal (MCP)
        synovectomy and soft tissue
        reconstruction, VI:390–391
      proximal interphalangeal (PIP)
        arthrodesis, VI:395
      proximal interphalangeal (PIP)
        arthroplasty, VI:394–395
      swan-neck deformity, VI:395–396
    proximal interphalangeal (PIP)
      arthrodesis
      basic procedure, VI:395
      K-wire and stainless steel wire
        configuration, VI:396f

Note: **Boldface** roman numerals indicate volume. Page numbers followed by f refer to figures; page numbers followed by t refer to tables; page numbers followed by b refer to boxes.

fingers (Continued)
outcomes and complicatons, **VI**:395
postoperative care and follow-up, **VI**:395
proximal interphalangeal (PIP) arthroplasty
basic procedure, **VI**:394–395
outcomes and complicatons, **VI**:395
postoperative care and follow-up, **VI**:395
secondary procedures, **VI**:395
surgical tips, **VI**:395b
scleroderma, **VI**:407t, 409
swan-neck deformity
basic procedure, **VI**:395–396, 397f–398f
patient presentation and diagnosis, **VI**:379f, 625f
postoperative care and follow-up, **VI**:396
surgical tips, **VI**:398b
thumb deformities, **VI**:399–400, 400f
ulnar deviation, **VI**:377f–378f
ring finger flexor digitorum superficialis transfer, **VI**:769
Smith extensor carpi radialis brevis transfer, **VI**:769–770, 770f
spastic hand surgery, **VI**:464, 465f
swan-neck deformity, **VI**:222–223, 222f–223f, 453f
thumb and finger reconstruction, **VI**:295–310
basic principles, **VI**:295–296
complications, **VI**:309
finger extension restoration, **VI**:774–775
finger flexion restoration, **VI**:775f, 776
fractures and joint injuries
acute ulnar collateral ligament (UCL) tear, **VI**:155, 155f
carpometacarpal (CMC) joint fractures, **VI**:156–158, 157f
chronic ulnar collateral ligament (UCL) tear, **VI**:155–156, 156f
general discussion, **VI**:153–158
metacarpal fractures, **VI**:156
metacarpophalangeal (MCP) joint, **VI**:153–154, 155f
pediatric fractures, **VI**:158, 158f
proximal phalanx neck fractures, **VI**:158, 159f
Stener lesion, **VI**:154–155, 154f
injury factors
finger reconstruction, **VI**:297–298
metacarpal hand, **VI**:298–300, 298t, 299f–300f
thumb reconstruction, **VI**:297
osteoarthritis
carpometacarpal (CMC) arthroscopy, **VI**:434–439
metacarpophalangeal (MCP) joint, **VI**:430
prevalence and characteristics, **VI**:430–441
prosthetic arthroplasty, **VI**:440–441, 440f
trapeziometacarpal arthritis, **VI**:430–434
trapeziometacarpal arthrodesis, **VI**:440–441, 441f
patient presentation and diagnosis
initial operation, **VI**:296–297
patient evaluation, **VI**:296–297, 296f

fingers (Continued)
patient selection
decision-making process, **VI**:297
injury factors, **VI**:297–300
primary versus secondary reconstruction, **VI**:297
postoperative care and follow-up
immediate postoperative period, **VI**:306
motor rehabilitation, **VI**:306–307
sensory rehabilitation, **VI**:307–308
prognosis and outcomes
appearance, **VI**:308
donor site outcome evaluation, **VI**:308, 309f
range of motion, **VI**:308
sensory recovery, **VI**:308
strength assessment, **VI**:308
success rates, **VI**:308
replantation and revascularization surgery
artery repair, **VI**:233–234, 234f
bone fixation, **VI**:232–233, 232b, 232f
complications, **VI**:248–249
ectopic replantation, **VI**:243, 244f
multiple digit replantations, **VI**:237–238, 237f–240f
nerve repair and grafting, **VI**:235
operative sequence, **VI**:231–232, 231f
outcome assessments, **VI**:247–248, 247t
patient selection indications and contraindications, **VI**:230–231, 230t–231t
postoperative monitoring, **VI**:245–246, 246b, 246t
postoperative therapy, **VI**:246
psychosocial aspects, **VI**:246–247
ring avulsion injuries, **VI**:242, 242b, 242t, 243f
secondary procedures, **VI**:248f, 249
single-digit amputation, **VI**:241f
skin closure, **VI**:235
tendon graft and repair, **VI**:233, 233b
thumb replantation, **VI**:235–237, 236f–237f
vein repair, **VI**:234–235, 235f
secondary procedures, **VI**:309, 309f
surgical technique and treatment
combined second- and third-toe transplantations, **VI**:305, 307f
donor closure guidelines, **VI**:301–302
first dorsal metatarsal artery (FDMA), **VI**:300, 301f
first-web neurosensory flap harvest, **VI**:305, 306f
flap inset guidelines, **VI**:302–303, 302b, 302f
great-toe wrap-around flap harvest, **VI**:304–305
pulp flap harvest, **VI**:305, 305f
recipient preparation, **VI**:300–301, 301b, 301f
total or partial second-toe harvest, **VI**:304, 304f
trimmed great toe harvest, **VI**:303–304, 303f
vascular dissection principles, **VI**:300, 300b, 301f
thumb adduction restoration, **VI**:768–769, 769f–770f

fingers (Continued)
thumb extension restoration, **VI**:773–774, 774f
thumb flexion restoration, **VI**:774f–775f, 775–776
thumb ulnar collateral ligament injuries, **VI**:85, 86f
toe-to-hand transplantations, **VI**:280–281, 280f, 295–296, 296f, 555, 555f, 642, 643f
thumb/digital dissections, **VI**:672, 673f, 673t
trigger finger
basic procedure, **VI**:402–404, 404f
occupational hand disorders, **VI**:367, 367f
outcomes and complicatons, **VI**:404
postoperative care and follow-up, **VI**:404
trigger thumb
etiology, **VI**:648
general discussion, **VI**:648–649
timing considerations, **VI**:546t
treatment strategies, **VI**:648–649
ulnar deviation of the small finger, **VI**:768
See also hands; nail and fingertip reconstruction
Finkelstein test, **VI**:56
Fioravanti, Leonardo, **I**:16, 17f
fire triad, **I**:132–133
first branchial cleft anomaly
disease process, **III**:886
patient presentation and diagnosis, **III**:886, 886f
surgical technique and treatment, **III**:886
first dorsal metatarsal artery (FDMA), **VI**:300, 301f
fish oil, **V**:33t–35t
Fitzpatrick skin phototype (SPT) system, **II**:13–14, 14t
5-fluorouracil (5-FU), **I**:309–310
5p-syndrome, **VI**:573t
flaps, **I**:512–586
Abbé flap
lip reconstruction, **III**:259–265, 261f–262f, 454
partial upper lid defects, **III**:450
secondary cleft deformities, **III**:637, 637f–638f
advancement flap
cheek reconstruction, **III**:271–272, 272f, 451–452, 453f
classifications, **I**:513f
anterior intercostal artery perforator (AICAP) flap, **V**:308, 488
anterolateral thigh flap
foot reconstruction, **IV**:211
lower extremity reconstructive surgery, **IV**:68–69, 69f, 75, 75f–76f, 81f, 88f
male genital reconstructive surgery, **IV**:304–310, 306f, 311f
mangled upper extremities, **VI**:274–275, 275f–276f
oral cavity and mouth reconstruction, **III**:321–322
perineal reconstruction, **IV**:388–389, 390f–391f
phalloplasty, **IV**:311f, 323, 324f–325f
pharyngoesophageal reconstruction
flap design and harvesting, **III**:339–341, 340f–342f
flap inset guidelines, **III**:342–347, 343f–348f
frozen neck, **III**:352–353

flaps (Continued)
  isolated cervical esophageal defects,
    III:354
  oral diet, III:356t
  postlaryngectomy pharyngocutaneous
    fistulas, III:353–354, 353f–354f
  selection guidelines, III:338–339
  scalp and forehead reconstruction, III:130
  tongue reconstruction, III:309t–310t
  applications
    advantages/disadvantages
      fascial/fasciocutaneous flaps, I:539
      muscle/musculocutaneous flaps,
        I:538–539
      perforator flaps, I:539
    arc of rotation, I:539–540, 540f
    donor site considerations, I:537
    flap transposition, I:539–540
    muscle function restoration, I:538
    patient safety, I:536
    reconstructive ladder analogy, I:534–541,
      536f
    reconstructive triangle, I:536, 536f
    skeletal support restoration, I:538
    skin territory considerations, I:540–541
    specialized functions, I:537
  arrow flap, V:503t, 507, 507f
  axial pattern flap, I:515, 515f
  back wounds
    flap closure
      adjacent tissue transfers, IV:268
      basic principles, IV:259–260
      erector spinae muscle flaps, IV:260–262,
        260f–267f
      external oblique flaps, IV:268–269
      latissimus muscle/myocutaneous flap,
        IV:262–263, 268f–270f, 272f–273f
      pedicled omental flap, IV:267–268
      perforator flaps, IV:268
      spine closure, IV:260–269
      superior gluteal artery flap, IV:264–265,
        277f
      trapezius muscle flap, IV:263–264,
        274f–276f
    free flap coverage
      bone grafts, IV:271
      soft tissue flaps, IV:270
    regional flap selection
      cervical spine area, IV:271
      lumbar area, IV:272
      lumbosacral region, IV:272–273
      thoracic area, IV:271–272
  bell flap, V:508, 508f, 508t
  biceps femoris muscle flap, IV:139–140
  bilobed flap, III:143–145, 144f–145f, 446f
  bipedicle flap delay, I:513f
  breast reconstruction
    autogenous breast reconstruction,
      V:457–471
      background information, V:457–458
      reconstruction population, V:458–470
      deep femoral artery perforator (DFAP)
        flap, V:464–467, 468f–469f
      deep inferior epigastric perforator (DIEP)
        flaps
        delayed reconstruction, V:291f
        immediate postmastectomy breast
          reconstruction, V:287–291, 288f

flaps (Continued)
      disease process, V:458
      expander-implants, V:367
      flap necrosis, V:243t, 246
      gluteus maximus muscle, V:292
      gracilis muscle, V:292
      inferior gluteal artery perforator (IGAP)
        flap
        advantages, V:459–464
        anatomical characteristics, V:461–463
        complications, V:464
        patient selection, V:460–461
        postoperative care, V:464
        surgical technique, V:463–464, 464b,
          467f–468f
      latissimus dorsi (LD) flap, V:306–308,
        309f, 311f, 485–489, 486f
      lumbar artery perforator (LAP) flap,
        V:467–470, 470b, 470f
      omentum reconstruction, V:472–481
        basic principles, V:472–473
        complications, V:480–481
        patient selection, V:473
        postoperative care and follow-up,
          V:480
        prognosis and outcomes, V:480–481
        secondary procedures, V:481
        skin preservation, V:472
        surgical technique and treatment,
          V:473–480, 473f–474f
      partial breast reconstruction, V:482–498
        basic principles, V:482–483
        batwing mastopexy, V:308f
        breast-conserving therapy (BCT), V:482
        complications, V:495
        decision-making process, V:483–485,
          485f
        donut type mastopexy, V:308f
        flap classification and vascular
          anatomy, V:485–489, 486f
        flap design, V:489–493
        inferior pedicle mastopexy, V:305f, 307f
        lateral quadrantectomy type defect,
          V:303f
        latissimus dorsi (LD) flap, V:82–83,
          306–308, 309f, 311f
        oncologic safety, V:310
        patient presentation and diagnosis,
          V:483–485
        patient selection, V:483
        pedicled flaps, V:489, 492f
        postoperative care and follow-up,
          V:493–495
        prognosis and outcomes, V:495
        secondary procedures, V:495–497,
          496f–497f
        superior pedicle mastopexy, V:304f
        surgical technique and treatment, V:485
        timing considerations, V:484–485
        volume displacement reconstruction,
          V:302–306, 304f–305f, 483–484
        volume replacement reconstruction,
          V:306–310, 309f, 483–484
      patient presentation and diagnosis
        deep femoral artery perforator (DFAP)
          flap, V:464–467, 468f–469f
        lumbar artery perforator (LAP) flap,
          V:467–470, 470b, 470f

flaps (Continued)
      reconstruction population, V:458–470
      superior/inferior gluteal artery
        perforator free flap (SGAP/IGAP),
        V:459–464
      transverse upper gracilis free flap
        (TUG), V:458–459, 460f–462f
      perforator surgery, V:326, 327f–329f
      secondary procedures, V:470–471
      superior gluteal artery perforator (SGAP)
        flap
        advantages, V:459–464
        anatomical characteristics, V:461–463
        complications, V:464
        patient selection, V:460–461
        postoperative care, V:464
        surgical technique, V:463–464, 464b,
          465f–467f
      transverse rectus abdominis
        myocutaneous (TRAM) flaps
        autogenous breast reconstruction,
          V:457–458
        bilateral pedicle TRAM flap, V:393–410
        free TRAM flap, V:411–434
        immediate postmastectomy breast
          reconstruction, V:288f
        patient selection, V:374–376
        surgical manipulation, I:578
      transverse upper gracilis free flap (TUG)
        anatomical characteristics, V:458–459,
          460f
        complications, V:459
        patient selection, V:458
        postoperative image, V:460f
        surgical technique and treatment,
          V:459, 459b, 461f–462f
  burn reconstruction
    fascial flaps, IV:503
    fasciocutaneous flaps, IV:449–450
    free flaps, IV:450
    local flaps, IV:502–503, 503f
    muscle flaps, IV:503
    myocutaneous flaps, IV:449–450
    rotation flaps, IV:448–449, 453f–454f
  cheek reconstruction
    anterolateral thigh flap, III:274
    cheek rotation advancement flap,
      III:271–272, 272f, 451, 451f–452f
    finger flap, III:452
    free tissue transfer, III:272
    island flap, III:452
    large cheek defects, III:452–453
    radial forearm flap, III:274
    scapular and parascapular flaps, III:273,
      275f
    selection guidelines, III:271–274
    soft tissue cheek reconstruction,
      III:272–273
    submental artery flap, III:272, 273f–274f
    transposition flap, III:452
  chest wall reconstruction
    latissimus dorsi (LD) flap, I:552–553,
      IV:241, 243f–244f
    muscle/musculocutaneous flaps,
      I:552–553
    omentum, I:553, IV:245, 246f–247f
    patient selection, IV:247
    pectoralis major muscle, IV:241, 241f–242f

*Note: **Boldface** roman numerals indicate volume. Page numbers followed by f refer to figures; page numbers followed by t refer to tables; page numbers followed by b refer to boxes.*

flaps (Continued)
rectus abdominis, I:552–553, IV:244–245, 245f
serratus anterior muscles, I:552, IV:244, 244f
chimeric flaps, I:612, 612f
circumflex iliac osteocutaneous flap, III:322, 323f
classifications
abdominal viscera classification, I:521, 521t
advancement flap, I:513f
axial pattern flap, I:515, 515f
background and general characteristics, I:512–521
bipedicle flap delay, I:513f
fascial/fasciocutaneous flaps
Mathes–Nahai Classification, I:517–519, 518f
type A fasciocutaneous flaps, I:518, 519t, 520f
type B fasciocutaneous flaps, I:518, 519t, 520f
type C fasciocutaneous flaps, I:519, 519t, 520f
muscle/musculocutaneous flaps
Mathes–Nahai Classification, I:516–517, 516f
Type I muscles (one vascular pedicle), I:516, 517t
Type II muscles (dominant vascular pedicle and minor pedicle), I:516, 517t
Type III muscles (two dominant pedicles), I:516–517, 517t
Type IV muscles (segmental vascular pedicles), I:517, 517t
Type V muscles (one dominant vascular pedicle and secondary segmental vascular pedicles), I:517, 517t
perforator flaps, I:519–521
rotation flaps, I:513f
standard delay flap, I:514, 514f
cleft palate surgery
buccal mucosal flaps, III:576–578, 578f
two-flap palatoplasty, III:578, 579f
Vomer flaps, III:578
craniofacial microsomia (CFM), III:786, 786f–787f
C–V flap, V:503t, 506–507, 506f, 514–515
deep femoral artery perforator (DFAP) flap, V:464–467, 468f–469f
deep inferior epigastric perforator (DIEP) flaps
anatomical characteristics, V:327f, 436–439, 437f–438f
breast reconstruction, V:287–291, 288f, 435–456
imaging methods, V:326, 327f–329f
definition, I:815
deltopectoral flaps, III:274f, 309t, 318–319, 319f
dorsal intercostal artery perforator (DICAP) flap, V:488
dorsal nasal flap, III:143, 144f–145f
double opposing peri-areolar/purse-string flap, V:508–510, 508t, 509f–510f
double-opposing tab flap, V:511t, 512–513, 512f–513f

flaps (Continued)
erector spinae muscle flaps
basic procedure, IV:260–262, 262f–267f
cadaver dissection, IV:261f
schematic diagram, IV:260f–261f
extensor digitorum brevis muscle flap, IV:205–206, 206f
external oblique muscle flap
abdominal wall reconstruction, I:553t, 554
back wounds, IV:268–269
eyebrow reconstruction, III:36–38, 37f
facial artery musculomucosal (FAMM) flap, III:163, 309t, 462–463, 463f, 643, 645f
facial burn wound treatment
basic principles, IV:480–481
indicators, IV:480b
trapeze-plasties, IV:481
Z-plasty technique, IV:481, 481f
facial reconstruction, III:440–460
basic principles, III:440–441
cheeks
advancement flap, III:451–452, 453f
finger flap, III:452
island flap, III:452
large cheek defects, III:452–453
rotation flaps, III:451, 451f–452f
transposition flap, III:452
ears
anterior concha, III:457, 458f
rim defects, III:456–457, 456f–457f
eyebrow reconstruction, III:441, 444f
eyelids
large defects, III:450
medial canthal defects, III:450
partial lower lid defects, III:449
partial upper lid defects, III:449–450
total lower lid defects, III:450
total upper lid defects, III:450
lips
commissure reconstruction, III:456
lower lip, III:454–456
total lower lip reconstruction, III:456
upper lip, III:453–454
nasal reconstruction
basic procedure, III:441–449
bilobed flap, III:143–145, 144f–145f, 446f
dorsal nasal flap, III:143, 144f–145f
forehead flaps, III:148–155, 149f
interpolated paramedian forehead flap, III:445f, 448f
lateral advancement flaps, III:445f
one-stage nasolabial flap, III:145–146
Rintala dorsal nasal advancement flap, III:447f
three stage full-thickness forehead flap, III:151–152, 152f
three stage full-thickness forehead flap (stage 1), III:152–153, 153f–159f
three stage full-thickness forehead flap (stage 2), III:153–155
three stage full-thickness forehead flap (stage 3), III:155, 155t
transoperative flap, III:447f
two-stage forehead flap, III:148, 150f–151f
two-stage forehead flap (stage 1), III:148–151
two-stage forehead flap (stage 2), III:151, 151t

flaps (Continued)
two-stage nasolabial flap, III:146–148, 146f–147f
two-stage nasolabial flap (stage 1), III:146
two-stage nasolabial flap (stage 2), III:146–148
V-Y advancement flap, III:446f
partial upper lid defects
Abbé flap, III:450
advancement flap, III:450
decision-making process, III:449–450
full-thickness skin graft, III:450
lower lid transposition, III:449f
perforator flaps, III:458–459
research summary, III:459
rhomboid flap, III:441, 442f–443f
scalp and forehead, III:123–127, 124f, 126f, 441, 442f–443f
skin expansion, III:457–458
skin viscoelasticity, III:441t
fan flaps, III:454
fascial flaps
lower extremity reconstructive surgery, IV:75
Mathes–Nahai Classification, I:517–519, 518f
reconstructive burn surgery, IV:503
tissue expansion, I:630
fasciocutaneous flaps
advantages/disadvantages, I:539
arc of rotation, I:539–540
extremity burn reconstruction, IV:449–450
lower extremity reconstructive surgery
anterolateral thigh perforator flap, IV:145, 145f–146f
characteristics, IV:143–147
foot reconstruction, IV:211–214, 215f–216f
groin/superficial circumflex iliac perforator flap, IV:143, 143f–144f
lateral thigh/profunda femoris perforator flap, IV:144–145, 144f
medial thigh septocutaneous flap, IV:143–144, 144f
sural flap, IV:146, 146f
thoracodorsal artery perforator, IV:147, 147f
trauma injuries, IV:81, 81f–82f
male genital reconstructive surgery, IV:307–310
mangled upper extremities, VI:254–255, 266–275
Mathes–Nahai Classification, I:517–519, 518f
oral cavity and mouth reconstruction, III:319–322
scalp and forehead reconstruction, III:130
selection guidelines, I:542
spina bifida, III:867–872, 868t–869t, 870f–871f
type A fasciocutaneous flaps, I:518, 519t, 520f
type B fasciocutaneous flaps, I:518, 519t, 520f
type C fasciocutaneous flaps, I:519, 519t, 520f
vascular anatomical research, I:504
vascularized bone flaps, I:526f
fibula flap, IV:323

flaps (Continued)
fibula osteoseptocutaneous flap, **III**:323, 324t
finger flap, **III**:452
fingertip reconstruction
  challenges, **VI**:128
  flap selection, **VI**:128, 129f
  reconstructive principles, **VI**:128
  skin grafts
    cross finger flaps, **VI**:130–131, 133f
    dorsal metacarpal artery flaps, **VI**:134, 135f
    heterodigital flaps, **VI**:130–134
    homodigital flaps, **VI**:130, 132f
    lateral V-Y advancement flaps, **VI**:130, 130f
    Littler neurovascular island flap, **VI**:132–134
    local flaps, **VI**:128–134
    patient selection, **VI**:128
    surgical technique and treatment, **VI**:128–134
    thenar crease flap, **VI**:132, 134f
    visor flaps, **VI**:130, 131f
    volar V-Y advancement flap, **VI**:128–130, 129f
flap fabrication, **I**:6
flap failure pathophysiology
  intracellular Ca^{2+} overload, **I**:576–577, 576f
  ischemia–reperfusion injury, **I**:575–576, 576f, 617–618
  ischemic tolerance, **I**:617–618
  myeloperoxidase (MPO) enzyme system, **I**:575–576
  nicotinamide adenine diphosphate (NADPH) enzyme system, **I**:575–576
  no-reflow phenomenon, **I**:577, 617–618
  thrombogenesis, **I**:615–617
  vasospasm and thrombosis, **I**:573–574, 574f, 615
  xanthine dehydrogenase/xanthine oxidase enzyme system, **I**:575, 575f
flap modifications
  background information, **I**:521–534
  circumflex scapular and thoracodorsal pedicles, **I**:530f
  combination flaps, **I**:528–530, 530f
  deep circumflex iliac artery composite flap, **I**:529f
  distally based flaps, **I**:531, 531t
  functional muscle flaps, **I**:528
  gluteus maximus muscle, **I**:523f–524f
  microvascular composite tissue transplantation, **I**:533–534
  pectoralis major muscle, **I**:524, 525f
  prelaminated and prefabricated flaps, **I**:530–531
  radial forearm flap, **I**:532f
  reverse-flow flaps, **I**:531, 532f
  reverse transposition flap, **I**:531–533, 533f
  segmental transposition flaps, **I**:522–524, 523f–524f
  sensory flaps, **I**:528
  tibialis anterior muscle flaps, **I**:526f
  tissue expansion, **I**:522
  vascularized bone flaps, **I**:524–525, 526f–528f, 528t
  venous flaps, **I**:533, 534f–535f

flaps (Continued)
flexor digitorum brevis flap, **I**:560–562, 562f
foot reconstruction
  anterolateral thigh flap, **IV**:211
  extensor digitorum brevis muscle flap, **IV**:205–206, 206f
  fasciocutaneous flaps, **IV**:211–214, 215f–216f
  gracilis muscle, **IV**:211
  heel pad flaps, **IV**:209
  intrinsic muscle flaps, **IV**:209, 210f
  lateral arm flap, **IV**:211, 213f
  lateral supramalleolar flap, **IV**:206–207
  medial plantar artery flap, **IV**:209
  microvascular free flap, **IV**:211–216
  midfoot amputations, **IV**:208
  neurovascular island flap, **IV**:207–208
  parascapular flap, **IV**:211, 212f
  pedicle flaps, **IV**:205–217
  radial forearm flap, **IV**:211, 214f
  rectus abdominis, **IV**:211
  rotation flaps, **IV**:205f
  serratus anterior muscles, **IV**:211
  suprafascial flaps, **IV**:208
  sural artery flap, **IV**:209–211
  toe fillet flap, **IV**:207
  transmetatarsal amputation, **IV**:207
  transposition flap, **IV**:201–205, 205f
  V-Y plantar flap, **IV**:207
forehead flaps, **III**:148–155, 149f
free flaps
  mangled upper extremities, **VI**:254–255, 266–275
  microvascular free-flap surgery
    advantages/disadvantages, **I**:608
    background information, **I**:607–611
    buried flaps, **I**:614
    chimeric flaps, **I**:612, 612f
    endoscopic harvests, **I**:611
    flap failure, **I**:614–618
    flap outcomes, **I**:614
    foot reconstruction, **IV**:211–216
    freestyle flaps, **I**:611
    perforator flaps, **I**:611, 612f
    postoperative management, **I**:613–620
    prefabricated/prelaminated flaps, **I**:612–613
    preoperative assessment, **I**:608–611
    thinned flaps, **I**:612, 612f
  perineal reconstruction, **IV**:390
  pressure sores, **IV**:368–369
  tissue expansion, **I**:630
  tongue reconstruction, **III**:309t
free flap viability augmentation
  causal factors, **I**:582–585
  drug therapy
    anticoagulant agents, **I**:582, **VI**:244–245
    antispasmodic agents, **I**:583
    general discussion, **I**:582–583
    thrombolytic agents, **I**:582–583
  ischemia–reperfusion injury
    background information, **I**:583–585
    postischemic conditioning, **I**:584–585
    preischemic conditioning, **I**:583
    remote preischemic conditioning, **I**:583–584, 584f
future trends, **I**:585

flaps (Continued)
gastrocnemius muscle flap, **I**:557–560, 559f–560f, **IV**:142, 142f
glandular correction flaps
  characteristics, **V**:529–531
  glandular flap Type I, **V**:530
  glandular flap Type II, **V**:530
  glandular flap Type III, **V**:530
  glandular flap Type IV, **V**:530–531
gluteus maximus muscle
  breast reconstruction, **V**:292
  characteristics, **I**:516f
  clinical applications, **I**:523f–524f
  perineal reconstruction, **I**:557
  pressure sores, **I**:562–565, 566f–568f
gracilis muscle
  breast reconstruction, **V**:292
  characteristics, **I**:516f
  foot reconstruction, **I**:563f, **IV**:211
  groin reconstruction, **I**:554–557
  lower extremity reconstructive surgery, **IV**:77, 80f, 89f–90f, 140–141, 140f
  male genital reconstructive surgery, **IV**:307–310
  microneurovascular muscle transplantation, **III**:295t
  perineal reconstruction, **I**:554–557, 556f, **IV**:388, 389f
  pressure sores, **I**:562–565, 564f–565f
groin flap, **IV**:143, 143f–144f, **VI**:264–266
hair-bearing flaps, **III**:463
heel pad flaps, **IV**:209
heterodigital flaps
  cross finger flaps, **VI**:130–131, 133f
  dorsal metacarpal artery flaps, **VI**:134, 135f
  Littler neurovascular island flap, **VI**:132–134
  thenar crease flap, **VI**:132, 134f
homodigital flaps, **VI**:130, 132f
inferior gluteal artery perforator (IGAP) flap
  advantages, **V**:459–464
  anatomical characteristics, **V**:461–463
  complications, **V**:464
  patient selection, **V**:460–461
  postoperative care, **V**:464
  surgical technique, **V**:463–464, 464b, 467f–468f
intercostal artery perforator (ICAP) flap, **V**:486f–488f, 487–488
intrinsic muscle flaps, **IV**:209, 210f
ischemic necrosis, **I**:573
island flap, **III**:452
jejunal flap
  pharyngoesophageal reconstruction
    flap harvesting, **III**:349–350, 349f–350f
    flap inset guidelines, **III**:350, 350f
    oral diet, **III**:356t
jumping man flap, **VI**:288f
Juri flap, **III**:123–124, 125f
lateral arm flap
  foot reconstruction, **IV**:211, 213f
  mangled upper extremities, **VI**:267, 269f–272f
  oral cavity and mouth reconstruction, **III**:321
  tongue reconstruction, **III**:309t

Note: **Boldface** roman numerals indicate volume. Page numbers followed by f refer to figures; page numbers followed by t refer to tables; page numbers followed by b refer to boxes.

flaps (Continued)
lateral intercostal artery perforator (LICAP) flap, **V:**487f–488f, 488
lateral supramalleolar flap, **IV:**206–207
lateral thoracodorsal flap (LTDF), **V:**306–308
latissimus dorsi (LD) flap
abdominal wall reconstruction, **I:**553t
back soft-tissue reconstruction, **IV:**262–263, 268f–270f, 272f–273f
breast reconstruction, **V:**288, 289f–290f
characteristics, **I:**516f
chest wall reconstruction, **I:**552–553, **IV:**241, 243f–244f
clinical applications, **I:**528
lower extremity reconstructive surgery, **IV:**77, 78f–79f
mangled upper extremities, **VI:**275, 277f
microneurovascular muscle transplantation, **III:**295t
scalp and forehead reconstruction, **III:**130, 130f
lip reconstruction
Abbé flap, **III:**259–265, 261f–262f
Estlander flap, **III:**259, 263f, 276f
Fujimori gate flaps, **III:**265–268, 266f
Gillies fan flap, **III:**261–262, 264f
Karapandzic flap, **III:**261–262, 264f
lip switch flaps, **III:**259b
radial forearm flap, **III:**267–268, 267f–268f
step flap, **III:**265f
local flaps
burn reconstruction, **IV:**502–503, 503f
cheek reconstruction
anterolateral thigh flap, **III:**274
cheek rotation advancement flap, **III:**271–272, 272f
free tissue transfer, **III:**272
radial forearm flap, **III:**274
scapular and parascapular flaps, **III:**273, 275f
selection guidelines, **III:**271–274
soft tissue cheek reconstruction, **III:**272–273
submental artery flap, **III:**272, 273f–274f
facial reconstruction, **III:**440–460
basic principles, **III:**440–441
cheeks, **III:**450–453
commissure reconstruction, **III:**456
ears, **III:**456–457
eyebrow reconstruction, **III:**441, 444f
eyelids, **III:**449–450
facial burn wound treatment, **IV:**474
lips, **III:**453–456
lower lip, **III:**454–456
nasal reconstruction, **III:**441–449
perforator flaps, **III:**458–459
research summary, **III:**459
rhomboid flap, **III:**441, 442f–443f
scalp and forehead, **III:**123–127, 124f, 126f, 441, 442f–443f
skin expansion, **III:**457–458
skin viscoelasticity, **III:**441t
total lower lip reconstruction, **III:**456
upper lip, **III:**453–454
fingertip reconstruction
local flaps, **VI:**128–134
volar V-Y advancement flap, **VI:**128–130
foot reconstruction, **IV:**201–205, 205f

flaps (Continued)
lower extremity reconstructive surgery, **IV:**68
mangled upper extremities, **VI:**254–255
nasal reconstruction
basic procedure, **III:**441–449
bilobed flap, **III:**143–145, 144f–145f, 446f
dorsal nasal flap, **III:**143, 144f–145f
forehead flaps, **III:**148–155, 149f
interpolated paramedian forehead flap, **III:**445f, 448f
lateral advancement flaps, **III:**445f
one-stage nasolabial flap, **III:**145–146
Rintala dorsal nasal advancement flap, **III:**447f
single-lobe transposition flap, **III:**143, 144f–145f
surgical guidelines, **III:**142–146
three stage full-thickness forehead flap, **III:**151–152, 152f
three stage full-thickness forehead flap (stage 1), **III:**152–153, 153f–159f
three stage full-thickness forehead flap (stage 2), **III:**153–155
three stage full-thickness forehead flap (stage 3), **III:**155, 155t
transoperative flap, **III:**447f
two-stage forehead flap, **III:**148, 150f–151f
two-stage forehead flap (stage 1), **III:**148–151
two-stage forehead flap (stage 2), **III:**151, 151t
two-stage nasolabial flap, **III:**146–148, 146f–147f
two-stage nasolabial flap (stage 1), **III:**146
two-stage nasolabial flap (stage 2), **III:**146–148
V-Y advancement flap, **III:**446f
oral cavity and mouth reconstruction, **III:**309t, 311
scalp and forehead reconstruction, **III:**123–127, 124f, 126f, 441, 442f–443f
lower extremity reconstructive surgery
anterolateral thigh flap, **IV:**68–69, 69f, 75, 75f–76f, 81f, 88f
compound flaps, **IV:**148, 148f
fasciocutaneous/perforator flap
anterolateral thigh perforator flap, **IV:**145, 145f–146f
characteristics, **IV:**143–147
groin/superficial circumflex iliac perforator flap, **IV:**143, 143f–144f
lateral thigh/profunda femoris perforator flap, **IV:**144–145, 144f
lower extremity reconstructive surgery, **IV:**81, 81f–82f
medial thigh septocutaneous flap, **IV:**143–144, 144f
sural flap, **IV:**146, 146f
thoracodorsal artery perforator, **IV:**147, 147f
gracilis muscle, **IV:**77, 80f, 89f–90f
latissimus dorsi (LD) flap, **IV:**77, 78f–79f
local flaps, **IV:**68
muscle/musculocutaneous flaps
biceps femoris muscle flap, **IV:**139–140
characteristics, **I:**557–560

flaps (Continued)
gastrocnemius muscle flap, **I:**557–560, 559f–560f, **IV:**142, 142f
gracilis muscle flap, **IV:**140–141, 140f
rectus femoris muscle flap, **IV:**139, 139f
soleus muscle flap, **I:**557–560, 561f, **IV:**141–142, 141f
tensor fascia lata, **IV:**138–139, 138f
trauma injuries, **IV:**72–75, 74f
perforator flaps
Achilles tendon exposure, **IV:**73f
anterior tibial artery pedicle perforator flap, **IV:**71f
basic procedure, **IV:**68–72
computed tomography angiography, **IV:**69f–70f, 73f
flap locations, **IV:**72f
pedicle perforator flap, **IV:**70f
peroneal artery perforator flaps, **IV:**73f
posterior tibial artery (PTA) flaps, **IV:**73f
rectus abdominis, **IV:**77, 79f
rectus femoris muscle flap, **IV:**82f
sarcoma-related reconstruction, **IV:**110–111
serratus anterior muscles, **IV:**77
supermicrosurgery technique, **IV:**149, 149f
sural artery flap, **IV:**75, 77f
thoracodorsal artery perforator (TDAP) flap, **IV:**77, 147, 147f
lumbar artery perforator (LAP) flap, **V:**467–470, 470b, 470f
male genital reconstructive surgery, **IV:**304–310, 306f, 311f
mangled upper extremities
anterolateral thigh flap, **VI:**274–275, 275f–276f
cutaneous versus muscle flaps, **VI:**263–279
fasciocutaneous flaps, **VI:**254–255, 266–275
free flaps, **VI:**254–255, 266–275
lateral arm flap, **VI:**267, 269f–272f
latissimus dorsi (LD) flap, **VI:**275, 277f
local flaps, **VI:**254–255
muscle/musculocutaneous flaps, **VI:**254–255, 275–279
pedicled groin flap, **VI:**264–266, 265f–266f
radial forearm flap, **VI:**266–267, 267f–269f
rectus abdominis, **VI:**275–277, 278f
scapular and parascapular flaps, **VI:**272, 273f
serratus anterior muscles, **VI:**277–279
temporoparietal fascia flaps, **VI:**272–274, 274f
medial plantar artery flap, **IV:**209
medial sural artery perforator (MSAP) flap, **III:**309t, 322
microvascular free flap, **III:**786, 786f–787f, **IV:**211–216
muscle/musculocutaneous flaps
advantages/disadvantages, **I:**538–539
burn reconstruction, **IV:**503
clinical application
background information, **I:**521–534
circumflex scapular and thoracodorsal pedicles, **I:**530f
combination flaps, **I:**528–530, 530f

flaps (Continued)
    deep circumflex iliac artery composite flap, **I**:529f
    distally based flaps, **I**:531, 531t
    functional muscle flaps, **I**:528
    gluteus maximus muscle, **I**:523f–524f
    microvascular composite tissue transplantation, **I**:533–534
    pectoralis major muscle, **I**:524, 525f
    prelaminated and prefabricated flaps, **I**:530–531
    radial forearm flap, **I**:532f
    reverse-flow flaps, **I**:531, 532f
    reverse transposition flap, **I**:531–533, 533f
    segmental transposition flaps, **I**:522–524, 523f–524f
    sensory flaps, **I**:528
    tibialis anterior muscle flaps, **I**:526f
    tissue expansion, **I**:522
    vascularized bone flaps, **I**:524–525, 526f–528f, 528t
    venous flaps, **I**:533, 534f–535f
  complications, **I**:571–572
  flap monitoring techniques, **I**:570
  lower extremity reconstructive surgery
    biceps femoris muscle flap, **IV**:139–140
    gastrocnemius muscle flap, **IV**:142, 142f
    gracilis muscle flap, **IV**:140–141, 140f
    rectus femoris muscle flap, **IV**:139, 139f
    soleus muscle flap, **IV**:141–142, 141f
    tensor fascia lata, **IV**:138–139, 138f
    trauma injuries, **IV**:72–75, 74f
  male genital reconstructive surgery, **IV**:307–310
  mangled upper extremities, **VI**:254–255, 275–279
  Mathes–Nahai Classification, **I**:516–517, 516f
  oral cavity and mouth reconstruction, **III**:319–322
  patient positioning, **I**:569–570
  preoperative and postoperative management, **I**:565–570
  pressure sores, **IV**:368
  regional applications
    abdominal wall, **I**:553–554, 553f, 553t, 555f
    breast reconstruction, **I**:546–549, 548f–549f
    chest wall reconstruction, **I**:552–553
    complications, **I**:571–572
    feet, **I**:560–562, 562f–563f
    flap monitoring techniques, **I**:570
    groin, **I**:554–557, 558f
    head and neck reconstruction, **I**:542–546, 543f–546f
    lower extremity reconstructive surgery, **I**:557–560, 559f–561f
    mediastinum, **I**:549–552, 550f–551f
    patient positioning, **I**:569–570
    perineal reconstruction, **I**:554–557, 556f–557f
    preoperative and postoperative management, **I**:565–570
    pressure sores, **I**:562–565, 564f–568f
    pulmonary cavity, **I**:552–553
  selection guidelines, **I**:541–542

flaps (Continued)
    spina bifida, **III**:867–872, 868t–869t
    Type I muscles (one vascular pedicle), **I**:516, 517t
    Type II muscles (dominant vascular pedicle and minor pedicle), **I**:516, 517t
    Type III muscles (two dominant pedicles), **I**:516–517, 517t
    Type IV muscles (segmental vascular pedicles), **I**:517, 517t
    Type V muscles (one dominant vascular pedicle and secondary segmental vascular pedicles), **I**:517, 517t
    vascular anatomical research, **I**:504–505
  Mustarde osteomuscular flaps, **III**:867–869, 872f
  myocutaneous flaps
    back soft-tissue reconstruction, **IV**:262–263, 268f–270f, 272f–273f
    burn reconstruction, **I**:630, **IV**:449–450
  myocutaneous gluteal rotation flap
    basic procedure, **IV**:370–375, 371f
    girdlestone arthroplasty, **IV**:376f
    ischial pressure sores, **IV**:372–373, 372t
    surgical guidelines, **IV**:372b
    trochanteric ulcers, **IV**:373–375, 375t, 376f
    V-Y hamstring advancement, **I**:562–565, 566f, 568f, **IV**:373, 374f
    V-Y tensor fasciae latae flap, **IV**:375, 377f
  nasolabial flaps, **III**:309t
  neurovascular island flap, **IV**:207–208
  nipple-areola complex reconstruction
    flap designs adjacent to scars
      double-opposing tab flap, **V**:511t, 512–513, 512f–513f
      general discussion, **V**:511–513
      S-flap, **V**:511–512, 511f, 511t
      spiral flap, **V**:513, 513f
    flaps with allograft augmentation, **V**:515–516, 516f
    flaps with alloplastic augmentation, **V**:515
    flaps with autologous graft augmentation
      cartilage grafts, **V**:514, 514f
      fat grafts, **V**:514–515, 514f
    flap techniques, **V**:501t
    pull-out/purse-string flap techniques
      bell flap, **V**:508, 508f, 508t
      double opposing peri-areolar/ purse-string flap, **V**:508–510, 508t, 509f–510f
      general discussion, **V**:507–510
      top-hat flap, **V**:510, 510f
    traditional flaps
      arrow flap, **V**:503t, 507, 507f
      C–V flap, **V**:503t, 506–507, 506f, 514–515
      general discussion, **V**:502–507
      skate flap, **V**:502–504, 503f–505f, 503t
      star flap, **V**:503t, 504–506, 505f
  nose reconstruction
    local flaps
      bilobed flap, **III**:143–145, 144f–145f, 446f
      dorsal nasal flap, **III**:143, 144f–145f
      forehead flaps, **III**:148–155, 149f
      one-stage nasolabial flap, **III**:145–146
      single-lobe transposition flap, **III**:143, 144f–145f

flaps (Continued)
      surgical guidelines, **III**:142–146
      three stage full-thickness forehead flap, **III**:151–152, 152f
      three stage full-thickness forehead flap (stage 1), **III**:152–153, 153f–159f
      three stage full-thickness forehead flap (stage 2), **III**:153–155
      three stage full-thickness forehead flap (stage 3), **III**:155, 155t
      two-stage forehead flap, **III**:148, 150f–151f
      two-stage forehead flap (stage 1), **III**:148–151
      two-stage forehead flap (stage 2), **III**:151, 151t
      two-stage nasolabial flap, **III**:146–148, 146f–147f
      two-stage nasolabial flap (stage 1), **III**:146
      two-stage nasolabial flap (stage 2), **III**:146–148
  oblique rectus abdominis myocutaneous (ORAM) flap, **IV**:387f
  omentum reconstruction
    breast reconstruction, **V**:472–481
    basic principles, **V**:472–473
    complications, **V**:480–481
    patient selection, **V**:473
    postoperative care and follow-up, **V**:480
    prognosis and outcomes, **V**:480–481
    secondary procedures, **V**:481
    skin preservation, **V**:472
    surgical technique and treatment, **V**:473–480, 473f–474f
  chest wall reconstruction, **I**:553, **IV**:245, 246f–247f
  one-stage nasolabial flap, **III**:145–146
  Orticochea three-flap technique, **III**:124f
  osteocutaneous flaps, **III**:317t
  palatal fistula repair, **III**:642–644, 645f
  parascapular flap, **IV**:211, 212f
  paraspinal flaps, **III**:872–874, 873f–875f
  pectoralis major muscle, **III**:274f, 309t, **IV**:241, 241f–242f
  pectoralis major myocutaneous flaps, **III**:319, 320f
  pectoralis major osteomusculocutaneous flap, **III**:322
  pedical flap viability augmentation
  pharmacologic therapy
    angiogenic cytokine proteins, **I**:581–582
    drug therapy, **I**:580–581
    gene therapy, **I**:581–582
    vasoconstriction and thrombosis reduction, **I**:580–581
  surgical delay procedures
    angiogenesis, **I**:580
    arteriovenous (AV) shunt flow reduction, **I**:578–579
    characteristics, **I**:577–578
    choke artery opening, **I**:579–580, 580f
    vascular territory expansion, **I**:579–580, 580f
    vasoconstriction and prothrombotic substance depletion, **I**:579

*Note: **Boldface** roman numerals indicate volume. Page numbers followed by f refer to figures; page numbers followed by t refer to tables; page numbers followed by b refer to boxes.*

flaps (Continued)
  surgical manipulation
    flap design, I:577, 577f
    surgical delay, I:577–578
    transverse rectus abdominis
      myocutaneous (TRAM) flaps, I:578
    vascular delay, I:578
pedicled groin flap, VI:264–266, 265f–266f
pedicled omental flap, IV:267–268
perforator flaps
  advantages/disadvantages, I:539
  back soft-tissue reconstruction, IV:268
  classifications, I:519–521
  facial reconstruction, III:458–459
  lower extremity reconstructive surgery
    Achilles tendon exposure, IV:73f
    anterior tibial artery pedicle perforator
      flap, IV:71f
    anterolateral thigh perforator flap,
      IV:145, 145f–146f
    basic procedure, IV:68–72
    characteristics, IV:143–147
    computed tomography angiography,
      IV:69f–70f, 73f
    flap locations, IV:72f
    groin/superficial circumflex iliac
      perforator flap, IV:143, 143f–144f
    lateral thigh/profunda femoris
      perforator flap, IV:144–145, 144f
    medial thigh septocutaneous flap,
      IV:143–144, 144f
    pedicle perforator flap, IV:70f
    peroneal artery perforator flaps, IV:73f
    posterior tibial artery (PTA) flaps,
      IV:73f
    sural flap, IV:146, 146f
    thoracodorsal artery perforator, IV:147,
      147f
  male genital reconstructive surgery,
    IV:304–306
  microvascular free-flap surgery, I:611,
    612f
  phalloplasty, IV:323
  pressure sores, IV:368
  vascular anatomical research, I:505–507,
    506f–507f
perineal reconstruction
  anterolateral thigh flap, IV:388–389,
    390f–391f
  free flaps, IV:390
  gracilis flaps, IV:388, 389f
  posterior thigh flap, IV:390
  rectus-based reconstruction, IV:386–388,
    387f–388f
  regional skin flaps, IV:385–386, 386f–387f
  Singapore flap, IV:387f, 389–390
pharyngoesophageal reconstruction
  anterolateral thigh flap
    flap design and harvesting, III:339–341,
      340f–342f
    flap inset guidelines, III:342–347,
      343f–348f
    frozen neck, III:352–353
    isolated cervical esophageal defects,
      III:354
    oral diet, III:356t
    postlaryngectomy pharyngocutaneous
      fistulas, III:353–354, 353f–354f
    selection guidelines, III:338–339
  flap debulking, III:358

flaps (Continued)
  jejunal flap
    flap harvesting, III:349–350, 349f–350f
    flap inset guidelines, III:350, 350f
    oral diet, III:356t
  preoperative assessment
    advantages/disadvantages, III:339t
    selection guidelines, III:338–339, 339f
  radial forearm flap
    flap design, III:347, 348f
    flap harvesting, III:347–349, 348f–349f
    oral diet, III:356t
  surgical technique and treatment
    anterolateral thigh flap, III:339–347
    jejunal flap, III:349–350
    radial forearm flap, III:347–349
    recipient vessel selection, III:351–352,
      351f–352f, 351t
    transverse cervical vessels, III:351–352,
      351f–352f
  posterior pharyngeal flap, III:625–626, 626f
  posterior thigh flap, IV:390
  prefabricated/prelaminated flaps, I:612–613
  pressure sores
    free flaps, IV:368–369
    gluteus maximus muscle, I:562–565,
      566f–568f
    gracilis muscle, I:562–565, 564f–565f
    muscle flaps, IV:368
    musculocutaneous flaps, I:562–565, IV:368
    myocutaneous gluteal rotation flap
      basic procedure, IV:370–375, 371f
      girdlestone arthroplasty, IV:376f
      ischial pressure sores, IV:372–373, 372t
      surgical guidelines, IV:372b
      trochanteric ulcers, IV:373–375, 375t,
        376f
      V-Y hamstring advancement, I:562–565,
        566f, 568f, IV:373, 374f
      V-Y tensor fasciae latae flap, IV:375,
        377f
    perforator flaps, IV:368
    superior gluteal artery perforator (SGAP)
      flap, I:562–565
    tensor fascia latae (TFL), I:562–565
  radial forearm flap
    burn wound treatment, IV:421f
    cheek reconstruction, III:274
    clinical application, I:532f
    foot reconstruction, IV:211, 214f
    lip reconstruction, III:267–268, 267f–268f
    mangled upper extremities, VI:266–267,
      267f–269f
    oral cavity and mouth reconstruction,
      III:311f, 319–320
    palatal fistula repair, III:644
    phalloplasty
      aesthetic phallus, IV:319, 320f
      donor site considerations, IV:321, 321f
      exstrophy and epispadias, IV:303f
      general discussion, IV:318–323
      minimal morbidity, IV:321
      normal scrotum, IV:321, 322f
      one-stage procedure, IV:319
      operative technique, IV:318, 319f–320f,
        324f–325f
      research summary, IV:322–323
      severe penile insufficiency, IV:304–306
      sexual intercourse, IV:321–322, 322f
      surgical goals, IV:318–322

flaps (Continued)
      tactile and erogenous sensation,
        IV:319–321
      voiding while standing, IV:321
    pharyngoesophageal reconstruction
      flap design, III:347, 348f
      flap harvesting, III:347–349, 348f–349f
      oral diet, III:356t
    scalp and forehead reconstruction,
      III:128–130, 129f
    tongue reconstruction, III:309t–310t
  reconstructive ladder analogy, I:534–541,
    536f
  reconstructive triangle, I:536, 536f
  rectus abdominis
    abdominal wall reconstruction, I:553t
    chest wall reconstruction, I:552–553,
      IV:244–245, 245f
    foot reconstruction, IV:211
    groin reconstruction, I:554–557, 558f
    lower extremity reconstructive surgery,
      IV:77, 79f
    male genital reconstructive surgery,
      IV:307–310
    mangled upper extremities, VI:275–277,
      278f
    microneurovascular muscle
      transplantation, III:295t
    oral cavity and mouth reconstruction,
      III:321, 321f
    perineal reconstruction, I:554–557, 557f
    tongue reconstruction, III:309t–310t
  rectus femoris muscle flap
    abdominal wall reconstruction, I:553t,
      554, 555f
    groin reconstruction, I:554–557
    lower extremity reconstructive surgery,
      IV:82f, 139, 139f
    male genital reconstructive surgery,
      IV:307–310
    microneurovascular muscle
      transplantation, III:295t
    perineal reconstruction, I:554–557
  research summary, I:585
  rotation flaps
    burn reconstruction, IV:448–449,
      453f–454f
    cheek reconstruction, III:451, 451f–452f
    classifications, I:513f
    foot reconstruction, IV:205, 205f
  sartorius muscle, I:516f, 554–557
  scalp and forehead reconstruction
    blood supply, III:128f
    cervical facial advancement flap, III:125,
      127f
    Juri flap, III:123–124, 125f
    latissimus dorsi (LD) flap, III:130, 130f
    local flaps, III:123–127, 126f
    microsurgical reconstruction, III:128–130
    Orticochea three-flap technique, III:124f
    pericranial flaps, III:125, 127f–128f
    radial forearm flap, III:128–130, 129f
    regional flaps, III:127–128, 129f
    scalp reduction techniques, III:124, 125f
    vertical trapezius flap, III:127–128, 129f
  scapular and parascapular flaps
    hemifacial atrophy, III:799–800, 800f
    mangled upper extremities, VI:272, 273f
  scapular osteomusculocutaneous flap,
    III:323, 323f

flaps (Continued)
  secondary facial reconstruction
    case study 1
      diagnosis, III:465
      patient description, III:464b–466b,
        464f–465f
      reconstructive plan, III:465–466
    case study 2
      diagnosis, III:466
      patient description, III:466b–467b,
        466f–467f
      reconstructive plan, III:467
    case study 3
      diagnosis, III:467
      patient description, III:467b–469b,
        468f
      reconstructive plan, III:467–469
    case study 4
      diagnosis, III:469
      patient description, III:469b–471b,
        469f–470f
      reconstructive plan, III:469–471
    flap prelamination, III:464–471
    hair-bearing flaps, III:463
    intraoral and intranasal lining, III:462–
      463, 463f
    planning guidelines, III:462–471
    prefabricated flaps, III:463
  segmental transposition flaps, I:522–524,
    523f–524f
  serratus anterior artery perforator (SAAP)
    flap, V:486f–488f, 488–489
  serratus anterior muscles
    chest wall reconstruction, I:552, IV:244,
      244f
    foot reconstruction, IV:211
    lower extremity reconstructive surgery,
      IV:77
    mangled upper extremities, VI:277–279
    microneurovascular muscle
      transplantation, III:295t
  S-flap, V:511–512, 511f, 511t
  Singapore flap, IV:387f, 389–390
  single-lobe transposition flap, III:143,
    144f–145f
  skate flap, V:502–504, 503f–505f, 503t
  soft tissue flaps, IV:270
  soleus muscle flap, I:557–560, 561f,
    IV:141–142, 141f
  spiral flap, V:513, 513f
  standard delay flap, I:514, 514f
  star flap, V:503t, 504–506, 505f
  submental artery flap, III:272, 273f–274f,
    309t
  superior epigastric artery perforator (SEAP)
    flap, V:308, 486f, 489
  superior gluteal artery flap, IV:264–265,
    277f
  superior gluteal artery perforator (SGAP)
    flap
    advantages, V:459–464
    anatomical characteristics, V:461–463
    complications, V:464
    imaging methods, V:327
    patient selection, V:460–461
    postoperative care, V:464
    pressure sores, I:562–565
    radiological protocol, V:330f, 333f–334f

flaps (Continued)
  spina bifida, III:867–872, 871f
  surgical technique, V:463–464, 464b,
    465f–467f
  suprafascial flaps, IV:208
  sural artery flap, IV:75, 77f, 209–211
  temporalis osteomuscular flap, III:322
  temporoparietal fascia flaps
    mangled upper extremities, VI:272–274,
      274f
    palatal fistula repair, III:643
  tensor fascia latae (TFL)
    abdominal wall reconstruction, I:553t, 554
    characteristics, I:516f
    groin reconstruction, I:554–557
    lower extremity reconstructive surgery,
      IV:138–139, 138f
    perineal reconstruction, I:554–557
    pressure sores, I:562–565, IV:375, 377f
    trochanteric ulcers, IV:375t
  thigh flaps, I:557
  thinned flaps, I:612, 612f
  thoracodorsal artery perforator (TDAP) flap
    breast reconstruction, V:308, 486–487,
      486f–488f
    lower extremity reconstructive surgery,
      IV:77, 147, 147f
    oral cavity and mouth reconstruction,
      III:322
    tongue reconstruction, III:309t
  three stage full-thickness forehead flap,
    III:151–152, 152f–153f
  thumb and finger reconstruction
    first-web neurosensory flap harvest,
      VI:305, 306f
    flap inset guidelines, VI:302–303, 302b,
      302f
    great-toe wrap-around flap, VI:304–305
    pulp flap harvest, VI:305, 305f
  tissue expansion
    fascial flaps, I:630
    free flaps, I:630
    myocutaneous flaps, I:630
  toe fillet flap, IV:207
  top-hat flap, V:510, 510f
  transposition flap, III:143, 452, IV:203, 205f
  transverse rectus abdominis myocutaneous
    (TRAM) flaps
    autogenous breast reconstruction,
      V:457–458
    bilateral pedicle TRAM flap, V:393–410
      background and general characteristics,
        V:393–394
      circulatory zones, V:395f
      external and internal oblique
        components, V:404f
      fascial and muscle strips, V:400f, 403f
      fascial closure, V:405f
      inferomedial dissection, V:402f
      lateral muscle dissection, V:401f
      markings, V:397f, 400f
      medial dissection, V:402f
      medial suprafascial dissection, V:399f
      muscle and fascial pedicle control,
        V:402f
      outcomes and complicatons, V:407–410
      patient selection, V:395–396
      pedicle arrangement, V:403f–404f

flaps (Continued)
    pedicle length, V:403f
    postoperative care and follow-up,
      V:406
    preoperative assessment, V:396
    Prolene mesh, V:405f
    secondary procedures, V:410
    shaping guidelines, V:405–406,
      406f–409f
    surgical procedures, V:396–405,
      397b–399b
    tunnel positions, V:398f
    vascular anatomy, V:394–395, 394f
  breast reconstruction, I:546–549, 548f–
    549f, V:288f
  free TRAM flap, V:411–434
    abdominal closure, V:426–428, 429f
    anatomical and physiological
      considerations, V:412
    complications, V:430, 431f
    delayed versus immediate
      reconstruction, V:414
    flap dissection, V:419–422, 420f–421f,
      423f
    flap inset guidelines, V:426, 427f–428f
    general discussion, V:411
    mastectomy planning, V:419, 419f
    nipple-areola complex reconstruction,
      V:430–432, 432f–433f
    patient presentation and diagnosis,
      V:414–416
    patient selection, V:416–418
    pedicled versus free TRAM, V:414–415
    postoperative care and follow-up,
      V:428–429
    procedure selection, V:417–418
    radiation therapy (RT), V:415–416
    recipient vessels, V:422–426, 424f–425f
    research summary, V:432
    risk factors, V:416–417
    surgical technique and treatment,
      V:418–428
    timing considerations, V:414
  patient selection, V:374–376
  perineal reconstruction, IV:387f
  surgical manipulation, I:578
  transverse upper gracilis free flap (TUG)
    anatomical characteristics, V:458–459,
      460f
    complications, V:459
    patient selection, V:458
    postoperative image, V:460f
    surgical technique and treatment, V:459,
      459b, 461f–462f
  trapezius muscle flap, III:127–128, 129f,
    IV:263–264, 274f–276f
  trapezius osteomusculocutaneous flap,
    III:322
  tuberous breast deformity
    glandular correction flaps
      characteristics, V:529–531
      glandular flap Type I, V:530
      glandular flap Type II, V:530
      glandular flap Type III, V:530
      glandular flap Type IV, V:530–531
  two-stage forehead flap, III:148, 150f–151f
  two-stage nasolabial flap, III:146–148,
    146f–147f

flaps (Continued)
    ulnar forearm flap, III:309t–310t, 312f,
        320–321
    vascular anatomical research
        anatomic concepts, I:492–500, 492b
        arterial radiation, I:494–495
        composite flaps, I:508
        connective tissue framework, I:493–494
        cutaneous perforators, I:496–497, 496f
        deep veins, I:499–500
        delay phenomenon, I:507–508, 507f–508f
        fasciocutaneous flaps, I:504
        law of equilibrium, I:498
        musculocutaneous flaps, I:504–505
        nerve–blood vessel relationship,
            I:495–496
        network interconnections
            arteries, I:497, 497f
            veins, I:497–498, 498f
        perforator flaps, I:505–507, 506f–507f
        preoperative assessment, I:500
        research summary, I:508
        skin flap axes
            characteristics, I:501–502
            distally based skin flaps, I:501–502,
                503f
            schematic diagram, I:503f
        skin flap dimensions, I:502–504
        superficial veins, I:499–500, 500f
        vein–muscle connection, I:499
        venous convergence, I:494–495
        venous networks
            directional veins, I:498f, 499
            general discussion, I:499
            oscillating avalvular veins, I:498f, 499
        vessel growth and orientation–tissue
            growth and differentiation
            relationship, I:496–497, 496f
        vessel origin and destination, I:499
    vascularized bone flaps
        advantages, I:455–459
        vacularized calvarium, I:457–459, 458f
        vacularized fibula, I:455, 457f
        vascularized iliac transfer, I:455, 456f
        vascularized rib, I:456–457
        vascularized scapula, I:455–456, 458f
    venous flaps, I:533, 534f–535f
    vertical trapezius flap, III:127–128, 129f
    visor flaps, VI:130, 131f
    Vomer flaps, III:578
    V-Y and Y-V advancement flaps
        fingertip reconstruction
            lateral V-Y advancement flaps, VI:130,
                130f
            volar V-Y advancement flap, VI:128–
                130, 129f
        foot reconstruction, IV:207
        ischial pressure sores, I:562–565, 566f,
            568f, IV:372–373, 374f
        pressure sores, IV:369–370
        reconstructive burn surgery, IV:502–503,
            503f
        scar revision, I:316, 316f
        spina bifida, III:867–872, 868t–869t,
            870f–871f, 875f
    V-Y plantar flap, IV:207
    V-Y plantar flap, IV:207
flash and flame burns, IV:394
flash freezing, IV:456–460
flavonoids, II:25

Fleming, Alexander, VI:xliii–xliv, 333
fleur-de-lis type abdominoplasty
    abdominal contouring, II:640–643, 640f–641f
    characteristics, II:548–549
    indicators, II:549
    markings, II:549–550, 550f
    operative technique, II:550
    outcome assessments, II:550–551, 551f
    patient selection, II:549
    postoperative care and follow-up, II:550
    preoperative procedures, II:550
FlexHD, V:69, 70t
flexor carpi radialis (FCR) muscle, VI:179–182
flexor carpi radialis transfer, VI:748t, 749–750,
    752f
flexor carpi ulnaris (FCU) muscle, VI:179–182
flexor digitorum brevis flap, I:560–562, 562f
flexor digitorum longus (FDL), IV:35f–36f
flexor digitorum profundus (FDP) muscle
    flexor tendon injuries, VI:179–182, 181f
    fractures and joint injuries, VI:138–139
    hand anatomy, VI:32b, 51
    tendon graft and repair, VI:233
flexor digitorum superficialis (FDS) muscle
    flexor tendon injuries, VI:179–182, 185f
    hand anatomy, VI:32b, 51, 181f
    leg anatomy, IV:35f–36f
    thumb hypoplasia, VI:588–590
flexor hallucis longus (FHL), IV:35f–36f
flexor pollicis brevis (FPB) muscle, VI:212
flexor pollicis longus (FPL) muscle
    flexor tendon injuries, VI:179–182, 196
    hand anatomy, VI:51
    tetraplegic restoration
        Brand–Moberg modification, VI:827–830,
            828f–829f
        key pinch restoration, VI:826–827, 827f,
            831f
        tenodesis, VI:827–830, 828f–829f
        wrist extension, VI:825f
flexor pulleys, VI:29–32, 29f–30f, 179–182,
    180f–181f
flexor retinaculum, IV:52–54, 52t, 54f
flexor sublimis test, VI:51, 53
flexor tendon injuries, VI:178–209
    anatomical considerations
        annular pulleys/cruciate pulleys, VI:180f
        flexor pulleys, VI:180f–181f
        general characteristics, VI:179–182
        tendon zones, VI:31–32, 31f, 181f
        vincula, VI:181f
    basic procedure, VI:402, 403f
    biomechanics
        gliding motions, VI:184
        linear versus bending forces, VI:183, 184f
        surgical repair strength, VI:182–184, 183f
        tendon–suture junctions, VI:182–184, 183f
    challenges, VI:178–179
    flexor tendon healing, VI:182
    mutilated/mangled hands, VI:253
    outcomes and complicatons, VI:199–201,
        201b, 201t, 402
    patient presentation and diagnosis,
        VI:184–185, 185f
    postoperative care and follow-up
        basic principles, VI:402
        care protocols, VI:197–199
        combined passive–active tendon motion
            protocol (Nantong regime), VI:199,
            200f, 202f

flexor tendon injuries (Continued)
        Duran–Houser method, VI:198–199, 198f
        early active motion, VI:199
        modified Kleinert method, VI:197–198,
            198f
    secondary procedures
        free tendon grafting
            donor tendons, VI:202f
            indications and contraindications,
                VI:201–202, 202b
            operative technique, VI:203–204,
                203f–205f
        general discussion, VI:201–208
        staged tendon reconstruction
            indications, VI:204
            operative technique (first stage),
                VI:204–206, 205f–207f
            operative technique (second stage),
                VI:206, 208f
        tenolysis
            anesthesia, VI:207
            indications, VI:206–207
            operative technique, VI:207–208, 208b
            postoperative treatment, VI:208
    surgical technique and treatment
        flexor pollicis longus (FPL) injuries,
            VI:196, 196f–197f
        indications and contraindications, VI:186,
            186b
        operative technique
            closed ruptures, VI:197
            flexor pollicis longus (FPL) injuries,
                VI:196, 196f–197f
            incisions, VI:187f
            partial tendon lacerations, VI:197
            pediatric injuries, VI:196–197
            surgical preparation, VI:186–197
            zone 1 injuries, VI:186–187, 188f
            zone 2 injuries, VI:187–194
            zone 3 injuries, VI:196
            zone 4 injuries, VI:196
            zone 5 injuries, VI:196
        primary and delayed primary repairs,
            VI:185–186, 186f
        surgical tips, VI:179b
        zone 1 injuries, VI:186–187, 188f
        zone 2 injuries
            A2 pulley, VI:194f
            A4 pulley, VI:193f
            core suture methods, VI:189f, 193f
            cruciate method, VI:189f
            extension ability, VI:192f, 194f
            flexion ability, VI:191f, 194f
            four-strand repair, VI:191f–192f
            modified Kessler method, VI:189f
            operative technique, VI:187–194, 190f
            peripheral sutures, VI:192f
            pulley–sheath complex, VI:195f
            ruptured primary repair, VI:193f
            simple running peripheral repair,
                VI:191f
            six-strand M-Tang tendon repair,
                VI:190f–191f, 194f
            surgical summary, VI:195t
            surgical tips, VI:190b
        zone 3 injuries, VI:196
        zone 4 injuries, VI:196
        zone 5 injuries, VI:196
flexor tenosynovitis, VI:339, 340f
floating digits, VI:546t

floor of mouth
  anatomical characteristics, **III:**422f
  cancer management
    diagnosis and treatment, **III:**427
    preoperative assessment, **III:**406
    surgical technique and treatment, **III:**406
fluidized beds, **IV:**364–366, 364f
Flumazenil, **I:**145
fluorescence-activated cell sorting (FACS), **I:**219f–220f, 389–390
fluorescent lights, **I:**107
fluorine (F) *See* hydrofluoric acid
fluoxetine, **I:**51
fluvoxamine, **I:**51
foams, **I:**289t
Fodor's Formula, **II:**516t
Fogarty catheter, **I:**842
Food and Drug Administration (FDA), **I:**847–849
forearm
  arterial system, **VI:**468–469
  burn reconstruction, **IV:**437f
  congenital transverse arrest, **VI:**550–551
  cross-section diagram, **VI:**268f
  functional role, **VI:**60–61
  melanoma excisions, **I:**766–768, 770f
  physical examination
    interosseous membrane
      distal membranous portion, **VI:**60, 60f
      middle ligamentous portion, **VI:**60, 60f
      proximal membranous portion, **VI:**60, 60f
    muscle strength measurement
      pronation, **VI:**61
      supination, **VI:**61
    rotation measurement, **VI:**61
  posterior interosseous nerve (PIN) compression
    anatomical considerations, **VI:**517
    posterior interosseous nerve (PIN) syndrome, **VI:**517
    radial tunnel syndrome
      nonsurgical management, **VI:**518
      outcomes and complicatons, **VI:**518
      patient presentation and diagnosis, **VI:**518
      surgical technique and treatment, **VI:**518, 519f
  pronators and supinators, **VI:**18–22, 21f
  replantation and revascularization surgery, **VI:**238–241, 239f–240f
  sequelae obstetric brachial plexus palsy, **VI:**815
  skeletal reconstruction, **IV:**181–183, 182f
  soft-tissue reconstruction, **VI:**262–263, 263f–264f
  spastic hand surgery, **VI:**460
  vascular anatomical research
    venous drainage channels, **VI:**39f
forehead
  aesthetic units, **III:**108–109, 109f
  aging process, **II:**88
  anatomical characteristics
    galea, **II:**94–95, 95f
    general characteristics, **III:**105–106
    medial zygomaticotemporal vein, **II:**94, 94f
    motor nerves, **II:**97–98, 97f

forehead *(Continued)*
    muscles
      characteristics, **II:**95–96
      frontalis, **II:**96f, 110–111, 110f–111f
      glabellar frown muscles, **II:**95f
      lateral orbicularis, **II:**96f
      orbital ligament, **II:**94f
      procerus, **II:**110–111, 110f
      sensory nerves, **II:**96–97, 96f–97f
      temporal fascia, **II:**94f
      temporal fossa, **II:**93–98, 94f
      temporal septum, **II:**94f
  anesthesia, **III:**26, 27f
  anthropometric analysis, **II:**356–358, 357f–358f
  Asian rhinoplasty, **II:**174f, 177
  congenital melanocytic nevi (CMN), **III:**844, 846f
  disorders
    basal cell carcinoma, **III:**117–118, 118f
    burns, **III:**119–120, 120f
    cicatricial alopecia, **III:**109–110, 111t
    cutaneous sarcoidosis, **III:**115–116, 116f
    discoid lupus erythematosus (DLE), **III:**115, 115f
    dysplastic nevus, **III:**113–114, 114f
    en coup de sabre (ECDS), **III:**114–115, 115f
    epidermoid cyst, **III:**116–117, 116f
    giant hair nevus/congenital nevomelanocytic nevus (CNN), **III:**112–113, 114f
    infections, **III:**119
    lipoma, **III:**116
    malignant melanomas, **III:**119, 119f
    neoplasms, **III:**116
    nevoid basal cell carcinoma syndrome (NBCCS), **III:**112, 112t, 113f
    nevus sebaceous of Jadassohn, **III:**111–112, 112f
    physical trauma, **III:**119–120
    squamous cell carcinomas (SCCs), **III:**118–119, 118f
    syringoma, **III:**117, 117f
    trichoepithelioma, **III:**117, 117f
    xeroderma pigmentosum (XP), **III:**112, 114f
  forehead lines
    botulinum toxin type-A (BoNT-A), **II:**33–34
    soft-tissue fillers, **II:**51, 52f
    subperiosteal facelift, **II:**268–270, 269f
  forehead rejuvenation, **II:**93–107
    aesthetic alterations, **II:**93
    complications, **II:**105–106, 105f–106f
    MACS (minimal access cranial suspension) lift, **II:**226
    patient presentation and diagnosis
      aesthetics, **II:**98f–100f, 99–100
      forehead aging, **II:**98–99, 98f–99f
    patient selection, **II:**100, 226
    postoperative care and follow-up, **II:**105
    prognosis and outcomes, **II:**105–106
    secondary procedures, **II:**106, 106f
    surgical technique
      anterior hairline approach, **II:**101–102, 102f
      direct suprabrow approach, **II:**104

forehead *(Continued)*
      endoscopic approach, **II:**102–103, 103f
      general discussion, **II:**100–105
      lateral brow approach, **II:**103–104, 104f
      open coronal approach, **II:**100–101, 101f
      suture suspension browplexy, **II:**105
      temple approach, **II:**103, 103f
      transpalpebral approach, **II:**103, 104f
      transpalpebral browplexy, **II:**104–105
    un-rejuvenated forehead, **II:**305–306, 306f
  forehead rhinoplasty
    forehead flaps, **III:**148–155
    full-thickness forehead skin graft, **III:**141, 142f
  nerves, **III:**107–108
  optimal brow positioning, **II:**122, 123f
  reconstructive surgeries, **III:**105–133
    anatomical considerations, **III:**105–106
    burn wound treatment, **IV:**485, 498–499
    complications, **III:**131–132
    nerves, **III:**107–108
    patient presentation and diagnosis, **III:**120
    patient selection, **III:**120–121, 121t
    postoperative care and follow-up, **III:**131
    secondary procedures, **III:**132
    surgical technique and treatment
      blood supply, **III:**128f
      cervical facial advancement flap, **III:**125, 127f
      closure by secondary intention, **III:**121
      facial transplantation, **III:**131
      Juri flap, **III:**123–124, 125f
      latissimus dorsi (LD) flap, **III:**130, 130f
      local flaps, **III:**123–127, 124f, 126f, 441
      microsurgical reconstruction, **III:**128–130, 129f
      Orticochea three-flap technique, **III:**124f
      pericranial flaps, **III:**125, 127f–128f
      primary closure, **III:**121
      radial forearm flap, **III:**128–130, 129f
      regional flaps, **III:**127–128, 129f
      rhomboid flap, **III:**441, 442f–443f
      scalp reduction techniques, **III:**124, 125f
      skin grafts, **III:**123, 123f
      tissue expansion, **III:**121–123, 122f
      vacuum-assisted closure (VAC), **III:**121, 122f
      vertical trapezius flap, **III:**127–128, 129f
    trauma-acquired defects, **III:**105
  tissue expansion, **I:**635
forehead flaps, **III:**148–155, 149f
foreign-body reactions, **I:**306, 375
Formacryl, **II:**48t
  See also soft-tissue fillers
formic acid, **IV:**461–463
for-profit corporations, **I:**85
four-flap Z-plasty
  hypoplastic thumb, **VI:**585f, 586–587
  thumb middle-third amputations, **VI:**287–291, 288f
Fournier disease, **IV:**312–313, 313f
fourth branchial cleft anomaly, **III:**887
FOXE1 (Forkhead box protein E1) mutation, **III:**510–511
fractional lasers, **IV:**454, 454t

Note: **Boldface** *roman numerals indicate volume. Page numbers followed by f refer to figures; page numbers followed by t refer to tables; page numbers followed by b refer to boxes.*

fractional photothermolysis, II:61, 61f, 65, 65f, 70–74, 71t
fracture fixation, VI:106–116
  Arbeitsgemeinschaft für Osteosynthesefragen (AO) principles, VI:106, 107t
  challenges, VI:106
  fixation options
    absolute versus relative stability, VI:108, 108b, 108f
    bridge plating, VI:113, 115f
    compression plating, VI:112–113, 114f
    external fixation, VI:110, 111f
    interfragmentary compression, VI:108
    interfragmentary lag screws, VI:111–112, 112f–113f
    Kirschner wires (K-wires), VI:107b, 108–109, 109f, 110t, 139
    locked plating, VI:115, 115f
    tension band constructs, VI:109–110, 109f–111f, 110t
  fluoroscopic imaging, VI:108–115
  patient selection
    fracture assessment, VI:106
    host factors, VI:106
  postoperative care and follow-up, VI:115
  preoperative imaging assessment, VI:107
  research summary, VI:115
  surgical technique and treatment
    fracture reduction
      basic procedure, VI:107
      Kapandji (intrafocal) pinning, VI:107b
      Kirschner wires (K-wires), VI:107b
      temporary/supplemental external fixation, VI:107b
    preoperative planning, VI:107
Franceschetti–Klein syndrome
  See Treacher Collins syndrome
Frankfort horizontal line, II:356t, 376f
fraud and abuse, I:95–96
Fraxel™ 1500 Re#store laser, II:70–74, 71t
Fraxel™ Re#pair laser, II:70–74, 71t
Fraxel™ SR laser, II:70–74, 71t
free flaps
  mangled upper extremities, VI:254–255, 266–275
  microvascular free-flap surgery
    advantages/disadvantages, I:608
    background information, I:607–611
    chimeric flaps, I:612, 612f
    endoscopic harvests, I:611
    flap failure
      anastomotic failure, I:614
      ischemia–reperfusion injury, I:617–618
      ischemic tolerance, I:617–618
      management approaches, I:618–620
      no-reflow phenomenon, I:617–618
      thrombogenesis, I:615–617
      vasospasm and thrombosis, I:615
    foot reconstruction, IV:211–216
    freestyle flaps, I:611
    outcomes and complicatons
      buried flaps, I:614
      donor site complications, I:618
      flap failure, I:614–618
      flap outcomes, I:614
      postoperative management, I:613–620
    perforator flaps, I:611, 612f
    prefabricated/prelaminated flaps, I:612–613

free flaps (Continued)
    preoperative assessment
      flap selection, I:609–610, 610f
      microvascular anesthesia, I:611
      patient evaluation, I:608–609
      recipient and donor site evaluation, I:609
      timing considerations, I:610–611
    thinned flaps, I:612, 612f
  perineal reconstruction, IV:390
  pressure sores, IV:368–369
  tissue expansion, I:630
  tongue reconstruction, III:309t
free-functioning muscle transfer, VI:777–788
  complications, VI:787
  muscle structure
    characteristics, VI:777–780
    length–tension relationship, VI:779f
    myosin cross-bridges, VI:778f
    schematic diagram, VI:778f
    strap and pennate muscles, VI:779f
  patient presentation and diagnosis, VI:780, 780f
  patient selection, VI:780–781, 781t
  secondary procedures, VI:787
  surgical technique and treatment
    basic principles, VI:781–787
    donor motor nerve, VI:783–785, 783b
    elbows, VI:787
    finger extension, VI:785–787
    flexor digitorum profundus (FDP) tendons, VI:782, 785f
    forearm dissection, VI:784–785, 784f
    gliding tendon path, VI:783f
    gracilis muscle, VI:781–787, 781f–782f
    insufficient coverage, VI:783f
    neurovascular structure alignment, VI:784f
    postoperative finger flexion, VI:786f
  tendon transfers, VI:780t
Freeman–Sheldon syndrome, VI:646, 646f
free radicals, I:573–574, 574f–575f
free TRAM flap, V:411–434
  anatomical and physiological considerations, V:412
  complications, V:430, 431f
  general discussion, V:411
  nipple-areola complex reconstruction, V:430–432, 432f–433f
  patient presentation and diagnosis
    delayed versus immediate reconstruction, V:414
    general discussion, V:414–416
    pedicled versus free TRAM, V:414–415
    radiation therapy (RT), V:415–416
    timing considerations, V:414
  patient selection
    procedure selection, V:417–418
    risk factors, V:416–417
  postoperative care and follow-up, V:428–429
  research summary, V:432
  surgical technique and treatment
    abdominal closure, V:426–428, 429f
    basic procedure, V:418–428, 418f
    flap dissection, V:419–422, 420f–421f, 423f
    flap inset guidelines, V:426, 427f–428f
    mastectomy planning, V:419, 419f
    preoperative assessment and marking, V:418–428
    recipient vessels, V:422–426, 424f–425f

Frey syndrome, III:377–378, 378f
Fricke, Johann, I:20
Fritillaria cirrhosa, V:33t–35t
Fritschi PF4T transfer, VI:767–768
Froment's test, VI:58, 58f, 514t, 762, 762f
frontal bone and sinus fractures
  clinical examination, III:51
  complications, III:53
  computed tomography (CT), III:51
  injury patterns, III:51
  nasofrontal duct, III:51, 52f
  surgical technique and treatment, III:52–53, 52f
frontalis, II:88, 96f, 110–111, 110f–111f, III:14
frontonasal prominence, III:508, 508f
frostbite
  upper extremities, IV:456–467
    classifications, IV:456–460
    complications, IV:459–460
    disease process
      freezing phase, IV:457
      pathophysiology, IV:456–457
      rewarming phase, IV:457
    nonsurgical interventions
      adjunctive therapy, IV:458
      field management, IV:458
      rapid rewarming, IV:458
      splinting, IV:458
    patient presentation and diagnosis
      clinical assessment, IV:457
      physical examination, IV:457–458
      radiographic imaging, IV:457–458
    patient selection, IV:458
    postoperative care and follow-up, IV:459
    prognosis and outcomes, IV:459–460
    research summary, IV:456
    secondary procedures
      hyperbaric oxygen therapy, IV:460
      sympathectomy, IV:460
      thrombolytics, IV:460
    surgical technique and treatment
      amputations, IV:458–459, 459f
      length salvage, IV:459
      nonsurgical interventions, IV:458
Froster contracture–torticollis syndrome, III:807t
frostnip, IV:456–460
frozen neck, III:352–353
Fry, William, I:21–22
Fujimori gate flaps, III:265–268, 266f
functional electrical stimulation (FES), VI:838
fundiform ligaments, II:656, IV:227–230, 227f
fungal infections, VI:343
funicular artery, IV:235, 238f
funnel chest, III:855–859
Furlow double-opposing z-palatoplasty
  palatoplasty, III:579, 580f
  velopharyngeal dysfunction (VPD), III:624–625, 624f
Furlow, Leonard T, Jr, VI:xlviii
Furnas sutures, II:487, 488f

G
gabapentin, IV:427
gadolinium contrast-enhanced MRI, IV:104
galea, II:94–95, 95f
galea aponeurotica, III:14
galeal fat pad, III:14
Galen, Claudius, VI:xliii–xliv
Gallaudet fascia, IV:230–235

ganglion cysts, **VI:**83, 84f, 318–319, 319f
ganglioside vaccine, **I:**781–782
Ganoderma lucidum, **II:**23
garlic, **V:**33t–35t
Garrod's nodules, **VI:**352f
gasoline, **IV:**395
gastric bypass surgery, **II:**636, 636t
gastrocnemius muscle flap
  lower extremity reconstructive surgery,
    I:557–560, 559f–560f, **IV:**142, 142f
  lower leg muscles, **IV:**35f–36f
gastroesophageal reflux, **III:**421
gastroschisis
  characteristics, **III:**865–866
  clinical presentation and evaluation, **III:**865,
    866f
  surgical indicators, **III:**865
  treatment strategies, **III:**865–866
gauze, **I:**289t
gelatinases, **I:**269–271
gender identity disorder, **IV:**336–351
  diagnosis, **IV:**339
  disorders of sex development (DSD),
    IV:336–338, 337t
  epidemiology, **IV:**336–338
  etiology, **IV:**338–339
  outcomes and complicatons, **IV:**348
  patient selection
    adolescents, **IV:**341
    hormonal therapies, **IV:**340, 341t
    preoperative assessment, **IV:**339–341
  postoperative care and follow-up,
    IV:347–348
  research summary, **IV:**350
  secondary procedures
    breast augmentation, **IV:**348–350
    female-to-male chest surgery, **IV:**349–350
  surgical management, **IV:**336–338
  surgical technique and treatment
    female-to-male transsexual surgery
      metaidoioplasty, **IV:**315–318, 317f, 346
      pars fixa of the urethra creation,
        IV:314–315, 316f–317f
      phalloplasty, **IV:**311f, 318–323
      vaginectomy, **IV:**314–315, 315f
    labiaplasty, **IV:**338f, 341–342, 342f
    preoperative depilation, **IV:**342f
    primary surgery
      basic procedure, **IV:**343–345, 343f–346f
      dorsal glans penis dissectiion, **IV:**347f
      labia minora formation, **IV:**348f
      neoclitoris, **IV:**347f–348f, 350f
      penile flap advancement, **IV:**347f
      perineal-scrotal flap, **IV:**343f–344f
      postoperative view, **IV:**349f–350f
      schematic diagram, **IV:**346f–347f
      second-stage labiaplasty, **IV:**350f
      single-stage vaginoplasty, **IV:**349f
      sigmoid vaginoplasty, **IV:**346–347
    surgical options, **IV:**341–342
    vaginoplasty, **IV:**338f, 341–342, 342f
    therapeutic goals, **IV:**338, 338f
generalized anxiety and panic disorders,
  I:48–49, 48b–49b
generalized plaque morphea, **III:**797, 797f
generalized skeletal abnormalities, **VI:**642–644
generally accepted accounting principles
  (GAAP), **I:**67–69

genetic engineering, **I:**6
genetics, **I:**176–200
  background information, **I:**176–177
  epigenetic mechanisms, **I:**181–182, 181f
  ethics, **I:**191–192
  future trends, **I:**199
  gene expression, **I:**179–180
  gene regulation, **I:**180–181, 180f
  gene therapy
    basic principles, **I:**185–191, 186f
    ethical issues, **I:**191–192
    gene delivery, **I:**186–187, 187f, 188t
    skin wound healing, **I:**295
    stem cell-mediated gene therapy, **I:**234,
      234f
    tissue repair, reconstruction, and
      regeneration
      biomaterial scaffolds, **I:**187–189, 189f
      tissue reconstruction and regeneration,
        I:190–191
      tissue repair, **I:**189–190
  genetically-caused disease
    characteristics, **I:**184–185, 192
    congenital defects
      characteristics, **I:**192–198
      craniosynostosis, **I:**195–196
      nomenclature, **I:**192–193
      nonsyndromic cleft lip and palate,
        I:193–194
      orofacial clefts, **I:**193
      syndromic cleft lip and palate,
        I:194–195
      syndromic craniosynostosis, **I:**196–198,
        197t
    inherited chromosomal abnormalities,
      I:185
    mutations, **I:**184–185
  inheritance
    Mendelian patterns
      autosomal inheritance, **I:**182–183, 182f
      sex-linked inheritance, **I:**183, 183f
    non-Mendelian patterns
      characteristics, **I:**183–184
      mitochondrial inheritance, **I:**183–184
      uniparental disomy, **I:**183
  molecular biology
    deoxyribonucleic acid (DNA)
      characteristics, **I:**177–182, 177f
      epigenetic mechanisms, **I:**181–182, 181f
      gene expression, **I:**179–180
      gene regulation, **I:**180–181, 180f
      genomic DNA organization, **I:**178–179,
        178f
  prenatal diagnosis
    functional role, **I:**198–199
    invasive testing, **I:**199
    ultrasonography, **I:**198
genetic sex, **IV:**297
genioglossus advancement, **III:**98, 98f
genioplasty
  Asian facial cosmetic surgery
    Asian rhinoplasty, **II:**177
    chin, **II:**178–179
    narrowing genioplasty, **II:**181, 181f
  orthognathic surgical procedures
    dentofacial deformities, **III:**662–663
    diagnostic tools, **II:**367–368, 368f
genital leiomyoma, **I:**731–732

genitals
  burn wound treatment, **IV:**407, 407f
  cutaneous and soft-tissue tumors
    clinical staging system, **I:**716t
    extramammary Paget's disease, **I:**739,
      739f
    TNM clinical classification system/pTNM
      pathologic classification system,
      I:715b
female genital aesthetic surgery, **II:**655–677
  aesthetic ideals, **II:**669
  labia majora reduction, **II:**673–674,
    674f–676f
  labia minora reduction
    characteristics, **II:**669–673
    outcomes and complicatons, **II:**672–673,
      672f–673f
    surgical technique, **II:**670–672,
      671f–672f
  lipodystrophy, **II:**674–676, 675f–677f
  mons correction, **II:**640, 641f–642f
  mons pubis descent, **II:**674–676, 675f–677f
  research summary, **II:**677
  self-esteem issues, **II:**655, 669
  vulvar anatomy, **II:**669
female perineum
  characteristics, **IV:**230–235
  cross-section diagram, **IV:**231f
  schematic diagram, **IV:**232f–233f
  urogenital triangle, **IV:**233f
  vascular anatomy, **IV:**232–235, 234f
gender identity disorder, **IV:**336–351
  diagnosis, **IV:**339
  disorders of sex development (DSD),
    IV:336–338, 337t
  epidemiology, **IV:**336–338
  etiology, **IV:**338–339
  outcomes and complicatons, **IV:**348
  patient selection
    adolescents, **IV:**341
    hormonal therapies, **IV:**340, 341t
    preoperative assessment, **IV:**339–341
  postoperative care and follow-up,
    IV:347–348
  research summary, **IV:**350
  secondary procedures
    breast augmentation, **IV:**348–350
    female-to-male chest surgery,
      IV:349–350
  surgical management, **IV:**336–338
  surgical technique and treatment
    female-to-male transsexual surgery,
      IV:311f, 314–323, 346
    labiaplasty, **IV:**338f, 341–342, 342f
    preoperative depilation, **IV:**342f
    primary surgery, **IV:**343–345
    sigmoid vaginoplasty, **IV:**346–347
    surgical options, **IV:**341–342
    vaginoplasty, **IV:**338f, 341–342, 342f
    therapeutic goals, **IV:**338, 338f
genital embryology
  genetic sex, **IV:**297
  gonadal sex, **IV:**297–298
  phenotypic sex, **IV:**298, 298f
male genital aesthetic surgery, **II:**655–677
  enhancement procedures, **II:**655
  flaccid versus erect penis measurements,
    II:655–656

genitals (Continued)
hidden penis
characteristics, II:665–668, 665f–666f
outcome assessments, II:668
post-bariatric surgery reconstruction, II:640, 643f
surgical technique, II:667–668, 667f–669f
patient selection and examination, II:656
penile anatomy, II:656
penile enlargement reconstruction
dermal fat graft and Alloderm removal, II:661–662, 661f
fat removal, II:660–661
outcomes and complicatons, II:662
postoperative care and follow-up, II:662
reconstructive issues, II:660–662
VY advancement flap reversal, II:658f, 660, 661f
penile girth enhancement
allograft dermal matrix grafts, II:660
challenges, II:659–660
dermal and dermal fat grafts, II:659–660
fat injections, II:658f–659f, 659
penile lengthening
basic procedure, II:656–658, 657f–658f
outcome assessments, II:657–658, 659f
VY advancement flap, II:656–658, 657f–658f
penoscrotal web, II:662, 663f
research summary, II:677
scrotal enlargement, II:662, 664f
self-esteem issues, II:655
male genital anatomy
blood supply, IV:299–301, 299f–301f
general discussion, IV:298–301
genital fascia, IV:298–299, 299f
lymphatic supply, IV:301
nerve supply, IV:301
male genital reconstructive surgery, IV:297–325
congenital defects
disorders of sex development (DSD), IV:303–304
exstrophy and epispadias, IV:301–303, 302f–303f
hidden penis, IV:304, 304f–305f
severe penile insufficiency, IV:304–306, 306f
female-to-male transsexual surgery
metaidoioplasty, IV:315–318, 317f, 346
pars fixa of the urethra creation, IV:314–315, 316f–317f
phalloplasty, IV:318–323
vaginectomy, IV:314–315, 315f
general discussion, IV:297
genital anatomy
blood supply, IV:299–301, 299f–301f
general discussion, IV:298–301
genital fascia, IV:298–299, 299f
lymphatic supply, IV:301
nerve supply, IV:301
genital embryology
genetic sex, IV:297
gonadal sex, IV:297–298
phenotypic sex, IV:298, 298f
microsurgical genital reconstruction
genital replantation, IV:310–312, 312f
phallic construction, IV:312

genitals (Continued)
multidisciplinary approach, IV:323
post-traumatic genital defects
basic principles, IV:306–313
genital flaps, IV:304–310, 306f, 311f
genital skin grafts, IV:307, 308f–309f
microsurgical genital reconstruction, IV:310–312
reconstructive indications, IV:312–313
reconstructive indications
Fournier disease, IV:312–313, 313f
penile cancer, IV:313, 314f
male perineum
characteristics, IV:235
cross-section diagram, IV:231f
schematic diagram, IV:236f–237f
vascular anatomy, IV:235, 238f
urogenital defect reconstruction, III:906–924
embryology, III:907–908
epidemiology, III:908
etiology, III:908
outcomes and complicatons, III:916–921
patient presentation and diagnosis, III:908–909
patient selection, III:909
postoperative care and follow-up, III:915
secondary procedures, III:921
surgical technique and treatment
meatoplasty and glanuloplasty, III:913–915, 914b, 916f
tubularized incised plate (TIP) repair, III:914, 917f
urethral reconstruction, III:913, 915f
vaginal reconstruction, III:909
geometric broken line, I:316, 317f
Geum japonicum, V:33t–35t
giant cell angioblastoma, VI:668t
giant cell tumors, I:736, VI:319, 319f
giant cell tumors of the bone, VI:329, 329f
giant cell tumors of the tendon sheath (GCTTS), VI:83, 84f
giant hair nevus/congenital nevomelanocytic nevus (CNN), III:112–113, 114f
giant pannus, II:640–643, 643f–644f
Gillies fan flap, III:261–262, 264f, 454
Gillies, Harold
nose reconstruction, VI:xlv
reconstructive and aesthetic surgery, I:24f
skin grafts, I:21–22
surgical innovation, I:4–5, 5f
Gillies near-far pulley, I:304
Gilula's lines, VI:10f, 161–162, 162f
ginger, V:33t–35t
gingival fibroma
patient presentation and diagnosis, III:881
surgical technique and treatment, III:881
gingivoperiosteoplasty (GPP), III:585, 586f, 588, 589f, 592–593
ginkgo, V:33t–35t
Ginkgo biloba, V:33t–35t
ginseng, II:22–23, V:33t–35t
glabella
anesthesia, III:26, 27f
anthropometric analysis, II:356t, 363f
botulinum toxin type-A (BoNT-A), II:33–34, 35f–36f
glabellar frown muscles, II:95f
photographic guidelines, I:108, 110f
glabellar lines, II:51
glabridin, II:25

glandular correction flaps
characteristics, V:529–531
glandular flap Type I, V:530
glandular flap Type II, V:530
glandular flap Type III, V:530
glandular flap Type IV, V:530–531
glandular hypomastia, V:13
glanuloplasty
basic procedure, III:913–915, 916f
onlay island flap repair, III:914–915, 918f
orthoplasty, III:915
surgical tips, III:914b–915b
tubularized incised plate (TIP) repair, III:914, 917f
two-stage repair, III:915, 919f–921f
Glasgow Coma Scale (GCS), IV:63, 64t
globe, II:120, 122, III:252–253, 252t
glomus tumors
characteristics, I:734, VI:325f
patient presentation and diagnosis, III:878
surgical technique and treatment, III:878, VI:324
glomuvenous malformation (GVM), I:677t, 693–694, VI:668t, 682–684
glossoptosis, III:803–804, 804f, 817f
glottic cancers, III:434–436, 436f
glucocorticosteroids, I:821
glucosamine, V:33t–35t
glues
See adhesives and glues
gluteal region
anatomical characteristics
fascial system, IV:5
innervation, IV:5–8, 7f
musculature, IV:5, 5t, 6f
skeletal structure, IV:2–5, 3f–4f
vascular supply, IV:5, 7f
gluteal aesthetic ideals, II:599–600, 600f, 603f
gluteus maximus muscle
breast reconstruction, V:292
characteristics, I:516f
clinical applications, I:523f–524f
gluteal aesthetic ideals, II:600, 600f
perineal reconstruction, I:557
pressure sores, I:562–565, 566f–568f
glycerin, II:17–18
glycolic acid, II:19
glycosaminoglycans, I:270–271, 320
glycyl-L-histidyl-L-lysine-Cu²⁺ (GHK-Cu), II:18
Glycyrrhiza glabra, II:23, 25, V:33t–35t
Glycyrrhiza inflata, II:23
GM2 ganglioside vaccine, I:781–782
gnathion, II:356t, 363f
Goes periareolar technique with mesh support
basic procedure, V:132–133
surgical technique
basic procedure, V:132–133
four cardinal points, V:132f
gland dissection, V:133f
mesh placement, V:134f
resection lines, V:134f
gold (Au)
gold alloys, I:787
radionuclides, I:656–657
Goldenhar syndrome, III:714–716
golden ratio, II:177, 354–355
golden ratio phi mask, II:354–355, 355f

gonadal sex, **IV**:297–298
Gore-Tex, **I**:790
　See also polytetrafluoroethylene (PTFE)
Gorham-Stout syndrome, **VI**:668, 668t
Gorlin's syndrome, **I**:194
Gorneygram, **I**:103, 103f
Gorney's patient selection graph, **II**:7–8, 7f
gout, **VI**:335, 335f, 407t, 409–410
gracilis muscle
　breast reconstruction, **V**:292
　characteristics, **I**:516f, **IV**:15t–16t, 18f–22f,
　　19t, 35f
　foot reconstruction, **I**:563f, **IV**:211
　free-functioning muscle transfer, **VI**:781–
　　787, 781f–782f
　groin reconstruction, **I**:554–557
　lower extremity reconstructive surgery,
　　IV:77, 80f, 89f–90f, 140–141, 140f
　male genital reconstructive surgery,
　　IV:307–310
　microneurovascular muscle transplantation,
　　III:295–297, 295t, 296f–298f
　perineal reconstruction, **I**:554–557, 556f,
　　IV:388, 389f
　pressure sores, **I**:562–565, 564f–565f
granulation tissue, **I**:253
granulocyte–macrophage colony-stimulating
　factor (GM-CSF), **I**:275, 369–371
granulocytes, **I**:817
granuloma annulare, **VI**:336
granulomas, **I**:733–734, 733f–734f
grape seed extract, **II**:27
gray (Gy) unit of measure, **I**:664
Grayson's ligaments, **VI**:5, 7f, 347, 348f,
　350f
greater trochanter harvests, **I**:452
Great Ormond Street ladder of functional
　ability, **VI**:549f
great-toe wrap-around flap, **VI**:304–305
Grebe syndrome, **VI**:573f
green tea, **II**:18, 21t, 27–28
Greig cephalopolysyndactyly syndrome,
　VI:537f, 617t
Grifola frondosa, **II**:23
groin flap, **IV**:143, 143f–144f, **VI**:264–266,
　265f–266f
groin reconstruction, **I**:554–557, 558f
gross tumor volumes (GTV), **I**:663
Grotting sculpted vertical pillar mastopexy
　basic procedure
　　characteristics, **V**:136–139
　　markings and incisions, **V**:138f
　　preferred technique, **V**:138f
　　preoperative markings, **V**:137f
　　surgical tips, **V**:136b
　operative technique
　　basic procedure, **V**:138–139
　　final closure, **V**:140f
　　flap detachment, **V**:139f
　　preferred technique, **V**:139f–140f
　　preoperative/postoperative comparisons,
　　　V:140f–141f
　　temporary breast closure, **V**:139f
growth factors
　bone tissue engineering, **I**:393
　Dupuytren's disease, **VI**:349
　fat grafting, **I**:345
　skin aging, **II**:15

growth factors (*Continued*)
　skin wound healing
　　fetal wound repair, **I**:278
　　regulation
　　　characteristics, **I**:273–275
　　　extra cellular matrix–growth factor
　　　　interactions, **I**:275
　　　fibroblast growth factor (FGF),
　　　　I:274–275
　　　heparin-binding epidermal growth
　　　　factor (HB–EGF), **I**:275
　　　platelet-derived growth factor (PDGF),
　　　　I:274
　　　transforming growth factor-β (TGF-β)
　　　　superfamily, **I**:274
　　　vascular endothelial growth factor
　　　　(VEGF), **I**:275
　　types and characteristics, **I**:270t
　tissue engineering, **I**:380–381, 381f
　wound healing, **I**:234
Grynfeltt triangle, **IV**:221
guanine, **I**:177–182, 177f
guanosine monophosphate (GMP), **I**:821–822
guanosine triphosphate (GTP), **I**:822–823
guilinggao, **V**:33t–35t
Guinea Pig club, **I**:5
Gulian knife, **I**:326–327, 327f
gunshot wounds
　delayed versus immediate reconstruction,
　　III:85
　immediate and high velocity gunshot
　　wounds, **III**:86–87
　low velocity gunshot wounds, **III**:85–87
　treatment strategies, **III**:86–87, 86f
Guy of Chauliac, **I**:15
Guyon's canal
　nerve compression syndromes
　　anatomical considerations, **VI**:511, 513f
　　etiology, **VI**:511
　　patient presentation and diagnosis,
　　　VI:511–512
　　surgical technique and treatment,
　　　VI:512–513
　occupational hand disorders, **VI**:368–369
gynecomastia
　adolescent aesthetic surgery, **I**:45t
　excision of gynecomastia with nipple
　　repositioning, **V**:575–579, 578f–580f
　outcomes and complicatons, **V**:579
　pathophysiology, **V**:573–574
　patient presentation and diagnosis, **V**:574
　patient selection, **V**:574–575, 575t
　postoperative care and follow-up, **V**:578
　pseudogynecomastia, **V**:575t, 576f–577f
　surgical markings, **V**:575–576, 576f–577f
　surgical technique and treatment, **V**:576–
　　578, 578f–580f
　surgical tips, **V**:578b

H

Haas syndrome, **VI**:645–646, 646f
Haber–Weiss (Fenton) reaction, **I**:575, 575f
haemoglobin, **I**:573–574, 574f
Hageman factor, **I**:268–269
hair
　anatomical characteristics
　　hair follicles, **II**:495–497, 495f
　　normal hairline, **II**:495–496, 496f

hair (*Continued*)
　general characteristics
　　hair growth cycles, **II**:496–497, 497f
　　hair types, **II**:496
　hair-bearing flaps, **III**:463
　hair follicles
　　anatomical characteristics, **II**:495–497,
　　　495f
　　growth cycles, **II**:496–497, 497f
　　skin grafts, **I**:321, 322f
　　skin wound healing, **I**:262–263, 262f
　　tissue expansion effects, **I**:631–633
　　tissue-specific stem cells, **I**:229, 229f
　hair restoration, **II**:494–506
　　anesthesia, **II**:503–504
　　background information, **II**:494
　　complications, **II**:504–505
　　facial burn wound treatment, **IV**:485
　　medical management, **II**:502
　　number of procedures, **II**:504–505
　　patient evaluation, **II**:498–502, 500f–501f
　　patient presentation and diagnosis
　　　baldness types and patterns, **II**:497–498
　　　hail loss classifications, **II**:498, 499f
　　prognosis and outcomes, **II**:504–505
　　secondary procedures, **II**:505–506
　　surgical technique, **II**:502–503, 503f–504f
　　unsatisfactory results, **II**:505–506
　hair structure and cycle, **III**:109, 110f
Hall-Findlay technique, **V**:159, 178t
Halsted radical mastectomy, **I**:202, **V**:280–286
hand-held Doppler ultrasound
　basic principles, **V**:327–328
hand injury severity scale (HISS), **VI**:247
hands
　aging process, **II**:329
　anatomical characteristics, **VI**:1–46
　　arterial system
　　　deep palmar arch, **VI**:469
　　　digital arteries, **VI**:469
　　　general discussion, **VI**:468–469
　　　superficial palmar arch, **VI**:468–469
　　blood flow physiology
　　　cellular control mechanisms,
　　　　VI:469–470
　　　hemodynamics, **VI**:469
　　　pathophysiology, **VI**:470
　　bones and joints
　　　bony anatomy, **VI**:12f
　　　carpal bones, **VI**:5–7, 7f
　　　check rein ligaments, **VI**:13b
　　　collateral ligaments, **VI**:13f
　　　functional elements, **VI**:5–7, 7f–8f
　　　joint motion, **VI**:11–13
　　　thumb, **VI**:13–14, 14f
　　　wrists, **VI**:7–11, 8f–11f, 10b
　　dorsal metacarpal artery flaps, **VI**:40b
　　embryology, **VI**:468
　　fascial system, **VI**:2–5, 4f, 6f–7f
　　functional dynamics, **VI**:36b
　　joint axes, **VI**:3f
　　joint motion
　　　biomechanics, **VI**:11b
　　　bony anatomy, **VI**:11–13, 12f
　　　check rein ligaments, **VI**:13b
　　　collateral ligaments, **VI**:13f
　　Kaplan's cardinal line, **VI**:2b, 2f
　　ligaments, **VI**:7f

hands (*Continued*)
  micro-arterial system, **VI:**469
  muscles and tendons
    biomechanics (extensor mechanism),
      VI:18b, 20f
    biomechanics (muscle structure),
      VI:18b, 19f
    extrinsic extensors, **VI:**14–18, 15f–17f
    extrinsic flexors, **VI:**22–29, 22b, 23f–27f,
      32b
    flexor tendon zones, **VI:**31–32, 31f
    intrinsic muscles, **VI:**32–35, 33f–36f, 35b
    pronators and supinators, **VI:**18–22, 21f
  palmar fascia, **VI:**2–5, 4f–5f
  peripheral nerves
    crowded areas with unyielding
      boundaries, **VI:**44b
    detailed characteristics, **VI:**40–44
    median and ulnar nerve lacerations,
      VI:44b
    median nerve, **VI:**43f
    proximal radial nerve, **VI:**41f
    radial nerve, **VI:**42f
    ulnar nerve, **VI:**45f
  radial and ulnar arteries, **VI:**40b
  research background, **VI:**1–2
  research summary, **VI:**46
  retinacular system
    annular pulleys, **VI:**29–32, 30f
    cruciate pulleys, **VI:**29–32, 30f
    flexor tendon zones, **VI:**31–32, 31f
    intrinsic muscles, **VI:**32–35, 33f–36f, 35b
    transverse carpal ligament, **VI:**29–32, 29f
    vincula, **VI:**29–32, 31f
  skin, **VI:**2–5, 2f
  subcutaneous tissue, **VI:**2–5
  vascular supply, **VI:**35–40, 37f–39f, 40b
  Apert syndrome
    characteristics, **VI:**610, 644–645, 645f
    complications, **VI:**614
    epidemiology, **VI:**610
    outcome assessments, **VI:**614
    pathogenesis, **VI:**610
    patient presentation and diagnosis,
      VI:611f, 611t, 613f, 682
    patient selection, **VI:**612
    postoperative care and follow-up, **VI:**614
    secondary procedures, **VI:**614
    surgical technique and treatment
      basic procedure, **VI:**612–614
      finger separation, **VI:**612
      metacarpal synostosis, **VI:**614
      preferred treatments, **VI:**611f, 612t–
        613t, 613f
      thumb and first web separation,
        VI:612–614
  biomechanics, **VI:**164–165
  brachydactyly
    brachymesophalangy, **VI:**637f, 639–640
    brachymetacarpia, **VI:**638f, 640, 640f
    causal factors, **VI:**637
    clinical manifestations, **VI:**635–641,
      636f–638f
    clinodactyly
      characteristics, **VI:**630, 636, 638f, 640
      outcomes and complicatons, **VI:**632
      pathogenesis, **VI:**630
      patient presentation and diagnosis,
        VI:630–631, 631f
      patient selection, **VI:**631

hands (*Continued*)
      postoperative care and follow-up,
        VI:632
      radiographic imaging, **VI:**637f
      secondary procedures, **VI:**632
      surgical technique and treatment,
        VI:546t, 631–632, 631f, 640
    Kirner's deformity, **VI:**639f
    Mohr–Wriedt syndrome, **VI:**636, 638f, 646
    polydactyly
      characteristics, **VI:**639f
      classification systems, **VI:**535–537,
        535f–536f
    symbrachydactyly
      classification systems, **VI:**537, 537f–538f
      patient presentation and diagnosis,
        VI:549–550, 550f, 609f, 640–641,
        640f–641f, 645f
      surgical technique and treatment,
        VI:546t
    syndactyly
      characteristics, **VI:**635f, 639f
      classification systems, **VI:**535–537, 535f,
        537f, 605f
      epidemiology, **VI:**604
      outcomes and complicatons, **VI:**608–
        609, 609f
      pathogenesis, **VI:**604
      patient presentation and diagnosis,
        VI:564–565, 604, 606f
      patient selection, **VI:**604–605
      postoperative care and follow-up,
        VI:608
      secondary procedures, **VI:**609
      surgical technique and treatment,
        VI:546t, 605–608, 605b, 608b
    treatment strategies, **VI:**637–639
  burn reconstruction, **IV:**507–509, 508f
  carpometacarpal (CMC) joints, **VI:**138–139,
    153, 153f, 434–439
  composite tissue allotransplantation (CTA),
    VI:843–854
    challenges, **VI:**852
    complications, **VI:**850–851
    donor and recipient selection, **VI:**845–846,
      846t
    emerging insights
      chronic rejection, **VI:**852–853, 853t
      cortical plasticity, **VI:**852
      future trends, **VI:**854
      immunomodulatory strategies,
        VI:853–854
      neural integration, **VI:**852
      tolerance approaches, **VI:**853–854
    epidemiology, **VI:**843–844
    evolutionary development
      chronology, **VI:**845
      experimental background, **VI:**844–845
      immunology, **VI:**844
    procedural aspects
      donor limb procurement, **VI:**846–847,
        847f
      recipient surgery, **VI:**847, 848f
    prognosis and outcomes, **VI:**850–851
    program establishment and
      implementation, **VI:**845
    protocol-related considerations
      immunomonitoring, **VI:**850
      maintenance immunosuppression,
        VI:847, 849f, 853–854

hands (*Continued*)
    rehabilitation and functional
      assessment, **I:**835–837, **VI:**848, 849f
    rejection assessments, **VI:**849–850,
      849f–851f, 849t
    upper extremity transplantation versus
      replantation, **VI:**851–852
  congenital deformities, **VI:**526–571, 603–650
    Apert syndrome
      characteristics, **VI:**610, 644–645, 645f
      complications, **VI:**614
      finger separation, **VI:**612
      outcome assessments, **VI:**614
      pathogenesis, **VI:**610
      patient presentation and diagnosis,
        VI:611f, 611t, 613f, 682
      patient selection, **VI:**612
      postoperative care and follow-up,
        VI:614
      preferred treatments, **VI:**611f, 612t–
        613t, 613f
      secondary procedures, **VI:**614
      surgical technique and treatment,
        VI:612–614
      thumb and first web separation,
        VI:612–614
    brachydactyly
      brachymesophalangy, **VI:**637f, 639–640
      brachymetacarpia, **VI:**638f, 640, 640f
      causal factors, **VI:**637
      clinical manifestations, **VI:**635–641,
        636f–638f
      clinodactyly, **VI:**546t, 636, 637f–638f,
        640
      Kirner's deformity, **VI:**639f
      Mohr–Wriedt syndrome, **VI:**636, 638f,
        646
      polydactyly, **VI:**535–537, 535f–536f, 639f
      symbrachydactyly, **VI:**537, 537f–538f,
        546t, 549–550, 550f, 609f, 640–641,
        640f–641f, 645f
      syndactyly, **VI:**535–537, 535f, 537f,
        604–609, 635f, 639f
      treatment strategies, **VI:**637–639
    camptodactyly
      characteristics, **VI:**628
      epidemiology, **VI:**628
      outcomes and complicatons, **VI:**630
      pathogenesis, **VI:**628
      patient presentation and diagnosis,
        VI:628–629
      patient selection, **VI:**629
      postoperative care and follow-up,
        VI:630
      secondary procedures, **VI:**630
      surgical technique and treatment,
        VI:546t, 629–630, 629f–630f
    central ray deficiency
      associated syndromes, **VI:**565t
      characteristics, **VI:**563–564, 563b, 564f
      classification systems, **VI:**565t
      outcomes and complicatons,
        VI:566–567
      pathogenesis, **VI:**564
      patient presentation and diagnosis,
        VI:564–565, 564f
      patient selection, **VI:**565
      postoperative care and follow-up,
        VI:566
      secondary procedures, **VI:**567

hands (*Continued*)

surgical technique and treatment, **VI:**565, 565f–566f

child and family assessments

diagnostic imaging, **VI:**543–544

hand control development, **VI:**541t, 542–543, 542f

ossification timing/growth plate closure, **VI:**543f

patient and family history, **VI:**541–542

physical examination, **VI:**541t, 542–543, 542f–543f

support systems, **VI:**539–544

surgical congenital hand clinic, **VI:**541

weight-bearing development, **VI:**543f

classification systems, **VI:**526–527

clinodactyly

characteristics, **VI:**630

outcomes and complicatons, **VI:**632

pathogenesis, **VI:**630

patient presentation and diagnosis, **VI:**630–631, 631f

patient selection, **VI:**631

postoperative care and follow-up, **VI:**632

secondary procedures, **VI:**632

surgical technique and treatment, **VI:**631–632, 631f

congenital alopecia, **VI:**646

congenital longitudinal arrest, **VI:**555–556

congenital transverse arrest

assessment strategies, **VI:**548, 549f

general considerations, **VI:**548b

outcomes and complicatons, **VI:**553–555

pathogenesis, **VI:**548–549

patient presentation and diagnosis, **VI:**549–550, 549f–550f

patient selection, **VI:**550–553

postoperative care and follow-up, **VI:**550–553

secondary procedures, **VI:**555

surgical technique and treatment, **VI:**550–553

constriction band syndrome

bone grafts, **VI:**642

clinical manifestations, **VI:**641–642, 642f

surgical treatment, **VI:**546t, 641–642, 642f–643f

toe-to-hand transplantations, **VI:**642, 643f

development anomalies

background information, **VI:**534–535

classification systems, **VI:**534–535

modified classification of congenital anomalies of the hand and upper limb, **VI:**537–539, 538f–541f, 538t

Swanson/IFSSH classification, **VI:**535–537

symbrachydactyly, **VI:**537, 537f–538f, 546t

syndactyly, **VI:**535–537, 535f, 537f

terminology, **VI:**534–535

diagnosis, **VI:**544

embryology, **VI:**526–534

Freeman–Sheldon syndrome, **VI:**646, 646f

general discussion, **VI:**634

hands (*Continued*)

generalized skeletal abnormalities, **VI:**642–644

Haas syndrome, **VI:**645–646, 646f

limb development

embryology, **VI:**526–534

hand development timing, **VI:**527t

molecular controls, **VI:**527–530, 529f–530f

upper limb morphogenesis, **VI:**527, 527t, 528f–529f

macrodactyly

classification systems, **VI:**541f

clinical manifestations, **VI:**634–635, 635f

Hong Kong survey, **VI:**635t

proteus syndrome, **VI:**635

surgical technique and treatment, **VI:**636f

Madelung's deformity, **VI:**646–647, 647f

metacarpal synostosis

characteristics, **VI:**614–615

outcomes and complicatons, **VI:**616

pathogenesis, **VI:**615

patient presentation and diagnosis, **VI:**615, 615f

patient selection, **VI:**615–616

postoperative care and follow-up, **VI:**616

secondary procedures, **VI:**616

surgical technique and treatment, **VI:**615–616

Mohr–Wriedt syndrome, **VI:**646

multiple exotoses, **VI:**642–644, 644f

phocomelia

characteristics, **VI:**556, 556b

outcomes and complicatons, **VI:**557

pathogenesis, **VI:**556

patient presentation and diagnosis, **VI:**556, 556f

patient selection, **VI:**556

postoperative care and follow-up, **VI:**557

secondary procedures, **VI:**557

surgical technique and treatment, **VI:**556–557

Pierre–Robin syndrome, **VI:**646, 646f

Poland syndrome

characteristics, **VI:**644–647, 644f

epidemiology, **VI:**609

outcomes and complicatons, **VI:**610

pathogenesis, **VI:**609

patient presentation and diagnosis, **VI:**609–610, 609f

patient selection, **VI:**610

postoperative care and follow-up, **VI:**610

secondary procedures, **VI:**610

surgical technique and treatment, **VI:**610

polydactyly

associated syndromes, **VI:**617t

central polydactyly, **VI:**546t, 618

characteristics, **VI:**616

classification systems, **VI:**535–537, 535f–536f

epidemiology, **VI:**616

genetic considerations, **VI:**616–617

hands (*Continued*)

outcomes and complicatons, **VI:**622–623, 623f, 623t

pathogenesis, **VI:**616–617

patient selection, **VI:**618

postaxial polydactyly, **VI:**546t

potassium titanium oxide phosphate (KTP) lasers, **VI:**622

radial polydactyly, **VI:**564–565, 617–618, 617f, 617t

secondary procedures, **VI:**623

surgical technique and treatment, **VI:**619–622

ulnar polydactyly, **VI:**617t, 618

radial hypoplasia/aplasia

characteristics, **VI:**557, 557b

classification systems, **VI:**558t, 559f

outcomes and complicatons, **VI:**563

pathogenesis, **VI:**557–558

patient presentation and diagnosis, **VI:**558–560, 558f–559f

patient selection, **VI:**560

postoperative care and follow-up, **VI:**563

secondary procedures, **VI:**563

surgical technique and treatment, **VI:**560–563, 560f–562f

timing considerations, **VI:**546t, 547f

research summary, **VI:**647–648

surgical indicators

appearance, **VI:**544–545, 545f

functionality, **VI:**544, 545f

timing considerations, **VI:**545–547, 546f–547f, 546t

symphalangism

characteristics, **VI:**614–615

outcomes and complicatons, **VI:**616

pathogenesis, **VI:**615

patient presentation and diagnosis, **VI:**615

patient selection, **VI:**615–616

postoperative care and follow-up, **VI:**616

secondary procedures, **VI:**616

surgical technique and treatment, **VI:**615–616

syndactyly

classification systems, **VI:**605f

differentiation and duplication, **VI:**604–609

epidemiology, **VI:**604

outcomes and complicatons, **VI:**608–609, 609f

pathogenesis, **VI:**604

patient presentation and diagnosis, **VI:**564–565, 604, 606f

patient selection, **VI:**604–605

postoperative care and follow-up, **VI:**608

secondary procedures, **VI:**609

surgical technique and treatment, **VI:**546t, 605–608, 605b, 608b

synostosis

characteristics, **VI:**614–615

outcomes and complicatons, **VI:**616

pathogenesis, **VI:**615

patient presentation and diagnosis, **VI:**615, 615f

Note: **Boldface** *roman numerals indicate volume. Page numbers followed by f refer to figures; page numbers followed by t refer to tables; page numbers followed by b refer to boxes.*

hands *(Continued)*
  patient selection, **VI:**615–616
  postoperative care and follow-up, **VI:**616
  secondary procedures, **VI:**616
  surgical technique and treatment, **VI:**615–616
  terminology, **VI:**527
  tissue development/differentiation
    general discussion, **VI:**530–534
    innervation, **VI:**534, 534f
    myogenesis, **VI:**532–534, 533f
    skeletogenesis, **VI:**531–532, 532f
    vasculogenesis, **VI:**530–531, 531f
  trigger thumb
    etiology, **VI:**648
    general discussion, **VI:**648–649
    timing considerations, **VI:**546t
    treatment strategies, **VI:**648–649
  triphalangeal thumb
    delta middle phalanx, **VI:**625–627, 626f–627f
    epidemiology, **VI:**623–624
    first web deficiency, **VI:**627, 628f
    five fingered hand, **VI:**627
    outcomes and complicatons, **VI:**627
    pathogenesis, **VI:**624
    patient presentation and diagnosis, **VI:**624, 625f
    patient selection, **VI:**624
    postoperative care and follow-up, **VI:**627
    preferred treatments, **VI:**625–627
    rectangular middle phalanx, **VI:**627
    secondary procedures, **VI:**627–628
    surgical technique and treatment, **VI:**624–627
  ulnar hypoplasia/aplasia
    associated syndromes, **VI:**567t
    characteristics, **VI:**567
    classification systems, **VI:**567, 568f, 568t–569t
    incidence, **VI:**567–570
    outcomes and complicatons, **VI:**570
    pathogenesis, **VI:**567
    patient presentation and diagnosis, **VI:**567–569, 567f–569f
    patient selection, **VI:**569
    postoperative care and follow-up, **VI:**570
    secondary procedures, **VI:**570
    surgical technique and treatment, **VI:**569–570, 570f
  constriction band syndrome
    bone grafts, **VI:**642
    clinical manifestations, **VI:**641–642, 642f
    surgical treatment, **VI:**546t, 641–642, 642f–643f
    toe-to-hand transplantations, **VI:**642, 643f
  diagnostic imaging, **VI:**68–91
    computed tomography (CT)
      advantages/disadvantages, **VI:**78–82, 81t
      bony tumors, **VI:**81–82
      fractures and dislocations, **VI:**78–79, 81f
      soft-tissue masses, **VI:**313
    general discussion, **VI:**68
    magnetic resonance imaging (MRI)
      advantages/disadvantages, **VI:**82–89, 82t
      basic principles, **VI:**82

hands *(Continued)*
      carpal fractures, **VI:**85
      enchondromas, **VI:**85
      fracture nonunion evaluations, **VI:**88
      ganglion cysts, **VI:**83, 84f
      giant cell tumors of the tendon sheath (GCTTS), **VI:**83, 84f
      hemangiomas, **VI:**83–85
      Kienbock's disease, **VI:**88, 89f
      ligamentous injuries, **VI:**85–86
      lipomas, **VI:**83
      occult scaphoid fractures, **VI:**85, 85f
      osteomyelitis, **VI:**88–89
      pulse sequences and enhancements, **VI:**83t
      scaphoid fracture nonunion evaluations, **VI:**88
      scapholunate interosseous ligament injury, **VI:**85–86, 87f
      signal intensities on weighted images, **VI:**82, 82t
      soft-tissue masses, **VI:**82–83
      thumb ulnar collateral ligament injuries, **VI:**85, 86f
      trauma-related injuries, **VI:**85
      tumors, **VI:**313
    radiographic imaging
      general discussion, **VI:**68–76
      hand evaluation, **VI:**69–70
    radionuclide imaging, **VI:**90
    vascular imaging techniques, **VI:**89–90, 90f
  distal interphalangeal (DIP) joint
    Dupuytren's disease, **VI:**350–353
    fractures and joint injuries, **VI:**138–139, 141–142, 142f
    osteoarthritis
      biomechanical effects, **VI:**414
      diagnosis, **VI:**414, 415f
      distal interphalangeal (DIP) arthrodesis, **VI:**414–416
      surgical indicators, **VI:**414
  Dupuytren's disease, **VI:**346–362
    arterial insufficiency, **VI:**360b
    clinical manifestations
      digital fascia, **VI:**347, 348f
      first webspace, **VI:**347–348, 348f
      Garrod's nodules, **VI:**352f
      general characteristics, **VI:**351–353
      general discussion, **VI:**346–348
      nodule formation, **VI:**351f
      palmar and palomodigital disease, **VI:**352f
      palmar fascia, **VI:**347, 347f
      plantar fibromatosis, **VI:**352, 352f
    complications, **VI:**359–360, 360b
    definition, **VI:**346–348
    digital anatomy, **VI:**349t, 350f–351f
    disease process, **VI:**349–351, 349t, 351f
    epidemiology, **VI:**346
    pathogenesis, **VI:**348–349
    patient presentation and diagnosis
      clinical manifestations, **VI:**351f–352f
      differential diagnoses, **VI:**353
      patient history, **VI:**351–353
      physical examination, **VI:**351–353
    patient selection, **VI:**353
    postoperative care and follow-up, **VI:**359
    prognosis and outcomes, **VI:**359–360

hands *(Continued)*
  research summary, **VI:**361
  secondary procedures
    amputation, **VI:**361
    indicators, **VI:**360–361
    proximal interphalangeal (PIP) arthrodesis, **VI:**361
    skeletal traction, **VI:**361
    total volar tenoarthrolysis, **VI:**361
    wedge osteotomy, **VI:**361
  surgical treatment
    check rein release technique, **VI:**358, 358f
    dermatofasciectomy, **VI:**355t, 359
    local fasciectomy, **VI:**355t, 356
    open fasciotomy, **VI:**355t, 356
    percutaneous (needle) aponeurotomy, **VI:**354–355, 355b, 355t, 356f
    radical fasciectomy, **VI:**355t, 358–359
    regional fasciectomy, **VI:**355t, 356–358, 357f–358f, 358b
    surgical options, **VI:**354–359, 355t
  treatment strategies
    general discussion, **VI:**353–359
    injection treatments, **VI:**353–354, 354f–355f
    modality therapy, **VI:**353
    surgical treatment, **VI:**354–359
fat grafting, **II:**332, 333f
flexor tendon injuries, **VI:**178–209
  anatomical considerations
    annular pulleys/cruciate pulleys, **VI:**180f
    flexor pulleys, **VI:**180f–181f
    general characteristics, **VI:**179–182
    tendon zones, **VI:**31–32, 31f, 181f
    vincula, **VI:**181f
  biomechanics
    gliding motions, **VI:**184
    linear versus bending forces, **VI:**183, 184f
    surgical repair strength, **VI:**182–184, 183f
    tendon–suture junctions, **VI:**182–184, 183f
  challenges, **VI:**178–179
  flexor pollicis longus (FPL) injuries, **VI:**196, 196f–197f
  flexor tendon healing, **VI:**182
  free tendon grafting
    donor tendons, **VI:**202f
    indications and contraindications, **VI:**201–202, 202b
    operative technique, **VI:**203–204, 203f–205f
  operative technique
    closed ruptures, **VI:**197
    flexor pollicis longus (FPL) injuries, **VI:**196, 196f–197f
    incisions, **VI:**187f
    partial tendon lacerations, **VI:**197
    pediatric injuries, **VI:**196–197
    surgical preparation, **VI:**186–197
    zone 1 injuries, **VI:**186–187, 188f
    zone 2 injuries, **VI:**187–194
    zone 3 injuries, **VI:**196
    zone 4 injuries, **VI:**196
    zone 5 injuries, **VI:**196
  outcomes and complicatons, **VI:**199–201, 201b, 201t

hands (Continued)
  patient presentation and diagnosis,
    VI:184–185, 185f
  postoperative care and follow-up
    care protocols, VI:197–199
    combined passive–active tendon
      motion protocol (Nantong regime),
      VI:199, 200f, 202f
    Duran–Houser method, VI:198–199,
      198f
    early active motion, VI:199
    modified Kleinert method, VI:197–198,
      198f
  secondary procedures
    free tendon grafting, VI:201–204
    general discussion, VI:201–208
    staged tendon reconstruction,
      VI:204–206
    tenolysis, VI:206–208
  staged tendon reconstruction
    indications, VI:204
    operative technique (first stage),
      VI:204–206, 205f–207f
    operative technique (second stage),
      VI:206, 208f
  surgical technique and treatment
    indications and contraindications,
      VI:186, 186b
    operative technique, VI:186–197
    primary and delayed primary repairs,
      VI:185–186, 186f
    surgical tips, VI:179b
  tenolysis
    anesthesia, VI:207
    indications, VI:206–207
    operative technique, VI:207–208, 208b
    postoperative treatment, VI:208
  zone 1 injuries, VI:186–187, 188f
  zone 2 injuries
    A2 pulley, VI:194f
    A4 pulley, VI:193f
    core suture methods, VI:189f, 193f
    cruciate method, VI:189f
    extension ability, VI:192f, 194f
    flexion ability, VI:191f, 194f
    four-strand repair, VI:191f–192f
    modified Kessler method, VI:189f
    operative technique, VI:187–194, 190f
    peripheral sutures, VI:192f
    pulley–sheath complex, VI:195f
    ruptured primary repair, VI:193f
    simple running peripheral repair,
      VI:191f
    six-strand M-Tang tendon repair,
      VI:190f–191f, 194f
    surgical summary, VI:195t
    surgical tips, VI:190b
  zone 3 injuries, VI:196
  zone 4 injuries, VI:196
  zone 5 injuries, VI:196
  fractures and joint injuries, VI:138–160
    anatomical considerations, VI:138–139
    associated deformities, VI:140f
    classification systems, VI:139, 139t, 141f
    complications, VI:158–159
    finger treatment strategies
      carpometacarpal (CMC) joints, VI:153,
        153f

hands (Continued)
    distal interphalangeal (DIP) joint,
      VI:141–142, 142f
    external fixation, VI:144, 145f
    hemi-hamate replacement arthroplasty
      (HHRA), VI:144–147, 146f–147f,
      147b
    internal fixation, VI:141–153
    metacarpal fractures, VI:150–153, 867
    metacarpal head fractures, VI:151
    metacarpal neck fractures, VI:151–152,
      151f
    metacarpal shaft fractures, VI:152, 152f
    metacarpophalangeal (MCP) joint,
      VI:150, 150f
    middle phalanx base articular fractures,
      VI:143–148, 143f
    middle phalanx shaft fractures, VI:142
    multiple metacarpal fractures, VI:152
    phalangeal fractures and dislocations,
      VI:141
    proximal interphalangeal (PIP) joint,
      VI:142–143, 143f, 144b
    proximal phalanx head fractures,
      VI:147
    proximal phalanx shaft and base
      fractures, VI:148, 149f
    surgical options, VI:141–153
    unicondylar fractures, VI:147–148, 148f
  fracture stabilization/fixation, VI:139
  open fractures, VI:139–140
  patient presentation and diagnosis,
    VI:140–141, 141f
  pediatric fractures, VI:139
  secondary procedures
    hardware removal, VI:159
    malunion correction, VI:159
    nonunion correction, VI:159
    tenolysis, VI:159
  surgical goals, VI:138
  thumb treatment strategies
    acute ulnar collateral ligament (UCL)
      tear, VI:155, 155f
    carpometacarpal (CMC) joint fractures,
      VI:156–158, 157f
    chronic ulnar collateral ligament (UCL)
      tear, VI:155–156, 156f
    general discussion, VI:153–158
    metacarpal fractures, VI:156
    metacarpophalangeal (MCP) joint,
      VI:153–154, 155f
    pediatric fractures, VI:158, 158f
    proximal phalanx neck fractures,
      VI:158, 159f
    Stener lesion, VI:154–155, 154f
Freeman–Sheldon syndrome, VI:646, 646f
generalized skeletal abnormalities,
  VI:642–644
Haas syndrome, VI:645–646, 646f
hand ischemia, VI:467–485
  acute ischemia
    acquired arteriovenous fistula,
      VI:473–474
    acute arterial injuries, VI:473, 473b
    arterial emboli, VI:473
    arterial injection injuries, VI:473
    cannulation injuries, VI:473
    iatrogenic injuries, VI:473

hands (Continued)
    aneurysms, VI:474, 479–481, 481f
    arteritis
      Buerger's disease, VI:474
      connective tissue disorders, VI:474
      Raynaud's phenomenon, VI:468, 474,
        474b, 475t, 479t
      vasospastic disease, VI:474
    chronic ischemia
      aneurysms, VI:474
      arterial thrombosis, VI:474
      treatment algorithms, VI:482–483
    complications, VI:484
    diagnostic tools
      angiography, VI:472, 472f
      capillaroscopy, VI:471
      computed tomography angiography,
        VI:472, 473f
      Duplex ultrasonography, VI:471, 472f
      infrared thermography, VI:472, 472f
      isolated cold stress tests, VI:471
      magnetic resonance angiography,
        VI:472
      pencil Doppler probe, VI:471
      ultrasound probes, VI:471
    etiology, VI:467, 468b
    medical management
      biofeedback, VI:476
      drug therapy, VI:475
      thrombolytic agents, VI:475–476
    nonsurgical interventions
      environmental modifications, VI:475
      medical management, VI:475–476
    occlusive/vasospastic/vaso-occlusive
      disease, VI:479t
    pathophysiology
      characteristics, VI:470
      emboli, VI:470
      systemic disease, VI:470
      traumatic causes, VI:470
    patient presentation and diagnosis
      evaluation examinations, VI:470
      patient history, VI:470–471
      physical examination, VI:470–471,
        471f
    patient selection, VI:473–474
    postoperative care and follow-up, VI:484
    prognosis and outcomes, VI:484
    Raynaud's phenomenon, VI:468, 474,
      474b, 475t, 479t
    secondary procedures, VI:484
    surgical treatment
      arterial reconstruction, VI:477–479,
        480f, 483f
      arteriectomy, VI:476
      characteristics, VI:476–479
      embolectomy, VI:476
      Leriche sympathectomy, VI:476
      limited digital sympathectomy, VI:478f
      periarterial sympathectomy, VI:476–
        477, 478f–479f
      radical digital sympathectomy, VI:479f
      sympathectomy, VI:476
    treatment strategies
      aneurysms, VI:479–481, 481f
      balloon angioplasty, VI:481, 482f
      evaluation examinations, VI:475–479
      nonsurgical interventions, VI:475–476

Note: **Boldface** roman numerals indicate volume. Page numbers followed by f refer to figures; page numbers followed by t refer to tables; page numbers followed by b refer to boxes.

hands (Continued)
    salvage options, **VI:**481–482
    surgical treatment, **VI:**476–479
    treatment algorithms, **VI:**482–483
    Wake Forest classifications, **VI:**479t
hand surgery, **VI:**xliii–xlix
    future directions, **VI:**xlviii
    historical background, **VI:**xlvf
    microsurgery, **II:**109
    modern hand surgery, **VI:**xlvi–xlvii
    origins, **VI:**xliii–xliv
    plastic surgery principles and
        applications, **VI:**xliv–xlvi
    post-World War II developments,
        II:108–109
    recent developments, **II:**110
hand therapy, **VI:**855–869
    basic principles, **VI:**855
    evaluative guidelines, **VI:**855–856
    nerve repair
        early postoperative care, **VI:**857–858
        general discussion, **VI:**857–859
        late rehabilitation, **VI:**858
        motor re-education, **VI:**858–859
        sensory re-education, **VI:**858, 858f
    post-nerve injury/surgery rehabilitation
        carpal tunnel syndrome, **VI:**856–857
        compression neuropathies, **VI:**856–857
        cubital tunnel syndrome, **VI:**857
        general discussion, **VI:**856–861
        nerve repair, **VI:**857–859
        nerve transfer, **VI:**859–861, 859f–860f
    post-skeletal injury/surgery rehabilitation
        metacarpal fractures, **VI:**150–153, 867,
            867f–868f
        proximal phalanx fractures, **VI:**866–867,
            867f
        thumb carpometacarpal osteoarthritis,
            VI:867–869, 868f
    post-tendon injury/surgery rehabilitation
        extensor tendon injuries, **VI:**862–865,
            865f
        flexor tendon injuries, **VI:**861–862,
            862f–864f, 862t
        tendon transfers, **VI:**865–866, 866f
        tenolysis, **VI:**159, 865
    research summary, **VI:**869
hand transplantation
    current status, **I:**834–837
    immunosuppression, **I:**834–835
    outcome assessments, **I:**835–837, **VI:**848
    transplant survival, **I:**834–835
    trauma-acquired defects, **I:**42
infections, **VI:**333–345
    antibiotics, **VI:**333
    bite wounds
        animal bites, **VI:**343
        characteristics, **VI:**343–344
        clenched-fist injuries, **VI:**343, 344f
        human bites, **VI:**343–344
    complications, **VI:**344
    disease process, **VI:**333–334
    infection mimics
        brown recluse spider bite, **VI:**336
        gout, **VI:**335, 335f
        granuloma annulare, **VI:**336
        pseudogout, **VI:**335
        pyoderma gangrenosum, **VI:**335–336,
            336f
        pyogenic granuloma, **VI:**335, 335f

hands (Continued)
        rheumatoid arthritis, **VI:**336
        treatment strategies, **VI:**335–336
    infection types
        cellulitis, **VI:**336
        deep space infections, **VI:**338–339, 338f
        felon, **VI:**337–338, 337f
        flexor tenosynovitis, **VI:**339, 340f
        fungal infections, **VI:**343
        herpetic whitlow, **VI:**342, 342f
        mycobacterial infections, **VI:**342–343
        necrotizing fasciitis, **VI:**341–342, 341f,
            342b
        noncholera *Vibrio* infections, **VI:**343
        osteomyelitis, **VI:**341
        paronychia, **VI:**336–337, 336f
        pyogenic flexor tenosynovitis, **VI:**339,
            340f
        septic arthritis, **VI:**339–341, 340f
    patient presentation and diagnosis
        bite wounds, **VI:**343–344
        hardware infections, **VI:**344
        infection classifications, **VI:**335, 335t
        infection mimics, **VI:**335–336
        infection types, **VI:**336–343
        methicillin-resistant Staphylococcus
            aureus (MRSA) infections, **VI:**334,
            334t
        patient history, **VI:**334–344
        physical examination, **VI:**334–344
    patient selection, **VI:**344
    prognosis and outcomes, **VI:**344
internal fracture fixation, **VI:**106–116
    Arbeitsgemeinschaft für
        Osteosynthesefragen (AO) principles,
        VI:106, 107t
    challenges, **VI:**106
    fixation options
        absolute versus relative stability,
            VI:108, 108b, 108f
        bridge plating, **VI:**113, 115f
        compression plating, **VI:**112–113, 114f
        external fixation, **VI:**110, 111f
        interfragmentary compression, **VI:**108
        interfragmentary lag screws, **VI:**111–
            112, 112f–113f
        Kirschner wires (K-wires), **VI:**107b,
            108–109, 109f, 110t, 139
        locked plating, **VI:**115, 115f
        tension band constructs, **VI:**109–110,
            109f–111f, 110t
    fluoroscopic imaging, **VI:**108–115
    fracture reduction
        basic procedure, **VI:**107
        Kapandji (intrafocal) pinning, **VI:**107b
        Kirschner wires (K-wires), **VI:**107b
        temporary/supplemental external
            fixation, **VI:**107b
    fractures and joint injuries, **VI:**138–160
        anatomical considerations, **VI:**138–139
        associated deformities, **VI:**140f
        classification systems, **VI:**139, 139t, 141f
        finger treatment strategies, **VI:**141–153
        fracture stabilization/fixation, **VI:**139
        hemi-hamate replacement arthroplasty
            (HHRA), **VI:**144–147, 146f–147f,
            147b
        open fractures, **VI:**139–140
        patient presentation and diagnosis,
            VI:140–141, 141f

hands (Continued)
        pediatric fractures, **VI:**139
        surgical goals, **VI:**138
    patient selection
        fracture assessment, **VI:**106
        host factors, **VI:**106
    postoperative care and follow-up, **VI:**115
    preoperative imaging assessment, **VI:**107
    research summary, **VI:**115
    surgical technique and treatment
        fracture reduction, **VI:**107
        preoperative planning, **VI:**107
    macrodactyly
        classification systems, **VI:**541f
        clinical manifestations, **VI:**634–635, 635f
        Hong Kong survey, **VI:**635t
        proteus syndrome, **VI:**635
        surgical technique and treatment, **VI:**636f
    Madelung's deformity, **VI:**646–647, 647f
    melanoma excisions, **I:**766–768
    metacarpal hand, **VI:**298–300, 298t,
        299f–300f
    metacarpophalangeal (MCP) joint
        Dupuytren's disease, **VI:**346–348, 349t,
            351–353, 355f
        fractures and joint injuries, **VI:**138–139,
            150, 150f, 153–154, 155f
        osteoarthritis
            anatomical considerations, **VI:**425
            arthrodesis, **VI:**429, 429f–430f
            biomechanics, **VI:**425
            implant arthroplasty, **VI:**426–429
            resurfacing arthroplasty, **VI:**425–426
            vascularized joint transfer/
                costochondral replacement,
                VI:429–430
    Mohr–Wriedt syndrome, **VI:**646
    multiple exotoses, **VI:**642–644, 644f
    mutilated/mangled hands, **VI:**250–281
        causal factors, **VI:**255, 256f
        flap reconstruction
            anterolateral thigh flap, **VI:**274–275,
                275f–276f
            cutaneous versus muscle flaps,
                VI:263–279
            fasciocutaneous flaps, **VI:**254–255,
                266–275
            free flaps, **VI:**254–255, 266–275
            lateral arm flap, **VI:**267, 269f–272f
            latissimus dorsi (LD) flap, **VI:**275,
                277f
            local flaps, **VI:**254–255
            muscle/musculocutaneous flaps,
                VI:254–255, 275–279
            pedicled groin flap, **VI:**264–266,
                265f–266f
            radial forearm flap, **VI:**266–267,
                267f–269f
            rectus abdominis, **VI:**275–277, 278f
            scapular and parascapular flaps,
                VI:272, 273f
            serratus anterior muscles, **VI:**277–279
            temporoparietal fascia flaps, **VI:**272–
                274, 274f
        initial evaluation and treatment
            debridement, **VI:**251, 251f
            guidelines, **VI:**250–255, 251b
            musculotendinous reconstruction,
                VI:253
            nerve repair, **VI:**253–254, 254f

hands (Continued)
  postoperative management, **VI**:255
  provisional revascularization, **VI**:251,
    252f
  skeletal stabilization, **VI**:251–252
  skin and soft-tissue reconstruction,
    VI:254–255
  vascular reconstruction, **VI**:252–253,
    253f
  injury impacts, **VI**:255–256
  injury types
    amputations, **VI**:256
    avulsion injuries, **VI**:256, 256f
    crush injuries, **VI**:256, 256f, 261f
    roller injuries, **VI**:256, 257f
  outcomes and complicatons, **VI**:279–281
  patient presentation and diagnosis
    emergency room evaluations,
      VI:256–257
    reconstruction planning, **VI**:257–259
  postoperative care and follow-up,
    VI:279
  reconstruction process
    amputation versus salvage decisions,
      VI:259
    delayed reconstruction, **VI**:259
    early (single-stage) reconstruction,
      VI:259
    emergency room evaluations,
      VI:257–259
    planning and preparation guidelines,
      VI:258
    spare-parts utilization, **VI**:259, 260f
    timing considerations, **VI**:258–259
  secondary procedures
    free fibula transfer, **VI**:279–280,
      280f
    innervated microvascular muscle
      transfer, **VI**:281
    microvascular toe transfer, **VI**:280–281,
      280f
  surgical technique and treatment
    bony reconstruction options, **VI**:259–
      261, 260f
    flap reconstruction, **VI**:263–279
    muscle reconstruction, **VI**:262
    nerve reconstruction, **VI**:262
    soft-tissue reconstruction, **VI**:262–263,
      263f–264f
    tendon graft and repair, **VI**:262
    vascular reconstruction options,
      VI:261–262, 261f
  occupational hand disorders, **VI**:363–370
    causal factors, **VI**:363–365
    clinical care
      chronic occupational injuries, **VI**:365–
        369, 365t
      de Quervain's tendonitis, **VI**:364–367,
        366f
      hand–arm vibration syndrome (HAVS),
        VI:368–369, 368t
      lateral epicondylitis, **VI**:366
      medial epicondylitis, **VI**:366
      nerve compression, **VI**:367–368
      patient management, **VI**:369
      tendinopathy, **VI**:366–368
      trigger finger, **VI**:367, 367f, 402–404
      vascular disorders, **VI**:368–369

hands (Continued)
  impairment measurement, **VI**:369–370
  patient presentation and diagnosis
    disease process, **VI**:364
    force, repetition, and vibration factors,
      VI:364–365, 366f
    patient history, **VI**:364
    physical examination, **VI**:364
  research summary, **VI**:370
  return to work, **VI**:369
  vascular disorders
    hand–arm vibration syndrome (HAVS),
      VI:368–369, 368t
    surgical treatment, **VI**:368–369
  work-related injuries, **VI**:363, 363b
  osteoarthritis, **VI**:411–448
    disease process, **VI**:412–413, 412f
    distal interphalangeal (DIP) joint
      biomechanical effects, **VI**:414
      diagnosis, **VI**:414, 415f
      distal interphalangeal (DIP)
        arthrodesis, **VI**:414–416
      surgical indicators, **VI**:414
    epidemiology, **VI**:411
    fingers, **VI**:414
    metacarpophalangeal (MCP) joint
      anatomical considerations, **VI**:425
      arthrodesis, **VI**:429, 429f–430f
      biomechanics, **VI**:425
      implant arthroplasty, **VI**:426–429
      resurfacing arthroplasty, **VI**:425–426
      vascularized joint transfer/
        costochondral replacement,
        VI:429–430
    pathophysiology, **VI**:413
    patient presentation and diagnosis,
      VI:413–414, 413f
    proximal interphalangeal (PIP) joint
      management approaches, **VI**:417–418
      prevalence and characteristics,
        VI:417–425
      proximal interphalangeal (PIP)
        arthrodesis, **VI**:418–419
    thumb
      carpometacarpal (CMC) arthroscopy,
        VI:434–439
      metacarpophalangeal (MCP) joint,
        VI:430
      prevalence and characteristics,
        VI:430–441
      prosthetic arthroplasty, **VI**:440–441,
        440f
      trapeziometacarpal arthritis,
        VI:430–434
      trapeziometacarpal arthrodesis,
        VI:440–441, 441f
  palmar dissections, **VI**:672, 672f, 672t
  partial hand, **VI**:872, 873f
  photographic guidelines, **I**:114, 118f
  physical examination
    examination guidelines, **VI**:48–60
    inspection process
      deformities, **VI**:48
      muscular atrophy, **VI**:48–49
      skin creases, **VI**:49
      skin discoloration, **VI**:48
      swelling, **VI**:49
      trophic changes, **VI**:49

hands (Continued)
  musculotendinous assessment
    dynamic tenodesis effect, **VI**:55–56
    Eichoff test, **VI**:56
    Finkelstein test, **VI**:56
    milking test, **VI**:56
    motion, **VI**:50
    posture, **VI**:50
    power, **VI**:50–51, 51t
    specific muscle tests, **VI**:51–52
  nerve assessment
    André–Thomas sign, **VI**:58–59
    Bouvier maneuver, **VI**:58–59
    "crossed fingers" sign, **VI**:58–59
    Duchenne's sign, **VI**:58–59
    Froment's test, **VI**:58, 58f
    Jeanne's sign, **VI**:58, 58f
    Moberg pick-up test, **VI**:59, 59f
    Phalen's test, **VI**:58, 58f
    Pitres–Testut sign, **VI**:58–59
    Semmes–Weinstein monofilament test,
      VI:53t, 59, 59t
    Tinel's sign, **VI**:56–58
    two-point discrimination (2 PD) testing,
      VI:52, 53t, 59
    Wartenberg's sign, **VI**:58, 58f
  palpation, **VI**:49
  range of motion assessment, **VI**:49
    extrinsic tightness test, **VI**:54
    flexor profundus test, **VI**:53
    flexor sublimis test, **VI**:53
    intrinsic tightness test, **VI**:53–54, 53f
    lumbrical muscle tightness test, **VI**:54,
      54f
  special provacative tests
    musculotendinous assessment,
      VI:55–56
    nerve assessment, **VI**:56–59
    range of motion assessment, **VI**:53–54
    stability assessment, **VI**:54–55
    vascular assessment, **VI**:60
  specific muscle tests
    extrinsic muscles, **VI**:51–52
    intrinsic muscles, **VI**:52
  stability assessment
    collateral ligaments, **VI**:49–50,
      49f–50f
    distal radioulnar joint instability test,
      VI:54–55, 56f
    extensor carpi ulnaris (ECU) synergy
      test, **VI**:55, 57f
    finger extension test, **VI**:54
    lunotriquetral shuck test, **VI**:54, 55f
    midcarpal instability test, **VI**:55
    pisiformis gliding test, **VI**:55, 57f
    scaphoid shift test, **VI**:54, 166f
    triquetrolunate ballottement test, **VI**:54,
      55f
    ulnocarpal abutment test, **VI**:55, 57f
  vascular assessment
    Allen's test, **VI**:52–53, 60
    digital Allen's test, **VI**:60
  Pierre–Robin syndrome, **VI**:646, 646f
  proximal interphalangeal (PIP) joint
    Dupuytren's disease, **VI**:346–348, 349t,
      351–353, 355f
    fractures and joint injuries, **VI**:138–139,
      142–143, 143f

hands (Continued)
  osteoarthritis
    management approaches, VI:417–418
    prevalence and characteristics,
      VI:417–425
    proximal interphalangeal (PIP)
      arthrodesis, VI:418–419
  radiographic imaging
    basic procedure, VI:69–70
    carpometacarpal joints (CMCJs),
      VI:69–70, 70f–71f
    osteoarthritis, VI:71f
    osteomyelitis, VI:70f
    pathological fractures, VI:70f
    pediatric hand radiographs, VI:71–72,
      72f–73f
    positioning, VI:69f
    soft-tissue mass, VI:69f
    special views, VI:70–71, 72b, 72f
    trapeziometacarpal joint (TMCJ),
      VI:70–71, 72b, 72f
  replantation and revascularization surgery
    complications, VI:248–249
    outcome assessments, VI:247–248, 247t
    proximal amputations, VI:238–241,
      238f–240f
    psychosocial aspects, VI:246–247
    secondary procedures, VI:248f, 249
  rheumatoid arthritis
    boutonnière deformity
      basic procedure, VI:396–398, 399f
      outcomes and complicatons, VI:398
      postoperative care and follow-up,
        VI:398
      surgical tips, VI:398b
      thumb deformities, VI:399–400, 400f
    crystalline arthropathy/gout, VI:407t,
      409–410
    infection mimics, VI:336
    metacarpophalangeal (MCP) arthrodesis
      basic procedure, VI:395
      outcomes and complicatons, VI:395
      postoperative care and follow-up,
        VI:395
    metacarpophalangeal (MCP)
        arthroplasty
      basic procedure, VI:392–394, 392f,
        394f
      entrance point, VI:392f
      final implant position, VI:394f
      osteotomy, VI:393f
      postoperative care and follow-up,
        VI:393–394
      PyroCarbon implants, VI:392f
    metacarpophalangeal (MCP)
        synovectomy and soft tissue
        reconstruction
      basic procedure, VI:390–391, 390f–391f
      outcomes and complicatons, VI:391,
        391f
      postoperative care and follow-up,
        VI:391
      secondary procedures, VI:391
      surgical tips, VI:395b
    operative procedures
      boutonnière deformity, VI:396–398
      metacarpophalangeal (MCP)
        arthrodesis, VI:395
      metacarpophalangeal (MCP)
        arthroplasty, VI:392–394

hands (Continued)
      metacarpophalangeal (MCP)
        synovectomy and soft tissue
        reconstruction, VI:390–391
      proximal interphalangeal (PIP)
        arthrodesis, VI:395
      proximal interphalangeal (PIP)
        arthroplasty, VI:394–395
      swan-neck deformity, VI:395–396
      thumb deformities, VI:399–400
    proximal interphalangeal (PIP)
        arthrodesis
      basic procedure, VI:395
      K-wire and stainless steel wire
        configuration, VI:396f
      outcomes and complicatons, VI:395
      postoperative care and follow-up,
        VI:395
    proximal interphalangeal (PIP)
        arthroplasty
      basic procedure, VI:394–395
      outcomes and complicatons, VI:395
      postoperative care and follow-up,
        VI:395
      secondary procedures, VI:395
      surgical tips, VI:395b
    scleroderma, VI:407t, 409
    seronegative spondyloarthropathies,
      VI:406–408, 407t
    swan-neck deformity
      basic procedure, VI:395–396,
        397f–398f
      postoperative care and follow-up,
        VI:396
      surgical tips, VI:398b
      thumb deformities, VI:399–400, 400f
    systemic lupus erythematosus (SLE),
      VI:407t, 408
    thumb deformities
      basic procedure, VI:399–400
      boutonnière deformity, VI:399–400,
        400f
      outcomes and complicatons, VI:400
      postoperative care and follow-up,
        VI:400
      swan-neck deformity, VI:400f
  sequelae obstetric brachial plexus palsy,
    VI:815
  soft-tissue fillers, II:57–58, 57f
  spastic hand, VI:449–466
    House functional classification for
      cerebral palsy, VI:459, 459t
    nonsurgical management, VI:459
    patient presentation and diagnosis,
      VI:459
    patient selection
      cerebral palsy, VI:459
      stroke/traumatic brain injury, VI:464
    research summary, VI:465
    surgical technique and treatment
      assessment strategies, VI:459–464
      elbows, VI:460, 461f
      forearm pronation, VI:460
      shoulder, VI:460
      stroke/traumatic brain injury, VI:464
      swan-neck deformity, VI:464, 465f
      thumb, VI:464, 464t
      typical spastic hemiplegic posture,
        VI:460f
      wrist flexion, VI:460–464, 462f–463f

hands (Continued)
    Zancolli classification of active finger
      and wrist extension, VI:461, 462t
  stiff hand, VI:449–466
    collateral ligament changes, VI:454, 454f
    extension contracture
      bone, VI:451–452, 451f
      capsular and pericapsular structures,
        VI:451
      collateral ligaments, VI:451
      dorsal capsule, VI:451
      flexor tendon adherence, VI:451
      intrinsic muscles, VI:451
      long extensors, VI:451
      patient presentation, VI:450–452, 450f
      skin, VI:450–451
      transverse retinacular ligaments, VI:451
      volar plate, VI:451
    flexion contracture
      accessory ligaments, VI:450
      bone, VI:450
      capsular and pericapsular structures,
        VI:449–450
      collateral ligaments, VI:449
      dorsal adhesions, VI:450
      intrinsic tendons, VI:450
      patient presentation, VI:449–450, 450f
      transverse retinacular ligaments, VI:450
      volar plate, VI:450
    general discussion, VI:449
    outcomes and complicatons, VI:458–459
    pathogenesis, VI:454–455, 457f
    patient presentation and diagnosis,
      VI:449–454
    patient selection, VI:455–456, 458f
    postoperative care and follow-up, VI:458
    secondary procedures, VI:459
    seesaw effect, VI:452–454, 452f–453f
    surgical technique and treatment
      metacarpophalangeal (MP) joint
        extension contracture, VI:457–458
      nonsurgical management, VI:456–458
      proximal interphalangeal (PIP) joint
        extension contracture, VI:457
      proximal interphalangeal (PIP) joint
        flexion contracture, VI:456–457
    volar plate changes, VI:454, 455f–456f
  tetraplegia
    biceps to triceps transfer
      advantages/disadvantages, VI:821–822
      postoperative care and follow-up,
        VI:822, 822f
      surgical technique, VI:821–822, 821f
    brachioradialis to flexor pollicis longus
      (FPL) transfer
      House intrinsic substitution procedure,
        VI:836f–837f
      IC group 2 and 3 patients, VI:830–832,
        831f
      operative procedures, VI:830–832,
        835f–837f, 839f–840f
      postoperative care and follow-up,
        VI:832, 841f
      surgical tips, VI:830b
      Zancolli "lasso" procedure, VI:835f
    carpometacarpal (CMC) joints
      IC group 4 and 5 patients, VI:834–838
      postoperative care and follow-up,
        VI:837–838
      stable thumb CMC joints, VI:837

hands (*Continued*)
 treatment strategies, **VI:**834–838
 unstable CMC joints, **VI:**837
 causal factors, **VI:**817
 classifications, **VI:**817–818, 818t
 deltoid to triceps transfer
  postoperative care and follow-up,
   VI:825
  surgical technique, **VI:**822–824, 822b,
   823f–824f
 elbow extension
  biceps to triceps transfer, **VI:**821–822
  deltoid to triceps transfer, **VI:**822–825
  hygiene considerations, **VI:**821f
  importance, **VI:**820–825
 grasp and release restoration
  extensor phase, **VI:**833
  flexor phase, **VI:**833, 833b
  House intrinsic substitution procedure,
   VI:834
  IC group 3 patients, **VI:**832–834
  IC groups 3, 4, and 5 patients,
   VI:832–834
  intrinsic stabilization, **VI:**833–834
  postoperative care and follow-up,
   VI:834
  Zancolli "lasso" procedure, **VI:**834
 IC group 0, 1 and 2 patients
  general considerations, **VI:**825–826
  postoperative care and follow-up,
   VI:826
  wrist extension, **VI:**825–826, 825f
 key pinch restoration
  brachioradialis to flexor pollicis longus
   (FPL) transfer, **VI:**830–832
  Brand–Moberg modification, **VI:**827–
   830, 828f–829f
  flexor pollicis longus (FPL) tenodesis,
   VI:827–830, 828f–829f
  IC group 1 and 2 patients, **VI:**826–830
  postoperative care and follow-up,
   VI:830
  split flexor pollicis longus (FPL) to
   extensor pollicis longus (EPL)
   interphalangeal stabilization,
   VI:826–827, 827f
  surgical technique and treatment,
   VI:826–830
  surgical tips, **VI:**826b
 reconstructive surgeries, **VI:**817–842
  general discussion, **VI:**817
  patient presentation, **VI:**818–820, 819f
  research summary, **VI:**840–841
  surgical team, **VI:**818–820
  surgical technique and treatment,
   VI:820–838
 surgical reconstruction
  elbow extension, **VI:**820–825
  functional electrical stimulation (FES),
   VI:838
  IC group 0, 1 and 2 patients,
   VI:825–826
  IC group 1 and 2 patients, **VI:**826–830,
   826b
  IC group 2 and 3 patients, **VI:**830–832
  IC group 4 and 5 patients, **VI:**834–838
  IC groups 3, 4, and 5 patients,
   VI:832–834

hands (*Continued*)
 IC groups 6, 7, and 8 patients, **VI:**838
 outcomes and complicatons, **VI:**838–
  840, 841f–842f
 strong grasp and refined pinch
  restoration, **VI:**838
 surgical guidelines, **VI:**820
 thumb and finger reconstruction,
  VI:295–310
 basic principles, **VI:**295–296
 complications, **VI:**309
 injury factors
  finger reconstruction, **VI:**297–298
  metacarpal hand, **VI:**298–300, 298t,
   299f–300f
  thumb reconstruction, **VI:**297
 patient presentation and diagnosis
  initial operation, **VI:**296–297
  patient evaluation, **VI:**296–297, 296f
 patient selection
  decision-making process, **VI:**297
  injury factors, **VI:**297–300
  primary versus secondary
   reconstruction, **VI:**297
 postoperative care and follow-up
  immediate postoperative period, **VI:**306
  motor rehabilitation, **VI:**306–307
  sensory rehabilitation, **VI:**307–308
 prognosis and outcomes
  appearance, **VI:**308
  donor site outcome evaluation, **VI:**308,
   309f
  range of motion, **VI:**308
  sensory recovery, **VI:**308
  strength assessment, **VI:**308
  success rates, **VI:**308
 secondary procedures, **VI:**309, 309f
 surgical technique and treatment
  combined second- and third-toe
   transplantations, **VI:**305, 307f
  donor closure guidelines, **VI:**301–302
  first dorsal metatarsal artery (FDMA),
   VI:300, 301f
  first-web neurosensory flap harvest,
   VI:305, 306f
  flap inset guidelines, **VI:**302–303, 302b,
   302f
  great-toe wrap-around flap harvest,
   VI:304–305
  pulp flap harvest, **VI:**305, 305f
  recipient preparation, **VI:**300–301, 301b,
   301f
  total or partial second-toe harvest,
   VI:304, 304f
  trimmed great toe harvest, **VI:**303–304,
   303f
  vascular dissection principles, **VI:**300,
   300b, 301f
 thumb hypoplasia, **VI:**572–602
  abductor digiti quinti minimi muscle
   (ADQM) transfer, **VI:**587–588, 589f
  associated conditions, **VI:**573–574, 573t
  characteristics, **VI:**572
  classification systems, **VI:**574, 574f
  clinical presentation, **VI:**574–583
  deficient first web space, **VI:**586–587
  etiology, **VI:**573
  Fanconi anemia (FA), **VI:**573t, 574

hands (*Continued*)
 flexor digitorum superficialis (FDS)
  transfer, **VI:**588–590
 four-flap Z-plasty, **VI:**585f, 586–587
 Holt–Oram syndrome, **VI:**573t, 574
 inadequate index finger, **VI:**599–600
 incidence, **VI:**572–573
 interphalangeal (IP) joint motion,
  VI:590
 metacarpophalangeal joint instability,
  VI:587, 588f
 outcomes and complicatons, **VI:**597–599
 patient presentation and diagnosis,
  VI:574–583
 patient selection, **VI:**583–584
 pollex abductus, **VI:**578f, 590
 pollicization technique, **VI:**590–594,
  591f–593f
 poor/absent palmar abduction
  (opposition), **VI:**587–590
 postoperative care and follow-up,
  VI:597
 secondary procedures, **VI:**599–600
 surgical technique and treatment,
  VI:586–594
 tendon graft stabilization, **VI:**587
 thrombocytopenia absent radius (TAR)
  syndrome, **VI:**573t, 574
 timing considerations, **VI:**546t, 583–584,
  583f
 Type I (mild hypoplasia), **VI:**574–575,
  575f, 584, 585f, 597
 Type II (moderate hypoplasia),
  VI:575–577, 576f, 578f, 584, 597
 Type III (severe hypoplasia), **VI:**577,
  579f–580f, 584, 587, 588f, 597
 Type IV (floating thumb), **VI:**577, 581f,
  586
 Type V (aplasia), **VI:**577, 582f, 586
 Type VI (cleft hand), **VI:**579–580,
  594–595, 598
 Type VI (symbrachydactyly thumb),
  VI:580–581, 595, 598
 Type VII (constriction ring syndrome),
  VI:581, 595–596, 599
 Type VIII (five-fingered hand),
  VI:581–582, 596, 599
 Type IX (radial polydactyly), **VI:**582–
  583, 596, 599
 Type X (syndromic short skeletal
  thumb ray), **VI:**583, 596–597, 599
 VACTERL association, **VI:**573t, 574
 toe-to-hand transplantations, **VI:**280–281,
  280f, 295–296, 296f, 555, 555f, 642,
  643f
tissue expansion, **I:**650
TNM clinical classification system/pTNM
 pathologic classification system, **I:**712f
trigger thumb
 etiology, **VI:**648
 general discussion, **VI:**648–649
 timing considerations, **VI:**546t
 treatment strategies, **VI:**648–649
tumors, **VI:**311–332
 background information, **VI:**311
 fibrous tissue lesions
  benign lesions, **VI:**321
  sarcomas, **VI:**321, 322f–323f

hands (Continued)
  lipoma, **VI:**321, 321f
  nerve tumors
    lipofibromatous hamartoma, **VI:**320–321, 320f
    neurofibromas, **VI:**320, 320f
    schwannomas, **I:**727, 728f, **VI:**320, 320f
  outcomes and complicatons, **VI:**331
  pathogenesis, **VI:**311–312
  patient presentation and diagnosis
    imaging methods, **VI:**312–313, 313f
    laboratory studies, **VI:**312
    patient history, **VI:**312
    physical examination, **VI:**312
  patient selection, **VI:**313
  postoperative care and follow-up, **VI:**331
  skin tumors
    actinic keratosis, **I:**736, 736f, **VI:**316–317, 317f
    basal cell carcinoma, **VI:**317, 317f
    benign pigmented nevus, **VI:**315, 315f
    characteristics, **VI:**313–318
    cutaneous horns, **VI:**314, 314f
    dermatofibroma, **I:**729, 729f, **VI:**316, 316f
    epidermal inclusion cysts, **VI:**314, 314f
    keratoacanthoma, **I:**719, 719f, **VI:**315–316, 316f
    melanoma, **VI:**318, 318f
    sebaceous cysts, **VI:**314, 314f
    seborrheic keratosis, **I:**719, 719f, **VI:**316
    squamous cell carcinomas (SCCs), **VI:**317, 317f
    verruca vulgaris, **VI:**314–315, 315f
  surgical technique and treatment
    aneurysmal bone cysts, **VI:**328–329, 328f
    benign fibrous lesions, **VI:**321
    chondrosarcoma, **I:**741, **VI:**329
    enchondromas, **VI:**327, 327f
    fibrous tissue lesions, **VI:**321
    giant cell tumors of the bone, **VI:**329, 329f
    glomus tumors, **VI:**324, 325f
    hemangiomas, **VI:**324, 324f
    leiomyoma, **VI:**326, 327f
    lipoma, **VI:**321, 321f
    metastatic lesions, **VI:**330–331, 330f
    musculoskeletal sarcomas, **VI:**329–330, 330t
    myositis ossificans, **VI:**326, 326f
    nerve tumors, **VI:**320–321
    osteochondroma, **VI:**328, 328f
    osteoid osteoma, **VI:**327, 327f
    osteosarcoma, **I:**741, 741f, **VI:**329
    pyogenic granuloma, **VI:**324–326, 325f
    rhabdomycosarcoma, **VI:**326
    sarcomas, **VI:**321, 322f–323f
    skin tumors, **VI:**313–318
    solitary unicameral bone cysts, **VI:**328, 328f
    synovial lesions, **VI:**318–319
    vascular lesions, **VI:**324–326
    vascular malformations, **VI:**324, 324f–325f
  synovial lesions
    ganglion cysts, **VI:**318–319, 319f
    giant cell tumors, **VI:**319, 319f
    pigmented villonodular synovitis, **VI:**319, 319f

hands (Continued)
  vascular lesions
    glomus tumors, **VI:**324, 325f
    hemangiomas, **VI:**324, 324f
    pyogenic granuloma, **VI:**324–326, 325f
    vascular malformations, **VI:**324, 324f–325f
Hand Transplantation Score System, **VI:**848
handwriting analyses, **I:**95–96
hanging fingertip, **VI:**221–222, 222f
Hanover Fracture Scale-97 (HFS-97), **IV:**63
hard palate
  anatomical characteristics, **III:**422f
  cancer management
    diagnosis and treatment, **III:**427
    preoperative assessment, **III:**408, 408f
    treatment strategies, **III:**408
hardware infections, **VI:**344
Harmony^XL laser, **II:**71t, 73
Harpagophytum procumbens, **V:**33t–35t
Hartrampf, Carl, **V:**393–394
hateful patients, **I:**36–37
haversian system, **I:**426, 426f
head
  acquired cranial and facial bone deformities, **III:**226–242
    access incisions
      coronal incisions, **III:**226–227, 227f
      intraoral incisions, **III:**227
      lower eyelid incisions, **III:**227
    background and general characteristics, **III:**226
    bone grafts
      donor site considerations, **III:**227, 228f–229f
      soft-tissue cover, **III:**227
    complications, **III:**242
    postoperative care and follow-up, **III:**240–242
    prognosis and outcomes, **III:**242
    secondary procedures, **III:**242
    surgical technique and treatment
      chin implants, **III:**240, 240f–241f
      cranium, **III:**228, 230f–231f
      irradiated orbit, **III:**235–238
      mandibular fractures, **III:**238–240, 239f
      mandibular reconstruction, **III:**240
      maxillary buttresses, **III:**236–238
      maxillary reconstructiion, **III:**238–240, 238f
      nasoethmoid area, **III:**232, 234f
      nose, **III:**228–229, 231f–233f
      orbitozygomatic region, **III:**232–234, 235f–236f
      posttraumatic enophthalmos, **III:**234–235, 237f
  anatomical characteristics, **III:**3–22
    adhesions, **III:**8–10
    buccal fat pad, **III:**10–11
    ears, **III:**19
    eyelids, **III:**19–21, 20f
    facial nerve
      buccal branch, **III:**12f, 13
      cervical branch, **III:**12f, 13–14
      deep fascia, **III:**6
      frontal/temporal branch, **III:**12–13, 12f
      general characteristics, **III:**11–14
      marginal mandibular nerve, **III:**12f, 13
      schematic diagram, **III:**9f, 12f

head (Continued)
  sensory nerve connections, **III:**14
  zygomatic branch, **III:**12f, 13
  fascial layers
    general characteristics, **III:**3–8, 4f–5f
    periorbital ligaments, **III:**9f
    superficial musculoaponeurotic system (SMAS), **III:**4f–5f, 5–6
    temporal region, **III:**6–7, 6f–8f, 106–107, 107f
  malar fat pad, **III:**10
  mastication muscles
    aesthetic importance, **III:**17
    general characteristics, **III:**16–17
    lateral pterygoid muscle, **III:**16
    masseter muscle, **III:**16
    medial pterygoid muscle, **III:**16
    muscle actions, **III:**16
    pterygomasseteric sling, **III:**16
    temporalis muscle, **III:**16
  musculature
    corrugators, **II:**110–111, 110f, **III:**15
    depressor supercilii, **III:**15–16
    frontalis, **III:**14
    galeal fat pad, **III:**14
    general discussion, **III:**14–16
    glide plane, **III:**14
    midfacial muscles, **III:**16
    procerus, **II:**110–111, 110f, **III:**15
    schematic diagram, **III:**15f
  nose, **III:**21
  retaining ligaments, **III:**8–10, 10f–11f
  sensory nerves, **III:**17–19, 17f–18f
head cancer
  cervical lymph nodes, **III:**415f
  complications
    dental follow-ups, **III:**418
    general discussion, **III:**416–418
    local recurrence, **III:**416
    osteoradionecrosis (ORN), **III:**417
    post-treatment surveillance, **III:**417–418
    regional recurrence, **III:**416–417
    wound infections, **III:**417
  epidemiology, **III:**399–400
  lymph node anatomy, **III:**399f
  medical challenges, **III:**398
  nodal status determination, **III:**429–431, 430f
  oral cavity/mouth/tongue/mandibular reconstruction, **III:**307–335
    acute complications, **III:**333
    challenges, **III:**307–308
    chronic complications, **III:**333–334
    decision-making process, **III:**311–313
    defect factors, **III:**310–311, 310t
    disease process, **III:**308
    flap options, **III:**310t
    free tissue transfer, **III:**311
    local/regional flaps, **III:**309t, 311
    patient factors, **III:**308–310, 310t
    patient presentation and diagnosis, **III:**308
    patient selection, **III:**308–316
    postoperative care and follow-up, **III:**332–333
    prognosis and outcomes, **III:**333–334
    secondary procedures, **III:**334
    skin grafts, **III:**311
    soft tissue flaps, **III:**309t
    surgical technique, **III:**316–332

head *(Continued)*
    pathogenesis, **III**:398–399
    patient presentation and diagnosis, **III**:400
    psychological aspects, **I**:43–44
    radiation treatment, **I**:668–669
    risk factors
        alcohol, **III**:421
        gastroesophageal reflux, **III**:421
        infectious agents, **III**:421
        pollution exposure, **III**:421–422
        tobacco, **III**:421
    surgical access, **III**:402, 403f–404f
    therapeutic choices, **III**:401–402
    TNM clinical classification system, **III**:308, 400–401, 401t
    upper aerodigestive tract, **III**:420–439
        anatomical considerations, **III**:422–424
        diagnosis and treatment, **III**:427–437
        epidemiology, **III**:420
        future trends, **III**:438
        incidence, **III**:421–427
        outcomes and complicatons, **III**:438
        patient evaluation, **III**:424–427
        postoperative care and follow-up, **III**:437–438
        prevalence, **III**:421–427
        risk factors, **III**:421–422
infantile hemangioma (IH), **I**:680
melanoma excisions, **I**:766, 767f
muscle/musculocutaneous flaps, **I**:542–546, 543f–546f
soft-tissue injuries
    systematic head and neck evaluations
        airway evaluation, **III**:25
        basic procedure, **III**:24–25
        cheek examination, **III**:25, 25f
        ear examination, **III**:25, 25f, 40
        eye examination, **III**:25
        nose examination, **III**:25
        oral cavity and mouth examination, **III**:25
tissue expansion
    basic principles, **I**:631–640
    ears, **I**:637–638
    forehead, **I**:635
    lateral face and neck, **I**:635–637, 636f, 638f
    male-pattern baldness, **I**:633–635
    nose, **I**:637, 639f
    periorbital area, **I**:638–640, 641f–642f
    scalp, **I**:631–633, 632f–634f
TNM clinical classification system/pTNM pathologic classification system, **I**:714f
healthcare–industrial complex, **I**:64–65
health information technology (HIT), **I**:171
Health Insurance Portability and Accountability Act (HIPAA, 1996), **I**:92–93, 121
Heberden's nodes, **VI**:414
Hedgehog signaling pathway, **I**:428–429
heel pad flaps, **IV**:209
Heister, Lorenz, **I**:18
helical rim, **III**:218–219, 219f
Helicobacter pylori, **II**:20–21, **III**:421
Heliodorus, **VI**:xliii–xliv
hemangioendothelioma, **I**:677t–678t, **VI**:668t

hemangiomas
    arteriovenous malformation (AVM)
        causal factors, **VI**:684–690
        pathogenesis, **VI**:685–686
        patient presentation and diagnosis, **VI**:686–687, 686f–688f
        Schobinger clinical staging system, **VI**:686t
        surgical technique and treatment, **VI**:687–690, 689f
    capillary malformation-arteriovenous malformation (CM-AVM)
        pathogenesis, **VI**:691
        patient presentation and diagnosis, **VI**:691
        surgical technique and treatment, **VI**:691
    capillary malformations (CM)
        pathogenesis, **VI**:675
        patient presentation and diagnosis, **VI**:675, 677f
    classification systems, **I**:677t, **VI**:667–669, 668t
    CLOVES syndrome
        pathogenesis, **VI**:691
        patient presentation and diagnosis, **VI**:692
        surgical technique and treatment, **VI**:692
    congenital hemangioma (CH)
        classification systems, **I**:677t
        clinical manifestations, **I**:687
        pathogenesis, **VI**:673–674
        patient presentation and diagnosis, **VI**:674, 676f
        surgical technique and treatment, **VI**:674
        treatment strategies, **I**:687
    diagnostic work-up, **VI**:670t
    hands, **VI**:83–85, 324, 324f
    historical background, **VI**:667–669
    infantile hemangioma (IH)
        classification systems, **I**:677t
        clinical manifestations
            characteristics, **I**:680–681
            head and neck hemangiomas, **I**:680
            hepatic hemangiomas, **I**:680–681
            multiple hemangiomas, **I**:680
            structural anomalies, **I**:681
        diagnosis, **I**:681
        nonoperative management
            embolic therapy, **I**:684
            intralesional corticosteroids, **I**:682
            laser therapy, **I**:684
            observation, **I**:681
            systemic corticosteroids, **I**:682–684
            topical corticosteroids, **I**:682
            wound care, **I**:682
        operative management
            involuted phase (late childhood), **I**:685
            involuting phase (early childhood), **I**:678f, 684–685
            proliferative phase (infancy), **I**:677f, 684
        pathogenesis, **I**:678–680, **VI**:672–673
        patient presentation and diagnosis, **VI**:672–673, 674f
        surgical technique and treatment, **VI**:673, 675f
        terminology, **I**:678t

hemangiomas *(Continued)*
    kaposiform hemangioendothelioma (KHE)
        classification systems, **I**:677t, **VI**:668t
        clinical manifestations, **I**:687
        treatment strategies, **I**:687–688
    Klippel–Trenaunay syndrome
        outcomes and complicatons, **VI**:691
        pathogenesis, **VI**:691
        patient presentation and diagnosis, **VI**:691
        surgical technique and treatment, **VI**:691
    lymphatic malformation (LM)
        outcomes and complicatons, **VI**:679–680
        pathogenesis, **VI**:675–677
        patient presentation and diagnosis, **VI**:677–679, 678f
        surgical technique and treatment, **VI**:679, 680f–681f
    palmar dissections, **VI**:672, 672f, 672t
    Parkes–Weber syndrome
        outcomes and complicatons, **VI**:690–691
        pathogenesis, **VI**:690
        patient presentation and diagnosis, **VI**:690
        surgical technique and treatment, **VI**:690
    patient presentation and diagnosis, **VI**:669, 670f
    PTEN (phosphatase and tensin homologue)-associated vascular anomaly (PTEN-AVA)
        classification systems, **I**:677t
        pathogenesis, **VI**:690
        patient presentation and diagnosis, **VI**:690
        surgical technique and treatment, **VI**:690
    pyogenic granuloma
        clinical manifestations, **I**:688
        pathogenesis, **VI**:674
        patient presentation and diagnosis, **I**:747–750, 748f, **VI**:675, 677f
        surgical technique and treatment, **VI**:675
    salivary gland tumors, **III**:364t–365t, 368, 369f, 373
    surgical technique and treatment, **VI**:669–672, 671t
    thumb/digital dissections, **VI**:672, 673f, 673t
    venous malformations (VM)
        associated syndromes, **VI**:682–684
        outcomes and complicatons, **VI**:684
        pathogenesis, **VI**:680–682
        patient presentation and diagnosis, **VI**:681f
        surgical technique and treatment, **VI**:682–684, 683f, 685f
    verrucous hemangioma (VH), **I**:677t, 695
hemangioma simplex, **I**:734, 734f–735f
hemangiomatosis, **I**:680, **VI**:668t
hemangiopericytoma, **VI**:668t
hematomas
    abdominal wall reconstruction, **IV**:293
    abdominoplasty, **II**:557–558
    brachioplasty, **II**:629t
    breast augmentation, **V**:32–37, 79t
    breast implants, **V**:359, 359f, 364t
    burn wound complications, **IV**:433t
    endoscopic augmentation mammaplasty, **V**:87–88
    endoscopic breast reconstruction, **V**:93–96

hematomas (Continued)
  facial aesthetic surgery, I:131–132
  facial skeletal augmentation, II:343
  lower extremity reconstructive surgery,
      IV:137
  male chest contouring, V:579
  mastopexy, V:150, 243t
  muscle/musculocutaneous flaps, I:571–572
  nails and fingertips, VI:119
  nasal fractures, III:60
  neck rejuvenation, II:324–325
  orbital fractures, III:53–54, 54f, 56
  periareolar surgical technique with mesh
      support, V:226, 226t
  postmastectomy breast reconstruction,
      V:359, 359f
  retrobulbar hematoma, III:56
  revisionary breast surgery, V:65–66, 66t, 79t,
      245–246, 246f
  rhinoplasty complications, II:411, 446
  scalp and forehead reconstruction,
      III:131–132
  sculpted pillar vertical reduction
      mammaplasty, V:236–239
  silicone gel implants, V:104–105, 104f–105f
  skin graft complications, I:334
  traumatic ear injuries, III:40–41, 41f
  upper extremity surgery, VI:102
  vertical scar reduction mammaplasty,
      V:191t
hematopoietic stem cells (HSCs), I:263,
    369–371
hemicorporectomy, IV:380, 381f–382f
hemifacial atrophy, III:792–802
  causal factors, III:792
  clinical manifestations
    central nervous system involvement,
        III:796
    cutaneous and subcutaneous tissue
        involvement, III:794–795, 795f
    general characteristics, III:794–797, 794f
    musculoskeletal involvement, III:795
    ocular involvement, III:796
    oral involvement, III:796–797, 796f
  complications, III:800–801
  differential diagnoses, III:797, 797f
  epidemiology, III:794
  etiopathogenesis
    autoimmune process, III:793
    general discussion, III:793–794
    histologic studies, III:793
    infection hypothesis, III:794
    neurogenic manifestations, III:793
    trauma-acquired defects, III:794
  laboratory studies, III:797
  patient selection and treatment, III:792–793
  prognosis and outcomes, III:800–801
  prognostic indicators, III:797
  secondary procedures, III:801–802
  surgical technique and treatment
    immunosuppressive therapy, III:797–798,
        798f
    nonsurgical interventions, III:798, 799f
    surgical intervention
      basic principles, III:798–800, 800f–802f
      scapular and parascapular flaps,
          III:799–800, 800f
hemi-hamate replacement arthroplasty
    (HHRA), VI:144–147, 146f–147f, 147b
hemopoietic markers (CDs), I:370

hemorrhage, II:371, 445, III:69, 74, IV:85
hemostasis
  facelift complications, II:205, 205f
  hair transplantation, II:503–504
  skin wound healing, I:268–269, 268f
  wound healing, I:242–245, 243f
hemothorax, IV:433t
Henry of Mondeville, I:15
heparin, I:582, 615–617, VI:244–245
heparin-binding epidermal growth factor
    (HB–EGF), I:270t, 275
heparin sulfate proteoglycan (HSPG), I:180f
hepatic hemangiomas, I:680–681
hepatitis B virus, I:459
hepatitis C virus, I:459
hepatocyte growth factor (HGF), III:837–838
HER2/neu oncoprotein, V:266–267
herbs/herbal extracts, V:33t–35t
hereditary hemorrhagic telangiectasia (HHT),
    I:677t, 696–698
hernia repair, IV:279–296
  background information, IV:279–280
  complications
    adhesions, IV:294
    pain management, IV:294–295
    recurrences, IV:294
    secondary hernias, IV:294
    seromas, IV:294
    wound breakdown, IV:294
  disease process, IV:280, 281f
  outcome assessments, IV:293
  patient presentation and diagnosis,
      IV:280–282
  patient selection, IV:282–283
  postoperative care and follow-up
    abdominal binders, IV:293
    analgesia, IV:293
    antibiotic therapy, IV:292–293
    drain management, IV:293
    limited physical activity, IV:293
    muscle relaxation, IV:293
    nutritional support, IV:292
    postoperative management, IV:291–292
  prognosis, IV:293–294
  research summary, IV:295
  secondary procedures, IV:295
  surgical technique and treatment
    abdominal wall transplantation, IV:290
    adjunctive techniques, IV:291, 292f
    autologous tissue repair, IV:289
    bioburden reduction, IV:283–284
    component separation method, IV:284–
        289, 285f–289f
    fascia lata grafts, IV:289, 290f
    negative-pressure wound therapy, IV:284
    parastomal hernia repair, IV:290
    primary suture technique, IV:284
    tissue expansion, IV:289–290, 291f
herpes simplex viruses, I:186–187, 188t
herpetic whitlow, VI:337, 342, 342f
Herring's law, II:145, 147f
heterodigital flaps
  cross finger flaps, VI:130–131, 133f
  dorsal metacarpal artery flaps, VI:134,
      135f
  Littler neurovascular island flap,
      VI:132–134
  thenar crease flap, VI:132, 134f
heterografts, I:325t
heterotopic ossification, IV:446

hidden penis
  characteristics, II:665–668, 665f–666f, IV:304,
      304f
  outcome assessments, II:668
  post-bariatric surgery reconstruction, II:640,
      643f
  surgical technique, II:667–668, 667f–669f,
      IV:305f
Highet Scale, VI:715, 716t
high median nerve palsy
  opposition tendon transfers, VI:761t
  outcomes and complicatons, VI:761
  patient selection, VI:759–761, 760f
  surgical technique and treatment, VI:759–
      761, 760f, 761t
high-molecular-weight kininogen, I:243f, 244
high ulnar nerve palsy
  outcome assessments, VI:771–772
  patient selection, VI:771
high velocity gunshot wounds, III:86–87
Hildanus, Fabricius, IV:393
Hippocrates
  burn wound treatment, IV:393
  hand surgery, VI:xliii–xliv
  reconstructive and aesthetic surgery, I:13
  wound healing, I:241
hips/flanks
  anatomical characteristics
    musculature, IV:6f, 13f
    skeletal structure, IV:8, 9f
  burn reconstruction, IV:443–444, 443t
  liposuctions, II:522–523, 522f–523f
hirudin, I:617
Hirudo medicinalis, I:617, VI:241–242
histamine, I:573–574, 574f
histiocystoma, I:736
histiocytic sarcoma, I:742
historical plastic surgery, I:11–29
  aesthetic surgery
    beauty doctors, I:26–27, 28f
    origins, I:25–26
    postwar aesthetic surgery, I:28
    rhinoplasty, I:26f
  ancient Egypt, I:11–12
  Byzantine Empire, I:14
  eighteenth century, I:18–19, 19f
  India, I:12–13, 13f
  Mesopotamia, I:12
  Middle Ages
    Arabian surgery, I:14–15
    printed textbooks, I:15
    universities, I:15, 15f
  nineteenth century, I:19–20
  Renaissance
    nose reconstruction, I:16–18, 18f
    surgeries, I:15–16, 16f–17f
    surgery decline, I:18
  Rome, I:13–14, 14f
  twentieth century
    modern plastic surgery, I:20–23, 22f–23f
    postwar plastic surgery, I:25, 25f–26f
    scientific journals, I:24–25, 25f
    scientific societies, I:24
    training programs, I:23–24
  wound management, I:11
histrionic personality, I:36
Hoffman–Tinel sign, VI:157, VI:796
holoprosencephaly (HPE), III:505, 506t
Holt–Oram syndrome, VI:538f, 573t, 574, 617t
homeopathic medicines, V:33t–35t

homodigital flaps, **VI:**130, 132f
homografts, **I:**325t
Hong Ge, **IV:**393
hooked nails
  characteristics, **VI:**124
  surgical technique and treatment,
    VI:124–125
horizontal advancement genioplasty, **II:**316,
    316f
hormone replacement therapy, **II:**194
Horner's syndrome, **IV:**433t, **VI:**796
Hospital Referral Regions (HRRs), **V:**315–316
Hospital Service Areas (HSAs), **V:**315–316
hot loop electrocoagulation, **II:**21t
hot tar burns, **IV:**395–396
hot water scalds, **IV:**394, 394f
House functional classification for cerebral
    palsy, **VI:**459, 459t
household bleach, **IV:**461–463
House intrinsic substitution procedure,
    VI:834, 836f–837f
Hoxa transcription factors, **VI:**531–532
Hox genes, **III:**518, 706, **VI:**530
Huber transfer, **VI:**758, 761t
Hueter–Volkmann principle, **VI:**658–659
human acellular dermal matrix (HADM), **I:**796
human bites, **VI:**219, 219f, 343–344
human embryonic stem cells (hESCs)
  clinical correlates, **I:**216–217
  current research and applications, **I:**215–216,
    215f
  definition, **I:**214–215
  research background, **I:**214–215
Human Genome Project, **I:**191–192
human growth hormone (hGH), **I:**189–190
human immunodeficiency virus (HIV), **I:**459
human leukocyte antigen (HLA), **I:**815–816
human papillomavirus-associated cyst, **I:**720
human papilloma virus (HPV), **III:**399, 421
human resource management, **I:**83–84
humectants
  characteristics, **II:**17–18
  glycerin, **II:**17–18
humerus, **IV:**181, 186f
humpback deformity, **VI:**165, 165f, 171
Hunstad's Formula, **II:**516t
Hunter's canal, **IV:**19–22
Hutchinson freckle, **I:**747–748, 749f
hyaline cartilage, **I:**397, 398f
HyalSkin, **II:**47t
Hyaluderm, **II:**47t
hyaluronic acid, **I:**270–271, 376f, **II:**47, 47t, 49t
  See also soft-tissue fillers
HydraFill, **II:**47t
hydrochloric acid, **IV:**461–463
hydrocolloids, **I:**289t
hydrofluoric acid, **IV:**461–462, 464
hydrogels, **I:**289t, 375–377, 377f, 627
hydrogen peroxide (H$_2$O$_2$), **I:**256, 256f, 575,
    575f, **VI:**228–229
hydroquinone, **II:**24
hydroxy acids
  alpha hydroxy acids (AHAs)
    characteristics, **II:**18–19
    glycolic acid, **II:**19
    lactic acid, **II:**18–19
    patient selection and treatment, **II:**66–67
  beta hydroxy acid (BHA), **II:**19

hydroxycoumarins, **II:**25
hydroxyl radical (OH), **I:**575, 575f, **VI:**228–229
hydroxyurea, **I:**779–781
Hylaform, **II:**49t
  See also soft-tissue fillers
hyperacute rejection, **I:**819
hyperbaric oxygen (HBO) therapy, **IV:**253
hypercellular-type fibrous dysplasia, **III:**381
hyperglycemia, **IV:**194–195
hyperhidrosis, **II:**42
hyperpigmentation/skin discoloration
  buttock augmentation, **II:**615
  liposuctions, **II:**526
hypertelorism
  characteristics, **III:**686
  oculomotor disorders, **III:**699
  outcomes and complicatons, **III:**698
  pathogenesis, **III:**686–689
  patient presentation and diagnosis
    faciocraniosynostosis
      Apert syndrome, **III:**689
      characteristics, **III:**688–689
      craniofrontonasal dysplasia, **III:**689
      Crouzon syndrome, **III:**688, 688f
      Pfeiffer syndrome, **III:**688–689
    median facial clefts, **III:**687
    Tessier cleft classification system,
      III:687–688, 687f
  patient selection, **III:**689
  postoperative care and follow-up,
    III:695–696
  recurrences, **III:**699–700
  secondary procedures, **III:**698f
    canthus correction, **III:**698f, 699
    eyebrows, **III:**699
    eyelids, **III:**699
    nose, **III:**699
    orbits, **III:**699
    scalp, **III:**699
    soft-tissue problems, **III:**698–700
  surgical technique and treatment
    asymmetrical cases, **III:**693–694
    basic principles, **III:**689–690, 690f
    bipartition surgery, **III:**693, 693f
    box-shift osteotomies
      basic procedure, **III:**692–693, 692f,
        694f
      frontal craniectomy, **III:**692–693
      orbit osteotomies, **III:**693
    indicators and timing
      face, **III:**694–695
      general discussion, **III:**694–695
      orbits, **III:**694, 694f
    infrafrontal correction, **III:**690–692,
      691f
    Le Fort III osteotomy–bipartition
      correction technique
      basic procedure, **III:**696f–697f
      bone grafts, **III:**695
      coronal approach, **III:**695
      general discussion, **III:**695
      osteosynthesis, **III:**695
      subcranial osteotomies, **III:**695
    surgical technique, **III:**690, 691f
hypertension
  local anesthesia, **I:**145
  rhinoplasty complications, **II:**410–411
hypertrophic rhinitis, **II:**454, 458

hypertrophic scars
  benign mesenchymal-origin tumors, **I:**730,
    731f
  brachioplasty, **V:**563–564
  laser treatments, **II:**69
  reconstructive burn surgery, **IV:**434, 497,
    501, 501f–502f
  wound healing, **I:**265, 283–284, 283t, 293f,
    302, 302t, 303f, 307–308
hypochlorous acid (HOCl), **I:**256, 256f
hypochondriasis, **I:**33
hypodermis, **IV:**397–402
hyponychial defects
  characteristics, **VI:**125
  surgical technique and treatment, **VI:**125
hypopharynx
  anatomical characteristics, **III:**337, 337f,
    432–433
  characteristics, **III:**432–433
  nodal status determination, **III:**432–433
  TNM clinical classification system,
    III:432–433
  See also pharyngoesophageal
    reconstruction
hypoplastic breast
  basic principles, **I:**647–648
  immature breast, **I:**648
  Poland syndrome, **I:**648, 649f
  tuberous breast, **I:**647
hypoplastic thumb, **VI:**572–602
  associated conditions, **VI:**573t
    Fanconi anemia (FA), **VI:**573t, 574
    general discussion, **VI:**573–574
    Holt–Oram syndrome, **VI:**573t, 574
    thrombocytopenia absent radius (TAR)
      syndrome, **VI:**573t, 574
    VACTERL association, **VI:**573t, 574
  characteristics, **VI:**572
  classification systems, **VI:**574, 574f
  clinical presentation
    general characteristics, **VI:**574–583
    Type I (mild hypoplasia), **VI:**574–575, 575f
    Type II (moderate hypoplasia), **VI:**575–
      577, 576f, 578f
    Type III (severe hypoplasia), **VI:**577,
      579f–580f
    Type IV (floating thumb), **VI:**577, 581f
    Type V (aplasia), **VI:**577, 582f
    Type VI (cleft hand), **VI:**579–580
    Type VI (symbrachydactyly thumb),
      VI:580–581
    Type VII (constriction ring syndrome),
      VI:581
    Type VIII (five-fingered hand),
      VI:581–582
    Type IX (radial polydactyly), **VI:**582–583
    Type X (syndromic short skeletal thumb
      ray), **VI:**583
  etiology, **VI:**573
  inadequate index finger, **VI:**599–600
  incidence, **VI:**572–573
  outcomes and complicatons
    Type I (mild hypoplasia), **VI:**597
    Type II (moderate hypoplasia), **VI:**597
    Type III (severe hypoplasia), **VI:**597
    Type VI (cleft hand), **VI:**598
    Type VI (symbrachydactyly thumb),
      VI:598

Note: **Boldface** *roman numerals indicate volume. Page numbers followed by f refer to figures; page numbers followed by t refer to tables; page numbers followed by b refer to boxes.*

hypoplastic thumb (Continued)
Type VII (constriction ring syndrome), **VI:**599
Type VIII (five-fingered hand), **VI:**599
Type IX (radial polydactyly), **VI:**599
Type X (syndromic short skeletal thumb ray), **VI:**599
patient presentation and diagnosis, **VI:**574–583
patient selection, **VI:**583
postoperative care and follow-up, **VI:**597
secondary procedures, **VI:**599–600
surgical technique and treatment
abductor digiti quinti minimi muscle (ADQM) transfer, **VI:**587–588, 589f
deficient first web space, **VI:**586–587
flexor digitorum superficialis (FDS) transfer, **VI:**588–590
four-flap Z-plasty, **VI:**585f, 586–587
interphalangeal (IP) joint motion, **VI:**590
metacarpophalangeal joint instability, **VI:**587, 588f
pollex abductus, **VI:**578f, 590
pollicization technique
basic principles, **VI:**590
dissection and exposure, **VI:**590
general discussion, **VI:**590–594
incisions, **VI:**590, 592f–593f
operative technique, **VI:**591f–593f
outcomes and complicatons, **VI:**598
skeletal shortening, **VI:**594
skin closure and web construction, **VI:**594
tendon and intrinsic muscle rebalancing, **VI:**594
poor/absent palmar abduction (opposition), **VI:**587–590
tendon graft stabilization, **VI:**587
Type III (severe hypoplasia), **VI:**587, 588f
Type VI (cleft hand), **VI:**594–595
Type VI (symbrachydactyly thumb), **VI:**595
Type VII (constriction ring syndrome), **VI:**595–596
Type VIII (five-fingered hand), **VI:**596
Type IX (radial polydactyly), **VI:**596
Type X (syndromic short skeletal thumb ray), **VI:**596–597
timing considerations, **VI:**546t, 583–584, 583f
treatment strategies
Type I (mild hypoplasia), **VI:**584, 585f
Type II (moderate hypoplasia), **VI:**584
Type III (severe hypoplasia), **VI:**584
Type IV (floating thumb), **VI:**586
Type V (aplasia), **VI:**586
hypospadia
defect occurrence, **III:**907f–908f
embryology, **III:**907–908
epidemiology, **III:**908
etiology, **III:**908
meatoplasty and glanuloplasty
basic procedure, **III:**913–915, 916f
onlay island flap repair, **III:**914–915, 918f
orthoplasty, **III:**915
surgical tips, **III:**914b–915b
tubularized incised plate (TIP) repair, **III:**914, 917f
two-stage repair, **III:**915, 919f–921f
outcomes and complicatons, **III:**916–921
hypospadia (Continued)
patient presentation and diagnosis, **III:**908–909
patient selection, **III:**909
postoperative care and follow-up, **III:**915
secondary procedures, **III:**921
urethral reconstruction, **III:**913, 915f
hypotension, **I:**145
hypothenar hammer syndrome, **VI:**368–369
hypothenar muscles, **VI:**52
hypothermia, **II:**638–639, **IV:**434
hypoxanthine, **I:**575, 575f
hypoxia
hypoxia-inducible factor-1α (HIF-1α), **I:**441–442
hypoxia-inducible factor 1 (HIF-1), **I:**260
wound healing, **I:**256–260, 257f

I
iatrogenic airway obstruction, **II:**444
ibuprofen, **II:**21–22
ice-pick scars, **II:**69
iliacus muscle, **IV:**15t–16t, 18f, 20f–22f
i-LIMB Pulse, **I:**858–861, 860f
ilioinguinal nerve, **IV:**230
ilium harvests, **I:**449–452, 450f–451f
Ilizarov technique, **IV:**179–180, 179f
image-guided core biopsy, **V:**271–272, 272f
imagined ugliness, **I:**50–51, 50b
imaging technology innovations, **I:**6, **V:**82
immature breast, **I:**648
immature scars, **I:**291t, 302t
immediate postmastectomy breast reconstruction
acellular allogenic dermal matrix (ADM), **I:**644–645, 644f
basic procedure, **V:**287–291
breast implants, **V:**353
deep inferior epigastric perforator (DIEP) flaps, **V:**288f
expander-implant insertion, **V:**353–354, 354f
latissimus dorsi (LD) flap, **V:**288, 289f–290f
muscle coverage, **I:**643–645
prosthesis insertion
basic procedure, **V:**356–358
capsulectomy, **V:**357f
contralateral adjustments, **V:**356–358
inframammary fold reconstruction, **V:**357f
large breast augmentation, **V:**358
medium breast augmentation, **V:**357–358
small breast augmentation, **V:**356–357
radiation therapy (RT), **V:**290
second-stage surgery, **V:**356, 357f
skin reducing mastectomy, **V:**354–356, 355f
submuscular position, **I:**643–644
subpectoral (dual-plane) position, **I:**644
transverse rectus abdominis myocutaneous (TRAM) flaps, **V:**288f
immediate velocity gunshot wounds, **III:**86–87
immune response cells
B lymphocytes, **I:**817
complement cascade, **I:**817
dendritic cells, **I:**818
general discussion, **I:**816–819
granulocytes, **I:**817
immunoglobulins, **I:**817
macrophages, **I:**816
natural killer (NK) cells, **I:**816–817
immune response cells (Continued)
T lymphocytes
anergy, **I:**827
antigen recognition and graft rejection, **I:**819
functional role, **I:**818–819
T-cell binding and activation, **I:**818
T-cell receptor (TCR), **I:**818–819, 826–827
immunoglobulins, **I:**817
immunomodulators, **II:**21t
immunotherapy, **I:**204–206, 205f–206f, 718
implants, **I:**786–797
adhesives and glues
characteristics, **I:**792b
cyanoacrylates, **I:**793
fibrin tissue adhesives, **I:**793
platelet gels, **I:**793
research background, **I:**792–793
biomaterial-based implants, **I:**786–797
bioprosthetic mesh, **I:**795–796, 795b
bovine fetal dermis, **I:**796
bovine pericardium, **I:**796
future trends, **I:**796–797
human acellular dermal matrix (HADM), **I:**796
porcine acellular dermal matrix (PADM), **I:**796
small intestinal mucosa, **I:**796
breast implants, **V:**336–369
applications, **V:**336
diagnostic imaging, **V:**270–271, 271f
evolutionary development
dimensions, **V:**352–353
filling material, **V:**352–353, 352f
shape, **V:**352, 352f
shell, **V:**352
expander-implants
adjustable, permanent expander-implants, **V:**366–367
average operative time, **V:**364t
basic procedure, **V:**338–340
breast envelope preservation, **V:**367–368
capsular contracture, **V:**362, 362t–364t
cellulitis, **V:**359, 360f
clinical studies, **V:**362, 363t
complication frequency, **V:**363–365, 364t
complications, **V:**359
cosmetic revision surgery, **V:**365, 366f
delayed reconstruction, **V:**342f, 358, 359f
erythema, **V:**359
evaluation studies, **V:**365
expander failure or malfunction, **V:**360–361, 360f–361f, 364t
fat injections, **V:**365, 368
flap-based reconstruction, **V:**367
hematomas, **V:**359, 359f, 364t
implant malposition, **V:**363t
implant removal, **V:**363t
implant rupture and deflation, **V:**361–362, 363t
infections, **V:**361–363, 363t–364t
insertion procedures, **V:**353–354
nipple reconstruction, **V:**365–366
outcome assessments, **V:**363–365
persistent serous drainage, **V:**359–360
postoperative care and follow-up, **V:**358–359

implants (Continued)
    preoperative/postoperative
        comparisons, **V:**340f–341f
    secondary procedures, **V:**365–366
    skin necrosis, **V:**360, 360f, 363t
    wrinkle formation, **V:**363t
  implant malposition
    clinical signs, **V:**79t
    double-bubble deformity, **V:**116, 116f
    inadequate muscle release, **V:**113, 114f
    incidence, **V:**79t
    plane of insertion, **V:**112–113, 113f
    submusculofascial plane, **V:**114–115,
        114f
    symmastia, **V:**115–116, 116f
    transaxillary dissection, **V:**115, 115f
  implant selection
    filling material, **V:**24–25
    implant shape, **V:**25–27, 28f–29f
    implant size determination, **V:**24–25, 25f
    implant surface texture, **V:**25, 26f–27f
  outcomes and complicatons
    capsular contracture, **V:**264, 336–340,
        362, 362t–364t
    cellulitis, **V:**359, 360f
    clinical studies, **V:**362, 363t
    erythema, **V:**359
    expander failure or malfunction,
        V:360–361, 360f–361f
    hematomas, **V:**359, 359f
    infections, **V:**361–363
    persistent serous drainage, **V:**359–360
    skin necrosis, **V:**360, 360f
  patient presentation and diagnosis
    exclusion criteria, **V:**345–346, 347f
    inclusion criteria, **V:**346
    large breast reconstruction, **V:**346, 350f
    medium breast reconstruction, **V:**346,
        349f
    small breast reconstruction, **V:**346, 348f
  perioperative complications
    delayed complications, **V:**36–37
    hematomas, **V:**32–37, 79t
    implant rupture and deflation, **V:**37, 79t
    medication and herbal supplement
        avoidance list, **V:**33t–35t
    Mondor's disease, **V:**35–36
    nipple sensitivity, **V:**32–37
    periprosthetic capsular contracture,
        V:36–37
    seromas, **V:**32–37, 79t
    wound infections, **V:**35, 79t
  postoperative care and follow-up, **V:**32,
    358–359
  prosthesis insertion
    basic procedure, **V:**356–358
    capsulectomy, **V:**357f
    contralateral adjustments, **V:**356–358
    inframammary fold reconstruction,
        V:357f
    large breast augmentation, **V:**358
    medium breast augmentation,
        V:357–358
    small breast augmentation, **V:**356–357
  reconstructive paradigms
    contralateral adjustments, **V:**343f
    cosmetic breast reconstruction,
        V:344f–345f

implants (Continued)
    indications and contraindications,
        V:343f
    mastectomy techniques, **V:**343f
    radiation therapy (RT), **V:**347f
    surgical strategy, **V:**340–344
  saline implants
    autoinflation, **V:**111–112, 112f
    capsular calcification, **V:**110, 110f
    decision guidelines, **V:**24–25
    deflation, **V:**110–111, 111f
    developmental background, **V:**13–14
    ripples and folds, **V:**111, 111f
  scientific research, **V:**336–340
  secondary procedures, **V:**37
  silicone gel implants
    capsular calcification, **V:**107–109,
        108f–109f
    capsular contracture, **V:**106–107,
        106f–107f
    characteristics, **I:**789–790, 790f
    closed capsulotomy, **V:**107, 107f–108f
    decision guidelines, **V:**24–25
    developmental background, **V:**14–15
    double-bubble deformity, **V:**116, 116f
    first generation implants, **V:**14–15, 103f
    fourth and fifth generation implants,
        V:15
    hematomas, **V:**104–105, 104f–105f
    historical background, **I:**789–790,
        V:102–109
    implant disruption, **V:**103–104, 103f
    implant malposition, **V:**112–113, 113f
    infections, **V:**105–106, 105f–106f
    second generation implants, **V:**14–15,
        104f
    third generation implants, **V:**14–15, 104f
  skin reducing mastectomy, **V:**354–356,
    355f
  sponges, **V:**101–102, 102f
  steroid atrophy, **V:**110, 110f
  surgical technique and treatment
    delayed reconstruction, **V:**358, 359f
    expander-implant insertion, **V:**353–354,
        354f
    immediate postmastectomy breast
        reconstruction, **V:**353
    inframammary incision, **V:**27–30
    periareolar incision, **V:**30–31
    preoperative markings, **V:**27–32
    preoperative project, **V:**346–352,
        350f–351f
    prosthesis insertion, **V:**356–358
    second-stage surgery, **V:**356, 357f
    skin reducing mastectomy, **V:**354–356,
        355f
    surgical guidelines, **V:**27b, 30b
    tissue preservation, **V:**353–358
    transaxillary incision, **V:**31
    transumbilical incision, **V:**32
  buttock augmentation
    complications
      capsular contracture, **II:**614
      implant exposure, **II:**614
      implant malposition, **II:**615, 615f
      implant rotation, **II:**615
      infections, **II:**614
      neuropraxia, **II:**614–615

implants (Continued)
      seromas, **II:**614
      wound dehiscence, **II:**614, 614f
    general discussion, **II:**599
    intramuscular implant surgical technique
      anesthesia, **II:**609
      drains, **II:**610
      expanders, **II:**610
      implant placement/closure, **II:**610–611
      incision design/selection, **II:**609–611,
        610f
      markings, **II:**609
      muscle dissection, **II:**610
      positioning, **II:**609
      preoperative preparations, **II:**609
      sizers/implant size, **II:**610
      skin flap dissection, **II:**610
    placement and selection
      general discussion, **II:**605–608
      implant shape selection, **II:**607
      implant size determination, **II:**607–608,
        608f
      implant size selection, **II:**608
      intramuscular implant surgical
        technique, **I:**806–808
      intramuscular plane, **II:**606–607
      lateral view, **II:**608
      muscle height to width ratio, **II:**607, 608f
      sciatic nerve, **II:**607f
      subcutaneous plane, **II:**606, 606f
      subfascial plane, **II:**607, 607f
      submuscular plane, **II:**606, 607f
    postoperative care and follow-up
      compressive garments, **II:**613
      drains, **II:**613
      pain management, **II:**613
      patient activity, **II:**613
    subfascial implant surgical technique
      markings, **II:**611, 611f
      surgical technique, **II:**611–612,
        611f–613f
  ceramics, **I:**792
  chin implants, **III:**240, 240f–241f
  craniofacial osteointegration
    bone bed, **I:**805
    bone preparation, **I:**805, 805f
    implant load, **I:**805
    implant materials, **I:**804
    implant–tissue interface, **I:**804–805
  facial skeletal augmentation
    chin augmentation
      characteristics, **II:**346, 349f–350f
      implant augmentation versus sliding
        genioplasty, **II:**348
      surgical technique, **II:**347–348,
        350f–351f
    guidelines, **II:**342
    hematoma prevention, **II:**343
    immobilization, **II:**343
    infraorbital rim
      Jelks and Jelks categorized globe–
        orbital rim relationships, **II:**343–
        344, 344f
      surgical technique, **II:**344, 345f
    malar region
      characteristics, **II:**345
      surgical technique, **II:**345–346,
        348f–349f

*Note: **Boldface** roman numerals indicate volume. Page numbers followed by f refer to figures; page numbers followed by t refer to tables; page numbers followed by b refer to boxes.*

implants (Continued)
   mandible implants
      chin augmentation, II:346
      general discussion, II:346–351
      ramus, angle, and body considerations,
         II:348, 351, 351f–352f
   midface implants
      general discussion, II:343–346
      infraorbital rim, II:343–344, 344f
      malar region, II:345
      pyriform aperture, II:344
      polyethylene, II:343
      positioning, II:343
      pyriform aperture
         characteristics, II:344, 346f
         surgical technique, II:344–345,
            346f–347f
      shape considerations, II:343
      silicone, II:342
   metals and alloys
      cobalt-chromium alloys, I:787
      composition, I:787t
      general discussion, I:786–788
      gold alloys, I:787
      platinum (Pt), I:788
      stainless steel, I:786–787
      titanium alloys, I:787, 788f
   omentum reconstruction, V:474–476, 476f
   orbital fractures, III:56
   osteoarthritis
      implant arthroplasty
         hinged prostheses, VI:426
         indications and contraindications,
            VI:426–429
         PyroCarbon arthroplasty, VI:427–429,
            440f
         silicone constrained prostheses, VI:426,
            427f
         surface replacement prostheses,
            VI:426–427
      proximal interphalangeal (PIP)
         arthroplasty
         developmental background, VI:420–422
         nonconstrained or semi-constrained
           techniques, VI:422, 422f–423f
         patient selection, VI:421–422
      thumb arthroplasty, VI:440–441, 440f
   pectus excavatum, III:856–859, 857f
   polymers
      biodegradable polymers, I:791–792
      characteristics, I:788–792
      polyester, I:791
      polyethylene, I:791, 791f
      polypropylene, I:791
      polytetrafluoroethylene (PTFE), I:790
      silicone, I:789–790, 789t, 790f, II:342
   revision breast augmentation, V:44–65, 44t,
      45f
   skin substitutes
      Apligraf, I:337, 794t, 795
      bioengineered skin substitutes, I:793–795
      commercial product comparisons, I:794t
      Dermagraft, I:338, 794t, 795
      Epicel, I:794t, 795
      Integra, I:794, 794t
   subperiosteal facelift, II:273
   tissue expansion
      characteristics, I:626–627
      differential expanders, I:627
      expanders with distal ports, I:627

implants (Continued)
      expanders with integrated ports, I:627
      implant and distal port positioning, I:628
      implant inflation strategy and technique,
         I:629
      implant selection, I:628
      self-inflating expanders, I:627
      textured silicone expanders, I:627
   unaesthetic facial implants, II:305
   See also breast augmentation
implied warranty, I:94–95
inadequate thumb, VI:546t
incisional biopsies, IV:107
incisional wounds, I:285–286, 286t
income statements, I:67, 70f
incomplete cleft palate, III:571
incontinence, IV:363–364
index finger abduction, VI:770–771, 771f
India, I:12–13, 13f
Indian hedgehog gene, I:428–429, VI:531–532
induced pluripotent stem cells
   characteristics, I:213f, 235–237, 235f
   in vitro applications
      clinical correlates, I:238–239
      fibroblast differentiation protocols, I:237
      in vitro differentiation protocols, I:237–238
      in vivo models, I:238–239
      lentivirus production and transduction,
         I:237
   potential risks, I:237, 237f–238f
   tissue engineering, I:370–371
   transcription factors, I:235f
   wound healing, I:264
infantile digital fibroma
   patient presentation and diagnosis, III:881,
      881f
   prognosis and outcomes, III:881
   surgical technique and treatment, III:881
infantile fibrosarcoma, VI:668t
infantile hemangioma (IH)
   classification systems, I:677t, VI:668t
   clinical manifestations
      characteristics, I:680–681
      head and neck hemangiomas, I:680
      hepatic hemangiomas, I:680–681
      multiple hemangiomas, I:680
      structural anomalies, I:681
   diagnosis, I:681
   nonoperative management
      embolic therapy, I:684
      intralesional corticosteroids, I:682
      laser therapy, I:684
      observation, I:681
      systemic corticosteroids, I:682–684
      topical corticosteroids, I:682
      wound care, I:682
   operative management
      involuted phase (late childhood), I:685
      involuting phase (early childhood), I:678f,
         684–685
      proliferative phase (infancy), I:677f, 684
   pathogenesis, I:678–680, VI:672–673
   patient presentation and diagnosis,
      VI:672–673, 674f
   surgical technique and treatment, VI:673,
      675f
   terminology, I:678t
infant obstetric brachial plexus palsy
   background information, VI:806–812
   clinical examination, VI:806–808, 808f–809f

infant obstetric brachial plexus palsy
   (Continued)
   clinical presentation, VI:806, 807f
   imaging methods, VI:809f
   injury type incidence, VI:810t
   intraoperative findings, VI:810t
   nerve graft results, VI:811–812, 812f–813f
   outcome assessments, VI:811, 812t
   postoperative care and follow-up, VI:810–
      811, 811f
   preoperative preparations, VI:808
   reconstructive strategies, VI:810, 810t
   rupture–avulsion injuries, VI:810, 810t–811t
   rupture injuries, VI:810, 810t
   surgical technique and treatment,
      VI:808–809
   surgical timing, VI:808
infections
   abdominoplasty, II:557–558
   brachioplasty, II:629t
   breast augmentation, V:35, 79t, 263–264
   breast implants, V:361–363, 363t–364t
   burn wound treatment, IV:427–428, 428f,
      432–434, 433t
   buttock augmentation, II:613–614
   diabetic foot ulcers, IV:194–195
   distal interphalangeal (DIP) fusion, VI:417
   face transplants, III:484
   fat-grafted breast reconstruction, V:602
   foot injuries, IV:196–197
   hands, VI:333–345
      antibiotics, VI:333
      bite wounds
         animal bites, VI:343
         characteristics, VI:343–344
         clenched-fist injuries, VI:343, 344f
         human bites, VI:343–344
      complications, VI:344
      disease process, VI:333–334
      infection mimics
         brown recluse spider bite, VI:336
         gout, VI:335, 335f
         granuloma annulare, VI:336
         pseudogout, VI:335
         pyoderma gangrenosum, VI:335–336,
           336f
         pyogenic granuloma, VI:335, 335f
         rheumatoid arthritis, VI:336
         treatment strategies, VI:335–336
      infection types
         cellulitis, VI:336
         deep space infections, VI:338–339, 338f
         felon, VI:337–338, 337f
         flexor tenosynovitis, VI:339, 340f
         fungal infections, VI:343
         herpetic whitlow, VI:342, 342f
         mycobacterial infections, VI:342–343
         necrotizing fasciitis, VI:341–342, 341f,
           342b
         noncholera Vibrio infections, VI:343
         osteomyelitis, VI:341
         paronychia, VI:336–337, 336f
         pyogenic flexor tenosynovitis, VI:339,
           340f
         septic arthritis, VI:339–341, 340f
      patient presentation and diagnosis
         bite wounds, VI:343–344
         hardware infections, VI:344
         infection classifications, VI:335, 335t
         infection mimics, VI:335–336

infections (Continued)
  infection types, **VI**:336–343
  methicillin-resistant Staphylococcus aureus (MRSA) infections, **VI**:334, 334t
  patient history, **VI**:334–344
  physical examination, **VI**:334–344
  patient selection, **VI**:344
  prognosis and outcomes, **VI**:344
  hardware infections, **VI**:344
  head and neck cancer, **III**:417
  lower bodylift/belt lipectomy surgery, **II**:592
  lower extremity reconstructive surgery, **IV**:137
  male chest contouring, **V**:579
  mastopexy, **V**:150, 243t
  maxillary fractures, **III**:74
  muscle/musculocutaneous flaps, **I**:571–572
  nasal fractures, **III**:60
  pressure sores, **IV**:366
  progressive hemifacial atrophy (PHA), **III**:794
  revisionary breast surgery, **V**:65–66, 66t, 79t, 263–264
  rhinoplasty complications, **II**:411, 445–446
  scalp and forehead reconstruction, **III**:119, 131–132
  silicone gel implants, **V**:105–106, 105f–106f
  tissue expansion complications, **I**:652
  toxic epidermal necrolysis (TEN), **IV**:513–514
  upper extremity surgery, **V**:102
  wound infections, **I**:249–250, 281–282, 306, **II**:526, **III**:417, **IV**:137, **V**:35
infectious agents, **III**:421
infectious rhinitis, **II**:454, 458
infective cicatricial alopecia, **III**:111t
inferior gluteal artery, **IV**:222f, 223, 224f
inferior gluteal artery perforator (IGAP) flap
  advantages, **V**:459–464
  anatomical characteristics, **V**:461–463
  complications, **V**:464
  patient selection, **V**:460–461
  postoperative care, **V**:464
  surgical technique, **V**:463–464, 464b, 467f–468f
inferior pedicle breast reduction, **V**:165–176
  background and general characteristics, **V**:154–156, 165–166
  case studies, **V**:172–175, 173f–174f
  complications, **V**:175
  patient selection, **V**:166
  planning and marking guidelines
    asymmetrical cases, **V**:168, 168f
    equilateral triangle marking, **V**:166–167, 167f
    inframammary fold, **V**:167
    preoperative markings, **V**:166, 167f
    symmetry assessments, **V**:168
    transverse incisions markings, **V**:167
  research summary, **V**:175
  surgical technique and treatment
    apical suture, **V**:171f
    basic procedure, **V**:168–172
    de-epithelialization, **V**:169f
    flap thickness evaluation, **V**:170f
    inferior pedicle with inverted-T skin closure, **V**:159f, 161f

inferior pedicle breast reduction (Continued)
    medial and lateral triangle excision, **V**:170f
    nipple-areola complex, **V**:168f, 171f–172f
    postoperative results, **V**:172f
    preoperative/postoperative comparisons, **V**:173f
    symmetry evaluation, **V**:172f
inferior retinacular lateral canthoplasty/canthopexy (IRLC), **II**:156–157, 160f
inferior temporal septum (ITS), **II**:83–85, 83f
infiltration
  abdominoplasties, **I**:143, 144f
  breast augmentation, **I**:142–143, 143f
  breast reduction, **I**:141–142, 141f–142f
  characteristics, **I**:140–144
  facelifts, **I**:140, 141f
  liposuctions
    infiltrating wetting solutions
      aspirated volumes, **II**:516t
      blood loss estimates, **II**:516t
      common formulations, **II**:516t
      epinephrine, **II**:516t, 517
      fluid requirement guidelines, **II**:517
      fluid resuscitation, **II**:517–518
      lidocaine, **II**:516t, 517
      perioperative fluid management, **II**:516–518
    local anesthesia, **I**:143–144, 144f
informed consent
  abdominal wall reconstruction, **IV**:283
  abdominoplasty, **II**:537
  breast augmentation, **V**:17–19
  cosmetic surgery, **II**:8
  informed consent versus informed choice, **V**:324
  liposuctions, **II**:513
  medico-legal issues, **I**:93–94, 105–106
  open rhinoplasty, **II**:389
  patient-centered health communication, **V**:324
  post-bariatric surgery reconstruction, **II**:637–638
infraclavicular block, **VI**:99, 100f
infraorbital nerve anesthesia, **III**:57
infraspinatus muscle, **IV**:221, 222f
infratrochlear nerve, **III**:26, 27f
infundibulum, **I**:321, 322f
inguinofemoral lymphadenectomy, **I**:772–777, 775f–777f
inherited chromosomal abnormalities, **I**:185
Injury Severity Scale (ISS), **IV**:63
inosine monophosphate (IMP), **I**:821–822
inositol 1,4,5-triphosphate (IP₃), **I**:626f
Institute for Healthcare Improvement, **I**:170
institutional review boards (IRBs), **I**:8–9
institutional technology transfer, **I**:847, 848t
insulin growth factor-1 (IGF1), **I**:189–190, 234, 270t, 275, 428, **VI**:412–413
Integra, **I**:794, 794t, **IV**:128–129, 415t, 448
integrins, **I**:270–271
intellectualization, **I**:33
intellectual property, **I**:846–847
intense pulsed light therapy, **II**:21t, 28, 67–70, **IV**:454, 454t
intensity-modulated radiation therapy (IMRT), **I**:658, 659f
Interactive Craniofacial Surgical Atlas, **I**:867

intercostal artery, **IV**:222f, 223
intercostal artery perforator (ICAP) flap, **V**:486f–488f, 487–488
intercostal muscles, **IV**:225
interferons
  interferon-regulatory factor 6 (IRF6), **I**:194
  melanoma treatment, **I**:777–778
  mesenchymal stem cells (MSCs), **I**:225–226
  scar treatment, **I**:294–295, 309–310
  wound healing, **I**:244–245
interfragmentary compression, **VI**:108
interfragmentary lag screws, **VI**:111–112, 112f–113f
interleukins
  Dupuytren's disease, **VI**:349
  inflammatory mediators, **I**:819–820
  macrophages, **I**:816
  melanoma treatment, **I**:782
  mesenchymal stem cells (MSCs), **I**:225–226
  radiation therapy (RT), **I**:662
  skin wound healing, **I**:270t, 275
  tissue transplantation, **I**:821t, 825
  wound healing, **I**:244–245
internal anterior scrotal artery, **IV**:235, 238f
internal fracture fixation, **VI**:106–116
  Arbeitsgemeinschaft für Osteosynthesefragen (AO) principles, **VI**:106, 107t
  challenges, **VI**:106
  fixation options
    absolute versus relative stability, **VI**:108, 108b, 108f
    bridge plating, **VI**:113, 115f
    compression plating, **VI**:112–113, 114f
    external fixation, **VI**:110, 111f
    interfragmentary compression, **VI**:108
    interfragmentary lag screws, **VI**:111–112, 112f–113f
    Kirschner wires (K-wires), **VI**:107b, 108–109, 109f, 110t, 139
    locked plating, **VI**:115, 115f
    tension band constructs, **VI**:109–110, 109f–111f, 110t
  fluoroscopic imaging, **VI**:108–115
  patient selection
    fracture assessment, **VI**:106
    host factors, **VI**:106
  postoperative care and follow-up, **VI**:115
  preoperative imaging assessment, **VI**:107
  research summary, **VI**:115
  surgical technique and treatment
    fracture reduction
      basic procedure, **VI**:107
      Kapandji (intrafocal) pinning, **VI**:107b
      Kirschner wires (K-wires), **VI**:107b
      temporary/supplemental external fixation, **VI**:107b
    preoperative planning, **VI**:107
internal mammary artery, **IV**:225–227
internal oblique muscle, **IV**:228–229, 229f
internal posterior scrotal artery, **IV**:235, 238f
International Clinic of Oto-Rhino-Laryngology and Facio-Maxillary Surgery, **I**:23–24
International Patient Decision Aid Standards (IPDAS), **V**:321
International Society for the Study of Vascular Anomalies (ISSVA), **VI**:667–669, 668t
Internet and blog defamation law, **I**:98–99

*Note: **Boldface** roman numerals indicate volume. Page numbers followed by f refer to figures; page numbers followed by t refer to tables; page numbers followed by b refer to boxes.*

interosseous (I-O) wire fixation, **VI**:232–233, 232b, 232f, 415
interosseous membrane
  distal membranous portion, **VI**:60, 60f
  leg anatomy, **IV**:34
  middle ligamentous portion, **VI**:60, 60f
  proximal membranous portion, **VI**:60, 60f
interosseous muscle, **VI**:52
interphalangeal (IP) joint, **VI**:590
Interplast, **I**:870
interscalene block, **VI**:97, 98f
intradermal nevi, **I**:744, 744f
intradural dermoids
  disease process, **III**:883
  patient presentation and diagnosis, **III**:883, 884f
  surgical technique and treatment, **III**:883–884
intraoral infracture technique with incomplete osteotomy, **II**:181
intraoral L-shaped ostectomy, **II**:181
intraoral vertical ramus osteotomy, **III**:662
intraosseous malignant fibrous histiocytomas, **IV**:103
intraplexus nerve transfer, **VI**:799
intravelar veloplasty, **III**:578–579, 580f
intravenous immune globulin (IVIG), **IV**:517
intravenous regional anesthesia, **VI**:97
intrinsic muscle flaps, **IV**:209, 210f
intrinsic tightness test, **VI**:53–54, 53f
involutional hypomastia, **V**:13
iodine (I), **I**:656–657
ionizing radiation, **I**:202–204
ipilimumab, **I**:782–783
irezumi, **I**:297–298
IRF6 (interferon regulatory factor) gene, **III**:511
iridium (Ir), **I**:656
iron (Fe) alloys, **I**:786–787
irradiated orbit, **III**:235–238
ischemia
  foot reconstruction, **IV**:193, 194f
  ischemia–reperfusion injury
    flap failure pathophysiology, **I**:575–576, 576f, 617–618
    free flap viability augmentation
      background information, **I**:583–585
      postischemic conditioning, **I**:584–585
      preischemic conditioning, **I**:583
      remote preischemic conditioning, **I**:583–584, 584f
  ischemia–reperfusion pathophysiology, **VI**:228–229
  ischemic necrosis, **I**:573
  Nerve injury, Ischemia, Soft-tissue Injury, Skeletal Injury, Shock, and Age of patient score (NISSSA), **IV**:63
  nipple areola ischemia, **V**:247–248, 248f–249f
  wound healing
    hypoxia, **I**:256–259
    nitric oxide (NO) synthesis, **I**:259
    oxygen imbalance, **I**:257–258
    redox signaling, **I**:258–259
    skin wound healing, **I**:279–281
    tissue oxygenation, **I**:256–259, 256f–257f
ischial pressure sores, **IV**:372–373, 372t
ischiopagus twins
  characteristics, **III**:898f
  classification systems, **III**:893–897, 894f–897f
  clinical case study, **III**:901b–903b, 901f–903f

ischiopagus twins (*Continued*)
  magnetic resonance imaging (MRI), **III**:899f
  prenatal evaluation, **III**:897–899
  preoperative planning, **III**:899–900, 900f
island flap, **III**:452
isografts, **I**:325t, 815
isotretinoin, **II**:21t
isthmus, **I**:321, 322f
item response theory (IRT), **I**:164
Ivy, Robert, **I**:23

J
Jackson–Weiss syndrome, **I**:197, 197f, 197t, **III**:749–750, 750t
Jadassohn, nevus sebaceous of, **III**:111–112, 112f
Jamshidi core needle bone biopsy, **IV**:358–360, 361f
Japanese honeysuckle, **V**:33t–35t
jaw
  anesthesia, **III**:27
  Asian facial bone surgery, **II**:181, 182f–183f
  jawline augmentation, **II**:54
Jeanne's sign, **VI**:58, 58f, 514t, 762, 762f
jejunal flap
  pharyngoesophageal reconstruction
    flap harvesting, **III**:349–350, 349f–350f
    flap inset guidelines, **III**:350, 350f
    oral diet, **III**:356t
Jelks and Jelks categorized globe–orbital rim relationships, **II**:343–344, 344f
Jeune's syndrome
  characteristics, **III**:860–861, 861f
  clinical presentation and evaluation, **III**:861
  surgical indicators, **III**:861
  treatment strategies, **III**:861, 862f
Jewer's and Boyd's defect classification, **III**:317t
Johns Hopkins University Applied Physics Laboratory (APL), **I**:860–861
joint cartilage repair and reconstruction, **I**:421–423
joint reconstruction, **IV**:441–442, 442f–443f, 445f
Joseph, Jacques, **I**:25–28, 26f
jumping man flap, **VI**:288f
c-jun amino-terminal kinase (JNK), **I**:626f
junctional nevi, **I**:744, 744f
Juri flap, **III**:123–124, 125f
Juvederm, **II**:47, 49t
  See also soft-tissue fillers
juvenile aggressive fibromatosis, **III**:880
juvenile melanoma, **I**:724–725, 726f
juvenile nasopharyngeal angiofibroma
  patient presentation and diagnosis, **III**:881
  prognosis and outcomes, **III**:881
  surgical technique and treatment, **III**:881
juvenile xanthogranuloma, **I**:729–730, 729f–730f
Juvia laser, **II**:71t, 74

K
Kabuki syndrome, **III**:805–807, 807t
kallikrein, **I**:243f, 244, **II**:20–21
Kallman's syndrome, **I**:194
Kanavel, Allen B, **VI**:0–2
kangen-karyu, **V**:33t–35t
Kapandji (intrafocal) pinning, **VI**:107b
Kaplan, Emmanuel B, **VI**:1–2, 2b
Kaplan's cardinal line, **VI**:2b, 2f

kaposiform hemangioendothelioma (KHE)
  classification systems, **I**:677t, **VI**:668t
  clinical manifestations, **I**:687
  treatment strategies, **I**:687–688
Kaposi's sarcoma, **I**:742
Karapandzic flap, **III**:261–262, 264f, 454, 455f
Kasabach–Merritt phenomenon (KMP), **I**:687, **VI**:324, 324f
Kazanjian, Varaztad, **I**:23
keloid scars
  characteristics, **I**:730, 730f
  wound healing, **I**:265, 283t, 284–285, 302–304, 302t, 303f, 308–309
Kentish, Edward, **IV**:393
keratinocytes
  aging process, **II**:44–45
  epidermis, **I**:319–320
  induced pluripotent stem cells, **I**:236
  keratinocyte cultures, **I**:336–337, 337f
  keratinocyte growth factor (KGF), **I**:189–190, 270t, 274–275
  skin wound healing, **I**:270t, 271f
keratoacanthoma, **I**:719, 719f, **VI**:315–316, 316f
keratocysts, **I**:720
kerosene, **IV**:395
Kessler tendon repair, **VI**:233
ketamine, **I**:138–139, **IV**:427
kickbacks, **I**:61–62
kidney transplants, **I**:2–3
Kienbock's disease, **VI**:88, 89f
Kilner, Pomfret, **I**:23, 24f
Kilner, Thomas, **III**:576–578
Kiloh–Nevin syndrome, **VI**:510–511
Kimura disease, **I**:736
Kirk, Norman T, **VI**:xlvi
Kirner's deformity, **VI**:639f
Kirschner wires (K-wires)
  distal interphalangeal (DIP) arthrodesis, **VI**:415
  hand and wrist fracture fixation, **VI**:107b, 108–109, 109f, 110t, 139, 145f
  mutilated/mangled hand reconstruction, **VI**:259–261, 260f
  nasal fracture fixation, **III**:59
  Pierre Robin sequence (PRS), **III**:817, 818f
  proximal interphalangeal (PIP) arthrodesis, **VI**:418
  radial hypoplasia/aplasia, **VI**:561f
  radioscapholunate arthrodesis, **VI**:385f, 386
  scaphoid fractures, **VI**:171f
  thumb and finger reconstruction, **VI**:232–233, 232f, 551–553
Kleinman shear test, **VI**:165–166, 166f
Klein's Formula, **II**:516t
Klippel–Feil syndrome, **VI**:567t
Klippel–Trenaunay syndrome
  benign mesenchymal-origin tumors
    hemangioma simplex, **I**:734
    venous malformation, **I**:735
  classification systems, **VI**:668, 668t
  outcomes and complicatons, **VI**:691
  pathogenesis, **I**:703, **VI**:691
  patient presentation and diagnosis, **VI**:691
  surgical technique and treatment, **VI**:691
Klumpke's palsy, **VI**:806, 807f
knees
  anatomical characteristics
    skeletal structure
      cruciate and collateral ligaments, **IV**:32f
      detailed characteristics, **IV**:30

knees (Continued)
  schematic diagram, IV:31f, 33f
  tibia and fibula, IV:34f
  vascular supply, IV:24f
  burn reconstruction, IV:443t, 444, 509
  liposuctions, II:525
  reconstructive surgeries, IV:131f, 137f
knowledge translation
  background information, I:168–169
  implementation barriers, I:169
  Knowledge To Action model, I:169, 169f
kojic acid, II:25
Kupffer cells, I:816

L
labia majora reduction, II:673–674,
    674f–676f
labia minora reduction
  characteristics, II:669–673
  outcomes and complicatons, II:672–673,
    672f–673f
  surgical technique, II:670–672, 671f–672f
labiaplasty, IV:338f, 341–342, 342f
lacerations
  acute wounds, I:241, 241f
  complex lacerations, III:31, 32f
  eyelid injuries, III:38–39, 40f
  nails and fingertips
    characteristics, VI:119–120
    postoperative care and follow-up,
      VI:120
    surgical technique and treatment, VI:120,
      120b, 121f–122f
  simple lacerations, III:30, 31f
  traumatic ear injuries, III:41, 41f
  traumatic nose injuries
    framework repair, III:43
    lining repair, III:43
    skin covering repair, III:43
La Chirurgie Esthétique pure, I:27, 28f
La Chirurgie Esthétique. Son Rôle Sociale, I:27
lacrimal system injury, III:63, 75
lactic acid, II:18–19
laminin, I:270–271
Langenbeck, Bernard von, I:19, III:576
Langerhans cell histiocytosis, I:736
Langerhans cells, I:320, 816
Langerhans cell sarcoma, I:742
Langer's lines, I:283–285, 306, 306f
lanolin, II:17
laparoscopic adjustable gastric banding
    (LAGB), I:636, 636f
Laresse Dermal Filler, II:48t
  See also soft-tissue fillers
large multicenter trials, I:154–155
Larsen syndrome, III:807t, VI:573t
larynx
  anatomical characteristics, III:423, 423f
  cancer management
    glottic cancers, III:434–436, 436f
    patient presentation and diagnosis,
      III:433–436
    subglottic cancers, III:434–436, 436f
    supraglottic cancers, III:434, 435f
    TNM clinical classification system,
      III:433–436
laser-assisted liposuction (LAL), II:507–508,
    519

lasers
  laser treatments
    burn reconstruction, IV:454, 454t, 484,
      484f
    cutaneous and soft-tissue tumors, I:718
    facial skin resurfacing, II:60–62
    infantile hemangioma (IH), I:684
    laser resurfacing, II:308
    laser–tissue interactions
      laser properties, II:63–64
      molecular bases, II:63–64
    liposuctions, II:527–528
    microvascular surgery, I:593
    nonablative facial skin rejuvenation
      (NSR), II:64–65
    patient selection and treatment, II:67–70,
      68f
    rosacea treatments, II:21t
    scar revision, I:308, II:67–70, IV:454t
    skin wound healing, I:293–294, 293f
    strawberry hemangioma, I:734–735
    traumatic tatoo, III:30
    turbinate disorders, II:461–462
Lassus, Claude, V:134–135
Lassus vertical scar technique, V:134–135,
    156–159, 177–180, 178t
latency-associated protein (LAP), I:275
lateral arm flap
  foot reconstruction, IV:211, 213f
  mangled upper extremities, VI:267,
    269f–272f
  oral cavity and mouth reconstruction,
    III:321
  tongue reconstruction, III:309t
lateral canthal tendon, II:109, 109f–110f
lateral canthoplasty, II:170, 171f–172f
lateral circumflex femoral arterial system,
    IV:23, 25f
lateral cutaneous nerve, VI:709, 711f–712f
lateral epicondylitis, VI:366
lateral femoral cutaneous nerve, VI:710
lateral intercostal artery perforator (LICAP)
    flap, V:487f–488f, 488
lateral nasal prominences, III:508, 509f
lateral orbicularis, II:96f
lateral pterygoid muscle, III:16
lateral retinaculum, II:109, 109f–110f
lateral supramalleolar flap, IV:206–207
lateral thigh/profunda femoris perforator
    flap, IV:144–145, 144f
lateral thoracic artery, IV:225–227, 226f
lateral thoracodorsal flap (LTDF), V:306–308
lateral V-Y advancement flaps, VI:130, 130f
Latham appliance, III:552–553, 553f
latissimus dorsi (LD) flap, V:370–392
  abdominal wall reconstruction, I:553t
  anatomical characteristics, V:370–372, 371f
  breast reconstruction
    contraindications, V:381
    immediate postmastectomy breast
      reconstruction, V:288, 289f–290f
    outcomes and complicatons
      donor site morbidity, V:390
      flap necrosis, V:390
      follow-up consultations, V:389–390
    partial breast reconstruction, V:306–308,
      309f, 311f, 485–489, 486f
    patient presentation and diagnosis, V:372

latissimus dorsi (LD) flap (Continued)
    patient selection and indicators, V:372–
      374, 373f–375f
    postoperative care and follow-up, V:389
    research summary, V:390
    secondary procedures
      secondary thoracodorsal nerve ligation,
        V:389
      timing considerations, V:389
      tissue expansion, V:389
    specific indicators
      augmentation mammaplasty, V:380
      large ptotic breasts, V:380–381
      partial mastectomy defects, V:380
      patient selection, V:374–376, 375f
      post-mastectomy defects, V:380
      prophylactic mastectomy, V:381
      radiation therapy (RT) history,
        V:376–378, 376f–379f
      thin or unreliable skin flaps, V:380, 380f
      transverse rectus abdominis
        myocutaneous (TRAM) flap
        candidates, V:374–376, 375f
    surgical technique
      basic procedure, V:381–387
      deep fat attachment, V:384f
      design guidelines, V:383f–384f
      elevation and transposition, V:385f
      flap shape, V:387f
      patient positioning, V:384f
      skin island placement, V:382f–383f, 386f
      surgical variants, V:387–389, 388f
  characteristics, I:516f
  chest wall reconstruction, I:552–553, IV:241,
    243f–244f
  clinical applications, I:528
  endoscopic approaches
    breast-conserving therapy (BCT), V:82–83
    outcomes and complicatons, V:93–96
    postoperative care and follow-up, V:93
    surgical technique and treatment
      basic procedure, V:89
      completed dissection, V:93f
      dissector instrumentation, V:91f
      hemostasis, V:94f
      instrumentation, V:90f
      laparotomy pad, V:91f
      markings, V:89f
      scissor dissection, V:92f–93f
      wetting solutions, V:90f
  general discussion, V:370
  head and neck reconstruction, I:545, 546f
  lower extremity reconstructive surgery,
    IV:77, 78f–79f
  mangled upper extremities, VI:275, 277f
  microneurovascular muscle transplantation,
    III:295t
  scalp and forehead reconstruction, III:130,
    130f
latissimus muscle, IV:222, 222f
LAVIV, II:46
leadership, I:88–90, 89f
Ledderhose's disease, VI:352, 352f
leeches, I:617, VI:241–242
Le Fort I osteotomy
  apertognathia, III:668f
  cleft lip surgery, III:610f–611f, 663–665, 663f,
    669t

Le Fort I osteotomy (Continued)
  craniofacial microsomia (CFM), III:782–786, 784f–785f
  dentofacial deformities, III:660–661, 661f
  mandibulomaxillary advancement (MMA), III:99f
  maxillary buttresses, III:236–238
  maxillary constriction, III:667f
Le Fort classification of facial fractures
  background information, III:71–75
  goals, III:71
  Le Fort I level fractures/transverse (Guerin) fractures, III:71, 72f, 73
  Le Fort II level fractures/pyramidal fractures, III:72f–73f, 73–74
  Le Fort III level fractures/craniofacial dysjunction, III:72f–73f, 73–74
Le Fort fracture patterns, III:672–674, 675f
Le Fort III advancement/distraction simulator, I:867
Le Fort III osteotomy
  acquired cranial and facial bone deformities, III:229, 233f
  faciocraniosynostosis, III:694–695
  Le Fort III osteotomy–bipartition correction technique
    basic procedure, III:696f–697f
    bone grafts, III:695
    coronal approach, III:695
    general discussion, III:695
    osteosynthesis, III:695
    subcranial osteotomies, III:695
  syndromic craniosynostosis, III:758f–759f
legs
  anatomical characteristics
    cross-section diagram, IV:36f
    fascial system
      compartment syndrome, IV:37
      components, IV:34–37, 36f
      deep fascia, IV:34
      interosseous membrane, IV:34
      lower leg compartments, IV:34–37
    innervation
      deep peroneal nerve, IV:48t
      lower leg cutaneous innervation, IV:48–50, 51f
      lower leg motor innervation, IV:48, 48t
      lower leg nerve topography, IV:48, 51f
      schematic diagram, IV:62f
      superficial peroneal nerve, IV:48t
      tibial nerve, IV:46f–47f, 48t
    knee skeletal structure
      cruciate and collateral ligaments, IV:32f
      detailed characteristics, IV:30
      schematic diagram, IV:31f, 33f
      tibia and fibula, IV:34f
    musculature
      anterior compartment, IV:37, 38t–39t, 40f–42f, 43t
      lateral compartment, IV:37–43, 38t–39t, 43t, 44f
      posterior compartment (deep layer), IV:38t–39t, 45, 45t, 46f
      posterior compartment (superficial layer), IV:38t–39t, 43, 43t, 45f
      schematic diagram, IV:62f
    redundant tissue, IV:30–50
    skeletal structure, IV:30–34, 34f–35f
    tibial nerve, IV:46f

legs (Continued)
  vascular supply
    detailed characteristics, IV:45–48
    fasciocutaneous perforators, IV:50f
    peroneal artery, IV:47f
    popliteal artery, IV:47f
    posterior tibial artery, IV:47f
    schematic diagram, IV:49f, 62f
  burn reconstruction, IV:509
  congenital melanocytic nevi (CMN), III:853f
  lower leg
    innervation
      cutaneous innervation, IV:48–50, 51f
      motor nerves, IV:48, 48t
      nerve topography, IV:48, 51f
    reconstructive surgeries, IV:130–131
    melanoma excisions, I:766–768, 770f
    tissue expansion, I:650
leiomyoma, I:731–732, VI:326, 327f
leiomyosarcoma, I:740, 740f, VI:326
Lejour, Madeleine, V:135–136
Lejour vertical scar technique, V:135–136, 159, 178t
Lemaître, Fernand, I:23–24, 24f
Lemperle classifications of nasolabial folds, II:53t
lentigo maligna melanoma, I:752–753, 754f
lentigo simplex, I:723–724, 724f
Lentinus edodes, II:23
lentivirus production and transduction, I:237
leopard's bane, V:33t–35t
Leriche sympathectomy, VI:476
Leser–Trélat syndrome, I:719
leukotrienes, I:573–574, 574f
levator scapulae, IV:221, 222f
leverage ratios, I:69
levobupivacaine, VI:96t
Levy–Hollister syndrome, VI:573t
liabilities, I:67–68, 71f
licochalcone, II:21t
licorice/licorice extract, II:21t, 23, 25, V:33t–35t
lid lamellae, III:57
lidocaine
  free flap viability augmentation, I:583
  infiltrating wetting solutions, II:516t, 517
  local anesthesia
    comparative pharmacology, VI:96t
    selection guidelines, I:139, 140f, VI:95–96
    toxicity, I:147–148
  patient safety, I:129–130
ligamentotaxis, VI:110
ligaments
  check rein ligaments, VI:13b, 456f
  Cleland's ligaments, VI:5, 7f, 347, 348f, 350f
  collateral ligaments
    hands and wrists, VI:13f
    hand stability assessment, VI:49–50, 49f–50f
    stiff hand, VI:449, 451, 454, 454f
  facial ligaments
    aging process, II:87
    anatomical characteristics, II:79f–80f, 189–191, 191f
    extended SMAS technique, II:239
    periorbital ligaments, III:9f
    retaining ligaments, II:112, 114f, III:8–10, 10f–11f
  femur, IV:11f
  Grayson's ligaments, VI:5, 7f, 347, 348f, 350f

ligaments (Continued)
  hands and wrists, VI:13f
  hips, IV:9f
  knees, IV:32f
  ligament of Grapow, VI:347f–348f
  ligament of Struthers, VI:510, 510f
  nasal anatomy, II:382f, 385f
  proximal commissural ligament, VI:347, 347f–348f
  thighs, IV:8
  transverse retinacular ligaments, VI:450–451
  wrists, VI:167f
lignocaine, IV:427
limb development (embryology)
  basic principles, VI:526
  development anomalies
    background information, VI:534–535
    classification systems, VI:534–535
    modified classification of congenital anomalies of the hand and upper limb
      acrosyndactyly, VI:540f
      anomaly characteristics, VI:537–539, 538t
      cleft hands, VI:540f
      constriction band syndrome, VI:540f
      dorsal dimelia, VI:540f
      macrodactyly, VI:541f
      radial and ulnar duplications, VI:539f
      radial longitudinal deficiency, VI:538f
      symbrachydactyly, VI:538f
      Swanson/IFSSH classification, VI:535–537
      symbrachydactyly, VI:537, 537f–538f, 546t
      syndactyly, VI:535–537, 535f, 537f
      terminology, VI:534–535
  hand development timing, VI:527t
  molecular controls, VI:527–530, 529f–530f
  tissue development/differentiation
    general discussion, VI:530–534
    innervation, VI:534, 534f
    myogenesis, VI:532–534, 533f
    skeletogenesis, VI:531–532, 532f
    vasculogenesis, VI:530–531, 531f
  upper limb morphogenesis, VI:527, 527t, 528f–529f
Limberg's four-flap Z-plasty, I:315
limbs, I:831–834
  See also lower extremities; upper extremities
Limb Salvage Index (LSI), IV:63
linea alba, IV:227–230, 227f
linear accelerator (linac), I:655
linear scleroderma, III:114–115, 115f
linea semilunaris, IV:227–230, 227f
LipiVage™ fat harvest system, V:598–599, 599f
lipoabdominoplasty, II:559–567
  anatomical principles, II:559–560, 560f
  background information, II:559
  complications, II:565–566, 566f
  dressings, II:565–566
  patient presentation and diagnosis
    patient selection, II:561
    preoperative ultrasound assessment, II:561
  postoperative care and follow-up, II:565–566
  prognosis and outcomes
    general discussion, II:565
    personal statistics, II:566t

lipoabdominoplasty (Continued)
  preoperative–postoperative comparisons, II:565f
  surgical revisions, II:566t
  surgical technique
    basic principles, II:560–561
    epigastric and subcostal liposuction
      infraumbilical tissue resection, II:563, 563f
      lower abdomen, II:561–562, 562f
      omphaloplasty, II:563–564, 564f
      rectus abdominal muscle plication, II:563, 563f
      Scarpa's fascia preservation, II:562–563, 563f
      selective undermining, II:562, 562f–563f
      superior abdominal liposuction, II:561–565, 562f
      suture layers and drain, II:564–565, 564f
    infiltration, II:561
    marking, II:561, 561f
    vascular perforators, II:559–560, 560f
lipodissolving treatments, II:527–528
lipodystrophy See liposuctions
lipofibromatous hamartomas, VI:320–321, 320f
lipofilling, IV:453–454, V:476
lipoma
  back soft-tissue reconstruction, IV:275–276
  characteristics, I:731
  diagnostic imaging, VI:83
  hand and wrist evaluations, VI:83, 321, 321f
  magnetic resonance imaging (MRI), III:364t
  scalp and forehead, III:116
  surgical technique and treatment, I:731, 731f–733f, VI:321, 321f
liposarcoma, I:740, 740f, VI:321
liposomes, I:186, 187f, 188t
liposuctions, II:507–529
  background information, II:507–508
  buttock augmentation, II:616
  classifications, II:508–509, 509f–511f
  complications, II:525–527, 526f, 527t
  emerging technologies, II:527–528
  epigastric and subcostal liposuction
    infraumbilical tissue resection, II:563, 563f
    lower abdomen, II:561–562, 562f
    omphaloplasty, II:563–564, 564f
    rectus abdominal muscle plication, II:563, 563f
    Scarpa's fascia preservation, II:562–563, 563f
    selective undermining, II:562, 562f–563f
    superior abdominal liposuction, II:561–565, 562f
    suture layers and drain, II:564–565, 564f
  fat grafting, II:332, 333f
  female genital aesthetic surgery, II:674–676, 675f–677f
  infiltration
    infiltrating wetting solutions
      aspirated volumes, II:516t
      blood loss estimates, II:516t
      common formulations, II:516t
      epinephrine, II:516t, 517
      fluid requirement guidelines, II:517
      fluid resuscitation, II:517–518

liposuctions (Continued)
    lidocaine, II:516t, 517
    perioperative fluid management, II:516–518
  local anesthesia, I:143–144, 144f
  informed consent, II:513
  lipoabdominoplasty, II:559
  lower bodylift (LBL)/buttock contouring, II:648f
  lymphedema, IV:94–95
  neck rejuvenation, II:320–321, 321f
  noninvasive body contouring, I:852–853
  operative procedures
    anesthesia, II:514–515
    core body temperature maintenance, II:515
    immediate preoperative care, II:515
    operation location, II:514–515
    patient positioning
      lateral decubitus position, II:516
      prone/supine position, II:515–516, 515f
    preoperative markings, II:513–514, 514f
  patient education, II:513
  patient presentation and diagnosis, II:509–511, 512f
  patient safety, I:129, 131
  patient selection, II:509–511
  postoperative care and follow-up, II:525
  power-assisted liposuction (PAL), II:507–508, 518, 520
  preoperative assessment
    initial evaluation, II:511–512
    physical examination, II:512–513, 513f–514f
  research summary, II:528
  subcutaneous fat
    characteristics, II:508–513, 508f
    zones of adherence, II:508, 508f
  suction-assisted lipectomy (SAL)
    adolescent aesthetic surgery, I:45t
    background information, II:507–508
    cannulas, II:520
    neck rejuvenation, II:320
    treatment options, II:518–525
  treatment options
    cannulas
      functional role, II:520
      injuries, II:525–526, 526f
      length, II:520
      power-assisted liposuction (PAL), II:520
      size and diameter, II:520, 520t
      suction-assisted lipectomy (SAL), II:520
      tip configuration, II:520
      ultrasound-assisted liposuction (UAL), II:520–521
    laser-assisted liposuction (LAL), II:519
    power-assisted liposuction (PAL), II:518
    suction-assisted lipectomy (SAL), II:518–525
    surgical endpoints, II:519–520, 520t
    treatment areas
      abdomen, II:521–522
      ankles, II:525
      arms, II:521
      buttocks, II:523, 524f
      hips/flanks, II:522–523, 522f–523f
      knees, II:525

liposuctions (Continued)
    neck, II:525
    thighs, II:524–525
    trunk/back, II:521, 521f
    ultrasound-assisted liposuction (UAL), II:518–519, 518f–519f
    vaser-assisted liposuction, II:519
  ultrasound-assisted liposuction (UAL)
    background information, II:507–508
    cannulas, II:520–521
    neck rejuvenation, II:320
    treatment options, II:518–519, 518f–519f
  vertical scar reduction mammaplasty, V:185
lips
  anatomical characteristics, III:422f, 633, 633f–634f
  anesthesia
    lower lip, III:27, 28f
    upper lip, III:27, 27f–28f
  anthropometric analysis, II:360, 360f
  burn wound treatment, IV:489, 490f–491f, 498–499
  facelift techniques, II:204–205, 204f
  facial paralysis
    soft-tissue rebalancing, III:302, 303f
    surgical management, III:287f, 291
  fat grafting, I:342–346, 344f–345f
  musculature, III:280–281, 282f, 282t
  photographic guidelines, I:110, 112f
  progressive hemifacial atrophy (PHA), III:796–797
  reconstructive surgeries, III:254–277
    algorithmic approach, III:271f
    anatomic considerations, III:255–256, 255f
    burn wound treatment, IV:489, 490f–491f, 498–499
    complications, III:270–271
    functional considerations, III:256
    importance, III:254–255
    lower lip
      decision-making process, III:454–456
      full-thickness defects, III:454, 455f
      Gillies fan flap, III:261–262, 264f, 454
      Karapandzic flap, III:261–262, 264f, 454, 455f
      tongue flaps, III:456
      total lower lip reconstruction, III:456
    nineteenth century, I:20, 20f
    operative technique
      Abbé flap, III:259–265, 261f–262f
      commissure reconstruction, III:456
      defect-specific reconstruction, III:257
      Estlander flap, III:259, 263f, 276f
      Fujimori gate flaps, III:265–268, 266f
      Gillies fan flap, III:261–262, 264f, 454
      intermediate full-thickness defects, III:259–265, 259b
      Karapandzic flap, III:261–262, 264f, 454, 455f
      large full-thickness defects, III:265–268, 454, 455f
      lip switch flaps, III:259b
      local flaps, III:453–456
      lower lip, III:454–456
      radial forearm flap, III:267–268, 267f–268f
      small full-thickness defects, III:258–259
      step flap, III:265f

Note: Boldface roman numerals indicate volume. Page numbers followed by f refer to figures; page numbers followed by t refer to tables; page numbers followed by b refer to boxes.

lips (Continued)
    tongue flaps, III:456
    total lower lip reconstruction, III:456
    upper lip, III:453–454
    vermillion defects, III:257–258, 258f
    wedge resection, III:258–259, 259b,
        259f–261f, 264f
    patient presentation and diagnosis
        goals, III:256–257, 256b
        patient selection, III:257
    postoperative care and follow-up,
        III:271
    reconstructive burn surgery, IV:505
    research summary, III:274–276
    secondary procedures, III:268–270,
        269f–270f
    surgical guidelines, III:254
    traumatic injuries, III:46, 47f–48f
    upper lip
        Abbé flap, III:454
        burn wound treatment, IV:489,
            490f–491f, 498–499
        decision-making process, III:453–454
        direct closure, III:453
        fan flaps, III:454
        large defects, III:453–454
    secondary cleft deformities
        cleft lip anatomy, III:633, 634f
        Cupid's bow, III:639
        long lip, III:637
        philtral column reconstruction, III:638–
            639, 639f
        short lateral lip, III:638
        short lip, III:635–637, 636f
        tight lip, III:637, 637f–638f
        wide lip, III:637–638
    soft-tissue fillers, II:55–56, 56f
    traumatic injuries, III:46, 47f–48f
    tumors, III:398–419
        cervical metastasis, III:405–406
        complications
            dental follow-ups, III:418
            general discussion, III:416–418
            local recurrence, III:416
            osteoradionecrosis (ORN), III:417
            post-treatment surveillance, III:417–418
            regional recurrence, III:416–417
            wound infections, III:417
        diagnosis and treatment, III:427
        epidemiology, III:399–400
        lymph node anatomy, III:399f
        medical challenges, III:398
        pathogenesis, III:398–399
        patient presentation and diagnosis,
            III:400
        preoperative assessment, III:402, 405f
        surgical access, III:402, 403f–404f
        surgical technique and treatment,
            III:402–405, 405f
        therapeutic choices, III:401–402
        TNM clinical classification system,
            III:400–401, 401t
        See also cleft lip surgery
liquidity ratios, I:69
liquid silicone injections, V:98–100, 99f–100f
liquid surfactants, II:16
Liquiritae officinalis, II:23
Lisch nodules
    patient presentation and diagnosis, III:878
    surgical technique and treatment, III:878

Lisfranc amputation, IV:208
Lister, Joseph, IV:393
Littler, J William, VI:xlvi, 224
Littler modification, VI:764–765
Littler neurovascular island flap, VI:132–134
Littler operation, VI:224, 224f
LIVINGSKIN, I:858–861, 861f
living skin replacements, I:336f
Lmx gene expression, VI:529f
local anesthesia, I:137–149
    absorption, I:147
    action variability, I:146–147
    carbonated anesthesia, I:140, 140f, 148
    comparative pharmacology, VI:96t
    complications
        adverse drug interactions, I:145
        allergic reactions, I:146
        bradycardia, I:145
        cardiovascular toxicity, I:146
        central nervous system toxicity, I:146
        hypertension, I:145
        hypotension, I:145
        nausea and vomiting, I:145
        respiration, I:144–145
        reversal effects, I:145
        tachycardia, I:145
        toxicity diagnosis and treatment, I:146,
            146b
    epinephrine, I:139, 140f, 147–148
    general discussion, I:137
    infiltration
        abdominoplasties, I:143, 144f
        breast augmentation, I:142–143, 143f
        breast reduction, I:141–142, 141f–142f
        characteristics, I:140–144
        facelifts, I:140, 141f
        liposuctions, I:143–144, 144f
    patient selection, I:137–138
    pharmacokinetics, VI:94
    pharmacology, VI:94–96
    pre-emptive effects, I:148–149
    premedication, I:138
    research summary, I:149
    sedation choice, I:138
    sedation drugs, I:138–139
    selection guidelines, VI:95–96, 95t
        anesthetic drugs, I:139
        carbonated anesthesia, I:140, 140f
        characteristics, I:139–140
        vasoconstricting agents, I:139–140
    toxicity, I:147–148, VI:94–95, 101–102
    vasoconstrictive effects, I:147
    vasoconstrictors, VI:95
locked plating, VI:115, 115f
Lockwood ligament, II:111f, 112
Lockwood technique, II:571–572, 573b, 579f
lomustine, I:779–781
long lip, III:637
long transhumeral amputation, VI:874–875
long, wide nose with a drooping tip and nasal
    airway obstruction
    outcome assessments, II:409
    surgical goals, II:409
    surgical plan, II:409
    systematic analysis, II:407–409, 407f–408f
Lonicera japonica, V:33t–35t
Lorazepam, I:138
loving cup ear, II:290–293, 292f
low air loss mattress concept, IV:364–366,
    364f

lower bodylift/belt lipectomy surgery,
    II:568–598
    anatomical considerations, II:568–569, 569f
    complications
        deep vein thrombosis (DVT), II:593–594
        dehiscence, II:591
        general discussion, II:589–595
        infections, II:592
        psychological difficulties, II:594–595
        pulmonary embolisms, II:593–594
        seromas, II:590
        tissue necrosis, II:592–593, 595f
        wound separation, II:590–591
    disease process
        massive weight loss patients, II:569, 570f
        normal weight patients group, II:570,
            572f–573f
        20–30 pounds overweight group, II:569,
            571f
    general discussion, II:568
    lower bodylift type II (Lockwood
        technique), II:571–572, 573b, 579f
    outcome assessments
        characteristics, II:588–595
        group I patients, II:589f–590f
        group II patients, II:591f–592f
        group III patients, II:593f–594f
    patient presentation and diagnosis
        back roll presentations, II:571, 578f
        body mass index (BMI), II:570, 574f
        buttocks variations, II:577f
        commonalities, II:570–571
        fat deposition pattern, II:570, 574f–575f
        hanging panniculi, II:576f
        skin/fat envelope, II:570, 574f–575f
    patient selection
        belt lipectomy/central bodylift, II:572–
            574, 574b
        general discussion, II:571–580
        lower bodylift type II (Lockwood
            technique), II:571–572, 573b, 579f
        preoperative assessment, II:577–580
        selection criteria, II:574–576, 577b
    postoperative care and follow-up, II:588,
        588b
    secondary procedures, II:595
    surgical technique and treatment
        circumferential excisional procedures,
            II:580–585, 580f–582f
        excisional tension, II:580–585, 580f–582f
        markings
            horizontal mons pubis marking,
                II:581–582, 583f
            inferior back marking, II:584, 584f
            lateral mons to anterior superior iliac
                spine (ASIS) marking, II:582, 583f
            posterior midline extent of resection
                marking, II:583–584, 584f
            posterior vertical midline marking,
                II:583
            superior back marking, II:584–585, 584f
            superior horizontal abdominal
                marking, II:582–583, 583f
            surgical guidelines, II:580–585
            vertical alignment marking, II:585
            vertical midline marking, II:581
        surgical procedures
            anesthesia, II:585–588
            dissection techniques, II:587f
            goals, II:580, 580b

lower bodylift/belt lipectomy surgery
    (Continued)
        markings, **II**:580–585, 583f–584f
        positioning, **II**:587f
        positioning sequence, **II**:585
        suturing techniques, **II**:585–588, 586f
    upper bodylift considerations, **II**:595, 596f–597f
    zones of adherence, **II**:568–569, 569f
lower bodylift (LBL)/buttock contouring, **II**:568–598
    major weight loss (MWL) patient, **II**:644b
    markings, **II**:645, 646f–647f, 649f
    operative technique, **II**:645, 647f–649f
    patient evaluation, **II**:644–645
    patient selection, **II**:645
    postoperative care and follow-up, **II**:645
lower extremities
    anatomical characteristics, **IV**:1–61
        ankles
            dorsalis pedis, **IV**:59, 60f
            extensor retinacula, **IV**:52, 52t, 54f
            fascial system, **IV**:52–56
            flexor retinaculum, **IV**:52–54, 52t, 54f
            functional role, **IV**:50–61
            innervation, **IV**:60f, 61
            peroneal artery, **IV**:47f, 59–61, 61f–62f
            peroneal retinaculum, **IV**:54, 54f, 54t
            posterior tibial artery, **IV**:47f, 59
            skeletal structure, **IV**:50, 52f
            vascular supply, **IV**:59–61
        embryology, **IV**:1, 2f
        feet
            cutaneous innervation, **IV**:46f, 51f, 61
            dorsalis pedis, **IV**:59, 60f
            extensor digitorum brevis muscle flap, **IV**:59f
            extensor retinacula, **IV**:52, 52t, 54f
            fascial compartments, **IV**:54–56, 56f–57f, 56t
            fascial system, **IV**:52–56
            flexor retinaculum, **IV**:52–54, 52t, 54f
            functional role, **IV**:50–61
            innervation, **IV**:46f, 51f, 60f
            motor nerves, **IV**:61
            musculature, **IV**:42f, 44f, 56–58, 56f–57f, 56t, 58t, 59f
            peroneal artery, **IV**:47f, 59–61, 61f–62f
            peroneal retinaculum, **IV**:54, 54f, 54t
            plantar fascia, **IV**:54, 55f
            posterior tibial artery, **IV**:47f, 59
            skeletal structure, **IV**:50, 53f
            vascular supply, **IV**:59–61
        gluteal region
            fascial system, **IV**:5
            innervation, **IV**:5–8, 7f
            musculature, **IV**:5, 5t, 6f
            skeletal structure, **IV**:2–5, 3f–4f
            vascular supply, **IV**:5, 7f
        legs
            anterior compartment musculature, **IV**:37, 38t–39t, 40f–42f, 43t
            compartment syndrome, **IV**:37
            cross-section diagram, **IV**:36f
            deep fascia, **IV**:34
            deep peroneal nerve, **IV**:48t
            fascial system, **IV**:34–37, 36f
            fasciocutaneous perforators, **IV**:50f

lower extremities (Continued)
        innervation, **IV**:48–50, 62f
        interosseous membrane, **IV**:34
        knee skeletal structure, **IV**:30, 31f–34f
        lateral compartment musculature, **IV**:37–43, 38t–39t, 43t, 44f
        lower leg compartments, **IV**:34–37
        lower leg cutaneous innervation, **IV**:48–50, 51f
        lower leg motor innervation, **IV**:48, 48t
        lower leg nerve topography, **IV**:48, 51f
        musculature, **IV**:62f
        peroneal artery, **IV**:47f
        popliteal artery, **IV**:47f
        posterior compartment musculature (deep layer), **IV**:38t–39t, 45, 45t, 46f
        posterior compartment musculature (superficial layer), **IV**:38t–39t, 43, 43t, 45f
        posterior tibial artery, **IV**:47f
        redundant tissue, **IV**:30–50
        skeletal structure, **IV**:30–34, 34f–35f
        superficial peroneal nerve, **IV**:48t
        tibial nerve, **IV**:46f–47f, 48t
        vascular supply, **IV**:45–48, 47f, 49f, 62f
    research summary, **IV**:61
    thighs
        adductor compartment musculature, **IV**:19t
        anterior thigh compartment musculature, **IV**:19t
        arteries and nerves, **IV**:18f
        cutaneous innervation, **IV**:26–30, 27f–29f
        fascial system, **IV**:8–11
        femur, **IV**:10f
        functional role, **IV**:8–30
        lateral circumflex femoral arterial system, **IV**:23, 25f
        medial circumflex femoral arterial system, **IV**:23–25, 26f
        medial femoral periosteal bone flap, **IV**:11f
        motor nerves, **IV**:26, 27f–28f
        musculature, **IV**:11–19, 13f, 15t–16t, 20f–22f
        obturator nerve, **IV**:29f
        pes anserinus, **IV**:19f
        posterior thigh compartment musculature, **IV**:19t
        profunda femoris, **IV**:22–23
        profunda femoris perforating branches, **IV**:25, 26f
        sciatic nerve, **IV**:28f
        serial cross-sections, **IV**:14f
        skeletal structure, **IV**:8, 9f–11f, 14f
        surface anatomy, **IV**:12f
        vascular supply, **IV**:19–25, 23f–24f
        vascular development, **IV**:2f
    burn reconstruction, **IV**:435–455
        acute phase surgery
            joint reconstruction, **IV**:441–442, 442f–443f, 445f
            skin grafts, **IV**:441
            skin substitutes, **IV**:441
        burn-related accidents, **IV**:435

lower extremities (Continued)
        complications
            axillary contractures, **IV**:445, 448f–449f
            bone exposure, **IV**:446, 450f
            elbow contractures, **IV**:445–446
            heterotopic ossification, **IV**:446
            scar retraction, **IV**:444–445
            skeletal-muscle complications, **IV**:446
            unstable healing, **IV**:444
        electrical burns, **IV**:435–436
        patient presentation and diagnosis
            compartment syndrome, **IV**:437–439, 437f–440f
            emergency surgical procedures, **IV**:437b
            escharotomy incisions, **IV**:429f–430f, 437–439, 437f–440f
            escharotomy lines, **IV**:428f
            extensive escharotomies, **IV**:431f
            fluid infusion and edema, **IV**:436–437
            full thickness burn escharotomies, **IV**:429f
            preoperative assessment, **IV**:436–440
            related trauma, **IV**:439–440
            zigzag escharotomies, **IV**:430f
        patient selection, **IV**:440
        postoperative care and follow-up
            active mobilization, **IV**:444
            ankles, **IV**:444
            compression garments, **IV**:447f
            hips/flanks, **IV**:443–444
            joint position, **IV**:443t
            knees, **IV**:444
            passive mobilization, **IV**:444
            patient positioning, **IV**:443
            physio-kinesitherapy tasks, **IV**:447f
            treatment strategies, **IV**:442–444
        prognosis and outcomes, **IV**:444–446
        secondary procedures
            amputations, **IV**:451–453
            fasciocutaneous flaps, **IV**:449–450
            free flaps, **IV**:450
            general characteristics, **IV**:446–454
            laser treatments, **IV**:454, 454t
            lipofilling, **IV**:453–454
            myocutaneous flaps, **IV**:449–450
            nerve repair and grafting, **IV**:450–451
            rotation flaps, **IV**:448–449, 453f–454f
            skin expansion, **IV**:450
            skin grafts, **IV**:447–448
            skin substitutes, **IV**:448
            tendon retraction, **IV**:451
            Z-plasty technique, **IV**:447, 451f–454f
        surgical technique and treatment
            acute phase surgery, **IV**:441
            basic procedure, **IV**:509
            characteristics, **IV**:440–442
    chronic nerve compression, **IV**:151–173
        numerical grading scale
            median nerve, **IV**:154t
            peripheral nerves, **IV**:154t
            tibial nerve, **IV**:155t
            ulnar nerve, **IV**:155t
        outcomes and complicatons, **IV**:172–173, 172t
        pathogenesis, **IV**:153–155
        patient presentation and diagnosis, **IV**:157

lower extremities (Continued)
  patient selection, **IV**:158
  postoperative care and follow-up, **IV**:170–172, 172f
  Pressure-Specified Sensory Device (PSSD), **IV**:154, 158f
  research background, **IV**:151–152
  surgical technique and treatment
    basic procedure, **IV**:164–170
    medial ankle tunnel release, **IV**:167f
    peroneal nerves, **IV**:168f–170f
    surgical tips, **IV**:164b, 166b
    tarsal tunnel, **IV**:167f
    tibial nerve, **IV**:171f
  tarsal tunnel decompression, **IV**:172t
congenital melanocytic nevi (CMN), **III**:848, 852f–853f
foot reconstruction, **IV**:189–219
  anatomic location-based reconstruction
    ankle and foot dorsum, **IV**:205–207, 206f
    anterolateral thigh flap, **IV**:211
    extensor digitorum brevis muscle flap, **IV**:205–206, 206f
    fasciocutaneous flaps, **IV**:211–214, 215f–216f
    gracilis muscle, **IV**:211
    heel pad flaps, **IV**:209
    hindfoot amputations, **IV**:216–217
    intrinsic muscle flaps, **IV**:209, 210f
    lateral arm flap, **IV**:211, 213f
    lateral supramalleolar flap, **IV**:206–207
    medial plantar artery flap, **IV**:209
    microvascular free flap, **IV**:211–216
    midfoot amputations, **IV**:208
    neurovascular island flap, **IV**:207–208
    parascapular flap, **IV**:211, 212f
    pedicle flaps, **IV**:205–217
    plantar forefoot, **IV**:207
    plantar hindfoot, **IV**:208–216, 210f, 212f–216f
    plantar midfoot, **IV**:208
    radial forearm flap, **IV**:211, 214f
    rectus abdominis, **IV**:211
    serratus anterior muscles, **IV**:211
    suprafascial flaps, **IV**:208
    sural artery flap, **IV**:209–211
    toe fillet flap, **IV**:207
    transmetatarsal amputation, **IV**:207
    V-Y plantar flap, **IV**:207
  disease process
    angiosomes, **IV**:189–190
    compartment pressure measurement, **IV**:190
    gait analysis, **IV**:190–191, 191f–192f
  outcome assessments, **IV**:217–218
  patient presentation and diagnosis
    antibiotic therapy, **IV**:196–197
    bone assessment, **IV**:196
    Charcot deformities, **IV**:195
    chronic wounds, **IV**:196
    clinical evaluations, **IV**:191–192
    connective tissue disorders, **IV**:192
    diabetic foot ulcers, **IV**:194–195
    hemorheologic abnormalities, **IV**:194f, 195–196
    infection identification, **IV**:196–197
    ischemia, **IV**:193, 194f
    neuropathic changes, **IV**:195
    venous stasis ulcers, **IV**:192–193

lower extremities (Continued)
  patient selection
    decision-making process, **IV**:197
    limb function, **IV**:197
  postoperative care and follow-up, **IV**:217
  research summary, **IV**:218
  soft tissue reconstruction
    angiosomes, **IV**:201
    closure techniques, **IV**:201–205, 202f–205f
  surgical technique and treatment
    anatomic location-based reconstruction, **IV**:205–217
    soft tissue reconstruction, **IV**:201–205
  trauma effects, **IV**:189
  treatment strategies
    debridement, **IV**:198–199, 200f
    external fixation, **IV**:199–201
    trauma and crush injuries, **IV**:198, 198f
    wound management, **IV**:199
lower extremity wounds
  diabetic ulcers, **I**:281
  ischemic wounds, **I**:279–281
  tissue expansion, **I**:650
  venous ulcers, **I**:279
lymphedema/lymphatic reconstruction, **IV**:92–100
  background information, **IV**:92
  classifications, **IV**:93
  complications, **IV**:98–99
  direct reconstruction
    lymphovenous bypass, **IV**:96, 97f, 98t
  disease process, **IV**:92–93
  etiology, **IV**:93
  patient presentation and diagnosis, **IV**:93
  patient selection
    nonsurgical therapy, **IV**:93–94
    reconstruction surgery, **IV**:94
  physiological operations
    Baumeister lymphatic vessel reconstruction technique, **IV**:95–96, 96f
    general discussion, **IV**:95–97
    lymphaticolymphatic bypass, **IV**:95
    lymphovenous bypass, **IV**:96, 97f, 98t
    lymphovenous shunts, **IV**:96–97, 99f
    microvascular lymph node transfer, **IV**:96, 96f
  postoperative care and follow-up, **IV**:97–98
  prognosis and outcomes, **IV**:98–99
  research summary, **IV**:99–100
  secondary procedures, **IV**:99
  surgical technique and treatment
    ablative operations, **IV**:94–95
    background information, **IV**:92
    goals, **IV**:94b
    liposuction, **IV**:94–95
    physiological operations, **IV**:95–97
melanoma excisions, **I**:767–768, 771f
painful neuroma, **IV**:151–173
  outcomes and complicatons, **IV**:172
  pathogenesis, **III**:441, **IV**:152f–153f
  patient presentation and diagnosis, **IV**:156–157, 156f
  patient selection, **IV**:157–158, 158f
  postoperative care and follow-up, **IV**:170, 172f
  research background, **IV**:151–152

lower extremities (Continued)
  surgical technique and treatment
    basic procedure, **IV**:159–164
    calcaneal nerve, **IV**:162f
    lateral knee denervation, **IV**:165f
    medial knee denervation, **IV**:165f
    plantar interdigital nerve, **IV**:163f
    saphenous nerve, **IV**:160f, 163f–164f
    superficial peroneal nerve, **IV**:160f
    sural nerve, **IV**:161f
    surgical tips, **IV**:159b
photographic guidelines, **I**:112, 117f
reconstructive surgeries, **IV**:127–150
  basic principles
    autologous tissue evaluation, **IV**:128, 129f
    goals, **IV**:127–131
    microvascular free tissue transfer, **IV**:131
    reconstructive ladder/reconstructive elevator analogy, **IV**:128, 130f
    skin grafts and substitutes, **IV**:128–129, 130f
  compound flaps, **IV**:148, 148f
  current perspectives, **IV**:127
  fasciocutaneous/perforator flap
    anterolateral thigh perforator flap, **IV**:145, 145f–146f
    characteristics, **IV**:143–147
    groin/superficial circumflex iliac perforator flap, **IV**:143, 143f–144f
    lateral thigh/profunda femoris perforator flap, **IV**:144–145, 144f
    medial thigh septocutaneous flap, **IV**:143–144, 144f
    sural flap, **IV**:146, 146f
    thoracodorsal artery perforator, **IV**:147, 147f
  foot reconstruction, **IV**:189–219
    anatomic location-based reconstruction, **IV**:205–217
    angiosomes, **IV**:189–190
    antibiotic therapy, **IV**:196–197
    bone assessment, **IV**:196
    Charcot deformities, **IV**:195
    chronic wound evaluation, **IV**:196
    clinical evaluations, **IV**:191–192
    closure techniques, **IV**:201–205, 202f–205f
    compartment pressure measurement, **IV**:190
    connective tissue disorders, **IV**:192
    debridement, **IV**:198–199, 200f
    diabetic foot ulcers, **IV**:194–195
    external fixation, **IV**:199–201
    gait analysis, **IV**:190–191, 191f–192f
    hemorheologic abnormalities, **IV**:194f, 195–196
    infection identification, **IV**:196–197
    ischemia, **IV**:193, 194f
    limb function, **IV**:197
    neuropathic changes, **IV**:195
    outcome assessments, **IV**:217–218
    patient presentation and diagnosis, **IV**:191–197
    patient selection, **IV**:197
    postoperative care and follow-up, **IV**:217
    research summary, **IV**:218
    soft tissue reconstruction, **IV**:201–205

lower extremities *(Continued)*
    surgical technique and treatment,
        IV:201–217
    trauma and crush injuries, **IV:**198, 198f
    trauma effects, **IV:**189
    treatment strategies, **IV:**198–201
    venous stasis ulcers, **IV:**192–193
    wound management, **IV:**199
muscle/musculocutaneous flaps
    biceps femoris muscle flap, **IV:**139–140
    characteristics, **I:**557–560
    gastrocnemius muscle flap, **I:**557–560,
        559f–560f, **IV:**142, 142f
    gracilis muscle flap, **IV:**140–141, 140f
    rectus femoris muscle flap, **IV:**139, 139f
    soleus muscle flap, **I:**557–560, 561f,
        IV:141–142, 141f
    tensor fascia lata, **IV:**138–139, 138f
postoperative care and follow-up
    flap complication management, **IV:**138
    postoperative monitoring, **IV:**137–138
    secondary operations, **IV:**138
sarcoma-related reconstruction,
    IV:101–126
    amputation indicators, **IV:**110
    bone sarcoma, **IV:**103
    chemotherapy, **IV:**106
    clinical manifestations, **IV:**102
    definitive resections, **IV:**108
    epidemiology, **IV:**102–103
    imaging methods, **IV:**104, 104f
    immediate postoperative care,
        IV:112–113
    lymph node dissection, **IV:**110
    Muskuloskeletal Tumor Society staging
        system, **IV:**105t
    nerve involvement, **IV:**109
    oncologic postoperative care and
        follow-up, **IV:**113
    osseous involvement, **IV:**109
    patient presentation and diagnosis,
        IV:103–104
    patient selection, **IV:**104
    preservation options, **IV:**110–112
    primary osseous sarcomas, **IV:**109
    prognosis and outcomes, **IV:**114
    radiation therapy (RT), **IV:**106
    recurrence management, **IV:**116–125
    secondary procedures, **IV:**113–114
    soft-tissue sarcomas, **IV:**102–103, 102t,
        103f
    specimen handling, **IV:**109
    surgical goals, **IV:**104–105
    surgical planning, **IV:**105, 105t
    surgical resection techniques,
        IV:106–110
    surgical treatment, **IV:**105–106
    TNM clinical classification system,
        IV:105t
    tumor growth and metastasis, **IV:**103
    vascular involvement, **IV:**108
    wound closure, **IV:**109
special considerations
    diabetes, **IV:**134, 134f–135f
    exposed prosthesis, **IV:**137, 137f
    osteomyelitis, **IV:**133–134, 134f
    soft-tissue expansion, **IV:**137
    tumor ablation, **IV:**136, 136f

lower extremities *(Continued)*
    specific location
        knees, **IV:**131f, 137f
        lower leg, **IV:**130–131
        thigh, **IV:**130, 131f
    supermicrosurgery technique, **IV:**149,
        149f
    surgical technique and treatment
        debridement, **IV:**133
        preoperative assessment, **IV:**131–132,
            131f–132f
        primary limb amputation, **IV:**83,
            132–133
        recipient vessels, **IV:**133
        timing considerations, **IV:**133
sarcoma-related reconstruction, **IV:**101–126
    biopsies
        core needle biopsy, **IV:**106
        excisional biopsies, **IV:**106–107
        fine-needle aspiration (FNA), **IV:**106
        incisional biopsies, **IV:**107
        reoperative biopsies, **IV:**107–108
    bone sarcoma
        characteristics, **IV:**101–102
        epidemiology, **IV:**103
        imaging methods, **IV:**104, 104f
        Muskuloskeletal Tumor Society staging
            system, **IV:**105t
        outcome assessments, **IV:**115–116
        patient presentation and diagnosis,
            IV:103–104, 104f
        patient selection, **IV:**104
        preservation options, **IV:**110–112
        recurrence management, **IV:**116–125
        surgical resection techniques,
            IV:106–108
        treatment strategies, **IV:**104
        tumor growth and metastasis, **IV:**103
    case studies
        case study 4.1, **IV:**116b–117b, 116f–117f
        case study 4.2, **IV:**117b, 118f
        case study 4.3, **IV:**117b–120b, 119f–120f
        case study 4.4, **IV:**120b, 121f
        case study 4.5, **IV:**120b–123b, 122f–123f
        case study 4.6, **IV:**123b–125b, 123f–124f
        case study 4.7, **IV:**124f–125f, 125b
    clinical manifestations, **IV:**102
    epidemiology, **IV:**102–103
    imaging methods, **IV:**104, 104f
    Muskuloskeletal Tumor Society staging
        system, **IV:**105t
    outcome assessments
        bone sarcoma, **IV:**115–116
        prognosis, **IV:**114
        soft-tissue sarcomas, **IV:**114–115, 115t
    patient presentation and diagnosis,
        IV:103–104
    patient selection, **IV:**104
    postoperative care and follow-up
        immediate postoperative care,
            IV:112–113
        oncologic postoperative care and
            follow-up, **IV:**113
    preservation options
        complex approaches, **IV:**112
        general discussion, **IV:**110–112
        neuromuscular units, **IV:**111
        skeletal reconstruction, **IV:**111–112, 111f

lower extremities *(Continued)*
    soft-tissue sarcomas, **IV:**110–111
    vascular surgery, **IV:**112
    recurrence management, **IV:**116–125
    secondary procedures
        late secondary procedures, **IV:**114
        skeletal reconstruction, **IV:**113–114
        soft tissue, **IV:**113
    soft-tissue sarcomas
        epidemiology, **IV:**102–103
        histopathologic types, **IV:**103f
        predisposing factors, **IV:**102t
        preservation options, **IV:**110–111
    surgical resection techniques
        amputation indicators, **IV:**110
        biopsies, **IV:**106–108
        definitive resections, **IV:**108
        lymph node dissection, **IV:**110
        nerve involvement, **IV:**109
        osseous involvement, **IV:**109
        primary osseous sarcomas, **IV:**109
        specimen handling, **IV:**109
        surgical revisions, **IV:**107–108, 108t
        vascular involvement, **IV:**108
        wound closure, **IV:**109
    TNM clinical classification system, **IV:**105t
    treatment strategies
        chemotherapy, **IV:**106
        radiation therapy (RT), **IV:**106
        surgical goals, **IV:**104–105
        surgical planning, **IV:**105, 105t
        surgical treatment, **IV:**105–106
    tumor growth and metastasis, **IV:**103
TNM clinical classification system/pTNM
    pathologic classification system, **I:**714f
trauma injuries, **IV:**63–91
    amputation versus salvage decisions,
        IV:65–66, 86
    associated complications
        compartment syndrome, **IV:**84–85
        fat embolism syndrome (FES), **IV:**84
        rhabdomyolysis, **IV:**83–84
    complications
        chronic pain, **IV:**87
        nonunion occurrences, **IV:**87
        osteomyelitis, **IV:**86–87
        wound complications, **IV:**86
    epidemiology, **IV:**63
    inflammatory response, **IV:**63–64
    Mangled Extremity Severity Score
        (MESS), **IV:**65–66, 66t
    outcome assessments
        amputation versus salvage decisions,
            IV:86
        cost-utility analysis, **IV:**86
        functional outcomes, **IV:**85–86
        patient satisfaction, **IV:**86
    patient presentation and diagnosis
        Glasgow Coma Scale (GCS), **IV:**64t
        injury assessments, **IV:**64–65
        injury classifications, **IV:**65t
        tetanus prophylaxis Immunization
            schedule, **IV:**65t
    patient selection, **IV:**65–66
    postoperative care and follow-up
        antibiotics, **IV:**85
        anticoagulant agents, **IV:**85
        hemorrhage, **IV:**85

Note: **Boldface** *roman numerals indicate volume. Page numbers followed by f refer to figures; page numbers followed by t refer to tables; page numbers followed by b refer to boxes.*

lower extremities (Continued)
  reconstruction options
    anterolateral thigh flap, **IV:**68–69, 69f, 75, 75f–76f, 81f, 88f
    complex defect and fracture, **IV:**77f–78f
    fasciocutaneous flaps, **IV:**81, 81f–82f
    gracilis muscle, **IV:**77, 80f, 89f–90f
    latissimus dorsi (LD) flap, **IV:**77, 78f–79f
    local flaps, **IV:**68
    muscle/musculocutaneous flaps, **IV:**72–75, 74f
    negative-pressure wound therapy (NPWT), **IV:**83
    perforator flaps, **IV:**68–72
    rectus abdominis, **IV:**77, 79f
    rectus femoris muscle flap, **IV:**82f
    serratus anterior muscles, **IV:**77
    skeletal reconstruction, **IV:**83, 83f
    soft-tissue destruction, **IV:**68–83, 68f
    sural artery flap, **IV:**75, 77f
    thoracodorsal artery perforator (TDAP) flap, **IV:**77, 147, 147f
  secondary cosmetic procedures
    anterolateral thigh flap, **IV:**88f
    basic procedure, **IV:**87
    debulking, **IV:**90f
    degloving injury, **IV:**88f
    gracilis muscle, **IV:**89f–90f
    liposuction, **IV:**89f
  secondary procedures
    characteristics, **IV:**87–91
    secondary cosmetic procedures, **IV:**87
    secondary functional procedures, **IV:**91
  surgical technique and treatment
    amputations, **IV:**83, 132–133
    fracture management strategies, **IV:**67
    reconstruction options, **IV:**68–83
    timing considerations, **IV:**66–67, 67t
    vascular injury, **IV:**67–68
Lower Extremity Assessment Project (LEAP), **IV:**65–66, 127
lower eyelid area
  access incisions, **III:**227
  anatomical characteristics, **II:**112
  anesthesia, **III:**27, 27f–28f
  facial paralysis, **III:**287–289, 287f, 290f
  lower eyelid surgery
    basic principles, **II:**127–131
    burn wound treatment, **IV:**486–488, 488f
    large defects, **III:**450
    orbicularis suspension, **II:**130–131
    orbital fat excision
      capsulopalpebral fascia plication, **II:**129–130, 132f
      general discussion, **II:**128–130
      orbital fat transposition, **II:**128
      orbital septum plication, **II:**128, 131f
      plication techniques, **II:**128
    partial lower lid defects, **III:**449
    total lower lid defects, **III:**450
    transconjunctival blepharoplasty, **II:**128, 129f–131f
    transcutaneous blepharoplasty, **II:**128
  lower eyelid tonicity, **II:**121
  secondary blepharoplasty
    anatomical analysis, **II:**148f, 151f
    canthoplasty techniques, **II:**151–160, 155f–156f, 155t

lower eyelid area (Continued)
  complications
    chemosis, **II:**162, 162f
    excessive fat resection, **II:**160–162, 161f
    inadequate fat resection, **II:**160–162, 161f
    persistent malar bags, **II:**161f, 162
  dermal orbicular pennant lateral canthoplasty (DOPLC), **II:**156, 158f–159f
  distraction test, **II:**150, 153f
  ectropion, **II:**150–151, 154f
  eyelid malposition, **II:**148–151, 152f
  inferior retinacular lateral canthoplasty/canthopexy (IRLC), **II:**156–157, 160f
  lateral bone-to-canthus relationship, **II:**149–150, 152f
  lower lid eversion, **II:**150–151, 154f
  medial canthus-to-lateral canthus relationship, **II:**150, 153f
  midface elevation and fixation, **II:**157, 161f
  midlamellar cicatricial retraction, **II:**150f
  patient evaluation, **II:**148–151, 149t
  snap test, **II:**150, 153f
  surgical procedures, **II:**151–160, 155t
  tarsal strip lateral canthoplasty, **II:**155–156, 156f–157f
subperiosteal facelift, **II:**270–273, 270f
vertical shortening, **III:**57
lower facial fractures
  mandibular fractures
    antibiotics, **III:**82
    characteristics, **III:**75
    classification systems, **III:**76–77
    clinical examination, **III:**76
    complications
      facial width, **III:**82
      hardware infection and migration, **III:**82
      malocclusion, **III:**82
      mandible rotation, **III:**82
      nonunion occurrences, **III:**82
      osteomyelitis, **III:**82–83
    dental wiring and fixation techniques
      arch-bars, **III:**75
      intermaxillary fixation (IMF) screws, **III:**75–76, 75f
    diagnosis, **III:**76
    displacement direction and extent
      fracture line direction and angulation, **III:**77, 77f
      general discussion, **III:**77
      teeth, **III:**77
    edentulous mandible fractures, **III:**83–84, 84f
    internal fixation devices
      Champy or miniplate system, **III:**80–81, 80f
      lag screw technique, **III:**81, 81f
      selection guidelines, **III:**80–83
    muscle function considerations, **III:**76
    temporomandibular joint, **III:**76–77
    third molar extraction, **III:**81, 81f
    treatment strategies
      basic principles, **III:**77
      Class I fractures, **III:**77–78
      Class II fractures, **III:**78
      Class III fractures, **III:**78–80
      comminuted fractures, **III:**78, 79f

lower facial fractures (Continued)
  intraoral approach, **III:**79
  open reduction treatment, **III:**78–79
  reduction and fixation principles, **III:**78, 78f
  surgical indicators, **III:**79–80
lower leg
  reconstructive surgeries, **IV:**130–131
lower plexus injuries
  examination findings, **VI:**732
  reconstruction techniques, **VI:**732, 732b
lower trunk, **I:**110, 115f–116f
low median nerve palsy
  pathogenesis, **VI:**753
  patient selection, **VI:**753–758
  surgical technique and treatment
    abductor digiti minimi (ADM) tendon, **VI:**758
    Bunnell ring finger flexor digitorum superficialis transfer, **VI:**755–756, 755f–757f, 761t
    Burkhalter extensor indicis proprius transfer, **VI:**754–755, 754f–755f
    Camitz palmaris longus transfer, **VI:**756–758, 757f–759f, 761t
    Huber transfer, **VI:**758, 761t
    opposition tendon transfers, **VI:**761t
low-molecular-weight heparin (LMWH), **VI:**244–245
low ulnar nerve palsy
  patient selection, **VI:**761–771, 762f, 762t
  surgical technique and treatment
    Bouvier maneuver, **VI:**764–765, 764f
    Brand EE4T transfer, **VI:**766–767, 766f
    Brand EF4T transfer, **VI:**767, 767f–768f
    donor muscle-tendon selection, **VI:**764–765, 765f
    Fritschi PF4T transfer, **VI:**767–768
    index finger abduction, **VI:**770–771, 771f
    Littler modification, **VI:**764–765
    modified Stiles–Bunnell technique, **VI:**764–766, 765f
    Neviaser accessory abductor pollicis longus and free tendon graft, **VI:**771, 771f
    pulley insertions, **VI:**764–765, 764f–765f
    ring finger flexor digitorum superficialis transfer, **VI:**769
    Smith extensor carpi radialis brevis transfer, **VI:**769–770, 770f
    static procedures, **VI:**763–764, 763f–764f
    thumb adduction restoration, **VI:**768–769, 769f–770f
    ulnar deviation of the small finger, **VI:**768
low velocity gunshot wounds, **III:**85–87
L short-scar mammaplasty, **V:**206–215
  background and general characteristics, **V:**206–207
  complications, **V:**213
  patient selection, **V:**206–207
  planning and marking guidelines, **V:**207, 208f–209f
  reduction results, **V:**210f–214f
  research summary, **V:**214–215
  surgical technique, **V:**207–210, 209f
Luer-to-Luer connector, **V:**598, 598f
lumbar artery, **IV:**222f, 223
lumbar artery perforator (LAP) flap, **V:**467–470, 470b, 470f
lumbocostoabdominal triangle, **IV:**221

lumbrical muscle, **VI**:52
lumbrical muscle tightness test, **VI**:54, 54f
lumpectomies, **I**:43, **V**:278f, 584t, 586–590, 590f
lunotriquetral shuck test, **VI**:54, 55f
Lux 1540 nm laser, **II**:71t, 73
Lux 2940 laser, **II**:73
Luzzi, Mondino de, **I**:15, 15f
lycopene, **II**:28
lymphadenectomy
  axillary lymphadenectomy, **I**:771–777, 775f
  cervical lymphadenectomy, **I**:771, 773f–774f
  decision-making process, **I**:768–777
  pelvic and inguinofemoral
    lymphadenectomy, **I**:772–777, 775f–777f
  research studies, **I**:768–777
lymphadenopathy
  atypical nontuberculous mycobacteria
    disease process, **III**:891
    patient presentation and diagnosis,
      III:891–892, 891f
    surgical technique and treatment, **III**:892
  bacterial lymphadenitis
    disease process, **III**:890
    patient presentation and diagnosis,
      III:891
    surgical technique and treatment, **III**:891
  cervical tuberculous adenitis (scrofula)
    disease process, **III**:891
    patient presentation and diagnosis,
      III:891
    surgical technique and treatment, **III**:891
  characteristics, **III**:890
  chronic regional lymphadenopathy
    complications, **III**:891
    disease process, **III**:891
    patient presentation and diagnosis,
      III:891
    prognosis and outcomes, **III**:891
lymphangioma, **I**:678t
lymphangiomatosis, **VI**:668, 668t
lymphatic malformation (LM)
  benign mesenchymal-origin tumors, **I**:736
  classification systems, **I**:676–677, 677t,
    VI:668t
  clinical manifestations, **I**:690–692
  diagnostic work-up, **VI**:670t
  outcomes and complicatons, **VI**:679–680
  pathogenesis, **I**:690, **VI**:675–677
  patient presentation and diagnosis, **VI**:669,
    670f, 677–679, 678f
  surgical technique and treatment, **VI**:669–
    672, 671t, 679, 680f–681f
  terminology, **I**:678t
  treatment strategies
    general discussion, **I**:692–693
    resection, **I**:693
    sclerotherapy, **I**:683f, 692–693
lymphatic system/abdominoplasty, **II**:533
lymphatic-venous malformation (LVM),
  I:677t
lymphedema/lymphatic reconstruction,
  IV:92–100
  background information, **IV**:92
  classifications, **IV**:93
  complications, **IV**:98–99
  disease process, **IV**:92–93
  etiology, **IV**:93
  patient presentation and diagnosis, **IV**:93

lymphedema/lymphatic reconstruction
  (Continued)
  patient selection
    nonsurgical therapy, **IV**:93–94
    reconstruction surgery, **IV**:94
  postoperative care and follow-up, **IV**:97–98
  prognosis and outcomes, **IV**:98–99
  radiation therapy (RT), **I**:288, 672
  research summary, **IV**:99–100
  secondary procedures, **IV**:99
  surgical technique and treatment
    ablative operations, **IV**:94–95
    background information, **IV**:92
    direct reconstruction
      lymphovenous bypass, **IV**:96, 97f, 98t
    goals, **IV**:94b
    liposuction, **IV**:94–95
    physiological operations
      Baumeister lymphatic vessel
        reconstruction technique, **IV**:95–96,
        96f
      general discussion, **IV**:95–97
      lymphaticolymphatic bypass, **IV**:95
      lymphovenous bypass, **IV**:96, 97f, 98t
      lymphovenous shunts, **IV**:96–97, 99f
      microvascular lymph node transfer,
        IV:96, 96f
lymph node anatomy, **III**:399f
lymph node drainage patterns, **III**:421
lymphoceles, **V**:563–564
lymphocytes, **I**:268–269, 268f
lymphoma, **III**:364t–365t, 370–371, 371f, 377
lympho-magnetic resonance imaging (MRI),
  V:334f
lymphoscintigraphy (lymphatic mapping),
  I:757–758, 758f–759f, 759t

M

MacDermol S/MacDermol R, **II**:47t
macrodactyly
  classification systems, **VI**:541f
  clinical manifestations, **VI**:634–635, 635f
  Hong Kong survey, **VI**:635t
  proteus syndrome, **VI**:635
  surgical technique and treatment, **VI**:636f
Macrolane, **II**:47t
macrolide inhibitors, **I**:822t
macromastia, **V**:152–153, 161–162, 240f–241f
macrophage colony-stimulating factor
  (M-CSF), **I**:431
macrophages
  functional role, **I**:816
  skin wound healing, **I**:268–269, 268f, 270t,
    271f
  wound healing, **I**:245f, 248, 256f–257f
MACS (minimal access cranial suspension)
  lift, **II**:223–231
  background information, **II**:223
  inappropriate skin shifts, **II**:300–301
  patient expectations, **II**:226–227
  patient selection
    evaluation examinations, **II**:225–226
    facial skeletal structure and asymmetry,
      II:226
    facial volume, **II**:226
    forehead rejuvenation, **II**:226
    glabellar rhytides, **II**:226
    jowls, **II**:226

MACS (minimal access cranial suspension) lift
  (Continued)
    medical history, **II**:226
    neck, **II**:226
    ocular region, **II**:226
    previous surgeries, **II**:226
    skin characteristics, **II**:226
  platysma-SMAS plication (PSP), **II**:216–217,
    217t
  research summary, **II**:231
  subcutaneous facelifts, **II**:209–210, 210f
  surgical foundation
    basic principles, **II**:224–225, 224f
    extended MACS procedure, **II**:225f
    facial nerves, **II**:226f
    microimbrication, **II**:225f
    short scar incision, **II**:225f, 228f
  surgical strategy
    anchor points, **II**:227, 228f
    basic guidelines, **II**:227–231
    cheek sutures, **II**:228
    malar sutures, **II**:228–229
    neck sutures, **II**:227–228, 228f, 316
    skin advancement and resection,
      II:229–231, 229f–231f
    skin incision and undermining, **II**:227
    surgical sequence, **II**:227
macular scars, **II**:69
Madelung's deformity, **VI**:646–647, 647f
mafenide acetate, **IV**:410
Maffucci's syndrome
  classification systems, **VI**:668, 668t
  hands, **VI**:324
  patient presentation and diagnosis, **I**:695
maggots, **IV**:366–367
magnetic resonance imaging (MRI)
  brachial plexus injuries, **VI**:796, 797f–798f
  breast cancer diagnoses, **V**:268–270, 270f
  breast reconstruction, **V**:326, 328–329, 329f
  conjoined twins, **III**:897–899, 899f
  craniofacial fibrous dysplasia, **III**:382
  cutaneous and soft-tissue tumors, **I**:710
  epiphyseal growth plate, **VI**:656
  fracture assessment, **VI**:107
  hand and wrist evaluations
    advantages/disadvantages, **VI**:82–89, 82t
    basic principles, **VI**:82
    clinical applications
      carpal fractures, **VI**:85
      distal radioulnar joint (DRUJ)
        instability, **VI**:86–88
      enchondromas, **VI**:85
      fracture nonunion evaluations, **VI**:88
      ganglion cysts, **VI**:83, 84f
      giant cell tumors of the tendon sheath
        (GCTTS), **VI**:83, 84f
      hemangiomas, **VI**:83–85
      Kienbock's disease, **VI**:88, 89f
      ligamentous injuries, **VI**:85–86
      lipomas, **VI**:83
      occult scaphoid fractures, **VI**:85, 85f
      osteomyelitis, **VI**:88–89
      right-sided wrist pain, **VI**:87f–88f
      scaphoid fracture nonunion
        evaluations, **VI**:88
      scapholunate interosseous ligament
        injury, **VI**:85–86, 87f
      soft-tissue masses, **VI**:82–83

magnetic resonance imaging (MRI) (Continued)
tendinopathies, **VI:**86–88
thumb ulnar collateral ligament injuries, **VI:**85, 86f
trauma-related injuries, **VI:**85
triangular fibrocartilage (TFCC) tears, **VI:**86, 87f
tumors, **VI:**313
ulnar-sided wrist pain, **VI:**86–88, 87f–88f
ulnocarpal abutment, **VI:**86, 88f
pulse sequences and enhancements, **VI:**83t
signal intensities on weighted images, **VI:**82, 82t
head and neck cancer detection, **III:**400, 417–418
infant obstetric brachial plexus palsy, **VI:**809f
lympho-magnetic resonance imaging (MRI), **V:**334f
magnetic resonance angiography, **VI:**90, 90f, 472
melanoma detection, **I:**762–764, 763f
noncontrast magnetic resonance imaging (MRI), **V:**329, 329f, 334f
occupational hand disorders, **VI:**368–369
osteomyelitis, **IV:**358
revision breast augmentation, **V:**37, 41
salivary gland tumors, **III:**364, 364t
sarcoma detection, **IV:**103–104
scalp and forehead reconstruction, **III:**120
temporomandibular joint (TMJ) dysfunction, **III:**92, 93f
vascular anomalies, **VI:**669
velopharyngeal dysfunction (VPD), **III:**623
venous malformations (VM), **I:**686f
wrist injuries, **VI:**166–169
maidenhair tree, **V:**33t–35t
major histocompatibility complex (MHC)
basic principles, **I:**815–816
composite tissue allotransplantation (CTA), **VI:**844
major histocompatibility (MHC) markers, **I:**370
major weight loss (MWL) patient
abdominoplasty, **II:**551
body contouring, **V:**558–581
arms
demand increases, **V:**558–564
outcomes and complicatons, **V:**563–564
pathophysiology, **V:**558–559
patient presentation and diagnosis, **V:**559–564
patient selection, **V:**559–560
Pittsburgh Rating Scale, **V:**559–560, 559t
postoperative care and follow-up, **V:**562–563
surgical technique and treatment, **V:**560–562, 561f–563f, 562b
back
back rolls, **V:**570–573
outcomes and complicatons, **V:**573
pathophysiology, **V:**570–571
patient presentation and diagnosis, **V:**571
patient selection, **V:**571–572
postoperative care and follow-up, **V:**573

major weight loss (MWL) patient (Continued)
surgical planning, **V:**571–572
surgical technique and treatment, **V:**572, 573f
surgical tips, **V:**572b
transverse excisional upper bodylift, **V:**570f, 572
gynecomastia/male chest contouring
excision of gynecomastia with nipple repositioning, **V:**575–579, 578f–580f
outcomes and complicatons, **V:**579
pathophysiology, **V:**573–574
patient presentation and diagnosis, **V:**574
patient selection, **V:**574–575, 575t
postoperative care and follow-up, **V:**578
pseudogynecomastia, **V:**575t, 576f–577f
surgical markings, **V:**575–576, 576f–577f
surgical technique and treatment, **V:**576–578, 578f–580f
surgical tips, **V:**578b
mastopexy
breast reshaping, **V:**564–570
dermal suspension, **V:**566–570, 568f
outcomes and complicatons, **V:**567–570
pathophysiology, **V:**564, 564b
patient presentation and diagnosis, **V:**564–565
patient selection, **V:**565–566
postoperative care and follow-up, **V:**567
surgical goals, **V:**565b
surgical planning, **V:**565–566, 566t, 569f–570f
surgical tips, **V:**567b
total parenchymal reshaping mastopexy, **V:**566–570
secondary procedures, **V:**579
total parenchymal reshaping mastopexy
surgical markings, **V:**566
surgical technique and treatment, **V:**566–567, 568f
lower bodylift/belt lipectomy surgery, **II:**568–598
anatomical considerations, **II:**568–569, 569f
complications
deep vein thrombosis (DVT), **II:**593–594
dehiscence, **II:**591
general discussion, **II:**589–595
infections, **II:**592
psychological difficulties, **II:**594–595
pulmonary embolisms, **II:**593–594
seromas, **II:**590
tissue necrosis, **II:**592–593, 595f
wound separation, **II:**590–591
disease process
massive weight loss patients, **II:**569, 570f
normal weight patients group, **II:**570, 572f–573f
20–30 pounds overweight group, **II:**569, 571f
general discussion, **II:**568
markings
horizontal mons pubis marking, **II:**581–582, 583f
inferior back marking, **II:**584, 584f

major weight loss (MWL) patient (Continued)
lateral mons to anterior superior iliac spine (ASIS) marking, **II:**582, 583f
posterior vertical midline marking, **II:**583–584, 584f
superior back marking, **II:**584–585, 584f
superior horizontal abdominal marking, **II:**582–583, 583f
surgical guidelines, **II:**580–585
vertical alignment marking, **II:**585
vertical midline marking, **II:**581
outcome assessments
characteristics, **II:**588–595
group I patients, **II:**589f–590f
group II patients, **II:**591f–592f
group III patients, **II:**593f–594f
patient presentation and diagnosis
back roll presentations, **II:**571, 578f
body mass index (BMI), **II:**570, 574f
buttocks variations, **II:**577f
commonalities, **II:**570–571
fat deposition pattern, **II:**570, 574f–575f
hanging panniculi, **II:**576f
skin/fat envelope, **II:**570, 574f–575f
patient selection
belt lipectomy/central bodylift, **II:**572–574, 574b
general discussion, **II:**571–580
lower bodylift type II (Lockwood technique), **II:**571–572, 573b, 579f
preoperative assessment, **II:**577–580
selection criteria, **II:**574–576, 577b
postoperative care and follow-up, **II:**588, 588b
secondary procedures, **II:**595
surgical procedures
anesthesia, **II:**585–588
dissection techniques, **II:**587f
goals, **II:**580, 580b
markings, **II:**580–585, 583f–584f
positioning, **II:**587f
positioning sequence, **II:**585
suturing techniques, **II:**585–588, 586f
surgical technique and treatment
belt lipectomy, **II:**580–585
circumferential excisional procedures, **II:**580–585, 580f–582f
excisional tension, **II:**580–585, 580f–582f
upper bodylift considerations, **II:**595, 596f–597f
zones of adherence, **II:**568–569, 569f
post-bariatric surgery reconstruction
abdominal contouring, **II:**639b
lower bodylift (LBL)/buttock contouring, **II:**644b
vertical thigh-lift, **II:**648b
malar augmentation, **II:**52f, 53, 54f
malar fat pad, **II:**186–188, 186f–188f, **III:**10
malar prominence, **II:**122
malar reduction
historical background, **II:**177–178
surgical technique
basic procedure, **II:**180–181, 180f
bicoronal approach, **II:**181
intraoral infracture technique with incomplete osteotomy, **II:**181
intraoral L-shaped ostectomy, **II:**181
malar region
Treacher Collins syndrome, **III:**828–830

male chest
  body contouring
    excision of gynecomastia with nipple
      repositioning, **V:**575–579, 578f–580f
    outcomes and complicatons, **V:**579
    pathophysiology, **V:**573–574
    patient presentation and diagnosis, **V:**574
    patient selection, **V:**574–575, 575t
    postoperative care and follow-up, **V:**578
    pseudogynecomastia, **V:**575t, 576f–577f
    surgical markings, **V:**575–576, 576f–577f
    surgical technique and treatment,
      V:576–578, 578f–580f
    surgical tips, **V:**578b
  post-bariatric surgery reconstruction, **II:**652
male cosmetic surgery patient, **II:**4, 4f
male genital aesthetic surgery, **II:**655–677
  enhancement procedures, **II:**655
  flaccid versus erect penis measurements,
    II:655–656
  hidden penis
    characteristics, **II:**665–668, 665f–666f
    outcome assessments, **II:**668
    post-bariatric surgery reconstruction,
      II:640, 643f
    surgical technique, **II:**667–668, 667f–669f
  patient selection and examination, **II:**656
  penile anatomy, **II:**656
  penile enlargement reconstruction
    dermal fat graft and Alloderm removal,
      II:661–662, 661f
    fat removal, **II:**660–661
    outcomes and complicatons, **II:**662
    postoperative care and follow-up, **II:**662
    reconstructive issues, **II:**660–662
    VY advancement flap reversal, **II:**658f,
      660, 661f
  penile girth enhancement
    allograft dermal matrix grafts, **II:**660
    challenges, **II:**659–660
    dermal and dermal fat grafts, **II:**659–660
    fat injections, **II:**658f–659f, 659
  penile lengthening
    basic procedure, **II:**656–658, 657f–658f
    outcome assessments, **II:**657–658, 659f
    VY advancement flap, **II:**656–658,
      657f–658f
  penoscrotal web, **II:**662, 663f
  research summary, **II:**677
  scrotal enlargement, **II:**662, 664f
  self-esteem issues, **II:**655
male genital reconstructive surgery,
  IV:297–325
  congenital defects
    disorders of sex development (DSD),
      IV:303–304
    exstrophy and epispadias, **IV:**301–303,
      302f–303f
    hidden penis, **IV:**304, 304f–305f
    severe penile insufficiency, **IV:**304–306, 306f
  female-to-male transsexual surgery
    metaidoioplasty, **IV:**315–318, 317f, 346
    pars fixa of the urethra creation,
      IV:314–315, 316f–317f
    phalloplasty
      anterolateral thigh flap, **IV:**311f, 323,
        324f–325f
      basic procedure, **IV:**318–323

male genital reconstructive surgery
  (*Continued*)
      fibula flap, **IV:**323
      perforator flaps, **IV:**323
      radial forearm flap, **IV:**318–323,
        319f–320f, 324f–325f
    vaginectomy, **IV:**314–315, 315f
  general discussion, **IV:**297
  genital anatomy
    blood supply, **IV:**299–301, 299f–301f
    general discussion, **IV:**298–301
    genital fascia, **IV:**298–299, 299f
    lymphatic supply, **IV:**301
    nerve supply, **IV:**301
  genital embryology
    genetic sex, **IV:**297
    gonadal sex, **IV:**297–298
    phenotypic sex, **IV:**298, 298f
  multidisciplinary approach, **IV:**323
  post-traumatic genital defects
    basic principles, **IV:**306–313
    microsurgical genital reconstruction
      genital replantation, **IV:**310–312, 312f
      phallic construction, **IV:**312
    reconstruction options
      genital flaps, **IV:**304–310, 306f, 311f
      genital skin grafts, **IV:**307, 308f–309f
      microsurgical genital reconstruction,
        IV:310–312
      reconstructive indications, **IV:**312–313
    reconstructive indications
      Fournier disease, **IV:**312–313, 313f
      penile cancer, **IV:**313, 314f
male-pattern baldness, **I:**633–635
male perineum
  characteristics, **IV:**235
  cross-section diagram, **IV:**231f
  schematic diagram, **IV:**236f–237f
  vascular anatomy, **IV:**235, 238f
male rhinoplasty, **II:**441
malformation, **I:**192–193
Malgaigne, Joseph, **I:**19
malignant appendage-origin tumors
  extramammary Paget's disease, **I:**739,
    739f
  Merkel cell carcinoma, **I:**716t, 739, 739f
  sebaceous carcinoma, **I:**738, 738f
  sweat gland carcinoma, **I:**738
  trichilemmal carcinoma, **I:**738, 738f
malignant cutaneous and soft-tissue tumors
  malignant appendage-origin tumors
    extramammary Paget's disease, **I:**739,
      739f
    Merkel cell carcinoma, **I:**716t, 739, 739f
    sebaceous carcinoma, **I:**738, 738f
    sweat gland carcinoma, **I:**738
    trichilemmal carcinoma, **I:**738, 738f
  malignant epithelial-origin tumors
    actinic keratosis, **I:**736, 736f, **VI:**316–317,
      317f
    basal cell carcinoma
      characteristics, **I:**737, 737f, **III:**117–118,
        118f, **VI:**317, 317f
      dermoscopic analysis, **I:**709, 709f
      histological classification, **I:**738b
      surgical margins, **I:**717
      tumor colors, **I:**709
    Bowen's disease, **I:**736–737

malignant cutaneous and soft-tissue tumors
  (*Continued*)
    squamous cell carcinomas (SCCs)
      characteristics, **I:**737, 737f, **III:**118–119,
        118f, **VI:**317, 317f
      epidermolysis bullosa, **IV:**520f, 521–522
      head and neck cancer, **I:**668–669
  malignant mesenchymal-origin tumors
    angiosarcomas, **I:**741–742, 741f
    chondrosarcoma, **I:**741, **VI:**329
    dermatofibrosarcoma protuberans
      (DFSP), **I:**739, 739f
    Kaposi's sarcoma, **I:**742
    leiomyosarcoma, **I:**740, 740f
    liposarcoma, **I:**740, 740f
    malignant fibrous histiocytoma (MFH),
      I:739–740, 740f, **VI:**321, 322f
    osteosarcoma, **I:**741, 741f, **VI:**329
    rhabdomyosarcoma, **I:**741
  malignant epithelial-origin tumors
    actinic keratosis, **I:**736, 736f, **VI:**316–317,
      317f
    basal cell carcinoma
      characteristics, **I:**737, 737f, **III:**117–118,
        118f, **VI:**317, 317f
      dermoscopic analysis, **I:**709, 709f
      histological classification, **I:**738b
      surgical margins, **I:**717
      tumor colors, **I:**709
    Bowen's disease, **I:**736–737
    scalp and forehead, **III:**118–119, 118f
    squamous cell carcinomas (SCCs)
      characteristics, **I:**737, 737f, **III:**118–119,
        118f, **VI:**317, 317f
      epidermolysis bullosa, **IV:**520f, 521–522
      head and neck cancer, **I:**668–669
  malignant fibrous histiocytoma (MFH),
    I:739–740, 740f, **VI:**321, 322f
  malignant melanomas, **I:**671
  malignant mesenchymal-origin tumors
    angiosarcomas, **I:**741–742, 741f
    chondrosarcoma, **I:**741, **VI:**329
    dermatofibrosarcoma protuberans (DFSP),
      I:739, 739f
    Kaposi's sarcoma, **I:**742
    leiomyosarcoma, **I:**740, 740f
    liposarcoma, **I:**740, 740f
    malignant fibrous histiocytoma (MFH),
      I:739–740, 740f, **VI:**321, 322f
    osteosarcoma, **I:**741, 741f, **VI:**329
    rhabdomyosarcoma, **I:**741
malignant mixed tumors
  characteristics, **III:**370
  classifications, **III:**365t
  incidence, **III:**376t
  outcomes and complicatons, **III:**377
  submandibular gland, **III:**370t
  surgical technique and treatment,
    III:376–377
Maliniak, Jacques, **I:**24, 27
mallet finger
  aluminum splint, **VI:**216f
  lateral view, **VI:**215f–216f
  posteroanterior view, **VI:**215f–216f
  postoperative doorstop, **VI:**217f
  stack splint, **VI:**216f
  surgical procedures, **VI:**214–216
malnutrition, **I:**282, **IV:**355, 362t–363t, 366

malpractice
  malpractice lawsuit guide, I:99–100
  tort law, I:93
Mammaprint 70 gene profile, V:267
mammary hypertrophy, V:152–153, 161–162,
  240f–241f, 455f
mammary hypoplasia, V:13, 83
mammography, V:268, 269f
managed care liabilities, I:101
Manchot, Carl, I:25f
mandible
  craniofacial microsomia (CFM), III:761–791
    disease process
      associated syndromes, III:769t
      auricular malformation, III:767, 771f
      embryology, III:763–764, 763f–764f
      etiopathogenesis, III:761–763, 762f
      extracraniofacial anatomy, III:768
      muscle function, III:766–767
      natural growth behavior, III:770–771
      nervous system anomalies, III:767
      nonskeletal (soft) tissue, III:765–766,
        770f
      pathology, III:764, 765f
      skeletal tissue, III:764–765, 766f–769f
      skin and subcutaneous tissue, III:767,
        771f
    incidence, III:761
    mandibular growth studies, III:790–791,
      790f
    occlusion management
      early intervention, III:787
      orthodontic management during active
        distraction, III:787–788, 788f
      postdistraction orthodontic
        management, III:788, 788f
      predistraction orthodontic
        management, III:787
    patient presentation and diagnosis
      cephalometrics, III:774–775, 776f
      classification systems, III:772–773, 772t,
        773f–774f, 774t–775t
      computed tomography (CT), III:775,
        777f
      differential diagnosis, III:771–772, 772f
      endoscopic approaches, III:775
      photographic documentation,
        III:773–774
      sleep studies, III:775
    patient selection, III:775–777
    surgical technique and treatment
      auricular reconstruction, III:786
      autogenous fat injections, III:786
      bone grafts, III:781–782, 783f
      commissuroplasty, III:777–779,
        778f–779f
      fronto-orbital advancement/cranial
        vault remodeling, III:786
      gastrostomy, III:777
      mandibular distraction, III:779–781,
        780f–782f
      maxillomandibular orthognathic
        surgery, III:782–786, 784f–785f
      microvascular free flap, III:786,
        786f–787f
      occlusion management, III:787–788
      tracheostomy, III:777
    treatment algorithms
      adolescence and adulthood, III:789–790
      childhood, III:789

mandible (Continued)
      early childhood, III:789
      neonatal period and infancy,
        III:788–789
mandible angle reduction, II:178–179,
  179f–180f, 182
mandibular fractures
  antibiotics, III:82
  characteristics, III:75
  classification systems, III:76–77
  clinical examination, III:76
  complications
    facial width, III:82
    hardware infection and migration, III:82
    malocclusion, III:82
    mandible rotation, III:82
    nonunion occurrences, III:82
    osteomyelitis, III:82–83
  dental wiring and fixation techniques
    arch-bars, III:75
    intermaxillary fixation (IMF) screws,
      III:75–76, 75f
  diagnosis, III:76
  displacement direction and extent
    fracture line direction and angulation,
      III:77, 77f
    general discussion, III:77
    teeth, III:77
  edentulous mandible fractures, III:83–84,
    84f
  internal fixation devices
    Champy or miniplate system, III:80–81,
      80f
    lag screw technique, III:81, 81f
    selection guidelines, III:80–83
  muscle function considerations, III:76
  surgical technique and treatment,
    III:238–240, 239f
  temporomandibular joint, III:76–77
  third molar extraction, III:81, 81f
  treatment strategies
    basic principles, III:77
    Class I fractures, III:77–78
    Class II fractures, III:78
    Class III fractures, III:78–80
    comminuted fractures, III:78, 79f
    intraoral approach, III:79
    open reduction treatment, III:78–79
    reduction and fixation principles,
      III:78, 78f
    surgical indicators, III:79–80
mandibular osteotomies, II:366–367, 367f
mandibular prominences, III:509
mandibular reconstruction
  acquired cranial and facial bone
    deformities, III:240
  mandibular fractures, III:75
  vascularized bone flaps, I:527f–528f
mandibulomaxillary advancement (MMA),
  III:99f–103f, 100–101
orthognathic surgery, III:655–670
  complications, III:667–670
  dentofacial deformities, III:655
  growth and development factors,
    III:655–656, 656f
  model surgery
    basic procedure, III:658
    isolated mandibular surgery, III:658
    isolated maxillary and two-jaw surgery,
      III:658

mandible (Continued)
    patient presentation and diagnosis
      cleft/craniofacial team, III:656
      patient history and examination,
        III:656–657
      preoperative assessment, III:656–657
    patient selection
      cephalometric and dental evaluation,
        III:657–658, 657f
      general discussion, III:657–660
      model surgery, III:658
      three-dimensional (3D) computed
        tomography (CT) models, III:658,
        659f
      treatment planning process, III:658–660
    postoperative care and follow-up, III:666
    prognosis and outcomes, III:667–670, 667t
    secondary procedures, III:670
    surgical technique and treatment
      apertognathia, III:666, 668f
      basic procedure, III:660
      bilateral sagittal split osteotomy,
        III:661–662
      cleft lip surgery, III:663–665, 663f–664f
      distraction osteogenesis, III:665
      genioplasty, III:662–663
      intraoral vertical ramus osteotomy,
        III:662
      Le Fort I osteotomy, III:610f–611f,
        660–661, 661f, 663f, 667f–668f, 669t
      maxillary constriction, III:665, 667f
      short lower face, III:666
      skeletal anatomy, III:660
      skeletal class II malocclusions, III:665,
        666f
      skeletal class III malocclusions, III:665
      surgically assisted rapid palatal
        expansion (SARPE) procedure,
        III:661
      two-jaw surgery, III:662
      vertical maxillary excess, III:666
    velopharyngeal insufficiency (VPI),
      III:667–670, 667t
  pediatric facial fractures, III:681f–682f, 682,
    684, 684f
  Pierre Robin sequence (PRS), III:808–809,
    809f
  reconstructive surgeries, III:307–335
    acquired cranial and facial bone
      deformities, III:240
    bone-carrying flaps
      circumflex iliac osteocutaneous flap,
        III:322, 323f
      fibula osteoseptocutaneous flap, III:323
      pectoralis major
        osteomusculocutaneous flap,
        III:322
      radius with radial forearm flap, III:323
      scapular osteomusculocutaneous flap,
        III:323, 323f
      temporalis osteomuscular flap, III:322
      trapezius osteomusculocutaneous flap,
        III:322
    challenges, III:307–308
    complications
      acute complications, III:334
      chronic complications, III:334
    decision-making process
      basic procedure, III:315–316
      defect classifications, III:317t

mandible (Continued)
    defect factors, III:310t
    osteocutaneous flaps, III:317t
    reconstruction options, III:318t
  disease process, III:308
  free tissue transfer, III:311
  local/regional flaps, III:309t, 311
  mandibular fractures, III:75
  patient presentation and diagnosis, III:308
  patient selection
    defect factors, III:310–311, 310t
    patient factors, III:308–310, 310t
  postoperative care and follow-up,
    III:332–333
  prognosis and outcomes, III:320–321
  surgical technique
    bone-carrying flaps, III:322–332
    custom-made templates, III:323–324
  defect assessment, III:323–324, 333–334
  secondary procedures, III:334
  skin grafts, III:311
  soft tissue flaps
    anterolateral thigh flap, III:321–322
    deltopectoral flaps, III:318–319, 319f
    lateral arm flap, III:321
    medial sural artery perforator (MSAP)
      flap, III:322
    pectoralis major myocutaneous flaps,
      III:319, 320f
    radial forearm flap, III:319–320
    rectus abdominis musculocutaneous
      flap, III:321, 321f
    submental flaps, III:316–318, 318f
    thoracodorsal artery perforator (TDAP)
      flap, III:322
  donor site selection, III:323f, 324–328,
    325f–326f
  fasciocutaneous flaps, III:319–322
  fibula osteocutaneous flap, III:327f–
    330f, 331
  fibula osteoseptocutaneous flap,
    III:323–332, 324t
  fibula segment fixation, III:326f–327f,
    329f–330f
  flap insets, III:331
  iliac bone grafts, III:327f
  ischemia time, III:331
  local flaps, III:316–318
  musculocutaneous flaps, III:319–322
  osseointegrated dental implants, III:332
  osteomusculocutaneous peroneal artery
    combined flap, III:325f
  osteomusculocutaneous peroneal artery
    combined flap harvest, III:328–331
  osteotomies, III:331
  patient follow-up, III:326f, 328f–330f
  pedicled osteocutaneous flaps, III:322
  recipient site preparation, III:324
  reconstruction plates and wiring,
    III:328f–329f, 331
  regional flaps, III:318–319
  segmental mandibulectomy, III:325f
  soft tissue flaps, III:316–322
  temporomandibular joint
    reconstruction, III:331–332,
    332f–333f
  vascularized osteocutaneous flaps,
    III:322–323

mandible (Continued)
  Treacher Collins syndrome, III:828–830,
    832–834, 832f–833f, 835f
  tumors, III:398–419
    complications
      dental follow-ups, III:418
      general discussion, III:416–418
      local recurrence, III:416
      osteoradionecrosis (ORN), III:417
      post-treatment surveillance, III:417–418
      regional recurrence, III:416–417
      wound infections, III:417
    diagnosis and treatment, III:427
    epidemiology, III:399–400
    lymph node anatomy, III:399f
    mandibulotomy, III:409–410, 411f, 414f,
      429f
    marginal resection, III:409, 410f
    medical challenges, III:398
    pathogenesis, III:398–399
    patient presentation and diagnosis,
      III:400
    surgical access, III:402, 403f–404f
    therapeutic choices, III:401–402
    TNM clinical classification system,
      III:400–401, 401t
manganese (Mn) alloys, I:786–787
Mangled Extremity Severity Score (MESS),
  IV:63, 65–66, 66t
mangled hands See mutilated/mangled hands
manipulative help-rejecting complainers,
  I:38–39
Mannerfelt lesion, VI:376, 376f, 402, 403f
Manske's classification of cleft hands, VI:565t
Manuzzi, Nicolò, I:12
MAPK kinase (MEK), I:626f
MAPK kinase (MEKK), I:626f
Marcaine, I:147–148
marginal mandibular nerve, II:314f, III:12f, 13
marionette lines, II:53–54, 53f–54f
Marjolin's ulcer, IV:379, 444
Marshall syndrome, III:805–807, 807t
Martin Gruber anastomosis, VI:697f
Martsolf syndrome, III:807t
Masquelet technique, IV:176–177
Masse's sign, VI:514t
masseter muscle, III:16
mast cells
  flap failure pathophysiology, I:573–574,
    574f
  skin wound healing, I:269–271
  wound healing, I:245f, 247–248
mastectomies
  breast reconstruction, V:411–412
  female-to-male chest surgery, IV:349–350
  planning and marking guidelines, V:419,
    419f
  postmastectomy breast reconstruction
    basic principles, I:640–647
    chest wall irradiated areas, I:645–647
    delayed reconstruction, V:291–292,
      291f–292f
    expander device, I:642–643, V:292f
    expander-implants
      adjustable, permanent expander-
        implants, V:366–367
      average operative time, V:364t
      basic procedure, V:338–340

mastectomies (Continued)
      breast envelope preservation,
        V:367–368
      capsular contracture, V:362, 362t–364t
      cellulitis, V:359, 360f
      clinical studies, V:362, 363t
      complication frequency, V:363–365,
        364t
      complications, V:359
      cosmetic revision surgery, V:365, 366f
      delayed reconstruction, V:342f, 358,
        359f
      erythema, V:359
      evaluation studies, V:365
      expander failure or malfunction,
        V:360–361, 360f–361f, 364t
      fat injections, V:365, 368
      flap-based reconstruction, V:367
      hematomas, V:359, 359f, 364t
      implant malposition, V:363t
      implant removal, V:363t
      implant rupture and deflation,
        V:361–362, 363t
      infections, V:361–363, 363t–364t
      insertion procedures, V:353–354
      nipple reconstruction, V:365–366
      outcome assessments, V:363–365
      persistent serous drainage, V:359–360
      postoperative care and follow-up,
        V:358–359
      preoperative/postoperative
        comparisons, V:340f–341f
      secondary procedures, V:365–366
      skin necrosis, V:360, 360f, 363t
      wrinkle formation, V:363t
  immediate postmastectomy breast
    reconstruction
    acellular allogenic dermal matrix
      (ADM), I:644–645, 644f
    basic procedure, V:287–291
    deep inferior epigastric perforator
      (DIEP) flaps, V:288f
    latissimus dorsi (LD) flap, V:288,
      289f–290f
    muscle coverage, I:643–645
    radiation therapy (RT), V:290
    submuscular position, I:643–644
    subpectoral (dual-plane) position, I:644
    transverse rectus abdominis
      myocutaneous (TRAM) flaps,
      V:288f
  patient presentation and diagnosis
    exclusion criteria, V:345–346, 347f
    inclusion criteria, V:346
    large breast reconstruction, V:346, 350f
    medium breast reconstruction, V:346,
      349f
    small breast reconstruction, V:346, 348f
  prosthesis insertion
    basic procedure, V:356–358
    capsulectomy, V:357f
    contralateral adjustments, V:356–358
    inframammary fold reconstruction,
      V:357f
    large breast augmentation, V:358
    medium breast augmentation,
      V:357–358
    small breast augmentation, V:356–357

mastectomies (Continued)
  reconstructive paradigms
    contralateral adjustments, **V:**343f
    cosmetic breast reconstruction,
      V:344f–345f
    indications and contraindications,
      V:343f
    mastectomy techniques, **V:**343f
    radiation therapy (RT), **V:**347f
    surgical strategy, **V:**340–344
  secondary breast reconstruction, **I:**645,
      646f
  skin reducing mastectomy, **V:**354–356, 355f
  surgical technique and treatment
    delayed reconstruction, **V:**358, 359f
    expander-implant insertion, **V:**353–354,
      354f
    immediate postmastectomy breast
      reconstruction, **V:**353
    prosthesis insertion, **V:**356–358
    second-stage surgery, **V:**356, 357f
    skin reducing mastectomy, **V:**354–356,
      355f
    tissue preservation, **V:**353–358
  postmastectomy radiation (PMRT), **I:**665
  psychological aspects, **I:**43
  surgical technique
    characteristics, **I:**202, 203f, **V:**280–286
    extended radical mastectomy, **V:**281f
    modified radical mastectomy, **V:**285, 285f
    nipple-sparing mastectomy, **V:**282–284,
      284f–285f
    nodal evaluation, **V:**286, 286f
    prophylactic mastectomy, **V:**284
    skin-sparing mastectomy, **V:**282,
      283f–284f, 288f
    total mastectomy, **V:**281–282, 281f
mastication muscles
  aesthetic importance, **III:**17
  general characteristics, **III:**16–17
  lateral pterygoid muscle, **III:**16
  masseter muscle, **III:**16
  medial pterygoid muscle, **III:**16
  muscle actions, **III:**16
  pterygomasseteric sling, **III:**16
  temporalis muscle, **III:**16
mastocytosis, **I:**736
mastopexy, **V:**119–151
  adolescent aesthetic surgery, **I:**45t
  breast ptosis
    background information, **V:**119–120
    pathophysiology
      basic principles, **V:**120–121
      breast anatomy, **V:**120f
      breast base anomaly classifications,
        V:123f
      breast development, **V:**123f
      classifications, **V:**122f
      Cooper's ligaments, **V:**120–121, 120f
      procedural guidelines, **V:**122t
      Regnault classification, **V:**121, 121f
      von Heimburg's tuberous breast
        classification, **V:**121, 124t
    ptosis types, **V:**122f
    Regnault classification, **V:**121f
  major weight loss (MWL) patient
    breast reshaping, **V:**564–570
    dermal suspension, **V:**566–570, 568f
    outcomes and complicatons, **V:**567–570
    pathophysiology, **V:**564, 564b

mastopexy (Continued)
    patient presentation and diagnosis,
      V:564–565
    patient selection, **V:**565–566
    postoperative care and follow-up, **V:**567
    surgical goals, **V:**565b
    surgical planning, **V:**565–566, 566t,
      569f–570f
    surgical tips, **V:**567b
    total parenchymal reshaping mastopexy
      surgical markings, **V:**566
      surgical technique and treatment,
        V:566–567, 568f
  McKissock procedure, **V:**117
  outcomes and complicatons
    cosmetic disappointments, **V:**149–150
    flap necrosis, **V:**149
    general discussion, **V:**148–150
    hematomas, **V:**150, 243t
    infections, **V:**150, 243t
    nipple loss, **V:**148, 243t
    nipple malposition, **V:**149, 243t, 252
    scars, **V:**149, 243t
  patient presentation and diagnosis,
    V:124–125
  patient selection, **V:**125
  revisionary surgery, **V:**242–265
    incidence, **V:**242
    outcomes and complicatons, **V:**245,
      263–264
    pathophysiology, **V:**244
    patient history, **V:**242–244
    patient presentation and diagnosis, **V:**244
    postoperative care and follow-up,
      V:244–245, 262
    preoperative assessment, **V:**244
    research summary, **V:**264
    surgical re-intervention
      areola deformities, **V:**248–249, 250f
      areola hypopigmentation, **V:**249–251
      asymmetries, **V:**251
      contour abnormalities, **V:**247
      fat necrosis, **V:**251
      flap necrosis, **V:**246
      hematomas, **V:**245–246, 246f
      mastopexy revision, **V:**254–261,
        258f–263f
      nipple areola ischemia, **V:**247–248,
        248f–249f
      nipple loss, **V:**148, 243t, 253–254, 255f
      nipple malposition, **V:**149, 243t, 252,
        252f–253f
      nipple retraction, **V:**252
      postoperative care and follow-up,
        V:246
      re-do breast reduction, **V:**254, 256f
      scars, **V:**246–247
      wound excision and re-closure,
        V:246–247
  secondary procedures, **V:**150
  surgical technique and treatment
    augmentation mammaplasty
      basic procedure, **V:**139–143
      operative technique, **V:**142–143
      preoperative/postoperative
        comparisons, **V:**143f
      surgical tips, **V:**142b
    Benelli mastopexy technique
      areola fixation, **V:**131f
      basic procedure, **V:**127–132

mastopexy (Continued)
    dissection techniques, **V:**128f
    flap attachment, **V:**129f–130f
    flap types, **V:**129f
    gland plication invagination, **V:**131f
    markings, **V:**128f
    round block suture, **V:**131f
    surgical technique, **V:**128–132
    U stitches, **V:**131f
  Goes periareolar technique with mesh
    support
    basic procedure, **V:**132–133
    surgical technique, **V:**132–133,
      132f–134f
  Grotting sculpted vertical pillar
    mastopexy
    basic procedure, **V:**136–139
    final closure, **V:**140f
    flap detachment, **V:**139f
    markings and incisions, **V:**138f
    operative technique, **V:**138–139
    preferred technique, **V:**138f–140f
    preoperative markings, **V:**137f
    preoperative/postoperative
      comparisons, **V:**140f–141f
    surgical tips, **V:**136b
    temporary breast closure, **V:**139f
  inverted-T technique
    basic procedure, **V:**146–147
    operative technique, **V:**146–147, 147f
  periareolar techniques
    basic procedure, **V:**126–133
    Benelli mastopexy technique,
      V:127–132
    concentric mastopexy without
      parenchymal reshaping, **V:**126–127
    Goes periareolar technique with mesh
      support, **V:**132–133
  postoperative care and follow-up,
    V:147–148
  scar pattern considerations, **V:**125–147
  vertical/short scar techniques
    augmentation mammaplasty, **V:**139–143
    general discussion, **V:**133–146
    Grotting sculpted vertical pillar
      mastopexy, **V:**136–139
    implant post-explantation, **V:**143–146,
      144f–145f, 145b
    Lassus vertical scar technique,
      V:134–135
    Lejour vertical scar technique,
      V:135–136
Mathes–Nahai classification system
  fascial/fasciocutaneous flaps, **I:**517–519,
    518f
  gluteus maximus muscle, **IV:**5, 5t
  muscle/musculocutaneous flaps, **I:**516–517,
    516f
Matriderm, **I:**336
Matridex, **II:**48t
  See also soft-tissue fillers
Matrigel, **I:**386f, 389–390, 389f
MatriStem, **V:**70t
matrix metalloproteinases (MMPs)
  osteoarthritis, **VI:**412–413
  rosacea, **II:**20–21
  scar biology and formation, **I:**300
  skin aging, **II:**86
  skin wound healing, **I:**269–273
mature scars, **I:**291t, 302t

maxilla
  mandibulomaxillary advancement (MMA), III:99f–103f, 100–101
  maxillary buttresses, III:236–238
  maxillary constriction, III:665, 667f
  maxillary incisor cross-section, II:366f
  maxillary osteotomy, II:368–370, 369b, 369f–370f
  maxillary prominences, III:508–509
  maxillary reconstructiion, III:238–240, 238f
  orthognathic surgery, III:655–670
    complications, III:667–670
    dentofacial deformities, III:655
    growth and development factors, III:655–656, 656f
    model surgery
      basic procedure, III:658
      isolated mandibular surgery, III:658
      isolated maxillary and two-jaw surgery, III:658
    patient presentation and diagnosis
      cleft/craniofacial team, III:656
      patient history and examination, III:656–657
      preoperative assessment, III:656–657
    patient selection
      cephalometric and dental evaluation, III:657–658, 657f
      general discussion, III:657–660
      model surgery, III:658
      three-dimensional (3D) computed tomography (CT) models, III:658, 659f
      treatment planning process, III:658–660
    postoperative care and follow-up, III:666
    prognosis and outcomes, III:667–670, 667t
    secondary procedures, III:670
    surgical technique and treatment
      apertognathia, III:666, 668f
      basic procedure, III:660
      bilateral sagittal split osteotomy, III:661–662
      cleft lip surgery, III:663–665, 663f–664f
      distraction osteogenesis, III:665
      genioplasty, III:662–663
      intraoral vertical ramus osteotomy, III:662
      Le Fort I osteotomy, III:610f–611f, 660–661, 661f, 663f, 667f–668f, 669t
      maxillary constriction, III:665, 667f
      short lower face, III:666
      skeletal anatomy, III:660
      skeletal class II malocclusions, III:665, 666f
      skeletal class III malocclusions, III:665
      surgically assisted rapid palatal expansion (SARPE) procedure, III:661
      two-jaw surgery, III:662
      vertical maxillary excess, III:666
      velopharyngeal insufficiency (VPI), III:667–670, 667t
  pediatric facial fractures, III:680, 681f, 684
  Pierre Robin sequence (PRS), III:808–809, 809f

maxilla (Continued)
  Treacher Collins syndrome, III:828–830
  tumors
    marginal resection, III:409, 410f
    maxillectomy, III:410–412, 412f–413f
maxillary fractures
  alveolar fractures, III:71
  characteristics, III:70–71, 70f
  clinical examination
    cerebral spinal rhinorrhea or otorrhea, III:71
    digital manipulation, III:71
    inspection process, III:70–71
    malocclusion of the teeth, III:71
    palpation, III:71
  complications
    airway management, III:74
    bleeding, III:74
    blindness, III:74
    cerebral spinal rhinorrhea or otorrhea, III:74
    infections, III:74
    late complications, III:74–75
    malocclusion, III:74–75
    malunion occurrences, III:74
    nasolacrimal duct injury, III:75
    nonunion occurrences, III:74
  computed tomography (CT), III:71
  Le Fort classification of facial fractures
    background information, III:71–75
    goals, III:71
    Le Fort I level fractures/transverse (Guerin) fractures, III:71, 72f, 73
    Le Fort II level fractures/pyramidal fractures, III:72f–73f, 73–74
    Le Fort III level fractures/craniofacial dysjunction, III:72f–73f, 73–74
  postoperative care and follow-up, III:74
  treatment strategies, III:71
maxillofacial injuries, III:23–48
  etiology, III:23–24, 24f
  general discussion, III:23
  patient presentation and diagnosis
    diagnostic studies
      computed tomography (CT), III:26
      general discussion, III:26
      X-ray analysis, III:26
    evaluation examinations
      diagnostic studies, III:26
      head and neck evaluations, III:24–25
      immediate life-threatening injuries, III:24
      provider consultations, III:26
    general discussion, III:24–26
    provider consultations
      dentists, III:26
      ophthalmologists, III:26
    systematic head and neck evaluations
      airway evaluation, III:25
      basic procedure, III:24–25
      cheek examination, III:25, 25f
      ear examination, III:25, 25f, 40
      eye examination, III:25
      nose examination, III:25
      oral cavity and mouth examination, III:25
  research summary, III:46
  skin considerations, III:23–24

maxillofacial injuries (Continued)
  surgical technique and treatment
    abrasions, III:29, 30f
    anesthesia
      auricular nerve, III:27
      cheeks, III:27, 27f–28f
      chin, III:27, 28f
      ears, III:27–29, 29f
      Erb's point, III:27
      facial field block, III:26–29
      forehead, III:26, 27f
      general discussion, III:26–29
      glabella, III:26, 27f
      jaw, III:27
      local infiltration, III:26
      lower eyelid area, III:27, 27f–28f
      lower lip, III:27, 28f
      neck, III:27
      nose, III:27, 27f–28f
      scalp, III:26, 27f
      teeth, III:27, 27f–28f
      topical anesthetics, III:26
      upper eyelid area, III:26, 27f
      upper lip, III:27, 27f–28f
    avulsions, III:31–32, 33f
    cheeks
      basic procedure, III:44–45
      facial nerve injury, III:45
      parotid duct repair, III:45, 45f
    complex lacerations, III:31, 32f
    ears
      anatomical considerations, III:40
      auditory canal stenosis, III:41–42
      causal factors, III:39–42
      complete amputation, III:42
      hematomas, III:40–41, 41f
      lacerations, III:41, 41f
      partial amputation with a narrow pedicle, III:42
      partial amputation with a wide pedicle, III:41f, 42
    eyebrows
      basic procedure, III:34–38
      Burow's triangles, III:37f
      local brow advancement flaps, III:36–38, 37f
      local grafts, III:38
    eyelids, III:38–39, 38f–40f
    irrigation and debridement, III:29
    neck, III:46
    nose
      abrasions, III:43
      amputations, III:44
      avulsions, III:43–44, 44f
      basic procedure, III:42–44
      lacerations, III:43
    oral cavity and mouth
      basic procedure, III:45–46
      lips, III:46, 47f–48f
      oral mucosa repair, III:46
      tongue, III:46
    scalp, III:33–34, 33f, 35f–37f
    secondary intention healing, III:32–33
    simple lacerations, III:30, 31f
    traumatic tatoo, III:29–30, 30f
Mayer–Rokitansky–Kuster–Hauser syndrome, III:906
mayonnaise, IV:395

MBA oath, **I:**88b
McCune–Albright syndrome, **III:**380–382
MCFONTZL classification system, **I:**299, 300t
McGill Pain Questionnaire (MPQ), **VI:**855–856
McIndoe, Archibald, **I:**5, 5f, **II:**108–109
McKissock procedure, **V:**117
meatoplasty
  basic procedure, **III:**913–915, 916f
  onlay island flap repair, **III:**914–915, 918f
  orthoplasty, **III:**915
  surgical tips, **III:**914b–915b
  tubularized incised plate (TIP) repair, **III:**914, 917f
  two-stage repair, **III:**915, 919f–921f
Medawar, Peter, **VI:**xlviii
medial canthal defects, **III:**450, **IV:**488
medial circumflex femoral arterial system, **IV:**23–25, 26f
medial cutaneous nerve, **VI:**709, 710f
medial epicanthoplasty, **II:**169, 170f–171f
medial epicondylitis, **VI:**366
medial orbital vault, **II:**110, 110f
medial plantar artery flap, **IV:**209
medial pterygoid muscle, **III:**16
medial sural artery perforator (MSAP) flap, **III:**309t, 322
medial thigh septocutaneous flap, **IV:**143–144, 144f
median craniofacial dysraphia
  anterior encephaloceles, **III:**703–704
  characteristics, **III:**703–704
  classifications, **III:**703t
  number 0 cleft, **III:**709
  true median cleft, **III:**703
median craniofacial hyperplasia (tissue excess or duplication), **III:**703t, 704
median craniofacial hypoplasia (tissue deficiency or agenesis)
  classifications, **III:**703t
  holoprosencephalic spectrum (alobar brain), **III:**702
  median cerebrofacial hypoplasia (lobar brain), **III:**702
  median facial hypoplasia, **III:**702
  microform variants, **III:**702–703
  number 0 cleft, **III:**703t, 708–709, 708f
mediastinum, **I:**549–552, 550f–551f
medical-grade silicone, **V:**98–100
medical sheepskin, **IV:**364–366
medical technology, **I:**854–874
  innovative nonbiological technologies, **I:**854–855
  robotics
    definition, **I:**855
    research summary, **I:**873
    surgical tools and prosthetics
      chest and abdominal surgery, **I:**863
      craniofacial surgery, **I:**862–863
      ear, nose, and throat surgery, **I:**862–863
      evidenced-based outcomes, **I:**864
      future trends, **I:**864–865
      limb and hand surgery, **I:**857–862
      next-generation devices, **I:**864–865
      operating rooms, **I:**855–857
      urologic/prostate surgery, **I:**863–864
  simulation
    basic principles, **I:**865
    functional role
      surgical planning simulators, **I:**868–869, 869f

medical technology *(Continued)*
      training simulators, **I:**865–868, 866f–868f, 867t
    future trends, **I:**869–870
    implementation, **I:**865
    physical–behavioral–genomics model, **I:**869–870, 869f
    research summary, **I:**873
    use rationale, **I:**865
  technological impacts, **I:**873
  telemedicine
    definition, **I:**870–871
    general discussion, **I:**870
    plastic surgery applications, **I:**871–872
    research summary, **I:**873
    social networks, **I:**871
    technologies, **I:**870, 871t
    telesurgery, **I:**871, 872f
    ubiquitous mobile telemedicine, **I:**872–873
medicinal leeches, **I:**617, **VI:**241–242
medico-legal issues, **I:**92–103
  aesthetic practice liabilities, **I:**100–101
  agency law, **I:**98
  background information, **I:**92
  contract law, **I:**97
  fraud and abuse, **I:**95–96
  Internet and blog defamation law, **I:**98–99
  legal areas
    general discussion, **I:**93–95
    informed consent, **I:**93–94, 105–106
    negligence and malpractice, **I:**93
    privacy law, **I:**94
    tort law, **I:**93
    warranty law, **I:**94–95
  legal interactions
    attorney–surgeon interactions, **I:**92–93
    depositions and narratives, **I:**93
  liability carrier's issues, **I:**101
  malpractice lawsuit guide, **I:**99–100
  managed care liabilities, **I:**101
  patient selection, **I:**102–103, 103f
  physician partnerships, **I:**101–102
  product liability, **I:**95
  regulatory issues, **I:**97–98
  research summary, **I:**103
Medpor, **I:**462
Meibomian gland carcinoma, **I:**738
melanocytes
  aging process, **II:**44–45
  induced pluripotent stem cells, **I:**236
  ontogenesis, **I:**707, 708f
  skin grafts, **I:**320
melanocytic lesions *See* cutaneous and soft-tissue tumors
melanoma, **I:**743–785
  acral lentiginous melanoma, **I:**752–753, 754f
  adjuvant treatment
    general discussion, **I:**777–779
    interferon-α, **I:**777–778
    isolated limb perfusion, **I:**778–779, 780f, 781t
    radiation therapy (RT), **I:**778
  amelanotic melanoma, **I:**753, 755f
  characteristics, **VI:**318, 318f
  classification/staging systems
    advantages, **I:**750–761
    histologic subtypes, **I:**752–753, 754f–755f
    melanoma stage/prognostic groups, **I:**753t
    TNM clinical classification system, **I:**750–761, 752t

melanoma *(Continued)*
  desmoplastic melanoma, **I:**753, 755f
  epidemiology, **I:**743–744
  evaluation examinations
    clinical diagnosis
      atypical (dysplastic) nevus, **I:**745–746, 747f
      atypical (dysplastic) nevus syndrome, **I:**746–747
      B-K mole syndrome, **I:**747
      blue nevi, **I:**744f, 745
      compound nevi, **I:**744, 744f
      congenital nevi, **I:**745, 745f–746f
      intradermal nevi, **I:**744, 744f
      junctional nevi, **I:**744, 744f
      nevi development, **I:**744–747
    differential diagnosis
      challenges, **I:**747–750
      Hutchinson freckle, **I:**747–748, 749f
      melanoma lesion characteristics, **I:**748–749, 750f–751f
      multiple primary melanomas, **I:**749–750
      pigmented basal cell carcinoma, **I:**747–750, 748f
      pigmented lesions, **I:**747–750
      pyogenic granuloma, **I:**747–750, 748f
      seborrheic keratosis, **I:**747–750, 748f
  in-transit and regional lymph node disease
    characteristics, **I:**756–761
    lymphoscintigraphy (lymphatic mapping), **I:**757–758, 758f–759f, 759t
    N category of TNM system, **I:**752t–753t, 760–761
    sentinel lymph node biopsy, **I:**758–760, 760f, 761t
  juvenile melanoma, **I:**724–725, 726f
  lentigo maligna melanoma, **I:**752–753, 754f
  malignant melanomas, **I:**671, **III:**119, 119f
  metastatic melanoma
    biochemotherapy, **I:**782
    chemotherapeutic agents, **I:**779–781
    interleukin-2 (IL-2), **I:**782
    ipilimumab, **I:**782–783
    molecularly targeted treatments, **I:**783
    outcome assessments, **I:**781t
    prognosis, **I:**779–783
    tumor vaccines, **I:**781–782
  nodular melanoma, **I:**752–753, 754f
  postoperative monitoring, **I:**783–784, 783t–784t
  recurrences, **I:**778–779, 779f, 779t, 783–784
  research summary, **I:**784
  scalp and forehead, **III:**119, 119f
  significant histopathologic factors
    depth classification and correlation, **I:**753–756, 756f
    T category of TNM staging system, **I:**752t–753t, 755–756
  superficial spreading melanoma, **I:**752–753, 754f
  surgical technique and treatment
    initial biopsy, **I:**764
    lymphadenectomy
      axillary lymphadenectomy, **I:**771–777, 775f
      cervical lymphadenectomy, **I:**771, 773f–774f
      decision-making process, **I:**768–777

melanoma (Continued)
    pelvic and inguinofemoral
        lymphadenectomy, I:772–777,
        775f–777f
    research studies, I:768–777
    wide local excision (WLE)
        extremities, I:766–768, 768f–771f
        head and neck region, I:766, 767f
        margin width, I:764–768, 765t
        prognosis, I:764–768
        scars, I:765–766, 766f
        trunk, I:768, 772f
    systemic disease evaluation
        computerized tomography (CT),
            I:762–764, 762f
        magnetic resonance imaging (MRI),
            I:762–764, 763f
        M category of TNM system, I:752t,
            763–764
        physical examination and tests, I:761–764,
            762t
        positron emission tomography (PET),
            I:762–764, 763f
melanosome transfer inhibitors
    niacinamide, II:25
    soy products, II:25–26
meloplasty See facelifts
Menick–Salibian surgical approach,
    III:176f
meningomyeloceles, III:868t–869t, 872–874,
    873f
mentalis, II:39f–40f, 41
mentum, I:110, 112f
mepivacaine, VI:95–96, 95t–96t
Merkel cell carcinoma, I:716t, 739, 739f
Merkel cells, I:320, 671
Mersilene, IV:239
mesenchymal stem cells (MSCs)
    bone homeostasis and turnover, I:425–434,
        434f
    bone marrow-derived mesenchymal stem
        cells (BMSC)
        clinical correlates, I:228
        current research and applications,
            I:224–226
        definitions, I:223–224
        gene therapy, I:190
        in vitro tissue harvest and differentiation
            protocols, I:226
        in vivo models, I:226–228
        wound healing, I:262, 262f
    skin wound healing, I:263, 296
    tissue engineering, I:369–371, 380f
Mesopotamia, I:12
messenger RNA (mRNA), I:179–180
metacarpal hand, VI:298–300, 298t,
    299f–300f
metacarpal synostosis
    characteristics, VI:614–615
    outcomes and complicatons, VI:616
    pathogenesis, VI:615
    patient presentation and diagnosis, VI:615,
        615f
    patient selection, VI:615–616
    postoperative care and follow-up, VI:616
    secondary procedures, VI:616
    surgical technique and treatment,
        VI:614–616

metacarpophalangeal (MCP) joint
    Dupuytren's disease, VI:346–348, 349t,
        351–353, 355f
    fractures and joint injuries, VI:138–139, 150,
        150f, 153–154, 155f
    osteoarthritis
        anatomical considerations, VI:425
        arthrodesis, VI:429, 429f–430f
        biomechanics, VI:425
        implant arthroplasty
            hinged prostheses, VI:426
            indications and contraindications,
                VI:426–429
            PyroCarbon arthroplasty, VI:427–429
            silicone constrained prostheses, VI:426,
                427f
            surface replacement prostheses,
                VI:426–427
        PyroCarbon arthroplasty
            basic principles, VI:427–429
            operative technique, VI:427–429,
                428f–429f
        resurfacing arthroplasty, VI:425–426
        vascularized joint transfer/costochondral
            replacement, VI:429–430
    spastic hand, VI:459, 464
    stiff hand
        collateral ligament changes, VI:454, 454f
        extension contracture
            bone, VI:451–452, 451f
            collateral ligaments, VI:451
            intrinsic muscles, VI:451
            volar plate, VI:451
        flexion contracture
            collateral ligaments, VI:449
            transverse retinacular ligaments, VI:450
        pathogenesis, VI:454–455, 457f
        patient presentation and diagnosis,
            VI:449–454
        seesaw effect, VI:452–454, 452f–453f
        surgical technique and treatment,
            VI:457–458
        volar plate changes, VI:454, 455f
Metacril, II:48t
    See also soft-tissue fillers
metaidoioplasty, IV:315–318, 317f, 346
metal alloys
    cobalt-chromium alloys, I:787
    composition, I:787t
    general discussion, I:786–788
    gold alloys, I:787
    stainless steel, I:786–787
    titanium alloys, I:787, 788f
metastatic lesions, VI:330–331, 330f
methicillin-resistant Staphylococcus aureus
    (MRSA), II:411, 526, III:119, IV:283–284,
    VI:334, 334t
methylmethacrylate, I:462, II:48t, IV:239
    See also soft-tissue fillers
methylparaben, I:146
metronidazole, II:21t
microdermabrasion, II:28
microform cleft lip
    pathology, III:542, 542f
    surgical correction techniques, III:542, 543f
micrognathia, III:832–834, 835f
micromastia, V:83
microribonucleic acid (miRNA), I:259–261

microseeding, I:186, 188t
microsurgery, I:8
microtia
    bilateral microtia, III:204
    clinical characteristics, III:190–191, 190f
    patient selection, III:191–192
    surgical technique and treatment
        preoperative assessment, III:192
        rib cartilage graft, III:194, 195f
        surgical planning and preparation,
            III:192–194
        surgical staging, III:192
microvascular composite tissue
    transplantation
    abdominal wall reconstruction, I:554
    clinical applications, I:533–534
    foot reconstruction, I:562, 563f
    head and neck reconstruction, I:545–546,
        546f
    lower extremity reconstructive surgery,
        I:559–560
microvascular free flap, III:786, 786f–787f,
    IV:211–216
microvascular free tissue transfer, IV:131
microvascular lymph node transfer, IV:96, 96f
microvascular surgery, I:587–621
    background information, I:587–588
    basic principles
        anastomotic sequence, I:598
        flap/flap inset surgery, I:594
        recipient vessels, I:594–596, 595f
        surgeon characteristics, I:593–594
        surgical planning and positioning, I:594
        vessel preparation
            adventitia trimming, I:597f
            artery forceps, I:598f
            basic procedure, I:596–597
            cross-section diagram, I:597f
            intraluminal irrigation, I:596f
            loose intima, I:596f
            luminal dilatation, I:598f
    definition, I:587–588
    flap modifications
        chimeric flaps, I:612, 612f
        endoscopic harvests, I:611
        freestyle flaps, I:611
        perforator flaps, I:611, 612f
        prefabricated/prelaminated flaps,
            I:612–613
        thinned flaps, I:612, 612f
    free-flap surgery
        advantages/disadvantages, I:608
        background information, I:607–611
        foot reconstruction, IV:211–216
        preoperative assessment
            flap selection, I:609–610, 610f
            microvascular anesthesia, I:611
            patient evaluation, I:608–609
            recipient and donor site evaluation,
                I:609
            timing considerations, I:610–611
    future outlook, I:620
    instrumentation
        anastomotic devices
            adhesives and glues, I:593
            lasers, I:593
            microsutures, I:591–592
            nonsuture devices, I:592–593

microvascular surgery (Continued)
  loupes
    characteristics, I:588–589
    selection guidelines, I:589
    types, I:589
  magnification, I:588–593
  microsurgical instruments
    bipolar coagulator, I:591
    characteristics, I:589–591
    forceps, I:590
    irrigation and suction, I:591
    needle holders, I:590
    scissors, I:590
    vascular clamps, I:590–591
  surgical microscopes, I:588, 589b
microvascular anastomosis techniques
  empty-and-refill test, I:607, 608f
  general discussion, I:598–607
  less commonly encountered
        microvascular anastomosis
    atherosclerotic vessels, I:605
    loose intima, I:605, 607f
    microvascular grafts, I:605–607
    size-discrepant vessels, I:604–605, 606f
    vertically oriented anastomosis, I:605
  patency testing, I:607, 608f
  suturing techniques
    anastomotic coupling device, I:604,
        604f
    continuous suture, I:601f–602f
    end-to-end anastomosis, I:598–601,
        599f–603f
    end-to-side anastomosis, I:601–604, 603f
    knot tying, I:599f
    open-loop suture, I:603f
    sleeve anastomosis, I:603f
outcomes and complicatons
  donor site complications, I:618
  flap failure
    anastomotic failure, I:614
    ischemia–reperfusion injury, I:617–618
    ischemic tolerance, I:617–618
    management approaches, I:618–620
    no-reflow phenomenon, I:617–618
    thrombogenesis, I:615–617
    vasospasm and thrombosis, I:615
  postoperative management, I:613–620
  postoperative monitoring
    basic procedure, I:613–618
    buried flaps, I:614
    flap failure, I:614–618
    flap outcomes, I:614
midazolam, I:138–139
midcarpal instability test, VI:55
Middle Ages
  Arabian surgery, I:14–15
  printed textbooks, I:15
  universities, I:15, 15f
midface buttress fractures
  alveolar fractures, III:71
  characteristics, III:70–71, 70f
  clinical examination
    cerebral spinal rhinorrhea or otorrhea,
        III:71
    digital manipulation, III:71
    inspection process, III:70–71
    malocclusion of the teeth, III:71
    palpation, III:71
  computed tomography (CT), III:71
  treatment strategies, III:71

midfacelift
  basic principles, II:204
  blepharoplasty, II:132–133, 135f–136f
  subperiosteal facelift, II:270–273, 271f–273f
midface reconstruction, III:243–253
  functional and aesthetic outcomes
    aesthetic results, III:252t, 253
    diet, III:252, 252t
    globe position and function, III:252–253,
        252t
    oral competence, III:252t, 253
    speech, III:252, 252t
  goals, III:243, 244f
  indicators, III:243
  maxilla structure, III:244f
  patient presentation and diagnosis
    limited maxillectomy defects (Type I),
        III:244, 244f–247f
    orbitomaxillectomy defects (Type IV),
        III:244f, 245, 250f–251f
    preoperative assessment, III:244–245,
        244f
    subtotal maxillectomy defects (Type II),
        III:244–245, 244f, 247f–248f
    total maxillectomy defects (Type III),
        III:244f, 245, 249f–250f
  pediatric facial fractures, III:680, 681f, 684
  research summary, III:253
midfacial fractures
  complications
    airway management, III:74
    bleeding, III:74
    blindness, III:74
    cerebral spinal rhinorrhea or otorrhea,
        III:74
    infections, III:74
    late complications, III:74–75
    malocclusion, III:74–75
    malunion occurrences, III:74
    nasolacrimal duct injury, III:75
    nonunion occurrences, III:74
  Le Fort classification of facial fractures
    background information, III:71–75
    goals, III:71
    Le Fort I level fractures/transverse
        (Guerin) fractures, III:71, 72f, 73
    Le Fort II level fractures/pyramidal
        fractures, III:72f–73f, 73–74
    Le Fort III level fractures/craniofacial
        dysjunction, III:72f–73f, 73–74
  midface buttresses
    alveolar fractures, III:71
    characteristics, III:70–71, 70f
    clinical examination
      cerebral spinal rhinorrhea or otorrhea,
          III:71
      digital manipulation, III:71
      inspection process, III:70–71
      malocclusion of the teeth, III:71
      palpation, III:71
    computed tomography (CT), III:71
    treatment strategies, III:71
  nasal fractures
    complications, III:60
    nasal septum fractures and dislocations
      characteristics, III:58–59, 58f
      treatment strategies, III:59–60
    treatment strategies
      closed reduction, III:59–60
      K-wire support, III:59

midfacial fractures (Continued)
    nasal septum fractures and
        dislocations, III:59–60
    open reduction, III:59
    soft tissue contracture, III:59–60, 59f
    types and locations, III:57, 58f
  nasoethmoidal orbital fractures
    characteristics, III:60–61
    classification systems, III:61–63, 62f
    clinical examination, III:60–61, 61f
    complications, III:63
    computed tomography (CT), III:61
    surgical pathology
      causal factors, III:60
      interorbital space, III:60
      traumatic orbital hypertelorism, III:60
      traumatic telecanthus, III:60
    treatment strategies
      basic procedure, III:61–63
      canthal reattachment, III:63
      central fragment considerations, III:63
      lacrimal system injury, III:63
  postoperative care and follow-up, III:74
  zygoma
    anterior treatment approach
      basic procedure, III:65–66
      endoscopic approaches, III:65
      minimalist approach, III:65
      preoperative/postoperative
          comparisons, III:66f
      Z-F suture diastasis, III:65–66
    characteristics, III:63–65
    classification systems
      anterior treatment approach, III:65–66
      posterior approach (coronal incisions),
          III:66
    complications
      bleeding, III:69
      late complications, III:69–70, 69f
      maxillary sinusitis, III:69
      numbness, III:69–70
      oral-antral fistula, III:70
      orbital complications, III:69, 69f
      plate complications, III:70
    compound comminuted fractures
      characteristics, III:69–70
      delayed treatment, III:69
    diagnosis, III:64–65
    high energy fractures
      characteristics, III:67–68, 68f
      intraoral approach, III:68
      maxillary sinus approach, III:68
    reduction methods
      Dingman approach, III:67
      maxillary sinus approach, III:67
      stability requirements, III:67
      temporal approach, III:67
    surgical pathology, III:64–65
    treatment strategies
      buttress articulations and alignment,
          III:66–67
      closed reduction, III:66
midfoot amputations, IV:208
migraine headaches, III:491–499
  corrugator supercilii muscle hypertrophy,
      III:492, 492f
  diagnostic criteria, III:491, 492b
  epidemiology, III:491
  migraine with aura, III:492
  migraine without aura, III:492

migraine headaches (Continued)
  patient presentation and diagnosis, III:492
  patient selection
    botulinum toxin type-A (BoNT-A),
        III:492–495, 494f
    trigger sites, III:492, 493t
  preoperative assessment, III:492, 492f, 494f
  research summary, III:498
  surgical technique and treatment
    endoscopic approach
      basic principles, III:495–496, 496f
      complications, III:496
    frontal trigger deactivation, III:495
    occipital trigger deactivation
      basic principles, III:496–498, 497f
      complications, III:498
    septonasal triggers
      basic principles, III:498
      complications, III:498
    temporal trigger deactivation
      basic principles, III:496
      complications, III:496
    transpalpebral approach
      basic principles, III:495
      complications, III:495
    zygomaticotemporal branch of the
        trigeminal nerve, III:492, 495–496,
        496f
milia, I:719–720, II:77
military combat injuries, IV:63
milking test, VI:56
Miller–Dieker syndrome, III:807t
Mimic dV-Trainer, I:865–868, 866f
minerals, IV:282–283
minimal defect rhinoplasty, I:40
minimally invasive repair of pectus
    excavatum (MIRPE), III:858, 859f
minimum erythema dose (MED), II:13–14
minocycline, II:21t
minor histocompatibility antigens, I:816
Mirault, Germanicus, I:19
mirror hand, VI:622
mitochondrial inheritance, I:183–184
mitogen-activated kinase (MAPK), I:626f
Miura–Komada technique, VI:565, 566f
mixed mesh See acellular dermal matrix
    (ADM)
Moberg pick-up test, VI:59, 59f
Möbius syndrome, III:284, 297–298, 300f, 305f,
    805–807, 807t
modern plastic surgery, I:20–23, 22f–23f
modified classification of congenital
    anomalies of the hand and upper limb
  acrosyndactyly, VI:540f
  anomaly characteristics, VI:537–539, 538t
  cleft hands, VI:540f
  constriction band syndrome, VI:540f
  dorsal dimelia, VI:540f
  macrodactyly, VI:541f
  radial and ulnar duplications, VI:539f
  radial longitudinal deficiency, VI:538f
  symbrachydactyly, VI:538f
modified House classification of thumb
    deformity, VI:464t
modified Kleinert method, VI:197–198, 198f
modified radical mastectomy, V:285, 285f
modified radical neck dissection, III:414f–416f,
    415–416

modified Stiles–Bunnell technique, VI:764–
    766, 765f
Mohr–Wriedt syndrome, VI:636, 638f, 646
Mohs surgery, IV:313
moisturizers
  characteristics, II:16–18
  emollients
    characteristics, II:18
    oatmeal, II:18
    shea butter, II:18
  humectants
    characteristics, II:17–18
    glycerin, II:17–18
  occlusives
    characteristics, II:17
    essential oils, II:17
    lanolin, II:17
molecular biology
  deoxyribonucleic acid (DNA)
    characteristics, I:177–182, 177f
    epigenetic mechanisms, I:181–182, 181f
    gene expression, I:179–180
    gene regulation, I:180–181, 180f
    genomic DNA organization, I:178–179,
        178f
molybdenum (Mo) alloys, I:786–787
Mondeville, Henry of, I:15
Mondor's disease, V:35–36
Mongolian spot, I:726–727, 728f
Monks, George H, VI:xlv
Monoblock advancement/distraction
    simulator, I:867
monoclonal antibodies, I:204–206, 205f
monoethylglycinexylidide (MEGX), II:517
monomorphic adenoma, III:365t, 367, 368f,
    372
monostotic fibrous dysplasia, III:380–382
mons pubis descent, II:674–676, 675f–677f
Montgomery glands, V:5
Montgomery's gland carcinoma, I:738
Morestin, Hippolyte, I:21
Morley's test, VI:66
morphine, IV:427
Morrison, Wayne, I:6
mortality rates, I:125–126, 157f
Morton's metatarsalgia, I:727
Morton's neuroma, I:727
Morton, William, VI:xliii
morula, III:504–505
Mosaic laser, II:71t, 74
motor nerves
  feet, IV:61
  forehead, II:97–98, 97f
  legs, IV:48, 48t
  thighs, IV:26, 27f–28f
motor vehicle accidents, III:49, IV:63
mouth
  anatomical characteristics, III:422, 422f
  reconstructive surgeries, III:307–335
    bone-carrying flaps
      circumflex iliac osteocutaneous flap,
          III:322, 323f
      fibula osteoseptocutaneous flap,
          III:323
      pectoralis major
          osteomusculocutaneous flap,
          III:322
      radius with radial forearm flap, III:323

mouth (Continued)
    scapular osteomusculocutaneous flap,
        III:323, 323f
    temporalis osteomuscular flap, III:322
    trapezius osteomusculocutaneous flap,
        III:322
  burn wound treatment, IV:473, 489–490,
      495f
  challenges, III:307–308
  complications
    acute complications, III:333
    chronic complications, III:333–334
  decision-making process
    basic procedure, III:311–313
    immediate postoperative appearance,
        III:314f
    myocutaneous perforator flap, III:313f
    patient follow-up, III:312f–314f
    radial forearm flap, III:311f
    squamous cell carcinomas (SCCs),
        III:311f–313f
    ulnar forearm flap, III:312f
  disease process, III:308
  evaluation examinations, III:25
  free tissue transfer, III:311
  lips, III:46, 47f–48f
  local/regional flaps, III:309t, 311
  oral mucosa repair, III:46
  patient presentation and diagnosis,
      III:308
  patient selection
    defect factors, III:310–311, 310t
    patient factors, III:308–310, 310t
  postoperative care and follow-up,
      III:332–333
  prognosis and outcomes, III:333–334
  secondary procedures, III:334
  skin grafts, III:311
  soft tissue flaps
    anterolateral thigh flap, III:321–322
    comparison studies, III:309t
    deltopectoral flaps, III:318–319, 319f
    lateral arm flap, III:321
    medial sural artery perforator (MSAP)
        flap, III:322
    pectoralis major myocutaneous flaps,
        III:319, 320f
    radial forearm flap, III:319–320
    rectus abdominis musculocutaneous
        flap, III:321, 321f
    selection guidelines, III:309t
    submental flaps, III:316–318, 318f
    thoracodorsal artery perforator (TDAP)
        flap, III:322
    ulnar forearm flap, III:320–321
  surgical technique
    bone-carrying flaps, III:322–332
    fasciocutaneous flaps, III:319–322
    local flaps, III:316–318
    musculocutaneous flaps, III:319–322
    pedicled osteocutaneous flaps, III:322
    regional flaps, III:318–319
    soft tissue flaps, III:316–322
    vascularized osteocutaneous flaps,
        III:322–323
  surgical technique and treatment,
      III:45–46
  tongue, III:46

mouth (Continued)
  tumors, III:398–419
    diagnosis and treatment, III:427
    floor of mouth tumors
      diagnosis and treatment, III:427
      preoperative assessment, III:406
      surgical technique and treatment, III:406
MSX gene family, I:180–181
mucocele, III:365
mucoepidermoid carcinoma
  characteristics, III:370
  classifications, III:365t
  incidence, III:376t
  outcomes and complicatons, III:377
  parotid gland, III:370t
  submandibular gland, III:370t
  surgical technique and treatment, III:373–374, 374f–376f
mucositis, I:668–669
mucous cyst of the oral mucosa, I:736, 736f
Muenke syndrome, I:197, 197f, 197t, III:749–750, 750t, 752f
Muir–Torre syndrome, VI:315–316
Müller's muscle, II:111f, 112
Multicenter Selective Lymphadenectomy Trial (MSLT), I:770
multidetector-row computed tomography (MDCT)
  breast reconstruction
    basic principles, V:328–329
    deep inferior epigastric perforator (DIEP) flaps, V:326, 327f–328f
    radiological protocol, V:329, 330f, 332f–334f
multileaf collimators (MLCs), I:658, 658f
multiple exotoses, VI:642–644, 644f
multiple-flap Z-plasty, I:315, 315f–316f
multiple piloleiomyoma, VI:731–732
multiple primary melanomas, I:749–750
multipotent stem cells, I:213f
MURCS association, VI:573t
Murray, Joseph, I:2–3, 3f, VI:xlviii
muscle dysmorphia, I:51
muscles
  abdomen, II:531–533, 532f
  aging process, II:86
  breast anatomy
    external oblique, V:10f, 11
    intercostal dissection, V:10f
    internal oblique, V:10f
    pectoralis major, V:9–11, 10f
    pectoralis minor, V:10f
    rectus abdominis, V:10f, 11
    serratus anterior, V:10–11, 10f
  facial muscles, II:34f, 189, 190f
  forehead muscles
    characteristics, II:95–96
    frontalis, II:96f
    glabellar frown muscles, II:95f
    lateral orbicularis, II:96f
  free-functioning muscle transfer, VI:777–788
    complications, VI:787
    muscle structure
      characteristics, VI:777–780
      length–tension relationship, VI:779f
      myosin cross-bridges, VI:778f
      schematic diagram, VI:778f
      strap and pennate muscles, VI:779f

muscles (Continued)
    patient presentation and diagnosis, VI:780, 780f
    patient selection, VI:780–781, 781t
    secondary procedures, VI:787
    surgical technique and treatment
      basic principles, VI:781–787
      donor motor nerve, VI:783–785, 783b
      elbows, VI:787
      finger extension, VI:785–787
      flexor digitorum profundus (FDP) tendons, VI:782, 785f
      forearm dissection, VI:784–785, 784f
      gliding tendon path, VI:783f
      gracilis muscle, VI:781–787, 781f–782f
      insufficient coverage, VI:783f
      neurovascular structure alignment, VI:784f
      postoperative finger flexion, VI:786f
    tendon transfers, VI:780t
  gluteus maximus muscle, II:600
    breast reconstruction, V:292
    characteristics, I:516f
    clinical applications, I:523f–524f
    gluteal aesthetic ideals, II:600, 600f
    perineal reconstruction, I:557
    pressure sores, I:562–565, 566f–568f
  hands
    biomechanics
      Blix curve, VI:28f
      extensor mechanism, VI:18b, 20f
      force–velocity curve, VI:28f
      moment arms, VI:28b, 29f
      muscle force production, VI:22b, 28f
      muscle shape, VI:22b
      muscle structure, VI:18b, 19f
    extrinsic extensors, VI:14–18, 15f–17f
    extrinsic flexors, VI:22–29, 22b, 23f–27f, 32b
    intrinsic muscles, VI:32–35, 33f–36f, 35b
    pronators and supinators, VI:18–22, 21f
  limb development (embryology), VI:532–534, 533f
  muscle graft and repair
    clinical application, I:364
    definition, I:364–366
    future trends, I:364–366, 365f
    mutilated/mangled hands, VI:253, 262
    surgical technique, I:364
  structure
    characteristics, VI:777–780
    length–tension relationship, VI:779f
    myosin cross-bridges, VI:778f
    schematic diagram, VI:778f
    strap and pennate muscles, VI:779f
  tissue engineering, I:390–391
  tissue expansion effects, I:623
  tissue-specific stem cells, I:230–232, 231f
  vascular anatomy
    classification systems, I:488–491, 489f, 489t
    innervation patterns, I:489f
    Type I muscles, I:489–491, 489f–490f, 489t
    Type II muscles, I:489f–490f, 489t, 491
    Type III muscles, I:489f–490f, 489t, 491
    Type IV muscles, I:489f–490f, 489t, 491
musculoaponeurotic fibrosarcoma oncogene homolog B (MafB), VI:348–349

musculocutaneous flaps
  advantages/disadvantages, I:538–539
  clinical application
    background information, I:521–534
    circumflex scapular and thoracodorsal pedicles, I:530f
    combination flaps, I:528–530, 530f
    deep circumflex iliac artery composite flap, I:529f
    distally based flaps, I:531, 531t
    functional muscle flaps, I:528
    gluteus maximus muscle, I:523f–524f
    microvascular composite tissue transplantation, I:533–534
    pectoralis major muscle, I:524, 525f
    prelaminated and prefabricated flaps, I:530–531
    radial forearm flap, I:532f
    reverse-flow flaps, I:531, 532f
    reverse transposition flap, I:531–533, 533f
    segmental transposition flaps, I:522–524, 523f–524f
    sensory flaps, I:528
    tibialis anterior muscle flaps, I:526f
    tissue expansion, I:522
    vascularized bone flaps, I:524–525, 526f–528f, 528t
    venous flaps, I:533, 534f–535f
  complications, I:571–572
  flap monitoring techniques, I:570
  lower extremity reconstructive surgery
    biceps femoris muscle flap, IV:139–140
    gastrocnemius muscle flap, IV:142, 142f
    gracilis muscle flap, IV:140–141, 140f
    rectus femoris muscle flap, IV:139, 139f
    soleus muscle flap, IV:141–142, 141f
    tensor fascia lata, IV:138–139, 138f
    trauma injuries, IV:72–75, 74f
  male genital reconstructive surgery, IV:307–310
  mangled upper extremities, VI:254–255, 275–279
  Mathes–Nahai Classification, I:516–517, 516f
  oral cavity and mouth reconstruction, III:319–322
  patient positioning, I:569–570
  preoperative and postoperative management, I:565–570
  pressure sores, I:562–565, IV:368
  regional applications
    abdominal wall, I:553–554, 553f, 553t, 555f
    breast reconstruction, I:546–549, 548f–549f
    chest wall reconstruction, I:552–553
    complications, I:571–572
    feet, I:560–562, 562f–563f
    flap monitoring techniques, I:570
    groin, I:554–557, 558f
    head and neck reconstruction, I:542–546, 543f–546f
    lower extremity reconstructive surgery, I:557–560, 559f–561f
    mediastinum, I:549–552, 550f–551f
    patient positioning, I:569–570
    perineal reconstruction, I:554–557, 556f–557f
    preoperative and postoperative management, I:565–570
    pressure sores, I:562–565, 564f–568f
    pulmonary cavity, I:552–553
  selection guidelines, I:541–542

musculocutaneous flaps *(Continued)*
  spina bifida, **III:**867–872, 868t–869t
  Type I muscles (one vascular pedicle), **I:**516, 517t
  Type II muscles (dominant vascular pedicle and minor pedicle), **I:**516, 517t
  Type III muscles (two dominant pedicles), **I:**516–517, 517t
  Type IV muscles (segmental vascular pedicles), **I:**517, 517t
  Type V muscles (one dominant vascular pedicle and secondary segmental vascular pedicles), **I:**517, 517t
  vascular anatomical research, **I:**504–505
musculoskeletal sarcomas, **VI:**329–330, 330t
mushrooms, **II:**23
Muskuloskeletal Tumor Society staging system, **IV:**105t
Mustardé expanded rotation flap, **I:**635–637, 636f
Mustarde osteomuscular flaps, **III:**867–869, 872f
Mustarde's "jumping man" five-flap Z-plasty, **I:**315
Mustarde sutures, **II:**487–488, 487f
mustard gas, **IV:**461–463
mutations, **I:**184–185
mutilated/mangled hands, **VI:**250–281
  causal factors, **VI:**255, 256f
  initial evaluation and treatment
    debridement, **VI:**251, 251f
    guidelines, **VI:**250–255, 251b
    musculotendinous reconstruction, **VI:**253
    nerve repair, **VI:**253–254, 254f
    postoperative management, **VI:**255
    provisional revascularization, **VI:**251, 252f
    skeletal stabilization, **VI:**251–252
    skin and soft-tissue reconstruction, **VI:**254–255
    vascular reconstruction, **VI:**252–253, 253f
  injury impacts, **VI:**255–256
  injury types
    amputations, **VI:**256
    avulsion injuries, **VI:**256, 256f
    crush injuries, **VI:**256, 256f, 261f
    roller injuries, **VI:**256, 257f
  outcomes and complicatons, **VI:**279–281
  patient presentation and diagnosis
    emergency room evaluations, **VI:**256–257
    reconstruction planning, **VI:**257–259
  postoperative care and follow-up, **VI:**279
  reconstruction process
    amputation versus salvage decisions, **VI:**259
    delayed reconstruction, **VI:**259
    early (single-stage) reconstruction, **VI:**259
    emergency room evaluations, **VI:**257–259
    planning and preparation guidelines, **VI:**258
    spare-parts utilization, **VI:**259, 260f
    timing considerations, **VI:**258–259
  secondary procedures
    free fibula transfer, **VI:**279–280, 280f
    innervated microvascular muscle transfer, **VI:**281
    microvascular toe transfer, **VI:**280–281, 280f

mutilated/mangled hands *(Continued)*
  surgical technique and treatment
    bony reconstruction options, **VI:**259–261, 260f
    flap reconstruction
      anterolateral thigh flap, **VI:**274–275, 275f–276f
      cutaneous versus muscle flaps, **VI:**263–279
      fasciocutaneous flaps, **VI:**254–255, 266–275
      free flaps, **VI:**254–255, 266–275
      lateral arm flap, **VI:**267, 269f–272f
      latissimus dorsi (LD) flap, **VI:**275, 277f
      local flaps, **VI:**254–255
      muscle/musculocutaneous flaps, **VI:**254–255, 275–279
      pedicled groin flap, **VI:**264–266, 265f–266f
      radial forearm flap, **VI:**266–267, 267f–269f
      rectus abdominis, **VI:**275–277, 278f
      scapular and parascapular flaps, **VI:**272, 273f
      serratus anterior muscles, **VI:**277–279
      temporoparietal fascia flaps, **VI:**272–274, 274f
    muscle reconstruction, **VI:**262
    nerve reconstruction, **VI:**262
    soft-tissue reconstruction, **VI:**262–263, 263f–264f
    tendon graft and repair, **VI:**262
    vascular reconstruction options, **VI:**261–262, 261f
mycobacterial infections, **VI:**342–343
Mycobacterium avium-intercellulare, **III:**891, **VI:**343
Mycobacterium marinum, **VI:**342–343
Mycobacterium scrofulaceum, **III:**891
Mycobacterium tuberculosis, **VI:**334–335
mycophenolate mofetil, **I:**822–823, 822t, 833t
myeloperoxidase (MPO) enzyme system, **I:**575–576
myocutaneous flaps, **I:**630, **IV:**449–450
myocutaneous gluteal rotation flap
  basic procedure, **IV:**370–375, 371f
  girdlestone arthroplasty, **IV:**376f
  ischial pressure sores, **IV:**372–373, 372t
  surgical guidelines, **IV:**372b
  trochanteric ulcers, **IV:**373–375, 375t, 376f
  V-Y hamstring advancement, **I:**562–565, 566f, 568f, **IV:**373, 374f
  V-Y tensor fasciae latae flap, **IV:**375, 377f
myoelectric prostheses, **VI:**870–871
myofibroblasts, **I:**271f, 272, **II:**63
myogenesis, **VI:**532–534, 533f
myoglobinuria, **IV:**436
myositis ossificans, **VI:**326, 326f

N
NADPH oxidase (nicotinamide adenine dinucleotide phosphate-oxidase), **I:**258–259
Nager syndrome, **III:**714, 805–807, 807t, **VI:**573t

nail and fingertip reconstruction, **VI:**117–137
  acute injuries
    cornified nail bed
      characteristics, **VI:**124
      surgical technique and treatment, **VI:**124
    distal phalanx fractures
      nail ridges, **VI:**121
      patient presentation and diagnosis, **VI:**120
      secondary procedures, **VI:**120–121
      surgical technique and treatment, **VI:**120, 141, 142f
    epidemiology, **VI:**119–128
    eponychial deformities
      characteristics, **VI:**125
      surgical technique and treatment, **VI:**125, 125f
    hooked nails
      characteristics, **VI:**124
      surgical technique and treatment, **VI:**124–125
    hyponychial defects
      characteristics, **VI:**125
      surgical technique and treatment, **VI:**125
    lacerations
      characteristics, **VI:**119–120
      postoperative care and follow-up, **VI:**120
      surgical technique and treatment, **VI:**120, 120b, 121f–122f
    nail absence
      characteristics, **VI:**123
      surgical technique and treatment, **VI:**123–124, 124f
    nail ridges, **VI:**121
    nail spikes and cysts
      characteristics, **VI:**124
      surgical technique and treatment, **VI:**124
    nonadherence (onycholysis)
      characteristics, **VI:**123
      surgical technique and treatment, **VI:**123
    pigmented lesions
      characteristics, **VI:**125
      patient presentation and diagnosis, **VI:**125–126, 126f–127f
    pincer nails
      characteristics, **VI:**126, 127f
      surgical technique and treatment, **VI:**126–128
    pterygium
      characteristics, **VI:**122–123
      surgical technique and treatment, **VI:**122–123
    split nails
      characteristics, **VI:**121
      surgical technique and treatment, **VI:**121–122, 123f
    subungual hematoma
      characteristics, **VI:**119
      surgical technique and treatment, **VI:**119, 119b
  burn reconstruction, **IV:**509
  flap reconstruction
    challenges, **VI:**128
    flap selection, **VI:**128, 129f
    reconstructive principles, **VI:**128

*Note: **Boldface** roman numerals indicate volume. Page numbers followed by f refer to figures; page numbers followed by t refer to tables; page numbers followed by b refer to boxes.*

nail and fingertip reconstruction (Continued)
  skin grafts
    cross finger flaps, VI:130–131, 133f
    dorsal metacarpal artery flaps, VI:134, 135f
    heterodigital flaps, VI:130–134
    homodigital flaps, VI:130, 132f
    lateral V-Y advancement flaps, VI:130, 130f
    Littler neurovascular island flap, VI:132–134
    local flaps, VI:128–134
    patient selection, VI:128
    surgical technique and treatment, VI:128–134
    thenar crease flap, VI:132, 134f
    visor flaps, VI:130, 131f
    volar V-Y advancement flap, VI:128–130, 129f
  nail/nail bed
    anatomical characteristics, VI:117, 118f
    embryology, VI:117
    functional role, VI:119
    nerve supply, VI:118
    physiology, VI:118–119
    vascular anatomy, VI:117–118
  nail ridges, VI:121
  split nails
    characteristics, VI:121
    surgical technique and treatment, VI:121–122, 123f
Najer syndrome, VI:573t
narcissistic personality, I:35
nasal reshaping, II:56, 57f
Nasenplastik und sonstige Gesichtsplastik (Rhinoplasty and other Facialplasties), I:25–28
nasion, II:356t, 363f
nasoalveolar molding (NAM), III:552–553
nasoethmoidal orbital fractures
  characteristics, III:60–61
  classification systems, III:61–63, 62f
  clinical examination, III:60–61, 61f
  complications, III:63
  computed tomography (CT), III:61
  surgical pathology
    causal factors, III:60
    interorbital space, III:60
    traumatic orbital hypertelorism, III:60
    traumatic telecanthus, III:60
  treatment strategies
    basic procedure, III:61–63
    canthal reattachment, III:63
    central fragment considerations, III:63
    lacrimal system injury, III:63
nasoethmoid injury, III:232, 234f
nasolabial adhesion cheiloplasty
  advantages/disadvantages, III:525–526
  surgical technique
    C flap mucosa elevation and insertion, III:527, 527f
    lateral lip incisions, III:527, 528f
    markings, III:526, 527f
    mucosal flaps, III:527, 528f
    muscle and skin closure, III:527
    nostril floor closure, III:527, 528f
    post-adhesion definitive cheiloplasty, III:527, 529f
    surgical indicators, III:526–527
  two-stage palate repair, III:525

nasolabial flaps, III:309t
nasolabial folds
  botulinum toxin type-A (BoNT-A), II:37–38, 38f
  Lemperle classifications, II:53t
  photographic guidelines, I:110, 112f
  soft-tissue fillers, II:53, 53f–54f
nasolacrimal duct injury, III:75
National Comprehensive Cancer Network (NCCN), I:158–159, 158t, 665, 777–778, V:286–287
National Pressure Ulcer Advisory Panel (NPUAP), IV:353, 356, 356f–358f
National Surgical Adjuvant Breast/Bowel Project (NSABP), V:274–280
National Surgical Quality Improvement Program (NSQIP), I:158t, 173
natural killer (NK) cells, I:816–817
nausea, I:145
neck
  aging process
    anatomical characteristics
      general discussion, II:313–315
      marginal mandibular nerve, II:314f
      platysma muscle, II:314f
      Type I interdigitation, II:314–315, 314f
      Type II interdigitation, II:314, 314f
      Type III noninterdigitation, II:314–315, 314f–315f
    disease process, II:315–316
  anatomical characteristics, III:3–8, 4f–5f, 8f, 424
  anesthesia, III:27
  botulinum toxin type-A (BoNT-A), II:37, 38f
  cervical lymph nodes, III:415f, 424, 427f
  congenital melanocytic nevi (CMN), III:844, 846f
  dermoid neck cysts
    disease process, III:885
    patient presentation and diagnosis, III:885
  facelifts
    basic surgical technique, II:202–203, 203f
    extended SMAS technique
      incisions, II:254–255
      platysma muscle release, II:252–255, 253f–254f
      SMAS fixation versus platysmaplasty, II:254, 255f
    horizontal advancement genioplasty, II:316, 316f
    lateral SMASectomy, II:234, 316
    MACS (minimal access cranial suspension) lift, II:226–228, 228f, 316
    neck and jowl defatting, II:234
    platysma-SMAS plication (PSP), II:219t, 220–221, 316
    secondary facelifts
      large digastric muscles, II:296–297, 297f
      over-excision of buccal fat, II:294, 295f
      over-excision of subcutaneous fat, II:293–294, 293f–294f
      over-excision of subplatysmal fat, II:294, 295f
      prominent submandibular glands, II:294–296, 296f
      residual platysma bands, II:297–299, 298f
    subperiosteal facelift, II:273–275, 274f
  fascial layers, III:3–8, 4f–5f, 8f

neck (Continued)
  infantile hemangioma (IH), I:680
  liposuctions, II:525
  lymph node drainage patterns, III:421
  melanoma excisions, I:766
  muscle/musculocutaneous flaps, I:542–546, 543f–546f
  neck cancer
    cervical lymph nodes, III:415f
    complications
      dental follow-ups, III:418
      general discussion, III:416–418
      local recurrence, III:416
      osteoradionecrosis (ORN), III:417
      post-treatment surveillance, III:417–418
      regional recurrence, III:416–417
      wound infections, III:417
    epidemiology, III:399–400
    lymph node anatomy, III:399f
    medical challenges, III:398
    neck dissection
      basic procedure, III:413–416, 427, 429f
      modified radical neck dissection, III:414f–416f, 415–416
      supraomohyoid neck dissection, III:413–415
    nodal status determination, III:429–431, 430f
    oral cavity/mouth/tongue/mandibular reconstruction, III:307–335
      acute complications, III:333
      challenges, III:307–308
      chronic complications, III:333–334
      decision-making process, III:311–313
      defect factors, III:310–311, 310t
      disease process, III:308
      flap options, III:310t
      free tissue transfer, III:311
      local/regional flaps, III:309t, 311
      patient factors, III:308–310, 310t
      patient presentation and diagnosis, III:308
      patient selection, III:308–316
      postoperative care and follow-up, III:332–333
      prognosis and outcomes, III:333–334
      secondary procedures, III:334
      skin grafts, III:311
      soft tissue flaps, III:309t
      surgical technique, III:316–332
    pathogenesis, III:398–399
    patient presentation and diagnosis, III:400
    psychological aspects, I:43–44
    radiation treatment, I:668–669
    risk factors
      alcohol, III:421
      gastroesophageal reflux, III:421
      infectious agents, III:421
      pollution exposure, III:421–422
      tobacco, III:421
    surgical access, III:402, 403f–404f
    therapeutic choices, III:401–402
    TNM clinical classification system, III:308, 400–401, 401t
    upper aerodigestive tract, III:420–439
      anatomical considerations, III:422–424
      diagnosis and treatment, III:427–437
      epidemiology, III:420
      future trends, III:438

neck (*Continued*)
  incidence, **III:**421–427
  outcomes and complicatons, **III:**438
  patient evaluation, **III:**424–427
  postoperative care and follow-up,
      III:437–438
  prevalence, **III:**421–427
  risk factors, **III:**421–422
neck rejuvenation, **II:**313–326
  complications, **II:**324–325
  general discussion, **II:**313
  minimally invasive options, **II:**319
  nonsurgical options, **II:**319
  postoperative care and follow-up, **II:**324
  preoperative assessment
      general discussion, **II:**316–318
      ideal facial proportion, **II:**317f
      ideal profile dimensions, **II:**317f
      preoperative–postoperative
          comparisons, **II:**317f–318f
      skin volume, **II:**319f
      transverse dimensions, **II:**317f
  submandibular gland care, **II:**324
  surgical options
      anterior/submental lipectomy and
          platysmaplasty, **II:**321–323, 322f
      characteristics, **II:**319–324
      Corset (Feldman) platysmaplasty,
          II:320f
      direct excision, **II:**323–324, 323f
      liposuction, **II:**320–321, 321f
      Z-plasty technique, **II:**323–324, 323f
  threadlift, **II:**319
platysmal bands, **II:**37, 38f
progressive hemifacial atrophy (PHA),
    III:797f
reconstructive burn surgery, **IV:**493–494,
    498–499, 506
soft-tissue injuries
  surgical technique and treatment, **III:**46
  systematic head and neck evaluations
      airway evaluation, **III:**25
      basic procedure, **III:**24–25
      cheek examination, **III:**25, 25f
      ear examination, **III:**25, 25f, 40
      eye examination, **III:**25
      nose examination, **III:**25
      oral cavity and mouth examination,
          III:25
tissue expansion
  basic principles, **I:**631–640
  lateral face and neck, **I:**635–637, 636f, 638f
TNM clinical classification system/pTNM
    pathologic classification system, **I:**714f
necrotizing fasciitis, **VI:**341–342, 341f, 342b
necrotizing sialometaplasia, **III:**366, 367f, 371
needle electromyography (EMG), **VI:**797–798
negative pressure devices (NPDs), **IV:**442
negative pressure wound therapy (NPWT),
    I:850–851, 850f, **IV:**83, 199, 367
negative transference, **I:**33–34
negligence, **I:**93
negotiation, **I:**86–87
neoadjuvant therapy, **I:**201–207
neoclassical canons, **II:**340, 356t
neodymium-doped yttrium aluminum garnet
    (YAG) lasers, **I:**718, 734–735, **II:**61, 67–70,
    461–462, **III:**30, **IV:**454, 454t

Neoform, **V:**69–71
neoplasms, **III:**116
neoplastic cicatricial alopecia, **III:**111t
neosporin, **IV:**395
neovascularization, **I:**230, 231f, 232
nerve compression syndromes, **VI:**503–525
  anterior interosseous nerve (AIN) syndrome
      characteristics, **VI:**510–511
      nonsurgical management, **VI:**511
      surgical technique and treatment, **VI:**511,
          512f–513f
  carpal tunnel syndrome
      American Academy of Orthopaedic
          Surgeons clinical practice guidelines
          for the treatment of carpal tunnel
          syndrome, **VI:**507t
      anatomical considerations, **VI:**505, 506f
      etiology, **VI:**505
      nonsurgical management, **VI:**507
      outcomes and complicatons, **VI:**509–510,
          509b
      patient presentation and diagnosis,
          VI:505–507, 507b
      patient selection, **VI:**507
      prevalence, **VI:**505–510
      surgical technique and treatment
          Agee endoscopic carpal tunnel release
              (ECTR), **VI:**509
          anesthesia, **VI:**507–509, 507b, 508f
          Chow technique, **VI:**509
          endoscopic carpal tunnel release
              (ECTR), **VI:**509
          open carpal tunnel release (OCTR),
              VI:507–509
          palmaris brevis/thenar muscle
              preservation, **VI:**509f
  cubital tunnel syndrome
      anatomical considerations, **VI:**513–514
      clinical signs, **VI:**514t
      outcomes and complicatons, **VI:**513b,
          515–516
      patient presentation and diagnosis,
          VI:514
      patient selection, **VI:**514
      surgical technique and treatment
          endoscopic decompression, **VI:**515
          intramuscular transposition, **VI:**515
          medial epicondylectomy technique,
              VI:515, 516f
          simple decompression, **VI:**514–515
          subcutaneous transposition, **VI:**515
          submuscular transposition, **VI:**515
  electrodiagnostic studies, **VI:**504–505, 504f
  general discussion, **VI:**503
  Guyon's canal
      anatomical considerations, **VI:**511, 513f
      etiology, **VI:**511
      patient presentation and diagnosis,
          VI:511–512
      surgical technique and treatment,
          VI:512–513
  median nerve compression
      anterior interosseous nerve (AIN)
          syndrome, **VI:**510–511
      carpal tunnel syndrome, **VI:**505–510
      pronator syndrome, **VI:**510
      proximal arm and elbow, **VI:**510, 510f
  pathophysiology, **VI:**503–504

nerve compression syndromes (*Continued*)
  posterior interosseous nerve (PIN)
      compression
      anatomical considerations, **VI:**517
  posterior interosseous nerve (PIN)
      syndrome, **VI:**517
  radial tunnel syndrome
      nonsurgical management, **VI:**518
      outcomes and complicatons, **VI:**518
      patient presentation and diagnosis,
          VI:518
      surgical technique and treatment,
          VI:518, 519f
  pronator syndrome, **VI:**510
  proximal arm and elbow, **VI:**510, 510f
  quadrilateral space syndrome
      anatomical considerations, **VI:**523, 523f
      etiology, **VI:**523
      patient presentation and diagnosis,
          VI:523
      patient selection, **VI:**523
      surgical technique and treatment, **VI:**524
  radial nerve compression
      incidence, **VI:**516–518
      posterior interosseous nerve (PIN)
          compression, **VI:**517
      Wartenberg's syndrome, **VI:**516–517
  suprascapular nerve compression
      anatomical considerations, **VI:**524, 524f
      etiology, **VI:**524
      patient presentation and diagnosis,
          VI:524
      patient selection, **VI:**524
      surgical technique and treatment,
          VI:524–525
  thoracic outlet syndrome (TOS)
      anatomical considerations, **VI:**64–65, 65f,
          519, 520f–521f
      classifications, **VI:**64
      definition, **VI:**63–66
      incidence, **VI:**518–522
      nonsurgical management, **VI:**521–522
      outcomes and complicatons, **VI:**522
      patient presentation and diagnosis,
          VI:520–521, 522f
      provocative maneuvers
          Adson test, **VI:**65, 66f
          costoclavicular compression test, **VI:**65,
              66f
          Morley's test, **VI:**66
          neck tilting test, **VI:**65
          Roos extended arm stress test, **VI:**66
          Wright test, **VI:**65, 66f
      surgical technique and treatment, **VI:**522
      Wright's hyperabduction test, **VI:**520–521,
          522f
  ulnar nerve compression
      cubital tunnel syndrome, **VI:**513–516
      Guyon's canal, **VI:**511–513
  Wartenberg's syndrome
      anatomical considerations, **VI:**516, 517f
      patient presentation and diagnosis,
          VI:516
      patient selection, **VI:**517
      surgical technique and treatment, **VI:**517
nerve conduction studies (NCSs), **VI:**504–505,
    504f, 797–798
nerve conduits, **I:**473, 473t, 474f

Note: **Boldface** *roman numerals indicate volume. Page numbers followed by f refer to figures; page numbers followed by t refer to tables; page numbers followed by b refer to boxes.*

Nerve injury, Ischemia, Soft-tissue Injury, Skeletal Injury, Shock, and Age of patient score (NISSSA), **IV:**63
nerve repair and grafting, **I:**464–478
  bioengineering techniques, **I:**476
  burn reconstruction, **IV:**450–451
  current grafting techniques
    allografts, **I:**473–474, 473t, 475f, 831
    autologous nerve grafts, **I:**472–474, 473t, 831
    autologous vein grafts, **I:**472–473, 473t
    nerve conduits, **I:**473, 473t, 474f
    nerve transfer, **I:**473t, 474–476, 475b
    nerve wraps, **I:**473, 473t, 475f
  hand therapy
    early postoperative care, **VI:**857–858
    general discussion, **VI:**857–859
    late rehabilitation, **VI:**858
    motor re-education, **VI:**858–859
    sensory re-education, **VI:**858, 858f
  intraoperative nerve stimulation, **I:**471
  mutilated/mangled hands, **VI:**253–254, 254f, 262
  nerve compression syndromes, **VI:**503–525
    anterior interosseous nerve (AIN) syndrome
      characteristics, **VI:**510–511
      nonsurgical management, **VI:**511
      surgical technique and treatment, **VI:**511, 512f–513f
    carpal tunnel syndrome
      American Academy of Orthopaedic Surgeons clinical practice guidelines for the treatment of carpal tunnel syndrome, **VI:**507t
      anatomical considerations, **VI:**505, 506f
      etiology, **VI:**505
      nonsurgical management, **VI:**507
      outcomes and complicatons, **VI:**509–510, 509b
      patient presentation and diagnosis, **VI:**505–507, 507b
      patient selection, **VI:**507
      prevalence, **VI:**505–510
      surgical technique and treatment, **VI:**507–509, 508f–509f
    cubital tunnel syndrome
      anatomical considerations, **VI:**513–514
      clinical signs, **VI:**514t
      endoscopic decompression technique, **VI:**515
      intramuscular transposition technique, **VI:**515
      medial epicondylectomy technique, **VI:**515, 516f
      outcomes and complicatons, **VI:**513b, 515–516
      patient presentation and diagnosis, **VI:**514
      patient selection, **VI:**514
      simple decompression technique, **VI:**514–515
      subcutaneous transposition technique, **VI:**515
      submuscular transposition technique, **VI:**515
    electrodiagnostic studies, **VI:**504–505, 504f
    general discussion, **VI:**503

nerve repair and grafting *(Continued)*
  Guyon's canal
    anatomical considerations, **VI:**511, 513f
    etiology, **VI:**511
    patient presentation and diagnosis, **VI:**511–512
    surgical technique and treatment, **VI:**512–513
  median nerve compression
    anterior interosseous nerve (AIN) syndrome, **VI:**510–511
    carpal tunnel syndrome, **VI:**505–510
    pronator syndrome, **VI:**510
    proximal arm and elbow, **VI:**510, 510f
  pathophysiology, **VI:**503–504
  posterior interosseous nerve (PIN) compression
    anatomical considerations, **VI:**517
    posterior interosseous nerve (PIN) syndrome, **VI:**517
    radial tunnel syndrome, **VI:**518
  pronator syndrome, **VI:**510
  proximal arm and elbow, **VI:**510, 510f
  quadrilateral space syndrome
    anatomical considerations, **VI:**523, 523f
    etiology, **VI:**523
    patient presentation and diagnosis, **VI:**523
    patient selection, **VI:**523
    surgical technique and treatment, **VI:**524
  radial nerve compression
    incidence, **VI:**516–518
    posterior interosseous nerve (PIN) compression, **VI:**517
    Wartenberg's syndrome, **VI:**516–517
  suprascapular nerve compression
    anatomical considerations, **VI:**524, 524f
    etiology, **VI:**524
    patient presentation and diagnosis, **VI:**524
    patient selection, **VI:**524
    surgical technique and treatment, **VI:**524–525
  thoracic outlet syndrome (TOS)
    anatomical considerations, **VI:**64–65, 65f, 519, 520f–521f
    classifications, **VI:**64
    definition, **VI:**63–66
    incidence, **VI:**518–522
    nonsurgical management, **VI:**521–522
    outcomes and complicatons, **VI:**522
    patient presentation and diagnosis, **VI:**520–521, 522f
    provocative maneuvers, **VI:**65–66
    surgical technique and treatment, **VI:**522
    Wright's hyperabduction test, **VI:**520–521, 522f
  ulnar nerve compression
    cubital tunnel syndrome, **VI:**513–516
    Guyon's canal, **VI:**511–513
  Wartenberg's syndrome
    anatomical considerations, **VI:**516, 517f
    patient presentation and diagnosis, **VI:**516
    patient selection, **VI:**517
    surgical technique and treatment, **VI:**517

nerve repair and grafting *(Continued)*
  nerve injuries
    avulsion injuries, **I:**466t, 467–468, 468f, **VI:**792, 792f–793f
    brachioplasty, **V:**563–564
    classifications, **I:**464–465, 465t–466t, **VI:**793
    crush/compression injuries, **I:**466–467, 466t
    evaluation examinations, **I:**468–469
    penetrating trauma, **I:**465–466, 466t, 467f
    stretch injuries, **I:**466t, 467–468, 468f
  nerve recovery, **I:**464
  nerve repair
    end-to-end versus end-to-side repair, **I:**470–471
    epineural versus fascicular repair, **I:**469–470, 470f
    mutilated/mangled hands, **VI:**253–254, 254f, 262
    surgical timing, **I:**469
    tension considerations, **I:**469
  nerve transfer, **VI:**719–744
    adult brachial plexus injury
      basic procedure, **VI:**799–800
      closed-target nerve transfer, **VI:**799
      end-to-side neurorrhaphy nerve transfer, **VI:**799–800
      extraplexus nerve transfer, **VI:**799
      functioning free muscle transplantation (FFMT), **VI:**801–802
      intraplexus nerve transfer, **VI:**799
      pedicled muscle transfer, **VI:**800–801
      proximal nerve transfer versus distal nerve transfer, **VI:**799t
      recommended induction exercises, **VI:**800t
      reconstructive strategies, **VI:**800, 801t
    complete/near-complete plexus injury
      contralateral C7 transfer, **VI:**732–733
      examination findings, **VI:**732
      phrenic nerve transfer, **VI:**732–733
      reconstruction techniques, **VI:**732–733, 732b
      spinal accessory and intercostal nerves, **VI:**732, 732f
    current grafting techniques, **I:**473t, 474–476, 475b
    end-to-side transfers, **VI:**719–720, 720b, 720f
    facial paralysis, **III:**291–292, 291f–292f
    general discussion, **VI:**719
    hand therapy, **VI:**859–861, 859f–860f
    lower plexus injuries
      examination findings, **VI:**732
      reconstruction techniques, **VI:**732, 732b
    median nerve injury
      adjunct tendon transfers, **VI:**733
      brachialis branch to anterior interosseous nerve (AIN) branch nerve transfer, **VI:**733, 735f
      examination findings, **VI:**733, 733b
      radial to median branch nerve transfers, **VI:**733, 734f
      reconstruction techniques, **VI:**733
    outcome assessments, **VI:**742–743
    patient presentation and diagnosis
      diagnostic imaging, **VI:**725
      electrodiagnostic testing, **VI:**725–726, 725b

nerve repair and grafting (Continued)
    pain questionnaire, **VI:**721f–724f
    patient history, **VI:**720, 721f–724f
    physical examination, **VI:**725, 725b
  patient selection, **VI:**726–727, 726t
  postoperative wound care
    basic procedure, **VI:**741–742
    complications, **VI:**742
    rehabilitation, **VI:**742
  radial nerve injury
    adjunct tendon transfers, **VI:**738–739
    examination findings, **VI:**737, 737b
    median to radial branch nerve
      transfers, **VI:**737–738, 738f
    reconstruction techniques, **VI:**737–739
  secondary procedures, **VI:**743, 743b
  sensory nerve injury
    first webspace sensation restoration,
      VI:740–741, 741f
    lateral antebrachial cutaneous nerve to
      radial nerve transfers, **VI:**741
    median to ulnar branch nerve transfers,
      VI:740, 740f
    radial to axillary nerve transfers,
      VI:741
    restoration techniques, **VI:**739–741
    ulnar to median branch nerve transfers,
      VI:739–740, 739f
  surgical procedures
    complete/near-complete plexus injury,
      VI:732–733
    lower plexus injuries, **VI:**732
    median nerve injury, **VI:**733
    radial nerve injury, **VI:**737–739
    sensory nerve injury, **VI:**739–741
    surgical tips, **VI:**727b
    ulnar nerve injury, **VI:**733–736
    upper plexus injuries, **VI:**727–731
  tubular repair, **VI:**713
  ulnar nerve injury
    adjunct tendon transfers, **VI:**736
    anterior interosseous nerve (AIN) to
      deep motor branch nerve transfer,
      VI:736, 736f–737f
    examination findings, **VI:**733–736, 736b
    median to ulnar branch nerve transfers,
      VI:736, 736f–737f
    reconstruction techniques, **VI:**736
  upper plexus injuries
    double fascicular nerve transfer, **VI:**731,
      731f
    examination findings, **VI:**727
    medial pectoral nerve and
      thoracodorsal nerve, **VI:**731, 731f
    reconstruction techniques, **VI:**727–731,
      727b
    spinal accessory to suprascapular nerve
      transfers, **VI:**727, 728f–729f
    triceps to axillary nerve transfer,
      VI:728, 729f–730f
    ulnar/median redundant branches to
      biceps brachii and brachialis
      branches nerve transfer, **VI:**731,
      731f
  outcome-related factors, **I:**471
  postoperative care and follow-up, **I:**476–477
  replantation and revascularization surgery,
    VI:235

nerve repair and grafting (Continued)
  research summary, **I:**477
  tissue engineering, **I:**391–392
  upper extremities, **VI:**694–718
    anatomical characteristics
      blood supply, **VI:**696, 697f
      brachial plexus nerves, **VI:**696f
      gross anatomy, **VI:**695, 695f–697f
      nerve trunk, **VI:**695–696, 697f
      neurons and supporting cells, **VI:**695,
        697f
      Riche–Cannieu anastomosis, **VI:**697f
      schematic diagram, **VI:**697f
    clinical examination
      correct diagnosis, **VI:**700–702, 701f
      electromyography/neurography,
        VI:700–701
      functional evaluation, **VI:**700
      wound inspection, **VI:**702
    donor nerves
      lateral cutaneous nerve, **VI:**709,
        711f–712f
      lateral femoral cutaneous nerve, **VI:**710
      medial cutaneous nerve, **VI:**709, 710f
      saphenous nerve, **VI:**710
      superficial sensory branch of the radial
        nerve, **VI:**710, 712f–713f
      sural nerve, **VI:**708–709, 709f
      terminal branch of the posterior
        interosseous nerve, **VI:**710
    epidemiology, **VI:**694
    future trends, **VI:**718
    immediate versus delayed repair
      basic principles, **VI:**703
      surgical approach, **VI:**703–704, 703f
      timing considerations, **VI:**703
    nerve reconstruction
      autografts, **VI:**707, 708f, 708t
      coaptation and maintenance, **VI:**708
      gap measurement, **VI:**708
      graft harvest, **VI:**708, 708t
      graft length, **VI:**708
      nerve ends, **VI:**708
      surgical approach and preparation,
        VI:707–708
    nerve repair principles
      basic principles, **VI:**704–705, 704f–706f
      end-to-side nerve repair, **VI:**707
      epineurial versus fascicular repair,
        VI:706–707, 706f–707f
      wound closure and immobilization,
        VI:707
    outcomes and complicatons
      age factors, **VI:**716
      British Medical Research Council
        (BMRC) Scale, **VI:**716, 716t
      digital nerves, **VI:**716
      Highet Scale, **VI:**715, 716t
      influencing factors, **VI:**716
      injury type, **VI:**717
      level of injury, **VI:**717
      nerve trunks, **VI:**716–717
      outcome assessments, **VI:**714
      repair type, **VI:**717
      Rosen score, **VI:**716
    patient presentation and diagnosis
      axonotmesis, **VI:**698–700, 699t
      fifth-degree injuries, **VI:**699t, 700

nerve repair and grafting (Continued)
      first-degree injuries, **VI:**698, 699t
      fourth-degree injuries, **VI:**699t, 700
      injury classifications, **VI:**698, 699f, 699t
      neuropraxia, **VI:**698, 699t
      neurotmesis, **VI:**699t, 700
      second-degree injuries, **VI:**698–700,
        699t
      sixth-degree injuries, **VI:**699t, 700
      third-degree injuries, **VI:**699t, 700
    patient selection
      correct diagnosis, **VI:**701f, 702–703
      nerve injury classifications, **VI:**702–703,
        702t
      wound condition, **VI:**703
    physiological characteristics
      degeneration/regeneration
        mechanisms, **VI:**697, 698f
      distal nerve segment, **VI:**697–698, 698f
      general characteristics, **VI:**696–698
      nodes of Ranvier, **VI:**696–698, 697f
    postoperative care and follow-up
      immobilization concerns, **VI:**713
      postoperative movement training,
        VI:713–714
      sensory re-education, **VI:**714
    postoperative dysfunction
      cold intolerance, **VI:**717–718
      complex regional pain syndrome
        (CRPS), **VI:**717
      general considerations, **VI:**717
    sensory re-education
      cortical reorganization, **VI:**714
      phase 1, **VI:**714
      phase 2, **VI:**714, 715f
    surgical technique and treatment
      artificial conduits, **VI:**710–713
      donor nerves, **VI:**708–710
      immediate versus delayed repair,
        VI:703–704
      nerve reconstruction, **VI:**707–708
      nerve repair principles, **VI:**704–707
      tubular repair, **VI:**710–713
    tubular repair
      artificial conduits, **VI:**710–713
      biodegradable conduits, **VI:**712
      biological conduits, **VI:**711
      fillers, **VI:**713
      longitudinal resorbable sutures,
        VI:713
      nerve transfers, **VI:**713
      nondegradable conduits, **VI:**712, 713f
nerve supply
  male genital anatomy, **IV:**301
  nail/nail bed, **VI:**118
nerve transfer, **VI:**719–744
  adult brachial plexus injury
    basic procedure, **VI:**799–800
    closed-target nerve transfer, **VI:**799
    end-to-side neurorrhaphy nerve transfer,
      VI:799–800
    extraplexus nerve transfer, **VI:**799
    functioning free muscle transplantation
      (FFMT), **VI:**801–802
    intraplexus nerve transfer, **VI:**799
    pedicled muscle transfer, **VI:**800–801
    proximal nerve transfer versus distal
      nerve transfer, **VI:**799t

nerve transfer (Continued)
  recommended induction exercises, VI:800t
  reconstructive strategies, VI:800
  current grafting techniques, I:473t, 474–476, 475b
  end-to-side transfers, VI:719–720, 720b, 720f
  facial paralysis, III:291–292, 291f–292f
  general discussion, VI:719
  hand therapy, VI:859–861, 859f–860f
  outcome assessments, VI:742–743
  patient presentation and diagnosis
    diagnostic imaging, VI:725
    electrodiagnostic testing, VI:725–726, 725b
    pain questionnaire, VI:721f–724f
    patient history, VI:720, 721f–724f
    physical examination, VI:725, 725b
    patient selection, VI:726–727, 726t
  postoperative wound care
    basic procedure, VI:741–742
    complications, VI:742
    rehabilitation, VI:742
  secondary procedures, VI:743, 743b
  surgical procedures
    complete/near-complete plexus injury
      contralateral C7 transfer, VI:732–733
      examination findings, VI:732
      phrenic nerve transfer, VI:732–733
      reconstruction techniques, VI:732–733, 732b
      spinal accessory and intercostal nerves, VI:732, 732f
    lower plexus injuries
      examination findings, VI:732
      reconstruction techniques, VI:732, 732b
    median nerve injury
      adjunct tendon transfers, VI:733
      brachialis branch to anterior interosseous nerve (AIN) branch nerve transfer, VI:733, 735f
      examination findings, VI:733, 733b
      radial to median branch nerve transfers, VI:733, 734f
      reconstruction techniques, VI:733
    radial nerve injury
      adjunct tendon transfers, VI:738–739
      examination findings, VI:737, 737b
      median to radial branch nerve transfers, VI:737–738, 738f
      reconstruction techniques, VI:737–739
    sensory nerve injury
      first webspace sensation restoration, VI:740–741, 741f
      lateral antebrachial cutaneous nerve to radial nerve transfers, VI:741
      median to ulnar branch nerve transfers, VI:740, 740f
      radial to axillary nerve transfers, VI:741
      restoration techniques, VI:739–741
      ulnar to median branch nerve transfers, VI:739–740, 739f
    surgical tips, VI:727b
    ulnar nerve injury
      adjunct tendon transfers, VI:736
      anterior interosseous nerve (AIN) to deep motor branch nerve transfer, VI:736, 736f–737f

nerve transfer (Continued)
      examination findings, VI:733–736, 736b
      median to ulnar branch nerve transfers, VI:736, 736f–737f
      reconstruction techniques, VI:736
    upper plexus injuries
      double fascicular nerve transfer, VI:731, 731f
      examination findings, VI:727
      medial pectoral nerve and thoracodorsal nerve, VI:731, 731f
      reconstruction techniques, VI:727–731, 727b
      spinal accessory to suprascapular nerve transfers, VI:727, 728f–729f
      triceps to axillary nerve transfer, VI:728, 729f–730f
      ulnar/median redundant branches to biceps brachii and brachialis branches nerve transfer, VI:731, 731f
  tubular repair, VI:713
nerve tumors
  lipofibromatous hamartoma, VI:320–321, 320f
  neurofibromas
    characteristics, I:728, 728f, VI:320, 320f
    patient presentation and diagnosis, III:880
    surgical technique and treatment, III:880
  schwannomas, I:727, 728f, VI:320, 320f
nerve wraps, I:473, 473t, 475f
net present value, I:72–73
Neumann–Morganstern utility theory, I:165
neurapraxia, I:464–465, 465t
neurilemmomas, I:727, VI:320, 320f
neurocutaneous melanosis (NCM), III:837–838, 838f
neuroendocrine carcinoma, III:436–437
neurofibromas
  characteristics, I:728, 728f, VI:320f
  patient presentation and diagnosis, III:880
  surgical technique and treatment, III:880, VI:320
neurofibromatoses
  café-au-lait spots
    patient presentation and diagnosis, III:878
    surgical technique and treatment, III:878
  congenital fibromatosis
    patient presentation and diagnosis, III:881
    surgical technique and treatment, III:881
  craniofacial manifestation
    patient presentation and diagnosis, III:878
    surgical technique and treatment, III:878, 879f
  definition, III:877
  disease process, III:877–878
  fibromatosis colli
    patient presentation and diagnosis, III:880–881
    surgical technique and treatment, III:881
  general discussion, III:877
  gingival fibroma
    patient presentation and diagnosis, III:881
    surgical technique and treatment, III:881

neurofibromatoses (Continued)
  glomus tumors
    patient presentation and diagnosis, III:878
    surgical technique and treatment, III:878
  infantile digital fibroma
    patient presentation and diagnosis, III:881, 881f
    prognosis and outcomes, III:881
    surgical technique and treatment, III:881
  juvenile aggressive fibromatosis, III:880
  juvenile nasopharyngeal angiofibroma
    patient presentation and diagnosis, III:881
    prognosis and outcomes, III:881
    surgical technique and treatment, III:881
  Lisch nodules
    patient presentation and diagnosis, III:878
    surgical technique and treatment, III:878
  neurofibromas
    patient presentation and diagnosis, III:880
    surgical technique and treatment, III:880
  neurofibrosarcomas
    patient presentation and diagnosis, III:880
    surgical technique and treatment, III:880
  optic nerve gliomas
    patient presentation and diagnosis, III:878
    surgical technique and treatment, III:878
  patient presentation and diagnosis
    café-au-lait spots, III:878
    congenital fibromatosis, III:881
    craniofacial manifestation, III:878
    fibromatosis colli, III:880–881
    gingival fibroma, III:881
    glomus tumors, III:878
    infantile digital fibroma, III:881, 881f
    juvenile nasopharyngeal angiofibroma, III:881
    Lisch nodules, III:878
    neurofibromas, III:880
    neurofibrosarcomas, III:880
    optic nerve gliomas, III:878
    peripheral nerve sheath malignancies, III:880
  peripheral nerve sheath malignancies
    patient presentation and diagnosis, III:880
    surgical technique and treatment, III:880
  surgical technique and treatment
    café-au-lait spots, III:878
    congenital fibromatosis, III:881
    craniofacial manifestation, III:878, 879f
    fibromatosis colli, III:881
    gingival fibroma, III:881
    glomus tumors, III:878
    infantile digital fibroma, III:881
    juvenile nasopharyngeal angiofibroma, III:881
    Lisch nodules, III:878
    neurofibromas, III:880
    neurofibrosarcomas, III:880
    optic nerve gliomas, III:878
    peripheral nerve sheath malignancies, III:880
neurofibrosarcomas
  patient presentation and diagnosis, III:880
  surgical technique and treatment, III:880

neuromas, **I:**727, **VI:**876
neuropraxia, **II:**614–615, **IV:**137, **VI:**698, 699t, 793
neurotmesis, **I:**464–465, 465t, **VI:**699t, 700, 793
neurotrophic growth factors (NGFs), **I:**232
neurotrophins, **I:**232
neurovascular island flap, **IV:**207–208
neutron therapy, **I:**656
neutrophils
  flap failure pathophysiology, **I:**573–576, 574f
  skin wound healing, **I:**268f–269f, 269, 270t, 271f
  wound healing, **I:**245f–246f, 246–247, 256f–257f
Neviaser accessory abductor pollicis longus and free tendon graft, **VI:**771, 771f
nevoid basal cell carcinoma syndrome (NBCCS), **III:**112, 112t, 113f
nevus/nevi
  benign pigmented nevus, **VI:**315, 315f
  dysplastic nevus, **III:**113–114, 114f
  evaluation examinations
    atypical (dysplastic) nevus, **I:**745–746, 747f
    atypical (dysplastic) nevus syndrome, **I:**746–747
    B-K mole syndrome, **I:**747
    blue nevi, **I:**744f, 745
    compound nevi, **I:**744, 744f
    congenital nevi, **I:**745, 745f–746f
    intradermal nevi, **I:**744, 744f
    junctional nevi, **I:**744, 744f
    nevi development, **I:**744–747
  eyebrow reconstruction, **III:**441, 444f
  giant hair nevus/congenital nevomelanocytic nevus (CNN), **III:**112–113, 114f
  nevus cartilagines, **I:**732–733
  nevus cell nevus, **I:**723–725
  nevus fuscoceruleus ophthalmomaxillaris, **I:**725–726
  nevus of Ito, **I:**726, 727f
  nevus of Ota, **I:**725–726, 726f
  nevus sebaceous, **I:**721, 721f
  nevus sebaceous of Jadassohn, **III:**111–112, 112f
  nevus spilus, **I:**725, 726f
  nevus Unna, **I:**734
  See also melanoma
niacinamide, **II:**18, 25
nickel (Ni) alloys, **I:**786–787
Nicoladoni, Carl, **VI:**xlv
nicotinamide adenine diphosphate (NADPH) enzyme system, **I:**575–576
nicotine, **IV:**283
nifedipine, **I:**583
Nikolsky sign, **IV:**513, 514f
nipple-areola complex
  anatomical characteristics, **V:**5, 10f
  characteristics, **V:**500f
  inferior pedicle breast reduction, **V:**168f, 171f–172f
  L short-scar mammaplasty, **V:**206–215
    background and general characteristics, **V:**206–207
    complications, **V:**213
    patient selection, **V:**206–207

nipple-areola complex *(Continued)*
    planning and marking guidelines, **V:**207, 208f–209f
    reduction results, **V:**210f–214f
    research summary, **V:**214–215
    surgical technique, **V:**207–210, 209f
  mastectomy planning, **V:**419, 419f
  mastopexy
    augmentation mammaplasty
     basic procedure, **V:**139–143
     operative technique, **V:**142–143
     preoperative/postoperative comparisons, **V:**143f
     surgical tips, **V:**142b
    Benelli mastopexy technique
     areola fixation, **V:**131f
     basic procedure, **V:**127–132
     dissection techniques, **V:**128f
     flap attachment, **V:**129f–130f
     flap types, **V:**129f
     gland plication invagination, **V:**131f
     markings, **V:**128f
     round block suture, **V:**131f
     surgical technique, **V:**128–132
     U stitches, **V:**131f
    Goes periareolar technique with mesh support
     basic procedure, **V:**132–133
     surgical technique, **V:**132–133, 132f–134f
    Grotting sculpted vertical pillar mastopexy
     basic procedure, **V:**136–139
     final closure, **V:**140f
     flap detachment, **V:**139f
     markings and incisions, **V:**138f
     operative technique, **V:**138–139
     preferred technique, **V:**138f–140f
     preoperative markings, **V:**137f
     preoperative/postoperative comparisons, **V:**140f–141f
     surgical tips, **V:**136b
     temporary breast closure, **V:**139f
    inverted-T technique
     basic procedure, **V:**146–147
     operative technique, **V:**146–147, 147f
    major weight loss (MWL) patient
     surgical markings, **V:**566
     surgical technique and treatment, **V:**566–567, 568f
    mastopexy revision, **V:**254–261, 258f–263f
    outcomes and complicatons
     cosmetic disappointments, **V:**149–150
     flap necrosis, **V:**149
     general discussion, **V:**148–150
     hematomas, **V:**150, 243t
     infections, **V:**150, 243t
     nipple loss, **V:**148, 243t, 253–254, 255f
     nipple malposition, **V:**149, 243t, 252, 252f–253f
     scars, **V:**149, 243t
    periareolar techniques
     basic procedure, **V:**126–133
     Benelli mastopexy technique, **V:**127–132
     concentric mastopexy without parenchymal reshaping, **V:**126–127

nipple-areola complex *(Continued)*
     Goes periareolar technique with mesh support, **V:**132–133
    postoperative care and follow-up, **V:**147–148
    secondary procedures, **V:**150
    vertical/short scar techniques
     augmentation mammaplasty, **V:**139–143
     general discussion, **V:**133–146
     Grotting sculpted vertical pillar mastopexy, **V:**136–139
     implant post-explantation, **V:**143–146, 144f–145f, 145b
     Lassus vertical scar technique, **V:**134–135
     Lejour vertical scar technique, **V:**135–136
  outcomes and complicatons, **V:**65–66, 66t, 245
  periareolar surgical technique with mesh support, **V:**216–227
    background and general characteristics, **V:**216–217
    complications, **V:**226, 226t
    patient selection, **V:**217
    planning and marking guidelines, **V:**217–218, 217f
    research summary, **V:**226
    surgical technique
     basic procedure, **V:**218–221, 218f–220f
     clinical results, **V:**222f–225f
     internal support system, **V:**217
     mesh application, **V:**219–221, 220f–221f
  post-mastectomy reconstructiion, **V:**430–432, 432f–433f
  reconstruction process
    areola deformities, **V:**248–249, 250f
    areola hypopigmentation, **V:**249–251
    areola reconstruction, **V:**516–518, 517b, 517f–518f
    asymmetries, **V:**251
    autologous fat grafts, **V:**407–410, 514–515, 514f
    batwing mastopexy, **V:**308f
    complications, **V:**245, 519, 519b
    deep inferior epigastric perforator (DIEP) flaps
     secondary procedures, **V:**453, 453f
     shaping guidelines, **V:**449f
    donut type mastopexy, **V:**308f
    flap designs adjacent to scars
     double-opposing tab flap, **V:**511t, 512–513, 512f–513f
     general discussion, **V:**511–513
     S-flap, **V:**511–512, 511f, 511t
     spiral flap, **V:**513, 513f
    flaps with autologous graft augmentation
     cartilage grafts, **V:**514, 514f
     fat grafts, **V:**514–515, 514f
    flap techniques, **V:**501t
    general discussion, **V:**499
    inferior pedicle mastopexy, **V:**307f
    latissimus dorsi (LD) flap, **V:**309f
    mastopexy revision, **V:**254–261, 258f–263f
    nipple areola ischemia, **V:**247–248, 248f–249f
    nipple loss, **V:**148, 243t, 253–254, 255f

nipple-areola complex *(Continued)*
  nipple malposition, **V:**149, 243t, 252, 252f–253f
  nipple retraction, **V:**252
  omentum reconstruction, **V:**476f–477f, 480
  outcome assessments, **V:**519
  patient presentation and diagnosis, **V:**499–500, 500f
  patient selection, **V:**500
  postmastectomy breast reconstruction, **V:**292–294, 293f
  postoperative care and follow-up, **V:**518, 518f
  pull-out/purse-string flap techniques
    bell flap, **V:**508, 508f, 508t
    double opposing peri-areolar/ purse-string flap, **V:**508–510, 508t, 509f–510f
    general discussion, **V:**507–510
    top-hat flap, **V:**510, 510f
  secondary/revisional procedures, **V:**519
  surgical technique and treatment
    composite nipple graft, **V:**500–502, 501f–502f
    flap designs adjacent to scars, **V:**511–513
    flaps with allograft augmentation, **V:**515–516, 516f
    flaps with alloplastic augmentation, **V:**515
    flaps with autologous graft augmentation, **V:**514–515
    general discussion, **V:**500–516
    pull-out/purse-string flap techniques, **V:**507–510
    surgical guidelines, **V:**502b, 504b, 506b–508b, 510b–516b
    traditional flaps, **V:**502–507
  symmetry, **V:**480
  traditional flaps
    arrow flap, **V:**503t, 507, 507f
    C-V flap, **V:**503t, 506–507, 506f, 514–515
    general discussion, **V:**502–507
    skate flap, **V:**502–504, 503f–505f, 503t
    star flap, **V:**503t, 504–506, 505f
reconstructive burn surgery, **IV:**506
revision breast augmentation, **V:**49f
sculpted pillar vertical reduction mammaplasty, **V:**228–241
  background and general characteristics, **V:**228
  complications, **V:**236–239, 239f–241f
  patient selection, **V:**228–229
  planning and marking guidelines, **V:**229, 229f–230f
  research summary, **V:**239
  surgical technique
    basic procedure, **V:**229–236
    large breast reduction, **V:**236, 238f
    moderate breast reduction, **V:**236, 237f
    small breast reduction, **V:**235, 236f
    wound closure, **V:**231–235, 232f–235f
short scar periareolar inferior pedicle reduction (SPAIR) mammaplasty, **V:**194–205
  background and general characteristics, **V:**159, 194–195
  complications
    areolar spreading, **V:**204
    fat necrosis, **V:**203–204

nipple-areola complex *(Continued)*
    general discussion, **V:**203–205
    hypertrophy recurrence, **V:**204–205
    polytetrafluoroethylene (PTFE) infection/exposure, **V:**204
    shape distortion, **V:**204
  patient selection, **V:**195–196
  planning and marking guidelines, **V:**196, 197f–198f
  reduction results
    large breast reduction, **V:**202–203, 203f
    modest breast reduction, **V:**202, 203f
    small breast reduction, **V:**201–203, 202f
  research summary, **V:**205
  surgical technique, **V:**196–201, 200f–201f
vertical scar reduction mammaplasty, **V:**177–193
  comparison studies, **V:**178t
  complications
    frequency, **V:**189–192, 191t
    scar healing, **V:**190, 191f
    under-resection, **V:**192
    wound dehiscence, **V:**191
  distance measurements, **V:**179f
  Hall-Findlay technique, **V:**159, 178t
  historical background, **V:**177–180
  Lassus technique, **V:**156–159, 178t
  Lejour technique, **V:**159, 178t
  Lista technique, **V:**178t
  medial pedicle breast reductions, **V:**189, 190f
  patient selection
    patient characteristics, **V:**180–181
    symptoms, **V:**180
  planning and marking guidelines
    perioperative care, **V:**181
    skin marking, **V:**181–182, 181f, 183f
  postoperative care and follow-up, **V:**188
  research summary, **V:**192
  superior pedicle breast reductions, **V:**188–189, 189f
  surgical technique and treatment
    anesthesia, **V:**182
    breast shaping, **V:**186–187, 187f
    de-epithelialization, **V:**184, 184f
    dressings and wound care, **V:**188
    infiltration, **V:**182–184
    liposuction, **V:**185
    patient positioning, **V:**182
    pedicle selection, **V:**182, 184f
    surgical excision, **V:**184–185, 185f–186f
    wound closure, **V:**187–188, 187f–188f
nipple-sparing mastectomy, **V:**282–284, 284f–285f
nitrogen (N)
  metal alloy compositions, **I:**786–787
  nitric oxide (NO)
    flap failure pathophysiology, **I:**573–574, 574f
    nitric oxide (NO) synthesis, **I:**256, 256f, 259
  nitrous oxide (NO), **I:**429–430
nodal evaluation, **V:**286, 286f
nodes of Ranvier, **VI:**696–698, 697f
nodular melanoma, **I:**752–753, 754f
Noël, Suzanne, **I:**27, 28f
Noggin gene, **III:**505, **VI:**615
nonablative facial skin rejuvenation (NSR), **II:**64–65
nonablative laser treatments, **IV:**454, 454t

nonaccidental burns, **IV:**397
nonanimal-stabilized hyaluronic acid (NASHA), **II:**47t
noncholera *Vibrio* infections, **VI:**343
noncontrast magnetic resonance imaging (MRI), **V:**329, 329f, 334f
non-FDA-approved biological fillers, **II:**47t
non-FDA-approved synthetic fillers, **II:**48t
nonhealing wounds
  characteristics, **I:**279–283
  influencing factors, **I:**280t
  lower-extremity wounds
    diabetic ulcers, **I:**281
    ischemic wounds, **I:**279–281
    venous ulcers, **I:**279
  malnutrition, **I:**282
  medical treatment, **I:**282–283
  obese patients, **I:**282
  pressure sores, **I:**279
  radiation injuries, **I:**281
  wound infections, **I:**281–282
noninvasive body contouring, **I:**852–853, 852f
noninvoluting congenital hemangioma (NICH), **I:**677t, 687, **VI:**668t, 673–674, 676f
nonmelanoma skin cancers, **I:**670–671
nonsinus tachycardia, **I:**145
nonsteroidal antiinflammatory drugs (NSAIDs)
  burn wound treatment, **IV:**427
  facelifts, **II:**194
  microvascular free-flap surgery, **I:**617
  nerve compression syndromes
    anterior interosseous nerve (AIN) syndrome, **VI:**511
    carpal tunnel syndrome, **VI:**507
    Guyon's canal, **VI:**512–513
    quadrilateral space syndrome, **VI:**523
    radial tunnel syndrome, **VI:**518
    suprascapular nerve compression, **VI:**524
    Wartenberg's syndrome, **VI:**517
  nonsurgical skin care and rejuvenation for sensitive skin, **II:**21–22
  rheumatoid arthritis, **VI:**372–373, 380b
  trapeziometacarpal arthritis, **VI:**433–434
  upper extremity surgery, **VI:**104
  wrist osteoarthritis, **VI:**442–443
nonsurgical skin care and rejuvenation, **II:**13–29
  aging process, **II:**15
  dry skin
    basic skin care formulations
      antioxidants, **II:**18
      characteristics, **II:**16–18
      cleansers, **II:**16
      moisturizers, **II:**16–18
    causal factors, **II:**15–19
    clinical signs, **II:**16
    hydroxy acids
      alpha hydroxy acids (AHAs), **II:**18–19
      beta hydroxy acid (BHA), **II:**19
  noninvasive procedures
    intense pulsed light therapy, **II:**28
    microdermabrasion, **II:**28
  pigmented skin
    care regimens, **II:**24
    general discussion, **II:**24–26
    melanosome transfer inhibitors
      niacinamide, **II:**25
      soy products, **II:**25–26

nonsurgical skin care and rejuvenation
(Continued)
tyrosinase inhibitors
aloesin, II:24
arbutin, II:24–25
emblicanin, II:25
flavonoids, II:25
general discussion, II:24–25
hydroquinone, II:24
hydroxycoumarins, II:25
kojic acid, II:25
licorice extract, II:25
research summary, II:28
sensitive skin
acne, II:19–20
classifications, II:19–24, 19t
rosacea, II:20–21, 21t
treatment strategies
aloe vera, II:22
chamomile, II:22
corticosteroids, II:21
curcumin, II:24
cyclooxygenase inhibitors, II:21–22
feverfew, II:22
food choices, II:24
ginseng, II:22–23
licorice extract, II:23
mushrooms, II:23
oatmeal, II:23
salicylic acid, II:22
selenium (Se), II:23–24
sulfur/sulfacetamide, II:22
turmeric, II:24
skin type determination
Baumann skin-typing system (BSTS),
II:14–15, 14t
Fitzpatrick skin phototype (SPT) system,
II:13–14, 14t
wrinkled skin
antioxidants
coenzyme Q10, II:27
general discussion, II:27–28
grape seed extract, II:27
green tea, II:27–28
lycopene, II:28
resveratrol, II:27
vitamin C, II:27
vitamin E, II:27
prevention and treatment, II:26–28
retinoids
action mechanisms, II:26
characteristics, II:26
side effects, II:26
usage guidelines, II:26
nonsyndromic cleft lip and palate, I:193–194
nonsyndromic craniosynostosis, III:726–748
definition, III:726
pathogenesis, III:726–728
patient presentation and diagnosis
anterior plagiocephaly, III:729, 730f, 730t
brachycephaly, III:729, 730f, 730t
cephalic index (CI), III:728t
characteristics, III:728–731
plagiocephaly, III:729, 729t
posterior plagiocephaly, III:729–731, 731f,
731t
scaphocephaly, III:728–729, 729f, 729t
skull shape, III:728f

nonsyndromic craniosynostosis (Continued)
synostotic versus deformational
plagiocephaly, III:729t
thumbprinting patterns, III:728, 730f
trigonocephaly, III:731, 731f, 731t
patient selection, III:731–732
nontuberous congenital breast asymmetry
bilateral but different surgical procedure,
V:537–538
bilateral but similar surgical procedure,
V:537–538
case studies
Case VII (volume asymmetry), V:538,
539f
Case VIII (volume asymmetry), V:538,
540f
Case IX (severe hypoplasia), V:538–541,
542f–543f
Case X (severe asymmetry), V:544
dermal apron, V:544, 545f
general considerations, V:537–538, 537b
monolateral operation, V:537
norepinephrine (NE), I:573–574, 574f, 580–581
Norian SRS/CRS, I:461
nose
aesthetic nasal reconstruction, III:134–186
defect classification
adversely located defects, III:139–140
composite defects, III:140
deep defects, III:140
large defects, III:140
small defects, III:139
superficial defects, III:139
disease process, III:134–135
false planning assumptions
donor site considerations, III:135
extra tissue transfer, III:135
flap design, III:135
scars, III:135
single flap approach, III:136
supportive frameworks, III:135–136
tissue expansion, III:135
tissue preservation, III:135
forehead donor site
expansion considerations, III:158–159
expansion delay, III:159–160
expansion technique, III:159–160
harvesting guidelines, III:160
primary closure, III:155
scars within the forehead territory,
III:156–157
surgical delay procedures, III:157–158
intranasal lining flaps
applications, III:166t
basic procedure, III:164f–166f
detailed characteristics, III:163–166
isolated unilateral mid-vault lining
loss, III:166–167
operative technique, III:166–170,
167f–169f
local flaps
bilobed flap, III:143–145, 144f–145f,
446f
dorsal nasal flap, III:143, 144f–145f
forehead flaps, III:148–155, 149f
one-stage nasolabial flap, III:145–146
single-lobe transposition flap, III:143,
144f–145f

nose (Continued)
surgical guidelines, III:142–146
three stage full-thickness forehead flap,
III:151–152, 152f
three stage full-thickness forehead flap
(stage 1), III:152–153, 153f–159f
three stage full-thickness forehead flap
(stage 2), III:153–155
three stage full-thickness forehead flap
(stage 3), III:155, 155t
two-stage forehead flap, III:148,
150f–151f
two-stage forehead flap (stage 1),
III:148–151
two-stage forehead flap (stage 2),
III:151, 151t
two-stage nasolabial flap, III:146–148,
146f–147f
two-stage nasolabial flap (stage 1),
III:146
two-stage nasolabial flap (stage 2),
III:146–148
nasal contour and support restoration
basic principles, III:160–179
composite grafts, III:161
design guidelines, III:160, 160t
facial artery myomucosal (FAMM) flap,
III:163
free flap nasal reconstruction,
III:173–174
graft fixation, III:161
hard-tissue support replacement,
III:160
harvesting guidelines, III:161
hingeover lining flaps, III:162
inadequate platforms, III:174
intranasal lining flaps, III:163–166,
164f–166f, 166t
lining restoration, III:161
material selection, III:160–161
microvascular transfer, III:173
modified folded forehead flap,
III:170–172, 170f–171f
nasal lining restoration, III:174–179
nasolabial flap, III:163
prelaminated flap technique, III:162
residual lining advancement,
III:161–162
second forehead flap, III:163
second lining flaps, III:162–163
skin graft linings, III:172–173
soft-tissue support and contouring,
III:161
timing considerations, III:160
nasal cover restoration
adversely located defects, III:146–148
deep defects, III:146–148
healing by secondary intention,
III:140–141
large defects, III:146–148
local flaps, III:142–146
primary repair procedures, III:141
skin grafts, III:141–142
small/superficial defects, III:140–141
nasal lining restoration
Burget–Walton approach, III:175f
Menick–Salibian approach, III:176f
mid-vault defects, III:174

Note: **Boldface** roman numerals indicate volume. Page numbers followed by f refer to figures; page numbers followed by t refer to tables; page numbers followed by b refer to boxes.

nose (*Continued*)
    operation 1, III:174–177
    operation 2, III:177
    operation 3, III:177–178
    operation 4, III:178
    operation 5, III:178–179
    subtotal and total nasal defects, III:174, 175f–181f
  outcomes and complicatons, III:179–181
  patient presentation and diagnosis, III:135
  regional unit repair
    basic principles, III:138–139
    contralateral normal, III:138
    donor site considerations, III:138
    exact dimensions and outline, III:138
    exact foil templates, III:138
    old scars, III:139
    preliminary operationa, III:139
    stable platforms, III:139
    subcutaneous framework restoration, III:139
    subunit principle, III:138
    surgical staging, III:139
    tissue transfer, III:138–139
    wound healing, III:138–139
  secondary procedures
    do-over revisions, III:184
    major revisions, III:184
    minor revisions, III:181–184
    secondary revisions, III:181–184, 182f–184f
  skin grafts
    basic principles, III:141–142
    full-thickness forehead skin graft, III:141, 142f
    operative technique, III:141–142
    preauricular and postauricular skin grafts, III:141
  surgical goals, III:134
  surgical planning and preparation
    central facial units, III:136–137, 137f
    defect classification, III:139–140
    false planning assumptions, III:135–136
    modern approach, III:136, 136t, 137f
    peripheral facial units, III:136, 137f
    regional unit repair principles, III:138–139
    traditional approach, III:135
  surgical technique and treatment
    challenges, III:140–179
    forehead donor site, III:155–160
    nasal contour and support restoration, III:160–179
    nasal cover restoration, III:140–155
    zones of nasal skin quality, III:140
  anthropometric analysis, II:358–359, 359f
  auricular cartilage graft, I:401f–402f, 405f
  bulbous nose, II:175, 176f
  cancer management, III:436–437, 436f
  contracted nose
    dermal fat graft, II:176
    derotation grafts, II:176, 176f
    rib cartilage graft, II:176
    septal extension grafts, II:176
    surgical technique and treatment, II:173–176
  craniofacial development
    frontonasal prominence, III:508, 508f
    lateral nasal prominences, III:508, 509f

nose (*Continued*)
  nasal airways, II:450–465
    airway outcome study results, II:420–421, 420f
    anatomical characteristics, II:450–452, 451f–452f
    clinical analysis, II:419–420
    disease and obstructions
      deviated septum, II:392–393, 454–455, 454f–456f
      external nasal valve, II:455–456
      internal nasal valve, II:455
      open rhinoplasty, II:392–394
      patient presentation and diagnosis, II:456–457
      patient selection, II:457–458
      rhinitis, II:453–454
    facial paralysis, III:287f, 291
    nasal valves, II:420f
    open rhinoplasty
      inferior turbinoplasty/outfracture/ submucous resection, II:393–394, 393f
      obstructions, II:392–394, 411
      septal reconstruction, II:392–393
    physiological characteristics
      humidification, II:453
      olfaction, II:453
      particulate filtration, II:453
      phonation, II:453
      secondary sex organ, II:453
      temperature regulation, II:453
      tubular flow, II:452–453
    preoperative assessment, II:450–453
    rhinitis, II:453–454, 458
    straight line strategy, II:420f
  nasal anatomy, II:373–386
    basic principles, II:414–419
    blood supply, II:379–380, 379f–380f
    bony base–alar base relationship, II:377f
    cartilage, II:382–386, 382f–385f
    characteristics and measurements, II:373–377
    cleft nose anatomy, III:646–647, 646f–647f
    crurae, II:373, 375f
    dorsal aesthetic lines, II:376f, 378f
    dorsum and tip
      alar cartilage malposition, II:418–419, 418f–419f
      anatomic variants, II:416–419
      characteristics, II:415–419, 416f
      inadequate tip projection, II:417, 418f–419f
      low radix/low dorsum, II:416, 418f–419f
      narrow middle vault, II:417, 417f–419f
    external nasal valve, II:455–456
    Frankfort horizontal line, II:376f
    general characteristics, III:20f, 423–424, 425f–426f
    internal nasal valve, II:455
    intrinsic and extrinsic nasal musculature, II:380–381, 381f
    middle and lower cartilaginous vaults, II:415
    nasal aesthetics guidelines, II:375f
    nasal airways, II:450–452, 451f–452f
    nasal bones, II:382–386, 382f–383f
    nasal length, II:377f
    nasal ligaments, II:381–382, 382f, 385f

nose (*Continued*)
    nasal symmetry guidelines, II:375f
    nasolabial measurements, II:378f
    normal anatomy, III:644–646, 646t
    osseocartilaginous skeleton, III:646t
    paranasal sinuses, III:423–424, 425f–426f
    schematic diagram, II:415f
    sensory nerves, II:380, 380f
    septum, II:382–386, 382f–385f, 450–452, 451f–452f
    standardized measurements, II:374f
    standardized terminology, II:374f
    tip projection, II:358–359, 373, 374f, 377f, 379f, 385f
    tip structure, III:646t
    turbinates, II:384, 386f, 450–452, 455–456, 457f
    upper cartilaginous vaults, II:414, 415f
  nasal and naso-orbital ethmoid fractures, III:681–682, 681t, 682f
  nasal dermoids
    complications, III:883
    disease process, III:882, 882f
    patient presentation and diagnosis, III:882
    prognosis and outcomes, III:883
    secondary procedures, III:883
    surgical technique and treatment, III:882–883, 882f–883f
  nasal disease and obstructions
    deviated septum, II:454–455, 454f–456f
    external nasal valve, II:455–456
    internal nasal valve, II:455
    patient presentation and diagnosis
      patient history, II:456
      physical examination, II:456–457, 457f
      radiologic scans, II:457, 457f
      rhinomanometry, II:457
    patient selection, II:457–458
    rhinitis, II:453–454
  nasal fractures
    complications, III:60
    nasal septum fractures and dislocations
      characteristics, III:58–59, 58f
      treatment strategies, III:59–60
    treatment strategies
      closed reduction, III:59–60
      K-wire support, III:59
      nasal septum fractures and dislocations, III:59–60
      open reduction, III:59
      soft tissue contracture, III:59–60, 59f
    types and locations, III:57, 58f
  nasoethmoidal orbital fractures
    characteristics, III:60–61
    classification systems, III:61–63, 62f
    clinical examination, III:60–61, 61f
    complications, III:63
    computed tomography (CT), III:61
    surgical pathology
      causal factors, III:60
      interorbital space, III:60
      traumatic orbital hypertelorism, III:60
      traumatic telecanthus, III:60
    treatment strategies
      basic procedure, III:61–63
      canthal reattachment, III:63
      central fragment considerations, III:63
      lacrimal system injury, III:63

nose *(Continued)*
nose reconstruction
acquired cranial and facial bone
deformities, **III:**228–229, 231f–233f
adolescent aesthetic surgery, **I:**45t
aesthetic nasal reconstruction, **III:**134–186
defect classification, **III:**139–140
disease process, **III:**134–135
false planning assumptions, **III:**135–136
outcomes and complicatons,
III:179–181
patient presentation and diagnosis,
III:135
postoperative care and follow-up,
III:140–179
secondary procedures, **III:**181–184
surgical goals, **III:**134
surgical planning and preparation,
III:135–140
surgical technique and treatment,
III:140–179
aesthetic surgery, **I:**25–28, 26f
ancient Egypt, **I:**11–12
Asian rhinoplasty
alar base surgery, **II:**177
blunt nasal tip, **II:**173
broad nasal dorsum, **II:**173
bulbous nose, **II:**175, 176f
capsular contractures, **II:**177
contracted nose, **II:**173–176
forehead augmentation, **II:**174f, 177
general discussion, **II:**172–173
genioplasty, **II:**177
historical background, **II:**173
implant deviation, **II:**176
implant exposure, **II:**176
implant infection, **II:**176
low profile nasal dorsum
augmentation, **II:**173–174, 174f
nasal skeleton, **II:**172–173
outcomes and complicatons, **II:**176–177
paranasal augmentation, **II:**177
patient presentation and diagnosis,
II:173
secondary procedures, **II:**177
septal extension grafts, **II:**175–176, 175f
short/contracted nose, **II:**173
short nose, **II:**175–176, 475–476,
478f–479f
soft tissue profile, **II:**172–173
surgical technique and treatment,
II:173–176
underprojected nasal tip, **II:**173–175
augmentation phase
columellar grafts, **II:**436
dorsum and radix, **II:**436
graft donor sites, **II:**439–440
graft selection, **II:**436–437
lateral wall grafts, **II:**436
spreader grafts, **II:**436
tip grafts, **II:**436–437, 437f–438f
autologous perichondrial grafts,
I:408–413, 412f
burn wound treatment, **IV:**473, 488–489,
498–499
closed rhinoplasty, **II:**413–449
augmentation phase, **II:**436–437
cleft lip nasal deformity, **II:**442

complications, **II:**444–446
dissatisfied patients, **II:**446–448
donor site-depleted patient, **II:**443
dressings, **II:**439
ethnic rhinoplasty, **II:**441–442
male rhinoplasty, **II:**441
nasal aesthetics, **II:**423–424
nasal deviation, **II:**441, 442f
older adults, **II:**442–443
open rhinoplasty-caused deformities,
II:448–449, 449f
patient selection, **II:**421–423
postoperative care and follow-up,
II:439–441
rhinophyma, **II:**443, 443f
secondary rhinoplasty, **II:**448–449
septal graft specimen, **II:**436–437
surgeon–patient relationship,
II:446–448
surgical planning, **II:**424–427
turbinectomy, **II:**435–436
complications
circulatory complications, **II:**445
general discussion, **II:**444–446
graft problems, **II:**444–445
hematomas, **II:**446
hemorrhage, **II:**445
iatrogenic airway obstruction, **II:**444
infections, **II:**445–446
lacrimal duct injury, **II:**446
red nose, **II:**446
rhinitis, **II:**445
septal collapse, **II:**446
septal perforation, **II:**445
skeletal problems, **II:**444
soft-tissue problems, **II:**444
dissatisfied patients
body dysmorphic disorder (BDD),
II:447–448
primary versus secondary candidates,
II:446–447
prior versus current surgeon, **II:**447
reoperations, **II:**448
surgeon–patient relationship,
II:446–448
dressings, **II:**439
eighteenth century, **I:**18–19, 19f
engineered cartilage, **I:**419–421, 422f
gender identity disorder surgery, **IV:**349
hypertelorism correction, **III:**699
India, **I:**12–13, 13f
local flaps
basic procedure, **III:**441–449
bilobed flap, **III:**143–145, 144f–145f,
446f
dorsal nasal flap, **III:**143, 144f–145f
interpolated paramedian forehead flap,
III:445f, 448f
lateral advancement flaps, **III:**445f
Rintala dorsal nasal advancement flap,
III:447f
transoperative flap, **III:**447f
V-Y advancement flap, **III:**446f
nasal aesthetics
potential complications and revisions,
II:424
preoperative photographs, **II:**423

surgical goals, **II:**423–424
surgical guidelines, **II:**423–424
nasal cartilage graft, **I:**404–407, 405f–407f
nineteenth century, **I:**19–20
open rhinoplasty, **II:**387–412
activity restrictions, **II:**410
advantages/disadvantages, **II:**388t
alar base surgery, **II:**404–405, 406f
alar–columellar relationship, **II:**401–
402, 403f
alar rim deformities, **II:**400–401
anesthesia, **II:**389–390
autologous cartilage harvesting,
II:394–396
closure, **II:**403
complications, **II:**410–411
component dorsal hump reduction,
II:391–392, 391f
depressor septi muscle translocation,
II:403–404, 405f
dorsal spreader grafts, **II:**392f
dressings and wound care, **II:**409
follow-up consultations, **II:**410
general discussion, **II:**387
general patient instructions, **II:**410
medications, **II:**409–410
nasal airway, **II:**392–394
nasal anatomy, **II:**387
nasal dorsum irregularities, **II:**391f
nasal tip, **II:**397–400
open rhinoplasty-caused deformities,
II:448–449, 449f
outcome assessments, **II:**410
patient presentation and diagnosis,
II:387–389
patient selection, **II:**389
percutaneous lateral nasal osteotomies,
II:402–403, 404f
postoperative care and follow-up,
II:409–410
preoperative management, **II:**389–390
prognosis, **II:**410
secondary procedures, **II:**412
surgical technique and treatment,
II:389–405
transcolumellar stair-step incision,
II:390–391, 390f
open rhinoplasty-caused deformities,
II:448–449, 449f
osseointegrated nasal reconstruction,
I:802, 802b, 802f–803f
patient selection, **II:**422–423
postoperative care and follow-up,
II:439–441
psychological aspects, **I:**39–40
reconstructive burn surgery, **IV:**473,
488–489, 498–499, 505
Renaissance, **I:**16–18, 18f
routine surgical order
alar cartilage resection, **II:**433–434
anesthesia, **II:**427–435
dorsal resection, **II:**428, 428f–433f
intracartilaginous incisions, **II:**428,
428f
nasal spine-caudal septum resection,
II:433
septoplasty, **II:**434–435

*Note: **Boldface** roman numerals indicate volume. Page numbers followed by f refer to figures; page numbers followed by t refer to tables; page numbers followed by b refer to boxes.*

nose *(Continued)*
  skeletonization, II:427–428
  spreader graft tunnels, II:434–435, 435f
  upper lateral cartilage resection, II:434
  secondary rhinoplasty, II:466–484
    anesthesia, II:468
    broad/bulbous/round tip, II:470
    cartilage grafts, II:470, 470f–471f
    challenges, II:466
    closed rhinoplasty, II:448–449
    columellar scars, II:481–482, 482f
    common problems, II:470–480
    complications, II:481–483
    definition, II:466
    difficult patients, II:482–483
    operative technique, II:467–470
    patient presentation and diagnosis, II:466
    patient selection, II:467–470
    postoperative care and follow-up, II:480–481
    post-rhinoplasty fibrotic syndrome, II:482, 483f
    skin necrosis, II:481, 482f
    suture-based tip plasty, II:471–480, 472f–473f
    suturing techniques, II:468–470, 534f
    untoward results, II:481–483
  septal graft specimen, II:436–437
  sixteenth century, VI:xlv
  surgical planning
    decision-making process, II:427
    endonasal rhinoplasty, II:425
    general discussion, II:424–427
    nasal base size–bridge height balance, II:425, 426f
    skin thickness and distribution, II:424, 424f
    teach-yourself concept, II:427
    tip lobular contour, II:424–425, 425f
  surgical technique and treatment
    general discussion, II:427–435
    local flaps, III:441–449
    routine order, II:427–435
  tissue expansion, I:637, 639f
  turbinectomy
    alar wedge resection, II:435–436
    characteristics, II:435–436
    graft placement, II:435–436
    osteotomy, II:435
    wound closure, II:435–436
  variants
    cleft lip nasal deformity, II:442
    donor site-depleted patient, II:443
    ethnic rhinoplasty, II:441–442
    male rhinoplasty, II:441
    nasal deviation, II:441, 442f
    older adults, II:442–443
    rhinophyma, II:443, 443f
  pediatric facial fractures, III:681–682, 681t, 682f
  photographic guidelines, I:108, 111f
  reconstructive burn surgery, IV:473, 488–489, 498–499, 505
  robotic surgery, I:862–863
secondary cleft deformities, III:631–654
  cleft nose
    cleft nose anatomy, III:646–647, 646f–647f

nose *(Continued)*
    decision-making process, III:653
    evaluation examinations, III:647–648
    normal anatomy, III:644–646, 646t
    patient selection, III:648
    surgical technique and treatment, III:648–653
    timing considerations, III:648
  etiology, III:631
  patient presentation and diagnosis, III:632
  wound healing and growth, III:631–632, 632f–633f
secondary rhinoplasty, II:466–484
  challenges, II:466
  common problems
    broad/bulbous/round tip, II:470
    suture-based tip plasty, II:471–480, 472f–473f
  complications
    columellar scars, II:481–482, 482f
    difficult patients, II:482–483
    post-rhinoplasty fibrotic syndrome, II:482, 483f
    skin necrosis, II:481, 482f
  definition, II:466
  operative technique
    anesthesia, II:468
    artistry, II:467, 467f
    cartilage grafts, II:470, 470f–471f
    open versus closed approach, II:467, 468f
    suturing techniques, II:468–470, 534f
  patient presentation and diagnosis, II:466
  patient selection, II:467
  postoperative care and follow-up
    corticosteroids, II:481
    early bad result, II:480–481, 481f
    early care, II:480
    fillers, II:481
  suture-based tip plasty
    alar rim deformities, II:473–475, 475f–478f
    broad nasal base, II:476–478, 479f–480f
    characteristics, II:471–480, 472f–473f
    closed approach, II:471–472
    deficient tip, II:472–473, 474f
    fascial graft and repair, II:477f–478f
    middle vault collapse, II:473
    nasal dorsum irregularities, II:478–479
    septoplasty, II:479–480, 480f
    short nose, II:475–476, 478f–479f
    thin skin tip, II:475, 477f–478f
  septum, II:450–452, 451f
  short nose, II:175–176, 475–476, 478f–479f
  surgical technique and treatment
    deviated nasal bones, II:458
    deviated septum
      characteristics, II:458–461
      complications, II:463
      C-shaped anteroposterior deviation, II:459, 460f
      C-shaped cephalocaudal deviation, II:459, 460f
      localized deviation, II:461
      postoperative care and follow-up, II:462–463
      prognosis and outcomes, II:463, 463f–464f

nose *(Continued)*
      secondary procedures, II:463
      septal tilt, II:459, 459f
      S-shaped anteroposterior deviation, II:459, 460f
      S-shaped cephalocaudal deviation, II:459, 460f
    incompetent external nasal valve, II:461, 462f
    incompetent internal nasal valve, II:461, 461f
    rhinitis
      allergic rhinitis, II:458
      atrophic rhinitis, II:458
      hypertrophic rhinitis, II:458
      infectious rhinitis, II:458
      rhinitis medicamentosa (RM), II:458
      vasomotor rhinitis, II:458
    turbinate disorders
      background information, II:461–462
      destructive procedures, II:461–462
      mechanical procedures, II:461
      turbinate resection procedures, II:462
  traumatic injuries
    abrasions, III:43
    amputations, III:44
    anesthesia, III:27, 27f–28f
    avulsions, III:43–44, 44f
    evaluation examinations, III:25
    lacerations
      framework repair, III:43
      lining repair, III:43
      skin covering repair, III:43
    surgical technique and treatment, III:42–44
  Treacher Collins syndrome, III:828–830
Notch signaling pathway, I:428–429
not-for-profit corporations, I:85
nuclear factor κ B, I:431
nude athymic mouse 4-mm calvarial defect, I:221–223, 222f
numbness, II:557–558, III:69–70, 76
Nuss repair, III:858, 859f

O
Oasis®, IV:412t–414t
oatmeal, II:18, 23
obesity
  body mass index (BMI), II:617, 634–635, 635t, 638–639
  definition, II:634–635
  epidemiology, II:634–635
  nonhealing wounds, I:282
  patient safety, I:126–128
  post-bariatric surgery reconstruction, II:634–654
    abdominal contouring
      giant pannus, II:640–643, 643f–644f
      hidden penis, II:640, 643f
      major weight loss (MWL) patient, II:639b
      mons correction, II:640, 641f–642f
      operative planning and technique, II:639–640
      patient evaluation, II:639
      surgical variations, II:640–643, 640f–641f
    body contouring centers of excellence, II:653
    complications, II:653

obesity (Continued)
  lower bodylift (LBL)/buttock contouring
    major weight loss (MWL) patient,
      II:644b
    markings, II:645, 646f–647f, 649f
    operative technique, II:645, 647f–649f
    patient evaluation, II:644–645
    patient selection, II:645
    postoperative care and follow-up,
      II:645
  patient presentation and diagnosis
    patient history, II:636–637
    physical examination, II:637
    preoperative assessment, II:637
    preoperative counseling and education,
      II:637–638
  patient selection
    body contouring, II:638, 638t
    body mass index (BMI), II:638–639
    intraoperative procedures, II:638–639,
      638t
    patient safety, II:638–639, 638t
    psychological considerations, II:638
  secondary procedures, II:653
  staging and combination procedures,
    II:653
  surgical technique
    abdominal contouring, II:639–643
    arms, II:652
    breast, II:652
    lower bodylift (LBL)/buttock
      contouring, II:644–645
    male chest, II:652
    trunk, II:652
    upper extremities, II:652
    vertical thigh-lift, II:645–652
  vertical thigh-lift
    complications, II:652
    major weight loss (MWL) patient,
      II:648b
    markings, II:649–652, 650f
    operative technique, II:651f–652f, 652
    patient evaluation, II:645–648
    patient selection, II:648–649
    postoperative care and follow-up,
      II:652
  weight loss methods
    advantages/disadvantages, II:636t
    bariatric surgery, II:635–636, 636t
    diet and exercise, II:635, 636t
    pharmacotherapy, II:635, 636t
obsessive-compulsive personality, I:34–35
obstetric brachial plexus palsy
  characteristics, VI:790t, 805, 805b
  infant obstetric brachial plexus palsy
    background information, VI:806–812
    clinical examination, VI:806–808,
      808f–809f
    clinical presentation, VI:806, 807f
    imaging methods, VI:809f
    injury type incidence, VI:810t
    intraoperative findings, VI:810t
    nerve graft results, VI:811–812, 812f–813f
    outcome assessments, VI:811, 812t
    postoperative care and follow-up,
      VI:810–811, 811f
    preoperative preparations, VI:808
    reconstructive strategies, VI:810, 810t

obstetric brachial plexus palsy (Continued)
    rupture–avulsion injuries, VI:810,
      810t–811t
    rupture injuries, VI:810, 810t
    surgical technique and treatment,
      VI:808–809
    surgical timing, VI:808
  injury type incidence, VI:810t
  intraoperative findings, VI:810t
  nerve graft results, VI:811–812, 812f–813f
  outcome assessments, VI:811, 812t
  postoperative care and follow-up, VI:810–
    811, 811f
  research summary, VI:815
  rupture–avulsion injuries, VI:810, 810t–811t
  rupture injuries, VI:810, 810t
  sequelae obstetric brachial plexus palsy
    characteristics, VI:812–815
    elbow deformity reconstruction, VI:815
    examination chart, VI:814t
    forearm and hand deformity
      reconstruction, VI:815
    shoulder deformity reconstruction,
      VI:813–815
obstructive sleep apnea (OSA), III:89–104
  characteristics, III:96
  disease process, III:96
  Epworth Sleepiness Scale (ESS), III:96–97
  patient presentation and diagnosis,
    III:96–97, 97f
  patient selection, III:97
  postoperative care and follow-up,
    III:101–102
  prognosis and outcomes, III:102–103
  secondary procedures, III:103
  surgical technique and treatment
    genioglossus advancement, III:98, 98f
    mandibulomaxillary advancement
      (MMA), III:99f–103f, 100–101
    nasal procedures, III:98
    surgical preparation, III:97–98
    uvulopalatopharyngoplasty (UVPP),
      III:97f–98f, 98
obturator nerve, IV:29f
occlusives
  characteristics, II:17
  essential oils, II:17
  lanolin, II:17
occlusive/vasospastic/vaso-occlusive disease,
  VI:479t
occult scaphoid fractures, VI:85, 85f
occupational hand disorders, VI:363–370
  causal factors, VI:363–365
  clinical care
    chronic occupational injuries, VI:365–369,
      365t
    hand–arm vibration syndrome (HAVS),
      VI:368–369, 368t
    patient management, VI:369
    tendinopathy
      de Quervain's tendonitis, VI:364–367,
        366f
      lateral epicondylitis, VI:366
      medial epicondylitis, VI:366
      nerve compression, VI:367–368
      trigger finger, VI:367, 367f, 402–404
      wrists, VI:366
    vascular disorders, VI:368–369

occupational hand disorders (Continued)
    impairment measurement, VI:369–370
    patient presentation and diagnosis
      disease process, VI:364
      force, repetition, and vibration factors,
        VI:364–365, 366f
      patient history
        course of illness, VI:364
        initial events, VI:364
      physical examination, VI:364
    research summary, VI:370
    return to work, VI:369
    vascular disorders
      hand–arm vibration syndrome (HAVS),
        VI:368–369, 368t
      surgical treatment, VI:368–369
    work-related injuries, VI:363, 363b
occupational pollution, III:421–422
occupational radiation exposure, I:673–674
Occupational Safety and Health
  Administration (OSHA), I:97–98
oculodermal melanocytosis, I:725–726
oculodigital complex, VI:565t
Ogee line, II:272
Ohngren's line, III:436
oil of wintergreen, V:33t–35t
ointments, IV:410
OK-432, I:692–693
OKT3, I:821t, 825
olecranon harvests, I:452
oligodendrocytes, I:217
Ollier, Louis Leopold, I:20
Ollier's disease, VI:327
OMENS classification of mandibular
  deformity, III:775t
omental flap, IV:267–268
omentum reconstruction, V:472–481
  acellular dermal matrix (ADM), V:474–476,
    477f
  basic principles, V:472–473
  bilateral reconstruction, V:476–477,
    478f–480f
  chest wall reconstruction, I:553, IV:245,
    246f–247f
  complications, V:480–481
  epigastric region closure, V:477–480
  implants, V:474–476, 476f
  laparoscopic harvesting, V:473, 473f–474f
  lipofilling, V:476
  nipple-areola complex
    reconstruction process, V:476f–477f, 480
    symmetry, V:480
  patient selection, V:473
  pectoralis major muscle, V:474–476
  postoperative care and follow-up, V:480
  prognosis and outcomes, V:480–481
  prostheses, V:474, 475f, 479f
  reconstruction process, V:473–474, 474f
  secondary procedures, V:481
  skin preservation, V:472
omphaloceles
  characteristics, III:865–866
  clinical presentation and evaluation, III:865,
    866f
  surgical indicators, III:865
  treatment strategies, III:865–866
omphalopagus twins, III:893–897, 894f,
    896f–897f, 901b–903b, 904f

omphaloplasty, **II:**563–564, 564f
oncocytic carcinoma, **III:**365t, 370, 377
oncocytoma, **III:**365t, 368, 373
Oncotype DX 21 gene recurrence score, **V:**267
1,25-dihydroxyvitamin D receptor
    (1,25-(OH)$_2$D$_3$-R), **I:**428
one-stage nasolabial flap, **III:**145–146
onlay cartilaginous grafts, **II:**175
open carpal tunnel release (OCTR),
    VI:507–509
open rhinoplasty, **II:**387–412
    advantages/disadvantages, **II:**388t
    complications
        bleeding, **II:**410–411
        deformities and deviations, **II:**411
        edema, **II:**411
        infections, **II:**411
        nasal airway obstructions, **II:**411
        open rhinoplasty-caused deformities,
            II:448–449, 449f
    deviated nose with dorsal hump
        outcome assessments, **II:**407
        surgical goals, **II:**406
        surgical plan, **II:**407
        systematic analysis, **II:**405–406, 406f
    general discussion, **II:**387
    long, wide nose with a drooping tip and
            nasal airway obstruction
        outcome assessments, **II:**409
        surgical goals, **II:**409
        surgical plan, **II:**409
        systematic analysis, **II:**407–409, 407f–408f
    nasal anatomy, **II:**387
    outcome assessments, **II:**410
    patient presentation and diagnosis
        anatomic examination, **II:**388–389
        external nasal examination, **II:**388t
        informed consent, **II:**389
        initial consultation, **II:**387–389
        internal nasal examination, **II:**389t
        nasal history, **II:**388
        patient expectations, **II:**389
        photographic documentation, **II:**389
    patient selection, **II:**389
    postoperative care and follow-up
        activity restrictions, **II:**410
        dressings and wound care, **II:**409
        follow-up consultations, **II:**410
        general patient instructions, **II:**410
        medications, **II:**409–410
        postoperative instructions, **II:**409–410
    prognosis, **II:**410
    secondary procedures, **II:**412
    surgical technique and treatment
        alar base surgery
            alar flaring, **II:**404
            alar flaring with modification of nostril
                shape, **II:**405
            characteristics, **II:**404–405, 406f
        alar–columellar relationship, **II:**401–402,
            403f
        alar rim deformities
            alar contour grafts, **II:**401, 401f
            characteristics, **II:**400–401
            lateral crural strut grafts, **II:**401, 402f
        anesthesia, **II:**389–390
        autologous cartilage harvesting
            background information, **II:**394–396
            costal cartilage, **II:**396, 397f
            ear cartilage, **II:**395–396, 396f

open rhinoplasty (Continued)
        septal cartilage, **II:**394–395, 394f
        septal L-strut, **II:**394–395, 395f
        submucoperichondrial dissection,
            II:394–395, 394f
        submucoperichondrial flaps, **II:**394–
            395, 395f
    closure, **II:**403
    component dorsal hump reduction,
        II:391–392, 391f
    depressor septi muscle translocation,
        II:403–404, 405f
    dorsal spreader grafts, **II:**392f
    nasal airway
        inferior turbinoplasty/outfracture/
            submucous resection, **II:**393–394,
            393f
        obstructions, **II:**392–394
        septal reconstruction, **II:**392–393
    nasal dorsum irregularities, **II:**391f
    nasal tip
        cephalic trim, **II:**397, 398f
        columellar strut graft, **II:**397–398, 398f
        grafting techniques, **II:**399–400, 400f
        surgical technique, **II:**397–400
        suturing techniques, **II:**398–399,
            399f–400f
    percutaneous lateral nasal osteotomies,
        II:402–403, 404f
    preoperative management, **II:**389–390
    transcolumellar stair-step incision,
        II:390–391, 390f
open wounds, **I:**241–242, 241f, 286–287
operating rooms
    ethics, **I:**61
    fire triad, **I:**132–133
    lighting, **I:**107
opioid analgesics, **IV:**427
opportunity cost, **I:**71–72
Opsite®, **IV:**412t–414t
optic nerve gliomas
    patient presentation and diagnosis, **III:**878
    surgical technique and treatment, **III:**878
oral antibiotics, **II:**21t
oral-antral fistula, **III:**70
oral cavity and mouth
    anatomical characteristics, **III:**422, 422f
    reconstructive surgeries, **III:**307–335
        bone-carrying flaps
            circumflex iliac osteocutaneous flap,
                III:322, 323f
            fibula osteoseptocutaneous flap, **III:**323
            pectoralis major
                osteomusculocutaneous flap,
                III:322
            radius with radial forearm flap, **III:**323
            scapular osteomusculocutaneous flap,
                III:323, 323f
            temporalis osteomuscular flap, **III:**322
            trapezius osteomusculocutaneous flap,
                III:322
        challenges, **III:**307–308
        complications
            acute complications, **III:**333
            chronic complications, **III:**333–334
        decision-making process
            basic procedure, **III:**311–313
            immediate postoperative appearance,
                III:314f
            myocutaneous perforator flap, **III:**313f

oral cavity and mouth (Continued)
        patient follow-up, **III:**312f–314f
        radial forearm flap, **III:**311f
        squamous cell carcinomas (SCCs),
            III:311f–313f
        ulnar forearm flap, **III:**312f
    disease process, **III:**308
    evaluation examinations, **III:**25
    free tissue transfer, **III:**311
    lips, **III:**46, 47f–48f
    local/regional flaps, **III:**309t, 311
    oral mucosa repair, **III:**46
    patient presentation and diagnosis,
        III:308
    patient selection
        defect factors, **III:**310–311, 310t
        patient factors, **III:**308–310, 310t
    postoperative care and follow-up,
        III:332–333
    prognosis and outcomes, **III:**333–334
    secondary procedures, **III:**334
    skin grafts, **III:**311
    soft tissue flaps
        anterolateral thigh flap, **III:**321–322
        comparison studies, **III:**309t
        deltopectoral flaps, **III:**318–319, 319f
        lateral arm flap, **III:**321
        medial sural artery perforator (MSAP)
            flap, **III:**322
        pectoralis major myocutaneous flaps,
            III:319, 320f
        radial forearm flap, **III:**319–320
        rectus abdominis musculocutaneous
            flap, **III:**321, 321f
        selection guidelines, **III:**309t
        submental flaps, **III:**316–318, 318f
        thoracodorsal artery perforator (TDAP)
            flap, **III:**322
        ulnar forearm flap, **III:**320–321
    surgical technique
        bone-carrying flaps, **III:**322–332
        fasciocutaneous flaps, **III:**319–322
        local flaps, **III:**316–318
        musculocutaneous flaps, **III:**319–322
        pedicled osteocutaneous flaps, **III:**322
        regional flaps, **III:**318–319
        soft tissue flaps, **III:**316–322
        vascularized osteocutaneous flaps,
            III:322–323
    surgical technique and treatment,
        III:45–46
    tongue, **III:**46
    tumors, **III:**398–419
        alveolar ridge lesions
            preoperative assessment, **III:**406
            treatment strategies, **III:**406–407, 407f,
                427
        buccal mucosa
            diagnosis and treatment, **III:**427
            preoperative assessment, **III:**406
            surgical technique and treatment,
                III:406
        complications
            dental follow-ups, **III:**418
            general discussion, **III:**416–418
            local recurrence, **III:**416
            osteoradionecrosis (ORN), **III:**417
            post-treatment surveillance, **III:**417–418
            regional recurrence, **III:**416–417
            wound infections, **III:**417

oral cavity and mouth *(Continued)*
  epidemiology, **III:**399–400
  floor of mouth
    diagnosis and treatment, **III:**427
    preoperative assessment, **III:**406
    surgical technique and treatment,
      III:406
  hard palate
    diagnosis and treatment, **III:**427
    preoperative assessment, **III:**408, 408f
    treatment strategies, **III:**408
  lips
    cervical metastasis, **III:**405–406
    diagnosis and treatment, **III:**427
    preoperative assessment, **III:**402, 405f
    surgical technique and treatment,
      III:402–405, 405f
  lymph node anatomy, **III:**399f
  medical challenges, **III:**398
  pathogenesis, **III:**398–399
  patient presentation and diagnosis,
    III:400, 427
  retromolar trigone, **III:**406, 427
  surgical access, **III:**402, 403f–404f
  therapeutic choices, **III:**401–402
  TNM clinical classification system,
    III:400–401, 401t
  tongue
    base of tongue, **III:**412, 428–432
    diagnosis and treatment, **III:**427
    preoperative assessment, **III:**408–409,
      408f
    treatment strategies, **III:**409
oral commissure, **III:**287f, 456, **IV:**489–490, 495f
oral contraceptives, **II:**21t
orbicularis muscle deformities, **III:**640–641
orbicularis oculi, **II:**110–111, 110f–111f
orbicularis retaining ligament (ORL), **II:**112,
  114f, **III:**9, 10f
orbicularis suspension, **II:**130–131
orbital apex syndrome, **III:**57
orbitale, **II:**356t, 363f
orbital fractures
  characteristics, **III:**53–57
  complications
    blindness, **III:**56
    diplopia, **III:**56
    enophthalmos, **III:**56
    implant migration or hemorrhage, **III:**56
    lid lamellae, **III:**57
    ocular globe injuries, **III:**56
    retrobulbar hematoma, **III:**56
    upper eyelid ptosis, **III:**57
    vertical shortening of the lower eyelid,
      III:57
  computed tomography (CT), **III:**54
  infraorbital nerve anesthesia, **III:**57
  nasoethmoidal orbital fractures
    characteristics, **III:**60–61
    classification systems, **III:**61–63, 62f
    clinical examination, **III:**60–61, 61f
    complications, **III:**63
    computed tomography (CT), **III:**61
    surgical pathology
      causal factors, **III:**60
      interorbital space, **III:**60
      traumatic orbital hypertelorism, **III:**60
      traumatic telecanthus, **III:**60

orbital fractures *(Continued)*
    treatment strategies
      basic procedure, **III:**61–63
      canthal reattachment, **III:**63
      central fragment considerations, **III:**63
      lacrimal system injury, **III:**63
  orbital apex syndrome, **III:**57
  physical examination, **III:**53–54, 54f
  postoperative care and follow-up, **III:**56
  schematic diagram, **III:**53f
  superior orbital fissure syndrome, **III:**57
  surgical anatomy, **III:**53
  surgical technique and treatment
    basic procedure, **III:**55–56
    bone grafts, **III:**55
    cutaneous exposures, **III:**55
    endoscopic approaches, **III:**55
    forced duction test, **III:**55, 55f
    goals, **III:**54–55
    inorganic implants, **III:**56
    orbital floor restoration, **III:**55, 56f
    timing considerations, **III:**55
  treatment indicators
    blow-out fractures (children), **III:**54, 54f
    blow-out fractures (floor of the orbit),
      III:54
    guidelines, **III:**54
orbital hypertelorism, **III:**226
  characteristics, **III:**686
  oculomotor disorders, **III:**699
  outcomes and complicatons, **III:**698
  pathogenesis, **III:**686–689
  patient presentation and diagnosis
    faciocraniosynostosis
      Apert syndrome, **III:**689
      characteristics, **III:**688–689
      craniofrontonasal dysplasia, **III:**689
      Crouzon syndrome, **III:**688, 688f
      Pfeiffer syndrome, **III:**688–689
    median facial clefts, **III:**687
    Tessier cleft classification system,
      III:687–688, 687f
  patient selection, **III:**689
  postoperative care and follow-up,
    III:695–696
  recurrences, **III:**699–700
  secondary procedures, **III:**698f
    canthus correction, **III:**698f, 699
    eyebrows, **III:**699
    eyelids, **III:**699
    nose, **III:**699
    orbits, **III:**699
    scalp, **III:**699
    soft-tissue problems, **III:**698–700
  surgical technique and treatment
    asymmetrical cases, **III:**693–694
    basic principles, **III:**689–690, 690f
    bipartition surgery, **III:**693, 693f
    box-shift osteotomies
      basic procedure, **III:**692–693, 692f,
        694f
      frontal craniectomy, **III:**692–693
      orbit osteotomies, **III:**693
    indicators and timing
      face, **III:**694–695
      general discussion, **III:**694–695
      orbits, **III:**694, 694f
    infrafrontal correction, **III:**690–692, 691f

orbital hypertelorism *(Continued)*
    Le Fort III osteotomy–bipartition
      correction technique
      basic procedure, **III:**696f–697f
      bone grafts, **III:**695
      coronal approach, **III:**695
      general discussion, **III:**695
      osteosynthesis, **III:**695
      subcranial osteotomies, **III:**695
      surgical technique, **III:**690, 691f
orbitozygomatic fracture, **III:**232–234,
  235f–236f
OrCel®, **IV:**415t
organic solvents, **IV:**395
organs at risk (OAR), **I:**663
Oribasius, **I:**14
Orlistat, **II:**635
ornipressin, **I:**140
orodigital complex, **VI:**565t
orofacial clefts, **I:**193
oropharynx
  tumors, **III:**398–419
    base of tongue, **III:**412, 428–432
    cervical lymph nodes, **III:**415f
    complications
      dental follow-ups, **III:**418
      general discussion, **III:**416–418
      local recurrence, **III:**416
      osteoradionecrosis (ORN), **III:**417
      post-treatment surveillance, **III:**417–418
      regional recurrence, **III:**416–417
      wound infections, **III:**417
    epidemiology, **III:**399–400, 412
    lymph node anatomy, **III:**399f
    medical challenges, **III:**398
    nodal status determination, **III:**429–431,
      430f
    pathogenesis, **III:**398–399
    patient presentation and diagnosis,
      III:400, 428–432
    pharyngeal wall, **III:**432
    soft palate, **III:**432
    surgical access, **III:**402, 403f–404f
    therapeutic choices, **III:**401–402
    TNM clinical classification system,
      III:400–401, 401t, 429–431
    tonsils, **III:**431
orthodontic treatment
  cleft lip and palate, **III:**595–613
    bilateral cleft lip
      distraction procedures, **III:**602–611,
        609f–611f
      growth considerations, **III:**611
      infants, **III:**596–597
      orthognathic surgery, **III:**602–611, 607f
      permanent dentition, **III:**602–611
      transitional dentition, **III:**597–602,
        601f
    distraction procedures, **III:**602–611,
      609f–611f
    growth considerations, **III:**611
    infants
      bilateral cleft lip, **III:**596–597
      treatment strategies, **III:**596–597
      unilateral cleft lip, **III:**596
    management goals, **III:**595–596
    orthognathic surgery, **III:**602–611,
      607f–608f

Note: **Boldface** *roman numerals indicate volume. Page numbers followed by f refer to figures; page numbers followed by t refer to tables; page numbers followed by b refer to boxes.*

orthodontic treatment (Continued)
permanent dentition, III:602–611,
603f–606f
primary dentition
anterior crossbite, III:597
posterior crossbite, III:597
research summary, III:611
transitional dentition, III:597–602,
598f–601f
unilateral cleft lip
Chang Gung Craniofacial Center
treatment plan, III:522–523
distraction procedures, III:602–611, 609f
growth considerations, III:611
infants, III:596
orthognathic surgery, III:602–611,
607f–608f
permanent dentition, III:602–611,
603f–606f
transitional dentition, III:597–602,
598f–601f
orthognathic surgery
Asian facial bone surgery, II:178, 181–182
cephalometrics
basic principles, II:360–363
bone landmarks, II:363f
craniofacial surgery, III:657–658, 657f
facial profile classifications, II:361f
malocclusions, II:362f
maxillary and mandibular dental arches,
II:362f
orthodontic considerations, II:363–364
software programs, II:363f
temporomandibular joint (TMJ),
II:364–365, 364f
cleft lip and palate orthodontic treatment,
III:602–611, 607f–608f
complications
avascular necrosis, II:371f, 372
dental and periodontal complications,
II:371
hemorrhage, II:371
neurosensory loss, II:371
unfavorable aesthetic outcomes, II:371
dentofacial deformities
complications, III:667–670
growth and development factors,
III:655–656, 656f
model surgery
basic procedure, III:658
isolated mandibular surgery, III:658
isolated maxillary and two-jaw surgery,
III:658
patient presentation and diagnosis
cleft/craniofacial team, III:656
patient history and examination,
III:656–657
preoperative assessment, III:656–657
patient selection
cephalometric and dental evaluation,
III:657–658, 657f
general discussion, III:657–660
model surgery, III:658
three-dimensional (3D) computed
tomography (CT) models, III:658,
659f
treatment planning process, III:658–660
postoperative care and follow-up, III:666
prognosis and outcomes, III:667–670,
667t

orthognathic surgery (Continued)
secondary procedures, III:670
surgical technique and treatment
apertognathia, III:666, 668f
basic procedure, III:660
bilateral sagittal split osteotomy,
III:661–662
cleft lip surgery, III:663–665, 663f–664f
distraction osteogenesis, III:665
genioplasty, III:662–663
intraoral vertical ramus osteotomy,
III:662
Le Fort I osteotomy, III:660–661, 661f,
663f, 667f–668f, 669t
maxillary constriction, III:665, 667f
short lower face, III:666
skeletal anatomy, III:660
skeletal class III malocclusions, III:665
skeletal class II malocclusions, III:665,
666f
surgically assisted rapid palatal
expansion (SARPE) procedure,
III:661
two-jaw surgery, III:662
vertical maxillary excess, III:666
velopharyngeal insufficiency (VPI),
III:667–670, 667t
facial skeletal augmentation
adjunct therapy, II:340, 341f
alternatives, II:340, 341f
genioplasty, II:367–368, 368f
mandibular osteotomies, II:366–367, 367f
maxillary osteotomy, II:368–370, 369b,
369f–370f
postoperative care and follow-up,
II:370–371
Treacher Collins syndrome, III:834f, 835
orthognathic surgical procedures
blood supply, II:366f
surgical technique, II:365–366
vascular networks, II:366f
orthoplasty, III:915
Orticochea three-flap technique, III:124f
ossoeintegration, I:445
osteoactive materials, I:461–462
osteoarthritis
disease process, VI:412–413, 412f
epidemiology, VI:411
hands and wrists, VI:411–448
disease process, VI:412–413, 412f
distal interphalangeal (DIP) joint
biomechanical effects, VI:414
diagnosis, VI:414, 415f
distal interphalangeal (DIP)
arthrodesis, VI:414–416
surgical indicators, VI:414
epidemiology, VI:411
fingers, VI:414
metacarpophalangeal (MCP) joint
anatomical considerations, VI:425
arthrodesis, VI:429, 429f–430f
biomechanics, VI:425
implant arthroplasty, VI:426–429
resurfacing arthroplasty, VI:425–426
vascularized joint transfer/
costochondral replacement,
VI:429–430
pathophysiology, VI:413
patient presentation and diagnosis,
VI:413–414, 413f

osteoarthritis (Continued)
proximal interphalangeal (PIP) joint
management approaches, VI:417–418
prevalence and characteristics,
VI:417–425
proximal interphalangeal (PIP)
arthrodesis, VI:418–419
thumb
carpometacarpal (CMC) arthroscopy,
VI:434–439
metacarpophalangeal (MCP) joint,
VI:430
prevalence and characteristics,
VI:430–441
prosthetic arthroplasty, VI:440–441,
440f
trapeziometacarpal arthritis,
VI:430–434
trapeziometacarpal arthrodesis,
VI:440–441, 441f
wrists
dorsal surgical approach, VI:443, 444f
etiology, VI:441–442
four-corner fusion, VI:445, 445f
neurectomy, VI:443–444
patient evaluation, VI:442–443
proximal row carpectomy (PRC),
VI:444–445, 444f
radial styloidectomy, VI:443
scaphoidectomy, VI:445, 445f
scaphoid nonunion advanced collapse
(SNAC) arthritis, VI:441–442, 443f
scapholunate advanced collapse
(SLAC) arthrtis, VI:441–442, 442f
surgical technique and treatment,
VI:443–446
total wrist arthrodesis/total wrist
arthroplasty, VI:445–446, 446f
pathophysiology, VI:413
patient presentation and diagnosis,
VI:413–414, 413f
temporomandibular joint (TMJ)
dysfunction, III:90, 91f
osteoblasts
characteristics and functional role, I:427t,
428
differentiation processes, I:230, 230f, 232
regulation mechanisms
major signaling pathways, I:428–429
transcriptional regulation, I:429
osteocalcin, I:428, 431–432, 432t, 434f
osteochondrogenic tumors, I:732, 733f
osteochondroma, IV:247, VI:328, 328f
osteoclasts
characteristics and functional role, I:427t,
430–431
differentiation mechanisms, I:431
osteoconduction, I:445
osteocutaneous flaps, III:317t
osteocytes
characteristics, I:427t, 429
functional role, I:427t, 429–430
histology, I:429
mechanotransduction, I:433
osteogenic sarcoma, IV:103
osteoid osteoma, VI:327, 327f
osteoinduction, I:444–445
osteomyelitis
foot reconstruction, IV:196
hand and wrist evaluations, VI:88–89

osteomyelitis (Continued)
  hand infections, VI:341
  lower extremity reconstructive surgery,
    IV:86–87, 133–134, 134f
  mandibular fractures, III:82–83
  pressure sores, IV:357–360, 359f–360f, 366
osteon, I:426, 426f
osteonectin, I:428, 431–432, 432t, 434f
osteopontin, I:428, 431–432, 432t, 434f
osteoprotegerin (OPG), I:431
osteoradionecrosis (ORN)
  head and neck cancer, III:417
  pathogenesis, IV:252–253, 254f
  radiation therapy (RT), I:671–672
  surgical technique and treatment, IV:253
osteosarcoma, I:741, 741f, VI:329, 655, 656f
Osterix (Osx) transcription factor, I:429, 434f,
    VI:531–532
otodigital complex, VI:565t
otohematoma, III:212, 215f
otoplasty, II:485–493
  adolescent aesthetic surgery, I:45t
  complications, II:492–493
  definition, II:485
  ear deformities, II:485
  patient dissatisfaction, II:493
  patient presentation and diagnosis
    anatomical structure, II:486f
    asymmetry, II:486
    lower third area, II:486
    main components, II:486f
    middle third area, II:486
    overall size and shape, II:485
    upper third area, II:485
  patient selection, II:486
  postoperative care and follow-up, II:492
  prognosis and outcomes, II:492–493
  secondary procedures, II:493
  surgical technique and treatment
    acquired deformities (loss of auricular
      tissue)
      amputated ears, III:209, 212, 213f–214f
      cartilage replantation, III:210, 212
      composite graft, III:210, 210f
      dermabraded amputated auricle
        replantation, III:211, 211f
      microsurgical ear replantation, III:212
      skin coverage considerations, III:207–
        212, 209f
      tissue attached by a narrow pedicle,
        III:209, 210f
    acquired partial defects, III:217
    aging, elongated ear lobes
      closure, II:491
      earlobe reduction, II:491
      incisions, II:491
    anatomic considerations, II:487–492
    constricted ears, II:489–490, III:204,
      205f–206f
    cryptotia, II:490, III:204, 206f–207f
    deformities with loss of auricular tissue
      auricular skin loss, III:214
      full-thickness defects, III:214
      prosthetics, III:217
      skin coverage considerations,
        III:215–217
      trauma-acquired defects, III:214–215,
        216f

otoplasty (Continued)
    deformities without loss of auricular
      tissue
      cauliflower ear, III:212, 215f
      contour irregularities, III:212
      external auditory canal stenosis,
        III:212, 215f
      otohematoma, III:212, 215f
    earring-related complications, II:491
    large ears
      closure, II:489
      correction, II:489, 490f
      dissection, II:488
      incisions, II:488
    near-ear facelift deformities
      classifications, II:491–492
      earlobe deformities, II:290–293, 292f,
        492
      retroauricular deformities, II:492
      scars, II:492
      tragal deformities, II:290, 291f, 492
    normal-sized prominent ears
      closure, II:488, 489f
      correction, II:487–488, 487f–488f
      dissection, II:487
      endpoint, II:488
      incisions, II:487
      lobule repositioning, II:487–488, 488f
    prominent ear
      antihelical fold restoration, III:206–207
      conchal alteration, III:206
      lateral cartilage surface alteration,
        III:207
      medial cartilage surface alteration,
        III:207
      pathology, III:204–206, 208f
      treatment strategies, III:206
    residual tissue utilization, III:217
    Stahl's ear deformity, II:490–491,
      490f–491f
outcomes research See evidence-based
    medicine and health service research
Outline, II:48t
    See also soft-tissue fillers
outpatient relationships, I:60–61
oxycodone, IV:427
oxygen-based alloys, I:786–787

P
P4P model, I:173–174
p53 (tumor suppressor gene), I:661–662, II:15
Padgett grafts, I:325–326
Paeoniae rubra, V:33t–35t
pagetoid-type fibrous dysplasia, III:381
Paget's disease, V:278f
Paget–von Schrotter syndrome, VI:520
painful neuroma
    outcomes and complicatons, IV:172
    pathogenesis, III:441, IV:152f–153f
    patient presentation and diagnosis,
      IV:156–157, 156f
    patient selection, IV:157–158, 158f
    postoperative care and follow-up, IV:170,
      172f
    research background, IV:151–152
    surgical technique and treatment
      basic procedure, IV:159–164
      calcaneal nerve, IV:162f

painful neuroma (Continued)
    lateral knee denervation, IV:165f
    medial knee denervation, IV:165f
    plantar interdigital nerve, IV:163f
    saphenous nerve, IV:160f, 163f–164f
    superficial peroneal nerve, IV:160f
    sural nerve, IV:161f
    surgical tips, IV:159b
palatoplasty, III:569–583
  nineteenth century, I:19–20
  palatal development
    anatomical characteristics, III:569, 570f
    ear pathology, III:570
    embryology, III:569
  patient presentation and diagnosis
    cleft palate with cleft lip and alveolus,
      III:570–571, 571f
    feeding and swallowing difficulties,
      III:573–574, 574f
    growth factors, III:573
    incomplete cleft palate, III:571
    multiple syndromes, III:572
    Pierre Robin sequence, III:572
    secondary palate clefts, III:571
    speech development, III:574, 575f
    submucous cleft palate, III:571–572, 571f
    22q chromosomal deletion, III:572–573,
      573f
  postoperative care and follow-up, III:581
  prognosis and outcomes
    fistula formation, III:581, 582f
    maxillary growth, III:581–582
    speech outcomes, III:581
  research summary, III:582
  surgical technique and treatment
    Furlow double-opposing z-palatoplasty,
      III:579, 580f
    hard versus soft palate closure, III:576
    intravelar veloplasty, III:578–579, 580f
    Langenbeck repair technique, III:576, 577f
    technical perioperative considerations,
      III:576
    timing considerations
      general discussion, III:574–576
      maxillary growth, III:575–576
      multiple syndromes, III:576
      speech development, III:574–575
    two-flap palatoplasty, III:578, 579f
    two-stage palate repair, III:579–581
    Vomer flaps, III:578
    V-Y palate repair (Veau–Wardill–Kilner),
      III:576–578, 577f–578f
Paley and Herzenberg classification and
    treatment algorithm, VI:569, 569t
Paley and Herzenberg classification of ulnar
    longitudinal deficiency, VI:567, 568t
palladium (Pd), I:656–657
palmar dissections, VI:672, 672f, 672t
palmar fascia, VI:2–5, 4f–5f, 347, 347f
palmaris longus (PL) muscle, VI:179–182
Panax ginseng, II:22–23, V:33t–35t
Paneth cells, I:262f
panfacial fractures
    complications, III:84–85, 85f
    definition, III:84–85
    postoperative care and follow-up, III:85
    surgical sequence, III:84
    treatment strategies, III:84

Note: **Boldface** roman numerals indicate volume. Page numbers followed by f refer to figures; page numbers followed by t refer to tables; page numbers followed by b refer to boxes.

panfacial volumetric augmentation, **II:**54, 55f
panic disorders, **I:**48–49, 48b
panniculectomy, **II:**639–640, **IV:**295
papillary cystadenoma lymphomatosum, **III:**365t, 367–368, 369f
papular scars, **II:**69
papverine, **I:**583
paracetamol, **IV:**427
paraffin injections, **I:**27, **V:**97–98, 98f
paralysis, facial *See* facial paralysis
paranasal augmentation, **II:**177
paranasal sinuses, **III:**423–424, 425f–426f, 436–437, 436f
paranoid personality disorder, **I:**35–36
parapagus twins, **III:**896f–898f
parascapular flap, **IV:**211, 212f
paraspinal flaps, **III:**872–874, 873f–875f
paraspinous muscles, **IV:**222–223, 222f
parastomal hernia repair, **IV:**290
parathyroid hormone receptor (PTH-R), **I:**428
PARC syndrome (poikilodermia, alopecia, retrognathism, cleft palate), **III:**807t
Paré, Ambroise
   burn wound treatment, **IV:**393
   hand surgery, **VI:**xlvf
   reconstructive and aesthetic surgery, **I:**15–16, 16f
parenteral nutrition, **IV:**292
paresthesias, **II:**526, 557–558
Parkes–Weber syndrome
   benign mesenchymal-origin tumors, **I:**735
   classification systems, **VI:**668, 668t
   outcomes and complicatons, **VI:**690–691
   pathogenesis, **I:**694f, 703, **VI:**690
   patient presentation and diagnosis, **VI:**690
   surgical technique and treatment, **VI:**690
paronychia, **VI:**126f, 336–337, 336f
parotid gland, **III:**360–361, 361f–362f
paroxetine, **I:**51
Parsonage–Turner syndrome, **VI:**520–521
partial hand, **VI:**872, 873f
partial trisomy 10q syndrome, **VI:**573t
partnerships, **I:**85
passive immunotherapy, **I:**204–206, 205f
Passot, Raymond, **I:**27, 28f, **V:**154
Pasteurella multocida, **VI:**334
Pasteur, Louis, **VI:**xliii–xliv
patents, **I:**846–847
pathogen-associated molecular patterns (PAMPs), **I:**249
Patient and Observer Scar Assessment Scale (POSAS), **I:**264–266, 299
patient-centered health communication, **V:**314–325
   evidence-based decision aids, **V:**321
   healthcare decisions, **V:**314
   high-quality decision-making methods, **V:**320–321
   informed consent versus informed choice, **V:**324
   medical practice variations
      evidence-based medicine and health service research, **V:**316–317
      geographic variations, **V:**315–316
      preference-sensitive decisions, **V:**315
      surgical decisions, **V:**315–316, 316f
      variation categories, **V:**315
   research summary, **V:**324

patient-centered health communication (*Continued*)
   risk communication
      absolute versus relative risk, **V:**318–319, 318f
      data presentation
         balanced framing, **V:**319
         teach-back method, **V:**320
         visual aids, **V:**319, 320f
      importance, **V:**317–320
      risk language and terminology, **V:**317–318, 318f
   shared decision-making (SDM)
      decision quality reports, **V:**322, 323b, 323f
      definition, **V:**321–323
      shared decision-making process, **V:**321, 322f
      value proposition
         general discussion, **V:**323
         patients' perception, **V:**323
         surgeons' acceptance, **V:**323
patient preference trials, **I:**154
patient problem, intervention, comparison, and outcome (PICO) approach, **I:**151
Patient Protection and Affordable Care Act (2010), **I:**86
patient safety, **I:**124–136
   breast surgery complications, **I:**132
   clinical outcomes, **I:**134–135
   facial aesthetic surgery, **I:**131–132
   intraoperative management, **I:**128–130
   liposuctions, **I:**129, 131
   mortality rates, **I:**125–126
   obese patients, **I:**126–128
   operating room fires, **I:**132–133
   policy failures, **I:**135
   sleep apnea patients, **I:**126–128, 127t
   surgical risk factors, **I:**124–126, 125t–126t
   venous thromboembolism, **I:**130–131
   wrong patient/wrong-sided surgery, **I:**133–134, 134b
pattern recognition receptors (PRRs), **I:**249
Paulus of Aegina, **I:**14
Pavilion for Facial Cripples, **I:**22–23, 23f
Pax6 gene expression, **III:**505, 505f–506f
Payne, Robert Lee, **II:**108–109
Peacock, Erle E, **II:**108–109
pectineus muscle, **IV:**15t–16t, 18f, 19t, 20f–22f
pectoralis major muscle
   anatomical characteristics, **IV:**224–225, 225f, 242f, **V:**10f
   chest wall reconstruction, **IV:**241, 241f
   head and neck reconstruction, **I:**543, 543f–544f
   mediastinum reconstruction, **I:**549–552, 550f–551f
   Poland syndrome, **V:**549, **VI:**609f
   revisionary breast surgery, **IV:**241, 241f, **V:**474–476
   segmental transposition flaps, **I:**524, 525f
   tongue reconstruction, **III:**274f, 309t
pectoralis major myocutaneous flaps, **III:**319, 320f
pectoralis major osteomusculocutaneous flap, **III:**322
pectoralis minor muscle, **III:**295t, **IV:**224–225, 225f, **V:**10f
pectus carinatum
   characteristics, **III:**859–860, 859f
   clinical presentation and evaluation, **III:**859

pectus carinatum (*Continued*)
   surgical indicators, **III:**859
   treatment strategies, **III:**859–860, 860f
pectus excavatum
   characteristics, **III:**855–859
   clinical presentation and evaluation, **III:**855–856, 856f
   minimally invasive repair of pectus excavatum (MIRPE), **III:**858, 859f
   Ravitch repair, **III:**857, 858f
   surgical indicators, **III:**856
   treatment strategies, **III:**856–859, 857f–858f
pediatric brachial plexus injury
   characteristics, **VI:**790t, 805, 805b
   infant obstetric brachial plexus palsy
      background information, **VI:**806–812
      clinical examination, **VI:**806–808, 808f–809f
      clinical presentation, **VI:**806, 807f
      imaging methods, **VI:**809f
      injury type incidence, **VI:**810t
      intraoperative findings, **VI:**810t
      nerve graft results, **VI:**811–812, 812f–813f
      outcome assessments, **VI:**811, 812t
      postoperative care and follow-up, **VI:**810–811, 811f
      preoperative preparations, **VI:**808
      reconstructive strategies, **VI:**810, 810t
      rupture–avulsion injuries, **VI:**810, 810t–811t
      rupture injuries, **VI:**810, 810t
      surgical technique and treatment, **VI:**808–809
      surgical timing, **VI:**808
   injury type incidence, **VI:**810t
   intraoperative findings, **VI:**810t
   nerve graft results, **VI:**811–812, 812f–813f
   outcome assessments, **VI:**811, 812t
   postoperative care and follow-up, **VI:**810–811, 811f
   research summary, **VI:**815
   rupture–avulsion injuries, **VI:**810, 810t–811t
   rupture injuries, **VI:**810, 810t
   sequelae obstetric brachial plexus palsy
      characteristics, **VI:**812–815
      elbow deformity reconstruction, **VI:**815
      examination chart, **VI:**814t
      forearm and hand deformity reconstruction, **VI:**815
      shoulder deformity reconstruction, **VI:**813–815
pediatric chest and trunk defects, **III:**855–876
   congenital defects, **III:**855
   embryology, **III:**855
   thoracic wall defects
      ectopia cordis
         characteristics, **III:**861–862, 862f
         clinical presentation and evaluation, **III:**861, 862f–863f
         surgical indicators, **III:**861
         treatment strategies, **III:**861–862
      Jeune's syndrome
         characteristics, **III:**860–861, 861f
         clinical presentation and evaluation, **III:**861
         surgical indicators, **III:**861
         treatment strategies, **III:**861, 862f
      pectus carinatum
         characteristics, **III:**859–860, 859f
         clinical presentation and evaluation, **III:**859

pediatric chest and trunk defects (Continued)
    surgical indicators, III:859
    treatment strategies, III:859–860, 860f
    pectus excavatum
        characteristics, III:855–859
        clinical presentation and evaluation,
            III:855–856, 856f
        minimally invasive repair of pectus
            excavatum (MIRPE), III:858, 859f
        Ravitch repair, III:857, 858f
        surgical indicators, III:856
        treatment strategies, III:856–859,
            857f–858f
    Poland syndrome
        characteristics, III:862–865
        clinical presentation and evaluation,
            III:863, 863f–864f
        surgical indicators, III:863
        treatment strategies, III:864–865,
            864f–865f
pediatric facial fractures, III:671–685
    associated injuries, III:672
    background information, III:671
    demographics, III:672
    growth and development factors
        basic principles, III:672–674
        condylar head fractures, III:678f
        cranial-to-facial ratio, III:672f
        Le Fort fracture patterns, III:675f
        mandibular condyle, III:677f
        oblique craniofacial fracture patterns,
            III:676f–677f
        orbital region, III:674f
        sinus development, III:673f
    incidence, III:671–672
    orbital fracture classification system, III:677t
    orbital fractures, III:54, 54f
    outcomes and complicatons
        adverse outcome classifications, III:683t
        basic principles, III:682–683
        cranial base/skull fractures, III:683
        mandible fractures, III:684, 684f
        maxillary and midface fractures, III:684
        metallic cranial hardware, III:683f–684f
        nasal fractures, III:684
        orbital fractures, III:683–684
        zygomaticomaxillary complex fractures,
            III:684
    patient presentation and diagnosis,
        III:674–675, 678f–679f
    patient selection, III:675–678
    postoperative care and follow-up, III:682
    research summary, III:685
    secondary procedures, III:684–685
    surgical technique and treatment
        basic procedure, III:678
        cranial base/frontal skull fractures,
            III:678–679, 679f–680f
        mandible fractures, III:681f–682f, 682
        maxillary and midface fractures, III:680,
            681f
        nasal and naso-orbital ethmoid fractures,
            III:681–682, 681t, 682f
        orbital fractures, III:679–680, 680f
        zygomaticomaxillary complex fractures,
            III:681
pediatric hand fractures, VI:139, 158, 158f
pediatric hand radiographs, VI:71–72, 72f–73f

pediatric plastic surgeries
    acquired and congenital defects, I:44
    adolescent aesthetic surgery, I:45–46, 45t
    craniofacial deformities, I:44–45
    tissue expansion, I:629
pediatric replantation, VI:244
pediatric tissue expansion, III:844
pediatric tumors, III:877–892
    background and general characteristics,
        III:877
    branchial cleft anomalies
        characteristics, III:885, 885f
        first branchial cleft anomaly
            disease process, III:886
            patient presentation and diagnosis,
                III:886, 886f
            surgical technique and treatment,
                III:886
        fourth branchial cleft anomaly, III:887
        second branchial cleft anomaly
            disease process, III:885, 885f
            patient presentation and diagnosis,
                III:885, 885f
            surgical technique and treatment,
                III:885–886, 886f
        third branchial cleft anomaly, III:886–887
    dermoids
        external angular dermoids
            disease process, III:884
            patient presentation and diagnosis,
                III:884
            surgical technique and treatment,
                III:884–885
        general characteristics, III:882
        intradural dermoids
            disease process, III:883
            patient presentation and diagnosis,
                III:883, 884f
            surgical technique and treatment,
                III:883–884
        nasal dermoids
            complications, III:883
            disease process, III:882, 882f
            patient presentation and diagnosis,
                III:882
            prognosis and outcomes, III:883
            secondary procedures, III:883
            surgical technique and treatment,
                III:882–883, 882f–883f
        neck cysts
            disease process, III:885
            patient presentation and diagnosis,
                III:885
    epiphyseal growth plate
        bone sarcoma, VI:655, 656f
        congenital chondrodysplasia, VI:655–656
    lymphadenopathy
        atypical nontuberculous mycobacteria
            disease process, III:891
            patient presentation and diagnosis,
                III:891–892, 891f
            surgical technique and treatment, III:892
        bacterial lymphadenitis
            disease process, III:890
            patient presentation and diagnosis,
                III:891
            surgical technique and treatment,
                III:891

pediatric tumors (Continued)
        cervical tuberculous adenitis (scrofula)
            disease process, III:891
            patient presentation and diagnosis,
                III:891
            surgical technique and treatment,
                III:891
        characteristics, III:890
        chronic regional lymphadenopathy
            complications, III:891
            disease process, III:891
            patient presentation and diagnosis,
                III:891
            prognosis and outcomes, III:891
            surgical technique and treatment,
                III:891
    neurofibromatoses
        café-au-lait spots
            patient presentation and diagnosis,
                III:878
            surgical technique and treatment,
                III:878
        congenital fibromatosis
            patient presentation and diagnosis,
                III:881
            surgical technique and treatment,
                III:881
        craniofacial manifestation
            patient presentation and diagnosis,
                III:878
            surgical technique and treatment,
                III:878, 879f
        definition, III:877
        disease process, III:877–878
        fibromatosis colli
            patient presentation and diagnosis,
                III:880–881
            surgical technique and treatment,
                III:881
        general discussion, III:877
        gingival fibroma
            patient presentation and diagnosis,
                III:881
            surgical technique and treatment,
                III:881
        glomus tumors
            patient presentation and diagnosis,
                III:878
            surgical technique and treatment,
                III:878
        infantile digital fibroma
            patient presentation and diagnosis,
                III:881, 881f
            prognosis and outcomes, III:881
            surgical technique and treatment,
                III:881
        juvenile aggressive fibromatosis, III:880
        juvenile nasopharyngeal angiofibroma
            patient presentation and diagnosis,
                III:881
            prognosis and outcomes, III:881
            surgical technique and treatment,
                III:881
        Lisch nodules
            patient presentation and diagnosis,
                III:878
            surgical technique and treatment,
                III:878

Note: **Boldface** roman numerals indicate volume. Page numbers followed by f refer to figures; page numbers followed by t refer to tables; page numbers followed by b refer to boxes.

pediatric tumors (Continued)
  neurofibromas
    patient presentation and diagnosis,
      III:880
    surgical technique and treatment,
      III:880
  neurofibrosarcomas
    patient presentation and diagnosis,
      III:880
    surgical technique and treatment,
      III:880
  optic nerve gliomas
    patient presentation and diagnosis,
      III:878
    surgical technique and treatment,
      III:878
  patient presentation and diagnosis
    café-au-lait spots, III:878
    congenital fibromatosis, III:881
    craniofacial manifestation, III:878
    fibromatosis colli, III:880–881
    gingival fibroma, III:881
    glomus tumors, III:878
    infantile digital fibroma, III:881, 881f
    juvenile nasopharyngeal angiofibroma,
      III:881
    Lisch nodules, III:878
    neurofibromas, III:880
    neurofibrosarcomas, III:880
    optic nerve gliomas, III:878
    peripheral nerve sheath malignancies,
      III:880
  peripheral nerve sheath malignancies
    patient presentation and diagnosis,
      III:880
    surgical technique and treatment,
      III:880
  surgical technique and treatment
    café-au-lait spots, III:878
    congenital fibromatosis, III:881
    craniofacial manifestation, III:878,
      879f
    fibromatosis colli, III:881
    gingival fibroma, III:881
    glomus tumors, III:878
    infantile digital fibroma, III:881
    juvenile nasopharyngeal angiofibroma,
      III:881
    Lisch nodules, III:878
    neurofibromas, III:880
    neurofibrosarcomas, III:880
    optic nerve gliomas, III:878
    peripheral nerve sheath malignancies,
      III:880
  pilomatrixoma
    characteristics, III:888
    complications, III:888
    disease process, III:888
    patient presentation and diagnosis,
      III:888, 888f
    postoperative care and follow-up, III:888
    prognosis and outcomes, III:888
    surgical technique and treatment, III:888
  soft-tissue sarcomas
    alveolar soft-part sarcoma
      characteristics, III:890
      complications, III:890
      disease process, III:890
      patient presentation and diagnosis,
        III:890

pediatric tumors (Continued)
      prognosis and outcomes, III:890
      surgical technique and treatment,
        III:890
    rhabdomycosarcoma
      characteristics, III:889
      complications, III:889
      disease process, III:889
      patient presentation and diagnosis,
        III:889, 889f
      postoperative care and follow-up,
        III:889
      prognosis and outcomes, III:889
      secondary procedures, III:889
      surgical technique and treatment,
        III:889
    synovial soft-tissue sarcoma
      characteristics, III:889
      complications, III:890
      disease process, III:889
      patient presentation and diagnosis,
        III:889–890
      prognosis and outcomes, III:890
      surgical technique and treatment,
        III:890
  thryoglossal duct cysts
    characteristics, III:887
    complications, III:887–888
    disease process, III:887
    patient presentation and diagnosis,
      III:887, 887f
    prognosis and outcomes, III:887–888
    surgical technique and treatment, III:887
pedicled groin flap, VI:264–266, 265f–266f
pedicled omental flap, IV:267–268
pelvis
  anatomical characteristics
    female perineum
      characteristics, IV:230–235
      cross-section diagram, IV:231f
      schematic diagram, IV:232f–233f
      urogenital triangle, IV:233f
      vascular anatomy, IV:232–235, 234f
    general characteristics, IV:230–235
    male perineum
      characteristics, IV:235
      cross-section diagram, IV:231f
      schematic diagram, IV:236f–237f
      vascular anatomy, IV:235, 238f
  fascial system, IV:5
  innervation, IV:5–8, 7f
  pelvic lymphadenectomy, I:772–777,
    775f–777f
  skeletal reconstruction, IV:184–185
  skeletal structure, IV:2–5, 3f–4f
  vascular supply, IV:5, 7f
penetrating injuries, I:465–466, 466t, 467f
penicillin, VI:333
Penicillium notatum, VI:xliii–xliv
penis
  anatomical characteristics, II:656, IV:235,
    236f–237f, 298–299, 299f
  blood supply, IV:299–301, 299f–301f
  cutaneous and soft-tissue tumors
    clinical staging system, I:716t
    extramammary Paget's disease, I:739
    TNM clinical classification system/pTNM
      pathologic classification system,
      I:715b
  lymphatic supply, IV:301

penis (Continued)
  male genital aesthetic surgery, II:655–677
    enhancement procedures, II:655
    flaccid versus erect penis measurements,
      II:655–656
    hidden penis
      characteristics, II:665–668, 665f–666f
      outcome assessments, II:668
      post-bariatric surgery reconstruction,
        II:640, 643f
      surgical technique, II:667–668,
        667f–669f
    patient selection and examination, II:656
    penile anatomy, II:656
    penile enlargement reconstruction
      dermal fat graft and Alloderm removal,
        II:661–662, 661f
      fat removal, II:660–661
      outcomes and complicatons, II:662
      postoperative care and follow-up,
        II:662
      reconstructive issues, II:660–662
      VY advancement flap reversal, II:658f,
        660, 661f
    penile girth enhancement
      allograft dermal matrix grafts, II:660
      challenges, II:659–660
      dermal and dermal fat grafts,
        II:659–660
      fat injections, II:658f–659f, 659
    penile lengthening
      basic procedure, II:656–658, 657f–658f
      outcome assessments, II:657–658, 659f
      VY advancement flap, II:656–658,
        657f–658f
    penoscrotal web, II:662, 663f
    scrotal enlargement, II:662, 664f
    self-esteem issues, II:655
  male genital reconstructive surgery,
    IV:297–325
    congenital defects
      disorders of sex development (DSD),
        IV:303–304
      exstrophy and epispadias, IV:301–303,
        302f–303f
      hidden penis, IV:304, 304f–305f
      severe penile insufficiency, IV:304–306,
        306f
    female-to-male transsexual surgery
      aesthetic phallus, IV:319, 320f
      metaidoioplasty, IV:315–318, 317f, 346
      pars fixa of the urethra creation,
        IV:314–315, 316f–317f
      phalloplasty, IV:318–323
      sexual intercourse, IV:321–322, 322f
      tactile and erogenous sensation,
        IV:319–321
      vaginectomy, IV:314–315, 315f
      voiding while standing, IV:321
    general discussion, IV:297
    genital anatomy
      blood supply, IV:299–301, 299f–301f
      general discussion, IV:298–301
      genital fascia, IV:298–299, 299f
      lymphatic supply, IV:301
      nerve supply, IV:301
    genital embryology
      genetic sex, IV:297
      gonadal sex, IV:297–298
      phenotypic sex, IV:298, 298f

penis (Continued)
    microsurgical genital reconstruction
        genital replantation, IV:310–312, 312f
        phallic construction, IV:312
    multidisciplinary approach, IV:323
    post-traumatic genital defects
        basic principles, IV:306–313
        genital flaps, IV:304–310, 306f, 311f
        genital skin grafts, IV:307, 308f–309f
        microsurgical genital reconstruction,
            IV:310–312
        reconstructive indications, IV:312–313
    reconstructive indications
        Fournier disease, IV:312–313, 313f
        penile cancer, IV:313, 314f
    nerve supply, IV:301
    reconstructive burn surgery, IV:506
    urogenital defect reconstruction, III:906–924
        embryology, III:907–908
        epidemiology, III:908
        etiology, III:908
        hypospadia
            defect occurrence, III:907f–908f
            embryology, III:907–908
            epidemiology, III:908
            etiology, III:908
            meatoplasty and glanuloplasty,
                III:913–915, 914b, 916f
            onlay island flap repair, III:914–915,
                918f
            orthoplasty, III:915
            outcomes and complicatons,
                III:916–921
            postoperative care and follow-up,
                III:915
            secondary procedures, III:921
            surgical tips, III:915b
            tubularized incised plate (TIP) repair,
                III:914, 917f
            two-stage repair, III:915, 919f–921f
            urethral reconstruction, III:913, 915f
        meatoplasty and glanuloplasty
            basic procedure, III:913–915, 916f
            onlay island flap repair, III:914–915,
                918f
            orthoplasty, III:915
            surgical tips, III:914b–915b
            tubularized incised plate (TIP) repair,
                III:914, 917f
            two-stage repair, III:915, 919f–921f
        outcomes and complicatons, III:916–921
        patient presentation and diagnosis,
            III:908–909
        patient selection, III:909
        postoperative care and follow-up,
            III:915
        secondary procedures, III:921
    vascular anatomy, IV:237f–238f
    See also gender identity disorder
penoscrotal web, II:662, 663f
pentoxifylline, I:617
percutaneous lateral nasal osteotomies,
    II:402–403, 404f
perforator flaps
    advantages/disadvantages, I:539
    back soft-tissue reconstruction, IV:268
    classifications, I:519–521
    facial reconstruction, III:458–459

perforator flaps (Continued)
    lower extremity reconstructive surgery
        anterolateral thigh perforator flap, IV:145,
            145f–146f
        characteristics, IV:143–147
        groin/superficial circumflex iliac
            perforator flap, IV:143, 143f–144f
        lateral thigh/profunda femoris perforator
            flap, IV:144–145, 144f
        medial thigh septocutaneous flap,
            IV:143–144, 144f
        sural flap, IV:146, 146f
        thoracodorsal artery perforator, IV:147,
            147f
    trauma injuries
        Achilles tendon exposure, IV:73f
        anterior tibial artery pedicle perforator
            flap, IV:71f
        basic procedure, IV:68–72
        computed tomography angiography,
            IV:69f–70f, 73f
        flap locations, IV:72f
        musculocutaneous perforator flaps,
            IV:70f
        pedicle perforator flap, IV:70f–71f
        peroneal artery perforator flaps, IV:73f
        posterior tibial artery (PTA) flaps,
            IV:73f
    male genital reconstructive surgery,
        IV:304–306
    microvascular free-flap surgery, I:611, 612f
    phalloplasty, IV:323
    pressure sores, IV:368
    vascular anatomical research, I:505–507,
        506f–507f
periareolar surgical technique with mesh
        support, V:216–227
    background and general characteristics,
        V:216–217
    complications, V:226, 226t
    patient selection, V:217
    planning and marking guidelines, V:217–
        218, 217f
    research summary, V:226
    surgical technique
        basic procedure, V:218–221, 218f–220f
        clinical results, V:222f–225f
        internal support system, V:217
        mesh application, V:219–221, 220f–221f
perichondrium, I:397
pericranium, III:14
perineum
    anatomical characteristics
        female perineum
            characteristics, IV:230–235
            cross-section diagram, IV:231f
            schematic diagram, IV:232f–233f
            urogenital triangle, IV:233f
            vascular anatomy, IV:232–235, 234f
        male perineum
            characteristics, IV:235
            cross-section diagram, IV:231f
            schematic diagram, IV:236f–237f
            vascular anatomy, IV:235, 238f
    perineal reconstruction, IV:383–392
        benign and malignant disease processes,
            IV:383, 384t
        challenges, IV:383

perineum (Continued)
        complications, IV:392
        muscle/musculocutaneous flaps,
            I:554–557, 556f–557f
        patient presentation and diagnosis,
            IV:383–384, 384f–385f
        patient selection, IV:384–385
        postoperative care and follow-up, IV:392
        prognosis and outcomes, IV:392
        reconstructive burn surgery, IV:506
        surgical technique and treatment
            anterolateral thigh flap, IV:388–389,
                390f–391f
            cutaneous paddle inserts, IV:388f
            free flaps, IV:390
            gracilis flaps, IV:388, 389f
            posterior thigh flap, IV:390
            rectus-based reconstruction, IV:386–
                388, 387f–388f
            regional skin flaps, IV:385–386,
                386f–387f
            Singapore flap, IV:387f, 389–390
            skin grafts, IV:385, 386f
            sphincter reconstruction, IV:390–392
perionychium, VI:117, 118f
perioperative psychological reactions, I:33
perioral lines
    botulinum toxin type-A (BoNT-A), II:39–41,
        39f–40f
    facial skin resurfacing, II:74–76, 74f–75f
periorbital anatomy
    blood supply, II:112, 114f
    eyelids, II:111, 111f
    facial nerve, II:112–115, 115f
    forehead, II:110–111, 110f–111f
    general discussion, II:108–115
    lateral retinaculum, II:109, 109f–110f
    lower eyelid area, II:112
    medial orbital vault, II:110, 110f
    orbital anatomy, II:108–109, 109f
    retaining ligaments, II:112, 114f
    sensory nerves, II:112–115, 114f
    septal extension, II:112, 114f
    temporal region, II:110–111, 110f
    trigeminal nerve, II:112–115
    upper eyelid area, II:111–112, 113f
periorbital ligaments, III:9f
peripheral arterial disease (PAD), I:257–258
peripheral nerve repair and grafting,
        I:464–478
    bioengineering techniques, I:476
    current grafting techniques
        allografts, I:473–474, 473t, 475f
        autologous nerve grafts, I:472–474, 473t
        autologous vein grafts, I:472–473, 473t
        nerve conduits, I:473, 473t, 474f
        nerve transfer, I:473t, 474–476, 475b
        nerve wraps, I:473, 473t, 475f
    intraoperative nerve stimulation, I:471
    lower extremities
        chronic nerve compression, IV:151–173
            numerical grading scale, IV:154t–155t
            outcomes and complicatons, IV:172–
                173, 172t
            pathogenesis, IV:153–155
            patient presentation and diagnosis,
                IV:157
            patient selection, IV:158

Note: **Boldface** roman numerals indicate volume. Page numbers followed by *f* refer to figures; page numbers followed by *t* refer to tables; page numbers followed by *b* refer to boxes.

peripheral nerve repair and grafting
(Continued)
  postoperative care and follow-up,
    IV:170–172, 172f
  Pressure-Specified Sensory Device
    (PSSD), IV:154, 158f
  research background, IV:151–152
  surgical technique and treatment,
    IV:164–170
  tarsal tunnel decompression, IV:172t
  painful neuroma, IV:151–173
    outcomes and complicatons, IV:172
    pathogenesis, III:441, IV:152f–153f
    patient presentation and diagnosis,
      IV:156–157, 156f
    patient selection, IV:157–158, 158f
    postoperative care and follow-up,
      IV:170, 172f
    research background, IV:151–152
    surgical technique and treatment,
      IV:159–164
nerve compression syndromes, VI:503–525
  anterior interosseous nerve (AIN)
    syndrome
    characteristics, VI:510–511
    nonsurgical management, VI:511
    surgical technique and treatment,
      VI:511, 512f–513f
  carpal tunnel syndrome
    American Academy of Orthopaedic
      Surgeons clinical practice
      guidelines for the treatment of
      carpal tunnel syndrome, VI:507t
    anatomical considerations, VI:505, 506f
    etiology, VI:505
    nonsurgical management, VI:507
    outcomes and complicatons, VI:509–
      510, 509b
    patient presentation and diagnosis,
      VI:505–507, 507b
    patient selection, VI:507
    prevalence, VI:505–510
    surgical technique and treatment,
      VI:507–509, 508f–509f
  cubital tunnel syndrome
    anatomical considerations, VI:513–514
    clinical signs, VI:514t
    endoscopic decompression technique,
      VI:515
    intramuscular transposition technique,
      VI:515
    medial epicondylectomy technique,
      VI:515, 516f
    outcomes and complicatons, VI:513b,
      515–516
    patient presentation and diagnosis,
      VI:514
    patient selection, VI:514
    simple decompression technique,
      VI:514–515
    subcutaneous transposition technique,
      VI:515
    submuscular transposition technique,
      VI:515
  electrodiagnostic studies, VI:504–505,
    504f
  general discussion, VI:503
  Guyon's canal
    anatomical considerations, VI:511, 513f
    etiology, VI:511

peripheral nerve repair and grafting
(Continued)
    patient presentation and diagnosis,
      VI:511–512
    surgical technique and treatment,
      VI:512–513
  median nerve compression
    anterior interosseous nerve (AIN)
      syndrome, VI:510–511
    carpal tunnel syndrome, VI:505–510
    pronator syndrome, VI:510
    proximal arm and elbow, VI:510, 510f
  pathophysiology, VI:503–504
  posterior interosseous nerve (PIN)
    compression
    anatomical considerations, VI:517
    posterior interosseous nerve (PIN)
      syndrome, VI:517
    radial tunnel syndrome, VI:518
  pronator syndrome, VI:510
  proximal arm and elbow, VI:510, 510f
  quadrilateral space syndrome
    anatomical considerations, VI:523, 523f
    etiology, VI:523
    patient presentation and diagnosis,
      VI:523
    patient selection, VI:523
    surgical technique and treatment,
      VI:524
  radial nerve compression
    incidence, VI:516–518
    posterior interosseous nerve (PIN)
      compression, VI:517
    Wartenberg's syndrome, VI:516–517
  suprascapular nerve compression
    anatomical considerations, VI:524, 524f
    etiology, VI:524
    patient presentation and diagnosis,
      VI:524
    patient selection, VI:524
    surgical technique and treatment,
      VI:524–525
  thoracic outlet syndrome (TOS)
    anatomical considerations, VI:64–65,
      65f, 519, 520f–521f
    classifications, VI:64
    definition, VI:63–66
    incidence, VI:518–522
    nonsurgical management, VI:521–522
    outcomes and complicatons, VI:522
    patient presentation and diagnosis,
      VI:520–521, 522f
    provocative maneuvers, VI:65–66
    surgical technique and treatment,
      VI:522
    Wright's hyperabduction test, VI:520–
      521, 522f
  ulnar nerve compression
    cubital tunnel syndrome, VI:513–516
    Guyon's canal, VI:511–513
  Wartenberg's syndrome
    anatomical considerations, VI:516, 517f
    patient presentation and diagnosis,
      VI:516
    patient selection, VI:517
    surgical technique and treatment,
      VI:517
nerve injuries
  avulsion injuries, I:466t, 467–468, 468f,
    VI:792, 792f–793f

peripheral nerve repair and grafting
(Continued)
  classifications, I:464–465, 465t–466t,
    VI:793
  crush/compression injuries, I:466–467,
    466t
  evaluation examinations, I:468–469
  penetrating trauma, I:465–466, 466t, 467f
  stretch injuries, I:466t, 467–468, 468f
nerve recovery, I:464
nerve repair
  end-to-end versus end-to-side repair,
    I:470–471
  epineural versus fascicular repair,
    I:469–470, 470f
  surgical timing, I:469
  tension considerations, I:469
nerve transfer, VI:719–744
  adult brachial plexus injury
    basic procedure, VI:799–800
    closed-target nerve transfer, VI:799
    end-to-side neurorrhaphy nerve
      transfer, VI:799–800
    extraplexus nerve transfer, VI:799
    functioning free muscle transplantation
      (FFMT), VI:801–802
    intraplexus nerve transfer, VI:799
    pedicled muscle transfer, VI:800–801
    proximal nerve transfer versus distal
      nerve transfer, VI:799t
    recommended induction exercises,
      VI:800t
    reconstructive strategies, VI:800
  complete/near-complete plexus injury
    contralateral C7 transfer, VI:732–733
    examination findings, VI:732
    phrenic nerve transfer, VI:732–733
    reconstruction techniques, VI:732–733,
      732b
    spinal accessory and intercostal nerves,
      VI:732, 732f
  current grafting techniques, I:473t,
    474–476, 475b
  end-to-side transfers, VI:719–720, 720b,
    720f
  facial paralysis, III:291–292, 291f–292f
  general discussion, VI:719
  hand therapy, VI:859–861, 859f–860f
  lower plexus injuries
    examination findings, VI:732
    reconstruction techniques, VI:732,
      732b
  median nerve injury
    adjunct tendon transfers, VI:733
    brachialis branch to anterior
      interosseous nerve (AIN) branch
      nerve transfer, VI:733, 735f
    examination findings, VI:733, 733b
    radial to median branch nerve
      transfers, VI:733, 734f
    reconstruction techniques, VI:733
  outcome assessments, VI:742–743
  patient presentation and diagnosis
    diagnostic imaging, VI:725
    electrodiagnostic testing, VI:725–726,
      725b
    pain questionnaire, VI:721f–724f
    patient history, VI:720, 721f–724f
    physical examination, VI:725, 725b
  patient selection, VI:726–727, 726t

peripheral nerve repair and grafting
  (Continued)
    postoperative wound care
      basic procedure, **VI:**741–742
      complications, **VI:**742
      rehabilitation, **VI:**742
    radial nerve injury
      adjunct tendon transfers, **VI:**738–739
      examination findings, **VI:**737, 737b
      median to radial branch nerve
        transfers, **VI:**737–738, 738f
      reconstruction techniques, **VI:**737–739
    secondary procedures, **VI:**743, 743b
    sensory nerve injury
      first webspace sensation restoration,
        VI:740–741, 741f
      lateral antebrachial cutaneous nerve to
        radial nerve transfers, **VI:**741
      median to ulnar branch nerve transfers,
        VI:740, 740f
      radial to axillary nerve transfers,
        VI:741
      restoration techniques, **VI:**739–741
      ulnar to median branch nerve transfers,
        VI:739–740, 739f
    surgical procedures
      complete/near-complete plexus injury,
        VI:732–733
      lower plexus injuries, **VI:**732
      median nerve injury, **VI:**733
      radial nerve injury, **VI:**737–739
      sensory nerve injury, **VI:**739–741
      surgical tips, **VI:**727b
      ulnar nerve injury, **VI:**733–736
      upper plexus injuries, **VI:**727–731
    tubular repair, **VI:**713
    ulnar nerve injury
      adjunct tendon transfers, **VI:**736
      anterior interosseous nerve (AIN) to
        deep motor branch nerve transfer,
        VI:736, 736f–737f
      examination findings, **VI:**733–736, 736b
      median to ulnar branch nerve transfers,
        VI:736, 736f–737f
      reconstruction techniques, **VI:**736
    upper plexus injuries
      double fascicular nerve transfer, **VI:**731,
        731f
      examination findings, **VI:**727
      medial pectoral nerve and
        thoracodorsal nerve, **VI:**731, 731f
      reconstruction techniques, **VI:**727–731,
        727b
      spinal accessory to suprascapular nerve
        transfers, **VI:**727, 728f–729f
      triceps to axillary nerve transfer,
        VI:728, 729f–730f
      ulnar/median redundant branches to
        biceps brachii and brachialis
        branches nerve transfer, **VI:**731,
        731f
  outcome-related factors, **I:**471
  peripheral nerve sheath malignancies
    patient presentation and diagnosis,
      III:880
    surgical technique and treatment, **III:**880
  postoperative care and follow-up, **I:**476–477
  research summary, **I:**477

peripheral nerve repair and grafting
  (Continued)
    tissue-specific stem cells, **I:**231–233, 231f
    upper extremities, **VI:**694–718
      anatomical characteristics
        blood supply, **VI:**696, 697f
        brachial plexus nerves, **VI:**696f
        gross anatomy, **VI:**695, 695f–697f
        nerve trunk, **VI:**695–696, 697f
        neurons and supporting cells, **VI:**695,
          697f
        Riche–Cannieu anastomosis, **VI:**697f
        schematic diagram, **VI:**697f
      clinical examination
        correct diagnosis, **VI:**700–702, 701f
        electromyography/neurography,
          VI:700–701
        functional evaluation, **VI:**700
        wound inspection, **VI:**702
      donor nerves
        lateral cutaneous nerve, **VI:**709,
          711f–712f
        lateral femoral cutaneous nerve, **VI:**710
        medial cutaneous nerve, **VI:**709, 710f
        saphenous nerve, **VI:**710
        superficial sensory branch of the radial
          nerve, **VI:**710, 712f–713f
        sural nerve, **VI:**708–709, 709f
        terminal branch of the posterior
          interosseous nerve, **VI:**710
      epidemiology, **VI:**694
      future trends, **VI:**718
      immediate versus delayed repair
        basic principles, **VI:**703
        surgical approach, **VI:**703–704, 703f
        timing considerations, **VI:**703
      nerve reconstruction
        autografts, **VI:**707, 708f, 708t
        coaptation and maintenance, **VI:**708
        gap measurement, **VI:**708
        graft harvest, **VI:**708, 708t
        graft length, **VI:**708
        nerve ends, **VI:**708
        surgical approach and preparation,
          VI:707–708
      nerve repair principles
        basic principles, **VI:**704–705, 704f–706f
        end-to-side nerve repair, **VI:**707
        epineurial versus fascicular repair,
          VI:706–707, 706f–707f
        wound closure and immobilization,
          VI:707
      outcomes and complicatons
        age factors, **VI:**716
        British Medical Research Council
          (BMRC) Scale, **VI:**716, 716t
        digital nerves, **VI:**716
        Highet Scale, **VI:**715, 716t
        influencing factors, **VI:**716
        injury type, **VI:**717
        level of injury, **VI:**717
        nerve trunks, **VI:**716–717
        outcome assessments, **VI:**714
        repair type, **VI:**717
        Rosen score, **VI:**716
      patient presentation and diagnosis
        axonotmesis, **VI:**698–700, 699t
        fifth-degree injuries, **VI:**699t, 700

peripheral nerve repair and grafting
  (Continued)
      first-degree injuries, **VI:**698, 699t
      fourth-degree injuries, **VI:**699t, 700
      injury classifications, **VI:**698, 699f, 699t
      neuropraxia, **VI:**698, 699t
      neurotmesis, **VI:**699t, 700
      second-degree injuries, **VI:**698–700,
        699t
      sixth-degree injuries, **VI:**699t, 700
      third-degree injuries, **VI:**699t, 700
    patient selection
      correct diagnosis, **VI:**701f, 702–703
      nerve injury classifications, **VI:**702–703,
        702t
      wound condition, **VI:**703
    physiological characteristics
      degeneration/regeneration
        mechanisms, **VI:**697, 698f
      distal nerve segment, **VI:**697–698, 698f
      general characteristics, **VI:**696–698
      nodes of Ranvier, **VI:**696–698, 697f
    postoperative care and follow-up
      immobilization concerns, **VI:**713
      postoperative movement training,
        VI:713–714
      sensory re-education, **VI:**714
    postoperative dysfunction
      cold intolerance, **VI:**248–249, 717–718
      complex regional pain syndrome
        (CRPS), **VI:**717
      general considerations, **VI:**717
    sensory re-education
      cortical reorganization, **VI:**714
      phase 1, **VI:**714
      phase 2, **VI:**714, 715f
    surgical technique and treatment
      artificial conduits, **VI:**710–713
      donor nerves, **VI:**708–710
      immediate versus delayed repair,
        VI:703–704
      nerve reconstruction, **VI:**707–708
      nerve repair principles, **VI:**704–707
      tubular repair, **VI:**710–713
    tubular repair
      artificial conduits, **VI:**710–713
      biodegradable conduits, **VI:**712
      biological conduits, **VI:**711
      fillers, **VI:**713
      longitudinal resorbable sutures, **VI:**713
      nerve transfers, **VI:**713
      nondegradable conduits, **VI:**712, 713f
peripheral neuropathy, **I:**254–255
Perlane, **II:**45t, 47, 49t
  See also soft-tissue fillers
peroneal artery, **IV:**47f, 59–61, 61f–62f
peroneal nerve, **IV:**48t, 51f
peroneal retinaculum, **IV:**54, 54f, 54t
peroneus brevis (PB), **IV:**35f–36f
peroneus longus (PL), **IV:**35f–36f
peroneus tertius (PT), **IV:**35f–36f
persistent left superior vena cava syndrome,
  III:807t
Peterson fracture classification, **VI:**655, 655f
Petit, Jean, **IV:**393
Pfeiffer syndrome
  characteristics, **I:**197, 197f, 197t, **III:**749–750,
    750t

Note: **Boldface** roman numerals indicate volume. Page numbers followed by f refer to figures; page numbers followed by t refer to tables; page numbers followed by b refer to boxes.

Pfeiffer syndrome (Continued)
  patient presentation and diagnosis,
    III:688–689
  patient selection, III:752f
  thumb hypoplasia, VI:573t
PHACE association, I:681
phagocytosis, I:816
Phalen's test, VI:58, 58f
pharyngeal wall, III:432
pharyngocutaneous fistula, III:357
pharyngoesophageal reconstruction,
    III:336–359
  anatomical considerations, III:337, 337f–338f
  complications
    anastomotic strictures, III:357–358, 357f
    neck wound infection, III:358
    pharyngocutaneous fistula, III:357
  defect types, III:337t
  guidelines, III:336
  outcome assessments, III:356–357
  patient selection, III:337–339
  postoperative care and follow-up
    general postoperative care, III:354–355
    oral diet, III:355–356, 355f, 356t
    voice rehabilitation, III:356, 356f
  preoperative assessment
    donor site evaluation, III:338
    flaps
      advantages/disadvantages, III:339t
      selection guidelines, III:338–339, 339f
    medical evaluation, III:337–338
    radiotherapy and surgery history, III:338
  secondary procedures
    flap debulking, III:358
    tracheal stomaplasty, III:358, 358f
  surgical technique and treatment
    anterolateral thigh flap
      flap design and harvesting, III:339–341,
        340f–342f
      flap inset guidelines, III:342–347,
        343f–348f
      frozen neck, III:352–353
      isolated cervical esophageal defects,
        III:354
      oral diet, III:356t
      postlaryngectomy pharyngocutaneous
        fistulas, III:353–354, 353f–354f
      selection guidelines, III:338–339
    frozen neck, III:352–353
    isolated cervical esophageal defects,
      III:354
    jejunal flap
      flap harvesting, III:349–350, 349f–350f
      flap inset guidelines, III:350, 350f
      oral diet, III:356t
    postlaryngectomy pharyngocutaneous
      fistulas, III:353–354, 353f–354f
    radial forearm flap
      flap design, III:347, 348f
      flap harvesting, III:347–349, 348f–349f
      oral diet, III:356t
    recipient vessel selection, III:351–352,
      351f–352f, 351t
pharynx
  anatomical characteristics, III:337, 337f,
    422–423, 422f
  tumors, III:398–419
    complications
      dental follow-ups, III:418
      general discussion, III:416–418

pharynx (Continued)
      local recurrence, III:416
      osteoradionecrosis (ORN), III:417
      post-treatment surveillance, III:417–418
      regional recurrence, III:416–417
      wound infections, III:417
    epidemiology, III:399–400
    lymph node anatomy, III:399f
    medical challenges, III:398
    pathogenesis, III:398–399
    patient presentation and diagnosis,
      III:400
    surgical access, III:402, 403f–404f
    therapeutic choices, III:401–402
    TNM clinical classification system,
      III:400–401, 401t
phenol
  chemical injuries, IV:461–463
  phenol peels, II:67
phenotypic sex, IV:298, 298f
phentermine, II:635
Philoderm, II:47t
philtral column reconstruction, III:533,
  638–639, 639f
philtral dimple, III:556–557, 558f
philtrum, IV:498
phocomelia
  characteristics, VI:556, 556b
  outcomes and complicatons, VI:557
  pathogenesis, VI:556
  patient presentation and diagnosis, VI:556,
    556f
  patient selection, VI:556
  postoperative care and follow-up, VI:557
  secondary procedures, VI:557
  surgical technique and treatment,
    VI:556–557
phospholipase C (PLC), I:626f
phospholipids, I:243f
phosphorus (P)
  calcium phosphate (CaP), I:445
  metal alloy compositions, I:786–787
  potassium titanium oxide phosphate (KTP)
    lasers, II:67–70, 68f
  tricalcium phosphate, II:48t.
  see also soft-tissue fillers
  white phosphorus, IV:461–463
photodynamic therapy, I:206–207, II:69–70, 70f
photography, I:104–123
  functional role, I:104–106
  future trends
    three-dimensional (3D) imaging,
      I:121–122
    video records, I:122
  image capture standards
    composition and positioning
      abdomen, I:110, 115f–116f
      buttocks, I:110, 115f–116f
      chest and breasts, I:110, 113f–114f
      dental occlusal views, I:110
      ears, I:110
      eyes, I:107–108, 109f
      full face view, I:107, 108f
      glabella, I:108, 110f
      hands and feet, I:114, 118f
      lips, I:110, 112f
      lower extremity, I:112, 117f
      lower trunk, I:110, 115f–116f
      mentum, I:110, 112f
      nasolabial folds, I:110, 112f

photography (Continued)
      nose, I:108, 111f
      standard views, I:107, 108f
    digital image characteristics
      backgrounds, I:107
      inconsistencies and variabilities,
        I:106–107
      white balance, I:107
    key principles, I:106–117, 106b
  image management
    cameras, I:117–119
    formats
      file formats, I:120
      image attributes, I:120–121
      memory cards, I:119–120
      metadata, I:120–121
      retrieval, I:120–121
  image processing
    measurement and analysis, I:121
    planning and simulation, I:121
  photographic documentation
    abdominoplasty, II:536–537
    bilateral cleft lip, III:563
    blepharoplasty, II:121, 121b
    closed rhinoplasty, II:423
    craniofacial microsomia (CFM),
      III:773–774
    open rhinoplasty, II:389
  storage and preservation, I:105
photon therapy, I:655–656
Physician Quality Reporting Initiative, I:173
physiological wound dressings, IV:415–416
Pickerill, Henry, I:21–22
PICO approach, I:151
Pierre Robin sequence (PRS), III:803–827
  cleft palate surgery, III:572
  congenital hand deformities, VI:646, 646f
  gene therapy, I:193
  historical background, III:803–804
  laryngeal mask airway (LMA), III:808, 808f
  pathogenesis
    associated syndromes, III:804–808, 805f,
      807t
    cleft palate, III:804–808, 805f
    epidemiology, III:804–808
    etiology, III:805
    glossoptosis-retrognathia-airway
      obstruction triad, III:804
    tongue and palate embryology, III:805,
      806f
  patient presentation and diagnosis, III:808
  patient selection
    airway obstruction, III:810, 810f–812f
    feeding assessment, III:809–810
    initial interaction, III:808–810
    maxillary–mandibular discrepancy
      (MMD), III:808–809, 809f
    respiratory assessment, III:809
  secondary procedures, III:826
  skeletal class II malocclusions, III:665
  treatment strategies
    algorithmic approach, III:825f
    decision-making process, III:811–826
    floor of the mouth musculature, III:818–
      819, 820f
    Kirschner wires (K-wires), III:817, 818f
    mandibular distraction osteogenesis,
      III:819–824, 821f, 823f–824f
    nonsurgical airway management, III:813,
      813f

Pierre Robin sequence (PRS) *(Continued)*
nutritional deficit, **III:**824–826
otologic conditions, **III:**826
skeletal techniques, **III:**819–824, 820f–821f
soft-tissue techniques, **III:**815–819, 815f–817f
steel wire technique, **III:**818, 819f
surgical airway management, **III:**813–815, 814f
tensor fascia latae sling, **III:**817, 818f
tongue lip adhesion (TLA), **III:**815–819, 815f–817f
tongue position, **III:**812f
pigment cell nevus
acquired pigment cell nevus, **I:**724, 724f
characteristics, **I:**723–725
congenital pigment cell nevus, **I:**724, 725f
dysplastic nevus, **I:**724, **III:**113–114, 114f
juvenile melanoma, **I:**724–725, 726f
lentigo simplex, **I:**723–724, 724f
pigmented basal cell carcinoma, **I:**747–750, 748f
pigmented lesions
characteristics, **VI:**125
evaluation examinations, **I:**747–750
patient presentation and diagnosis, **VI:**125–126, 126f–127f
pigmented skin
care regimens, **II:**24
general discussion, **II:**24–26
melanosome transfer inhibitors
niacinamide, **II:**25
soy products, **II:**25–26
tyrosinase inhibitors
aloesin, **II:**24
arbutin, **II:**24–25
emblicanin, **II:**25
flavonoids, **II:**25
general discussion, **II:**24–25
hydroquinone, **II:**24
hydroxycoumarins, **II:**25
kojic acid, **II:**25
licorice extract, **II:**25
pigmented villonodular synovitis, **VI:**319, 319f
pilomatricoma, **I:**721–722, 721f
pilomatrixoma
characteristics, **I:**721–722, 721f, **III:**888
complications, **III:**888
disease process, **III:**888
patient presentation and diagnosis, **III:**888, 888f
postoperative care and follow-up, **III:**888
prognosis and outcomes, **III:**888
surgical technique and treatment, **III:**888
pimecrolimus, **II:**21t
pincer nails
characteristics, **VI:**126, 127f
surgical technique and treatment, **VI:**126–128
pisiformis gliding test, **VI:**55, 57f
Pitres–Testut sign, **VI:**58–59
Pittsburgh fistula classification system, **III:**642, 642t
Pittsburgh Rating Scale, **II:**535, **V:**559–560, 559t
pivot shift test maneuver, **VI:**63, 64f
Pixel CO₂ Omnifit™ laser, **II:**71t, 73
pixy ear, **II:**290–293, 292f
plagiocephaly, **III:**729, 729t

planimetric Z-plasty, **I:**314, 314f
plantar fascia, **IV:**54, 55f
plantar fibromatosis, **VI:**352, 352f
plasmacytosis, **I:**736
plasma factor, **I:**242–245, 243f
Plastic and Reconstructive Surgery Journal, **I:**24
platelet-derived growth factor (PDGF)
bone regeneration, **I:**435t, 438, 443t–444t
Dupuytren's disease, **VI:**349
gene therapy, **I:**189–190
osteoblasts, **I:**428
pedical flap viability augmentation, **I:**581–582
skin wound healing, **I:**268–269, 270t, 274
tissue expansion effects, **I:**625f
wound healing, **I:**234, **II:**62
platelet gels, **I:**793
platelet-rich fibrin matrix (PRFM), **II:**46
platelet-rich plasma (PRP), **I:**793
platinum (Pt), **I:**788
platysmal bands, **II:**37, 38f
pleomorphic adenomas
characteristics, **III:**366–367
classifications, **III:**365f
magnetic resonance imaging (MRI), **III:**364t
surgical technique and treatment, **III:**371–372, 372f–373f
pleural effusion, **IV:**433t
Pliny, the Elder, **IV:**393
Plummer–Vinson syndrome, **III:**398–399
pluripotent stem cells, **I:**213f, 261–264, 261f
PLX4032, **I:**783
pneumothorax, **IV:**433t
pogonion, **II:**356t, 363f
Poiseuille's law, **II:**452–453
Poland syndrome, **V:**548–557
breast reconstruction
congenital deformities, **V:**591
hypoplastic breast, **I:**648, 649f
skeletal support, **V:**5–6
characteristics, **III:**862–865, **V:**548
chest deformity classifications
general characteristics, **V:**550–554
group I patients
case study 1, **V:**550–551, 551f
general discussion, **V:**550–551
group II patients
basic procedure, **V:**551–552
case study 2, **V:**552, 553f–554f
group III patients
basic procedure, **V:**552–554
case study 3, **V:**552–554, 555f
clinical presentation and evaluation, **III:**863, 863f–864f
congenital deformities
breast reconstruction, **V:**591
hands, **VI:**644–647, 644f
epidemiology, **VI:**609
outcomes and complicatons, **VI:**610
pathogenesis, **V:**549, **VI:**609
patient presentation and diagnosis, **V:**549, **VI:**609–610, 609f
patient selection, **VI:**610
pectoralis major muscle, **V:**549, **VI:**609f
postoperative care and follow-up, **VI:**610
secondary procedures
alternative correction methods, **V:**557
general discussion, **VI:**610

Poland syndrome *(Continued)*
long-term adjustments, **V:**554–557
thoracic anomaly correction, **V:**556–557
surgical indicators, **III:**863
surgical technique and treatment
chest deformity classifications, **V:**550–554
general discussion, **VI:**610
long-term results, **V:**554
reconstruction options, **III:**864–865, 864f–865f
thoracic anomaly correction, **V:**549–550
thumb hypoplasia, **VI:**573t
pollex abductus, **VI:**578f, 590
pollicization technique
basic principles, **VI:**590
dissection and exposure, **VI:**590
general discussion, **VI:**590–594
incisions, **VI:**590, 592f–593f
operative technique, **VI:**591f–593f
outcomes and complicatons, **VI:**598
skeletal shortening, **VI:**594
skin closure and web construction, **VI:**594
tendon and intrinsic muscle rebalancing, **VI:**594
pollution exposure, **III:**421–422
polyacrylamide, **II:**48t
See also soft-tissue fillers
polyacrylamide hydrogel injections, **V:**100–101, 100f–101f
poly(β-hydroxybutyrate), **I:**376f
Polycleitus, **II:**354–365, 355f
polydactyly
associated syndromes, **VI:**617t
characteristics, **VI:**616, 639f
classification systems, **VI:**535–537, 535f–536f
epidemiology, **VI:**616
genetic considerations, **VI:**616–617
outcomes and complicatons, **VI:**622–623, 623f, 623t
pathogenesis, **VI:**616–617
patient presentation and diagnosis
central polydactyly, **VI:**546t, 618
radial polydactyly, **VI:**564–565, 617–618, 617f, 617t
ulnar polydactyly, **VI:**617t, 618
patient selection, **VI:**618
postaxial polydactyly, **VI:**546t
potassium titanium oxide phosphate (KTP) lasers, **VI:**622
secondary procedures, **VI:**623
surgical technique and treatment
central polydactyly, **VI:**622, 622f
mirror hand, **VI:**622
radial polydactyly
basic procedure, **VI:**619, 619b
Wassel type II technique, **VI:**619, 620f
Wassel type IV technique, **VI:**619, 621f
timing considerations, **VI:**619–622
ulnar polydactyly, **VI:**619–622, 621f
polydimethylsiloxane (PDMS), **I:**789t
polydioxanone, **I:**376f
poly(ε-caprolactone), **I:**376f
polyester, **I:**791
polyethylene, **I:**791, 791f, **II:**343
polyethylene-terephthalate, **IV:**239
poly(glycolic acid) (PGA)
cartilage engineering, **I:**413–419, 421–423
implant materials, **I:**791–792

*Note: **Boldface** roman numerals indicate volume. Page numbers followed by f refer to figures; page numbers followed by t refer to tables; page numbers followed by b refer to boxes.*

poly(glycolic acid) (PGA) (Continued)
 tendon substitutes/engineered tendons,
  I:352–353, 358f, 360f
 tissue engineering materials, I:375, 376f
poly(hydroxyvalerate), I:376f
poly(lactic acid) (PLA), I:375, 376f, 421–423,
  791–792
poly(lactic-co-glycolic acid) (PLGA), I:375,
  791–792
poly-L-lactic acid (PLLA), II:47t, 48
polymer implants
 biodegradable polymers, I:791–792
 characteristics, I:788–792
 polyester, I:791
 polyethylene, I:791, 791f
 polypropylene, I:791
 polytetrafluoroethylene (PTFE), I:790
 silicone, I:789–790, 789t, 790f, II:342
polymethylmethacrylate (PMMA), II:47t
poly(PCPP-SA anhydride), I:376f
Poly[(p-methyl phenoxy) (ethyl glycinato)
  phosphazene], I:376f
polypropylene, I:791, IV:239, 240f
polysorbate, IV:395
polytetrafluoroethylene (PTFE), I:790, II:305,
  IV:239, 240f, V:204, 515
polyvinyl alcohol, II:48t
 See also soft-tissue fillers
Poncirus trifoliate, V:33t–35t
poncitrin, V:33t–35t
popliteal artery, IV:45–48, 47f
popliteal pterygium syndrome, III:805–807,
  807t
popliteus, IV:35f–36f
porcine acellular dermal matrix (PADM), I:796
porcine skin xenografts, IV:410–415, 412t–414t
porion, II:356t, 363f
poroma folliculare, I:723
Porter's 5-Forces model of competition, I:66,
  66f
portwine stain, I:678t, 734, 734f–735f, VI:668t
 See also capillary malformations (CM)
positive transference, I:33
positron emission tomography (PET)
 cutaneous and soft-tissue tumors, I:710
 head and neck cancer detection, III:418
 melanoma detection, I:762–764, 763f
postanal pits, III:874
postaxial acrofacial dysostosis, III:807t
postaxial polydactyly, VI:546t
post-bariatric surgery reconstruction,
  II:634–654
 arm contouring
  demand increases, V:558–564
  outcomes and complicatons, V:563–564
  pathophysiology, V:558–559
  patient presentation and diagnosis,
   V:559–564
  patient selection, V:559–560
  Pittsburgh Rating Scale, V:559–560, 559t
  postoperative care and follow-up,
   V:562–563
  surgical technique and treatment,
   V:560–562, 561f–563f, 562b
 back contouring
  back rolls, V:570–573
  outcomes and complicatons, V:573
  pathophysiology, V:570–571
  patient presentation and diagnosis, V:571
  patient selection, V:571–572

post-bariatric surgery reconstruction
  (Continued)
  postoperative care and follow-up, V:573
  surgical planning, V:571–572
  surgical technique and treatment, V:572,
   573f
  surgical tips, V:572b
  transverse excisional upper bodylift,
   V:570f, 572
 body contouring centers of excellence,
  II:653
 complications, II:653
 gynecomastia/male chest contouring
  excision of gynecomastia with nipple
   repositioning, V:575–579, 578f–580f
  outcomes and complicatons, V:579
  pathophysiology, V:573–574
  patient presentation and diagnosis, V:574
  patient selection, V:574–575, 575t
  postoperative care and follow-up, V:578
  pseudogynecomastia, V:575t, 576f–577f
  surgical markings, V:575–576, 576f–577f
  surgical technique and treatment,
   V:576–578, 578f–580f
  surgical tips, V:578b
 mastopexy
  breast reshaping, V:564–570
  dermal suspension, V:566–570, 568f
  outcomes and complicatons, V:567–570
  pathophysiology, V:564, 564b
  patient presentation and diagnosis,
   V:564–565
  patient selection, V:565–566
  postoperative care and follow-up, V:567
  surgical goals, V:565b
  surgical planning, V:565–566, 566t,
   569f–570f
  surgical tips, V:567b
  total parenchymal reshaping mastopexy
   surgical markings, V:566
   surgical technique and treatment,
    V:566–567, 568f
 patient presentation and diagnosis
  patient history, II:636–637
  physical examination, II:637
  preoperative assessment, II:637
  preoperative counseling and education,
   II:637–638
 patient selection
  body contouring, II:638, 638t
  body mass index (BMI), II:638–639
  intraoperative procedures, II:638–639,
   638t
  patient safety, II:638–639, 638t
  psychological considerations, II:638
 secondary procedures, II:653
 staging and combination procedures, II:653
 surgical technique
  abdominal contouring
   giant pannus, II:640–643, 643f–644f
   hidden penis, II:640, 643f
   major weight loss (MWL) patient,
    II:639b
   mons correction, II:640, 641f–642f
   operative planning and technique,
    II:639–640
   patient evaluation, II:639
   surgical variations, II:640–643,
    640f–641f
  arms, II:652

post-bariatric surgery reconstruction
  (Continued)
  breast, II:652
  lower bodylift (LBL)/buttock contouring
   major weight loss (MWL) patient,
    II:644b
   markings, II:645, 646f–647f, 649f
   operative technique, II:645, 647f–649f
   patient evaluation, II:644–645
   patient selection, II:645
   postoperative care and follow-up,
    II:645
  male chest, II:652
  trunk, II:652
  upper extremities, II:652
  vertical thigh-lift
   complications, II:652
   major weight loss (MWL) patient,
    II:648b
   markings, II:649–652, 650f
   operative technique, II:651f–652f, 652
   patient evaluation, II:645–648
   patient selection, II:648–649
   postoperative care and follow-up,
    II:652
posterior circumflex humeral artery, IV:225–
  227, 226f
posterior interosseous nerve (PIN)
  compression
  anatomical considerations, VI:517
  posterior interosseous nerve (PIN)
   syndrome, VI:517
  radial tunnel syndrome
   nonsurgical management, VI:518
   outcomes and complicatons, VI:518
   patient presentation and diagnosis,
    VI:518
   surgical technique and treatment, VI:518,
    519f
posterior interosseous nerve (PIN) syndrome,
  VI:517
posterior pharyngeal flap, III:625–626, 626f
posterior pharyngeal wall augmentation,
  III:628
posterior plagiocephaly, III:729–731, 731f, 731t
posterior thigh flap, IV:390
posterior tibial artery, IV:47f, 59
posterolateral rotatory instability (PLRI),
  VI:63
postlaryngectomy pharyngocutaneous
  fistulas, III:353–354, 353f–354f
postmastectomy breast reconstruction
  basic principles, I:640–647
  chest wall irradiated areas, I:645–647
  complications
   clinical studies, V:362, 363t
   expander failure or malfunction, V:360f
   infections, V:361–363
   skin necrosis, V:360f
  expander device, I:642–643, V:292f
  expander-implants
   adjustable, permanent expander-implants,
    V:366–367
   average operative time, V:364t
   basic procedure, V:338–340
   breast envelope preservation, V:367–368
   capsular contracture, V:362, 362t–364t
   cellulitis, V:359, 360f
   clinical studies, V:362, 363t
   complication frequency, V:363–365, 364t

postmastectomy breast reconstruction (Continued)
  complications, **V:**359
  delayed reconstruction, **V:**342f, 358, 359f
  erythema, **V:**359
  evaluation studies, **V:**365
  expander failure or malfunction, **V:**360–361, 360f–361f, 364t
  fat injections, **V:**365, 368
  flap-based reconstruction, **V:**367
  hematomas, **V:**359, 359f, 364t
  implant malposition, **V:**363t
  implant removal, **V:**363t
  implant rupture and deflation, **V:**361–362, 363t
  infections, **V:**361–363, 363t–364t
  insertion procedures, **V:**353–354
  outcome assessments, **V:**363–365
  persistent serous drainage, **V:**359–360
  postoperative care and follow-up, **V:**358–359
  preoperative/postoperative comparisons, **V:**340f–341f
  secondary procedures
    cosmetic revision surgery, **V:**365, 366f
    fat injections, **V:**365, 368
    nipple reconstruction, **V:**365–366
  skin necrosis, **V:**360, 360f, 363t
  wrinkle formation, **V:**363t
immediate postmastectomy breast reconstruction
  acellular allogenic dermal matrix (ADM), **I:**644–645, 644f
  basic procedure, **V:**287–291
  breast implants, **V:**353
  deep inferior epigastric perforator (DIEP) flaps, **V:**288f
  expander-implant insertion, **V:**353–354, 354f
  latissimus dorsi (LD) flap, **V:**288, 289f–290f
  muscle coverage, **I:**643–645
  prosthesis insertion
    basic procedure, **V:**356–358
    capsulectomy, **V:**357f
    contralateral adjustments, **V:**356–358
    inframammary fold reconstruction, **V:**357f
    large breast augmentation, **V:**358
    medium breast augmentation, **V:**357–358
    small breast augmentation, **V:**356–357
  radiation therapy (RT), **V:**290
  second-stage surgery, **V:**356, 357f
  skin reducing mastectomy, **V:**354–356, 355f
  submuscular position, **I:**643–644
  subpectoral (dual-plane) position, **I:**644
  transverse rectus abdominis myocutaneous (TRAM) flaps, **V:**288f
outcomes and complicatons
  cellulitis, **V:**359, 360f
  erythema, **V:**359
  expander failure or malfunction, **V:**360–361, 361f
  hematomas, **V:**359, 359f
  persistent serous drainage, **V:**359–360
  skin necrosis, **V:**360

postmastectomy breast reconstruction (Continued)
  patient presentation and diagnosis
    exclusion criteria, **V:**345–346, 347f
    inclusion criteria
      contralateral adjustments, **V:**346
      large breast reconstruction, **V:**346, 350f
      medium breast reconstruction, **V:**346, 349f
      small breast reconstruction, **V:**346, 348f
  postoperative care and follow-up, **V:**358–359
  reconstructive paradigms
    contralateral adjustments, **V:**343f
    cosmetic breast reconstruction, **V:**344f–345f
    indications and contraindications, **V:**343f
    mastectomy techniques, **V:**343f
    radiation therapy (RT), **V:**347f
    surgical strategy, **V:**340–344
  secondary breast reconstruction, **I:**645, 646f
  surgical technique and treatment
    delayed reconstruction, **V:**291–292, 291f–292f, 358, 359f
    expander-implant insertion, **V:**353–354, 354f
    immediate postmastectomy breast reconstruction, **V:**353
    prosthesis insertion
      basic procedure, **V:**356–358
      capsulectomy, **V:**357f
      contralateral adjustments, **V:**356–358
      inframammary fold reconstruction, **V:**357f
      large breast augmentation, **V:**358
      medium breast augmentation, **V:**357–358
      small breast augmentation, **V:**356–357
    second-stage surgery, **V:**356, 357f
    skin reducing mastectomy, **V:**354–356, 355f
    tissue preservation, **V:**353–358
postnatal and somatic stem cells
  adipose-derived stem/stromal cells (ASCs)
    cell surface receptors, **I:**219–220, 219f–220f
    characteristics, **I:**217–218, 217f
    delivery methods, **I:**220
    fat grafting, **I:**345f–347f, 346–347, **II:**327–328
    harvesting methods, **I:**218–219, 218f
    induced pluripotent stem cells, **I:**236
    in vitro differentiation protocols
      adipogenic differentiation, **I:**221, 222f
      chondrogenic differentiation, **I:**221
      osteogenic differentiation, **I:**220–221, 221f
    in vivo model
      clinical correlates, **I:**223
      future trends, **I:**223, 224f–225f
      nude athymic mouse 4-mm calvarial defect, **I:**221–223, 222f
    mouse versus human ASCs, **I:**219
    tissue engineering, **I:**369–371
  bone marrow-derived mesenchymal stem cells (BMSC)
    clinical correlates, **I:**228
    current research and applications, **I:**224–226
    definitions, **I:**223–224

postnatal and somatic stem cells (Continued)
    in vitro tissue harvest and differentiation protocols, **I:**226
    in vivo models, **I:**226–228
    current research
      cell surface receptors, **I:**219–220, 219f–220f
      delivery methods, **I:**220
      mouse versus human ASCs, **I:**219
    in vitro differentiation protocols
      adipogenic differentiation, **I:**221, 222f
      chondrogenic differentiation, **I:**221
      osteogenic differentiation, **I:**220–221, 221f
    in vivo model
      clinical correlates, **I:**223
      future trends, **I:**223, 224f–225f
      nude athymic mouse 4-mm calvarial defect, **I:**221–223, 222f
    tissue-specific stem cells
      clinical correlates
        blood vessels, **I:**232
        muscles, **I:**232
        osteoblast differentiation, **I:**232
        peripheral nerve repair, **I:**233
        skin regeneration, **I:**232
      current research and applications
        blood vessels, **I:**230, 231f
        muscles, **I:**230–231, 231f
        osteoblast differentiation, **I:**230, 230f
        peripheral nerve repair, **I:**231–232, 231f
        skin regeneration, **I:**229, 229f
      definitions, **I:**228–229
postoperative rhinitis, **II:**454
post-rhinoplasty fibrotic syndrome, **II:**482, 483f
post-rhinoplasty red nose, **II:**446
posttraumatic enophthalmos, **III:**234–235, 237f
posttraumatic stress disorder (PTSD), **VI:**246
postwar aesthetic surgery, **I:**28
postwar plastic surgery, **I:**25, 25f–26f
potassium titanium oxide phosphate (KTP) lasers, **II:**67–70, 68f
power-assisted liposuction (PAL), **II:**507–508, 518, 520
Prader–Willi syndrome, **I:**183
Predictive Salvage Index (PSI), **IV:**63
prefabricated/prelaminated flaps, **I:**612–613
prekallikrein, **I:**243f, 244
prelaminated and prefabricated flaps, **I:**530–531
pre-market approval application (PMA), **I:**847–849
pre-market notification (PMN), **I:**847–849
premasseter space, **II:**84, 84f, 90f
prenatal diagnosis
  functional role, **I:**198–199
  invasive testing, **I:**199
  ultrasonography, **I:**198
pressure garments, **IV:**426f, 509
pressure sores, **IV:**352–382
  anatomic distribution, **IV:**353
  basic principles
    excess moisture effects, **IV:**355, 362t–363t
    friction effects, **IV:**354, 355f, 362t–363t
    malnutrition, **IV:**355, 362t–363t
    neurological injuries, **IV:**355–356
    pressure effects, **IV:**353–354, 354f–355f
    shear, **IV:**354–355, 355f, 362t–363t
    spinal cord injuries, **IV:**355–356

pressure sores *(Continued)*
  complications, **IV:**379
  diagnosis
    classification systems, **IV:**356, 356f–358f
    Jamshidi core needle bone biopsy,
      IV:358–360, 361f
    osteomyelitis, **IV:**357–360, 359f–360f
    patient evaluation, **IV:**356–357
    psychological evaluation, **IV:**360
  economic factors, **IV:**353
  epidemiology, **IV:**352–353
  ischial pressure sores, **IV:**372t
  myocutaneous gluteal rotation flap
    basic procedure, **IV:**370–375, 371f
    girdlestone arthroplasty, **IV:**376f
    ischial pressure sores, **IV:**372–373, 372t
    surgical guidelines, **IV:**372b
    trochanteric ulcers, **IV:**373–375, 375t,
      376f
    V-Y hamstring advancement, **I:**562–565,
      566f, 568f, **IV:**373, 374f
    V-Y tensor fasciae latae flap, **IV:**375, 377f
  nonhealing wounds, **I:**279
  outcome assessments, **IV:**379
  patient selection, **IV:**360–361
  postoperative care and follow-up, **IV:**378,
    378f
  seat mapping, **IV:**378f
  secondary procedures, **IV:**380, 380f–382f
  terminology, **IV:**352
  treatment strategies
    incontinence, **IV:**363–364
    muscle/musculocutaneous flaps,
      I:562–565, 564f–568f
    myocutaneous gluteal rotation flap
      basic procedure, **IV:**370–375, 371f
      girdlestone arthroplasty, **IV:**376f
      ischial pressure sores, **IV:**372–373,
        372t
      surgical guidelines, **IV:**372b
      trochanteric ulcers, **IV:**373–375, 375t,
        376f
      V-Y hamstring advancement, **I:**562–565,
        566f, 568f, **IV:**373, 374f
      V-Y tensor fasciae latae flap, **IV:**375,
        377f
    nonsurgical management
      dressings and wound care, **IV:**366–367,
        367f
      infection, **IV:**366
      malnutrition, **IV:**366
      negative pressure wound therapy
        (NPWT), **IV:**367
      osteomyelitis, **IV:**366
      pressure relief, **IV:**366
      spasticity, **IV:**366
      spontaneous healing, **IV:**366–367
    nutrition, **IV:**362t–363t, 366
    pressure relief
      buttock–cushion interface, **IV:**365f
      fluidized beds, **IV:**364f
      low air loss mattress concept, **IV:**364f
      low-pressure/alternating-pressure
        surfaces, **IV:**364f
      support surfaces, **IV:**364–366, 378, 378f
      wheelchairs, **IV:**365f
    prevention, **IV:**361
    procedure selection
      free flaps, **IV:**368–369
      muscle flaps, **IV:**368

pressure sores *(Continued)*
      musculocutaneous flaps, **I:**562–565,
        IV:368
      perforator flaps, **IV:**368
      selection guidelines, **IV:**368–369
      tissue expansion, **IV:**369
    risk assessments, **IV:**361, 362t–363t
    skin care, **IV:**362–363, 362b
    spasticity, **IV:**364
    surgical treatment
      anatomic site-based reconstruction,
        IV:369–370, 370t
      bone resection, **IV:**375–376
      debridement, **IV:**367–368, 368f
      myocutaneous gluteal rotation flap,
        IV:370–375
      procedure selection, **IV:**368–369
      single- versus multiple-stage
        reconstruction, **IV:**369
      surgical guidelines, **IV:**367
Pressure-Specified Sensory Device (PSSD),
  IV:154, 158f
pressure ulcers, **I:**255–256, 279
Prevelle Silk, **II:**47
prezygomatic space, **II:**84, 84f, 90f
prilocaine, **VI:**96t
primary bone repair, **I:**439, 439f–440f
printed textbooks, **I:**15
privacy law, **I:**94
procaine, **VI:**96t
procerus, **II:**110–111, 110f, **III:**15
ProDigits, **I:**858–861, 861f
product liability, **I:**95
professional associations
  Code of Ethics, **I:**57–58
  ethics complaints, **I:**57t
profitability ratios, **I:**69
profit/loss statements, **I:**67, 70f
PROfractional™ laser, **II:**71t, 73
profunda femoris, **IV:**22–23
profunda femoris perforating branches, **IV:**25,
  26f
progesterone receptor (PR), **V:**266–267
progressive hemifacial atrophy (PHA),
  III:792–802
  causal factors, **III:**792
  clinical manifestations
    central nervous system involvement,
      III:796
    cutaneous and subcutaneous tissue
      involvement, **III:**794–795, 795f
    general characteristics, **III:**794–797, 794f
    musculoskeletal involvement, **III:**795
    ocular involvement, **III:**796
    oral involvement, **III:**796–797, 796f
  complications, **III:**800–801
  differential diagnoses, **III:**797, 797f
  epidemiology, **III:**794
  etiopathogenesis
    autoimmune process, **III:**793
    general discussion, **III:**793–794
    histologic studies, **III:**793
    infection hypothesis, **III:**794
    neurogenic manifestations, **III:**793
    trauma-acquired defects, **III:**794
  laboratory studies, **III:**797
  patient selection and treatment, **III:**792–793
  prognosis and outcomes, **III:**800–801
  prognostic indicators, **III:**797
  secondary procedures, **III:**801–802

progressive hemifacial atrophy (PHA)
  (Continued)
  surgical technique and treatment
    immunosuppressive therapy, **III:**797–798,
      798f
    nonsurgical interventions, **III:**798
    surgical intervention
      basic principles, **III:**798–800, 800f–802f
      scapular and parascapular flaps,
        III:799–800, 800f
progress zone (PZ), **VI:**527, 529f
projection, **I:**32
Prolene mesh, **V:**404–405, 405f
proliferating epidermal cyst, **I:**720
prolonged edema, **II:**411
prolonged erythema, **II:**77
prominent ear
  antihelical fold restoration, **III:**206–207
  conchal alteration, **III:**206
  lateral cartilage surface alteration, **III:**207
  medial cartilage surface alteration, **III:**207
  pathology, **III:**204–206, 208f
  treatment strategies, **III:**206
pronasale, **II:**356t
pronator syndrome, **VI:**510
pro-opiomelanocortin (POMC), **I:**284–285
prophylactic mastectomy, **V:**284
propofol, **I:**139
prostacyclin, **I:**573–574, 574f
prostaglandin E_1 (PGE$_1$), **I:**433, 617
prostaglandin E_2 (PGE$_2$), **I:**626f
prostate surgery, **I:**863–864
prosthetics
  congenital transverse arrest, **VI:**553
  ear reconstruction, **III:**217
  facial burn wound treatment, **IV:**485
  metacarpophalangeal (MCP) joint arthritis
    hinged prostheses, **VI:**426
    silicone constrained prostheses, **VI:**426,
      427f
    surface replacement prostheses,
      VI:426–427
  thumb arthroplasty, **VI:**440–441, 440f
  upper extremity amputees, **VI:**870–880
    aesthetic prostheses, **VI:**870, 871f
    body-powered prostheses, **VI:**870–871
    control mechanisms, **VI:**870–871
    general characteristics, **VI:**870
    prosthetics–composite tissue
      allotransplantation (CTA)
      comparisons, **VI:**879–880
    residual limb surgery
      neuroma management, **VI:**876
      soft-tissue improvement, **VI:**875–876,
        875f–876f
      targeted muscle reinnervation (TMR),
        VI:871, 876–879
    surgery–prosthesis considerations
      elbow disarticulation/long
        transhumeral amputation,
        VI:874–875
      finger amputation, **VI:**872, 872f
      general discussion, **VI:**872–875
      partial hand, **VI:**872, 873f
      shoulder disarticulation/proximal
        transhumeral amputation,
        VI:875
      wrist disarticulation/transradial
        amputation, **VI:**873–874,
        873f–874f

prosthetics (Continued)
  targeted muscle reinnervation (TMR)
    characteristics, VI:876–879
    myoelectric prostheses, VI:871
    shoulder disarticulation level,
      VI:877–879, 878f–879f, 879t
    transhumeral level, VI:876–877,
      876f–877f
    transradial level, VI:879
proteases, I:269–271
Protected Health Information (PHI), I:121
protein kinase A (PKA), I:626f
protein kinase C (PKC), I:624–626
Proteus spp., I:249–250
Proteus syndrome
  characteristics, VI:635
  classification systems, VI:668–669, 668t
prothrombin, I:243f, 268–269
proton therapy, I:655–656
providers and third-party payers, I:61–62
provisionally unique vascular anomalies
  (PUVA), VI:668–669
provisional patents, I:846–847
proximal amputations, VI:238–241, 238f–240f
proximal commissural ligament, VI:347,
  347f–348f
proximal interphalangeal (PIP) joint
  Dupuytren's disease, VI:346–348, 349t,
    351–353, 355f
  fractures and joint injuries, VI:138–139,
    142–143, 143f
  osteoarthritis
    management approaches, VI:417–418
    prevalence and characteristics,
      VI:417–425
    proximal interphalangeal (PIP)
      arthrodesis
      fixation techniques, VI:418–419
      fusion approach, VI:418–419, 418f
  proximal interphalangeal (PIP) arthrodesis
    fixation techniques
      basic procedure, VI:418–419
      compression screws, VI:419, 419f–420f
      crossed K-wire technique, VI:418
      mini-plates, VI:419, 419f
      tension band wire technique,
        VI:418–419
    fusion approach, VI:418–419, 418f
  proximal interphalangeal (PIP) arthroplasty
    basic principles, VI:419–422
    outcomes and complicatons, VI:424–425
    postoperative therapy, VI:422–424, 424f
    silicone interposition arthroplasty, VI:420,
      421f
    surface replacement arthroplasty with
      nonconstrained implants
      developmental background, VI:420–422
      nonconstrained or semi-constrained
        techniques, VI:422, 422f–423f
      patient selection, VI:421–422
  stiff hand, VI:449–466
    collateral ligament changes, VI:454, 454f
    extension contracture
      bone, VI:451–452, 451f
      capsular and pericapsular structures,
        VI:451
      collateral ligaments, VI:451
      dorsal capsule, VI:451

proximal interphalangeal (PIP) joint
  (Continued)
    flexor tendon adherence, VI:451
    intrinsic muscles, VI:451
    long extensors, VI:451
    patient presentation, VI:450–452, 450f
    skin, VI:450–451
    transverse retinacular ligaments, VI:451
    volar plate, VI:451
  flexion contracture
    accessory ligaments, VI:450
    bone, VI:450
    capsular and pericapsular structures,
      VI:449–450
    collateral ligaments, VI:449
    dorsal adhesions, VI:450
    intrinsic tendons, VI:450
    patient presentation, VI:449–450, 450f
    transverse retinacular ligaments,
      VI:450
    volar plate, VI:450
  general discussion, VI:449
  outcomes and complicatons, VI:458–459
  pathogenesis, VI:454–455, 457f
  patient presentation and diagnosis,
    VI:449–454
  patient selection, VI:455–456, 458f
  postoperative care and follow-up, VI:458
  secondary procedures, VI:459
  seesaw effect, VI:452–454, 452f–453f
  surgical technique and treatment
    nonsurgical management, VI:456–458
    proximal interphalangeal (PIP) joint
      extension contracture, VI:457
    proximal interphalangeal (PIP) joint
      flexion contracture, VI:456–457
    volar plate changes, VI:454, 455f–456f
proximal transhumeral amputation, VI:875
Pruzansky classification of mandibular
  deformity, III:772–773, 772t, 773f
psaos major muscle, IV:15t–16t, 18f, 20f–22f
pseudoaneurysms, IV:433t, VI:324, 325f
pseudogout, VI:335
pseudogynecomastia, V:575t, 576f–577f
Pseudomonas aeruginosa, I:249–250, IV:86–87,
  428f, 513–514
psoriasis, VI:337
psoriatic arthritis, VI:406–408, 407t
psychological aspects, I:30–54
  body image
    definition, I:30–31
    developmental stages
      adolescence, I:31
      early childhood, I:31
      older adults, I:31
      school-age children, I:31
    emotional response and behavior, I:31
    plastic surgery effects, I:31–32
  character formation, I:32–33
  childhood plastic surgeries
    acquired and congenital defects, I:44
    adolescent aesthetic surgery, I:45–46, 45t
    craniofacial deformities, I:44–45
  defense mechanisms, I:32–33
  difficult patients
    dependent clingers, I:37
    entitled demanders, I:38
    hateful patients, I:36–37

psychological aspects (Continued)
    manipulative help-rejecting complainers,
      I:38–39
    self-destructive deniers, I:37–38
  dissatisfied patients, I:52, 53b
  patient selection
    general risk factors, I:46–47
    psychiatric syndromes
      body dysmorphic disorder (BDD),
        I:50–51, 50b
      depressive disorders, I:47–48, 48b
      eating disorders, I:49–50
      generalized anxiety and panic
        disorders, I:48–49, 48b–49b
      substance abuse, I:50
      violent behavior, I:51–52
    risk assessments, I:47b
  perioperative psychological reactions, I:33
  personality styles/personality disorders
    borderline personality disorder, I:36
    characteristics, I:34–36
    dependent personality, I:35
    histrionic personality, I:36
    narcissistic personality, I:35
    obsessive-compulsive personality, I:34–35
    paranoid personality disorder, I:35–36
  personality traits, I:32–33
  physician–patient relationship, I:33–34
  psychological contraindications, I:52, 52b
  research summary, I:53
  surgical procedures
    aesthetic facial surgery, I:39
    augmentation mammaplasty, I:40–41
    cancer and reconstruction
      breast cancer, I:43
      head and neck cancer, I:43–44
      reduction mammaplasty, I:41–42
    rhinoplasty, I:39–40
    trauma-acquired defects
      burns, I:42–43
      hand transplantation, I:42
PTEN hamartoma-tumor syndrome (PHTS),
  I:704–705, VI:669, 690
PTEN (phosphatase and tensin homologue)-
  associated vascular anomaly (PTEN-AVA)
  classification systems, I:677t
  pathogenesis, I:697f, 704–705, VI:690
  patient presentation and diagnosis, VI:690
  surgical technique and treatment, VI:690
pterygium, VI:122–123
pterygium syndrome (PPS), I:195
pterygomasseteric sling, III:16
pTNM clinical classification system, I:711,
  712f–714f, 715b
PubMed, I:151
pulmonary cavity, I:552–553
pulmonary embolisms, I:781t, II:525–527, 591,
  593–594, IV:433t
pulsed dye lasers, II:21t, 67–70, IV:484, 484f
punctures, I:241, 241f
Puragen, II:47t, 49t
  See also soft-tissue fillers
pygopagus twins, III:893–897, 894f, 896f–898f
pyoderma gangrenosum, VI:335–336, 336f
pyogenic flexor tenosynovitis, VI:339, 340f
pyogenic granuloma
  classification systems, I:677t, VI:668t
  clinical manifestations, I:688

pyogenic granuloma *(Continued)*
  hands
    infection mimics, **VI:**335, 335f
    surgical technique and treatment,
      VI:324–326, 325f
  pathogenesis, **VI:**674
  patient presentation and diagnosis,
    I:747–750, 748f, **VI:**675, 677f
  surgical technique and treatment, **VI:**675
pyridoxine, **I:**282
PyroCarbon arthroplasty, **VI:**427–429, 440f

Q

Q-switched alexandrite laser, **I:**718, 725–726,
  II:68, **III:**30, **IV:**454, 454t
quadrilateral space syndrome
  anatomical considerations, **VI:**523, 523f
  etiology, **VI:**523
  patient presentation and diagnosis, **VI:**523
  patient selection, **VI:**523
  surgical technique and treatment, **VI:**524
quality-adjusted life years (QALYs), **I:**164–165
quality of life (QoL) measures, **I:**161–162

R

rachipagus twins, **III:**896f–898f
radial forearm flap
  burn wound treatment, **IV:**421f
  cheek reconstruction, **III:**274
  clinical application, **I:**532f
  foot reconstruction, **IV:**211, 214f
  lip reconstruction, **III:**267–268, 267f–268f
  mangled upper extremities, **VI:**266–267,
    267f–269f
  oral cavity and mouth reconstruction,
    III:311f, 319–320
  palatal fistula repair, **III:**644
  phalloplasty
    exstrophy and epispadias, **IV:**303f
    general discussion, **IV:**318–323
    operative technique, **IV:**318, 319f–320f,
      324f–325f
    research summary, **IV:**322–323
    severe penile insufficiency, **IV:**304–306
    surgical goals
      aesthetic phallus, **IV:**319, 320f
      donor site considerations, **IV:**321, 321f
      ideal goals, **IV:**318–322
      minimal morbidity, **IV:**321
      normal scrotum, **IV:**321, 322f
      one-stage procedure, **IV:**319
      sexual intercourse, **IV:**321–322, 322f
      tactile and erogenous sensation,
        IV:319–321
      voiding while standing, **IV:**321
  pharyngoesophageal reconstruction
    flap design, **III:**347, 348f
    flap harvesting, **III:**347–349, 348f–349f
    oral diet, **III:**356t
  scalp and forehead reconstruction,
    III:128–130, 129f
  tongue reconstruction, **III:**309t–310t
radial hypoplasia/aplasia
  characteristics, **VI:**557, 557b
  classification systems, **VI:**558t, 559f
  outcomes and complicatons, **VI:**563
  pathogenesis, **VI:**557–558
  patient presentation and diagnosis,
    VI:558–560, 558f–559f
  patient selection, **VI:**560

radial hypoplasia/aplasia *(Continued)*
  postoperative care and follow-up, **VI:**563
  secondary procedures, **VI:**563
  surgical technique and treatment
    basic procedure, **VI:**560–563
    carpal tunnel slot, **VI:**560f, 562f
    centralization, **VI:**562f
    dorsoradial muscle transfer, **VI:**561f
    growth discrepancies, **VI:**562f
    K-wire fixation, **VI:**561f
    post-wrist stabilization, **VI:**562f
    radialization, **VI:**562f
    soft tissue distraction, **VI:**560f
    soft tissue release, **VI:**561f
    timing considerations, **VI:**546t, 547f
radial longitudinal deficiency, **VI:**546t, 547f
radial nerve palsy
  outcomes and complicatons, **VI:**752–753
  patient selection, **VI:**747–752, 747f
  surgical technique and treatment
    basic procedure, **VI:**748, 748t
    Boyes superficialis transfer, **VI:**748t,
      750–752, 752f
    flexor carpi radialis transfer, **VI:**748t,
      749–750, 752f
    standard flexor carpi ulnaris transfer,
      VI:748–749, 748f–751f, 748t
radial polydactyly
  characteristics, **VI:**616, 617t
  patient presentation and diagnosis,
    VI:564–565, 617–618, 617f
  surgical technique and treatment
    basic procedure, **VI:**619, 619b
    Wassel type II technique, **VI:**619, 620f
    Wassel type IV technique, **VI:**619, 621f
radial tunnel syndrome
  nonsurgical management, **VI:**518
  outcomes and complicatons, **VI:**518
  patient presentation and diagnosis, **VI:**518
  surgical technique and treatment, **VI:**518,
    519f
radiation injuries, **I:**281
radiation therapy (RT), **I:**654–675
  basic principles
    brachytherapy, **I:**656–657
    particle therapy, **I:**655–656
    physics concepts
      characteristics, **I:**657–659
      depth dose distribution, **I:**657f
      intensity-modulated radiation therapy
        (IMRT), **I:**658, 659f
      multileaf collimators (MLCs), **I:**658,
        658f
      photon interactions, **I:**657f
    radiation technology, **I:**655
    radiobiology
      normal tissue complications, **I:**659–662,
        660f
      radiation toxicity, **I:**660, 661f–662f
      tumor response, **I:**659–662, 660f
    voltage therapy, **I:**655
  bone remodeling effects, **I:**448
  breast reconstruction considerations
    breast implants, **V:**347f
    free TRAM flap, **V:**415–416
    immediate postmastectomy breast
      reconstruction, **V:**290
    latissimus dorsi (LD) flap, **V:**376–378,
      376f–379f
  cutaneous and soft-tissue tumors, **I:**717

radiation therapy (RT) *(Continued)*
  future trends, **I:**674
  general discussion, **I:**654–655
  radiation treatment
    benign disorders, **I:**671
    breast cancer
      breast conservation, **I:**665
      chemotherapy sequencing, **I:**668
      immediate postmastectomy breast
        reconstruction, **V:**290
      nodal draining area irradiation,
        I:665–666
      postmastectomy radiation (PMRT),
        I:665
      radiotherapy techniques, **I:**666–668,
        666f–667f
      research background, **I:**664–668
    clinical applications
      patient selection, **I:**664, 664b
      treatment intent, **I:**664
      units of radiation, **I:**664
    head and neck cancer, **I:**668–669
    melanoma, **I:**778
    nonmelanoma skin cancers, **I:**670–671
    planning and process, **I:**662–664, 663f
    sarcomas, **IV:**106
    soft-tissue sarcomas, **I:**669–670
  research summary, **I:**674
  toxicities and complications
    accidental and occupational radiation
      exposure, **I:**673–674
    bony injuries, **I:**671–672
    lymphedema, **I:**672
    pediatric bone development, **I:**672
    radiation-induced malignancies, **I:**673
radical mastectomies, **I:**202, 203f
Radiesse, **II:**47–48, 47t, 49t
  See also soft-tissue fillers
radiobiology
  normal tissue complications, **I:**659–662,
    660f
  radiation toxicity, **I:**660, 661f–662f
  tumor response, **I:**659–662, 660f
radiographic imaging
  general discussion, **VI:**68
  hands and wrists
    general discussion, **VI:**68–76
    hand evaluation
      basic procedure, **VI:**69–70
      carpometacarpal joints (CMCJs),
        VI:69–70, 70f–71f
      osteoarthritis, **VI:**71f
      osteomyelitis, **VI:**70f
      pathological fractures, **VI:**70f
      pediatric hand radiographs, **VI:**71–72,
        72f–73f
      positioning, **VI:**69f
      soft-tissue mass, **VI:**69f
      special views, **VI:**70–71, 72b, 72f
      trapeziometacarpal joint (TMCJ),
        VI:70–71, 72b, 72f
    wrist evaluation
      assessment criteria, **VI:**73b
      basic procedure, **VI:**72–76
      carpal height ratio, **VI:**74f
      carpal indices, **VI:**79f
      carpal tunnel view, **VI:**78f
      distal radioulnar joint (DRUJ)
        instability, **VI:**75f
      distal radius fracture, **VI:**75f

radiographic imaging (Continued)
    dorsal intercalated segmental
        instability, **VI:**78f
    dynamic scapholunate instability,
        VI:79f
    normal distal radius indices, **VI:**75f
    normal posteroanterior radiograph,
        VI:73f
    perilunate dislocation, **VI:**74f
    positioning, **VI:**69f, 73f–74f, 76f
    scaphoid fractures, **VI:**76b, 77f
    ulnar abutment syndrome, **VI:**76b, 80f
    ulnar variance, **VI:**74f
    pharyngoesophageal reconstruction, **III:**338
    temporomandibular joint (TMJ)
        dysfunction, **III:**92
radiohumeral synostosis, **III:**807t
radionuclides
    brachytherapy, **I:**656
    diagnostic imaging, **VI:**90
radio-ulnar synostosis, **VI:**614–615, 615f
radius, **IV:**181–183, 182f
randomized controlled clinical trials,
    I:153–154, 154t, 307
RANK, **I:**431
RANKL, **I:**431
rapamycin, **I:**822t, 824
rapidly involuting congenital hemangioma
    (RICH), **I:**677t, 687, **VI:**668t, 673–674, 676f
Rasch measurement, **I:**164
rationalization, **I:**33
Ravitch repair, **III:**857, 858f
Raynaud's phenomenon, **VI:**409, 468, 474,
    474b, 475t, 479t
    See also hands
reactive oxygen species (ROS), **I:**256, **II:**86,
    VI:228–229
receptor activator for nuclear factor κ B
    (RANK), **I:**431
receptor activator for nuclear factor κ B
    (RANK) ligand (RANKL), **I:**431
reconstructive and aesthetic surgical history,
    I:11–29
    aesthetic surgery
        beauty doctors, **I:**26–27, 28f
        origins, **I:**25–26
        postwar aesthetic surgery, **I:**28
        rhinoplasty, **I:**26f
    ancient Egypt, **I:**11–12
    Byzantine Empire, **I:**14
    eighteenth century, **I:**18–19, 19f
    Greece, **I:**13
    India, **I:**12–13, 13f
    Mesopotamia, **I:**12
    Middle Ages
        Arabian surgery, **I:**14–15
        printed textbooks, **I:**15
        universities, **I:**15, 15f
    nineteenth century, **I:**19–20
    Renaissance
        nose reconstruction, **I:**16–18, 18f
        surgeries, **I:**15–16, 16f–17f
        surgery decline, **I:**18
    Rome, **I:**13–14, 14f
    twentieth century
        modern plastic surgery, **I:**20–23, 22f–23f
        postwar plastic surgery, **I:**25, 25f–26f
        scientific journals, **I:**24–25, 25f

reconstructive and aesthetic surgical history
        (Continued)
    scientific societies, **I:**24
    training programs, **I:**23–24
    wound management, **I:**11
reconstructive burn surgery, **IV:**500–510
    breast reconstruction, **IV:**506
    extremity burn reconstruction, **IV:**435–455
        acute phase surgery
            joint reconstruction, **IV:**441–442,
                442f–443f, 445f
            skin grafts, **IV:**441
            skin substitutes, **IV:**441
        burn-related accidents, **IV:**435
        complications
            axillary contractures, **IV:**445,
                448f–449f
            bone exposure, **IV:**446, 450f
            elbow contractures, **IV:**445–446
            heterotopic ossification, **IV:**446
            scar retraction, **IV:**444–445
            skeletal-muscle complications, **IV:**446
            unstable healing, **IV:**444
        electrical burns, **IV:**435–436
        patient presentation and diagnosis
            compartment syndrome, **IV:**437–439,
                437f–440f
            emergency surgical procedures,
                IV:437b
            escharotomy incisions, **IV:**437–439,
                437f–440f
            fluid infusion and edema, **IV:**436–437
            preoperative assessment, **IV:**436–440
            related trauma, **IV:**439–440
        patient selection, **IV:**440
        postoperative care and follow-up
            active mobilization, **IV:**444
            ankles, **IV:**444
            compression garments, **IV:**447f
            elbows, **IV:**443
            hips/flanks, **IV:**443–444
            joint position, **IV:**443t
            knees, **IV:**444
            passive mobilization, **IV:**444
            patient positioning, **IV:**443
            physio-kinesitherapy tasks, **IV:**447f
            shoulder, **IV:**443
            treatment strategies, **IV:**442–444
            wrists, **IV:**443
        prognosis and outcomes, **IV:**444–446
        secondary procedures
            amputations, **IV:**451–453
            fasciocutaneous flaps, **IV:**449–450
            free flaps, **IV:**450
            general characteristics, **IV:**446–454
            laser treatments, **IV:**454, 454t
            lipofilling, **IV:**453–454
            myocutaneous flaps, **IV:**449–450
            nerve repair and grafting, **IV:**450–451
            rotation flaps, **IV:**448–449, 453f–454f
            skin expansion, **IV:**450
            skin grafts, **IV:**447–448
            skin substitutes, **IV:**448
            tendon retraction, **IV:**451
            Z-plasty technique, **IV:**447, 451f–454f
        surgical technique and treatment
            acute phase surgery, **IV:**441
            characteristics, **IV:**440–442

reconstructive burn surgery (Continued)
    facial burn wound treatment, **IV:**468–499
        acute facial burns
            ears, **IV:**473
            eyes/eyelids, **IV:**470–473
            mouth, **IV:**473
            nose, **IV:**473
            treatment strategies, **IV:**470–473,
                471f–472f
        complications, **IV:**497
        damage process
            acute facial burns, **IV:**470–473
            damage assessments, **IV:**468–473, 469f
            depth of burn determination, **IV:**470
        epidemiology, **IV:**468
        flaps
            basic principles, **IV:**480–481
            indicators, **IV:**480b
            trapeze-plasties, **IV:**481
            Z-plasty technique, **IV:**481, 481f
        inadequate donor-site skin
            dermal substitutes, **IV:**480, 482–484
            general discussion, **IV:**482–484
            tissue expansion, **IV:**482, 483f
        nonoperative facial reconstructive adjunct
            techniques
            corrective cosmetics, **IV:**485
            fat transplantation, **IV:**485
            hair transplantation, **IV:**485
            laser therapy, **IV:**484, 484f
            prosthetics, **IV:**485
            steroid treatments, **IV:**485
        nonsurgical management, **IV:**473
        outcome assessments, **IV:**497–498
        postoperative care and follow-up, **IV:**497
        secondary procedures, **IV:**498–499
        skin grafts
            advantages, **IV:**474
            basic principles, **IV:**479
            composite grafts, **IV:**480
            full-thickness skin graft, **IV:**479–480
            skin substitutes, **IV:**480, 482–484
            split-thickness skin graft, **IV:**479
        specific areas
            cheeks, **IV:**490–491, 506
            commissure, **IV:**473, 489–490, 495f
            ears, **IV:**473, 491–492, 496f, 498–499,
                505–506
            eyebrows, **IV:**485, 498–499
            eyelids, **IV:**470–473, 485–488, 486f–487f,
                498–499, 504–505, 504f
            forehead, **IV:**485, 498–499
            lower eyelids, **IV:**486–488, 488f
            lower lip and chin, **IV:**489, 492f–494f,
                498–499
            medial canthus scars, **IV:**488
            neck, **IV:**493–494, 498–499, 506
            nose, **IV:**473, 488–489, 498–499, 505
            scalp, **IV:**492–493, 498–499, 504, 504f
            severe cervical burn scars and
                contractures, **IV:**494
            upper eyelids, **IV:**486, 487f
            upper lip, **IV:**489, 490f–491f, 498–499
        specific surgical techniques
            scar replacement with local skin,
                IV:478, 478f
            serial excision, **IV:**478
            W-plasty technique, **IV:**478–479, 478f

*Note: **Boldface** roman numerals indicate volume. Page numbers followed by f refer to figures; page numbers followed by t refer to tables; page numbers followed by b refer to boxes.*

reconstructive burn surgery *(Continued)*
  surgical management
    algorithmic approach, **IV:**475–477, 476f–477f
    basic principles, **IV:**474–475
    flaps, **IV:**480–481
    inadequate donor-site skin, **IV:**482–484
    skin grafts, **IV:**479–480
    specific techniques, **IV:**478–479
    surgical techniques, **IV:**473
    total wound healing/scar maturation, **IV:**474–475, 474f
  total wound healing/scar maturation
    aesthetic units, **IV:**474, 475f
    ancillary techniques, **IV:**475, 475b, 476f
    diagnosis, **IV:**474
    functional restoration, **IV:**474, 475f
    local flaps, **IV:**474
    reconstruction planning, **IV:**474
    skin grafts, **IV:**474
    skin-matching considerations, **IV:**475
    surgical goals, **IV:**475
    timing considerations, **IV:**474–475, 474f
  general discussion, **IV:**500
  historical background, **IV:**500–501
  hypertrophic scars, **IV:**501, 501f–502f
  outcome assessments, **IV:**509
  postoperative care and follow-up, **IV:**509
  research summary, **IV:**509
  surgical technique
    cheeks, **IV:**490–491, 506
    ears, **IV:**473, 491–492, 496f, 498–499, 505–506
    eyebrows, **IV:**504–505
    eyelids, **IV:**470–473, 485–488, 486f–487f, 498–499, 504–505, 504f
    lips, **IV:**505
    lower extremities, **IV:**509
    neck, **IV:**506
    nose, **IV:**473, 488–489, 498–499, 505
    perineum, **IV:**506–507
    scalp, **III:**119–120, 120f, **IV:**492–493, 498–499, 504, 504f
    scar release, **IV:**501–502, 502f
    upper extremities
      axillary contractures, **IV:**507, 507f
      elbows, **IV:**507
      fingers, **IV:**508, 508f
      hands, **IV:**507–509, 508f
      nail deformities, **IV:**509
      web space contractures, **IV:**508
      wrists, **IV:**508, 508f
    wound closure
      fascial flaps, **IV:**503
      local flaps, **IV:**502–503, 503f
      muscle flaps, **IV:**503
      reconstructive ladder analogy, **IV:**502–503
      skin grafts, **IV:**502
      skin substitutes, **IV:**502
      tissue expansion, **IV:**503
    timing considerations, **IV:**500–501
  wound contraction, **IV:**501
reconstructive ladder analogy
  congenital transverse arrest, **VI:**549f
  flap applications, **I:**534–541, 536f
  Great Ormond Street ladder of functional ability, **VI:**549f
  limb and hand surgery, **I:**857–862, 857f, **IV:**128

reconstructive ladder analogy *(Continued)*
  lower extremity reconstructive surgery, **IV:**128, 130f
  reconstructive burn surgery, **I:**857–862, **IV:**502–503
reconstructive triangle, **I:**536, 536f
record alterations, **I:**95–96
rectus abdominis
  abdominal wall reconstruction, **I:**553t
  anatomical characteristics, **IV:**228–229, 229f
  chest wall reconstruction, **I:**552–553, **IV:**244–245, 245f
  foot reconstruction, **IV:**211
  groin reconstruction, **I:**554–557, 558f
  lower extremity reconstructive surgery, **IV:**77, 79f
  male genital reconstructive surgery, **IV:**307–310
  mangled upper extremies, **VI:**275–277, 278f
  microneurovascular muscle transplantation, **III:**295t
  oral cavity and mouth reconstruction, **III:**321, 321f
  perineal reconstruction, **I:**554–557, 557f
  tongue reconstruction, **III:**309t–310t
rectus-based reconstruction, **IV:**386–388, 387f–388f
rectus diastases, **IV:**280, 281f
rectus femoris muscle, **IV:**15t–16t, 18f, 19t, 20f–22f, 25f
rectus femoris muscle flap
  abdominal wall reconstruction, **I:**553t, 554, 555f
  groin reconstruction, **I:**554–557
  lower extremity reconstructive surgery, **IV:**82f, 139, 139f
  male genital reconstructive surgery, **IV:**307–310
  microneurovascular muscle transplantation, **III:**295t
  perineal reconstruction, **I:**554–557
rectus sheath, **IV:**227–230, 227f
red chili pepper, **V:**33t–35t
Red Flag Rules, **I:**94, 97–98
red nose, **II:**446
reduction mammaplasty, **V:**152–164
  adolescent aesthetic surgery, **I:**45t
  Biesenberger technique, **V:**154, 155f
  central mound technique, **V:**156–159, 160f
  complications, **V:**243t
  evaluation examinations, **V:**162–163
  evidence-based medicine and health service research, **I:**160–161, 161f
  historical background, **V:**153–159
  inferior pedicle breast reduction, **V:**165–176
    background and general characteristics, **V:**154–156, 165–166
    case studies, **V:**172–175, 173f–174f
    complications, **V:**175
    inferior pedicle technique with Wise-pattern skin excision, **V:**156, 159f, 161f
    patient selection, **V:**166
    planning and marking guidelines
      asymmetrical cases, **V:**168, 168f
      equilateral triangle marking, **V:**166–167, 167f
      inframammary fold, **V:**167
      preoperative markings, **V:**166, 167f

reduction mammaplasty *(Continued)*
    symmetry assessments, **V:**168
    transverse incisions markings, **V:**167
    research summary, **V:**175
    surgical technique and treatment
      apical suture, **V:**171f
      basic procedure, **V:**168–172
      de-epithelialization, **V:**169f
      flap thickness evaluation, **V:**170f
      inferior pedicle with inverted-T skin closure, **V:**159f, 161f
      medial and lateral triangle excision, **V:**170f
      nipple-areola complex, **V:**168f, 171f–172f
      postoperative results, **V:**172f
      preoperative/postoperative comparisons, **V:**173f
      symmetry evaluation, **V:**172f
  infiltration, **I:**141–142, 141f–142f
  L short-scar mammaplasty, **V:**206–215
    background and general characteristics, **V:**206–207
    complications, **V:**213
    patient selection, **V:**206–207
    planning and marking guidelines, **V:**207, 208f–209f
    reduction results, **V:**210f–214f
    research summary, **V:**214–215
    surgical technique, **V:**207–210, 209f
  mammary hypertrophy, **V:**152–153, 161–162, 240f–241f
  McKissock vertical bipedicled dermoglandular flap with Wise-pattern skin excision, **V:**156, 157f–158f
  McKissock vertical dermoglandular flap with Wise-pattern skin excision, **V:**156, 159f
  Passot technique, **V:**154, 154f
  patient presentation and diagnosis, **V:**162–163
  psychological aspects, **I:**41–42
  revisionary surgery, **V:**242–265
    incidence, **V:**242
    outcomes and complicatons, **V:**245
    pathophysiology, **V:**244
    patient history, **V:**242–244
    patient presentation and diagnosis, **V:**244
    postoperative care and follow-up, **V:**244–245, 262
    preoperative assessment, **V:**244
    research summary, **V:**264
    surgical re-intervention
      areola deformities, **V:**248–249, 250f
      areola hypopigmentation, **V:**249–251
      asymmetries, **V:**251
      contour abnormalities, **V:**247
      fat necrosis, **V:**251
      flap necrosis, **V:**246
      hematomas, **V:**245–246, 246f
      mastopexy revision, **V:**254–261, 258f–263f
      nipple areola ischemia, **V:**247–248, 248f–249f
      nipple loss, **V:**148, 243t, 253–254, 255f
      nipple malposition, **V:**149, 243t, 252, 252f–253f
      nipple retraction, **V:**252
      postoperative care and follow-up, **V:**246
      re-do breast reduction, **V:**254, 256f

reduction mammaplasty *(Continued)*
scars, **V:**246–247
wound excision and re-closure,
V:246–247
Schwarzmann technique, **V:**154, 155f
sculpted pillar vertical reduction
mammaplasty, **V:**228–241
background and general characteristics,
V:228
complications, **V:**236–239, 239f–241f
patient selection, **V:**228–229
planning and marking guidelines, **V:**229,
229f–230f
research summary, **V:**239
surgical technique
basic procedure, **V:**229–236
large breast reduction, **V:**236, 238f
moderate breast reduction, **V:**236, 237f
small breast reduction, **V:**235, 236f
wound closure, **V:**231–235, 232f–235f
short scar periareolar inferior pedicle
reduction (SPAIR) mammaplasty,
V:194–205
background and general characteristics,
V:159, 194–195
complications
areolar spreading, **V:**204
fat necrosis, **V:**203–204
general discussion, **V:**203–205
hypertrophy recurrence, **V:**204–205
polytetrafluoroethylene (PTFE)
infection/exposure, **V:**204
shape distortion, **V:**204
patient selection, **V:**195–196
planning and marking guidelines, **V:**196,
197f–198f
reduction results
large breast reduction, **V:**202–203, 203f
modest breast reduction, **V:**202, 203f
small breast reduction, **V:**201–203, 202f
research summary, **V:**205
surgical technique, **V:**196–201, 200f–201f
Strombeck horizontal bipedicle technique,
V:156, 156f
superomedial pedicle with Wise-pattern
skin closure, **V:**156–159, 161f
vertical scar reduction mammaplasty,
V:177–193
comparison studies, **V:**178t
complications
frequency, **V:**189–192, 191t
scar healing, **V:**190, 191f
under-resection, **V:**192
wound dehiscence, **V:**191
Hall-Findlay technique, **V:**159, 178t
historical background, **V:**177–180
Lassus technique, **V:**156–159, 178t
Lejour technique, **V:**159, 178t
Lista technique, **V:**178t
medial pedicle breast reductions, **V:**189,
190f
nipple-areola complex, **V:**179f
patient selection
patient characteristics, **V:**180–181
symptoms, **V:**180
planning and marking guidelines
perioperative care, **V:**181
skin marking, **V:**181–182, 181f, 183f

reduction mammaplasty *(Continued)*
postoperative care and follow-up, **V:**188
research summary, **V:**192
superior pedicle breast reductions,
V:188–189, 189f
surgical technique and treatment
anesthesia, **V:**182
breast shaping, **V:**186–187, 187f
de-epithelialization, **V:**184, 184f
dressings and wound care, **V:**188
infiltration, **V:**182–184
liposuction, **V:**185
patient positioning, **V:**182
pedicle selection, **V:**182, 184f
surgical excision, **V:**184–185, 185f–186f
wound closure, **V:**187–188, 187f–188f
reduction thyroid chondroplasty, **IV:**349
refining technology, **I:**843
reflex sympathetic dystrophy (RSD) *See*
complex regional pain syndrome (CRPS)
regenerative fetal healing, **I:**265–266
regenerative medicine, **I:**367–368
regional anesthesia techniques
axillary block, **VI:**99–100, 101f
Bier block, **VI:**97
characteristics, **VI:**96–100
digital blockade, **VI:**96–97
infraclavicular block, **VI:**99, 100f
interscalene block, **VI:**97, 98f
intravenous regional anesthesia, **VI:**97
supraclavicular block, **VI:**97–99, 99f
wrist block, **VI:**97
Regnault classification, **V:**121, 121f
regression, **I:**32
Reiter's syndrome, **VI:**337, 406–408
remifentanil, **IV:**427
Renaissance
nose reconstruction, **I:**16–18, 18f
surgeries, **I:**15–16, 16f–17f
surgery decline, **I:**18
reoperative biopsies, **IV:**107–108
replantation and revascularization surgery,
VI:228–249
complications, **VI:**248–249
general discussion, **VI:**228
ischemia–reperfusion pathophysiology,
VI:228–229
outcome assessments, **VI:**247–248, 247t
patient presentation and diagnosis
replantation centers, **VI:**229–230, 229t,
230f
transportation considerations, **VI:**229,
229f
patient selection indications and
contraindications, **VI:**230–231,
230t–231t
postoperative care and follow-up
anticoagulant agents, **VI:**244–245
postoperative monitoring, **VI:**245–246,
246b, 246t
postoperative therapy, **VI:**246
psychosocial aspects, **VI:**246–247
secondary procedures, **VI:**248f, 249
surgical technique and treatment
artery repair, **VI:**233–234, 234f
bone fixation, **VI:**232–233, 232b, 232f
distal amputations, **VI:**241–242, 241f
ectopic replantation, **VI:**243, 244f

replantation and revascularization surgery
(Continued)
multiple digit replantations, **VI:**237–238,
237f–240f
nerve repair and grafting, **VI:**235
operative sequence, **VI:**231–232, 231f
pediatric replantation, **VI:**244
proximal amputations, **VI:**238–241,
238f–240f
ring avulsion injuries, **VI:**242, 242b, 242t,
243f
single-digit amputation, **VI:**241f
skin closure, **VI:**235
tendon graft and repair, **VI:**233, 233b
thumb replantation, **VI:**235–237,
236f–237f
vein repair, **VI:**234–235, 235f
repression, **I:**33
respiration, **I:**144–145
Restylane, **II:**45t, 47, 49t
See also soft-tissue fillers
Restylane Touch, **II:**47
resuscitation formulae, **IV:**409, 409t
resveratrol, **II:**25, 27
retaining ligaments
aging process, **II:**87
anatomical characteristics, **II:**79f–80f, 112,
114f, 189–191, 191f
characteristics, **III:**8–10, 10f–11f
extended SMAS technique, **II:**239
orbicularis retaining ligament (ORL), **III:**9,
10f
reticular hemangioma, **I:**681
reticulohistiocystoma, **I:**736
retinoic acid, **I:**282, **II:**26, **III:**514–515
retinoic acid receptor-α (RARA), **III:**518
retinoids
action mechanisms, **II:**26
characteristics, **II:**26
craniofacial development, **III:**514–515
side effects, **II:**26
usage guidelines, **II:**26
retroauricular deformities, **II:**492
retrobulbar hematoma, **III:**56
retromolar trigone, **III:**406, 422f, 427
retroviral gene delivery, **I:**186–187, 188f, 188t
return on investment, **I:**73
Revanesse/ReDexis, **II:**47t
Reverdin, Jacques, **I:**20
reverse-flow flaps, **I:**531, 532f
reverse Phalen's test, **VI:**505–507
reverse transposition flap, **I:**531–533, 533f
Reviderm, **II:**48t
See also soft-tissue fillers
revisionary breast surgery, **V:**39–80, 242–265
acellular dermal matrix (ADM)
basic principles, **V:**68–69
capsular contracture, **V:**52–53, 52f
comparison studies, **V:**70t
omentum reconstruction, **V:**474–476, 477f
patient presentation and diagnosis, **V:**71
patient selection, **V:**71, 72t
surgical technique and treatment, **V:**71–78
background and challenges, **V:**39–40
biological responses, **V:**40
body responses
encapsulation processes, **V:**71
published research, **V:**69–71

Note: **Boldface** *roman numerals indicate volume. Page numbers followed by f refer to figures; page numbers followed by t refer to tables; page numbers followed by b refer to boxes.*

revisionary breast surgery (Continued)
    regeneration processes, **V:**69
    resorption processes, **V:**69
causal factors, **V:**67–68, 68b
clinical signs, **V:**79t
incidence, **V:**242
outcomes and complicatons, **V:**65–66, 66t,
        78–79, 79t, 243t, 245, 263–264
pathophysiology, **V:**244
patient history, **V:**242–244
patient presentation and diagnosis, **V:**244
    acellular dermal matrix (ADM), **V:**71
    classifications, **V:**41–42, 42f
    indicators, **V:**42–44
    patient history, **V:**40–44, 41t
    physical examination, **V:**40
patient selection, **V:**42–44, 71, 72t
postoperative care and follow-up, **V:**65,
        244–245, 262
preoperative assessment, **V:**244
preoperative/postoperative Baker
        classifications, **V:**79, 79t
prognosis and outcomes, **V:**78–79
published research, **V:**69–71
research summary, **V:**264
secondary procedures, **V:**37
surgical re-intervention
    areola deformities, **V:**248–249, 250f
    areola hypopigmentation, **V:**249–251
    asymmetries, **V:**251
    contour abnormalities, **V:**247
    fat necrosis, **V:**251
    flap necrosis, **V:**246
    hematomas, **V:**245–246, 246f
    mastopexy revision, **V:**254–261, 258f–263f
    nipple areola ischemia, **V:**247–248,
            248f–249f
    nipple loss, **V:**148, 243t, 253–254, 255f
    nipple malposition, **V:**149, 243t, 252,
            252f–253f
    nipple retraction, **V:**252
    postoperative care and follow-up, **V:**246
    re-do breast reduction, **V:**254, 256f
    scars, **V:**246–247
    wound excision and re-closure, **V:**246–247
surgical technique and treatment
    augmentation versus augmentation
            mastopexy, **V:**79t
    breast asymmetry, **V:**61–63, 62f–63f
    capsular contracture
        acellular dermal matrix (ADM),
                V:52–53, 52f, 336–340
        Baker classifications, **V:**36t, 46–53
        blood supply, **V:**49f
        capsulectomy, **V:**47, 48f–49f
        capsulotomies, **V:**47
        clinical signs, **V:**79t
        etiology, **V:**46t
        mastopexy, **V:**47, 48f
        neo subpectoral pocket conversion,
                V:50–52, 51f
        nipple-areola complex, **V:**49f
        subglandular to subpectoral
                conversion, **V:**50, 50f–51f
        surgical options, **V:**47t
        treatment strategies, **V:**77–78, 77f, 264
    implant failure, **V:**58–59
    implant malposition
        characteristics, **V:**53, 53f–54f
        etiology, **V:**53–55, 54f

revisionary breast surgery (Continued)
        incidence, **V:**79t
        treatment strategies, **V:**55–58, 55t,
                56f–57f
    implant pocket options, **V:**44–65, 44t, 45f
    implant stabilization, **V:**75–76, 75f–76f
    lamellar separation, **V:**73–75, 73f
    lower pole coverage, **V:**73–75, 73f–76f
    placement indicators, **V:**71–78, 72f, 73b
    preoperative assessment, **V:**44–65
    rippling/implant edge palpability,
            V:59–61, 61f
    size changes, **V:**64–65
    soft tissue changes, **V:**63–64, 64f
    surgical tips, **V:**44b
    tissue thickeners, **V:**76–77
    tissue changes, **V:**68–69
Revue de Chirurgie Plastique, **I:**24–25, 25f
R-fine, **II:**47t
rhabdomycosarcoma
    characteristics, **III:**889
    complications, **III:**889
    disease process, **III:**889
    patient presentation and diagnosis, **III:**889,
            889f
    postoperative care and follow-up, **III:**889
    prognosis and outcomes, **III:**889
    secondary procedures, **III:**889
    surgical technique and treatment, **III:**889,
            VI:326
rhabdomyolysis, **IV:**83–84
rhabdomyoma, **I:**732
rhabdomyosarcoma, **I:**741
Rhazes, **IV:**393
Rhegecoll, **II:**48t
    See also soft-tissue fillers
rheumatoid arthritis, **VI:**371–410
    characteristics, **VI:**371
    etiology, **VI:**371–372
    hands
        boutonnière deformity
            basic procedure, **VI:**396–398, 399f
            outcomes and complicatons, **VI:**398
            postoperative care and follow-up,
                    VI:398
            surgical tips, **VI:**398b
            thumb deformities, **VI:**399–400, 400f
        crystalline arthropathy/gout, **VI:**407t,
                409–410
        infection mimics, **VI:**336
        metacarpophalangeal (MCP) arthrodesis
            basic procedure, **VI:**395
            outcomes and complicatons, **VI:**395
            postoperative care and follow-up,
                    VI:395
        metacarpophalangeal (MCP) arthroplasty
            basic procedure, **VI:**392–394, 392f,
                    394f
            entrance point, **VI:**392f
            final implant position, **VI:**394f
            osteotomy, **VI:**393f
            postoperative care and follow-up,
                    VI:393–394
            PyroCarbon implants, **VI:**392f
        metacarpophalangeal (MCP)
                synovectomy and soft tissue
                reconstruction
            basic procedure, **VI:**390–391, 390f–391f
            outcomes and complicatons, **VI:**391,
                    391f

rheumatoid arthritis (Continued)
            postoperative care and follow-up,
                    VI:391
            secondary procedures, **VI:**391
            surgical tips, **VI:**395b
        operative procedures
            boutonnière deformity, **VI:**396–398
            metacarpophalangeal (MCP)
                    arthrodesis, **VI:**395
            metacarpophalangeal (MCP)
                    arthroplasty, **VI:**392–394
            metacarpophalangeal (MCP)
                    synovectomy and soft tissue
                    reconstruction, **VI:**390–391
            proximal interphalangeal (PIP)
                    arthrodesis, **VI:**395
            proximal interphalangeal (PIP)
                    arthroplasty, **VI:**394–395
            swan-neck deformity, **VI:**395–396
            thumb deformities, **VI:**399–400
        proximal interphalangeal (PIP)
                arthrodesis
            basic procedure, **VI:**395
            K-wire and stainless steel wire
                    configuration, **VI:**396f
            outcomes and complicatons, **VI:**395
            postoperative care and follow-up,
                    VI:395
        proximal interphalangeal (PIP)
                arthroplasty
            basic procedure, **VI:**394–395
            outcomes and complicatons, **VI:**395
            postoperative care and follow-up,
                    VI:395
            secondary procedures, **VI:**395
            surgical tips, **VI:**395b
        scleroderma, **VI:**407t, 409
        seronegative spondyloarthropathies,
                VI:406–408, 407t
        swan-neck deformity
            basic procedure, **VI:**395–396, 397f–398f
            postoperative care and follow-up,
                    VI:396
            surgical tips, **VI:**398b
            thumb deformities, **VI:**399–400, 400f
        systemic lupus erythematosus (SLE),
                VI:407t, 408
        thumb deformities
            basic procedure, **VI:**399–400
            boutonnière deformity, **VI:**399–400,
                    400f
            outcomes and complicatons, **VI:**400
            postoperative care and follow-up,
                    VI:400
            swan-neck deformity, **VI:**400f
    medical management, **VI:**372–373, 380b
    pathogenesis, **VI:**372, 372f
    patient presentation and diagnosis
        diagnostic criteria, **VI:**373–379, 374b
        finger and thumb involvement
            basic principles, **VI:**376–379
            boutonnière deformity, **VI:**378f–380f
            flexion and volar subluxation,
                    VI:377f
            swan-neck deformity, **VI:**379f, 625f
            ulnar deviation, **VI:**377f–378f
        wrist involvement
            basic principles, **VI:**374–376
            caput ulnae, **VI:**375f
            extensor tenosynovitis, **VI:**376, 376f

rheumatoid arthritis (Continued)
    large proliferative flexor tendon
        tenosynovitis, **VI**:376f
    Mannerfelt lesion, **VI**:376, 376f
    radiographic imaging, **VI**:374f–375f
    Vaughn–Jackson syndrome, **VI**:376,
        376f
patient selection
    perioperative considerations, **VI**:380,
        380b
    surgical goals, **VI**:380
    surgical sequence, **VI**:380–381
research summary, **VI**:410
surgical technique and treatment
    complete wrist arthrodesis
        basic procedure, **VI**:386–388, 386f–387f
        intramedullary pin, **VI**:388f
        outcomes and complicatons, **VI**:388
        postoperative care and follow-up,
            VI:388
        radiographic imaging, **VI**:388f
        secondary procedures, **VI**:388
        Steinmann pin, **VI**:387f–388f
        surgical tips, **VI**:388b
    crystalline arthropathy/gout, **VI**:407t,
        409–410
    distal ulna resection (Darrach procedure)
        basic procedure, **VI**:382–384
        chevron incision, **VI**:382f
        outcomes and complicatons,
            VI:383–384
        postoperative care and follow-up,
            VI:383
        pronator quadratus release, **VI**:383f
        radiographic imaging, **VI**:384f
        secondary procedures, **VI**:384
        surgical tips, **VI**:384b
        ulnar head exposure, **VI**:382f
        ulnar head removal, **VI**:383f
        ulnar stump stabilization, **VI**:384f
    hand and finger operations
        boutonnière deformity, **VI**:396–398
        metacarpophalangeal (MCP)
            arthrodesis, **VI**:395
        metacarpophalangeal (MCP)
            arthroplasty, **VI**:392–394
        metacarpophalangeal (MCP)
            synovectomy and soft tissue
            reconstruction, **VI**:390–391
        proximal interphalangeal (PIP)
            arthrodesis, **VI**:395
        proximal interphalangeal (PIP)
            arthroplasty, **VI**:394–395
        swan-neck deformity, **VI**:395–396
        thumb deformities, **VI**:399–400
    metacarpophalangeal (MCP) arthrodesis
        basic procedure, **VI**:395
        outcomes and complicatons, **VI**:395
        postoperative care and follow-up,
            VI:395
    metacarpophalangeal (MCP) arthroplasty
        basic procedure, **VI**:392–394, 392f, 394f
        entrance point, **VI**:392f
        final implant position, **VI**:394f
        osteotomy, **VI**:393f
        postoperative care and follow-up,
            VI:393–394
        PyroCarbon implants, **VI**:392f

rheumatoid arthritis (Continued)
    metacarpophalangeal (MCP)
        synovectomy and soft tissue
        reconstruction
        basic procedure, **VI**:390–391, 390f–391f
        outcomes and complicatons, **VI**:391,
            391f
        postoperative care and follow-up,
            VI:391
        secondary procedures, **VI**:391
        surgical tips, **VI**:395b
    proximal interphalangeal (PIP)
        arthrodesis
        basic procedure, **VI**:395
        K-wire and stainless steel wire
            configuration, **VI**:396f
        outcomes and complicatons, **VI**:395
        postoperative care and follow-up,
            VI:395
    proximal interphalangeal (PIP)
        arthroplasty
        basic procedure, **VI**:394–395
        outcomes and complicatons, **VI**:395
        postoperative care and follow-up,
            VI:395
        secondary procedures, **VI**:395
        surgical tips, **VI**:395b
    radioscapholunate arthrodesis
        basic procedure, **VI**:384–386
        compression screws, **VI**:385f
        K-wire fixation, **VI**:385f
        postoperative care and follow-up,
            VI:386
        radiographic imaging, **VI**:385f
    scleroderma, **VI**:407t, 409
    seronegative spondyloarthropathies,
        VI:406–408, 407t
    systemic lupus erythematosus (SLE),
        VI:407t, 408
    tendon surgery
        carpal tunnel syndrome, **VI**:401–402
        extensor tendon ruptures, **VI**:404–406
        flexor tendon injuries, **VI**:402
        trigger finger, **VI**:402–404
    thumb deformities
        basic procedure, **VI**:399–400
        boutonnière deformity, **VI**:399–400,
            400f
        outcomes and complicatons, **VI**:400
        postoperative care and follow-up,
            VI:400
        swan-neck deformity, **VI**:400f
    total wrist arthroplasty
        basic procedure, **VI**:388–390
        capsulotomy, **VI**:389f
        carpal component placement, **VI**:389f
        extensor tendon exposure, **VI**:389f
        osteotomy, **VI**:389f
        outcomes and complicatons, **VI**:390
        postoperative care and follow-up,
            VI:390
        radiographic imaging, **VI**:390f
        secondary procedures, **VI**:390
        surgical tips, **VI**:390b
    wrist operations
        complete wrist arthrodesis, **VI**:386–388
        distal ulna resection (Darrach
            procedure), **VI**:382–384

rheumatoid arthritis (Continued)
    radioscapholunate arthrodesis,
        VI:384–386
    total wrist arthroplasty, **VI**:388–390
    wrist synovectomy/dorsal
        tenosynovectomy, **VI**:381–382
    wrist synovectomy/dorsal
        tenosynovectomy
        basic procedure, **VI**:381–382, 381f–382f
        outcomes and complicatons, **VI**:382
        postoperative care and follow-up,
            VI:381–382
        secondary procedures, **VI**:382
        surgical tips, **VI**:382b
temporomandibular joint (TMJ)
    dysfunction, **III**:90
rhinitis
    nasal airways, **II**:453–454
    rhinoplasty complications, **II**:445
    surgical technique and treatment
        allergic rhinitis, **II**:458
        atrophic rhinitis, **II**:458
        hypertrophic rhinitis, **II**:458
        infectious rhinitis, **II**:458
        rhinitis medicamentosa (RM), **II**:458
        vasomotor rhinitis, **II**:458
rhinitis medicamentosa (RM), **II**:454, 458
rhinomanometry, **II**:457
rhinophyma, **II**:443, 443f
rhinoplasty
    acquired cranial and facial bone
        deformities, **III**:228–229, 231f–233f
    adolescent aesthetic surgery, **I**:45t
    aesthetic nasal reconstruction, **III**:134–186
        defect classification
            adversely located defects, **III**:139–140
            composite defects, **III**:140
            deep defects, **III**:140
            large defects, **III**:140
            small defects, **III**:139
            superficial defects, **III**:139
        disease process, **III**:134–135
        false planning assumptions
            donor site considerations, **III**:135
            extra tissue transfer, **III**:135
            flap design, **III**:135
            scars, **III**:135
            single flap approach, **III**:136
            supportive frameworks, **III**:135–136
            tissue expansion, **III**:135
            tissue preservation, **III**:135
        forehead donor site
            expansion considerations, **III**:158–159
            expansion delay, **III**:159–160
            expansion technique, **III**:159–160
            harvesting guidelines, **III**:160
            primary closure, **III**:155
            scars within the forehead territory,
                III:156–157
            surgical delay procedures, **III**:157–158
        intranasal lining flaps
            applications, **III**:166t
            basic procedure, **III**:164f–166f
            detailed characteristics, **III**:163–166
            isolated unilateral mid-vault lining
                loss, **III**:166–167
            operative technique, **III**:166–170,
                167f–169f

Note: **Boldface** *roman numerals indicate volume. Page numbers followed by* f *refer to figures; page numbers followed by* t *refer to tables; page numbers followed by* b *refer to boxes.*

rhinoplasty *(Continued)*
  local flaps
    bilobed flap, **III:**143–145, 144f–145f, 446f
    dorsal nasal flap, **III:**143, 144f–145f
    forehead flaps, **III:**148–155, 149f
    one-stage nasolabial flap, **III:**145–146
    single-lobe transposition flap, **III:**143, 144f–145f
    surgical guidelines, **III:**142–146
    three stage full-thickness forehead flap, **III:**151–152, 152f
    three stage full-thickness forehead flap (stage 1), **III:**152–153, 153f–159f
    three stage full-thickness forehead flap (stage 2), **III:**153–155
    three stage full-thickness forehead flap (stage 3), **III:**155, 155t
    two-stage forehead flap, **III:**148, 150f–151f
    two-stage forehead flap (stage 1), **III:**148–151
    two-stage forehead flap (stage 2), **III:**151, 151t
    two-stage nasolabial flap, **III:**146–148, 146f–147f
    two-stage nasolabial flap (stage 1), **III:**146
    two-stage nasolabial flap (stage 2), **III:**146–148
  nasal contour and support restoration
    basic principles, **III:**160–179
    composite grafts, **III:**161
    design guidelines, **III:**160, 160t
    facial artery myomucosal (FAMM) flap, **III:**163
    free flap nasal reconstruction, **III:**173–174
    graft fixation, **III:**161
    hard-tissue support replacement, **III:**160
    harvesting guidelines, **III:**161
    hingeover lining flaps, **III:**162
    inadequate platforms, **III:**174
    intranasal lining flaps, **III:**163–166, 164f–166f, 166t
    lining restoration, **III:**161
    material selection, **III:**160–161
    microvascular transfer, **III:**173
    modified folded forehead flap, **III:**170–172, 170f–171f
    nasal lining restoration, **III:**174–179
    nasolabial flap, **III:**163
    prelaminated flap technique, **III:**162
    residual lining advancement, **III:**161–162
    second forehead flap, **III:**163
    second lining flaps, **III:**162–163
    skin graft linings, **III:**172–173
    soft-tissue support and contouring, **III:**161
    timing considerations, **III:**160
  nasal cover restoration
    adversely located defects, **III:**146–148
    deep defects, **III:**146–148
    healing by secondary intention, **III:**140–141
    large defects, **III:**146–148
    local flaps, **III:**142–146
    primary repair procedures, **III:**141

rhinoplasty *(Continued)*
    skin grafts, **III:**141–142
    small/superficial defects, **III:**140–141
  nasal lining restoration
    Burget–Walton approach, **III:**175f
    Menick–Salibian approach, **III:**176f
    mid-vault defects, **III:**174
    operation 1, **III:**174–177
    operation 2, **III:**177
    operation 3, **III:**177–178
    operation 4, **III:**178
    operation 5, **III:**178–179
    subtotal and total nasal defects, **III:**174, 175f–181f
  outcomes and complicatons, **III:**179–181
  patient presentation and diagnosis, **III:**135
  regional unit repair
    basic principles, **III:**138–139
    contralateral normal, **III:**138
    donor site considerations, **III:**138
    exact dimensions and outline, **III:**138
    exact foil templates, **III:**138
    old scars, **III:**139
    preliminary operationa, **III:**139
    stable platforms, **III:**139
    subcutaneous framework restoration, **III:**139
    subunit principle, **III:**138
    surgical staging, **III:**139
    tissue transfer, **III:**138–139
    wound healing, **III:**138–139
  secondary procedures
    do-over revisions, **III:**184
    major revisions, **III:**184
    minor revisions, **III:**181–184
    secondary revisions, **III:**181–184, 182f–184f
  skin grafts
    basic principles, **III:**141–142
    full-thickness forehead skin graft, **III:**141, 142f
    operative technique, **III:**141–142
    preauricular and postauricular skin grafts, **III:**141
  surgical goals, **III:**134
  surgical planning and preparation
    central facial units, **III:**136–137, 137f
    defect classification, **III:**139–140
    false planning assumptions, **III:**135–136
    modern approach, **III:**136, 136t, 137f
    peripheral facial units, **III:**136, 137f
    regional unit repair principles, **III:**138–139
    traditional approach, **III:**135
  surgical technique and treatment
    challenges, **III:**140–179
    forehead donor site, **III:**155–160
    nasal contour and support restoration, **III:**160–179
    nasal cover restoration, **III:**140–155
    zones of nasal skin quality, **III:**140
  aesthetic surgery, **I:**25–28, 26f
  ancient Egypt, **I:**11–12
  Asian rhinoplasty
    contracted nose
      dermal fat graft, **II:**176
      derotation grafts, **II:**176, 176f
      rib cartilage graft, **II:**176

rhinoplasty *(Continued)*
    septal extension grafts, **II:**176
    surgical technique and treatment, **II:**173–176
    general discussion, **II:**172–173
    historical background, **II:**173
    low profile nasal dorsum augmentation
      implant materials, **II:**173–174
      one-piece augmentation rhinoplasty, **II:**174
      preoperative view, **II:**174f
      two-piece augmentation rhinoplasty, **II:**174, 174f
    nasal skeleton, **II:**172–173
    outcomes and complicatons
      capsular contractures, **II:**177
      implant deviation, **II:**176
      implant exposure, **II:**176
      implant infection, **II:**176
    patient presentation and diagnosis
      blunt nasal tip, **II:**173
      broad nasal dorsum, **II:**173
      general discussion, **II:**173
      short/contracted nose, **II:**173
      underprojected nasal tip, **II:**173
    secondary procedures
      alar base surgery, **II:**177
      forehead augmentation, **II:**174f, 177
      genioplasty, **II:**177
      paranasal augmentation, **II:**177
    soft tissue profile, **II:**172–173
    surgical technique and treatment
      bulbous nose, **II:**175, 176f
      contracted nose, **II:**173–176
      low profile nasal dorsum augmentation, **II:**173–174, 174f
      septal extension grafts, **II:**175–176, 175f
      short nose, **II:**175–176, 475–476, 478f–479f
      underprojected nasal tip, **II:**174–175
    underprojected nasal tip
      alloplastic materials, **II:**175
      cartilage grafts, **II:**175
      general discussion, **II:**174–175
      onlay cartilaginous grafts, **II:**175
      septal extension grafts, **II:**175, 175f
  augmentation phase
    columellar grafts, **II:**436
    dorsum and radix, **II:**436
    graft donor sites
      alloplastic materials, **II:**439–440
      calvarial bone, **II:**439
      conchal cartilage, **II:**439
      costal cartilage, **II:**439
      general discussion, **II:**439–440
      maxillary augmentation, **II:**440
    graft selection, **II:**436–437
    lateral wall grafts, **II:**436
    spreader grafts, **II:**436
    tip grafts, **II:**436–437, 437f–438f
  autologous perichondrial grafts, **I:**408–413, 412f
  burn wound treatment, **IV:**473, 488–489, 498–499, 505
  challenges, **II:**413
  closed rhinoplasty, **II:**413–449
    augmentation phase
      columellar grafts, **II:**436
      dorsum and radix, **II:**436
      graft donor sites, **II:**439–440

rhinoplasty *(Continued)*
  graft selection, II:436–437
  lateral wall grafts, II:436
  spreader grafts, II:436
  tip grafts, II:436–437, 437f–438f
complications
  circulatory complications, II:445
  general discussion, II:444–446
  graft problems, II:444–445
  hematomas, II:446
  hemorrhage, II:445
  iatrogenic airway obstruction, II:444
  infections, II:445–446
  lacrimal duct injury, II:446
  red nose, II:446
  rhinitis, II:445
  septal collapse, II:446
  septal perforation, II:445
  skeletal problems, II:444
  soft-tissue problems, II:444
dissatisfied patients
  body dysmorphic disorder (BDD),
    II:447–448
  primary versus secondary candidates,
    II:446–447
  prior versus current surgeon, II:447
  reoperations, II:448
  surgeon–patient relationship,
    II:446–448
dressings, II:439
graft donor sites
  alloplastic materials, II:439–440
  calvarial bone, II:439
  conchal cartilage, II:439
  costal cartilage, II:439
  general discussion, II:439–440
  maxillary augmentation, II:440
nasal aesthetics
  potential complications and revisions,
    II:424
  preoperative photographs, II:423
  surgical goals, II:423–424
  surgical guidelines, II:423–424
open rhinoplasty-caused deformities,
  II:448–449, 449f
patient selection
  false planning assumptions, II:421–422
  patient interview, II:422
  preoperative assessment, II:422–423
  primary versus secondary candidates,
    II:422
postoperative care and follow-up,
  II:439–441
preoperative assessment
  evaluation examinations, II:422–423
  external nose, II:423
  septum, II:423
  turbinates, II:423
  valves, II:423
routine surgical order
  alar cartilage resection, II:433–434
  anesthesia, II:427–435
  dorsal resection, II:428, 428f–433f
  intracartilaginous incisions, II:428, 428f
  nasal spine-caudal septum resection,
    II:433
  septoplasty, II:434–435
  skeletonization, II:427–428

rhinoplasty *(Continued)*
  spreader graft tunnels, II:434–435,
    435f
  upper lateral cartilage resection, II:434
secondary rhinoplasty, II:448–449
septal graft specimen, II:436–437
surgical planning
  decision-making process, II:427
  endonasal rhinoplasty, II:425
  general discussion, II:424–427
  nasal base size–bridge height balance,
    II:425, 426f
  skin thickness and distribution, II:424,
    424f
  teach-yourself concept, II:427
  tip lobular contour, II:424–425, 425f
surgical technique and treatment
  general discussion, II:427–435
  routine order, II:427–435
turbinectomy
  alar wedge resection, II:435–436
  characteristics, II:435–436
  graft placement, II:435–436
  osteotomy, II:435
  wound closure, II:435–436
variants
  cleft lip nasal deformity, II:442
  donor site-depleted patient, II:443
  ethnic rhinoplasty, II:441–442
  male rhinoplasty, II:441
  nasal deviation, II:441, 442f
  older adults, II:442–443
  rhinophyma, II:443, 443f
complications
  circulatory complications, II:445
  general discussion, II:444–446
  graft problems, II:444–445
  hematomas, II:446
  hemorrhage, II:445
  iatrogenic airway obstruction, II:444
  infections, II:445–446
  lacrimal duct injury, II:446
  red nose, II:446
  rhinitis, II:445
  septal collapse, II:446
  septal perforation, II:445
  skeletal problems, II:444
  soft-tissue problems, II:444
dissatisfied patients
  body dysmorphic disorder (BDD),
    II:447–448
  primary versus secondary candidates,
    II:446–447
  prior versus current surgeon, II:447
  reoperations, II:448
  surgeon–patient relationship, II:446–448
dressings, II:439
dynamic equilibrium concept, II:414, 414f
eighteenth century, I:18–19, 19f
engineered cartilage, II:419–421, 422f
general discussion, II:413
India, I:12–13, 13f
nasal aesthetics
  potential complications and revisions,
    II:424
  preoperative photographs, II:423
  surgical goals, II:423–424
  surgical guidelines, II:423–424

rhinoplasty *(Continued)*
  nasal airways, II:450–465
    airway outcome study results, II:420–421,
      420f
    anatomical characteristics, II:450–452,
      451f–452f
    clinical analysis, II:419–420
    disease and obstructions
      deviated septum, II:392–393, 454–455,
        454f–456f
      external nasal valve, II:455–456
      internal nasal valve, II:455
      open rhinoplasty, II:392–394
      patient presentation and diagnosis,
        II:456–457
      patient selection, II:457–458
      rhinitis, II:453–454
    nasal valves, II:420f
    physiological characteristics
      humidification, II:453
      olfaction, II:453
      particulate filtration, II:453
      phonation, II:453
      secondary sex organ, II:453
      temperature regulation, II:453
      tubular flow, II:452–453
    preoperative assessment, II:450–453
    rhinitis, II:453–454, 458
    straight line strategy, II:420f
  nasal anatomy
    basic principles, II:414–419
    dorsum and tip
      alar cartilage malposition, II:418–419,
        418f–419f
      anatomic variants, II:416–419
      characteristics, II:415–419, 416f
      inadequate tip projection, II:417,
        418f–419f
      low radix/low dorsum, II:416, 418f–419f
      narrow middle vault, II:417, 417f–419f
      middle and lower cartilaginous vaults,
        II:415
      schematic diagram, II:415f
      upper cartilaginous vaults, II:414, 415f
  nasal cartilage graft, I:404–407, 405f–407f
  nasal disease and obstructions
    deviated septum, II:454–455, 454f–456f
    external nasal valve, II:455–456
    internal nasal valve, II:455
    patient presentation and diagnosis
      patient history, II:456
      physical examination, II:456–457, 457f
      radiologic scans, II:457, 457f
      rhinomanometry, II:457
    patient selection, II:457–458
    rhinitis, II:453–454
  nineteenth century, I:19–20
  open rhinoplasty, II:387–412
    advantages/disadvantages, II:388t
    alar base surgery
      alar flaring, II:404
      alar flaring with modification of nostril
        shape, II:405
      characteristics, II:404–405, 406f
    alar rim deformities
      alar contour grafts, II:401, 401f
      characteristics, II:400–401
      lateral crural strut grafts, II:401, 402f

Note: **Boldface** *roman numerals indicate volume. Page numbers followed by f refer to figures; page numbers followed by t refer to tables; page numbers followed by b refer to boxes.*

rhinoplasty (Continued)
   autologous cartilage harvesting
     background information, **II:**394–396
     costal cartilage, **II:**396, 397f
     ear cartilage, **II:**395–396, 396f
     septal cartilage, **II:**394–395, 394f
     septal L-strut, **II:**394–395, 395f
     submucoperichondrial dissection,
       II:394–395, 394f
     submucoperichondrial flaps, **II:**394–
       395, 395f
   complications
     bleeding, **II:**410–411
     deformities and deviations, **II:**411
     edema, **II:**411
     infections, **II:**411
     nasal airway obstructions, **II:**411
     open rhinoplasty-caused deformities,
       II:448–449, 449f
   deviated nose with dorsal hump
     outcome assessments, **II:**407
     surgical goals, **II:**406
     surgical plan, **II:**407
     systematic analysis, **II:**405–406, 406f
   general discussion, **II:**387
   long, wide nose with a drooping tip and
     nasal airway obstruction
     outcome assessments, **II:**409
     surgical goals, **II:**409
     surgical plan, **II:**409
     systematic analysis, **II:**407–409,
       407f–408f
   nasal airway
     inferior turbinoplasty/outfracture/
       submucous resection, **II:**393–394,
       393f
     obstructions, **II:**392–394
     septal reconstruction, **II:**392–393
   nasal anatomy, **II:**387
   nasal tip
     cephalic trim, **II:**397, 398f
     columellar strut graft, **II:**397–398, 398f
     grafting techniques, **II:**399–400, 400f
     surgical technique, **II:**397–400
     suturing techniques, **II:**398–399,
       399f–400f
   outcome assessments, **II:**410
   patient presentation and diagnosis
     anatomic examination, **II:**388–389
     external nasal exammination, **II:**388t
     informed consent, **II:**389
     initial consultation, **II:**387–389
     internal nasal exammination, **II:**389t
     nasal history, **II:**388
     patient expectations, **II:**389
     photographic documentation, **II:**389
   patient selection, **II:**389
   postoperative care and follow-up
     activity restrictions, **II:**410
     dressings and wound care, **II:**409
     follow-up consultations, **II:**410
     general patient instructions, **II:**410
     medications, **II:**409–410
     postoperative instructions, **II:**409–410
   prognosis, **II:**410
   secondary procedures, **II:**412
   surgical technique and treatment
     alar base surgery, **II:**404–405, 406f
     alar–columellar relationship, **II:**401–
       402, 403f

rhinoplasty (Continued)
     alar rim deformities, **II:**400–401
     anesthesia, **II:**389–390
     autologous cartilage harvesting,
       II:394–396
     closure, **II:**403
     component dorsal hump reduction,
       II:391–392, 391f
     depressor septi muscle translocation,
       II:403–404, 405f
     dorsal spreader grafts, **II:**392f
     nasal airway, **II:**392–394
     nasal dorsum irregularities, **II:**391f
     nasal tip, **II:**397–400
     percutaneous lateral nasal osteotomies,
       II:402–403, 404f
     preoperative management, **II:**389–390
     transcolumellar stair-step incision,
       II:390–391, 390f
   open rhinoplasty-caused deformities,
     II:448–449, 449f
   osseointegrated nasal reconstruction, **I:**802,
     802b, 802f–803f
   patient selection
     false planning assumptions, **II:**421–422
     patient interview, **II:**422
     preoperative assessment
       evaluation examinations, **II:**422–423
       external nose, **II:**423
       septum, **II:**423
       turbinates, **II:**423
       valves, **II:**423
     primary versus secondary candidates,
       II:422
   postoperative care and follow-up,
     II:439–441
   psychological aspects, **I:**39–40
   reconstructive burn surgery, **IV:**473,
     488–489, 498–499, 505
   Renaissance, **I:**16–18, 18f
   right-brain operation concept, **II:**413–414
   secondary rhinoplasty, **II:**466–484
     challenges, **II:**466
     characteristics, **II:**448
     common problems
       broad/bulbous/round tip, **II:**470
       open rhinoplasty-caused deformities,
         II:448–449, 449f
       suture-based tip plasty, **II:**471–480,
         472f–473f
     complications
       columellar scars, **II:**481–482, 482f
       difficult patients, **II:**482–483
       post-rhinoplasty fibrotic syndrome,
         II:482, 483f
       skin necrosis, **II:**481, 482f
     definition, **II:**466
     general discussion, **II:**448–449
     operative technique
       anesthesia, **II:**468
       artistry, **II:**467, 467f
       cartilage grafts, **II:**470, 470f–471f
       open versus closed approach, **II:**467,
         468f
       suturing techniques, **II:**468–470, 534f
     patient presentation and diagnosis, **II:**466
     patient selection, **II:**467
     postoperative care and follow-up
       corticosteroids, **II:**481
       early bad result, **II:**480–481, 481f

rhinoplasty (Continued)
     early care, **II:**480
     fillers, **II:**481
     suture-based tip plasty
       alar rim deformities, **II:**473–475,
         475f–478f
       broad nasal base, **II:**476–478, 479f–480f
       characteristics, **II:**471–480, 472f–473f
       closed approach, **II:**471–472
       deficient tip, **II:**472–473, 474f
       fascial graft and repair, **II:**477f–478f
       middle vault collapse, **II:**473
       nasal dorsum irregularities, **II:**478–479
       septoplasty, **II:**479–480, 480f
       short nose, **II:**475–476, 478f–479f
       thin skin tip, **II:**475, 477f–478f
   semi-open rhinoplasty
     alar base positioning, **III:**536–537
     alar-facial groove creation, **III:**537,
       538f–539f
     background information, **III:**535–537
     excessive skin trimming, **III:**536, 537f
     fibrofatty tissue release, **III:**536, 537f
     incisions, **III:**536, 537f
     lower lateral cartilage repositioning,
       III:536, 537f
   septal graft specimen, **II:**436–437
   sixteenth century, **VI:**xlv
   surgical planning
     decision-making process, **II:**427
     endonasal rhinoplasty, **II:**425
     general discussion, **II:**424–427
     nasal base size–bridge height balance,
       II:425, 426f
     skin thickness and distribution, **II:**424,
       424f
     teach-yourself concept, **II:**427
     tip lobular contour, **II:**424–425, 425f
   surgical technique and treatment
     deviated nasal bones, **II:**458
     deviated septum
       characteristics, **II:**458–461
       complications, **II:**463
       C-shaped anteroposterior deviation,
         II:459, 460f
       C-shaped cephalocaudal deviation,
         II:459, 460f
       localized deviation, **II:**461
       postoperative care and follow-up,
         II:462–463
       prognosis and outcomes, **II:**463,
         463f–464f
       secondary procedures, **II:**463
       septal tilt, **II:**459, 459f
       S-shaped anteroposterior deviation,
         II:459, 460f
       S-shaped cephalocaudal deviation,
         II:459, 460f
     general discussion, **II:**427–435
     incompetent external nasal valve, **II:**461,
       462f
     incompetent internal nasal valve, **II:**461,
       461f
     local flaps
       basic procedure, **III:**441–449
       bilobed flap, **III:**143–145, 144f–145f, 446f
       dorsal nasal flap, **III:**143, 144f–145f
       forehead flaps, **III:**148–155, 149f
       interpolated paramedian forehead flap,
         III:445f, 448f

rhinoplasty (Continued)
  lateral advancement flaps, **III**:445f
  one-stage nasolabial flap, **III**:145–146
  Rintala dorsal nasal advancement flap,
    III:447f
  three stage full-thickness forehead flap,
    III:151–152, 152f
  three stage full-thickness forehead flap
    (stage 1), **III**:152–153, 153f–159f
  three stage full-thickness forehead flap
    (stage 2), **III**:153–155
  three stage full-thickness forehead flap
    (stage 3), **III**:155, 155t
  transoperative flap, **III**:447f
  two-stage forehead flap, **III**:148,
    150f–151f
  two-stage forehead flap (stage 1),
    III:148–151
  two-stage forehead flap (stage 2),
    III:151, 151t
  two-stage nasolabial flap, **III**:146–148,
    146f–147f
  two-stage nasolabial flap (stage 1),
    III:146
  two-stage nasolabial flap (stage 2),
    III:146–148
  V-Y advancement flap, **III**:446f
rhinitis
  allergic rhinitis, **II**:458
  atrophic rhinitis, **II**:458
  hypertrophic rhinitis, **II**:458
  infectious rhinitis, **II**:458
  rhinitis medicamentosa (RM), **II**:458
  vasomotor rhinitis, **II**:458
routine order
  alar cartilage resection, **II**:433–434
  anesthesia, **II**:427–435
  dorsal resection, **II**:428, 428f–433f
  intracartilaginous incisions, **II**:428, 428f
  nasal spine-caudal septum resection,
    II:433
  septoplasty, **II**:434–435
  skeletonization, **II**:427–428
  spreader graft tunnels, **II**:434–435, 435f
  upper lateral cartilage resection, **II**:434
turbinate disorders
  background information, **II**:461–462
  destructive procedures, **II**:461–462
  mechanical procedures, **II**:461
  turbinate resection procedures, **II**:462
tissue expansion, **I**:637, 639f
turbinectomy
  alar wedge resection, **II**:435–436
  characteristics, **II**:435–436
  graft placement, **II**:435–436
  osteotomy
    basic procedure, **II**:435
    goals, **II**:435
  wound closure, **II**:435–436
variants
  cleft lip nasal deformity, **II**:442
  donor site-depleted patient, **II**:443
  ethnic rhinoplasty, **II**:441–442
  male rhinoplasty, **II**:441
  nasal deviation, **II**:441, 442f
  older adults, **II**:442–443
  rhinophyma, **II**:443, 443f
rhomboid flap, **III**:441, 442f–443f

Rhomboid muscles, **IV**:221, 222f
rhytidectomy
  hypertelorism correction, **III**:699
  See also facelifts
rhytides, **II**:15
rhytidoplasty See facelifts
ribbon sign, **VI**:252–253, 253f
rib cartilage graft, **I**:407–408, 408f–411f
rib harvests, **I**:452–454, 453f
riboflavin, **I**:282
ribonucleic acid (RNA), **I**:179–180
ribosomal RNA (rRNA), **I**:179–180
Riche–Cannieu anastomosis, **VI**:697f
Richieri–Costa syndrome, **III**:807t
ring avulsion injuries, **VI**:242, 242b, 242t, 243f
ring finger flexor digitorum superficialis
  transfer, **VI**:769
Risser'sign, **VI**:653, 653f
ritual scarring, **I**:297–298
Roberts–SC phocomelia syndrome, **VI**:556,
  573t
Robin–oligodactyly syndrome, **III**:807t
Robinow syndrome, **VI**:573t
Robin, Pierre, **III**:803–804
Robin sequence See Pierre Robin sequence
  (PRS)
robotics
  definition, **I**:855
  research summary, **I**:873
  surgical tools and prosthetics
    chest and abdominal surgery, **I**:863
    craniofacial surgery, **I**:862–863
    ear, nose, and throat surgery, **I**:862–863
    evidenced-based outcomes, **I**:864
    future trends, **I**:864–865
    limb and hand surgery
      lower limb prostheses, **I**:862
      neural arm–hand prostheses, **I**:858–861
      reconstructive ladder analogy,
        I:857–862, 857f
      reconstructive surgeries, **I**:857–862
      robotic hand prostheses, **I**:858–861
      upper extremity prosthetic options,
        I:857–858, 858f–860f
    next-generation devices, **I**:864–865
    operating rooms
      advantages/disadvantages, **I**:856
      da Vinci system, **I**:855–857, 856f
      design features, **I**:855–856
      future trends, **I**:857
    robotic-assisted laparoscopic
      prostatectomy (RALP), **I**:864
    robotic hand prostheses
      advantages/disadvantages, **I**:861–862,
        862f
      i-LIMB Pulse, **I**:860f
      LIVINGSKIN, **I**:861f
      ProDigits, **I**:861f
      state-of-the-art robotic hands, **I**:858–861
    urologic/prostate surgery, **I**:863–864
Roe, John Orlando, **I**:25–28
Rolando's fracture, **VI**:158
Rolifan, **II**:47t
roller injuries, **VI**:256, 257f
rolling scars, **II**:69
Rome, **I**:13–14, 14f
Roos extended arm stress test, **VI**:66
ropivacaine, **VI**:95–96, 95t–96t

rosacea, **II**:20–21, 21t
Rosen score, **VI**:716
Rosselli, Gustavo Sanvenero, **I**:22–23, 24f
rotation advancement cheiloplasty (complete
  clefts)
  adequate rotation, **III**:530–531, 531f, 535,
    536f
  alar base mobilization, **III**:532
  alar base repositioning, **III**:532, 533f
  basic principles, **III**:527–539
  C flap incisions, **III**:531, 531f–532f
  final skin closure, **III**:535, 536f
  free border of the lip closure, **III**:534, 535f
  inferior turbinate flap, **III**:532, 532f
  lateral lip incisions, **III**:530f, 531, 532f
  medial incisions, **III**:530, 530f
  muscle reconstruction, **III**:533, 534f
  nasal floor incisions, **III**:534–535, 535f
  nasal floor reconstruction, **III**:532, 533f
  orbicularis marginalis flap elevation, **III**:532,
    533f
  orbicularis muscle dissection, **III**:532
  philtral column reconstruction, **III**:533
  piriform deficiency correction, **III**:532, 533f
  preoperative markings, **III**:530f
  semi-open rhinoplasty
    alar base positioning, **III**:536–537
    alar-facial groove creation, **III**:537,
      538f–539f
    background information, **III**:535–537
    excessive skin trimming, **III**:536, 537f
    fibrofatty tissue release, **III**:536, 537f
    incisions, **III**:536, 537f
    lower lateral cartilage repositioning,
      III:536, 537f
    triangular vermillion flap incisions,
      III:533–534, 534f
rotation advancement cheiloplasty
  (incomplete clefts)
  basic principles, **III**:539–542
  excessive skin trimming, **III**:540–542
  markings and incisions, **III**:539, 540f
  muscle dissection and release, **III**:540
  muscle reconstruction, **III**:540
  nasal correction, **III**:540, 541f
  nasal floor incisions, **III**:540, 541f
  nasal floor reconstruction, **III**:540, 541f
  orbicularis marginalis flap elevation, **III**:540
rotation flaps
  cheek reconstruction, **III**:451, 451f–452f
  classifications, **I**:513f
  foot reconstruction, **IV**:205, 205f
Rothmund–Thomson syndrome, **VI**:573t
roux-en-Y gastric bypass (RYGB), **II**:636, 636t
Roux, Philibert, **I**:19
Rubinstein–Tabyi syndrome, **VI**:573t
ruby lasers, **III**:30
Runt-related transcription factor 2 (Runx2),
  I:429, 434f, **VI**:531–532
Ruvalcaba syndrome, **VI**:573t

S
Sabattini, Pietro, **I**:20
saber mark, **III**:792
sacral pressure ulcers, **IV**:370t
sacrococcygeal teratoma
  characteristics, **III**:874
  clinical presentation and evaluation, **III**:874

Note: **Boldface** roman numerals indicate volume. Page numbers followed by f refer to figures; page numbers followed by t refer to tables; page numbers followed by b refer to boxes.

sacrococcygeal teratoma (Continued)
  surgical indicators, III:874
  treatment strategies, III:874
Saethre–Chotzen syndrome, I:196–198, 197t,
    III:512, 749–750, VI:573t
sagittal band injuries, VI:219, 225, 225b, 225f
Saldanha's retractor, II:563f
Saliceto, William of, I:15
salicylic acid, II:22
saline implants
  autoinflation, V:111–112, 112f
  capsular calcification, V:110, 110f
  decision guidelines, V:24–25
  deflation, V:110–111, 111f
  developmental background, V:13–14
  ripples and folds, V:111, 111f
salivary glands
  anatomical characteristics
    facial nerve, III:362f
    general discussion, III:360–361
    minor salivary glands, III:361
    parotid gland, III:360–361, 361f–362f
    sublingual gland, III:361, 361f
    submandibular gland, III:361, 361f
  tumors, III:360–379
    benign neoplastic lesions
      hemangiomas, III:364t–365t, 368, 369f
      monomorphic adenoma, III:365t, 367,
        368f
      oncocytoma, III:365t, 368
      pleomorphic adenoma, III:364t–365t,
        366–367
      Warthin's tumor, III:364t–365t, 367–368,
        369f
    benign versus malignant tumors,
      III:364t–365t
    classifications
      benign neoplastic lesions, III:366–368
      malignant neoplastic lesions, III:365t,
        370–371, 370t
      nonneoplastic lesions, III:365–366
    epidemiology, III:361–362, 362t
    imaging methods
      benign versus malignant tumors,
        III:364t
      computed tomography (CT),
        III:363–364
      magnetic resonance imaging (MRI),
        III:364, 364t
      sialography, III:364
      technetium scans, III:364
      ultrasound imaging, III:364
    malignant neoplastic lesions
      acinic cell carcinoma, III:365t, 370, 370t
      adenocarcinoma, III:365t, 370, 370t
      adenoid cystic carcinoma (cylindroma),
        III:365t, 370, 370f, 370t
      lymphoma, III:365t, 370–371, 371f
      malignant mixed tumors, III:365t, 370,
        370t
      metastatic tumors, III:365t, 371
      mucoepidermoid carcinoma, III:365t,
        370, 370t
      oncocytic carcinoma, III:365t, 370
      squamous cell carcinomas (SCCs),
        III:365t, 370, 370t
    nonneoplastic lesions
      mucocele, III:365
      necrotizing sialometaplasia, III:366,
        367f

salivary glands (Continued)
    sialadenitis, III:365, 365f
    sialadenosis, III:365
    sialolithiasis, III:365, 366f–367f
  outcomes and complicatons
    acinic cell carcinoma, III:377
    adenocarcinoma, III:377, 377f
    adenoid cystic carcinoma (cylindroma),
      III:377
    Frey syndrome, III:377–378, 378f
    malignant mixed tumors, III:377
    mucoepidermoid carcinoma, III:377
    squamous cell carcinomas (SCCs),
      III:377
  patient presentation and diagnosis
    challenges, III:362–371
    fine-needle aspiration (FNA), III:363,
      363f
    imaging methods, III:363–364
  surgical technique and treatment
    acinic cell carcinoma, III:375–376, 376t
    adenocarcinoma, III:376, 376t
    adenoid cystic carcinoma (cylindroma),
      III:374–375, 376t
    benign neoplastic lesions, III:371–373
    hemangiomas, III:373
    lymphoma, III:377
    malignant mixed tumors, III:376–377,
      376t
    malignant neoplastic lesions,
      III:373–377
    monomorphic adenoma, III:372
    mucoepidermoid carcinoma, III:373–
      374, 374f–376f, 376t
    necrotizing sialometaplasia, III:371
    nonneoplastic lesions, III:371
    oncocytic carcinoma, III:377
    oncocytoma, III:373
    pleomorphic adenoma, III:371–372,
      372f–373f
    squamous cell carcinomas (SCCs),
      III:376t
    Warthin's tumor, III:372–373
Salmon, Michel, I:482–484
salmon patch, I:734
Salter–Harris fracture classification, VI:73f,
    139t, 141f, 654–655, 654f
Salvia miltiorrhiza, V:33t–35t
Sanderson–Fraser syndrome, III:807t
saphenous nerve, VI:710
saponification, II:16
Sappey's lines, I:757–758, 758f
Sarbanes–Oxley Act (SOX, 2002), I:85
sarcoidosis, III:115–116, 116f
sarcomas
  bone sarcoma
    biopsies
      core needle biopsy, IV:106
      excisional biopsies, IV:106–107
      fine-needle aspiration (FNA), IV:106
      incisional biopsies, IV:107
      reoperative biopsies, IV:107–108
    characteristics, IV:101–102
    epidemiology, IV:103
    imaging methods, IV:104, 104f
    Muskuloskeletal Tumor Society staging
      system, IV:105t
    outcome assessments, IV:115–116
    patient presentation and diagnosis,
      IV:103–104, 104f

sarcomas (Continued)
    patient selection, IV:104
    pediatric tumors, VI:655, 656f
    preservation options
      complex approaches, IV:112
      general discussion, IV:110–112
      neuromuscular units, IV:111
      skeletal reconstruction, IV:111–112, 111f
      vascular surgery, IV:112
    recurrence management, IV:116–125
    surgical resection techniques
      amputation indicators, IV:110
      biopsies, IV:106–108
      lymph node dissection, IV:110
      nerve involvement, IV:109
      osseous involvement, IV:109
      primary osseous sarcomas, IV:109
      specimen handling, IV:109
      surgical revisions, IV:107–108, 108t
      vascular involvement, IV:108
      wound closure, IV:109
    treatment strategies
      chemotherapy, IV:106
      radiation therapy (RT), IV:106
      surgical goals, IV:104–105
      surgical planning, IV:105
      surgical treatment, IV:105–106
    tumor growth and metastasis, IV:103
  chest wall tumors, IV:247
  hand tumors, VI:321, 322f–323f
  lower extremity reconstructive surgery,
    IV:101–126
  biopsies
    core needle biopsy, IV:106
    excisional biopsies, IV:106–107
    fine-needle aspiration (FNA), IV:106
    incisional biopsies, IV:107
    reoperative biopsies, IV:107–108
  bone sarcoma
    characteristics, IV:101–102
    epidemiology, IV:103
    imaging methods, IV:104, 104f
    Muskuloskeletal Tumor Society staging
      system, IV:105t
    outcome assessments, IV:115–116
    patient presentation and diagnosis,
      IV:103–104, 104f
    patient selection, IV:104
    preservation options, IV:110–112
    recurrence management, IV:116–125
    surgical resection techniques, IV:106–108
    treatment strategies, IV:104
    tumor growth and metastasis, IV:103
  case studies
    case study 4.1, IV:116b–117b, 116f–117f
    case study 4.2, IV:117b, 118f
    case study 4.3, IV:117b–120b, 119f–120f
    case study 4.4, IV:120b, 121f
    case study 4.5, IV:120b–123b, 122f–123f
    case study 4.6, IV:123b–125b, 123f–124f
    case study 4.7, IV:124f–125f, 125b
  clinical manifestations, IV:102
  epidemiology, IV:102–103
  imaging methods, IV:104, 104f
  Muskuloskeletal Tumor Society staging
    system, IV:105t
  outcome assessments
    bone sarcoma, IV:115–116
    prognosis, IV:114
    soft-tissue sarcomas, IV:114–115, 115t

sarcomas (Continued)
patient presentation and diagnosis, IV:103–104
patient selection, IV:104
postoperative care and follow-up
immediate postoperative care, IV:112–113
oncologic postoperative care and follow-up, IV:113
preservation options
complex approaches, IV:112
general discussion, IV:110–112
neuromuscular units, IV:111
skeletal reconstruction, IV:111–112, 111f
soft-tissue sarcomas, IV:110–111
vascular surgery, IV:112
recurrence management, IV:116–125
secondary procedures
late secondary procedures, IV:114
skeletal reconstruction, IV:113–114
soft tissue, IV:113
soft-tissue sarcomas
epidemiology, IV:102–103
histopathologic types, IV:103f
predisposing factors, IV:102t
preservation options, IV:110–111
surgical resection techniques
amputation indicators, IV:110
biopsies, IV:106–108
definitive resections, IV:108
lymph node dissection, IV:110
nerve involvement, IV:109
osseous involvement, IV:109
primary osseous sarcomas, IV:109
specimen handling, IV:109
surgical revisions, IV:107–108, 108t
vascular involvement, IV:108
wound closure, IV:109
TNM clinical classification system, IV:105t
treatment strategies
chemotherapy, IV:106
radiation therapy (RT), IV:106
surgical goals, IV:104–105
surgical planning, IV:105, 105t
surgical treatment, IV:105–106
tumor growth and metastasis, IV:103
soft-tissue sarcomas
biopsies
core needle biopsy, IV:106
excisional biopsies, IV:106–107
fine-needle aspiration (FNA), IV:106
incisional biopsies, IV:107
reoperative biopsies, IV:107–108
characteristics, IV:101–102
epidemiology, IV:102–103
histopathologic types, IV:103f
imaging methods, IV:104, 104f
Muskuloskeletal Tumor Society staging system, IV:105t
outcome assessments, IV:114–115, 115t
patient presentation and diagnosis, IV:103–104, 104f
patient selection, IV:104
predisposing factors, IV:102t
preservation options
complex approaches, IV:112
flaps, IV:110–111

sarcomas (Continued)
general discussion, IV:110–112
neuromuscular units, IV:111
skeletal reconstruction, IV:111–112, 111f
vascular surgery, IV:112
recurrence management, IV:116–125
surgical resection techniques
amputation indicators, IV:110
biopsies, IV:106–108
definitive resections, IV:108
lymph node dissection, IV:110
nerve involvement, IV:109
osseous involvement, IV:109
primary osseous sarcomas, IV:109
specimen handling, IV:109
surgical revisions, IV:107–108, 108t
vascular involvement, IV:108
wound closure, IV:109
TNM clinical classification system, IV:105t
treatment strategies
chemotherapy, IV:106
radiation therapy (RT), IV:106
surgical goals, IV:104–105
surgical planning, IV:105, 105t
surgical treatment, IV:105–106
tumor growth and metastasis, IV:103
sartorius muscle, I:516f, 554–557, IV:15t–16t, 18f–22f, 19t, 35f
SAT classification of mandibular deformity, III:774t
satellite nevi, III:848–851, 849f
saw palmetto, V:33t–35t
scalds, IV:394, 394f
scalp
aesthetic units, III:108–109, 109f
anatomical characteristics, III:14
aesthetic units, III:108–109, 109f
auricular muscles, III:107f
blood supply, III:107, 108f
general characteristics, III:105–106
hair structure and cycle, III:109, 110f
nerves, III:107–108, 108f
schematic diagram, III:106f
temporal region, III:106–107, 107f
congenital melanocytic nevi (CMN), III:844, 845f
disorders
aplasia cutis congenita (ACC), III:110–111, 111f
basal cell carcinoma, III:117–118, 118f
burns, III:119–120, 120f
cicatricial alopecia, III:109–110, 111t
cutaneous sarcoidosis, III:115–116, 116f
discoid lupus erythematosus (DLE), III:115, 115f
dysplastic nevus, III:113–114, 114f
en coup de sabre (ECDS), III:114–115, 115f
epidermoid cyst, III:116–117, 116f
giant hair nevus/congenital nevomelanocytic nevus (CNN), III:112–113, 114f
infections, III:119
lipoma, III:116
malignant melanomas, III:119, 119f
neoplasms, III:116

scalp (Continued)
nevoid basal cell carcinoma syndrome (NBCCS), III:112, 112t, 113f
nevus sebaceous of Jadassohn, III:111–112, 112f
physical trauma, III:119–120
squamous cell carcinomas (SCCs), III:118–119, 118f
syringoma, III:117, 117f
trichoepithelioma, III:117, 117f
xeroderma pigmentosum (XP), III:112, 114f
fascial layers, III:3–8, 4f
hair structure and cycle, III:109, 110f
hypertelorism correction, III:699
reconstructive surgeries, III:105–133
anatomical considerations
auricular muscles, III:107f
blood supply, III:107, 108f
general characteristics, III:105–106
nerves, III:107–108, 108f
schematic diagram, III:106f
temporal region, III:106–107, 107f
burn wound treatment, III:119–120, 120f, IV:492–493, 498–499, 504, 504f
complications, III:131–132
patient presentation and diagnosis, III:120
patient selection, III:120–121, 121t
postoperative care and follow-up, III:131
secondary procedures, III:132
surgical technique and treatment
blood supply, III:128f
cervical facial advancement flap, III:125, 127f
closure by secondary intention, III:121
Juri flap, III:123–124, 125f
latissimus dorsi (LD) flap, III:130, 130f
local flaps, III:123–127, 124f, 126f, 441
microsurgical reconstruction, III:128–130, 129f
Orticochea three-flap technique, III:124f
pericranial flaps, III:125, 127f–128f
primary closure, III:121
radial forearm flap, III:128–130, 129f
regional flaps, III:127–128, 129f
rhomboid flap, III:441, 442f–443f
scalp reduction techniques, III:124, 125f
scalp replantation, III:130–131, 131f
skin grafts, III:123, 123f
tissue expansion, III:121–123, 122f
vacuum-assisted closure (VAC), III:121, 122f
vertical trapezius flap, III:127–128, 129f
trauma-acquired defects, III:105
soft-tissue injuries
anesthesia, III:26, 27f
surgical technique and treatment, III:33–34, 33f, 35f–37f
tissue expansion, I:631–633, 632f–634f
scaphocephaly, III:728–729, 729f, 729t
scaphoid bone, VI:163–164
scaphoid nonunion advanced collapse (SNAC) arthritis, VI:441–442, 443f
scaphoid shift test, VI:54, 166f
scapholunate advanced collapse (SLAC) arthrtis, VI:441–442, 442f

scapholunate interosseous ligament injury, **VI:**85–86, 87f
scapular and parascapular flaps
  hemifacial atrophy, **III:**799–800, 800f
  mangled upper extremities, **VI:**272, 273f
scapular and thoracodorsal pedicles, **I:**530f
scapular osteomusculocutaneous flap, **III:**323, 323f
Scarpa's fascia
  abdominoplasty
    characteristics, **II:**551
    indicators, **II:**551
    operative technique, **II:**551
    outcome assessments, **II:**551, 552f–553f
  anatomical characteristics, **IV:**227–230, 227f, 298–299
  lipoabdominoplasty, **II:**561–563, 562f–563f
  lower bodylift/belt lipectomy surgery, **II:**585–588, 586f
  male genital aesthetic surgery, **II:**656
  male perineum, **IV:**235, 236f–237f
scars, **I:**297–318
  abdominoplasty, **II:**554–555, 556f
  brachioplasty, **II:**630f–632f, 632–633
  burn reconstruction, **IV:**444–445, 497
  buttock augmentation, **II:**616
  characteristics and functional role, **I:**250–252, 301–304, 302t
  cicatricial alopecia, **III:**109–110, 111t
  clinical evaluations, **I:**264–266, 298–299, 299t–300t
  etiological determination, **I:**298, 298b
  facelift complications, **II:**206
  facial skin resurfacing, **II:**77
  hypertrophic scars
    benign mesenchymal-origin tumors, **I:**730, 731f
    brachioplasty, **V:**563–564
    laser treatments, **II:**69
    reconstructive burn surgery, **IV:**434, 497, 501, 501f–502f
    wound healing, **I:**265, 283–284, 283t, 293f, 302, 302t, 303f, 307–308
  keloid scars, **I:**730, 730f
  mastopexy, **V:**125–147, 149, 243t
  melanoma excisions, **I:**765–766, 766f
  near-ear facelift deformities, **II:**492
  personal and social significance, **I:**297–298
  physical examination, **I:**298, 298b
  postoperative care and follow-up, **I:**316–317
  prevention
    adjunct therapy, **I:**306–307
    foreign-body reactions, **I:**306
    patient-specific factors, **I:**306
    surgical technique, **I:**304–306, 304b, 305f–306f
    wound infections, **I:**306
  revisionary breast surgery, **V:**65–66, 66t, 246–247
  scar biology and formation, **I:**300, 301f–302f
  scar retraction, **IV:**444–445
  scar revision
    abdominal wall reconstruction, **IV:**295
    basic principles, **I:**310
    buttock augmentation, **II:**616
    indicators, **I:**310
    laser treatments, **I:**308, **II:**67–70, **IV:**454t
    planning strategies, **I:**311
    scar release, **I:**311–312, **IV:**501–502, 502f
    serial excision, **I:**311, 311f

scars (Continued)
    surgical timing, **I:**310
    tissue rearrangement, **I:**312
    Z-plasty technique
      basic principles, **I:**312–316, 313b
      gains in length, **I:**312t
      geometric broken line, **I:**316, 317f
      lip reconstruction, **III:**268–270, 269f–270f
      multiple-flap Z-plasty, **I:**315, 315f–316f
      planimetric Z-plasty, **I:**314, 314f
      simple Z-plasty, **I:**313–314, 313f
      skew Z-plasty, **I:**314–315, 314f
      V-Y and Y-V advancement flaps, **I:**316, 316f
      W-plasty, **I:**316, 317f, **III:**268–270
  secondary cleft deformities, **III:**635, 636f
  secondary facelifts
    cross-hatched scars, **II:**288–290, 290f
    poorly situated scars, **II:**284–288, 285f–289f
    wide scars, **II:**288, 289f
  skeletal reconstruction, **IV:**187–188
  soft-tissue fillers, **II:**57
  treatment strategies
    clinical wound management
      closed wounds, **I:**285–286, 286t
      engineered skin replacements, **I:**289t, 290
      excessive scar treatment, **I:**290–291
      excisional wounds, **I:**286–287
      general discussion, **I:**285–295
      incisional wounds, **I:**285–286, 286t
      open wounds, **I:**286–287
      pharmacologic treatment, **I:**290
      wound dressings, **I:**287–288, 289t
      wound treatment, **I:**287
    emerging treatments, **I:**294–295, 309–310
    excessive scars
      prevention and reduction therapies, **I:**291, 292t
      scar classification, **I:**290, 291t
      therapies, **I:**290–291
    hypertrophic scars, **I:**307–308
    keloid scars, **I:**308–309
    proper diagnosis, **I:**307–310
  wound healing
    characteristics and functional role, **I:**264–266, 301–304, 302t
    hypertrophic scars, **I:**265, 283–284, 283t, 302, 302t, 303f, 307–308
    immature scars, **I:**302t
    keloid scars, **I:**265, 283t, 284–285, 302–304, 302t, 303f, 308–309
    mature scars, **I:**302t
    regenerative fetal healing, **I:**265–266
    scar biology and formation, **I:**273, 276f, 300, 301f–302f
    vertical scar reduction mammaplasty, **V:**190, 191f
Schinzel syndrome, **VI:**567t
Schireson, Henry J, **I:**27
Schobinger clinical staging system, **VI:**686t
Schobinger staging system, **I:**698–699, 699t
Schwann cells, **I:**231–232, 707, **VI:**697, 698f
schwannomas, **I:**727, 728f, **VI:**320, 320f
schwannomatosis, **III:**877–878
sciatic nerve, **II:**607f, **IV:**28f
scientific journals (twentieth century), **I:**24–25, 25f

scientific societies (twentieth century), **I:**24
scintigraphy, **I:**710, **VI:**312
scleroderma, **VI:**407t, 409
sclerotherapy, **I:**683f, 692–693, 696, 718
S-corporations, **I:**85
scratch collapse test, **VI:**514
scrofula
  disease process, **III:**891
  patient presentation and diagnosis, **III:**891
  surgical technique and treatment, **III:**891
scrotum
  anatomical characteristics, **IV:**235, 236f–237f, 298–299, 299f
  blood supply, **IV:**299–301, 299f–301f
  hypospadia
    defect occurrence, **III:**907f–908f
    embryology, **III:**907–908
    epidemiology, **III:**908
    etiology, **III:**908
    meatoplasty and glanuloplasty
      basic procedure, **III:**913–915, 916f
      onlay island flap repair, **III:**914–915, 918f
      orthoplasty, **III:**915
      surgical tips, **III:**914b–915b
      tubularized incised plate (TIP) repair, **III:**914, 917f
      two-stage repair, **III:**915, 919f–921f
    outcomes and complicatons, **III:**916–921
    postoperative care and follow-up, **III:**915
    secondary procedures, **III:**921
    urethral reconstruction, **III:**913, 915f
  lymphatic supply, **IV:**301
  male genital aesthetic surgery
    penoscrotal web, **II:**662, 663f
    scrotal enlargement, **II:**662, 664f
  male genital reconstructive surgery, **IV:**297–325
    congenital defects
      disorders of sex development (DSD), **IV:**303–304
      exstrophy and epispadias, **IV:**301–303, 302f–303f
      hidden penis, **IV:**304, 304f–305f
      severe penile insufficiency, **IV:**304–306, 306f
    female-to-male transsexual surgery
      metaidoioplasty, **IV:**315–318, 317f, 346
      normal scrotum, **IV:**321, 322f
      pars fixa of the urethra creation, **IV:**314–315, 316f–317f
      phalloplasty, **IV:**318–323
      vaginectomy, **IV:**314–315, 315f
    general discussion, **IV:**297
    genital anatomy
      blood supply, **IV:**299–301, 299f–301f
      general discussion, **IV:**298–301
      genital fascia, **IV:**298–299, 299f
      lymphatic supply, **IV:**301
      nerve supply, **IV:**301
    genital embryology
      genetic sex, **IV:**297
      gonadal sex, **IV:**297–298
      phenotypic sex, **IV:**298, 298f
    microsurgical genital reconstruction
      genital replantation, **IV:**310–312, 312f
      phallic construction, **IV:**312
    multidisciplinary approach, **IV:**323
    post-traumatic genital defects
      basic principles, **IV:**306–313
      genital flaps, **IV:**304–310, 306f, 311f

scrotum (Continued)
    genital skin grafts, IV:307, 308f–309f
    microsurgical genital reconstruction,
        IV:310–312
    reconstructive indications, IV:312–313
    reconstructive indications
        Fournier disease, IV:312–313, 313f
        penile cancer, IV:313, 314f
    meatoplasty and glanuloplasty
        basic procedure, III:913–915, 916f
        onlay island flap repair, III:914–915, 918f
        orthoplasty, III:915
        surgical tips, III:914b–915b
        tubularized incised plate (TIP) repair,
            III:914, 917f
        two-stage repair, III:915, 919f–921f
    nerve supply, IV:301
    reconstructive burn surgery, IV:506
    scrotoplasty, III:913, IV:314–315, 315f–317f,
        346
    vascular anatomy, IV:237f–238f
    See also gender identity disorder
sculpted pillar vertical reduction
    mammaplasty, V:228–241
    background and general characteristics,
        V:228
    complications, V:236–239, 239f–241f
    patient selection, V:228–229
    planning and marking guidelines, V:229,
        229f–230f
    research summary, V:239
    surgical technique
        basic procedure, V:229–236
        large breast reduction, V:236, 238f
        moderate breast reduction, V:236, 237f
        small breast reduction, V:235, 236f
        wound closure, V:231–235, 232f–235f
Sculptra (New-Fill), II:47–48, 47t, 49t
    See also soft-tissue fillers
Scutellaria baicalensis, V:33t–35t
seasonal tonics, V:33t–35t
seat mapping, IV:378f
sebaceous adenoma, I:723
sebaceous carcinoma, I:738, 738f
sebaceous cysts, VI:314, 314f
sebaceous glands, I:321–323, 322f, II:44–45
seborrheic keratosis, I:719, 719f, 747–750, 748f,
    VI:316
    See also cutaneous and soft-tissue tumors
Seckel syndrome, VI:573t
secondary breast augmentation See
    revisionary breast surgery
secondary breast reconstruction, I:645, 646f
secondary (callus) bone repair, I:439–441, 439f,
    441f
secondary cleft deformities, III:631–654
    cleft lip
        cleft lip anatomy, III:633, 634f
        evaluation examinations, III:634–635, 635f
        lips
            Cupid's bow, III:639
            long lip, III:637
            philtral column reconstruction,
                III:638–639, 639f
            short lateral lip, III:638
            short lip, III:635–637, 636f
            tight lip, III:637, 637f–638f
            wide lip, III:637–638

secondary cleft deformities (Continued)
        normal lip anatomy, III:633, 633f–634f
        patient selection, III:635
        scarring considerations, III:635, 636f
        timing considerations, III:635
        vermillion
            buccal sulcus deformities, III:641–642,
                641f
            orbicularis muscle deformities,
                III:640–641
            thick lip, III:639
            thin lip, III:639, 640f
            vermillion mismatch, III:639–640
            vermillion notching/vermillion border
                malalignment, III:640
            whistle deformity, III:640
    cleft nose
        cleft nose anatomy, III:646–647, 646f–647f
        decision-making process, III:653
        evaluation examinations, III:647–648
        normal anatomy, III:644–646, 646t
        patient selection, III:648
        surgical technique and treatment
            goals, III:648–653, 648f
            operative technique, III:649–650,
                649f–651f
            preoperative/postoperative
                comparisons, III:648f
            skeletal access, III:648–649
            supporting grafts, III:650–653,
                652f–653f
            suturing techniques, III:649–650,
                649f–652f
            Weir excision, III:650f
        timing considerations, III:648
    cleft palate
        evaluation examinations, III:642
        palatal fistulas, III:642, 643f
        patient selection, III:642
        Pittsburgh fistula classification system,
            III:642, 642t
        surgical technique and treatment,
            III:642–644, 643f–646f
        timing considerations, III:642
    etiology, III:631
    patient presentation and diagnosis, III:632
    wound healing and growth, III:631–632,
        632f–633f
secondary facelifts, II:277–312
    patient considerations, II:308–309
    planning considerations, II:311
    secondary deformities
        general discussion, II:278
        secondary aging deformities, II:278, 278f
        secondary surgical deformities
            characteristics, II:278–308
            cross-hatched scars, II:288–290, 290f
            drapery lines, II:303f
            earlobe deformities, II:290–293, 292f
            eyelid skin deficiencies/eyelid
                malposition, II:308
            facial atrophy, II:306–308, 307f
            fat injections, II:306–308, 307f
            hairline displacement and disruption,
                II:279–282, 279f–283f
            hair loss, II:282–284, 283f–284f
            inappropriate skin shifts, II:300–301,
                301f–302f

secondary facelifts (Continued)
        inappropriate SMAS shifts/SMAS
            injury, II:304, 304f
        large digastric muscles, II:296–297, 297f
        laser resurfacing, II:308
        over-excision of buccal fat, II:294, 295f
        over-excision of subcutaneous fat,
            II:293–294, 293f–294f
        over-excision of subplatysmal fat,
            II:294, 295f
        poorly situated scars, II:284–288,
            285f–289f
        prominent submandibular glands,
            II:294–296, 296f
        residual jowl, II:300, 300f
        residual platysma bands, II:297–299,
            298f
        skin deficiencies, II:301–303
        skin slough, II:303
        smile block, II:304–305, 304f
        temporal face compression, II:301
        tightness and wrinkling, II:301–303,
            302f–303f
        tragal deformities, II:290, 291f, 492
        unaesthetic facial implants, II:305
        uncorrected and under-corrected
            mid-face deformities, II:299–300,
            299f–300f
        un-rejuvenated forehead, II:305–306,
            306f
        un-rejuvenated peri-oral region, II:306
        wide scars, II:288, 289f
    technical considerations, II:309
secondary facial reconstruction, III:461–472
    complications, III:471
    etiology, III:461
    goals, III:461
    patient presentation and diagnosis,
        III:461–462
    patient selection, III:462
    postoperative care and follow-up, III:471
    prognosis and outcomes, III:471
    surgical technique and treatment
        case study 1
            diagnosis, III:465
            patient description, III:464b–466b,
                464f–465f
            reconstructive plan, III:465–466
        case study 2
            diagnosis, III:466
            patient description, III:466b–467b,
                466f–467f
            reconstructive plan, III:467
        case study 3
            diagnosis, III:467
            patient description, III:467b–469b, 468f
            reconstructive plan, III:467–469
        case study 4
            diagnosis, III:469
            patient description, III:469b–471b,
                469f–470f
            reconstructive plan, III:469–471
        flap prelamination, III:464–471
        hair-bearing flaps, III:463
        intraoral and intranasal lining, III:462–
            463, 463f
        planning guidelines, III:462–471
        prefabricated flaps, III:463

Note: **Boldface** roman numerals indicate volume. Page numbers followed by f refer to figures; page numbers followed by t refer to tables; page numbers followed by b refer to boxes.

secondary hernias, **IV**:294
secondary intention healing, **III**:32–33
secondary palate clefts, **III**:571
secondary rhinoplasty, **II**:466–484
    challenges, **II**:466
    characteristics, **II**:448
    common problems
        broad/bulbous/round tip, **II**:470
        open rhinoplasty-caused deformities,
            II:448–449, 449f
        suture-based tip plasty
            alar rim deformities, **II**:473–475,
                475f–478f
            broad nasal base, **II**:476–478, 479f–480f
            characteristics, **II**:471–480, 472f–473f
            closed approach, **II**:471–472
            deficient tip, **II**:472–473, 474f
            fascial graft and repair, **II**:477f–478f
            middle vault collapse, **II**:473
            nasal dorsum irregularities, **II**:478–479
            septoplasty, **II**:479–480, 480f
            short nose, **II**:475–476, 478f–479f
            thin skin tip, **II**:475, 477f–478f
    complications
        columellar scars, **II**:481–482, 482f
        difficult patients, **II**:482–483
        post-rhinoplasty fibrotic syndrome,
            II:482, 483f
        skin necrosis, **II**:481, 482f
    definition, **II**:466
    general discussion, **II**:448–449
    nasal evaluation, **II**:467
    operative technique
        anesthesia, **II**:468
        artistry, **II**:467, 467f
        cartilage grafts, **II**:470, 470f–471f
        open versus closed approach, **II**:467, 468f
        suturing techniques, **II**:468–470, 534f
    patient presentation and diagnosis, **II**:466
    patient selection, **II**:467
    postoperative care and follow-up
        corticosteroids, **II**:481
        early bad result, **II**:480–481, 481f
        early care, **II**:480
        fillers, **II**:481
secondary sclerosing cholangitis (SSC), **IV**:434
second branchial cleft anomaly
    disease process, **III**:885, 885f
    patient presentation and diagnosis, **III**:885,
        885f
    surgical technique and treatment, **III**:885–
        886, 886f
seed money, **I**:845–846, 845f
segmental transposition flaps, **I**:522–524,
    523f–524f
selective norepinephrine reuptake inhibitors,
    I:51
selective photothermolysis (SPT)
    characteristics, **II**:64
    reaction types
        biostimulation, **II**:64
        photochemical reactions, **II**:64
        photothermal reactions, **II**:64
        surface cooling, **II**:64
selective serotonin reuptake inhibitors, **II**:21t
selenium (Se), **II**:23–24
self-destructive deniers, **I**:37–38
Selphyl, **II**:46
semimembranosus muscle, **IV**:15t–16t, 18f–22f,
    19t

semi-open rhinoplasty
    alar base positioning, **III**:536–537
    alar-facial groove creation, **III**:537, 538f–539f
    background information, **III**:535–537
    excessive skin trimming, **III**:536, 537f
    fibrofatty tissue release, **III**:536, 537f
    incisions, **III**:536, 537f
    lower lateral cartilage repositioning, **III**:536,
        537f
semitendinosus muscle, **IV**:15t–16t, 18f–22f,
    19t, 35f
Semmes–Weinstein monofilament test, **VI**:53t,
    59, 59t, 505–507
senile wart, **I**:719, 719f
sensitive nerves, **I**:320
sensitive skin
    acne, **II**:19–20
    classifications, **II**:19–24, 19t
    rosacea, **II**:20–21, 21t
    treatment strategies
        aloe vera, **II**:22
        chamomile, **II**:22
        corticosteroids, **II**:21
        curcumin, **II**:24
        cyclooxygenase inhibitors, **II**:21–22
        feverfew, **II**:22
        food choices, **II**:24
        ginseng, **II**:22–23
        licorice extract, **II**:23
        mushrooms, **II**:23
        oatmeal, **II**:23
        salicylic acid, **II**:22
        selenium (Se), **II**:23–24
        sulfur/sulfacetamide, **II**:22
        turmeric, **II**:24
sensory nerve action potential (SNAP),
    VI:504
sensory nerves
    anatomical characteristics, **III**:17–19,
        17f–18f
    brachial plexus injuries, **VI**:796, 796t
    breast anatomy, **V**:9
    facial nerve connections, **III**:14
    forehead, **II**:96–97, 96f–97f
    sensory nerve action potentials (SNAPs),
        VI:797–798
sentinel lymph node biopsy (SNLB), **I**:758–
    760, 760f, 761t
septal extension, **II**:112, 114f, 175, 175f
septic arthritis, **VI**:339–341, 340f
septum
    anatomical characteristics, **II**:382–386,
        382f–385f, 450–452, 451f–452f
    autologous cartilage harvesting
        basic procedure, **II**:394–395
        septal L-strut, **II**:395f
        submucoperichondrial dissection, **II**:394f
        submucoperichondrial flaps, **II**:395f
    deviated septum, **II**:392–393, 454–455,
        454f–456f
    fractures and dislocations
        characteristics, **III**:58–59, 58f
        complications, **III**:60
        treatment strategies, **III**:59–60
    pediatric facial fractures, **III**:681–682
    preoperative assessment, **II**:423
    septal collapse, **II**:446
    septal perforation, **II**:445
    septoplasty, **II**:434–435, 479–480, 480f
    traumatic injuries, **III**:43

sequelae obstetric brachial plexus palsy
    characteristics, **VI**:812–815
    elbow deformity reconstruction, **VI**:815
    examination chart, **VI**:814t
    forearm and hand deformity reconstruction,
        VI:815
    shoulder deformity reconstruction,
        VI:813–815
Serenoa repens, **V**:33t–35t
serine, **I**:269–271
seromas
    abdominal wall reconstruction, **IV**:293–294
    abdominoplasty, **II**:557–558
    bilateral pedicle TRAM flap reconstruction,
        V:407–410
    brachioplasty, **II**:629t, **V**:563–564
    breast augmentation, **V**:32–37, 79t
    breast reduction, **V**:243t
    buttock augmentation, **II**:614
    liposuctions, **II**:526
    lower bodylift/belt lipectomy surgery,
        II:590
    male chest contouring, **V**:579
    melanoma treatment, **I**:781t
    muscle/musculocutaneous flaps, **I**:571–572
    periareolar surgical technique with mesh
        support, **V**:226, 226t
    post-bariatric surgery reconstruction, **II**:653
    revisionary breast surgery, **V**:65–66, 66t, 79t,
        243t
    scalp and forehead reconstruction,
        III:131–132
    sculpted pillar vertical reduction
        mammaplasty, **V**:237–238
    skin grafts, **I**:334
    vertical scar reduction mammaplasty, **V**:191t
seronegative spondyloarthropathies, **VI**:406–
    408, 407t
serotonin, **I**:573–574, 574f, 580–581
serous drainage, **V**:359–360
serratus anterior artery perforator (SAAP)
    flap, **V**:486f–488f, 488–489
serratus anterior muscles
    anatomical characteristics, **IV**:224–225,
        V:10–11, 10f
    chest wall reconstruction, **I**:552, **IV**:244, 244f
    foot reconstruction, **IV**:211
    lower extremity reconstructive surgery,
        IV:77
    mangled upper extremities, **VI**:277–279
    microneurovascular muscle transplantation,
        III:295t
serratus posterior muscles, **IV**:222, 222f
sertraline, **I**:51
17β-estradiol, **IV**:341t
severe penile insufficiency, **IV**:304–306, 306f
sex-linked inheritance, **I**:183, 183f
Seymour fracture, **VI**:158, 158f
S-flap, **V**:511–512, 511f, 511t
Shaw, Darrel T, **II**:108–109
shea butter, **II**:18
Sheehan, Eastman, **I**:23–24, 24f, 27
sheepskin, medical, **IV**:364–366
Short-Form McGill Pain Questionnaire
    (SF-MPQ), **VI**:855–856
short lateral lip, **III**:638
short lip, **III**:635–637, 636f
short lower face, **III**:666
short nose, **II**:175–176, 475–476, 478f–479f
short rib-polydactyly, Majewski type, **VI**:573t

short rib-polydactyly, non-Majewski type, **VI:**573t
short scar periareolar inferior pedicle reduction (SPAIR) mammaplasty, **V:**194–205
    background and general characteristics, **V:**159, 194–195
    complications
        areolar spreading, **V:**204
        fat necrosis, **V:**203–204
        general discussion, **V:**203–205
        hypertrophy recurrence, **V:**204–205
        polytetrafluoroethylene (PTFE) infection/exposure, **V:**204
        shape distortion, **V:**204
    patient selection, **V:**195–196
    planning and marking guidelines, **V:**196, 197f–198f
    reduction results
        large breast reduction, **V:**202–203, 203f
        modest breast reduction, **V:**202, 203f
        small breast reduction, **V:**201–203, 202f
    research summary, **V:**205
    surgical technique, **V:**196–201, 200f–201f
shoulder
    adult brachial plexus injury reconstructive strategies, **VI:**800, 801t
    burn reconstruction, **IV:**443, 443t
    joint denervation surgery, **VI:**497t
    sequelae obstetric brachial plexus palsy, **VI:**813–815
    shoulder disarticulation/proximal transhumeral amputation, **VI:**875
    spastic hand surgery, **VI:**460
    targeted muscle reinnervation (TMR), **VI:**877–879, 878f–879f, 879t
Shprintzen syndrome, **III:**807
sialadenitis, **III:**365, 365f
sialadenosis, **III:**365
sialography, **III:**364
sialolithiasis, **III:**365, 366f–367f
Siamese twins *See* conjoined twins
Sibutramine, **II:**635
Sickler syndrome, **III:**665
Sickness Impact Profile (SIP) questionnaire, **IV:**85–86
sigmoid vaginoplasty, **IV:**346–347
silicone
    facial skeletal augmentation, **II:**342
    implants, **I:**789–790, 790f, **II:**342
    liquid silicone injections, **V:**98–100, 99f–100f
    nomenclature, **I:**789t
    physicochemical properties, **V:**14
    pressure garments, **IV:**426f
    silicone constrained prostheses, **VI:**426, 427f
    silicone gel implants
        capsular calcification, **V:**107–109, 108f–109f
        capsular contracture, **V:**106–107, 106f–107f
        characteristics, **I:**789–790, 790f
        closed capsulotomy, **V:**107, 107f–108f
        decision guidelines, **V:**24–25
        developmental background, **V:**14–15
        double-bubble deformity, **V:**116, 116f
        first generation implants, **V:**14–15, 103f
        fourth and fifth generation implants, **V:**15
        hematomas, **V:**104–105, 104f–105f

silicone *(Continued)*
        historical background, **I:**789–790, **V:**102–109
        implant disruption, **V:**103–104, 103f
        implant malposition, **V:**112–113, 113f
        infections, **V:**105–106, 105f–106f
        pectus excavatum, **III:**856–859, 857f
        second generation implants, **V:**14–15, 104f
        third generation implants, **V:**14–15, 104f
    silicone gel sheeting, **I:**289t, 292t, 293f, 307
    synthetic fillers, **II:**47t
    textured silicone expanders, **I:**627
silicon (Si)
    metal alloy compositions, **I:**786–787
    nomenclature, **I:**789t
    silica, **I:**789t
    silicates, **I:**789t
Silikon 1000, **II:**47–48, 47t
    See also soft-tissue fillers
siloxane, **I:**789t
silver nitrate, **IV:**410
Silver–Russell syndrome, **VI:**565t
silver sulfadiazine, **IV:**395, 410
simple analgesics, **IV:**427
simple lacerations, **III:**30, 31f
simple Z-plasty, **I:**313–314, 313f
simulation
    basic principles, **I:**865
    functional role
        surgical planning simulators, **I:**868–869, 869f
        training simulators, **I:**865–868, 866f–868f, 867t
    future trends, **I:**869–870
    implementation, **I:**865
    physical–behavioral–genomics model, **I:**869–870, 869f
    research summary, **I:**873
    use rationale, **I:**865
Singapore flap, **IV:**387f, 389–390
single-lobe transposition flap, **III:**143, 144f–145f
single nucleotide polymorphism (SNPs), **I:**184–185
single-photon emission computed tomography (SPECT), **III:**382
sinonasal undifferentiated carcinoma (SNUC), **III:**436–437
sinus pericranii, **I:**695
SIPOC analysis (suppliers, inputs, process, outputs, and customers), **I:**77–78
sirolimus, **I:**822t
Six Sigma program case study, **I:**78b
skate flap, **V:**502–504, 503f–505f, 503t
skeletal reconstruction, **IV:**174–188
    bone grafts, **I:**425–463
        acquired cranial and facial bone deformities, **III:**227, 228f–229f
        allogeneic bone grafts
            advantages, **I:**459–460
            allograft bone incorporation, **I:**460
            bone graft formulations, **I:**460
            disease transmission risk, **I:**459
            immunogenicity, **I:**460
            processing and preservation techniques, **I:**459
        allografts, **IV:**174–175
        back soft-tissue reconstruction, **IV:**271

skeletal reconstruction *(Continued)*
    bone morphogenetic proteins (BMPs), **IV:**174–175, 186–187
    bone remodeling
        age factors, **I:**448
        blood supply, **I:**448
        distraction osteogenesis, **I:**446–447, 447f
        influencing factors, **I:**447–448
        ossoeintegration, **I:**445
        osteoconduction, **I:**445
        osteoinduction, **I:**444–445
        patient factors, **I:**448
        radiation therapy (RT), **I:**448
    bone transfers
        allogeneic bone grafts, **I:**459–460
        basic principles, **I:**459
        bone graft healing and graft survival, **I:**448–449
        bone substitutes, **I:**460
        calvarium harvests, **I:**454–455, 454f
        cement pastes, **I:**460–462
        clinical considerations, **I:**449
        cortical versus cancellous bone grafts, **I:**449
        fibula harvests, **I:**452
        greater trochanter harvests, **I:**452
        harvesting methods, **I:**449–455
        ilium harvests, **I:**449–452, 450f–451f
        indicators, **I:**448
        olecranon harvests, **I:**452
        prefabricated polymers, **I:**462
        rib harvests, **I:**452–454, 453f
        tibia harvests, **I:**452, 452f
        vascularized bone flaps, **I:**455–459
        xenogeneic bone grafts, **I:**460
    cement pastes
        BoneSource, **I:**461
        calcium phosphate (CaP), **I:**460–461
        Norian SRS/CRS, **I:**461
        osteoactive materials, **I:**461–462
    constriction band syndrome, **VI:**642
    craniofacial microsomia (CFM), **III:**781–782, 783f
    distraction osteogenesis
        basic principles, **I:**446–447
        histology, **I:**446–447, 447f
    donor site considerations, **III:**227, 228f–229f
    fracture healing
        age factors, **I:**444
        blood supply, **I:**441–442, 442f
        characteristics, **I:**438–444
        fracture fixation, **I:**442
        primary bone repair, **I:**439, 439f–440f
        secondary (callus) bone repair, **I:**439–441, 439f, 441f
    Le Fort III osteotomy–bipartition correction technique, **III:**695
    orbital fractures, **III:**55
    prefabricated polymers
        Medpor, **I:**462
        methylmethacrylate, **I:**462
    soft-tissue cover, **III:**227
    surgical technique and treatment, **IV:**176–177
    vascularized bone flaps, **IV:**175, 175f
        advantages, **I:**455–459
        vacularized calvarium, **I:**457–459, 458f

Note: **Boldface** roman numerals indicate volume. Page numbers followed by f refer to figures; page numbers followed by t refer to tables; page numbers followed by b refer to boxes.

skeletal reconstruction (Continued)
vacularized fibula, I:455, 457f
vascularized iliac transfer, I:455, 456f
vascularized rib, I:456–457
vascularized scapula, I:455–456, 458f
facial injuries, III:49–88
causal factors, III:49
condylar and subcondylar fractures, III:83, 83f
edentulous mandible fractures, III:83–84, 84f
frontal bone and sinus fractures
clinical examination, III:51
complications, III:53
computed tomography (CT), III:51
injury patterns, III:51
nasofrontal duct, III:51, 52f
surgical technique and treatment, III:52–53, 52f
gunshot wounds
delayed versus immediate reconstruction, III:85
immediate and high velocity gunshot wounds, III:86–87
low velocity gunshot wounds, III:85–87
treatment strategies, III:86–87, 86f
initial assessment
blunt trauma craniofacial injuries, III:50–51
clinical examination, III:50–51
computed tomography (CT), III:51
general discussion, III:49–51
timing considerations, III:49–50
lower facial fractures, III:75
mandibular fractures
antibiotics, III:82
characteristics, III:75
Class I fractures, III:77–78
Class II fractures, III:78
Class III fractures, III:78–80
classification systems, III:76–77
clinical examination, III:76
comminuted fractures, III:78, 79f
complications, III:82–83
dental wiring and fixation techniques, III:75–76
diagnosis, III:76
displacement direction and extent, III:77
edentulous mandible fractures, III:83–84, 84f
fracture line direction and angulation, III:77, 77f
internal fixation devices, III:80–83
intraoral approach, III:79
muscle function considerations, III:76
open reduction treatment, III:78–79
reduction and fixation principles, III:78, 78f
surgical indicators, III:79–80
teeth, III:77
temporomandibular joint, III:76–77
third molar extraction, III:81, 81f
treatment strategies, III:77
midfacial fractures
complications, III:74
Le Fort classification of facial fractures, III:71–75, 72f
midface buttresses, III:70–71, 70f
nasal fractures, III:57–59, 58f

skeletal reconstruction (Continued)
nasoethmoidal orbital fractures, III:60–61
postoperative care and follow-up, III:74
zygoma, III:63–65
orbital fractures
blow-out fractures (children), III:54, 54f
blow-out fractures (floor of the orbit), III:54
characteristics, III:53–57
complications, III:56–57
computed tomography (CT), III:54
infraorbital nerve anesthesia, III:57
operative technique, III:55
orbital apex syndrome, III:57
physical examination, III:53–54, 54f
postoperative care and follow-up, III:56
schematic diagram, III:53f
superior orbital fissure syndrome, III:57
surgical anatomy, III:53
surgical technique and treatment, III:54–55
timing considerations, III:55
treatment indicators, III:54
panfacial fractures
complications, III:84–85, 85f
definition, III:84–85
postoperative care and follow-up, III:85
surgical sequence, III:84
treatment strategies, III:84
upper facial fractures
frontal bone and sinus injury patterns, III:51
orbital fractures, III:53–57
foot reconstruction, IV:196
generalized skeletal abnormalities, VI:642–644
lower extremity reconstructive surgery, IV:83, 83f
patient presentation and diagnosis, IV:175–176
postoperative care and follow-up
adjunct therapy, IV:186–187
postoperative aesthetic conditions, IV:187–188
postoperative monitoring, IV:186
research summary, IV:188
sarcoma-related reconstruction, IV:111–112, 111f
skeletal defects, IV:174
surgical technique and treatment
allograft reconstruction, IV:180–181, 180f
bone grafts, IV:176–177
distraction osteogenesis, IV:179–180, 179f
Ilizarov technique, IV:179–180, 179f
periosteal and osteoperiosteal grafts, IV:178–179
reconstruction methods, IV:176
upper extremities
clavicle, IV:185
femur, IV:183
forearm, IV:181–183, 182f
humerus, IV:181, 186f
pelvis, IV:184–185
spine, IV:184–185, 184f–185f
tibia, IV:183–184

skeletal reconstruction (Continued)
vascularized bone transfer, IV:177–178, 177f–178f
vascularized epiphyseal reconstruction, IV:185–186, 186f–187f
skeletogenesis, VI:531–532, 532f
skew Z-plasty, I:314–315, 314f
skin
abdomen, II:531–533
acute wounds, I:241–242, 241f
aging process, II:44–45, 86, 185–186, 185f
Banff grading scale, VI:849t, 850f
characteristics, IV:397–402
craniofacial microsomia (CFM), III:767, 771f
craniofacial osteointegration, I:812, 812f
cutaneous and soft-tissue tumors, I:707–742
basal cell carcinoma
characteristics, I:737, 737f, III:117–118, 118f, VI:317, 317f
dermoscopic analysis, I:709, 709f
histological classification, I:738b
surgical margins, I:717
tumor colors, I:709
benign appendage-origin tumors
apocrine cystadenoma, I:722–723, 723f
chondroid syringoma, I:723, 723f
nevus sebaceous, I:721, 721f
pilomatricoma, I:721–722, 721f
steatocystoma multiplex, I:723, 724f
syringoma, I:722, III:117, 117f
trichilemmal cyst, I:722, 722f
benign epithelial-origin tumors
dermoid cyst, I:720, 721f
epidermal nevus, I:718, 718f
epidermoid cyst, I:719, 720f
keratoacanthoma, I:719, 719f, VI:315–316, 316f
milia, I:719–720
seborrheic keratosis, I:719, 719f, VI:316
benign mesenchymal-origin tumors
accessory auricles, I:732–733, 733f
acrochordon, I:730, 730f
arteriovenous fistula and arteriovenous malformation (AVM), I:735, 736f
capillary malformation, I:734–735
cavernous hemangioma, I:735, 735f
dermatofibroma, I:729, 729f, VI:316, 316f
fibroma pendulum, I:730, 730f
glomus tumors, I:734
granulomas, I:733–734, 733f–734f
hemangioma simplex, I:734, 734f–735f
hypertrophic scars, I:730, 731f
juvenile xanthogranuloma, I:729–730, 729f–730f
keloid scars, I:730, 730f
leiomyoma, I:731–732
lipoma, I:731, 731f–733f
lymphatic malformation, I:736
mucous cyst of the oral mucosa, I:736, 736f
osteochondrogenic tumors, I:732, 733f
rhabdomyoma, I:732
soft fibroma, I:730
strawberry hemangioma, I:734–735, 735f
venous malformation, I:735, 735f
xanthoma, I:729, 729f
benign neural crest-origin tumors
acquired pigment cell nevus, I:724, 724f
Becker's melanosis, I:725
blue nevus, I:727

skin (Continued)
 congenital pigment cell nevus, I:724, 725f
 dysplastic nevus, I:724, III:113–114, 114f
 juvenile melanoma, I:724–725, 726f
 lentigo simplex, I:723–724, 724f
 Mongolian spot, I:726–727, 728f
 neurofibroma, I:728, 728f, VI:320, 320f
 neuromas, I:727
 nevus of Ito, I:726, 727f
 nevus of Ota, I:725–726, 726f
 nevus spilus, I:725, 726f
 pigment cell nevus, I:723–725
 schwannoma, I:727, 728f, VI:320, 320f
 lymph node dissection
 axillary lymph node dissection, I:714–715
 inguinal lymph node dissection, I:715
 malignant appendage-origin tumors
 extramammary Paget's disease, I:739, 739f
 Merkel cell carcinoma, I:716t, 739, 739f
 sebaceous carcinoma, I:738, 738f
 sweat gland carcinoma, I:738
 trichilemmal carcinoma, I:738, 738f
 malignant epithelial-origin tumors
 actinic keratosis, I:736, 736f, VI:316–317, 317f
 basal cell carcinoma, I:709f
 Bowen's disease, I:736–737
 squamous cell carcinomas (SCCs), I:737, 737f, III:118–119, 118f, VI:317, 317f
 malignant mesenchymal-origin tumors
 angiosarcomas, I:741–742, 741f
 chondrosarcoma, I:741, VI:329
 dermatofibrosarcoma protuberans (DFSP), I:739, 739f
 Kaposi's sarcoma, I:742
 leiomyosarcoma, I:740, 740f
 liposarcoma, I:740, 740f
 malignant fibrous histiocytoma (MFH), I:739–740, 740f, VI:321, 322f
 osteosarcoma, I:741, 741f, VI:329
 rhabdomyosarcoma, I:741
 patient presentation and diagnosis
 angiography, I:710
 clinical staging system, I:711, 716t
 computed tomography (CT), I:710
 dermoscopic analysis, I:709, 709b, 709f
 Doppler imaging, I:709–710
 inspection and palpation, I:707–709
 magnetic resonance imaging (MRI), I:710
 pathogenic diagnosis, I:710–711
 positron emission tomography (PET), I:710
 scintigraphy, I:710
 TNM clinical classification system/pTNM pathologic classification system, I:711, 712f–714f, 715b, 750–761, 752t
 tumor colors, I:709b
 ultrasound imaging, I:709–710
 X-ray analysis, I:710
 treatment strategies
 chemotherapy, I:717–718
 cryotherapy, I:718

skin (Continued)
 electrocoagulation therapy, I:718
 immunotherapy, I:718
 laser treatments, I:718
 lymph node dissection, I:714–715
 radiation therapy (RT), I:717
 reconstructive surgeries, I:717
 sclerotherapy, I:718
 wide excision, I:711–712, 717b
 epidermal stem cells, I:262–263, 262f
 epidermolysis bullosa, IV:511–525
 general discussion, IV:511
 mitten hand deformity, IV:523f–524f
 outcomes and complicatons, IV:522
 pathogenesis, IV:517–518, 518t
 patient presentation and diagnosis
 biopsies, IV:520, 521f
 blistering, IV:518f–520f, 519–520
 characteristics, IV:518–520, 518f–519f
 hyperkeratosis, IV:519f
 squamous cell carcinoma, IV:520f
 syndactyly, IV:519f
 patient selection, IV:521
 postoperative care and follow-up, IV:522
 surgical technique and treatment
 skin substitutes, IV:522, 523f–524f
 surgical care, IV:521–522
 wound care, IV:521–522
 facial anatomy, II:79–80, 79f–80f
 facial burn wound treatment, IV:468–499
 acute facial burns
 ears, IV:473
 eyes/eyelids, IV:470–473
 mouth, IV:473
 nose, IV:473
 treatment strategies, IV:470–473, 471f–472f
 complications, IV:497
 damage process
 acute facial burns, IV:470–473
 damage assessments, IV:468–473, 469f
 depth of burn determination, IV:470
 epidemiology, IV:468
 flaps
 basic principles, IV:480–481
 indicators, IV:480b
 trapeze-plasties, IV:481
 Z-plasty technique, IV:481, 481f
 inadequate donor-site skin
 dermal substitutes, IV:480, 482–484
 general discussion, IV:482–484
 tissue expansion, IV:482, 483f
 nonoperative facial reconstructive adjunct techniques
 corrective cosmetics, IV:485
 fat transplantation, IV:485
 hair transplantation, IV:485
 laser therapy, IV:484, 484f
 prosthetics, IV:485
 steroid treatments, IV:485
 nonsurgical management, IV:473
 outcome assessments, IV:497–498
 postoperative care and follow-up, IV:497
 secondary procedures, IV:498–499
 skin grafts
 advantages, IV:474
 basic principles, IV:479
 composite grafts, IV:480

skin (Continued)
 full-thickness skin graft, IV:479–480
 skin substitutes, IV:480, 482–484
 split-thickness skin graft, IV:479
 specific areas
 cheeks, IV:490–491, 506
 commissure, IV:473, 489–490, 495f
 ears, IV:473, 491–492, 496f, 498–499, 505–506
 eyebrows, IV:485, 498–499
 eyelids, IV:470–473, 485–488, 486f–487f, 498–499, 504–505, 504f
 forehead, IV:485, 498–499
 lower eyelids, IV:486–488, 488f
 lower lip and chin, IV:489, 492f–494f, 498–499
 medial canthus scars, IV:488
 neck, IV:493–494, 498–499, 506
 nose, IV:473, 488–489, 498–499, 505
 scalp, III:119–120, 120f, IV:492–493, 498–499, 504, 504f
 severe cervical burn scars and contractures, IV:494
 upper eyelids, IV:486, 487f
 upper lip, IV:489, 490f–491f, 498–499
 specific surgical techniques
 scar replacement with local skin, IV:478, 478f
 serial excision, IV:478
 W-plasty technique, IV:478–479, 478f
 surgical management
 algorithmic approach, IV:475–477, 476f–477f
 basic principles, IV:474–475
 flaps, IV:480–481
 inadequate donor-site skin, IV:482–484
 skin grafts, IV:479–480
 specific techniques, IV:478–479
 surgical techniques, IV:473
 total wound healing/scar maturation, IV:474–475, 474f
 total wound healing/scar maturation
 aesthetic units, IV:474, 475f
 ancillary techniques, IV:475, 475b, 476f
 diagnosis, IV:474
 functional restoration, IV:474, 475f
 local flaps, IV:474
 reconstruction planning, IV:474
 skin grafts, IV:474
 skin-matching considerations, IV:475
 surgical goals, IV:475
 timing considerations, IV:474–475, 474f
 facial skin resurfacing, II:60–77
 chemical peeling methods
 characteristics, II:62
 patient selection and treatment, II:66–67
 wound healing biology, II:62–63
 complications
 acne, II:77
 characteristics, II:76
 infections, II:77
 milia, II:77
 pigmentary changes, II:77
 prolonged erythema, II:77
 scarring, II:77
 fractional photothermolysis, II:61, 61f, 65, 65f

skin *(Continued)*
  laser–tissue interactions
    laser properties, **II**:63–64
    molecular bases, **II**:63–64
  nonablative facial skin rejuvenation (NSR), **II**:64–65
  patient presentation and diagnosis, **II**:65–66
  patient selection and treatment
    acne scars, **II**:75f
    chemical peeling methods, **II**:66–67
    complications, **II**:76
    deeper heating long pulse skin tightening procedures, **II**:70, 71f
    facelifts, **II**:76f
    fractional photothermolysis, **II**:70–74, 71t
    laser treatments, **II**:67–70, 68f
    perioral lines, **II**:74–76, 74f–75f
    photodynamic therapy, **II**:69–70, 70f
  postoperative care and follow-up, **II**:76
  selective photothermolysis (SPT)
    biostimulation, **II**:64
    characteristics, **II**:64
    photochemical reactions, **II**:64
    photothermal reactions, **II**:64
    surface cooling, **II**:64
  treatment strategies
    chemical peeling methods, **II**:62, 66–67
    fractional photothermolysis, **II**:61, 61f, 70–74, 71t
    laser treatments, **II**:60–62
  facial soft-tissue injuries, **III**:23–24
  hands, **VI**:2–5, 2f
  mutilated/mangled hands, **VI**:254–255
  nonsurgical skin care and rejuvenation, **II**:13–29
    aging process, **II**:15
    dry skin
      antioxidants, **II**:18
      basic skin care formulations, **II**:16–18
      causal factors, **II**:15–19
      cleansers, **II**:16
      clinical signs, **II**:16
      hydroxy acids, **II**:18–19
      moisturizers, **II**:16–18
    noninvasive procedures
      intense pulsed light therapy, **II**:28
      microdermabrasion, **II**:28
    pigmented skin
      care regimens, **II**:24
      general discussion, **II**:24–26
      melanosome transfer inhibitors, **II**:25–26
      tyrosinase inhibitors, **II**:24–25
    research summary, **II**:28
    sensitive skin
      acne, **II**:19–20
      classifications, **II**:19–24, 19t
      rosacea, **II**:20–21, 21f
      treatment strategies, **II**:21–24
    skin type determination
      Baumann skin-typing system (BSTS), **II**:14–15, 14t
      Fitzpatrick skin phototype (SPT) system, **II**:13–14, 14t
    wrinkled skin
      antioxidants, **II**:27–28
      prevention and treatment, **II**:26–28
      retinoids, **II**:26

skin *(Continued)*
  ontogenesis, **I**:707, 708f
  skin-only facelifts, **II**:208–210, 209f
  skin-specific antigens, **I**:816
  skin substitutes
    Apligraf, **I**:337, 794t, 795
    bioengineered skin substitutes, **I**:793–795
    burn reconstruction, **IV**:441, 448, 502
    burn wound treatment, **IV**:411b, 412t–415t
    commercial product comparisons, **I**:794t
    Dermagraft, **I**:338, 794t, 795
    Epicel, **I**:794t, 795
    epidermolysis bullosa, **IV**:522, 523f–524f
    facial burn wound treatment, **IV**:480, 482–484
    Integra, **I**:794, 794t, **IV**:448
    lower extremity reconstructive surgery, **IV**:128–129, 130f
  skin wound healing, **I**:267–296
    adult wound pathology
      excessive healing, **I**:283–285
      nonhealing wounds, **I**:279–283
    adult wound repair
      characteristics, **I**:268–273, 268f
      fetal wound repair comparisons, **I**:277–278
      inflammatory phase, **I**:268–269, 268f
      proliferation phase, **I**:268f, 269–273
      remodeling phase, **I**:268f, 273, 276f
      scar formation, **I**:276f
    adult wound repair–fetal wound repair comparisons
      cellular differences, **I**:277
      extracellular matrix (ECM) differences, **I**:278
      gene expression differences, **I**:278
      growth factor expression, **I**:278
      repair differences, **I**:277–278
    clinical wound management
      closed wounds, **I**:285–286, 286t
      engineered skin replacements, **I**:289t, 290
      excessive scar treatment, **I**:290–291
      excisional wounds, **I**:286–287
      general discussion, **I**:285–295
      incisional wounds, **I**:285–286, 286t
      open wounds, **I**:286–287
      pharmacologic treatment, **I**:290
      wound dressings, **I**:287–288, 289t, **IV**:410–416
      wound treatment, **I**:287
    excessive healing
      characteristics, **I**:283–285
      hypertrophic scars, **I**:283–284, 283t
      keloid scars, **I**:283t, 284–285
    excessive scar treatment
      prevention and reduction therapies, **I**:291, 292t
      scar classification, **I**:290, 291t
      therapies, **I**:290–291
    fetal wound repair
      adult wound repair comparisons, **I**:277–278
      growth factor expression, **I**:278
      scar-free healing–scar formation transition, **I**:277
      scarless wound healing, **I**:276–278, 277f
    future trends
      gene therapy, **I**:295
      growth factor therapy, **I**:295

skin *(Continued)*
      protease-scavenging therapy, **I**:295
      stem cell therapy, **I**:296
    growth factor regulation
      characteristics, **I**:273–275
      extra cellular matrix–growth factor interactions, **I**:275
      fibroblast growth factor (FGF), **I**:274–275
      heparin-binding epidermal growth factor (HB–EGF), **I**:275
      platelet-derived growth factor (PDGF), **I**:274
      transforming growth factor-β (TGF-β) superfamily, **I**:274
      vascular endothelial growth factor (VEGF), **I**:275
    historical background, **I**:267
    mutilated/mangled hands, **VI**:254–255
    nonhealing wounds
      characteristics, **I**:279–283
      diabetic ulcers, **I**:281
      influencing factors, **I**:280t
      ischemic wounds, **I**:279–281
      lower extremity wounds, **I**:279–281
      malnutrition, **I**:282
      medical treatment, **I**:282–283
      obese patients, **I**:282
      pressure sores, **I**:279
      radiation injuries, **I**:281
      venous ulcers, **I**:279
      wound infections, **I**:281–282
    proliferation phase
      angiogenesis, **I**:271
      epithelial resurfacing, **I**:272–273
      extracellular matrix (ECM) formation, **I**:269–271, 271f
      granulation tissue formation, **I**:271
      wound contraction, **I**:271–272, 272f
    toxic epidermal necrolysis (TEN), **IV**:515, 516f
    treatment strategies
      chronic open wounds, **I**:287
      emerging treatments, **I**:294–295
      future trends, **I**:295–296
      immature hypertrophic scars, **I**:291–292, 293f
      linear hypertrophic scars, **I**:292–293, 293f
      major keloids, **I**:293f, 294
      minor keloids, **I**:293f, 294
      necrotic tissue, **I**:287
      plastic surgery effects, **I**:294–295
      treatment algorithms, **I**:290–291, 293f
      widespread burn hypertrophic scars, **I**:293–294, 293f
    wound dressings
      classifications, **I**:287–288, 289t
      compression therapy, **I**:288, 289t
      subatmospheric dressing device, **I**:288, 289t
  stiff hand, **VI**:450–451
  tissue engineering, **I**:388–389
  tissue expansion effects, **I**:623
  toxic epidermal necrolysis (TEN), **IV**:511–525
    dermatologic exfoliative disorders, **IV**:511–517
    general discussion, **IV**:511
    outcomes and complicatons, **IV**:517
    pathogenesis, **IV**:511–512

skin (Continued)
  patient presentation and diagnosis
    epidermal detachment, IV:513f–514f
    etiology and epidemiology, IV:512–514, 512t
    mucosal involvement, IV:513, 514f
    Nikolsky sign, IV:513, 514f
  patient selection, IV:514–515
  postoperative care and follow-up
    general care, IV:516
    novel pharmacologic therapy, IV:517
    ocular care, IV:516
  secondary procedures, IV:517
  surgical technique and treatment
    basic procedure, IV:515
    corticosteroid therapy, IV:515–516
    drug withdrawal, IV:515–516
    wound care, IV:515, 516f
  tumors
    actinic keratosis, I:736, 736f, VI:316–317, 317f
    basal cell carcinoma, VI:317, 317f
      characteristics, I:737, 737f, III:117–118, 118f, VI:317, 317f
      dermoscopic analysis, I:709, 709f
      histological classification, I:738b
      surgical margins, I:717
      tumor colors, I:709
    benign pigmented nevus, VI:315, 315f
    characteristics, VI:313–318
    cutaneous horns, VI:314, 314f
    dermatofibroma, I:729, 729f, VI:316, 316f
    epidermal inclusion cysts, VI:314, 314f
    keratoacanthoma, I:719, 719f, VI:315–316, 316f
    melanoma, VI:318, 318f
    sebaceous cysts, VI:314, 314f
    seborrheic keratosis, I:719, 719f, VI:316
    squamous cell carcinomas (SCCs), VI:317, 317f
    verruca vulgaris, VI:314–315, 315f
  viscoelasticity, III:441t
  See also burns; wound healing
skin adnexal structures, I:320
skin cancers, I:670–671
skin grafts, I:319–338
  aesthetic nasal reconstruction
    basic principles, III:141–142
    full-thickness forehead skin graft, III:141, 142f
    operative technique, III:141–142
    preauricular and postauricular skin grafts, III:141
  anatomy and physiology
    blood vessel supply, I:321
    dermis, I:320, 322f
    epidermis, I:319–320, 322f
    glandular structures, I:322–323
    hair follicles, I:321, 322f
    sebaceous glands, I:322–323
    skin functions, I:319–323
    skin regeneration, I:321
    stem cells, I:321
  burn reconstruction
    debridement, IV:441
    secondary procedures, IV:447–448
    skin graft loss, IV:427

skin grafts (Continued)
    skin substitutes, IV:441, 502
    wound closure, IV:502
  clinical application
    composite graft, I:329, IV:480
    deep wound healing, I:325–334
    donor site considerations
      common regions, I:325f, 329f, 333–334
      donor site dressings, I:333
      skin graft storage, I:334
    full-thickness skin graft, I:322f, 326t, 329, 329f–330f, IV:307, 479–480
    meshed skin graft, I:327–329, 328f, IV:307, 309f
    recent developments, I:340–342
    recipient site considerations
      aesthetic considerations, I:332–333
      functional considerations, I:332
      general discussion, I:331–333
      wound bed preparation, I:331–332
    skin fixation and dressing
      basic principles, I:323f, 329–330, 331f
      first dressing change, I:330
      sealants, I:330
    skin graft origins and classifications, I:325–334, 325t
    split-thickness skin graft, I:322f, 325f, 326–327, 326t, 327f–328f, IV:307, 308f
    facial burn wound treatment, IV:479
  complications
    cosmetic issues, I:334–335
    donor site infections, I:335
    hematomas, I:334
    infection, I:334
    instability, I:334
    nontake conditions, I:334
    seromas, I:334
    wound contraction, I:334
  congenital melanocytic nevi (CMN), III:840–842, 842f–843f
  conjoined twins, III:900–901
  cutaneous and soft-tissue tumors, I:717
  definition, I:319, 339–342, 815
  expanded full-thickness skin grafts, I:630
  facial burn wound treatment
    advantages, IV:474
    basic principles, IV:479
    composite grafts, IV:480
    full-thickness skin graft, IV:479–480
    skin substitutes, IV:480, 482–484
    split-thickness skin graft, IV:479
  fingertip reconstruction
    patient selection, VI:128
    surgical technique and treatment
      cross finger flaps, VI:130–131, 133f
      dorsal metacarpal artery flaps, VI:134, 135f
      heterodigital flaps, VI:130–134
      homodigital flaps, VI:130, 132f
      lateral V-Y advancement flaps, VI:130, 130f
      Littler neurovascular island flap, VI:132–134
      local flaps, VI:128–134
      thenar crease flap, VI:134f
      visor flaps, VI:130, 131f
      volar V-Y advancement flap, VI:128–130, 129f

skin grafts (Continued)
    foot reconstruction, IV:201–205
    future trends
      bioengineered cultured allogenicbilayered constructs, I:337–338
      cell cultures, I:336–337, 337f
      dermal substitutes, I:335–336, 335t, 336f, 342, 342f
      engineered skin replacements, I:289t, 290
    genital skin grafts, IV:307, 308f–309f
    lower extremity reconstructive surgery, IV:128–129, 130f
    nineteenth century, I:20, 21f
    nose reconstruction
      basic principles, III:141–142
      full-thickness forehead skin graft, III:141, 142f
      operative technique, III:141–142
      preauricular and postauricular skin grafts, III:141
    oral cavity and mouth reconstruction, III:311
    penile girth enhancement, II:659–660
    perineal reconstruction, IV:385, 386f
    periorbital area, I:638–640, 641f–642f
    post-traumatic genital defects, IV:307, 308f–309f
    postwar plastic surgery, I:26f
    scalp and forehead reconstruction, III:123, 123f
    schematic diagram, I:340f
    skin graft mechanisms
      maturation, I:325f
      revascularization, I:325f
      serum imbibition, I:325f
    skin graft process
      functional structures, I:325
      maturation, I:324
      operative procedures, I:323–325
      revascularization, I:323–324
      serum imbibition, I:323
      skin appendages, I:325
    spina bifida, III:872
    surgical technique
      general requirements, I:340
      split-thickness skin graft, I:326–327, 327f–328f
    survival rates, I:340, 341f
    tissue expansion, I:630, 638–640, 641f–642f
    tissue transplantation
      allografts, I:829
      autografts, I:828–829
      xenografts, I:829
  skin necrosis
    brachioplasty, II:629t
    breast implants, V:360, 360f, 363t
    muscle/musculocutaneous flaps, I:571–572
    scalp and forehead reconstruction, III:131–132
    secondary rhinoplasty, II:481, 482f
  skin-sparing mastectomy, V:282, 283f–284f, 288f
  skin tags, I:730, 730f
  sleep apnea patients, I:126–128, 127t
  small business innovation research (SBIR), I:845–846
  small intestinal mucosa, I:796
  smile analysis, III:292, 293f

Note: **Boldface** roman numerals indicate volume. Page numbers followed by f refer to figures; page numbers followed by t refer to tables; page numbers followed by b refer to boxes.

Smith extensor carpi radialis brevis transfer, **VI:**769–770, 770f
Smith, Ferris, **I:**27
Smith–Lemli–Opitz syndrome, **VI:**617t
smoke inhalation, **IV:**407–408
  See also burns
smokers, **II:**194, **IV:**283
Smyth papyrus, **I:**11–12
Snow–Littler technique, **VI:**565, 566f
soap
  characteristics, **II:**16
  combination bars, **II:**16
  superfatted soaps, **II:**16
  transparent soaps, **II:**16
social networks, **I:**98–99, 871
Société Européenne de Chirurgie Structive, **I:**24, 24f
Société Française de Chirurgie Réparatrice Plastique et Esthétique, **I:**24
sodium (Na)
  intracellular Na^{2+} overload, **I:**576–577, 576f
  sodium hypochlorite, **IV:**461–463
  Na$^+$/H$^+$ exchange isoform-1 (NHE-1) antiporter, **I:**576–577, 576f
  sodium sulfacetamide, **II:**21t, 22
  sodium tetradecyl sulfate (STS), **I:**692–693, 696
soft fibroma, **I:**730
soft palate, **III:**432
soft tissue facial analysis, **II:**355–356, 356b, 356f–357f, 356t
soft-tissue fillers, **II:**44–59
  classifications
    autologous fillers, **II:**45b, 46
    biologic fillers, **II:**45t, 46–47, 47t, 49t
    general discussion, **II:**45–48
    synthetic fillers, **II:**47–48, 47t–49t
  complications, **II:**58–59
  contraindications, **II:**58
  cross-hatcing, **II:**50, 51f
  general discussion, **II:**44
  ideal filler characteristics, **II:**45b
  indicators and applications
    deformities, **II:**57
    eyebrows, **II:**51
    facial lipoatrophy, **II:**54–55
    forehead lines, **II:**51, 52f
    general discussion, **II:**50–58
    glabellar lines, **II:**51
    hand rejuvenation, **II:**57–58, 57f
    jawline augmentation, **II:**54
    lips, **II:**55–56, 56f
    malar augmentation, **II:**52f, 53, 54f
    marionette lines, **II:**53–54, 53f–54f
    nasal reshaping, **II:**56, 57f
    nasolabial folds, **II:**53, 53f–54f, 53t
    panfacial volumetric augmentation, **II:**54, 55f
    scars, **II:**57
    tear troughs, **II:**51–52, 52f
  injection techniques, **II:**48–50, 50f–51f
  linear threading, **II:**48–50, 50f
  radial fanning, **II:**50, 51f
  wrinkle formation, **II:**44–45
soft-tissue sarcomas
  alveolar soft-part sarcoma
    characteristics, **III:**890
    complications, **III:**890
    disease process, **III:**890
    patient presentation and diagnosis, **III:**890

soft-tissue sarcomas *(Continued)*
    prognosis and outcomes, **III:**890
    surgical technique and treatment, **III:**890
  biopsies
    core needle biopsy, **IV:**106
    excisional biopsies, **IV:**106–107
    fine-needle aspiration (FNA), **IV:**106
    incisional biopsies, **IV:**107
    reoperative biopsies, **IV:**107–108
  characteristics, **IV:**101–102
  clinical staging system, **I:**716t
  epidemiology, **IV:**102–103
  histopathologic types, **IV:**103f
  imaging methods, **IV:**104, 104f
  Muskuloskeletal Tumor Society staging system, **IV:**105t
  outcome assessments, **IV:**114–115, 115t
  patient presentation and diagnosis, **IV:**103–104, 104f
  patient selection, **IV:**104
  predisposing factors, **IV:**102t
  preservation options
    complex approaches, **IV:**112
    flaps, **IV:**110–111
    general discussion, **IV:**110–112
    neuromuscular units, **IV:**111
    skeletal reconstruction, **IV:**111–112, 111f
    vascular surgery, **IV:**112
  radiation treatment, **I:**669–670
  recurrence management, **IV:**116–125
  rhabdomyosarcoma
    characteristics, **III:**889
    complications, **III:**889
    disease process, **III:**889
    patient presentation and diagnosis, **III:**889, 889f
    postoperative care and follow-up, **III:**889
    prognosis and outcomes, **III:**889
    secondary procedures, **III:**889
    surgical technique and treatment, **III:**889
  surgical resection techniques
    amputation indicators, **IV:**110
    biopsies, **IV:**106–108
    definitive resections, **IV:**108
    lymph node dissection, **IV:**110
    nerve involvement, **IV:**109
    osseous involvement, **IV:**109
    primary osseous sarcomas, **IV:**109
    specimen handling, **IV:**109
    surgical revisions, **IV:**107–108, 108t
    vascular involvement, **IV:**108
    wound closure, **IV:**109
  synovial soft-tissue sarcoma
    characteristics, **III:**889
    complications, **III:**890
    disease process, **III:**889
    patient presentation and diagnosis, **III:**889–890
    prognosis and outcomes, **III:**890
    surgical technique and treatment, **III:**890
  TNM clinical classification system, **IV:**105t
  TNM clinical classification system/pTNM pathologic classification system, **I:**715b
  treatment strategies
    chemotherapy, **IV:**106
    radiation therapy (RT), **IV:**106
    surgical goals, **IV:**104–105
    surgical planning, **IV:**105, 105t
    surgical treatment, **IV:**105–106
  tumor growth and metastasis, **IV:**103

sole proprietorship, **I:**85
soleus muscle flap
  lower extremity reconstructive surgery, **I:**557–560, 561f, **IV:**141–142, 141f
  lower leg muscles, **IV:**35f–36f
solitary piloleiomyoma, **I:**731–732
solitary unicameral bone cysts, **VI:**328, 328f
solvents, **IV:**395
somatization, **I:**33
somatostatin C (Sm-C), **I:**270t
Sonic hedgehog (Shh) gene
  craniofacial clefts, **III:**706
  craniofacial development, **III:**505, 505f–506f, 506t
  hand plate development, **VI:**528–530, 529f
  osteoblasts, **I:**428–429
Sox gene expression, **VI:**530–532
soy products, **II:**18, 25–26
SPAIR mammoplasty *See* short scar periareolar inferior pedicle reduction (SPAIR) mammaplasty
spastic hand, **VI:**449–466
  cerebral palsy
    House functional classification for cerebral palsy, **VI:**459, 459t
    nonsurgical management, **VI:**459
    patient presentation and diagnosis, **VI:**459
    patient selection, **VI:**459
    surgical technique and treatment
      assessment strategies, **VI:**459–464
      elbows, **VI:**460, 461f
      forearm pronation, **VI:**460
      shoulder, **VI:**460
      swan-neck deformity, **VI:**464, 465f
      thumb, **VI:**464, 464t
      typical spastic hemiplegic posture, **VI:**460f
      wrist flexion, **VI:**460–464, 462f–463f
      Zancolli classification of active finger and wrist extension, **VI:**461, 462t
  research summary, **VI:**465
  stroke/traumatic brain injury
    patient selection, **VI:**464
    surgical technique and treatment, **VI:**464
spasticity, **IV:**364, 366
speech pathology terminology, **III:**620b
sphincter pharyngoplasty, **III:**626–628, 627f
sphincter reconstruction, **IV:**390–392
spider bites, **VI:**336
spina bifida
  characteristics, **III:**866–874
  clinical presentation and evaluation, **III:**867
  meningomyeloceles, **III:**868t–869t, 872–874, 873f
  paraspinal flap method, **III:**872–874, 873f–875f
  surgical indicators, **III:**867
  treatment strategies, **III:**867–872, 868t–869t, 870f–872f
spinal cord injuries, **IV:**355–356, **VI:**817
spinal fusion, **I:**227
spindle cell mesenchymal sarcoma, **IV:**103
spine, **IV:**184–185, 184f–185f
spiral flap, **V:**513, 513f
spironolactone, **IV:**341t
Spitz nevus, **I:**724–725, 726f
splints, **IV:**509

split nails
   characteristics, **VI**:121
   surgical technique and treatment, **VI**:121–122, 123f
spondyloepiphyseal dysplasia congenital, **III**:807t
sponge implants, **V**:101–102, 102f
squamous cell carcinomas (SCCs)
   buccal mucosa, **III**:311f–313f, 406
   characteristics, **I**:737, 737f, **III**:118–119, 118f, **VI**:317, 317f
   epidermolysis bullosa, **IV**:520f, 521–522
   head and neck cancer
      epidemiology, **III**:420
      hard palate, **III**:408, 408f
      incidence, **III**:421–427
      nose and paranasal sinuses, **III**:436–437, 436f
      outcomes and complicatons, **III**:438
      postoperative care and follow-up, **III**:437–438
      preoperative assessment, **III**:402, 405f
      prevalence, **III**:421–427
      radiation treatment, **I**:668–669
      risk factors
         alcohol, **III**:421
         gastroesophageal reflux, **III**:421
         infectious agents, **III**:421
         pollution exposure, **III**:421–422
         tobacco, **III**:421
      surgical technique and treatment, **III**:402–405, 405f
      tongue, **III**:408–409, 408f
   pharyngoesophageal reconstruction, **III**:337t
   salivary gland tumors
      characteristics, **III**:370
      classifications, **III**:365t
      incidence, **III**:376t
      outcomes and complicatons, **III**:377
      parotid gland, **III**:370t
Stahl's ear deformity, **II**:490–491, 490f–491f
stainless steel, **I**:786–787
Stal–Feldman alar facial rotation excision, **III**:651f
standard delay flap, **I**:514, 514f
standard flexor carpi ulnaris transfer, **VI**:748–749, 748f–751f, 748t
Staphylococcus aureus, **I**:249–250, **II**:411, **III**:890, **IV**:86–87, 513–514, **VI**:334
Staphylococcus epidermidis, **IV**:275, **V**:35
star flap, **V**:503t, 504–506, 505f
stasis ulcers, **I**:253
steatocystoma multiplex, **I**:723, 724f
stem cells, **I**:212–239
   breast cancer, **V**:267
   characteristics and classifications, **I**:212–214, 213f
   hemangioma-derived-stem cell (HemSC), **I**:678–680
   human embryonic stem cells (hESCs)
      clinical correlates, **I**:216–217
      current research and applications, **I**:215–216, 215f
      definition, **I**:214–215
      research background, **I**:214–215
   mesenchymal stem cells (MSCs)
      bone homeostasis and turnover, **I**:425–434, 434f

stem cells (*Continued*)
   bone marrow-derived mesenchymal stem cells (BMSC)
      clinical correlates, **I**:228
      current research and applications, **I**:224–226
      definitions, **I**:223–224
      gene therapy, **I**:190
      in vitro tissue harvest and differentiation protocols, **I**:226
      in vivo models, **I**:226–228
      wound healing, **I**:262, 262f
   skin wound healing, **I**:263, 296
   tissue engineering, **I**:369–371, 380f
postnatal and somatic stem cells
   adipose-derived stem/stromal cells (ASCs)
      adipogenic differentiation, **I**:221, 222f
      cell surface receptors, **I**:219–220, 219f–220f
      characteristics, **I**:217–218, 217f
      chondrogenic differentiation, **I**:221
      delivery methods, **I**:220
      fat grafting, **II**:327–328
      harvesting methods, **I**:218–219, 218f
      induced pluripotent stem cells, **I**:236
      in vitro differentiation protocols, **I**:220–221
      in vivo model, **I**:221–223, 224f–225f
      mouse versus human ASCs, **I**:219
      nude athymic mouse 4-mm calvarial defect, **I**:221–223, 222f
      osteogenic differentiation, **I**:220–221, 221f
      regenerative qualities, **V**:583–584
      tissue engineering, **I**:369–371
   bone marrow-derived mesenchymal stem cells (BMSC)
      clinical correlates, **I**:228
      current research and applications, **I**:224–226
      definitions, **I**:223–224
      in vitro tissue harvest and differentiation protocols, **I**:226
      in vivo models, **I**:226–228
   current research
      cell surface receptors, **I**:219–220, 219f–220f
      delivery methods, **I**:220
      mouse versus human ASCs, **I**:219
   in vitro differentiation protocols
      adipogenic differentiation, **I**:221, 222f
      chondrogenic differentiation, **I**:221
      osteogenic differentiation, **I**:220–221, 221f
   in vivo model
      clinical correlates, **I**:223
      future trends, **I**:223, 224f–225f
      nude athymic mouse 4-mm calvarial defect, **I**:221–223, 222f
   tissue-specific stem cells
      blood vessels, **I**:230, 231f, 232
      clinical correlates, **I**:232–233
      current research and applications, **I**:229–232
      definitions, **I**:228–229
      muscles, **I**:230–232, 231f

stem cells (*Continued*)
      osteoblast differentiation, **I**:230, 230f, 232
      peripheral nerve repair, **I**:231–233, 231f
      skin regeneration, **I**:229, 229f, 232
   potential applications, **I**:213–214
   prospective clinical applications
      biomaterial scaffolds, **I**:233–234, 233f
      genetic induction therapies, **I**:234, 234f
      induced pluripotent stem cells
         characteristics, **I**:235–237, 235f
         clinical correlates, **I**:238–239
         fibroblast differentiation protocols, **I**:237
         in vitro applications, **I**:237–238
         in vitro differentiation protocols, **I**:237–238
         in vivo models, **I**:238–239
         lentivirus production and transduction, **I**:237
         potential risks, **I**:237, 237f–238f
         transcription factors, **I**:235f
   skin regeneration, **I**:229, 229f, 232, 321
   stem cell-based cartilage engineering, **I**:423
   tissue engineering, **I**:369–371, 394–395
   wound healing
      characteristics, **I**:261–264, 261f–262f
      induced pluripotent stem cells, **I**:264
      microribonucleic acid (miRNA), **I**:260–261
      regeneration processes, **I**:261–264, 261f
      skin wound healing, **I**:296
Stener lesion, **VI**:49–50, 154–155, 154f
stenosis, **I**:677t
stereotactic biopsy, **V**:271–272, 272f
steroid atrophy, **V**:110, 110f
steroid treatments, **IV**:485
Stevens–Johnson syndrome (SJS)
   See toxic epidernal necrolysis (TEN)
Stickler syndrome, **III**:805, 805f, 807t
stiff hand, **VI**:449–466
   collateral ligament changes, **VI**:454, 454f
   extension contracture
      bone, **VI**:451–452, 451f
      capsular and pericapsular structures
         collateral ligaments, **VI**:451
         dorsal capsule, **VI**:451
         flexor tendon adherence, **VI**:451
         transverse retinacular ligaments, **VI**:451
         volar plate, **VI**:451
      intrinsic muscles, **VI**:451
      long extensors, **VI**:451
      patient presentation, **VI**:450–452, 450f
      skin, **VI**:450–451
   flexion contracture
      bone, **VI**:450
      capsular and pericapsular structures
         accessory ligaments, **VI**:450
         collateral ligaments, **VI**:449
         dorsal adhesions, **VI**:450
         intrinsic tendons, **VI**:450
         transverse retinacular ligaments, **VI**:450
         volar plate, **VI**:450
      patient presentation, **VI**:449–450, 450f
   general discussion, **VI**:449
   outcomes and complicatons, **VI**:458–459
   pathogenesis, **VI**:454–455, 457f
   patient presentation and diagnosis, **VI**:449–454

Note: **Boldface** roman numerals indicate volume. Page numbers followed by f refer to figures; page numbers followed by t refer to tables; page numbers followed by b refer to boxes.

stiff hand *(Continued)*
  patient selection, **VI:**455–456, 458f
  postoperative care and follow-up, **VI:**458
  secondary procedures, **VI:**459
  seesaw effect, **VI:**452–454, 452f–453f
  surgical technique and treatment
    metacarpophalangeal (MP) joint
      extension contracture, **VI:**457–458
    nonsurgical management, **VI:**456–458
    proximal interphalangeal (PIP) joint
      extension contracture, **VI:**457
    proximal interphalangeal (PIP) joint
      flexion contracture, **VI:**456–457
  volar plate changes, **VI:**454, 455f–456f
Stockholm Workshop Scale, **VI:**368–369, 368t
Stoll syndrome, **III:**807t
stomelysins, **I:**269–271
stomion, **II:**356t
Stony Brook Scar Evaluation Scale (SBSES),
  I:264–266, 299
store-and-forward technology, **I:**870, 871t
strainers/straining methods, **V:**598–599
Strattice, **V:**69, 70t
stratum corneum, **I:**320
strawberry hemangioma, **I:**678t, 734–735,
  735f
Streptococcus, **VI:**334
Streptococcus agalactiae, **III:**890
Streptococcus pyogenes, **II:**411, **III:**890
streptokinase, **I:**617
Streptomyces hygroscopicus, **I:**824
Streptomyces tsukubaensis, **I:**823–824
stretch injuries, **I:**466t, 467–468, 468f
Sturge–Weber syndrome, **I:**679f, 688–689,
  701–702, 734
subcondylar fractures, **III:**83, 83f
subglottic cancers, **III:**434–436, 436f
sublabial, **II:**356t
sublimation, **I:**33
sublingual gland, **III:**361, 361f
submandibular gland, **III:**361f
submental artery flap, **III:**272, 273f–274f, 309t
submucous cleft palate, **III:**571–572, 571f
submusculofascial plane, **V:**114–115, 114f
subnasale, **II:**356t
suborbicularis oculi fat (SOOF), **II:**132–133,
  270–272, 271f, 273f
subscapular artery, **IV:**222f, 223, 225–227, 226f
subscapularis muscle, **IV:**221, 222f
substance abuse, **I:**50
suction-assisted lipectomy (SAL)
  adolescent aesthetic surgery, **I:**45t
  background information, **II:**507–508
  cannulas, **II:**520
  neck rejuvenation, **II:**320
  treatment options, **II:**518–525
sulfur (S)
  metal alloy compositions, **I:**786–787
  rosacea treatments, **II:**21t
  sodium sulfacetamide, **II:**21t, 22
  sulfamethoxazole, **II:**21t
  sulfuric acid, **IV:**461–463
sun exposure, **II:**45
sunflower seed oil, **IV:**395
superfatted soaps, **II:**16
superficial cervical artery, **IV:**222f, 223
superficial circumflex iliac artery, **IV:**229–230,
  229f, **VI:**265f
superficial circumflex iliac perforator flap,
  IV:143, 143f–144f

superficial inferior epigastric artery (SIEA),
  IV:229–230, 229f, **V:**436–437, 437f–438f,
  VI:265f
superficial palmar arch, **VI:**468–469
superficial perineal artery, **IV:**232–235, 234f,
  238f
superficial peroneal nerve, **IV:**48t
superficial sensory branch of the radial nerve,
  VI:710, 712f–713f
superficial spreading melanoma, **I:**752–753,
  754f
superior epigastric artery, **IV:**229–230, 229f
superior epigastric artery perforator (SEAP)
  flap, **V:**308, 486f, 489
superior gluteal artery, **IV:**222f, 223, 224f
superior gluteal artery flap, **IV:**264–265, 277f
superior gluteal artery perforator (SGAP)
  flap
  advantages, **V:**459–464
  anatomical characteristics, **V:**461–463
  complications, **V:**464
  imaging methods, **V:**327
  patient selection, **V:**460–461
  postoperative care, **V:**464
  pressure sores, **I:**562–565
  radiological protocol, **V:**330f, 333f–334f
  spina bifida, **III:**867–872, 871f
  surgical technique, **V:**463–464, 464b,
    465f–467f
superior orbital fissure syndrome, **III:**57
superior temporal septum (STS), **II:**83–85, 83f
superior thoracic artery, **IV:**225–227, 226f
supermicrosurgery technique, **IV:**149, 149f
superoxide (O₂), **I:**575, 575f, **VI:**228–229
supraclavicular block, **VI:**97–99, 99f
suprafascial flaps, **IV:**208
supraglottic cancers, **III:**434, 435f
supra muscle, **IV:**221, 222f
supraomohyoid neck dissection, **III:**413–415
supraorbital nerve, **III:**26, 27f
suprascapular artery, **IV:**222f, 223
suprascapular nerve compression
  anatomical considerations, **VI:**524, 524f
  etiology, **VI:**524
  patient presentation and diagnosis, **VI:**524
  patient selection, **VI:**524
  surgical technique and treatment,
    VI:524–525
Suprathel®, **IV:**412t–414t, 418f
supratrochlear nerve, **III:**26, 27f
supraventricular tachycardia, **I:**145
sural flap, **IV:**75, 77f, 146, 146f, 209–211
sural nerve, **VI:**708–709, 709f
Surgical Care Improvement Project (SCIP),
  I:172–173
surgical endoscopy, **V:**81–96
  background and general characteristics
    general discussion, **V:**81–82
    illumination and imaging technology,
      V:82
    latissimus dorsi (LD) flap, **V:**82–83
    optical cavities, **V:**81–82
    support systems, **V:**82
  breast reconstruction
    breast anatomy, **V:**88
    outcomes and complicatons, **V:**93–96
    patient presentation and diagnosis,
      V:88–89
    patient selection, **V:**89
    postoperative care and follow-up, **V:**93

surgical endoscopy *(Continued)*
  surgical technique and treatment
    basic procedure, **V:**89–93
    completed dissection, **V:**93f
    dissector instrumentation, **V:**91f
    hemostasis, **V:**94f
    instrumentation, **V:**90f
    laparotomy pad, **V:**91f
    markings, **V:**89f
    scissor dissection, **V:**92f–93f
    wetting solutions, **V:**90f
  endoscopic augmentation mammaplasty
    breast anatomy, **V:**83
    outcomes and complicatons, **V:**87–88, 88f
    patient presentation and diagnosis, **V:**83
    patient selection, **V:**83–84
    postoperative care and follow-up,
      V:87–88
    surgical technique and treatment,
      V:84–87, 84f–87f
surgical innovation, **I:**1–10, 841–853
  acellular dermal matrix (ADM), **I:**851–852,
    851f
  background information, **I:**841–842
  basic principles, **I:**5–7
  Center for Devices and Radiological Health
    (CDRH), **I:**847–849
  collaborations, **I:**3–4
  composite tissue allotransplantation (CTA),
    I:2–3
  conflict of interest, **I:**849
  documentation and data gathering, **I:**8–9
  driving forces, **I:**4–5
  external influences, **I:**8
  funding processes, **I:**845–846, 845f
  general discussion, **I:**1
  innovative ideas, **I:**842–843
  institutional technology transfer, **I:**847, 848t
  intellectual property, **I:**846–847
  noninvasive body contouring, **I:**852–853,
    852f
  plastic surgery–innovation relationship, **I:**2
  plastic surgery innovations, **I:**850
  regulatory approval processes, **I:**847–849
  regulatory issues, **I:**8–9
  research–innovation relationship, **I:**2
  technological impacts, **I:**843, 844f
  value determinations, **I:**843–844, 844f
surgically assisted rapid palatal expansion
  (SARPE) procedure, **III:**661
SurgiMend, **V:**69, 70t
Surgisis, **II:**45t, 47, **V:**70t
Surveillance Epidemiology and End Results
  (SEER) registry, **I:**158–159, 158t
Sushruta
  hand surgery, **VI:**xliv–xlvi
sustainable enterprise, **I:**82–83
sustaining technology, **I:**843–844, 844f
swan-neck deformity, **VI:**222–223, 222f–223f,
  453f, 464, 465f
Swanson/IFSSH classification, **VI:**535–537
sweat glands, **I:**322–323, 322f, 738
swine leukocyte antigen (SLA), **I:**815–816
symbrachydactyly
  classification systems, **VI:**537, 537f–538f
  patient presentation and diagnosis,
    VI:549–550, 550f, 609f, 640–641,
    640f–641f, 645f
  surgical technique and treatment, **VI:**546t
symmastia, **V:**79t, 115–116, 116f

sympathetically independent pain (SIP), **VI**:487f
sympathetically maintained pain (SMP), **VI**:487f
symphalangism
    characteristics, **VI**:614–615
    outcomes and complicatons, **VI**:616
    pathogenesis, **VI**:615
    patient presentation and diagnosis, **VI**:615
    patient selection, **VI**:615–616
    postoperative care and follow-up, **VI**:616
    secondary procedures, **VI**:616
    surgical technique and treatment, **VI**:615–616
syndactyly
    characteristics, **VI**:635f, 639f
    classification systems, **VI**:535–537, 535f, 537f, 605f
    epidemiology, **VI**:604
    epidermolysis bullosa, **IV**:519f
    outcomes and complicatons, **VI**:608–609, 609f
    pathogenesis, **VI**:604
    patient presentation and diagnosis, **VI**:564–565, 604, 606f
    patient selection, **VI**:604–605
    postoperative care and follow-up, **VI**:608
    secondary procedures, **VI**:609
    surgical technique and treatment
        basic procedure, **VI**:605–608, 605b, 608b
        complete and complex syndactyly, **VI**:608
        fingertip separation, **VI**:608
        incomplete syndactyly, **VI**:608
        lateral soft tissue defects, **VI**:606–607, 608f
        timing considerations, **VI**:546t
        web creation, **VI**:606, 607f
syndromic cleft lip and palate, **I**:194–195
syndromic craniosynostosis, **III**:749–760
    characteristics, **I**:196–198, 197t, **III**:749
    complications, **III**:759–760
    disease characteristics, **III**:749–750, 750t
    fibroblast growth factor receptor (FGFR)-related mutations, **III**:749–750, 750t
    patient presentation and diagnosis, **III**:750–751, 750t
    patient selection, **III**:751–752, 752f
    postoperative care and follow-up, **III**:757–759
    prognosis and outcomes, **III**:759–760
    secondary procedures, **III**:760
    surgical technique and treatment
        anterior fossa enlargement, **III**:753f
        bandeau design, **III**:754f
        basic techniques, **III**:752–757
        facial bipartition, **III**:758f
        Le Fort III osteotomy, **III**:758f–759f
        low frontal osteotomy, **III**:755f
        low posteriorly draining enlarged transcranial veins, **III**:756f
        midvault cranioplasty, **III**:756f
        monobloc frontofacial advancement procedure, **III**:757f
        posterior keels of bone, **III**:757f
        skull base osteotomies, **III**:755f
        stair-step osteotomy, **III**:754f
synovial sheath, **VI**:179–182

synovial soft-tissue sarcoma
    characteristics, **I**:742, **III**:889
    complications, **III**:890
    disease process, **III**:889
    hands and wrists, **VI**:321
    patient presentation and diagnosis, **III**:889–890
    prognosis and outcomes, **III**:890
    surgical technique and treatment, **III**:890, **VI**:321
synthetic detergent bars, **II**:16
synthetic fillers, **II**:47–48, 47t–49t
syringoma, **I**:722, **III**:117, 117f
systemic lupus erythematosus (SLE), **VI**:407t, 408

T
tachycardia, **I**:145
tacrolimus, **I**:822t, 823–824, 833t, **II**:21t
Tagliacozzi, Gaspare
    nose reconstruction, **I**:11, 17–18, **VI**:xlv
tallow, **II**:16
Tamai scale, **VI**:247
Tanacetum parthenium, **V**:33t–35t
Tansini, Iginio, **I**:26f
tar burns, **IV**:395–396
targeted muscle reinnervation (TMR)
    characteristics, **VI**:876–879
    myoelectric prostheses, **VI**:871
    shoulder disarticulation level, **VI**:877–879, 878f–879f, 879t
    transhumeral level, **VI**:876–877, 876f–877f
    transradial level, **VI**:879
tarsal strip lateral canthoplasty, **II**:155–156, 156f–157f
tartrate-resistant acid protease (TRAP), **I**:430–431
tattoos, **I**:297–298, **V**:517, 518f
Taylor, Ian, **VI**:xlvii
Taylor spatial frame, **IV**:179–180
Tbx5 gene expression, **VI**:527–530
tear troughs
    ocular examination, **II**:120, 120f
    soft-tissue fillers, **II**:51–52, 52f
    tear trough deformities, **II**:122, 123f
teas, herbal, **V**:33t–35t
technetium scans, **III**:364, **IV**:104
technology-licensing offices (TLO), **I**:847, 848t
technology transfer, **I**:845–847, 848t
teeth
    anesthesia, **III**:27, 27f–28f
    mandibular fractures, **III**:77
    progressive hemifacial atrophy (PHA), **III**:796–797
Teflon, **I**:790
Tegaderm®, **IV**:412t–414t
te gastronol, **V**:33t–35t
telangiectasias, **I**:677t, **VI**:668t, 673–674, 676f
telemedicine
    definition, **I**:870–871
    general discussion, **I**:870
    plastic surgery applications, **I**:871–872
    research summary, **I**:873
    social networks, **I**:871
    technologies, **I**:870, 871t
    telesurgery, **I**:871, 872f
    ubiquitous mobile telemedicine, **I**:872–873
telesurgery, **I**:871, 872f

temozolomide, **I**:779–781
temporal fossa, **II**:93–98, 94f
temporalis muscle, **III**:16
temporalis osteomuscular flap, **III**:322
temporomandibular joint, **III**:76–77
temporomandibular joint (TMJ) dysfunction, **III**:89–104
    cartilage engineering, **I**:421–423
    cephalometrics, **II**:364–365, 364f
    complications, **III**:95
    disease process
        anatomical characteristics, **III**:89–90
        condylar fractures, **III**:90–91
        inflammation
            causal factors, **III**:90
            osteoarthritis, **III**:90, 91f
            rheumatoid arthritis, **III**:90
        internal derangement, **III**:91–92, 91f
        myofascial pain and dysfunction (MPD), **III**:90
    general discussion, **III**:89
    patient presentation and diagnosis
        diagnostic imaging, **III**:92, 93f
        patient history, **III**:92
        physical examination, **III**:92
    patient selection, **III**:92–93
    postoperative care and follow-up, **III**:94–95
    prognosis and outcomes, **III**:95
    secondary procedures, **III**:95–96, 95f–96f
    surgical technique and treatment
        noninvasive management, **III**:93–94
        surgical management, **III**:94, 94f–95f
temporoparietal fascia flaps
    mangled upper extremities, **VI**:272–274, 274f
    palatal fistula repair, **III**:643
tenascin, **I**:270–271, **VI**:348–349
tendinopathy
    de Quervain's tendonitis, **VI**:364–367, 366f
    lateral epicondylitis, **VI**:366
    medial epicondylitis, **VI**:366
    nerve compression, **VI**:367–368
    trigger finger
        basic procedure, **VI**:402–404, 404f
        occupational hand disorders, **VI**:367, 367f
        outcomes and complicatons, **VI**:404
        postoperative care and follow-up, **VI**:404
    wrists, **VI**:366
tendon graft and repair
    burn reconstruction, **IV**:451
    carpal tunnel syndrome
        basic procedure, **VI**:401–402, 401f
        outcomes and complicatons, **VI**:401
        patient presentation and diagnosis, **VI**:364–365
        post-nerve injury/surgery rehabilitation, **VI**:856–857
        postoperative care and follow-up, **VI**:401
        secondary procedures, **VI**:401–402
        surgical tips, **VI**:402b
    clinical application, **I**:353f–354f
    definition, **I**:350–364
    extensor tendon injuries, **VI**:210–227
        anatomical characteristics
            extrinsic muscles, **VI**:211, 211f
            functional anatomy, **VI**:212–213
            general discussion, **VI**:211–212
            intrinsic muscles, **VI**:211–212, 212f

*Note: **Boldface** roman numerals indicate volume. Page numbers followed by f refer to figures; page numbers followed by t refer to tables; page numbers followed by b refer to boxes.*

tendon graft and repair (Continued)
complications, VI:221
functional anatomy
extrinsic muscles, VI:213
intrinsic muscles, VI:212–213
joint extension mechanisms, VI:213
linked chains, VI:212, 212f
hand therapy, VI:862–865, 865f
outcome assessments, VI:221
patient presentation and diagnosis,
VI:213, 213f–214f
patient selection, VI:213–214, 214b
postoperative care and follow-up,
VI:220–221, 221f
research summary, VI:227
secondary procedures
boutonnière deformity, VI:223–224, 223f
challenges, VI:221b
delayed sagittal band reconstruction,
VI:225, 225b, 225f
hanging fingertip, VI:221–222, 222f
missing tendons, VI:225
soft-tissue management/staged
reconstruction, VI:226–227,
226f–227f
swan-neck deformity, VI:222–223,
222f–223f
tendon transfers versus tendon grafts,
VI:225
surgical technique and treatment
suturing techniques, VI:214, 214f, 215b
zone I, VI:214–216
zone II, VI:217, 217f
zone III, VI:217–218
zone IV, VI:218–219
zone V, VI:219
zone VI, VI:219
zone VII, VI:219–220
zone VIII, VI:220
zone IX, VI:220
treatment challenges, VI:210
zone I surgical technique
chronic injuries, VI:216
mallet finger, VI:214–216, 215f–217f
open injuries, VI:216
zone II surgical technique, VI:217, 217f
zone III surgical technique
characteristics, VI:217–218
closed injuries, VI:217, 218f
open lacerations, VI:218, 218f
zone IV surgical technique, VI:218–219
zone V surgical technique
human bites, VI:219, 219f
partial lacerations, VI:219
sagittal band, VI:219
zone VI surgical technique, VI:219
zone VII surgical technique, VI:219–220
zone VIII surgical technique, VI:220
zone IX surgical technique, VI:220
extensor tendon ruptures
basic procedure, VI:404–406, 405f–408f
outcomes and complicatons, VI:405–406
postoperative care and follow-up, VI:405
surgical tips, VI:406b
flexor tendon injuries, VI:178–209
anatomical considerations
annular pulleys/cruciate pulleys,
VI:180f
flexor pulleys, VI:180f–181f
general characteristics, VI:179–182

tendon graft and repair (Continued)
tendon zones, VI:31–32, 31f, 181f
vincula, VI:181f
basic procedure, VI:402, 403f
biomechanics
gliding motions, VI:184
linear versus bending forces, VI:183,
184f
surgical repair strength, VI:182–184,
183f
tendon–suture junctions, VI:182–184,
183f
challenges, VI:178–179
flexor pollicis longus (FPL) injuries,
VI:196, 196f–197f
flexor tendon healing, VI:182
free tendon grafting
donor tendons, VI:202f
indications and contraindications,
VI:201–202, 202b
operative technique, VI:203–204,
203f–205f
mutilated/mangled hands, VI:253
operative technique
closed ruptures, VI:197
flexor pollicis longus (FPL) injuries,
VI:196, 196f–197f
incisions, VI:187f
partial tendon lacerations, VI:197
pediatric injuries, VI:196–197
surgical preparation, VI:186–197
zone 1 injuries, VI:186–187, 188f
zone 2 injuries, VI:187–194
zone 3 injuries, VI:196
zone 4 injuries, VI:196
zone 5 injuries, VI:196
outcomes and complicatons, VI:199–201,
201b, 201t, 402
patient presentation and diagnosis,
VI:184–185, 185f
postoperative care and follow-up
basic principles, VI:402
care protocols, VI:197–199
combined passive–active tendon
motion protocol (Nantong regime),
VI:199, 200f, 202f
Duran–Houser method, VI:198–199,
198f
early active motion, VI:199
modified Kleinert method, VI:197–198,
198f
secondary procedures
free tendon grafting, VI:201–204
general discussion, VI:201–208
staged tendon reconstruction,
VI:204–206
tenolysis, VI:206–208
staged tendon reconstruction
indications, VI:204
operative technique (first stage),
VI:204–206, 205f–207f
operative technique (second stage),
VI:206, 208f
surgical technique and treatment
indications and contraindications,
VI:186, 186b
operative technique, VI:186–197
primary and delayed primary repairs,
VI:185–186, 186f
surgical tips, VI:179b

tendon graft and repair (Continued)
tenolysis
anesthesia, VI:207
indications, VI:206–207
operative technique, VI:207–208,
208b
postoperative treatment, VI:208
zone 1 injuries, VI:186–187, 188f
zone 2 injuries
A2 pulley, VI:194f
A4 pulley, VI:193f
core suture methods, VI:189f, 193f
cruciate method, VI:189f
extension ability, VI:192f, 194f
flexion ability, VI:191f, 194f
four-strand repair, VI:191f–192f
modified Kessler method, VI:189f
operative technique, VI:187–194,
190f
peripheral sutures, VI:192f
pulley–sheath complex, VI:195f
ruptured primary repair, VI:193f
simple running peripheral repair,
VI:191f
six-strand M-Tang tendon repair,
VI:190f–191f, 194f
surgical summary, VI:195t
surgical tips, VI:190b
zone 3 injuries, VI:196
zone 4 injuries, VI:196
zone 5 injuries, VI:196
future trends, I:364
mutilated/mangled hands, VI:253, 262
replantation and revascularization surgery,
VI:233, 233b
rheumatoid arthritis
carpal tunnel syndrome
basic procedure, VI:401–402, 401f
outcomes and complicatons, VI:401
postoperative care and follow-up,
VI:401
secondary procedures, VI:401–402
surgical tips, VI:402b
extensor tendon ruptures
basic procedure, VI:404–406,
405f–408f
outcomes and complicatons,
VI:405–406
postoperative care and follow-up,
VI:405
surgical tips, VI:406b
flexor tendon injuries
basic procedure, VI:402, 403f
outcomes and complicatons, VI:402
postoperative care and follow-up,
VI:402
trigger finger
basic procedure, VI:402–404, 404f
outcomes and complicatons, VI:404
postoperative care and follow-up,
VI:404
surgical technique, I:352f–354f
tendon characteristics, I:351f
tendon substitutes/engineered tendons
basic principles, I:351–364
engineered sheath, I:362f
gross views, I:355f, 358f, 360f
histologic studies, I:356f–357f, 359f–361f,
363f
in vivo model, I:355f

tendon graft and repair (Continued)
  tendon transfers, **VI:**745–776
    basic principles, **VI:**745, 746t
    clawing of the fingers
      Bouvier maneuver, **VI:**764–765, 764f
      Brand EE4T transfer, **VI:**766–767, 766f
      Brand EF4T transfer, **VI:**767, 767f–768f
      donor muscle-tendon selection, **VI:**764–765, 765f
      Fritschi PF4T transfer, **VI:**767–768
      Littler modification, **VI:**764–765
      modified Stiles–Bunnell technique, **VI:**764–766, 765f
      pulley insertions, **VI:**764–765, 764f–765f
      static procedures, **VI:**763–764, 763f–764f
    combined nerve injuries
      finger extension restoration, **VI:**774–775
      finger flexion restoration, **VI:**775f, 776
      high median-high ulnar nerve palsy, **VI:**773
      low median-low ulnar nerve palsy, **VI:**772–773
      patient selection, **VI:**772–776
      post-trauma reconstruction, **VI:**773
      thumb extension restoration, **VI:**773–774, 774f
      thumb flexion restoration, **VI:**774f–775f, 775–776
    donor muscle-tendon selection
      expendability, **VI:**746
      muscle integrity, **VI:**746–747
      strength assessment, **VI:**746, 746f
      transfer direction, **VI:**746–747
    extensor tendon injuries, **VI:**225
    high median nerve palsy
      opposition tendon transfers, **VI:**761t
      outcomes and complicatons, **VI:**761
      patient selection, **VI:**759–761, 760f
      surgical technique and treatment, **VI:**759–761, 760f, 761t
    high ulnar nerve palsy
      outcome assessments, **VI:**771–772
      patient selection, **VI:**771
    low median nerve palsy
      abductor digiti minimi (ADM) tendon, **VI:**758
      Bunnell ring finger flexor digitorum superficialis transfer, **VI:**755–756, 755f–757f, 761t
      Burkhalter extensor indicis proprius transfer, **VI:**754–755, 754f–755f
      Camitz palmaris longus transfer, **VI:**756–758, 757f–759f, 761t
      Huber transfer, **VI:**758, 761t
      opposition tendon transfers, **VI:**761t
      pathogenesis, **VI:**753
      patient selection, **VI:**753–758
    low ulnar nerve palsy
      Bouvier maneuver, **VI:**764–765, 764f
      Brand EE4T transfer, **VI:**766–767, 766f
      Brand EF4T transfer, **VI:**767, 767f–768f
      donor muscle-tendon selection, **VI:**764–765, 765f
      Fritschi PF4T transfer, **VI:**767–768
      index finger abduction, **VI:**770–771, 771f
      Littler modification, **VI:**764–765

tendon graft and repair (Continued)
      modified Stiles–Bunnell technique, **VI:**764–766, 765f
      Neviaser accessory abductor pollicis longus and free tendon graft, **VI:**771, 771f
      patient selection, **VI:**761–771, 762f, 762t
      pulley insertions, **VI:**764–765, 764f–765f
      ring finger flexor digitorum superficialis transfer, **VI:**769
      Smith extensor carpi radialis brevis transfer, **VI:**769–770, 770f
      static procedures, **VI:**763–764, 763f–764f
      thumb adduction restoration, **VI:**768–769, 769f–770f
      ulnar deviation of the small finger, **VI:**768
    postoperative care and follow-up, **VI:**749
    radial nerve palsy
      Boyes superficialis transfer, **VI:**748t, 750–752, 752f
      flexor carpi radialis transfer, **VI:**748t, 749–750, 752f
      outcomes and complicatons, **VI:**752–753
      patient selection, **VI:**747–752, 747f
      standard flexor carpi ulnaris transfer, **VI:**748–749, 748f–751f, 748t
      surgical technique and treatment, **VI:**748, 748t
    research summary, **VI:**776
    standard flexor carpi ulnaris transfer, **VI:**749
    surgical approach
      bone and soft tissue healing, **VI:**745–746
      donor muscle-tendon selection, **VI:**746–747
      timing considerations, **VI:**747
    surgical technique and treatment
      combined nerve injuries, **VI:**772–776
      finger extension restoration, **VI:**774–775
      finger flexion restoration, **VI:**775f, 776
      high median-high ulnar nerve palsy, **VI:**773
      high median nerve palsy, **VI:**759–761
      high ulnar nerve palsy, **VI:**771–772
      low median-low ulnar nerve palsy, **VI:**772–773
      low median nerve palsy, **VI:**753–758
      low ulnar nerve palsy, **VI:**761–771
      planning guidelines, **VI:**747
      post-trauma reconstruction, **VI:**773
      radial nerve palsy, **VI:**747–753
      thumb extension restoration, **VI:**773–774, 774f
      thumb flexion restoration, **VI:**774f–775f, 775–776
  trigger finger
    basic procedure, **VI:**402–404, 404f
    outcomes and complicatons, **VI:**404
    postoperative care and follow-up, **VI:**404
tendonitis, **VI:**364–365, 366f
tennis elbow, **VI:**366
tenolysis
  flexor tendon injuries
    anesthesia, **VI:**207
    indications, **VI:**206–207

tenolysis (Continued)
    operative technique, **VI:**207–208, 208b
    postoperative treatment, **VI:**208
  hand therapy, **VI:**159, 865
tensor fascia latae (TFL)
  abdominal wall reconstruction, **I:**553t, 554
  characteristics, **I:**516f, **IV:**15t–16t, 18f, 20f–22f, 25f
  groin reconstruction, **I:**554–557
  lower extremity reconstructive surgery, **IV:**138–139, 138f
  perineal reconstruction, **I:**554–557
  Pierre Robin sequence (PRS), **III:**817, 818f
  pressure sores, **I:**562–565, **IV:**375, 377f
  trochanteric ulcers, **IV:**375t
Teosyal, **II:**47t
teres major muscle, **IV:**221–222, 222f
teres minor muscle, **IV:**221, 222f
terminal branch of the posterior interosseous nerve, **VI:**710
Tessier cleft classification system, **III:**687–688, 687f, 706, 707f
Tessier, Paul, **I:**3–4, 4f, 25, 862–863, **III:**226
testes, **IV:**235, 236f–237f
tetanus prophylaxis Immunization schedule, **IV:**65t
tetracaine, **VI:**96t
tetracyclines, **II:**21–22, 21t
tetraplegia
  causal factors, **VI:**817
  classifications, **VI:**817–818, 818t
  reconstructive surgeries, **VI:**817–842
    general discussion, **VI:**817
    patient presentation, **VI:**818–820, 819f
    research summary, **VI:**840–841
    surgical team, **VI:**818–820
  surgical reconstruction
    biceps to triceps transfer
      advantages/disadvantages, **VI:**821–822
      postoperative care and follow-up, **VI:**822, 822f
      surgical technique, **VI:**821–822, 821f
    brachioradialis to flexor pollicis longus (FPL) transfer
      House intrinsic substitution procedure, **VI:**836f–837f
      IC group 2 and 3 patients, **VI:**830–832, 831f
      operative procedures, **VI:**830–832, 835f–837f, 839f–840f
      postoperative care and follow-up, **VI:**832, 841f
      surgical tips, **VI:**830b
      Zancolli "lasso" procedure, **VI:**835f
    carpometacarpal (CMC) joints
      IC group 4 and 5 patients, **VI:**834–838
      postoperative care and follow-up, **VI:**837–838
      stable thumb CMC joints, **VI:**837
      treatment strategies, **VI:**834–838
      unstable CMC joints, **VI:**837
    deltoid to triceps transfer
      postoperative care and follow-up, **VI:**825
      surgical technique, **VI:**822–824, 822b, 823f–824f

Note: **Boldface** roman numerals indicate volume. Page numbers followed by f refer to figures; page numbers followed by t refer to tables; page numbers followed by b refer to boxes.

tetraplegia (Continued)
  elbow extension
    biceps to triceps transfer, VI:821–822
    deltoid to triceps transfer, VI:821–822
    hygiene considerations, VI:821f
    importance, VI:820–825
  functional electrical stimulation (FES),
      VI:838
  grasp and release restoration
    extensor phase, VI:833
    flexor phase, VI:833, 833b
    House intrinsic substitution procedure,
        VI:834
    IC group 3 patients, VI:832–834
    IC groups 3, 4, and 5 patients,
        VI:832–834
    intrinsic stabilization, VI:833–834
    postoperative care and follow-up,
        VI:834
    Zancolli "lasso" procedure, VI:834
  IC group 0, 1 and 2 patients
    general considerations, VI:825–826
    postoperative care and follow-up,
        VI:826
    wrist extension, VI:825–826, 825f
  IC group 1 and 2 patients, VI:826–830,
      826b
  IC group 2 and 3 patients, VI:830–832
  IC group 4 and 5 patients, VI:834–838
  IC groups 3, 4, and 5 patients,
      VI:832–834
  IC groups 6, 7, and 8 patients, VI:838
  key pinch restoration
    brachioradialis to flexor pollicis longus
        (FPL) transfer, VI:830–832
    Brand–Moberg modification, VI:827–
        830, 828f–829f
    flexor pollicis longus (FPL) tenodesis,
        VI:827–830, 828f–829f
    IC group 1 and 2 patients, VI:826–830
    postoperative care and follow-up,
        VI:830
    split flexor pollicis longus (FPL) to
        extensor pollicis longus (EPL)
        interphalangeal stabilization,
        VI:826–827, 827f
    surgical technique and treatment,
        VI:826–830
    surgical tips, VI:826b
  outcomes and complicatons, VI:838–840,
      841f–842f
  strong grasp and refined pinch
      restoration, VI:838
  surgical guidelines, VI:820
thenar crease flap, VI:132, 134f
thenar muscles, VI:52
therapeutic radiation, I:654–675
  basic principles
    brachytherapy, I:656–657
    particle therapy, I:655–656
    physics concepts
      characteristics, I:657–659
      depth dose distribution, I:657f
      intensity-modulated radiation therapy
          (IMRT), I:658, 659f
      multileaf collimators (MLCs), I:658,
          658f
      photon interactions, I:657f
    radiation technology, I:655
    radiobiology

therapeutic radiation (Continued)
      normal tissue complications, I:659–662,
          660f
        radiation toxicity, I:660, 661f–662f
        tumor response, I:659–662, 660f
    voltage therapy, I:655
  future trends, I:674
  general discussion, I:654–655
  radiation treatment
    benign disorders, I:671
    breast cancer
      breast conservation, I:665
      chemotherapy sequencing, I:668
      nodal draining area irradiation,
          I:665–666
      postmastectomy radiation (PMRT),
          I:665
      radiotherapy techniques, I:666–668,
          666f–667f
      research background, I:664–668
    clinical applications
      patient selection, I:664, 664b
      treatment intent, I:664
      units of radiation, I:664
    head and neck cancer, I:668–669
    nonmelanoma skin cancers, I:670–671
    planning and process, I:662–664, 663f
    soft-tissue sarcomas, I:669–670
  research summary, I:674
  toxicities and complications
    accidental and occupational radiation
        exposure, I:673–674
    bony injuries, I:671–672
    lymphedema, I:672
    pediatric bone development, I:672
    radiation-induced malignancies, I:673
thermal burns
  contact burns, IV:394–395, 395f
  flash and flame burns, IV:394
  scalds, IV:394, 394f
  tar, IV:395–396
thiamine, I:282
thick lip, III:639
Thiersch, Carl, I:20
Thiersch–Ollier grafts, I:325–326
thighs
  anatomical characteristics
    fascial system, IV:8–11
    functional role, IV:8–30
    innervation, IV:5–8, 7f
      cutaneous innervation, IV:26–30,
          27f–29f
      motor nerves, IV:26, 27f–28f
      obturator nerve, IV:29f
      sciatic nerve, IV:28f
    musculature, IV:6f
      adductor compartment musculature,
          IV:19t
      anterior thigh compartment
          musculature, IV:19t
      anterior view, IV:21f–22f
      arteries and nerves, IV:18f
      detailed characteristics, IV:11–19, 15t–16t
      pes anserinus, IV:19f
      posterior thigh compartment
          musculature, IV:19t
      schematic diagram, IV:20f
    skeletal structure
      bony attachments, IV:4f
      characteristics, IV:8

thighs (Continued)
    femur, IV:10f
    joints and ligaments, IV:9f
    medial femoral periosteal bone flap,
        IV:11f
    musculature, IV:13f
    serial cross-sections, IV:14f
    surface anatomy, IV:12f
  vascular supply, IV:5, 7f
    arteries, IV:24f
    detailed characteristics, IV:19–25
    femoral and profunda arteries, IV:23f
    lateral circumflex femoral arterial
        system, IV:23, 25f
    medial circumflex femoral arterial
        system, IV:23–25, 26f
    profunda femoris, IV:22–23
    profunda femoris perforating branches,
        IV:25, 26f
  burn reconstruction, IV:509
  congenital melanocytic nevi (CMN), III:848,
      852f
  functional role, IV:8–30
  liposuctions
    anterior thigh, II:525
    cellulite, II:524–525
    lateral and posterior thighs, II:524
    medial thigh, II:525
  reconstructive surgeries
    anterolateral thigh perforator flap, IV:145,
        145f–146f
    basic procedure, IV:130
    lateral thigh/profunda femoris perforator
        flap, IV:144–145, 144f
    medial thigh septocutaneous flap,
        IV:143–144, 144f
    perforator flaps, IV:131f
  thigh flaps, I:557
  vertical thigh-lift
    complications, II:652
    major weight loss (MWL) patient, II:648b
    markings, II:649–652, 650f
    operative technique, II:651f–652f, 652
    patient evaluation, II:645–648
    patient selection, II:648–649
    postoperative care and follow-up, II:652
thin lip, III:639, 640f
thinned flaps, I:612, 612f
third branchial cleft anomaly, III:886–887
third-party payers, I:61–62
13q-syndrome, VI:573t
thoracic hypoplasia, V:591, 591f
thoracic outlet syndrome (TOS)
  anatomical considerations, VI:64–65, 65f,
      519, 520f–521f
  classifications, VI:64
  definition, VI:63–66
  incidence, VI:518–522
  nonsurgical management, VI:521–522
  outcomes and complicatons, VI:522
  patient presentation and diagnosis,
      VI:520–521, 522f
  provocative maneuvers
    Adson test, VI:65, 66f
    costoclavicular compression test, VI:65,
        66f
    Morley's test, VI:66
    neck tilting test, VI:65
    Roos extended arm stress test, VI:66
    Wright test, VI:65, 66f

thoracic outlet syndrome (TOS) (Continued)
surgical technique and treatment, VI:522
Wright's hyperabduction test, VI:520–521,
522f
thoracoacromial trunk artery, IV:225–227, 226f
thoracodorsal artery, IV:222f, 223
thoracodorsal artery perforator (TDAP) flap
breast reconstruction, V:308, 486–487,
486f–488f
lower extremity reconstructive surgery,
IV:77, 147, 147f
oral cavity and mouth reconstruction,
III:322
tongue reconstruction, III:309t
thoracodorsal pedicle, I:530f
thoracolumbar fascia, IV:221
thoracopagus twins, III:893–897, 894f–898f,
901b, 901f
three-dimensional (3D) computed
tomography (CT), I:662–664
three stage full-thickness forehead flap,
III:151–152, 152f–153f
throat surgery, I:862–863
thrombin, I:242–245, 243f, 268–269
thrombocytopenia absent radius (TAR)
syndrome, VI:573t, 574
thrombophlebitis, IV:433t
thrombosis, IV:433t
thrombospondin, I:244
thromboxane A₂ (TXA₂), I:573–574, 574f,
580–581
thryoglossal duct cysts
characteristics, III:887
complications, III:887–888
disease process, III:887
patient presentation and diagnosis, III:887,
887f
prognosis and outcomes, III:887–888
surgical technique and treatment, III:887
thumb
absent thumb, VI:546t
anatomical characteristics, VI:13–14, 14f
flexor pulleys, VI:29–32, 29f–30f, 179–182,
180f
inadequate thumb, VI:546t
modified House classification of thumb
deformity, VI:464t
osteoarthritis
carpometacarpal (CMC) arthroscopy
basic principles, VI:434–439
Burton–Pelligrini procedure, VI:437–
439, 438f
dorsal wedge extension osteotomy,
VI:435
Eaton–Littler procedure, VI:435–437,
436f
simple trapeziectomy, VI:437
stage II-IV surgical procedures, VI:437
trapeziectomy with ligament
reconstruction and/or tendon
interposition, VI:437–439,
438f–439f
volar ligament reconstruction,
VI:435–437
Weilby suspensionplasty, VI:438, 439f
metacarpophalangeal (MCP) joint, VI:430
prevalence and characteristics,
VI:430–441

thumb (Continued)
prosthetic arthroplasty, VI:440–441, 440f
trapeziometacarpal arthritis
anatomy and biomechanics, VI:431,
431f
Burton–Pelligrini procedure, VI:437–
439, 438f
diagnosis and classification, VI:431–
433, 432t, 433f
etiology and epidemiology, VI:430–431
nonsurgical treatments, VI:433–434
simple trapeziectomy, VI:437
stage I surgical procedures, VI:434
stage II-IV surgical procedures, VI:437
trapeziectomy with ligament
reconstruction and/or tendon
interposition, VI:437–439,
438f–439f
trapeziometacarpal arthrodesis,
VI:440–441, 441f
Weilby suspensionplasty, VI:438, 439f
trapeziometacarpal arthrodesis, VI:440–
441, 441f
reconstructive surgeries, VI:282–294
distal-third amputations
avulsion injuries, VI:287f
basic procedure, VI:283–287
cross-finger flap, VI:285f
dorsal metacarpal artery flap,
VI:286f–287f
kite flap, VI:286f
Moberg thumb volar advancement
flap, VI:284f–285f
neurovascular island flap, VI:286f
surgical guidelines, VI:287b
thumb tip closure via volar V-Y
advancement flap, VI:284f
general discussion, VI:282
injury factors, VI:282–283
middle-third amputations
basic procedure, VI:287–291
dorsal hand flap, VI:289f
first webspace, VI:287f–288f
iliac crest bone graft, VI:291f
metacarpal lengthening, VI:290f
pedicled radial forearm fascia flap,
VI:290f
severe dorsal thumb injury, VI:289f
surgical guidelines, VI:291b
Z-plasty technique, VI:287–291, 288f
outcomes and complicatons, VI:293
patient presentation and diagnosis,
VI:283
patient selection, VI:283, 297
postoperative care and follow-up, VI:293
secondary procedures, VI:293–294
surgical technique and treatment
distal-third amputations, VI:283–287
middle-third amputations, VI:287–291
prosthetics, VI:293
proximal-third amputations, VI:292–
293, 292f–293f, 293b
thumb loss classification, VI:283, 283f
rheumatoid arthritis
basic principles, VI:376–379
boutonnière deformity, VI:378f–380f
flexion and volar subluxation, VI:377f
scleroderma, VI:407t, 409

thumb (Continued)
swan-neck deformity, VI:379f, 625f
thumb deformities
basic procedure, VI:399–400
boutonnière deformity, VI:378f–380f,
399–400, 400f
outcomes and complicatons, VI:400
postoperative care and follow-up,
VI:400
swan-neck deformity, VI:400f
ulnar deviation, VI:377f–378f
spastic hand surgery, VI:464, 464t
thumb duplication, VI:546t
thumb hypoplasia, VI:572–602
associated conditions, VI:573t
Fanconi anemia (FA), VI:573t, 574
general discussion, VI:573–574
Holt–Oram syndrome, VI:573t, 574
thrombocytopenia absent radius (TAR)
syndrome, VI:573t, 574
VACTERL association, VI:573t, 574
characteristics, VI:572
classification systems, VI:574, 574f
clinical presentation
general characteristics, VI:574–583
Type I (mild hypoplasia), VI:574–575,
575f
Type II (moderate hypoplasia),
VI:575–577, 576f, 578f
Type III (severe hypoplasia), VI:577,
579f–580f
Type IV (floating thumb), VI:577, 581f
Type V (aplasia), VI:577, 582f
Type VI (cleft hand), VI:579–580
Type VI (symbrachydactyly thumb),
VI:580–581
Type VII (constriction ring syndrome),
VI:581
Type VIII (five-fingered hand),
VI:581–582
Type IX (radial polydactyly),
VI:582–583
Type X (syndromic short skeletal
thumb ray), VI:583
etiology, VI:573
inadequate index finger, VI:599–600
incidence, VI:572–573
outcomes and complicatons
Type I (mild hypoplasia), VI:597
Type II (moderate hypoplasia), VI:597
Type III (severe hypoplasia), VI:597
Type VI (cleft hand), VI:598
Type VI (symbrachydactyly thumb),
VI:598
Type VII (constriction ring syndrome),
VI:599
Type VIII (five-fingered hand), VI:599
Type IX (radial polydactyly), VI:599
Type X (syndromic short skeletal
thumb ray), VI:599
patient presentation and diagnosis,
VI:574–583
patient selection, VI:583
pollicization technique
basic principles, VI:590
dissection and exposure, VI:590
general discussion, VI:590–594
incisions, VI:590, 592f–593f

Note: **Boldface** roman numerals indicate volume. Page numbers followed by f refer to figures; page numbers followed by t refer to tables; page numbers followed by b refer to boxes.

thumb (Continued)
  operative technique, **VI:**591f–593f
  outcomes and complicatons, **VI:**598
  skeletal shortening, **VI:**594
  skin closure and web construction, **VI:**594
  tendon and intrinsic muscle rebalancing, **VI:**594
postoperative care and follow-up, **VI:**597
secondary procedures, **VI:**599–600
surgical technique and treatment
  abductor digiti quinti minimi muscle (ADQM) transfer, **VI:**587–588, 589f
  deficient first web space, **VI:**586–587
  flexor digitorum superficialis (FDS) transfer, **VI:**588–590
  four-flap Z-plasty, **VI:**585f, 586–587
  interphalangeal (IP) joint motion, **VI:**590
  metacarpophalangeal joint instability, **VI:**587, 588f
  pollex abductus, **VI:**578f, 590
  pollicization technique, **VI:**590–594, 591f–593f
  poor/absent palmar abduction (opposition), **VI:**587–590
  tendon graft stabilization, **VI:**587
  Type III (severe hypoplasia), **VI:**587, 588f
  Type VI (cleft hand), **VI:**594–595
  Type VI (symbrachydactyly thumb), **VI:**595
  Type VII (constriction ring syndrome), **VI:**595–596
  Type VIII (five-fingered hand), **VI:**596
  Type IX (radial polydactyly), **VI:**596
  Type X (syndromic short skeletal thumb ray), **VI:**596–597
  timing considerations, **VI:**546t, 583–584, 583f
treatment strategies
  Type I (mild hypoplasia), **VI:**584, 585f
  Type II (moderate hypoplasia), **VI:**584
  Type III (severe hypoplasia), **VI:**584
  Type IV (floating thumb), **VI:**586
  Type V (aplasia), **VI:**586
trigger thumb
  etiology, **VI:**648
  general discussion, **VI:**648–649
  timing considerations, **VI:**546t
  treatment strategies, **VI:**648–649
triphalangeal thumb
  epidemiology, **VI:**623–624
  outcomes and complicatons, **VI:**627
  pathogenesis, **VI:**624
  patient presentation and diagnosis, **VI:**624, 625f
  patient selection, **VI:**624
  postoperative care and follow-up, **VI:**627
  preferred treatments
    delta middle phalanx, **VI:**625–627, 626f–627f
    first web deficiency, **VI:**627, 628f
    five fingered hand, **VI:**627
    rectangular middle phalanx, **VI:**627
  secondary procedures, **VI:**627–628
  surgical technique and treatment, **VI:**624–627

thumb and finger reconstruction, **VI:**282–310
  basic principles, **VI:**295–296
  clinodactyly, **VI:**631f
  complications, **VI:**309
  fractures and joint injuries
    acute ulnar collateral ligament (UCL) tear, **VI:**155, 155f
    carpometacarpal (CMC) joint fractures, **VI:**156–158, 157f
    chronic ulnar collateral ligament (UCL) tear, **VI:**155–156, 156f
    general discussion, **VI:**153–158
    metacarpal fractures, **VI:**156
    metacarpophalangeal (MCP) joint, **VI:**153–154, 155f
    pediatric fractures, **VI:**158, 158f
    proximal phalanx neck fractures, **VI:**158, 159f
    Stener lesion, **VI:**154–155, 154f
  general discussion, **VI:**282
  injury factors, **VI:**282–283
  patient presentation and diagnosis
    initial operation, **VI:**296–297
    patient evaluation, **VI:**296–297, 296f
    thumb trauma diagnosis, **VI:**283
  patient selection
    decision-making process, **VI:**283, 297
    injury factors
      finger reconstruction, **VI:**297–298
      metacarpal hand, **VI:**298–300, 298t, 299f–300f
      thumb reconstruction, **VI:**297
    primary versus secondary reconstruction, **VI:**297
    thumb loss classification, **VI:**283, 283f
  postoperative care and follow-up
    immediate postoperative period, **VI:**306
    motor rehabilitation, **VI:**306–307
    sensory rehabilitation, **VI:**307–308
    thumb reconstruction, **VI:**293
  prognosis and outcomes
    appearance, **VI:**308
    donor site outcome evaluation, **VI:**308, 309f
    range of motion, **VI:**308
    sensory recovery, **VI:**308
    strength assessment, **VI:**308
    success rates, **VI:**308
    thumb reconstruction, **VI:**293
  replantation and revascularization surgery
    artery repair, **VI:**233–234, 234f
    bone fixation, **VI:**232–233, 232b, 232f
    complications, **VI:**248–249
    ectopic replantation, **VI:**243, 244f
    multiple digit replantations, **VI:**237–238, 237f–240f
    nerve repair and grafting, **VI:**235
    operative sequence, **VI:**231–232, 231f
    outcome assessments, **VI:**247–248, 247t
    patient selection indications and contraindications, **VI:**230–231, 230t–231t
    postoperative monitoring, **VI:**245–246, 246b, 246t
    postoperative therapy, **VI:**246
    psychosocial aspects, **VI:**246–247
    ring avulsion injuries, **VI:**242, 242b, 242t, 243f
    secondary procedures, **VI:**248f, 249
    single-digit amputation, **VI:**241f

thumb and finger reconstruction (Continued)
    skin closure, **VI:**235
    tendon graft and repair, **VI:**233, 233b
    thumb replantation, **VI:**235–237, 236f–237f
    vein repair, **VI:**234–235, 235f
  secondary procedures, **VI:**293–294, 309, 309f
  surgical technique and treatment
    donor closure guidelines, **VI:**301–302
    first dorsal metatarsal artery (FDMA), **VI:**300, 301f
    flap inset guidelines, **VI:**302–303, 302b, 302f
    prosthetics, **VI:**293
    recipient preparation, **VI:**300–301, 301b, 301f
    specific operations
      combined second- and third-toe transplantations, **VI:**305, 307f
      first-web neurosensory flap harvest, **VI:**305, 306f
      great-toe wrap-around flap harvest, **VI:**304–305
      pulp flap harvest, **VI:**305, 305f
      total or partial second-toe harvest, **VI:**304, 304f
      trimmed great toe harvest, **VI:**303–304, 303f
    thumb distal-third amputations
      avulsion injuries, **VI:**287f
      basic procedure, **VI:**283–287
      cross-finger flap, **VI:**285f
      dorsal metacarpal artery flap, **VI:**286f–287f
      kite flap, **VI:**286f
      Moberg thumb volar advancement flap, **VI:**284f–285f
      neurovascular island flap, **VI:**286f
      surgical guidelines, **VI:**287b
      thumb tip closure via volar V-Y advancement flap, **VI:**284f
    thumb middle-third amputations
      basic procedure, **VI:**287–291
      dorsal hand flap, **VI:**289f
      first webspace, **VI:**287f–288f
      iliac crest bone graft, **VI:**291f
      metacarpal lengthening, **VI:**290f
      pedicled radial forearm fascia flap, **VI:**290f
      severe dorsal thumb injury, **VI:**289f
      surgical guidelines, **VI:**291b
      Z-plasty technique, **VI:**287–291, 288f
    thumb proximal-third amputations, **VI:**292–293, 292f–293f, 293b
    vascular dissection principles, **VI:**300, 300b, 301f
thumb adduction restoration, **VI:**768–769, 769f–770f
thumb/digital dissections, **VI:**672, 673f, 673t
thumb extension restoration, **VI:**773–774, 774f
thumb flexion restoration, **VI:**774f–775f, 775–776
thumb reconstruction, **VI:**282–294
  distal-third amputations
    avulsion injuries, **VI:**287f
    basic procedure, **VI:**283–287
    cross-finger flap, **VI:**285f
    dorsal metacarpal artery flap, **VI:**286f–287f

thumb and finger reconstruction (Continued)
    kite flap, **VI:**286f
    Moberg thumb volar advancement
        flap, **VI:**284f–285f
    neurovascular island flap, **VI:**286f
    surgical guidelines, **VI:**287b
    thumb tip closure via volar V-Y
        advancement flap, **VI:**284f
general discussion, **VI:**282
injury factors, **VI:**282–283
middle-third amputations
    basic procedure, **VI:**287–291
    dorsal hand flap, **VI:**289f
    first webspace, **VI:**287f–288f
    iliac crest bone graft, **VI:**291f
    metacarpal lengthening, **VI:**290f
    pedicled radial forearm fascia flap,
        VI:290f
    severe dorsal thumb injury, **VI:**289f
    surgical guidelines, **VI:**291b
    Z-plasty technique, **VI:**287–291, 288f
outcomes and complicatons, **VI:**293
patient presentation and diagnosis,
    VI:283
patient selection, **VI:**283, 297
postoperative care and follow-up, **VI:**293
secondary procedures, **VI:**293–294
surgical technique and treatment
    distal-third amputations, **VI:**283–287
    middle-third amputations, **VI:**287–291
    prosthetics, **VI:**293
    proximal-third amputations, **VI:**292–
        293, 292f–293f, 293b
thumb loss classification, **VI:**283, 283f
thumb ulnar collateral ligament injuries,
    VI:85, 86f
toe-to-hand transplantations, **VI:**280–281,
    280f, 295–296, 296f, 555, 555f, 642, 643f
thymine, **I:**177–182, 177f
thyroid chondroplasty, **IV:**349
tibia, **IV:**34f, 183–184
tibia harvests, **I:**452, 452f
tibialis anterior muscle flaps, **I:**526f, **IV:**35f–36f
tibialis posterior muscle, **IV:**35f–36f
tibial nerve, **IV:**46f–47f, 48t, 155t, 171f
ticlopidine, **I:**617
tight lip, **III:**637, 637f–638f
Time Trade Off (TTO), **III:**475
time value of money, **I:**70–71
Tinel's sign, **VI:**56–58, 505–507, 514, 796,
    876–877
tissue engineering, **I:**367–396
    basic principles, **I:**367b
    biomedical burden, **I:**212–213, 213f
    cartilage engineering
        auricular cartilage
            chondrocyte seeding, **I:**414f
            construct appearance, **I:**415f
            ear-shaped scaffolds, **I:**416f
            external stents, **I:**415f
            generation techniques and tests,
                I:413–419, 420f–421f
            gross mechanical tests, **I:**419f
            gross views, **I:**416f
            histologic studies, **I:**418f
            shape evaluation, **I:**417f
        basic principles, **I:**413
        facial contouring, **I:**419–421

tissue engineering (Continued)
    future trends
        general discussion, **I:**423–424
        in vitro cartilage engineering, **I:**423–424
        stem cell-based cartilage engineering,
            I:423
        three-dimensional (3D) structural
            control, **I:**424
    joint cartilage repair and reconstruction,
        I:421–423
    research background, **I:**413
    rhinoplasty, **I:**419–421, 422f
components
    biomaterials
        ceramic biomaterials, **I:**375
        general criteria, **I:**374–377, 375f
        hydrogels, **I:**375–377, 377f
        natural biomaterials, **I:**375
        synthetic biomaterials, **I:**375, 376f
    cells
        applications, **I:**373–374
        biochemical signaling, **I:**371
        bioreactors, **I:**372–373, 373f
        cell sources, **I:**369–371
        co-cultures, **I:**372
        two-dimensional/three-dimensional
            (2D/3D) cultures, **I:**371–372, 371f
    characteristics, **I:**369–386
    matrix
        biomaterials, **I:**374–377
        tailored delivery systems, **I:**380–381,
            381f
        tissue-engineering construct fabric,
            I:377–380, 378f–380f, 380t
    definition, **I:**367
    embryology, **I:**368–369
    ethics, **I:**388
    general discussion, **I:**367–369
    natural examples, **I:**369, 369f
    regenerative medicine, **I:**367–368
    regulatory approval processes, **I:**388
    risk management, **I:**388
    specific tissues
        adipose tissue engineering, **I:**387f,
            389–390, 389f
        bladder, **I:**394–395
        blood vessels, **I:**392
        bone tissue engineering, **I:**392–393
        cartilage, **I:**393–394, 394f
        muscle tissue engineering, **I:**390–391
        nerve tissue engineering, **I:**391–392
        organ regeneration, **I:**394–395
        skin tissue engineering, **I:**388–389
    testing and characterization, **I:**386–388
    vascularization model
        cellular and tissue nutrition, **I:**381
        extrinsic vascularization model, **I:**381–382
        intrinsic vascularization model/in vivo
            bioreactors
            angiogenic sprouting, **I:**385f
            basic principles, **I:**382–386
            human angioblast, **I:**385f
            Matrigel-based vascularization, **I:**386f
            neonatal cardiomyocytes, **I:**386f
            pig model chambers, **I:**387f
            polycarbonate chamber, **I:**384f–385f
            prefabricated flaps, **I:**383f
            silicon tube chamber, **I:**385f

tissue expansion, **I:**622–653
    aesthetic nasal reconstruction, **III:**135
    background information, **I:**622
    back soft-tissue reconstruction, **IV:**269–270
    basic principles
        general discussion, **I:**627–629
        implant and distal port positioning, **I:**628
        implant inflation strategy and technique,
            I:629
        implant selection, **I:**628
        incision planning, **I:**628
    biological characteristics
        bone, **I:**623–624
        cellular and molecular bases, **I:**624–626,
            625f–626f
        fibrous capsules, **I:**623
        general discussion, **I:**623–626
        muscle atrophy, **I:**623
        signal transduction pathways, **I:**626f
        skin, **I:**623
        vascularity, **I:**624, 624f–625f
    breast reconstruction, **V:**338–340, 389
    burn reconstruction
        extremity burn reconstruction, **IV:**450
        facial burn wound treatment, **IV:**482,
            483f, 497
        wound closure, **IV:**503
    complications
        flap tissue compromise and loss, **I:**652
        implant exposure, **I:**652
        implant failure, **I:**652
        infections, **I:**652
        rate incidence, **I:**651–652
    congenital melanocytic nevi (CMN),
        III:842–844
    conjoined twins, **III:**900–901
    extremities expansion, **I:**650
    facial reconstruction, **III:**457–458
    head and neck reconstruction
        basic principles, **I:**631–640
        ears, **I:**637–638
        forehead, **I:**635
        lateral face and neck, **I:**635–637, 636f,
            638f
        male-pattern baldness, **I:**633–635
        nose, **I:**637, 639f
        periorbital area, **I:**638–640, 641f–642f
        scalp, **I:**631–633, 632f–634f
    hernia repair, **IV:**289–290, 291f
    hypoplastic breast
        basic principles, **I:**647–648
        immature breast, **I:**648
        Poland syndrome, **I:**648, 649f
        tuberous breast, **I:**647
    implant types
        characteristics, **I:**626–627
        differential expanders, **I:**627
        expanders with distal ports, **I:**627
        expanders with integrated ports, **I:**627
        self-inflating expanders, **I:**627
        textured silicone expanders, **I:**627
    lower extremity reconstructive surgery,
        IV:137
    muscle/musculocutaneous flaps, **I:**522
    nose reconstruction, **III:**135
    postmastectomy breast reconstruction
        basic principles, **I:**640–647
        chest wall irradiated areas, **I:**645–647

*Note: **Boldface** roman numerals indicate volume. Page numbers followed by f refer to figures; page numbers followed by t refer to tables; page numbers followed by b refer to boxes.*

tissue expansion (Continued)
  complications
    clinical studies, **V:**362, 363t
    expander failure or malfunction,
      V:360f–361f
    infections, **V:**361–363
    skin necrosis, **V:**360f
  expander device, **I:**642–643, **V:**292f
  expander-implants
    adjustable, permanent expander-
      implants, **V:**366–367
    average operative time, **V:**364t
    basic procedure, **V:**338–340
    breast envelope preservation,
      V:367–368
    capsular contracture, **V:**362, 362t–364t
    cellulitis, **V:**359, 360f
    clinical studies, **V:**362, 363t
    complication frequency, **V:**363–365, 364t
    complications, **V:**359
    cosmetic revision surgery, **V:**365, 366f
    delayed reconstruction, **V:**342f, 358,
      359f
    erythema, **V:**359
    evaluation studies, **V:**365
    expander failure or malfunction,
      V:360–361, 360f–361f, 364t
    fat injections, **V:**365, 368
    flap-based reconstruction, **V:**367
    hematomas, **V:**359, 359f, 364t
    implant malposition, **V:**363t
    implant removal, **V:**363t
    implant rupture and deflation,
      V:361–362, 363t
    infections, **V:**361–363, 363t–364t
    insertion procedures, **V:**353–354
    nipple reconstruction, **V:**365–366
    outcome assessments, **V:**363–365
    persistent serous drainage, **V:**359–360
    postoperative care and follow-up,
      V:358–359
    preoperative/postoperative
      comparisons, **V:**340f–341f
    secondary procedures, **V:**365–366
    skin necrosis, **V:**360, 360f, 363t
    wrinkle formation, **V:**363t
  immediate postmastectomy breast
    reconstruction
    acellular allogenic dermal matrix
      (ADM), **I:**644–645, 644f
    muscle coverage, **I:**643–645
    submuscular position, **I:**643–644
    subpectoral (dual-plane) position, **I:**644
  outcomes and complicatons
    cellulitis, **V:**359, 360f
    erythema, **V:**359
    expander failure or malfunction,
      V:360–361
    hematomas, **V:**359, 359f
    persistent serous drainage, **V:**359–360
    skin necrosis, **V:**360
  patient presentation and diagnosis
    exclusion criteria, **V:**345–346, 347f
    inclusion criteria, **V:**346
    large breast reconstruction, **V:**346, 350f
    medium breast reconstruction, **V:**346,
      349f
    small breast reconstruction, **V:**346, 348f
  postoperative care and follow-up,
    V:358–359

tissue expansion (Continued)
  prosthesis insertion
    basic procedure, **V:**356–358
    capsulectomy, **V:**357f
    contralateral adjustments, **V:**356–358
    inframammary fold reconstruction,
      V:357f
    large breast augmentation, **V:**358
    medium breast augmentation,
      V:357–358
    small breast augmentation, **V:**356–357
  reconstructive paradigms
    contralateral adjustments, **V:**343f
    cosmetic breast reconstruction,
      V:344f–345f
    indications and contraindications,
      V:343f
    mastectomy techniques, **V:**343f
    radiation therapy (RT), **V:**347f
    surgical strategy, **V:**340–344
  secondary breast reconstruction, **I:**645,
    646f
  skin reducing mastectomy, **V:**354–356,
    355f
  surgical technique and treatment
    delayed reconstruction, **V:**358, 359f
    expander-implant insertion, **V:**353–354,
      354f
    immediate postmastectomy breast
      reconstruction, **V:**353
    prosthesis insertion, **V:**356–358
    second-stage surgery, **V:**356, 357f
    skin reducing mastectomy, **V:**354–356,
      355f
    tissue preservation, **V:**353–358
  pressure sore treatment, **IV:**369
  scalp and forehead reconstruction,
    III:121–123, 122f, 441, 443f
  special cases
    burns, **I:**629
    children, **I:**629–630
    expanded full-thickness skin grafts,
      I:630
    fascial flaps, **I:**630
    free flaps, **I:**630
    myocutaneous flaps, **I:**630
  surgical innovation, **I:**6–7
  trunk expansion, **I:**648–650, 650f–651f
tissue factor, **I:**242–245, 243f
tissue grafts, **I:**339–366
  background information, **I:**339
  composite tissue grafts, **I:**365f, 366
  dermal graft and repair
    clinical application, **I:**340–342
    definition, **I:**339–342
    dermal substitutes, **I:**342, 342f
    future trends, **I:**342
    schematic diagram, **I:**340f
    surgical technique, **I:**340
    survival rates, **I:**340, 341f
  fascial graft and repair
    clinical application, **I:**348, 349f–350f
    definition, **I:**348–350
    future trends, **I:**348–350
    surgical technique, **I:**348
  fat grafts
    clinical application, **I:**342–346, 344f–347f
    definition, **I:**342–347
    future trends, **I:**346–347, 348f
    harvesting methods, **I:**342f–343f

tissue grafts (Continued)
  muscle graft and repair
    clinical application, **I:**364
    definition, **I:**364–366
    future trends, **I:**364–366, 365f
    surgical technique, **I:**364
  tendon graft and repair
    clinical application, **I:**353f–354f
    definition, **I:**350–364
    future trends, **I:**364
    surgical technique, **I:**352f–354f
    tendon characteristics, **I:**351f
    tendon substitutes/engineered tendons
      basic principles, **I:**351–364
      engineered sheath, **I:**362f
      gross views, **I:**355f, 358f, 360f
      histologic studies, **I:**356f–357f,
        359f–361f, 363f
      in vivo model, **I:**355f
tissue inhibitors of metalloproteinases
  (TIMPs), **I:**300
tissue oxygenation, **I:**256–259, 256f–257f
tissue rearrangement, **I:**312
tissue repair, reconstruction, and
  regeneration
  biomaterial scaffolds, **I:**187–189, 189f
  biomedical burden, **I:**212–213, 213f
  tissue grafts, **I:**339–366
    background information, **I:**339
    composite tissue grafts, **I:**365f, 366
    dermal graft and repair
      clinical application, **I:**340–342
      definition, **I:**339–342
      dermal substitutes, **I:**342, 342f
      future trends, **I:**342
      schematic diagram, **I:**340f
      surgical technique, **I:**340
      survival rates, **I:**340, 341f
    fascial graft and repair
      clinical application, **I:**348, 349f–350f
      definition, **I:**348–350
      future trends, **I:**348–350
      surgical technique, **I:**348
    fat grafts
      clinical application, **I:**342–346, 344f–347f
      definition, **I:**342–347
      future trends, **I:**346–347, 348f
      harvesting methods, **I:**342f–343f
    muscle graft and repair
      clinical application, **I:**364
      definition, **I:**364–366
      future trends, **I:**364–366, 365f
      surgical technique, **I:**364
    tendon graft and repair
      clinical application, **I:**353f–354f
      definition, **I:**350–364
      future trends, **I:**364
      surgical technique, **I:**352f–354f
      tendon characteristics, **I:**351f
      tendon substitutes/engineered tendons,
        I:351–364, 355f–363f
  tissue reconstruction and regeneration,
    I:190–191
  tissue repair, **I:**189–190
tissue-specific stem cells
  clinical correlates
    blood vessels, **I:**232
    muscles, **I:**232
    osteoblast differentiation, **I:**232

tissue-specific stem cells (Continued)
    peripheral nerve repair, I:233
    skin regeneration, I:232
    current research and applications
        blood vessels, I:230, 231f
        muscles, I:230–231, 231f
        osteoblast differentiation, I:230, 230f
        peripheral nerve repair, I:231–232, 231f
        skin regeneration, I:229, 229f
    definitions, I:228–229
tissue transplantation, I:814–840
    background information, I:814
    challenges, I:814
    clonal deletion, I:826–827
    corticosteroids, I:821, 822t
    future outlook, I:837–839
    nomenclature, I:815
    plastic surgery applications
        bone
            allografts, I:830
            autografts, I:829–830
        cartilage
            allografts, I:831
            autografts, I:830–831
            xenografts, I:831
        hand transplantation
            current status, I:834–837
            immunosuppression, I:834–835
            outcome assessments, I:835–837, VI:848
            transplant survival, I:834–835
        limb and composite tissue
            experimental limb transplantation,
                I:832–834, 833t
            functional considerations, I:832
            general discussion, I:831–834
            immunologic considerations, I:832
            technical considerations, I:832
        nerve
            allografts, I:831
            autografts, I:831
        skin
            allografts, I:829
            autografts, I:828–829
            xenografts, I:829
    transplantation immunology
        anergy, I:827
        antilymphocyte preparations
            alemtuzumab, I:821t, 825–826
            anti-IL-2, I:821t, 825
            antilymphocyte globulin, I:821t, 824
            antithymocyte globulin, I:821t, 824
            immunologic tolerance, I:826
            OKT3, I:821t, 825
        antiproliferative agents
            azathioprine, I:821–822, 822t, 833t
            mycophenolate mofetil, I:822–823, 822t,
                833t
        blood group antigens, I:816
        calcineurin inhibitors
            cyclosporine, I:822t, 823
            rapamycin, I:822t, 824
            tacrolimus, I:822t, 823–824
        current immunosuppressive methods,
            I:820–821, 821t–822t
        immune response cells
            B lymphocytes, I:817
            complement cascade, I:817
            dendritic cells, I:818

tissue transplantation (Continued)
        general discussion, I:816–819
        granulocytes, I:817
        immunoglobulins, I:817
        macrophages, I:816
        natural killer (NK) cells, I:816–817
        T lymphocytes, I:818–819
    immunologic rejection cascade, I:816–819
    immunologic screening, I:820
    inflammatory mediators, I:819–820
    major histocompatibility complex (MHC),
        I:815–816
    minor histocompatibility antigens, I:816
    regulatory cells, I:827–828
    skin-specific antigens, I:816
titanium (Ti)
    craniofacial osteointegration
        bone–titanium interface, I:805, 805f
        implant–tissue interface, I:804
    metal alloy compositions, I:786–787
    potassium titanium oxide phosphate (KTP)
        lasers, II:67–70, 68f
    titanium alloys, I:787, 788f
T lymphocytes
    anergy, I:827
    antigen recognition and graft rejection, I:819
    bone marrow-derived mesenchymal stem
        cells (BMSC), I:225–226
    CD4/CD8 T lymphocytes, I:47–48, 818–819,
        827–828
    CD25 T lymphocytes, I:827–828
    clonal deletion, I:826–827
    functional role, I:818–819
    future research outlook, I:837–839
    skin wound healing, I:268–269, 268f
    T-cell binding and activation, I:818
    T-cell receptor (TCR), I:818–819, 826–827
TNF receptor-associated factor (TRAF) family,
    I:431
TNM clinical classification system
    cutaneous and soft-tissue tumors, I:711,
        712f–714f, 715b
    head and neck cancer, III:308, 400–401, 401t
    larynx cancer, III:433–436
    melanoma, I:750–761, 752t
    oropharynx cancer, III:429–431
    soft-tissue sarcomas, IV:105t
tobacco/tobacco smoke, III:398–399, 421
tocopherol, II:27
toes
    burn reconstruction, IV:509
    melanoma excisions, I:767–768
    microvascular toe transfer, VI:280–281, 280f
    toe fillet flap, IV:207
    toe-to-hand transplantations, VI:280–281,
        280f, 295–296, 296f, 555, 555f, 642, 643f
Toll-like receptors (TLRs), I:247, 247f, 249
Tolypocladium inflatum gams, I:823
tongue
    anatomical characteristics, III:422f
    cancer management
        base of tongue, III:412, 428–432
        diagnosis and treatment, III:427
        preoperative assessment, III:408–409, 408f
        treatment strategies, III:409
    palatal fistula repair, III:643, 646f
    progressive hemifacial atrophy (PHA),
        III:796–797

tongue (Continued)
    reconstructive surgeries, III:307–335
        bone-carrying flaps
            circumflex iliac osteocutaneous flap,
                III:322, 323f
            fibula osteoseptocutaneous flap, III:323
            pectoralis major
                osteomusculocutaneous flap,
                III:322
            radius with radial forearm flap, III:323
            scapular osteomusculocutaneous flap,
                III:323, 323f
            temporalis osteomuscular flap, III:322
            trapezius osteomusculocutaneous flap,
                III:322
        challenges, III:307–308
        complications
            acute complications, III:333
            chronic complications, III:333–334
        decision-making process
            anterolateral thigh flap, III:315f–316f
            basic procedure, III:313–315
            defect factors, III:310t, 315f
            neotongue reconstruction, III:316f
            tongue cancer, III:316f
        disease process, III:308
        flap options, III:310t
        free tissue transfer, III:311
        historical background
        local/regional flaps, III:309t, 311
        patient presentation and diagnosis, III:308
        patient selection
            defect factors, III:310–311, 310t
            patient factors, III:308–310, 310t
        postoperative care and follow-up,
            III:332–333
        prognosis and outcomes, III:333–334
        secondary procedures, III:334
        skin grafts, III:311
        soft-tissue flaps, III:309t
        soft tissue flaps
            anterolateral thigh flap, III:321–322
            deltopectoral flaps, III:318–319, 319f
            lateral arm flap, III:321
            medial sural artery perforator (MSAP)
                flap, III:322
            pectoralis major myocutaneous flaps,
                III:319, 320f
            radial forearm flap, III:319–320
            rectus abdominis musculocutaneous
                flap, III:321, 321f
            submental flaps, III:316–318, 318f
            thoracodorsal artery perforator (TDAP)
                flap, III:322
            ulnar forearm flap, III:320–321
        surgical technique
            bone-carrying flaps, III:322–332
            fasciocutaneous flaps, III:319–322
            local flaps, III:316–318
            musculocutaneous flaps, III:319–322
            pedicled osteocutaneous flaps, III:322
            regional flaps, III:318–319
            soft tissue flaps, III:316–322
            vascularized osteocutaneous flaps,
                III:322–323
    traumatic injuries, III:46
tongue lip adhesion (TLA), III:803–804,
    815–819, 815f–817f

Note: **Boldface** roman numerals indicate volume. Page numbers followed by f refer to figures; page numbers followed by t refer to tables; page numbers followed by b refer to boxes.

tonsils, **III:**431
top-hat flap, **V:**510, 510f
topical ointments, **IV:**410
topical treatments for rosacea, **II:**21t
Toriello–Carey syndrome, **III:**807t
tort law, **I:**93
tortoise jelly, **V:**33t–35t
total breast reconstruction, **V:**595
total mastectomy, **V:**281–282, 281f
total or partial second-toe harvest, **VI:**304, 304f
total parenteral nutrition (TPN), **IV:**292
totipotent stem cells, **I:**261–264, 261f
Touch Bionics, **I:**858–861, 860f–861f
tourniquet tests, **VI:**505–507
Townes–Brocks syndrome, **VI:**617t
Townes syndrome, **VI:**573t
toxic epidermal necrolysis (TEN), **IV:**511–525
    dermatologic exfoliative disorders, **IV:**511–517
    general discussion, **IV:**511
    outcomes and complicatons, **IV:**517
    pathogenesis, **IV:**511–512
    patient presentation and diagnosis
        epidermal detachment, **IV:**513f–514f
        etiology and epidemiology, **IV:**512–514, 512t
        mucosal involvement, **IV:**513, 514f
        Nikolsky sign, **IV:**513, 514f
    patient selection, **IV:**514–515
    postoperative care and follow-up
        general care, **IV:**516
        novel pharmacologic therapy, **IV:**517
        ocular care, **IV:**516
    secondary procedures, **IV:**517
    surgical technique and treatment
        basic procedure, **IV:**515
        corticosteroid therapy, **IV:**515–516
        drug withdrawal, **IV:**515–516
        wound care, **IV:**515, 516f
toxic shock syndrome, **II:**411
trace metal deficiencies, **I:**282
trachea
    tracheal stomaplasty, **III:**358, 358f
Tracking Operations and Outcomes for Plastic Surgeons (TOPS), **I:**158–159, 158t
tragal deformities, **II:**290, 291f, 492
training programs, **I:**23–24
transaxillary dissection, **V:**115, 115f
transconjunctival blepharoplasty, **II:**128, 129f–131f
transcutaneous blepharoplasty, **II:**128
Transcyte®, **IV:**412t–414t
transdifferentiation processes, **I:**261–264, 261f
transepidermal water loss (TEWL), **II:**15–19
transference, **I:**33
transfer RNA (tRNA), **I:**179–180
transforming growth factor (TGF)
    transforming growth factor-α (TGF-α), **I:**270t, 275, **III:**518
    transforming growth factor-β (TGF-β) superfamily
        bone regeneration, **I:**435t, 436–437, 443t–444t
        craniofacial clefts, **III:**509, 509f–510f
        Dupuytren's disease, **VI:**348–349
        gene regulation, **I:**180–181
        osteoarthritis, **VI:**412–413
        osteoblasts, **I:**428
        radiation therapy (RT), **I:**662

transforming growth factor (TGF) (*Continued*)
        scar treatment, **I:**309–310
        skin wound healing, **I:**270t, 274, 294–295
        tissue expansion effects, **I:**625f
        unilateral cleft lip, **III:**518
        wound healing, **I:**244–245
transit amplifying (TA) cells, **I:**262f
transmetatarsal amputation, **IV:**207
transparent soaps, **II:**16
transperineal arteries, **IV:**235, 238f
transport distraction osteogenesis (TDO), **III:**587–588
transposition flap, **III:**143, 452, **IV:**203, 205f
transradial amputation, **VI:**873–874, 873f–874f
transverse carpal ligament (TCL), **VI:**505, 506f
transverse cervical artery, **IV:**222f, 223
transverse rectus abdominis myocutaneous (TRAM) flaps
    autogenous breast reconstruction, **V:**457–458
    bilateral pedicle TRAM flap, **V:**393–410
        background and general characteristics, **V:**393–394
        circulatory zones, **V:**395f
        outcomes and complicatons, **V:**407–410
        patient selection, **V:**395–396
        postoperative care and follow-up, **V:**406
        secondary procedures, **V:**410
        surgical technique and treatment
            external and internal oblique components, **V:**404f
            fascial and muscle strips, **V:**400f, 403f
            fascial closure, **V:**405f
            inferomedial dissection, **V:**402f
            lateral muscle dissection, **V:**401f
            markings, **V:**397f, 400f
            medial dissection, **V:**402f
            medial suprafascial dissection, **V:**399f
            muscle and fascial pedicle control, **V:**402f
            pedicle arrangement, **V:**403f–404f
            pedicle length, **V:**403f
            preoperative assessment, **V:**396
            Prolene mesh, **V:**405f
            shaping guidelines, **V:**405–406, 406f–409f
            surgical procedures, **V:**396–405, 397b–399b
            tunnel positions, **V:**398f
        vascular anatomy, **V:**394–395, 394f
    breast reconstruction, **I:**546–549, 548f–549f, **V:**288f
    free TRAM flap, **V:**411–434
        anatomical and physiological considerations, **V:**412
        complications, **V:**430, 431f
        general discussion, **V:**411
        nipple-areola complex reconstruction, **V:**430–432, 432f–433f
        patient presentation and diagnosis
            delayed versus immediate reconstruction, **V:**414
            general discussion, **V:**414–416
            pedicled versus free TRAM, **V:**414–415
            radiation therapy (RT), **V:**415–416
            timing considerations, **V:**414
        patient selection
            procedure selection, **V:**417–418
            risk factors, **V:**416–417
        postoperative care and follow-up, **V:**428–429

transverse rectus abdominis myocutaneous (TRAM) flaps (*Continued*)
        research summary, **V:**432
        surgical technique and treatment
            abdominal closure, **V:**426–428, 429f
            basic procedure, **V:**418–428, 418f
            flap dissection, **V:**419–422, 420f–421f, 423f
            flap inset guidelines, **V:**426, 427f–428f
            mastectomy planning, **V:**419, 419f
            preoperative assessment and marking, **V:**418–428
            recipient vessels, **V:**422–426, 424f–425f
    patient selection, **V:**374–376
    perineal reconstruction, **IV:**387f
    surgical manipulation, **I:**578
transverse retinacular ligaments, **VI:**450–451
transverse upper gracilis free flap (TUG)
    anatomical characteristics, **V:**458–459, 460f
    complications, **V:**459
    patient selection, **V:**458
    postoperative image, **V:**460f
    surgical technique and treatment, **V:**459, 459b, 461f–462f
transversus abdominis muscle, **IV:**228–229, 229f
trapeze-plasties, **IV:**481
trapeziometacarpal arthritis
    anatomy and biomechanics, **VI:**431, 431f
    Burton–Pelligrini procedure, **VI:**437–439, 438f
    diagnosis and classification, **VI:**431–433, 432t, 433f
    etiology and epidemiology, **VI:**430–431
    nonsurgical treatments, **VI:**433–434
    simple trapeziectomy, **VI:**437
    stage I surgical procedures, **VI:**434
    stage II-IV surgical procedures, **VI:**437
    trapeziectomy with ligament reconstruction and/or tendon interposition, **VI:**437–439, 438f–439f
    trapeziometacarpal arthrodesis, **VI:**440–441, 441f
    Weilby suspensionplasty, **VI:**438, 439f
trapeziometacarpal joint (TMCJ), **VI:**70–71, 72b, 72f
trapezius muscle
    anatomical characteristics, **IV:**221–223, 222f
    back wounds, **IV:**263–264, 274f–276f
    head and neck reconstruction, **I:**544, 544f–545f
    scalp and forehead reconstruction, **III:**127–128, 129f
trapezius osteomusculocutaneous flap, **III:**322
trauma-acquired defects
    burns, **I:**42–43
    ear reconstruction, **III:**214–215, 216f
    facial injuries, **III:**49–88
        causal factors, **III:**49
        condylar and subcondylar fractures, **III:**83, 83f
        edentulous mandible fractures, **III:**83–84, 84f
        frontal bone and sinus fractures
            clinical examination, **III:**51
            complications, **III:**53
            computed tomography (CT), **III:**51
            injury patterns, **III:**51
            nasofrontal duct, **III:**51, 52f

trauma-acquired defects *(Continued)*
  surgical technique and treatment,
    III:52–53, 52f
  gunshot wounds
    delayed versus immediate
      reconstruction, **III:**85
    immediate and high velocity gunshot
      wounds, **III:**86–87
    low velocity gunshot wounds, **III:**85–87
    treatment strategies, **III:**86–87, 86f
  initial assessment
    blunt trauma craniofacial injuries,
      III:50–51
    clinical examination, **III:**50–51
    computed tomography (CT), **III:**51
    general discussion, **III:**49–51
    timing considerations, **III:**49–50
  lower facial fractures, **III:**75
  mandibular fractures
    antibiotics, **III:**82
    characteristics, **III:**75
    Class I fractures, **III:**77–78
    Class II fractures, **III:**78
    Class III fractures, **III:**78–80
    classification systems, **III:**76–77
    clinical examination, **III:**76
    comminuted fractures, **III:**78, 79f
    complications, **III:**82–83
    dental wiring and fixation techniques,
      III:75–76
    diagnosis, **III:**76
    displacement direction and extent,
      III:77
    edentulous mandible fractures,
      III:83–84, 84f
    fracture line direction and angulation,
      III:77, 77f
    internal fixation devices, **III:**80–83
    intraoral approach, **III:**79
    muscle function considerations, **III:**76
    open reduction treatment, **III:**78–79
    reduction and fixation principles,
      III:78, 78f
    surgical indicators, **III:**79–80
    teeth, **III:**77
    temporomandibular joint, **III:**76–77
    third molar extraction, **III:**81, 81f
    treatment strategies, **III:**77
  midfacial fractures
    complications, **III:**74
    Le Fort classification of facial fractures,
      III:71–75, 72f
    midface buttresses, **III:**70–71, 70f
    nasal fractures, **III:**57–59, 58f
    nasoethmoidal orbital fractures,
      III:60–61
    postoperative care and follow-up,
      III:74
    zygoma, **III:**63–65
  orbital fractures
    blow-out fractures (children), **III:**54, 54f
    blow-out fractures (floor of the orbit),
      III:54
    characteristics, **III:**53–57
    complications, **III:**56–57
    computed tomography (CT), **III:**54
    infraorbital nerve anesthesia, **III:**57
    operative technique, **III:**55

trauma-acquired defects *(Continued)*
    orbital apex syndrome, **III:**57
    physical examination, **III:**53–54, 54f
    postoperative care and follow-up,
      III:56
    schematic diagram, **III:**53f
    superior orbital fissure syndrome,
      III:57
    surgical anatomy, **III:**53
    surgical technique and treatment,
      III:54–55
    timing considerations, **III:**55
    treatment indicators, **III:**54
  panfacial fractures
    complications, **III:**84–85, 85f
    definition, **III:**84–85
    postoperative care and follow-up,
      III:85
    surgical sequence, **III:**84
    treatment strategies, **III:**84
  upper facial fractures
    frontal bone and sinus injury patterns,
      III:51
    orbital fractures, **III:**53–57
foot reconstruction, **IV:**198, 198f
hand transplantation, **I:**42
lower extremities, **IV:**63–91
  amputation versus salvage decisions,
    IV:65–66, 86
  associated complications
    compartment syndrome, **IV:**84–85
    fat embolism syndrome (FES), **IV:**84
    rhabdomyolysis, **IV:**83–84
  complications
    chronic pain, **IV:**87
    nonunion occurrences, **IV:**87
    osteomyelitis, **IV:**86–87
    wound complications, **IV:**86
  epidemiology, **IV:**63
  inflammatory response, **IV:**63–64
  Mangled Extremity Severity Score
    (MESS), **IV:**65–66, 66t
  outcome assessments
    amputation versus salvage decisions,
      IV:86
    cost-utility analysis, **IV:**86
    functional outcomes, **IV:**85–86
    patient satisfaction, **IV:**86
  patient presentation and diagnosis
    Glasgow Coma Scale (GCS), **IV:**64t
    injury assessments, **IV:**64–65
    injury classifications, **IV:**65t
    tetanus prophylaxis Immunization
      schedule, **IV:**65t
  patient selection, **IV:**65–66
  postoperative care and follow-up
    antibiotics, **IV:**85
    anticoagulant agents, **IV:**85
    hemorrhage, **IV:**85
  reconstruction options
    anterolateral thigh flap, **IV:**68–69, 69f,
      75, 75f–76f, 81f, 88f
    complex defect and fracture, **IV:**77f–78f
    fasciocutaneous flaps, **IV:**81, 81f–82f
    gracilis muscle, **IV:**77, 80f, 89f–90f
    latissimus dorsi (LD) flap, **IV:**77,
      78f–79f
    local flaps, **IV:**68

trauma-acquired defects *(Continued)*
    muscle/musculocutaneous flaps,
      IV:72–75, 74f
    negative-pressure wound therapy
      (NPWT), **IV:**83
    perforator flaps, **IV:**68–72
    rectus abdominis, **IV:**77, 79f
    rectus femoris muscle flap, **IV:**82f
    serratus anterior muscles, **IV:**77
    skeletal reconstruction, **IV:**83, 83f
    soft-tissue destruction, **IV:**68–83, 68f
    sural artery flap, **IV:**75, 77f
    thoracodorsal artery perforator (TDAP)
      flap, **IV:**77, 147, 147f
  secondary cosmetic procedures
    anterolateral thigh flap, **IV:**88f
    basic procedure, **IV:**87
    debulking, **IV:**90f
    degloving injury, **IV:**88f
    gracilis muscle, **IV:**89f–90f
    liposuction, **IV:**89f
  secondary procedures
    characteristics, **IV:**87–91
    secondary cosmetic procedures, **IV:**87
    secondary functional procedures, **IV:**91
  surgical technique and treatment
    amputations, **IV:**83, 132–133
    fracture management strategies, **IV:**67
    reconstruction options, **IV:**68–83
    timing considerations, **IV:**66–67, 67t
    vascular injury, **IV:**67–68
pediatric facial fractures, **III:**671–685
  associated injuries, **III:**672
  background information, **III:**671
  demographics, **III:**672
  growth and development factors
    basic principles, **III:**672–674
    condylar head fractures, **III:**678f
    cranial-to-facial ratio, **III:**672f
    Le Fort fracture patterns, **III:**675f
    mandibular condyle, **III:**677f
    oblique craniofacial fracture patterns,
      III:676f–677f
    orbital region, **III:**674f
    sinus development, **III:**673f
  incidence, **III:**671–672
  orbital fracture classification system,
    III:677t
  orbital fractures, **III:**54, 54f
  outcomes and complicatons
    adverse outcome classifications,
      III:683t
    basic principles, **III:**682–683
    cranial base/skull fractures, **III:**683
    mandible fractures, **III:**684, 684f
    maxillary and midface fractures,
      III:684
    metallic cranial hardware, **III:**683f–684f
    nasal fractures, **III:**684
    orbital fractures, **III:**683–684
    zygomaticomaxillary complex
      fractures, **III:**684
  patient presentation and diagnosis,
    III:674–675, 678f–679f
  patient selection, **III:**675–678
  postoperative care and follow-up, **III:**682
  research summary, **III:**685
  secondary procedures, **III:**684–685

Note: **Boldface** *roman numerals indicate volume. Page numbers followed by f refer to figures; page numbers followed by t refer to tables; page numbers followed by b refer to boxes.*

trauma-acquired defects (Continued)
surgical technique and treatment
basic procedure, III:678
cranial base/frontal skull fractures, III:678–679, 679f–680f
mandible fractures, III:681f–682f, 682
maxillary and midface fractures, III:680, 681f
nasal and naso-orbital ethmoid fractures, III:681–682, 681t, 682f
orbital fractures, III:679–680, 680f
zygomaticomaxillary complex fractures, III:681
progressive hemifacial atrophy (PHA), III:794
scalp and forehead, III:119–120
Trauma and Injury Severity Score (TRISS), IV:63
traumatic alopecia, II:498
traumatic chest wall deformities
occurrence, IV:253
outcome assessments, IV:255
patient presentation and diagnosis, IV:253
patient selection, IV:253–255
surgical technique and treatment, IV:253–255, 255f
traumatic inclusion cyst, I:720
traumatic tatoo, III:29–30, 30f
Treacher Collins–Franceschetti syndrome, III:226
Treacher Collins syndrome, III:828–836
associated syndromes, III:805–807, 807t
craniofacial clefts
number 6 cleft, III:714, 714f, 829–830, 830f
number 7 cleft, III:829–830, 830f
number 8 cleft, III:715–716, 829–830, 830f
eyelid repair, II:332f
fat grafting, II:330
general discussion, III:828
pathogenesis, III:828
patient presentation and diagnosis, III:828–830, 829b, 829f–830f
patient selection, III:830
postoperative care and follow-up, III:835
secondary procedures, III:835, 835f
skeletal class II malocclusions, III:665
surgical technique and treatment
basic procedure, III:830–835
colobomas, III:830, 831f, 833f, 835f
mandible, III:832–834, 832f–833f, 835f
orthognathic surgery, III:834f, 835
zygoma, III:830–832, 831f–832f
zygomaticomaxillary region distraction, III:833f, 835, 835f
tretinoin, II:26
triangular fibrocartilage complex (TFCC), VI:211, 211f
triangularis, III:282
tricalcium phosphate, II:48t
See also soft-tissue fillers
trichilemmal carcinoma, I:738, 738f
trichilemmal cyst, I:722, 722f
trichilemmoma, I:723
trichion, II:356t
trichloroacetic acid (TCA), II:67
trichoepithelioma, I:723, III:117, 117f
trichofolliculoma, I:723
tricho-rhino-phalangeal syndrome, VI:573t

trigger finger
basic procedure, VI:402–404, 404f
occupational hand disorders, VI:367, 367f
outcomes and complicatons, VI:404
postoperative care and follow-up, VI:404
trigger thumb
etiology, VI:648
general discussion, VI:648–649
timing considerations, VI:546t
treatment strategies, VI:648–649
trigonocephaly, III:731, 731f, 731t
trimethoprim, II:21t
trimmed great toe harvest, VI:303–304, 303f
triphalangeal thumb
epidemiology, VI:623–624
outcomes and complicatons, VI:627
pathogenesis, VI:624
patient presentation and diagnosis, VI:624, 625f
patient selection, VI:624
postoperative care and follow-up, VI:627
preferred treatments
delta middle phalanx, VI:625–627, 626f–627f
first web deficiency, VI:627, 628f
five fingered hand, VI:627
rectangular middle phalanx, VI:627
secondary procedures, VI:627–628
surgical technique and treatment, VI:624–627
triploidy syndrome, VI:573t
triquetrolunate ballottement test, VI:54, 55f
trismus, II:76
trisomies
inherited chromosomal abnormalities, I:185
trisomy 9p syndrome, VI:573t
trisomy 13 syndrome, VI:573t, 617t
trisomy 18 syndrome, VI:573t
trochanteric ulcers, IV:373–375, 375t, 376f
trophoblast, III:504–505
trunk
anatomical characteristics, IV:220–238
abdomen
general characteristics, IV:227–230, 227f, V:412, 413f
musculature, IV:228–229, 229f, V:412, 413f
nerves, IV:230, V:412, 413f
vascular anatomy, IV:229–230, 229f, V:412, 413f
back
general characteristics, IV:220–223, 221f
musculature, IV:221–223, 222f, 224f
vascular anatomy, IV:222f, 223, 224f
chest
general characteristics, IV:223–227, 225f
musculature, IV:224–225
vascular anatomy, IV:225–227, 226f
embryology, IV:220
pelvis
female perineum, IV:230–235, 231f–234f
general characteristics, IV:230–235
male perineum, IV:231f, 235, 236f–237f
brachial plexus, VI:92–94, 93f
congenital melanocytic nevi (CMN), III:844–848, 847f–850f
liposuctions, II:521, 521f
melanoma excisions, I:768, 772f

trunk (Continued)
pediatric chest and trunk defects, III:855–876
abdominal wall defects, III:865–866
congenital defects, III:855
ectopia cordis
characteristics, III:861–862, 862f
clinical presentation and evaluation, III:861, 862f–863f
surgical indicators, III:861
treatment strategies, III:861–862
embryology, III:855
Jeune's syndrome
characteristics, III:860–861, 861f
clinical presentation and evaluation, III:861
surgical indicators, III:861
treatment strategies, III:861, 862f
omphalocele and gastroschisis
characteristics, III:865–866
clinical presentation and evaluation, III:865, 866f
surgical indicators, III:865
treatment strategies, III:865–866
pectus carinatum
characteristics, III:859–860, 859f
clinical presentation and evaluation, III:859
surgical indicators, III:859
treatment strategies, III:859–860, 860f
pectus excavatum
characteristics, III:855–859
clinical presentation and evaluation, III:855–856, 856f
minimally invasive repair of pectus excavatum (MIRPE), III:858, 859f
Ravitch repair, III:857, 858f
surgical indicators, III:856
treatment strategies, III:856–859, 857f–858f
Poland syndrome
characteristics, III:862–865
clinical presentation and evaluation, III:863, 863f–864f
surgical indicators, III:863
treatment strategies, III:864–865, 864f–865f
posterior defects
dermal sinuses, III:874
diastematomyelia, III:874
embryology, III:866
postanal pits, III:874
sacrococcygeal teratoma, III:874
spina bifida, III:866–874
sacrococcygeal teratoma
characteristics, III:874
clinical presentation and evaluation, III:874
surgical indicators, III:874
treatment strategies, III:874
spina bifida
characteristics, III:866–874
clinical presentation and evaluation, III:867
meningomyeloceles, III:868t–869t, 872–874, 873f
paraspinal flap method, III:872–874, 873f–875f
surgical indicators, III:867
treatment strategies, III:867–872, 868t–869t, 870f–872f

trunk (Continued)
  thoracic wall defects
    ectopia cordis, **III**:861–862
    Jeune's syndrome, **III**:860–861
    pectus carinatum, **III**:859–860
    pectus excavatum, **III**:855–859
    Poland syndrome, **III**:862–865
  post-bariatric surgery reconstruction,
    II:652
  tissue expansion, **I**:648–650, 650f–651f
  TNM clinical classification system/pTNM
    pathologic classification system,
    I:713f–714f
  Wesseling trunk adiposity classification,
    II:535f
tuberous breast deformity, **V**:521–547
  asymmetric tuberous breast deformity
    Case III (asymmetric tuberous breast
      deformity)
      patient presentation and diagnosis,
        V:533
      preoperative assessment, **V**:533
      surgical procedures, **V**:533
    Case IV (Type II tuberous breast)
      operative sequence, **V**:533–534
      patient presentation and diagnosis,
        V:533–534, 534f–535f
      postoperative result, **V**:534
      preoperative assessment, **V**:533
    Case VI (Type III flap), **V**:534–537
    Case V (severe bilateral mammary
      hypoplasia and tuberous deformity)
      patient presentation and diagnosis,
        V:534, 536f
      post-lipostructure result, **V**:534
    general considerations, **V**:532
  autologous fat grafts, **V**:591
  background information, **V**:521–522
  classifications
    background information, **V**:526–529
    Type I tuberous breast, **V**:523f–526f, 526
    Type II tuberous breast, **V**:526–527,
      527f–528f, 529b
    Type III tuberous breast, **V**:529, 529b
  pathogenesis, **V**:522
  patient presentation and diagnosis
    diagnosis, **V**:522–529, 523b
    evaluation examinations, **V**:526–529
  postoperative care and follow-up,
    V:544–545
  reconstructive surgeries, **I**:647
  surgical technique and treatment
    case studies
      asymmetric tuberous breast deformity,
        V:533–537, 534f–536f
      Case I (bilateral symmetric tuberous
        breast), **V**:523f–524f, 531
      Case III (asymmetric tuberous breast
        deformity), **V**:533
      Case II (severe tuberous breast
        deformity), **V**:524f–526f, 531–532
      Case IV (Type II tuberous breast),
        V:533–534, 534f–535f
      Case VI (Type III flap), **V**:534–537
      Case V (severe bilateral mammary
        hypoplasia and tuberous
        deformity), **V**:534, 536f
      glandular flap Type III, **V**:534–537

tuberous breast deformity (Continued)
      severe tuberous breast deformity,
        V:524f–526f, 531–532
    general considerations, **V**:529, 529b
    glandular correction flaps
      characteristics, **V**:529–531
      glandular flap Type I, **V**:530
      glandular flap Type II, **V**:530
      glandular flap Type III, **V**:530
      glandular flap Type IV, **V**:530–531
    intraoperative sequence, **V**:532
    suturing techniques, **V**:544–545
  terminology, **V**:521–522
  See also Poland syndrome
tulles, **I**:289t
tumescence, **I**:140–144
tumor necrosis factor (TNF)
  inflammatory mediators, **I**:819–820
  mesenchymal stem cells (MSCs), **I**:225–226
  osteoarthritis, **VI**:412–413
  radiation therapy (RT), **I**:662
  skin wound healing, **I**:270t, 275
  wound healing, **I**:244–245
tumors
  buccal mucosa
    preoperative assessment, **III**:406
    surgical technique and treatment, **III**:406
  chest wall tumors
    outcome assessments, **IV**:249
    pathogenesis, **IV**:247
    patient presentation and diagnosis,
      IV:247, 247f
    patient selection, **IV**:247
    surgical technique and treatment, **IV**:248f,
      249
  clinical target volumes (CTV), **I**:663
  craniofacial fibrous dysplasia, **III**:380–397
    assessment and diagnosis considerations,
      III:380
    complications, **III**:392–393
    disease process, **III**:380–382
    pathogenesis, **III**:380–382
    patient presentation and diagnosis,
      III:382
    patient selection, **III**:382–383, 384f
    postoperative care and follow-up, **III**:389
    research summary, **III**:395–396
    secondary procedures, **III**:393–395,
      395f–396f
    surgical approach
      optic nerve decompression, **III**:384f,
        386
      zonal procedure, **III**:385–389, 385f
      zone 1, **III**:385–386, 386f–393f
      zone 2, **III**:387
      zone 3, **III**:387
      zone 4, **III**:387–389, 394f
    surgical technique and treatment
      nonsurgical treatments, **III**:383
      operation timing, **III**:383–385
      preoperative assessment, **III**:383
      surgical approach, **III**:385–389
  cutaneous and soft-tissue tumors, **I**:707–742
    basal cell carcinoma
      characteristics, **I**:737, 737f, **III**:117–118,
        118f, **VI**:317, 317f
      dermoscopic analysis, **I**:709, 709f
      histological classification, **I**:738b

tumors (Continued)
    surgical margins, **I**:717
    tumor colors, **I**:709
  benign appendage-origin tumors
    apocrine cystadenoma, **I**:722–723, 723f
    chondroid syringoma, **I**:723, 723f
    nevus sebaceous, **I**:721, 721f
    pilomatricoma, **I**:721–722, 721f
    steatocystoma multiplex, **I**:723, 724f
    syringoma, **I**:722, **III**:117, 117f
    trichilemmal cyst, **I**:722, 722f
  benign epithelial-origin tumors
    dermoid cyst, **I**:720, 721f
    epidermal nevus, **I**:718, 718f
    epidermoid cyst, **I**:719, 720f
    keratoacanthoma, **I**:719, 719f, **VI**:315–
      316, 316f
    milia, **I**:719–720
    seborrheic keratosis, **I**:719, 719f, **VI**:316
  benign mesenchymal-origin tumors
    accessory auricles, **I**:732–733, 733f
    acrochordon, **I**:730, 730f
    arteriovenous fistula and arteriovenous
      malformation (AVM), **I**:735, 736f
    capillary malformation, **I**:734–735
    cavernous hemangioma, **I**:735, 735f
    dermatofibroma, **I**:729, 729f, **VI**:316,
      316f
    fibroma pendulum, **I**:730, 730f
    glomus tumors, **I**:734
    granulomas, **I**:733–734, 733f–734f
    hemangioma simplex, **I**:734, 734f–735f
    hypertrophic scars, **I**:730, 731f
    juvenile xanthogranuloma, **I**:729–730,
      729f–730f
    keloid scars, **I**:730, 730f
    leiomyoma, **I**:731–732
    lipoma, **I**:731, 731f–733f
    lymphatic malformation, **I**:736
    mucous cyst of the oral mucosa, **I**:736,
      736f
    osteochondrogenic tumors, **I**:732, 733f
    rhabdomyoma, **I**:732
    soft fibroma, **I**:730
    strawberry hemangioma, **I**:734–735, 735f
    venous malformation, **I**:735, 735f
    xanthoma, **I**:729, 729f
  benign neural crest-origin tumors
    acquired pigment cell nevus, **I**:724, 724f
    Becker's melanosis, **I**:725
    blue nevus, **I**:727
    congenital pigment cell nevus, **I**:724,
      725f
    dysplastic nevus, **I**:724, **III**:113–114, 114f
    juvenile melanoma, **I**:724–725, 726f
    lentigo simplex, **I**:723–724, 724f
    Mongolian spot, **I**:726–727, 728f
    neurofibroma, **I**:728, 728f, **VI**:320, 320f
    neuromas, **I**:727
    nevus of Ito, **I**:726, 727f
    nevus of Ota, **I**:725–726, 726f
    nevus spilus, **I**:725, 726f
    pigment cell nevus, **I**:723–725
    schwannoma, **I**:727, 728f, **VI**:320, 320f
  lymph node dissection
    axillary lymph node dissection,
      I:714–715
    inguinal lymph node dissection, **I**:715

tumors (Continued)
  malignant appendage-origin tumors
    extramammary Paget's disease, I:739, 739f
    Merkel cell carcinoma, I:716t, 739, 739f
    sebaceous carcinoma, I:738, 738f
    sweat gland carcinoma, I:738
    trichilemmal carcinoma, I:738, 738f
  malignant epithelial-origin tumors
    actinic keratosis, I:736, 736f, VI:316–317, 317f
    basal cell carcinoma, I:709f
    Bowen's disease, I:736–737
    squamous cell carcinomas (SCCs), I:737, 737f, III:118–119, 118f, VI:317, 317f
  malignant mesenchymal-origin tumors
    angiosarcomas, I:741–742, 741f
    chondrosarcoma, I:741, VI:329
    dermatofibrosarcoma protuberans (DFSP), I:739, 739f
    Kaposi's sarcoma, I:742
    leiomyosarcoma, I:740, 740f
    liposarcoma, I:740, 740f
    malignant fibrous histiocytoma (MFH), I:739–740, 740f, VI:321, 322f
    osteosarcoma, I:741, 741f, VI:329
    rhabdomyosarcoma, I:741
  patient presentation and diagnosis
    angiography, I:710
    clinical staging system, I:711, 716t
    computed tomography (CT), I:710
    dermoscopic analysis, I:709, 709b, 709f
    Doppler imaging, I:709–710
    inspection and palpation, I:707–709
    magnetic resonance imaging (MRI), I:710
    pathogenic diagnosis, I:710–711
    positron emission tomography (PET), I:710
    scintigraphy, I:710
    TNM clinical classification system/ pTNM pathologic classification system, I:711, 712f–714f, 715b, 750–761, 752t
    tumor colors, I:709b
    ultrasound imaging, I:709–710
    X-ray analysis, I:710
  treatment strategies
    chemotherapy, I:717–718
    cryotherapy, I:718
    electrocoagulation therapy, I:718
    immunotherapy, I:718
    laser treatments, I:718
    lymph node dissection, I:714–715
    radiation therapy (RT), I:717
    reconstructive surgeries, I:717
    sclerotherapy, I:718
    wide excision, I:711–712, 717b
  ears
    benign tumors, III:221
    malignant tumors, III:221–222
  gross tumor volumes (GTV), I:663
  hands, VI:311–332
    background information, VI:311
    fibrous tissue lesions
      benign lesions, VI:321
      sarcomas, VI:321, 322f–323f

tumors (Continued)
  lipoma, VI:321, 321f
  nerve tumors
    lipofibromatous hamartoma, VI:320–321, 320f
    neurofibromas, VI:320, 320f
    schwannomas, I:727, 728f, VI:320, 320f
  outcomes and complicatons, VI:331
  pathogenesis, VI:311–312
  patient presentation and diagnosis
    imaging methods, VI:312–313, 313f
    laboratory studies, VI:312
    patient history, VI:312
    physical examination, VI:312
  patient selection, VI:313
  postoperative care and follow-up, VI:331
  skin tumors
    actinic keratosis, I:736, 736f, VI:316–317, 317f
    basal cell carcinoma, VI:317, 317f
    benign pigmented nevus, VI:315, 315f
    characteristics, VI:313–318
    cutaneous horns, VI:314, 314f
    dermatofibroma, I:729, 729f, VI:316, 316f
    epidermal inclusion cysts, VI:314, 314f
    keratoacanthoma, I:719, 719f, VI:315–316, 316f
    melanoma, VI:318, 318f
    sebaceous cysts, VI:314, 314f
    seborrheic keratosis, I:719, 719f, VI:316
    squamous cell carcinomas (SCCs), VI:317, 317f
    verruca vulgaris, VI:314–315, 315f
  surgical technique and treatment
    aneurysmal bone cysts, VI:328–329, 328f
    benign fibrous lesions, VI:321
    chondrosarcoma, I:741, VI:329
    enchondromas, VI:327, 327f
    fibrous tissue lesions, VI:321
    giant cell tumors of the bone, VI:329, 329f
    glomus tumors, VI:324, 325f
    hemangiomas, VI:324, 324f
    leiomyoma, VI:326, 327f
    lipoma, VI:321, 321f
    metastatic lesions, VI:330–331, 330f
    musculoskeletal sarcomas, VI:329–330, 330t
    myositis ossificans, VI:326, 326f
    nerve tumors, VI:320–321
    osteochondroma, VI:328, 328f
    osteoid osteoma, VI:327, 327f
    osteosarcoma, I:741, 741f, VI:329
    pyogenic granuloma, VI:324–326, 325f
    rhabdomycosarcoma, VI:326
    sarcomas, VI:321, 322f–323f
    skin tumors, VI:313–318
    solitary unicameral bone cysts, VI:328, 328f
    synovial lesions, VI:318–319
    vascular lesions, VI:324–326
    vascular malformations, VI:324, 324f–325f
  synovial lesions
    ganglion cysts, VI:318–319, 319f
    giant cell tumors, VI:319, 319f
    pigmented villonodular synovitis, VI:319, 319f

tumors (Continued)
  vascular lesions
    glomus tumors, VI:324, 325f
    hemangiomas, VI:324, 324f
    pyogenic granuloma, VI:324–326, 325f
    vascular malformations, VI:324, 324f–325f
  lips, III:398–419
    cervical metastasis, III:405–406
    complications
      dental follow-ups, III:418
      general discussion, III:416–418
      local recurrence, III:416
      osteoradionecrosis (ORN), III:417
      post-treatment surveillance, III:417–418
      regional recurrence, III:416–417
      wound infections, III:417
    diagnosis and treatment, III:427
    epidemiology, III:399–400
    lymph node anatomy, III:399f
    medical challenges, III:398
    pathogenesis, III:398–399
    patient presentation and diagnosis, III:400
    preoperative assessment, III:402, 405f
    surgical access, III:402, 403f–404f
    surgical technique and treatment, III:402–405, 405f
    therapeutic choices, III:401–402
    TNM clinical classification system, III:400–401, 401t
  lower extremity reconstructive surgery, IV:136, 136f
  mandible, III:398–419
    complications
      dental follow-ups, III:418
      general discussion, III:416–418
      local recurrence, III:416
      osteoradionecrosis (ORN), III:417
      post-treatment surveillance, III:417–418
      regional recurrence, III:416–417
      wound infections, III:417
    diagnosis and treatment, III:427
    epidemiology, III:399–400
    lymph node anatomy, III:399f
    mandibulotomy, III:409–410, 411f, 414f, 429f
    marginal resection, III:409, 410f
    medical challenges, III:398
    pathogenesis, III:398–399
    patient presentation and diagnosis, III:400
    surgical access, III:402, 403f–404f
    therapeutic choices, III:401–402
    TNM clinical classification system, III:400–401, 401t
  maxilla
    marginal resection, III:409, 410f
    maxillectomy, III:410–412, 412f–413f
  oral cavity and mouth, III:398–419
    alveolar ridge lesions
      preoperative assessment, III:406
      treatment strategies, III:406–407, 407f, 427
    buccal mucosa
      diagnosis and treatment, III:427
      preoperative assessment, III:406
      surgical technique and treatment, III:406

tumors (Continued)
   complications
      dental follow-ups, III:418
      general discussion, III:416–418
      local recurrence, III:416
      osteoradionecrosis (ORN), III:417
      post-treatment surveillance, III:417–418
      regional recurrence, III:416–417
      wound infections, III:417
   epidemiology, III:399–400
   floor of mouth
      diagnosis and treatment, III:427
      preoperative assessment, III:406
      surgical technique and treatment, III:406
   hard palate
      diagnosis and treatment, III:427
      preoperative assessment, III:408, 408f
      treatment strategies, III:408
   lips
      cervical metastasis, III:405–406
      diagnosis and treatment, III:427
      preoperative assessment, III:402, 405f
      surgical technique and treatment, III:402–405, 405f
   lymph node anatomy, III:399f
   medical challenges, III:398
   pathogenesis, III:398–399
   patient presentation and diagnosis, III:400, 427
   retromolar trigone, III:406, 427
   surgical access, III:402, 403f–404f
   therapeutic choices, III:401–402
   TNM clinical classification system, III:400–401, 401t
   tongue
      base of tongue, III:412, 428–432
      diagnosis and treatment, III:427
      preoperative assessment, III:408–409, 408f
      treatment strategies, III:409
   oropharynx, III:398–419
      base of tongue, III:412, 428–432
      cervical lymph nodes, III:415f
      complications
         dental follow-ups, III:418
         general discussion, III:416–418
         local recurrence, III:416
         osteoradionecrosis (ORN), III:417
         post-treatment surveillance, III:417–418
         regional recurrence, III:416–417
         wound infections, III:417
      epidemiology, III:399–400, 412
      lymph node anatomy, III:399f
      medical challenges, III:398
      nodal status determination, III:429–431, 430f
      pathogenesis, III:398–399
      patient presentation and diagnosis, III:400, 428–432
      pharyngeal wall, III:432
      soft palate, III:432
      surgical access, III:402, 403f–404f
      therapeutic choices, III:401–402
      TNM clinical classification system, III:400–401, 401t, 429–431
      tonsils, III:431

tumors (Continued)
   pediatric tumors, III:877–892
      background and general characteristics, III:877
      branchial cleft anomalies
         characteristics, III:885, 885f
         first branchial cleft anomaly, III:886
         fourth branchial cleft anomaly, III:887
         second branchial cleft anomaly, III:885–886, 885f
         third branchial cleft anomaly, III:886–887
      dermoids
         dermal sinus tracts, III:883–884
         external angular dermoids, III:884–885
         general characteristics, III:882
         intradural dermoids, III:883–884
         nasal dermoids, III:882–883, 882f
         neck cysts, III:885
      epiphyseal growth plate
         bone sarcoma, VI:655, 656f
         congenital chondrodysplasia, VI:655–656
      lymphadenopathy
         atypical nontuberculous mycobacteria, III:891–892
         bacterial lymphadenitis, III:890–891
         cervical tuberculous adenitis (scrofula), III:891
         characteristics, III:890
         chronic regional lymphadenopathy, III:891
      neurofibromatoses
         café-au-lait spots, III:878
         congenital fibromatosis, III:881
         craniofacial manifestation, III:878, 879f
         definition, III:877
         disease process, III:877–878
         fibromatosis colli, III:880–881
         general discussion, III:877
         gingival fibroma, III:881
         glomus tumors, III:878
         infantile digital fibroma, III:881, 881f
         juvenile aggressive fibromatosis, III:880
         juvenile nasopharyngeal angiofibroma, III:881
         Lisch nodules, III:878
         neurofibromas, III:880
         neurofibrosarcomas, III:880
         optic nerve gliomas, III:878
         peripheral nerve sheath malignancies, III:880
      pilomatrixoma
         characteristics, III:888
         complications, III:888
         disease process, III:888
         patient presentation and diagnosis, III:888, 888f
         postoperative care and follow-up, III:888
         prognosis and outcomes, III:888
         surgical technique and treatment, III:888
      soft-tissue sarcomas
         alveolar soft-part sarcoma, III:890
         rhabdomycosarcoma, III:888–889
         synovial soft-tissue sarcoma, III:889–890

tumors (Continued)
   thryoglossal duct cysts
      characteristics, III:887
      complications, III:887–888
      disease process, III:887
      patient presentation and diagnosis, III:887, 887f
      prognosis and outcomes, III:887–888
      surgical technique and treatment, III:887
   salivary gland tumors, III:360–379
      benign neoplastic lesions
         hemangiomas, III:364t–365t, 368, 369f
         monomorphic adenoma, III:365t, 367, 368f
         oncocytoma, III:365t, 368
         pleomorphic adenoma, III:364t–365t, 366–367
         Warthin's tumor, III:364t–365t, 367–368, 369f
      benign versus malignant tumors, III:364t–365t
      classifications
         benign neoplastic lesions, III:366–368
         malignant neoplastic lesions, III:365t, 370–371, 370t
         nonneoplastic lesions, III:365–366
      epidemiology, III:361–362, 362t
      imaging methods
         benign versus malignant tumors, III:364t
         computed tomography (CT), III:363–364
         magnetic resonance imaging (MRI), III:364, 364t
         sialography, III:364
         technetium scans, III:364
         ultrasound imaging, III:364
      malignant neoplastic lesions
         acinic cell carcinoma, III:365t, 370, 370t
         adenocarcinoma, III:365t, 370, 370t
         adenoid cystic carcinoma (cylindroma), III:365t, 370, 370f, 370t
         lymphoma, III:365t, 370–371, 371f
         malignant mixed tumors, III:365t, 370, 370t
         metastatic tumors, III:365t, 371
         mucoepidermoid carcinoma, III:365t, 370, 370t
         oncocytic carcinoma, III:365t, 370
         squamous cell carcinomas (SCCs), III:365t, 370, 370t
      nonneoplastic lesions
         mucocele, III:365
         necrotizing sialometaplasia, III:366, 367f
         sialadenitis, III:365, 365f
         sialadenosis, III:365
         sialolithiasis, III:365, 366f–367f
      outcomes and complicatons
         acinic cell carcinoma, III:377
         adenocarcinoma, III:377, 377f
         adenoid cystic carcinoma (cylindroma), III:377
         Frey syndrome, III:377–378, 378f
         malignant mixed tumors, III:377
         mucoepidermoid carcinoma, III:377
         squamous cell carcinomas (SCCs), III:377

tumors (Continued)
  patient presentation and diagnosis
    challenges, III:362–371
      fine-needle aspiration (FNA), III:363,
        363f
      imaging methods, III:363–364
  surgical technique and treatment
    acinic cell carcinoma, III:375–376, 376t
    adenocarcinoma, III:376, 376t
    adenoid cystic carcinoma (cylindroma),
      III:374–375, 376t
    benign neoplastic lesions, III:371–373
    hemangiomas, III:373
    lymphoma, III:377
    malignant mixed tumors, III:376–377,
      376t
    malignant neoplastic lesions,
      III:373–377
    monomorphic adenoma, III:372
    mucoepidermoid carcinoma, III:373–
      374, 374f–376f, 376t
    necrotizing sialometaplasia, III:371
    nonneoplastic lesions, III:371
    oncocytic carcinoma, III:377
    oncocytoma, III:373
    pleomorphic adenoma, III:371–372,
      372f–373f
    squamous cell carcinomas (SCCs),
      III:376t
    Warthin's tumor, III:372–373
tumor management, I:201–211
  background information, I:201
  cancer treatments
    biologics, I:206
    chemotherapy, I:204
    historical background, I:201–207
    immunotherapy, I:204–206
    ionizing radiation, I:202–204
    photodynamic therapy, I:206–207
    surgery, I:202
  clinical target volumes (CTV), I:663
  gross tumor volumes (GTV), I:663
  management approaches, I:208–210
  pathobiology
    critical mass, I:207
    tumor classifications, I:208
    tumor margins, I:207–208
  research summary, I:210
  See also sarcomas
tumor suppressor gene p53, I:661–662, II:15
turbinectomy
  alar wedge resection, II:435–436
  characteristics, II:435–436
  graft placement, II:435–436
  osteotomy
    basic procedure, II:435
    goals, II:435
  wound closure, II:435–436
turmeric, II:24
turnip plots, V:315–316, 316f
twentieth century
  modern plastic surgery, I:20–23, 22f–23f
  postwar plastic surgery, I:25, 25f–26f
  scientific journals, I:24–25, 25f
  scientific societies, I:24
  training programs, I:23–24
22q chromosomal deletion, III:572–573, 573f
Twist1 transcription factor, III:749–750,
  VI:531–532
Twitter, I:98–99

two-stage forehead flap, III:148, 150f–151f
two-stage nasolabial flap, III:146–148,
  146f–147f
two-stage palate repair, III:579–581
two-way interactive television, I:870–871, 871t
tyrosinase inhibitors
  aloesin, II:24
  arbutin, II:24–25
  emblicanin, II:25
  flavonoids, II:25
  general discussion, II:24–25
  hydroquinone, II:24
  hydroxycoumarins, II:25
  kojic acid, II:25
  licorice extract, II:25

U
ubiquinone, II:27
ubiquitous mobile telemedicine, I:872–873
ulcers
  arterial ulcers, I:253–254
  diabetic ulcers, I:254–255, 254f
  pressure ulcers, I:255–256
  venous ulcers, I:253, 279
ulna, IV:182f
ulnar club hand See ulnar hypoplasia/aplasia
ulnar deviation of the small finger, VI:768
ulnar fibula dysplasia, VI:567t
ulnar forearm flap, III:309t–310t, 312f, 320–321
ulnar hypoplasia/aplasia
  associated syndromes, VI:567t
  characteristics, VI:567
  classification systems, VI:567, 568f,
    568t–569t
  incidence, VI:567–570
  outcomes and complicatons, VI:570
  pathogenesis, VI:567
  patient presentation and diagnosis,
    VI:567–569, 567f–569f
  patient selection, VI:569
  postoperative care and follow-up, VI:570
  secondary procedures, VI:570
  surgical technique and treatment, VI:569–
    570, 570f
ulnar mammary syndrome, VI:567t
ulnar polydactyly
  characteristics, VI:616, 617t
  patient presentation and diagnosis, VI:618
  surgical technique and treatment, VI:619–
    622, 621f
ulnocarpal abutment test, VI:55, 57f
Ultra Plus, II:49t
  See also soft-tissue fillers
ultrasonography, I:198
ultrasound-assisted liposuction (UAL)
  background information, II:507–508
  cannulas, II:520–521
  neck rejuvenation, II:320
  treatment options, II:518–519, 518f–519f
ultrasound imaging
  advantages/disadvantages, VI:77t
  basic principles, VI:76–78
  breast cancer diagnoses, V:268, 269f
  finger tendon tears, VI:80f
  hand tumors, VI:312–313
  salivary gland tumors, III:364
  sarcoma detection, IV:104
  ultrasound guidance biopsy, V:271–272,
    272f–273f
ultraviolet (UV) radiation, II:15

umbilical cord blood, I:236
umbilicoplasty, II:553–554, 554f–555f
unaesthetic facial implants, II:305
unethical advertising, I:59–60, 59f–60f
unilateral cleft lip, III:517–549
  characteristics, III:519f–521f
  classification systems, III:518–519, 519f
  complications, III:545
  general discussion, III:517
  genetic considerations, III:517–518, 518t
  incidence, III:517–518, 518t
  orthodontic treatment
    Chang Gung Craniofacial Center
      treatment plan, III:522–523
    distraction procedures, III:602–611, 609f
    growth considerations, III:611
    infants, III:596
    orthognathic surgery, III:602–611,
      607f–608f
    permanent dentition, III:602–611,
      603f–606f
    transitional dentition, III:597–602,
      598f–601f
  outcome assessments
    long-term lip morphology, III:542–543,
      544f
    long-term nasal morphology, III:543–544,
      545f
    patient and parental satisfaction, III:545
  pathological diversity, III:519, 519f–521f
  patient presentation and diagnosis
    anthropometrics
      general discussion, III:519–522
      lip measurements and markings,
        III:520–522, 521f
    lip measurements and markings
      base of the cleft-side philtral column
        (CPHL'), III:520–521, 521f
      columella, III:522
      Cupid's bow, III:520, 521f
      Cupid's bow peaking, III:522
      lateral lip length and height, III:522
      nasal floor skin, III:522
      tissue deficiency/excess evaluation,
        III:521
      vermillion, III:520, 521f
      vermillion deficiency, III:522
  prenatal diagnosis, III:517
  research summary, III:548
  secondary procedures
    Cupid's bow, III:545, 546f
    flared ala-facial groove, III:547
    free border repair, III:546, 546f–547f
    horizontal shortness of the lateral lip,
      III:546
    infrasill depression, III:547
    lower lateral cartilage correction, III:547
    secondary rhinoplasty, III:547–548, 548f
    soft triangle of nostril hood, III:547
    vermillion repair, III:546
    vertical discrepancy of the lateral lip,
      III:545–546
    vestibular webbing, III:547
    wide nostril repair, III:546
  surgical technique and treatment
    adjustment surgeries
      free border of the lateral lip, III:539, 540f
      general discussion, III:537–539
      long horizontal length of cleft side lip,
        III:539

unilateral cleft lip (Continued)
    long vertical height of cleft side lip,
      III:539
    long vertical length of cleft side lip,
      III:537
    short horizontal length of cleft side lip,
      III:539
    short vertical length of cleft side lip,
      III:539
  alveolar molding, III:523–524, 523f–524f
  Chang Gung Craniofacial Center
    treatment plan
    orthodontic treatment, III:522–523
    patient presentation and diagnosis,
      III:522–523, 522f
    surgical approach, III:522, 523f
  microform cleft lip
    pathology, III:542, 542f
    surgical correction techniques, III:542,
      543f
  nasoalveolar molding
    Grayson's method, III:524, 526f
    Liou's method, III:524, 524f–525f
  nasolabial adhesion cheiloplasty
    advantages/disadvantages, III:525–526
    C flap mucosa elevation and insertion,
      III:527, 527f
    lateral lip incisions, III:527, 528f
    markings, III:526, 527f
    mucosal flaps, III:527, 528f
    muscle and skin closure, III:527
    nostril floor closure, III:527, 528f
    post-adhesion definitive cheiloplasty,
      III:527, 529f
    surgical indicators, III:526–527
    two-stage palate repair, III:525
  postoperative care and follow-up, III:542,
    543f
  postoperative management of nasal
    shape, III:542, 544f
  presurgical orthopedics, III:523f, 525
  rotation advancement cheiloplasty
    (complete clefts)
    adequate rotation, III:530–531, 531f,
      535, 536f
    alar base mobilization, III:532
    alar base repositioning, III:532, 533f
    basic principles, III:527–539
    C flap incisions, III:531, 531f–532f
    final skin closure, III:535, 536f
    free border of the lip closure, III:534,
      535f
    inferior turbinate flap, III:532, 532f
    lateral lip incisions, III:530f, 531, 532f
    medial incisions, III:530, 530f
    muscle reconstruction, III:533, 534f
    nasal floor incisions, III:534–535, 535f
    nasal floor reconstruction, III:532, 533f
    orbicularis marginalis flap elevation,
      III:532, 533f
    orbicularis muscle dissection, III:532
    philtral column reconstruction, III:533
    piriform deficiency correction, III:532,
      533f
    preoperative markings, III:530f
    semi-open rhinoplasty, III:535–537
    triangular vermillion flap incisions,
      III:533–534, 534f

unilateral cleft lip (Continued)
  rotation advancement cheiloplasty
    (incomplete clefts)
    basic principles, III:539–542
    excessive skin trimming, III:540–542
    markings and incisions, III:539, 540f
    muscle dissection and release, III:540
    muscle reconstruction, III:540
    nasal correction, III:540, 541f
    nasal floor incisions, III:540, 541f
    nasal floor reconstruction, III:540, 541f
    orbicularis marginalis flap elevation,
      III:540
  semi-open rhinoplasty
    alar base positioning, III:536–537
    alar-facial groove creation, III:537,
      538f–539f
    background information, III:535–537
    excessive skin trimming, III:536, 537f
    fibrofatty tissue release, III:536, 537f
    incisions, III:536, 537f
    lower lateral cartilage repositioning,
      III:536, 537f
Union Internationale Contre le Cancer
  (UICC), III:400–401
uniparental disomy, I:183
universities, I:15, 15f
un-rejuvenated forehead, II:305–306, 306f
un-rejuvenated peri-oral region, II:306
upper aerodigestive tract carcinoma,
  III:420–439
  anatomical considerations
    cervical lymph nodes, III:424, 427f
    hypopharynx, III:432–433
    larynx, III:423, 423f
    lymph node drainage patterns, III:421
    neck, III:424
    nose, III:423–424, 425f–426f
    oral cavity and mouth, III:422, 422f
    paranasal sinuses, III:423–424, 425f–426f
    pharynx, III:422–423, 422f
  diagnosis and treatment
    hypopharynx
      characteristics, III:432–433
      nodal status determination, III:432–433
      TNM clinical classification system,
        III:432–433
    larynx
      glottic cancers, III:434–436, 436f
      patient presentation and diagnosis,
        III:433–436
      subglottic cancers, III:434–436, 436f
      supraglottic cancers, III:434, 435f
      TNM clinical classification system,
        III:433–436
    nose, III:436–437, 436f
    oral cavity and mouth, III:427
    oropharynx
      base of tongue, III:431
      patient presentation and diagnosis,
        III:428–432
      pharyngeal wall, III:432
      soft palate, III:432
      TNM clinical classification system,
        III:429–431
      tonsils, III:431
    paranasal sinuses, III:436–437, 436f
  epidemiology, III:420

upper aerodigestive tract carcinoma
  (Continued)
  future trends, III:438
  incidence, III:421–427
  outcomes and complicatons, III:438
  patient evaluation, III:424–427
  postoperative care and follow-up,
    III:437–438
  prevalence, III:421–427
  risk factors
    alcohol, III:421
    gastroesophageal reflux, III:421
    infectious agents, III:421
    pollution exposure, III:421–422
    tobacco, III:421
upper extremities
  body contouring, V:558–581
    arms
      demand increases, V:558–564
      outcomes and complicatons, V:563–564
      pathophysiology, V:558–559
      patient presentation and diagnosis,
        V:559–564
      patient selection, V:559–560
      Pittsburgh Rating Scale, V:559–560,
        559t
      postoperative care and follow-up,
        V:562–563
      surgical technique and treatment,
        V:560–562, 561f–563f, 562b
    back
      back rolls, V:570–573
      outcomes and complicatons, V:573
      pathophysiology, V:570–571
      patient presentation and diagnosis,
        V:571
      patient selection, V:571–572
      postoperative care and follow-up,
        V:573
      surgical planning, V:571–572
      surgical technique and treatment,
        V:572, 573f
      surgical tips, V:572b
      transverse excisional upper bodylift,
        V:570f, 572
    gynecomastia/male chest contouring
      excision of gynecomastia with nipple
        repositioning, V:575–579, 578f–580f
      outcomes and complicatons, V:579
      pathophysiology, V:573–574
      patient presentation and diagnosis,
        V:574
      patient selection, V:574–575, 575t
      postoperative care and follow-up,
        V:578
      pseudogynecomastia, V:575t, 576f–577f
      surgical markings, V:575–576, 576f–577f
      surgical technique and treatment,
        V:576–578, 578f–580f
      surgical tips, V:578b
    mastopexy
      breast reshaping, V:564–570
      dermal suspension, V:566–570, 568f
      outcomes and complicatons, V:567–570
      pathophysiology, V:564, 564b
      patient presentation and diagnosis,
        V:564–565
      patient selection, V:565–566

Note: **Boldface** *roman numerals indicate volume. Page numbers followed by f refer to figures; page numbers followed by t refer to tables; page numbers followed by b refer to boxes.*

upper extremities *(Continued)*
    postoperative care and follow-up,
        V:567
    surgical goals, **V:**565b
    surgical planning, **V:**565–566, 566t,
        569f–570f
    surgical tips, **V:**567b
    total parenchymal reshaping
        mastopexy, **V:**566–570
    secondary procedures, **V:**579
    total parenchymal reshaping mastopexy
        surgical markings, **V:**566
        surgical technique and treatment,
            V:566–567, 568f
burn reconstruction, **IV:**435–455
    acute phase surgery
        joint reconstruction, **IV:**441–442,
            442f–443f, 445f
        skin grafts, **IV:**441
        skin substitutes, **IV:**441
    axillary contractures, **IV:**507, 507f
    burn-related accidents, **IV:**435
    complications
        axillary contractures, **IV:**445, 448f–449f
        bone exposure, **IV:**446, 450f
        elbow contractures, **IV:**445–446
        heterotopic ossification, **IV:**446
        scar retraction, **IV:**444–445
        skeletal-muscle complications, **IV:**446
        unstable healing, **IV:**444
    elbows, **IV:**507
    electrical burns, **IV:**435–436
    fingers, **IV:**508, 508f
    hands, **IV:**507–509, 508f
    nail deformities, **IV:**509
    patient presentation and diagnosis
        compartment syndrome, **IV:**437–439,
            437f–440f
        emergency surgical procedures, **IV:**437b
        escharotomy incisions, **IV:**429f,
            437–439, 437f–440f
        escharotomy lines, **IV:**428f
        extensive escharotomies, **IV:**431f
        fluid infusion and edema, **IV:**436–437
        full thickness burn escharotomies,
            IV:429f
        hand escharotomies, **IV:**429f
        preoperative assessment, **IV:**436–440
        related trauma, **IV:**439–440
        zigzag escharotomies, **IV:**430f
    patient selection, **IV:**440
    postoperative care and follow-up
        active mobilization, **IV:**444
        compression garments, **IV:**447f
        elbows, **IV:**443
        joint position, **IV:**443t
        passive mobilization, **IV:**444
        patient positioning, **IV:**443
        physio-kinesitherapy tasks, **IV:**447f
        shoulder, **IV:**443
        treatment strategies, **IV:**442–444
        wrists, **IV:**443
    prognosis and outcomes, **IV:**444–446
    secondary procedures
        amputations, **IV:**451–453
        fasciocutaneous flaps, **IV:**449–450
        free flaps, **IV:**450
        general characteristics, **IV:**446–454
        laser treatments, **IV:**454, 454t
        lipofilling, **IV:**453–454

upper extremities *(Continued)*
        myocutaneous flaps, **IV:**449–450
        nerve repair and grafting, **IV:**450–451
        rotation flaps, **IV:**448–449, 453f–454f
        skin expansion, **IV:**450
        skin grafts, **IV:**447–448
        skin substitutes, **IV:**448
        tendon retraction, **IV:**451
        Z-plasty technique, **III:**269f, **IV:**447,
            451f–454f
    surgical technique and treatment
        acute phase surgery, **IV:**441
        characteristics, **IV:**440–442
    web space contractures, **IV:**508
    wrists, **IV:**508, 508f
chemical injury, **IV:**456–467
    characteristics, **IV:**460–464
    complications, **IV:**464
    corrosive agents
        characteristics, **IV:**461
        patient presentation and diagnosis,
            IV:462
        phenol, **IV:**461–463
        secondary surgical treatment, **IV:**463
        white phosphorus, **IV:**461–463
    desiccants
        characteristics, **IV:**461
        patient presentation and diagnosis,
            IV:462
        secondary surgical treatment, **IV:**463
        sulfuric acid, **IV:**461–463
    disease process
        classifications, **IV:**460–461
        corrosive agents, **IV:**461
        desiccants, **IV:**461
        oxidizing agents, **IV:**460–461
        pathophysiology, **IV:**460
        protoplasmic poisons, **IV:**461
        reducing agents, **IV:**461
        vesicants, **IV:**461
    oxidizing agents
        characteristics, **IV:**460–461
        chromic acid, **IV:**460–461, 463
        patient presentation and diagnosis,
            IV:461–462
        secondary surgical treatment, **IV:**463
        sodium hypochlorite, **IV:**461–463
    patient presentation and diagnosis
        characteristics, **IV:**461–462
        corrosive agents, **IV:**462
        desiccants, **IV:**462
        oxidizing agents, **IV:**461–462
        protoplasmic poisons, **IV:**462
        reducing agents, **IV:**462
        vesicants, **IV:**462
    patient selection, **IV:**462
    postoperative care and follow-up,
        IV:464
    prognosis and outcomes, **IV:**464
    protoplasmic poisons
        characteristics, **IV:**461
        formic acid, **IV:**461–463
        hydrofluoric acid, **IV:**461–462, 464
        patient presentation and diagnosis,
            IV:462
        secondary surgical treatment,
            IV:463–464
    reducing agents
        characteristics, **IV:**461
        hydrochloric acid, **IV:**461–463

upper extremities *(Continued)*
        patient presentation and diagnosis,
            IV:462
        secondary surgical treatment, **IV:**463
    research summary, **IV:**456
    secondary procedures, **IV:**464
    secondary surgical treatment
        characteristics, **IV:**463–464
        corrosive agents, **IV:**463
        desiccants, **IV:**463
        oxidizing agents, **IV:**463
        protoplasmic poisons, **IV:**463–464
        reducing agents, **IV:**463
        vesicants, **IV:**463
    surgical technique and treatment
        primary treatment, **IV:**462–463
        secondary treatment, **IV:**463–464
    vesicants
        characteristics, **IV:**461
        mustard gas, **IV:**461–463
        patient presentation and diagnosis,
            IV:462
        secondary surgical treatment, **IV:**463
cold injury/frostbite, **IV:**456–467
    classifications, **IV:**456–460
    complications, **IV:**459–460
    disease process
        freezing phase, **IV:**457
        pathophysiology, **IV:**456–457
        rewarming phase, **IV:**457
    nonsurgical interventions
        adjunctive therapy, **IV:**458
        field management, **IV:**458
        rapid rewarming, **IV:**458
        splinting, **IV:**458
    patient presentation and diagnosis
        clinical assessment, **IV:**457
        physical examination, **IV:**457–458
        radiographic imaging, **IV:**457–458
    patient selection, **IV:**458
    postoperative care and follow-up, **IV:**459
    prognosis and outcomes, **IV:**459–460
    research summary, **IV:**456
    secondary procedures
        hyperbaric oxygen therapy, **IV:**460
        sympathectomy, **IV:**460
        thrombolytics, **IV:**460
    surgical technique and treatment
        amputations, **IV:**458–459, 459f
        length salvage, **IV:**459
        nonsurgical interventions, **IV:**458
complex regional pain syndrome (CRPS),
    VI:486–502
    background and general characteristics,
        VI:486–487, 487f, 488t
    nerve compression syndromes, **VI:**497t,
        498f, 503–525
    pathophysiology, **VI:**487–490, 488f–489f
    patient presentation and diagnosis
        adjunctive diagnostic measures,
            VI:492–493
        clinical diagnosis, **VI:**488t, 491–493,
            491f–492f
        epidemiology, **VI:**490
        patient characteristics, **VI:**490–491
        precipitating events, **VI:**490
    peripheral nerve surgery
        joint denervation surgery, **VI:**497t
        nerve compression syndromes, **VI:**497t,
            498f

upper extremities (Continued)
  patient selection, **VI**:495, 496f
  perioperative pain management,
    VI:495–497
  surgical technique, **VI**:489f, 497,
    498f–500f
postoperative care and follow-up, **VI**:497
prognosis and outcomes, **VI**:497–499
research summary, **VI**:501
secondary procedures, **VI**:499–501
treatment strategies
  basic principles, **VI**:493–495, 493f
  botulinum toxin (BTX), **VI**:495
  drug therapy, **VI**:494
  interventional therapies, **VI**:494
  intravenous ketamine infusion therapy,
    VI:494–495
  invasive pain management therapies,
    VI:495
  peripheral nerve surgery, **VI**:495–499
  physical therapy and rehabilitation,
    VI:493
  psychological support, **VI**:493–494
  spinal cord stimulation, **VI**:495
congenital melanocytic nevi (CMN), **III**:848,
    849f–851f
extravasation injury, **IV**:456–467
  causal factors, **IV**:464–467
  complications, **IV**:466–467, 467f
  disease process
    characteristics, **IV**:464–465
    cytotoxic agents, **IV**:464–465
    osmotically active agents, **IV**:464
    vasoconstrictive agents, **IV**:464
  patient presentation and diagnosis,
    IV:465, 465f
  patient selection, **IV**:465
  postoperative care and follow-up, **IV**:466
  prognosis and outcomes, **IV**:466–467
  research summary, **IV**:456
  secondary procedures, **IV**:467
  surgical technique and treatment
    cytotoxic agents, **IV**:466
    osmotically active agents, **IV**:466
    treatment strategies, **IV**:465–466
    vasoconstrictive agents, **IV**:466
lymphedema/lymphatic reconstruction,
    IV:92–100
  background information, **IV**:92
  classifications, **IV**:93
  complications, **IV**:98–99
  direct reconstruction
    lymphovenous bypass, **IV**:96, 97f, 98t
  disease process, **IV**:92–93
  etiology, **IV**:93
  patient presentation and diagnosis,
    IV:93
  patient selection
    nonsurgical therapy, **IV**:93–94
    reconstruction surgery, **IV**:94
  physiological operations
    Baumeister lymphatic vessel
      reconstruction technique, **IV**:95–96,
      96f
    general discussion, **IV**:95–97
    lymphaticolymphatic bypass, **IV**:95
    lymphovenous bypass, **IV**:96, 97f, 98t
    lymphovenous shunts, **IV**:96–97, 99f

upper extremities (Continued)
  microvascular lymph node transfer,
    IV:96, 96f
  postoperative care and follow-up,
    IV:97–98
  prognosis and outcomes, **IV**:98–99
  research summary, **IV**:99–100
  secondary procedures, **IV**:99
  surgical technique and treatment
    ablative operations, **IV**:94–95
    background information, **IV**:92
    goals, **IV**:94b
    liposuction, **IV**:94–95
    physiological operations, **IV**:95–97
mangled upper extremities, **VI**:250–281
  causal factors, **VI**:255, 256f
  flap reconstruction
    anterolateral thigh flap, **VI**:274–275,
      275f–276f
    cutaneous versus muscle flaps,
      VI:263–279
    fasciocutaneous flaps, **VI**:254–255,
      266–275
    free flaps, **VI**:254–255, 266–275
    lateral arm flap, **VI**:267, 269f–272f
    latissimus dorsi (LD) flap, **VI**:275, 277f
    local flaps, **VI**:254–255
    muscle/musculocutaneous flaps,
      VI:254–255, 275–279
    pedicled groin flap, **VI**:264–266,
      265f–266f
    radial forearm flap, **VI**:266–267,
      267f–269f
    rectus abdominis, **VI**:275–277, 278f
    scapular and parascapular flaps,
      VI:272, 273f
    serratus anterior muscles, **VI**:277–279
    temporoparietal fascia flaps, **VI**:272–
      274, 274f
  initial evaluation and treatment
    debridement, **VI**:251, 251f
    guidelines, **VI**:250–255, 251b
    musculotendinous reconstruction,
      VI:253
    nerve repair, **VI**:253–254, 254f
    postoperative management, **VI**:255
    provisional revascularization, **VI**:251,
      252f
    skeletal stabilization, **VI**:251–252
    skin and soft-tissue reconstruction,
      VI:254–255
    vascular reconstruction, **VI**:252–253,
      253f
  injury impacts, **VI**:255–256
  injury types
    amputations, **VI**:256
    avulsion injuries, **VI**:256, 256f
    crush injuries, **VI**:256, 256f, 261f
    roller injuries, **VI**:256, 257f
  outcomes and complicatons, **VI**:279–281
  patient presentation and diagnosis
    emergency room evaluations,
      VI:256–257
    reconstruction planning, **VI**:257–259
  postoperative care and follow-up, **VI**:279
  reconstruction process
    amputation versus salvage decisions,
      VI:259

upper extremities (Continued)
  delayed reconstruction, **VI**:259
  early (single-stage) reconstruction,
    VI:259
  emergency room evaluations,
    VI:257–259
  planning and preparation guidelines,
    VI:258
  spare-parts utilization, **VI**:259, 260f
  timing considerations, **VI**:258–259
secondary procedures
  free fibula transfer, **VI**:279–280, 280f
  innervated microvascular muscle
    transfer, **VI**:281
  microvascular toe transfer, **VI**:280–281,
    280f
surgical technique and treatment
  bony reconstruction options, **VI**:259–
    261, 260f
  flap reconstruction, **VI**:263–279
  muscle reconstruction, **VI**:262
  nerve reconstruction, **VI**:262
  soft-tissue reconstruction, **VI**:262–263,
    263f–264f
  tendon graft and repair, **VI**:262
  vascular reconstruction options,
    VI:261–262, 261f
melanoma excisions, **I**:766–768, 768f–770f
nerve compression syndromes, **VI**:503–525
  anterior interosseous nerve (AIN)
    syndrome
    characteristics, **VI**:510–511
    nonsurgical management, **VI**:511
    surgical technique and treatment,
      VI:511, 512f–513f
  carpal tunnel syndrome
    American Academy of Orthopaedic
      Surgeons clinical practice
      guidelines for the treatment of
      carpal tunnel syndrome, **VI**:507t
    anatomical considerations, **VI**:505,
      506f
    etiology, **VI**:505
    nonsurgical management, **VI**:507
    outcomes and complicatons, **VI**:509–
      510, 509b
    patient presentation and diagnosis,
      VI:505–507, 507b
    patient selection, **VI**:507
    prevalence, **VI**:505–510
    surgical technique and treatment,
      VI:507–509, 508f–509f
  cubital tunnel syndrome
    anatomical considerations, **VI**:513–514
    clinical signs, **VI**:514t
    endoscopic decompression technique,
      VI:515
    intramuscular transposition technique,
      VI:515
    medial epicondylectomy technique,
      VI:515, 516f
    outcomes and complicatons, **VI**:513b,
      515–516
    patient presentation and diagnosis,
      VI:514
    patient selection, **VI**:514
    simple decompression technique,
      VI:514–515

*Note: **Boldface** roman numerals indicate volume. Page numbers followed by f refer to figures; page numbers followed by t refer to tables; page numbers followed by b refer to boxes.*

upper extremities (Continued)
    subcutaneous transposition technique, **VI:**515
    submuscular transposition technique, **VI:**515
  electrodiagnostic studies, **VI:**504–505, 504f
  general discussion, **VI:**503
  Guyon's canal
    anatomical considerations, **VI:**511, 513f
    etiology, **VI:**511
    patient presentation and diagnosis, **VI:**511–512
    surgical technique and treatment, **VI:**512–513
  median nerve compression
    anterior interosseous nerve (AIN) syndrome, **VI:**510–511
    carpal tunnel syndrome, **VI:**505–510
    pronator syndrome, **VI:**510
    proximal arm and elbow, **VI:**510, 510f
  pathophysiology, **VI:**503–504
  posterior interosseous nerve (PIN) compression
    anatomical considerations, **VI:**517
    posterior interosseous nerve (PIN) syndrome, **VI:**517
    radial tunnel syndrome, **VI:**518
  pronator syndrome, **VI:**510
  proximal arm and elbow, **VI:**510, 510f
  quadrilateral space syndrome
    anatomical considerations, **VI:**523, 523f
    etiology, **VI:**523
    patient presentation and diagnosis, **VI:**523
    patient selection, **VI:**523
    surgical technique and treatment, **VI:**524
  radial nerve compression
    incidence, **VI:**516–518
    posterior interosseous nerve (PIN) compression, **VI:**517
    Wartenberg's syndrome, **VI:**516–517
  suprascapular nerve compression
    anatomical considerations, **VI:**524, 524f
    etiology, **VI:**524
    patient presentation and diagnosis, **VI:**524
    patient selection, **VI:**524
    surgical technique and treatment, **VI:**524–525
  thoracic outlet syndrome (TOS)
    anatomical considerations, **VI:**64–65, 65f, 519, 520f–521f
    classifications, **VI:**64
    definition, **VI:**63–66
    incidence, **VI:**518–522
    nonsurgical management, **VI:**521–522
    outcomes and complicatons, **VI:**522
    patient presentation and diagnosis, **VI:**520–521, 522f
    provocative maneuvers, **VI:**65–66
    surgical technique and treatment, **VI:**522
    Wright's hyperabduction test, **VI:**520–521, 522f
  ulnar nerve compression
    cubital tunnel syndrome, **VI:**513–516
    Guyon's canal, **VI:**511–513

upper extremities (Continued)
  Wartenberg's syndrome
    anatomical considerations, **VI:**516, 517f
    patient presentation and diagnosis, **VI:**516
    patient selection, **VI:**517
    surgical technique and treatment, **VI:**517
pediatric patients
  epiphyseal growth plate, **VI:**651–666
    anatomical characteristics, **VI:**651–652, 652f
    growth plate closure, **VI:**652–654
    outcomes and complicatons, **VI:**664–665, 665f
    patient presentation and diagnosis, **VI:**654–656
    patient selection, **VI:**656, 656f
    postoperative care and follow-up, **VI:**664
    puberty-related skeletal assessments, **VI:**652–654, 653f
    secondary procedures, **VI:**665
    surgical technique and treatment, **VI:**656–664
    vascular anatomy, **VI:**652
  physical examinations, **VI:**67
  surgical technique and treatment
    anesthesia, **VI:**103
    epiphyseal growth plate, **VI:**651–666
peripheral nerve injuries, **VI:**694–718
  anatomical characteristics
    blood supply, **VI:**696, 697f
    brachial plexus nerves, **VI:**696f
    gross anatomy, **VI:**695, 695f–697f
    nerve trunk, **VI:**695–696, 697f
    neurons and supporting cells, **VI:**695, 697f
    Riche–Cannieu anastomosis, **VI:**697f
    schematic diagram, **VI:**697f
  clinical examination
    correct diagnosis, **VI:**700–702, 701f
    electromyography/neurography, **VI:**700–701
    functional evaluation, **VI:**700
    wound inspection, **VI:**702
  donor nerves
    lateral cutaneous nerve, **VI:**709, 711f–712f
    lateral femoral cutaneous nerve, **VI:**710
    medial cutaneous nerve, **VI:**709, 710f
    saphenous nerve, **VI:**710
    superficial sensory branch of the radial nerve, **VI:**710, 712f–713f
    sural nerve, **VI:**708–709, 709f
    terminal branch of the posterior interosseous nerve, **VI:**710
  epidemiology, **VI:**694
  future trends, **VI:**718
  immediate versus delayed repair
    basic principles, **VI:**703
    surgical approach, **VI:**703–704, 703f
    timing considerations, **VI:**703
  nerve reconstruction
    autografts, **VI:**707, 708f, 708t
    coaptation and maintenance, **VI:**708
    gap measurement, **VI:**708
    graft harvest, **VI:**708, 708t
    graft length, **VI:**708
    nerve ends, **VI:**708

upper extremities (Continued)
    surgical approach and preparation, **VI:**707–708
  nerve repair principles
    basic principles, **VI:**704–705, 704f–706f
    end-to-side nerve repair, **VI:**707
    epineurial versus fascicular repair, **VI:**706–707, 706f–707f
    wound closure and immobilization, **VI:**707
  outcomes and complicatons
    age factors, **VI:**716
    British Medical Research Council (BMRC) Scale, **VI:**716, 716t
    digital nerves, **VI:**716
    Highet Scale, **VI:**715, 716t
    influencing factors, **VI:**716
    injury type, **VI:**717
    level of injury, **VI:**717
    nerve trunks, **VI:**716–717
    outcome assessments, **VI:**714
    repair type, **VI:**717
    Rosen score, **VI:**716
  patient presentation and diagnosis
    axonotmesis, **VI:**698–700, 699t
    fifth-degree injuries, **VI:**699t, 700
    first-degree injuries, **VI:**698, 699t
    fourth-degree injuries, **VI:**699t, 700
    injury classifications, **VI:**698, 699f, 699t
    neuropraxia, **VI:**698, 699t
    neurotmesis, **VI:**699t, 700
    second-degree injuries, **VI:**698–700, 699t
    sixth-degree injuries, **VI:**699t, 700
    third-degree injuries, **VI:**699t, 700
  patient selection
    correct diagnosis, **VI:**701f, 702–703
    nerve injury classifications, **VI:**702–703, 702t
    wound condition, **VI:**703
  physiological characteristics
    degeneration/regeneration mechanisms, **VI:**697, 698f
    distal nerve segment, **VI:**697–698, 698f
    general characteristics, **VI:**696–698
    nodes of Ranvier, **VI:**696–698, 697f
  postoperative care and follow-up
    immobilization concerns, **VI:**713
    postoperative movement training, **VI:**713–714
    sensory re-education, **VI:**714
  postoperative dysfunction
    cold intolerance, **VI:**248–249, 717–718
    complex regional pain syndrome (CRPS), **VI:**717
    general considerations, **VI:**717
  sensory re-education
    cortical reorganization, **VI:**714
    phase 1, **VI:**714
    phase 2, **VI:**714, 715f
  surgical technique and treatment
    artificial conduits, **VI:**710–713
    donor nerves, **VI:**708–710
    immediate versus delayed repair, **VI:**703–704
    nerve reconstruction, **VI:**707–708
    nerve repair principles, **VI:**704–707
    tubular repair, **VI:**710–713
  tubular repair
    artificial conduits, **VI:**710–713
    biodegradable conduits, **VI:**712

upper extremities (Continued)
- biological conduits, **VI:**711
- fillers, **VI:**713
- longitudinal resorbable sutures, **VI:**713
- nerve transfers, **VI:**713
- nondegradable conduits, **VI:**712, 713f
- physical examination, **VI:**47–67
  - elbows
    - bony landmarks, **VI:**61, 62f
    - distal humerus malrotation measurement, **VI:**63, 64f
    - joint instability, **VI:**61–63, 63f
    - lateral ligament complex, **VI:**61
    - medial collateral ligament complex, **VI:**61, 62f
    - pivot shift test maneuver, **VI:**63, 64f
    - posterolateral rotatory instability (PLRI), **VI:**63
  - forearm
    - functional role, **VI:**60–61
    - interosseous membrane, **VI:**60, 60f
    - muscle strength measurement, **VI:**61
    - rotation measurement, **VI:**61
  - hands
    - deformities, **VI:**48
    - examination guidelines, **VI:**48–60
    - muscular atrophy, **VI:**48–49
    - musculotendinous assessment, **VI:**50–52
    - nerve assessment, **VI:**52, 53t
    - palpation, **VI:**49
    - range of motion assessment, **VI:**49
    - skin creases, **VI:**49
    - skin discoloration, **VI:**48
    - special provacative tests, **VI:**53–60
    - stability assessment, **VI:**49–50, 49f–50f
    - swelling, **VI:**49
    - trophic changes, **VI:**49
    - vascular assessment, **VI:**52–53
  - patient history
    - allergies, **VI:**48
    - current complaint, **VI:**47–48
    - importance, **VI:**47–48
    - medical history, **VI:**48
    - medications, **VI:**48
    - patient demographics, **VI:**47
    - social history, **VI:**48
  - pediatric patients, **VI:**67
  - thoracic outlet syndrome (TOS)
    - Adson test, **VI:**65, 66f
    - anatomical characteristics, **VI:**64–65, 65f
    - classifications, **VI:**64
    - costoclavicular compression test, **VI:**65, 66f
    - definition, **VI:**63–66
    - Morley's test, **VI:**66
    - neck tilting test, **VI:**65
    - provocative maneuvers, **VI:**65–66
    - Roos extended arm stress test, **VI:**66
    - Wright test, **VI:**65, 66f
- post-bariatric surgery reconstruction, **II:**652
- tendon transfers, **VI:**745–776
  - basic principles, **VI:**745, 746t
  - clawing of the fingers
    - Bouvier maneuver, **VI:**764–765, 764f
    - Brand EE4T transfer, **VI:**766–767, 766f
    - Brand EF4T transfer, **VI:**767, 767f–768f

upper extremities (Continued)
  - donor muscle-tendon selection, **VI:**764–765, 765f
  - Fritschi PF4T transfer, **VI:**767–768
  - Littler modification, **VI:**764–765
  - modified Stiles–Bunnell technique, **VI:**764–766, 765f
  - pulley insertions, **VI:**764–765, 764f–765f
  - static procedures, **VI:**763–764, 763f–764f
  - combined nerve injuries
    - finger extension restoration, **VI:**774–775
    - finger flexion restoration, **VI:**775f, 776
    - high median-high ulnar nerve palsy, **VI:**773
    - low median-low ulnar nerve palsy, **VI:**772–773
    - patient selection, **VI:**772–776
    - post-trauma reconstruction, **VI:**773
    - thumb extension restoration, **VI:**773–774, 774f
    - thumb flexion restoration, **VI:**774f–775f, 775–776
  - donor muscle-tendon selection
    - expendability, **VI:**746
    - muscle integrity, **VI:**746–747
    - strength assessment, **VI:**746, 746f
    - transfer direction, **VI:**746–747
  - high median nerve palsy
    - opposition tendon transfers, **VI:**761t
    - outcomes and complicatons, **VI:**761
    - patient selection, **VI:**759–761, 760f
    - surgical technique and treatment, **VI:**759–761, 760f, 761t
  - high ulnar nerve palsy
    - outcome assessments, **VI:**771–772
    - patient selection, **VI:**771
  - low median nerve palsy
    - abductor digiti minimi (ADM) tendon, **VI:**758
    - Bunnell ring finger flexor digitorum superficialis transfer, **VI:**755–756, 755f–757f, 761t
    - Burkhalter extensor indicis proprius transfer, **VI:**754–755, 754f–755f
    - Camitz palmaris longus transfer, **VI:**756–758, 757f–759f, 761t
    - Huber transfer, **VI:**758, 761t
    - opposition tendon transfers, **VI:**761t
    - pathogenesis, **VI:**753
    - patient selection, **VI:**753–758
  - low ulnar nerve palsy
    - Bouvier maneuver, **VI:**764–765, 764f
    - Brand EE4T transfer, **VI:**766–767, 766f
    - Brand EF4T transfer, **VI:**767, 767f–768f
    - donor muscle-tendon selection, **VI:**764–765, 765f
    - Fritschi PF4T transfer, **VI:**767–768
    - index finger abduction, **VI:**770–771, 771f
    - Littler modification, **VI:**764–765
    - modified Stiles–Bunnell technique, **VI:**764–766, 765f
    - Neviaser accessory abductor pollicis longus and free tendon graft, **VI:**771, 771f
    - patient selection, **VI:**761–771, 762f, 762t
    - pulley insertions, **VI:**764–765, 764f–765f

upper extremities (Continued)
  - ring finger flexor digitorum superficialis transfer, **VI:**769
  - Smith extensor carpi radialis brevis transfer, **VI:**769–770, 770f
  - static procedures, **VI:**763–764, 763f–764f
  - thumb adduction restoration, **VI:**768–769, 769f–770f
  - ulnar deviation of the small finger, **VI:**768
  - postoperative care and follow-up, **VI:**749
  - radial nerve palsy
    - Boyes superficialis transfer, **VI:**748t, 750–752, 752f
    - flexor carpi radialis transfer, **VI:**748t, 749–750, 752f
    - outcomes and complicatons, **VI:**752–753
    - patient selection, **VI:**747–752, 747f
    - standard flexor carpi ulnaris transfer, **VI:**748–749, 748f–751f, 748t
    - surgical technique and treatment, **VI:**748, 748t
  - research summary, **VI:**776
  - standard flexor carpi ulnaris transfer, **VI:**749
  - surgical approach
    - bone and soft tissue healing, **VI:**745–746
    - donor muscle-tendon selection, **VI:**746–747
    - timing considerations, **VI:**747
  - surgical technique and treatment
    - combined nerve injuries, **VI:**772–776
    - finger extension restoration, **VI:**774–775
    - finger flexion restoration, **VI:**775f, 776
    - high median-high ulnar nerve palsy, **VI:**773
    - high median nerve palsy, **VI:**759–761
    - high ulnar nerve palsy, **VI:**771–772
    - low median-low ulnar nerve palsy, **VI:**772–773
    - low median nerve palsy, **VI:**753–758
    - low ulnar nerve palsy, **VI:**761–771
    - planning guidelines, **VI:**747
    - post-trauma reconstruction, **VI:**773
    - radial nerve palsy, **VI:**747–753
    - thumb extension restoration, **VI:**773–774, 774f
    - thumb flexion restoration, **VI:**774f–775f, 775–776
- tetraplegia
  - biceps to triceps transfer
    - advantages/disadvantages, **VI:**821–822
    - postoperative care and follow-up, **VI:**822, 822f
    - surgical technique, **VI:**821–822, 821f
  - brachioradialis to flexor pollicis longus (FPL) transfer
    - House intrinsic substitution procedure, **VI:**836f–837f
    - IC group 2 and 3 patients, **VI:**830–832, 831f
    - operative procedures, **VI:**830–832, 835f–837f, 839f–840f
    - postoperative care and follow-up, **VI:**832, 841f

Note: **Boldface** *roman numerals indicate volume. Page numbers followed by f refer to figures; page numbers followed by t refer to tables; page numbers followed by b refer to boxes.*

upper extremities (Continued)
    surgical tips, **VI:**830b
    Zancolli "lasso" procedure, **VI:**835f
  carpometacarpal (CMC) joints
    IC group 4 and 5 patients, **VI:**834–838
    postoperative care and follow-up,
      VI:837–838
    stable thumb CMC joints, **VI:**837
    treatment strategies, **VI:**834–838
    unstable CMC joints, **VI:**837
  causal factors, **VI:**817
  classifications, **VI:**817–818, 818t
  deltoid to triceps transfer
    postoperative care and follow-up,
      VI:825
    surgical technique, **VI:**822–824, 822b,
      823f–824f
  elbow extension
    biceps to triceps transfer, **VI:**821–822
    deltoid to triceps transfer, **VI:**821–822
    hygiene considerations, **VI:**821f
    importance, **VI:**820–825
  grasp and release restoration
    extensor phase, **VI:**833
    flexor phase, **VI:**833, 833b
    House intrinsic substitution procedure,
      VI:834
    IC group 3 patients, **VI:**832–834
    IC groups 3, 4, and 5 patients,
      VI:832–834
    intrinsic stabilization, **VI:**833–834
    postoperative care and follow-up,
      VI:834
    Zancolli "lasso" procedure, **VI:**834
  IC group 0, 1 and 2 patients
    general considerations, **VI:**825–826
    postoperative care and follow-up,
      VI:826
    wrist extension, **VI:**825–826, 825f
  key pinch restoration
    brachioradialis to flexor pollicis longus
      (FPL) transfer, **VI:**830–832
    Brand–Moberg modification, **VI:**827–
      830, 828f–829f
    flexor pollicis longus (FPL) tenodesis,
      VI:827–830, 828f–829f
    IC group 1 and 2 patients, **VI:**826–830
    postoperative care and follow-up,
      VI:830
    split flexor pollicis longus (FPL) to
      extensor pollicis longus (EPL)
      interphalangeal stabilization,
      VI:826–827, 827f
    surgical technique and treatment,
      VI:826–830
    surgical tips, **VI:**826b
  reconstructive surgeries, **VI:**817–842
    general discussion, **VI:**817
    patient presentation, **VI:**818–820,
      819f
    research summary, **VI:**840–841
    surgical team, **VI:**818–820
    surgical technique and treatment,
      VI:820–838
  surgical reconstruction
    elbow extension, **VI:**820–825
    functional electrical stimulation (FES),
      VI:838
    IC group 0, 1 and 2 patients,
      VI:825–826

upper extremities (Continued)
    IC group 1 and 2 patients, **VI:**826–830,
      826b
    IC group 2 and 3 patients, **VI:**830–832
    IC group 4 and 5 patients, **VI:**834–838
    IC groups 3, 4, and 5 patients,
      VI:832–834
    IC groups 6, 7, and 8 patients, **VI:**838
    outcomes and complicatons, **VI:**838–
      840, 841f–842f
    strong grasp and refined pinch
      restoration, **VI:**838
    surgical guidelines, **VI:**820
  TNM clinical classification system/pTNM
    pathologic classification system, **I:**714f
upper extremity amputees, **VI:**870–880
  aesthetic prostheses, **VI:**870, 871f
  body-powered prostheses, **VI:**870–871
  control mechanisms, **VI:**870–871
  general characteristics, **VI:**870
  prosthetics–composite tissue
    allotransplantation (CTA)
    comparisons, **VI:**879–880
  residual limb surgery
    neuroma management, **VI:**876
    soft-tissue improvement, **VI:**875–876,
      875f–876f
    targeted muscle reinnervation (TMR),
      VI:871, 876–879
  surgery–prosthesis considerations
    elbow disarticulation/long
      transhumeral amputation,
      VI:874–875
    finger amputation, **VI:**872, 872f
    general discussion, **VI:**872–875
    partial hand, **VI:**872, 873f
    shoulder disarticulation/proximal
      transhumeral amputation, **VI:**875
    wrist disarticulation/transradial
      amputation, **VI:**873–874, 873f–874f
  targeted muscle reinnervation (TMR)
    characteristics, **VI:**876–879
    myoelectric prostheses, **VI:**871
    shoulder disarticulation level,
      VI:877–879, 878f–879f, 879t
    transhumeral level, **VI:**876–877,
      876f–877f
    transradial level, **VI:**879
vascular anomalies, **VI:**667–693
  arteriovenous malformation (AVM)
    causal factors, **VI:**684–690
    pathogenesis, **VI:**685–686
    patient presentation and diagnosis,
      VI:686–687, 686f–688f
    Schobinger clinical staging system,
      VI:686t
    surgical technique and treatment,
      VI:687–690, 689f
  capillary malformation-arteriovenous
    malformation (CM-AVM)
    pathogenesis, **VI:**691
    patient presentation and diagnosis,
      VI:691
    surgical technique and treatment,
      VI:691
  capillary malformations (CM)
    pathogenesis, **VI:**675
    patient presentation and diagnosis,
      VI:675, 677f
  classification systems, **VI:**667–669, 668t

upper extremities (Continued)
  CLOVES syndrome
    pathogenesis, **VI:**691
    patient presentation and diagnosis,
      VI:692
    surgical technique and treatment,
      VI:692
  congenital hemangioma (CH)
    pathogenesis, **VI:**673–674
    patient presentation and diagnosis,
      VI:674, 676f
    surgical technique and treatment,
      VI:674
  diagnostic work-up, **VI:**670t
  general discussion, **VI:**667
  hemangiomas
    arteriovenous malformation (AVM),
      VI:684–690, 686f–688f
    capillary malformation-arteriovenous
      malformation (CM-AVM), **VI:**691
    capillary malformations (CM), **VI:**675,
      677f
    classification systems, **VI:**667–669, 668t
    CLOVES syndrome, **VI:**691–692
    congenital hemangioma (CH),
      VI:673–674, 676f
    diagnostic work-up, **VI:**670t
    historical background, **VI:**667–669
    infantile hemangioma (IH), **VI:**672–673,
      674f–675f
    Klippel–Trenaunay syndrome, **VI:**691
    lymphatic malformation (LM),
      VI:675–680, 678f
    palmar dissections, **VI:**672, 672f, 672t
    Parkes–Weber syndrome, **VI:**690–691
    patient presentation and diagnosis,
      VI:669, 670f
    PTEN (phosphatase and tensin
      homologue)-associated vascular
      anomaly (PTEN-AVA), **VI:**690
    pyogenic granuloma, **I:**747–750, 748f,
      VI:674–675, 677f
    surgical technique and treatment,
      VI:669–672, 671t
    thumb/digital dissections, **VI:**672, 673f,
      673t
    venous malformations (VM), **VI:**680–
      682, 681f
  historical background, **VI:**667–669
  infantile hemangioma (IH)
    pathogenesis, **VI:**672–673
    patient presentation and diagnosis,
      VI:672–673, 674f
    surgical technique and treatment,
      VI:673, 675f
  Klippel–Trenaunay syndrome
    outcomes and complicatons, **VI:**691
    pathogenesis, **VI:**691
    patient presentation and diagnosis,
      VI:691
    surgical technique and treatment,
      VI:691
  lymphatic malformation (LM)
    outcomes and complicatons,
      VI:679–680
    pathogenesis, **VI:**675–677
    patient presentation and diagnosis,
      VI:677–679, 678f
    surgical technique and treatment,
      VI:679, 680f–681f

upper extremities (Continued)
  palmar dissections, **VI**:672, 672f, 672t
  Parkes–Weber syndrome
    outcomes and complicatons,
      VI:690–691
    pathogenesis, **VI**:690
    patient presentation and diagnosis,
      VI:690
    surgical technique and treatment,
      VI:690
  patient presentation and diagnosis,
    VI:669
  PTEN (phosphatase and tensin
    homologue)-associated vascular
    anomaly (PTEN-AVA)
    pathogenesis, **VI**:690
    patient presentation and diagnosis,
      VI:690
    surgical technique and treatment,
      VI:690
  pyogenic granuloma
    pathogenesis, **VI**:674
    patient presentation and diagnosis,
      I:747–750, 748f, **VI**:675, 677f
    surgical technique and treatment, **VI**:675
  surgical technique and treatment,
    VI:669–672, 671t
  thumb/digital dissections, **VI**:672, 673f,
    673t
  vascular malformations
    diagnostic work-up, **VI**:670t
    historical background, **VI**:667–669
    palmar dissections, **VI**:672, 672f, 672t
    patient presentation and diagnosis,
      VI:669
    surgical technique and treatment,
      VI:669–672, 671t
    thumb/digital dissections, **VI**:672, 673f,
      673t
  venous malformations (VM)
    associated syndromes, **VI**:682–684
    outcomes and complicatons, **VI**:684
    pathogenesis, **VI**:680–682
    patient presentation and diagnosis,
      VI:681f
    surgical technique and treatment,
      VI:682–684, 683f, 685f
  vascular imaging techniques, **VI**:89–90, 90f
  See also arms; elbows; hands
upper extremity functional test (UEFT),
  VI:247
upper extremity surgery
  anesthesia, **VI**:92–105
    anatomical characteristics
      axillary sheath, **VI**:92–94
      brachial plexus, **VI**:92–94, 93f
      microneuroanatomy, **VI**:94
      nerve innervation, **VI**:93f
      perineurial environment, **VI**:92–94
      sonoanatomy, **VI**:94
    complications
      characteristics, **VI**:100–102
      evaluation and management, **VI**:101
      infections, **VI**:102
      local anesthetic toxicity, **VI**:94–95,
        101–102
      peripheral nerve injury, **VI**:100
      vascular injury, **VI**:102

upper extremity surgery (Continued)
  goals, **VI**:92
  local anesthesia
    comparative pharmacology, **VI**:96t
    pharmacokinetics, **VI**:94
    pharmacology, **VI**:94–96
    selection guidelines, **VI**:95–96, 95t
    toxicity, **VI**:94–95, 101–102
    vasoconstrictors, **VI**:95
  outcome assessments
    anesthetic types, **VI**:102–103
    clinical outcomes, **VI**:102
    operating room cost and efficiency,
      VI:103
    patient satisfaction, **VI**:102
  perioperative pain management
    chronic postoperative pain, **VI**:104, 104t
    general discussion, **VI**:103–104
    peripheral catheters, **VI**:103
    preemptive analgesia, **VI**:103–104
    risk factors, **VI**:104t
  regional anesthesia techniques
    axillary block, **VI**:99–100, 101f
    Bier block, **VI**:97
    characteristics, **VI**:96–100
    digital blockade, **VI**:96–97
    infraclavicular block, **VI**:99, 100f
    interscalene block, **VI**:97, 98f
    intravenous regional anesthesia, **VI**:97
    supraclavicular block, **VI**:97–99, 99f
    wrist block, **VI**:97
  special cases
    cardiac patients, **VI**:103
    pediatric patients, **VI**:103
composite tissue allotransplantation (CTA),
  VI:843–854
  challenges, **VI**:852
  complications, **VI**:850–851
  donor and recipient selection, **VI**:845–846,
    846t
  emerging insights
    chronic rejection, **VI**:852–853, 853t
    cortical plasticity, **VI**:852
    future trends, **VI**:854
    immunomodulatory strategies,
      VI:853–854
    neural integration, **VI**:852
    tolerance approaches, **VI**:853–854
  epidemiology, **VI**:843–844
  evolutionary development
    chronology, **VI**:845
    experimental background, **VI**:844–845
    immunology, **VI**:844
  procedural aspects
    donor limb procurement, **VI**:846–847,
      847f
    recipient surgery, **VI**:847, 848f
  prognosis and outcomes, **VI**:850–851
  program establishment and
    implementation, **VI**:845
  protocol-related considerations
    immunomonitoring, **VI**:850
    maintenance immunosuppression,
      VI:847, 849f, 853–854
    rehabilitation and functional
      assessment, **I**:835–837, **VI**:848, 849f
    rejection assessments, **VI**:849–850,
      849f–851f, 849t

upper extremity surgery (Continued)
    upper extremity transplantation versus
      replantation, **VI**:851–852
  epidemiology, **VI**:843–844
  free-functioning muscle transfer, **VI**:777–788
    complications, **VI**:787
    muscle structure
      characteristics, **VI**:777–780
      length–tension relationship, **VI**:779f
      myosin cross-bridges, **VI**:778f
      schematic diagram, **VI**:778f
      strap and pennate muscles, **VI**:779f
    patient presentation and diagnosis,
      VI:780, 780f
    patient selection, **VI**:780–781, 781t
    secondary procedures, **VI**:787
    surgical technique and treatment
      basic principles, **VI**:781–787
      donor motor nerve, **VI**:783–785, 783b
      elbows, **VI**:787
      finger extension, **VI**:785–787
      flexor digitorum profundus (FDP)
        tendons, **VI**:782, 785f
      forearm dissection, **VI**:784–785, 784f
      gliding tendon path, **VI**:783f
      gracilis muscle, **VI**:781–787, 781f–782f
      insufficient coverage, **VI**:783f
      neurovascular structure alignment,
        VI:784f
      postoperative finger flexion, **VI**:786f
    tendon transfers, **VI**:780t
  skeletal reconstruction
    clavicle, **IV**:185
    femur, **IV**:183
    forearm, **IV**:181–183, 182f
    humerus, **IV**:181, 186f
    pelvis, **IV**:184–185
    spine, **IV**:184–185, 184f–185f
    tibia, **IV**:183–184
  work-related injuries, **VI**:363, 363b
  See also hands
upper eyelid area
  anatomical characteristics, **II**:111–112, 113f
  anatomic-directed therapy, **II**:121
  anesthesia, **III**:26, 27f
  epicanthal fold, **II**:164–165
  facial paralysis, **III**:287–289, 287f–289f
  partial upper lid defects
    Abbé flap, **III**:450
    advancement flap, **III**:450
    decision-making process, **III**:449–450
    full-thickness skin graft, **III**:450
    lower lid transposition, **III**:449f
  ptosis, **III**:57
  secondary blepharoplasty
    Fasanella–Servat operation, **II**:146f
    Herring's law, **II**:145, 147f
    patient evaluation, **II**:142–145, 142t,
      143f–144f
    ptosis, **II**:143–145, 144f–146f
    retraction, **II**:145, 147f
  subperiosteal facelift, **II**:268–270, 269f
upper eyelid surgery
  anchor/invagination blepharoplasty,
    II:124, 126f
  burn wound treatment, **IV**:486, 487f
  general discussion, **II**:123–124
  orbital fat excision, **II**:124, 126f

Note: **Boldface** *roman numerals indicate volume. Page numbers followed by f refer to figures; page numbers followed by t refer to tables; page numbers followed by b refer to boxes.*

upper eyelid area *(Continued)*
  partial upper lid defects
    Abbé flap, **III:**450
    advancement flap, **III:**450
    decision-making process, **III:**449–450
    full-thickness skin graft, **III:**450
    lower lid transposition, **III:**449f
  simple skin blepharoplasty, **II:**124, 125f
  total upper lid defects, **III:**450
upper facial fractures
  frontal bone and sinus fractures
    clinical examination, **III:**51
    complications, **III:**53
    computed tomography (CT), **III:**51
    injury patterns, **III:**51
    nasofrontal duct, **III:**51, 52f
    surgical technique and treatment,
      III:52–53, 52f
  orbital fractures
    characteristics, **III:**53–57
    complications
      blindness, **III:**56
      diplopia, **III:**56
      enophthalmos, **III:**56
      implant migration or hemorrhage,
        III:56
      lid lamellae, **III:**57
      ocular globe injuries, **III:**56
      retrobulbar hematoma, **III:**56
      upper eyelid ptosis, **III:**57
      vertical shortening of the lower eyelid,
        III:57
    computed tomography (CT), **III:**54
    infraorbital nerve anesthesia, **III:**57
    orbital apex syndrome, **III:**57
    physical examination, **III:**53–54, 54f
    postoperative care and follow-up, **III:**56
    schematic diagram, **III:**53f
    superior orbital fissure syndrome, **III:**57
    surgical anatomy, **III:**53
    surgical technique and treatment
      basic procedure, **III:**55–56
      bone grafts, **III:**55
      cutaneous exposures, **III:**55
      endoscopic approaches, **III:**55
      forced duction test, **III:**55, 55f
      goals, **III:**54–55
      inorganic implants, **III:**56
      orbital floor restoration, **III:**55, 56f
      timing considerations, **III:**55
    treatment indicators
      blow-out fractures (children), **III:**54, 54f
      blow-out fractures (floor of the orbit),
        III:54
      guidelines, **III:**54
upper limb contouring, **II:**617–633, **V:**558–581
  arms
    demand increases, **V:**558–564
    outcomes and complicatons, **V:**563–564
    pathophysiology, **V:**558–559
    patient presentation and diagnosis,
      V:559–564
    patient selection, **V:**559–560
    Pittsburgh Rating Scale, **V:**559–560, 559t
    postoperative care and follow-up,
      V:562–563
    surgical technique and treatment,
      V:560–562, 561f–563f, 562b
  causal factors, **II:**617, 618f–620f
  complications, **II:**629–631, 629t

upper limb contouring *(Continued)*
  demand increases, **II:**617
  patient presentation and diagnosis,
    II:617–620
  patient selection
    arm surface anatomy, **II:**624f
    laboratory work-up, **II:**623
    marking, **II:**624–626, 627f
    operative procedures, **II:**626–629,
      627f–629f
    physical examination, **II:**620–624,
      621f–622f
    plan formulation, **II:**622–623
    preoperative assessment, **II:**623
    sagittal view of arm anatomy, **II:**625f
    surface anatomy, **II:**624, 624f–626f
    thromboembolic disease prophylaxis,
      II:623–624
  postoperative care and follow-up, **II:**629
  prognosis and outcomes, **II:**629–631,
    630f–632f
  secondary procedures, **II:**632–633, 632f
upper plexus injuries
  examination findings, **VI:**727
  reconstruction techniques
    spinal accessory to suprascapular nerve
      transfers, **VI:**727, 728f–729f
    surgical tips, **VI:**727b
  reconstructive surgeries
    double fascicular nerve transfer, **VI:**731,
      731f
    medial pectoral nerve and thoracodorsal
      nerve, **VI:**731, 731f
    triceps to axillary nerve transfer, **VI:**728,
      729f–730f
    ulnar/median redundant branches to
      biceps brachii and brachialis
      branches nerve transfer, **VI:**731, 731f
uracil, **I:**179–180
urogenital defect reconstruction, **III:**906–924
  embryology, **III:**907–908
  epidemiology, **III:**908
  etiology, **III:**908
  outcomes and complicatons, **III:**916–921
  patient presentation and diagnosis,
    III:908–909
  patient selection, **III:**909
  postoperative care and follow-up, **III:**915
  secondary procedures, **III:**921
  surgical technique and treatment
    bladder exstrophy, **III:**912–913, 913f
    female epispadias repair, **III:**912–913, 914f
    meatoplasty and glanuloplasty
      basic procedure, **III:**913–915, 916f
      onlay island flap repair, **III:**914–915,
        918f
      orthoplasty, **III:**915
      surgical tips, **III:**914b–915b
      tubularized incised plate (TIP) repair,
        III:914, 917f
      two-stage repair, **III:**915, 919f–921f
    urethral reconstruction, **III:**913, 915f
    vaginal reconstruction
      bowel vaginoplasty, **III:**910f
      clitoromegaly, **III:**910–912
      cloacal exstrophy repair, **III:**912, 913f
      urogenital sinus abnormalities,
        III:910–912, 911f–912f, 912b
      vaginal agenesis, **III:**909, 909b, 910f
urokinase, **I:**617

urologic/prostate surgery, **I:**863–864
US Patent and Trademark Office (USPTO),
  I:846–847
UT Southwestern Formula, **II:**516t, 527t
uvulopalatopharyngoplasty (UVPP),
  III:97f–98f, 98

V
VACTERL association, **VI:**573t, 574
vacuum-assisted closure (VAC), **I:**7, 622,
  III:121, 122f, **IV:**367
vagina
  anatomical characteristics, **IV:**326, 327f
  sigmoid vaginoplasty, **IV:**346–347
  urogenital defect reconstruction, **III:**906–924
    embryology, **III:**907–908
    epidemiology, **III:**908
    etiology, **III:**908
    outcomes and complicatons, **III:**916–921
    patient presentation and diagnosis,
      III:908–909
    patient selection, **III:**909
    postoperative care and follow-up, **III:**915
    secondary procedures, **III:**921
    vaginal reconstruction
      bowel vaginoplasty, **III:**910f
      clitoromegaly, **III:**910–912
      cloacal exstrophy repair, **III:**912, 913f
      urogenital sinus abnormalities,
        III:910–912, 911f–912f, 912b
      vaginal agenesis, **III:**909, 909b, 910f
  vaginectomy, **IV:**314–315, 315f
  vaginoplasty, **IV:**338f, 341–342, 342f
    See also gender identity disorder
vagus nerve, **III:**27–29, 29f
Valadier, Charles Auguste, **I:**21
vanadium (V) alloys, **I:**786–787
Vancouver Scar Scale (VSS), **I:**264–266,
  298–299, 299t
Van der Woude syndrome (VWS), **I:**194–195
varicose ulcers, **I:**253
Varioderm, **II:**47t
vascular anatomy, **I:**479–511
  bilateral pedicle TRAM flap, **V:**394–395,
    394f
  breast-conserving therapy (BCT)
    anterior intercostal artery perforator
      (AICAP) flap, **V:**308, 488
    dorsal intercostal artery perforator
      (DICAP) flap, **V:**488
    intercostal artery perforator (ICAP) flap,
      V:486f–488f, 487–488
    lateral intercostal artery perforator
      (LICAP) flap, **V:**487f–488f, 488
    lateral thoracodorsal flap (LTDF),
      V:306–308
    latissimus dorsi (LD) flap, **V:**82–83,
      306–308, 309f, 311f, 485–489, 486f
    pedicled flaps, **V:**489, 492f
    serratus anterior artery perforator (SAAP)
      flap, **V:**486f–488f, 488–489
    superior epigastric artery perforator
      (SEAP) flap, **V:**308, 486f, 489
    thoracodorsal artery perforator (TDAP)
      flap, **V:**308, 486–487, 486f–488f
  forearm, **VI:**37f
  hands, **VI:**35–40, 37f–39f, 40b
  lower extremities, **IV:**2f, 45–48, 47f
  male genital anatomy, **IV:**299–301, 299f–301f
  nail/nail bed, **VI:**117–118

vascular anatomy *(Continued)*
  orthognathic surgical procedures, **II:**366f
  scalp, **III:**107, 108f
  trunk
    abdomen, **IV:**229–230, 229f
    back, **IV:**222f, 223, 224f
    chest, **IV:**225–227, 226f
    embryology, **IV:**220
    female perineum, **IV:**232–235, 234f
    male perineum, **IV:**235, 238f
vascular anatomical research
  angiosome
    arterial perforators, **I:**482, 483f
    characteristics, **I:**480–482
    computed tomography angiography,
      I:483f
    cutaneous arteries, **I:**482f
    vessel networks, **I:**483f
  angiosome concept, **I:**491, 492f–494f,
    500–508
  arterial territories, **I:**482–484, 484f
  arteriosomes, **I:**491
  clinical applications
    angiosome concept, **I:**500–508
    composite flaps, **I:**508
    delay phenomenon, **I:**507–508,
      507f–508f
    distally based skin flaps, **I:**501–502,
      503f
    fasciocutaneous flaps, **I:**504
    musculocutaneous flaps, **I:**504–505
    perforator flaps, **I:**505–507, 506f–507f
    preoperative assessment, **I:**500–501
    skin flap axes, **I:**501–502, 503f
    skin flap dimensions, **I:**502–504
  flap design
    anatomic concepts, **I:**492–500, 492b
    arterial radiation, **I:**494–495
    connective tissue framework, **I:**493–494
    cutaneous perforators, **I:**496–497, 496f
    deep veins, **I:**499–500
    directional veins, **I:**498f, 499
    law of equilibrium, **I:**498
    nerve–blood vessel relationship,
      I:495–496
    network interconnections, **I:**497–498
    oscillating avalvular veins, **I:**498f, 499
    preoperative assessment, **I:**500
    superficial veins, **I:**499–500, 500f
    vein–muscle connection, **I:**499
    venous convergence, **I:**494–495
    venous networks, **I:**499
    vessel growth and orientation–tissue
      growth and differentiation
      relationship, **I:**496–497, 496f
    vessel origin and destination, **I:**499
  musculature
    classification systems, **I:**488–491, 489f,
      489t
    innervation patterns, **I:**489f
    Type I muscles, **I:**489–491, 489f–490f,
      489t
    Type II muscles, **I:**489f–490f, 489t, 491
    Type III muscles, **I:**489f–490f, 489t, 491
    Type IV muscles, **I:**489f–490f, 489t, 491
  network interconnections
    arteries, **I:**497, 497f
    veins, **I:**497–498, 498f

vascular anatomy *(Continued)*
  neurovascular territories, **I:**487–488, 488f
  preoperative assessment
    color duplex Doppler imaging, **I:**501
    computed tomography (CT), **I:**501, 502f
    Doppler imaging, **I:**500–501
    flap design, **I:**500
  research summary, **I:**508
  skin flap axes
    characteristics, **I:**501–502
    schematic diagram, **I:**503f
  venosomes, **I:**491, 494f
  venous drainage channels, **I:**484–487,
    485f–487f
  vascular architecture, **I:**479–480, 480f
vascular anomalies, **I:**676–706
  arteriovenous malformation (AVM)
    causal factors, **VI:**684–690
    classification systems, **I:**676–677, 677t
    clinical manifestations, **I:**698–699
    pathogenesis, **I:**696–698, **VI:**685–686
    patient presentation and diagnosis,
      VI:686–687, 686f–688f
    Schobinger clinical staging system,
      VI:686t
    Schobinger staging system, **I:**698–699,
      699t
    surgical technique and treatment,
      VI:687–690, 689f
    terminology, **I:**678t
    treatment strategies
      embolization, **I:**700
      intervention guidelines, **I:**699–700
      resection, **I:**689f, 700
  capillary-arteriovenous malformation
    (CAVM), **I:**677t
  capillary-lymphatic arteriovenous
    malformation (CLAVM), **I:**677t
  capillary-lymphatic malformation (CLM),
    I:677t
  capillary-lymphatic-venous malformation
    (CLVM), **I:**677t
  capillary malformation-arteriovenous
    malformation (CM-AVM)
    classification systems, **I:**677t
    pathogenesis, **I:**692f, 696–698, 700, **VI:**691
    patient presentation and diagnosis,
      VI:691
    surgical technique and treatment, **VI:**691
  capillary malformations (CM)
    classification systems, **I:**676–677, 677t
    clinical manifestations, **I:**688–689
    pathogenesis, **I:**688, **VI:**675
    patient presentation and diagnosis,
      VI:675, 677f
    terminology, **I:**678t
    treatment strategies, **I:**679f, 689–690
  capillary-venous malformation (CVM),
    I:677t
  cerebral cavernous malformation (CCM),
    I:677t, 693–694
  classification systems, **I:**676–678, 677t,
    VI:667–669, 668t
  CLOVES syndrome
    pathogenesis, **I:**698f, 705, **VI:**691
    patient presentation and diagnosis,
      VI:692
    surgical technique and treatment, **VI:**692

vascular anomalies *(Continued)*
  congenital hemangioma (CH)
    pathogenesis, **VI:**673–674
    patient presentation and diagnosis,
      VI:674, 676f
    surgical technique and treatment, **VI:**674
  cutaneomucosal venous malformation
    (CMVM), **I:**677t, 693–694
  diagnostic work-up, **VI:**670t
  general discussion, **VI:**667
  glomuvenous malformation (GVM), **I:**677t,
    693–694, **VI:**668t, 682–684
  hemangiomas
    arteriovenous malformation (AVM),
      I:677t, **VI:**684–690, 686f–688f
    capillary malformation-arteriovenous
      malformation (CM-AVM), **I:**677t,
      VI:691
    capillary malformations (CM), **I:**677t,
      VI:675, 677f
    classification systems, **VI:**667–669, 668t
    CLOVES syndrome, **VI:**691–692
    congenital hemangioma (CH)
      clinical manifestations, **I:**687
      pathogenesis, **VI:**673–674
      patient presentation and diagnosis,
        VI:674, 676f
      surgical technique and treatment,
        VI:674
      treatment strategies, **I:**687
    diagnostic work-up, **VI:**670t
    historical background, **VI:**667–669
    infantile hemangioma (IH)
      classification systems, **I:**677t
      clinical manifestations, **I:**680–681
      diagnosis, **I:**681
      nonoperative management, **I:**681–684
      operative management, **I:**684–685
      pathogenesis, **I:**678–680, **VI:**672–673
      patient presentation and diagnosis,
        VI:672–673, 674f
      surgical technique and treatment,
        VI:673, 675f
      terminology, **I:**678t
    kaposiform hemangioendothelioma
      (KHE)
      classification systems, **I:**677t, **VI:**668t
      clinical manifestations, **I:**687
      treatment strategies, **I:**687–688
    Klippel–Trenaunay syndrome, **VI:**691
    lymphatic malformation (LM), **I:**677t,
      VI:675–680, 678f
    palmar dissections, **VI:**672, 672f, 672t
    Parkes–Weber syndrome, **VI:**690–691
    patient presentation and diagnosis,
      VI:669, 670f
    PTEN (phosphatase and tensin
      homologue)-associated vascular
      anomaly (PTEN-AVA), **I:**677t, **VI:**690
    pyogenic granuloma, **I:**688, **VI:**674–675,
      677f
    surgical technique and treatment,
      VI:669–672, 671t
    thumb/digital dissections, **VI:**672, 673f,
      673t
    venous malformations (VM), **VI:**680–682,
      681f
    verrucous hemangioma (VH), **I:**677t, 695

*Note: **Boldface** roman numerals indicate volume. Page numbers followed by f refer to figures; page numbers followed by t refer to tables; page numbers followed by b refer to boxes.*

vascular anomalies (Continued)
  hereditary hemorrhagic telangiectasia (HHT), I:677t, 696–698
  historical background, I:676–678, VI:667–669
  infantile hemangioma (IH)
    pathogenesis, VI:672–673
    patient presentation and diagnosis, VI:672–673, 674f
    surgical technique and treatment, VI:673, 675f
  Klippel–Trenaunay syndrome
    benign mesenchymal-origin tumors
      hemangioma simplex, I:734
      venous malformation, I:735
    classification systems, VI:668, 668t
    outcomes and complicatons, VI:691
    pathogenesis, I:703, VI:691
    patient presentation and diagnosis, VI:691
    surgical technique and treatment, VI:691
  lymphatic malformation (LM)
    classification systems, I:676–677, 677t
    clinical manifestations, I:690–692
    outcomes and complicatons, VI:679–680
    pathogenesis, I:690, VI:675–677
    patient presentation and diagnosis, VI:677–679, 678f
    surgical technique and treatment, VI:679, 680f–681f
    terminology, I:678t
    treatment strategies
      general discussion, I:692–693
      resection, I:693
      sclerotherapy, I:683f, 692–693
  lymphatic-venous malformation (LVM), I:677t
  palmar dissections, VI:672, 672f, 672t
  Parkes–Weber syndrome
    outcomes and complicatons, VI:690–691
    pathogenesis, I:694f, 703, VI:690
    patient presentation and diagnosis, VI:690
    surgical technique and treatment, VI:690
  patient presentation and diagnosis, VI:669
  PTEN (phosphatase and tensin homologue)-associated vascular anomaly (PTEN-AVA)
    pathogenesis, I:697f, 704–705, VI:690
    patient presentation and diagnosis, VI:690
    surgical technique and treatment, VI:690
  pyogenic granuloma
    pathogenesis, VI:674
    patient presentation and diagnosis, VI:675, 677f
    surgical technique and treatment, VI:675
  Sturge–Weber syndrome, I:701–702
  thumb/digital dissections, VI:672, 673f, 673t
  vascular malformations
    arteriovenous malformation (AVM)
      clinical manifestations, I:698–699
      pathogenesis, I:696–698
      Schobinger staging system, I:698–699, 699t
      treatment strategies, I:699–700
    capillary malformation-arteriovenous malformation (CM-AVM), I:692f, 700
    capillary malformations (CM)
      classification systems, I:676–677, 677t
      clinical manifestations, I:688–689

vascular anomalies (Continued)
    pathogenesis, I:688, VI:675
    patient presentation and diagnosis, VI:675, 677f
    terminology, I:678t
    treatment strategies, I:679f, 689–690
  classification systems, I:676–677, 677t
  CLOVES syndrome, I:698f, 705
  cutis marmorata telangiectatica congenita (CMTC), I:677t, 690
  diagnostic work-up, VI:670t
  historical background, VI:667–669
  Klippel–Trenaunay syndrome, I:703
  lymphatic malformation (LM)
    clinical manifestations, I:690–692
    pathogenesis, I:690
    treatment strategies, I:692–693
  palmar dissections, VI:672, 672f, 672t
  Parkes–Weber syndrome, I:694f, 703
  patient presentation and diagnosis, VI:669
  PTEN (phosphatase and tensin homologue)-associated vascular anomaly (PTEN-AVA), I:697f, 704–705
  research summary, I:705
  Sturge–Weber syndrome, I:701–702
  surgical technique and treatment, VI:669–672, 671t
  thumb/digital dissections, VI:672, 673f, 673t
  venous malformations (VM)
    clinical manifestations, I:685f–686f, 694–695
    pathogenesis, I:693–694
    treatment strategies, I:695–696
  vascular tumors
    congenital hemangioma (CH)
      clinical manifestations, I:687
      treatment strategies, I:687
    infantile hemangioma (IH)
      clinical manifestations, I:680–681
      diagnosis, I:681
      nonoperative management, I:681–684
      operative management, I:684–685
      pathogenesis, I:678–680
    kaposiform hemangioendothelioma (KHE)
      classification systems, I:677t, VI:668t
      clinical manifestations, I:687
      treatment strategies, I:687–688
    pyogenic granuloma, I:688
  venous malformations (VM)
    associated syndromes, VI:682–684
    classification systems, I:676–677, 677t
    clinical manifestations, I:685f–686f, 694–695
    outcomes and complicatons, VI:684
    pathogenesis, I:693–694, VI:680–682
    patient presentation and diagnosis, VI:681f
    surgical technique and treatment, VI:682–684, 683f, 685f
    terminology, I:678t
    treatment strategies
      anticoagulant agents, I:695–696
      resection, I:696
      sclerotherapy, I:696
  verrucous hemangioma (VH), I:677t, 695

vascular endothelial growth factor (VEGF)
  bone regeneration, I:435t, 438, 441–442, 443t–444t
  fat grafting, I:345
  gene therapy, I:189–190
  limb development (embryology), VI:530–531
  pedical flap viability augmentation, I:580–582
  rosacea, II:20–21
  skin wound healing, I:270t, 275
  tissue engineering, I:373–374
  wound healing, I:234, 244, 250–252, 251f
vascular imaging techniques, VI:89–90, 90f
vascularized bone flaps
  advantages, I:455–459
  classifications, I:528t
  clinical applications, I:524–525, 526f–528f
  vacularized calvarium, I:457–459, 458f
  vacularized fibula, I:455, 457f
  vascularized iliac transfer, I:455, 456f
  vascularized rib, I:456–457
  vascularized scapula, I:455–456, 458f
vascular lasers, II:21t
vascular lesions See cutaneous and soft-tissue tumors
vascular malformations
  arteriovenous malformation (AVM)
    causal factors, VI:684–690
    classification systems, I:676–677, 677t, VI:668t
    clinical manifestations, I:698–699
    diagnostic work-up, VI:670t
    pathogenesis, I:696–698, VI:685–686
    patient presentation and diagnosis, VI:669, 670f, 686–687, 686f–688f
    Schobinger clinical staging system, VI:686t
    Schobinger staging system, I:698–699, 699t
    surgical technique and treatment, VI:669–672, 671t, 687–690, 689f
    terminology, I:678t
    treatment strategies
      embolization, I:700
      intervention guidelines, I:699–700
      resection, I:689f, 700
  capillary malformation-arteriovenous malformation (CM-AVM), I:692f, 700
  capillary malformations (CM)
    clinical manifestations, I:688–689
    pathogenesis, I:688
    treatment strategies, I:679f, 689–690
  classification systems, I:676–677, 677t, VI:667–669, 668t
  CLOVES syndrome
    classification systems, VI:668, 668t
    pathogenesis, I:698f, 705, VI:691
    patient presentation and diagnosis, VI:688f, 692
    surgical technique and treatment, VI:692
  cutis marmorata telangiectatica congenita (CMTC), I:677t, 690
  diagnostic work-up, VI:670t
  historical background, VI:667–669
  Klippel–Trenaunay syndrome
    benign mesenchymal-origin tumors
      hemangioma simplex, I:734
      venous malformation, I:735
    classification systems, VI:668, 668t

vascular malformations (Continued)
outcomes and complicatons, **VI:**691
pathogenesis, **I:**703, **VI:**691
patient presentation and diagnosis, **VI:**691
surgical technique and treatment, **VI:**691
lymphatic malformation (LM)
classification systems, **I:**676–677, 677t
clinical manifestations, **I:**690–692
outcomes and complicatons, **VI:**679–680
pathogenesis, **I:**690, **VI:**675–677
patient presentation and diagnosis, **VI:**677–679, 678f
surgical technique and treatment, **VI:**679, 680f–681f
treatment strategies
general discussion, **I:**692–693
resection, **I:**693
sclerotherapy, **I:**683f, 692–693
palmar dissections, **VI:**672, 672f, 672t
Parkes–Weber syndrome
benign mesenchymal-origin tumors, **I:**735
classification systems, **VI:**668, 668t
outcomes and complicatons, **VI:**690–691
pathogenesis, **I:**694f, 703, **VI:**690
patient presentation and diagnosis, **VI:**690
surgical technique and treatment, **VI:**690
patient presentation and diagnosis, **VI:**669
PTEN (phosphatase and tensin homologue)-associated vascular anomaly (PTEN-AVA)
classification systems, **I:**677t
pathogenesis, **I:**697f, 704–705, **VI:**690
patient presentation and diagnosis, **VI:**690
surgical technique and treatment, **VI:**690
research summary, **I:**705
Sturge–Weber syndrome, **I:**701–702
surgical technique and treatment, **VI:**669–672, 671t
thumb/digital dissections, **VI:**672, 673f, 673t
venous malformations (VM)
associated syndromes, **VI:**682–684
classification systems, **I:**676–677, 677t
clinical manifestations, **I:**685f–686f, 694–695
outcomes and complicatons, **VI:**684
pathogenesis, **I:**693–694, **VI:**680–682
patient presentation and diagnosis, **VI:**681f
surgical technique and treatment, **VI:**682–684, 683f, 685f
terminology, **I:**678t
treatment strategies
anticoagulant agents, **I:**695–696
resection, **I:**696
sclerotherapy, **I:**696
vasculogenesis, **I:**250–252, 251f, **VI:**530–531, 531f
vaser-assisted liposuction, **II:**507–508, 519
vasoconstricting agents, **I:**139–140, **VI:**95
vasomotor rhinitis, **II:**454, 458
vastus intermedialis muscle, **IV:**15t–16t, 18f, 19t, 20f–22f, 25f
vastus lateralis muscle, **IV:**15t–16t, 18f, 19t, 20f–22f, 25f

vastus medialis muscle, **IV:**15t–16t, 18f–22f, 19t
Vaughn–Jackson syndrome, **VI:**376, 376f
Veau, Victor, **III:**576–578
Veau–Wardill–Kilner palate repair technique, **III:**576–578, 577f–578f
vegetable oils, **II:**16
vein repair, **VI:**234–235, 235f
velocardiofacial syndrome, **III:**807, 807t
velopharyngeal dysfunction (VPD), **III:**614–630
background information, **III:**614
disease process
combined conditions, **III:**619
velopharyngeal incompetence, **III:**618
velopharyngeal insufficiency, **III:**616–618, 618f
velopharyngeal mislearning, **III:**619
patient presentation and diagnosis
imaging methods
characteristics, **III:**621–623
multiview videofluoroscopy, **III:**622
nasopharyngoscopy, **III:**622–623, 623f
static radiographs, **III:**622, 622f
patient history, **III:**619
perceptual speech assessment, **III:**619–620
physical examination, **III:**619
speech pathology terminology, **III:**620b
velopharyngeal closure measures
general discussion, **III:**620–621
nasometer, **III:**621f
pressure–flow instrumentation, **III:**621f
surgical technique and treatment
Furlow double-opposing z-palatoplasty, **III:**624–625, 624f
goals, **III:**623–630
nonsurgical treatments
behavioral speech therapy, **III:**629–630
general discussion, **III:**628–630
prosthetic treatments, **III:**629, 629f
posterior pharyngeal flap, **III:**625–626, 626f
posterior pharyngeal wall augmentation, **III:**628
preoperative assessment, **III:**623–624
sphincter pharyngoplasty, **III:**626–628, 627f
velopharynx
anatomical characteristics, **III:**614–616, 615f
physiological characteristics, **III:**616, 616f–617f
velopharyngeal insufficiency (VPI), **III:**667–670, 667t
venous flaps, **I:**533, 534f–535f
venous insufficiency, **I:**258
venous laceration, **IV:**433t
venous malformations (VM)
associated syndromes, **VI:**682–684
benign mesenchymal-origin tumors, **I:**735, 735f
classification systems, **I:**676–677, 677t, **VI:**668t
clinical manifestations, **I:**685f–686f, 694–695
diagnostic work-up, **VI:**670t
outcomes and complicatons, **VI:**684
pathogenesis, **I:**693–694, **VI:**680–682

venous malformations (VM) (Continued)
patient presentation and diagnosis, **VI:**669, 670f, 681f
surgical technique and treatment, **VI:**669–672, 671t, 682–684, 683f, 685f
terminology, **I:**678t
treatment strategies
anticoagulant agents, **I:**695–696
resection, **I:**696
sclerotherapy, **I:**696
venous repair, **VI:**234–235, 235f
venous thromboembolism (VTE)
lower extremity injuries, **IV:**85
patient safety, **I:**130–131
Venous Thromboembolism Prevention Study, **I:**168
venous ulcers, **I:**253, 279
venture capital, **I:**845
Veratrum californicum, **III:**515
Veritas, **V:**70t
vermillion
lip reconstruction, **III:**257–258, 258f
secondary cleft deformities
buccal sulcus deformities, **III:**641–642, 641f
orbicularis muscle deformities, **III:**640–641
thick lip, **III:**639
thin lip, **III:**639, 640f
vermillion mismatch, **III:**639–640
vermillion notching/vermillion border malalignment, **III:**640
whistle deformity, **III:**640
verruca vulgaris, **VI:**314–315, 315f
verrucous hemangioma (VH), **I:**677t, 695
Vertebral malformations–Anal atresia or hypoplasias–Cardiovascular anomalies–all degrees of Tracheoesophageal fistuli–Esophageal atresia–Renal malformations, and Limb (VACTERL) abnormalities *See* VACTERL association
vertex, **II:**356t
vertical banded gastroplasty (VBG), **II:**635–636, 636t
vertical maxillary excess, **III:**666
vertical orbital dystopias, **III:**226
vertical scar reduction mammaplasty, **V:**177–193
comparison studies, **V:**178t
complications
frequency, **V:**189–192, 191t
scar healing, **V:**190, 191f
under-resection, **V:**192
wound dehiscence, **V:**191
Hall-Findlay technique, **V:**159, 178t
historical background, **V:**177–180
Lassus technique, **V:**156–159, 178t
Lejour technique, **V:**159, 178t
Lista technique, **V:**178t
medial pedicle breast reductions, **V:**189, 190f
nipple-areola complex, **V:**179f
patient selection
patient characteristics, **V:**180–181
symptoms, **V:**180
planning and marking guidelines
perioperative care, **V:**181
skin marking, **V:**181–182, 181f, 183f

*Note: **Boldface** roman numerals indicate volume. Page numbers followed by f refer to figures; page numbers followed by t refer to tables; page numbers followed by b refer to boxes.*

vertical scar reduction mammaplasty
    (Continued)
  postoperative care and follow-up, **V:**188
  research summary, **V:**192
  superior pedicle breast reductions,
      V:188–189, 189f
  surgical technique and treatment
    anesthesia, **V:**182
    breast shaping, **V:**186–187, 187f
    de-epithelialization, **V:**184, 184f
    dressings and wound care, **V:**188
    infiltration, **V:**182–184
    liposuction, **V:**185
    patient positioning, **V:**182
    pedicle selection, **V:**182, 184f
    surgical excision, **V:**184–185, 185f–186f
    wound closure, **V:**187–188, 187f–188f
vertical thigh-lift
  complications, **II:**652
  major weight loss (MWL) patient, **II:**648b
  markings, **II:**649–652, 650f
  operative technique, **II:**651f–652f, 652
  patient evaluation, **II:**645–648
  patient selection, **II:**648–649
  postoperative care and follow-up, **II:**652
vertical trapezius flap, **III:**127–128, 129f
Vesalius, Andreas, **I:**15–16, –**VI:**2, 161–163
Vianeo, Vincenzo, **I:**16
Vibrio vulnificus, **VI:**343
ViKY surgical robot system, **I:**856
vincula, **VI:**29–32, 31f, 180, 181f
violent behavior, **I:**51–52
viral gene delivery, **I:**186–187, 188f, 188t
viscerocranium development, **III:**512
visor flaps, **VI:**130, 131f
Visual Analog Scale (VAS), **I:**299
vitallium, **I:**787
vitamin A, **I:**282
vitamin B₁, **I:**282
vitamin B₂, **I:**282
vitamin B₆, **I:**282
vitamin C, **I:**282, **II:**18, 27
vitamin E, **II:**18, 27, **V:**33t–35t
vitamins
  abdominal wall reconstruction, **IV:**282–283
  dry skin care, **II:**18
  medication avoidance list, **V:**33t–35t
  skin wound healing, **I:**282
Vitis vinifera, **II:**27
vitronectin, **I:**244
VOC (voice of the customer), **I:**78b
voice surgery, **IV:**349
volar V-Y advancement flap, **VI:**128–130, 129f
Volkmann test, **VI:**460–464, 462f
Vomer flaps, **III:**578
vomiting, **I:**145
von Bruns, Victor, **I:**20
von Gräfe, Carl Ferdinand, **I:**19–20
von Heimburg's tuberous breast classification,
    V:121, 124t
von Langenbeck, Bernard, **I:**19, **III:**576
von Recklinghausen's disease, **I:**725, 726f
vulva
  anatomical characteristics, **II:**669
  cutaneous and soft-tissue tumors
    clinical staging system, **I:**716t
    extramammary Paget's disease, **I:**739, 739f
    TNM clinical classification system/pTNM
        pathologic classification system,
        I:715b

V-Y and Y-V advancement flaps
  fingertip reconstruction
    lateral V-Y advancement flaps, **VI:**130,
        130f
    volar V-Y advancement flap, **VI:**128–130,
        129f
  foot reconstruction, **IV:**207
  ischial pressure sores, **I:**562–565, 566f, 568f,
      IV:372–373, 374f
  pressure sores, **IV:**369–370
  reconstructive burn surgery, **IV:**502–503,
      503f
  scar revision, **I:**316, 316f
  spina bifida, **III:**867–872, 868t–869t,
      870f–871f, 875f
  V-Y plantar flap, **IV:**207
V-Y palate repair (Veau–Wardill–Kilner),
    III:576–578, 577f–578f

W
Wake Forest classifications of occlusive/
    vasospastic/vaso-occlusive disease,
    VI:479t
Wallace's rule of nines, **IV:**402f
Wardill, William, **III:**576–578
warfare, **IV:**63
warranty law, **I:**94–95
Warren, John Collins, **VI:**xliii
Wartenberg's sign, **VI:**58, 58f, 514t, 762
Wartenberg's syndrome
  anatomical considerations, **VI:**516, 517f
  patient presentation and diagnosis, **VI:**516
  patient selection, **VI:**517
  surgical technique and treatment, **VI:**517
Warthin's tumor, **III:**364t–365t, 367–368, 369f,
    372–373
warts, **VI:**314–315, 315f
warty dyskeratoma, **I:**720
Wassel classification, **VI:**617–618, 617f
Watson scaphoid shift test, **VI:**54, 166f
Weber–Ferguson technique, **III:**402, 403f–404f,
    436f
web space contractures, **IV:**508
Webster, Jerome P, **I:**27
weight loss methods
  abdominal wall reconstruction, **IV:**282
  advantages/disadvantages, **II:**636t
  bariatric surgery, **II:**635–636, 636t
  diet and exercise, **II:**635, 636t
  pharmacotherapy, **II:**635, 636t
Weilby suspensionplasty, **VI:**438, 439f
Weir excision, **III:**650f
Weir, Robert, **I:**25–28
Weissenbacher–Zweymuller syndrome,
    III:805–807, 807t
Wesseling trunk adiposity classification,
    II:535f
Weyer ulnar ray oligodactyly syndrome,
    VI:567t
wheelchairs, **IV:**365, 365f
whistle deformity, **III:**640
white phosphorus, **IV:**461–463
white space, **I:**66
Whitnall tubercle, **II:**109, 109f–110f
wide lip, **III:**637–638
wild oats, **II:**18
William of Saliceto, **I:**15
"wind-blown" hand, **VI:**646, 646f
Wingless (Wnt) gene, **III:**509–510, 512, 706,
    VI:527–530, 529f

wintergreen, oil of, **V:**33t–35t
Wnt signaling pathway, **I:**428–429, **VI:**527–530,
    529f
Wolfe, John Reissberg, **I:**20
Wolfe–Krause grafts, **I:**325–326
Wolff's law, **I:**433
wolf's bane, **V:**33t–35t
World Health Organization (WHO) patient
    safety considerations, **I:**134, 134b
World War I facial mutilations, **I:**20–23, 22f
wound dehiscence
  abdominoplasty, **II:**557–558
  buttock augmentation, **II:**614, 614f
  lower bodylift/belt lipectomy surgery,
      II:591
  reduction mammaplasty, **V:**191
  scalp and forehead reconstruction,
      III:131–132
wound healing, **I:**240–266
  acute wounds, **I:**241–242, 241f
  aesthetic nasal reconstruction, **III:**138–139
  back
    patient presentation and diagnosis
      midline back wounds, **IV:**256–257
      nonmidline back wounds, **IV:**257
    treatment strategies
      local wound care, **IV:**257, 257f–258f
      operative debridement, **IV:**258–259,
          259f–260f
  biofilms, **I:**250
  breast augmentation, **V:**263–264
  chemical peeling methods
    characteristics, **II:**62–63
    inflammatory response, **II:**62
    proliferation phase, **II:**62
    remodeling phase, **II:**63
  chronic wounds
    arterial ulcers, **I:**253–254
    definition, **I:**253–256
    diabetic ulcers, **I:**254–255, 254f
    foot injuries, **IV:**196
    pressure ulcers, **I:**255–256
    treatment strategies, **I:**287
    venous ulcers, **I:**253
    wound infection, **I:**249–250
  facial burn wound treatment, **IV:**468–499
    acute facial burns
      ears, **IV:**473
      eyes/eyelids, **IV:**470–473
      mouth, **IV:**473
      nose, **IV:**473
      treatment strategies, **IV:**470–473,
          471f–472f
    complications, **IV:**497
    damage process
      acute facial burns, **IV:**470–473
      damage assessments, **IV:**468–473,
          469f
      depth of burn determination,
          IV:470
    epidemiology, **IV:**468
    flaps
      basic principles, **IV:**480–481
      indicators, **IV:**480b
      trapeze-plasties, **IV:**481
      Z-plasty technique, **IV:**481, 481f
    inadequate donor-site skin
      dermal substitutes, **IV:**480, 482–484
      general discussion, **IV:**482–484
      tissue expansion, **IV:**482, 483f

wound healing (Continued)
    nonoperative facial reconstructive adjunct
            techniques
        corrective cosmetics, **IV:**485
        fat transplantation, **IV:**485
        hair transplantation, **IV:**485
        laser therapy, **IV:**484, 484f
        prosthetics, **IV:**485
        steroid treatments, **IV:**485
    nonsurgical management, **IV:**473
    outcome assessments, **IV:**497–498
    postoperative care and follow-up,
            IV:497
    secondary procedures, **IV:**498–499
    skin grafts
        advantages, **IV:**474
        basic principles, **IV:**479
        composite grafts, **IV:**480
        full-thickness skin graft, **IV:**479–480
        skin substitutes, **IV:**480, 482–484
        split-thickness skin graft, **IV:**479
    specific areas
        cheeks, **IV:**490–491, 506
        commissure, **IV:**473, 489–490, 495f
        ears, **IV:**473, 491–492, 496f, 498–499,
            505–506
        eyebrows, **IV:**485, 498–499
        eyelids, **IV:**470–473, 485–488, 486f–487f,
            498–499, 504–505, 504f
        forehead, **IV:**485, 498–499
        lower eyelids, **IV:**486–488, 488f
        lower lip and chin, **IV:**489, 492f–494f,
            498–499
        medial canthus scars, **IV:**488
        neck, **IV:**493–494, 498–499, 506
        nose, **IV:**473, 488–489, 498–499, 505
        scalp, **III:**119–120, 120f, **IV:**492–493,
            498–499, 504, 504f
        severe cervical burn scars and
            contractures, **IV:**494
        upper eyelids, **IV:**486, 487f
        upper lip, **IV:**489, 490f–491f, 498–499
    specific surgical techniques
        scar replacement with local skin,
            IV:478, 478f
        serial excision, **IV:**478
        W-plasty technique, **IV:**478–479, 478f
    surgical management
        algorithmic approach, **IV:**475–477,
            476f–477f
        basic principles, **IV:**474–475
        flaps, **IV:**480–481
        inadequate donor-site skin, **IV:**482–484
        skin grafts, **IV:**479–480
        specific techniques, **IV:**478–479
        surgical techniques, **IV:**473
        total wound healing/scar maturation,
            IV:474–475, 474f
    total wound healing/scar maturation
        aesthetic units, **IV:**474, 475f
        ancillary techniques, **IV:**475, 475b,
            476f
        diagnosis, **IV:**474
        functional restoration, **IV:**474, 475f
        local flaps, **IV:**474
        reconstruction planning, **IV:**474
        skin grafts, **IV:**474
        skin-matching considerations, **IV:**475

wound healing (Continued)
        surgical goals, **IV:**475
        timing considerations, **IV:**474–475, 474f
    hemostasis, **I:**242–245, 243f
    historical background, **I:**241
    hypoxia, **I:**257f
    infantile hemangioma (IH), **I:**682
    inflammatory response
        characteristics, **I:**245–249, 245f
        chemical peeling methods, **II:**62
        diapedesis, **I:**245, 246f
        inflammation resolution, **I:**248–249
        leukocyte migration, **I:**245, 246f
        macrophages, **I:**245f, 248, 256f–257f,
            268–269, 268f, 271f
        mast cells, **I:**245f, 247–248
        microribonucleic acid (miRNA),
            I:259–260
        neutrophil infiltration, **I:**245f–246f,
            246–247, 256f–257f, 268–269,
            268f–269f, 271f
        platelet activation, **I:**245, 245f
        Toll-like receptors (TLRs), **I:**247, 247f
    lower extremity injuries, **IV:**86
    male chest contouring, **V:**579
    microribonucleic acid (miRNA)
        angiogenesis, **I:**260
        characteristics, **I:**259–261
        hypoxia response, **I:**260
        inflammatory response, **I:**259–260
        stem cells, **I:**260–261
    muscle/musculocutaneous flaps,
            I:571–572
    negative pressure wound therapy (NPWT),
            I:850–851, 850f
    nose reconstruction, **III:**138–139
    postoperative care and follow-up, **I:**316–317
    pressure sores, **IV:**366–367, 367f
    revisionary breast surgery, **V:**263–264
    scalp and forehead reconstruction,
            III:131–132
    scars
        characteristics and functional role,
            I:264–266, 301–304, 302t
        hypertrophic scars, **I:**265, 283–284, 283t,
            302, 302t, 303f, 307–308
        immature scars, **I:**302t
        keloid scars, **I:**265, 283t, 284–285, 302–304,
            302t, 303f, 308–309
        mature scars, **I:**302t
        regenerative fetal healing, **I:**265–266
        revisionary breast surgery, **V:**246–247
        scar biology and formation, **I:**300,
            301f–302f
    secondary cleft deformities, **III:**631–632,
            632f–633f
    skin wound healing, **I:**267–296
        adult wound pathology
            excessive healing, **I:**283–285
            nonhealing wounds, **I:**279–283
        adult wound repair
            characteristics, **I:**268–273, 268f
            fetal wound repair comparisons,
                I:277–278
            inflammatory phase, **I:**268–269, 268f
            proliferation phase, **I:**268f, 269–273
            remodeling phase, **I:**268f, 273, 276f
            scar formation, **I:**276f

wound healing (Continued)
        adult wound repair–fetal wound repair
                comparisons
            cellular differences, **I:**277
            extracellular matrix (ECM) differences,
                I:278
            gene expression differences, **I:**278
            growth factor expression, **I:**278
            repair differences, **I:**277–278
        clinical wound management
            closed wounds, **I:**285–286, 286t
            engineered skin replacements, **I:**289t,
                290
            excessive scar treatment, **I:**290–291
            excisional wounds, **I:**286–287
            general discussion, **I:**285–295
            incisional wounds, **I:**285–286, 286t
            open wounds, **I:**286–287
            pharmacologic treatment, **I:**290
            wound dressings, **I:**287–288, 289t,
                IV:410–416
            wound treatment, **I:**287
        excessive healing
            characteristics, **I:**283–285
            hypertrophic scars, **I:**283–284, 283t
            keloid scars, **I:**283t, 284–285
        excessive scar treatment
            prevention and reduction therapies,
                I:291, 292t
            scar classification, **I:**290, 291t
            therapies, **I:**290–291
        fetal wound repair
            adult wound repair comparisons,
                I:277–278
            growth factor expression, **I:**278
            scar-free healing–scar formation
                transition, **I:**277
            scarless wound healing, **I:**276–278, 277f
        future trends
            gene therapy, **I:**295
            growth factor therapy, **I:**295
            protease-scavenging therapy, **I:**295
            stem cell therapy, **I:**296
        growth factor regulation
            characteristics, **I:**273–275
            extra cellular matrix–growth factor
                interactions, **I:**275
            fibroblast growth factor (FGF),
                I:274–275
            heparin-binding epidermal growth
                factor (HB–EGF), **I:**275
            platelet-derived growth factor (PDGF),
                I:274
            transforming growth factor-β (TGF-β)
                superfamily, **I:**274
            vascular endothelial growth factor
                (VEGF), **I:**275
        historical background, **I:**267
        mutilated/mangled hands, **VI:**254–255
        nonhealing wounds
            characteristics, **I:**279–283
            diabetic ulcers, **I:**281
            influencing factors, **I:**280t
            ischemic wounds, **I:**279–281
            lower extremity wounds, **I:**279–281
            malnutrition, **I:**282
            medical treatment, **I:**282–283
            obese patients, **I:**282

Note: Boldface *roman numerals indicate volume. Page numbers followed by f refer to figures; page numbers followed by t refer to tables; page numbers followed by b refer to boxes.*

wound healing (*Continued*)
  pressure sores, **I:**279
  radiation injuries, **I:**281
  venous ulcers, **I:**279
  wound infections, **I:**281–282
  proliferation phase
    angiogenesis, **I:**271
    epithelial resurfacing, **I:**272–273
    extracellular matrix (ECM) formation, **I:**269–271, 271f
    granulation tissue formation, **I:**271
    wound contraction, **I:**271–272, 272f
  toxic epidermal necrolysis (TEN), **IV:**515, 516f
  treatment strategies
    chronic open wounds, **I:**287
    emerging treatments, **I:**294–295
    future trends, **I:**295–296
    immature hypertrophic scars, **I:**291–292, 293f
    linear hypertrophic scars, **I:**292–293, 293f
    major keloids, **I:**293f, 294
    minor keloids, **I:**293f, 294
    necrotic tissue, **I:**287
    plastic surgery effects, **I:**294–295
    treatment algorithms, **I:**290–291, 293f
    widespread burn hypertrophic scars, **I:**293–294, 293f
  wound dressings
    classifications, **I:**287–288, 289t
    compression therapy, **I:**288, 289t
    subatmospheric dressing device, **I:**288, 289t
  stem cells
    characteristics, **I:**261–264, 261f–262f
    induced pluripotent stem cells, **I:**264
    microribonucleic acid (miRNA), **I:**260–261
    regeneration processes, **I:**261–264, 261f
    skin wound healing, **I:**296
  tissue repair, **I:**189–190
  vascularization, **I:**250–252, 251f
  warfare, **IV:**63
  wound closure
    abdominoplasty, **II:**538–539, 539f
    contraction and re-epithelialization, **I:**252–253
    granulation tissue, **I:**253
    proliferative phase, **I:**253
    sculpted pillar vertical reduction mammaplasty, **V:**231–235, 232f–235f
    vertical scar reduction mammaplasty, **V:**187–188, 187f–188f
  wound-healing process, **I:**242, 242f
  wound infections, **I:**249–250, 281–282, 306, **II:**526, **III:**417, **IV:**137, **V:**35
  wound ischemia
    hypoxia, **I:**256–259
    nitric oxide (NO) synthesis, **I:**259
    oxygen imbalance, **I:**257–258
    redox signaling, **I:**258–259
    tissue oxygenation, **I:**256–259, 256f–257f
  wound management
    historical background, **I:**11
    tissue repair, **I:**189–190
W-plasty technique
  burn reconstruction, **IV:**502–503
  facial burn wound treatment, **IV:**478–479, 478f
  labia minora reduction, **II:**669–673

W-plasty technique (*Continued*)
  lip reconstruction, **III:**268–270
  scar revision, **I:**316, 317f, **III:**268–270
  triphalangeal thumb, **VI:**624–627
Wright's hyperabduction test, **VI:**520–521, 522f
Wright test, **VI:**65, 66f
wrinkled skin
  classic aging characteristics, **II:**185f
  nonsurgical skin care and rejuvenation
    antioxidants
      coenzyme Q10, **II:**27
      general discussion, **II:**27–28
      grape seed extract, **II:**27
      green tea, **II:**27–28
      lycopene, **II:**28
      resveratrol, **II:**27
      vitamin C, **II:**27
      vitamin E, **II:**27
    prevention and treatment, **II:**26–28
    retinoids
      action mechanisms, **II:**26
      characteristics, **II:**26
      side effects, **II:**26
      usage guidelines, **II:**26
  wrinkle formation
    fat grafting, **II:**328, 329f
    soft-tissue fillers, **II:**44–45
wrists
  anatomical characteristics, **VI:**163–164, 164f, 167f
  bones and joints
    alignment points, **VI:**11f
    blood supply, **VI:**10b
    bony anatomy, **VI:**12f
    check rein ligaments, **VI:**13b
    collateral ligaments, **VI:**13f
    detailed characteristics, **VI:**7–11
    Gilula's lines, **VI:**10f
    malrotations, **VI:**10b
    palmar and dorsal views, **VI:**8f
    radius and ulna, **VI:**9f
    ulnar positive variance, **VI:**10f
  biomechanics, **VI:**164–165
  burn reconstruction, **IV:**443, 443t, 508, 508f
  carpal bones, **VI:**161–163, 162f
  carpal instability, **VI:**164–165, 164t
  diagnostic imaging, **VI:**68–91
    computed tomography (CT)
      advantages/disadvantages, **VI:**78–82, 81t
      bony tumors, **VI:**81–82
      fractures and dislocations, **VI:**78–79, 81f
      general discussion, **VI:**68
    magnetic resonance imaging (MRI)
      advantages/disadvantages, **VI:**82–89, 82t
      basic principles, **VI:**82
      carpal fractures, **VI:**85
      distal radioulnar joint (DRUJ) instability, **VI:**86–88
      enchondromas, **VI:**85
      fracture nonunion evaluations, **VI:**88
      ganglion cysts, **VI:**83, 84f
      giant cell tumors of the tendon sheath (GCTTS), **VI:**83, 84f
      hemangiomas, **VI:**83–85
      Kienbock's disease, **VI:**88, 89f
      ligamentous injuries, **VI:**85–86
      lipomas, **VI:**83

wrists (*Continued*)
      occult scaphoid fractures, **VI:**85, 85f
      osteomyelitis, **VI:**88–89
      pulse sequences and enhancements, **VI:**83t
      right-sided wrist pain, **VI:**87f–88f
      scaphoid fracture nonunion evaluations, **VI:**88
      scapholunate interosseous ligament injury, **VI:**85–86, 87f
      signal intensities on weighted images, **VI:**82, 82t
      soft-tissue masses, **VI:**82–83
      tendinopathies, **VI:**86–88
      thumb ulnar collateral ligament injuries, **VI:**85, 86f
      trauma-related injuries, **VI:**85
      triangular fibrocartilage (TFCC) tears, **VI:**86, 87f
      ulnar-sided wrist pain, **VI:**86–88, 87f–88f
      ulnocarpal abutment, **VI:**86, 88f
    radiographic imaging
      basic procedure, **VI:**72–76
      general discussion, **VI:**68–76
    radionuclide imaging, **VI:**90
    vascular imaging techniques, **VI:**89–90, 90f
  fractures and dislocations
    carpal fractures
      epidemiology, **VI:**161, 162f
      magnetic resonance imaging (MRI), **VI:**85
    distal radius fracture, **VI:**161–177
      anatomical considerations, **VI:**163–164, 164f
      classifications, **VI:**163, 163f
      epidemiology, **VI:**161, 162f
      future trends, **VI:**177
      historical background, **VI:**161–163
      patient selection, **VI:**169–170
      radiographic imaging, **VI:**75f
      surgical technique and treatment, **VI:**175–176, 176f
    dorsal intercalated segment instability (DISI)/volar intercalated segment instability (VISI) deformities, **VI:**166–168, 168f
    humpback deformity, **VI:**165, 165f, 171
    injury mechanisms, **VI:**165
    lunotriquetral (LT) ligament tears, **VI:**174, 174f
    patient presentation and diagnosis
      diagnostic imaging, **VI:**166–169, 168f–169f
      Kleinman shear test, **VI:**165–166, 166f
      patient history, **VI:**165
      physical examination, **VI:**165–166
      Watson scaphoid shift test, **VI:**54, 166f
    patient selection, **VI:**169–170
    perilunate dislocation, **VI:**174–175, 175f
    scaphoid fractures
      humpback deformity, **VI:**165, 165f, 171
      scaphoid nonunion occurrences, **VI:**170–171, 172f
      surgical technique and treatment, **VI:**170, 171f
    scapholunate (SL) ligament injury, **VI:**171–174, 172f–174f

wrists (Continued)
    surgical technique and treatment
        distal radius fracture, VI:175–176, 176f
        lunotriquetral (LT) ligament tears,
            VI:174, 174f
        perilunate dislocation, VI:174–175, 175f
        scaphoid fractures, VI:170, 171f
        scapholunate (SL) ligament injury,
            VI:171–174, 172f–174f
        ulnar styloid fracture, VI:176–177
    ulnar styloid fracture, VI:176–177
infections, VI:333–334
internal fracture fixation, VI:106–116
    Arbeitsgemeinschaft für
        Osteosynthesefragen (AO) principles,
        VI:106, 107t
    challenges, VI:106
    fixation options
        absolute versus relative stability,
            VI:108, 108b, 108f
        bridge plating, VI:113, 115f
        compression plating, VI:112–113, 114f
        external fixation, VI:110, 111f
        interfragmentary compression, VI:108
        interfragmentary lag screws, VI:111–
            112, 112f–113f
        Kirschner wires (K-wires), VI:107b,
            108–109, 109f, 110t, 139
        locked plating, VI:115, 115f
        tension band constructs, VI:109–110,
            109f–111f, 110t
    fluoroscopic imaging, VI:108–115
    fracture reduction
        basic procedure, VI:107
        Kapandji (intrafocal) pinning, VI:107b
        Kirschner wires (K-wires), VI:107b
        temporary/supplemental external
            fixation, VI:107b
    patient selection
        fracture assessment, VI:106
        host factors, VI:106
    postoperative care and follow-up, VI:115
    preoperative imaging assessment, VI:107
    research summary, VI:115
    surgical technique and treatment
        fracture reduction, VI:107
        preoperative planning, VI:107
joint denervation surgery, VI:497t
ligaments, VI:167f
osteoarthritis, VI:411–448
    disease process, VI:412–413, 412f
    epidemiology, VI:411
    etiology, VI:441–442
    pathophysiology, VI:413
    patient evaluation, VI:442–443
    patient presentation and diagnosis,
        VI:413–414, 413f
    scaphoid nonunion advanced collapse
        (SNAC) arthritis, VI:441–442, 443f
    scapholunate advanced collapse (SLAC)
        arthrtis, VI:441–442, 442f
    surgical technique and treatment
        basic procedure, VI:443–446
        dorsal surgical approach, VI:443, 444f
        four-corner fusion, VI:445, 445f
        neurectomy, VI:443–444
        proximal row carpectomy (PRC),
            VI:444–445, 444f

wrists (Continued)
        radial styloidectomy, VI:443
        scaphoidectomy, VI:445, 445f
        total wrist arthrodesis/total wrist
            arthroplasty, VI:445–446, 446f
pseudogout, VI:335
radiographic imaging
    assessment criteria, VI:73b
    basic procedure, VI:72–76
    carpal height ratio, VI:74f
    carpal indices, VI:79f
    carpal tunnel view, VI:78f
    distal radioulnar joint (DRUJ) instability,
        VI:75f
    distal radius fracture, VI:75f
    dorsal intercalated segmental instability,
        VI:78f
    dynamic scapholunate instability,
        VI:79f
    normal distal radius indices, VI:75f
    normal posteroanterior radiograph,
        VI:73f
    perilunate dislocation, VI:74f
    positioning, VI:69f, 73f–74f, 76f
    scaphoid fractures, VI:76b, 77f
    ulnar abutment syndrome, VI:76b, 80f
    ulnar variance, VI:74f
replantation and revascularization surgery,
    VI:238–241, 239f–240f
rheumatoid arthritis
    basic principles, VI:374–376
    caput ulnae, VI:375f
    complete wrist arthrodesis
        basic procedure, VI:386–388, 386f–387f
        intramedullary pin, VI:388f
        outcomes and complicatons, VI:388
        postoperative care and follow-up,
            VI:388
        radiographic imaging, VI:388f
        secondary procedures, VI:388
        Steinmann pin, VI:387f–388f
        surgical tips, VI:388b
    crystalline arthropathy/gout, VI:407t,
        409–410
    distal ulna resection (Darrach procedure)
        basic procedure, VI:382–384
        chevron incision, VI:382f
        outcomes and complicatons,
            VI:383–384
        postoperative care and follow-up,
            VI:383
        pronator quadratus release, VI:383f
        radiographic imaging, VI:384f
        secondary procedures, VI:384
        surgical tips, VI:384b
        ulnar head exposure, VI:382f
        ulnar head removal, VI:383f
        ulnar stump stabilization, VI:384f
    extensor tenosynovitis, VI:376, 376f
    large proliferative flexor tendon
        tenosynovitis, VI:376f
    Mannerfelt lesion, VI:376, 376f
    operative procedures
        complete wrist arthrodesis, VI:386–388
        distal ulna resection (Darrach
            procedure), VI:382–384
        radioscapholunate arthrodesis,
            VI:384–386

wrists (Continued)
        total wrist arthroplasty, VI:388–390
        wrist synovectomy/dorsal
            tenosynovectomy, VI:381–382
    radiographic imaging, VI:374f–375f
    radioscapholunate arthrodesis
        basic procedure, VI:384–386
        compression screws, VI:385f
        K-wire fixation, VI:385f
        postoperative care and follow-up,
            VI:386
        radiographic imaging, VI:385f
    scleroderma, VI:407t, 409
    seronegative spondyloarthropathies,
        VI:406–408, 407t
    systemic lupus erythematosus (SLE),
        VI:407t, 408
    total wrist arthroplasty
        basic procedure, VI:388–390
        capsulotomy, VI:389f
        carpal component placement, VI:389f
        extensor tendon exposure, VI:389f
        osteotomy, VI:389f
        outcomes and complicatons, VI:390
        postoperative care and follow-up,
            VI:390
        radiographic imaging, VI:390f
        secondary procedures, VI:390
        surgical tips, VI:390b
    Vaughn–Jackson syndrome, VI:376,
        376f
    wrist synovectomy/dorsal
        tenosynovectomy
        basic procedure, VI:381–382, 381f–382f
        outcomes and complicatons, VI:382
        postoperative care and follow-up,
            VI:381–382
        secondary procedures, VI:382
        surgical tips, VI:382b
spastic hand surgery, VI:460–464, 462f–463f
tendinopathy, VI:366
tetraplegic restoration, VI:825–826
wrist disarticulation/transradial
    amputation, VI:873–874, 873f–874f

X
xanthogranuloma, juvenile, I:729–730,
    729f–730f
xanthoma, I:729, 729f
X chromosome inactivation, I:181–182
xenogeneic bone grafts, I:460
xenogenic acellular dermal matrix (ADM),
    I:342
xenografts
    cartilage, I:831
    characteristics, IV:412t–414t
    definition, I:815
    skin grafts, I:325t, 829
xeroderma pigmentosum (XP), III:112, 114f
X-ray analysis
    brachial plexus injuries, VI:796
    congenital hand deformities, VI:543–544
    cutaneous and soft-tissue tumors, I:710
    facial soft-tissue injuries, III:26
    hand tumors, VI:312–313, 313f
    osteoarthritis, VI:413–414, 413f
    sarcoma detection, IV:104, 104f
    wrist injuries, VI:166–169, 168f–169f

Note: **Boldface** roman numerals indicate volume. Page numbers followed by f refer to figures; page numbers followed by t refer to tables; page numbers followed by b refer to boxes.

Y

young cosmetic surgery patient, **II:**4–5, 4f–5f
youthful and beautiful eyes characteristics,
    II:115–116, 115f

Z

Zancolli capsulodesis, **VI:**763–764, 763f
Zancolli classification of active finger and
    wrist extension, **VI:**461, 462t
Zancolli "lasso" procedure, **VI:**834, 835f
Zeis gland carcinoma, **I:**738
Zetaderm/Zetavisc, **II:**47t
zinc (Zn) deficiencies, **I:**282
Zingiber officinale, **V:**33t–35t
Zocor, **V:**318–319, 318f
zone of polarizing activity (ZPA), **VI:**527, 529f
Z-plasty technique
    Apert syndrome, **VI:**612–614
    axillary contractures, **IV:**507
    basic principles, **I:**312–316, 313b
    burn reconstruction
        extremity burn reconstruction, **III:**269f,
            IV:447, 451f–454f
        facial burn wound treatment, **IV:**481, 481f
        local flaps, **IV:**502–503, 503f
    constriction band syndrome, **VI:**641–642
    double-opposing Z-plasty, **VI:**288f
    four-flap Z-plasty
        thumb hypoplasia, **VI:**585f
        thumb middle-third amputations,
            VI:287–291, 288f
    Furlow double-opposing z-palatoplasty,
        III:579, 580f, 624–625, 624f
    gains in length, **I:**312t
    geometric broken line, **I:**316, 317f
    labia minora reduction, **II:**669–673
    lip reconstruction, **III:**268–270, 269f–270f

Z-plasty technique (*Continued*)
    male genital reconstructive surgery, **IV:**302f
    multiple-flap Z-plasty, **I:**315, 315f–316f
    neck rejuvenation, **II:**323–324, 323f
    planimetric Z-plasty, **I:**314, 314f
    simple Z-plasty, **I:**313–314, 313f
    skew Z-plasty, **I:**314–315, 314f
    spina bifida, **III:**867–872, 868t–869t,
        870f–871f
    syndactyly surgery, **VI:**606, 607f
    thumb reconstruction, **VI:**287–291, 288f
    triphalangeal thumb, **VI:**624–627
    V-Y and Y-V advancement flaps, **I:**316, 316f
    widespread burn hypertrophic scars,
        I:293–294
    W-plasty, **I:**316, 317f, **III:**268–270
Zyderm/Zyplast, **II:**45t, 47, 49t
    See also soft-tissue fillers
zygoma
    Asian facial cosmetic surgery, **II:**178
    characteristics, **III:**63–65
    facial fractures
        anterior treatment approach
            basic procedure, **III:**65–66
            endoscopic approaches, **III:**65
            minimalist approach, **III:**65
            preoperative/postoperative
                comparisons, **III:**66f
            Z-F suture diastasis, **III:**65–66
        characteristics, **III:**63–65
        classification systems
            anterior treatment approach, **III:**65–66
            posterior approach (coronal incisions),
                III:66
        complications
            bleeding, **III:**69
            late complications, **III:**69–70, 69f

zygoma (*Continued*)
        maxillary sinusitis, **III:**69
        numbness, **III:**69–70
        oral-antral fistula, **III:**70
        orbital complications, **III:**69, 69f
        plate complications, **III:**70
    compound comminuted fractures
        characteristics, **III:**69–70
        delayed treatment, **III:**69
    diagnosis, **III:**64–65
    high energy fractures
        characteristics, **III:**67–68, 68f
        intraoral approach, **III:**68
        maxillary sinus approach, **III:**68
    reduction methods
        Dingman approach, **III:**67
        maxillary sinus approach, **III:**67
        stability requirements, **III:**67
        temporal approach, **III:**67
    surgical pathology, **III:**64–65
    treatment strategies
        buttress articulations and alignment,
            III:66–67
        closed reduction, **III:**66
    musculature, **III:**280–282, 281f
    Treacher Collins syndrome, **III:**830–832,
        831f–832f
zygomatic arch, **III:**6–7, 6f, 830–832
zygomaticomaxillary complex
    pediatric facial fractures, **III:**681, 684
    Treacher Collins syndrome, **III:**714, 714f,
        833f, 835, 835f
zygomaticotemporal branch of the trigeminal
    nerve, **III:**492, 495–496, 496f
zygomaticus major muscle, **II:**240, 241f,
    259f, **III:**255–256, 280–282, 281f,
    282t